For all that CMDT has to offer, visit AccessMedicine.com/CMDT

You will have access to all the great content found in the book, as well as online-only chapters and the CMDT Media Library—all in a convenient online format that can be accessed on your desktop or mobile device.

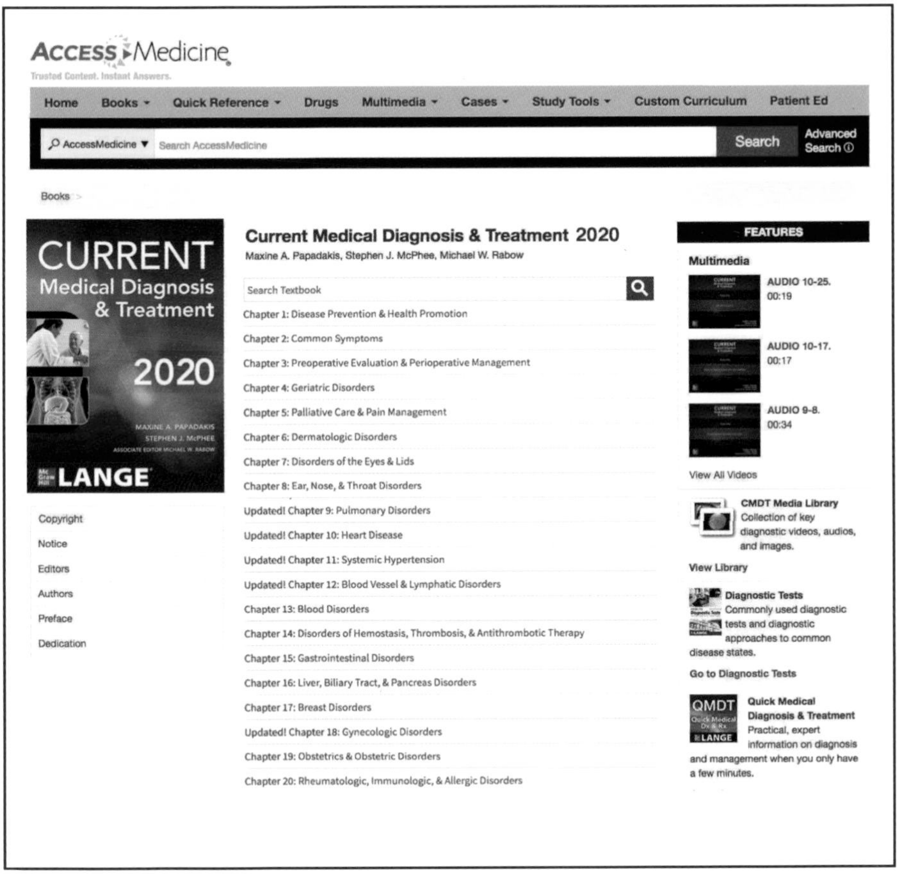

ACCESS▸Medicine
Trusted Content. Instant Answers.

| Home | Books ▾ | Quick Reference ▾ | Drugs | Multimedia ▾ | Cases ▾ | Study Tools ▾ | Custom Curriculum | Patient Ed |

🔍 AccessMedicine ▾ | Search AccessMedicine | **Search** | Advanced Search ⓘ

Books ⊳

CURRENT Medical Diagnosis & Treatment 2020

MAXINE A. PAPADAKIS
STEPHEN J. McPHEE
ASSOCIATE EDITOR MICHAEL W. RABOW

LANGE

Copyright
Notice
Editors
Authors
Preface
Dedication

Current Medical Diagnosis & Treatment 2020
Maxine A. Papadakis, Stephen J. McPhee, Michael W. Rabow

Search Textbook 🔍

Chapter 1: Disease Prevention & Health Promotion
Chapter 2: Common Symptoms
Chapter 3: Preoperative Evaluation & Perioperative Management
Chapter 4: Geriatric Disorders
Chapter 5: Palliative Care & Pain Management
Chapter 6: Dermatologic Disorders
Chapter 7: Disorders of the Eyes & Lids
Chapter 8: Ear, Nose, & Throat Disorders
Updated! Chapter 9: Pulmonary Disorders
Updated! Chapter 10: Heart Disease
Updated! Chapter 11: Systemic Hypertension
Updated! Chapter 12: Blood Vessel & Lymphatic Disorders
Chapter 13: Blood Disorders
Chapter 14: Disorders of Hemostasis, Thrombosis, & Antithrombotic Therapy
Chapter 15: Gastrointestinal Disorders
Chapter 16: Liver, Biliary Tract, & Pancreas Disorders
Chapter 17: Breast Disorders
Updated! Chapter 18: Gynecologic Disorders
Chapter 19: Obstetrics & Obstetric Disorders
Chapter 20: Rheumatologic, Immunologic, & Allergic Disorders

FEATURES

Multimedia

AUDIO 10-25.
00:19

AUDIO 10-17.
00:17

AUDIO 9-8.
00:34

View All Videos

CMDT Media Library
Collection of key diagnostic videos, audios, and images.
View Library

Diagnostic Tests
Commonly used diagnostic tests and diagnostic approaches to common disease states.
Go to Diagnostic Tests

QMDT Quick Medical Diagnosis & Treatment
Practical, expert information on diagnosis and management when you only have a few minutes.

Immediate access to evidence-based diagnosis and treatment information

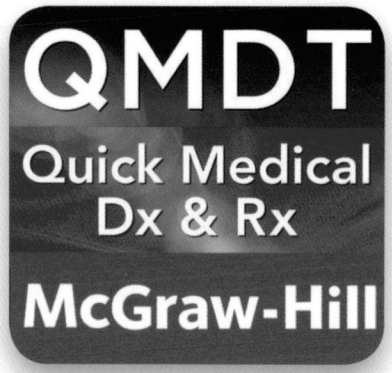

Quick Medical Diagnosis & Treatment (QMDT) provides practical, expert information on the diagnosis and management of over 950 disorders.

Structured alphabetically, topics include easy-to-read bulleted information that promotes rapid comprehension and immediate access in any clinical setting.

Each disease entry includes:

- **Key Features:** Essentials of diagnosis and general considerations

- **Clinical Findings:** Symptoms and signs and differential diagnosis

- **Diagnosis:** Laboratory tests, imaging studies and diagnostic procedures with most also including:

    - **Treatment:** Medications, surgery, and therapeutic procedures

    - **Outcomes:** Complications, prognosis, when to refer, and when to admit

    - **Evidence:** Up to date clinical guidelines, targeted references, and web sites for clinicians and patients

You will also find pertinent tables and figures to help quickly pinpoint individual drugs and dosages, as well as solutions to other clinical problems.

Available online at AccessMedicine.com or download it from the App store

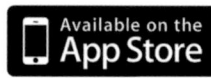 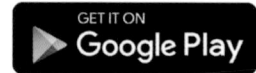

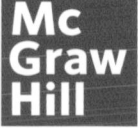

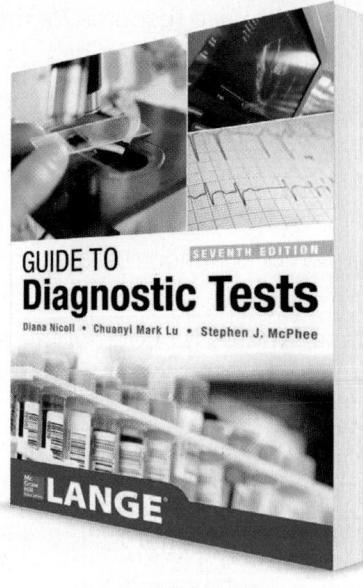
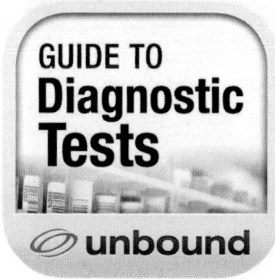
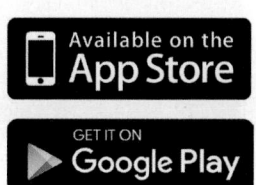
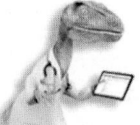
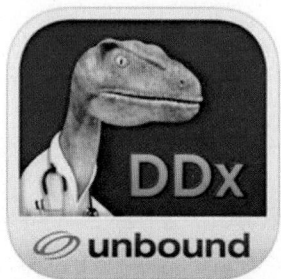
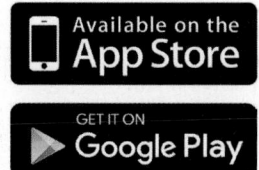
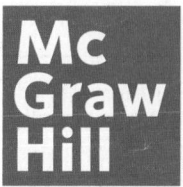

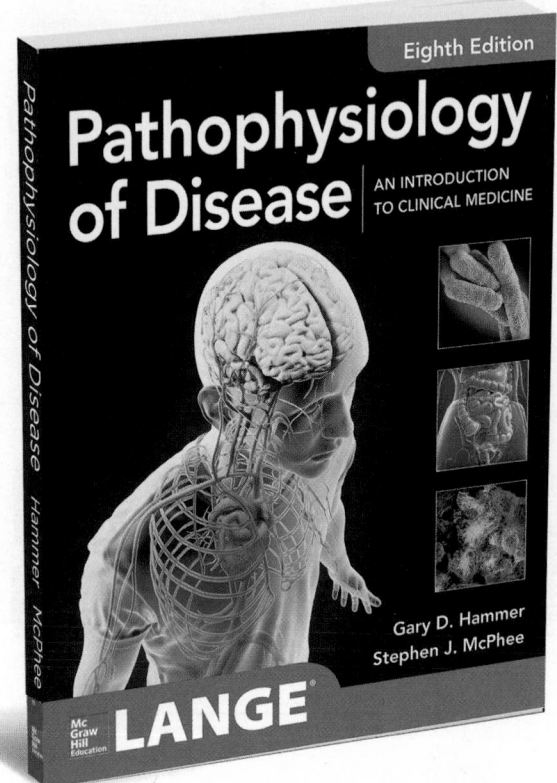
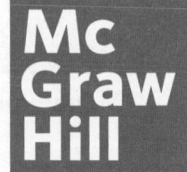

2020

CURRENT
Medical Diagnosis
& Treatment

FIFTY-NINTH EDITION

Edited by

Maxine A. Papadakis, MD
Professor of Medicine, Emeritus
Department of Medicine
University of California, San Francisco

Stephen J. McPhee, MD
Professor of Medicine, Emeritus
Division of General Internal Medicine
Department of Medicine
University of California, San Francisco

Associate Editor

Michael W. Rabow, MD
Professor of Medicine and Urology
Division of Palliative Medicine
Department of Medicine
University of California, San Francisco

With Associate Authors

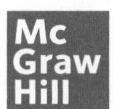

New York   Chicago   San Francisco   Athens   London   Madrid   Mexico City
Milan   New Delhi   Singapore   Sydney   Toronto

Current Medical Diagnosis & Treatment 2020, Fifty-Ninth Edition

Previous editions copyright 2000 through 2019 by McGraw-Hill Education; copyright © 1987 through 1999 by Appleton & Lange; copyright 1962 through 1986 by Lange Medical Publications.

2 3 4 5 6 7 8 9 0   LWI   24 23 22 21 20

ISBN 978-1-26-045528-1
MHID 1-26-045528-9
ISSN 0092-8682

Notice

Medicine is an ever-changing science. As new research and clinical experience broaden our knowledge, changes in treatment and drug therapy are required. The authors and the publisher of this work have checked with sources believed to be reliable in their efforts to provide information that is complete and generally in accord with the standards accepted at the time of publication. However, in view of the possibility of human error or changes in medical sciences, neither the authors nor the publisher nor any other party who has been involved in the preparation or publication of this work warrants that the information contained herein is in every respect accurate or complete, and they disclaim all responsibility for any errors or omissions or for the results obtained from use of the information contained in this work. Readers are encouraged to confirm the information contained herein with other sources. For example and in particular, readers are advised to check the product information sheet included in the package of each medication they plan to administer to be certain that the information contained in this work is accurate and that changes have not been made in the recommended dose or in the contraindications for administration. This recommendation is of particular importance in connection with new or infrequently used medications.

This book was set by Cenveo® Publisher Services.
The editors were Amanda Fielding, Kay Conerly, and Harriet Lebowitz.
The production supervisor was Jeffrey Herzich.
Project management was provided by Radhika Jolly at Cenveo Publisher Services.
The copyeditor was Jennifer Bernstein.
Design modified from original by Alan Barnett.
The index was prepared by Katherine Pitcoff.

This book is printed on acid-free paper.

McGraw-Hill Education books are available at special quantity discounts to use as premiums and sales promotions, or for use in corporate training programs. To contact a representative, please visit the Contact Us pages at www.mhprofessional.com.

Contents

*Free access to online chapters at www.accessmedicine.com/cmdt

Authors

N. Franklin Adkinson Jr., MD
Professor of Medicine, Johns Hopkins Asthma &
Allergy Center, Baltimore, Maryland
fadkinso@jhmi.edu
Allergic & Immunologic Disorders (in Chapter 20)

Michael J. Aminoff, MD, DSc, FRCP
Distinguished Professor and Executive Vice Chair,
Department of Neurology, University of California,
San Francisco; Attending Physician, University of
California Medical Center, San Francisco
michael.aminoff@ucsf.edu
Nervous System Disorders

Charalambos Babis Andreadis, MD, MSCE
Associate Professor of Clinical Medicine, Division of
Hematology/Oncology, University of California,
San Francisco
Charalambos.Andreadis@ucsf.edu
Blood Disorders

Naomi B. Anker, MD
Assistant Professor of Medicine, Division of Nephrology,
Veterans Affairs Health Care System, San Francisco,
California, Department of Medicine, University of
California, San Francisco
Naomi.Anker@ucsf.edu
Electrolyte & Acid-Base Disorders

Kevin L. Ard, MD, MPH
Faculty, Division of Infectious Diseases, Massachusetts
General Hospital; Medical Director, National LGBT
Health Education Center, Fenway Institute; Instructor
in Medicine, Harvard Medical School, Boston,
Massachusetts
kard@mgh.harvard.edu
Lesbian, Gay, Bisexual, & Transgender Health

Antoine Azar, MD
Assistant Professor of Medicine, Division of Allergy &
Clinical Immunology, Johns Hopkins Asthma &
Allergy Center, Baltimore, Maryland
aazar4@jhmi.edu
Allergic & Immunologic Disorders (in Chapter 20)

David M. Barbour, PharmD, BCPS
Pharmacist, Denver, Colorado
dbarbour99@gmail.com
Drug References

Robert B. Baron, MD, MS
Professor of Medicine; Associate Dean for Graduate and
Continuing Medical Education; University of
California, San Francisco
baron@medicine.ucsf.edu
Lipid Disorders; Nutritional Disorders

Thomas M. Bashore, MD
Professor of Medicine; Senior Vice Chief, Division of
Cardiology, Duke University Medical Center, Durham,
North Carolina
thomas.bashore@duke.edu
Heart Disease

Aaron Baugh, MD
Pulmonary & Critical Care Fellow, University of
California, San Francisco
References

Michael J. Blaha, MD, MPH
Director of Clinical Research, Ciccarone Center for the
Prevention of Cardiovascular Disease; Associate
Professor of Medicine, Johns Hopkins University
School of Medicine, Baltimore, Maryland
mblaha1@jhmi.edu
Lipid Disorders

Bryn A. Boslett, MD
Assistant Professor, Division of Infectious Diseases,
Department of Medicine, University of California,
San Francisco
Bryn.Boslett@ucsf.edu
Bacterial & Chlamydial Infections

Hugo Q. Cheng, MD
Clinical Professor of Medicine, University of California,
San Francisco
quinny.cheng@ucsf.edu
Preoperative Evaluation & Perioperative Management

Asha N. Chesnutt, MD
Clinical Assistant Professor, Division of Pulmonary &
Critical Care Medicine, Department of Medicine,
Oregon Health & Science University, Portland, Oregon
Asha.Chesnutt2@providence.org
Pulmonary Disorders

Mark S. Chesnutt, MD
Professor, Pulmonary & Critical Care Medicine, Dotter
Interventional Institute, Oregon Health & Science
University, Portland, Oregon; Director, Critical Care,
Portland Veterans Affairs Health Care System
chesnutm@ohsu.edu
Pulmonary Disorders

Peter V. Chin-Hong, MD
Professor, Division of Infectious Diseases, Department of
Medicine, University of California, San Francisco
peter.chin-hong@ucsf.edu
*Common Problems in Infectious Diseases & Antimicrobial
Therapy*

Kerry C. Cho, MD
Clinical Professor of Medicine, Division of Nephrology, University of California, San Francisco
kerry.cho@ucsf.edu
Electrolyte & Acid-Base Disorders

Eva Clark, MD, PhD
Infectious Diseases Fellow, Baylor College of Medicine, Houston, Texas
eva.clark@bcm.edu
Viral & Rickettsial Infections

Patricia A. Cornett, MD
Professor of Medicine, Division of Hematology/Oncology, University of California, San Francisco
patricia.cornett@ucsf.edu
Cancer

Russ Cucina, MD, MS
Professor of Hospital Medicine; Chief Health Information Officer, UCSF Health System; University of California, San Francisco
russ.cucina@ucsf.edu
CMDT Online—Information Technology in Patient Care

Lloyd E. Damon, MD
Professor of Clinical Medicine, Department of Medicine, Division of Hematology/Oncology; Director of Adult Hematologic Malignancies and Blood and Marrow Transplantation, Deputy Chief of the Division of Hematology and Medical Oncology, University of California, San Francisco
lloyd.damon@ucsf.edu
Blood Disorders

Tiffany O. Dea, PharmD, BCOP
Oncology Pharmacist, Veterans Affairs Health Care System, San Francisco, California; Adjunct Professor, Thomas J. Long School of Pharmacy and Health Sciences, Stockton, California
tiffany.dea@va.gov
Cancer

Charles DeBattista, DMH, MD
Professor of Psychiatry and Behavioral Sciences; Director, Depression Clinic and Research Program; Director of Medical Student Education in Psychiatry, Stanford University School of Medicine, Stanford, California
debattista@stanford.edu
Psychiatric Disorders

Madeline B. Deutsch, MD, MPH
Associate Professor of Clinical Family & Community Medicine; Director, UCSF Transgender Care; Center of Excellence for Transgender Health, University of California, San Francisco
Madeline.Deutsch@ucsf.edu
Lesbian, Gay, Bisexual, & Transgender Health

Monara Dini, DPM
Assistant Clinical Professor, Chief of Podiatric Surgery Division, Department of Orthopedic Surgery, University of California, San Francisco
monara.dini@ucsf.edu
CMDT Online—Podiatric Disorders

Tonja C. Dirkx, MD
Associate Professor of Medicine, Division of Nephrology, Department of Medicine, Oregon Health & Science University, Portland, Oregon; Acting Nephrology Division Chief, Portland Veterans Affairs Health Care System
dirkxt@ohsu.edu
Kidney Disease

Vanja C. Douglas, MD
Sara & Evan Williams Foundation Endowed Neurohospitalist Chair, Associate Professor of Clinical Neurology, Department of Neurology, University of California, San Francisco
Vanja.Douglas@ucsf.edu
Nervous System Disorders

Jacque L. Duncan, MD
Professor of Clinical Ophthalmology, University of California, San Francisco
jacque.duncan@ucsf.edu
Disorders of the Eyes & Lids

Paul A. Fitzgerald, MD
Clinical Professor of Medicine, Department of Medicine, Division of Endocrinology, University of California, San Francisco
paul.fitzgerald@ucsf.edu
Endocrine Disorders

Lindy P. Fox, MD
Associate Professor, Department of Dermatology, University of California, San Francisco
Lindy.Fox@ucsf.edu
Dermatologic Disorders

Lawrence S. Friedman, MD
Professor of Medicine, Harvard Medical School; Professor of Medicine, Tufts University School of Medicine, Boston, Massachusetts; The Anton R. Fried, MD, Chair, Department of Medicine, Newton-Wellesley Hospital, Newton, Massachusetts; Assistant Chief of Medicine, Massachusetts General Hospital, Boston
lfriedman@partners.org
Liver, Biliary Tract, & Pancreas Disorders; Hepatobiliary Cancers (in Chapter 39)

Warren J. Gasper, MD
Assistant Professor of Clinical Surgery, Division of Vascular and Endovascular Surgery, Department of Surgery, University of California, San Francisco
warren.gasper@ucsf.edu
Blood Vessel & Lymphatic Disorders

Armando E. Giuliano, MD, FACS, FRCSEd
Executive Vice Chair of Surgery, Associate Director of
    Surgical Oncology, Cedars-Sinai Medical Center,
    Los Angeles, California
armando.giuliano@cshs.org
Breast Disorders

Ralph Gonzales, MD, MSPH
Associate Dean, Clinical Innovation and Chief Innovation
    Officer, UCSF Health; Professor of Medicine, Division
    of General Internal Medicine, Department of Medicine,
    University of California, San Francisco
ralph.gonzales@ucsf.edu
Common Symptoms

Christopher B. Granger, MD
Professor of Medicine; Director, Cardiac Care Unit, Duke
    University Medical Center, Duke Clinical Research
    Institute, Durham, North Carolina
christopher.granger@dm.duke.edu
Heart Disease

Katherine Gruenberg, PharmD
Assistant Professor, School of Pharmacy, University of
    California, San Francisco
Katherine.Gruenberg@ucsf.edu
CMDT Online—Anti-Infective Chemotherapeutic &
    Antibiotic Agents

B. Joseph Guglielmo, PharmD
Professor and Dean, School of Pharmacy, University of
    California, San Francisco
BJoseph.Guglielmo@ucsf.edu
Common Problems in Infectious Diseases & Antimicrobial
    Therapy; CMDT Online—Anti-Infective
    Chemotherapeutic & Antibiotic Agents

Richard J. Hamill, MD
Professor, Division of Infectious Diseases, Departments of
    Medicine and Molecular Virology & Microbiology,
    Baylor College of Medicine, Houston, Texas
rhamill@bcm.edu
Mycotic Infections

G. Michael Harper, MD
Professor, Division of Geriatrics, Department of Medicine,
    University of California San Francisco School of
    Medicine; San Francisco Veterans Affairs Health Care
    System, San Francisco, California
Michael.Harper@ucsf.edu
Geriatric Disorders

David B. Hellmann, MD, MACP
Aliki Perroti Professor of Medicine; Vice Dean for Johns
    Hopkins Bayview; Chairman, Department of Medicine,
    Johns Hopkins Bayview Medical Center, Johns Hopkins
    University School of Medicine, Baltimore, Maryland
hellmann@jhmi.edu
Rheumatologic, Immunologic, & Allergic Disorders

Ruth Hsu, MD
Chief Resident, Department of Psychiatry and Behavioral
    Sciences, Stanford University, Stanford, California
References

Sara A. Hurvitz, MD, FACP
Associate Professor; Director, Breast Oncology Program,
    Division of Hematology/Oncology, Department of
    Internal Medicine, University of California, Los Angeles
shurvitz@mednet.ucla.edu
Breast Disorders

Leon I. Igel, MD, FACP, FTOS
Assistant Professor of Clinical Medicine, Division of
    Endocrinology, Diabetes and Metabolism, Weill
    Cornell Medical College, New York, New York
lei9004@med.cornell.edu
Nutritional Disorders

John B. Imboden Jr., MD
Alice Betts Endowed Chair for Arthritis Research;
    Professor of Medicine, University of California,
    San Francisco; Chief, Division of Rheumatology,
    Zuckerberg San Francisco General Hospital
John.Imboden@ucsf.edu
Rheumatologic, Immunologic, & Allergic Disorders

Kevin P. Jackson, MD
Assistant Professor of Medicine, Director of
    Electrophysiology, Duke Raleigh Hospital, Duke
    University Medical Center, Durham, North Carolina
k.j@duke.edu
Heart Disease

Jane Jih, MD, MPH, MAS
Assistant Professor of Medicine, Division of General
    Internal Medicine, Department of Medicine, University
    of California, San Francisco
References

Meshell D. Johnson, MD
Associate Professor of Medicine, Division of Pulmonary
    and Critical Care Medicine; Director of Faculty
    Diversity, Department of Medicine, University of
    California, San Francisco
meshell.johnson@ucsf.edu
Blood Vessel & Lymphatic Disorders; Alcohol Use Disorder
    (Alcoholism) (in Chapter 25)

C. Bree Johnston, MD, MPH
Medical Director of Palliative and Supportive Care,
    PeaceHealth St. Joseph Medical Center, Bellingham,
    Washington; Clinical Professor of Medicine, University
    of Washington
bjohnston@peacehealth.org
Geriatric Disorders

Marianne A. Juarez, MD
Assistant Clinical Professor, Department of Emergency
    Medicine, University of California, San Francisco
Marianne.Juarez@ucsf.edu
Disorders Related to Environmental Emergencies

Mitchell H. Katz, MD
President and Chief Executive Officer of NYC Health + Hospitals, New York, New York
mitchell.katz@nychhc.org
HIV Infection & AIDS

Julia Knypinski, MD
Resident Physician, Department of Obstetrics and Gynecology, University of Texas Southwestern Medical Center, Dallas, Texas
References

Tejaswi Kompala, MD
Clinical Fellow, Endocrinology, Department of Medicine, University of California, San Francisco
References

C. Seth Landefeld, MD
Professor of Medicine; Chair, Department of Medicine and Spencer Chair in Medical Science Leadership, University of Alabama at Birmingham
sethlandefeld@uab.edu
Geriatric Disorders

Andrew D. Leavitt, MD
Professor, Departments of Medicine (Hematology) and Laboratory Medicine; Medical Director, UCSF Adult Hemophilia Treatment Center, University of California, San Francisco
andrew.leavitt@ucsf.edu
Disorders of Hemostasis, Thrombosis, & Antithrombotic Therapy

Chuanyi Mark Lu, MD
Professor and Vice Chair, Department of Laboratory Medicine, University of California, San Francisco; Chief, Lab Medicine Service, Veterans Affairs Health Care System, San Francisco, California
mark.lu@va.gov
CMDT Online—Diagnostic Testing & Medical Decision Making; CMDT Online—Appendix: Therapeutic Drug Monitoring, Laboratory Reference Intervals, & Pharmacogenetic Tests

Anthony Luke, MD, MPH
Professor of Clinical Orthopaedics, Department of Orthopaedics; Director, UCSF Primary Care Sports Medicine; Director, Human Performance Center at the Orthopaedic Institute, University of California, San Francisco
anthony.luke@ucsf.edu
Sports Medicine & Outpatient Orthopedics

Lawrence R. Lustig, MD
Howard W. Smith Professor and Chair, Department of Otolaryngology—Head & Neck Surgery, Columbia University Medical Center & New York Presbyterian Hospital, New York, New York
lrl2125@cumc.columbia.edu
Ear, Nose, & Throat Disorders

C. Benjamin Ma, MD
Professor, Department of Orthopaedic Surgery; Chief, Sports Medicine and Shoulder Service, University of California, San Francisco
MaBen@orthosurg.ucsf.edu
Sports Medicine & Outpatient Orthopedics

Umesh Masharani, MB, BS, MRCP (UK)
Professor of Medicine, Division of Endocrinology and Metabolism, Department of Medicine, University of California, San Francisco
umesh.masharani@ucsf.edu
Diabetes Mellitus & Hypoglycemia

Kenneth H. Mayer, MD
Co-Chair and Medical Research Director, The Fenway Institute; Director of HIV Prevention Research, Beth Israel Deaconess Medical Center; Professor of Medicine, Harvard Medical School, Boston, Massachusetts
kmayer@fenwayhealth.org
Lesbian, Gay, Bisexual, & Transgender Health

Megan McNamara, MD, MSc
Associate Professor of Medicine, Case Western Reserve University School of Medicine; Louis Stokes Cleveland Veterans Affairs Medical Center, Cleveland, Ohio
Megan.Mcnamara@va.gov
CMDT Online—Women's Health Issues

Kenneth R. McQuaid, MD
Chief, Gastroenterology and Medical Service, San Francisco Veterans Affairs Medical Center; Professor of Clinical Medicine, Marvin H. Sleisenger Endowed Chair and Vice-Chairman, Department of Medicine, University of California, San Francisco
Kenneth.Mcquaid@va.gov
Gastrointestinal Disorders; Alimentary Tract Cancers (in Chapter 39)

Darshan Mehta, MD, MPH
Medical Director, Benson-Henry Institute for Mind Body Medicine, Massachusetts General Hospital; Associate Director of Education, Osher Center for Integrative Medicine, Harvard Medical School and Brigham and Women's Hospital, Boston
dmehta@mgh.harvard.edu
CMDT Online—Integrative Medicine

Tracy Minichiello, MD
Clinical Professor of Medicine, University of California, San Francisco; Chief, Anticoagulation and Thrombosis Services, San Francisco Veterans Affairs Medical Center
Tracy.Minichiello@ucsf.edu
Disorders of Hemostasis, Thrombosis, & Antithrombotic Therapy

Paul L. Nadler, MD
Clinical Professor of Medicine; Director, Screening and
Acute Care Clinic, Division of General Internal
Medicine, Department of Medicine, University of
California, San Francisco
Paul.Nadler@ucsf.edu
Common Symptoms

Jacqueline A. Nemer, MD, FACEP
Professor of Emergency Medicine, Director of Quality &
Safety, Director of Advanced Clinical Skills,
Department of Emergency Medicine, University of
California, San Francisco
jacqueline.nemer@ucsf.edu
Disorders Related to Environmental Emergencies

Juno Obedin-Maliver, MD, MPH, MAS
Assistant Professor, Department of Obstetrics and
Gynecology; Founder and Investigator, Lesbian, Gay,
Bisexual, and Transgender Medical Education Research
Group, Stanford University School of Medicine,
Stanford, California
junoom@stanford.edu
Lesbian, Gay, Bisexual, & Transgender Health

Kent R. Olson, MD
Clinical Professor of Medicine, Pediatrics, and Pharmacy,
University of California, San Francisco; Medical
Director, San Francisco Division, California Poison
Control System
kent.olson@ucsf.edu
Poisoning

Kevin A. Ostrowski, MD
Assistant Professor of Urology, University of Washington
School of Medicine, Seattle, Washington
ostrowsk@uw.edu
Urologic Disorders

Steven Z. Pantilat, MD
Professor of Medicine, Department of Medicine;
Kates-Burnard and Hellman Distinguished Professor of
Palliative Care; Director, Palliative Care Program,
University of California, San Francisco
steve.pantilat@ucsf.edu
Palliative Care & Pain Management

Neeti B. Parikh, MD
Assistant Professor, Department of Ophthalmology,
University of California, San Francisco
Neeti.Parikh@ucsf.edu
Disorders of the Eyes & Lids

Charles B. Parks, DPM
Assistant Clinical Professor, Chief of Podiatric Surgery
Division, Department of Orthopedic Surgery,
University of California, San Francisco
Charles.Parks@ucsf.edu
CMDT Online—Podiatric Disorders

Manesh R. Patel, MD
Associate Professor of Medicine, Division of Cardiology,
Department of Medicine; Director of Interventional
Cardiology, Duke University Medical Center, Durham,
North Carolina
manesh.patel@duke.edu
Heart Disease

Susan S. Philip, MD, MPH
Assistant Clinical Professor, Division of Infectious
Diseases, Department of Medicine, University of
California, San Francisco; Disease Prevention and
Control Branch, Population Health Division,
San Francisco Department of Public Health,
San Francisco, California
susan.philip@sfdph.org
Spirochetal Infections

Michael Pignone, MD, MPH
Professor of Medicine; Chair, Department of Medicine,
Dell Medical School, The University of Texas at Austin
pignone@austin.utexas.edu
Disease Prevention & Health Promotion

Lawrence Poree, MD, MPH, PhD
Professor, Department of Anesthesia & Perioperative
Care, University of California, San Francisco
Lawrence.Poree@ucsf.edu
Palliative Care & Pain Management

Toya Pratt, MD
Clinical Fellow, Female Pelvic Medicine & Reconstructive
Surgery, Kaiser Permanente-University of California,
San Francisco
References

Niall T. Prendergast, MD
Fellow, Division of Pulmonary, Allergy and Critical Care
Medicine, Department of Medicine, University of
Pittsburgh School of Medicine, Pittsburgh,
Pennsylvania
niall.prendergast@gmail.com
Pulmonary Disorders

Thomas J. Prendergast, MD
Clinical Professor of Medicine, Oregon Health & Science
University; Pulmonary Critical Care Section Chief,
Portland Veterans Affairs Health Care System,
Portland, Oregon
thomas.prendergast@va.gov
Pulmonary Disorders

Reed E. Pyeritz, MD, PhD
William Smilow Professor of Medicine and Genetics,
Raymond and Ruth Perelman School of Medicine of
the University of Pennsylvania, Philadelphia
reed.pyeritz@uphs.upenn.edu
Genetic & Genomic Disorders

Michael W. Rabow, MD, FAAHPM
Helen Diller Family Chair in Palliative Care, Professor of Clinical Medicine and Urology, Division of Palliative Medicine, Department of Medicine; Director, Symptom Management Service, Helen Diller Family Comprehensive Cancer Center, University of California, San Francisco
Mike.Rabow@ucsf.edu
Palliative Care & Pain Management

Kristin S. Raj, MD
Clinical Instructor, Department of Psychiatry and Behavioral Sciences, Stanford University School of Medicine, Stanford, California
kraj@stanford.edu
Psychiatric Disorders

Julia Goodnough Ramos, MD, PhD
Hematology Fellow, Division of Hematology and Oncology, Department of Medicine, University of California, San Francisco
References

Joseph H. Rapp, MD
Professor of Surgery, Emeritus, Division of Vascular and Endovascular Surgery, University of California, San Francisco
Joseph.Rapp@ucsf.edu
Blood Vessel & Lymphatic Disorders

Paul Riordan-Eva, FRCOphth
Consultant Ophthalmologist, King's College Hospital, London, United Kingdom
paulreva@doctors.org.uk
Disorders of the Eyes & Lids

Scott W. Roberts, MD
Associate Professor, Obstetrics and Gynecology, University of Texas Southwestern Medical Center, Dallas, Texas
scott.roberts@utsouthwestern.edu
Obstetrics & Obstetric Disorders

Patricia A. Robertson, MD
Professor, Department of Obstetrics, Gynecology, and Reproductive Sciences, University of California, San Francisco
Patricia.Robertson@ucsf.edu
Lesbian, Gay, Bisexual, & Transgender Health

Vanessa L. Rogers, MD
Associate Professor, Obstetrics and Gynecology, University of Texas Southwestern Medical Center, Dallas, Texas
vanessa.rogers@utsouthwestern.edu
Obstetrics & Obstetric Disorders

Stacey R. Rose, MD, FACP
Assistant Professor of Internal Medicine, Division of Infectious Diseases; Director of Clinical Sciences Curriculum; Wellness Director, Residency Program in Internal Medicine, Baylor College of Medicine, Houston, Texas
srrose@bcm.edu
Mycotic Infections

Philip J. Rosenthal, MD
Professor, Department of Medicine, University of California, San Francisco; Associate Chief, Division of HIV, Infectious Diseases, and Global Health, Zuckerberg San Francisco General Hospital
philip.rosenthal@ucsf.edu
Protozoal & Helminthic Infections

René Salazar, MD
Professor of Medical Education, Assistant Dean for Diversity, Dell Medical School, The University of Texas at Austin
rene.salazar@austin.utexas.edu
Disease Prevention & Health Promotion

Katherine H. Saunders, MD
Assistant Professor of Clinical Medicine, Weill Cornell Medicine, New York, New York
kph2001@med.cornell.edu
Nutritional Disorders

George Schade, MD
Assistant Professor, Department of Urology, University of Washington, Seattle
grschade@uw.edu
Cancers of the Genitourinary Tract (in Chapter 39)

Joshua S. Schindler, MD
Associate Professor, Department of Otolaryngology, Oregon Health & Science University, Portland, Oregon; Medical Director, OHSU-Northwest Clinic for Voice and Swallowing
schindlj@ohsu.edu
Ear, Nose, & Throat Disorders

Brian S. Schwartz, MD
Associate Professor, Division of Infectious Diseases, Department of Medicine, University of California, San Francisco
brian.schwartz@ucsf.edu
Bacterial & Chlamydial Infections

Rachel K. Scott, MD, MPH, FACOG
Scientific Director of Women's Health Research, MedStar Health Research Institute Director, Women's Center for Positive Living, MedStar Washington Hospital Center, Department of Women's and Infants' Services; Assistant Professor of Obstetrics and Gynecology, Georgetown University School of Medicine, Washington, D.C.
Rachel.K.Scott@Medstar.net
Gynecologic Disorders

Gerami D. Seitzman, MD
Associate Professor, Department of Ophthalmology, Francis I. Proctor Foundation, University of California, San Francisco
gerami.seitzman@ucsf.edu
Disorders of the Eyes & Lids

J.D. Serfas, MD
Cardiology Fellow, Department of Medicine, Duke University, Durham, North Carolina
References

Ann Cai Shah, MD
Assistant Clinical Professor, Anesthesia and Pain Medicine, Department of Anesthesia and Perioperative Care, University of California, San Francisco
Palliative Care & Pain Management

Wayne X. Shandera, MD
Assistant Professor, Department of Medicine, Baylor College of Medicine, Houston, Texas
shandera@bcm.tmc.edu
Viral & Rickettsial Infections

Kanade Shinkai, MD, PhD
Associate Professor, Department of Dermatology, University of California, San Francisco
Kanade.Shinkai@ucsf.edu
Dermatologic Disorders

Craig Smollin, MD
Professor, Emergency Medicine, School of Medicine, University of California, San Francisco
Craig.Smollin@ucsf.edu
Poisoning

Mathew Sorensen, MD, MS, FACS
Associate Professor, Residency Program Director, Department of Urology, University of Washington, Seattle; Director, Comprehensive Metabolic Stone Clinic, Puget Sound Veteran's Affairs Health Care System
mathews@uw.edu
Urologic Disorders

Scott Steiger, MD
Associate Professor of Clinical Medicine and Psychiatry, Division of General Internal Medicine, Department of Medicine, University of California, San Francisco; Deputy Medical Director, Opiate Treatment Outpatient Program, Division of Substance Abuse and Addiction Medicine, Department of Psychiatry, Zuckerberg San Francisco General Hospital
scott.steiger@ucsf.edu
Palliative Care & Pain Management

Leslie Suen, MD
Primary Care Internal Medicine Resident, Department of Medicine, University of California, San Francisco
References

Michael Sutters, MD, MRCP (UK)
Attending Nephrologist, Virginia Mason Medical Center, Seattle, Washington; Affiliate Assistant Professor of Medicine, Division of Nephrology, University of Washington School of Medicine, Seattle, Washington
michael.sutters@vmmc.org
Systemic Hypertension

Diana Thiara, MD
General Medicine Clinician Educator Fellow, Division of General Internal Medicine, Department of Medicine, University of California, San Francisco
References

Philip Tiso
Principal Editor, Division of General Internal Medicine, University of California, San Francisco
References

Vaibhav Upadhyay, MD, PhD
Pulmonary and Critical Care Medicine Fellow, Department of Medicine, University of California, San Francisco
References

Carling Ursem, MD
Assistant Professor, Division of Hematology and Oncology, Department of Medicine, University of California, San Francisco; Staff Physician, Veterans Affairs Health Care System, San Francisco
Carling.Ursem@ucsf.edu
Alimentary Tract Cancers (in Chapter 39)

Jessica Valente, MD, MPH
Ambulatory Chief Resident, Department of Medicine, University of California, San Francisco
References

Evan J. Walker, MD
Hematology/Oncology Fellow, University of California San Francisco
References

Judith Walsh, MD, MPH
Professor of Clinical Medicine, Division of General Internal Medicine, Women's Health Center of Excellence, University of California, San Francisco
Judith.Walsh@ucsf.edu
CMDT Online—Women's Health Issues

Thomas J. Walsh, MD, MS
Associate Professor, Department of Urology, University of Washington School of Medicine, Seattle, Washington
walsht@uw.edu
Urologic Disorders

Sunny Wang, MD
Associate Professor of Medicine, Division of Hematology/
Oncology, University of California,
San Francisco; San Francisco Veterans Affairs Health
Care System
sunny.wang@ucsf.edu
Lung Cancer (in Chapter 39)

Nolan Williams, MD
Assistant Professor of Psychiatry and Behavioral Sciences;
Director of Brain Stimulation Laboratory,
Department of Psychiatry, Stanford University School
of Medicine, Stanford, California
nolanw@stanford.edu
Psychiatric Disorders

Andrew D. Wisneski, MD
Surgery Resident, Department of Surgery, University of
California, San Francisco
References

CAPT Jason Woo, MD, MPH, FACOG
Medical Officer, Office of Generic Drugs, Center for Drug
Evaluation and Research, U.S. Food and Drug
Administration, Silver Spring, Maryland
woojjmd@gmail.com
Gynecologic Disorders

Tyler Woodell, MD, MCR
Assistant Professor of Medicine, Division of Nephrology-
Hypertension, University of California, San Diego
twoodell@ucsd.edu
Kidney Disease

Wesley Y. Yu, MD
Chief Resident, Dermatology, University of California,
San Francisco
References

Preface

Current Medical Diagnosis & Treatment 2020 (CMDT 2020) is the 59th edition of this single-source reference for practitioners in both hospital and ambulatory settings. The book emphasizes the practical features of clinical diagnosis and patient management in all fields of internal medicine and in specialties of interest to primary care practitioners and to subspecialists who provide general care.

Our students have inspired us to look at issues of race and justice, which surely impact people's health. We have therefore reviewed the content of our work to ensure that it contains the dignity and equality that every patient deserves.

INTENDED AUDIENCE FOR *CMDT*

House officers, medical students, and all other health professions students will find the descriptions of diagnostic and therapeutic modalities, with citations to the current literature, of everyday usefulness in patient care.

Internists, family physicians, hospitalists, nurse practitioners, physician assistants, and all primary care providers will appreciate *CMDT* as a ready reference and refresher text. Physicians in other specialties, pharmacists, and dentists will find the book a useful basic medical reference text. Nurses, nurse practitioners, and physician assistants will welcome the format and scope of the book as a means of referencing medical diagnosis and treatment.

Patients and their family members who seek information about the nature of specific diseases and their diagnosis and treatment may also find this book to be a valuable resource.

NEW IN THIS EDITION OF *CMDT*

- Extensive updating of images
- FDA designates esketamine as breakthrough medication for resistant depression
- New FDA-approved medication for multiple sclerosis
- Extensive revision of Viral & Rickettsial Infections chapter, including updates on measles, polio, and acute flaccid paralysis outbreaks; immunizations; as well as preventing and treating Epstein-Barr virus and cytomegalovirus infections in transplant patients
- FDA re-approval of tegaserod for irritable bowel syndrome with constipation
- Treatment options for prevention of opioid overdose and substance abuse disorders
- Clarification of the appropriate role of opioids and buprenorphine formulations in chronic pain management
- Information on new biologic agents for asthma
- Evolving treatment for chronic lymphocytic leukemia
- Differentiation of patients with celiac disease from patients intolerant of short-chain carbohydrates (fermentable oligosaccharides, disaccharides, monosaccharides, and polyols or "FODMAPS")
- New treatment recommendations for bacterial peritonitis
- Recommendations regarding use of tofacitinib to treat moderate to severe ulcerative colitis
- New model for acetaminophen-induced acute liver failure
- New table summarizing recommended FDA-approved oral direct-acting antiviral treatment regimens for hepatitis C
- New minimally invasive procedures for benign prostatic hyperplasia
- Rewritten Lipid Disorders chapter
- New table summarizing pharmacologic options for treatment of obesity
- Recommendations for treatment of fever during neutropenia following chemotherapy
- Update on biologic markers for breast cancer and their use in staging
- US Preventive Services Task Force screening recommendations for osteoporosis, prostate cancer, ovarian cancer, and cervical cancer
- Targeted therapies in advanced non-small cell lung cancers
- New immunotherapies for esophageal cancer, bladder cancer, and hepatocellular carcinoma
- Inclusion of most recent adult congenital heart disease guideline recommendations

- Detailed recommendations for the treatment of pulmonary stenosis
- Important update on cardiac amyloidosis treatment
- New discussion about management of subclinical atrial fibrillation
- Extensive update of immune modulation therapy and adjuvant treatments in breast cancer
- Approval of transcutaneous supraorbital neurostimulation and use of monoclonal antibodies for migraine
- Recommendations for thrombolysis and endovascular therapies in stroke as well as dual antiplatelet therapy in transient ischemic attack and stroke
- Novel treatments for posttraumatic stress disorder
- Revised table showing how to initiate and subsequently titrate antihypertensive medications
- Addition of angiotensin II in vasodilatory shock that is refractory to catecholamines and vasopressin
- Rewritten section on Health Care for Sexual and Gender Minority Patients

OUTSTANDING FEATURES OF *CMDT*

- Medical advances up to time of annual publication
- Detailed presentation of internal medicine disciplines, plus primary care topics including gynecology, obstetrics, dermatology, ophthalmology, otolaryngology, psychiatry, neurology, toxicology, urology, geriatrics, orthopedics, women's health, LGBT health, preventive medicine, and palliative care
- Concise format, facilitating efficient use in any practice setting
- More than 1000 diseases and disorders
- Annual update on HIV/AIDS and other newly emerging infections
- Specific disease prevention information
- Easy access to medication dosages, with trade names indexed and costs updated in each edition
- Recent references, with unique identifiers (PubMed, PMID numbers) for rapid downloading of article abstracts and, in some instances, full-text reference articles

E-CHAPTERS, *CMDT ONLINE*, & AVAILABLE APPS

Seven *e-chapters* mentioned in the Table of Contents can be accessed at www.AccessMedicine.com/CMDT. These online-only chapters (available without need for subscription) include

- Anti-Infective Chemotherapeutic & Antibiotic Agents
- Diagnostic Testing & Medical Decision Making
- Information Technology in Patient Care
- Integrative Medicine
- Podiatric Disorders
- Women's Health Issues
- Appendix: Therapeutic Drug Monitoring, Laboratory Reference Intervals, & Pharmacogenetic Tests

Institutional or individual subscriptions to AccessMedicine also have full electronic access to *CMDT 2020*. Subscribers to **CMDT Online** receive full electronic access to *CMDT 2020* as well as

- An expanded, dedicated media gallery
- *Quick Medical Diagnosis & Treatment (QMDT)*—a concise, bulleted version of *CMDT 2020*
- *Guide to Diagnostic Tests*—for quick reference to the selection and interpretation of commonly used diagnostic tests
- CURRENT Practice Guidelines in Primary Care—delivering concise summaries of the most relevant guidelines in primary care
- *Diagnosaurus*—consisting of 1000+ differential diagnoses

CMDT 2020, QMDT, Guide to Diagnostic Tests, and *Diagnosaurus* are also available as individual apps for your smartphone or tablet and can be found in the Apple App Store and Google Play.

SPECIAL RECOGNITION

With this 2020 edition, Dr. Robert Baron will be retiring from *CMDT* after more than 30 years of contributions. Dr. Baron has authored *CMDT's* Nutritional Disorders chapter for 31 years (since 1989) and its Lipid Disorders chapter for 22 years (since 1998).

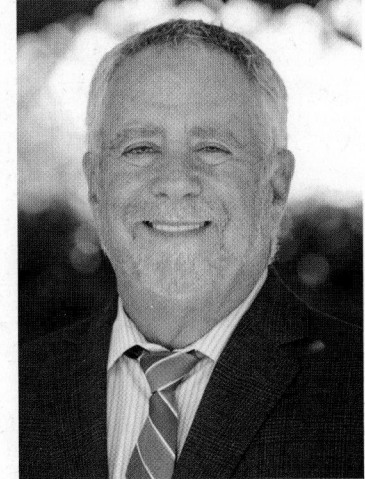

Dr. Baron has had a distinguished career in internal medicine. He received his BA in anthropology and sociology from Princeton University, his MS in nutrition from the University of Wisconsin, Madison, and his MD from the University of California, San Francisco (UCSF). After his residency training in UCSF's Primary Care Internal Medicine Residency Program, he joined the UCSF faculty in 1981. He directed that residency from 1989 until 2006. In 2000, he became Associate Dean for Continuing Medical Education (CME) and continues to lead UCSF's extensive CME program. Since 2006, Dr. Baron has also been serving as Associate Dean for Graduate Medical Education and Designated Institutional Official for UCSF, overseeing its 92 Accreditation Council for Graduate Medical Education (ACGME)-accredited residency and fellowship training programs and 50 non-ACGME programs.

A practicing primary care general internist, Dr. Baron has been recognized as one of America's Top Doctors and as one of its Outstanding Primary Care Physicians. He has received numerous other teaching and service awards. Focusing his scholarship on graduate and continuing medical education and on nutrition, preventive medicine, and chronic disease, he has published 69 peer-reviewed papers and 99 book chapters and reviews.

Dr. Baron lives in San Francisco with his wife, Randie Bencanann. Their daughter, Micki, is a practicing obstetrician-gynecologist and daughter, Haley, recently obtained her master's degree in food studies.

As his editors, we offer our immense gratitude to Dr. Baron for 30 years of work on *CMDT*. It has been a genuine pleasure to edit his two chapters each year. We will miss working with you, Bobby!

ACKNOWLEDGMENTS

We wish to thank our authors for participating once again in the annual updating of this important book. We are especially grateful to Kevin Barrows, MD, Thomas D. Chi, MD, Pelin Cinar, MD, MS, Dima Dandachi, MD, Maxwell V. Meng, MD, FACS, Ramana K. Naidu, MD, Charles J. Ryan, MD, and Samuel A. Shelburne III, MD, PhD, who are leaving *CMDT* this year. We have all benefited from their clinical wisdom and commitment.

Many students and physicians also have contributed useful suggestions to this and previous editions, and we are grateful. We continue to welcome comments and recommendations for future editions in writing or via electronic mail. The editors' e-mail addresses are below and author e-mail addresses are included in the Authors section.

Maxine A. Papadakis, MD
Maxine.Papadakis@ucsf.edu
Stephen J. McPhee, MD
Stephen.McPhee@ucsf.edu

Michael W. Rabow, MD
Mike.Rabow@ucsf.edu

San Francisco, California

From inability to let well alone; from too much zeal for the new and contempt for what is old; from putting knowledge before wisdom, science before art and cleverness before common sense; from treating patients as cases; and from making the cure of the disease more grievous than the endurance of the same, Good Lord, deliver us.

—Sir Robert Hutchison

Disease Prevention & Health Promotion

Michael Pignone, MD, MPH[1]

René Salazar, MD

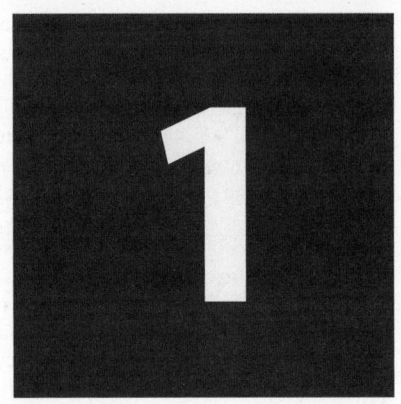

▼ GENERAL APPROACH TO THE PATIENT

The medical interview serves several functions. It is used to collect information to assist in diagnosis (the "history" of the present illness), to understand patient values, to assess and communicate prognosis, to establish a therapeutic relationship, and to reach agreement with the patient about further diagnostic procedures and therapeutic options. It also serves as an opportunity to influence patient behavior, such as in motivational discussions about smoking cessation or medication adherence. Interviewing techniques that avoid domination by the clinician increase patient involvement in care and patient satisfaction. Effective clinician-patient communication and increased patient involvement can improve health outcomes.

► Patient Adherence

For many illnesses, treatment depends on difficult fundamental behavioral changes, including alterating diet, taking up exercise, giving up smoking, cutting down drinking, and adhering to medication regimens that are often complex. Adherence is a problem in every practice; up to 50% of patients fail to achieve full adherence, and one-third never take their medicines. Many patients with medical problems, even those with access to care, do not seek appropriate care or may drop out of care prematurely. Adherence rates for short-term, self-administered therapies are higher than for long-term therapies and are inversely correlated with the number of interventions, their complexity and cost, and the patient's perception of overmedication.

As an example, in HIV-infected patients, adherence to antiretroviral therapy is a crucial determinant of treatment success. Studies have unequivocally demonstrated a close relationship between patient adherence and plasma HIV RNA levels, CD4 cell counts, and mortality. Adherence levels of more than 95% are needed to maintain virologic suppression. However, studies show that over 60% of patients are less than 90% adherent and that adherence tends to decrease over time.

Patient reasons for nonadherence include simple forgetfulness, being away from home, being busy, and changing daily routine. Other reasons include psychiatric disorders (depression or substance misuse), uncertainty about the effectiveness of treatment, lack of knowledge about the consequences of poor adherence, regimen complexity, and treatment side effects. The rising costs of medications, including generic drugs, and the increase in patient cost-sharing burden, has made adherence even more difficult, particularly for those with lower incomes.

Patients seem better able to take prescribed medications than to adhere to recommendations to change their diet, exercise habits, or alcohol intake or to perform various self-care activities (such as monitoring blood glucose levels at home). For short-term regimens, adherence to medications can be improved by giving clear instructions. Writing out advice to patients, including changes in medication, may be helpful. Because low functional health literacy is common (almost half of English-speaking US patients are unable to read and understand standard health education materials), other forms of communication—such as illustrated simple text, videotapes, or oral instructions—may be more effective. For non–English-speaking patients, clinicians and health care delivery systems can work to provide culturally and linguistically appropriate health services.

To help improve adherence to long-term regimens, clinicians can work with patients to reach agreement on the goals for therapy, provide information about the regimen, ensure understanding by using the "teach-back" method, counsel about the importance of adherence and how to organize medication-taking, reinforce self-monitoring, provide more convenient care, prescribe a simple dosage regimen for all medications (preferably one or two doses daily), suggest ways to help in remembering to take doses (time of day, mealtime, alarms) and to keep appointments, and provide ways to simplify dosing (medication boxes). Single-unit doses supplied in foil wrappers can increase adherence but should be avoided for patients who have difficulty opening them. Medication boxes with compartments (eg, Medisets) that are filled weekly are useful. Microelectronic devices can provide feedback to show

[1]Dr. Pignone is a former member of the US Preventive Services Task Force (USPSTF). The views expressed in this chapter are his and Dr. Salazar's and not necessarily those of the USPSTF.

patients whether they have taken doses as scheduled or to notify patients within a day if doses are skipped. Reminders, including cell phone text messages, are another effective means of encouraging adherence. The clinician can also enlist social support from family and friends, recruit an adherence monitor, provide a more convenient care environment, and provide rewards and recognition for the patient's efforts to follow the regimen. Collaborative programs that utilize pharmacists to help ensure adherence are also effective.

Adherence is also improved when a trusting doctor-patient relationship has been established and when patients actively participate in their care. Clinicians can improve patient adherence by inquiring specifically about the behaviors in question. When asked, many patients admit to incomplete adherence with medication regimens, with advice about giving up cigarettes, or with engaging only in "safer sex" practices. Although difficult, sufficient time must be made available for communication of health messages.

Medication adherence can be assessed generally with a single question: "In the past month, how often did you take your medications as the doctor prescribed?" Other ways of assessing medication adherence include pill counts and refill records; monitoring serum, urine, or saliva levels of drugs or metabolites; watching for appointment nonattendance and treatment nonresponse; and assessing predictable drug effects, such as weight changes with diuretics or bradycardia from beta-blockers. In some conditions, even partial adherence, as with drug treatment of hypertension and diabetes mellitus, improves outcomes compared with nonadherence; in other cases, such as HIV antiretroviral therapy or tuberculosis treatment, partial adherence may be worse than complete nonadherence.

Guiding Principles of Care

Ethical decisions are often called for in medical practice, at both the "micro" level of the individual patient-clinician relationship and at the "macro" level of the allocation of resources. Ethical principles that guide the successful approach to diagnosis and treatment are honesty, beneficence, justice, avoidance of conflict of interest, and the pledge to do no harm. Increasingly, Western medicine involves patients in important decisions about medical care, eg, which colorectal screening test to obtain or which modality of therapy for breast cancer or how far to proceed with treatment of patients who have terminal illnesses (see Chapter 5).

The clinician's role does not end with diagnosis and treatment. The importance of the empathic clinician in helping patients and their families bear the burden of serious illness and death cannot be overemphasized. "To cure sometimes, to relieve often, and to comfort always" is a French saying as apt today as it was five centuries ago—as is Francis Peabody's admonition: "The secret of the care of the patient is in caring for the patient." Training to improve mindfulness and enhance patient-centered communication increases patient satisfaction and may also improve clinician satisfaction.

Choudhry NK et al. Improving adherence to therapy and clinical outcomes while containing costs: opportunities from the greater use of generic medications: best practice advice from the Clinical Guidelines Committee of the American College of Physicians. Ann Intern Med. 2016 Jan 5;164(1):41–9. [PMID: 26594818]

Cutler RL et al. Economic impact of medication non-adherence by disease groups: a systematic review. BMJ Open. 2018 Jan 21; 8(1):e016982. [PMID: 29358417]

Kini V et al. Interventions to improve medication adherence: a review. JAMA. 2018 Dec 18;320(23):2461–73. [PMID: 30561486]

HEALTH MAINTENANCE & DISEASE PREVENTION

Preventive medicine can be categorized as primary, secondary, or tertiary. Primary prevention aims to remove or reduce disease risk factors (eg, immunization, giving up or not starting smoking). Secondary prevention techniques promote early detection of disease or precursor states (eg, routine cervical Papanicolaou screening to detect carcinoma or dysplasia of the cervix). Tertiary prevention measures are aimed at limiting the impact of established disease (eg, partial mastectomy and radiation therapy to remove and control localized breast cancer).

Tables 1–1 and 1–2 give leading causes of death in the United States and estimates of deaths from preventable causes. Recent data suggest increased rates of death, mainly from suicide and substance misuse. Unintentional injuries, including deaths from opioid-related overdoses, have become the third leading cause of death in the United States.

Many effective preventive services are underutilized, and few adults receive all of the most strongly recommended services. Several methods, including the use of provider or patient reminder systems (including interactive patient health records), reorganization of care environments, and

Table 1–1. Leading causes of death in the United States, 2016.

Category	Estimate
All causes	**2,744,248**
1. Diseases of the heart	635,260
2. Malignant neoplasms	598,038
3. Unintentional injuries	161,374
4. Chronic lower respiratory diseases	154,596
5. Cerebrovascular diseases	142,142
6. Alzheimer disease	116,103
7. Diabetes mellitus	80,058
8. Influenza and pneumonia	51,537
9. Nephritis, nephrotic syndrome, and nephrosis	50,046
10. Intentional self-harm (suicide)	44,965

Data from National Center for Health Statistics 2018.

Table 1–2. Deaths from all causes attributable to common preventable risk factors. (Numbers given in the thousands.)

Risk Factor	Male (95% CI)	Female (95% CI)	Both Sexes (95% CI)
Tobacco smoking	248 (226–269)	219 (196–244)	467 (436–500)
High blood pressure	164 (153–175)	231 (213–249)	395 (372–414)
Overweight–obesity (high BMI)	114 (95–128)	102 (80–119)	216 (188–237)
Physical inactivity	88 (72–105)	103 (80–128)	191 (164–222)
High blood glucose	102 (80–122)	89 (69–108)	190 (163–217)
High LDL cholesterol	60 (42–70)	53 (44–59)	113 (94–124)
High dietary salt (sodium)	49 (46–51)	54 (50–57)	102 (97–107)
Low dietary omega-3 fatty acids (seafood)	45 (37–52)	39 (31–47)	84 (72–96)
High dietary trans fatty acids	46 (33–58)	35 (23–46)	82 (63–97)
Alcohol use	45 (32–49)	20 (17–22)	64 (51–69)
Low intake of fruits and vegetables	33 (23–45)	24 (15–36)	58 (44–74)
Low dietary polyunsaturated fatty acids (in place of saturated fatty acids)	9 (6–12)	6 (3–9)	15 (11–20)

BMI, body mass index; CI, confidence interval; LDL, low-density lipoprotein.
Note: Numbers of deaths cannot be summed across categories.
Used, with permission, from Danaei G et al. The preventable causes of death in the United States: comparative risk assessment of dietary, lifestyle, and metabolic risk factors. PLoS Med. 2009 Apr 28;6(4):e1000058.

possibly provision of financial incentives to clinicians (though this remains controversial), can increase utilization of preventive services, but such methods have not been widely adopted.

Borsky A et al. Few Americans receive all high-priority, appropriate clinical preventive services. Health Aff. (Millwood). 2018 Jun;37(6):925–8. [PMID: 29863918]

García MC et al. Potentially preventable deaths among the five leading causes of death—United States, 2010 and 2014. MMWR Morb Mortal Wkly Rep. 2016 Nov 18;65(45):1245–55. [PMID: 27855145]

Levine DM et al. The quality of outpatient care delivered to adults in the United States, 2002 to 2013. JAMA Intern Med. 2016 Dec 1;176(12):1778–90. [PMID: 27749962]

US Burden of Disease Collaborators. The state of US health, 1990–2016: burden of diseases, injuries, and risk factors among US states. JAMA. 2018 Apr 10;319(14):1444–72. [PMID: 29634829]

Xu J et al. Deaths: Final data for 2016. Natl Vital Stat Rep. 2018 Jul; 67(5):1–76. [PMID: 30248015]

PREVENTION OF INFECTIOUS DISEASES

Much of the decline in the incidence and fatality rates of infectious diseases is attributable to public health measures—especially immunization, improved sanitation, and better nutrition.

Immunization remains the best means of preventing many infectious diseases. Recommended immunization schedules for children and adolescents can be found online at http://www.cdc.gov/vaccines/schedules/hcp/child-adolescent.html, and the schedule for adults is at http://www.cdc.gov/vaccines/schedules/hcp/adult.html (see also Chapter 30). Substantial morbidity and mortality from vaccine-preventable diseases, such as hepatitis A, hepatitis B, influenza, and pneumococcal infections, continue to occur among adults. Increases in the number of vaccine-preventable diseases in the United States (eg, regional epidemics) highlight the need to understand the association of vaccine refusal and disease epidemiology.

Evidence suggests annual **influenza vaccination** is safe and effective with potential benefit in all age groups, and the Advisory Committee on Immunization Practices (ACIP) recommends routine influenza vaccination for all persons aged 6 months and older, including all adults. When vaccine supply is limited, certain groups should be given priority, such as adults 50 years and older, individuals with chronic illness or immunosuppression, and pregnant women. An alternative high-dose inactivated vaccine is available for adults 65 years and older. Adults 65 years and older can receive either the standard-dose or high-dose vaccine, whereas those younger than 65 years should receive a standard-dose preparation.

The ACIP recommends two doses of **measles, mumps, and rubella (MMR) vaccine** in adults at high risk for exposure and transmission (eg, college students, health care workers). Otherwise, one dose is recommended for adults aged 18 years and older. Physician documentation of disease is not acceptable evidence of MMR immunity.

Routine use of **13-valent pneumococcal conjugate vaccine (PCV13)** is recommended among adults aged 65 and older. Individuals 65 years of age or older who have never received a pneumococcal vaccine should first receive PCV13 followed by a dose of **23-valent pneumococcal** polysaccharide vaccine (PPSV23) 6–12 months later. Individuals who have received more than one dose of PPSV23 should receive a dose of PCV13 more than 1 year after the last dose of PPSV23 was administered.

The ACIP recommends routine use of a single dose of **tetanus, diphtheria,** and 5-component **acellular pertussis vaccine (Tdap)** for adults aged 19–64 years to replace the next booster dose of **tetanus and diphtheria toxoids vaccine (Td).** Due to increasing reports of pertussis in the United States, clinicians may choose to give Tdap to persons aged 65 years and older (particularly to those who might risk transmission to at-risk infants who are most susceptible to complications, including death), despite limited published data on the safety and efficacy of the vaccine in this age group.

Both **hepatitis A vaccine** and **immune globulin** provide protection against hepatitis A; however, administration of immune globulin may provide a modest benefit over vaccination in some settings. Hepatitis B vaccine administered as a three-dose series is recommended for all children aged 0–18 years and high-risk individuals (ie, health care workers, injection drug users, people with end-stage renal disease). Adults with diabetes are also at increased risk for hepatitis B infection. The ACIP recommends **vaccination for hepatitis B** in diabetic patients aged 19–59 years. The hepatitis B vaccine should also be considered in diabetic persons age 60 and older.

Human papillomavirus (HPV) virus-like particle (VLP) vaccines have demonstrated effectiveness in preventing persistent HPV infections and thus may impact the rate of cervical intraepithelial neoplasia (CIN) II–III. The ACIP recommends routine HPV vaccination (three doses) for girls aged 11–12 years. The ACIP also recommends that all unvaccinated girls and women through age 26 years receive the three-dose HPV vaccination. Some studies suggest that one dose of vaccine may be as effective as three. The ACIP also recommends the routine vaccination with three doses of the vaccine for boys aged 11 or 12 years, males through age 21 years, and men who have sex with men and immunocompromised men (including those with HPV infection) through age 26 years. Vaccination of males with HPV may lead to indirect protection of women by reducing transmission of HPV and may prevent anal intraepithelial neoplasia and squamous cell carcinoma in men who have sex with men. In October 2018, the US Food and Drug Administration (FDA) approved the expanded use of the vaccine to include women and men age 27–45. After 2016, only the 9-valent HPV vaccine is being distributed in the U.S.

Persons traveling to countries where infections are endemic should take the precautions described in Chapter 30 and at http://wwwnc.cdc.gov/travel/destinations/list. Immunization registries—confidential, population-based, computerized information systems that collect vaccination data about all residents of a geographic area—can be used to increase and sustain high vaccination coverage.

The US Preventive Services Task Force (USPSTF) recommends behavioral counseling for adolescents and adults who are sexually active and at increased risk for sexually transmitted infections. Sexually active women aged 24 years or younger and older women who are at increased risk for infection should be screened for chlamydia and gonorrhea. Screening HIV-positive men or men who have sex with men for syphilis every 3 months is associated with improved syphilis detection.

HIV infection remains a major infectious disease problem in the world. The CDC recommends universal HIV screening of all patients aged 13–64, and the USPSTF recommends that clinicians screen adolescents and adults aged 15 to 65 years. Clinicians should integrate biomedical and behavioral approaches for HIV prevention. In addition to reducing sexual transmission of HIV, initiation of antiretroviral therapy reduces the risk for AIDS-defining events and death among patients with less immunologically advanced disease.

Daily **preexposure prophylaxis (PrEP)** with the fixed-dose combination of tenofovir disoproxil 300 mg and emtricitabine 200 mg (Truvada) should be considered for people who are HIV-negative but at substantial of risk for HIV infection. Studies of men who have sex with men suggest that PrEP is very effective in reducing the risk of contracting HIV. Patients taking PrEP should be encouraged to use other prevention strategies, such as consistent condom use and choosing less risky sexual behaviors (eg, oral sex), to maximally reduce their risk. **Postexposure prophylaxis (PEP)** with combinations of antiretroviral drugs is widely used after occupational and nonoccupational contact, and may reduce the risk of transmission by approximately 80%. PEP should be initiated within 72 hours of exposure.

In immunocompromised patients, live vaccines are contraindicated, but many killed or component vaccines are safe and recommended. *Asymptomatic* HIV-infected patients have not shown adverse consequences when given live MMR and influenza vaccinations as well as tetanus, hepatitis B, *Haemophilus influenzae* type b, and pneumococcal vaccinations—all should be given. However, if poliomyelitis immunization is required, the inactivated poliomyelitis vaccine is indicated. In *symptomatic* HIV-infected patients, live-virus vaccines, such as MMR, should generally be avoided, but annual influenza vaccination is safe.

Herpes zoster, caused by reactivation from previous varicella zoster virus infection, affects many older adults and people with immune system dysfunction. It can cause postherpetic neuralgia, a potentially debilitating chronic pain syndrome. Two vaccines are available for the prevention of herpes zoster, a live virus vaccine (Zostavax) and a herpes zoster subunit vaccine (HZ/su; Shingrix) (approved by the FDA in October 2017). The ACIP recommends the HZ/su vaccine be used for the prevention of herpes zoster and related complications in immunocompetent adults age 50 and older and in individuals who previously received Zostavax. The ACIP prefers the use of the new HZ/su vaccine over the older live virus vaccine.

In May 2015, the World Health Organization reported the first local transmission of Zika virus in the Western Hemisphere. Zika virus spreads to people primarily through mosquito bites but can also spread during sex by a person infected with Zika to his or her partner. Although clinical disease is usually mild, Zika virus infections in women infected during pregnancy have been linked to fetal microcephaly and loss, and newborn and infant blindness and other neurologic problems (see Chapter 32). Pregnant women should consider postponing travel to areas where Zika virus transmission is ongoing.

American Academy of Family Practitioners. ACIP recommends new herpes zoster subunit vaccine. 2017 Oct 31. http://www.aafp.org/news/health-of-the-public/20171031acipmeeting.html

Basta NE et al. Immunogenicity of a meningococcal B vaccine during a university outbreak. N Engl J Med. 2016 Jul 21; 375(3):220–8. [PMID: 27468058]

Blackstock OJ et al. A cross-sectional online survey of HIV pre-exposure prophylaxis adoption among primary care physicians. J Gen Intern Med. 2017 Jan;32(1):62–70. [PMID: 27778215]

Cantor AG et al. Screening for syphilis: updated evidence report and systematic review for the US Preventive Services Task Force. JAMA. 2016 Jun 7;315(21):2328–37. [PMID: 27272584]

Centers for Disease Control and Prevention (CDC). Adult Immunization Schedules: United States, 2018. http://www.cdc.gov/vaccines/schedules/hcp/adult.html

Centers for Disease Control and Prevention (CDC). Pertussis outbreak trends, 2015. http://www.cdc.gov/pertussis/outbreaks/trends.html

Centers for Disease Control and Prevention (CDC). HIV/AIDS, 2017. http://www.cdc.gov/hiv/basics/index.html

Centers for Disease Control and Prevention (CDC). Zika virus. http://www.cdc.gov/zika/index.html

Food and Drug Administration (FDA). FDA News Release, October 5, 2018. FDA approves expanded use of Gardasil 9 to include individuals 27 through 45 years old. https://www.fda.gov/NewsEvents/Newsroom/PressAnnouncements/ucm622715.htm

Jin J. JAMA patient page. Screening for syphilis. JAMA. 2016 Jun 7; 315(21):2367. [PMID: 27272600]

Phadke VK et al. Association between vaccine refusal and vaccine-preventable diseases in the United States: a review of measles and pertussis. JAMA. 2016 Mar 15;315(11):1149–58. Erratum in: JAMA. 2016 May 17;315(19):2125. [PMID: 26978210]

PEP (postexposure prophylaxis), 2017. http://www.cdc.gov/hiv/basics//pep.html.

PrEP (preexposure prophylaxis), 2017. http://www.cdc.gov/hiv/basics/prep.html

Riddell J 4th et al. HIV preexposure prophylaxis: a review. JAMA. 2018 Mar 27;319(12):1261–8. [PMID: 29584848]

PREVENTION OF CARDIOVASCULAR DISEASE

Cardiovascular diseases, including coronary heart disease (CHD) and stroke, represent two of the most important causes of morbidity and mortality in developed countries. Several risk factors increase the risk for coronary disease and stroke. These risk factors can be divided into those that are modifiable (eg, lipid disorders, hypertension, cigarette smoking) and those that are not (eg, age, sex, family history of early coronary disease). Impressive declines in age-specific mortality rates from heart disease and stroke have been achieved in all age groups in North America during the past two decades, in large part through improvement of modifiable risk factors: reductions in cigarette smoking, improvements in lipid levels, and more aggressive detection and treatment of hypertension. This section considers the role of screening for cardiovascular risk and the use of

effective therapies to reduce such risk. Key recommendations for cardiovascular prevention are shown in Table 1–3. Guidelines encourage regular assessment of global cardiovascular risk in adults 40–79 years of age without known cardiovascular disease, using standard cardiovascular risk factors. The role of nontraditional risk factors for improving risk estimation remains unclear.

Lin JS et al. Nontraditional risk factors in cardiovascular disease risk assessment: a systematic evidence report for the US Preventive Services Task Force [Internet]. Rockville, MD: Agency for Healthcare Research and Quality (US); 2018 Jul. http://www.ncbi.nlm.nih.gov/books/NBK525925/ [PMID: 30234933]

US Preventive Services Task Force. Behavioral counseling to promote a healthful diet and physical activity for cardiovascular disease prevention in adults without cardiovascular risk factors: US Preventive Services Task Force Recommendation Statement. JAMA. 2017 Jul 11;318(2):167–74. [PMID: 28697260]

Wall HK et al. Vital signs: prevalence of key cardiovascular disease risk factors for Million Hearts 2022—United States, 2011–2016. MMWR Morb Mortal Wkly Rep. 2018 Sep 7; 67(35):983–91. [PMID: 30188885]

Yadlowsky S et al. Clinical implications of revised pooled cohort equations for estimating atherosclerotic cardiovascular disease risk. Ann Intern Med. 2018 Jul 3;169(1):20–9. [PMID: 29868850]

▶ Abdominal Aortic Aneurysm

One-time screening for abdominal aortic aneurysm (AAA) by ultrasonography in men aged 65–75 years is associated with a relative reduction in odds of AAA-related mortality of almost 50% and possibly a small reduction in all-cause mortality. Women do not appear to benefit from screening, and most of the benefit in men appears to accrue among current or former smokers. Screening men aged 65 years and older is highly cost effective.

Canadian Task Force on Preventive Health Care. Recommendations on screening for abdominal aortic aneurysm in primary care. CMAJ. 2017 Sep 11;189(36):E1137–45. [PMID: 28893876]

Wanhainen A et al; Swedish Aneurysm Screening Study Group (SASS). Outcome of the Swedish nationwide abdominal aortic aneurysm screening program. Circulation. 2016 Oct 18; 134(16):1141–8. [PMID: 27630132]

Ying AJ et al. Abdominal aortic aneurysm screening: a systematic review and meta-analysis of efficacy and cost. Ann Vasc Surg. 2019 Jan;54:298–303.e3. [PMID: 30081169]

▶ Cigarette Smoking

Cigarette smoking remains the most important cause of preventable morbidity and early mortality. In 2015, there were an estimated 6.4 million premature deaths in the world attributable to smoking and tobacco use; smoking is the second leading cause of disability-adjusted life-years lost. Cigarettes are responsible for one in every five deaths in the United States. In 2014, approximately 450,000 deaths (258,456 in men and 190,409 in women) resulted from active cigarette smoking, accounting for almost 18% of all

Table 1–3. Expert recommendations for cardiovascular risk prevention methods: US Preventive Services Task Force (USPSTF).[1]

Prevention Method	Recommendation/[Year Issued]
Screening for abdominal aortic aneurysm (AAA)	Recommends one-time screening for AAA by ultrasonography in men aged 65–75 years who have ever smoked. (B) Selectively offer screening for AAA in men aged 65–75 years who have never smoked. (C) Current evidence is insufficient to assess the balance of benefits and harms of screening for AAA in women aged 65–75 years who have ever smoked. (I) Recommends against routine screening for AAA in women who have never smoked. (D) [2014]
Aspirin use	Recommends initiating low-dose aspirin use for the primary prevention of cardiovascular disease (CVD) and colorectal cancer (CRC) in adults aged 50–59 years who have a 10% or greater 10-year CVD risk, are not at increased risk for bleeding, have a life expectancy of at least 10 years, and are willing to take low-dose aspirin daily for at least 10 years. (B) The decision to initiate low-dose aspirin use for the primary prevention of CVD and CRC in adults aged 60–69 years who have a 10% or greater 10-year CVD risk should be an individual one. Persons who are not at increased risk for bleeding, have a life expectancy of at least 10 years, and are willing to take low-dose aspirin daily for at least 10 years are more likely to benefit. Persons who place a higher value on the potential benefits than the potential harms may choose to initiate low-dose aspirin. (C) The current evidence is insufficient to assess the balance of benefits and harms of initiating aspirin use for the primary prevention of CVD and CRC in adults younger than 50 years or older than age 70. (I) [2016]
Blood pressure screening	The USPSTF recommends screening for high blood pressure in adults aged 18 years or older. The USPSTF recommends obtaining measurements outside of the clinical setting for diagnostic confirmation before starting treatment. (A) [2015]
Serum lipid screening and use of statins for prevention	The USPSTF recommends that adults without a history of CVD use a low- to moderate-dose statin for the prevention of CVD events and mortality when all of the following criteria are met: (1) they are aged 40–75 years; (2) they have one or more CVD risk factors (ie, dyslipidemia, diabetes mellitus, hypertension, or smoking); and (3) they have a calculated 10-year risk of a cardiovascular event of 10% or greater. Identification of dyslipidemia and calculation of 10-year CVD event risk requires universal lipids screening in adults aged 40–75 years. See the "Clinical Considerations" section of the USPSTF recommendations[1] for more information on lipids screening and the assessment of cardiovascular risk. (B) The USPSTF concludes that the current evidence is insufficient to assess the balance of benefits and harms of initiating statin use for the primary prevention of CVD events and mortality in adults aged 76 years and older without a history of heart attack or stroke. (I) [2016]
Counseling about healthful diet and physical activity for CVD prevention	Recommends offering or referring adults who are overweight or obese and have additional CVD risk factors to intensive behavioral counseling interventions to promote a healthful diet and physical activity for CVD prevention. (B) [2014] Recommends that primary care professionals individualize the decision to offer or refer adults without obesity who do not have hypertension, dyslipidemia, abnormal blood glucose levels, or diabetes to behavioral counseling to promote a healthful diet and physical activity. (C) [2017]
Screening for diabetes mellitus	Recommends screening for abnormal blood glucose as part of cardiovascular risk assessment in adults aged 40–70 years who are overweight or obese. Clinicians should offer or refer patients with abnormal blood glucose to intensive behavioral counseling interventions to promote a healthful diet and physical activity. (B) [2015]
Screening for smoking and counseling to promote cessation	Recommends that clinicians ask all adults about tobacco use, advise them to stop using tobacco, and provide behavioral interventions and US Food and Drug Administration (FDA)–approved pharmacotherapy for cessation to adults who use tobacco. (A) [2015]

[1]US Preventive Services Task Force recommendations available at http://www.uspreventiveservicestaskforce.org/BrowseRec/Index/browse-recommendations.

Recommendation A: The USPSTF strongly recommends that clinicians routinely provide the service to eligible patients. (The USPSTF found good evidence that the service improves important health outcomes and concludes that benefits substantially outweigh harms.)

Recommendation B: The USPSTF recommends that clinicians routinely provide the service to eligible patients. (The USPSTF found at least fair evidence that the service improves important health outcomes and concludes that benefits substantially outweigh harms.)

Recommendation C: The USPSTF makes no recommendation for or against routine provision of the service.

Recommendation D: The USPSTF recommends against routinely providing the service to asymptomatic patients. (The USPSTF found at least fair evidence that the service is ineffective or that harms outweigh benefits.)

Recommendation I: The USPSTF concludes that the evidence is insufficient to recommend for or against routinely providing the service.

deaths in adults over age 35 in the United States. Annual cost of smoking-related health care is approximately $130 billion in the United States, with another $150 billion in productivity losses. Fortunately, US smoking rates have been declining; in 2015, 15.1% of US adults were smokers, and by 2017, 14% were smokers. Global direct health care costs from smoking in 2012 were estimated at $422 billion, with total costs of over $1.4 trillion.

Over 41,000 deaths per year in the United States are attributable to environmental tobacco smoke.

Smoking cessation reduces the risks of death and of myocardial infarction in people with coronary artery disease; reduces the rate of death and acute myocardial infarction in patients who have undergone percutaneous coronary revascularization; lessens the risk of stroke; and is associated with improvement of chronic obstructive pulmonary disease symptoms. On average, women smokers who quit smoking by age 35 add about 3 years to their life expectancy, and men add more than 2 years to theirs. Smoking cessation can increase life expectancy even for those who stop after the age of 65.

Although tobacco use constitutes the most serious common medical problem, it is undertreated. Almost 40% of smokers attempt to quit each year, but only 4% are successful. Persons whose clinicians advise them to quit are 1.6 times as likely to attempt quitting. Over 70% of smokers see a physician each year, but only 20% of them receive any medical quitting advice or assistance.

Factors associated with successful cessation include having a rule against smoking in the home, being older, and having greater education. Several effective clinical interventions are available to promote smoking cessation, including counseling, pharmacotherapy, and combinations of the two. The five steps for helping smokers quit are summarized in Table 1–4.

Common elements of supportive smoking cessation treatments are reviewed in Table 1–5. A system should be implemented to identify smokers, and advice to quit should be tailored to the patient's level of readiness to change. All patients trying to quit should be offered pharmacotherapy except those with medical contraindications, women who are pregnant or breast-feeding, and adolescents. Weight gain occurs in most patients (80%) following smoking cessation. Average weight gain is 2 kg, but for some (10–15%), major weight gain—over 13 kg—may occur. Planning for the possibility of weight gain, and means of mitigating it, may help with maintenance of cessation.

Several pharmacologic therapies have been shown to be effective in promoting cessation. Nicotine replacement therapy doubles the chance of successful quitting. The nicotine patch, gum, and lozenges are available over the counter and nicotine nasal spray and inhalers by prescription. The sustained-release antidepressant drug bupropion (150–300 mg/day orally) is an effective smoking cessation agent and is associated with minimal weight gain, although seizures are a contraindication. It acts by boosting brain levels of dopamine and norepinephrine, mimicking the effect of nicotine. More recently, varenicline, a partial nicotinic acetylcholine-receptor agonist, has been shown to improve cessation rates; however, its adverse effects, particularly its

effects on mood, are not completely understood and warrant careful consideration. No single pharmacotherapy is clearly more effective than others, so patient preferences and data on adverse effects should be taken into account in selecting a treatment. Combination therapy is more effective than a single pharmacologic modality. The efficacy of e-cigarettes in smoking cessation has not been well evaluated, and some users may find them addictive.

Clinicians should not show disapproval of patients who failed to stop smoking or who are not ready to make a quit attempt. Thoughtful advice that emphasizes the benefits of cessation and recognizes common barriers to success can increase motivation to quit and quit rates. An intercurrent illness or hospitalization may motivate even the most addicted smoker to quit.

Individualized or group counseling is very cost effective, even more so than treating hypertension. Smoking cessation counseling by telephone ("quitlines") and text messaging–based interventions have both proved effective. An additional strategy is to recommend that any smoking take place outdoors to limit the effects of passive smoke on housemates and coworkers. This can lead to smoking reduction and quitting.

The clinician's role in smoking cessation is summarized in Tables 1–4 and 1–5. Public policies, including higher cigarette taxes and more restrictive public smoking laws, have also been shown to encourage cessation, as have financial incentives directed to patients.

Centers for Disease Control and Prevention (CDC). Current cigarette smoking among adults in the United States in 2017. 2019 February 4. https://www.cdc.gov/tobacco/data_statistics/fact_sheets/adult_data/cig_smoking/index.htm
Goodchild M et al. Global economic cost of smoking-attributable diseases. Tob Control. 2018 Jan;27(1):58–64. [PMID: 28138063]
Ma J et al. Smoking-attributable mortality by state in 2014, US Am J Prev Med. 2018 May;54(5):661–70. [PMID: 29551325]
Stead LF et al. Combined pharmacotherapy and behavioural interventions for smoking cessation. Cochrane Database Syst Rev. 2016 Mar 24;3:CD008286. [PMID: 27009521]

▶ Lipid Disorders

Higher low-density lipoprotein (LDL) cholesterol concentrations and lower high-density lipoprotein (HDL) levels are associated with an increased risk of CHD (see Chapter 28). Measurement of total and high-density lipoprotein cholesterol levels can help assess the degree of CHD risk. The best age to start screening is controversial, as is its frequency. Cholesterol-lowering therapy reduces the relative risk of CHD events, with the degree of reduction proportional to the reduction in LDL cholesterol achieved, at least at LDL levels greater than 100 mg/dL. The absolute benefits of screening for—and treating—abnormal lipid levels depend on the presence and level of other cardiovascular risk factors, including hypertension, diabetes mellitus, smoking, age, and sex. If other risk factors are present, atherosclerotic cardiovascular disease risk is higher and the potential benefits of therapy are greater. Patients with known cardiovascular disease are at higher risk and have larger benefits from reduction in LDL cholesterol. The optimal risk threshold for initiating statins for primary prevention

Table 1–4. Actions and strategies for the primary care clinician to help patients quit smoking.

Action	Strategies for Implementation
Step 1. Ask—Systematically Identify All Tobacco Users at Every Visit	
Implement an officewide system that ensures that for *every* patient at *every* clinic visit, tobacco-use status is queried and documented[1]	Expand the vital signs to include tobacco use. Data should be collected by the health care team. The action should be implemented using preprinted progress note paper that includes the expanded vital signs, a vital signs stamp or, for computerized records, an item assessing tobacco-use status. Alternatives to the vital signs stamp are to place tobacco-use status stickers on all patients' charts or to indicate smoking status using computerized reminder systems.
Step 2. Advise—Strongly Urge All Smokers to Quit	
In a clear, strong, and personalized manner, urge every smoker to quit	Advice should be **Clear:** "I think it is important for you to quit smoking now, and I will help you. Cutting down while you are ill is not enough." **Strong:** "As your clinician, I need you to know that quitting smoking is the most important thing you can do to protect your current and future health." **Personalized:** Tie smoking to current health or illness and/or the social and economic costs of tobacco use, motivational level/readiness to quit, and the impact of smoking on children and others in the household. Encourage clinic staff to reinforce the cessation message and support the patient's quit attempt.
Step 3. Attempt—Identify Smokers Willing to Make a Quit Attempt	
Ask every smoker if he or she is willing to make a quit attempt at this time	If the patient is willing to make a quit attempt at this time, provide assistance (see step 4). If the patient prefers a more intensive treatment or the clinician believes more intensive treatment is appropriate, refer the patient to interventions administered by a smoking cessation specialist and follow up with him or her regarding quitting (see step 5). If the patient clearly states he or she is not willing to make a quit attempt at this time, provide a motivational intervention.
Step 4. Assist—Aid the Patient in Quitting	

A. Help the patient with a quit plan	**Set a quit date.** Ideally, the quit date should be within 2 weeks, taking patient preference into account.
	Help the patient prepare for quitting. The patient must:
	  Inform family, friends, and coworkers of quitting and request understanding and support.
	  Prepare the environment prior to quitting by removing cigarettes from it and ask the patient to avoid smoking wherever he or she spends a lot of time (eg, home, car).
	  Review previous quit attempts. What helped? What led to relapse?
	  Anticipate challenges to the planned quit attempt, particularly during the critical first few weeks.

B. Encourage nicotine replacement therapy except in special circumstances	Encourage the use of the nicotine patch or nicotine gum therapy for smoking cessation.
C. Give key advice on successful quitting	**Abstinence:** Total abstinence is essential. Not even a single puff after the quit date. **Alcohol:** Drinking alcohol is highly associated with relapse. Those who stop smoking should review their alcohol use and consider limiting or abstaining from alcohol use during the quit process. **Other smokers in the household:** The presence of other smokers in the household, particularly a spouse, is associated with lower success rates. Patients should consider quitting along with their significant others and/or developing specific plans to maintain abstinence in a household where others still smoke.
D. Provide supplementary materials	**Source:** Federal agencies, including the National Cancer Institute and the Agency for Health Care Policy and Research; nonprofit agencies (American Cancer Society, American Lung Association, American Heart Association); or local or state health departments. **Selection concerns:** The material must be culturally, racially, educationally, and age appropriate for the patient. **Location:** Readily available in every clinic office.

(continued)

Table 1–4. Actions and strategies for the primary care clinician to help patients quit smoking. (continued)

Action	Strategies for Implementation
Step 5. Arrange—Schedule Follow-Up Contact	
Schedule follow-up contact, either in person or via telephone	**Timing:** Follow-up contact should occur soon after the quit date, preferably during the first week. A second follow-up contact is recommended within the first month. Schedule further follow-up contacts as indicated. **Actions during follow-up:** Congratulate success. If smoking occurred, review the circumstances and elicit recommitment to total abstinence. Remind the patient that a lapse can be used as a learning experience and is not a sign of failure. Identify the problems already encountered and anticipate challenges in the immediate future. Assess nicotine replacement therapy use and problems. Consider referral to a more intense or specialized program.

[1]Repeated assessment is not necessary in the case of the adult who has never smoked or not smoked for many years and for whom the information is clearly documented in the medical record.

remains somewhat controversial, although most guidelines now suggest statin therapy when the 10-year atherosclerotic cardiovascular risk is greater than 10%.

Evidence for the effectiveness of statin-type drugs is better than for the other classes of lipid-lowering agents or dietary changes specifically for improving lipid levels. Multiple large, randomized, placebo-controlled trials have demonstrated important reductions in total mortality, major coronary events, and strokes with lowering levels of LDL cholesterol by statin therapy for patients with known cardiovascular disease. Statins also reduce cardiovascular events for patients with diabetes mellitus. For patients with no previous history of cardiovascular events or diabetes, meta-analyses have shown important reductions of cardiovascular events.

Newer antilipidemic monoclonal antibody agents (eg, evolocumab and alirocumab) lower LDL cholesterol by 50–60% by binding proprotein convertase subtilisin kexin type 9 (PCSK9), which decreases the degradation of LDL receptors. PCSK9 inhibitors also decrease Lp(a) levels. These newer agents are very expensive so are often used mainly in high-risk patients when statin therapy does not reduce the LDL cholesterol sufficiently at maximally tolerated doses or when patients are intolerant of statins. So far, few side effects have been reported with PCSK9 inhibitor use.

Guidelines for statin and PCSK9 therapy are discussed in Chapter 28.

Table 1–5. Common elements of supportive smoking treatments.

Component	Examples
Encouragement of the patient in the quit attempt	Note that effective cessation treatments are now available. Note that half the people who have *ever* smoked have now quit. Communicate belief in the patient's ability to quit.
Communication of caring and concern	Ask how the patient feels about quitting. Directly express concern and a willingness to help. Be open to the patient's expression of fears of quitting, difficulties experienced, and ambivalent feelings.
Encouragement of the patient to talk about the quitting process	Ask about: Reasons that the patient wants to quit. Difficulties encountered while quitting. Success the patient has achieved. Concerns or worries about quitting.
Provision of basic information about smoking and successful quitting	Inform the patient about: The nature and time course of withdrawal. The addictive nature of smoking. The fact that any smoking (even a single puff) increases the likelihood of full relapse.

Cholesterol Treatment Trialists' (CTT) Collaboration; Fulcher J et al. Efficacy and safety of LDL-lowering therapy among men and women: meta-analysis of individual data from 174,000 participants in 27 randomised trials. Lancet. 2015 Apr 11; 385(9976):1397–405. [PMID: 25579834]

Navarese EP et al. Association between baseline LDL-C level and total and cardiovascular mortality after LDL-C lowering: a systematic review and meta-analysis. JAMA. 2018 Apr 17; 319(15):1566–79. [PMID: 29677301]

Pagidipati NJ et al. Comparison of recommended eligibility for primary prevention statin therapy based on the US Preventive Services Task Force Recommendations vs the ACC/AHA Guidelines. JAMA. 2017 Apr 18;317(15):1563–7. [PMID: 28418481]

US Preventive Services Task Force. Statin use for the primary prevention of cardiovascular disease in adults: US Preventive Services Task Force Recommendation Statement. JAMA. 2016 Nov 15;316(19):1997–2007. [PMID: 27838723]

Hypertension

Over 67 million adults in the United States have hypertension, representing 29% of the adult US population (see Chapter 11). Hypertension in nearly half of these adults is not controlled (ie, less than 140/90 mm Hg). Among those whose hypertension is not well controlled, nearly 40% are not aware of their elevated blood pressure; almost 16% are aware but not being treated; and 45% are being treated but the hypertension is not controlled. In every adult age group, higher values of systolic and diastolic blood pressure carry greater risks of stroke and heart failure. Systolic blood pressure is a better predictor of morbid events than diastolic blood pressure. Home monitoring is better correlated with target organ damage than clinic-based values. Clinicians can apply specific blood pressure criteria, such as those of the Joint National Committee or American Heart Association guidelines, along with consideration of the patient's cardiovascular risk and personal values, to decide at what levels treatment should be considered in individual cases.

Primary prevention of hypertension can be accomplished by strategies aimed at both the general population and special high-risk populations. The latter include persons with high-normal blood pressure or a family history of hypertension, blacks, and individuals with various behavioral risk factors, such as physical inactivity; excessive consumption of salt, alcohol, or calories; and deficient intake of potassium. Effective interventions for primary prevention of hypertension include reduced sodium and alcohol consumption, weight loss, and regular exercise. Potassium supplementation lowers blood pressure modestly, and a diet high in fresh fruits and vegetables and low in fat, red meats, and sugar-containing beverages also reduces blood pressure. Interventions of unproven efficacy include pill supplementation of potassium, calcium, magnesium, fish oil, or fiber; macronutrient alteration; and stress management.

Improved identification and treatment of hypertension is a major cause of the recent decline in stroke deaths as well as the reduction in incidence of heart failure–related hospitalizations. Because hypertension is usually asymptomatic, screening is strongly recommended to identify patients for treatment. Elevated office readings should be confirmed with repeated measurements, ideally from ambulatory monitoring or home measurements. Despite strong recommendations in favor of screening and treatment, hypertension control remains suboptimal. An intervention that included both patient and provider education was more effective than provider education alone in achieving control of hypertension, suggesting the benefits of patient participation; another trial found that home monitoring combined with telephone-based nurse support was more effective than home monitoring alone for blood pressure control. Pharmacologic management of hypertension is discussed in Chapter 11.

Ettehad D et al. Blood pressure lowering for prevention of cardiovascular disease and death: a systematic review and meta-analysis. Lancet. 2016 Mar 5;387(10022):957–67. [PMID: 26724178]

Fryar CD et al. Hypertension prevalence and control among adults: United States, 2015-2016. NCHS Data Brief. 2017 Oct; (289):1–8. [PMID: 29155682]

Piper MA et al. Diagnostic and predictive accuracy of blood pressure screening methods with consideration of rescreening intervals: a systematic review for the US Preventive Services Task Force. Ann Intern Med. 2015 Feb 3;162(3):192–204. [PMID: 25531400]

Weiss J et al. Benefits and harms of intensive blood pressure treatment in adults aged 60 years or older: a systematic review and meta-analysis. Ann Intern Med. 2017 Mar 21;166(6): 419–29. [PMID: 28114673]

Whelton PK et al. ACC/AHA/AAPA/ABC/ACPM/AGS/APhA/ ASH/ASPC/NMA/PCNA guideline for the prevention, detection, evaluation, and management of high blood pressure in adults: a report of the American College of Cardiology/ American Heart Association Task Force on Clinical Practice Guidelines. Hypertension. 2018 Jun;71(6):1269–324. [PMID: 29133354]

Chemoprevention

Regular use of low-dose aspirin (81–325 mg) can reduce cardiovascular events but increases gastrointestinal bleeding. Aspirin may also reduce the risk of death from several common types of cancer (colorectal, esophageal, gastric, breast, prostate, and possibly lung). The potential benefits of aspirin appear to exceed the harms for middle-aged adults who are at increased cardiovascular risk, which can be defined as a 10-year risk of greater than 10%, and who do not have an increased risk of bleeding. A newer trial in older healthy adults did not find clear benefit from aspirin for reduction of cardiovascular events and saw an increase in all-cause mortality with aspirin. Therefore, aspirin should not be routinely initiated in healthy adults over age 70.

Nonsteroidal anti-inflammatory drugs may reduce the incidence of colorectal adenomas and polyps but may also increase heart disease and gastrointestinal bleeding, and thus are not recommended for colon cancer prevention in average-risk patients.

Antioxidant vitamin (vitamin E, vitamin C, and beta-carotene) supplementation produced no significant reductions in the 5-year incidence of—or mortality from—vascular disease, cancer, or other major outcomes in high-risk individuals with coronary artery disease, other occlusive arterial disease, or diabetes mellitus.

Gaziano JM. Aspirin for primary prevention: clinical considerations in 2019. JAMA. 2019 Jan 22;321(3):253–55. [PMID: 30667488]

Guirguis-Blake JM et al. Aspirin for the primary prevention of cardiovascular events: a systematic evidence review for the US Preventive Services Task Force. Ann Intern Med. 2016 Jun 21;164(12):804–13. [PMID: 27064410]

McNeil JJ et al; ASPREE Investigator Group. Effect of aspirin on cardiovascular events and bleeding in the healthy elderly. N Engl J Med. 2018 Oct 18;379(16):1509–18. [PMID: 30221597]

Zheng SL et al. Association of aspirin use for primary prevention with cardiovascular events and bleeding events: a systematic review and meta-analysis. JAMA. 2019 Jan 22;321(3):277–87. [PMID: 30667501]

PREVENTION OF OSTEOPOROSIS

See Chapter 26.

Osteoporosis, characterized by low bone mineral density, is common and associated with an increased risk of fracture. The lifetime risk of an osteoporotic fracture is approximately 50% for women and 30% for men. Osteoporotic fractures can cause significant pain and disability. As such, research has focused on means of preventing osteoporosis and related fractures. Primary prevention strategies include calcium supplementation, vitamin D supplementation, and exercise programs. The effectiveness of calcium and vitamin D for fracture prevention remain controversial, particularly in noninstitutionalized individuals.

Screening for osteoporosis on the basis of low bone mineral density is recommended for women over age 65, based on indirect evidence that screening can identify women with low bone mineral density and that treatment of women with low bone density with bisphosphonates is effective in reducing fractures. However, real-world adherence to pharmacologic therapy for osteoporosis is low: one-third to one-half of patients do not take their medication as directed. Screening for osteoporosis is also recommended in younger women who are at increased risk. The effectiveness of screening in men has not been established. Concern has been raised that bisphosphonates may increase the risk of certain uncommon atypical types of femoral fractures and rare osteonecrosis of the jaw, making consideration of the benefits and risks of therapy important when considering osteoporosis screening.

Black DM et al. Clinical Practice. Postmenopausal osteoporosis. N Engl J Med. 2016 Jan 21;374(3):254–62. [PMID: 26789873]

US Preventive Services Task Force. Screening for osteoporosis to prevent fractures: US Preventive Services Task Force recommendation statement. JAMA. 2018 Jun 26;319(24):2521–31. [PMID: 29946735]

US Preventive Services Task Force. Vitamin D, calcium, or combined supplementation for the primary prevention of fractures in community-dwelling adults: US Preventive Services Task Force recommendation statement. JAMA. 2018 Apr 17; 319(15):1592–9. [PMID: 29677309]

PREVENTION OF PHYSICAL INACTIVITY

Lack of sufficient physical activity is the second most important contributor to preventable deaths, trailing only tobacco use.

The US Department of Health and Human Services and the CDC recommend that adults (including older adults) engage in 150 minutes of moderate-intensity (such as brisk walking) or 75 minutes of vigorous-intensity (such as jogging or running) aerobic activity or an equivalent mix of moderate- and vigorous-intensity aerobic activity each week. In addition to activity recommendations, the CDC recommends activities to strengthen all major muscle groups (abdomen, arms, back, chest, hips, legs, and shoulders) at least twice a week.

Patients who engage in regular moderate to vigorous exercise have a lower risk of myocardial infarction, stroke, hypertension, hyperlipidemia, type 2 diabetes mellitus, diverticular disease, and osteoporosis. Evidence supports the recommended guidelines of 30 minutes of moderate physical activity on most days of the week in both the primary and secondary prevention of CHD.

In longitudinal cohort studies, individuals who report higher levels of leisure-time physical activity are less likely to gain weight. Conversely, individuals who are overweight are less likely to stay active. However, at least 60 minutes of daily moderate-intensity physical activity may be necessary to maximize weight loss and prevent significant weight regain. Moreover, adequate levels of physical activity appear to be important for the prevention of weight gain and the development of obesity. Physical activity also appears to have an independent effect on health-related outcomes, such as development of type 2 diabetes mellitus in patients with impaired glucose tolerance when compared with body weight, suggesting that adequate levels of activity may counteract the negative influence of body weight on health outcomes.

Physical activity can be incorporated into any person's daily routine. For example, the clinician can advise a patient to take the stairs instead of the elevator, to walk or bike instead of driving, to do housework or yard work, to get off the bus one or two stops earlier and walk the rest of the way, to park at the far end of the parking lot, or to walk during the lunch hour. The basic message should be the more the better, and anything is better than nothing.

To be more effective in counseling about exercise, clinicians can also incorporate motivational interviewing techniques, adopt a whole-practice approach (eg, use practice nurses to assist), and establish linkages with community agencies. Clinicians can incorporate the "5 As" approach:

1. Ask (identify those who can benefit).

2. Assess (current activity level).

3. Advise (individualize plan).

4. Assist (provide a written exercise prescription and support material).

5. Arrange (appropriate referral and follow-up).

Such interventions have a moderate effect on self-reported physical activity and cardiorespiratory fitness, even if they do not always help patients achieve a predetermined level of physical activity. In their counseling, clinicians should advise patients about both the benefits and risks of exercise, prescribe an exercise program appropriate for each patient, and provide advice to help prevent injuries and cardiovascular complications.

Although primary care providers regularly ask patients about physical activity and advise them with verbal counseling, few providers provide written prescriptions or perform fitness assessments. Tailored interventions may potentially help increase physical activity in individuals. Exercise counseling with a prescription, eg, for walking at either a hard intensity or a moderate intensity with a high frequency, can produce significant long-term improvements in cardiorespiratory fitness. To be effective, exercise prescriptions must include recommendations on type, frequency, intensity, time, and progression of exercise and must follow disease-specific guidelines. Several factors influence physical activity behavior, including personal, social (eg, family and work), and environmental (eg, access to exercise facilities and well-lit parks) factors. Walkable neighborhoods around workplaces support physical activity such as walking and bicycling. A community-based volunteer intervention resulted in increased walking activity among older women, who were at elevated risk for both inactivity and adverse health outcomes.

Broad-based interventions targeting various factors are often the most successful, and interventions to promote physical activity are more effective when health agencies work with community partners, such as schools, businesses, and health care organizations. Enhanced community awareness through mass media campaigns, school-based strategies, and policy approaches are proven strategies to increase physical activity.

Adlakha D et al. Home and workplace built environment supports for physical activity. Am J Prev Med. 2015 Jan;48(1):104–7. [PMID: 25442233]

Centers for Disease Control and Prevention (CDC). How much physical activity do adults need? 2015 Jun 4. https://www.cdc.gov/physicalactivity/basics/adults/index.htm

Giroir BP et al. Physical activity guidelines for health and prosperity in the United States [Viewpoint]. JAMA. 2018 Nov 20;320(19):1971–2. [PMID: 30418473]

Hoang TD et al. Effect of early adult patterns of physical activity and television viewing on midlife cognitive function. JAMA Psychiatry. 2016 Jan;73(1):73–9. [PMID: 26629780]

Kennedy AB et al. Tools clinicians can use to help get patients active. Curr Sports Med Rep. 2018 Aug;17(8):271–6. [PMID: 30095547]

Piercy KL et al. The physical activity guidelines for Americans. JAMA. 2018 Nov 20;320(19):2020–8. [PMID: 30418471]

Thompson PD et al. New physical activity guidelines: a call to activity for clinicians and patients [Editorial]. JAMA. 2018 Nov 20;320(19):1983–4. [PMID: 30418469]

Varma VR et al. Effect of community volunteering on physical activity: a randomized controlled trial. Am J Prev Med. 2016 Jan;50(1):106–10. [PMID: 26340864]

PREVENTION OF OVERWEIGHT & OBESITY

Obesity is now a true epidemic and public health crisis that both clinicians and patients must face. Normal body weight is defined as a body mass index (BMI), calculated as the weight in kilograms divided by the height in meters squared, of less than 25; overweight is defined as a BMI = 25.0–29.9, and obesity as a BMI greater than 30.

Risk assessment of the overweight and obese patient begins with determination of BMI, waist circumference for those with a BMI of 35 or less, presence of comorbid conditions, and a fasting blood glucose and lipid panel. Obesity is clearly associated with type 2 diabetes mellitus, hypertension, hyperlipidemia, cancer, osteoarthritis, cardiovascular disease, obstructive sleep apnea, and asthma. In addition, almost one-quarter of the US population currently has the metabolic syndrome.

Obesity is associated with a higher all-cause mortality rate. Data suggest an increase among those with grades 2 and 3 obesity (BMI more than 35); however, the impact on all-cause mortality among overweight (BMI 25–30) and grade 1 obesity (BMI 30–35) is questionable. Persons with a BMI of 40 or higher have death rates from cancers that are 52% higher for men and 62% higher for women than the rates in men and women of normal weight.

Prevention of overweight and obesity involves both increasing physical activity and dietary modification to reduce caloric intake. Adequate levels of physical activity appear to be important for the prevention of weight gain and the development of obesity. Physical activity programs consistent with public health recommendations may promote modest weight loss (~2 kg); however, the amount of weight loss for any one individual is highly variable.

Clinicians can help guide patients to develop personalized eating plans to reduce energy intake, particularly by recognizing the contributions of fat, concentrated carbohydrates, and large portion sizes (see Chapter 29). Patients typically underestimate caloric content, especially when consuming food away from home. Providing patients with caloric and nutritional information may help address the current obesity epidemic. To prevent the long-term chronic disease sequelae of overweight and obesity, clinicians must work with patients to modify other risk factors, eg, by smoking cessation (see previous section on cigarette smoking) and strict blood pressure and glycemic control (see Chapters 11 and 27).

Lifestyle modification, including diet, physical activity, and behavior therapy, has been shown to induce clinically significant weight loss. Other treatment options for obesity include pharmacotherapy and surgery (see Chapter 29). Counseling interventions or pharmacotherapy can produce modest (3–5 kg) sustained weight loss over 6–12 months. Counseling appears to be most effective when intensive and combined with behavioral therapy. Pharmacotherapy appears safe in the short term; long-term safety is still not established.

Commercial weight loss programs are effective in promoting weight loss and weight loss management. A randomized controlled trial of over 400 overweight or obese women demonstrated the effectiveness of a free prepared meal and incentivized structured weight loss program compared with usual care.

Weight loss strategies using dietary, physical activity, or behavioral interventions can produce significant improvements in weight among persons with prediabetes and a significant decrease in diabetes incidence. Lifestyle interventions including diet combined with physical activity are effective in achieving weight loss and reducing cardiometabolic risk factors among patients with severe obesity.

Bariatric surgical procedures, eg, adjustable gastric band, sleeve gastrectomy, and Roux-en-Y gastric bypass, are reserved for patients with morbid obesity whose BMI exceeds 40, or for less severely obese patients (with BMIs between 35 and 40) with high-risk comorbid conditions such as life-threatening cardiopulmonary problems (eg, severe sleep apnea, Pickwickian syndrome, and obesity-related cardiomyopathy) or severe diabetes mellitus. In selected patients, surgery can produce substantial weight loss (10–159 kg) over 1–5 years, with rare but sometimes severe complications. Nutritional deficiencies are one complication of bariatric surgical procedures and close monitoring of a patient's metabolic and nutritional status is essential.

Finally, clinicians seem to share a general perception that almost no one succeeds in long-term maintenance of weight loss. However, research demonstrates that approximately 20% of overweight individuals are successful at long-term weight loss (defined as losing 10% or more of initial body weight and maintaining the loss for 1 year or longer).

Clinicians must work to identify and provide the best prevention and treatment strategies for patients who are overweight and obese. Clinician advice on weight loss can have a significant impact on patient attempts to adjust weight-related behaviors. Unfortunately, many clinicians are poorly prepared to address obesity. Clinician bias and lack of training in behavior-change strategies impair the care of obese patients. Strategies to address these issues should be incorporated into innovative treatment and care-delivery strategies (see Chapter 29).

Dietz WH et al. Management of obesity: improvement of health-care training and systems for prevention and care. Lancet. 2015 Jun 20;385(9986):2521–33. [PMID: 25703112]

Evert AB et al. Lifestyle intervention: nutrition therapy and physical activity. Med Clin North Am. 2015 Jan;99(1):69–85. [PMID: 25456644]

Guth E. JAMA patient page. Healthy weight loss. JAMA. 2014 Sep 3;312(9):974. [PMID: 25182116]

Hartmann-Boyce J et al. Self-help for weight loss in overweight and obese adults: systematic review and meta-analysis. Am J Public Health. 2015 Mar;105(3):e43–57. [PMID: 25602873]

Ogden CL et al. Prevalence of childhood and adult obesity in the United States, 2011–2012. JAMA. 2014 Feb 26;311(8):806–14. [PMID: 24570244]

Ryan DH et al. Guideline recommendations for obesity management. Med Clin North Am. 2018 Jan;102(1):49–63. [PMID: 29156187]

Swift DL et al. The role of exercise and physical activity in weight loss and maintenance. Prog Cardiovasc Dis. 2014 Jan–Feb; 56(4):441–7. [PMID: 24438736]

CANCER PREVENTION

Primary Prevention

Cancer mortality rates continue to decrease in the United States; part of this decrease results from reductions in tobacco use, since cigarette smoking is the most important preventable cause of cancer. Primary prevention of skin cancer consists of restricting exposure to ultraviolet light by wearing appropriate clothing, and use of sunscreens. Persons who engage in regular physical exercise and avoid obesity have lower rates of breast and colon cancer. Prevention of occupationally induced cancers involves minimizing exposure to carcinogenic substances, such as asbestos, ionizing radiation, and benzene compounds. Chemoprevention has been widely studied for primary cancer prevention (see earlier Chemoprevention section and Chapter 39). Use of tamoxifen, raloxifene, and aromatase inhibitors for breast cancer prevention is discussed in Chapters 17 and 39. Hepatitis B vaccination can prevent hepatocellular carcinoma (HCC), and screening and vaccination programs may be cost effective and useful in preventing HCC in high-risk groups, such as Asians and Pacific Islanders. Screening and treatment of hepatitis C is another strategy to prevent HCC (see Chapter 16). The use of HPV vaccine to prevent cervical and possibly anal cancer is discussed earlier in this chapter. HPV vaccines may also have a role in the prevention of HPV-related head and neck cancers. Guidelines for optimal cancer screening in adults over the age of 75 are unsettled; thus, an individualized approach that considers differences in disease risk rather than chronological age alone is recommended.

Breslau ES et al. An individualized approach to cancer screening decisions in older adults: a multilevel framework. J Gen Intern Med. 2016 May;31(5):539–47. [PMID: 26941042]

Salzman B et al. Cancer screening in older patients. Am Fam Physician. 2016 Apr 15;93(8):659–67. [PMID: 27175838]

Smith RA et al. Cancer screening in the United States, 2016: a review of current American Cancer Society guidelines and current issues in cancer screening. CA Cancer J Clin. 2016 Mar–Apr;66(2):96–114. [PMID: 26797525]

Wernli KJ et al. Screening for skin cancer in adults: updated evidence report and systematic review for the US Preventive Services Task Force. JAMA. 2016 Jul 26;316(4):436–47. [PMID: 27458949]

Screening & Early Detection

Screening prevents death from cancers of the breast, colon, and cervix. Current cancer screening recommendations from the USPSTF are shown in Table 1–6. Despite an increase in rates of screening for breast, cervical, and colon cancer over the last decade, overall screening for these cancers is suboptimal. Interventions effective in promoting recommended cancer screening include group education, one-on-one education, patient reminders, reduction of structural barriers, reduction of out-of-pocket costs, and provider assessment and feedback.

Though breast cancer mortality is generally reduced with mammography screening, evidence from randomized trials suggests that screening mammography has both benefits and downsides. Clinicians should discuss the risks and benefits with each patient and consider individual patient preferences when deciding when to begin screening (see Chapters 17 and e6).

Digital mammography is more sensitive in women with dense breasts and in younger women; however, studies exploring outcomes are lacking. MRI is not currently recommended for general screening, and its impact on breast cancer mortality is uncertain; nevertheless, the American Cancer Society recommends it for women at high risk (20–25% or more), including those with a strong family history of breast or ovarian cancer. Screening with both MRI and mammography might be superior to mammography alone in ruling out cancerous lesions in women with an inherited predisposition to breast cancer. Digital breast tomosynthesis (three-dimensional mammography) integrated with digital mammography increases cancer detection rates compared to digital mammography alone; however, the extent of improved detection and impact on assessment outcomes need further exploration.

All current recommendations call for cervical and colorectal cancer screening. Screening for testicular cancers among asymptomatic adolescent or adult males is not recommended by the USPSTF. Prostate cancer screening remains controversial, since no completed trials have answered the question of whether early detection and treatment after screen detection produce sufficient benefits

Table 1–6. Cancer screening recommendations for average-risk adults: US Preventive Services Task Force (USPSTF).[1]

Type of Screening	USPSTF Recommendation/[Year Issued]
Breast cancer screening	Recommends biennial screening mammography for women aged 50–74 years. (B) The decision to start screening mammography in women prior to age 50 years should be an individual one. Women who place a higher value on the potential benefit than the potential harms may choose to begin biennial screening between the ages of 40 and 49 years. (C) [2016]
Cervical cancer screening	Recommends screening for cervical cancer in women aged 21–65 years with cytology (Pap smear) every 3 years or, for women aged 30–65 years who want to lengthen the screening interval, screening with a combination of cytology and human papillomavirus (HPV) testing every 5 years. (A) Recommends against screening for cervical cancer in women younger than 21 years. (D) Recommends against screening for cervical cancer in women older than 65 years who have had adequate prior screening and are not otherwise at high risk for cervical cancer. (D) Recommends against screening for cervical cancer in women who have had a hysterectomy with removal of the cervix and who do not have a history of a high-grade precancerous lesion (ie, cervical intraepithelial neoplasia [CIN] grade 2 or 3) or cervical cancer. (D) [2018]
Colorectal cancer (CRC) screening	Recommends screening for CRC starting at age 50 years and continuing until age 75 years. (A) The decision to screen for CRC in adults aged 76–85 years should be an individual one, taking into account the patient's overall health and prior screening history. (C) [2016] Available tests include fecal occult blood tests (gFOBT, FIT) every year; FIT-DNA every 1 or 3 years; colonoscopy every 10 years; CT colonography every 5 years; flexible sigmoidoscopy every 5 years; flexible sigmoidoscopy every 10 years plus FIT every 1 year.
Lung cancer screening	Recommends annual lung cancer screening using low-dose CT in current smokers aged 55–80 years with a 30-pack-year smoking history, or in smokers who quit within the past 15 years. (B) Recommends stopping screening once a person has not smoked for 15 years or a health problem that significantly limits life expectancy has developed. [2013]
Prostate cancer screening	Recommends that clinicians individualize the decision to inform men aged 55–69 years about the potential benefits and harms of prostate-specific antigen (PSA)–based screening for prostate cancer. (C) Recommends against PSA–based screening for prostate cancer in men age 70 years and older. (D) [2018]
Testicular cancer screening	Recommends against screening for testicular cancer in adolescent or adult males. (D) [2011]

[1]US Preventive Services Task Force recommendations available at https://www.uspreventiveservicestaskforce.org/BrowseRec/Index/browse-recommendations.

Recommendation A: The USPSTF strongly recommends that clinicians routinely provide the service to eligible patients. (The USPSTF found good evidence that the service improves important health outcomes and concludes that benefits substantially outweigh harms.)
Recommendation B: The USPSTF recommends that clinicians routinely provide the service to eligible patients. (The USPSTF found at least fair evidence that the service improves important health outcomes and concludes that benefits substantially outweigh harms.)
Recommendation C: The USPSTF recommends against routinely providing the service. There may be considerations that support providing the service in an individual patient. There is at least moderate certainty that the net benefit is small.
Recommendation D: The USPSTF recommends against routinely providing the service to asymptomatic patients. (The USPSTF found at least fair evidence that the service is ineffective or that harms outweigh benefits.)
Recommendation I: The USPSTF concludes that the evidence is insufficient to recommend for or against routinely providing the service.

to outweigh harms of treatment. For men between the ages of 55 and 69, the decision to screen should be individualized and include a discussion of its risks and benefits with a clinician. The USPSTF recommends against PSA-based prostate cancer screening for men older than age 70 years (grade D recommendation).

Annual or biennial fecal occult blood testing reduces mortality from colorectal cancer by 16–33%. Fecal immunochemical tests (FIT) are superior to guaiac-based fecal occult blood tests (gFOBT) in detecting advanced adenomatous polyps and colorectal cancer, and patients are more likely to favor FIT over gFOBT. Randomized trials using sigmoidoscopy as the screening method found 20–30% reductions in mortality from colorectal cancer. Colonoscopy has also been advocated as a screening examination. It is more accurate than flexible sigmoidoscopy for detecting cancer and polyps, but its value in reducing colon cancer mortality has not been studied directly. CT colonography (virtual colonoscopy) is a noninvasive option in screening for colorectal cancer. It has been shown to have a high safety profile and performance similar to colonoscopy. The American College of Physicians (ACP) recommends clinicians stop screening for colorectal cancer in individuals over the age of 75 years or with a life expectancy of less than 10 years. The USPSTF recommends screening for colorectal cancer starting at age 50 years and continuing until age 75 years (grade A recommendation) but says that the decision to screen for colorectal cancer in adults aged 76–85 years should be an individual one, taking into account the patient's overall health and prior screening history (grade C recommendation).

The USPSTF recommends screening for cervical cancer in women aged 21–65 years with a Papanicolaou smear (cytology) every 3 years or, for women aged 30–65 years who desire longer intervals, screening with cytology and HPV testing every 5 years. The USPSTF recommends against screening in women younger than 21 years of age and average-risk women over 65 with adequate negative prior screenings. Receipt of HPV vaccination has no impact on screening intervals.

Women whose cervical specimen HPV tests are positive but cytology results are otherwise negative should repeat cotesting in 12 months (option 1) or undergo HPV-genotype–specific testing for types 16 or 16/18 (option 2). Colposcopy is recommended in women who test positive for types 16 or 16/18. Women with atypical squamous cells of undetermined significance (ASCUS) on cytology and a negative HPV test result should continue routine screening as per age-specific guidelines.

In a randomized, controlled trial, transvaginal ultrasound combined with serum cancer antigen 125 (CA-125) as screening tools to detect ovarian cancer did not reduce mortality. Furthermore, complications were associated with diagnostic evaluations to follow up false-positive screening test results. Thus, screening for ovarian cancer with transvaginal ultrasound and CA-125 is not recommended.

Evidence suggests that chest CT is significantly more sensitive than chest radiography in identifying small asymptomatic lung cancers; however, controversy exists regarding the efficacy and cost-effectiveness of low-dose CT screening in high-risk individuals.

The USPSTF recommends annual lung cancer screening with low-dose CT in current smokers aged 55 to 80 years with a 30-pack-year smoking history or smokers who quit within the past 15 years. Screening should stop once a person has not smoked for 15 years or a health problem that significantly limits life expectancy has developed. Screening should not be viewed as an alternative to smoking cessation.

Jin J. JAMA patient page. Screening tests for colorectal cancer. JAMA. 2016 Jun 21;315(23):2636. [PMID: 27305292]

Li T et al. Digital breast tomosynthesis (3D mammography) for breast cancer screening and for assessment of screen-recalled findings: review of the evidence. Expert Rev Anticancer Ther. 2018 Aug;18(8):785–91. [PMID: 29847744]

Lieberman D et al. Screening for colorectal cancer and evolving issues for physicians and patients: a review. JAMA. 2016 Nov 22; 316(20):2135–45. [PMID: 27893135]

Melnikow J et al. Supplemental screening for breast cancer in women with dense breasts: a systematic review for the US Preventive Services Task Force. Ann Intern Med. 2016 Feb 16; 164(4):268–78. [PMID: 26757021]

Moyer VA; US Preventive Services Task Force. Screening for lung cancer: US Preventive Services Task Force recommendation statement. Ann Intern Med. 2014 Mar 4;160(5):330–8. [PMID: 24378917]

Nelson HD et al. Effectiveness of breast cancer screening: systematic review and meta-analysis to update the 2009 US Preventive Services Task Force Recommendation. Ann Intern Med. 2016 Feb 16;164(4):244–55. [PMID: 26756588]

Tanoue LT et al. Lung cancer screening. Am J Respir Crit Care Med. 2015 Jan 1;191(1):19–33. [PMID: 25369325]

US Preventive Services Task Force; Grossman DC et al. Screening for prostate cancer: US Preventive Services Task Force recommendation statement. JAMA. 2018 May 8;319(18):1901–13. Erratum in: JAMA. 2018 Jun 19;319(23):2443. [PMID: 29801017]

US Preventive Services Task Force; Grossman DC et al. Screening for ovarian cancer: US Preventive Services Task Force recommendation statement. JAMA. 2018 Feb 13;319(6):588–94. [PMID: 29450531]

US Preventive Services Task Force; Curry SJ et al. Screening for cervical cancer: US Preventive Services Task Force recommendation statement. JAMA. 2018 Aug 21;320(7):674–86. [PMID: 30140884]

Wood DE. National Comprehensive Cancer Network (NCCN) clinical practice guidelines for lung cancer screening. Thorac Surg Clin. 2015 May;25(2):185–97. [PMID: 25901562]

PREVENTION OF INJURIES & VIOLENCE

Injuries remain the most important cause of loss of potential years of life before age 65. Homicide and motor vehicle accidents are a major cause of injury-related deaths among young adults, and accidental falls are the most common cause of injury-related death in older adults. Approximately one-third of all injury deaths include a diagnosis of traumatic brain injury, which has been associated with an increased risk of suicide.

Although motor vehicle accident deaths per miles driven have declined in the United States, there has been an increase in motor vehicle accidents related to distracted driving (using a cell phone, texting, eating). Evidence also suggests that motorists' use of sleeping medications (such as zolpidem) almost doubles the risk of motor vehicle accidents. Clinicians should discuss this risk when selecting a sleeping medication. For 16- and 17-year-old drivers, the risk of fatal crashes increases with the number of passengers.

Men ages 16–35 are at especially high risk for serious injury and death from accidents and violence, with blacks and Latinos at greatest risk. Deaths from firearms have reached epidemic levels in the United States. In 2015, a total of 13,286 people were killed in the United States in a gun homicide, unintentional shooting, or murder/suicide. Having a gun in the home increases the likelihood of homicide nearly threefold and of suicide fivefold. Educating clinicians to recognize and treat depression as well as restricting access to lethal methods have been found to reduce suicide rates.

In addition, clinicians should try to educate their patients about always wearing seat belts and safety helmets, about the risks of using cellular telephones or texting while driving and of drinking and driving—or of using other intoxicants (including marijuana) or long-acting benzodiazepines and then driving—and about the risks of having guns in the home.

Clinicians have a critical role in the detection, prevention, and management of intimate partner violence (see Chapter e6). The USPSTF recommends screening women of childbearing age for intimate partner violence and providing or referring women to intervention services when needed. Inclusion of a single question in the medical history—"At any time, has a partner ever hit you, kicked you, or otherwise physically hurt you?"—can increase identification of this common problem. Assessment for abuse and offering of referrals to community resources create the potential to interrupt and prevent recurrence of domestic violence and associated trauma. Clinicians should take an active role in following up with patients whenever possible, since intimate partner violence screening with passive referrals to services may not be adequate. Evaluation of services available to patients after identification of intimate partner violence should be a priority.

Physical and psychological abuse, exploitation, and neglect of older adults are serious, underrecognized problems; they may occur in up to 10% of elders. Risk factors for elder abuse include a culture of violence in the family; a demented, debilitated, or depressed and socially isolated victim; and a perpetrator profile of mental illness, alcohol or drug abuse, or emotional and/or financial dependence on the victim. Clues to elder mistreatment include the patient's ill-kempt appearance, recurrent urgent-care visits, missed appointments, suspicious physical findings, and implausible explanations for injuries.

Dicola D et al. Intimate partner violence. Am Fam Physician. 2016 Oct 15;94(8):646–51. [PMID: 27929227]

Jin J. JAMA Patient Page. Screening for intimate partner violence, elder abuse, and abuse of vulnerable adults. JAMA. 2018 Oct 23;320(16):1718. [PMID: 30357300]

Riley CL et al; Society of Critical Care Medicine. Critical violent injury in the United States: a review and call to action. Crit Care Med. 2015 Nov;43(11):2460–7. [PMID: 26327199]

Sumner SA et al. Violence in the United States: status, challenges, and opportunities. JAMA. 2015 Aug 4;314(5):478–88. [PMID: 26241599]

PREVENTION OF SUBSTANCE USE DISORDER: ALCOHOL & ILLICIT DRUGS

Alcohol misuse is a major public health problem in the United States, where approximately 51% of adults 18 years and older are current regular drinkers (at least 12 drinks in the past year). Maximum recommended consumption for adult women and those older than 65 years is 3 or fewer drinks in any day (and less than 7 per week), and for adult men, 4 or fewer drinks in any day (and less than 14 per week). The spectrum of alcohol misuse includes risky drinking (alcohol consumption above the recommended daily, weekly, or per-occasion amounts), harmful use (a pattern causing damage to health), alcohol abuse (a pattern leading to clinically significant impairment or distress), and alcohol dependence (defined as three or more of the following: tolerance, withdrawal, increased consumption, desire to cut down use, giving up social activities, increased time using alcohol or recovering from use, continued use despite known adverse effects). Underdiagnosis and undertreatment of alcohol misuse is substantial, both because of patient denial and lack of detection of clinical clues.

As with cigarette use, clinician identification and counseling about alcohol misuse are essential. The USPSTF recommends screening adults aged 18 years and older for alcohol misuse.

The Alcohol Use Disorder Identification Test (AUDIT) consists of questions on the quantity and frequency of alcohol consumption, on alcohol dependence symptoms, and on alcohol-related problems (Table 1–7). The AUDIT questionnaire is a cost-effective and efficient diagnostic tool for routine screening of alcohol use disorders in primary care settings. Brief advice and counseling without regular follow-up and reinforcement cannot sustain significant long-term reductions in unhealthy drinking behaviors.

Time restraints may prevent clinicians from using the AUDIT to screen patients, but single-question screening tests for unhealthy alcohol use may help increase the frequency of subsequent AUDIT screening in primary care settings. The National Institute on Alcohol Abuse and Alcoholism recommends the following single-question screening test (validated in primary care settings): "How many times in the past year have you had X or more drinks in a day?" (X is 5 for men and 4 for women, and a response of more than 1 time is considered positive.)

Clinicians should provide those who screen positive for hazardous or risky drinking with brief behavioral counseling interventions to reduce alcohol misuse. Use of screening procedures and brief intervention methods (see Chapter 25) can produce a 10–30% reduction in long-term alcohol use and alcohol-related problems.

Several pharmacologic agents are effective in reducing alcohol consumption. In acute alcohol detoxification, long-acting benzodiazepines are preferred because they can be given on a fixed schedule or through "front-loading" or "symptom-triggered" regimens. Adjuvant sympatholytic medications can be used to treat hyperadrenergic symptoms that persist despite adequate sedation. Three drugs are FDA approved for treatment of alcohol dependence: disulfiram, naltrexone, and acamprosate. Topiramate is a promising treatment for alcohol dependence. A 6-month randomized trial of topiramate versus naltrexone revealed a greater reduction of alcohol intake and cravings in participants receiving topiramate. Topiramate's side effect profile is favorable, and its benefits appear to increase over time. Clinicians should be aware that although topiramate appears to be an effective treatment for alcohol dependence, the manufacturer has not pursued FDA approval for this indication.

Prescription and nonprescription opioid-based drug abuse, misuse, and overdose has reached epidemic proportions in the United States. Deaths due to opioid overdose have dramatically increased. Opioid risk mitigation

Table 1–7. Screening for alcohol abuse using the Alcohol Use Disorder Identification Test (AUDIT).

(Scores for response categories are given in parentheses. Scores range from 0 to 40, with a cutoff score of 5 or more indicating hazardous drinking, harmful drinking, or alcohol dependence.)				
1. How often do you have a drink containing alcohol?				
(0) Never	(1) Monthly or less	(2) Two to four times a month	(3) Two or three times a week	(4) Four or more times a week
2. How many drinks containing alcohol do you have on a typical day when you are drinking?				
(0) 1 or 2	(1) 3 or 4	(2) 5 or 6	(3) 7 to 9	(4) 10 or more
3. How often do you have six or more drinks on one occasion?				
(0) Never	(1) Less than monthly	(2) Monthly	(3) Weekly	(4) Daily or almost daily
4. How often during the past year have you found that you were not able to stop drinking once you had started?				
(0) Never	(1) Less than monthly	(2) Monthly	(3) Weekly	(4) Daily or almost daily
5. How often during the past year have you failed to do what was normally expected of you because of drinking?				
(0) Never	(1) Less than monthly	(2) Monthly	(3) Weekly	(4) Daily or almost daily
6. How often during the past year have you needed a first drink in the morning to get yourself going after a heavy drinking session?				
(0) Never	(1) Less than monthly	(2) Monthly	(3) Weekly	(4) Daily or almost daily
7. How often during the past year have you had a feeling of guilt or remorse after drinking?				
(0) Never	(1) Less than monthly	(2) Monthly	(3) Weekly	(4) Daily or almost daily
8. How often during the past year have you been unable to remember what happened the night before because you had been drinking?				
(0) Never	(1) Less than monthly	(2) Monthly	(3) Weekly	(4) Daily or almost daily
9. Have you or has someone else been injured as a result of your drinking?				
(0) No		(2) Yes, but not in the past year		(4) Yes, during the past year
10. Has a relative or friend or a doctor or other health worker been concerned about your drinking or suggested you cut down?				
(0) No		(2) Yes, but not in the past year		(4) Yes, during the past year

Adapted, with permission, from BMJ Publishing Group Ltd. and Piccinelli M et al. Efficacy of the alcohol use disorders identification test as a screening tool for hazardous alcohol intake and related disorders in primary care: a validity study. BMJ. 1997 Feb 8;314 (7078):420–4.

strategies include use of risk assessment tools, treatment agreements (contracts), and urine drug testing. Additional strategies include establishing and strengthening prescription drug monitoring programs, regulating pain management facilities, and establishing dosage thresholds requiring consultation with pain specialists. Medication-assisted treatment, the use of medications with counseling and behavioral therapy, is effective in the prevention of opioid overdose and substance abuse disorders. Methadone, buprenorphine, and naltrexone are FDA approved for use in medication-assisted treatment. Buprenorphine has potential as a medication to ameliorate the symptoms and signs of withdrawal from opioids and is effective in reducing concomitant cocaine and opioid abuse. The risk of overdose is lower with buprenorphine than methadone, and it is preferred for patients at high risk for methadone toxicity (see Chapter 5). The FDA supports greater access to naloxone and is currently exploring options to make naloxone more available to treat opioid overdose. (See Chapter 5.)

Use of illegal drugs—including cocaine, methamphetamine, and so-called designer drugs—either sporadically or episodically remains an important problem. Lifetime prevalence of drug abuse is approximately 8% and is generally greater among men, young and unmarried individuals, Native Americans, and those of lower socioeconomic status. As with alcohol, drug abuse disorders often coexist with personality, anxiety, and other substance abuse disorders. Abuse of anabolic-androgenic steroids has been associated with use of other illicit drugs, alcohol, and cigarettes and with violence and criminal behavior.

As with alcohol abuse, the lifetime treatment rate for drug abuse is low (8%). The recognition of drug abuse presents special problems and requires that the clinician actively consider the diagnosis. Clinical aspects of substance abuse are discussed in Chapter 25.

Delker E et al. Alcohol consumption in demographic subpopulations: an epidemiologic overview. Alcohol Res. 2016;38(1): 7–15. [PMID: 27159807]

Denny CH et al. Self-reported prevalence of alcohol screening among U.S. adults. Am J Prev Med. 2016 Mar;50(3):380–3. [PMID: 26520573]

Dowell D et al. CDC guideline for prescribing opioids for chronic pain—United States, 2016. JAMA. 2016 Apr 19; 315(15):1624–45. [PMID: 26977696]

Kaner EF et al. Effectiveness of brief alcohol interventions in primary care populations. Cochrane Database Syst Rev. 2018 Feb 24;2:CD004148. [PMID: 29476653]

Pace CA et al. Addressing unhealthy substance use in primary care. Med Clin North Am. 2018 Jul;102(4):567–86. [PMID: 29933816]

Peglow SL et al. Preventing opioid overdose in the clinic and hospital: analgesia and opioid antagonists. Med Clin North Am. 2018 Jul;102(4):621–34. [PMID: 29933819]

Substance Abuse and Mental Health Services Administration (SAMHSA). Medication-Assisted Treatment (MAT). https://www.samhsa.gov/medication-assisted-treatment

US Food and Drug Administration. Statement from FDA Commissioner Scott Gottlieb, MD, on unprecedented efforts to make naloxone available over-the-counter to help reduce deaths from opioid overdose. 2019 January 17. https://www.fda.gov/NewsEvents/Newsroom/PressAnnouncements/ucm629571.htm

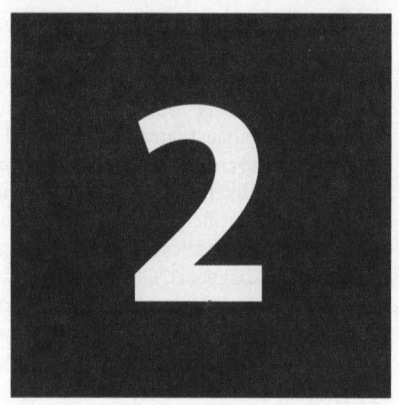

Common Symptoms

Paul L. Nadler, MD
Ralph Gonzales, MD, MSPH

COUGH

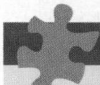

ESSENTIAL INQUIRIES

▶ Age, tobacco or cannabis use, occupational history, environmental exposures, and duration of cough.

▶ Dyspnea (at rest or with exertion).

▶ Vital signs (heart rate, respiratory rate, body temperature).

▶ Chest examination.

▶ Chest radiography when unexplained cough lasts more than 3–6 weeks.

▶ General Considerations

Cough is the most common symptom for which patients seek medical attention. Cough adversely affects personal and work-related interactions, disrupts sleep, and often causes discomfort of the throat and chest wall. Most people seeking medical attention for acute cough desire symptom relief; few are worried about serious illness. Cough results from stimulation of mechanical or chemical afferent nerve receptors in the bronchial tree. Effective cough depends on an intact afferent–efferent reflex arc, adequate expiratory and chest wall muscle strength, and normal mucociliary production and clearance.

▶ Clinical Findings

A. Symptoms

Distinguishing **acute** (less than 3 weeks), **persistent** (3–8 weeks), and **chronic** (more than 8 weeks) cough illness syndromes is a useful first step in evaluation. Postinfectious cough lasting 3–8 weeks has also been referred to as **subacute** cough to distinguish this common, distinct clinical entity from acute and chronic cough.

1. Acute cough—In healthy adults, most acute cough syndromes are due to viral respiratory tract infections. Additional features of infection such as fever, nasal congestion, and sore throat help confirm this diagnosis. Dyspnea (at rest or with exertion) may reflect a more serious condition, and further evaluation should include assessment of oxygenation (pulse oximetry or arterial blood gas measurement), airflow (peak flow or spirometry), and pulmonary parenchymal disease (chest radiography). The timing and character of the cough are not very useful in establishing the cause of acute cough syndromes, although cough-variant asthma should be considered in adults with prominent nocturnal cough, and persistent cough with phlegm increases the likelihood of chronic obstructive pulmonary disease (COPD). The presence of posttussive emesis or inspiratory whoop in adults modestly increases the likelihood of pertussis, and the absence of paroxysmal cough and the presence of fever decrease its likelihood. Uncommon causes of acute cough should be suspected in those with heart disease (heart failure [HF]) or hay fever (allergic rhinitis) and those with occupational risk factors (such as farmworkers).

2. Persistent and chronic cough—Cough due to acute respiratory tract infection resolves within 3 weeks in the vast majority (more than 90%) of patients. Pertussis should be considered in adolescents and adults with persistent or severe cough lasting more than 3 weeks, and in selected geographic areas where its prevalence approaches 20% (although its exact prevalence is difficult to ascertain due to the limited sensitivity of diagnostic tests).

When angiotensin-converting enzyme (ACE) inhibitor therapy, acute respiratory tract infection, and chest radiograph abnormalities are absent, most cases of persistent and chronic cough are due to (or exacerbated by) postnasal drip (upper airway cough syndrome), asthma, or gastroesophageal reflux disease (GERD), or some combination of these three entities. Approximately 10% of cases are caused by nonasthmatic eosinophilic bronchitis. A history of nasal or sinus congestion, wheezing, or heartburn should direct subsequent evaluation and treatment, though these conditions frequently cause persistent cough in the absence of typical symptoms. Dyspnea at rest or with exertion is not commonly reported among patients with persistent cough; dyspnea requires assessment for chronic lung disease, HF, anemia, pulmonary embolism, or pulmonary hypertension.

Bronchogenic carcinoma is suspected when cough is accompanied by unexplained weight loss, hemoptysis, and fevers with night sweats, particularly in persons with significant tobacco or occupational exposures (asbestos, radon, diesel exhaust, and metals). Persistent and chronic cough accompanied by excessive mucus secretions increases the likelihood of COPD, particularly among smokers, or of bronchiectasis if accompanied by a history of recurrent or complicated pneumonia; chest radiographs are helpful in diagnosis. Chronic cough with dry eyes may represent Sjögren syndrome. A chronic dry cough may be the first symptom of idiopathic pulmonary fibrosis.

B. Physical Examination

Examination can direct subsequent diagnostic testing for acute cough. Pneumonia is suspected when acute cough is accompanied by vital sign abnormalities (tachycardia, tachypnea, fever). Findings suggestive of airspace consolidation (rales, decreased breath sounds, fremitus, egophony) are significant predictors of community-acquired pneumonia but are present in the minority of cases. Purulent sputum is associated with bacterial infections in patients with structural lung disease (eg, COPD, cystic fibrosis), but it is a poor predictor of pneumonia in the otherwise healthy adult. Wheezing and rhonchi are frequent findings in adults with acute bronchitis and do not indicate consolidation or adult-onset asthma in most cases.

Examination of patients with persistent cough should look for evidence of chronic sinusitis, contributing to postnasal drip syndrome or asthma. Chest and cardiac signs may help distinguish COPD from HF. In patients with cough and dyspnea, a normal match test (ability to blow out a match from 25 cm away) and maximum laryngeal height greater than 4 cm (measured from the sternal notch to the cricoid cartilage at end expiration) substantially decrease the likelihood of COPD. Similarly, normal jugular venous pressure and no hepatojugular reflux decrease the likelihood of biventricular HF.

C. Diagnostic Studies

1. Acute cough—Chest radiography should be considered for any adult with acute cough whose vital signs are abnormal or whose chest examination suggests pneumonia. The relationship between specific clinical findings and the probability of pneumonia is shown in Table 2–1. A large, multicenter randomized clinical trial found that elevated serum C-reactive protein (levels greater than 30 mg/dL) improves diagnostic accuracy of clinical prediction rules for pneumonia in adults with acute cough; procalcitonin added no clinically relevant information. A meta-analysis found that lung ultrasonography had better accuracy than chest radiography for the diagnosis of adult community-acquired pneumonia. Lung ultrasonography had a pooled sensitivity of 0.95 (95% confidence interval [CI], 0.93–0.97) and a specificity of 0.90 (95% CI, 0.86–0.94). Chest radiography had a pooled sensitivity of 0.77 (95% CI, 0.73–0.80) and a specificity of 0.91 (95% CI, 0.87–0.94). In patients with dyspnea, pulse oximetry and peak flow help

Table 2–1. Positive and negative likelihood ratios for history, physical examination, and laboratory findings in the diagnosis of pneumonia.

Finding	Positive Likelihood Ratio	Negative Likelihood Ratio
Medical history		
Fever	1.7–2.1	0.6–0.7
Chills	1.3–1.7	0.7–0.9
Physical examination		
Tachypnea (RR > 25 breaths/min)	1.5–3.4	0.8
Tachycardia (> 100 beats/min in two studies or > 120 beats/min in one study)	1.6–2.3	0.5–0.7
Hyperthermia (> 37.8°C)	1.4–4.4	0.6–0.8
Chest examination		
Dullness to percussion	2.2–4.3	0.8–0.9
Decreased breath sounds	2.3–2.5	0.6–0.8
Crackles	1.6–2.7	0.6–0.9
Rhonchi	1.4–1.5	0.8–0.9
Egophony	2.0–8.6	0.8–1.0
Laboratory findings		
Leukocytosis (> 11 × 10^9/L in one study or ≥ 10.4 × 10^9/L in another study)	1.9–3.7	0.3–0.6

RR, respiratory rate.

exclude hypoxemia or obstructive airway disease. However, a normal pulse oximetry value (eg, greater than 93%) does not rule out a significant alveolar–arterial (A–a) gradient when patients have effective respiratory compensation. During documented outbreaks, clinical diagnosis of influenza has a positive predictive value of ~70%; this usually obviates the need for rapid diagnostic tests. No evidence exists to assess whether the initial evaluation of cough in immunocompromised patients should differ from immunocompetent patients, but expert recommendations suggest that tuberculosis be considered in HIV-infected patients in areas with a high prevalence of tuberculosis regardless of radiographic findings.

2. Persistent and chronic cough—Chest radiography is indicated when ACE inhibitor therapy–related and postinfectious cough are excluded. If pertussis is suspected, polymerase chain reaction testing should be performed on a nasopharyngeal swab or nasal wash specimen—although the ability to detect pertussis decreases as the duration of cough increases. When the chest film is normal, postnasal drip, asthma, or GERD are the most likely causes. The presence of typical symptoms of these conditions directs further evaluation or empiric therapy, though typical symptoms are often absent. Definitive tests for determining the presence

Table 2–2. Empiric therapy or definitive testing for persistent cough.

Suspected Condition	Step 1 (Empiric Therapy)	Step 2 (Definitive Testing)
Postnasal drip	Therapy for allergy or chronic sinusitis	Sinus CT scan; ENT referral
Asthma	Beta-2-agonist	Spirometry; consider methacholine challenge if normal
GERD	Lifestyle and diet modifications with or without proton pump inhibitors	Esophageal pH monitoring

ENT, ear, nose, and throat; GERD, gastroesophageal reflux disease.

of each are available (Table 2–2). However, empiric treatment with a maximum-strength regimen for postnasal drip, asthma, or GERD for 2–4 weeks is one recommended approach since documenting the presence of postnasal drip, asthma, or GERD does not mean they are the cause of the cough. Alternative approaches to identifying patients who have asthma with its corticosteroid-responsive cough include examining induced sputum for increased eosinophil counts (greater than 3%) or providing an empiric trial of prednisone, 30 mg daily orally for 2 weeks. Spirometry may help identify large airway obstruction in patients who have persistent cough and wheezing and who are not responding to asthma treatment. When empiric treatment trials are not successful, additional evaluation with pH manometry, endoscopy, barium swallow, sinus CT, or high-resolution chest CT may identify the cause.

▶ **Differential Diagnosis**

A. Acute Cough

Acute cough may be a symptom of acute respiratory tract infection, asthma, allergic rhinitis, and HF, as well as many less common causes.

B. Persistent and Chronic Cough

Causes of persistent cough include environmental exposures (cigarette smoke, air pollution), occupational exposures, pertussis, postnasal drip, asthma (including cough-variant asthma), GERD, COPD, bronchiectasis, eosinophilic bronchitis, tuberculosis or other chronic infection, interstitial lung disease, and bronchogenic carcinoma. COPD is a common cause of persistent cough among patients older than 50 years. Persistent cough may also be due to somatic cough syndrome (previously called "psychogenic cough") or tic cough (previously called "habit cough").

▶ **Treatment**

A. Acute Cough

Treatment of acute cough should target the underlying etiology of the illness, the cough reflex itself, and any additional factors that exacerbate the cough. Cough duration is typically 1–3 weeks, yet patients frequently expect cough to last fewer than 10 days. Limited studies on the use of dextromethorphan suggest a minor or modest benefit.

When influenza is diagnosed (including H1N1 influenza), oral oseltamivir or zanamivir or intravenous peramivir are equally effective (1 less day of illness) when initiated within 30–48 hours of illness onset; treatment is recommended regardless of illness duration when patients have severe influenza requiring hospitalization. In *Chlamydophila*- or *Mycoplasma*-documented infection or outbreaks, first-line antibiotics include erythromycin or doxycycline. Antibiotics do not improve cough severity or duration in patients with uncomplicated acute bronchitis. In patients with bronchitis and wheezing, inhaled beta-2-agonist therapy reduces severity and duration of cough. In patients with acute cough, treating the accompanying postnasal drip (with antihistamines, decongestants, or nasal corticosteroids) can be helpful. A Cochrane review (n = 163) found codeine to be no more effective than placebo in reducing cough symptoms.

B. Persistent and Chronic Cough

Evaluation and management of persistent cough often require multiple visits and therapeutic trials, which frequently lead to frustration, anger, and anxiety. When pertussis infection is suspected early in its course, treatment with a macrolide antibiotic (see Chapter 33) is appropriate to reduce organism shedding and transmission. When pertussis has lasted more than 7–10 days, antibiotic treatment does not affect the duration of cough, which can last up to 6 months. Early identification, revaccination with Tdap, and treatment of adult patients who work or live with persons at high risk for complications from pertussis (pregnant women, infants [particularly younger than 1 year], and immunosuppressed individuals) are encouraged.

Table 2–2 outlines empiric treatments for persistent cough. There is no evidence to guide how long to continue treatment for persistent cough due to postnasal drip, asthma, or GERD. Studies have not found a consistent benefit of inhaled corticosteroid therapy in adults with persistent cough. Eight weeks of thrice-weekly azithromycin did not improve cough in patients without asthma.

When empiric treatment trials fail, consider other causes of chronic cough such as obstructive sleep apnea, tonsillar or uvular enlargement, and environmental fungi. The small percentage of patients with idiopathic chronic cough should be managed in consultation with an otolaryngologist or a pulmonologist; consider a high-resolution CT scan of the lungs. Treatment options include nebulized lidocaine therapy and morphine sulfate, 5–10 mg orally twice daily. Sensory dysfunction of the laryngeal branches of the vagus nerve may contribute to persistent cough syndromes and may help explain the effectiveness of gabapentin in patients with chronic cough. Speech pathology therapy combined with pregabalin has some benefit in chronic refractory cough. In patients with reflex cough syndrome, therapy aimed at shifting the patient's attentional focus from internal stimuli to external focal points can be helpful. Proton pump inhibitors are not effective on their own; most benefit appears to come from lifestyle modifications and weight reduction.

When to Refer

- Failure to control persistent or chronic cough following empiric treatment trials.
- Patients with recurrent symptoms should be referred to an otolaryngologist, pulmonologist, or gastroenterologist.

When to Admit

- Patient at high risk for tuberculosis for whom compliance with respiratory precautions is uncertain.
- Need for urgent bronchoscopy, such as suspected foreign body.
- Smoke or toxic fume inhalational injury.
- Gas exchanged is impaired by cough.
- Patients at high risk for barotrauma (eg, recent pneumothorax).

Gibson P et al; CHEST Expert Cough Panel. Treatment of unexplained chronic cough: CHEST Guideline and Expert Panel Report. Chest. 2016 Jan;149(1):27–44. [PMID: 26426314]

Kahrilas PJ et al; CHEST Expert Cough Panel. Chronic cough due to gastroesophageal reflux in adults: CHEST guideline and expert panel report. Chest. 2016 Dec;150(6):1341–60. [PMID: 27614002]

Michaudet C et al. Chronic cough: evaluation and management. Am Fam Physician. 2017 Nov 1;96(9):575–80. [PMID: 29094873]

Moore A et al. Clinical characteristics of pertussis-associated cough in adults and children: a diagnostic systematic review and meta-analysis. Chest. 2017 Aug;152(2):353–67. [PMID: 28511929]

Nguyen VTN et al. Pertussis: the whooping cough. Prim Care. 2018 Sep;45(3):423–31. [PMID: 30115332]

Smith JA et al. Chronic cough. N Engl J Med. 2016 Oct 20; 375(16):1544–51. [PMID: 27797316]

Smith SM et al. Antibiotics for acute bronchitis. Cochrane Database Syst Rev. 2017 Jun 19;6:CD000245. [PMID: 28626858]

Teepe J et al; GRACE Consortium. Predicting the presence of bacterial pathogens in the airways of primary care patients with acute cough. CMAJ. 2017 Jan 16;189(2):E50–5. [PMID: 27777252]

DYSPNEA

> ### ESSENTIAL INQUIRIES
>
> ▶ Fever, cough, and chest pain.
> ▶ Vital sign measurements; pulse oximetry.
> ▶ Cardiac and chest examination.
> ▶ Chest radiography and arterial blood gas measurement in selected patients.

General Considerations

Dyspnea is a subjective experience or perception of uncomfortable breathing. There is a lack of empiric evidence on the prevalence, etiology, and prognosis of dyspnea in general practice. The relationship between level of dyspnea and the severity of underlying disease varies widely among individuals. Dyspnea can result from conditions that increase the mechanical effort of breathing (eg, asthma, COPD, restrictive lung disease, respiratory muscle weakness), conditions that produce compensatory tachypnea (eg, hypoxemia, acidosis), primary pulmonary vasculopathy (pulmonary hypertension), or psychogenic conditions. The following factors play a role in how and when dyspnea presents in patients: rate of onset, previous dyspnea, medications, comorbidities, psychological profile, and severity of underlying disorder.

Clinical Findings

A. Symptoms

The duration, severity, and periodicity of dyspnea influence the tempo of the clinical evaluation. Rapid onset or severe dyspnea in the absence of other clinical features should raise concern for pneumothorax, pulmonary embolism, or increased left ventricular end-diastolic pressure (LVEDP). Spontaneous pneumothorax is usually accompanied by chest pain and occurs most often in thin, young males and in those with underlying lung disease. Pulmonary embolism should always be suspected when a patient with new dyspnea reports a recent history (previous 4 weeks) of prolonged immobilization or surgery, estrogen therapy, or other risk factors for deep venous thrombosis (DVT) (eg, previous history of thromboembolism, cancer, obesity, lower extremity trauma) and when the cause of dyspnea is not apparent. Silent myocardial infarction, which occurs more frequently in diabetic persons and women, can result in increased LVEDP, acute HF, and dyspnea.

Accompanying symptoms provide important clues to causes of dyspnea. When cough and fever are present, pulmonary disease (particularly infection) is the primary concern; myocarditis, pericarditis, and septic emboli can present in this manner. Chest pain should be further characterized as acute or chronic, pleuritic or exertional. Although acute pleuritic chest pain is the rule in acute pericarditis and pneumothorax, most patients with pleuritic chest pain in the outpatient clinic have pleurisy due to acute viral respiratory tract infection. Periodic chest pain that precedes the onset of dyspnea suggests myocardial ischemia or pulmonary embolism. When associated with wheezing, most cases of dyspnea are due to acute bronchitis; however, other causes include new-onset asthma, foreign body, and vocal cord dysfunction. Interstitial lung disease and pulmonary hypertension should be considered in patients with symptoms (or history) of connective tissue disease.

When a patient reports prominent dyspnea with mild or no accompanying features, consider noncardiopulmonary causes of impaired oxygen delivery (anemia, methemoglobinemia, cyanide ingestion, carbon monoxide), metabolic acidosis, panic disorder, neuromuscular disorders, and chronic pulmonary embolism.

Platypnea-orthodeoxia syndrome is characterized by dyspnea and hypoxemia on sitting or standing that improves in the recumbent position. It may be caused by an intracardiac shunt, pulmonary vascular shunt, or ventilation-perfusion mismatch. Hyperthyroidism can cause dyspnea from increased ventilatory drive, respiratory muscle weakness, or pulmonary hypertension.

B. Physical Examination

A focused physical examination should include evaluation of the head and neck, chest, heart, and lower extremities. Visual inspection of the patient can suggest obstructive airway disease (pursed-lip breathing, use of accessory respiratory muscles, barrel-shaped chest), pneumothorax (asymmetric excursion), or metabolic acidosis (Kussmaul respirations). Patients with impending upper airway obstruction (eg, epiglottitis, foreign body) or severe asthma exacerbation sometimes assume a tripod position. Focal wheezing raises the suspicion for a foreign body or other bronchial obstruction. Maximum laryngeal height (the distance between the top of the thyroid cartilage and the suprasternal notch at end expiration) is a measure of hyperinflation. Obstructive airway disease is virtually nonexistent when a nonsmoking patient younger than 45 years has a maximum laryngeal height greater than 4 cm (Table 2–3). Absent breath sounds suggest a pneumothorax. An accentuated pulmonic component of the second heart sound (loud P2) is a sign of pulmonary hypertension and pulmonary embolism.

Table 2–4 shows clinical predictors of increased LVEDP in dyspneic patients with no prior history of HF. When none is present, there is a very low probability (less than 10%) of increased LVEDP, but when two or more are present, there is a very high probability (greater than 90%) of increased LVEDP.

C. Diagnostic Studies

Causes of dyspnea that can be managed without chest radiography are few: ingestions causing lactic acidosis, anemia, methemoglobinemia, and carbon monoxide poisoning. The diagnosis of pneumonia should be confirmed by chest

Table 2–3. Clinical findings suggesting obstructive airway disease.

Factor	Adjusted Likelihood Ratios	
	Factor Present	Factor Absent
> 40 pack-years smoking	11.6	0.9
Age ≥ 45 years	1.4	0.5
Maximum laryngeal height ≤ 4 cm	3.6	0.7
All three factors	58.5	0.3

Table 2–4. Clinical findings suggesting increased left ventricular end-diastolic pressure.

Tachycardia
Systolic hypotension
Jugular venous distention (> 5–7 cm H_2O)[1]
Hepatojugular reflux (> 1 cm)[2]
Crackles, especially bibasilar
Third heart sound[3]
Lower extremity edema
Radiographic pulmonary vascular redistribution or cardiomegaly[1]

[1]These findings are particularly helpful.
[2]Proper abdominal compression for evaluating hepatojugular reflux requires > 30 seconds of sustained right upper quadrant abdominal compression.
[3]Auscultation of the heart at 45-degree angle in left lateral decubitus position doubles the detection rate of third heart sounds.
Data from Badgett RG et al. Can the clinical examination diagnose left-sided heart failure in adults? JAMA. 1997 Jun 4;277(21):1712–9.

radiography in most patients, and elevated blood levels of procalcitonin or C-reactive protein can support the diagnosis of pneumonia in equivocal cases or in the presence of interstitial lung disease. Conversely, a low procalcitonin can help exclude pneumonia in dyspneic patients presenting with HF. Chest radiography is fairly sensitive and specific for new-onset HF (represented by redistribution of pulmonary venous circulation) and can help guide treatment of patients with other cardiac diseases. NT-proBNP can assist in the diagnosis of HF. End-expiratory chest radiography enhances detection of small pneumothoraces.

A normal chest radiograph has substantial diagnostic value. When there is no physical examination evidence of COPD or HF and the chest radiograph is normal, the major remaining causes of dyspnea include pulmonary embolism, *Pneumocystis jirovecii* infection (initial radiograph may be normal in up to 25%), upper airway obstruction, foreign body, anemia, and metabolic acidosis. If a patient has tachycardia and hypoxemia but a normal chest radiograph and electrocardiogram (ECG), then tests to exclude pulmonary emboli, anemia, or metabolic acidosis are warranted. High-resolution chest CT is particularly useful in the evaluation of interstitial and alveolar lung disease. Helical ("spiral") CT is useful to diagnose pulmonary embolism since the images are high resolution and require only one breathhold by the patient, but to minimize unnecessary testing and radiation exposure, the clinician should first consider a clinical decision rule (with or without D-dimer testing) to estimate the pretest probability of a pulmonary embolism. It is appropriate to forego CT scanning in patients with very low probability of pulmonary embolus when other causes of dyspnea are more likely (see Chapter 9).

Table 2–4 shows clinical findings suggesting increased LVEDP. Elevated serum B-type natriuretic peptide (BNP or NT-proBNP) levels are both sensitive and specific for increased LVEDP in symptomatic persons. BNP has been shown to reliably diagnose severe dyspnea caused by HF and to differentiate it from dyspnea due to other conditions.

Arterial blood gas measurement may be considered if clinical examination and routine diagnostic testing are equivocal. With two notable exceptions (carbon monoxide poisoning and cyanide toxicity), arterial blood gas measurement distinguishes increased mechanical effort causes of dyspnea (respiratory acidosis with or without hypoxemia) from compensatory tachypnea (respiratory alkalosis with or without hypoxemia or metabolic acidosis) and from psychogenic dyspnea (respiratory alkalosis). An observational study, however, found that arterial blood gas measurement had little value in determining the cause of dyspnea in patients presenting to the emergency department. Carbon monoxide and cyanide impair oxygen delivery with minimal alterations in Po_2; percent carboxyhemoglobin identifies carbon monoxide toxicity. Cyanide poisoning should be considered in a patient with profound lactic acidosis following exposure to burning vinyl (such as a theater fire or industrial accident). Suspected carbon monoxide poisoning or methemoglobinemia can also be confirmed with venous carboxyhemoglobin or methemoglobin levels. Venous blood gas testing is also an option for assessing respiratory and acid-base status by measuring venous pH and Pco_2 but is unable to provide information on oxygenation status. To correlate with arterial blood gas values, venous pH is typically 0.03–0.05 units lower, and venous Pco_2 is typically 4–5 mm Hg higher than arterial samples.

Because arterial blood gas testing is impractical in most outpatient settings, **pulse oximetry** has assumed a central role in the office evaluation of dyspnea. Oxygen saturation values above 96% almost always correspond with a Po_2 greater than 70 mm Hg, whereas values less than 94% may represent clinically significant hypoxemia. Important exceptions to this rule include carbon monoxide toxicity, which leads to a normal oxygen saturation (due to the similar wavelengths of oxyhemoglobin and carboxyhemoglobin), and methemoglobinemia, which results in an oxygen saturation of about 85% that fails to increase with supplemental oxygen. A delirious or obtunded patient with obstructive lung disease warrants immediate measurement of arterial blood gases to exclude hypercapnia and the need for intubation, regardless of the oxygen saturation. If a patient reports dyspnea with exertion, but resting oximetry is normal, assessment of desaturation with ambulation (eg, a brisk walk around the clinic) can be useful for confirming impaired gas exchange.

A study found that for adults without known cardiac or pulmonary disease reporting dyspnea on exertion, spirometry, NT-proBNP, and CT imaging were the most informative tests.

Episodic dyspnea can be challenging if an evaluation cannot be performed during symptoms. Life-threatening causes include recurrent pulmonary embolism, myocardial ischemia, and reactive airway disease. When associated with audible wheezing, vocal cord dysfunction should be considered, particularly in a young woman who does not respond to asthma therapy. Spirometry is very helpful in further classifying patients with obstructive airway disease but is rarely needed in the initial or emergent evaluation of patients with acute dyspnea.

► Differential Diagnosis

Urgent and emergent conditions causing acute dyspnea include pneumonia, COPD, asthma, pneumothorax, pulmonary embolism, cardiac disease (eg, HF, acute myocardial infarction, valvular dysfunction, arrhythmia, intracardiac shunt), pleural effusion, diffuse alveolar hemorrhage, metabolic acidosis, cyanide toxicity, methemoglobinemia, and carbon monoxide poisoning. Chronic dyspnea may be caused by interstitial lung disease and pulmonary hypertension.

► Treatment

The treatment of urgent or emergent causes of dyspnea should aim to relieve the underlying cause. Pending diagnosis, patients with hypoxemia should be immediately provided supplemental oxygen unless significant hypercapnia is present or strongly suspected pending arterial blood gas measurement. Dyspnea frequently occurs in patients nearing the end of life. Opioid therapy, anxiolytics, and corticosteroids can provide substantial relief independent of the severity of hypoxemia. However, inhaled opioids are not effective. Oxygen therapy is most beneficial to patients with significant hypoxemia (Pao_2 less than 55 mm Hg) (see Chapter 5). In patients with severe COPD and hypoxemia, oxygen therapy improves exercise performance and mortality. Pulmonary rehabilitation programs are another therapeutic option for patients with moderate to severe COPD or interstitial pulmonary fibrosis. Noninvasive ventilation may be considered for patients with dyspnea caused by an acute COPD exacerbation, but the efficacy of this treatment is still uncertain.

► When to Refer

- Following acute stabilization, patients with advanced COPD should be referred to a pulmonologist, and patients with HF or valvular heart disease should be referred to a cardiologist.

- Cyanide toxicity or carbon monoxide poisoning should be managed in conjunction with a toxicologist.

- Lung transplantation can be considered for patients with advanced interstitial lung disease.

► When to Admit

- Impaired gas exchange from any cause or high risk of pulmonary embolism pending definitive diagnosis.

- Suspected cyanide toxicity or carbon monoxide poisoning.

Freund Y et al; PROPER Investigator Group. Effect of the Pulmonary Embolism Rule-Out Criteria on subsequent thromboembolic events among low-risk emergency department patients: the PROPER randomized clinical trial. JAMA. 2018 Feb 13;319(6):559–66. [PMID: 29450523]

Mahler DA. Evaluation of dyspnea in the elderly. Clin Geriatr Med. 2017 Nov;33(4):503–21. [PMID: 28991647]

Pisani L et al. Management of dyspnea in the terminally ill. Chest. 2018 Oct;154(4):925–34. [PMID: 29679597]

Taggart C. Shortness of breath: looking beyond the usual suspects. J Fam Pract. 2016 Aug;65(8):526–33. [PMID: 27660836]

HEMOPTYSIS

ESSENTIAL INQUIRIES

▶ Fever, cough, and other symptoms of lower respiratory tract infection.

▶ Smoking history.

▶ Nasopharyngeal or gastrointestinal bleeding.

▶ Chest radiography and complete blood count (and, in some cases, INR).

General Considerations

Hemoptysis is the expectoration of blood that originates below the vocal cords. It is commonly classified as trivial, mild, or massive—the latter defined as more than 200–600 mL (about 1–2 cups) in 24 hours. Massive hemoptysis can be usefully defined as any amount that is hemodynamically significant or threatens ventilation. Its in-hospital mortality was 6.5% in one study. The initial goal of management of massive hemoptysis is therapeutic, not diagnostic.

The causes of hemoptysis can be classified anatomically. Blood may arise from the airways in COPD, bronchiectasis, and bronchogenic carcinoma; from the pulmonary vasculature in left ventricular failure, mitral stenosis, pulmonary embolism, pulmonary arterial hypertension, and arteriovenous malformations; or from the pulmonary parenchyma in pneumonia, fungal infections, inhalation of crack cocaine, or granulomatosis with polyangiitis (formerly Wegener granulomatosis). Diffuse alveolar hemorrhage—manifested by alveolar infiltrates on chest radiography—is due to small vessel bleeding usually caused by autoimmune or hematologic disorders, or rarely precipitated by warfarin. Most cases of hemoptysis presenting in the outpatient setting are due to infection (eg, acute or chronic bronchitis, pneumonia, tuberculosis, aspergillosis). Hemoptysis due to lung cancer increases with age, causing up to 20% of cases among older adults. Less commonly (less than 10% of cases), pulmonary venous hypertension (eg, mitral stenosis, pulmonary embolism) causes hemoptysis. Most cases of hemoptysis that have no visible cause on CT scan or bronchoscopy will resolve within 6 months without treatment, with the notable exception of patients at high risk for lung cancer (smokers older than 40 years). Iatrogenic hemorrhage may follow transbronchial lung biopsies, anticoagulation, or pulmonary artery rupture due to distal placement of a balloon-tipped catheter. Obstructive sleep apnea may be a risk factor for hemoptysis. Amyloidosis of the lung can cause hemoptysis. No cause is identified in up to 15–30% of cases.

Clinical Findings

A. Symptoms

Blood-tinged sputum in the setting of an upper respiratory tract infection in an otherwise healthy, young (age under 40 years) nonsmoker does not warrant an extensive diagnostic evaluation if the hemoptysis subsides with resolution of the infection. However, hemoptysis is frequently a sign of serious disease, especially in patients with a high prior probability of underlying pulmonary pathology. Hemoptysis is the only symptom found to be a specific predictor of lung cancer. There is no value in distinguishing blood-streaked sputum and cough productive of blood during evaluation; the goal of the history is to identify patients at risk for one of the disorders listed earlier. Pertinent features include duration of symptoms, presence of respiratory infection, and past or current tobacco use. Nonpulmonary sources of hemorrhage—from the sinuses or the gastrointestinal tract—must be excluded.

B. Physical Examination

Elevated pulse, hypotension, and decreased oxygen saturation suggest large-volume hemorrhage that warrants emergent evaluation and stabilization. The nares and oropharynx should be carefully inspected to identify a potential upper airway source of bleeding. Chest and cardiac examination may reveal evidence of HF or mitral stenosis.

C. Diagnostic Studies

Diagnostic evaluation should include a chest radiograph and complete blood count. Kidney function tests, urinalysis, and coagulation studies are appropriate in specific circumstances. Hematuria that accompanies hemoptysis may be a clue to Goodpasture syndrome or vasculitis. Flexible bronchoscopy reveals endobronchial cancer in 3–6% of patients with hemoptysis who have a normal (non-lateralizing) chest radiograph. Nearly all of these patients are smokers over the age of 40, and most will have had symptoms for more than 1 week. High-resolution chest CT scan complements bronchoscopy; it can visualize unsuspected bronchiectasis and arteriovenous malformations and will show central endobronchial cancers in many cases. It is the test of choice for suspected small peripheral malignancies. Helical CT pulmonary angiography is the initial test of choice for evaluating patients with suspected pulmonary embolism, although caution should be taken to avoid large contrast loads in patients with even mild chronic kidney disease (serum creatinine greater than 2.0 g/dL or rapidly rising creatinine in normal range). Helical CT scanning can be avoided in patients who are at "unlikely" risk for pulmonary embolism using the Wells score or PERC rule for pulmonary embolism and the sensitive D-dimer test. Echocardiography may reveal evidence of HF or mitral stenosis.

Treatment

Management of mild hemoptysis consists of identifying and treating the specific cause. Massive hemoptysis is life-threatening. The airway should be protected with endotracheal intubation, ventilation ensured, and effective circulation maintained. If the location of the bleeding site is known, the patient should be placed in the decubitus position with the involved lung dependent. Uncontrollable hemorrhage warrants rigid bronchoscopy and surgical consultation. In stable patients, flexible bronchoscopy may localize the site of bleeding, and angiography can embolize the involved bronchial arteries. Embolization is effective initially in 85% of cases, although rebleeding may occur in up to 20% of patients during the following year. The anterior spinal artery arises from the bronchial artery in up to 5% of people, and paraplegia may result if it is inadvertently cannulated and embolized. There is some evidence that antifibrinolytics may reduce the duration of bleeding.

▶ When to Refer

- Patients should be referred to a pulmonologist when bronchoscopy of the lower respiratory tract is needed.
- Patients should be referred to an otolaryngologist when an upper respiratory tract bleeding source is identified.
- Patients with severe coagulopathy complicating management should be referred to a hematologist.

▶ When to Admit

- To stabilize bleeding process in patients at risk for or experiencing massive hemoptysis.
- To correct disordered coagulation (using clotting factors or platelets, or both) or to reverse anticoagulation.
- To stabilize gas exchange.

Freund Y et al; PROPER Investigator Group. Effect of the Pulmonary Embolism Rule-Out Criteria on subsequent thromboembolic events among low-risk emergency department patients: the PROPER randomized clinical trial. JAMA. 2018 Feb 13;319(6):559–66. [PMID: 29450523]

Ittrich H et al. The diagnosis and treatment of hemoptysis. Dtsch Arztebl Int. 2017 Jun 5;114(21):371–81. [PMID: 28625277]

Uyar M et al. Obstructive sleep apnea is the triggering factor for massive hemoptysis: obstructive sleep apnea and hemoptysis. Sleep Breath. 2017 May;21(2):475–8. [PMID: 27995436]

CHEST PAIN

ESSENTIAL INQUIRIES

- ▶ Pain onset, character, location/size, duration, periodicity, and exacerbators; shortness of breath.
- ▶ Vital signs; chest and cardiac examination.
- ▶ Electrocardiography and biomarkers of myocardial necrosis in selected patients.

▶ General Considerations

Chest pain (or chest discomfort) is a common symptom that can occur as a result of cardiovascular, pulmonary, pleural, or musculoskeletal disease; esophageal or other gastrointestinal disorders; herpes zoster; cocaine use; or anxiety states. The frequency and distribution of life-threatening causes of chest pain, such as acute coronary syndrome (ACS), pericarditis, aortic dissection, vasospastic angina, pulmonary embolism, pneumonia, and esophageal perforation, vary substantially between clinical settings. Systemic lupus erythematosus, rheumatoid arthritis, reduced estimated glomerular filtration rate, and HIV infection are conditions that confer a strong risk of coronary artery disease. Precocious ACS may represent acute thrombosis independent of underlying atherosclerotic disease. In patients aged 35 years or younger, risk factors for ACS are obesity, hyperlipidemia, and smoking.

Chest pain characteristics that can lead to early diagnosis of acute myocardial infarction do not differ in frequency or strength of association between men and women. Because pulmonary embolism can present with a wide variety of symptoms, consideration of the diagnosis and rigorous risk factor assessment for venous thromboembolism (VTE) is critical. Classic VTE risk factors include cancer, trauma, recent surgery, prolonged immobilization, pregnancy, oral contraceptives, and family history and prior history of VTE. Other conditions associated with increased risk of pulmonary embolism include HF and COPD. Sickle cell anemia can cause acute chest syndrome. Patients with this syndrome often have chest pain, fever, and cough.

▶ Clinical Findings

A. Symptoms

Myocardial ischemia is usually described as a dull, aching sensation of "pressure," "tightness," "squeezing," or "gas," rather than as sharp or spasmodic. Ischemic symptoms usually subside within 5–20 minutes but may last longer. Progressive symptoms or symptoms at rest may represent unstable angina. Prolonged chest pain episodes might represent myocardial infarction, although up to one-third of patients with acute myocardial infarction do not report chest pain. When present, pain due to myocardial ischemia is commonly accompanied by a sense of anxiety or uneasiness. The location is usually retrosternal or left precordial. Because the heart lacks somatic innervation, precise localization of pain due to cardiac ischemia is difficult; the pain is commonly referred to the throat, lower jaw, shoulders, inner arms, upper abdomen, or back. Ischemic pain may be precipitated or exacerbated by exertion, cold temperature, meals, stress, or combinations of these factors and is usually relieved by rest. However, many episodes do not conform to these patterns, and atypical presentations of ACS are more common in older adults, women, and persons with diabetes mellitus. Other symptoms that are associated with ACS include shortness of breath; dizziness; a feeling of impending doom; and vagal symptoms, such as nausea and diaphoresis. In older persons, fatigue is a common presenting complaint of ACS. Likelihood ratios (LRs) for cardinal symptoms considered in the evaluation of acute myocardial infarction are summarized in Table 2–5.

A meta-analysis found the clinical findings and risk factors most suggestive of ACS were prior abnormal stress test (specificity, 96%; LR, 3.1 [95% CI, 2.0–4.7]), peripheral arterial disease (specificity, 97%; LR, 2.7 [95% CI, 1.5–4.8]), and pain radiation to both arms (specificity, 96%; LR, 2.6 [95% CI, 1.8–3.7]). The ECG findings associated with ACS were ST-segment depression (specificity, 95%; LR, 5.3 [95%

Table 2–5. Likelihood ratios (LRs) for clinical features associated with acute myocardial infarction.

Clinical Feature	LR+ (95% CI)
History	
Chest pain that radiates to the left arm	2.3 (1.7–3.1)
Chest pain that radiates to the right shoulder	2.9 (1.4–3.0)
Chest pain that radiates to both arms	7.1 (3.6–14.2)
Pleuritic chest pain	0.2 (0.2–0.3)
Sharp or stabbing chest pain	0.3 (0.2–0.5)
Positional chest pain	0.3 (0.2–0.4)
Nausea or vomiting	1.9 (1.7–2.3)
Diaphoresis	2.0 (1.9–2.2)
Physical examination	
Systolic blood pressure ≤ 80 mm Hg	3.1 (1.8–5.2)
Chest pain reproduced by palpation	0.2–0.41
Pulmonary crackles	2.1 (1.4–3.1)
Third heart sound	3.2 (1.6–6.5)
Electrocardiogram	
Any ST-segment elevation (≥ 1 mm)	11.2 (7.1–17.8)
Any ST-segment depression	3.2 (2.5–4.1)
Any Q wave	3.9 (2.7–7.7)
Any conduction defect	2.7 (1.4–5.4)
New ST-segment elevation (≥ 1 mm)	(5.7–53.9)[1]
New ST-segment depression	(3.0–5.2)[1]
New Q wave	(5.3–24.8)[1]
New conduction defect	6.3 (2.5–15.7)

CI, confidence interval.

[1]Heterogeneous studies do not allow for calculation of a point estimate.

Adapted, with permission, from Panju AA et al. The rational clinical examination. Is this patient having a myocardial infarction? JAMA. 1998 Oct 14;280(14):1256–63. © 1998 American Medical Association. All rights reserved.

CI, 2.1–8.6]) and any evidence of ischemia (specificity, 91%; LR, 3.6 [95% CI, 1.6–5.7]). Risk scores derived from both the History, Electrocardiogram, Age, Risk Factors, Troponin (HEART) and Thrombolysis in Myocardial Infarction (TIMI) trials performed well in detecting ACS (LR, 13 [95% CI, 7.0–24] for HEART score of 7–10, and LR, 6.8 [95% CI, 5.2–8.9] for TIMI score of 5–7).

Hypertrophy of either ventricle or aortic stenosis may also give rise to chest pain with less typical features. Pericarditis produces pain that may be greater when supine than upright and increases with respiration, coughing, or swallowing. Pleuritic chest pain is usually not ischemic, and pain on palpation may indicate a musculoskeletal cause. Aortic dissection classically produces an abrupt onset of tearing pain of great intensity that often radiates to the back; however, this classic presentation occurs in a small proportion of cases. Anterior aortic dissection can also lead to myocardial or cerebrovascular ischemia.

Pulmonary embolism has a wide range of clinical presentations, with chest pain present in about 75% of cases. The chief objective in evaluating patients with suspected pulmonary embolism is to assess the patient's clinical risk for VTE based on medical history and associated symptoms and signs (see above and Chapter 9). Rupture of the thoracic esophagus iatrogenically or secondary to vomiting is another cause of chest pain.

B. Physical Examination

Findings on physical examination can occasionally yield important clues to the underlying cause of chest pain; however, a normal physical examination should never be used as the sole basis for ruling out most diagnoses, particularly ACS and aortic dissection. Vital signs (including pulse oximetry) and cardiopulmonary examination are always the first steps for assessing the urgency and tempo of the subsequent examination and diagnostic workup.

Findings that increase the likelihood of ACS include diaphoresis, hypotension, S_3 or S_4 gallop, pulmonary crackles, or elevated jugular venous pressure (see Table 2–5). Although chest pain that is reproducible or worsened with palpation strongly suggests a musculoskeletal cause, up to 15% of patients with ACS will have reproducible chest wall tenderness. Pointing to the location of the pain with one finger has been shown to be highly correlated with nonischemic chest pain. Aortic dissection can result in differential blood pressures (greater than 20 mm Hg), pulse amplitude deficits, and new diastolic murmurs. Although hypertension is considered the rule in patients with aortic dissection, systolic blood pressure less than 100 mm Hg is present in up to 25% of patients.

A cardiac friction rub represents pericarditis until proven otherwise. It can best be heard with the patient sitting forward at end-expiration. Tamponade should be excluded in all patients with a clinical diagnosis of pericarditis by assessing pulsus paradoxus (a decrease in systolic blood pressure during inspiration greater than 10 mm Hg) and inspection of jugular venous pulsations. Subcutaneous emphysema is common following cervical esophageal perforation but present in only about one-third of thoracic perforations (ie, those most commonly presenting with chest pain).

The absence of abnormal physical examination findings in patients with suspected pulmonary embolism usually serves to *increase* the likelihood of pulmonary embolism, although a normal physical examination is also compatible with the much more common conditions of panic/anxiety disorder and musculoskeletal disease.

C. Diagnostic Studies

Unless a competing diagnosis can be confirmed, an ECG is warranted in the initial evaluation of most patients with acute chest pain to help exclude ACS. ST-segment elevation is the ECG finding that is the strongest predictor of acute myocardial infarction (see Table 2–5); however, up to 20% of patients with ACS can have a normal ECG. In the emergency department, patients with suspected ACS can be safely removed from cardiac monitoring if they are pain-free at initial physician assessment and have a normal or nonspecific ECG. This decision rule had 100% sensitivity for serious arrhythmia (95% CI, 80–100%). Clinically stable patients with cardiovascular disease risk factors, normal ECG, normal cardiac biomarkers, and no alternative diagnoses (such as typical GERD or costochondritis) should be followed up with a timely exercise stress test that includes perfusion imaging. However, more than 25% of patients with stable chest pain referred for noninvasive testing will have normal coronary arteries and no long-term clinical events. The ECG can also provide evidence for alternative diagnoses, such as pericarditis and pulmonary embolism. Chest radiography is often useful in the evaluation of chest pain, and is always indicated when cough or shortness of breath accompanies chest pain. Findings of pneumomediastinum or new pleural effusion are consistent with esophageal perforation. Stress echocardiography is useful in risk stratifying patients with chest pain, even among those with significant obesity.

Diagnostic protocols using a single high-sensitivity troponin assay combined with a standardized clinical assessment are an efficient strategy to rapidly determine whether patients with chest pain are at low risk and may be discharged from the emergency department. Five established risk scores are (1) the modified Goldman Risk Score, (2) TIMI Risk Score, (3) Global Registry of Acute Cardiac Events (GRACE) Risk Score, (4) HEART Risk Score, and (5) Vancouver Chest Pain Rule. A study compared these risk scores for predicting acute myocardial infarction within 30 days and reported a sensitivity of 98% (which correlates with a negative predictive value of greater than or equal to 99.5%). Patients eligible for discharge (about 30%) were those with a TIMI score of less than or equal to 1, modified Goldman score of less than or equal to 1 with normal high-sensitivity troponin T, TIMI score of 0, or HEART score of less than or equal to 3 with normal high-sensitivity troponin I.

While some studies of high-sensitivity cardiac troponin suggest that it may be the best cardiac biomarker, it may not outperform conventional troponin assays if an appropriate cutoff is used.

Patients who arrive at the emergency department with chest pain of intermediate or high probability for ACS without electrocardiographic or biomarker evidence of a myocardial infarction can be safely discharged from an observation unit after stress cardiac MRI. Sixty-four–slice CT coronary angiography (CTA) is an alternative to stress testing in the emergency department for detecting ACS among patients with normal or nonspecific ECG and normal biomarkers. A meta-analysis of nine studies found ACS in 10% of patients, and an estimated sensitivity of CTA for ACS of 95% and specificity of 87%, yielding a negative LR of 0.06 and a positive LR of 7.4. Coronary CTA applied early in the evaluation of suspected ACS does not identify more patients with significant coronary artery disease requiring coronary revascularization, shorten hospital stay, or allow for more direct discharge from the emergency department compared to high-sensitivity troponins. Thus, functional testing appears to be the best initial noninvasive test in symptomatic patients with suspected coronary artery disease. CTA is an option for patients who do not have access to functional testing.

For patients at low risk for ACS, an initial diagnostic strategy of stress echocardiography or cardiovascular magnetic resonance is associated with similar cardiac event rates, but a substantially lower invasive testing rate.

A minimal-risk model developed by the PROMISE investigators includes 10 clinical variables that correlate with normal coronary CTA results and no clinical events (C statistic = 0.725 for the derivation and validation subsets; 95% CI, 0.705–0.746). These variables include (1) younger age; (2) female sex; (3) racial or ethnic minority; (4–6) no history of hypertension, diabetes, or dyslipidemia; (7) no family history of premature coronary artery disease; (8) never smoking; (9) symptoms unrelated to physical or mental stress; and (10) higher high-density lipoprotein cholesterol level.

In the evaluation of pulmonary embolism, diagnostic test decisions and results must be interpreted in the context of the clinical likelihood of VTE. A negative D-dimer test is helpful for excluding pulmonary embolism in patients with low clinical probability of VTE (3-month incidence = 0.5%); however, the 3-month risk of VTE among patients with intermediate and high risk of VTE is sufficiently high in the setting of a negative D-dimer test (3.5% and 21.4%, respectively) to warrant further imaging given the life-threatening nature of this condition if left untreated. CTA (with helical or multidetector CT imaging) has replaced ventilation-perfusion scanning as the preferred initial diagnostic test, having approximately 90–95% sensitivity and 95% specificity for detecting pulmonary embolism (compared with pulmonary angiography). However, for patients with high clinical probability of VTE, lower extremity ultrasound or pulmonary angiogram may be indicated even with a normal helical CT.

Panic disorder is a common cause of chest pain, accounting for up to 25% of cases that present to emergency departments and a higher proportion of cases presenting in primary care office practices. Features that correlate with an increased likelihood of panic disorder include absence of coronary artery disease, atypical quality of chest pain, female sex, younger age, and a high level of self-reported anxiety. Depression is associated with recurrent chest pain with or without coronary artery disease (odds ratio [OR], 2.11; 95% CI, 1.18–3.79).

▶ **Treatment**

Treatment of chest pain should be guided by the underlying etiology. The term "noncardiac chest pain" is used when a diagnosis remains elusive after patients have undergone an extensive workup. Almost half reported symptom improvement with high-dose proton-pump inhibitor therapy. A meta-analysis of 15 trials suggested modest to moderate benefit for psychological (especially cognitive-behavioral) interventions. It is unclear whether tricyclic or selective serotonin reuptake inhibitor antidepressants have benefit in noncardiac chest pain. Hypnotherapy may offer some benefit.

When to Refer

- Refer patients with poorly controlled, noncardiac chest pain to a pain specialist.
- Refer patients with sickle cell anemia to a hematologist.

When to Admit

- Failure to adequately exclude life-threatening causes of chest pain, particularly myocardial infarction, dissecting aortic aneurysm, pulmonary embolism, and esophageal rupture.
- High risk of pulmonary embolism and a positive sensitive D-dimer test.
- TIMI score of 1 or more, HEART score greater than 3, abnormal ECG, and abnormal 0- and 2-hour troponin tests.
- Pain control for rib fracture that impairs gas exchange.

Berko EH et al. Behavioral health consult: ensuring prompt recognition and treatment of panic disorder. J Fam Pract. 2017 Dec;66(12):750–3. [PMID: 29202148]

Budoff MJ et al; PROMISE Investigators. Prognostic value of coronary artery calcium in the PROMISE Study (Prospective Multicenter Imaging Study for Evaluation of Chest Pain). Circulation. 2017 Nov 21;136(21):1993–2005. [PMID: 28847895]

Dedic A et al. Coronary CT angiography for suspected ACS in the era of high-sensitivity troponins: randomized multicenter study. J Am Coll Cardiol. 2016 Jan 5;67(1):16–26. [PMID: 26764061]

Fordyce CB et al; Prospective Multicenter Imaging Study for Evaluation of Chest Pain (PROMISE) Investigators. Identification of patients with stable chest pain deriving minimal value from noninvasive testing: the PROMISE minimal-risk tool, a secondary analysis of a randomized clinical trial. JAMA Cardiol. 2017 Apr 1;2(4):400–8. [PMID: 28199464]

Frieling T. Non-cardiac chest pain. Visc Med. 2018 Apr;34(2): 92–6. [PMID: 29888236]

Hoorweg BB et al. Frequency of chest pain in primary care, diagnostic tests performed and final diagnoses. Heart. 2017 Nov; 103(21):1727–32. [PMID: 28634285]

Kim Y et al. Depression is associated with recurrent chest pain with or without coronary artery disease: a prospective cohort study in the emergency department. Am Heart J. 2017 Sep; 191:47–54. [PMID: 28888269]

Maroules CD et al. Growing evidence for coronary computed tomography angiography as a first-line test in stable chest pain. J Thorac Imaging. 2019 Jan;34(1):4–11. [PMID: 30157094]

Reinhardt SW et al. Noninvasive cardiac testing vs clinical evaluation alone in acute chest pain: a secondary analysis of the ROMICAT-II randomized clinical trial. JAMA Intern Med. 2018 Feb 1;178(2):212–19. [PMID: 29138794]

Rushton S et al. Chest pain: if it is not the heart, what is it? Nurs Clin North Am. 2018 Sep;53(3):421–31. [PMID: 30100007]

Syed S et al. Prospective validation of a clinical decision rule to identify patients presenting to the emergency department with chest pain who can safely be removed from cardiac monitoring. CMAJ. 2017 Jan 30;189(4):E139–145. [PMID: 28246315]

PALPITATIONS

ESSENTIAL INQUIRIES

- ▶ Forceful, rapid, or irregular beating of the heart.
- ▶ Rate, duration, and degree of regularity of heartbeat; age at first episode.
- ▶ Factors that precipitate or terminate episodes.
- ▶ Light-headedness or syncope; neck pounding.
- ▶ Chest pain; history of myocardial infarction or structural heart disease.

General Considerations

Palpitations are defined as an unpleasant awareness of the forceful, rapid, or irregular beating of the heart. They are the primary symptom for approximately 16% of patients presenting to an outpatient clinic with a cardiac complaint. In an observational cohort study of palpitations at an outpatient cardiac unit, cardiac arrhythmias were the cause of palpitations in 81% of cases. Palpitations represent 5.8 of every 1000 emergency department visits, with an admission rate of 24.6%. While palpitations are usually benign, they are occasionally the symptom of a life-threatening arrhythmia. To avoid missing a dangerous cause of the patient's symptom, clinicians sometimes pursue expensive and invasive testing when a conservative diagnostic evaluation is sufficient. The converse is also true; in one study, 54% of patients with supraventricular tachycardia were initially wrongly diagnosed with panic, stress, or anxiety disorder. A disproportionate number of these misdiagnosed patients are women. Table 2–6 lists history, physical examination, and ECG findings suggesting a cardiovascular cause for the palpitations.

Table 2–6. Palpitations: Patients at high risk for a cardiovascular cause.

Historical risk factors
Family history of significant arrhythmias
Personal or family history of syncope or resuscitated sudden death
History of myocardial infarction (and likely scarred myocardium)
Palpitations that occur during sleep
Anatomic abnormalities
Structural heart disease such as dilated or hypertrophic cardiomyopathies
Valvular disease (stenotic or regurgitant)
ECG findings
Long QT syndrome
Bradycardia
Second- or third-degree heart block
Sustained ventricular arrhythmias

► Clinical Findings

A. Symptoms

Although described by patients in a myriad of ways, guiding the patient through a careful description of their palpitations may indicate a mechanism and narrow the differential diagnosis. Pertinent questions include the age at first episode; precipitants; and rate, duration, and degree of regularity of the heartbeat during the subjective palpitations. Palpitations lasting less than 5 minutes and a family history of panic disorder reduce the likelihood of an arrhythmic cause (LR = 0.38 and LR = 0.26, respectively). To better understand the symptom, the examiner can ask the patient to "tap out" the rhythm with his or her fingers. The circumstances associated with onset and termination can also be helpful in determining the cause. Palpitations that start and stop abruptly suggest supraventricular or ventricular tachycardias. Termination of palpitations using vagal maneuvers (eg, Valsalva maneuver) suggests supraventricular tachycardia.

Three common descriptions of palpitations are (1) "flip-flopping" (or "stop and start"), often caused by premature contraction of the atrium or ventricle, with the perceived "stop" from the pause following the contraction, and the "start" from the subsequent forceful contraction; (2) rapid "fluttering in the chest," with regular "fluttering" suggesting supraventricular or ventricular arrhythmias (including sinus tachycardia) and irregular "fluttering" suggesting atrial fibrillation, atrial flutter, or tachycardia with variable block; and (3) "pounding in the neck" or neck pulsations, often due to "cannon" A waves in the jugular venous pulsations that occur when the right atrium contracts against a closed tricuspid valve.

Palpitations associated with chest pain suggest ischemic heart disease, or if the chest pain is relieved by leaning forward, pericardial disease is suspected. Palpitations associated with light-headedness, presyncope, or syncope suggest hypotension and may signify a life-threatening cardiac arrhythmia. Palpitations that occur regularly with exertion suggest a rate-dependent bypass tract or hypertrophic cardiomyopathy. If a benign etiology for these concerning symptoms cannot be ascertained at the initial visit, then ambulatory monitoring or prolonged cardiac monitoring in the hospital might be warranted.

Noncardiac symptoms should also be elicited since the palpitations may be caused by a normal heart responding to a metabolic or inflammatory condition. Weight loss suggests hyperthyroidism. Palpitations can be precipitated by vomiting or diarrhea that leads to electrolyte disorders and hypovolemia. Hyperventilation, hand tingling, and nervousness are common when anxiety or panic disorder is the cause of the palpitations. Palpitations associated with flushing, episodic hypertension, headaches, anxiety, and diaphoresis may be caused by a pheochromocytoma or paraganglioma. In patients with suspected pheochromocytoma or paraganglioma, fractionated plasma or urinary metanephrine and normetanephrine (metanephrines) should be measured.

A family history of palpitations or sudden death suggests an inherited etiology such as long QT syndrome or Brugada syndrome. Chagas disease may cause palpitations and acute myocarditis.

B. Physical Examination

Rarely does the clinician have the opportunity to examine a patient during an episode of palpitations. However, careful cardiovascular examination can find abnormalities that can increase the likelihood of specific cardiac arrhythmias. The midsystolic click of mitral valve prolapse can suggest the diagnosis of a supraventricular arrhythmia. The harsh holosystolic murmur of hypertrophic cardiomyopathy, which occurs along the left sternal border and increases with the Valsalva maneuver, suggests atrial fibrillation or ventricular tachycardia. A crescendo mid-diastolic murmur may be caused by an atrial myxoma. The presence of dilated cardiomyopathy, suggested on examination by a displaced and enlarged cardiac point-of-maximal impulse, increases the likelihood of ventricular tachycardia and atrial fibrillation. In patients with chronic atrial fibrillation, in-office exercise (eg, a brisk walk in the hallway) may reveal an intermittent accelerated ventricular response as the cause of the palpitations. The clinician should also look for signs of hyperthyroidism (eg, tremulousness, brisk deep tendon reflexes, or fine hand tremor), or signs of stimulant drug use (eg, dilated pupils or skin or nasal septal perforations). Visible neck pulsations (LR, 2.68; 95% CI, 1.25–5.78) in association with palpitations increases the likelihood of atrioventricular nodal reentry tachycardia.

C. Diagnostic Studies

1. ECG—A 12-lead ECG should be performed on all patients reporting palpitations because it can provide evidence for a wide variety of causes. Although in most instances a specific arrhythmia will not be detected on the tracing, a careful evaluation of the ECG can help the clinician deduce a likely etiology in certain circumstances.

For instance, bradyarrhythmias and heart block can be associated with ventricular ectopy or escape beats that may be experienced as palpitations by the patient. Evidence of prior myocardial infarction on ECG (eg, Q waves) increases the patient's risk for nonsustained or sustained ventricular tachycardia. Ventricular preexcitation (Wolff-Parkinson-White syndrome) is suggested by a short PR interval (less than 0.20 ms) and delta waves (upsloping PR segments). Left ventricular hypertrophy with deep septal Q waves in I, AVL, and V4 through V6 is seen in patients with hypertrophic obstructive cardiomyopathy. The presence of left atrial enlargement as suggested by a terminal P-wave force in V1 more negative than 0.04 msec and notching in lead II reflects a patient at increased risk for atrial fibrillation. A prolonged QT interval and abnormal T-wave morphology suggest the long QT syndrome, which puts patients at increased risk for ventricular tachycardia. Persistent ST-segment elevations in ECG leads V1–V3 (particularly with a coved or saddle-back pattern) suggest Brugada syndrome.

2. Monitoring devices—For high-risk patients (Table 2–6), further diagnostic studies are warranted. A step-wise approach has been suggested—starting with ambulatory monitoring devices (ambulatory ECG [Holter] monitoring if the palpitations are expected to occur within the subsequent 72-hour period, event monitoring if less frequent). An implantable loop recorder can be used for extended monitoring if clinical suspicion is high, especially if there is syncope. A single-lead, lightweight, continuously recording ambulatory adhesive patch monitor (Zio Patch) worn for 14 days has been shown to be superior to 24-hour ambulatory ECG (Holter) monitoring. This is then followed by inpatient continuous monitoring if serious arrhythmias are strongly suspected despite normal findings on the ambulatory monitoring, and by invasive electrophysiologic testing if the ambulatory or inpatient monitor records a worrisome arrhythmia.

In patients with a prior myocardial infarction, ambulatory cardiac monitoring or signal-averaged ECG is an appropriate next step to help exclude ventricular tachycardia. ECG exercise testing is appropriate in patients with suspected coronary artery disease and in patients who have palpitations with physical exertion. Echocardiography is useful when physical examination or ECG suggests structural abnormalities or decreased ventricular function.

▶ Differential Diagnosis

When assessing a patient with palpitations in an urgent care setting, the clinician must ascertain whether the symptoms represent (1) an arrhythmia that is minor and transient, (2) a significant cardiovascular disease, (3) a cardiac manifestation of a systemic disease such as thyrotoxicosis, or (4) a benign somatic symptom that is amplified by the patient's underlying psychological state.

Patients with palpitations who seek medical attention in an emergency department instead of a medical clinic are more likely to have a cardiac cause (47% versus 21%), whereas psychiatric causes are more common among those who seek attention in office practices (45% versus 27%). In a study of patients who went to a university medical clinic with the chief complaint of palpitations, causes were cardiac in 43%, psychiatric in 31%, and miscellaneous in 10%.

The most common psychiatric causes of palpitations are anxiety and panic disorder. The release of catecholamines during a significant stress or panic attack can trigger an arrhythmia. Asking a single question, "Have you experienced brief periods, for seconds or minutes, of an overwhelming panic or terror that was accompanied by racing heartbeats, shortness of breath, or dizziness?" can help identify patients with panic disorder.

Miscellaneous causes of palpitations include fever, dehydration, hypoglycemia, anemia, thyrotoxicosis, mastocytosis, and pheochromocytoma. Drugs such as cocaine, alcohol, caffeine, pseudoephedrine, and illicit ephedra can precipitate palpitations, as can prescription medications, including digoxin, amitriptyline, erythromycin and other drugs that prolong the QT interval, class 1 antiarrhythmics, dihydropyridine calcium channel blockers, phenothiazines, theophylline, and beta-agonists.

▶ Treatment

After ambulatory monitoring, most patients with palpitations are found to have benign atrial or ventricular ectopy or nonsustained ventricular tachycardia. In patients with structurally normal hearts, these arrhythmias are not associated with adverse outcomes. Abstention from caffeine and tobacco may help. Often, reassurance suffices. If not, or in very symptomatic patients, a trial of a beta-blocker may be prescribed. A three-session course of cognitive-behavioral therapy that includes some physical activity has proven effective for patients with benign palpitations with or without chest pain. For treatment of specific atrial or ventricular arrhythmias, see Chapter 10.

▶ When to Refer

- For electrophysiologic studies.
- For advice regarding treatment of atrial or ventricular arrhythmias.

▶ When to Admit

- Palpitations associated with syncope or near-syncope, particularly when the patient is aged 75 years or older and has an abnormal ECG, hematocrit less than 30%, shortness of breath, respiratory rate higher than 24/min, or a history of HF.
- Patients with risk factors for a serious arrhythmia.

Abi Khalil C et al. Investigating palpitations: the role of Holter monitoring and loop recorders. BMJ. 2017 Jul 27;358:j3123. [PMID: 28751495]

Clementy N et al. Benefits of an early management of palpitations. Medicine (Baltimore). 2018 Jul;97(28):e11466. [PMID: 29995805]

Francisco-Pascual J et al. Diagnostic yield and economic assessment of a diagnostic protocol with systematic use of an external loop recorder for patients with palpitations. Rev Esp Cardiol (Engl Ed). 2018 May 24. [Epub ahead of print] [PMID: 29805092]

Gale CP et al. Assessment of palpitations. BMJ. 2016 Jan 6; 352:h5649. [PMID: 26739319]

Giada F et al. Clinical approach to patients with palpitations. Card Electrophysiol Clin. 2018 Jun;10(2):387–96. [PMID: 29784490]

Wexler RK et al. Palpitations: evaluation in the primary care setting. Am Fam Physician. 2017 Dec 15;96(12):784–9. [PMID: 29431371]

LOWER EXTREMITY EDEMA

ESSENTIAL INQUIRIES

- ▶ History of venous thromboembolism.
- ▶ Symmetry of swelling.
- ▶ Pain.
- ▶ Change with dependence.
- ▶ Skin findings: hyperpigmentation, stasis dermatitis, lipodermatosclerosis, atrophie blanche, ulceration.

General Considerations

Acute and chronic lower extremity edema present important diagnostic and treatment challenges. Lower extremities can swell in response to increased venous or lymphatic pressures, decreased intravascular oncotic pressure, increased capillary leak, and local injury or infection. **Chronic venous insufficiency** is by far the most common cause, affecting up to 2% of the population, and the incidence of venous insufficiency has not changed over the past 25 years. Venous insufficiency is a common complication of DVT; however, only a small number of patients with chronic venous insufficiency report a history of this disorder. Venous ulceration commonly affects patients with chronic venous insufficiency, and its management is labor-intensive and expensive. Normal lower extremity venous pressure (in the erect position: 80 mm Hg in deep veins, 20–30 mm Hg in superficial veins) and cephalad venous blood flow require competent bicuspid venous valves, effective muscle contractions, normal ankle range of motion, and normal respirations. When one or more of these components fail, venous hypertension may result. Chronic exposure to elevated venous pressure by the post-capillary venules in the legs leads to leakage of fibrinogen and growth factors into the interstitial space, leukocyte aggregation and activation, and obliteration of the cutaneous lymphatic network.

Clinical Findings

A. Symptoms and Signs

1. Unilateral lower extremity edema—Among common causes of unilateral lower extremity swelling, DVT is the most life-threatening. Clues suggesting DVT include a history of cancer, recent limb immobilization, or confinement to bed for at least 3 days following major surgery within the past month (Table 2–7). Adults with varicose veins have a significantly increased risk of DVT. Lower extremity swelling and inflammation in a limb recently affected by DVT could represent anticoagulation failure and thrombus recurrence but more often are caused by **postphlebitic syndrome** with valvular incompetence. A search for alternative explanations is equally important in excluding DVT. Other causes of a painful, swollen calf include cellulitis, musculoskeletal disorders (Baker cyst rupture ["pseudothrombophlebitis"]), gastrocnemius tear or rupture, calf strain or trauma, and left common iliac vein compression (May-Thurner syndrome), as well as other sites of non-thrombotic venous outflow obstruction, such as the inguinal ligament, iliac bifurcation, and popliteal fossa.

2. Bilateral lower extremity edema—Bilateral involvement and significant improvement upon awakening favor systemic causes (eg, venous insufficiency) and can be presenting symptoms of volume overload (HF, cirrhosis, kidney disease [eg, nephrotic syndrome]). The sensation of "heavy legs" is the most frequent symptom of chronic venous insufficiency, followed by itching. Chronic exposure to elevated venous pressure accounts for the brawny, fibrotic skin changes observed in patients with chronic venous insufficiency as well as the predisposition toward

Table 2–7. Risk stratification of adults referred for ultrasound to rule out DVT.

Step 1:
Score 1 point for each
Untreated malignancy
Paralysis, paresis, or recent plaster immobilization
Recently bedridden for > 3 days due to major surgery within 4 weeks
Localized tenderness along distribution of deep venous system
Entire leg swelling
Swelling of one calf > 3 cm more than the other (measured 10 cm below tibial tuberosity)
Ipsilateral pitting edema
Collateral superficial (nonvaricose) veins
Previously documented DVT
Step 2:
Subtract 2 points if alternative diagnosis has equal or greater likelihood than DVT
Step 3:
Obtain sensitive D-dimer for score ≥ 0

Score	D-Dimer Positive[1]	D-Dimer Negative[1]
0–1	Obtain ultrasound	Ultrasound not required
≥ 2	Obtain ultrasound	

DVT, deep venous thrombosis.
[1]"Positive" is above local laboratory threshold based on specific test and patient age.

skin ulceration, particularly in the medial malleolar area. Pain, particularly if severe, is uncommon in uncomplicated venous insufficiency.

Lower extremity swelling is a familiar complication of therapy with calcium channel blockers (particularly felodipine and amlodipine), pioglitazone, gabapentin, and minoxidil. Prolonged airline flights (longer than 10 hours) are associated with edema even in the absence of DVT. Lymphedema and lipedema are other causes of bilateral lower extremity edema.

B. Physical Examination

Physical examination should include assessment of the heart, lungs, and abdomen for evidence of pulmonary hypertension (primary or secondary to chronic lung disease), HF, or cirrhosis. Some patients with cirrhosis have pulmonary hypertension without lung disease. There is a spectrum of skin findings related to chronic venous insufficiency that depends on the severity and chronicity of the disease, ranging from hyperpigmentation and stasis dermatitis to abnormalities highly specific for chronic venous insufficiency: lipodermatosclerosis (thick, brawny skin; in advanced cases, the lower leg resembles an inverted champagne bottle) and atrophie blanche (small depigmented macules within areas of heavy pigmentation). The size of both calves should be measured 10 cm below the tibial tuberosity and pitting and tenderness elicited. Leg edema may also be measured by ultrasonography with a gel pad if physical examination is equivocal. Swelling of the entire leg or of one leg 3 cm more than the other suggests deep venous obstruction. The left calf is normally slightly larger than the right as a result of the left common iliac vein coursing under the aorta.

An ulcer located over the medial malleolus is a hallmark of chronic venous insufficiency but can be due to other causes. Shallow, large, modestly painful ulcers are characteristic of venous insufficiency, whereas small, deep, and more painful ulcers are more apt to be due to arterial insufficiency, vasculitis, or infection (including cutaneous diphtheria). Diabetic vascular ulcers, however, may be painless. When an ulcer is on the foot or above the mid-calf, causes other than venous insufficiency should be considered.

C. Diagnostic Studies

Patients without an obvious cause of acute lower extremity swelling (eg, calf strain) should have an ultrasound performed, since DVT is difficult to exclude on clinical grounds. A prediction rule allows a clinician to exclude a lower extremity DVT in patients without an ultrasound if the patient has low pretest probability for DVT and a negative sensitive D-dimer test (the "Wells prediction rule"). Assessment of the ankle-brachial pressure index (ABPI) is important in the management of chronic venous insufficiency, since peripheral arterial disease may be exacerbated by compression therapy. This can be performed at the same time as ultrasound. Caution is required in interpreting the results of ABPI in older patients and diabetics due to the decreased compressibility of their arteries. A urine dipstick test that is strongly positive for protein can suggest nephrotic syndrome, and a serum creatinine can help estimate kidney function.

▶ Treatment

Treatment of lower extremity edema should be guided by the underlying cause. See relevant chapters for treatment of edema in patients with HF (Chapter 10), nephrosis (Chapter 22), cirrhosis (Chapter 16), and lymphedema and venous stasis ulcers (Chapter 12). Edema resulting from calcium channel blocker therapy responds to concomitant therapy with ACE inhibitors or angiotensin receptor blockers.

In patients with chronic venous insufficiency without a comorbid volume overload state (eg, HF), it is best to avoid diuretic therapy. These patients have relatively decreased intravascular volume, and administration of diuretics may first enhance sodium retention through increased secretion of renin and angiotensin and then result in acute kidney injury and oliguria. Instead, the most effective treatment involves (1) leg elevation, above the level of the heart, for 30 minutes three to four times daily, and during sleep; (2) compression therapy; and (3) ambulatory exercise to increase venous return through calf muscle contractions. There is no evidence for benefit or harm of valvuloplasty in the treatment of patients with deep venous insufficiency secondary to primary valvular incompetence.

A wide variety of stockings and devices are effective in decreasing swelling and preventing ulcer formation. They should be put on with awakening, before hydrostatic forces result in edema. To control simple edema, 20–30 mm Hg compression is usually sufficient, whereas 30–40 mm Hg compression is usually required to control moderate to severe edema associated with ulcer formation. To maintain improvement, consider switching from an elastic stocking to one made of inelastic grosgrain material. Patients with decreased ABPI should be managed in concert with a vascular surgeon. Compression stockings (12–18 mm Hg at the ankle) are effective in preventing edema and asymptomatic thrombosis associated with long airline flights in low- to medium-risk persons. For lymphedema, bandaging systems applied twice weekly can be effective. Short-term manual lymphatic drainage treatment may improve chronic venous insufficiency severity, symptoms, and quality of life. For patients with reduced mobility and leg edema, intermittent pneumatic compression treatment can reduce edema and improve ankle range of motion.

▶ When to Refer

- Chronic lower extremity ulcerations requiring specialist wound care.
- Refer patients with nephrotic syndrome to a nephrologist.
- Refer patients with coexisting severe arterial insufficiency (claudication) that would complicate treatment with compression stockings to a vascular surgeon.

▶ When to Admit

- Pending definitive diagnosis in patients at high risk for DVT despite normal lower extremity ultrasound.
- Severe, acute swelling raising concern for an impending compartment syndrome.
- Severe edema that impairs ability to ambulate or perform activities of daily living.

Chang SL et al. Association of varicose veins with incident venous thromboembolism and peripheral artery disease. JAMA. 2018 Feb 27;319(8):807–17. [PMID: 29486040]

Clarke MJ et al. Compression stockings for preventing deep vein thrombosis in airline passengers. Cochrane Database Syst Rev. 2016 Sep 14;9:CD004002. [PMID: 27624857]

Dean SM. Cutaneous manifestations of chronic vascular disease. Prog Cardiovasc Dis. 2018 Mar–Apr;60(6):567–79. [PMID: 29534983]

Fox JD et al. Ankle range of motion, leg pain, and leg edema improvement in patients with venous leg ulcers. JAMA Dermatol. 2016 Apr;152(4):472–4. [PMID: 26818102]

Garcia R et al. Duplex ultrasound for the diagnosis of acute and chronic venous diseases. Surg Clin North Am. 2018 Apr; 98(2):201–18. [PMID: 29502767]

Raffetto JD. Pathophysiology of chronic venous disease and venous ulcers. Surg Clin North Am. 2018 Apr;98(2):337–47. [PMID: 29502775]

Tessari M et al. Effects of intermittent pneumatic compression treatment on clinical outcomes and biochemical markers in patients at low mobility with lower limb edema. J Vasc Surg Venous Lymphat Disord. 2018 Jul;6(4):500–10. [PMID: 29909855]

FEVER & HYPERTHERMIA

▶ Age; injection substance use.

▶ Localizing symptoms; weight loss; joint pain.

▶ Immunosuppression or neutropenia; history of cancer.

▶ Medications.

▶ Travel.

▶ General Considerations

The average normal oral body temperature taken in mid-morning is 36.7°C (range 36–37.4°C). This range includes a mean and 2 standard deviations, thus encompassing 95% of a normal population (normal diurnal temperature variation is 0.5–1°C). The normal rectal or vaginal temperature is 0.5°C higher than the oral temperature, and the axillary temperature is 0.5°C lower. Interestingly, in a pooled meta-analysis comparing peripheral with central body temperature measurement, peripheral thermometers (tympanic membrane, temporal artery, axillary, oral) showed low sensitivity but high specificity. This suggests that a normal body temperature based on a peripheral measurement does not always exclude the presence of a fever. Thus, to exclude a fever, a rectal temperature is more reliable than an oral temperature (particularly in patients who breathe through their mouth or are tachypneic or who are in an intensive care unit setting where a rectal temperature probe can be placed to detect fever). Wearable digital thermometers may detect early mild increased temperature in patients with low white blood cell counts.

Fever is a regulated rise to a new "set point" of body temperature in the hypothalamus induced by pyrogenic cytokines. The elevation in temperature results from either increased heat production (eg, shivering) or decreased heat loss (eg, peripheral vasoconstriction). Body temperature in cytokine-induced fever seldom exceeds 41.1°C unless there is structural damage to hypothalamic regulatory centers.

▶ Clinical Findings

A. Fever

Fever as a symptom provides important information about the presence of illness—particularly infections—and about changes in the clinical status of the patient. Fever may be more predictive of bacteremia in elderly patients. The fever pattern, however, is of marginal value for most specific diagnoses except for the relapsing fever of malaria, borreliosis, and occasional cases of lymphoma, especially Hodgkin disease. Furthermore, the degree of temperature elevation does not necessarily correspond to the severity of the illness. Contrary to common perceptions, a Swedish study found that increased body temperature in the emergency department was strongly associated with lower mortality and shorter hospital stays in patients with severe sepsis or septic shock subsequently admitted to the intensive care unit even after adjustment for quality of care measures. Fever, with rash and eosinophilia, define the **d**rug **r**eaction with **e**osinophilia and **s**ystemic **s**ymptoms (DRESS) syndrome.

In general, the febrile response tends to be greater in children than in adults. In older persons, neonates, and persons receiving certain medications (eg, nonsteroidal anti-inflammatory drugs [NSAIDs], corticosteroids), a normal temperature or even hypothermia may be observed. Markedly elevated body temperature may result in profound metabolic disturbances. High temperature during the first trimester of pregnancy may cause birth defects, such as anencephaly. Fever increases insulin requirements and alters the metabolism and disposition of drugs used for the treatment of the diverse diseases associated with fever.

The source of fever varies by population and setting. In a study involving patients who underwent shoulder arthroplasty, fever was documented in 92 patients. Among these 92 patients, an infectious cause was found in only 6 patients. In the neurointensive care unit, fever can occur directly from brain injury (called "central fever"). One model predicted "central fever" with 90% probability if a patient met all of the following criteria: (1) less than 72 hours of neurologic intensive care unit admission, (2) presence of subarachnoid hemorrhage, intraventricular hemorrhage or brain tumor, (3) absence of infiltrate on chest radiograph, and (4) negative cultures. Finally, among pregnant women, the prevalence of intrapartum fever of 38°C or greater in pregnancies of 36 weeks' gestation or more is 6.8% (or 1 in 15 women in labor). And the neonatal sepsis rate among affected mothers is 0.24% (or less than 1 in 400 babies). This finding calls into question the need for universal laboratory work, cultures, and antibiotic treatment pending culture results for this newborn population.

B. Hyperthermia

Hyperthermia—not mediated by cytokines—occurs when body metabolic heat production (as in thyroid storm) or environmental heat load exceeds normal heat loss capacity or when there is impaired heat loss; heat stroke is an example. Body temperature may rise to levels (more than 41.1°C) capable of producing irreversible protein denaturation and resultant brain damage; no diurnal variation is observed.

Malignant catatonia is a disorder consisting of catatonic symptoms, hyperthermia, autonomic instability, and altered mental status.

Neuroleptic malignant syndrome, a variant of malignant catatonia, is a rare and potentially lethal idiosyncratic reaction to neuroleptic medications, particularly haloperidol and fluphenazine; however, it has also been reported with the atypical neuroleptics (such as olanzapine or risperidone) (see Chapter 25). **Serotonin syndrome** resembles neuroleptic malignant syndrome but occurs within hours of ingestion of agents that increase levels of serotonin in the central nervous system, including serotonin reuptake inhibitors, monoamine oxidase inhibitors, tricyclic antidepressants, meperidine, dextromethorphan, bromocriptine, tramadol, lithium, and psychostimulants (such as cocaine, methamphetamine, and MDMA) (see Chapter 38).

Clonus and hyperreflexia are more common in serotonin syndrome, whereas "lead pipe" rigidity is more common in neuroleptic malignant syndrome. Neuroleptic malignant and serotonin syndromes share common clinical and pathophysiologic features with **malignant hyperthermia of anesthesia** (see Chapter 38).

C. Fever of Undetermined Origin

See Fever of Unknown Origin, Chapter 30.

▶ Treatment

Most fever is well tolerated. When the temperature is less than 40°C, symptomatic treatment only is required. A temperature greater than 41°C is likely to be hyperthermia rather than cytokine mediated, and *emergent management is indicated*. (See Heat Stroke, Chapter 37.) The treatment of fever with antipyretics does not appear to affect mortality of critically ill patients or affect the number of intensive care unit–free days.

A. General Measures for Removal of Heat

Regardless of the cause of the fever, alcohol sponges, cold sponges, ice bags, ice-water enemas, and ice baths will lower body temperature (see Chapter 37). They are more useful in hyperthermia, since patients with cytokine-related fever will attempt to override these therapies.

B. Pharmacologic Treatment of Fever

1. Antipyretic drugs—Antipyretic therapy is not needed except for patients with marginal hemodynamic status. Early administration of acetaminophen to treat fever due to probable infection did not affect the number of intensive care unit–free days. Aspirin or acetaminophen, 325–650 mg every 4 hours, is effective in reducing fever. These drugs are best administered around the clock, rather than as needed, since "as needed" dosing results in periodic chills and sweats due to fluctuations in temperature caused by varying levels of drug.

2. Antimicrobial therapy—Antibacterial and antifungal prophylactic regimens are recommended only for patients expected to have less than 100 neutrophils/mcL for more than 7 days, unless other factors increase risks for complications or mortality. In most febrile patients, empiric antibiotic therapy should be deferred pending further evaluation. However, empiric antibiotic therapy is sometimes warranted. Prompt broad-spectrum antimicrobials are indicated for febrile patients who are clinically unstable, even before infection can be documented. These include patients with hemodynamic instability, those with neutropenia (neutrophils less than 500/mcL), others who are asplenic (surgically or secondary to sickle cell disease) or immunosuppressed (including individuals taking systemic corticosteroids, azathioprine, cyclosporine, or other immunosuppressive medications) (Tables 30–4 and 30–5), and those who are HIV infected (see Chapter 31).

Febrile neutropenic patients should receive initial doses of empiric antibacterial therapy within an hour of triage and should either be monitored for at least 4 hours to determine suitability for outpatient management or be admitted to the hospital (see Infections in the Immunocompromised Patient, Chapter 30). Inpatient treatment is standard to manage febrile neutropenic episodes, although carefully selected patients may be managed as outpatients after systematic assessment beginning with a validated risk index (eg, Multinational Association for Supportive Care in Cancer [MASCC] score or Talcott rules). In the MASCC index calculation, low-risk factors include the following: age under 60 years (2 points), burden of illness (5 points for no or mild symptoms and 3 points for moderate symptoms), outpatient status (3 points), solid tumor or hematologic malignancy with no previous fungal infection (4 points), no COPD (4 points), no dehydration requiring parenteral fluids (3 points), and systolic blood pressure greater than 90 mm Hg (5 points). Patients with MASCC scores 21 or higher or in Talcott group 4 (presentation as an outpatient without significant comorbidity or uncontrolled cancer), and without other risk factors, can be managed safely as outpatients.

The carefully selected outpatients determined to be at low risk by MASCC score (particularly in combination with a normal serum C-reactive protein level) or by Talcott rules can be managed with an oral fluoroquinolone plus amoxicillin/clavulanate (or clindamycin, if penicillin allergic), unless fluoroquinolone prophylaxis was used before fever developed. For treatment of fever during neutropenia following chemotherapy, outpatient parenteral antimicrobial therapy can be provided effectively and safely in low-risk patients with a single agent such as cefepime, piperacillin/tazobactam, imipenem, meropenem, or doripenem. High-risk patients should be referred for inpatient management with combination parenteral antimicrobial therapy based on specific risk factors such as pneumonia-causing pathogens or central line–associated bloodstream infections (see Infections in the Immunocompromised Patient and Table 30–5 in Chapter 30, and see Infections in Chapter 39).

If a fungal infection is suspected in patients with prolonged fever and neutropenia, fluconazole is an equally effective but less toxic alternative to amphotericin B.

C. Treatment of Hyperthermia

Discontinuation of the offending agent is mandatory. Treatment of neuroleptic malignant syndrome includes dantrolene in combination with bromocriptine or levodopa (see Chapter 25). Treatment of serotonin syndrome includes administration of a central serotonin receptor antagonist—cyproheptadine or chlorpromazine—alone or in combination with a benzodiazepine (see Chapter 38). In patients for whom it is difficult to distinguish which syndrome is present, treatment with a benzodiazepine may be the safest therapeutic option.

▶ When to Admit

- Presence of additional vital sign abnormalities or evidence of end-organ dysfunction in clinical cases when early sepsis is suspected.

- For measures to control a temperature higher than 41°C or when fever is associated with seizure or other mental status changes.
- Heat stroke (see Chapter 37).
- Malignant catatonia; neuroleptic malignant syndrome; serotonin syndrome; malignant hyperthermia of anesthesia.

Abbasi J. Wearable digital thermometer improves fever detection. JAMA. 2017 Aug 8;318(6):510. [PMID: 28787489]

DeWitt S et al. Evaluation of fever in the emergency department. Am J Emerg Med. 2017 Nov;35(11):1755–8. [PMID: 28822610]

Sundén-Cullberg J et al. Fever in the emergency department predicts survival of patients with severe sepsis and septic shock admitted to the ICU. Crit Care Med. 2017 Apr;45(4):591–9. [PMID: 28141683]

INVOLUNTARY WEIGHT LOSS

ESSENTIAL INQUIRIES

- ▶ Age; caloric intake; secondary confirmation (eg, changes in clothing size).
- ▶ Fever; change in bowel habits.
- ▶ Substance abuse.
- ▶ Age-appropriate cancer screening history.

General Considerations

Body weight is determined by a person's caloric intake, absorptive capacity, metabolic rate, and energy losses. Body weight normally peaks by the fifth or sixth decade and then gradually declines at a rate of 1–2 kg per decade. In NHANES II, a national survey of community-dwelling elders (aged 50–80 years), recent involuntary weight loss (more than 5% usual body weight) was reported by 7% of respondents, and this was associated with a 24% higher mortality. In contrast, one study found that a body mass index of 33 or less is not associated with an increased mortality in adults aged 65 years or older. In postmenopausal women, unintentional weight loss was associated with increased rates of hip and vertebral fractures.

Etiology

Involuntary weight loss is regarded as clinically significant when it exceeds 5% or more of usual body weight over a 6- to 12-month period. It often indicates serious physical or psychological illness. Physical causes are usually evident during the initial evaluation. The most common causes are cancer (about 30%), gastrointestinal disorders (about 15%), and dementia or depression (about 15%). When an adequately nourished–appearing patient complains of weight loss, inquiry should be made about exact weight changes (with approximate dates) and about changes in clothing size. Family members can provide confirmation of weight loss, as can old documents such as driver's licenses. A mild, gradual weight loss occurs in some older individuals because of decreased energy requirements. However, rapid involuntary weight loss is predictive of morbidity and mortality. In addition to various disease states, causes in older individuals include loss of teeth and consequent difficulty with chewing, medications interfering with taste or causing nausea, alcoholism, and social isolation.

Clinical Findings

Once the weight loss is established, the history, medication profile, physical examination, and conventional laboratory and radiologic investigations (eg, complete blood count, liver biochemical tests, kidney panel, serologic tests including HIV, thyroid-stimulating hormone [TSH] level, urinalysis, fecal occult blood test, chest radiography, and upper gastrointestinal series) usually reveal the cause. Whole-body CT imaging is increasingly used for diagnosis; one study found its diagnostic yield to be 33.5%. When these tests are normal, the second phase of evaluation should focus on more definitive gastrointestinal investigation (eg, tests for malabsorption, endoscopy) and cancer screening (eg, Papanicolaou smear, mammography, prostate-specific antigen [PSA]). However, one prospective case study in patients with unintentional weight loss showed that colonoscopy did not find colorectal cancer if weight loss was the sole indication for the test.

If the initial evaluation is unrevealing, follow-up is preferable to further diagnostic testing. Death at 2-year follow-up was not nearly as common in patients with unexplained involuntary weight loss (8%) as in those with weight loss due to malignant (79%) and established nonmalignant diseases (19%). Psychiatric consultation should be considered when there is evidence of depression, dementia, anorexia nervosa, or other emotional problems. Ultimately, in approximately 15–25% of cases, no cause for the weight loss can be found.

Differential Diagnosis

Malignancy, gastrointestinal disorders (poorly fitting dentures, cavities, swallowing or malabsorption disorders, pancreatic insufficiency), HF, psychological problems (dementia, depression, paranoia), endocrine disorders (hyperthyroidism, hypothyroidism, hyperparathyroidism, hypoadrenalism), eating problems (dietary restrictions, lack of money for food), social problems (alcohol use disorder, social isolation), and medication side effects are all established causes.

Treatment

Weight stabilization occurs in most surviving patients with both established and unknown causes of weight loss through treatment of the underlying disorder and caloric supplementation. Nutrient intake goals are established in relation to the severity of weight loss, in general ranging from 30 to 40 kcal/kg/day. In order of preference, route of administration options include oral, temporary nasojejunal tube, or percutaneous gastric or jejunal tube. Parenteral nutrition is reserved for patients with serious associated problems. A variety of pharmacologic agents have been proposed for the treatment of weight loss. These can be categorized into appetite stimulants (corticosteroids, progestational agents, dronabinol, and serotonin antagonists); anabolic agents (growth hormone and testosterone derivatives); and anticatabolic agents (omega-3 fatty acids, pentoxifylline, hydrazine sulfate, and thalidomide). There is no evidence that appetite stimulants decrease mortality, and they may have severe adverse side effects. Exercise training may prevent or even reverse the process of muscle wasting in HF ("cardiac cachexia"). Protein supplementation combined with resistance exercise training and aerobic activity may prevent aging-related muscle mass attenuation and functional performance.

When to Refer

- Weight loss caused by malabsorption.
- Persistent nutritional deficiencies despite adequate supplementation.
- Weight loss as a result of anorexia or bulimia.

When to Admit

- Severe protein-energy malnutrition, including the syndromes of kwashiorkor and marasmus.
- Vitamin deficiency syndromes.
- Cachexia with anticipated progressive weight loss secondary to unmanageable psychiatric disease.
- Careful electrolyte and fluid replacement in protein-energy malnutrition and avoidance of "re-feeding syndrome."

Bradlee ML et al. High-protein foods and physical activity protect against age-related muscle loss and functional decline. J Gerontol A Biol Sci Med Sci. 2017 Dec 12;73(1):88–94. [PMID: 28549098]

Garcia JM et al. Nonsteroidal anti-inflammatory drugs in patients with anorexia-cachexia syndrome associated with malignancy and its treatments. Am J Med. 2017 Sep;130(9):1033–6. [PMID: 29016346]

Goh Y et al. Diagnostic utility of whole body CT scanning in patients with unexplained weight loss. PLoS One. 2018 Jul 27; 13(7):e0200686. [PMID: 30052642]

Venturelli M et al. Possible predictors of involuntary weight loss in patients with Alzheimer's disease. PLoS One. 2016 Jun 27; 11(6):e0157384. [PMID: 27347878]

Villareal DT et al. Aerobic or resistance exercise, or both, in dieting obese older adults. N Engl J Med. 2017 May 18;376(20): 1943–55. [PMID: 28514618]

FATIGUE & CHRONIC FATIGUE SYNDROME

ESSENTIAL INQUIRIES

- Weight loss; fever.
- Sleep-disordered breathing.
- Medications; substance use.

General Considerations

Fatigue, as an isolated symptom, accounts for 1–3% of visits to generalists. The symptom of fatigue is often poorly described and less well defined by patients than symptoms associated with specific dysfunction of organ systems. Fatigue or lassitude and the closely related complaints of weakness, tiredness, and lethargy are often attributed to overexertion, poor physical conditioning, sleep disturbance, obesity, undernutrition, and emotional problems. A history of the patient's daily living and working habits may obviate the need for extensive and unproductive diagnostic studies.

The diagnosis of chronic fatigue syndrome remains hotly debated because of the lack of a gold standard. Persons with chronic fatigue syndrome meeting specific criteria (such as those from the CDC) report a greater frequency of childhood trauma and psychopathology and demonstrate higher levels of emotional instability and self-reported stress than persons who do not have chronic fatigue. Neuropsychological and neuroendocrine studies reveal abnormalities in most patients but no consistent pattern. Sleep disorders have been reported in 40–80% of patients with chronic fatigue syndrome, but polysomnographic studies have not shown a greater incidence of primary sleep disorders in those with chronic fatigue syndrome than in controls, suggesting that the sleep disorders are comorbid rather than causative. Older patients with chronic fatigue syndrome demonstrate a greater disease impact than younger patients. A retrospective cohort study in Germany found an increased risk of chronic fatigue syndrome after a first-time diagnosis of gastrointestinal infection (hazard ratio, 1.35–1.82).

Clinical Findings

A. Fatigue

Clinically relevant fatigue is composed of three major components: generalized weakness (difficulty in initiating activities); easy fatigability (difficulty in completing activities); and mental fatigue (difficulty with concentration and memory). Important diseases that can cause fatigue include hyperthyroidism and hypothyroidism, HF, infections (endocarditis, hepatitis), COPD, sleep apnea, anemia, autoimmune disorders, multiple sclerosis, irritable bowel syndrome, Parkinson disease, cerebral vascular accident, and cancer. Solution-focused therapy has a significant initial beneficial effect on the severity of fatigue and quality of life in patients with quiescent inflammatory bowel disease.

Alcohol use disorder, vitamin C deficiency (scurvy), side effects from medications (eg, sedatives and beta-blockers), and psychological conditions (eg, insomnia, depression, anxiety, panic attacks, dysthmia, and somatization disorder) may be the cause. Common outpatient infectious causes include mononucleosis and sinusitis. These conditions are usually associated with other characteristic signs, but patients may emphasize fatigue and not reveal their other symptoms unless directly asked. The lifetime prevalence of significant fatigue (present for at least 2 weeks) is about 25%. Fatigue of unknown cause or related to psychiatric illness exceeds that due to physical illness, injury, alcohol, or medications.

Although frequently associated with Lyme disease, severe fatigue as a long-term sequela is rare.

B. Chronic Fatigue Syndrome

A working case definition of chronic fatigue syndrome indicates that it is not a homogeneous abnormality, there is no single pathogenic mechanism (Figure 2–1), and no physical finding or laboratory test can be used to confirm the diagnosis.

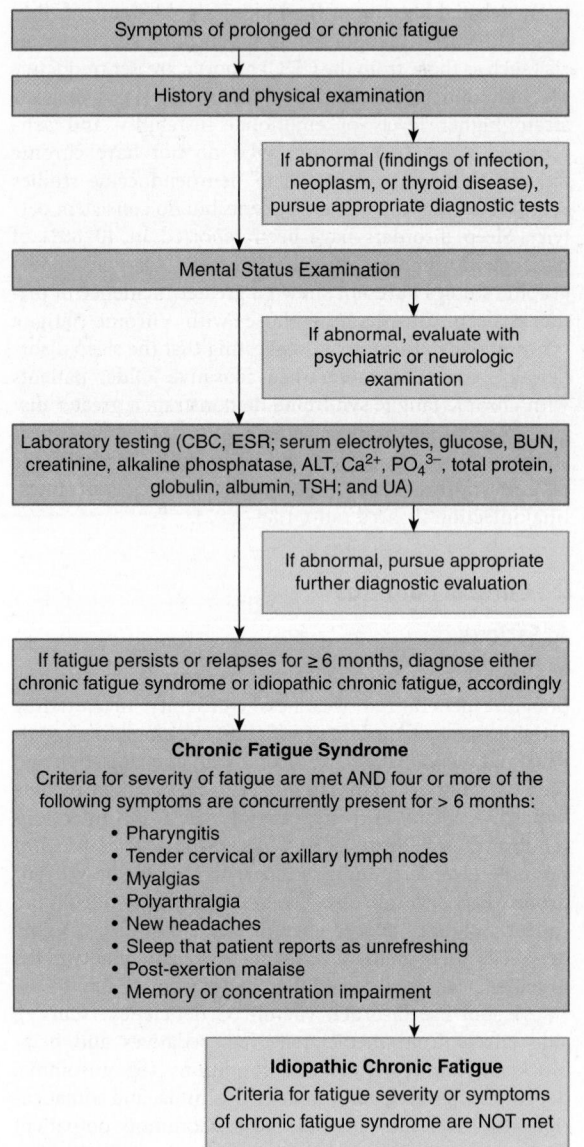

▲ **Figure 2–1.** Classification of chronic fatigue patients. ALT, alanine aminotransferase; BUN, blood urea nitrogen; Ca^{2+}, calcium; CBC, complete blood count; ESR, erythrocyte sedimentation rate; PO_4^{3-}, phosphate; TSH, thyroid-stimulating hormone; UA, urinalysis.

The evaluation of chronic fatigue syndrome includes a history and physical examination as well as complete blood count, erythrocyte sedimentation rate, chemistries (blood urea nitrogen [BUN], serum electrolytes, glucose, creatinine, calcium, liver biochemical tests, and thyroid function tests), urinalysis, tuberculin skin test, and screening questionnaires for psychiatric disorders. Other tests to be performed as clinically indicated are serum cortisol, antinuclear antibody, rheumatoid factor, immunoglobulin levels, Lyme serology in endemic areas (although rarely a long-term complication of this infection), and HIV antibody. More extensive testing is usually unhelpful, including antibody to Epstein-Barr virus. There may be an abnormally high rate of postural hypotension. Brain MRI is not routinely recommended.

▶ Treatment

A. Fatigue

Management of fatigue involves identification and treatment of conditions that contribute to fatigue, such as cancer, pain, depression, disordered sleep, weight loss, and anemia. Resistance training and aerobic exercise lessens fatigue and improves performance for a number of chronic conditions associated with a high prevalence of fatigue, including HF, COPD, arthritis, and cancer. Continuous positive airway pressure is an effective treatment for obstructive sleep apnea. Psychostimulants such as methylphenidate have shown inconsistent results in randomized trials of treatment of cancer-related fatigue. Modafinil and armodafinil appear to be effective, well-tolerated agents in HIV-positive patients with fatigue and as adjunctive agents in patients with depression or bipolar disorder with fatigue. Testosterone replacement in hypoandrogenic men over age 65 had no significant benefit with respect to walking distance or vitality, as assessed by the Functional Assessment of Chronic Illness Therapy-Fatigue scale, but men who received the testosterone reported slightly better mood and lower severity of depressive symptoms than those who received placebo.

Therapeutic Care (a complementary medicine modality that uses acupressure) reduces fatigue in some patients with breast cancer receiving chemotherapy, and Internet-based cognitive-behavioral therapy is effective in reducing severe fatigue in breast cancer survivors.

Methylphenidate, as well as cognitive-behavioral therapy, may improve mental fatigue and cognitive functions in patients with traumatic brain injury. The TRUST study found that treatment of subclinical hypothyroidism did not improve symptoms of fatigue as measured by the Tiredness score (3.2±17.7 and 3.8±18.4, respectively; between-group difference, 0.4; 95% CI, –2.1–2.9). Vitamin D treatment significantly improved fatigue in kidney transplantation patients as well as in otherwise healthy persons with vitamin D deficiency.

B. Chronic Fatigue Syndrome

A variety of agents and modalities have been tried for the treatment of chronic fatigue syndrome. Acyclovir, intravenous immunoglobulin, nystatin, clonidine (in adolescent chronic fatigue syndrome), peripheral IL-1 inhibition with anakinra, and low-dose hydrocortisone do not improve symptoms. Inhibition of cytokine IL-1 with anakinra for 4 weeks does not result in a clinically significant reduction in fatigue severity in women with chronic fatigue syndrome. Some patients with postural hypotension report response to increases in dietary sodium as well as fludrocortisone, 0.1 mg orally daily. The immune modulator rintatolimod improved some measures of exercise performance compared with placebo in two trials (low strength of evidence). There is very limited evidence that dietary modification is beneficial.

There is a greater prevalence of past and current psychiatric diagnoses in patients with this syndrome. Affective disorders are especially common. Patients with chronic fatigue syndrome have benefited from a comprehensive multidisciplinary intervention, including optimal medical management, treating any ongoing affective or anxiety disorder pharmacologically, and implementing a comprehensive cognitive-behavioral treatment program. At present, cognitive-behavioral therapy and graded exercise are the treatments of choice for patients with chronic fatigue syndrome. **Cognitive-behavioral therapy,** a form of non-pharmacologic treatment emphasizing self-help and aiming to change perceptions and behaviors that may perpetuate symptoms and disability, may be helpful in some patients. Response to cognitive-behavioral therapy is not predictable on the basis of severity or duration of chronic fatigue syndrome. Patients with high neuroticism or low acceptance show more improvement in mental quality of life with cognitive-behavioral therapy.

Graded exercise may result in mild-to-moderate improvements in functional work capacity and physical function in some patients but may prove risky in others. A 2011 randomized trial (PACE trial) confirmed the independent benefits of cognitive-behavioral therapy and graded exercise, but recent meta-analyses and re-analysis of PACE are calling into question the magnitude of the benefit and safety of graded exercise. Physiologic studies find an altered immune response to exercise in patients with chronic fatigue syndrome. A self-help booklet describing a six-step graded exercise program over 12 weeks and up to four guidance sessions with a physiotherapist over 8 weeks may be as helpful as specialist medical care alone.

In addition, the clinician's sympathetic listening and explanatory responses can help overcome the patient's frustrations and debilitation by this still mysterious illness. All patients should be encouraged to engage in normal activities to the extent possible and should be reassured that full recovery is eventually possible in most cases. Chronic fatigue syndrome is not associated with increased all-cause mortality, but one study showed a substantially increased risk of completed suicide.

▶ **When to Refer**

- Infections not responsive to standard treatment.
- Difficult-to-control hyperthyroidism or hypothyroidism.
- Severe psychological illness.
- Malignancy.

▶ **When to Admit**

- Failure to thrive.
- Fatigue severe enough to impair activities of daily living.

Abrahams HJG et al. The efficacy of Internet-based cognitive behavioral therapy for severely fatigued survivors of breast cancer compared with care as usual: a randomized controlled trial. Cancer. 2017 Oct 1;123(19):3825–34. [PMID: 28621820]

Clark LV et al. Guided graded exercise self-help plus specialist medical care versus specialist medical care alone for chronic fatigue syndrome (GETSET): a pragmatic randomised controlled trial. Lancet. 2017 Jul 22;390(10092):363–73. [PMID: 28648402]

Donnachie E et al. Incidence of irritable bowel syndrome and chronic fatigue following GI infection: a population-level study using routinely collected claims data. Gut. 2018 Jun; 67(6):1078–86. [PMID: 28601847]

Larun L et al. Exercise therapy for chronic fatigue syndrome. Cochrane Database Syst Rev. 2017 Apr 25;4:CD003200. [PMID: 28444695]

Nguyen S et al. Cognitive behavior therapy to treat sleep disturbance and fatigue after traumatic brain injury: a pilot randomized controlled trial. Arch Phys Med Rehabil. 2017 Aug; 98(8):1508–17.e2. [PMID: 28400181]

Nowak A et al. Effect of vitamin D3 on self-perceived fatigue: a double-blind randomized placebo-controlled trial. Medicine (Baltimore). 2016 Dec;95(52):e5353. [PMID: 28033244]

Roberts E et al. Mortality of people with chronic fatigue syndrome: a retrospective cohort study in England and Wales from the South London and Maudsley NHS Foundation Trust Biomedical Research Centre (SLaM BRC) Clinical Record Interactive Search (CRIS) Register. Lancet. 2016 Apr 16; 387(10028):1638–43. [PMID: 26873808]

Roerink ME et al. Cytokine inhibition in patients with chronic fatigue syndrome: a randomized trial. Ann Intern Med. 2017 Apr 18;166(8):557–64. [PMID: 28265678]

Snyder PJ et al; Testosterone Trials Investigators. Effects of testosterone treatment in older men. N Engl J Med. 2016 Feb 18; 374(7):611–24. [PMID: 26886521]

Stott DJ et al; TRUST Study Group. Thyroid hormone therapy for older adults with subclinical hypothyroidism. N Engl J Med. 2017 Jun 29;376(26):2534–44. [PMID: 28402245]

Unger ER et al. CDC Grand Rounds: chronic fatigue syndrome—advancing research and clinical education. MMWR Morb Mortal Wkly Rep. 2016 Dec 30;65(5051):1434–8. [PMID: 28033311]

Vink M et al. Graded exercise therapy for myalgic encephalomyelitis/chronic fatigue syndrome is not effective and unsafe. Re-analysis of a Cochrane review. Health Psychol Open. 2018 Oct 8;5(2):2055102918805187. [PMID: 30305916]

Vink M et al. Multidisciplinary rehabilitation treatment is not effective for myalgic encephalomyelitis/chronic fatigue syndrome: a review of the FatiGo trial. Health Psychol Open. 2018 Aug 6;5(2):2055102918792648. [PMID: 30094055]

Wilshire CE et al. Rethinking the treatment of chronic fatigue syndrome-a reanalysis and evaluation of findings from a recent major trial of graded exercise and CBT. BMC Psychol. 2018 Mar 22;6(1):6. [PMID: 29562932]

Zhang B et al. Effect of therapeutic care for treating fatigue in patients with breast cancer receiving chemotherapy. Medicine (Baltimore). 2017 Aug;96(33):e7750. [PMID: 28816951]

ACUTE HEADACHE

ESSENTIAL INQUIRIES

▶ Age older than 40 years.

▶ Rapid onset and severe intensity (ie, "thunderclap" headache), trauma, onset during exertion.

▶ Fever, vision changes, neck stiffness.

▶ HIV infection.

▶ Current or past history of hypertension.

▶ Neurologic findings (mental status changes, motor or sensory deficits, loss of consciousness).

▶ General Considerations

Headache is a common reason that adults seek medical care, accounting for approximately 13 million visits each year in the United States to physicians' offices, urgent care clinics, and emergency departments. It is the fifth most common reason for emergency department visits, and second most common reason for neurologic consultation in the emergency department. A broad range of disorders can cause headache (see Chapter 24). This section deals only with acute nontraumatic headache in adults and adolescents. The challenge in the initial evaluation of acute headache is to identify which patients are presenting with an uncommon but life-threatening condition; approximately 1% of patients seeking care in emergency department settings and considerably less in office practice settings fall into this category.

Diminution of headache in response to typical migraine therapies (such as serotonin receptor antagonists or ketorolac) does not rule out critical conditions such as subarachnoid hemorrhage or meningitis as the underlying cause.

▶ Clinical Findings

A. Symptoms

A careful history and physical examination should aim to identify causes of acute headache that require immediate treatment. These causes can be broadly classified as imminent or completed **vascular events** (intracranial hemorrhage, thrombosis, cavernous sinus thrombosis, vasculitis, malignant hypertension, arterial dissection, cerebral venous thrombosis, transient ischemic attack, or aneurysm), **infections** (abscess, encephalitis, or meningitis), **intracranial masses** causing intracranial hypertension, **preeclampsia,** and **carbon monoxide poisoning.** Having the patient carefully describe the onset of headache can be helpful in diagnosing a serious cause. Report of a sudden-onset headache that reaches maximal and severe intensity within seconds or a few minutes is the classic description of a "thunderclap" headache; it should precipitate workup for subarachnoid hemorrhage, since the estimated prevalence of subarachnoid hemorrhage in patients with thunderclap headache is 43%. Thunderclap headache during the

Table 2–8. Clinical features associated with acute headache that warrant urgent or emergent neuroimaging.

Prior to lumbar puncture
Abnormal neurologic examination
Abnormal mental status
Abnormal funduscopic examination (papilledema; loss of venous pulsations)
Meningeal signs
Emergent (conduct prior to leaving office or emergency department)
Abnormal neurologic examination
Abnormal mental status
"Thunderclap" headache
Urgent (scheduled prior to leaving office or emergency department)
HIV-positive patient[1]
Age > 50 years (normal neurologic examination)

[1]Use CT with or without contrast or MRI if HIV positive.
Data from American College of Emergency Physicians. Clinical policy: critical issues in the evaluation and management of patients presenting to the emergency department with acute headache. Ann Emerg Med. 2002 Jan;39(1):108–22.

postpartum period precipitated by the Valsalva maneuver or recumbent positioning may indicate reversible cerebral vasoconstriction syndrome. Other historical features that raise the need for diagnostic testing include headache brought on by the Valsalva maneuver, cough, exertion, or sexual activity.

The medical history can also guide the need for additional workup. Under most circumstances (including a normal neurologic examination), new headache in a patient older than 50 years or with HIV infection warrants immediate neuroimaging (Table 2–8). When the patient has a history of hypertension—particularly uncontrolled hypertension—a complete search for other features of "malignant hypertension" is appropriate to determine the urgency of control of hypertension (see Chapter 11). Headache and hypertension associated with pregnancy may be due to preeclampsia. Episodic headache associated with the triad of hypertension, palpitations, and sweats is suggestive of pheochromocytoma. In the absence of thunderclap headache, advanced age, and HIV infection, a careful physical examination and detailed neurologic examination will usually determine acuity of the workup and need for further diagnostic testing. A history consistent with hypercoagulability is associated with an increased risk of cerebral venous thrombosis.

Symptoms can also be useful for diagnosing migraine headache in the absence of the "classic" migraine pattern of scintillating scotoma followed by unilateral headache, photophobia, and nausea and vomiting (Table 2–9). The presence of three or more of these symptoms (nausea, photophobia, phonophobia, and exacerbation by physical activity) can establish the diagnosis of migraine (in the absence of other clinical features that warrant neuroimaging studies), and the presence of only one or two symptoms (provided one is not nausea) can help rule out migraine.

Table 2–9. Summary likelihood ratios (LRs) for individual clinical features associated with migraine diagnosis.

Clinical Feature	LR+ (95% CI)	LR− (95% CI)
Nausea	19 (15–25)	0.19 (0.18–0.20)
Photophobia	5.8 (5.1–6.6)	0.24 (0.23–0.26)
Phonophobia	5.2 (4.5–5.9)	0.38 (0.36–0.40)
Exacerbation by physical activity	3.7 (3.4–4.0)	0.24 (0.23–0.26)

CI, confidence interval.

B. Physical Examination

Critical components of the physical examination of the patient with acute headache include vital signs, neurologic examination, and vision testing with funduscopic examination. The finding of fever with acute headache warrants additional maneuvers to elicit evidence of meningeal inflammation, such as Kernig and Brudzinski signs. The absence of jolt accentuation of headache cannot accurately rule out meningitis. Patients older than 60 years should be examined for scalp or temporal artery tenderness.

Careful assessment of visual acuity, ocular gaze, visual fields, pupillary defects, optic disks, and retinal vein pulsations is crucial. Diminished visual acuity is suggestive of glaucoma, temporal arteritis, or optic neuritis. Ophthalmoplegia or visual field defects may be signs of venous sinus thrombosis, tumor, or aneurysm. Afferent pupillary defects can be due to intracranial masses or optic neuritis. In the setting of headache and hypertension, retinal cotton wool spots, flame hemorrhages, and disk swelling indicate acute severe hypertensive retinopathy. Ipsilateral ptosis and miosis suggest Horner syndrome and in conjunction with acute headache may signify carotid artery dissection. Finally, papilledema or absent retinal venous pulsations are signs of elevated intracranial pressure—findings that should be followed by neuroimaging prior to performing lumbar puncture (Table 2–8). On nonmydriatic fundoscopy, up to 8.5% of patients who arrive at the emergency department complaining of headache had abnormalities; although few had other significant physical examination findings, 59% of them had abnormal neuroimaging studies.

Complete neurologic evaluations are also critical and should include assessment of mental status, motor and sensory systems, reflexes, gait, cerebellar function, and pronator drift. Any abnormality on neurologic evaluation (especially mental status) warrants emergent neuroimaging (Table 2–8).

C. Diagnostic Studies

Neuroimaging is summarized in Table 2–8. Under most circumstances, a noncontrast head CT is sufficient to exclude intracranial hypertension with impending herniation, intracranial hemorrhage, and many types of intracranial masses (notable exceptions include lymphoma and toxoplasmosis in HIV-positive patients, herpes simplex encephalitis, and brain abscess). When needed, a contrast study can be ordered to follow a normal noncontrast study. A normal neuroimaging study does not exclude subarachnoid hemorrhage and should be followed by lumbar puncture. One study supported a change of practice wherein a lumbar puncture can be withheld when a head CT scan was performed less than 6 hours after headache onset and showed no evidence of subarachnoid hemorrhage (negative predictive value 99.9% [95% CI, 99.3–100.0%]).

In patients for whom there is a high level of suspicion for subarachnoid hemorrhage or aneurysm, a normal CT and lumbar puncture should be followed by angiography within the next few days (provided the patient is medically stable). Lumbar puncture is also indicated to exclude infectious causes of acute headache, particularly in patients with fever or meningeal signs. Cerebrospinal fluid tests should routinely include Gram stain, white blood cell count with differential, red blood cell count, glucose, total protein, and bacterial culture. In appropriate patients, also consider testing cerebrospinal fluid for VDRL (syphilis), cryptococcal antigen (HIV-positive patients), acid-fast bacillus stain and culture, and complement fixation and culture for coccidioidomycosis. Storage of an extra tube with 5 mL of cerebrospinal fluid is also prudent for conducting unanticipated tests in the immediate future. Polymerase chain reaction tests for specific infectious pathogens (eg, herpes simplex 2) should also be considered in patients with evidence of central nervous system infection but no identifiable pathogen.

The Ottawa subarachnoid hemorrhage clinical decision rule had 100% sensitivity (and 13–15% specificity in different studies) in predicting subarachnoid hemorrhage. According to it, patients who seek medical attention in an emergency department complaining of an acute nontraumatic headache should be evaluated for subarachnoid hemorrhage if they have one or more of the following factors: age 40 years or older, neck pain or stiffness, witnessed loss of consciousness, onset during exertion, thunderclap headache (instantly peaking pain), or limited neck flexion on examination.

In addition to neuroimaging and lumbar puncture, additional diagnostic tests for exclusion of life-threatening causes of acute headache include erythrocyte sedimentation rate (temporal arteritis; endocarditis), urinalysis (malignant hypertension; preeclampsia), and sinus CT (bacterial sinusitis, independently or as a cause of venous sinus thrombosis).

▶ Treatment

Treatment should be directed at the cause of acute headache. In patients in whom migraine or migraine-like headache has been diagnosed, early treatment with NSAIDs (oral, nasal, or intramuscular ketorolac), metoclopramide, dihydroergotamine, or triptans (oral, nasal, subcutaneous) can often abort or provide significant relief of symptoms (see Chapter 24). Intravenous prochlorperazine plus diphenhydramine was more effective for migraine pain relief than intravenous hydromorphone in the emergency department. There appears to be no benefit of adding intravenous diphenhydramine to intravenous metoclopramide. Sumatriptan may be less effective as immediate therapy for migraine attacks with aura compared to attacks without aura. Parenteral morphine and hydromorphone are best avoided as first-line therapy.

Subanesthetic ketamine infusions may be beneficial in individuals with chronic migraine and new daily persistent headache that has not responded to other aggressive treatments. Peripheral nerve blocks may be a safe and effective way to treat headaches in older adults. Surgical decompression of peripheral cranial and spinal nerves at trigger sites have been used to treat migraine. Noninvasive vagus nerve stimulation has shown promise in the management of migraine and acute cluster headaches.

High-flow oxygen therapy may also provide effective treatment for all headache types in the emergency department setting. Peripheral nerve blocks for treatment-refractory migraine may be an effective therapeutic option in pregnancy. The oral 5-HT$_{1F}$ receptor agonist, lasmiditan, is currently in clinical trials and awaiting US Food and Drug Administration (FDA) approval for the treatment of acute migraine.

Regular exercise may have a prophylactic effect on migraine frequency; however, new, intense exercise can trigger migraine.

▶ When to Refer

- Frequent migraines not responsive to standard therapy.
- Migraines with atypical features.
- Chronic daily headaches due to medication overuse.

▶ When to Admit

- Need for repeated doses of parenteral pain medication.
- To facilitate an expedited workup requiring a sequence of neuroimaging and procedures.
- To monitor for progression of symptoms and to obtain neurologic consultation when the initial emergency department workup is inconclusive.
- Pain severe enough to impair activities of daily living or impede follow-up appointments or consultations.
- Patients with subarachnoid hemorrhage, intracranial mass, or meningitis.

Amin FM et al; European Headache Federation School of Advanced Studies (EHF-SAS). The association between migraine and physical exercise. J Headache Pain. 2018 Sep 10; 19(1):83. [PMID: 30203180]

Avcu N et al. Intranasal lidocaine in acute treatment of migraine: a randomized controlled trial. Ann Emerg Med. 2017 Jun; 69(6):743–51. [PMID: 27889366]

Buttgereit F et al. Polymyalgia rheumatica and giant cell arteritis: a systematic review. JAMA. 2016 Jun 14;315(22):2442–58. [PMID: 27299619]

Chessman AW. IV prochlorperazine + diphenhydramine improved migraine pain relief more than IV hydromorphone in the ED. Ann Intern Med. 2018 Mar 20;168(6):JC28. [PMID: 29554666]

Chinthapalli K et al. Assessment of acute headache in adults—what the general physician needs to know. Clin Med (Lond). 2018 Oct;18(5):422–7. [PMID: 30287441]

Dagenais R et al. Intranasal lidocaine for acute management of primary headaches: a systematic review. Pharmacotherapy. 2018 Oct;38(10):1038–50. [PMID: 30098024]

Dodick DW. Migraine. Lancet. 2018 Mar 31;391(10127):1315–30. [PMID: 29523342]

Friedman BW et al. Randomized study of IV prochlorperazine plus diphenhydramine vs IV hydromorphone for migraine. Neurology. 2017 Nov 14;89(20):2075–82. [PMID: 29046364]

Lawton MT et al. Subarachnoid hemorrhage. N Engl J Med. 2017 Jul 20;377(3):257–66. [PMID: 28723321]

Mayans L et al. Acute migraine headache: treatment strategies. Am Fam Physician. 2018 Feb 15;97(4):243–51. [PMID: 29671521]

Orr SL et al. Management of adults with acute migraine in the emergency department: the American Headache Society evidence assessment of parenteral pharmacotherapies. Headache. 2016 Jun;56(6):911–40. [PMID: 27300483]

Pringsheim T et al. How to apply the AHS evidence assessment of the acute treatment of migraine in adults to your patient with migraine. Headache. 2016 Jul;56(7):1194–200. [PMID: 27322907]

DYSURIA

ESSENTIAL INQUIRIES

- ▶ Fever; new back or flank pain; nausea or vomiting.
- ▶ Vaginal discharge.
- ▶ Pregnancy risk.
- ▶ Structural abnormalities.
- ▶ Instrumentation of urethra or bladder.

▶ General Considerations

Dysuria (painful urination) is a common reason for adults and adolescents to seek urgent medical attention. An inflammatory process (eg, urinary tract infection [UTI], autoimmune disorder) underlies most causes of dysuria. In women, cystitis will be diagnosed in up to 50–60% of cases. Cystitis has an incidence of 0.5–0.7% per year in sexually active young women. The key objective in evaluating women with dysuria is to exclude serious upper urinary tract disease, such as acute pyelonephritis, and sexually transmitted diseases. In elderly men, dysuria may be a symptom of prostatitis. In contrast, in younger men, urethritis accounts for the vast majority of cases of dysuria.

▶ Clinical Findings

A. Symptoms

Well-designed cohort studies have shown that some women can be reliably diagnosed with uncomplicated cystitis without a physical examination or urinalysis, and randomized controlled trials show that telephone management of uncomplicated cystitis is safe and effective. An increased likelihood of cystitis is present when women report multiple irritative voiding symptoms (dysuria, urgency, frequency), fever, or back pain (LRs = 1.6–2.0). A cohort study found that the symptom of dysuria most reliably predicted a culture-positive UTI. Inquiring about symptoms of vulvovaginitis is imperative. When women report dysuria and urinary frequency, and deny vaginal discharge and irritation, the LR for culture-confirmed cystitis is 24.5. In contrast, when vaginal discharge or irritation is present, as well as dysuria or urinary frequency, the LR is 0.7. Gross hematuria in women with voiding symptoms usually represents hemorrhagic cystitis but can also be a sign of bladder cancer (particularly in older patients) or upper tract disease. Failure of hematuria to resolve with antibiotic treatment should prompt further evaluation of the bladder and kidneys. Chlamydial infection should be strongly considered among women aged 25 years or younger who are sexually active and seeking medical attention for a suspected UTI for the first time or who have a new partner.

Because fever and back pain, as well as nausea and vomiting, are considered harbingers of (or clinical criteria for) acute pyelonephritis, women with these symptoms should usually be examined by a clinician prior to treatment in order to exclude coexistent urosepsis, hydronephrosis, or nephrolithiasis that would affect management decisions. Risk factors for acute pyelonephritis among women 18–49 years of age relate to sexual behaviors (frequent sexual intercourse (3 times per week or more), new sexual partner in previous year, recent spermicide use), as well as diabetes mellitus and recent UTI or incontinence. Finally, pregnancy, underlying structural factors (polycystic kidney disease, nephrolithiasis, neurogenic bladder), immunosuppression, diabetes mellitus, and a history of recent bladder or urethral instrumentation usually alter the treatment regimen (antibiotic choice or duration of treatment, or both) of cystitis. Presence of UTI during pregnancy is strongly associated with preeclampsia (particularly during the third trimester).

B. Physical Examination

Fever, tachycardia, or hypotension suggests, the possibility of urosepsis and potential need for hospitalization. A focused examination in women, in uncomplicated circumstances, could be limited to ascertainment of costovertebral angle tenderness and to a lower abdominal and pelvic examination if the history suggests vulvovaginitis or cervicitis.

C. Diagnostic Studies

1. Urinalysis—Urinalysis is probably overutilized in the evaluation of dysuria. The probability of culture-confirmed UTI among women with a history and physical examination compatible with uncomplicated cystitis is about 70–90%. Urinalysis is most helpful in atypical presentations of cystitis. Dipstick detection (greater than trace) of leukocytes, nitrites, or blood supports a diagnosis of cystitis. When both leukocyte and nitrite tests are positive, the LR is 4.2, and when both are negative, the LR is 0.3. The negative predictive value of urinalysis is not sufficient to exclude culture-confirmed UTI in women with multiple and typical symptoms, and randomized trial evidence shows that antibiotic treatment is beneficial to women with typical symptoms and negative urinalysis dipstick tests.

Microscopy of unspun urine may also be helpful in diagnosis and reduces unnecessary use of antibiotics. The combination of urgency, dysuria, and pyuria, assessed with the high-power objective (40 ×) for pus cells (more than 1 pus cell/7 high-power fields) had a positive predictive value of 71 and LR of 2.97.

2. Urine culture—Urine culture should be considered for all women with upper tract symptoms (prior to initiating antibiotic therapy), as well as those with dysuria and a negative urine dipstick test. In symptomatic women, a clean-catch urine culture is considered positive when 10^2–10^3 colony-forming units/mL of a uropathogenic organism is detected.

3. Renal imaging—When severe flank or back pain is present, the possibility of complicated kidney infection (perinephric abscess, nephrolithiasis) or of hydronephrosis should be considered. Renal ultrasound or CT scanning should be done to rule out abscess and hydronephrosis. To exclude nephrolithiasis, noncontrast helical CT scanning is more accurate than intravenous urography and is the diagnostic test of choice. In a meta-analysis, the positive and negative LRs of helical CT scanning for diagnosis of nephrolithiasis were 23.2 and 0.05, respectively.

▶ Differential Diagnosis

The differential diagnosis of dysuria in women includes acute cystitis, acute pyelonephritis, vaginitis (*Candida*, bacterial vaginosis, *Trichomonas*, herpes simplex), urethritis/cervicitis (*Chlamydia*, gonorrhea), and interstitial cystitis/painful bladder syndrome. Nucleic acid amplification tests from first-void urine or vaginal swab specimens are highly sensitive for detecting chlamydial infection. Other infectious pathogens associated with dysuria and urethritis in men include *Mycoplasma genitalium* and Enterobacteriaceae.

▶ Treatment

Definitive treatment is directed to the underlying cause of the dysuria. An evidence-informed algorithm for managing suspected UTI in women is shown in Figure 2–2. This algorithm supports antibiotic treatment of most women with multiple and typical symptoms of UTI without performing urinalysis or urine culture. Antibiotic selection should be guided by local resistance patterns and expert-panel clinical practice guidelines; major options for uncomplicated cystitis include nitrofurantoin, cephalosporins, ciprofloxacin, fosfomycin, and trimethoprim-sulfamethoxazole. Five days of nitrofurantoin resulted in a significantly greater likelihood of clinical and microbiologic resolution than single-dose fosfomycin. According to the American Academy of Pediatrics' Committee on Drugs, antibiotics that are usually acceptable when treating women who are breastfeeding include trimethoprim-sulfamethoxazole (unless G6PD deficiency is present), amoxicillin, nitrofurantoin, ciprofloxacin, and ofloxacin.

In men, prolonged treatment of UTIs (more than 7 days) out of concern for delayed clearance of infection within the prostate does not appear to reduce early or late

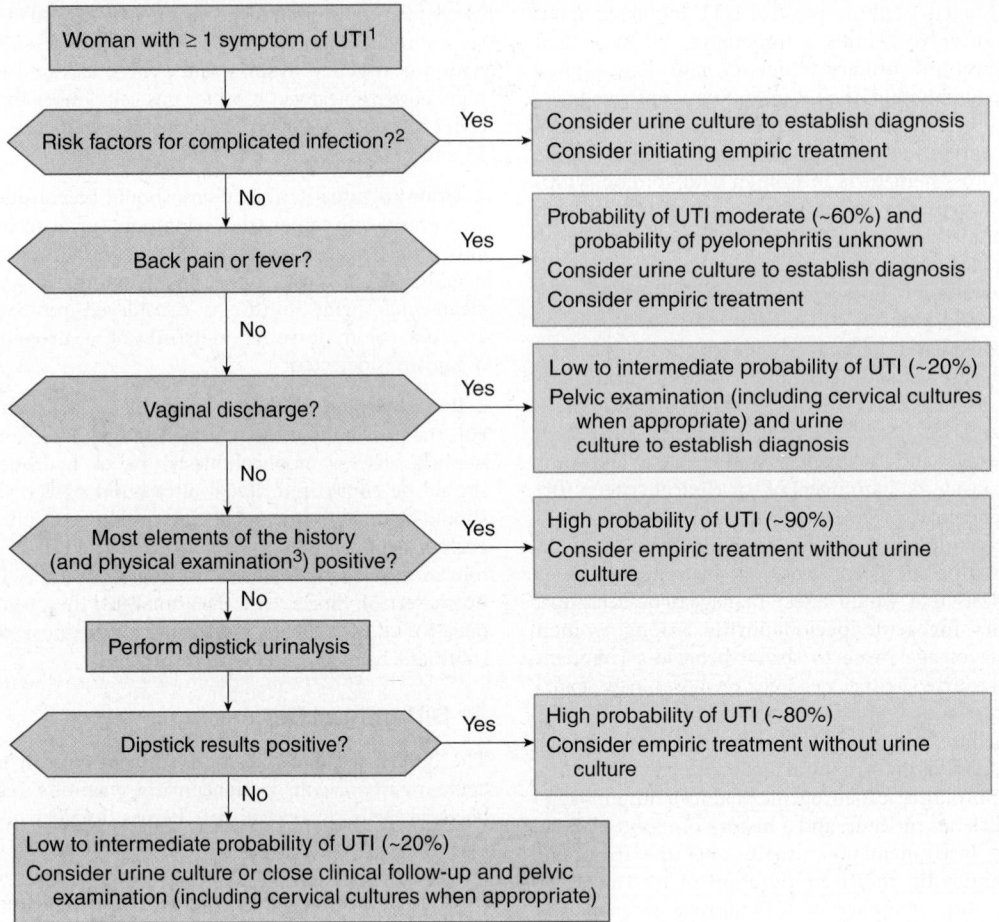

▲ **Figure 2–2.** Proposed algorithm for evaluating women with symptoms of acute urinary tract infection (UTI). (Modified and reproduced, with permission, from Bent S et al. Does this woman have an acute uncomplicated urinary tract infection? JAMA. 2002 May 22–29;287(20):2701–10. © 2002 American Medical Association. All rights reserved.)

recurrences. A 5-day course of fluoroquinolones in outpatient men with UTI is as effective as a 10-day course.

Symptomatic relief can be provided with phenazopyridine, a urinary analgesic that is available over the counter; it is used in combination with antibiotic therapy (when a UTI has been confirmed) but for no more than 2 days. Patients should be informed that phenazopyridine will cause orange/red discoloration of their urine and other body fluids (eg, some contact lens wearers have reported discoloration of their lenses). Rare cases of methemoglobinemia and hemolytic anemia have been reported, usually with overdoses or underlying kidney dysfunction. NSAIDs have also been shown to be of symptomatic benefit, but less effective than antibiotic therapy. Although some women recover from uncomplicated UTI when treated with NSAIDs alone (53% in a Norwegian study), the rate of progression to pyelonephritis was substantial. If a broad-spectrum antibiotic was initially prescribed empirically for UTI and urine culture results return establishing efficacy of a narrow-spectrum antibiotic, treatment should be "de-escalated" to the narrow-spectrum antimicrobial. In patients with recurrent UTIs and asymptomatic renal calculi, 50% may be rendered infection-free following stone extraction.

In cases of interstitial cystitis/painful bladder syndrome (see Chapter 23), patients will often respond to a multimodal approach that may include urethral/vesicular dilation, biofeedback, cognitive-behavioral therapy, antidepressants, dietary changes, vaginal emollients, and other supportive measures. Vaginal estrogen effectively relieves urinary urgency and frequency as well as recurrent UTIs related to vulvovaginal atrophy of menopause (also known as genitourinary syndrome of menopause).

A meta-analysis found that for most people with asymptomatic bacteriuria, antibiotic treatment is not beneficial and may be harmful. Antibiotic treatment does provide benefit to women in pregnancy with asymptomatic bacteriuria and to those about to undergo urologic surgery.

There were no differences in the prevalence of postoperative UTI in women who had preoperative mixed-flora urine cultures compared to no-growth preoperative urine cultures.

When to Refer

- Anatomic abnormalities leading to repeated urinary infections.
- Infections associated with nephrolithiasis.
- Persistent interstitial cystitis/painful bladder syndrome.

When to Admit

- Severe pain requiring parenteral medication or impairing ambulation or urination (such as severe primary herpes simplex genitalis).

- Dysuria associated with urinary retention or obstruction.
- Pyelonephritis with ureteral obstruction.
- Symptoms and signs suggesting urosepsis.

Crellin E et al. Trimethoprim use for urinary tract infection and risk of adverse outcomes in older patients: cohort study. BMJ. 2018 Feb 9;360:k341. [PMID: 29438980]

Dune TJ et al. Urinary symptoms and their associations with urinary tract infections in urogynecologic patients. Obstet Gynecol. 2017 Oct;130(4):718–25. [PMID: 28885414]

Fox MT et al. A seven-day course of TMP-SMX may be as effective as a seven-day course of ciprofloxacin for the treatment of pyelonephritis. Am J Med. 2017 Jul;130(7):842–5. [PMID: 28216442]

Gupta K et al. Urinary tract infection. Ann Intern Med. 2017 Oct 3; 167(7):ITC49–64. [PMID: 28973215]

Huttner A et al. Effect of 5-day nitrofurantoin vs single-dose fosfomycin on clinical resolution of uncomplicated lower urinary tract infection in women: a randomized clinical trial. JAMA. 2018 May 1;319(17):1781–9. [PMID: 29710295]

Köves B et al. Benefits and harms of treatment of asymptomatic bacteriuria: a systematic review and meta-analysis by the European Association of Urology Urological Infection Guidelines Panel. Eur Urol. 2017 Dec;72(6):865–8. [PMID: 28754533]

Kronenberg A et al. Symptomatic treatment of uncomplicated lower urinary tract infections in the ambulatory setting: randomised, double blind trial. BMJ. 2017 Nov 7;359:j4784. Erratum in: BMJ. 2017 Nov 13;359:j5268. [PMID: 29113968]

Polin MR et al. Do mixed-flora preoperative urine cultures matter? South Med J. 2017 Jun;110(6):426–9. [PMID: 28575903]

Schaeffer AJ et al. Clinical Practice. Urinary tract infections in older men. N Engl J Med. 2016 Feb 11;374(6):562–71. [PMID: 26863357]

Vik I et al. Ibuprofen versus pivmecillinam for uncomplicated urinary tract infection in women—a double-blind, randomized non-inferiority trial. PLoS Med. 2018 May 15;15(5):e1002569. [PMID: 29763434]

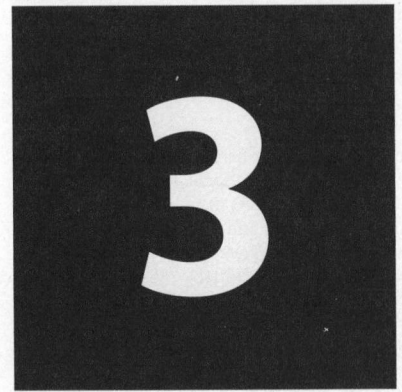

3

Preoperative Evaluation & Perioperative Management

Hugo Q. Cheng, MD

EVALUATION OF THE ASYMPTOMATIC PATIENT

Patients without significant medical problems—especially those under age 50—are at very low risk for perioperative complications. Their preoperative evaluation should include a history and physical examination. Special emphasis is placed on obtaining a careful pharmacologic history and assessment of functional status, exercise tolerance, and cardiopulmonary symptoms and signs in an effort to reveal previously unrecognized disease that may require further evaluation prior to surgery. In addition, a directed bleeding history (Table 3–1) should be taken to uncover coagulopathy that could contribute to excessive surgical blood loss. Routine preoperative laboratory tests in asymptomatic healthy patients under age 50 have *not* been found to help predict or prevent complications. Even elderly patients undergoing minor or minimally invasive procedures (such as cataract surgery) are unlikely to benefit from preoperative screening tests.

Mohanty S et al. Optimal perioperative management of the geriatric patient: a best practices guideline from the American College of Surgeons NSQIP and the American Geriatrics Society. J Am Coll Surg. 2016 May;222(5):930–47. [PMID: 27049783]

O'Neill F et al. Routine preoperative tests for elective surgery: summary of updated NICE guidance. BMJ. 2016 Jul 14;354: i3292. [PMID: 27418436]

Table 3–1. Directed bleeding history: Findings suggestive of a bleeding disorder.

Unprovoked bruising on the trunk of > 5 cm in diameter
Frequent unprovoked epistaxis or gingival bleeding
Menorrhagia with iron deficiency
Hemarthrosis with mild trauma
Prior excessive surgical blood loss or reoperation for bleeding
Family history of abnormal bleeding
Presence of severe kidney or liver disease
Use of medications that impair coagulation, including nutritional supplements and herbal remedies

CARDIAC RISK ASSESSMENT & REDUCTION IN NONCARDIAC SURGERY

The most important perioperative cardiac complications are myocardial infarction (MI) and cardiac death. Other complications include heart failure (HF), arrhythmias, and unstable angina. The principal patient-specific risk factor is the presence of end-organ cardiovascular disease. This includes not only coronary artery disease and HF but also cerebrovascular disease and chronic kidney disease. Diabetes mellitus, especially if treated with insulin, is considered a cardiovascular disease equivalent that increases the risk of cardiac complications. Major abdominal, thoracic, and vascular surgical procedures (especially abdominal aortic aneurysm repair) carry a higher risk of postoperative cardiac complications, likely due to their associated major fluid shifts, hemorrhage, and hypoxemia. These risk factors were identified in a validated, multifactorial risk prediction tool: the Revised Cardiac Risk Index (RCRI) (Table 3–2). Another risk prediction tool, derived from the American College of Surgeons' National Surgical Quality Improvement Program (NSQIP) patient database, identified patient age, the location or type of operation, serum creatinine greater than 1.5 mg/dL (132.6 mcmol/L), dependency in activities of daily living, and the patient's American Society of Anesthesiologists physical status classification as predictors for postoperative MI or cardiac arrest. An online risk calculator using the NSQIP tool can be found at http:// www.qxmd.com/calculate-online/cardiology/gupta-perioperative-cardiac-risk. The American College of Cardiology and American Heart Association endorse both prediction tools. Patients with two or more RCRI predictors or a risk of perioperative MI or cardiac arrest in excess of 1% as calculated by the NSQIP prediction tool are deemed to be at elevated risk for cardiac complications.

Limited exercise capacity (eg, the inability to walk for two blocks at a normal pace or climb a flight of stairs without resting) also predicts higher cardiac risk. Emergency operations are also associated with greater cardiac risk, but should not be delayed for extensive cardiac evaluation. Instead, patients facing emergency surgery should be medically optimized for surgery as quickly as possible and closely monitored for cardiac complications during the perioperative period.

Table 3–2. Revised Cardiac Risk Index.

Independent Predictors of Postoperative Cardiac Complications
1. Intrathoracic, intraperitoneal, or suprainguinal vascular surgery
2. History of ischemic heart disease
3. History of heart failure
4. Insulin treatment for diabetes mellitus
5. Serum creatinine level > 2 mg/dL [> 176.8 mcmol/L]
6. History of cerebrovascular disease

Scoring (Number of Predictors Present)	Risk of Major Cardiac Complications[1]
None	0.4%
One	1%
Two	2.4%
More than two	5.4%

[1]Cardiac death, myocardial infarction, or nonfatal cardiac arrest.
Data from Devereaux PJ et al. Perioperative cardiac events in patients undergoing noncardiac surgery: a review of the magnitude of the problem, the pathophysiology of the events and methods to estimate and communicate risk. CMAJ. 2005 Sept 13; 173(6):627–34.

► Role of Preoperative Noninvasive Ischemia Testing

Most patients can be accurately risk-stratified by history and physical examination. A resting electrocardiogram (ECG) should also be obtained in patients with at least one RCRI predictor prior to major surgery but generally omitted in asymptomatic patients undergoing minor operations. Additional noninvasive stress testing rarely improves risk stratification or management, especially in patients without cardiovascular disease undergoing minor operations, or who have at least fair functional capacity. Stress testing has more utility in patients with elevated risk-based clinical prediction tools, especially if they also have poor functional status. The absence of ischemia on dipyridamole scintigraphy or dobutamine stress echocardiography is reassuring in these patients. In contrast, extensive inducible ischemia in this population predicts a high risk of cardiac complications, particularly with vascular surgery, which may not be modifiable by either medical management or coronary revascularization. The predictive value of an abnormal stress test result for nonvascular surgery patients is less well established. An approach to perioperative cardiac risk assessment and management in patients with known or suspected stable coronary artery disease is shown in Figure 3–1.

► Role of Cardiac Biomarkers

Preoperative B-type natriuretic peptide (BNP) or N-terminal fragment of proBNP (NT-proBNP) levels directly correlate with the risk for perioperative cardiac complications, and their measurement may improve risk assessment.

In vascular surgery patients, the addition of BNP level measurement reclassified many intermediate-risk patients (based on RCRI score) as high or low risk. Postoperative troponin levels also correlate directly with mortality risk, even in patients without symptoms or signs of myocardial ischemia. However, it remains unclear how to incorporate biomarker measurements into the overall approach to risk assessment and reduction. Presently, American and European society guidelines do not recommend their routine use, whereas the Canadian guideline encourages it for patients who have elevated clinical risk.

► Perioperative Management of Patients with Coronary Artery Disease

Patients with acute coronary syndromes require immediate management of their cardiac disease prior to any preoperative evaluation (see Chapter 10). In a large cohort study, postoperative MI typically occurred within 3 days of surgery and was associated with a 30-day mortality rate of 11.6%. Postoperative MI often presents without chest pain. Symptoms and signs that should prompt consideration of postoperative MI include unexplained hypotension, hypoxemia, and delirium. Screening asymptomatic patients for postoperative MI monitoring remains controversial, since it has not yet been demonstrated to improve outcomes.

A. Medications

Preoperative antianginal medications, including beta-blockers, calcium channel blockers, and nitrates, should be continued throughout the perioperative period. Several trials have shown that initiation of beta-blockers reduces the risk of nonfatal myocardial infarction. However, in the largest trial, a high, fixed dose of metoprolol succinate *increased* total mortality and the risk of stroke. Because of the uncertain benefit-to-risk ratio, initiation of perioperative beta-blockade should be considered only in patients with a high risk of cardiac complications. If used, beta-blockers should be started well in advance of surgery, to allow time to gradually titrate up the dose without causing excessive bradycardia or hypotension. They should not be started on the day of surgery. Possible indications and starting doses for prophylactic beta-blockade are presented in Table 3–3. See Hypertension section, below, regarding perioperatively holding some antihypertensive medications for patients with hypertension who do not have coronary artery disease.

Several randomized trials and retrospective studies found that HMG-CoA reductase inhibitors (statins) prevent MI in patients undergoing noncardiac surgery. Safety concerns, such as liver failure or rhabdomyolysis, have not materialized in these studies. It is unclear how far in advance of surgery statins must be started and what doses are needed to see benefits. However, based on treatment protocols used in clinical trials, at least a moderate statin dose (eg, atorvastatin 20 mg or fluvastatin 80 mg orally daily) should be considered in all patients undergoing vascular surgery and other patients deemed to be at high risk for cardiac complications, regardless of lipid levels, and

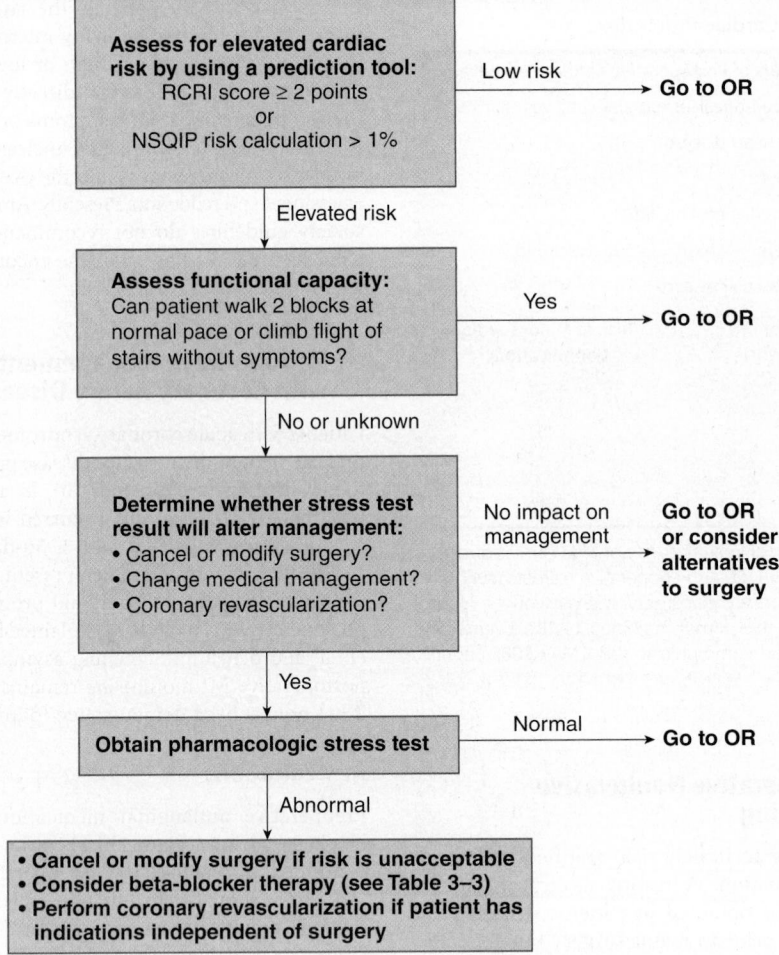

▲ **Figure 3–1.** Assessment and management of patients with known or suspected stable coronary artery disease (CAD) undergoing major elective noncardiac surgery. (OR, operating room; RCRI, Revised Cardiac Risk Index [Table 3–2]; NSQIP, National Surgical Quality Improvement Program: http://www.qxmd.com/calculate-online/cardiology/gupta-perioperative-cardiac-risk)

initiated as early as possible. Patients already taking statins should continue these agents during the perioperative period. In patients without coronary stents, initiation of aspirin therapy before noncardiac surgery is not

recommended because it did not reduce cardiac risk and caused increased bleeding in a large randomized trial. Holding long-term prophylactic aspirin therapy in such patients does not increase cardiac risk.

B. Coronary Revascularization

Patients who have previously had coronary artery bypass grafting (CABG) surgery or percutaneous coronary interventions (PCI) have a relatively low risk of cardiac complications when undergoing subsequent noncardiac surgery. However, a trial that randomized over 500 patients with angiographically proven coronary artery disease to either coronary revascularization (with either CABG or PCI) or medical management alone before vascular surgery found no difference in postoperative MI, 30-day mortality, and long-term mortality. Thus, **preoperative CABG or PCI should be performed only on patients who have guideline-concordant indications independent of the planned noncardiac operation.** In addition, surgical patients who

Table 3–3. Indications for prophylactic perioperative beta-blockade.[1]

Strong indications	Patient already taking beta-blocker to treat ischemia, arrhythmia, or hypertension
Possible indications	Patient with myocardial ischemia detected on preoperative stress testing Patient with 3 or more Revised Cardiac Risk Index predictors (see Table 3–2)

[1]Initial dose recommendations: atenolol 25 mg orally daily, bisoprolol 2.5 mg orally daily, or metoprolol tartrate 25 mg orally twice daily. The dose of beta-blocker should be carefully titrated to keep heart rate < 70 beats per minute and systolic blood pressure > 100 mm Hg. Avoid initiating beta-blockade on the day of surgery.

have undergone recent coronary stenting are at high risk for stent thrombosis, especially if antiplatelet therapy is stopped prematurely. Therefore, elective surgery should be deferred for at least 30 days after placement of a bare-metal stent and ideally for 6 months after placement of a drug-eluting stent. If this delay poses significant risks, such as in patients undergoing an operation for cancer, surgery could be considered 3 months after drug-eluting stent implantation. Antiplatelet agents should be continued perioperatively if possible or resumed as soon as possible after surgery.

Heart Failure & Left Ventricular Dysfunction

Decompensated HF, manifested by an elevated jugular venous pressure, an audible third heart sound, or evidence of pulmonary edema on physical examination or chest radiography, significantly increases the risk of perioperative cardiac complications. The risk of perioperative cardiac complications is similar in patients with ischemic or nonischemic cardiomyopathy. HF with reduced ejection fraction likely confers more risk than HF with preserved ejection fraction. Patients who have had symptomatic HF are at higher risk than those with asymptomatic left ventricular systolic dysfunction.

Elective surgery should be postponed in patients with decompensated HF until it can be evaluated and brought under control. Guidelines recommend preoperative echocardiography in patients without known HF with unexplained dyspnea and in patients with known HF with clinical deterioration. A small observational study found that routine echocardiography in patients with suspected heart disease or those aged 65 years or older prior to emergency noncardiac surgery frequently led to a change in diagnosis or management plan. While this is not an established practice, **preoperative echocardiography should be considered when there is uncertainty about the patient's cardiac status.**

Patients receiving diuretics and digoxin should have serum electrolyte and digoxin levels measured prior to surgery because abnormalities in these levels may increase the risk of perioperative arrhythmias. Clinicians must be cautious not to give too much diuretic, since the volume-depleted patient will be much more susceptible to intraoperative hypotension. The surgeon and anesthesiologist should be made aware of the presence and severity of left ventricular dysfunction so that appropriate decisions can be made regarding perioperative fluid management and intraoperative monitoring.

Valvular Heart Disease

If the nature or severity of valvular lesions is unknown, or if there has been a recent change in clinical status, echocardiography should be performed prior to noncardiac surgery. Candidates for valve replacement or repair independent of the planned noncardiac surgery should have the valve correction procedure performed first. Patients with uncorrected severe or symptomatic aortic stenosis are at particular risk for cardiac complications. They should undergo surgery only after consultation with a cardiologist and anesthesiologist. Patients with mitral stenosis require heart rate control to prolong diastolic filling time. Regurgitant valvular lesions are generally less problematic during surgery because the vasodilatory effect of anesthetics promotes forward flow. Patients with aortic or mitral regurgitation likely benefit from afterload reduction and careful attention to volume status, but negative chronotropes should be avoided to reduce the regurgitant volume.

Arrhythmias

The finding of a rhythm disturbance on preoperative evaluation should prompt consideration of further cardiac evaluation, particularly when the finding of structural heart disease would alter perioperative management. **Patients with a rhythm disturbance without evidence of underlying heart disease are at low risk for perioperative cardiac complications.** There is no evidence that the use of antiarrhythmic medications to suppress an asymptomatic arrhythmia alters perioperative risk.

Patients with symptomatic arrhythmias should not undergo elective surgery until their cardiac condition has been addressed. Thus, in patients with atrial fibrillation or other supraventricular arrhythmias, adequate rate control should be established prior to surgery. Symptomatic ventricular tachycardia must be thoroughly evaluated and controlled prior to surgery. Patients who have independent indications for a permanent pacemaker or implanted defibrillator should have it placed prior to noncardiac surgery. The anesthesiologist must be notified that a patient has an implanted pacemaker or defibrillator so that steps may be taken to prevent device malfunction caused by electromagnetic interference from the intraoperative use of electrocautery.

Hypertension

Mild to moderate hypertension (systolic blood pressure below 180 mm Hg and diastolic blood pressure below 110 mm Hg) does not appear to be an independent risk factor for postoperative MI or cardiac death. No evidence supports delaying surgery in order to better control mild to moderate hypertension. Most medications for chronic hypertension should generally be continued up to and including the day of surgery. Consideration should be given to holding angiotensin-converting enzyme inhibitors and angiotensin receptor blockers on the day of surgery in the absence of HF, since these agents may increase the risk of intraoperative hypotension and potentiate postoperative acute kidney injury. Diuretic agents are also frequently held on the day of surgery to prevent hypovolemia and electrolyte disorders if they are not needed to control HF; however, the benefit of this practice is uncertain.

Severe hypertension, defined as a systolic pressure greater than 180 mm Hg or diastolic pressure greater than 110 mm Hg, does appear to be an independent predictor of perioperative cardiac complications, including MI and HF. It is reasonable to consider delaying surgery in patients with such severe hypertension until blood pressure can be controlled, although it is not known whether the risk of cardiac complications is reduced with this approach.

Devereaux PJ et al. Cardiac complications in patients undergoing major noncardiac surgery. N Engl J Med. 2015 Dec 3;373(23): 2258–69. [PMID: 26630144]

Fleisher LA et al. 2014 ACC/AHA guideline on perioperative cardiovascular evaluation and management of patients undergoing noncardiac surgery: a report of the American College of Cardiology/American Heart Association Task Force on Practice Guidelines. J Am Coll Cardiol. 2014 Dec 9; 64(22):e77–137. [PMID: 25091544]

Levine GN et al. 2016 ACC/AHA guideline focused update on duration of dual antiplatelet therapy in patients with coronary artery disease: a report of the American College of Cardiology/ American Heart Association Task Force on Clinical Practice Guidelines. J Am Coll Cardiol. 2016 Sep;68(10):1082–115. [PMID: 27036918]

PULMONARY EVALUATION IN NON–LUNG RESECTION SURGERY

Pneumonia and respiratory failure requiring prolonged mechanical ventilation are the most important postoperative pulmonary complications. The occurrence of these complications has been associated with a significant increase in mortality and hospital length of stay. Pulmonary thromboembolism is another serious complication; prophylaxis against venous thromboembolic disease is described in Chapter 14.

► Risk Factors for the Development of Postoperative Pulmonary Complications

Procedure-related risk factors for postoperative pulmonary complications include location of surgery (with highest rates occurring in cardiac, thoracic, and upper abdominal cases), prolonged anesthesia, and emergency cases. Operations not requiring general anesthesia tend to have lower rates of postoperative pulmonary complications, and laparoscopic procedures tend to have lower risk than comparable open procedures.

It remains unclear which of the many patient-specific risk factors that have been identified are independent predictors. Advanced age appears to confer increased risk. The presence and severity of systemic disease of any type is associated with pulmonary complications. In particular, patients with chronic obstructive pulmonary disease (COPD) or HF have at least twice the risk of postoperative pulmonary complications compared with patients without these conditions. As with preoperative cardiac risk assessment, physical debility and poor functional capacity predict higher risk of postoperative pulmonary complications. A summary of risk factors for pulmonary complications is presented in Table 3–4. A risk calculator for predicting postoperative respiratory failure derived from the NSQIP patient database (http://www.qxmd.com/calculate-online/ respirology/postoperative-respiratory-failure-risk-calculator) includes the type of surgery, emergency surgery, preoperative sepsis, dependency in activities of daily living, and the patient's American Society of Anesthesiologists physical status classification.

Table 3–4. Clinical risk factors for postoperative pulmonary complications.

Upper abdominal or cardiothoracic surgery
Prolonged anesthesia time (> 4 hours)
Emergency surgery
Age > 60 years
Chronic obstructive pulmonary disease
Heart failure
Severe systemic disease
Tobacco use (> 20 pack-years)
Impaired cognition or sensorium
Functional dependency or prior stroke
Preoperative sepsis
Low serum albumin level
Obstructive sleep apnea

► Pulmonary Function Testing & Laboratory Studies

The main role for preoperative pulmonary function tests (PFTs) is to identify and characterize pulmonary disease in patients with unexplained symptoms prior to major abdominal or cardiothoracic surgery. In patients with diagnosed lung disease, PFTs often add little information above clinical assessment. Furthermore, there is no clear degree of PFT abnormality that can be used as an absolute contraindication to non–lung resection surgery. Chest radiographs in unselected patients also rarely add clinically useful information. Some experts have advocated polysomnography to diagnose obstructive sleep apnea prior to bariatric surgery, but the benefits of this approach are unproven. Arterial blood gas measurement is not routinely recommended except in patients with known lung disease and suspected hypoxemia or hypercapnia.

► Perioperative Management

Retrospective studies have shown that smoking cessation reduced the incidence of pulmonary complications, but only if it was initiated at least 1–2 months before surgery. A meta-analysis of randomized trials found that preoperative smoking cessation programs reduced both pulmonary and surgical wound complications, especially if smoking cessation was initiated at least 4 weeks prior to surgery. **The preoperative period may be an optimal time to initiate smoking cessation efforts.** A systematic review found that smoking cessation programs started in a preoperative evaluation clinic increased the odds of abstinence at 3–6 months by nearly 60%.

Postoperative risk reduction strategies have centered on promoting lung expansion through the use of incentive spirometry, continuous positive airway pressure (CPAP), intermittent positive-pressure breathing (IPPB), and deep breathing exercises. Although trial results have been mixed, all these techniques have been shown to reduce the incidence of postoperative atelectasis and, in a few studies, to reduce the incidence of other postoperative pulmonary complications. In most comparative trials, these methods were equally effective. Given the higher cost of CPAP and IPPB, **incentive spirometry and deep breathing exercises are the preferred methods for most patients.** Multicomponent respiratory care programs may be particularly beneficial. One program termed "I COUGH"—an acronym for *I*ncentive spirometry, *C*oughing and deep breathing, *O*ral care, *U*nderstanding (patient education), *G*et out of bed (early ambulation), and *H*ead of bed elevation—reduced the rates of pneumonia and unplanned intubation after general and vascular surgery.

Lee SM et al. Long-term quit rates after a perioperative smoking cessation randomized controlled trial. Anesth Analg. 2015 Mar; 120(3):582–7. [PMID: 25695576]
Marseu K et al. Peri-operative pulmonary dysfunction and protection. Anaesthesia. 2016 Jan;71(Suppl 1):46–50. [PMID: 26620146]
Taylor A et al. Prevention of postoperative pulmonary complications. Surg Clin North Am. 2015 Apr;95(2):237–54. [PMID: 25814104]

EVALUATION OF THE PATIENT WITH LIVER DISEASE

Patients with serious liver disease are at increased risk for perioperative morbidity and demise. Appropriate preoperative evaluation requires consideration of the effects of anesthesia and surgery on postoperative liver function and of the complications associated with anesthesia and surgery in patients with preexisting liver disease.

▶ Risk Assessment in Surgical Patients with Liver Disease

Screening unselected patients with liver biochemical tests has a low yield and is not recommended. Patients with suspected or known liver disease based on history or physical examination, however, should have measurement of liver enzyme levels as well as tests of hepatic synthetic function performed prior to surgery.

Elective surgery in patients with acute viral or alcoholic hepatitis should be delayed until the acute episode has resolved. In three small series of patients with acute viral hepatitis who underwent abdominal surgery, the mortality rate was roughly 10%. Similarly, patients with undiagnosed alcoholic hepatitis had high mortality rates when undergoing abdominal surgery. In the absence of cirrhosis or synthetic dysfunction, chronic viral hepatitis is unlikely to increase risk significantly. Similarly, nonalcoholic fatty liver disease without cirrhosis probably does not pose a serious risk in surgical patients.

In patients with cirrhosis, postoperative complication rates correlate with the severity of liver dysfunction. Traditionally, severity of dysfunction has been assessed with the Child-Pugh score (see Chapter 16). A conservative approach would be to avoid elective surgery in patients with Child-Pugh class C cirrhosis and pursue it with great caution in class B patients. The Model for End-stage Liver Disease (MELD) score, based on serum bilirubin and creatinine levels, and the prothrombin time expressed as the international normalized ratio (INR), also predicted surgical mortality and outperformed the Child-Pugh classification in some studies. A web-based risk assessment calculator incorporating age and MELD score can predict both perioperative and long-term mortality (https://www.mayoclinic.org/medical-professionals/model-end-stage-liver-disease/post-operative-mortality-risk-patients-cirrhosis). Generally, a MELD score less than 10 predicts low risk, whereas a score greater than 16 portends high mortality after elective surgery.

When surgery is elective, controlling ascites, encephalopathy, and coagulopathy preoperatively is prudent. Ascites is a particular problem in abdominal operations, where it can lead to wound dehiscence, hernias, or both. Great care should be taken when using analgesics and sedatives, since these can worsen hepatic encephalopathy. In general, short-acting agents and lower doses should be used. Patients with coagulopathy should receive vitamin K and may need fresh frozen plasma transfusion at the time of surgery; however, transfusing to a specific INR target for cirrhosis is discouraged.

Abbas N et al. Perioperative care of patients with liver cirrhosis: a review. Health Serv Insights. 2017 Feb 24;10:1–12. [PMID: 28469455]
Northup PG et al. AGA Clinical Practice Update: surgical risk assessment and perioperative management in cirrhosis. Clin Gastroenterol Hepatol. 2019 Mar;17(4):595–606. [PMID: 30273751]

PREOPERATIVE HEMATOLOGIC EVALUATION

Three of the more common clinical situations faced by the medical consultant are the patient with anemia, the assessment of bleeding risk, and the perioperative management of long-term anticoagulation.

Preoperative anemia is common, with a prevalence of 43% in a large cohort of elderly veterans undergoing surgery. The main goals of the preoperative evaluation of the anemic patient are to determine the need for preoperative diagnostic evaluation and the need for transfusion. **When feasible, the diagnostic evaluation of the patient with previously unrecognized anemia should be done prior to surgery because certain types of anemia (particularly those due to sickle cell disease, hemolysis, and acute blood loss) have implications for perioperative management.** These types of anemia are typically associated with an elevated reticulocyte count. Preoperative anemia is associated with higher perioperative morbidity and mortality. It is not known whether raising preoperative hemoglobin level to specific targets will improve postoperative outcomes. The clinician determining the need for preoperative transfusion in an individual patient must consider factors other than the absolute hemoglobin level, including the presence of cardiopulmonary disease, the type of surgery, and the likely severity of surgical blood loss. The few studies that have compared different postoperative transfusion thresholds failed to demonstrate improved outcomes with a more aggressive transfusion strategy.

Table 3–5. Recommendations for management of perioperative anticoagulation with warfarin.

Thromboembolic Risk without Anticoagulation	Recommendation
Low (eg, atrial fibrillation with CHADS$_2$ score 0–4[1], mechanical bileaflet aortic valve prosthesis, or single venous thromboembolism > 3 months ago without hypercoagulability condition[2])	Stop warfarin 5 days before surgery Measure INR the day before surgery to confirm that it is acceptable (< 1.6 for most operations) Resume warfarin when hemostasis permits No bridging with parenteral anticoagulants before or after surgery
High (eg, atrial fibrillation or mechanical heart valve with stroke < 3 months prior, atrial fibrillation with CHADS$_2$ score 5 or 6, mechanical mitral valve prosthesis, caged-ball or tilting disk valve prosthesis, or venous thrombosis < 3 months ago or associated with hypercoagulability condition[2])	Stop warfarin 5 days before surgery Begin bridging with therapeutic dose UFH infusion or LMWH 2 days after stopping oral anticoagulation Administer last dose of LMWH 24 hours before surgery; discontinue UFH 4–6 hours before surgery Measure INR the day before surgery to confirm that it is acceptable (< 1.6 for most operations) Resume warfarin when hemostasis permits If hemostasis permits, resume bridging with therapeutic dose UFH infusion or LMWH beginning 48–72 hours after surgery and continuing until the INR is therapeutic

[1]1 point each for heart failure, hypertension, diabetes mellitus, age > 75 years, and 2 points for stroke or transient ischemic attack.
[2]Patients should receive venous thromboembolism prophylaxis after surgery (see Chapter 14).
INR, international normalized ratio; LMWH, low-molecular-weight heparin; UFH, unfractionated heparin.

Based on available evidence, the AABB (formerly American Association of Blood Banks) recommends transfusion for a hemoglobin level less than 8 g/dL (80 g/L) or for symptomatic anemia in patients undergoing orthopedic or cardiac surgery.

The most important component of the bleeding risk assessment is a directed bleeding history (see Table 3–1). Patients who provide a reliable history of no abnormal bleeding on directed bleeding history and have no suggestion of abnormal bleeding on physical examination are at very low risk for having an occult bleeding disorder. Laboratory tests of hemostatic parameters in these patients are generally not needed. When the directed bleeding history is unreliable or incomplete, or when abnormal bleeding is suggested, a formal evaluation of hemostasis should be done prior to surgery and should include measurement of the prothrombin time, activated partial thromboplastin time, and platelet count (see Chapter 13).

Patients receiving long-term oral anticoagulation are at risk for thromboembolic complications when an operation requires interruption of this therapy. "Bridging anticoagulation," where unfractionated or low-molecular-weight heparin is administered parenterally while oral anticoagulants are held, is commonly practiced, but its benefit is unproven and there is the potential for harm. A randomized trial of bridging anticoagulation in surgical patients taking warfarin for atrial fibrillation demonstrated no difference in thromboembolism. Bleeding complications were twice as common in patients who received bridging anticoagulation. **Most experts recommend bridging therapy only in patients at high risk for thromboembolism.** An approach to perioperative anticoagulation management is shown in Table 3–5, but the recommendations must be considered in the context of patient preference and hemorrhagic risk. Direct-acting oral anticoagulants should be withheld several days prior to surgery, based on the patient's kidney function (Table 3–6). Because these agents take effect immediately, bridging is generally not needed when they are resumed, but they should be restarted after surgery only when adequate hemostasis is ensured (see Chapter 14).

Doherty JU et al. 2017 ACC Expert consensus decision pathway for periprocedural management of anticoagulation in patients with nonvalvular atrial fibrillation. A report of the American College of Cardiology Clinical Expert Consensus Document Task Force. J Am Coll Cardiol. 2017 Feb 21;69(7):871–98. [PMID: 28081965]

Table 3–6. Recommendations for preoperative management of direct-acting oral anticoagulants.[1]

Creatinine Clearance	Dabigatran	Rivaroxaban	Apixaban	Edoxaban
> 50 mL/min/1.73 m^2 (0.83 mL/s/m^2)	Hold 4–6 doses	Hold 2 doses	Hold 4 doses	Hold 2 doses
30–50 mL/min/1.73 m^2 (0.5–0.83 mL/s/m^2)	Hold 6–8 doses	Hold 2 doses	Hold 6 doses	Hold 2 doses

[1]Recommendations are for the number of doses to hold before the day of surgery for complete reversal of anticoagulant effect. If mild to moderate anticoagulant effect at time of procedure is desired, the number of held doses should be reduced by 50%.

Muñoz M et al. Pre-operative haematological assessment in patients scheduled for major surgery. Anaesthesia. 2016 Jan; 71(Suppl 1):19–28. [PMID: 26620143]

NEUROLOGIC EVALUATION

Delirium can occur after any major operation but is particularly common after hip fracture repair and cardiovascular surgery, where the incidence is 30–60%. **Postoperative delirium has been associated with higher rates of major postoperative cardiac and pulmonary complications, poor functional recovery, increased length of hospital stay, increased risk of subsequent dementia and functional decline, and increased mortality.** The American Geriatrics Society recommends screening preoperative patients for these delirium risk factors: age greater than 65 years, chronic cognitive impairment or dementia, severe illness, poor vision or hearing, and the presence of infection. Patients with any of these risk factors should be enrolled in a multi-component, nonpharmacologic delirium prevention program after surgery, which includes interventions such as reorientation, sleep hygiene, bowel and bladder care, mobilization and physical therapy, and the elimination of unnecessary medications. Moderate-quality evidence supports the use of these nonpharmacologic interventions.

Only a minority of patients with postoperative delirium will have a single, reversible etiology for their condition. Evaluation of delirious patients should exclude electrolyte derangements, occult urinary tract infection, and adverse effects from psychotropic medications such as opioids, benzodiazepines, anticholinergic agents, and antispasmodics. Conservative management includes reassuring and reorienting the patient; eliminating unneeded medications, intravenous lines, and urinary catheters; and keeping the patient active during the day while allowing uninterrupted sleep at night. When agitation jeopardizes patient or provider safety, neuroleptic agents, given at the lowest effective dose for the shortest duration needed, are preferred over the use of benzodiazepines or physical restraints.

Stroke complicates less than 1% of all surgical procedures but may occur in 1–6% of patients undergoing cardiac or carotid artery surgery. Most of the strokes in cardiac surgery patients are embolic in origin, and about half occur within the first postoperative day. Stroke after cardiac surgery is associated with significantly increased mortality, up to 22% in some studies. A retrospective analysis found that patients who had previously suffered a stroke had an 18% risk of MI, recurrent stroke, or cardiac death if they underwent noncardiac surgery within 3 months of the stroke. This risk declined over time and reached its nadir 9 months after the stroke, suggesting a benefit to delaying elective surgery.

Symptomatic carotid artery stenosis is associated with a high risk of stroke in patients undergoing cardiac surgery. In general, patients with independent indications for correction of carotid stenosis should have the procedure done prior to elective surgery. In contrast, most studies suggest that asymptomatic carotid bruits and asymptomatic carotid stenosis are associated with little or no increased risk of stroke in surgical patients.

American Geriatrics Society Expert Panel on Postoperative Delirium in Older Adults. Postoperative delirium in older adults: best practice statement from the American Geriatrics Society. J Am Coll Surg. 2015 Feb;220(2):136–48. [PMID: 25535170]

Mashour GA et al. Neurological complications of surgery and anaesthesia. Br J Anaesth. 2015 Feb;114(2):194–203. [PMID: 25204699]

MANAGEMENT OF ENDOCRINE DISEASES

▶ Diabetes Mellitus

The most challenging issue in diabetic patients is the maintenance of glucose control during the perioperative period. The increased secretion of cortisol, epinephrine, glucagon, and growth hormone during surgery is associated with insulin resistance and hyperglycemia in diabetic patients. **The goal of management is the prevention of severe hyperglycemia or hypoglycemia in the perioperative period.**

Poor preoperative glycemic control, as indicated by an elevated hemoglobin A_{1c} level, is associated with a greater risk of surgical complications, particularly infections. However, a strategy of delaying surgery until glycemic control improves has not been rigorously studied. The ideal postoperative blood glucose target is also unknown. Based on trials that showed increased mortality in hospitalized patients randomized to tight control, the American College of Physicians recommends maintaining serum glucose between 140 mg/dL and 200 mg/dL (7.8–11.1 mmol/L), whereas the British National Health Service guidelines recommend a range of 108–180 mg/dL (6–10 mmol/L).

The specific pharmacologic management of diabetes during the perioperative period depends on the type of diabetes (insulin-dependent or not), the level of glycemic control, and the type and length of surgery. Oral hypoglycemic agents should be held on the day of surgery. They should not be restarted after surgery until oral intake is adequate and unlikely to be interrupted. For patients taking insulin, a common practice is to reduce the last preoperative dose of long-acting, basal insulin by 30–50% and hold short-acting nutritional insulin (Table 27–11). Use of correctional insulin only (without basal or nutritional insulin after surgery) is discouraged. A trial comparing correctional insulin with basal-bolus dosing found that the latter strategy led to fewer postoperative complications. Most patients with type 1 diabetes and some with type 2 diabetes will need an intravenous insulin infusion perioperatively. Consultation with an endocrinologist should be strongly considered when patients with type 1 diabetes mellitus undergo major surgery (also see Diabetes Management in the Hospital, Chapter 27). All diabetic patients require frequent blood glucose monitoring to prevent hypoglycemia and to ensure prompt treatment of hyperglycemia. Perioperative use of corticosteroids, common in neurosurgical and organ transplant procedures, increases glucose intolerance. Patients receiving corticosteroids often require additional short-acting insulin with meals, while their fasting glucose levels and basal insulin requirements may remain relatively unchanged.

Corticosteroid Replacement

Hypotension or shock resulting from primary or secondary adrenocortical insufficiency is rare. The common practice of administering high-dose corticosteroids during the perioperative period in patients at risk for adrenocortical insufficiency has not been rigorously studied. While definitive recommendations regarding perioperative corticosteroid therapy cannot be made, a conservative approach would be to **consider any patient who has received the equivalent of at least 7.5 mg of prednisone daily for 3 weeks within the past year to be at risk for having adrenocortical insufficiency.** Patients who have been taking less than 5 mg of prednisone daily and those receiving alternate-day corticosteroid dosing are unlikely to require supplemental coverage. A commonly used regimen is 100 mg of hydrocortisone given intravenously daily, divided every 8 hours, beginning before induction of anesthesia and continuing for 24–48 hours. Tapering the dose is not necessary. Patients receiving long-term maintenance corticosteroid therapy should also continue their usual dose throughout the perioperative period.

Thyroid Disease

Severe symptomatic hypothyroidism has been associated with perioperative complications, including intraoperative hypotension, HF, cardiac arrest, and death. Elective surgery should be delayed in patients with severe hypothyroidism until adequate thyroid hormone replacement can be achieved. Similarly, patients with symptomatic hyperthyroidism are at risk for perioperative thyroid storm and should not undergo elective surgery until their thyrotoxicosis is controlled. An endocrinologist should be consulted if emergency surgery is needed in such patients. Conversely, a study found that patients with mild hypothyroidism (median thyroid-stimulating hormone level 8.6 milli-international units/L) tolerated surgery well, with only a slight increase in the incidence of intraoperative hypotension; surgery need not be delayed for the month or more required to ensure adequate thyroid hormone replacement.

Komatsu R et al. The effect of hypothyroidism on a composite of mortality, cardiovascular and wound complications after noncardiac surgery: a retrospective cohort analysis. Anesth Analg. 2015 Sep;121(3):716–26. [PMID: 26287300]
MacKenzie CR et al. Stress dose steroids: myths and perioperative medicine. Curr Rheumatol Rep. 2016 Jul;18(7):47. [PMID: 27351679]

KIDNEY DISEASE

Approximately one-third of patients undergoing general surgery will suffer some degree of acute kidney injury, and 3% of patients will develop a creatinine elevation greater

Table 3–7. Risk factors for the development of acute kidney injury after general surgery.[1]

Age > 55 years
Male sex
Chronic kidney disease
Heart failure
Diabetes mellitus
Hypertension
Ascites
Intraperitoneal surgery
Emergency surgery

[1]Presence of 5 or more risk factors associated with > 3% risk of creatinine elevation > 2 mg/dL (176.8 mcmol/L) above baseline or requirement for dialysis.
Reproduced, with permission, from Kheterpal S et al. Development and validation of an acute kidney injury risk index for patients undergoing general surgery: results from a national data set. Anesthesiology. 2009;110(3):505–15.

than 2 mg/dL (176.8 mcmol/L) above baseline or require renal replacement therapy. **The development of acute kidney injury is an independent predictor of mortality, even if mild or if kidney dysfunction resolves.** The mortality associated with the development of perioperative acute kidney injury that requires dialysis exceeds 50%. Risk factors associated with postoperative deterioration in kidney function are shown in Table 3–7. Several medications, including "renal-dose" dopamine, mannitol, *N*-acetylcysteine, and clonidine, have been evaluated in an attempt to preserve kidney function during the perioperative period. None of these has proved effective in clinical trials and should not be used for this indication. **Maintenance of adequate intravascular volume is likely to be the most effective method to reduce the risk of perioperative deterioration in kidney function.** Exposure to renal-toxic agents, such as nonsteroidal anti-inflammatory drugs and intravenous contrast, should be minimized or avoided. Angiotensin-converting enzyme inhibitors and angiotensin receptor blockers reduce renal perfusion and may increase the risk of perioperative acute kidney injury. Although firm evidence is lacking, it may be useful to temporarily discontinue these medications in patients at risk for perioperative acute kidney injury.

Although the mortality rate for elective major surgery is low (1–4%) in patients with dialysis-dependent chronic kidney disease, the risk for perioperative complications, including postoperative hyperkalemia, pneumonia, fluid overload, and bleeding, is substantially increased. Postoperative hyperkalemia requiring emergent hemodialysis has been reported to occur in 20–30% of patients. Patients should undergo dialysis preoperatively within 24 hours before surgery, and their serum electrolyte levels should be measured just prior to surgery and monitored closely during the postoperative period.

Golden D et al. Peri-operative renal dysfunction: prevention and management. Anaesthesia. 2016 Jan;71(Suppl 1):51–7. [PMID: 26620147]

ANTIBIOTIC PROPHYLAXIS OF SURGICAL SITE INFECTIONS

Surgical site infection is estimated to occur in roughly 4% of general or vascular operations. Although the type of procedure is the main factor determining the risk of developing a surgical site infection, certain patient factors have been associated with increased risk, including diabetes mellitus, older age, obesity, heavy alcohol consumption, admission from a long-term care facility, and multiple medical comorbidities. **For most major procedures, the use of prophylactic antibiotics has been demonstrated to reduce the incidence of surgical site infections significantly.** Several general conclusions can be drawn from studies of different antibiotic regimens for surgical procedures. First, substantial evidence suggests that a single dose of an appropriate intravenous antibiotic—or combination of antibiotics—is as effective as multiple-dose regimens that extend into the postoperative period. Second, for most procedures, a first-generation cephalosporin is as effective as later-generation agents. Third, prophylactic antibiotics should be given intravenously at induction of anesthesia or roughly 30–60 minutes prior to the skin incision.

Guidelines for antibiotic prophylaxis against infective endocarditis in patients undergoing invasive procedures are presented in Chapter 33. Given the lack of evidence for antibiotic prophylaxis against prosthetic joint infection before dental procedures, guidelines from the American Academy of Orthopedic Surgeons and the American Dental Association recommend against this practice.

Berríos-Torres SI et al; Healthcare Infection Control Practices Advisory Committee. Centers for Disease Control and Prevention guideline for the prevention of surgical site infection, 2017. JAMA Surg. 2017 Aug 1;152(8):784–91. [PMID: 28467526]

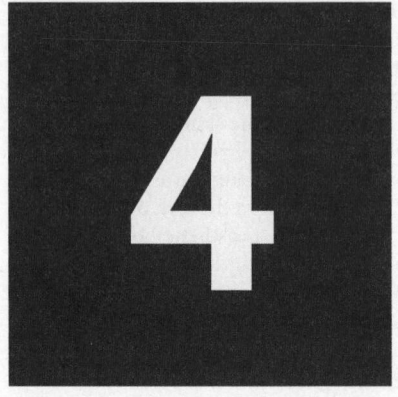

Geriatric Disorders

G. Michael Harper, MD
C. Bree Johnston, MD, MPH
C. Seth Landefeld, MD

GENERAL PRINCIPLES OF GERIATRIC CARE

The following principles help in caring for older adults:

1. Many disorders are multifactorial in origin and are best managed by multifactorial interventions.
2. Diseases often present atypically or with nonspecific symptoms (eg, confusion, functional decline).
3. Not all abnormalities require evaluation and treatment.
4. Complex medication regimens, adherence problems, and polypharmacy are common challenges.
5. Multiple chronic conditions often coexist and should be managed in concert with one another.

COMPREHENSIVE ASSESSMENT OF THE OLDER ADULT

In addition to conventional assessment of symptoms and diseases, comprehensive assessment addresses three topics: **prognosis, values and preferences**, and **ability to function independently**. Comprehensive assessment is warranted before major clinical decisions are made.

▶ Assessment of Prognosis

When an older person's life expectancy is longer than 10 years (ie, 50% of similar persons live longer than 10 years), it is reasonable to consider effective tests and treatments much as they are considered in younger persons. When life expectancy is less than 10 years (and especially when it is much less), choices of tests and treatments should be made based on their ability to improve that patient's prognosis and quality of life given that patient's shorter life expectancy. The relative benefits and harms of tests and treatments often change as prognosis worsens, and net benefit often worsens.

When an older patient's clinical situation is dominated by a single disease process (eg, lung cancer metastatic to brain), prognosis can be estimated well with a disease-specific instrument. Even in this situation, however, prognosis generally worsens with age (especially over age 90 years) and with the presence of serious age-related conditions, such as dementia, malnutrition, or impaired ability to walk.

When an older patient's clinical situation is not dominated by a single disease process, prognosis can be estimated initially by considering basic demographic and health elements (Figure 4–1). For example, less than 25% of men aged 95 will live 5 years, whereas nearly 75% of women aged 70 will live 10 years. The prognosis of older persons living at home can be estimated by considering age, sex, comorbid conditions, and function (Table 4–1). The prognosis of older persons discharged from the hospital is worse than that of those living at home and can be estimated by considering sex, comorbid conditions, and function at discharge (Table 4–2).

▶ Assessment of Values & Preferences

Although patients vary in their values and preferences, most frail older patients prioritize maintaining their independence over prolonging survival. Values and preferences are determined by speaking directly with a patient or, when the patient cannot express preferences reliably, with the patient's surrogate.

In assessing values and preferences, it is important to keep in mind the following:

1. Patients are experts about their preferences for outcomes and experiences; however, they often do not have adequate information to make and express informed preferences for specific tests or treatments.
2. Patients' preferences often change over time. For example, some patients find living with a disability more acceptable than they thought before experiencing it.

▶ Assessment of Function

People often lose function in multiple domains as they age, with the result that they may not be able to do some activities as quickly or capably and may need assistance with other activities. Assessment of function improves prognostic estimates. **Assessment of function is essential to determining an individual's needs in the context of his or her values and preferences and the possible effects of prescribed treatment.**

About one-fourth of patients over age 65 and half of persons older than 85 need help performing their **basic**

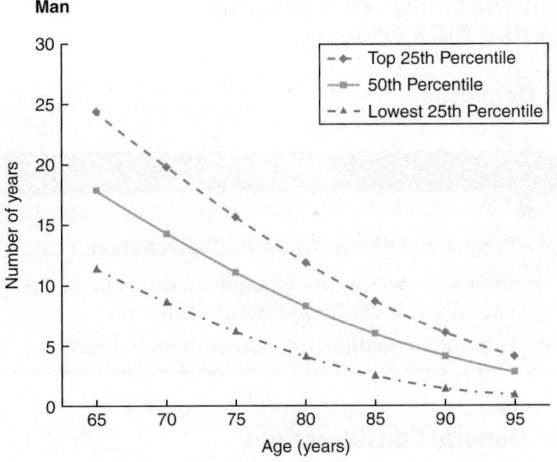

Man

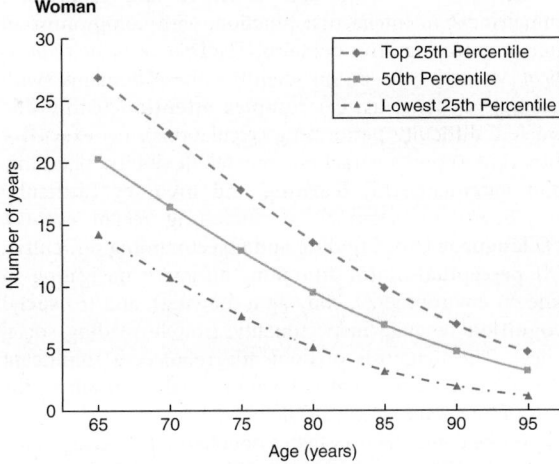

Woman

▲ **Figure 4–1.** Median life expectancy of older men and women. (Data derived from Arias E. United States Life Tables, 2011. Natl Vital Stat Rep. 2015 Sep 22; 64(11):1–63.)

Table 4–1. Prognostic factors, "risk points," and 4-year mortality rates for older persons living at home.

Prognostic Factor	Risk Points
Age	
60–64 years	1
65–69 years	2
70–74 years	3
75–79 years	4
80–84 years	5
85 years and older	7
Male sex	2
Comorbid conditions reported by patients	
Diabetes mellitus	1
Cancer	2
Lung disease	2
Heart failure	2
Body mass index < 25	1
Current smoker	2
Function	
Bathing difficulty	2
Difficulty handling finances	2
Difficulty walking several blocks	2
Sum of Risk Points	**4-Year Mortality Rate**
1–2	2%
3–6	7%
7–10	19%
> 10	53%

activities of daily living (ADLs; eg, bathing, dressing, eating, transferring from bed to chair, continence, toileting) or instrumental activities of daily living (IADLs; eg, transportation, shopping, cooking, using the telephone, managing money, taking medications, housecleaning, laundry).

Functional screening should include assessment of ADLs and IADLs and questions to detect weight loss, falls, incontinence, depressed mood, self-neglect, fear for personal safety, and common serious impairments (eg, hearing, vision, cognition, and mobility). Standard functional screening measures may not be useful in capturing subtle impairments in highly functional independent elders. One technique for these patients is to identify and regularly ask about a target activity, such as bowling or gardening. If the patient begins to have trouble with or discontinues such an **"advanced" ADL**, it may indicate early impairment, such as onset of cognitive impairment, incontinence, or worsening hearing loss, which may be uncovered with additional gentle questioning or assessment.

► Frailty

Frailty is a syndrome characterized by loss of physiologic reserve and dysregulation across multiple systems, ultimately resulting in greater risk of poor health outcomes. One well-recognized model defines frailty as a phenotype that includes **weakness, slow gait speed, decreased physical activity, weight loss,** and **exhaustion or low energy**. While there is not one universally agreed upon definition or assessment tool for frailty, generally an individual is defined as frail when three or more of the above features are present. Persons with frailty are at increased risk for falls, hospitalization, functional decline, and death. Frailty is also recognized as a risk for worse outcomes following surgery and complications from chemotherapy. The ideal strategies for preventing and treating the frailty syndrome are largely unknown. Higher levels of protein and mono-unsaturated fatty acid intake are

Table 4–2. Prognostic factors, "risk points," and 1-year mortality rates for older patients discharged from the hospital after an acute medical illness.

Prognostic Factor	Risk Points
Male sex	1
Comorbid conditions reported by patients	
Cancer, metastatic	8
Cancer, not metastatic	3
Serum creatinine > 3 mg/dL	2
Albumin < 3 mg/dL	2
Albumin 3.0–3.4 mg/dL	1
Function	
Dependent in 1–4 ADL[1]	2
Dependent in 5 ADL[1]	5
Sum of Risk Points	**1-Year Mortality Rate**
0–1	4%
2–3	19%
4–6	34%
> 6	64%

[1]ADL refers to five activities of daily living: bathing, dressing, transferring, using the toilet, and eating.
Reprinted, with permission, from Walter LC et al. Development and validation of a prognostic index for 1-year mortality in older adults after hospitalization. JAMA. 2001 Jun 20;285(23):2987–94. Copyright © 2001 American Medical Association. All rights reserved.

inversely associated with incident frailty, and are reasonable to encourage for patients at risk. At present, treatment is largely supportive, multifactorial, and individualized based on patient goals, life expectancy, and comorbidities. **Evidence shows that exercise, particularly strength and resistance training, can increase walking speed and improve function.** Sometimes, transitioning a patient to a comfort-focused or hospice approach is the most appropriate clinical intervention when efforts to prevent functional decline fail.

Bleijenberg N et al. Difficulty managing medications and finances in older adults: a 10-year cohort study. J Am Geriatr Soc. 2017 Jul;65(7):1455–61. [PMID: 28378345]

Ellis G et al. Comprehensive geriatric assessment for older adults admitted to hospital. Cochrane Database Syst Rev. 2017 Sep 12;9:CD006211. [PMID: 28898390]

Kim DH et al. Preoperative frailty assessment and outcomes at 6 months or later in older adults undergoing cardiac surgical procedures: a systematic review. Ann Intern Med. 2016 Nov 1; 165(9):650–60. [PMID: 27548070]

Parker SG et al. What is Comprehensive Geriatric Assessment (CGA)? An umbrella review. Age Ageing. 2018 Jan 1;47(1): 149–55. [PMID: 29206906]

Sandoval-Insausti H et al. Macronutrients intake and incident frailty in older adults: a prospective cohort study. J Gerontol A Biol Sci Med Sci. 2016 Oct;71(10):1329–34. [PMID: 26946103]

MANAGEMENT OF COMMON GERIATRIC PROBLEMS

1. Dementia

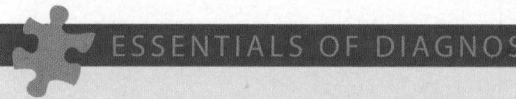

ESSENTIALS OF DIAGNOSIS

▶ Progressive decline of intellectual function.
▶ Deficits in one or more cognitive domains severe enough to cause impairment of function.
▶ Not due to delirium or another mental disorder.

▶ General Considerations

Dementia is an acquired, persistent, and progressive impairment in intellectual function, with compromise of one or more cognitive domains. *The Diagnostic and Statistical Manual,* 5th edition identifies these domains (with example deficits) as: (1) **complex attention** (easily distracted, difficulty performing calculations), (2) **executive function** (poor abstraction, mental flexibility, planning, and judgment), (3) **learning and memory** (difficulty recalling items from a list, forgetting recent events), (4) **language** (word finding and object naming difficulty), (5) **perceptual-motor function** (difficulty navigating in known environments, copying a drawing), and (6) **social cognition** (change in personality, trouble reading social cues). The diagnosis of dementia requires a significant decline in function that is severe enough to result in the loss of independence in IADLs.

While dementia prevalence doubles every 5 years in the older population, reaching 30–50% at age 85, the prevalence among US adults 65 years or older has been declining. This improvement has been attributed to higher education levels and better control of cardiovascular risk factors. Alzheimer disease accounts for roughly two-thirds of dementia cases in the United States, with vascular dementia (either alone or combined with Alzheimer disease) and dementia with Lewy bodies accounting for much of the rest.

Depression and delirium are also common in elders, may coexist with dementia, and may also present with cognitive impairment. Depression is a common concomitant of early dementia. A patient with depression and cognitive impairment whose intellectual function improves with treatment of the mood disorder has an almost fivefold greater risk of suffering irreversible dementia later in life. Delirium, characterized by acute confusion, occurs much more commonly in patients with underlying dementia.

▶ Clinical Findings

A. Screening

1. Cognitive impairment—According to the US Preventive Services Task Force (USPSTF), there is insufficient evidence to recommend for or against screening all older adults for cognitive impairment. While there is logic in the argument that early detection may improve future planning and patient outcomes, empiric evidence that demonstrates a clear benefit for either patients or caregivers is lacking. It is important to note, however, that the Medicare Annual Wellness Visit mandates that clinicians assess patients for cognitive impairment based on the clinician's observations and reports from others.

At-home genetic testing for a susceptibility gene that is associated with late-onset Alzheimer disease (APOE-e4) has US Food and Drug Administration approval. While the presence of the APOE-e4 allele increases the risk of developing Alzheimer disease, quantifying such risk for an individual is difficult. Because it is possible to have one or two copies of the APOE-e4 allele and not develop Alzheimer disease or to have no copies and yet still become stricken, genetic testing is not widely recommended and, if considered, should not proceed without genetic counseling.

When there is suspicion of cognitive impairment, several cognitive tests have been validated for clinical use. The **mini-cog** is a combination of a three-item word recall with a clock drawing task, and it can be completed in 3 minutes. When a patient fails this simple test, further cognitive evaluation with a standardized instrument is warranted. The **Montreal Cognitive Assessment (MoCA©)** is a 30-point test that takes about 10 minutes to administer and examines several areas of cognitive function. A score below 26 has a sensitivity of 0.94 or more and a specificity of 0.60 or less. Free downloadable versions in multiple languages are available at http://www.mocatest.org.

2. Decision-making capacity—Older adults with cognitive impairment commonly face serious medical decisions, and the clinicians involved in their care must ascertain whether the capacity exists to make medical decisions. While no single test of capacity exists, the following five elements should be considered in a thorough assessment: (1) ability to express a choice; (2) understanding relevant information about the risks and benefits of planned therapy and the alternatives (including no treatment), in the context of one's values; (3) comprehension of the problem and its consequences; (4) ability to reason; and (5) consistency of choice. A patient's choice should follow from an understanding of the consequences.

Sensitivity must be used in applying these five components to people of various cultural backgrounds. Decision-making capacity varies over time. Furthermore, the capacity to make a decision is **a function of the decision in question.** A woman with mild dementia may lack the capacity to consent to coronary artery bypass grafting yet retain the capacity to designate a surrogate decision maker.

B. Symptoms and Signs

The clinician can gather important information about the type of dementia by asking about (1) the rate of progression of the deficits as well as their nature (including any personality or behavioral change); (2) the presence of other neurologic and psychiatric symptoms, particularly motor problems and psychotic symptoms; (3) risk factors for HIV; (4) family history of dementia; and (5) medications, with particular attention to recent changes.

Workup is directed at identifying any potentially reversible causes of dementia. However, such cases are rare. For a detailed description of the symptoms and signs of different forms of dementia, see Chapter 24.

C. Physical Examination

The neurologic examination emphasizes assessment of mental status but should also include evaluation for sensory deficits, previous strokes, parkinsonism, or peripheral neuropathy. The remainder of the physical examination should focus on identifying comorbid conditions that may aggravate the individual's disability. For a detailed description of the neuropsychological assessment, see Chapter 24.

D. Laboratory Findings

Laboratory studies should include a complete blood count and serum electrolytes, calcium, creatinine, glucose, thyroid-stimulating hormone (TSH), and vitamin B_{12} levels. While hypothyroidism or vitamin B_{12} deficiency may contribute to the cognitive impairment, treating these conditions typically does not completely reverse the dementia. HIV and rapid plasma reagin (RPR) tests, a heavy metal screen, and liver biochemical tests may be informative in selected patients but are not part of routine testing. For a detailed description of laboratory findings, see Chapter 24.

E. Imaging

Most patients should receive neuroimaging as part of the workup to rule out subdural hematoma, tumor, previous stroke, and hydrocephalus (usually normal pressure). Those who are younger; those who have focal neurologic symptoms or signs, seizures, or gait abnormalities; and those with an acute or subacute onset are most likely to have positive findings and most likely to benefit from MRI scanning. In older patients with a more classic picture of Alzheimer disease for whom neuroimaging is desired, a noncontrast CT scan is sufficient. For a detailed description of imaging, see Chapter 24.

▶ Differential Diagnosis

Older individuals experience occasional difficulty retrieving items from memory (usually word-finding difficulty) and experience a slowing in their rate of information processing. In the amnestic type of **mild cognitive impairment,** a patient complains of memory problems, demonstrates mild deficits (most commonly in short-term memory) on formal testing, but the impairment does not significantly impact function. Annual dementia conversion rates vary from less than 5% to 20%. No medications have been demonstrated to delay the progression of mild cognitive impairment to Alzheimer disease. An elderly patient with intact cognition but with severe impairments in vision or hearing commonly becomes confused in an unfamiliar medical setting and consequently may be falsely labeled as demented.

Delirium can be distinguished from dementia by its acute onset, fluctuating course, and deficits in attention rather than memory. Many medications have been associated with delirium and other types of cognitive impairment in older patients. Anticholinergic agents, hypnotics, neuroleptics, opioids, nonsteroidal anti-inflammatory drugs (NSAIDs), antihistamines (both H_1- and H_2-antagonists), and corticosteroids are just some of the medications that have been associated with cognitive impairment in elders.

► Treatment

Patients and families should be made aware of the Alzheimer's Association (http://www.alz.org) as well as the wealth of helpful community and online resources and publications available. Caregiver support, education, and counseling may prevent or delay nursing home placement. Education should include the manifestations and natural history of dementia as well as the availability of local support services, such as respite care. Exercise should be a component of treatment as evidence suggests physical activity may have beneficial effects on cognition and physical function.

A. Cognitive Impairment

1. Acetylcholinesterase inhibitors—Many experts recommend a trial of acetylcholinesterase inhibitors (eg, donepezil, galantamine, rivastigmine) in most patients with mild to moderate Alzheimer disease. These medications produce a modest improvement in cognitive function that is *not* likely to be detected in routine clinical encounters. Acetylcholinesterase inhibitors have not convincingly been shown to delay functional decline or institutionalization. There is insufficient evidence to recommend their use in mild cognitive impairment to slow the progression toward dementia.

Starting (and maximum) doses are donepezil, 5 mg orally once daily (maximum 10 mg once daily); galantamine, 4 mg orally twice daily (maximum 12 mg twice daily); and rivastigmine, 1.5 mg orally twice daily (maximum 6 mg twice daily). Dosages are increased gradually as tolerated. The most bothersome side effects include diarrhea, nausea, anorexia, weight loss, and syncope. While some patients with moderate to severe cognitive impairment may experience benefits from acetylcholinesterase inhibitors, the medication should be discontinued in those patients who have had no apparent benefit, who experience side effects, or for whom the financial outlay is a burden. While there are no published guidelines that describe what constitutes an adequate treatment trial, evaluation after 2 months at the highest tolerated dose is reasonable.

2. Memantine—In clinical trials, patients with more advanced disease have been shown to have statistical benefit from the use of memantine (5 mg orally daily to 10 mg twice daily), an *N*-methyl-D-aspartate (NMDA) antagonist, with or without concomitant use of an acetylcholinesterase inhibitor. Long-term and meaningful functional outcomes have yet to be demonstrated and evidence suggests there is no benefit to giving memantine in addition to an acetylcholinesterase inhibitor.

B. Behavioral Problems

1. Nonpharmacologic approaches—Behavioral problems in patients with dementia are often best managed nonpharmacologically. Initially, it should be established that the

problem is not unrecognized delirium, pain, urinary obstruction, or fecal impaction. Determining whether the caregiver or institutional staff can tolerate the behavior is also helpful, since it is often easier to find ways to accommodate the behavior than to modify it. If not, the caregiver should keep a brief log in which the behavior is described along with antecedent events and consequences. This may uncover patterns that delineate precipitants of the behavior or perhaps that the behavior is being rewarded. Caregivers are taught to use simple language when communicating with the patient, to break down activities into simple component tasks, and to use a "distract, not confront" approach when the patient seems disturbed by a troublesome issue. Additional steps to address behavioral problems include providing structure and routine, discontinuing all medications except those considered absolutely necessary, and correcting, if possible, sensory deficits.

2. Pharmacologic approaches—There is no clear consensus about pharmacologic approaches to the treatment of behavioral problems in patients who have not benefited from nonpharmacologic therapies. Pharmacologic treatment should be reserved for those patients who pose an imminent danger to others or themselves or when symptoms are substantially distressing to the patient.

Despite the lack of strong evidence, antipsychotic medications have remained a mainstay for the treatment of behavioral disturbances, particularly agitation and aggression, largely because of the lack of alternatives. The atypical antipsychotic agents (eg, risperidone, olanzapine, quetiapine, aripiprazole) are increasingly becoming the first choice because of an overall better side-effect profile compared to typical agents (eg, haloperidol) but should be used with caution in patients with vascular risk factors due to an increased risk of stroke; they can also cause weight gain and are also associated with hyperglycemia in diabetic patients and are considerably more expensive. **Both typical and atypical antipsychotics increase mortality compared with placebo when used to treat elderly patients with dementia and behavioral disturbances.** Starting and target dosages should be much lower than those used in schizophrenia (eg, haloperidol, 0.5–2 mg orally; risperidone, 0.25–2 mg orally).

Citalopram at a dose of 30 mg daily may improve symptoms of agitation. However, the US Food and Drug Administration has issued a warning against using doses greater than 40 mg daily because of the risk of dysrhythmia from QT interval prolongation. For patients older than age 60, the maximum recommended dose is 20 mg daily. Thus, while citalopram may be used to treat agitation, safe and effective dosing for patients older than age 60 has not been established. In the specific instance of patients with dementia with Lewy bodies, treatment with acetylcholinesterase inhibitors has been shown to improve behavioral symptoms. Valproate medications have been used in the treatment of agitated and physically aggressive behavior, but evidence demonstrates no identifiable benefit.

C. Driving

Although drivers with dementia are at an increased risk for motor vehicle accidents, many patients continue to drive safely well beyond the time of initial diagnosis, making the timing of when to recommend that a patient stop driving particularly challenging.

There is no clear-cut evidence to suggest a single best approach to determining an individual patient's capability, and there is no accepted "gold-standard" test. The result is that clinicians must consider several factors upon which to base their judgment. For example, determining the severity of dementia can be useful. Patients with very mild or mild dementia according to the Clinical Dementia Rating Scale were able to pass formal road tests at rates of 88% and 69%, respectively. **Experts agree that patients with moderately severe or more advanced dementia should be counseled to stop driving.** Although not well studied, clinicians should also consider the effects of comorbid conditions and medications and the role each may play in contributing to the risk of driving by a patient with dementia. Assessment of the ability to carry out IADLs may also assist in the determination of risk. Finally, in some cases of mild dementia, referral may be needed to a driver rehabilitation specialist for evaluation. Although not standardized, this evaluation often consists of both off- and on-road testing. Experts recommend such an evaluation for patients with mild dementia, for those with dementia for whom new impairment in driving skills is observed, and for those with significant deficits in cognitive domains, such as attention, executive function, and visuospatial skills.

Clinicians must also be aware of the reporting requirements in their individual jurisdictions. When a clinician has made the decision to report an unsafe driver to the Department of Motor Vehicles, he or she must consider the impact of a potential breach in confidentiality and must weigh and address, in advance when possible, the consequences of the loss of driving independence.

D. Advance Financial Planning

Difficulty in managing financial affairs often develops early in the course of dementia. Although expertise is not expected, clinicians should have some proficiency to address financial concerns. Just as clinicians counsel patients and families about advance care planning, the same should be done to educate about the need for advance financial planning and to recommend that patients complete a durable power of attorney for finance matters (DPOAF) when the capacity to do so still exists. Other options to assist in managing and monitoring finances include online banking, automatic bill payments, direct deposits, and joint bank accounts.

No gold-standard test is available to identify when a patient with dementia no longer has financial capacity. However, the clinician should be on the lookout for signs that a patient is either at risk for or actually experiencing financial incapacity. Because financial impairment can occur when dementia is mild, making that diagnosis should alone be enough to warrant further investigation. Questioning patients and caregivers about late, missed, or repeated bill payments, unusual or uncharacteristic purchases or gifts, overdrawn bank accounts, or reports of missing funds can provide evidence of suspected financial impairment. Patients with dementia are also at increased risk for becoming victims of financial abuse, and some answers to these same questions might also be signs of potential financial abuse. When financial abuse is suspected, clinicians should be aware of the reporting requirements in their local jurisdictions.

▶ Prognosis

Life expectancy after a diagnosis of Alzheimer disease is typically 3–15 years; it may be shorter than previously reported. Other neurodegenerative dementias, such as dementia with Lewy bodies, show more rapid decline. Hospice care is often appropriate for patients with end-stage dementia.

▶ When to Refer

Referral for neuropsychological testing may be helpful to distinguish dementia from depression, to diagnose dementia in persons of very poor education or very high premorbid intellect, and to aid diagnosis when impairment is mild.

Baillon SF et al. Valproate preparations for agitation in dementia. Cochrane Database Syst Rev. 2018 Oct 5;10:CD003945. [PMID: 30293233]

Fink HA et al. Pharmacologic interventions to prevent cognitive decline, mild cognitive impairment, and clinical Alzheimer-type dementia: a systematic review. Ann Intern Med. 2018 Jan 2; 168(1):39–51. [PMID: 29255847]

Panza GA et al. Can exercise improve cognitive symptoms of Alzheimer's disease? J Am Geriatr Soc. 2018 Mar;66(3): 487–95. [PMID: 29363108]

Yohanna D et al. Antipsychotics to treat agitation or psychosis in patients with dementia. JAMA. 2017 Sep 19;318(11):1057–58. [PMID: 28975291]

2. Depression

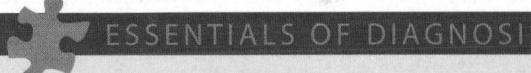

ESSENTIALS OF DIAGNOSIS

▶ Some depressed elders may not admit to depressed mood.

▶ Depression screening in elders should include a question about anhedonia.

▶ General Considerations

Major depressive disorder has prevalence rates of 0.3–10% among community-dwelling adults aged 55 years and older, with most studies reporting a prevalence rate of less than 3%. While major depressive disorder appears to be less common in older adults than younger adults, clinically significant depressive symptoms and subclinical depression are more common, being present in up to 16% of younger adults but 50% of older adults. Among older adults, depressive symptoms are often related to loss, illness, or bereavement. Depression rates rise as illness burden increases. Depression is more common among hospitalized and institutionalized elders. Older single men have the highest rate of completed suicides of any demographic group.

New incidence of depressive symptoms may be an early sign of a dementing illness. Older patients with depression and depressive symptoms who have comorbid conditions (eg, heart failure) are at higher risk for hospitalization, tend to have longer hospital stays, and have worse outcomes than their nondepressed counterparts.

Clinical Findings

The Patient Health Questionnaire-2 (PHQ-2) is highly sensitive for detecting major depression in persons over age 65. Positive responses should be followed up with more comprehensive, structured interviews, such as the Geriatric Depression Scale (http://www.stanford.edu/~yesavage/GDS.html) or the PHQ-9.

Elderly patients with depressive symptoms should be questioned about use of alcohol and medications (eg, benzodiazepines, corticosteroids), since these may contribute to the clinical picture. Similarly, many medical problems can cause fatigue, lethargy, or hypoactive delirium, all of which may be mistaken for depression.

Treatment

Treatment may involve psychosocial interventions, increased physical activity, psychotherapy, problem-solving therapy, cognitive-behavioral therapy, reduction of alcohol or medication intake, antidepressant medications, or a combination approach. Depressed elders may do better with a collaborative or multidisciplinary care model that includes socialization and other support elements than with usual care. In older patients with depressive symptoms who do not meet criteria for major depressive disorder, nonpharmacologic treatment approaches should be used.

Choice of antidepressant agent is usually based on side-effect profile, cost, and patient-specific factors, such as presenting symptoms and comorbidities. Selective serotonin reuptake inhibitors (SSRIs) are often used as first-line agents because they are relatively well-tolerated (see Table 25–7). Paroxetine and fluoxetine are often more poorly tolerated by elders than other SSRIs, so they are usually avoided as first-line agents. Mirtazapine is often used for patients with weight loss, anorexia, or insomnia. Duloxetine is useful in patients who also have neuropathic pain. Regardless of the medication chosen, many experts recommend starting elders at a relatively low dose, titrating to full dose slowly, and continuing for a longer trial (at least 8 weeks) before trying a different medication. Augmentation therapy (eg, with lithium, methylphenidate, or aripiprazole) can enhance clinical response in treatment-resistant depression. For patients with severe or catatonic depression, electroconvulsive therapy should be considered.

For patients experiencing their first episode of depression, pharmacologic treatment should continue for at least 6 months after remission of the depression. Recurrence of major depression is common enough among elders that long-term maintenance medication therapy should be considered.

When to Refer

Any patient who might be considered for electroconvulsive therapy should be referred for psychiatric evaluation. Consider referral for patients who have mania, psychosis, catatonia, or treatment-resistant depression.

When to Admit

Consider psychiatric evaluation and admission for patients who are psychotic, suicidal, homicidal, catatonic, or gravely disabled.

Dham P et al. Collaborative care for psychiatric disorders in older adults: a systematic review. Can J Psychiatry. 2017 Nov;62(11):761–71. [PMID: 28718325]

Haigh EAP et al. Depression among older adults: a 20-year update on five common myths and misconceptions. Am J Geriatr Psychiatry. 2018 Jan;26(1):107–22. [PMID: 28735658]

Kok RM et al. Management of depression in older adults: a review. JAMA. 2017 May 23;317(20):2114–22. [PMID: 28535241]

3. Delirium

ESSENTIALS OF DIAGNOSIS

▶ Rapid onset and fluctuating course.
▶ Primary deficit in attention rather than memory.
▶ May be hypoactive or hyperactive.
▶ Dementia frequently coexists.

General Considerations

Delirium is an acute, fluctuating disturbance of consciousness, associated with a change in cognition or development of perceptual disturbances (see also Chapter 25). It is the pathophysiologic consequence of an underlying general medical condition, such as infection, coronary ischemia, hypoxemia, or metabolic derangement. Delirium occurs in 29–64% of hospitalized older adults, persists in 25% or more, and is associated with worse clinical outcomes (higher in-hospital and postdischarge mortality, longer lengths of stay, delayed and limited recovery of physical function, greater probability of placement in a nursing facility).

Although the acutely agitated elderly patient often comes to mind when considering delirium, many episodes are subtler. Such **hypoactive delirium** may be suspected only if one notices new cognitive slowing or inattention.

Cognitive impairment is an important risk factor for delirium. Other risk factors include severe illness, polypharmacy, use of psychoactive medications, sensory impairment, depression, and alcoholism.

Clinical Findings

Several bedside instruments are available for the assessment of delirium (http://www.hospitalelderlifeprogram.org/delirium-instruments/). The **confusion assessment method (CAM)** requires (1) acute onset and fluctuating course and (2) inattention and *either* (3) disorganized thinking *or* (4) altered level of consciousness. The 3D CAM (3-minute diagnostic CAM) is particularly useful for clinical assessment of delirium.

A key component of a delirium workup is review of medications because many medications, the addition of a new medication, an increase in dose of a medication, or the discontinuation of a medication known to cause withdrawal symptoms are all associated with the development of delirium. Medications that are particularly likely to increase the risk of delirium include sedative/hypnotics, anticholinergics, opioids, benzodiazepines, and H_1- and H_2-antihistamines.

Evaluation of most patients should include a complete blood count; blood urea nitrogen (BUN); serum electrolytes, creatinine, glucose, calcium, albumin, and liver biochemical tests; urinalysis; and ECG. In selected cases, serum magnesium, medication levels, arterial blood gas measurements, blood cultures, chest radiography, urinary toxin screen, and lumbar puncture may be helpful. When delirium develops during a hospitalization in the absence of trauma or new localizing neurologic signs, a head CT is rarely revealing.

▶ Prevention

The best evidence for prevention comes from nonpharmacologic multicomponent interventions. These components include improving cognition (frequent reorientation, activities, socialization with family and friends when possible), sleep (massage, noise reduction, minimizing interruptions at night), mobility, vision (visual aids and adaptive equipment), hearing (portable amplifiers, cerumen disimpaction), and hydration status (volume repletion). No medications, including antipsychotics, have been consistently shown to prevent delirium or improve outcomes such as length of stay or mortality should delirium develop.

▶ Treatment

Management of established episodes of delirium combines the elements of preventive interventions with reassurance and reorientation, treatment of underlying causes, eliminating unnecessary medications, and avoidance of indwelling catheters and restraints. The role of antipsychotic agents (eg, haloperidol, 0.5–1 mg orally, or quetiapine, 25 mg orally, at bedtime or twice daily) is uncertain because the evidence of benefit has been inconsistent. While these agents may reduce distressing symptoms of hyperactive delirium, improvements in complication rates, length of stay, or mortality have not been shown. As with dementia, caution should be used when prescribing antipsychotic medications, including checking the QTc interval on the ECG, eliminating other QTc-prolonging medications, and correcting any electrolyte abnormalities. Benzodiazepines should be avoided except in the circumstance of alcohol or benzodiazepine withdrawal. In ventilated patients in the intensive care unit setting, dexmedetomidine or propofol (or both) may also be useful alternatives or adjuncts to antipsychotic therapy in patients with delirium.

Most episodes of delirium clear in a matter of days after correction of the precipitant, but some patients suffer episodes of much longer duration, and a significant percentage never return to their former baseline level of functioning.

▶ When to Refer

If an initial evaluation does not reveal the cause of delirium or if entities other than delirium are in the differential diagnosis, referral to a neuropsychologist, neurologist, or geropsychiatrist should be considered.

▶ When to Admit

Patients with delirium of unknown cause should be admitted for an expedited workup if consistent with the patient's goals of care.

Neufeld KJ et al. Antipsychotic medication for prevention and treatment of delirium in hospitalized adults: a systematic review and meta-analysis. J Am Geriatr Soc. 2016 Apr;64(4):705–14. [PMID: 27004732]

4. Immobility

Physical activity is associated with a myriad of health benefits in older adults. Unfortunately, mobility limitation is common in older adults and is associated with increased rates of morbidity, hospitalization, disability, and mortality. Structured physical activity programs may help reduce mobility-related disability among community-dwelling elders. Hospital-associated bed rest is a common precipitant of immobility and functional decline. Among hospitalized medical patients over age 70, about 10% experience a decline in function, and those who experience critical illness are at particularly high risk.

The hazards of bed rest in older adults are multiple, serious, quick to develop, and slow to reverse. Within days after being confined to bed, deconditioning of the cardiovascular system occurs and involves fluid shifts, decreased cardiac output, decreased peak oxygen uptake, increased resting heart rate, and postural hypotension. More striking changes occur in skeletal muscle, with a resulting loss of strength and function. Pressure injuries (previously called "pressure ulcers"), deep venous thrombosis, pulmonary embolism, and falls are additional serious risks. Recovery from these changes usually takes weeks to months, and is frequently only partial.

▶ Prevention & Treatment

Physical activity should be encouraged for all elders, particularly sedentary elders. Protocols for hospitalized elders that promote walking two to three times daily and sitting upright for much of the day can minimize unnecessary immobility. When immobilization cannot be avoided, several measures can be used to minimize its consequences. To reduce the risks of contracture and weakness, range-of-motion and strengthening exercises should be started immediately and continued as long as the patient is in bed. Avoiding restraints and discontinuing intravenous lines and urinary catheters will increase opportunities for early mobility. Graduated ambulation should begin as soon as it is feasible. Prior to discharge, physical therapists can recommend appropriate exercises and assistive devices; after discharge, they can recommend safety modifications and maintenance exercises.

McPhee JS et al. Physical activity in older age: perspectives for healthy ageing and frailty. Biogerontology. 2016 Jun;17(3): 567–80. [PMID: 26936444]

Olanrewaju O et al. Physical activity in community dwelling older people: a systematic review of reviews of interventions and context. PLoS One. 2016 Dec 20;11(12):e0168614. [PMID: 27997604]

5. Falls & Gait Disorders

Annually, about one-third of people over age 65 fall, and the frequency of falls increases markedly with advancing age. About 10% of falls result in serious injuries, such as fractures, soft tissue injuries, and traumatic brain injuries. **Complications from falls are the leading cause of death from injury in persons over age 65.** Hip fractures are common precursors to functional impairment, nursing home placement, and death.

Every older person should be asked about falls. Assessment of patients who fall should include postural blood pressure and pulse; cardiac examination; evaluations of strength, range of motion, cognition, and proprioception; and examination of feet and footwear. A thorough gait assessment should be performed in all older people. Gait and balance can be readily assessed by the **"Up and Go Test,"** in which the patient is asked to stand up from a sitting position without use of hands, walk 10 feet, turn around, walk back, and sit down. Patients who take less than 10 seconds are usually normal, while patients who take longer than 13.5 seconds are considered at increased risk for falling. The ability to recognize common patterns of gait disorders is an extremely useful clinical skill to develop. Examples of gait abnormalities and their causes are listed in Table 4–3.

▶ Causes of Falls

Balance and ambulation require a complex interplay of cognitive, neuromuscular, and cardiovascular function. With age, balance mechanisms can become compromised, reaction time slows, and postural sway increases. These changes predispose the older person to a fall when challenged by an additional insult to any of these systems.

Falls in older people are rarely due to a single cause, and effective intervention entails a comprehensive assessment of the patient's intrinsic deficits (eg, diseases and medications), the activity engaged in at the time of the fall, and environmental obstacles (Table 4–4).

Intrinsic deficits are those that impair sensory input, judgment, blood pressure regulation, reaction time, and balance and gait. Dizziness may be closely related to the deficits associated with falls and gait abnormalities. While it may be impossible to isolate a sole "cause" or a "cure" for falls, gait abnormalities, or dizziness, it is often possible to identify and ameliorate some of the underlying contributory conditions and improve the patient's overall function.

Medication use is one of the most common, significant, and reversible causes of falling. A meta-analysis found that sedative/hypnotics, antidepressants, and benzodiazepines were the classes of medications most likely to be associated with falling. The use of multiple medications simultaneously has also been associated with an increased fall risk. Other often overlooked but treatable contributors include postural hypotension (including postprandial, which peaks 30–60 minutes after a meal), insomnia, use of multifocal lenses, and urinary urgency.

Since most falls occur in or around the home, a visit by a visiting nurse, physical therapist, or health care provider

Table 4–3. Evaluation of gait abnormalities.

Gait Abnormality	Possible Cause
Inability to stand without use of hands	Deconditioning Myopathy (hyperthyroidism, alcohol, statin-induced) Hip or knee pain
Unsteadiness upon standing	Orthostatic hypotension Balance problem (peripheral neuropathy, vision problem, vestibular, other central nervous system causes) Generalized weakness
Stagger with eyes closed	Often indicates that vision is compensating for another deficit
Short steps	Weakness Parkinson disease or related condition
Asymmetry	Cerebrovascular accident Focal pain or arthritis
Wide-based gait	Fear, balance problems
Flexed knees	Contractures, quadriceps weakness
Slow gait	Fear of falling, weakness, deconditioning, peripheral vascular disease, chronic obstructive pulmonary disease, heart failure, angina pectoris

for a **home safety evaluation** may be beneficial in identifying environmental obstacles and is generally reimbursed by third-party payers, including Medicare.

Complications of Falls

The most common fractures resulting from falls are of the wrist, hip, and vertebrae. There is a high mortality rate (approximately 20% in 1 year) in elderly women with hip fractures, particularly if they were debilitated prior to the time of the fracture. Fear of falling again is a common, serious, but treatable factor in the elderly person's loss of confidence and independence. Referral to a physical therapist for gait training with special devices is often all that is required.

Chronic subdural hematoma is an easily overlooked complication of falls that must be considered in any elderly patient presenting with new neurologic symptoms or signs. Headache and known history of trauma may both be absent.

Patients who are unable to get up from a fall are at risk for dehydration, electrolyte imbalance, pressure injuries, rhabdomyolysis, and hypothermia.

Prevention & Management

Exercise is the intervention that is most consistently reported to reduce the risk of falls. Balance focused exercises (eg, Tai Chi), gait, and strength training appear to be more effective for fall prevention than general exercise programs (Table 4–4).

Multifactorial interventions appear to have a small benefit in preventing falls. These interventions include an assessment of potentially modifiable risk factors and tailored interventions to reduce risk. Emphasis is placed on treating all contributory medical conditions, minimizing environmental hazards, and eliminating medications where the harms may outweigh the benefits—particularly those that induce orthostasis (eg, alpha-blockers, nitrates, antipsychotics).

The USPSTF recommends against vitamin D supplementation to prevent falls in community-dwelling adults. Vitamin D supplementation might be considered for high-risk individuals (eg, institutionalized elders) on a case-by-case basis. High-dose vitamin D (60,000 international units per month) has been shown to *increase* the incidence of falls.

Assistive devices, such as canes and walkers, are useful for many older adults but are often used incorrectly. Canes should be used on the "good" side. The height of walkers and canes should generally be about the level of the wrist. Physical therapists are invaluable in assessing the need for an assistive device, selecting the best device, and training a patient in its correct use.

Eyeglasses, particularly bifocal or graduated lenses, may increase the risk of falls, particularly in the early weeks of use. Patients should be counseled about the need to take extra care when new eyeglasses are being used.

Patients with repeated falls are often reassured by the availability of telephones at floor level, a mobile telephone on their person, or a lightweight radio call system. Their therapy should also include training in techniques for arising after a fall.

Table 4–4. Fall risk factors, targeted interventions, and best evidence for fall prevention.

To Consider for All Patients	
Exercise or physical therapy	Tai Chi, gait training, balance training, strength training
Multifactorial intervention	Home safety assessment, medication review, review of specific conditions (below), advice on appropriate footwear, vision check, adaptive aids as appropriate, physical therapy or exercise as appropriate
Condition	**Targeted Intervention**
Postural hypotension (> 20 mm Hg drop in systolic blood pressure, or systolic blood pressure < 90 mm Hg)	Behavioral recommendations, such as hand clenching, elevation of head of bed; discontinuation or substitution of high-risk medications
Use of benzodiazepine or sedative/hypnotic agent	Education about sleep hygiene; discontinuation or substitution of medications
Use of multiple prescription medications	Review of medications
Environmental hazards	Appropriate changes; installation of safety equipment (eg, grab bars)
Gait impairment	Gait training, assistive devices, balance or strengthening exercises
Impairment in transfer or balance	Balance exercises, training in transfers, environmental alterations (eg, grab bars)
Impairment in leg or arm muscle strength or limb range of motion	Exercise with resistance bands or putty, with graduated increases in resistance
Vision impairment	Cataract surgery or other interventions as appropriate
Inability to get up after a fall	Medic-alert system, physical therapy training for strategies
High-risk footwear	Education on appropriate footwear (eg, avoid slippers, high heels)

When to Refer

Patients with a recent history of falls should be referred for physical therapy, eye examination, and home safety evaluation.

When to Admit

If the patient has new falls that are unexplained, particularly in combination with a change in the physical examination or an injury requiring surgery, hospitalization should be considered.

Li F et al. Effectiveness of a therapeutic Tai Ji Quan intervention vs a multimodal exercise intervention to prevent falls among older adults at high risk of falling: a randomized clinical trial. JAMA Intern Med. 2018 Oct 1;178(10):1301–10. [PMID: 30208396]

US Preventive Services Task Force; Grossman DC et al. Interventions to prevent falls in community-dwelling older adults: US Preventive Services Task Force recommendation statement. JAMA. 2018 Apr 24;319(16):1696–704. [PMID: 29710141]

6. Urinary Incontinence

ESSENTIALS OF DIAGNOSIS

- ▶ Involuntary loss of urine.
- ▶ *Stress* incontinence: leakage of urine upon coughing, sneezing, or standing.
- ▶ *Urge* incontinence: urgency and inability to delay urination.
- ▶ *Overflow* incontinence: variable presentation.

General Considerations

Urinary incontinence in older adults is common, and interventions can improve most patients. Many patients fail to tell their providers about it. A simple question about involuntary leakage of urine is a reasonable annual screen: "Do you have a problem with urine leaks or accidents?"

Classification

A. Transient Causes

Use of the mnemonic "DIAPPERS" may be helpful in remembering the categories of "transient" urinary incontinence.

1. Delirium—A clouded sensorium impedes recognition of both the need to void and the location of the nearest toilet. Delirium is the most common cause of incontinence in hospitalized patients; once it clears, incontinence usually resolves.

2. Infection—Symptomatic urinary tract infection commonly causes or contributes to urgency and incontinence. Asymptomatic bacteriuria does not.

3. Atrophic urethritis and vaginitis—Atrophic urethritis and vaginitis can usually be diagnosed presumptively by the presence of vaginal mucosal telangiectasia, petechiae, erosions, erythema, or friability. Urethral inflammation, if symptomatic, may contribute to incontinence in some women. Some experts suggest a trial of topical estrogen in these cases.

4. Pharmaceuticals—Medications are one of the most common causes of transient incontinence. Typical offending agents include potent diuretics, anticholinergics, psychotropics, opioid analgesics, alpha-blockers (in women), alpha-agonists (in men), and calcium channel blockers.

5. Psychological factors—Severe depression with psychomotor retardation may impede the ability or motivation to reach a toilet.

6. Excess urinary output—Excess urinary output may overwhelm the ability of an older person to reach a toilet in time. In addition to diuretics, common causes include excess fluid intake; metabolic abnormalities (eg, hyperglycemia, hypercalcemia, diabetes insipidus); and disorders associated with peripheral edema, with its associated heavy nocturia when previously dependent legs assume a horizontal position in bed.

7. Restricted mobility—(See Immobility, above.) If mobility cannot be improved, access to a urinal or commode (eg, at the bedside) may improve continence.

8. Stool impaction—This is a common cause of urinary incontinence in hospitalized or immobile patients. Although the mechanism is still unknown, a clinical clue to its presence is the onset of both urinary and fecal incontinence. Disimpaction usually restores urinary continence.

B. Established Causes

Causes of "established" incontinence should be addressed after the "transient" causes have been uncovered and managed appropriately.

1. Detrusor overactivity (urge incontinence)—Detrusor overactivity refers to uninhibited bladder contractions that cause leakage. It is the most common cause of established geriatric incontinence, accounting for two-thirds of cases, and is usually idiopathic. Women will complain of urinary leakage after the onset of an intense urge to urinate that cannot be forestalled. In men, the symptoms are similar, but detrusor overactivity commonly coexists with urethral obstruction from benign prostatic hyperplasia. Because detrusor overactivity also may be due to bladder stones or tumor, the abrupt onset of otherwise unexplained urge incontinence—especially if accompanied by perineal or suprapubic discomfort or sterile hematuria—should be investigated by cystoscopy and cytologic examination of a urine specimen.

2. Urethral incompetence (stress incontinence)—Urethral incompetence is the second most common cause of established urinary incontinence in older women. Stress incontinence is most commonly seen in men after radical prostatectomy. Stress incontinence is characterized by instantaneous leakage of urine in response to a stress maneuver. It commonly coexists with detrusor overactivity. Typically, urinary loss occurs with laughing, coughing, or lifting heavy objects. Leakage is worse or occurs only during the day, unless another abnormality (eg, detrusor overactivity) is also present. To test for stress incontinence, have the patient relax her perineum and cough vigorously (a single cough) while standing with a full bladder. Instantaneous leakage indicates stress incontinence (if urinary retention has been excluded by postvoiding residual determination using ultrasound). A delay of several seconds or persistent leakage suggests that the problem is instead caused by an uninhibited bladder contraction induced by coughing.

3. Urethral obstruction—Urethral obstruction (due to prostatic enlargement, urethral stricture, bladder neck contracture, or prostatic cancer) is a common cause of established incontinence in older men but is rare in older women. It can present as dribbling incontinence after voiding, urge incontinence due to detrusor overactivity (which coexists in two-thirds of cases), or overflow incontinence due to urinary retention.

4. Detrusor underactivity (overflow incontinence)—Detrusor underactivity is the least common cause of incontinence. It may be idiopathic or due to sacral lower motor nerve dysfunction. When it causes incontinence, detrusor underactivity is associated with urinary frequency, nocturia, and frequent leakage of small amounts. The elevated postvoiding residual urine (generally over 450 mL) distinguishes it from detrusor overactivity and stress incontinence, but only urodynamic testing differentiates it from urethral obstruction in men. Such testing usually is not required in women, in whom obstruction is rarely present.

▶ **Treatment**

A. Transient Causes

Each identified transient cause should be treated regardless of whether an established cause coexists. For patients with urinary retention induced by an anticholinergic agent, discontinuation of the medication should first be considered. If this is not feasible, substituting a less anticholinergic agent may be useful.

B. Established Causes

1. Detrusor overactivity—The cornerstone of treatment is **bladder training**. Patients start by voiding on a schedule based on the shortest interval recorded on a bladder record. They then gradually lengthen the interval between voids by 30 minutes each week using relaxation techniques to postpone the urge to void. Lifestyle modifications, including weight loss and caffeine reduction, may also improve incontinence symptoms. For cognitively impaired patients and nursing home residents who are unable to manage on their own, **timed and prompted voiding** initiated by caregivers is effective. **Pelvic floor muscle ("Kegel") exercises** can reduce the frequency of incontinence episodes when performed correctly and sustained.

If behavioral approaches prove insufficient, **antimuscarinic agents** may provide additional benefit. Tolterodine and oxybutynin are the two oral medications for which there is the most experience. Available regimens of these agents include short-acting tolterodine, 1–2 mg orally twice a day; long-acting tolterodine, 2–4 mg orally daily; short-acting oxybutynin, 2.5–5 mg orally twice or three times a day; long-acting oxybutynin, 5–15 mg orally daily; and oxybutynin transdermal patch, 3.9 mg/day applied twice weekly. All of these agents can produce delirium, dry mouth, or urinary retention; long-acting preparations may be better tolerated. Agents such as fesoterodine (4–8 mg orally once daily), trospium chloride (20 mg orally once or twice daily), long-acting trospium chloride (60 mg orally daily), darifenacin (7.5–15 mg orally daily), and solifenacin (5–10 mg orally daily) appear to have similar efficacy, but only fesoterodine has been demonstrated to have tolerability in medically complex older adults that is comparable to younger adults.

The beta-3-agonist **mirabegron,** 25–50 mg orally daily, is approved for overactive bladder symptoms, which include urge urinary incontinence. In trials comparing mirabegron with antimuscarinic agents, the efficacy and safety profiles have been comparable, with less dry mouth reported in persons who received mirabegron. While its potential cardiac effects warrant ongoing surveillance, the experience accruing among adults over the age of 70 shows that adherence rates may be superior to the antimuscarinic medications. For frail older adults and those with hypertension or cardiac conditions, the long-term safety remains to be determined.

An alternative to oral agents is an injection of **onabotulinum toxin A** into the detrusor muscle. While effective, it can lead to urinary retention and the need for self-catheterization.

The combination of behavioral therapy and antimuscarinics appears to be more effective than either alone, although one study in a group of younger women showed that adding behavioral therapy to individually titrated doses of extended-release oxybutynin was no better than with medication treatment alone.

In men with both benign prostatic hyperplasia and detrusor overactivity and with postvoiding residual volumes of 150 mL or less, an antimuscarinic agent added to an alpha-blocker may provide additional relief of lower urinary tract symptoms.

2. Urethral incompetence (stress incontinence)—Lifestyle modifications, including limiting caffeine and fluid intake, may be helpful for some women, particularly women with mixed stress/urge incontinence; strong evidence supports weight loss in obese women. **Pelvic floor muscle exercises** are effective for women with mild to moderate stress incontinence. Instruct the patient to pull in the pelvic floor muscles and hold for 6–10 seconds and to perform three sets of 8–12 contractions daily. Benefits may not be seen for 6 weeks. **Pessaries** or **vaginal cones** may be helpful in some women but should be prescribed only by providers who are experienced with using these modalities.

No medications are approved for the treatment of stress incontinence, and a clinical practice guideline from the

American College of Physicians recommends against pharmacologic treatment. Although a last resort, **surgery** is the most effective treatment for stress incontinence; cure rates as high as 96% can result, even in older women.

3. Urethral obstruction—**Surgical decompression** is the most effective treatment for obstruction, especially in the setting of urinary retention due to benign prostatic hyperplasia. A variety of nonsurgical techniques make decompression feasible even for frail men. For the nonoperative candidate with urinary retention, intermittent or **indwelling catheterization** is used. For a man with prostatic obstruction who does not require or desire immediate surgery, treatment with **alpha-blocking agents** (eg, terazosin, 1–10 mg orally daily; prazosin, 1–5 mg orally twice daily; tamsulosin, 0.4–0.8 mg orally daily taken 30 minutes after the same meal) can improve symptoms and delay obstruction. **Finasteride,** 5 mg orally daily, can provide additional benefit to an alpha-blocking agent in men with an enlarged prostate.

4. Detrusor underactivity—For the patient with a poorly contractile bladder, **augmented voiding techniques** (eg, double voiding, suprapubic pressure) can prove effective. If further emptying is needed, intermittent or indwelling **catheterization** is the only option. Antibiotics should be used only for symptomatic urinary tract infection or as prophylaxis against recurrent symptomatic infections in a patient using intermittent catheterization; they should not be used as prophylaxis in a patient with an indwelling catheter.

When to Refer

- Men with urinary obstruction who do not respond to medical therapy should be referred to a urologist.
- Women who do not respond to medical and behavioral therapy should be referred to a urogynecologist or urologist.

Culbertson S et al. Nonsurgical management of urinary incontinence in women. JAMA. 2017 Jan 3;317(1):79–80. [PMID: 28030686]

Lukacz ES et al. Urinary incontinence in women: a review. JAMA. 2017 Oct 24;318(16):1592–604. [PMID: 29067433]

7. Involuntary Weight Loss

General Considerations

Aging, even in the absence of disease, is associated with reduced appetite. Involuntary weight loss affects substantial numbers of elders. Most studies of involuntary weight loss in community-dwelling older adults define it as loss of 5% of body weight in 6 months or 10% of body weight in 1 year.

Clinical Findings

The causes of involuntary weight loss are many but generally break down along medical (60–70%) and psychiatric (10–20%) causes, while up to 25% of the time a cause will not be identified. Social factors such as access to food and dental health should also be explored. The history and physical examination should guide the evaluation looking for symptoms and signs that could point to a potential cause (eg, abdominal pain—peptic ulcer disease, tachycardia—hyperthyroidism). When the history, physical examination, and basic laboratory studies do not suggest a possible diagnosis, additional evaluation (eg, total body CT scan) is usually low yield. When no other cause is identified, the frailty syndrome should be considered in the differential diagnosis.

Treatment

Initial treatment should focus on any identified causes of involuntary weight loss while also addressing social barriers that may impact the patient's access to food. Oral nutritional supplements of 200–1000 kcal/day can increase weight and improve outcomes in malnourished hospitalized elders but have *not* been shown to have benefits in community-dwelling older adults. Sodium-containing flavor enhancers (eg, iodized salt) can improve food intake without adverse health effects when there is no contraindication to their use. Megestrol acetate as an appetite stimulant has *not* been shown to increase lean body mass or lengthen life among elders and has significant side effects. For those patients with advanced dementia, percutaneous tube feeding is *not* recommended, but rather assiduous hand feeding may allow maintenance of weight and provide more comfort.

Abu RA et al. PEG insertion in patients with dementia does not improve nutritional status and has worse outcomes as compared with PEG insertion for other indications. J Clin Gastroenterol. 2017 May/Jun;51(5):417–20. [PMID: 27505401]

8. Pressure Injury

ESSENTIALS OF DIAGNOSIS

▶ Examine at-risk patients on admission to the hospital and daily thereafter.

▶ Pressure injury is classified into one of six categories:
  - Stage 1: Non-blanchable erythema of intact skin
  - Stage 2: Partial-thickness skin loss with exposed dermis
  - Stage 3: Full-thickness skin loss
  - Stage 4: Full-thickness skin and tissue loss
  - Unstageable: Obscured full-thickness skin and tissue loss
  - Deep tissue: Persistent non-blanchable deep red, maroon, or purple discoloration

General Considerations

In 2016, the National Pressure Ulcer Advisory Panel changed the term "pressure ulcer" to "pressure injury" to more accurately reflect the fact that stage 1 and deep tissue injury describe injuries to intact skin, compared to the ulcers described in the other four stages. Most pressure injuries develop during a hospital stay for an acute illness. The primary risk factor for pressure injuries is immobility. Other contributing risk factors include reduced sensory perception, moisture (urinary and fecal incontinence), poor nutritional status, and friction and shear forces.

Deep tissue and unstageable pressure injury are included in the six pressure injury stages. An area of purple or maroon discolored intact skin or blood-filled blister is characteristic of deep tissue injury. The area may be preceded by tissue that is painful, firm, mushy, boggy, warmer, or cooler compared with adjacent tissue. Ulcers in which the base is covered by slough (yellow, tan, gray, green, or brown) or eschar (tan, brown, or black) are considered unstageable.

Older adults admitted to hospitals and nursing homes should be assessed for their risk of developing pressure injuries, and several risk assessment instruments can be used, including the Braden Scale and the Norton score.

While Medicare does not reimburse for hospital-acquired pressure injury, there is a higher reimbursement for pressure injury present on admission. Clinicians should include a full skin assessment on every admission evaluation.

▶ Prevention

Using specialized support surfaces (including mattresses, beds, and cushions), patient repositioning, optimizing nutritional status, and moisturizing sacral skin are strategies that have been shown to reduce pressure injury. For moderate- to high-risk patients, mattresses or overlays that reduce tissue pressure below that of a standard mattress appear to be superior to standard mattresses.

▶ Evaluation

Evaluation of pressure injuries should include patient's risk factors and goals of care; injury stage, size, and depth; absence or presence (and type) of exudate; appearance of the wound bed and possible surrounding infection; and sinus tracking, or cellulitis.

▶ Treatment

Treatment is aimed toward pressure reduction, removing necrotic debris, and maintaining a moist wound bed that will promote healing and formation of granulation tissue. The type of dressing that is recommended depends on the location and depth of the wound, whether necrotic tissue or dead space is present, and the amount of exudate (Table 4–5). Pressure-reducing devices (eg, air-fluid beds and low-air-loss beds) are associated with improved healing rates. Although poor nutritional status is a risk factor for the development of pressure injury, the evidence that nutritional supplementation helps correct pressure injury is limited.

Table 4–5. Treatment of pressure injury.

Injury Type	Dressing Type and Considerations
Stage 1 and deep tissue injury	Polyurethane film Hydrocolloid wafer Semipermeable foam dressing
Stage 2	Hydrocolloid wafers Semipermeable foam dressing Polyurethane film
Stages 3 and 4	For highly exudative wounds, use highly absorptive dressing or packing, such as calcium alginate Wounds with necrotic debris must be debrided Debridement can be autolytic, enzymatic, or surgical Shallow, clean wounds can be dressed with hydrocolloid wafers, semipermeable foam, or polyurethane film Deep wounds can be packed with gauze; if the wound is deep and highly exudative, an absorptive packing should be used
Heel injury	Do not remove eschar on heel ulcers because it can help promote healing (eschar in other locations should be debrided)
Unstageable	Debride before deciding on further therapy
Deep tissue injury	Avoid pressure to the area

Providers can become easily overwhelmed by the array of products available for the treatment of established pressure injuries. Most institutions should designate a wound care expert or team to select a streamlined wound care product line that has simple guidelines. In a patient with end-stage disease who is receiving end-of-life care, appropriate treatment might be directed toward palliation (including minimizing dressing changes and odors) rather than efforts directed at healing.

▶ Complications

Bacteria contaminate all chronic pressure injuries with skin loss, but it can be difficult to identify those wounds that are infected. Suspicion for infection should rise if there is pain, increased or foul-smelling wound drainage, erythema of the skin around the wound, or if the wound will not heal. Fever and leukocytosis are other indicators of systemic infection but are not always present. Culture from a superficial swab adds little valuable diagnostic information. For nonhealing infected wounds without evidence of systemic involvement, topical antiseptics (eg, silver sulfadiazine) are recommended and may need to be accompanied by debridement of necrotic tissue. When systemic infections such as cellulitis and osteomyelitis are present, oral or parenteral antibiotics are warranted and medication choice should be guided by tissue culture, but this can be painful and is not always readily available.

When to Refer

Pressure injuries that are large or nonhealing should be referred to a plastic or general surgeon or dermatologist for biopsy, debridement, and possible skin grafting.

When to Admit

Patients with pressure injury should be admitted if the primary residence is unable to provide adequate wound care or pressure reduction, or if the wound is infected or requires complex or surgical care.

Qaseem A et al. Treatment of pressure ulcers: a clinical practice guideline from the American College of Physicians. Ann Intern Med. 2015 Mar 3;162(5):370–9. [PMID: 25732279]
Ricci JA et al. Evidence-based medicine: the evaluation and treatment of pressure injuries. Plast Reconstr Surg. 2017 Jan;139(1):275–86. [PMID: 28027261]
Tran JP et al. Prevention of pressure ulcers in the acute care setting: new innovations and technologies. Plast Reconstr Surg. 2016 Sep;138(3 Suppl):232–40S. [PMID: 27556767]

9. Pharmacotherapy & Polypharmacy

There are several reasons for the greater incidence of iatrogenic medication reactions in the elderly population, the most important of which is the large number of medications that many elders take. Medication metabolism is often impaired in elders due to a decrease in glomerular filtration rate, reduced hepatic clearance, and changes in body composition. Older individuals often have varying responses to a given serum medication level. Most emergency hospitalizations for recognized adverse medication events among older persons result from only a few common medications used alone or in combination.

Precautions in Administering Medications

Nonpharmacologic interventions can often be a first-line alternative to medications (eg, diet for mild hypertension or type 2 diabetes mellitus). Pharmacologic therapy often should begin with less than the medication's usual adult dosage, with slow increases in dosage until a therapeutic level is reached or intolerable side effects develop. Despite the importance of beginning new medications in a slow, measured fashion, medical trials are often inadequate in terms of duration or dose before discontinuation. Antidepressants, in particular, are frequently stopped before therapeutic dosages are reached for sufficient durations.

A number of simple interventions can help improve adherence to the prescribed medical regimen. When possible, the clinician should keep the dosing schedule simple, the number of pills low, the medication changes as infrequent as possible, and encourage the patient to use a single pharmacy. Pillboxes or "medi-sets" help some patients with adherence.

Having the patient or caregiver bring in all medications at each visit can help the clinician perform **medication reconciliation** and reinforce reasons for medication use, dosage, frequency of administration, and possible adverse effects. Medication reconciliation is particularly important if the patient sees multiple providers.

The risk of toxicity goes up with the number of medications prescribed. Certain combinations of medications (eg, warfarin and many types of antibiotics, angiotensin-converting enzyme inhibitors and NSAIDs, opioids and sedative-hypnotics) are particularly likely to cause drug-drug interactions and should be watched carefully.

Trials of individual medication discontinuation should be considered when the original indication is unclear, the goals of care have changed, or the patient might be experiencing side effects. Medication discontinuation is particularly important in patients with limited life expectancy who may experience increasing burdens and modest, if any, benefits from many classes of medications (eg, bisphosphonates, cholesterol-lowering medications). Utilization of clinical tools such as "STOPP/START" and the Beers Criteria can improve medication prescribing and clinical outcomes.

When to Refer

Patients with poor or uncertain adherence may benefit from referral to a pharmacist or a home health nurse.

Morin L et al. Choosing wisely? Measuring the burden of medications in older adults near the end of life: nationwide, longitudinal cohort study. Am J Med. 2017 Aug;130(8):927–36.e9. [PMID: 28454668]
Zullo AR et al. Screening for medication appropriateness in older adults. Clin Geriatr Med. 2018 Feb;34(1):39–54. [PMID: 29129216]

10. Vision Impairment

Visual impairment due to age-related refractive error ("presbyopia"), macular degeneration, cataracts, glaucoma, and diabetic retinopathy is associated with significant physical and mental health comorbidities, falls, mobility impairment, and reduced quality of life. High-quality evidence does *not* support routine screening for vision impairment in elders. However, the authors of this chapter believe that serious and correctable vision disorders are prevalent and morbid enough that it is reasonable for most elders to undergo periodic eye examination by an ophthalmologist or optometrist. Many patients with visual loss benefit from a referral to a low-vision program.

Clarke EL et al. Community screening for visual impairment in older people. Cochrane Database Syst Rev. 2018 Feb 20;2: CD001054. [PMID: 29460275]
Naël V et al. Visual impairment, undercorrected refractive errors, and activity limitations in older adults: findings from the three-city alienor study. Invest Ophthalmol Vis Sci. 2017 Apr 1;58(4):2359–65. [PMID: 28437525]

11. Hearing Impairment

Over one-third of persons over age 65 and half of those over age 85 have some hearing loss. Hearing loss is associated with social isolation, depression, disability, cognitive impairment, and excess risk of hospitalization and nursing home placement. A reasonable screen is to ask patients if they have hearing impairment. Those who answer "yes" should be referred for audiometry. Those who answer "no" may still have hearing impairment and can be screened by a handheld audioscope or the whispered voice test. The whispered voice test is administered by standing 2 feet behind the subject, whispering three random numbers while simultaneously rubbing the external auditory canal of the non-tested ear to mask the sound. If the patient is unable to identify all three numbers, the test should be repeated with different numbers, and if still abnormal, a referral should be made for an audiogram. To determine the degree to which hearing impairment interferes with functioning, the provider may ask if the patient becomes frustrated when conversing with family members, is embarrassed when meeting new people, has difficulty watching TV, or has problems understanding conversations. Caregivers or family members often have important information on the impact of hearing loss on the patient's social interactions.

Hearing amplification or cochlear implantation can improve hearing-related quality of life and reduce depressive symptoms in patients with hearing loss. Compliance with hearing amplification can be a challenge because of dissatisfaction with performance, stigma associated with hearing aid use, and cost. Newer digital devices may perform better but are considerably more expensive. Cochlear implantation is increasingly being recommended for selected elders with profound sensory hearing loss. Special telephones, amplifiers for the television, and other devices are helpful to many patients. Portable amplifiers are pager-sized units with earphones attached; they can be purchased inexpensively at many electronics stores and can be useful in health care settings for improving communication with hearing-impaired patients. A US federal law signed in 2017 designed to lower the cost of hearing aids and increase accessibility will allow for the sale of over-the-counter devices. In general, facing the patient and speaking slowly in a low tone is a more effective communication strategy than shouting.

Choi JS et al. Association of using hearing aids or cochlear implants with changes in depressive symptoms in older adults. JAMA Otolaryngol Head Neck Surg. 2016 Jul 1; 142(7):652–7. [PMID: 27258813]

Goman AM et al. Prevalence of hearing loss by severity in the United States. Am J Public Health. 2016 Oct;106(10):1820–2. [PMID: 27552261]

12. Elder Mistreatment & Self-Neglect

Elder mistreatment is defined as "actions that cause harm or create a serious risk of harm to an older adult by a caregiver or other person who stands in a trust relationship to the older adult, or failure by a caregiver to satisfy the elder's basic needs or to protect the elder from harm." **Self-neglect** is the most common form of elder mistreatment

and occurs among all demographic strata of the aging population. In the United States, about 14% of adults over age 70 experience some sort of mistreatment annually, with about 12% experiencing psychological mistreatment and almost 2% experiencing physical mistreatment. Each year, 5–7% of elders may be victims of financial abuse or scams.

Clues to the possibility of elder mistreatment include behavioral changes in the presence of the caregiver, delays between occurrences of injuries and when treatment was sought, inconsistencies between an observed injury and its associated explanation, lack of appropriate clothing or hygiene, and not filling prescriptions. Many elders with cognitive impairment become targets of financial abuse. Both elder mistreatment and self-neglect are associated with an increased risk of mortality.

It is helpful to observe and talk with every older person alone for at least part of a visit to ask questions directly about possible mistreatment and neglect (Table 4–6). When self-neglect is suspected, it is critical to establish whether a patient has decision-making capacity in order to determine what course of action needs to be taken. A patient who has full decision-making capacity should be provided with help and support but can choose to live in conditions of self-neglect, providing that the public is not endangered by the actions of the person. In contrast, a patient who lacks decision-making capacity who lives in conditions of self-neglect will require more aggressive intervention, which may include guardianship, in-home help, or placement in a supervised setting. Mental state scores, such as the MoCA, may provide some insight into the patient's cognitive status but are not designed to assess decision-making capacity. A standardized tool, such as the "Aid to Capacity Evaluation," is easy to administer, has good performance characteristics for determining decision-making capacity, and is available free online at http://www.jcb.utoronto.ca/tools/documents/ace.pdf.

Table 4–6. Phrases and actions that may be helpful in situations of suspected abuse or neglect.

Questions for the Elder
1. Has anyone hurt you?
2. Are you afraid of anybody?
3. Is anyone taking or using your money without your permission?
Questions for the Caregiver
1. Are your relative's needs more than you can handle?
2. Are you worried that you might hit your relative?
3. Have you hit your relative?
If abuse is suspected
Tell the patient that you are concerned, want to help, and will call Adult Protective Services to see if there is anything that they can do to help
Document any injuries
Document the patient's words
Document whether the patient has decision-making capacity using a tool such as "Aid to Capacity Evaluation"

When to Refer

- Refer elders with suspected mistreatment or self-neglect to Adult Protective Services, as required by law in most states (consult the National Center on Elder Abuse at http://www.ncea.aoa.gov).

- Refer elders to a mental health professional when it is unclear whether they have decision-making capacity after an initial assessment or whether an untreated mental health disorder is contributing to their problem.

When to Admit

- Admit elders who would be unsafe in the community when an alternative plan cannot be put into place in a timely manner.

Burnes D et al. Prevalence of financial fraud and scams among older adults in the United States: a systematic review and meta-analysis. Am J Public Health. 2017 Aug;107(8):1295. [PMID: 28700284]

Friedman LS et al. Physical abuse of elderly adults: victim characteristics and determinants of revictimization. J Am Geriatr Soc. 2017 Jul;65(7):1420–6. [PMID: 28485492]

Rosay AB. Prevalence estimates and correlates of elder abuse in the United States: the National Intimate Partner and Sexual Violence Survey. J Elder Abuse Negl. 2017 Jan–Feb;29(1): 1–14. [PMID: 27782784]

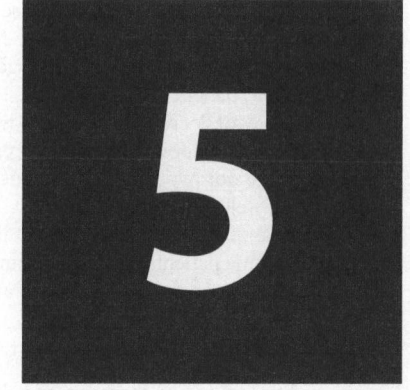

Palliative Care & Pain Management

Michael W. Rabow, MD   Steven Z. Pantilat, MD

Ann Cai Shah, MD   Scott Steiger, MD

Lawrence Poree, MD, MPH, PhD

PALLIATIVE CARE

DEFINITION & SCOPE

Palliative care is medical care focused on improving quality of life for people living with serious illness. Serious illness is defined as "a condition that carries a high risk of mortality, negatively impacts quality of life and daily function, and/or is burdensome in symptoms, treatments or caregiver stress." Palliative care addresses and treats symptoms, supports patients' families and loved ones, and through clear communication helps ensure that care aligns with patients' preferences, values, and goals. Near the end of life, palliative care may become the sole focus of care, but palliative care *alongside cure-focused treatment or disease management* is beneficial throughout the course of a serious illness, regardless of its prognosis.

Palliative care includes management of physical symptoms, such as pain, dyspnea, nausea and vomiting, constipation, delirium, and agitation; emotional distress, such as depression, anxiety, and interpersonal strain; and existential distress, such as spiritual crisis. While palliative care is a medical subspecialty recognized by the American Board of Medical Specialties ("specialty palliative care") and is typically provided by an interdisciplinary team of experts, *all* clinicians should have the skills to provide "primary palliative care" including managing pain; treating dyspnea; identifying mood disorders; communicating about prognosis and patient preferences for care; and helping address spiritual distress. The fourth edition of the National Consensus Project's Clinical Practice Guidelines for Quality Palliative Care emphasizes that palliative care is the responsibility of all clinicians and disciplines caring for people with serious illness, in all health care settings (including hospitals, primary care and specialty clinics, nursing homes, and the community).

During any stage of illness, patients should be screened routinely for symptoms. Any symptoms that cause significant suffering are a medical emergency that should be managed aggressively with frequent elicitation and reassessment as well as individualized treatment. While patients at the end of life may experience a host of distressing symptoms, pain,

dyspnea, and delirium are among the most feared and burdensome. Management of these common symptoms is described later in this chapter. Randomized studies have shown that palliative care provided alongside disease-focused treatment can improve quality of life, promote symptom management, and even prolong life.

Ahluwalia SC et al. A systematic review in support of the National Consensus Project Clinical Practice Guidelines for Quality Palliative Care, 4th edition. J Pain Symptom Manage. 2018 Dec;56(6):831–70. [PMID: 30391049]

Basch E et al. Overall survival results of a trial assessing patient-reported outcomes for symptom monitoring during routine cancer treatment. JAMA. 2017 Jul 11;318(2):197–8. [PMID: 28586821]

Ferrell BR et al. Integration of palliative care into standard oncology care: American Society of Clinical Oncology Clinical Practice Guideline Update. J Clin Oncol. 2017 Jan;35(1):96–112. [PMID: 28034065]

Kelley AS et al. Identifying older adults with serious illness: a critical step toward improving the value of health care. Health Serv Res. 2017 Feb;52(1):113–31. [PMID: 26990009]

Zhou K et al. Palliative care in heart failure: a meta-analysis of randomized controlled trials. Herz. 2018 Feb 21. [Epub ahead of print] [PMID: 29468259]

PALLIATION OF COMMON NONPAIN SYMPTOMS

DYSPNEA

Dyspnea is the subjective experience of difficulty breathing and may be characterized by patients as tightness in the chest, shortness of breath, breathlessness, or a feeling of suffocation. Up to half of people at the end of life may experience severe dyspnea.

Treatment of dyspnea is usually first directed at the cause (see Chapter 9). At the end of life, dyspnea is often treated nonspecifically with opioids, which are the single best class of medications for dyspnea with demonstrated effectiveness in multiple randomized trials. Starting doses are typically lower than would be necessary for the relief of moderate pain. Immediate-release morphine given orally (2–4 mg every 4 hours) or intravenously (1–2 mg every 4 hours) treats dyspnea effectively. Sustained-release morphine given orally at 10 mg daily is safe and effective for most patients with ongoing dyspnea. Supplemental oxygen may be useful for the dyspneic patient *who is hypoxic.* However, a nasal cannula and face mask are sometimes not well tolerated, and fresh air from a window or fan may provide relief for patients who are not hypoxic. Judicious use of noninvasive ventilation as well as nonpharmacologic relaxation techniques, such as meditation and guided imagery, may be beneficial for some patients. Benzodiazepines may be useful adjuncts for treatment of dyspnea-related anxiety.

NAUSEA & VOMITING

Nausea and vomiting are common and distressing symptoms. As with pain, the management of nausea may be optimized by regular dosing and often requires multiple medications targeting the four major inputs to the vomiting center (see Chapter 15).

Vomiting associated with opioids is discussed below. Nasogastric suction may provide rapid, short-term relief for vomiting associated with constipation (in addition to laxatives), gastroparesis, or gastric outlet or bowel obstruction. Prokinetic agents, such as metoclopramide (5–20 mg orally or intravenously four times a day), can be helpful in the setting of partial gastric outlet obstruction. Transdermal scopolamine (1.5-mg patch every 3 days) can reduce peristalsis and cramping pain, and ranitidine (50 mg intravenously every 6 hours) can reduce gastric secretions. High-dose corticosteroids (eg, dexamethasone, 20 mg orally or intravenously daily in divided doses) can be used in refractory cases of nausea or vomiting or when it is due to bowel obstruction or increased intracranial pressure. Malignant bowel obstruction in people with advanced cancer is a poor prognostic sign and surgery is rarely helpful.

Vomiting due to disturbance of the vestibular apparatus may be treated with anticholinergic and antihistaminic agents (including diphenhydramine, 25 mg orally or intravenously every 8 hours, or scopolamine, 1.5-mg patch every 3 days).

Benzodiazepines (eg, lorazepam, 0.5–1.0 mg given orally every 6–8 hours) can be effective in preventing the *anticipatory* nausea associated with chemotherapy. For emetogenic chemotherapy, therapy includes combinations of 5-HT$_3$-antagonists (eg, ondansetron, granisetron, dolasetron, or palonosetron), neurokinin-1 receptor antagonists (eg, aprepitant, fosaprepitant, or rolapitant), the N-receptor antagonist netupitant combined with palonosetron (NEPA), olanzapine, dexamethasone, and prochlorperazine. In addition to its effect on mood, mirtazepine, 15–45 mg orally nightly, may help with nausea and improve appetite. Finally, dronabinol (2.5–20 mg orally every 4–6 hours) can be helpful in the management of nausea and vomiting. Patients report relief from medical cannabis, especially strains high in tetrahydrocannabinol (THC).

CONSTIPATION

Given the frequent use of opioids, poor dietary intake, physical inactivity, and lack of privacy, constipation is a common problem in seriously ill and dying patients.

Clinicians must inquire about any difficulty with hard or infrequent stools. Constipation is an easily preventable and treatable cause of discomfort, distress, and nausea and vomiting (see Chapter 15).

Constipation may be prevented or relieved if patients can increase their activity and their intake of fluids. Simple considerations, such as privacy, undisturbed toilet time, and a bedside commode rather than a bedpan may be important for some patients.

A prophylactic bowel regimen with a stimulant laxative (senna or bisacodyl) should be started when opioid treatment is begun. Table 15–4 lists other agents (including osmotic laxatives such as polyethylene glycol) that can be added as needed. Docusate, a stool softener, is not recommended because it does not add benefit beyond stimulant laxatives in well-hydrated patients. Naloxegol, an oral peripherally acting receptor antagonist, and lubiprostone are FDA approved to treat opioid-induced constipation in patients with chronic noncancer pain. Methylnaltrexone, a subcutaneous medication, is a peripherally acting mu-receptor antagonist and is available for severe, unrelieved, opioid-induced constipation. Patients who report being constipated and then have diarrhea typically are passing liquid stool around impacted stool.

FATIGUE

Fatigue is a distressing symptom and is the most common complaint among people with cancer. Specific abnormalities that can contribute to fatigue, including anemia, hypothyroidism, hypogonadism, cognitive and functional impairment, and malnutrition, should be corrected. Because pain, depression, and fatigue often coexist in patients with cancer, pain and depression should be managed appropriately in patients with fatigue. Fatigue from medication adverse effects and polypharmacy is common and should be addressed. For nonspecific fatigue, exercise and physical rehabilitation may be most effective. Although commonly used, strong evidence for psychostimulants, such as methylphenidate, 5–10 mg orally in the morning and afternoon, or modafinil, 200 mg orally in the morning, for cancer-related fatigue is lacking. American Ginseng (*Panax quinquefolius*) has been shown to be effective for cancer-related fatigue but may have an estrogenic effect. Corticosteroids may have a short-term benefit. Caffeinated beverages can help.

DELIRIUM & AGITATION

Many patients die in a state of delirium—a waxing and waning in level of consciousness and a change in cognition that develops over a short time and is manifested by misinterpretations, illusions, hallucinations, sleep-wake cycle disruptions, psychomotor disturbances (eg, lethargy, restlessness), and mood disturbances (eg, fear, anxiety). Delirium may be hyperactive, hypoactive, or mixed. Agitated delirium at the end of life has been called **terminal restlessness.**

Some delirious patients may appear "pleasantly confused," although it is difficult to know what patients experience. In the absence of obvious distress in the patient, a decision by the patient's family and the clinician not to treat delirium may be considered. More commonly, however, agitated delirium at the end of life is distressing to patients and family and requires treatment. Delirium may interfere with the family's ability to interact with or feel comforting to the patient and may prevent a patient from being able to recognize and report important symptoms. Reversible causes of delirium include urinary retention, constipation, anticholinergic medications, and pain; these should be addressed whenever possible. There is no evidence that hydration relieves or dehydration causes delirium. Careful attention to patient safety and nonpharmacologic strategies to help the patient remain oriented (clock, calendar, familiar environment, reassurance and redirection from caregivers) may be sufficient to prevent or manage mild delirium. A randomized trial of placebo compared to risperidone or haloperidol in delirious patients demonstrated increased mortality with neuroleptics. Thus, neuroleptic agents (eg, haloperidol, 1–10 mg orally, subcutaneously, intramuscularly, or intravenously twice or three times a day, or risperidone, 1–3 mg orally twice a day) should generally be avoided and used cautiously, if at all, for agitated delirium at the very end of life. When delirium is refractory to treatment and remains intolerable, sedation may be required to provide relief.

Agar M. Medicinal cannabinoids in palliative care. Br J Clin Pharmacol. 2018 Nov;84(11):2491–4. [PMID: 29923616]

Agar MR et al. Efficacy of oral risperidone, haloperidol, or placebo for symptoms of delirium among patients in palliative care: a randomized clinical trial. JAMA Intern Med. 2017 Jan 1; 177(1):34–42. [PMID: 27918778]

Hui D et al. Effect of lorazepam with haloperidol vs haloperidol alone on agitated delirium in patients with advanced cancer receiving palliative care: a randomized clinical trial. JAMA. 2017 Sep 19;318(11):1047–56. [PMID: 28975307]

Mitchell GK et al. The effect of methylphenidate on fatigue in advanced cancer: an aggregated N-of-1 trial. J Pain Symptom Manage. 2015 Sep;50(3):289–96. [PMID: 25896104]

Singer AE et al. Symptom trends in the last year of life from 1998 to 2010: a cohort study. Ann Intern Med. 2015 Feb 3; 162(3):175–83. [PMID: 25643305]

CARE OF PATIENTS AT THE END OF LIFE

In the United States, nearly 2.5 million people die each year. Caring for patients at the end of life is an important responsibility and a rewarding opportunity for clinicians. From the medical perspective, the end of life may be defined as that time when death—whether due to terminal illness or acute or chronic illness—is expected within hours to months and can no longer be reasonably forestalled by medical intervention. Palliative care at the end of life focuses on relieving distressing symptoms and promoting quality of life (as in all other stages of illness). For patients at the end of life, palliative care may become the sole focus of care.

Emanuel EJ. The status of end-of-life care in the United States: the glass is half full. JAMA. 2018 Jul 17;320(3):239–41. [PMID: 30027232]

Razmaria AA. JAMA patient page. End-of-life care. JAMA. 2016 Jul 5;316(1):115. [PMID: 27380364]

Prognosis at the End of Life

Clinicians must help patients understand when they are approaching the end of life. Most patients, and their family caregivers, want accurate prognostic information. This information influences patients' treatment decisions, may change how they spend their remaining time, and does not negatively impact patient survival. One-half or more of cancer patients do not understand that many treatments they might be offered are palliative and not curative.

While certain diseases, such as cancer, are more amenable to prognostic estimates regarding the time course to death, the other common causes of mortality—including heart disease, stroke, chronic lung disease, and dementia—have more variable trajectories and difficult-to-predict prognoses. Even for patients with cancer, clinician estimates of prognosis are often inaccurate and generally overly optimistic. The advent of new anticancer treatments including immunotherapy and targeted therapies has made prognosis more challenging in some cancers. Nonetheless, clinical experience, epidemiologic data, guidelines from professional organizations, and computer modeling and prediction tools (eg, the Palliative Performance Scale or http://eprognosis.ucsf.edu/index.php) may be used to help offer patients more realistic estimates of prognosis. Clinicians can also ask themselves "Would I be surprised if this patient died in the next year?" to determine whether a discussion of prognosis would be appropriate. If the answer is "no," then the clinician should initiate a discussion. Recognizing that patients may have different levels of comfort with prognostic information, clinicians can introduce the topic by simply saying, "I have information about the likely time course of your illness. Would you like to talk about it?"

Liu Y et al. The application of the palliative prognostic index in predicting the life expectancy of patients in palliative care: a systematic review and meta-analysis. Aging Clin Exp Res. 2018 Dec;30(12):1417–28. [PMID: 29572610]

White DB et al. Prevalence of and factors related to discordance about prognosis between physicians and surrogate decision makers of critically ill patients. JAMA. 2016 May 17; 315(19):2086–94. [PMID: 27187301]

Expectations About the End of Life

Death is often regarded by clinicians, patients, and families as a failure of medical science. This attitude can create or heighten a sense of guilt about the failure to prevent dying. Both the general public and clinicians often view death as an enemy to be battled furiously in hospitals rather than as an inevitable outcome to be experienced as a part of life at home. As a result, most people in the United States die in hospitals or long-term care facilities, but over time there is a trend of fewer deaths in hospitals and more deaths at home or in other community settings.

Even when the clinician and patient continue to pursue cure of potentially reversible disease, relieving suffering, providing support, and helping the patient make the most of their life should be foremost considerations. Patients at the end of life and their families identify a number of elements as important to quality end-of-life care: managing pain and other symptoms adequately, avoiding inappropriate prolongation of dying, communicating clearly, preserving dignity, preparing for death, achieving a sense of control, relieving the burden on others, and strengthening relationships with loved ones.

Keating NL et al. Factors contributing to geographic variation in end-of-life expenditures for cancer patients. Health Aff (Millwood). 2018 Jul;37(7):1136–43. [PMID: 29985699]

Teno JM et al. Site of death, place of care, and health care transitions among US Medicare beneficiaries, 2000–2015. JAMA. 2018 Jul 17;320(3):264–71. [PMID: 29946682]

▶ Communication & Care of the Patient

Caring for patients at the end of life requires the same skills clinicians use in other tasks of medical care: diagnosing treatable conditions, providing patient education, facilitating decision making, and expressing understanding and caring. Communication skills are vitally important and can be improved through training. Higher-quality communication is associated with greater satisfaction and awareness of patient wishes. Clinicians must become proficient at delivering serious news and then dealing with its consequences (Table 5–1). Smartphone and Internet communication resources are available to support clinicians (www.vitaltalk.org), and evidence suggests that communication checklists and guides can be effective. When the clinician and patient do not share a common language, the use of a professional interpreter is needed to facilitate clear communication and help broker cultural issues.

Three further obligations are central to the clinician's role at this time. First, he or she must work to identify, understand, and relieve physical, psychological, social, and spiritual distress or suffering. Second, clinicians can serve as facilitators or catalysts for hope. While hope for a particular outcome such as cure may fade, it can be refocused on what is *still* possible. Although a patient may hope for a "miracle," other more likely hopes can be encouraged and supported, including hope for relief of pain, for reconciliation with loved ones, for discovery of meaning, and for spiritual growth. With such questions as "What is still possible now for you?" and "When you look to the future, what do you hope for?" clinicians can help patients uncover hope, explore meaningful and realistic goals, and develop strategies to achieve them.

Table 5–1. Suggestions for the delivery of serious news.

Prepare an appropriate place and time.
Address basic information needs.
Be direct; avoid jargon and euphemisms.
Allow for silence and emotional ventilation.
Assess and validate patient reactions.
Respond to immediate discomforts and risks.
Listen actively and express empathy.
Achieve a common perception of the problem.
Reassure about pain relief.
Ensure follow-up and make specific plans for the future.

Finally, dying patients' feelings of isolation and fear demand that clinicians assert that they will care for the patient throughout the final stage of life. The promise of *nonabandonment* is the central principle of end-of-life care and is a clinician's pledge to serve as a caring partner, a resource for creative problem solving and relief of suffering, a guide during uncertain times, and a witness to the patient's experiences—no matter what happens. Clinicians can say to a patient, "I will care for you whatever happens."

Rodenbach RA et al. Promoting end-of-life discussions in advanced cancer: effects of patient coaching and question prompt lists. J Clin Oncol. 2017 Mar 10;35(8):842–51. [PMID: 28135140]

▶ Caring for the Family

Clinicians must be attuned to the potential impact of illness on the patient's family: greater physical caregiving responsibilities and financial burdens as well as higher rates of anxiety, depression, chronic illness, and even mortality. The threatened loss of a loved one may create or reveal dysfunctional or painful family dynamics. Family caregivers, typically women, commonly provide the bulk of care for patients at the end of life, yet their work is often not acknowledged, supported, or compensated. Clinicians should recognize that patients and their families are the unit of care. Simply acknowledging and praising the caregiver can provide much needed and appreciated support.

Clinicians can help families confront the imminent loss of a loved one (Table 5–2) and often must negotiate amid complex and changing family needs. Identifying a spokesperson for the family, conducting family meetings, allowing all to be heard, and providing time for consensus may

Table 5–2. Clinician interventions helpful to families of dying patients.

Excellent communication, including clinician willingness to talk about death, to supply timely and clear information, to give proactive guidance, to listen, and to provide empathic responses

Advance care planning and clear decision making, including ensuring culturally sensitive communication, and achieving consensus among family members and an understanding that surrogate decision makers are trying to determine what the *patient* would have wanted, not what the surrogate would want

Support for home care, including orienting family members to the scope and details of family caregiving, providing clear direction about how to contact professional caregivers, and informing patients and families of the benefits of hospice care

Empathy for family emotions and relationships, including recognizing and validating common positive and negative feelings

Attention to grief and bereavement, including support for anticipatory grief and follow-up with the family after the patient's death

Data from Rabow MW et al. Supporting family caregivers at the end of life: "they don't know what they don't know." JAMA. 2004 Jan 28; 291(4):483–91.

help the clinician work effectively with the family. Providing good palliative care to the patient can reduce the risk of depression and complicated grief in loved ones after the patient's death. Palliative care support directly for caregivers improves caregiver depression.

Dionne-Odom JN et al. Benefits of early versus delayed palliative care to informal family caregivers of patients with advanced cancer: outcomes from the ENABLE III randomized controlled trial. J Clin Oncol. 2015 May 1;33(13):1446–52. [PMID: 25800762]

Wright AA et al. Family perspectives on aggressive cancer care near the end of life. JAMA. 2016 Jan 19;315(3):284–92. [PMID: 26784776]

▶ Clinician Self-Care

Many clinicians find caring for patients at the end of life to be one of the most rewarding aspects of practice. However, working with the dying is also sad and can invoke feelings of grief and loss in clinicians. Clinicians must be able to tolerate its uncertainty, ambiguity, and existential challenges. Clinicians also need to recognize and respect their own limitations and attend to their own needs in order to avoid being overburdened, overly distressed, or emotionally depleted.

Back AL et al. Building resilience for palliative care clinicians: an approach to burnout prevention based on individual skills and workplace factors. J Pain Symptom Manage. 2016 Aug; 52(2):284–91. [PMID: 26921494]

Kamal AH et al. Prevalence and predictors of burnout among hospice and palliative care clinicians in the U.S. J Pain Symptom Manage. 2016 Apr;51(4):690–6. [PMID: 26620234]

▶ Decision Making, Advance Care Planning, & Advance Directives

The idea that patients must choose between quality and quantity of life is an outmoded concept that presents patients with a false choice. Clinicians should discuss with patients that an approach that provides concurrent palliative and disease-focused care is the one most likely to achieve improvements in both quality *and* quantity of life. Patients deserve to have their health care be consistent with their values, preferences, and goals of care. Unfortunately, some evidence suggests that end-of-life care for some patients is determined more by local availability of services and physician comfort than by patient wishes. Well-informed, competent adults have a right to refuse life-sustaining interventions even if this would result in death. In order to promote patient autonomy, clinicians are obligated to inform patients about the risks, benefits, alternatives, and expected outcomes of medical interventions, such as cardiopulmonary resuscitation (CPR), mechanical ventilation, hospitalization and ICU care, and artificial nutrition and hydration. **Advance directives** are oral or written statements made by patients when they are competent that project their autonomy into the future and are intended to guide care should they lose the ability to make and communicate their own decisions. Advance directives are an important part of **advance care planning**—defined by an international Delphi panel as "a process that supports adults at any age or stage of

health in understanding and sharing their personal values, life goals, and preferences regarding future medical care. The goal of advance care planning is to help ensure that people receive medical care that is consistent with their values, goals and preferences during serious and chronic illness." Advance directives take effect when the patient can no longer communicate his or her preferences directly. While oral statements about these matters are ethically binding, they are not legally binding in all states. State-specific advance directive forms are available from a number of sources, including http://www.caringinfo.org.

Clinicians should facilitate the process for all patients—ideally, well before the end of life—to consider their preferences, to appoint a surrogate, to talk to that person about their preferences, and to complete a formal advance directive. Most patients with a serious illness have already thought about end-of-life issues, want to discuss them with their clinician, want the clinician to bring up the subject, and feel better for having had the discussion. Patients who have such discussions with their clinicians are more satisfied with their clinician, perceived by their family as having a better quality of life at the end of life, less likely to die in the hospital, and more likely to utilize hospice care. The loved ones of patients who engage in advance care planning discussions are less likely to suffer from depression during bereavement. In the United States, Medicare provides payment to clinicians for having advance care planning discussions with patients.

One type of advance directive is the **Durable Power of Attorney for Health Care (DPOA-HC)** that allows the patient to designate a surrogate decision maker. The DPOA-HC is particularly useful because it is often difficult to anticipate what specific decisions will need to be made. The responsibility of the surrogate is to provide "substituted judgment"—to decide as the *patient* would, not as the *surrogate* wants. Clinicians should encourage patients to talk with their surrogates about their preferences generally and about scenarios that are likely to arise, such as the need for mechanical ventilation in a patient with end-stage emphysema. Clear clinician communication is important to correct misunderstandings and address biases. In the absence of a designated surrogate, clinicians usually turn to family members or next of kin. Regulations require health care institutions to inform patients of their rights to formulate an advance directive. **Physician (or Medical) Orders for Life-Sustaining Treatment (POLST or MOLST) or Physician (or Medical) Orders for Scope of Treatment (POST or MOST)** forms are clinician orders that document patient preferences and accompany patients wherever they are cared for—home, hospital, or nursing home. They are available in most states and used to complement advance directives for patients approaching the end of life.

Bischoff KE et al. Care planning for inpatients referred for palliative care consultation. JAMA Intern Med. 2018 Jan 1; 178(1):48–54. [PMID: 29159371]

Dixon J et al. The effectiveness of advance care planning in improving end-of-life outcomes for people with dementia and their carers: a systematic review and critical discussion. J Pain Symptom Manage. 2018 Jan;55(1):132–50.e1. [PMID: 28827062]

Hanson LC et al. Effect of the goals of care intervention for advanced dementia: a randomized clinical trial. JAMA Intern Med. 2017 Jan 1;177(1):24–31. [PMID: 27893884]

Sudore RL et al. Defining advance care planning for adults: a consensus definition from a multidisciplinary Delphi panel. J Pain Symptom Manage. 2017 May;53(5):821–32.e1. [PMID: 28062339]

Sudore RL et al. Engaging diverse English- and Spanish-speaking older adults in advance care planning: the PREPARE randomized clinical trial. JAMA Intern Med. 2018 Dec 1; 178(12):1616–25. [PMID: 30383086]

► Do Not Attempt Resuscitation Orders

Because the "default" in US hospitals is that patients will undergo CPR in the event of cardiopulmonary arrest, as part of advance care planning, clinicians should elicit patient preferences about CPR. Most patients and many clinicians overestimate the chances of success of CPR. Only about 17% of all patients who undergo CPR in the hospital survive to hospital discharge and, among people with multisystem organ failure, metastatic cancer, and sepsis, the likelihood of survival to hospital discharge following CPR is virtually nil. Patients may ask their clinician to write an order that CPR not be attempted on them. Although this order initially was referred to as a **"DNR" (do not resuscitate)** order, many clinicians prefer the term **"DNAR" (do not attempt resuscitation)** to emphasize the low likelihood of success. Some clinicians and institutions use an order to "Allow Natural Death" for situations in which death is imminent and the patient wishes to receive only those interventions that will promote comfort.

For most patients at the end of life, decisions about CPR may not be about *whether* they will live but about *how* they will die. Clinicians should correct the misconception that withholding CPR in appropriate circumstances is tantamount to "not doing everything" or "just letting someone die." While respecting the patient's right ultimately to make the decision—and keeping in mind their own biases and prejudices—clinicians should offer explicit recommendations about DNAR orders and protect dying patients and their families from feelings of guilt and from the sorrow associated with vain hopes. Clinicians should discuss what interventions will be continued and started to promote quality of life rather than focusing only on what is *not* to be done. For patients with implantable cardioverter defibrillators (ICDs), clinicians must also address issues of turning off these devices, while leaving the pacemaker function on, as death approaches to prevent the uncommon but distressing situation of the ICD discharging during the dying process.

► Hospice & Other Palliative Care Services

In the United States, hospice is a specific type of palliative care service that comprehensively addresses the needs of the dying, focusing on their comfort while not attempting to prolong their life or hasten their death. In the United States, about 45% of people who die use hospice, and about 78% of hospice patients die at home or in a nursing home where they can be cared for by their family, other caregivers, and visiting hospice staff. Hospice care can also be provided in institutional residences and hospitals. As is true of all types of palliative care, hospice emphasizes individualized attention and human contact, and uses an interdisciplinary team approach. Hospice care can include arranging for respite for family caregivers and assisting with referrals for legal, financial, and other services. Patients in hospice require a physician, preferably their primary care clinician or specialist, to oversee their care.

Hospice care was used by 1.43 million Medicare beneficiaries in 2016 (the most recent year for which there are published data), a plurality of whom had cancer, is rated highly by families and has been shown to increase patient satisfaction and to decrease family caregiver mortality. In 2016, 45% of hospice patients died at home; 33% died in a nursing home. Despite evidence that suggests that hospice care does not shorten, and may even extend, length of life, hospice care tends to be used very late, often near the very end of life. In 2016, the mean average length of stay in hospice care in the United States was 71 days, but the median length of stay was 24 days, and 28% of patients died within 7 days of starting hospice services.

In the United States, most hospice organizations require clinicians to estimate the patient's prognosis to be less than 6 months, since this is a criterion for eligibility under the Medicare hospice benefit that is typically the same for other insurance coverage.

► Cultural Issues

The individual patient's experience of dying occurs in the context of a complex interaction of personal, philosophic, and cultural values. Various religious, ethnic, gender, class, and cultural traditions influence a patient's style of communication, comfort in discussing particular topics, expectations about dying and medical interventions, and attitudes about the appropriate disposition of dead bodies. While there are differences in beliefs regarding advance directives, autopsy, organ donation, hospice care, and withdrawal of life-sustaining interventions among patients of different ethnic groups, clinicians should be careful not to make assumptions about individual patients. Clinicians must appreciate that palliative care is susceptible to the same explicit and implicit biases documented in other medical disciplines. Being sensitive to a person's cultural beliefs and respecting traditions are important responsibilities of the clinician caring for a patient at the end of life. A clinician may ask a patient, "What do I need to know about you and your beliefs that will help me take care of you?" and "How do you deal with these issues in your family?"

► Nutrition & Hydration

People approaching the end of life often lose their appetite and most stop eating and drinking in their last days. Clinicians should explain to families that the dying patient is not suffering from hunger or thirst; rather, the discontinuation of eating and drinking is part of dying. The anorexia-cachexia syndrome frequently occurs in patients with advanced cancer, and cachexia is common and a poor prognostic sign in patients with heart failure. Seriously ill people often have no hunger despite not eating at all and the associated ketonemia can produce a sense of well-being, analgesia, and mild euphoria. Although it is unclear to what extent withholding hydration at the end of life creates an uncomfortable sensation of thirst, any such sensation is usually relieved by simply moistening the dry mouth. Ice chips, hard candy, swabs, popsicles, or minted mouthwash may be effective. Although this normal process of diminishing oral intake and accompanying weight loss is very common, it can be distressing to patients and families who may associate the offering of food with compassion and love and lack of eating with distressing images of starvation. In response, patients and families often ask about supplemental enteral or parenteral nutrition.

Supplemental artificial nutrition and hydration offer no benefit to those at the end of life and rarely achieve patient and family goals. The American Geriatrics Society recommends against liquid artificial nutrition ("tube feeding") in people with advanced dementia because it does not provide any benefit. Furthermore, enteral feeding may cause nausea and vomiting in ill patients and can lead to diarrhea in the setting of malabsorption. Artificial nutrition and hydration may increase oral and airway secretions as well as increase the risk of choking, aspiration, and dyspnea; ascites, edema, and effusions may be worsened. In addition, liquid artificial nutrition by nasogastric and gastrostomy tubes and parenteral nutrition impose risks of infection, epistaxis, pneumothorax, electrolyte imbalance, and aspiration—as well as the need to physically restrain the delirious patient to prevent dislodgment of tubes and catheters. A randomized trial of intravenous fluids similarly found no benefit.

Individuals at the end of life have a right to voluntarily refuse all nutrition and hydration. Because they may have deep social and cultural significance for patients, families, and clinicians themselves, decisions about artificial nutrition and hydration are not simply medical. Eliciting perceived goals of artificial nutrition and hydration and correcting misperceptions can help patients and families make clear decisions.

Flaschner E et al. American Geriatrics Society Position Statement on feeding tubes in advanced dementia. J Am Geriatr Soc. 2015;63(7):1490–1. [PMID: 26189864]

▶ Withdrawal of Curative Efforts

Requests from appropriately informed and competent patients or their surrogates for withdrawal of life-sustaining interventions must be respected. Limitation of life-sustaining interventions prior to death is common practice in ICUs. The withdrawal of life-sustaining interventions, such as mechanical ventilation, must be approached carefully to avoid patient suffering and distress for those in attendance. Clinicians should educate the patient and family about the expected course of events and the difficulty of determining the precise timing of death after withdrawal of interventions. Sedative and analgesic agents should be administered to ensure patient comfort even at the risk of respiratory depression or hypotension. While "death rattle," the sound of air flowing over airway secretions, is common

in actively dying patients and can be distressing to families, it is doubtful that it causes discomfort to the patient. Turning the patient can decrease the sound of death rattle. There is no evidence that any medications reduce death rattle, and suctioning should be avoided as it can cause patient discomfort.

▶ Physician-Assisted Death

Physician-assisted death is the legally sanctioned process by which patients who have a terminal illness may request and receive a prescription from a physician for a lethal dose of medication that they themselves would self-administer for the purpose of ending their own life. Terminology for this practice varies. "Physician-assisted death" is used here to clarify that a willing physician provides assistance in accordance with the law (by writing a prescription for a lethal medication) to a patient who makes a request for it and who meets specific criteria. Patients, family members, nonmedical and medical organizations, clinicians, lawmakers, and the public frequently use other terms, namely, "physician or medical aid in dying," "aid in dying," "death with dignity," "compassionate death," or "physician-assisted suicide." This latter term is not preferred because when this action is taken according to the law, it is not considered suicide and people who are actively suicidal are not eligible for this process.

Although public and state support for physician-assisted death has grown in the United States, physician-assisted death remains an area of active and intense debate. To date, no state court has recognized physician-assisted death as a fundamental "right." As of 2018, physician-assisted death has been legalized with careful restriction and specific procedures for residents in seven US states (Oregon, Washington, Montana, Vermont, Colorado, Hawaii, and California) and in the District of Columbia. Physician-assisted death remains illegal in all other states. Other state legislatures or courts are still considering its legalization while others have rejected it. Internationally, physician-assisted death (and/or euthanasia, the administration a lethal dose of medication by a clinician) is legal in nine countries (the Netherlands, Belgium, Luxembourg, Switzerland, Colombia, Canada, Germany, Japan, and the Australian state of Victoria). There are no universal standards about whether patients who request lethal medication for self-administration require a particular prognosis or about what types and levels of suffering qualify them for it, although the current US state laws permitting it generally require physician certification of a terminal disease with a prognosis of 6 months or less. These laws generally also require the individual to be an adult resident of the state, to be physically capable of self-administering the medication, and to be mentally competent (eg, physician or mental health professional certification that they are capable of making and communicating their own healthcare decisions). Laws in the United States authorizing physician-assisted death distinguish it from euthanasia, which is illegal in the United States.

Most requests for physician-assisted death come from patients with cancer. In the United States, most patients requesting it are male, well-educated, and receiving hospice care. Requests for physician-assisted death are relatively rare. Internationally, less than 5% of deaths are due to either physician-assisted death or euthanasia in locales where one or both of these are legal. In Oregon, the first US state to legalize physician-assisted death, approximately 0.39% of deaths in 2015 resulted from this practice. Patient motivations for physician-assisted death generally revolve around preserving dignity, self-respect, and autonomy (control), and maintaining personal connections at the end of life rather than experiencing intolerable pain or suffering. Notably, despite initial concerns, there has been no evidence of greater use or abuse of physician-assisted death in vulnerable populations compared with the general population. Some patients who have requested medication to self-administer for a physician-assisted death later withdraw their request when provided palliative care interventions.

Each clinician must decide his or her personal approach in caring for patients who ask about physician-assisted death. Regardless of the clinician's personal feelings about the process, the clinician can respond initially by exploring the patient's reasons and concerns that prompted the request (Table 5–3). During the dialog, the clinician should inform the patient about palliative options, including hospice care; access to expert symptom management; and psychological, social, and spiritual support, as needed, and provide reassurance and commitment to address future problems that may arise. For clinicians who object to physician-assisted death on moral or ethical grounds, referral to another clinician may be necessary and may help the patient avoid feeling abandoned. That clinician must be willing to provide the prescription for lethal medication, to care for the patient until death (though it is not necessary to be present at the death), to sign the death certificate listing the underlying terminal condition as the cause of death, and in some jurisdictions to complete a mandatory follow-up form.

Table 5–3. Exploring inquiries about physician-assisted death.

Patient Concerns	Useful Clinician Questions
Patient is worried about future suffering: "I can see what's going to happen and I don't like it."	• "What are you most worried about?" • "Tell me more about exactly what frightens you." • "What kinds of deaths have you seen in your family?" • "How are you hoping I can help you?"
Patient feels quality of life is intolerable: "I've suffered enough."	• "What makes your situation most intolerable right now?" • "Tell me more about the worst part." • "How do you think your family feels or would feel about your wish to end your own life?" • "Exactly how are you hoping I can help you?"

Blanke C et al. Characterizing 18 years of the Death With Dignity Act in Oregon. JAMA Oncol. 2017 Oct 1;3(10):1403–6. [PMID: 28384683]

Emanuel EJ et al. Attitudes and practices of euthanasia and physician-assisted suicide in the United States, Canada, and Europe. JAMA. 2016 Jul 5;316(1):79–90. [PMID: 27380345]

Gostin LO et al. Physician-assisted dying: a turning point? JAMA. 2016 Jan 19;315(3):249–50. [PMID: 26784764]

Quill TE et al. Responding to patients requesting physician-assisted death: physician involvement at the very end of life. JAMA. 2016 Jan 19;315(3):245–6. [PMID: 26784762]

► Ethical & Legal Issues

Clinicians' care of patients at the end of life is guided by the same ethical and legal principles that inform other types of medical care. Foremost among these are (1) truthtelling, (2) nonmaleficence, (3) beneficence, (4) autonomy, (5) confidentiality, and (6) procedural and distributive justice. Important ethical principles may come into conflict when caring for patients. For example, many treatments that promote beneficence and autonomy, such as surgery or bone marrow transplant, may violate the clinician's obligation for nonmaleficence; thus, balancing the benefits and risks of treatments is a fundamental ethical responsibility. Similarly, while a patient may express his or her autonomy as a desire for a particular medical intervention such as CPR in the setting of multisystem organ failure, the clinician may decline to provide the intervention because it is futile (ie, of no therapeutic benefit and thus violates both beneficence and nonmaleficence). However, clinicians must use caution in invoking futility, since strict futility is rare and what constitutes futility is often a matter of controversy and subject to bias. While in the vast majority of cases clinicians and patients and families will agree on the appropriateness of and decisions to withdraw life-sustaining interventions, in rare cases, such as CPR in multisystem organ failure, clinicians may determine *unilaterally* that a particular intervention is medically inappropriate. In such cases, the clinician's intention to withhold CPR should be communicated to the patient and family and documented, and the clinician must consult with another clinician not involved in the care of the patient. If differences of opinion persist about the appropriateness of particular care decisions, the assistance of an institutional ethics committee should be sought. Because such unilateral actions violate the autonomy of the patient, clinicians should rarely resort to such unilateral actions. Studies confirm that most disagreements between patients and families and clinicians can be resolved with good communication. Although clinicians and family members often feel differently about withholding versus withdrawing life-sustaining interventions, there is consensus among ethicists, supported by legal precedent, of their ethical equivalence.

The ethical principle of **"double effect"** argues that the potential to hasten imminent death is acceptable if it comes as the known but unintended consequence of a primary intention to provide comfort and relieve suffering. For example, it is acceptable to provide high doses of opioids if needed to control pain even if there is the known and unintended effect of depressing respiration.

Rodrigues P et al. Palliative sedation for existential suffering: a systematic review of argument-based ethics literature. J Pain Symptom Manage. 2018 Jun;55(6):1577–90. [PMID: 29382541]

Psychological, Social, & Spiritual Issues

Dying is not exclusively or even primarily a biomedical event. It is an intimate personal experience with profound psychological, interpersonal, and existential meanings. For many people at the end of life, the prospect of impending death stimulates a deep and urgent assessment of their identity, the quality of their relationships, the meaning and purpose of their life, and their legacy.

A. Psychological Challenges

In 1969, Dr. Elisabeth Kübler-Ross identified five psychological reactions or patterns of emotions that patients at the end of life may experience: denial and isolation, anger, bargaining, depression, and acceptance. Most patients will experience these reactions throughout the course of illness and not in an orderly progression. In addition to these five reactions are the perpetual challenges of anxiety and fear of the unknown. Simple information, listening, assurance, and support may help patients with these psychological challenges. In fact, patients and families rank emotional support as one of the most important aspects of good end-of-life care. Psychotherapy and group support may be beneficial as well.

Despite the significant emotional stress of facing death, clinical depression is *not* normal at the end of life and should be treated. Cognitive and affective signs of depression, such as feelings of worthlessness, hopelessness, or helplessness, may help distinguish depression from the low energy and other vegetative signs common with advanced illness. Although traditional antidepressant treatments such as selective serotonin reuptake inhibitors are effective, more rapidly acting medications, such as dextroamphetamine (2.5–7.5 mg orally at 8 AM and noon) or methylphenidate (2.5–10 mg orally at 8 AM and noon), may be particularly useful when the end of life is near or while waiting for another antidepressant medication to take effect. Oral ketamine and psychedelics are being explored as rapid-onset treatment for anxiety and depression at the end of life. Some research suggests a mortality benefit from treating depression in the setting of serious illness.

B. Social Challenges

At the end of life, patients should be encouraged to take care of personal, professional, and business obligations. These tasks include completing important work or personal projects, distributing possessions, writing a will, and making funeral and burial arrangements. The prospect of death often prompts patients to examine the quality of their interpersonal relationships and to begin the process of saying goodbye (Table 5–4). Concern about estranged relationships or "unfinished business" with significant others and interest in reconciliation may become paramount at this time.

Table 5–4. Five statements often necessary for the completion of important interpersonal relationships.

1. "Forgive me."	(An expression of regret)
2. "I forgive you."	(An expression of acceptance)
3. "Thank you."	(An expression of gratitude)
4. "I love you."	(An expression of affection)
5. "Goodbye."	(Leave-taking)

Source: Byock I. *Dying Well: Peace and Possibilities at the End of Life.* New York: Riverhead Books, an imprint of Penguin Group (USA) LLC, 1997.

C. Spiritual Challenges

Spirituality includes the attempt to understand or accept the underlying meaning of life, one's relationships to oneself and other people, one's place in the universe, one's legacy, and the possibility of a "higher power" in the universe. People may experience spirituality as part of or distinct from particular religious practices or beliefs.

Unlike physical ailments, such as infections and fractures, which usually require a clinician's intervention to be treated, the patient's spiritual concerns often require only a clinician's attention, listening, and witness. Clinicians can inquire about the patient's spiritual concerns and ask whether the patient wishes to discuss them. For example, asking, "How are you within yourself?" or "Are you at peace?" communicates that the clinician is interested in the patient's whole experience and provides an opportunity for the patient to share perceptions about his or her inner life. Questions that might constitute an existential "review of systems" are presented in Table 5–5. Formal legacy work and dignity therapy have been shown to be effective in improving quality of life and spiritual well-being.

Attending to the spiritual concerns of patients calls for listening to their stories. Storytelling gives patients the opportunity to verbalize what is meaningful to them and to

Table 5–5. An existential review of systems.

Intrapersonal
"What does your illness/dying mean to you?"
"What do you think caused your illness?"
"How have you been healed in the past?"
"What do you think is needed for you to be healed now?"
"What is right with you now?"
"What do you hope for?"
"Are you at peace?"
Interpersonal
"Who is important to you?"
"To whom does your illness/dying matter?"
"Do you have any unfinished business with significant others?"
Transpersonal
"What is your source of strength, help, or hope?"
"Do you have spiritual concerns or a spiritual practice?"
"If so, how does your spirituality relate to your illness/dying, and how can I help integrate your spirituality into your health care?"
"What do you think happens after we die?"
"What purpose might your illness/dying serve?"
"What do you think is trying to happen here?"

leave something of themselves behind—a legacy, the promise of being remembered. Storytelling may be facilitated by suggesting that the patient share his or her life story with family members, make an audio or video recording, assemble a photo album, organize a scrapbook, or write or dictate an autobiography.

The end of life offers an opportunity for psychological, interpersonal, and spiritual development and to experience and achieve important goals. Individuals may grow—even experience a heightened sense of well-being or transcendence—in the process of dying. Through listening, support, and presence, clinicians may help foster this learning and be a catalyst for this transformation. Rather than thinking of dying simply as the termination of life, clinicians and patients may be guided by a developmental model of life that recognizes a series of lifelong developmental tasks and landmarks and allows for growth at the end of life.

Best M et al. Doctors discussing religion and spirituality: a systematic literature review. Palliat Med. 2016 Apr;30(4):327–37. [PMID: 26269325]

Egan R et al. Spiritual beliefs, practices, and needs at the end of life: results from a New Zealand national hospice study. Palliat Support Care. 2017 Feb; 31(2):140–6. [PMID: 27572901]

Johnson J et al. The impact of faith beliefs on perceptions of end-of-life care and decision making among African American church members. J Palliat Med. 2016 Feb;19(2):143–8. [PMID: 26840849]

Puchalski CM et al. Spiritual considerations. Hematol Oncol Clin North Am. 2018 Jun;32(3):505–17. [PMID: 29729785]

Sun A et al. Efficacy of a church-based, culturally-tailored program to promote completion of advance directives among Asian Americans. J Immigr Minor Health. 2017 Apr;19(2):381–91. [PMID: 27103618]

TASKS AFTER DEATH

After the death of a patient, the clinician is called upon to perform a number of tasks, both required and recommended. The clinician must plainly and directly inform the family of the death, complete a death certificate, contact an organ procurement organization, and request an autopsy. Providing words of sympathy and reassurance, time for questions and initial grief and, for people who die in the hospital or other health care facility, a quiet private room for the family to grieve is appropriate and much appreciated.

► The Pronouncement & Death Certificate

In the United States, state policies direct clinicians to confirm the death of a patient in a formal process called "pronouncement." The diagnosis of death is typically easy to make, and the clinician need only verify the absence of spontaneous respirations and cardiac activity by auscultating for each for 1 minute. Attempting to elicit pain in a patient who has died is unnecessary and disrespectful and should be avoided. A note describing these findings, the time of death, and that the family has been notified is entered in the patient's medical record. In many states, when a patient whose death is expected dies outside of the hospital (at home or in prison, for example), nurses may be authorized to report the death over the telephone to a physician who assumes responsibility for signing the death certificate within 24 hours. For traumatic deaths, some states allow emergency medical technicians to pronounce a patient dead at the scene based on clearly defined criteria and with physician telephonic or radio supervision.

While the pronouncement may often seem like an awkward and unnecessary formality, clinicians may use this time to reassure the patient's loved ones at the bedside that the patient died peacefully and that all appropriate care had been given. Both clinicians and families may use the ritual of the pronouncement as an opportunity to begin to process emotionally the death of the patient.

Physicians are legally required to report certain deaths to the coroner and to accurately report the underlying cause of death on the death certificate. This reporting is important both for patients' families (for insurance purposes and the need for an accurate family medical history) and for the epidemiologic study of disease and public health. The physician should be specific about the major cause of death being the condition without which the patient would not have died (eg, "decompensated cirrhosis") and its contributory cause (eg, "hepatitis B and hepatitis C infections, chronic alcoholic hepatitis, and alcoholism") as well as any associated conditions (eg, "acute kidney injury")—and not simply put down "cardiac arrest" as the cause of death.

► Autopsy & Organ Donation

Discussing the options and obtaining consent for autopsy and organ donation with patients prior to death is a good practice as it advances the principle of patient autonomy and lessens the responsibilities of distressed family members during the period immediately following the death. In the case of brain death, designated organ transplant personnel are more successful than treating clinicians at obtaining consent for organ donation from surviving family members. In the United States, federal regulations require that a designated representative of an organ procurement organization approach the family about organ donation if the organs are appropriate for transplantation. Most people in the United States support the donation of organs for transplants. However, organ transplantation is severely limited by the availability of donor organs. The families of donors experience a sense of reward in contributing, even through death, to the lives of others.

Clinicians must be sensitive to ethnic and cultural differences in attitudes about autopsy and organ donation. Patients or their families should be reminded of their right to limit autopsy or organ donation in any way they choose, although such restriction may limit the utility of autopsy. Pathologists can perform autopsies without interfering with funeral plans or the appearance of the deceased.

The results of an autopsy may help surviving family members and clinicians understand the exact cause of a patient's death and foster a sense of closure. Despite the use of more sophisticated diagnostic tests, the rate of unexpected findings at autopsy has remained stable, and thus, an autopsy can provide important health information to families. A clinician–family conference to review the results of the autopsy provides a good opportunity for clinicians to assess how well families are grieving and to answer questions.

Follow-Up & Grieving

Proper care of patients at the end of life includes following up with surviving family members after the patient has died. Contacting loved ones by telephone enables the clinician to assuage any guilt about decisions the family may have made, assess how families are grieving, reassure them about the nature of normal grieving, and identify complicated grief or depression. Clinicians can recommend support groups and counseling as needed. A card or telephone call from the clinician to the family days to weeks after the patient's death (and perhaps on the anniversary of the death) allows the clinician to express concern for the family and the deceased.

After a patient dies, clinicians also grieve. Although clinicians may be relatively unaffected by the deaths of some patients, other deaths may cause feelings of sadness, loss, and guilt. These emotions should be recognized as the first step toward processing and healing them. Each clinician may find personal or communal resources that help with the process of grieving. Shedding tears, sharing with colleagues, taking time for reflection, and engaging in traditional or personal mourning rituals all may be effective. Attending the funeral of a patient who has died can be a satisfying personal experience that is almost universally appreciated by families and that may be the final element in caring well for people at the end of life.

Morris SE et al. Adding value to palliative care services: the development of an institutional bereavement program. J Palliat Med. 2015 Nov;18(11):915–22. [PMID: 26275079]

PAIN MANAGEMENT

TAXONOMY OF PAIN

The International Association for the Study of Pain (IASP) defines **pain** as an unpleasant sensory and emotional experience associated with actual or potential tissue damage, or described in terms of such damage. **Acute pain** resolves within the expected period of healing and is self-limited. **Chronic pain** persists beyond the expected period of healing and is itself a disease state. In general, chronic pain is defined as extending beyond 3–6 months, although definitions vary in terms of the time period from initial onset of nociception. **Cancer pain** is in its own special category because of the unique ways neoplasia and its therapies (such as surgery, chemotherapy, or radiation therapy) can lead to burdensome pain. Finally, related to cancer pain, there is **pain at the end of life**, for which measures to alleviate suffering may take priority over promoting restoration of function.

Pain is a worldwide burden; across the globe, one in five adults suffers from pain. In 2010, members from 130 countries signed the Declaration of Montreal stating that access to pain management is a fundamental human right. The first CDC guidelines on opioid prescribing for chronic pain, including chronic noncancer pain, cancer pain, and pain at the end of life, were published in March of 2016.

Centers for Disease Control and Prevention (CDC). CDC guideline for prescribing opioids for chronic pain. 2017 Aug 29. http://www.cdc.gov/drugoverdose/prescribing/guideline.html

Dowell D et al. CDC guideline for prescribing opioids for chronic pain—United States, 2016. JAMA. 2016 Apr 19; 315(15):1624–45. [PMID: 26977696]

Henschke N et al. The epidemiology and economic consequences of pain. Mayo Clin Proc. 2015 Jan;90(1):139–47. [PMID: 25572198]

Williams AC et al. Updating the definition of pain. Pain. 2016 Nov; 157(11):2420–23. [PMID: 27200490]

ACUTE PAIN

Acute pain resolves within the expected period of healing and is self-limited. Common examples include pain from dental caries, kidney stones, surgery, or trauma. Management of acute pain depends on comprehending the type of pain (somatic, visceral, or neuropathic) and on understanding the risks and benefits of potential therapies. At times, treating the underlying cause of the pain (eg, dental caries) may be all that is needed, and pharmacologic therapies may not be required for additional analgesia. On the other hand, not relieving acute pain can have consequences beyond the immediate suffering. Inadequately treated acute pain can develop into chronic pain in some patients. This transition from acute to chronic pain (so-called "chronification" of pain) depends on the pain's cause, type, and severity and on the patient's age, psychological status, and genetics, among other factors. This transition is an area of increasing study because chronic pain leads to significant societal costs beyond the individual's experiences of suffering, helplessness, and depression. Emerging studies have shown that increased intensity and duration of acute pain may be correlated with a higher incidence of chronic pain, and regional anesthesia, ketamine, gabapentinoids, and cyclooxygenase (COX) inhibitors may be helpful for prevention of chronic postsurgical pain. These approaches are particularly important given concerns that exposure to opioids in the perioperative period can lead to chronic opioid dependence beyond the immediate postoperative period.

The Oxford League Table of Analgesics is a useful guide; for example, it lists the number-needed-to-treat for specific doses of various medications to relieve acute pain. Nonsteroidal anti-inflammatory drugs (NSAIDs) or COX inhibitors are at the top of the list, with the lowest number-needed-to-treat. These medications can be delivered via oral, intramuscular, intravenous, intranasal, rectal, and other routes of administration. They generally work by inhibiting COX-1 and -2 and therefore reduce the levels of prostaglandins involved in inflammatory nociception (eg, PGI2 and PGE2). These oxygenase enzymes also determine levels of other breakdown products such as other prostaglandins, thromboxane, and prostacyclins that play a role in renal, gastrointestinal, and cardiovascular homeostasis. For this reason, the primary limitation of the COX inhibitors is their side effect profile of gastritis, kidney dysfunction, bleeding, hypertension, and cardiovascular adverse events such as myocardial infarction or stroke. Ketorolac is primarily a COX-1 inhibitor that has an analgesic effect as potent as morphine at the appropriate dosage. Like most pharmacologic therapies, the limitation of COX inhibitors is that they have a "ceiling" effect, meaning that beyond a certain dose, there is no additional benefit.

Acetaminophen (paracetamol) is effective as a sole agent, or in combination with a COX inhibitor or an opioid in acute pain. Its mechanism of action remains undetermined but is thought to act centrally through mechanisms such as the prostaglandin, serotonergic, and opioid pathways. It is one of the most widely used and best tolerated analgesics; its primary limitation is hepatoxicity when given in high doses or to patients with underlying impaired liver function.

Postoperatively, **patient-controlled analgesia (PCA)** with intravenous morphine, hydromorphone, or another opioid can achieve analgesia faster and with less daily medication requirement than with standard "as needed" or even scheduled intermittent dosing. PCA has been adapted for use with oral analgesic opioid medications and for neuraxial delivery of both opioids and local anesthetics in the epidural and intrathecal spaces. The goal of PCA is to maintain a patient's plasma concentration of opioid in the "therapeutic window," between the minimum effective analgesic concentration and a toxic dose.

Chou R et al. Management of postoperative pain: a clinical practice guideline from the American Pain Society, the American Society of Regional Anesthesia and Pain Medicine, and the American Society of Anesthesiologists' Committee on Regional Anesthesia, Executive Committee, and Administrative Council. J Pain. 2016 Feb;17(2):131–57. Erratum in: J Pain. 2016 Apr;17(4):508–10. Dosage error in article text. [PMID: 26827847]

Helander EM et al. Multimodal analgesia, current concepts, and acute pain considerations. Curr Pain Headache Rep. 2017 Jan; 21(1):3. [PMID: 28132136]

Koepke EJ et al. The rising tide of opioid use and abuse: the role of the anesthesiologist. Perioper Med (Lond). 2018 Jul 3;7:16. [PMID: 29988696]

Pak DJ et al. Chronification of pain: mechanisms, current understanding, and clinical implications. Curr Pain Headache Rep. 2018 Feb 5;22(2):9. [PMID: 29404791]

Polomano RC et al. Multimodal analgesia for acute postoperative and trauma-related pain. Am J Nurs. 2017 Mar; 117(3 Suppl 1):S12–26. [PMID: 28212146]

CHRONIC NONCANCER PAIN

Chronic noncancer pain may begin as acute pain that then fails to resolve and extends beyond the expected period of healing or it may be a primary disease state, rather than the symptom residual from another condition. Common examples of chronic noncancer pain include chronic low-back pain and arthralgias (often somatic in origin), chronic abdominal pain and pelvic pain (often visceral in origin), and chronic headaches, peripheral neuropathy, and postherpetic neuralgia (neuropathic origin) as well as other less common but debilitating syndromes such as chronic trigeminal neuralgia (neuropathic origin) and complex regional pain syndrome (mixed origin). Chronic noncancer pain is common, with the World Health Organization estimating a worldwide prevalence of 20%. In the United States, 11% of adults suffer from chronic noncancer pain, and the

Institute of Medicine estimates that it costs $635 billion annually in treatment and lost productivity costs.

Chronic noncancer pain requires interdisciplinary management. Generally, no one therapy by itself is sufficient to manage such chronic pain. Physical or functional therapy and cognitive behavioral therapy have been shown to be the most effective for treating chronic noncancer pain, but other modalities including pharmacologic therapy, interventional modalities, and complementary/integrative approaches are useful in caring for affected patients.

Chronic low-back pain is one example of a common chronic noncancer pain. It causes more disability globally than any other condition. Chronic low-back pain includes spondylosis, spondylolisthesis, and spinal canal stenosis (Chapter 24), and the "failed back surgical syndrome," a term used to refer to patients in whom chronic pain develops and persists after lumbar spine surgery. Also referred to as the post-laminectomy pain syndrome, it can affect 10–40% of patients after lumbar spine surgery.

The importance of clinicians knowing the many causes of chronic low-back pain and, in particular, understanding how anatomic structures relate to one another and how they can cause the different types of low-back pain, has been highlighted by the epidemic of opioid abuse in the United States since the year 2000. In fact, current evidence-based practice does *not* support the use of prolonged opioid therapy for chronic low-back pain.

Ashburn MA et al. Increasing evidence for the limited role of opioids to treat chronic noncancer pain. JAMA. 2018 Dec 18; 320(23):2427–28. [PMID: 30561463]

Beal BR et al. An overview of pharmacologic management of chronic pain. Med Clin North Am. 2016 Jan;100(1):65–79. [PMID: 26614720]

Busse JW et al. Opioids for chronic noncancer pain: a systematic review and meta-analysis. JAMA. 2018 Dec 18;320(23): 2448–60. [PMID: 30561481]

Centers for Disease Control and Prevention (CDC). CDC Guidelines for Prescribing Opioids for Chronic Pain. 2017 Aug 29. https://www.cdc.gov/drugoverdose/prescribing/guideline.html

Chapman CR et al. The transition of acute postoperative pain to chronic pain: an integrative overview of research on mechanisms. J Pain. 2017 Apr;18(4):359.e1–38. [PMID: 27908839]

Enthoven WT et al. Non-steroidal anti-inflammatory drugs for chronic low back pain. Cochrane Database Syst Rev. 2016 Feb 10;2:CD012087. [PMID: 26863524]

Manchikanti L et al. Responsible, safe, and effective prescription of opioids for chronic non-cancer pain: American Society of Interventional Pain Physicians (ASIPP) guidelines. Pain Physician. 2017 Feb;20(2S):S3–92. [PMID: 28226332]

Qaseem A et al. Clinical Guidelines Committee of the American College of Physicians. Noninvasive treatments for acute, subacute, and chronic low back pain: a clinical practice guideline from the American College of Physicians. Ann Intern Med. 2017 Apr 4;166(7):514–30. [PMID: 28192789]

Ray WA et al. Prescription of long-acting opioids and mortality in patients with chronic noncancer pain. JAMA. 2016 Jun 14; 315(22):2415–23. [PMID: 27299617]

CANCER PAIN

Cancer pain deserves its own category because it is unique in cause and in therapies. Cancer pain consists of both acute pain and chronic pain from the neoplasm itself and from the therapies associated with it, such as surgery, chemotherapy, radiation, and immunotherapy. In addition, patients with cancer pain may also have acute or chronic non–cancer-related pain, and this possibility should not be overlooked when taking care of cancer patients.

Cancer pain includes somatic pain (eg, neoplastic invasion of tissue such as painful fungating chest wall masses in breast cancer), visceral pain (eg, painful hepatomegaly from liver metastases, stretching the liver capsule), neuropathic pain (eg, neoplastic invasion of sacral nerve roots), or pain from a paraneoplastic syndrome (eg, peripheral neuropathy related to anti-Hu antibody production). Chemotherapy can cause peripheral neuropathies, radiation can cause neuritis or skin allodynia, and surgery can cause persistent postsurgical pain syndromes such as post-mastectomy or post-thoracotomy pain syndromes.

Generally, patients with cancer pain do not exhibit a single type of pain—they may have multiple reasons for pain and thus benefit from a comprehensive and multimodal strategy. The WHO Analgesic Ladder, first published in 1986, suggests starting medication treatment with nonopioid analgesics, then weak opioid agonists, followed by strong opioid agonists. While opioid therapy can be helpful for a majority of patients living with cancer pain, therapy must be individualized depending on the individual patient, their family, and the clinician. For example, if one of the goals of care is to have a lucid and coherent patient, opioids may not be the optimal choice; interventional therapies such as implantable devices may be an option, weighing their risks and costs against their potential benefits. Alternatively, in dying patients, provided there is careful documentation of continued, renewed, or accelerating pain, use of opioid doses exceeding those recommended as standard for acute (postoperative) pain is acceptable.

One of the unique challenges in treating cancer pain is that it is often a "moving target," with disease progression and improvements from chemotherapy, radiation, or immunotherapy. Therefore, frequent adjustments may be required to any pharmacologic regimen. Interventional approaches such as celiac plexus neurolysis and intrathecal therapy are well-studied and may be appropriate both for analgesia as well as reduction of side effects from systemic medications. Radiation therapy (including single-fraction external beam treatments) or radionuclide therapy (eg, strontium-89), which aims to decrease the size of both primary and metastatic disease, is one of the unique options for patients with pain from cancer.

Careskey H et al. Interventional anesthetic methods for pain in hematology/oncology patients. Hematol Oncol Clin North Am. 2018 Jun;32(3):433–45. [PMID: 29729779]

Neufeld NJ et al. Cancer pain: a review of epidemiology, clinical quality and value impact. Future Oncol. 2017 Apr;13(9):833–41. [PMID: 27875910]

Paice JA. Under pressure: the tension between access and abuse of opioids in cancer pain management. J Oncol Pract. 2017 Sep; 13(9):595–6. [PMID: 28813190]

PAIN AT THE END OF LIFE

Pain is what many people say they fear most about dying, and pain at the end of life is consistently undertreated. Up to 75% of patients dying of cancer, heart failure, chronic obstructive pulmonary disease, AIDS, or other diseases experience pain. In the United States, the Joint Commission includes pain management standards in its reviews of health care organizations and, in 2018, it began mandating that each hospital have a designated leader in pain management.

The ratio of risk versus benefit changes in end-of-life pain management. Harms from the use of opioid analgesics, including death, eg, from respiratory depression (rare), are perhaps less of a concern in patients approaching the end of life. In all cases, clinicians must be prepared to use appropriate doses of opioids in order to relieve this distressing symptom for these patients. Typically, for ongoing cancer pain, a long-acting opioid analgesic can be given around the clock with a short-acting opioid medication as needed for "breakthrough" pain.

PRINCIPLES OF PAIN MANAGEMENT

The experience of pain is unique to each person and influenced by many factors, including the patient's prior experiences with pain, meaning given to the pain, emotional stresses, and family and cultural influences. Pain is a subjective and multi-faceted phenomenon, and clinicians cannot reliably detect its existence or quantify its severity without asking the patient directly. A brief means of assessing pain and evaluating the effectiveness of analgesia is to ask the patient to rate the degree of pain along a numeric or visual pain scale (Table 5–6), assessing trends over time. Clinicians should ask about the nature, severity, timing, location, quality, and aggravating and relieving factors of the pain.

General guidelines for diagnosis and management of pain are recommended for the treatment of all patients with pain but clinicians must comprehend that such guidelines may not be suited for every individual. Because of pain's complexity, it is important to understand benefits and risks of treatment with growing evidence for each patient. Distinguishing between nociceptive (somatic or visceral) and neuropathic pain is essential to proper management.

In addition, while clinicians should seek to diagnose the underlying cause of pain and then treat it, they must balance the burden of diagnostic tests or therapeutic interventions with the patient's suffering. For example, single-fraction radiation therapy for painful bone metastases or nerve blocks for neuropathic pain may obviate the need for ongoing treatment with analgesics and their side effects. Regardless of decisions about seeking and treating the underlying cause of pain, every patient should be offered prompt pain relief.

The aim of effective pain management is to meet specific goals, such as preservation or restoration of function or quality of life, and this aim must be discussed between provider and patient, as well as their family. For example, some patients may wish to be completely free of pain even at the cost of significant sedation, while others will wish to control pain to a level that still allows maximal cognitive

Table 5–6. Pain assessment scales.

A. Numeric Rating Scale		
No pain Worst pain 0 1 2 3 4 5 6 7 8 9 10		None, mild, moderate, severe

B. Numeric Rating Scale Translated into Word and Behavior Scales		
Pain Intensity	**Word Scale**	**Nonverbal Behaviors**
0	No pain	Relaxed, calm expression
1–2	Least pain	Stressed, tense expression
3–4	Mild pain	Guarded movement, grimacing
5–6	Moderate pain	Moaning, restlessness
7–8	Severe pain	Crying out
9–10	Excruciating pain	Increased intensity of above

C. Wong-Baker FACES Pain Rating Scale[1]

0	1	2	3	4	5
No hurt	Hurts Little Bit	Hurts Little More	Hurts Even More	Hurts Whole Lot	Hurts Worst

[1]Especially useful for patients who cannot read English (and for pediatric patients).
© 1983 Wong-Baker FACES Foundation. www.WongBakerFACES.org. Used with permission. Originally published in *Whaley & Wong's Nursing Care of Infants and Children* (Mosby Elsevier).

functioning. Therefore, opioids may not be the optimal option for every patient because not all pain is responsive to opioids; additionally, opioids may pose significant risks or side effects (eg, sedation) that the patient finds intolerable.

Whenever possible, the oral route of analgesic administration is preferred because it is easier to manage at home, is not itself painful, and imposes no risk from needle exposure. In unique situations, or near the end of life, transdermal, subcutaneous, rectal, and intravenous routes of administration are used; intrathecal administration is used when necessary.

Finally, pain management should not automatically indicate opioid therapy. While many individuals fare better with opioid therapy in specific situations, this does not mean that opioids are the answer for every patient. There are situations where opioids actually make the quality of life worse for individuals, due to a lack of adequate analgesic effect or due to their side effects.

Barriers to Good Care

One barrier to good pain control is that many clinicians have limited training and clinical experience with pain management and thus are reluctant to attempt to manage severe pain. Lack of knowledge about the proper selection and dosing of analgesic medications carries with it attendant and typically exaggerated fears about the side effects of pain medications, such as the possibility of respiratory depression from opioids. Most clinicians, however, can develop good pain management skills, and nearly all pain, even at the end of life, can be managed without necessarily hastening death through respiratory depression. However, consultation with a palliative care or a pain management specialist may provide additional expertise.

PHARMACOLOGIC PAIN MANAGEMENT STRATEGIES

Pain generally can be well controlled with nonopioid and opioid analgesic medications, complemented by nonpharmacologic adjunctive and interventional treatments. For mild to moderate pain, acetaminophen, aspirin, and NSAIDs (also known as COX inhibitors) may be sufficient. For moderate to severe pain, especially for those with acute pain, short courses of opioids are sometimes necessary; for those with cancer pain or pain from advanced, progressive serious illness, opioids are generally required and interventional modalities should be considered. In all cases, the choice of an analgesic medication must be guided by careful attention to the physiology of the pain and the benefits and risks of the particular analgesic being considered.

Acetaminophen, Aspirin, Celecoxib, & NSAIDs (COX Inhibitors)

Table 5–7 provides comparison information for acetaminophen, aspirin, the COX-2 inhibitor celecoxib and the

Table 5–7. Acetaminophen, aspirin, and useful nonsteroidal anti-inflammatory drugs and COX inhibitors.

Medication (alphabetic order)	Usual Dose for Adults ≥ 50 kg	Usual Dose for Adults < 50 kg[1]	Cost per Unit	Cost for 30 Days[2]	Comments[3]
Acetaminophen (Ofirmev)	1000 mg intravenously every 6–8 hours		$45.02 per vial of 1000 mg	$5402.40	
Acetaminophen or paracetamol[4] (Tylenol, Datril, etc)	325–500 mg orally every 4 hours or 500–1000 mg orally every 6 hours, up to 2000–4000 mg/day	10–15 mg/kg every 4 hours orally; 15–20 mg/kg every 4 hours rectally, up to 2000–3000 mg/day	$0.02/500 mg (oral) OTC; $0.43/650 mg (rectal) OTC	$3.60 (oral); $77.40 (rectal)	Not an NSAID because it lacks peripheral anti-inflammatory effects. Equivalent to aspirin as analgesic and antipyretic agent. Limit dose to 4000 mg/day in acute pain, and to 3000 mg/day in chronic pain. Limit doses to 2000 mg/day in older patients and those with liver disease. Be mindful of multiple sources of acetaminophen as in combination analgesics, cold remedies, and sleep aids.
Aspirin[5]	325–650 mg orally every 4 hours	10–15 mg/kg every 4 hours orally; 15–20 mg/kg every 4 hours rectally	$0.02/325 mg OTC; $1.51/600 mg (rectal) OTC	$7.20 (oral); $271.80 (rectal)	Available also in enteric-coated oral form that is more slowly absorbed but better tolerated.
Celecoxib[4] (Celebrex)	200 mg orally once daily (osteoarthritis); 100–200 mg orally twice daily (RA)	100 mg orally once or twice daily	$4.37/100 mg; $7.58/200 mg	$227.40 OA; $454.80 RA	Cyclooxygenase-2 inhibitor. No antiplatelet effects. Lower doses for elderly who weigh < 50 kg. Lower incidence of endoscopic gastrointestinal ulceration than NSAIDs. Not known if true lower incidence of gastrointestinal bleeding. Celecoxib is contraindicated in sulfonamide allergy.
Choline magnesium salicylate[6] (Trilasate, others)	1000–1500 mg orally three times daily	25 mg/kg orally three times daily	$0.46/500 mg	$124.20	Salicylates cause less gastrointestinal distress and kidney impairment than NSAIDs but are probably less effective in pain management than NSAIDs.
Diclofenac (Flector)	1.3% topical patch applied twice daily		$13.43/patch	$805.80	Apply patch to most painful area.
Diclofenac (Voltaren, Cataflam, others)	50–75 mg orally two or three times daily; 1% gel 2–4 g four times daily		$0.95/50 mg; $1.14/75 mg; $0.52/g gel	$85.50; $102.60; $249.60 gel	May impose higher risk of hepatotoxicity. Enteric-coated product; slow onset. Topical formulations may result in fewer side effects than oral formulations.
Diclofenac sustained release (Voltaren-XR, others)	100–200 mg orally once daily		$2.70/100 mg	$162.00	
Diflunisal[7] (Dolobid, others)	500 mg orally every 12 hours		$2.07/500 mg	$124.20	Fluorinated acetylsalicylic acid derivative.
Etodolac (Lodine, others)	200–400 mg orally every 6–8 hours		$1.32/400 mg	$158.40	
Fenoprofen calcium (Nalfon, others)	300–600 mg orally every 6 hours		$3.40/600 mg	$408.00	Perhaps more side effects than others, including tubulointerstitial nephritis.

(continued)

Table 5–7. Acetaminophen, aspirin, and useful nonsteroidal anti-inflammatory drugs and COX inhibitors. (continued)

Medication (alphabetic order)	Usual Dose for Adults ≥ 50 kg	Usual Dose for Adults < 50 kg[1]	Cost per Unit	Cost for 30 Days[2]	Comments[3]
Flurbiprofen (Ansaid)	50–100 mg orally three or four times daily		$0.78/50 mg; $1.18/100 mg	$93.60; $141.60	Adverse gastrointestinal effects may be more common among elderly.
Ibuprofen (Caldolor)	400–800 mg intravenously every 6 hours		$20.08/800 mg vial	$2410.00	
Ibuprofen (Motrin, Advil, Rufen, others)	400–800 mg orally every 6 hours	10 mg/kg orally every 6–8 hours	$0.28/600 mg Rx; $0.05/200 mg OTC	$33.60; $9.00	Relatively well tolerated and inexpensive.
Indomethacin (Indocin, Indo-meth, others)	25–50 mg orally two to four times daily		$0.38/25 mg; $0.64/50 mg	$45.60; $76.80	Higher incidence of dose-related toxic effects, especially gastrointestinal and bone marrow effects.
Ketoprofen (Orudis, Oruvail, others)	25–75 mg orally every 6–8 hours (max 300 mg/day)		$1.12/50 mg Rx; $1.24/75 mg Rx	$134.40; $148.80	Lower doses for elderly.
Ketorolac tromethamine	10 mg orally every 4–6 hours to a maximum of 40 mg/day orally		$2.16/10 mg	Not recommended	Short-term use (< 5 days) only; otherwise, increased risk of gastrointestinal side effects.
Ketorolac tromethamine[8]	60 mg intramuscularly or 30 mg intravenously initially, then 30 mg every 6 hours intramuscularly or intravenously		$1.45/30 mg	Not recommended	Intramuscular or intravenous NSAID as alternative to opioid. Lower doses for elderly. Short-term use (< 5 days) only.
Magnesium salicylate (various)	325–650 mg orally every 6 hours		$0.25/325 mg OTC	$60.00	
Meclofenamate sodium[9] (Meclomen)	50–100 mg orally every 6 hours		$7.74/100 mg	$928.80	Diarrhea more common.
Mefenamic acid (Ponstel)	250 mg orally every 6 hours		$17.41/250 mg	$2089.20	
Meloxicam (Mobic)	7.5 mg orally every 12 hours		$3.16/7.5 mg	$189.60	Intermediate COX-2/COX-1 ratio similar to diclofenac.
Nabumetone (Relafen)	500–1000 mg orally once daily (max dose 2000 mg/day)		$1.30/500 mg; $1.53/750 mg	$78.00; $91.80	May be less ulcerogenic than ibuprofen, but overall side effects may not be less.
Naproxen (Naprosyn, Anaprox, Aleve [OTC], others)	250–500 mg orally every 6–8 hours	5 mg/kg every 8 hours	$1.29/500 mg Rx; $0.09/220 mg OTC	$154.80; $8.10 OTC	Generally well tolerated. Lower doses for elderly.
Oxaprozin (Daypro, others)	600–1200 mg orally once daily		$1.50/600 mg	$90.00	Similar to ibuprofen. May cause rash, pruritus, photosensitivity.
Piroxicam (Feldene, others)	20 mg orally once daily		$4.39/20 mg	$131.70	Not recommended in the elderly due to high adverse drug reaction rate. Single daily dose convenient. Long half-life. May cause higher rate of gastrointestinal bleeding and dermatologic side effects.

(continued)

Table 5–7. Acetaminophen, aspirin, and useful nonsteroidal anti-inflammatory drugs and COX inhibitors. (continued)

Medication (alphabetic order)	Usual Dose for Adults ≥ 50 kg	Usual Dose for Adults < 50 kg[1]	Cost per Unit	Cost for 30 Days[2]	Comments[3]
Sulindac (Clinoril, others)	150–200 mg orally twice daily		$0.98/150 mg; $1.21/200 mg	$58.80; $72.60	May cause higher rate of gastrointestinal bleeding. May have less nephrotoxic potential.
Tolmetin (Tolectin)	200–600 mg orally four times daily		$0.75/200 mg; $3.98/600 mg	$90.00; $477.60	Perhaps more side effects than others, including anaphylactic reactions.

[1]Acetaminophen and NSAID dosages for adults weighing < 50 kg should be adjusted for weight.
[2]Average wholesale price (AWP, for AB-rated generic when available) for quantity listed. Source: IBM Micromedex Red Book (electronic version) IBM Watson Health. Greenwood Village, CO, USA. Available at https://www.micromedexsolutions.com, accessed March 12, 2019. AWP may not accurately represent the actual pharmacy cost because wide contractual variations exist among institutions.
[3]The adverse effects of headache, tinnitus, dizziness, confusion, rashes, anorexia, nausea, vomiting, gastrointestinal bleeding, diarrhea, nephrotoxicity, visual disturbances, etc, can occur with any of these drugs. Tolerance and efficacy are subject to great individual variations among patients. Note: All NSAIDs can increase serum lithium levels.
[4]Acetaminophen and celecoxib lack antiplatelet effects.
[5]May inhibit platelet aggregation for 1 week or more and may cause bleeding.
[6]May have minimal antiplatelet activity.
[7]Administration with antacids may decrease absorption.
[8]Has the same gastrointestinal toxicities as oral NSAIDs.
[9]Coombs-positive autoimmune hemolytic anemia has been associated with prolonged use.
COX, cyclooxygenase; OA, osteoarthritis; OTC, over the counter; RA, rheumatoid arthritis; Rx, prescription.

NSAIDs. An appropriate dose of acetaminophen may be just as effective an analgesic and antipyretic as an NSAID but without the risk of gastrointestinal bleeding or ulceration. Acetaminophen can be given at a dosage of 500–1000 mg orally every 6 hours, not to exceed 4000 mg/day maximum for short-term use. Total acetaminophen doses should not exceed 3000 mg/day for long-term use or 2000 mg/day for older patients and for those with liver disease. Hepatotoxicity is of particular concern because of how commonly acetaminophen is also an ingredient in various over-the-counter medications and because of failure to account for the acetaminophen dose in combination acetaminophen-opioid medications such as Vicodin or Norco. The FDA has limited the amount of acetaminophen available in some combination analgesics (eg, in acetaminophen plus codeine preparations).

Aspirin (325–650 mg orally every 4 hours) is an effective analgesic, antipyretic, and anti-inflammatory medication. Gastrointestinal irritation and bleeding are side effects that are lessened with enteric-coated formulations and by concomitant use of proton pump inhibitor medication. Bleeding, allergy, and an association with Reye syndrome in children and adolescents further limit its use.

NSAIDs are antipyretic, analgesic, and anti-inflammatory. Treatment with NSAIDs increases the risk of gastrointestinal bleeding 1.5 times; the risks of bleeding and nephrotoxicity are both increased in elders. Gastrointestinal bleeding and ulceration may be prevented with the concurrent use of proton pump inhibitors (eg, omeprazole, 20–40 mg orally daily) or with use of celecoxib (100 mg orally daily to 200 mg orally twice daily), the only COX-2 inhibitor available. Celecoxib and the

NSAIDs can lead to fluid retention, kidney injury, and exacerbations of heart failure and should be used with caution in patients with that condition. Topical formulations of NSAIDs (such as diclofenac 1.3% patch or 1% gel), placed over the painful body part for treatment of musculoskeletal pain, are associated with less systemic absorption and fewer side effects than oral administration and are likely underutilized in patients at risk for gastrointestinal bleeding.

Chang AK et al. Effect of a single dose of oral opioid and nonopioid analgesics on acute extremity pain in the emergency department: a randomized clinical trial. JAMA. 2017 Nov 7; 318(17):1661–7. [PMID: 29114833]
Wiffen PJ et al. Oral paracetamol (acetaminophen) for cancer pain. Cochrane Database Syst Rev. 2017 Jul 12;7:CD012637. [PMID: 28700092]

▶ Opioids

A. Formulations and Regimens

For many patients, opioids are the mainstay of pain management (Table 5–8). Opioids are appropriate for managing severe pain at the end of life due to any cause, including the following: neuropathic pain, cancer pain, and pain from other serious illnesses. Full opioid agonists such as morphine, hydromorphone, oxycodone, methadone, fentanyl, hydrocodone, tramadol, and codeine are used most commonly. Hydrocodone and codeine are typically combined with acetaminophen or an NSAID, although acetaminophen in these combinations is restricted to 300–325 mg per unit dose due to the risk of hepatotoxicity.

Table 5–8. Opioids.

Medication	Approximate Equianalgesic Dose (compared to morphine 30 mg orally or 10 mg intravenously/subcutaneously)[1]		Usual Starting Dose				Potential Advantages	Potential Disadvantages
			Adults ≥ 50 kg Body Weight		Adults < 50 kg Body Weight			
	Oral	Parenteral	Oral	Parenteral	Oral	Parenteral		
Opioid Agonists[2,3]								
Buprenorphine parenteral (Buprenex)	Not available	300 mcg intravenously slowly once, may be repeated after 30–60 minutes once; or 600 mcg intramuscularly once		300 mcg intravenously slowly once, may be repeated after 30–60 minutes once; or 600 mcg intramuscularly once; $18.20/300 mcg	Not available	Not available		
Buprenorphine transdermal (BuTrans)	Not available	Not available orally. Transdermal doses available: 5, 10, and 20 mcg/h. Initiate 5 mcg/h patch for opioid-naïve patients (may currently be using nonopioid analgesics); $114.77/10 mcg/h.		Not available	Not available	Not available	7-day analgesia; may be initiated in opioid-naïve patients with 5 mcg/h. Can titrate up dose by 5 mcg/h after 72 hours, to a maximum dose of 20 mcg/h.	Concomitant use of other opioids for acute pain could be difficult due to strong receptor binding of buprenorphine, although this is often not found in clinical practice. QT prolongation.

Opioid	Approximate Equianalgesic Dose (Oral)	Approximate Equianalgesic Dose (Parenteral)	Usual Starting Dose, Adults (Oral)	Usual Starting Dose, Adults (Parenteral)	Usual Starting Dose, Children (Oral)	Usual Starting Dose, Children (Parenteral)	Potential Advantages	Potential Disadvantages
Buprenorphine sublingual (Belbuca)	Sublingual strip approved for pain	Not available	In opioid-naive or opioid-intolerant patients, individualize dose every 12 h. Start: 75 mcg buccally every 12–24 h for at least 4 days, then increase to 150 mcg buccally every 12 h, then may increase by no more than 150 mcg buccally every 12 h no more frequently than every 4 days. Maximum: 900 mcg/12 h; $6.07/75 mcg.					Used by pain management specialists. Do no cut, chew, swallow strip. Taper slowly to discontinue. Use lowest effective dose, shortest effective treatment duration. Titrate slowly in patients age > 65 yrs. See footnote[4] for dosing in opioid-experienced patients.
Fentanyl	Not available	100 mcg every hour	Not available	50–100 mcg intravenously/intramuscularly every hour or 0.5–1.5 mcg/kg/h intravenous infusion; $1.51/100 mcg	Not available	0.5–1 mcg/kg intravenously every 1–4 hours or 1–2 mcg/kg intravenously × 1, then 0.5–1 mcg/kg/h infusion	Possibly less neuroexcitatory effects, including in kidney failure.	
Fentanyl oral transmucosal (Actiq); buccal (Fentora)	Not available	Not available	200 mcg transmucosal; 100 mcg buccal; $18.80/200 mcg transmucosal; $81.60/200 mcg buccal	Not available	Not available	Not available	For pain breaking through long-acting opioid medication.	Transmucosal and buccal formulations are not bioequivalent; there is higher bioavailability in buccal formulation.

(continued)

Table 5–8. Opioids. (continued)

Medication	Approximate Equianalgesic Dose (compared to morphine 30 mg orally or 10 mg intravenously/subcutaneously)[1]		Usual Starting Dose				Potential Advantages	Potential Disadvantages
			Adults ≥ 50 kg Body Weight		Adults < 50 kg Body Weight			
	Oral	Parenteral	Oral	Parenteral	Oral	Parenteral		
Fentanyl transdermal	Conversion to fentanyl patch is based on total daily dose of oral morphine:[2] morphine 60–134 mg/day orally = fentanyl 25 mcg/h patch; morphine 135–224 mg/day orally = fentanyl 50 mcg/h patch; morphine 225–314 mg/day orally = fentanyl 75 mcg/h patch; and morphine 315–404 mg/day orally = fentanyl 100 mcg/h patch	Not available	Not available orally 12.5–25 mcg/h patch every 72 hours; $14.43/25 mcg/h	Not available	12.5–25 mcg/h patch every 72 hours	Not available	Stable medication blood levels.	Not for use in opioid-naive patients. Minimum starting dose is 25 mcg/h patch in patients who have been taking stable dose of opioids for at least 1 week at the equivalent of at least 60 mg/day of oral morphine.
Hydrocodone, extended release (Zohydro ER)	20 mg[1]	Not available	10 mg every 12 hours; $11.11/10 mg	Not available	Not available	Not available	Available as an extended-release formulation without acetaminophen.	
Hydromorphone[5] (Dilaudid)	7.5 mg every 3–4 hours	1.5 mg every 3–4 hours	1–2 mg every 3–4 hours; $0.48/2 mg	1.5 mg every 3–4 hours; $1.80/2 mg	0.06/every 3–4 hours	0.015 mg/kg every 3–4 hours	Similar to morphine. Available in injectable high-potency preparation, rectal suppository.	Short duration.
Hydromorphone extended release (Exalgo)	45–60 mg every 24 hours	Not available	8 mg every 24 hours; $16.73/8 mg	Not available	Not available	Not available	Similar to morphine.	Taper dose 25–50% every 2–3 days to 8 mg/day to discontinue.
Levorphanol (Levo-Dromoran)	4 mg every 6–8 hours	Not available	4 mg every 6–8 hours; $53.40/2 mg	Not available	0.04 mg/kg every 6–8 hours	Not available	Longer acting than morphine sulfate.	

Drug							Potential Advantages	Potential Disadvantages
Meperidine[6] (Demerol)	300 mg every 2–3 hours; usual dose 50–150 mg every 3–4 hours	100 mg every 3 hours	Not recommended	100 mg every 3 hours; $2.72/100 mg	Not recommended	0.75 mg/kg every 2–3 hours	Use only when single-dose, short-duration analgesia is needed, as for outpatient procedures like colonoscopy. Not recommended for chronic pain or for repeated dosing.	Short duration. Normeperidine metabolite accumulates in kidney failure and other situations, and in high concentrations may cause irritability and seizures.
Methadone (Dolophine, others)	10–20 mg every 6–8 hours (when converting from < 100 mg long-term daily oral morphine[7])	5–10 mg every 6–8 hours	5–20 mg every 6–8 hours; $0.31/10 mg	2.5–10 mg every 6–8 hours; $21.00/10 mg	0.2 mg/kg every 6–8 hours	0.1 mg/kg every 6–8 hours	Somewhat longer acting than morphine. Useful in cases of intolerance to morphine. May be particularly useful for neuropathic pain. Available in liquid formulation.	Analgesic duration shorter than plasma duration. May accumulate, requiring close monitoring during first weeks of treatment. Equianalgesic ratios vary with opioid dose. Risk of QT prolongation at doses > 100–150 mg/day. Baseline ECG recommended.
Morphine[5] immediate release (Morphine sulfate tablets, Roxanol liquid)	30 mg every 3–4 hours (around-the-clock dosing); 60 mg every 3–4 hours (single or intermittent dosing)	10 mg every 3–4 hours	4–8 mg every 3–4 hours; used for breakthrough pain in patients already taking controlled-release preparations; $0.52/15 mg tab; $0.84/20 mg liquid	10 mg every 3–4 hours; $11.90/10 mg	0.3 mg/kg every 3–4 hours	0.1 mg/kg every 3–4 hours	Standard of comparison; multiple dosage forms available.	No unique problems when compared with other opioids. Active metabolite accumulates in kidney dysfunction.

(continued)

Table 5–8. Opioids. (continued)

Medication	Approximate Equianalgesic Dose (compared to morphine 30 mg orally or 10 mg intravenously/subcutaneously)[1]		Usual Starting Dose				Potential Advantages	Potential Disadvantages
			Adults ≥ 50 kg Body Weight		Adults < 50 kg Body Weight			
	Oral	Parenteral	Oral	Parenteral	Oral	Parenteral		
Morphine controlled release (MS Contin, Oramorph)	90–120 mg every 12 hours	Not available	15–60 mg every 12 hours; $1.50/30 mg	Not available	Not available	Not available		
Morphine extended release (Kadian, Avinza)	180–240 mg every 24 hours	Not available	20–30 mg every 24 hours; $5.69/30 mg	Not available	Not available	Not available	Once-daily dosing possible.	
Oxycodone (Roxicodone, OxyIR)	20–30 mg every 3–4 hours	Not available	5–10 mg every 3–4 hours; $0.48/5 mg	Not available	0.2 mg/kg every 3–4 hours	Not available	Similar to morphine.	
Oxycodone controlled release (Oxycontin)	40 mg every 12 hours	Not available	20–40 mg every 12 hours; $9.00/20 mg	Not available				Physical and chemical pill formulation to deter misuse (injection or intranasal administration).
Oxymorphone[5,8] oral, immediate release (Opana)	10 mg every 6 hours	Not available	5–10 mg every 6 hours; $2.95/5 mg	Not available				Taking with food can increase serum levels by 50%. Equianalgesic dosing conversion range is wide.

Drug	Approximate Equivalent Dose (Oral)	Approximate Equivalent Dose (Parenteral)	Usual Starting Dose (Adults) Oral	Usual Starting Dose (Adults) Parenteral	Usual Starting Dose (Children) Oral	Usual Starting Dose (Children) Parenteral	Potency	Comments
Combination Opioid Agonist–Nonopioid Preparations								
Codeine[9,10] (with aspirin or acetaminophen)[11]	180–200 mg every 3–4 hours; commonly available dose in combination with acetaminophen, 15–60 mg of codeine every 4–6 hours	130 mg every 3–4 hours	60 mg every 4–6 hours; $0.64/60 mg	60 mg every 2 hours intramuscularly/subcutaneously; not available in the United States	0.5–1 mg/kg every 3–4 hours	Not recommended	Similar to morphine.	Closely monitor for efficacy as patients vary in their ability to convert the prodrug codeine to morphine.
Hydrocodone[8] (in Lorcet, Lortab, Vicodin, others)[11]	30 mg every 3–4 hours	Not available	10 mg every 3–4 hours; $0.54/5 mg	Not available	0.2 mg/kg every 3–4 hours	Not available		Combination with acetaminophen limits dosage titration.
Oxycodone[10] (in Percodan, Tylox, others)[11]	30 mg every 3–4 hours	Not available	10 mg every 3–4 hours; $1.37/5 mg	Not available	0.2 mg/kg every 3–4 hours	Not available	Similar to morphine.	Combination with acetaminophen and aspirin limits dosage titration.
Combination Opioid Agonist–Norepinephrine Reuptake Inhibitor Preparations								
Tapentadol (Nucynta)	Not known		Start 50–100 mg once, may repeat dose in 1 hour. Can increase to 50–100 mg every 4 hours. Maximum daily dose 600 mg; $11.89/100 mg.	Not available			Not available	Avoid in severe kidney or liver impairment.
Tapentadol, extended release (Nucynta ER)	Not known		Start 50 mg orally every 12 hours. Can increase by 50-mg increments twice daily every 3 days to dose of 100–250 mg twice daily; $15.20/100 mg.	Not available			Not available	Avoid in severe kidney or liver impairment.

(continued)

Table 5–8. Opioids. (continued)

Medication	Approximate Equianalgesic Dose (compared to morphine 30 mg orally or 10 mg intravenously/subcutaneously)[1]		Usual Starting Dose				Potential Advantages	Potential Disadvantages
			Adults ≥ 50 kg Body Weight		Adults < 50 kg Body Weight			
	Oral	Parenteral	Oral	Parenteral	Oral	Parenteral		
Tramadol (Ultram)	Not known	Not known	Start 25 mg orally daily. Can increase by 25 mg every 3 days to 25 mg orally 4 times daily, then may increase by 50 mg/day every 3 days to 100 mg orally 4 times daily. Limit of 300 mg/day in patients > 75 years old; $0.83/50 mg.	Not available		Not available		If creatinine clearance less than 30, limit to 200 mg/day; with cirrhosis, limit to 100 mg/day.

[1]Published tables vary in the suggested doses that are equianalgesic to morphine. Clinical response is the criterion that must be applied for each patient; titration to clinical efficacy is necessary. Because there is not complete cross-tolerance among these drugs, it is usually necessary to use a lower than equianalgesic dose initially when changing drugs and to retitrate to response.

[2]Conversion is conservative; therefore, do not use these equianalgesic doses for converting back from fentanyl patch to other opioids because they may lead to inadvertent overdose. Patients may require breakthrough doses of short-acting opioids during conversion to transdermal fentanyl.

[3]Several significantly more potent formulations of buprenorphine are available but generally reserved for the treatment of opioid use disorder with or without comorbid constant pain, most often by pain management specialists: a sublingual tablet (Subutex and others) or a sublingual film (Suboxone and others) in which the buprenorphine is combined with naloxone; a subdermal implant of buprenorphine alone (Probuphine); and a subcutaneous depot injection (Sublocade). Each of these is used in maintenance treatment to reduce problematic use of other opioids. See text.

[4]In opioid-experienced patients, taper current opioids to 30 mg/day oral morphine equivalent prior to starting buprenorphine. Thereafter, buprenorphine dosing schedule depends on prior current oral morphine equivalent:

< 30 mg/day, 75 mcg buccally every 12 h;

30–89 mg/day, 150 mcg buccally every 12 h;

90–160 mg/ day, 300 mcg buccally every 12 h;

In all patients, use same dose escalation and maximum dose as shown for opioid-naive patients.

[5]*Caution:* For morphine, hydromorphone, and oxymorphone, rectal administration is an alternative route for patients unable to take oral medications. Equianalgesic doses may differ from oral and parenteral doses. A short-acting opioid should normally be used for initial therapy.

[6]Not recommended for chronic pain. Doses listed are for brief therapy of acute pain only. Switch to another opioid for long-term therapy.

[7]Methadone conversion varies depending on the equivalent total daily dose of morphine. Consult with a pain management or palliative care expert for conversion.

[8]*Caution:* Recommended doses do not apply to adult patients with kidney or liver impairment or other conditions affecting drug metabolism.

[9]*Caution:* Individual doses of codeine above 60 mg often are not appropriate because of diminishing incremental analgesia with increasing doses but continually increasing nausea, constipation, and other side effects.

[10]*Caution:* Doses of aspirin and acetaminophen in combination products must also be adjusted to the patient's body weight.

[11]*Caution:* Monitor total acetaminophen dose carefully, including any OTC use. Total acetaminophen dose maximum 3 g/day. If liver impairment or heavy alcohol use, maximum is 2 g/day. Available dosing formulations of these combination medications are being adjusted to reflect increased caution about acetaminophen toxicity. Acetaminophen doses in a single combination tablet or capsule will be limited to no more than 325 mg.

Note: Average wholesale price (AWP, generic when available) for quantity listed. Source: IBM Micromedex Red Book (electronic version) IBM Watson Health. Greenwood Village, CO, USA. Available at https://www.micromedexsolutions.com, accessed March 12, 2019. AWP may not accurately represent the actual pharmacy cost because wide contractual variations exist among institutions.

Extended-release hydrocodone without acetaminophen is also available. **Short-acting formulations** of oral morphine sulfate (starting dosage 4–8 mg orally every 3–4 hours), hydromorphone (1–2 mg orally every 3–4 hours), or oxycodone (5 mg orally every 3–4 hours) are useful for severe acute pain not controlled with other analgesics. The transmucosal intermediate-release fentanyl products, such as oral transmucosal fentanyl (200 mcg oralet dissolved in the mouth) or buccal fentanyl (100 mcg dissolved in the mouth), can be used for treating patients with cancer pain that breaks through long-acting medications, or it can be administered before activity known to cause more pain (such as burn wound dressing changes). Buprenorphine as a short-acting analgesic generally should be reserved for use by pain management specialists.

For chronic stable cancer pain, **long-acting medications** are preferred, such as oral sustained-release formulations of morphine (one to three times a day), hydromorphone (once daily), oxymorphone (two times a day), oxycodone (two or three times a day), or hydrocodone (two times a day), or the long-acting medication, methadone (three or four times a day) (Table 5–8).

Clinicians prescribing opioids must understand the concept of **equianalgesic dosing.** The dosages of any full opioid agonists used to control pain can be converted into an equivalent dose of any other opioid. This approach is helpful in estimating the appropriate dose of a long-acting opioid based on the amount of short-acting opioid required over the preceding days. For example, 24-hour opioid requirements established using short-acting opioid medications can be converted into equivalent dosages of long-acting medications or formulations. Cross-tolerance is often incomplete, however, so generally only two-thirds to three-quarters of the full, calculated equianalgesic dosage is administered initially when switching between opioid formulations.

Methadone deserves special consideration among the long-acting opioids because it is inexpensive, available in a liquid formulation, and may have added efficacy for neuropathic pain. However, equianalgesic dosing is complex because it varies with the patient's opioid dose, and caution must be exercised at higher methadone doses (generally more than 100–150 mg/day) because of the risk of QT prolongation. Baseline electrocardiography is recommended before starting methadone and repeated up to monthly except at the end of life where comfort is the only goal. Given the complexities of management, consultation with a palliative medicine or pain specialist may be appropriate.

Transdermal fentanyl is appropriate for patients already tolerant to other opioids for at least 1 week at a dose equivalent to at least 60 mg/day of oral morphine (equivalent to a transdermal fentanyl 25 mcg/h patch applied topically every 72 hours) and therefore should not be used in the postoperative setting or be the first opioid used. Since transdermal fentanyl can require 24–48 hours to achieve pharmacologic "steady state," patients should be weaned off their current opioid and given short-acting opioids while awaiting the full analgesic effect of a new transdermal fentanyl patch, and changes in dose of transdermal fentanyl should be made no more frequently than every 6 days.

Buprenorphine has been FDA-approved for treatment of moderate to severe chronic pain and is available in parenteral, transdermal, and buccal formulations. The usual dosages of the **parenteral** formulation (Buprenex) are 300 mcg intravenously once (may be repeated once after 30–60 minutes) or as 600 mcg intramuscularly once. The **transdermal patch** (BuTrans) is available in dosages of 5, 10, and 20 mcg/h. The benefits of transdermal buprenorphine include its long half-life, once-weekly change of patch, lower risk of respiratory depression during treatment, and lower likelihood of withdrawal upon discontinuation than with other opioids. The **buccal buprenorphine** strip formulation (Belbuca) is sometimes used by pain management specialists for moderate to severe constant pain. It can be more frequently uptitrated since it is given twice daily. Depending on the patient's current opioid usage, it can be started at 75–300 mcg once or twice daily, then escalated by 150- to 450-mcg doses twice daily to a maximum of 900 mcg twice daily. Although there is a theoretical concern about decreased efficacy of short-acting opioid agents unable to compete with buprenorphine at the opioid receptor, this is not a major issue with the formulations available in the United States.

In addition, buprenorphine comes in significantly more potent formulations generally reserved for the treatment of opioid use disorder with or without comorbid constant pain: a **sublingual tablet** (Subutex and others), a **sublingual film** (Suboxone and others) in which the buprenorphine is combined with naloxone, a **subdermal implant** of buprenorphine alone (Probuphine), and a **subcutaneous depot injection** (Sublocade), each of which is used in maintenance treatment to reduce problematic use of other opioids.

While some clinicians and patients inexperienced with the management of severe pain may feel more comfortable with combined nonopioid-opioid agents, full agonist opioids are typically a better choice in patients with severe pain because the dose of opioid is not limited by the toxicities of the acetaminophen, aspirin, or NSAID component of combination preparations. There may be no maximal allowable or effective dose for full opioid agonists. Generally, the dose can be gradually increased to whatever is necessary to relieve pain, as long as the side effects are tolerable. Clinicians should confirm that increasing doses of opioid provide additional pain relief and remember that not all pain is opioid sensitive and that certain types of pain, such as neuropathic pain, may respond better to agents other than opioids, or to combinations of opioids with co-analgesic medications for neuropathic pain (see below).

While physiologic tolerance is possible with opioids, failure of a previously effective opioid dose to adequately relieve pain in a patient with cancer is usually due to worsening of the underlying condition causing pain, such as tumor growth or new metastasis. In this case, for moderate unrelieved pain, the dose of opioid can be increased by 25–50%. For severe unrelieved pain, a dose increase of 50–100% may be appropriate. The frequency of dosing should be adjusted so that pain control is continuous.

Long-term dosing may then be adjusted by adding the average daily amount of short-acting opioid necessary for breakthrough pain over the preceding 72–96 hours to the long-acting medication dose. In establishing or reestablishing adequate dosing, frequent reassessments of the patient's pain and medication side effects are necessary.

B. Assessing Benefits of Opioids

The potential benefits and harms of daily opioid therapy for patients with chronic noncancer pain differ than for patients with cancer pain and for patients receiving palliative care or end-of-life care. For example, research demonstrates that the beneficial effect of opioids for chronic noncancer pain is modest at best, and no measures have been identified to predict a good response. The improvements are generally measured in terms of a reduction in the analog pain score of 2–3 points on a 10-point scale (see Table 5–6) or in improvements in the important but less precise outcome of function. Prior to considering a trial of daily opioids, clinicians should discuss these modest possible benefits with patients to help set realistic goals of therapy (eg, moving from an average pain level of a "7" to a "4"). Clinicians should also set a deadline for reaching the patient's goals. Since the published trials have generally lasted less than 16 weeks, it is reasonable to set a deadline before that, with some experts advocating a 90-day trial period. Limiting the time of a trial also helps prevent dose escalation to levels associated with increased risk of adverse effects, including overdose.

For the many patients who do not have specific, measurable goals—or who come to the clinician already taking daily opioid medication—monitoring response to treatment over time can be difficult. A useful tracking measure derived from the Brief Pain Inventory and validated for use in primary care is the "PEG," which directs patients to quantify on a scale of 0–10 the following three outcomes over the last week: average **p**ain intensity, how much the pain has affected their **e**njoyment of life, and how much their pain has impacted their **g**eneral activity. Patients who do not progress toward their goal or whose PEG scores remain high over time may have pain that is unresponsive to opioids, and clinicians should reconsider the original diagnosis and use other modalities (both pharmacologic and nonpharmacologic) to provide analgesia. Without a clear analgesic benefit from opioids for chronic noncancer pain, the risks may predominate, and the ineffective therapy should be discontinued in a patient-centered manner.

C. Common Side Effects of Opioids

At higher doses or with long-term use of opioids, patients may experience increasing difficulty with the side effects. Opioid-related **constipation** should be anticipated and prevented in all patients. Constipation is common at any dose of opioid, and tolerance to this side effect does not develop over time. Prescribing a bowel regimen (see Chapter 15) to a patient taking opioids long term is a quality of care measure supported by the National Quality Forum.

Sedation can be expected with opioids, although tolerance to this effect and to side effects other than constipation typically develops within 24–72 hours at a stable dose. Sedation typically appears well before significant respiratory depression. If treatment for sedation is desired, dextroamphetamine (2.5–7.5 mg orally at 8 AM and noon) or methylphenidate (2.5–10 mg orally at 8 AM and noon) may be helpful. Caffeinated beverages can also ameliorate minor opioid sedation.

Opioid-induced **neurotoxicity,** including myoclonus, hyperalgesia, delirium with hallucinosis, and seizures, may develop in patients who take high doses of opioids for a prolonged period. Opioid-induced hyperalgesia appears to be a result of changes in both the peripheral and central nervous systems such that typically benign or even soothing stimuli (eg, light massage) may be perceived as painful (allodynia); increasing the opioid dose may exacerbate the problem. Opioid-induced neurotoxicity symptoms typically resolve after lowering the dose or switching opioids ("opioid rotation"), especially to opioids that do not have active metabolites (such as fentanyl or methadone). While waiting for the level of the offending opioid to fall, low doses of clonazepam, baclofen, or gabapentin may be helpful for treating myoclonus; haloperidol may be useful for treating delirium. Avoiding or correcting dehydration may be helpful for avoiding opioid-induced neurotoxicity.

Nausea may occur with initiation of opioid therapy and resolve after a few days. Notably, unrelieved constipation may be a more likely cause of nausea in the setting of opioid use than opioid-induced nausea. Severe or persistent nausea despite treatment of constipation can be managed by switching opioids or by giving haloperidol, 0.5–4 mg orally, subcutaneously, or intravenously every 6 hours or prochlorperazine, 10 mg orally or intravenously or 25 mg rectally every 6 hours. Ondansetron, 4–8 mg orally or intravenously every 6 hours, also relieves nausea but can contribute to constipation. Mirtazapine and medical cannabis may each have a role in treating opioid-induced nausea. Most antiemetic treatments can contribute to sedation.

The risk of **respiratory depression** with opioids may be decreased by initiating at a low dose and titrating upward slowly, taking advantage of physiologic **tolerance**. Patients at particular risk for respiratory depression include those with obstructive sleep apnea or central sleep apnea, chronic obstructive pulmonary disease, and baseline CO_2 retention; those with liver or kidney or combined liver-kidney failure; and those with adrenal insufficiency or frank myxedema. Yet, even patients with severe pulmonary disease and obstructive sleep apnea can tolerate low-dose opioids, although these patients should be monitored carefully. Hospitalized patients with these conditions who require increased doses of opioids should be monitored with continuous pulse oximetry.

While physiologic **tolerance** (requiring increasing dosage to achieve the same analgesic effect) and **dependence** (requiring continued dosing to prevent symptoms of medication withdrawal) are expected with regular opioid use, the use of opioids at the end of life for relief of pain and dyspnea is not generally associated with a risk of psychological addiction (use of a substance despite negative health or social consequences, cravings to use a substance, compulsive use or loss of control over level or time of use). Except in end-of-life care situations, the risk of addiction increases the longer the duration and the higher the dose of opioid exposure. If a patient is diagnosed with an opioid use disorder, then the appropriate treatment is opioid agonist therapy with either methadone or buprenorphine, often accompanied by psychosocial interventions. Patients with opioid use disorder or other substance use disorders may need pain relief and may benefit from additional opioids, but their pain control will be inadequate without proper treatment of the substance use disorder.

D. Adverse Effects and Risks of Opioids

In an effort to treat chronic pain more aggressively, clinicians in the United States dramatically increased the prescription of opioids beginning in the mid-1990s and peaking in 2010. After a modest decline, the amount of opioids prescribed per capita in 2015 remained triple the amount prescribed in 1999. The increased attention to treating chronic noncancer pain undoubtedly improved the lives of many patients, but the increase in prescribed opioids also had a deleterious effect on the health of the population as a whole. The increased population exposure to prescription opioids appears to have expanded the market for illicit opioids (heroin, fentanyl and its derivatives), with concomitant increase in opioid use disorder and opioid overdoses, which caused nearly 50,000 deaths in 2017. The CDC named both misuse of prescription medications and opioid overdoses as epidemics in the United States and released guidelines in 2016 to limit the risks of prescribed opioids (https://www.cdc.gov/drugoverdose/prescribing/guideline.html). Also in 2016, the US Surgeon General directly appealed to prescribing physicians to focus on combating the opioid epidemic and issued a report titled "Facing Addiction in America" (https://www.surgeongeneral.gov/library/2016alcoholdrugshealth/index.html).

In addition to the grave risks of **addiction** and **overdose** and the common side effects of constipation and sedation, long-term opioid use leads to increased risk of many other problems, including hypogonadism, fracture, hyperalgesia, psychosocial problems, and fraught interactions with the health care system. When considering whether to initiate or continue opioids for chronic noncancer pain, clinicians should delineate these specific risks for patients so that an informed decision can be made.

Finally, **diversion** of medication from patients to whom they are prescribed into other hands is an additional risk that must be considered when prescribing long-term opioids for chronic noncancer pain. Diversion can represent opportunism, eg, when a patient sells medication in order to make money. Family members (including children), acquaintances, or strangers may steal or extort medication for their own use or monetary gain.

E. Limiting Risks of Opioids

A number of interventions have been used in an effort to limit the risks of opioids for patients with chronic noncancer pain. Data demonstrating the effectiveness of such measures are limited, but nearly all medical society consensus panels and expert guidelines recommend using a risk assessment tool, patient-provider agreements, urine drug testing, dose limitations, limits on the use of some medications, and medication treatment of opioid use disorder.

1. Risk assessment tool—There are no highly predictive models for who will benefit from long-term opioids for chronic noncancer pain, and no models adequately predict harms. Some models can identify patients most likely to exhibit aberrant or addictive behaviors. Most published guidelines recommend using an instrument like the Opioid Risk Tool (available at https://www.drugabuse.gov/sites/default/files/files/OpioidRiskTool.pdf) to determine how closely to monitor patients who are receiving opioids long term, or whether to offer long-term opioids at all.

2. Patient-provider agreements—Also known as "pain contracts," these agreements have a modest effect, with a 7–23% reduction in aberrant behaviors reported. They do represent an opportunity for the clinician to discuss explicitly the risks and benefits of opioids for chronic noncancer pain, protocols and procedural requirements for refills and monitoring, and consequences of worrisome behaviors.

3. Urine drug testing—Toxicology testing is a tool borrowed from addiction treatment with goals of limiting diversion and identifying risky secondary drug use. Guidelines recommend more frequent testing with any increased risk as determined by dose, risk assessment tool, or recent behavior. It is imperative that clinicians choose the tests appropriately and understand the limitations of toxicology testing when using this tool. Universal testing is recommended, given provider inability to judge misuse of medication and documented racial biases in monitoring.

4. Dose limitations—Risk of overdose increases approximately linearly with dose in observational studies. The CDC considers doses above the equivalent of 50 mg of morphine per day to be risky, and specifically recommends against prescribing more than 120 mg of morphine per day. Clinicians must be cautious when tapering a patient's long-term dose to meet these limits in order to avoid withdrawal. No data support one tapering regimen over another, but for patients taking opioids for years, the CDC recommends no more than a monthly decrease of 10% of the original daily dose. Tapering too quickly may result in dissolution of the therapeutic relationship or risky patient behavior, such as use of nonprescribed prescription medications or heroin. It is notable that the most rapid rise of opioid overdose deaths in the United States occurred following the institution of restrictions on prescription opioids.

5. Special medication limitations—The FDA requires companies making extended-release opioid formulations to provide trainings for prescribers, although these trainings have not reduced the increase in opioid overdoses. Many guidelines recommend that the prescription of methadone and fentanyl be limited to specialists, and because of the increased incidence of opioid overdose, the CDC recommends against concurrent prescription of opioids and benzodiazepines.

6. Antidote to overdose—Distributing naloxone, a quick-onset opioid-receptor antagonist, has long been known to reduce overdose deaths in people who use heroin. More recently, prescribing naloxone to patients taking opioids for chronic noncancer pain has been demonstrated to reduce rates of opioid overdose death. Educating both patients and their caregivers on the use of rescue naloxone is important, since those experiencing sedation and respiratory suppression from opioid overdose will not be able to self-administer the naloxone. In addition to preloaded needle-tipped syringes, intranasal and intramuscular auto-injector naloxone preparations are approved for sale in the United States, where an increasing number of states authorize pharmacies to dispense naloxone in the absence of a prescription. CDC guidelines recommend prescribing naloxone for any patient with history of overdose, substance use disorder, concomitant benzodiazepine use, or daily doses above 50 mg morphine equivalent.

7. Medication treatment of opioid use disorder—Some patients who have been treated with long-term opioids will develop an opioid use disorder, and when this diagnosis is made, their opioid management should transition to appropriate treatment with methadone or buprenorphine maintenance. Both of these options have demonstrated a mortality benefit for patients with opioid addiction. Depending on jurisdiction, restrictions on how these—or other opioid agonist—treatments are delivered will apply.

Coffin PO et al. Nonrandomized intervention study of naloxone coprescription for primary care patients receiving long-term opioid therapy for pain. Ann Intern Med. 2016 Aug 16;165(4): 245–52. [PMID: 27366987]

Frank JW et al. Patient outcomes in dose reduction or discontinuation of long-term opioid therapy: a systematic review. Ann Intern Med. 2017 Aug 1;167(3):181–91. [PMID: 28715848]

Manchikanti L et al. Responsible, safe, and effective prescription of opioids for chronic non-cancer pain: American Society of Interventional Pain Physicians (ASIPP) guidelines. Pain Physician. 2017 Feb;20(2S):S3–92. [PMID: 28226332]

Ray WA et al. Prescription of long-acting opioids and mortality in patients with chronic noncancer pain. JAMA. 2016 Jun 14; 315(22):2415–23. [PMID: 27299617]

Sordo L et al. Mortality risk during and after opioid substitution treatment: systematic review and meta-analysis of cohort studies. BMJ 2017 Apr 26;357:j1550. [PMID: 28446428]

F. A Shared Decision-Making Approach to Opioid Use

As opposed to using opioids in patients with cancer or at the end of life, prescribing opioids for patients with chronic noncancer pain is fraught with challenges for clinicians. But taking the approach of carefully evaluating benefits and risks in individual cases allows the opportunity for shared decision making between patient and clinician. Clinical trials do not suggest that the majority of people with chronic noncancer pain benefit significantly from daily opioid therapy, and the dramatic increase in morbidity and mortality witnessed with the increased availability of these medications warrants very careful patient selection. It is incumbent upon the clinician to provide frank advice to patients prescribed long-term opioids for chronic noncancer pain and to offer safer alternatives when the benefit is insufficient or the risks are too high.

Gaither JR et al. The association between receipt of guideline-concordant long-term opioid therapy and all-cause mortality. J Gen Intern Med. 2016 May;31(5):492–501. [PMID: 26847447]

Garg RK et al. Patterns of opioid use and risk of opioid overdose death among Medicaid patients. Med Care. 2017 Jul;55(7): 661–8. [PMID: 28614178]

▶ Medications for Neuropathic Pain

When taking a patient's history, listening for pain descriptions such as "burning," "shooting," "pins and needles," or "electricity," and for pain associated with numbness is essential because such a history suggests neuropathic pain. Studies are mixed with regard to efficacy of opioids for neuropathic pain. However, a number of nonopioid medications have also been found to be effective in randomized trials (Table 5–9). Successful management of neuropathic pain often requires the use of more than one effective medication.

The calcium channel alpha2-delta ligands, gabapentin and pregabalin, are first-line therapies for neuropathic pain. Both medications have no significant medication interactions but can cause sedation, dizziness, ataxia, and gastrointestinal side effects. Both medications require dose adjustments in patients with kidney dysfunction. Gabapentin should be started at low dosages of 100–300 mg orally once daily and titrated upward by 300 mg/day every 4–7 days by adding additional doses throughout the day with a typical effective dose of 1800–3600 mg/day in three divided doses. Pregabalin should be started at 40–150 mg/day in two or three divided doses. If necessary, the dose of pregabalin can be titrated upward to 300–600 mg/day in two or three divided doses. Both medications are relatively safe in accidental overdose and may be preferred over tricyclic antidepressants (TCAs) for a patient with a history of heart failure or arrhythmia or if there is a risk of suicide. Prescribing both gabapentin and an opioid for neuropathic pain may provide better analgesia at lower doses than if each is used as a single agent.

The serotonin norepinephrine reuptake inhibitors (SNRIs) duloxetine and venlafaxine are also first-line treatments for neuropathic pain. Patients should be advised to take duloxetine on a full stomach because nausea is a common side effect. Duloxetine may provide increased benefit for neuropathic pain up to a total daily dose of 120 mg, beyond the 60-mg limit used for depression. Duloxetine generally should not be combined with other serotonin or norepinephrine uptake inhibitors, but it can be combined with gabapentin or pregabalin. Lower doses of venlafaxine have more serotonin than norepinephrine activity; therefore, higher doses may be required to treat neuropathic pain. Because venlafaxine can cause hypertension and induce ECG changes, patients with cardiovascular risk factors should be carefully monitored when starting this medication. Desvenlafaxine, the active metabolite of

Table 5–9. Pharmacologic management of neuropathic pain.

Medication[1]	Starting Dose	Typical Dose
Antidepressants[2]		
Nortriptyline	10 mg orally at bedtime	10–150 mg orally at bedtime
Amitriptyline	10 mg orally at bedtime	10–150 mg orally at bedtime
Desipramine	12.5 mg orally at bedtime	12.5–250 mg orally at bedtime (can be divided into two doses)
Calcium-channel Alpha2-delta Ligands		
Gabapentin[3]	100–300 mg orally once to three times daily	300–1200 mg orally three times daily
Pregabalin[4]	50 mg orally three times daily	50–150 mg orally three times daily
Selective Serotonin Norepinephrine Reuptake Inhibitors		
Duloxetine	30–60 mg orally daily or 20 mg orally twice daily in elders	60–120 mg orally daily
Venlafaxine[5]	75 mg orally daily divided into two or three doses	150–225 mg orally daily divided into two or three doses
Opioids	(see Table 5–8)	(see Table 5–8)
Other Medications		
Lidocaine transdermal	5% patch applied daily, for a maximum of 12 hours	1–3 patches applied daily for a maximum of 12 hours
Tramadol hydrochloride[6]	50 mg orally four times daily	100 mg orally two to four times daily

[1]Begin at the starting dose and titrate up every 4 or 5 days. Within each category, drugs listed in order of prescribing preference.
[2]Begin with a low dose. Use the lowest effective dose. Pain relief may be achieved at doses below antidepressant doses, thereby minimizing adverse side effects. Do not combine with serotonin or norepinephrine uptake inhibitors.
[3]Common side effects include nausea, somnolence, and dizziness. Must adjust dose for kidney impairment.
[4]Common side effects include dizziness, somnolence, peripheral edema, and weight gain. Must adjust dose for kidney impairment.
[5]*Caution:* Can cause hypertension and ECG changes. Consider obtaining baseline ECG and monitor.
[6]Tramadol is classified by the DEA as a Schedule IV controlled substance.

venlafaxine, is also available and may be tolerated better than venlafaxine.

TCAs are another class of medications for neuropathic pain that work through the norepinephrine and serotonin pathways. Among the TCAs that are effective for neuropathic pain, nortriptyline and desipramine are preferred over amitriptyline because they cause less orthostatic hypotension and have fewer anticholinergic effects. Start with a low dosage (10–25 mg orally daily) and titrate upward in 10-mg increments every 4 or 5 days aiming to use the lowest effective dose and to titrate up to a maximum of no greater than 100 mg daily. It may take several weeks for a TCA to have its full analgesic effect for neuropathic pain. Because TCAs and SNRIs both work through the serotonin and norepinephrine pathways, they generally should not be co-prescribed, particularly due to concerns for the serotonin syndrome.

Topical medications, such as 5% lidocaine patch and capsaicin 8% patches, are considered second-line therapies. The 5% lidocaine patch is particularly effective in postherpetic neuralgia and may be effective in other types of localized neuropathic pain. Due to its relatively minimal adverse effects, it is commonly used despite being considered second-line. The 4% lidocaine patch is available over the counter. Other medications effective for neuropathic pain include tramadol and tapentadol, both of which are opioids with norepinephrine activity. Medical cannabis strains

high in cannabidiol have proven efficacy for some types of neuropathic pain.

Alles SRA et al. Etiology and pharmacology of neuropathic pain. Pharmacol Rev. 2018 Apr;70(2):315–47. [PMID: 29500312]
Fornasari D. Pharmacotherapy for neuropathic pain: a review. Pain Ther. 2017 Dec;6(Suppl 1):25–33. [PMID: 29178034]

▶ **Adjuvant Pain Medications & Treatments**

If pain cannot be controlled without intolerable medication side effects, clinicians should consider using lower doses of multiple medications, which is done commonly for neuropathic pain, rather than larger doses of one or two medications.

For metastatic bone pain, the anti-inflammatory effect of NSAIDs can be helpful. Furthermore, bisphosphonates (such as pamidronate and zoledronic acid) and receptor activator of NF-kappa-B ligand (RANKL) inhibitors (such as denosumab) may relieve such bone pain, although they are generally more useful for prevention of bone metastases than for analgesia.

Corticosteroids, such as dexamethasone, prednisone, and methylprednisolone, can be helpful for patients with headache due to increased intracranial pressure, pain from spinal cord compression, metastatic bone pain, and neuropathic pain due to invasion or infiltration of nerves by tumor. Because of the side effects of long-term corticosteroid administration, they are most appropriate for short-term use and in patients with end-stage disease. Low-dose intravenous, oral, buccal, and nasal ketamine has been used successfully for neuropathic and other pain syndromes refractory to opioids, although research data are limited.

Chen F et al. Safety of denosumab versus zoledronic acid in patients with bone metastases: a meta-analysis of randomized controlled trials. Oncol Res Treat. 2016;39(7–8):453–9. [PMID: 27487236]

Michelet D et al. Ketamine for chronic non-cancer pain: a meta-analysis and trial sequential analysis of randomized controlled trials. Eur J Pain. 2018 Apr;22(4):632–46. [PMID: 29178663]

Rasu RS et al. Assessing prescribing trends of adjuvant medication therapy in outpatients with a diagnosis of noncancer chronic pain. Clin J Pain. 2017 Sep;33(9):786–92. [PMID: 28002095]

INTEGRATIVE THERAPIES & OTHER PAIN MANAGEMENT

Nonpharmacologic and noninterventional therapies are valuable in treating pain. In fact, physical or functional therapy and cognitive behavioral therapy have been shown to be the most effective for management of chronic pain. In particular, cognitive behavioral therapy has been proven effective in multiple randomized controlled studies as a primary evidence-based treatment for chronic pain. Hot or cold packs, massage, and physical therapy can be helpful for musculoskeletal pain. Similarly, integrative medicine therapies of acupuncture, chiropractic care, biofeedback, meditation, music therapy, guided imagery, cognitive distraction, and framing may be of help in treating pain. Because mood and psychological issues play an important role in the patient's perception of and response to pain, psychotherapy, support groups, prayer, and pastoral counseling can also help in pain management. Depression and anxiety, which may be instigated by chronic pain or may alter the response to pain, should be treated aggressively with antidepressants and anxiolytics.

Martorella G et al. Tailored web-based interventions for pain: systematic review and meta-analysis. J Med Internet Res. 2017 Nov 10;19(11):e385. [PMID: 29127076]

Polatin P et al. Pharmacological treatment of depression in geriatric chronic pain patients: a biopsychosocial approach integrating functional restoration. Expert Rev Clin Pharmacol. 2017 Sep;10(9):957–63. [PMID: 28590144]

Zhao M et al. Acupressure therapy for acute ankle sprains: a randomized clinical trial. PM R Phys Med Rehab. 2018 Jan; 10(1):36–44. [PMID: 28634002]

SELECTED INTERVENTIONAL MODALITIES FOR PAIN RELIEF

Pain management specialists are physicians who have completed a residency in anesthesiology, physical medicine and rehabilitation, neurology, internal medicine, emergency medicine, or psychiatry and usually also a fellowship in pain management to learn medication management and interventional techniques for acute, chronic, and cancer pain. Interventional pain management modalities performed by pain management specialists involve neuromodulation of specific targets to alleviate pain. The procedures they perform include percutaneous needle injection of local anesthetics and/or corticosteroids, radiofrequency (thermal) lesioning, cryotherapy, chemical neurolysis, or surgical implantation of intrathecal medication delivery pump systems or neurostimulation devices. While invasive procedures carry their own inherent risks such as bleeding or infection, they can drastically reduce or even obviate the need for conventional pharmacological therapies that may have side effects or be burdensome to the individual.

For some patients, a nerve block, such as a celiac plexus block for pain from pancreatic cancer, can provide substantial relief. Intrathecal pumps may be most useful for patients with severe pain responsive to opioids but who require such large doses that systemic side effects (eg, sedation, urinary retention, and constipation) become limiting. In the palliative care setting, these pumps are appropriate when life expectancy is long enough to justify the discomfort and cost of surgical implantation.

Clinicians do not need to know all the details of interventional pain procedures but should consider referring their patients to pain management specialists if such procedures may be beneficial. For example, a common question is whether prolonged opioid therapy with its inherent risks is better than an injection or an implanted device. Beyond knowing the benefits and risks, fiscal considerations may be key.

Tables 5–10 and 5–11 list the procedures and the agents typically used in interventional pain modalities.

INTRATHECAL DRUG DELIVERY SYSTEM

A. Indications

Intrathecal drug delivery therapy is indicated for patients with both malignant and nonmalignant pain and has been shown to be effective, cost-effective, and safe. It is generally accepted that intrathecal opioids have a 100- to 300-fold efficacy compared with oral opioids; therefore, the best candidates may be patients with good analgesic benefit from opioids but burdensome side effects. Common indications include cancer pain, chronic low-back pain (in particular, post-laminectomy syndrome), complex regional pain syndrome, and other causes of neuropathic pain. In a randomized controlled trial comparing intrathecal therapy with comprehensive medication management in cancer pain, intrathecal therapy was shown to be superior in both analgesia as well as to have fewer side effects. Due to the cost of implanting the device as well as the recovery time needed from surgical implantation, it is recommended that patients have a life expectancy of at least 2–3 months.

B. Procedure

Intrathecal drug delivery systems consist of a pump with a drug reservoir, typically implanted in the abdominal wall,

Table 5–10. Interventional techniques for chronic pain by anatomic location.

Neuraxial
  Intrathecal
  Epidural (caudal, lumbar, thoracic, cervical; interlaminar vs. transforaminal)
Paraneuraxial (planar blockade)
  Paravertebral (intercostal)
  Transversus abdominis plane/quadratus lumborum
  Pectoralis and serratus anterior
Peripheral nerve (perineural blockade)
  Brachial plexus and branches
  Lumbar plexus and branches
Joints
  Intra-articular injections
  Joint denervation procedures
Sympathetic ganglion
  Gasserian ganglion
  Sphenopalatine ganglion
  Cervical sympathetic blockade (stellate ganglion)
  Lumbar sympathetic blockade
  Celiac plexus
  Superior hypogastric plexus
  Ganglion impar
Continuous neuraxial drug delivery
  Epidural (tunneled catheter, port)
  Intrathecal (implanted intrathecal pump)
Neurostimulation
  Dorsal column stimulation (spinal cord stimulation)
  Dorsal root ganglion stimulation
  Peripheral nerve or field stimulation

Table 5–11. Agents used[1] in neuromodulatory therapies.

Voltage-gated sodium channel blockade—local anesthetics
  Lidocaine
  Mepivacaine
  Bupivacaine
  Ropivacaine
Corticosteroids
  Triamcinolone
  Methylprednisolone
  Dexamethasone
Opioids
  Morphine
  Hydromorphone
  Fentanyl
Adjuvants
  Clonidine
  Dexmedetomidine
  Others
Chemical neurolysis
  Alcohol
  Phenol
  Glycerol
Thermal neurolysis
  Radiofrequency ablation
  Cryoanalgesia
Neurostimulation
  Various patterns, frequency, amplitude, pulse width

[1]Injected or applied.
List is not comprehensive but includes most commonly used agents.

connected to a catheter that delivers medications into the intrathecal space. Initial percutaneous trialing is indicated for patients with noncancer or cancer pain; such percutaneous trialing may consist of either epidural or intrathecal delivery of bolus or continuous medication to determine efficacy and side effect profiles of planned therapeutic agent(s). Some cancer patients may not undergo a trial to avoid delaying final implantation. Subsequent implantation of an intrathecal drug delivery system involves two incisions: one in the spine to accommodate the catheter and anchor, and another in the lower abdominal region to create a pocket to hold the pump. The catheter is tunneled through the lower abdominal and flank subcutaneous tissues to connect to the pump. Both trial and implantation are typically performed under sedation with local anesthetic infiltration; spinal anesthesia delivered from the pump itself can also be utilized for pump implantation. Some patients may require general anesthesia to tolerate the implantation procedure.

C. Medications Used

According to the Polyanalgesic Conference Consensus (PACC) guidelines for both malignant and nonmalignant pain, first-line intrathecal delivery medications include monotherapy with either morphine or ziconotide, a calcium channel inhibitor. However, the PACC guidelines also state that de facto practice includes combination therapy with opioids (eg, fentanyl, hydromorphone) and local anesthetic (eg, bupivacaine) and may include other medications (eg, baclofen or clonidine). Respiratory depression and sedation are two of the most concerning side effects of many intrathecal medications. Ziconotide may cause myositis and polyarthralgias as well as psychiatric and neurologic adverse effects (it is contraindicated in patients with preexisting psychosis). Side effects of morphine and fentanyl include nausea, edema, constipation, urinary retention, and pruritus.

D. Advantages and Disadvantages

The main advantage of intrathecal delivery therapy is targeted delivery of medication to the spinal cord with increased efficacy and diminished side effects compared with systemic analgesic medications. The increased efficacy is due to the 100- to 300-fold increased concentration of intrathecal drug compared with systemic medication. However, intrathecal therapy requires regular pump refills and may be complicated by infections, catheter or pump malfunctions requiring surgical revision, or development of catheter tip granulomas, potentially leading to inadequate analgesia or neurologic deficits. Pump batteries may last from 5 years to 10 years depending on usage. Fatalities surrounding intrathecal therapy have been linked to respiratory depression; patients must be monitored for respiratory depression or sedation when initiating or increasing intrathecal therapeutic agents.

E. Alternatives

For patients with limited life expectancy, continuous epidural drug delivery via an external pump or subcutaneous port may be more appropriate. Systemic medication delivered orally, intravenously, topically, or even by a subcutaneous infusion (as in palliative care settings) are alternatives to intrathecal therapy.

SPINAL STIMULATION

A. Indications

Spinal stimulation targets lower body neuropathic pain, such as failed back surgery syndrome, complex regional pain syndrome, and radiculopathy. There is also growing literature around its use for neuropathic pain associated with cancer.

B. Procedure

Neurostimulation devices consist of an implantable pulse generator typically placed in the flank or abdomen just under the skin and an array of electrical contacts on small cylindrical or paddle leads placed in the epidural space. **Neurostimulation** devices transmit electrical pulses to the spinal cord or dorsal root ganglion to block pain transmission. Paddle leads require neurosurgical implantation with laminotomy (and general anesthesia), while percutaneous wire leads may be implanted under sedation. Patients undergo a 3- to 7-day trial during which the leads are attached to an external battery source and undergo programming with different pulse waveforms to assess therapeutic efficacy prior to surgical implantation of permanent leads and implantable pulse generator.

C. Frequencies Used

Traditional neurostimulation resulted in paresthesias that were used to mask pain. It was presumed that these paresthesias were the result of stimulation of the dorsal column axons. More recent studies have revealed that analgesia can be obtained independent of paresthesias by altering a variety of spinal cord stimulation parameters, including constant high-frequency stimulation, burst high-frequency stimulation, and closed-loop evoked compound action potential stimulation, and by stimulating targets other than the spinal cord, including stimulation of the dorsal root ganglion. These newer, more versatile systems deliver paresthesia-free analgesia with analgesic response rates that have steadily increased from about 50% with the traditional devices to about 80%. The newer devices also have greater longevity and are MRI compatible.

D. Advantages and Disadvantages

Spinal cord stimulation is a reversible technology that may provide superior analgesic efficacy while eliminating the need for systemic medications. In fact, spinal cord stimulation has now advanced to a higher position in the treatment continuum; it can be considered before using chronic moderate doses of systemic opioids. However, because it is a surgical procedure, it may be associated with complications, including infection, lead migration, device malfunction, or neurologic deficits. While MRIs were contraindicated with some older systems, most newer systems allow for limited MRI imaging. Batteries may require daily charging but typically do not require replacement for 5–10 years.

E. Alternatives

Peripheral nerve stimulation is an emerging field that targets peripheral nerves using a similar system of a lead connected to a pulse generator. It may be most appropriate when there is a very specific neurologic target. Transcutaneous electrical nerve stimulators (TENS) and systemic pharmacologic therapies are alternatives.

CELIAC PLEXUS BLOCK & NEUROLYSIS

A. Indications

A celiac plexus block refers to injection of a long-acting anesthetic (eg, bupivacaine) with or without a corticosteroid (eg, methylprednisolone); with steroids, the block can provide relief for a few weeks to months. Celiac plexus neurolysis involves injection of a neurolytic agent (eg, alcohol or phenol); it may provide pain relief more consistently for 2–6 months. The most common indication is pancreatic cancer pain, but it can be used for pain from other malignancies (eg, stomach, liver, spleen, kidney, and gastrointestinal tract) or from chronic pancreatitis. Multiple randomized controlled trials and meta-analyses have shown superiority of celiac plexus neurolysis to medication management for pancreatic cancer, but evidence of its efficacy for chronic pancreatitis is more mixed.

B. Procedure

The most common approach is a percutaneous posterior approach under fluoroscopy guidance, with bilateral needles targeted to the celiac plexus at the level of T12–L1. Alternatively, ultrasound, CT, or endoscopic guidance can be used. Minimal sedation is required for the percutaneous approaches, while heavy sedation or general anesthesia may be required for endoscopic guidance.

C. Medications Used

Chemical neurolysis with alcohol or phenol is used to extend the duration of the analgesia to 2 or more months compared to a block with local anesthetic (eg, bupivacaine) and corticosteroid (eg, methylprednisolone), which produces an analgesic duration of weeks to months. For chemical neurolysis, alcohol is used most often because it does not require compounding, and importantly has a lower chance of permanent neurologic damage compared with phenol; however, it is more painful on injection.

D. Advantages and Disadvantages

The primary advantage is improved analgesia without need for systemic medications and their untoward effects. Common side effects of celiac plexus interventions include transient hypotension and transient diarrhea. Transient or permanent spinal cord damage is rare, although there is an increased risk of its occurrence with plexus (chemical) neurolysis compared with plexus (anesthetic) block.

E. Alternatives

Standard pain management is with oral or transdermal systemic medication. Intrathecal therapy is also an alternative, especially for cancer pain.

▶ When to Refer

Patients should be referred to pain management specialists if they have:

- Pain that does not respond to opioids at typical doses or causes major adverse effects at typical doses.
- Pain that cannot be controlled expeditiously or safely by other clinicians.
- Neuropathic pain that does not respond to first-line treatments.
- Complex medication management that uses buprenorphine or methadone.
- Severe pain from malignancy, including primary disease (eg, pancreatic cancer) or metastatic disease (eg, bony metastases).

▶ When to Admit

Patients should be hospitalized if they have:

- Severe exacerbation of pain not responsive to previous stable oral opioids given around-the-clock plus breakthrough doses.
- Pain that is so severe that it cannot be controlled at home.
- Uncontrollable side effects from opioids, including nausea, vomiting, myoclonus, and altered mental status.
- Need for a surgical procedure, such as implantation of an intrathecal drug delivery pump or neurostimulation device.

Careskey H et al. Interventional anesthetic methods for pain in hematology/oncology patients. Hematol Oncol Clin North Am. 2018 Jun;32(3):433–45. [PMID: 29729779]

Deer TR et al. The Polyanalgesic Consensus Conference (PACC): recommendations on intrathecal drug infusion systems best practices and guidelines. Neuromodulation. 2017 Feb;20(2): 96–132. Erratum in: Neuromodulation. 2017 Jun;20(4):405–6. [PMID: 28042904]

Deer TR et al. The neuromodulation appropriateness consensus committee on best practices for dorsal root ganglion stimulation. Neuromodulation. 2019 Jan;22(1):1–35. [PMID: 30246899]

Sharan A et al. An overview of chronic spinal pain: revisiting diagnostic categories and exploring an evolving role for neurostimulation. Spine (Phila Pa 1976). 2017 Jul 15;42 (Suppl 14):S35–40. [PMID: 28441315]

Zheng S et al. Evaluation of intrathecal drug delivery system for intractable pain in advanced malignancies: a prospective cohort study. Medicine (Baltimore). 2017 Mar;96(11):e6354. [PMID: 28296770]

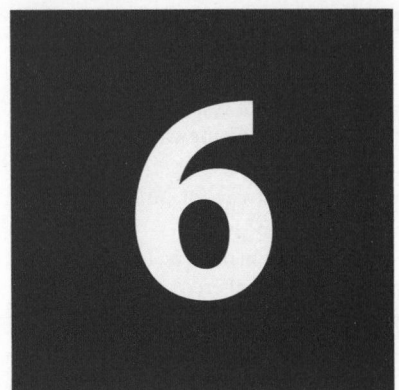

Dermatologic Disorders

Kanade Shinkai, MD, PhD

Lindy P. Fox, MD

INTRODUCTION

Dermatologic diseases are diagnosed by the types of lesions they cause. To make a diagnosis: (1) identify the type of lesion(s) the patient exhibits by morphology establishing a differential diagnosis (Table 6–1); and (2) obtain the elements of the history, physical examination, and appropriate laboratory tests to confirm the diagnosis. Specific clinical situations, such as an immunocompromised or critically ill patient, lead to different diagnostic considerations.

PRINCIPLES OF DERMATOLOGIC THERAPY

▶ Frequently Used Treatment Measures

A. Bathing

Soap should be used only in the axillae and groin and on the feet by persons with dry or inflamed skin. Soaking in water for 10–15 minutes before applying topical corticosteroids or emollient enhances their efficacy (Soak and Smear).

B. Topical Therapy

Nondermatologists should become familiar with a representative agent in each category for each indication (eg, topical corticosteroid, topical retinoid, etc).

1. Corticosteroids—Topical corticosteroid creams, lotions, ointments, gels, foams, and sprays are presented in Table 6–2. Topical corticosteroids are divided into classes based on potency. Agents within the same class are equivalent therapies; however, prices of even generic topical corticosteroids vary dramatically. **For a given agent, an ointment is more potent than a cream**. The potency of a topical corticosteroid may be dramatically increased by occlusion (covering with a water-impermeable barrier) for at least 4 hours. Depending on the location of the skin condition, gloves, plastic wrap, moist pajamas covered by dry pajamas (wet wraps), or plastic occlusive suits for patients can be used. Caution should be used in applying topical corticosteroids to areas of thin skin (face, scrotum, vulva, skin folds). Topical corticosteroid use on the eyelids may result in glaucoma or cataracts. One may estimate the amount of topical corticosteroid needed by using the "rule of nines" (as in burn evaluation; see Figure 37–2). Approximately 20–30 g is needed to cover the entire body surface of an adult. Systemic absorption does occur, but adrenal suppression, diabetes mellitus, hypertension, osteoporosis, and other complications of systemic corticosteroids are very rare with topical corticosteroid therapy.

2. Emollients for dry skin ("moisturizers")—Dry skin is a result of abnormal function of the epidermis. Emollients restore the epidermis by promoting keratinocyte differentiation and production of innate antimicrobials in skin. Many types of emollients are available. Petrolatum, mineral oil, Aquaphor, CeraVe, Cetaphil, and Eucerin cream are the heaviest and best. **Emollients are most effective when applied to wet skin but can also be used on dry skin.** If the skin is too greasy after application, pat dry with a damp towel. Vanicream is relatively allergen-free and can be used if allergic contact dermatitis to topical products is suspected.

The scaly appearance of dry skin may be improved by emollients with concomitant use of keratolytics including urea, lactic acid, or glycolic acid–containing products provided no inflammation (erythema or pruritus) is present.

3. Drying agents for weepy dermatoses—If the skin is weepy from infection or inflammation, drying agents may be beneficial. The best drying agent is water, applied as repeated compresses for 15–30 minutes, alone or with aluminum salts (Burow solution, Domeboro tablets).

4. Topical antipruritics—Lotions that contain 0.5% each of camphor and menthol (Sarna) or pramoxine hydrochloride 1% (with or without 0.5% menthol, eg, Prax, PrameGel, Aveeno Anti-Itch lotion) are effective antipruritic agents. Hydrocortisone, 1% or 2.5%, may be incorporated for its anti-inflammatory effect (Pramosone cream, lotion, or ointment). Doxepin cream 5% may reduce pruritus but may cause drowsiness. Pramoxine and doxepin are most effective when applied with topical corticosteroids. Topical capsaicin can be effective in some forms of neuropathic itch.

C. Systemic Antipruritic Drugs

1. Antihistamines and antidepressants—H_1-blockers are the agents of choice for pruritus when due to histamine, such as in urticaria. Otherwise, they appear to benefit itchy

Table 6–1. Morphologic categorization of skin lesions and diseases.

Pigmented	Freckle, lentigo, seborrheic keratosis, nevus, blue nevus, halo nevus, atypical nevus, melanoma
Scaly	Psoriasis, dermatitis (atopic, stasis, seborrheic, chronic allergic contact or irritant contact), xerosis (dry skin), lichen simplex chronicus, tinea pedis/cruris/corporis, tinea versicolor, secondary syphilis, pityriasis rosea, discoid lupus erythematosus, exfoliative dermatitis, actinic keratoses, Bowen disease, Paget disease, drug eruption
Vesicular	Herpes simplex, varicella, herpes zoster, pompholyx (vesicular dermatitis of palms and soles), vesicular tinea, autoeczematization, dermatitis herpetiformis, miliaria crystallina, scabies, photosensitivity, acute contact allergic dermatitis, drug eruption
Weepy or encrusted	Impetigo, acute contact allergic dermatitis, any vesicular dermatitis
Pustular	Acne vulgaris, acne rosacea, folliculitis, candidiasis, miliaria pustulosa, pustular psoriasis, any vesicular dermatitis, drug eruption
Figurate ("shaped") erythema	Urticaria, erythema multiforme, erythema migrans, cellulitis, erysipelas, erysipeloid, arthropod bites
Bullous	Impetigo, blistering dactylitis, pemphigus, pemphigoid, porphyria cutanea tarda, drug eruptions, erythema multiforme, toxic epidermal necrolysis
Papular	Hyperkeratotic: warts, corns, seborrheic keratoses Purple-violet: lichen planus, drug eruptions, Kaposi sarcoma, lymphoma cutis, Sweet syndrome Flesh-colored, umbilicated: molluscum contagiosum Pearly: basal cell carcinoma, intradermal nevi Small, red, inflammatory: acne, rosacea, miliaria rubra, candidiasis, scabies, folliculitis
Pruritus[1]	Xerosis, scabies, pediculosis, lichen planus, lichen simplex chronicus, bites, systemic causes, anogenital pruritus
Nodular, cystic	Erythema nodosum, furuncle, cystic acne, follicular (epidermal) inclusion cyst, metastatic tumor to skin
Photodermatitis (photodistributed rashes)	Drug eruption, polymorphic light eruption, lupus erythematosus
Morbilliform	Drug eruption, viral infection, secondary syphilis
Erosive	Any vesicular dermatitis, impetigo, aphthae, lichen planus, erythema multiforme, intertrigo
Ulcerated	Decubiti, herpes simplex, skin cancers, parasitic infections, syphilis (chancre), chancroid, vasculitis, stasis, arterial disease, pyoderma gangrenosum

[1]Not a morphologic class but included because it is one of the most common dermatologic presentations.

Table 6–2. Useful topical dermatologic therapeutic agents.

Agent	Formulations, Strengths, and Prices[1]	Frequency of Application	Potency Class	Common Indications	Comments
Corticosteroids (Listed in Order of Increasing Potency)					
Hydrocortisone acetate	Cream 1%: $1.38/30 g Ointment 1%: $3.91/40 g Solution 1%: $7.49/44 mL	Twice daily	Low	Seborrheic dermatitis Pruritus ani Intertrigo	Not the same as hydrocortisone butyrate or valerate Not for poison oak OTC lotion (Aquanil HC), OTC solution (Scalpicin)
	Cream 2.5%: $3.09/4 g			As for 1% hydrocortisone	Perhaps better for pruritus ani Not clearly better than 1% More expensive Not OTC
Alclometasone dipropionate (Aclovate)	Cream 0.05%: $48.08/15 g Ointment 0.05%: $20.00/15 g	Twice daily	Low	As for hydrocortisone	More efficacious than hydrocortisone Perhaps causes less atrophy
Desonide	Cream 0.05%: $80.29/15 g Ointment 0.05%: $60.10/15 g Lotion 0.05%: $296.10/60 mL	Twice daily	Low	As for hydrocortisone For lesions on face or body folds resistant to hydrocortisone	More efficacious than hydrocortisone Can cause rosacea or atrophy Not fluorinated

(continued)

Table 6–2. Useful topical dermatologic therapeutic agents. (continued)

Agent	Formulations, Strengths, and Prices[1]	Frequency of Application	Potency Class	Common Indications	Comments
Clocortolone (Cloderm)	Cream 0.1%: $410.06/45 g	Three times daily	Medium	Contact dermatitis Atopic dermatitis	Does not cross-react with other corticosteroids chemically and can be used in patients allergic to other corticosteroids
Prednicarbate (Dermatop)	Emollient cream 0.1%: $137.10/60 g Ointment 0.1%: $30.00/15 g	Twice daily	Medium	As for triamcinolone	May cause less atrophy No generic formulations Preservative-free
Triamcinolone acetonide	Cream 0.1%: $5.55/15 g Ointment 0.1%: $5.55/15 g Lotion 0.1%: $90.00/60 mL	Twice daily	Medium	Eczema on extensor areas Used for psoriasis with tar Seborrheic dermatitis and psoriasis on scalp	Caution in body folds, face Economical in 0.5-lb and 1-lb sizes for treatment of large body surfaces Economical as solution for scalp
	Cream 0.025%: $4.45/15 g Ointment 0.025%: $10.11/80 g	Twice daily	Medium	As for 0.1% strength	Possibly less efficacy and few advantages over 0.1% formulation
Fluocinolone acetonide	Cream 0.025%: $33.77/15 g Ointment 0.025%: $33.77/15 g	Twice daily	Medium	As for triamcinolone	
	Solution 0.01%: $180.00/60 mL	Twice daily	Medium	As for triamcinolone solution	
Mometasone furoate (Elocon)	Cream 0.1%: $6.05/15 g Ointment 0.1%: $24.30/15 g Lotion 0.1%: $57.04/60 mL	Once daily	Medium	As for triamcinolone	Often used inappropriately on the face or on children Not fluorinated
Diflorasone diacetate	Cream 0.05%: $209.68/15 g Ointment 0.05%: $209.68/15 g	Twice daily	High	Nummular dermatitis Allergic contact dermatitis Lichen simplex chronicus	
Fluocinonide (Lidex)	Cream 0.05%: $45.55/15 g Gel 0.05%: $59.56/15 g Ointment 0.05%: $28.53/15 g Solution 0.05%: $97.19/60 mL	Twice daily	High	As for betamethasone Gel useful for poison oak	Economical generics Lidex cream can cause stinging on eczema Lidex emollient cream preferred
Betamethasone dipropionate (Diprolene)	Cream 0.05%: $41.60/15 g Ointment 0.05%: $50.45/15 g Lotion 0.05%: $45.00/60 mL	Twice daily	Ultra-high	For lesions resistant to high-potency corticosteroids Lichen planus Insect bites	Economical generics available
Clobetasol propionate (Temovate)	Cream 0.05%: $68.10/15 g Ointment 0.05%: $155.45/15 g Lotion 0.05%: $289.28/60 mL	Twice daily	Ultra-high	As for betamethasone dipropionate	Somewhat more potent than diflorasone Limited to 2 continuous weeks of use Limited to 50 g or less per week Cream may cause stinging; use "emollient cream" formulation Generic available

(continued)

Table 6–2. Useful topical dermatologic therapeutic agents. (continued)

Agent	Formulations, Strengths, and Prices[1]	Frequency of Application	Potency Class	Common Indications	Comments
Halobetasol propionate (Ultravate)	Cream 0.05%: $79.58/15 g Ointment 0.05%: $79.58/15 g	Twice daily	Ultra-high	As for clobetasol	Same restrictions as clobetasol Cream does not cause stinging Compatible with calcipotriene (Dovonex)
Desoximetasone	Cream 0.05%: $62.43/15 g Cream 0.25%: $58.28/15 g Gel 0.05%: $298.38/60 g Ointment 0.25%: $18.00/15 g	Twice daily	High	As for triamcinolone	Comparable potency to fluocinonide Suggested for use when allergic contact dermatitis to topical corticosteroid is suspected; ointment useful when allergic contact dermatitis to propylene glycol is suspected
Flurandrenolide (Cordran)	Tape: $816.46/24" × 3" roll Lotion 0.05%: $394.68/60 mL	Every 12 hours	Ultra-high	Lichen simplex chronicus	Tape version protects the skin and prevents scratching
Nonsteroidal Anti-inflammatory Agents (Listed Alphabetically)					
Crisaborole (Eucrisa)	Ointment 2%: $759.89/60 g	Twice daily	N/A	Atopic dermatitis	Steroid substitute not causing atrophy or striae May sting or burn on initial application
Pimecrolimus[2] (Elidel)	Cream 1%: $643.25/60 g	Twice daily	N/A	Atopic dermatitis	Steroid substitute not causing atrophy or striae
Tacrolimus[2] (Protopic)	Ointment 0.1%: $520.90/60 g Ointment 0.03%: $520.90/60 g	Twice daily	N/A	Atopic dermatitis	Steroid substitute not causing atrophy or striae Burns in ≥ 40% of patients with eczema
Antibiotics (for Acne) (Listed Alphabetically)					
Clindamycin phosphate	Solution 1%: $28.94/30 mL Gel 1%: $86.38/30 mL Lotion 1%: $120.18/60 mL Pledget 1%: $46.40/60	Twice daily	N/A	Mild papular acne	Lotion is less drying for patients with sensitive skin Recommend use with benzoyl peroxide to avoid antibiotic resistance from monotherapy
Clindamycin/Benzoyl peroxide (BenzaClin)	Gel: $204.19/25 g Gel: $408.35/50 g	Twice daily	N/A	As for benzamycin	No generic More effective than either agent alone
Dapsone	Gel 5%: $585.50/60 g	Once daily	N/A	Mild papulopustular acne	More expensive, well tolerated Recommend use with benzoyl peroxide to avoid antibiotic resistance from monotherapy
Erythromycin	Solution 2%: $47.63/60 mL Gel 2%: $60.48/30 g Pledget 2%: $92.65/60	Twice daily	N/A	As for clindamycin	Many different manufacturers Economical Recommend use with benzoyl peroxide to avoid antibiotic resistance from monotherapy
Erythromycin/ Benzoyl peroxide (Benzamycin)	Gel: $199.08/23.3 g Gel: $90.00/46.6 g	Twice daily	N/A	As for clindamycin Can help treat comedonal acne	No generics More expensive More effective than other topical antibiotics Main jar requires refrigeration

(continued)

Table 6–2. Useful topical dermatologic therapeutic agents. (continued)

Agent	Formulations, Strengths, and Prices[1]	Frequency of Application	Potency Class	Common Indications	Comments
Antibiotics (for Impetigo)					
Mupirocin (Bactroban)	Ointment 2%: $11.25/22 g Cream 2%: $245.16/15 g	Three times daily	N/A	Impetigo, folliculitis	Because of cost, use limited to tiny areas of impetigo Used in the nose twice daily for 5 days to reduce staphylococcal carriage
Retapamulin (Altabax)	Ointment 1%: $360.04/15 g	Twice daily	N/A	Impetigo	For *Staphylococcus aureus* or *Streptococcus pyogenes* infection Typically reserved for mupirocin-resistant infections
Antifungals: Imidazoles (Listed Alphabetically)					
Clotrimazole	Cream 1%: $5.29/15 g OTC Solution 1%: $36.06/10 mL	Twice daily	N/A	Dermatophyte and *Candida* infections	Available OTC Inexpensive generic cream available
Econazole (Spectazole)	Cream 1%: $30.04/15 g	Once daily	N/A	As for clotrimazole	Somewhat more effective than clotrimazole and miconazole
Ketoconazole	Cream 2%: $30.90/15 g	Once daily	N/A	As for clotrimazole	Somewhat more effective than clotrimazole and miconazole
Miconazole	Cream 2%: $3.30/30 g OTC	Twice daily	N/A	As for clotrimazole	As for clotrimazole
Oxiconazole (Oxistat)	Cream 1%: $614.73/30 g Lotion 1%: $771.91/30 mL	Twice daily	N/A	As for clotrimazole	
Sertaconazole (Ertaczo)	Cream 2%: $1079.41/60 g	Twice daily	N/A	Refractory tinea pedis	By prescription More expensive
Sulconazole (Exelderm)	Cream 1%: $72.38/15 g Solution 1%: $449.72/30 mL	Twice daily	N/A	As for clotrimazole	No generic Somewhat more effective than clotrimazole and miconazole
Other Antifungals (Listed Alphabetically)					
Butenafine (Mentax)	Cream 1%: $117.68/15 g	Once daily	N/A	Dermatophytes	Fast response; high cure rate; expensive Available OTC
Ciclopirox (Loprox) (Penlac)	Cream 0.77%: $51.10/30 g Lotion 0.77%: $80.68/30 g Solution 8%: $52.95/6.6 mL	Twice daily	N/A	As for clotrimazole	No generic Somewhat more effective than clotrimazole and miconazole
Efinaconazole (Jublia)	Solution 10%: $687.38/4 mL	Once daily for 48 weeks	N/A	Onychomycosis	No generic; more effective than ciclopirox for nail disease
Naftifine (Naftin)	Cream 1%: $375.38/60 g Gel 1%: $497.51/60 mL	Once daily	N/A	Dermatophytes	No generic Somewhat more effective than clotrimazole and miconazole
Tavaborole (Kerydin)	Solution 5%: $725.21/4 mL	Once daily for 48 weeks	N/A	Onychomycosis	No generic available
Terbinafine (Lamisil)	Cream 1%: $8.72/12 g OTC	Once daily	N/A	Dermatophytes	Fast clinical response OTC
Antipruritics (Listed Alphabetically)					
Camphor/menthol (Sarna)	Lotion 0.5%/0.5%: $7.80/222 mL	Two to three times daily	N/A	Mild eczema, xerosis, mild contact dermatitis	

(continued)

Table 6–2. Useful topical dermatologic therapeutic agents. (continued)

Agent	Formulations, Strengths, and Prices[1]	Frequency of Application	Potency Class	Common Indications	Comments
Capsaicin (various)	Cream 0.025–0.1% Cream 0.025%: $9.95/60 g Cream 0.075%: $10.39/56 g	Three to four times daily	N/A	Topical antipruritic, best used for neuropathic itching	Burning/stinging with initial application that subsides with consistent ongoing use
Doxepin (Zonalon)	Cream 5%: $722.32/45 g	Four times daily	N/A	Topical antipruritic, best used in combination with appropriate topical corticosteroid to enhance efficacy	Can cause sedation
Pramoxine hydrochloride (Prax)	Lotion 1%: $17.86/120 mL OTC	Four times daily	N/A	Dry skin, varicella, mild eczema, pruritus ani	OTC formulations (Prax, Aveeno Anti-Itch Cream or Lotion; Itch-X Gel) By prescription mixed with 1% or 2% hydrocortisone
Emollients (Listed Alphabetically)					
Aqua glycolic	Cream, lotion, shampoo, others: $17.94/177 mL	Once to three times daily	N/A	Xerosis, ichthyosis, keratosis pilaris Mild facial wrinkles Mild acne or seborrheic dermatitis	Contains 8% glycolic acid Available from other makers, eg, Alpha Hydrox, or generic 8% glycolic acid lotion May cause stinging on eczematous skin
Aquaphor	Ointment: $5.49/50 g	Once to three times daily	N/A	Xerosis, eczema For protection of area in pruritus ani	Not as greasy as petrolatum
Aveeno	Cream, lotion, cleanser, others: $7.18/354 mL	Once to three times daily	N/A	Xerosis, eczema	Many formulations made Some facial and body moisturizers contain sunscreen
Ceratopic cream	Cream: $35.00/2 oz	Twice daily	N/A	Xerosis, eczema	Contains ceramide; anti-inflammatory and nongreasy moisturizer
CeraVe	Cream, lotion, cleanser, others: $13.29/453 g	Once to three times daily	N/A	Xerosis, eczema	Many formulations made CeraVe SA formulation contains salicylic acid, ammonium lactate as keratolytics Some facial and body moisturizers contain sunscreen
Cetaphil	$10.50/480 mL	Once to three times daily	N/A	Xerosis, eczema	Many formulations made Some facial and body moisturizers contain sunscreen
Complex 15[3]	Lotion: $6.48/240 mL Cream: $4.82/75 g	Once to three times daily	N/A	Xerosis Lotion or cream recommended for split or dry nails	Active ingredient is a phospholipid
DML	Cream, lotion, facial moisturizer: $5.95/240 mL	Once to three times daily	N/A	As for Complex 15	Face cream has sunscreen
Eucerin	Cream: $9.45/454 g Lotion: $3.75/120 mL	Once to three times daily	N/A	Xerosis, eczema	Many formulations made Eucerin Plus contains alphahydroxy acid and may cause stinging on eczematous skin Facial moisturizer has SPF 25 sunscreen
Lac-Hydrin-Five	Lotion: $13.25/226 g OTC	Twice daily	N/A	Xerosis, ichthyosis, keratosis pilaris	Most effective strength is 12% May sting on eczematous skin
Lubriderm	Lotion: $6.13/473 mL	Once to three times daily	N/A	Xerosis, eczema	Unscented usually preferred

(continued)

Table 6–2. Useful topical dermatologic therapeutic agents. (continued)

Agent	Formulations, Strengths, and Prices[1]	Frequency of Application	Potency Class	Common Indications	Comments
Neutrogena	Cream, lotion, facial moisturizer: $8.05/240 mL	Once to three times daily	N/A	Xerosis, eczema	Face cream has titanium-based sunscreen
U-Lactin	Lotion: $16.73/480 mL OTC	Once daily	N/A	Hyperkeratotic heels	Moisturizes and removes keratin May sting on eczematous skin
Urea (various)	Cream 20%: $10.37/85 g Lotion 10%: $8.64/240 mL	Twice daily	N/A	Xerosis	Contains urea as humectant Nongreasy hydrating agent (10%); debrides keratin (20%, 40%)
Vanicream	Lotion, cream, cleanser, others: $12.99/453 g	Once to three times daily	N/A	Xerosis, eczema	Many formulations available Branded as hypoallergenic

[1]Average wholesale price (AWP, for AB-rated generic when available) for quantity listed. AWP may not accurately represent the actual pharmacy cost because wide contractual variations exist among institutions. Source: IBM Micromedex. Red Book (electronic version). Watson Health, Greenwood Village, CO, USA. Available at https://www.micromedexsolutions.com/ (cited March 12, 2019.)
[2]Topical tacrolimus and pimecrolimus should be used only when other topical treatments are ineffective. Treatment should be limited to an area and duration to be as brief as possible. Treatment with these agents should be avoided in persons with known immunosuppression, HIV infection, bone marrow and organ transplantation, lymphoma, at high risk for lymphoma, and those with a prior history of lymphoma.
[3]Discontinued in the United States; available in Canada.
N/A, not applicable; OTC, over-the-counter.

patients only by their sedating effects. Hydroxyzine 25–50 mg orally at night is a typical dose. Sedating and nonsedating antihistamines are of limited value for the treatment of pruritus associated with inflammatory skin disease. Agents that may treat pruritus better include antidepressants (such as doxepin, mirtazapine, and paroxetine) as well as agents that may act either centrally or peripherally directly on the neurons that perceive or modulate pruritus (such as gabapentin, pregabalin, and duloxetine). Aprepitant and opioid antagonists, such as naltrexone and butorphanol, can be very effective in select patients, but their exact role in the management of the pruritic patient is not yet defined.

2. Systemic corticosteroids—(See Chapter 26.)

American Academy of Dermatology. Medical student core curriculum. http://www.aad.org/education-and-quality-care/medical-student-core-curriculum
Jewell JR et al. Topical therapy primer for nondermatologists. Med Clin North Am. 2015 Nov;99(6):1167–82. [PMID: 26476246]
McEwen MW et al. Drugs on the horizon for chronic pruritus. Dermatol Clin. 2018 Jul;36(3):335–44. [PMID: 29929605]
van Zuuren EJ et al. Emollients and moisturisers for eczema: abridged Cochrane systematic review including GRADE assessments. Br J Dermatol. 2017 Nov;177(5):1256–71. [PMID: 28432721]

Sunscreens

Protection from ultraviolet light should begin at birth and will reduce the incidence of actinic keratoses, melanoma, and some nonmelanoma skin cancers when initiated at any age and in any skin type. The best protection is shade, but protective clothing, avoidance of direct sun exposure during the peak hours of the day, and daily use of sunscreens are important.

Fair-complexioned persons should use a sunscreen with a sun protective factor (SPF) of at least 30 every day. Clinicians should reinforce regular sunscreen use. Sunscreens with protection against UVA as well as UVB are helpful in managing photosensitivity disorders. The actual SPF achieved relies on adequate application compared with the amount used in tests to determine the listed SPF. Repeated daily applications enhance sunscreen efficacy. Aggressive sunscreen use should be accompanied by vitamin D supplementation in persons at risk for osteopenia.

Henrikson NB et al. Behavioral counseling for skin cancer prevention: evidence report and systematic review for the US Preventive Services Task Force. JAMA. 2018 Mar 20;319(11):1143–57. [PMID: 29558557]
Mancuso JB et al. Sunscreens: an update. Am J Clin Dermatol. 2017 Oct;18(5):643–50. [PMID: 28510141]
Sánchez G et al. Sun protection for preventing basal cell and squamous cell skin cancers. Cochrane Database Syst Rev. 2016 Jul 25;7:CD011161. [PMID: 27455163]

Complications of Topical Dermatologic Therapy

Complications of topical therapy can be largely avoided. They fall into several categories: allergy, irritation, and other side effects. Reactions may result from the active or inactive ingredients, including fragrances and preservatives.

A. Allergy

Of the topical antibiotics, neomycin and bacitracin have the greatest potential for sensitization. Diphenhydramine, benzocaine, vitamin E, aromatic oils, preservatives, fragrances, tea tree oil, and even the topical corticosteroids themselves can cause allergic contact dermatitis.

B. Irritation

Preparations of tretinoin, benzoyl peroxide, and other acne medications should be applied sparingly to the skin.

C. Other Side Effects

Topical corticosteroids may induce acne-like lesions on the face (steroid rosacea) and atrophic striae in body folds.

▼ COMMON DERMATOSES

PIGMENTED LESIONS

MELANOCYTIC NEVI (Normal Moles)

In general, a benign mole is a small (less than 6 mm) macule or papule with a well-defined border and homogeneous beige or pink to dark brown pigment. They represent benign melanocytic growths.

Moles have a typical natural history. Early in life, moles often appear as flat, small, brown lesions and are termed "junctional nevi" because the nevus cells are at the junction of the epidermis and dermis. Over time, these moles enlarge and often become raised, reflecting the appearance of a dermal component, giving rise to "compound nevi" (Figure 6–1). Moles may darken and grow during pregnancy. As white patients enter their eighth decade, most moles have lost their junctional component and dark pigmentation. At every stage of life, normal moles should be well demarcated, symmetric, and uniform in contour and color. Regular mole screening is not an evidence-based recommendation for all adults although rates of screening continue to rise.

Linos E et al. Skin cancer—the importance of prevention. JAMA Intern Med. 2016 Oct 1;176(10):1435–6. [PMID: 27459394]
Livingston EH. JAMA patient page. Screening for skin cancer. JAMA. 2016 Jul 26;316(4):470. [PMID: 27458970]

Watts CG et al. Clinical practice guidelines for identification, screening and follow-up of individuals at high risk of primary cutaneous melanoma: a systematic review. Br J Dermatol. 2015 Jan;172(1):33–47. [PMID: 25204572]

ATYPICAL NEVI

The term "atypical nevus" or "atypical mole" has supplanted "dysplastic nevus." The diagnosis of atypical moles is made clinically and not histologically, and moles should be removed only if they are suspected to be melanomas. Dermoscopy by a trained clinician may be a useful tool in the evaluation of atypical nevi. Clinically, these moles are large (6 mm or more in diameter), with an ill-defined, irregular border and irregularly distributed pigmentation (Figure 6–2). It is estimated that 5–10% of the white population in the United States has one or more atypical nevi, and recreational sun exposure is a primary risk for the development of atypical nevi in nonfamilial settings. Studies have defined an increased risk of melanoma in the following populations: patients with 50 or more nevi with one or more atypical moles and one mole at least 8 mm or larger, and patients with any number of definitely atypical moles. These patients should be educated in how to recognize changes in moles and be monitored regularly (every 6–12 months) by a clinician. Kindreds with familial melanoma (numerous atypical nevi and a family history of two first-degree relatives with melanoma) deserve even closer attention, as the risk of developing single or even multiple melanomas in these individuals approaches 50% by age 50.

Kim CC et al. Addressing the knowledge gap in clinical recommendations for management and complete excision of clinically atypical nevi/dysplastic nevi: Pigmented Lesion Subcommittee consensus statement. JAMA Dermatol. 2015 Feb 1;151(2):212–8. [PMID: 25409291]

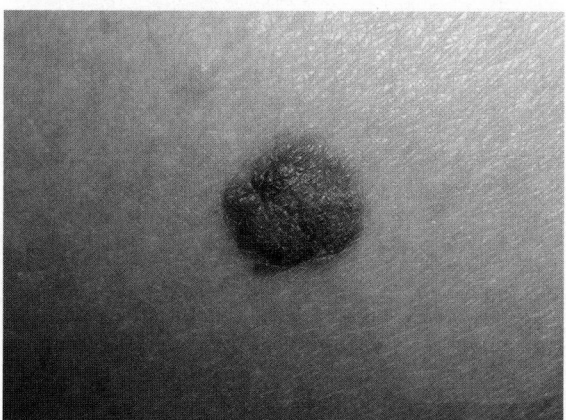

▲ **Figure 6–1.** Benign, compound nevus on the back. (Used, with permission, from Richard P. Usatine, MD, in Usatine RP, Smith MA, Mayeaux EJ Jr, Chumley H. *The Color Atlas of Family Medicine,* 2nd ed. McGraw-Hill, 2013.)

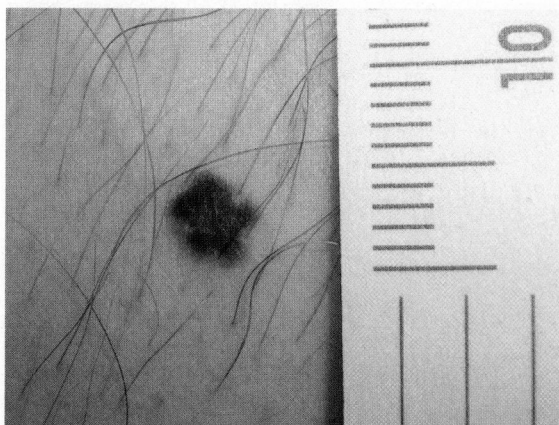

▲ **Figure 6–2.** Atypical (dysplastic) nevus on the chest. Note irregular border and variegation in color. (Used, with permission, from Richard P. Usatine, MD, in Usatine RP, Smith MA, Mayeaux EJ Jr, Chumley H. *The Color Atlas of Family Medicine,* 2nd ed. McGraw-Hill, 2013.)

BLUE NEVI

Blue nevi are small, slightly elevated, blue-black lesions (Figure 6–3) that favor the dorsal hands. They are common in persons of Asian descent, and an individual patient may have several of them. If the lesion has remained unchanged for years, it may be considered benign, since malignant blue nevi are rare. However, blue-black papules and nodules that are new or growing must be evaluated to rule out nodular melanoma.

Borgenvik TL et al. Blue nevus-like and blue nevus-associated melanoma: a comprehensive review of the literature. ANZ J Surg. 2017 May;87(5):345–9. [PMID: 28318130]

Zembowicz A. Blue nevi and related tumors. Clin Lab Med. 2017 Sep;37(3):401–15. [PMID: 28802492]

FRECKLES & LENTIGINES

Freckles (ephelides) and lentigines are flat brown macules, typically between 3 mm and 5 mm in diameter. Freckles first appear in young children, darken with ultraviolet exposure, and fade with cessation of sun exposure. They

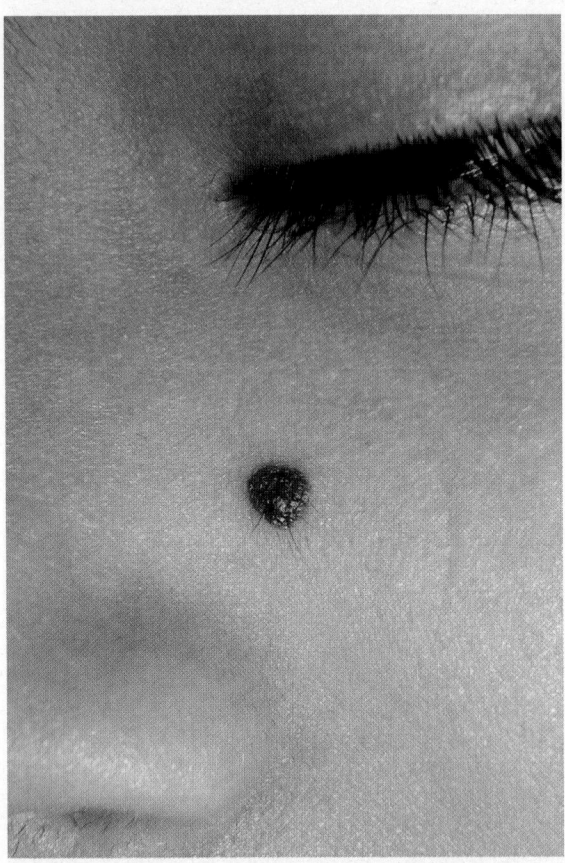

▲ **Figure 6–3.** Blue nevus on the left cheek, a darkly pigmented blue-black macule with some resemblance to a melanoma due to its dark pigmentation. (Used, with permission, from Richard P. Usatine, MD, in Usatine RP, Smith MA, Mayeaux EJ Jr, Chumley H, Tysinger J. *The Color Atlas of Family Medicine.* McGraw-Hill, 2009.)

are determined by genetic factors. In adults, lentigines gradually appear in sun-exposed areas, particularly the face, dorsal hands, upper back, and upper chest, starting in the fourth to fifth decade of life, and are associated with photoaging as well as estrogen and progesterone use. On the upper back, they may have a very irregular border (inkspot lentigines). They do not fade with cessation of sun exposure. They should be evaluated like all pigmented lesions: if the pigmentation is homogeneous and they are symmetric and flat, they are most likely benign. They can be treated with topical retinoids such as 0.1% tretinoin or 0.1% tazarotene, hydroquinone, laser/light therapy, or cryotherapy.

Hexsel D et al. Triple combination as adjuvant to cryotherapy in the treatment of solar lentigines: investigator-blinded, randomized clinical trial. J Eur Acad Dermatol Venereol. 2015 Jan;29(1):128–33. [PMID: 24684165]

SEBORRHEIC KERATOSES

Seborrheic keratoses are benign papules and plaques, beige to brown or even black, 3–20 mm in diameter, with a velvety or warty surface (Figure 6–4). They appear to be stuck or pasted onto the skin. They are extremely common—especially in older adults—and may be mistaken for melanomas or other types of cutaneous neoplasms. Although they may be frozen with liquid nitrogen or curetted if they itch or are inflamed, no treatment is needed.

Jackson JM et al. Current understanding of seborrheic keratosis: prevalence, etiology, clinical presentation, diagnosis, and management. J Drugs Dermatol. 2015 Oct;14(10):1119–25. [PMID: 26461823]

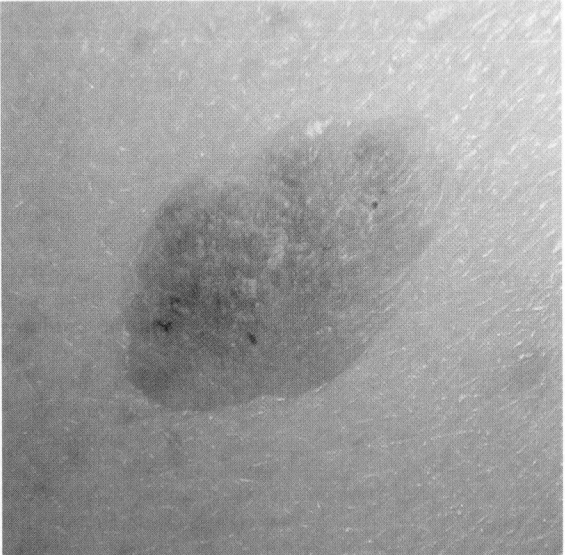

▲ **Figure 6–4.** Seborrheic keratosis with light pigmentation, with waxy, dry, "stuck-on appearance." (Used, with permission, from Richard P. Usatine, MD, in Usatine RP, Smith MA, Mayeaux EJ Jr, Chumley H. *The Color Atlas of Family Medicine,* 2nd ed. McGraw-Hill, 2013.)

MALIGNANT MELANOMA

ESSENTIALS OF DIAGNOSIS

▸ May be flat or raised.

▸ Should be suspected in any pigmented skin lesion with recent change in appearance.

▸ Examination with good light may show varying colors, including red, white, black, and blue.

▸ Borders typically irregular.

General Considerations

Malignant melanoma is the leading cause of death due to skin disease and the fifth most common cancer. The reported incidence of melanoma has doubled over the past 30 years. In 2017, approximately 87,110 new melanomas were diagnosed in the United States, with approximately 60% of cases in men. Each year melanoma causes an estimated 9730 deaths (two-thirds in men). One in four cases of melanoma occurs before the age of 40. Increased detection of early melanomas has led to increased survival, but melanoma fatalities continue to increase, especially in men older than 70 years. The lifetime risk of melanoma is 2% in whites, and 0.1–0.5% in nonwhites.

Tumor thickness is the single most important prognostic factor. Ten-year survival rates—related to thickness in millimeters—are as follows: less than 1 mm, 95%; 1–2 mm, 80%; 2–4 mm, 55%; and greater than 4 mm, 30%. With lymph node involvement, the 5-year survival rate is 62%; with distant metastases, it is 16%.

Clinical Findings

Primary malignant melanomas may be classified into various clinicohistologic types, including lentigo maligna melanoma (arising on chronically sun-exposed skin of older individuals); superficial spreading malignant melanoma (two-thirds of all melanomas arising on intermittently sun-exposed skin); nodular malignant melanoma; acral-lentiginous melanomas (arising on palms, soles, and nail beds); ocular melanoma; and malignant melanomas on mucous membranes. These different clinical types of melanoma appear to have different oncogenic mutations, which may be important in the treatment of patients with advanced disease. Clinical features of pigmented lesions suspicious for melanoma are an irregular, notched border where the pigment appears to be spreading into the normal surrounding skin, and surface topography that may be irregular, ie, partly raised and partly flat (Figure 6–5). Color variegation is present and is an important indication for referral. A useful mnemonic is the ABCDE rule: "ABCDE = Asymmetry, Border irregularity, Color variegation, Diameter greater than 6 mm, and Evolution." **The history of a changing mole (evolution) is the single most important historical reason for close evaluation and possible referral.** Bleeding and ulceration are

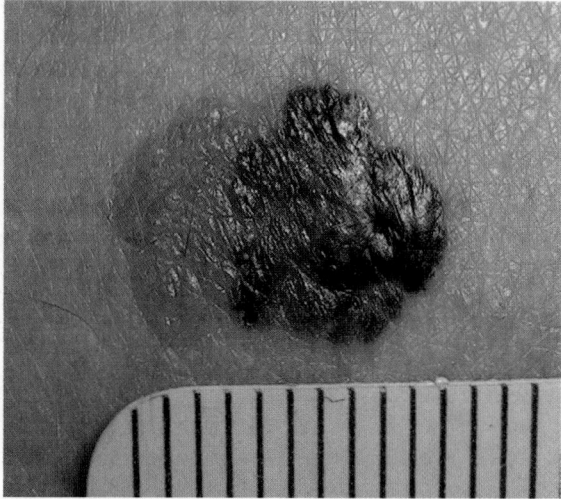

▲ **Figure 6–5.** Malignant melanoma. Note the classic "ABCDE" features: asymmetry, irregular border, multiple colors, diameter greater than 6 mm, and evolution or change. (Used, with permission, from Richard P. Usatine, MD, in Usatine RP, Smith MA, Mayeaux EJ Jr, Chumley H. *The Color Atlas of Family Medicine,* 2nd ed. McGraw-Hill, 2013.)

ominous signs. A mole that appears distinct from the patient's other moles deserves special scrutiny—the "ugly duckling sign." A patient with a large number of moles is statistically at increased risk for melanoma and deserves annual total body skin examination by a primary care clinician or dermatologist, particularly if the lesions are atypical. Referral of suspicious pigmented lesions is always appropriate.

While superficial spreading melanoma is largely a disease of whites, persons of other races are at risk for this and other types of melanoma, particularly acral lentiginous melanomas. These occur as dark, irregularly shaped lesions on the palms and soles and as new, often broad and solitary, darkly pigmented, longitudinal streaks in the nails, typically with involvement of the proximal nail fold. Acral lentiginous melanoma may be a difficult or delayed diagnosis because benign pigmented lesions of the hands, feet, and nails occur commonly in more darkly pigmented persons, and clinicians may hesitate to biopsy these sites. Clinicians should give special attention to new or changing lesions in these areas.

Treatment

Treatment of melanoma starts with excision. After histologic diagnosis, reexcision is recommended with margins dictated by the thickness of the tumor. Surgical margins of 0.5–1 cm for melanoma in situ and 1 cm for lesions less than 1 mm in thickness are recommended.

Sentinel lymph node biopsy (selective lymphadenectomy) using preoperative lymphoscintigraphy and intraoperative lymphatic mapping is effective for staging melanoma patients with intermediate risk without clinical adenopathy and is recommended for all patients with lesions over 1 mm in thickness or with high-risk histologic features (ulceration). This procedure may not confer a survival advantage. Referral of intermediate-risk and high-risk patients to centers with expertise in melanoma is strongly recommended. Identifying the oncogenic mutations in patients with advanced melanoma may dictate targeted therapy, most commonly to specific BRAF mutations. Additionally, immunotherapy treatments directed toward immune costimulatory molecules such as PD-1 can activate systemic immune-directed destruction of metastatic melanoma.

Faries MB et al. Completion dissection or observation for sentinel-node metastasis in melanoma. N Engl J Med. 2017 Jun 8;376(23):2211–22. [PMID: 28591523]

Higgins HW 2nd et al. Melanoma in situ: Part I. Epidemiology, screening, and clinical features. J Am Acad Dermatol. 2015 Aug; 73(2):181–90. [PMID: 26183967]

Higgins HW 2nd et al. Melanoma in situ: Part II. Histopathology, treatment, and clinical management. J Am Acad Dermatol. 2015Aug;73(2):193–203. [PMID: 26183968]

Luke JJ et al. Targeted agents and immunotherapies: optimizing outcomes in melanoma. Nat Rev Clin Oncol. 2017 Aug; 14(8):463–82. [PMID: 28374786]

SCALING DISORDERS

ATOPIC DERMATITIS

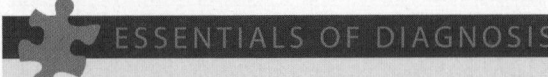

ESSENTIALS OF DIAGNOSIS

▶ Pruritic, xerotic, exudative, or lichenified eruption on face, neck, upper trunk, wrists, and hands and in the antecubital and popliteal folds.

▶ Personal or family history of atopy (eg, asthma, allergic rhinitis, atopic dermatitis).

▶ Tendency to recur.

▶ Onset in childhood in most patients. Onset after age 30 is very uncommon.

General Considerations

Atopic dermatitis (also known as eczema) has distinct presentations in people of different ages and races. Diagnostic criteria for atopic dermatitis must include pruritus, typical morphology and distribution (flexural lichenification, hand eczema, nipple eczema, and eyelid eczema in adults), onset in childhood, and chronicity. Also helpful are (1) a personal or family history of atopy (asthma, allergic rhinitis, atopic dermatitis), (2) xerosis-ichthyosis, (3) facial pallor with infraorbital darkening, (4) elevated serum IgE, and (5) repeated skin infections.

Clinical Findings

A. Symptoms and Signs

Itching is a key clinical feature and may be severe and prolonged. Ill-defined, scaly, red plaques affect the face, neck,

and upper trunk. The flexural surfaces of elbows and knees are often involved. In chronic cases, the skin is dry and lichenified. In dark-skinned patients with severe disease, pigmentation may be lost in lichenified areas. During acute flares, widespread redness with weeping, either diffusely or in discrete plaques, is common. Since virtually all patients with atopic dermatitis have skin disease before age 5, a new diagnosis of atopic dermatitis in an adult over age 30 should be made only after consultation with a dermatologist.

B. Laboratory Findings

Food allergy is an uncommon cause of flares of atopic dermatitis in adults. Eosinophilia and increased serum IgE levels may be present.

▶ Differential Diagnosis

Atopic dermatitis must be distinguished from seborrheic dermatitis (less pruritic, frequent scalp and central face involvement, greasy and scaly lesions, and quick response to therapy). Psoriasis is marked by sharply demarcated thickly scaled plaques on elbows, knees, scalp, and intergluteal cleft. Secondary staphylococcal or herpetic infections may exacerbate atopic dermatitis and should be considered during hyperacute, weeping flares of atopic dermatitis. An infra-auricular fissure is a cardinal sign of secondary infection.

▶ Treatment

Patient education regarding gentle skin care and exactly how to use medications is critical to successful management of atopic dermatitis.

A. General Measures

Atopic patients have hyperirritable skin. Anything that dries or irritates the skin will potentially trigger dermatitis. Atopic individuals are sensitive to low humidity and often flare in the winter. Adults with atopic disorders should not bathe more than once daily. Soap should be confined to the armpits, groin, scalp, and feet. Washcloths and brushes should not be used. After rinsing, the skin should be patted dry (not rubbed) and then immediately—within minutes—covered with a thin film of an emollient or a corticosteroid as needed. Vanicream can be used if contact dermatitis resulting from additives in medication is suspected. Atopic patients may be irritated by rough fabrics, including wools and acrylics. Cottons are preferable, but synthetic blends also are tolerated. Other triggers of atopic dermatitis in some patients include sweating, ointments, and heat.

B. Local Treatment

Corticosteroids should be applied sparingly to the dermatitis once or twice daily and rubbed in well. Their potency should be appropriate to the severity of the dermatitis. In general, for treatment of lesions on the body (excluding genitalia, axillary or crural folds), one should begin with triamcinolone 0.1% or a stronger corticosteroid, then taper to hydrocortisone or another slightly stronger mild corticosteroid (alclometasone, desonide). **It is vital that** patients taper off corticosteroids and substitute emol-lients as the dermatitis clears to avoid side effects of corticosteroids. Tapering is also important to avoid rebound flares of the dermatitis that may follow their abrupt cessation. Tacrolimus ointment (Protopic 0.03% or 0.1%), pimecrolimus cream (Elidel 1%), and crisaborole (Eucrisa 2%) can be effective in managing atopic dermatitis when applied twice daily. Burning on application occurs in about 50% of patients using Protopic and in 10–25% of Elidel users, but it may resolve with continued treatment. These noncorticosteroid medications do not cause skin atrophy or striae, avoiding the complications of long-term topical corticosteroid use. They are safe for application on the face and even the eyelids but are more expensive than generic topical corticosteroids.

There is a Food and Drug Administration (FDA) black box warning for both topical tacrolimus and pimecrolimus due to concerns about the development of T-cell lym-phoma. The agents should be used sparingly and only in locations where less expensive corticosteroids cannot be used. They should be avoided in patients at high risk for lymphoma (ie, those with HIV, iatrogenic immunosup-pression, or prior lymphoma).

The treatment of atopic dermatitis is dictated by the pattern and stage of the dermatitis—acute/weepy, sub-acute/scaly, or chronic/lichenified.

1. Acute weeping lesions—Staphylococcal or herpetic superinfection should be formally excluded. Use water or aluminum subacetate solution (Domeboro or burow solu-tion), or colloidal oatmeal as a bath or as wet dressings for 10–30 minutes two to four times daily. Lesions on extremi-ties may be bandaged for protection at night. Use high-potency corticosteroids after soaking, but spare the face and body folds. Tacrolimus is usually not tolerated at this stage. Systemic corticosteroids may be required.

2. Subacute or scaly lesions—At this stage, the lesions are dry but still red and pruritic. Mid- to high-potency corticosteroids in ointment form should be continued until skin lesions are cleared and itching is decreased substantially. At that point, patients should begin a 2- to 4-week taper from twice-daily to daily dosing with topical corticosteroids to reliance on emollients, with occasional use of corticosteroids only to inflamed areas. It is prefer-able to switch to daily use of a low-potency corticosteroid instead of further tapering the frequency of usage of a more potent corticosteroid. Tacrolimus and pimecroli-mus may be substituted if corticosteroids cannot be stopped completely.

3. Chronic, dry, lichenified lesions—Thickened and usu-ally well demarcated, they are best treated with high-potency to ultra–high-potency corticosteroid ointments. Nightly occlusion for 2–6 weeks may enhance the initial response. Adding tar preparations, such as liquor carbonis detergens (LCD) 10% in Aquaphor or 2% crude coal tar may be beneficial.

4. Maintenance treatment—Once symptoms have improved, constant application of effective moisturizers is recommended to prevent flares. In patients with moderate disease, use of topical anti-inflammatories only on week-ends or three times weekly can prevent flares.

C. Systemic and Adjuvant Therapy

Systemic corticosteroids are indicated only for severe acute exacerbations. Oral prednisone dosages should be high enough to suppress the dermatitis quickly, usually starting with 1 mg/kg daily. The dosage is then tapered off over a period of 2–4 weeks. Owing to the chronic nature of atopic dermatitis and the side effects of long-term systemic corti-costeroids, ongoing use of these agents is not recom-mended for maintenance therapy. Bedtime doses of hydroxyzine, diphenhydramine, or doxepin may be helpful via their sedative properties to mitigate perceived pruritus. Dupilumab is a targeted immunomodulator with minimal systemic adverse effects and requires minimal laboratory monitoring. Oral cyclosporine, mycophenolate mofetil, methotrexate, tofacitinib, or azathioprine may also be used for the most severe and recalcitrant cases.

▶ Complications of Treatment

The clinician should monitor for skin atrophy. Eczema herpeticum, a generalized herpes simplex infection mani-fested by monomorphic vesicles, crusts, or scalloped erosions superimposed on atopic dermatitis or other extensive eczematous processes, is treated successfully with oral acyclovir, 200 mg five times daily, or intravenous acy-clovir in a dose of 10 mg/kg intravenously every 8 hours (500 mg/m^2 every 8 hours). Fissures, crusts, erosions, or pustules indicate staphylococcal or herpetic infection clini-cally. Systemic antistaphylococcal antibiotics—such as a first-generation cephalosporin or doxycycline if methicil-lin-resistant *Staphylococcus aureus* is suspected—should be given only if indicated and guided by bacterial culture. Cultures to exclude methicillin-resistant *S aureus* are rec-ommended. In this setting, continuing and augmenting the topical anti-inflammatory treatment often improves the dermatitis despite the presence of infection.

▶ Prognosis

Atopic dermatitis runs a chronic or intermittent course. Affected adults may have only hand dermatitis. Poor prog-nostic factors for persistence into adulthood in atopic der-matitis include generalized disease or onset early in childhood and asthma. Only 40–60% of these patients have lasting remissions.

Blauvelt A et al. Long-term management of moderate-to-severe atopic dermatitis with dupilumab and concomitant topical corticosteroids (LIBERTY AD CHRONOS): a 1-year, randomised, double-blinded, placebo-controlled, phase 3 trial. Lancet. 2017 Jun 10;389(10086):2287–303. [PMID: 28478972]

Stein SL et al. Management of atopic dermatitis. JAMA. 2016 Apr 12;315(14):1510–1. [PMID: 27115267]

Weidinger S et al. Atopic dermatitis. Lancet. 2016 Mar 12; 387(10023):1109–22. [PMID: 26377142]

LICHEN SIMPLEX CHRONICUS (Circumscribed Neurodermatitis)

ESSENTIALS OF DIAGNOSIS

▶ Chronic itching and scratching.

▶ Lichenified lesions with exaggerated skin lines overlying a thickened, well-circumscribed, scaly plaque.

▶ Predilection for nape of neck, wrists, external surfaces of forearms, lower legs, scrotum, and vulva.

General Considerations

Lichen simplex chronicus represents a self-perpetuating scratch-itch cycle that is hard to disrupt.

Clinical Findings

Intermittent itching incites the patient to scratch the lesions. Itching may be so intense as to interfere with sleep. Dry, hypertrophic, lichenified plaques appear on the neck, wrists, ankles, or perineum (Figure 6–6). The patches are rectangular, thickened, and hyperpigmented. The skin lines are exaggerated.

Differential Diagnosis

This disorder can be differentiated from plaque-like lesions such as psoriasis (redder lesions having whiter scales on the elbows, knees, and scalp and nail findings), lichen planus (violaceous, usually smaller polygonal papules), and nummular (coin-shaped) dermatitis. Lichen simplex chronicus may complicate chronic atopic dermatitis or scabetic infestation.

Treatment

For lesions in extragenital regions, superpotent topical corticosteroids are effective, with or without occlusion, when used twice daily for several weeks. In some patients,

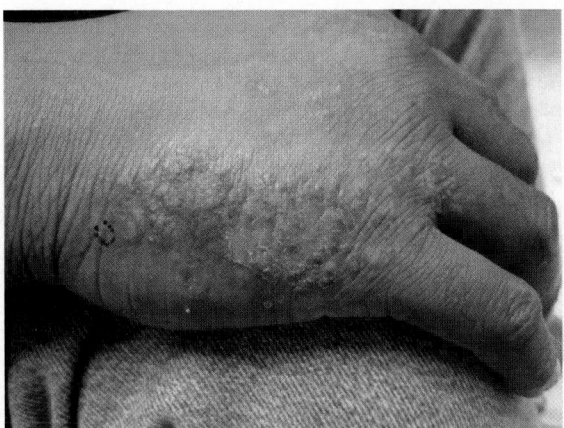

▲ **Figure 6–6.** Lichen simplex chronicus on the hand. (Used, with permission, from Lindy Fox, MD.)

flurandrenolide (Cordran) tape may be effective, since it prevents scratching and rubbing of the lesion. The injection of triamcinolone acetonide suspension (5–10 mg/mL) into the lesions may occasionally be curative. Continuous occlusion with a flexible hydrocolloid dressing for 7 days at a time for 1–2 months may also be helpful. For genital lesions, see the section Pruritus Ani.

Prognosis

The disease tends to remit during treatment but may recur or develop at another site.

Chibnall R. Vulvar pruritus and lichen chronic simplex. Obstet Gynecol Clin North Am. 2017 Sep;44(3):379–88. [PMID: 28778638]

Jung HM et al. Less painful and effective intralesional injection method for lichen simplex chronicus. J Am Acad Dermatol. 2018 Dec;79(6):e105–e106. [PMID: 30025827]

PSORIASIS

ESSENTIALS OF DIAGNOSIS

▶ Silvery scales on bright red, well-demarcated plaques, usually on the knees, elbows, and scalp.

▶ Nails: pitting and onycholysis (separation of the nail plate from the bed).

▶ Mild itching is common.

▶ May be associated with psoriatic arthritis.

▶ Increased risk of cardiovascular events, type 2 diabetes mellitus, metabolic syndrome, and lymphoma.

▶ Histopathology helpful.

General Considerations

Psoriasis is a common benign, chronic inflammatory skin disease with both a genetic basis and known environmental triggers. Injury or irritation of normal skin tends to induce lesions of psoriasis at the site (Koebner phenomenon). Obesity worsens psoriasis, and significant weight loss in obese persons may lead to substantial improvement of their psoriasis. Psoriasis has several variants—the most common is the plaque type. Eruptive (guttate) psoriasis consisting of myriad lesions 3–10 mm in diameter occurs occasionally after streptococcal pharyngitis. Rarely, grave, occasionally life-threatening forms (generalized pustular and erythrodermic psoriasis) may occur.

Clinical Findings

There are often no symptoms, but itching may occur and be severe. Favored sites include the scalp, elbows, knees, palms and soles, and nails. The lesions are red, sharply defined plaques covered with silvery scale (Figure 6–7).

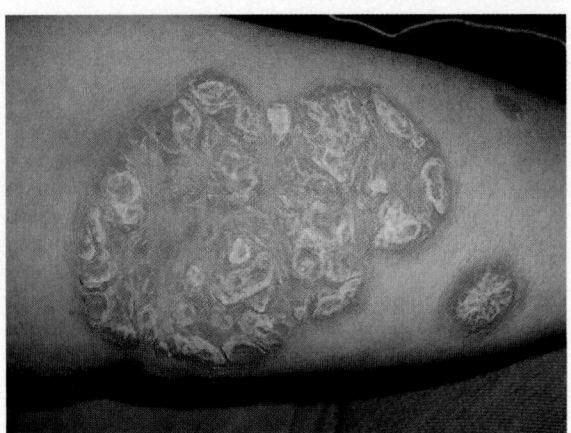

▲ **Figure 6–7.** Plaque—psoriatic plaque. (Used, with permission, from Richard P. Usatine, MD, in Usatine RP, Smith MA, Mayeaux EJ Jr, Chumley H. *The Color Atlas of Family Medicine*, 3rd ed. McGraw-Hill, 2018.)

The glans penis and vulva may be affected. The combination of red plaques with silvery scales on elbows and knees, with scaliness in the scalp or nail findings, is diagnostic. Occasionally, only the flexures (axillae, inguinal areas) are involved (termed inverse psoriasis). Fine stippling ("pitting") in the nails is highly suggestive of psoriasis (Figure 6–8). Patients with psoriasis often have a pink or red intergluteal fold. Not all patients have findings in all locations, but the occurrence of a few may help make the diagnosis when other lesions are not typical. Some patients have mainly hand or foot dermatitis and only minimal findings elsewhere. There may be associated arthritis that is most commonly distal and oligoarticular, although the rheumatoid variety with a negative rheumatoid factor may occur. The psychosocial impact of psoriasis is a major factor in determining the treatment of the patient.

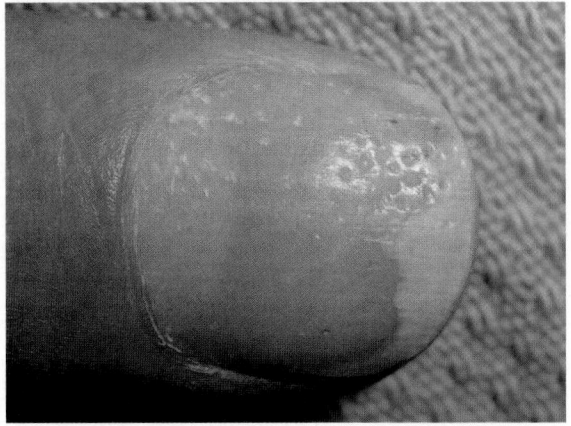

▲ **Figure 6–8.** Nail pitting due to psoriasis. (Used, with permission, from Richard P. Usatine, MD, in Usatine RP, Smith MA, Mayeaux EJ Jr, Chumley H. *The Color Atlas of Family Medicine*, 2nd ed. McGraw-Hill, 2013.)

▶ Differential Diagnosis

Psoriasis lesions are well demarcated and affect extensor surfaces—in contrast to atopic dermatitis, with poorly demarcated plaques in flexural distribution. In body folds, scraping and culture for *Candida* and examination of scalp and nails will distinguish inverse psoriasis from intertrigo and candidiasis. Dystrophic changes in nails may mimic onychomycosis, and a potassium hydroxide (KOH) preparation or fungal culture is valuable in diagnosis. The cutaneous features of reactive arthritis, pityriasis rosea, systemic lupus erythematosus, and syphilis mimic psoriasis.

▶ Treatment

There are many therapeutic options in psoriasis to be chosen according to the extent (body surface area [BSA] affected) and the presence of other findings (for example, arthritis). **Systemic corticosteroids should never be used to treat flares of psoriasis** because they may lead to severe rebound flares of the disease when they are tapered. Certain medications, such as beta-blockers, antimalarials, statins, and lithium, may flare or worsen psoriasis. Patients with moderate to severe psoriasis should be managed by or in conjunction with a dermatologist.

A. Limited Disease

For patients with large plaques and less than 10% of the BSA involved, the easiest regimen is to use a high-potency to ultra–high-potency topical corticosteroid cream or ointment. It is best to restrict the ultra–high-potency corticosteroids to 2–3 weeks of twice-daily use and then use them in a pulse fashion three or four times on weekends or switch to a mid-potency corticosteroid. Topical corticosteroids rarely induce a lasting remission. Additional measures are therefore commonly added to topical corticosteroid therapy. Calcipotriene ointment 0.005% or calcitriol ointment 0.003%, both vitamin D analogs, are used twice daily for plaque psoriasis. Initially, patients are treated with twice-daily topical corticosteroids plus a vitamin D analog twice daily. This rapidly clears the lesions; eventually, the topical corticosteroids are stopped, and once- or twice-daily application of the vitamin D analog is continued long-term. Calcipotriene usually cannot be applied to the groin or face because of irritation. Treatment of extensive psoriasis with vitamin D analogs may result in hypercalcemia, so that the maximum dose for calcipotriene is 100 g/week and for calcitriol it is 200 g/week. Calcipotriene is incompatible with many topical corticosteroids (but not halobetasol), so if used concurrently, it must be applied at a different time. For patients with numerous small plaques, phototherapy is the best therapy.

For thick plaques on the scalp, start with a tar shampoo, used daily if possible. Additional treatments include 6% salicylic acid gel (eg, Keralyt), P & S solution (phenol, mineral oil, and glycerin), or fluocinolone acetonide 0.01% in oil (Derma-Smoothe/FS) under a shower cap at night, and shampoo in the morning. In order of increasing potency, triamcinolone 0.1%, fluocinolone, betamethasone dipropionate, amcinonide, and clobetasol are available in solution form for use on the scalp twice daily. Tacrolimus ointment 0.1% or 0.03% or pimecrolimus cream 1% may be effective in intertriginous, genital, and facial psoriasis, since potent corticosteroids are not recommended due to skin atrophy.

B. Moderate Disease

Psoriasis affecting 10–30% of the patient's BSA is frequently treated with UV phototherapy, either in a medical office or via a home light unit. Systemic agents listed below may also be used.

C. Generalized Disease

If psoriasis involves more than 30% of the body surface, it is difficult to treat with topical agents. The treatment of choice is outpatient narrowband UVB (NB-UVB) three times weekly. Clearing occurs in an average of 7 weeks, and maintenance may be required.

Psoralen plus UVA (PUVA) photochemotherapy may be effective even in patients who have not responded to standard NB-UVB treatment. Long-term use of PUVA (greater than 250 doses) is associated with an increased risk of skin cancer (especially squamous cell carcinoma and perhaps melanoma) in persons with fair complexions. Thus, periodic examination (every 3–6 months) of the skin is imperative. Atypical lentigines are a common complication. There can be rapid aging of the skin in fair individuals. Cataracts have not been reported with proper use of protective glasses. PUVA may be used in combination with other therapy, such as acitretin or methotrexate.

Methotrexate is very effective for severe psoriasis in doses up to 25 mg once weekly according to published protocols. Long-term methotrexate use may be associated with cirrhosis. After receiving a 3.5–4-g cumulative dose, the patient should be referred to a hepatologist for evaluation. Administration of folic acid, 1–2 mg daily, can eliminate nausea caused by methotrexate without compromising efficacy.

Acitretin, a synthetic retinoid, is most effective for pustular psoriasis in oral dosages of 0.5–0.75 mg/kg/day. Liver enzymes and serum lipids must be checked periodically. Because acitretin is a teratogen and persists for 2–3 years in fat, women of childbearing age must wait at least 3 years after completing acitretin treatment before considering pregnancy. When used as single agents, retinoids will flatten psoriatic plaques, but will rarely result in complete clearing. Retinoids find their greatest use when combined with phototherapy—either UVB or PUVA, with which they are synergistic.

Cyclosporine dramatically improves psoriasis and may be used to control severe cases. Rapid relapse (rebound) frequently occurs after cessation of therapy, so another agent must be added if cyclosporine is stopped. The tumor necrosis factor (TNF) inhibitors etanercept (Enbrel), infliximab (Remicade), and adalimumab (Humira) are effective in pustular and chronic plaque psoriasis and are also effective for the associated arthritis. Infliximab provides the most rapid response and can be used for severe pustular or erythrodermic flares. Etanercept is used more frequently for long-term treatment at a dose of 50 mg subcutaneously twice weekly for 3 months, then 50 mg once weekly. All three TNF inhibitors can also induce or worsen psoriasis. IL-12/23 monoclonal antibodies (ustekinumab [Stelara], guselkumab), Janus kinase inhibitors (tofacitinib, approved for use in rheumatoid arthritis but with strong data supporting its use in psoriasis), and IL-17 monoclonal antibodies (secukinumab, brodalumab, and ixekizumab) are also highly effective treatments. The oral phosphodiesterase 4 inhibitor apremilast is an approved option for plaque-type psoriasis with minimal immunosuppressive effects and requires no laboratory monitoring. Given the large number of psoriasis treatments available, consultation with a dermatologist is recommended when considering systemic treatment for moderate to severe psoriasis.

▶ Prognosis

The course tends to be chronic and unpredictable, and the disease may be refractory to treatment. Patients (especially those older than 40 years) should be monitored for metabolic syndrome, which correlates with the severity of their skin disease.

Boehncke WH et al. Psoriasis. Lancet. 2015 Sep 5;386(9997): 983–94. [PMID: 26025581]

Nast A et al. Efficacy and safety of systemic long-term treatments for moderate-to-severe psoriasis: a systematic review and meta-analysis. J Invest Dermatol. 2015 Nov;135(11):2641–8. [PMID: 26046458]

Sbidian E et al. Systemic pharmacological treatments for chronic plaque psoriasis: a network meta-analysis. Cochrane Database Syst Rev. 2017 Dec 22;12:CD011535. [PMID: 29271481]

PITYRIASIS ROSEA

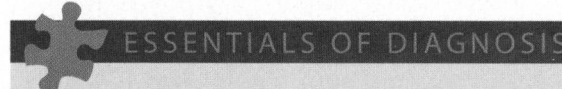
ESSENTIALS OF DIAGNOSIS

▶ Oval, fawn-colored, scaly eruption following cleavage lines of trunk.

▶ Herald patch precedes eruption by 1–2 weeks.

▶ Occasional pruritus.

▶ General Considerations

Pityriasis rosea is a common mild, acute inflammatory disease that is 50% more common in females. Young adults are principally affected, mostly in the spring or fall. Concurrent household cases have been reported.

▶ Clinical Findings

Itching is common but is usually mild. The diagnosis is made by finding one or more classic lesions. The lesions

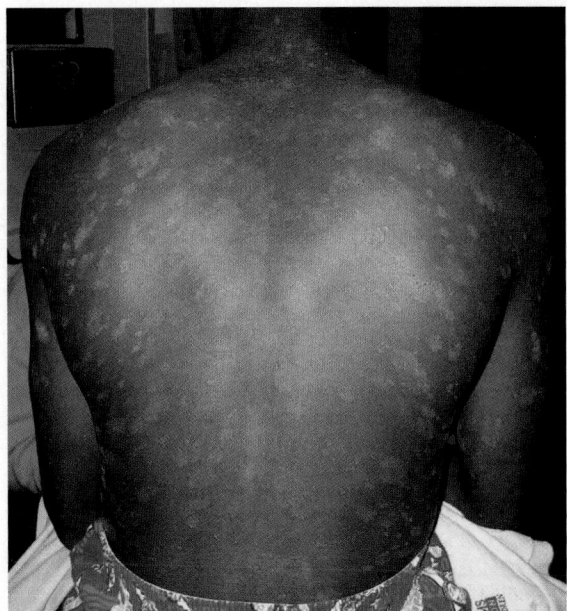

▲ **Figure 6–9.** Pityriasis rosea with scaling lesions following skin lines and resembling a Christmas tree. (Used, with permission, from EJ Mayeaux, MD in Usatine RP, Smith MA, Mayeaux EJ Jr, Chumley H, Tysinger J. *The Color Atlas of Family Medicine.* McGraw-Hill, 2009.)

consist of oval, fawn-colored plaques up to 2 cm in diameter. The centers of the lesions have a crinkled or "cigarette paper" appearance and a collarette scale, ie, a thin bit of scale that is bound at the periphery and free in the center. Only a few lesions in the eruption may have this characteristic appearance, however. Lesions follow cleavage lines on the trunk (so-called Christmas tree pattern, Figure 6–9), and the proximal portions of the extremities are often involved. A variant that affects the flexures (axillae and groin), so-called inverse pityriasis rosea, and a papular variant, especially in black patients, also occur. An initial lesion ("herald patch") that is often larger than the later lesions often precedes the general eruption by 1–2 weeks. The eruption usually lasts 6–8 weeks and heals without scarring.

► Differential Diagnosis

Serologic testing for syphilis should be performed if at least a few perfectly typical lesions are not present and especially if there are palmar and plantar or mucous membrane lesions or adenopathy, features that are suggestive of secondary syphilis. Tinea corporis may present with red, slightly scaly plaques, but rarely are there more than a few lesions of tinea corporis compared to the many lesions of pityriasis rosea. A potassium hydroxide examination should be performed to exclude a fungal cause. Seborrheic dermatitis on occasion presents on the body with poorly demarcated patches over the sternum, in the pubic area, and in the axillae. Tinea versicolor lacks the typical collarette rimmed lesions. Certain medications (eg, angiotensin-converting enzyme [ACE] inhibitors and metronidazole)

and immunizations rarely may induce a skin eruption mimicking pityriasis rosea.

► Treatment

Pityriasis rosea often requires no treatment. In darker-skinned individuals, more aggressive management may be indicated because dyspigmentation of lesions may remain for some time. Treatment is, otherwise, indicated only if the patient is symptomatic. While adequately controlled and reproduced trials have not demonstrated widely effective treatments, most dermatologists recommend UVB treatments or a short course of prednisone for severe or severely symptomatic cases. For mild to moderate cases, topical corticosteroids of medium strength (triamcinolone 0.1%) and oral antihistamines may also be used if pruritus is bothersome. The role of macrolide antibiotics is not evidence based.

► Prognosis

Pityriasis rosea is usually an acute self-limiting illness that typically disappears in about 6 weeks, although prolonged variants have been reported.

Chuh A et al. A position statement on the management of patients with pityriasis rosea. J Eur Acad Dermatol Venereol. 2016 Oct;30(10):1670–81. [PMID: 27406919]

Urbina F et al. Clinical variants of pityriasis rosea. World J Clin Cases. 2017 Jun 16;5(6):203–11. [PMID: 28685133]

SEBORRHEIC DERMATITIS

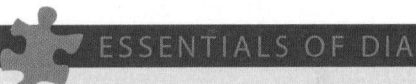

ESSENTIALS OF DIAGNOSIS

► Dry scales and underlying erythema.
► Scalp, central face, presternal, interscapular areas, umbilicus, and body folds.

► General Considerations

Seborrheic dermatitis is an acute or chronic papulosquamous dermatitis that often coexists with psoriasis.

► Clinical Findings

The scalp, face, chest, back, umbilicus, eyelid margins, genitalia, and body folds have dry scales (dandruff) or oily yellowish scurf (Figure 6–10). Pruritus is a variable finding. Patients with Parkinson disease, HIV-infected patients, and patients who become acutely ill often have seborrheic dermatitis.

► Differential Diagnosis

There is a spectrum from seborrheic dermatitis to scalp psoriasis. Extensive seborrheic dermatitis may simulate intertrigo in flexural areas, but scalp, face, and sternal involvement suggests seborrheic dermatitis.

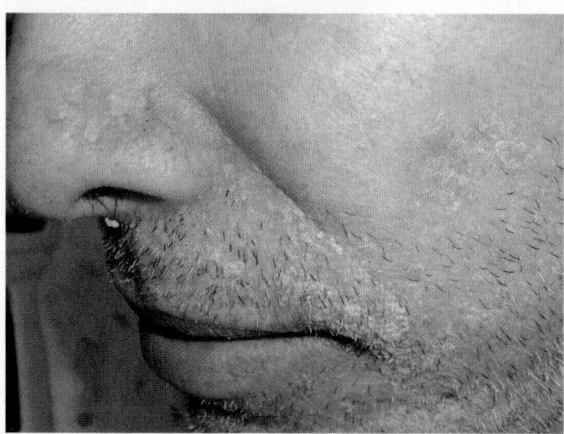

▲ **Figure 6–10.** Seborrheic dermatitis with classic crusting in the nasolabial crease and beard area. (Used, with permission, from Richard P. Usatine, MD, in Usatine RP, Smith MA, Mayeaux EJ Jr, Chumley H. *The Color Atlas of Family Medicine,* 2nd ed. McGraw-Hill, 2013.)

▶ Treatment

A. Seborrhea of the Scalp

Shampoos that contain zinc pyrithione or selenium are used daily if possible. These may be alternated with ketoconazole shampoo (1% or 2%) used twice weekly. A combination of shampoos is used in refractory cases. Tar shampoos are also effective for milder cases and for scalp psoriasis. Topical corticosteroid solutions or lotions are then added if necessary and are used twice daily. (See treatment for scalp psoriasis, above.)

B. Facial Seborrheic Dermatitis

The mainstay of therapy is a mild corticosteroid (hydrocortisone 1%, alclometasone, desonide) used intermittently and not near the eyes. If the disorder cannot be controlled with intermittent use of a mild topical corticosteroid alone, ketoconazole (Nizoral) 2% cream is added twice daily. Topical tacrolimus (Protopic) and pimecrolimus (Elidel) are steroid-sparing alternatives.

C. Seborrheic Dermatitis of Nonhairy Areas

Low-potency corticosteroid creams—ie, 1% or 2.5% hydrocortisone, desonide, or alclometasone dipropionate—are highly effective.

D. Seborrhea of Intertriginous Areas

Apply low-potency corticosteroid lotions or creams twice daily for 5–7 days and then once or twice weekly for maintenance as necessary. Selenium lotion, ketoconazole, or clotrimazole gel or cream may be a useful adjunct. Tacrolimus or pimecrolimus topically may avoid corticosteroid atrophy in chronic cases.

E. Involvement of Eyelid Margins

"Marginal blepharitis" usually responds to gentle cleaning of the lid margins nightly as needed, with undiluted Johnson & Johnson Baby Shampoo using a cotton swab.

▶ Prognosis

The tendency is for lifelong recurrences. Individual outbreaks may last weeks, months, or years.

Clark GW et al. Diagnosis and treatment of seborrheic dermatitis. Am Fam Physician. 2015 Feb 1;91(3):185–90. [PMID: 25822272]
Gupta AK et al. Topical treatment of facial seborrheic dermatitis: a systematic review. Am J Clin Dermatol. 2017 Apr;18(2): 193–213. [PMID: 27804089]

FUNGAL INFECTIONS OF THE SKIN

The diagnosis of fungal infections of the skin is usually based on the location and characteristics of the lesions and on the following laboratory examinations: (1) Direct demonstration of fungi in 10% KOH evaluation of suspected lesions. **"If it's scaly, scrape it" is a time-honored maxim** (Figure 6–11). (2) Cultures of organisms from skin scrapings. (3) Histologic sections of biopsies stained with periodic acid-Schiff technique may be diagnostic if scrapings and cultures are falsely negative.

▶ Principles of Treatment

A diagnosis should always be confirmed by KOH preparation, culture, or biopsy. Many other diseases cause scaling,

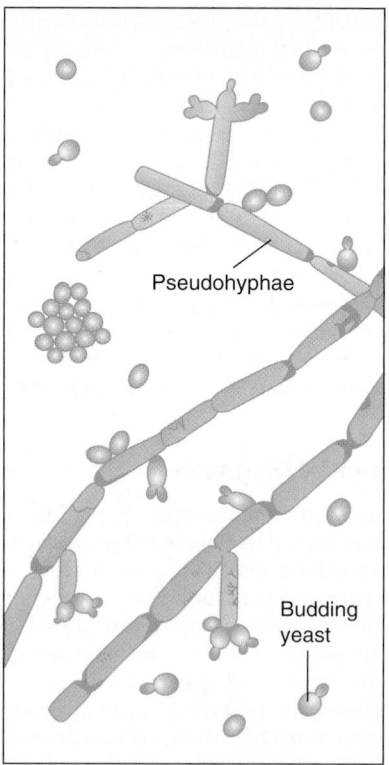

▲ **Figure 6–11.** KOH preparation of fungus demonstrating pseudohyphae and budding yeast forms. (Reproduced, with permission, from Nicoll D et al. *Pocket Guide to Diagnostic Tests,* 6th ed. McGraw-Hill, 2012.)

and use of an antifungal agent without a firm diagnosis makes subsequent diagnosis more difficult. In general, fungal infections are treated topically except for those with extensive involvement or involving the nails or hair follicles. In these situations, oral agents may be useful, with special attention to their side effects and complications, including hepatic toxicity.

General Measures & Prevention

Since moist skin favors the growth of fungi, dry the skin carefully after bathing or after perspiring heavily. Talc or other drying powders may be useful with the exception of powders containing corn starch, which may exacerbate fungal infections. The use of topical corticosteroids for other diseases may be complicated by intercurrent tinea or candidal infection, and topical antifungals are often used in intertriginous areas with corticosteroids to prevent this.

1. Tinea Corporis or Tinea Circinata

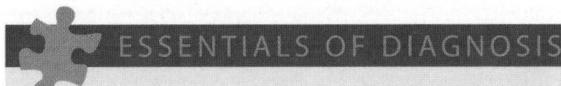

> ► Ring-shaped lesions with an advancing scaly border and central clearing or scaly patches with a distinct border.
>
> ► Microscopic examination of scrapings or culture confirms the diagnosis.

General Considerations

The lesions are often on exposed areas of the body such as the face and arms. A history of exposure to an infected pet (who may have scaly rash or patches of alopecia) may occasionally be obtained, usually indicating *Microsporum* infection. *Trichophyton rubrum* is the most common pathogen, usually representing extension onto the trunk or extremities of tinea cruris, pedis, or manuum.

Clinical Findings

A. Symptoms and Signs

Itching may be present. In classic lesions, rings of erythema have an advancing scaly border and central clearing.

B. Laboratory Findings

The diagnosis should be confirmed by KOH preparation or culture.

Differential Diagnosis

Positive fungal studies distinguish tinea corporis from other skin lesions with annular configuration, such as the annular lesions of psoriasis, lupus erythematosus, syphilis, granuloma annulare, and pityriasis rosea. Psoriasis has typical lesions on elbows, knees, scalp, and nails. Secondary syphilis is often manifested by characteristic palmar,

plantar, and mucous membrane lesions. Tinea corporis rarely has the large number of symmetric lesions seen in pityriasis rosea. Granuloma annulare lacks scale.

Complications

Complications include extension of the disease down the hair follicles (which presents as papules and pustules and is more difficult to cure) and pyoderma.

Prevention

Treat infected household pets (*Microsporum* infections). To prevent recurrences, the use of foot powder and keeping feet dry by wearing sandals, or changing socks can be useful.

Treatment

A. Local Measures

Tinea corporis responds to most topical antifungals, including terbinafine, butenafine, econazole, miconazole, and clotrimazole, most of which are available over the counter in the United States (see Table 6–2). Terbinafine and butenafine require shorter courses and lead to the most rapid response. **Treatment should be continued for 1–2 weeks after clinical clearing**. Betamethasone dipropionate with clotrimazole (Lotrisone) is not recommended. Long-term improper use may result in side effects from the high-potency corticosteroid component, especially in body folds.

B. Systemic Measures

Itraconazole as a single weeklong pulse of 200 mg orally daily is effective in tinea corporis. Terbinafine, 250 mg orally daily for 1 month, is an alternative.

Prognosis

Tinea corporis usually responds promptly to conservative topical therapy or to an oral agent within 4 weeks.

van Zuuren EJ et al. Evidence-based topical treatments for tinea cruris and tinea corporis: a summary of a Cochrane systematic review. Br J Dermatol. 2015 Mar;172(3):616–41. [PMID: 25294700]

2. Tinea Cruris (Jock Itch)

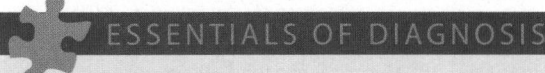

> ► Marked itching in intertriginous areas, usually sparing the scrotum.
>
> ► Peripherally spreading, sharply demarcated, centrally clearing erythematous lesions.
>
> ► May have associated tinea infection of feet or toenails.
>
> ► Laboratory examination with microscope or culture confirms diagnosis.

General Considerations

Tinea cruris lesions are confined to the groin and gluteal cleft. Intractable pruritus ani may occasionally be caused by a tinea infection.

Clinical Findings

A. Symptoms and Signs

Itching may be severe, or the rash may be asymptomatic. The lesions have sharp margins, cleared centers, and active, spreading scaly peripheries. Follicular pustules are sometimes encountered. The area may be hyperpigmented on resolution.

B. Laboratory Findings

Hyphae can be demonstrated microscopically in KOH preparations or skin biopsy. The organism may be cultured.

Differential Diagnosis

Tinea cruris must be distinguished from other lesions involving the intertriginous areas, such as candidiasis, seborrheic dermatitis, intertrigo, psoriasis of body folds ("inverse psoriasis"), and erythrasma (corynebacterial infection of intertriginous areas). Candidiasis is generally bright red and marked by satellite papules and pustules outside of the main border of the lesion. *Candida* typically involves the scrotum. Seborrheic dermatitis also often involves the face, sternum, and axillae. Intertrigo tends to be less red, less scaly, and present in obese individuals in moist body folds with less extension onto the thigh. "Inverse psoriasis" is characterized by distinct plaques. Other areas of typical psoriatic involvement should be checked, and the KOH examination will be negative. Erythrasma is best diagnosed with Wood (ultraviolet) light—a brilliant coral-red fluorescence is seen.

Treatment

A. General Measures

Drying powder (eg, miconazole nitrate [Zeasorb-AF]) can be dusted into the involved area in patients with excessive perspiration or occlusion of skin due to obesity as a preventive measure.

B. Local Measures

Any of the topical antifungal preparations listed in Table 6–2 may be used. Terbinafine cream is curative in over 80% of cases after once-daily use for 7 days.

C. Systemic Measures

One week of either itraconazole, 200 mg orally daily, or terbinafine, 250 mg orally daily, can be effective.

Prognosis

Tinea cruris usually responds promptly to topical or systemic treatment but often recurs.

van Zuuren EJ et al. Evidence-based topical treatments for tinea cruris and tinea corporis: a summary of a Cochrane systematic review. Br J Dermatol. 2015 Mar;172(3):616–41. [PMID: 25294700]

3. Tinea Manuum & Tinea Pedis (Tinea of Palms & Soles)

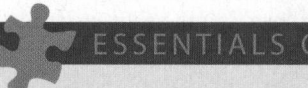

ESSENTIALS OF DIAGNOSIS

▸ Most often presents with asymptomatic scaling.

▸ May progress to fissuring or maceration in toe web spaces.

▸ May be a portal of entry for bacteria causing lower extremity cellulitis.

▸ Itching, burning, and stinging of interdigital web; scaling palms and soles; vesicles on soles in inflammatory cases.

▸ The fungus is shown in skin scrapings examined microscopically or by culture of scrapings.

General Considerations

Tinea of the feet (athlete's foot) is an extremely common acute or chronic dermatosis. Most infections are caused by *Trichophyton* species.

Clinical Findings

A. Symptoms and Signs

The presenting symptom may be itching, burning, or stinging. Pain may indicate secondary infection with complicating cellulitis. Interdigital tinea pedis is the most common predisposing cause of lower extremity cellulitis in healthy individuals. Regular examination of the feet of diabetic patients for evidence of scaling and fissuring and treatment of any identified tinea pedis may prevent complications. Tinea pedis has several presentations that vary with the location. On the sole and heel, tinea may appear as chronic noninflammatory scaling, occasionally with thickening and fissuring. This may extend over the sides of the feet in a "moccasin" distribution (Figure 6–12). The

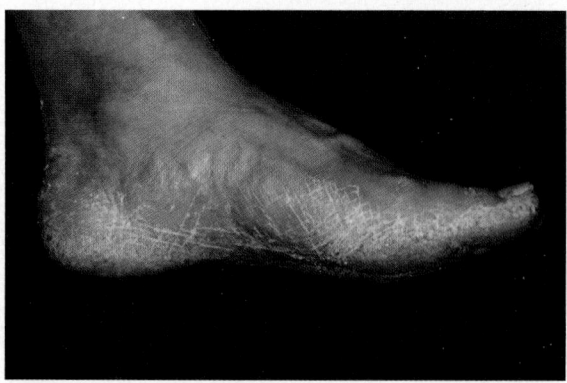

▲ **Figure 6–12.** Tinea pedis in the moccasin distribution. (Used, with permission, from Richard P. Usatine, MD, in Usatine RP, Smith MA, Mayeaux EJ Jr, Chumley H. *The Color Atlas of Family Medicine,* 2nd ed. McGraw-Hill, 2013.)

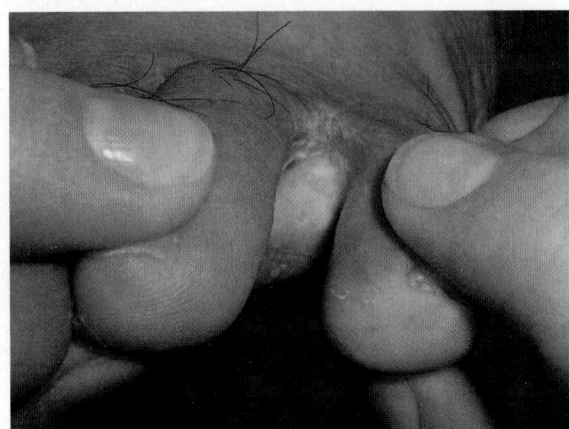

▲ **Figure 6–13.** Tinea pedis in the interdigital space between fourth and fifth digits. The differential diagnosis includes a bacterial primary or secondary infection with gram-negative organisms. (Used, with permission, from Richard P. Usatine, MD, in Usatine RP, Smith MA, Mayeaux EJ Jr, Chumley H, Tysinger J. *The Color Atlas of Family Medicine.* McGraw-Hill, 2009.)

KOH preparation is usually positive. Tinea pedis often appears as a scaling or fissuring of the toe webs, often with maceration (Figure 6–13). As the web spaces become more macerated, the KOH preparation and fungal culture are less often positive because bacterial species begin to dominate. Finally, there may also be vesicles, bullae, or generalized exfoliation of the skin of the soles, or nail involvement in the form of discoloration, friability, and thickening of the nail plate.

B. Laboratory Findings

KOH and culture do not always demonstrate pathogenic fungi from macerated areas.

▶ Differential Diagnosis

Another skin condition involving the same areas is interdigital erythrasma (use Wood light). Psoriasis may be a cause of chronic scaling on the palms or soles and may cause nail changes. Repeated fungal cultures should be negative, and the condition will not respond to antifungal therapy. Contact dermatitis will often involve the dorsal surfaces and will respond to topical or systemic corticosteroids. Vesicular lesions should be differentiated from pompholyx (dyshidrosis) and scabies by proper scraping of the roofs of individual vesicles. Rarely, gram-negative organisms may cause toe web infections, manifested as an acute erosive flare of interdigital disease. This entity is treated with aluminum salts and imidazole antifungal agents or ciclopirox. *Candida* may also cause erosive interdigital disease.

▶ Prevention

The essential factor in prevention is personal hygiene. Wear open-toed sandals if possible. Use of sandals in community showers and bathing places is often recommended,

though the effectiveness of this practice has not been studied. Careful drying between the toes after showering is essential. A hair dryer used on low setting may be used. Socks should be changed frequently, and absorbent nonsynthetic socks are preferred. Apply dusting and drying powders as necessary. The use of powders containing antifungal agents (eg, Zeasorb-AF) or long-term use of antifungal creams may prevent recurrences of tinea pedis.

▶ Treatment

A. Local Measures

1. Macerated stage—Treat with aluminum subacetate solution soaks for 20 minutes twice daily. Broad-spectrum antifungal creams and solutions (containing imidazoles or ciclopirox) (Table 6–2) will help combat diphtheroids and other gram-positive organisms present at this stage and alone may be adequate therapy. If topical imidazoles fail, 1 week of once-daily topical allylamine treatment (terbinafine or butenafine) will often result in clearing.

2. Dry and scaly stage—Use any of the antifungal agents listed in Table 6–2. The addition of urea 10–20% lotion or cream may increase the efficacy of topical treatments in thick ("moccasin") tinea of the soles.

B. Systemic Measures

Itraconazole, 200 mg orally daily for 2 weeks or 400 mg daily for 1 week, or terbinafine, 250 mg orally daily for 2–4 weeks, may be used in refractory cases. If the infection is cleared by systemic therapy, the patient should be encouraged to begin maintenance with topical therapy, since recurrence is common.

▶ Prognosis

For many individuals, tinea pedis is a chronic affliction, temporarily cleared by therapy only to recur.

Canavan TN et al. Identifying signs of tinea pedis: a key to understanding clinical variables. J Drugs Dermatol. 2015 Oct; 14(10):s42–7. [PMID: 26461834]
Kaushik N et al. Superficial fungal infections. Prim Care. 2015 Dec;42(4):501–16. [PMID: 26612371]

4. Tinea Versicolor (Pityriasis Versicolor)

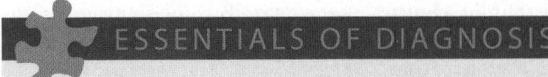
ESSENTIALS OF DIAGNOSIS

▶ Velvety, tan, pink, or white macules or white macules that do not tan with sun exposure.

▶ Fine scales that are not visible but are seen by scraping the lesion.

▶ Central upper trunk the most frequent site.

▶ Yeast and short hyphae observed on microscopic examination of scales.

General Considerations

Tinea versicolor is a mild, superficial *Malassezia* infection of the skin (usually of the upper trunk). This yeast is a colonizer of all humans, which accounts for the high recurrence rate after treatment. The eruption is often called to patients' attention by the fact that the involved areas will not tan, and the resulting hypopigmentation may be mistaken for vitiligo. A hyperpigmented form is not uncommon.

Clinical Findings

A. Symptoms and Signs

Lesions are asymptomatic, but a few patients note itching. The lesions are velvety, tan, pink, or white macules or thin papules that vary from 4 mm to 5 mm in diameter to large confluent areas. The lesions initially do not look scaly, but scales may be readily obtained by scraping the area. Lesions may appear on the trunk, upper arms, neck, and groin.

B. Laboratory Findings

Large, blunt hyphae and thick-walled budding spores ("spaghetti and meatballs") are seen on KOH. Fungal culture is not useful.

Differential Diagnosis

Vitiligo usually presents with larger periorificial and acral lesions and is also characterized by total (not partial) depigmentation. Vitiligo does not scale. Pink and red-brown lesions on the chest are differentiated from seborrheic dermatitis of the same areas by the KOH preparation.

Treatment & Prognosis

A. Initial Treatment

Topical treatments include selenium sulfide lotion, which may be applied from neck to waist daily and left on for 5–15 minutes for 7 days; this treatment is repeated weekly for a month. Ketoconazole shampoo, 1% or 2%, lathered on the chest and back and left on for 5 minutes may also be used weekly for treatment. Clinicians must stress to the patient that the raised and scaly aspects of the rash are being treated; the alterations in pigmentation may take months to fade or fill in.

A regimen of two doses of oral fluconazole, 300 mg, 14 days apart, is first-line treatment; the risk of hepatitis is minimal. Additional doses may be required in severe cases or humid climates. Ketoconazole is no longer recommended as first-line treatment because of the risk of drug-induced hepatitis.

B. Maintenance Therapy

Topical treatments as described above can be used for maintenance therapy. Selenium sulfide lotion should be used monthly, and ketoconazole shampoo, 1% or 2%, may be used to prevent recurrence. Imidazole creams, solutions, and lotions (eg, clotrimazole or miconazole) are quite effective for localized areas but are too expensive for use over large areas, such as the chest and back. Without maintenance therapy, recurrences will occur in over 80% of "cured" cases over the subsequent 2 years.

Gupta AK et al. Systematic review of systemic treatments for tinea versicolor and evidence-based dosing regimen recommendations. J Cutan Med Surg. 2014 Mar–Apr;18(2):79–90. [PMID: 24636433]

Hudson A et al. JAMA patient page. Tinea versicolor. JAMA. 2018 Oct 2;320(13):1396. [PMID: 30285180]

CUTANEOUS LUPUS ERYTHEMATOSUS

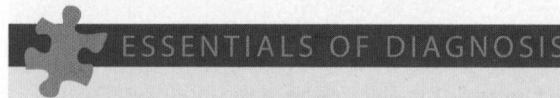

ESSENTIALS OF DIAGNOSIS

- ▶ Localized violaceous red plaques, usually on the face and scalp.
- ▶ Scaling, follicular plugging, atrophy, dyspigmentation, and telangiectasia of involved areas.
- ▶ Distinctive histology.
- ▶ Photosensitivity.

General Considerations

Common forms of cutaneous lupus include chronic cutaneous lupus erythematosus (CCLE), typically chronic scarring (discoid) lupus erythematosus (DLE), and erythematous nonscarring red plaques of subacute cutaneous LE (SCLE). All occur most frequently in photoexposed areas. Permanent hair loss and loss of pigmentation are common sequelae of discoid lesions. Systemic lupus erythematosus (SLE) is discussed in Chapter 20. Patients with SLE may have DLE or SCLE lesions.

Clinical Findings

A. Symptoms and Signs

Symptoms are usually mild. The lesions consist of violaceous red, well-localized, single or multiple plaques, 5–20 mm in diameter, usually on the head in DLE and the trunk in SCLE. In DLE, the scalp, face, and external ears (conchal bowl) may be involved. In discoid lesions, there is atrophy, telangiectasia, central depigmentation, a hyperpigmented rim, and follicular plugging. On the scalp, significant permanent hair loss may occur in lesions of DLE. In SCLE, the lesions are erythematous annular or psoriasiform plaques up to several centimeters in diameter and favor the upper chest and back.

B. Laboratory Findings

In patients with DLE, the possibility of SLE should be considered if the following findings are present: positive antinuclear antibody (ANA), other positive serologic studies (eg, anti-double-stranded DNA or anti-Smith antibody), high erythrocyte sedimentation rate, arthralgias/arthritis, hypocomplementemia, widespread lesions (not localized to the head), or nailfold changes (dilated or thrombosed nailfold capillary loops). Patients with marked photosensitivity and a picture otherwise suggestive of lupus may have negative ANA tests but are positive for antibodies against Ro/SSA or La/SSB (SCLE).

Differential Diagnosis

The diagnosis is based on the clinical appearance confirmed by skin biopsy in all cases. In DLE, the scales are dry and "thumbtack-like" and can thus be distinguished from those of seborrheic dermatitis and psoriasis. Older lesions that have left depigmented scarring or areas of hair loss will also differentiate lupus from these diseases. Ten percent of patients with SLE have discoid skin lesions, and 5% of patients with discoid lesions have SLE. Medications (most commonly, hydrochlorothiazide, calcium channel blockers, H_2-blockers and proton pump inhibitors, ACE inhibitors, TNF inhibitors, and terbinafine) may induce SCLE with a positive Ro/SSA.

Treatment

A. General Measures

Use photoprotective clothing and sunblock with UVB and UVA coverage daily. Avoid using radiation therapy or medications that are potentially photosensitizing when possible.

B. Local Treatment

For limited lesions, the following should be tried before systemic therapy: high-potency corticosteroid creams applied each night and covered with airtight, thin, pliable plastic film (eg, Saran Wrap); Cordran tape; or ultra–high-potency corticosteroid cream or ointment applied twice daily without occlusion.

C. Local Infiltration

Triamcinolone acetonide suspension, 2.5–10 mg/mL, may be injected into the lesions of DLE once a month.

D. Systemic Treatment

1. Antimalarials—These medications should be used only when the diagnosis is secure because they have been associated with flares of psoriasis, which may be in the differential diagnosis.

A. HYDROXYCHLOROQUINE SULFATE—0.2–0.4 g orally daily for several months may be effective and is often used prior to chloroquine. A minimum 3-month trial is recommended. Screening for ocular toxicity is needed.

B. CHLOROQUINE SULFATE—250 mg orally daily may be effective in some cases when hydroxychloroquine is not.

C. QUINACRINE (ATABRINE)—100 mg orally daily may be the safest of the antimalarials, since ocular toxicity has not been reported. It colors the skin yellow and is therefore not acceptable to some patients. It may be added to the other antimalarials for patients with incomplete responses.

2. Isotretinoin—Isotretinoin, 1 mg/kg/day orally, is effective in hypertrophic DLE lesions.

3. Thalidomide—Thalidomide is effective in refractory cases in doses of 50–300 mg orally daily. Monitor for neuropathy. Lenalidomide (5–10 mg orally daily) may also be effective with less risk for neuropathy.

Isotretinoin, thalidomide, and lenalidomide are teratogens and should be used with appropriate contraception and monitoring in women of childbearing age.

Prognosis

The disease is persistent but not life-endangering unless systemic lupus is present. Treatment with one or more antimalarials is effective in more than half of cases. Although the only morbidity may be cosmetic, this can be of overwhelming significance in more darkly pigmented patients with widespread disease. Scarring alopecia can be prevented or lessened with close attention and aggressive therapy. Over years, DLE tends to become inactive. Drug-induced SCLE usually resolves over months when the inciting medication is stopped.

Chasset F et al. Efficacy and comparison of antimalarials in cutaneous lupus erythematosus subtypes: a systematic review and meta-analysis. Br J Dermatol. 2017 Jul;177(1):188–96. [PMID: 28112801]

Hejazi EZ et al. Cutaneous lupus erythematosus: an update on pathogenesis, diagnosis and treatment. Am J Clin Dermatol. 2016 Apr;17(2):135–46. [PMID: 26872954]

CUTANEOUS T-CELL LYMPHOMA (Mycosis Fungoides)

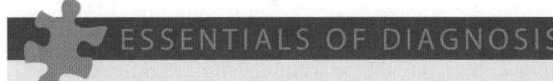
ESSENTIALS OF DIAGNOSIS

▶ Localized or generalized erythematous scaling patches that progress to plaques and nodules.

▶ Pruritus.

▶ Lymphadenopathy.

▶ Distinctive histology.

General Considerations

Mycosis fungoides is a cutaneous T-cell lymphoma that begins on the skin and may involve only the skin for years or decades. It may progress to systemic disease, including Sézary syndrome (erythroderma with circulating malignant T cells).

Clinical Findings

A. Symptoms and Signs

Localized or generalized erythematous scaly patches or plaques are present usually on the trunk. Plaques are almost always over 5 cm in diameter. Pruritus is a frequent complaint and can be severe. The lesions often begin as nondescript or nondiagnostic patches, and it is not unusual for the patient to have skin lesions for more than a decade before the diagnosis can be confirmed. Follicular involvement with hair loss is characteristic of mycosis fungoides, and its presence should raise the suspicion of mycosis fungoides for any pruritic eruption. In more advanced cases, tumors appear. Lymphadenopathy may occur locally or widely. Lymph node enlargement may be due to benign expansion of the node (dermatopathic lymphadenopathy) or by specific involvement with mycosis fungoides.

B. Laboratory Findings

The skin biopsy remains the basis of diagnosis, though at times numerous biopsies are required before the diagnosis can be confirmed. In more advanced disease, circulating malignant T cells (Sézary cells) can be detected in the blood (T-cell gene rearrangement test). Eosinophilia may be present.

► Differential Diagnosis

Mycosis fungoides may be confused with psoriasis, a drug eruption (including to serotonin reuptake inhibitors), photoallergy, an eczematous dermatitis, or tinea corporis. Histologic examination can distinguish these conditions.

► Treatment

The treatment of mycosis fungoides is complex. Early and aggressive treatment has not been proven to cure or prevent disease progression. Skin-directed therapies, including topical corticosteroids, topical mechlorethamine, bexarotene gel, and UV phototherapy, are used initially. If the disease progresses, PUVA plus retinoids, PUVA plus interferon, extracorporeal photophoresis, bexarotene, alpha-interferon with or without retinoids, interleukin-12, denileukin, targeted immunomodulators, and total skin electron beam treatment are used.

► Prognosis

Mycosis fungoides is usually slowly progressive (over decades). Prognosis is better in patients with patch or plaque stage disease and worse in patients with erythroderma, tumors, and lymphadenopathy. Survival is not reduced in patients with limited patch disease. Elderly patients with limited patch and plaque stage disease commonly die of other causes. Overly aggressive treatment may lead to complications and premature demise.

Devata S et al. Cutaneous T-cell lymphoma: a review with a focus on targeted agents. Am J Clin Dermatol. 2016 Jun;17(3):225–37. [PMID: 26923912]

Olsen EA et al. Guidelines for phototherapy of mycosis fungoides and Sézary syndrome: a consensus statement of the United States Cutaneous Lymphoma Consortium. J Am Acad Dermatol. 2016 Jan;74(1):27–58. [PMID: 26547257]

Wilcox RA. Cutaneous T-cell lymphoma: 2016 update on diagnosis, risk-stratification, and management. Am J Hematol. 2016 Jan;91(1):151–65. [PMID: 26607183]

EXFOLIATIVE DERMATITIS
(Exfoliative Erythroderma)

 ESSENTIALS OF DIAGNOSIS

► Scaling and erythema over most of the body.
► Itching, malaise, fever, chills, weight loss.

► General Considerations

Erythroderma describes generalized redness and scaling of the skin of more than 30% BSA. A preexisting dermatosis is the cause of exfoliative dermatitis in two-thirds of cases, including psoriasis, atopic dermatitis, contact dermatitis, pityriasis rubra pilaris, and seborrheic dermatitis. Reactions to topical or systemic medications account for about 15% of cases, cancer (underlying lymphoma, solid tumors and, most commonly, cutaneous T-cell lymphoma) for about 10%, and 10% are idiopathic. Widespread scabies is an important diagnostic consideration since patients with erythrodermic presentation are highly contagious. At the time of acute presentation, without a clear-cut prior history of skin disease or medication exposure, it may be impossible to make a specific diagnosis of the underlying condition, and diagnosis may require continued observation.

► Clinical Findings

A. Symptoms and Signs

Symptoms may include itching, weakness, malaise, fever, and weight loss. Chills are prominent. Erythema and scaling are widespread. Loss of hair and nails can occur. Generalized lymphadenopathy may be due to lymphoma or leukemia or may be reactive. The mucosae are typically spared.

B. Laboratory Findings

A skin biopsy is required and may show changes of a specific inflammatory dermatitis or cutaneous T-cell lymphoma. Peripheral leukocytes may show clonal rearrangements of the T-cell receptor in Sézary syndrome.

► Complications

Protein and electrolyte loss as well as dehydration may develop in patients with generalized inflammatory exfoliative erythroderma; sepsis may occur.

► Treatment

A. Topical Therapy

Home treatment is with cool to tepid baths and application of mid-potency corticosteroids under wet dressings or with the use of an occlusive plastic suit. If the exfoliative erythroderma becomes chronic and is not manageable in an outpatient setting, the patient should be hospitalized. Keep the room at a constant warm temperature and provide the same topical treatment as for an outpatient.

B. Specific Measures

Stop all medications, if possible. Systemic corticosteroids may provide marked improvement in severe or fulminant exfoliative dermatitis, but long-term therapy should be avoided (see Chapter 26). In addition, systemic corticosteroids must be used with caution because some patients with erythroderma have psoriasis and could develop pustular flare. For cases of psoriatic erythroderma and pityriasis rubra pilaris, acitretin, methotrexate, cyclosporine, or a TNF inhibitor may be indicated. Erythroderma secondary to lymphoma or leukemia requires specific topical or systemic chemotherapy. Suitable antibiotic medications with coverage for *Staphylococcus* should be given when there is evidence of bacterial infection.

▶ Prognosis

Careful follow-up is necessary because identifying the cause of exfoliative erythroderma early in the course of the disease may be impossible. Most patients recover completely or improve greatly over time but may require long-term therapy. Deaths are rare in the absence of cutaneous T-cell lymphoma. A minority of patients will suffer from undiminished erythroderma for indefinite periods.

César A et al. Erythroderma. A clinical and etiological study of 103 patients. J Dermatol Case Rep. 2016 Mar 31;10(1):1–9. [PMID: 27119000]

MISCELLANEOUS SCALING DERMATOSES

Isolated scaly patches may represent actinic (solar) keratoses, nonpigmented seborrheic keratoses, or Bowen or Paget disease.

1. Actinic Keratoses

Actinic keratoses are small (0.2–0.6 cm) macules or papules—flesh-colored, pink, or slightly hyperpigmented—that feel like sandpaper and are tender to palpation. They occur on sun-exposed parts of the body in persons of fair complexion. Actinic keratoses are considered premalignant, but only 1:1000 lesions per year progress to become squamous cell carcinomas.

Application of liquid nitrogen is a rapid method of eradication. The lesions crust and disappear in 10–14 days. "Field treatment" with a topical agent to the anatomic area where the actinic keratoses are most prevalent (eg, forehead, dorsal hands, etc) can be considered in patients with multiple lesions in one region. The topical agents used for field treatment include fluorouracil, imiquimod, and ingenol mebutate. Photodynamic therapy can be effective in cases refractory to topical treatment. Any lesions that persist should be evaluated for possible biopsy.

Arenberger P et al. New and current preventive treatment options in actinic keratosis. J Eur Acad Dermatol Venereol. 2017 Sep;31(Suppl 5):13–7. [PMID: 28805940]

Siegel JA et al. Current perspective on actinic keratosis: a review. Br J Dermatol. 2017 Aug;177(2):350–8. [PMID: 27500794]

Werner RN et al. Evidence- and consensus-based (S3) guidelines for the treatment of actinic keratosis—International League of Dermatological Societies in cooperation with the European Dermatology Forum—short version. J Eur Acad Dermatol Venereol. 2015 Nov;29(11):2069–79. [PMID: 26370093]

2. Bowen Disease & Paget Disease

Bowen disease (intraepidermal squamous cell carcinoma) can develop on both sun-exposed and non–sun-exposed skin. The lesion is usually a small (0.5–3 cm), well-demarcated, slightly raised, pink to red, scaly plaque and may resemble psoriasis or a large actinic keratosis. These lesions may progress to invasive squamous cell carcinoma. Excision or other definitive treatment is indicated.

Extramammary Paget disease, a manifestation of intraepidermal carcinoma or underlying genitourinary or gastrointestinal cancer, resembles chronic eczema and usually involves apocrine areas such as the genitalia. Mammary Paget disease of the nipple, a unilateral or rarely bilateral red scaling plaque that may ooze, is associated with an underlying intraductal mammary carcinoma (Figure 17–4). While these lesions appear as red patches and plaques in fair-skinned persons, in darker-skinned individuals, hyperpigmentation may be prominent.

Cohen JM et al. Risk stratification in extramammary Paget disease. Clin Exp Dermatol. 2015 Jul;40(5):473–8. [PMID: 26011765]

Morton CA et al. British Association of Dermatologists' guidelines for the management of squamous cell carcinoma in situ (Bowen's disease) 2014. Br J Dermatol. 2014 Feb;170(2):245–60. [PMID: 24313974]

INTERTRIGO

Intertrigo is caused by the macerating effect of heat, moisture, and friction. It is especially likely to occur in obese persons and in humid climates. The symptoms are itching, stinging, and burning. The body folds develop fissures, erythema, maceration, and superficial denudation. Candidiasis may complicate intertrigo. "Inverse psoriasis," seborrheic dermatitis, tinea cruris, erythrasma, and candidiasis must be ruled out.

Maintain hygiene in the area, and keep it dry. Compresses may be useful acutely. Hydrocortisone 1% cream plus an imidazole or clotrimazole 1% cream is effective. Recurrences are common.

Metin A et al. Recurrent candida intertrigo: challenges and solutions. Clin Cosmet Investig Dermatol. 2018 Apr 17; 11:175–85. [PMID: 29713190]

VESICULAR DERMATOSES

HERPES SIMPLEX
(Cold or Fever Sore; Genital Herpes)

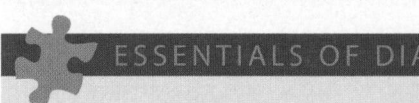

ESSENTIALS OF DIAGNOSIS

▸ Recurrent small grouped vesicles (especially orolabial and genital) on an erythematous base.

▸ May follow minor infections, trauma, stress, or sun exposure; regional lymph nodes may be swollen and tender.

▸ Direct fluorescent antibody tests are positive.

▸ General Considerations

Over 85% of adults have serologic evidence of herpes simplex type 1 (HSV-1) infections, most often acquired asymptomatically in childhood. Occasionally, primary infections may be manifested as severe gingivostomatitis. Thereafter, the patient may have recurrent self-limited attacks, provoked by sun exposure, orofacial surgery, fever, or a viral infection.

About 25% of the US population has serologic evidence of infection with herpes simplex type 2 (HSV-2). HSV-2 causes lesions whose morphology and natural history are similar to those caused by HSV-1 but are typically located on the genitalia of both sexes. The infection is acquired by sexual contact. In monogamous heterosexual couples where one partner has HSV-2 infection, seroconversion of the noninfected partner occurs in 10% over a 1-year period. Up to 70% of such infections appeared to be transmitted during periods of asymptomatic shedding. Genital herpes may also be due to HSV-1.

▸ Clinical Findings

A. Symptoms and Signs

The principal symptoms are burning and stinging. Neuralgia may precede or accompany attacks. The lesions consist of small, grouped vesicles on an erythematous base that can occur anywhere but that most often occur on the vermilion border of the lips (Figure 6–14), the penile shaft, the labia, the perianal skin, and the buttocks. Any erosion or fissure in the anogenital region can be due to herpes simplex. Regional lymph nodes may be swollen and tender. The lesions usually crust and heal in 1 week. Immunosuppressed patients may have unusual variants, including verrucous or nodular herpes lesions at typical sites of involvement. Lesions of herpes simplex must be distinguished from chancroid, syphilis, pyoderma, or trauma.

B. Laboratory Findings

Direct fluorescent antibody slide tests offer rapid, sensitive diagnosis. Viral culture or polymerase chain reaction (PCR) may also be helpful. Herpes serology is not used in the diagnosis of an acute genital ulcer. However, specific HSV-2 serology by Western blot assay or enzyme-linked immunosorbent assay (ELISA) can determine who is

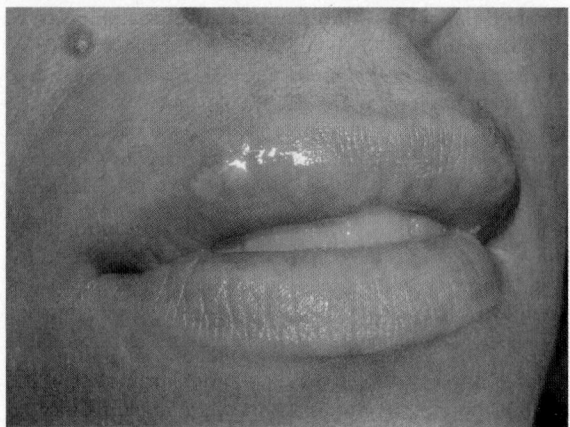

▲ **Figure 6–14.** Orolabial herpes simplex showing deroofed blisters (ulcer). (Used, with permission, from Richard P. Usatine, MD, in Usatine RP, Smith MA, Mayeaux EJ Jr, Chumley H. *The Color Atlas of Family Medicine,* 2nd ed. McGraw-Hill, 2013.)

HSV-infected and potentially infectious, but routine HSV-2 screening is not recommended.

▸ Complications

Complications include pyoderma, eczema herpeticum, herpetic whitlow, herpes gladiatorum (epidemic herpes in wrestlers transmitted by contact), proctitis, esophagitis, neonatal infection, keratitis, and encephalitis.

▸ Treatment

A. Systemic Therapy

Three systemic agents are available for the treatment of acute herpes infections: acyclovir, its valine analog valacyclovir, and famciclovir. All three agents are very effective, and when used properly, virtually nontoxic. Only acyclovir is available for intravenous administration. In the immunocompetent, with the exception of severe orolabial herpes, only genital disease is treated.

1. For first clinical episode—For first clinical episodes of herpes simplex, the dosage of acyclovir is 400 mg orally five times daily (or 800 mg three times daily); of valacyclovir, 1000 mg orally twice daily; and of famciclovir, 250 mg orally three times daily. The duration of treatment is from 7 to 10 days depending on the severity of the outbreak.

2. For mild recurrences—Most cases do not require therapy. In addition, pharmacotherapy of recurrent HSV is of limited benefit, with studies finding a reduction in the average outbreak by only 12–24 hours. **To be effective, the treatment must be initiated by the patient at the first sign of recurrence.** If treatment is desired, recurrent genital herpes outbreaks may be treated with 3 days of valacyclovir, 500 mg orally twice daily, 5 days of acyclovir, 200 mg orally five times a day, or 5 days of famciclovir, 125 mg orally twice daily. Valacyclovir, 2 g twice daily for 1 day, or famciclovir, 1 g once or twice in 1 day, are equally effective short-course alternatives and can abort impending recurrences of both orolabial and genital herpes. The addition of a potent topical corticosteroid three times daily reduces the duration, size, and pain of orolabial herpes treated with an oral antiviral agent.

3. For frequent or severe recurrences—Suppressive treatment will reduce outbreaks by 85% and reduces viral shedding by more than 90%. This results in about a 50% reduced risk of transmission. The recommended suppressive doses, taken continuously, are acyclovir, 400 mg orally twice daily; valacyclovir, 500 mg orally once daily; or famciclovir, 125–250 mg orally twice daily. Pritelivir, 100 mg orally once daily, may have superior reduction of viral shedding in HSV-2 compared to valacyclovir, 500 mg orally once daily. Long-term suppression appears very safe, and after 5–7 years a substantial proportion of patients can discontinue treatment.

The use of latex condoms and patient education have proved effective in reducing genital herpes transmission in some studies but have not proved beneficial in others. No single or combination intervention absolutely prevents transmission. Sunscreens are useful adjuncts in preventing sun-induced HSV-1 recurrences. A preventive antiviral medication should be started beginning 24 hours prior to ultraviolet light exposure, dental surgery, or orolabial cosmetic surgery.

B. Local Measures

In general, topical therapy has only limited efficacy and is generally not recommended because evidence shows that it only minimally reduces skin healing time.

▶ Prognosis

Aside from the complications described above, recurrent attacks last several days, and patients recover without sequelae.

Chi CC et al. Interventions for prevention of herpes simplex labialis (cold sores on the lips). Cochrane Database Syst Rev. 2015 Aug 7;(8):CD010095. [PMID: 26252373]
Feltner C et al. Serologic screening for genital herpes: an updated evidence report and systematic review for the US Preventive Services Task Force. JAMA. 2016 Dec 20;316(23):2531–43. [PMID: 27997660]
Sauerbrei A. Optimal management of genital herpes: current perspectives. Infect Drug Resist. 2016 Jun 13;9:129–41. [PMID: 27358569]

HERPES ZOSTER (Shingles)

See Chapter 32.

POMPHOLYX

ESSENTIALS OF DIAGNOSIS

▶ Pruritic "tapioca" vesicles of 1–2 mm on the palms, soles, and sides of fingers.

▶ Vesicles may coalesce to form multiloculated blisters.

▶ Scaling and fissuring may follow drying of the blisters.

▶ Appearance in the third decade, with lifelong recurrences.

▶ General Considerations

Pompholyx, or vesiculobullous dermatitis of the palms and soles, is formerly known as dyshidrosis or dyshidrotic eczema. About half of patients have an atopic background, and many patients report flares with stress. Patients with widespread dermatitis due to any cause may develop pompholyx-like eruptions as a part of an autoeczematization response.

▶ Clinical Findings

Small clear vesicles resembling grains of tapioca stud the skin at the sides of the fingers and on the palms (Figure 6–15) and may also affect the soles, albeit less frequently. They may be associated with intense itching. Later, the vesicles dry and the area becomes scaly and fissured.

▶ Differential Diagnosis

Unroofing the vesicles and examining the blister roof with a KOH preparation will reveal hyphae in cases of bullous tinea. Always examine the feet of a patient with a hand eruption because patients with inflammatory tinea pedis may have a vesicular autoeczematization of the palms. Nonsteroidal anti-inflammatory drugs (NSAIDs) may produce an eruption very similar to that of vesiculobullous dermatitis on the hands.

▶ Prevention

There is no known way to prevent attacks if the condition is idiopathic. About one-third to one-half of patients with

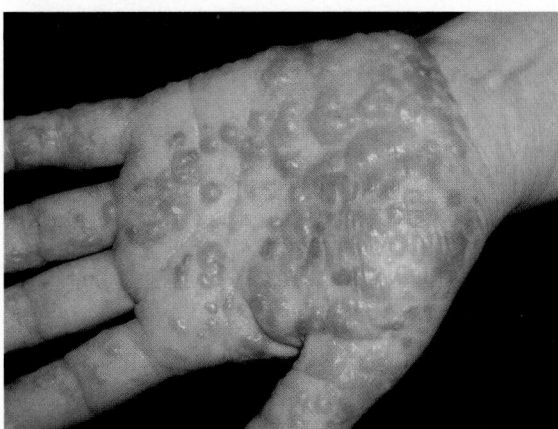

▲ **Figure 6–15.** Severe pompholyx. (Used, with permission, from Richard P. Usatine, MD, in Usatine RP, Smith MA, Mayeaux EJ Jr, Chumley H. *The Color Atlas of Family Medicine,* 2nd ed. McGraw-Hill, 2013.)

vesiculobullous hand dermatitis have a relevant contact allergen, especially nickel. Patch testing and avoidance of identified allergens can lead to improvement.

Treatment

Topical and systemic corticosteroids help some patients dramatically. Since this is a chronic problem, systemic corticosteroids are generally not appropriate therapy. A high-potency topical corticosteroid used early in the attack may help abort the flare and ameliorate pruritus. Topical corticosteroids are also important in treating the scaling and fissuring that are seen after the vesicular phase. It is essential that patients avoid anything that irritates the skin; they should wear cotton gloves inside vinyl gloves when doing dishes or other wet chores and use a hand cream after washing the hands. Patients respond to PUVA therapy and injection of botulinum toxin into the palms as for hyperhidrosis.

Prognosis

For most patients, the disease is an inconvenience. For some, vesiculobullous hand eczema can be incapacitating.

Brans R et al. Clinical patterns and associated factors in patients with hand eczema of primarily occupational origin. J Eur Acad Dermatol Venereol. 2016 May;30(5):798–805. [PMID: 26660508]
Crane MM et al. Hand eczema and steroid-refractory chronic hand eczema in general practice: prevalence and initial treatment. Br J Dermatol. 2017 Apr;176(4):955–64. [PMID: 27534443]
Halling-Overgaard AS et al. Management of atopic hand dermatitis. Dermatol Clin. 2017 Jul;35(3):365–72. [PMID: 28577805]

PORPHYRIA CUTANEA TARDA

> ### ESSENTIALS OF DIAGNOSIS
>
> ▸ Noninflammatory blisters on sun-exposed sites, especially the dorsal surfaces of the hands.
> ▸ Hypertrichosis, skin fragility.
> ▸ Associated liver disease.
> ▸ Elevated urine porphyrins.

General Considerations

Porphyria cutanea tarda is the most common type of porphyria. Cases are sporadic or hereditary. The disease is associated with ingestion of certain medications (eg, estrogens) and alcoholic liver disease, hemochromatosis, or hepatitis C.

Clinical Findings

A. Symptoms and Signs

Patients complain of painless blistering and fragility of the skin of the dorsal surfaces of the hands (Figure 6–16). Facial hypertrichosis and hyperpigmentation are common.

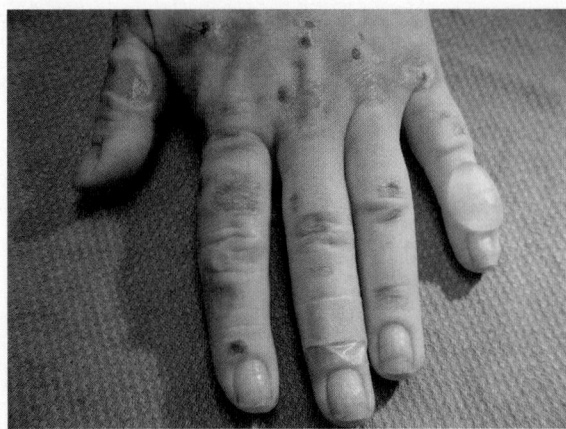

▲ **Figure 6–16.** Porphyria cutanea tarda. (Used, with permission, from Lewis Rose, MD, in Usatine RP, Smith MA, Mayeaux EJ Jr, Chumley H, Tysinger J. *The Color Atlas of Family Medicine*. McGraw-Hill, 2009.)

B. Laboratory Findings

Urinary uroporphyrins are elevated twofold to fivefold above coproporphyrins. Patients may also have abnormal liver biochemical tests, evidence of hepatitis C infection, increased liver iron stores, and hemochromatosis gene mutations.

Differential Diagnosis

Skin lesions identical to those of porphyria cutanea tarda may be seen in patients who undergo dialysis and in those who take certain medications (tetracyclines, voriconazole, and NSAIDs, especially naproxen). In this so-called pseudoporphyria, the biopsy results are the same as those associated with porphyria cutanea tarda, but urine porphyrins are normal.

Prevention

Barrier sun protection with clothing is required. Although the lesions are triggered by sun exposure, the wavelength of light triggering the lesions is beyond that absorbed by sunscreens.

Treatment

Stopping all triggering medications and substantially reducing or stopping alcohol consumption may alone lead to improvement in most cases. Phlebotomy without oral iron supplementation at a rate of 1 unit every 2–4 weeks will gradually lead to improvement. Very low-dose antimalarial medication (as low as 200 mg of hydroxychloroquine orally twice weekly), alone or in combination with phlebotomy, will increase the excretion of porphyrins, improving the skin disease. Deferasirox, an iron chelator, can also improve porphyria cutanea tarda. Treatment is continued until the patient is asymptomatic. Urine porphyrins may be monitored.

Prognosis

Most patients improve with treatment. Sclerodermoid skin lesions may develop on the trunk, scalp, and face.

Handler NS et al. Porphyria cutanea tarda: an intriguing genetic disease and marker. Int J Dermatol. 2017 Jun;56(6):e106–17. [PMID: 28321838]

DERMATITIS HERPETIFORMIS

Dermatitis herpetiformis is an uncommon disease manifested by pruritic papules, vesicles, and papulovesicles mainly on the elbows, knees, buttocks, posterior neck, and scalp. It appears to have its highest prevalence in Northern Europe and is associated with HLA antigens -B8, -DR3, and -DQ2. The histopathology is distinctive. Circulating antibodies to tissue transglutaminase are present in 90% of cases. NSAIDs may cause flares. Patients have gluten-sensitive enteropathy, but it is subclinical in the great majority. However, ingestion of gluten is the cause of the disease, and strict long-term avoidance of dietary gluten has been shown to decrease the dose of dapsone (usually 100–200 mg orally daily) required to control the disease and may even eliminate the need for treatment. Patients with dermatitis herpetiformis are at increased risk for development of gastrointestinal lymphoma, and this risk is reduced by a gluten-free diet.

Collin P et al. Dermatitis herpetiformis: a cutaneous manifestation of coeliac disease. Ann Med. 2017 Feb;49(1):23–31. [PMID: 27499257]

WEEPING OR CRUSTED LESIONS

IMPETIGO

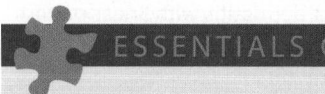

> ESSENTIALS OF DIAGNOSIS

- ▶ Superficial blisters filled with purulent material that rupture easily.
- ▶ Crusted superficial erosions.
- ▶ Positive Gram stain and bacterial culture.

General Considerations

Impetigo is a contagious and autoinoculable infection of the skin (epidermis) caused by staphylococci or streptococci.

Clinical Findings

A. Symptoms and Signs

The lesions consist of macules, vesicles, bullae, pustules, and honey-colored crusts that when removed leave denuded red areas (Figure 6–17). The face and other exposed parts are most often involved. Ecthyma is a deeper form of impetigo caused by staphylococci or streptococci, with ulceration and scarring that occurs frequently on the extremities.

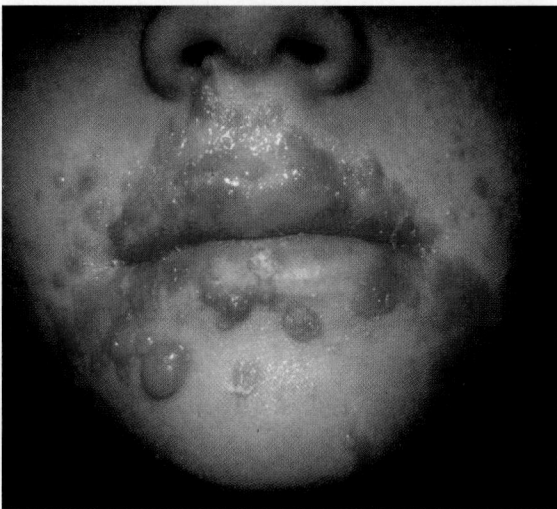

▲ **Figure 6–17.** Bullous impetigo. (Used, with permission, from Jack Resneck, Sr, MD, in Usatine RP, Smith MA, Mayeaux EJ Jr, Chumley H. *The Color Atlas of Family Medicine,* 2nd ed. McGraw-Hill, 2013.)

B. Laboratory Findings

Gram stain and culture confirm the diagnosis. In temperate climates, most cases are associated with *S aureus* infection. *Streptococcus* species are more common in tropical infections.

Differential Diagnosis

The main differential diagnoses are acute allergic contact dermatitis and herpes simplex. Contact dermatitis may be suggested by the history or by linear distribution of the lesions, and culture should be negative for staphylococci and streptococci. Herpes simplex infection usually presents with grouped vesicles or discrete erosions and may be associated with a history of recurrences. Viral cultures are positive.

Treatment

Soaks and scrubbing can be beneficial, especially in unroofing lakes of pus under thick crusts. Topical agents, such as bacitracin, mupirocin, and retapamulin, are first-line treatment options for infections limited to small areas. In widespread cases, or in immunosuppressed individuals, systemic antibiotics are indicated. Cephalexin, 250 mg orally four times daily, is usually effective. Doxycycline, 100 mg orally twice daily, is a reasonable alternative. Community-associated methicillin-resistant *S aureus* (CA-MRSA) may cause impetigo, and initial coverage for MRSA could include doxycycline (100 mg orally twice daily) or trimethoprim-sulfamethoxazole (TMP-SMZ, double-strength tablet orally twice daily). About 50% of CA-MRSA cases are quinolone resistant. Recurrent impetigo is associated with nasal carriage of *S aureus* and is treated with rifampin, 300 mg orally twice daily for 5 days. Intranasal mupirocin ointment twice daily for 5 days clears the carriage of 40% of MRSA strains. Bleach baths (¼ to ½ cup per 20 liters of bathwater for 15 minutes 3–5 times weekly) for all family members, and the use of dilute household bleach to clean showers and other bath surfaces may help reduce the spread. Individuals should not share towels if there is a case of impetigo in the household.

Hartman-Adams H et al. Impetigo: diagnosis and treatment. Am Fam Physician. 2014 Aug 15;90(4):229–35. [PMID: 25250996]

CONTACT DERMATITIS

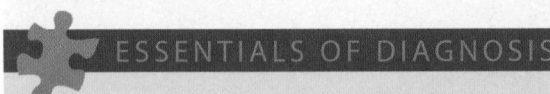

ESSENTIALS OF DIAGNOSIS

▶ Erythema and edema, with pruritus, vesicles, bullae, weeping or crusting.

▶ **Irritant contact dermatitis:** occurs only in area of direct contact with irritant.

▶ **Allergic contact dermatitis:** extends beyond area of direct contact with allergen; positive patch test.

▶ General Considerations

Contact dermatitis (irritant or allergic) is an acute or chronic dermatitis that results from direct skin contact with chemicals or allergens. Eighty percent of cases are due to excessive exposure to or additive effects of universal irritants (eg, soaps, detergents, organic solvents) and are called **irritant contact dermatitis**. The most common causes of **allergic contact dermatitis** are poison ivy or poison oak, topically applied antimicrobials (especially bacitracin and neomycin), anesthetics (benzocaine), preservatives, jewelry (nickel), rubber, essential oils, propolis (from bees), vitamin E, and adhesive tape. Occupational exposure is an important cause of allergic contact dermatitis.

▶ Clinical Findings

A. Symptoms and Signs

1. Allergic contact dermatitis—The acute phase is characterized by intense pruritus, tiny vesicles and weepy and crusted lesions. The lesions, distributed on exposed parts or in bizarre asymmetric patterns, consist of erythematous macules, papules, and vesicles and may occur beyond the contact area, distinguishing it from irritant dermatitis. The affected area may also be edematous and warm, simulating—and at times complicated by—infection. The pattern of the eruption may be diagnostic (eg, typical linear streaked vesicles on the extremities in poison oak or ivy dermatitis [Figure 6–18]). The location will often suggest the cause: scalp involvement suggests hair dyes or shampoos; face involvement, creams, cosmetics, soaps, shaving materials, nail polish; and neck involvement, jewelry, hair dyes. Reactions may not develop for 48–72 hours after exposure.

2. Irritant contact dermatitis—The rash is erythematous and scaly (but less likely vesicular) and occurs only in the

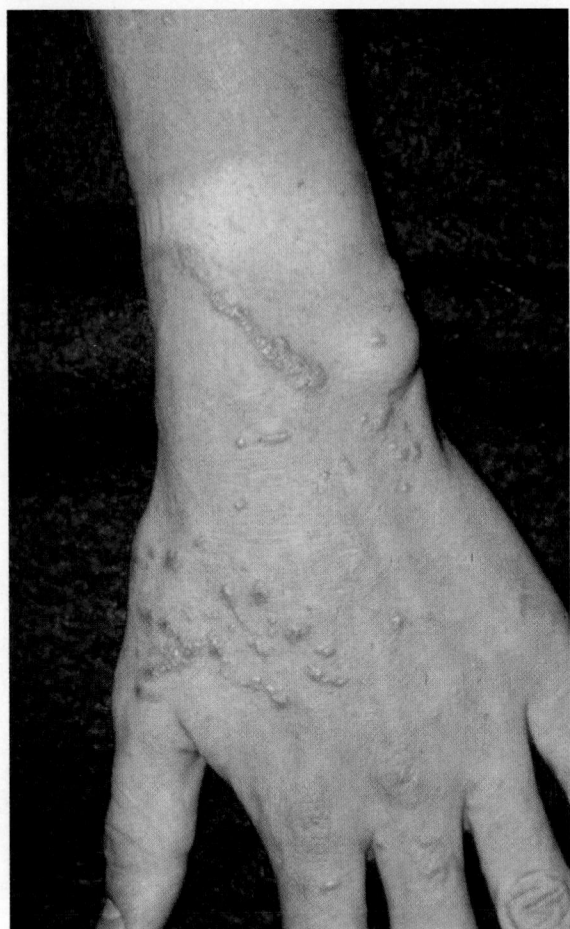

▲ **Figure 6–18.** Contact dermatitis with linear pattern due to poison ivy. (Used, with permission, from TG Berger, MD, Dept Dermatology, UCSF.)

direct sites of contact with the irritant. Resolving or chronic contact dermatitis presents with scaling, erythema, and possibly thickened skin. Itching, burning, and stinging may be severe in both allergic and irritant contact dermatitis. Reactions may develop within 24 hours of contact exposure.

B. Laboratory Findings

Gram stain and culture will rule out impetigo or secondary infection (impetiginization). After the episode of allergic contact dermatitis has cleared, patch testing may be useful if the triggering allergen is not known.

▶ Differential Diagnosis

Asymmetric distribution, blotchy erythema around the face, linear lesions, and a history of exposure help distinguish acute contact dermatitis from other skin lesions. The most commonly mistaken diagnosis is impetigo or cellulitis. Chronic allergic contact dermatitis must be differentiated from scabies, particularly if itching is generalized; atopic dermatitis; and pompholyx.

Prevention

Prompt and thorough removal of the causative oil by washing with liquid soap may be effective if done within 30 minutes after exposure to poison oak or ivy. Goop and Tecnu are also effective but much more expensive without increased efficacy. Over-the-counter barrier creams may be effective when applied prior to exposure and prevent/reduce the severity of the dermatitis.

The mainstay of prevention is identification of the agent causing the dermatitis and strict avoidance of exposure or use of protective clothing and gloves. In industry-related cases, prevention may be accomplished by moving or retraining the worker.

Treatment

A. Overview

While local measures are important, severe or widespread involvement is difficult to manage without systemic corticosteroids because even the highest-potency topical corticosteroids seem not to work well on vesicular and weepy lesions. Localized involvement (except on the face) can often be managed solely with topical agents. Irritant contact dermatitis is treated by protection from the irritant and use of topical corticosteroids as for atopic dermatitis (described above). The treatment of allergic contact dermatitis is detailed below.

B. Local Measures

1. Acute weeping dermatitis—Gentle cleansing and drying compresses (such as Domeboro) are recommended. Calamine lotion or zinc oxide paste may be used between wet dressings, especially for involvement of intertriginous areas or when oozing is not marked. Lesions on the extremities may be bandaged with wet dressings for 30–60 minutes several times a day. High-potency topical corticosteroids in gel or cream form (eg, fluocinonide, clobetasol, or halobetasol) may help suppress acute contact dermatitis and relieve itching. This treatment should be followed by tapering of the number of applications per day or use of a mid-potency corticosteroid, such as triamcinolone 0.1% cream to prevent rebound of the dermatitis. A soothing formulation is 2 oz of 0.1% triamcinolone acetonide cream in 7.5 oz Sarna lotion (0.5% camphor, 0.5% menthol, 0.5% phenol) mixed by the patient.

2. Subacute dermatitis (subsiding)—Mid-potency (triamcinolone 0.1%) to high-potency corticosteroids (clobetasol, fluocinonide, desoximetasone) are the mainstays of therapy.

3. Chronic dermatitis (dry and lichenified)—High-potency to superpotency corticosteroids are used in ointment form. Occlusion may be helpful on the hands.

C. Systemic Therapy

For acute severe cases, prednisone may be given orally for 12–21 days. Prednisone, 60 mg for 4–7 days, 40 mg for 4–7 days, and 20 mg for 4–7 days without a further taper is one useful regimen. The key is to use enough corticosteroid (and as early as possible) to achieve a clinical effect and to taper slowly over 2–3 weeks to avoid rebound.

Prognosis

Allergic contact dermatitis is self-limited if reexposure is prevented but often takes 2–3 weeks for full resolution. Removal of the causative agent is paramount to avoid recurrences.

Mowad CM. Contact dermatitis: practice gaps and challenges. Dermatol Clin. 2016 Jul;34(3):263–7. [PMID: 27363882]

Mowad CM et al. Allergic contact dermatitis: patient diagnosis and evaluation. J Am Acad Dermatol. 2016 Jun;74(6):1029–40. [PMID: 27185421]

Mowad CM et al. Allergic contact dermatitis: patient management and education. J Am Acad Dermatol. 2016 Jun;74(6):1043–54. [PMID: 27185422]

PUSTULAR DISORDERS

ACNE VULGARIS

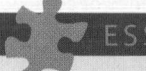

ESSENTIALS OF DIAGNOSIS

► Almost universal in puberty, though may begin in premenarchal girls and present or persist into the fourth or fifth decade.

► Comedones are the hallmark. Severity varies from purely comedonal to papular or pustular inflammatory acne to cysts or nodules.

► Face, neck, and upper trunk may be affected.

► Scarring may be a sequela of the disease or picking by the patient.

General Considerations

Acne vulgaris is polymorphic. Open and closed comedones, papules, pustules, and cysts are found.

In younger persons, acne vulgaris is more common and more severe in males. It does not always clear spontaneously when maturity is reached. Twelve percent of women and 3% of men over age 25 have acne vulgaris. This rate does not decrease until the fourth or fifth decade of life. The skin lesions parallel sebaceous activity. Pathogenic events include plugging of the infundibulum of the follicles, retention of sebum, overgrowth of the acne bacillus (*Propionibacterium acnes*) with resultant release of and irritation by accumulated fatty acids, and foreign-body reaction to extrafollicular sebum. Antibiotics may help control acne because of their antibacterial or anti-inflammatory properties.

Hyperandrogenism may be a cause of acne in women and may or may not be accompanied by hirsutism or irregular menses. Polycystic ovary syndrome (PCOS) is the most common identifiable cause. Acne may develop in patients who use systemic corticosteroids or topical fluorinated corticosteroids on the face. Acne may be exacerbated or caused by cosmetic creams or oils.

Clinical Findings

There may be mild tenderness, pain, or itching. The lesions occur mainly over the face, neck, upper chest, back, and shoulders. Comedones (tiny, flesh-colored, white or black noninflamed superficial papules that give the skin a rough texture or appearance) are the hallmark of acne vulgaris. Inflammatory papules, pustules, ectatic pores, acne cysts, and scarring are also seen (Figure 6–19).

Acne may have different presentations at different ages. Preteens often present with comedones as their first lesions. Inflammatory lesions in young teenagers are often found in the middle of the face, extending outward as the patient becomes older. Women in their third and fourth decades (often with no prior history of acne) commonly present with papular lesions on the chin and jawline.

Differential Diagnosis

In adults, rosacea presents with papules and pustules in the middle third of the face, but absence of truncal involvement, telangiectasia, flushing, and the absence of comedones distinguish rosacea from acne vulgaris. A pustular eruption on the face in patients receiving antibiotics or with otitis externa should be investigated with culture to

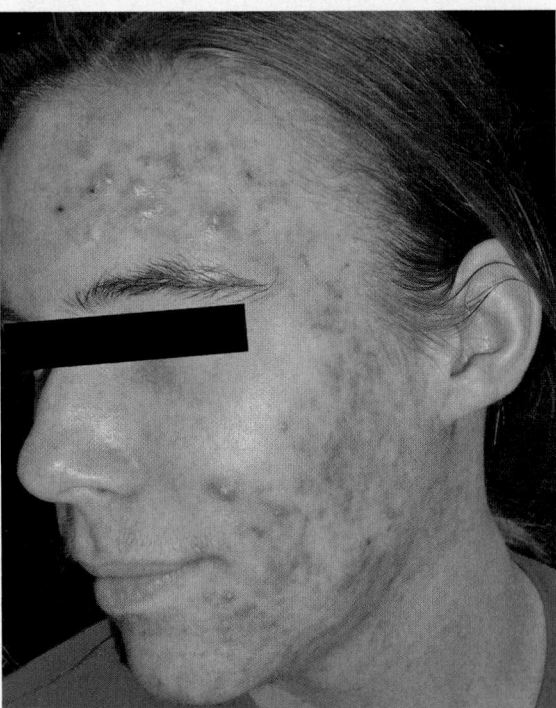

▲ **Figure 6–19.** Acne vulgaris, severe papulopustular and nodular cystic form with scarring. (Used, with permission, from Richard P. Usatine, MD, in Usatine RP, Smith MA, Mayeaux EJ Jr, Chumley H, Tysinger J. *The Color Atlas of Family Medicine*. McGraw-Hill, 2009.)

rule out a gram-negative folliculitis. Pustules on the face can also be caused by tinea infections. Lesions on the back are more problematic. When they occur alone, staphylococcal folliculitis, miliaria ("heat rash") or, uncommonly, *Malassezia (Pityrosporum)* folliculitis should be suspected. Bacterial culture, trial of an antistaphylococcal antibiotic, and observing the response to therapy will help in the differential diagnosis. In patients with HIV infection, folliculitis is common and may be either staphylococcal folliculitis or eosinophilic folliculitis (typically pruritic tumid papules on the face and neck).

Complications

Cyst formation, pigmentary changes, scarring, and poor quality of life may result.

Treatment

A. General Measures

1. Education of the patient—Education on proper use of medications and cosmetics is paramount. Because lesions take 4–6 weeks to improve, clinical improvement should be measured by the number of new lesions forming after 6–8 weeks of therapy. Additional time (3–4 months) will be required to see improvement on the back and chest, as these areas are slowest to respond. Avoid topical exposure to oils, cocoa butter (theobroma oil), and greases in cosmetics, including hair products. Scarring may occur with or without the patient manipulating the lesions. It is essential that the patient be educated in a supportive way about this complication. Anxiety and depression are common in patients with excoriated acne.

2. Diet—A low glycemic diet has been associated with improvement and lower incidence of acne. This improvement was associated with a reduction in insulin resistance. Hyperinsulinemia has also been associated with acne in both eumenorrheic women and individuals with PCOS.

B. Comedonal Acne

Treatment of acne is based on the type and severity of lesions. Comedones require treatment different from that of pustules and cystic lesions. In assessing severity, take the sequelae of the lesions into account. An individual who gets only a few new lesions per month that scar or leave postinflammatory hyperpigmentation must be treated much more aggressively than a comparable patient whose lesions clear without sequelae. Hygiene plays little role in acne treatment, and a mild soap is almost always recommended. The agents effective in comedonal acne are listed below in the order in which they should be tried.

1. Topical retinoids—Tretinoin is very effective for comedonal acne or for treatment of the comedonal component of more severe acne, but its usefulness is limited by irritation. Start with 0.025% cream (not gel) and have the patient use it at first twice weekly at night, increasing frequency to nightly as tolerated. A few patients cannot use even this low-strength preparation more than three times weekly but even that may cause improvement. A lentil-sized amount is sufficient to cover the entire face. To avoid irritation, have the patient wait 20 minutes after washing to apply. Adapalene gel 0.1% and reformulated tretinoin (Renova, Retin A Micro, Avita) are other options for patients irritated by standard tretinoin preparations. Although the absorption of tretinoin is minimal, its use during pregnancy is contraindicated. Patients should be warned that their acne may flare in the first 4 weeks of treatment.

2. Benzoyl peroxide—Benzoyl peroxide products are available in concentrations of 2.5%, 4%, 5%, 8%, and 10%, but 2.5% is as effective as 10% and less irritating. In general, water-based and not alcohol-based gels should be used to decrease irritation. Single formulations of benzoyl peroxide in combination with several other topical agents, including adapalene and topical antibiotics (erythromycin, clindamycin phosphate), are available.

C. Papular or Cystic Inflammatory Acne

Brief treatment (3 weeks to 3 months) with topical or oral antibiotics is the mainstay for treatment of inflammatory acne that does not respond to topical therapy with retinoids or benzoyl peroxide. Topical clindamycin phosphate and erythromycin are used only for mild papular acne that can be controlled by topicals alone or for patients who refuse or cannot tolerate oral antibiotics. To decrease resistance, benzoyl peroxide should be used in combination with the topical antibiotic.

1. Mild acne—The first choice of topical antibiotics in terms of efficacy and relative lack of induction of resistant *P acnes* is the combination of erythromycin or clindamycin with benzoyl peroxide topical gel or wash. These may be used once or twice daily. The addition of tretinoin cream or gel at night may increase improvement, since it works via a different mechanism. Topical retinoids ideally are used after acne clearance is achieved as a long-term maintenance therapy.

2. Moderate acne—Common oral antibiotics used for acne include doxycycline (100 mg twice daily), minocycline (50–100 mg once or twice daily), TMP-SMZ (one double-strength tablet twice daily), or a cephalosporin (cefadroxil or cephalexin 500 mg twice daily), which should be used in combination with benzoyl peroxide to minimize development of antibiotic resistance. Once the patient's skin is clear, instructions should be given for tapering the dose by 50% every 6–8 weeks—while treating with topical antibiotics or retinoids—to arrive at the lowest systemic dose needed to maintain clearing. In general, discontinuing antibiotics immediately without adjunctive topical therapy results in prompt recurrence. Topical retinoids are excellent for long-term maintenance following antibiotics. Subantimicrobial dosing of doxycycline (40–50 mg orally daily) can be used in patients who require long-term systemic therapy. Combination oral contraceptives or spironolactone (50–200 mg orally daily) are highly effective alternatives in women with treatment-resistant acne. Tetracycline, minocycline, and doxycycline are contraindicated in pregnancy, but certain oral erythromycins or cephalosporins may be used.

3. Severe acne—

A. ISOTRETINOIN—A vitamin A analog, isotretinoin is used for the treatment of severe acne that has not responded to conventional therapy. An oral dosage of 0.5–1 mg/kg/day for 20 weeks for a cumulative dose of at least 120 mg/kg is usually adequate for severe cystic acne. Patients should be offered isotretinoin therapy before they experience significant scarring if they are not promptly and adequately controlled by antibiotics. **The medication is absolutely contraindicated during pregnancy because of its teratogenicity.** Two forms of effective contraception must be used; abstinence is an acceptable alternative. Informed consent must be obtained before its use, and patients must be enrolled in a monitoring program (iPledge). In addition to its teratogenicity, isotretinoin has numerous serious side effects and should only be prescribed by clinicians (usually dermatologists) well aware of these issues. Consider ordering laboratory tests, including total cholesterol levels, triglyceride levels, and liver enzyme tests (particularly alanine aminotransferase, which is the most liver-specific enzyme), in patients before treatment and after achieving therapeutic dosing; monitoring through the entire treatment may not be high value.

Abnormal laboratory tests, especially elevated liver enzymes and triglyceride levels, return to normal quickly upon conclusion of therapy. The medication may induce long-term remissions in 40–60%, or acne may recur that is more easily controlled with conventional therapy. Occasionally, a second course is needed if acne does not respond or recurs.

B. INTRALESIONAL INJECTION—Intralesional injection of dilute suspensions of triamcinolone acetonide (2.5 mg/mL, 0.05 mL per lesion) will often hasten the resolution of deeper papules and occasional cysts.

C. SCAR REVISION—Cosmetic improvement may be achieved by excision and punch-grafting of deep scars and by physical or chemical abrasion of inactive acne lesions, particularly flat, superficial scars.

▶ **Prognosis**

Acne vulgaris eventually remits spontaneously, but when this will occur cannot be predicted. The condition may persist throughout adulthood and may lead to severe scarring if left untreated. Patients treated with antibiotics continue to improve for the first 3–6 months of therapy. Relapse during treatment may suggest the emergence of resistant *P acnes*. The disease is chronic and tends to flare intermittently in spite of treatment. Remissions following systemic treatment with isotretinoin may be lasting in up to 60% of cases. Relapses after isotretinoin usually occur within 3 years and require a second course in up to 20% of patients. Immediate relapse after isotretinoin discontinuation may suggest hyperandrogenism or other underlying hormonal disorders in a female patient.

Bienenfeld A et al. Oral antibacterial therapy for acne vulgaris: an evidence-based review. Am J Clin Dermatol. 2017 Aug; 18(4):469–90. [PMID: 28255924]

Zaenglein AL. Acne vulgaris. N Engl J Med. 2018 Oct 4;379(14): 1343–52. [PMID: 30281982]

ROSACEA

▶ A chronic disorder affecting the face.

▶ Neurovascular component: erythema and telangi-
ectasis and a tendency to flush easily.

▶ Acneiform component: papules and pustules may
be present.

▶ Glandular component: sebaceous hyperplasia and
fibrosis of affected areas (eg, rhinophyma).

▶ General Considerations

Rosacea is a common condition that presents in adulthood.
The pathogenesis of this chronic disorder is not known.
Topical corticosteroids applied to the face can induce
rosacea-like conditions.

▶ Clinical Findings

Patients frequently report flushing or exacerbation of their
rosacea due to heat, hot drinks, spicy food, sunlight, exercise, alcohol, emotions, or menopausal flushing. The
cheeks, nose, chin, and ears —at times the entire face—may
be affected. No comedones are seen. In its mildest form,
erythema and telangiectasias are seen on the cheeks.
Inflammatory papules may be superimposed on this background and may evolve to pustules (Figure 6–20). Associated seborrhea may be found. The patient often complains
of burning or stinging with episodes of flushing and
extremely cosmetic-intolerant skin. Patients may have
associated ophthalmic disease, including blepharitis, keratitis, and chalazion, which often requires topical or systemic antibiotic or immunosuppressive therapy.

▶ Differential Diagnosis

Rosacea is distinguished from acne by the presence of the
neurovascular component and the absence of comedones.
Lupus is often misdiagnosed, but the presence of pustules
excludes that diagnosis.

▶ Treatment

Educating patients to avoid the factors they know to produce
exacerbations is important. Patients should wear a broad-
spectrum mineral-based sunscreen; zinc- or titanium-based
sunscreens are tolerated best. Medical management is most
effective for the inflammatory papules and pustules and the
erythema that surrounds them. Rosacea is usually a lifelong
condition, so maintenance therapy is required. Telangiectases are benefited by laser therapy, and phymatous overgrowth of the nose can be treated by surgical reduction.

A. Local Therapy

Avoidance of triggers (especially alcohol and spicy or hot
foods) and drinking ice water may be effective in reducing

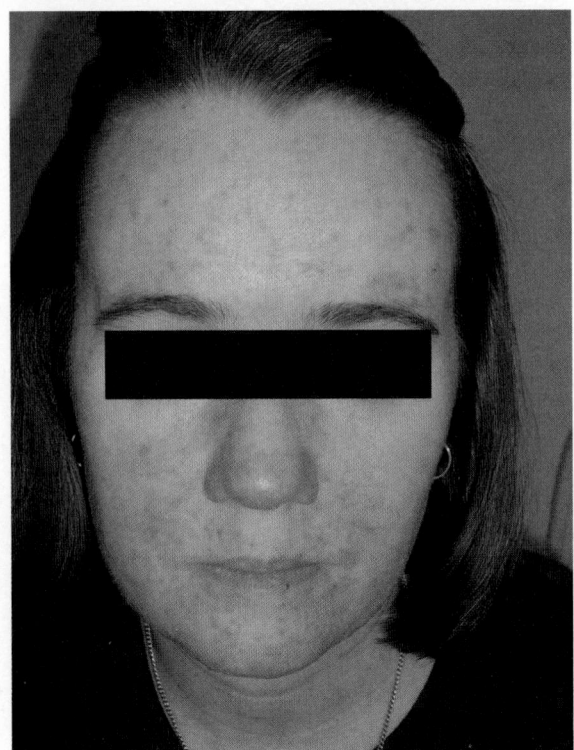

▲ **Figure 6–20.** Rosacea in a 34-year-old woman showing erythema, papules, and pustules covering much of
the face. (Used, with permission, from Richard P. Usatine,
MD, in Usatine RP, Smith MA, Mayeaux EJ Jr, Chumley H.
The Color Atlas of Family Medicine, 2nd ed. McGraw-Hill,
2013.)

facial erythema and flushing. Metronidazole (available as
creams, gels, or lotions), 0.75% applied twice daily or 1%
applied once daily, and ivermectin 1% cream applied once
daily are effective topical treatments. Another effective treatment includes topical clindamycin (solution, gel, or lotion)
1% applied twice daily. Response is noted in 4–8 weeks.
Sulfur-sodium sulfacetamide-containing topicals are helpful
in patients only partially responsive to topical antibiotics.
Topical retinoids can be carefully added for maintenance.
Topical brimonidine tartrate gel 0.33% or oxymetazoline 1%
cream can temporarily reduce the erythema.

B. Systemic Therapy

Oral tetracyclines should be used when topical therapy is
inadequate. Minocycline or doxycycline, 50–100 mg orally
once or twice daily, is effective. Metronidazole or amoxicillin, 250–500 mg orally twice daily, or rifaximin, 400 mg
orally three times daily (for 10 days), may be used in refractory cases. Side effects are few, although metronidazole
may produce a disulfiram-like effect when the patient
ingests alcohol, and it may cause neuropathy with long-term
use. Long-term maintenance with subantimicrobial dosing
of minocycline or doxycycline is recommended once the
initial flare of rosacea has resolved. Isotretinoin may suc-
ceed where other measures fail. A dosage of 0.5 mg/kg/day

orally for 12–28 weeks is recommended, although very low-dose isotretinoin may also be effective. See precautions above.

Prognosis

Rosacea tends to be a persistent process. With the regimens described above, it can usually be controlled adequately.

Two AM et al. Rosacea: part I. Introduction, categorization, histology, pathogenesis, and risk factors. J Am Acad Dermatol. 2015 May;72(5):749–58. [PMID: 25890455]

Two AM et al. Rosacea: part II. Topical and systemic therapies in the treatment of rosacea. J Am Acad Dermatol. 2015 May; 72(5):761–70. [PMID: 25890456]

Van Zuuren EJ et al. Interventions for rosacea: abridged updated Cochrane systematic review including GRADE assessments. Br J Dermatol. 2015 Sep;173(3):651–62. [PMID: 26099423]

FOLLICULITIS (Including Sycosis)

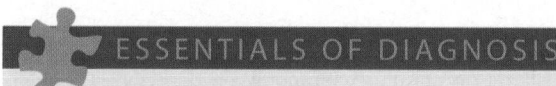

ESSENTIALS OF DIAGNOSIS

- ▶ Itching and burning in hairy areas.
- ▶ Pustule surrounding and including the hair follicle.

General Considerations

Folliculitis has multiple causes. It is frequently caused by staphylococcal infection and may be more common in the diabetic patient. When the lesion is deep-seated, chronic, and recalcitrant on the head and neck, it is called **sycosis.**

Gram-negative folliculitis, which may develop during antibiotic treatment of acne, may present as a flare of acne pustules or nodules. *Klebsiella, Enterobacter, Escherichia coli,* and *Proteus* have been isolated from these lesions.

Hot tub folliculitis (*Pseudomonas* folliculitis), caused by *Pseudomonas aeruginosa,* is characterized by pruritic or tender follicular, pustular lesions occurring within 1–4 days after bathing in a contaminated hot tub, whirlpool, or swimming pool. Systemic flu-like symptoms may be present. Rarely, systemic infections may result. Neutropenic patients should avoid these exposures.

Nonbacterial folliculitis may also be caused by friction and oils. Occlusion, perspiration, and chronic rubbing (eg, from tight jeans or other heavy fabrics on the buttocks and thighs) can worsen this type of folliculitis.

Steroid acne may be seen during topical or systemic corticosteroid therapy and presents as eruptive monomorphous papules and papulopustules on the face and trunk. It responds to topical benzoyl peroxide.

Eosinophilic folliculitis is a sterile folliculitis that presents with urticarial papules with prominent eosinophilic infiltration. It is common in patients with AIDS. It may appear first with institution of highly active antiretroviral therapy (ART) and be mistaken for a drug eruption.

Pseudofolliculitis is caused by ingrowing hairs in the beard area. It occurs in men and women with tightly curled beard hair. In this entity, the papules and pustules are located at the side of and not in follicles. It may be treated by growing a beard, by using chemical depilatories, or by shaving with a foil-guard razor. Medically indicated laser hair removal is dramatically beneficial in patients with pseudofolliculitis and can be done on patients of any skin color.

Malassezia (Pityrosporum) folliculitis presents as 1–2-mm pruritic pink papulopustules on the upper trunk and arms. It is often pruritic and tends to develop during periods of excessive sweating.

Demodex folliculitis is caused by the mite *Demodex folliculorum* and presents as 1–2 mm papules and pustules on an erythematous base, often on the background of rosacea-like changes, in patients who have not responded to conventional treatment for rosacea. It is more common in immunosuppressed patients. KOH from the pustules will demonstrate *Demodex folliculorum* mites.

Clinical Findings

The symptoms range from slight burning and tenderness to intense itching. The lesions consist of pustules of hair follicles (Figure 6–21).

Differential Diagnosis

It is important to differentiate bacterial from nonbacterial folliculitis. The history is important for pinpointing the causes of nonbacterial folliculitis, and a Gram stain and culture are indispensable. One must differentiate folliculitis from acne vulgaris or pustular miliaria (heat rash) and from infections of the skin, such as impetigo or fungal infections, especially *Malassezia (Pityrosporum)* folliculitis. *Pseudomonas* folliculitis is often suggested by the history of hot tub use. Eosinophilic folliculitis in AIDS often requires biopsy for diagnosis.

Complications

Abscess formation is the major complication of bacterial folliculitis.

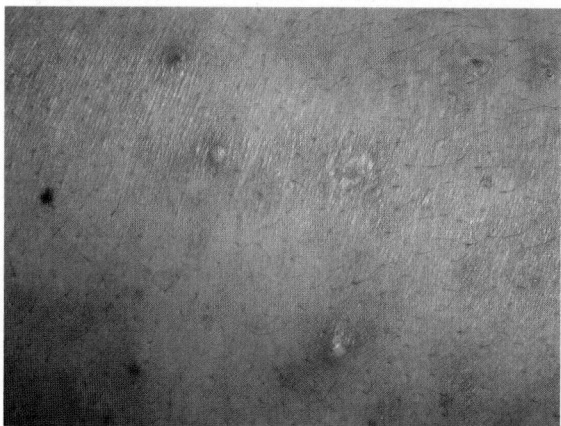

▲ **Figure 6–21.** Bacterial folliculitis. Hair eminating from the center of the pustule is the clinical hallmark of folliculitis. (Used, with permission, from Richard P. Usatine, MD, in Usatine RP, Smith MA, Mayeaux EJ Jr, Chumley H. *The Color Atlas of Family Medicine,* 2nd ed. McGraw-Hill, 2013.)

Prevention

Correct any predisposing local causes, such as oils or friction. Be sure that the water in hot tubs and spas is treated properly. If staphylococcal folliculitis is persistent, treatment of nasal or perineal carriage with rifampin, 600 mg daily for 5 days, or with topical mupirocin ointment 2% twice daily for 5 days, may help. Prolonged oral clindamycin, 150–300 mg/day for 4–6 weeks, or oral TMP-SMZ given 1 week per month for 6 months can be effective in preventing recurrent staphylococcal folliculitis and furunculosis. Bleach baths (¼ to ½ cup per 20 liters of bathwater for 15 minutes 3–5 times weekly) may reduce cutaneous staphylococcal carriage and not contribute to antibiotic resistance. Control of blood glucose in diabetes may reduce the number of these infections.

Treatment

A. Local Measures

Anhydrous ethyl alcohol containing 6.25% aluminum chloride (Xerac AC), applied three to seven times weekly to lesions, may be helpful, especially for chronic frictional folliculitis of the buttocks. Topical antibiotics are generally ineffective if bacteria have invaded the hair follicle but may be prophylactic if used as an aftershave in patients with recurrent folliculitis after shaving.

B. Specific Measures

Pseudomonas folliculitis will clear spontaneously in non-neutropenic patients if the lesions are superficial. It may be treated with ciprofloxacin, 500 mg orally twice daily for 5 days.

Systemic antibiotics are recommended for bacterial folliculitis due to other organisms. Extended periods of treatment (4–8 weeks or more) with antistaphylococcal antibiotics are required if infection has involved the scalp or densely hairy areas, such as the axilla, beard, or groin (see Table 30–4).

Gram-negative folliculitis in acne patients may be treated with isotretinoin in compliance with all precautions discussed above (see Acne Vulgaris).

Eosinophilic folliculitis may be treated initially by the combination of potent topical corticosteroids and oral antihistamines. In more severe cases, treatment is with one of the following: topical permethrin (application for 12 hours every other night for 6 weeks); itraconazole, 200–400 mg orally daily; UVB or PUVA phototherapy; or isotretinoin, 0.5 mg/kg/day orally for up to 5 months. A remission may be induced by some of these therapies, but long-term treatment may be required.

Malassezia (Pityrosporum) folliculitis is treated with topical sulfacetamide lotion twice a day, alone or in combination with itraconazole or fluconazole.

Demodex folliculitis is treated with topical 5% permethrin applied every other night or ivermectin either by daily topical or weekly oral administration.

Prognosis

Bacterial folliculitis is occasionally stubborn and persistent, requiring prolonged or intermittent courses of antibiotics.

Bachmeyer C et al. Demodex folliculitis. CMAJ. 2017 Jun 26; 189(25):E865. [PMID: 28652482]

Laureano AC et al. Facial bacterial infections: folliculitis. Clin Dermatol. 2014 Nov–Dec;32(6):711–4. [PMID: 25441463]

MILIARIA (Heat Rash)

ESSENTIALS OF DIAGNOSIS

▶ Burning, itching, superficial aggregated small vesicles, papules, or pustules on covered areas of the skin, usually the trunk.

▶ More common in hot, moist climates.

▶ Rare forms associated with fever and even heat prostration.

General Considerations

Miliaria occurs most commonly on the trunk and intertriginous areas. A hot, moist environment is the most frequent cause. Occlusive clothing, fever while bedridden, and medications that enhance sweat gland function (eg, clonidine, beta-blockers, opioids) may increase the risk. Plugging of the ostia of sweat ducts occurs, with ultimate rupture of the sweat duct, producing an irritating, stinging reaction. Increase in numbers of resident aerobes, notably cocci, plays a role.

Clinical Findings

The usual symptoms are burning and itching. The histologic depth of sweat gland obstruction determines the clinical presentation: miliaria crystallina in the superficial (subcorneal) epidermis, miliaria rubra in the deep epidermis, and miliaria profunda in the dermis. The lesions consist of small (1–3 mm) nonfollicular lesions. Subcorneal thin-walled, discrete clear fluid-filled vesicles are termed "miliaria crystallina." When fluid is turbid and lesions present as vesicopustules or pustules, they are called miliaria pustulosa. Miliaria rubra (prickly heat) presents as pink papules. Miliaria profunda presents as nonfollicular skin-colored papules that develop after multiple bouts of miliaria rubra. In a hospitalized patient, the reaction virtually always affects the back.

Differential Diagnosis

Miliaria is to be distinguished from a drug eruption and folliculitis.

Prevention

Use of a topical antibacterial preparation, such as chlorhexidine, prior to exposure to heat and humidity may help prevent the condition. Frequent turning or sitting of the hospitalized patient may reduce miliaria on the back.

Treatment

The patient should keep cool and wear light clothing. Triamcinolone acetonide, 0.1% in Sarna lotion, or a mid-potency corticosteroid in a lotion or cream may be applied two to four times daily. Secondary infections (superficial pyoderma) are treated with appropriate anti-staphylococcal antibiotics. Anticholinergic medications (eg, glycopyrrolate 1 mg orally twice a day) may be helpful in severe cases.

Prognosis

Miliaria is usually a mild disorder, but severe forms (tropical anhidrosis and asthenia) result from interference with the heat-regulating mechanism.

Tey HL et al. In vivo imaging of miliaria profunda using high-definition optical coherence tomography: diagnosis, pathogenesis, and treatment. JAMA Dermatol. 2015 Mar 1;151(3):346–8. [PMID: 25390622]

Yanamandra U et al. Miliaria crystallina: relevance in patients with hemato-oncological febrile neutropenia. BMJ Case Rep. 2015 Nov 26;5:212231. [PMID: 26611484]

MUCOCUTANEOUS CANDIDIASIS

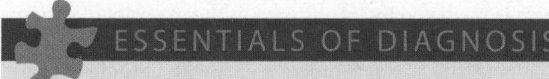

ESSENTIALS OF DIAGNOSIS

▶ Severe pruritus of vulva, anus, or body folds.

▶ Superficial denuded, beefy-red areas with or without satellite vesicopustules.

▶ Whitish curd-like concretions on the oral and vaginal mucous membranes.

▶ Yeast and pseudohyphae on microscopic examination of scales or curd.

General Considerations

Mucocutaneous candidiasis is a superficial fungal infection that may involve almost any cutaneous or mucous surface of the body. It is particularly likely to occur in diabetic patients, during pregnancy, in obese persons, and in the setting of immunosuppression. Systemic antibiotics, oral corticosteroids, hormone replacement therapy, and oral contraceptive agents may be contributory. Oral and inter-digital candidiasis may be the first sign of HIV infection (see Chapter 31). Denture use predisposes the elderly to infection.

Clinical Findings

A. Symptoms and Signs

Itching may be intense. Burning is reported, particularly around the vulva and anus. The lesions consist of

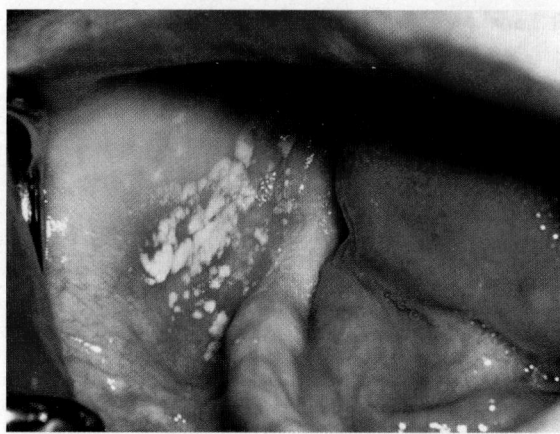

▲ **Figure 6–22.** Oral mucosal candidiasis. (Used with permission from Sol Silverman, Jr, DDS, Public Health Image Library, CDC.)

superficially denuded, beefy-red areas in the depths of the body folds, such as in the groin and the intergluteal cleft, beneath the breasts, at the angles of the mouth, in the webspaces of digits, and in the umbilicus. The peripheries of these denuded lesions are superficially undermined, and there may be satellite vesicopustules. Whitish, curd-like concretions may be present on mucosal lesions (Figure 6–22). Paronychia may occur.

B. Laboratory Findings

Clusters of budding yeast and pseudohyphae can be seen under high power (400×) when skin scales or curd-like lesions are mounted in 10% KOH. Culture can confirm the diagnosis.

Differential Diagnosis

Intertrigo, seborrheic dermatitis, tinea cruris, "inverse psoriasis", and erythrasma involving the same areas may mimic mucocutaneous candidiasis.

Complications

Systemic invasive candidiasis with candidemia may be seen with immunosuppression and in patients receiving broad-spectrum antibiotic and hypertonic glucose solutions, as in hyperalimentation. There may or may not be clinically evident mucocutaneous candidiasis.

Treatment

A. General Measures

Affected parts should be kept dry and exposed to air as much as possible. Water immersion should be minimized and gloves should be worn for those with infected nails or digital skin. If possible, discontinue systemic antibiotics. For treatment of systemic invasive candidiasis, see Chapter 36.

B. Local Measures

1. Nails and paronychia—Apply clotrimazole solution 1% twice daily. Thymol 4% in ethanol applied once daily is an alternative.

2. Skin—Apply either nystatin ointment or clotrimazole cream 1%, with hydrocortisone cream 1%, twice daily. Gentian violet 0.5% solution is economical and highly effective in treating mucocutaneous candidiasis, but the purple discoloration may represent a cosmetic issue. Severe or widespread cutaneous disease responds to fluconazole, 100–200 mg orally daily, for 1 week.

3. Vulvar and anal mucous membranes—For vaginal candidiasis, single-dose fluconazole (150 mg orally) is effective. Intravaginal clotrimazole, miconazole, terconazole, or nystatin may also be used. Long-term suppressive therapy may be required for recurrent or "intractable" cases. Non-albicans candidal species may be identified by culture in some refractory cases and may respond to oral itraconazole, 200 mg twice daily for 2–4 weeks.

4. Balanitis—This is most frequent in uncircumcised men, and *Candida* usually plays a role. Topical nystatin ointment is the initial treatment if the lesions are mildly erythematous or superficially erosive. Soaking with dilute aluminum acetate for 15 minutes twice daily may quickly relieve burning or itching. Chronicity and relapses, especially after sexual contact, suggest reinfection from a sexual partner who should be treated. Severe purulent balanitis is usually due to bacteria. If it is so severe that phimosis occurs, oral antibiotics—some with activity against anaerobes—are required; if rapid improvement does not occur, urologic consultation is indicated.

5. Mastitis—Lancinating breast pain and nipple dermatitis in breast-feeding women may be a manifestation of *Candida* colonization/infection of the breast ducts. Topical nystatin cream and clotrimazole 0.1% cream are safe during lactation. Topical gentian violet 0.5% daily for 7 days is also useful. Oral fluconazole, 200 mg daily for 2 weeks, can be dramatically effective.

▶ Prognosis

Cases of cutaneous candidiasis range from the easily cured to the intractable and prolonged.

Gonçalves B et al. Vulvovaginal candidiasis: epidemiology, microbiology and risk factors. Crit Rev Microbiol. 2016 Nov; 42(6):905–27. [PMID: 26690853]

Millsop JW et al. Oral candidiasis. Clin Dermatol. 2016 Jul–Aug; 34(4):487–94. [PMID: 27343964]

Pappas PG et al. Executive summary: clinical practice guideline for the management of candidiasis: 2016 update by the Infectious Diseases Society of America. Clin Infect Dis. 2016 Feb 15; 62(4):409–17. [PMID: 26810419]

Pichard DC et al. Primary immunodeficiency update: part II. Syndromes associated with mucocutaneous candidiasis and noninfectious cutaneous manifestations. J Am Acad Dermatol. 2015 Sep;73(3):367–81. [PMID: 26282795]

Sobel JD. Recurrent vulvovaginal candidiasis. Am J Obstet Gynecol. 2016 Jan;214(1):15–21. [PMID: 26164695]

ERYTHEMAS

REACTIVE ERYTHEMAS

1. Urticaria & Angioedema

ESSENTIALS OF DIAGNOSIS

▶ Eruptions of evanescent wheals or hives.

▶ Itching is intense but, rarely, may be absent.

▶ Special forms of urticaria have special features (dermatographism, cholinergic urticaria, solar urticaria, or cold urticaria).

▶ Most incidents are acute and self-limited (1–2 weeks).

▶ Chronic urticaria (episodes lasting longer than 6 weeks) may have an autoimmune basis.

▶ General Considerations

Urticaria is defined as acute (less than 6 weeks' duration) or chronic (more than 6 weeks' duration). Urticaria can result from many different stimuli on an immunologic or nonimmunologic basis. The most common immunologic mechanism is mediated by IgE, as seen in the majority of patients with acute urticaria; another involves activation of the complement cascade. Some patients with chronic urticaria demonstrate autoantibodies directed against mast cell IgE receptors. ACE inhibitor and angiotensin receptor blocker therapy may be complicated by urticaria or angioedema. In general, extensive costly workups are not indicated in patients who have urticaria. A careful history and physical examination are more helpful.

▶ Clinical Findings

A. Symptoms and Signs

Lesions are itchy, red swellings of a few millimeters to many centimeters (Figure 6–23). The morphology of the lesions may vary over a period of minutes to hours, resulting in geographic or bizarre patterns. Individual lesions in true urticaria last less than 24 hours, and often only 2–4 hours. Angioedema is involvement of deeper subcutaneous tissue with swelling of the lips, eyelids, palms, soles, and genitalia. **Angioedema is no more likely than urticaria to be associated with systemic complications, such as laryngeal edema or hypotension.** In cholinergic urticaria, which is triggered by a rise in core body temperature (hot showers, exercise), wheals are 2–3 mm in diameter with a large surrounding red flare. Cold urticaria is acquired or inherited and triggered by exposure to cold and wind (see Chapter 37).

B. Laboratory Findings

The most common causes of acute urticaria are foods, upper respiratory infections, and medications. The cause of

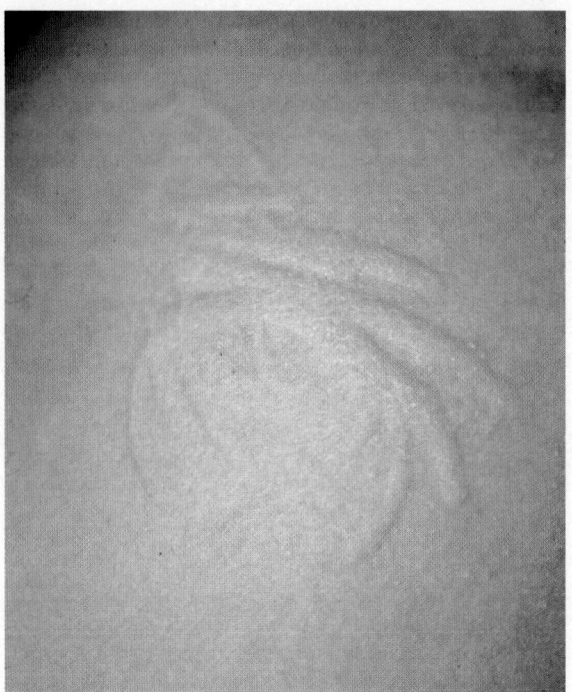

▲ **Figure 6–23.** Urticaria. (Used, with permission, from TG Berger, MD, Dept Dermatology, UCSF.)

chronic urticaria is often not found. Although laboratory studies are not likely to be helpful in the evaluation of acute or chronic urticaria, a complete blood count with differential, erythrocyte sedimentation rate, C-reactive protein, thyroid-stimulating hormone, and liver biochemical tests might be appropriate for some patients with chronic urticaria. In patients with individual lesions that persist past 24 hours, skin biopsy may confirm neutrophilic urticaria or urticarial vasculitis. A functional ELISA test looking for antibodies against the high-affinity receptor for IgE (Fc-Epislon RI) can detect patients with an autoimmune basis for their chronic urticaria.

► Differential Diagnosis

Papular urticaria resulting from insect bites persists for days. A central punctum can usually be seen. Streaked urticarial lesions may be seen in the 24–48 hours before blisters appear in acute allergic plant dermatitis, eg, poison ivy, oak, or sumac. Urticarial responses to heat, sun, water, and pressure are quite rare. Urticarial vasculitis is defined as cutaneous vasculitis where the skin lesions clinically mimic urticaria. Lesions last longer than 24 hours and often sting or burn rather than itch. Patients do not respond to antihistamines. Urticarial vasculitis may be caused by viral hepatitis and may be seen as part of serum sickness. In hereditary angioedema, there is generally a positive family history and gastrointestinal or respiratory symptoms. Urticaria is not part of the syndrome, and lesions are not pruritic.

► Treatment

A. General Measures

A detailed search by history for a cause of urticaria should be undertaken, and treatment may then be tailored to include the provocative condition. The etiology of acute urticaria is found in less than half of cases. The etiology of chronic urticaria is found in even fewer cases. Patients with chronic autoimmune urticaria may have other autoimmune diseases and may be more difficult to treat. In cases of chronic inducible urticaria, exposure to physical factors, such as heat, cold, sunlight, pressure, heat induced by exercise, excitement, and hot showers, should be modulated.

B. Systemic Treatment

The mainstay of treatment initially includes H_1-antihistamines. Initial therapy is hydroxyzine, 10 mg orally twice daily to 25 mg three times daily, or as a single nightly dose of 50–75 mg to reduce daytime sedation. Cyproheptadine, 4 mg orally four times daily, may be especially useful for cold urticaria. Second-generation H_1-antihistamines are added if the generic sedating antihistamines are not effective. Options include fexofenadine, 180 mg orally once daily; or cetirizine or loratadine, 10 mg orally daily. Higher doses of these second-generation antihistamines may be required to suppress urticaria (up to four times the standard recommended dose) and increase the likelihood of response to therapy to 60%. Combining antihistamines (eg, fexofenadine plus cetirizine) at these higher doses can be done safely to achieve remission in refractory cases, since less than 40% of cases of chronic urticaria respond to standard to H_1 blockade.

Doxepin (a tricyclic antidepressant with potent antihistaminic properties), 10–75 mg orally at bedtime, can be very effective in chronic urticaria. It has anticholinergic side effects.

H_2-antihistamines in combination with H_1-blockers may be helpful in patients with symptomatic dermatographism and to a lesser degree in chronic urticaria. UVB phototherapy can suppress some cases of chronic urticaria. If a skin biopsy of a lesion of chronic urticaria identifies neutrophils as a significant component of the inflammatory infiltrate, dapsone or colchicine (or both) may be useful.

A few patients with chronic urticaria may respond to elimination of salicylates and tartrazine (a coloring agent). Asymptomatic foci of infection—sinusitis, vaginal candidiasis, cholecystitis, and intestinal parasites—may rarely cause chronic urticaria. Although systemic corticosteroids in a dose of about 40 mg daily will usually suppress acute and chronic urticaria, the use of corticosteroids is rarely indicated and, once withdrawn, the urticaria virtually always returns. Instead of instituting systemic corticosteroids, consultation should be sought from a dermatologist or an allergist with experience in managing severe urticaria. Omalizumab is approved for the treatment of refractory chronic urticaria and should be considered when severe chronic urticaria fails to respond to high-dose antihistamines. Cyclosporine (3–5 mg/kg/day), mycophenolate mofetil, and other immunosuppressives may be effective in severe cases of chronic urticaria.

C. Local Treatment

Local treatment is rarely rewarding.

▶ Prognosis

Acute urticaria usually lasts only a few days to weeks. Half of patients whose urticaria persists for longer than 6 weeks will have it for years. Patients in whom angioedema develops with an ACE inhibitor may be switched to an angiotensin receptor blocker with caution (estimated cross-reaction about 10%).

Antia C et al. Urticaria: a comprehensive review: epidemiology, diagnosis, and work-up. J Am Acad Dermatol. 2018 Oct;79(4):599–614. [PMID: 30241623]

Antia C et al. Urticaria: a comprehensive review: treatment of chronic urticaria, special populations, and disease outcomes. J Am Acad Dermatol. 2018 Oct;79(4):617–33. [PMID: 30241624]

Fine LM et al. Guideline of chronic urticaria beyond. Allergy Asthma Immunol Res. 2016 Sep;8(5):396–403. [PMID: 27334777]

Gill P et al. The clinical evaluation of angioedema. Immunol Allergy Clin North Am. 2017 Aug;37(3):449–66. [PMID: 28687102]

Guillén-Aguinaga S et al. Updosing nonsedating antihistamines in patients with chronic spontaneous urticaria: a systematic review and meta-analysis. Br J Dermatol. 2016 Dec;175(6):1153–65. [PMID: 27237730]

Larenas-Linnemann DES et al. Update on omalizumab for urticaria: what's new in the literature from mechanisms to clinic. Curr Allergy Asthma Rep. 2018 May 9;18(5):33. [PMID: 29744661]

Rutkowski K et al. How to manage chronic urticaria 'beyond' guidelines: a practical algorithm. Clin Exp Allergy. 2017 Jun; 47(6):710–8. [PMID: 28452145]

2. Erythema Multiforme/Stevens-Johnson Syndrome/Toxic Epidermal Necrolysis

ESSENTIALS OF DIAGNOSIS

Erythema multiforme

▶ Herpes simplex is most common cause.

▶ Cutaneous lesions are true three ring targets.

▶ Presents on the extensor surfaces, palms, soles, or mucous membranes.

▶ Disease remains localized.

Stevens-Johnson syndrome and toxic epidermal necrolysis

▶ **Stevens-Johnson syndrome:** Less than 10% BSA detachment

▶ **Stevens-Johnson syndrome/toxic epidermal necrolysis overlap:** 10–30% BSA detachment

▶ **Toxic epidermal necrolysis:** Greater than 30% BSA detachment

▶ Medications are most common cause.

▶ Cutaneous lesions are targetoid but often not true three ring targets.

▶ Favors the trunk.

▶ Involves two or more mucous membranes.

▶ May progress so that significant BSA is involved and may be life-threatening.

▶ General Considerations

Erythema multiforme is an acute inflammatory skin disease that was traditionally divided clinically into minor and major types based on the clinical findings. Approximately 90% of cases of erythema multiforme minor follow outbreaks of herpes simplex, and so it is preferably termed "herpes-associated erythema multiforme." The term "erythema multiforme major" has largely been abandoned.

Stevens-Johnson syndrome (SJS) is defined as atypical target lesions with less than 10% BSA detachment; toxic epidermal necrolysis (TEN) is defined as lesions with greater than 30% BSA detachment; and patients with SJS/TEN overlap have between 10% and 30% BSA detachment. The abbreviation SJS/TEN is often used to refer to these three variants of what is considered one syndrome. SJS/TEN is characterized by toxicity and involvement of two or more mucosal surfaces (often oral and conjunctival but can involve any mucosal surface, including respiratory epithelium). SJS/TEN is most often caused by medications, especially sulfonamides, NSAIDs, allopurinol, and anticonvulsants. In certain races, polymorphisms of antigen-presenting major histocompatibility (MHC) loci increase the risk for the development of SJS/TEN; for example, screening for HLA-B*5801, which is associated with allopurinol-induced SJS/TEN, is recommended in Han Chinese, those of Thai descent, and Koreans with stage 3 or worse chronic kidney disease before initiation of allopurinol (see Chapter 20). The exposure to medications associated with SJS/TEN may be systemic or, less commonly, topical (eg, eyedrops). *Mycoplasma pneumoniae* may trigger a mucocutaneous reaction with skin and oral lesions closely resembling SJS in up to 50% of children/young adults in some series. This syndrome, *M pneumoniae*-induced rash and mucositis, tends not to progress to TEN-like disease and carries an overall good prognosis.

▶ Clinical Findings

A. Symptoms and Signs

A classic target lesion, as in herpes-associated erythema multiforme, consists of three concentric zones of color change, most often found acrally on the hands and feet (Figure 6–24). SJS/TEN presents with raised purpuric target-like lesions, with only two zones of color change and a central blister, or nondescript reddish or purpuric macules favoring the trunk and proximal upper extremities (Figure 6–25). Pain on eating, swallowing, and urination can occur if relevant mucosae are involved.

B. Laboratory Findings

Blood tests are not useful for diagnosis. Skin biopsy is diagnostic. Direct immunofluorescence studies are negative.

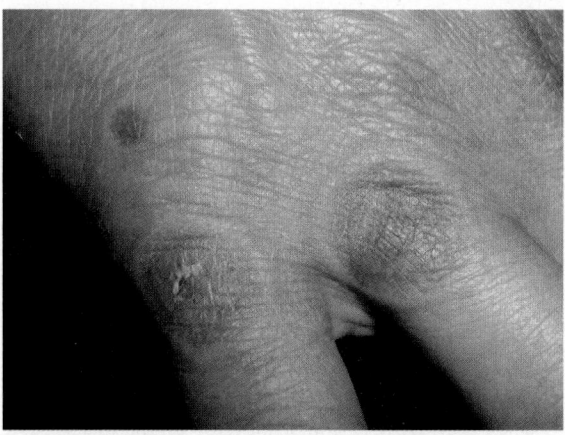

▲ **Figure 6–24.** Erythema multiforme with classic target lesions. Note the three zones of color change. (Used, with permission, from Richard P. Usatine, MD, in Usatine RP, Smith MA, Mayeaux EJ Jr, Chumley H. *The Color Atlas of Family Medicine,* 2nd ed. McGraw-Hill, 2013.)

▶ Differential Diagnosis

Urticaria and drug eruptions are the chief entities that must be differentiated from erythema multiforme minor. In true urticaria, lesions are not purpuric or bullous, last less than 24 hours, and respond to antihistamines. The differential diagnosis of SJS/TEN includes autoimmune bullous diseases (eg, pemphigus, pemphigoid, and linear IgA bullous dermatosis), acute systemic lupus erythematosus, vasculitis, and Sweet syndrome. The presence of a blistering eruption requires biopsy and consultation for appropriate diagnosis and treatment.

▶ Complications

The tracheobronchial mucosa, conjunctiva, and urethral mucosa may be involved, and severe cases result in scarring. *Ophthalmologic consultation is required if ocular involvement is present because vision loss is the major consequence of SJS/TEN.*

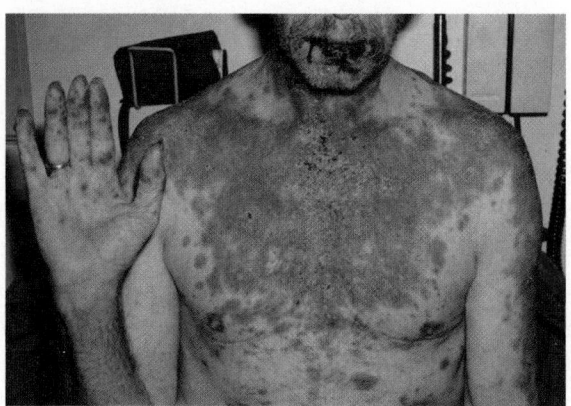

▲ **Figure 6–25.** Stevens-Johnson syndrome. (Used, with permission, from TG Berger, MD, Dept Dermatology, UCSF.)

▶ Treatment

A. General Measures

Toxic epidermal necrolysis is best treated in an acute care environment, which may include an ICU or a burn unit. Patients should be admitted if mucosal involvement interferes with hydration and nutrition or extensive blistering develops. Open lesions should be managed like second-degree burns. Immediate discontinuation of the inciting medication (before blistering occurs) is a significant predictor of outcome. Delay in establishing the diagnosis and inadvertently continuing the offending medication results in higher morbidity and mortality.

B. Specific Measures

The most important aspect of treatment is to stop the offending medication and to move patients with greater than 25–30% BSA involvement to an appropriate acute care environment. Nutritional and fluid support and high vigilance for infection are the most important aspects of care. Reviews of systemic treatments for SJS and TEN have been conflicting. Some data support the use of high-dose corticosteroids. If corticosteroids are to be tried, they should be used early, before blistering occurs, and in high doses (prednisone, 1–2 mg/kg/day). Intravenous immunoglobulin (IVIG) (1 g/kg/day for 4 days) has become standard of care at some centers for toxic epidermal necrolysis cases. IVIG used early in the course and at a total dose of at least 2 g/kg may result in decreased mortality, although not all studies support this finding. Cyclosporine (3–5 mg/kg/day for 7 days) may also be effective. Etanercept is being used more frequently and may be a promising therapy for SJS/TEN. Oral and topical corticosteroids are useful in the oral variant of erythema multiforme. Oral acyclovir prophylaxis of herpes simplex infections may be effective in preventing recurrent herpes-associated erythema multiforme minor.

C. Local Measures

Topical therapy is not very effective in this disease.

▶ Prognosis

Erythema multiforme minor usually lasts 2–6 weeks and may recur. SJS/TEN may be serious with a mortality of about 30% in cases with greater than 30% BSA involvement. SCORTEN (a severity of illness scale) predicts mortality in SJS/TEN.

Barron SJ et al. Intravenous immunoglobulin in the treatment of Stevens-Johnson syndrome and toxic epidermal necrolysis: a meta-analysis with meta-regression of observational studies. Int J Dermatol. 2015 Jan;54(1):108–15. [PMID: 24697283]

Cheng L et al. HLA-B*58:01 is strongly associated with allopurinol-induced severe cutaneous adverse reactions in Han Chinese patients: a multicentre retrospective case-control clinical study. Br J Dermatol. 2015 Aug;173(2):555–8. [PMID: 26104483]

Creamer D et al. U.K. guidelines for the management of Stevens-Johnson syndrome/toxic epidermal necrolysis in adults 2016. Br J Dermatol. 2016 Jun;174(6):1194–227. [PMID: 27317286]

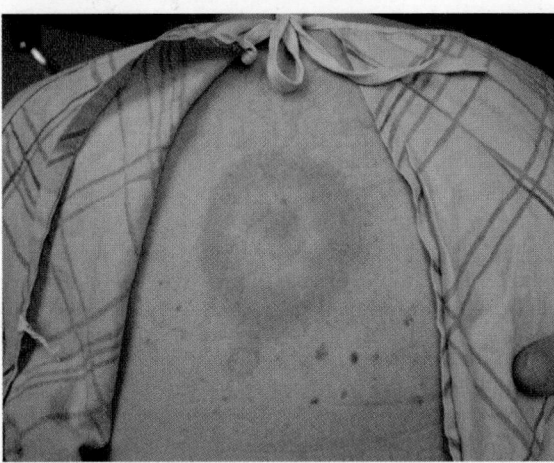

▲ **Figure 6–26.** Erythema migrans due to *Borrelia burgdorferi* (Lyme disease). (Used, with permission, from Thomas Corson, MD, in Usatine RP, Smith MA, Mayeaux EJ Jr, Chumley H. *The Color Atlas of Family Medicine,* 2nd ed. McGraw-Hill, 2013.)

Law EH et al. Corticosteroids in Stevens-Johnson syndrome/ toxic epidermal necrolysis: current evidence and implications for future research. Ann Pharmacother. 2015 Mar;49(3):335–42. [PMID: 25406459]

Lee HY et al. Long-term complications of Stevens-Johnson syndrome/toxic epidermal necrolysis (SJS/TEN): the spectrum of chronic problems in patients who survive an episode of SJS/ TEN necessitates multidisciplinary follow-up. Br J Dermatol. 2017 Oct;177(4):924–35. [PMID: 28144971]

Wang CW et al; Taiwan Severe Cutaneous Adverse Reaction (TSCAR) Consortium. Randomized, controlled trial of TNF-α antagonist in CTL-mediated severe cutaneous adverse reactions. J Clin Invest. 2018 Mar 1;128(3):985–96. [PMID: 29400697]

Zimmermann S et al. Systemic immunomodulating therapies for Stevens-Johnson syndrome and toxic epidermal necrolysis: a systematic review and meta-analysis. JAMA Dermatol. 2017 Jun 1;153(6):514–22. [PMID: 28329382]

3. Erythema Migrans (See also Chapter 34)

Erythema migrans is a unique cutaneous eruption that characterizes the localized or generalized early stage of Lyme disease (caused by *Borrelia burgdorferi*) (Figure 6–26).

INFECTIOUS ERYTHEMAS

1. Erysipelas

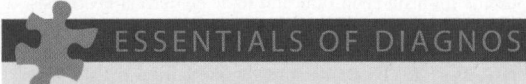

ESSENTIALS OF DIAGNOSIS

▶ Edematous, circumscribed, hot, erythematous area, with raised advancing border.

▶ Central face or lower extremity frequently involved.

▶ Pain and systemic toxicity may be striking.

▶ General Considerations

Erysipelas is a superficial form of cellulitis that is caused by beta-hemolytic streptococci.

▶ Clinical Findings

A. Symptoms and Signs

The symptoms are pain, malaise, chills, and moderate fever. A bright red spot appears and then spreads to form a tense, sharply demarcated, glistening, smooth, hot plaque. The margin characteristically makes noticeable advances in days or even hours. The lesion is edematous with a raised edge and may pit slightly with the finger. Vesicles or bullae occasionally develop on the surface. The lesion does not usually become pustular or gangrenous and heals without scar formation. The disease may complicate any break in the skin that provides a portal of entry for the organism. On the face, erysipelas begins near a fissure at the angle of the nose. On the lower extremity, tinea pedis with interdigital fissuring is a common portal of entry.

B. Laboratory Findings

Leukocytosis is almost invariably present; blood cultures may be positive.

▶ Differential Diagnosis

Erysipeloid is a benign bacillary infection producing cellulitis of the skin of the fingers or the backs of the hands in fishermen and meat handlers.

▶ Complications

Unless erysipelas is promptly treated, death may result from bacterial dissemination, particularly in older adults.

▶ Treatment

Intravenous antibiotics effective against group A beta-hemolytic streptococci and staphylococci should be considered, but outpatient treatment with oral antibiotics has demonstrated equal efficacy. Oral regimens include a 7-day course with penicillin VK (250 mg), dicloxacillin (250 mg), or a first-generation cephalosporin (250 mg) orally four times a day. Alternatives in penicillin-allergic patients are clindamycin (250 mg twice daily orally for 7–14 days) or erythromycin (250 mg four times daily orally for 7–14 days), the latter only if the infection is known to be due to streptococci.

▶ Prognosis

With appropriate treatment, rapid improvement is expected. The presence of lymphedema carries the greatest risk of recurrence.

2. Cellulitis

▶ Edematous, expanding, erythematous, warm plaque with or without vesicles or bullae.

▶ Lower leg is frequently involved.

▶ Pain, chills, and fever are commonly present.

▶ Septicemia may develop.

General Considerations

Cellulitis, a diffuse spreading infection of the dermis and subcutaneous tissue, is usually on the lower leg (Figure 6–27) and most commonly due to gram-positive cocci, especially group A beta-hemolytic streptococci and *S aureus*. Rarely, gram-negative rods or even fungi can produce a similar picture. In otherwise healthy persons, the most common portal of entry for lower leg cellulitis is toe web intertrigo with fissuring, usually a complication of interdigital tinea pedis. Other diseases that predispose to cellulitis are prior episodes of cellulitis, chronic edema, venous insufficiency with secondary edema, lymphatic obstruction, saphenectomy, and other perturbations of the skin barrier. Bacterial cellulitis is almost never bilateral.

Clinical Findings

A. Symptoms and Signs

Cellulitis begins as a tender small patch. Swelling, erythema, and pain are often present. The lesion expands over hours, so that from onset to presentation is usually 6 to 36 hours. As the lesion grows, the patient becomes more ill with progressive chills, fever, and malaise. Lymphangitis and lymphadenopathy are often present. If septicemia develops, hypotension may develop, followed by shock.

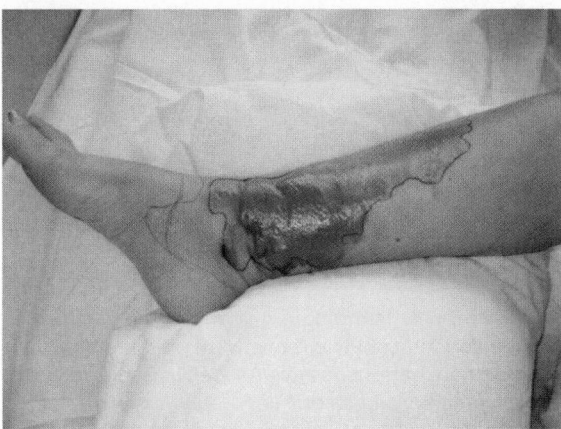

▲ **Figure 6–27.** **Cellulitis.** (Used, with permission, from Lindy Fox, MD.)

B. Laboratory Findings

Leukocytosis or at least a neutrophilia (left shift) may be present from early in the course. Blood cultures are positive in only 8% of patients. If a central ulceration, pustule, or abscess is present, culture may be of value. Aspiration of the advancing edge has a low yield (less than 20%) and is usually not performed. In immunosuppressed patients, or if an unusual organism is suspected and there is no loculated site to culture, a full-thickness skin biopsy taken before antibiotics are given can be useful. Either two specimens or one divided in half should be sent for routine histologic evaluation and for culture (bacterial, fungal, and mycobacterial). Skin biopsy is particularly important in the immunocompromised patient in whom cellulitis may be due to an uncommon organism. If a primary source for the infection is identified (wound, leg ulcer, toe web intertrigo), cultures from these sites isolate the causative pathogen in half of cases and can be used to guide antibiotic therapy.

Differential Diagnosis

Two potentially life-threatening entities that can mimic cellulitis (ie, present with a painful, red, swollen lower extremity) include deep venous thrombosis and necrotizing fasciitis. The diagnosis of necrotizing fasciitis should be suspected in a patient who has a very toxic appearance, bullae, crepitus or anesthesia of the involved skin, overlying skin necrosis, and laboratory evidence of rhabdomyolysis (elevated creatine kinase) or disseminated intravascular coagulation. While these findings may be present with severe cellulitis and bacteremia, it is essential to rule out necrotizing fasciitis because rapid surgical debridement is essential. Other noninfectious skin lesions that may resemble cellulitis (termed "pseudocellulitis") include sclerosing panniculitis, an acute, exquisitely tender red plaque on the medial lower legs above the malleolus in patients with venous stasis or varicosities, and acute severe contact dermatitis on a limb, which produces erythema, vesiculation, and edema, as seen in cellulitis, but with itching instead of pain. Bilateral lower leg bacterial cellulitis is exceedingly rare, and other diagnoses, especially severe stasis dermatitis (see Figure 12–2), should be considered in this setting. Severe lower extremity stasis dermatitis usually develops over days to weeks rather than the hours of cellulitis. It is also not as tender to palpation as cellulitis. Cryptococcal cellulitis in the organ transplant recipient is often bilateral.

Treatment

Intravenous or parenteral antibiotics may be required for the first 2–5 days, with adequate coverage for *Streptococcus* and *Staphylococcus*. Methicillin-susceptible *S aureus* (MSSA) can be treated with nafcillin, cefazolin, clindamycin, dicloxacillin, cephalexin, doxycycline, or TMP-SMZ. If MRSA is suspected or proven, treatment options include vancomycin, linezolid, clindamycin, daptomycin, doxycycline, or TMP-SMZ. In mild cases or following the initial parenteral therapy, oral dicloxacillin or cephalexin, 250–500 mg four times daily for 5–10 days, is usually adequate. In patients in whom intravenous treatment is not instituted, the first dose of oral antibiotic can be doubled to achieve high blood levels rapidly. In patients with recurrent lower leg cellulitis (three to four episodes per year), oral penicillin 250 mg twice daily or erythromycin can delay the appearance of the next episode. Prior episodes of cellulitis, lymphedema, chronic venous insufficiency, peripheral vascular disease, and deep venous thrombosis are associated with an increased risk of recurrent cellulitis.

When to Admit

- Severe local symptoms and signs.
- Systemic inflammatory response syndrome (SIRS) criteria are met.
- Elevated white blood cell count with marked left shift.
- Failure to respond to oral antibiotics.

Dalal A et al. Interventions for the prevention of recurrent erysipelas and cellulitis. Cochrane Database Syst Rev. 2017 Jun 20;6:CD009758. [PMID: 28631307]

Ko LN et al. Clinical usefulness of imaging and blood cultures in cellulitis evaluation. JAMA Intern Med. 2018 Jul 1;178(7): 994–6. [PMID: 29610842]

Patel M et al. The red leg dilemma: a scoping review of the challenges of diagnosing lower limb cellulitis. Br J Dermatol. 2018 Nov 13. [Epub ahead of print] [PMID: 30422315]

Quirke M et al. Risk factors for nonpurulent leg cellulitis: a systematic review and meta-analysis. Br J Dermatol. 2017 Aug; 177(2):382–94. [PMID: 27864837]

Raff AB et al. Cellulitis: a review. JAMA. 2016 Jul 19;316(3):325–37. [PMID: 27434444]

Stevens DL et al. Practice guidelines for the diagnosis and management of skin and soft tissue infections: 2014 update by the Infectious Diseases Society of America. Clin Infect Dis. 2014 Jul 15;59(2):147–59. [PMID: 24947530]

Talan DA et al. Factors associated with decision to hospitalize emergency department patients with skin and soft tissue infection. West J Emerg Med. 2015 Jan;16(1):89–97. [PMID: 25671016]

BLISTERING DISEASES

PEMPHIGUS

ESSENTIALS OF DIAGNOSIS

- ▶ Relapsing crops of bullae, often fragile and leading to erosions.
- ▶ Often preceded by mucous membrane bullae, erosions, and ulcerations.
- ▶ Superficial detachment of the skin after pressure or trauma variably present (Nikolsky sign).
- ▶ Acantholysis on biopsy.
- ▶ Immunofluorescence studies and serum ELISA for pathogenic antibodies are confirmatory.

General Considerations

Pemphigus is an uncommon intraepidermal blistering disease occurring on skin and mucous membranes. It is caused by autoantibodies to adhesion molecules expressed in the skin and mucous membranes. The cause is unknown, and in the preantibiotic, presteroid era, the condition was usually fatal within 5 years. The bullae appear spontaneously and are tender and painful when they rupture. Drug-induced pemphigus from penicillamine, captopril, and others has been reported. There are several forms of pemphigus: pemphigus vulgaris and its variant, pemphigus vegetans; and the more superficially blistering pemphigus foliaceus and its variant, pemphigus erythematosus. All forms may occur at any age, but most present in middle age. The vulgaris form begins in the mouth in over 50% of cases. The foliaceus form is especially apt to be associated with other autoimmune diseases, or it may be drug-induced. Paraneoplastic pemphigus, a unique form of the disorder, is associated with numerous types of benign and malignant neoplasms but most frequently non-Hodgkin lymphoma.

Clinical Findings

A. Symptoms and Signs

Pemphigus is characterized by an insidious onset of flaccid bullae, crusts, and erosions in crops or waves (Figure 6–28). In pemphigus vulgaris, lesions often appear first on the oral mucous membranes. These rapidly become erosive. The scalp is another site of early involvement. Rubbing a cotton swab or finger laterally on the surface of uninvolved skin may cause easy separation of the epidermis (Nikolsky sign). Pemphigus vegetans presents as erosive vegetating

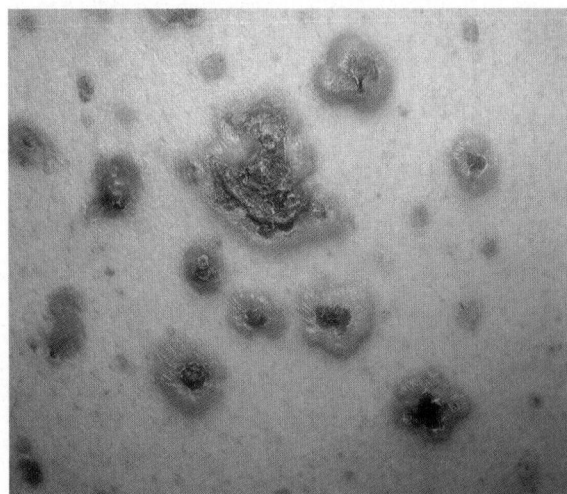

▲ **Figure 6–28.** Pemphigus vulgaris on the back with crusted and intact bullae. Downward pressure on a bulla demonstrates a positive Asboe-Hansen sign with lateral spread of a fresh bullae. (Used, with permission, from Eric Kraus, MD, in Usatine RP, Smith MA, Mayeaux EJ Jr, Chumley H. *The Color Atlas of Family Medicine,* 2nd ed. McGraw-Hill, 2013.)

plaques, most often in intertriginous areas. Pemphigus foliaceus is a superficial form of pemphigus where cutaneous lesions present as flaccid bullae that quickly evolve into superficial erosions and thin pink plaques with overlying scale. Mucosal lesions are rare in pemphigus foliaceus. Pemphigus erythematosus has overlapping features of pemphigus foliaceus and lupus erythematosus. It presents with flaccid bullae that develop overlying scale and crust in a photodistributed area. Again, mucosal lesions are rare. Paraneoplastic pemphigus is histologically, and immunologically distinct from other forms of the disease. While clinical lesions may not be distinct from pemphigus vulgaris, oral lesions predominate and cutaneous erythematous plaques resembling erythema multiforme are characteristic. Survival rates are low because of the underlying malignancy.

B. Laboratory Findings

The diagnosis is made by light microscopy and by direct and indirect immunofluorescence (IIF) microscopy. Autoantibodies to intercellular adhesion molecules (desmoglien 3 and 1) can be detected with ELISA assays and have replaced the use of IIF in some centers.

▶ Differential Diagnosis

Blistering diseases include erythema multiforme (Figure 6–24), SJS/TEN, drug eruptions, bullous impetigo, contact dermatitis, dermatitis herpetiformis, and bullous pemphigoid, but flaccid blisters are not typical of these diseases, and acantholysis is not seen on biopsy. All of these diseases have clinical characteristics and different immunofluorescence test results that distinguish them from pemphigus. Pemphigus foliaceus must be distinguished from subacute cutaneous lupus erythematosus.

▶ Complications

Secondary infection commonly occurs; this is a major cause of morbidity and mortality. Disturbances of fluid, electrolyte, and nutritional intake can occur as a result of painful oral ulcers.

▶ Treatment

A. General Measures

When the disease is severe, hospitalize the patient at bed rest and provide antibiotics and intravenous feedings as indicated. Anesthetic troches used before eating ease painful oral lesions.

B. Systemic Measures

Pemphigus requires systemic therapy as early in its course as possible. However, the main morbidity in this disease is due to the side effects of such therapy. Initial therapy is with prednisone, 60–80 mg orally daily. In all but the mildest cases, a steroid-sparing agent is added from the beginning, since the course of the disease is long and the steroid-sparing agents take several weeks to exert their activity. Azathioprine (100–200 mg orally daily) or mycophenolate

mofetil (1–1.5 g orally twice daily) are often used. Rituximab treatment (1 g intravenously on days 1 and 15), especially early in the course, appears to be associated with therapeutic induction of a complete remission and is increasingly being used as first-line therapy. Repeated courses are efficacious and well tolerated in patients who do not achieve complete remission or relapse. Monthly IVIG at 2 g/kg intravenously over 3–4 days frequently is beneficial. In refractory cases, cyclophosphamide, pulse intravenous corticosteroids, and plasmapheresis can be used. Other anti-CD20 medications may be future therapeutic options.

C. Local Measures

In patients with limited disease, skin and mucous membrane lesions should be treated with topical corticosteroids. Complicating infection requires appropriate systemic and local antibiotic therapy.

▶ Prognosis

The course tends to be chronic in most patients, though about one-third appear to experience remission. Infection is the most frequent cause of death, usually from *S aureus* septicemia.

Cholera M et al. Management of pemphigus vulgaris. Adv Ther. 2016 Jun;33(6):910–58. [PMID: 27287854]

Huang A et al. Future therapies for pemphigus vulgaris: rituximab and beyond. J Am Acad Dermatol. 2016 Apr;74(4): 746–53. [PMID: 26792592]

Ishii K. Importance of serological tests in diagnosis of autoimmune blistering diseases. J Dermatol. 2015 Jan;42(1):3–10. [PMID: 25558946]

Joly P et al; French study group on autoimmune bullous skin diseases. First-line rituximab combined with short-term prednisone versus prednisone alone for the treatment of pemphigus (Ritux 3): a prospective, multicentre, parallel-group, open-label randomised trial. Lancet. 2017 May 20;389(10083):2031–40. [PMID: 28342637]

Kasperkiewicz M et al. Pemphigus. Nat Rev Dis Primers. 2017 May 11;3:17026. [PMID: 28492232]

BULLOUS PEMPHIGOID

Many autoimmune skin disorders are characterized by formation of bullae, or blisters. These include bullous pemphigoid, cicatricial pemphigoid, dermatitis herpetiformis, and pemphigoid gestationis.

Bullous pemphigoid is a relatively benign pruritic disease characterized by tense blisters in flexural areas, usually remitting in 5 or 6 years, with a course characterized by exacerbations and remissions. Most affected persons are over the age of 60 (often in their 70s or 80s), and men are affected twice as frequently as women. The appearance of blisters may be preceded by pruritic urticarial or edematous lesions for months. Oral lesions are present in about one-third of affected persons. The disease may occur in various forms, including localized, vesicular, vegetating, erythematous, erythrodermic, and nodular. Drugs may induce bullous pemphigoid. The most common offender is furosemide. PD-1 inhibitors are an emerging cause of drug-induced bullous pemphigoid in patients receiving this immunotherapy for malignancies.

The diagnosis is made by biopsy and direct immuno-fluorescence examination. Light microscopy shows a sub-epidermal blister. With direct immunofluorescence, IgG and C3 are found at the dermal-epidermal junction. ELISA tests for bullous pemphigoid antibodies (BP 180 or BP 230) are 87% sensitive and 95% specific. If the patient has mild disease, ultrapotent topical corticosteroids may be adequate. Prednisone at a dosage of 0.75 mg/kg orally daily is often used to achieve rapid control of more widespread disease. Tetracycline (500 mg orally three times daily) or doxycycline (100 mg orally twice a day), alone or combined with nicotinamide—not nicotinic acid or niacin—(up to 1.5 g orally daily), may control the disease in patients who cannot use corticosteroids or may allow for decreasing or eliminating corticosteroids after control is achieved. Dapsone is particularly effective in mucous membrane pemphigoid. If these medications are not effective, methotrexate (5–25 mg orally weekly), azathioprine (50 mg one to three times orally daily), or mycophenolate mofetil (1–1.5 g orally twice daily) may be used as steroid-sparing agents. Intravenous immunoglobulin, rituximab, and omalizumab have been used with success in refractory cases.

Bağcı IS et al. Bullous pemphigoid. Autoimmun Rev. 2017 May; 16(5):445–55. [PMID: 28286109]

Bernard P et al. Bullous pemphigoid: a review of its diagnosis, associations and treatment. Am J Clin Dermatol. 2017 Aug; 18(4):513–28. [PMID: 28247089]

Cho YT et al. First-line combination therapy with rituximab and corticosteroids provides a high complete remission rate in moderate-to-severe bullous pemphigoid. Br J Dermatol. 2015 Jul; 173(1):302–4. [PMID: 25529394]

Kremer N et al. Rituximab and omalizumab for the treatment of bullous pemphigoid: a systematic review of the literature. Am J Clin Dermatol. 2018 Nov 13. [Epub ahead of print] [PMID: 30421306]

PAPULES

WARWS

ESSENTIALS OF DIAGNOSIS

► Verrucous papules anywhere on the skin or mucous membranes, usually no larger than 1 cm in diameter.

► Prolonged incubation period (average 2–18 months).

► Spontaneous "cures" of common warts in 50% at 2 years.

► "Recurrences" (new lesions) are frequent.

▶ General Considerations

Warts (common, plantar, and genital) are caused by human papillomaviruses (HPVs). Typing of HPV lesions is not a

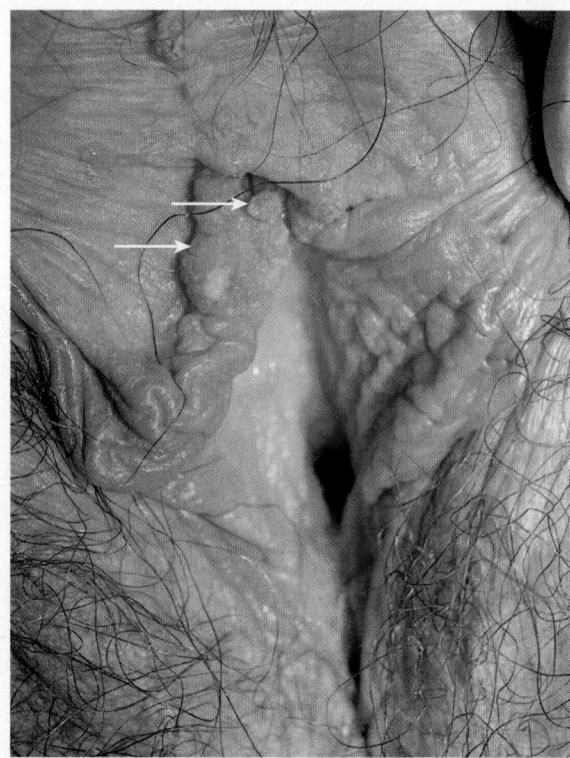

▲ **Figure 6–29.** Condyloma around the clitoris, labia minor, and opening of the vagina. (Used, with permission, from Richard P. Usatine, MD, in Usatine RP, Smith MA, Mayeaux EJ Jr, Chumley H. *The Color Atlas of Family Medicine,* 2nd ed. McGraw-Hill, 2013.)

part of standard medical evaluation except in the case of anogenital dysplasia.

▶ Clinical Findings

There are usually no symptoms. Tenderness on pressure occurs with plantar warts; itching occurs with anogenital warts (Figure 6–29). Flat warts are most evident under oblique illumination. Periungual warts may be dry, fissured, and hyperkeratotic and may resemble hangnails. Plantar warts resemble plantar corns or calluses.

▶ Differential Diagnosis

Some warty-looking lesions are actually hypertrophic actinic keratoses or squamous cell carcinomas. Some genital warty lesions are condylomata lata of secondary syphilis. Molluscum contagiosum lesions are pearly with a central dell. In AIDS, wart-like lesions may be caused by varicella zoster virus.

▶ Prevention

Administration of a vaccine against certain anogenital HPV types (including 6, 11, 16, 18, 31, 33, 45, 52, and 58) can prevent infection with these wart types and reduce anogenital, oropharyngeal, and cervical cancer. It is recommended for teenagers and young adults, men who have sex with men, and immunocompromised patients (see Chapters 1 and 18). There may be a role for adjuvant vaccination in HPV-infected patients.

► Treatment

Treatment is aimed at inducing "wart-free" intervals for as long as possible without scarring, since no treatment can guarantee a remission or prevent recurrences. In immuno-compromised patients, the goal is even more modest, ie, to control the size and number of lesions present.

A. Treatment of Nongenital Warts

For common warts of the hands, patients are usually offered liquid nitrogen or keratolytic agents. The former may work in fewer treatments but requires office visits and is painful.

1. Liquid nitrogen—Liquid nitrogen cryotherapy is applied to achieve a thaw time of 30–45 seconds. Two freeze-thaw cycles are given every 2–4 weeks for several visits. Scarring will occur if it is used incorrectly. Liquid nitrogen may cause permanent depigmentation in pigmented individuals.

2. Keratolytic agents and occlusion—Salicylic acid products may be used against common warts or plantar warts. They are applied, then occluded. Plantar warts may be treated by applying a 40% salicylic acid plaster after paring. The plaster may be left on for 5–6 days, then removed, the lesion pared down, and another plaster applied. Although it may take weeks or months to eradicate the wart, the method is safe and effective with almost no side effects. Chronic occlusion alone with water-impermeable tape (duct tape, adhesive tape) is less effective than cryotherapy.

3. Operative removal—Plantar warts may be removed by blunt dissection.

4. Laser therapy—The CO_2 laser can be effective for treating recurrent warts, periungual warts, plantar warts, and condylomata acuminata. It leaves open wounds that must fill in with granulation tissue over 4–6 weeks and is best reserved for warts resistant to all other modalities. Lasers with emissions of 585, 595, or 532 nm may also be used every 3–4 weeks to gradually ablate common, plantar, facial, and anogenital warts. This is no more effective than cryotherapy in controlled trials. Photodynamic therapy can be considered in refractory widespread flat warts.

5. Immunotherapy—Squaric acid dibutylester may be applied in a concentration of 0.2–2% directly to the warts from once weekly to five times weekly to induce a mild contact dermatitis. Between 60% and 80% of warts clear over 10–20 weeks. Injection of *Candida* antigen starting at 1:50 dilution and repeated every 3–4 weeks may be similarly effective in stimulating immunologic regression of common and plantar warts.

6. Other agents—Bleomycin, diluted to 1 unit/mL, injected into common and plantar warts has been shown to have a high cure rate. It should be used with caution on digital warts because of the potential complications of Raynaud phenomenon, nail loss, and terminal digital necrosis. 5-Fluorouracil 5% cream applied once or twice daily, usually with occlusion, may be applied to warts with similar efficacy to other treatment methods.

7. Physical modalities—Soaking warts in hot (42.2°C) water for 10–30 minutes daily for 6 weeks has resulted in involution in some cases.

B. Treatment of Genital Warts

1. Liquid nitrogen—Cryotherapy is first-line clinician-applied surgical treatment for genital warts (condyloma acuminata). Liquid nitrogen cryotherapy is applied to achieve a thaw time of 30–45 seconds. Two freeze-thaw cycles are given every 2–4 weeks for several visits. Scarring will occur if it is used incorrectly. Liquid nitrogen may cause permanent depigmentation in pigmented individuals.

2. Podophyllum resin—For genital warts, the purified active component of the podophyllum resin, podofilox, is applied by the patient twice daily 3 consecutive days a week for cycles of 4–6 weeks. It is less irritating and more effective than "clinician-applied" podophyllum resin. After a single 4-week cycle, 45% of patients were wart-free; but of these, 60% relapsed at 6 weeks. Thus, multiple cycles of treatment are often necessary. Patients unable to obtain the take-home podofilox may be treated in the clinician's office by painting each wart carefully (protecting normal skin) every 2–3 weeks with 25% podophyllum resin (podophyllin) in compound tincture of benzoin.

3. Imiquimod—A 5% cream of this local interferon inducer has moderate activity in clearing external genital warts. Treatment is once daily on 3 alternate days per week. Response may be slow, with patients who eventually cleared having responses at 8 weeks (44%) or 12 weeks (69%). There is a marked difference between the sexes with respect to response, with 77% of women and 40% of men having complete clearing of their lesions. Once cleared, about 13% have recurrences in the short term.

Although imiquimod is considerably more expensive than podophyllotoxin, its high rate of response in women and its safety make it the "patient-administered" treatment of choice for external genital warts in women. In men, the more rapid response, lower cost, and similar efficacy make podophyllotoxin the initial treatment of choice, with imiquimod used for recurrences or refractory cases. Imiquimod has no demonstrated efficacy for—and should not be used to treat—plantar or common warts.

4. Operative removal—For pedunculated or large genital warts, snip biopsy (scissors) removal followed by light electrocautery is more effective than cryotherapy.

5. Laser therapy—See Treatment of Nongenital Warts, above. For genital warts, it has not been shown that laser therapy is more effective than electrosurgical removal. Photodynamic therapy can be considered in refractory genital warts.

► Prognosis

There is a striking tendency to develop new lesions. Warts may disappear spontaneously or may be unresponsive to treatment. Combining therapies (eg, liquid nitrogen plus immunotherapy) may improve therapeutic response.

Aldahan AS et al. Efficacy of intralesional immunotherapy for the treatment of warts: a review of the literature. Dermatol Ther. 2016 May;29(3):197–207. [PMID: 26991521]

Alikhan A et al. Use of *Candida* antigen injections for the treatment of verruca vulgaris: a two-year Mayo Clinic experience. J Dermatolog Treat. 2016 Aug;27(4):355–8. [PMID: 26558635]

Bertolotti A et al. Cryotherapy to treat anogenital warts in non-immunocompromised adults: systematic review and meta-analysis. J Am Acad Dermatol. 2017 Sep;77(3):518–26. [PMID: 28651824]

Grillo-Ardila CF et al. Imiquimod for anogenital warts in non-immunocompromised adults. Cochrane Database Syst Rev. 2014 Nov 1;1:CD010389. [PMID: 25362229]

Veitch D et al. Pulsed dye laser therapy in the treatment of warts: a review of the literature. Dermatol Surg. 2017 Apr;43(4):485–93. [PMID: 28272080]

MOLLUSCUM CONTAGIOSUM

Molluscum contagiosum, caused by a poxvirus, presents as single or multiple dome-shaped, waxy papules 2–5 mm in diameter that are umbilicated (Figure 6–30). Lesions at first are firm, solid, and flesh-colored but upon reaching maturity become soft, whitish, or pearly gray and may suppurate. The principal sites of involvement are the face, lower abdomen, and genitals.

The lesions are autoinoculable and spread by wet skin-to-skin contact. In sexually active individuals, they may be confined to the penis, pubis, and inner thighs and are considered a sexually transmitted infection.

Molluscum contagiosum is common in patients with AIDS, usually with a helper T-cell count less than 100/mcL. Extensive lesions tend to develop over the face and neck as well as in the genital area.

The diagnosis is easily established in most instances because of the distinctive central umbilication of the dome-shaped lesion. Estimated time to remission is 13 months. The best treatment is by curettage or applications of liquid nitrogen as for warts—but more briefly. When lesions are frozen, the central umbilication often becomes more apparent. Light electrosurgery with a fine needle is also effective. Cantharadin (applied in the office and then washed off by the patient 4 hours later) is a safe and effective option. Ten percent potassium hydroxide solution applied twice daily until lesions clear is another treatment option. Salicylic acid, podophyllotoxin, tretinoin, imiquimod, and pulsed dye laser are additional treatment options. Lesions are difficult to eradicate in patients with AIDS unless immunity improves; however, with highly effective antiretroviral treatment, molluscum will usually spontaneously clear.

Martin P. Interventions for molluscum contagiosum in people infected with human immunodeficiency virus: a systematic review. Int J Dermatol. 2016 Sep;55(9):956–66. [PMID: 26991246]

Vakharia PP et al. Efficacy and safety of topical cantharidin treatment for molluscum contagiosum and warts: a systematic review. Am J Clin Dermatol. 2018 Dec;19(6):791–803. [PMID: 30097988]

van der Wouden JC et al. Interventions for cutaneous molluscum contagiosum. Cochrane Database Syst Rev. 2017 May 17;5:CD004767. [PMID: 28513067]

BASAL CELL CARCINOMA

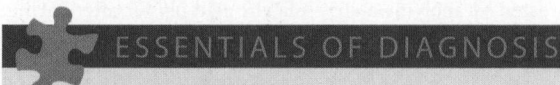

ESSENTIALS OF DIAGNOSIS

► Pearly papule, erythematous patch greater than 6 mm, or nonhealing ulcer in sun-exposed areas (face, trunk, lower legs).

► History of bleeding.

► Fair-skinned person with a history of sun exposure (often intense, intermittent).

► General Considerations

Basal cell carcinomas are the most common form of cancer. They occur on sun-exposed skin in otherwise normal, fair-skinned individuals; ultraviolet light is the cause. Basal cell carcinomas can be divided into clinical and histologic subtypes, which determine both clinical behavior and treatment. The clinical subtypes include superficial, nodular, pigmented, and morpheaform. The histologic subtypes include superficial, nodular, micronodular, and infiltrative. Morpheaform, micronodular, and infiltrative basal cell carcinomas are not amenable to topical therapy or electrodesiccation and curettage and typically require surgical excision or Mohs micrographic surgery.

► Clinical Findings

The most common presentation is a papule or nodule that may have a central scab or erosion (Figure 6–31). Occasionally the nodules have stippled pigment (pigmented basal cell carcinoma). Intradermal nevi without pigment on the face of older white individuals may resemble basal

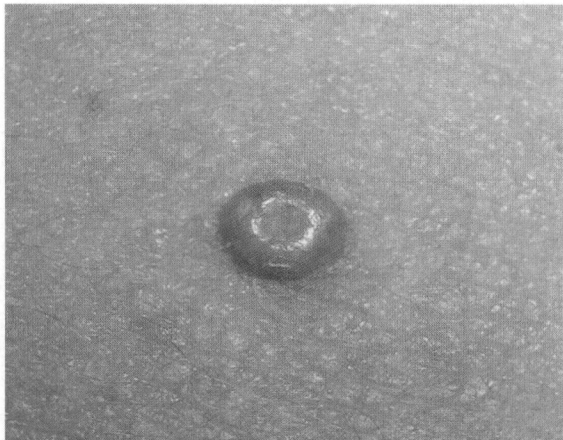

▲ **Figure 6–30.** Umbilicated—molluscum. (Used, with permission, from Richard P. Usatine, MD, in Usatine RP, Smith MA, Mayeaux EJ Jr, Chumley H. *The Color Atlas of Family Medicine,* 3rd ed. McGraw-Hill, 2018.)

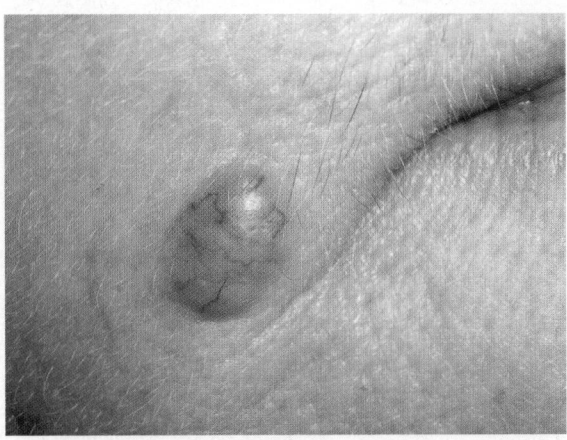

▲ **Figure 6–31.** Pearly nodular basal cell carcinoma on the face of a 52-year-old woman present for 5 years. (Used, with permission, from Richard P. Usatine, MD, in Usatine RP, Smith MA, Mayeaux EJ Jr, Chumley H. *The Color Atlas of Family Medicine,* 2nd ed. McGraw-Hill, 2013.)

cell carcinomas. Basal cell carcinomas grow slowly, attaining a size of 1–2 cm or more in diameter, usually only after years of growth. There is a waxy, "pearly" appearance, with telangiectatic vessels easily visible. It is the pearly or translucent quality of these lesions that is most diagnostic, a feature best appreciated if the skin is stretched. On the back and chest, basal cell carcinomas appear as reddish, somewhat shiny, scaly patches. Morpheaform basal cell carcinomas are scar-like in appearance. Basal cell carcinomas are more common and more likely to recur in immunosuppressed patients, including those with non-Hodgkin lymphoma and those who have undergone solid organ or allogeneic hematopoietic stem cell transplantation.

▶ Treatment

Lesions suspected to be basal cell carcinomas should be biopsied by shave or punch biopsy. Therapy is then aimed at eradication with minimal cosmetic deformity. The histopathologic classification of basal cell carcinomas determines therapy. Imiquimod (applied topically 5 nights per week for 6–10 weeks depending on patient reaction) and 5-fluorouracil (applied topically twice daily for up to 12 weeks) may be appropriate for select patients with superficial basal cell carcinomas, but the treated area must be observed for evidence of complete cure. Superficial or nodular type lesions can be treated with curettage and electrodesiccation, excision, or Mohs micrographic surgery, while those that are classified as micronodular or infiltrative should be treated with excision or Mohs micrographic surgery depending on the size and location of the lesion.

Excision and suturing have a recurrence rate of 5% or less. The technique of three cycles of curettage and electrodesiccation depends on the skill of the operator and is not recommended for head and neck lesions or basal cell carcinomas with morpheaform, infiltrative, or micronodular histopathology. After 4–6 weeks of healing, it leaves a broad, hypopigmented, at times hypertrophic scar.

Radiotherapy is effective and sometimes appropriate for older individuals (over age 65), but recurrent tumors after radiation therapy are more difficult to treat and may be more aggressive. Radiation therapy is the most expensive method to treat basal cell carcinoma and should be used only if other treatment options are not appropriate. Mohs micrographic surgery—removal of the tumor followed by immediate frozen section histopathologic examination of margins with subsequent reexcision of tumor-positive areas and final closure of the defect—gives the highest cure rates (98%) and results in least tissue loss. It is an appropriate therapy for tumors of the eyelids, nasolabial folds, canthi, external ear, and temple; for recurrent lesions; where tissue sparing is needed for cosmesis; and for those with morpheaform, infiltrative, or micronodular histopathology in certain locations.

Photodynamic therapy is approved in Europe, Australia, and New Zealand for the treatment of superficial and nodular basal cell carcinomas.

Hedgehog pathway inhibitors (vismodegib, sonidegib) are reserved for the treatment of advanced or metastatic basal cell carcinoma or in patients with extensive tumor burden (eg, basal cell nevus syndrome). Since a second lesion will develop in up to half of patients with a basal cell carcinoma, patients with basal cell carcinomas must be monitored at least yearly to detect new or recurrent lesions.

Danhof R et al. Small molecule inhibitors of the hedgehog pathway in the treatment of basal cell carcinoma of the skin. Am J Clin Dermatol. 2018 Apr;19(2):195–207. [PMID: 28887802]

Kauvar AN et al; American Society for Dermatologic Surgery. Consensus for nonmelanoma skin cancer treatment: basal cell carcinoma, including a cost analysis of treatment methods. Dermatol Surg. 2015 May;41(5):550–71. [PMID: 25868035]

Kim JYS et al. Guidelines of care for the management of basal cell carcinoma. J Am Acad Dermatol. 2018 Mar;78(3):540–59. [PMID: 29331385]

Nehal KS et al. Update on keratinocyte carcinomas. N Engl J Med. 2018 Jul 26;379(4):363–74. [PMID: 30044931]

Tolkachjov SN et al. Understanding Mohs micrographic surgery: a review and practical guide for the nondermatologist. Mayo Clin Proc. 2017 Aug;92(8):1261–71. [PMID: 28778259]

Williams HC et al; Surgery Versus Imiquimod for Nodular and Superficial Basal Cell Carcinoma (SINS) Study Group. Surgery versus 5% imiquimod for nodular and superficial basal cell carcinoma: 5-year results of the SINS randomized controlled trial. J Invest Dermatol. 2017 Mar;137(3):614–9. [PMID: 27932240]

SQUAMOUS CELL CARCINOMA

 ESSENTIALS OF DIAGNOSIS

▶ Nonhealing ulcer or warty nodule.

▶ Skin damage due to long-term sun exposure.

▶ Common in fair-skinned organ transplant recipients.

Squamous cell carcinoma usually occurs subsequent to prolonged sun exposure on exposed parts in fair-skinned

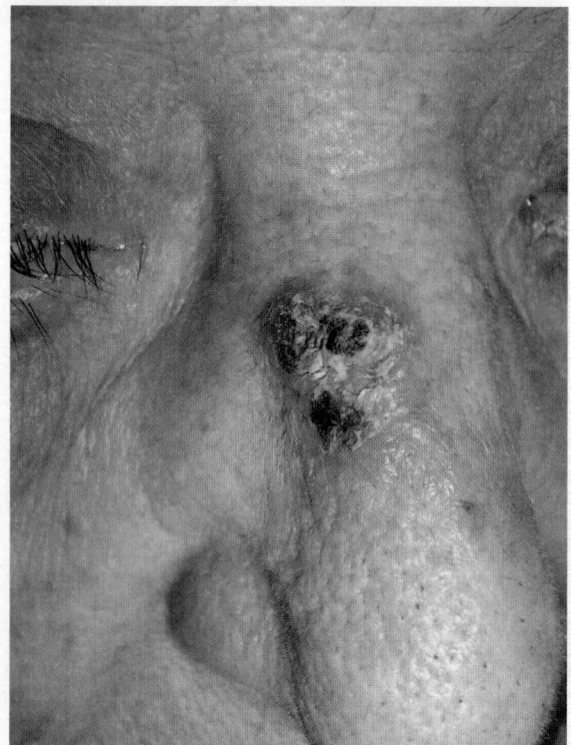

▲ **Figure 6–32.** Squamous cell carcinoma: an irregular shaped pink plaque with overlong hemorrhagic crust in a chronically sun exposed area. (Used, with permission, from Richard P. Usatine, MD, in Usatine RP, Smith MA, Mayeaux EJ Jr, Chumley H. *The Color Atlas of Family Medicine,* 2nd ed. McGraw-Hill, 2013.)

individuals who sunburn easily and tan poorly. It may arise from an actinic keratosis. The lesions appear as small red, conical, hard nodules that occasionally ulcerate (Figure 6–32). In actinically induced squamous cell cancers, rates of metastasis are estimated from retrospective studies to be 3–7%. Squamous cell carcinomas of the ear, temple, lip, oral cavity, tongue, and genitalia have much higher rates of recurrence or metastasis and require special management. Patients with multiple squamous cell carcinomas (especially more than 10) have higher rates of local recurrence and nodal metastases.

Examination of the skin and therapy are essentially the same as for basal cell carcinoma. The preferred treatment of squamous cell carcinoma is excision. Electrodesiccation and curettage and x-ray radiation may be used for some lesions. Mohs micrographic surgery is recommended for high-risk lesions (lips, temples, ears, nose), recurrent tumors, aggressive histologic subtypes (perineural or perivascular invasion), large lesions (greater than 1.0 cm face, greater than 2.0 cm trunk or extremities), immunosuppressed patients, lesions developing within a scar, and for tumors arising in the setting of genetic diseases. Follow-up for squamous cell carcinoma must be more frequent and thorough than for basal cell carcinoma, starting at every 3 months, with careful examination of lymph nodes for

1 year, then twice yearly thereafter. In addition, palpation of the lips is essential to detect hard or indurated areas that represent early squamous cell carcinoma. All such cases must be biopsied.

Transplant patients with squamous cell carcinomas represent a highly specialized patient population. Biologic behavior of skin cancer in organ transplant recipients may be aggressive, and careful management is required. Multiple squamous cell carcinomas are very common on the sun-exposed skin of organ transplant patients. The intensity of immunosuppression, not the use of any particular immunosuppressive agent, is the primary risk factor in determining the development of skin cancer after transplant. The tumors begin to appear after 5 years of immunosuppression. Voriconazole treatment appears to increase the risk of development of squamous cell carcinoma, especially in lung transplant patients. Regular dermatologic evaluation in at-risk organ transplant recipients is recommended. Other forms of immunosuppression, such as allogeneic hematopoietic stem cell transplants, chronic lymphocytic leukemia, HIV/AIDS, and chronic iatrogenic immunosuppression, may also increase skin cancer risk and be associated with more aggressive skin cancer behavior.

Burton KA et al. Cutaneous squamous cell carcinoma: a review of high-risk and metastatic disease. Am J Clin Dermatol. 2016 Oct;17(5):491–508. [PMID: 27358187]

Eigentler TK et al. Survival of patients with cutaneous squamous cell carcinoma: results of a prospective cohort study. J Invest Dermatol. 2017 Nov;137(11):2309–15. [PMID: 28736229]

Kauvar AN et al. Consensus for nonmelanoma skin cancer treatment, part II: squamous cell carcinoma, including a cost analysis of treatment methods. Dermatol Surg. 2015 Nov; 41(11):1214–40. [PMID: 26445288]

Kim JYS et al. Guidelines of care for the management of cutaneous squamous cell carcinoma. J Am Acad Dermatol. 2018 Mar; 78(3):560–78. [PMID: 29331386]

Stratigos A et al; European Dermatology Forum (EDF); European Association of Dermato-Oncology (EADO); European Organization for Research and Treatment of Cancer (EORTC). Diagnosis and treatment of invasive squamous cell carcinoma of the skin: European consensus-based interdisciplinary guideline. Eur J Cancer. 2015 Sep;51(14):1989–2007. [PMID: 26219687]

VIOLACEOUS TO PURPLE PAPULES & NODULES

LICHEN PLANUS

 ESSENTIALS OF DIAGNOSIS

► Pruritic, violaceous, flat-topped papules with fine white streaks and symmetric distribution.

► Lacy or erosive lesions of the buccal, vulvar, and vaginal mucosa; nail dystrophy.

► Commonly seen along linear scratch marks (Koebner phenomenon) on anterior wrists, penis, and legs.

► Histopathologic examination is diagnostic.

General Considerations

Lichen planus is an inflammatory pruritic disease of the skin and mucous membranes characterized by distinctive papules with a predilection for the flexor surfaces and trunk. The three cardinal findings are typical skin lesions, mucosal lesions, and histopathologic features of band-like infiltration of lymphocytes in the upper dermis. The most common medications causing lichen planus–like reactions include sulfonamides, tetracyclines, quinidine, NSAIDs, beta-blockers, and hydrochlorothiazide. Lichenoid drug eruptions can resemble lichen planus clinically and histologically. Hepatitis C infection is found with greater frequency in lichen planus patients than in controls. Allergy to mercury and other metal-containing amalgams can trigger oral lesions identical to lichen planus.

Clinical Findings

The lesions are violaceous, flat-topped, angulated papules, up to 1 cm in diameter, discrete or in clusters, with very fine white streaks (Wickham striae) on the flexor surfaces of the wrists and on the penis, lips, tongue as well as buccal, vulvar, vaginal, esophageal, and anorectal mucous membranes (Figure 6–33). Itching is mild to severe. The papules

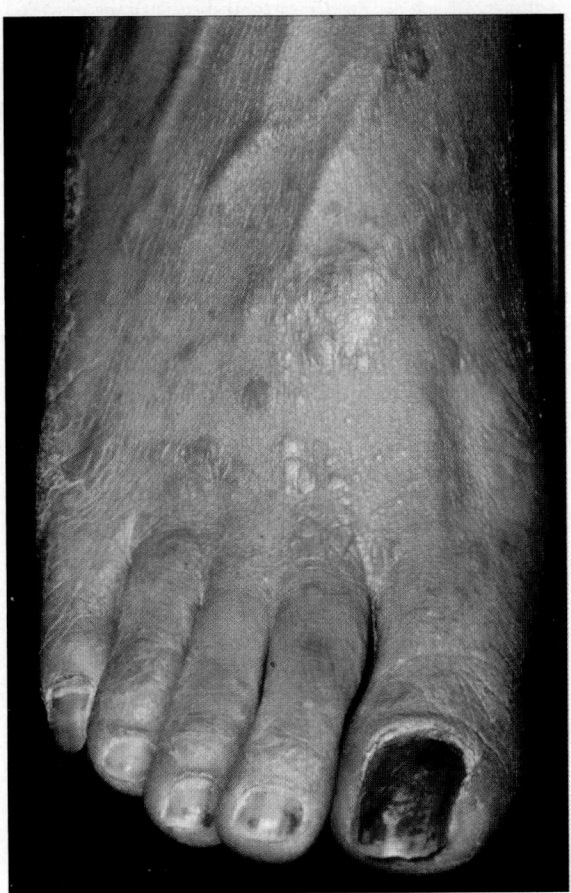

▲ **Figure 6–33.** Lichen planus. (Used, with permission, from TG Berger, MD, Dept Dermatology, UCSF.)

may become bullous or eroded. The disease may be generalized. Mucous membrane lesions have a lacy white network overlying them that may be confused with leukoplakia. The presence of oral and vulvo-vaginal lichen planus in the same patient is common. Patients with both these mucous membranes involved are at much higher risk for esophageal lichen planus. The Koebner phenomenon (appearance of lesions in areas of trauma) may be seen.

A special form of lichen planus is the erosive or ulcerative variety, a major problem in the mouth or genitalia. Squamous cell carcinoma develops in up to 5% of patients with erosive oral or genital lichen planus and may occur in esophageal lichen planus. There is also an increased risk of squamous cell carcinoma developing in lesions of hypertrophic lichen on the lower extremities.

Differential Diagnosis

Lichen planus must be distinguished from similar lesions produced by medications and other papular lesions, such as psoriasis, lichen simplex chronicus, graft-versus-host disease, and syphilis. Lichen planus on the mucous membranes must be differentiated from leukoplakia. Erosive oral lesions require biopsy and often direct immunofluorescence for diagnosis since lichen planus may simulate other erosive diseases.

Treatment

A. Topical Therapy

Superpotent topical corticosteroids applied twice daily are most helpful for localized disease in nonflexural areas. Alternatively, high-potency corticosteroid cream or ointment may be used nightly under thin, pliable plastic film.

Topical tacrolimus appears effective in oral and vaginal erosive lichen planus, but long-term therapy is required to prevent relapse. If tacrolimus is used, lesions must be observed carefully for development of squamous cell carcinoma. Since absorption can occur through mucous membranes, serum tacrolimus levels should be checked at least once if widespread mucosal application (more than 5–10 cm^2) is used. If the erosive oral lichen planus lesions are adjacent to a metal-containing amalgam, removal of the amalgam may result in clearing of the erosions.

B. Systemic Therapy

NB-UVB, bath PUVA, oral PUVA, and the combination of an oral retinoid plus PUVA (re-PUVA) are all forms of phototherapy that can improve lichen planus. Hydroxychloroquine, 200 mg orally twice daily, acitretin 10–25 mg orally daily, cyclosporine 3–5 mg/kg orally, and mycophenolate mofetil, 1 g orally twice daily, can also be effective in mucosal and cutaneous lichen planus. Apremilast has reported efficacy in case series. Corticosteroids may be required in severe cases or in circumstances where the most rapid response to treatment is desired. Unfortunately, relapse almost always occurs as the corticosteroids are tapered, making systemic corticosteroid therapy an impractical option for the management of chronic lichen planus.

Prognosis

Lichen planus is a benign disease, but it may persist for months or years and may be recurrent. Hypertrophic lichen planus and oral lesions tend to be especially persistent, and neoplastic degeneration has been described in chronically eroded lesions.

García-Pola MJ et al. Treatment of oral lichen planus. Systematic review and therapeutic guide. Med Clin (Barc). 2017 Oct 23; 149(8):351–62. [PMID: 28756997]

Gupta S et al. Interventions for the management of oral lichen planus: a review of the conventional and novel therapies. Oral Dis. 2017 Nov;23(8):1029–42. [PMID: 28055124]

Mauskar M. Erosive lichen planus. Obstet Gynecol Clin North Am. 2017 Sep;44(3):407–20. [PMID: 28778640]

Tziotzios C et al. Lichen planus and lichenoid dermatoses: clinical overview and molecular basis. J Am Acad Dermatol. 2018 Nov; 79(5):789–804. [PMID: 30318136]

Tziotzios C et al. Lichen planus and lichenoid dermatoses: conventional and emerging therapeutic strategies. J Am Acad Dermatol. 2018 Nov;79(5):807–18. [PMID: 30318137]

KAPOSI SARCOMA

General Considerations

Human herpes virus 8 (HHV-8), or Kaposi sarcoma–associated herpes virus, is the cause of all forms of Kaposi sarcoma.

Before 1980 in the United States, this rare, malignant skin lesion was seen mostly in elderly men, had a chronic clinical course, and was rarely fatal. Kaposi sarcoma occurs endemically in an often aggressive form in young black men of equatorial Africa, but it is rare in American blacks. Kaposi sarcoma continues to occur largely in homosexual men with HIV infection. Kaposi sarcoma may complicate immunosuppressive therapy, and stopping the immunosuppression may result in improvement.

Red or purple plaques or nodules on cutaneous or mucosal surfaces are characteristic. Marked edema may occur with few or no skin lesions. Kaposi sarcoma commonly involves the gastrointestinal tract and can be screened for by fecal occult blood testing. In asymptomatic patients, these lesions are not sought or treated. Pulmonary Kaposi sarcoma can present with shortness of breath, cough, hemoptysis, or chest pain; it may be asymptomatic, appearing only on chest radiograph. Bronchoscopy may be indicated. The incidence of AIDS-associated Kaposi sarcoma is diminishing. However, chronic Kaposi sarcoma can develop in patients with HIV infection, high CD4 counts, and low viral loads. In this setting, the Kaposi sarcoma usually resembles the endemic form, being indolent and localized. At times, however, it can be clinically aggressive. The presence of Kaposi sarcoma at the time of antiretroviral initiation is associated with Kaposi sarcoma–immune reconstitution inflammatory syndrome (KS-IRIS), which has an especially aggressive course in patients with visceral disease.

Treatment

For Kaposi sarcoma in elders, palliative local therapy with intralesional chemotherapy or radiation is usually all that is required. In the setting of iatrogenic immunosuppression, the treatment of Kaposi sarcoma is primarily reduction of doses of immunosuppressive medications. In AIDS-associated Kaposi sarcoma, the patient should first be given ART. Other therapeutic options include cryotherapy or intralesional vinblastine (0.1–0.5 mg/mL) for cosmetically objectionable lesions; radiation therapy for accessible and space-occupying lesions; and laser surgery for certain intraoral and pharyngeal lesions. Systemic therapy is indicated in patients with rapidly progressive skin disease (more than 10 new lesions per month), with edema or pain, and with symptomatic visceral disease or pulmonary disease. ART plus chemotherapy appears to be more effective than ART alone (see Table 39–3). Liposomal doxorubicin is highly effective in severe cases and may be used alone or in combination with bleomycin and vincristine. Alpha-interferon may also be used. Paclitaxel and other taxanes can be effective even in patients who do not respond to anthracycline treatment. Targeted immunotherapy is under active investigation.

Cancer Project Working Group for the Collaboration of Observational HIV Epidemiological Research Europe (COHERE) study in EuroCoord. Changing incidence and risk factors for Kaposi sarcoma by time since starting antiretroviral therapy: collaborative analysis of 21 European cohort studies. Clin Infect Dis. 2016 Nov 15;63(10):1373–9. [PMID: 27535953]

Dittmer DP et al. Kaposi sarcoma-associated herpesvirus: immunobiology, oncogenesis, and therapy. J Clin Invest. 2016 Sep 1;126(9):3165–75. [PMID: 27584730]

Gbabe OF et al. Treatment of severe or progressive Kaposi's sarcoma in HIV-infected adults. Cochrane Database Syst Rev. 2014 Aug 13;8:CD003256. [PMID: 25221796]

Schneider JW et al. Diagnosis and treatment of Kaposi sarcoma. Am J Clin Dermatol. 2017 Aug;18(4):529–39. [PMID: 28324233]

PRURITUS (ITCHING)

Pruritus is the sensation that provokes a desire to scratch. Pruritus as a medical complaint is 40% as common as low back pain. Elderly Asian men are most significantly affected, with 20% of all health care visits in Asian men over the age of 65 involving the complaint of itch. The quality of life of a patient with chronic pruritus is the same as a patient undergoing hemodialysis. Evidence suggests that increased interleukin-31 (IL-31) signaling through the IL-31 receptor on epithelial cells and keratinocytes is associated with itch, especially in allergic skin disease. It also appears that Il-4 and Il-13 (via binding to the Il-4R) lower the itch threshold of sensory neurons. Janus kinase signaling (which occurs downstream from the Il-4R) is also emerging as important in the pathophysiology of itch.

Dry skin is the first cause of itch that should be sought, since it is common and easily treated. The next step in physical evaluation of the itchy patient is deciding whether a primary skin lesion is present or absent. If a primary skin lesion is present, then the patient has a primary cutaneous disease with associated pruritus. Examples of primary cutaneous pruritic diseases include scabies, atopic dermatitis, insect bites, pediculosis, contact dermatitis, drug reactions, urticaria, psoriasis, lichen planus, and fiberglass dermatitis. These conditions all present with recognizable cutaneous morphologies, and the treatment of the skin condition usually results in control of the associated pruritus.

Persistent pruritus not explained by cutaneous disease or association with a primary skin eruption should prompt a staged workup for systemic causes. Common causes of pruritus associated with systemic diseases include endocrine disorders (eg, hypothyroidism, hyperthyroidism, or hyperparathyroidism), psychiatric disturbances, lymphoma, leukemia, and other internal malignant disorders, iron deficiency anemia, HIV, hypercalcemia, cholestasis, and certain neurologic disorders. Calcium channel blockers can cause pruritus with or without eczema, even years after they have been started, and it may take up to 1 year for the pruritus to resolve after the calcium channel blocker has been stopped.

Treatment

The treatment of chronic pruritus can be frustrating. Most cases of pruritus are not mediated by histamine, hence the poor response of many pruritic patients to antihistamines. Emollients for dry skin are listed in Table 6–2. Emollient creams (preferred over lotions) should be generously applied from neck to toe immediately after towel drying and again one more time per day. Neuropathic disease, especially in diabetic patients, is associated with pruritus, making neurally acting agents, such as gabapentin (starting at 300 mg orally at around 4 PM and a second dose of 600 mg orally at bedtime) or pregabalin (150 mg orally daily), attractive approaches to the management of pruritus. Combinations of antihistamines, sinequan, gabapentin, pregabalin, mirtazapine, and opioid antagonists can be attempted in refractory cases. In cancer-associated and other forms of pruritus, aprepitant (Emend) 80 mg orally daily for several days can be dramatically effective. The uremia in conjunction with hemodialysis and to a lesser degree the pruritus of liver disease may be helped by phototherapy with ultraviolet B or PUVA. Naltrexone and nalmefene have been shown to relieve the pruritus of liver disease. Naltrexone is not effective in pruritus associated with advanced chronic kidney disease, but gabapentin or mirtazapine may be effective. Il-31 blockade (nemolizumab), Il-4 blockade (dupilumab), and inhibition of the Janus kinase pathway (tofacitinib) are demonstrating some efficacy in the treatment of chronic pruritus.

Prognosis

Elimination of external factors and irritating agents may give complete relief. Pruritus accompanying a specific skin disease will subside when the skin disease is controlled. Pruritus accompanying serious internal disease may not respond to any type of therapy.

Leslie TA. Itch management in the elderly. Curr Probl Dermatol. 2016;0:192–201. [PMID: 27578088]

Matsuda KM et al. Gabapentin and pregabalin for the treatment of chronic pruritus. J Am Acad Dermatol. 2016 Sep;75(3):619–25.e6. [PMID: 27206757]

Metz M et al. Itch management: topical agents. Curr Probl Dermatol. 2016;0:40–5. [PMID: 27578070]

Patel JM et al. Chronic pruritus: a review of neurophysiology and associated immune neuromodulatory treatments. Skin Therapy Lett. 2018 Sep;23(5):5–9. [PMID: 30248162]

Pereira MP et al. Chronic pruritus in the absence of skin disease: pathophysiology, diagnosis and treatment. Am J Clin Dermatol. 2016 Aug;17(4):337–48. [PMID: 27216284]

Ruzicka T et al; XCIMA Study Group. Anti-interleukin-31 receptor A antibody for atopic dermatitis. N Engl J Med. 2017 Mar 2;376(9):826–35. [PMID: 28249150]

Şavk E. Neurologic itch management. Curr Probl Dermatol. 2016;50:116–23. [PMID: 27578080]

Silverberg JI. Practice gaps in pruritus. Dermatol Clin. 2016 Jul; 34(3):257–61. [PMID: 27363881]

Ständer S et al. Validation of the itch severity item as a measurement tool for pruritus in patients with psoriasis: results from a phase 3 tofacitinib program. Acta Derm Venereol. 2018 Mar 13;98(3):340–5. [PMID: 29182790]

Stull C et al. Advances in therapeutic strategies for the treatment of pruritus. Expert Opin Pharmacother. 2016;17(5):671–87. [PMID: 26630350]

ANOGENITAL PRURITUS

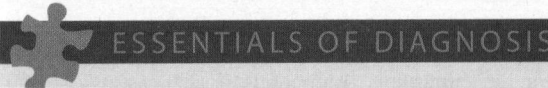

ESSENTIALS OF DIAGNOSIS

► Itching, chiefly nocturnal, of the anogenital area.

► Examination is highly variable, ranging from no skin findings to excoriations and inflammation of any degree, including lichenification.

General Considerations

Anogenital pruritus may be due to a primary inflammatory skin disease (intertrigo, psoriasis, lichen simplex chronicus, seborrheic dermatitis, lichen sclerosus), contact dermatitis (soaps, colognes, douches, and topical treatments), irritating secretions (diarrhea, leukorrhea, or trichomoniasis), infections (candidiasis, dermatophytosis, erythrasma), or oxyuriasis (pinworms). Erythrasma (Figure 6–34) is

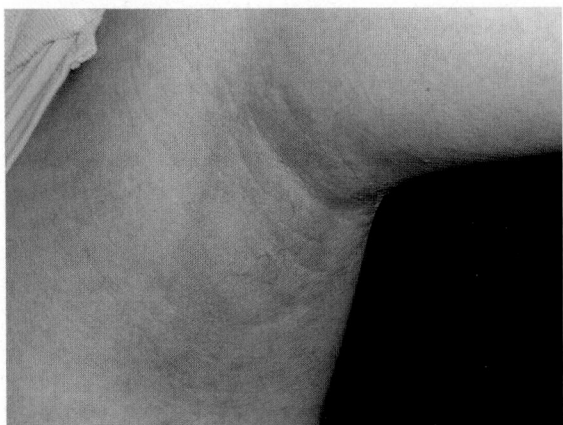

▲ **Figure 6–34.** Erythrasma of the axilla. (Used, with permission, from Richard P. Usatine, MD, in Usatine RP, Smith MA, Mayeaux EJ Jr, Chumley H, Tysinger J. *The Color Atlas of Family Medicine*. McGraw-Hill, 2009.)

diagnosed by coral-red fluorescence with Wood light and cured with erythromycin. Squamous cell carcinoma of the anus and extramammary Paget disease are rare causes of genital pruritus.

In pruritus ani, hemorrhoids are often found, and leakage of mucus and bacteria from the distal rectum onto the perianal skin may be important in cases in which no other skin abnormality is found.

Many women experience pruritus vulvae. Pruritus vulvae does not usually involve the anal area, though anal itching may spread to the vulva. In men, pruritus of the scrotum is most commonly seen in the absence of pruritus ani.

Up to one-third of unidentified causes of anogenital pruritus may be due to nerve impingements of the lumbosacral spine, so evaluation of lumbosacral spine disease is appropriate if no skin disorder is identified and topical therapy is ineffective.

Clinical Findings

A. Symptoms and Signs

The only symptom is itching. Physical findings are usually not present, but there may be erythema, fissuring, maceration, lichenification, excoriations, or changes suggestive of candidiasis or tinea.

B. Laboratory Findings

Microscopic examination or culture of tissue scrapings may reveal yeasts or fungi. Stool examination may show pinworms. Radiologic studies may demonstrate spinal disease.

Differential Diagnosis

The etiologic differential diagnosis consists of *Candida* infection, parasitosis, local irritation from contactants or irritants, nerve impingement, and other primary skin disorders of the genital area, such as psoriasis, seborrhea, intertrigo, or lichen sclerosus.

Prevention

Instruct the patient in proper anogenital hygiene after treating systemic or local conditions.

Treatment

Treating constipation, preferably with high-fiber management (psyllium), may help. Instruct the patient to use very soft or moistened tissue or cotton after bowel movements and to clean the perianal area thoroughly with cool water if possible. Women should use similar precautions after urinating. Patch testing most commonly reveals clinically relevant allergy in about 20% of patients, often to methylchloroisothiazolinone or methylisothiazolinone, preservatives commonly found in "baby wipes" and other personal care products.

Pramoxine cream or lotion or hydrocortisone-pramoxine (Pramosone), 1% or 2.5% cream, lotion, or ointment, is helpful for anogenital pruritus and should be applied after a bowel movement. Topical doxepin cream 5% is similarly effective, but it may be sedating. Topical calcineurin inhibitors (tacrolimus 0.03%) improve pruritus ani in patients with atopic dermatitis. Underclothing should be changed daily, and in men, the seam of their "boxers" should not rub against or contact the scrotum. Balneol Perianal Cleansing Lotion or Tucks premoistened pads, ointment, or cream may be very useful for pruritus ani. About one-third of patients with scrotal or anal pruritus will respond to capsaicin cream 0.006%. In cases where underlying spinal neurologic disease is suspected, gabapentin or pregabalin may be helpful. The use of high-potency topical corticosteroids should be avoided in the genital area.

Prognosis

Although benign, anogenital pruritus is often persistent and recurrent.

Abu-Asi MJ et al. Patch testing is clinically important for patients with peri-anal dermatoses and pruritus ani. Contact Dermatitis. 2016 May;74(5):298–300. [PMID: 27040873]

Ansari P. Pruritus ani. Clin Colon Rectal Surg. 2016 Mar;29(1):38–42. [PMID: 26929750]

Chibnall R. Vulvar pruritus and lichen simplex chronicus. Obstet Gynecol Clin North Am. 2017 Sep;44(3):379–88. [PMID: 28778638]

Şavk E. Neurologic itch management. Curr Probl Dermatol. 2016;0:116–23. [PMID: 27578080]

SCABIES

ESSENTIALS OF DIAGNOSIS

- ▶ Generalized very severe itching but infestation usually spares the head and neck.
- ▶ Burrows, vesicles, and pustules, especially on finger webs and in wrist creases.
- ▶ Mites, ova, and brown dots of feces (scybala) visible microscopically.
- ▶ Red papules or nodules on the scrotum and on the penile glans and shaft are pathognomonic.

General Considerations

Scabies is caused by infestation with *Sarcoptes scabiei*, affecting over 200 million people worldwide. Close physical contact for 15–20 minutes with an infected person is the typical mode of transmission. However, scabies may be acquired by contact with the bedding of an infested individual. Facility-associated scabies is common, primarily in long-term care facilities, and misdiagnosis is common. Index patients are usually elderly and immunosuppressed. When these patients are hospitalized, hospital-based epidemics can occur. These epidemics are difficult to eradicate since many health care workers become infected and spread the infestation to other patients.

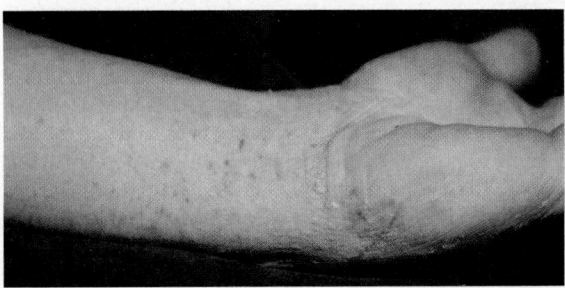

▲ **Figure 6–35.** Scabies. (Used, with permission, from TG Berger, MD, Dept Dermatology, UCSF.)

► Clinical Findings

A. Symptoms and Signs

Itching is almost always present and can be severe. The lesions consist of more or less generalized excoriations with small pruritic vesicles, pustules, and "burrows" in the interdigital spaces of the hands and feet, on the heels of the palms, wrists (Figure 6–35), elbows, umbilicus, around the axillae, on the areolae in women, or on the penile shaft and scrotum in men. The burrow appears as a short irregular mark, 2–3 mm long and the width of a hair. Characteristic nodular lesions may occur on the scrotum or penis and along the posterior axillary line. The infestation usually spares the head and neck (though these areas may be involved in infants, older adults, and patients with AIDS).

Hyperkeratotic or crusted scabies presents as thick flaking scale. These areas contain millions of mites, and these patients are highly infectious. Pruritus is often absent. Patients with widespread hyperkeratotic scabies are at risk for superinfection with *S aureus*, which in some cases progresses to sepsis if left untreated. Crusted scabies is the cause of 83% of scabies outbreaks in institutions.

B. Laboratory Findings

The diagnosis should be confirmed by microscopic demonstration of the organism, ova, or feces in a mounted specimen, examined with tap water, mineral oil, or KOH. Best results are obtained when multiple lesions are scraped, choosing the best unexcoriated lesions from interdigital webs, wrists, elbows, or feet. A No. 15 blade is used to scrape each lesion until it is flat. Patients with crusted/hyperkeratotic scabies must be evaluated for immunosuppression (especially HIV and HTLV-1 infections) if no iatrogenic cause of immunosuppression is present. Patients with hyperkeratotic scabies and associated bacterial superinfection may have laboratory findings consistent with infection and, if severe, sepsis.

► Differential Diagnosis

Scabies must be distinguished from the various forms of pediculosis, from bedbug and flea bites, and from other causes of pruritus.

► Treatment & Prognosis

Treatment is aimed at killing scabies mites and controlling the dermatitis, which can persist for months after effective eradication of the mites. Bedding and clothing should be laundered or cleaned or set aside for 14 days in plastic bags. High heat (60°C) is required to kill the mites and ova. Treatment is aimed at all infected persons in a family or institutionalized group. Otherwise, reinfestations will likely occur, which is why scabies in nursing home patients, institutionalized or mentally impaired patients, and AIDS patients may be much more difficult to treat.

1. Permethrin 5% cream—Treatment with permethrin, a highly effective and safe agent, consists of a single application from the neck down for 8–12 hours then washed off, repeated in 1 week. Patients often continue to itch for several weeks after treatment. Use of triamcinolone 0.1% cream helps resolve the dermatitis.

Pregnant patients should be treated only if they have documented scabies themselves. Permethrin 5% cream once for 12 hours—or 5% or 6% sulfur in petrolatum applied nightly for 3 nights from the collarbones down—may be used.

Most failures in normal persons are related to incorrect use or incomplete treatment of the housing unit. In these cases, repeat treatment with permethrin once weekly for 2 weeks, with re-education regarding the method and extent of application, is suggested.

2. Ivermectin—In immunocompetent individuals, 200 mcg/kg orally is effective in about 75% of cases with a single dose and 95% of cases with two doses 2 weeks apart. A single dose (versus two doses) of ivermectin was associated with treatment failure in one study, but this not substantiated by a Cochrane review.

Ivermectin is often used in combination with permethrin. In immunosuppressed persons and those with crusted (hyperkeratotic) scabies, multiple doses of ivermectin (every 2 weeks for 2 or 3 doses) plus topical therapy with permethrin every 3 days to once weekly, depending on degree of involvement, may be effective when topical treatment and oral therapy alone fail. A topical keratolytic (urea) should be used to help remove the scale, thereby decreasing the mite load, of hyperkeratotic scabies.

Ivermectin can be very beneficial in mass treatment to eradicate infections in institutions or villages. In endemic areas, mass intervention with ivermectin is effective in controlling both scabies and associated bacterial infections.

If secondary pyoderma is present, it is treated with systemic antibiotics. Staphylococcal superinfection may lead to sepsis. In areas where nephritogenic streptococcal strains are prevalent, infestation with scabies or exposure to scabies-infested dogs may be followed by acute poststreptococcal glomerulonephritis.

Persistent pruritic postscabietic papules may be treated with mid- to high-potency corticosteroids or with intralesional triamcinolone acetonide (2.5–5 mg/mL).

Anderson KL et al. Epidemiology, diagnosis, and treatment of scabies in a dermatology office. J Am Board Fam Med. 2017 1/2; 30(1):78–84. [PMID: 28062820]

Aussy A et al; investigators from the Normandy association of medical education in dermatology. Risk factors for treatment failure in scabies: a cohort study. Br J Dermatol. 2019 Apr; 180(4):888–93. [PMID: 30376179]

Goldust M. Treatment of scabies, comparing the different medications. Ann Parasitol. 2016 Oct 1;62(3):243. [PMID: 27770765]

Hardy M et al. Scabies: a clinical update. Aust Fam Physician. 2017;46(5):264–68. [PMID: 28472570]

Rosumeck S et al. Ivermectin and permethrin for treating scabies. Cochrane Database Syst Rev. 2018 Apr 2;4:CD012994. [PMID: 29608022]

Thean LJ et al. Scabies: new opportunities for management and population control. Pediatr Infect Dis J. 2019 Feb;38(2):211–3. [PMID: 30299425]

White LC et al. The management of scabies outbreaks in residential care facilities for the elderly in England: a review of current health protection guidelines. Epidemiol Infect. 2016 Nov; 144(15):3121–30. [PMID: 27734781]

PEDICULOSIS

ESSENTIALS OF DIAGNOSIS

► Pruritus with excoriation.

► Nits on hair shafts; lice on skin or clothes.

► Occasionally, sky-blue macules (maculae ceruleae) on the inner thighs or lower abdomen in pubic louse infestation.

General Considerations

Pediculosis is a parasitic infestation of the skin of the scalp, trunk, or pubic areas. Body lice usually occur among people who live in overcrowded dwellings with inadequate hygiene facilities. Pubic lice may be sexually transmitted. Head lice may be transmitted by shared use of hats or combs. Adults in contact with children with head lice frequently acquire the infestation.

There are three different varieties (1) **pediculosis capitis,** caused by *Pediculus humanus* var *capitis* (head louse); (2) **pediculosis corporis,** caused by *Pediculus humanus* var *corporis* (body louse); and (3) **pediculosis pubis,** caused by *Phthirus pubis* (pubic louse, "crabs").

Head and body lice are similar in appearance and are 3–4 mm long. The body louse can seldom be found on the body, because the insect comes onto the skin only to feed and must be looked for in the seams of the clothing. Trench fever, relapsing fever, and typhus are transmitted by the body louse in countries where those diseases are endemic. In the United States, *Bartonella quintana*, the organism that causes trench fever, has been found in lice infesting the homeless population.

Clinical Findings

In body louse infestations, itching may be very intense, and scratching may result in deep excoriations, especially over the upper shoulders, posterior flanks, and neck. In some cases, only itching is present, with few excoriations seen. Pyoderma may be the presenting sign. Diagnosis is made by examining the seams of clothing for nits and lice. Head lice presents as scalp pruritus often accompanied by erosions on the occipital scalp, posterior neck, and upper back. Diagnosis is made by finding lice on the scalp or small nits resembling pussy willow buds on the scalp hairs close to the skin. Nits are easiest to see above the ears and at the nape of the neck. Pubic louse infestations are occasionally generalized, particularly in hairy individuals; the lice may even be found on the eyelashes and in the scalp. Diagnosis is made by finding lice or nits on pubic hair, body hair, or eyelashes.

Differential Diagnosis

Head louse infestation must be distinguished from seborrheic dermatitis, body louse infestation from scabies and bedbug bites, and pubic louse infestation from anogenital pruritus and eczema.

Treatment

1. Pediculosis capitis—Permethrin 1% cream rinse (Nix) is a topical over-the-counter pediculicide and ovicide. It is applied to the scalp and hair and left on for 8 hours before being rinsed off. Although it is the treatment of choice for head lice, permethrin resistance is common. Malathion lotion 1% (Ovide) is very effective, but it is highly volatile and flammable, so application must be done in a well-ventilated room or out of doors. Topical ivermectin 0.5% lotion, benzyl alcohol 5%, Oxyphthirine® lotion, spinosad 0.9% suspension, dimethicone, and abametapir 0.74% lotion are additional agents that appear to have efficacy against pediculosis capitis; of these agents, topical ivermectin is the most effective. All infested persons in a household, school, or other facility should ideally be treated at the same time. Other than topical ivermectin, topical therapies should be repeated 7–9 days after the initial treatment. For involvement of eyelashes, petrolatum is applied thickly twice daily for 8 days, and remaining nits are then plucked off. Systemic treatment options, often used in combination with topical agents, are oral ivermectin (200 mcg/kg orally, repeated in 7 days) (for children older than 5 years and more than 15 kg) and oral TMP-SMZ (10 mg TMP/kg/day and 50 mg SMZ/kg/day divided twice daily for 10 days).

2. Pediculosis corporis—Body lice are treated by disposing of the infested clothing and addressing the patient's social situation.

3. Pediculosis pubis—Application of permethrin rinse 1% for 10 minutes or permethrin cream 5% for 8 hours to the pubis is effective. Sexual contacts should be treated. Clothes and bedclothes should be washed and dried at high temperature.

Bowles VM et al. Clinical studies evaluating abametapir lotion, 0.74%, for the treatment of head louse infestation. Pediatr Dermatol. 2018 Sep;35(5):616–21. [PMID: 29999197]

Dadabhoy I et al. Parasitic skin infections for primary care physicians. Prim Care. 2015 Dec;42(4):661–75. [PMID: 26612378]

Devore CD et al; Council on School Health and Committee on Infectious Diseases, American Academy of Pediatrics. Head lice. Pediatrics. 2015 May;135(5):e1355–65. [PMID: 25917986]

Koch E et al. Management of head louse infestations in the United States—a literature review. Pediatr Dermatol. 2016 Sep; 33(5):466–72. [PMID: 27595869]

Salavastru CM et al. European guideline for the management of pediculosis pubis. J Eur Acad Dermatol Venereol. 2017 Sep; 31(9):1425–8. [PMID: 28714128]

Sangaré AK et al. Management and treatment of human lice. Biomed Res Int. 2016;6:8962685. [PMID: 27529073]

SKIN LESIONS DUE TO OTHER ARTHROPODS

ESSENTIALS OF DIAGNOSIS

► Localized urticarial papules with pruritus.

► Lesions in linear groups of three ("breakfast, lunch, and dinner") are characteristic of bedbugs.

► Furuncle-like lesions containing live arthropods.

► Tender erythematous patches that migrate ("larva migrans").

General Considerations

Some arthropods (eg, mosquitoes and biting flies) are readily detected as they bite. Many others are not because they are too small, because there is no immediate reaction, or because they bite during sleep. Reactions are allergic and may be delayed for hours to days. Patients are most apt to consult a clinician when the lesions are multiple and pruritus is intense.

Many persons will react severely only to their earliest contacts with an arthropod, thus presenting with pruritic lesions when traveling, moving into new quarters, etc. Body lice, fleas, bedbugs, and mosquitoes should be considered. Bedbug exposure typically occurs in hotels and in housing with inadequate hygiene but also may occur in stable domiciles. Spiders are often incorrectly believed to be the source of bites; they rarely attack humans, though the brown recluse spider (*Loxosceles laeta, L reclusa*) may cause severe necrotic reactions and death due to intravascular hemolysis, and the black widow spider (*Latrodectus mactans*) may cause severe systemic symptoms and death. (See also Chapter 38.) The majority of patient-diagnosed, clinician-diagnosed, and even published cases of brown recluse spider bites (or loxoscelism) are incorrect, especially if made in areas where these spiders are not endemic. Many of these lesions are actually due to CA-MRSA.

In addition to arthropod bites, the most common lesions are venomous stings (wasps, hornets, bees, ants, scorpions) or bites (centipedes), furuncle-like lesions due to fly maggots or sand fleas in the skin, and a linear creeping eruption due to a migrating larva.

Clinical Findings

The diagnosis may be difficult when the patient has not noticed the initial attack but suffers a delayed reaction. Individual bites are often in clusters and tend to occur either on exposed parts (eg, midges and gnats) or under clothing, especially around the waist or at flexures (eg, small mites or insects in bedding or clothing). The reaction is often delayed for 1–24 hours or more. Pruritus is almost always present and may be all but intolerable once the patient starts to scratch. Secondary infection may follow scratching. Urticarial wheals are common. Papules may become vesicular. The diagnosis is aided by searching for exposure to arthropods and by considering the patient's occupation and recent activities.

The principal arthropods are as follows:

1. **Fleas:** Fleas are bloodsucking ectoparasites that feed on dogs, cats, humans, and other species. Flea saliva produces papular urticaria in sensitized individuals. To break the life cycle of the flea, one must treat the home and pets, using quick-kill insecticides, residual insecticides, and a growth regulator.

2. **Bedbugs:** In crevices of beds or furniture; bites tend to occur in lines or clusters. Papular urticaria is a characteristic lesion of bedbug (*Cimex lectularius*) bites. Bedbugs are not restricted to any socioeconomic group and are a major health problem in some major metropolitan areas, especially in commercial and residential hotels.

3. **Ticks:** Usually picked up by brushing against low vegetation.

4. **Chiggers or red bugs:** These are larvae of trombiculid mites. A few species confined to particular regions and locally recognized habitats (eg, berry patches, woodland edges, lawns, brush turkey mounds in Australia, poultry farms) attack humans, often around the waist, on the ankles, or in flexures, raising intensely itching erythematous papules after a delay of many hours. The red chiggers may sometimes be seen in the center of papules that have not yet been scratched.

5. **Bird and rodent mites:** Larger than chiggers, bird mites infest birds and their nests. Bites are multiple anywhere on the body. Room air conditioning units may suck in bird mites and infest the inhabitants of the room. Rodent mites from mice or rats may cause similar effects. If the domicile has evidence of rodent activity, then rodent mite dermatitis should be suspected, as the mites are rarely found. Pet rodents or birds may be infested with mites, maintaining the infestation.

6. **Mites in stored products:** These are white and almost invisible and infest products, such as copra, vanilla pods, sugar, straw, cottonseeds, and cereals. Persons who handle these products may be attacked, especially on the hands and forearms and sometimes on the feet.

7. **Caterpillars of moths with urticating hairs:** The hairs are blown from cocoons or carried by emergent moths, causing severe and often seasonally recurrent outbreaks after mass emergence. The gypsy moth is a cause in the eastern United States.

8. **Tungiasis:** Tungiasis is due to the burrowing flea known as *Tunga penetrans* and is found in Africa, the

West Indies, and South and Central America. The female burrows under the skin, sucks blood, swells to 0.5 cm, and then ejects her eggs onto the ground. Ulceration, lymphangitis, gangrene, and septicemia may result, in some cases with lethal effect. Simple surgical removal is usually performed.

▶ Prevention

Arthropod infestations are best prevented by avoidance of contaminated areas, personal cleanliness, and disinfection of clothing, bedclothes, and furniture as indicated. Chiggers and mites can be repelled by permethrin applied to the head and clothing. (It is not necessary to remove clothing.) Bedbugs are no longer repelled by permethrin and can survive for up to 1 year without feeding. Aggressive cleaning, usually requiring removal of the affected occupant from the domicile, may be necessary to eradicate bedbug infestation in a residence.

▶ Treatment

Living arthropods should be removed carefully with tweezers after application of alcohol and preserved in alcohol for identification. In endemic Rocky Mountain spotted fever areas, ticks should not be removed with the bare fingers.

Corticosteroid lotions or creams are helpful. Topical antibiotics may be applied if secondary infection is suspected. Localized persistent lesions may be treated with intralesional corticosteroids.

Stings produced by many arthropods may be alleviated by applying papain powder (Adolph's Meat Tenderizer) mixed with water, or aluminum chloride hexahydrate (Xerac AC).

Extracts from venom sacs of bees, wasps, yellow jackets, and hornets are available for immunotherapy of patients at risk for anaphylaxis.

McMenaman KS et al. *Cimex lectularius* ("bed bugs"): recognition, management, and eradication. Pediatr Emerg Care. 2016 Nov; 32(11):801–6. [PMID: 27811535]
Vasievich MP et al. Got the travel bug? A review of common infections, infestations, bites, and stings among returning travelers. Am J Clin Dermatol. 2016 Oct;17(5):451–62. [PMID: 27344566]

INFLAMMATORY NODULES

ERYTHEMA NODOSUM

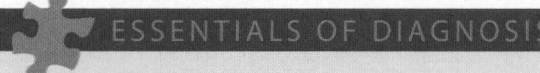

ESSENTIALS OF DIAGNOSIS

▶ Painful nodules without ulceration on anterior aspects of legs.

▶ Slow regression over several weeks to resemble contusions.

▶ Women are predominantly affected by a ratio of 10:1 compared to men.

▶ Some cases associated with infection, inflammatory bowel disease, or medication exposure.

▶ General Considerations

Erythema nodosum is a symptom complex characterized by tender, erythematous nodules that appear most commonly on the extensor surfaces of the lower legs. It usually lasts about 6 weeks and may recur. Most cases are idiopathic in nature. However, erythema nodosum can be considered a skin sign of systemic disease. Evaluation and management includes making the diagnosis, treating the symptoms, and searching for an underlying cause. The disease may be associated with various infections—streptococcosis, primary coccidioidomycosis, other deep fungal infections, tuberculosis, *Yersinia pseudotuberculosis* and *Y enterocolitica* infection, diverticulitis, or syphilis. It may accompany sarcoidosis, Behçet disease, and inflammatory bowel disease. Erythema nodosum may be associated with pregnancy or with use of oral contraceptives.

▶ Clinical Findings

A. Symptoms and Signs

The subcutaneous swellings are exquisitely tender and may be preceded by fever, malaise, and arthralgia. They are most often located on the anterior surfaces of the legs below the knees but may occur on the arms, trunk, and face. The lesions, 1–10 cm in diameter, are at first pink to red; with regression, all the various hues seen in a contusion can be observed (Figure 6–36) but, as a rule, the lesions do not ulcerate.

B. Laboratory Findings

Evaluation of patients presenting with acute erythema nodosum should include a careful history (including medication exposures) and physical examination. Significant findings include a history of prior upper respiratory infection or diarrheal illness or symptoms of any deep fungal infection endemic to the area. All patients should get a chest radiograph, a purified protein derivative or blood interferon gamma release assay (such as QuantiFERON) (see Pulmonary Tuberculosis in Chapter 9), and two consecutive ASO/DNAse B titers at 2- to 4-week intervals. Coccidioidomycosis should be looked for in patients from endemic areas. If no underlying cause is found, only a small percentage of patients will go on to develop a significant underlying illness (usually sarcoidosis) over the next year.

▶ Differential Diagnosis

Unlike other forms of panniculitis, a defining feature of erythema nodosum is that it does not ulcerate. Erythema induratum from tuberculosis is seen on the posterior surfaces of the legs and may ulcerate. Lupus panniculitis presents as tender nodules in fatty areas of the buttocks and posterior arms and heals with depressed scars. In polyarteritis nodosa, the subcutaneous nodules are often associated with fixed livedo reticularis. In its late stages, erythema nodosum must be distinguished from simple bruises and contusions.

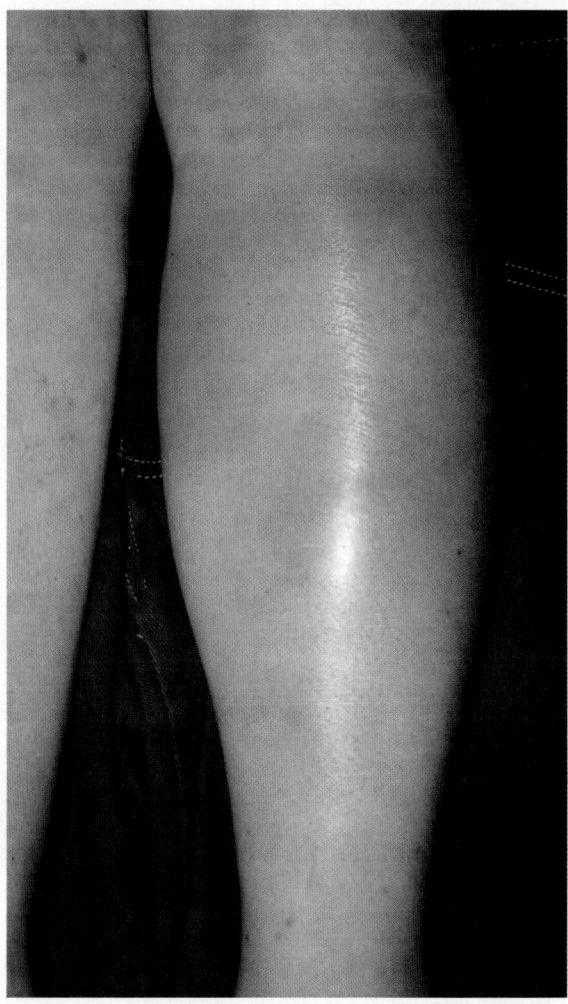

▲ **Figure 6–36.** Erythema nodosum. (Used, with permission, from TG Berger, MD, Dept Dermatology, UCSF.)

Treatment

First, the underlying cause should be identified and treated. Primary therapy is with NSAIDs in usual doses. Saturated solution of potassium iodide, 5–15 drops three times daily, results in prompt involution in many cases. Complete bed rest may be advisable if the lesions are painful. Systemic therapy directed against the lesions themselves may include corticosteroid therapy (see Chapter 26) (unless contraindicated by associated infection), dapsone, colchicine, or hydroxychloroquine.

Prognosis

The lesions usually disappear after about 6 weeks, but they may recur.

Chen S et al. *Mycobacterium tuberculosis* infection is associated with the development of erythema nodosum and nodular vasculitis. PLoS One. 2013 May 1;8(5):e62653. [PMID: 23650522]

Chowaniec M et al. Erythema nodosum—review of the literature. Reumatologia. 2016;54(2):79–82. [PMID: 27407284]
De Simone C et al. Clinical, histopathological, and immunological evaluation of a series of patients with erythema nodosum. Int J Dermatol. 2016 May;55(5):e289–94. [PMID: 26917228]

FURUNCULOSIS (Boils) & CARBUNCLES

ESSENTIALS OF DIAGNOSIS

► Extremely painful inflammatory swelling based on a hair follicle that forms an abscess.

► Coagulase-positive *S aureus* is the causative organism.

► Predisposing condition (diabetes mellitus, HIV disease, injection drug use) sometimes present.

General Considerations

A **furuncle (boil)** is a deep-seated infection (abscess) caused by *S aureus* and involving the entire hair follicle and adjacent subcutaneous tissue. The most common sites of occurrence are the hairy parts exposed to irritation and friction, pressure, or moisture. Because the lesions are autoinoculable, they are often multiple. Diabetes mellitus (especially if using insulin injections), injection drug use, allergy injections, and HIV disease all increase the risk of staphylococcal infections by increasing the rate of carriage. Certain other exposures including hospitalization, athletic teams, prisons, military service, and homelessness may also increase the risk of infection.

A **carbuncle** consists of several furuncles developing in adjoining hair follicles and coalescing to form a conglomerate, deeply situated mass with multiple drainage points.

Recurrent furunculosis (three or more episodes in 12 months) tends to occur in those with direct contact with other infected individuals, especially family members.

Clinical Findings

A. Symptoms and Signs

Pain and tenderness may be prominent. The abscess is either rounded or conical. It gradually enlarges, becomes fluctuant, and then softens and opens spontaneously after a few days to 1–2 weeks to discharge a core of necrotic tissue and pus. The inflammation occasionally subsides before necrosis occurs.

B. Laboratory Findings

There may be slight leukocytosis, but a white blood cell count is rarely required. Pus can be cultured to rule out MRSA or other bacteria. Culture of the anterior nares and anogenital area (including the rectum to test for gastrointestinal carriage) may identify chronic staphylococcal carriage in cases of recurrent cutaneous infection.

Differential Diagnosis

The most common entity in the differential is an inflamed **epidermal inclusion cyst** that suddenly becomes red, tender, and expands greatly in size over one to a few days. The history of a prior cyst in the same location, the presence of a clearly visible cyst orifice, and the extrusion of malodorous cheesy material (rather than purulent material) helps in the diagnosis. Tinea profunda (deep dermatophyte infection of the hair follicle) may simulate recurrent furunculosis. Furuncle is also to be distinguished from deep mycotic infections, such as sporotrichosis; from other bacterial infections, such as anthrax and tularemia (rare); from atypical mycobacterial infections; and from acne cysts. Hidradenitis suppurativa (acne inversa) presents with recurrent tender, sterile abscesses in the axillae and groin, on the buttocks, or below the breasts. The presence of old scars or sinus tracts plus negative cultures suggests this diagnosis.

Complications

Serious and sometimes fatal complications of staphylococcal infection such as septicemia can occur.

Prevention

Identifying and eliminating the source of infection is critical to prevent recurrences after treatment. The source individual may have chronic dermatitis or be an asymptomatic carrier. Nasal carriage of MRSA and the number of children in a household are risk factors for transmission between household members. Local measures, such as meticulous handwashing; no sharing of towels, clothing, and personal hygiene products; avoiding loofas or sponges in the bath or shower; changing underwear, sleepwear, towels, and washcloths daily; aggressive scrubbing of showers, bathrooms, and surfaces with bleach; bleach baths (¼–½ cup per 20 liters of bathwater for 15 minutes 3–5 times weekly), 4% chlorhexidine washes, and isolation of infected patients who reside in institutions to prevent spread are all effective measures.

Treatment

A. Specific Measures

Incision and drainage is recommended for all loculated suppurations and is the mainstay of therapy. Systemic antibiotics are usually given. Patients who receive antibiotics (specifically, TMP-SMZ [160/800 or 320/1600 mg orally twice a day for 10 days or 7 days, respectively] or clindamycin [300 mg orally three times daily for 10 days]) at the time of drainage have higher cure rates and lower new infection rates. Other oral antibiotic options include dicloxacillin or cephalexin, 1 g daily in divided doses for 10 days. For suspected MRSA, doxycycline 100 mg twice daily, TMP-SMZ double-strength one tablet twice daily, clindamycin 150–300 mg twice daily, and linezolid 400 mg twice daily for 7–10 days are effective. Recurrent furunculosis may be effectively treated with a combination of cephalexin (250–500 mg four times daily) or doxycycline

(100 mg twice daily) for 2–4 weeks plus either rifampin (300 mg twice daily for 5 days) or long-term clindamycin (150–300 mg daily for 1–2 months). Shorter courses of antibiotics (7–14 days) plus longer-term daily 4% chlorhexidine whole body washing and intranasal, axilla, and anogenital mupirocin or retapamulin may also cure recurrent furunculosis. Oral vancomycin (1 g twice daily for 5 days) can treat gastrointestinal carriage of *S aureus*. Family members, pets, and intimate contacts may need evaluation for staphylococcal carrier state and perhaps concomitant treatment. Stopping high-risk behavior, such as injection drug use, can also prevent recurrence of furunculosis.

B. Local Measures

Immobilize the part and avoid overmanipulation of inflamed areas. Use moist heat to help larger lesions "localize." Use surgical incision and drainage after the lesions are "mature."

Prognosis

Recurrent crops may harass the patient for months or years.

Creech CB et al. Prevention of recurrent staphylococcal skin infections. Infect Dis Clin North Am. 2015 Sep;29(3):429–64. [PMID: 26311356]

Daum RS et al; DMID 07-0051 Team. A placebo-controlled trial of antibiotics for smaller skin abscesses. N Engl J Med. 2017 Jun 29;376(26):2545–55. [PMID: 28657870]

Ibler KS et al. Recurrent furunculosis—challenges and management: a review. Clin Cosmet Investig Dermatol. 2014 Feb 18;7: 59–64. [PMID: 24591845]

Talan DA et al. Trimethoprim-sulfamethoxazole versus placebo for uncomplicated skin abscess. N Engl J Med. 2016 Mar 3; 374(9):823–32. [PMID: 26962903]

EPIDERMAL INCLUSION CYST

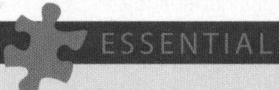

ESSENTIALS OF DIAGNOSIS

► Firm dermal papule or nodule.
► Overlying black comedone or "punctum."
► Expressible foul-smelling cheesy material.
► May become red and drain, mimicking an abscess.

General Considerations

Epidermal inclusion cysts (EICs) are common, benign growths of the upper portion of the hair follicle. They are common in Gardner syndrome and may be the first stigmata of the condition.

EICs favor the face and trunk and may complicate nodulocystic acne vulgaris. Individual lesions range in size from 0.3 cm to several centimeters. An overlying pore or punctum is characteristic. Dermoscopy can aid in observing a tiny punctum when not visible to the naked eye. Lateral pressure may lead to extrusion of a foul-smelling, cheesy material.

Differential Diagnosis

EICs are distinguished from lipomas by being more superficial (in the dermis, not the subcutaneous fat) and by their overlying punctum. Many other benign and malignant tumors may superficially resemble EICs, but all lack the punctum.

Complications

EICs may rupture, creating an acute inflammatory nodule very similar to an abscess. Cultures of the expressed material will be sterile.

Treatment

Treatment is not required if asymptomatic. Inflamed lesions may be treated with incision and drainage or intralesional triamcinolone acetomide 5–10 mg/mL. For large or symptomatic cysts, surgical excision is curative.

Mun JH et al. Importance of keen observation for the diagnosis of epidermal cysts: dermoscopy can be a useful adjuvant tool. J Am Acad Dermatol. 2014 Oct;71(4):e138–40. [PMID: 25219733]

PHOTODERMATITIS

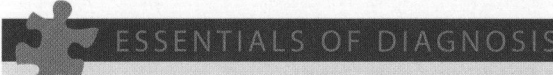

ESSENTIALS OF DIAGNOSIS

- ► Painful or pruritic erythema, edema, or vesiculation on sun-exposed surfaces (face, neck, hands, and "V" of the chest).
- ► Inner upper eyelids and area under the chin are spared.

General Considerations

Photodermatitis is a cutaneous reaction to ultraviolet radiation. Photodermatitis is classified into four groups: (1) primary photodermatoses that are immunologically mediated but are idiopathic in etiology; (2) drug- or chemical-induced photodermatoses; (3) dermatoses that are worsened or aggravated by ultraviolet exposure; and (4) genetic diseases with mutations predisposing to photodermatitis.

Primary photodermatoses include polymorphic light eruption, chronic actinic dermatitis, and actinic prurigo. Drug- or chemical-induced photodermatitis may be either exogenous or endogenous in origin. Porphyria cutanea tarda and pellagra are examples of endogenous phototoxic dermatoses. Exogenous drug- or chemical-induced photodermatitis manifests either as phototoxicity (a tendency for the individual to sunburn more easily than expected) or as photoallergy (a true immunologic reaction that presents with dermatitis). Drug-induced phototoxicity is triggered by UVA. Contact photosensitivity may occur with plants, perfumes, and sunscreens. The sunscreen oxybenzone (a benzophenone) is a common cause of photoallergic dermatitis. Dermatoses that are worsened or aggravated by ultraviolet exposure include systemic lupus erythematosus and dermatomyositis. Three percent of persons with atopic dermatitis, especially middle-aged women, are photosensitive.

Clinical Findings

A. Symptoms and Signs

The acute inflammatory phase of phototoxicity, if severe enough, is accompanied by pain, fever, gastrointestinal symptoms, malaise, and even prostration. Signs include erythema, edema, and possibly vesiculation and oozing on exposed surfaces. Peeling of the epidermis and pigmentary changes often result. The key to diagnosis is localization of the rash to photoexposed areas, though these eruptions may become generalized with time to involve even photoprotected areas. The lower lip may be affected.

B. Laboratory Findings

Blood and urine tests are generally not helpful unless porphyria cutanea tarda is suggested by the presence of blistering, scarring, milia (white cysts 1–2 mm in diameter) and skin fragility of the dorsal hands, and facial hypertrichosis. Eosinophilia may be present in chronic photoallergic responses.

Differential Diagnosis

The differential diagnosis is long. If a clear history of the use of a topical or systemic photosensitizer is not available and if the eruption is persistent, then a workup including biopsy and light testing may be required. Photodermatitis must be differentiated from contact dermatitis that may develop from one of the many substances in suntan lotions and oils, as these may often have a similar distribution. Sensitivity to actinic rays may also be part of a more serious condition, such as porphyria cutanea tarda or lupus erythematosus. These disorders are diagnosed by appropriate blood or urine tests. The most common medications causing a phototoxic reaction are tetracyclines, quinolones, and TMP-SMZ. The most common medications causing a photoallergic reaction are hydrochlorothiazide, amiodarone, and chlorpromazine. Other potent photosensitizers include quinine or quinidine, griseofulvin, NSAIDs, voriconazole, eculizumab, topical and systemic retinoids (tretinoin, isotretinoin, acitretin), and calcium channel blockers. Polymorphous light eruption (PMLE) is a very common idiopathic photodermatitis and often has its onset in the third to fourth decades, except in Native Americans and Latinos, in whom it may present in childhood. PMLE is chronic in nature. Transitory periods of spontaneous remission do occur.

Complications

Some individuals continue to be chronic light reactors even when they apparently are no longer exposed to photosensitizing medications.

Prevention

While sunscreens are useful agents in general and should be used by persons with photosensitivity, patients may react to such low amounts of energy that sunscreens alone may not be sufficient. Sunscreens with an SPF of 30–60 and broad UVA coverage, containing dicamphor sulfonic acid (Mexoryl SX), avobenzone (Parasol 1789), titanium dioxide, and micronized zinc oxide, are especially useful in patients with photoallergic dermatitis. Photosensitivity due to porphyria is not prevented by sunscreens and requires barrier protection (clothing) to prevent outbreaks.

Treatment

A. Specific Measures

Medications should be suspected in cases of photosensitivity even if the particular medication (such as hydrochlorothiazide) has been used for months.

B. Local Measures

When the eruption is vesicular or weepy, treatment is similar to that of any acute dermatitis, using cooling and soothing wet dressings.

Sunscreens should be used as described above. Mid-potency to high-potency topical corticosteroids are of limited benefit in phototoxic reactions but may help in PMLE and photoallergic reactions. Since the face is often involved, close monitoring for corticosteroid side effects is recommended.

C. Systemic Measures

Aspirin may have some value for fever and pain of acute sunburn. Systemic corticosteroids in doses as described for acute contact dermatitis may be required for severe photosensitivity reactions. Otherwise, different photodermatoses are treated in specific ways.

Patients with severe photoallergy may require immunosuppressives, such as azathioprine, in the range of 50–300 mg/day, or cyclosporine, 3–5 mg/kg/day.

Prognosis

The most common phototoxic sunburn reactions are usually benign and self-limited. PMLE and some cases of photoallergy can persist for years.

Choi D et al. Evaluation of patients with photodermatoses. Dermatol Clin. 2014 Jul;32(3):267–75. [PMID: 24891050]

Coffin SL et al. Photodermatitis for the allergist. Curr Allergy Asthma Rep. 2017 Jun;17(6):36. [PMID: 28477263]

Dawe RS et al. Drug-induced photosensitivity. Dermatol Clin. 2014 Jul;32(3):363–8. [PMID: 24891058]

Gozali MV et al. Update on treatment of photodermatosis. Dermatol Online J. 2016 Feb 17;22(2). pii: 13030/qt1rx7d228. [PMID: 27267185]

Gutierrez D et al. Photodermatoses in skin of colour. J Eur Acad Dermatol Venereol. 2018 Nov;32(11):1879–86. [PMID: 29888465]

ULCERS

LEG ULCERS SECONDARY TO VENOUS INSUFFICIENCY

ESSENTIALS OF DIAGNOSIS

▶ History of varicosities, thrombophlebitis, or postphlebitic syndrome.

▶ Irregular ulceration, often on the medial lower legs above the malleolus.

▶ Edema of the legs, varicosities, hyperpigmentation, red and scaly areas (stasis dermatitis), and scars from old ulcers support the diagnosis.

General Considerations

Patients at risk may have a history of venous insufficiency, either with obvious varicosities or with a past history of thrombophlebitis, or with immobility of the calf muscle group (paraplegics, etc) (see Chronic Venous Insufficiency, Chapter 12). The left leg is usually more severely affected than the right.

Clinical Findings

A. Symptoms and Signs

Classically, chronic edema is followed by a dermatitis, which is often pruritic. These changes are followed by hyperpigmentation, skin breakdown, and eventually sclerosis of the skin of the lower leg (Figure 6–37). Red, pruritic patches of stasis dermatitis often precede ulceration (Figure 12–2). The ulcer base may be clean, but it often has a yellow fibrin eschar that may require surgical removal. Ulcers that appear on the feet, toes, or above the knees should be approached with other diagnoses in mind.

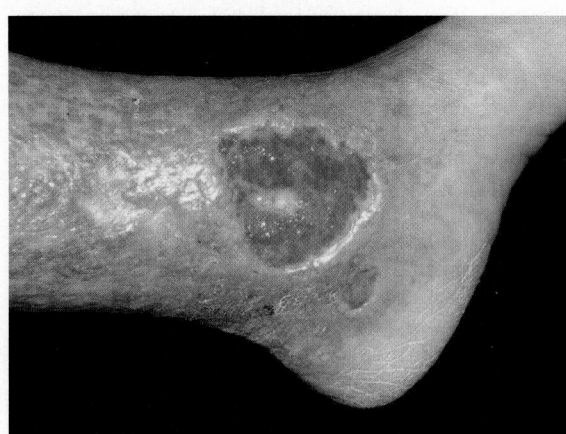

▲ **Figure 6–37.** Ulcer—venous stasis ulcer. (Used, with permission, from Richard P. Usatine, MD, in Usatine RP, Smith MA, Mayeaux EJ Jr, Chumley H. *The Color Atlas of Family Medicine*, 3rd ed. McGraw-Hill, 2018.)

B. Laboratory Findings

Because venous insufficiency plays a role in 75–90% of lower leg ulcerations, testing of venous competence is a required part of a leg ulcer evaluation even when no changes of venous insufficiency are present (see Chapter 12). Doppler examination is usually sufficient (except in the diabetic patient) to evaluate venous competence. Arterial insufficiency may coexist with venous disease. An ankle/brachial index (ABI) less than 0.7 indicates the presence of significant arterial disease and therefore requires vascular surgery consultation to address the component of arterial insufficiency.

▶ Differential Diagnosis

The differential includes vasculitis, pyoderma gangrenosum, arterial ulcerations, infection, trauma, skin cancer, arachnid bites, and sickle cell anemia. When the diagnosis is in doubt, a punch biopsy from the border (not base) of the lesion may be helpful.

▶ Prevention

Compression stockings to reduce edema are the most important means of prevention. Compression should achieve a pressure of 30 mm Hg below the knee and 40 mm Hg at the ankle. The stockings should not be used in patients with arterial insufficiency with an ABI less than 0.7. Pneumatic sequential compression devices may be of great benefit when edema is refractory to standard compression dressings.

▶ Treatment

A. Local Measures

Clean the base of the ulcer with saline or cleansers, such as Saf-Clens®. A curette or small scissors can be used to remove the yellow fibrin eschar; local anesthesia may be used if the areas are very tender.

Overall, there is little evidence to support topical antibiotics other than cadexomer iodine for the treatment of venous insufficiency ulcerations. In dermatology clinics, metronidazole gel is used to reduce bacterial growth and odor. Red dermatitic skin is treated with a medium- to high-potency corticosteroid ointment such as triamcinolone acetonide 0.1% ointment. The ulcer is then covered with an occlusive hydroactive dressing (DuoDerm® or Cutinova®) or a polyurethane foam (Allevyn) followed by an Unna zinc paste boot. This is changed weekly. The ulcer should begin to heal within weeks, and healing should be complete within 4–6 months. If the patient is diabetic, becaplermin (Regranex) may be applied to those ulcers that are not becoming smaller or developing a granulating base. Some ulcerations require grafting. Full- or split-thickness grafts often do not take, and pinch grafts (small shaves of skin laid onto the bed) may be effective. Cultured epidermal cell grafts may accelerate wound healing, but they are very expensive. They should be considered in refractory ulcers, especially those that have not healed after a year or more of conservative therapy.

No topical intervention has evidence to suggest that it will improve healing of arterial leg ulcers.

B. Systemic Therapy

Pentoxifylline, 400 mg orally three times daily administered with compression dressings, is beneficial in accelerating healing of venous insufficiency leg ulcers. Zinc supplementation is occasionally beneficial in patients with low serum zinc levels.

In the absence of cellulitis, there is no role for systemic antibiotics in the treatment of venous insufficiency ulcers. The diagnosis of cellulitis in the setting of a venous insufficiency ulcer can be very difficult. Surface cultures are of limited value. The diagnosis of cellulitis should be considered in the following settings: (1) expanding warmth and erythema surrounding the ulceration, with or without (2) increasing pain of the ulceration. The patient may also report increased exudate from the ulceration, but this without the other cardinal findings of cellulitis does not confirm the diagnosis of cellulitis. If cellulitis accompanies the ulcer, oral antibiotics are recommended: dicloxacillin, 250 mg four times a day, or levofloxacin, 500 mg once daily for 1–2 weeks, is usually adequate. Routine use of antibiotics and treating bacteria isolated from a chronic ulcer without clinical evidence of infection is discouraged. If the ulcer fails to heal or there is a persistent draining tract in the ulcer, an underlying osteomyelitis should be sought.

▶ Prognosis

The combination of limited debridement, compression dressings or stockings, and moist dressings will heal the majority of venous stasis ulcers within an average of 18 months. These modalities need to be applied at least 80% of the time to optimize ulcer healing. Topical growth factors, antibiotics, debriding agents, and xenografts and autografts can be considered in recalcitrant cases, but they are usually not required in most patients. The failure of venous insufficiency ulcerations to heal is most often related to not using the basic treatment methods consistently, rather than failure to use these specific modalities. Ongoing control of edema is essential to prevent recurrent ulceration. The use of compression stockings following ulcer healing is critical to prevent recurrence, with recurrence rates 2–20 times higher if patients do not comply with compression stocking use. If the ABI is less than 0.5, the prognosis for healing is poor. Patients with an ABI below 0.5 or refractory ulcerations (or both) should be considered for surgical procedure (artery-opening procedures or ablation of the incompetent superficial vein).

Attaran RR et al. Compression therapy for venous disease. Phlebology. 2017 Mar;32(2):81–8. [PMID: 26908640]

Couch KS et al. The international consolidated venous ulcer guideline update 2015: process improvement, evidence analysis, and future goals. Ostomy Wound Manage. 2017 May;63(5): 42–6. [PMID: 28570248]

Neumann HA et al. Evidence-based (S3) guidelines for diagnostics and treatment of venous leg ulcers. J Eur Acad Dermatol Venereol. 2016 Nov;30(11):1843–75. [PMID: 27558268]

Sundaresan S et al. Stasis dermatitis: pathophysiology, evaluation, and management. Am J Clin Dermatol. 2017 Jun;18(3): 383–90. [PMID: 28063094]

MISCELLANEOUS DERMATOLOGIC DISORDERS[1]

PIGMENTARY DISORDERS

Although the color of skin may be altered by many diseases and agents, the vast majority of patients have either an increase or decrease in pigment secondary to an inflammatory disease, such as acne or atopic dermatitis.

Other pigmentary disorders include those resulting from exposure to exogenous pigments, such as carotenemia, argyria, and tattooing. Other endogenous pigmentary disorders are attributable to metabolic substances (eg, hemosiderin [iron]) in purpuric processes, to homogentisic acid in ochronosis, and bile pigments.

► Classification

First, determine whether the disorder is hyperpigmentation or hypopigmentation, ie, an increase or decrease in normal skin colors. Each may be considered to be primary or to be secondary to other disorders. Depigmentation, the absence of all pigment, should also be differentiated from hypopigmentation, in which the affected skin is lighter than baseline skin color, but not completely devoid of pigment.

The evaluation of pigmentary disorders is helped by Wood light, which accentuates epidermal pigmentation in hyperpigmented disorders and highlights depigmentation. Depigmentation, as seen in vitiligo, enhances with Wood light examination, whereas postinflammatory hypopigmentation does not.

A. Primary Pigmentary Disorders

1. Hyperpigmentation—The disorders in this category are nevoid, congenital or acquired, and include pigmented nevi, mosaic hyperpigmentation, ephelides (juvenile freckles), and lentigines (senile freckles). Hyperpigmentation occurs also in association with Addison disease. Melasma (chloasma) occurs as patterned hyperpigmentation of the face, most commonly as a direct effect of estrogens. It may occur during pregnancy, exposure to oral contraceptives, or be idiopathic. Although more common in women, melasma affects both sexes and all races.

2. Hypopigmentation and depigmentation—The disorders in this category are vitiligo, albinism, and piebaldism. In vitiligo, pigment cells (melanocytes) are destroyed (Figure 6–38). Vitiligo, present in approximately 1% of the population, may be associated with other autoimmune disorders, such as autoimmune thyroid disease, pernicious anemia, diabetes mellitus, and Addison disease.

B. Secondary Pigmentary Disorders

Any damage to the skin (irritation, allergy, infection, excoriation, burns, or dermatologic therapy, such as chemical peels and freezing with liquid nitrogen) may result in hyperpigmentation or hypopigmentation. Several disorders of clinical importance are described below.

---

[1]Hirsutism is discussed in Chapter 26.

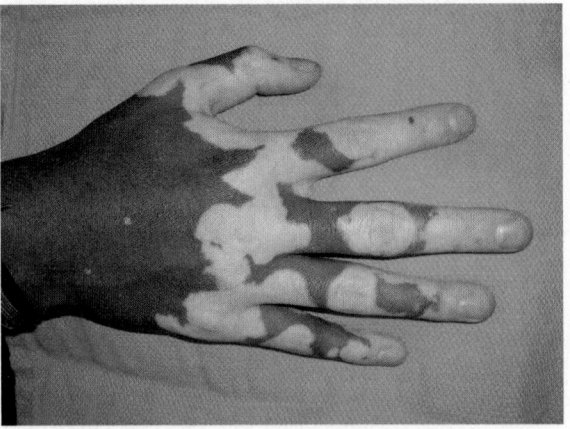

▲ **Figure 6–38.** Depigmented—vitiligo. (Used, with permission, from Richard P. Usatine, MD, in Usatine RP, Smith MA, Mayeaux EJ Jr, Chumley H. *The Color Atlas of Family Medicine*, 3rd ed. McGraw-Hill, 2018.)

1. Hyperpigmentation—The most common type of secondary hyperpigmentation occurs after another inflammatory dermatologic condition, such as acne, lichen planus, or eczema, and is most commonly seen in moderately complexioned persons (Asians, Hispanics, and light-skinned black individuals). It is called post-inflammatory hyperpigmentation. Hemosiderin deposition, as in stasis dermatitis, may lead to hyperpigmentation that is red-brown in color.

Pigmentation may be produced by certain medications, eg, chloroquine, chlorpromazine, minocycline (Figure 6–39), and amiodarone. Fixed drug eruptions to phenolphthalein (in laxatives), TMP-SMZ, NSAIDs, and tetracyclines also lead to hyperpigmentation, typically in annular patches.

2. Hypopigmentation—Hypopigmentation may complicate atopic dermatitis, lichen planus, psoriasis, discoid lupus, and lichen simplex chronicus. It may also be posttraumatic or iatrogenic or both. *Clinicians must exercise special care in using liquid nitrogen on any patient with olive or darker complexions, since doing so may result in hypopigmentation or depigmentation, at times permanent.* Intralesional or intra-articular injections of high concentrations of corticosteroids may also cause localized temporary hypopigmentation.

► Complications

Actinic keratoses and skin cancers are more likely to develop in persons with vitiligo. Severe emotional trauma may occur in extensive vitiligo and other types of hypopigmentation and hyperpigmentation, particularly in naturally dark-skinned persons.

► Treatment & Prognosis

A. Hyperpigmentation

Therapeutic bleaching preparations generally contain hydroquinone. Hydroquinone has occasionally caused unexpected hypopigmentation, hyperpigmentation, or

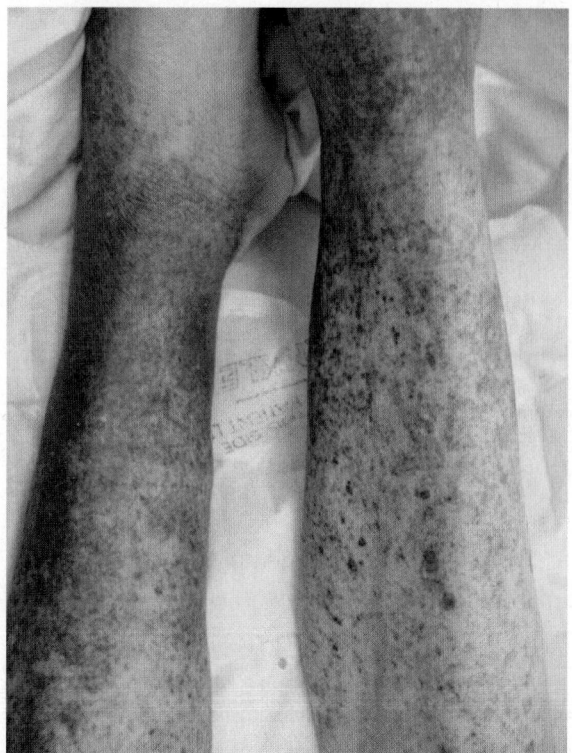

▲ **Figure 6–39.** Minocycline hyperpigmentation. (Used, with permission, from Lindy Fox, MD.)

even secondary ochronosis and pigmented milia, particularly with prolonged use.

The role of exposure to ultraviolet light cannot be overstressed as a factor promoting or contributing to most disorders of hyperpigmentation, and such exposure should be minimized. Melasma, ephelides, and postinflammatory hyperpigmentation may be treated with varying success with 4% hydroquinone and a sunscreen containing UVA photoprotectants (Avobenzone, Mexoryl, zinc oxide, titanium dioxide). Tretinoin cream, 0.025–0.05%, may be added. Adjuvant topical options for melasma include kojic acid, ascorbic acid, niacinamide, and azelaic acid. Superficial melasma responds well to topical therapy, but if there is predominantly dermal deposition of pigment (does not enhance with Wood light), the prognosis is poor. Response to therapy may take months and requires avoidance of sunlight. Hyperpigmentation often recurs after treatment if the skin is exposed to ultraviolet light. Oral tranexamic acid, 250 mg twice a day for 8–12 weeks, is an emerging treatment for melasma. Tranexamic acid should not be used in patients with hypercoagulability. Acne with postinflammatory hyperpigmentation responds well to azelaic acid and tretinoin, since both address acne and hyperpigmentation. Solar lentigines respond to liquid nitrogen application. Tretinoin 0.1% cream or tazarotene 0.1% used over 10 months can fade solar lentigines, facial hyperpigmentation, and postinflammatory hyperpigmentation. Lasers are available for the removal of epidermal and dermal pigment, and referral should be considered for patients whose responses to medical treatment are inadequate.

B. Hypopigmentation

In secondary hypopigmentation, repigmentation may occur spontaneously. Cosmetics such as Covermark and Dermablend are highly effective for concealing disfiguring patches. Therapy of vitiligo is long and tedious, and the patient must be strongly motivated. If less than 20% of the skin is involved (most cases), topical tacrolimus 0.1% twice daily is the first-line therapy. A superpotent corticosteroid may also be used, but local skin atrophy from prolonged use may ensue. With 20–25% involvement, narrowband UVB or oral PUVA is the best option. Severe phototoxic response (sunburn) may occur with PUVA. The face and upper chest respond best, and the fingertips and the genital areas do not respond as well to treatment. Years of treatment may be required. There is some emerging evidence that topical or systemic JAK inhibitors (tofactinib) may have a role in the treatment of vitiligo.

Bala HR et al. Oral tranexamic acid for the treatment of melasma: a review. Dermatol Surg. 2018 Jun;44(6):814–25. [PMID: 29677015]

Bastonini E et al. Skin pigmentation and pigmentary disorders: focus on epidermal/dermal cross-talk. Ann Dermatol. 2016 Jun; 28(3):279–89. [PMID: 27274625]

Gill L et al. Comorbid autoimmune diseases in patients with vitiligo: a cross-sectional study. J Am Acad Dermatol. 2016 Feb; 74(2):295–302. [PMID: 26518171]

Hosking AM et al. Topical Janus kinase inhibitors: a review of applications in dermatology. J Am Acad Dermatol. 2018 Sep; 79(3):535–44. [PMID: 29673776]

Kwon SH et al. Melasma: updates and perspectives. Exp Dermatol. 2018 Nov 13. [Epub ahead of print] [PMID: 30422338]

Mohammad TF et al. Practice and educational gaps in abnormal pigmentation. Dermatol Clin. 2016 Jul;34(3):291–301. [PMID: 27363886]

Ogbechie-Godec OA et al. Melasma: an up-to-date comprehensive review. Dermatol Ther (Heidelb). 2017 Sep;7(3):305–18. [PMID: 28726212]

Passeron T. Medical and maintenance treatments for vitiligo. Dermatol Clin. 2017 Apr;35(2):163–70. [PMID: 28317526]

Rodrigues M et al; Vitiligo Working Group. Current and emerging treatments for vitiligo. J Am Acad Dermatol. 2017 Jul;77(1): 17–29. [PMID: 28619557]

ALOPECIA

► Classification

Alopecias are divided into scarring and nonscarring forms. When first evaluating a patient who complains of hair loss, it is most important on physical examination to determine if follicular markings (the opening where hair exits the skin) are present or absent. Present follicular markings suggest a nonscarring alopecia; absent follicular markings suggest a scarring alopecia.

► Nonscarring Alopecia

Nonscarring alopecia may occur in association with various systemic diseases, such as SLE, secondary syphilis, hyperthyroidism or hypothyroidism, iron deficiency anemia, vitamin D deficiency, and pituitary insufficiency. The only treatment necessary is prompt and adequate control of the underlying disorder, which usually leads to regrowth of the hair.

Androgenetic alopecia, the most common form of alopecia, is of genetic predetermination. In men, the earliest changes occur at the anterior portions of the calvarium on either side of the "widow's peak" and on the crown (vertex). The extent of hair loss is variable and unpredictable. Minoxidil 5% is available over the counter and can be specifically recommended for persons with recent onset (less than 5 years) and smaller areas of alopecia. Approximately 40% of patients treated twice daily for a year will have moderate to dense growth. Finasteride (Propecia), 1 mg orally daily, has similar efficacy and may be additive to minoxidil.

Androgenetic alopecia also occurs in women. Classically, there is retention of the anterior hairline while there is diffuse thinning of the vertex scalp hair and a widening of the part. Treatment includes topical minoxidil and, in women not of childbearing potential, finasteride at doses up to 2.5 mg/day. A workup consisting of determination of serum testosterone, DHEAS, iron, total iron-binding capacity, thyroid function tests, vitamin D level, and a complete blood count will identify most other causes of hair thinning in premenopausal women. Women who complain of thin hair but show little evidence of alopecia need follow-up, because more than 50% of the scalp hair can be lost before the clinician can perceive it.

Telogen effluvium is a transitory increase in the number of hairs in the telogen (resting) phase of the hair growth cycle. This may occur spontaneously; may appear at the termination of pregnancy; may be precipitated by "crash dieting," high fever, stress from surgery, shock, or malnutrition; or may be provoked by hormonal contraceptives. Whatever the cause, telogen effluvium usually has a latent period of 4 months. The prognosis is generally good. The condition is diagnosed by the presence of large numbers of hairs with white bulbs coming out upon gentle tugging of the hair. Counts of hairs lost by the patient on combing or shampooing often exceed 150 per day, compared to an average of 70–100. In one study, a major cause of telogen effluvium was found to be iron deficiency, and the hair counts bore a clear relationship to serum iron levels. If iron deficiency is suspected, a serum ferritin should be obtained, and any value less than 40 ng/mL followed with supplementation.

Alopecia areata is of unknown cause but is believed to be an immunologic process. Typically, there are patches that are perfectly smooth and without scarring. Tiny hairs 2–3 mm in length, called "exclamation hairs," may be seen. Telogen hairs are easily dislodged from the periphery of active lesions. The beard, brows, and lashes may be involved. Involvement may extend to all of the scalp hair (**alopecia totalis**) or to all scalp and body hair (**alopecia universalis**). Severe forms may be treated by systemic corticosteroid therapy, although recurrences follow discontinuation of therapy. Alopecia areata is occasionally associated with autoimmune disorders, including Hashimoto thyroiditis, pernicious anemia, Addison disease, and vitiligo. Additional comorbidities may include SLE, atopy, and mental health disease.

Intralesional corticosteroids are frequently effective for alopecia areata. Triamcinolone acetonide in a concentration of 2.5–10 mg/mL is injected in aliquots of 0.1 mL at approximately 1- to 2-cm intervals, not exceeding a total dose of 30 mg per month for adults. Alopecia areata is usually self-limiting, with complete regrowth of hair in 80% of patients with focal disease. Some mild cases are resistant to treatment, as are the extensive totalis and universalis types. Support groups for patients with extensive alopecia areata are very beneficial. Oral JAK inhibitors (ruxolitinib, tofacitinib) are therapeutic options for patients with highly morbid disease, although relapse is the rule once the medication has been stopped.

In **trichotillomania** (the pulling out of one's own hair), the patches of hair loss are irregular, with short, growing hairs almost always present, since they cannot be pulled out until they are long enough. The patches are often unilateral, occurring on the same side as the patient's dominant hand. The patient may be unaware of the habit. N-acetylcysteine (1200–2400 mg orally per day for 12 weeks) may be effective.

▶ Scarring (Cicatricial) Alopecia

Cicatricial alopecia may occur following any type of trauma or inflammation that may scar hair follicles. Examples include chemical or physical trauma, lichen planopilaris, bacterial or fungal infections, severe herpes zoster, chronic discoid lupus erythematosus (DLE), scleroderma, and excessive ionizing radiation. The specific cause is often suggested by the history, the distribution of hair loss, and the appearance of the skin, as in DLE. Biopsy is useful in the diagnosis of scarring alopecia, but specimens must be taken from the active border and not from the scarred central zone. Scarring alopecias are irreversible and permanent. It is important to diagnose and treat the scarring process as early in its course as possible.

Adil A et al. The effectiveness of treatments for androgenetic alopecia: a systematic review and meta-analysis. J Am Acad Dermatol. 2017 Jul;77(1):136–41.e5. [PMID: 28396101]

Bolduc C et al. Primary cicatricial alopecia: lymphocytic primary cicatricial alopecias, including chronic cutaneous lupus erythematosus, lichen planopilaris, frontal fibrosing alopecia, and Graham-Little syndrome. J Am Acad Dermatol. 2016 Dec; 75(6):1081–99. [PMID: 27846944]

Jones G et al. Assessment and treatment of trichotillomania (hair pulling disorder) and excoriation (skin picking) disorder. Clin Dermatol. 2018 Nov–Dec;36(6):728–36. [PMID: 30446196]

Kennedy Crispin M et al. Safety and efficacy of the JAK inhibitor tofacitinib citrate in patients with alopecia areata. JCI Insight. 2016 Sep 22;1(15):e89776. [PMID: 27699252]

Lee S et al. Management of alopecia areata: updates and algorithmic approach. J Dermatol. 2017 Nov;44(11):1199–211. [PMID: 28635045]

Mackay-Wiggan J et al. Oral ruxolitinib induces hair regrowth in patients with moderate-to-severe alopecia areata. JCI Insight. 2016 Sep 22;1(15):e89790. [PMID: 27699253]

Pratt CH et al. Alopecia areata. Nat Rev Dis Primers. 2017 Mar 16; 3:17011. [PMID: 28300084]

Strazzulla LC et al. Alopecia areata: disease characteristics, clinical evaluation, and new perspectives on pathogenesis. J Am Acad Dermatol. 2018 Jan;78(1):1–12. [PMID: 29241771]

van Zuuren EJ et al. Interventions for female pattern hair loss. Cochrane Database Syst Rev. 2016 May 26;(5):CD007628. [PMID: 27225981]

NAIL DISORDERS

1. Morphologic Abnormalities of the Nails

▶ Classification

Acquired nail disorders may be classified as local or those associated with systemic or generalized skin diseases.

A. Local Nail Disorders

1. Onycholysis (distal separation of the nail plate from the nail bed, usually of the fingers) is caused by excessive exposure to water, soaps, detergents, alkalies, and industrial cleaning agents. Candidal infection of the nail folds and subungual area, nail hardeners, drug-induced photosensitivity, hyperthyroidism, hypothyroidism, and psoriasis may cause onycholysis.

2. Distortion of the nail, including nail splitting, occurs as a result of chronic inflammation or infiltration of the nail matrix underlying the eponychial fold. Such changes may be caused by impingement on the nail matrix by inflammatory diseases (eg, psoriasis, lichen planus, eczema), warts, tumors, or cysts.

3. Discoloration and crumbly thickened nails are noted in dermatophyte infection and psoriasis.

4. Allergic reactions (to resins in undercoats and polishes or to nail glues) are characterized by onycholysis or by grossly distorted, hypertrophic, and misshapen nails.

5. Paronychia is inflammation of the lateral or proximal nail folds. It is divided into acute or chronic forms. Acute paronychia presents as a painful erythematous papulonodule or frank abscess of the nail fold and is most commonly due to infection with *S aureus* (Figure 6–40). Chronic paronychia is most often caused by irritation from water or chemicals with resultant inflammation and possible *Candida* superinfection.

B. Nail Changes Associated with Systemic or Generalized Skin Diseases

1. Beau lines (transverse furrows) affect all nails and classically develop after a serious systemic illness.

2. Atrophy of the nails may be related to trauma or to vascular or neurologic disease.

3. Clubbed fingers may be due to the prolonged hypoxemia associated with cardiopulmonary disorders (Figure 6–41) (See Chapter 9).

4. Spoon nails may be seen in anemic patients.

5. Stippling or pitting of the nails is seen in psoriasis, alopecia areata, and hand eczema.

6. Nail hyperpigmentation may be caused by many chemotherapeutic agents, but especially the taxanes.

▶ Differential Diagnosis

Onychomycosis may cause nail changes identical to those seen in psoriasis. Careful examination for more characteristic lesions elsewhere on the body is essential to the diagnosis of the nail disorders. Cancer should be suspected (eg, Bowen disease or squamous cell carcinoma) as the cause of any persistent solitary subungual or periungual lesion.

▶ Complications

Toenail changes may lead to an ingrown nail—in turn often complicated by bacterial infection and occasionally by exuberant granulation tissue. Poor manicuring and

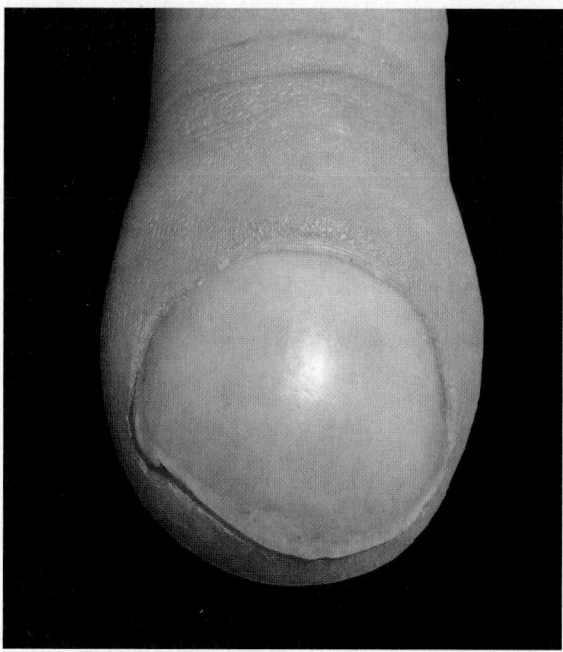

▲ **Figure 6–41.** Clubbing of the finger in a 31-year-old man with congenital heart disease. Note the thickening around the proximal nail folds. (Used, with permission, from Richard P. Usatine, MD, in Usatine RP, Smith MA, Mayeaux EJ Jr, Chumley H. *The Color Atlas of Family Medicine*, 3rd ed. McGraw-Hill, 2018.)

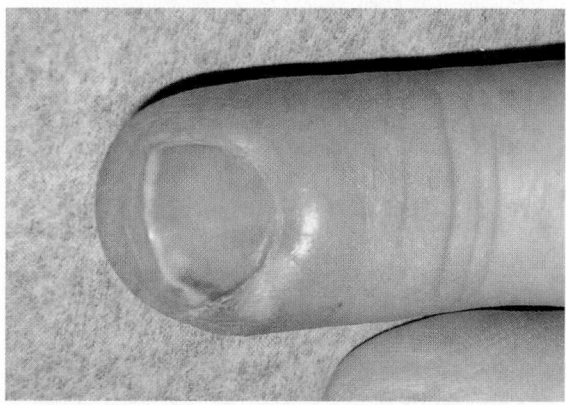

▲ **Figure 6–40.** Acute paronychia. (Used, with permission, from E.J. Mayeaux Jr, MD, in Usatine RP, Smith MA, Mayeaux EJ Jr, Chumley H. *The Color Atlas of Family Medicine*, 2nd ed. McGraw-Hill, 2013.)

poorly fitting shoes may contribute to this complication. Cellulitis may result.

▶ Treatment & Prognosis

Treatment consists usually of careful debridement and manicuring and, above all, reduction of exposure to irritants (soaps, detergents, alkali, bleaches, solvents, etc). Longitudinal grooving due to temporary lesions of the matrix, such as warts, synovial cysts, and other impingements, may be cured by removal of the offending lesion.

Acute paronychia is treated with topical antibiotics and drainage of the abscess, if present. To incise and drain an acute staphylococcal paronychia, insert a flat metal spatula or sharpened hardwood stick into the nail fold where it adjoins the nail. This will release pus from a mature lesion.

Treatment of chronic paronychia includes minimizing wetwork and toxic contactants, wearing gloves while performing tasks that expose the skin to water, minimizing trauma to the nailfolds, and a combination of topical corticosteroids and an anticandidal twice daily to the affected area.

2. Tinea Unguium (Onychomycosis)

Tinea unguium is a trichophyton infection of one or more (but rarely all) fingernails or toenails. The species most commonly found is *T rubrum*. "Saprophytic" fungi may rarely cause onychomycosis (less than 5% of cases). Evidence supporting a genetic defect in the innate and adaptive immune system may explain why some people suffer from chronic tinea pedis and onychomycosis.

The nails are lusterless, brittle, and hypertrophic, and the substance of the nail is friable. Laboratory diagnosis is mandatory since only 50% of dystrophic nails are due to dermatophytosis. Portions of the nail should be clipped, digested with 10% KOH, and examined under the microscope for hyphae. Fungi may also be cultured from debris collected from underneath the nail plate. Periodic acid-Schiff stain of a histologic section of the nail plate will also demonstrate the fungus readily. Each technique is positive in only 50% of cases so several different tests may need to be performed. Periodic acid-Schiff staining of nail plate coupled with fungal culture has a sensitivity of 96%.

Onychomycosis is difficult to treat because of the long duration of therapy required and the frequency of recurrences. Fingernails respond more readily than toenails. For toenails, treatment is indicated for patients with discomfort, inability to exercise, diabetes, and immune compromise.

In general, systemic therapy is required to effectively treat nail onychomycosis. Although historically topical therapy has had limited value, efinaconazole 10% has been approved as a topical therapy; evidence suggests that it performs better than prior topical treatment options. Tavaborole 5% solution is also approved for the treatment of onychomycosis, but its clearance rates do not appear to be as good as those of efinaconazole. Adjunctive value of surgical procedures is unproven, and the efficacy of laser treatments is lacking, especially with regard to long-term cures.

Fingernails can virtually always be cured, and toenails are cured 35–50% of the time and are clinically improved about 75% of the time. In all cases, before treatment, the diagnosis should be confirmed. The costs of the various treatment options should be known and the most cost-effective treatment chosen. Medication interactions must be avoided. Ketoconazole, due to its higher risk for hepatotoxicity, is not recommended to treat any form of onychomycosis. For fingernails, ultramicronized griseofulvin 250 mg orally three times daily for 6 months can be effective. Alternative treatments are (in order of preference) oral terbinafine 250 mg daily for 6 weeks, oral itraconazole 400 mg daily for 7 days each month for 2 months, and oral itraconazole 200 mg daily for 2 months. Off-label use of fluconazole, 400 mg once weekly for 6 months, can also be effective, but there is limited evidence for this option. Once clear, fingernails usually remain free of disease for some years.

Onychomycosis of the toenails does not respond to griseofulvin therapy. The best treatment, which is also FDA approved, is oral terbinafine 250 mg daily for 12 weeks. Liver biochemical tests and a complete blood count with platelets are performed 4–6 weeks after starting treatment, although because the risk of idiosyncratic injury is very low (transaminitis occurs in less than 0.5% of patients) and the presentation of drug-induced liver injury is usually symptomatic (jaundice, malaise, abdominal pain), routine monitoring is falling out of favor. Pulse oral itraconazole 200 mg twice daily for 1 week per month for 3 months is inferior to standard terbinafine treatments, but it is an acceptable alternative for those unable to take terbinafine. The courses of terbinafine or itraconazole may need to be repeated 6 months after the first treatment cycle if fungal cultures of the nail are still positive.

Elewski BE et al. Topical treatment for onychomycosis: is it more effective than the clinical data suggests? J Clin Aesthet Dermatol. 2016 Nov;9(11):34–9. [PMID: 28210388]

Ghannoum M et al. Examining the importance of laboratory and diagnostic testing when treating and diagnosing onychomycosis. Int J Dermatol. 2018 Feb;57(2):131–8. [PMID: 28653769]

Iorizzo M. Tips to treat the 5 most common nail disorders: brittle nails, onycholysis, paronychia, psoriasis, onychomycosis. Dermatol Clin. 2015 Apr;33(2):175–83. [PMID: 25828710]

Kramer ON et al. Clinical presentation of terbinafine-induced severe liver injury and the value of laboratory monitoring: a critically appraised topic. Br J Dermatol. 2017 Nov; 177(5):1279–84. [PMID: 28762471]

Kreijkamp-Kaspers S et al. Oral antifungal medication for toenail onychomycosis. Cochrane Database Syst Rev. 2017 Jul 14; 7:CD010031. [PMID: 28707751]

Leggit JC. Acute and chronic paronychia. Am Fam Physician. 2017 Jul 1;96(1):44–51. [PMID: 28671378]

DRUG ERUPTION (Dermatitis Medicamentosa)

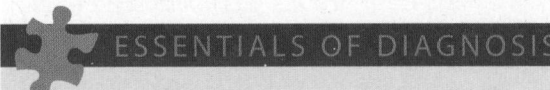

ESSENTIALS OF DIAGNOSIS

► Usually, abrupt onset of widespread, symmetric erythematous eruption.

► May mimic any inflammatory skin condition.

► Constitutional symptoms (malaise, arthralgia, headache, and fever) may be present.

General Considerations

Rashes are among the most common adverse reactions to medications and occur in 2–3% of hospitalized patients. There are multiple different types of cutaneous reactions to medications. Penicillin and other beta-lactam antibiotics and TMP-SMZ are the most common causes of urticarial and maculopapular reactions. Drug-induced hypersensitivity reaction (DIHS) (also known as drug eruption with eosinophilia and systemic symptoms [DRESS]) is most often caused by anticonvulsants, allopurinol, and sulfonamides. SJS and TEN most commonly occur in response to antibiotics, sulfonamides, anticonvulsants, allopurinol, and NSAIDs. Phenolphthalein, pyrazolone derivatives, tetracyclines, NSAIDs, TMP-SMZ, and barbiturates are the major causes of fixed drug eruptions. Calcium channel blockers are a common cause of pruritus and eczemas in older adults.

Certain genetic polymorphisms of antigen-presenting major histocompatibility (MHC) loci increase the risk for the development of severe drug eruptions, including SJS/TEN and DIHS. Pharmacogenetic testing is increasingly utilized to predict who is at risk for and therefore should avoid certain medication exposures. For example, in Han Chinese, HLA typing is indicated before institution of carbamazepine treatment.

Clinical Findings

A. Symptoms and Signs

Drug eruptions are generally classified as "simple" or "complex," referring to the risk of morbidity and mortality associated with the specific eruption. Simple drug eruptions involve an exanthem, usually appear in the second week of medication therapy, and have no associated constitutional symptoms or abnormal laboratory findings. Antibiotics, including the penicillins and quinolones, are the most common causes. Complex drug eruptions include DIHS and SJS/TEN.

DIHS occurs later than the simple morbilliform drug eruptions with signs and symptoms developing 2–6 weeks after the medication has been started and has associated constitutional symptoms and abnormal laboratory findings. These may include fevers, chills, hematologic abnormalities (especially eosinophilia and atypical lymphocystosis), and abnormal liver or kidney function. Coexistent reactivation of certain viruses, especially HHV-6, but also Epstein-Barr virus, cytomegalovirus, HHV-7, and parvovirus B19, may be present and may be important in the pathogenesis of these complex drug eruptions. Table 6–3 summarizes the types of skin reactions, their appearance and distribution, and the common offenders in each case.

Table 6–3. Skin reactions due to systemic medications.

Reaction	Appearance	Distribution and Comments	Common Offenders
Allergic vasculitis	The primary lesion is typically a 2–3 mm purpuric papule. Other morphologies include urticaria that lasts over 24 hours, vesicles, bullae, or necrotic ulcers.	Most severe on the legs.	Sulfonamides, phenytoin, propylthiouracil.
Drug exanthem	Morbilliform, maculopapular, exanthematous reactions.	The most common skin reaction to medications. Initially begins on trunk 7–10 days after the medication has been started. Spreads to extremities and begins to clear on the trunk over 3–5 days. In previously exposed patients, the rash may start in 2–3 days. Fever may be present.	Antibiotics (especially ampicillin and TMP-SMZ), sulfonamides and related compounds (including thiazide diuretics, furosemide, and sulfonylurea hypoglycemic agents), and barbiturates.
Drug-related subacute cutaneous lupus erythematosus (Drug-induced SLE rarely produces a skin reaction)	May present with a photosensitive rash, annular lesions, or psoriasis on upper trunk.	Less severe than SLE, sparing the kidneys and central nervous system. Recovery often follows medication withdrawal.	Diltiazem, etanercept, hydrochlorothiazide, infliximab, lisinopril, terbinafine.
Erythema nodosum	Inflammatory cutaneous nodules.	Usually limited to the extensor aspects of the legs. May be accompanied by fever, arthralgias, and pain.	Oral contraceptives.
Exfoliative dermatitis and erythroderma (Drug-induced hypersensitivity syndrome)	Red and scaly.	Entire skin surface. Typically associated with elevated liver biochemical tests, eosinophilia, and acute kidney injury. Eruption begins between 2 and 6 weeks after first dose of medication.	Allopurinol, sulfonamides, isoniazid, anticonvulsants, or carbamazepine.

(continued)

Table 6–3. Skin reactions due to systemic medications. (continued)

Reaction	Appearance	Distribution and Comments	Common Offenders
Fixed drug eruptions	Single or multiple demarcated, round, erythematous plaques that often become hyperpigmented.	Recur at the same site when the medication is repeated. Hyperpigmentation, if present, remains after healing.	Antimicrobials, analgesics (acetaminophen, ibuprofen, and naproxen), barbiturates, cardiovascular drugs, heavy metals, antiparasitic agents, antihistamines, phenolphthalein.
Lichenoid and lichen planus–like eruptions	Pruritic, erythematous to violaceous polygonal papules that coalesce or expand to form plaques.	May be in photo- or nonphotodistributed pattern.	Carbamazepine, furosemide, hydroxychloroquine, phenothiazines, beta-blockers, quinidine, quinine, sulfonylureas, tetracyclines, thiazides, and triprolidine.
Photosensitivity: increased sensitivity to light, often of ultraviolet A wavelengths, but may be due to UVB or visible light as well	Sunburn, vesicles, papules in photodistributed pattern.	Exposed skin of the face, the neck, and the backs of the hands and, in women, the lower legs. Exaggerated response to ultraviolet light.	Sulfonamides and sulfonamide-related compounds (thiazide diuretics, furosemide, sulfonylureas), tetracyclines, phenothiazines, sulindac, amiodarone, voriconazole, and NSAIDs.
Pigmentary changes	Flat hyperpigmented areas.	Forehead and cheeks (chloasma, melasma). The most common pigmentary disorder associated with drug ingestion. Improvement is slow despite stopping the medication.	Oral contraceptives are the usual cause. Diltiazem causes facial hyperpigmentation that may be difficult to distinguish from melasma.
	Blue-gray discoloration.	Light-exposed areas.	Chlorpromazine and related phenothiazines.
	Brown or blue-gray pigmentation.	Generalized.	Heavy metals (silver, gold, bismuth, and arsenic).
	Yellow color.	Generalized.	Quinacrine.
	Blue-black patches on the shins.		Minocycline, chloroquine.
	Blue-black pigmentation of the nails and palate and depigmentation of the hair.		Chloroquine.
	Slate-gray color.	Primarily in photoexposed areas.	Amiodarone.
	Brown discoloration of the nails.	Especially in more darkly pigmented patients.	Hydroxyurea.
Pityriasis rosea–like eruptions	Oval, red, slightly raised patches with central scale.	Mainly on the trunk.	Barbiturates, bismuth, captopril, clonidine, methopromazine, metoprolol, metronidazole, and tripelennamine.
Psoriasiform eruptions	Scaly red plaques.	May be located on trunk and extremities. Palms and soles may be hyperkeratotic. May cause psoriasiform eruption or worsen psoriasis.	Antimalarials, lithium, beta-blockers, and TNF inhibitors.
SJS/TEN	Target-like lesions. Bullae may occur. Mucosal involvement.	Usually trunk and proximal extremities.	Sulfonamides, anticonvulsants, allopurinol, NSAIDs, lamotrigine.
Urticaria	Red, itchy wheals that vary in size from less than 1 cm to many centimeters. May be accompanied by angioedema.	Chronic urticaria is rarely caused by medications.	Acute urticaria: penicillins, NSAIDs, sulfonamides, opioids, and salicylates. Angioedema is common in patients receiving ACE inhibitors and angiotensin receptor blockers.

ACE, angiotensin-converting enzyme; NSAIDs, nonsteroidal anti-inflammatory drugs; SJS/TEN, Stevens-Johnson syndrome/toxic epidermal necrolysis; SLE, systemic lupus erythematosus; TMP-SMZ, trimethoprim-sulfamethoxazole; TNF, tumor necrosis factor.

B. Laboratory Findings

Routinely ordered blood work is of no value in the diagnosis of simple drug eruptions, except upon initial evaluation to ensure that there is no systemic involvement. In complex drug eruptions, the complete blood count, liver biochemical tests, and kidney function tests should be monitored. Skin biopsies may be helpful in making the diagnosis. Serum PCR for HHV-6, HHV-7, Epstein-Barr virus, cytomegalovirus, and parvovirus B19 is performed in some centers.

► Differential Diagnosis

Observation after discontinuation, which may be a slow process, helps establish the diagnosis. Rechallenge, though of theoretical value, may pose a danger to the patient and is best avoided.

► Complications

Some cutaneous drug reactions may be associated with visceral involvement. The organ systems involved depend on the individual medication or drug class. Most common is an infectious mononucleosis-like illness and hepatitis associated with administration of anticonvulsants. Myocarditis may be a serious complication of drug-induced hypersensitivity syndrome and may present acutely or months after initial rash onset. Months after recovering from DIHS, patients may suffer hypothyroidism.

► Treatment

A. General Measures

Systemic manifestations are treated as they arise (eg, anemia, icterus, purpura). Antihistamines may be of value in urticarial and angioneurotic reactions. Epinephrine 1:1000, 0.5–1 mL intravenously or subcutaneously, should be used as an emergency measure. In DIHS, corticosteroids are typically required, most commonly oral prednisone at a dose of 1–1.5 mg/kg/day and tapering very slowly over a minimum of 6 weeks, since rapid taper leads to rebound and more recalcitrant disease. In the case of allopurinol-induced DIHS, starting a steroid-sparing agent (eg, mycophenolate mofetil) at the time of prednisone initiation is recommended because allopurinol-induced DIHS tends to rebound after corticosteroid discontinuation. Treatment in this special case often takes up to 12 months.

B. Local Measures

SJS/TEN with extensive blistering eruptions resulting in erosions and superficial ulcerations demands hospitalization and nursing care as for burn patients. See Erythema Multiforme/Stevens-Johnson Syndrome/Toxic Epidermal Necrolysis, above.

► Prognosis

Drug rash usually disappears upon withdrawal of the medication and proper treatment. DIHS may be associated with autoimmune phenomena, including abnormal thyroid function. This can occur months after the hypersensitivity syndrome has resolved.

Cheng CY et al. HLA associations and clinical implications in T-cell mediated drug hypersensitivity reactions: an updated review. J Immunol Res. 2014;4:565320. [PMID: 24901010]

Chung WH et al. Severe cutaneous adverse drug reactions. J Dermatol. 2016 Jul;43(7):758–66. [PMID: 27154258]

Duong TA et al. Severe cutaneous adverse reactions to drugs. Lancet. 2017 Oct 28;390(10106):1996–2011. [PMID: 28476287]

Gerogianni K et al. Drug-induced skin adverse reactions: the role of pharmacogenomics in their prevention. Mol Diagn Ther. 2018 Jun;22(3):297–314. [PMID: 29564734]

Mockenhaupt M. Epidemiology of cutaneous adverse drug reactions. Allergol Select. 2017 Aug 4;1(1):96–108. [PMID: 30402608]

Wolverton SE. Practice gaps: drug reactions. Dermatol Clin. 2016 Jul;34(3):311–8. [PMID: 27363888]

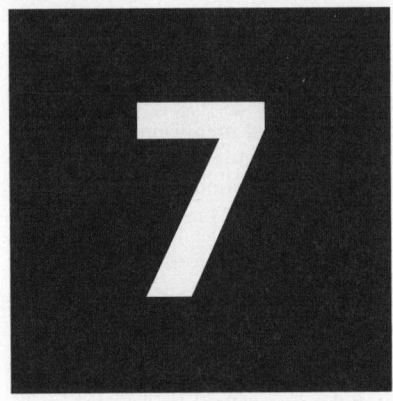

7

Disorders of the Eyes & Lids

Jacque L. Duncan, MD

Neeti B. Parikh, MD

Gerami D. Seitzman, MD

Paul Riordan-Eva, FRCOphth

REFRACTIVE ERRORS

Refractive error is the most common cause of reduced clarity of vision (visual acuity) and may be a readily treatable component of poor vision in patients with other diagnoses.

Use of a pinhole will overcome most refractive errors and thus allows their identification as a cause of reduced visual acuity. Refractive error can be treated with glasses, contact lenses, or surgery.

► Treatment

A. Contact Lenses

An estimated 40.9 million US adults wear contact lenses, mostly for correction of refractive errors, though decorative-colored contact lenses are increasingly being used.

The major risk from contact lens wear is corneal infection, potentially a blinding condition. Such infections occur more often with soft lenses, particularly extended wear, for which there is at least a fivefold increase in risk of corneal infection compared with daily wear. Decorative contact lenses have a high prevalence of microbial contamination. Contact lens wearers should be made aware of the risks they face and ways to minimize them, such as avoiding overnight wear or use of lenses past their replacement date and maintaining meticulous lens hygiene, including not using tap water or saliva for lens cleaning. Contact lenses should be removed whenever there is ocular discomfort or redness.

Cope JR et al. Risk behaviors for contact lens-related eye infections among adults and adolescents—United States, 2016. MMWR Morb Mortal Wkly Rep. 2017 Aug 18;66(32):841–5. [PMID: 28817556]

Razmaria AA. JAMA patient page. Proper care of contact lenses. JAMA. 2015 Oct 13;314(14):1534. [PMID: 26462011]

B. Surgery

Various surgical techniques are available to reduce refractive errors, particularly nearsightedness. Laser corneal refractive surgery reshapes the middle layer (stroma) of the cornea with an excimer laser. Other refractive surgery techniques are extraction of the clear crystalline lens with insertion of a single vision, multifocal, or accommodative intraocular lens; insertion of an intraocular lens without removal of the crystalline lens (phakic intraocular lens); intrastromal corneal ring segments (INTACS); collagen cross-linking; laser thermal keratoplasty; and conductive keratoplasty (CK).

Wilkinson JM et al. Refractive eye surgery: helping patients make informed decisions about LASIK. Am Fam Physician. 2017 May 15;95(10):637–44. [PMID: 28671403]

C. Reduction of Rate of Progression of Nearsightedness

Topical atropine and pirenzepine, a selective muscarinic antagonist; rigid contact lens wear during sleep (orthokeratology); and various types of soft contact lenses and spectacles reduce the rate of progression of nearsightedness, but their long-term efficacy and safety are uncertain.

► When to Refer

Any contact lens wearer with an acute painful red eye must be referred emergently for ophthalmologic evaluation.

DISORDERS OF THE LIDS & LACRIMAL APPARATUS

1. Hordeolum

Hordeolum is an acute infection that is commonly due to *Staphylococcus aureus*. It is characterized by a localized red, swollen, acutely tender area on the upper or lower lid. Internal hordeolum is a meibomian gland abscess that usually points onto the conjunctival surface of the lid; external hordeolum, or stye, is usually smaller and on the lid margin and is an abscess of the gland of Zeis.

Warm compresses are helpful. Incision may be indicated if resolution does not begin within 48 hours. An antibiotic ointment (bacitracin or erythromycin) applied to the lid every 3 hours may be beneficial during the acute stage. Internal hordeolum may lead to generalized cellulitis of the lid.

Willmann D et al. Stye. StatPearls [Internet]. Treasure Island (FL): StatPearls Publishing; 2017 Oct 13. [PMID: 29083787]

2. Chalazion

Chalazion is a common granulomatous inflammation of a meibomian gland that may follow an internal hordeolum. It is characterized by a hard, nontender swelling on the upper or lower lid with redness and swelling of the adjacent conjunctiva. Initial treatment is with warm compresses. If resolution has not occurred by 2–3 weeks, incision and curettage is indicated. Corticosteroid injection may also be effective.

3. Blepharitis

Blepharitis is a common chronic bilateral inflammatory condition of the lid margins. **Anterior blepharitis** involves the lid skin, eyelashes, and associated glands. It may be ulcerative, because of infection by staphylococci, or seborrheic in association with seborrhea of the scalp, brows, and ears. **Posterior blepharitis** results from inflammation of the meibomian glands. There may be bacterial infection, particularly with staphylococci, or primary glandular dysfunction, in which there is a strong association with acne rosacea.

▶ Clinical Findings

Symptoms are irritation, burning, and itching. In **anterior blepharitis,** the eyes are "red-rimmed" and scales or collerettes can be seen clinging to the lashes. In **posterior blepharitis,** the lid margins are hyperemic with telangiectasias, and the meibomian glands and their orifices are inflamed. The lid margin is frequently rolled inward to produce a mild entropion, and the tear film may be frothy or abnormally greasy.

Blepharitis is a common cause of recurrent conjunctivitis. Both anterior and, more particularly, posterior blepharitis may be complicated by hordeola or chalazia; abnormal lid or lash positions, producing trichiasis; epithelial keratitis of the lower third of the cornea; marginal corneal infiltrates; and inferior corneal vascularization and thinning.

▶ Treatment

Anterior blepharitis is usually controlled by eyelid hygiene. Warm compresses help soften the scales and warm the meibomian gland secretions. Eyelid cleansing can be achieved by gentle eyelid massage and lid scrubs with baby shampoo or 0.01% hypochlorous acid. In acute exacerbations, an antibiotic eye ointment, such as bacitracin or erythromycin, is applied daily to the lid margins.

In mild **posterior blepharitis**, regular meibomian gland expression and warm compresses may be sufficient to control symptoms. Inflammation of the conjunctiva and cornea indicates a need for more active treatment, including long-term low-dose oral antibiotic therapy, usually with tetracycline (250 mg twice daily), doxycycline (100 mg daily), minocycline (50–100 mg daily), erythromycin (250 mg three times daily), or azithromycin (500 mg daily for 3 days in three cycles with 7-day intervals). Short-term topical corticosteroids, eg, prednisolone, 0.125% twice daily, may also be indicated. Topical therapy with antibiotics, such as ciprofloxacin 0.3% ophthalmic solution twice daily, may be helpful but should be restricted to short courses.

Amescua G et al; American Academy of Ophthalmology Preferred Practice Pattern Cornea and External Disease Panel. Blepharitis Preferred Practice Pattern®. Ophthalmology. 2019 Jan;126(1):P56–P93. [PMID: 30366800]
Eberhardt M et al. Blepharitis. StatPearls [Internet]. Treasure Island (FL): StatPearls Publishing; 2017 Oct 17. [PMID: 29083763] http://www.ncbi.nlm.nih.gov/books/NBK459305/

4. Entropion & Ectropion

Entropion (inward turning of usually the lower lid) occurs occasionally in older people as a result of degeneration of the lid fascia, or may follow extensive scarring of the conjunctiva and tarsus. Surgery is indicated if the lashes rub on the cornea. Botulinum toxin injections may also be used for temporary correction of the involutional lower lid entropion of older people.

Ectropion (outward turning of the lower lid) is common with advanced age. Surgery is indicated if there is excessive tearing, exposure keratitis, or a cosmetic problem.

Hahn S et al. Lower lid malposition: causes and correction. Facial Plast Surg Clin North Am. 2016 May;24(2):163–71. [PMID: 27105802]

5. Tumors

Lid tumors are usually benign. Basal cell carcinoma is the most common malignant tumor. Squamous cell carcinoma, meibomian gland carcinoma, and malignant melanoma also occur. Surgery for any lesion involving the lid margin should be performed by an ophthalmologist or suitably trained plastic surgeon to avoid deformity of the lid. Histopathologic examination of eyelid tumors should be routine, since 2% of lesions thought to be benign clinically are found to be malignant. The Mohs technique of intraoperative examination of excised tissue is particularly valuable in ensuring complete excision so that the risk of recurrence is reduced. Medications such as vismodegib (an oral inhibitor of the hedgehog pathway), imiquimod (an immunomodulator), and 5-fluorouracil occasionally are used instead of or as an adjunct to surgery.

Silverman N et al. What's new in eyelid tumors. Asia Pac J Ophthalmol (Phila). 2017 Mar–Apr;6(2):143–52. [PMID: 28399340]

6. Dacryocystitis

Dacryocystitis is infection of the lacrimal sac usually due to congenital or acquired obstruction of the nasolacrimal system. It may be acute or chronic and occurs most often in infants and in persons over 40 years. It is usually unilateral. The usual infectious organisms are *S aureus* and streptococci in acute dacryocystitis and *Staphylococcus epidermidis*, streptococci, or gram-negative bacilli in chronic dacryocystitis.

Acute dacryocystitis is characterized by pain, swelling, tenderness, and redness in the tear sac area; purulent material may be expressed. In chronic dacryocystitis, tearing and discharge are the principal signs, and mucus or pus may also be expressed.

Acute dacryocystitis responds well to systemic antibiotic therapy. To relieve the underlying obstruction, surgery is usually done electively but may be performed urgently in acute cases. The chronic form may be kept latent with antibiotics, but relief of the obstruction is the only cure. In adults, the standard procedure is dacryocystorhinostomy, which involves surgical exploration of the lacrimal sac and formation of a fistula into the nasal cavity and, if necessary, supplemented by nasolacrimal intubation. Congenital nasolacrimal duct obstruction is common and often resolves spontaneously. It can be treated by probing the nasolacrimal system, supplemented by nasolacrimal intubation or balloon catheter dilation, if necessary. Dacryocystorhinostomy is rarely required.

CONJUNCTIVITIS

Conjunctivitis is inflammation of the mucous membrane that lines the surface of the eyeball and inner eyelids. It may be acute or chronic. Most cases are due to viral or bacterial (including gonococcal and chlamydial) infection. Other causes include keratoconjunctivitis sicca, allergy, chemical irritants, and trauma. The mode of transmission of infectious conjunctivitis is usually via direct contact of contaminated fingers or objects to the fellow eye or to other persons. It may also be spread through respiratory secretions or contaminated eye drops.

Conjunctivitis must be differentiated from acute uveitis, acute glaucoma, and corneal disorders (Table 7–1).

1. Viral Conjunctivitis

Adenovirus is the most common cause of viral conjunctivitis. There is usually sequential bilateral disease with copious watery discharge and a follicular conjunctivitis. Infection spreads easily. Epidemic keratoconjunctivitis, which may result in decreased vision from corneal subepithelial infiltrates, is usually caused by adenovirus types 8, 19, and 37. The active viral conjunctivitis lasts up to 2 weeks, with the immune-mediated keratitis occurring later. Infection with adenovirus types 3, 4, 7, and 11 is typically associated with pharyngitis, fever, malaise, and preauricular adenopathy (pharyngoconjunctival fever). The disease usually lasts 10 days. Contagious acute hemorrhagic conjunctivitis (see Chapter 32) may be caused by enterovirus 70 or coxsackievirus A24. Viral conjunctivitis from herpes simplex virus (HSV) is typically unilateral and may be associated with lid vesicles.

Except for HSV infection for which treatment with topical (eg, ganciclovir 0.15% gel) and/or systemic (eg, oral acyclovir, valacyclovir) antivirals is recommended (Table 32–1), there is no specific treatment for contagious viral conjunctivitis. Artificial tears and cold compresses may help reduce discomfort. The use of topical antibiotics and steroids in the acute infection is discouraged. Frequent hand and linen hygiene is encouraged to minimize spread.

Jhanji V et al. Adenoviral keratoconjunctivitis. Surv Ophthalmol. 2015 Sep–Oct;60(5):435–43. [PMID: 26077630]
Varu DM et al; American Academy of Ophthalmology Preferred Practice Pattern Cornea and External Disease Panel. Conjunctivitis Preferred Practice Pattern®. Ophthalmology. 2019 Jan; 126(1):P94–P169. [PMID: 30366797]

2. Bacterial Conjunctivitis

The organisms isolated most commonly in bacterial conjunctivitis are staphylococci, including methicillin-resistant *S aureus* (MRSA); streptococci, particularly *Streptococcus pneumoniae*; *Haemophilus* species; *Pseudomonas*; and *Moraxella*. All may produce a copious purulent discharge. There is no blurring of vision and only mild discomfort. In severe (hyperpurulent) cases, examination of stained conjunctival scrapings and cultures is recommended, particularly to identify gonococcal infection that requires emergent treatment.

Table 7–1. The inflamed eye: differential diagnosis of common causes.

	Acute Conjunctivitis	Acute Anterior Uveitis (Iritis)	Acute Angle-Closure Glaucoma	Corneal Trauma or Infection
Incidence	Extremely common	Common	Uncommon	Common
Discharge	Moderate to copious	None	None	Watery or purulent
Vision	No effect on vision	Often blurred	Markedly blurred	Usually blurred
Pain	Mild	Moderate	Severe	Moderate to severe
Conjunctival injection	Diffuse; more toward fornices	Mainly circumcorneal	Mainly circumcorneal	Mainly circumcorneal
Cornea	Clear	Usually clear	Cloudy	Clarity change related to cause
Pupil size	Normal	Small	Moderately dilated	Normal or small
Pupillary light response	Normal	Poor	None	Normal
Intraocular pressure	Normal	Usually normal but may be elevated	Markedly elevated	Normal
Smear	Causative organisms	No organisms	No organisms	Organisms found only in corneal infection

The disease is usually self-limited, lasting about 10–14 days if untreated. Most topical antibiotics hasten clinical remission. This infection is typically self-limited and benign, and no topical antibiotic has proven superiority over another.

A. Gonococcal Conjunctivitis

Gonococcal conjunctivitis, usually acquired through contact with infected genital secretions, typically causes copious purulent discharge. It is an ophthalmologic emergency because corneal involvement may rapidly lead to perforation. The diagnosis should be confirmed by stained smear and culture of the discharge. Systemic treatment is required. A single 1-g dose of intramuscular ceftriaxone is usually adequate. (Fluoroquinolone resistance is common.) Eye irrigation with saline may promote resolution of conjunctivitis. Topical antibiotics such as erythromycin and bacitracin may be added. Other sexually transmitted diseases, including chlamydiosis, syphilis, and HIV infection, should be considered. Routine treatment for chlamydial infection is recommended.

Costumbrado J et al. Conjunctivitis, gonococcal. StatPearls [Internet]. Treasure Island (FL): StatPearls Publishing; 2017 Oct 11. [PMID: 29083770]

B. Chlamydial Keratoconjunctivitis

1. Trachoma—Trachoma is the most common infectious cause of blindness worldwide, with approximately 40 million people affected and 1.2 million blind. Recurrent episodes of infection in childhood manifest as bilateral follicular conjunctivitis, epithelial keratitis, and corneal vascularization (pannus). Scarring (cicatrization) of the tarsal conjunctiva leads to entropion and trichiasis in adulthood with secondary central corneal scarring.

Immunologic tests or polymerase chain reaction on conjunctival samples will confirm the diagnosis but treatment should be started on the basis of clinical findings. A single 1-g dose of oral azithromycin is the preferred drug for mass treatment campaigns, but improvements in hygiene and living conditions probably have contributed more to the marked reduction in the prevalence of trachoma during the past 25 years. Local treatment is not necessary. Surgical treatment includes correction of lid deformities and corneal transplantation.

Amza A et al. A cluster-randomized trial to assess the efficacy of targeting trachoma treatment to children. Clin Infect Dis. 2017 Mar 15;64(6):743–50. [PMID: 27956455]

2. Inclusion conjunctivitis—The eye becomes infected after contact with infected genital secretions. The disease starts with acute redness, discharge, and irritation. The eye findings consist of follicular conjunctivitis with mild keratitis. A nontender preauricular lymph node can often be palpated. Healing usually leaves no sequelae. Diagnosis can be rapidly confirmed by immunologic tests or polymerase chain reaction on conjunctival samples. Treatment is with a single dose of azithromycin, 1 g orally. All cases should be assessed for genital tract infection and other sexually transmitted diseases.

Satpathy G et al. Chlamydial eye infections: current perspectives. Indian J Ophthalmol. 2017 Feb;65(2):97–102. [PMID: 28345563]

3. Dry Eyes

This is a common and chronic disorder. Dry eye is an umbrella diagnostic term that describes a condition of tear film instability and associated ocular and visual complaints. Dry eye is more common in women than men and increases with age. Hypofunction of the lacrimal glands, causing loss of the aqueous component of tears (keratoconjunctivitis sicca), may be due to aging, hereditary disorders, systemic disease (eg, Sjögren syndrome), or systemic drugs. Excessive evaporation of tears may be due to environmental factors (eg, a hot, dry, or windy climate) or abnormalities of the lipid component of the tear film, as in blepharitis. Mucin deficiency may be due to vitamin A deficiency or conjunctival scarring from trachoma, Stevens-Johnson syndrome and related conditions, mucous membrane pemphigoid, graft-versus-host disease, chemical burns, or topical drug toxicity.

► Clinical Findings

The patient complains of dryness, redness, foreign body sensation, and variable vision. In severe cases, there is persistent marked discomfort, with photophobia, difficulty in moving the lids, and excessive mucus secretion. In many cases, gross inspection reveals no abnormality, but on slit-lamp examination there are abnormalities of tear film stability and reduced tear volume. In more severe cases, damaged corneal and conjunctival cells stain with the vital stains rose bengal and lissamine green. In the most severe cases, there is marked conjunctival injection, mucoid discharge, loss of the normal conjunctival and corneal luster, and epithelial keratitis that stains with fluorescein and may progress to frank ulceration. The Schirmer test, which measures the rate of production of the aqueous component of tears, may be helpful.

► Treatment

Aqueous deficiency can be treated with various types of artificial tears drops or ointments. The simplest preparations are physiologic (0.9%) or hypo-osmotic (0.45%) solutions of sodium chloride, which can be used as frequently as every half-hour, but in most cases are needed only three or four times a day. More prolonged duration of action can be achieved with drop preparations containing a mucomimetic such as hydroxypropyl methylcellulose (HPMC) or carboxymethylcellulose (carmellose). If there is tenacious mucus, mucolytic agents (eg, acetylcysteine 10% or 20%, one drop six times daily) may be helpful.

Artificial tear preparations are generally very safe, without side effects and in most cases are used three or four times a day. However, preservatives included in some preparations to maintain sterility are potentially toxic and allergenic and may cause ocular surface toxicity in frequent users. The development of such reactions may be misinterpreted as a worsening of the dry eye state requiring more frequent use of the artificial tears and leading in turn to further deterioration, rather than being recognized as a need to change to a preservative-free preparation. Preservative-free preparations are recommended for any frequency of use greater than four times a day. Eye drops claiming to "get the red out" are not recommended as they cause toxicity and rebound hyperemia with prolonged use.

Dry eye is generally thought of as an inflammatory ocular surface disease. Accordingly, disease modification may require episodic treatment with low potency corticosteroid drops. All patients using topical corticosteroids should have their intraocular pressure monitored by eye care professionals. Corticosteroid-sparing anti-inflammatory drops such as the calcineurin inhibitor cyclosporine 0.05% ophthalmic emulsion (Restasis) and the integrin antagonist lifitegrast 5% are commonly used. Increased dietary intake of omega-3 fatty acids has not been shown to have a meaningful effect on dry eye syndrome. Lacrimal punctal occlusion by canalicular plugs or cautery is useful in severe cases.

Blepharitis is treated as described above.

Dry Eye Assessment and Management Study Research Group; Asbell PA et al. n-3 fatty acid supplementation for the treatment of dry eye disease. N Engl J Med. 2018 May 3;378(18):1681–90. [PMID: 29652551]

Mathews PM et al. Functional impairment of reading in patients with dry eye. Br J Ophthalmol. 2017 Apr;101(4):481–6. [PMID: 27450145]

Pflugfelder SC et al. The pathophysiology of dry eye disease: what we know and future directions for research. Ophthalmology. 2017 Nov;124(11S):S4–13. [PMID: 29055361]

4. Allergic Eye Disease

Allergic eye disease is common and takes a number of different forms but all are expressions of atopy, which may also manifest as atopic asthma, atopic dermatitis, or allergic rhinitis.

▶ Clinical Findings

Symptoms include itching, tearing, redness, stringy discharge, and occasionally, photophobia and visual loss.

Allergic conjunctivitis is a benign disease, occurring usually in late childhood and early adulthood. It may be seasonal (hay fever), developing usually during the spring or summer, or perennial. Clinical signs include conjunctival hyperemia and edema (chemosis), the latter at times being marked and sudden in onset. **Vernal keratoconjunctivitis** also tends to occur in late childhood and early adulthood. It is usually seasonal, with a predilection for the spring. Large "cobblestone" papillae are noted on the upper tarsal conjunctiva. There may be lymphoid follicles at the limbus. **Atopic keratoconjunctivitis** is a more chronic disorder of adulthood. Both the upper and the lower tarsal conjunctivas exhibit a papillary conjunctivitis. Severe cases demonstrate conjunctival fibrosis, resulting in forniceal shortening and entropion with trichiasis. Corneal involvement, including refractory ulceration, is frequent during exacerbations of both vernal and atopic keratoconjunctivitis. The latter may be complicated by herpes simplex keratitis.

▶ Treatment

A. Mild and Moderately Severe Allergic Eye Disease

Anti-inflammatory agents for topical treatment include mast cell stabilizers and antihistamines (Table 7–2). Mast cell stabilization takes longer to act than antihistamines but can be useful for prophylaxis. Topical vasoconstrictors, such as ephedrine, naphazoline, tetrahydrozoline, and phenylephrine, alone or in combination with antihistamines, are available as over-the-counter medications and not typically used because of limited efficacy, rebound hyperemia, and follicular conjunctivitis. Systemic antihistamines (eg, loratadine 10 mg orally daily) may be useful in prolonged atopic keratoconjunctivitis. In allergic conjunctivitis, specific allergens may be avoidable. In vernal keratoconjunctivitis, a cooler climate often provides significant benefit.

B. Acute Exacerbations and Severe Allergic Eye Disease

Topical corticosteroids (Table 7–2) are essential to control acute exacerbations of both vernal and atopic keratoconjunctivitis. Corticosteroid-induced side effects should be monitored by eye care professionals and include cataracts, glaucoma, and exacerbation of herpes simplex keratitis. The lowest potency corticosteroid that controls ocular inflammation should be used. Topical cyclosporine or tacrolimus is also effective. Systemic corticosteroid or other immunosuppressant therapy may be required in severe atopic keratoconjunctivitis.

Castillo M et al. Topical antihistamines and mast cell stabilisers for treating seasonal and perennial allergic conjunctivitis. Cochrane Database Syst Rev. 2015 Jun 1;6:CD009566. [PMID: 26028608]

Mounsey AL et al. Topical antihistamines and mast cell stabilizers for treating allergic conjunctivitis. Am Fam Physician. 2016 Jun 1;93(11):915–6. [PMID: 27281835]

PINGUECULA & PTERYGIUM

Pinguecula is a yellowish, elevated conjunctival nodule in the area of the palpebral fissure. It is common in persons over age 35 years. Pterygium is a fleshy, triangular encroachment of the conjunctiva onto the cornea and is usually associated with prolonged exposure to wind, sun, sand, and dust. Pinguecula and pterygium are often bilateral and occur more frequently on the nasal side of the conjunctiva.

Pingueculae rarely grow but may become inflamed (pingueculitis). Pterygia become inflamed and may grow. Treatment is rarely required for inflammation of pinguecula or pterygium, and artificial tears are often beneficial.

The indications for excision of pterygium are growth that threatens vision by encroaching on the visual axis, marked induced astigmatism, or severe ocular irritation.

Clearfield E et al. Conjunctival autograft for pterygium. Cochrane Database Syst Rev. 2016 Feb 11;2:CD011349. [PMID: 26867004]

Hovanesian JA et al; ASCRS Cornea Clinical Committee. Surgical techniques and adjuvants for the management of primary and recurrent pterygia. J Cataract Refract Surg. 2017 Mar; 43(3):405–19. [PMID: 28410726]

Table 7–2. Topical ophthalmic agents.

Agent	Cost/Size[1]	Recommended Regimen	Indications
Antibiotics[2]			
Amikacin 2.5% (fortified) solution	Compounding pharmacy		
Azithromycin (AzaSite)	$213.41/2.5 mL	1 drop two times daily for 2 days, then once daily for 5 days	Bacterial conjunctivitis
Bacitracin 500 units/g ointment (various)[3]	$118.44/3.5 g	Apply small amount (0.5 inch) into lower conjunctival sac or to eyelids three to four times daily for 7–10 days	Bacterial conjunctivitis, blepharitis, sty
Bacitracin/Polymyxin ointment (Polysporin, AK-Poly)	$25.70/3.5 g	Apply small amount (0.5 inch) into lower conjunctival sac and then three to four times daily, then as required	Corneal abrasion Following corneal foreign body removal
Besifloxacin ophthalmic suspension, 0.6% (Besivance)	$203.23/5 mL	1–2 drops every 2 hours while awake for 2 days, then every 4 hours for 5 days 1 drop every hour during the day and every 2 hours during the night for 48 hours, then gradually reducing	Bacterial conjunctivitis Bacterial keratitis
Cefazolin 5–10% (fortified) solution	Compounding pharmacy		
Ceftazidime 5% (fortified) solution	Compounding pharmacy		
Cefuroxime 5% (fortified) solution	Compounding pharmacy		
Chloramphenicol 1% ointment[4]	Compounding pharmacy		
Chloramphenicol 0.5% solution[4]	Compounding pharmacy		
Ciprofloxacin HCl 0.3% solution (Ciloxan)	$47.31/5 mL	1–2 drops every 2 hours while awake for 2 days, then every 4 hours for 5 days 1 drop every hour during the day and every 2 hours during the night for 48 hours, then gradually reducing	Bacterial conjunctivitis Bacterial keratitis
Ciprofloxacin HCl 0.3% ointment	$257.23/3.5 g	Apply small amount (0.5 inch) into lower conjunctival sac three times daily for 2 days, then two times daily for 5 days	Bacterial conjunctivitis
Erythromycin 0.5% ointment (various)[5]	$17.96/3.5 g	1-cm ribbon up to six times daily (depending on severity of infection)	Bacterial infection of the eye
Fusidic acid 1% gel (Fucithalmic)	Not available in United States	1 drop two times daily	Bacterial conjunctivitis, blepharitis, sty, keratitis
Gatifloxacin 0.5% solution (Zymaxid)	$118.16/2.5 mL	1 drop every 2 hours while awake, up to eight times on day 1, then two to four times daily while awake, days 2–7 1 drop every hour during the day and every 2 hours during the night for 48 hours, then gradually reducing	Bacterial conjunctivitis Bacterial keratitis
Gentamicin sulfate 0.3% solution (various)	$19.18/5 mL	1–2 drops every 4 hours up to 2 drops every hour for severe infections	Ocular surface infection
Gentamicin sulfate 0.3% ointment (various)	$35.44/3.5 g	Apply small amount (0.5 inch) into lower conjunctival sac two to three times daily	Ocular surface infection

(continued)

Table 7–2. Topical ophthalmic agents. (continued)

Agent	Cost/Size[1]	Recommended Regimen	Indications
Gentamicin sulfate 1.5% (fortified preparation)	Compounding pharmacy	1 drop every hour during the day and every 2 hours during the night for 48 hours, then gradually reducing	Bacterial keratitis
Levofloxacin 0.5% solution (various)	$74.76/5 mL	1–2 drops every 2 hours while awake for 2 days (maximum eight times per day), then every 4 hours for 5 days (maximum four times per day) 1 drop every hour during the day and every 2 hours during the night for 48 hours, then gradually reducing	Bacterial conjunctivitis Bacterial keratitis
Moxifloxacin 0.5% solution (Vigamox)	$167.35/3 mL	1 drop three times daily for 7 days 1 drop every hour during the day and every 2 hours during the night for 48 hours, then gradually reducing	Bacterial conjunctivitis Bacterial keratitis
Neomycin/Polymyxin B/Gramicidin (Neosporin)	$61.26/10 mL	1–2 drops every 4 hours for 7–10 days or more frequently, as required	Ocular surface infection
Norfloxacin 0.3% solution	Not available in United States	1 drop every hour during the day and every 2 hours during the night for 48 hours, then gradually reducing	Ocular surface infection Bacterial keratitis
Ofloxacin 0.3% solution (Ocuflox)	$20.94/5 mL	1–2 drops every 2–4 hours for 2 days, then four times daily for 5 days 1 drop every hour during the day and every 2 hours during the night for 48 hours, then gradually reducing	Bacterial conjunctivitis Bacterial keratitis
Polymyxin B 10,000 U/mL/ Trimethoprim sulfate 1 mg/mL (Polytrim)[6]	$12.90/10 mL	1 drop every 3 hours for 7–10 days (maximum of 6 doses per day)	Ocular surface infection
Propamidine isethionate 0.1% solution	Not available in the United States	1–2 drops every 2–4 hours for 2 days, then four times daily for 5 days	Ocular surface infection (including Acanthamoeba keratitis)
Propamidine isethionate 0.1% ointment	Not available in the United States	Apply small amount (0.5 inch) into lower conjunctival sac up to four times daily	
Sulfacetamide sodium 10% solution (various)	$55.65/15 mL	1 or 2 drops every 2–3 hours initially; taper by increasing time intervals as condition responds; usual duration 7–10 days	Bacterial infection of the eye
Sulfacetamide sodium 10% ointment (various)	$65.86/3.5 g	Apply small amount (0.5 inch) into lower conjunctival sac once every 3–4 hours and at bedtime; taper by increasing time intervals as condition responds; usual duration 7–10 days	Bacterial infections of the eye
Tobramycin 0.3% solution (various)	$14.10/5 mL	1–2 drops every 4 hours for a mild to moderate infection or hourly until improvement (then reduce prior to discontinuation) for a severe infection	
Tobramycin 1.5% (fortified) solution	Compounding pharmacy	1 drop every hour during the day and every 2 hours during the night for 48 hours, then gradually reducing	Bacterial keratitis

(continued)

Table 7–2. Topical ophthalmic agents. (continued)

Agent	Cost/Size[1]	Recommended Regimen	Indications
Tobramycin 0.3% ointment (Tobrex)	$257.23/3.5 g	Apply small amount (0.5 inch) into lower conjunctival sac two to three times daily for a mild to moderate infection or every 3–4 hours until improvement (then reduce prior to discontinuation) for a severe infection	
Antifungal Agents			
Amphotericin 0.1–0.5% solution	Compounding pharmacy		
Natamycin 5% suspension (Natacyn)	$395.00/15 mL	1 drop every 1–2 hours initially; see prescribing information for further recommendations	Fungal blepharitis, conjunctivitis, keratitis
Voriconazole 1% solution	Compounding pharmacy		
Antiviral Agents			
Acyclovir 3% ointment (Zovirax)	Not available in United States	Five times daily	Herpes simplex virus keratitis
Ganciclovir 0.15% gel (Zirgan)	$421.51/5 g	Five times daily	Herpetic keratitis
Trifluridine 1% solution (Viroptic)	$178.28/7.5 mL	1 drop onto cornea every 2 hours while awake for a maximum daily dose of 9 drops until resolution occurs; then an additional 7 days of 1 drop every 4 hours while awake (minimum five times daily)	Herpes simplex virus keratitis
Anti-Inflammatory Agents			
Antihistamines[7]			
Emedastine difumarate 0.05% solution (Emadine)	$159.20/5 mL	1 drop four times daily	Allergic eye disease
Levocabastine (Livostin)	Not available in United States	1 drop twice daily	
Mast cell stabilizers			
Cromolyn sodium 4% solution (Crolom)	$37.20/10 mL	1 drop four to six times daily	
Lodoxamide tromethamine 0.1% solution (Alomide)	$205.28/10 mL	1 or 2 drops four times daily (up to 3 months)	
Nedocromil sodium 2% solution (Alocril)	$256.58/5 mL	1 drop twice daily	
Pemirolast potassium 0.1% solution (Alamast)	Not available in the United States	1 drop four times daily	
Combined antihistamines and mast cell stabilizers			
Alcaftadine 0.25% ophthalmic solution (Lastacaft)	$270.47/3 mL	1 drop once daily	
Azelastine HCl 0.05% ophthalmic solution (Optivar)	$104.06/6 mL	1 drop two to four times daily (up to 6 weeks)	
Bepotastine besilate 1.5% solution (Bepreve)	$498.22/10 mL	1 drop twice daily	
Epinastine hydrochloride 0.05% ophthalmic solution (Elestat)	$106.99/5 mL	1 drop twice daily (up to 8 weeks)	
Ketotifen fumarate 0.025% solution (Zaditor)	OTC $10.36/5 mL	1 drop two to four times daily	
Olopatadine hydrochloride 0.1% solution (Patanol)	$256.50/5 mL	1 drop twice daily	

(continued)

Table 7–2. Topical ophthalmic agents. (continued)

Agent	Cost/Size[1]	Recommended Regimen	Indications
Nonsteroidal anti-inflammatory agents[8]			
Bromfenac 0.09% solution (Xibrom)	$202.52/1.7 mL	1 drop to operated eye twice daily beginning 24 hours after cataract surgery and continuing through first 2 postoperative weeks	Treatment of postoperative inflammation following cataract extraction
Diclofenac sodium 0.1% solution (Voltaren)	$17.50/5 mL	1 drop to operated eye four times daily beginning 24 hours after surgery and continuing through first 2 postoperative weeks.	Treatment of postoperative inflammation following cataract extraction and laser corneal surgery
Flurbiprofen sodium 0.03% solution (various)	$8.73/2.5 mL	1 drop every half hour beginning 2 hours before surgery; 1 drop to operated eye four times daily beginning 24 hours after cataract surgery	Inhibition of intraoperative miosis; treatment of cystoid macular edema and inflammation after cataract surgery
Indomethacin 1% solution (Indocid)	Not available in United States	1 drop four times daily	Treatment of allergic eye disease, postoperative inflammation following cataract extraction and laser corneal surgery
Ketorolac tromethamine 0.5% solution (Acular)	$105.50/5 mL	1 drop four times daily	Treatment of allergic eye disease, postoperative inflammation following cataract extraction and laser corneal surgery
Nepafenac 0.1% suspension (Nevanac)	$325.96/3 mL	1 drop to operated eye three times daily beginning 24 hours after cataract surgery and continuing through first 2 postoperative weeks	Treatment of postoperative inflammation following cataract extraction
Corticosteroids[9]			
Dexamethasone sodium phosphate 0.1% solution (various)	$21.10/5 mL	1 or 2 drops as often as indicated by severity; use every hour during the day and every 2 hours during the night in severe inflammation; taper off as inflammation decreases	Treatment of steroid-responsive inflammatory conditions
Dexamethasone sodium phosphate 0.05% ointment	Compounding pharmacy	Apply thin coating on lower conjunctival sac three or four times daily	
Fluorometholone 0.1% suspension (various)[10]	$170.50/10 mL	1 or 2 drops as often as indicated by severity; use every hour during the day and every 2 hours during the night in severe inflammation; taper off as inflammation decreases	
Fluorometholone 0.25% suspension (FML Forte)[10]	$366.64/10 mL	1 drop two to four times daily	
Fluorometholone 0.1% ointment (FML S.O.P.)	$183.31/3.5 g	Apply thin coating on lower conjunctival sac three or four times daily	
Loteprednol etabonate 0.5% (Lotemax)	$570.47/10 mL	1 or 2 drops four times daily	
Prednisolone acetate 0.12% suspension (Pred Mild)	$349.18/10 mL	1 or 2 drops as often as indicated by severity of inflammation; use every hour during the day and every 2 hours during the night in severe inflammation; taper off as inflammation decreases	

(continued)

Table 7–2. Topical ophthalmic agents. (continued)

Agent	Cost/Size[1]	Recommended Regimen	Indications
Prednisolone sodium phosphate 0.125% solution	Compounding pharmacy		
Prednisolone acetate 1% suspension (various)	$105.60/10 mL	2 drops four times daily	
Prednisolone sodium phosphate 1% solution (various)	$63.25/10 mL	1–2 drops two to four times daily	
Immunomodulators			
Cyclosporine 0.05% emulsion (Restasis) 0.4 mL/container	$334.62/30 containers	1 drop twice daily	Dry eyes and severe allergic eye disease
Tacrolimus 0.1% ointment	$260.45/30 g tube	Not yet established (no label to support)	Severe allergic eye disease; no indication in United States
Agents for Glaucoma and Ocular Hypertension			
Sympathomimetics			
Apraclonidine HCl 0.5% solution (Iopidine)	$86.77/5 mL	1 drop three times daily	Reduction of intraocular pressure; expensive; reserve for treatment of resistant cases
Apraclonidine HCl 1% solution (Iopidine)	$33.27/unit dose	1 drop 1 hour before and immediately after anterior segment laser surgery	To control or prevent elevations of intraocular pressure after laser trabeculoplasty or iridotomy
Brimonidine tartrate 0.2% solution (Alphagan, Alphagan P [benzalkonium chloride-free])	$18.13/5 mL	1 drop two or three times daily	Reduction of intraocular pressure
Beta-adrenergic blocking agents			
Betaxolol HCl 0.5% solution (Betoptic) and 0.25% suspension (Betoptic S)[11]	0.5%: $117.91/10 mL 0.25%: $372.64/10 mL	1 drop twice daily	Reduction of intraocular pressure
Carteolol HCl 1% and 2% solution (various, Teoptic)[12]	1%: $40.10/10 mL	1 drop twice daily	
Levobunolol HCl 0.25% and 0.5% solution (Betagan)[13]	0.5%: $11.94/10 mL	1 drop once or twice daily	
Metipranolol HCl 0.3% solution (OptiPranolol)[13]	$50.17/10 mL	1 drop twice daily	
Timolol 0.25% and 0.5% solution (Betimol)[13]	0.5%: $155.40/10 mL	1 drop once or twice daily	
Timolol maleate 0.25% and 0.5% solution (Istalol, Ocudose [preservative-free], Timoptic) and 0.1%, 0.25% and 0.5% gel (Timoptic-XE, Timoptic GFS)[13]	0.5% solution: $8.80/10 mL 0.5% gel: $217.27/5 mL	1 drop once or twice daily	
Miotics			
Pilocarpine HCl 1–4% solution[14]	1% solution: $98.56/15 mL	1 drop up to four times daily for elevated intraocular pressure	Reduction of intraocular pressure, treatment of acute or chronic angle-closure glaucoma, and pupillary constriction
Carbonic anhydrase inhibitors			
Brinzolamide 1% suspension (Azopt)	$370.06/10 mL	1 drop three times daily	Reduction of intraocular pressure
Dorzolamide HCl 2% solution (Trusopt)	$45.89/10 mL	1 drop three times daily	

(continued)

Table 7–2. Topical ophthalmic agents. (continued)

Agent	Cost/Size[1]	Recommended Regimen	Indications
Prostaglandin analogs			
Bimatoprost 0.03% solution (Lumigan)	$144.65/3 mL	1 drop once daily at night	Reduction of intraocular pressure
Latanoprost 0.005% solution (Xalatan, Monopost [preservative-free])	$21.60/2.5 mL (Monopost not available in United States)	1 drop once or twice daily at night	
Tafluprost 0.0015% solution (Saflutan [preservative-free], Taflotan, Zioptan [preservative-free])	$220.45/30 units (Saflutan not available in United States)	1 drop once daily at night	
Travoprost 0.004% solution (Travatan, Travatan Z [benzalkonium chloride-free])	$220.64/2.5 mL	1 drop once daily at night	
Unoprostone isopropyl 0.15% solution (Rescula)	$153.84/5 mL	1 drop twice daily	
Combined preparations			
Bimatoprost 0.03% and timolol 0.5% (Ganfort)	Not available in United States	1 drop daily in the morning	Reduction of intraocular pressure
Brimonidine 0.2% and timolol 0.5% (Combigan)	$423.22/10 mL	1 drop twice daily	
Brimonidine 0.2% and brinzolamide 1% (Simbrinza)	$195.28/8 mL	1 drop three times a day	
Brinzolamide 1% and timolol 0.5% (Azarga)	Not available in United States	1 drop twice daily	
Dorzolamide 2% and timolol 0.5% (Cosopt, Cosopt PF [preservative-free])	$67.49/10 mL	1 drop twice daily	
Latanoprost 0.005% and timolol 0.5% (Xalacom)	Not available in United States	1 drop daily in the morning	
Tafluprost 0.0015% and timolol 0.5% (Taptiqom [preservative-free])	Not available in United States	1 drop daily	
Travoprost 0.004% and timolol 0.5% (DuoTrav)	Not available in United States	1 drop daily	

[1]Average wholesale price (AWP, for AB-rated generic when available) for quantity listed. Source: IBM Micromedex Red Book (electronic version) IBM Watson Health. Greenwood Village, CO, USA. Available at https://www.micromedexsolutions.com, accessed March 12, 2019. AWP may not accurately represent the actual pharmacy cost because wide contractual variations exist among institutions.

[2]Many combination products containing antibiotics or antibiotics and corticosteroids are available.

[3]Little efficacy against gram-negative organisms (except *Neisseria*).

[4]Aplastic anemia has been reported with prolonged ophthalmic use.

[5]Also indicated for prophylaxis of neonatal conjunctivitis due to *Neisseria gonorrhoeae* or *Chlamydia trachomatis*.

[6]No gram-positive coverage.

[7]May produce rebound hyperemia and local reactions.

[8]Cross-sensitivity to aspirin and other nonsteroidal anti-inflammatory drugs.

[9]Long-term use increases intraocular pressure, causes cataracts, and predisposes to bacterial, herpes simplex virus, and fungal keratitis. These problems may be attenuated by the ester corticosteroid, loteprednol.

[10]Less likely to elevate intraocular pressure.

[11]Cardioselective (beta-1) beta-blocker.

[12]Teoptic is not available in the United States.

[13]Nonselective (beta-1 and beta-2) beta-blocker. Monitor all patients for systemic side effects, particularly exacerbation of asthma.

[14]Decreased night vision and headaches possible.

CORNEAL ULCER

Corneal ulcers are most commonly due to infection by bacteria, viruses, fungi, or amoebas. Noninfectious causes—all of which may be complicated by infection—include neurotrophic keratitis (resulting from loss of corneal sensation), exposure keratitis (due to inadequate lid closure), severe dry eye, severe allergic eye disease, and various inflammatory disorders that may be purely ocular or part of a systemic vasculitis. Delayed or ineffective treatment of corneal ulceration may lead to devastating consequences with corneal scarring and rarely intraocular infection. Prompt referral is essential.

Patients complain of pain, photophobia, tearing, and reduced vision. The conjunctiva is injected, and there may be purulent or watery discharge. The corneal appearance varies according to the underlying cause.

▶ When to Refer

Any patient with an acute painful red eye and corneal abnormality should be referred emergently to an ophthalmologist. Contact lens wearers with acute eye pain, redness, and decreased vision should be referred immediately.

Austin A et al. Update on the management of infectious keratitis. Ophthalmology. 2017 Nov;124(11):1678–89. [PMID: 28942073]

Gomes BA et al. Corneal involvement in systemic inflammatory diseases. Eye Contact Lens. 2015 May;41(3):141–4. [PMID: 25794330]

INFECTIOUS KERATITIS

1. Bacterial Keratitis

Risk factors for bacterial keratitis include contact lens wear—especially overnight wear—and corneal trauma, including refractive surgery. The pathogens most commonly isolated are staphylococci, including MRSA; streptococci; and *Pseudomonas aeruginosa, Moraxella* species, and other gram-negative bacilli. The cornea has an epithelial defect and an underlying opacity. Hypopyon may be present. Topical fluoroquinolones, such as levofloxacin 0.5%, ofloxacin 0.3%, norfloxacin 0.3%, or ciprofloxacin 0.3%, are commonly used as first-line agents as long as local prevalence of resistant organisms is low (Table 7–2). For severe central ulcers, diagnostic scrapings can be sent for Gram stain and culture. Treatment may include compounded high-concentration topical antibiotic drops applied hourly day and night for at least the first 48 hours. Fourth-generation fluoroquinolones (moxifloxacin 0.5% and gatifloxacin 0.3%) are also frequently used in this setting. Although early adjunctive topical corticosteroid therapy may improve visual outcome, it should be prescribed only by an ophthalmologist.

▶ When to Refer

Any patient with suspected bacterial keratitis must be referred emergently to an ophthalmologist.

Herretes S et al. Topical corticosteroids as adjunctive therapy for bacterial keratitis. Cochrane Database Syst Rev. 2014 Oct 16;10:CD005430. [PMID: 25321340]

Lin A et al; American Academy of Ophthalmology Preferred Practice Pattern Cornea and External Disease Panel. Bacterial Preferred Practice Pattern®. Ophthalmology. 2019 Jan;126(1): P1–P55. [PMID: 30366799]

Peng MY et al. Bacterial keratitis: isolated organisms and antibiotic resistance patterns in San Francisco. Cornea. 2018 Jan; 37(1):84–7. [PMID: 29053557]

Tam ALC et al. Bacterial keratitis in Toronto: a 16-year review of the microorganisms isolated and the resistance patterns observed. Cornea. 2017 Dec;36(12):1528–34. [PMID: 28938380]

2. Herpes Simplex Keratitis

Primary ocular herpes simplex virus infection may manifest as lid, conjunctival, or corneal ulceration. The ability of the virus to colonize the trigeminal ganglion leads to recurrences that may be precipitated by fever, excessive exposure to sunlight, or immunodeficiency. Herpetic corneal disease is typically unilateral but can be seen bilaterally in the setting of atopy or immunocompromise. The dendritic (branching) corneal ulcer is the most characteristic manifestation of herpetic corneal disease. More extensive ("geographic") ulcers also occur, particularly if topical corticosteroids have been used. The corneal ulcers are most easily seen after instillation of fluorescein and examination with a blue light. Resolution of corneal herpetic disease is hastened by treatment with topical antiviral agents (eg, trifluridine drops, ganciclovir gel, acyclovir ointment) or oral antiviral agents (eg, acyclovir, 400–800 mg five times daily or valacyclovir 500–1000 mg three times daily for 7–14 days). Topical antiviral agents may cause corneal toxicity after approximately 10–14 days of therapy and for that reason are not commonly used for long-term suppressive therapy.

Stromal herpes simplex keratitis produces increasingly severe corneal opacity with each recurrence. Antiviral agents alone are insufficient to control stromal disease, so topical corticosteroids are also used, but they may enhance viral replication and steroid dependence frequently occurs. Severe stromal scarring may require corneal transplantation; recurrence in the new cornea is common and long-term oral antiviral agents are required.

The rate of recurrent corneal herpetic disease is reduced by using long-term oral acyclovir, 400 mg twice daily; famciclovir, 250 mg once daily; or valacyclovir, 500 mg once daily. Long-term oral antiviral dosing may be adjusted if the disease breaks through suppressive dosing or if kidney dysfunction is present. **Caution:** For patients with known or possible herpetic disease, topical corticosteroids should be prescribed only with ophthalmologic supervision.

▶ When to Refer

Any patient with a history of herpes simplex keratitis and an acute red eye should be referred urgently to an ophthalmologist.

Azher TN et al. Herpes simplex keratitis: challenges in diagnosis and clinical management. Clin Ophthalmol. 2017 Jan 19;11: 185–91. [PMID: 28176902]

Prakash G et al. The three faces of herpes simplex epithelial keratitis: a steroid-induced situation. BMJ Case Rep. 2015 Apr 2;2015. [PMID: 25837655]

Tsatsos M et al. Herpes simplex virus keratitis: an update of the pathogenesis and current treatment with oral and topical antiviral agents. Clin Exp Ophthalmol. 2016 Dec;44(9):824–37. [PMID: 27273328]

3. Herpes Zoster Ophthalmicus

Herpes zoster frequently involves the ophthalmic division of the trigeminal nerve. It presents with malaise, fever, headache, and periorbital burning and itching. These symptoms may precede the eruption by a day or more. The rash is initially vesicular, quickly becoming pustular and then crusting. Involvement of the tip of the nose or the lid margin predicts involvement of the eye. Ocular signs include conjunctivitis, keratitis, episcleritis, and anterior uveitis, often with elevated intraocular pressure. Recurrent anterior segment inflammation, neurotrophic keratitis, and posterior subcapsular cataract are long-term complications. Optic neuropathy, cranial nerve palsies, acute retinal necrosis, and cerebral angiitis occur infrequently. HIV infection is an important risk factor for herpes zoster ophthalmicus and increases the likelihood of complications.

High-dose oral acyclovir (800 mg five times a day), valacyclovir (1 g three times a day), or famciclovir (500 mg three times a day) for 7–10 days started within 72 hours after the appearance of the rash reduces the incidence of ocular complications but not of postherpetic neuralgia. Acute keratitis, or a "pseudo-dendrite," can be treated with a topical antiviral such as ganciclovir 0.15% gel. Anterior uveitis requires additional treatment with topical corticosteroids and cycloplegics. Topical corticosteroids, which promote viral replication, may have to be delayed until the keratitis has resolved. Neurotrophic keratitis is an important cause of long-term morbidity.

▶ When to Refer

Any patient with herpes zoster ophthalmicus and ocular symptoms or signs should be referred urgently to an ophthalmologist.

Cohen EJ. Management and prevention of herpes zoster ocular disease. Cornea. 2015 Oct;34(Suppl 10):S3–8. [PMID: 26114827]

Jastrzebski A et al. Reactivation of herpes zoster keratitis with corneal perforation after zoster vaccination. Cornea. 2017 Jun; 36(6):740–2. [PMID: 28410358]

Johnson JL et al. Herpes zoster ophthalmicus. Prim Care. 2015 Sep; 42(3):285–303. [PMID: 26319339]

Vrcek I et al. Herpes zoster ophthalmicus: a review for the internist. Am J Med. 2017 Jan;130(1):21–6. [PMID: 27644149]

4. Fungal Keratitis

Fungal keratitis tends to occur after corneal injury involving plant material or in an agricultural setting, in eyes with chronic ocular surface disease, and increasingly in contact lens wearers. It may be an indolent process. The corneal infiltrate my have feathery edges and multiple "satellite" lesions. A hypopyon may be present. Unlike bacterial keratitis, an epithelial defect may or may not be present. Corneal scrapings should be cultured on media suitable for fungi whenever the history or corneal appearance is suggestive of fungal disease. Diagnosis is often delayed and treatment is difficult, commonly requiring 6 months or longer for severe disease. Natamycin 5%, amphotericin 0.1–0.5%, and voriconazole 0.2–1% are the most frequently used topical agents. Systemic azoles are probably not helpful unless there is scleritis or intraocular infection. Corneal grafting is often required.

Maharana PK et al. Recent advances in diagnosis and management of mycotic keratitis. Indian J Ophthalmol. 2016 May;64(5): 346–57. [PMID: 27380973]

Prajna NV et al. Effect of oral voriconazole on fungal keratitis in the Mycotic Ulcer Treatment Trial II (MUTT II): a randomized clinical trial. JAMA Ophthalmol. 2016 Dec 1;134(12): 1365–72. [PMID: 27787540]

Prajna NV et al. Predictors of corneal perforation or need for therapeutic keratoplasty in severe fungal keratitis: a secondary analysis of the Mycotic Ulcer Treatment Trial II. JAMA Ophthalmol. 2017 Sep 1;135(9):987–91. [PMID: 28817744]

Prajna VN et al. Fungal keratitis: the Aravind experience. Indian J Ophthalmol. 2017 Oct;65(10):912–9. [PMID: 29044053]

5. Amoebic Keratitis

Amoebic infection, usually due to *Acanthamoeba*, is an important cause of keratitis. The two greatest risk factors in developed countries are contact lens wear and fresh-water or hot-tub exposure. Although severe pain with perineural and ring infiltrates in the corneal stroma is characteristic, it is not specific and earlier forms with changes confined to the corneal epithelium are identifiable. Diagnosis is facilitated by confocal microscopy and Giemsa staining of cornea smears. Culture requires specialized media. Intensive topical compounded biguanide (polyhexamethylene or chlorhexidine) is initiated immediately, and long-term treatment is required. Diamidine (propamidine or hexamidine) may be added. Oral miltefosine is FDA approved for the treatment of *Acanthamoeba* keratitis, but indications and efficacy have yet to be established. There should be close monitoring for systemic toxicity (vomiting, diarrhea, elevation of transaminases, and kidney function studies) during its use. Delayed diagnosis and prior treatment with topical corticosteroids adversely affect the visual outcome. Corneal grafting may be required after resolution of infection to restore vision. If there is scleral involvement, systemic anti-inflammatory and immunosuppressant medication is helpful in controlling pain, but the prognosis is poor.

Carrijo-Carvalho LC et al. Therapeutic agents and biocides for ocular infections by free-living amoebae of *Acanthamoeba* genus. Surv Ophthalmol. 2017 Mar–Apr;62(2):203–18.

Pinna A et al. Free-living amoebae keratitis. Cornea. 2017 Jul; 36(7):785–90. [PMID: 28486311]

ACUTE ANGLE-CLOSURE GLAUCOMA

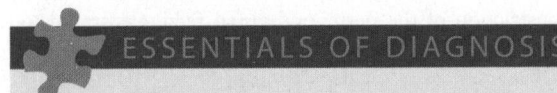

> ## ESSENTIALS OF DIAGNOSIS
>
> ▶ Older age group, particularly farsighted individuals.
> ▶ Rapid onset of severe pain and profound visual loss with "halos around lights."
> ▶ Red eye, cloudy cornea, dilated pupil.
> ▶ Hard eye on palpation.

General Considerations

Primary acute angle-closure glaucoma (acute angle-closure crisis) results from closure of a preexisting narrow anterior chamber angle. The predisposing factors are shallow anterior chamber, which may be associated with farsightedness or a small eye (short axial length); enlargement of the crystalline lens with age; and inheritance, such as among Inuits and Asians. Closure of the angle is precipitated by pupillary dilation and thus can occur from sitting in a darkened theater, during times of stress, following nonocular administration of anticholinergic or sympathomimetic agents (eg, nebulized bronchodilators, atropine for preoperative medication, antidepressants, bowel or bladder antispasmodics, nasal decongestants, or tocolytics), or, rarely, from pharmacologic mydriasis (see Precautions in Management of Ocular Disorders, below). Subacute primary angle-closure glaucoma may present as recurrent headache.

Secondary acute angle-closure glaucoma, which does not require a preexisting narrow angle, may occur in anterior uveitis, with dislocation of the lens, or due to various drugs (see Adverse Ocular Effects of Systemic Drugs, below). Symptoms are the same as in primary acute angle-closure glaucoma, but differentiation is important because of differences in management. Acute angle-closure glaucoma, for which the mechanism may not be the same in all cases, can occur in association with hemodialysis.

Clinical Findings

Patients with acute glaucoma usually seek treatment immediately because of extreme pain and blurred vision, though there are subacute cases. Typically, the blurred vision is associated with halos around lights. Nausea and abdominal pain may occur. The eye is red, the cornea cloudy, and the pupil moderately dilated and nonreactive to light. Intraocular pressure is usually over 50 mm Hg, producing a hard eye on palpation.

Differential Diagnosis

Acute glaucoma must be differentiated from conjunctivitis, acute uveitis, and corneal disorders (Table 7–1).

Treatment

Initial treatment, regardless of mechanism, is reduction of intraocular pressure. A single 500-mg intravenous dose of acetazolamide, followed by 250 mg orally four times a day, together with topical medications that lower intraocular pressure is usually sufficient. Osmotic diuretics, such as oral glycerin and intravenous urea or mannitol—the dosage of all three being 1–2 g/kg—may be necessary if there is no response to acetazolamide. Definitive treatment depends on the mechanism.

A. Primary

In primary acute angle-closure glaucoma, once the intraocular pressure has started to fall, topical 4% pilocarpine, 1 drop every 15 minutes for 1 hour and then four times a day, is used to reverse the underlying angle closure. The definitive treatment is laser peripheral iridotomy or surgical peripheral iridectomy. Cataract extraction is a possible alternative. If it is not possible to control the intraocular pressure medically, the angle closure may be overcome by corneal indentation, laser treatment (argon laser peripheral iridoplasty), cyclodiode laser treatment, or paracentesis; or by glaucoma drainage surgery as for uncontrolled openangle glaucoma.

All patients with primary acute angle closure should undergo prophylactic laser peripheral iridotomy to the unaffected eye, unless that eye has already undergone cataract or glaucoma surgery. Whether prophylactic laser peripheral iridotomy should be undertaken in asymptomatic patients with narrow anterior chamber angles is mainly influenced by the risk of the more common chronic angle closure.

B. Secondary

In secondary acute angle-closure glaucoma, additional treatment is determined by the cause.

Prognosis

Untreated acute angle-closure glaucoma results in severe and permanent visual loss within 2–5 days after onset of symptoms. Affected patients need to be monitored for development of chronic glaucoma.

When to Refer

Any patient with suspected acute angle-closure glaucoma must be referred emergently to an ophthalmologist.

Ah-Kee EY et al. A review of drug-induced acute angle closure glaucoma for non-ophthalmologists. Qatar Med J. 2015 May 10; 2015(1):6. [PMID: 26535174]

Gracitelli CP et al. Ability of non-ophthalmologist doctors to detect eyes with occludable angles using the flashlight test. Int Ophthalmol. 2014 Jun; 34(3):557–61. [PMID: 24081914]

Khazaeni B et al. Glaucoma, acute closed angle. StatPearls [Internet]. Treasure Island (FL): StatPearls Publishing; 2017 Apr 9. [PMID: 28613607]

Zhang X et al. Why does acute primary angle closure happen? Potential risk factors for acute primary angle closure. Surv Ophthalmol. 2017 Sep–Oct;62(5):635–47. [PMID: 28428109]

CHRONIC GLAUCOMA

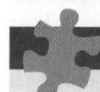

ESSENTIALS OF DIAGNOSIS

► No symptoms in early stages.

► Insidious progressive bilateral loss of peripheral vision, resulting in tunnel vision but preserved visual acuities until advanced disease.

► Pathologic cupping of the optic disks.

► Intraocular pressure is usually elevated.

General Considerations

Chronic glaucoma is characterized by gradually progressive excavation ("cupping") of the optic disk with loss of vision progressing from slight visual field loss to complete blindness. In chronic open-angle glaucoma, primary or secondary, intraocular pressure is elevated due to reduced drainage of aqueous fluid through the trabecular meshwork. In chronic angle-closure glaucoma, which is particularly common in Inuits and eastern Asians, flow of aqueous fluid into the anterior chamber angle is obstructed. In normal-tension glaucoma, intraocular pressure is not elevated but the same pattern of optic nerve damage occurs.

Primary (chronic) open-angle glaucoma is usually bilateral. There is an increased prevalence in first-degree relatives of affected individuals and in diabetic patients. In Afro-Caribbean and African persons, and probably in Hispanic persons, it is more frequent, occurs at an earlier age, and results in more severe optic nerve damage. Secondary open-angle glaucoma may result from ocular disease, eg, pigment dispersion, pseudoexfoliation, uveitis, or trauma; or corticosteroid therapy, whether it is intraocular, topical, inhaled, intranasal, or systemic.

In the United States, it is estimated that 2% of people over 40 years of age have glaucoma, affecting over 2.5 million individuals. At least 25% of cases are undetected. Over 90% of cases are of the open-angle type. Worldwide, about 45 million people have open-angle glaucoma, of whom about 4.5 million are bilaterally blind. About 4 million people, of whom approximately 50% live in China, are bilaterally blind from chronic angle-closure glaucoma.

Clinical Findings

Because initially there are no symptoms, chronic glaucoma is often first suspected at a routine eye test. Diagnosis requires consistent and reproducible abnormalities in at least two of three parameters—optic disk or retinal nerve fiber layer (or both), visual field, and intraocular pressure. Optic disk cupping is identified as an absolute increase or an asymmetry between the two eyes of the ratio of the diameter of the optic cup to the diameter of the whole optic disk (cup-disk ratio). (Cup-disk ratio greater than 0.5 or asymmetry between eyes of 0.2 or more is suggestive.) Detection of optic disk cupping and associated abnormalities of the retinal nerve fiber layer is facilitated by optical coherence tomography scans. Visual field abnormalities initially develop in the paracentral region, followed by constriction of the peripheral visual field. Central vision remains good until late in the disease. The normal range of intraocular pressure is 10–21 mm Hg.

In many individuals (about 4.5 million in the United States), elevated intraocular pressure is not associated with optic disk or visual field abnormalities (ocular hypertension). Treatment to reduce intraocular pressure is justified if there is a moderate to high risk of progression to glaucoma, but monitoring for development of glaucoma is required in all cases. A significant proportion of eyes with primary open-angle glaucoma have normal intraocular pressure when it is first measured, and only repeated measurements identify the abnormally high pressure. In normal-tension glaucoma, intraocular pressure is always within the normal range.

Prevention

There are many causes of optic disk abnormalities or visual field changes that mimic glaucoma, and visual field testing may prove unreliable in some patients, particularly in the older age group. Hence, the diagnosis of glaucoma is not always straightforward and screening programs need to involve eye care professionals.

Although all persons over age 50 years may benefit from intraocular pressure measurement and optic disk examination every 3–5 years, screening for chronic open-angle glaucoma should be targeted at individuals with an affected first-degree relative, at persons who have diabetes mellitus, and at older individuals with African or Hispanic ancestry. Screening may also be warranted in patients taking long-term oral or combined intranasal and inhaled corticosteroid therapy. Screening for chronic angle-closure glaucoma should be targeted at Inuits and Asians.

Treatment

A. Medications

Medical treatment is directed toward lowering intraocular pressure. Prostaglandin analog eye drops are commonly used as first-line therapy because of their efficacy, lack of systemic side effects, and convenient once-daily dose, (except unoprostone) (Table 7–2). All may produce conjunctival hyperemia, permanent darkening of the iris and eyebrow color, increased eyelash growth, and reduction of periorbital fat (prostaglandin-associated periorbitopathy). Topical beta-adrenergic blocking agents may be used alone or in combination with a prostaglandin analog. They may be contraindicated in patients with reactive airway disease or heart failure. Betaxolol is theoretically safer in reactive airway disease but less effective at reducing intraocular pressure. Brimonidine 0.2%, a selective alpha-2-agonist, and topical carbonic anhydrase inhibitors also can be used in addition to a prostaglandin analog or a beta-blocker (twice daily) or as initial therapy when prostaglandin analogs and beta-blockers are contraindicated (brimonidine twice daily, carbonic anhydrase inhibitors three times daily). All three are associated with allergic reactions.

Brimonidine may cause uveitis. Apraclonidine, 0.5–1%, another alpha-2-agonist, can be used three times a day to postpone the need for surgery in patients receiving maximal medical therapy, but long-term use is limited by adverse reactions. It is more commonly used to control acute rise in intraocular pressure, such as after laser therapy. Pilocarpine 1–4% is rarely used because of adverse effects. A newer topical agent is netarsudil ophthalmic solution 0.02%, a rho kinase inhibitor, which has once a day dosing. Oral carbonic anhydrase inhibitors (acetazolamide [Diamox], methazolamide [Neptazane], and dichlorphenamide [Daranide]) may be used on a long-term basis if topical therapy is inadequate and surgical or laser therapy is inappropriate.

Various eye drop preparations combining two agents out of the prostaglandin analogs, beta-adrenergic blocking agents, brimonidine, and topical carbonic anhydrase inhibitors are available to improve compliance when multiple medications are required. Formulations of one or two agents without preservative or not including benzalkonium chloride as the preservative are preferred to reduce adverse effects on the ocular surface for patients with allergies or severe dry eyes.

B. Laser Therapy and Surgery

Laser trabeculoplasty is used as an adjunct to topical therapy to defer surgery and is also advocated as primary treatment, especially when compliance with medications is an issue. Surgery is generally undertaken when intraocular pressure is inadequately controlled by medical and laser therapy, but it may also be used as primary treatment in advanced cases. Trabeculectomy remains the standard procedure. Adjunctive treatment with subconjunctival mitomycin or fluorouracil is used perioperatively or postoperatively in worse prognosis cases. Viscocanalostomy, deep sclerectomy with collagen implant and Trabectome—alternative procedures that avoid a full-thickness incision into the eye—are associated with fewer complications but can be more difficult to perform.

In chronic angle-closure glaucoma, laser peripheral iridotomy or surgical peripheral iridectomy may be helpful. In patients with asymptomatic narrow anterior chamber angles, which includes about 10% of Chinese adults, prophylactic laser peripheral iridotomy can be performed to reduce the risk of acute and chronic angle-closure glaucoma. However, there are concerns about the efficacy of such treatment and the risk of cataract progression and corneal decompensation. In the United States, about 1% of people over age 35 years have narrow anterior chamber angles, but acute and chronic angle closure are sufficiently uncommon that prophylactic therapy is not generally advised.

▶ Prognosis

Untreated chronic glaucoma that begins at age 40–45 years will probably cause complete blindness by age 60–65. Early diagnosis and treatment can preserve useful vision throughout life. In primary open-angle glaucoma and if treatment is required in ocular hypertension, the aim is to reduce intraocular pressure to a level that will adequately reduce progression of visual field loss. In eyes with marked visual field or optic disk changes, intraocular pressure must be reduced to less than 16 mm Hg. In normal-tension glaucoma with progressive visual field loss, it is necessary to achieve even lower intraocular pressure such that surgery is often required.

▶ When to Refer

All patients with suspected chronic glaucoma should be referred to an ophthalmologist.

Feroze KB et al. Glaucoma, secondary glaucoma, steroid. StatPearls [Internet]. Treasure Island (FL): StatPearls Publishing; 2017 Apr 16. [PMID: 28613653]

Foris LA et al. Glaucoma, open angle. StatPearls [Internet]. Treasure Island (FL): StatPearls Publishing; 2017 Oct 13. [PMID: 28722917]

Jonas JB et al. Glaucoma. Lancet. 2017 Nov 11;390(10108): 2183–93. [PMID: 28577860]

Prum BE Jr et al. Primary Open-Angle Glaucoma Preferred Practice Pattern(*) guidelines. Ophthalmology. 2016 Jan; 123(1):P41–111. [PMID: 26581556]

Prum BE Jr et al. Primary Open-Angle Glaucoma Suspect Preferred Practice Pattern(*) guidelines. Ophthalmology. 2016 Jan; 123(1):P112–51. [PMID: 26581560]

UVEITIS

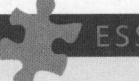

ESSENTIALS OF DIAGNOSIS

▶ Usually immunologic but possibly infective or neoplastic.

▶ Inflammation may be confined to the eye or may be systemic.

▶ **Acute nongranulomatous anterior uveitis:** pain, redness, photophobia, and visual loss.

▶ **Granulomatous anterior uveitis:** blurred vision in a variably painful and inflamed eye.

▶ **Posterior uveitis:** gradual loss of vision in a variably inflamed eye.

▶ General Considerations

Intraocular inflammation (uveitis) is classified as acute or chronic and as nongranulomatous or granulomatous, according to the clinical signs, and by its involvement of the anterior, intermediate, posterior, or all (panuveitis) segments of the eye. The common types are acute nongranulomatous anterior, granulomatous anterior, and posterior.

In most cases the pathogenesis of uveitis is primarily immunologic, but infection may be the cause, particularly in immunodeficiency states. The systemic disorders associated with acute nongranulomatous anterior uveitis are the HLA-B27-related conditions (ankylosing spondylitis, reactive arthritis, psoriasis, ulcerative colitis, and Crohn disease). Chronic nongranulomatous anterior uveitis occurs in juvenile idiopathic arthritis. Behçet syndrome produces both anterior uveitis, with recurrent hypopyon but little discomfort, and posterior uveitis, characteristically with branch retinal vein occlusions. Both herpes simplex and herpes zoster infections may cause nongranulomatous and granulomatous anterior uveitis as well as retinitis (acute retinal necrosis).

Diseases producing granulomatous anterior uveitis also tend to be causes of posterior uveitis. These include sarcoidosis, toxoplasmosis, tuberculosis, syphilis, Vogt-Koyanagi-Harada disease (bilateral uveitis associated with alopecia, poliosis [depigmented eyelashes, eyebrows, or hair], vitiligo, and hearing loss) (Figure 7–1), and sympathetic ophthalmia that occurs after penetrating ocular trauma. In toxoplasmosis, there may be evidence of previous episodes of retinochoroiditis. Syphilis characteristically produces a "salt and pepper" fundus but may present with a wide variety of clinical manifestations. The other principal pathogens responsible for ocular inflammation in HIV infection are cytomegalovirus (CMV), herpes simplex and herpes zoster viruses, mycobacteria, *Cryptococcus, Toxoplasma,* and *Candida.*

Retinal vasculitis and intermediate uveitis predominantly manifest as posterior uveitis with central or peripheral retinal abnormalities in retinal vasculitis and far peripheral retinal abnormalities (pars planitis) in intermediate uveitis. Retinal vasculitis can be caused by a wide variety of infectious agents and noninfectious systemic conditions but also may be idiopathic. Intermediate uveitis is often idiopathic but can be due to multiple sclerosis or sarcoidosis.

▶ Clinical Findings

Anterior uveitis is characterized by inflammatory cells and flare within the aqueous. In severe cases, there may be hypopyon (layered collection of white cells) and fibrin within the anterior chamber. Cells may also be seen on the corneal endothelium as keratic precipitates (KPs). In granulomatous uveitis, there are large "mutton-fat" KPs, and sometimes iris nodules. In nongranulomatous uveitis the KPs are smaller with no iris nodules. The pupil is usually small, and with the development of posterior synechiae (adhesions between the iris and anterior lens capsule) it also becomes irregular.

Nongranulomatous anterior uveitis tends to present acutely with unilateral pain, redness, photophobia, and visual loss. However, in juvenile idiopathic arthritis there tends to be an indolent, often initially asymptomatic process with a high risk of sight-threatening complications. Granulomatous anterior uveitis is more frequently indolent, causing blurred vision in a variably inflamed eye.

In **posterior uveitis,** there are cells in the vitreous and there may be inflammatory retinal or choroidal lesions. New retinal lesions are yellow with indistinct margins and there may be retinal hemorrhages, whereas older lesions have more definite margins and are commonly pigmented. Retinal vessel sheathing may occur adjacent to such lesions or more diffusely. In severe cases, vitreous opacity precludes visualization of retinal details.

Posterior uveitis tends to present with floaters and visual loss. Symptoms are commonly slower in onset, though acute presentations can occur. Bilateral involvement is common. Visual loss may be due to vitreous haze and opacities, inflammatory lesions involving the macula, macular edema, retinal vein occlusion, or rarely, optic neuropathy.

▶ Differential Diagnosis

Retinal detachment, intraocular tumors, and central nervous system lymphoma may all masquerade as uveitis.

▶ Treatment

Anterior uveitis usually responds to topical corticosteroids. Occasionally, periocular or intraocular corticosteroid injections or even systemic corticosteroids are required. Dilation of the pupil is important to relieve discomfort and prevent permanent posterior synechiae. **Posterior uveitis** more commonly requires systemic, periocular, or intravitreal

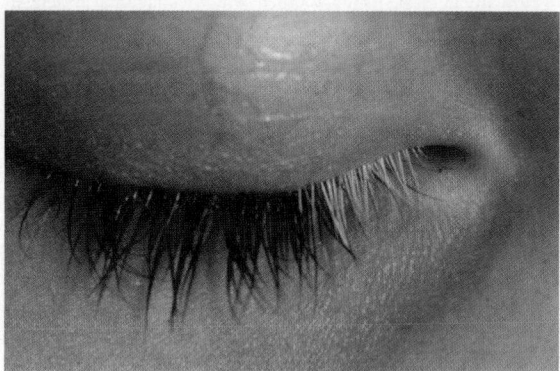

A

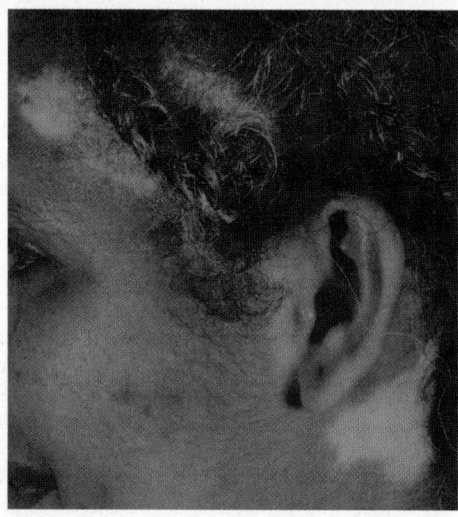

B

▲ **Figure 7–1.** Vogt–Koyanagi–Harada (VKH) disease. **A:** Poliosis of the eyelashes. **B:** Alopecia, vitiligo, and poliosis of the hair. (Reproduced, with permission, from A: Lueder GT. *Pediatric Practice: Ophthalmology.* McGraw-Hill, 2011; B: Riordan-Eva P, Augsburger JJ. *Vaughan & Asbury's General Ophthalmology,* 19th ed. McGraw-Hill, 2018.)

corticosteroid therapy. In chronic cases, systemic corticosteroid-sparing immunomodulatory therapy with agents such as azathioprine, cyclosporine, mycophenolate, methotrexate, tacrolimus, or sirolimus is commonly required. The use of biologic therapies is rapidly increasing. Pupillary dilation is not usually necessary.

If an infectious cause is identified, specific antimicrobial therapy is often needed. In general, the prognosis for anterior uveitis, particularly the nongranulomatous type, is better than for posterior uveitis.

When to Refer

- Any patient with suspected acute uveitis should be referred urgently to an ophthalmologist or emergently if visual loss or pain is severe.
- Any patient with suspected chronic uveitis should be referred to an ophthalmologist, urgently if there is more than mild visual loss.

When to Admit

Patients with severe uveitis, particularly those requiring intravenous therapy, may require hospital admission.

Foster CS et al. The Ocular Immunology and Uveitis Foundation preferred practice patterns of uveitis management. Surv Ophthalmol. 2016 Jan–Feb;61(1):1–17. [PMID: 26164736]

Jabs DA. Immunosuppression for the uveitides. Ophthalmology. 2018 Feb;125(2):193–202. [PMID: 28942074]

Krishna U et al. Uveitis: a sight-threatening disease which can impact all systems. Postgrad Med J. 2017 Dec;93(1106):766–73. [PMID: 28942431]

Sève P et al. Uveitis: diagnostic work-up. A literature review and recommendations from an expert committee. Autoimmun Rev. 2017 Dec;16(12):1254–64. [PMID: 29037906]

CATARACT

> ### ESSENTIALS OF DIAGNOSIS
>
> ▶ Gradually progressive blurred vision.
> ▶ No pain or redness.
> ▶ Lens opacities (may be grossly visible).

General Considerations

Cataracts are opacities of the crystalline lens and are usually bilateral. They are the leading cause of blindness worldwide. Age-related cataract is by far the most common cause. Other causes include (1) congenital (owing to intrauterine infections, such as rubella and CMV, or inborn errors of metabolism, such as galactosemia); (2) traumatic; (3) secondary to systemic disease (diabetes mellitus, myotonic dystrophy, atopic dermatitis); (4) topical, systemic, or inhaled corticosteroid treatment; (5) uveitis; or (6) radiation exposure. Most persons over age 60 have some degree of lens opacity. Cigarette smoking increases the risk of cataract formation. Multivitamin/mineral supplements and high dietary antioxidants may prevent the development of age-related cataract.

Clinical Findings

The predominant symptom is progressive blurring of vision. Glare, especially in bright light or when driving at night; change of focusing, particularly development of nearsightedness; and monocular double vision may also occur.

Even in its early stages, a cataract can be seen through a dilated pupil with an ophthalmoscope or slit lamp. As the cataract matures, the retina will become increasingly difficult to visualize, until finally the fundus reflection is absent and the pupil is white.

Treatment

Functional visual impairment, specifically its effect on daily activities such as increased falls, is the prime criterion for surgery. The cataract is usually removed by one of the techniques in which the posterior lens capsule remains (extracapsular), thus providing support for a prosthetic intraocular lens. Ultrasonic fragmentation (phacoemulsification) of the lens nucleus and foldable intraocular lenses allow cataract surgery to be performed through a small incision without the need for sutures, thus reducing the postoperative complication rate and accelerating visual rehabilitation. The standard monofocal prosthetic intraocular lens can correct near or far vision. Multifocal, extended depth of focus, and accommodative intraocular lenses reduce the need for both distance and near vision correction. In the developing world, manual small-incision surgery, in which the lens nucleus is removed intact, is popular because less equipment is required. Laser treatment may be required subsequently if the posterior capsule opacifies.

Prognosis

Cataract surgery is cost-effective in improving survival and quality of life. In the developed world, it improves visual acuity in 95% of cases. In the other 5%, there is preexisting retinal damage or operative or postoperative complications. In less developed areas, the improvement in visual acuity is not as high, in part due to uncorrected refractive error postoperatively. A large number of drugs, such as alpha-1-antagonists for benign prostatic hyperplasia or systemic hypertension and antipsychotics, increase the risk of complications during surgery (floppy iris syndrome) and in the early postoperative period. Nasolacrimal duct obstruction increases the risk of intraocular infection (endophthalmitis).

Tamsulosin has been shown to have the greatest risk of floppy iris syndrome. There is no consensus about whether to stop alpha-blockers before surgery because the effects of the drug on the iris can persist for months to years. The surgeon must know if the patient is taking an alpha-blocker to prepare for iris issues during surgery. If the patient has not yet started an alpha-blocker and is planning to have cataract surgery shortly, it is best to wait until after surgery to begin the medication, if possible.

When to Refer

Patients with cataracts should be referred to an ophthalmologist when their visual impairment adversely affects their everyday activities.

Breyer DRH et al. Multifocal intraocular lenses and extended depth of focus intraocular lenses. Asia Pac J Ophthalmol (Phila). 2017 Jul–Aug;6(4):339–49. [PMID: 28780781]

Enright JM et al. Floppy iris syndrome and cataract surgery. Curr Opin Ophthalmol. 2017 Jan;28(1):29–34. [PMID: 27653607]

Nanji KC et al. Preventing adverse events in cataract surgery: recommendations from a Massachusetts expert panel. Anesth Analg. 2018 May;126(5):1537–47. [PMID: 28991115]

Roberto SA et al. Patient harm in cataract surgery: a series of adverse events in Massachusetts. Anesth Analg. 2018 May; 126(5):1548–50. [PMID: 28991108]

Thompson J et al. Cataracts. Prim Care. 2015 Sep;42(3):409–23. [PMID: 26319346]

RETINAL DETACHMENT

ESSENTIALS OF DIAGNOSIS

▸ Loss of vision in one eye that is usually rapid, possibly with "curtain" spreading across field of vision.

▸ No pain or redness.

▸ Detachment seen by ophthalmoscopy.

General Considerations

Most cases of retinal detachment are due to development of one or more peripheral retinal tears or holes (rhegmatogenous retinal detachment). This usually results from posterior vitreous detachment, related to degenerative changes in the vitreous, and generally occurs in persons over 50 years of age. Nearsightedness and cataract extraction are the two most common predisposing causes. It may also be caused by penetrating or blunt ocular trauma.

Tractional retinal detachment occurs when there is preretinal fibrosis, such as in proliferative retinopathy due to diabetic retinopathy or retinal vein occlusion, or as a complication of rhegmatogenous retinal detachment. Exudative retinal detachment results from accumulation of subretinal fluid, such as in neovascular age-related macular degeneration or secondary to choroidal tumor.

Clinical Findings

Rhegmatogenous retinal detachment usually starts in the superior temporal area, spreading rapidly to cause visual field loss that starts inferiorly and expands upward but can occur at other locations. Premonitory symptoms of the predisposing vitreous degeneration and vitreo-retinal traction include recent onset of or increase in floaters (moving spots or strands like cobwebs in the visual field) and photopsias (flashes of light). Central vision remains intact until the central macula becomes detached. On ophthalmoscopic examination, the retina may be seen elevated

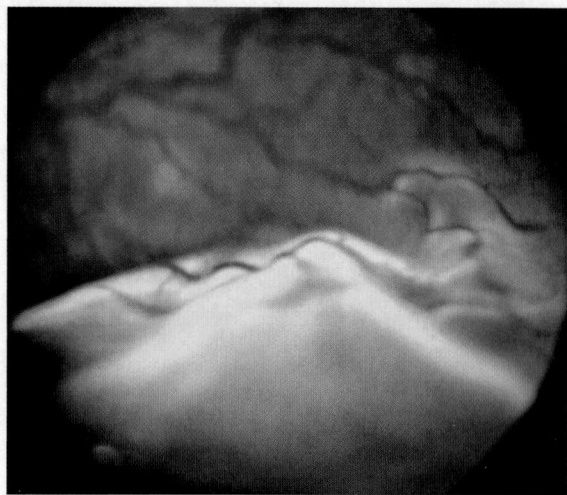

▲ **Figure 7–2.** Inferior retinal detachment as seen on direct or indirect ophthalmoscopy.

in the vitreous cavity with an irregular surface (Figure 7–2). One or more retinal tears or holes can usually be found on retinal examination with scleral depression, which is a technique to examine the peripheral retina using a cotton tip swab or blunt instrument to push on, or depress, the external eye to evaluate the peripheral retina through a dilated pupil. In tractional retinal detachment, there is irregular retinal elevation adherent to scar tissue on the retinal surface, sometimes extending into the vitreous. In exudative retinal detachment, the retina is dome-shaped and the subretinal fluid shifts position with changes in posture. Ocular ultrasonography assists the detection and characterization of retinal detachment.

Treatment

Treatment of rhegmatogenous retinal detachments requires closing all of the retinal tears and holes by forming a permanent adhesion between the neurosensory retina, the retinal pigment epithelium, and the choroid with laser photocoagulation to the retina or cryotherapy to the sclera. The following may be required to achieve apposition of the neurosensory retina to the retinal pigment epithelium while the adhesion is developing: (1) indentation of the sclera with a silicone sponge or buckle, (2) subretinal fluid drainage via an incision in the sclera or internally through a retinal break or hole, or (3) injection of an expansile gas or silicone oil into the vitreous cavity following intraocular surgery to remove the vitreous (pars plana vitrectomy). Certain types of uncomplicated retinal detachment may be treated by pneumatic retinopexy, in which an expansile gas is injected into the vitreous cavity followed by positioning of the patient's head to facilitate apposition between the gas and the hole to permit reattachment of the retina. Once the retina is reattached, the defects are surrounded by laser photocoagulation or cryotherapy scars; these two methods are also used to seal retinal defects without associated detachment.

In complicated retinal detachments, particularly traction retinal detachments, retinal reattachment can be accomplished only by pars plana vitrectomy, direct manipulation of the retina, and internal tamponade of the retina with air, expansile gas, or silicone oil. The presence of an expansile gas within the eye is a contraindication to air travel, mountaineering at high altitude, and nitrous oxide anesthesia. Such gases persist in the globe for weeks after surgery. (See Chapter 37.) Treatment of exudative retinal detachments is determined by the underlying cause.

► Prognosis

About 90% of uncomplicated rhegmatogenous retinal detachments can be cured with one operation. The visual prognosis is worse if the macula is detached or if the detachment is of long duration.

► When to Refer

All cases of retinal detachment must be referred urgently to an ophthalmologist, and emergently if central vision is good because this indicates that the macula has not detached. During transportation, the patient's head is positioned so that the retinal tear is placed at the lowest point of the eye. If the inferior retina is detached, the patient should keep the head upright so that the tear is located at the lowest point, whereas if the temporal retina is detached, the patient should keep the temporal part of the eye with the temporal side of the head down to reduce the chances that the fluid will extend beneath the central retina, causing the macula to detach. If vision is good and the macula is attached, patients should minimize eye motion; in some patients, patching both eyes can be helpful in preventing the eyes from moving rapidly around until surgery can be performed to repair the retinal detachment.

Bond-Taylor M et al. Posterior vitreous detachment—prevalence of and risk factors for retinal tears. Clin Ophthalmol. 2017 Sep 18;11:1689–95. [PMID: 29075095]
Park DH et al. Factors associated with visual outcome after macula-off rhegmatogenous retinal detachment surgery. Retina. 2018 Jan;38(1):137–47. [PMID: 28099315]

VITREOUS HEMORRHAGE

Patients with vitreous hemorrhage complain of sudden visual loss, abrupt onset of floaters that may progressively increase in severity, or occasionally, "bleeding within the eye." Visual acuity ranges from 20/20 (6/6) to light perception. The eye is not inflamed, red, or painful, and clues to diagnosis are inability to see fundus details or localized collection of blood in the vitreous, in front of the retina. Causes of vitreous hemorrhage include retinal tear (with or without detachment), diabetic or sickle cell retinopathy, retinal vein occlusion, retinal vasculitis, neovascular age-related macular degeneration, retinal arterial macroaneurysm, blood dyscrasia, therapeutic anticoagulation, trauma, subarachnoid hemorrhage, and severe straining (Valsalva retinopathy).

► When to Refer

All patients with suspected vitreous hemorrhage must be referred urgently to an ophthalmologist to determine the etiology. If the vitreous hemorrhage is caused by a retinal tear or detachment, it must be repaired urgently to prevent permanent vision loss.

Shieh WS et al. Ophthalmic complications associated with direct oral anticoagulant medications. Semin Ophthalmol. 2017;32(5):614–9. [PMID: 27367495]
Zhang T et al. Early vitrectomy for dense vitreous hemorrhage in adults with non-traumatic and non-diabetic retinopathy. J Int Med Res. 2017 Dec;45(6):2065–71. [PMID: 28627981]

AGE-RELATED MACULAR DEGENERATION

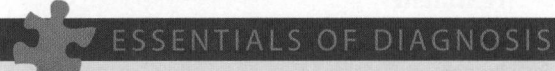

ESSENTIALS OF DIAGNOSIS

- ► Older age group.
- ► Acute or chronic deterioration of central vision in one or both eyes.
- ► Distortion or abnormal size of images in one or both eyes, sometimes developing acutely.
- ► No pain or redness.
- ► Macular abnormalities seen by ophthalmoscopy.

► General Considerations

In developed countries, age-related macular degeneration is the leading cause of permanent visual loss in the older population. Its prevalence progressively increases over age 50 years (to almost 30% by age 75). Its occurrence and response to treatment are likely influenced by genetically determined variations, many of which involve the complement pathway. Other associated factors are race (usually white), sex (slight female predominance), family history, hypertension, hypercholesterolemia, cardiovascular disease, farsightedness, light iris color, and cigarette smoking (the most readily modifiable risk factor).

Age-related macular degeneration is classified into dry ("atrophic," "geographic") and wet ("neovascular," "exudative"). Although both are progressive and usually bilateral, they differ in manifestations, prognosis, and management.

► Clinical Findings

The precursor to age-related macular degeneration is age-related maculopathy that is characterized by retinal drusen. Hard drusen appear ophthalmoscopically as discrete yellow subretinal deposits. Soft drusen are larger, paler, and less distinct. Large, confluent soft drusen are risk factors for neovascular (wet) age-related macular degeneration. Age-related macular degeneration results in loss of central field of vision only in most patients. Peripheral fields, and hence navigational vision, are maintained, except in patients with severe neovascular age-related macular degeneration.

"Dry" age-related macular degeneration is characterized by gradually progressive bilateral visual loss of moderate severity due to atrophy of the outer retina, the retinal pigment epithelium, and the choriocapillaris, which supplies blood to both the outer retina and the retinal pigment epithelium. In "wet" age-related macular degeneration, choroidal new vessels grow under either the retina or the retinal pigment epithelial cells, leading to accumulation of exudative fluid, hemorrhage, and fibrosis. The onset of visual loss is more rapid and more severe than in atrophic degeneration. The two eyes are frequently affected sequentially over a period of a few years. Although "dry" age-related macular degeneration is much more common, "wet" age-related macular degeneration accounts for about 90% of all cases of legal blindness due to age-related macular degeneration.

► Treatment

No dietary modification has been shown to prevent the development of age-related maculopathy, but its progression may be reduced by oral treatment with antioxidants (vitamins C and E), zinc, copper, and carotenoids (lutein and zeaxanthin, rather than vitamin A [beta-carotene]). Oral omega-3 fatty acids do not provide additional benefit.

In wet age-related macular degeneration, inhibitors of vascular endothelial growth factors (VEGF), such as ranibizumab (Lucentis), bevacizumab (Avastin), and aflibercept (VEGF Trap-Eye, Eylea), cause regression of choroidal neovascularization with resorption of subretinal fluid and improvement or stabilization of vision. Long-term repeated intraocular injections are required and must be administered in the eye clinic several times a year, if not monthly. Treatment is well tolerated with minimal adverse effects, but there is a risk of infection (1/2000), retinal detachment (1/10,000), vitreous hemorrhage, and cataract. A certain percentage of patients do not respond to anti-VEGF injections and up to one-third of eyes lose vision despite regular treatment.

There is no specific treatment for dry age-related macular degeneration but, as for wet degeneration, rehabilitation including low-vision aids is important. In addition, patients should be advised to stop smoking and to take vitamin supplements as described above.

► When to Refer

Older patients with sudden visual loss due to macular disease, particularly paracentral or central distortion or scotoma with preservation of central acuity, should be referred urgently to an ophthalmologist.

Evans JR et al. Antioxidant vitamin and mineral supplements for preventing age-related macular degeneration. Cochrane Database Syst Rev. 2017 Jul 30;7:CD000253. [PMID: 28756617]

Evans JR et al. Antioxidant vitamin and mineral supplements for slowing the progression of age-related macular degeneration. Cochrane Database Syst Rev. 2017 Jul 31;7:CD000254. [PMID: 28756618]

Kataja M et al. Outcome of anti-vascular endothelial growth factor therapy for neovascular age-related macular degeneration in real-life setting. Br J Ophthalmol. 2018 Jul;102(7):959–65. [PMID: 29074495]

Mehta S. Age-related macular degeneration. Prim Care. 2015 Sep; 42(3):377–91. [PMID: 26319344]

CENTRAL & BRANCH RETINAL VEIN OCCLUSIONS

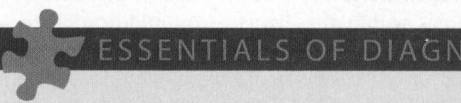

ESSENTIALS OF DIAGNOSIS

- ► Sudden monocular loss of vision.
- ► No pain or redness.
- ► Widespread or sectoral retinal hemorrhages.

► General Considerations

Central and branch retinal vein occlusion are common causes of acute loss of vision, with branch vein occlusions being four times more common. The major predisposing factors are the etiologic factors associated with arteriosclerosis, but glaucoma is also a major risk factor for central and branch retinal vein occlusion.

► Clinical Findings

A. Symptoms and Signs

Ophthalmoscopic signs of **central retinal vein occlusion** include widespread retinal hemorrhages, retinal venous dilation and tortuosity, retinal cotton-wool spots, and optic disk swelling (Figure 7–3).

Branch retinal vein occlusion may present in a variety of ways. Sudden loss of vision may occur at the time of occlusion if the fovea is involved, or some time afterward from vitreous hemorrhage due to retinal new vessels. More gradual visual loss may occur with development of macular edema. In acute branch retinal vein occlusion, the retinal abnormalities (hemorrhages, venous dilation and tortuosity, and cotton-wool spots) are confined to the area drained by the obstructed vein.

To assess possible reversible risk factors, check blood pressure and ask about tobacco smoking in all patients, and ask women about estrogen therapy (including combined oral contraceptives). Patients should also be asked about a history of glaucoma and should undergo a comprehensive

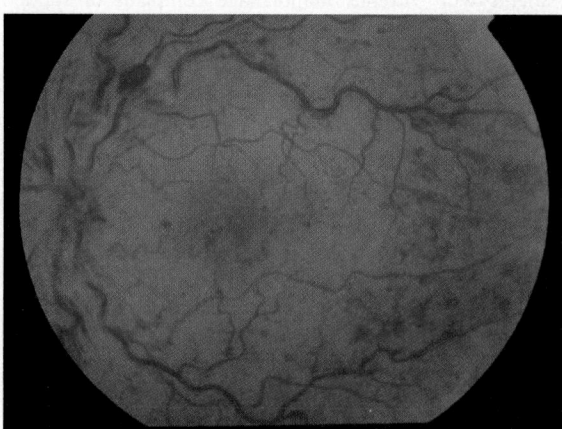

▲ **Figure 7–3.** Central retinal vein occlusion.

eye examination to check intraocular pressure and for signs of open- or narrow-angle glaucoma.

B. Laboratory Findings

Obtain screening laboratory studies for diabetes mellitus, hyperlipidemia, and hyperviscosity (especially in simultaneous bilateral disease), including serum protein electrophoresis for paraproteinemia. Particularly in younger patients, consider obtaining antiphospholipid antibodies, lupus anticoagulant, tests for inherited thrombophilia, and plasma homocysteine levels.

Complications

If central retinal vein occlusion is associated with widespread retinal ischemia, manifesting as poor visual acuity (20/200 [6/60] or worse), florid retinal abnormalities, and extensive areas of capillary closure on fluorescein angiography, there is a high risk of development of neovascular (rubeotic) glaucoma, typically within the first 3 months after the occlusion. Branch retinal vein occlusion may be complicated by peripheral retinal neovascularization or chronic macular edema.

Treatment

Eyes at risk for neovascular glaucoma following ischemic central retinal vein occlusion can be treated with panretinal laser photocoagulation prophylactically or as soon as there is evidence of neovascularization, with the latter approach necessitating frequent monitoring. Regression of iris neovascularization can be achieved with intravitreal injections of bevacizumab. In branch retinal vein occlusion complicated by retinal neovascularization, the ischemic retina should be laser photocoagulated.

Intravitreal injection of antibodies with activity against VEGF, including ranibizumab (Lucentis), bevacizumab (Avastin), or aflibercept (VEGF Trap-Eye, Eylea), is beneficial in patients with macular edema due to either branch or central retinal vein occlusion. Intravitreal triamcinolone improves vision in chronic macular edema due to nonischemic central retinal vein occlusion, whereas an intravitreal implant containing dexamethasone is beneficial in both central and branch retinal vein occlusion, but carries the risk of glaucoma in 20–65% of patients, and will cause cataract in all patients who have not already had cataract surgery. Retinal laser photocoagulation may be indicated in chronic macular edema due to branch, but not central, retinal vein occlusion, but most patients are managed with anti-VEGF antibody injections rather than laser.

Prognosis

In central retinal vein occlusion, severity of visual loss initially is a good guide to visual outcome. Initial visual acuity of 20/60 (6/18) or better indicates a good prognosis. Visual prognosis is poor for eyes with neovascular glaucoma. In branch retinal vein occlusion, visual outcome is determined by the severity of glaucoma and macular damage from hemorrhage, ischemia, or edema.

When to Refer

All patients with retinal vein occlusion should be referred urgently to an ophthalmologist.

Ehlers JP et al. Therapies for macular edema associated with branch retinal vein occlusion: a report by the American Academy of Ophthalmology. Ophthalmology. 2017 Sep;124(9):1412–23. [PMID: 28551163]
Jonas JB et al. Retinal vein occlusions. Dev Ophthalmol. 2017;58:139–67. [PMID: 28351046]
Li J et al. New developments in the classification, pathogenesis, risk factors, natural history, and treatment of branch retinal vein occlusion. J Ophthalmol. 2017;2017:4936924. [PMID: 28386476]
Sinawat S et al. Systemic abnormalities associated with retinal vein occlusion in young patients. Clin Ophthalmol. 2017 Feb 23;11:441–7. [PMID: 28260858]

CENTRAL & BRANCH RETINAL ARTERY OCCLUSIONS

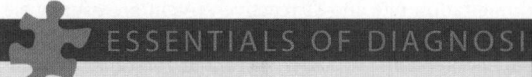

ESSENTIALS OF DIAGNOSIS

► Sudden monocular loss of vision.
► No pain or redness.
► Widespread or sectoral pallid retinal swelling.

General Considerations

In patients 50 years of age or older with central retinal artery occlusion, giant cell arteritis must be considered (see Ischemic Optic Neuropathy and Chapter 20). Otherwise, even if no retinal emboli are identified on ophthalmoscopy, urgent investigation for carotid and cardiac sources of emboli must be undertaken in central and branch retinal artery occlusion so that timely treatment can be given to reduce the risk of stroke (see Chapters 12, 14, and 24). Diabetes mellitus, hyperlipidemia, and systemic hypertension are common etiologic factors. Migraine, oral contraceptives, systemic vasculitis, congenital or acquired thrombophilia, and hyperhomocysteinemia are also causes, particularly in young patients. Internal carotid artery dissection should be considered especially when there is neck pain or a recent history of neck trauma.

Clinical Findings

A. Symptoms and Signs

Central retinal artery occlusion presents as sudden profound monocular visual loss. Visual acuity is usually reduced to counting fingers or worse, and visual field is restricted to an island of vision in the temporal field. Ophthalmoscopy reveals pallid swelling of the retina with a cherry-red spot at the fovea. The retinal arteries are attenuated, and "box-car" segmentation of blood in the veins may be seen. Occasionally, emboli are seen in the central retinal artery or its branches. The retinal swelling subsides over a period of 4–6 weeks, leaving a pale optic disk with thinning of the inner retina on optical coherence tomography scans.

Branch retinal artery occlusion may also present with sudden loss of vision if the fovea is involved, but more commonly sudden loss of a discrete area in the visual field in one eye is the presenting complaint. Fundus signs of retinal swelling and sometimes adjacent cotton-wool spots are limited to the area of retina supplied by the occluded artery.

Identify risk factors for cardiac source of emboli including arrhythmia, particularly atrial fibrillation, and cardiac valvular disease, and check the blood pressure. Nonocular clinical features of giant cell arteritis are age 50 years or older, headache, scalp tenderness, jaw claudication, general malaise, weight loss, symptoms of polymyalgia rheumatica, and tenderness, thickening, or absence of pulse of the superficial temporal arteries. Table 20–12 lists the clinical manifestations of vasculitis.

B. Laboratory Findings

Giant cell arteritis should be considered in cases of central retinal artery occlusion without visible emboli. Erythrocyte sedimentation rate and C-reactive protein are usually elevated in giant cell arteritis but one or both may be normal (see Chapter 20). Consider screening for other types of vasculitis (see Table 20–11). Screen for diabetes mellitus and hyperlipidemia in all patients. Particularly in younger patients, consider testing for antiphospholipid antibodies, lupus anticoagulant, inherited thrombophilia, and elevated plasma homocysteine.

C. Imaging

To identify carotid and cardiac sources of emboli, obtain duplex ultrasonography of the carotid arteries, ECG, and echocardiography, with transesophageal studies (if necessary). When indicated, obtain CT or MR studies for internal carotid artery dissection.

▶ Treatment

If the patient is seen within a few hours after onset, emergency treatment, comprising laying the patient flat, ocular massage, intravenous acetazolamide, and anterior chamber paracentesis, may influence the visual outcome. Early thrombolysis, particularly by local intra-arterial injection, but also intravenously, has shown good results in central retinal artery occlusion not due to giant cell arteritis. However, intra-arterial injection of thrombolytic agents has a high incidence of adverse effects and may be difficult to accomplish quickly enough after the occlusion develops to prevent permanent vision loss due to inner retinal ischemia, which non-human primate studies suggest occurs within 90 minutes of occlusion.

In giant cell arteritis, there is risk of involvement of the other eye without prompt treatment. Recommended initial empiric treatment is intravenous methylprednisolone 0.5–1 g/day for 1–3 days, but intravenous hydrocortisone 250–500 mg may be easier to administer. Whether oral methylprednisolone is similarly effective is unknown. All patients require subsequent long-term corticosteroid therapy (eg, oral prednisolone 1–1.5 mg/kg/day) and possibly low-dose aspirin (~81 mg/day orally). There must be close monitoring to ensure that symptoms resolve and do not recur. Temporal artery biopsy should be performed promptly, and if necessary, assistance sought from a rheumatologist (see Polymyalgia Rheumatica & Giant Cell Arteritis, Chapter 20).

Patients with embolic retinal artery occlusion and 70–99% ipsilateral carotid artery stenosis and possibly those with 50–69% stenosis should be considered for carotid endarterectomy or possibly angioplasty with stenting to be performed within 2 weeks (see Chapters 12 and 24). Retinal embolization due to cardiac disease such as atrial fibrillation or a hypercoagulable state usually requires anticoagulation. Cardiac valvular disease and patent foramen ovale may require surgical treatment.

▶ When to Refer

- Patients with central retinal artery occlusion should be referred emergently to an ophthalmologist.
- Patients with branch retinal artery occlusion should be referred urgently.
- Patients with retinal artery occlusions should be referred urgently to an emergency department to evaluate the patient for stroke manifestations and treatment.

▶ When to Admit

Patients with visual loss due to giant cell arteritis may require emergency admission for high-dose corticosteroid therapy and close monitoring to ensure that treatment is adequate.

Abel AS et al. Practice patterns after acute embolic retinal artery occlusion. Asia Pac J Ophthalmol (Phila). 2017 Jan–Feb; 6(1):37–9. [PMID: 28161924]

Hayreh SS et al. Ocular arterial occlusive disorders and carotid artery disease. Ophthalmol Retina. 2017 Jan–Feb;1(1):12–8. [PMID: 28547004]

Mehta N et al. Central retinal artery occlusion: acute management and treatment. Curr Ophthalmol Rep. 2017 Jun;5(2):149–59. [PMID: 29051845]

Soriano A et al. Visual loss and other cranial ischaemic complications in giant cell arteritis. Nat Rev Rheumatol. 2017 Aug; 13(8):476–84. [PMID: 28680132]

Vodopivec I et al. Management of transient monocular vision loss and retinal artery occlusions. Semin Ophthalmol. 2017; 32(1):125–33. [PMID: 27780399]

TRANSIENT MONOCULAR VISUAL LOSS

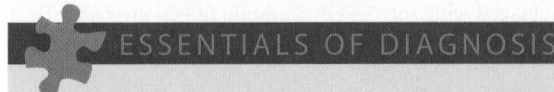

ESSENTIALS OF DIAGNOSIS

▶ Sudden-onset, monocular loss of vision usually lasting a few minutes with complete recovery.

Transient monocular visual loss ("ocular transient ischemic attack [TIA]") is usually caused by a retinal embolus from ipsilateral carotid disease or the heart. The visual loss is characteristically described as a curtain passing vertically across the visual field with complete monocular visual loss lasting a few minutes and a similar curtain effect as the episode passes (amaurosis fugax; also called "fleeting blindness"). An embolus is rarely seen on ophthalmoscopy. Other causes of transient, often recurrent, visual loss due to ocular ischemia are giant cell arteritis, hypercoagulable state (such as antiphospholipid syndrome), hyperviscosity, and severe occlusive carotid disease. More transient visual loss, lasting only a few seconds to 1 minute, usually recurrent, and affecting one or both eyes, occurs in patients with optic disk swelling, for example in those with raised intracranial pressure.

▶ Diagnostic Studies

In most cases, clinical assessment and investigations are much the same as for retinal artery occlusion with emphasis on identification of a source of emboli, since patients with embolic transient vision loss are at increased risk for stroke, myocardial infarction, and other vascular events. Optic disk swelling requires different investigations.

▶ Treatment

All patients with possible embolic transient visual loss should be treated immediately with oral aspirin (at least 81 mg daily), or another antiplatelet drug, until the cause has been determined. Affected patients with 70–99% (and possibly those with 50–69%) ipsilateral carotid artery stenosis should be considered for urgent carotid endarterectomy or possibly angioplasty with stenting (see Chapters 12 and 24). In all patients, vascular risk factors (eg, hypertension) need to be controlled. Retinal embolization due to cardiac arrhythmia, such as atrial fibrillation, or hypercoagulable state usually requires anticoagulation. Cardiac valvular disease and patent foramen ovale may require surgical treatment.

▶ When to Refer

In all cases of episodic visual loss, early ophthalmologic consultation is advisable.

▶ When to Admit

Referral to a stroke center or hospital admission is recommended in embolic transient visual loss if there have been two or more episodes in the preceding week ("crescendo TIA") or the underlying cause is cardiac or a hypercoagulable state.

Bagheri N et al. Acute vision loss. Prim Care. 2015 Sep; 42(3):347–61. [PMID: 26319342]

Biousse V et al. Management of acute retinal ischemia: follow the guidelines! Ophthalmology. 2018 Oct;125(10):1597–607. [PMID: 29716787]

Pula JH et al. Update on the evaluation of transient vision loss. Clin Ophthalmol. 2016 Feb 11;10:297–303. [PMID: 26929593]

Vodopivec I et al. Management of transient monocular vision loss and retinal artery occlusions. Semin Ophthalmol. 2017;32(1):125–33. [PMID: 27780399]

RETINAL DISORDERS ASSOCIATED WITH SYSTEMIC DISEASES

1. Diabetic Retinopathy

ESSENTIALS OF DIAGNOSIS

▶ Present in about 35% of all diagnosed diabetic patients.

▶ Present in about 20% of type 2 diabetic patients at diagnosis of diabetes.

▶ By 20 years after diagnosis of diabetes, 99% of type 1 diabetic patients and 60% of type 2 diabetic patients will have diabetic retinopathy.

▶ **Nonproliferative diabetic retinopathy:** can be mild, moderate, or severe. Microvascular changes are limited to the retina.

▶ **Mild nonproliferative diabetic retinopathy:** mild retinal abnormalities without visual loss.

▶ **Proliferative diabetic retinopathy:** new blood vessels grow on the surface of the retina, optic nerve, or iris.

▶ **Diabetic macular edema:** central retinal swelling; can occur with any severity level of diabetic retinopathy; reduces visual acuity if center involved.

▶ General Considerations

Diabetic retinopathy is broadly classified as **nonproliferative,** which is subclassified as mild, moderate, or severe, or **proliferative,** which is less common but causes more severe visual loss. Diabetic retinopathy is present in about one-third of patients in whom diabetes has been diagnosed, and about one-third of those have sight-threatening disease. In the United States, it affects about 4 million people; it is the leading cause of new blindness among adults aged 20–65 years; and the number of affected individuals aged 65 years or older is increasing. Worldwide, there are approximately 93 million people with diabetic retinopathy, including 28 million with vision-threatening disease. Retinopathy increases in prevalence and severity with increasing duration and poorer control of diabetes. In type 1 diabetes, retinopathy is not detectable for the first 5 years after diagnosis. In type 2 diabetes, retinopathy is present in about 20% of patients at diagnosis and may be the presenting feature.

▶ Clinical Findings

Clinical assessment comprises visual acuity testing, stereoscopic examination of the retina, retinal imaging with optical coherence tomography, and sometimes fluorescein angiography.

Nonproliferative retinopathy manifests as microaneurysms, retinal hemorrhages, venous beading, retinal edema, and hard exudates. Reduction of vision is most commonly due to diabetic macular edema, which may be focal or diffuse, but it can also be due to macular ischemia. Macular involvement is the most common cause of legal blindness in type 2 diabetes. Macular edema may be associated with treatment with thiazolidinediones (glitazones).

Proliferative retinopathy is characterized by neovascularization, arising from either the optic disk or the major vascular arcades. Vitreous hemorrhage is a common sequela. Proliferation into the vitreous of blood vessels, with associated fibrosis, may lead to vitreous hemorrhage and tractional retinal detachment.

Screening

Visual symptoms and visual acuity are poor guides to the presence of diabetic retinopathy. Adult and adolescent patients with diabetes mellitus should undergo regular screening by fundus photography, which can be performed using telemedicine that may involve computer detection software programs or dilated slit-lamp examination of the retina. More frequent monitoring is required in women with type 1 or 2 diabetes during pregnancy and in those planning pregnancy. Patients with type 2 diabetes mellitus should be screened at or shortly after diagnosis of diabetes. Diabetic retinopathy may worsen after bariatric surgery or in patients with long-standing hyperglycemia that is rapidly brought under tight control, such as after receiving an insulin pump with continuous glucose monitoring.

Treatment

Treatment includes optimizing blood glucose, blood pressure, kidney function, and serum lipids. Glycemic control is the most important modifiable factor in treating patients with diabetic retinopathy, but intensive blood pressure control also slows retinopathy progression.

Macular edema and exudates, but not ischemia, may respond to laser photocoagulation; to intravitreal administration of a VEGF inhibitor (ranibizumab [Lucentis], bevacizumab [Avastin], or aflibercept [VEGF Trap-Eye, Eylea]) or corticosteroid (triamcinolone, dexamethasone implant [Ozurdex], or fluocinolone implant [Retisert, Iluvien]) or to vitrectomy. However, VEGF inhibitor therapy improves diabetic retinopathy severity in eyes at all levels of nonproliferative diabetic retinopathy and is the mainstay of treatment for diabetic macular edema.

Proliferative retinopathy is usually treated by intravitreal injection of a VEGF inhibitor or panretinal laser photocoagulation, preferably before vitreous hemorrhage or tractional detachment has occurred. In patients with **severe nonproliferative retinopathy** (defined as having any one of the following: severe intraretinal hemorrhages and microaneurysms in four quadrants, venous beading in two or more quadrants, or intraretinal microvascular abnormalities in at least one quadrant), fluorescein angiography can help determine whether panretinal laser photocoagulation should be undertaken prophylactically by determining the extent of retinal ischemia. Vitrectomy is necessary for removal of persistent vitreous hemorrhage, to improve vision and allow panretinal laser photocoagulation for the underlying retinal neovascularization, for treatment of tractional retinal detachment involving the macula, and for management of rapidly progressive proliferative disease.

Proliferative diabetic retinopathy, especially after successful laser treatment, is not a contraindication to treatment with thrombolytic agents, aspirin, or warfarin unless there has been recent intraocular hemorrhage.

When to Refer

- All diabetic patients with sudden loss of vision or retinal detachment should be referred emergently to an ophthalmologist.
- Proliferative retinopathy or macular involvement requires urgent referral to an ophthalmologist.
- Severe nonproliferative retinopathy or unexplained reduction of visual acuity requires early referral to an ophthalmologist.

Gross JG et al; Diabetic Retinopathy Clinical Research Network. Five-year outcomes of panretinal photocoagulation vs intravitreous ranibizumab for proliferative diabetic retinopathy: a randomized clinical trial. JAMA Ophthalmol. 2018 Oct 1; 136(10):1138–48. [PMID: 30043039]

Hendrick AM et al. Diabetic retinopathy. Prim Care. 2015 Sep; 42(3):451–64. [PMID: 26319349]

Liu Y et al. Risk factors of diabetic retinopathy and sight-threatening diabetic retinopathy: a cross-sectional study of 13 473 patients with type 2 diabetes mellitus in mainland China. BMJ Open. 2017 Sep 1;7(9):e016280. [PMID: 28864696]

Mbata O et al. Obesity, metabolic syndrome and diabetic retinopathy: beyond hyperglycemia. World J Diabetes. 2017 Jul 15;8(7):317–29. [PMID: 28751954]

National Collaborating Centre for Women's and Children's Health (UK). Diabetes in pregnancy: management of diabetes and its complications from preconception to the postnatal period. 2015 Feb. [PMID: 25950069]

Shah AR et al. Diabetic retinopathy: research to clinical practice. Clin Diabetes Endocrinol. 2017 Oct 19;3:9. [PMID: 29075511]

2. Hypertensive Retinochoroidopathy

Systemic hypertension affects both the retinal and choroidal circulations. The clinical manifestations vary according to the degree and rapidity of rise in blood pressure and the underlying state of the ocular circulation. The most florid ocular changes occur in young patients with abrupt elevations of blood pressure, such as may occur in pheochromocytoma, malignant hypertension, or preeclampsia-eclampsia. Hypertensive retinopathy can be a surrogate marker for current and future nonocular end-organ damage. Its detection is aided by nonmydriatic fundus photography.

Chronic hypertension accelerates the development of atherosclerosis. The retinal arterioles become more tortuous and narrower and develop abnormal light reflexes ("silver-wiring" and "copper-wiring") (Figure 11–2). There is increased venous compression at the retinal arteriovenous crossings ("arteriovenous nicking"), predisposing to branch retinal vein occlusions. Flame-shaped hemorrhages occur in the nerve fiber layer of the retina.

Acute elevations of blood pressure result in loss of autoregulation in the retinal circulation, leading to breakdown of endothelial integrity and occlusion of precapillary arterioles and capillaries that manifest as cotton-wool spots, retinal hemorrhages, retinal edema, and retinal exudates, often in a stellate appearance at the macula. Vasoconstriction and ischemia in the choroid result in exudative retinal detachments and retinal pigment epithelial infarcts that later develop into pigmented lesions that may be focal, linear, or wedge-shaped. The abnormalities in the choroidal circulation may also affect the optic nerve head, producing ischemic optic neuropathy with optic disk swelling. Fundus abnormalities are the hallmark of hypertensive crisis with retinopathy (previously known as malignant hypertension) that requires emergency treatment. Marked fundus abnormalities are likely to be associated with permanent retinal, choroidal, or optic nerve damage. Precipitous reduction of blood pressure may exacerbate such damage.

Fraser-Bell S et al. Hypertensive eye disease: a review. Clin Exp Ophthalmol. 2017 Jan;45(1):45–53. [PMID: 27990740]

Kolman SA et al. Consideration of hypertensive retinopathy as an important end-organ damage in patients with hypertension. J Hum Hypertens. 2017 Feb;31(2):121–5.

Omotoso AB et al. Relationship between retinopathy and renal abnormalities in black hypertensive patients. Clin Hypertens. 2016 Oct 21;22:19. [PMID: 28828178]

Shantsila A et al. Malignant hypertension revisited—does this still exist? Am J Hypertens. 2017 Jun 1;30(6):543–9. [PMID: 28200072]

3. Blood Dyscrasias

Severe thrombocytopenia or anemia may result in various types of retinal or choroidal hemorrhages, including white centered retinal hemorrhages (Roth spots) that occur in leukemia and other situations (eg, bacterial endocarditis). Involvement of the macula may result in permanent visual loss.

Sickle cell retinopathy is particularly common in hemoglobin SC disease but may also occur with other hemoglobin S variants. Manifestations include "salmon-patch" preretinal/intraretinal hemorrhages, "black sunbursts" resulting from intraretinal hemorrhage, and new vessels. Severe visual loss is rare but more common in patients with pulmonary hypertension. Retinal laser photocoagulation reduces the frequency of vitreous hemorrhage from new vessels. Surgery is occasionally needed for persistent vitreous hemorrhage or tractional retinal detachment.

Do BK et al. Sickle cell disease and the eye. Curr Opin Ophthalmol. 2017 Nov;28(6):623–8. [PMID: 28984727]

Talcott KE et al. Ophthalmic manifestations of leukemia. Curr Opin Ophthalmol. 2016 Nov;27(6):545–51. [PMID: 27585213]

4. HIV Infection/AIDS

HIV retinopathy causes cotton-wool spots, retinal hemorrhages, and microaneurysms but may also lead to reduced contrast sensitivity and retinal nerve fiber layer and outer retinal damage (HIV neuroretinal disorder).

CMV retinitis is less common since the availability of antiretroviral therapy (ART) but continues to be prevalent where resources are limited. It usually occurs when CD4 counts are below 50/mcL (or 0.05×10^9/L) and is characterized by progressively enlarging yellowish-white patches of retinal opacification, accompanied by retinal hemorrhages, and usually beginning adjacent to the major retinal vascular arcades. Patients are often asymptomatic until there is involvement of the fovea or optic nerve, or until retinal detachment develops. Choices for initial therapy are (1) valganciclovir 900 mg orally twice daily for 3 weeks; (2) ganciclovir 5 mg/kg intravenously twice a day, foscarnet 60 mg/kg intravenously three times a day, or cidofovir 5 mg/kg intravenously once weekly, for 2–3 weeks; or (3) local administration, using either intravitreal injection of ganciclovir or foscarnet, or the sustained-release ganciclovir intravitreal implant. All available agents are virostatic. Maintenance therapy can be achieved with lower-dose therapy (oral valganciclovir 900 mg once daily, intravenous ganciclovir 5 mg/kg/day, intravenous foscarnet 90 mg/kg/day, or intravenous cidofovir 5 mg/kg once every 2 weeks) or with intravitreal therapy. Systemic therapy has a greater risk of nonocular adverse effects but reduces mortality, incidence of nonocular CMV disease (but this is less common with ART), and incidence of retinitis in the fellow eye and avoids intraocular complications of intravitreal administration. Pharmacologic prophylaxis against CMV retinitis in patients with low CD4 counts or high CMV burdens has not been found to be worthwhile. In all patients with CMV retinitis, ART needs to be instituted or adjusted. This may lead to the immune reconstitution inflammatory syndrome (IRIS), of which the immune recovery uveitis may lead to visual loss, predominantly due to cystoid macular edema. It may be possible to reduce the likelihood of IRIS by using immunomodulatory therapy to suppress the immune response causing the inflammation. If the CD4 count is maintained above 100/mcL (0.1×10^9/L), it may be possible to discontinue maintenance anti-CMV therapy.

Other ophthalmic manifestations of opportunistic infections occurring in AIDS patients include herpes simplex retinitis, which usually manifests as acute retinal necrosis; toxoplasmic and candidal chorioretinitis possibly progressing to endophthalmitis; herpes zoster ophthalmicus and herpes zoster retinitis, which can manifest as acute retinal necrosis or progressive outer retinal necrosis; and various entities due to syphilis, tuberculosis, or cryptococcosis. Kaposi sarcoma of the conjunctiva (see Chapter 31) and orbital lymphoma may also be seen on rare occasions.

Chang CC et al. Immune reconstitution disorders in patients with HIV infection: from pathogenesis to prevention and treatment. Curr HIV/AIDS Rep. 2014 Sep;11(3):223–32. [PMID: 24950732]

Hassan-Moosa R et al. Cytomegalovirus retinitis and HIV: case reviews from KwaZulu-Natal Province, South Africa. S Afr Med J. 2017 Sep 22;107(10):843–6. [PMID: 29022526]

Kim DY et al. Comparison of visual prognosis and clinical features of cytomegalovirus retinitis in HIV and non-HIV patients. Retina. 2017 Feb;37(2):376–81. [PMID: 28118285]

ISCHEMIC OPTIC NEUROPATHY

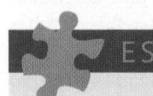

> ## ESSENTIALS OF DIAGNOSIS

> ▶ Sudden painless visual loss with signs of optic nerve dysfunction.
>
> ▶ Optic disk swelling in anterior ischemic optic neuropathy.

Anterior ischemic optic neuropathy—due to inadequate perfusion of the posterior ciliary arteries that supply the anterior portion of the optic nerve—produces sudden visual loss, usually with an altitudinal field defect, and optic disk swelling. In older patients, it may be caused by giant cell arteritis (arteritic anterior ischemic optic neuropathy). The predominant factor predisposing to nonarteritic anterior ischemic optic neuropathy, which subsequently affects the fellow eye in around 15% of cases, is a congenitally crowded optic disk, compromising optic disk circulation. Other predisposing factors are systemic hypertension, diabetes mellitus, hyperlipidemia, systemic vasculitis, inherited or acquired thrombophilia, interferon-alpha therapy, obstructive sleep apnea, and phosphodiesterase type 5 inhibitors.

Ischemic optic neuropathy, usually involving the retrobulbar optic nerve and thus not causing any optic disk swelling (**posterior ischemic optic neuropathy**), may occur with severe blood loss; nonocular surgery, particularly prolonged lumbar spine surgery in the prone position; severe burns; or in association with dialysis. In all such situations, there may be several contributory factors.

▶ Treatment

Arteritic anterior ischemic optic neuropathy necessitates emergency high-dose systemic corticosteroid treatment to prevent visual loss in the other eye. (See Central & Branch Retinal Artery Occlusions, above, and Polymyalgia Rheumatica & Giant Cell Arteritis, Chapter 20.) It is uncertain whether systemic or intravitreal corticosteroid therapy influences the outcome in nonarteritic anterior ischemic optic neuropathy or whether oral low-dose (~81 mg daily) aspirin reduces the risk of fellow eye involvement. In ischemic optic neuropathy after nonocular surgery, treatment of marked anemia by blood transfusion may be beneficial.

▶ When to Refer

Patients with ischemic optic neuropathy should be referred urgently to an ophthalmologist.

▶ When to Admit

Patients with ischemic optic neuropathy due to giant cell arteritis or other vasculitis may require emergency admission for high-dose corticosteroid therapy and close monitoring to ensure that treatment is adequate.

Berry S et al. Nonarteritic anterior ischemic optic neuropathy: cause, effect, and management. Eye Brain. 2017 Sep 27;9:23–8. [PMID: 29033621]

Fandino W. Strategies to prevent ischemic optic neuropathy following major spine surgery: a narrative review. J Clin Anesth. 2017 Oct 3;43:50–8. [PMID: 28985584]

Mendel E et al. Revisiting postoperative vision loss following non-ocular surgery: a short review of etiology and legal considerations. Front Surg. 2017 Jun 26;4:34. [PMID: 28695122]

OPTIC NEURITIS

> ## ESSENTIALS OF DIAGNOSIS

> ▶ Subacute usually unilateral visual loss.
>
> ▶ Pain exacerbated by eye movements.
>
> ▶ Optic disk usually normal in acute stage but subsequently develops pallor.

▶ General Considerations

Inflammatory optic neuropathy is strongly associated with demyelinating disease (typical optic neuritis), particularly multiple sclerosis but also acute disseminated encephalomyelitis. It also occurs in sarcoidosis; in neuromyelitis optica spectrum disorder, which is characterized by serum antibodies to aquaporin-4; in association with serum antibodies to myelin oligodendrocyte glycoprotein; following viral infection (usually in children); in varicella zoster virus infection; in various autoimmune disorders, particularly systemic lupus erythematosus and Sjögren syndrome; during treatment with biologics; and by spread of inflammation from the meninges, orbital tissues, or paranasal sinuses.

▶ Clinical Findings

Optic neuritis in demyelinating disease is characterized by unilateral loss of vision developing over a few days. Visual acuity ranges from 20/30 (6/9) to no perception of light, with more severe visual loss being associated with low serum vitamin D. In almost all cases there is pain behind the eye, exacerbated by eye movements. Field loss is usually central. There is particular loss of color vision and a relative afferent pupillary defect. In about two-thirds of cases, the optic nerve is normal during the acute stage (retrobulbar optic neuritis). In the remainder, the optic disk is swollen (papillitis) with occasional flame-shaped peripapillary hemorrhages. Visual acuity usually improves within 2–3 weeks and returns to 20/40 (6/12) or better in 95% of previously unaffected eyes. Optic atrophy subsequently develops if there has been damage to sufficient optic nerve fibers. Any patient without a known diagnosis of multiple sclerosis with presumed demyelinating optic neuritis in which visual recovery does not occur or there are other atypical features, including continuing deterioration of vision or persisting pain after 2 weeks, should undergo further investigation; MRI of the head and orbits can look for periventricular white matter demyelination, examine for a lesion compressing the optic nerve, and identify atypical optic neuritis.

Treatment

In acute demyelinating optic neuritis, intravenous methylprednisolone (1 g daily for 3 days followed by a tapering course of oral prednisolone) has been shown to accelerate visual recovery, although in clinical practice, the oral taper is not often prescribed and oral methylprednisolone may be used. Use in an individual patient is determined by the degree of visual loss, the state of the fellow eye, and the patient's visual requirements. Phenytoin may be neuroprotective in typical optic neuritis.

Atypical optic neuritis due to sarcoidosis, neuromyelitis optica, herpes zoster, or systemic lupus erythematosus generally has a poorer prognosis, requires immediate and more prolonged corticosteroid therapy, may require plasma exchange, and may necessitate long-term immunosuppression.

Prognosis

Among patients with a first episode of clinically isolated optic neuritis, multiple sclerosis will develop in 50% within 15 years but the visual and neurologic prognoses are good. The major risk factors are female sex and multiple white matter lesions on brain MRI. Many disease-modifying drugs are available to reduce the risk of further neurologic episodes and potentially the accumulation of disability, but each has adverse effects that in some instances are life-threatening. Fingolimod is associated with macular edema. Retinal nerve fiber layer optical coherence tomography quantifies axonal damage that can be used to monitor disease progression.

When to Refer

All patients with optic neuritis should be referred urgently for ophthalmologic or neurologic assessment.

Deschamps R et al. Etiologies of acute demyelinating optic neuritis: an observational study of 110 patients. Eur J Neurol. 2017 Jun;24(6):875–9. [PMID: 28477397]
Morrow MJ et al. Should oral corticosteroids be used to treat demyelinating optic neuritis? J Neuroophthalmol. 2017 Dec; 37(4):444–50. [PMID: 28857910]
Patterson SL et al. Neuromyelitis optica. Rheum Dis Clin North Am. 2017 Nov;43(4):579–91. [PMID: 29061244]

OPTIC DISK SWELLING

Optic disk swelling may result from intraocular disease, orbital and optic nerve lesions, severe hypertensive retinochoroidopathy, or raised intracranial pressure, the last necessitating urgent imaging to exclude an intracranial mass or cerebral venous sinus occlusion. Intraocular causes include central retinal vein occlusion, posterior uveitis, and posterior scleritis. Optic nerve lesions causing disk swelling include anterior ischemic optic neuropathy; optic neuritis; optic nerve sheath meningioma; and infiltration by sarcoidosis, leukemia, or lymphoma. Any orbital lesion causing nerve compression may produce disk swelling.

Papilledema (optic disk swelling due to raised intracranial pressure) is usually bilateral and most commonly produces enlargement of the blind spot without loss of acuity. Chronic papilledema, as in idiopathic intracranial hypertension and cerebral venous sinus occlusion, or severe acute papilledema may be associated with visual field loss and occasionally with profound loss of acuity. All patients with chronic papilledema must be monitored carefully—especially their visual fields—and cerebrospinal fluid shunt or optic nerve sheath fenestration should be considered in those with progressive visual failure not controlled by medical therapy (weight loss where appropriate and usually acetazolamide in patients with idiopathic intracranial hypertension). In idiopathic intracranial hypertension, transverse venous sinus stenting is also an option.

Optic disk drusen and congenitally crowded optic disks, which are associated with farsightedness, cause optic disk elevation that may be mistaken for swelling (pseudopapilledema). Exposed optic disk drusen may be obvious clinically or can be demonstrated by their autofluorescence. Buried drusen are best detected by orbital ultrasound or CT scanning. Other family members may be similarly affected.

Chan JW. Current concepts and strategies in the diagnosis and management of idiopathic intracranial hypertension in adults. J Neurol. 2017 Aug;264(8):1622–33. [PMID: 28144922]
Ottridge R et al. Randomised controlled trial of bariatric surgery versus a community weight loss programme for the sustained treatment of idiopathic intracranial hypertension: the Idiopathic Intracranial Hypertension Weight Trial (IIH:WT) protocol. BMJ Open. 2017 Sep 27;7(9):e017426. [PMID: 28963303]
Wall M. Update on idiopathic intracranial hypertension. Neurol Clin. 2017 Feb;35(1):45–57. [PMID: 27886895]
Wall M et al; NORDIC Idiopathic Intracranial Hypertension Study Group. The longitudinal Idiopathic Intracranial Hypertension Trial: outcomes from months 6–12. Am J Ophthalmol. 2017 Apr;176:102–7. [PMID: 28104417]

CRANIAL NERVE PALSIES

A cranial nerve palsy of any of the three cranial nerves that supply the extraocular muscles can cause double vision.

In a complete **third nerve palsy,** there is ptosis with a divergent and slightly depressed eye (Figure 7–4). Extraocular movements are restricted in all directions except laterally (preserved lateral rectus function). Intact fourth nerve (superior oblique) function is detected by inward rotation on attempted depression of the eye. Pupillary involvement, manifesting as a relatively dilated pupil that does not constrict normally to light, usually means compression, which may be due to aneurysm of the posterior communicating artery or uncal herniation due to a supratentorial mass lesion. In acute painful isolated third nerve palsy with pupillary involvement, posterior communicating artery aneurysm must be excluded. Pituitary apoplexy is a rarer cause. Causes of isolated third nerve palsy without pupillary involvement include diabetes mellitus, hypertension, giant cell arteritis, and herpes zoster.

Fourth nerve palsy causes upward deviation of the eye with failure of depression on adduction. In acquired cases, there is vertical and torsional diplopia that is most apparent

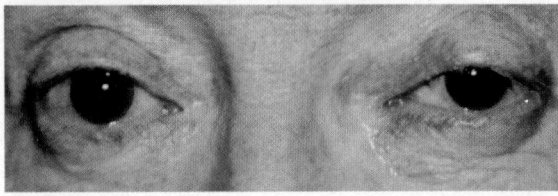

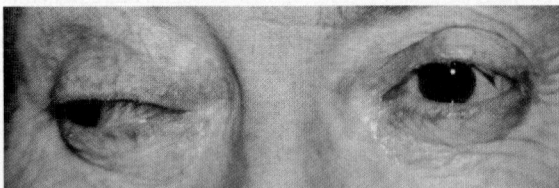

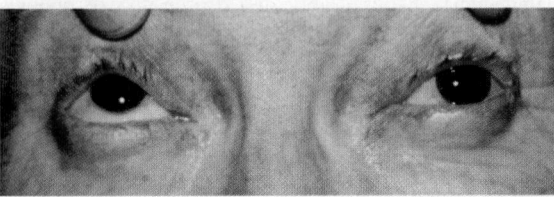

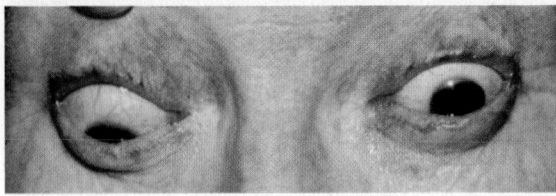

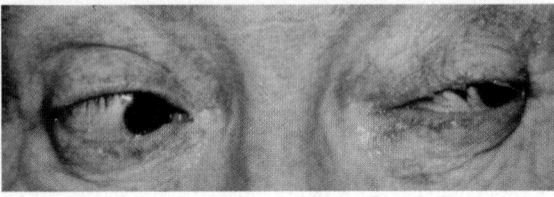

▲ **Figure 7–4.** Left partial third nerve palsy with ptosis **(A)**, reduced adduction **(B)**, elevation **(C)**, and depression **(D)** but normal abduction **(E)** of the left eye.

on looking down. Trauma is a major cause of acquired—particularly bilateral—fourth nerve palsy, but posterior fossa tumor and medical causes, such as in third nerve palsy, should also be considered. Similar clinical features are seen in congenital cases due to developmental anomaly of the nerve, muscle, or tendon.

Sixth nerve palsy causes convergent squint in the primary position with failure of abduction of the affected eye, producing horizontal diplopia that increases on gaze to the affected side and on looking into the distance. It is an important sign of raised intracranial pressure and may also be due to trauma, neoplasms, brainstem lesions, petrous

apex lesions, or medical causes (such as diabetes mellitus, hypertension, giant cell arteritis, and herpes zoster).

In an isolated cranial nerve palsy presumed to be due a medical cause, brain MRI is not always required initially, but it is necessary if recovery has not begun within 3 months.

A cranial nerve palsy accompanied by other neurologic signs may be due to lesions in the brainstem, cavernous sinus, or orbit. Lesions around the cavernous sinus involve the first and second divisions of the trigeminal nerve, the third, fourth, and sixth cranial nerves, and occasionally the optic chiasm. Orbital apex lesions involve the optic nerve and the three cranial nerves supplying the extraocular muscles.

Myasthenia gravis and thyroid eye disease (Graves ophthalmopathy) should be considered in the differential diagnosis of disordered extraocular movements.

▶ When to Refer

- In recent-onset isolated third nerve palsy, especially if there is pupillary involvement or pain, emergency referral is required for neurologic assessment and possibly CT, MRI, or catheter angiography for intracranial aneurysm.

- All patients with recent onset double vision should be referred urgently to a neurologist or ophthalmologist, particularly if there are multiple cranial nerve dysfunctions or other neurologic abnormalities.

▶ When to Admit

Patients with double vision due to giant cell arteritis may require emergency admission for high-dose corticosteroid therapy and close monitoring to ensure that treatment is adequate. (See Central & Branch Retinal Artery Occlusions and Chapter 20.)

Huff JS et al. Neuro-ophthalmology in emergency medicine. Emerg Med Clin North Am. 2016 Nov;34(4):967–86. [PMID: 27741997]

Klein Hesselink T et al. Neurological imaging in acquired cranial nerve palsy: ophthalmologists vs. neurologists. Strabismus. 2017 Sep;25(3):134–9. [PMID: 28759288]

Kung NH et al. Isolated ocular motor nerve palsies. Semin Neurol. 2015 Oct;35(5):539–48. [PMID: 26444399]

Prasad S. A window to the brain: neuro-ophthalmology for the primary care practitioner. Am J Med. 2018 Feb;131(2):120–8. [PMID: 29079403]

THYROID EYE DISEASE
(Graves Ophthalmopathy)

Thyroid eye disease is a syndrome of clinical and orbital imaging abnormalities caused by deposition of mucopolysaccharides and infiltration with chronic inflammatory cells of the orbital tissues, particularly the extraocular muscles. It usually occurs in association with autoimmune hyperthyroidism. Clinical or laboratory evidence of thyroid dysfunction and thyroid antibodies may not be detectable at presentation or even on long-term follow-up, but their absence requires consideration of other disease entities. Radioiodine therapy, possibly indirectly due to induction of hypothyroidism, and cigarette smoking increase the severity of thyroid eye disease, and ethanol injection of thyroid nodules have been reported to be followed by severe disease (see Chapter 26). Ocular myasthenia and thyroid eye disease are associated and may coexist, the presence of ptosis rather than lid retraction being more characteristic of the former.

Clinical Findings

The primary clinical features are proptosis, lid retraction and lid lag, conjunctival chemosis and episcleral inflammation, and extraocular muscle dysfunction (Figure 7–5). Resulting symptoms are cosmetic abnormalities, surface irritation, which usually responds to artificial tears, and diplopia, which should be treated conservatively (eg, with prisms) in the active stages of the disease and only by surgery when the disease has been static for at least 6 months. The important complications are corneal exposure and optic nerve compression, both of which may lead to marked visual loss. The primary imaging features are enlargement of the extraocular muscles, usually affecting both orbits. The clinical and imaging abnormalities of thyroid eye disease may be mimicked by dural caroticocavernous sinus fistula.

Treatment

See Graves Ophthalmopathy, Chapter 26.

When to Refer

All patients with thyroid eye disease should be referred to an ophthalmologist, urgently if there is reduced vision.

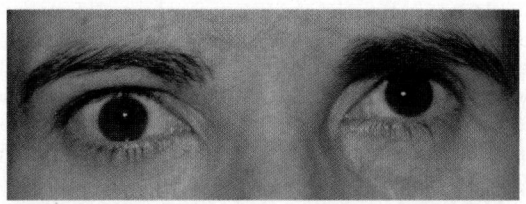

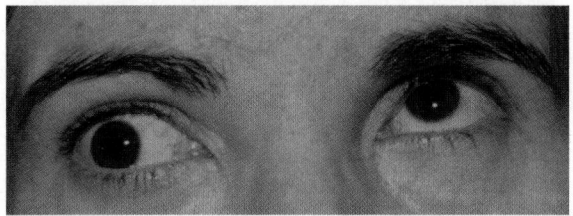

▲ **Figure 7–5.** Thyroid eye disease. Inferior rectus fibrosis causing **(A)** downward deviation and **(B)** limitation of elevation of right eye. (Reproduced, with permission, from Riordan-Eva P, Augsburger JJ. *Vaughan & Asbury's General Ophthalmology*, 19th ed. McGraw-Hill, 2018.)

Blandford AD et al. Dysthyroid optic neuropathy: update on pathogenesis, diagnosis, and management. Expert Rev Ophthalmol. 2017;12(2):111–21. [PMID: 28775762]

Smith TJ et al. Graves' disease. N Engl J Med. 2016 Oct 20; 375(16):1552–65. [PMID: 27797318]

Strianese D. Update on Graves disease: advances in treatment of mild, moderate and severe thyroid eye disease. Curr Opin Ophthalmol. 2017 Sep;28(5):505–13. [PMID: 28700384]

Wiersinga WM. Advances in treatment of active, moderate-to-severe Graves' ophthalmopathy. Lancet Diabetes Endocrinol. 2017 Feb;5(2):134–42. [PMID: 27346786]

ORBITAL CELLULITIS

Orbital cellulitis is characterized by fever, proptosis, restriction of extraocular movements, and swelling with redness of the lids. Immediate treatment with intravenous antibiotics is necessary to prevent optic nerve damage and spread of infection to the cavernous sinuses, meninges, and brain. Infection of the paranasal sinuses is the usual underlying cause. Infecting organisms include *S pneumoniae*, the incidence of which has been reduced by the administration of pneumococcal vaccine; other streptococci, such as the anginosus group; *H influenzae*; and, less commonly, *S aureus* including MRSA. Penicillinase-resistant penicillin, such as nafcillin, is recommended, possibly together with metronidazole or clindamycin to treat anaerobic infections. If trauma is the underlying cause, a cephalosporin, such as cefazolin or ceftriaxone, should be added to ensure coverage for *S aureus* and group A beta-hemolytic streptococci. If MRSA infection is a concern, vancomycin or clindamycin may be required. For patients with penicillin hypersensitivity, vancomycin, levofloxacin, and metronidazole are recommended. The response to antibiotics is usually excellent, but surgery may be required to drain the paranasal sinuses or orbital abscess. In immunocompromised patients, zygomycosis must be considered.

When to Refer

All patients with suspected orbital cellulitis must be referred emergently to an ophthalmologist.

Amin N et al. Assessment and management of orbital cellulitis. Br J Hosp Med (Lond). 2016 Apr;77(4):216–20. [PMID: 27071427]

Marchiano E et al. Characteristics of patients treated for orbital cellulitis: an analysis of inpatient data. Laryngoscope. 2016 Mar; 126(3):554–9. [PMID: 26307941]

OCULAR TRAUMA

Ocular trauma, which occurs in many different circumstances and by a variety of mechanisms, is an important cause of avoidable severe visual impairment at all ages but particularly in young adult males and is the leading cause of monocular blindness in the United States. Thorough but safe clinical assessment, supplemented when necessary by imaging, is crucial to effective management. Ocular damage and the possible need for early assessment by an ophthalmologist need to be borne in mind in the assessment of any patient with mid-facial injury.

1. Conjunctival & Corneal Foreign Bodies

If a patient complains of "something in my eye" and gives a consistent history, a foreign body is usually present on the cornea or under the upper lid even though it may not be visible. Visual acuity should be tested before treatment is instituted, to assess the severity of the injury and as a basis for comparison in the event of complications.

After a local anesthetic (eg, proparacaine, 0.5%) is instilled, the eye is examined with a slit lamp or with a hand flashlight, using oblique illumination, and loupe. Corneal foreign bodies may be made more apparent by the instillation of sterile fluorescein. They are then removed with a sterile wet cotton-tipped applicator or hypodermic needle. Bacitracin-polymyxin ophthalmic ointment should be instilled. It is not necessary to patch the eye. All patients need to be advised to return promptly for reassessment if there is any increase in pain, redness, or impairment of vision.

Iron foreign bodies usually leave a diffuse rust ring. This requires excision and is best done under local anesthesia using a slit lamp. **Caution:** Anesthetic drops should not be given to the patient for self-administration.

If there is no infection, a layer of corneal epithelial cells will line the crater within 24 hours. While the epithelium is defective, the cornea is extremely susceptible to infection. Early infection is manifested by a white necrotic area around the crater and a small amount of gray exudate.

In the case of a foreign body under the upper lid, a local anesthetic is instilled and the lid is everted by grasping the lashes gently and exerting pressure on the mid portion of the outer surface of the upper lid with an applicator (Figure 7–6). If a foreign body is present, it can easily be removed by passing a wet sterile cotton-tipped applicator across the conjunctival surface.

▶ When to Refer

Urgent referral to an ophthalmologist should be arranged if a corneal foreign body cannot be removed or if there is suspicion of corneal infection.

Fraenkel A et al. Managing corneal foreign bodies in office-based general practice. Aust Fam Physician. 2017 Mar; 46(3):89–93. [PMID: 28260265]

2. Intraocular Foreign Body

Intraocular foreign body requires emergency treatment by an ophthalmologist. Patients giving a history of "something hitting the eye"—particularly while hammering on metal or using grinding equipment—must be assessed for this possibility, especially when no corneal foreign body is seen, a corneal or scleral wound is apparent, or there is marked visual loss or media opacity. Such patients must be treated as for open globe injury and referred without delay. Intraocular foreign bodies significantly increase the risk of intraocular infection.

▶ When to Refer

Patients with suspected intraocular foreign body must be referred emergently to an ophthalmologist.

Loporchio D et al. Intraocular foreign bodies: a review. Surv Ophthalmol. 2016 Sep–Oct;61(5):582–96. [PMID: 26994871]

3. Corneal Abrasions

A patient with a corneal abrasion complains of severe pain and photophobia. There is often a history of trauma to the eye, commonly involving a fingernail, piece of paper, or contact lens. Visual acuity is recorded, and the cornea and conjunctiva are examined with a light and loupe to rule out a foreign body. If an abrasion is suspected but cannot be seen, sterile fluorescein is instilled into the conjunctival sac: the area of corneal abrasion will stain because fluorescein stains areas that are devoid of epithelium.

Treatment includes bacitracin-polymyxin ophthalmic ointment or drops, or a fluoroquinolone topical antibiotic in contact lens wearers, as prophylaxis against infection. A mydriatic (cyclopentolate 1%) and either topical or oral nonsteroidal anti-inflammatory agents can be used for pain control. Patching the eye is probably not helpful for small abrasions. Corneal abrasions heal more slowly in persons who smoke cigarettes. Recurrent corneal erosion may follow corneal abrasions.

Although topical tetracaine for 24 hours in the treatment of corneal abrasion has been reported to be safe and effective, there is a risk of severe corneal disease from misuse of topical anesthetics, so it is not recommended.

Ahmed F et al. Corneal abrasions and corneal foreign bodies. Prim Care. 2015 Sep;42(3):363–75. [PMID: 26319343]
Wakai A et al. Topical non-steroidal anti-inflammatory drugs for analgesia in traumatic corneal abrasions. Cochrane Database Syst Rev. 2017 May 18;5:CD009781. [PMID: 28516471]

4. Contusions

Contusion injury of the eye (closed globe injury) and surrounding structures may cause ecchymosis ("black eye"), subconjunctival hemorrhage, edema of the cornea, hemorrhage into the anterior chamber (hyphema), rupture of the root of the iris (iridodialysis), paralysis of the pupillary sphincter, paralysis of the muscles of accommodation, cataract, dislocation of the lens, vitreous hemorrhage, retinal hemorrhage and edema (most common in the macular area), detachment of the retina, rupture of the choroid, fracture of the orbital floor ("blowout fracture"), or optic nerve injury. Many of these injuries are immediately obvious; others may not become apparent for days or weeks. The possibility of globe injury must always be considered in patients with facial injury, particularly if there is an orbital fracture. Patients with moderate to severe contusions should be seen by an ophthalmologist.

Any injury causing hyphema involves the danger of secondary hemorrhage, which may cause intractable glaucoma with permanent visual loss. The patient should be advised to rest until complete resolution has occurred. Frequent ophthalmologic assessment is essential. Aspirin and any drugs inhibiting coagulation increase the risk of secondary hemorrhage and are to be avoided. Sickle cell anemia or trait adversely affects outcome.

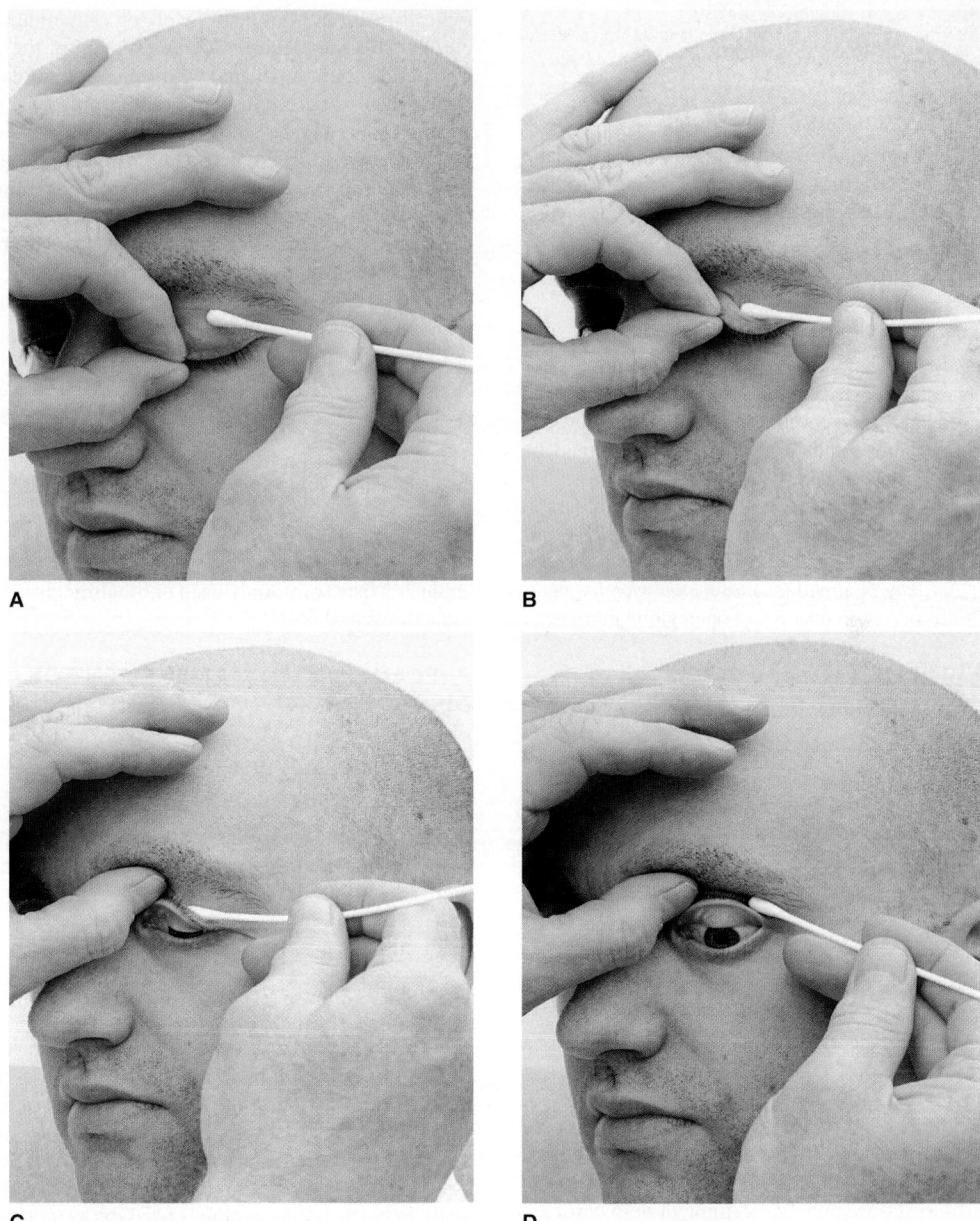

▲ **Figure 7–6.** Technique of lid eversion. **A:** With the patient looking down, the upper lashes are grasped with one hand as an applicator stick is positioned at the superior edge of the upper tarsus (at the upper lid crease). **B** and **C:** As the lashes are lifted, slight downward pressure is simultaneously applied with the applicator stick. **D:** The thumb pins the lashes against the superior orbital rim, allowing examination of the undersurface of the tarsus. (Photos by Richard Leung and Matthew Richardson. Used with permission from King's College Hospital, London in Riordan-Eva P, Augsburger JJ. *Vaughan & Asbury's General Ophthalmology*, 19th ed. McGraw-Hill, 2018.)

▶ When to Refer

Patients with moderate or severe ocular contusion should be referred to an ophthalmologist, emergently if there is hyphema.

Bansal S et al. Controversies in the pathophysiology and management of hyphema. Surv Ophthalmol. 2016 May–Jun;61(3): 297–308. [PMID: 26632664]

5. Lacerations

A. Lids

If the lid margin is lacerated, the patient should be referred for specialized care, since permanent notching may result. Lacerations of the lower eyelid near the inner canthus often sever the lower canaliculus, for which canalicular intubation is likely to be required. Lid lacerations not involving the margin may be sutured like any skin laceration.

Ko AC et al. Eyelid and periorbital soft tissue trauma. Facial Plast Surg Clin North Am. 2017 Nov;25(4):605–16. [PMID: 28941512]

B. Conjunctiva

In lacerations of the conjunctiva, sutures are not necessary. To prevent infection, topical sulfonamide or other antibiotic is used until the laceration is healed.

C. Cornea or Sclera

Patients with suspected corneal or scleral laceration or rupture (open globe injury) must be seen emergently by an ophthalmologist. Manipulation is kept to a minimum, since pressure may result in extrusion of intraocular contents. The eye is bandaged lightly and covered with a shield that rests on the orbital bones above and below. The patient should be instructed not to squeeze the eye shut and to remain still. If there may be a metallic intraocular foreign body, a radiograph or CT scan is obtained to identify and localize it. *MRI is contraindicated because of the risk of movement of any metallic foreign body but may be useful for non-metallic foreign body.* Endophthalmitis occurs in over 5% of open globe injuries.

► When to Refer

Patients with suspected open globe injury must be referred emergently to an ophthalmologist.

Beshay N et al. The epidemiology of open globe injuries presenting to a tertiary referral eye hospital in Australia. Injury. 2017 Jul; 48(7):1348–54. [PMID: 28438416]
Page RD et al. Risk factors for poor outcomes in patients with open-globe injuries. Clin Ophthalmol. 2016 Aug 1;10:1461–6. [PMID: 27536059]

ULTRAVIOLET KERATITIS (Actinic Keratitis)

Ultraviolet burns of the cornea are usually caused by use of a sunlamp without eye protection, exposure to a welding arc, or exposure to the sun when skiing ("snow blindness"). There are no immediate symptoms, but about 6–12 hours later the patient complains of agonizing pain and severe photophobia. Slit-lamp examination after instillation of sterile fluorescein shows diffuse punctate staining of both corneas.

Treatment consists of binocular patching and instillation of 1–2 drops of 1% cyclopentolate (to relieve the discomfort of ciliary spasm). Patients typically recover within 24–48 hours without complications. Local anesthetics should not be prescribed because they delay corneal epithelial healing.

CHEMICAL CONJUNCTIVITIS & KERATITIS

Chemical burns are treated by copious irrigation of the eyes as soon as possible after exposure, with tap water, saline solution, or buffering solution if available. Neutralization of an acid with an alkali or vice versa may cause further damage. Alkali injuries are more serious and require prolonged irrigation, since alkalies are not precipitated by the proteins of the eye as are acids. It is important to remove any retained particulate matter, such as is typically present in injuries involving cement and building plaster. This may require double eversion of the upper lid. The pupil should be dilated with 1% cyclopentolate, 1 drop twice a day, to relieve discomfort, and prophylactic topical antibiotics should be started. In moderate to severe injuries, intensive topical corticosteroids and topical and systemic vitamin C are also necessary. Complications include mucus deficiency, scarring of the cornea and conjunctiva, symblepharon (adhesions between the tarsal and bulbar conjunctiva), tear duct obstruction, and secondary infection. It is difficult to assess severity of chemical burns without slit-lamp examination.

Haring RS et al. Epidemiologic trends of chemical ocular burns in the United States. JAMA Ophthalmol. 2016 Oct 1; 134(10):1119–24. [PMID: 27490908]
Sharma N et al. Treatment of acute ocular chemical burns. Surv Ophthalmol. 2018 Mar–Apr; 63(2):214–35. [PMID: 28935121]

TREATMENT OF OCULAR DISORDERS

Table 7–2 lists commonly used ophthalmic drugs and their indications and costs.

PRECAUTIONS IN MANAGEMENT OF OCULAR DISORDERS

1. Use of Local Anesthetics

Unsupervised self-administration of local anesthetics is dangerous because they are toxic to the corneal epithelium, delay healing, and the patient may further injure an anesthetized eye without knowing it.

2. Pupillary Dilation

Dilating the pupil can very occasionally precipitate acute glaucoma if the patient has a narrow anterior chamber angle and should be undertaken with caution if the anterior chamber is obviously shallow (readily determined by oblique illumination of the anterior segment of the eye). A short-acting mydriatic, such as tropicamide, should be used and the patient warned to report immediately if ocular discomfort or redness develops. Angle closure is more likely to occur if pilocarpine is used to overcome pupillary dilation than if the pupil is allowed to constrict naturally.

Ah-Kee EY et al. A review of drug-induced acute angle closure glaucoma for non-ophthalmologists. Qatar Med J. 2015 May 10; 2015(1):6. [PMID: 26535174]

3. Corticosteroid Therapy

Comanagement with eye specialists is strongly recommended to monitor for ocular complications of corticosteroid therapy. Long-term use of local corticosteroids presents several hazards: ocular hypertension leading to open-angle glaucoma; cataract formation; and exacerbation of ocular infections, such as herpes simplex (dendritic) and fungal keratitis. Furthermore, perforation of the cornea may occur when corticosteroids are used indiscriminately for infectious keratitis. The potential for causing or exacerbating systemic hypertension, diabetes mellitus, gastritis, osteoporosis, or glaucoma must always be borne in mind when systemic corticosteroids are prescribed for such conditions as uveitis or giant cell arteritis.

4. Contaminated Eye Medications

Ophthalmic solutions are prepared with the same degree of care as fluids intended for intravenous administration, but once bottles are opened there is always a risk of contamination, particularly with solutions of tetracaine, proparacaine, fluorescein, and any preservative-free preparations. Single-use fluorescein eye drops or sterile fluorescein filter paper strips are recommended for use in place of multiple-use fluorescein solutions.

Whether in plastic or glass containers, eye solutions should not remain in use for long periods after the bottle is opened. Four weeks after opening is the usual maximum time for use of a solution containing preservatives before discarding. Preservative-free preparations should be kept refrigerated and usually discarded within 1 week after opening. Single-use products should not be reused.

If the eye has been injured by accident or by surgical trauma, it is of the greatest importance to use freshly opened bottles of sterile medications or single-use products.

5. Toxic & Hypersensitivity Reactions to Topical Therapy

In patients receiving long-term topical therapy, local toxic or hypersensitivity reactions to the active agent or preservatives may develop (Figure 7–7), especially if there is inadequate tear secretion. Preservatives in contact lens cleaning solutions may produce similar problems. Burning and soreness are exacerbated by drop instillation or contact lens insertion; occasionally, fibrosis and scarring of the conjunctiva and cornea may occur. Preservative-free topical medications, increasingly used in the treatment of glaucoma, and preservative-free contact lens solutions are available.

An antibiotic instilled into the eye can sensitize the patient to that drug and cause an allergic reaction upon subsequent systemic administration. Potentially fatal

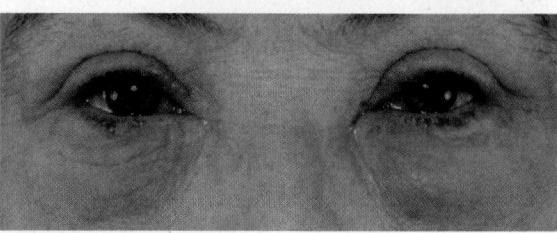

▲ **Figure 7–7.** Periocular contact dermatitis due to eye drop preservative.

anaphylaxis is known to occur in up to 0.3% of patients after intravenous fluorescein for fluorescein angiography. Anaphylaxis also has been reported after topical fluorescein.

6. Systemic Effects of Ocular Drugs

The systemic absorption of certain topical drugs (through the conjunctival vessels and lacrimal drainage system) must be considered when there is a systemic medical contraindication to the use of the drug. Ophthalmic solutions of the nonselective beta-blockers, eg, timolol, may worsen bradycardia, heart failure, or asthma. Phenylephrine eye drops may precipitate hypertensive crises and angina. Adverse interactions between systemically administered and ocular drugs should also be considered. Using only 1 or 2 drops at a time and a few minutes of nasolacrimal occlusion or eyelid closure ensures maximum ocular efficacy and decreases systemic side effects of topical agents.

ADVERSE OCULAR EFFECTS OF SYSTEMIC DRUGS

Systemically administered drugs produce a wide variety of adverse effects on the visual system. Table 7–3 lists the major examples. The likelihood of most complications is rare, but if visual changes develop while the patient is being treated with these medications, the patient should be referred to an eye care professional for an eye examination. Repeated screening for toxic retinopathy is recommended

Table 7–3. Adverse ophthalmic effects of systemic drugs.

Drug	Possible Side Effects
Ophthalmic drugs	
Carbonic anhydrase inhibitors (eg, acetazolamide, methazolamide)	Epidermal necrolysis, nearsightedness, angle-closure glaucoma due to ciliary body swelling, hypokalemia, aplastic anemia
Respiratory drugs	
Anticholinergic bronchodilators (eg, ipratropium)	Angle-closure glaucoma due to mydriasis, blurring of vision due to cycloplegia, dry eyes
Oxygen delivery to preterm infants < 36 weeks	Retinopathy of prematurity
Sympathomimetic bronchodilators (eg, salbutamol) and decongestants (eg, ephedrine)	Angle-closure glaucoma due to mydriasis

(continued)

Table 7–3. Adverse ophthalmic effects of systemic drugs. (continued)

Drug	Possible Side Effects
Cardiovascular system drugs	
Amiodarone	Corneal deposits (vortex keratopathy), optic neuropathy, thyroid eye disease
Amlodipine	Chemosis (conjunctival edema)
Anticoagulants	Conjunctival, retinal and vitreous hemorrhage Warfarin taken during pregnancy may cause fetal facial deformity with nasolacrimal duct obstruction, microphthalmos, cataract, optic atrophy
Chlorthalidone	Angle-closure glaucoma due to ciliary body swelling
Digitalis	Disturbance of color vision, photopsia
Furosemide	Angle-closure glaucoma due to ciliary body swelling
Phosphodiesterase type 5 inhibitors (eg, sildenafil, tadalafil, vardenafil)	Disturbance of color vision, ischemic optic neuropathy
Statins	Extraocular muscle palsy (myasthenic syndrome)
Thiazides (eg, indapamide)	Angle-closure glaucoma due to ciliary body swelling, nearsightedness, xanthopsia (yellow vision)
Gastrointestinal drugs	
Anticholinergic agents	Angle-closure glaucoma due to mydriasis, blurring of vision due to cycloplegia, dry eyes
Urinary tract drugs	
Alpha-2-antagonists (eg, alfuzosin, doxazosin, prazosin, tamsulosin, terazosin, silodosin)	Complications during (floppy iris syndrome) and after cataract surgery
Anticholinergic agents	Angle-closure glaucoma due to mydriasis, blurring of vision due to cycloplegia, dry eyes
Finasteride	Complications during (floppy iris syndrome) and after cataract surgery
Central nervous system drugs	
Amphetamines	Widening of palpebral fissure, blurring of vision due to mydriasis, elevated intraocular pressure
Anticholinergic agents including preoperative medications	Angle-closure glaucoma due to mydriasis, blurring of vision due to cycloplegia, dry eyes
Aripiprazole	Nearsightedness
Diazepam	Nystagmus
Haloperidol	Capsular cataract
Lithium carbonate	Proptosis, oculogyric crisis, nystagmus
Monoamine oxidase inhibitors	Nystagmus
Morphine	Miosis
Neostigmine	Nystagmus, miosis
Olanzapine	Angle-closure glaucoma due to mydriasis
Phenothiazines (eg, chlorpromazine)	Pigmentary deposits in conjunctiva, cornea, lens, and retina, oculogyric crisis Chlorpromazine causes complications during (floppy iris syndrome) and after cataract surgery
Phenytoin	Nystagmus
Quetiapine	Complications during (floppy iris syndrome) and after cataract surgery
Retigabine	Ocular pigmentation and retinopathy
Risperidone, paliperidone	Complications during (floppy iris syndrome) and after cataract surgery
Selective serotonin reuptake inhibitors (SSRIs) (eg, paroxetine, sertraline)	Angle-closure glaucoma, optic neuropathy
Serotonin and noradrenaline reuptake inhibitors (eg, venlafaxine)	Angle-closure glaucoma
Thioridazine	Corneal and lens deposits, retinopathy, oculogyric crisis

(continued)

Table 7–3. Adverse ophthalmic effects of systemic drugs. (continued)

Drug	Possible Side Effects
Topiramate	Angle-closure glaucoma due to ciliary body swelling, nearsightedness, macular folds, anterior uveitis
Tricyclic agents (eg, imipramine)	Angle-closure glaucoma due to mydriasis, blurring of vision due to cycloplegia
Triptans (sumatriptan, zolmitriptan)	Angle-closure glaucoma due to ciliary body swelling, nearsightedness
Vigabatrin	Visual field constriction
Zonisamide	Angle-closure glaucoma due to ciliary body swelling, nearsightedness
Obstetric drugs	
Sympathomimetic tocolytics	Angle-closure glaucoma due to mydriasis
Hormonal agents	
Aromatase inhibitors (eg, anastozole)	Dry eye, vitreo-retinal traction, retinal hemorrhages
Cabergoline	Angle-closure glaucoma
Female sex hormones	Retinal artery occlusion, retinal vein occlusion, papilledema, cranial nerve palsies, ischemic optic neuropathy
Tamoxifen	Crystalline retinal and corneal deposits, altered color perception, cataract, optic neuropathy
Immunomodulators	
Alpha-interferon	Retinopathy, keratoconjunctivitis, dry eyes, optic neuropathy
Corticosteroids	Cataract (posterior subcapsular); susceptibility to viral (herpes simplex), bacterial, and fungal infections; steroid-induced glaucoma
Cyclosporine	Posterior reversible leukoencephalopathy
Fingolimod	Macular edema
Tacrolimus	Optic neuropathy, posterior reversible leukoencephalopathy
Antibiotics	
Chloramphenicol	Optic neuropathy
Clofazimine	Crystalline deposits (conjunctiva, cornea, iris)
Ethambutol	Optic neuropathy
Fluoroquinolones	Diplopia, retinal detachment
Isoniazid	Optic neuropathy
Linezolid	Optic neuropathy
Rifabutin	Uveitis
Streptomycin	Optic neuropathy, epidermal necrolysis
Sulfonamides	Epidermal necrolysis, nearsightedness, angle-closure glaucoma due to ciliary body swelling
Tetracycline, doxycycline, minocycline	Papilledema
Antivirals	
Cidofovir	Uveitis
Antimalarial agents	
Chloroquine, hydroxychloroquine	Retinal degeneration principally involving the macula, keratopathy
Quinine	Retinal toxicity, pupillary abnormalities
Amebicides	
Iodochlorhydroxyquin	Optic neuropathy
Chemotherapeutic agents	
Bortezomib	Chalazia
Chlorambucil	Optic neuropathy
Cisplatin	Optic neuropathy

(continued)

Table 7–3. Adverse ophthalmic effects of systemic drugs. (continued)

Drug	Possible Side Effects
Docetaxel	Lacrimal (canalicular) obstruction
Fluorouracil	Lacrimal (canalicular) obstruction
MEK inhibitors: trametinib, selumetinib, cobimetinib, pimasertib	Multifocal serous retinal detachment, retinal vein occlusion, cystoid macular edema
Vincristine	Optic neuropathy
Chelating agents	
Deferoxamine, deferasirox	Retinopathy, optic neuropathy, lens opacity
Penicillamine	Ocular pemphigoid, optic neuropathy, extraocular muscle palsy (myasthenic syndrome)
Oral hypoglycemic agents	
Chlorpropamide	Refractive error, epidermal necrolysis, optic neuropathy
Thiazolidinediones (glitazones)	Increase in diabetic macular edema
Vitamins	
Vitamin A	Papilledema
Vitamin D	Band-shaped keratopathy
Antirheumatic agents	
Allopurinol	Epidermal necrolysis
Chloroquine, hydroxychloroquine	Retinal degeneration principally involving the macula, vortex keratopathy
Gold salts	Deposits in the cornea, conjunctiva, and lens
Nonsteroidal anti-inflammatory drugs (NSAIDs) (eg, ibuprofen, naproxen, indomethacin)	Vortex keratopathy (ibuprofen, naproxen), corneal deposits (indomethacin), retinal degeneration principally involving the macula (indomethacin)
Penicillamine	Ocular pemphigoid, optic neuropathy, extraocular muscle palsy (myasthenic syndrome)
Phenylbutazone	Retinal hemorrhages
Salicylates	Subconjunctival and retinal hemorrhages, nystagmus
Dermatologic agents	
Retinoids (eg, isotretinoin, tretinoin, acitretin, and etretinate)	Papilledema, blepharoconjunctivitis, corneal opacities, decreased contact lens tolerance, decreased dark adaptation, teratogenic ocular abnormalities
Bisphosphonates	
Alendronate, pamidronate	Scleritis, episcleritis, uveitis

in patients receiving long-term chloroquine or hydroxychloroquine therapy. If no baseline abnormalities are present, screening should be repeated annually beginning after 5 years. More frequent screening is necessary in patients treated with doses greater than 5.0 mg/kg real weight/day of hydroxychloroquine or greater than 2.3 mg/kg/day of chloroquine, or in patients with kidney disease or in those taking tamoxifen. Patients receiving long-term systemic corticosteroids are at increased risk for several ocular complications, including glaucoma, cataract, and central serous retinopathy. They should be referred to an eye care professional for an eye examination at baseline before starting corticosteroids and at any time if reduced or blurry vision develops. It is important that an ophthalmologist is made aware before cataract surgery that a patient is taking a medication associated with floppy iris syndrome because the medication can make cataract surgery more challenging.

The chemotherapeutic MEK inhibitors are associated with ocular complications including serous retinal detachment, cystoid macular edema, and retinal vein occlusion. Patients receiving MEK inhibitors should have a complete eye examination at baseline before the initiation of these medications, and should be referred for an eye examination if blurred or reduced vision develops while taking MEK inhibitors.

Alves C et al. Risk of ophthalmic adverse effects in patients treated with MEK inhibitors: a systematic review and meta-analysis. Ophthalmic Res. 2017;57(1):60–9. [PMID: 27404571]

Chatziralli IP et al. Risk factors for intraoperative floppy iris syndrome: a prospective study. Eye (Lond). 2016 Aug; 30(8):1039–44. [PMID: 27367744]

Fraunfelder FW et al. Ocular & systemic side effects of drugs. In: Riordan-Eva P, Augsburger JJ. *Vaughan & Asbury's General Ophthalmology*, 19th ed. McGraw-Hill, 2018.

Raizman MB et al. Drug-induced corneal epithelial changes. Surv Ophthalmol. 2017 May–Jun;62(3):286–301. [PMID: 27890620]

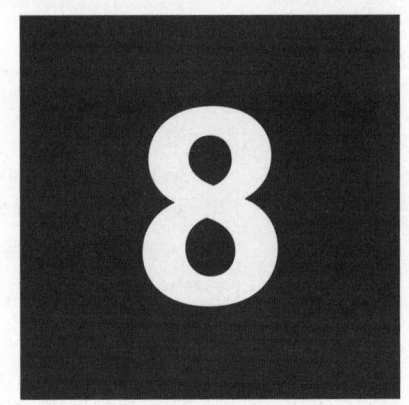

Ear, Nose, & Throat Disorders

Lawrence R. Lustig, MD

Joshua S. Schindler, MD

DISEASES OF THE EAR

HEARING LOSS

 ESSENTIALS OF DIAGNOSIS

► Two main types of hearing loss: conductive and sensorineural.

► Most commonly due to cerumen impaction, transient eustachian tube dysfunction from upper respiratory tract infection, or age-related hearing loss.

Classification & Epidemiology

Table 8–1 categorizes hearing loss as normal, mild, moderate, severe, and profound and outlines the vocal equivalent as well as the decibel range.

A. Conductive Hearing Loss

Conductive hearing loss results from external or middle ear dysfunction. Four mechanisms each result in impairment of the passage of sound vibrations to the inner ear: (1) obstruction (eg, cerumen impaction), (2) mass loading (eg, middle ear effusion), (3) stiffness (eg, otosclerosis), and (4) discontinuity (eg, ossicular disruption). Conductive losses in adults are most commonly due to cerumen impaction or transient eustachian tube dysfunction from upper respiratory tract infection. Persistent conductive losses usually result from chronic ear infection, trauma, or otosclerosis. Conductive hearing loss is often correctable with medical or surgical therapy, or both.

B. Sensorineural Hearing Loss

Sensory and neural causes of hearing loss are difficult to differentiate due to testing methodology, thus often referred to as "sensorineural." Sensorineural hearing losses are common in adults.

Sensory hearing loss results from deterioration of the cochlea, usually due to loss of hair cells from the organ of Corti. The most common form is a gradually progressive, predominantly high-frequency loss with advancing age (presbyacusis); other causes include excessive noise exposure, head trauma, and systemic diseases. Sensory hearing loss is usually not correctable with medical or surgical therapy but often may be prevented or stabilized. An exception is a sudden sensory hearing loss, which may respond to corticosteroids if delivered within several weeks of onset.

Neural hearing loss lesions involve the eighth cranial nerve, auditory nuclei, ascending tracts, or auditory cortex. Neural hearing loss is much less commonly recognized. Causes include acoustic neuroma, multiple sclerosis, and auditory neuropathy.

Cunningham LL et al. Hearing loss in adults. N Engl J Med. 2017 Dec 21;377(25):2465–73. [PMID: 29262274]

Kaga K. Auditory nerve disease and auditory neuropathy spectrum disorders. Auris Nasus Larynx. 2016 Feb;43(1): 10–20. [PMID: 26209259]

Roberts B et al. What can 35 years and over 700,000 measurements tell us about noise exposure in the mining industry? Int J Audiol. 2016 Nov 22:1–9. [PMID: 27871188]

Evaluation of Hearing (Audiology)

In a quiet room, the hearing level may be estimated by having the patient repeat aloud words presented in a soft whisper, a normal spoken voice, or a shout. A 512-Hz tuning fork is useful in differentiating conductive from sensorineural losses. In the **Weber test,** the tuning fork is placed on the forehead or front teeth. In conductive losses, the sound appears louder in the poorer-hearing ear, whereas in sensorineural losses it radiates to the better side. In the **Rinne test,** the tuning fork is placed alternately on the mastoid bone and in front of the ear canal. In conductive losses greater than 25 dB, bone conduction exceeds air conduction; in sensorineural losses, the opposite is true.

Formal audiometric studies are performed in a soundproofed room. Pure-tone thresholds in decibels (dB) are obtained over the range of 250–8000 Hz for both air and bone conduction. Conductive losses create a gap between

Table 8–1. Hearing loss classification.

Classification	Vocal Equivalent	Decibel (dB) Range
Normal	Soft whisper	0–20 dB
Mild	Soft spoken voice	20–40 dB
Moderate	Normal spoken voice	40–60 dB
Severe	Loud spoken voice	60–80 dB
Profound	Shout	> 80 dB

the air and bone thresholds, whereas in sensorineural losses, both air and bone thresholds are equally diminished. Speech discrimination measures the clarity of hearing, reported as percentage correct (90–100% is normal). Auditory brainstem-evoked responses may determine whether the lesion is sensory (cochlea) or neural (central). However, MRI scanning is more sensitive and specific in detecting central lesions.

Every patient who complains of a hearing loss should be referred for audiologic evaluation unless the cause is easily remediable (eg, cerumen impaction, otitis media). Immediate audiometric referral is indicated for patients with idiopathic sudden sensorineural hearing loss because it requires treatment (corticosteroids) within a limited several-week time period. Routine audiologic screening is recommended for adults with prior exposure to potentially injurious noise levels of noise or in adults at age 65, and every few years thereafter.

Musiek FE et al. Perspectives on the pure-tone audiogram. J Am Acad Audiol. 2017 Jul/Aug;28(7):655–71. [PMID: 28722648]

Phan NT et al. Diagnosis and management of hearing loss in elderly patients. Aust Fam Physician. 2016 Jun;45(6):366–9. [PMID: 27622223]

▶ **Hearing Amplification**

Patients with hearing loss not correctable by medical therapy may benefit from hearing amplification. Contemporary hearing aids are comparatively free of distortion and have been miniaturized to the point where they often may be contained entirely within the ear canal or lie inconspicuously behind the ear.

For patients with conductive loss or unilateral profound sensorineural loss, bone-conducting hearing aids directly stimulate the ipsilateral cochlea (for conductive losses) or contralateral ear (profound unilateral sensorineural loss).

In most adults with severe to profound sensory hearing loss, the cochlear implant—an electronic device that is surgically implanted into the cochlea to stimulate the auditory nerve—offers socially beneficial auditory rehabilitation.

Barker F et al. Interventions to improve hearing aid use in adult auditory rehabilitation. Cochrane Database Syst Rev. 2016 Aug 18;(8):CD010342. [PMID: 27537242]

Johnson CE et al. Benefits from, satisfaction with, and self-efficacy for advanced digital hearing aids in users with mild sensorineural hearing loss. Semin Hear. 2018 May;39(2):158–71. [PMID: 29915453]

McRackan TR et al. Meta-analysis of quality-of-life improvement after cochlear implantation and associations with speech recognition abilities. Laryngoscope. 2018 Apr;128(4):982–990. [PMID: 28731538]

Michaud HN et al. Aural rehabilitation for older adults with hearing loss: impacts on quality of life—a systematic review of randomized controlled trials. J Am Acad Audiol. 2017 Jul/Aug;28(7):596–609. [PMID: 28722643]

DISEASES OF THE AURICLE

Disorders of the auricle include skin cancers due to sun exposure. Traumatic auricular hematoma must be drained to prevent significant cosmetic deformity (cauliflower ear) or canal blockage resulting from dissolution of supporting cartilage. Similarly, cellulitis of the auricle must be treated promptly to prevent perichondritis and resultant deformity. Relapsing polychondritis is characterized by recurrent, frequently bilateral, painful episodes of auricular erythema and edema and sometimes progressive involvement of the cartilaginous tracheobronchial tree. Treatment with corticosteroids may help forestall cartilage dissolution. Polychondritis and perichondritis may be differentiated from cellulitis by sparing of involvement of the lobule, which does not contain cartilage.

Shakeel M et al. Open surgical management of auricular haematoma: incision, evacuation and mattress sutures. J Laryngol Otol. 2015 May;129(5):496–501. [PMID: 25994384]

DISEASES OF THE EAR CANAL

1. Cerumen Impaction

Cerumen is a protective secretion produced by the outer portion of the ear canal. In most persons, the ear canal is self-cleansing. Recommended hygiene consists of cleaning the external opening only with a washcloth over the index finger. Cerumen impaction is most often self-induced through ill-advised cleansing attempts by entering the canal itself. It may be relieved by the patient using detergent ear drops (eg, 3% hydrogen peroxide; 6.5% carbamide peroxide) and irrigation, or by the clinician using mechanical removal, suction, or irrigation. Irrigation is performed with water at body temperature to avoid a vestibular caloric response. The stream should be directed at the posterior ear canal wall adjacent to the cerumen plug. Irrigation should be performed only when the tympanic membrane is known to be intact.

Use of jet irrigators (eg, WaterPik) should be avoided since they may result in tympanic membrane perforations. Following irrigation, the ear canal should be thoroughly dried (eg, by the patient using a hair blow-dryer on low-power setting or by the clinician instilling isopropyl alcohol) to reduce the likelihood of external otitis. Specialty referral is indicated if impaction is frequently recurrent, if it has not responded to routine measures, or if there is tympanic membrane perforation or chronic otitis media.

Schwartz SR et al. Clinical Practice Guideline (Update): Earwax (cerumen impaction). Otolaryngol Head Neck Surg. 2017 Jan;156(1 Suppl):S1–29. [PMID: 28045591]

2. Foreign Bodies

Foreign bodies in the ear canal are more frequent in children than in adults. Firm materials may be removed with a loop or a hook, taking care not to displace the object medially toward the tympanic membrane; microscopic guidance is helpful. Aqueous irrigation should not be performed for organic foreign bodies (eg, beans, insects), because water may cause them to swell. Living insects are best immobilized before removal by filling the ear canal with lidocaine.

Friedman EM. Videos in clinical medicine. Removal of foreign bodies from the ear and nose. N Engl J Med. 2016 Feb 18; 374(7):e7. [PMID: 26886547]

Karimnejad K et al. External auditory canal foreign body extraction outcomes. Ann Otol Rhinol Laryngol. 2017 Nov;126(11): 755–61. [PMID: 28954532]

Shunyu NB et al. Ear, nose and throat foreign bodies removed under general anaesthesia: a retrospective study. J Clin Diagn Res. 2017 Feb;11(2):MC01–4. [PMID: 28384894]

3. External Otitis

ESSENTIALS OF DIAGNOSIS

▶ Painful erythema and edema of the ear canal skin.

▶ Purulent exudate.

▶ In diabetic or immunocompromised patients, osteomyelitis of the skull base ("malignant external otitis") may occur.

▶ General Considerations

External otitis presents with otalgia, frequently accompanied by pruritus and purulent discharge. There is often a history of recent water exposure (ie, swimmer's ear) or mechanical trauma (eg, scratching, cotton applicators). External otitis is usually caused by gram-negative rods (eg, *Pseudomonas, Proteus*) or fungi (eg, *Aspergillus*), which grow in the presence of excessive moisture. In diabetic or immunocompromised patients, persistent external otitis may evolve into osteomyelitis of the skull base (so-called malignant external otitis). Usually caused by *Pseudomonas aeruginosa*, osteomyelitis begins in the floor of the ear canal and may extend into the middle fossa floor, the clivus, and even the contralateral skull base.

▶ Clinical Findings

Examination reveals erythema and edema of the ear canal skin, often with a purulent exudate (Figure 8–1). Manipulation of the auricle elicits pain. Because the lateral surface of the tympanic membrane is ear canal skin, it is often erythematous. However, in contrast to acute otitis media, it moves normally with pneumatic otoscopy. When the canal skin is very edematous, it may be impossible to visualize the tympanic membrane. Malignant external otitis typically presents with persistent foul aural discharge, granulations in the ear canal, deep otalgia, and in advanced cases, progressive palsies of cranial nerves VI, VII, IX, X, XI, or XII.

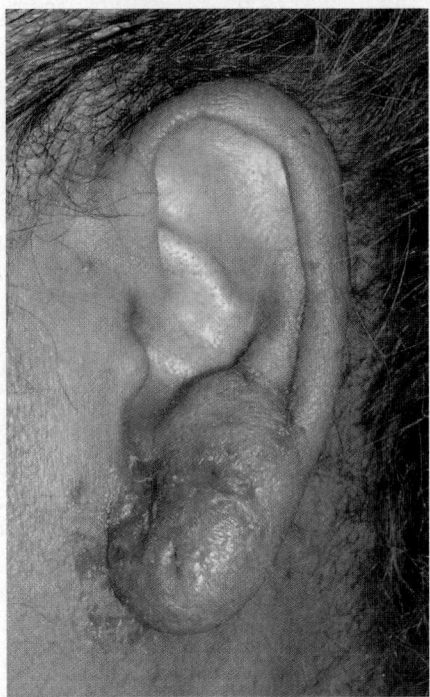

▲ **Figure 8–1.** Malignant external otitis in a 40-year-old woman with diabetes mellitus, with typical swelling and honey-colored crusting of the pinna. Both the external auditory canal and temporal bone were involved in the pseudomonal infection. (Used, with permission, from E.J. Mayeaux Jr, MD, in Usatine RP, Smith MA, Mayeaux EJ Jr, Chumley H. *The Color Atlas of Family Medicine*, 2nd ed. McGraw-Hill, 2013.)

Diagnosis is confirmed by the demonstration of osseous erosion on CT scanning.

▶ Treatment

Treatment of external otitis involves protection of the ear from additional moisture and avoidance of further mechanical injury by scratching. In cases of moisture in the ear (eg, swimmer's ear), acidification with a drying agent (ie, a 50/50 mixture of isopropyl alcohol/white vinegar) is often helpful. When infected, an otic antibiotic solution or suspension of an aminoglycoside (eg, neomycin/polymyxin B) or fluoroquinolone (eg, ciprofloxacin), with or without a corticosteroid (eg, hydrocortisone), is usually effective. Purulent debris filling the ear canal should be gently removed to permit entry of the topical medication. Drops should be used abundantly (five or more drops three or four times a day) to penetrate the depths of the canal. When substantial edema of the canal wall prevents entry of drops into the ear canal, a wick is placed to facilitate their entry. In recalcitrant cases—particularly when cellulitis of the periauricular tissue has developed—oral fluoroquinolones (eg, ciprofloxacin, 500 mg twice daily for 1 week) are used because of their effectiveness against *Pseudomonas*. Any case of persistent otitis externa in an immunocompromised or diabetic individual must be referred for specialty evaluation.

Treatment of "malignant external otitis" requires prolonged antipseudomonal antibiotic administration, often for several months. Although intravenous therapy is often required initially (eg, ciprofloxacin 200–400 mg every 12 hours), selected patients may be graduated to oral ciprofloxacin (500–1000 mg twice daily). To avoid relapse, antibiotic therapy should be continued, even in the asymptomatic patient, until gallium scanning indicates marked reduction or resolution of the inflammation. Surgical debridement of infected bone is reserved for cases of deterioration despite medical therapy.

Chawdhary G et al. Current management of necrotising otitis externa in the UK: survey of 221 UK otolaryngologists. Acta Otolaryngol. 2017 Aug;137(8):818–22. [PMID: 28301961]

Peled C et al. Necrotizing otitis externa-analysis of 83 cases: clinical findings and course of disease. Otol Neurotol. 2019 Jan;40(1):56–62. [PMID: 30239427]

Wang X et al. Use of systemic antibiotics for acute otitis externa: impact of a clinical practice guideline. Otol Neurotol. 2018 Oct;39(9):1088–94. [PMID: 30124617]

4. Pruritus

Pruritus of the external auditory canal, particularly at the meatus, is common. While it may be associated with external otitis or with seborrheic dermatitis or psoriasis, most cases are self-induced from excoriation or overly zealous ear cleaning. To permit regeneration of the protective cerumen blanket, patients should be instructed to avoid use of soap and water or cotton swabs in the ear canal and avoid any scratching. Patients with excessively dry canal skin may benefit from application of mineral oil, which helps counteract dryness and repel moisture. When an inflammatory component is present, topical application of a corticosteroid (eg, 0.1% triamcinolone) may be beneficial.

Babakurban ST et al. Therapeutic effect of Castellani's paint in patients with an itchy ear canal. J Laryngol Otol. 2016 Oct; 130(10):934–8. [PMID: 27774921]

5. Exostoses & Osteomas

Bony overgrowths of the ear canal are a frequent incidental finding and occasionally have clinical significance. Clinically, they present as skin-covered bony mounds in the medial ear canal obscuring the tympanic membrane to a variable degree. Solitary osteomas are of no significance as long as they do not cause obstruction or infection. Multiple exostoses, which are generally acquired from repeated exposure to cold water (eg, "surfer's ear"), may progress and require surgical removal.

Grinblat G et al. Outcomes of drill canalplasty in exostoses and osteoma: analysis of 256 cases and literature review. Otol Neurotol. 2016 Dec;37(10):1565–72. [PMID: 27755370]

Kim SH. Exostoses of the external auditory canals. Br J Hosp Med (Lond). 2017 Mar 2;78(3):174. [PMID: 28277770]

Morris S et al. Awareness and attitudes towards external auditory canal exostosis and its preventability in surfers in the UK: cross-sectional study. J Laryngol Otol. 2016 Jul;130(7):628–34. [PMID: 2726234]

6. Neoplasia

The most common neoplasm of the ear canal is squamous cell carcinoma. When an apparent otitis externa does not resolve on therapy, a malignancy should be suspected and biopsy performed. This disease carries a very high 5-year mortality rate because the tumor tends to invade the lymphatics of the cranial base and must be treated with wide surgical resection and radiation therapy. Adenomatous tumors, originating from the ceruminous glands, generally follow a more indolent course.

Mazzoni A et al. En bloc temporal bone resections in squamous cell carcinoma of the ear. Technique, principles, and limits. Acta Otolaryngol. 2016;136(5):425–32. [PMID: 26824405]

Oya R et al. Surgery with or without postoperative radiation therapy for early-stage external auditory canal squamous cell carcinoma: a meta-analysis. Otol Neurotol. 2017 Oct; 38(9):1333–8. [PMID: 28796084]

Wang Z et al. The contribution of CT and MRI in staging, treatment planning and prognosis prediction of malignant tumors of external auditory canal. Clin Imaging. 2016 Nov–Dec; 40(6):1262–8. [PMID: 27639864]

DISEASES OF THE EUSTACHIAN TUBE

1. Eustachian Tube Dysfunction

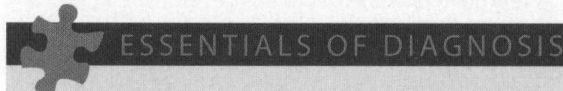

ESSENTIALS OF DIAGNOSIS

► Aural fullness.

► Fluctuating hearing.

► Discomfort with barometric pressure change.

► At risk for serous otitis media.

The tube that connects the middle ear to the nasopharynx—the eustachian tube—provides ventilation and drainage for the middle ear cleft. It is normally closed, opening only during swallowing or yawning. When eustachian tube function is compromised, air trapped within the middle ear becomes absorbed and negative pressure results. The most common causes of eustachian tube dysfunction are diseases associated with edema of the tubal lining, such as viral upper respiratory tract infections and allergy. The patient usually reports a sense of fullness in the ear and mild to moderate impairment of hearing. When the tube is only partially blocked, swallowing or yawning may elicit a popping or crackling sound. Examination may reveal retraction of the tympanic membrane and decreased mobility on pneumatic otoscopy. Following a viral illness, this disorder is usually transient, lasting days to weeks. Treatment with systemic and intranasal decongestants (eg, pseudoephedrine, 60 mg orally every 4–6 hours; oxymetazoline, 0.05% spray every 8–12 hours) combined with autoinflation by forced exhalation against closed nostrils may hasten relief. Autoinflation should not be recommended to patients with active intranasal infection, since this maneuver may precipitate middle ear infection.

Allergic patients may also benefit from intranasal cortico-steroids (eg, beclomethasone dipropionate, two sprays in each nostril twice daily for 2–6 weeks). Air travel, rapid altitudinal change, and underwater diving should be avoided until resolution.

Conversely, an overly patent eustachian tube ("patu-lous eustachian tube") is a relatively uncommon, though quite distressing problem. Typical complaints include full-ness in the ear and autophony, an exaggerated ability to hear oneself breathe and speak. A patulous eustachian tube may develop during rapid weight loss, or it may be idiopathic. In contrast to eustachian tube dysfunction, the aural pressure is often made worse by exertion and may diminish during an upper respiratory tract infection. Although physical examination is usually normal, respira-tory excursions of the tympanic membrane may occasion-ally be detected during vigorous breathing. Treatment includes avoidance of decongestant products, insertion of a ventilating tube to reduce the outward stretch of the eardrum during phonation, and rarely, surgery on the eustachian tube itself.

Huisman JML et al. Treatment of eustachian tube dysfunction with balloon dilation: a systematic review. Laryngoscope. 2018 Jan;128(1):237–47. [PMID: 28799657]

Meyer TA et al. A randomized controlled trial of balloon dilation as a treatment for persistent Eustachian tube dysfunction with 1-year follow-up. Otol Neurotol. 2018 Aug;39(7):894–902. [PMID: 29912819]

Ward BK et al. Patulous eustachian tube dysfunction: patient demographics and comorbidities. Otol Neurotol. 2017 Oct; 38(9):1362–9. [PMID: 28796094]

2. Serous Otitis Media

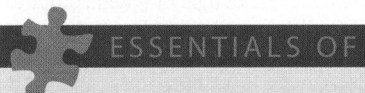

ESSENTIALS OF DIAGNOSIS

▶ Eustachian tube remains blocked for a prolonged period.

▶ Resultant negative pressure results in transudation of fluid.

Prolonged eustachian tube dysfunction with resultant negative middle ear pressure may cause a transudation of fluid. In adults, serous otitis media usually occurs with an upper respiratory tract infection, with barotrauma, or with chronic allergic rhinitis, but when persistent and unilateral, nasopharyngeal carcinoma must be excluded. The tym-panic membrane is dull and hypomobile, occasionally accompanied by air bubbles in the middle ear and conduc-tive hearing loss. The treatment of serous otitis media is similar to that for eustachian tube dysfunction. When medication fails to bring relief after several months, a ven-tilating tube placed through the tympanic membrane may restore hearing and alleviate the sense of aural fullness. Endoscopically guided laser expansion of the nasopharyn-geal orifice of the eustachian tube or balloon dilation may improve function in recalcitrant cases.

Roditi RE et al. Otitis media with effusion: our national practice. Otolaryngol Head Neck Surg. 2017 Aug;157(2):171–2. [PMID: 28535139]

Schilder AG et al. Otitis media. Nat Rev Dis Primers. 2016 Sep 8;2: 16063. [PMID: 27604644]

3. Barotrauma

Persons with poor eustachian tube function (eg, congeni-tal narrowness or acquired mucosal edema) may be unable to equalize the barometric stress exerted on the middle ear by air travel, rapid altitudinal change, or underwater diving. The problem is generally most acute during airplane descent, since the negative middle ear pressure tends to collapse and block the eustachian tube, causing pain. Several measures are useful to enhance eustachian tube function and avoid otic barotrauma. The patient should be advised to swallow, yawn, and auto-inflate frequently during descent. Oral decongestants (eg, pseudoephedrine, 60–120 mg) should be taken several hours before anticipated arrival time so that they will be maximally effective during descent. Topical decongestants such as 1% phenylephrine nasal spray should be adminis-tered 1 hour before arrival.

For acute negative middle ear pressure that persists on the ground, treatment includes decongestants and attempts at autoinflation. Myringotomy (creation of a small eardrum perforation) provides immediate relief and is appropriate in the setting of severe otalgia and hearing loss. Repeated epi-sodes of barotrauma in persons who must fly frequently may be alleviated by insertion of ventilating tubes.

Underwater diving may represent an even greater baro-metric stress to the ear than flying. Patients should be warned to avoid diving when they have an upper respira-tory infection or episode of nasal allergy. During the descent phase of the dive, if inflation of the middle ear via the eustachian tube has not occurred, pain will develop within the first 15 feet; the dive must be aborted. In all cases, divers must descend slowly and equilibrate in stages to avoid the development of severely negative pressures in the tympanum that may result in hemorrhage (hemo-tympanum) or in perilymphatic fistula. In the latter, the oval or round window ruptures, resulting in sensory hearing loss and acute vertigo. During the ascent phase of a saturation dive, sensory hearing loss or vertigo may develop as the first (or only) symptom of decompression sickness. Immediate recompression will return intravascu-lar gas bubbles to solution and restore the inner ear microcirculation.

Tympanic membrane perforation is an absolute contra-indication to diving, as the patient will experience an unbal-anced thermal stimulus to the semicircular canals and may experience vertigo, disorientation, and even emesis.

Rozycki SW et al. Inner ear barotrauma in divers: an evidence-based tool for evaluation and treatment. Diving Hyperb Med. 2018 Sep 30;48(3):186–93. [PMID: 30199891]

Ryan P et al. Prevention of otic barotrauma in aviation: a system-atic review. Otol Neurotol. 2018 Jun;39(5):539–49. [PMID: 29595579]

DISEASES OF THE MIDDLE EAR

1. Acute Otitis Media

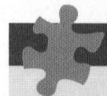

▶ Otalgia, often with an upper respiratory tract infection.

▶ Erythema and hypomobility of tympanic membrane.

General Considerations

Acute otitis media is a bacterial infection of the mucosally lined air-containing spaces of the temporal bone. Purulent material forms not only within the middle ear cleft but also within the pneumatized mastoid air cells and petrous apex. Acute otitis media is usually precipitated by a viral upper respiratory tract infection that causes eustachian tube obstruction. This results in accumulation of fluid and mucus, which becomes secondarily infected by bacteria. The most common pathogens are *Streptococcus pneumoniae,* *Haemophilus influenzae,* and *Streptococcus pyogenes.*

Clinical Findings

Acute otitis media may occur at any age. Presenting symptoms and signs include otalgia, aural pressure, decreased hearing, and often fever. The typical physical findings are erythema and decreased mobility of the tympanic membrane (Figure 8–2). Occasionally, bullae will appear on the tympanic membrane.

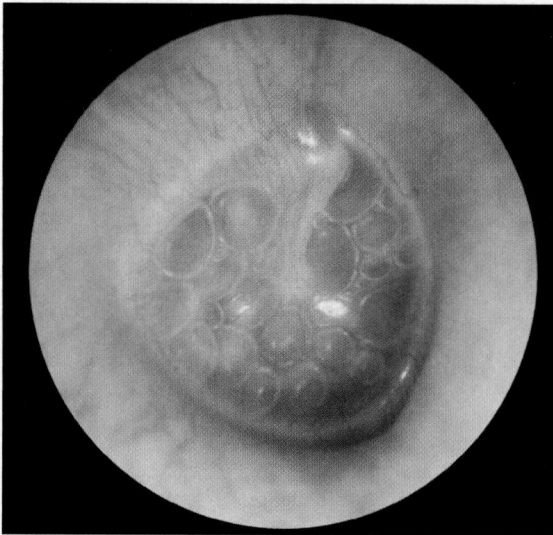

▲ **Figure 8–2.** Acute otitis media with effusion of right ear, with multiple air-fluid levels visible through a translucent, slightly retracted, nonerythematous tympanic membrane. (Used, with permission, from Frank Miller, MD, in Usatine RP, Smith MA, Mayeaux EJ Jr, Chumley H. *The Color Atlas of Family Medicine,* 2nd ed. McGraw-Hill, 2013.)

Rarely, when middle ear empyema is severe, the tympanic membrane bulges outward. In such cases, tympanic membrane rupture is imminent. Rupture is accompanied by a sudden decrease in pain, followed by the onset of otorrhea. With appropriate therapy, spontaneous healing of the tympanic membrane occurs in most cases. When perforation persists, chronic otitis media may develop. Mastoid tenderness often accompanies acute otitis media and is due to the presence of pus within the mastoid air cells. This alone does not indicate suppurative (surgical) mastoiditis. Frank swelling over the mastoid bone or the association of cranial neuropathies or central findings indicates severe disease requiring urgent care.

Treatment

The treatment of acute otitis media is specific antibiotic therapy, often combined with nasal decongestants. The first-choice oral antibiotic treatment is amoxicillin (80–90 mg/kg/day divided twice daily) (*or* erythromycin [50 mg/kg/day]) plus sulfonamide (150 mg/kg/day) for 10 days. Alternatives useful in resistant cases are cefaclor (20–40 mg/kg/day) or amoxicillin-clavulanate (20–40 mg/kg/day).

Tympanocentesis for bacterial (aerobic and anaerobic) and fungal culture may be performed by any experienced physician. A 20-gauge spinal needle bent 90 degrees to the hub attached to a 3-mL syringe is inserted through the inferior portion of the tympanic membrane. Interposition of a pliable connecting tube between the needle and syringe permits an assistant to aspirate without inducing movement of the needle. Tympanocentesis is useful for otitis media in immunocompromised patients and when infection persists or recurs despite multiple courses of antibiotics.

Surgical drainage of the middle ear (myringotomy) is reserved for patients with severe otalgia or when complications of otitis (eg, mastoiditis, meningitis) have occurred.

Recurrent acute otitis media may be managed with long-term antibiotic prophylaxis. Single daily oral doses of sulfamethoxazole (500 mg) or amoxicillin (250 or 500 mg) are given over a period of 1–3 months. Failure of this regimen to control infection is an indication for insertion of ventilating tubes.

Hutz MJ et al. Neurological complications of acute and chronic otitis media. Curr Neurol Neurosci Rep. 2018 Feb 14;18(3):11. [PMID: 29445883]

Schilder AG et al. Panel 7: Otitis media: treatment and complications. Otolaryngol Head Neck Surg. 2017 Apr;156(4 Suppl): S88–105. [PMID: 28372534]

2. Chronic Otitis Media

▶ Chronic otorrhea with or without otalgia.

▶ Tympanic membrane perforation with conductive hearing loss.

▶ Often amenable to surgical correction.

General Considerations

Chronic infection of the middle ear and mastoid generally develops as a consequence of recurrent acute otitis media, although it may follow other diseases and trauma. Perforation of the tympanic membrane is usually present. The bacteriology of chronic otitis media differs from that of acute otitis media. Common organisms include *P aeruginosa*, *Proteus* species, *Staphylococcus aureus*, and mixed anaerobic infections.

Clinical Findings

The clinical hallmark of chronic otitis media is purulent aural discharge. Drainage may be continuous or intermittent, with increased severity during upper respiratory tract infection or following water exposure. Pain is uncommon except during acute exacerbations. Conductive hearing loss results from destruction of the tympanic membrane or ossicular chain, or both.

Treatment

The medical treatment of chronic otitis media includes regular removal of infected debris, use of earplugs to protect against water exposure, and topical antibiotic drops (ofloxacin 0.3% or ciprofloxacin with dexamethasone) for exacerbations. Oral ciprofloxacin, active against *Pseudomonas*, 500 mg twice a day for 1–6 weeks may help dry a chronically discharging ear.

Definitive management is surgical in most cases. Successful reconstruction of the tympanic membrane may be achieved in about 90% of cases, often with elimination of infection and significant improvement in hearing. When the mastoid air cells are involved by irreversible infection, they should be exenterated at the same time through a mastoidectomy.

Harris AS et al. Why are ototopical aminoglycosides still first-line therapy for chronic suppurative otitis media? A systematic review and discussion of aminoglycosides versus quinolones. J Laryngol Otol. 2016 Jan;130(1):2–7. [PMID: 26584651]

Master A et al. Management of chronic suppurative otitis media and otosclerosis in developing countries. Otolaryngol Clin North Am. 2018 Jun;51(3):593–605. [PMID: 29525390]

Schilder AG et al. Otitis media. Nat Rev Dis Primers. 2016 Sep 8; 2:16063. [PMID: 27604644]

Complications of Otitis Media

A. Cholesteatoma

Cholesteatoma is a special variety of chronic otitis media (Figure 8–3). The most common cause is prolonged eustachian tube dysfunction, with inward migration of the upper flaccid portion of the tympanic membrane. This creates a squamous epithelium-lined sac, which—when its neck becomes obstructed—may fill with desquamated keratin and become chronically infected. Cholesteatomas typically erode bone, with early penetration of the mastoid and destruction of the ossicular chain. Over time they may

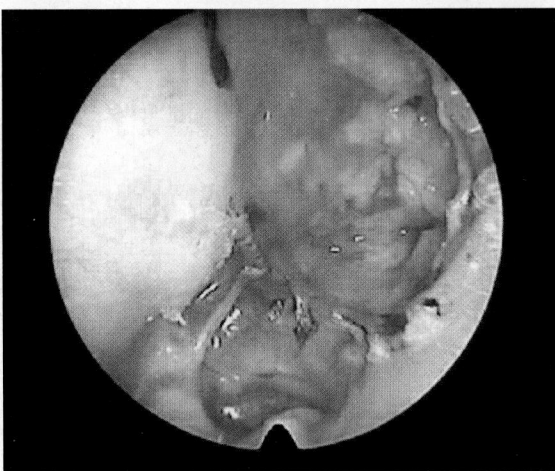

▲ **Figure 8–3.** Cholesteatoma. (Used, with permission, from Vladimir Zlinsky, MD, in Roy F. Sullivan, PhD: Audiology Forum: Video Otoscopy, www.RCSullivan.com; from Usatine RP, Smith MA, Mayeaux EJ Jr, Chumley H, Tysinger J. *The Color Atlas of Family Medicine.* McGraw-Hill, 2009.)

erode into the inner ear, involve the facial nerve, and on rare occasions spread intracranially. Otoscopic examination may reveal an epitympanic retraction pocket or a marginal tympanic membrane perforation that exudes keratin debris, or granulation tissue. The treatment of cholesteatoma is surgical marsupialization of the sac or its complete removal. This may require the creation of a "mastoid bowl" in which the ear canal and mastoid are joined into a large common cavity that must be periodically cleaned.

Kao R et al. Outpatient management of cholesteatoma with canal wall reconstruction tympanomastoidectomy. Laryngoscope Investig Otolaryngol. 2017 Oct 31;2(6):351–7. [PMID: 29299507]

Rutkowska J et al. Cholesteatoma definition and classification: a literature review. J Int Adv Otol. 2017 Aug;13(2):266–71. [PMID: 28274903]

B. Mastoiditis

Acute suppurative mastoiditis usually evolves following several weeks of inadequately treated acute otitis media. It is characterized by postauricular pain and erythema accompanied by a spiking fever. CT scan reveals coalescence of the mastoid air cells due to destruction of their bony septa. Initial treatment consists of intravenous antibiotics (eg, cefazolin 0.5–1.5 g every 6–8 hours) directed against the most common offending organisms (*S pneumoniae*, *H influenzae*, and *S pyogenes*), and myringotomy for culture and drainage. Failure of medical therapy indicates the need for surgical drainage (mastoidectomy).

C. Petrous Apicitis

The medial portion of the petrous bone between the inner ear and clivus may become a site of persistent infection when the drainage of its pneumatic cell tracts becomes blocked. This may cause foul discharge, deep ear and retro-orbital pain, and sixth nerve palsy (Gradenigo syndrome); meningitis may be a complication. Treatment is with prolonged antibiotic therapy (based on culture results) and surgical drainage via petrous apicectomy.

Gadre AK et al. The changing face of petrous apicitis—a 40-year experience. Laryngoscope. 2018 Jan;128(1):195–201. [PMID: 28378370]

Vitale M et al. Gradenigo's syndrome: a common infection with uncommon consequences. Am J Emerg Med. 2017 Sep; 35(9):1388.e1–2. [PMID: 28720403]

D. Facial Paralysis

Facial palsy may be associated with either acute or chronic otitis media. In the acute setting, it results from inflammation of the seventh nerve in its middle ear segment. Treatment consists of myringotomy for drainage and culture, followed by intravenous antibiotics (based on culture results). The use of corticosteroids is controversial. The prognosis is excellent, with complete recovery in most cases.

Facial palsy associated with chronic otitis media usually evolves slowly due to chronic pressure on the seventh nerve in the middle ear or mastoid by cholesteatoma. Treatment requires surgical correction of the underlying disease. The prognosis is less favorable than for facial palsy associated with acute otitis media.

Prasad S et al. Facial nerve paralysis in acute suppurative otitis media—management. Indian J Otolaryngol Head Neck Surg. 2017 Mar;69(1):58–61. [PMID: 28239580]

E. Sigmoid Sinus Thrombosis

Trapped infection within the mastoid air cells adjacent to the sigmoid sinus may cause septic thrombophlebitis. This is heralded by signs of systemic sepsis (spiking fevers, chills), at times accompanied by signs of increased intracranial pressure (headache, lethargy, nausea and vomiting, papilledema). Diagnosis can be made noninvasively by magnetic resonance venography (MRV). Primary treatment is with intravenous antibiotics (based on culture results). Surgical drainage with ligation of the internal jugular vein may be indicated when embolization is suspected.

F. Central Nervous System Infection

Otogenic meningitis is by far the most common intracranial complication of ear infection. In the setting of acute suppurative otitis media, it arises from hematogenous spread of bacteria, most commonly *H influenzae* and *S pneumoniae*. In chronic otitis media, it results either from passage of infection along preformed pathways, such as the petrosquamous suture line, or from direct extension of disease through the dural plates of the petrous pyramid.

Epidural abscesses arise from direct extension of disease in the setting of chronic infection. They are usually asymptomatic but may present with deep local pain, headache, and low-grade fever. They are often discovered as an incidental finding at surgery. Brain abscess may arise in the temporal lobe or cerebellum as a result of septic thrombophlebitis adjacent to an epidural abscess. The predominant causative organisms are *S aureus*, *S pyogenes*, and *S pneumoniae*. Rupture into the subarachnoid space results in meningitis and often death. (See Chapter 30.)

Hutz MJ et al. Neurological complications of acute and chronic otitis media. Curr Neurol Neurosci Rep. 2018 Feb 14;18(3):11. [PMID: 29445883]

Laulajainen Hongisto A et al. Otogenic intracranial abscesses, our experience over the last four decades. J Int Adv Otol. 2017 Apr;13(1):40–6. [PMID: 28084999]

3. Otosclerosis

Otosclerosis is a progressive disease with a marked familial tendency that affects the bony otic capsule. Lesions involving the footplate of the stapes result in increased impedance to the passage of sound through the ossicular chain, producing conductive hearing loss. This may be treated either through the use of a hearing aid or surgical replacement of the stapes with a prosthesis (stapedectomy). When otosclerotic lesions impinge on the cochlea ("cochlear otosclerosis"), permanent sensory hearing loss occurs.

Master A et al. Management of chronic suppurative otitis media and otosclerosis in developing countries. Otolaryngol Clin North Am. 2018 Jun;51(3):593–605. [PMID: 29525390]

McElveen JT Jr et al. Controversies in the evaluation and management of otosclerosis. Otolaryngol Clin North Am. 2018 Apr;51(2):487–99. [PMID: 29502731]

4. Trauma to the Middle Ear

Tympanic membrane perforation may result from impact injury or explosive acoustic trauma (Figure 8–4). Spontaneous healing occurs in most cases. Persistent perforation may result from secondary infection brought on by exposure to water. During the healing period, patients should be

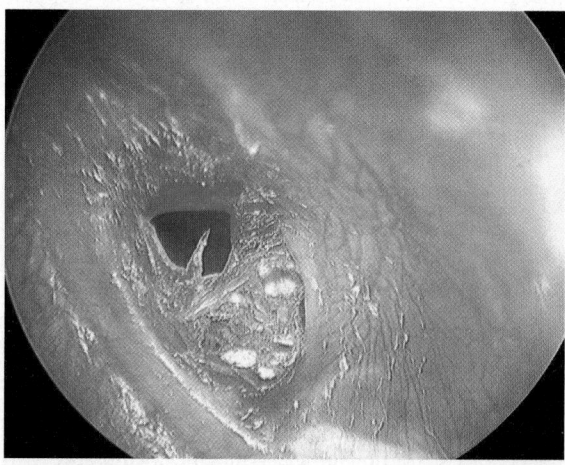

▲ **Figure 8–4.** Traumatic perforation of the left tympanic membrane. (Used, with permission, from William Clark, MD, in Usatine RP, Smith MA, Mayeaux EJ Jr, Chumley H, Tysinger J. *The Color Atlas of Family Medicine.* McGraw-Hill, 2009.)

advised to wear earplugs while swimming or bathing. Hemorrhage behind an intact tympanic membrane (hemotympanum) may follow blunt trauma or extreme barotrauma. Spontaneous resolution over several weeks is the usual course. When a conductive hearing loss greater than 30 dB persists for more than 3 months following trauma, disruption of the ossicular chain should be suspected. Middle ear exploration with reconstruction of the ossicular chain, combined with repair of the tympanic membrane when required, will usually restore hearing.

Sagiv D et al. Traumatic perforation of the tympanic membrane: a review of 80 cases. J Emerg Med. 2018 Feb;54(2):186–90. [PMID: 29110975]

5. Middle Ear Neoplasia

Primary middle ear tumors are rare. Glomus tumors arise either in the middle ear (glomus tympanicum) or in the jugular bulb with upward erosion into the hypotympanum (glomus jugulare). They present clinically with pulsatile tinnitus and hearing loss. A vascular mass may be visible behind an intact tympanic membrane. Large glomus jugulare tumors are often associated with multiple cranial neuropathies, especially involving nerves VII, IX, X, XI, and XII. Treatment usually requires surgery, radiotherapy, or both. Pulsatile tinnitus thus warrants magnetic resonance angiography (MRA) and MRV to rule out a vascular mass.

Killeen DE et al. Endoscopic management of middle ear paragangliomas: a case series. Otol Neurotol. 2017 Mar;38(3):408–15. [PMID: 28192382]
Marinelli JP et al. Adenomatous neuroendocrine tumors of the middle ear: a multi-institutional investigation of 32 cases and development of a staging system. Otol Neurotol. 2018 Sep; 39(8):e712–21. [PMID: 30001283]

EARACHE

Earache can be caused by a variety of otologic problems, but external otitis and acute otitis media are the most common. Differentiation of the two should be apparent by pneumatic otoscopy. Pain out of proportion to the physical findings may be due to herpes zoster oticus, especially when vesicles appear in the ear canal or concha. Persistent pain and discharge from the ear suggest osteomyelitis of the skull base or cancer, and patients with these complaints should be referred for specialty evaluation.

Nonotologic causes of otalgia are numerous. The sensory innervation of the ear is derived from the trigeminal, facial, glossopharyngeal, vagal, and upper cervical nerves. Because of this rich innervation, referred otalgia is quite frequent. Temporomandibular joint dysfunction is a common cause of referred ear pain. Pain is exacerbated by chewing or psychogenic grinding of the teeth (bruxism) and may be associated with dental malocclusion. Repeated episodes of severe lancinating otalgia may occur in glossopharyngeal neuralgia. Infections and neoplasia that involve the oropharynx, hypopharynx, and larynx frequently cause otalgia. Persistent earache demands specialty referral to exclude cancer of the upper aerodigestive tract.

Harrison E et al. Otalgia. Aust Fam Physician. 2016 Jul; 45(7):493–7. [PMID: 27610432]

DISEASES OF THE INNER EAR

1. Sensory Hearing Loss

Diseases of the cochlea result in sensory hearing loss, a condition that is usually irreversible. Most cochlear diseases result in bilateral symmetric hearing loss. The presence of unilateral or asymmetric sensorineural hearing loss suggests a lesion proximal to the cochlea. The primary goals in the management of sensory hearing loss are prevention of further losses and functional improvement with amplification and auditory rehabilitation.

A. Presbyacusis

Presbyacusis, or age-related hearing loss, is the most frequent cause of sensory hearing loss and is progressive, predominantly high-frequency, and symmetrical. Various etiologic factors (eg, prior noise trauma, drug exposure, genetic predisposition) may contribute to presbyacusis. Most patients notice a loss of speech discrimination that is especially pronounced in noisy environments. About 25% of people between the ages of 65 and 75 years and almost 50% of those over 75 experience hearing difficulties.

Golub JS. Brain changes associated with age-related hearing loss. Curr Opin Otolaryngol Head Neck Surg. 2017 Oct;25(5): 347–52. [PMID: 28661962]
Tu NC et al. Age-related hearing loss: unraveling the pieces. Laryngoscope Investig Otolaryngol. 2018 Feb 21;3(2):68–72. [PMID: 29721536]
Vaisbuch Y et al. Age-related hearing loss: innovations in hearing augmentation. Otolaryngol Clin North Am. 2018 Aug; 51(4):705–23. [PMID: 29735277]

B. Noise Trauma

Noise trauma is the second most common cause of sensory hearing loss. Sounds exceeding 85 dB are potentially injurious to the cochlea, especially with prolonged exposures. The loss typically begins in the high frequencies (especially 4000 Hz) and, with continuing exposure, progresses to involve the speech frequencies. Among the more common sources of injurious noise are industrial machinery, weapons, and excessively loud music. Personal music devices used at excessive loudness levels may also be injurious. Monitoring noise levels in the workplace by regulatory agencies has led to preventive programs that have reduced the frequency of occupational losses. Individuals of all ages, especially those with existing hearing losses, should wear earplugs when exposed to moderately loud noises and specially designed earmuffs when exposed to explosive noises.

Le TN et al. Current insights in noise-induced hearing loss: a literature review of the underlying mechanism, pathophysiology, asymmetry, and management options. J Otolaryngol Head Neck Surg. 2017 May 23;46(1):41. [PMID: 28535812]

C. Physical Trauma

Head trauma (eg, deployment of air bags during an automobile accident) has effects on the inner ear similar to those of severe acoustic trauma. Some degree of sensory hearing loss may occur following simple concussion and is frequent after skull fracture.

Ballivet de Régloix S et al. Blast injury of the ear by massive explosion: a review of 41 cases. J R Army Med Corps. 2017 Oct;163(5):333–38. [PMID: 28209807]
Honeybrook A et al. Hearing and mortality outcomes following temporal bone fractures. Craniomaxillofac Trauma Reconstr. 2017 Dec;10(4):281–5. [PMID: 29109839]

D. Ototoxicity

Ototoxic substances may affect both the auditory and vestibular systems. The most commonly used ototoxic medications are aminoglycosides; loop diuretics; and several antineoplastic agents, notably cisplatin. These medications may cause irreversible hearing loss even when administered in therapeutic doses. When using these medications, it is important to identify high-risk patients, such as those with preexisting hearing losses or kidney disease. Patients simultaneously receiving multiple ototoxic agents are at particular risk owing to ototoxic synergy. Useful measures to reduce the risk of ototoxic injury include serial audiometry, monitoring of serum peak and trough levels, and substitution of equivalent nonototoxic drugs whenever possible.

It is possible for topical agents that enter the middle ear to be absorbed into the inner ear via the round window. When the tympanic membrane is perforated, use of potentially ototoxic ear drops (eg, neomycin, gentamicin) is best avoided.

Jiang M et al. Aminoglycoside-induced cochleotoxicity: a review. Front Cell Neurosci. 2017 Oct 9;11:308. [PMID: 29062271]

E. Sudden Sensory Hearing Loss

Idiopathic sudden loss of hearing in one ear may occur at any age, but typically it occurs in persons over age 20 years. The cause is unknown; however, one hypothesis is that it results from a viral infection or a sudden vascular occlusion of the internal auditory artery. Prognosis is mixed, with many patients suffering permanent deafness in the involved ear, while others have complete recovery. Prompt treatment with corticosteroids has been shown to improve the odds of recovery. A common regimen is oral prednisone, 1 mg/kg/day, followed by a tapering dose over a 10-day period. Intratympanic administration of corticosteroids alone or in association with oral corticosteroids has been associated with an equal or more favorable prognosis. Because treatment appears to be most effective as close to the onset of the loss as possible, and appears not to be effective after 6 weeks, a prompt audiogram should be obtained in all patients who present with sudden hearing loss without obvious middle ear pathology.

El Sabbagh NG et al. Intratympanic dexamethasone in sudden sensorineural hearing loss: a systematic review and meta-analysis. Laryngoscope. 2017 Aug;127(8):1897–1908. [PMID: 27861924]

Plontke SK. Diagnostics and therapy of sudden hearing loss. GMS Curr Top Otorhinolaryngol Head Neck Surg. 2018 Feb 19;16:Doc05. [PMID: 29503670]

F. Autoimmune Hearing Loss

Sensory hearing loss may be associated with a wide array of systemic autoimmune disorders, such as systemic lupus erythematosus, granulomatosis with polyangiitis (formerly Wegener granulomatosis), and Cogan syndrome (hearing loss, keratitis, aortitis). The loss is most often bilateral and progressive. The hearing level often fluctuates, with periods of deterioration alternating with partial or even complete remission. Usually, there is the gradual evolution of permanent hearing loss, which often stabilizes with some remaining auditory function but occasionally proceeds to complete deafness. Vestibular dysfunction, particularly dysequilibrium and postural instability, may accompany the auditory symptoms.

In many cases, the autoimmune pattern of audiovestibular dysfunction presents in the absence of recognized systemic autoimmune disease. Responsiveness to oral corticosteroid treatment is helpful in making the diagnosis and constitutes first-line therapy. If stabilization of hearing becomes dependent on long-term corticosteroid use, steroid-sparing immunosuppressive regimens may become necessary.

Atturo F et al. Can unilateral, progressive or sudden hearing loss be immune-mediated in origin? Acta Otolaryngol. 2017 Aug; 137(8):823–8. [PMID: 28296514]
Mancini P et al. Hearing loss in autoimmune disorders: prevalence and therapeutic options. Autoimmun Rev. 2018 Jul; 17(7):644–52. [PMID: 29729446]

2. Tinnitus

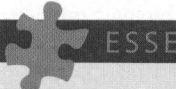

ESSENTIALS OF DIAGNOSIS

▶ Perception of abnormal ear or head noises.

▶ Persistent tinnitus often, though not always, indicates the presence of sensory hearing loss.

▶ Intermittent periods of mild, high-pitched tinnitus lasting seconds to minutes are common in normal-hearing persons.

▶ General Considerations

Tinnitus is defined as the sensation of sound in the absence of an exogenous sound source. Tinnitus can accompany any form of hearing loss, and its presence provides no diagnostic value in determining the cause of a hearing loss. Approximately 15% of the general population experiences some type of tinnitus, with prevalence beyond 20% in aging populations.

Clinical Findings

A. Symptoms and Signs

Though tinnitus is commonly associated with hearing loss, tinnitus severity correlates poorly with the degree of hearing loss. About one in seven tinnitus sufferers experiences severe annoyance, and 4% are severely disabled. When severe and persistent, tinnitus may interfere with sleep and ability to concentrate, resulting in considerable psychological distress.

Pulsatile tinnitus—often described by the patient as listening to one's own heartbeat—should be distinguished from tonal tinnitus. Although often ascribed to conductive hearing loss, pulsatile tinnitus may be far more serious and may indicate a vascular abnormality, such as glomus tumor, venous sinus stenosis, carotid vaso-occlusive disease, arteriovenous malformation, or aneurysm. In contrast, a staccato "clicking" tinnitus may result from middle ear muscle spasm, sometimes associated with palatal myoclonus. The patient typically perceives a rapid series of popping noises, lasting seconds to a few minutes, accompanied by a fluttering feeling in the ear.

B. Diagnostic Testing

For routine, nonpulsatile tinnitus, audiometry should be ordered to rule out an associated hearing loss. For unilateral tinnitus, particularly associated with hearing loss in the absence of an obvious causative factor (ie, noise trauma), an MRI should be obtained to rule out a retrocochlear lesion, such as vestibular schwannoma. MRA and MRV and temporal bone computed tomography (CT) should be considered for patients who have pulsatile tinnitus to exclude a causative vascular lesion or sigmoid sinus abnormality.

Treatment

The most important treatment of tinnitus is avoidance of exposure to excessive noise, ototoxic agents, and other factors that may cause cochlear damage. Masking the tinnitus with music or through amplification of normal sounds with a hearing aid may also bring some relief. Among the numerous drugs that have been tried, oral antidepressants (eg, nortriptyline at an initial dosage of 50 mg orally at bedtime) have proved to be the most effective. In addition to masking techniques, habituation techniques, such as tinnitus retraining therapy, may prove beneficial in those with refractory symptoms.

McCormack A et al. A systematic review of the reporting of tinnitus prevalence and severity. Hear Res. 2016 Jul;337:70–9. [PMID: 27246985]

Wu V et al. Approach to tinnitus management. Can Fam Physician. 2018 Jul;64(7):491–5. [PMID: 30002023]

Zenner HP et al. A multidisciplinary systematic review of the treatment for chronic idiopathic tinnitus. Eur Arch Otorhinolaryngol. 2017 May;274(5):2079–91. [PMID: 27995315]

3. Hyperacusis

Excessive sensitivity to sound may occur in normal-hearing individuals, either in association with ear disease, following noise trauma, in patients susceptible to migraines, or for psychological reasons. Patients with cochlear dysfunction commonly experience "recruitment," an abnormal sensitivity to loud sounds despite a reduced sensitivity to softer ones. Fitting hearing aids and other amplification devices to patients with recruitment requires use of compression circuitry to avoid uncomfortable overamplification. For normal-hearing individuals with hyperacusis, use of an earplug in noisy environments may be beneficial, though attempts should be made at habituation.

Baguley DM et al. Hyperacusis: major research questions. HNO. 2018 May;66(5):358–63. [PMID: 29392341]

4. Vertigo

> **ESSENTIALS OF DIAGNOSIS**
>
> ► Either a sensation of motion when there is no motion or an exaggerated sense of motion in response to movement.
> ► Duration of vertigo episodes and association with hearing loss are the keys to diagnosis.
> ► Must differentiate peripheral from central etiologies of vestibular dysfunction.
> ► **Peripheral:** Onset is sudden; often associated with tinnitus and hearing loss; horizontal nystagmus may be present.
> ► **Central:** Onset is gradual; no associated auditory symptoms.
> ► Evaluation includes audiogram and electronystagmography (ENG) or videonystagmography (VNG) and head MRI.

General Considerations

Vertigo can be caused by either a peripheral or central etiology, or both (Table 8–2).

Clinical Findings

A. Symptoms and Signs

Vertigo is the cardinal symptom of vestibular disease. Vertigo is typically experienced as a distinct "spinning" sensation or a sense of tumbling or of falling forward or backward. It should be distinguished from imbalance, light-headedness, and syncope, all of which are nonvestibular in origin (Table 8–3).

1. Peripheral vestibular disease—Peripheral vestibulopathy usually causes vertigo of sudden onset, may be so severe that the patient is unable to walk or stand, and is frequently accompanied by nausea and vomiting. Tinnitus and hearing loss may be associated and provide strong support for a peripheral (ie, otologic) origin.

Table 8–2. Causes of vertigo.

Peripheral causes
Vestibular neuritis/labyrinthitis
Ménière disease
Benign paroxysmal positioning vertigo
Ethanol intoxication
Inner ear barotraumas
Semicircular canal dehiscence
Central causes
Seizure
Multiple sclerosis
Wernicke encephalopathy
Chiari malformation
Cerebellar ataxia syndromes
Mixed central and peripheral causes
Migraine
Stroke and vascular insufficiency
Posterior inferior cerebellar artery stroke
Anterior inferior cerebellar artery stroke
Vertebral artery insufficiency
Vasculitides
Cogan syndrome
Susac syndrome
Granulomatosis with polyangiitis (formerly Wegener granulomatosis)
Behçet disease
Cerebellopontine angle tumors
Vestibular schwannoma
Meningioma
Infections
Lyme disease
Syphilis
Vascular compression
Hyperviscosity syndromes
Waldenström macroglobulinemia
Endocrinopathies
Hypothyroidism
Pendred syndrome

Critical elements of the history include the duration of the discrete vertiginous episodes (seconds, minutes to hours, or days), and associated symptoms. Triggers should be sought, including diet (eg, high salt in the case of Ménière disease), stress, fatigue, and bright lights (eg, migraine-associated dizziness).

The physical examination of the patient with vertigo includes evaluation of the ears, observation of eye motion

Table 8–3. Common vestibular disorders: differential diagnosis based on classic presentations.

Duration of Typical Vertiginous Episodes	Auditory Symptoms Present	Auditory Symptoms Absent
Seconds	Perilymphatic fistula	Benign paroxysmal positioning vertigo (cupulolithiasis), vertebrobasilar insufficiency, migraine-associated vertigo
Hours	Endolymphatic hydrops (Ménière syndrome, syphilis)	Migraine-associated vertigo
Days	Labyrinthitis, labyrinthine concussion, autoimmune inner ear disease	Vestibular neuronitis, migraine-associated vertigo
Months	Acoustic neuroma, ototoxicity	Multiple sclerosis, cerebellar degeneration

and nystagmus in response to head turning, cranial nerve examination, and Romberg testing. In acute peripheral lesions, nystagmus is usually horizontal with a rotatory component; the fast phase usually beats away from the diseased side. Visual fixation tends to inhibit nystagmus except in very acute peripheral lesions or with CNS disease. In benign paroxysmal positioning vertigo, Dix-Hallpike testing (quickly lowering the patient to the supine position with the head extending over the edge and placed 30 degrees lower than the body, turned either to the left or right) will elicit a delayed onset (~10 sec) fatiguable nystagmus. Nonfatigable nystagmus in this position indicates CNS disease.

Since visual fixation often suppresses observed nystagmus, many of these maneuvers are performed with Frenzel goggles, which prevent visual fixation, and often bring out subtle forms of nystagmus. The Fukuda test can demonstrate vestibular asymmetry when the patient steps in place with eyes closed and consistently rotates in one direction.

2. Central disease—In contrast, vertigo arising from CNS disease (Table 8–2) tends to develop gradually and then becomes progressively more severe and debilitating. Nystagmus is not always present but can occur in any direction, may be dissociated in the two eyes, and is often nonfatigable, vertical rather than horizontal in orientation, without latency, and unsuppressed by visual fixation. ENG is useful in documenting these characteristics. Evaluation of central audiovestibular dysfunction requires MRI of the brain.

Episodic vertigo can occur in patients with diplopia from external ophthalmoplegia and is maximal when the patient looks in the direction where the separation of images is greatest. Cerebral lesions involving the temporal cortex may also produce vertigo; it is sometimes the initial symptom of a seizure. Finally, vertigo may be a feature of a number of systemic disorders and can occur as a side effect of certain anticonvulsant, antibiotic, hypnotic, analgesic, and tranquilizer medications or of alcohol.

B. Laboratory Findings

Laboratory investigations, such as audiologic evaluation, caloric stimulation, ENG, VNG, vestibular-evoked myogenic potentials (VEMPs), and MRI, are indicated in patients with persistent vertigo or when CNS disease is suspected. These studies help distinguish between central and peripheral lesions and identify causes requiring specific therapy. ENG consists of objective recording of the nystagmus induced by head and body movements, gaze, and caloric stimulation. It is helpful in quantifying the degree of vestibular hypofunction.

Sandhu JS et al. Clinical examination and management of the dizzy patient. Br J Hosp Med (Lond). 2016 Dec 2;77(12):692–8. [PMID: 27937029]
Whitman GT. Dizziness. Am J Med. 2018 Dec;131(12):1431–7. [PMID: 29859806]

▶ Vertigo Syndromes Due to Peripheral Lesions

A. Endolymphatic Hydrops (Ménière Syndrome)

The cause of Ménière syndrome is unknown. The classic syndrome consists of episodic vertigo, with discrete vertigo spells lasting 20 minutes to several hours in association with fluctuating low-frequency sensorineural hearing loss, tinnitus (usually low-tone and "blowing" in quality), and a sensation of unilateral aural pressure (Table 8–3). These symptoms in the absence of hearing fluctuations suggest migraine-associated dizziness. Symptoms wax and wane as the endolymphatic pressure rises and falls. Caloric testing commonly reveals loss or impairment of thermally induced nystagmus on the involved side. Primary treatment involves a low-salt diet and diuretics (eg, acetazolamide). For symptomatic relief of acute vertigo attacks, oral meclizine (25 mg) or diazepam (2–5 mg) can be used. In refractory cases, patients may undergo intratympanic corticosteroid injections, endolymphatic sac decompression, or vestibular ablation, either through transtympanic gentamicin, vestibular nerve section, or surgical labyrinthectomy.

Tabet P et al. Meniere's disease and vestibular migraine: updates and review of the literature. J Clin Med Res. 2017 Sep;9(9): 733–44. [PMID: 28811849]

B. Labyrinthitis

Patients with labyrinthitis suffer from acute onset of continuous, usually severe vertigo lasting several days to a week, accompanied by hearing loss and tinnitus. During a recovery period that lasts for several weeks, the vertigo gradually improves. Hearing may return to normal or remain permanently impaired in the involved ear. The cause of labyrinthitis is unknown. Treatment consists of antibiotics if the patient is febrile or has symptoms of a bacterial infection, and supportive care. Vestibular

suppressants are useful during the acute phase of the attack (eg, diazepam or meclizine) but should be discontinued as soon as feasible to avoid long-term dysequilibrium from inadequate compensation.

C. Benign Paroxysmal Positioning Vertigo

Patients suffering from recurrent spells of vertigo, lasting a few minutes per spell, associated with changes in head position (often provoked by rolling over in bed), usually have benign paroxysmal positioning vertigo (BPPV). The term "positioning vertigo" is more accurate than "positional vertigo" because it is provoked by changes in head position rather than by the maintenance of a particular posture.

The typical symptoms of BPPV occur in clusters that persist for several days. There is a brief (10–15 sec) latency period following a head movement before symptoms develop, and the acute vertigo subsides within 10–60 seconds, though the patient may remain imbalanced for several hours. Constant repetition of the positional change leads to habituation. Since some CNS disorders can mimic BPPV (eg, vertebrobasilar insufficiency), recurrent cases warrant head MRI/MRA. In central lesions, there is no latent period, fatigability, or habituation of the symptoms and signs. Treatment of BPPV involves physical therapy protocols (eg, the Epley maneuver or Brandt-Daroff exercises), based on the theory that it results from cupulolithiasis (free-floating statoconia, also known as otoconia) within a semicircular canal.

Balatsouras DG et al. Benign paroxysmal positional vertigo secondary to mild head trauma. Ann Otol Rhinol Laryngol. 2017 Jan;126(1):54–60. [PMID: 27780909]
von Brevern M et al. Benign paroxysmal positional vertigo: diagnostic criteria consensus document of the Committee for the Classification of Vestibular Disorders of the Bárány Society. Acta Otorrinolaringol Esp. 2017 Nov–Dec;68(6):349–60. [PMID: 29056234]

D. Vestibular Neuronitis

In vestibular neuronitis, a paroxysmal, usually single attack of vertigo occurs without accompanying impairment of auditory function and will persist for several days to a week before gradually abating. During the acute phase, examination reveals nystagmus and absent responses to caloric stimulation on one or both sides. The cause of the disorder is unclear though presumed to be viral. Treatment consists of supportive care, including oral diazepam, 2–5 mg every 6–12 hours, or meclizine, 25–100 mg divided 2–3 times daily, during the acute phases of the vertigo only, followed by vestibular therapy if the patient does not completely compensate.

van Esch BF et al. Clinical characteristics of benign recurrent vestibulopathy: clearly distinctive from vestibular migraine and Menière's disease? Otol Neurotol. 2017 Oct;38(9):e357–63. [PMID: 28834943]

E. Traumatic Vertigo

Labyrinthine concussion is the most common cause of vertigo following head injury. Symptoms generally diminish within several days but may linger for a month or more.

Basilar skull fractures that traverse the inner ear usually result in severe vertigo lasting several days to a week and deafness in the involved ear. Chronic posttraumatic vertigo may result from cupulolithiasis. This occurs when traumatically detached statoconia (otoconia) settle on the ampulla of the posterior semicircular canal and cause an excessive degree of cupular deflection in response to head motion. Clinically, this presents as episodic positioning vertigo. Treatment consists of supportive care and vestibular suppressant medication (diazepam or meclizine) during the acute phase of the attack, and vestibular therapy.

Szczupak M et al. Posttraumatic dizziness and vertigo. Handb Clin Neurol. 2016;137:295–300. [PMID: 27638079]

F. Perilymphatic Fistula

Leakage of perilymphatic fluid from the inner ear into the tympanic cavity via the round or oval window is a rare cause of vertigo and sensory hearing loss. Most cases result from either physical injury (eg, blunt head trauma, hand slap to ear); extreme barotrauma during airflight, scuba diving, etc; or vigorous Valsalva maneuvers (eg, during weight lifting). Treatment may require middle ear exploration and window sealing with a tissue graft.

Deveze A et al. Diagnosis and treatment of perilymphatic fistula. Adv Otorhinolaryngol. 2018;81:133–45. [PMID: 29794455]

G. Cervical Vertigo

Position receptors located in the facets of the cervical spine are important physiologically in the coordination of head and eye movements. Cervical proprioceptive dysfunction is a common cause of vertigo triggered by neck movements. This disturbance often commences after neck injury, particularly hyperextension; it is also associated with degenerative cervical spine disease. Although symptoms vary, vertigo may be triggered by assuming a particular head position as opposed to moving to a new head position (the latter typical of labyrinthine dysfunction). Cervical vertigo may often be confused with migraine-associated vertigo, which is also associated with head movement. Management consists of neck movement exercises to the extent permitted by orthopedic considerations.

Devaraja K. Approach to cervicogenic dizziness: a comprehensive review of its aetiopathology and management. Eur Arch Otorhinolaryngol. 2018 Oct;275(10):2421–33. [PMID: 30094486]
Peng B. Cervical vertigo: historical reviews and advances. World Neurosurg. 2018 Jan;109:347–50. [PMID: 29061460]

H. Migrainous Vertigo

Episodic vertigo is frequently associated with migraine headache. Head trauma may also be a precipitating feature. The vertigo may be temporally related to the headache and last up to several hours, or it may also occur in the absence of any headache. Migrainous vertigo may resemble Ménière disease but without associated hearing loss or tinnitus. Accompanying symptoms may include head pressure;

visual, motion, or auditory sensitivity; and photosensitivity. Symptoms typically worsen with lack of sleep and anxiety or stress. Food triggers include caffeine, chocolate, and alcohol, among others. There is often a history of motion intolerance (easily carsick as a child). Migrainous vertigo may be familial. Treatment includes dietary and lifestyle changes (improved sleep pattern, avoidance of stress) and antimigraine prophylactic medication.

Sohn JH. Recent advances in the understanding of vestibular migraine. Behav Neurol. 2016;2016:1801845. [PMID: 27821976]
Tabet P et al. Meniere's disease and vestibular migraine: updates and review of the literature. J Clin Med Res. 2017 Sep;9(9): 733–44. [PMID: 28811849]
von Brevern M et al. Vestibular migraine. Handb Clin Neurol. 2016;137:301–16. [PMID: 27638080]

I. Superior Semicircular Canal Dehiscence

Deficiency in the bony covering of the superior semicircular canal may be associated with vertigo triggered by loud noise exposure, straining, and an apparent conductive hearing loss. Autophony is also a common feature. Diagnosis is with coronal high-resolution CT scan and VEMPs. Surgically resurfacing or plugging the dehiscent canal can improve symptoms.

Naert L et al. Aggregating the symptoms of superior semicircular canal dehiscence syndrome. Laryngoscope. 2018 Aug;128(8): 1932–8. [PMID: 29280497]
Ziylan F et al. A comparison of surgical treatments for superior semicircular canal dehiscence: a systematic review. Otol Neurotol. 2017 Jan;38(1):1–10. [PMID: 27861193]

▶ Vertigo Syndromes Due to Central Lesions

CNS causes of vertigo include brainstem vascular disease, arteriovenous malformations, tumors of the brainstem and cerebellum, multiple sclerosis, and vertebrobasilar migraine (Table 8–2). Vertigo of central origin often becomes unremitting and disabling. The associated nystagmus is often nonfatigable, vertical rather than horizontal in orientation, without latency, and unsuppressed by visual fixation. ENG is useful in documenting these characteristics. There are commonly other signs of brainstem dysfunction (eg, cranial nerve palsies; motor, sensory, or cerebellar deficits in the limbs) or of increased intracranial pressure. Auditory function is generally spared. The underlying cause should be treated.

Choi JY et al. Central vertigo. Curr Opin Neurol. 2018 Feb; 31(1):81–9. [PMID: 29084063]
Tsang BK et al. Acute evaluation of the acute vestibular syndrome—differentiating posterior circulation stroke from acute peripheral vestibulopathies. Intern Med J. 2017 Dec; 47(12):1352–60. [PMID: 28696571]

DISEASES OF THE CENTRAL AUDITORY & VESTIBULAR SYSTEMS

Lesions of the eighth cranial nerve and central audiovestibular pathways produce neural hearing loss and vertigo (Table 8–3). One characteristic of neural hearing loss is deterioration of speech discrimination out of proportion to the decrease in pure tone thresholds. Another is auditory adaptation, wherein a steady tone appears to the listener to decay and eventually disappear. Auditory evoked responses are useful in distinguishing cochlear from neural losses and may give insight into the site of lesion within the central pathways.

The evaluation of central audiovestibular disorders usually requires imaging of the internal auditory canal, cerebellopontine angle, and brain with enhanced MRI.

1. Vestibular Schwannoma (Acoustic Neuroma)

Eighth cranial nerve schwannomas are among the most common intracranial tumors. Most are unilateral, but about 5% are associated with the hereditary syndrome neurofibromatosis type 2, in which bilateral eighth nerve tumors may be accompanied by meningiomas and other intracranial and spinal tumors. These benign lesions arise within the internal auditory canal and gradually grow to involve the cerebellopontine angle, eventually compressing the pons and resulting in hydrocephalus. Their typical auditory symptoms are unilateral hearing loss with a deterioration of speech discrimination exceeding that predicted by the degree of pure tone loss. Nonclassic presentations, such as sudden unilateral hearing loss, are fairly common. Any individual with a unilateral or asymmetric sensorineural hearing loss should be evaluated for an intracranial mass lesion. Vestibular dysfunction more often takes the form of continuous dysequilibrium than episodic vertigo. Diagnosis is made by enhanced MRI. Treatment consists of observation, microsurgical excision, or stereotactic radiotherapy, depending on such factors as patient age, underlying health, and size of the tumor. Bevacizumab (vascular endothelial growth factor blocker) has shown promise for treatment of tumors in neurofibromatosis type 2.

Apicella G et al. Radiotherapy for vestibular schwannoma: review of recent literature results. Rep Pract Oncol Radiother. 2016 Jul–Aug;21(4):399–406. [PMID: 27330427]
Kirchmann M et al. Ten-year follow-up on tumor growth and hearing in patients observed with an intracanalicular vestibular schwannoma. Neurosurgery. 2017 Jan 1;80(1):49–56. [PMID: 27571523]

2. Vascular Compromise

Vertebrobasilar insufficiency is a common cause of vertigo in the elderly. It is often triggered by changes in posture or extension of the neck. Reduced flow in the vertebrobasilar system may be demonstrated noninvasively through MRA. Empiric treatment is with vasodilators and aspirin.

Choi KD et al. Ischemic syndromes causing dizziness and vertigo. Handb Clin Neurol. 2016;137:317–40. [PMID: 27638081]

3. Multiple Sclerosis

Patients with multiple sclerosis may suffer from episodic vertigo and chronic imbalance. Hearing loss in this disease is most commonly unilateral and of rapid onset. Spontaneous recovery may occur.

Kim HA et al. Recent advances in understanding audiovestibular loss of a vascular cause. J Stroke. 2017 Jan;19(1):61–6. [PMID: 28030893]

OTOLOGIC MANIFESTATIONS OF AIDS

The otologic manifestations of AIDS are protean. The pinna and external auditory canal may be affected by Kaposi sarcoma and by persistent and potentially invasive fungal infections (particularly *Aspergillus fumigatus*). Serous otitis media due to eustachian tube dysfunction may arise from adenoidal hypertrophy (HIV lymphadenopathy), recurrent mucosal viral infections, or an obstructing nasopharyngeal tumor (eg, lymphoma). Unfortunately, ventilating tubes are seldom helpful and may trigger profuse watery otorrhea. Acute otitis media is usually caused by typical bacterial organisms, including *Proteus, Staphylococcus,* and *Pseudomonas,* and rarely, by *Pneumocystis jirovecii.* Sensorineural hearing loss is common and, in some cases, results from viral CNS infection. In cases of progressive hearing loss, cryptococcal meningitis and syphilis must be excluded. Acute facial paralysis due to herpes zoster infection (Ramsay Hunt syndrome) occurs commonly and follows a clinical course similar to that in nonimmunocompromised patients. Treatment is with high-dose acyclovir (see Chapter 32). Corticosteroids may also be effective as an adjunct.

Matas CG et al. Audiological and electrophysiological alterations in HIV-infected individuals subjected or not to antiretroviral therapy. Braz J Otorhinolaryngol. 2018 Sep–Oct;84(5): 574–82. [PMID: 28823692]
Sathirapanya P et al. Peripheral facial paralysis associated with HIV infection: a case series and literature review. Clin Neurol Neurosurg. 2018 Sep;172:124–9. [PMID: 29990960]

DISEASES OF THE NOSE & PARANASAL SINUSES

INFECTIONS OF THE NOSE & PARANASAL SINUSES

1. Acute Viral Rhinosinusitis (Common Cold)

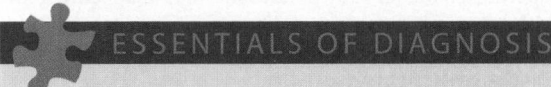

ESSENTIALS OF DIAGNOSIS

► Nasal congestion, clear rhinorrhea, and hyposmia.

► Associated malaise, headache, and cough.

► Erythematous, engorged nasal mucosa without intranasal purulence.

► Symptoms are self-limited, lasting less than 4 weeks and typically less than 10 days.

► Clinical Findings

Because there are numerous serologic types of rhinoviruses, adenoviruses, and other viruses, patients remain susceptible to the common cold throughout life. These infections, while generally quite benign and self-limited, have been implicated in the development or exacerbation of more serious conditions, such as acute bacterial sinusitis and acute otitis media, asthma, cystic fibrosis, and bronchitis. Nasal congestion, decreased sense of smell, watery rhinorrhea, and sneezing, accompanied by general malaise, throat discomfort and, occasionally, headache are typical in viral infections. Nasal examination usually shows erythematous, edematous mucosa and a watery discharge. The presence of purulent nasal discharge suggests bacterial rhinosinusitis.

▶ Treatment

There are no effective antiviral therapies for either the prevention or treatment of most viral rhinitis despite a common misperception among patients that antibiotics are helpful. Prevention of influenza virus infection by boosting the immune system using the annually created vaccine may be the most effective management strategy. Oseltamivir is the first neuramidase inhibitor approved for the treatment and prevention of influenza virus infection, but its use is generally limited to those patients considered high risk. These high-risk patients include young children, pregnant women, and adults older than 65 years of age. Oseltamivir is hard to use because it must be started within 48 hours for optimal effect. Buffered hypertonic saline (3–5%) nasal irrigation has been shown to improve symptoms and reduce the need for nonsteroidal anti-inflammatory drugs (NSAIDs). Other supportive measures, such as oral decongestants (pseudoephedrine, 30–60 mg every 4–6 hours or 120 mg twice daily), may provide some relief of rhinorrhea and nasal obstruction. Nasal sprays, such as oxymetazoline or phenylephrine, are rapidly effective but should not be used for more than a few days to prevent rebound congestion. Withdrawal of the drug after prolonged use leads to **rhinitis medicamentosa,** an almost addictive need for continuous usage. Treatment of rhinitis medicamentosa requires mandatory cessation of the sprays, and this is often extremely frustrating for patients. Topical intranasal corticosteroids (eg, flunisolide, 2 sprays in each nostril twice daily), intranasal anticholinergic (ipratropium 0.06% nasal spray, 2–3 sprays every 8 hours as needed), or a short tapering course of oral prednisone may help during the withdrawal process.

▶ Complications

Other than mild eustachian tube dysfunction or transient middle ear effusion, complications of viral rhinitis are unusual. Secondary acute bacterial rhinosinusitis is a well-accepted complication of acute viral rhinitis and is suggested by persistence of symptoms beyond 10 days with purulent green or yellow nasal secretions and unilateral facial or tooth pain.

Bergmark RW et al. Diagnosis and first-line treatment of chronic sinusitis. JAMA. 2017 Dec 19;318(23):2344–5. [PMID: 29260210]

Harris AM et al; High Value Care Task Force of the American College of Physicians and for the Centers for Disease Control and Prevention. Appropriate antibiotic use for acute respiratory tract infection in adults: advice for high-value care from the American College of Physicians and the Centers for Disease Control and Prevention. Ann Intern Med. 2016 Mar 15; 164(6):425–34. [PMID: 26785402]

King D et al. Saline nasal irrigation for acute upper respiratory tract infections. Cochrane Database Syst Rev. 2015 Apr 20;(4): CD006821. [PMID: 25892369]

Tan KS et al. Impact of respiratory virus infections in exacerbation of acute and chronic rhinosinusitis. Curr Allergy Asthma Rep. 2017 Apr;17(4):24. [PMID: 28389843]

2. Acute Bacterial Rhinosinusitis (Sinusitis)

ESSENTIALS OF DIAGNOSIS

- ▶ Purulent yellow-green nasal discharge or expectoration.
- ▶ Facial pain or pressure over the affected sinus or sinuses.
- ▶ Nasal obstruction.
- ▶ Acute onset of symptoms (between 1 and 4 weeks' duration).
- ▶ Associated cough, malaise, fever, and headache.

▶ General Considerations

Compared with viral rhinitis, acute bacterial rhinosinusitis infections are uncommon, but they still affect nearly 20 million Americans annually and account for over 2 billion dollars in health care expenditures.

Acute bacterial rhinosinusitis is believed to be the result of impaired mucociliary clearance, inflammation of the nasal cavity mucosa, and obstruction of the ostiomeatal complex, or sinus "pore." Edematous mucosa causes obstruction of the complex, resulting in the accumulation of mucus in the sinus cavity that becomes secondarily infected by bacteria. The largest of these ostiomeatal complexes is deep to the middle turbinate in the middle meatus. This complex is actually a confluence of complexes draining the maxillary, ethmoid, and frontal sinuses. The sphenoid drains from a separate complex between the septum and superior turbinate.

The typical pathogens of bacterial rhinosinusitis are *S pneumoniae*, other streptococci, *H influenzae,* and less commonly, *S aureus* and *Moraxella catarrhalis*. Pathogens vary regionally in both prevalence and drug resistance; about 25% of healthy asymptomatic individuals may, if sinus aspirates are cultured, harbor such bacteria as well.

▶ Clinical Findings

A. Symptoms and Signs

There are no agreed-upon criteria for the diagnosis of acute bacterial rhinosinusitis in adults. Major symptoms include purulent nasal drainage, nasal obstruction or congestion, facial pain/pressure, altered smell, cough, and fever. Minor symptoms include headache, otalgia, halitosis, dental pain, and fatigue. Many of the more specific symptoms and signs relate to the affected sinus(es). Bacterial rhinosinusitis can be distinguished from viral rhinitis by persistence of symptoms for more than 10 days after onset or worsening of symptoms within 10 days after initial improvement. Acute rhinosinusitis is defined as lasting less than 4 weeks, and subacute rhinosinusitis, as lasting 4–12 weeks.

Acute maxillary sinusitis is the most common form of acute bacterial rhinosinusitis because the maxillary is the largest sinus with a single drainage pathway that is easily obstructed. Unilateral facial fullness, pressure, and tenderness over the cheek are common symptoms, but may not always be present. Pain may refer to the upper incisor and canine teeth via branches of the trigeminal nerve, which traverse the floor of the sinus. Purulent nasal drainage should be noted with nasal airway obstruction or facial pain (pressure). Maxillary sinusitis may result from dental infection, and teeth that are tender should be carefully examined for signs of abscess. Drainage of the periapical abscess or removal of the diseased tooth typically resolves the sinus infection.

Acute ethmoiditis in adults is often accompanied by maxillary sinusitis, and symptoms are similar to those described above. Localized ethmoid sinusitis may present with pain and pressure over the high lateral wall of the nose between the eyes that may radiate to the orbit.

Sphenoid sinusitis is usually seen in the setting of pansinusitis or infection of all the paranasal sinuses on at least one side. The patient may complain of a headache "in the middle of the head" and often points to the vertex.

Acute frontal sinusitis may cause pain and tenderness of the forehead. This is most easily elicited by palpation of the orbital roof just below the medial end of the eyebrow.

Hospital-associated sinusitis is a form of acute bacterial rhinosinusitis that may present without the usual symptoms. Instead, it may be a cause of fever in critically ill patients. It is often associated with prolonged presence of a nasogastric or, rarely, nasotracheal tube causing nasal mucosal inflammation and ostiomeatal complex obstruction. Pansinusitis on the side of the tube is common on imaging studies.

B. Imaging

The diagnosis of acute bacterial rhinosinusitis can usually be made on clinical grounds alone. Although more sensitive than clinical examination, routine radiographs are not cost-effective and are not recommended by the Agency for Health Care Policy and Research or American Association of Otolaryngology Guidelines. Consensus guidelines recommend imaging when clinical criteria are difficult to evaluate, when the patient does not respond to appropriate therapy or has been treated repeatedly with antibiotics, when intracranial involvement or cerebrospinal fluid rhinorrhea is suspected, when complicated dental infection is suspected, or when symptoms of more serious infection are noted.

When necessary, noncontrast screening coronal CT scans are more cost-effective and provide more information than conventional sinus films. CT provides a rapid and effective means to assess all of the paranasal sinuses,

identify areas of greater concern (such as bony dehiscence, periosteal elevation or maxillary tooth root exposure within the sinus), and speed appropriate therapy.

CT scans are reasonably sensitive but are not specific. Swollen soft tissue and fluid may be difficult to distinguish when opacification of the sinus is due to other conditions, such as chronic rhinosinusitis, nasal polyposis, or mucus retention cysts. Sinus abnormalities can be seen in most patients with an upper respiratory infection, while bacterial rhinosinusitis develops in only 2%.

If malignancy, intracranial extension, or opportunistic infection is suspected, MRI with gadolinium should be ordered instead of, or in addition to, CT. MRI will distinguish tumor from fluid, inflammation, and inspissated mucus far better than CT, and will better delineate tumor extent (eg, involvement of adjacent structures, such as the orbit, skull base, and palate). Bone destruction can be demonstrated as well by MRI as by CT.

▶ Treatment

All patients with acute bacterial rhinosinusitis should have careful evaluation of pain. The European Position Paper on Rhinosinusitis and Nasal Polyps (EPOS) 2012 recommends NSAIDs, saline nasal sprays, and nasal decongestants (pseudoephedrine, 30–60 mg every 6 hours, up to 240 mg/day; nasal oxymetazoline, 0.05% or oxymetazoline, 0.05–0.1%, one or two sprays in each nostril every 6–8 hours for up to 3 days) for symptom reduction in viral rhinitis and bacterial rhinosinusitis without complication. In cases of suspected bacterial rhinosinusitis, intranasal corticosteroids (eg, high-dose mometasone furoate 200 mcg each nostril twice daily for 21 days) have demonstrated efficacy in reducing nasal symptoms and are recommended. Other medications, such as mucolytics, vitamin C, probiotics, and antihistamines, have not demonstrated efficacy in the management of acute rhinosinusitis.

Antibiotic therapy should be reserved for complicated or protracted acute bacterial rhinosinusitis. Between 40% and 69% of patients with acute bacterial rhinosinusitis improve symptomatically within 2 weeks without antibiotic therapy. Antibiotic treatment is controversial in uncomplicated cases of clinically diagnosed acute bacterial rhinosinusitis because only 5% of patients will note a shorter duration of illness with treatment, and antibiotic treatment is associated with nearly twice the number of adverse events compared with placebo. Antibiotics may be considered when symptoms last more than 10 days or when symptoms (including fever, facial pain, and swelling of the face) are severe or when cases are complicated (such as immunodeficiency). In these patients, administration of antibiotics does reduce the incidence of clinical failure by 50% and represents the most cost-effective treatment strategy.

Selection of antibiotics is usually empiric and based on a number of factors, including regional patterns of antibiotic resistance, antibiotic allergy, cost, and patient tolerance. For adults younger than 65 years with mild to moderate acute bacterial rhinosinusitis, the recommended first-line therapy is amoxicillin-clavulanate (500 mg/125 mg orally three times daily or 875 mg/125 mg orally twice daily for 5–7 days), or in those with severe sinusitis, high-dose amoxicillin-clavulanate (2000 mg/125 mg extended-release orally twice daily for 7–10 days). In patients with a high risk for penicillin-resistant *S pneumoniae* (age over 65 years, hospitalization in the prior 5 days, antibiotic use in the prior month, immunocompromised status, multiple comorbidities, or severe sinus infection), the recommended first-line therapy is the high-dose amoxicillin-clavulanate option (2000 mg/125 mg extended-release orally twice daily for 7–10 days). For those with penicillin allergy or hepatic impairment, then doxycycline (100 mg orally twice daily or 200 mg orally once daily for 5–7 days), or clindamycin (150–300 mg every 6 hours) plus a cephalosporin (cefixime 400 mg orally once daily or cefpodoxime proxetil 200 mg orally twice daily) for 10 days are options. Macrolides, trimethoprim-sulfamethoxazole, and second- or third-generation cephalosporins are not recommended for empiric therapy.

Hospital-associated infections in critically ill patients are treated differently from community-acquired infections. Removal of a nasogastric tube and improved nasal hygiene (nasal saline sprays, humidification of supplemental nasal oxygen, and nasal decongestants) are critical interventions and often curative in mild cases without aggressive antibiotic use. Endoscopic or transantral cultures may help direct medical therapy in complicated cases. In addition, broad-spectrum antibiotic coverage directed at *P aeruginosa, S aureus* (including methicillin-resistant strains), and anaerobes may be required.

► Complications

Local complications of acute bacterial rhinosinusitis include orbital cellulitis and abscess, osteomyelitis, cavernous sinus thrombosis, and intracranial extension.

Orbital complications typically occur by extension of ethmoid sinusitis through the lamina papyracea, a thin layer of bone that comprises the medial orbital wall. Any change in the ocular examination necessitates immediate CT imaging. Extension in this area may cause orbital cellulitis leading to proptosis, gaze restriction, and orbital pain. Select cases are responsive to intravenous antibiotics, with or without corticosteroids, and should be managed in close conjunction with an ophthalmologist or otolaryngologist, or both. Extension through the lamina papyracea can also lead to subperiosteal abscess formation (orbital abscess). Such abscesses cause marked proptosis, ophthalmoplegia, and pain with medial gaze. While some cases respond to antibiotics, such findings should prompt an immediate referral to a specialist for consideration of decompression and evacuation. Failure to intervene quickly may lead to permanent visual impairment and a "frozen globe."

Osteomyelitis requires prolonged antibiotics as well as removal of necrotic bone. The frontal sinus is most commonly affected, with bone involvement suggested by a tender swelling of the forehead (Pott puffy tumor). Following treatment, secondary cosmetic reconstructive procedures may be necessary.

Intracranial complications of sinusitis can occur either through hematogenous spread, as in cavernous sinus thrombosis and meningitis, or by direct extension, as in epidural and intraparenchymal brain abscesses. Fortunately, they are rare today. Cavernous sinus thrombosis is heralded by ophthalmoplegia, chemosis, and visual loss; the diagnosis is most commonly confirmed by MRI. When identified early, cavernous sinus thrombosis typically responds to intravenous antibiotics. Frontal epidural and intracranial abscesses are often clinically silent, but may present with altered mental status, persistent fever, or severe headache.

► When to Refer

Failure of acute bacterial rhinosinusitis to resolve after an adequate course of oral antibiotics necessitates referral to an otolaryngologist for evaluation. Endoscopic cultures may direct further treatment choices. Nasal endoscopy and CT scan are indicated when symptoms persist longer than 4–12 weeks. Any patients with suspected extension of disease outside the sinuses should be evaluated urgently by an otolaryngologist and imaging should be obtained.

► When to Admit

- Facial swelling and erythema indicative of facial cellulitis.
- Proptosis.
- Vision change or gaze abnormality indicative of orbital cellulitis.
- Abscess or cavernous sinus involvement.
- Mental status changes suggestive of intracranial extension.
- Immunocompromised status.
- Failure to respond to appropriate first-line treatment or symptoms persisting longer than 4 weeks.

Ahovuo-Saloranta A et al. Antibiotics for acute maxillary sinusitis in adults. Cochrane Database Syst Rev. 2014 Feb 11;(2):CD000243. Update in: Cochrane Database Syst Rev. 2015;(10):CD000243. [PMID: 24515610]

Carr TF. Complications of sinusitis. Am J Rhinol Allergy. 2016 Jul;30(4):241–5. [PMID: 27456592]

Dass K et al. Diagnosis and management of rhinosinusitis: highlights from the 2015 Practice Parameter. Curr Allergy Asthma Rep. 2016 Apr;16(4):29. [PMID: 26949223]

Harris AM et al; High Value Care Task Force of the American College of Physicians and for the Centers for Disease Control and Prevention. Appropriate antibiotic use for acute respiratory tract infection in adults: advice for high-value care from the American College of Physicians and the Centers for Disease Control and Prevention. Ann Intern Med. 2016 Mar 15;164(6):425–34. [PMID: 26785402]

Jaume F et al. Overuse of diagnostic tools and medications in acute rhinosinusitis in Spain: a population-based study (the PROSINUS study). BMJ Open. 2018 Jan 31;8(1):e018788. [PMID: 29391364]

Rosenfeld RM et al. Clinical practice guideline (update): adult sinusitis. Otolaryngol Head Neck Surg. 2015 Apr;152(Suppl 2):S1–39. [PMID: 25832968]

Smith SS et al. The prevalence of bacterial infection in acute rhinosinusitis: a systematic review and meta-analysis. Laryngoscope. 2015 Jan;125(1):57–69. [PMID: 24723427]

Snidvongs K et al. Update on intranasal medications in rhinosinusitis. Curr Allergy Asthma Rep. 2017 Jul;17(7):47. [PMID: 28602009]

3. Nasal Vestibulitis & *S aureus* Nasal Colonization

Inflammation of the nasal vestibule may result from folliculitis of the hairs that line this orifice and is usually the result of nasal manipulation or hair trimming. Systemic antibiotics effective against *S aureus* (such as dicloxacillin, 250 mg orally four times daily for 7–10 days) are indicated. Topical mupirocin 2% nasal ointment (applied two or three times daily) may be a helpful addition and may prevent future occurrences. If recurrent, the addition of rifampin (10 mg/kg orally twice daily for the last 4 days of dicloxacillin treatment) may eliminate the *S aureus* carrier state. If a furuncle exists, it should be incised and drained, preferably intranasally. Adequate treatment of these infections is important to prevent retrograde spread of infection through valveless veins into the cavernous sinus and intracranial structures.

S aureus is the leading nosocomial pathogen, and nasal carriage is a well-defined risk factor in the development and spread of nosocomial infections. Nasal and extranasal methicillin-resistant *S aureus* (MRSA) colonization are associated with a 30% risk of developing an invasive MRSA infection during hospital stays. While the vast majority have no vestibulitis symptoms, screening by nasal swabs and PCR-based assays has demonstrated a 30% rate of *S aureus* colonization in hospital patients and an 11% rate of MRSA colonization in intensive care unit patients. Elimination of the carrier state is challenging, but studies of mupirocin 2% nasal ointment application with chlorhexidine facial washing (40 mg/mL) twice daily for 5 days have demonstrated decolonization in 39% of patients.

Lipschitz N et al. Nasal vestibulitis: etiology, risk factors, and clinical characteristics: a retrospective study of 118 cases. Diagn Microbiol Infect Dis. 2017 Oct;89(2):131–4. [PMID: 28780999]

Sai N et al. Efficacy of the decolonization of methicillin-resistant *Staphylococcus aureus* carriers in clinical practice. Antimicrob Resist Infect Control. 2015 Dec 18;4:56. [PMID: 26688720]

4. Invasive Fungal Sinusitis

Invasive fungal sinusitis is rare and includes both rhinocerebral mucormycosis (*Mucor, Absidia,* and *Rhizopus* sp.) and other invasive fungal infections, such as *Aspergillus*. The fungus spreads rapidly through vascular channels and may be lethal if not detected early. Patients with mucormycosis almost invariably have some degree of immunocompromise, such as diabetes mellitus, long-term corticosteroid therapy, neutropenia associated with chemotherapy for hematologic malignancy, or end-stage renal disease. Occasional cases of sinonasal infection with *Aspergillus* sp. have been reported in patients with untreated HIV/AIDS. The initial symptoms may be similar to those of acute bacterial rhinosinusitis, although facial pain is often more severe. Nasal drainage is typically clear or straw-colored, rather than purulent, and visual symptoms may be noted at presentation in the absence of significant nasal findings. On examination, the classic finding of mucormycosis is a black eschar on the middle turbinate, but this finding is not universal and may not be apparent if the infection is deep or

high within the nasal bones. Often the mucosa appears normal or simply pale and dry. Early diagnosis requires suspicion of the disease and nasal biopsy with silver stains, revealing broad nonseptate hyphae within tissues and necrosis with vascular occlusion. Because CT or MRI may initially show only soft tissue changes, biopsy and ultimate debridement should be based on the clinical setting rather than radiographic demonstration of bony destruction or intracranial changes.

Invasive fungal sinusitis represents a medical and surgical emergency. Once recognized, amphotericin B by intravenous infusion and prompt wide surgical debridement are indicated for patients with reversible immune deficiency (eg, poorly controlled hyperglycemia in diabetes). Lipid-based amphotericin B (Ambisome) may be used in patients who have kidney disease or in whom nephrotoxicity from nonlipid amphotericin develops. Other antifungals, including voriconazole and caspofungin, may be appropriate therapy depending on the fungus. Surgical management, while necessary for any possibility of cure, often results in tremendous disfigurement and functional deficits (eg, often resulting in the loss of at least one eye). Even with early diagnosis and immediate appropriate intervention, the prognosis is guarded. In persons with diabetes, the mortality rate is about 20%. If kidney disease is present or develops, mortality is over 50%; in the setting of AIDS or hematologic malignancy with neutropenia, mortality approaches 100%. Whether to undertake aggressive surgical management should be considered carefully because many patients are gravely ill at the time of diagnosis, and overall disease-specific survival is only about 57%.

Ergun O et al. Acute invasive fungal rhinosinusitis: presentation of 19 cases, review of the literature, and a new classification system. J Oral Maxillofac Surg. 2017 Apr;75(4):767.e1–9. [PMID: 27918884]

Kashkouli MB et al. Outcomes and factors affecting them in patients with rhino-orbito-cerebral mucormycosis. Br J Ophthalmol. 2018 Dec 4. [Epub ahead of print] [PMID: 30514712]

Steve AK et al. Orbitomaxillofacial mucormycosis requiring complex multifactorial management. Plast Reconstr Surg Glob Open. 2018 Oct 2;6(10):e1927. [PMID: 30534490]

ALLERGIC RHINITIS

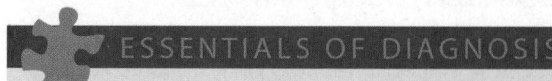

ESSENTIALS OF DIAGNOSIS

► Clear rhinorrhea, sneezing, tearing, eye irritation, and pruritus.

► Associated symptoms include cough, bronchospasm, and eczematous dermatitis.

► Environmental allergen exposure in the presence of allergen-specific IgE.

► General Considerations

Allergic rhinitis is very common in the United States with population studies reporting a prevalence of 20–30% of adults and up to 40% of children. Allergic rhinitis adversely affects school and work performance, costing about $6 billion annually in the United States through direct costs of therapy as well as the indirect costs of sleep deprivation, fatigue and reduced productivity, or absenteeism. Seasonal allergic rhinitis is most commonly caused by pollens and spores. Flowering shrub and tree pollens are most common in the spring, flowering plants and grasses in the summer, and ragweed and molds in the fall. Interestingly, climate change may have an impact on the occurrence of allergic rhinitis since increased temperature and carbon dioxide exposure cause increased pollen production in ragweed plants and since the extended duration of summer correlates with longer periods of pollen production in these and other flowering weeds. Dust, household mites, air pollution, and pet dander may produce year-round symptoms, termed "perennial rhinitis."

▶ **Clinical Findings**

The symptoms of "hay fever" are similar to those of viral rhinitis but are usually persistent and may show seasonal variation. Nasal symptoms are often accompanied by eye irritation, pruritus, conjunctival erythema, and excessive tearing. Many patients have a strong family history of atopy or allergy.

The clinician should be careful to distinguish allergic rhinitis from other types of nonallergic rhinitis. **Vasomotor rhinitis** (sometimes called **senile rhinitis**) is caused by increased sensitivity of the vidian nerve and is a common cause of clear rhinorrhea in elderly persons. Often patients will report that they have troubling rhinorrhea in response to numerous nasal stimuli, including warm or cold air, odors or scents, light, or particulate matter. Other types of rhinitis, including gustatory, atrophic, and drug-induced rhinorrhea, have also been described.

On physical examination, the mucosa of the turbinates is usually pale or violaceous because of venous engorgement. This is in contrast to the erythema of viral rhinitis. Nasal polyps, which are yellowish boggy masses of hypertrophic mucosa, are associated with long-standing allergic rhinitis.

▶ **Treatment**

A. Intranasal Corticosteroids

Intranasal corticosteroid sprays remain the mainstay of treatment of allergic rhinitis. They are more effective—and frequently less expensive—than nonsedating antihistamines, though patients should be reminded that there may be a delay in onset of relief of 2 or more weeks. Corticosteroid sprays may also shrink hypertrophic nasal mucosa and nasal polyps, thereby providing an improved nasal airway and ostiomeatal complex drainage. Because of this effect, intranasal corticosteroids are critical in treating allergy in patients prone to recurrent acute bacterial rhinosinusitis or chronic rhinosinusitis. Available preparations include beclomethasone (42 mcg/spray twice daily per nostril), flunisolide (25 mcg/spray twice daily per nostril), mometasone furoate (200 mcg once daily per

nostril), budesonide (100 mcg twice daily per nostril), and fluticasone propionate (200 mcg once daily per nostril). All are considered equally effective. Probably the most critical factors are compliance with regular use and proper introduction into the nasal cavity. In order to deliver medication to the region of the middle meatus, proper application involves holding the bottle straight up with the head tilted forward and pointing the bottle toward the ipsilateral ear when spraying. Side effects are limited, the most annoying being epistaxis (perhaps related to incorrect delivery of the drug toward the nasal septum).

B. Antihistamines

Antihistamines offer temporary, but immediate, control of many of the most troubling symptoms of allergic rhinitis. Effective oral antihistamines include nonsedating loratadine (10 mg once daily), desloratadine (5 mg once daily), and fexofenadine (60 mg twice daily or 120 mg once daily), and minimally sedating cetirizine (10 mg once daily). Brompheniramine or chlorpheniramine (4 mg orally every 6–8 hours, or 8–12 mg orally every 8–12 hours as a sustained-release tablet) and clemastine (1.34–2.68 mg orally twice daily) may be less expensive but are usually associated with some drowsiness. The H_1-receptor antagonist nasal spray azelastine (1–2 sprays per nostril daily) is also effective and now included in the treatment guidelines of many consensus statements, but some patients object to its bitter taste. Other side effects of oral antihistamines besides sedation include xerostomia and antihistamine tolerance (with eventual return of allergy symptoms despite initial benefit after several months of use). In such patients, typically those with perennial allergy, alternating effective antihistamines periodically can control symptoms over the long term.

C. Adjunctive Treatment Measures

Antileukotriene medications, such as montelukast (10 mg/day orally), alone or with cetirizine (10 mg/day orally) or loratadine (10 mg/day orally), may improve nasal rhinorrhea, sneezing, and congestion. Cromolyn sodium and sodium nedocromil are also useful adjunct agents for allergic rhinitis. They work by stabilizing mast cells and preventing proinflammatory mediator release. Topical agents, they have very few side effects. The most useful form of cromolyn is probably the ophthalmologic preparation. Intranasal cromolyn is cleared rapidly and must be administered four times daily for continued symptom relief, and it is not nearly as effective as inhaled corticosteroid.

Intranasal anticholinergic agents, such as ipratropium bromide 0.03% or 0.06% sprays (42–84 mcg per nostril three times daily), may be helpful adjuncts when rhinorrhea is a major symptom. They are not as effective for treating allergic rhinitis but are more useful for treating vasomotor rhinitis.

Avoiding or reducing exposure to airborne allergens is the most effective means of alleviating symptoms of allergic rhinitis. Depending on the allergen, this can be extremely difficult. Maintaining an allergen-free environment by covering pillows and mattresses with plastic covers, substituting synthetic materials (foam mattress, acrylics) for animal products (wool, horsehair), and removing dust-collecting household fixtures (carpets, drapes, bedspreads, wicker) is worth the attempt to help more troubled patients. Air purifiers and dust filters may also aid in maintaining an allergen-free environment. Nasal saline irrigations are a useful adjunct in the treatment of allergic rhinitis to mechanically flush the allergens from the nasal cavity. When symptoms are extremely bothersome, a search for offending allergens may prove helpful. This can either be done by serum radioallergosorbent test (RAST) testing or skin testing by an allergist.

In some cases, allergic rhinitis symptoms are inadequately relieved by medication and avoidance measures. Often, such patients have a strong family history of atopy and may also have lower respiratory manifestations, such as allergic asthma. Referral to an allergist for immunotherapy may be appropriate. Such treatment involves proper identification of offending allergens, progressively increasing doses of allergen(s), and eventual maintenance dose administration over a period of 3–5 years. Immunotherapy has been proven to reduce circulating IgE levels in patients with allergic rhinitis and reduce the need for allergy medications. Both subcutaneous and topical immunotherapy have been shown to be effective in the long-term treatment of refractory allergic rhinitis. Emerging evidence demonstrating the safety and efficacy of sublingual and intranasal immunotherapy may allow these outpatient treatment options to replace more traditional parenteral allergen desensitization for allergic rhinitis in the near future.

Hoyte FCL et al. Recent advances in allergic rhinitis. F1000Res. 2018 Aug 23;7. [PMID: 30210782]
May JR et al. Management of allergic rhinitis: a review for the community pharmacist. Clin Ther. 2017 Dec;39(12):2410–9. [PMID: 29079387]
Reitsma S et al. Recent developments and highlights in rhinitis and allergen immunotherapy. Allergy. 2018 Dec;73(12):2306–13. [PMID: 30260494]
Singh AK et al. Fungal rhinosinusitis: microbiological and histopathological perspective. J Clin Diagn Res. 2017 Jul;11(7):DC10–12. [PMID: 28892889]
Small P et al. Allergic rhinitis. Allergy Asthma Clin Immunol. 2018 Sep 12;14(Suppl 2):51. [PMID: 30263033]

OLFACTORY DYSFUNCTION

ESSENTIALS OF DIAGNOSIS

▸ Subjective diminished smell or taste sensation.

▸ Lack of objective nasal obstruction.

▸ Objective decrease in olfaction demonstrated by testing.

▸ General Considerations

Anatomic blockage of the nasal cavity with subsequent airflow disruption is the most common cause of olfactory dysfunction (hyposmia or anosmia). Polyps, septal deformities, and nasal tumors may be the cause. Transient olfactory dysfunction often accompanies the common cold, nasal allergies, and perennial rhinitis through changes in the nasal and olfactory epithelium. About 20% of olfactory dysfunction is idiopathic, although it often follows a viral illness. Central nervous system neoplasms, especially those that involve the olfactory groove or temporal lobe, may affect olfaction and must be considered in patients with no other explanation for their hyposmia or for other neurologic signs. Head trauma is a rare but severe cause of olfactory dysfunction. Shearing of the olfactory neurites is more commonly associated with anosmia. Absent, diminished, or distorted smell or taste has been reported in a wide variety of endocrine, nutritional, and nervous disorders (eg, Parkinson disease and Alzheimer disease).

▸ Clinical Findings

Evaluation of olfactory dysfunction should include a thorough history of systemic illnesses and medication use as well as a physical examination focusing on the nose and nervous system. Nasal obstruction (from polyps, trauma, foreign bodies, or nasal masses) can cause functional hyposmia. Most clinical offices are not set up to test olfaction, but such tests may at times be worthwhile if only to assess whether a patient possesses any sense of smell at all. The University of Pennsylvania Smell Identification Test (UPSIT) is available commercially and is a simple, self-administered "scratch-and-sniff" test that is useful in differentiating hyposmia, anosmia, and malingering.

▸ Treatment

Hyposmia secondary to nasal polyposis, obstruction, and chronic rhinosinusitis may respond to endoscopic sinus surgery. Unfortunately, there is no specific treatment for primary disruption of olfaction; some disturbances spontaneously resolve. The degree of hyposmia is the greatest predictor of recovery, with less severe hyposmia recovering at a much higher rate. In permanent hyposmia, counseling should be offered about seasoning foods (such as using pepper that stimulates the trigeminal as well as olfactory chemoreceptors, rather than table salt) and safety issues (such as installing home smoke alarms and using electric rather than gas appliances).

Doty RL. Age-related deficits in taste and smell. Otolaryngol Clin North Am. 2018 Aug;51(4):815–25. [PMID: 30001793]
Howell J et al. Head trauma and olfactory function. World J Otorhinolaryngol Head Neck Surg. 2018 Mar 14;4(1):39–45. [PMID: 30035260]
Werner S et al. Olfactory dysfunction revisited: a reappraisal of work-related olfactory dysfunction caused by chemicals. J Occup Med Toxicol. 2018 Sep 4;13:28. [PMID: 30202422]

EPISTAXIS

ESSENTIALS OF DIAGNOSIS

► Bleeding from a unilateral anterior nasal cavity most common.

► Most cases may be successfully treated by direct pressure on the bleeding site for 15 minutes. When this is inadequate, topical sympathomimetics and various nasal tamponade methods are usually effective.

► Posterior, bilateral, or large-volume epistaxis should be triaged immediately to a specialist in a critical care setting.

General Considerations

Epistaxis is an extremely common problem in the primary care setting. Bleeding is most common in the anterior septum where a confluence of veins creates a superficial venous plexus (Kiesselbach plexus). Predisposing factors include nasal trauma (nose picking, foreign bodies, forceful nose blowing), rhinitis, nasal mucosal drying from low humidity or supplemental nasal oxygen, deviation of the nasal septum, atherosclerotic disease, hereditary hemorrhagic telangiectasia (Osler-Weber-Rendu syndrome), inhaled nasal cocaine (or other illicit drug), and alcohol abuse. Poorly controlled hypertension is associated with epistaxis. Anticoagulation or antiplatelet medications may be associated with a higher incidence, more frequent recurrence, and greater difficulty in control of epistaxis, but they do not cause it.

Clinical Findings

Laboratory assessment of bleeding parameters may be indicated, especially in recurrent epistaxis. Once the acute episode has passed, careful examination of the nose and paranasal sinuses is indicated to rule out neoplasia and hereditary hemorrhagic telangiectasia.

Repeated evaluation for diagnosis and treatment of clinically significant hypertension should be performed following control of epistaxis and removal of any packing.

Treatment

Most cases of anterior epistaxis may be successfully treated by direct pressure on the site by compression of the nares continuously for 15 minutes. Venous pressure is reduced in the sitting position, and slight leaning forward lessens the swallowing of blood. Short-acting topical nasal decongestants (eg, phenylephrine, 0.125–1% solution, one or two sprays), which act as vasoconstrictors, may also help. When the bleeding does not readily subside, the nose should be examined, using good illumination and suction, in an attempt to locate the bleeding site. Topical 4% cocaine applied either as a spray or on a cotton strip serves both as an anesthetic and a vasoconstrictor. If cocaine is unavailable, a topical decongestant (eg, oxymetazoline) and a topical anesthetic (eg, tetracaine or lidocaine) provide similar results. When visible, the bleeding site may be cauterized with silver nitrate, diathermy, or electrocautery. A supplemental patch of Surgicel or Gelfoam may be helpful with a moisture barrier, such as petroleum-based ointment, to prevent drying and crusting. Warfarin may be continued in the setting of controlled epistaxis, although resorbable packing may be preferable in these patients.

Occasionally, a site of bleeding may be inaccessible to direct control, or attempts at direct control may be unsuccessful. In such cases, there are a number of alternatives. When the site of bleeding is anterior, a hemostatic sealant, pneumatic or other nasal tamponade, or anterior packing may suffice as the latter may be accomplished with several feet of lubricated iodoform packing systematically placed in the floor of the nose and then the vault of the nose.

About 5% of nasal bleeding originates in the posterior nasal cavity, commonly associated with atherosclerotic disease and hypertension. In such cases, it may be necessary to consult an otolaryngologist for a pack to occlude the choana before placing a pack anteriorly. In emergency settings, double balloon packs (Epistat) may facilitate rapid control of bleeding with little or no mucosal trauma. Because such packing is uncomfortable, bleeding may persist, and vasovagal syncope is possible, hospitalization for monitoring and stabilization is indicated. Opioid analgesics are needed to reduce the considerable discomfort and elevated blood pressure caused by a posterior pack.

Surgical management of epistaxis, through ligation of the nasal arterial supply (internal maxillary artery and ethmoid arteries) is indicated when direct pressure and nasal packing fail. The most common approach to surgical treatment is endoscopic sphenopalatine artery ligation. This method has a reported efficacy of 73–100% in studies; however, it may miss bleeds caused by the ethmoid arterial supply and it will leave an external scar beside the lateral canthus. Alternatively, endovascular epistaxis control is highly effective (75–92%) and can address all potential sources of intranasal bleeding. Its use may be reserved for when a surgical approach fails because it is associated with a 1.1–1.5% risk of stroke.

After control of epistaxis, the patient is advised to avoid straining and vigorous exercise for several days. Nasal saline should be applied to the packing frequently to keep the packing moist. Avoidance of hot or spicy foods and tobacco is also advisable, since these may cause nasal vasodilation. Avoiding nasal trauma, including nose picking, is an obvious necessity. Lubrication with petroleum jelly or bacitracin ointment and increased home humidity may also be useful ancillary measures. Finally, antistaphylococcal antibiotics (eg, cephalexin, 500 mg orally four times daily, or clindamycin, 150 mg orally four times daily) are indicated to reduce the risk of toxic shock syndrome developing while the packing remains in place (at least 5 days).

When to Refer

- Patients with recurrent epistaxis, large-volume epistaxis, and episodic epistaxis with associated nasal obstruction should be referred to an otolaryngologist for endoscopic evaluation and possible imaging.

- Those with ongoing bleeding beyond 15 minutes should be taken to a local emergency department if the clinician is not prepared to manage acute epistaxis.

Khan M et al. Initial assessment in the management of adult epistaxis: systematic review. J Laryngol Otol. 2017 Dec; 131(12):1035–55. [PMID: 29280694]

Min HJ et al. Association between hypertension and epistaxis: systematic review and meta-analysis. Otolaryngol Head Neck Surg. 2017 Dec;157(6):921–7. [PMID: 28742425]

Swords C et al. Surgical and interventional radiological management of adult epistaxis: systematic review. J Laryngol Otol. 2017 Dec;131(12):1108–30. [PMID: 29280696]

Williams A et al. Haematological factors in the management of adult epistaxis: systematic review. J Laryngol Otol. 2017 Dec; 131(12):1093–107. [PMID: 29280698]

NASAL TRAUMA

The nasal pyramid is the most frequently fractured bone in the body. Fracture is suggested by crepitance or palpably mobile bony segments. Epistaxis and pain are common, as are soft-tissue hematomas ("black eye"). It is important to make certain that there is no palpable step-off of the infraorbital rim, which would indicate the presence of a zygomatic complex fracture. Radiologic confirmation may at times be helpful but is not necessary in uncomplicated nasal fractures. It is also important to assess for possible concomitant additional facial, spine, pulmonary, or intracranial injuries when the circumstances of injury are suggestive, as in the case of automobile and motorcycle accidents.

Treatment is aimed at maintaining long-term nasal airway patency and cosmesis. Closed reduction can be performed under local or general anesthesia; closed reduction under general anesthesia appears to afford better patient satisfaction and decreased need for subsequent revision septoplasty or rhinoplasty.

Intranasal examination should be performed in all cases to rule out septal hematoma, which appears as a widening of the anterior septum, visible just posterior to the columella. The septal cartilage receives its only nutrition from its closely adherent mucoperichondrium. An untreated subperichondrial hematoma will result in loss of the nasal cartilage with resultant saddle nose deformity. Septal hematomas may become infected, with *S aureus* most commonly, and should be drained with an incision in the inferior mucoperichondrium on both sides. The drained fluid should be sent for culture.

Packing for 2–5 days is often helpful to help prevent re-formation of the hematoma. Antibiotics with antistaphylococcal efficacy (eg, cephalexin, 500 mg four times daily, or clindamycin, 150 mg four times daily) should be given for 3–5 days or the duration of the packing to reduce the risk of toxic shock syndrome.

Lu GN et al. Correction of nasal fractures. Facial Plast Surg Clin North Am. 2017 Nov;25(4):537–46. [PMID: 28941506]

TUMORS & GRANULOMATOUS DISEASE

1. Benign Nasal Tumors

A. Nasal Polyps

Nasal polyps are pale, edematous, mucosally covered masses commonly seen in patients with allergic rhinitis. They may result in chronic nasal obstruction and a diminished sense of smell. In patients with nasal polyps and a history of asthma, aspirin should be avoided as it may precipitate a severe episode of bronchospasm, known as **triad asthma** (Samter triad). Such patients may have an immunologic salicylate sensitivity.

Use of topical intranasal corticosteroids improves the quality of life in patients with nasal polyposis and chronic rhinosinusitis. Initial treatment with topical nasal corticosteroids (see Allergic Rhinitis section for specific drugs) for 1–3 months is usually successful for small polyps and may reduce the need for operation. A short course of oral corticosteroids (eg, prednisone, 6-day course using 21 [5-mg] tablets: 6 tablets [30 mg] on day 1 and tapering by 1 tablet [5 mg] each day) may also be of benefit. When polyps are massive or medical management is unsuccessful, polyps may be removed surgically. In healthy persons, this is a minor outpatient procedure. In recurrent cases or when surgery itself is associated with increased risk (such as in patients with asthma), a more complete procedure, such as ethmoidectomy, may be advisable. In recurrent polyposis, it may be necessary to remove polyps from the ethmoid, sphenoid, and maxillary sinuses to provide longer-lasting relief. Intranasal corticosteroids should be continued following polyp removal to prevent recurrence, and the clinician should consider allergen testing to determine the offending allergen and avoidance measures.

Brescia G et al. Nasal polyposis pathophysiology: endotype and phenotype open issues. Am J Otolaryngol. 2018 Jul–Aug;39(4): 441–4. [PMID: 29550078]

Rivero A et al. Anti-IgE and anti-IL5 biologic therapy in the treatment of nasal polyposis: a systematic review and meta-analysis. Ann Otol Rhinol Laryngol. 2017 Nov;126(11):739–47. [PMID: 28918644]

B. Inverted Papillomas

Inverted papillomas are benign tumors caused by human papillomavirus (HPV) that usually arise on the lateral nasal wall. They present with unilateral nasal obstruction and occasionally hemorrhage. They are often easily seen on anterior rhinoscopy as cauliflower-like growths in or around the middle meatus. Because squamous cell carcinoma is seen in about 10% of inverted or schneiderian papillomas, complete excision is strongly recommended. This usually requires a medial maxillectomy, but in selected cases an endoscopic approach may be possible. Because recurrence rates for inverted papillomas are reported to be as high as 20%, subsequent clinical and radiologic follow-up is imperative. All excised tissue (not just a portion) should be carefully reviewed by the pathologist to be sure no carcinoma is present.

Bugter O et al. Surgical management of inverted papilloma; a single-center analysis of 247 patients with long follow-up. J Otolaryngol Head Neck Surg. 2017 Dec 20;46(1):67. [PMID: 29262865]

Gamrot-Wrzoł M et al. Risk factors of recurrence and malignant transformation of sinonasal inverted papilloma. Biomed Res Int. 2017;2017:9195163. [PMID: 29250552]

2. Malignant Nasopharyngeal & Paranasal Sinus Tumors

Though rare, malignant tumors of the nose, nasopharynx, and paranasal sinuses are quite problematic because they tend to remain asymptomatic until late in their course. Squamous cell carcinoma is the most common cancer found in the sinuses and nasopharynx. It is especially common in the nasopharynx, where it obstructs the eustachian tube and results in serous otitis media. Nasopharyngeal carcinoma (nonkeratinizing squamous cell carcinoma or lymphoepithelioma) is usually associated with elevated IgA antibody to the viral capsid antigen of the Epstein-Barr virus (EBV). It is particularly common in patients of southern Chinese descent and has a weaker association with tobacco exposure than other head and neck squamous cell carcinomas. Adenocarcinomas, mucosal melanomas, sarcomas, and non-Hodgkin lymphomas are less commonly encountered neoplasms of this area.

Early symptoms are nonspecific, mimicking those of rhinitis or sinusitis. Unilateral nasal obstruction, otitis media, and discharge are common, with pain and recurrent hemorrhage often clues to the diagnosis of cancer. Any adult with persistent unilateral nasal symptoms or new otitis media should be thoroughly evaluated with nasal endoscopy and nasopharyngoscopy. A high index of suspicion remains a key to early diagnosis of these tumors. Patients often present with advanced symptoms, such as proptosis, expansion of a cheek, or ill-fitting maxillary dentures. Malar hypesthesia, due to involvement of the infraorbital nerve, is common in maxillary sinus tumors. Biopsy is necessary for definitive diagnosis, and MRI is the best imaging study to delineate the extent of disease and plan appropriate surgery and radiation.

Treatment depends on the tumor type and the extent of disease. Very early stage disease may be treated with megavoltage radiation therapy alone, but advanced nasopharyngeal carcinoma is best treated with concurrent radiation and cisplatin followed by adjuvant chemotherapy with cisplatin and fluorouracil. This chemoradiation therapy protocol significantly decreases local, nodal, and distant failures and increases progression-free and overall survival in advanced stage disease. Locally recurrent nasopharyngeal carcinoma may in selected cases be treated with repeat irradiation protocols or surgery with moderate success and a high degree of concern about local wound healing. Other squamous cell carcinomas are best treated—when resectable—with a combination of surgery and irradiation. Cranial base surgery, which can be done endoscopically using image navigation, appears to be an effective modality in improving the overall prognosis in paranasal sinus malignancies eroding the ethmoid roof. Although the prognosis is poor for advanced tumors, the results of treating resectable tumors of paranasal sinus origin have improved with the wider use of skull base resections and intensity-modulated radiation therapy. Cure rates are often 45–60%.

El-Sharkawy A et al. Epstein-Barr virus-associated malignancies: roles of viral oncoproteins in carcinogenesis. Front Oncol. 2018 Aug 2;8:265. [PMID: 30116721]

Lee AW et al. Management of nasopharyngeal carcinoma: current practice and future perspective. J Clin Oncol. 2015 Oct 10; 33(29):3356–64. [PMID: 26351355]

Vartanian JG et al. Orbital exenteration for sinonasal malignancies: indications, rehabilitation and oncologic outcomes. Curr Opin Otolaryngol Head Neck Surg. 2018 Apr;26(2):122–6. [PMID: 29465436]

3. Sinonasal Inflammatory Disease (Granulomatosis with Polyangiitis & Sarcoidosis)

The nose and paranasal sinuses are involved in over 90% of cases of **granulomatosis with polyangiitis**. It is often not realized that involvement at these sites is more common than involvement of lungs or kidneys. Examination shows bloodstained crusts and friable mucosa. Biopsy, when positive, shows necrotizing granulomas and vasculitis. Other recognized sites of granulomatosis with polyangiitis in the head and neck include the subglottis and the middle ear. For treatment of granulomatosis with polyangiitis, see Chapter 20.

Sarcoidosis commonly involves the paranasal sinuses and is clinically similar to other chronic sinonasal inflammatory processes. Sinonasal symptoms, including rhinorrhea, nasal obstruction, and hyposmia or anosmia may precede diagnosis of sarcoidosis in other organ systems. Clinically, the turbinates appear engorged with small white granulomas. Biopsy shows classic noncaseating granulomas. Notably, patients with sinonasal involvement generally have more trouble managing sarcoidosis in other organ systems.

Polymorphic reticulosis (midline malignant reticulosis, idiopathic midline destructive disease, lethal midline granuloma)—as the multitude of apt descriptive terms suggests—is not well understood but appears to be a nasal T-cell or NK-cell lymphoma. In contrast to granulomatosis with polyangiitis, involvement is limited to the mid-face, and there may be extensive bone destruction. Many destructive lesions of the mucosa and nasal structures labeled as polymorphic reticulosis are in fact non-Hodgkin lymphoma of either NK-cell or T-cell origin. Immunophenotyping, especially for CD56 expression, is essential in the histologic evaluation. Even when apparently localized, these lymphomas have a poor prognosis, with progression and death within a year the rule.

Chapman MN et al. Sarcoidosis in the head and neck: an illustrative review of clinical presentations and imaging findings. AJR Am J Roentgenol. 2017 Jan;208(1):66–75. [PMID: 27657552]

D'Anza B et al. Sinonasal imaging findings in granulomatosis with polyangiitis (Wegener granulomatosis): a systematic review. Am J Rhinol Allergy. 2017 Jan 1;31(1):16–21. [PMID: 28234146]

Hintze JM et al. Sarcoidosis presenting as bilateral vocal fold immobility. J Voice. 2018 May;32(3):359–62. [PMID: 28684250]

Kühn D et al. Manifestation of granulomatosis with polyangiitis in head and neck. Clin Exp Rheumatol. 2018 Mar–Apr; 36 Suppl 111(2):78–84. [PMID: 29799391]

DISEASES OF THE ORAL CAVITY & PHARYNX

LEUKOPLAKIA, ERYTHROPLAKIA, ORAL LICHEN PLANUS, & ORAL CANCER

ESSENTIALS OF DIAGNOSIS

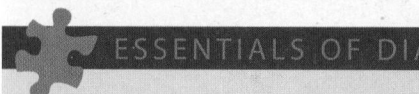

- ► **Leukoplakia:** A white lesion that cannot be removed by rubbing the mucosal surface.
- ► **Erythroplakia:** Similar to leukoplakia except that it has a definite erythematous component.
- ► **Oral Lichen Planus:** Most commonly presents as lacy leukoplakia but may be erosive; definitive diagnosis requires biopsy.
- ► **Oral Cancer:** Early lesions appear as leukoplakia or erythroplakia; more advanced lesions will be larger, with invasion into the tongue such that a mass lesion is palpable. Ulceration may be present.
- ► **Oropharynx Cancer:** Unilateral throat masses, typically presenting with painful swallowing and weight loss.

Leukoplakic regions range from small to several centimeters in diameter (Figure 8–5). Histologically, they are often hyperkeratoses occurring in response to chronic irritation (eg, from dentures, tobacco, lichen planus); about 2–6%, however, represent either dysplasia or early invasive squamous cell carcinoma. Distinguishing between **leukoplakia** and **erythroplakia** is important because about 90% of cases of erythroplakia are either dysplasia or carcinoma. **Squamous cell carcinoma** accounts for 90% of oral cancer. Alcohol and tobacco use are the major epidemiologic risk factors.

The differential diagnosis may include oral candidiasis, necrotizing sialometaplasia, pseudoepitheliomatous hyperplasia, median rhomboid glossitis, and vesiculoerosive inflammatory disease, such as erosive lichen planus. This should not be confused with the brown-black gingival melanin pigmentation—diffuse or speckled—common in nonwhites, blue-black embedded fragments of dental amalgam, or other systemic disorders associated with general pigmentation (neurofibromatosis, familial polyposis, Addison disease). Intraoral melanoma is extremely rare and carries a dismal prognosis.

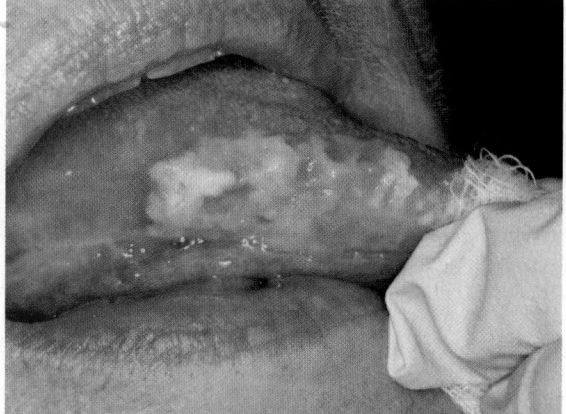

▲ **Figure 8–5.** Leukoplakia with moderate dysplasia on the lateral border of the tongue. (Used, with permission, from Ellen Eisenberg, DMD, in Usatine RP, Smith MA, Mayeaux EJ Jr, Chumley H, Tysinger J. *The Color Atlas of Family Medicine.* McGraw-Hill, 2009.)

Any area of **erythroplakia**, enlarging area of **leukoplakia**, or a lesion that has submucosal depth on palpation should have an incisional biopsy or an exfoliative cytologic examination. Ulcerative lesions are particularly suspicious and worrisome. Specialty referral should be sought early both for diagnosis and treatment. A systematic intraoral examination—including the lateral tongue, floor of the mouth, gingiva, buccal area, palate, and tonsillar fossae—and palpation of the neck for enlarged lymph nodes should be part of any general physical examination, especially in patients over the age of 45 who smoke tobacco or drink immoderately. Indirect or fiberoptic examination of the nasopharynx, oropharynx, hypopharynx, and larynx by an otolaryngologist, head and neck surgeon, or radiation oncologist should also be considered for such patients when there is unexplained or persistent throat or ear pain, oral or nasal bleeding, or oral erythroplakia. Fine-needle aspiration (FNA) biopsy may expedite the diagnosis if an enlarged lymph node is found.

To date, there remain no approved therapies for reversing or stabilizing leukoplakia or erythroplakia. Clinical trials have suggested a role for beta-carotene, celecoxib, vitamin E, and retinoids in producing regression of leukoplakia and reducing the incidence of recurrent squamous cell carcinomas. None have demonstrated benefit in large studies and these agents are not in general use today. The mainstays of management are surveillance following elimination of carcinogenic irritants (eg, smoking tobacco, chewing tobacco or betel nut, drinking alcohol) along with serial biopsies and excisions.

Oral lichen planus is a relatively common (0.5–2% of the population) chronic inflammatory autoimmune disease that may be difficult to diagnose clinically because of its numerous distinct phenotypic subtypes. For example, the reticular pattern may mimic candidiasis or hyperkeratosis, while the erosive pattern may mimic squamous cell carcinoma. Management begins with distinguishing it from other oral lesions. Exfoliative cytology or a small incisional or excisional biopsy is indicated, especially if squamous cell carcinoma is suspected. Therapy of lichen planus is aimed at managing pain and discomfort. Daily topical corticosteroid remains the most effective treatment for symptomatic lichen planus, but cyclosporines, retinoids, and tacrolimus have also been used. Many experts think there is a low rate (1%) of squamous cell carcinoma arising within lichen planus (in addition to the possibility of clinical misdiagnosis) and prevention of malignant transformation remains a goal of treatment. Photodynamic therapy is being studied as an approach to both treatment of symptomatic lichen planus as well as prevention of malignant transformation, but there is no compelling evidence to argue for widespread application of this technique at this time.

Hairy leukoplakia occurs on the lateral border of the tongue and is a common early finding in HIV infection (see Chapter 31). It often develops quickly and appears as slightly raised leukoplakic areas with a corrugated or "hairy" surface (Figure 8–6). While much more prevalent in HIV-positive patients, hairy leukoplakia can occur following solid organ transplantation and is associated with Epstein-Barr virus infection and long-term systemic corticosteroid use. Hairy leukoplakia waxes and wanes over time with generally modest irritative symptoms. Acyclovir, valacyclovir, and famciclovir have all been used for treatment but produce only temporary resolution of the condition. It does not appear to predispose to malignant transformation.

Oral cavity squamous cell carcinoma can be hard to distinguish from other oral lesions, but early detection is the key to successful management (Figure 8–7). Raised, firm, white lesions with ulcers at the base are highly suspicious and generally quite painful on even gentle palpation. Lesions less than 4 mm in depth have a low propensity to metastasize. Most patients in whom the tumor is detected before it is 2 cm in diameter are cured by local resection. Radiation is reserved for patients with positive margins or metastatic disease. Large tumors are usually treated with a combination of resection, neck dissection, and external

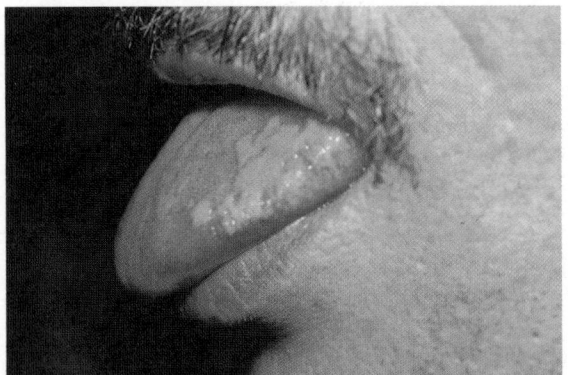

▲ **Figure 8–6.** Oral hairy leukoplakia on the side of the tongue in AIDS. (Used, with permission, from Richard P. Usatine, MD, in Usatine RP, Smith MA, Mayeaux EJ Jr, Chumley H, Tysinger J. *The Color Atlas of Family Medicine.* McGraw-Hill, 2009.)

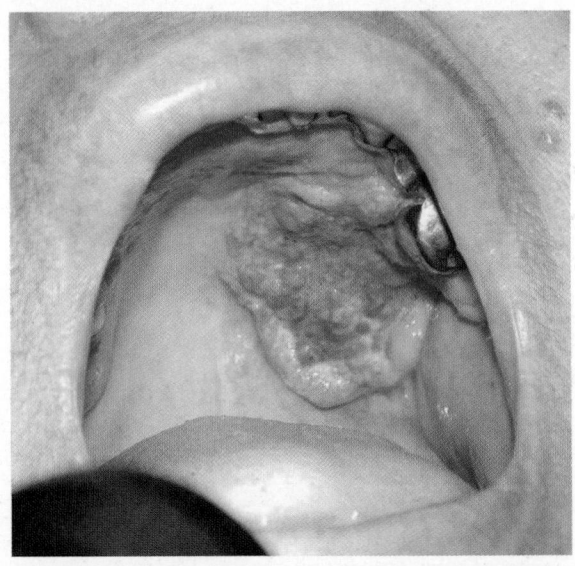

▲ **Figure 8–7.** Squamous cell carcinoma of the palate. (Used, with permission, from Frank Miller, MD, in Usatine RP, Smith MA, Mayeaux EJ Jr, Chumley H, Tysinger J. *The Color Atlas of Family Medicine.* McGraw-Hill, 2009.)

beam radiation. Reconstruction, if required, is done at the time of resection and can involve the use of myocutaneous flaps or vascularized free flaps with or without bone.

Oropharyngeal squamous cell carcinoma generally presents later than oral cavity squamous cell carcinoma. The lesions tend to be larger and are often buried within the lymphoid tissue of the palatine or lingual tonsils. Most patients note only unilateral odynophagia and weight loss, but ipsilateral cervical lymphadenopathy is often identified by the careful clinician. While these tumors are typically associated with known carcinogens such as tobacco and alcohol, their epidemiology has changed dramatically over the past 20 years. Despite demonstrated reductions in tobacco and alcohol use within developed nations, the incidence of oropharyngeal squamous cell carcinoma has not declined over this period. Known as a possible cause of head and neck cancer since 1983, the human papillomavirus (HPV)—most commonly, type 16—is now believed to be the cause of up to 70% of all oropharyngeal squamous cell carcinoma. HPV-positive tumors are readily distinguished by immunostaining of primary tumor or fine-needle aspiration biopsy specimens for the p16 protein, a tumor suppressor protein that is highly correlated with the presence of HPV. These tumors often present in advanced stages of the disease with regional cervical lymph node metastases (stages III and IV), but have a better prognosis than similarly staged lesions in tobacco and alcohol users. This difference in disease control is so apparent in multicenter studies that, based on the presence or absence of the p16 protein, two distinct staging systems for oropharyngeal squamous cell carcinoma were introduced in 2018. Ongoing clinical trials are trying to determine if a reduction in treatment intensity is warranted for HPV-associated cancers.

Awadallah M et al. Management update of potentially premalignant oral epithelial lesions. Oral Surg Oral Med Oral Pathol Oral Radiol. 2018 Jun;125(6):628–36. [PMID: 29656948]

Chera BS et al. Current status and future directions of treatment deintensification in human papilloma virus–associated oropharyngeal squamous cell carcinoma. Semin Radiat Oncol. 2018 Jan;28(1):27–34. [PMID: 29173753]

Giannetti L et al. Oral lichen planus. J Biol Regul Homeost Agents. 2018 Mar–Apr;32(2):391–5. [PMID: 29685024]

Gooi Z et al. The epidemiology of the human papillomavirus related to oropharyngeal head and neck cancer. Laryngoscope. 2016 Apr;126(4):894–900. [PMID: 26845348]

Gupta S et al. Interventions for the management of oral lichen planus: a review of the conventional and novel therapies. Oral Dis. 2017 Nov;23(8):1029–42. [PMID: 28055124]

Huang SH et al. Overview of the 8th edition TNM classification for head and neck cancer. Curr Treat Options Oncol. 2017 Jul;18(7):40. [PMID: 28555375]

Lowy DR et al. Preventing cancer and other diseases caused by human papillomavirus infection: 2017 Lasker-DeBakey Clinical Research Award. JAMA. 2017 Sept 12;318(10):901–2. [PMID: 28876435]

Mello FW et al. Prevalence of oral potentially malignant disorders: a systematic review and meta-analysis. J Oral Pathol Med. 2018 Aug;47(7):633–40. [PMID: 29738071]

Nadeau C et al. Evaluation and management of oral potentially malignant disorders. Dent Clin North Am. 2018 Jan;62(1):1–27. [PMID: 29126487]

Staines K et al. Oral leukoplakia and proliferative verrucous leukoplakia: a review for dental practitioners. Br Dent J. 2017 Dec;223(9):655–61. [PMID: 29097794]

ORAL CANDIDIASIS

ESSENTIALS OF DIAGNOSIS

- ▶ Fluctuating throat or mouth discomfort.
- ▶ Systemic or local immunosuppression, such as recent corticosteroid, chemotherapy, or antibiotic use.
- ▶ Erythema of the oral cavity or oropharynx with creamy-white, curd-like patches.
- ▶ Rapid resolution of symptoms with appropriate treatment.

▶ Clinical Findings

A. Symptoms and Signs

Oral candidiasis (thrush) is usually painful and looks like creamy-white curd-like patches overlying erythematous mucosa (see Figure 6–22). Because these white areas are easily rubbed off (eg, by a tongue depressor)—unlike leukoplakia or lichen planus—only the underlying irregular erythema may be seen. Oral candidiasis is commonly associated with the following risk factors: (1) use of dentures, (2) debilitated state with poor oral hygiene, (3) diabetes mellitus, (4) anemia, (5) chemotherapy or local irradiation, (6) corticosteroid use (oral or systemic), or (7) broad-spectrum antibiotics. Another manifestation of candidiasis is angular cheilitis (also seen in nutritional deficiencies) (Figure 8–8).

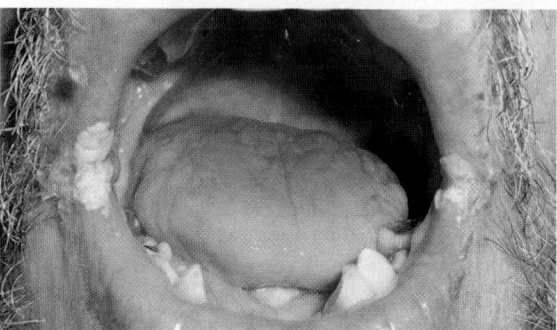

▲ **Figure 8–8.** Severe angular cheilitis in HIV-positive man with oral thrush. (Used, with permission, from Richard P. Usatine, MD, in Usatine RP, Smith MA, Mayeaux EJ Jr, Chumley H, Tysinger J. *The Color Atlas of Family Medicine.* McGraw-Hill, 2009.)

B. Diagnostic Studies

The diagnosis is made clinically. A wet preparation using potassium hydroxide will reveal spores and may show non-septate mycelia. Biopsy will show intraepithelial pseudomycelia of *Candida albicans*.

Candidiasis is often the first manifestation of HIV infection, and HIV testing should be considered in patients with no known predisposing cause for *Candida* overgrowth (see also Chapter 31). The US Department of Health Services Clinical Practice Guideline for Evaluation and Management of Early HIV Infection recommends examination of the oral mucosa with each clinician visit as well as at a dental examination every 6 months for individuals infected with HIV.

▶ Treatment

Effective antifungal therapy may be achieved with any of the following: fluconazole (100 mg orally daily for 7 days), ketoconazole (200–400 mg orally with breakfast [requires acidic gastric environment for absorption] for 7–14 days), clotrimazole troches (10 mg dissolved orally five times daily), or nystatin mouth rinses (500,000 units [5 mL of 100,000 units/mL] held in the mouth before swallowing three times daily). In patients with HIV infection, however, longer courses of therapy with fluconazole may be needed, and oral itraconazole (200 mg/day) may be indicated in fluconazole-refractory cases. Many of the *Candida* species in these patients are resistant to first-line azoles and may require newer drugs, such as voriconazole. In addition, 0.12% chlorhexidine or half-strength hydrogen peroxide mouth rinses may provide local relief. Nystatin powder (100,000 units/g) applied to dentures three or four times daily and rinsed off for several weeks may help denture wearers.

Lewis MAO et al. Diagnosis and management of oral candidosis. Br Dent J. 2017 Nov 10;223(9):675–81. [PMID: 29123282]

Patton LL. Current strategies for prevention of oral manifestations of human immunodeficiency virus. Oral Surg Oral Med Oral Pathol Oral Radiol. 2016 Jan;121(1):29–38. [PMID: 26679357]

GLOSSITIS, GLOSSODYNIA, DYSGEUSIA, & BURNING MOUTH SYNDROME

Inflammation of the tongue with loss of filiform papillae leads to a red, smooth-surfaced tongue (glossitis). Rarely painful, it may be secondary to nutritional deficiencies (eg, niacin, riboflavin, iron, or vitamin E), drug reactions, dehydration, irritants, or foods and liquids, and possibly to autoimmune reactions or psoriasis. If the primary cause cannot be identified and corrected, empiric nutritional replacement therapy may be of value.

Glossodynia is burning and pain of the tongue, which may occur with or without glossitis. In the absence of any clinical findings, it has been termed "burning mouth syndrome." Glossodynia with glossitis has been associated with diabetes mellitus, drugs (eg, diuretics), tobacco, xerostomia, and candidiasis as well as the listed causes of glossitis. The burning mouth syndrome typically has no identifiable associated risk factors and seems to be most common in postmenopausal women. Treating possible underlying causes, changing long-term medications to alternative ones, and smoking cessation may resolve symptoms of glossitis. Effective treatments for the burning mouth syndrome include alpha-lipoic acid and clonazepam. Clonazepam is most effective as a rapid-dissolving tablet placed on the tongue in doses from 0.25 mg to 0.5 mg every 8–12 hours. Both glossodynia and the burning mouth syndrome are benign, and reassurance that there is no infection or tumor is likely to be appreciated. Unilateral symptoms, symptoms that cannot be related to a specific medication, and symptoms and signs involving regions supplied by other cranial nerves all may suggest neuropathology, and imaging of the brain, brainstem, and skull base with MRI should be considered.

Klasser GD et al. Burning mouth syndrome. Oral Maxillofac Surg Clin North Am. 2016 Aug;28(3):381–96. [PMID: 27475513]

Salerno C et al. An overview of burning mouth syndrome. Front Biosci (Elite Ed). 2016 Jan 1;8:213–8. [PMID: 26709657]

Silvestre FJ et al. Burning mouth syndrome: a review and update. Rev Neurol. 2015 May 16;60(10):457–63. [PMID: 25952601]

Syed Q et al. The impact of aging and medical status on dysgeusia. Am J Med. 2016 Jul;129(7):753.e1–6. [PMID: 26899755]

INTRAORAL ULCERATIVE LESIONS

1. Necrotizing Ulcerative Gingivitis (Trench Mouth, Vincent Angina)

Necrotizing ulcerative gingivitis, often caused by an infection with both spirochetes and fusiform bacilli, is common in young adults under stress (classically in students at examination time). Underlying systemic diseases may also predispose to this disorder. Clinically, there is painful acute gingival inflammation and necrosis, often with bleeding, halitosis, fever, and cervical lymphadenopathy. Warm half-strength peroxide rinses and oral penicillin (250 mg three times daily for 10 days) may help. Dental gingival curettage may prove necessary.

Dufty J et al. Necrotising ulcerative gingivitis: a literature review. Oral Health Prev Dent. 2017;15(4):321–7. [PMID: 28761942]

2. Aphthous Ulcer (Canker Sore, Ulcerative Stomatitis)

Aphthous ulcers are very common and easy to recognize. Their cause remains uncertain, although an association with human herpesvirus 6 has been suggested. Found on freely moving, nonkeratinized mucosa (eg, buccal and labial mucosa and not attached gingiva or palate), they may be single or multiple, are usually recurrent, and appear as painful small round ulcerations with yellow-gray fibrinoid centers surrounded by red halos. Minor aphthous ulcers are less than 1 cm in diameter and generally heal in 10–14 days. Major aphthous ulcers are greater than 1 cm in diameter and can be disabling due to the degree of associated oral pain. Stress seems to be a major predisposing factor to the eruptions of aphthous ulcers. A study found that the frequency of viral rhinitis and bedtime after 11 PM were independent predictors of aphthous ulcer frequency and severity in college students.

Treatment is challenging because no single systemic treatment has proven effective. Topical corticosteroids (triamcinolone acetonide, 0.1%, or fluocinonide ointment, 0.05%) in an adhesive base (Orabase Plain) do appear to provide symptomatic relief in many patients. Other topical therapies shown to be effective in controlled studies include diclofenac 3% in hyaluronan 2.5%, doxymycine-cyanoacrylate, mouthwashes containing the enzymes amyloglucosidase and glucose oxidase, and amlexanox 5% oral paste. A 1-week tapering course of prednisone (40–60 mg/day) has also been used successfully. Cimetidine maintenance therapy may be useful in patients with recurrent aphthous ulcers. Thalidomide has been used selectively in recurrent aphthous ulcerations in HIV-positive patients.

Large or persistent areas of ulcerative stomatitis may be secondary to erythema multiforme or drug allergies, acute herpes simplex, pemphigus, pemphigoid, epidermolysis bullosa acquisita, bullous lichen planus, Behçet disease, or inflammatory bowel disease. Squamous cell carcinoma may occasionally present in this fashion. When the diagnosis is not clear, incisional biopsy is indicated.

Cui RZ et al. Recurrent aphthous stomatitis. Clin Dermatol. 2016 Jul–Aug;34(4):475–81. [PMID: 27343962]

Ranganath SP et al. Is optimal management of recurrent aphthous stomatitis possible? A reality check. J Clin Diagn Res. 2016 Oct;10(10):ZE08–13. [PMID: 27891490]

3. Herpes Stomatitis

Herpes gingivostomatitis is common, mild, and short-lived and requires no intervention in most adults. In immunocompromised persons, however, reactivation of herpes simplex virus infection is frequent and may be severe. Clinically, there is initial burning, followed by typical small vesicles that rupture and form scabs. Lesions are most commonly found on the attached gingiva and mucocutaneous junction of the lip, but lesions can also form on the tongue, buccal mucosa, and soft palate. Acyclovir (200–800 mg orally five times daily for 7–10 days) or valacyclovir (1000 mg orally twice daily for 7–10 days) may shorten the course and reduce postherpetic pain. These treatments may be effective only when started within 24–48 hours of the onset of initial symptoms (pain, itching, burning) and are not effective once vesicles have erupted. Differential diagnosis includes aphthous stomatitis, erythema multiforme, syphilitic chancre, and carcinoma.

Chi CC et al. Interventions for prevention of herpes simplex labialis (cold sores on the lips). Cochrane Database Syst Rev. 2015 Aug 7;(8):CD010095. [PMID: 26252373]

Hargitai IA. Painful oral lesions. Dent Clin North Am. 2018 Oct; 62(4):597–609. [PMID: 30189985]

PHARYNGITIS & TONSILLITIS

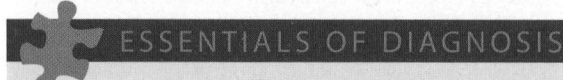

ESSENTIALS OF DIAGNOSIS

- ▶ Sore throat.
- ▶ Fever.
- ▶ Anterior cervical adenopathy.
- ▶ Tonsillar exudate.
- ▶ Focus is to treat group A beta-hemolytic *Streptococcus* infection to prevent rheumatic sequelae.

▶ General Considerations

Pharyngitis and tonsillitis account for over 10% of all office visits to primary care clinicians and 50% of outpatient antibiotic use. The main concern is determining who is likely to have a group A beta-hemolytic streptococcal (GABHS) infection, since this can lead to subsequent complications, such as rheumatic fever and glomerulonephritis. A second public health policy concern is reducing the extraordinary cost (both in dollars and in the development of antibiotic-resistant *S pneumoniae*) in the United States associated with unnecessary antibiotic use. Questions being asked include: Have the rapid antigen tests supplanted the need to culture a throat under most circumstances? Are clinical criteria alone a sufficient basis for decisions about which patients should be given antibiotics? Should any patient receive any antibiotic other than penicillin (or erythromycin if penicillin-allergic)? For how long should treatment be continued? Numerous well-done studies and experience with rapid laboratory tests for detection of streptococci (eliminating the delay caused by culturing) informed a consensus experience.

▶ Clinical Findings

A. Symptoms and Signs

The clinical features most suggestive of GABHS pharyngitis include fever over 38°C, tender anterior cervical adenopathy, lack of a cough, and pharyngotonsillar exudate (Figure 8–9). These four features (the Centor criteria), when present, strongly suggest GABHS. When two or three

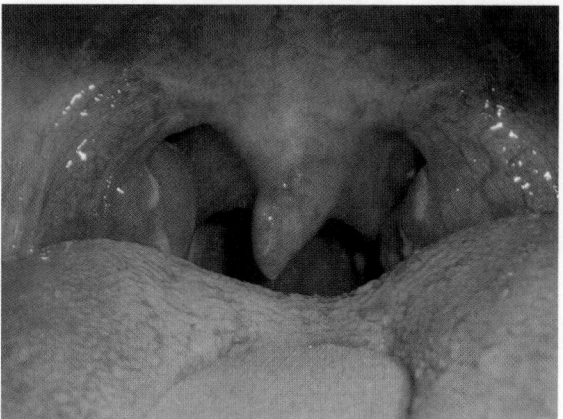

▲ **Figure 8–9.** Streptococcal pharyngitis showing tonsillar exudate and erythema. (From Michael Nguyen, MD; reproduced, with permission, from Usatine RP, Smith MA, Mayeaux EJ Jr, Chumley H, Tysinger J. *The Color Atlas of Family Medicine.* McGraw-Hill, 2009.)

of the four are present, there is an intermediate likelihood of GABHS. When only one criterion is present, GABHS is unlikely. Sore throat may be severe, with odynophagia, tender adenopathy, and a scarlatiniform rash. An elevated white count and left shift are also possible. Hoarseness, cough, and coryza are not suggestive of this disease.

Marked lymphadenopathy and a shaggy, white-purple tonsillar exudate, often extending into the nasopharynx, suggest mononucleosis, especially if present in a young adult. With about 90% sensitivity, lymphocyte-to-white-blood-cell ratios of greater than 35% suggest EBV infection and not tonsillitis. Hepatosplenomegaly and a positive heterophile agglutination test or elevated anti-EBV titer are corroborative. However, about one-third of patients with infectious mononucleosis have secondary streptococcal tonsillitis, requiring treatment. Ampicillin should routinely be avoided if mononucleosis is suspected because it induces a rash that might be misinterpreted by the patient as a penicillin allergy. Diphtheria (extremely rare but described in the alcoholic population) presents with low-grade fever and an ill patient with a gray tonsillar pseudomembrane.

The most common pathogens other than GABHS in the differential diagnosis of "sore throat" are viruses, *Neisseria gonorrhoeae*, *Mycoplasma*, and *Chlamydia trachomatis*. Rhinorrhea and lack of exudate would suggest a virus, but in practice it is not possible to confidently distinguish viral upper respiratory infection from GABHS on clinical grounds alone. Infections with *Corynebacterium diphtheria*, anaerobic streptococci, and *Corynebacterium haemolyticum* (which responds better to erythromycin than penicillin) may also mimic pharyngitis due to GABHS.

B. Laboratory Findings

A single-swab throat culture is 90–95% sensitive and the rapid antigen detection testing (RADT) is 90–99% sensitive for GABHS. Results from the RADT are available in about 15 minutes.

► Treatment

The Infectious Diseases Society of America recommends laboratory confirmation of the clinical diagnosis by means of either throat culture or RADT of the throat swab. The American College of Physicians–American Society of Internal Medicine (ACP-ASIM), in collaboration with the Centers for Disease Control and Prevention, advocates use of a clinical algorithm alone—in lieu of microbiologic testing—for confirmation of the diagnosis in adults for whom the suspicion of streptococcal infection is high. Others examine the assumptions of the ACP-ASIM guideline for using a clinical algorithm alone and question whether those recommendations will achieve the stated objective of dramatically decreasing excess antibiotic use. A reasonable strategy to follow is that patients with zero or one Centor criteria are at very low risk for GABHS and therefore do not need throat cultures or RADT of the throat swab and should not receive antibiotics. Patients with two or three Centor criteria need throat cultures or RADT of the throat swab, since positive results would warrant antibiotic treatment. Patients who have four Centor criteria are likely to have GABHS and can receive empiric therapy without throat culture or RADT.

A single intramuscular injection of benzathine penicillin or procaine penicillin, 1.2 million units is an effective antibiotic treatment, but the injection is painful. It is now used for patients if compliance with an oral regimen is an issue. Currently, oral treatment is effective and preferred. Penicillin V potassium (250 mg orally three times daily or 500 mg twice daily for 10 days) or cefuroxime axetil (250 mg orally twice daily for 5–10 days) are both effective. The efficacy of a 5-day regimen of penicillin V potassium appears to be similar to that of a 10-day course, with a 94% clinical response rate and an 84% streptococcal eradication rate. Erythromycin (also active against *Mycoplasma* and *Chlamydia*) is a reasonable alternative to penicillin in allergic patients. Cephalosporins are somewhat more effective than penicillin in producing bacteriologic cures; 5-day courses of cefpodoxime and cefuroxime have been successful. The macrolide antibiotics have also been reported to be successful in shorter-duration regimens. Azithromycin (500 mg once daily), because of its long half-life, need be taken for only 3 days.

Adequate antibiotic treatment usually avoids the streptococcal complications of scarlet fever, glomerulonephritis, rheumatic myocarditis, and local abscess formation.

Antibiotics for treatment failures are also somewhat controversial. Surprisingly, penicillin-tolerant strains are not isolated more frequently in those who fail treatment than in those treated successfully with penicillin. The reasons for failure appear to be complex, and a second course of treatment with the same drug is reasonable. Alternatives to penicillin include cefuroxime and other cephalosporins, dicloxacillin (which is beta-lactamase–resistant), and amoxicillin with clavulanate. When there is a history of penicillin allergy, alternatives should be used, such as erythromycin. Erythromycin resistance—with failure rates of about 25%—is an increasing problem in many areas. In cases of severe penicillin allergy, cephalosporins should be avoided since cross-reaction occurs in > 8% of cases.

Ancillary treatment of pharyngitis includes analgesics and anti-inflammatory agents, such as aspirin, acetaminophen, and corticosteroids. In meta-analysis, corticosteroids increased the likelihood of complete pain resolution at 24 hours by threefold without an increase in recurrence or adverse events. Some patients find that salt water gargling is soothing. In severe cases, anesthetic gargles and lozenges (eg, benzocaine) may provide additional symptomatic relief. Occasionally, odynophagia is so intense that hospitalization for intravenous hydration and antibiotics is necessary. (See Chapter 33.)

Patients who have had rheumatic fever should be treated with a continuous course of antimicrobial prophylaxis (penicillin G, 500 mg once daily orally or erythromycin, 250 mg twice daily orally) for at least 5 years.

Berkley J. Management of pharyngitis. Circulation. 2018 Oct 30; 138(18):1920–2. [PMID: 30372134]

Brook I. Treatment challenges of group A beta-hemolytic streptococcal pharyngo-tonsillitis. Int Arch Otorhinolaryngol. 2017 Jul;21(3):286–96. [PMID: 28680500]

Harris AM et al; High Value Care Task Force of the American College of Physicians and for the Centers for Disease Control and Prevention. Appropriate antibiotic use for acute respiratory tract infection in adults: advice for high-value care from the American College of Physicians and the Centers for Disease Control and Prevention. Ann Intern Med. 2016 Mar 15; 164(6):425–34. [PMID: 26785402]

Klein MR. Infections of the oropharynx. Emerg Med Clin North Am. 2019 Feb;37(1):69–80. [PMID: 30454781]

Munck H et al. Antibiotics for recurrent acute pharyngo-tonsillitis: systematic review. Eur J Clin Microbiol Infect Dis. 2018 Jul; 37(7):1221–30. [PMID: 29651614]

PERITONSILLAR ABSCESS & CELLULITIS

When infection penetrates the tonsillar capsule and involves the surrounding tissues, peritonsillar cellulitis results. Peritonsillar abscess (**quinsy**) and cellulitis present with severe sore throat, odynophagia, trismus, medial deviation of the soft palate and peritonsillar fold, and an abnormal muffled ("hot potato") voice. Following therapy, peritonsillar cellulitis usually either resolves over several days or evolves into peritonsillar abscess. Ultrasound may be a useful adjunct to clinical suspicion, but imaging is not required for the diagnosis. The existence of an abscess may be confirmed by aspirating pus from the peritonsillar fold just superior and medial to the upper pole of the tonsil. A 19-gauge or 21-gauge needle should be passed medial to the molar and no deeper than 1 cm, because the internal carotid artery may lie more medially than its usual location and pass posterior and deep to the tonsillar fossa. Most commonly, patients with peritonsillar abscess present to the emergency department and receive a dose of parenteral amoxicillin (1 g), amoxicillin-sulbactam (3 g), or clindamycin (600–900 mg). Less severe cases and patients who are able to tolerate oral intake may be treated for 7–10 days with oral antibiotics, including amoxicillin, 500 mg three times a day; amoxicillin-clavulanate, 875 mg twice a day; or clindamycin, 300 mg four times daily. Although antibiotic treatment is generally undisputed, there is controversy regarding the surgical management of peritonsillar abscess. Methods include needle aspiration, incision and drainage, and tonsillectomy. Some clinicians incise and drain the area and continue with parenteral antibiotics, whereas others aspirate only and monitor as an outpatient. To drain the abscess and avoid recurrence, it may be appropriate to consider immediate tonsillectomy (quinsy tonsillectomy). About 10% of patients with peritonsillar abscess exhibit relative indications for tonsillectomy. All three approaches are effective. Regardless of the method used, one must be sure the abscess is adequately treated, since complications such as extension to the retropharyngeal, deep neck, and posterior mediastinal spaces are possible. Bacteria may also be aspirated into the lungs, resulting in pneumonia. There is controversy about whether a single abscess is a sufficient indication for tonsillectomy; about 30% of patients aged 17–30 who do not undergo early planned tonsillectomy following peritonsillar abscess ultimately undergo surgery, and only about 13% of those over 30 have their tonsils removed.

Blair AB et al. A unifying theory of tonsillitis, intratonsillar abscess and peritonsillar abscess. Am J Otolaryngol. 2015 Jul–Aug;36(4):517–20. [PMID: 25865201]

Galioto NJ. Peritonsillar abscess. Am Fam Physician. 2017 Apr 15;95(8):501–6. [PMID: 28409615]

Holm K et al. The role of *Fusobacterium necrophorum* in pharyngotonsillitis—a review. Anaerobe. 2016 Sep 28;42:89–97. [PMID: 27693542]

Klein MR. Infections of the oropharynx. Emerg Med Clin North Am. 2019 Feb;37(1):69–80. [PMID: 30454781]

Lee YJ et al. The efficacy of corticosteroids in the treatment of peritonsillar abscess: a meta-analysis. Clin Exp Otorhinolaryngol. 2016 Jun;9(2):89–97. [PMID: 27090283]

DEEP NECK INFECTIONS

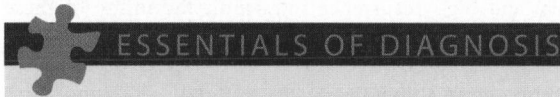

ESSENTIALS OF DIAGNOSIS

▶ Marked acute neck pain and swelling.

▶ Abscesses are emergencies because rapid airway compromise may occur.

▶ May spread to the mediastinum or cause sepsis.

General Considerations

Ludwig angina is the most commonly encountered neck space infection. It is a cellulitis of the sublingual and submaxillary spaces, often arising from infection of the mandibular dentition. **Deep neck abscesses** most commonly originate from odontogenic infections. Other causes include suppurative lymphadenitis, direct spread of pharyngeal infection, penetrating trauma, pharyngoesophageal foreign bodies, cervical osteomyelitis, and intravenous injection of the internal jugular vein, especially in drug abusers. Recurrent deep neck infection may suggest an underlying congenital lesion, such as a branchial cleft cyst. Suppurative lymphadenopathy in middle-aged persons

who smoke and drink alcohol regularly should be considered a manifestation of malignancy (typically metastatic squamous cell carcinoma) until proven otherwise.

Clinical Findings

Patients with **Ludwig angina** have edema and erythema of the upper neck under the chin and often of the floor of the mouth. The tongue may be displaced upward and backward by the posterior spread of cellulitis, and coalescence of pus is often present in the floor of mouth. This may lead to occlusion of the airway. Microbiologic isolates include streptococci, staphylococci, *Bacteroides,* and *Fusobacterium.* Patients with diabetes may have different flora, including *Klebsiella*, and a more aggressive clinical course.

Patients with **deep neck abscesses** usually present with marked neck pain and swelling. Fever is common but not always present. *Deep neck abscesses are emergencies because they may rapidly compromise the airway.* Untreated or inadequately treated, they may spread to the mediastinum or cause sepsis.

Contrast-enhanced CT usually augments the clinical examination in defining the extent of the infection. It often will distinguish inflammation and phlegmon (requiring antibiotics) from abscess (requiring drainage) and define for the surgeon the extent of an abscess. CT with MRI may also identify thrombophlebitis of the internal jugular vein secondary to oropharyngeal inflammation. This condition, known as **Lemierre syndrome**, is rare and usually associated with severe headache. The presence of pulmonary infiltrates consistent with septic emboli in the setting of a neck abscess should lead one to suspect Lemierre syndrome or injection drug use, or both.

Treatment

Usual doses of penicillin plus metronidazole, ampicillin-sulbactam, clindamycin, or selective cephalosporins are good initial choices for treatment of **Ludwig angina**. Culture and sensitivity data are then used to refine the choice. Dental consultation is advisable to address the offending tooth or teeth. External drainage via bilateral submental incisions is required if the airway is threatened or when medical therapy has not reversed the process.

Treatment of **deep neck abscesses** includes securing the airway, intravenous antibiotics, and incision and drainage. When the infection involves the floor of the mouth, base of the tongue, or the supraglottic or paraglottic space, the airway may be secured either by intubation or tracheotomy. Tracheotomy is preferable in the patients with substantial pharyngeal edema, since attempts at intubation may precipitate acute airway obstruction. Bleeding in association with a deep neck abscess is very rare but suggests carotid artery or internal jugular vein involvement and requires prompt neck exploration both for drainage of pus and for vascular control.

Patients with **Lemierre syndrome** require prompt institution of antibiotics appropriate for *Fusobacterium necrophorum* as well as the more usual upper airway pathogens. The use of anticoagulation in treatment is of no proven benefit.

Brito TP et al. Deep neck abscesses: study of 101 cases. Braz J Otorhinolaryngol. 2017 May–Jun;83(3):341–8. [PMID: 27236632]

Li RM et al. Infections of the neck. Emerg Med Clin North Am. 2019 Feb;37(1):95–107. [PMID: 30454783]

Mejzlik J et al. Univariate and multivariate models for the prediction of life-threatening complications in 586 cases of deep neck space infections: retrospective multi-institutional study. J Laryngol Otol. 2017 Sep;131(9):779–84. [PMID: 28578716]

SNORING

ESSENTIALS OF DIAGNOSIS

▶ Noise produced on inspiration during sleep.

▶ Snoring is associated with obstructive sleep apnea (OSA) but has no disruption of sleep on clinical sleep evaluation.

▶ General Considerations

Ventilation disorders during sleep are extremely common. While OSA occurs in 5–10% of Americans, clinically relevant snoring may occur in as many as 59%. In general, sleep-disordered breathing problems are attributed to narrowing of the upper aerodigestive tract during sleep due to changes in position, muscle tone, and soft tissue hypertrophy or laxity. The most common sites of obstruction are the oropharynx and the base of the tongue. The spectrum of the problem ranges from simple snoring without cessation of airflow to OSA with long periods of apnea and life-threatening physiologic sequelae. OSA is discussed in Chapter 9. In contrast to OSA, snoring is almost exclusively a social problem, and despite its prevalence and association with OSA, there is comparatively little known about the management of this problem.

▶ Clinical Findings

A. Symptoms and Signs

All patients who complain of snoring should be evaluated for OSA as discussed in Chapter 9. Symptoms of OSA (including snoring, excessive daytime somnolence, daytime headaches, and weight gain) may be present in as many as 30% of patients without demonstrable apnea or hypopnea on formal testing. Clinical examination should include examination of the nasal cavity, nasopharynx, oropharynx, and larynx to help exclude other causes of dynamic airway obstruction. In many cases of isolated snoring, the palate and uvula appear enlarged and elongated with excessive mucosa hanging below the muscular portion of the soft palate.

B. Imaging and Diagnostic Testing

Sleep examination with polysomnography is strongly advised in the evaluation of a patient with complaints of snoring. Radiographic imaging of the head or neck is generally not necessary.

▶ Treatment

Expeditious and inexpensive management solutions of snoring are sought, often with little or no benefit. Diet modification and physical exercise can lead to improvement in snoring through the weight loss and improvement in pharyngeal tone that accompanies overall physical conditioning. Position change during sleep can be effective, and time-honored treatments, such as placing a golf or tennis ball into a pocket sewn on the back of the pajama top worn during sleep, may satisfactorily eliminate symptoms by ensuring recumbency on one side. Although numerous pharmacologic therapies have been endorsed, none demonstrate any significant utility when scrutinized.

Anatomic management of snoring can be challenging. As with OSA, snoring can come from a number of sites in the upper aerodigestive tract. While medical or surgical correction of nasal obstruction may help alleviate snoring problems, most interventions aim to improve airflow through the nasopharynx and oropharynx. Nonsurgical options include mandibular advancement appliances designed to pull the base of the tongue forward and continuous positive airway pressure via face or nasal mask. Compliance with both of these treatment options is problematic because snorers without OSA do not notice the physiologic benefits of these devices noted by patients with sleep apnea.

Surgical correction of snoring is most commonly directed at the soft palate. Historical approaches involved resection of redundant mucosa and the uvula similar to uvulopalatopharyngoplasty that is used for OSA. Regardless of how limited the procedure or what technique was used, postoperative pain, the expense of general anesthesia, and high recurrence rates limit the utility of these procedures. Office-based approaches are more widely used because of these limitations. Most of these procedures aim to stiffen the palate to prevent vibration rather than remove it. A series of procedures, including injection snoreplasty, radiofrequency thermal fibrosis, and an implantable palatal device, have been used with variable success and patient tolerance. The techniques can be technically challenging. Persistent symptoms may occur following initial treatment necessitating costly (and sometimes painful) repeat procedures. The durability of these procedures in alleviating symptoms is also poorly understood, and late failures can lead to patient and clinician frustration.

Bratton DJ et al. CPAP vs mandibular advancement devices and blood pressure in patients with obstructive sleep apnea: a systematic review and meta-analysis. JAMA. 2015 Dec 1;314(21):2280–93. [PMID: 26624827]

Chang ET et al. The relationship of the uvula with snoring and obstructive sleep apnea: a systematic review. Sleep Breath. 2018 Dec;22(4):955–61. [PMID: 29524092]

Rivas M et al. Obstructive sleep apnea and its effects on cardiovascular diseases: a narrative review. Anatol J Cardiol. 2015 Nov;15(11):944–50. [PMID: 26574763]

DISEASES OF THE SALIVARY GLANDS

ACUTE INFLAMMATORY SALIVARY GLAND DISORDERS

1. Sialadenitis

Acute bacterial sialadenitis most commonly affects either the parotid or submandibular gland. It typically presents with acute swelling of the gland, increased pain and swelling with meals, and tenderness and erythema of the duct opening. Pus often can be massaged from the duct. Sialadenitis often occurs in the setting of dehydration or in association with chronic illness. Underlying Sjögren syndrome and chronic periodontitis may contribute. Ductal obstruction, often by an inspissated mucous plug, is followed by salivary stasis and secondary infection. The most common organism recovered from purulent draining saliva is *S aureus*. Treatment consists of intravenous antibiotics, such as nafcillin (1 g intravenously every 4–6 hours), and measures to increase salivary flow, including hydration, warm compresses, sialagogues (eg, lemon drops), and massage of the gland. Treatment can usually then be switched to an oral agent based on clinical improvement and microbiologic results to complete a 10-day treatment course. Less severe cases can often be treated with oral antibiotics with similar spectrum. Complete resolution of parotid swelling and pain can take 2–3 weeks. Failure of the process to improve and ultimately resolve on this regimen suggests abscess formation, ductal stricture, stone, or tumor causing obstruction. Ultrasound or CT scan may be helpful in establishing the diagnosis. In the setting of acute illness, a severe and potentially life-threatening form of sialadenitis, sometimes called **suppurative sialadenitis**, may develop. The causative organism is usually *S aureus*, but often no pus will drain from Stensen papilla. These patients often do not respond to rehydration and intravenous antibiotics and thus may require operative incision and drainage to resolve the infection.

2. Sialolithiasis

Calculus formation is more common in the Wharton duct (draining the submandibular glands) than in the Stensen duct (draining the parotid glands). Clinically, a patient may note postprandial pain and local swelling, often with a history of recurrent acute sialadenitis. Stones in the Wharton duct are usually large and radiopaque, whereas those in the Stensen duct are usually radiolucent and smaller. Those very close to the orifice of the Wharton duct may be palpated manually in the anterior floor of the mouth and removed intraorally by dilating or incising the distal duct. Those more than 1.5–2 cm from the duct are too close to the lingual nerve to be removed safely in this manner. Similarly, dilation of the Stensen duct, located on the buccal surface opposite the second maxillary molar, may relieve distal stricture or allow a small stone to pass. Sialoendoscopy for the management of chronic sialolithiasis is superior to extracorporeal shock-wave lithotripsy and fluoroscopically guided basket retrieval. Repeated episodes of sialadenitis are usually associated with stricture and chronic infection. If the obstruction cannot be safely removed or dilated, excision of the gland may be necessary to relieve recurrent symptoms.

Delagnes EA et al. Sialadenitis without sialolithiasis: prospective outcomes after sialendoscopy-assisted salivary duct surgery. Laryngoscope. 2017 May;127(5):1073–9. [PMID: 27701754]

Xiao JQ et al. Evaluation of sialendoscopy-assisted treatment of submandibular gland stones. J Oral Maxillofac Surg. 2017 Feb; 75(2):309–16. [PMID: 27663537]

CHRONIC INFLAMMATORY & INFILTRATIVE DISORDERS OF THE SALIVARY GLANDS

Numerous infiltrative disorders may cause unilateral or bilateral parotid gland enlargement. Sjögren syndrome and sarcoidosis are examples of lymphoepithelial and granulomatous diseases that may affect the salivary glands. Metabolic disorders, including alcoholism, diabetes mellitus, and vitamin deficiencies, may also cause diffuse enlargement. Several drugs have been associated with parotid enlargement, including thioureas, iodine, and drugs with cholinergic effects (eg, phenothiazines), which stimulate salivary flow and cause more viscous saliva.

SALIVARY GLAND TUMORS

Approximately 80% of salivary gland tumors occur in the parotid gland. In adults, about 80% of these are benign. In the submandibular triangle, it is sometimes difficult to distinguish a primary submandibular gland tumor from a metastatic submandibular space node. Only 50–60% of primary submandibular tumors are benign. Tumors of the minor salivary glands are most likely to be malignant, with adenoid cystic carcinoma predominating, and may be found throughout the oral cavity or oropharynx.

Most parotid tumors present as an asymptomatic mass in the superficial part of the gland. Their presence may have been noted by the patient for months or years. Facial nerve involvement correlates strongly with malignancy. Tumors may extend deep to the plane of the facial nerve or may originate in the parapharyngeal space. In such cases, medial deviation of the soft palate is visible on intraoral examination. MRI and CT scans have largely replaced sialography in defining the extent of tumor. At least one new study demonstrates the potential benefit of enhanced MRI imaging in distinguishing among Warthin tumors and pleomorphic adenomas and malignant salivary gland tumors.

When the clinician encounters a patient with an otherwise asymptomatic salivary gland mass where tumor is the most likely diagnosis, the choice is whether to simply excise the mass via a parotidectomy with facial nerve dissection or submandibular gland excision or to first obtain an FNA biopsy. Although the accuracy of FNA biopsy for malignancy has been reported to be quite high, results vary among institutions. If a negative FNA biopsy would lead to a decision not to proceed to surgery, then it should be considered. Poor overall health of the patient and the possibility of inflammatory disease as the cause of the mass are situations where FNA biopsy might be helpful. In otherwise straightforward nonrecurrent cases, excision is indicated. In benign and small, low-grade malignant tumors, no additional treatment is needed. Postoperative irradiation is indicated for larger and high-grade cancers.

D'heygere E et al. Salivary duct carcinoma. Curr Opin Otolaryngol Head Neck Surg. 2018 Apr;26(2):142–51. [PMID: 29373327]
Ogawa T et al. Clinical utility of dynamic-enhanced MRI in salivary gland tumors: retrospective study and literature review. Eur Arch Otorhinolaryngol. 2018 Jun;275(6):1613–21. [PMID: 29623392]
Sood S et al. Management of salivary gland tumours: United Kingdom national multidisciplinary guidelines. J Laryngol Otol. 2016 May;130(S2):S142–9. [PMID: 27841127]

▼ DISEASES OF THE LARYNX

DYSPHONIA, HOARSENESS, & STRIDOR

The primary symptoms of laryngeal disease are hoarseness and stridor. Hoarseness is caused by an abnormal vibration of the vocal folds. The voice is breathy when too much air passes incompletely apposed vocal folds, as in unilateral vocal fold paralysis or vocal fold mass. The voice is harsh when the vocal folds are stiff and vibrate irregularly, as is the case in laryngitis or malignancy. Heavy, edematous vocal folds produce a rough, low-pitched vocal quality. Stridor (a high-pitched, typically inspiratory, sound) is the result of turbulent airflow from a narrowed upper airway. Airway narrowing at or above the vocal folds produces inspiratory stridor. Airway narrowing below the vocal fold level produces either expiratory or biphasic stridor. The timing and rapidity of onset of stridor are critically important in determining the seriousness of the airway problem. All cases of stridor should be evaluated by a specialist and rapid-onset stridor should be evaluated emergently.

Evaluation of an abnormal voice begins with obtaining a history of the circumstances preceding its onset and an examination of the airway. Any patient with hoarseness that has persisted beyond 2 weeks should be evaluated by an otolaryngologist with laryngoscopy. Especially when the patient has a history of tobacco use, laryngeal cancer or lung cancer (leading to paralysis of a recurrent laryngeal nerve) must be strongly considered. In addition to structural causes of dysphonia, laryngoscopy can help identify functional problems with the voice, including vocal fold paralysis, muscle tension dysphonia, and spasmodic dysphonia.

Andreassen ML et al. Emerging techniques in assessment and treatment of muscle tension dysphonia. Curr Opin Otolaryngol Head Neck Surg. 2017 Dec;25(6):447–52. [PMID: 28984699]
van Esch BF et al. Effect of botulinum toxin and surgery among spasmodic dysphonia patients: a systematic review. Otolaryngol Head Neck Surg. 2017 Feb;156(2):238–54. [PMID: 27803079]

COMMON LARYNGEAL DISORDERS

1. Acute Laryngitis

Acute laryngitis is probably the most common cause of hoarseness, which may persist for a week or so after other symptoms of an upper respiratory infection have cleared.

The patient should be warned to avoid vigorous use of the voice (singing, shouting) until their voice returns to normal, since persistent use may lead to the formation of traumatic vocal fold hemorrhage, polyps, and cysts. Although thought to be usually viral in origin, both *M catarrhalis* and *H influenzae* may be isolated from the nasopharynx at higher than expected frequencies. Despite this finding, a meta-analysis has failed to demonstrate any convincing evidence that antibiotics significantly alter the natural resolution of acute laryngitis. Erythromycin may speed improvement of hoarseness at 1 week and cough at 2 weeks when measured subjectively. Oral or intramuscular corticosteroids may be used in highly selected cases of professional vocalists to speed recovery and allow scheduled performances. Examination of the vocal folds and assessment of vocal technique are mandatory prior to corticosteroid initiation, since inflamed vocal folds are at greater risk for hemorrhage and the subsequent development of traumatic vocal fold pathology.

Jaworek AJ et al. Acute infectious laryngitis: a case series. Ear Nose Throat J. 2018 Sep;97(9):306–13. [PMID: 30273430]

2. Laryngopharyngeal Reflux

ESSENTIALS OF DIAGNOSIS

- ► Commonly associated with hoarseness, throat irritation, and chronic cough.
- ► Symptoms typically occur when upright, and half of patients do not experience heartburn.
- ► Laryngoscopy is critical to exclude other causes of hoarseness.
- ► Diagnosis is made based following response to proton-pump inhibitor therapy.
- ► Treatment failure with proton-pump inhibitors is common and suggests other etiologies.

Gastroesophageal reflux into the larynx (laryngopharyngeal reflux) is considered a cause of chronic hoarseness when other causes of abnormal vocal fold vibration (such as tumor or nodules) have been excluded by laryngoscopy. Gastroesophageal reflux disease (GERD) has also been suggested as a contributing factor to other symptoms, such as throat clearing, throat discomfort, chronic cough, a sensation of postnasal drip, esophageal spasm, and some cases of asthma. Since less than half of patients with laryngeal acid exposure have typical symptoms of heartburn and regurgitation, the lack of such symptoms should not be construed as eliminating this cause. Indeed, most patients with symptomatic laryngopharyngeal reflux, as it is now called, do not meet criteria for GERD by pH probe testing and these entities must be considered separately. The prevalence of this condition is hotly debated in the literature, and laryngopharyngeal reflux may not be as common as once thought.

Evaluation should initially exclude other causes of dysphonia through laryngoscopy; consultation with an otolaryngologist is advisable. Many clinicians opt for an empiric trial of a proton-pump inhibitor since no gold standard exists for diagnosing this condition. Such an empiric trial should not precede visualization of the vocal folds to exclude other causes of hoarseness. When used, the American Academy of Otolaryngology—Head and Neck Surgery recommends twice-daily therapy with full-strength proton-pump inhibitor (eg, omeprazole 40 mg orally twice daily, or equivalent) for a minimum of 3 months. Patients may note improvement in symptoms after 3 months, but the changes in the larynx often take 6 months to resolve. If symptoms improve and cessation of therapy leads to symptoms again, then a proton-pump inhibitor is resumed at the lowest dose effective for remission, usually daily but at times on a demand basis. Although H_2-receptor antagonists are an alternative to proton-pump inhibitors, they are generally both less clinically effective and less cost-effective. Nonresponders should undergo pH testing and manometry. Twenty-four-hour pH monitoring of the pharynx should best document laryngopharyngeal reflux and is advocated by some as the initial management step, but it is costly, more difficult, and less available than lower esophageal monitoring alone. Double pH probe (proximal and distal esophageal probes) testing is the best option for evaluation, since lower esophageal pH monitoring alone does not correlate well with laryngopharyngeal reflux symptoms. Oropharyngeal pH probe testing is available, but its ability to predict response to reflux treatment in patients with laryngopharyngeal reflux is not known.

Lechien JR et al. Laryngopharyngeal reflux and voice disorders: a multifactorial model of etiology and pathophysiology. J Voice. 2017 Nov;31(6):733–52. [PMID: 28438489]
Lechien JR et al. Voice outcomes of laryngopharyngeal reflux treatment: a systematic review of 1483 patients. Eur Arch Otorhinolaryngol. 2017 Jan;274(1):1–23. [PMID: 27007132]
Wei C. A meta-analysis for the role of proton pump inhibitor therapy in patients with laryngopharyngeal reflux. Eur Arch Otorhinolaryngol. 2016 Nov;273(11):3795–801. [PMID: 27312992]

3. Recurrent Respiratory Papillomatosis

Papillomas are common lesions of the larynx and other sites where ciliated and squamous epithelia meet. Unlike oral papillomas, recurrent respiratory papillomatosis typically becomes symptomatic, with hoarseness that occasionally progresses over weeks to months. These papillomas are almost always due to HPV types 6 and 11. Repeated laser vaporizations or cold knife resections via operative laryngoscopy are the mainstay of treatment. Severe cases can cause airway compromise in adults and may require treatment as often as every 6 weeks to maintain airway patency. Extension can occur into the trachea and lungs. Tracheotomy should be avoided, if possible, since it introduces an additional squamociliary junction for which papillomas appear to have an affinity. Interferon treatment has been under investigation for many years but is only indicated in severe cases with pulmonary involvement. Rarely, cases of malignant transformation have been reported (often in

smokers), but recurrent respiratory papillomatosis should generally be thought of as a benign condition. Cidofovir (a cytosine nucleotide analog in use to treat cytomegalovirus retinitis) has been used with success as intralesional therapy for recurrent respiratory papillomatosis. Because cidofovir causes adenocarcinomas in laboratory animals, its potential for carcinogenesis is being monitored. The quadrivalent and new 9 serotype recombinant human HPV vaccines (Gardasil and Gardasil 9) offer hope for the eventual prevention of this benign, but terribly morbid, disease.

Donne A et al. Prevalence and management of recurrent respiratory papillomatosis (RRP) in the UK: cross sectional study. Clin Otolaryngol. 2017 Feb;42(1):86–91. [PMID: 27208548]
Ivancic R et al. Current and future management of recurrent respiratory papillomatosis. Laryngoscope Investig Otolaryngol. 2018 Jan 14;3(1):22–34. [PMID: 29492465]

4. Epiglottitis

Epiglottitis (or, more correctly, supraglottitis) should be suspected when a patient presents with a rapidly developing sore throat or when odynophagia (pain on swallowing) is out of proportion to apparently minimal oropharyngeal findings on examination. It is more common in diabetic patients and may be viral or bacterial in origin. Rarely in the era of *H influenzae* type b vaccine is this bacterium isolated in adults. Unlike in children, indirect laryngoscopy is generally safe and may demonstrate a swollen, erythematous epiglottis. Lateral plain radiographs may demonstrate an enlarged epiglottis (the epiglottis "thumb sign"). Initial treatment is hospitalization for intravenous antibiotics—eg, ceftizoxime, 1–2 g intravenously every 8–12 hours; or cefuroxime, 750–1500 mg intravenously every 8 hours; and dexamethasone, usually 4–10 mg as initial bolus, then 4 mg intravenously every 6 hours—and observation of the airway. Corticosteroids may be tapered as symptoms and signs resolve. Similarly, substitution of oral antibiotics may be appropriate to complete a 10-day course. Less than 10% of adults require intubation. Indications for intubation are dyspnea, rapid pace of sore throat (where progression to airway compromise may occur before the effects of corticosteroids and antibiotics), and endolaryngeal abscess noted on CT imaging. If the patient is not intubated, prudence suggests monitoring oxygen saturation with continuous pulse oximetry and initial admission to a monitored unit.

Chen C et al. Acute epiglottitis in the immunocompromised host: case report and review of the literature. Open Forum Infect Dis. 2018 Feb 17;5(3):ofy038. [PMID: 29564363]
Lee SH et al. Do we need a change in ED diagnostic strategy for adult acute epiglottitis? Am J Emerg Med. 2017 Oct;35(10):1519–24. [PMID: 28460811]

MASSES OF THE LARYNX

1. Traumatic Lesions of the Vocal Folds

Vocal fold nodules are smooth, paired lesions that form at the junction of the anterior one-third and posterior two-thirds of the vocal folds. They are a common cause of hoarseness resulting from vocal abuse. In adults, they are referred to as "singer's nodules" and in children as "screamer's nodules." Treatment requires modification of voice habits, and referral to a speech therapist is indicated. While nearly all true nodules will resolve with behavior modification, recalcitrant nodules may require surgical excision. Often, additional pathology, such as a polyp or cyst, may be encountered.

Vocal fold polyps are unilateral masses that form within the superficial lamina propria of the vocal fold. They are related to vocal trauma and seem to follow resolution of vocal fold hemorrhage. Small, sessile polyps may resolve with conservative measures, such as voice rest and corticosteroids, but larger polyps are often irreversible and require operative removal to restore normal voice.

Vocal fold cysts are also considered traumatic lesions of the vocal folds and are either true cysts with an epithelial lining or pseudocysts. They typically form from mucus-secreting glands on the inferior aspect of the vocal folds. Cysts may fluctuate in size from week to week and cause a variable degree of hoarseness. They rarely, if ever, resolve completely and may leave behind a sulcus, or vocal fold scar, if they decompress or are marsupialized. Such scarring can be a frustrating cause of permanent dysphonia.

Polypoid corditis is different from vocal fold polyps and may form from loss of elastin fibers and loosening of the intracellular junctions within the lamina propria. This loss allows swelling of the gelatinous matrix of the superficial lamina propria (called **Reinke edema**). These changes in the vocal folds are strongly associated with smoking, but also with vocal abuse, chemical industrial irritants, and hypothyroidism. While this problem is common in both male and female smokers, women seem more troubled by the characteristic decline in modal pitch caused by the increased mass of the vocal folds. If the patient stops smoking or the lesions cause stridor and airway obstruction, surgical resection of the hyperplastic vocal fold mucosa may be indicated to improve the voice or airway, or both.

A common but often unrecognized cause of hoarseness and odynophonia are **contact ulcers** or their close relatives, **granulomas**. Both lesions form on the vocal processes of the arytenoid cartilages, and patients often can correctly inform the clinician which side is affected. The cause of these ulcers and granulomas is disputed, but they are clearly related to trauma and may be related to exposure of the underlying perichondrium. They are common following intubation and generally resolve quite quickly. Chronic ulceration or granuloma formation has been associated with gastroesophageal reflux but is also common in patients with muscle tension dysphonia. Treatment is often multimodal, and an inhaled corticosteroid (eg, fluticasone 440 mcg twice daily) may be the most effective pharmacologic therapy. Adjunctive treatment measures include proton-pump inhibitor therapy (omeprazole 40 mg orally twice daily, or equivalent) and voice therapy with special attention to vocal hygiene. Rare cases can be quite stubborn and persistent without adequate therapy. Surgical removal is rarely, if ever, required for nonobstructive lesions.

Ogawa M et al. Is voice therapy effective for the treatment of dysphonic patients with benign vocal fold lesions? Auris Nasus Larynx. 2018 Aug;45(4):661–6. [PMID: 28844607]

Zhukhovitskaya A et al. Gender and age in benign vocal fold lesions. Laryngoscope. 2015 Jan;125(1):191–6. [PMID: 25216037]

2. Laryngeal Leukoplakia

Leukoplakia of the vocal folds is commonly found in association with hoarseness in smokers. Direct laryngoscopy with biopsy is advised in almost all cases. Histologic examination usually demonstrates mild, moderate, or severe dysplasia. In some cases, invasive squamous cell carcinoma is present in the initial biopsy specimen. Cessation of smoking may reverse or stabilize mild or moderate dysplasia. Some patients—estimated to be less than 5% of those with mild dysplasia and about 35–60% of those with severe dysplasia—will subsequently develop squamous cell carcinoma. Treatment options include proton-pump inhibitor therapy, close follow-up with laryngovideostroboscopy, serial resection, and external beam radiation therapy.

Parker NP. Vocal fold leukoplakia: incidence, management, and prevention. Curr Opin Otolaryngol Head Neck Surg. 2017 Dec;25(6):464–8. [PMID: 28857841]

3. Squamous Cell Carcinoma of the Larynx

ESSENTIALS OF DIAGNOSIS

- ▶ New and persistent (more than 2 weeks' duration) hoarseness in a smoker.
- ▶ Persistent throat or ear pain, especially with swallowing.
- ▶ Neck mass.
- ▶ Hemoptysis.
- ▶ Stridor or other symptoms of a compromised airway.

▶ General Considerations

Squamous cell carcinoma of the larynx, the most common malignancy of the larynx, occurs almost exclusively in patients with a history of significant tobacco use. Squamous cell carcinoma is usually seen in men aged 50–70 years; an estimated 13,150 new cases in both sexes (10,490 in men) will be seen in United States in 2018. There may be an association between laryngeal cancer and HPV type 16 or 18 infection, but this association is much less strong than that between HPV 16 or 18 and oropharyngeal cancer. In both cancer types, the association with HPV seems to be strongest in nonsmokers. Laryngeal cancer is very treatable and early detection is the key to maximizing posttreatment voice, swallowing, and breathing function.

Clinical Findings

A. Symptoms and Signs

A change in voice quality is most often the presenting complaint, although throat or ear pain, hemoptysis, dysphagia, weight loss, and airway compromise may occur. Because of their early impact on vocal quality, glottic cancers are among the smallest detectable human malignancies and treatment success is very high with early lesions. Neck metastases are not common in early glottic (true vocal fold) cancer in which the vocal folds are mobile, but a third of patients in whom there is impaired fold mobility will also have involved lymph nodes at neck dissection. Supraglottic carcinoma (false vocal folds, aryepiglottic folds, epiglottis), on the other hand, often metastasizes to both sides of the neck early in the disease. Complete head and neck examination, including laryngoscopy, by an experienced clinician is mandated for any person with the concerning symptoms listed under Essentials of Diagnosis.

B. Imaging and Laboratory Studies

Radiologic evaluation by CT or MRI is helpful in assessing tumor extent. Imaging evaluates neck nodes, tumor volume, and cartilage sclerosis or destruction. A chest CT scan is indicated if there are level VI enlarged nodes (around the trachea and the thyroid gland) or level IV enlarged nodes (inferior to the cricoid cartilage along the internal jugular vein), or if a chest film is concerning for a second primary lesion or metastases. Laboratory evaluation includes complete blood count and liver biochemical tests. Formal cardiopulmonary evaluation may be indicated, especially if partial laryngeal surgery is being considered. All partial laryngectomy candidates should have good to excellent lung function and exercise tolerance because chronic microaspiration may be expected following the procedure. A positron emission tomography (PET) scan or CT-PET scan may be indicated to assess for distant metastases when there appears to be advanced local or regional disease.

C. Biopsy

Diagnosis is made by biopsy at the time of laryngoscopy when true fold mobility and arytenoid fixation, as well as surface tumor extent, can be evaluated. Most otolaryngologists recommend esophagoscopy and bronchoscopy at the same time to exclude synchronous primary tumor. Although an FNA biopsy of an enlarged neck node may have already been done, it is generally acceptable to assume radiographically enlarged neck nodes (greater than 1–1.5 cm) or nodes with necrotic centers are neck metastases. Open biopsies of nodal metastases should be discouraged because they may lead to higher rates of tumor treatment failure.

D. Tumor Staging

The American Joint Committee on Cancer (AJCC) staging of laryngeal cancers uses the TNM system to describe tumor extent and can be used for prognosis. Early laryngeal cancers, T1 and T2 (stage I and II) lesions, involve 1–2 laryngeal subsites locally and have no nodal metastases or profound functional abnormalities. T3 and T4 lesions may involve multiple laryngeal subsites with limitation of laryngeal mobility. These locally advanced lesions are stage III or IV cancers, and any size tumor with regional nodal metastases is at least a stage III tumor. Stage I and II lesions are generally treated with single-modality therapy (surgery or radiation), while multimodality therapy, usually including chemotherapy with radiation therapy, is reserved for more advanced stage III and IV lesions.

Treatment

Treatment of laryngeal carcinoma has four goals: cure, preservation of safe and effective swallowing, preservation of useful voice, and avoidance of a permanent tracheostoma. For early glottic and supraglottic cancers, radiation therapy is the standard of care since cure rates are greater than 95% and 80%, respectively. That said, radiation therapy carries substantial morbidity, and many early tumors (T1 and T2 lesions, without involved nodes) and selected advanced tumors (T3 and T4) may be treated with partial laryngectomy if at least one cricoarytenoid unit can be preserved. Five-year locoregional cure rates exceed 80–90% with surgery, and patient-reported satisfaction is excellent. In supraglottic tumors, even when clinically N0, elective limited neck dissection is indicated following surgical resection because of the high risk of neck node involvement.

Advanced stage III and IV tumors represent a challenging and ever-changing treatment dilemma. Twenty-five years ago, total laryngectomy was often recommended for such patients. However, the 1994 VA study (with induction cisplatin and 5-fluorouracil followed by irradiation alone in responders) demonstrated that two-thirds of patients could preserve their larynx. Subsequent studies have further defined multimodal therapy. Cisplatin-based chemotherapy concomitant with radiation therapy has been shown to be superior to either irradiation alone or induction chemotherapy followed by radiation. The same benefits have been demonstrated with the epidermal growth factor receptor blocker cetuximab with lower overall systemic toxicity and better patient tolerance. However, chemoradiation using either cetuximab or cisplatin is associated with prolonged gastrostomy-dependent dysphagia.

The high rate of dysphagia and morbidity associated with severe laryngeal stenosis following chemoradiation has prompted a reevaluation of the role of extended, but less-than-total, laryngeal resection for selected advanced laryngeal carcinoma in which at least one cricoarytenoid unit is intact (organ preservation surgery). In addition to the late complications, clinicians have noted that the overall success in the treatment of larynx cancer has declined in parallel with the increase in organ preservation chemoradiation therapy over the past 20 years. Some experts have proposed that this decline is the direct result of the shift in management of advanced laryngeal cancer away from surgery. Organ preservation surgery should be considered and discussed as an alternative to chemoradiation but may require referral to an appropriate regional center where such techniques are offered. After thorough evaluation of candidacy and discussion of the treatment options, patient choice plays a critical role in the ultimate decision to pursue surgery or chemoradiation as a definitive treatment modality. The patient and treating clinicians must carefully consider different early and late side effects and complications associated with different treatment modalities.

The presence of malignant adenopathy in the neck affects the prognosis greatly. Supraglottic tumors metastasize early and bilaterally to the neck, and this must be included in the treatment plans even when the neck is apparently uninvolved. Glottic tumors in which the true vocal folds are mobile (T1 or T2) have less than a 5% rate of nodal involvement; when a fold is immobile, the rate of ipsilateral nodal involvement climbs to about 30%. An involved neck is treated by surgery or chemoradiation, or both. This decision will depend on the treatment chosen for the larynx and the extent of neck involvement.

Total laryngectomy is largely reserved for patients with advanced resectable tumors with extralaryngeal spread or cartilage involvement, for those with persistent tumor following chemoradiation, and for patients with recurrent or second primary tumor following previous radiation therapy. Voice rehabilitation via a primary (or at times secondary) tracheoesophageal puncture produces intelligible and serviceable speech in about 75–85% of patients. Indwelling prostheses that are changed every 3–6 months are a common alternative to patient-inserted prostheses, which need changing more frequently.

Long-term follow-up is critical in head and neck cancer patients. In addition to the 3–4% annual rate of second tumors and monitoring for recurrence, psychosocial aspects of treatment are common. Dysphagia, impaired communication, and altered appearance may result in patient difficulties adapting to the workplace and to social interactions. In addition, smoking cessation and alcohol abatement are common challenges. Nevertheless, about 65% of patients with larynx cancer are cured, most have useful speech, and many resume their prior livelihoods with adaptations.

Castellsagué X et al; ICO International HPV in Head and Neck Cancer Study Group. HPV involvement in head and neck cancers: comprehensive assessment of biomarkers in 3680 patients. J Natl Cancer Inst. 2016 Jan 28;108(6):djv403. [PMID: 26823521]

Marchiano E et al. Subglottic squamous cell carcinoma: a population-based study of 889 cases. Otolaryngol Head Neck Surg. 2016 Feb;154(2):315–21. [PMID: 26607281]

Marur S et al. Head and neck squamous cell carcinoma: update on epidemiology, diagnosis, and treatment. Mayo Clin Proc. 2016 Mar;91(3):386–96. [PMID: 26944243]

Patel KB et al. Treatment of early stage supraglottic squamous cell carcinoma: meta-analysis comparing primary surgery versus primary radiotherapy. J Otolaryngol Head Neck Surg. 2018 Mar 5;47(1):19. [PMID: 29506564]

VOCAL FOLD PARALYSIS

Vocal fold paralysis can result from a lesion or damage to either the vagus or recurrent laryngeal nerve and usually results in breathy dysphonia and effortful voicing. Common causes of **unilateral recurrent laryngeal nerve** involvement include thyroid surgery (and occasionally thyroid cancer), other neck surgery (anterior discectomy and carotid endarterectomy), and mediastinal or apical involvement by lung cancer. Skull base tumors often involve or abut upon lower cranial nerves and may affect the vagus nerve directly, or the vagus nerve may be damaged during surgical management of the lesion. While iatrogenic injury is the most common cause of unilateral vocal fold paralysis, the second most common cause is idiopathic. However, before deciding whether the paralysis is due to iatrogenic injury or is idiopathic, the clinician must exclude other causes, such as malignancy. In the absence of other cranial neuropathies, a CT scan with contrast from the skull base to the aortopulmonary window (the span of the recurrent laryngeal nerve) should be performed. If other cranial nerve deficits or high vagal weakness with palate paralysis is noted, an MRI scan of the brain and brainstem is warranted.

Unlike unilateral fold paralysis, **bilateral fold paralysis** usually causes inspiratory stridor with deep inspiration. If the onset of bilateral fold paralysis is insidious, it may be asymptomatic at rest, and the patient may have a normal voice. However, the acute onset of bilateral vocal fold paralysis with inspiratory stridor at rest should be managed by a specialist immediately in a critical care environment. Causes of bilateral fold paralysis include thyroid surgery, esophageal cancer, and ventricular shunt malfunction. Unilateral or bilateral fold immobility may also be seen in cricoarytenoid arthritis secondary to advanced rheumatoid arthritis, intubation injuries, glottic and subglottic stenosis, and, of course, laryngeal cancer. The goal of intervention is the creation of a safe airway with minimal reduction in voice quality and airway protection from aspiration. A number of fold lateralization procedures for bilateral paralysis have been advocated as a means of removing the tracheotomy tube.

Unilateral vocal fold paralysis is occasionally temporary and may take over a year to resolve spontaneously. Surgical management of persistent or irrecoverable symptomatic unilateral vocal fold paralysis has evolved over the last several decades. The primary goal is medialization of the paralyzed fold in order to create a stable platform for vocal fold vibration. Additional goals include advancing diet and improving pulmonary toilet by facilitating cough. Success has been reported for years with injection laryngoplasty using Teflon, Gelfoam, fat, and collagen. Teflon is the only permanent injectable material, but its use is discouraged because of granuloma formation within the vocal folds of some patients. Temporary injectable materials, such as collagen or fat, provide excellent temporary restoration of voice and can be placed under local or general anesthesia. Once the paralysis is determined to be permanent, formal medialization thyroplasty may be performed by creating a small window in the thyroid cartilage and placing an implant between the thyroarytenoid muscle and inner table of the thyroid cartilage. This procedure moves the vocal fold medially and creates a stable platform for bilateral, symmetric mucosal vibration.

Desuter G et al. Voice outcome indicators for unilateral vocal fold paralysis surgery: a review of the literature. Eur Arch Otorhinolaryngol. 2018 Feb;275(2):459–68. [PMID: 29264655]

Kandil E et al. Assessment of vocal fold function using transcutaneous laryngeal ultrasonography and flexible laryngoscopy. JAMA Otolaryngol Head Neck Surg. 2016 Jan;142(1):74–8. [PMID: 26632676]

Paddle PM et al. Diagnostic yield of computed tomography in the evaluation of idiopathic vocal fold paresis. Otolaryngol Head Neck Surg. 2015 Sep;153(3):414–9. [PMID: 26156423]

TRACHEOSTOMY & CRICOTHYROTOMY

There are two primary indications for tracheotomy: airway obstruction at or above the level of the larynx and respiratory failure requiring prolonged mechanical ventilation. In an acute emergency, cricothyrotomy secures an airway more rapidly than tracheotomy, with fewer potential immediate complications, such as pneumothorax and hemorrhage. Percutaneous dilatational tracheotomy as an elective bedside (or intensive care unit) procedure has undergone scrutiny in recent years as an alternative to tracheotomy. In experienced hands, the various methods of percutaneous tracheotomy have been documented to be safe in carefully selected patients. Simultaneous videobronchoscopy can reduce the incidence of major complications. The major cost reduction comes from avoiding the operating room. Bedside tracheotomy (in the intensive care unit) achieves similar cost reduction and is advocated by some experts as slightly less costly than the percutaneous procedures.

The most common indication for elective tracheotomy is the need for prolonged mechanical ventilation. There is no firm rule about how many days a patient must be intubated before conversion to tracheotomy should be advised. The incidence of serious complications, such as subglottic stenosis, increases with extended endotracheal intubation. As soon as it is apparent that the patient will require protracted ventilatory support, tracheotomy should replace the endotracheal tube. Less frequent indications for tracheostomy are life-threatening aspiration pneumonia, the need to improve pulmonary toilet to correct problems related to insufficient clearing of tracheobronchial secretions, and sleep apnea.

Posttracheotomy care requires humidified air to prevent secretions from crusting and occluding the inner cannula of the tracheotomy tube. The tracheotomy tube should be cleaned several times daily. The most frequent early complication of tracheotomy is dislodgment of the tracheotomy tube. Surgical creation of an inferiorly based tracheal flap sutured to the inferior neck skin may make reinsertion of a dislodged tube easier. It should be recalled that the act of swallowing requires elevation of the larynx, which is limited by tracheotomy. Therefore, frequent tracheal and bronchial suctioning is often required to clear the aspirated saliva as well as the increased tracheobronchial secretions. Care of the skin around the stoma is important to prevent maceration and secondary infection.

Adly A et al. Timing of tracheostomy in patients with prolonged endotracheal intubation: a systematic review. Eur Arch Otorhinolaryngol. 2018 Mar;275(3):679–90. [PMID: 29255970]

Cooper JD. Tracheal injuries complicating prolonged intubation and tracheostomy. Thorac Surg Clin. 2018 May;28(2):139–44. [PMID: 29627046]

Lerner AD et al. Percutaneous dilational tracheostomy. Clin Chest Med. 2018 Mar;39(1):211–22. [PMID: 29433716]

Yildirim E. Principles of urgent management of acute airway obstruction. Thorac Surg Clin. 2018 Aug;28(3):415–28. [PMID: 30054079]

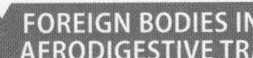

FOREIGN BODIES IN THE UPPER AERODIGESTIVE TRACT

FOREIGN BODIES OF THE TRACHEA & BRONCHI

Aspiration of foreign bodies occurs much less frequently in adults than in children. Older adults and denture wearers appear to be at greatest risk. Wider familiarity with the Heimlich maneuver has reduced deaths. If the maneuver is unsuccessful, cricothyrotomy may be necessary. Plain chest radiographs may reveal a radiopaque foreign body. Detection of radiolucent foreign bodies may be aided by inspiration-expiration films that demonstrate air trapping distal to the obstructed segment. Atelectasis and pneumonia may occur later.

Tracheal and bronchial foreign bodies should be removed under general anesthesia with rigid bronchoscopy by a skilled endoscopist working with an experienced anesthesiologist.

Altuntas B et al. Foreign bodies in trachea: 25 years of experience. Eurasian J Med. 2016 Jun;48(2):119–23. [PMID: 27551175]

ESOPHAGEAL FOREIGN BODIES

Foreign bodies in the esophagus create urgent but not life-threatening situations as long as the airway is not compromised. There is probably time to consult an experienced clinician for management. It is a useful diagnostic sign of complete obstruction if the patient is drooling or cannot handle secretions. Patients may often point to the exact level of the obstruction. Indirect laryngoscopy often shows pooling of saliva at the esophageal inlet. Plain films may detect radiopaque foreign bodies, such as chicken bones. Coins tend to align in the coronal plane in the esophagus and sagittally in the trachea. If a foreign body is suspected, a barium swallow may help make the diagnosis.

The treatment of an esophageal foreign body depends very much on identification of its nature. In children, swallowed nonfood objects are common. In adults, however, food foreign bodies are more common, and there is the greater possibility of underlying esophageal pathology. Endoscopic removal and examination are usually best via flexible esophagoscopy or rigid laryngoscopy and esophagoscopy. If there is nothing sharp, such as a bone, some clinicians advocate a hospitalized 24-hour observation period prior to esophagoscopy, noting that spontaneous passage of the foreign body will occur in 50% of adult patients. In the management of meat obstruction, the use of papain (meat tenderizer) should be discouraged because it can damage the esophageal mucosa and lead to stenosis or perforation.

Bekkerman M et al. Endoscopic management of foreign bodies in the gastrointestinal tract: a review of the literature. Gastroenterol Res Pract. 2016;2016:8520767. [PMID: 27807447]

Geraci G et al. Retrospective analysis of management of ingested foreign bodies and food impactions in emergency endoscopic setting in adults. BMC Emerg Med. 2016 Nov 4;16(1):42. [PMID: 27809769]

Zhong Q et al. Esophageal foreign body ingestion in adults on weekdays and holidays: a retrospective study of 1058 patients. Medicine (Baltimore). 2017 Oct;96(43):e8409. [PMID: 29069038]

DISEASES PRESENTING AS NECK MASSES

The differential diagnosis of neck masses is heavily dependent on the location in the neck, the age of the patient, and the presence of associated disease processes. Rapid growth and tenderness suggest an inflammatory process, while firm, painless, and slowly enlarging masses are often neoplastic. In young adults, most neck masses are benign (branchial cleft cyst, thyroglossal duct cyst, reactive lymphadenitis), although malignancy should always be considered (lymphoma, metastatic thyroid carcinoma). Lymphadenopathy is common in HIV-positive persons, but a growing or dominant mass may well represent lymphoma. In adults over age 40, cancer is the most common cause of persistent neck mass. A metastasis from squamous cell carcinoma arising within the mouth, pharynx, larynx, or upper esophagus should be suspected, especially if there is a history of tobacco or significant alcohol use. Especially among patients younger than 30 or older than 70, lymphoma should be considered. In any case, a comprehensive otolaryngologic examination is needed. Cytologic evaluation of the neck mass via FNA biopsy is likely to be the next step if a primary tumor is not obvious on physical examination.

CONGENITAL LESIONS PRESENTING AS NECK MASSES IN ADULTS

1. Branchial Cleft Cysts

Branchial cleft cysts usually present as a soft cystic mass along the anterior border of the sternocleidomastoid muscle. These lesions are usually recognized in the second or third decades of life, often when they suddenly swell or become infected. To prevent recurrent infection and possible carcinoma, they should be completely excised, along with their fistulous tracts.

First branchial cleft cysts present high in the neck, sometimes just below the ear. A fistulous connection with the floor of the external auditory canal may be present. Second branchial cleft cysts, which are far more common, may communicate with the tonsillar fossa. Third branchial cleft cysts, which may communicate with the piriform sinus, are rare and present low in the neck.

Derks LS et al. Surgery versus endoscopic cauterization in patients with third or fourth branchial pouch sinuses: a systematic review. Laryngoscope. 2016 Jan;126(1):212–7. [PMID: 26372400]

Ha EJ et al. Efficacy and safety of ethanol ablation for branchial cleft cysts. AJNR Am J Neuroradiol. 2017 Dec;38(12):2351–6. [PMID: 28970243]

2. Thyroglossal Duct Cysts

Thyroglossal duct cysts occur along the embryologic course of the thyroid's descent from the tuberculum impar of the tongue base to its usual position in the low neck. Although they may occur at any age, they are most common before age 20. They present as a midline neck mass, often just below the hyoid bone, which moves with swallowing. Surgical excision is recommended to prevent recurrent infection. This requires removal of the entire fistulous tract along with the middle portion of the hyoid bone through which many of the fistulas pass. Preoperative evaluation should include a thyroid ultrasound to confirm anatomic position of the thyroid.

Ross J et al. Thyroglossal duct cyst surgery: a ten-year single institution experience. Int J Pediatr Otorhinolaryngol. 2017 Oct; 101:132–6. [PMID: 28964283]

INFECTIOUS & INFLAMMATORY NECK MASSES

1. Reactive Cervical Lymphadenopathy

Normal lymph nodes in the neck are usually less than 1 cm in length. Infections involving the pharynx, salivary glands, and scalp often cause tender enlargement of neck nodes. Enlarged nodes are common in HIV-infected persons. Except for the occasional node that suppurates and requires incision and drainage, treatment is directed against the underlying infection. An enlarged node (larger than 1.5 cm) or node with a necrotic center that is not associated with an obvious infection should be further evaluated, especially if the patient has a history of smoking, alcohol use, or prior cancer. Other common indications for FNA biopsy of a node include its persistence or continued enlargement. Common causes of cervical adenopathy include tumor (squamous cell carcinoma, lymphoma, occasional metastases from non-head and neck sites) and infection (eg, reactive nodes, mycobacteria, and cat-scratch disease). Rare causes of adenopathy include Kikuchi disease (histiocytic necrotizing lymphadenitis) and autoimmune adenopathy.

Białek EJ et al. Mistakes in ultrasound diagnosis of superficial lymph nodes. J Ultrason. 2017 Mar;17(68):59–65. [PMID: 28439430]

Celenk F et al. Predictive factors for malignancy in patients with persistent cervical lymphadenopathy. Eur Arch Otorhinolaryngol. 2016 Jan;273(1):251–6. [PMID: 26187739]

2. Tuberculous & Nontuberculous Mycobacterial Lymphadenitis

Granulomatous neck masses are not uncommon. The differential diagnosis includes mycobacterial adenitis, sarcoidosis, and cat-scratch disease due to *Bartonella henselae*. The incidence of mycobacterial lymphadenitis is on the rise both in immunocompromised and immunocompetent individuals. The usual presentation of granulomatous disease in the neck is simply single or matted nodes. Although mycobacterial adenitis can extend to the skin and drain externally (as described for atypical mycobacteria and referred to as scrofula), this late presentation is no longer common.

FNA biopsy is usually the best initial diagnostic approach: cytology, smear for acid-fast bacilli, mycobacterial culture, and a sensitivity test can all be done. PCR from FNA (or from excised tissue) is the most sensitive test and is particularly useful when conventional methods have not been diagnostic but clinical impression remains consistent for tuberculous infection. While FNA has a high sensitivity (about 88%), its specificity is low (49%); thus, an excisional biopsy is often required to confirm the diagnosis.

See Table 9–15 for current recommended treatment of tuberculosis infection, which includes infection of the lymph nodes (tuberculous lymphadenopathy). For atypical (nontuberculous) infection of the lymph nodes, treatment depends on the sensitivity results of culture, but antibiotics likely to be useful include 6 months of isoniazid and rifampin and, for at least the first 2 months, ethambutol—all in standard dosages. Some would totally excise the involved nodes prior to chemotherapy, depending on location and other factors, but this can lead to chronic draining fistulas.

Białek EJ et al. Mistakes in ultrasound diagnosis of superficial lymph nodes. J Ultrason. 2017 Mar;17(68):59–65. [PMID: 28439430]

Gonzalez CD et al. Complex nontuberculous mycobacterial cervicofacial lymphadenitis: what is the optimal approach? Laryngoscope. 2016 Jul;126(7):1677–80. [PMID: 26372159]

Kim KH et al. The efficacy of the interferon-γ release assay for diagnosing cervical tuberculous lymphadenitis: a prospective controlled study. Laryngoscope. 2016 Feb;126(2):378–84. [PMID: 26267599]

Meghji S et al. What is the optimal diagnostic pathway in tuberculous lymphadenitis in the face of increasing resistance: cytology or histology? Am J Otolaryngol. 2015 Nov–Dec;36(6):781–5. [PMID: 26545471]

3. Lyme Disease

Lyme disease, caused by the spirochete *Borrelia burgdorferi* and transmitted by ticks of the *Ixodes* genus, may have protean manifestations, but over 75% of patients have symptoms involving the head and neck. Facial paralysis, dysesthesias, dysgeusia, or other cranial neuropathies are most common. Headache, pain, and cervical lymphadenopathy may occur. See Chapter 34 for a more detailed discussion.

Bush LM et al. Tick-borne illness–Lyme disease. Dis Mon. 2018 May;64(5):195–212. [PMID: 29402399]

Cruickshank M et al; Guideline Committee. Lyme disease: summary of NICE guidance. BMJ. 2018 Apr 12;361:k1261. [PMID: 29650513]

Shapiro ED et al. Lyme disease in 2018: what is new (and what is not). JAMA. 2018 Aug 21;320(7):635–36. [PMID: 30073279]

TUMOR METASTASES

In older adults, 80% of firm, persistent, and enlarging neck masses are metastatic in origin. The great majority of these arise from squamous cell carcinoma of the upper aerodigestive tract. A complete head and neck examination may reveal the tumor of origin, but examination under anesthesia with direct laryngoscopy, esophagoscopy, and bronchoscopy is usually required to fully evaluate the tumor and exclude second primaries.

It is often helpful to obtain a cytologic diagnosis if initial head and neck examination fails to reveal the primary tumor. An open biopsy should be done only when neither physical examination by an experienced clinician specializing in head and neck cancer nor FNA biopsy performed by an experienced cytopathologist yields a diagnosis. In such a setting, one should strongly consider obtaining an MRI or PET scan prior to open biopsy, as these methods may yield valuable information about a possible presumed primary site or another site for FNA.

With the exception of papillary thyroid carcinoma, non–squamous cell metastases to the neck are infrequent. While tumors that are not primary in the head or neck seldom metastasize to the cervical lymph nodes, the supraclavicular lymph nodes are quite often involved by lung, gastroesophageal, and breast tumors. Infradiaphragmatic tumors, with the exception of renal cell carcinoma and testicular cancer, rarely metastasize to the neck.

Bochtler T et al. Diagnosis and management of metastatic neoplasms with unknown primary. Semin Diagn Pathol. 2018 May;35(3):199–206. [PMID: 29203116]

Green B et al. Current surgical management of metastases in the neck from mucosal squamous cell carcinoma of the head and neck. Br J Oral Maxillofac Surg. 2016 Feb;54(2):135–40. [PMID: 26432197]

Liang L et al. A meta-analysis on selective versus comprehensive neck dissection in oral squamous cell carcinoma patients with clinically node-positive neck. Oral Oncol. 2015 Dec;51(12):1076–81. [PMID: 26500065]

LYMPHOMA

About 10% of lymphomas present in the head and neck. Multiple rubbery nodes, especially in young adults or in patients who have AIDS, are suggestive of this disease. A thorough physical examination may demonstrate other sites of nodal or organ involvement. FNA biopsy may be diagnostic, but open biopsy is often required to determine architecture and an appropriate treatment course.

Oishi N et al. Head and neck lymphomas in HIV patients: a clinical perspective. Int Arch Otorhinolaryngol. 2017 Oct; 21(4):399–407. [PMID: 29018505]

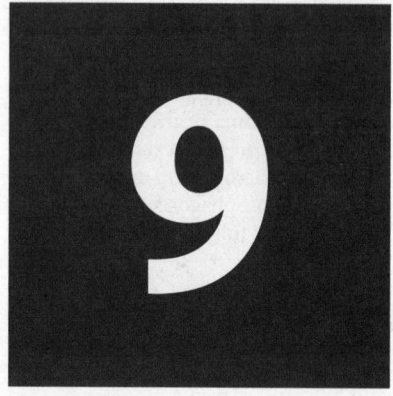

Pulmonary Disorders

Asha N. Chesnutt, MD

Mark S. Chesnutt, MD

Niall T. Prendergast, MD

Thomas J. Prendergast, MD

DISORDERS OF THE AIRWAYS

Airway disorders have diverse causes but share certain common pathophysiologic and clinical features. Airflow limitation is characteristic and frequently causes dyspnea and cough. Other symptoms are typically disease-specific. Disorders of the airways can be classified as those that involve the upper airways—loosely defined as those above and including the vocal folds—and those that involve the lower airways.

DISORDERS OF THE UPPER AIRWAYS

Acute obstruction of the upper airway can be immediately life-threatening and must be relieved promptly to avoid asphyxia. Causes of acute upper airway obstruction include trauma to the larynx or pharynx, foreign body aspiration, laryngospasm, laryngeal edema from thermal injury or angioedema, infections (acute epiglottitis, Ludwig angina, pharyngeal or retropharyngeal abscess), and acute allergic laryngitis.

Chronic obstruction of the upper airway may be caused by carcinoma of the pharynx or larynx, laryngeal or subglottic stenosis, laryngeal granulomas or webs, or bilateral vocal fold paralysis. Laryngeal or subglottic stenosis may become evident weeks or months after translaryngeal endotracheal intubation. Inspiratory stridor, intercostal retractions on inspiration, a palpable inspiratory thrill over the larynx, and wheezing localized to the neck or trachea on auscultation are characteristic findings. Flow-volume loops may show characteristic flow limitations. Soft-tissue radiographs of the neck may show supraglottic or infraglottic narrowing. CT and MRI scans can reveal exact sites of obstruction. Flexible endoscopy may be diagnostic, but caution is necessary to avoid exacerbating upper airway edema and precipitating critical airway narrowing.

Vocal fold dysfunction syndrome is characterized by paradoxical vocal fold adduction, resulting in both acute and chronic upper airway obstruction. It can cause dyspnea and wheezing that may be distinguished from asthma or exercise-induced asthma by the lack of response to bronchodilator therapy, normal spirometry immediately after an attack, spirometric evidence of upper airway obstruction, a negative bronchial provocation test, or direct visualization of adduction of the vocal folds on both inspiration and expiration. The condition appears to be psychogenic in nature. Treatment consists of speech therapy, which uses breathing, voice, and neck relaxation exercises to abort the symptoms.

Denipah N et al. Acute management of paradoxical vocal fold motion (vocal cord dysfunction). Ann Emerg Med. 2017 Jan; 69(1):18–23. [PMID: 27522309]

Fretzayas A et al. Differentiating vocal cord dysfunction from asthma. J Asthma Allergy. 2017 Oct 12;10:277–83. [PMID: 29066919]

DISORDERS OF THE LOWER AIRWAYS

Tracheal obstruction may be intrathoracic (below the suprasternal notch) or extrathoracic. Fixed tracheal obstruction may be caused by acquired or congenital tracheal stenosis, primary or secondary tracheal neoplasms, extrinsic compression (tumors of the lung, thymus, or thyroid; lymphadenopathy; congenital vascular rings; aneurysms; etc), foreign body aspiration, tracheal granulomas and papillomas, and tracheal trauma. Tracheomalacia, foreign body aspiration, and retained secretions may cause variable tracheal obstruction.

Acquired **tracheal stenosis** is usually secondary to previous tracheotomy or endotracheal intubation. Dyspnea, cough, and inability to clear pulmonary secretions occur weeks to months after tracheal decannulation or extubation. Physical findings may be absent until tracheal diameter is reduced 50% or more, when wheezing, a palpable tracheal thrill, and harsh breath sounds may be detected. The diagnosis is usually confirmed by plain films or CT of the trachea. Complications include recurring pulmonary infection and life-threatening respiratory failure. Management is directed toward ensuring adequate ventilation and oxygenation and avoiding manipulative procedures that may increase edema of the tracheal mucosa. Surgical reconstruction, endotracheal stent placement, or laser photoresection may be required.

Bronchial obstruction may be caused by retained pulmonary secretions, aspiration, foreign bodies, bronchomalacia, bronchogenic carcinoma, compression by extrinsic masses, and tumors metastatic to the airway. Clinical and radiographic findings vary depending on the location of the obstruction and the degree of airway narrowing. Symptoms include dyspnea, cough, wheezing, and, if infection is present, fever and chills. A history of recurrent pneumonia in the same lobe or segment or slow resolution (more than 3 months) of pneumonia on successive radiographs suggests the possibility of bronchial obstruction and the need for bronchoscopy.

Radiographic findings include **atelectasis** (local parenchymal collapse), postobstructive infiltrates, and air trapping caused by unidirectional expiratory obstruction. CT scanning may demonstrate the nature and exact location of obstruction of the central bronchi. MRI may be superior to CT for delineating the extent of underlying disease in the hilum, but it is usually reserved for cases in which CT findings are equivocal. Bronchoscopy is the definitive diagnostic study, particularly if tumor or foreign body aspiration is suspected. The finding of bronchial breath sounds on physical examination or an air bronchogram on chest radiograph in an area of atelectasis rules out complete airway obstruction. Bronchoscopy is unlikely to be of therapeutic benefit in this situation.

Murgu SD et al. Central airway obstruction: benign strictures, tracheobronchomalacia, and malignancy-related obstruction. Chest. 2016;150(2):426–41. [PMID: 26874192]
Shroff GS et al. Pathology of the trachea and central bronchi. Semin Ultrasound CT MR. 2016 Jun;37(3):177–89. [PMID: 27261343]

ASTHMA

ESSENTIALS OF DIAGNOSIS

- ▶ Episodic or chronic symptoms of wheezing, dyspnea, or cough.
- ▶ Symptoms frequently worse at night or in the early morning.
- ▶ Prolonged expiration and diffuse wheezes on physical examination.
- ▶ Limitation of airflow on pulmonary function testing or positive bronchoprovocation challenge.
- ▶ Reversibility of airflow obstruction, either spontaneously or following bronchodilator therapy.

▶ General Considerations

Asthma is a common disease, affecting approximately 8–10% of the population. It is slightly more common in male children (younger than 14 years) and in female adults. There is a genetic predisposition to asthma. Prevalence, hospitalizations, and fatal asthma have all increased in the United States over the past 20 years. Each year, approximately 10 million office visits, 1.8 million emergency department visits, and more than 3500 deaths in the United States are attributed to asthma. Hospitalization rates have been highest among blacks and children, and death rates are consistently highest among blacks aged 15–24 years.

▶ Definition & Pathogenesis

Asthma is a chronic disorder of the airways characterized by variable airway obstruction, airway hyperresponsiveness, and airway inflammation. No single histopathologic feature is pathognomonic but common findings include airway inflammatory cell infiltration with eosinophils, neutrophils, and lymphocytes (especially T cells); goblet cell hyperplasia, sometimes plugging of small airways with mucus; collagen deposition beneath the basement membrane; hypertrophy of bronchial smooth muscle; airway edema; mast cell activation; and denudation of airway epithelium. IgE plays a central role in the pathogenesis of allergic asthma. Interleukin-5 is important in promoting eosinophilic inflammation.

The strongest identifiable predisposing factor for the development of asthma is atopy, but obesity is increasingly recognized as a risk factor. Exposure of sensitive patients to inhaled allergens increases airway inflammation, airway hyper-responsiveness, and symptoms. Symptoms may develop immediately (immediate asthmatic response) or 4–6 hours after allergen exposure (late asthmatic response). Common allergens include house dust mites (often found in pillows, mattresses, upholstered furniture, carpets, and drapes), cockroaches, cat dander, and seasonal pollens. Substantially reducing exposure reduces pathologic findings and clinical symptoms.

Nonspecific precipitants of asthma include exercise, upper respiratory tract infections, rhinosinusitis, postnasal drip, aspiration, gastroesophageal reflux, changes in the weather, and stress. Exposure to **products of combustion** (eg, from tobacco, crack cocaine, methamphetamines, and other agents) increases asthma symptoms and the need for medications and reduces lung function. **Air pollution** (increased air levels of respirable particles, ozone, SO_2, and NO_2) precipitate asthma symptoms and increase emergency department visits and hospitalizations. Selected individuals may experience asthma symptoms after exposure to aspirin (aspirin-exacerbated respiratory disease), nonsteroidal anti-inflammatory drugs, or tartrazine dyes. Other **medications** may precipitate asthma symptoms (see Table 9–24). **Occupational asthma** is triggered by various agents in the workplace and may occur weeks to years after initial exposure and sensitization. Women may experience **catamenial asthma** at predictable times during the menstrual cycle. **Exercise-induced bronchoconstriction** begins during exercise or within 3 minutes after its end, peaks within 10–15 minutes, and then resolves by 60 minutes. This phenomenon is thought to be a consequence of the airways' attempt to warm and humidify an increased volume of expired air during exercise. **"Cardiac asthma"** is wheezing precipitated by decompensated heart failure. Cough-variant asthma has cough instead of wheezing as the predominant symptom of bronchial hyperreactivity.

Clinical Findings

Symptoms and signs vary widely among patients as well as individually over time. General clinical findings in stable asthma patients are listed in Figure 9–1 and Table 9–1; Table 9–2 lists findings seen during asthma exacerbations.

A. Symptoms and Signs

Asthma is characterized by episodic wheezing, difficulty in breathing, chest tightness, and cough. Excess sputum production is common. The frequency of asthma symptoms is highly variable. Some patients have infrequent, brief attacks of asthma while others may suffer nearly continuous

Components of Severity		Classification of Asthma Severity ≥ 12 years of age			
			Persistent		
		Intermittent	**Mild**	**Moderate**	**Severe**
Impairment Normal FEV₁/FVC: 8–19 yr 85% 20–39 yr 80% 40–59 yr 75% 60–80 yr 70%	Symptoms	≤ 2 days/week	> 2 days/week but not daily	Daily	Throughout the day
	Nighttime awakenings	≤ 2×/month	3–4×/month	> 1×/week but not nightly	Often 7×/week
	Short-acting β₂-agonist use for symptom control (not prevention of EIB)	≤ 2 days/week	> 2 days/week but not daily, and not more than 1× on any day	Daily	Several times per day
	Interference with normal activity	None	Minor limitation	Some limitation	Extremely limited
	Lung function	• Normal FEV₁ between exacerbations • FEV₁ > 80% predicted • FEV₁/FVC normal	• FEV₁ > 80% predicted • FEV₁/FVC normal	• FEV₁ > 60% but < 80% predicted • FEV₁/FVC reduced 5%	• FEV₁ < 60% predicted • FEV₁/FVC reduced > 5%
Risk	Exacerbations requiring oral systemic corticosteroids	0–1/year (see note)	≥ 2/year (see note) ———————————→		
		Consider severity and interval since last exacerbation. ←——————→ Frequency and severity may fluctuate over time for patients in any severity category. Relative annual risk of exacerbations may be related to FEV₁.			
Recommended Step for Initiating Treatment (See Figure 9–2 for treatment steps.)		Step 1	Step 2	Step 3	Step 4 or 5 and consider short course of oral systemic corticosteroids
		In 2–6 weeks, evaluate level of asthma control that is achieved and adjust therapy accordingly.			

EIB, exercise-induced bronchospasm; FEV₁, forced expiratory volume in 1 second; FVC, forced vital capacity; ICU, intensive care unit.

Notes:
- The stepwise approach is meant to assist, not replace, the clinical decision-making required to meet individual patient needs.

- Level of severity is determined by assessment of both impairment and risk. Assess impairment domain by patient's/caregiver's recall of previous 2–4 weeks and spirometry. Assign severity to the most severe category in which any feature occurs.

- At present, there are inadequate data to correspond frequencies of exacerbations with different levels of asthma severity. In general, more frequent and intense exacerbations (eg, requiring urgent, unscheduled care, hospitalization, or ICU admission) indicate greater underlying disease severity. For treatment purposes, patients who had ≥ 2 exacerbations requiring oral systemic corticosteroids in the past year may be considered the same as patients who have persistent asthma, even in the absence of impairment levels consistent with persistent asthma.

▲ **Figure 9–1.** Classifying asthma severity and initiating treatment. (Adapted from National Asthma Education and Prevention Program. Expert Panel Report 3: Guidelines for the Diagnosis and Management of Asthma. National Institutes of Health Pub. No. 08-4051. Bethesda, MD, 2007.)

Table 9–1. Assessing asthma control.

Components of Control		Classification of Asthma Control (≥ 12 years of age)		
		Well Controlled	Not Well Controlled	Very Poorly Controlled
Impairment	Symptoms	≤ 2 days/week	> 2 days/week	Throughout the day
	Nighttime awakenings	≤ 2×/month	1–3×/week	≥ 4×/week
	Interference with normal activity	None	Some limitation	Extremely limited
	Short-acting beta-2-agonist use for symptom control (not prevention of EIB)	≤ 2 days/week	> 2 days/week	Several times/day
	FEV_1 or peak flow	> 80% predicted/ personal best	60–80% predicted/ personal best	< 60% predicted/ personal best
	Validated Questionnaires			
	ATAQ[1]	0	1–2	3–4
	ACQ[1]	≤ 0.75	≥ 1.5	N/A
	ACT[1]	≥ 20	16–19	≤ 15
Risk	Exacerbations requiring oral systemic corticosteroids	0–1/year	≥ 2/year (see note)	
		Consider severity and interval since last exacerbation		
	Loss of lung function	Evaluation requires long-term follow-up care.		
	Treatment-related adverse effects	Medication side effects can vary in intensity from none to very troublesome and worrisome. The level of intensity does not correlate to specific levels of control but should be considered in the overall assessment of risk.		
Recommended Action for Treatment (see Figure 9–2 for steps)		• Maintain current step. • Regular follow-ups every 1–6 months to maintain control. • Consider step down if well controlled for at least 3 months.	• Step up 1 step, and • Reevaluate in 2–6 weeks. • For side effects, consider alternative treatment options.	• Consider short course of oral systemic corticosteroids. • Step up 1–2 steps, and • Reevaluate in 2 weeks. • For side effects, consider alternative options.

[1]Minimal importance differences: 1.0 for the ATAQ; 0.5 for the ACQ with values of 0.76–1.4 considered indeterminate; not determined for the ACT.

ACQ, Asthma Control Questionnaire©; ACT, Asthma Control Test™; ATAQ = Asthma Therapy Assessment Questionnaire©; EIB, exercise-induced bronchospasm; FEV_1, forced expiratory volume in 1 second; ICU, intensive care unit.

Notes:
- The stepwise approach is meant to assist, not replace, the clinical decision making required to meet individual patient needs.
- The level of control is based on the most severe impairment or risk category. Assess impairment domain by patient's recall of previous 2–4 weeks and by spirometry or peak flow measures. Symptom assessment for longer periods should reflect a global assessment, such as inquiring whether the patient's asthma is better or worse since the last visit.
- Inadequate data to correspond frequencies of exacerbations with different levels of asthma control. In general, more frequent and intense exacerbations (eg, requiring urgent, unscheduled care, hospitalization, or ICU admission) indicate poorer control. For therapy purposes, patients with ≥ 2 exacerbations requiring oral systemic corticosteroids in the past year may be considered the same as patients who have not-well-controlled asthma, even in the absence of impairment levels consistent with not-well-controlled asthma.
- Before step up in therapy:
  —Review adherence to medication, inhaler.
  —If an alternative treatment option was used in a step, discontinue and use the preferred treatment for that step.

Adapted from National Asthma Education and Prevention Program. Expert Panel Report 3: Guidelines for the Diagnosis and Management of Asthma. National Institutes of Health Pub. No. 08-4051. Bethesda, MD, 2007.

symptoms. Asthma symptoms may occur spontaneously or be precipitated or exacerbated by many different triggers as discussed above. Asthma symptoms are frequently worse at night; circadian variations in bronchomotor tone and bronchial reactivity reach their nadir between 3 AM and 4 AM, increasing symptoms of bronchoconstriction.

Some physical examination findings increase the probability of asthma. Nasal mucosal swelling, increased secretions, and polyps are often seen in patients with allergic asthma. Eczema, atopic dermatitis, or other allergic skin disorders may also be present. Wheezing or a prolonged expiratory phase during normal breathing correlates well with the presence of airflow obstruction. (Wheezing during forced expiration does not.) Chest examination may be normal between exacerbations in patients with mild asthma. During severe asthma exacerbations, airflow may be too limited to produce

Table 9–2. Evaluation and classification of severity of asthma exacerbations.

	Mild	Moderate	Severe	Respiratory Arrest Imminent
Symptoms				
Breathlessness	While walking	At rest, limits activity	At rest, interferes with conversation	While at rest, mute
Talks in	Sentences	Phrases	Words	Silent
Alertness	May be agitated	Usually agitated	Usually agitated	Drowsy or confused
Signs				
Respiratory rate	Increased	Increased	Often > 30/minute	> 30/minute
Body position	Can lie down	Prefers sitting	Sits upright	Unable to recline
Use of accessory muscles; suprasternal retractions	Usually not	Commonly	Usually	Paradoxical thoracoabdominal movement
Wheeze	Moderate, often only end expiratory	Loud; throughout exhalation	Usually loud; throughout inhalation and exhalation	Absent
Pulse/minute	< 100	100–120	> 120	Bradycardia
Pulsus paradoxus	Absent < 10 mm Hg	May be present 10–25 mm Hg	Often present > 25 mm Hg	Absence suggests respiratory muscle fatigue
Functional Assessment				
PEF or FEV_1 % predicted or % personal best	≥ 70%	40–69%	< 40%	< 25%
Pao_2 (on air, mm Hg)	Normal[1]	≥ 60[1]	< 60: possible cyanosis	< 60: possible cyanosis
Pco_2 (mm Hg)	< 42 mm Hg[1]	< 42 mm Hg[1]	≥ 42[1]	≥ 42[1]
Sao_2 (on air, %)	> 95%[1]	90–95%[1]	< 90%[1]	< 90%[1]

[1]Test not usually necessary.
FEV_1, forced expiratory volume in 1 second; PEF, peak expiratory flow; Sao_2, oxygen saturation.
Adapted from National Asthma Education and Prevention Program. Expert Panel Report 3: Guidelines for the Diagnosis and Management of Asthma. National Institutes of Health Pub. No. 08-4051. Bethesda, MD, 2007.

wheezing, and the only diagnostic clue on auscultation may be globally reduced breath sounds with prolonged expiration. Hunched shoulders and use of accessory muscles of respiration suggest an increased work of breathing.

B. Laboratory Findings

Arterial blood gas measurements may be normal during a mild asthma exacerbation, but respiratory alkalosis and an increase in the alveolar-arterial oxygen difference ($A–a–Do_2$) are common. During severe exacerbations, hypoxemia develops and the $Paco_2$ returns to normal. The combination of an increased $Paco_2$ and respiratory acidosis may indicate impending respiratory failure and the need for mechanical ventilation.

C. Pulmonary Function Testing

Clinicians are able to identify airflow obstruction on examination, but they have limited ability to assess its severity or to predict whether it is reversible. The evaluation for asthma should therefore include **spirometry** (forced expiratory volume in 1 second [FEV_1], forced vital capacity [FVC], FEV_1/FVC) before and after the administration of a short-acting bronchodilator. These measurements help determine the presence and extent of airflow obstruction and whether

it is immediately reversible. Airflow obstruction is indicated by a reduced FEV_1/FVC ratio. Significant reversibility of airflow obstruction is defined by an increase of 12% or more and 200 mL in FEV_1 or FVC after inhaling a short-acting bronchodilator. A positive bronchodilator response strongly confirms the diagnosis of asthma but a lack of responsiveness in the pulmonary function laboratory does not preclude success in a clinical trial of bronchodilator therapy. Severe airflow obstruction results in significant air trapping, with an increase in residual volume and consequent reduction in FVC, resulting in a pattern that may mimic a restrictive ventilatory defect.

Bronchial provocation testing with inhaled histamine or methacholine may be useful when asthma is suspected but spirometry is nondiagnostic. Bronchial provocation is not recommended if the FEV_1 is less than 65% of predicted. A positive methacholine test is defined as a fall in the FEV_1 of 20% or more at exposure to a concentration of less than or equal to 8 mg/mL. A negative test has a negative predictive value for asthma of 95%. Exercise challenge testing may be useful in patients with symptoms of exercise-induced bronchospasm.

Peak expiratory flow (PEF) meters are handheld devices designed as personal monitoring tools. PEF monitoring can establish peak flow variability, quantify asthma severity, and provide both patient and clinician with objective measurements on which to base treatment decisions. There are conflicting data about whether measuring PEF improves asthma outcomes, but doing so is recommended to help confirm the diagnosis of asthma, to improve asthma control in patients with poor perception of airflow obstruction, and to identify environmental and occupational causes of symptoms. Predicted values for PEF vary with age, height, and sex but are poorly standardized. Comparison with reference values is less helpful than comparison with the patient's own baseline. PEF shows diurnal variation. It is generally lowest on first awakening and highest several hours before the midpoint of the waking day. PEF should be measured in the morning before the administration of a bronchodilator and in the afternoon after taking a bronchodilator. A 20% change in PEF values from morning to afternoon or from day to day suggests inadequately controlled asthma. PEF values less than 200 L/min indicate severe airflow obstruction.

D. Additional Testing

Routine chest radiographs in patients with asthma are usually normal or show only hyperinflation. Other findings may include bronchial wall thickening and diminished peripheral lung vascular shadows. Chest imaging is indicated when pneumonia, another disorder mimicking asthma, or a complication of asthma such as pneumothorax is suspected.

Skin testing or in vitro testing, including total serum IgE and allergen-specific IgE, to assess sensitivity to environmental allergens can identify atopy in patients with persistent asthma who may benefit from therapies directed at their allergic diathesis. Evaluations for paranasal sinus disease or gastroesophageal reflux should be considered in patients with pertinent, severe, or refractory asthma symptoms. An absolute eosinophil count can identify patients eligible for anti–interleukin-5 therapy to manage eosinophilic airway disease.

▶ Complications

Complications of asthma include exhaustion, dehydration, airway infection, and tussive syncope. Pneumothorax occurs but is rare. Acute hypercapnic and hypoxemic respiratory failure occurs in severe disease.

▶ Differential Diagnosis

Patients who have atypical symptoms or poor response to therapy may have a condition that mimics asthma. These disorders typically fall into one of five categories: upper airway disorders, lower airway disorders, systemic vasculitides, cardiac disorders, and psychiatric disorders. **Upper airway disorders** that mimic asthma include vocal fold paralysis, vocal fold dysfunction syndrome, foreign body aspiration, laryngotracheal masses, tracheal narrowing, tracheobronchomalacia, and airway edema (eg, angioedema or inhalation injury). **Lower airway disorders** include nonasthmatic chronic obstructive pulmonary disease (COPD) (chronic bronchitis or emphysema), bronchiectasis, allergic bronchopulmonary mycosis, cystic fibrosis, eosinophilic pneumonia, hypersensitivity pneumonitis, sarcoidosis, and bronchiolitis obliterans. **Systemic vasculitides** with pulmonary involvement may have an asthmatic component, such as eosinophilic granulomatosis with polyangiitis. **Cardiac disorders** include heart failure and pulmonary hypertension. **Psychiatric causes** include conversion disorders ("functional" asthma), emotional laryngeal wheezing, vocal fold dysfunction, or episodic laryngeal dyskinesis. Rarely, Münchausen syndrome or malingering may explain a patient's complaints.

▶ NAEPP 3 Diagnosis & Management Guidelines

The third Expert Panel Report of the National Asthma Education and Prevention Program (NAEPP), in conjunction with the Global Initiative for Asthma, a collaboration between the National Institutes of Health/National Heart, Lung, and Blood Institute and the World Health Organization, provides guidelines for diagnosis and management of asthma (NAEPP 3) (Figure 9–2). This report identifies four components of chronic asthma diagnosis and management: (1) assessing and monitoring asthma severity and asthma control, (2) patient education designed to foster a partnership for care, (3) control of environmental factors and comorbid conditions that affect asthma, and (4) pharmacologic therapy for asthma.

1. Assessing and monitoring asthma severity and asthma control—**Severity** is the intrinsic intensity of the disease process. **Control** is the degree to which symptoms and limitations on activity are minimized by therapy. **Responsiveness** is the ease with which control is achieved with therapy. NAEPP 3 guidelines emphasize control over classifications of severity, since the latter is variable over time and in response to therapy. A measure of severity on initial presentation (Figure 9–1) is helpful, however, in guiding the initiation of therapy. Control of asthma is assessed in terms of **impairment** (frequency and intensity of symptoms and functional limitations) and **risk** (the likelihood of acute exacerbations or chronic decline in lung function). A key insight is that these two domains of control may respond differently to treatment: some patients may have minimal impairment yet remain at risk for severe exacerbations, for example, in the setting of an upper respiratory tract infection. Table 9–1 is used to assess the adequacy of asthma control and is used in conjunction with Figure 9–2 to guide adjustments in therapy based on the level of control.

2. Patient education designed to foster a partnership for care—Active self-management reduces urgent care visits and hospitalizations and improves perceived control of asthma. Therefore, an outpatient preventive approach that includes self-management education is an integral part of effective asthma care.

All patients, but particularly those with poorly controlled symptoms or history of severe exacerbations, should have a written **asthma action plan** that includes instructions for daily management and measures to take in response to specific changes in status. Patients should be taught to recognize symptoms—especially patterns indicating inadequate asthma control or predicting the need for additional therapy.

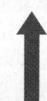

Intermittent Asthma	**Persistent Asthma: Daily Medication** Consult with asthma specialist if step 4 care or higher is required. Consider consultation at step 3.

Step 6
Preferred:
High-dose ICS + LABA + oral corticosteroid

AND

Consider omalizumab for patients who have allergies

Step 5
Preferred:
High-dose ICS + LABA

AND

Consider omalizumab for patients who have allergies

Step 4
Preferred:
Medium-dose ICS + LABA

Alternative:
Low-dose ICS + either LTRA, theophylline, or zileuton

Step 3
Preferred:
Low-dose ICS + LABA
OR
Medium-dose ICS

Alternative:
Low-dose ICS + either LTRA, theophylline, or zileuton

Step 2
Preferred:
Low-dose ICS

Alternative:
Cromolyn, LTRA, nedocromil, or theophylline

Step 1
Preferred:
SABA PRN

Step up if needed
(first, check adherence, environmental control, and comorbid conditions)

Assess control

Step down if possible
(and asthma is well controlled at least 3 months)

Each step: Patient education, environmental control, and management of comorbidities.

Steps 2–4: Consider subcutaneous allergen immunotherapy for patients who have allergic asthma (see notes).

Quick-Relief Medication for All Patients

- SABA as needed for symptoms. Intensity of treatment depends on severity of symptoms: up to three treatments at 20-minute intervals as needed. Short course of oral systemic corticosteroids may be needed.
- Use of SABA > 2 days a week for symptom relief (not prevention of EIB) generally indicates inadequate control and the need to step up treatment.

Key: *Alphabetical order is used when more than one treatment option is listed within either preferred or alternative therapy.* EIB, exercise-induced bronchospasm; ICS, inhaled corticosteroid; LABA, inhaled long-acting beta-2-agonist; LTRA, leukotriene receptor antagonist; SABA, inhaled short-acting beta-2-agonist.

Notes:

- The stepwise approach is meant to assist, not replace, the clinical decision making required to meet individual patient needs.
- If alternative treatment is used and response is inadequate, discontinue it and use the preferred treatment before stepping up.
- Zileuton is a less desirable alternative as adjunctive therapy due to limited studies and the need to monitor liver function. Theophylline requires monitoring of serum concentration levels.
- In step 6, before oral systemic corticosteroids are introduced, a trial of high-dose ICS + LABA + either LTRA, theophylline, or zileuton may be considered, although this approach has not been studied in clinical trials.
- Step 1, 2, and 3 preferred therapies are based on Evidence A; step 3 alternative therapy is based on Evidence A for LTRA, Evidence B for theophylline, and Evidence D for zileuton. Step 4 preferred therapy is based on Evidence B, and alternative therapy is based on Evidence B for LTRA and theophylline and Evidence D for zileuton. Step 5 preferred therapy is based on Evidence B. Step 6 preferred therapy is based on NAEPP Expert Panel Report 2, 1997 and Evidence B for omalizumab.
- Immunotherapy for steps 2–4 is based on Evidence B for house-dust mites, animal danders, and pollens; evidence is weak or lacking for molds and cockroaches. Evidence is strongest for immunotherapy with single allergens. The role of allergy in asthma is greater in children than in adults.
- Clinicians who administer immunotherapy or omalizumab should be prepared and equipped to identify and treat anaphylaxis that may occur.

▲ **Figure 9–2.** Stepwise approach to managing asthma. (Adapted from National Asthma Education and Prevention Program. Expert Panel Report 3: Guidelines for the Diagnosis and Management of Asthma. National Institutes of Health Pub. No. 08-4051. Bethesda, MD, 2007.)

3. Control of environmental factors and comorbid conditions that affect asthma

—Significant reduction in exposure to nonspecific airway irritants or to inhaled allergens in atopic patients may reduce symptoms and medication needs. Comorbid conditions that impair asthma management, such as rhinosinusitis, gastroesophageal reflux, obesity, and obstructive sleep apnea, should be identified and treated. This search for complicating conditions is particularly crucial in the initial evaluation of new asthma, and in patients who have difficult-to-control symptoms or frequent exacerbations.

4. Pharmacotherapy for asthma

—The goals of pharmacologic therapy are to minimize chronic symptoms that interfere with normal activity (including exercise), to prevent recurrent exacerbations, to reduce or eliminate the need for emergency department visits or hospitalizations, and to maintain normal or near-normal pulmonary function. These goals should be met while providing therapeutic agents with the fewest adverse effects and while satisfying patients' and families' expectations of asthma care.

 Treatment

A. Pharmacologic Agents

Asthma medications can be divided into two categories: (1) quick-relief (**reliever**) medications that act principally by direct relaxation of bronchial smooth muscle, thereby promoting prompt reversal of acute airflow obstruction to relieve accompanying symptom; and (2) long-term control (**controller**) medications that act primarily to attenuate airway inflammation and that are taken daily independent of symptoms to achieve and maintain control of persistent asthma. Anti-inflammatory agents, long-acting bronchodilators, and leukotriene modifiers comprise the important long-term control medications (Tables 9–3 and 9–4). Other classes of agents are mentioned briefly below.

Table 9–3. Quick-relief medications for asthma.

Medication	Dosage Form	Adult Dose	Comments
Inhaled Short-Acting Beta-2-Agonists			
	MDI		
Albuterol CFC Albuterol HFA Pirbuterol CFC Levalbuterol HFA	90 mcg/puff, 200 puffs/canister 90 mcg/puff, 200 puffs/canister 200 mcg/puff, 400 puffs/canister 45 mcg/puff, 200 puffs/canister	2 puffs 5 minutes before exercise 2 puffs every 4–6 hours as needed	• An increasing use or lack of expected effect indicates diminished control of asthma. • Not recommended for long-term daily treatment. Regular use exceeding 2 days/week for symptom control (not prevention of EIB) indicates the need to step up therapy. • Differences in potency exist, but all products are essentially comparable on a per-puff basis. • May double usual dose for mild exacerbations. • Prime the inhaler by releasing four actuations prior to use. • Periodically clean HFA activator, as drug may block/plug orifice.
	Nebulizer solution		
Albuterol	0.63 mg/3 mL 1.25 mg/3 mL 2.5 mg/3 mL 5 mg/mL (0.5%)	1.25–5 mg in 3 mL of saline every 4–8 hours as needed	• May mix with budesonide inhalant suspension, cromolyn, or ipratropium nebulizer solutions. • May double dose for severe exacerbations.
Levalbuterol (R-albuterol)	0.31 mg/3 mL 0.63 mg/3 mL 1.25 mg/0.5 mL 1.25 mg/3 mL	0.63–1.25 mg every 8 hours as needed	• Compatible with budesonide inhalant suspension. The product is a sterile-filled, preservative-free, unit dose vial.
Anticholinergics			
	MDI		
Ipratropium HFA	17 mcg/puff, 200 puffs/canister	2–3 puffs every 6 hours	• Evidence is lacking for anticholinergics producing added benefit to beta-2-agonists in long-term asthma control therapy.
	Nebulizer solution		
	0.25 mg/mL (0.025%)	0.25 mg every 6 hours	

(continued)

Table 9–3. Quick-relief medications for asthma. (continued)

Medication	Dosage Form	Adult Dose	Comments
Anticholinergics			
	MDI		
Ipratropium with albuterol	18 mcg/puff of ipratropium bromide and 90 mcg/puff of albuterol, 200 puffs/canister	2–3 puffs every 6 hours	
	Nebulizer solution		
	0.5 mg/3 mL ipratropium bromide and 2.5 mg/3 mL albuterol	3 mL every 4–6 hours	• Contains EDTA to prevent discolorations of the solution. This additive does not induce bronchospasm.
Systemic Corticosteroids			
Methylprednisolone	2-, 4-, 6-, 8-, 16-, 32-mg tablets	40–60 mg/day as single or 2 divided doses	• Short courses or "bursts" are effective for establishing control when initiating therapy or during a period of gradual deterioration. • The burst should be continued until symptoms resolve and the PEF is at least 80% of personal best. This usually requires 3–10 days but may require longer. There is no evidence that tapering the dose following improvements prevents relapse.
Prednisolone	5-mg tablets; 5 mg/5 mL, 15 mg/5 mL oral solution	40–60 mg/day as single or 2 divided doses	
Prednisone	1-, 2.5-, 5-, 10-, 20-, 50-mg tablets; 5 mg/mL oral solution	40–60 mg/day as single or 2 divided doses	
	Repository injection		
Methylprednisolone acetate	40 mg/mL 80 mg/mL	240 mg intramuscularly once	• May be used in place of a short burst of oral corticosteroids in patients who are vomiting or if adherence is a problem.

CFC, chlorofluorocarbon; EIB, exercise-induced bronchospasm; HFA, hydrofluoroalkane; MDI, metered-dose inhaler; PEF, peak expiratory flow.
Adapted from National Asthma Education and Prevention Program. Expert Panel Report 3: Guidelines for the Diagnosis and Management of Asthma. National Institutes of Health Pub. No. 08-4051. Bethesda, MD, 2007.

Most asthma medications are administered by inhalation or orally. Inhalation of an appropriate agent results in a more rapid onset of pulmonary effects as well as fewer systemic effects compared with oral administration of the same dose. Proper inhaler technique and the use of an inhalation chamber (a "spacer") with metered-dose inhalers (MDIs) decrease oropharyngeal deposition and improve drug delivery to the lung. Nebulizer therapy is reserved for patients who are acutely ill and those who cannot use inhalers because of difficulties with coordination, understanding, or cooperation.

1. Beta-adrenergic agonists—Beta-agonists are divided into **short-acting beta-agonists** (SABAs) and **long-acting beta-agonists** (LABAs). SABAs, including albuterol, levalbuterol, bitolterol, pirbuterol, and terbutaline (Table 9–3), are the mainstays of reliever or rescue therapy for asthma patients; all asthmatics should have immediate access to a SABA. SABAs are the most effective bronchodilators during exacerbations and provide immediate relief of symptoms. There is no convincing evidence to support the use of one agent over another. Administration before exercise effectively prevents exercise-induced bronchoconstriction.

Inhaled SABA therapy is as effective as oral or parenteral therapy in relaxing airway smooth muscle and improving acute asthma and offers the advantages of rapid onset of action (less than 5 minutes) with fewer systemic side effects. Repetitive administration produces incremental bronchodilation. One or two inhalations of a SABA from an MDI are usually sufficient for mild to moderate symptoms. Severe exacerbations frequently require higher doses: 6–12 puffs every 30–60 minutes of albuterol by MDI with an inhalation chamber or 2.5 mg by nebulizer provide equivalent bronchodilation. Administration by nebulization does not offer more effective delivery than MDIs used correctly but does provide higher doses. With most SABAs, the recommended dose by nebulizer for acute asthma (albuterol, 2.5 mg) is 25–30 times that delivered by a single activation of the MDI (albuterol, 0.09 mg). This difference suggests that standard dosing of inhalations from an MDI are often insufficient in the setting of an acute exacerbation. Independent of dose, nebulizer therapy may be more effective in patients who are unable to coordinate inhalation of medication from an MDI because of age, agitation, or severity of the exacerbation.

Scheduled daily use of SABAs is not recommended. Increased use (more than one canister a month) or lack of expected effect indicates diminished asthma control and the need for additional long-term control therapy.

Table 9–4. Estimated comparative daily dosages for inhaled corticosteroids for asthma.

Medication	Low Daily Dose Adult	Medium Daily Dose Adult	High Daily Dose Adult
Beclomethasone HFA 40 or 80 mcg/puff	80–240 mcg	> 240–480 mcg	> 480 mcg
Budesonide DPI 90, 180, or 200 mcg/inhalation	180–600 mcg	> 600–1200 mcg	> 1200 mcg
Flunisolide 250 mcg/puff	500–1000 mcg	> 1000–2000 mcg	> 2000 mcg
Flunisolide HFA 80 mcg/puff	320 mcg	> 320–640 mcg	> 640 mcg
Fluticasone HFA/MDI: 44, 110, or 220 mcg/puff DPI: 50, 100, or 250 mcg/inhalation	88–264 mcg 100–300 mcg	> 264–440 mcg > 300–500 mcg	> 440 mcg > 500 mcg
Mometasone DPI 200 mcg/puff	200 mcg	400 mcg	> 400 mcg
Triamcinolone acetonide 75 mcg/puff	300–750 mcg	> 750–1500 mcg	> 1500 mcg

DPI, dry powder inhaler; HFA, hydrofluoroalkaline; MDI, metered-dose inhaler.
Notes:
• The most important determinant of appropriate dosing is the clinician's judgment of the patient's response to therapy.
• Potential drug interactions:
  A number of the inhaled corticosteroids, including fluticasone, budesonide, and mometasone, are metabolized in the gastrointestinal tract and liver by CYP 3A4 isoenzymes. Potent inhibitors of CYP 3A4, such as ritonavir and ketoconazole, have the potential for increasing systemic concentrations of these inhaled corticosteroids by increasing oral availability and decreasing systemic clearance. Some cases of clinically significant Cushing syndrome and secondary adrenal insufficiency have been reported.
Adapted from National Asthma Education and Prevention Program. Expert Panel Report 3: Guidelines for the Diagnosis and Management of Asthma. National Institutes of Health Pub. No. 08-4051. Bethesda, MD, 2007.

LABAs provide bronchodilation for up to 12 hours after a single dose. Salmeterol and formoterol are the LABAs available for asthma in the United States. They are administered via dry powder delivery devices. They are indicated for long-term prevention of asthma symptoms (including nocturnal symptoms) and for prevention of exercise-induced bronchospasm. When added to low and medium daily doses of inhaled corticosteroids (Table 9–4), LABAs provide control equivalent to what is achieved by doubling the inhaled corticosteroid dose. Side effects are minimal at standard doses. LABAs should not be used as monotherapy since they have no anti-inflammatory effect and since monotherapy has been associated with a small but statistically significant increased risk of severe or fatal asthma attacks in two large studies. This increased risk has not been fully explained but may relate to genetic variation in the beta-adrenergic receptor; it remains an area of controversy. The efficacy of combined inhaled corticosteroid and LABA therapy has led to the marketing of combination medications that deliver both agents simultaneously (Table 9–5). Combination inhalers containing formoterol and budesonide have shown efficacy in both rescue (given formoterol's short time to onset) and maintenance (budesonide).

2. Corticosteroids—Corticosteroids are the most potent and consistently effective anti-inflammatory agents currently available. They decrease both acute and chronic inflammation, resulting in reduced symptoms and improved lung function. These agents may also potentiate the action of beta-adrenergic agonists.

Inhaled corticosteroids are preferred, first-line agents for all patients with persistent asthma. Patients with persistent symptoms or asthma exacerbations who are not taking an inhaled corticosteroid should be started on one. The most important determinants of agent selection and appropriate dosing are the patient's status and response to treatment. Dosages for inhaled corticosteroids vary depending on the specific agent and delivery device (Table 9–4). For most patients, twice-daily dosing provides adequate control of asthma. Once-daily dosing may be sufficient in selected patients. Maximum responses from inhaled corticosteroids may not be observed for months. The use of an inhalation chamber coupled with mouth washing after inhaled corticosteroid use decreases local side effects (cough, dysphonia, oropharyngeal candidiasis) and systemic absorption. Dry powder inhalers (DPIs) are not used with an inhalation chamber. Systemic effects (adrenal suppression, osteoporosis, skin thinning, easy bruising, and cataracts) may occur with high-dose inhaled corticosteroid therapy. Many combination inhalers with inhaled corticosteroid/LABA offer convenient treatment of persistent asthma.

Systemic corticosteroids (oral or parenteral) are most effective in achieving prompt control of asthma during exacerbations. Systemic corticosteroids are effective primary treatment for patients with moderate to severe asthma

Table 9–5. Long-term control medications for asthma.

Medication	Dosage Form	Adult Dose	Comments
Inhaled Corticosteroids			(See Table 9–4)
Systemic Corticosteroids			(Applies to all three corticosteroids)
Methylprednisolone Prednisolone Prednisone	2-, 4-, 6-, 8-, 16-, 32-mg tablets 5-mg tablets; 5 mg/5 mL, 15 mg/5 mL oral solution 1-, 2.5-, 5-, 10-, 20-, 50-mg tablets; 5 mg/mL oral solution	7.5–60 mg 40–60 mg	• Administer single dose in AM either daily or on alternate days (alternate-day therapy may produce less adrenal suppression) as needed for control. • Short courses or "bursts" as single or 2 divided doses for 3–10 days are effective for establishing control when initiating therapy or during a period of gradual deterioration. • There is no evidence that tapering the dose following improvement in symptom control and pulmonary function prevents relapse.
Inhaled Long-Acting Beta-2-Agonists			Should not be used for symptom relief or exacerbations. Use with inhaled corticosteroids.
Formoterol Salmeterol	Inhalation 20 mcg/2 mL neb (DPI discontinued by FDA in United States) DPI 50 mcg/actuation	20 mcg every 12 hours 1 blister every 12 hours	• Additional doses should not be administered for at least 12 hours. • Agents should be used only with their specific inhaler and should not be taken orally. • Decreased duration of protection against EIB may occur with regular use.
Combined Medication			
Budesonide/formoterol	HFA MDI 80 mcg/4.5 mcg 160 mcg/4.5 mcg	2 inhalations twice daily; dose depends on severity of asthma	• 80/4.5 for asthma not controlled on low- to medium-dose inhaled corticosteroids. • 160/4.5 for asthma not controlled on medium- to high-dose inhaled corticosteroids.
Fluticasone/salmeterol	DPI 100 mcg/50 mcg 250 mcg/50 mcg, or 500 mcg/50 mcg HFA 45 mcg/21 mcg 115 mcg/21 mcg 230 mcg/21 mcg	1 inhalation twice daily; dose depends on severity of asthma	• 100/50 DPI or 45/21 HFA for patient not controlled on low- to medium-dose inhaled corticosteroids. • 250/50 DPI or 115/21 HFA for patients not controlled on medium- to high-dose inhaled corticosteroids.
Fluticasone furoate/ vilanterol	100 mcg/25 mcg, 200 mcg/ 25 mcg per blister DPI	1 puff inhaled daily	• Once-daily asthma maintenance.
Mometasone/formoterol	100 mcg/5 mcg/spray 200 mcg/5 mcg/spray	2 inhalations twice daily	
Cromolyn and Nedocromil			
Cromolyn Nedocromil	MDI 0.8 mg/puff Nebulizer 20 mg/ampule MDI 1.75 mg/puff	2 puffs four times daily 1 ampule four times daily 2 puffs four times daily	• 4–6 week trial may be needed to determine maximum benefit. • Dose by MDI may be inadequate to affect hyperresponsiveness. • One dose before exercise or allergen exposure provides effective prophylaxis for 1–2 hours. Not as effective for EIB as SABA. • Once control is achieved, the frequency of dosing may be reduced.
Inhaled Long-Acting Anticholinergic			Should not be used for symptom relief or exacerbations. Use with inhaled corticosteroids.
Tiotropium	DPI 18 mcg/blister	1 blister daily	
Leukotriene Modifiers			
Leukotriene Receptor Antagonists			
Montelukast	4- or 5-mg chewable tablet; 10-mg tablet	10 mg daily at bedtime	• Exhibits a flat dose-response curve. Doses > 10 mg will not produce a greater response in adults.

(continued)

Table 9–5. Long-term control medications for asthma. (continued)

Medication	Dosage Form	Adult Dose	Comments
Zafirlukast	10- or 20-mg tablet	20-mg tablet twice daily	• Administration with meals decreases bioavailability; take at least 1 hour before or 2 hours after meals. • Monitor for symptoms and signs of hepatic dysfunction.
5-Lipoxygenase Inhibitor			
Zileuton	600-mg tablet	600 mg four times daily	• Monitor hepatic enzyme (ALT).
Methylxanthines			
Theophylline	Liquids, sustained-release tablets, and capsules	Starting dose 10 mg/kg/day up to 300 mg maximum; usual maximum dose 800 mg/day	• Adjust dose to achieve serum concentration of 5–15 mcg/mL after at least 48 hours on same dose. • Due to wide interpatient variability in theophylline metabolic clearance, routine serum theophylline level monitoring is important.

ALT, alanine aminotransferase; DPI, dry powder inhaler; EIB, exercise-induced bronchospasm; FDA, US Food and Drug Administration; HFA, hydrofluoroalkaline; MDI, metered-dose inhaler; SABA, short-acting beta-2-agonist.

exacerbations and for patients with exacerbations who do not respond promptly and completely to inhaled SABA therapy. These medications speed the resolution of airflow obstruction and reduce the rate of relapse. Delays in administering corticosteroids may result in delayed benefits from these important agents. Therefore, oral corticosteroids should generally be prescribed to have available at home for early administration in patients with moderate to severe asthma. The minimal effective dose of systemic corticosteroids for asthma patients has not been identified. Outpatient prednisone "burst" therapy is 0.5–1 mg/kg/day (typically 40–60 mg) in 1–2 doses for 3–10 days. Severe exacerbations requiring hospitalization typically require 1 mg/kg of prednisone or methylprednisolone every 6–12 hours for 48 hours or until the FEV_1 (or PEF rate) returns to 50% of predicted (or 50% of baseline). The dose is then decreased to 60–80 mg/day until the PEF reaches 70% of predicted or personal best. No clear advantage has been found for higher doses of corticosteroids. It may be prudent to administer corticosteroids intravenously to critically ill patients to avoid concerns about altered gastrointestinal absorption.

In patients with refractory, poorly controlled asthma, systemic corticosteroids may be required for the long-term suppression of symptoms. Repeated efforts should be made to reduce the dose to the minimum needed to control symptoms. Alternate-day treatment is preferred to daily treatment. Concurrent treatment with calcium supplements and vitamin D should be initiated to prevent corticosteroid-induced bone mineral loss in long-term administration. Bone mineral density testing after 3 or more months of systemic corticosteroid lifetime use can guide the use of bisphosphonates for treatment of steroid-induced osteoporosis. Rapid discontinuation of systemic corticosteroids after long-term use may precipitate adrenal insufficiency.

3. Anticholinergics—Anticholinergic agents reverse vagally mediated bronchospasm but not allergen- or exercise-induced bronchospasm. They may decrease mucus gland hypersecretion. Both **short-acting muscarinic agents** (SAMAs) and **long-acting muscarinic agents** (LAMAs) are available. Ipratropium bromide, a SAMA, is less effective than SABA for relief of acute bronchospasm, but it is the inhaled drug of choice for patients with intolerance to SABA or with bronchospasm due to beta-blocker medications. Ipratropium bromide reduces the rate of hospital admissions when added to inhaled SABAs in patients with moderate to severe asthma exacerbations. Although LAMAs have long been the cornerstone of therapy for COPD, their role in asthma continues to evolve. Studies have shown that the addition of tiotropium to medium-dose inhaled corticosteroid and salmeterol improve lung function and reduce the frequency of asthma exacerbations. One study showed that the addition of once-daily tiotropium to an inhaled corticosteroid is as effective as twice-daily salmeterol.

4. Leukotriene modifiers—Leukotrienes are potent mediators that contribute to airway obstruction and asthma symptoms by contracting airway smooth muscle, increasing vascular permeability and mucus secretion, and attracting and activating airway inflammatory cells. Zileuton is a 5-lipoxygenase inhibitor that decreases leukotriene production, and zafirlukast and montelukast are cysteinyl leukotriene receptor antagonists. In randomized controlled trials, these agents caused modest improvements in lung function and reductions in asthma symptoms and lessened the need for SABA rescue therapy. These agents are alternatives to low-dose inhaled corticosteroids in patients with mild persistent asthma, although, as monotherapy, their effect is generally less than inhaled corticosteroids. In real-life community trials, leukotriene receptor antagonists were equivalent in efficacy to an inhaled corticosteroid as first-line long-term controller medication or to a LABA as add-on therapy. Zileuton can cause reversible elevations in plasma aminotransferase levels. Eosinophilic granulomatosis with polyangiitis has been diagnosed in a small number of patients who have taken montelukast or zafirlukast, perhaps due to corticosteroid withdrawal rather than a direct drug effect.

5. Phosphodiesterase inhibitor—Theophylline provides mild bronchodilation in asthmatic patients. Theophylline also has anti-inflammatory and immunomodulatory properties, enhances mucociliary clearance, and strengthens diaphragmatic contractility. Sustained-release theophylline preparations are effective in controlling nocturnal symptoms and as added therapy in patients with moderate or severe persistent asthma whose symptoms are inadequately controlled by inhaled corticosteroids. When added to an inhaled corticosteroid, theophylline may allow equivalent control at lower corticosteroid doses.

Theophylline serum concentrations need to be monitored closely owing to the medication's narrow therapeutic-toxic range, individual differences in metabolism, and the effects of many factors on drug absorption and metabolism. At therapeutic doses, potential adverse effects include insomnia, aggravation of dyspepsia and gastroesophageal reflux, and urination difficulties in men with prostatic hyperplasia. Dose-related toxicities include nausea, vomiting, tachyarrhythmias, headache, seizures, hyperglycemia, and hypokalemia.

6. Mediator inhibitors—Cromolyn sodium and nedocromil are long-term control medications that prevent asthma symptoms and improve airway function in patients with mild persistent or exercise-induced asthma. These agents modulate mast cell mediator release and eosinophil recruitment and inhibit both early and late asthmatic responses to allergen challenge and exercise-induced bronchospasm. They can be effective when taken before an exposure or exercise but do not relieve asthmatic symptoms once present. The clinical response to these agents is less predictable than to inhaled corticosteroids. Nedocromil may help reduce the dose requirements for inhaled corticosteroids. Both agents have excellent safety profiles.

7. Other agents—Asthmatic patients who require other therapies should be evaluated by either a pulmonologist or allergist experienced with their use. Omalizumab is a recombinant antibody that binds IgE without activating mast cells. In clinical trials in patients with moderate to severe asthma and elevated serum IgE levels, omalizumab reduced the need for corticosteroids. Reslizumab, mepoluzimab, and benralizumab are interleukin-5 antagonist monoclonal antibodies that are approved for the treatment of severe asthma with peripheral blood eosinophilia that has not responded to other standard treatments. Dupilumab is a self-administered biologic agent that inhibits overactive signaling of interleukin-4 and interleukin-13.

B. Desensitization

Immunotherapy for specific allergens may be considered in selected asthma patients who have exacerbations when exposed to allergens to which they are sensitive and when unresponsive to environmental control measures or other therapies. Studies show a reduction in asthma symptoms in patients treated with single-allergen immunotherapy. Because of the risk of immunotherapy-induced bronchoconstriction, it should be administered only in a setting where such complications can be immediately treated.

C. Vaccination

Patients with asthma should receive pneumococcal vaccination (Pneumovax 23) and annual influenza vaccinations.

Inactive vaccines (Pneumovax) are associated with few side effects, but the use of the live attenuated influenza vaccine intranasally may be associated with asthma exacerbations in young children.

▶ Treatment of Asthma Exacerbations

NAEPP 3 asthma treatment algorithms begin with an assessment of the severity of a patient's baseline asthma. Adjustments to that algorithm follow a stepwise approach based on a careful assessment of asthma control. Educating patients to recognize symptoms of an exacerbation and use their action plan is an important aspect of asthma management. Symptoms of exacerbations include progressive breathlessness, increasing chest tightness, decreased peak flow, and lack of improvement after SABA therapy. Most instances of uncontrolled asthma are mild and can be managed successfully by patients at home with the telephone assistance of a clinician (Figure 9–3). More severe exacerbations require evaluation and management in an urgent care or emergency department setting (Figure 9–4).

A. Mild Exacerbations

Mild asthma exacerbations are characterized by only minor changes in airway function (PEF more than 80%) and minimal symptoms and signs of airway dysfunction (see Table 9–2). Many such patients respond quickly and fully to an inhaled SABA alone. However, an inhaled SABA may need to be continued at increased doses, eg, every 3–4 hours for 24–48 hours. In patients not taking an inhaled corticosteroid, initiating one should be considered during the mild exacerbation. In patients already taking an inhaled corticosteroid, a 7-day course of oral corticosteroids (0.5–1.0 mg/kg/day) may be necessary. Doubling the dose of inhaled corticosteroid is not effective and is not recommended in the NAEPP 3 guidelines.

B. Moderate Exacerbations

The principal goals of treatment of moderate asthma exacerbations are correction of hypoxemia, reversal of airflow obstruction, and reduction of the likelihood of recurrence of obstruction. Early intervention may lessen the severity and shorten the duration of an exacerbation. Airflow obstruction is treated with continuous administration of an inhaled SABA and the early administration of systemic corticosteroids. Systemic corticosteroids should be given to patients with a peak flow of less than 70% of baseline or who do not respond to several treatments of SABA. Serial measurements of lung function to quantify the severity of airflow obstruction and its response to treatment are useful. The improvement in FEV_1 after 30 minutes of treatment correlates significantly with the severity of the asthma exacerbation. Serial measurement of airflow in the emergency department may reduce the rate of hospital admissions for asthma exacerbations. The post-exacerbation care plan is important. Regardless of the severity, all patients should be provided with necessary medications and education in how to use them, instruction in self-assessment, a follow-up appointment, and an action plan for managing recurrence.

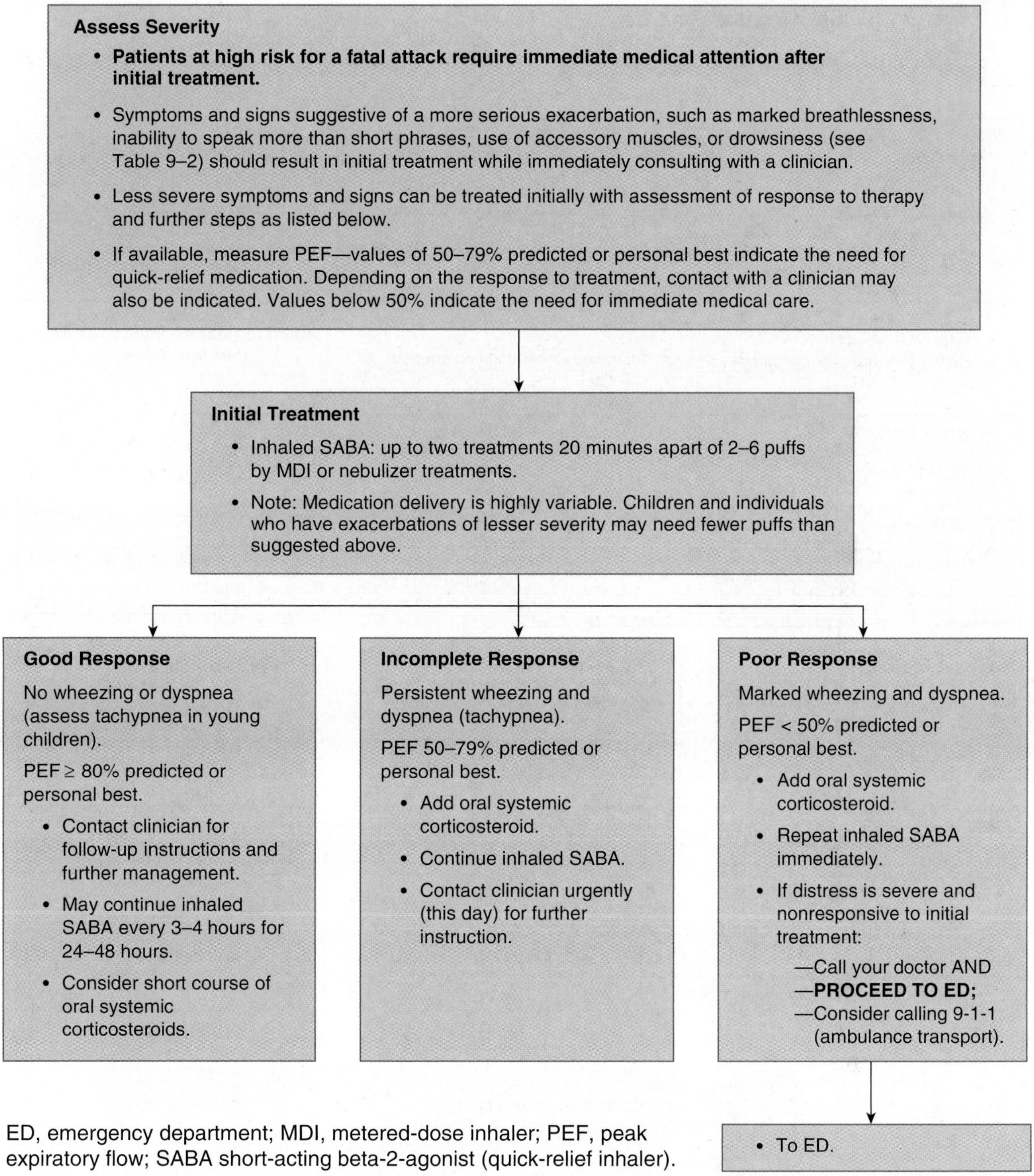

Assess Severity

- **Patients at high risk for a fatal attack require immediate medical attention after initial treatment.**

- Symptoms and signs suggestive of a more serious exacerbation, such as marked breathlessness, inability to speak more than short phrases, use of accessory muscles, or drowsiness (see Table 9–2) should result in initial treatment while immediately consulting with a clinician.

- Less severe symptoms and signs can be treated initially with assessment of response to therapy and further steps as listed below.

- If available, measure PEF—values of 50–79% predicted or personal best indicate the need for quick-relief medication. Depending on the response to treatment, contact with a clinician may also be indicated. Values below 50% indicate the need for immediate medical care.

Initial Treatment

- Inhaled SABA: up to two treatments 20 minutes apart of 2–6 puffs by MDI or nebulizer treatments.

- Note: Medication delivery is highly variable. Children and individuals who have exacerbations of lesser severity may need fewer puffs than suggested above.

Good Response

No wheezing or dyspnea (assess tachypnea in young children).

PEF ≥ 80% predicted or personal best.

- Contact clinician for follow-up instructions and further management.

- May continue inhaled SABA every 3–4 hours for 24–48 hours.

- Consider short course of oral systemic corticosteroids.

Incomplete Response

Persistent wheezing and dyspnea (tachypnea).

PEF 50–79% predicted or personal best.

- Add oral systemic corticosteroid.

- Continue inhaled SABA.

- Contact clinician urgently (this day) for further instruction.

Poor Response

Marked wheezing and dyspnea.

PEF < 50% predicted or personal best.

- Add oral systemic corticosteroid.

- Repeat inhaled SABA immediately.

- If distress is severe and nonresponsive to initial treatment:
  —Call your doctor AND
  —**PROCEED TO ED;**
  —Consider calling 9-1-1 (ambulance transport).

- To ED.

ED, emergency department; MDI, metered-dose inhaler; PEF, peak expiratory flow; SABA short-acting beta-2-agonist (quick-relief inhaler).

▲ **Figure 9–3.** Management of asthma exacerbations: home treatment. (Adapted from National Asthma Education and Prevention Program. Expert Panel Report 3: Guidelines for the Diagnosis and Management of Asthma. National Institutes of Health Pub. No. 08-4051. Bethesda, MD, 2007.)

C. Severe Exacerbations

Severe exacerbations of asthma can be life-threatening, so treatment should be started immediately. All patients with a severe exacerbation should immediately receive oxygen, high doses of an inhaled SABA, and systemic corticosteroids. A brief history pertinent to the exacerbation can be completed while such treatment is being initiated. More detailed assessments, including laboratory studies, usually add little early on and so should be postponed until after therapy is instituted. Early initiation of **oxygen therapy** is paramount because asphyxia is a common cause of asthma deaths. Supplemental oxygen should be given to maintain an Sao_2 greater than 90% or a Pao_2 greater than 60 mm Hg. Oxygen-induced hypoventilation is extremely rare, and concern for hypercapnia should never delay correction of hypoxemia.

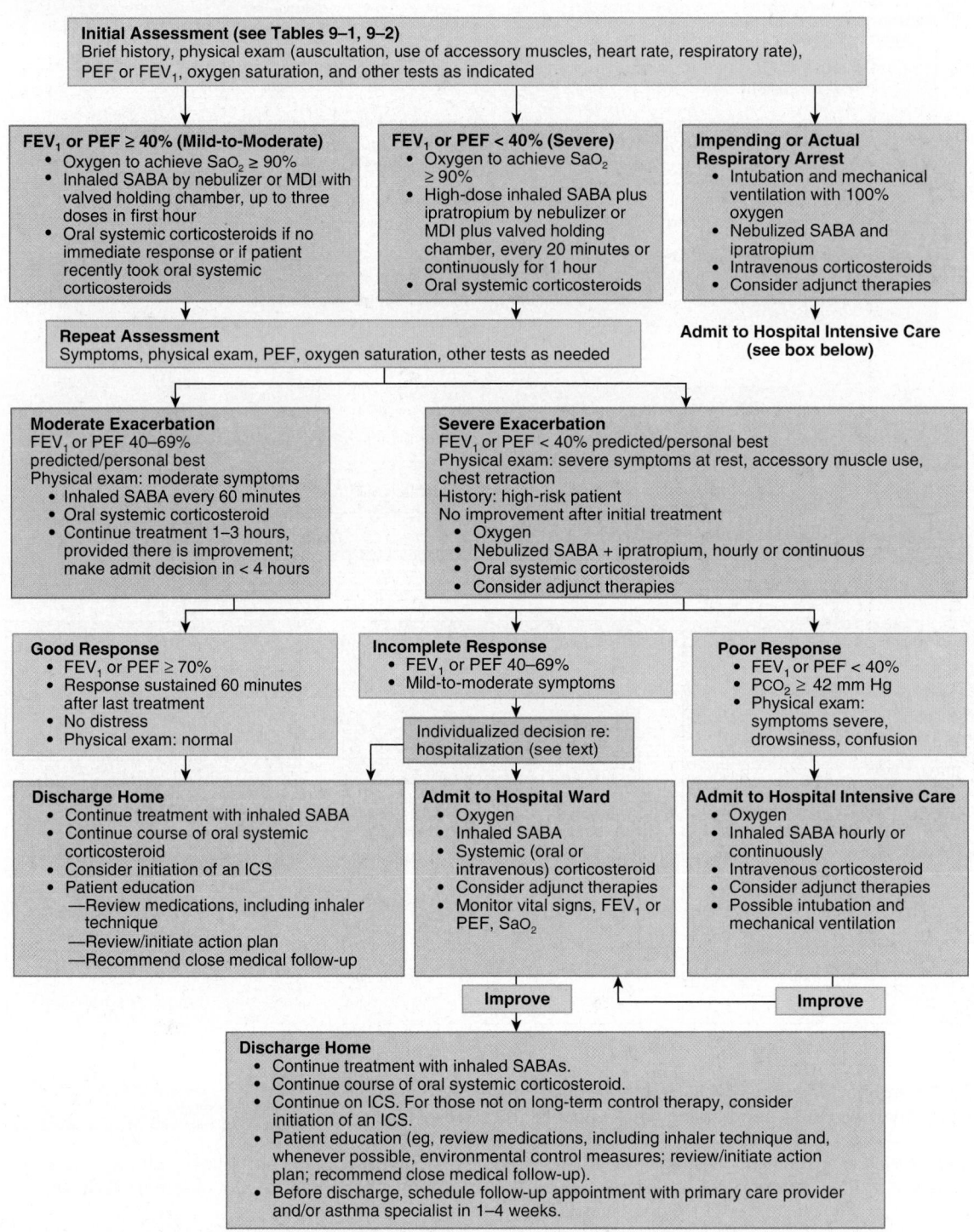

FEV$_1$, forced expiratory volume in 1 second; ICS, inhaled corticosteroid; MDI, metered-dose inhaler; PEF, peak expiratory flow; SABA, short-acting beta-2-agonist; SaO$_2$, oxygen saturation.

▲ **Figure 9–4.** Management of asthma exacerbations: emergency department and hospital-based treatment. (Adapted from National Asthma Education and Prevention Program. Expert Panel Report 3: Guidelines for the Diagnosis and Management of Asthma. National Institutes of Health Pub. No. 08-4051. Bethesda, MD, 2007.)

Frequent high-dose delivery of an **inhaled SABA** is indicated and usually well tolerated in severe airway obstruction. Some studies suggest that continuous therapy is more effective than intermittent administration of these agents, but there is no clear consensus as long as similar doses are administered. At least three MDI or nebulizer treatments should be given in the first hour of therapy. Thereafter, the frequency of administration varies according to the improvement in airflow and symptoms and the occurrence of side effects. Ipratropium bromide reduces the rate of hospital admissions when added to inhaled SABAs in patients with moderate to severe asthma exacerbations.

Systemic corticosteroids are administered as detailed above. **Intravenous magnesium sulfate** (2 g intravenously over 20 minutes) produces a detectable improvement in airflow and may reduce hospitalization rates in acute severe asthma (FEV_1 less than 25% of predicted on presentation or failure to respond to initial treatment).

Mucolytic agents (eg, acetylcysteine, potassium iodide) may worsen cough or airflow obstruction. Anxiolytic and hypnotic drugs are generally contraindicated in severe asthma exacerbations because of their potential respiratory depressant effects.

Multiple studies suggest that infections with viruses (rhinovirus) and bacteria (*Mycoplasma pneumoniae*, *Chlamydophila pneumoniae*) predispose to acute exacerbations of asthma and may underlie chronic, severe asthma. The use of empiric antibiotics is, however, not recommended in routine asthma exacerbations because there is no consistent evidence to support improved clinical outcomes. Antibiotics should be considered when there is a high likelihood of acute bacterial respiratory tract infection, such as patients with fever or purulent sputum and evidence of pneumonia or bacterial sinusitis.

In the **emergency department setting,** repeat assessment of patients with severe exacerbations should be done after the initial dose of an inhaled SABA and again after three doses of an inhaled SABA (60–90 minutes after initiating treatment). The response to initial treatment is a better predictor of the need for hospitalization than is the severity of an exacerbation on presentation. The decision to hospitalize a patient should be based on the duration and severity of symptoms, severity of airflow obstruction, arterial blood gas results (if available), course and severity of prior exacerbations, medication use at the time of the exacerbation, access to medical care and medications, adequacy of social support and home conditions, and presence of psychiatric illness. In general, discharge to home is appropriate if the PEF or FEV_1 has returned to 60% or more of predicted or personal best and symptoms are minimal or absent. Patients with a rapid response to treatment should be observed for 30 minutes after the most recent dose of bronchodilator to ensure stability of response before discharge.

In the **intensive care setting,** a small subset of patients will not respond to treatment and will progress to impending respiratory failure due to a combination of worsening airflow obstruction and respiratory muscle fatigue (see Table 9–2). Since such patients can deteriorate rapidly, they must be monitored in a critical care setting. Intubation of an acutely ill asthma patient is technically difficult and is best done semi-electively, before the crisis of a respiratory arrest. At the time of intubation, the patient's intravascular volume should be closely monitored because hypotension commonly follows the administration of sedative medications and the initiation of positive-pressure ventilation; these patients are often dehydrated due to poor recent oral intake and high insensible losses.

The main goals of mechanical ventilation are to ensure adequate oxygenation and to avoid barotrauma. Controlled hypoventilation with permissive hypercapnia is often required to limit airway pressures. Frequent high-dose delivery of inhaled SABAs should be continued along with anti-inflammatory agents as discussed above. Many questions remain regarding the optimal delivery of inhaled SABAs to intubated, mechanically ventilated patients.

▶ **When to Refer**

- Atypical presentation or uncertain diagnosis of asthma, particularly if additional diagnostic testing is required (bronchoprovocation challenge, allergy skin testing, rhinoscopy, consideration of occupational exposure).
- Complicating comorbid problems, such as rhinosinusitis, tobacco use, multiple environmental allergies, suspected allergic bronchopulmonary mycosis.
- Uncontrolled symptoms despite LABA and high-dose inhaled corticosteroid.
- Patient not meeting goals of asthma therapy after 3–6 months of treatment.
- More than two courses of oral prednisone therapy in the past 12 months.
- Any life-threatening asthma exacerbation or exacerbation requiring hospitalization in the past 12 months.
- Presence of social or psychological issues interfering with asthma management.

Bateman ED et al. As-needed budesonide-formoterol versus maintenance budesonide in mild asthma. N Engl J Med. 2018 May 17;378(20):1877–87. [PMID: 29768147]

Benralizumab (Fasenra) for severe eosinophilic asthma. JAMA. 2018 Apr 10;319(14):1501–2. [Corrected and republished from Med Lett Drugs Ther. 2018] [PMID: 29634828]

Drazen JE et al. New biologics for asthma. N Engl J Med. 2018 Jun 28;378(26):2533–4. [PMID: 29782236]

Israel E et al. Severe and difficult-to-treat asthma in adults. N Engl J Med. 2017 Sep 7;377(10):965–76. [PMID: 28877019]

McCracken J et al. Diagnosis and management of asthma in adults: a review. JAMA. 2017 Jul 18;318(3):279–90. [PMID: 28719697]

Rabe KF et al. Efficacy and safety of dupilumab in glucocorticoid-dependent severe asthma. N Engl J Med. 2018 Jun 28; 378(26):2475–85. [PMID: 29782224]

Sobieraj DM et al. Association of inhaled corticosteroids and long-acting β-agonists as controller and quick relief therapy with exacerbations and symptom control in persistent asthma: a systematic review and meta-analysis. JAMA. 2018 Apr 10; 319(14):1485–96. [PMID: 29554195]

Sobieraj DM et al. Association of inhaled corticosteroids and long-acting muscarinic antagonists with asthma control in patients with uncontrolled, persistent asthma: a systematic review and meta-analysis. JAMA. 2018 Apr 10;319(14): 1473–84. [PMID: 29554174]

Sobieraj DM et al. Medications for asthma. JAMA. 2018 Apr 10; 319(14):1520. [PMID: 29634830]

CHRONIC OBSTRUCTIVE PULMONARY DISEASE

ESSENTIALS OF DIAGNOSIS

▶ History of cigarette smoking or other chronic inhalational exposure.

▶ Chronic cough, dyspnea, and sputum production.

▶ Rhonchi, decreased intensity of breath sounds, and prolonged expiration on physical examination.

▶ Airflow limitation on pulmonary function testing that is not fully reversible and is most often progressive.

General Considerations

The Global Initiative for Chronic Obstructive Lung Disease (GOLD) defines COPD as a common, preventable, and treatable disease state characterized by persistent respiratory symptoms and airflow limitation due to airway and alveolar abnormalities usually caused by significant exposure to noxious particles or gases. Symptoms include cough, dyspnea, and sputum production. COPD is a major cause of chronic morbidity and mortality worldwide.

Most patients with COPD have features of both emphysema and chronic bronchitis. **Chronic bronchitis** is a clinical diagnosis defined by excessive secretion of bronchial mucus and is manifested by daily productive cough for 3 months or more in at least 2 consecutive years. **Emphysema** is a pathologic diagnosis that denotes abnormal permanent enlargement of air spaces distal to the terminal bronchiole, with destruction of alveolar walls and without obvious fibrosis. Both of these definitions are no longer included in GOLD because they comprise a minority of patients. Chronic respiratory symptoms also exist in people with normal spirometry, and a number of smokers without airflow limitation will have varying degrees of emphysema.

Cigarette smoking is by far the most important cause of COPD in North America and Western Europe. Nearly all smokers suffer an accelerated decline in lung function that is dose- and duration-dependent. One major study reported yearly decreases in FEV_1 of 66.1 mL per year in men and 54.2 mL per year in women who continued to smoke, compared to 30.2 mL per year in men and 21.5 mL per year in women who sustained smoking cessation. Fifteen percent develop progressively disabling symptoms in their 40s and 50s. Approximately 80% of patients seen for COPD have significant exposure to tobacco smoke. The remaining 20% frequently have a combination of exposures to environmental tobacco smoke, occupational dusts and chemicals, and indoor air pollution from biomass fuel used for cooking and heating in poorly ventilated buildings. Outdoor air pollution, airway infection, environmental factors, and allergy have also been implicated in chronic bronchitis, and hereditary factors (most notably, deficiency of alpha-1-antiprotease [alpha-1-antitrypsin]) have been implicated in emphysema. Atopy and the tendency for bronchoconstriction to develop in response to nonspecific airway stimuli may be important risks. Evidence suggests that lung exposures to pollution and allergens early in life can lead to poor lung growth in childhood and expiratory airflow limitation, resulting in lower than predicted spirometric values in midlife.

Clinical Findings

A. Symptoms and Signs

Patients with COPD characteristically present in the fifth or sixth decade of life complaining of excessive cough, sputum production, and shortness of breath. Symptoms have often been present for 10 years or more. Dyspnea is noted initially only on heavy exertion, but as the condition progresses it occurs with mild activity. In severe disease, dyspnea occurs at rest. As the disease progresses, two symptom patterns tend to emerge, historically referred to as "pink puffers" and "blue bloaters" (Table 9–6). Most COPD patients have pathologic evidence of both disorders, and their clinical course may involve other factors, such as central control of ventilation and concomitant sleep-disordered breathing.

Pneumonia, pulmonary hypertension, cor pulmonale, and chronic respiratory failure characterize the late stage of COPD. A hallmark of COPD is the periodic exacerbation of symptoms beyond normal day-to-day variation, often including increased dyspnea, an increased frequency or severity of cough, and increased sputum volume or change in sputum character. These exacerbations are commonly precipitated by infection (more often viral than bacterial) or environmental factors. Exacerbations of COPD vary widely in severity but typically require a change in regular therapy.

B. Laboratory Findings

Spirometry provides objective information about pulmonary function and assesses the response to therapy. Pulmonary function tests early in the course of COPD reveal only evidence of abnormal closing volume and reduced midexpiratory flow rates. Reductions in FEV_1 and in the ratio of forced expiratory volume to vital capacity ($FEV_1\%$ or FEV_1/FVC ratio) (Table 9–6) occur later. Post-bronchodilator FEV_1/FVC less than 0.70 establishes the presence of airflow obstruction (GOLD definition). In severe disease, the FVC is markedly reduced. Lung volume measurements reveal a marked increase in residual volume (RV), an increase in total lung capacity (TLC), and an elevation of the RV/TLC ratio, indicative of air trapping, particularly in emphysema.

Arterial blood gas measurements characteristically show no abnormalities early in COPD other than an increased $A–a–Do_2$. Indeed, measurement is unnecessary unless (1) hypoxemia or hypercapnia is suspected, (2) the FEV_1 is less than 40% of predicted, or (3) there are clinical signs of right heart failure. Hypoxemia occurs in advanced disease, particularly when chronic bronchitis predominates. Compensated respiratory acidosis occurs in patients with chronic respiratory failure, particularly in chronic bronchitis, with worsening of acidemia during acute exacerbations.

Positive sputum cultures are poorly correlated with acute exacerbations, and research techniques demonstrate evidence of preceding viral infection in a majority of

Table 9–6. Patterns of disease in advanced COPD.

	Type A: Pink Puffer (Emphysema Predominant)	Type B: Blue Bloater (Bronchitis Predominant)
History and physical examination	Major complaint is dyspnea, often severe, usually presenting after age 50. Cough is rare, with scant clear, mucoid sputum. Patients are thin, with recent weight loss common. They appear uncomfortable, with evident use of accessory muscles of respiration. Chest is very quiet without adventitious sounds. No peripheral edema.	Major complaint is chronic cough, productive of mucopurulent sputum, with frequent exacerbations due to chest infections. Often presents in late 30s and 40s. Dyspnea usually mild, though patients may note limitations to exercise. Patients frequently overweight and cyanotic but seem comfortable at rest. Peripheral edema is common. Chest is noisy, with rhonchi invariably present; wheezes are common.
Laboratory studies	Hemoglobin usually normal (12–15 g/dL). PaO_2 normal to slightly reduced (65–75 mm Hg) but SaO_2 normal at rest. $PaCO_2$ normal to slightly reduced (35–40 mm Hg). Chest radiograph shows hyperinflation with flattened diaphragms. Vascular markings are diminished, particularly at the apices.	Hemoglobin usually elevated (15–18 g/dL). PaO_2 reduced (45–60 mm Hg) and $PaCO_2$ slightly to markedly elevated (50–60 mm Hg). Chest radiograph shows increased interstitial markings ("dirty lungs"), especially at bases. Diaphragms are not flattened.
Pulmonary function tests	Airflow obstruction ubiquitous. Total lung capacity increased, sometimes markedly so. DL_{CO} reduced. Static lung compliance increased.	Airflow obstruction ubiquitous. Total lung capacity generally normal but may be slightly increased. DL_{CO} normal. Static lung compliance normal.
Special Evaluations		
Ventilation-perfusion testing	Increased ventilation to high $\dot{V}/\dot{Q}$ areas, ie, high dead space ventilation.	Increased perfusion to low $\dot{V}/\dot{Q}$ areas.
Hemodynamics	Cardiac output normal to slightly low. Pulmonary artery pressures mildly elevated and increase with exercise.	Cardiac output normal. Pulmonary artery pressures elevated, sometimes markedly so, and worsen with exercise.
Nocturnal ventilation	Mild to moderate degree of oxygen desaturation not usually associated with obstructive sleep apnea.	Severe oxygen desaturation, frequently associated with obstructive sleep apnea.
Exercise ventilation	Increased minute ventilation for level of oxygen consumption; PaO_2 tends to fall; $PaCO_2$ rises slightly.	Decreased minute ventilation for level of oxygen consumption. PaO_2 may rise; $PaCO_2$ may rise significantly.

DL_{CO}, single-breath diffusing capacity for carbon monoxide; $\dot{V}/\dot{Q}$, ventilation-perfusion.

patients with exacerbations. The ECG may show sinus tachycardia and, in advanced disease, chronic pulmonary hypertension may produce electrocardiographic abnormalities typical of cor pulmonale. Supraventricular arrhythmias (multifocal atrial tachycardia, atrial flutter, and atrial fibrillation) and ventricular irritability also occur.

C. Imaging

Radiographs of patients with chronic bronchitis typically show only nonspecific peribronchial and perivascular markings. Plain radiographs are insensitive for the diagnosis of emphysema; they show hyperinflation with flattening of the diaphragm or peripheral arterial deficiency in about half of cases. CT of the chest, particularly using high-resolution CT, is more sensitive and specific than plain radiographs for its diagnosis. In advanced disease, pulmonary hypertension may be suggested by enlargement of central pulmonary arteries on radiographs, and Doppler echocardiography provides an estimate of pulmonary artery pressure.

▶ Differential Diagnosis

Clinical, imaging, and laboratory findings should enable the clinician to distinguish COPD from other obstructive pulmonary disorders, such as asthma, bronchiectasis,

cystic fibrosis, bronchopulmonary mycosis, and central airflow obstruction. Asthma is characterized by complete or near-complete reversibility of airflow obstruction. Bronchiectasis is distinguished from COPD by recurrent pneumonia and hemoptysis, digital clubbing, and characteristic imaging abnormalities. Cystic fibrosis occurs in children, adolescents, and young adults and has characteristic imaging as well as endocrine and hepatic abnormalities. Bronchopulmonary mycosis is characterized by eosinophilia; elevated levels of immunoglobulin E; and episodic worsening marked by fever, malaise, productive cough, and radiographic infiltrates. Mechanical obstruction of the central airways can be distinguished from COPD by flow-volume loops.

▶ Complications

Acute bronchitis, pneumonia, pulmonary thromboembolism, atrial dysrhythmias (such as atrial fibrillation, atrial flutter, and multifocal atrial tachycardia), and concomitant left ventricular failure may worsen otherwise stable COPD. Pulmonary hypertension, cor pulmonale, and chronic respiratory failure are common in advanced COPD. Spontaneous pneumothorax occurs in a small fraction of patients with emphysema. Hemoptysis may result from chronic bronchitis or may signal bronchogenic carcinoma.

▶ Prevention

COPD is largely preventable through elimination of long-term exposure to tobacco smoke, combustion of biomass fuels, and other inhaled toxins. Smokers with early evidence of airflow limitation can significantly alter their disease by smoking cessation. Smoking cessation slows the decline in FEV_1 in middle-aged smokers with mild airway obstruction. Influenza vaccination reduces the frequency and severity of influenza-like illness as well as the number of COPD exacerbations. Pneumococcal vaccination appears to reduce both the frequency of community-acquired pneumonia and the number of COPD exacerbations.

▶ Treatment

The treatment of COPD is guided by the severity of symptoms or the presence of an exacerbation of stable symptoms. Standards for the management of patients with stable COPD and COPD exacerbations from the American Thoracic Society and GOLD, a joint expert committee of the National Heart, Lung, and Blood Institute and the World Health Organization, are incorporated in the recommendations below. There are three commonly used ways to identify high-risk COPD patients who may require more intense treatment: (1) FEV_1 less than 50% (GOLD III/IV), (2) more than two exacerbations within the previous 12 months, and (3) one or more hospitalizations for COPD exacerbation in the previous year.

See Chapter 37 for a discussion of air travel in patients with lung disease.

A. Ambulatory Patients

1. Smoking cessation—The single most important intervention in smokers with COPD is to encourage smoking cessation (see Chapter 1). Simply telling a patient to quit succeeds 5% of the time. Behavioral approaches, ranging from clinician advice to intensive group programs, may improve cessation rates. Pharmacologic therapy includes bupropion, nicotine replacement (transdermal patch, gum, lozenge, inhaler, or nasal spray), varenicline (a partial agonist of nicotinic acetylcholine receptors), and cytisine. Combined pharmacotherapies (two forms of nicotine replacement, or nicotine replacement and bupropion), with or without behavioral approaches, have been recommended. Varenicline is effective but use has been limited by concerns of neuropsychiatric side effects. Electronic cigarettes are being aggressively marketed as an aid for tobacco cigarette cessation. One randomized controlled trial (RCT) showed electronic cigarettes to be noninferior to nicotine transdermal patches. Most pulmonologists do not recommend electronic cigarettes as a tobacco cessation aid, based on safety concerns (they are not regulated and contain a variety of chemicals) and limited clinical trial data, although some clinicians will not discourage motivated smokers who refuse to consider standard approaches from trying electronic cigarettes.

2. Oxygen therapy—Supplemental oxygen for patients with resting hypoxemia ($Pao_2 < 56$ mm Hg) is the only therapy with evidence of improvement in the natural history of COPD. Proved benefits of home oxygen therapy in hypoxemic patients include longer survival, reduced hospitalizations, and better quality of life. Survival in hypoxemic patients with COPD treated with supplemental oxygen therapy is directly proportionate to the number of hours per day oxygen is administered: in COPD hypoxemic patients treated with continuous oxygen for 24 hours daily, the survival after 36 months is about 65%—significantly better than the survival rate of about 45% in those treated with only nocturnal oxygen. Oxygen by nasal prongs must be given for at least 15 hours a day unless therapy is specifically intended only for exercise or sleep. However, several studies of supplemental oxygen therapy showed no survival benefit in COPD patients with borderline low-normal resting oxygen levels (Pao_2 between 56 mm Hg and 69 mm Hg). In a study of patients with stable COPD and resting or exercise-induced moderate desaturation, the prescription of long-term supplemental oxygen did not result in a longer time to first hospitalization or death than no long-term supplemental oxygen, nor did it provide sustained benefit with regard to any of the other measured outcomes. Requirements for US Medicare coverage for a patient's home use of oxygen and oxygen equipment are listed in Table 9–7. Arterial blood gas analysis is preferred over oximetry to guide initial oxygen therapy. Hypoxemic patients with pulmonary hypertension, chronic cor pulmonale, erythrocytosis, impaired cognitive function, exercise intolerance, nocturnal restlessness, or morning headache are particularly likely to benefit from home oxygen therapy.

Home oxygen may be supplied by liquid oxygen systems, compressed gas cylinders, or oxygen concentrators. Most patients benefit from having both stationary and

Table 9–7. Home oxygen therapy: requirements for Medicare coverage.[1]

Group I (any of the following):
1. $Pao_2 \leq 55$ mm Hg or $Sao_2 \leq 88\%$ taken while awake, at rest, breathing room air.
2. During sleep (prescription for nocturnal oxygen use only): $Pao_2 \leq 55$ mm Hg or $Sao_2 \leq 88\%$ for a patient whose awake, resting, room air Pao_2 is ≥ 56 mm Hg or $Sao_2 \geq 89\%$, or Decrease in $Pao_2 > 10$ mm Hg or decrease in $Sao_2 > 5\%$ associated with symptoms or signs reasonably attributed to hypoxemia (eg, impaired cognitive processes, nocturnal restlessness, insomnia).
3. During exercise (prescription for oxygen use only during exercise): $Pao_2 \leq 55$ mg Hg or $Sao_2 \leq 88\%$ taken during exercise for a patient whose awake, resting, room air Pao_2 is ≥ 56 mm Hg or $Sao_2 \geq 89\%$, and there is evidence that the use of supplemental oxygen during exercise improves the hypoxemia that was demonstrated during exercise while breathing room air.
Group II[2]:
$Pao_2 = 56–59$ mm Hg or $Sao_2 = 89\%$ if there is evidence of any of the following:
1. Dependent edema suggesting heart failure.
2. P pulmonale on ECG (P wave > 3 mm in standard leads II, III, or aVF).
3. Hematocrit > 56%.

[1]Centers for Medicare & Medicaid Services, 2003.
[2]Patients in this group must have a second oxygen test 3 months after the initial oxygen setup.

portable systems. For most patients, a flow rate of 1–3 L/min achieves a PaO_2 greater than 55 mm Hg. The monthly cost of home oxygen therapy ranges from $300 to $500 or more, higher for liquid oxygen systems. Medicare covers approximately 80% of home oxygen expenses. Reservoir nasal cannulas or "pendants" and demand (pulse) oxygen delivery systems are also available to conserve oxygen.

3. Inhaled bronchodilators—Bronchodilators do not alter the inexorable decline in lung function that is a hallmark of COPD, but they improve symptoms, exercise tolerance, FEV_1, and overall health status. Aggressiveness of bronchodilator therapy should be matched to the severity of the patient's disease. In patients who experience no symptomatic improvement, bronchodilators should be discontinued.

The most commonly prescribed short-acting bronchodilators are the anticholinergic ipratropium bromide and SABAs (eg, albuterol, metaproterenol), delivered by MDI or as an inhalation solution by nebulizer. Some clinicians prefer ipratropium as a first-line agent because of its longer duration of action and absence of sympathomimetic side effects. Some studies have suggested that ipratropium achieves superior bronchodilation in COPD patients. Typical doses are two to four puffs (36–72 mcg) every 6 hours. Other clinicians prefer SABAs because they are less expensive and have a more rapid onset of action, commonly leading to greater patient satisfaction. At maximal doses, beta-2-agonists have bronchodilator action equivalent to that of ipratropium but may cause tachycardia, tremor, or hypokalemia. There does not appear to be any advantage of scheduled use of SABAs compared with as-needed administration. There has been no consistent difference in efficacy demonstrated between SABAs and SAMAs. Use of both SABAs and anticholinergics at submaximal doses leads to improved bronchodilation compared with either agent alone but does not improve dyspnea.

LAMAs (eg, tiotropium, aclidinium, umeclidinium) and LABAs (eg, formoterol, salmeterol, indacaterol, arformoterol, vilanterol) appear to achieve bronchodilation that is equivalent or superior to what is experienced with ipratropium, in addition to similar improvements in health status. Although more expensive than short-acting agents, long-acting bronchodilators may have superior clinical efficacy in persons with advanced disease. One RCT of long-term administration of tiotropium added to standard therapy reported fewer exacerbations or hospitalizations, and improved dyspnea scores, in the tiotropium group. Tiotropium had no effect on long-term decline in lung function, however. Another RCT comparing the effects of tiotropium with those of salmeterol-fluticasone over 2 years reported no difference in the risk of COPD exacerbation. The incidence of pneumonia was higher in the salmeterol-fluticasone group, yet dyspnea scores were lower and there was a mortality benefit compared with tiotropium. The combination of tiotropium and formoterol (LAMA/LABA) has been shown to improve FEV_1 and FVC more than the inhaled corticosteroid/LABA combination salmeterol and fluticasone in patients with a baseline FEV_1 of less than 55% predicted.

The symptomatic benefits of long-acting bronchodilators are firmly established. Increased exacerbations and mortality in asthmatic patients treated with salmeterol have not been observed in COPD patients, and several studies report a trend toward lower mortality in patients treated with salmeterol alone, compared with placebo. In addition, a 4-year tiotropium trial reported fewer cardiovascular events in the intervention group. Subsequent meta-analyses that include the 4-year tiotropium trial did not find an increase in cardiovascular events in treated patients. Most practitioners believe that the documented benefits of anticholinergic therapy outweigh any potential risks.

4. Corticosteroids—Multiple large clinical trials have reported a reduction in the frequency of COPD exacerbations and an increase in self-reported functional status in COPD patients treated with inhaled corticosteroids. These same trials demonstrate no effect of inhaled corticosteroids on mortality or the characteristic decline in lung function experienced by COPD patients. Thus, inhaled corticosteroids alone should not be considered first-line therapy in stable COPD patients.

However, combination therapy with an inhaled corticosteroid and a LABA reduces the frequency of exacerbations and improves self-reported functional status in COPD patients, compared with placebo or with sole use of inhaled corticosteroids, LABAs, or anticholinergics. In one RCT, addition of an inhaled corticosteroid/LABA to tiotropium therapy in COPD patients did not reduce the frequency of exacerbations but did improve hospitalization rates and functional status.

Apart from acute exacerbations, COPD is not generally responsive to oral corticosteroid therapy. Given the risks of adverse side effects, oral corticosteroids are not recommended for the long-term treatment of COPD.

5. Theophylline—Oral theophylline is a fourth-line agent for treating COPD patients who do not achieve adequate symptom control with inhaled anticholinergic, beta-2-agonist, and corticosteroid therapies. Sustained-release theophylline improves hemoglobin saturation during sleep in COPD patients and is a first-line agent for those with sleep-related breathing disorders. Theophylline improves dyspnea ratings, exercise performance, and pulmonary function in many patients with stable COPD. Its benefits result from bronchodilation; anti-inflammatory properties; and extrapulmonary effects on diaphragm strength, myocardial contractility, and kidney function. Theophylline toxicity is a significant concern due to the medication's narrow therapeutic window, and long-term administration requires careful monitoring of serum levels. Despite potential for adverse effects, theophylline continues to have a beneficial role in carefully selected patients.

6. Antibiotics—Antibiotics are commonly prescribed to outpatients with COPD for the following indications: (1) to treat an acute exacerbation, (2) to treat acute bronchitis, and (3) to prevent acute exacerbations of chronic bronchitis (prophylactic antibiotics). In patients with COPD, antibiotics appear to improve outcomes slightly in all three situations. Patients with a COPD exacerbation associated with increased sputum purulence accompanied by dyspnea or an increase in the quantity of sputum are thought to benefit the most from antibiotic therapy. The choice of antibiotic depends on local bacterial resistance patterns and individual risk of *Pseudomonas aeruginosa* infection (history of *Pseudomonas* isolation, FEV_1 less than 50% of predicted, recent hospitalization [2 or more days in the past 3 months], more than three courses of antibiotics within the past year, use of systemic corticosteroids). Oral antibiotic options include doxycycline (100 mg every 12 hours), trimethoprim-sulfamethoxazole (160/800 mg every 12 hours), a cephalosporin (eg, cefpodoxime 200 mg every 12 hours or cefprozil 500 mg every 12 hours), a macrolide (eg, azithromycin 500 mg followed by 250 mg daily for 5 days), a fluoroquinolone (eg, ciprofloxacin 500 mg every 12 hours), and amoxicillin-clavulanate (875/125 mg every 12 hours). Suggested duration of therapy is 3–7 days and depends on response to therapy; some studies suggest that 5 days is as effective as 7 days but with fewer adverse effects. There are few controlled trials of antibiotics in severe COPD exacerbations, but prompt administration is appropriate, particularly in persons with risk factors for poor outcomes (age older than 65 years, FEV_1 less than 50% of predicted, three or more exacerbations in the past year, antibiotic therapy within the past 3 months, comorbid conditions, such as cardiac disease). In COPD patients subject to frequent exacerbations despite optimal medical therapy, azithromycin (daily or three times weekly) and moxifloxacin (a 5-day course 1 week in 8 over 48 weeks) were modestly effective in clinical trials at reducing the frequency of exacerbations; monitoring for hearing loss and QT prolongation is essential.

7. Pulmonary rehabilitation—Graded aerobic physical exercise programs (eg, walking 20 minutes three times weekly or bicycling) are helpful to prevent deterioration of physical condition and to improve patients' ability to carry out daily activities. Training of inspiratory muscles by inspiring against progressively larger resistive loads reduces dyspnea and improves exercise tolerance, health status, and respiratory muscle strength in some but not all patients. Pursed-lip breathing to slow the rate of breathing and abdominal breathing exercises to relieve fatigue of accessory muscles of respiration may reduce dyspnea in some patients. Many patients undergo these exercise and educational interventions in a structured rehabilitation program. In a number of studies, pulmonary rehabilitation has been shown to improve exercise capacity, decrease hospitalizations, and enhance quality of life. Referral to a comprehensive rehabilitation program is recommended in patients who have severe dyspnea, reduced quality of life, or frequent hospitalizations despite optimal medical therapy.

8. Phosphodiesterase 4 inhibitor—Roflumilast has been shown to reduce exacerbation frequency in patients who have moderate or severe (FEV_1 less than 50% of predicted) COPD and chronic bronchitis, with frequent exacerbations and are taking LABA/inhaled corticosteroid with or without a LAMA.

9. Other measures—In patients with chronic bronchitis, increased mobilization of secretions may be accomplished through the use of adequate systemic hydration, effective cough training methods, or the use of a handheld flutter device and postural drainage, sometimes with chest percussion or vibration. Postural drainage and chest percussion should be used only in selected patients with excessive amounts of retained secretions that cannot be cleared by coughing and other methods; these measures are of no benefit in pure emphysema. Expectorant-mucolytic therapy has generally been regarded as unhelpful in patients with chronic bronchitis. Cough suppressants and sedatives should be avoided. Morphine can reduce chronic dyspnea in patients with very severe COPD.

Human alpha-1-antitrypsin is available for replacement therapy in emphysema due to congenital deficiency (PiZZ or null genotype) of alpha-1-antiprotease (alpha-1-antitrypsin). Patients over 18 years of age with airflow obstruction by spirometry and serum levels less than 11 mcmol/L (~50 mg/dL) are potential candidates for replacement therapy. Alpha-1-antitrypsin is administered intravenously in a dose of 60 mg/kg body weight once weekly.

Severe dyspnea in spite of optimal medical management may warrant a clinical trial of an opioid (eg, morphine 5–10 mg orally every 3–4 hours, oxycodone 5–10 mg orally every 4–6 hours, sustained-release morphine 10 mg orally once daily). Sedative-hypnotic drugs (eg, diazepam, 5 mg three times daily) marginally improve intractable dyspnea but cause significant drowsiness; they may benefit very anxious patients. Transnasal positive-pressure ventilation at home to rest the respiratory muscles is an approach to improve respiratory muscle function and reduce dyspnea in patients with severe COPD.

B. Hospitalized Patients

Management of the hospitalized patient with an acute exacerbation of COPD includes (1) supplemental oxygen (titrated to maintain Sao_2 between 90% and 94% or Pao_2 between 60 mm Hg and 70 mm Hg); (2) inhaled ipratropium bromide (500 mcg by nebulizer, or 36 mcg by MDI with spacer, every 4 hours as needed) plus beta-2-agonists (eg, albuterol 2.5 mg diluted with saline to a total of 3 mL by nebulizer, or MDI, 90 mcg per puff, four to eight puffs via spacer, every 1–4 hours as needed); (3) corticosteroids (prednisone 30–40 mg orally per day for 7–10 days is usually sufficient, even 5 days may be adequate); (4) broad-spectrum antibiotics; and (5) in selected cases, chest physiotherapy.

For patients without risk factors for *Pseudomonas*, management options include a fluoroquinolone (eg, levofloxacin 750 mg orally or intravenously per day, or moxifloxacin 400 mg orally or intravenously every 24 hours) or a third-generation cephalosporin (eg, ceftriaxone 1 g intravenously per day, or cefotaxime 1 g intravenously every 8 hours).

For patients with risk factors for *Pseudomonas*, therapeutic options include piperacillin-tazobactam (4.5 g intravenously every 6 hours), ceftazidime (1 g intravenously every 8 hours), cefepime (1 g intravenously every 12 hours), or levofloxacin (750 mg orally or intravenously per day for 3–7 days).

Theophylline should not be initiated in the acute setting, but patients taking theophylline prior to acute hospitalization should have their theophylline serum levels measured and maintained in the therapeutic range. Oxygen therapy should *not* be withheld for fear of worsening respiratory acidemia; hypoxemia is more detrimental than hypercapnia. Cor pulmonale usually responds to measures that reduce pulmonary artery pressure, such as supplemental oxygen and correction of acidemia; bed rest, salt restriction, and diuretics may add some benefit. Cardiac dysrhythmias, particularly multifocal atrial tachycardia, usually respond to aggressive treatment of COPD itself. Atrial fibrillation and flutter may require DC cardioversion after initiation of the above therapy. If progressive respiratory failure ensues, tracheal intubation and mechanical ventilation are necessary. In clinical trials of COPD patients with hypercapnic acute respiratory failure, **noninvasive positive-pressure ventilation (NIPPV)** delivered via face mask reduced the need for intubation and shortened lengths of stay in the intensive care unit (ICU). Other studies have suggested a lower risk of nosocomial infections and less use of antibiotics in COPD patients treated with NIPPV. These benefits do not appear to extend to hypoxemic respiratory failure or to patients with acute lung injury or acute respiratory distress syndrome (ARDS).

C. Procedures for COPD

1. Lung transplantation—Requirements for lung transplantation are severe lung disease, limited activities of daily living, exhaustion of medical therapy, ambulatory status, potential for pulmonary rehabilitation, limited life expectancy without transplantation, adequate function of other organ systems, and a good social support system. Average total charges for lung transplantation through the end of the first postoperative year exceed $250,000. The 2-year survival rate after lung transplantation for COPD is 75%. Complications include acute rejection, opportunistic infection, and obliterative bronchiolitis. Substantial improvements in pulmonary function and exercise performance have been noted after transplantation.

2. Lung volume reduction surgery—Lung volume reduction surgery (LVRS), or reduction pneumoplasty, is a surgical approach to relieve dyspnea and improve exercise tolerance in patients with advanced diffuse emphysema and lung hyperinflation. Bilateral resection of 20–30% of lung volume in selected patients results in modest improvements in pulmonary function, exercise performance, and dyspnea. The duration of any improvement as well as any mortality benefit remains uncertain. Prolonged air leaks occur in up to 50% of patients postoperatively. Mortality rates in centers with the largest experience with LVRS range from 4% to 10%.

The National Emphysema Treatment Trial compared LVRS with medical treatment in a randomized, multicenter clinical trial of 1218 patients with severe emphysema. Overall, surgery improved exercise capacity but not mortality when compared with medical therapy. The persistence of this benefit remains to be defined. Subgroup analysis suggested that patients with upper lobe–predominant emphysema and low exercise capacity might have improved survival, while other groups suffered excess mortality when randomized to surgery.

3. Bullectomy—Bullectomy is an older surgical procedure for palliation of dyspnea in patients with severe bullous emphysema. Bullectomy is most commonly pursued when a single bulla occupies at least 30–50% of the hemithorax.

► Prognosis

The outlook for patients with clinically significant COPD is poor. The degree of pulmonary dysfunction at the time the patient is first seen is an important predictor of survival: median survival of patients with FEV_1 1 L or less is about 4 years. A multidimensional index (the BODE index), which includes **b**ody mass index, airway **o**bstruction (FEV_1), **d**yspnea (modified Medical Research Council dyspnea score), and **e**xercise capacity, is a tool that predicts death and hospitalization better than FEV_1 alone. Comprehensive care programs, cessation of smoking, and supplemental oxygen may reduce the rate of decline of pulmonary function, but therapy with bronchodilators and other approaches probably have little, if any, impact on the natural course of COPD.

Dyspnea at the end of life can be extremely uncomfortable and distressing to the patient and family. As patients near the end of life, meticulous attention to palliative care is essential to effectively manage dyspnea (see Chapter 5).

► When to Refer

- COPD onset occurs before the age of 40.
- Frequent exacerbations (two or more a year) despite optimal treatment.
- Severe or rapidly progressive COPD.
- Symptoms disproportionate to the severity of airflow obstruction.
- Need for long-term oxygen therapy.
- Onset of comorbid illnesses (eg, bronchiectasis, heart failure, or lung cancer).

► When to Admit

- Severe symptoms or acute worsening that fails to respond to outpatient management.
- Acute or worsening hypoxemia, hypercapnia, peripheral edema, or change in mental status.
- Inadequate home care, or inability to sleep or maintain nutrition/hydration due to symptoms.
- The presence of high-risk comorbid conditions.

Global Initiative for Chronic Obstructive Lung Disease (GOLD). Global strategy for the diagnosis, management, and prevention of chronic obstructive lung disease 2019 report. https://goldcopd.org/gold-reports/

Hurley K et al. Serum α1-antitrypsin concentration in the diagnosis of α1-antitrypsin deficiency. JAMA. 2018 May 15;319(19):2034–5. [PMID: 29800192]

Lipson DA et al. FULFIL trial: once-daily triple therapy for patients with chronic obstructive pulmonary disease. Am J Respir Crit Care Med. 2017 Aug 15;196(4):438–46. [PMID: 28375647]

Mackay AJ et al. Randomized double-blind controlled trial of roflumilast at acute exacerbations of chronic obstructive pulmonary disease. Am J Respir Crit Care Med. 2017 Sep 1;196(5):656–9. [PMID: 28146642]

Pavord ID et al. Mepolizumab for eosinophilic chronic obstructive pulmonary disease. N Engl J Med. 2017 Oct 26;377(17):1613–29. [PMID: 28893134]

The Global Initiative for Chronic Obstructive Lung Disease (GOLD). https://goldcopd.org/

The Long-Term Oxygen Treatment Trial Research Group. A randomized trial of long-term oxygen for COPD with moderate desaturation. N Engl J Med. 2016 Oct 27;375(17):1617–27. [PMID: 27783918]

Vogelmeier CF et al. Global strategy for the diagnosis, management, and prevention of chronic obstructive lung disease 2017 report. GOLD executive summary. Am J Respir Crit Care Med. 2017 Mar 1;195(5):557–82. [PMID: 28128970]

Wedzicha JA et al. Management of COPD exacerbations: a European Respiratory Society/American Thoracic Society guideline. Eur Respir J. 2017 Mar 15;49(3):1600791. [PMID: 28298398]

Wedzicha JA et al. Prevention of COPD exacerbations: a European Respiratory Society/American Thoracic Society guideline. Eur Respir J. 2017 Sept 9 50(3):1602265. [PMID: 28889106]

Zhou Y et al. Tiotropium in early-stage chronic obstructive pulmonary disease. N Engl J Med. 2017 Sep 7;377(10):923–35. [PMID: 28877027]

BRONCHIECTASIS

ESSENTIALS OF DIAGNOSIS

▶ Chronic productive cough with dyspnea and wheezing.

▶ Radiographic findings of dilated, thickened airways and scattered, irregular opacities.

▶ General Considerations

Bronchiectasis is a congenital or acquired disorder of the large bronchi characterized by permanent, abnormal dilation and destruction of bronchial walls. It may be caused by recurrent inflammation or infection of the airways and may be localized or diffuse. Cystic fibrosis causes about half of all cases of bronchiectasis. Other causes include lung infection (tuberculosis, fungal infections, lung abscess, pneumonia), abnormal lung defense mechanisms (humoral immunodeficiency, alpha-1-antitrypsin deficiency with cigarette smoking, mucociliary clearance disorders, rheumatic diseases), and localized airway obstruction (foreign body, tumor, mucoid impaction). Immunodeficiency states that may lead to bronchiectasis include congenital or acquired panhypogammaglobulinemia; common variable immunodeficiency; selective IgA, IgM, and IgG subclass deficiencies; and acquired immunodeficiency from cytotoxic therapy, AIDS, lymphoma, plasma cell myeloma (previously called multiple myeloma), and leukemia. Most patients with bronchiectasis have panhypergammaglobulinemia, however, presumably reflecting an immune system response to chronic airway infection.

▶ Clinical Findings

A. Symptoms and Signs

Symptoms of bronchiectasis include chronic cough with production of copious amounts of purulent sputum, hemoptysis, and pleuritic chest pain. Dyspnea and wheezing occur in 75% of patients. Weight loss, anemia, and other systemic manifestations are common. Physical findings are nonspecific, but persistent crackles at the lung bases are common. Clubbing is infrequent in mild cases but is common in severe disease (Figure 6–41). Copious, foul-smelling, purulent sputum is characteristic. Obstructive pulmonary dysfunction with hypoxemia is seen in moderate or severe disease.

B. Imaging

Radiographic abnormalities include dilated and thickened bronchi that may appear as "tram tracks" or as ring-like markings. Scattered irregular opacities, atelectasis, and focal consolidation may be present. High-resolution CT is the diagnostic study of choice.

C. Microbiology

H influenzae is the most common organism recovered from non–cystic fibrosis patients with bronchiectasis. *P aeruginosa, S pneumoniae*, and *Staphylococcus aureus* are commonly identified. Nontuberculous mycobacteria are seen less commonly. Patients with *Pseudomonas* infection experience an accelerated course, with more frequent exacerbations and more rapid decline in lung function.

▶ Treatment

Treatment of acute exacerbations consists of antibiotics, daily chest physiotherapy with postural drainage and chest percussion, and inhaled bronchodilators. Handheld flutter valve devices may be as effective as chest physiotherapy in clearing secretions. Antibiotic therapy should be guided by sputum smears and prior cultures. If a specific bacterial pathogen cannot be isolated, then empiric oral antibiotic therapy for 10–14 days is appropriate. Common regimens include amoxicillin or amoxicillin-clavulanate (500 mg every 8 hours), ampicillin (250–500 mg four times daily), doxycycline (100 mg twice daily), trimethoprim-sulfamethoxazole (160/800 mg every 12 hours), or ciprofloxacin (500–750 mg twice daily). It is important to screen patients for infection with nontuberculous mycobacteria because these organisms may underlie a lack of treatment response. Preventive or suppressive treatment is sometimes given to stable outpatients with bronchiectasis who have copious purulent sputum. Prolonged macrolide therapy (azithromycin 500 mg three times a week for 6 months or 250 mg daily for 12 months) has been found to decrease the frequency of exacerbations compared to placebo. Alternating cycles of the antibiotics listed above given orally for 2–4 weeks are also used in patients who are not colonized with *Pseudomonas*, although this practice is not supported by clinical trial data. In patients with underlying cystic fibrosis, inhaled aerosolized aminoglycosides reduce colonization by *Pseudomonas* species, improve FEV_1, and reduce hospitalizations; in patients with non–cystic fibrosis bronchiectasis, the role of inhaled aerosolized aminoglycosides is unclear. Complications of bronchiectasis include hemoptysis, cor pulmonale, amyloidosis, and secondary visceral abscesses at distant sites (eg, brain). Bronchoscopy is sometimes necessary to evaluate hemoptysis, remove retained secretions, and rule out obstructing airway lesions. Massive hemoptysis may require embolization of bronchial arteries or surgical resection. Surgical resection is otherwise reserved for the few patients with localized bronchiectasis and adequate pulmonary function in whom conservative management fails.

Fjaellegaard K et al. Antibiotic therapy for stable non-CF bronchiectasis in adults—a systematic review. Chron Respir Dis. 2017 May;14(2):174–86. [PMID: 27507832]

Tarrant BJ et al. Mucoactive agents for chronic, non-cystic fibrosis lung disease: a systematic review and meta-analysis. Respirology. 2017 Aug;22(6):1084–92. [PMID: 28397992]

Wilson R et al. Challenges in managing *Pseudomonas aeruginosa* in non-cystic fibrosis bronchiectasis. Respir Med. 2016 Aug; 117:179–89. [PMID: 27492530]

ALLERGIC BRONCHOPULMONARY MYCOSIS

Allergic bronchopulmonary mycosis is a pulmonary hypersensitivity disorder caused by allergy to fungal antigens that colonize the tracheobronchial tree. It usually occurs in atopic asthmatic individuals who are 20–40 years of age or those with cystic fibrosis, in response to antigens of *Aspergillus* species. For this reason, the disorder is commonly referred to as allergic bronchopulmonary aspergillosis (ABPA). Primary criteria for the diagnosis of ABPA include (1) a clinical history of asthma or cystic fibrosis; (2) elevated serum total IgE levels (typically greater than 1000 international units/mL; a value less than 1000 international units/mL may be acceptable if all other criteria are met); (3) immediate cutaneous hypersensitivity to *Aspergillus* antigens or elevated serum IgE levels specific to *Aspergillus fumigatus;* and (4) at least two of the following: (a) precipitating serum antibodies to *Aspergillus* antigen or elevated serum *Aspergillus* IgG by immunoassay, (b) radiographic pulmonary opacities consistent with ABPA, or (c) peripheral blood eosinophil count greater than 500 cells/mcL. High-dose prednisone (0.5–1 mg/kg orally per day) for at least 2 weeks is the initial treatment of choice. Depending on the clinical situation, prednisone dose can then be reduced or converted to every other day and slowly tapered over 3–6 months. Relapses are frequent, and protracted or repeated treatment with corticosteroids is not uncommon. Patients with corticosteroid-dependent disease may benefit from itraconazole (200 mg orally three times a day for 3 days, followed by twice daily [with food if the capsule formulation is used] for at least 16 weeks) without added toxicity. Bronchodilators (see Table 9–3) are also helpful. Complications include hemoptysis, severe bronchiectasis, and pulmonary fibrosis.

Muldoon EG et al. Allergic and noninvasive infectious pulmonary aspergillosis syndromes. Clin Chest Med. 2017 Sep; 38(3):521–34. [PMID: 28797493]

Shah A et al. Allergic bronchopulmonary aspergillosis: a perplexing clinical entity. Allergy Asthma Immunol Res. 2016 Jul;8(4):282–97. [PMID: 27126721]

CYSTIC FIBROSIS

ESSENTIALS OF DIAGNOSIS

▶ Pulmonary problems: chronic or recurrent productive cough, dyspnea, and wheezing; recurrent airway infections or chronic colonization of the airways with *H influenzae, P aeruginosa, S aureus,* or *Burkholderia cepacia*; bronchiectasis and scarring on chest radiographs; airflow obstruction on spirometry.

▶ Gastrointestinal problems: pancreatic insufficiency, recurrent pancreatitis, distal intestinal obstruction syndrome, or chronic liver disease.

▶ Genitourinary problems: male infertility and urogenital abnormalities.

▶ Sweat chloride concentration greater than 60 mEq/L on two occasions.

▶ Presence of two (one from each parent) gene mutations known to cause cystic fibrosis.

▶ Abnormal nasal potential difference.

▶ General Considerations

Cystic fibrosis is the most common cause of severe chronic lung disease in young adults and the most common fatal hereditary disorder of whites in the United States. It is an autosomal-recessive disorder affecting about 1 in 3000 whites; 1 in 25 is a carrier. Cystic fibrosis is caused by abnormalities in a membrane chloride channel (the cystic fibrosis transmembrane conductance regulator [CFTR] protein) that results in altered chloride transport and water flux across the apical surface of epithelial cells. Almost all exocrine glands produce an abnormal mucus that obstructs glands and ducts and leads to tissue damage. In the respiratory tract, inadequate hydration of the tracheobronchial epithelium impairs mucociliary function. High concentration of extracellular DNA in airway secretions (due to chronic airway inflammation and autolysis of neutrophils) increases sputum viscosity.

Over one-third of the nearly 30,000 cystic fibrosis patients in the United States are adults. Adult patients with cystic fibrosis have an increased risk of osteopenia, arthropathies, and malignancies of the gastrointestinal tract.

▶ Clinical Findings

A. Symptoms and Signs

Cystic fibrosis should be suspected in an adult with a history of chronic lung disease (especially bronchiectasis), pancreatitis, or infertility. Cough, sputum production, decreased exercise tolerance, and recurrent hemoptysis are typical complaints. Patients also often complain of chronic rhinosinusitis symptoms, steatorrhea, diarrhea, and abdominal pain. Patients with cystic fibrosis are often malnourished with low body mass index. Digital clubbing (Figure 6–41), increased anteroposterior chest diameter, hyperresonance to percussion, and apical crackles are noted on physical examination. Sinus tenderness, purulent nasal secretions, and nasal polyps may also be seen. Nearly all men with cystic fibrosis have congenital bilateral absence of the vas deferens with azoospermia. Biliary cirrhosis and gallstones may occur.

B. Laboratory Findings

Arterial blood gas studies often reveal hypoxemia and, in advanced disease, a chronic, compensated respiratory acidosis. Pulmonary function studies show a mixed obstructive and restrictive pattern. There is a reduction in FVC, airflow rates, and TLC. Air trapping (high ratio of RV to TLC) and reduction in pulmonary diffusing capacity are common.

C. Imaging

Hyperinflation is seen early in the disease process. Peribronchial cuffing, mucus plugging, bronchiectasis (ring shadows and cysts), increased interstitial markings, small rounded peripheral opacities, and focal atelectasis are common findings. Pneumothorax can also be seen. Thin-section CT scanning often confirms the presence of bronchiectasis.

D. Diagnosis

The **quantitative pilocarpine iontophoresis sweat test** reveals elevated sodium and chloride levels (greater than 60 mEq/L) in the sweat of patients with cystic fibrosis. Two tests on different days performed in experienced laboratories are required for accurate diagnosis. A normal sweat chloride test does not exclude the diagnosis, in which case genotyping or other alternative diagnostic studies (such as measurement of nasal membrane potential difference, semen analysis, or assessment of pancreatic function) should be pursued, especially if there is a high clinical suspicion of cystic fibrosis. All patients with cystic fibrosis should undergo *CFTR* genotyping.

▶ Treatment

Early recognition and comprehensive multidisciplinary therapy improve symptom control and the chances of survival. Referral to a regional cystic fibrosis center is strongly recommended. Conventional treatment programs focus on the following areas: clearance and reduction of lower airway secretions, reversal of bronchoconstriction, treatment of respiratory tract infections and airway bacterial burden, pancreatic enzyme replacement, and nutritional and psychosocial support (including genetic and occupational counseling). Oral CFTR modulator drugs, alone or in combination, are available for patients with specific genetic mutations. The Pulmonary Therapies Committee, established by the Cystic Fibrosis Foundation, has issued evidenced-based recommendations regarding long-term use of medications for maintenance of lung function and reduction of exacerbations in patients with cystic fibrosis.

Clearance of lower airway secretions can be promoted by postural drainage, chest percussion or vibration techniques, positive expiratory pressure (PEP) or flutter valve breathing devices, directed cough, and other breathing techniques; these approaches require detailed patient instruction by experienced personnel. **Inhaled recombinant human deoxyribonuclease (rhDNase, dornase alpha)** cleaves extracellular DNA in sputum, decreasing sputum viscosity; when administered long-term at a daily nebulized dose of 2.5 mg, this therapy leads to improved FEV_1 and reduces the risk of cystic fibrosis–related respiratory exacerbations and the need for intravenous antibiotics. Inhalation of hypertonic (7%) saline twice daily has been associated with small improvements in pulmonary function and fewer pulmonary exacerbations. The beneficial effects of hypertonic saline may derive from improved airway mucous clearance.

Short-term antibiotics are used to treat active airway infections based on results of culture and susceptibility testing of sputum. *S aureus* (including methicillin-resistant strains) and a mucoid variant of *P aeruginosa* are commonly present. *H influenzae, Stenotrophomonas maltophilia*, and *B cepacia* (a highly drug-resistant organism) are occasionally isolated. **Long-term antibiotic therapy** is helpful in slowing disease progression and reducing exacerbations in patients with sputum cultures positive for *P aeruginosa*. These antibiotics include azithromycin 500 mg orally three times a week, which has immunomodulatory properties, and various inhaled antibiotics (eg, tobramycin, aztreonam, colistin, and levofloxacin) taken two to three times a day. The length of therapy depends on the persistent presence of *P aeruginosa* in the sputum. The incidence of atypical mycobacterial colonization is higher in cystic fibrosis patients, and directed antibiotic treatment is recommended for frequent exacerbations, progressive decline in lung function, or failure to thrive. Yearly screening with sputum acid-fast bacilli cultures is advised.

Inhaled bronchodilators (eg, albuterol, two puffs every 4 hours as needed) should be considered in patients who demonstrate an increase of at least 12% in FEV_1 after an inhaled bronchodilator. An inhaled corticosteroid should be added to the treatment regimen for patients who have cystic fibrosis with persistent asthma or allergic bronchopulmonary mycosis.

Lung transplantation is the only definitive treatment for advanced cystic fibrosis. Double-lung or heart-lung transplantation is required. A few transplant centers offer living lobar lung transplantation to selected patients. The median survival following transplantation for cystic fibrosis is 7.8 years.

Vaccination against pneumococcal infection and annual influenza vaccination are advised. **Screening** of family members and genetic counseling are suggested.

▶ Prognosis

The longevity of patients with cystic fibrosis is increasing, and the median survival age is over 39 years. Death occurs from pulmonary complications (eg, pneumonia, pneumothorax, or hemoptysis) or as a result of terminal chronic respiratory failure and cor pulmonale.

Farrell PM et al. Diagnosis of cystic fibrosis: consensus guidelines from the Cystic Fibrosis Foundation. J Pediatr. 2017 Feb;181S:S4–15. [PMID: 28129811]

Langton Hewer SC et al. Antibiotic strategies for eradicating *Pseudomonas aeruginosa* in people with cystic fibrosis. Cochrane Database Syst Rev. 2017 Apr 25;4:CD004197. [PMID: 28440853]

Quon BS et al. New and emerging targeted therapies for cystic fibrosis. BMJ. 2016 Mar 30;352:i859. [PMID: 27030675]

BRONCHIOLITIS

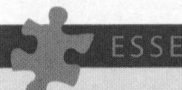

ESSENTIALS OF DIAGNOSIS

- ▶ Insidious onset of cough and dyspnea.
- ▶ Irreversible airflow obstruction on pulmonary function testing.
- ▶ Minimal findings on chest radiograph.
- ▶ Relevant exposure or risk factors: toxic fumes, viral infections, organ transplantation, connective tissue disease.

▶ General Considerations

Bronchiolitis is a generic term applied to varied inflammatory processes that affect the bronchioles, which are small conducting airways less than 2 mm in diameter. Disorders associated with bronchiolitis include organ transplantation, connective tissue diseases, and hypersensitivity pneumonitis. Inhalational injuries as well as postinfectious and drug-induced causes are identified by association with a known exposure or illness prior to the onset of symptoms. Idiopathic cases are characterized by the insidious onset of dyspnea or cough.

▶ Clinical Findings

Acute bronchiolitis can be seen following viral infections.

Constrictive bronchiolitis (also referred to as obliterative bronchiolitis, or bronchiolitis obliterans) is relatively infrequent although it is the most common finding following inhalation injury. It may also be seen in rheumatoid arthritis; medication reactions; and chronic rejection following heart-lung, lung, or bone marrow transplant. Patients with constrictive bronchiolitis have airflow obstruction on spirometry; minimal radiographic abnormalities; and a progressive, deteriorating clinical course.

Proliferative bronchiolitis is associated with diverse pulmonary disorders, including infection, aspiration, ARDS, hypersensitivity pneumonitis, connective tissue diseases, and organ transplantation. Compared with constrictive bronchiolitis, proliferative bronchiolitis is more likely to have an abnormal chest radiograph.

Cryptogenic organizing pneumonitis (COP) formerly referred to as **bronchiolitis obliterans with organizing pneumonia (BOOP)** affects men and women between the ages of 50 and 70 years, typically with a dry cough, dyspnea, and constitutional symptoms that may be present for weeks to months prior to seeking medical attention. A history of a preceding viral illness is present in half of cases. Pulmonary function testing typically reveals a restrictive ventilatory defect and impaired oxygenation. The chest radiograph frequently shows bilateral patchy, ground-glass or alveolar infiltrates, although other patterns have been described.

Follicular bronchiolitis is most commonly associated with connective tissue disease, especially rheumatoid arthritis and Sjögren syndrome, and with immunodeficiency states.

Respiratory bronchiolitis usually occurs without symptoms or physiologic evidence of lung impairment.

Diffuse panbronchiolitis is most frequently diagnosed in Japan. Men are affected about twice as often as women, two-thirds are nonsmokers, and most patients have a history of chronic pansinusitis. Patients complain of dyspnea, cough, and sputum production, and chest examination shows crackles and rhonchi. Pulmonary function tests reveal obstructive abnormalities, and the chest radiograph shows a distinct pattern of diffuse, small, nodular shadows with hyperinflation.

▶ Treatment

Constrictive bronchiolitis is relatively unresponsive to corticosteroids and is frequently progressive. Corticosteroids are effective in two-thirds of patients with **proliferative bronchiolitis,** and improvement can be prompt. Therapy is initiated with prednisone at 1 mg/kg/day orally for 1–3 months. The dose is then tapered slowly to 20–40 mg/day, depending on the response, and weaned over the subsequent 3–6 months as tolerated. Relapses are common if corticosteroids are stopped prematurely or tapered too quickly. Most patients with **COP** recover following corticosteroid treatment. **Diffuse panbronchiolitis** is effectively treated with azithromycin.

Bergeron A et al. Budesonide/formoterol for bronchiolitis obliterans after hematopoietic stem cell transplantation. Am J Respir Crit Care Med. 2015 Jun 1;191(11):1242–9. [PMID: 25835160]

Ruttens D et al. Montelukast for bronchiolitis obliterans syndrome after lung transplantation: a randomized controlled trial. PLoS One. 2018 Apr 6;13(4):e0193564. [PMID: 29624575]

PULMONARY INFECTIONS

PNEUMONIA

Pneumonia has classically been considered in terms of the infecting organism (Table 9–8). This approach facilitates discussion of characteristic clinical presentations but is a limited guide to patient management since specific microbiologic information is rarely available at initial presentation. More recent classification schemes emphasize epidemiologic factors that predict etiology and guide initial therapy. Pneumonia may be classified as **community-acquired (CAP)** or **nosocomial** and, within the latter, as **hospital-acquired (HAP)** or **ventilator-associated (VAP).** These categories are based on differing settings and infectious agents and require different diagnostic and

Table 9–8. Characteristics of selected pneumonias.

Organism; Appearance on Smear of Sputum	Clinical Setting	Complications
Streptococcus pneumoniae (pneumococcus). Gram-positive diplococci.	Chronic cardiopulmonary disease; follows upper respiratory tract infection	Bacteremia, meningitis, endocarditis, pericarditis, empyema
Haemophilus influenzae. Pleomorphic gram-negative coccobacilli.	Chronic cardiopulmonary disease; follows upper respiratory tract infection	Empyema, endocarditis
Staphylococcus aureus. Plump gram-positive cocci in clumps.	Residence in chronic care facility, hospital-associated, influenza epidemics, cystic fibrosis, bronchiectasis, injection drug use	Empyema, cavitation
Klebsiella pneumoniae. Plump gram-negative encapsulated rods.	Alcohol abuse, diabetes mellitus; hospital-associated	Cavitation, empyema
Escherichia coli. Gram-negative rods.	Hospital-associated; rarely, community-acquired	Empyema
Pseudomonas aeruginosa. Gram-negative rods.	Hospital-associated; cystic fibrosis, bronchiectasis	Cavitation
Anaerobes. Mixed flora.	Aspiration, poor dental hygiene	Necrotizing pneumonia, abscess, empyema
Mycoplasma pneumoniae. PMNs and monocytes; no bacteria.	Young adults; summer and fall	Skin rashes, bullous myringitis; hemolytic anemia
Legionella species. Few PMNs; no bacteria.	Summer and fall; exposure to contaminated construction site, water source, air conditioner; community-acquired or hospital-associated	Empyema, cavitation, endocarditis, pericarditis
Chlamydophila pneumoniae. Nonspecific.	Clinically similar to *M pneumoniae*, but prodromal symptoms last longer (up to 2 weeks); sore throat with hoarseness common; mild pneumonia in teenagers and young adults	Reinfection in older adults with underlying COPD or heart failure may be severe or even fatal
Moraxella catarrhalis. Gram-negative diplococci.	Preexisting lung disease; elderly patients; corticosteroid or immunosuppressive therapy	Rarely, pleural effusions and bacteremia
Pneumocystis jirovecii. Nonspecific.	AIDS, immunosuppressive or cytotoxic drug therapy, cancer	Pneumothorax, respiratory failure, ARDS, death

ARDS, acute respiratory distress syndrome; COPD, chronic obstructive pulmonary disease; PMN, polymorphonuclear leukocyte.

therapeutic interventions. **Anaerobic pneumonia** and **lung abscess** can occur in both hospital and community settings and warrant separate consideration.

This section sets forth the evaluation and management of pulmonary infiltrates in immunocompetent persons separately from the approach to immunocompromised persons—defined as those with HIV disease, absolute neutrophil counts less than 1000/mcL (1.0×10^9/L), current or recent exposure to myelosuppressive or immunosuppressive medications, or those currently taking prednisone in a dosage greater than 5 mg/day.

1. Community-Acquired Pneumonia

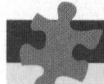
ESSENTIALS OF DIAGNOSIS

▶ Fever or hypothermia, tachypnea, cough with or without sputum, dyspnea, chest discomfort, sweats or rigors (or both).

▶ Bronchial breath sounds or inspiratory crackles on chest auscultation.

▶ Parenchymal opacity on chest radiograph.

▶ Occurs outside of the hospital or within 48 hours of hospital admission in a patient not residing in a long-term care facility.

▶ General Considerations

Community-acquired pneumonia (CAP) is a common disorder, with approximately 4–5 million cases diagnosed each year in the United States, 25% of which require hospitalization. It is the deadliest infectious disease in the United States and the eighth leading cause of death. Mortality in milder cases treated as outpatients is less than 1%. Among patients hospitalized for CAP, in-hospital mortality is approximately 10–12% and 1-year mortality (in those over age 65) is greater than 40%. Risk factors for the development of CAP include advanced age; alcoholism; tobacco use; comorbid medical conditions, especially asthma or COPD; and immunosuppression.

The patient's history, physical examination, and imaging studies are essential to establishing a diagnosis of CAP.

Table 9–9. Recommended empiric antibiotics for community-acquired pneumonia.

Outpatient management

1. For previously healthy patients who have not taken antibiotics within the past 3 months:
   a. A macrolide (clarithromycin, 500 mg orally twice a day; or azithromycin, 500 mg orally as a first dose and then 250 mg orally daily for 4 days, or 500 mg orally daily for 3 days), or
   b. Doxycycline, 100 mg orally twice a day.
2. For patients with comorbid medical conditions such as chronic heart, lung, liver, or kidney disease; diabetes mellitus; alcoholism; malignancy; asplenia; immunosuppressant conditions or use of immunosuppressive drugs; or use of antibiotics within the previous 3 months (in which case an alternative from a different antibiotic class should be selected):
   a. A respiratory fluoroquinolone (moxifloxacin, 400 mg orally daily; gemifloxacin, 320 mg orally daily; levofloxacin, 750 mg orally daily) or
   b. A macrolide (as above) plus a beta-lactam (amoxicillin, 1 g orally three times a day; amoxicillin-clavulanate, 2 g orally twice a day are preferred to cefpodoxime, 200 mg orally twice a day; cefuroxime, 500 mg orally twice a day).
3. In regions with a high rate (> 25%) of infection with high level (MIC ≥ 16 mcg/mL) macrolide-resistant *Streptococcus pneumoniae*, consider use of alternative agents listed above in (2) for patients with comorbidities.

Inpatient management not requiring intensive care

1. A respiratory fluoroquinolone. See above for oral therapy. For intravenous therapy, moxifloxacin, 400 mg daily; levofloxacin, 750 mg daily; ciprofloxacin, 400 mg every 8–12 hours, or
2. A macrolide plus a beta-lactam. See above for oral therapy. For intravenous therapy, ampicillin, 1–2 g every 4–6 hours; cefotaxime, 1–2 g every 4–12 hours; ceftriaxone, 1–2 g every 12–24 hours.

Inpatient management requiring intensive care (all agents administered intravenously, except as noted)

1. Azithromycin (500 mg orally as a first dose and then 250 mg orally daily for 4 days, or 500 mg orally daily for 3 days) or a respiratory fluoroquinolone plus an anti-pneumococcal beta-lactam (cefotaxime, ceftriaxone, or ampicillin-sulbactam, 1.5–3 g every 6 hours).
2. For patients allergic to beta-lactam antibiotics, a fluoroquinolone plus aztreonam (1–2 g every 6–12 hours).
3. For routine patients at risk for *Pseudomonas* infection:
   a. An anti-pneumococcal, anti-pseudomonal beta-lactam (piperacillin-tazobactam, 3.375–4.5 g every 6 hours; cefepime, 1–2 g twice a day; imipenem, 0.5–1 g every 6–8 hours; meropenem, 1 g every 8 hours) plus azithromycin (500 mg orally as a first dose and then 250 mg orally daily for 4 days, or 500 mg orally daily for 3 days) or a respiratory fluoroquinolone.
4. For patients who are at risk for *Pseudomonas* infection AND are critically ill, at increased risk for drug resistance, or if the unit incidence of monotherapy-resistant *Pseudomonas* is > 10%:
   a. An anti-pneumococcal, anti-pseudomonal beta-lactam (piperacillin-tazobactam, 3.375–4.5 g every 6 hours; cefepime, 1–2 g twice a day; imipenem, 0.5–1 g every 6–8 hours; meropenem, 1 g every 8 hours) plus ciprofloxacin (400 mg every 8–12 hours) or levofloxacin, or
   b. The above beta-lactam plus an aminoglycoside (gentamicin, tobramycin, amikacin, all weight-based dosing administered daily adjusted to appropriate trough levels) plus azithromycin or a respiratory fluoroquinolone.
5. For patients at risk for methicillin-resistant *Staphylococcus aureus* infection, add vancomycin (interval dosing based on kidney function to achieve serum trough concentration 15–20 mcg/mL) or linezolid (600 mg twice a day).

MIC, minimum inhibitory concentration.
Recommendations assembled from Mandell LA et al. Infectious Diseases Society of America/American Thoracic Society consensus guidelines on the management of community-acquired pneumonia in adults. Clin Infect Dis. 2007;44:S27–72.

None of these efforts identifies a specific microbiologic cause, however. Sputum examination may be helpful in selected patients but 40% of patients cannot produce an evaluable sputum sample and Gram stain and culture lack sensitivity for the most common causes of pneumonia. Since patient outcomes improve when the initial antibiotic choice is appropriate for the infecting organism, the American Thoracic Society and the Infectious Diseases Society of America recommend empiric treatment based on epidemiologic data (Table 9–9). Such treatment improves initial antibiotic coverage, reduces unnecessary hospitalization, and appears to improve 30-day survival.

Decisions regarding hospitalization and ICU care should be based on prognostic criteria.

▶ Definition & Pathogenesis

CAP is diagnosed outside of the hospital in ambulatory patients who are not residents of nursing homes or other long-term care facilities. It may also be diagnosed in a previously ambulatory patient within 48 hours after admission to the hospital.

Pulmonary defense mechanisms (cough reflex, mucociliary clearance system, immune responses) normally prevent the development of lower respiratory tract infections following aspiration of oropharyngeal secretions containing bacteria or inhalation of infected aerosols. CAP occurs when there is a defect in one or more of these normal defense mechanisms or when a large infectious inoculum or a virulent pathogen overwhelms the immune response.

Prospective studies fail to identify the cause of CAP in 30–60% of cases; two or more causes are identified in up to 26% of cases. Bacteria are more commonly identified than viruses. The most common bacterial pathogen identified in most studies of CAP is *S pneumoniae*, accounting for approximately two-thirds of bacterial isolates. Other common bacterial pathogens include *H influenzae*, *Mycoplasma pneumoniae*, *C pneumoniae*, *S aureus*, *Neisseria meningitidis*, *M catarrhalis*, *Klebsiella pneumoniae*, other gram-negative rods, and *Legionella* species. Common viral causes of CAP include influenza virus, respiratory syncytial virus, adenovirus, and parainfluenza virus. A detailed assessment of epidemiologic risk factors may aid in diagnosing pneumonias due to the following uncommon causes: *Chlamydophila psittaci* (psittacosis), *Coxiella burnetii* (Q fever), *Francisella tularensis* (tularemia), endemic fungi (*Blastomyces, Coccidioides, Histoplasma*), and sin nombre virus (hantavirus pulmonary syndrome).

▶ Clinical Findings

A. Symptoms and Signs

Most patients with CAP experience an acute or subacute onset of fever, cough with or without sputum production, and dyspnea. Other common symptoms include sweats, chills, rigors, chest discomfort, pleurisy, hemoptysis, fatigue, myalgias, anorexia, headache, and abdominal pain.

Common physical findings include fever or hypothermia, tachypnea, tachycardia, and arterial oxygen desaturation. Many patients appear acutely ill. Chest examination often reveals inspiratory crackles and bronchial breath sounds. Dullness to percussion may be observed if lobar consolidation or a parapneumonic pleural effusion is present. The clinical evaluation is less than 50% sensitive compared to chest imaging for the diagnosis of CAP (see Imaging section below). In most patients, therefore, a chest radiograph is essential to the evaluation of suspected CAP.

B. Diagnostic Testing

Diagnostic testing for a specific infectious cause of CAP is not generally indicated in ambulatory patients treated as outpatients because empiric antibiotic therapy is almost always effective in this population. In ambulatory outpatients whose presentation (travel history, exposure) suggests an etiology not covered by standard therapy (eg, *Coccidioides*) or public health concerns (eg, *Mycobacterium tuberculosis*, influenza), diagnostic testing is appropriate. Diagnostic testing is recommended in hospitalized CAP patients for multiple reasons: the likelihood of an infectious cause unresponsive to standard therapy is higher in more severe illness, the inpatient setting allows narrowing of antibiotic coverage as specific diagnostic information is available, and the yield of testing is improved in more acutely ill patients.

Diagnostic tests are used to guide initial antibiotic therapy, permit adjustment of empirically chosen therapy to a specific infectious cause or resistance pattern, and facilitate epidemiologic analysis. Three widely available, rapid point-of-care diagnostic tests may guide initial therapy: the sputum Gram stain, urinary antigen tests for *S pneumoniae* and *Legionella* species, and rapid antigen detection tests for influenza. Sputum Gram stain is neither sensitive nor specific for *S pneumoniae*, the most common cause of CAP. The usefulness of a sputum Gram stain lies in broadening initial coverage in patients to be hospitalized for CAP, most commonly to cover *S aureus* (including community-acquired methicillin-resistant strains, CA-MRSA) or gram-negative rods. Urinary antigen assays for *Legionella pneumophilia* and *S pneumoniae* are at least as sensitive and specific as sputum Gram stain and culture. Results are available immediately and are not affected by early initiation of antibiotic therapy. Positive tests may allow narrowing of initial antibiotic coverage. Urinary antigen assay for *S pneumoniae* should be ordered for patients

with leukopenia, asplenia, active alcohol use, chronic severe liver disease, pleural effusion, and those requiring ICU admission. Urinary antigen assay for *L pneumophilia* should be ordered for patients with active alcohol use, travel within previous 2 weeks, pleural effusion, and those requiring ICU admission. Rapid influenza testing has intermediate sensitivity but high specificity. Positive tests may reduce unnecessary antibacterial use and direct isolation of hospitalized patients.

Rapid turnaround multiplex-polymerase chain reaction (PCR) amplification is clinically available. Different commercial products can identify multiple strains of bacteria and viruses, in addition to genes that encode for antibiotic resistance, with results available in 60–90 minutes. Early experience with multiplex-PCR shows improved overall diagnostic yield, particularly for viral infections, and a higher incidence of bacterial/viral coinfection than previously recognized. Given the lack of effective treatment for most respiratory viral infections, the value of multiplex-PCR may be to avoid antibacterial therapy in viral infections, and early adjustment of empiric antibiotic therapy according to resistance patterns. Limitations of multiplex-PCR include cost and lack of availability, in addition to the challenge of interpreting potentially false-positive results from a highly sensitive test.

Additional microbiologic testing including pre-antibiotic sputum and blood cultures (at least two sets with needle sticks at separate sites) has been standard practice for patients with CAP who require hospitalization. The yield of blood and sputum cultures is low, however; false-positive results are common, and the impact of culture results on patient outcomes is small. As a result, targeted testing based on specific indications is recommended. Culture results are not available prior to initiation of antibiotic therapy. Their role is to allow narrowing of initial empiric antibiotic coverage, adjustment of coverage based on specific antibiotic resistance patterns, to identify unsuspected pathogens not covered by initial therapy, and to provide information for epidemiologic analysis.

Apart from microbiologic testing, hospitalized patients should undergo complete blood count with differential and a chemistry panel (including serum glucose, electrolytes, urea nitrogen, creatinine, bilirubin, and liver enzymes). Hypoxemic patients should have arterial blood gases sampled. Test results help assess severity of illness and guide evaluation and management. HIV testing should be considered in all adult patients, and performed in those with risk factors.

C. Imaging

A pulmonary opacity on chest radiography or CT scan is required to establish a diagnosis of CAP. Chest CT scan is more sensitive and specific than chest radiography and may be indicated in selected cases. Radiographic findings range from patchy airspace opacities to lobar consolidation with air bronchograms to diffuse alveolar or interstitial opacities. Additional findings can include pleural effusions and cavitation. Chest imaging cannot identify a specific microbiologic cause of CAP, however. No pattern of radiographic abnormalities is pathognomonic of any infectious cause.

Chest imaging may help assess severity and response to therapy over time. Progression of pulmonary opacities during antibiotic therapy or lack of radiographic improvement over time are poor prognostic signs and also raise concerns about secondary or alternative pulmonary processes. Clearing of pulmonary opacities in patients with CAP can take 6 weeks or longer. Clearance is usually quickest in younger patients, nonsmokers, and those with only single-lobe involvement.

D. Special Examinations

Patients with CAP who have significant pleural fluid collections may require diagnostic thoracentesis (glucose, lactate dehydrogenase [LD], and total protein levels; leukocyte count with differential; pH determination) with pleural fluid Gram stain and culture. Positive pleural cultures indicate the need for tube thoracostomy drainage.

Patients with cavitary opacities should have sputum fungal and mycobacterial cultures.

Sputum induction and fiberoptic bronchoscopy to obtain samples of lower respiratory secretions are indicated in patients who cannot provide expectorated sputum samples or who may have *P jirovecii* or *M tuberculosis* pneumonia.

Procalcitonin is a calcitonin precursor released in response to bacterial toxins and inhibited by viral infections. This divergent response to bacterial and viral infections offers laboratory support for a clinical judgment of a viral process in patients with lower respiratory symptoms. Multiple clinical trials have shown that procalcitonin measurement allows clinicians to reduce both initial administration of antibiotics and the duration of antibiotic therapy in CAP without compromising patient outcomes.

► Differential Diagnosis

The differential diagnosis of lower respiratory tract infection is extensive and includes upper respiratory tract infections, reactive airway diseases, heart failure, cryptogenic organizing pneumonitis, lung cancer, pulmonary vasculitis, pulmonary thromboembolic disease, and atelectasis.

► Treatment

Two general principles guide antibiotic therapy once the diagnosis of CAP is established: **prompt** initiation of a medication to which the etiologic pathogen is **susceptible.**

In patients who require specific diagnostic evaluation, sputum and blood culture specimens should be obtained prior to initiation of antibiotics. Since early administration of antibiotics to acutely ill patients is associated with improved outcomes; obtaining other diagnostic specimens or test results should not delay the initial dose of antibiotics.

Optimal antibiotic therapy would be pathogen directed, but a definitive microbiologic diagnosis is rarely available on presentation. A syndromic approach to therapy, based on clinical presentation and chest imaging, does not reliably predict the microbiology of CAP. Therefore, initial antibiotic choices are typically empiric, based on acuity (treatment as an outpatient, inpatient, or in the ICU), patient risk factors for specific pathogens, and local antibiotic resistance patterns (Table 9–9).

Since *S pneumoniae* remains a common cause of CAP in all patient groups, local prevalence of drug-resistant *S pneumoniae* significantly affects initial antibiotic choice. Prior treatment with one antibiotic in a pharmacologic class (eg, beta-lactam, macrolide, fluoroquinolone) predisposes the emergence of drug-resistant *S pneumoniae*, with resistance developing against that class of antibiotics to which the pathogen was previously exposed. Definitions of resistance have shifted based on observations of continued clinical efficacy at achievable serum levels. In CAP, for parenteral penicillin G or oral amoxicillin, susceptible strains have a minimum inhibitory concentration (MIC) 2 mcg/mL or less; intermediate resistance is defined as an MIC between 2 mcg/mL and 4 mcg/mL because treatment failures are uncommon with MIC 4 mcg/mL or less. Macrolide resistance has increased; approximately one-third of *S pneumoniae* isolates now show in vitro resistance to macrolides. Treatment failures have been reported but remain rare compared to the number of patients treated. Current in vivo efficacy appears to justify maintaining macrolides as first-line therapy except in areas where there is a high prevalence of resistant strains. *S pneumoniae* resistant to fluoroquinolones is rare in the United States (1% to levofloxacin, 2% to ciprofloxacin) but is increasing.

Community-acquired methicillin-resistant *S aureus* (CA-MRSA) is genetically and phenotypically different from hospital-acquired MRSA strains. CA-MRSA is a rare cause of necrotizing pneumonia, empyema, respiratory failure, and shock; it appears to be associated with prior influenza infection. Linezolid may be preferred to vancomycin in treatment of CA-MRSA pulmonary infection. For expanded discussions of specific antibiotics, see Chapters 30 and e1.

A. Treatment of Outpatients

See Table 9–9 for specific medication dosages. The most common etiologies of CAP in outpatients who do not require hospitalization are *S pneumoniae; M pneumoniae; C pneumoniae;* and respiratory viruses, including influenza. For previously healthy patients with no recent (90 days) use of antibiotics, the recommended treatment is a macrolide (clarithromycin or azithromycin) or doxycycline.

In patients at risk for drug resistance (antibiotic therapy within the past 90 days, age greater than 65 years, comorbid illness, immunosuppression, exposure to a child in daycare), the recommended treatment is a macrolide plus a beta-lactam (high-dose amoxicillin and amoxicillin-clavulanate are preferred to cefpodoxime and cefuroxime) or a respiratory fluoroquinolone (moxifloxacin, gemifloxacin, or levofloxacin).

In regions where there is a high incidence of macrolide-resistant *S pneumoniae*, initial therapy in patients with no comorbidities may include the combination of a beta-lactam added to a macrolide or a respiratory fluoroquinolone.

There are limited data to guide recommendations for duration of treatment. The decision should be influenced by severity of illness, etiology, response to therapy, comorbid medical problems, and complications. Infectious Diseases Society of America/American Thoracic Society guidelines recommend administering a minimum of 5 days of therapy and continuing antibiotics until the patient is afebrile for 48–72 hours.

B. Treatment of Hospitalized and ICU Patients

The most common etiologies of CAP in patients who require hospitalization but not intensive care are *S pneumoniae, M pneumoniae, C pneumoniae, H influenzae, Legionella* species, and respiratory viruses. Some patients have aspiration as an immediate precipitant to the CAP without a specific bacterial etiology. First-line therapy in hospitalized patients is the combination of a macrolide (clarithromycin or azithromycin) plus a beta-lactam (cefotaxime, ceftriaxone, or ampicillin) or a respiratory fluoroquinolone (eg, moxifloxacin, gemifloxacin, or levofloxacin) (see Table 9–9).

Almost all patients admitted to a hospital for treatment of CAP receive intravenous antibiotics. However, no studies in hospitalized patients demonstrated superior outcomes with intravenous antibiotics compared with oral antibiotics, provided patients were able to tolerate oral therapy and the medication was well absorbed. Duration of inpatient antibiotic treatment is the same as for outpatients.

The most common etiologies of CAP in patients who require admission to intensive care are *S pneumoniae, Legionella* species, *H influenzae, Enterobacteriaceae* species, *S aureus, Pseudomonas* species, and respiratory viruses. First-line therapy in ICU patients with CAP is an anti-pneumococcal beta-lactam (cefotaxime, ceftriaxone, or ampicillin-sulbactam) combined with either azithromycin or a respiratory fluoroquinolone (moxifloxacin, gemifloxacin, or levofloxacin). In patients with specific risk factors for *Pseudomonas* infection, combine an anti-pneumococcal, anti-pseudomonal beta-lactam (piperacillin-tazobactam, cefepime, imipenem, meropenem) with either azithromycin or a respiratory fluoroquinolone (moxifloxacin, gemifloxacin, or levofloxacin). In critically ill patients, in those at increased risk for drug resistance, or if the unit incidence of monotherapy-resistant *Pseudomonas* is greater than 10%, then use two agents with anti-pseudomonal efficacy: either ciprofloxacin or levofloxacin plus the above anti-pneumococcal, anti-pseudomonal beta-lactam **or** an anti-pneumococcal, anti-pseudomonal beta-lactam plus an aminoglycoside (gentamicin, tobramycin, amikacin) plus either azithromycin or a respiratory fluoroquinolone. Patients with specific risk factors for methicillin-resistant *S aureus* (MRSA) and those with severe disease (respiratory failure requiring mechanical ventilation or septic shock) also should be treated with vancomycin or linezolid.

Prevention

Pneumococcal vaccines have the potential to prevent or lessen the severity of pneumococcal infections in immunocompetent patients. Two pneumococcal vaccines for adults are available and approved for use in the United States: one containing capsular polysaccharide antigens of 23 common strains of *S pneumoniae* in use for many years (Pneumovax 23) and a conjugate vaccine containing 13 common strains approved for adult use in 2011 (Prevnar-13). Current recommendations are for sequential administration of the two vaccines in those aged 65 years or older and in immunocompromised persons, starting with Prevnar-13. Adults with chronic illness that increases the risk of CAP (see Chapter 30) should receive the 23-valent vaccine regardless of age. Immunocompromised patients and those at highest risk for fatal pneumococcal infections should receive a single revaccination of the 23-valent vaccine 5 years after the first vaccination regardless of age. Immunocompetent persons 65 years of age or older should receive a second dose of the 23-valent vaccine if the patient first received the vaccine 6 or more years previously and was under 65 years old at the time of first vaccination.

The seasonal influenza vaccine is effective in preventing severe disease due to influenza virus with a resulting positive impact on both primary influenza pneumonia and secondary bacterial pneumonias. The seasonal influenza vaccine is administered annually to persons at risk for complications of influenza infection (aged 65 years or older, residents of long-term care facilities, patients with pulmonary or cardiovascular disorders, patients recently hospitalized with chronic metabolic disorders) as well as health care workers and others who are able to transmit influenza to high-risk patients.

Hospitalized patients who would benefit from pneumococcal and influenza vaccines should be vaccinated during hospitalization. The vaccines can be given simultaneously, and may be administered as soon as the patient has stabilized.

When to Admit

Once a diagnosis of CAP is made, the first management decision is to determine the site of care: Is it safe to treat the patient at home or does he or she require hospital or intensive care admission? There are two widely used clinical prediction rules available to guide admission and triage decisions, the **Pneumonia Severity Index (PSI)** and the **CURB-65.**

A. Hospital Admission Decision

The PSI is a validated prediction model that uses 20 items from demographics, medical history, physical examination, laboratory results, and imaging to stratify patients into five risk groups. The PSI is weighted toward discrimination at low predicted mortality. In conjunction with clinical judgment, it facilitates safe decisions to treat CAP in the outpatient setting. An online PSI risk calculator is available at https://www.thecalculator.co/health/Pneumonia-Severity-Index-(PSI)-Calculator-977.html. The CURB-65 assesses five simple, independent predictors of increased mortality (**c**onfusion, **u**remia, **r**espiratory rate, **b**lood pressure, and age greater than **65**) to calculate a 30-day predicted mortality (https://www.mdcalc.com/curb-65-score-pneumonia-severity). Compared with the PSI, the simpler CURB-65 is less discriminating at low mortality but excellent at identifying patients with high mortality who may benefit from ICU-level care. A modified version (CRB-65) dispenses with serum blood urea nitrogen and eliminates the need for laboratory testing. Both have the advantage of simplicity: Patients with zero CRB-65 predictors have a low predicted mortality (less than 1%) and usually do not need hospitalization;

hospitalization should be considered for those with one or two predictors, since they have an increased risk of death; and urgent hospitalization (with consideration of ICU admission) is required for those with three or four predictors.

B. Intensive Care Unit Admission Decision

Expert opinion has defined major and minor criteria to identify patients at high risk for death. Major criteria are septic shock with need for vasopressor support and respiratory failure with need for mechanical ventilation. Minor criteria are respiratory rate 30 breaths or more per minute, hypoxemia (defined as Pao_2/Fio_2 250 or less), hypothermia (core temperature less than $36.0°C$), hypotension requiring aggressive fluid resuscitation, confusion/disorientation, multilobar pulmonary opacities, leukopenia due to infection with WBC less than 4000/mcL (less than $4.0 \times 10^9/L$), thrombocytopenia with platelet count less than 100,000/mcL (less than $100 \times 10^9/L$), uremia with blood urea nitrogen 20 mg/dL or more (7.1 mmol/L or more), metabolic acidosis, or elevated lactate level. Either one major criterion or three or more minor criteria of illness severity generally require ICU-level care.

In addition to pneumonia-specific issues, good clinical practice always makes an admission decision in light of the whole patient. Additional factors suggesting need for inpatient hospitalization include the following:

- Exacerbations of underlying disease (eg, heart failure) that would benefit from hospitalization.

- Other medical or psychosocial needs (such as cognitive dysfunction, psychiatric disease, homelessness, drug abuse, lack of outpatient resources, or poor overall functional status).

- Failure of outpatient therapy, including inability to maintain oral intake and medications.

Lee JS et al. Antibiotic therapy for adults hospitalized with community-acquired pneumonia: a systematic review. JAMA. 2016 Feb 9;315(6):593–602. [PMID: 26864413]

Masiá M et al. Procalcitonin for selecting the antibiotic regimen in outpatients with low-risk community-acquired pneumonia using a rapid point-of-care testing: a single-arm clinical trial. PLoS One. 2017 Apr 20;12(4):e0175634. [PMID: 28426811]

Noguchi S et al. Pneumonia severity assessment tools for predicting mortality in patients with healthcare-associated pneumonia: a systematic review and meta-analysis. Respiration. 2017;93(6):441–50. [PMID: 28449003]

Stern A et al. Corticosteroids for pneumonia. Cochrane Database Syst Rev. 2017 Dec 13;12:CD007720. [PMID: 29236286]

Uranga A et al. Duration of antibiotic treatment in community-acquired pneumonia: a multicenter randomized clinical trial. JAMA Intern Med. 2016 Sep 1;176(9):1257–65. [PMID: 27455166]

van Deursen AMM et al. Immunogenicity of the 13-valent pneumococcal conjugate vaccine in older adults with and without comorbidities in the Community-Acquired Pneumonia Immunization Trial in Adults (CAPiTA). Clin Infect Dis. 2017 Sep 1;65(5):787–95. [PMID: 29017280]

Wunderink RG et al. Advances in the causes and management of community acquired pneumonia in adults. BMJ. 2017 Jul 10; 358:j2471. [PMID: 28694251]

2. Nosocomial Pneumonia (Hospital-Acquired & Ventilator-Associated)

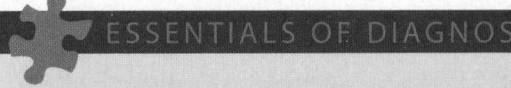

ESSENTIALS OF DIAGNOSIS

- ► **Hospital-acquired pneumonia (HAP)** occurs more than 48 hours after admission to the hospital or other health care facility and excludes any infection present at the time of admission.

- ► **Ventilator-associated pneumonia (VAP)** develops more than 48 hours following endotracheal intubation and mechanical ventilation.

- ► At least two of the following: fever, leukocytosis, purulent sputum.

- ► New or progressive parenchymal opacities on chest radiograph.

- ► Especially common in patients requiring intensive care or mechanical ventilation.

► General Considerations

Hospitalized patients carry different flora with different resistance patterns than healthy patients in the community, and their health status may place them at higher risk for more severe infection. The diagnostic approach and antibiotic treatment of patients with HAP is, therefore, different from patients with CAP. Similarly, management of patients in whom VAP develops following endotracheal intubation and mechanical ventilation should address issues specific to this group of patients.

Considered together, these nosocomial pneumonias (HAP or VAP) represent an important cause of morbidity and mortality despite widespread use of preventive measures, advances in diagnostic testing, and potent new antimicrobial agents. HAP is the second most common cause of infection among hospital inpatients and is the leading cause of death due to infection, with mortality rates ranging from 20% to 50%. While a minority of cases occur in ICU patients, the highest-risk patients are those who are in ICUs or who are being mechanically ventilated; these patients also experience higher morbidity and mortality from HAP. Definitive identification of the infectious cause of a lower respiratory infection is rarely available on presentation; initial antibiotic treatment is therefore empiric and informed by epidemiologic and patient data rather than pathogen-directed.

► Definition & Pathogenesis

HAP develops more than 48 hours after admission to the hospital and VAP develops in a mechanically ventilated patient more than 48 hours after endotracheal intubation.

Three factors distinguish nosocomial pneumonia from CAP: (1) different infectious causes; (2) different antibiotic susceptibility patterns, specifically, a higher incidence of drug resistance; and (3) poorer underlying health status of patients putting them at risk for more severe infections.

Since access to the lower respiratory tract occurs primarily through microaspiration, nosocomial pneumonia starts with a change in upper respiratory tract flora. Colonization of the pharynx and possibly the stomach with bacteria is the most important step in the pathogenesis of nosocomial pneumonia. Pharyngeal colonization is promoted by exogenous factors (eg, instrumentation of the upper airway with nasogastric and endotracheal tubes; contamination by dirty hands, equipment, and contaminated aerosols; and treatment with broad-spectrum antibiotics that promote the emergence of drug-resistant organisms) and patient factors (eg, malnutrition, advanced age, altered consciousness, swallowing disorders, and underlying pulmonary and systemic diseases). Within 48 hours of admission, 75% of seriously ill hospitalized patients have their upper airway colonized with organisms from the hospital environment. Impaired cellular and mechanical defense mechanisms in the lungs of hospitalized patients raise the risk of infection after aspiration has occurred.

Gastric acid may play a role in protection against nosocomial pneumonias. Observational studies have suggested that elevation of gastric pH due to antacids, H_2-receptor antagonists, proton-pump inhibitors (PPIs), or enteral feeding is associated with gastric microbial overgrowth, tracheobronchial colonization, and HAP/VAP. Sucralfate, a cytoprotective agent that does not alter gastric pH, is associated with a trend toward a lower incidence of VAP. The Infectious Diseases Society of America and other professional organizations recommend that acid-suppressive medications (H_2-receptor antagonists and PPIs) be given only to patients at high risk for stress gastritis.

The microbiology of the nosocomial pneumonias differs from CAP but is substantially the same among HAP and VAP. The most common organisms responsible for HAP include *S aureus* (both methicillin-sensitive *S aureus* and MRSA), *P aeruginosa*, gram-negative rods, including non-extended spectrum beta-lactamase (non-ESBL)–producing and ESBL-producing (*Enterobacter* species, *K pneumoniae*, and *Escherichia coli*) organisms. VAP patients may be infected with *Acinetobacter* species and *S maltophilia*. Anaerobic organisms (bacteroides, anaerobic streptococci, fusobacterium) may also cause pneumonia in the hospitalized patient; when isolated, they are commonly part of a polymicrobial flora. Mycobacteria, fungi, chlamydiae, viruses, rickettsiae, and protozoal organisms are uncommon causes of nosocomial pneumonias.

► Clinical Findings

A. Symptoms and Signs

The symptoms and signs associated with nosocomial pneumonias are nonspecific; however, two or more clinical findings (fever, leukocytosis, purulent sputum) in the setting of a new or progressive pulmonary opacity on chest radiograph were approximately 70% sensitive and 75% specific for the diagnosis of VAP in one study. Other findings include those listed above for CAP.

The differential diagnosis of new lower respiratory tract symptoms and signs in hospitalized patients includes heart failure, atelectasis, aspiration, ARDS, pulmonary thromboembolism, pulmonary hemorrhage, and medication reactions.

B. Laboratory Findings

Diagnostic evaluation for suspected nosocomial pneumonia includes blood cultures from two different sites. Blood cultures can identify the pathogen in up to 20% of all patients with nosocomial pneumonias; positivity is associated with increased risk of complications and other sites of infection. Blood counts and clinical chemistry tests do not establish a specific diagnosis; however, they help define the severity of illness and identify complications. The assessment of oxygenation by an arterial blood gas or pulse oximetry determination helps define the severity of illness and determines the need for assisted ventilation. Thoracentesis for pleural fluid analysis should be considered in patients with pleural effusions.

Examination of lower respiratory tract secretions is attended by the same disadvantages as in CAP. Gram stains and cultures of sputum are neither sensitive nor specific in the diagnosis of nosocomial pneumonias. The identification of a bacterial organism by culture of lower respiratory tract secretions does not prove that the organism is a lower respiratory tract pathogen. However, it can be used to help identify bacterial antibiotic sensitivity patterns and as a guide to adjusting empiric therapy.

C. Imaging

Radiographic findings in HAP/VAP are nonspecific and often confounded by other processes that led initially to hospitalization or ICU admission. (See CAP above.)

D. Special Examinations

When HAP is suspected in a patient who subsequently requires mechanical ventilation, secretions obtained by spontaneous expectoration, sputum induction, nasotracheal suctioning, and endotracheal aspiration should be cultured. For patients with suspected VAP, endotracheal aspiration using a sterile suction catheter with semiquantitative cultures of lower respiratory tract secretions is the recommended method of evaluation.

► Treatment

The initial treatment of HAP and VAP is usually empiric, based on risk factors for MRSA and multiple drug-resistant pathogens (Table 9–10) as well as local antibiograms and mortality risk (Table 9–11). Each hospital should generate antibiograms to guide the optimal choice of antibiotics with the goals of reducing exposure to unnecessary antibiotics and the development of antibiotic resistance, thus minimizing patient harm. Because of the high mortality rate, therapy should be started as soon as HAP or VAP is suspected. After results of sputum, blood, and pleural fluid cultures are available, it may be possible to change initially broad to more specific therapy. Endotracheal aspiration cultures have significant negative predictive value but limited positive predictive value in the diagnosis of specific infectious causes of HAP/VAP. If an invasive diagnostic

Table 9–10. Risk factors for multidrug-resistant (MDR) pathogens, methicillin-resistant *Staphylococcus aureus* (MRSA), and *Pseudomonas* and other gram-negative bacilli in patients with hospital-acquired pneumonia (HAP) and ventilator-associated pneumonia (VAP).

Risk factors for MDR pathogens
Antibiotic therapy in the preceding 90 days
Septic shock
Acute respiratory distress syndrome preceding VAP
5 or more days in hospital prior to occurrence of HAP/VAP
Acute renal replacement therapy prior to HAP/VAP onset
Treatment in a unit where > 10% of gram-negative isolates are resistant to an agent being considered for monotherapy
Treatment in a unit where local antibiotic susceptibility rates are not known

Risk factors for MRSA
Antibiotic therapy in the preceding 90 days
Renal replacement therapy in the preceding 30 days
Use of gastric acid suppressive agents
Positive culture or prior MRSA colonization, especially in the preceding 90 days
Hospitalization in a unit where > 20% of *S aureus* isolates are MRSA
Hospitalization in a unit where prevalence of MRSA is not known

Risk factors for *Pseudomonas aeruginosa* and other gram-negative bacilli
Antibiotic therapy in the preceding 90 days
Structural lung disease (COPD, especially with recurrent exacerbations; bronchiectasis; or cystic fibrosis)
Recent hospitalizations, especially with manipulation of the aerodigestive tract (nasoenteric nutrition, intubation)
High-quality Gram stain of respiratory secretions with numerous and predominant gram-negative bacilli
Positive culture for *P aeruginosa* in the past year

COPD, chronic obstructive lung disease.
Data from Kalil AC et al. Management of adults with hospital-acquired and ventilator-associated pneumonia: 2016 Clinical Practice Guidelines by the Infectious Diseases Society of America and the American Thoracic Society. Clin Infect Dis. 2016 Sept 1;63(5):e61–111.

approach to suspected VAP using quantitative culture of bronchoalveolar lavage (BAL), protected specimen brush (PSB), or blind bronchial sampling (BBS) is used, antibiotics can be withheld when results are below a diagnostic threshold (BAL less than 10^4 CFU/mL, PSB or BBS less than 10^3 CFU/mL). Duration of antibiotic therapy should be individualized based on the pathogen, severity of illness, response to therapy, and comorbid conditions. Data from one large trial assessing treatment outcomes in VAP suggested that 8 days of antibiotics is as effective as 15 days.

For expanded discussions of specific antibiotics, see Chapter 30.

Kalil AC et al. Management of adults with hospital-acquired and ventilator-associated pneumonia: 2016 Clinical Practice Guidelines by the Infectious Diseases Society of America and the American Thoracic Society. Clin Infect Dis. 2016 Sept 1; 63(5):e61–111. [PMID: 27418577]

Kollef MH et al. Ventilator-associated pneumonia: the role of emerging diagnostic technologies. Semin Respir Crit Care Med. 2017 Jun;38(3):253–63. [PMID: 28578550]
Spalding MC et al. Ventilator-associated pneumonia: new definitions. Crit Care Clin. 2017 Apr;33(2):277–92. [PMID: 28284295]
Timsit JF et al. Update on ventilator-associated pneumonia. F1000Res. 2017 Nov 29;6:2061. [PMID: 29225790]

3. Anaerobic Pneumonia & Lung Abscess

ESSENTIALS OF DIAGNOSIS

▸ History of or predisposition to aspiration.

▸ Indolent symptoms, including fever, weight loss, and malaise.

▸ Poor dentition.

▸ Foul-smelling purulent sputum (in many patients).

▸ Infiltrate in dependent lung zone, with single or multiple areas of cavitation or pleural effusion.

General Considerations

Aspiration of small amounts of oropharyngeal secretions occurs during sleep in normal individuals but rarely causes disease. Sequelae of aspiration of larger amounts of material include nocturnal asthma, chemical pneumonitis, mechanical obstruction of airways by particulate matter, bronchiectasis, and pleuropulmonary infection. Individuals predisposed to disease induced by aspiration include those with depressed levels of consciousness due to drug or alcohol use, seizures, general anesthesia, or central nervous system disease; those with impaired deglutition due to esophageal disease or neurologic disorders; and those with tracheal or nasogastric tubes, which disrupt the mechanical defenses of the airways.

Periodontal disease and poor dental hygiene, which increase the number of anaerobic bacteria in aspirated material, are associated with a greater likelihood of anaerobic pleuropulmonary infection. Aspiration of infected oropharyngeal contents initially leads to pneumonia in dependent lung zones, such as the posterior segments of the upper lobes and superior and basilar segments of the lower lobes. Body position at the time of aspiration determines which lung zones are dependent. The onset of symptoms is insidious. By the time the patient seeks medical attention, necrotizing pneumonia, lung abscess, or empyema may be apparent.

In most cases of aspiration and necrotizing pneumonia, lung abscess, and empyema, multiple species of anaerobic bacteria are causing the infection. Most of the remaining cases are caused by infection with both anaerobic and aerobic bacteria. *Prevotella melaninogenica*, *Peptostreptococcus*, *Fusobacterium nucleatum*, and *Bacteroides* species are commonly isolated anaerobic bacteria.

Table 9–11. Recommended initial empiric antibiotics for hospital-acquired pneumonia (HAP) and ventilator-associated pneumonia (VAP).

HAP not at high risk for mortality, or VAP with no risk factors for MDR, MRSA, or *Pseudomonas* and other gram-negative bacilli
USE **one** of the following:
Piperacillin-tazobactam, 4.5 g intravenously every 6 hours[1]
Cefepime, 2 g intravenously every 8 hours[1]
Levofloxacin, 750 mg intravenously daily
Imipenem, 500 mg intravenously every 6 hours[1]
Meropenem, 1 g intravenously every 8 hours[1]
HAP or VAP with risk factors for MRSA but no risk factors for MDR, *Pseudomonas*, and other gram-negative bacilli
USE **one** of the following:
Piperacillin-tazobactam, 4.5 g intravenously every 6 hours[1]
Cefepime, 2 g intravenously every 8 hours[1]
Ceftazidime, 2 g intravenously every 8 hours
Levofloxacin, 750 mg intravenously daily
Ciprofloxacin, 400 mg intravenously every 8 hours
Imipenem, 500 mg intravenously every 6 hours[1]
Meropenem, 1 g intravenously every 8 hours[1]
Aztreonam, 2 g intravenously every 8 hours
PLUS **one** of the following:
Vancomycin, 15 mg/kg intravenously every 8–12 hours with goal to target trough level = 15–20 mg/mL (consider a loading dose of 25–30 mg/kg once for severe illness)[2]
Linezolid, 600 mg intravenously every 12 hours
HAP with risk factors for *Pseudomonas* and other gram-negative bacilli, but no risk factors for MRSA and not at high risk for mortality
USE **one** of the following:
Piperacillin-tazobactam, 4.5 g intravenously every 6 hours[1]
Cefepime, 2 g intravenously every 8 hours[1]
Ceftazidime, 2 g intravenously every 8 hours
Imipenem, 500 mg intravenously every 6 hours[1]
Meropenem, 1 g intravenously every 8 hours[1]
Aztreonam, 2 g intravenously every 8 hours
PLUS **one** of the following:
Levofloxacin, 750 mg intravenously daily
Ciprofloxacin, 400 mg intravenously every 8 hours
Gentamicin, 5–7 mg/kg intravenously daily[2]
Tobramycin, 5–7 mg/kg intravenously daily[2]
Aztreonam, 2 g intravenously every 8 hours
HAP at high risk for mortality or VAP with risk factors for MRSA *and* risk factors for MDR, *Pseudomonas*, and other gram-negative bacilli
USE **one** of the following:
Piperacillin-tazobactam, 4.5 g intravenously every 6 hours[1]
Cefepime, 2 g intravenously every 8 hours[1]
Ceftazidime, 2 g intravenously every 8 hours
Imipenem, 500 mg intravenously every 6 hours[1]
Meropenem, 1 g intravenously every 8 hours[1]
Aztreonam, 2 g intravenously every 8 hours
PLUS **one** of the following:
Levofloxacin, 750 mg intravenously daily
Ciprofloxacin, 400 mg intravenously every 8 hours
Amikacin, 15–20 mg/kg intravenously daily[2]
Gentamicin, 5–7 mg/kg intravenously daily[2]
Tobramycin, 5–7 mg/kg intravenously daily[2]
Meropenem, 1 g intravenously every 8 hours[1]
Polymyxin B, 2.5–3.0 mg/kg per day divided in 2 daily intravenous doses
Colistin: consult clinical pharmacist for assistance with dosing
PLUS **one** of the following:
Vancomycin, 15 mg/kg intravenously every 8–12 hours with goal to target trough level = 15–20 mg/mL (consider a loading dose of 25–30 mg/kg once for severe illness)[2]
Linezolid, 600 mg intravenously every 12 hours

CrCl, creatinine clearance; MDR, multidrug resistant; MRSA, methicillin-resistant *Staphylococcus aureus*.
[1]Extended infusions may be appropriate.
[2]Drug level monitoring and adjustment of dosing are required.
Data from Kalil AC et al. Management of adults with hospital-acquired and ventilator-associated pneumonia: 2016 Clinical Practice Guidelines by the Infectious Diseases Society of America and the American Thoracic Society. Clin Infect Dis. 2016 Sept 1;63(5):e61–111.

Clinical Findings

A. Symptoms and Signs

Patients with anaerobic pleuropulmonary infection usually present with constitutional symptoms, such as fever, weight loss, and malaise. Cough with expectoration of foul-smelling purulent sputum suggests anaerobic infection, though the absence of productive cough does not rule out such an infection. Dentition is often poor. Patients are rarely edentulous; if so, an obstructing bronchial lesion may be present.

B. Laboratory Findings

Expectorated sputum is inappropriate for culture of anaerobic organisms because of contaminating mouth flora. Representative material for culture can be obtained only by transthoracic aspiration, thoracentesis, or bronchoscopy with a protected brush. Transthoracic aspiration is rarely indicated, because drainage occurs via the bronchus and anaerobic pleuropulmonary infections usually respond well to empiric therapy.

C. Imaging

The different types of anaerobic pleuropulmonary infection are distinguished on the basis of their radiographic appearance. **Lung abscess** appears as a thick-walled solitary cavity surrounded by consolidation. An air-fluid level is usually present. Other causes of cavitary lung disease (tuberculosis, mycosis, cancer, infarction, granulomatosis with polyangiitis [formerly Wegener granulomatosis]) should be excluded. **Necrotizing pneumonia** is distinguished by multiple areas of cavitation within an area of consolidation. **Empyema** is characterized by the presence of purulent pleural fluid and may accompany either of the other two radiographic findings. Ultrasonography is of value in locating fluid and may also reveal pleural loculations.

Treatment

Medications of choice are clindamycin (600 mg intravenously every 8 hours until improvement, then 300 mg orally every 6 hours) or amoxicillin-clavulanate (875 mg/125 mg orally every 12 hours). Penicillin (amoxicillin, 500 mg every 8 hours, or penicillin G, 1–2 million units intravenously every 4–6 hours) plus metronidazole (500 mg orally or intravenously every 8–12 hours) is another option. Penicillin alone is inadequate treatment for anaerobic pleuropulmonary infections because an increasing number of anaerobic organisms produce beta-lactamases, and up to 20% of patients do not respond to penicillin or amoxicillin. Antibiotic therapy for anaerobic pneumonia should be continued until the chest radiograph improves, a process that may take a month or more; patients with lung abscesses have traditionally been treated until resolution of the abscess cavity is demonstrated by chest radiograph. In both cases, optimal duration of therapy is unknown, and prolonged courses (more than 4 weeks) of therapy are controversial. Anaerobic pleuropulmonary disease requires adequate drainage with tube thoracostomy for the treatment of empyema. Open pleural drainage is sometimes necessary because of the propensity of these infections to produce loculations in the pleural space.

DiBardino DM et al. Aspiration pneumonia: a review of modern trends. J Crit Care. 2015 Feb;30(1):40–8. [PMID: 25129577]
Rolston KVI et al. Post-obstructive pneumonia in patients with cancer: a review. Infect Dis Ther. 2018 Mar;7(1):29–38. [PMID: 29392577]

PULMONARY INFILTRATES IN THE IMMUNOCOMPROMISED HOST

Pulmonary infiltrates in immunocompromised patients (patients with HIV disease, absolute neutrophil counts less than 1000/mcL [less than 1.0×10^9/L], current or recent exposure to myelosuppressive or immunosuppressive medications, or those currently taking more than 5 mg/day of prednisone) may arise from infectious or noninfectious causes. Infection may be due to bacterial, mycobacterial, fungal, protozoal, helminthic, or viral pathogens. Noninfectious processes, such as pulmonary edema, alveolar hemorrhage, medication reactions, pulmonary thromboembolic disease, malignancy, and radiation pneumonitis, may mimic infection.

Although almost any pathogen can cause pneumonia in an immunocompromised host, two clinical tools help the clinician narrow the differential diagnosis. The first is knowledge of the underlying immunologic defect. Specific immunologic defects are associated with particular infections. Defects in humoral immunity predispose to bacterial infections; defects in cellular immunity lead to infections with viruses, fungi, mycobacteria, and protozoa. Neutropenia and impaired granulocyte function predispose to infections from *S aureus*, *Aspergillus*, gram-negative bacilli, and *Candida*. Second, the time course of infection also provides clues to the etiology of pneumonia in immunocompromised patients. A fulminant pneumonia is often caused by bacterial infection, whereas an insidious pneumonia is more apt to be caused by viral, fungal, protozoal, or mycobacterial infection. Pneumonia occurring within 2–4 weeks after organ transplantation is usually bacterial, whereas several months or more after transplantation *P jirovecii*, viruses (eg, cytomegalovirus) and fungi (eg, *Aspergillus*) are encountered more often.

Clinical Findings

Chest radiography is rarely helpful in narrowing the differential diagnosis. Examination of expectorated sputum for bacteria, fungi, mycobacteria, *Legionella*, and *P jirovecii* is important and may preclude the need for expensive, invasive diagnostic procedures. Sputum induction is often necessary for diagnosis. The sensitivity of induced sputum for detection of *P jirovecii* depends on institutional expertise, number of specimens analyzed, and detection methods.

Routine evaluation frequently fails to identify a causative organism. The clinician may begin empiric antimicrobial therapy before proceeding to invasive procedures, such as bronchoscopy, transthoracic needle aspiration, or open lung biopsy. The approach to management must be based on the severity of the pulmonary infection, the underlying disease, the risks of empiric therapy, and local expertise and experience with diagnostic procedures. BAL using the flexible bronchoscope is a safe and effective method for obtaining representative pulmonary secretions for microbiologic studies. It involves less risk of bleeding and other complications than bronchial brushing and transbronchial biopsy. BAL is especially suitable for the diagnosis of *P jirovecii* pneumonia in patients with HIV/AIDS when induced sputum analysis is negative. Surgical lung biopsy, now often performed by video-assisted thoracoscopy, provides the definitive option for diagnosis of pulmonary infiltrates in the immunocompromised host. However, a specific diagnosis is obtained in only about two-thirds of cases, and the information obtained may not affect the outcome.

Alanio A et al; 5th European Conference on Infections in Leukemia (ECIL-5), a joint venture of The European Group for Blood and Marrow Transplantation (EBMT), The European Organization for Research and Treatment of Cancer (EORTC), the Immunocompromised Host Society (ICHS) and The European LeukemiaNet (ELN). ECIL guidelines for the diagnosis of *Pneumocystis jirovecii* pneumonia in patients with haematological malignancies and stem cell transplant recipients. J Antimicrob Chemother. 2016 Sep;71(9):2386–96. [PMID: 27550991]

Bassetti M et al. Overview of fungal infections—the Italian experience. Semin Respir Crit Care Med. 2015 Oct;36(5):796–805. [PMID: 26398544]

Maschmeyer G et al; 6th European Conference on Infections in Leukemia (ECIL-6), a joint venture of The European Group for Blood and Marrow Transplantation (EBMT), The European Organization for Research and Treatment of Cancer (EORTC), the International Immunocompromised Host Society (ICHS) and The European LeukemiaNet (ELN). ECIL guidelines for treatment of *Pneumocystis jirovecii* pneumonia in non-HIV-infected haematology patients. J Antimicrob Chemother. 2016 Sep;71(9):2405–13. [PMID: 27550993]

Vakil E et al. Viral pneumonia in patients with hematologic malignancy or hematopoietic stem cell transplantation. Clin Chest Med. 2017 Mar;38(1):97–111. [PMID: 28159165]

PULMONARY TUBERCULOSIS

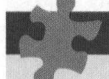

ESSENTIALS OF DIAGNOSIS

► Fatigue, weight loss, fever, night sweats, and productive cough.

► Risk factors for acquisition of infection: household exposure, incarceration, drug use, travel to an endemic area.

► Chest radiograph: pulmonary opacities, most often apical.

► Acid-fast bacilli on smear of sputum or sputum culture positive for *M tuberculosis*.

► General Considerations

Tuberculosis is one of the world's most widespread and deadly illnesses. *M tuberculosis*, the organism that causes tuberculosis infection and disease, infects one-third of the world's population. In 2014, there were 9.6 million new cases of tuberculosis worldwide with 1.5 million people dying of the disease. In the United States, an estimated 11 million people are infected with *M tuberculosis*, and in 2014, there were 9421 active cases. By 2015, the number of cases of tuberculosis increased for the first time in 23 years in 29 US states, particularly in Texas, California, Florida, and New York. Tuberculosis occurs disproportionately among disadvantaged populations, such as the malnourished, homeless, and those living in overcrowded and substandard housing. There is an increased occurrence of tuberculosis among HIV-positive individuals.

Infection with *M tuberculosis* begins when a susceptible person inhales airborne droplet nuclei containing viable organisms. Tubercle bacilli that reach the alveoli are ingested by alveolar macrophages. Infection follows if the inoculum escapes alveolar macrophage microbicidal activity. Once infection is established, lymphatic and hematogenous dissemination of tuberculosis typically occurs before the development of an effective immune response. This stage of infection, **primary tuberculosis,** is usually clinically and radiographically silent. In most persons with intact cell-mediated immunity, T-cells and macrophages surround the organisms in granulomas that limit their multiplication and spread. The infection is contained but not eradicated, since viable organisms may lie dormant within granulomas for years to decades.

Individuals with **latent tuberculosis infection** do not have active disease and cannot transmit the organism to others. However, reactivation of disease may occur if the host's immune defenses are impaired. **Active tuberculosis** will develop in approximately 6% of individuals with latent tuberculosis infection who are not given preventive therapy; half of these cases occur in the 2 years following primary infection. Diverse conditions such as gastrectomy, silicosis, diabetes mellitus, and an impaired immune response (eg, HIV infection; therapy with corticosteroids, tumor necrosis factor inhibitors or other immunosuppressive drugs) are associated with an increased risk of reactivation.

In approximately 5% of cases, the immune response is inadequate to contain the primary infection and **progressive primary tuberculosis** develops, accompanied by both pulmonary and constitutional symptoms as described below. The clinical presentation does not definitively distinguish primary disease from reactivation of latent tuberculosis infection. Standard teaching has held that 90% of tuberculosis in adults represents activation of latent disease. However, DNA fingerprinting of the bacillus suggests that as many as one-third of new cases of tuberculosis in urban populations are primary infections resulting from person-to-person transmission.

The prevalence of drug-resistant strains is increasing worldwide; however, in the United States, the rate of drug-resistant isolates has fallen to less than 1.3%. Risk factors for drug resistance include immigration from countries with a high prevalence of drug-resistant tuberculosis, close and prolonged contact with individuals with drug-resistant tuberculosis, unsuccessful previous therapy, and nonadherence to treatment. Drug resistance may be single or multiple. **Drug-resistant tuberculosis** is resistant to one first-line antituberculous drug, either isoniazid or rifampin. **Multidrug-resistant tuberculosis** is resistant to isoniazid and rifampin, and possibly additional agents. **Extensively drug-resistant tuberculosis** is resistant to isoniazid, rifampin, fluoroquinolones, and either aminoglycosides or capreomycin or both. Outcomes of drug-resistant tuberculosis treatment are worse than when the isolate is drug-sensitive, but outcomes appear to vary with HIV status. In a review of extensively drug-resistant tuberculosis cases in the United States, mortality was 10% and 68% in HIV-negative and HIV-positive patients, respectively.

▶ Clinical Findings

A. Symptoms and Signs

The patient with pulmonary tuberculosis typically presents with slowly progressive constitutional symptoms of malaise, anorexia, weight loss, fever, and night sweats. Chronic cough is the most common pulmonary symptom. It may be dry at first but typically becomes productive of purulent sputum as the disease progresses. Blood-streaked sputum is common, but significant hemoptysis is rarely a presenting symptom; life-threatening hemoptysis may occur in advanced disease. Dyspnea is unusual unless there is extensive disease. On physical examination, the patient appears chronically ill and malnourished. On chest examination, there are no physical findings specific for tuberculosis infection. The examination may be normal or may reveal classic findings such as posttussive apical rales.

B. Laboratory Findings

Definitive diagnosis depends on recovery of *M tuberculosis* from cultures or identification of the organism by DNA or RNA amplification techniques. Three consecutive morning sputum specimens are advised. Fluorochrome staining with rhodamine-auramine of concentrated, digested sputum specimens is performed initially as a screening method, with confirmation by the Kinyoun or Ziehl-Neelsen stains. Demonstration of acid-fast bacilli on sputum smear does not establish a diagnosis of *M tuberculosis*, since nontuberculous mycobacteria may colonize the airways and are increasingly recognized to cause clinical illness in patients with underlying structural lung disease.

In patients thought to have tuberculosis who cannot produce satisfactory specimens or when the smear of the spontaneously expectorated sputum is negative for acid-fast bacilli, sputum induction with 3% hypertonic saline should be performed. Flexible bronchoscopy with bronchial washings has similar diagnostic yield to induced sputum; transbronchial lung biopsies do not significantly increase the diagnostic yield but may lead to earlier diagnosis by identifying tissue granulomas. Post-bronchoscopy expectorated sputum specimens should be collected. Positive blood cultures for *M tuberculosis* are uncommon in patients with normal CD4 cell counts, but the organism may be cultured from blood in up to 50% of HIV-seropositive patients with tuberculosis whose CD4 cell counts are less than 100/mcL (less than 0.1×10^9/L).

Traditional light-microscopic examination of stained sputum for acid-fast bacilli and culture of sputum specimens remain the mainstay of tuberculosis diagnosis. The slow rate of mycobacterial growth, the urgency to provide early, appropriate treatment to patients to improve their outcomes and limit community spread, and concerns about potential drug toxicities in patients treated empirically who do not have tuberculosis infection have fostered the use of rapid diagnostic techniques (Table 9–12). Molecular diagnostics offer multiple options and many advantages at significantly increased expense. Nucleic acid amplification testing not only detects *M tuberculosis* (NAAT-TB) but it also identifies resistance markers (NAAT-R). NAAT-TB can identify *M tuberculosis* within hours of sputum processing, allowing early isolation and treatment, but the negative predictive value is low in smear-negative patients. NAAT-R allows rapid identification of primary drug resistance and is indicated in the following patients: (1) those treated previously for tuberculosis, (2) those born (or who lived for more than 1 year) in a country with moderate tuberculosis incidence or a high incidence of multiple drug-resistant isolates, (3) contacts of patients with multidrug-resistant tuberculosis, or (4) those who are HIV seropositive. Clinical suspicion remains the critical factor in interpreting all these studies. Standard drug susceptibility testing of culture isolates is considered routine for the first isolate of *M tuberculosis*, when a treatment regimen is failing, and when sputum cultures remain positive after 2 months of therapy.

Needle biopsy of the pleura reveals granulomatous inflammation in approximately 60% of patients with pleural effusions caused by *M tuberculosis*. Pleural fluid cultures are positive for *M tuberculosis* in 23–58% of cases of pleural tuberculosis. Culture of three pleural biopsy specimens combined with microscopic examination of a pleural biopsy yields a diagnosis in up to 90% of patients with pleural tuberculosis. Tests for pleural fluid adenosine deaminase (approximately 90% sensitivity and specificity for pleural tuberculosis at levels greater than 70 units/L) and interferon-gamma (89% sensitivity, 97% specificity in a recent meta-analysis) can be extremely helpful diagnostic aids, particularly in making decisions to pursue invasive testing in complex cases.

C. Imaging

Contrary to traditional teaching, molecular analysis demonstrates that radiographic abnormalities in pulmonary tuberculosis do not distinguish primary disease from reactivation of latent tuberculosis (Figure 9–5). The only independent predictor of an atypical pattern on chest radiograph—that is, not associated with upper lobe or cavitary disease—is an impaired host immune response. In elderly patients, lower lobe infiltrates with or without pleural effusion are frequently encountered. Lower lung tuberculosis may masquerade as pneumonia or lung cancer. A "miliary" pattern (diffuse small nodular densities) can be seen with hematologic or lymphatic dissemination of the organism. Immunocompromised patients—particularly those with late-stage HIV infection—often display lower lung zone, diffuse, or miliary

Table 9–12. Essential laboratory tests for the detection of *Mycobacterium tuberculosis*.[1]

Test	Time to Result	Test Characteristics
Acid-fast bacilli light microscopy	1 day	Three morning specimens recommended. Combined sensitivity of 70% (54% for the first specimen, 11% for the second specimen, and 5% for the third specimen). First morning specimen increased yield by 12% compared to spot specimen.
Nucleic acid amplification test, detection (NAAT-TB)	1 day	Sensitivity/specificity high for smear-positive specimens, 85–97% for both; sensitivity falls in smear-negative specimens to ~66%. A positive NAAT in smear-negative patients with intermediate to high (> 30%) pretest probability of *M tuberculosis* infection is helpful while a negative NAAT is not. Should not be ordered in patients with low pretest probability of *M tuberculosis* infection.
Nucleic acid amplification test, resistance markers (NAAT-R)	1–2 days	Multiple assays for rifampin and isoniazid are available. Specificity uniformly high, > 98%. Sensitivity varies from about 84% to 96%, increases with multiple specimens. See text for indications for testing.
Mycobacterial growth detection Liquid (broth based) medium Solid (agar or egg based) medium	Up to 6–8 weeks Avg 10–14 days Avg 3–4 weeks	Liquid culture methods are more sensitive than solid culture methods (~90% and 76%, respectively) with shorter time to detection but higher contamination with bacterial growth. Specificity exceeds 99% for all methods.
Identification of *M tuberculosis* complex by DNA probe or high-performance liquid chromatography	1 day[1]	May be useful in areas of low *M tuberculosis* incidence where nontuberculous mycobacteria are commonly isolated.
First-line drug susceptibility testing (liquid medium)	1–2 weeks[1]	Gold standard. Should be performed routinely on the initial isolate.
Second-line and novel compound drug susceptibility testing Liquid (broth based) medium Solid (agar or egg based) medium	 1–2 weeks[1] 3–4 weeks[1]	

[1]Following detection of mycobacterial growth.

Adapted from Diagnostic Standards and Classification of Tuberculosis in Adults and Children. This official statement of the American Thoracic Society and the Centers for Disease Control and Prevention was adopted by the ATS Board of Directors, July 1999. This statement was endorsed by the Council of the Infectious Disease Society of America, September 1999. Am J Respir Crit Care Med. 2000 Apr; 161(4 Pt 1): 1376–95.

infiltrates; pleural effusions; and involvement of hilar and, in particular, mediastinal lymph nodes.

Resolution of active tuberculosis leaves characteristic radiographic findings. Dense nodules in the pulmonary hila, with or without obvious calcification, upper lobe fibronodular scarring, and bronchiectasis with volume loss are common findings. Ghon (calcified primary focus) and Ranke (calcified primary focus and calcified hilar lymph node) complexes are seen in a minority of patients.

D. Special Examinations

Testing for latent tuberculosis infection is used to evaluate an asymptomatic person in whom *M tuberculosis* infection is suspected (eg, following contact exposure) or to establish the prevalence of tuberculosis infection in a population. Testing may be used in a person with symptoms of active tuberculosis, but a positive test does not distinguish between active and latent infection. Routine testing of individuals at low risk for tuberculosis is not recommended.

The traditional approach to testing for latent tuberculosis infection is the **tuberculin skin test.** The Mantoux test is the preferred method: 0.1 mL of purified protein derivative (PPD) containing 5 tuberculin units is injected intradermally on the volar surface of the forearm using a 27-gauge needle on a tuberculin syringe. The **transverse width in millimeters of induration** at the skin test site is measured after 48–72 hours. To optimize test performance, criteria for determining a positive reaction vary depending on the likelihood of infection. Table 9–13 summarizes the criteria established by the Centers for Disease Control and Prevention (CDC) for interpretation of the Mantoux tuberculin skin test. Sensitivity and specificity of the tuberculin skin test are high: 77% and 97%, respectively. Specificity falls to 59% in populations previously vaccinated with bacillus Calmette-Guérin (BCG, an attenuated form of *Mycobacterium bovis*). False-negative tuberculin skin test reactions may result from improper testing technique; concurrent infections, including fulminant tuberculosis; malnutrition; advanced age; immunologic disorders; malignancy; corticosteroid therapy; chronic kidney disease; and HIV infection. Some individuals with latent tuberculosis infection may have a negative tuberculin skin test when tested many years after exposure. Anergy testing is not recommended for routine use to distinguish a true-negative result from anergy. Poor anergy

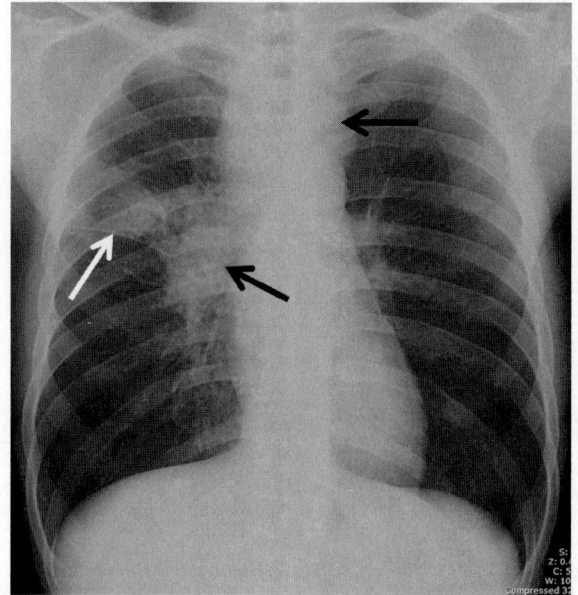

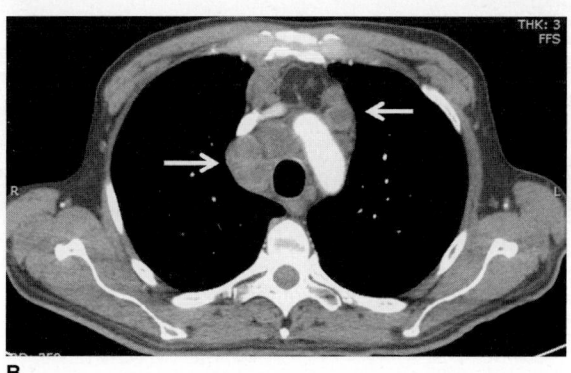

▲ **Figure 9–5.** Pulmonary tuberculosis. Primary pulmonary tuberculosis in a 20-year-old man with chest radiograph **(A)** showing right upper lobe consolidation (white arrow) and right hilar and mediastinal lymphadenopathy (black arrows) and contrast-enhanced CT scan **(B)** showing mediastinal lymphadenopathy (arrows). (Used, with permission, from Carlos Santiago Restrepo, MD, in Usatine RP, Smith MA, Mayeaux EJ Jr, Chumley H. *The Color Atlas of Family Medicine*, 2nd ed. McGraw-Hill, 2013.)

test standardization and lack of outcome data limit the evaluation of its effectiveness. Interpretation of the tuberculin skin test in persons who have previously received BCG vaccination is the same as in those who have not had BCG.

Interferon gamma release assays (including the QuantiFERON and T-SPOT tests) are in vitro assays of CD4+ T-cell–mediated interferon gamma release in response to stimulation by specific *M tuberculosis* antigens. The antigens are absent from all BCG strains and most nontuberculous mycobacteria; therefore, in whole blood, the specificity of interferon gamma release assays is superior to the tuberculin skin test in BGC-vaccinated individuals.

Sensitivity is comparable to the tuberculin skin test: 60–90% depending on the specific assay and study population. Sensitivity is reduced by HIV infection, particularly in patients with low CD4 counts. Specificity is high, greater than 95%. Potential advantages of interferon gamma release assay testing include fewer false-positive results from prior BCG vaccination, better discrimination of positive responses due to nontuberculous mycobacteria, and the requirement for only one patient contact (ie, no need for the patient to return to have the tuberculin skin test read 48–72 hours later). Disadvantages include the need for specialized laboratory equipment and personnel, and the substantially increased cost compared to the tuberculin skin test.

In endemic areas, interferon gamma release assays are no more sensitive than the tuberculin skin test in active tuberculosis (20–40% false-negative rate) and cannot distinguish active from latent disease. Interferon gamma release assays should not be used to exclude active tuberculosis.

Guidelines established by the CDC allow interferon gamma release assays to be used interchangeably with the tuberculin skin testing in the diagnosis of latent tuberculosis infection. Interferon gamma release assays are preferred in patients with prior BCG vaccination; the tuberculin skin test is preferred in children under 5 years old. Routine use of both tests is not recommended. In individuals with a positive tuberculin skin test but a low prior probability of latent tuberculosis infection and low-risk for progression to active disease, the interferon gamma release assay may be helpful as a confirmatory test to exclude a false-positive tuberculin skin test.

► **Treatment**

A. General Measures

The goals of therapy are to cure the individual patient, minimize risk of morbidity and mortality related to treatment, reduce transmission of *M tuberculosis* to other persons, and prevent the emergence of clinically significant drug resistance in tubercle bacilli. The basic principles of antituberculous treatment are (1) to administer multiple medications to which the organisms are susceptible; (2) to provide the safest, most effective therapy in the shortest period of time; (3) to ensure adherence to therapy; and (4) to add at least two new antituberculous agents to a regimen when treatment failure is suspected.

All suspected and confirmed cases of tuberculosis should be reported promptly to local and state public health authorities. Public health departments will perform case investigations on sources and patient contacts to determine if other individuals with untreated, infectious tuberculosis are present in the community. They can identify infected contacts eligible for treatment of latent tuberculous infection and ensure that a plan for monitoring adherence to therapy is established for each patient with tuberculosis. Patients with tuberculosis should be treated by clinicians who are skilled in the management of this infection. Clinical expertise is especially important in cases of drug-resistant tuberculosis.

Table 9–13. Classification of positive tuberculin skin test reactions.[1]

Induration Size	Group
≥ 5 mm	1. HIV-positive persons. 2. Recent contacts of a person with infectious tuberculosis disease. 3. Persons with fibrotic changes on chest radiographs suggestive of prior tuberculosis. 4. Patients with organ transplants and other immunosuppressed patients (receiving the equivalent of > 15 mg/day of prednisone for 1 month or more, or those taking TNF-alpha antagonists).
≥ 10 mm	1. Recent immigrants (< 5 years) from countries with a high prevalence of tuberculosis (eg, Asia, Africa, Latin America). 2. HIV-negative injection drug users. 3. Mycobacteriology laboratory personnel. 4. Residents of and employees in high-risk congregate settings: correctional institutions; long-term care facilities; hospitals and other health care facilities; residential facilities for HIV/AIDS patients; and homeless shelters. 5. Persons with medical conditions that increase the risk of progression to tuberculosis disease: gastrectomy, ≥ 10% below ideal body weight, jejunoileal bypass, diabetes mellitus, silicosis, advanced chronic kidney disease, some hematologic disorders, (eg, leukemias, lymphomas), and other specific malignancies (eg, carcinoma of the head or neck and lung). 6. Children younger than 4 years or infants, children, and adolescents exposed to adults at high risk.
≥ 15 mm	1. Persons with no known risk factors for tuberculosis.

[1]A tuberculin skin test reaction is considered positive if the transverse diameter of the *indurated* area reaches the size required for the specific group. All other reactions are considered negative.
Data from Latent Tuberculosis Infection: A Guide for Primary Health Care Providers. Centers for Disease Control and Prevention. https://www.cdc.gov/tb/publications/ltbi/pdf/targetedltbi.pdf

Nonadherence to antituberculous treatment is a major cause of treatment failure, continued transmission of tuberculosis, and the development of medication resistance. Adherence to treatment can be improved by providing detailed patient education about tuberculosis and its treatment in addition to a case manager who oversees all aspects of an individual patient's care. **Directly observed therapy (DOT),** which requires that a health care worker physically observe the patient ingest antituberculous medications in the home, clinic, hospital, or elsewhere, also improves adherence to treatment. The importance of direct observation of therapy cannot be overemphasized. The CDC recommends DOT for all patients with drug-resistant tuberculosis and for those receiving intermittent (twice- or thrice-weekly) therapy.

Hospitalization for initial therapy of tuberculosis is not necessary for most patients. It should be considered if a patient is incapable of self-care or is likely to expose new, susceptible individuals to tuberculosis. Hospitalized patients with active disease require a private room with negative-pressure ventilation until tubercle bacilli are no longer found in their sputum ("smear-negative") on three consecutive smears taken on separate days.

Characteristics of antituberculous drugs are provided in Table 9–14. Additional treatment considerations can be found in Chapter 33. More complete information can be obtained from the CDC's Division of Tuberculosis Elimination Web site at https://www.cdc.gov/tb/.

B. Treatment of Tuberculosis in HIV-Negative Persons

Most patients with previously untreated pulmonary tuberculosis can be effectively treated with either a 6-month or a 9-month regimen, though the 6-month regimen is preferred. The initial phase of a 6-month regimen consists of 2 months of daily isoniazid, rifampin, pyrazinamide, and ethambutol. Once the isolate is determined to be isoniazid-sensitive, ethambutol may be discontinued. If the *M tuberculosis* isolate is susceptible to isoniazid and rifampin, the second phase of therapy consists of isoniazid and rifampin for a minimum of 4 additional months, with treatment to extend at least 3 months beyond documentation of conversion of sputum cultures to negative for *M tuberculosis*. If DOT is used, medications may be given intermittently using one of three regimens: (1) Daily isoniazid, rifampin, pyrazinamide, and ethambutol for 2 months, followed by isoniazid and rifampin two or three times each week for 4 months if susceptibility to isoniazid and rifampin is demonstrated. (2) Daily isoniazid, rifampin, pyrazinamide, and ethambutol for 2 weeks, then administration of the same agents twice a week for 6 weeks followed by administration of isoniazid and rifampin twice each week for 4 months if susceptibility to isoniazid and rifampin is demonstrated. (3) Isoniazid, rifampin, pyrazinamide, and ethambutol three times a week for 6 months.

Patients who cannot or should not (eg, pregnant women) take pyrazinamide should receive daily isoniazid and rifampin along with ethambutol for 4–8 weeks. If susceptibility to isoniazid and rifampin is demonstrated or drug resistance is unlikely, ethambutol can be discontinued and isoniazid and rifampin may be given twice a week for a total of 9 months of therapy. If drug resistance is a concern, patients should receive isoniazid, rifampin, and ethambutol for 9 months. Patients with smear- and culture-negative disease (eg, pulmonary tuberculosis diagnosed on clinical grounds) and patients for whom drug susceptibility testing is not available can be treated with

Table 9–14. Characteristics of antituberculous medications.

Medication	Most Common Side Effects	Tests for Side Effects	Drug Interactions	Remarks
Isoniazid	Peripheral neuropathy, hepatitis, rash, mild CNS effects.	AST and ALT; neurologic examination.	Phenytoin (synergistic); disulfiram.	Bactericidal to both extracellular and intracellular organisms. Pyridoxine, 25–50 mg orally daily as prophylaxis for neuritis; 50–100 mg orally daily as treatment.
Rifampin	Hepatitis, fever, rash, flu-like illness, gastrointestinal upset, bleeding problems, kidney failure.	CBC, platelets, AST and ALT.	Rifampin inhibits the effect of oral contraceptives, quinidine, corticosteroids, warfarin, methadone, digoxin, oral hypoglycemics; aminosalicylic acid may interfere with absorption of rifampin. Significant interactions with protease inhibitors and nonnucleoside reverse transcriptase inhibitors.	Bactericidal to all populations of organisms. Colors urine and other body secretions orange. Discoloring of contact lenses.
Rifapentine	Bone marrow suppression, hematuria/pyuria, hepatitis, gastrointestinal upset, flu-like illness.	CBC, platelets, AST and ALT.	Strong cytochrome P450 inducer with multiple drug interactions. Use in HIV patients receiving antiretroviral therapy should be limited to experts in antiretroviral therapy.	Bactericidal to both extracellular and intracellular organisms. Colors urine and other body secretions orange. Long half-life, can be administered weekly in LTBI prophylaxis. Not for use in induction phase of therapy.
Pyrazinamide	Hyperuricemia, hepatotoxicity, rash, gastrointestinal upset, joint aches.	Uric acid, AST, ALT.	Rare.	Bactericidal to intracellular organisms.
Ethambutol	Optic neuritis (reversible with discontinuance of drug; rare at 15 mg/kg); rash.	Red-green color discrimination and visual acuity.	Rare.	Bacteriostatic to both intracellular and extracellular organisms. Mainly used to inhibit development of resistant mutants. Use with caution in kidney disease or when ophthalmologic testing is not feasible.
Streptomycin	Eighth nerve damage, nephrotoxicity.	Vestibular function (audiograms); BUN and creatinine.	Neuromuscular blocking agents may be potentiated and cause prolonged paralysis.	Bactericidal to extracellular organisms. Use with caution in older patients or those with kidney disease.

ALT, alanine aminotransferase; AST, aspartate aminotransferase; BUN, blood urea nitrogen; CBC, complete blood count; LTBI, latent tuberculosis infection.

6 months of isoniazid and rifampin combined with pyrazinamide for the first 2 months. This regimen assumes low prevalence of drug resistance. Previous guidelines have used streptomycin interchangeably with ethambutol. Increasing worldwide streptomycin resistance has made this medication less useful as empiric therapy.

When a twice-weekly or thrice-weekly regimen is used instead of a daily regimen, the dosages of isoniazid, pyrazinamide, and ethambutol or streptomycin must be increased. Recommended dosages for the initial treatment of tuberculosis are listed in Table 9–15. Fixed-dose combinations of isoniazid and rifampin (Rifamate) and of isoniazid, rifampin, and pyrazinamide (Rifater) are available to simplify treatment. Single tablets improve compliance but are more expensive than the individual medications purchased separately.

C. Treatment of Tuberculosis in HIV-Positive Persons

Management of tuberculosis is complex in patients with concomitant HIV disease. Experts in the management of both tuberculosis and HIV disease should be involved in the care of such patients. The CDC has published detailed recommendations for the treatment of tuberculosis in HIV-positive patients (www.cdc.gov/tb/topic/basics/tbhiv-coinfection.htm).

The basic approach to HIV-positive patients with tuberculosis is similar to that detailed above for patients without HIV disease. Additional considerations in HIV-positive patients include (1) longer duration of therapy and (2) drug interactions between rifamycin derivatives such as rifampin and rifabutin used to treat tuberculosis

Table 9–15. Recommended dosages for the initial treatment of tuberculosis.[1]

Medication	Daily[2]	Cost[3]/Day	Twice a Week[2]	Cost[3]/Wk	Three Times a Week[2]	Cost[3]/Wk
Isoniazid	5 mg/kg Max: 300 mg/dose	$0.31/300 mg	15 mg/kg Max: 900 mg/dose	$1.86	15 mg/kg Max: 900 mg/dose	$2.79
Rifampin	10 mg/kg Max: 600 mg/dose	$2.66/600 mg	10 mg/kg Max: 600 mg/dose	$5.32	10 mg/kg Max: 600 mg/dose	$7.98
Pyrazinamide	18.2–26.3 mg/kg Max: 2 g/dose	$11.44/2 g	Weight-based dosing: see references below[1]	—	Weight-based dosing: see references below[1]	—
Ethambutol	14.5–21.1 mg/kg Max: 1.6 g/dose	$3.76/1.6 g	Weight-based dosing: see references below[1]	—	Weight-based dosing: see references below[1]	—

[1]Data from Nahid P et al. Official American Thoracic Society/Centers for Disease Control and Prevention/Infectious Diseases Society of America Clinical Practice Guidelines: Treatment of drug-susceptible tuberculosis. Clin Infect Dis. 2016 Oct 1;63(7):e147–95.
[2]All dosing regimens should be used with directly observed therapy.
[3]Average wholesale price (AWP, for AB-rated generic when available) for quantity listed. Source: IBM Micromedex. Red Book (electronic version). IBM Watson Health, Greenwood Village, CO, USA. Available at https://www.micromedexsolutions.com/ (cited March 12, 2019). AWP may not accurately represent the actual pharmacy cost because wide contractual variations exist among institutions.
Also available at www.cdc.gov/tb/topic/treatment/guidelinehighlights.htm

and some of the protease inhibitors and nonnucleoside reverse transcriptase inhibitors (NNRTIs) used to treat HIV (see www.cdc.gov/tb/topic/basics/tbhivcoinfection.htm). DOT should be used for all HIV-positive tuberculosis patients. Pyridoxine (vitamin B$_6$), 25–50 mg orally each day, should be administered to all HIV-positive patients being treated with isoniazid to reduce central and peripheral nervous system side effects.

D. Treatment of Drug-Resistant Tuberculosis

Patients with drug-resistant *M tuberculosis* infection require careful supervision and management. Clinicians who are unfamiliar with the treatment of drug-resistant tuberculosis should seek expert advice. Tuberculosis resistant only to isoniazid can be successfully treated with a 6-month regimen of rifampin, pyrazinamide, and ethambutol or streptomycin or a 12-month regimen of rifampin and ethambutol. When isoniazid resistance is documented during a 9-month regimen without pyrazinamide, isoniazid should be discontinued. If ethambutol was part of the initial regimen, rifampin and ethambutol should be continued for a minimum of 12 months. If ethambutol was not part of the initial regimen, susceptibility tests should be repeated and two other medications to which the organism is susceptible should be added. Treatment of *M tuberculosis* isolates resistant to agents other than isoniazid and treatment of drug resistance in HIV-infected patients require expert consultation.

Multidrug-resistant tuberculosis and extensively drug-resistant tuberculosis call for an individualized daily DOT plan under the supervision of an experienced clinician. Treatment regimens are based on the patient's overall status and the results of susceptibility studies. Most drug-resistant isolates are resistant to at least isoniazid and rifampin and require a minimum of three drugs to which the organism is susceptible. These regimens are continued until culture conversion is documented, and then a two-drug regimen is

continued for at least another 12 months. Some experts recommend at least 18–24 months of a three-drug regimen.

E. Treatment of Extrapulmonary Tuberculosis

In most cases, regimens that are effective for treating pulmonary tuberculosis are also effective for treating extrapulmonary disease. However, many experts recommend 9–12 months of therapy when miliary, meningeal, or bone and joint disease is present. Treatment of skeletal tuberculosis is enhanced by early surgical drainage and debridement of necrotic bone. Corticosteroid therapy has been shown to help prevent constrictive pericarditis from tuberculous pericarditis and to reduce neurologic complications from tuberculous meningitis (Chapter 33).

F. Treatment of Pregnant or Lactating Women

Tuberculosis in pregnancy is usually treated with isoniazid, rifampin, and ethambutol for 2 months, followed by isoniazid and rifampin for an additional 7 months. Ethambutol can be stopped after the first month if isoniazid and rifampin susceptibility is confirmed. Since the risk of teratogenicity with pyrazinamide has not been clearly defined, pyrazinamide should be used only if resistance to other drugs is documented and susceptibility to pyrazinamide is likely. Streptomycin is contraindicated in pregnancy because it may cause congenital deafness. Pregnant women taking isoniazid should receive pyridoxine (vitamin B$_6$), 10–25 mg orally once a day, to prevent peripheral neuropathy.

Small concentrations of antituberculous drugs are present in breast milk. First-line therapy is not known to be harmful to nursing newborns at these concentrations. Therefore, breastfeeding is not contraindicated while receiving first-line antituberculous therapy. Lactating women receiving other agents should consult a tuberculosis expert.

G. Treatment Monitoring

Adults should have measurements of a complete blood count (including platelets) and serum bilirubin, hepatic enzymes, urea nitrogen, and creatinine before starting therapy for tuberculosis. Visual acuity and red-green color vision tests are recommended before initiation of ethambutol and serum uric acid before starting pyrazinamide. Audiometry should be performed if streptomycin therapy is initiated.

Routine monitoring of laboratory tests for evidence of medication toxicity during therapy is not recommended, unless baseline results are abnormal or liver disease is suspected. Monthly questioning for symptoms of medication toxicity is advised. Patients should be educated about common side effects of antituberculous medications and instructed to seek medical attention should these symptoms occur. Monthly follow-up of outpatients is recommended, including sputum smear and culture for *M tuberculosis*, until cultures convert to negative. Patients with negative sputum cultures after 2 months of treatment should have at least one additional sputum smear and culture performed at the end of therapy. Patients with drug-resistant isolates should have sputum cultures performed monthly during the entire course of treatment. A chest radiograph at the end of therapy provides a useful baseline for any future films.

Patients whose cultures do not become negative or whose symptoms do not resolve despite 3 months of therapy should be evaluated for nonadherence to the regimen and for drug-resistant organisms. DOT is required for the remainder of the treatment regimen, and the addition of at least two drugs not previously given should be considered pending repeat drug susceptibility testing. The clinician should seek expert assistance if drug resistance is newly found, if the patient remains symptomatic, or if smears or cultures remain positive.

Patients with only a clinical diagnosis of pulmonary tuberculosis (smears and cultures negative for *M tuberculosis*) whose symptoms and radiographic abnormalities are unchanged after 3 months of treatment usually either have another process or have had tuberculosis in the past.

H. Treatment of Latent Tuberculosis

Treatment of latent tuberculous infection is essential to controlling and eliminating tuberculosis. Treatment of latent tuberculous infection substantially reduces the risk that infection will progress to active disease. Targeted testing with the tuberculin skin test or interferon gamma release assays is used to identify persons who are at high risk for tuberculosis and who stand to benefit from treatment of latent infection. Table 9–13 gives the tuberculin skin test criteria for treatment of latent tuberculous infection. In general, patients with a positive tuberculin skin test or interferon gamma release assay who are at increased risk for exposure or disease are treated. It is essential that each person who meets the criteria for treatment of latent tuberculous infection undergo a careful assessment to exclude active disease. A history of past treatment for tuberculosis and contraindications to treatment should be sought. All patients at risk for HIV infection should have an HIV test. Patients suspected of having tuberculosis should receive one of the recommended multidrug regimens for active disease until the diagnosis is confirmed or excluded.

Some close contacts of persons with active tuberculosis should be evaluated for treatment of latent tuberculous infection despite a negative tuberculin skin test reaction (less than 5 mm induration). These include immunosuppressed persons and those who may develop disease quickly after tuberculous infection. Close contacts who have a negative tuberculin skin test reaction on initial testing should be retested 10–12 weeks later.

Several treatment regimens for both HIV-negative and HIV-positive persons are available for the treatment of latent tuberculous infection: (1) **Isoniazid:** A 9-month oral regimen (minimum of 270 doses administered within 12 months) is preferable to 6 months of therapy. Dosing options include a daily dose of 300 mg or twice-weekly doses of 15 mg/kg. Persons at risk for developing isoniazid-associated peripheral neuropathy (those with diabetes mellitus, uremia, malnutrition, alcoholism, HIV infection, pregnancy, or seizure disorder) may be given supplemental pyridoxine (vitamin B_6), 10–50 mg/day. (2) **Isoniazid and rifampin:** A 3-month oral regimen of daily isoniazid (300 mg) and rifampin (600 mg). (3) **Isoniazid and rifapentine:** A 3-month oral regimen of once weekly isoniazid at 15 mg/kg and rifapentine at 15–30 mg/kg. (4) **Rifampin:** Patients who cannot tolerate isoniazid can be considered for a 4-month oral regimen of rifampin at 600 mg daily. HIV-positive patients receiving protease inhibitors or NNRTIs who are given rifampin or rifapentine require management by experts in both tuberculosis and HIV disease (see Treatment of Tuberculosis in HIV-Positive Persons, above).

Contacts of persons with isoniazid-resistant, rifampin-sensitive tuberculosis should receive a 2-month regimen of rifampin and pyrazinamide or a 4-month regimen of daily rifampin alone. Contacts of persons with drug-resistant tuberculosis should receive two drugs to which the infecting organism has demonstrated susceptibility. Contacts in whom the tuberculin skin test or interferon gamma release assay is negative and contacts who are HIV seronegative may be observed without treatment or treated for 6 months. HIV-positive contacts should be treated for 12 months. All contacts of persons with multidrug-resistant tuberculosis or extensively drug-resistant tuberculosis should have 2 years of follow-up regardless of type of treatment.

Persons with a positive tuberculin skin test (5 mm or more of induration) and fibrotic lesions suggestive of old tuberculosis on chest radiographs who have no evidence of active disease and no history of treatment for tuberculosis should receive 9 months of isoniazid or 4 months of rifampin (with or without isoniazid). Pregnant or breastfeeding women with latent tuberculosis should receive either daily or twice-weekly isoniazid with pyridoxine (vitamin B_6).

Baseline laboratory testing is indicated for patients at risk for liver disease, patients with HIV infection, women who are pregnant or within 3 months of delivery, and persons who use alcohol regularly. Patients receiving treatment for latent tuberculous infection should be evaluated once a month to assess for symptoms and signs of active tuberculosis and hepatitis and for adherence to their treatment regimen. Routine laboratory testing during treatment is indicated for those with abnormal baseline laboratory tests and for those at risk for developing liver disease.

BCG vaccine is an antimycobacterial vaccine developed from an attenuated strain of *M bovis*. Millions of individuals worldwide have been vaccinated with BCG. However, it is not generally recommended in the United States because of the low prevalence of tuberculous infection, the vaccine's interference with the ability to determine latent tuberculous infection using tuberculin skin test reactivity, and its variable effectiveness in prophylaxis of pulmonary tuberculosis. BCG vaccination in the United States should be undertaken only after consultation with local health officials and tuberculosis experts. Vaccination of health care workers should be considered on an individual basis in settings in which a high percentage of tuberculosis patients are infected with strains resistant to both isoniazid and rifampin, in which transmission of such drug-resistant *M tuberculosis* and subsequent infection are likely, and in which comprehensive tuberculous infection-control precautions have been implemented but have not been successful. The BCG vaccine is contraindicated in persons with impaired immune responses due to disease or medications.

Prognosis

Almost all properly treated immunocompetent patients with tuberculosis can be cured. Relapse rates are less than 5% with current regimens. The main cause of treatment failure is nonadherence to therapy.

Getahun H et al. Latent *Mycobacterium tuberculosis* infection. N Engl J Med. 2015 May 28;372(22):2127–35. [PMID: 26017823]

Horsburgh CR Jr et al. Treatment of tuberculosis. N Engl J Med. 2015 Nov 26;373(22):2149–60. [PMID: 26605929]

Lewinsohn DM et al. Official American Thoracic Society/Infectious Diseases Society of America/Centers for Disease Control and Prevention Clinical Practice Guidelines: diagnosis of tuberculosis in adults and children. Clin Infect Dis. 2017 Jan 15;64(2):111–5. [PMID: 28052967]

Manosuthi W et al. Integrated therapy for HIV and tuberculosis. AIDS research and therapy. 2016 May 12;13;22. [PMID: 27182275]

Menzies D et al. Four months of rifampin or nine months of isoniazid for latent tuberculosis in adults. N Engl J Med. 2018 Aug 2;379(5):440–53. [PMID: 30067931]

Nahid P et al. Official American Thoracic Society/Centers for Disease Control and Prevention/Infectious Diseases Society of America Clinical Practice Guidelines: treatment of drug-susceptible tuberculosis. Clin Infect Dis. 2016 Oct 1;63(7):e147–95. [PMID: 27516382]

Nemes E et al; C-040-404 Study Team. Prevention of *M. tuberculosis* infection with H4:IC31 vaccine or BCG revaccination. N Engl J Med. 2018 Jul 12;379(2):138–49. [PMID: 29996082]

Ruhwald M et al; TESEC Working Group. Safety and efficacy of the C-Tb skin test to diagnose *Mycobacterium tuberculosis* infection, compared with an interferon γ release assay and the tuberculin skin test: a phase 3, double-blind, randomised, controlled trial. Lancet Respir Med. 2017 Apr;5(4):259–68. [PMID: 28159608]

Wilson JW et al. Extensively drug-resistant tuberculosis: principles of resistance, diagnosis, and management. Mayo Clin Proc. 2016 Apr;91(4):482–95. [PMID: 26906649]

PULMONARY DISEASE CAUSED BY NONTUBERCULOUS MYCOBACTERIA

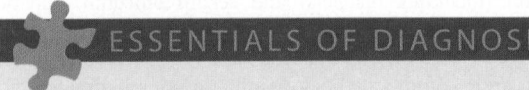

ESSENTIALS OF DIAGNOSIS

▸ Chronic cough, sputum production, and fatigue; less commonly: malaise, dyspnea, fever, hemoptysis, and weight loss.

▸ Parenchymal opacities on chest radiograph, most often thin-walled cavities or multiple small nodules associated with bronchiectasis.

▸ Isolation of nontuberculous mycobacteria in a sputum culture.

General Considerations

Mycobacteria other than *M tuberculosis*—nontuberculous mycobacteria (NTM), sometimes referred to as "atypical" mycobacteria—are ubiquitous in water and soil and have been isolated from tap water. Marked geographic variability exists, both in the NTM species responsible for disease and in the prevalence of disease. These organisms are not considered communicable from person to person, have distinct laboratory characteristics, and are often resistant to most antituberculous medications (Chapter 33). Long-term epidemiologic data suggest that NTM disease has been increasing in the United States.

Definition & Pathogenesis

The diagnosis of lung disease caused by NTM is based on a combination of clinical, radiographic, and bacteriologic criteria and the exclusion of other diseases that can resemble the condition. Specific diagnostic criteria are discussed below. Complementary data are important for diagnosis because NTM organisms can reside in or colonize the airways without causing clinical disease.

Mycobacterium avium complex (MAC) is the most frequent cause of NTM pulmonary disease in humans in the United States. *Mycobacterium kansasii* is the next most frequent pulmonary pathogen. Other NTM causes of pulmonary disease include *Mycobacterium abscessus*, *Mycobacterium xenopi*, and *Mycobacterium malmoense*; the list of more unusual etiologic NTM species is long. Most NTM cause a chronic pulmonary infection that resembles tuberculosis, but tends to progress more slowly. Disseminated disease is rare in immunocompetent hosts; however, disseminated MAC disease is common in patients with AIDS.

Clinical Findings

A. Symptoms and Signs

NTM infection among immunocompetent hosts frequently presents in one of three prototypical patterns: cavitary, upper lobe lesions in older male smokers that may mimic *M tuberculosis*; nodular bronchiectasis affecting the mid lung zones in middle-aged women with chronic cough; and hypersensitivity pneumonitis following environmental exposure. Most patients with NTM infection experience a chronic cough, sputum production, and fatigue. Less common symptoms include malaise, dyspnea, fever, hemoptysis, and weight loss. Symptoms from coexisting lung disease (COPD, bronchiectasis, previous mycobacterial disease, cystic fibrosis, and pneumoconiosis) may confound the evaluation. In patients with bronchiectasis, coinfection with NTM and *Aspergillus* is a negative prognostic factor. New or worsening infiltrates as well as adenopathy or pleural effusion (or both) are described in HIV-positive patients with NTM infection as part of the immune reconstitution inflammatory syndrome following institution of antiretroviral therapy.

B. Laboratory Findings

The diagnosis of NTM infection rests on recovery of the pathogen from cultures. Sputum cultures positive for atypical mycobacteria do not prove infection because NTM may exist as saprophytes colonizing the airways or may be environmental contaminants. Bronchial washings are considered to be more sensitive than expectorated sputum samples; however, their specificity for clinical disease is not known.

Bacteriologic criteria have been proposed based on studies of patients with cavitary disease with MAC or *M kansasii*. Diagnostic criteria in immunocompetent persons include the following: positive culture results from at least two separate expectorated sputum samples; or positive culture from at least one bronchial wash; or a positive culture from pleural fluid or any other normally sterile site. The diagnosis can also be established by demonstrating NTM cultured from a lung biopsy, bronchial wash, or sputum plus histopathologic changes, such as granulomatous inflammation in a lung biopsy. Rapid species identification of some NTM is possible using DNA probes or high-pressure liquid chromatography.

Diagnostic criteria are less stringent for patients with severe immunosuppression. HIV-infected patients may show significant MAC growth on culture of bronchial washings without clinical infection; therefore, HIV patients being evaluated for MAC infection must be considered individually.

Medication susceptibility testing on cultures of NTM is recommended for the following NTM: (1) *Mycobacterium avium intracellulare* to macrolides only (clarithromycin and azithromycin); (2) *M kansasii* to rifampin; and (3) rapid growers (such as *Mycobacterium fortuitum, Mycobacterium chelonae,* and *M abscessus*) to amikacin, doxycycline, imipenem, fluoroquinolones, clarithromycin, cefoxitin, and sulfonamides.

C. Imaging

Chest radiographic findings include infiltrates that are progressive or persist for at least 2 months, cavitary lesions, and multiple nodular densities. The cavities are often thinwalled and have less surrounding parenchymal infiltrate than is commonly seen with MTB infections. Evidence of contiguous spread and pleural involvement is often present. High-resolution CT of the chest may show multiple small nodules with or without multifocal bronchiectasis. Progression of pulmonary infiltrates during therapy or lack of radiographic improvement over time are poor prognostic signs and also raise concerns about secondary or alternative pulmonary processes. Clearing of pulmonary infiltrates due to NTM is slow.

▶ Treatment

Establishing NTM infection does not mandate treatment in all cases, for two reasons. First, clinical disease may never develop in some patients, particularly asymptomatic patients with few organisms isolated from single specimens. Second, the spectrum of clinical disease severity is very wide; in patients with mild or slowly progressive symptoms, traditional chemotherapeutic regimens using a combination of agents may lead to drug-induced side effects worse than the disease itself.

Specific treatment regimens and responses to therapy vary with the species of NTM. HIV-seronegative patients with MAC pulmonary disease usually receive a combination of daily clarithromycin or azithromycin, rifampin or rifabutin, and ethambutol (Table 9–15). For patients with severe fibrocavitary disease, streptomycin or amikacin is added for the first 2 months. The optimal duration of treatment is unknown, but therapy should be continued for 12 months after sputum conversion. Medical treatment is initially successful in about two-thirds of cases, but relapses after treatment are common; long-term benefit is demonstrated in about half of all patients. Those who do not respond favorably generally have active but stable disease. Surgical resection is an alternative for the patient with progressive disease that responds poorly to chemotherapy; the success rate with surgical therapy is good. Disease caused by *M kansasii* responds well to drug therapy. A daily regimen of rifampin, isoniazid, and ethambutol for at least 18 months with a minimum of 12 months of negative cultures is usually successful. Rapidly growing mycobacteria (*M abscessus, M fortuitum, M chelonae*) are generally resistant to standard antituberculous therapy.

▶ When to Refer

Patients with rapidly growing mycobacteria infection should be referred for expert management.

Cowman S et al. The antimicrobial susceptibility of non-tuberculous mycobacteria. J Infect. 2016 Mar;72(3):324–31. [PMID: 26723913]

Diel R et al. Microbiological and clinical outcomes of treating non-*Mycobacterium avium* complex nontuberculous mycobacterial pulmonary disease: a systematic review and meta-analysis. Chest. 2017 Jul;152(1):120–42. [PMID: 28461147]

Wassilew N et al. Pulmonary disease caused by non-tuberculous mycobacteria. Respiration. 2016;91(5):386–402. [PMID: 27207809]

▼ PULMONARY NEOPLASMS

See Chapter 39 for discussions of Lung Cancer, Secondary Lung Cancer, and Mesothelioma.

SCREENING FOR LUNG CANCER

Two large RCTs reported findings in 2011 regarding the utility of lung cancer screening. The Prostate, Lung, Colorectal and Ovarian Randomized Trial (PLCO) randomized 154,901 adults (52% current or former smokers) between the ages of 55 and 74 years to receive either no screening or annual posterior-anterior chest radiographs for 4 consecutive years. The investigators monitored the participants after screening for an average of 12 years. Results showed no mortality benefit from four annual chest radiographs either in the whole cohort or in a subset of heavy smokers who met the entry criteria for the other major trial, the National Lung Screening Trial (NLST). The NLST enrolled 53,454 current or former smokers (minimum 30-pack year exposure history) between the ages of 55 and 74 years who were randomly assigned to one of two screening modalities: three annual posterior-anterior chest radiographs or three annual low-dose chest CT scans. They were monitored for an additional 6.5 years after screening. Compared with chest radiography, low-dose chest CT detected more early-stage lung cancers and fewer advanced-stage lung cancers, indicating that CT screening systematically shifted the time of diagnosis to earlier stages, thereby providing more persons the opportunity for effective treatment. Furthermore, compared with chest radiographs, the cohort that received three annual CT scans had a statistically significant mortality benefit, with reductions in both lung cancer deaths (20.0%) and all-cause mortality (6.7%). This is the first time that evidence from an RCT demonstrated that lung cancer screening reduces all-cause mortality.

Additional information from PLCO, the NLST, and multiple other ongoing randomized trials is available. Trials in the Netherlands and Belgium (NELSON), Germany (LUSI), Denmark (DLCST), the United Kingdom (UKLS), and Italy (MILD) have been completed. These have revealed variable findings depending on the risk profile of the included patients, but the broad results are that screening is most likely to be effective if performed at short intervals in a high-risk population, as was done in NLST.

Salient issues that temper enthusiasm for widespread screening at this time include the following: **(1) Generalizability to community practice:** NLST-participating institutions demonstrated a high level of expertise in imaging interpretation and diagnostic evaluation. Ninety-six percent of findings on CT were false positives but the vast majority of patients were monitored with serial imaging. Invasive diagnostic evaluations were uncommon and were associated with a low complication rate (1.4%). **(2) Duration of screening:** The rate of detection of new lung cancers did not fall with each subsequent annual screening over 3 years. Since new lung cancers become detectable during each year-long screening interval, the optimal number of annual CT scans is unknown as is the optimal screening interval. **(3) Overdiagnosis:** After 6.4 years of post-screening observation, there were more lung cancers in the NLST CT cohort than the chest radiography cohort (1089 and 969, respectively). Since the groups were randomized and well matched, lung cancer incidence should have been identical. Therefore, 18.5% of the lung cancers detected by CT remained clinically silent and invisible on chest radiograph for 6.4 years. Many, perhaps most, of these lung cancers will never cause clinical disease and represent overdiagnosis. **(4) Cost effectiveness:** The number needed to screen with three annual chest CT scans to prevent one death from lung cancer was 320.

Given the level of evidence from US studies showing benefit, the US Preventive Services Task Force has been recommending screening with low-dose chest CT in high-risk individuals since late 2013. There is no evidence of benefit in a mixed population screened with chest radiography.

Infante M et al. Lung cancer screening with low-dose spiral computed tomography: evidence from a pooled analysis of two Italian randomized trials. Eur J Cancer Prev. 2017 Jul; 26(4):324–29. [PMID: 27222939]

Pinsky PF et al. Nodules in the National Lung Screening Trial. AJR Am J Roentgenol. 2017 Nov;209(5):1009–14. [PMID: 28898131]

Ruparel M et al. Pulmonary nodules and CT screening: the past, present and future. Thorax. 2016 Apr;71(4):367–75. [PMID: 26921304]

Tanoue LT. Lung cancer screening. Curr Opin Pulm Med. 2016 Jul;22(4):327–35. [PMID: 27159896]

SOLITARY PULMONARY NODULE

A solitary pulmonary nodule, sometimes referred to as a "coin lesion," is a less-than-3-cm isolated, rounded opacity on chest imaging outlined by normal lung and not associated with infiltrate, atelectasis, or adenopathy. Most are asymptomatic and represent an unexpected finding on chest radiography or CT scanning. The finding is important because it carries a significant risk of malignancy. The frequency of malignancy in surgical series ranges from 10% to 68% depending on patient population. Benign neoplasms, such as hamartomas, account for less than 5% of solitary nodules. Most benign nodules are infectious granulomas.

The goals of evaluation are to identify and resect malignant tumors in patients who will benefit from resection while avoiding invasive procedures in benign disease. The task is to identify nodules with a sufficiently high probability of malignancy to warrant biopsy or resection or a sufficiently low probability of malignancy to justify observation.

Symptoms alone rarely establish the cause, but clinical and imaging data can be used to assess the probability of malignancy. Malignant nodules are rare in persons under age 30. Above age 30, the likelihood of malignancy increases with age. Smokers are at increased risk, and the likelihood of malignancy increases with the number of cigarettes smoked daily. Patients with a prior malignancy have a higher likelihood of having a malignant solitary nodule.

The first and most important step in the imaging evaluation is to review old imaging studies. Comparison with prior studies allows estimation of doubling time, which is an important marker for malignancy. Rapid progression (doubling time less than 30 days) suggests infection, while long-term stability (doubling time greater than 465 days) suggests benignity. Certain radiographic features help in estimating the probability of malignancy. Size is correlated with malignancy. A study of solitary nodules identified by CT scan showed a 1% malignancy rate in those measuring 2–5 mm, and 24% in 6–10 mm, 33% in 11–20 mm, and 80% in 21–45 mm nodules. The appearance of a smooth, well-defined edge is characteristic of a benign process. Ill-defined margins or a lobular appearance suggest malignancy. A high-resolution CT finding of spiculated margins and a peripheral halo are both highly associated with malignancy. Calcification and its pattern are also helpful clues. Benign lesions tend to have dense calcification in a central or laminated pattern. Malignant lesions are associated with sparser calcification that is typically stippled or eccentric. Cavitary lesions with thick (greater than 16 mm) walls are much more likely to be malignant. High-resolution CT offers better resolution of these characteristics than chest radiography and is more likely to detect lymphadenopathy or the presence of multiple lesions. Chest CT is indicated for any suspicious solitary pulmonary nodule.

▶ Treatment

Based on clinical and radiologic data, the clinician should assign a specific probability of malignancy to the lesion. The decision whether to recommend a biopsy or surgical excision depends on the interpretation of this probability in light of the patient's unique clinical situation. The probabilities in parentheses below represent guidelines only and should not be interpreted as prescriptive.

In the case of solitary pulmonary nodules, a continuous probability function may be grouped into three categories. In patients with a **low probability (less than 5%) of malignancy** (eg, age under 30, lesions stable for more than 2 years, characteristic pattern of benign calcification), watchful waiting is appropriate. Management consists of serial imaging studies (CT scans or chest radiographs) at intervals that could identify growth suggestive of malignancy. Three-dimensional reconstruction of high-resolution CT images provides a more sensitive test for growth.

Patients with a **high probability (greater than 60%) of malignancy** should proceed directly to resection following staging, provided the surgical risk is acceptable. Biopsies rarely yield a specific benign diagnosis and are not indicated.

Optimal management of patients with an **intermediate probability of malignancy (5–60%)** remains controversial. The traditional approach is to obtain a diagnostic biopsy, either through transthoracic needle aspiration (TTNA) or bronchoscopy. Bronchoscopy yields a diagnosis in 10–80% of procedures depending on the size of the nodule and its location. In general, the bronchoscopic yield for nodules that are less than 2 cm and peripheral is low, although complications are generally rare. Newer bronchoscopic modalities, such as electromagnetic navigation and ultrathin bronchoscopy are being studied, although their impact upon diagnostic yield remains uncertain. TTNA has a higher diagnostic yield, reported to be between 50% and 97%. The yield is strongly operator-dependent, however, and is affected by the location and size of the lesion. Complications are higher than bronchoscopy, with pneumothorax occurring in up to 30% of patients, with up to one-third of these patients requiring placement of a chest tube.

Disappointing diagnostic yields and a high false-negative rate (up to 20–30% in TTNA) have prompted alternative approaches. **Positron emission tomography (PET)** detects increased glucose metabolism within malignant lesions with high sensitivity (85–97%) and specificity (70–85%). Many diagnostic algorithms have incorporated PET into the assessment of patients with inconclusive high-resolution CT findings. A positive PET increases the likelihood of malignancy, and a negative PET correctly excludes cancer in most cases. False-negative PET scans can occur with tumors with low metabolic activity (most notably, carcinoid tumors and adenocarcinomas, particularly minimally invasive or in situ adenocarcinomas), and follow-up CT imaging is typically performed at discrete intervals to ensure absence of growth. PET has several drawbacks, however: resolution below 1 cm is poor, the test is expensive, and availability remains limited.

Sputum cytology is highly specific but lacks sensitivity. It is used in central lesions and in patients who are poor candidates for invasive diagnostic procedures.

Some centers recommend **video-assisted thoracoscopic surgery (VATS)** resection of all solitary pulmonary nodules with intermediate probability of malignancy. In some cases, the surgeon will remove the nodule and evaluate it in the operating room with frozen section. If the nodule is malignant, he or she will proceed to lobectomy and lymph node sampling, either thoracoscopically or through conversion to standard thoracotomy. This approach is less common when PET scanning is available.

All patients should be provided with an estimate of the likelihood of malignancy, and their preferences should be used to help guide diagnostic and therapeutic decisions. A strategy that recommends observation may not be preferred by a patient who desires a definitive diagnosis. Similarly, a surgical approach may not be agreeable to all patients unless the presence of cancer is definitive. Patient preferences should be elicited, and patients should be well informed regarding the specific risks and benefits associated with the recommended approach as well as the alternative strategies.

Alpert JB et al. Imaging the solitary pulmonary nodule. Clin Chest Med. 2015 Jun;36(2):161–78. [PMID: 26024598]

Dobbins JT 3rd et al. Multi-institutional evaluation of digital tomosynthesis, dual-energy radiography, and conventional chest radiography for the detection and management of pulmonary nodules. Radiology. 2017 Jan;282(1):236–50. [PMID: 27439324]

MacMahon H et al. Guidelines for management of incidental pulmonary nodules detected on CT images: from the Fleischner Society 2017. Radiology. 2017 Jul;284(1):228–43. [PMID: 28240562]

Ruparel M et al. Pulmonary nodules and CT screening: the past, present and future. Thorax. 2016 Apr;71(4):367–75. [PMID: 26921304]

RIGHT MIDDLE LOBE SYNDROME

Right middle lobe syndrome is recurrent or persistent atelectasis of the right middle lobe. This collapse is related to the relatively long length and narrow diameter of the right middle lobe bronchus and the oval ("fish mouth") opening to the lobe, in the setting of impaired collateral ventilation. Fiberoptic bronchoscopy or CT scan is often necessary to rule out obstructing tumor. Foreign body or other benign causes are common.

BRONCHIAL CARCINOID TUMORS

Carcinoid and bronchial gland tumors are sometimes termed "bronchial adenomas." This term should be avoided because it implies that the lesions are benign when, in fact, carcinoid tumors and bronchial gland carcinomas are low-grade malignant neoplasms.

Carcinoid tumors are about six times more common than bronchial gland carcinomas, and most of them occur as pedunculated or sessile growths in central bronchi. Men and women are equally affected. Most patients are under 60 years of age. Common symptoms of bronchial carcinoid tumors are hemoptysis, cough, focal wheezing, and recurrent pneumonia. Peripherally located bronchial carcinoid tumors are rare and present as asymptomatic solitary pulmonary nodules. **Carcinoid syndrome** (flushing, diarrhea, wheezing, hypotension) is rare. Fiberoptic bronchoscopy may reveal a pink or purple tumor in a central airway. These lesions have a well-vascularized stroma, and biopsy may be complicated by significant bleeding. CT scanning is helpful to localize the lesion and to follow its growth over time. Octreotide scintigraphy is also available for localization of these tumors.

Bronchial carcinoid tumors grow slowly and rarely metastasize. Complications involve bleeding and airway obstruction rather than invasion by tumor and metastases. Surgical excision of clinically symptomatic lesions is often necessary, and the prognosis is generally favorable. Most bronchial carcinoid tumors are resistant to radiation and chemotherapy (see Chapter 39).

Caplin ME et al; ENETS consensus conference participants. Pulmonary neuroendocrine (carcinoid) tumors: European Neuroendocrine Tumor Society expert consensus and recommendations for best practice for typical and atypical pulmonary carcinoids. Ann Oncol. 2015 Aug;26(8):1604–20. [PMID: 25646366]

Pusceddu S et al. Diagnosis and management of typical and atypical lung carcinoids. Crit Rev Oncol Hematol. 2016 Apr; 100:167–76. [PMID: 26917456]

Reuling EMBP et al. Endobronchial treatment for bronchial carcinoid: patient selection and predictors of outcome. Respiration. 2018;95(4):220–7. [PMID: 29433123]

MEDIASTINAL MASSES

Various developmental, neoplastic, infectious, traumatic, and cardiovascular disorders may cause masses that appear in the mediastinum on chest radiograph. A useful convention arbitrarily divides the mediastinum into three compartments—anterior, middle, and posterior—in order to classify mediastinal masses and assist in differential diagnosis. Specific mediastinal masses have a predilection for one or more of these compartments; most are located in the anterior or middle compartment. The differential diagnosis of an **anterior mediastinal mass** includes thymoma, teratoma, thyroid lesions, lymphoma, and mesenchymal tumors (lipoma, fibroma). The differential diagnosis of a **middle mediastinal mass** includes lymphadenopathy, pulmonary artery enlargement, aneurysm of the aorta or innominate artery, developmental cyst (bronchogenic, enteric, pleuropericardial), dilated azygous or hemiazygous vein, and foramen of Morgagni hernia. The differential diagnosis of a **posterior mediastinal mass** includes hiatal hernia, neurogenic tumor, meningocele, esophageal tumor, foramen of Bochdalek hernia, thoracic spine disease, and extramedullary hematopoiesis. The neurogenic tumor group includes neurilemmoma, neurofibroma, neurosarcoma, ganglioneuroma, and pheochromocytoma.

Symptoms and signs of mediastinal masses are nonspecific and are usually caused by the effects of the mass on surrounding structures. Insidious onset of retrosternal chest pain, dysphagia, or dyspnea is often an important clue to the presence of a mediastinal mass. In about half of cases, symptoms are absent, and the mass is detected on routine chest radiograph. Physical findings vary depending on the nature and location of the mass.

CT scanning is helpful in management; additional radiographic studies of benefit include barium swallow if esophageal disease is suspected, Doppler sonography or venography of brachiocephalic veins and the superior vena cava, and angiography. MRI is useful; its advantages include better delineation of hilar structures and distinction between vessels and masses. MRI also allows imaging in multiple planes, whereas CT permits only axial imaging. Tissue diagnosis is necessary if a neoplastic disorder is suspected. Treatment and prognosis depend on the underlying cause of the mediastinal mass.

Azizad S et al. Solid tumors of the mediastinum in adults. Semin Ultrasound CT MR. 2016 Jun;37(3):196–211. [PMID: 27261345]

Carter BW et al. MR imaging of mediastinal masses. Top Magn Reson Imaging. 2017 Aug;26(4):153–65. [PMID: 28777164]

Sakka D et al. Mediastinal masses: clinical, radiological and pathological analysis. Eur Respir J. 2018;52 (Suppl 62):PA2579.

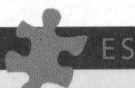

INTERSTITIAL LUNG DISEASE
(Diffuse Parenchymal Lung Disease)

ESSENTIALS OF DIAGNOSIS

▸ Insidious onset of progressive dyspnea and non-productive chronic cough; extrapulmonary findings may accompany specific diagnoses.

▸ Tachypnea, small lung volumes, bibasilar dry rales; digital clubbing and right heart failure with advanced disease.

▸ Chest radiographs with low lung volumes and patchy distribution of ground glass, reticular, nodular, reticulonodular, or cystic opacities.

▸ Reduced lung volumes, pulmonary diffusing capacity and 6-minute walk distance; hypoxemia with exercise.

Table 9–16. Differential diagnosis of interstitial lung disease (listed alphabetically within category).

Medication-related
    Antiarrhythmic agents (amiodarone)
    Antibacterial agents (nitrofurantoin, sulfonamides)
    Antineoplastic agents (bleomycin, cyclophosphamide, methotrexate, nitrosoureas)
    Antirheumatic agents (gold salts, penicillamine)
    Phenytoin
Environmental and occupational (inhalation exposures)
    Dust, inorganic (asbestos, silica, hard metals, beryllium)
    Dust, organic (thermophilic actinomycetes, avian antigens, *Aspergillus* species)
    Gases, fumes, and vapors (chlorine, isocyanates, paraquat, sulfur dioxide)
    Ionizing radiation
    Talc (injection drug users)
Infections
    Fungus, disseminated (*Coccidioides immitis, Blastomyces dermatitidis, Histoplasma capsulatum*)
    Mycobacteria, disseminated
    Pneumocystis jirovecii
    Viruses
Primary pulmonary disorders
    Cryptogenic organizing pneumonia
    Idiopathic interstitial pneumonia: acute interstitial pneumonia, desquamative interstitial pneumonia, nonspecific interstitial pneumonia,
       usual interstitial pneumonia, respiratory bronchiolitis-associated interstitial lung disease
    Pulmonary alveolar proteinosis
Systemic disorders
    Acute respiratory distress syndrome
    Amyloidosis
    Ankylosing spondylitis
    Autoimmune disease: dermatomyositis, polymyositis, rheumatoid arthritis, systemic sclerosis (scleroderma), systemic lupus erythematosus
    Chronic eosinophilic pneumonia
    Goodpasture syndrome
    Idiopathic pulmonary hemosiderosis
    Inflammatory bowel disease
    Langerhans cell histiocytosis (eosinophilic granuloma)
    Lymphangitic spread of cancer (lymphangitic carcinomatosis)
    Lymphangioleiomyomatosis
    Pulmonary edema
    Pulmonary venous hypertension, chronic
    Sarcoidosis
    Granulomatosis polyangiitis (formerly Wegener granulomatosis)

Interstitial lung disease, or diffuse parenchymal lung disease, comprises a heterogeneous group of disorders that share common presentations (dyspnea), physical findings (late inspiratory crackles), and chest radiographs (septal thickening and reticulonodular changes).

The term "interstitial" is misleading since the pathologic process usually begins with injury to the alveolar epithelial or capillary endothelial cells (alveolitis). Persistent alveolitis may lead to obliteration of alveolar capillaries and reorganization of the lung parenchyma, accompanied by irreversible fibrosis. The process does not affect the airways proximal to the respiratory bronchioles. At least 180 disease entities may present as interstitial lung disease. Table 9–16 outlines a selected list of differential diagnoses of interstitial lung disease. In most patients, no specific cause can be identified. In the remainder, medications, a variety of organic and inorganic dusts, and connective tissue disease are the principal causes. The history—particularly the occupational and medication history—may provide evidence of a specific cause.

The presence of diffuse parenchymal lung disease in the setting of an established connective tissue disease, such as rheumatoid arthritis, systemic lupus erythematosus, scleroderma, polymyositis-dermatomyositis, Sjögren syndrome, and other overlap conditions, is suggestive of the etiology. In some cases, lung disease precedes the more typical manifestations of the underlying connective tissue disease by months or years.

Known causes of interstitial lung disease are dealt with in their specific sections. The important idiopathic forms are discussed below.

DIFFUSE INTERSTITIAL PNEUMONIAS

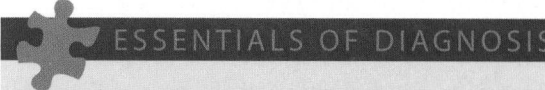

ESSENTIALS OF DIAGNOSIS

▶ Important to identify specific fibrosing disorders.

▶ Idiopathic disease may require biopsy for diagnosis.

▶ Accurate diagnosis identifies patients most likely to benefit from therapy.

General Considerations

The most common diagnosis among patients with diffuse interstitial lung disease is one of the interstitial pneumonias, including all the entities described in Table 9–17. Historically, a diagnosis of interstitial lung disease was based on clinical and radiographic criteria with only a small number of patients undergoing surgical lung biopsy. When biopsies were obtained, the common element of fibrosis led to the grouping together of several histologic patterns under the category of interstitial pneumonia or idiopathic pulmonary fibrosis (IPF). Distinct histopathologic features are now understood to represent different natural histories and responses to therapy (Table 9–17). Therefore, in the evaluation of patients with diffuse interstitial lung disease, clinicians should attempt to identify specific disorders.

Patients with diffuse interstitial pneumonia may have any of the histologic patterns described in Table 9–17. The first step in evaluation is to identify patients whose disease is truly idiopathic. As indicated in Table 9–16, most identifiable causes of diffuse interstitial pneumonia are medication-related, environmental or occupational agent exposure, or infectious. Interstitial lung diseases associated with other systemic disorders (pulmonary renal syndromes, autoimmune disease) may be identified through a careful medical history. Apart from acute interstitial pneumonia, the clinical presentations of the diffuse interstitial pneumonias are sufficiently similar to preclude a specific diagnosis. Chest radiographs and high-resolution CT scans are diagnostic in some patients. Ultimately, many patients with apparently idiopathic disease require surgical lung biopsy to make a definitive diagnosis. The importance of accurate diagnosis is twofold. First, it allows the clinician to provide accurate information about the cause and natural history of the illness. Second, accurate diagnosis helps distinguish patients most likely to benefit from therapy.

Clinical Findings

A. Symptoms, Signs, and Imaging

The most common of the diffuse interstitial pneumonias is pulmonary fibrosis associated with the histopathologic pattern of **usual interstitial pneumonia (UIP).** When no associated cause is evident, this is **IPF.** A diagnosis of IPF/UIP can be made with 90% confidence in patients over 65 years of age who have (1) idiopathic disease by history and inspiratory crackles on physical examination (2) restrictive physiology on pulmonary function testing; (3) characteristic radiographic evidence of progressive fibrosis over several years; and (4) diffuse, patchy fibrosis with pleural-based honeycombing on high-resolution CT scan (Figure 9–6). Such patients do not need surgical lung biopsy.

B. Special Studies

Three diagnostic techniques are in common use: BAL, transbronchial biopsy, and surgical lung biopsy, either through an open procedure or using VATS.

BAL may provide a specific diagnosis in cases of infection, particularly with *P jirovecii* or mycobacteria, or when cytologic examination reveals the presence of malignant cells. The findings may be suggestive and sometimes diagnostic of eosinophilic pneumonia, Langerhans cell histiocytosis, or alveolar proteinosis.

Transbronchial biopsy through the flexible bronchoscope is easily performed in most patients. The risks of pneumothorax (5%) and hemorrhage (1–10%) are low. However, the tissue specimens recovered are small, sampling error is common, and crush artifact may complicate diagnosis. Transbronchial biopsy can make a definitive diagnosis of sarcoidosis, lymphangitic spread of carcinoma, pulmonary alveolar proteinosis, miliary tuberculosis, and Langerhans cell histiocytosis. Note that the diagnosis of IPF cannot be confirmed on transbronchial lung biopsy since the histologic diagnosis requires a pattern of changes rather than a single pathognomonic finding. Transbronchial biopsy may exclude IPF by confirming a specific alternative diagnosis. Transbronchial biopsy also cannot establish a specific diagnosis of idiopathic interstitial pneumonia. These patients generally require surgical lung biopsy.

Surgical lung biopsy is the standard for diagnosis of diffuse interstitial lung disease. Two or three biopsies taken from multiple sites in the same lung, including apparently normal tissue, may yield a specific diagnosis as well as prognostic information regarding the extent of fibrosis versus active inflammation. Patients under age 60 without a specific diagnosis generally should undergo surgical lung biopsy. In older and sicker patients, the risks and benefits must be weighed carefully for three reasons: (1) the morbidity of the procedure can be significant; (2) a definitive diagnosis may not be possible even with surgical lung biopsy; and (3) when a specific diagnosis is made, there may be no effective treatment. Empiric therapy or no treatment may be preferable to surgical lung biopsy in some patients.

Treatment

Patients with diffuse interstitial pneumonia should be treated by a pulmonologist. Clinical experience suggests that patients with RB-ILD, nonspecific interstitial pneumonia (NSIP), or COP (Table 9–17) frequently respond to corticosteroids and should be given a trial of therapy—typically prednisone, 1–2 mg/kg/day for a minimum of 2 months. The same therapy is ineffective in patients with IPF. Since this therapy carries significant morbidity, experts do not recommend routine use of corticosteroids in patients with IPF. Nintedanib and pirfenidone are approved for the treatment of IPF based on controlled trials in highly selected patients showing a significant reduction in their rate of decline in lung function. Neither agent improved survival or quality of life compared with no treatment, however. The only definitive treatment for IPF is lung transplantation, with a 5-year survival rate estimated at 50%.

When to Refer

Patients with diffuse interstitial pneumonia should be referred early to a pulmonologist for expert diagnosis and management. Patients with IPF should be referred early to a lung transplant program for evaluation.

Table 9–17. Idiopathic interstitial pneumonias.

Name and Clinical Presentation	Histopathology	Radiographic Pattern	Response to Therapy and Prognosis
Usual interstitial pneumonia (UIP)[1] Age 55–60, slight male predominance. Insidious dry cough and dyspnea lasting months to years. Clubbing present at diagnosis in 25–50%. Diffuse fine late inspiratory crackles on lung auscultation. Restrictive ventilatory defect and reduced diffusing capacity on pulmonary function tests. ANA and RF positive in ~25% in the absence of documented collagen-vascular disease.	Patchy, temporally and geographically nonuniform distribution of fibrosis, honeycomb change, and normal lung. Type I pneumocytes are lost, and there is proliferation of alveolar type II cells. "Fibroblast foci" of actively proliferating fibroblasts and myofibroblasts. Inflammation is generally mild and consists of small lymphocytes. Intra-alveolar macrophage accumulation is present but is not a prominent feature.	Diminished lung volume. Increased linear or reticular bibasilar and subpleural opacities. Unilateral disease is rare. High-resolution CT scanning shows minimal ground-glass and variable honeycomb change. Areas of normal lung may be adjacent to areas of advanced fibrosis. Between 2% and 10% have normal chest radiographs and high-resolution CT scans on diagnosis.	No randomized study has demonstrated improved survival compared with untreated patients. Inexorably progressive. Median survival approximately 3 years, depending on stage at presentation. Nintedanib and pirfenidone reduce rate of decline in lung function.
Respiratory bronchiolitis-associated interstitial lung disease (RB-ILD)[1] Age 40–45. Presentation similar to that of UIP though in younger patients. Similar results on pulmonary function tests, but less severe abnormalities. Patients with respiratory bronchiolitis are invariably heavy smokers.	Increased numbers of macrophages evenly dispersed within the alveolar spaces. Rare fibroblast foci, little fibrosis, minimal honeycomb change. In RB-ILD the accumulation of macrophages is localized within the peribronchiolar air spaces; in DIP[1], it is diffuse. Alveolar architecture is preserved.	May be indistinguishable from UIP. More often presents with a nodular or reticulonodular pattern. Honeycombing rare. High-resolution CT more likely to reveal diffuse ground-glass opacities and upper lobe emphysema.	Spontaneous remission occurs in up to 20% of patients, so natural history unclear. Smoking cessation is essential. Prognosis clearly better than that of UIP: median survival greater than 10 years. Corticosteroids thought to be effective, but there are no randomized clinical trials to support this view.
Acute interstitial pneumonia (AIP) Clinically known as Hamman-Rich syndrome. Wide age range, many young patients. Acute onset of dyspnea followed by rapid development of respiratory failure. Half of patients report a viral syndrome preceding lung disease. Clinical course indistinguishable from that of idiopathic ARDS.	Pathologic changes reflect acute response to injury within days to weeks. Resembles organizing phase of diffuse alveolar damage. Fibrosis and minimal collagen deposition. May appear similar to UIP but more homogeneous and there is no honeycomb change—though this may appear if the process persists for more than a month in a patient on mechanical ventilation.	Diffuse bilateral airspace consolidation with areas of ground-glass attenuation on high-resolution CT scan.	Supportive care (mechanical ventilation) critical but effect of specific therapies unclear. High initial mortality: 50–90% die within 2 months after diagnosis. Not progressive if patient survives. Lung function may return to normal or may be permanently impaired.
Nonspecific interstitial pneumonia (NSIP) Age 45–55. Slight female predominance. Similar to UIP but onset of cough and dyspnea over months, not years.	Nonspecific in that histopathology does not fit into better-established categories. Varying degrees of inflammation and fibrosis, patchy in distribution but uniform in time, suggesting response to single injury. Most have lymphocytic and plasma cell inflammation without fibrosis. Honeycombing present but scant. Some have advocated division into cellular and fibrotic subtypes.	May be indistinguishable from UIP. Most typical picture is bilateral areas of ground-glass attenuation and fibrosis on high-resolution CT. Honeycombing is rare.	Treatment thought to be effective, but no prospective clinical studies have been published. Prognosis overall good but depends on the extent of fibrosis at diagnosis. Median survival greater than 10 years.
Cryptogenic organizing pneumonia (COP; formerly bronchiolitis obliterans organizing pneumonia [BOOP]) Typically age 50–60 but wide variation. Abrupt onset, frequently weeks to a few months following a flu-like illness. Dyspnea and dry cough prominent, but constitutional symptoms are common: fatigue, fever, and weight loss. Pulmonary function tests usually show restriction, but up to 25% show concomitant obstruction.	Included in the idiopathic interstitial pneumonias on clinical grounds. Buds of loose connective tissue (Masson bodies) and inflammatory cells fill alveoli and distal bronchioles.	Lung volumes normal. Chest radiograph typically shows interstitial and parenchymal disease with discrete, peripheral alveolar and ground-glass infiltrates. Nodular opacities common. High-resolution CT shows subpleural consolidation and bronchial wall thickening and dilation.	Rapid response to corticosteroids in two-thirds of patients. Long-term prognosis generally good for those who respond. Relapses are common.

[1]Includes desquamative interstitial pneumonia (DIP).
ANA, antinuclear antibody; ARDS, acute respiratory distress syndrome; RF, rheumatoid factor; UIP, usual interstitial pneumonia.

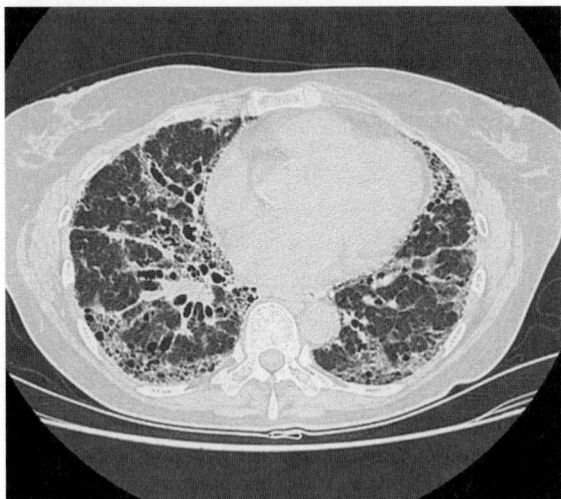

▲ **Figure 9–6.** Idiopathic pulmonary fibrosis. CT scan of the lungs showing the typical radiographic pattern of idiopathic pulmonary fibrosis, with a predominantly basilar, peripheral pattern of traction bronchiectasis, reticulation, and early honeycombing.

Barratt SL et al. Idiopathic pulmonary fibrosis (IPF): an overview. J Clin Med. 2018 Aug 6;7(8). [Epub ahead of print] [PMID: 30082599]

Lederer DJ et al. Idiopathic pulmonary fibrosis. N Engl J Med. 2018 May 10;378(19):1811–23. [PMID: 29742380]

Sverzellati N et al. American Thoracic Society-European Respiratory Society classification of the idiopathic interstitial pneumonias: advances in knowledge since 2002. Radiographics. 2015 Nov–Dec;35(7):1849–71. [PMID: 26452110]

SARCOIDOSIS

ESSENTIALS OF DIAGNOSIS

► Symptoms related to the lung, skin, eyes, peripheral nerves, liver, kidney, heart, and other tissues.

► Demonstration of noncaseating granulomas in a biopsy specimen.

► Exclusion of other granulomatous disorders.

▶ General Considerations

Sarcoidosis is a systemic disease of unknown etiology characterized in about 90% of patients by granulomatous inflammation of the lung. The incidence is highest in North American blacks and northern European whites; among blacks, women are more frequently affected than men. Onset of disease is usually in the third or fourth decade.

▶ Clinical Findings

A. Symptoms and Signs

Patients may have malaise, fever, and dyspnea of insidious onset. Symptoms from skin involvement (erythema

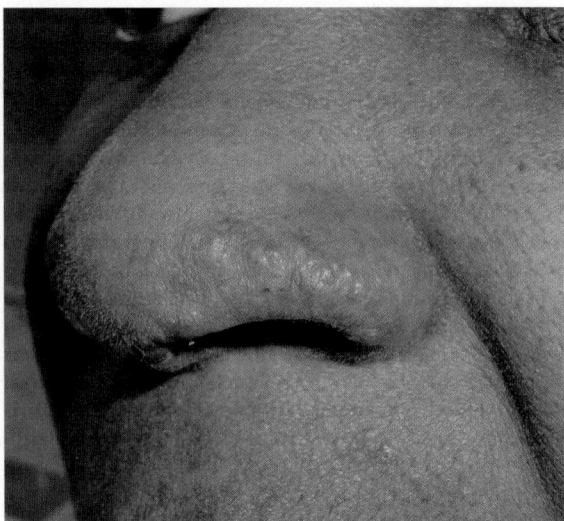

▲ **Figure 9–7.** Skin involvement in sarcoidosis (lupus pernio), here involving the nasal rim. (Used, with permission, from Richard P. Usatine, MD, in Usatine RP, Smith MA, Mayeaux EJ Jr, Chumley H, Tysinger J. *The Color Atlas of Family Medicine.* McGraw-Hill, 2009.)

nodosum, lupus pernio [Figure 9–7]), iritis, peripheral neuropathy, arthritis (Chapter 20), or cardiomyopathy may also cause the patient to seek care. Some individuals are asymptomatic and come to medical attention after abnormal findings (typically bilateral hilar and right paratracheal lymphadenopathy) on chest radiographs. Physical findings are atypical of interstitial lung disease in that crackles are uncommon on chest examination. Other symptoms and findings may include parotid gland enlargement, hepatosplenomegaly, and lymphadenopathy.

B. Laboratory Findings

Laboratory tests may show leukopenia, an elevated erythrocyte sedimentation rate, and hypercalcemia (about 5% of patients) or hypercalciuria (20%). Angiotensin-converting enzyme (ACE) levels are elevated in 40–80% of patients with active disease. This finding is neither sensitive nor specific enough to have diagnostic significance. Physiologic testing may reveal evidence of airflow obstruction, but restrictive changes with decreased lung volumes and diffusing capacity are more common. Skin test anergy is present in 70%. ECG may show conduction disturbances and dysrhythmias.

C. Imaging

Radiographic findings are variable and include bilateral hilar adenopathy alone (radiographic stage I), hilar adenopathy and parenchymal involvement (radiographic stage II), or parenchymal involvement alone (radiographic stage III). Parenchymal involvement is usually manifested radiographically by diffuse reticular infiltrates, but focal infiltrates, acinar shadows, nodules, and, rarely, cavitation may be seen. Pleural effusion is noted in less than 10% of patients. Stage IV disease refers to advanced fibrotic changes principally in the upper lobes.

D. Special Examinations

The diagnosis of sarcoidosis generally requires histologic demonstration of noncaseating granulomas in biopsies from a patient with other typical associated manifestations. Other granulomatous diseases (eg, berylliosis, tuberculosis, fungal infections) and lymphoma must be excluded. Biopsy of easily accessible sites (eg, palpable lymph nodes, skin lesions, or salivary glands) is likely to be positive. Transbronchial lung biopsy has a high yield (75–90%) as well, especially in patients with radiographic evidence of parenchymal involvement. Some clinicians believe that tissue biopsy is not necessary when stage I radiographic findings are detected in a clinical situation that strongly favors the diagnosis of sarcoidosis (eg, a young black woman with erythema nodosum). Biopsy is essential whenever clinical and radiographic findings suggest the possibility of an alternative diagnosis, such as lymphoma. BAL fluid in sarcoidosis is usually characterized by an increase in lymphocytes and a high CD4/CD8 cell ratio. BAL does not establish a diagnosis but may be useful in following the activity of sarcoidosis in selected patients. All patients require a complete ophthalmologic evaluation.

▶ Treatment

Indications for treatment with oral corticosteroids (prednisone, 0.5–1.0 mg/kg/day) include disabling constitutional symptoms, hypercalcemia, iritis, uveitis, arthritis, central nervous system involvement, cardiac involvement, granulomatous hepatitis, cutaneous lesions other than erythema nodosum, and progressive pulmonary lesions. Long-term therapy is usually required over months to years. Immunosuppressive medications, most commonly methotrexate, azathioprine, or infliximab, are used in patients who are intolerant of corticosteroids or who have corticosteroid-refractory disease, but sound clinical research to support specific agents is lacking.

▶ Prognosis

The outlook is best for patients with hilar adenopathy alone; radiographic involvement of the lung parenchyma is associated with a worse prognosis. Erythema nodosum portends a good outcome. About 20% of patients with lung involvement suffer irreversible lung impairment, characterized by progressive fibrosis, bronchiectasis, and cavitation. Pneumothorax, hemoptysis, mycetoma formation in lung cavities, and respiratory failure often complicate this advanced stage. Myocardial sarcoidosis occurs in about 5% of patients, sometimes leading to restrictive cardiomyopathy, cardiac dysrhythmias, and conduction disturbances. Death from respiratory insufficiency occurs in about 5% of patients.

Patients require long-term follow-up: at a minimum, yearly physical examination, pulmonary function tests, chemistry panel, ophthalmologic evaluation, chest radiograph, and ECG.

Baughman RP et al. New treatment strategies for pulmonary sarcoidosis: antimetabolites, biological drugs, and other treatment approaches. Lancet Respir Med. 2015 Oct;3(10):813–22. [PMID: 26204816]

Birnie DH et al. Cardiac manifestations of sarcoidosis: diagnosis and management. Eur Heart J. 2017 Sep 14;38(35):2663–70. [PMID: 27469375]
Judson MA. Corticosteroids in sarcoidosis. Rheum Dis Clin North Am. 2016 Feb;42(1):119–35. [PMID: 26611555]
Spagnolo P et al. Pulmonary sarcoidosis. Lancet Respir Med. 2018 May;6(5):389–402. [PMID: 29625772]

PULMONARY ALVEOLAR PROTEINOSIS

Pulmonary alveolar proteinosis is a rare disease in which phospholipids accumulate within alveolar spaces. The condition may be primary (idiopathic) or secondary (occurring in immunodeficiency; hematologic malignancies; inhalation of mineral dusts; or following lung infections, including tuberculosis and viral infections). Progressive dyspnea is the usual presenting symptom, and chest radiograph shows bilateral alveolar infiltrates suggestive of pulmonary edema. The diagnosis is based on demonstration of characteristic findings on BAL (milky appearance and PAS-positive lipoproteinaceous material) in association with typical clinical and radiographic features. In secondary disease, an elevated anti-GM-CSF (anti-granulocyte-macrophage colony-stimulating factor) titer in serum or BAL fluid is highly sensitive and specific. In some cases, transbronchial or surgical lung biopsy (revealing amorphous intra-alveolar phospholipid) is necessary.

The course of the disease varies. Some patients experience spontaneous remission; others develop progressive respiratory insufficiency. Pulmonary infection with *Nocardia* or fungi may occur. Therapy for alveolar proteinosis consists of periodic whole-lung lavage. Patients who cannot tolerate whole lung lavage or who fail to respond may benefit from inhalational or subcutaneous GM-CSF.

Kumar A et al. Pulmonary alveolar proteinosis in adults: pathophysiology and clinical approach. Lancet Respir Med. 2018 Jul;6(7):554–65. [PMID: 29397349]
Suzuki T et al. Pulmonary alveolar proteinosis syndrome. Clin Chest Med. 2016 Sep;37(3):431–40. [PMID: 27514590]

EOSINOPHILIC PULMONARY SYNDROMES

Eosinophilic pulmonary syndromes are a diverse group of disorders typically characterized by eosinophilic pulmonary infiltrates, dyspnea, and cough. Many patients have constitutional symptoms, including fever. Common causes include exposure to medications (nitrofurantoin, phenytoin, ampicillin, acetaminophen, ranitidine) or infection with helminths (eg, *Ascaris*, hookworms, *Strongyloides*) or filariae (eg, *Wuchereria bancrofti*, *Brugia malayi*, tropical pulmonary eosinophilia). **Löffler syndrome** refers to acute eosinophilic pulmonary infiltrates in response to transpulmonary passage of helminth larvae. Pulmonary eosinophilia can also be a feature of other illnesses, including allergic bronchopulmonary mycosis, eosinophilic granulomatosis with polyangiitis, systemic hypereosinophilic syndromes, eosinophilic granuloma of the lung (properly referred to as pulmonary Langerhans cell histiocytosis), neoplasms, and numerous interstitial lung diseases. If an extrinsic cause is identified, therapy consists of removal of the offending medication or treatment of the underlying parasitic infection.

One-third of cases are idiopathic, and there are two common syndromes. **Chronic eosinophilic pneumonia** is seen predominantly in women and is characterized by fever, night sweats, weight loss, and dyspnea. Asthma is present in half of cases. Chest radiographs often show peripheral infiltrates, the "photographic negative" of pulmonary edema. BAL typically has a marked eosinophilia; peripheral blood eosinophilia is present in greater than 80%. Therapy with oral prednisone (1 mg/kg/day for 1–2 weeks, followed by a gradual taper over many months) usually results in dramatic improvement; however, most patients require at least 10–15 mg of prednisone every other day for a year or more (sometimes indefinitely) to prevent relapses. **Acute eosinophilic pneumonia** is an acute, febrile illness characterized by cough and dyspnea, sometimes rapidly progressing to respiratory failure. The chest radiograph is abnormal but nonspecific. BAL frequently shows eosinophilia but peripheral blood eosinophilia is rare at the onset of symptoms. The response to corticosteroids is usually dramatic.

Sergew A et al. Current approach to diagnosis and management of pulmonary eosinophilic syndromes: eosinophilic pneumonias, eosinophilic granulomatosis with polyangiitis, and hypereosinophilic syndrome. Semin Respir Crit Care Med. 2016 Jun;37(3):441–56. [PMID: 27231866]

Weissler JC. Eosinophilic lung disease. Am J Med Sci. 2017 Oct; 354(4):339–49. [PMID: 29078837]

DISORDERS OF THE PULMONARY CIRCULATION

PULMONARY VENOUS THROMBOEMBOLISM

ESSENTIALS OF DIAGNOSIS

- ▶ Predisposition to venous thrombosis, usually of the lower extremities.
- ▶ One or more of the following: dyspnea, chest pain, hemoptysis, syncope.
- ▶ Tachypnea and a widened alveolar-arterial P_{O_2} difference.
- ▶ Elevated rapid D-dimer and characteristic defects on CT pulmonary angiography, ventilation-perfusion lung scan, or pulmonary angiogram.

▶ General Considerations

Pulmonary venous thromboembolism, often referred to as pulmonary embolism (PE), is a common, serious, and potentially fatal complication of thrombus formation within the deep venous circulation. PE is the third leading cause of death among hospitalized patients. Despite this prevalence, most cases are not recognized antemortem, and less than 10% of patients with fatal emboli have received specific treatment for the condition. Management demands a vigilant systematic approach to diagnosis and an understanding of risk factors so that appropriate preventive therapy can be given.

Many substances can embolize to the pulmonary circulation, including air (during neurosurgery, from central venous catheters), amniotic fluid (during active labor), fat (long bone fractures), foreign bodies (talc in injection drug users), parasite eggs (schistosomiasis), septic emboli (acute infective endocarditis), and tumor cells (renal cell carcinoma). The most common embolus is thrombus, which may arise anywhere in the venous circulation or heart but most often originates in the deep veins of the lower extremities. Thrombi confined to the calf rarely embolize to the pulmonary circulation. However, about 20% of calf vein thrombi propagate proximally to the popliteal and iliofemoral veins, at which point they may break off and embolize to the pulmonary circulation. Pulmonary emboli will develop in 50–60% of patients with proximal deep venous thrombosis (DVT); half of these embolic events will be asymptomatic. Approximately 50–70% of patients who have symptomatic pulmonary emboli will have lower extremity DVT when evaluated.

PE and DVT are two manifestations of the same disease. The risk factors for PE are the risk factors for thrombus formation within the venous circulation: venous stasis, injury to the vessel wall, and hypercoagulability (Virchow triad). Venous stasis increases with immobility (bed rest—especially postoperative—obesity, stroke), hyperviscosity (polycythemia), and increased central venous pressures (low cardiac output states, pregnancy). Vessels may be damaged by prior episodes of thrombosis, orthopedic surgery, or trauma. Hypercoagulability can be caused by medications (oral contraceptives, hormonal replacement therapy) or disease (malignancy, surgery) or may be the result of inherited gene defects. The most common inherited cause in white populations is resistance to activated protein C, also known as factor V Leiden. The trait is present in approximately 3% of healthy American men and in 20–40% of patients with idiopathic venous thrombosis. Other major risks for hypercoagulability include the following: deficiencies or dysfunction of protein C, protein S, and antithrombin; prothrombin gene mutation; hyperhomocysteinemia and the presence of antiphospholipid antibodies (lupus anticoagulant and anticardiolipin antibody).

PE has multiple physiologic effects. Physical obstruction of the vascular bed and vasoconstriction from neurohumoral reflexes both increase pulmonary vascular resistance. Massive thrombus may cause right ventricular failure. Vascular obstruction increases physiologic dead space (wasted ventilation) and leads to hypoxemia through right-to-left shunting, decreased cardiac output, and surfactant depletion causing atelectasis. Reflex bronchoconstriction promotes wheezing and increased work of breathing.

▶ Clinical Findings

A. Symptoms and Signs

The clinical diagnosis of PE is notoriously difficult for two reasons. First, the clinical findings depend on both the size of the embolus and the patient's preexisting cardiopulmonary status. Second, common symptoms and signs of pulmonary emboli are not specific to this disorder (Table 9–18).

Table 9–18. Frequency of specific symptoms and signs in patients at risk for pulmonary thromboembolism.

	UPET[1] PE+ (n = 327)	PIOPED I[2] PE+ (n = 117)	PIOPED I[2] PE− (n = 248)
Symptoms			
Dyspnea	84%	73%	72%
Respirophasic chest pain	74%	66%	59%
Cough	53%	37%	36%
Leg pain	NR	26%	24%
Hemoptysis	30%	13%	8%
Palpitations	NR	10%	18%
Wheezing	NR	9%	11%
Anginal pain	14%	4%	6%
Signs			
Respiratory rate ≥ 16 UPET, ≥ 20 PIOPED I	92%	70%	68%
Crackles (rales)	58%	51%	40%[3]
Heart rate ≥ 100/min	44%	30%	24%
Fourth heart sound (S_4)	NR	24%	13%[3]
Accentuated pulmonary component of second heart sound (S_2P)	53%	23%	13%[3]
T ≥ 37.5°C UPET, ≥ 38.5°C PIOPED	43%	7%	12%
Homans sign	NR	4%	2%
Pleural friction rub	NR	3%	2%
Third heart sound (S_3)	NR	3%	4%
Cyanosis	19%	1%	2%

[1]Data from the Urokinase-Streptokinase Pulmonary Embolism Trial (UPET), as reported in Bell WR et al. The clinical features of submassive and massive pulmonary emboli. Am J Med. 1977 Mar;62(3):355–60.
[2]Data from patients enrolled in the PIOPED I study, as reported in Stein PD et al. Clinical, laboratory, roentgenographic, and electrocardiographic findings in patients with acute pulmonary embolism and no preexisting cardiac or pulmonary disease. Chest. 1991 Sep; 100(3):598–603.
[3]$P < 0.05$ comparing patients in the PIOPED I study.
PE+, confirmed diagnosis of pulmonary embolism; PE−, diagnosis of pulmonary embolism ruled out; NR, not reported.

Indeed, no single symptom or sign or combination of clinical findings is specific to PE. Some findings are fairly sensitive: dyspnea and pain on inspiration occur in 75–85% and 65–75% of patients, respectively. Tachypnea is the only sign reliably found in more than half of patients. A common clinical strategy is to use combinations of clinical findings to identify patients' risk for PE. For example, 97% of patients in the original Prospective Investigation of Pulmonary Embolism Diagnosis (PIOPED I) study with angiographically proved pulmonary emboli had one or more of three findings: dyspnea, chest pain with breathing, or tachypnea. Wells and colleagues have published and validated a simple clinical decision rule that quantifies and dichotomizes this clinical risk assessment, allowing diversion of patients deemed unlikely to have PE to a simpler diagnostic algorithm (see Integrated Approach to Diagnosis of Pulmonary Embolism).

B. Laboratory Findings

The **ECG** is abnormal in 70% of patients with PE. However, the most common abnormalities are sinus tachycardia and nonspecific ST and T wave changes, each seen in approximately 40% of patients. Five percent or less of patients in the PIOPED I study had P pulmonale, right ventricular hypertrophy, right axis deviation, and right bundle branch block.

Arterial blood gases usually reveal acute respiratory alkalosis due to hyperventilation. The arterial Po_2 and the alveolar-arterial oxygen difference ($A–a–Do_2$) are usually abnormal in patients with PE compared with healthy, age-matched controls. However, arterial blood gases are not diagnostic: among patients who were evaluated in the PIOPED I study; neither the Po_2 nor the $A–a–Do_2$ differentiated between those with and those without pulmonary emboli. Profound hypoxia with a normal chest radiograph in the absence of preexisting lung disease is highly suspicious for PE.

Plasma levels of **D-dimer,** a degradation product of cross-linked fibrin, are elevated in the presence of thrombus. Its value is as a diagnostic tool to exclude PE. Using a D-dimer threshold between 300 and 500 ng/mL (300 and 500 mcg/L), a rapid quantitative enzyme-linked immunosorbent assay (ELISA) has shown a sensitivity for venous thromboembolism of 95–97% and a specificity of 45%. Therefore, a D-dimer less than 500 ng/mL (less than 500 mcg/L) using a rapid quantitative ELISA provides strong evidence against venous thromboembolism, with a likelihood ratio of 0.11–0.13. D-dimer, is not useful in the hospital setting.

Serum troponin I, troponin T, and plasma B-type natriuretic peptide (BNP) levels are typically higher in patients with PE compared with those without embolism; the presence and magnitude of the elevation are not useful in diagnosis, but correlate with adverse outcomes, including mechanical ventilation, prolonged hospitalization, and death.

C. Imaging and Special Examinations

1. Chest radiography—The chest radiograph is necessary to exclude other common lung diseases and to permit interpretation of the ventilation-perfusion ($\dot{V}/\dot{Q}$) scan, but it does not establish the diagnosis by itself. The chest radiograph was normal in only 12% of patients with confirmed PE in the PIOPED I study. The most frequent findings were atelectasis, parenchymal infiltrates, and pleural effusions. However, the prevalence of these findings was the same in hospitalized patients without PE. A prominent central pulmonary artery with local oligemia (Westermark sign) or pleural-based areas of increased opacity that represent intraparenchymal hemorrhage (Hampton hump) are uncommon. Paradoxically, the chest radiograph may be most suggestive of PE when normal in the setting of hypoxemia.

2. CT-pulmonary angiography (PA)—Helical CT-PA is used as the initial diagnostic study in North America for suspected PE. CT-PA requires administration of intravenous radiocontrast dye but is otherwise noninvasive. A high-quality study is very sensitive for the detection of thrombus in the proximal pulmonary arteries. Comparing CT-PA to the $\dot{V}/\dot{Q}$ scan as the initial test for PE, detection of thrombi is roughly comparable, although more alternative pulmonary diagnoses are made with CT-PA scanning.

Test characteristics of CT-PA vary widely by study and facility. Factors influencing results include patient size and cooperation, the type and quality of the scanner, the imaging protocol, and the experience of the interpreting radiologist. The 2006 PIOPED II study, using multi-detector (four-row) helical CT and excluding the 6% of patients whose studies were "inconclusive," reported sensitivity of 83% and specificity of 96%.

A 15–20% false-negative rate is high for a screening test, and raises the practical question whether it is safe to withhold anticoagulation in patients with a negative CT-PA. Research data provide two complementary answers. The insight of PIOPED I, that the clinical assessment of pretest probability improves the performance of the $\dot{V}/\dot{Q}$ scan, was confirmed with CT-PA in PIOPED II, where positive and negative predictive values were highest in patients with concordant clinical assessments but poor with conflicting assessments. The negative predictive value of a normal CT-PA in patients with a high pretest probability was only 60%. Therefore, a normal CT-PA alone does not exclude PE in high-risk patients, and either empiric therapy or further testing is indicated.

A large, prospective trial, the Christopher Study, incorporated objective, validated pretest clinical assessment into diagnostic algorithms using D-dimer measurement. In this study, patients with a high pretest probability and a negative CT-PA who were not receiving anticoagulation had a low (less than 2%) 3-month incidence of subsequent PE. This low rate of complications supports the contention that many false-negative studies represent clinically insignificant, small distal thrombi and provides support for monitoring most patients with a high-quality negative CT-PA off therapy (see Integrated Approach to Diagnosis of Pulmonary Embolism below). The rate of false-positive CT-PA and overtreatment of PE has not been as well studied to date.

3. Ventilation-perfusion lung scanning—A perfusion scan is performed by injecting radiolabeled microaggregated albumin into the venous system, allowing the particles to embolize to the pulmonary capillary bed. To perform a ventilation scan, the patient breathes a radioactive gas or aerosol while the distribution of radioactivity in the lungs is recorded. A defect on perfusion scanning represents diminished blood flow to that region of the lung. This finding is not specific for PE. Defects in the perfusion scan are interpreted in conjunction with the ventilation scan to give a high, low, or intermediate (indeterminate) probability that PE is the cause of the abnormalities. Criteria for the combined interpretation of ventilation and perfusion scans (commonly referred to as a single test, the $\dot{V}/\dot{Q}$ scan) are complex, confusing, and not completely standardized. A normal perfusion scan excludes the diagnosis of clinically significant PE (negative predictive value of 91% in the PIOPED I study). A high-probability $\dot{V}/\dot{Q}$ scan is most often defined as having two or more segmental perfusion defects in the presence of normal ventilation and is sufficient to make the diagnosis of PE in most instances (positive predictive value of 88% among PIOPED I patients). $\dot{V}/\dot{Q}$ scans are most helpful when they are either normal or indicate a high probability of PE. Such readings are reliable—interobserver agreement is best for normal and high-probability scans—and they carry predictive power. The likelihood ratios associated with normal and high-probability scans are 0.10 and 18, respectively, indicating significant and frequently conclusive changes from pretest to posttest probability.

However, 75% of PIOPED I $\dot{V}/\dot{Q}$ scans were nondiagnostic, ie, of low or intermediate probability. At angiography, these patients had an overall incidence of PE of 14% and 30%, respectively.

One of the most important findings of PIOPED I was that the clinical assessment of pretest probability could be used to aid the interpretation of the $\dot{V}/\dot{Q}$ scan. For patients with low-probability $\dot{V}/\dot{Q}$ scans and a low (20% or less) clinical pretest probability of PE, the diagnosis was confirmed in only 4%. Such patients may reasonably be observed off therapy without angiography. All other patients with nondiagnostic $\dot{V}/\dot{Q}$ scans require further testing to determine the presence of venous thromboembolism.

4. Venous thrombosis studies—Seventy percent of patients with PE will have DVT on evaluation, and approximately half of patients with DVT will have PE on angiography. Since the history and physical examination are neither sensitive nor specific for PE and since the results of $\dot{V}/\dot{Q}$ scanning are frequently equivocal, documentation of

DVT in a patient with suspected PE establishes the need for treatment and may preclude further testing.

Commonly available diagnostic techniques include venous ultrasonography, impedance plethysmography, and contrast venography. In most centers, **venous ultrasonography** is the test of choice to detect proximal DVT. Inability to compress the common femoral or popliteal veins in symptomatic patients is diagnostic of first-episode DVT (positive predictive value of 97%); full compressibility of both sites excludes proximal DVT (negative predictive value of 98%). The test is less accurate in distal thrombi, recurrent thrombi, or in asymptomatic patients. Impedance plethysmography relies on changes in electrical impedance between patent and obstructed veins to determine the presence of thrombus. Accuracy is comparable though not quite as high as ultrasonography. Both ultrasonography and impedance plethysmography are useful in the serial examination of patients with high clinical suspicion of venous thromboembolism but negative leg studies. In patients with suspected first-episode DVT and a negative ultrasound or impedance plethysmography examination, multiple studies have confirmed the safety of withholding anticoagulation while conducting two sequential studies on days 1–3 and 7–10. Similarly, patients with nondiagnostic $\dot{V}/\dot{Q}$ scans and an initial negative venous ultrasound or impedance plethysmography examination may be monitored off therapy with serial leg studies over 2 weeks. When serial examinations are negative for proximal DVT, the risk of subsequent venous thromboembolism over the following 6 months is less than 2%.

Contrast venography remains the reference standard for the diagnosis of DVT. An intraluminal filling defect is diagnostic of venous thrombosis. However, venography has significant shortcomings and has been replaced by venous ultrasound as the diagnostic procedure of choice. Venography may be useful in complex situations where there is discrepancy between clinical suspicion and noninvasive testing.

5. Pulmonary angiography—Pulmonary angiography is the historical reference standard for the diagnosis of PE.

It is a safe but invasive procedure with well-defined morbidity and mortality data. Minor complications occur in approximately 5% of patients. Most are allergic contrast reactions, transient kidney injury, or percutaneous catheter–related injuries; cardiac perforation and arrhythmias are reported but rare.

Pulmonary angiography is indicated in any patient in whom the diagnosis is in doubt when there is a high clinical pretest probability of PE or when the diagnosis of PE must be established with certainty, as when anticoagulation is contraindicated or placement of an inferior vena cava filter is contemplated.

▶ Integrated Approach to Diagnosis of Pulmonary Embolism

An integrated approach to the diagnosis of PE uses the clinical likelihood of venous thromboembolism derived from a clinical prediction rule (Table 9–19) along with the results of diagnostic tests to come to one of three decision

Table 9–19. Clinical prediction rule for pulmonary embolism (PE).

Variable	Points
Clinical symptoms and signs of deep venous thrombosis (DVT) (leg swelling and pain with palpation of deep veins)	3.0
Alternative diagnosis less likely than PE	3.0
Heart rate > 100 beats/min	1.5
Immobilization for more than 3 days or surgery in previous 4 weeks	1.5
Previous PE or DVT	1.5
Hemoptysis	1.0
Cancer (with treatment within past 6 months or palliative care)	1.0
Three-tiered clinical probability assessment (Wells criteria)	**Score**
High	> 6.0
Moderate	2.0 to 6.0
Low	< 2.0
Dichotomous clinical probability assessment (Modified Wells criteria)	**Score**
PE likely	> 4.0
PE unlikely	< or = 4.0

Data from Wells PS et al. Derivation of a simple clinical model to categorize patients' probability of pulmonary embolism: increasing the models' utility with the SimpliRED D-dimer. Thromb Haemost. 2000 Mar;83(3):416–20.

points: to establish venous thromboembolism (PE or DVT) as the diagnosis, to exclude venous thromboembolism with sufficient confidence to discontinue anticoagulation therapy and monitor the patient, or to refer the patient for additional testing. An ideal diagnostic algorithm would proceed in a cost-effective, stepwise fashion to come to these decision points at minimal risk to the patient. Most North American centers use Wells' clinical prediction rule (Table 9–19) or something similar to guide a rapid D-dimer and CT-PA–based diagnostic algorithm (Figure 9–8). This approach is highly effective when applied correctly. The Christopher Study, a rigorous study that used the Wells' approach, found the incidence of venous thromboembolism was 1.3% and fatal PE occurred in 0.5% of persons who stopped anticoagulation therapy and were monitored for 3 months. The incidence of PE following a negative integrated clinical, D-dimer, and CT-PA evaluation that excludes PE is comparable to that seen following the traditional gold standard of a negative pulmonary angiography.

Concern over false-positive D-dimer measurements in low-risk patients that prompt unnecessary CT-PA has led researchers to develop the Pulmonary Embolism Rule-Out Criteria (PERC, Table 9–20). In a prospective analysis of 8138 emergency department patients at risk for PE, researchers identified 20% (1666) who had *both* a low (less than 20%) pretest probability of PE *and* met all eight PERC

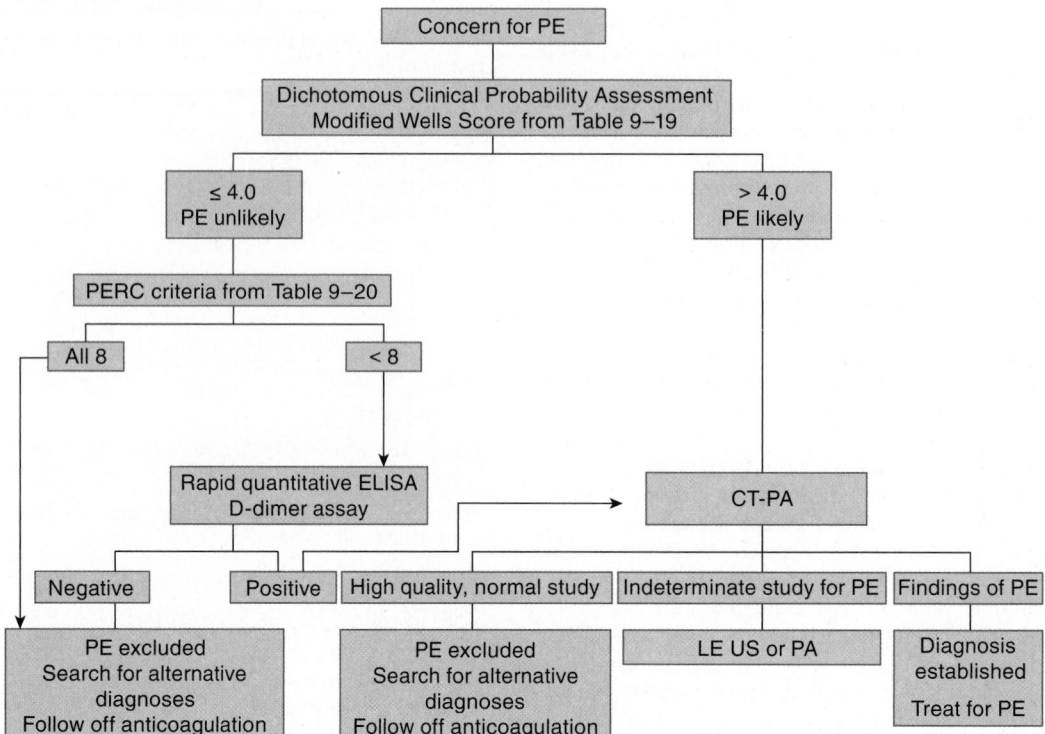

▲ **Figure 9–8.** D-dimer and helical CT-PA–based diagnostic algorithm for PE. CT-PA, CT pulmonary angiogram; PE, pulmonary embolism; ELISA, enzyme-linked immunosorbent assay; PERC, pulmonary embolism rule-out criteria; VTE, venous thromboembolic disease; LE US, lower extremity venous ultrasound for deep venous thrombosis; PA, pulmonary angiogram. (Adapted, with permission, from van Belle A et al. Effectiveness of managing suspected pulmonary embolism using an algorithm combining clinical probability, D-dimer testing, and computed tomography. JAMA. 2006 Jan 11;295(2): 172–9. Copyright © 2006 American Medical Association. All rights reserved.)

criteria. This group had a 1.0% incidence of PE, with one fatality. Using the algorithm in Figure 9–8, patients with a Modified Wells Score of 4 or less who meet all eight PERC criteria do not need to undergo D-dimer testing and may be monitored clinically.

Table 9–20. Pulmonary embolism rule-out criteria (PERC) for low-risk patients.

For patients with a Modified Wells Score ≤ 4[1] who meet ALL of the following criteria, PE is excluded, follow off anticoagulation, and search for alternative diagnoses.
• Age < 50 years
• Heart rate < 100 bpm
• Oxyhemoglobin saturation on room air ≥ 95%
• No prior history of venous thromboembolism
• No recent (within 4 weeks) trauma or surgery requiring hospitalization
• No presenting hemoptysis
• No estrogen therapy
• No unilateral leg swelling

[1]See Table 9–19.
Data from: Kline JA et al. Impact of a rapid rule-out protocol for pulmonary embolism on the rate of screening, missed cases, and pulmonary vascular imaging in an urban US emergency room. Ann Emerg Med. 2004 Nov;44(5):490–502.

The standard $\dot{V}/\dot{Q}$ scan-based algorithm (Table 9–21) remains useful in many patients, especially those who are not able to undergo CT-PA (eg, those with advanced chronic kidney disease).

Clinical prediction scores, D-dimers, and other diagnostic tests have not been well validated during pregnancy. An 8-year European study of 395 pregnant women using a diagnostic algorithm, a sensitive D-dimer, venous ultrasonography, and CT-PA excluded PE if the diagnostic workup was negative; follow-up at 3 months resulted in a 0.0% rate of venous thromboembolism events among untreated participants. The overall incidence of PE in this population was 7.1%.

► **Prevention**

Venous thromboembolism is often clinically silent until it presents with significant morbidity or mortality. It is a prevalent disease, clearly associated with identifiable risk factors. For example, the incidence of proximal DVT, PE, and fatal PE in untreated patients undergoing hip fracture surgery is reported to be 10–20%, 4–10%, and 0.2–5%, respectively. There is unambiguous evidence of the efficacy of prophylactic therapy in this and other clinical situations, yet it remains underused. Only about 50% of surgical deaths from PE had received any form of preventive therapy. Discussion of strategies for the prevention of venous thromboembolism can be found in Chapter 14.

Table 9–21. Pulmonary ventilation-perfusion scan based diagnostic algorithm for PE.

Clinical concern for PE:			
1. Analyze by three-tiered clinical probability assessment (Table 9–19)			
2. Obtain scan			
3. Match results in the following table			

	Clinical suspicion for PE by clinical probability assessment		
	HIGH	**MODERATE**	**LOW**
High Probability scan	STOP. Diagnosis established. Treat for PE.	STOP. Diagnosis established. Treat for PE.	Diagnosis likely (56% in PIOPED I, but small number of patients). Treat for PE or evaluate further with LE US or CT-PA.
Indeterminate Probability scan	Diagnosis highly likely (66% in PIOPED I). Treat for PE or evaluate further with LE US or CT-PA.	Uncertain diagnosis. Evaluate further with LE US or CT-PA.	Uncertain diagnosis. Evaluate further with LE US or CT-PA.
Low Probability scan	Uncertain diagnosis. Evaluate further with LE US or CT-PA.	Uncertain diagnosis. Evaluate further with LE US or CT-PA.	STOP. Diagnosis excluded; monitor off anticoagulation. Consider alternative diagnoses.
Normal scan	STOP. Diagnosis excluded; monitor off anticoagulation. Consider alternative diagnoses.	STOP. Diagnosis excluded; monitor off anticoagulation. Consider alternative diagnoses.	STOP. Diagnosis excluded; monitor off anticoagulation. Consider alternative diagnoses.

CT-PA, helical CT pulmonary angiography; LE US, lower extremity venous ultrasound for DVT; PE, pulmonary embolism.
Data from The PIOPED Investigators. Value of the ventilation/perfusion scan in acute pulmonary embolism: results of the Prospective Investigation of Pulmonary Embolism Diagnosis (PIOPED). JAMA. 1990 May 23–30;263(20):2753–9.

▶ Treatment

A. Anticoagulation

Anticoagulation is not definitive therapy but a form of secondary prevention. Heparin binds to and accelerates the ability of antithrombin to inactivate thrombin, factor Xa, and factor IXa. It thus retards additional thrombus formation, allowing endogenous fibrinolytic mechanisms to lyse-existing clot. The standard regimen of heparin followed by 6 months of oral warfarin results in an 80–90% reduction in the risk of both recurrent venous thrombosis and death from PE (see Tables 14–16, 14–19, 14–20). Low-molecular-weight heparins (LMWHs) are as effective as unfractionated heparin in the treatment of venous thromboembolism. The 2016 CHEST Guideline and Expert Panel Report recommends direct oral anticoagulants over vitamin K antagonist (warfarin) and LMWH in all patients with venous thromboembolism without a cancer diagnosis and recommends LMWH for patients with cancer.

The optimal duration of anticoagulation therapy for venous thromboembolism is unknown. There appears to be a protective benefit to continued anticoagulation in first-episode venous thromboembolism (twice the rate of recurrence in 6 weeks compared with 6 months of therapy) and recurrent disease (eightfold risk of recurrence in 6 months compared with 4 years of therapy). These studies did not distinguish patients with reversible risk factors, such as surgery or transient immobility, from patients who have a nonreversible hypercoagulable state, such as factor V Leiden, antithrombin deficiency, antiphospholipid syndrome, or malignancy. An RCT of low-dose warfarin (INR 1.5–2.0) versus no therapy following 6 months of standard therapy in patients with idiopathic DVT was stopped early. The protective benefits of continued anticoagulation include fewer DVTs in addition to a trend toward lower mortality despite more hemorrhage in the warfarin group. Risk reductions were consistent across groups with and without inherited thrombophilia.

For many patients, venous thrombosis is a recurrent disease, and continued therapy results in a lower rate of recurrence at the cost of an increased risk of hemorrhage. Therefore, the appropriate duration of therapy needs to take into consideration the patient's age, potentially reversible risk factors, likelihood and potential consequences of hemorrhage, and preferences for continued therapy. The 2016 CHEST Guideline and Expert Panel

Report recommends 3 months of anticoagulation after a first episode provoked by a surgery or a transient nonsurgical risk factor. Extended therapy (no scheduled stop date) is recommended for an unprovoked episode with a low to moderate risk of bleeding. Patient sex and D-dimer level measured a month after stopping anticoagulant therapy may influence this treatment decision. Patients who continue to receive anticoagulation long term should be reassessed for venous thrombosis periodically (at least annually). For patients with cancer, extended therapy with LMWH is recommended regardless of bleeding risk. D-dimer testing has been suggested to identify those who may benefit from continued anticoagulation after 3 months of therapy but clinical data have not supported its utility in this regard.

The major complication of anticoagulation is hemorrhage. Risk factors for hemorrhage include the intensity of the anticoagulation; duration of therapy; concomitant administration of medications, such as aspirin, that interfere with platelet function; and patient characteristics, particularly increased age, previous gastrointestinal hemorrhage, and coexistent chronic kidney disease.

The reported incidence of major hemorrhage following intravenous administration of unfractionated heparin is nil to 7%; that of fatal hemorrhage is nil to 2%. The incidence with LMWHs is not statistically different. There is no information comparing hemorrhage rates at different doses of heparin. The risk of death from another pulmonary embolism during subtherapeutic heparin administration in the first 24–48 hours after diagnosis is significant; it appears to outweigh the risk of short-term supratherapeutic heparin levels. The incidence of hemorrhage during therapy with warfarin is reported to be between 3% and 4% per patient year. The frequency varies with the target INR and is consistently higher when the INR exceeds 4.0. There is no apparent additional antithrombotic benefit in venous thromboembolism with a target INR above 2.0–3.0 (see Chapter 14).

B. Thrombolytic Therapy

Streptokinase, urokinase, and recombinant tissue plasminogen activator (rt-PA; alteplase) increase plasmin levels and thereby directly lyse intravascular thrombi. In patients with established PE, thrombolytic therapy accelerates resolution of emboli within the first 24 hours compared with standard heparin therapy. This is a consistent finding using angiography, $\dot{V}/\dot{Q}$ scanning, echocardiography, and direct measurement of pulmonary artery pressures. However, at 1 week and 1 month after diagnosis, these agents show no difference in outcome compared with heparin and warfarin. Hemodynamically stable patients with echocardiographic evidence of right heart strain from acute PE show no long-term improvement in function or mortality when given thrombolytic therapy. Indeed, clinical research shows no improvements in mortality in any patient population. Subtle improvements in pulmonary function, including improved single-breath diffusing capacity and a lower incidence of exercise-induced pulmonary hypertension, have been observed. The reliability and clinical importance of these findings is unclear. The major disadvantages of thrombolytic therapy compared with

heparin are its greater cost and significant increase in major hemorrhagic complications. The incidence of intracranial hemorrhage in patients with PE treated with alteplase is 2.1% compared with 0.2% in patients treated with heparin. Current practice supports thrombolytic therapy for PE in patients at high risk for death from refractory hypotension or hypoxemia despite heparin therapy, patients in whom the more rapid resolution of thrombus may be lifesaving.

Absolute contraindications to thrombolytic therapy include active internal bleeding and stroke within the past 2 months. Major contraindications include uncontrolled hypertension and surgery or trauma within the past 6 weeks.

C. Additional Measures

Interruption of the inferior vena cava may be indicated in patients with a major contraindication to anticoagulation who have or are at high risk for development of proximal DVT or PE. Placement of an inferior vena cava filter is also recommended for recurrent thromboembolism despite adequate anticoagulation, for chronic recurrent embolism with a compromised pulmonary vascular bed (eg, in pulmonary hypertension), and with the concurrent performance of surgical pulmonary embolectomy or pulmonary thromboendarterectomy. Percutaneous transjugular placement of a mechanical filter is the preferred mode of inferior vena cava interruption. These devices reduce the short-term incidence of PE in patients presenting with proximal lower extremity DVT. However, they are associated with a twofold increased risk of recurrent DVT in the first 2 years following placement so plans must be usually made for their subsequent removal.

In rare critically ill patients for whom thrombolytic therapy is contraindicated or unsuccessful, mechanical or surgical extraction of thrombus may be indicated. Pulmonary embolectomy is an emergency procedure of last resort with a very high mortality rate. It is performed only in a few specialized centers.

▶ Prognosis

PE is estimated to cause more than 50,000 deaths annually. In the majority of deaths, PE is not recognized antemortem or death occurs before specific treatment can be initiated. These statistics highlight the importance of preventive therapy in high-risk patients (Chapter 14). The outlook for patients with diagnosed and appropriately treated PE is generally good. Overall prognosis depends on the underlying disease rather than the PE itself. Death from recurrent thromboemboli is uncommon, occurring in less than 3% of cases. Perfusion defects resolve in most survivors. Chronic thromboembolic pulmonary hypertension develops in approximately 1% of patients. Selected patients may benefit from pulmonary endarterectomy.

▶ When to Admit

Most patients with acute PE require hospitalization. The decision to admit patients with acute PE requires assessment of factors placing them at high risk, including their severity of illness (eg, severe hypoxemia), comorbidities (eg, DVT, cardiac dysfunction), educational needs (eg, lack of knowledge about PE and its management), and/or problematic social situations (eg, prior noncompliance with follow-up care). Some institutions and healthcare systems have demonstrated that carefully selected low-risk patients with acute PE can be safely and effectively managed as outpatients with the aid of integrated clinical decision support systems.

Anderson DR et al. Aspirin or rivaroxaban for VTE prophylaxis after hip or knee arthroplasty. N Engl J Med. 2018 Feb 22; 378(8):699–707. [PMID: 29466159]

Freund Y et al; PROPER Investigator Group. Effect of the Pulmonary Embolism Rule-Out criteria on subsequent thromboembolic events among low-risk emergency department patients: the PROPER Randomized Clinical Trial. JAMA. 2018 Feb 13; 319(6):559–66. [PMID: 29450523]

Kahale LA et al. Anticoagulation for people with cancer and central venous catheters. Cochrane Database Syst Rev. 2018 Jun 1;6:CD006468. [PMID: 29856471]

Kahn SR et al. Interventions for implementation of thromboprophylaxis in hospitalized patients at risk for venous thromboembolism. Cochrane Database Syst Rev. 2018 Apr 24;4: CD008201. [PMID: 29687454]

Kearon C et al. Antithrombotic therapy for VTE disease: CHEST Guideline and Expert Panel Report. Chest. 2016 Feb; 149(2):315–52. [PMID: 26867832]

Kline JA. Utility of a clinical prediction rule to exclude pulmonary embolism among low-risk emergency department patients: reason to PERC up. JAMA. 2018 Feb 13;319(6): 551–3. [PMID: 29450510]

Meinel FG et al. Predictive value of computed tomography in acute pulmonary embolism: systematic review and meta-analysis. Am J Med. 2015 Jul;128(7):747–59. [PMID: 25680885]

Raja AS et al. Evaluation of patients with suspected acute pulmonary embolism: best practice advice from the Clinical Guidelines Committee of the American College of Physicians. Ann Intern Med. 2015 Nov 3;163(9):701–11. [PMID: 26414967]

Righini M et al. Diagnosis of pulmonary embolism during pregnancy: a multicenter prospective management outcome study. Ann Intern Med. 2018 Dec 4;169(11):766–73. [PMID: 30357273]

van der Hulle T et al; YEARS study group. Simplified diagnostic management of suspected pulmonary embolism (the YEARS study): a prospective, multicentre, cohort study. Lancet. 2017 Jul 15;390(10091):289–97. Erratum in: Lancet. 2017 Jul 15; 390(10091):230. [PMID: 28549662]

Vinson DR et al; eSPEED Investigators of the KP CREST Network. Increasing safe outpatient management of emergency department patients with pulmonary embolism: a controlled pragmatic trial. Ann Intern Med. 2018 Dec 18; 169(12):855–65. [PMID: 30422263]

Wells PS et al. Diagnosis of venous thromboembolism: 20 years of progress. Ann Intern Med. 2018 Jan 16;168(2):131–40. [PMID: 29310137]

PULMONARY HYPERTENSION

ESSENTIALS OF DIAGNOSIS

▸ Dyspnea, fatigue, chest pain, and syncope on exertion.

▸ Narrow splitting of second heart sound with loud pulmonary component; findings of right ventricular hypertrophy and heart failure in advanced disease.

▸ Electrocardiographic evidence of right ventricular strain or hypertrophy and right atrial enlargement.

▸ Enlarged central pulmonary arteries on chest radiograph.

▸ Elevated right ventricular systolic pressure on two-dimensional echocardiography with Doppler flow studies.

▸ General Considerations

Pulmonary hypertension is a complex problem characterized by pathologic elevation in pulmonary arterial pressure. Normal pulmonary artery systolic pressure at rest is 15–30 mm Hg, with a mean pressure between 10 mm Hg and 18 mm Hg. The pulmonary circulation is a low-pressure, low-resistance system due to its large cross-sectional area, and it can accommodate significant increase in blood flow during exercise. The primary pathologic mechanism in pulmonary hypertension is an increase in pulmonary vascular resistance that leads to an increase in the pulmonary systolic pressure greater than 30 mm Hg or the mean pressure greater than 25 mm Hg.

The World Health Organization currently classifies pulmonary hypertension based on similarities in pathologic mechanisms and includes the following five groups.

Group 1 (pulmonary arterial hypertension secondary to various disorders): This group gathers diseases that localize directly to the pulmonary arteries leading to structural changes, smooth muscle hypertrophy, and endothelial dysfunction. This group includes idiopathic (formerly primary) pulmonary arterial hypertension, heritable pulmonary arterial hypertension, HIV infection, portal hypertension, drugs and toxins, connective tissue disorders, congenital heart disease, schistosomiasis, primary veno-occlusive disease, and pulmonary capillary hemangiomatosis.

Group 2 (pulmonary venous hypertension secondary to left heart disease): Often referred to as pulmonary venous hypertension or "post-capillary" pulmonary hypertension, this group includes left ventricular systolic or diastolic dysfunction and valvular heart disease.

Group 3 (pulmonary hypertension secondary to lung disease or hypoxemia): This group is caused by advanced obstructive and restrictive lung disease, including COPD, interstitial lung disease, pulmonary fibrosis, bronchiectasis, as well as other causes of chronic hypoxemia, such as sleep-disordered breathing, alveolar hypoventilation syndromes, and high-altitude exposure.

Group 4 (pulmonary hypertension secondary to chronic thromboembolism): This group consists of patients with pulmonary hypertension due to thromboembolic occlusion of the proximal and distal pulmonary arteries. (This classification no longer includes patients with nonthrombotic occlusion, such as tumors or foreign objects.)

Group 5 (pulmonary arterial hypertension secondary to hematologic, systemic, metabolic, or miscellaneous causes): These patients have pulmonary hypertension secondary to hematologic disorders (eg, chronic hemolytic anemia, myeloproliferative disorders, splenectomy), systemic disorders (eg, sarcoidosis, vasculitis, pulmonary Langerhans cell histiocytosis, neurofibromatosis type 1), metabolic disorders (eg, glycogen storage disease, Gaucher disease, thyroid disease), and miscellaneous causes (tumor embolization, external compression of the pulmonary vasculature, end-stage renal disease on dialysis).

The clinical severity of pulmonary hypertension is classified according to the New York Heart Association (NYHA) classification system, which was originally developed for heart failure but subsequently modified by the World Health Organization; it is based primarily on symptoms and functional status.

Class I: Pulmonary hypertension without limitation of physical activity. No dyspnea, fatigue, chest pain, or near syncope with exertion.

Class II: Pulmonary hypertension resulting in slight limitation of physical activity. No symptoms at rest but ordinary physical activity causes dyspnea, fatigue, chest pain, or near syncope.

Class III: Pulmonary hypertension resulting in marked limitation of physical activity. No symptoms at rest but less than ordinary activity causes dyspnea, fatigue, chest pain, or near syncope.

Class IV: Pulmonary hypertension with inability to perform any physical activity without symptoms. Evidence of right heart failure. Dyspnea and fatigue at rest and worsening of symptoms with any activity.

▶ Clinical Findings

A. Symptoms and Signs

There are no specific symptoms or signs but patients with pulmonary hypertension typically experience dyspnea with exertion and even, with advanced disease, at rest. Anginal pain, nonproductive cough, malaise, and fatigue may be present. Syncope occurs with exertion when there is insufficient cardiac output or if there is an arrhythmia. Hemoptysis is a rare but life-threatening event in pulmonary hypertension usually caused by the rupture of a pulmonary artery.

Findings on physical examination can include jugular venous distention, accentuated pulmonary valve component of the second heart sound, right-sided third heart sound, tricuspid regurgitation murmur, hepatomegaly, and lower extremity edema. Cyanosis can occur in patients with an open patent foramen ovale and right-to-left shunt due to increased right atrial pressure.

B. Laboratory Findings

Routine blood work is often normal; any abnormalities noted are usually related to the underlying disease in secondary pulmonary hypertension. On arterial blood gas analysis, patients with idiopathic pulmonary arterial hypertension often have normal Pao_2 at rest but show evidence of hyperventilation with a decrease in $Paco_2$. All patients should be evaluated for HIV and collagen vascular disease.

The ECG is typically normal except in advanced disease, where right ventricular hypertrophy (right axis deviation, incomplete right bundle branch block) and right atrial enlargement (peaked P wave in the inferior and right-sided leads) can be noted.

C. Imaging and Special Examinations

Radiographs and CT scans of the chest are useful in diagnosis. Enlargement of the right and left main pulmonary arteries is common; right ventricular and right atrial enlargement is seen in advanced disease. Chest imaging and pulmonary function testing are also useful in determining the cause of pulmonary hypertension for patients in Group 3 (pulmonary hypertension due to lung disease). On pulmonary function testing, the combination of decreased single-breath diffusing capacity, normal FVC on spirometry, normal TLC on lung volume measurement, and increased wasted ventilation on cardiopulmonary exercise testing is suggestive of pathologically increased pulmonary arterial pressures.

Patients in whom pulmonary hypertension is suspected should undergo echocardiography with Doppler flow. The echocardiogram is useful in the assessment of underlying cardiac disease, while Doppler flow can estimate the right ventricular systolic pressure. Right ventricular systolic pressure can be estimated based on tricuspid jet velocity and right atrial pressure. The severity of pulmonary hypertension can also be assessed based on the right ventricular size and function. Right-sided cardiac catheterization remains the gold standard for the diagnosis and quantification of pulmonary hypertension and should be performed prior to initiation of advanced therapies. Estimated pressures on echocardiogram correlate with right heart catheterization measurement but can vary by at least 10 mm Hg in more than 50% of cases so should not be used to direct therapy. Cardiac catheterization is particularly helpful in differentiating pulmonary arterial hypertension from pulmonary venous hypertension by assessment of the drop in pressure across the pulmonary circulation, also known as the transpulmonary gradient. Vasodilator challenge is often performed during right heart catheterization and a significant acute vasodilator response consists of a drop in mean pulmonary pressure of greater than 10 mm Hg (or 20%) to less than 40 mm Hg.

In patients with unexplained pulmonary hypertension who have a history of PE or risk factors for thromboembolic disease, chronic thromboembolic disease (Group 4 pulmonary hypertension) should be excluded prior to diagnosing idiopathic pulmonary hypertension. V̇/Q̇ lung scanning is a very sensitive test that can differentiate chronic thromboembolic pulmonary hypertension from idiopathic pulmonary arterial hypertension. Currently, pulmonary angiography is considered the most definitive diagnostic procedure for defining the distribution and extent of disease in chronic thromboembolic pulmonary hypertension.

▶ Treatment

Primary therapy refers to treatment directed at the underlying cause of pulmonary hypertension. Currently, there are no primary therapies available targeting the underlying lesion for patients in Group 1 (pulmonary arterial hypertension) but advanced therapies are available directly targeting the pulmonary hypertension itself. The advanced therapy chosen is typically based on patient symptoms and functional status according to the NYHA/WHO classification. Based on observational studies showing improved functional status and possible decreased mortality, first-line therapy consists of oral calcium channel blockers. However, these medications should be given only to patients with positive acute vasodilator response when tested in the cardiac catheterization laboratory because they may be harmful to nonresponders. Preferred treatments for Group 1 patients in functional class II include oral endothelin receptor antagonists (ambrisentan, bosentan, macitentan), phosphodiesterase inhibitors (sildenafil, tadalafil), and soluble guanylate cyclase stimulators (riociguat). RCTs using either endothelin receptor antagonists or phosphodiesterase inhibitors have shown improvement in symptoms, 6-minute walk distance, WHO functional status, and hemodynamic measurements. For Group 1 patients in functional classes III and IV or Group 1 patients who are not responsive to previous therapies, prostanoid agents (intravenous epoprostenol, intravenous or subcutaneous treprostinil) are available. Continuous long-term intravenous epoprostenol infusion improved mortality in a prospective RCT. Limitations to intravenous prostacyclins include short medication half-life requiring a reliable continuous infusion, difficulty in titration, and high cost of therapy. Inhaled prostanoids (iloprost, treprostinil) and subcutaneous prostanoids (treprostinil) are available for patients unable to tolerate continuous intravenous infusion. Generally, monotherapy is started with either a phosphodiesterase inhibitor or an endothelin receptor antagonist; with clinical worsening, a second agent is usually added to achieve combination therapy of both phosphodiesterase inhibitor and endothelin receptor antagonist.

Treatment of patients with Group 2 pulmonary hypertension (secondary to left heart failure) is discussed in Chapter 10. The main goal is to decrease pulmonary venous pressure by treating heart failure and volume overload.

Patients with Group 3 pulmonary hypertension (due to lung disease) and hypoxemia at rest or with physical activity should receive supplemental oxygen. In patients with COPD and hypoxemia, administration of supplemental oxygen for 15 hours or more per day has been shown to slow the progression of pulmonary hypertension.

For patients with Group 1 pulmonary hypertension and Group 4 pulmonary hypertension (due to thromboembolic disease), long-term anticoagulation is recommended and generally accepted, based solely on observational studies suggesting improvement in survival. For Group 4 patients in functional class IV and no response to other advanced therapies, thromboendarterectomy is recommended. Only patients with surgically accessible lesions and acceptable perioperative risk should undergo this procedure.

Lung transplantation is a treatment option for selected patients with pulmonary hypertension when medical therapy is no longer effective. Double-lung transplant is the preferred method, although single-lung transplant is routinely done as well. In some cases, transplantation of the heart and both lungs is needed.

Prognosis

The prognosis of idiopathic (some Group 1) pulmonary hypertension is poor and is not affected by therapies primarily used to treat symptoms. Conversely, the prognosis for patients with secondary pulmonary hypertension (some Group 1 and Groups 2–5) depends on the underlying disease and its response to treatment. In all cases, right ventricular function is one of the most important prognostic factors. The presence of cor pulmonale carries a poor survival outcome regardless of the underlying cause.

When to Refer

Patients with pulmonary arterial hypertension and symptoms of dyspnea, fatigue, chest pain, or near syncope should be referred to a pulmonologist or cardiologist at a specialized center for expert management.

When to Admit

- Patients with pulmonary hypertension, severe symptoms, and evidence of decompensated right heart failure with volume overload should be admitted to the hospital for aggressive diuresis.
- Patients with Group 1 pulmonary hypertension and functional class III or IV symptoms should be admitted to a specialized center for initiation of advanced therapies, such as intravenous prostacyclins.

Ghofrani HA et al; MERIT study investigators. Macitentan for the treatment of inoperable chronic thromboembolic pulmonary hypertension (MERIT-1): results from the multicentre, phase 2, randomised, double-blind, placebo-controlled study. Lancet Respir Med. 2017 Oct;5(10):785–94. [PMID: 28919201]

Hill NS et al. New therapeutic paradigms and guidelines in the management of pulmonary arterial hypertension. J Manag Care Spec Pharm. 2016 Mar;22(3 Suppl A):S3–21. [PMID: 27003666]

Mehta S et al. Macitentan improves health-related quality of life for patients with pulmonary arterial hypertension: results from the randomized controlled SERAPHIN Trial. Chest. 2017 Jan; 151(1):106–18. Erratum in: Chest. 2018 May;153(5):1287. [PMID: 27671974]

Thenappan T et al. Pulmonary arterial hypertension: pathogenesis and clinical management. BMJ. 2018 Mar 14;360:j5492. [PMID: 29540357]

Westerhof BE et al. Treatment strategies for the right heart in pulmonary hypertension. Cardiovasc Res. 2017 Oct 1;113(12): 1465–73. [PMID: 28957540]

PULMONARY VASCULITIS

Granulomatosis with polyangiitis is an idiopathic disease manifested by a combination of glomerulonephritis, necrotizing granulomatous vasculitis of the upper and lower respiratory tracts, and varying degrees of small-vessel vasculitis. Chronic sinusitis, arthralgias, fever, skin rash, and weight loss are frequent presenting symptoms. Specific pulmonary complaints occur less often. The most common sign of lung disease is nodular pulmonary infiltrates, often with cavitation, seen on chest radiography. Tracheal stenosis and endobronchial disease are sometimes seen.

The diagnosis is most often based on serologic testing and biopsy of lung, sinus tissue, or kidney with demonstration of necrotizing granulomatous vasculitis (Chapter 20).

Eosinophilic granulomatosis with polyangiitis is an idiopathic multisystem vasculitis of small and medium-sized arteries that occurs in patients with asthma. The skin and lungs are most often involved, but other organs, including the paranasal sinuses, the heart, gastrointestinal tract, liver, and peripheral nerves, may also be affected. Peripheral eosinophilia greater than 1500 cells/mcL (greater than 1.5×10^9/L) or greater than 10% of peripheral WBCs is the rule. Abnormalities on chest radiographs range from transient opacities to multiple nodules. This illness may be part of a spectrum that includes polyarteritis nodosa. The diagnosis requires demonstration of histologic features, including fibrinoid necrotizing epithelioid and eosinophilic granulomas.

▶ **Treatment**

Treatment of pulmonary vasculitis usually requires corticosteroids and cyclophosphamide. Oral prednisone (1 mg/kg ideal body weight per day initially, tapering slowly to alternate-day therapy over 3–6 months) is the corticosteroid of choice; in granulomatosis with polyangiitis, some clinicians may use cyclophosphamide alone. For fulminant vasculitis, therapy may be initiated with intravenous methylprednisolone (up to 1 g intravenously per day) for several days. Cyclophosphamide (1–2 mg/kg ideal body weight orally per day initially, with dosage adjustments to avoid neutropenia) is given until complete remission is obtained and then is slowly tapered, and often replaced with methotrexate or azathioprine for maintenance therapy.

▶ **Prognosis**

Five-year survival rates in patients with these vasculitis syndromes have been improved by combination therapy. Complete remission can be achieved in over 90% of patients with granulomatosis with polyangiitis. The addition of trimethoprim-sulfamethoxazole (one double-strength tablet by mouth twice daily) to standard therapy may help prevent relapses.

Flores-Suárez LF et al. Pulmonary involvement in systemic vasculitis. Curr Rheumatol Rep. 2017 Sep;19(9):56. [PMID: 28752492]
Greco A et al. Churg-Strauss syndrome. Autoimmun Rev. 2015 Apr;14(4):341–8. [PMID: 25500434]
Greco A et al. Goodpasture's syndrome: a clinical update. Autoimmun Rev. 2015 Mar;14(3):246–53. [PMID: 25462583]
Talarico R et al. Systemic vasculitis and the lung. Curr Opin Rheumatol. 2017 Jan;29(1):45–50. [PMID: 27755177]
Wechsler ME et al; EGPA Mepolizumab Study Team. Mepolizumab or placebo for eosinophilic granulomatosis with polyangiitis. N Engl J Med. 2017 May 18;376(20):1921–32. [PMID: 28514601]

ALVEOLAR HEMORRHAGE SYNDROMES

Diffuse alveolar hemorrhage may occur in a variety of immune and nonimmune disorders. Alveolar infiltrates on chest radiograph, dyspnea, anemia, hemoptysis, and occasionally fever are characteristic. Rapid clearing of diffuse lung infiltrates within 2 days is a clue to the diagnosis of diffuse alveolar hemorrhage. Pulmonary hemorrhage can be associated with an increased single-breath diffusing capacity for carbon monoxide ($D_{L_{CO}}$).

Causes of diffuse **immune alveolar hemorrhage** include anti-basement membrane antibody disease (Goodpasture syndrome), granulomatosis with polyangiitis, systemic necrotizing vasculitis, pulmonary capillaritis associated with idiopathic rapidly progressive glomerulonephritis, systemic lupus erythematosus, and other vasculitic and collagen vascular diseases. **Nonimmune causes** of diffuse hemorrhage include coagulopathy, mitral stenosis, necrotizing pulmonary infection, drugs (penicillamine), toxins (trimellitic anhydride), and idiopathic pulmonary hemosiderosis.

Goodpasture syndrome is idiopathic recurrent alveolar hemorrhage and rapidly progressive glomerulonephritis. The disease is mediated by anti-glomerular basement membrane antibodies. Goodpasture syndrome occurs mainly in men who are in their 30s and 40s. Hemoptysis is the usual presenting symptom, but pulmonary hemorrhage may be occult. Dyspnea, cough, hypoxemia, and diffuse bilateral alveolar infiltrates are typical features. Iron deficiency anemia and microscopic hematuria are usually present. The diagnosis is based on characteristic linear IgG deposits detected by immunofluorescence in glomeruli or alveoli and on the presence of anti-glomerular basement membrane antibody in serum. Combinations of immunosuppressive drugs (initially methylprednisolone, 30 mg/kg intravenously over 20 minutes every other day for three doses, followed by daily oral prednisone, 1 mg/kg/day, with cyclophosphamide, 2 mg/kg orally per day) and plasmapheresis have yielded excellent results.

Idiopathic pulmonary hemosiderosis is a disease of children or young adults characterized by recurrent pulmonary hemorrhage; in contrast to Goodpasture syndrome, renal involvement and anti-glomerular basement membrane antibodies are absent, but iron deficiency is typical. It is frequently associated with celiac disease. Treatment of acute episodes of hemorrhage with corticosteroids may be useful. Recurrent episodes of pulmonary hemorrhage may result in interstitial fibrosis and pulmonary failure.

Martínez-Martínez MU et al. Diffuse alveolar hemorrhage in autoimmune diseases. Curr Rheumatol Rep. 2017 May; 19(5):27. [PMID: 28397125]
McAdoo SP et al. Anti-glomerular basement membrane disease. Clin J Am Soc Nephrol. 2017 Jul 7;12(7):1162–72. [PMID: 28515156]
Xi-Yuan C et al. Idiopathic pulmonary hemosiderosis in adults: review of cases reported in the latest 15 years. Clin Respir J. 2017 Nov;11(6):677–81. [PMID: 26692115]

ENVIRONMENTAL & OCCUPATIONAL LUNG DISORDERS

SMOKE INHALATION

The inhalation of products of combustion may cause serious respiratory complications. As many as one-third of patients admitted to burn treatment units have pulmonary injury from smoke inhalation. Morbidity and mortality due to smoke inhalation may exceed those attributed to the burns themselves. The death rate of patients with both severe burns and smoke inhalation exceeds 50%.

All patients in whom significant smoke inhalation is suspected must be assessed for three consequences of smoke inhalation: impaired tissue oxygenation, thermal injury to the upper airway, and injury to the lower airways and lung parenchyma. Impaired tissue oxygenation may result from inhalation of a hypoxic gas mixture, carbon monoxide or cyanide, or from alterations in $\dot{V}/\dot{Q}$ matching, and is an immediate threat to life. Immediate treatment with 100% oxygen is essential. The management of patients with carbon monoxide and cyanide poisoning is discussed in Chapter 38. The clinician must recognize that patients with carbon monoxide poisoning display a normal partial pressure of oxygen in arterial blood (Pao_2), but have a low *measured* (ie, not oximetric) hemoglobin saturation (Sao_2). Treatment with 100% oxygen should be continued until the measured carboxyhemoglobin level falls to less than 10% and concomitant metabolic acidosis has resolved.

Thermal injury to the mucosal surfaces of the upper airway occurs from inhalation of super-heated gases. Complications, including mucosal edema, upper airway obstruction, and impaired ability to clear oral secretions, usually become evident by 18–24 hours and produce inspiratory stridor. Respiratory failure occurs in severe cases. Early management (Chapter 37) includes the use of a high-humidity face mask with supplemental oxygen, gentle suctioning to evacuate oral secretions, elevation of the head 30 degrees to promote clearing of secretions, and topical epinephrine to reduce edema of the oropharyngeal mucous membrane. Helium-oxygen gas mixtures (Heliox) may reduce labored breathing due to critical upper airway narrowing. Close monitoring with arterial blood gases and later with oximetry is important. Examination of the upper airway with a fiberoptic laryngoscope or bronchoscope is superior to routine physical examination. Endotracheal intubation is often necessary to maintain airway patency and is likely to be necessary in patients with deep facial burns or oropharyngeal or laryngeal edema. Tracheotomy should be avoided if possible because of an increased risk of pneumonia and death from sepsis.

Injury to the lower airways and lung parenchyma results from inhalation of toxic gases and products of combustion, including aldehydes and organic acids. The site of lung injury depends on the solubility of the gases inhaled, the duration of exposure, and the size of inhaled particles that transport noxious gases to distal lung units. Bronchorrhea and bronchospasm are seen early after exposure along with dyspnea, tachypnea, and tachycardia. Labored breathing and cyanosis may follow. Physical examination at this stage reveals diffuse wheezing and rhonchi. Bronchiolar and alveolar edema (eg, ARDS) may develop within 1–2 days after exposure. Sloughing of the bronchiolar mucosa may occur within 2–3 days, leading to airway obstruction, atelectasis, and worsening hypoxemia. Bacterial colonization and pneumonia are common by 5–7 days after the exposure.

Treatment of smoke inhalation consists of supplemental oxygen, bronchodilators, suctioning of mucosal debris and mucopurulent secretions via an indwelling endotracheal tube, chest physical therapy to aid clearance of secretions, and adequate humidification of inspired gases. Positive end-expiratory pressure (PEEP) has been advocated to treat bronchiolar edema. Judicious fluid management and close monitoring for secondary bacterial infection round out the management protocol.

The routine use of corticosteroids for lung injury from smoke inhalation has been shown to be ineffective and may even be harmful. Routine or prophylactic use of antibiotics is not recommended.

Patients who survive should be watched for the late development of bronchiolitis obliterans.

Enkhbaatar P et al. Pathophysiology, research challenges, and clinical management of smoke inhalation injury. Lancet. 2016 Oct 1;388(10052):1437–46. [PMID: 27707500]

Walker PF et al. Diagnosis and management of inhalation injury: an updated review. Crit Care. 2015 Oct 28;19:351. [PMID: 26507130]

PULMONARY ASPIRATION SYNDROMES

Aspiration of material into the tracheobronchial tree results from various disorders that impair normal deglutition, especially disturbances of consciousness and esophageal dysfunction.

1. Acute Aspiration of Gastric Contents (Mendelson Syndrome)

Acute aspiration of gastric contents may be catastrophic. The pulmonary response depends on the characteristics and amount of gastric contents aspirated. The more acidic the material, the greater the degree of chemical pneumonitis. Aspiration of pure gastric acid (pH < 2.5) causes extensive desquamation of the bronchial epithelium, bronchiolitis, hemorrhage, and pulmonary edema. Acute gastric aspiration is one of the most common causes of ARDS. The clinical picture is one of abrupt onset of respiratory distress, with cough, wheezing, fever, and tachypnea. Crackles may be audible at the bases of the lungs. Hypoxemia may be noted immediately after aspiration occurs. Radiographic abnormalities, consisting of patchy alveolar opacities in dependent lung zones, appear within a few hours. If particulate food matter has been aspirated along with gastric acid, radiographic features of bronchial obstruction may be observed. Fever and leukocytosis are common even in the absence of infection.

Treatment of acute aspiration of gastric contents consists of supplemental oxygen, measures to maintain the airway, and the usual measures for treatment of acute respiratory failure. There is no evidence to support the routine use of prophylactic antibiotics or corticosteroids after gastric aspiration. Secondary pulmonary infection, which occurs in about one-fourth of patients, typically appears 2–3 days after aspiration. Management of infection depends on the observed flora of the tracheobronchial tree. Hypotension secondary to alveolar capillary membrane injury and intravascular volume depletion is common and is managed with the judicious administration of intravenous fluids.

2. Chronic Aspiration of Gastric Contents

Chronic aspiration of gastric contents may result from primary disorders of the larynx or the esophagus, such as achalasia, esophageal stricture, systemic sclerosis (scleroderma), esophageal carcinoma, esophagitis, and gastroesophageal reflux. In the last condition, relaxation of the tone of the lower esophageal sphincter allows reflux of gastric contents into the esophagus and predisposes to chronic pulmonary aspiration, especially at night. Cigarette smoking, consumption of alcohol or caffeine, and use of theophylline are known to relax the lower esophageal sphincter. Pulmonary disorders linked to gastroesophageal reflux and chronic aspiration include asthma, chronic cough, bronchiectasis, and pulmonary fibrosis. Even in the absence of aspiration, acid in the esophagus may trigger bronchospasm or bronchial hyperreactivity through reflex mechanisms.

The diagnosis and management of gastroesophageal reflux and chronic aspiration are challenging. A discussion of strategies for the evaluation, prevention, and management of extraesophageal reflux manifestations can be found in Chapter 15.

3. "Café Coronary"

Acute obstruction of the upper airway by food is associated with difficulty swallowing, old age, dental problems that impair chewing, and use of alcohol and sedative drugs. The Heimlich procedure is lifesaving in many cases.

4. Retention of an Aspirated Foreign Body

Retention of an aspirated foreign body in the tracheobronchial tree may produce both acute and chronic conditions, including atelectasis, postobstructive hyperinflation, both acute and recurrent pneumonia, bronchiectasis, and lung abscess. Occasionally, a misdiagnosis of asthma, COPD, or lung cancer is made in adult patients who have aspirated a foreign body. The plain chest radiograph usually suggests the site of the foreign body. In some cases, an expiratory film, demonstrating regional hyperinflation due to a check-valve effect, is helpful. Bronchoscopy is usually necessary to establish the diagnosis and attempt removal of the foreign body.

5. Aspiration of Inert Material

Most patients suffer no serious sequelae from aspiration of inert material. However, it may cause asphyxia if the amount aspirated is massive and if cough is impaired, in which case immediate tracheobronchial suctioning is necessary.

6. Aspiration of Toxic Material

Aspiration of toxic material into the lung usually results in clinically evident pneumonia. **Hydrocarbon pneumonitis** is caused by aspiration of ingested petroleum distillates, eg, gasoline, kerosene, furniture polish, and other household petroleum products. Lung injury results mainly from vomiting of ingested products and secondary aspiration. Therapy is supportive. The lung should be protected from repeated aspiration with a cuffed endotracheal tube if necessary. **Lipoid pneumonia** is a chronic syndrome related to the repeated aspiration of oily materials, eg, mineral oil, cod liver oil, and oily nose drops; it usually occurs in elderly patients with impaired swallowing. Patchy opacities in dependent lung zones and lipid-laden macrophages in expectorated sputum are characteristic findings.

DiBardino DM et al. Aspiration pneumonia: a review of modern trends. J Crit Care. 2015 Feb;30(1):40–8. [PMID: 25129577]

OCCUPATIONAL PULMONARY DISEASES

Many acute and chronic pulmonary diseases are directly related to inhalation of noxious substances encountered in the workplace. Disorders that are linked to occupational exposures may be classified as follows: (1) pneumoconioses, (2) hypersensitivity pneumonitis, (3) obstructive airway disorders, (4) toxic lung injury, (5) lung cancer, (6) pleural diseases, and (7) other occupational pulmonary diseases.

1. Pneumoconioses

Pneumoconioses are chronic fibrotic lung diseases caused by the inhalation of inert inorganic dusts. Pneumoconioses may be asymptomatic disorders with diffuse nodular opacities on chest radiograph or may be severe, symptomatic, life-shortening disorders. Clinically important pneumoconioses include coal worker's pneumoconiosis, silicosis, and asbestosis (Table 9–22). Treatment for each is supportive.

A. Coal Worker's Pneumoconiosis

In coal worker's pneumoconiosis, ingestion of inhaled coal dust by alveolar macrophages leads to the formation of coal macules, usually 2–5 mm in diameter, that appear on chest radiograph as diffuse small opacities that are especially prominent in the upper lung. Simple coal worker's pneumoconiosis is usually asymptomatic; pulmonary function abnormalities are unimpressive. Cigarette smoking does not increase the prevalence of coal worker's pneumoconiosis but may have an additive detrimental effect on ventilatory function. In complicated coal worker's pneumoconiosis (**"progressive massive fibrosis"**), conglomeration and contraction in the upper lung zones occur, with radiographic features resembling complicated silicosis. **Caplan syndrome** is a rare condition characterized by the presence of necrobiotic rheumatoid nodules (1–5 cm in diameter) in the periphery of the lung in coal workers with rheumatoid arthritis.

B. Silicosis

In silicosis, extensive or prolonged inhalation of free silica (silicon dioxide) particles in the respirable range (0.3–5 mcm) causes the formation of small rounded opacities (silicotic nodules) throughout the lung. Calcification of the periphery of hilar lymph nodes ("eggshell" calcification) is an unusual radiographic finding that strongly suggests silicosis. Simple silicosis is usually asymptomatic and has no effect on routine pulmonary function tests; in complicated silicosis, large conglomerate densities appear in the upper lung and are

Table 9–22. Selected pneumoconioses.

Disease	Agent	Occupations
Asbestosis	Asbestos	Mining, insulation, construction, shipbuilding
Baritosis	Barium salts	Glass and insecticide manufacturing
Coal worker's pneumoconiosis	Coal dust	Coal mining
Kaolin pneumoconiosis	Sand, mica, aluminum silicate	Mining of china clay; pottery and cement work
Shaver disease	Aluminum powder	Manufacture of corundum
Siderosis	Metallic iron or iron oxide	Mining, welding, foundry work
Silicosis	Free silica (silicon dioxide)	Rock mining, quarrying, stone cutting, tunneling, sandblasting, pottery, diatomaceous earth
Stannosis	Tin, tin oxide	Mining, tin-working, smelting
Talcosis	Magnesium silicate	Mining, insulation, construction, shipbuilding

accompanied by dyspnea and obstructive and restrictive pulmonary dysfunction. The incidence of pulmonary tuberculosis is increased in patients with silicosis. All patients with silicosis should have a tuberculin skin test and a current chest radiograph. If old, healed pulmonary tuberculosis is suspected, multidrug treatment for tuberculosis (not single-agent preventive therapy) should be instituted.

C. Asbestosis

Asbestosis is a nodular interstitial fibrosis occurring in workers exposed to asbestos fibers (shipyard and construction workers, pipe fitters, insulators) over many years (typically 10–20 years). Patients with asbestosis usually first seek medical attention at least 15 years after exposure with the following symptoms and signs: progressive dyspnea, inspiratory crackles, and in some cases, clubbing and cyanosis. The radiographic features of asbestosis include linear streaking at the lung bases, opacities of various shapes and sizes, and honeycomb changes in advanced cases. The presence of pleural calcifications may be a clue to diagnosis. High-resolution CT scanning is the best imaging method for asbestosis because of its ability to detect parenchymal fibrosis and define the presence of coexisting pleural plaques. Cigarette smoking in asbestos workers increases the prevalence of radiographic pleural and parenchymal changes and markedly increases the incidence of lung carcinoma. It may also interfere with the clearance of short asbestos fibers from the lung. Pulmonary function studies show restrictive dysfunction and reduced diffusing capacity. The presence of a ferruginous body in tissue suggests significant asbestos exposure; however, other histologic features must be present for diagnosis. There is no specific treatment.

Cohen RA et al. Lung pathology in U.S. coal workers with rapidly progressive pneumoconiosis implicates silica and silicates. Am J Respir Crit Care Med. 2016 Mar 15;193(6):673–80. [PMID: 26513613]

Fell AKM et al. Association between exposure in the cement production industry and non-malignant respiratory effects: a systematic review. BMJ Open. 2017 Apr 24;7(4):e012381. [PMID: 28442577]

Go LH et al. Lung disease and coal mining: what pulmonologists need to know. Curr Opin Pulm Med. 2016 Mar;22(2):170–8. [PMID: 26761630]

2. Hypersensitivity Pneumonitis

Hypersensitivity pneumonitis (also called extrinsic allergic alveolitis) is a nonatopic, nonasthmatic inflammatory pulmonary disease. It is manifested mainly as an occupational disease (Table 9–23), in which exposure to inhaled organic antigens leads to an acute illness. Prompt

Table 9–23. Selected causes of hypersensitivity pneumonitis.

Disease	Antigen	Source
Farmer's lung	*Micropolyspora faeni, Thermoactinomyces vulgaris*	Moldy hay
"Humidifier" lung	Thermophilic actinomycetes	Contaminated humidifiers, heating systems, or air conditioners
Bird fancier's lung	Avian proteins	Bird serum and excreta
Bagassosis	*Thermoactinomyces sacchari* and *T vulgaris*	Moldy sugar cane fiber (bagasse)
Sequoiosis	*Graphium, Aureobasidium,* and other fungi	Moldy redwood sawdust
Maple bark stripper's disease	*Cryptostroma (Coniosporium) corticale*	Rotting maple tree logs or bark
Mushroom picker's disease	Same as farmer's lung	Moldy compost
Suberosis	*Penicillium frequentans*	Moldy cork dust
Detergent worker's lung	*Bacillus subtilis* enzyme	Enzyme additives

diagnosis is essential since symptoms are usually reversible if the offending antigen is removed from the patient's environment early in the course of illness. Continued exposure may lead to progressive disease. The histopathology of acute hypersensitivity pneumonitis is characterized by interstitial infiltrates of lymphocytes and plasma cells, with noncaseating granulomas in the interstitium and air spaces.

▶ Clinical Findings

A. Acute Illness

The symptoms are characterized by sudden onset of malaise, chills, fever, cough, dyspnea, and nausea 4–8 hours after exposure to the offending antigen. This may occur after the patient has left work or even at night and thus may mimic paroxysmal nocturnal dyspnea. Bibasilar crackles, tachypnea, tachycardia, and (occasionally) cyanosis are noted. Small nodular densities sparing the apices and bases of the lungs are noted on chest radiograph. Laboratory studies reveal an increase in the white blood cell count with a shift to the left, hypoxemia, and the presence of precipitating antibodies to the offending agent in serum. Hypersensitivity pneumonitis antibody panels against common offending antigens are available; positive results, while supportive, do not establish a definitive diagnosis. Pulmonary function studies reveal restrictive dysfunction and reduced diffusing capacity.

B. Subacute and Chronic Illness

A subacute hypersensitivity pneumonitis syndrome (15% of cases) is characterized by the insidious onset of chronic cough and slowly progressive dyspnea, anorexia, and weight loss. Chronic exposure leads to progressive respiratory insufficiency and the appearance of pulmonary fibrosis on chest imaging. Surgical lung biopsy may be necessary for the diagnosis of subacute and chronic hypersensitivity pneumonitis. Even with surgical lung biopsy, however, chronic hypersensitivity pneumonitis may be difficult to diagnose because histopathologic patterns overlap with several idiopathic interstitial pneumonias.

▶ Treatment

Treatment of acute hypersensitivity pneumonitis consists of identification of the offending agent and avoidance of further exposure. In severe acute or protracted cases, oral corticosteroids (prednisone, 0.5 mg/kg daily as a single morning dose for 2 weeks, tapered to nil over 4–6 weeks) may be given. Change in occupation is often unavoidable.

Elicker BM et al. Multidisciplinary approach to hypersensitivity pneumonitis. J Thorac Imaging. 2016 Mar;31(2):92–103. [PMID: 26479131]
Raj R et al. Surgical lung biopsy for interstitial lung diseases. Chest. 2017 May;151(5):1131–40. [PMID: 27471113]
Spagnolo P et al. Hypersensitivity pneumonitis: a comprehensive review. J Investig Allergol Clin Immunol. 2015;25(4):237–50. [PMID: 26310038]

3. Obstructive Airway Disorders

Occupational pulmonary diseases manifested as obstructive airway disorders include occupational asthma, industrial bronchitis, and byssinosis.

A. Occupational Asthma

It has been estimated that from 2% to 5% of all cases of asthma are related to occupation. Offending agents in the workplace are numerous; they include grain dust, wood dust, tobacco, pollens, enzymes, gum arabic, synthetic dyes, isocyanates (particularly toluene diisocyanate), rosin (soldering flux), inorganic chemicals (salts of nickel, platinum, and chromium), trimellitic anhydride, phthalic anhydride, formaldehyde, and various pharmaceutical agents. Diagnosis of occupational asthma depends on a high index of suspicion, an appropriate history, spirometric studies before and after exposure to the offending substance, and peak flow rate measurements in the workplace. Bronchial provocation testing may be helpful in some cases. Treatment consists of avoidance of further exposure to the offending agent and bronchodilators, but symptoms may persist for years after workplace exposure has been terminated.

Cullinan P et al. Occupational lung diseases: from old and novel exposures to effective preventive strategies. Lancet Respir Med. 2017 May;5(5):445–55. Erratum in: Lancet Respir Med. 2017 Jun;5(6):e22. [PMID: 28089118]
Ojanguren I et al. Clinical and inflammatory characteristics of asthma—COPD overlap in workers with occupational asthma. PLoS One. 2018 Mar 2;13(3):e0193144. Erratum in: PLoS One. 2018 Apr 4;13(4):e0195648. [PMID: 29499062]
Pralong JA et al. Review of diagnostic challenges in occupational asthma. Curr Allergy Asthma Rep. 2017 Jan;17(1):1. [PMID: 28091866]

B. Industrial Bronchitis

Industrial bronchitis is chronic bronchitis found in coal miners and others exposed to cotton, flax, or hemp dust. Chronic disability from industrial bronchitis is infrequent.

C. Byssinosis

Byssinosis is an asthma-like disorder in textile workers caused by inhalation of cotton dust. The pathogenesis is obscure. Chest tightness, cough, and dyspnea are characteristically worse on Mondays or the first day back at work, with symptoms subsiding later in the week. Repeated exposure leads to chronic bronchitis.

4. Toxic Lung Injury

Toxic lung injury from inhalation of irritant gases is discussed in the section on smoke inhalation. **Silo-filler's disease** is acute toxic high-permeability pulmonary edema caused by inhalation of nitrogen dioxide encountered in recently filled silos. Bronchiolitis obliterans is a common late complication, which may be prevented by early treatment of the acute reaction with corticosteroids. Extensive exposure to silage gas may be fatal. Inhalation of the compound diacetyl, a constituent of butter-flavoring, has been linked to the development of bronchiolitis obliterans among microwave popcorn production workers.

5. Lung Cancer

Many industrial pulmonary carcinogens have been identified, including asbestos, radon gas, arsenic, iron, chromium, nickel, coal tar fumes, petroleum oil mists, isopropyl oil, mustard gas, and printing ink. Almost all histologic types of lung cancer have been associated with these carcinogens. Cigarette smoking acts as a cocarcinogen with asbestos and radon gas to cause bronchogenic carcinoma. Asbestos alone causes malignant mesothelioma. Chloromethyl methyl ether specifically causes small-cell carcinoma of the lung.

6. Pleural Diseases

Occupational diseases of the pleura may result from exposure to asbestos or talc. Inhalation of talc causes pleural plaques that are similar to those caused by asbestos. Benign asbestos pleural effusion occurs in some asbestos workers and may cause chronic blunting of the costophrenic angle on chest radiograph.

7. Other Occupational Pulmonary Diseases

Occupational agents are also responsible for other pulmonary disorders. These include exposure to beryllium, which now occurs in machining and handling of beryllium products and alloys. Beryllium miners are not at risk for berylliosis and beryllium is no longer used in fluorescent lamp production, which was a source of exposure before 1950. **Berylliosis,** an acute or chronic pulmonary disorder, occurs from absorption of beryllium through the lungs or skin and wide dissemination throughout the body. Acute berylliosis is a toxic, ulcerative tracheobronchitis and chemical pneumonitis following intense and severe exposure to beryllium. Chronic berylliosis, a systemic disease closely resembling sarcoidosis, is more common. Chronic pulmonary beryllium disease is an alveolitis mediated by the proliferation of beryllium-specific CD4 T-cells in the lung.

Markowitz S. Asbestos-related lung cancer and malignant mesothelioma of the pleura: selected current issues. Semin Respir Crit Care Med. 2015 Jun;36(3):334–46. Erratum in: Semin Respir Crit Care Med. 2016 Feb;37(1):143–4. [PMID: 26024342]

MEDICATION-INDUCED LUNG DISEASE

Typical patterns of pulmonary response to medications implicated in medication-induced respiratory disease are summarized in Table 9–24. Pulmonary injury due to medications occurs as a result of allergic reactions, idiosyncratic reactions, overdose, or undesirable side effects. In most patients, the mechanism of pulmonary injury is unknown.

Precise diagnosis of medication-induced pulmonary disease is often difficult because results of routine laboratory studies are not helpful and radiographic findings are not specific. A high index of suspicion and a thorough history of medication usage are critical to establishing the

Table 9–24. Pulmonary manifestations of selected medication toxicities.

Asthma	**Pulmonary edema**
Beta-blockers	Noncardiogenic
Aspirin	Aspirin
Nonsteroidal anti-inflammatory drugs	Chlordiazepoxide
	Cocaine
Histamine	Ethchlorvynol
Methacholine	Heroin
Acetylcysteine	Cardiogenic
Aerosolized pentamidine	Beta-blockers
Any nebulized medication	**Pleural effusion**
Chronic cough	Bromocriptine
Angiotensin-converting enzyme inhibitors	Nitrofurantoin
	Any drug inducing systemic lupus erythematosus
Pulmonary infiltration	Methysergide
Without eosinophilia	Chemotherapeutic agents (eg, carmustine, cyclophosphamide, dasatinib, docetaxel, GM-CSF, methotrexate)
Amitriptyline	
Azathioprine	
Amiodarone	
With eosinophilia	
Sulfonamides	**Mediastinal widening**
L-Tryptophan	Phenytoin
Nitrofurantoin	Corticosteroids
Penicillin	Methotrexate
Methotrexate	**Respiratory failure**
Crack cocaine	Neuromuscular blockade
Drug-induced systemic lupus erythematosus	Aminoglycosides
	Paralytic agents
Hydralazine	Central nervous system
Procainamide	Depression
Isoniazid	Sedatives
Chlorpromazine	Hypnotics
Phenytoin	Opioids
Interstitial pneumonitis/fibrosis	Alcohol
	Tricyclic antidepressants
Nitrofurantoin	Oxygen
Bleomycin	
Busulfan	
Cyclophosphamide	
Methysergide	
Phenytoin	

GM-CSF, granulocyte-macrophage colony-stimulating factor.

diagnosis of medication-induced lung disease. The clinical response to cessation of the suspected offending agent is also helpful. Acute episodes of medication-induced pulmonary disease usually disappear 24–48 hours after the medication has been discontinued, but chronic syndromes may take longer to resolve. Challenge tests to confirm the diagnosis are risky and rarely performed.

Treatment of medication-induced lung disease consists of discontinuing the offending agent immediately and managing the pulmonary symptoms appropriately.

Inhalation of crack cocaine may cause a spectrum of acute pulmonary syndromes, including pulmonary infiltration with eosinophilia, pneumothorax and pneumomediastinum, bronchiolitis obliterans, and acute respiratory failure associated with diffuse alveolar damage and alveolar hemorrhage. Corticosteroids have been used with variable success to treat alveolar hemorrhage.

Leger P et al. Pulmonary toxicities from conventional chemotherapy. Clin Chest Med. 2017 Jun;38(2):209–22. [PMID: 28477634]

RADIATION LUNG INJURY

The lung is an exquisitely radiosensitive organ that can be damaged by external beam radiation therapy. The degree of pulmonary injury is determined by the volume of lung irradiated, the dose and rate of exposure, and potentiating factors (eg, concurrent chemotherapy, previous radiation therapy in the same area, and simultaneous withdrawal of corticosteroid therapy). Symptomatic radiation lung injury occurs in about 10% of patients treated for carcinoma of the breast, 5–15% of patients treated for carcinoma of the lung, and 5–35% of patients treated for lymphoma. Two phases of the pulmonary response to radiation are apparent: an acute phase (radiation pneumonitis) and a chronic phase (radiation fibrosis).

1. Radiation Pneumonitis

Acute radiation pneumonitis usually occurs 2–3 months (range 1–6 months) after completion of radiotherapy and is characterized by insidious onset of dyspnea, intractable dry cough, chest fullness or pain, weakness, and fever. Late radiation pneumonitis may develop 6–12 months after completion of radiation. The pathogenesis of acute radiation pneumonitis is unknown, but there is speculation that hypersensitivity mechanisms are involved. The dominant histopathologic findings are a lymphocytic interstitial pneumonitis progressing to an exudative alveolitis. Inspiratory crackles may be heard in the involved area. In severe disease, respiratory distress and cyanosis occur that are characteristic of ARDS. An increased white blood cell count and elevated sedimentation rate are common. Pulmonary function studies reveal reduced lung volumes, reduced lung compliance, hypoxemia, reduced diffusing capacity, and reduced maximum voluntary ventilation. Chest radiography, which correlates poorly with the presence of symptoms, usually demonstrates alveolar or nodular opacities limited to the irradiated area. Air bronchograms are often observed. Sharp borders of an opacity may help distinguish radiation pneumonitis from other conditions, such as infectious pneumonia, lymphangitic spread of carcinoma, and recurrent tumor; however, the opacity may extend beyond the radiation field. No specific therapy is proved to be effective in radiation pneumonitis, but prednisone (1 mg/kg/day orally) is commonly given immediately for about 1 week. The dose is reduced and maintained at 20–40 mg/day for several weeks, then slowly tapered. Radiation pneumonitis may improve in 2–3 weeks following onset of symptoms as the exudative phase resolves. Acute respiratory failure, if present, is treated supportively. Death from ARDS is unusual in radiation pneumonitis.

Bledsoe TJ et al. Radiation pneumonitis. Clin Chest Med. 2017 Jun;38(2):201–8. [PMID: 28477633]

2. Pulmonary Radiation Fibrosis

Radiation fibrosis may occur with or without antecedent radiation pneumonitis. Cor pulmonale and chronic respiratory failure are rare. Radiographic findings include obliteration of normal lung markings, dense interstitial and pleural fibrosis, reduced lung volumes, tenting of the diaphragm, and sharp delineation of the irradiated area. No specific therapy is proven effective, and corticosteroids have no value. Pulmonary fibrosis may develop after an intervening period (6–12 months) of well-being in patients who experience radiation pneumonitis. Pulmonary radiation fibrosis occurs in most patients who receive a full course of radiation therapy for cancer of the lung or breast. Most patients are asymptomatic, although slowly progressive dyspnea may occur.

3. Other Complications of Radiation Therapy

Other complications of radiation therapy directed to the thorax include pericardial effusion, constrictive pericarditis, tracheoesophageal fistula, esophageal candidiasis, radiation dermatitis, and rib fractures. Small pleural effusions, radiation pneumonitis outside the irradiated area, spontaneous pneumothorax, and complete obstruction of central airways are unusual occurrences.

Giridhar P et al. Radiation induced lung injury: prediction, assessment and management. Asian Pac J Cancer Prev. 2015;16(7):2613–7. [PMID: 25854336]

▼ PLEURAL DISEASES

PLEURITIS

Pain due to acute pleural inflammation is caused by irritation of the parietal pleura. Such pain is localized, sharp, and fleeting; it is made worse by coughing, sneezing, deep breathing, or movement. When the central portion of the diaphragmatic parietal pleura is irritated, pain may be referred to the ipsilateral shoulder. There are numerous causes of pleuritis. The setting in which pleuritic pain develops helps narrow the differential diagnosis. In young, otherwise healthy individuals, pleuritis is usually caused by viral respiratory infections or pneumonia. The presence of pleural effusion, pleural thickening, or air in the pleural space requires further diagnostic and therapeutic measures. Simple rib fracture may cause severe pleurisy.

Treatment of pleuritis consists of treating the underlying disease. Analgesics and anti-inflammatory medications (eg, indomethacin, 25 mg orally two or three times daily) are often helpful for pain relief. Codeine (30–60 mg orally every 8 hours) or other opioids may be used to control cough associated with pleuritic chest pain if retention of airway secretions is not a likely complication. Intercostal nerve blocks are sometimes helpful but the benefit is usually transient.

PLEURAL EFFUSION

ESSENTIALS OF DIAGNOSIS

▶ May be asymptomatic; chest pain frequently seen in the setting of pleuritis, trauma, or infection; dyspnea is common with large effusions.

▶ Dullness to percussion and decreased breath sounds over the effusion.

▶ Radiographic evidence of pleural effusion.

▶ Diagnostic findings on thoracentesis.

General Considerations

There is constant movement of fluid from parietal pleural capillaries into the pleural space at a rate of 0.01 mL/kg body weight/h. Absorption of pleural fluid occurs through parietal pleural lymphatics. The resultant homeostasis leaves 5–15 mL of fluid in the normal pleural space. A pleural effusion is an abnormal accumulation of fluid in the pleural space. Pleural effusions may be classified by differential diagnosis (Table 9–25) or by underlying pathophysiology. Five pathophysiologic processes account for most pleural effusions: increased production of fluid in the setting of normal capillaries due to increased hydrostatic or decreased oncotic pressures **(transudates);** increased production of fluid due to abnormal capillary permeability **(exudates);** decreased lymphatic clearance of fluid from the pleural space **(exudates);** infection in the pleural space **(empyema);** and bleeding into the pleural space **(hemothorax). Parapneumonic pleural effusions** are exudates that accompany bacterial pneumonias.

Diagnostic thoracentesis should be performed whenever there is a new pleural effusion and no clinically apparent cause. Observation is appropriate in some situations (eg, symmetric bilateral pleural effusions in the setting of heart failure), but an atypical presentation or failure of an effusion to resolve as expected warrants thoracentesis. Sampling allows visualization of the fluid in addition to chemical and microbiologic analyses to identify the underlying pathophysiologic process.

Clinical Findings

A. Symptoms and Signs

Patients with pleural effusions most often report dyspnea, cough, or respirophasic chest pain. Symptoms are more common in patients with existing cardiopulmonary disease. Small pleural effusions are less likely to be symptomatic than larger effusions. Physical findings are usually absent in small effusions. Larger effusions may present with dullness to percussion and diminished or absent breath sounds over the effusion. Compressive atelectasis may cause bronchial breath sounds and egophony just above the effusion. A massive effusion with increased intrapleural pressure may cause contralateral shift of the trachea and bulging of the intercostal spaces. A pleural friction rub indicates pulmonary infarction or pleuritis.

B. Laboratory Findings

The gross appearance of pleural fluid helps identify several types of pleural effusion. Grossly purulent fluid signifies empyema. Milky white pleural fluid should be centrifuged. A clear supernatant above a pellet of white cells indicates empyema, whereas a persistently turbid supernatant suggests a **chylous effusion;** analysis of this supernatant reveals chylomicrons and a high triglyceride level (greater than 100 mg/dL [1 mmol/L]), often from disruption of the thoracic duct. **Hemorrhagic pleural effusion** is a mixture of blood and pleural fluid. Ten thousand red cells per microliter create blood-tinged pleural fluid; 100,000 red cells/mcL create grossly bloody pleural fluid. **Hemothorax** is the presence of gross blood in the pleural space, usually following chest trauma or instrumentation. It is defined as a ratio of pleural fluid hematocrit to peripheral blood hematocrit greater than 0.5.

Pleural fluid samples should be sent for measurement of protein, glucose, and LD in addition to total and differential white blood cell counts. Chemistry determinations are used to classify effusions as transudates or exudates. This classification is important because the differential diagnosis and subsequent evaluation for each entity is vastly different (Table 9–25). A **pleural exudate** is an effusion that has one or more of the following laboratory features: (1) ratio of pleural fluid protein to serum protein

Table 9–25. Causes of pleural fluid transudates and exudates.

Transudates	Exudates
Heart failure (> 90% of cases)	Pneumonia (parapneumonic effusion, including empyema)
Cirrhosis with ascites	Cancer
Nephrotic syndrome	Pulmonary embolism
Peritoneal dialysis	Bacterial infection (including empyema)
Myxedema	Tuberculosis
Atelectasis (acute)	Connective tissue disease
Constrictive pericarditis	Viral infection
Superior vena cava obstruction	Fungal infection
Pulmonary embolism	Rickettsial infection
	Parasitic infection
	Asbestos
	Meigs syndrome
	Pancreatic disease
	Uremia
	Chronic atelectasis
	Trapped lung
	Chylothorax
	Sarcoidosis
	Drug reaction
	Post–myocardial injury syndrome

greater than 0.5; (2) ratio of pleural fluid LD to serum LD greater than 0.6; (3) pleural fluid LD greater than two-thirds the upper limit of normal serum LD. **Pleural transudates** occur in the setting of normal capillary integrity and demonstrate none of the laboratory features of exudates. A transudate suggests the absence of local pleural disease; characteristic laboratory findings include a glucose equal to serum glucose, pH between 7.40 and 7.55, and fewer than 1000 white blood cells/mcL (1.0×10^9/L) with a predominance of mononuclear cells.

Heart failure accounts for 90% of transudates. Bacterial pneumonia and cancer are the most common causes of exudative effusion. Other causes of exudates with characteristic laboratory findings are summarized in Table 9–26.

Pleural fluid pH is useful in the assessment of parapneumonic effusions. A pH < 7.30 suggests the need for drainage of the pleural space. An elevated amylase level in pleural fluid suggests pancreatitis, pancreatic pseudocyst, adenocarcinoma of the lung or pancreas, or esophageal rupture.

Suspected tuberculous pleural effusion should be evaluated by thoracentesis with culture along with pleural biopsy, since pleural fluid culture positivity for *M tuberculosis* is low (less than 23–58% of cases). Closed pleural biopsy reveals granulomatous inflammation in approximately 60% of patients, and culture of three pleural biopsy specimens combined with histologic examination of a pleural biopsy for granulomas yields a diagnosis in up to 90% of patients. Tests for pleural fluid adenosine deaminase (approximately 90% sensitivity and specificity for pleural tuberculosis at levels greater than 70 units/L) and interferon-gamma (89% sensitivity, 97% specificity in a meta-analysis) can be extremely helpful diagnostic aids, particularly in making decisions to pursue invasive testing in complex patients.

Between 40% and 80% of exudative pleural effusions are malignant, while over 90% of malignant pleural effusions are exudative. Almost any form of cancer may cause effusions, but the most common causes are lung cancer (one-third of cases) and breast cancer. In 5–10% of malignant pleural effusions, no primary tumor is identified.

Pleural fluid specimens should be sent for cytologic examination in all cases of exudative effusions in patients suspected of harboring an underlying malignancy. The diagnostic yield depends on the nature and extent of the

Table 9–26. Characteristics of important exudative pleural effusions.

Etiology or Type of Effusion	Gross Appearance	White Blood Cell Count (cells/mcL)	Red Blood Cell Count (cells/mcL)	Glucose	Comments
Malignancy	Turbid to bloody; occasionally serous	1000–100,000 M	100 to several hundred thousand	Equal to serum levels; < 60 mg/dL in 15% of cases	Eosinophilia uncommon; positive results on cytologic examination
Uncomplicated parapneumonic	Clear to turbid	5000–25,000 P	< 5000	Equal to serum levels	Tube thoracostomy unnecessary
Empyema	Turbid to purulent	25,000–100,000 P	< 5000	Less than serum levels; often very low	Drainage necessary; putrid odor suggests anaerobic infection
Tuberculosis	Serous to serosanguineous	5000–10,000 M	< 10,000	Equal to serum levels; occasionally < 60 mg/dL	Protein > 4.0 g/dL (may exceed 5 g/dL); eosinophils (> 10%) or mesothelial cells (> 5%) make diagnosis unlikely; see text for additional diagnostic tests
Rheumatoid	Turbid; greenish yellow	1000–20,000 M or P	< 1000	< 40 mg/dL	Secondary empyema common; high LD, low complement, high rheumatoid factor, cholesterol crystals are characteristic
Pulmonary infarction	Serous to grossly bloody	1000–50,000 M or P	100 to > 100,000	Equal to serum levels	Variable findings; no pathognomonic features
Esophageal rupture	Turbid to purulent; red-brown	< 5000 to > 50,000 P	1000–10,000	Usually low	High amylase level (salivary origin); pneumothorax in 25% of cases; effusion usually on left side; pH < 6.0 strongly suggests diagnosis
Pancreatitis	Turbid to serosanguineous	1000–50,000 P	1000–10,000	Equal to serum levels	Usually left-sided; high amylase level

LD, lactate dehydrogenase; M, mononuclear cell predominance; P, polymorphonuclear leukocyte predominance.

underlying malignancy. Sensitivity is between 50% and 65%. A negative cytologic examination in a patient with a high prior probability of malignancy should be followed by one repeat thoracentesis. If that examination is negative, thoracoscopy is preferred to closed pleural biopsy. The sensitivity of thoracoscopy is 92–96%.

The term **paramalignant** pleural effusion refers to an effusion in a patient with cancer when repeated attempts to identify tumor cells in the pleura or pleural fluid are non-diagnostic but when there is a presumptive relation to the underlying malignancy. For example, superior vena cava syndrome with elevated systemic venous pressures causing a transudative effusion would be "paramalignant."

C. Imaging

The lung is less dense than water and floats on pleural fluid that accumulates in dependent regions. Subpulmonary fluid may appear as lateral displacement of the apex of the diaphragm with an abrupt slope to the costophrenic sulcus or a greater than 2-cm separation between the gastric air bubble and the lung. On a standard upright chest radio-graph (Figure 9–9), approximately 75–100 mL of pleural fluid must accumulate in the posterior costophrenic sulcus to be visible on the lateral view, and 175–200 mL must be present in the lateral costophrenic sulcus to be visible on the frontal view. Chest CT scans may identify as little as 10 mL of fluid. At least 1 cm of fluid on the decubitus view is necessary to permit blind thoracentesis. Ultrasonography is useful to guide thoracentesis in the setting of smaller effusions.

Pleural fluid may become trapped (loculated) by pleural adhesions, thereby forming unusual collections along the lateral chest wall or within lung fissures. Round or oval

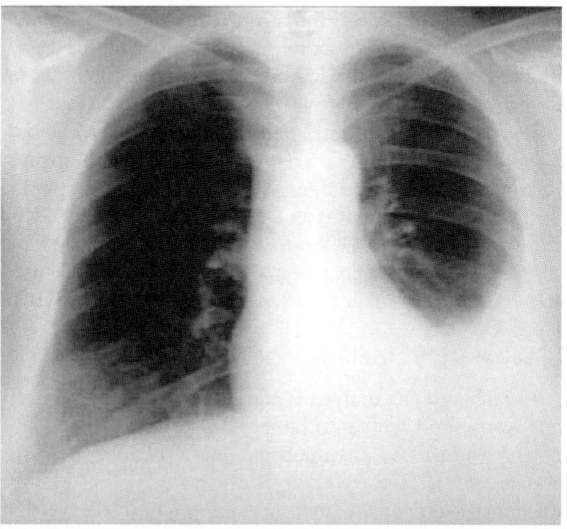

▲ **Figure 9–9.** Left pleural effusion. Frontal chest radiograph showing a meniscus-shaped density at the left costophrenic angle sulcus indicative of a moderate-sized pleural effusion. (Reproduced, with permission, from Lechner AJ, Matuschak GM, Brink DS. *Respiratory: An Integrated Approach to Disease.* McGraw-Hill, 2012.)

fluid collections in fissures that resemble intraparenchymal masses are called pseudotumors. Massive pleural effusion causing opacification of an entire hemithorax is most commonly caused by cancer but may be seen in tuberculosis and other diseases.

▶ Treatment

A. Transudative Pleural Effusion

Transudative pleural effusions characteristically occur in the absence of pleural disease. Therefore, treatment is directed at the underlying condition. Therapeutic thoracentesis for severe dyspnea typically offers only transient benefit. Pleurodesis and tube thoracostomy are rarely indicated.

B. Malignant Pleural Effusion

Chemotherapy or radiation therapy or both offer temporary control in some malignant effusions but are generally ineffective in lung cancer in the pleural space except for small-cell lung cancer. Asymptomatic malignant effusions usually do not require specific treatment. Symptomatic patients should have a therapeutic thoracentesis. If symptoms are relieved but the effusion returns, the options are serial thoracenteses, attempted pleurodesis, or placement of an indwelling drainage catheter that the patient can access at home. Choice among these options depends on the rate of reaccumulation in addition to the functional status, tolerance for discomfort, and life expectancy of the patient. Consultation with a thoracic specialist is advised (Chapter 39).

C. Parapneumonic Pleural Effusion

Parapneumonic pleural effusions are divided into three categories: simple or uncomplicated, complicated, and empyema. **Uncomplicated parapneumonic effusions** are free-flowing sterile exudates of modest size that resolve quickly with antibiotic treatment of pneumonia. They do not need drainage. **Empyema** is gross infection of the pleural space indicated by positive Gram stain or culture. Empyema should always be drained by tube thoracostomy to facilitate clearance of infection and to reduce the probability of fibrous encasement of the lung, causing permanent pulmonary impairment.

Complicated parapneumonic effusions present the most difficult management decisions. They tend to be larger than simple parapneumonic effusions and to show more evidence of inflammatory stimuli, such as low glucose level, low pH, or evidence of loculation. Inflammation probably reflects ongoing bacterial invasion of the pleural space despite rare positive bacterial cultures. The morbidity associated with complicated effusions is due to their tendency to form a fibropurulent pleural "peel," trapping otherwise functional lung and leading to permanent impairment. Tube thoracostomy is indicated when pleural fluid glucose is less than 60 mg/dL (less than 3.3 mmol/L) or the pH is < 7.2. These thresholds have not been prospectively validated and should not be interpreted strictly. The clinician should consider drainage of a complicated effusion if the pleural fluid pH is between 7.2 and 7.3 or the LD is greater than 1000 units/L (greater than 20 mckat/L). Pleural fluid cell count and protein have little diagnostic value in this setting.

Tube thoracostomy drainage of empyema or complicated parapneumonic effusions is frequently complicated by loculation that prevents adequate drainage. Intrapleural instillation of fibrinolytic agents has not been shown in controlled trials to improve drainage. The combination of intrapleural tissue plasminogen activator and deoxyribonuclease (DNase), an enzyme that catalyses extracellular DNA and degrades biofilm formation within the pleural cavity, has been found to improve clinical outcome (increased drainage, decreased length of stay and surgical referral) compared with placebo or either agent alone.

D. Hemothorax

A small-volume hemothorax that is stable or improving on chest radiographs may be managed by close observation. In all other cases, hemothorax is treated by immediate insertion of a thoracostomy tube to (1) drain existing blood and clot, (2) quantify the amount of bleeding, (3) reduce the risk of fibrothorax, and (4) permit apposition of the pleural surfaces in an attempt to reduce hemorrhage. Thoracic surgery consultation is indicated. Thoracotomy may be required to control hemorrhage, remove clot, and treat complications such as bronchopleural fistula formation.

Bhatnagar R et al. Outpatient talc administration by indwelling pleural catheter for malignant effusion. N Engl J Med. 2018 Apr 5;378(14):1313–22. [PMID: 29617585]

Feller-Kopman D et al. Pleural disease. N Engl J Med. 2018 Feb 22;378(8):740–51. [PMID: 29466146]

Patil M et al. Management of benign pleural effusions using indwelling pleural catheters: a systematic review and meta-analysis. Chest. 2017 Mar;151(3):626–35. [PMID: 27845052]

PNEUMOTHORAX

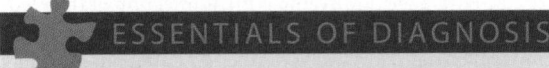

ESSENTIALS OF DIAGNOSIS

- ▶ Acute onset of unilateral chest pain and dyspnea.
- ▶ Minimal physical findings in mild cases; unilateral chest expansion, decreased tactile fremitus, hyperresonance, diminished breath sounds, mediastinal shift, cyanosis and hypotension in tension pneumothorax.
- ▶ Presence of pleural air on chest radiograph.

▶ General Considerations

Pneumothorax, or accumulation of air in the pleural space, is classified as spontaneous (primary or secondary), traumatic, or iatrogenic. Primary spontaneous pneumothorax occurs in the absence of an underlying lung disease, whereas secondary spontaneous pneumothorax is a complication of preexisting pulmonary disease. Traumatic pneumothorax results from penetrating or blunt trauma.

Iatrogenic pneumothorax may follow procedures such as thoracentesis, pleural biopsy, subclavian or internal jugular vein catheter placement, percutaneous lung biopsy, bronchoscopy with transbronchial biopsy, and positive-pressure mechanical ventilation. Tension pneumothorax usually occurs in the setting of penetrating trauma, lung infection, cardiopulmonary resuscitation, or positive-pressure mechanical ventilation. In tension pneumothorax, the pressure of air in the pleural space exceeds ambient pressure throughout the respiratory cycle. A check-valve mechanism allows air to enter the pleural space on inspiration and prevents egress of air on expiration.

Primary pneumothorax affects mainly tall, thin boys and men between the ages of 10 and 30 years. It is thought to occur from rupture of subpleural apical blebs in response to high negative intrapleural pressures. Family history and cigarette smoking may also be important factors.

Secondary pneumothorax occurs as a complication of COPD, asthma, cystic fibrosis, tuberculosis, *Pneumocystis* pneumonia, menstruation (catamenial pneumothorax), and a wide variety of interstitial lung diseases, including sarcoidosis, lymphangioleiomyomatosis, Langerhans cell histiocytosis, and tuberous sclerosis. A history of *Pneumocystis* pneumonia is a risk factor for the development of pneumothorax. One-half of patients with pneumothorax in the setting of recurrent (but not primary) *Pneumocystis* pneumonia will develop pneumothorax on the contralateral side. The mortality rate of pneumothorax in *Pneumocystis* pneumonia is high.

▶ Clinical Findings

A. Symptoms and Signs

Chest pain ranging from minimal to severe on the affected side and dyspnea occur in nearly all patients. Symptoms usually begin during rest and usually resolve within 24 hours even if the pneumothorax persists. Alternatively, pneumothorax may present with life-threatening respiratory failure if underlying lung disease is present.

If pneumothorax is small (less than 15% of a hemithorax), physical findings, other than mild tachycardia, are normal. If pneumothorax is large, diminished breath sounds, decreased tactile fremitus, and decreased movement of the chest are often noted. Tension pneumothorax should be suspected in the presence of marked tachycardia, hypotension, and mediastinal or tracheal shift.

B. Laboratory Findings

Arterial blood gas analysis is often unnecessary but reveals hypoxemia and acute respiratory alkalosis in most patients. Left-sided primary pneumothorax may produce QRS axis and precordial T-wave changes on the ECG that may be misinterpreted as acute myocardial infarction.

C. Imaging

Demonstration of a visceral pleural line on chest radiograph is diagnostic and may be seen only on an expiratory film. A few patients have secondary pleural effusion that demonstrates a characteristic air-fluid level on chest radiography. In supine patients, pneumothorax on a conventional chest radiograph may appear as an abnormally radiolucent costophrenic sulcus (the "deep sulcus" sign). In patients with tension pneumothorax, chest radiographs show a large amount of air in the affected hemithorax and contralateral shift of the mediastinum.

▶ Differential Diagnosis

If the patient is a young, tall, thin, cigarette-smoking man, the diagnosis of primary spontaneous pneumothorax is usually obvious and can be confirmed by chest radiograph. In secondary pneumothorax, it is sometimes difficult to distinguish loculated pneumothorax from an emphysematous bleb. Occasionally, pneumothorax may mimic myocardial infarction, pulmonary embolism, or pneumonia.

▶ Complications

Tension pneumothorax may be life-threatening. Pneumomediastinum and subcutaneous emphysema may occur as complications of spontaneous pneumothorax. If pneumomediastinum is detected, rupture of the esophagus or a bronchus should be considered in the differential diagnosis.

▶ Treatment

Treatment depends on the severity of the pneumothorax and the nature of the underlying disease. In a reliable patient with a small (less than 15% of a hemithorax), stable, spontaneous primary pneumothorax, observation alone may be appropriate. Many small pneumothoraces resolve spontaneously as air is absorbed from the pleural space; supplemental oxygen therapy may increase the rate of reabsorption. Simple aspiration drainage of pleural air with a small-bore catheter (eg, 16-gauge angiocatheter or larger drainage catheter) can be performed for spontaneous primary pneumothoraces that are large or progressive. Placement of a small-bore chest tube (7F to 14F) attached to a one-way Heimlich valve provides protection against development of tension pneumothorax and may permit observation from home. The patient should be treated symptomatically for cough and chest pain, and followed with serial chest radiographs every 24 hours.

Patients with secondary pneumothorax, large pneumothorax, tension pneumothorax, or severe symptoms or those who have a pneumothorax on mechanical ventilation should undergo chest tube placement (tube thoracostomy). The chest tube is placed under water-seal drainage, and suction is applied until the lung expands. The chest tube can be removed after the air leak subsides.

All patients who smoke should be advised to discontinue smoking and warned that the risk of recurrence is 50% if cigarette smoking is continued. Future exposure to high altitudes, flying in unpressurized aircraft, and scuba diving should be avoided.

Indications for thoracoscopy or open thoracotomy include recurrences of spontaneous pneumothorax, any occurrence of bilateral pneumothorax, and failure of tube thoracostomy for the first episode (failure of lung to reexpand or persistent air leak). Surgery permits resection of blebs responsible for the pneumothorax and pleurodesis by mechanical abrasion and insufflation of talc.

Management of pneumothorax in patients with *Pneumocystis* pneumonia is challenging because of a tendency toward recurrence, and there is no consensus on the best approach. Use of a small chest tube attached to a Heimlich valve has been proposed to allow the patient to leave the hospital. Some clinicians favor its insertion early in the course.

▶ Prognosis

An average of 30% of patients with spontaneous pneumothorax experience recurrence of the disorder after either observation or tube thoracostomy for the first episode. Recurrence after surgical therapy is less frequent. Following successful therapy, there are no long-term complications.

Hsu HH et al. The etiology and therapy of primary spontaneous pneumothoraces. Expert Rev Respir Med. 2015 Oct;9(5): 655–65. [PMID: 26366808]

Imran JB et al. JAMA patient page. Pneumothorax. JAMA. 2017 Sep 12;318(10):974. [PMID: 28898380]

Novoa NM et al. When to remove a chest tube. Thorac Surg Clin. 2017 Feb;27(1):41–6. [PMID: 27865326]

Pompili C et al. Chest tube management after surgery for pneumothorax. Thorac Surg Clin. 2017 Feb;27(1):25–8. [PMID: 27865323]

Thelle A et al. Randomised comparison of needle aspiration and chest tube drainage in spontaneous pneumothorax. Eur Respir J. 2017 Apr 12;49(4). [PMID: 28404647]

▼ DISORDERS OF CONTROL OF VENTILATION

The principal influences on ventilatory control are arterial P_{CO_2}, pH, P_{O_2}, and brainstem tissue pH. These variables are monitored by peripheral and central chemoreceptors. Under normal conditions, the ventilatory control system maintains arterial pH and P_{CO_2} within narrow limits; arterial P_{O_2} is more loosely controlled.

Abnormal control of ventilation can be seen with a variety of conditions ranging from rare disorders, such as central alveolar hypoventilation, Ondine curse, neuromuscular disorders, myxedema, starvation, and carotid body resection to more common disorders, such as asthma, COPD, obesity, heart failure, and sleep-related breathing disorders. A few of these disorders will be discussed in this section.

HYPERVENTILATION SYNDROMES

Hyperventilation is an increase in alveolar minute ventilation that leads to hypocapnia. It may be caused by a variety of conditions, such as pregnancy, hypoxemia, obstructive and infiltrative lung diseases, sepsis, liver dysfunction, fever, and pain. Functional hyperventilation may be acute or chronic. **Acute hyperventilation** presents with hyperpnea, paresthesias, carpopedal spasm, tetany, and anxiety. **Chronic hyperventilation** may present with various nonspecific symptoms, including fatigue, dyspnea, anxiety, palpitations, and dizziness. The diagnosis of chronic hyperventilation syndrome is established if symptoms are reproduced during voluntary hyperventilation. Once organic causes of hyperventilation have been excluded, treatment of acute hyperventilation consists of breathing through pursed lips or through the nose with one nostril pinched, or rebreathing expired gas from a paper bag held over the face in order to decrease respiratory alkalemia and its associated symptoms. Anxiolytic drugs may also be useful.

Boulding R et al. Dysfunctional breathing: a review of the literature and proposal for classification. Eur Respir Rev. 2016 Sep;25(141):287–94. [PMID: 27581828]

OBESITY-HYPOVENTILATION SYNDROME (Pickwickian Syndrome)

In obesity-hypoventilation syndrome, awake alveolar hypoventilation appears to result from a combination of blunted ventilatory drive and increased mechanical load imposed upon the chest by obesity. Voluntary hyperventilation returns the PCO_2 and the PO_2 toward normal values, a correction not seen in lung diseases causing chronic respiratory failure, such as COPD. Diagnostic criteria include a body mass index greater than 30, an arterial partial pressure of carbon dioxide greater than 45 mm Hg, and exclusion of other causes of alveolar hypoventilation. Most patients with obesity-hypoventilation syndrome also suffer from obstructive sleep apnea, which must be treated aggressively if identified as a comorbid disorder. Therapy of obesity-hypoventilation syndrome consists mainly of weight loss, which improves hypercapnia and hypoxemia as well as the ventilatory responses to hypoxia and hypercapnia. Avoidance of sedative hypnotics, opioids, and alcohol is also recommended. NIPPV is helpful in many patients. Patients with obesity-hypoventilation syndrome have a higher risk of complications in the perioperative period, including respiratory failure, intubation, and cardiac failure. Recognition of these patients in the perioperative period is an important safety measure.

Böing S et al. Chronic hypoventilation syndromes and sleep-related hypoventilation. J Thorac Dis. 2015 Aug;7(8): 1273–85. [PMID: 26380756]

Howard ME et al. A randomised controlled trial of CPAP versus non-invasive ventilation for initial treatment of obesity hypoventilation syndrome. Thorax. 2017 May;72(5):437–44. [PMID: 27852952]

Piper A. Obesity hypoventilation syndrome: weighing in on therapy options. Chest. 2016 Mar;149(3):856–68. [PMID: 26292036]

SLEEP-RELATED BREATHING DISORDERS

Abnormal ventilation during sleep is manifested by apnea (breath cessation for at least 10 seconds) or hypopnea (decrement in airflow with drop in hemoglobin saturation of at least 4%). Episodes of apnea are **central** if ventilatory effort is absent for the duration of the apneic episode, **obstructive** if ventilatory effort persists throughout the apneic episode but no airflow occurs because of transient obstruction of the upper airway, and **mixed** if absent ventilatory effort precedes upper airway obstruction during the apneic episode. Pure central sleep apnea is uncommon; it may be an isolated finding or may occur in patients with primary alveolar hypoventilation or with lesions of the brainstem. Obstructive and mixed sleep apneas are more common and may be associated with life-threatening cardiac arrhythmias, severe hypoxemia during sleep, daytime somnolence, pulmonary hypertension, cor pulmonale, systemic hypertension, and secondary erythrocytosis.

OBSTRUCTIVE SLEEP APNEA

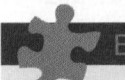

ESSENTIALS OF DIAGNOSIS

▶ Daytime somnolence or fatigue.

▶ A history of loud snoring with witnessed apneic events.

▶ Overnight polysomnography demonstrating apneic episodes with hypoxemia.

▶ General Considerations

Upper airway obstruction during sleep occurs when loss of normal pharyngeal muscle tone allows the pharynx to collapse passively during inspiration. Patients with anatomically narrowed upper airways (eg, micrognathia, macroglossia, obesity, tonsillar hypertrophy) are predisposed to the development of obstructive sleep apnea. Ingestion of alcohol or sedatives before sleeping or nasal obstruction of any type, including the common cold, may precipitate or worsen the condition. Hypothyroidism and cigarette smoking are additional risk factors for obstructive sleep apnea. Before making the diagnosis of obstructive sleep apnea, a drug history should be obtained and a seizure disorder, narcolepsy, and depression should be excluded.

▶ Clinical Findings

A. Symptoms and Signs

Most patients with obstructive or mixed sleep apnea are obese, middle-aged men. Arterial hypertension is common. Patients may complain of excessive daytime somnolence, morning sluggishness and headaches, daytime fatigue, cognitive impairment, recent weight gain, and impotence. Bed partners usually report loud cyclical snoring, breath cessation, witnessed apneas, restlessness, and thrashing movements of the extremities during sleep. Personality changes, poor judgment, work-related problems, depression, and intellectual deterioration (memory impairment, inability to concentrate) may also be observed. The US Preventive Services Task Force does not recommend screening asymptomatic adults for sleep apnea.

Physical examination may be normal or may reveal systemic and pulmonary hypertension with cor pulmonale. The patient may appear sleepy or even fall asleep during the evaluation. The oropharynx is frequently found to be narrowed by excessive soft tissue folds, large tonsils, elongated uvula, or prominent tongue. Nasal obstruction by a deviated nasal septum, poor nasal airflow, and a nasal twang to the speech may be observed. A "bull neck" appearance is common.

B. Laboratory Findings

Erythrocytosis is common. Thyroid function tests (serum TSH, FT_4) should be obtained to exclude hypothyroidism.

C. Other Studies

Observation of the sleeping patient may reveal loud snoring interrupted by episodes of increasingly strong ventilatory effort that fail to produce airflow. A loud snort often accompanies the first breath following an apneic episode. Definitive diagnostic evaluation for suspected sleep apnea includes otorhinolaryngologic examination and overnight polysomnography (the monitoring of multiple physiologic factors during sleep). A complete **polysomnography** examination includes electroencephalography, electrooculography, electromyography, ECG, pulse oximetry, and measurement of respiratory effort and airflow. Polysomnography reveals apneic episodes lasting as long as 60 seconds. Oxygen saturation falls, often to very low levels. Bradydysrhythmias, such as sinus bradycardia, sinus arrest, or atrioventricular block, may occur. Tachydysrhythmias, including paroxysmal supraventricular tachycardia, atrial fibrillation, and ventricular tachycardia, may be seen once airflow is reestablished. Home sleep studies can be done for the person without comorbidities and a moderate to high pretest probability of obstructive sleep apnea. While home studies cannot quantify the stages of sleep, they can provide a reliable index of respiratory and desaturation events.

Treatment

Weight loss and strict avoidance of alcohol and hypnotic medications are the first steps in management. Weight loss may be curative, but most patients are unable to lose the 10–20% of body weight required. **Nasal continuous positive airway pressure (nasal CPAP)** at night is curative in many patients. Auto-titrating CPAP machines allow a range of pressures to be prescribed (5–15 cm H_2O). Polysomnography is frequently necessary to optimize the level of CPAP necessary to abolish obstructive apneas and manage hypoxemia. Unfortunately, only about 75% of patients continue to use nasal CPAP after 1 year. Pharmacologic therapy for obstructive sleep apnea is disappointing. Supplemental oxygen may lessen the severity of nocturnal desaturation but may also lengthen apneas; it should not be routinely prescribed without polysomnography to assess the effects of oxygen therapy. Mechanical devices inserted into the mouth at bedtime to hold the jaw forward and prevent pharyngeal occlusion have modest effectiveness in relieving apnea; however, patient compliance is not optimal.

Uvulopalatopharyngoplasty (UPPP), a procedure consisting of resection of pharyngeal soft tissue and amputation of approximately 15 mm of the free edge of the soft palate and uvula, is helpful in approximately 50% of selected patients. It is more effective in eliminating snoring than apneic episodes. UPPP may be performed on an outpatient basis with a laser. **Nasal septoplasty** is performed if gross anatomic nasal septal deformity is present. **Tracheostomy** relieves upper airway obstruction and its physiologic consequences and represents the definitive treatment for obstructive sleep apnea. However, it has numerous adverse effects, including granuloma formation, difficulty with speech, and stoma and airway infection. Furthermore, the long-term care of the tracheostomy, especially in obese patients, can be difficult. Tracheostomy and other maxillofacial surgery approaches are reserved for patients with life-threatening arrhythmias or severe disability who have not responded to conservative therapy. Hypoglossal nerve stimulation can be an option for select patients who do not respond to CPAP and have certain anatomic features, including nonconcentric airway collapse; a 5-year follow-up study showed improvement in sleepiness, quality of life, and respiratory outcomes in the treatment cohort. A randomized trial of adaptive servo-ventilation in sleep apnea patients with predominant central apnea and impaired left ventricular ejection fraction (less than 45%) reported increased cardiovascular and all-cause mortality in the treatment group.

Jun JC et al. Sleep apnoea. Eur Respir Rev. 2016 Mar;25(139): 12–8. [PMID: 26929416]

Lim DC et al. Obstructive sleep apnea: update and future. Annu Rev Med. 2017 Jan 14;68:99–112. [PMID: 27732789]

Mokhlesi B et al. Diagnostic testing for obstructive sleep apnea in adults. JAMA. 2017 Nov 28;318(20):2035–6. [PMID: 29183053]

Woodson BT et al. Upper airway stimulation for obstructive sleep apnea: 5-year outcomes. Otolaryngol Head Neck Surg 2018 Jul;159(1):194–202. [PMID: 29582703]

ACUTE RESPIRATORY FAILURE

Respiratory failure is defined as respiratory dysfunction resulting in abnormalities of oxygenation or ventilation (CO_2 elimination) severe enough to threaten the function of vital organs. Arterial blood gas criteria for respiratory failure are not absolute but may be arbitrarily established as a PO_2 under 60 mm Hg (7.8 kPa) or a PCO_2 over 50 mm Hg (6.5 kPa). Acute respiratory failure may occur in a variety of pulmonary and nonpulmonary disorders (Table 9–27). Only a few selected general principles of management will be reviewed here.

Clinical Findings

Symptoms and signs of acute respiratory failure are those of the underlying disease combined with those of hypoxemia or hypercapnia. The chief symptom of hypoxemia is dyspnea, though profound hypoxemia may exist in the absence of complaints. Signs of hypoxemia include cyanosis, restlessness, confusion, anxiety, delirium, tachypnea, bradycardia or tachycardia, hypertension, cardiac dysrhythmias, and tremor. Dyspnea and headache are the cardinal symptoms of hypercapnia. Signs of hypercapnia include peripheral and conjunctival hyperemia, hypertension, tachycardia, tachypnea, impaired consciousness,

Table 9–27. Selected causes of acute respiratory failure in adults.

Airway disorders	Neuromuscular and related disorders
Asthma	Primary neuromuscular diseases
Acute exacerbation of chronic bronchitis or emphysema	Guillain-Barré syndrome
Obstruction of pharynx, larynx, trachea, mainstem bronchus, or lobar bronchus by edema, mucus, mass, or foreign body	Myasthenia gravis
	Poliomyelitis
	Polymyositis
	Drug- or toxin-induced
	Botulism
Pulmonary edema	Organophosphates
Increased hydrostatic pressure	Neuromuscular blocking agents
Left ventricular dysfunction (eg, myocardial ischemia, heart failure)	Aminoglycosides
Mitral regurgitation	Spinal cord injury
Left atrial outflow obstruction (eg, mitral stenosis)	Phrenic nerve injury or dysfunction
Volume overload states	Electrolyte disturbances
Increased pulmonary capillary permeability	Hypokalemia
	Hypophosphatemia
Acute respiratory distress syndrome	Myxedema
Acute lung injury	**Central nervous system disorders**
Unclear etiology	Drugs: sedatives, hypnotics, opioids, anesthetics
Neurogenic	Brainstem respiratory center disorders: trauma, tumor, vascular disorders, hypothyroidism
Negative pressure (inspiratory airway obstruction)	
Re-expansion	Intracranial hypertension
Tocolytic-associated	Central nervous system infections
Parenchymal lung disorders	**Increased CO$_2$ production**
Pneumonia	Fever
Interstitial lung diseases	Infection
Diffuse alveolar hemorrhage syndromes	Hyperalimentation with excess caloric and carbohydrate intake
Aspiration	Hyperthyroidism
Lung contusion	Seizures
Pulmonary vascular disorders	Rigors
Thromboembolism	Drugs
Air embolism	
Amniotic fluid embolism	
Chest wall, diaphragm, and pleural disorders	
Rib fracture	
Flail chest	
Pneumothorax	
Pleural effusion	
Massive ascites	
Abdominal distention and abdominal compartment syndrome	

papilledema, and asterixis. The symptoms and signs of acute respiratory failure are both insensitive and nonspecific; therefore, the clinician must maintain a high index of suspicion and obtain arterial blood gas analysis if respiratory failure is suspected.

▶ **Treatment**

Treatment of the patient with acute respiratory failure consists of (1) specific therapy directed toward the underlying disease, (2) respiratory supportive care directed toward the maintenance of adequate gas exchange, and (3) general supportive care. Only the last two aspects are discussed below.

A. Respiratory Support

Respiratory support has both nonventilatory and ventilatory aspects.

1. Nonventilatory aspects—The main therapeutic goal in acute hypoxemic respiratory failure is to ensure adequate oxygenation of vital organs. Inspired oxygen concentration should be the lowest value that results in an arterial hemoglobin saturation of 88% or more (PO$_2$ 55 mm Hg or more [7.3 kPa or more]). Higher arterial oxygen tensions are of no proven benefit and may be deleterious. Restoration of normoxia may rarely cause hypoventilation in patients with chronic hypercapnia; however, oxygen therapy should not be withheld for fear of causing progressive respiratory acidemia. Hypoxemia in patients with obstructive airway disease is usually easily corrected by administering low-flow oxygen by nasal cannula (1–3 L/min) or Venturi mask (24–40%). Higher concentrations of oxygen are necessary to correct hypoxemia in patients with ARDS, pneumonia, and other parenchymal lung diseases. The high flow nasal cannula provides adjustable oxygen delivery and flow-dependent clearance of carbon dioxide from the upper airway resulting in reduced work of breathing and better matching of respiratory demand during respiratory distress. In hypoxemia due to acute respiratory failure, oxygenation with use of a high flow nasal cannula has been shown to be similar, and in some cases superior, to conventional low flow oxygen supplementation and to noninvasive positive pressure ventilation.

2. Ventilatory aspects—Ventilatory support consists of maintaining patency of the airway and ensuring adequate alveolar ventilation. Mechanical ventilation may be provided via mask (noninvasive) or through tracheal intubation.

A. NONINVASIVE POSITIVE-PRESSURE VENTILATION—NIPPV delivered via a full face mask or nasal mask is first-line therapy in COPD patients with hypercapnic respiratory failure who can protect and maintain the patency of their airway, handle their own secretions, and tolerate the mask apparatus. Several studies have demonstrated the effectiveness of this therapy in reducing intubation rates and ICU stays in patients with ventilatory failure. A bilevel positive-pressure ventilation mode is preferred for most patients. Patients with acute lung injury or ARDS or those who suffer from severely impaired oxygenation are less likely to benefit and should be intubated if they require mechanical ventilation.

B. TRACHEAL INTUBATION—Indications for tracheal intubation include (1) hypoxemia despite supplemental oxygen; (2) upper airway obstruction; (3) impaired airway protection; (4) inability to clear secretions; (5) respiratory acidosis; (6) progressive general fatigue, tachypnea, use of accessory respiratory muscles, or mental status deterioration; and (7) apnea. Patients in respiratory failure who undergo a trial of NIPPV and do not improve within 30–90 minutes should be intubated. In general, orotracheal intubation is preferred to nasotracheal intubation in urgent or emergency situations because it is easier, faster, and less traumatic. The tip of the endotracheal tube should be positioned 2–4 cm above the carina and be verified by chest radiograph immediately following intubation. Only tracheal tubes with high-volume, low-pressure air-filled cuffs should be used. Cuff inflation pressure should be kept below 20 mm Hg if possible to minimize tracheal mucosal injury.

C. MECHANICAL VENTILATION—Indications for mechanical ventilation include (1) apnea, (2) acute hypercapnia that is not quickly reversed by appropriate specific therapy, (3) severe hypoxemia, and (4) progressive patient fatigue despite appropriate treatment.

Several modes of positive-pressure ventilation are available. Controlled mechanical ventilation (CMV; also known as assist-control [A-C]) and synchronized intermittent mandatory ventilation (SIMV) are ventilatory modes in which the ventilator delivers a minimum number of breaths of a specified tidal volume each minute. In both CMV and SIMV, the patient may trigger the ventilator to deliver additional breaths. In CMV, the ventilator responds to breaths initiated by the patient above the set rate by delivering additional full tidal volume breaths. In SIMV, additional breaths are not supported by the ventilator unless the pressure support mode is added. Numerous alternative modes of mechanical ventilation now exist, the most popular being pressure support ventilation (PSV), pressure control ventilation (PCV), and CPAP.

PEEP is useful in improving oxygenation in patients with diffuse parenchymal lung disease, such as ARDS. It should be used cautiously in patients with localized parenchymal disease, emphysema, hyperinflation, or very high airway pressure requirements during mechanical ventilation.

D. COMPLICATIONS OF MECHANICAL VENTILATION—Potential complications of mechanical ventilation are numerous. Migration of the tip of the endotracheal tube into a main bronchus can cause atelectasis of the contralateral lung and overdistention of the intubated lung. Barotrauma refers to rupture and loss of integrity of the alveolar space secondary to high transmural pressures applied during positive pressure ventilation. Barotrauma is manifested by subcutaneous emphysema, pneumomediastinum, subpleural air cysts, pneumothorax, or systemic gas embolism. Volutrauma is sometimes used to refer to subtle parenchymal injury due to overdistention of alveoli from excessive tidal volumes without alveolar rupture, mediated through inflammatory rather than physical mechanisms. The principal strategy to avoid volutrauma is the use of low tidal volume ventilation.

Acute respiratory alkalosis caused by overventilation is common. Hypotension induced by elevated intrathoracic pressure that results in decreased return of systemic venous blood to the heart may occur in patients treated with PEEP, particularly those with intravascular volume depletion, and in patients with severe airflow obstruction at high respiratory rates that promote "breath stacking" (dynamic hyperinflation). Ventilator-associated pneumonia is another serious complication of mechanical ventilation.

B. General Supportive Care

Hypokalemia and hypophosphatemia may worsen hypoventilation due to respiratory muscle weakness. Sedative-hypnotics and opioid analgesics should be titrated carefully to avoid oversedation, leading to prolongation of intubation. Temporary paralysis with a nondepolarizing neuromuscular blocking agent is used to facilitate mechanical ventilation and to lower oxygen consumption. Prolonged muscle weakness due to an acute myopathy is a potential complication of these agents. Myopathy is more common in patients with kidney injury and in those given concomitant corticosteroids.

Psychological and emotional support of the patient and family, skin care to avoid pressure injuries (previously called pressure ulcers), and meticulous avoidance of health care–associated infection and complications of tracheal tubes are vital aspects of comprehensive care for patients with acute respiratory failure.

Attention must also be paid to preventing complications associated with serious illness. Stress gastritis and ulcers may be avoided by administering sucralfate (1 g orally twice a day), histamine H_2-receptor antagonists, or PPIs. There is some concern that the latter two agents, which raise gastric pH, may permit increased growth of gram-negative bacteria in the stomach, predisposing to pharyngeal colonization and ultimately HCAP; many clinicians therefore prefer sucralfate. The risk of DVT and PE may be reduced by subcutaneous administration of heparin (5000 units every 12 hours), the use of LMWH (see Table 14–14), or placement of sequential compression devices on the lower extremities.

▶ Course & Prognosis

The course and prognosis of acute respiratory failure vary and depend on the underlying disease. The prognosis of acute respiratory failure caused by uncomplicated sedative or opioid overdose is excellent. Acute respiratory failure in patients with COPD who do not require intubation and mechanical ventilation has a good immediate prognosis. On the other hand, ARDS and respiratory failure associated with sepsis have a poor prognosis.

Drake MG. High flow nasal cannula oxygen in adults: an evidence-based assessment. Ann Am Thorac Soc. 2018 Feb;15(2): 145–55. [PMID: 29144160]

Li Z et al. Efficacy of non-invasive ventilation and oxygen therapy on immunocompromised patients with acute hypoxaemic respiratory failure: protocol for a systematic review and meta-analysis of randomised controlled trials. BMJ Open. 2017 Jun 30;7(6):e015335. [PMID: 28667214]

Meeder AM et al. Noninvasive and invasive positive pressure ventilation for acute respiratory failure in critically ill patients: a comparative cohort study. J Thorac Dis. 2016 May;8(5): 813–25. [PMID: 27162654]

Ni YN et al. Can high-flow nasal cannula reduce the rate of endotracheal intubation in adult patients with acute respiratory failure compared with conventional oxygen therapy and noninvasive positive pressure ventilation? A systematic review and meta-analysis. Chest. 2017 Apr;151(4):764–75. [PMID: 28089816]

Rochwerg B et al. Official ERS/ATS clinical practice guidelines: noninvasive ventilation for acute respiratory failure. Eur Respir J. 2017 Aug 31;50(2). [PMID: 28860265]

ACUTE RESPIRATORY DISTRESS SYNDROME

ESSENTIALS OF DIAGNOSIS

▶ Onset of respiratory distress, often progressing to respiratory failure, within 7 days of a known clinical insult.

▶ New, bilateral radiographic pulmonary opacities not explained by pleural effusion, atelectasis, or nodules.

▶ Respiratory failure not fully explained by heart failure or volume overload.

▶ Impaired oxygenation, with ratio of partial pressure of oxygen in arterial blood (Pao_2) to fractional concentration of inspired oxygen (Fio_2) less than 300 mm Hg, with PEEP 5 cm H_2O or more.

General Considerations

Acute respiratory distress syndrome (ARDS) as a clinical syndrome is based on three inclusion criteria plus one exclusion criterion, as detailed above. The severity of ARDS is based on the level of oxygenation impairment: **mild,** Pao_2/Fio_2 ratio between 200 and 300 mm Hg; **moderate,** Pao_2/Fio_2 ratio between 100 and 200 mm Hg; and **severe,** Pao_2/Fio_2 ratio less than 100 mm Hg.

ARDS may follow a wide variety of clinical events (Table 9–28). Common risk factors for ARDS include sepsis, aspiration of gastric contents, shock, infection, lung contusion, nonthoracic trauma, toxic inhalation, near-drowning, and multiple blood transfusions. About one-third of ARDS patients initially have sepsis syndrome. Damage to capillary endothelial cells and alveolar epithelial cells is common to ARDS regardless of cause or mechanism of lung injury, resulting in increased vascular permeability and decreased production and activity of surfactant; these abnormalities lead to interstitial and alveolar pulmonary edema, alveolar collapse, and hypoxemia.

Clinical Findings

ARDS is marked by the rapid onset of profound dyspnea that usually occurs 12–48 hours after the initiating event. Labored breathing, tachypnea, intercostal retractions, and crackles are noted on physical examination.

Table 9–28. Selected disorders associated with ARDS.

Systemic Insults	Pulmonary Insults
Trauma	Aspiration of gastric contents
Sepsis	Embolism of thrombus, fat, air, or amniotic fluid
Pancreatitis	
Shock	Miliary tuberculosis
Multiple transfusions	Diffuse pneumonia (eg, SARS)
Disseminated intravascular coagulation	Acute eosinophilic pneumonia
	Cryptogenic organizing pneumonitis
Burns	
Drugs and drug overdose	Upper airway obstruction
Opioids	Free-base cocaine smoking
Aspirin	Near-drowning
Phenothiazines	Toxic gas inhalation
Tricyclic antidepressants	Nitrogen dioxide
Amiodarone	Chlorine
Chemotherapeutic agents	Sulfur dioxide
Nitrofurantoin	Ammonia
Protamine	Smoke
Thrombotic thrombocytopenic purpura	Oxygen toxicity
	Lung contusion
Cardiopulmonary bypass	Radiation exposure
Head injury	High-altitude exposure
Paraquat	Lung reexpansion or reperfusion

ARDS, acute respiratory distress syndrome; SARS, severe acute respiratory syndrome.

Chest radiography shows diffuse or patchy bilateral infiltrates that rapidly become confluent; these characteristically spare the costophrenic angles. Air bronchograms occur in about 80% of cases. Heart size is usually normal, and pleural effusions are small or nonexistent. Marked hypoxemia occurs that is refractory to treatment with supplemental oxygen. Many patients with ARDS demonstrate multiple organ failure, particularly involving the kidneys, liver, gut, central nervous system, and cardiovascular system.

Differential Diagnosis

Since ARDS is a physiologic and radiographic syndrome rather than a specific disease, the concept of differential diagnosis does not strictly apply. Normal-permeability ("cardiogenic" or hydrostatic) pulmonary edema must be excluded, however, because specific therapy is available for that disorder. Emergent echocardiogram or measurement of pulmonary capillary wedge pressure by means of a flow-directed pulmonary artery catheter may be required in selected patients with suspected cardiac dysfunction; routine use in ARDS is discouraged.

Prevention

No measures that effectively prevent ARDS have been identified. Specifically, neither PEEP nor aspirin when used prophylactically has been shown to be effective in patients at risk for ARDS. Intravenous methylprednisolone does not prevent ARDS when given early to patients with sepsis syndrome or septic shock.

► **Treatment**

The first principle in management is to identify and treat the primary condition that has led to ARDS. Meticulous supportive care must then be provided to compensate for the severe dysfunction of the respiratory system associated with ARDS and to prevent complications.

Treatment of the hypoxemia seen in ARDS usually requires tracheal intubation and positive-pressure mechanical ventilation. The lowest levels of PEEP (used to recruit atelectatic alveoli) and supplemental oxygen required to maintain the Pao_2 above 55 mm Hg (7.13 kPa) or the Sao_2 above 88% should be used. Efforts should be made to decrease Fio_2 as soon as possible in order to avoid oxygen toxicity. PEEP can be increased as needed as long as cardiac output and oxygen delivery do not decrease and airway pressures do not increase excessively (ie, plateau pressures remain below 30 cm H_2O). Prone positioning frequently improves oxygenation by helping recruit atelectatic alveoli and has been shown in some (although not all) trials to provide a mortality benefit in severe ARDS. In one placebo-controlled randomized trial, neuromuscular blockade (by continuous infusion of cisatracurium at 37.5 mg/h) for 48 hours upon initiation of mechanical ventilation was associated with improved mortality and more ventilator-free days in patients with Pao_2/Fio_2 ratio less than 120 mm Hg.

A variety of mechanical ventilation strategies are available. The most significant advance in the treatment of ARDS over the past 20 years has been the recognition of the potential for excessive alveolar stretch to cause lung injury, and the widespread adoption of low tidal volume ventilation. A multicenter study of 800 patients demonstrated that a protocol using volume-control ventilation with low tidal volumes (6 mL/kg of ideal body weight) resulted in an 8.8% absolute mortality reduction over therapy with standard tidal volumes (defined as 12 mL/kg of ideal body weight). Varying ventilator modes have been used; conventional modes of ventilation are essentially equivalent, while high-frequency oscillatory ventilation should not be used an as initial mode. Some early data support the use of airway pressure-release ventilation as an initial mode but are not yet convincing enough to change general practice.

Approaches to hemodynamic monitoring and fluid management in patients with acute lung injury have been carefully studied. A prospective RCT comparing hemodynamic management guided either by a pulmonary artery catheter or a central venous catheter using an explicit management protocol demonstrated that a pulmonary artery catheter should not be routinely used for the management of acute lung injury. A subsequent randomized, prospective clinical study of restrictive fluid intake and diuresis as needed to maintain central venous pressure less than 4 mm Hg or pulmonary artery occlusion pressure less than 8 mm Hg (conservative strategy group) versus a fluid management protocol to target a central venous pressure of 10–14 mm Hg or a pulmonary artery occlusion pressure 14–18 mm Hg (liberal strategy group) showed that patients in the conservative strategy group experienced faster improvement in lung function and spent significantly fewer days on mechanical ventilation and in the ICU

without an improvement in death by 60 days or worsening nonpulmonary organ failure at 28 days. Oxygen delivery can be increased in anemic patients by ensuring that hemoglobin concentrations are at least 7 g/dL (70 g/L); patients are not likely to benefit from higher levels. Increasing oxygen delivery to supranormal levels through the use of inotropes and high hemoglobin concentrations is not clinically useful and may be harmful. Strategies to decrease oxygen consumption include the appropriate use of sedatives, analgesics, and antipyretics.

A large number of innovative therapeutic interventions to improve outcomes in ARDS patients have been or are being investigated. Unfortunately, to date, none have consistently shown benefit in clinical trials. Systemic corticosteroids have been studied extensively with variable and inconsistent results. While a few small studies suggest some specific improved outcomes when given within the first 2 weeks after the onset of ARDS, mortality appears increased when corticosteroids are started more than 2 weeks after the onset of ARDS. Therefore, routine use of corticosteroids is not recommended.

Another therapeutic intervention is extracorporeal membrane oxygenation (ECMO). The technique has been in use since the 1970s but has been gaining wider acceptance. The EOLIA trial, published in May 2018, compared the early use of ECMO in very severe ARDS with conventional strategies built on low-tidal-volume ventilation. Results failed to show a difference in 60-day mortality; however, 28% of the control group crossed over to receive ECMO. As a result, ECMO seems unlikely to become a standard first-line therapy but is likely to remain a salvage option for patients with very severe ARDS.

► **Course & Prognosis**

Overall, ARDS mortality with low tidal volume ventilation is around 30% in ARDSnet studies. The major causes of death are the primary illness and secondary complications, such as multiple organ system failure or sepsis. Many patients who die of ARDS and its complications die after withdrawal of mechanical ventilation (see Chapter 5). One troubling aspect of ARDS care is that the actual mortality of ARDS in community hospitals continues to be higher than at academic hospitals. This may reflect the fact that a significant number of community hospital–based clinicians have not adopted low lung volume ventilation.

Different clinical syndromes that lead to ARDS carry different prognoses. For example, patients with trauma-associated ARDS have better prognosis, with a mortality rate close to 20%, whereas those with end-stage liver disease have an 80% mortality rate. This likely reflects both the effects of significant comorbidities (trauma patients tend to be younger and healthier) as well as phenotypic differences within ARDS associated with different precipitants. Post-hoc analyses of data from several major trials have shown that a hyperinflammatory phenotype associated with high levels of interleukin-6 and soluble tumor necrosis factor receptor in ARDS patients precipitated by sepsis is associated with more multiorgan dysfunction and higher mortality. This may have implications for precision-medicine treatment of ARDS. Reanalysis of data from the HARP-2 trial studying the use of simvastatin in ARDS found it to have a mortality benefit in the hyperinflammatory patient.

Failure to improve in the first week of treatment is a poor prognostic sign. Survivors tend to be young and pulmonary function generally recovers over 6–12 months, although residual abnormalities often remain, including restrictive or obstructive defects, low diffusion capacity, and impaired gas exchange with exercise. Survivors of ARDS also have diminished health-related and pulmonary disease–specific quality of life as well as systemic effects, such as muscle wasting, weakness, and fatigue.

Calfee C et al. Acute respiratory distress syndrome subphenotypes and differential response to simvastatin: secondary analysis of a randomised controlled trial. Lancet Respir Med. 2018 Sep;6(9):691–8. [PMID: 30078618]

Combes A et al; EOLIA Trial Group, REVA, and ECMONet. Extracorporeal membrane oxygenation for severe acute respiratory distress syndrome. N Engl J Med. 2018 May 24; 378(21):1965–75. [PMID: 29791822]

Fan E et al. Acute respiratory distress syndrome: advances in diagnosis and treatment. JAMA. 2018 Feb 20;319(7):698–710. [PMID: 29466596]

Gattinoni L et al. Time to rethink the approach to treating acute respiratory distress syndrome. JAMA. 2018 Feb 20;319(7): 664–6. [PMID: 29466572]

Howell MD et al. Management of ARDS in adults. JAMA. 2018 Feb 20;319(7):711–2. [PMID: 29466577]

Matthay MA et al. Clinical trials in acute respiratory distress syndrome: challenges and opportunities. Lancet Respir Med. 2017 Jun;5(6):524–34. [PMID: 28664851]

Thompson BT et al. Acute respiratory distress syndrome. N Engl J Med. 2017 Aug 10;377(6):562–72. [PMID: 28792873]

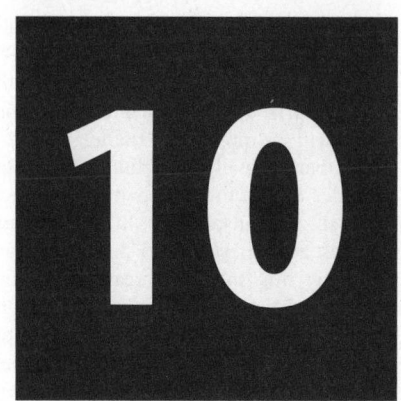

Heart Disease

Thomas M. Bashore, MD
Christopher B. Granger, MD
Kevin P. Jackson, MD
Manesh R. Patel, MD

ADULT CONGENITAL HEART DISEASE

In the United States, there are many more adults with congenital heart disease than children, with an estimated 2 million adults in the United States surviving with congenital heart disease.

Bhatt AB et al. Congenital heart disease in the older adult: a scientific statement from the American Heart Association. Circulation. 2015 May 26;131(21):1884–931. [PMID: 25896865]

Canobbio MM et al; American Heart Association Council on Cardiovascular and Stroke Nursing; Council on Clinical Cardiology; Council on Cardiovascular Disease in the Young; Council on Functional Genomics and Translational Biology; and Council on Quality of Care and Outcomes Research. Management of pregnancy in patients with complex congenital heart disease: a scientific statement for healthcare professionals from the American Heart Association. Circulation. 2017 Feb 21;135(8):e50–87. [PMID: 28082385]

Lui GK et al; American Heart Association Adult Congenital Heart Disease Committee of the Council on Clinical Cardiology and Council on Cardiovascular Disease in the Young; Council on Cardiovascular Radiology and Intervention; and Council on Quality of Care and Outcomes Research. Diagnosis and management of noncardiac complications in adults with congenital heart disease: a scientific statement from the American Heart Association. Circulation. 2017 Nov 14; 136(20):e348–92. [PMID: 28993401]

Stout KK et al. 2018 AHA/ACC guideline for the management of adults with congenital heart disease: a report of the American College of Cardiology/American Heart Association Task Force on Clinical Practice Guidelines. J Am Coll Cardiol. 2019 Apr 2; 73(12):e81–e192. [PMID: 30121239]

Warnes CA. Adult congenital heart disease: the challenges of a lifetime. Eur Heart J. 2017 Jul 7;38(26):2041–7. [PMID: 28011704]

PULMONARY VALVE STENOSIS

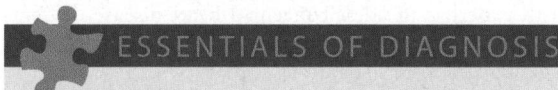

ESSENTIALS OF DIAGNOSIS

▶ Severe cases may present with right-sided heart failure.

▶ P_2 delayed and soft or absent.

▶ Pulmonary ejection click often present and decreases with inspiration—the only right heart sound that *decreases* with inspiration; all other right heart sounds increase.

▶ Echocardiography/Doppler is diagnostic.

▶ Patients with peak pulmonic valve gradients greater than 60 mm Hg or a mean of 40 mm Hg by echocardiography/Doppler should undergo intervention regardless of symptoms. Otherwise, operate for symptoms or evidence for right ventricular dysfunction.

General Considerations

Stenosis of the pulmonary valve or right ventricular (RV) infundibulum increases the resistance to RV outflow, raises the RV pressure, and limits pulmonary blood flow. Pulmonic stenosis is often congenital and associated with other cardiac lesions. Pulmonary blood flow preferentially goes to the left lung in valvular pulmonic stenosis. In the absence of associated shunts, arterial saturation is normal. Peripheral pulmonic stenosis can accompany valvular pulmonic stenosis and may be part of a variety of clinical syndromes, including the congenital rubella syndrome. Patients who have had the **Ross procedure** for aortic valve disease (transfer of the pulmonary valve to the aortic position with a homograft pulmonary valve placed in the pulmonary position) may experience noncongenital postoperative pulmonic valvular or main pulmonary artery (PA) stenosis due to an immune response in the homograft. RV outflow obstructions can also occur when there is a conduit from the RV to the pulmonary artery that becomes stenotic from degenerative changes over time or when there is degeneration of a bioprosthetic replacement pulmonary valve.

Clinical Findings

A. Symptoms and Signs

Mild cases of pulmonic stenosis are asymptomatic; moderate to severe pulmonic stenosis may cause symptoms of dyspnea on exertion, syncope, chest pain, and eventually RV failure.

On examination, there is often a palpable parasternal lift due to right ventricular hypertrophy (RVH) and the pulmonary outflow tract may be palpable if the PA is enlarged. A loud, harsh systolic murmur and occasionally a prominent thrill are present in the left second and third interspaces parasternally. The murmur radiates toward the left shoulder due to the flow pattern within the main PA and increases with inspiration. In mild to moderate pulmonic stenosis, a loud ejection click can be heard to precede the murmur; this sound decreases with inspiration as the increased RV filling from inspiration prematurely opens the valve during atrial systole when inspiratory increased blood flow to the right heart occurs. The valve excursion during systole is thus less with inspiration than with expiration, and the click is therefore less audible with inspiration. **This is the only right-sided auscultatory event that** *decreases* **with inspiration.** All of the other auscultatory events increase with the increased right heart output that occurs with inspiration. In severe pulmonic stenosis, the second sound is obscured by the murmur and the pulmonary component of S_2 may be diminished, delayed, or absent. A right-sided S_4 and a prominent *a* wave in the venous pulse are present when there is RV diastolic dysfunction or a *c-v* wave may be observed in the jugular venous pressure if tricuspid regurgitation is present. Pulmonary valve regurgitation is relatively uncommon in primary pulmonic stenosis and may be very difficult to hear, as the gradient between the reduced PA diastolic pressure and the elevated RV diastolic pressure may be quite small (low-pressure pulmonary valve regurgitation).

B. ECG and Chest Radiography

Right axis deviation or RVH is noted; peaked P waves provide evidence of right atrial (RA) overload. Heart size may be normal on radiographs, or there may be a prominent RV and RA or gross cardiac enlargement, depending on the severity. There is often poststenotic dilation of the main and left pulmonary arteries. Pulmonary vascularity is usually normal, although there tends to be preferential flow to the left lung.

C. Diagnostic Studies

Echocardiography/Doppler is the diagnostic tool of choice, can provide evidence for a doming valve versus a dysplastic valve, can determine the gradient across the valve, and can provide information regarding subvalvular obstruction and the presence or absence of tricuspid or pulmonic valvular regurgitation. Mild pulmonic stenosis is present if the peak gradient by echocardiography/Doppler is less than 30 mm Hg, moderate pulmonic stenosis is present if the peak gradient is between 30 mm Hg and 60 mm Hg, and severe pulmonic stenosis is present if the peak gradient is greater than 60 mm Hg or the mean gradient is greater than 40 mm Hg. A lower gradient may be evident if there is RV dysfunction. Catheterization is usually unnecessary for the diagnosis; it should be used only if the data are unclear or in preparation for either percutaneous intervention or surgery.

Prognosis & Treatment

Patients with mild pulmonic stenosis have a normal life span with no intervention. Moderate stenosis may be asymptomatic in childhood and adolescence, but symptoms often appear as patients grow older. The degree of stenosis does worsen with time in a few patients, so serial follow-up is important. Severe stenosis is rarely associated with sudden death but can cause right heart failure in patients as early as in their 20s and 30s. Pregnancy and exercise tend to be well tolerated except in severe stenosis.

Class I (definitive) indications for intervention include all symptomatic patients and all those with a resting peak-to-peak gradient greater than 60 mm Hg or a mean greater than 40 mm Hg, regardless of symptoms. Percutaneous balloon valvuloplasty is highly successful in domed valve patients and is the treatment of choice. Surgical commissurotomy can also be done, or pulmonary valve replacement (with either a bioprosthetic valve or homograft) when pulmonary valve regurgitation is too severe or the valve is dysplastic. Pulmonary outflow tract obstruction due to RV to PA conduit obstruction or to homograft pulmonary valve stenosis can often be relieved with a percutaneously implanted pulmonary valve (both the Medtronic Melody valve and the Edwards Sapien XT valve are FDA approved). Frequently the seating of these valves is facilitated by placing a stent within the pulmonary artery first, then the transcatheter device within this stent. Because the new catheter valve may result in compression of the coronary artery, it is a Class I requirement to assess the effect of the device on the coronary by use of a temporary balloon inflation prior to delivery of the device. Percutaneous pulmonary valve replacement is also FDA approved for those with conduit stenosis or following the Ross procedure. Percutaneous valve replacements have also been performed off-label for patients with native pulmonary valve disease, including those who have had tetralogy of Fallot repair (assuming the PA root size is small enough to seat a percutaneous valve).

Endocarditis prophylaxis is unnecessary for native valves even after valvuloplasty unless there has been prior pulmonary valve endocarditis (an unusual occurrence) (see Table 33–3). It should be used if surgical or percutaneous valve replacement has occurred. There appears to be more pulmonary valve endocarditis following percutaneous pulmonary valve replacement with the Melody valve than expected, and this is being closely monitored by the FDA.

When to Refer

All symptomatic patients (regardless of gradient) and all asymptomatic patients whose peak pulmonary valve gradient is greater than 64 mm Hg or whose mean gradient is greater than 35 mm Hg should be referred to a cardiologist with expertise in adult congenital heart disease. Patients also require intervention if cyanosis occurs due to patent foramen ovale (PFO) or atrial septal defect (ASD) or if there is exercise intolerance.

Boudjemline Y. Percutaneous pulmonary valve implantation: what have we learned over the years? EuroIntervention. 2017 Sep 24;13(AA):AA60–7. [PMID: 28942387]

Fathallah M et al. Pulmonic valve disease: review of pathology and current treatment options. Curr Cardiol Rep. 2017 Sep 16;19(11):108. [PMID: 28916901]

Hascoet S et al. Infective endocarditis risk after percutaneous pulmonary valve replacement with the Melody and Sapien valves. JACC Cardiovasc Interv. 2017 Mar 13;10(5):510–7. [PMID: 28279319]

Stout KK et al. 2018 AHA/ACC guideline for the management of adults with congenital heart disease: a report of the American College of Cardiology/American Heart Association Task Force on Clinical Practice Guidelines. J Am Coll Cardiol. 2019 Apr 2;73(12):e81–e192. [PMID: 30121239]

COARCTATION OF THE AORTA

 ESSENTIALS OF DIAGNOSIS

► Usual presentation is systemic hypertension.

► Echocardiography/Doppler is diagnostic; a peak gradient of more than 20 mm Hg may be significant due to collaterals around the coarctation reducing gradient despite severe obstruction.

► Associated bicuspid aortic valve in 50–80% of patients.

► Delayed pulse in femoral artery compared to brachial artery.

► Systolic pressure is higher in upper extremities than in lower extremities; diastolic pressures are similar.

General Considerations

Coarctation of the aorta consists of localized narrowing of the aortic arch just distal to the origin of the left subclavian artery. If the stenosis is severe, collateral circulation develops around the coarctation site through the intercostal arteries and the branches of the subclavian arteries and can result in a lower transcoarctation gradient by enabling blood flow to bypass the obstruction. **Coarctation is a cause of secondary hypertension and should be considered in young patients with elevated blood pressure (BP).** The renin-angiotensin system is often abnormal, however, and contributes to the hypertension occasionally seen even after coarctation repair. A bicuspid valve is seen in approximately 50–80% of the cases, and there is an increased incidence of cerebral berry aneurysms. Significant native or recurrent aortic coarctation has been defined as follows: upper extremity/lower extremity resting peak-to-peak gradient greater than 20 mm Hg or mean Doppler systolic gradient greater than 20 mm Hg; upper extremity/lower extremity gradient greater than 10 mm Hg or mean Doppler gradient greater than 10 mm Hg when there is either decreased left ventricular (LV) systolic function or aortic regurgitation (AR); or upper extremity/lower extremity gradient greater than 10 mm Hg or mean Doppler gradient greater than 10 mm Hg when there is evidence for collateral flow around the coarctation. This should be coupled with anatomic evidence for coarctation of the aorta, typically defined by advanced imaging (cardiac magnetic resonance, CT angiography).

Clinical Findings

A. Symptoms and Signs

If cardiac failure does not occur in infancy, there are usually no symptoms until the hypertension produces LV failure. Cerebral hemorrhage, though rare, may occur. Multiple studies have demonstrated an increased frequency of intracranial aneurysm in adults with coarctation of the aorta. Approximately 10% of patients with coarctation of the aorta have intracranial aneurysms identified on magnetic resonance angiography or CT angiography. Increasing age has been identified as a risk factor. Strong arterial pulsations are seen in the neck and suprasternal notch. Hypertension is present in the arms, but the pressure is normal or low in the legs. This difference is exaggerated by exercise. Femoral pulsations are weak and are delayed in comparison with the brachial or radial pulse. A continuous murmur heard superiorly and midline in the back or over the left anterior chest may be present when large collaterals are present and is a clue that the coarctation is severe. The coarctation itself may result in systolic ejection murmurs heard in the left upper lung field anteriorly and near the spine on the left side posteriorly. There may be an aortic regurgitation or stenosis murmur due to an associated bicuspid aortic valve. Coarctation is associated with Turner syndrome (a sex chromosomal abnormality [XO]); a webbed neck may be present in these patients.

B. ECG and Chest Radiography

The ECG usually shows LV hypertrophy (LVH). Radiography may show scalloping of the inferior portion of the ribs (rib notching) due to enlarged collateral intercostal arteries. Dilation of the left subclavian artery and poststenotic aortic dilation along with LV enlargement may be present. The coarctation region and the poststenotic dilation of the descending aorta may result in a **"3" sign** along the aortic shadow on the PA chest radiograph (the notch in the "3" representing the area of coarctation).

C. Diagnostic Studies

Echocardiography/Doppler is usually diagnostic and may provide additional evidence for a bicuspid aortic valve. Both MRI and CT can provide excellent images of the coarctation anatomy, and one or the other should always be done to define the coarctation anatomic structure. MRI and echocardiography/Doppler can also provide estimates of the gradient across the lesion. Cardiac catheterization provides definitive gradient information and is necessary if percutaneous stenting is to be considered.

Prognosis & Treatment

Cardiac failure is common in infancy and in older untreated patients when the coarctation is severe. Patients with a demonstrated peak gradient of greater than 20 mm Hg should be considered for intervention, especially if there is evidence of collateral blood vessels. Many untreated patients with severe coarctation die of hypertension, rupture of the aorta, infective endarteritis, or cerebral hemorrhage before the age of 50. Aortic dissection also occurs with increased frequency. Coarctation of any significance may be poorly tolerated in pregnancy because of the inability to support the placental flow.

Resection of the coarctation site has a surgical mortality rate of 1–4% and includes risk of spinal cord injury. The percutaneous interventional procedure of choice is endovascular stenting; when anatomically feasible, self-expanding and balloon-expandable covered stents have been shown to be advantageous over bare metal stents. These covered stents are FDA approved. Most coarctation repair in adults is percutaneous. Otherwise, surgical resection (usually with end-to-end anastomosis) should be performed. About 25% of surgically corrected patients continue to be hypertensive years after surgery because of permanent changes in the renin-angiotensin system, endothelial dysfunction, aortic stiffness, altered arch morphology, and increased ventricular stiffness. Recurrence of the coarctation stenosis following intervention requires long-term follow-up.

► When to Refer

All patients with aortic coarctation and any detectable gradient should be referred to a cardiologist with expertise in adult congenital heart disease.

Haji Zeinali AM et al. Midterm to long-term safety and efficacy of self-expandable nitinol stent implantation for coarctation of aorta in adults. Catheter Cardiovasc Interv. 2017 Sep 1; 90(3):425–31. [PMID: 28707350]

Morgan GJ et al. Optimus covered stent: advanced covered stent technology for complex congenital heart disease. Congenit Heart Dis. 2018 May;13(3):458–62. [PMID: 29468813]

Rinnström D et al. Hypertension in adults with repaired coarctation of the aorta. Am Heart J. 2016 Nov;181:10–5. [PMID: 27823680]

Schneider H. Modern management of coarctation of the aorta: transcatheter and surgical options. J Cardiovasc Surg (Torino). 2016 Aug;57(4):557–68. [PMID: 27243624]

Stout KK et al. 2018 AHA/ACC guideline for the management of adults with congenital heart disease: a report of the American College of Cardiology/American Heart Association Task Force on Clinical Practice Guidelines. J Am Coll Cardiol. 2019 Apr 2;73(12):e81–e192. [PMID: 30121239]

ATRIAL SEPTAL DEFECT & PATENT FORAMEN OVALE

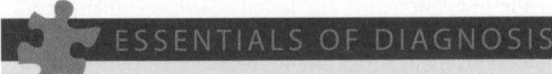

ESSENTIALS OF DIAGNOSIS

► Often asymptomatic and discovered on routine physical examination.

► With an atrial septal defect (ASD) and left to right shunt: RV lift; S_2 widely split and fixed.

► Echocardiography/Doppler is diagnostic.

► ASDs should be closed if there is evidence of an RV volume overload regardless of symptoms.

► A patent foramen ovale (PFO), present in 25% of the population, rarely can lead to paradoxic emboli.

► General Considerations

The most common form of ASD (80% of cases) is persistence of the ostium secundum in the mid-septum. A less common abnormality is persistence of the ostium primum (low in the septum). In most patients with an ostium primum defect, there are mitral or tricuspid valve "clefts" as well as a ventricular septal defect (VSD) as part of the atrioventricular (AV) septal defect. A sinus venosus defect is a hole, usually at the upper (or rarely the lower) part of the atrial septum, due to failure of the embryonic superior vena cava or the inferior vena cava to merge with the atria properly. The superior vena cava sinus venosus defect is usually associated with an anomalous connection of the right upper pulmonary vein into the superior vena cava. The coronary sinus ASD is rare and is basically an unroofed coronary sinus that results in shunting from the left atrium (LA) to the coronary sinus and then to the RA.

In all cases, normally oxygenated blood from the higher-pressure LA shunts into the RA, increasing RV output and pulmonary blood flow. In children, the degree of shunting across these defects may be quite large (pulmonary to systemic blood flow ratios of 3:1 or so). As the RV compliance worsens from the chronic volume overload, the RA pressure may rise and the degree of left-to-right shunting may decrease over time. Eventually, if the RA pressure exceeds the LA, the shunt may reverse and be primarily right-to-left. When this happens, systemic cyanosis appears. The major factor in the direction of shunt flow is thus the compliance of the respective atrial chambers.

The pulmonary pressures are modestly elevated in most patients with an ASD due to the high pulmonary blood flow, but severe pulmonary hypertension with cyanosis (**Eisenmenger physiology**) is actually unusual, occurring in only about 15% of the patients with an ASD alone. Increased pulmonary vascular resistance (PVR) and pulmonary hypertension secondary to pulmonary vascular disease rarely occur in childhood or young adult life in secundum defects and are more common in primum defects, especially if there is an associated VSD. Eventual RV failure may occur with any atrial shunt of significant size, and most shunts should be corrected unless they are quite small (less than 1.5:1 left-to-right shunt). In adults, a large left-to-right shunt may have begun to reverse, so the absolute left-to-right shunt measurement (Qp/Qs, where Qp = pulmonary flow and Qs = systemic flow) at the time the patient is studied may underestimate the original shunt size. In addition, in most people the LV and LA compliance normally declines more over time than the RV and RA compliance; for this reason, the natural history of small atrial septal shunts is to increase the left-to-right shunting as the patient ages. There is generally only trivial shunting with a PFO compared to a true ASD. ASDs predispose to atrial fibrillation due to RA enlargement, and paradoxic right-to-left emboli do occur. If pulmonary hypertension does occur, the 2018 guidelines recommend that the shunt should still be closed as long as the left-to-right shunt is still greater than 1.5:1 and the systolic PA pressure is less than one-half the systemic arterial pressure and the PVR calculation is less than one-third systemic vascular resistance.

Interestingly, paradoxic emboli may be more common in patients with a PFO than a true ASD, especially when there is an atrial septal aneurysm. An aneurysm of the atrial septum is not a true aneurysm but rather simply a redundancy of the atrial septum that causes it to swing back and forth (greater than 10 mm). When present with a PFO, the back-and-forth swinging tends to pull open the PFO, encouraging shunting. This may help explain why more right-to-left shunting occurs in patients with an atrial septal aneurysm and PFO than in those with a PFO alone. This creates the anatomic substrate for the occurrence of paradoxical emboli. Other factors may distort the atrial septum (such as an enlarged aorta) and result in an increase shunting in patients with a PFO. Right-to-left PFO shunting may be more prominent upright than supine, creating orthostatic hypoxemia **(platypnea orthodeoxia)**. There may also be increased shunting in patients with a PFO and sleep apnea as the RA compliance may worsen during apneic spells when pulmonary pressures increase.

▶ Clinical Findings

A. Symptoms and Signs

Patients with a small or moderate ASD or with a PFO are asymptomatic unless a complication occurs. There is only trivial shunting in a PFO unless the RA pressure increases for some other reason or the atrial septum is distorted. With larger ASD shunts, exertional dyspnea or heart failure may develop, most commonly in the fourth decade of life or later. Prominent RV and PA pulsations are then readily visible and palpable. A moderately loud systolic ejection murmur can be heard in the second and third interspaces parasternally as a result of increased flow through the pulmonary valve. S_2 is widely split and does not vary with respiration. The left-to-right shunt across the defect decreases with inspiration (as the RA pressure increases) and then increases with expiration (as the RA pressure decreases), thus keeping the RV stroke volume relatively constant in inspiration and expiration. A **"fixed" splitting** of the second sound results. In very large left-to-right shunts, a tricuspid rumble may be heard due to the high flow across the tricuspid valve in diastole.

B. ECG and Chest Radiography

Right axis deviation or RVH may be present depending on the size of the RV volume overload. Incomplete or complete right bundle branch block is present in nearly all cases of ASD, and superior axis deviation (left anterior fascicular block) is noted in the complete AV septal defect, where complete heart block is often seen as well. With sinus venosus defects, the P axis is leftward of +15° due to abnormal atrial activation with loss of the upper RA tissue from around the sinus node. This creates the negative P waves in the inferior leads. The chest radiograph shows large pulmonary arteries, increased pulmonary vascularity, an enlarged RA and RV, and a small aortic knob, as with all pre-tricuspid valve cardiac left-to-right shunts. The LA is not traditionally enlarged due to an ASD shunt because the chamber is being decompressed.

C. Diagnostic Studies

Echocardiography demonstrates evidence of RA and RV volume overload. The atrial defect is usually observed by echocardiography, although sinus venosus defects may be elusive since they are high in the atrial septum. Many patients with a PFO also have an atrial septal aneurysm (defined as greater than 10-mm excursion of the septum from the static position). Echocardiography with saline injection (bubble contrast) can demonstrate the right-to-left component of the shunt, and both pulsed and color flow Doppler flow studies can demonstrate shunting in either direction. In platypnea orthodeoxia, the shunt may primarily result from inferior vena cava blood, and a femoral vein saline injection may be required to demonstrate the shunt. Transesophageal echocardiography (TEE) is helpful when transthoracic echocardiography quality is not optimal because it improves the sensitivity for detection of small shunts and provides a better assessment of PFO or ASD anatomy. Both CT and MRI can elucidate the atrial septal anatomy, better detect multiple fenestrations, and demonstrate associated lesions such as anomalous pulmonary venous connections. Atrial septal anatomy can be complex, and either MRI, TEE, or CT can reveal whether there is an adequate rim around the defect to allow for safe positioning of an atrial septal occluder device. These studies can also help identify any anomalous pulmonary venous connections. Cardiac catheterization can define the size and location of the shunt and determine the pulmonary pressure and PVR.

▶ Prognosis & Treatment

Patients with small atrial shunts live a normal life span with no intervention. Large shunts usually cause disability by age 40 years. Because left-to-right shunts and RV overload tend to increase with normal age-related reduction in LV (and subsequently LA) compliance, guidelines suggest that closure of all left-to-right shunts greater than 1.5:1 should be accomplished either by a percutaneous device or by surgery. This situation always results in RV volume overload if the lesion is left untreated. If the pulmonary systolic pressure is more than two-thirds the systemic systolic pressure, then pulmonary hypertension may preclude ASD closure. Testing with transient balloon occlusion of the shunt and with pulmonary vasodilators may be required in the presence of pulmonary hypertension. Preservation of the cardiac output after transient balloon occlusion and evidence for preserved pulmonary vasoreactivity with pulmonary vasodilator testing all favor closure when pulmonary hypertension and at least a 1.5:1 left-to-right shunt are present. After age 40 years, cardiac arrhythmias (especially atrial fibrillation) and heart failure occur with increased frequency due to the chronic right heart volume overload. Paradoxical systemic arterial embolization also becomes more of a concern as RV compliance is lost and the left-to-right shunt begins to reverse.

PFOs are usually not associated with significant shunting, and therefore the patients are hemodynamically asymptomatic and the heart size is normal. However, PFOs can be responsible for paradoxical emboli and are a possible cause of cryptogenic strokes in patients under age 55 years. Interestingly, the risk of *recurrent* paradoxical emboli is low regardless of whether the PFO is closed or not, and that observation has reduced the value of closing these defects in cryptogenic stroke. Further confounding the advantage of PFO closure for cryptogenic stroke or transient ischemic attack (TIA) has been the discovery of frequent bouts of paroxysmal atrial fibrillation using 30-day monitoring in these patients, suggesting atrial fibrillation is the real stroke/TIA risk factor in some patients.

Occasionally, a PFO that has not been pathologic may become responsible for cyanosis, especially if the RA pressure is elevated from pulmonary or RV hypertension or from severe tricuspid regurgitation.

Surgery involves stitching or patching of the foramen. For ostium secundum ASDs, percutaneous closure by use of a variety of devices is preferred over surgery when the anatomy is appropriate (usually this means there must bean adequate atrial septal rim around the defect to secure the occluder device).

Patients who have hypoxemia (especially upon standing or with exercise) should have the PFO closed if no other cause for hypoxemia is evident and there is right-to-left shunting demonstrated through the PFO. For patients with cryptogenic stroke or TIA, it remains uncertain whether closure of the PFO, either by open surgical or percutaneous techniques, has any advantage over anticoagulation with either warfarin, one of the direct-acting oral anticoagulants (DOACs), or aspirin. As of 2017, there were five major randomized clinical trials evaluating the advantage of PFO closure in cryptogenic stroke (at ages greater than 55 years). Three of the five trials did not show an advantage of device closure over medical therapy with antiplatelet or anticoagulation medication; however, two of the five suggested there may be a role. The FDA has approved one device for use when both a cardiologist and neurologist feel the PFO contributed to a TIA or stroke.

From a practical standpoint, patients younger than 55 years with cryptogenic stroke/TIA and no other identifiable cause except for the presence of a PFO should still be considered for PFO closure, albeit some of the data suggest medical therapy remains an equally viable option. A workup for any causes for hypercoagulability and a 30-day monitor should also be part of the clinical assessment to exclude other potential causes for cryptogenic stroke/TIA. As of 2018, the major neurologic and cardiologic governing bodies had yet to rule on an appropriate strategy following the publication of the Gore REDUCE and the CLOSE trials. However, in meta-analysis of data in patients with cryptogenic stroke/TIA and PFO who have their PFO closed, ischemic stroke recurrence is less frequent compared with patients receiving medical treatment. Atrial fibrillation is more frequent but mostly transient in patients who have device closure. There is no difference in TIA, all-cause mortality, or myocardial infarction (MI) between those treated with medicine versus a closure device. In a large, multicenter trial in France among patients who had had a recent cryptogenic stroke attributed to PFO with an associated atrial septal aneurysm or large interatrial shunt, the rate of stroke recurrence was lower among those assigned to PFO closure combined with antiplatelet therapy than among those assigned to antiplatelet therapy alone. PFO closure was associated with an increased risk of atrial fibrillation.

▶ When to Refer

- All patients with an ASD should be evaluated by a cardiologist with expertise in adult congenital disease to ensure no other structural disease is present and to investigate whether the RV is enlarged.

- If the RA and RV sizes remain normal, serial echocardiography should be performed every 3–5 years.

- If the RA and RV volumes are increased, then referral to a cardiologist who performs percutaneous closure is warranted.

- Patients younger than 55 years with cryptogenic stroke when no other source is identified except for a PFO with right-to-left shunting should be considered for PFO closure or medical therapy. The indication for PFO closure in younger patients with either a TIA or stroke is changing as newer data become available. Aspirin alone appears not to be effective. DOACs with or without device closure of the PFO may have a role in preventing recurrent stroke.

- Patients with cyanosis and a PFO with evidence of a right-to-left shunt by agitated saline bubble contrast on echocardiography, especially if the cyanosis is worsened upon assuming the upright posture.

Mas JL et al; CLOSE Investigators. Patent foramen ovale closure or anticoagulation vs. antiplatelets after stroke. N Engl J Med. 2017 Sep 14;377(11):1011–21. [PMID: 28902593]

Ntaios G et al. Closure of patent foramen ovale versus medical therapy in patients with cryptogenic stroke or transient ischemic attack: updated systematic review and meta-analysis. Stroke. 2018 Feb;49(2):412–8. [PMID: 29335335]

Saver JL et al; RESPECT Investigators. Long-term outcomes of patent foramen ovale closure or medical therapy after stroke. N Engl J Med. 2017 Sep 14;377(11):1022–32. [PMID: 28902590]

Søndergaard L et al; Gore REDUCE Clinical Study Investigators. Patent foramen ovale closure or antiplatelet therapy for cryptogenic stroke. N Engl J Med. 2017 Sep 14;377(11):1033–42. [PMID: 28902580]

Stout KK et al. 2018 AHA/ACC guideline for the management of adults with congenital heart disease: a report of the American College of Cardiology/American Heart Association Task Force on Clinical Practice Guidelines. J Am Coll Cardiol. 2019 Apr 2;73(12):e81–e192. [PMID: 30121239]

VENTRICULAR SEPTAL DEFECT

ESSENTIALS OF DIAGNOSIS

- ▶ A restrictive VSD is small and makes a louder murmur than an unrestricted one, often with an accompanying thrill. The higher the gradient across the septum, the smaller the left-to-right shunt.
- ▶ Small defects may be asymptomatic.
- ▶ Larger defects result in pulmonary hypertension (Eisenmenger physiology) if not repaired or if the pulmonary circuit is not protected by RV outflow tract obstruction.
- ▶ Echocardiography/Doppler is diagnostic.

▶ General Considerations

Congenital VSDs occur in various parts of the ventricular septum. Membranous and muscular septal defects may spontaneously close in childhood as the septum grows and hypertrophies. A left-to-right shunt is present, with the degree depending on associated RV pressure. The smaller the defect, the greater is the gradient from the LV to the RV and the louder the murmur. The presentation in adults depends on the size of the shunt and whether there is associated pulmonic or subpulmonic stenosis that has protected the lung from the systemic pressure and volume. Unprotected lungs with large shunts invariably lead to pulmonary vascular disease and severe pulmonary hypertension (Eisenmenger physiology). VSD sizes are defined by comparison to the aortic root size; a small or restrictive VSD diameter is less than 25% of the aortic root diameter, a moderately restrictive VSD diameter is 25–75% of the aorta, and an unrestricted VSD size is greater than 75% of the aortic diameter. The size can also be quantitated based on the Qp/Qs (left-to-right shunt), with a restrictive lesion being less than 1.5:1, moderately restrictive VSD being 1.5–2.2:1, and an unrestricted lesion being greater than 2.2:1.

▶ Clinical Findings

A. Symptoms and Signs

The clinical features depend on the size of the defect and the presence or absence of RV outflow obstruction or increased PVR. Small shunts are associated with loud, harsh holosystolic murmurs in the left third and fourth interspaces along the sternum. A systolic thrill is common. Larger shunts may create both LV and RV volume and pressure overload. If pulmonary hypertension occurs, high-pressure pulmonary valve regurgitation may result. Right heart failure may gradually become evident late in the course, and the shunt will begin to balance or reverse as RV and LV systolic pressures equalize with the advent of pulmonary hypertension. Cyanosis from a developing right-to-left shunt may then occur. Cyanosis with pulmonary hypertension and an intracardiac shunt define the **Eisenmenger syndrome.**

B. ECG and Chest Radiography

The ECG may be normal or may show right, left, or biventricular hypertrophy, depending on the size of the defect and the PVR. With large shunts, the LV, the LA, and the pulmonary arteries are enlarged and pulmonary vascularity is increased on chest radiographs. The RV is often normal until late in the process. If an increased PVR (pulmonary hypertension) evolves, an enlarged PA with pruning of the distal pulmonary vascular bed is seen. In rare cases of a VSD high in the ventricular septum, an aortic cusp (right coronary cusp) may prolapse into the VSD and reduce the VSD shunt but result in acute aortic regurgitation and acute heart failure.

C. Diagnostic Studies

Echocardiography can demonstrate the size of the overloaded chambers and can usually define the defect anatomy. Doppler can qualitatively assess the magnitude of shunting by noting the gradient from LV to RV and, if some tricuspid regurgitation is present, the RV systolic pressure can be estimated. The septal leaflet of the tricuspid valve may be part of the VSD anatomy and the complex appears as a ventricular septal "aneurysm." These membranous septal aneurysms resemble a "windsock" and may fenestrate and result in a VSD shunt being present or they may remain intact. Color flow Doppler helps delineate the shunt severity and the presence of valvular regurgitation. MRI and cardiac CT can often visualize the defect and describe any other anatomic abnormalities. MRI can provide quantitative shunt data as well.

Cardiac catheterization is usually reserved for those with at least moderate shunting, to quantitate the PVR and the degree of pulmonary hypertension. The 2018 adult congenital heart disease guidelines suggest that if there is still at least a 1.5:1 left-to-right shunt and if the PVR is less than one-third that of the systemic vascular resistance, and the PA systolic pressure is more than one-half of the aortic systolic pressure, then the risk of VSD closure despite some pulmonary hypertension is acceptable and it should be done. If the systemic vascular resistance and ratios of the PVR, systemic vascular resistance, or PA systolic/aortic systolic pressure are greater than two-thirds or there is a net right-to-left shunt, then closure is contraindicated.

The vasoreactivity of the pulmonary circuit may be tested at catheterization using agents such as inhaled nitric oxide, and if the pulmonary pressures can be lowered enough that the above ratios fall below the two-thirds value, then repair is reasonable as long as the left-to-right VSD shunt is greater than 1.5:1. Bosentan, an endothelial receptor blocker that reduces pulmonary pressure in Eisenmenger syndrome, has been given a class I indication in these patients.

Prognosis & Treatment

Patients with a small VSD have a normal life expectancy except for the small risk of infective endocarditis. Antibiotic prophylaxis after dental work is recommended only when the VSD is residual from a prior patch closure or when there is associated pulmonary hypertension and cyanosis (see Tables 33–3, 33–4, and 33–5). With large VSD shunts, heart failure may develop early in life, and survival beyond age 40 years is unusual without intervention.

Small shunts (pulmonary-to-systemic flow ratio less than 1.5) in asymptomatic patients do not require surgery or other intervention. The presence of RV infundibular stenosis or pulmonary valve stenosis may protect the pulmonary circuit such that some patients, even with a large VSD, may still be surgical candidates as adults if there is no pulmonary hypertension.

Surgical repair of a VSD is generally a low-risk procedure unless there is significant Eisenmenger physiology. Devices for nonsurgical closure of muscular VSDs are approved and those for membranous VSDs are being implanted with promising results; however, conduction disturbance is a major complication. The percutaneous devices are also approved for closure of a VSD related to acute MI, although the results in this very high-risk patient population have not been encouraging. The medications used to treat pulmonary hypertension secondary to VSD are similar to those used to treat idiopathic ("primary") pulmonary hypertension and at times can be quite effective in relieving symptoms and cyanosis. **All patients who have a right-to-left shunt present should have filters placed on any intravenous lines to avoid any contamination or air bubbles from becoming systemic.**

When to Refer

All patients with a VSD should be referred to a cardiologist with expertise in adult congenital disease to decide if long-term follow-up is warranted.

Bhatt AB et al. Congenital heart disease in the older adult: a scientific statement from the American Heart Association. Circulation. 2015 May 26;131(21):1884–931. [PMID: 25896865]

Hamilton MCK et al. The in vivo morphology of post-infarct ventricular septal defect and the implications for closure. JACC Cardiovasc Interv. 2017 Jun 26;10(12):1233–43. [PMID: 28641844]

Menting ME et al. The unnatural history of the ventricular septal defect: outcome up to 40 years after surgical closure. J Am Coll Cardiol. 2015 May 12;65(18):1941–51. [PMID: 25953746]

Saurav A et al. Comparison of percutaneous device closure versus surgical closure of peri-membranous ventricular septal defects: a systematic review and meta-analysis. Catheter Cardiovasc Interv. 2015 Nov 15;86(6):1048–56. [PMID: 26257085]

Stout KK et al. 2018 AHA/ACC guideline for the management of adults with congenital heart disease: a report of the American College of Cardiology/American Heart Association Task Force on Clinical Practice Guidelines. J Am Coll Cardiol. 2019 Apr 2;73(12):e81–e192. [PMID: 30121239]

TETRALOGY OF FALLOT

ESSENTIALS OF DIAGNOSIS

▶ Five features are characteristic:
- VSD.
- Concentric RVH.
- RV outflow obstruction due to infundibular stenosis.
- Overriding aorta in half (requires less than 50% of the aorta to override the septum).
- A right-sided aortic arch in 25%.

▶ Most adult patients with tetralogy of Fallot have been operated on, usually with an RV outflow patch and VSD closure.

▶ Physical examination may be deceptive after classic tetralogy repair, with severe pulmonary valve regurgitation often present if a transannular patch was used.

▶ Echocardiography/Doppler may underestimate significant pulmonary valve regurgitation. Be wary if the RV is enlarged.

▶ Arrhythmias are common; periodic ambulatory monitoring is recommended.

▶ Serious arrhythmias and sudden death may occur if the QRS is wide or the RV becomes quite large, or both.

General Considerations

Patients with tetralogy of Fallot have a VSD, RV infundibular stenosis, RVH, and a dilated aorta (in about half of patients it overrides the septum). If there is an associated ASD, the complex is referred to as pentalogy of Fallot. There may or may not be pulmonary valve stenosis as well, usually due to a bicuspid pulmonary valve or RV outflow hypoplasia. The aorta can be quite enlarged and aortic regurgitation may occur. If more than 50% of the aorta overrides into the RV outflow tract, the anatomy is referred to as a "double outlet RV." Two vascular abnormalities are common: a right-sided aortic arch (in 25%) and an anomalous left anterior descending coronary artery from the right cusp (7–9%). The latter is important in that surgical correction must avoid injuring the coronary artery when repairing the RV outflow obstruction. Pulmonary branch stenosis may also be present.

Most adult patients have undergone prior surgery. If significant RV outflow obstruction is present in the neonatal period, a systemic arterial to pulmonary artery shunt may be the initial surgical procedure to improve pulmonary blood flow, though many infants undergo repair without this first step. Most adults will have had this initial palliative repair, however. The palliative procedure enables blood to reach the underperfused lung either by directly attaching one of the subclavian arteries to a main PA branch (**classic Blalock shunt**) or, more likely, by creating a conduit between the two (**modified Blalock shunt**). In the adult, there may be a reduced upper extremity pulse on the side used for the classic Blalock procedure. Total repair of the tetralogy of Fallot generally includes a VSD patch and usually an enlarging RV outflow tract patch, as well as a take-down of any prior arterial-pulmonary artery shunt. If the RV outflow tract patch extends through the pulmonary valve into the PA (transannular patch), varying degrees of pulmonary valve regurgitation often develop. Most surgeons approach the inside of the RV via the right atrium and through the tricuspid valve. Over the years, the volume overload from any severe pulmonary valve regurgitation becomes the major hemodynamic problem to deal with in adults. Ventricular arrhythmias can also originate from the edge of either the VSD or outflow tract and tend to increase in frequency as the size of the RV increases.

▶ Clinical Findings

Most adult patients in whom tetralogy of Fallot has been repaired are relatively asymptomatic unless right heart failure occurs or arrhythmias become an issue. Patients can be active and generally require no specific therapy.

A. Symptoms and Signs

Physical examination should include checking both arms for any loss of pulse from a prior shunt procedure in infancy. The jugular venous pulsations (JVP) may reveal an increased *a* wave from poor RV compliance or rarely a *c-v* wave due to tricuspid regurgitation. The right-sided arch has no consequence. The precordium may be active, often with a persistent pulmonary outflow murmur. P_2 may or may not be audible. A right-sided gallop may be heard. A residual VSD or an aortic regurgitation murmur may be present. At times, the insertion site of a prior Blalock or other shunt may create a stenotic area in the branch PA and a continuous murmur occurs as a result.

B. ECG and Chest Radiography

The ECG reveals RVH and right axis deviation; in repaired tetralogy, there is often a right bundle branch block pattern. The chest radiograph shows a classic boot-shaped heart with prominence of the RV and a concavity in the RV outflow tract. This may be less impressive following repair. The aorta may be enlarged and right-sided. Importantly, the width of the QRS should be examined yearly because persons at greatest risk for sudden death are traditionally those with a QRS width of more than 180 msec, although more recent data have suggested that this cutoff is not as specific as once thought. Most experts recommend ambulatory monitoring periodically as well, especially if the patient experiences palpitations. Other identified risk factors for ventricular arrhythmias include having multiple prior cardiac surgeries, an elevated LV end-diastolic pressure (LVEDP), and older age at time of repair. In fact, it appears that the more the left side of the heart is involved, the higher the risk of sudden death.

C. Diagnostic Studies

Echocardiography/Doppler usually establishes the diagnosis by noting the unrestricted (large) VSD, the RV infundibular stenosis, and the enlarged aorta. In patients who have had tetralogy of Fallot repaired, echocardiography/Doppler also provides data regarding the amount of residual pulmonary valve regurgitation if a transannular patch is present, RV and LV function, and the presence of aortic regurgitation. Elevated N-terminal pro B-type natriuretic peptide (NT-proBNP) blood levels have also been correlated with increasing RV enlargement.

Cardiac MRI and CT can quantitate both the pulmonary regurgitation and the RV volumes. In addition, cardiac MRI and CT can identify whether there is either a native pulmonary arterial branch stenosis or a stenosis at the distal site of a prior arterial-to-PA shunt or other anomalies, such as an ASD. The ability of cardiac MRI to accurately quantitate the pulmonary regurgitation severity and provide more accurate RV volume measurements than other modalities has resulted in it having an advantage over other imaging studies. Cardiac catheterization may be required to document the degree of pulmonary valve regurgitation because noninvasive studies depend on velocity gradients. Pulmonary angiography demonstrates the degree of pulmonary valve regurgitation, and RV angiography helps assess any postoperative outflow tract aneurysm.

The need for electrophysiologic studies with ventricular stimulation and potential ventricular tachycardia ablation has been suggested by some experts for patients who have had evidence for ventricular tachycardia, unexplained syncope, a wide QRS, are older, or who are about to undergo pulmonary valve replacement.

▶ Prognosis & Treatment

A few patients with "just the right amount" of subpulmonic stenosis enter adulthood without having had surgical correction. However, most adult patients have had surgical repair, including VSD closure, resection of infundibular muscle, and insertion of an outflow tract patch to relieve the subpulmonic obstruction. Many have a transannular patch resulting in pulmonary valve regurgitation. Patients with pulmonary valve regurgitation should be monitored to ensure the RV volume does not progressively increase. Low-pressure pulmonary valve regurgitation is difficult to diagnose due to the fact that the RV diastolic pressures tend to be high and the pulmonary arterial diastolic pressure low. This means there is little gradient between the PA and the RV in diastole, so that there may be little murmur or evidence of turbulence on color flow Doppler. If the RV begins to enlarge, it must be assumed that this is due to pulmonary valve regurgitation until proven otherwise. Early surgical pulmonary valve replacement is increasingly being favored. A percutaneous approach to pulmonary valve regurgitation remains limited as the available percutaneous valve diameters are frequently too small for the size of the pulmonary annulus. The Melody valve is a bovine jugular vein prosthesis with the largest size being 22 mm in diameter. Percutaneous stented valves, particularly the Edwards SAPIEN XT, have been used successfully and can be used in patients with larger pulmonary root sizes. Often, a stent is placed within the vessel first with the stented valve placed within the stent. The expansion of the PA must not impede flow down any coronary artery; this is tested by a trial balloon expansion while imaging the coronary artery at the same time (class I requirement). There has been an increase in stented valve endocarditis noted after the placement of the Melody valve; this is being closely monitored.

If an anomalous coronary artery is present, then an extracardiac conduit around it from the RV to the PA may be necessary. By 20-year follow-up, reoperation of the common tetralogy repair is needed in about 10–15%, not only for severe pulmonary valve regurgitation but also for residual infundibular stenosis. Usually the pulmonary valve is replaced with a pulmonary homograft, although a porcine bioprosthetic valve is also suitable. Percutaneous valve-in-valve bioprosthetic valves have successfully been used when there is surgical bioprosthetic valve dysfunction. Cryoablation of tissue giving rise to arrhythmias is sometimes performed at the time of reoperation. Branch pulmonary stenosis may be percutaneously opened by stenting. If a conduit has been used already for repair of the RV outflow obstruction, a percutaneous approach with a stented pulmonary valve may be possible. All patients require endocarditis prophylaxis (see Tables 33–3, 33–4, and 33–5). Most adults with stable hemodynamics can be quite active, and most women can carry a pregnancy adequately if RV function is preserved.

Atrial fibrillation, reentrant atrial arrhythmias, and ventricular ectopy are common, especially after the age of 45. Left heart disease appears to cause these arrhythmias more often than right heart disease. Biventricular dysfunction is not an uncommon consequence as the patient ages. The cause of associated LV dysfunction is often multifactorial and frequently unclear. Similarly, the aorta may enlarge with accompanying aortic regurgitation, and these lesions can become severe enough to warrant surgical intervention. Patients with RV or LV dysfunction or with dysfunction of both ventricles may require a prophylactic defibrillator.

▶ When to Refer

All patients with tetralogy of Fallot should be referred to a cardiologist with expertise in adult congenital heart disease.

Bhatt AB et al. Congenital heart disease in the older adult: a scientific statement from the American Heart Association. Circulation. 2015 May 26;131(21):1884–931. [PMID: 25896865]

Downing TE et al. Tetralolgy of Fallot: general principles of management. Cardiol Clin. 2015 Nov;33(4):531–41. [PMID: 26471818]

Fraser CD et al. Tetralogy of Fallot. Semin Thorac Cardiovasc Surg. 2015 Summer;27(2):189–204. [PMID: 26686447]

Haas NA et al. Early outcomes of percutaneous pulmonary valve implantation using the Edwards SAPIEN XT transcatheter heart valve system. Int J Cardiol. 2018 Jan 1;250:86–91. [PMID: 29017776]

Paolino A et al. NT-proBNP as marker of ventricular dilatation and pulmonary regurgitation after surgical correction of tetralogy of Fallot: a MRI validation study. Pediatr Cardiol. 2017 Feb;38(2):324–31. [PMID: 27872995]

Stout KK et al. 2018 AHA/ACC guideline for the management of adults with congenital heart disease: a report of the American College of Cardiology/American Heart Association Task Force on Clinical Practice Guidelines. J Am Coll Cardiol. 2019 Apr 2;73(12):e81–e192. [PMID: 30121239]

▼ VALVULAR HEART DISEASE

The 2014 American Heart Association (AHA)/American College of Cardiology (ACC) guidelines provide information on valvular heart disease diagnosis and treatment. The typical findings of each native valve lesion are described in Table 10–1. Table 10–2 outlines bedside maneuvers to distinguish among the various systolic murmurs. These guidelines were updated in 2017 to reflect the remarkable increase in the use of percutaneous valvular devices, some of the newer information regarding anticoagulation usage, and when to intervene.

The updated AHA/ACC valvular guidelines suggests all lesions may be best classified clinically into one of six categories based on anatomy and symptoms.

Stage A: Patients at risk for valvular heart disease.

Stage B: Patients with progressive valvular heart disease (mild to moderate severity) and asymptomatic.

Stage C: Asymptomatic patients who have reached criteria for severe valvular heart disease.

    C1: Severe valve lesion. Asymptomatic. Normal LV function.

    C2: Severe valve lesion. Asymptomatic. Abnormal LV function.

Stage D: Symptomatic patients as a result of valvular heart disease.

Nishimura RA et al. 2014 AHA/ACC guideline for the management of patients with valvular heart disease: executive summary: a report of the American College of Cardiology/American Heart Association Task Force on Practice Guidelines. J Am Coll Cardiol. 2014 Jun 10;63(22):2438–88. Erratum in: J Am Coll Cardiol. 2014 Jun 10;63(22):2489. [PMID: 24603192]

Nishimura RA et al. 2017 AHA/ACC focused update of the 2014 AHA/ACC guideline for the management of patients with valvular heart disease: a report of the American College of Cardiology/American Heart Association Task Force on Practice Guidelines. Circulation. 2017 Jun 20;135(25):e1159–95. [PMID: 28298458]

MITRAL STENOSIS

ESSENTIALS OF DIAGNOSIS

▶ Fatigue, exertional dyspnea, and orthopnea when the stenosis becomes severe.

▶ Symptoms often precipitated by onset of atrial fibrillation or pregnancy.

▶ Intervention indicated for symptoms, atrial fibrillation, or evidence of pulmonary hypertension. Most symptomatic patients have a mitral valve area of less than 1.5 cm².

Table 10–1. Differential diagnosis of valvular heart disease.

	Mitral Stenosis	Mitral Regurgitation	Aortic Stenosis	Aortic Regurgitation	Tricuspid Stenosis	Tricuspid Regurgitation
Inspection	Malar flush, precordial bulge, and diffuse pulsation in young patients.	Usually prominent and hyperdynamic apical impulse to left of MCL.	Sustained PMI, prominent atrial filling wave.	Hyperdynamic PMI to left of MCL and downward. Visible carotid pulsations. Pulsating nailbeds (Quincke sign), head bob (deMusset sign).	Giant a wave in jugular pulse with sinus rhythm. Peripheral edema or ascites, or both.	Large v wave in jugular pulse; time with carotid pulsation. Peripheral edema or ascites, or both.
Palpation	"Tapping" sensation over area of expected PMI. Right ventricular pulsation in left third to fifth ICS parasternally when pulmonary hypertension is present. P_2 may be palpable.	Forceful, brisk PMI; systolic thrill over PMI. Pulse normal, small, or slightly collapsing.	Powerful, heaving PMI to left and slightly below MCL. Systolic thrill over aortic area, sternal notch, or carotid arteries in severe disease. Small and slowly rising carotid pulse. If bicuspid AS, check for delay at femoral artery to exclude coarctation.	Apical impulse forceful and displaced significantly to left and downward. Prominent carotid pulses. Rapidly rising and collapsing pulses (Corrigan pulse).	Pulsating, enlarged liver in ventricular systole.	Right ventricular pulsation. Systolic pulsation of liver.
Heart sounds, rhythm, and blood pressure	S_1 loud if valve mobile. Opening snap following S_2. The worse the disease, the closer the S_2-opening snap interval.	S_1 normal or buried in early part of murmur (exception in mitral prolapse where murmur may be late). Prominent third heart sound when severe MR. Atrial fibrillation common. Blood pressure normal. Midsystolic clicks may be present and may be multiple.	A_2 normal, soft, or absent. Prominent S_4. Blood pressure normal, or systolic pressure normal with high diastolic pressure.	S_1 normal or reduced, A_2 loud. Wide pulse pressure with diastolic pressure < 60 mm Hg. When severe, gentle compression of femoral artery with diaphragm of stethoscope may reveal diastolic flow (Duroziez) and pressure in leg on palpation > 40 mm Hg than arm (Hill).	S_1 often loud.	Atrial fibrillation may be present.
Murmurs						
Location and transmission	Localized at or near apex. Diastolic rumble best heard in left lateral position; may be accentuated by having patient do sit-ups. Rarely, short diastolic murmur along lower left sternal border (Graham Steell) in severe pulmonary hypertension.	Loudest over PMI; posteriorly directed jets (ie, anterior mitral prolapse) transmitted to left axilla, left infrascapular area; anteriorly directed jets (ie, posterior mitral prolapse) heard over anterior precordium. Murmur unchanged after premature beat.	Right second ICS parasternally or at apex, heard in carotid arteries and occasionally in upper interscapular area. May sound like MR at apex (Gallaverdin phenomenon), but murmur occurs after S_1 and stops before S_2.	Diastolic: louder along left sternal border in third to fourth interspace. Heard over aortic area and apex. May be associated with low-pitched middiastolic murmur at apex (Austin Flint) due to functional mitral stenosis. If due to an enlarged aorta, murmur may radiate to right sternal border.	Third to fifth ICS along left sternal border out to apex. Murmur increases with inspiration.	Third to fifth ICS along left sternal border. Murmur hard to hear but increases with inspiration. Sit-ups can increase cardiac output and accentuate murmur.

(continued)

Table 10–1. Differential diagnosis of valvular heart disease. (continued)

	Mitral Stenosis	Mitral Regurgitation	Aortic Stenosis	Aortic Regurgitation	Tricuspid Stenosis	Tricuspid Regurgitation
Timing	Relation of opening snap to A_2 important. The higher the LA pressure, the earlier the opening snap. Presystolic accentuation before S_1 if in sinus rhythm. Graham Steell begins with P_2 (early diastole) if associated pulmonary hypertension.	Pansystolic: begins with S_1 and ends at or after A_2. May be late systolic in mitral valve prolapse.	Begins after S_1, ends before A_2. The more severe the stenosis, the later the murmur peaks.	Begins immediately after aortic second sound and ends before first sound (blurring both); helps distinguish from MR.	Rumble often follows audible opening snap.	At times, hard to hear. Begins with S_1 and fills systole. Increases with inspiration.
Character	Low-pitched, rumbling; presystolic murmur merges with loud S_1.	Blowing, high-pitched; occasionally harsh or musical.	Harsh, rough.	Blowing, often faint.	As for mitral stenosis.	Blowing, coarse, or musical.
Optimum auscultatory conditions	After exercise, left lateral recumbency. Use stethoscope bell, lightly applied.	After exercise; use stethoscope diaphragm. In prolapse, findings may be more evident while standing.	Use stethoscope diaphragm. Patient resting, leaning forward, breath held in full expiration.	Use stethoscope diaphragm. Patient leaning forward, breath held in expiration.	Use stethoscope bell. Murmur usually louder and at peak during inspiration. Patient recumbent.	Use stethoscope diaphragm. Murmur usually becomes louder during inspiration.
Radiography	Straight left heart border from enlarged LA appendage. Elevation of left mainstem bronchus. Large right ventricle and pulmonary artery if pulmonary hypertension is present. Calcification in mitral valve in rheumatic mitral stenosis or in annulus in calcific mitral stenosis.	Enlarged left ventricle and LA.	Concentric left ventricular hypertrophy. Prominent ascending aorta. Calcified aortic valve common.	Moderate to severe left ventricular enlargement. Aortic root often dilated.	Enlarged right atrium with prominent SVC and azygous shadow.	Enlarged right atrium and right ventricle.
ECG	Broad P waves in standard leads; broad negative phase of diphasic P in V_1. If pulmonary hypertension is present, tall peaked P waves, right axis deviation, or right ventricular hypertrophy appears.	Left axis deviation or frank left ventricular hypertrophy. P waves broad, tall, or notched in standard leads. Broad negative phase of diphasic P in V_1.	Left ventricular hypertrophy.	Left ventricular hypertrophy.	Tall, peaked P waves. Possible right ventricular hypertrophy.	Right axis usual.

Echocardiography

Two-dimensional echocardiography	Thickened, immobile mitral valve with anterior and posterior leaflets moving together. "Hockey stick" shape to opened anterior leaflet in rheumatic mitral stenosis. Annular calcium with thin leaflets in calcific mitral stenosis. LA enlargement, normal to small left ventricle. Orifice can be traced to approximate mitral valve orifice area.	Thickened mitral valve in rheumatic disease; mitral valve prolapse; flail leaflet or vegetations may be seen. Dilated left ventricle in volume overload. Operate for left ventricular end-systolic dimension < 4.5 cm.	Dense persistent echoes from the aortic valve with poor leaflet excursion. Left ventricular hypertrophy late in the disease. Bicuspid valve in younger patients.	Abnormal aortic valve or dilated aortic root. Diastolic vibrations of the anterior leaflet of the mitral valve and septum. In acute aortic regurgitation, premature closure of the mitral valve before the QRS. When severe, dilated left ventricle with normal or decreased contractility. Operate when left ventricular end-systolic dimension > 5.0 cm.	In rheumatic disease, tricuspid valve thickening, decreased early diastolic filling slope of the tricuspid valve. In carcinoid, leaflets fixed, but no significant thickening.	Enlarged right ventricle with paradoxical septal motion. Tricuspid valve often pulled open by displaced chordae.
Continuous and color flow-Doppler and TEE	Prolonged pressure half-time across mitral valve allows estimation of gradient. MVA estimated from pressure half-time. Indirect evidence of pulmonary hypertension by noting elevated right ventricular systolic pressure measured from the tricuspid regurgitation jet.	Regurgitant flow mapped into LA. Use of PISA helps assess MR severity. TEE important in prosthetic mitral valve regurgitation.	Increased transvalvular flow velocity; severe AS when peak jet > 4 m/sec (64 mm Hg). Valve area estimate using continuity equation is poorly reproducible.	Demonstrates regurgitation and qualitatively estimates severity based on percentage of left ventricular outflow filled with jet and distance jet penetrates into left ventricle. TEE important in aortic valve endocarditis to exclude abscess. Mitral inflow pattern describes diastolic dysfunction.	Prolonged pressure half-time across tricuspid valve can be used to estimate mean gradient. Severe tricuspid stenosis present when mean gradient > 5 mm Hg.	Regurgitant flow mapped into right atrium and venae cavae. Right ventricular systolic pressure estimated by tricuspid jet regurgitation velocity.

A_2, aortic second sound; AS, aortic stenosis; ICS, intercostal space; LA, left atrial; MCL, midclavicular line; MR, mitral regurgitation; MVA, measured valve area; P_2, pulmonary second sound; PISA, proximal isovelocity surface area; PMI, point of maximal impulse; S_1, first heart sound; S_2, second heart sound; S_4, fourth heart sound; SVC, superior vena cava; TEE, transesophageal echocardiography; V_1, chest ECG lead 1.

Table 10–2. Effect of various interventions on systolic murmurs.

Intervention	Hypertrophic Cardiomyopathy	Aortic Stenosis	Mitral Regurgitation	Mitral Prolapse
Valsalva	↑	↓	↓ or ×	↑ or ↓
Standing	↑	↑ or ×	↓ or ×	↑
Handgrip or squatting	↓	↓ or ×	↑	↓
Supine position with legs elevated	↓	↑ or ×	×	↓
Exercise	↑	↑ or ×	↓	↑

↑, increased; ↓, decreased; ×, unchanged.
Modified, with permission, from Paraskos JA. Combined valvular disease. In: *Valvular Heart Disease*, 3e. Dalen JE, Alpert JS, Rahimtoola SH (editors). Philadelphia: Lippincott Williams & Wilkins, 2000.

General Considerations

Most patients with native valve mitral stenosis are presumed to have had rheumatic heart disease, although a history of rheumatic fever is noted in only about one-third. (Also see section on Rheumatic Fever.) Rheumatic mitral stenosis results in thickening of the leaflets, fusion of the mitral commissures, retraction, thickening and fusion of the chordae, and calcium deposition in the valve. Mitral stenosis can also occur due to congenital disease with chordal fusion or papillary muscle malposition. The papillary muscles may be abnormally close together, sometimes so close that they merge into a single papillary muscle (the **"parachute mitral valve"**). In these patients, the chordae or valvular tissue (or both) may also be fused. In older patients and in those undergoing dialysis, mitral annular calcification may stiffen the mitral valve and reduce its motion to the point where a mitral gradient is present. Calcium in the mitral annulus virtually invades the mitral leaflet from the annulus inward as opposed to the calcium buildup in the leaflets and commissures as seen in rheumatic heart disease. Mitral valve obstruction may also develop in patients who have had mitral valve repair with a mitral annular ring that is too small, or in patients who have had a surgical valve replacement (prosthetic valve-patient mismatch or degeneration of the prosthetic valve over time).

Clinical Findings

A. Symptoms and Signs

Two clinical syndromes classically occur in patients with mitral stenosis. In mild to moderate mitral stenosis, LA pressure and cardiac output may be essentially normal, and the patient is either asymptomatic or symptomatic only with extreme exertion. The measured valve area is usually between 1.5 cm^2 and 1.0 cm^2. In severe mitral stenosis (valve area less than 1.0 cm^2), severe pulmonary hypertension develops due to a "secondary stenosis" of the pulmonary vasculature. In this condition, pulmonary edema is uncommon, but symptoms of low cardiac output and right heart failure predominate.

A characteristic finding of rheumatic mitral stenosis is an **opening snap** following A$_2$ due to the stiff mitral valve. The interval between the opening snap and aortic closure sound is long when the LA pressure is low, but shortens as the LA pressure rises and approaches the aortic diastolic pressure. As mitral stenosis worsens, there is a localized low-pitched diastolic murmur whose duration increases with the severity of the stenosis when the mitral gradient continues throughout more of diastole. The diastolic murmur is best heard at the apex with the patient in the left lateral position (Table 10–1). Mitral regurgitation may be present as well.

Paroxysmal or chronic atrial fibrillation eventually develops in 50–80% of patients. Any increase in the heart rate reduces diastolic filling time and increases the mitral gradient. A sudden increase in heart rate may precipitate pulmonary edema. Therefore, heart rate control is important, with slow heart rates allowing for more diastolic filling of the LV.

B. Diagnostic Studies

Echocardiography is the most valuable technique for assessing mitral stenosis (Table 10–1). LA size can also be determined by echocardiography; increased size denotes an increased likelihood of atrial fibrillation and thrombus formation.

Because echocardiography and careful symptom evaluation provide most of the needed information, cardiac catheterization is used primarily to detect associated coronary or myocardial disease—usually after the decision to intervene has been made.

Treatment & Prognosis

In most cases, there is a long asymptomatic phase after the initial rheumatic infection, followed by subtle limitation of activity. Pregnancy and its associated increase in stroke volume and heart rate result in an increased transmitral pressure gradient and may precipitate symptoms. In particular, toward the end of pregnancy, the cardiac output continues to be maintained by an increase in heart rate, increasing the mitral gradient by shortening diastolic time.

Patients with moderate to severe mitral stenosis should have the condition corrected prior to becoming pregnant if possible (when the measured valve area is less than 2.0 cm²). Pregnant patients who become symptomatic can undergo successful surgery, preferably in the third trimester, although balloon valvuloplasty is the treatment of choice if the echocardiography valve score is low enough.

The onset of atrial fibrillation often precipitates symptoms, which improve with control of the ventricular rate or restoration of sinus rhythm. Conversion to and subsequent maintenance of sinus rhythm are most commonly successful when the duration of atrial fibrillation is brief (less than 6–12 months) and the LA is not severely dilated (diameter less than 4.5 cm). Once atrial fibrillation occurs, the patient should receive warfarin anticoagulation therapy even if sinus rhythm is restored, since atrial fibrillation often recurs even with antiarrhythmic therapy and 20–30% of these patients will have systemic embolization if untreated. Systemic embolization in the presence of only mild to moderate disease is not an indication for surgery but should be treated with warfarin anticoagulation. DOACs (dabigatran, apixaban, rivaroxaban, edoxaban) have not

been studied for the prevention of stroke and non–central nervous system embolism in patients with moderate or severe mitral stenosis and atrial fibrillation, and the 2017 valvular guidelines do not recommend them as an anticoagulant option for these patients.

Indications for intervention focus on symptoms such as an episode of pulmonary edema, a decline in exercise capacity, or any evidence of pulmonary hypertension (peak systolic pulmonary pressure greater than 50 mm Hg). Some experts believe that the presence of atrial fibrillation should also be a consideration for an intervention. Most interventions are not pursued until the patient is symptomatic (stage D) (Figure 10–1). In some patients, symptoms develop with calculated mitral valve areas between 1.5 cm² and 1.0 cm². Symptoms or evidence of pulmonary hypertension should drive the decision to intervene in these patients, not the estimated valve area.

Open mitral commissurotomy is now rarely performed and has given way to percutaneous balloon valvuloplasty. Ten-year follow-up data comparing surgery to balloon valvuloplasty suggest no real difference in outcome between the two modalities. Replacement of the valve is

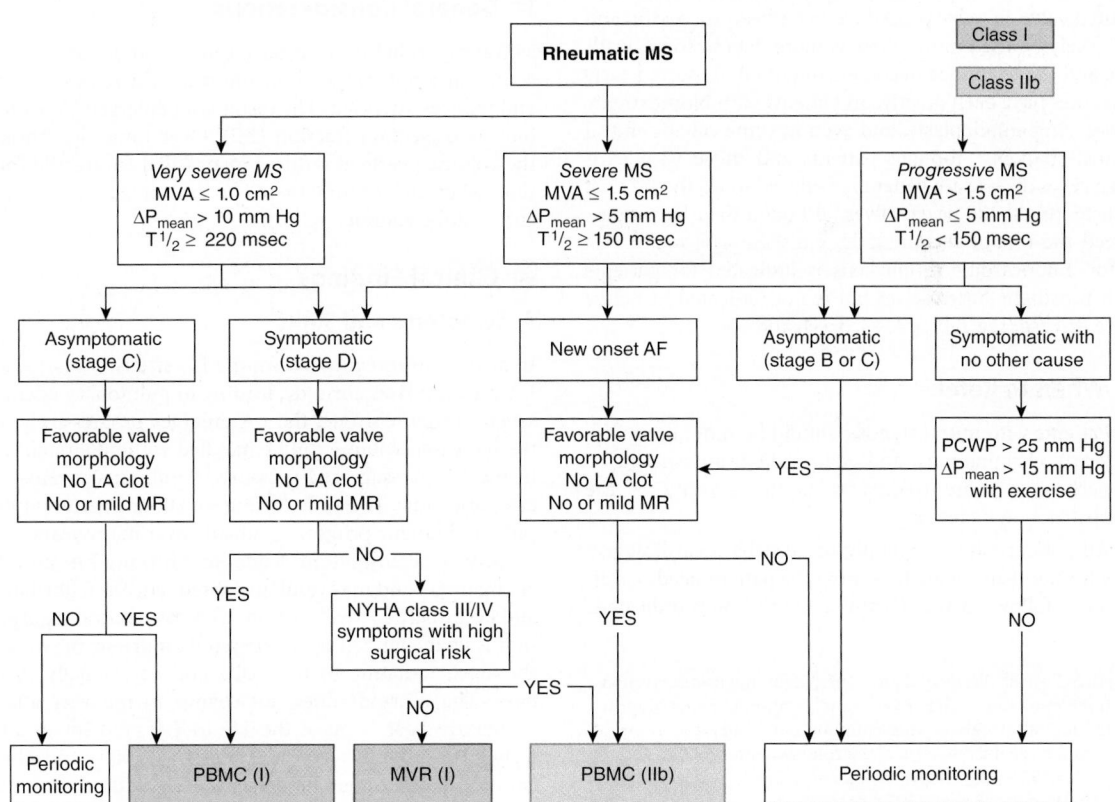

▲ **Figure 10–1.** The 2014 AHA/ACC guidelines for intervention in mitral stenosis. (Reproduced, with permission, from Nishimura RA et al. 2014 AHA/ACC Guideline for the Management of Patients With Valvular Heart Disease: A Report of the American College of Cardiology/American Heart Association Task Force on Practice Guidelines. Circulation. 2014 Jun 10;129(23):e521–643. © 2014 American Heart Association, Inc.)

indicated when combined stenosis and regurgitation are present or when the mitral valve echo score is much greater than 8–10. To determine the valve score, numbers 1 to 4 are assigned to four valve characteristics: mobility, calcification, thickening and submitral scar. Thus, a maximum score is 16. Percutaneous balloon valvuloplasty has a very low mortality rate (less than 0.5%) and a low morbidity rate (3–5%). Operative mortality rates are also low: 1–3% in most institutions. Repeat balloon valvuloplasty can be done if the morphology of the valve remains suitable. At surgery, a **Maze procedure** may be done at the same time to reduce recurrent atrial arrhythmias. It involves a number of endocardial incisions across the right and left atria to disrupt the electrical activity that sustains atrial arrhythmias.

Mechanical mitral prosthetic valves are more prone to thrombosis than mechanical aortic prosthetic valves. **The recommended INR range is thus higher (INR 2.5–3.5) and low-dose aspirin should be used in conjunction.** It is a IIa recommendation that warfarin be used for up to 6 months after implantation of a bioprosthetic mitral valve. Bioprosthetic valves tend to degenerate after about 10–15 years. Percutaneous balloon valvuloplasty is not effective when bioprosthetic valve stenosis occurs, but stented valve-in-valve procedures have been successful and will likely be used more often as more data become available and the technique becomes simplified. Reported early outcomes have been positive in patients with bioprosthetic valves, ring annuloplasty, and even in some calcific mitral stenosis patients. Younger patients and those with end-stage renal disease are generally believed to do the poorest with bioprosthetic heart valves, although data have questioned the role of chronic kidney disease as a major risk factor. Endocarditis prophylaxis is indicated for patients with prosthetic heart valves but is not indicated in native valve disease (see Tables 33–3, 33–4, and 33–5).

▶ When to Refer

- Patients with mitral stenosis should be monitored with yearly examinations, and echocardiograms should be performed more frequently as the severity of the obstruction increases.

- All patients should initially be seen by a cardiologist, who can then decide how often the patient needs cardiology follow-up and whether intervention is indicated.

Eleid MF et al. Early outcomes of percutaneous transvenous transseptal transcatheter valve implantation in failed bioprosthetic mitral valves, ring annuloplasty, and severe mitral annular calcification. JACC Cardiovasc Interv. 2017 Oct 9; 10(19):1932–42. [PMID: 28982556]

Ghosh-Dastidar M et al. Mitral valve-in-valve and valve-in-ring for failing surgical bioprosthetic valves and rings. J Cardiovasc Surg (Torino). 2016 Jun;57(3):372–80. [PMID: 26923547]

Nishimura RA et al. 2017 AHA/ACC focused update of the 2014 AHA/ACC guideline for the management of patients with valvular heart disease: a report of the American College of Cardiology/American Heart Association Task Force on Practice Guidelines. Circulation. 2017 Jun 20;135(25):e1159–95. [PMID: 28298458]

MITRAL REGURGITATION

 ESSENTIALS OF DIAGNOSIS

- ▶ May be asymptomatic for years (or for life).
- ▶ Severe mitral regurgitation may cause left-sided heart failure.
- ▶ For chronic primary mitral regurgitation, surgery is indicated for symptoms or when the LV ejection fraction (LVEF) is less than 60% or the echocardiographic LV end-systolic dimension is greater than 4.0 cm.
- ▶ In patients with mitral prolapse and severe mitral regurgitation, earlier surgery is indicated if mitral repair can be performed.
- ▶ Patients with functional mitral regurgitation may improve with biventricular pacing. Some may benefit from surgical intervention or percutaneous repair.

▶ General Considerations

Mitral regurgitation (formerly called mitral insufficiency) results in a volume load on the heart (increases preload) and reduces afterload. The result is an enlarged LV with an increased ejection fraction (EF). Over time, the stress of the volume overload reduces myocardial contractile function; when this occurs, there is a drop in EF and a rise in end-systolic volume.

▶ Clinical Findings

A. Symptoms and Signs

In acute mitral regurgitation, the LA size is not large, and LA pressure rises abruptly, leading to pulmonary edema if severe. When chronic, the LA enlarges progressively and the increased volume can be handled without a major rise in the LA pressure; the pressure in pulmonary veins and capillaries may rise only during exertion. Exertional dyspnea and fatigue progress gradually over many years.

Mitral regurgitation leads to chronic LA and LV enlargement and may result in subsequent atrial fibrillation and eventually LV dysfunction. Clinically, mitral regurgitation is characterized by a pansystolic murmur maximal at the apex, radiating to the axilla and occasionally to the base. The murmur does not change in intensity after a premature beat because the LV to LA gradient is unaffected. In addition, a hyperdynamic LV impulse and a brisk carotid upstroke may be present along with a prominent third heart sound due to the increased volume returning to the LV in early diastole (Tables 10–1 and 10–2). In acute mitral regurgitation, the murmur intensity may be modest due to little difference between the LA and LV systolic pressures during ventricular systole. The mitral regurgitation murmur due to mitral valve prolapse tends to radiate anteriorly in the presence of posterior leaflet prolapse and posteriorly when the prolapse is primarily of the anterior leaflet. Mitral regurgitation may not be pansystolic in these patients but occur only after the mitral click (until late in the disease process when it then becomes progressively more holosystolic).

B. Diagnostic Studies

Echocardiographic information demonstrating the underlying pathologic process (rheumatic, calcific, prolapse, flail leaflet, endocarditis, cardiomyopathy), LV size and function, LA size, PA pressure, and RV function can be invaluable in planning treatment as well as in recognizing associated lesions. The 2014 and 2017 updated guidelines for valvular heart disease from the AHA/ACC provide details of the classification and measures of severity for primary and secondary mitral valve regurgitation. Doppler techniques provide qualitative and semiquantitative estimates of the severity of mitral regurgitation. TEE may help reveal the cause of regurgitation and is especially useful in patients who have had mitral valve replacement, in suspected endocarditis, and in identifying candidates for valvular repair. Echocardiographic dimensions and measures of systolic function are critical in deciding the timing of surgery. Asymptomatic patients with severe mitral regurgitation (stage C1) but preserved LV dimensions should undergo at least yearly echocardiography. Exercise hemodynamics with either Doppler echocardiography or cardiac catheterization may be useful when the symptoms do not fit the anatomic severity of mitral regurgitation. B-type natriuretic peptide (BNP or NT-proBNP) is useful in the early identification of LV dysfunction in the presence of mitral regurgitation and asymptomatic patients, and values that trend upward over time appear to have prognostic importance.

Cardiac MRI is occasionally useful, especially if specific myocardial causes are being sought (such as amyloid or myocarditis) or if myocardial viability assessment is needed prior to deciding whether to add coronary artery bypass grafting to mitral valve surgery.

Cardiac catheterization provides a further assessment of regurgitation and its hemodynamic impact along with LV function, resting cardiac output, and PA pressure. **The 2014 AHA/ACC guidelines on valvular disease recommend coronary angiography to determine the presence of incidental coronary artery disease (CAD) prior to valve surgery in all men over age 40 years and in menopausal women with coronary risk factors.** In younger patients, cardiac multidetector coronary CT may be adequate to screen patients with valvular heart disease for asymptomatic CAD. A normal CT coronary angiogram has a high predictive value for patients with normal or insignificant disease.

▶ Treatment & Prognosis

A. Primary Mitral Regurgitation

The degree of LV enlargement reflects the severity and chronicity of regurgitation. LV volume overload may ultimately lead to LV failure and reduced cardiac output. LA enlargement may be considerable in **chronic mitral regurgitation** and a large amount of mitral regurgitant

regurgitant volume may be tolerated. Patients with chronic lesions may thus remain asymptomatic for many years. Surgery is necessary when symptoms develop or when there is evidence for LV dysfunction, since progressive and irreversible deterioration of LV function can occur prior to the onset of symptoms. Early surgery is indicated even in asymptomatic patients with a reduced EF (less than 60%) or marked LV dilation with reduced contractility (end-systolic dimension greater than 4.0 cm) (Figure 10–2). The 2017 update of the valvular guidelines has added a IIa indication for mitral valve surgery when the LVEF is greater than 60% and the LV end-systolic dimension is still less than 4.0 cm. The new guidelines suggest that mitral valve replacement should be done if serial imaging reveals a progressive increase in the LV end-systolic dimension or a serial decrease in the EF. This latter recommendation is based on information that LV function is more likely to return to normal when the LVEF is greater than 64% and the LV end-systolic dimension is less than 3.7 cm. Pulmonary hypertension development suggests the mitral regurgitation is severe and should prompt intervention.

Acute mitral regurgitation may develop abruptly, such as with papillary muscle dysfunction following MI, valve perforation in infective endocarditis, in patients with hypertrophic cardiomyopathy, or when there are ruptured chordae tendineae in patients with mitral valve prolapse. Emergency surgery may be required.

Some patients may become hemodynamically unstable and require treatment with vasodilators or intra-aortic balloon counterpulsation that reduce the amount of retrograde regurgitant flow by lowering systemic vascular resistance and improving forward stroke volume. There is controversy regarding the role of afterload reduction in chronic mitral regurgitation, since the lesion inherently results in a reduction in afterload, and there are no data that chronic afterload reduction is effective in avoiding LV dysfunction or surgical intervention. A heightened sympathetic state has led some experts to suggest that beta-blockade be considered routinely, though this also remains speculative. The mitral regurgitation in patients with tachycardia-related cardiomyopathy may improve with normalization of the heart rate.

B. Myocardial Disease and Mitral Regurgitation

When mitral regurgitation is due to papillary dysfunction, it may subside as the infarction heals or LV dilation diminishes. The cause of the regurgitation in most of these situations is displacement of the papillary muscles and an enlarged mitral annulus rather than papillary muscle ischemia. The fundamental problem is the lack of leaflet coaptation during systole (due to either leaflet prolapse or retraction). In acute MI, rupture of the papillary muscle may occur with catastrophic results. Transient—but sometimes severe—mitral regurgitation may occur during episodes of myocardial ischemia and contribute to flash pulmonary edema. Patients with dilated cardiomyopathies of any origin may have **secondary mitral regurgitation** due to the papillary muscle displacement or dilation of the mitral annulus, or both. If mitral valve replacement is performed, preservation of the chordae to the native valve

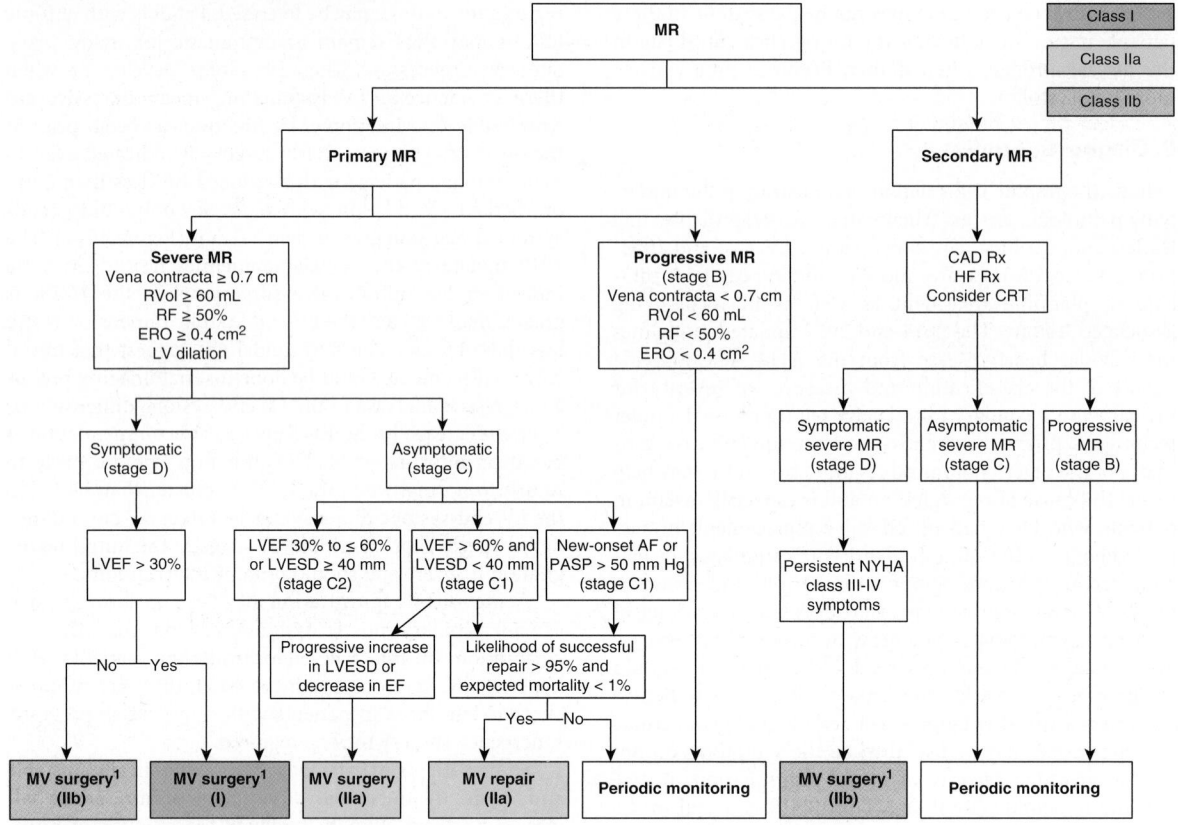

¹MV repair is preferred over MV replacement when possible.
AF, atrial fibrillation; CAD, coronary artery disease; CRT, cardiac resynchronization therapy; EF, ejection fraction; ERO, effective regurgitant orifice; HF, heart failure; LV, left ventricular; LVEF, left ventricular ejection fraction; LVESD, left ventricular end-systolic diameter; MR, mitral regurgitation; MV, mitral valve; NYHA, New York Heart Association; PASP, pulmonary artery systolic pressure; RF, regurgitant fraction; RVol, regurgitant volume; Rx, therapy.

▲ **Figure 10–2.** The 2017 focused update of the AHA/ACC guidelines for intervention in mitral regurgitation. (Reproduced, with permission, Nishimura RA et al. 2017 AHA/ACC focused update of the 2014 AHA/ACC guideline for the management of patients with valvular heart disease: a report of the American College of Cardiology/American Heart Association Task Force on Practice Guidelines. Circulation. 2017 Jun 20;135(25):e1159–95. © 2017 American Heart Association, Inc.)

helps prevent further ventricular dilation following surgery. Initially, several groups reported good results with mitral valve repair in patients with LVEF less than 30% and secondary mitral regurgitation. The 2014 AHA/ACC guidelines advise that mitral valve repair/replacement can be attempted in severe mitral regurgitation patients with an EF less than 30% or an LV end-systolic dimension greater than 5.5 cm, or both, as long as repair and preservation of the chordae are possible. The 2017 update of these guidelines (Figure 10–2) suggests the latest data favor mitral valve replacement with chordal preservation over mitral valve repair in patients with chronic ischemic cardiomyopathy. There may also be a role for cardiac resynchronization therapy with biventricular pacemaker insertion, which has been found to reduce mitral regurgitation related to cardiomyopathy in many patients. Guidelines recommend biventricular pacing prior to surgical repair in symptomatic patients who have functional mitral regurgitation as long as other criteria (eg, a QRS of greater than 150 msec or left bundle branch block or both) are present.

There are several ongoing trials of percutaneous approaches to reducing mitral regurgitation. These approaches include the use of a **mitral clip** device to create a double orifice mitral valve, various coronary catheter devices to reduce the mitral annular area, and devices to reduce the septal-lateral ventricular size and consequent mitral orifice size. Of these devices, the most success has been noted with the mitral clip device. The device, however, is reserved for patients in whom surgical risk is considered excessive and there is primary mitral valve disease with at least 3+ mitral regurgitation. Two major trials addressing the advantage of the percutaneous MitraClip reported findings in 2018. In the COAPT (Clinical Outcomes Assessment of MitraClip) trial among patients with heart failure and moderate-to-severe or severe secondary mitral regurgitation who remained symptomatic despite the use of maximum doses of guideline-directed medical therapy, transcatheter mitral-valve repair resulted in a lower rate of hospitalization for heart failure and lower all-cause mortality within 24 months of follow-up than medical therapy alone. The absolute risk reduction in all-cause mortality in patients receiving the MitraClip in the COAPT trial was 17%, which translated to a number needed to treat (NNT) of 6 to prevent 1 death over 2 years. This rather remarkably positive result, however, was tempered by another MitraClip randomized trial in a similar population that had a rather neutral result, the MITRA-FR (Percutaneous Repair with MitraClip Device for Severe Functional/Secondary Mitral Regurgitation) study, in which the MitraClip therapy failed to show any survival benefit over medical therapy during the 1-year follow-up period. One suggestion to reconcile the differences in outcome has been suggested wherein the MitraClip is ineffective if the regurgitant orifice size is consistent with the size of the dilated LV, but the device is effective if the regurgitant orifice size is large compared to the size of the LV. This seemed to be verified by the results of the two trials. The acceptance of the results from the COAPT trial is awaiting further confirmation. In addition, vascular plugging and occluder devices are being used in selected patients to occlude perivalvular leaks around prosthetic mitral valves. A transcatheter stented valve, which is used as a **transcatheter aortic valve replacement (TAVR)** device, can be used to open a degenerated mitral bioprosthetic valve in any position (aortic, mitral, tricuspid, or pulmonary). Transcatheter valve replacement has also been attempted in small series to repair mitral regurgitation following mitral valve repair with mixed results. Finally, the first cases of a stented mitral valve prosthesis to replace the entire mitral valve have been reported. Abbott has initiated the SUMMIT trial, a US-based pivotal trial utilizing the Tendyne percutaneous mitral valve replacement device.

▶ When to Refer

- All patients with more than mild mitral regurgitation should be referred to a cardiologist for an evaluation.
- Serial examinations and echocardiograms should be obtained and surgical referral made if there is an increase in the LV end-systolic dimensions, a fall in the LVEF to less than 60%, symptoms, evidence for pulmonary hypertension, or the new onset of atrial fibrillation.
- There is growing evidence that mitral valve repair should be done early in the course of the disease to improve mortality and morbidity.
- Treatment in the presence of mitral regurgitation in a dilated cardiomyopathy remains controversial, though biventricular pacing may improve mitral regurgitation in patients with left bundle branch block, and percutaneous MitraClip valve repair may have a role in selected patients.

Grayburn PA et al. Proportionate and disproportionate functional mitral regurgitation: a new conceptual framework that reconciles the results of the MITRA-FR and COAPT trials. JACC Cardiovasc Imaging. 2019 Feb;12(2):353–62. [PMID: 30553663]

Nishimura RA et al. 2017 AHA/ACC focused update of the 2014 AHA/ACC guideline for the management of patients with valvular heart disease: a report of the American College of Cardiology/American Heart Association Task Force on Practice Guidelines. Circulation. 2017 Jun 20;135(25):e1159–95. [PMID: 28298458]

Obadia JF et al; MITRA-FR Investigators. Percutaneous repair or medical treatment for secondary mitral regurgitation. N Engl J Med. 2018 Dec 13;379(24):2297–306. [PMID: 30145927]

O'Gara PT et al. 2017 ACC expert consensus decision pathway on the management of mitral regurgitation: a report of the American College of Cardiology Task Force on Expert Consensus Decision Pathways. J Am Coll Cardiol. 2017 Nov 7;70(19):2421–49. [PMID: 29055505]

Praz F et al. Expanding indications of transcatheter heart valve interventions. JACC Cardiovasc Interv. 2015 Dec 21;8(14):1777–96. [PMID: 26718509]

Stone GW et al; COAPT Investigators. Transcatheter mitral-valve repair in patients with heart failure. N Engl J Med. 2018 Dec 13;379(24):2307–18. [PMID: 30280640]

MITRAL VALVE PROLAPSE SYNDROME

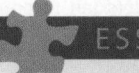

ESSENTIALS OF DIAGNOSIS

▶ Single or multiple mid-systolic clicks often heard on auscultation.

▶ Murmur may be pansystolic or only late in systole.

▶ Often associated with skeletal changes (straight back, pectus excavatum, and scoliosis) or hyperflexibility of joints.

▶ Echocardiography is confirmatory with prolapse of mitral leaflets in systole into the LA.

▶ Chest pain and palpitations are common symptoms in the young adult.

▶ General Considerations

The significance of mild mitral valve prolapse ("floppy" or myxomatous mitral valve), also commonly referred to as **"degenerative" mitral valve disease,** has been in dispute because of the frequency with which it is diagnosed by echocardiography in even healthy young women (up to 10%). A controversial hyperadrenergic syndrome not too dissimilar to the **postural orthostatic tachycardia syndrome** has also been described (especially in young females) that may be responsible for some of the noncardiac symptoms observed. Fortunately, this hyperadrenergic component attenuates with age and is infrequent in persons older than 40–45 years. Some patients with mitral prolapse have findings of a systemic collagen abnormality (Marfan or Ehlers-Danlos syndrome). In these conditions, a dilated aortic root and aortic regurgitation may coexist. In many persons, the "degenerative" myxomatous mitral valve clearly leads to long-term sequelae and is the most common cause of mitral regurgitation in developed countries. Recent MRI-derived data suggest an increase in myocardial fibrosis in patients with mitral regurgitation and prolapse compared to those with mitral regurgitation without prolapse.

Patients who have only a mid-systolic click usually have no immediate clinical issues, but significant mitral regurgitation may develop, occasionally suddenly due to rupture of chordae tendineae (flail leaflet) or gradually due to progressive annular and LV dilation. The need for valve repair or replacement increases with age, so that approximately 2% per year of patients with mitral valve prolapse with clinically significant regurgitation over age 60 years will eventually require surgery.

Clinical Findings

A. Symptoms and Signs

Mitral valve prolapse without significant mitral regurgitation is usually asymptomatic but may be associated with a syndrome of nonspecific chest pain, dyspnea, fatigue, or palpitations. Most patients are young, female, thin, and some have skeletal deformities, such as pectus excavatum or scoliosis. On auscultation, there are characteristic mid-systolic clicks that may be multiple and emanate from the chordae or redundant valve tissue. If leaflets fail to come together properly, the clicks will be followed by a late systolic murmur. As the mitral regurgitation worsens, the murmur is heard more and more throughout systole. The smaller the LV chamber, the greater the degree of leaflet prolapse, and thus auscultatory findings are often accentuated in the standing position or during the Valsalva maneuver. Whether sudden cardiac death presumably due to ventricular arrhythmias is more frequent in patients with mitral valve prolapse remains controversial. Mitral prolapse progresses to significant mitral regurgitation over 3–16 years in about one-fourth of individuals.

B. Diagnostic Studies

The diagnosis is primarily clinical and confirmed echocardiographically. Mitral prolapse is often associated with aortic root disease, and any evidence for a dilated aorta by chest radiography should prompt either CT or MRI angiography. If palpitations are an issue, an ambulatory monitor is often helpful to distinguish atrial from ventricular tachyarrhythmias.

Treatment

Beta-blockers in low doses are used to treat the hyperadrenergic state when present and are usually satisfactory for treatment of arrhythmias (see Table 11–9). Selective serotonin reuptake inhibitors have also been used, especially if orthostatic hypotension or anxiety is associated with mitral valve prolapse; results have been mixed. Some patients have associated postural orthostatic tachycardia syndrome. Afterload reduction has not been shown to change prognosis when mitral regurgitation is present.

Mitral valve repair is strongly favored over valve replacement, and its efficacy has led many to recommend intervention earlier and earlier in the course of the disease process. Mitral repair may include shortening of chordae, chordae transfers, wedge resection of redundant valve tissue, the insertion of a mitral annular ring to reduce the annular size, or some combination of these techniques. Stitching the middle of the leaflets together to create a double-orifice mitral valve is also used at times (**Alfieri procedure**) and can be performed percutaneously (**MitraClip**). Mitral repair or replacement can usually

be achieved through a right minithoracotomy with or without the use of a robotic device. Endocarditis prophylaxis is not recommended for most patients with mitral valve prolapse regardless of the degree of mitral regurgitation. A variety of percutaneous techniques and devices have been tried with some success, although results suggest that surgical repair is generally more durable.

When to Refer

- All patients with mitral valve prolapse and audible mitral regurgitation should be seen at least once by a cardiologist.
- Periodic echocardiography is warranted to assess LV size (especially end-systolic dimensions) and EF when mitral regurgitation is present. If only mitral clicks are audible, then serial echocardiography is not warranted.

Basso C et al. Arrhythmic mitral valve prolapse and sudden cardiac death. Circulation. 2015 Aug 18;132(7):556–66. [PMID: 26160859]

Delling FN et al. Evolution of mitral valve prolapse: insights from the Framingham Heart Study. Circulation. 2016 Apr 26; 133(17):1688–95. [PMID: 27006478]

Kitkungvan D et al. Myocardial fibrosis in patients with primary mitral regurgitation with and without prolapse. J Am Coll Cardiol. 2018 Aug 21;72(8):823–34. [PMID: 30115220]

Theofilogiannakos EK et al. Floppy mitral valve/mitral valve prolapse syndrome: beta-adrenergic receptor polymorphism may contribute to the pathogenesis of symptoms. J Cardiol. 2015 May;65(5):434–8. [PMID: 25172623]

AORTIC STENOSIS

ESSENTIALS OF DIAGNOSIS

▶ Congenital bicuspid aortic valve (usually asymptomatic until middle or old age).

▶ "Degenerative" or calcific aortic stenosis; similar risk factors as atherosclerosis.

▶ Visual observation of immobile aortic valve plus a valve area of less than 1.0 cm^2 define severe disease; low-gradient but severe aortic stenosis can thus be recognized.

▶ Echocardiography/Doppler is diagnostic.

▶ Surgery typically indicated for symptoms. Percutaneous valve replacement is being used increasingly.

▶ Surgery considered for asymptomatic patients with severe aortic stenosis (mean gradient greater than 55 mm Hg) or when undergoing heart surgery for other reasons (eg, coronary artery bypass grafting [CABG]).

▶ BNP is a marker of early LV myocardial failure, and high levels suggest poor prognosis.

General Considerations

There are two common clinical scenarios in which aortic stenosis is prevalent. The first is due to a congenitally abnormal **unicuspid** or **bicuspid valve,** rather than tricuspid. Symptoms can occur in young or adolescent individuals if the stenosis is severe, but more often emerge at age 50–65 years when calcification and degeneration of the valve become manifest. A dilated ascending aorta, due to an intrinsic defect in the aortic root media and the hemodynamic effects of the eccentric aortic jet, may accompany the bicuspid valve in about half of these patients. Coarctation of the aorta is also seen in a number of patients with congenital aortic stenosis. Offspring of patients with a bicuspid valve have a much higher incidence of the disease in either the valve, the aorta, or both (up to 30% in some series).

A second pathologic process, **degenerative** or **calcific aortic stenosis**, is thought to be related to calcium deposition due to processes similar to those that occur in atherosclerotic vascular disease. Approximately 25% of patients over age 65 years and 35% of those over age 70 years have echocardiographic evidence of aortic valve thickening (sclerosis). About 10–20% of these will progress to hemodynamically significant aortic stenosis over a period of 10–15 years. Certain genetic markers are associated with aortic stenosis (most notably Notch 1), so a genetic component appears a likely contributor, at least in some patients. Other associated genetic markers have also been described.

Aortic stenosis has become the most common surgical valve lesion in developed countries, and many patients are elderly. The risk factors include hypertension, hypercholesterolemia, and smoking. Hypertrophic cardiomyopathy may also coexist with valvular aortic stenosis.

Clinical Findings

A. Symptoms and Signs

Slightly narrowed, thickened, or roughened valves (**aortic sclerosis**) or aortic dilation may contribute to the typical ejection murmur of aortic stenosis. In mild or moderate cases where the valve is still pliable, an ejection click may precede the murmur and the closure of the valve (S_2) is preserved. The characteristic systolic ejection murmur is heard at the aortic area and is usually transmitted to the neck and apex. In severe aortic stenosis, a palpable LV heave or thrill, a weak to absent aortic second sound, or reversed splitting of the second sound is present (see Table 10–1). In some cases, only the high-pitched components of the murmur are heard at the apex, and the murmur may sound like mitral regurgitation (the so-called Gallaverdin phenomenon). When the valve area is less than 0.8–1.0 cm^2 (normal, 3–4 cm^2), ventricular systole becomes prolonged and the typical carotid pulse pattern of delayed upstroke and low amplitude is present. A delayed upstroke, though, is an unreliable finding in older patients with extensive arteriosclerotic vascular disease and a stiff, noncompliant aorta. LVH increases progressively due to the pressure overload, eventually resulting in elevation of ventricular end-diastolic pressure. Cardiac output is maintained until the stenosis is severe. LV failure, angina pectoris, or syncope may be presenting symptoms of significant aortic stenosis; importantly, all symptoms tend to first occur with exertion.

B. Redefining Severe Aortic Stenosis

There are four different anatomic syndromes that occur in patients with severe aortic stenosis. The common underlying measure of **severe aortic stenosis** is an aortic valve area of less than 1.0 cm^2 and echocardiographic evidence of an immobile aortic valve. In patients with a normal LVEF and normal cardiac output, the threshold for intervention is a peak aortic gradient of greater than 64 mm Hg and mean aortic gradient of greater than 40 mm Hg. In the same situation, **super-severe aortic stenosis** is defined as a mean gradient of greater than 55 mm Hg or peak aortic velocity greater than 5 m/sec by Doppler.

In some patients with an aortic valve area of less than 1.0 cm^2 with a low cardiac output and stroke volume, the mean gradient may be less than 40 mm Hg. This can occur when the LV systolic function is poor (**low-gradient severe aortic stenosis with low LVEF**) or when the LV systolic function is normal (*paradoxical* **low-flow severe aortic stenosis with a normal LVEF).** Low flow (low output) in these situations is defined by an echocardiographic stroke volume index of less than 35 mL/min/m^2. Prognosis in patients with low gradient, low valve area, low output, and a normal LVEF aortic stenosis may actually be worse than in patients with the traditional high gradient, low valve area, normal output, and normal LVEF aortic stenosis. If low-flow severe aortic stenosis is present in the face of a low LVEF, provocative testing with dobutamine or nitroprusside is warranted to increase the stroke volume to discover if a mean aortic valve gradient of at least 40 mm Hg can be demonstrated without increasing the aortic valve area. If the aortic valve area can be made to increase and a mean gradient of greater than 40 mm Hg cannot be demonstrated by inotropic challenge, the presumption is that the low gradient is due to an associated cardiomyopathy and not the aortic valve stenosis. In this latter situation intervention is not indicated. The 2014 AHA/ACC guidelines acknowledge these four situations (Table 10–3). Intervention is indicated in super-severe aortic stenosis even without demonstrable symptoms (grade C) and in any of the other situations when symptoms are present: D1 defines the symptomatic high gradient patient; D2 the

Table 10–3. Summary of 2014 AHA/ACC guideline definitions of symptomatic severe aortic stenosis.

Category of Severe Aortic Stenosis[1]	Properties
High Gradient	
High gradient	> 4.0 m/sec Doppler jet velocity > 40 mm Hg mean gradient
Super-severe	> 5.0 m/sec Doppler jet velocity > 55 mm Hg mean gradient
Low Gradient	
Low flow	Reduced LVEF (< 50%)
Low flow	Paradoxical with normal LVEF (> 50%)

[1]All categories of severe aortic stenosis have abnormal systolic opening of the aortic valve and an aortic valve area < 1.0 cm^2. LVEF, left ventricular ejection fraction.

symptomatic low-flow, low-gradient patient with low LVEF; and D3 the symptomatic low-flow, low-gradient patient with normal LVEF.

Symptoms of LV failure may be sudden in onset or may progress gradually. Angina pectoris frequently occurs in aortic stenosis due to underperfusion of the endocardium. Of patients with calcific aortic stenosis and angina, half have significant associated CAD. Syncope, a late finding, occurs with exertion as the LV pressure rises, stimulating the LV baroreceptors to cause peripheral vasodilation. This vasodilation results in the need for an increase in stroke volume, which increases the LV systolic pressure again, creating a cycle of vasodilation and stimulation of the baroreceptors that eventually results in a drop in systemic BP, as the stenotic valve prevents further increase in stroke volume. Less commonly, syncope may be due to arrhythmias (usually ventricular tachycardia but sometimes AV block as calcific invasion of the conduction system from the aortic valve may occur).

C. Diagnostic Studies

The ECG reveals LVH or secondary repolarization changes in most patients but can be normal in up to 10%. The chest radiograph may show (1) a normal or enlarged cardiac silhouette, (2) calcification of the aortic valve, and (3) dilation or calcification (or both) of the ascending aorta. The echocardiogram provides useful data about aortic valve calcification and leaflet opening, the severity of LV wall thickness, and overall ventricular function, while Doppler can provide an excellent estimate of the aortic valve gradient. Valve area estimation by echocardiography is less reliable but is a critical component of the diagnosis of aortic

stenosis due to issues such as paradoxical low-flow aortic stenosis (low-gradient, low-flow, normal LVEF patients). Likewise, the echocardiography/Doppler can estimate the stroke volume index used to define the low-flow state when the valve area is small but the gradient is less than 40 mm Hg. Cardiac catheterization mostly provides an assessment of the hemodynamic consequence of the aortic stenosis, and the anatomy of the coronary arteries. Catheterization data can be important when there is a discrepancy between symptoms and the echocardiography/Dopper information of aortic stenosis severity. In younger patients and in patients with high aortic gradients, the aortic valve need not be crossed at catheterization. Aortic regurgitation can be semiquantified by aortic root angiography. Some authors have suggested the use of BNP (or NT-proBNP) may provide additional prognostic data in the setting of poor LV function and aortic stenosis. A BNP greater than 550 pg/mL has been associated with a poor outcome in these patients regardless of the results of dobutamine testing. Stress testing can be done cautiously in patients in whom the aortic stenosis severity does not match the reported symptoms in order to confirm the reported clinical status. It should *not* be done in patients with super-severe aortic stenosis.

▶ Prognosis & Treatment

Table 10–4 outlines the 2014 guidelines for surgical intervention in aortic stenosis. Valve intervention is warranted in all patients who have symptomatic severe aortic stenosis. There are also times when asymptomatic aortic stenosis should undergo intervention. Asymptomatic patients with severe aortic stenosis (aortic valve area less than 1.0 cm^2)

Table 10–4. 2014 AHA/ACC guidelines for surgical indications in aortic stenosis.

Recommendations	COR	LOE
AVR is recommended in symptomatic patients with severe AS (stage D)	I	B
AVR is recommended for asymptomatic patients with severe AS (stage C2 or D) and LVEF < 50%	I	B
AVR is indicated for patients with severe AS (stage C or D) when undergoing other cardiac surgery	I	B
AVR is reasonable for asymptomatic patients with very severe AS (aortic velocity ≥ 5 m/s) (stage C2) and low surgical risk	IIa	B
AVR is reasonable in asymptomatic patients (stage C1) with severe AS and an abnormal exercise test	IIa	B
AVR is reasonable in symptomatic patients with low-flow/low-gradient severe AS with reduced LVEF (stage S1) with a low-dose dobutamine stress study that shows an aortic velocity ≥ 4 m/s (or mean gradient ≥ 40 mm Hg) with a valve area ≤ 1.0 cm^2 at any dobutamine dose	IIa	B
AVR is reasonable for patients with moderate AS (stage B) (velocity 3.0–3.9 m/s) who are undergoing other cardiac surgery	IIa	C
AVR may be considered for asymptomatic patients with severe AS (stage C1) and rapid disease progression and low surgical risk	IIb	C
AVR may be considered in symptomatic patients who have low-flow/low-gradient severe AS (stage S2) who are normotensive and have an LVEF ≥ 50% if clinical, hemodynamic, and anatomic data support valve obstruction as the most likely cause of symptoms	IIb	C

AS, aortic stenosis; AVR, aortic valve replacement; COR, class of recommendation; LOE, level of evidence; LVEF, left ventricular ejection fraction.
Reproduced, with permission, from Nishimura RA et al. 2014 AHA/ACC Guideline for the Management of Patients With Valvular Heart Disease: A Report of the American College of Cardiology/American Heart Association Task Force on Practice Guidelines. Circulation. 2014 Jun 10;129(23):e521–643. © 2014 American Heart Association, Inc.

should generally undergo intervention according to the following guidelines: (1) they are undergoing other cardiac surgery (ie, CABG), (2) there is evidence for a reduced LVEF (less than 50%), (3) when the mean gradient exceeds 55 mm Hg (peak velocity greater than 5 m/sec), (4) when there is failure of the BP to rise more than 20 mm Hg with exercise, (5) when there is severe valvular calcium, or (6) when there is evidence of a rapid increase in the peak aortic gradient (more than 0.3 m/sec/year). Following the onset of heart failure, angina, or syncope, the prognosis without surgery is poor (50% 3-year mortality rate). Medical treatment may stabilize patients in heart failure, but intervention is indicated for all symptomatic patients with evidence of significant aortic stenosis.

The surgical mortality rate for valve replacement is low, even in older adults, and ranges from 2% to 5%. This low risk is due to the dramatic hemodynamic improvement that occurs with relief of the increased afterload. Mortality rates are substantially higher when there is an associated ischemic cardiomyopathy. Severe coronary lesions are usually bypassed at the same time as aortic valve replacement (AVR), although there are few data to suggest this practice affects outcome. In some cases, a staged procedure with stenting of the coronaries prior to surgery may be considered, especially if a percutaneous AVR approach is being considered. Around one-third to one-half of all patients with aortic stenosis have significant CAD, so this is a common concern. With the success of **transcatheter aortic valve replacement (TAVR)**, the treatment options have greatly expanded for many patients with severe aortic stenosis. For this reason, a **Heart Valve Team** approach bringing together invasive and noninvasive cardiologists, radiologists, anesthesiologists, and cardiac surgeons is mandatory; clinical factors (such as frailty) and anatomic features (such as a calcified aorta, vascular access, etc) can affect the decision making.

Medical therapy to reduce the progression of disease has *not* been effective to date. Statins have been assessed in four major clinical trials. None revealed any benefit on the the progression of aortic stenosis or on clinical outcomes despite the association of aortic stenosis with atherosclerosis. If patients with aortic stenosis have concomitant CAD, the guidelines for the use of statins should be followed. Efforts to reduce stenosis progression by blockage of the renin-angiotensin system have also been ineffective. Control of systemic hypertension, though, is an important adjunct, and inadequate systemic BP control is all too common due to unreasonable concerns about providing too much afterload reduction in patients with aortic stenosis. Normal systemic BP is important to maintain as the LV is affected by the total afterload (systemic BP plus the aortic valve gradient).

The interventional options in patients with aortic valve stenosis has expanded with the use of TAVR and depend on the patient's lifestyle and age. The algorithm to decide when an AVR is appropriate in various situations is outlined in Figure 10–3. The 2017 ACC/AHA valvular guidelines modify this only in that surgical AVR can be considered for any of the indications outlined in the figure, whether asymptomatic or not. TAVR should be reserved only for those patients with symptoms. These newest guidelines point out that TAVR is equivalent to surgical AVR in all of the randomized trials of symptomatic patients. As of 2017, TAVR for aortic stenosis can be applied to all except the lowest risk (less than 4%). The lowest risk patients are being studied in trials randomizing between TAVR and surgical AVR.

In young and adolescent patients, percutaneous balloon valvuloplasty still has a small role. Balloon valvuloplasty is associated with early restenosis in the elderly population, and thus is rarely used except as a temporizing measure. Data suggest aortic balloon valvuloplasty in elderly people has an advantage only in those with preserved LV function, and such patients are usually excellent candidates for surgical AVR. Middle-aged adults generally can tolerate the anticoagulation therapy necessary for the use of mechanical aortic valves, so patients younger than 60 years generally undergo AVR with a bileaflet mechanical valve. If the aortic root is severely dilated as well (greater than 4.5 cm), then the valve may be housed in a Dacron sheath (**Bentall procedure**) and the root replaced along with the aortic valve. Alternatively, a human homograft root and valve replacement can be used. In patients older than 60 years, bioprosthetic (either porcine or bovine pericardial) valves with a life expectancy of about 10–15 years are routinely used instead of mechanical valves to avoid need for anticoagulation. Data favor the bovine pericardial valve over the porcine aortic valve. As it is becoming clearer that bioprosthetic valve degeneration in the larger valves can be potentially repaired by percutaneous valve-in-valve TAVR, it is likely that the use of mechanical valves will continue to decline. If the aortic annulus is small, a bioprosthetic valve with a short sheath can be sewn to the aortic wall (the stentless AVR) rather than sewing the prosthetic annulus to the aortic annulus. (Annulus is a relative term when speaking of the aortic valve, since there is no true annulus.) Another popular surgical option when the aorta is enlarged is the use of the **Wheat procedure;** it involves aortic root replacement above the coronary arteries and replacement of the aortic valve below the coronary arteries. The coronary arteries thus remain attached to the native aorta between the new graft and prosthetic valve rather than being reimplanted onto an artificial sheath or homograft.

In patients with a bicuspid aortic valve, there is an associated ascending aortic aneurysm in about half. If the maximal dimension of the aortic root is greater than 5.5 cm, it is recommended to proceed with root replacement regardless of the severity of the aortic valve disease. It is also appropriate to intervene when the maximal aortic root size is greater than 5.0 cm in diameter if there is a family history of aortic dissection or the aortic root size increases by more than 0.5 cm in 1 year. The aortic valve may be replaced at the same time if at least moderate aortic stenosis is present or may be either left alone or repaired (valve sparing operation). If there is an indication for AVR and the root is greater than 4.5 cm in diameter, root replacement is also recommended.

The use of mechanical versus bioprosthetic AVR has changed over time. A bioprosthetic valve is acceptable for patients at any age for whom anticoagulant therapy is

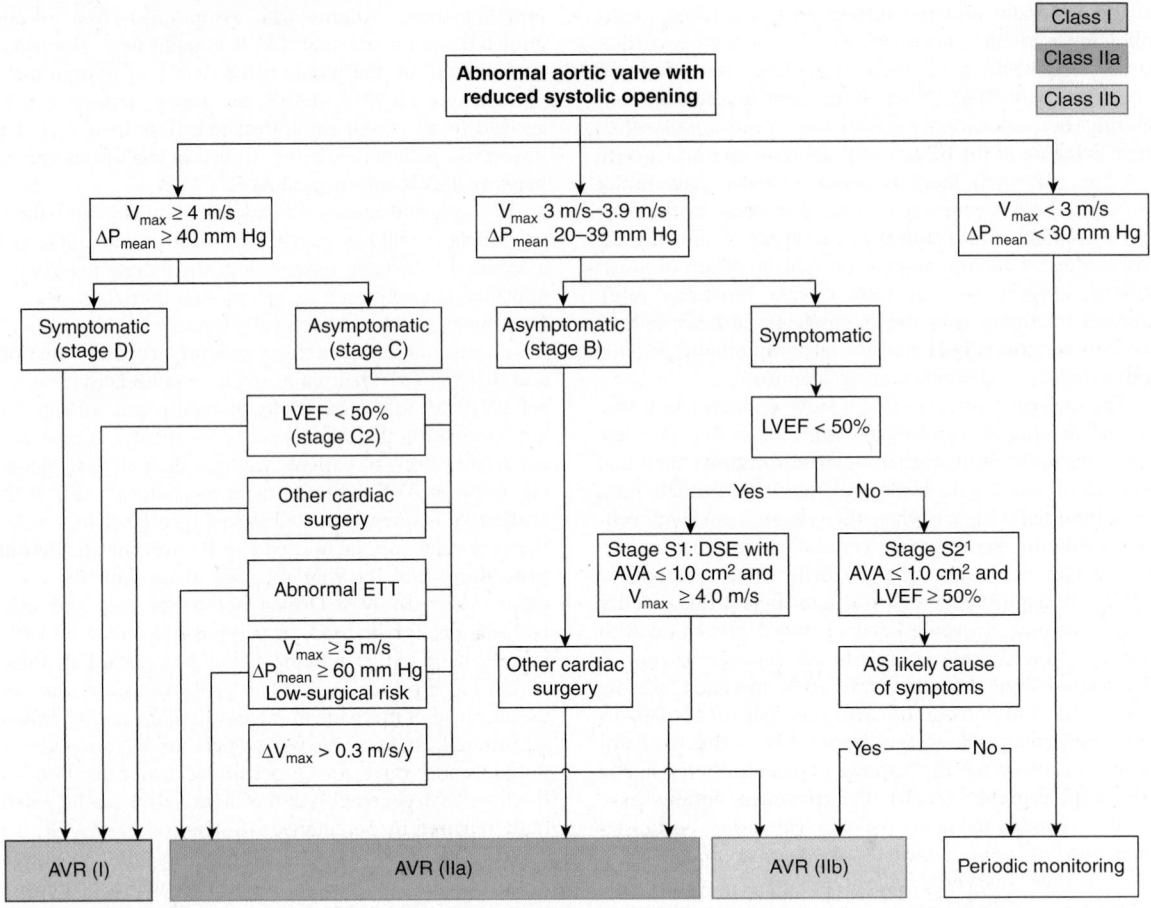

Figure 10–3. Algorithm for the management of aortic valve stenosis. (Reproduced, with permission, from Nishimura RA et al. 2014 AHA/ACC Guideline for the Management of Patients With Valvular Heart Disease: A Report of the American College of Cardiology/American Heart Association Task Force on Practice Guidelines. Circulation. 2014 Jun 10; 129(23):e521–643. © 2014 American Heart Association, Inc.)

contraindicated, not desired, or cannot be managed, and is preferred in patients over the age of 70. An aortic mechanical valve should be used in patients younger than 50 years of age who can take warfarin (this recommendation is a decrease from age 60 in the recent updated guidelines). Either type of valve is acceptable between the ages of 50 and 70 years depending on patient preference and any issues with warfarin usage.

Anticoagulation is required with the use of mechanical aortic valves, and the international normalized ratio (INR) should be maintained between 2.0 and 3.0 for bileaflet valves. In general, mechanical aortic valves are less subject to thrombosis than mechanical mitral valves and do not need bridging with anticoagulation unless there are other thromboembolic risk factors or there is an older generation AVR. Low-dose aspirin is recommended as well. Some

newer bileaflet mechanical valves (On-X) allow for a lower INR range from 1.5 to 2.0. Clopidogrel is recommended for the first 6 months after TAVR in combination with lifelong aspirin therapy. DOACs are *not* recommended for any mechanical valves but may be used in patients with a bioprosthetic AVR if treating atrial fibrillation or venous thrombosis.

The estimated use of TAVR has grown dramatically, with a gross estimate of over 500,000 implants worldwide. In the United States, the Food and Drug Administration (FDA) has granted approval for two devices, the Edwards SAPIEN and the Medtronic CoreValve, for use in patients with at least a 4% surgical risk (intermediate risk) as measured by the Society of Thoracic Surgeons. These devices are fundamentally stents with a trileaflet bioprosthetic valve constructed within them. There are a variety of implantation approaches, though most valves are placed via a femoral artery approach. Other options include an antegrade approach via transseptal across the atrial septum, via the LV apex with a small surgical incision, via the subclavian arteries, via the carotid, or via a minithoracotomy. The Edwards SAPIEN valve is a balloon-expandable valvular stent, while the CoreValve is a valvular stent that self-expands when pushed out of the catheter sheath. Multiple other devices are in trials, many with excellent early results. These devices will allow for a wider range of aortic valve sizes to be treated; can be delivered with smaller catheters, eliminating the need for femoral artery cutdowns; will allow for repositioning before permanent implantation; and appear to result in less paravalvular regurgitation and less injury to the conduction system. Cost remains a major issue. All of the professional societies stress the importance of a Heart Valve Team when considering aortic stenosis intervention. This is critically important because many patients referred for TAVR have serious comorbid conditions that will not improve with alleviation of the aortic stenosis. A 2017 consensus document from the ACC provides a decision pathway for the use of TAVR. This document summarizes background information and provides a checklist of items to consider when deciding between surgical AVR and TAVR. The importance of quality of life and frailty is emphasized because some of the most elderly or most debilitated patients may not benefit from any procedure. Frailty is a risk factor for death and disability following TAVR and surgical aortic valve replacement. A brief four-item scale encompassing lower-extremity weakness, cognitive impairment, anemia, and hypoalbuminemia outperformed other frailty scales.

Figure 10–4 outlines the suggested indications for TAVR based on the 2017 updated AHA/ACC guidelines.

TAVR is also being used more frequently in "valve-in-valve" procedures to reduce the gradient in patients with prosthetic valve dysfunction (regardless of whether in the aortic, mitral, tricuspid, or pulmonary position). While the results of TAVR in patients with bicuspid aortic valves (as opposed to tricuspid) have been less impressive, newer modifications have improved the success rates in these anatomic situations as well.

► When to Refer

- All patients with echocardiographic evidence for mild-to-moderate aortic stenosis (estimated peak valve gradient greater than 30 mm Hg by echocardiography/ Doppler) should be referred to a cardiologist for evaluation and to determine the frequency of follow-up.

- Any patients with symptoms suggestive of aortic stenosis (ie, exertional symptoms of chest pressure, shortness of breath, or presyncope) should be seen by a cardiologist.

Babaliarois V. Innovation in intervention: transcatheter aortic valve replacement focus issue. JACC Cardiol Interv. 2015 Apr 27;8(5):758–9. [PMID: 25946454]

Bonow RO et al. 2017 appropriate use criteria for the treatment of patients with severe aortic stenosis: a report of the American College of Cardiology Appropriate Use Criteria Task Force, American Association for Thoracic Surgery, American Heart Association, American Society of Echocardiography, European Association for Cardio-Thoracic Surgery, Heart Valve Society, Society of Cardiovascular Anesthesiologists, Society for Cardiovascular Angiography and Interventions, Society of Cardiovascular Computed Tomography, Society for Cardiovascular Magnetic Resonance, and Society of Thoracic Surgeons. J Am Coll Cardiol. 2017 Nov 14;70(20): 2566–98. [PMID: 29054308]

Hakeem A et al. Outcomes of TAVR in bicuspid aortic valve stenosis. J Am Coll Cardiol. 2017 Sep 26;70(13):1684–5. [PMID: 28935046]

Moat NE. Will TAVR become the predominant method for treating severe aortic stenosis? N Engl J Med. 2016 Apr 28; 374(17):1682–3. [PMID: 27040006]

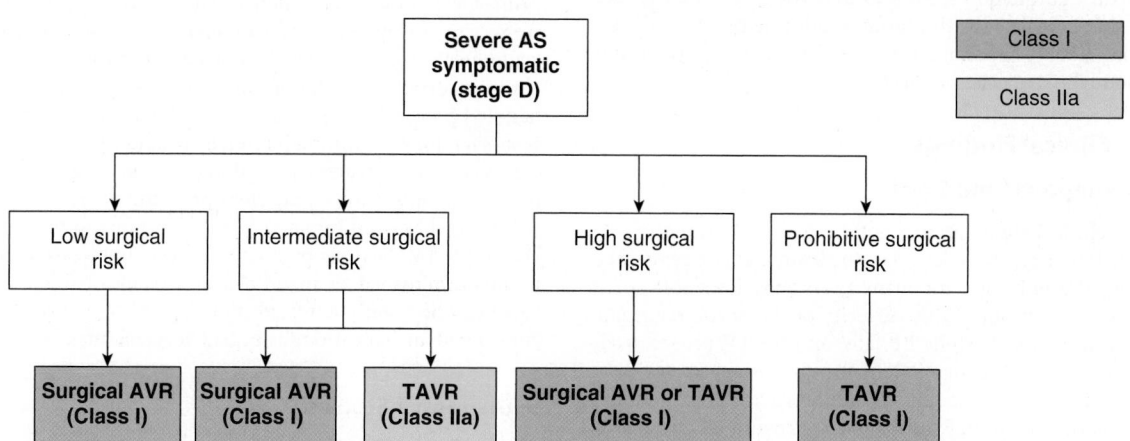

AS, aortic stenosis; AVR, aortic valve replacement; TAVR, transcatheter aortic valve replacement.

▲ **Figure 10–4.** Choice of TAVR versus surgical AVR in patients with severe symptomatic AS. (Reproduced, with permission, from Nishimura RA et al. 2017 AHA/ACC focused update of the 2014 AHA/ACC guideline for the management of patients with valvular heart disease: a report of the American College of Cardiology/American Heart Association Task Force on Practice Guidelines. Circulation. 2017 Jun 20;135(25):e1159–95. © 2017 American Heart Association, Inc.)

Nishimura RA et al. 2017 AHA/ACC focused update of the 2014 AHA/ACC guideline for the management of patients with valvular heart disease: a report of the American College of Cardiology/American Heart Association Task Force on Practice Guidelines. Circulation. 2017 Jun 20;135(25):e1159–95. [PMID: 28298458]

Otto CM et al. 2017 ACC expert consensus decision pathway for transcatheter aortic valve replacement in the management of adults with aortic stenosis: a report of the American College of Cardiology Task Force on Clinical Expert Consensus Documents. J Am Coll Cardiol. 2017 Mar 14;69(10):1313–46. [PMID: 28063810]

Reardon MJ et al; SURTAVI Investigators. Surgical or transcatheter aortic-valve replacement in intermediate-risk patients. N Engl J Med. 2017 Apr 6;376(14):1321–31. [PMID: 28304219]

AORTIC REGURGITATION

 ESSENTIALS OF DIAGNOSIS

- ► Usually asymptomatic until middle age; presents with left-sided failure or rarely chest pain.
- ► Echocardiography/Doppler is diagnostic.
- ► Surgery for symptoms, EF less than 50%, LV end-systolic dimension greater than 50 mm, or LV end-diastolic dimension greater than 65 mm.

► General Considerations

Of all patients with isolated aortic valve disease, about 13% have predominately aortic regurgitation. Rheumatic aortic regurgitation has become much less common than in the preantibiotic era, and nonrheumatic causes now predominate. These include congenitally bicuspid valves, infective endocarditis, and hypertension. Many patients also have aortic regurgitation secondary to aortic root diseases, such as that associated with Marfan syndrome or aortic dissection. Rarely, inflammatory diseases, such as ankylosing spondylitis, may be implicated.

► Clinical Findings

A. Symptoms and Signs

The clinical presentation is determined by the rapidity with which regurgitation develops. In **chronic aortic regurgitation,** the only sign for many years may be a soft aortic diastolic murmur. As the severity of the aortic regurgitation increases, diastolic BP falls, and the LV progressively enlarges. Most patients remain asymptomatic for long periods even at this point. LV failure is a late event and may be sudden in onset. Exertional dyspnea and fatigue are the most frequent symptoms, but paroxysmal nocturnal dyspnea and pulmonary edema may also occur. Angina pectoris or atypical chest pain may occasionally be present. Associated CAD and presyncope or syncope are less common than in aortic stenosis.

Hemodynamically, because of compensatory LV dilation, patients eject a large stroke volume, which is adequate to maintain forward cardiac output until late in the course of the disease. LV diastolic pressure may rise when heart failure occurs. Abnormal LV systolic function as manifested by reduced EF (less than 50%) and increasing end-systolic LV volume (greater than 5.0 cm) are signs that surgical intervention is warranted.

The major physical findings in chronic aortic regurgitation relate to the high stroke volume being ejected into the systemic vascular system with rapid runoff as the regurgitation takes place (see Table 10–1). This results in a **wide arterial pulse pressure.** The pulse has a rapid rise and fall (**water-hammer pulse** or **Corrigan pulse**), with an elevated systolic and low diastolic pressure. The large stroke volume and flow back into the heart are also responsible for characteristic findings, such as **Quincke pulses** (nailbed capillary pulsations), **Duroziez sign** (to-and-fro murmur over a partially compressed femoral peripheral artery), and **Musset sign** (head bob with each pulse). In younger patients, the increased stroke volume may summate with the pressure wave reflected from the periphery and create a higher than expected systolic pressure in the lower extremities compared with the central aorta. Since the peripheral bed is much larger in the leg than the arm, the BP in the leg may be over 40 mm Hg higher than in the arm (**Hill sign**) in severe aortic regurgitation. The apical impulse is prominent, laterally displaced, usually hyperdynamic, and may be sustained. A systolic flow murmur is usually present and may be quite soft and localized; the aortic diastolic murmur is usually high-pitched and decrescendo. A mid or late diastolic low-pitched mitral murmur (**Austin Flint murmur**) may be heard in advanced aortic regurgitation, owing to relative obstruction of mitral inflow produced by partial closure of the mitral valve by the rapidly rising LV diastolic pressure due to the aortic regurgitation.

In **acute aortic regurgitation** (usually from aortic dissection or infective endocarditis), LV failure is manifested primarily as pulmonary edema and may develop rapidly; surgery is urgently required in such cases. Patients with acute aortic regurgitation do not have the dilated LV of chronic aortic regurgitation and the extra LV volume is handled poorly. For the same reason, the diastolic murmur is shorter, may be minimal in intensity, and the pulse pressure may not be widened—making clinical diagnosis difficult. The mitral valve may close prematurely even before LV systole has been initiated (preclosure) due to the rapid rise in the LV diastolic pressure, and the first heart sound is thus diminished or inaudible. Preclosure of the mitral valve can be readily detected on echocardiography and is considered an indication for urgent surgical intervention.

B. Diagnostic Studies

The ECG usually shows moderate to severe LVH. Radiographs show cardiomegaly with LV prominence and sometimes a dilated aorta.

Echocardiography demonstrates the major diagnostic features, including whether the lesion includes the proximal aortic root and what valvular pathology is present. Annual assessments of LV size and function are critical in determining the timing for valve replacement when the aortic regurgitation is severe. The 2014 AHA/ACC valvular guideline provides criteria for assessing the severity of aortic regurgitation. Cardiac MRI and CT can estimate aortic root size, particularly when there is concern for an ascending aneurysm. MRI can provide a regurgitant fraction to help confirm severity. Cardiac catheterization may be unnecessary in younger patients, particularly those with acute aortic regurgitation, but can help define hemodynamics, aortic root abnormalities, and associated CAD preoperatively in older patients. Increasing data are emerging that serum BNP or NT-proBNP may be an early sign of LV dysfunction, and it is possible that these data will be added to recommendations for surgical intervention in the future.

▶ Treatment & Prognosis

Aortic regurgitation that appears or worsens during or after an episode of infective endocarditis or aortic dissection may lead to acute severe LV failure or subacute progression over weeks or months. The former usually presents as pulmonary edema; surgical replacement of the valve is indicated even during active infection. These patients may be transiently improved or stabilized by vasodilators.

Chronic aortic regurgitation may be tolerated for many years, but the prognosis without surgery becomes poor when symptoms occur. Since aortic regurgitation places both a preload (volume) and afterload increase on the LV, medications that decrease afterload can reduce regurgitation severity, although there are no convincing data that afterload reduction alters mortality. **Recommendations advocate afterload reduction in aortic regurgitation only when there is associated systolic hypertension (systolic BP greater than 140 mm Hg).** Afterload reduction in normotensive patients does not appear warranted. Angiotensin receptor blockers (ARBs), rather than beta-blockers, are the preferred additions to the medical therapy in patients with an enlarged aorta, such as in Marfan syndrome, because of the theoretical ability of an ARB to reduce aortic stiffness (by blocking TGF-beta) and to slow the rate of aortic dilation. However, clinical trials evaluating the efficacy of ARBs to reduce aortic stiffness and slow the rate of aortic dilation have not yielded a positive outcome to support their use at this time.

Surgery is indicated once symptoms emerge or for any evidence of LV dysfunction (as exhibited by a reduction in the LVEF or increase in the LV end-systolic diameter). In addition, it is suggested that surgery should be considered when the LV becomes excessively enlarged (LV end-diastolic diameter greater than 65 mm) (Table 10–5).

The issues with AVR covered in the above section concerning aortic stenosis pertain here. Early trials of TAVR had a high incidence of postprocedural residual aortic regurgitation (18.8% in one trial). Newer TAVR valves have greatly reduced residual aortic regurgitation when used in patients with pure native aortic regurgitation (4.2%). In multivariable analysis, postprocedural at least moderate

Table 10–5. When to operate in chronic severe aortic regurgitation (AR).

Indication for Surgery	Class and Level of Evidence (LOE)
Symptomatic	Class I LOE B
Asymptomatic	
Abnormal LVEF < 50%	Class I LOE B
Undergoing other heart surgery	Class I LOE C
Normal LVEF, but LVESD > 50 mm	Class IIa LOE B
Moderate AR and other heart surgery	Class IIa LOE C
Normal LVEF, but LVEDD > 65 mm	Class IIb LOE C

LVEDD, left ventricular end-diastolic dimension; LVEF, left ventricular ejection fraction; LVESD, left ventricular end-systolic dimension.

aortic regurgitation was independently associated with 1-year all-cause mortality (hazard ratio: 2.85; 95% confidence interval: 1.52 to 5.35; $P = 0.001$). Compared with the early-generation devices, TAVR using the new-generation devices was associated with improved procedural outcomes in treating patients with pure native aortic regurgitation. In patients with pure native aortic regurgitation, significant postprocedural aortic regurgitation was independently associated with increased mortality.

Aortic regurgitation due to a paravalvular prosthetic valve defect can occasionally be occluded with percutaneous occluder devices. The choice of prosthetic valve for AVR depends on the patient's age and compatibility with warfarin anticoagulation similar to the choices for AVR in aortic stenosis.

The operative mortality for AVR is usually in the 3–5% range. Aortic regurgitation due to aortic root disease requires repair or replacement of the root as well as surgical treatment of the aortic valve. Though valve-sparing operations have improved recently, most patients with root replacement undergo valve replacement at the same time. Root replacement in association with valve replacement may require reanastomosis of the coronary arteries, and thus the procedure is more complex than valve replacement alone. The Wheat procedure replaces the aortic root but spares the area where the coronaries attach to avoid the necessity for their reimplantation. Following any aortic valve surgery, LV size usually decreases and LV function generally improves even when the baseline EF is depressed.

The AHA/ACC 2014 valvular guidelines and a 2015 consensus document recommend the "cutoff" diameter that indicates repair of the aortic root in patients with a bicuspid valve should be 5.5 cm regardless of aortic valve disease severity. There are data that dissection is much more prevalent when the aortic root diameter exceeds 6.0 cm, and the general sense is not to let it approach that size. Patients with risk factors (family history of dissection or an increase in the diameter of the root greater than 0.5 cm in 1 year) should have the aorta repaired when the maximal dimension exceeds 5.0 cm. The following classifications summarize when to operate on the aortic root in patients with a bicuspid aortic valve based on the guidelines:

Class I indication (LOE C): aortic root diameter at sinuses or ascending aorta greater than 5.5 cm (regardless of need for AVR).

Class IIa indication (LOE C): aortic root diameter at sinuses or ascending aorta greater than 5.0 cm when there are associated risk factors (family history of dissection or increase in size more than 0.5 cm in 1 year).

Class IIa indication (LOE C): aortic root diameter greater than 4.5 cm if patient undergoing AVR for valvular reasons.

► When to Refer

- Patients with audible aortic regurgitation should be seen, at least initially, by a cardiologist who can determine whether the patient needs follow-up.

- Patients with a dilated aortic root should be monitored by a cardiologist, since imaging studies other than the chest radiograph or echocardiogram may be required to decide surgical timing.

Franzone A et al. Transcatheter aortic valve replacement for the treatment of pure native aortic valve regurgitation: a systematic review. JACC Cardiovasc Interv. 2016 Nov 28;9(22): 2308–17. [PMID: 28026742]

Hiratzka LF et al. Surgery for aortic dilatation in patients with bicuspid aortic valves: a statement of clarification from the American College of Cardiology/American Heart Association Task Force on Clinical Practice Guidelines. J Am Coll Cardiol. 2016 Feb 16;67(6):724–31. [PMID: 26658475]

Nishimura RA et al. 2017 AHA/ACC focused update of the 2014 AHA/ACC guideline for the management of patients with valvular heart disease: a report of the American College of Cardiology/American Heart Association Task Force on Practice Guidelines. Circulation. 2017 Jun 20;135(25):e1159–95. [PMID: 28298458]

Yoon SH et al. Transcatheter aortic valve replacement in pure native aortic valve regurgitation. J Am Coll Cardiol. 2017 Dec 5;70(22):2752–63. [PMID: 29191323]

TRICUSPID STENOSIS

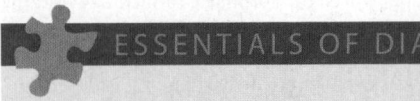

ESSENTIALS OF DIAGNOSIS

▶ Female predominance.

▶ History of rheumatic heart disease most likely. Carcinoid disease and prosthetic valve degeneration are the most common etiologies in the United States.

▶ Echocardiography/Doppler is diagnostic.

► General Considerations

Tricuspid stenosis is rare, affecting less than 1% of the population in developed countries and less than 3% worldwide. Native valve tricuspid valve stenosis is usually rheumatic in origin. In the United States, tricuspid stenosis is more commonly due to prior tricuspid valve repair or replacement or to the carcinoid syndrome. Tricuspid regurgitation frequently accompanies the lesion. It should be suspected when right heart failure appears in the course of mitral valve disease or in the postoperative period after tricuspid valve repair or replacement. Congenital forms of tricuspid stenosis may also be rarely observed, as have case reports of multiple pacemaker leads creating RV inflow obstruction at the tricuspid valve.

► Clinical Findings

A. Symptoms and Signs

Tricuspid stenosis is characterized by right heart failure with hepatomegaly, ascites, and dependent edema. In sinus rhythm, a giant *a* wave is seen in the JVP, which is also elevated (see Table 10–1). The typical diastolic rumble along the lower left sternal border mimics mitral stenosis, though in tricuspid stenosis the rumble increases with inspiration. In sinus rhythm, a presystolic liver pulsation may be found. It should be considered when patients exhibit signs of carcinoid syndrome.

B. Diagnostic Studies

In the absence of atrial fibrillation, the ECG reveals RA enlargement. The chest radiograph may show marked cardiomegaly with a normal PA size. A dilated superior vena cava and azygous vein may be evident.

The normal valve area of the tricuspid valve is 10 cm^2, so significant stenosis must be present to produce a gradient. Hemodynamically, a mean diastolic pressure gradient greater than 5 mm Hg is considered significant, although even a 2 mm Hg gradient can be considered abnormal. This can be demonstrated by echocardiography or cardiac catheterization. The 2017 update of the 2014 AHA/ACC guidelines suggests a tricuspid valve area of less than 1.0 cm^2 and a pressure half-time longer than 190 msec should be considered significant.

► Treatment & Prognosis

Tricuspid stenosis may be progressive, eventually causing severe right-sided heart failure. Initial therapy is directed at reducing the fluid congestion, with diuretics the mainstay (see Treatment, Heart Failure). When there is considerable bowel edema, torsemide or bumetanide may have an advantage over other loop diuretics, such as furosemide, because they are better absorbed from the gut. Aldosterone inhibitors also help, particularly if there is liver engorgement or ascites. Neither surgical nor percutaneous valvuloplasty is particularly effective for relief of tricuspid stenosis, as residual tricuspid regurgitation is common. Tricuspid valve replacement is the preferred surgical approach. Mechanical tricuspid valve replacement is rarely done because the low flow predisposes to thrombosis and because the mechanical valve cannot be crossed should the need arise for right heart catheterization or pacemaker implantation. Therefore, bioprosthetic valves are almost always preferred. Often tricuspid valve replacement is performed in conjunction with mitral valve replacement for rheumatic mitral stenosis or regurgitation. Percutaneous transcatheter valve replacement (stented valve) has been used in degenerative prosthetic valve stenosis and a percutaneous tricuspid valve replacement device is being investigated. The indications for valve replacement in severe tricuspid stenosis are straightforward:

Class I indication (LOE C): at time of operation for left-sided valve disease.

Class I indication (LOE C): if symptomatic.

Class IIb indication (LOE C): rarely percutaneous balloon commissurotomy for isolated tricuspid stenosis in high-risk patients with no significant tricuspid regurgitation.

► When to Refer

All patients with any evidence for tricuspid stenosis on an echocardiogram should be seen and monitored by a cardiologist to assess when intervention may be required.

Al-Hijii M et al. The forgotten valve: isolated severe tricuspid valve stenosis. Circulation. 2015 Aug 18;132(7):e123–5. [PMID: 26283605]

Cevasco M et al. Surgical management of tricuspid stenosis. Ann Cardiothorac Surg. 2017 May;6(3):275–82. [PMID: 28706872]

TRICUSPID REGURGITATION

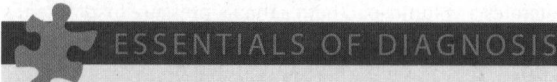

ESSENTIALS OF DIAGNOSIS

► Frequently occurs in patients with pulmonary or cardiac disease with pressure or volume overload on the right ventricle.

► Tricuspid valve regurgitation from pacemaker lead placement is becoming more common.

► Echocardiography useful in determining cause (low- or high-pressure tricuspid regurgitation).

► General Considerations

Tricuspid valvular regurgitation often occurs whenever there is RV dilation from any cause. As tricuspid regurgitation increases, the RV size increases further pulling the valve open due to chordal and papillary muscle displacement. This, in turn, worsens the severity of the tricuspid regurgitation. In addition, the tricuspid annulus is shaped like a horse's saddle. With RV failure, the annulus flattens and becomes elliptical, further distorting the relationship between the leaflets and chordal attachments. In most cases, the cause of the tricuspid regurgitation is the RV geometry (functional) and not primary tricuspid valve disease. An enlarged, dilated RV may be present if there is RV systolic hypertension from valvular or subvalvular pulmonary valve stenosis, pulmonary hypertension for

any reason, in severe pulmonary valve regurgitation, or in cardiomyopathy. The RV may also be injured from MI or may be inherently dilated due to infiltrative diseases (RV dysplasia or sarcoidosis). RV dilation often occurs secondary to left heart failure. Inherent abnormalities of the tricuspid valve include Ebstein anomaly (displacement of the septal and posterior, but not the anterior, leaflets into the RV), tricuspid valve prolapse, carcinoid plaque formation, collagen disease inflammation, valvular tumors, or tricuspid endocarditis. In addition, pacemaker lead valvular injury is becoming an increasingly frequent iatrogenic cause.

► Clinical Findings

A. Symptoms and Signs

The symptoms and signs of tricuspid regurgitation are identical to those resulting from RV failure due to any cause. As a generality, the diagnosis can be made by careful inspection of the JVP. The JVP waveform should decline during ventricular systole (the x descent). The timing of this decline can be observed by palpating the opposite carotid artery. As tricuspid regurgitation worsens, more and more of this x descent valley in the JVP is filled with the regurgitant wave until all of the x descent is obliterated and a positive systolic waveform will be noted in the JVP. An associated tricuspid regurgitation murmur may or may not be audible and can be distinguished from mitral regurgitation by the left parasternal location and an increase with inspiration (**Carvallo sign**). An S_3 may accompany the murmur and is related to the high flow returning to the RV from the RA. Cyanosis may be present if the increased RA pressure stretches the atrial septum and opens a PFO or there is a true ASD (eg, in about 50% of patients with Ebstein anomaly). Severe tricuspid regurgitation results in hepatomegaly, edema, and ascites.

B. Diagnostic Studies

The ECG is usually nonspecific, though atrial flutter or atrial fibrillation is common. The chest radiograph may reveal evidence of an enlarged RA or dilated azygous vein and pleural effusion. The echocardiogram helps assess severity of tricuspid regurgitation (see the 2014 AHA/ACC valvular heart disease guidelines for definitions). In addition, echocardiography/Doppler provides RV systolic pressure as well as RV size and function. A paradoxically moving interventricular septum may be present due to the volume overload on the RV. Catheterization confirms the presence of the regurgitant wave in the RA and elevated RA pressures. If the PA or RV systolic pressure is less than 40 mm Hg, primary valvular tricuspid regurgitation should be suspected. In addition, in patients with severe tricuspid regurgitation and ascites, a hepatic wedge pressure can be performed at the time of the right heart catheterization. If there is a high gradient between the mean RA pressure and mean hepatic wedge, then cirrhosis is likely present. Normally, the gradient across the liver is less than 5 mm Hg. Mild cirrhosis is suspected if gradient is 5–10 mm Hg, moderate disease if 10–15 mm Hg, and significant cirrhosis if greater than 15 mm Hg.

Treatment & Prognosis

Mild tricuspid regurgitation is common and generally can be well managed with diuretics. When severe tricuspid regurgitation is present, bowel edema may reduce the effectiveness of diuretics, such as furosemide, and intravenous diuretics should be used initially. Torsemide or bumetanide is better absorbed in this situation when oral diuretics are added. Aldosterone antagonists have a role as well, particularly if ascites is present. At times, the efficacy of loop diuretics can be enhanced by adding a thiazide diuretic (see Treatment, Heart Failure).

Since most tricuspid regurgitation is secondary, definitive treatment usually requires elimination of the cause of the RV dysfunction. Surgical valve replacement in secondary (functional) tricuspid regurgitation is rarely if ever indicated until the cause of the RV dysfunction is resolved. If the problem is left heart disease, then treatment of the left heart issues may lower pulmonary pressures, reduce RV size, and resolve the tricuspid regurgitation. Treatment for primary and secondary causes of pulmonary hypertension will generally reduce the tricuspid regurgitation. It is a class I recommendation that tricuspid annuloplasty be performed when significant tricuspid regurgitation is present and mitral valve replacement or repair is being performed for mitral regurgitation. Annuloplasty without insertion of a prosthetic ring (**DeVega annuloplasty**) may also be effective in reducing the tricuspid annular dilation. The valve leaflet itself can occasionally be primarily repaired in tricuspid valve endocarditis. If there is an inherent defect in the tricuspid valve apparatus that cannot be repaired, then replacement of the tricuspid valve is warranted. A bioprosthetic valve rather than a mechanical valve, is almost always used because the risk of mechanical valve thrombosis is increased if the INR is not stable. Anticoagulation is not required for bioprosthetic valves unless there is associated atrial fibrillation or flutter. Tricuspid regurgitation due to bioprosthetic degeneration has been shown to respond to transcatheter valve replacement. There are early reports of percutaneous tricuspid valve replacement for native valve tricuspid regurgitation being successful, so this may emerge as a treatment option in the future.

When to Refer

- Anyone with moderate or severe tricuspid regurgitation should be seen at least once by a cardiologist to determine whether studies and intervention are needed.
- Severe tricuspid regurgitation requires regular follow-up by a cardiologist.

Arsalan M et al. Tricuspid regurgitation diagnosis and treatment. Eur Heart J. 2017 Mar 1;38(9):634–8. [PMID: 26358570]

Asmarats L et al. Transcatheter tricuspid valve interventions: landscape, challenges, and future directions. J Am Coll Cardiol. 2018 Jun 26;71(25):2935–56. [PMID: 29929618]

Nishimura RA et al. 2014 AHA/ACC guideline for the management of patients with valvular heart disease: executive summary: a report of the American College of Cardiology/American Heart Association Task Force on Practice Guidelines. J Am Coll Cardiol. 2014 Jun 10;63(22):2438–88. Erratum in: J Am Coll Cardiol. 2014 Jun 10;63(22):2489. [PMID: 24603192]

Taramasso M et al. The International Multicenter TriValve Registry: which patients are undergoing transcatheter tricuspid repair? JACC Cardiovasc Interv. 2017 Oct 9;10(19):1982–90. [PMID: 28982563]

PULMONARY VALVE REGURGITATION

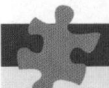

ESSENTIALS OF DIAGNOSIS

- ► Most cases are due to pulmonary hypertension resulting in high-pressure pulmonary valve regurgitation.
- ► Echocardiogram is definitive in high-pressure, but may be less definitive in low-pressure pulmonary valve regurgitation.
- ► Low-pressure pulmonary valve regurgitation is well tolerated.

General Considerations

Pulmonary valve regurgitation can be divided into **high-pressure causes** (due to pulmonary hypertension) and **low-pressure causes** (usually due to a dilated pulmonary annulus, a congenitally abnormal [bicuspid or dysplastic] pulmonary valve, plaque from carcinoid disease, surgical pulmonary valve replacement, or the residual physiology following a surgical transannular patch used to reduce the outflow gradient in tetralogy of Fallot). Because the RV tolerates a volume load better than a pressure load, it tends to tolerate low-pressure pulmonary valve regurgitation for long periods of time without dysfunction.

Clinical Findings

Most patients are asymptomatic. Those with marked PR may exhibit symptoms of right heart volume overload. On examination, a hyperdynamic RV can usually be palpated (RV lift). If the PA is enlarged, it also may be palpated along the left sternal border. P_2 will be palpable in pulmonary hypertension and both systolic and diastolic thrills are occasionally noted. On auscultation, the second heart sound may be widely split due to prolonged RV systole or an associated right bundle branch block. A pulmonary valve systolic click may be noted as well as a right-sided gallop. If pulmonic stenosis is also present, the ejection click may decline with inspiration, while any associated systolic pulmonary murmur will increase. In high-pressure pulmonary valve regurgitation, the pulmonary diastolic (**Graham Steell**) murmur is readily audible. It is often contributed to by a dilated pulmonary annulus. The murmur increases with inspiration and diminishes with the Valsalva maneuver. In low-pressure pulmonary valve regurgitation, the PA diastolic pressure may be only a few mm Hg higher than the RV diastolic pressure, and there is little diastolic gradient to produce a murmur or characteristic echocardiography/Doppler findings. At times, only contrast angiography or MRI of the main PA will show the free-flowing pulmonary valve regurgitation in low-pressure pulmonary valve regurgitation. This situation is common in patients following repair of tetralogy of Fallot where, despite little murmur, there may effectively be no pulmonary valve present. This can be suspected by noting an enlarging right ventricle.

The ECG is generally of little value, although right bundle branch block is common, and there may be ECG criteria for RVH. The chest radiograph may show only the enlarged RV and PA. Echocardiography may demonstrate evidence of RV volume overload (paradoxic septal motion and an enlarged RV), and Doppler can determine peak systolic RV pressure and reveal any associated tricuspid regurgitation. The interventricular septum may appear flattened if there is pulmonary hypertension. The size of the main PA can be determined and color flow Doppler can demonstrate the pulmonary valve regurgitation, particularly in the high-pressure situation. Cardiac MRI and CT can be useful for assessing the size of the PA, for estimating regurgitant flow, for excluding other causes of pulmonary hypertension (eg, thromboembolic disease, peripheral PA stenosis), and for evaluating RV function. Cardiac catheterization is confirmatory only.

▶ Treatment & Prognosis

Pulmonary valve regurgitation rarely needs specific therapy other than treatment of the primary cause. In low-pressure pulmonary valve regurgitation due to surgical transannular patch repair of tetralogy of Fallot, pulmonary valve replacement may be indicated if RV enlargement or dysfunction is present. In tetralogy of Fallot, the QRS will widen as RV function declines (a QRS greater than 180 msec suggests a higher risk for sudden death) and increasing RV volumes should trigger an evaluation for potential severe pulmonary valve regurgitation. In carcinoid heart disease, pulmonary valve replacement with a porcine bioprosthesis may be undertaken, though the plaque from this disorder eventually coats the prosthetic pulmonary valve, which tends to limit the life span of these valves. In high-pressure pulmonary valve regurgitation, treatment to control the cause of the pulmonary hypertension is key. High-pressure pulmonary valve regurgitation is poorly tolerated and is a serious condition that needs a thorough evaluation for cause and choice of therapy. Pulmonary valve replacement requires a bioprosthetic valve in most cases. Pulmonary valve regurgitation due to an RV to PA conduit or due to a pulmonary autograft replacement as part of the Ross procedure can be repaired with a percutaneous pulmonary valve (Melody valve). Bioprosthetic pulmonary valve regurgitation has also been treated using a percutaneous valve (Edwards Sapien).

▶ When to Refer

- Patients with pulmonary valve regurgitation that results in RV enlargement should be referred to a cardiologist regardless of the estimated pulmonary pressures.

Bhatt AB et al. Congenital heart disease in the older adult: a scientific statement from the American Heart Association. Circulation. 2015 May 26;131(21):1884–931. [PMID: 25896865]

Boudjemline Y. Percutaneous pulmonary valve implantation: what have we learned over the years? EuroIntervention. 2017 Sep 24;13(AA):AA60–7. [PMID: 28942387]

Hascoet S et al. Infective endocarditis risk after percutaneous pulmonary valve implantation with Melody and Sapien valves. JACC Cardiovasc Interv. 2017 Mar 13;10(5):510–7. [PMID: 28279319]

Martin MH et al. Safety and feasibility of Melody transcatheter pulmonary valve replacement in the native right ventricular outflow tract: a multicenter pediatric heart network scholar study. JACC Cardiovasc Interv. 2018 Aug 27;11(16):1642–50. [PMID: 30077685]

MANAGEMENT OF ANTICOAGULATION FOR PATIENTS WITH PROSTHETIC HEART VALVES

The risk of thromboembolism is much lower with bioprosthetic valves than mechanical prosthetic valves. Mechanical mitral valve prostheses also pose a greater risk for thrombosis than mechanical aortic valves. For that reason, the INR should be kept between 2.5 and 3.5 for mechanical mitral prosthetic valves but can be kept between 2.0 and 2.5 for most mechanical aortic prosthetic valves. Several changes were recommended regarding anticoagulation use in valvular heart disease with the publication of the 2017 update to the 2014 ACC/AHA valve guidelines, including (1) a recommendation (class IIa) to expand the use of vitamin K antagonists (VKAs), such as warfarin, for up to 6 months after initial bioprosthetic valve replacement; (2) a lower target INR of 1.5–2.0 for a mechanical AVR using the On-X valve (class IIb); and (3) a consideration of VKA use with an INR of 2.5 for 3 months after TAVR (class IIa). Data from 2018 suggest that antiplatelet medications are inferior to warfarin for the prevention of thrombus in patients with the On-X mechanical valve. The concern regarding thrombus formation on bioprosthetic valves (including TAVR valves) also led to a class I recommendation to use multimodality imaging to identify such thrombus (class I).

In 2015 the European Registry of Pregnancy and Cardiac Disease (ROPAC) reported on a registry that compared pregnant women who had undergone mechanical and bioprosthetic valve replacement to pregnant women who had not. Maternal mortality was similar between the mechanical and bioprosthetic valve patients (1.5% and 1.4%, respectively) but was much higher than those without an artificial valve (0.2%). When patients with either mechanical or bioprosthetic valves were further assessed, it was found that pregnant women with mechanical valves were more likely to suffer adverse events than women with bioprosthetic valves. Hemorraghic events occurred in 23.1% versus 9.2%, miscarriage on warfarin occurred in 28.6% versus 9.2%, and late fetal death was noted in 7.1% versus 0.7%, respectively. These data suggest **a high risk for mortality and morbidity for pregnant patients with mechanical heart valves,** and in the WHO Classification of Maternal Cardiac Risk, the presence of a mechanical valve is considered a class III (out of IV) risk for pregnancy complications.

Stoppage of warfarin for noncardiac surgery is likewise dependent on which mechanical valve is involved, the patient-specific risk factors, and the procedure contemplated. The risk of thromboembolism is highest in the first few months after valve replacement. While the interruption of warfarin therapy is generally safe, most cases of valve thrombosis occur during periods of inadequate anticoagulation, so the time interval without coverage should be kept as short as possible. High-risk features include atrial fibrillation, a prior history of thromboembolism, heart failure or low LVEF, a hypercoagualable state, a mechanical valve in the mitral position, a known high-risk valve (ball-in-cage), or concomitant hypercoagulable state (such as with an associated cancer). The use of bridging VKAs, unfractionated heparin, low-molecular-weight heparin (LMWH), and antifibrinolytics in various clinical situations in patients with valvular heart disease is summarized in Table 10–6 and the issues are covered in more depth in both the 2012 European Society of Cardiology (ESC) guidelines

and the 2017 update to the 2014 AHA/ACC valvular heart disease guidelines. In general, low-risk procedures (eg, pacemaker implantation and routine dental work) require no stoppage of VKAs, while in other situations the warfarin can be stopped 3 days ahead of the procedure and resumed the night after the procedure (ie, in patients with bileaflet aortic valves) without any bridging unfractionated heparin or LMWH. In high-risk patients, though, the warfarin should be stopped and *bridging with either unfractionated heparin or LMWH* begun once the INR falls below therapeutic levels. Fresh frozen plasma or prothrombin complex concentrate is reasonable in an emergency situation for acute reversal if serious bleeding occurs. Most patients with a mechanical valve should not have the warfarin reversed with vitamin K, if it can be avoided, because this

Table 10–6. Recommendations for administering vitamin K antagonist (VKA) therapy in patients undergoing procedures or patients with certain clinical conditions.

Procedures	Recommendations
General	Stop VKA 5 days prior and resume 12–24 hours after procedure
Bridging for mechanical heart valves	Required only for those at high risk for thromboembolism Bridge with UFH or LMWH and stop UFH 4–6 hours before procedure or stop LMWH 24 hours before procedure Resume 48–72 hours after the procedure
Clinical Situations	**Recommendations**
Atrial fibrillation and moderate or severe mitral stenosis	VKA (target INR 2.0–3.0) If patient refuses, aspirin (50–100 mg) plus clopidogrel (75 mg)
Sinus rhythm and mitral stenosis	If left atrial size > 5.5 cm, then consider VKA (target 2.0–3.0)
Intermittent atrial fibrillation or history of systemic embolus and mitral stenosis	VKA (target INR 2.0–3.0)

Endocarditis
   Native valve or bioprosthetic valve endocarditis
   Mechanical valve endocarditis
	
	No anticoagulation recommended
	Hold VKA until "safe to resume" (generally when mycotic aneurysm is ruled out or there is no need for urgent surgery)

First 3 months following valve replacement
   Bioprosthetic aortic valve replacement
   Transcatheter valve replacement
   Mitral or aortic repair
   Bioprosthetic mitral valve
	
	Aspirin (50–100 mg)
	Aspirin (50–100 mg) plus clopidogrel (75 mg)
	Aspirin (50–100 mg)
	VKA (target INR 2.0–3.0)

Long-term anticoagulation after valve replacement
   Bioprosthetic valve in normal sinus rhythm
   Mechanical valve replacement
	
	Aspirin (50–100 mg)
	VKA (target INR 2.0–3.0 for aortic, target INR 2.5–3.5 for mitral) plus aspirin (50–100 mg)

Prosthetic valve thrombosis
   Right-sided valve
   Left-sided valve
	
	Fibrinolytic therapy
	Early surgery if thrombus large (> 0.8 cm^2 area), otherwise either fibrinolytic therapy or UFH

Pregnancy and a mechanical heart valve	Add aspirin (50–100 mg) for high risk Adjusted dose LMWH twice daily throughout pregnancy (follow anti-Xa 4 hours after dose) *or* Adjusted dose UFH every 12 hours throughout pregnancy (aPTT > 2 times control or anti-Xa between 0.35 and 0.70) *or* Adjusted dose UFH or LMWH until 13th week of pregnancy then VKA until close to delivery, then resume UFH or LMWH

aPTT, activated partial thromboplastin time; INR, international normalized ratio; LMWH, low-molecular-weight heparin; UFH, unfractionated heparin.

Data from Holbrook A et al. Evidence-Based Management of Anticoagulant Therapy: Antithrombotic Therapy and Prevention of Thrombosis, 9th ed: American College of Chest Physicians Evidence-Based Clinical Practice Guidelines. Chest. 2012;141(Suppl 2):e152S–84S.

can result in a transient hypercoagulable state, and it may take many days to reach a therapeutic INR again.

Warfarin causes fetal skeletal abnormalities in up to 2% of women who become pregnant while taking the medication, so every effort is made to defer valve replacement in women until after childbearing age. However, if a woman with a mechanical valve becomes pregnant while taking warfarin, the risk of stopping warfarin may be higher for the mother than the risk of continuing warfarin for the fetus. The risk of warfarin to the fetal skeleton is greatest during the first trimester and, remarkably, is more related to dose than to the INR level. Guidelines suggest it is reasonable to continue warfarin for the first trimester if the dose is 5 mg/day or less. If the dose is more than 5 mg/day, it is appropriate to consider either LMWH (as long as the anti-Xa is being monitored [range: 0.8 unit/mL to 1.2 units/mL 4–6 hours post-dose]) or continuous intravenous unfractionated heparin (if the activated partial thromboplastin time [aPTT] can be monitored and is at least two times control). Guidelines suggest warfarin and low-dose aspirin are safe during the second and third trimester, and then should be stopped upon anticipation of delivery. At time of vaginal delivery, unfractionated intravenous heparin with aPTT at least two times control is desirable. DOACs (antithrombin or Xa inhibitors) should *not* be used in place of warfarin for mechanical prosthetic valves since there are no data they are safe during pregnancy.

Management of suspected mechanical valve thrombosis depends on whether a left-sided or right-sided valve is involved, the size of the thrombus, and the patient's clinical condition. Simple fluoroscopy can help assess mechanical valve motion, although a TEE is indicated to assess thrombus size. Therapeutic unfractionated heparin should be given to all patients with a thrombosed valve, and this alone is generally effective. Fibrinolytic therapy is indicated if heparin therapy is ineffective and the clinical onset has been less than 2 weeks, the thrombus is smaller than 0.8 cm^2, New York Heart Association (NYHA) class symptoms are mild (functional class I or II), or the valve is right-sided. Surgery is rarely indicated, and reserved for those with left-sided mechanical valves in NYHA functional class III or IV heart failure or in whom TEE demonstrates a mobile thrombus larger than 0.8 cm^2. The 2017 updated valvular heart disease guidelines added (class I) the use of urgent initial therapy for a thrombosed mechanical valve to include low-dose, slow-infusion fibrinolytic therapy or urgent surgery if the patient is symptomatic.

Alshawabkeh L et al. Anticoagulation during pregnancy: evolving strategies with a focus on mechanical valves. J Am Coll Cardiol. 2016 Oct 18;68(16):1804–13. [PMID: 27737747]

Nishimura RA et al. 2017 AHA/ACC focused update of the 2014 AHA/ACC guideline for the management of patients with valvular heart disease: a report of the American College of Cardiology/American Heart Association Task Force on Practice Guidelines. Circulation. 2017 Jun 20;135(25):e1159–95. [PMID: 28298458]

Puskas JD et al; PROACT Investigators. Anticoagulation and antiplatelet strategies after On-X mechanical aortic valve replacement. J Am Coll Cardiol. 2018 Jun 19;71(24):2717–26. [PMID: 29903344]

Van Hagen IM et al. Pregnancy in women with a mechanical heart valve: data from the ESC Registry of Pregnancy and Cardiac Diseases (ROPAC). Circulation. 2015 Jul 14; 132(2):132–42. [PMID: 26100109]

CORONARY HEART DISEASE (Atherosclerotic CAD, Ischemic Heart Disease)

Coronary heart disease (CHD), or atherosclerotic CAD, is the number one cause of death in the United States and worldwide. Every minute, an American dies of CHD. About 37% of people who experience an acute coronary event, either angina or MI, will die of it in the same year. Death rates of CHD have declined every year since 1968, with about half of the decline from 1980 to 2000 due to treatments and half due to improved risk factors. CHD is still responsible for approximately one of five deaths and over 600,000 deaths per year in the United States. CHD afflicts nearly 16 million Americans and the prevalence rises steadily with age; thus, the aging of the US population promises to increase the overall burden of CHD.

▶ Risk Factors for CAD

Most patients with CHD have some identifiable risk factor. These include a **positive family history** (the younger the onset in a first-degree relative, the greater the risk), **male sex, blood lipid abnormalities, diabetes mellitus, hypertension, physical inactivity, abdominal obesity, cigarette smoking, psychosocial factors,** and consumption of **too few fruits and vegetables** and **too much alcohol**. Many of these risk factors are modifiable. **Smoking remains the number one preventable cause of death and illness in the United States.** Although smoking rates have declined in the United States in recent decades, 18% of women and 21% of men still smoke. According to the World Health Organization, 1 year after quitting, the risk of CHD decreases by 50%. Various interventions have been shown to increase the likelihood of successful smoking cessation (see Chapter 1).

Hypercholesterolemia is an important modifiable risk factor for CHD. Risk increases progressively with higher levels of low-density lipoprotein (LDL) cholesterol and declines with higher levels of high-density lipoprotein (HDL) cholesterol. Composite risk scores, such as the Framingham score and the 10-year atherosclerotic cardiovascular disease risk calculator (http://my.americanheart .org/cvriskcalculator), provide estimates of the 10-year probability of development of CHD that can guide primary prevention strategies. The 2018 ACC/AHA Guideline on the Treatment of Blood Cholesterol to Reduce Atherosclerotic Cardiovascular Risk in Adults suggests statin therapy in four populations: patients with (1) clinical atherosclerotic disease, (2) LDL cholesterol 190 mg/dL or higher, (3) diabetes who are aged 40–75 years, and (4) an estimated 10-year atherosclotic risk of 7.5% or more aged 40–75 years (Figure 10–5). Importantly, **the guidelines do not recommend treating to a *target* LDL cholesterol.** Patients in these categories should be treated with

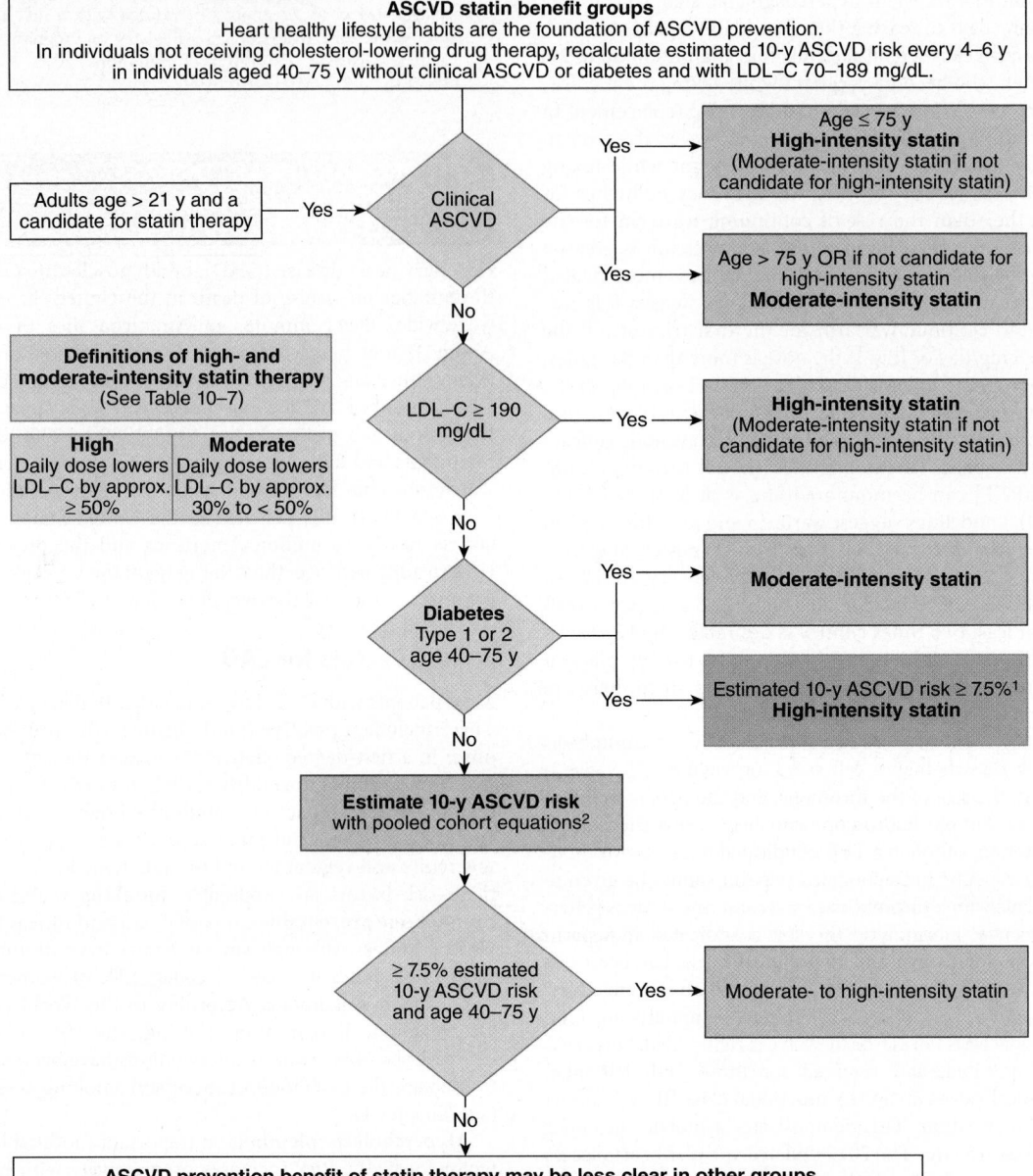

ASCVD statin benefit groups
Heart healthy lifestyle habits are the foundation of ASCVD prevention.
In individuals not receiving cholesterol-lowering drug therapy, recalculate estimated 10-y ASCVD risk every 4–6 y in individuals aged 40–75 y without clinical ASCVD or diabetes and with LDL–C 70–189 mg/dL.

Adults age > 21 y and a candidate for statin therapy → **Yes** →

Clinical ASCVD
- Yes → Age ≤ 75 y **High-intensity statin** (Moderate-intensity statin if not candidate for high-intensity statin)
- Yes → Age > 75 y OR if not candidate for high-intensity statin **Moderate-intensity statin**

Definitions of high- and moderate-intensity statin therapy
(See Table 10–7)

High	Moderate
Daily dose lowers LDL–C by approx. ≥ 50%	Daily dose lowers LDL–C by approx. 30% to < 50%

LDL–C ≥ 190 mg/dL
- Yes → **High-intensity statin** (Moderate-intensity statin if not candidate for high-intensity statin)

Diabetes Type 1 or 2 age 40–75 y
- Yes → **Moderate-intensity statin**
- Yes → Estimated 10-y ASCVD risk ≥ 7.5%[1] **High-intensity statin**

Estimate 10-y ASCVD risk with pooled cohort equations[2]

≥ 7.5% estimated 10-y ASCVD risk and age 40–75 y
- Yes → Moderate- to high-intensity statin

ASCVD prevention benefit of statin therapy may be less clear in other groups.
In selected individuals, consider additional factors influencing ASCVD risk[3] and potential ASCVD risk benefits and adverse effects, drug-drug interactions, and patient preferences for statin treatment.

[1]Percent reduction in LDL–C can be used as an indication of response and adherence to therapy but is not in itself a treatment goal.

[2]The Pooled Cohort Equations can be used to estimate 10-year ASCVD risk in individuals with and without diabetes. A downloadable spreadsheet enabling estimation of 10-year and lifetime risk for ASCVD and a web-based calculator are available at http://my.americanheart.org/cvriskcalculator and http://www.cardiosource.org/science-and-quality/practice-guidelines-and-quality-standards/2013-prevention-guideline-tools.aspx.

[3]Primary LDL–C ≥ 160 mg/dL or other evidence of genetic hyperlipidemias, family history of premature ASCVD with onset < 55 years of age in a first-degree male relative or < 65 years of age in a first-degree female relative, high-sensitivity C-reactive protein > 2 mg/L, CAC score ≥ 300 Agatston units or ≥ 75 percentile for age, sex, and ethnicity, ankle-brachial index < 0.9, or elevated lifetime risk of ASCVD.

ASCVD, atherosclerotic cardiovascular disease; CAC, coronary artery calcium; LDL–C, low-density lipoprotein cholesterol.

▲ **Figure 10–5.** Major recommendations for statin therapy for atherosclerotic cardiovascular disease prevention. (Adapted from Stone NJ et al. 2013 ACC/AHA Guideline on the Treatment of Blood Cholesterol to Reduce Atherosclerotic Cardiovascular Risk in Adults: A Report of the American College of Cardiology/American Heart Association Task Force on Practice Guidelines. Circulation. 2014 Jun 24;129(25 Suppl 2):S1–45.)

Table 10–7. High-, moderate-, and low-intensity statin therapy (used in the RCTs reviewed by the expert panel).[1,2]

High-Intensity Statin Therapy	Moderate-Intensity Statin Therapy	Low-Intensity Statin Therapy
Daily dose lowers LDL–C on average by approximately ≥ 50%	Daily dose lowers LDL–C on average by approximately 30% to < 50%	Daily dose lowers LDL–C on average by < 30%
Atorvastatin (40[3])–80 mg Rosuvastatin 20 (40) mg	Atorvastatin 10 (20) mg Rosuvastatin (5) 10 mg Simvastatin 20–40 mg[4] Pravastatin 40 (80) mg Lovastatin 40 mg *Fluvastatin XL 80 mg* Fluvastatin 40 mg twice daily *Pitavastatin 2–4 mg*	*Simvastatin 10 mg* Pravastatin 10–20 mg Lovastatin 20 mg *Fluvastatin 20–40 mg* *Pitavastatin 1 mg*

[1]Statins and doses in **boldface** were evaluated in RCTs; all demonstrated a reduction in major cardiovascular events. Statins and doses that are approved by the US FDA but were not tested in the RCTs reviewed are listed in *italics*.
[2]Individual responses to statin therapy varied in the RCTs and should be expected to vary in clinical practice. There might be a biologic basis for a less-than-average response.
[3]Evidence from one RCT only: down-titration if unable to tolerate atorvastatin 80 mg in IDEAL.
[4]Although simvastatin 80 mg was evaluated in RCTs, initiation of simvastatin 80 mg or titration to 80 mg is not recommended by the FDA due to the increased risk of myopathy, including rhabdomyolysis.
FDA, Food and Drug Administration; IDEAL, Incremental Decrease through Aggressive Lipid Lowering study; LDL–C, low-density lipoprotein cholesterol; RCTs, randomized controlled trials.
Modified, with permission, from Stone NJ et al. 2013 ACC/AHA Guideline on the Treatment of Blood Cholesterol to Reduce Atherosclerotic Cardiovascular Risk in Adults: A Report of the American College of Cardiology/American Heart Association Task Force on Practice Guidelines. Circulation. 2014 Jun 24;129(25 Suppl 2):S1–45. © 2014 American Heart Association, Inc.

a moderate- or high-intensity statin, with high-intensity statin for the higher-risk populations (Table 10–7). The ACC/AHA atherosclerotic cardiovascular disease risk estimator allows clinicians to determine the 10-year CHD risk to determine treatment decisions (http://tools.acc.org/ascvd-risk-estimator-plus/).

The **metabolic syndrome** is defined as a constellation of three or more of the following: abdominal obesity, triglycerides 150 mg/dL or higher, HDL cholesterol less than 40 mg/dL for men or less than 50 mg/dL for women, fasting glucose 110 mg/dL or higher, and hypertension. This syndrome is increasing in prevalence at an alarming rate. Related to the metabolic syndrome, the epidemic of **obesity** in the United States is likewise a major factor contributing to CHD risk.

Myocardial Hibernation & Stunning

Areas of myocardium that are persistently underperfused but still viable may develop sustained contractile dysfunction. This phenomenon, which is termed **myocardial hibernation,** appears to represent an adaptive response that may be associated with depressed LV function. It is important to recognize this phenomenon, since this form of dysfunction is reversible following coronary revascularization. Hibernating myocardium can be identified by radionuclide testing, positron emission tomography (PET), contrast-enhanced MRI, or its retained response to inotropic stimulation with dobutamine. A related phenomenon, termed **myocardial stunning,** is the occurrence of persistent contractile dysfunction following prolonged or repetitive episodes of myocardial ischemia. Clinically, myocardial stunning is often seen after reperfusion of acute MI and is defined with improvement following revascularization.

Ridker PM et al. CANTOS Trial Group. Antiinflammatory therapy with canakinumab for atherosclerotic disease. N Engl J Med. 2017 Sep 21;377(12):1119–31. [PMID: 28845751]
Yu Y. Four decades of obesity trends among non-hispanic whites and blacks in the United States: analyzing the influences of educational inequalities in obesity and population improvements in education. PLoS One. 2016 Nov 28;11(11):e0167193. [PMID: 27893853]

Primary & Secondary Prevention of CHD

Although many risk factors for CHD are not modifiable, it is now clear that interventions, such as smoking cessation, treatment of dyslipidemia, and lowering of BP can both prevent coronary disease and delay its progression and complications after it is manifest.

Lowering LDL levels delays the progression of atherosclerosis and in some cases may produce regression. Even in the absence of regression, fewer new lesions develop, endothelial function may be restored, and coronary event rates are markedly reduced in patients with clinical evidence of vascular disease.

A series of clinical trials has demonstrated the efficacy of hydroxymethylglutaryl coenzyme A (HMG-CoA) reductase inhibitors (statins) in preventing death, coronary events, and strokes. Beneficial results have been found in patients who have already experienced coronary events (secondary prevention), those at particularly high risk for events (patients with diabetes and patients with peripheral artery disease), those with elevated cholesterol without multiple risk factors, and those without vascular disease or diabetes with elevated high-sensitivity C-reactive protein (hsCRP) with normal LDL levels. The benefits of statin therapy at moderate and high doses (Table 10–7) are recommended by the cholesterol treatment guidelines. The IMPROVE-IT study showed that ezetimibe, 10 mg daily, combined with simvastatin was modestly better than simvastatin alone in reducing the risk of MI and ischemic stroke, but not mortality, in stabilized patients following an acute coronary syndrome. This was associated with a reduction of LDL to 53.7 mg/dL compared to 69.7 mg/dL. With this data, ezetimibe can be used in combination with statin therapy in patients who are not at target cholesterol level or cannot tolerate high-dose statin therapy.

Benefits occurred regardless of age, race, baseline cholesterol levels, or the presence of hypertension. It is clear that for patients with vascular disease, statins provide benefit for those with normal cholesterol levels, and that more aggressive statin use is associated with greater benefits. **All patients at significant risk for vascular events should receive a statin regardless of their cholesterol levels,** and many recommend that with those who have prior cardiovascular events should have their LDL lowered below 70 mg/dL.

Novel monoclonal antibodies that inhibit proprotein convertase subtilisin/kexin type 9 (PCSK9) have been developed and have shown to reduce LDL cholesterol levels significantly beyond levels associated with traditional statin therapy. These therapies have been studied in initial randomized trials of patients with maximally tolerated statin therapy (and for patients with statin intolerance) and have lowered LDL with signals of improved cardiovascular outcomes. The FOURIER trial showed that the PCSK9 inhibitor evolocumab, on top of statin, reduced the composite of atherothrombotic outcomes by 20% but did not reduce mortality. The ODYSSEY Outcomes trial demonstrated alirocumab reduced cardiovascular events in patients with acute coronary syndromes. Alirocumab and evolocumab have been approved by the FDA for patients on maximally tolerated statin therapy with familial hypercholesterolemia and atherosclerotic vascular disease, or both, and who require additional lowering of LDL. These medications cost approximately $10,000 per year in the United States.

While fish oil supplements have *not* been shown to provide benefit for reducing risk, icosapent ethyl, a concentrated eicosapentaenoic acid at a high dose, was shown to be beneficial in the REDUCE-IT trial. Patients with established cardiovascular disease or with diabetes and other risk factors, with fasting triglyceride level of 135–499 mg/dL, who were on statins were randomized to 2 g of icosapent ethyl twice daily or placebo. There was a 26% relative risk reduction in cardiovascular death, MI, and stroke, as well as a 20% relative risk reduction in cardiovascular death.

The CANTOS trial has demonstrated as a proof of concept that canakinumab (antibody targeting IL-1 and leading to IL-6 inhibition) can modestly reduce cardiovascular events by targeting inflammation—patients with controlled LDL cholesterol and elevated hsCRP. This agent has not been approved by the FDA for use in patients with CAD.

Treatment to raise HDL levels has failed to show benefit. The AIM High trial found no benefit from the addition of niacin in patients with vascular disease and a serum LDL near 70 mg/dL who were receiving statin therapy. The HPS2-THRIVE trial found no benefit but rather substantial harm of extended-release niacin (2 g) plus laropiprant

(an antiflushing agent) for preventing vascular events in a population of over 25,000 patients with vascular disease who were taking simvastatin.

The value of medications that reduce elevated triglyceride levels is less clear, unless triglycerides are elevated to greater than 500 mg/dL despite diet intervention.

Antiplatelet therapy is another very effective measure for secondary prevention and **patients with established vascular disease should be treated with aspirin. For primary prevention, aspirin has little overall benefit, including for patients with established diabetes, and as of 2019, is no longer recommended for most patients.** The exact dose of aspirin in chronic CAD (81 mg vs 325 mg) is being evaluated in a large ongoing pragmatic trial (ADAPTABLE). While clopidogrel was found to be effective at preventing vascular events for 9–12 months after acute coronary syndromes, and there are some benefits in prolonging dual antiplatelet therapy after coronary stenting, clopidogrel was *not* found to be effective at preventing vascular events in combination with aspirin with longer-term treatment in the CHARISMA trial. This trial included patients with clinically evident stable atherothrombosis or with multiple risk factors; all were treated with aspirin and observed for a median of 28 months.

In the COMPASS trial, rivaroxaban, a direct factor Xa inhibitor, at a dose of 2.5 mg twice daily in addition to 100 mg of aspirin, was shown to reduce cardiovascular death, MI, and stroke by a relative risk reduction of 24% compared to 100 mg aspirin monotherapy in stable patients with CAD and peripheral artery disease. Bleeding was modestly increased. All cause mortality was also reduced by 18%. This regimen is approved by the FDA and is used for long-term management of patients with CAD and peripheral artery disease.

The HOPE and the EUROPA trials demonstrated that angiotensin-converting enzyme (ACE) inhibitors (ramipril 10 mg/day and perindopril 8 mg/day, respectively) reduced fatal and nonfatal vascular events (cardiovascular deaths, nonfatal MIs, and nonfatal strokes) by 20–25% in patients at high risk, including patients with diabetes with additional risk factors or patients with clinical coronary, cerebral, or peripheral arterial atherosclerotic disease. An overview of these trials has demonstrated that while low-risk patients may *not* derive substantial benefits from ACE inhibitors, **most patients with vascular disease, even in the absence of heart failure or LV dysfunction, should be treated with an ACE inhibitor.**

ASCEND Study Collaborative Group et al. Effects of aspirin for primary prevention in persons with diabetes mellitus. N Engl J Med. 2018 Oct 18;379(16):1529–39. [PMID: 30146931]

Bhatt DL et al; REDUCE-IT Investigators. Cardiovascular risk reduction with icosapent ethyl for hypertriglyceridemia. N Engl J Med. 2019 Jan 3;380(1):11–22. [PMID: 30415628]

Cannon CP et al; IMPROVE-IT Investigators. Ezetimibe added to statin therapy after acute coronary syndromes. N Engl J Med. 2015 Jun 18;372(25):2387–97. [PMID: 26039521]

Donadini MP et al. Aspirin plus clopidogrel vs aspirin alone for preventing cardiovascular events among patients at high risk for cardiovascular events. JAMA. 2018 Aug 14;320(6):593–4. [PMID: 30054611]

Eikelboom JW et al; COMPASS Investigators. Rivaroxaban with or without aspirin in stable cardiovascular disease. N Engl J Med. 2017 Oct 5;377(14):1319–30. [PMID: 28844192]

Gaziano JM. Aspirin for primary prevention: clinical considerations in 2019. JAMA. 2019 Jan 22;321(3):253–55. [PMID: 30667488]

Gaziano JM et al; ARRIVE Executive Committee. Use of aspirin to reduce risk of initial vascular events in patients at moderate risk of cardiovascular disease (ARRIVE): a randomised, double-blind, placebo-controlled trial. Lancet. 2018 Sep 22; 392(10152):1036–46. [PMID: 30158069]

Lloyd-Jones DM et al. 2017 focused update of the 2016 ACC expert consensus decision pathway on the role of non-statin therapies for LDL-cholesterol lowering in the management of atherosclerotic cardiovascular disease risk: a report of the American College of Cardiology Task Force on Expert Consensus Decision Pathways. J Am Coll Cardiol. 2017 Oct 3; 70(14):1785–822. [PMID: 28886926]

McNeil JJ et al; ASPREE Investigator Group. Effect of aspirin on cardiovascular events and bleeding in the healthy elderly. N Engl J Med. 2018 Oct 18;379(16):1509–18. [PMID: 30221597]

Ramos R et al. Statins for primary prevention of cardiovascular events and mortality in old and very old adults with and without type 2 diabetes: retrospective cohort study. BMJ. 2018 Sep 5;362:k3359. [PMID: 30185425]

Ridker PM et al; CANTOS Trial Group. Antiinflammatory therapy with canakinumab for atherosclerotic disease. N Engl J Med. 2017 Sep 21;377(12):1119–31. [PMID: 28845751]

Sabatine MS et al; FOURIER Steering Committee and Investigators. Evolocumab and clinical outcomes in patients with cardiovascular disease. N Engl J Med. 2017 May 4;376(18): 1713–22. [PMID: 28304224]

Schwartz GG et al; ODYSSEY OUTCOMES Committees and Investigators. Alirocumab and cardiovascular outcomes after acute coronary syndrome. N Engl J Med. 2018 Nov 29; 379(22):2097–107. [PMID: 30403574]

Zheng SL et al. Association of aspirin use for primary prevention with cardiovascular events and bleeding events: a systematic review and meta-analysis. JAMA. 2019 Jan 22;321(3):277–87. [PMID: 30667501]

CHRONIC STABLE ANGINA PECTORIS

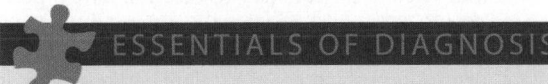

ESSENTIALS OF DIAGNOSIS

- ► Precordial chest pain, usually precipitated by stress or exertion, relieved rapidly by rest or nitrates.
- ► ECG or scintigraphic evidence of ischemia during pain or stress testing.
- ► Angiographic demonstration of significant obstruction of major coronary vessels.

General Considerations

Angina pectoris is usually due to atherosclerotic heart disease. Coronary vasospasm may occur at the site of a lesion or, less frequently, in apparently normal vessels. Other unusual causes of coronary artery obstruction, such as congenital anomalies, emboli, arteritis, or dissection may cause ischemia or infarction. Angina may also occur in the absence of coronary artery obstruction as a result of severe myocardial hypertrophy, severe aortic stenosis or regurgitation, or in response to increased metabolic demands, as in hyperthyroidism, marked anemia, or paroxysmal tachycardias with rapid ventricular rates.

Clinical Findings

A. Symptoms

The diagnosis of angina pectoris principally depends on the history, which should specifically include the following information: circumstances that precipitate and relieve angina, characteristics of the discomfort, location and radiation, duration of attacks, and effect of nitroglycerin.

1. Circumstances that precipitate and relieve angina— Angina occurs most commonly during activity and is relieved by resting. Patients may prefer to remain upright rather than lie down, as increased preload in recumbency increases myocardial work. The amount of activity required to produce angina may be relatively consistent under comparable physical and emotional circumstances or may vary from day to day. The threshold for angina is usually lower after meals, during excitement, or on exposure to cold. It is often lower in the morning or after strong emotion; the latter can provoke attacks in the absence of exertion. In addition, discomfort may occur during sexual activity, at rest, or at night as a result of coronary spasm.

2. Characteristics of the discomfort—Patients often do not refer to angina as "pain" but as a sensation of tightness, squeezing, burning, pressing, choking, aching, bursting, "gas," indigestion, or an ill-characterized discomfort. It is often characterized by clenching a fist over the mid chest. The distress of angina is rarely sharply localized and is not spasmodic.

3. Location and radiation—The distribution of the distress may vary widely in different patients but is usually the same for each patient unless unstable angina or MI supervenes. In most cases, the discomfort is felt behind or slightly to the left of the mid sternum. When it begins farther to the left or, uncommonly, on the right, it characteristically moves centrally substernally. Although angina may radiate to any dermatome from C8 to T4, it radiates most often to the left shoulder and upper arm, frequently moving down the inner volar aspect of the arm to the elbow, forearm, wrist, or fourth and fifth fingers. It may also radiate to the right shoulder or arm, the lower jaw, the neck, or even the back.

4. Duration of attacks—Angina is generally of short duration and subsides completely without residual discomfort. If the attack is precipitated by exertion and the patient promptly stops to rest, it usually lasts under 3 minutes. Attacks following a heavy meal or brought on by anger often last 15–20 minutes. Attacks lasting more than 30 minutes are unusual and suggest the development of an acute coronary syndrome with unstable angina, MI, or an alternative diagnosis.

5. Effect of nitroglycerin—The diagnosis of angina pectoris is supported if sublingual nitroglycerin promptly and invariably shortens an attack and if prophylactic nitrates permit greater exertion or prevent angina entirely.

B. Signs

Examination during angina frequently reveals a significant elevation in systolic and diastolic BP, although hypotension may also occur, and may reflect more severe ischemia or inferior ischemia (especially with bradycardia) due to a Bezold-Jarisch reflex. Occasionally, a gallop rhythm and an apical systolic murmur due to transient mitral regurgitation from papillary muscle dysfunction are present during pain only. Supraventricular or ventricular arrhythmias may be present, either as the precipitating factor or as a result of ischemia.

It is important to detect signs of diseases that may contribute to or accompany atherosclerotic heart disease, eg, diabetes mellitus (retinopathy or neuropathy), xanthelasma tendinous xanthomas, hypertension, thyrotoxicosis, myxedema, or peripheral artery disease. Aortic stenosis or regurgitation, hypertrophic cardiomyopathy, and mitral valve prolapse should be sought, since they may produce angina or other forms of chest pain.

C. Laboratory Findings

Other than standard laboratory tests to evaluate for acute coronary syndrome (troponin and CK-MB), factors contributing to ischemia (such as anemia), and to screen for risk factors that may increase the probability of true CHD (such as hyperlipidemia and diabetes mellitus), blood tests are not helpful to diagnose chronic angina.

D. ECG

The resting ECG is often normal in patients with angina. In the remainder, abnormalities include old MI, nonspecific ST–T changes, and changes of LVH. During anginal episodes, as well as during asymptomatic ischemia, the characteristic ECG change is **horizontal or downsloping ST-segment depression that reverses after the ischemia disappears.** T wave flattening or inversion may also occur. Less frequently, transient ST-segment elevation is observed; this finding suggests severe (transmural) ischemia from coronary occlusion, and it can occur with coronary spasm.

E. Pretest Probability

The history as detailed above, the physical examination findings, and laboratory and ECG findings are used to develop a pretest probability of CAD as the cause of the clinical symptoms. Other important factors to include in calculating the pretest probability of CAD are patient age, sex, and clinical symptoms. Patients with low to intermediate pretest probability for CAD should undergo noninvasive stress testing whereas patients with high pretest probability are generally referred for cardiac catheterization. National review of diagnostic cardiac catheterization findings in patients without known CAD undergoing angiography has shown that between 38% and 40% of patients do not have obstructive disease.

F. Exercise ECG

Exercise ECG testing is the most commonly used noninvasive procedure for evaluating for inducible ischemia in the patient with angina. Exercise ECG testing is often combined with imaging studies (nuclear or echocardiography),

but in low-risk patients without baseline ST-segment abnormalities or in whom anatomic localization is not necessary, the exercise ECG remains the recommended initial procedure because of considerations of cost, convenience, and longstanding prognostic data.

Exercise testing can be done on a motorized treadmill or with a bicycle ergometer. A variety of exercise protocols are utilized, the most common being the **Bruce protocol,** which increases the treadmill speed and elevation every 3 minutes until limited by symptoms. At least two ECG leads should be monitored continuously.

1. Precautions and risks—The risk of exercise testing is about one infarction or death per 1000 tests, but individuals who have pain at rest or minimal activity are at higher risk and should not be tested. **Many of the traditional exclusions, such as recent MI or heart failure, are no longer used if the patient is stable and ambulatory, but symptomatic aortic stenosis remains a relative contraindication.**

2. Indications—Exercise testing is used (1) to confirm the diagnosis of angina; (2) to determine the severity of limitation of activity due to angina; (3) to assess prognosis in patients with known coronary disease, including those recovering from MI, by detecting groups at high or low risk; and (4) to evaluate responses to therapy. Because false-positive tests often exceed true positives, leading to much patient anxiety and self-imposed or mandated disability, exercise testing of asymptomatic individuals should be done only for those whose occupations place them or others at special risk (eg, airline pilots).

3. Interpretation—The usual ECG criterion for a positive test is 1-mm (0.1-mV) horizontal or downsloping ST-segment depression (beyond baseline) measured 80 msec after the J point. By this criterion, 60–80% of patients with anatomically significant coronary disease will have a positive test, but 10–30% of those without significant disease will also be positive. False positives are uncommon when a 2-mm depression is present. Additional information is inferred from the time of onset and duration of the ECG changes, their magnitude and configuration, BP and heart rate changes, the duration of exercise, and the presence of associated symptoms. In general, patients exhibiting more severe ST-segment depression (more than 2 mm) at low workloads (less than 6 minutes on the Bruce protocol) or heart rates (less than 70% of age-predicted maximum)—especially when the duration of exercise and rise in BP are limited or when hypotension occurs during the test—have more severe disease and a poorer prognosis. Depending on symptom status, age, and other factors, such patients should be referred for coronary arteriography and possible revascularization. On the other hand, less impressive positive tests in asymptomatic patients are often "false positives." Therefore, exercise testing results that do not conform to the clinical suspicion should be confirmed by stress imaging.

G. Myocardial Stress Imaging

Myocardial stress imaging (scintigraphy, echocardiography, or MRI) is indicated (1) when the resting ECG makes an exercise ECG difficult to interpret (eg, left bundle branch block, baseline ST–T changes, low voltage); (2) for confirmation of the results of the exercise ECG when they are contrary to the clinical impression (eg, a positive test in an asymptomatic patient); (3) to localize the region of ischemia; (4) to distinguish ischemic from infarcted myocardium; (5) to assess the completeness of revascularization following bypass surgery or coronary angioplasty; or (6) as a prognostic indicator in patients with known coronary disease. Published criteria summarize these indications for stress testing.

1. Myocardial perfusion scintigraphy—This test, also known as **radionuclide imaging,** provides images in which radionuclide uptake is proportionate to blood flow at the time of injection.

Stress imaging is positive in about 75–90% of patients with anatomically significant coronary disease and in 20–30% of those without it. Occasionally, other conditions, including infiltrative diseases (sarcoidosis, amyloidosis), left bundle branch block, and dilated cardiomyopathy, may produce resting or persistent perfusion defects. False-positive radionuclide tests may occur as a result of diaphragmatic attenuation or, in women, attenuation through breast tissue. Tomographic imaging (single-photon emission computed tomography, SPECT) can reduce the severity of artifacts.

2. Radionuclide angiography—This procedure, also known as **multi-gated acquisition scan,** or **MUGA scan,** uses radionuclide tracers to image the LV and measures its EF and wall motion. In coronary disease, resting abnormalities usually represent infarction, and those that occur only with exercise usually indicate stress-induced ischemia. Exercise radionuclide angiography has approximately the same sensitivity as myocardial perfusion scintigraphy, but it is less specific in older individuals and those with other forms of heart disease. In addition, because of the precision around LVEF, the test is also used for monitoring patients exposed to cardiotoxic therapies (such as chemotherapeutic agents).

3. Stress echocardiography—Echocardiograms performed during supine exercise or immediately following upright exercise may demonstrate exercise-induced segmental wall motion abnormalities as an indicator of ischemia. In experienced laboratories, the test accuracy is comparable to that obtained with scintigraphy—though a higher proportion of tests is technically inadequate. While exercise is the preferred stress because of other information derived, pharmacologic stress with high-dose dobutamine (20–40 mcg/kg/min) can be used as an alternative to exercise.

H. Other Imaging

1. Positron emission tomography—PET and SPECT scanning can accurately distinguish transiently dysfunctional ("stunned") myocardium from scar tissue.

2. CT and MRI scanning—CT scanning can image the heart and, with contrast medium and multislice technology, the coronary arteries. **Multislice CT angiography may be useful in evaluating patients with low likelihood of significant**

CAD to rule out disease. Its use has been associated with lower 5-year mortality compared to standard care in patients with stable chest pain in one study, and this finding is being confirmed. With lower radiation exposure than radionuclide SPECT imaging, CT angiography may also be useful for evaluating chest pain and suspected acute coronary syndrome. In the large randomized comparative effectiveness PROMISE trial, patients with stable chest pain undergoing anatomic imaging with CT angiography had similar outcomes to patients undergoing functional testing (stress ECG, stress radionuclide, or stress echocardiography). CT angiography with noninvasive functional assessment of coronary stenosis (fractional flow reserve), termed **CT-FFR,** has also been evaluated in patients with low-intermediate likelihood of CAD. CT-FFR has been shown to reduce the number of patients without coronary disease requiring invasive angiography. CT-FFR has been approved for clinical use and is being used in clinical practice in the United States and Europe.

Electron beam CT (EBCT) (Coronary Calcium Score) can quantify coronary artery calcification, which is highly correlated with atheromatous plaque and has high sensitivity, but low specificity, for obstructive coronary disease. This test has not traditionally been used in symptomatic patients. According to the AHA, persons who are at low risk (less than 10% 10-year risk) or at high risk (greater than 20% 10-year risk) for obstructive coronary disease do not benefit from coronary calcium assessment (class III, level of evidence: B). However, in clinically selected, intermediate-risk patients (5–7.5% atherosclerotic cardiovascular disease), it may be reasonable to determine the atherosclerosis burden using EBCT in order to refine clinical risk prediction and to select patients for more aggressive target values for lipid-lowering therapies (class IIb, level of evidence: B).

Cardiac MRI using gadolinium provides high-resolution images of the heart and great vessels without radiation exposure or use of iodinated contrast media. Gadolinium has been associated with a rare but fatal complication in patients with severe kidney disease, called **necrotizing systemic fibrosis.** Gadolinium can demonstrate perfusion using dobutamine or adenosine to produce pharmacologic stress. Advances have been made in imaging the proximal coronary arteries. Perhaps the most clinically used indication of cardiac MRI is for identification of myocardial fibrosis, either from MI or infiltration, done with gadolinium contrast. This allows high-resolution imaging of myocardial viability and infiltrative cardiomyopathies.

I. Ambulatory ECG Monitoring

Ambulatory ECG recorders can monitor for ischemic ST-segment depression, but this modality is rarely used for ischemia detection. In patients with CAD, these episodes usually signify ischemia, even when asymptomatic ("silent").

J. Coronary Angiography

Selective coronary arteriography is the definitive diagnostic procedure for CAD. It can be performed with low mortality (about 0.1%) and morbidity (1–5%), but due to the invasive nature and cost, it is recommended only in patients with a high pretest probability of CAD.

Coronary arteriography should be performed in the following circumstances if percutaneous transluminal coronary angioplasty or bypass surgery is a consideration:

1. Life-limiting stable angina despite an adequate medical regimen.

2. Clinical presentation (unstable angina, postinfarction angina, etc) or noninvasive testing suggests high-risk disease (see Indications for Revascularization).

3. Concomitant aortic valve disease and angina pectoris, to determine whether the angina is due to accompanying coronary disease.

4. Asymptomatic older patients undergoing valve surgery so that concomitant bypass may be done if the anatomy is propitious.

5. Recurrence of symptoms after coronary revascularization to determine whether bypass grafts or native vessels are occluded.

6. Cardiac failure where a surgically correctable lesion, such as LV aneurysm, mitral regurgitation, or reversible ischemic dysfunction, is suspected.

7. Survivors of sudden death, symptomatic, or life-threatening arrhythmias when CAD may be a correctable cause.

8. Chest pain of uncertain cause or cardiomyopathy of unknown cause.

9. Emergently performed cardiac catheterization with intention to perform primary PCI in patients with suspected acute MI.

A narrowing of more than 50% of the luminal diameter is considered hemodynamically (and clinically) significant, although most lesions producing ischemia are associated with narrowing in excess of 70%. In those with strongly positive exercise ECGs or scintigraphic studies, three-vessel or left main disease may be present in 75–95% depending on the criteria used. **Intravascular ultrasound (IVUS)** is useful as an adjunct for assessing the results of angioplasty or stenting. In addition, IVUS is the invasive diagnostic method of choice for ostial left main lesions and coronary dissections. In **fractional flow reserve (FFR),** a pressure wire is used to measure the relative change in pressure across a coronary lesion after adenosine-induced hyperemia. Revascularization based on abnormal FFR improves clinical outcomes compared to revascularization of all angiographically stenotic lesions. FFR is an important invasive tool to aid with ischemia-driven revascularization and has become the standard tool to evaluate borderline lesions in cases in which the clinical team is evaluating the clinical and hemodynamic significance of a coronary stenosis. Additionally, pressures distally/pressures proximally during a wave-free period in diastole have been shown to demonstrate similar clinical outcomes to FFR, without the use of adenosine.

LV angiography is usually performed at the same time as coronary arteriography. Global and regional LV function are visualized, as well as mitral regurgitation if present. LV function is a major determinant of prognosis in CHD.

▶ **Differential Diagnosis**

When atypical features are present—such as prolonged duration (hours or days) or darting, or knifelike pains at the apex or over the precordium—ischemia is less likely.

Anterior chest wall syndrome is characterized by a sharply localized tenderness of the intercostal muscles. Inflammation of the chondrocostal junctions may result in diffuse chest pain that is also reproduced by local pressure (Tietze syndrome). Intercostal neuritis (due to herpes zoster or diabetes mellitus, for example) also mimics angina.

Cervical or thoracic spine disease involving the dorsal roots produces sudden sharp, severe chest pain suggesting angina in location and "radiation" but related to specific movements of the neck or spine, recumbency, and straining or lifting. Pain due to cervical or thoracic disk disease involves the outer or dorsal aspect of the arm and the thumb and index fingers rather than the ring and little fingers.

Reflux esophagitis, peptic ulcer, chronic cholecystitis, esophageal spasm, and functional gastrointestinal disease may produce pain suggestive of angina pectoris. The picture may be especially confusing because ischemic pain may also be associated with upper gastrointestinal symptoms, and esophageal motility disorders may be improved by nitrates and calcium channel blockers. Assessment of esophageal motility may be helpful.

Degenerative and inflammatory lesions of the left shoulder and thoracic outlet syndromes may cause chest pain due to nerve irritation or muscular compression; the symptoms are usually precipitated by movement of the arm and shoulder and are associated with paresthesias.

Pneumonia, pulmonary embolism, and spontaneous pneumothorax may cause chest pain as well as dyspnea. Dissection of the thoracic aorta can cause severe chest pain that is commonly felt in the back; it is sudden in onset, reaches maximum intensity immediately, and may be associated with changes in pulses. Other cardiac disorders, such as mitral valve prolapse, hypertrophic cardiomyopathy, myocarditis, pericarditis, aortic valve disease, or RVH, may cause atypical chest pain or even myocardial ischemia.

▶ **Treatment**

Sublingual nitroglycerin is the medication of choice for acute management; it acts in about 1–2 minutes. As soon as the attack begins, one fresh tablet is placed under the tongue. This may be repeated at 3- to 5-minute intervals, but if pain is not relieved or improving after 5 minutes, the patient should call 9-1-1; pain not responding to three tablets or lasting more than 20 minutes may represent evolving infarction. The dosage (0.3, 0.4, or 0.6 mg) and the number of tablets to be used before seeking further medical attention must be individualized. Nitroglycerin buccal spray is also available as a metered (0.4 mg) delivery system. It has the advantage of being more convenient for patients who have difficulty handling the pills and of being more stable.

▶ **Prevention of Further Attacks**

A. Aggravating Factors

Angina may be aggravated by hypertension, LV failure, arrhythmia (usually tachycardias), strenuous activity, cold temperatures, and emotional states. These factors should be identified and treated when possible.

B. Nitroglycerin

Nitroglycerin, 0.3–0.6 mg sublingually or 0.4–0.8 mg translingually by spray, should be taken 5 minutes before any activity likely to precipitate angina. Sublingual isosorbide dinitrate (2.5–5 mg) is only slightly longer-acting than sublingual nitroglycerin.

C. Long-Acting Nitrates

Longer-acting nitrate preparations include isosorbide dinitrate, 10–40 mg orally three times daily; isosorbide mononitrate, 10–40 mg orally twice daily or 60–120 mg once daily in a sustained-release preparation; oral sustained-release nitroglycerin preparations, 6.25–12.5 mg two to four times daily; nitroglycerin ointment, 2% ointment, 0.5 to 2 inches (7.5 to 30 mg in the morning and six hours later); and transdermal nitroglycerin patches that deliver nitroglycerin at rates of 0.2, 0.4, and 0.6 mg/h rate (0.1–0.8 mg/h), and should be taken off after 12–14 hours of use for a 10–12 hour patch-free interval daily. The main limitation to long-term nitrate therapy is tolerance, which can be limited by using a regimen that includes a minimum 8- to 10-hour period per day without nitrates. Isosorbide dinitrate can be given three times daily, with the last dose after dinner, or longer-acting isosorbide mononitrate once daily. Transdermal nitrate preparations should be removed overnight in most patients.

Nitrate therapy is often limited by headache. Other side effects include nausea, light-headedness, and hypotension. Importantly, phosphodiesterase inhibitors used commonly for erectile dysfunction should not be taken within 24 hours of nitrate use.

D. Beta-Blockers

Beta-blockers are the only antianginal agents that have been demonstrated to prolong life in patients with coronary disease (post-MI). Beta-blockers should be considered for first-line therapy in most patients with chronic angina and are recommended as such by the stable ischemic heart disease guidelines (Figure 10–6).

Beta-blockers with intrinsic sympathomimetic activity, such as pindolol, are less desirable because they may exacerbate angina in some individuals and have not been effective in secondary prevention trials. The pharmacology and side effects of the beta-blockers are discussed in Chapter 11 (see Table 11–9). The dosages of all these medications when given for angina are similar. The major contraindications are severe bronchospastic disease, bradyarrhythmias, and decompensated heart failure.

E. Ranolazine

Ranolazine is indicated for chronic angina. Ranolazine has no effect on heart rate and BP, and it has been shown in clinical trials to prolong exercise duration and time to angina, both as monotherapy and when administered with conventional antianginal therapy. It is safe to use with erectile dysfunction medications. The usual dose is 500 mg orally twice a day. Because it can cause QT prolongation, it is contraindicated in patients with existing QT prolongation; in patients taking QT prolonging medications, such as class I or III antiarrhythmics (eg, quinidine, dofetilide, sotalol); and in those taking potent and moderate CYP450 3A inhibitors (eg, clarithromycin and rifampin). Of interest, in spite of the QT prolongation, there is a significantly lower rate of ventricular arrhythmias with its use following acute coronary syndromes, as shown in the MERLIN trial.

F. Calcium Channel Blocking Agents

Unlike the beta-blockers, calcium channel blockers have *not* been shown to reduce mortality postinfarction and in some cases have increased ischemia and mortality rates. This appears to be the case with some dihydropyridines (eg, nifedipine) and with diltiazem and verapamil in patients with clinical heart failure or moderate to severe LV dysfunction. Meta-analyses have suggested that short-acting nifedipine in moderate to high doses causes an *increase* in mortality. It is uncertain whether these findings are relevant to longer-acting dihydropyridines. Nevertheless, considering the uncertainties and the lack of demonstrated favorable effect on outcomes, calcium channel blockers should be considered third-line anti-ischemic medications in the postinfarction patient. Similarly, these agents, with the exception of amlodipine (which proved safe in patients with heart failure in the PRAISE-2 trial), should be avoided in patients with heart failure or low EFs.

The pharmacologic effects and side effects of the calcium channel blockers are discussed in Chapter 11 and summarized in Table 11–7. Diltiazem, amlodipine, and verapamil are preferable because they produce less reflex tachycardia and because the former, at least, may cause fewer side effects. Nifedipine, nicardipine, and amlodipine are also approved agents for angina. Isradipine, felodipine, and nisoldipine are not approved for angina but probably are as effective as the other dihydropyridines.

G. Ivabradine

Ivabradine selectively blocks the I_f current and specifically lowers heart rate. It has been shown to reduce angina in patients with chronic stable angina and is approved in Europe. However, the SIGNIFY trial found no overall difference in clinical outcomes in patients without heart failure and angina and that there may have been harm for patients with significant angina with regard to outcomes of cardiovascular death and MI.

H. Alternative and Combination Therapies

Patients who do not respond to one class of antianginal medication often respond to another. It may, therefore, be worthwhile to use an alternative agent before progressing to combinations. The stable ischemic heart disease guidelines recommend starting with a beta-blocker as initial therapy, followed by calcium channel blockers, long-acting nitrates, or ranolazine. A few patients will have further response to a regimen including all four agents.

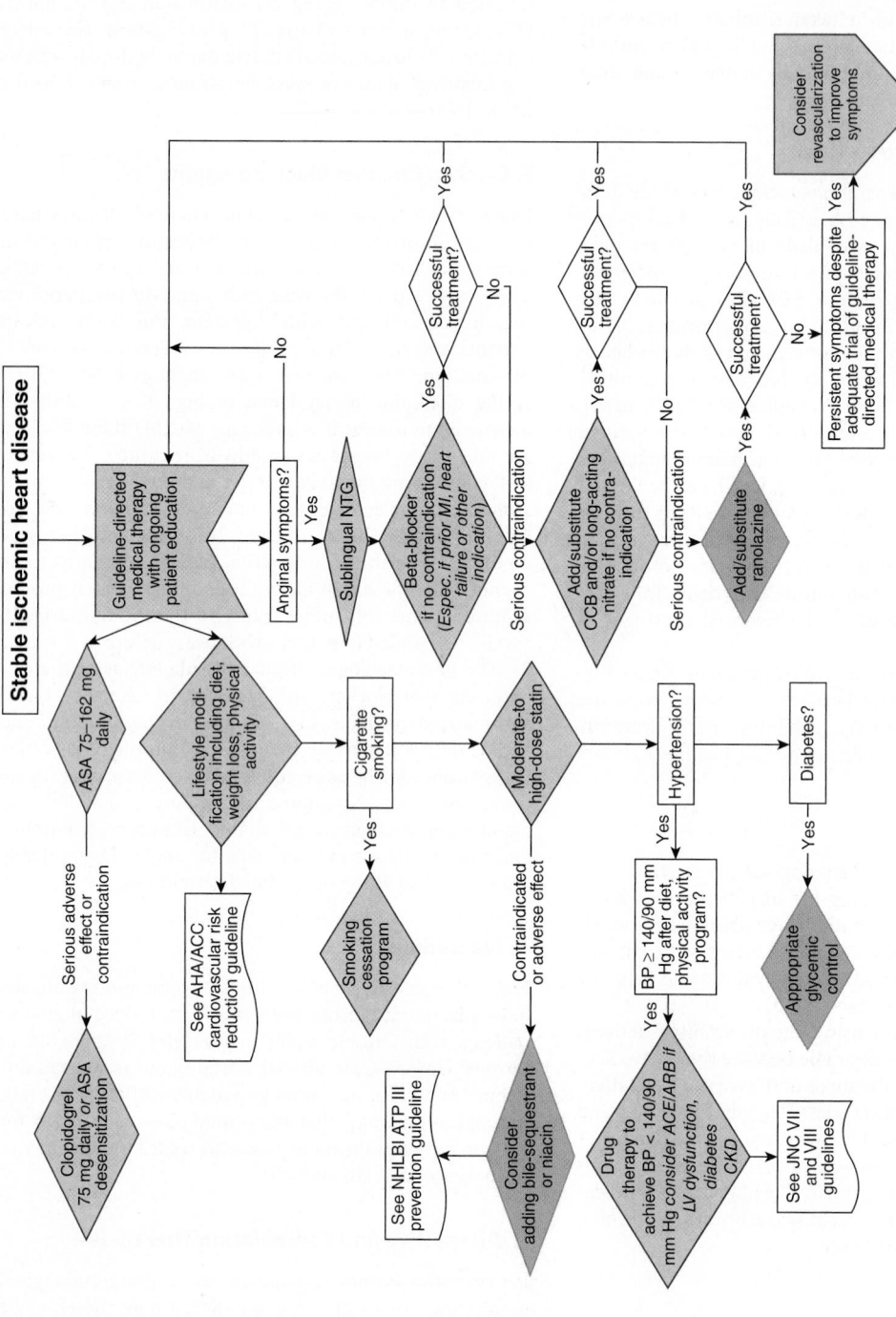

▲ **Figure 10–6.** Algorithm for guideline-directed medical therapy for patients with stable ischemic heart disease. The use of bile acid sequestrant is relatively contraindicated when triglycerides are 200 mg/dL or higher and contraindicated when triglycerides are 500 mg/dL or higher. Dietary supplement niacin must not be used as a substitute for prescription niacin. (Reproduced, with permission, from Fihn SD et al; American College of Cardiology Foundation/American Heart Association Task Force. 2012 ACCF/AHA/ACP/AATS/PCNA/SCAI/STS guideline for the diagnosis and management of patients with stable ischemic heart disease. Circulation. 2012 Dec 18;126(25):e354–471. © 2012 American Heart Association, Inc.)

ACE/ARB, angiotensin-converting enzyme/angiotensin receptor blocker; AHA/ACC, American Heart Association/American College of Cardiology; ASA, aspirin; BP, blood pressure; CCB, calcium channel blocker; CKD, chronic kidney disease; MI, myocardial infarction; NTG, nitroglycerin.

I. Platelet-Inhibiting Agents

Several studies have demonstrated the benefit of antiplatelet medications for patients with stable and unstable vascular disease. Therefore, unless contraindicated, **aspirin** (81–325 mg orally daily) should be prescribed for all patients with angina. **Clopidogrel,** 75 mg orally daily, reduces vascular events in patients with stable vascular disease (as an alternative to aspirin) and in patients with acute coronary syndromes (in addition to aspirin). Thus, it is also a good alternative in aspirin-intolerant patients. Clopidogrel in addition to aspirin did not reduce MI, stroke, or cardiovascular death in the CHARISMA trial of patients with cardiovascular disease or multiple risk factors, with about a 50% increase in bleeding. However, it might be reasonable to use combination clopidogrel and aspirin for certain high-risk patients with established coronary disease, as tested in the DAPT trial. Specifically, **prolonged used of dual antiplatelet therapy with aspirin and clopidogrel may be beneficial in patients post–percutaneous stenting with drug-eluting stents, in patients with low bleeding risk.**

Ticagrelor, a P2Y12 inhibitor, has been shown to reduce cardiovascular events in patients with acute coronary syndromes. Additionally, in patients with prior MI, long-term treatment with ticagrelor plus aspirin reduced cardiovascular events compared to aspirin alone. In patients with peripheral artery disease, ticagrelor monotherapy did not reduce cardiovascular events compared to clopidogrel.

The latest antiplatelet agent to be approved by the FDA, **vorapaxar,** is an inhibitor of the protease-activated receptor-1. It was shown to reduce cardiovascular events for patients with stable atherosclerosis with a history of MI or peripheral artery disease in the TRA 2P trial. It is contraindicated for patients with a history of stroke or TIA due to increased risk of intracranial hemorrhage.

Rivaroxaban, a direct factor Xa inhibitor, when used at a dose of 2.5 mg twice daily in addition to low-dose aspirin was found to reduce cardiovascular events including cardiovascular death, MI, or stroke when compared to aspirin monotherapy in patients with known CAD or peripheral artery disease. This agent is approved and provides another option for patients.

Current guidelines recommend **dual antiplatelet therapy (aspirin and P2Y12 therapy) in patients with recent MI (within 1 year) or recent stenting (within 6 months) and for prolonged therapy (more than 1 year) in patients at high ischemic risk (multivessel coronary disease or polyvascular disease) and low bleeding risk.**

J. Risk Reduction

Patients with coronary disease should undergo aggressive **risk factor modification.** This approach, with a particular focus on statin treatment, treating hypertension, stopping smoking, and exercise and weight control (especially for patients with metabolic syndrome or at risk for diabetes), may markedly improve outcomes. For patients with diabetes and cardiovascular disease, there is uncertainty about the optimal target blood sugar control. The ADVANCE trial suggested some benefit for tight blood sugar control with target HbA_{1C} of 6.5% or less, but the ACCORD trial found that routine aggressive targeting for blood sugar control to HbA_{1C} to less than 6.0% in patients with diabetes and coronary disease was associated with increased mortality. Therefore, tight blood sugar control should be avoided particularly in patients with a history of severe hypoglycemia, long-standing diabetes, and advanced vascular disease. Aggressive BP control (target systolic BP less than 120 mm Hg) in the ACCORD trial was not associated with reduction in CHD events despite reducing stroke. In contrast, the SPRINT trial, which did not include diabetic patients, demonstrated a reduction in cardiovascular events in patients with a reduction in death from any cause and reduction in MI with a goal systolic BP of less than 120 mm Hg versus of goal of less than 140 mm Hg. Some increase in adverse events was noted. Based on this and the totality of results, the AHA has recommended defining hypertension at the 130 mm Hg level.

K. Revascularization

1. Indications—There is general agreement that otherwise healthy patients in the following groups should undergo revascularization: (1) patients with unacceptable symptoms despite medical therapy to its tolerable limits; (2) patients with left main coronary artery stenosis greater than 50% with or without symptoms; (3) patients with three-vessel disease with LV dysfunction (EF less than 50% or previous transmural infarction); (4) patients with unstable angina who after symptom control by medical therapy continue to exhibit ischemia on exercise testing or monitoring and; (5) post-MI patients with continuing angina or severe ischemia on noninvasive testing. The use of revascularization for patients with acute coronary syndromes and acute ST-segment elevation MI (STEMI) is discussed below.

Data from the COURAGE trial have shown that for patients with chronic angina and disease suitable for PCI, PCI in addition to stringent guideline-directed medical therapy aimed at both risk reduction and anti-anginal care offers no mortality benefit beyond excellent medical therapy alone, and relatively moderate long-term symptomatic improvement. Therefore, for patients with mild to moderate CAD and limited symptoms, revascularization may not provide significant functional status quality-of-life benefit. For patients with moderate to significant coronary stenosis, such as those who have two-vessel disease associated with underlying LV dysfunction, anatomically critical lesions (greater than 90% proximal stenoses, especially of the proximal left anterior descending artery), or physiologic evidence of severe ischemia (early positive exercise tests, large exercise-induced thallium scintigraphic defects, or frequent episodes of ischemia on ambulatory monitoring), a heart team consisting of revascularization physicians (interventional cardiologists and surgeons) may be required to review and provide patients with the best revascularization options.

2. Type of procedure

A. PERCUTANEOUS CORONARY INTERVENTION INCLUDING STENTING—PCI, including balloon angioplasty and coronary stenting, can effectively open stenotic coronary arteries. Coronary stenting, with either bare metal stents or drug-eluting stents, has substantially reduced restenosis. Stenting can also be used selectively for left main coronary stenosis, particularly when CABG is contraindicated or deemed high risk.

PCI is possible but often less successful in bypass graft stenoses. Experienced operators are able to successfully dilate more than 90% of lesions attempted. The major early complication is intimal dissection with vessel occlusion, although this is rare with coronary stenting. The use of intravenous platelet glycoprotein IIb/IIIa inhibitors (abciximab, eptifibatide, tirofiban) substantially reduces the rate of periprocedural MI, and placement of intracoronary stents markedly improves initial and long-term angiographic results, especially with complex and long lesions. After percutaneous coronary intervention, all patients should have CK-MB and troponin measured. The definition of a periprocedural infarction has been debated, with many experts advocating for a clinical definition that incorporates different enzyme cutpoints, angiographic findings, and electrocardiographic evidence. Acute thrombosis after stent placement can largely be prevented by aggressive antithrombotic therapy (long-term aspirin, 81–325 mg, plus clopidogrel, 300–600 mg loading dose followed by 75 mg daily, for between 30 days and 1 year, and with acute use of platelet glycoprotein IIb/IIIa inhibitors).

A major limitation with PCI has been **restenosis,** which occurs in the first 6 months in less than 10% of vessels treated with drug-eluting stents, 15–30% of vessels treated with bare metal stents, and 30–40% of vessels without stenting. Factors associated with higher restenosis rates include diabetes, small luminal diameter, longer and more complex lesions, and lesions at coronary ostia or in the left anterior descending coronary artery. Drug-eluting stents that elute antiproliferative agents, such as sirolimus, everolimus, zotarolimus, or paclitaxel, have substantially reduced restenosis. In-stent restenosis is often treated with restenting with drug-eluting stents, and rarely with brachytherapy. The nearly 2 million PCIs performed worldwide per year far exceed the number of CABG operations, but the rationale for many of the procedures performed in patients with stable angina should be for angina symptom reduction. The COURAGE trial and the ORBITA sham-controlled trial have confirmed earlier studies in showing that, even for patients with moderate anginal symptoms and positive stress tests, PCI provides no benefit over medical therapy with respect to death or MI. PCI was more effective at relieving angina, although most patients in the medical group had improvement in symptoms. PCI was also not more effective than optimal medical therapy for exercise time in patients with one vessel coronary disease. Thus, **in patients with mild or moderate stable symptoms, aggressive lipid-lowering and antianginal therapy may be a preferable initial strategy, reserving PCI for patients with significant and refractory symptoms or for those who are unable to take the prescribed medicines.**

Several studies of PCI, including those with drug-eluting stents, versus CABG in patients with multivessel disease have been reported. The SYNTAX trial as well as previously performed trials with drug-eluting stent use in PCI patients show comparable mortality and infarction rates over follow-up periods of 1–3 years but a high rate (approximately 40%) of repeat procedures following PCI. Stroke rates are higher with CABG. As a result, the choice of revascularization procedure may depend on details of coronary anatomy and is often a matter of patient preference. However, it should be noted that less than 20% of patients with multivessel disease meet the entry criteria for the clinical trials, so these results cannot be generalized to all multivessel disease patients. Outcomes with percutaneous revascularization in patients with diabetes have generally been inferior to those with CABG. The FREEDOM trial demonstrated that CABG surgery was superior to PCI with regards to death, MI, and stroke for patients with diabetes and multivessel coronary disease at 5 years across all subgroups of SYNTAX score anatomy.

B. Coronary artery bypass grafting—CABG can be accomplished with a very low mortality rate (1–3%) in otherwise healthy patients with preserved cardiac function. However, the mortality rate of this procedure rises to 4–8% in older individuals and in patients who have had a prior CABG.

Grafts using one or both internal mammary arteries (usually to the left anterior descending artery or its branches) provide the best long-term results in terms of patency and flow. Segments of the saphenous vein (or, less optimally, other veins) or the radial artery interposed between the aorta and the coronary arteries distal to the obstructions are also used. One to five distal anastomoses are commonly performed.

Minimally invasive surgical techniques may involve a limited sternotomy, lateral thoracotomy (MIDCAB), or thoracoscopy (port-access). They are more technically demanding, usually not suitable for more than two grafts, and do not have established durability. Bypass surgery can be performed both on circulatory support (on-pump) and without direct circulatory support (off-pump). Randomized trial data have not shown a benefit with off-pump bypass surgery, but minimally invasive surgical techniques allow earlier postoperative mobilization and discharge.

The operative mortality rate is increased in patients with poor LV function (LVEF less than 35%) or those requiring additional procedures (valve replacement or ventricular aneurysmectomy). Patients over 70 years of age, patients undergoing repeat procedures, or those with important noncardiac disease (especially chronic kidney disease and diabetes) or poor general health also have higher operative mortality and morbidity rates, and full recovery is slow. Thus, CABG should be reserved for more severely symptomatic patients in this group. Early (1–6 months) graft patency rates average 85–90% (higher for internal mammary grafts), and subsequent graft closure rates are about 4% annually. Early graft failure is common in vessels with poor distal flow, while late closure is more frequent in patients who continue smoking and those with untreated hyperlipidemia. Antiplatelet therapy with aspirin improves graft patency rates. Smoking cessation and vigorous treatment of blood lipid abnormalities (particularly with statins) are necessary. Repeat revascularization may be necessitated because of recurrent symptoms due to progressive native vessel disease and graft occlusions. Reoperation is technically demanding and less often fully successful than the initial operation. In addition, in patients with ischemic mitral regurgitation, mitral repair at the time of a CABG does not offer any clinical benefit.

L. Mechanical Extracorporeal Counterpulsation

Extracorporeal counterpulsation entails repetitive inflation of a high-pressure chamber surrounding the lower half of the body during the diastolic phase of the cardiac cycle for daily 1-hour sessions over a period of 7 weeks. Randomized trials have shown that extracorporeal counterpulsation reduces angina, thus it may be considered for relief of refractory angina in patients with stable coronary disease.

M. Neuromodulation

Spinal cord stimulation can be used to relieve chronic refractory angina. Spinal cord stimulators are subcutaneously implantable via a minimally invasive procedure under local anesthesia.

► Prognosis

The prognosis of angina pectoris has improved with development of therapies aimed at secondary prevention. Mortality rates vary depending on the number of vessels diseased, the severity of obstruction, the status of LV function, and the presence of complex arrhythmias. Mortality rates are progressively higher in patients with one-, two-, and three-vessel disease and those with left main coronary artery obstruction (ranging from 1% per year to 25% per year). The outlook in individual patients is unpredictable, and nearly half of the deaths are sudden. Therefore, risk stratification is attempted. Patients with accelerating symptoms have a poorer outlook. Among stable patients, those whose exercise tolerance is severely limited by ischemia (less than 6 minutes on the Bruce treadmill protocol) and those with extensive ischemia by exercise ECG or scintigraphy have more severe anatomic disease and a poorer prognosis. The Duke Treadmill Score, based on a standard Bruce protocol exercise treadmill test, provides an estimate of risk of death at 1 year. The score uses time on the treadmill, amount of ST-segment depression, and presence of angina (Table 10–8).

► When to Refer

All patients with new or worsening symptoms believed to represent progressive angina or a positive stress test for myocardial ischemia with continued angina despite medical therapy (or both) should be referred to a cardiologist.

Table 10–8. Duke Treadmill Score: calculation and interpretation.

Time in minutes on Bruce protocol	= _____		
−5 × amount of depression (in mm)	= _____		
−4 × angina index 0 = no angina on test 1 = angina, not limiting 2 = limiting angina	= _____		
Total Summed Score	**Risk Group**	**Annual Mortality**	
≥ 5	Low	0.25%	
−10 to 4	Intermediate	1.25%	
≤ −11	High	5.25%	

► When to Admit

- Patients with elevated cardiac biomarkers, ischemic ECG findings, or hemodynamic instability.
- Patients with new or worsened symptoms, possibly thought to be ischemic, but who lack high-risk features can be observed with serial ECGs and biomarkers, and discharged if stress testing shows low-risk findings.

Al-Lamee R et al; ORBITA Investigators. Percutaneous coronary intervention in stable angina (ORBITA): a double-blind, randomised controlled trial. Lancet. 2018 Jan 6;391(10115):31–40. [PMID: 29103656]

Davies JE et al. Use of the instantaneous wave-free ratio or fractional flow reserve in PCI. N Engl J Med. 2017 May 11;376(19):1824–34. [PMID: 28317458]

Douglas PS et al; PLATFORM Investigators. Clinical outcomes of fractional flow reserve by computed tomographic angiography-guided diagnostic strategies vs. usual care in patients with suspected coronary artery disease: the prospective longitudinal trial of FFRCT: outcome and resource impacts study. Eur Heart J. 2015 Dec 14;36(47):3359–67. [PMID: 26330417]

Douglas PS et al; PROMISE Investigators. Outcomes of anatomical versus functional testing for coronary artery disease. N Engl J Med. 2015 Apr 2;372(14):1291–300. [PMID: 25773919]

Eikelboom JW et al; COMPASS Investigators. Rivaroxaban with or without aspirin in stable cardiovascular disease. N Engl J Med. 2017 Oct 5;377(14):1319–30. [PMID: 28844192]

Fihn SD et al. 2012 ACCF/AHA/ACP/AATS/PCNA/SCAI/STS guideline for the diagnosis and management of patients with stable ischemic heart disease: a report of the American College of Cardiology Foundation/American Heart Association Task Force on Practice Guidelines, and the American College of Physicians, American Association for Thoracic Surgery, Preventive Cardiovascular Nurses Association, Society for Cardiovascular Angiography and Interventions, and Society of Thoracic Surgeons. Circulation. 2012 Dec 18;126(25):e354–471. [PMID: 23166211]

Götberg M et al; iFR-SWEDEHEART Investigators. Instantaneous wave-free ratio versus fractional flow reserve to guide PCI. N Engl J Med. 2017 May 11;376(19):1813–23. [PMID: 28317438]

Hiatt WR et al; EUCLID Trial Steering Committee and Investigators. Ticagrelor versus clopidogrel in symptomatic peripheral artery disease. N Engl J Med. 2017 Jan 5;376(1):32–40. [PMID: 27959717]

Levine GN et al. 2016 ACC/AHA guideline focused update on duration of dual antiplatelet therapy in patients with coronary artery disease: a report of the American College of Cardiology/American Heart Association Task Force on Clinical Practice Guidelines: an update of the 2011 ACCF/AHA/SCAI guideline for percutaneous coronary intervention, 2011 ACCF/AHA guideline for coronary artery bypass graft surgery, 2012 ACC/AHA/ACP/AATS/PCNA/SCAI/STS guideline for the diagnosis and management of patients with stable ischemic heart disease, 2013 ACCF/AHA guideline for the management of ST-elevation myocardial infarction, 2014 AHA/ACC guideline for the management of patients with non-ST-elevation acute coronary syndromes, and 2014 ACC/AHA guideline on perioperative cardiovascular evaluation and management of patients undergoing noncardiac surgery. Circulation. 2016 Sep 6;134(10):e123–55. Erratum in: Circulation. 2016 Sep 6;134(10):e192–4. [PMID: 27026020]

SCOT-HEART Investigators et al. Coronary CT angiography and 5-year risk of myocardial infarction. N Engl J Med. 2018 Sep 6;379(10):924–33. [PMID: 30145934]

SPRINT Research Group; Wright JT Jr et al. A randomized trial of intensive versus standard blood-pressure control. N Engl J Med. 2015 Nov 26;373(22):2103–16. Erratum in: N Engl J Med. 2017 Dec 21;377(25):2506. [PMID: 26551272]

Stone GW et al; EXCEL Trial Investigators. Everolimus-eluting stents or bypass surgery for left main coronary artery disease. N Engl J Med. 2016 Dec 8;375(23):2223–35. [PMID: 27797291]

Weisz G et al; RIVER-PCI investigators. Ranolazine in patients with incomplete revascularisation after percutaneous coronary intervention (RIVER-PCI): a multicentre, randomised, double-blind, placebo-controlled trial. Lancet. 2016 Jan 9;387(10014):136–45.

CORONARY VASOSPASM & ANGINA WITH NORMAL CORONARY ARTERIOGRAMS

ESSENTIALS OF DIAGNOSIS

▸ Precordial chest pain, often occurring at rest during stress or without known precipitant, relieved rapidly by nitrates.

▸ ECG evidence of ischemia during pain, sometimes with ST-segment elevation.

▸ Angiographic demonstration of:

  – No significant obstruction of major coronary vessels.

  – Coronary spasm that responds to intracoronary nitroglycerin or calcium channel blockers.

General Considerations

Although most symptoms of myocardial ischemia result from fixed stenosis of the coronary arteries, intraplaque hemorrhage, or thrombosis at the site of lesions, some ischemic events may be precipitated or exacerbated by coronary vasoconstriction.

Spasm of the large coronary arteries with resulting decreased coronary blood flow may occur spontaneously or may be induced by exposure to cold, emotional stress, or vasoconstricting medications, such as ergot-derivative medications. Spasm may occur both in normal and in stenosed coronary arteries. Even MI may occur as a result of spasm in the absence of visible obstructive CHD, although most instances of such coronary spasm occur in the presence of coronary stenosis.

Cocaine can induce myocardial ischemia and infarction by causing coronary artery vasoconstriction or by increasing myocardial energy requirements. It also may contribute to accelerated atherosclerosis and thrombosis. The ischemia in **Prinzmetal (variant) angina** usually results from coronary vasoconstriction. It tends to involve the right coronary artery and there may be no fixed stenoses. Myocardial ischemia may also occur in patients with normal coronary arteries as a result of disease of the coronary microcirculation or abnormal vascular reactivity. This has been termed "**syndrome X.**"

Clinical Findings

Ischemia may be silent or result in angina pectoris.

Prinzmetal (variant) angina is a clinical syndrome in which chest pain occurs without the usual precipitating factors and is associated with ST-segment elevation rather than depression. It often affects women under 50 years of age. It characteristically occurs in the early morning, awakening patients from sleep, and is apt to be associated with arrhythmias or conduction defects. It may be diagnosed by challenge with ergonovine (a vasoconstrictor), although the results of such provocation are not specific and it entails risk.

Treatment

Patients with chest pain associated with ST-segment elevation should undergo coronary arteriography to determine whether fixed stenotic lesions are present. If they are, aggressive medical therapy or revascularization is indicated, since this may represent an unstable phase of the disease. If significant lesions are not seen and spasm is suspected, avoidance of precipitants, such as cigarette smoking and cocaine, is the top priority. Episodes of coronary spasm generally respond well to nitrates, and both nitrates and calcium channel blockers (including long-acting nifedipine, diltiazem, or amlodipine [see Table 11–7]) are effective prophylactically. By allowing unopposed alpha-1-mediated vasoconstriction, beta-blockers have exacerbated coronary vasospasm, but they may have a role in management of patients in whom spasm is associated with fixed stenoses.

When to Refer

All patients with persistent symptoms of chest pain that may represent spasm should be referred to a cardiologist.

ACUTE CORONARY SYNDROMES WITHOUT ST-SEGMENT ELEVATION

ESSENTIALS OF DIAGNOSIS

▸ Distinction in acute coronary syndrome between patients with and without ST-segment elevation at presentation is essential to determine need for reperfusion therapy.

▸ Fibrinolytic therapy is harmful in acute coronary syndrome without ST-segment elevation, unlike with ST-segment elevation, where acute reperfusion saves lives.

▸ Antiplatelet and anticoagulation therapies and coronary intervention are mainstays of treatment.

General Considerations

Acute coronary syndromes comprise the spectrum of unstable cardiac ischemia from unstable angina to acute MI. Acute coronary syndromes are classified based on the presenting ECG as either **STEMI** or **non–ST-segment elevation MI (NSTEMI)**. This allows for immediate classification and guides determination of whether patients should be considered for acute reperfusion therapy. The evolution of cardiac biomarkers then allows determination of whether MI has occurred.

Acute coronary syndromes represent a dynamic state in which patients frequently shift from one category to another, as new ST elevation can develop after presentation and cardiac biomarkers can become abnormal with recurrent ischemic episodes.

▶ Clinical Findings

A. Symptoms and Signs

Patients with acute coronary syndromes generally have symptoms and signs of myocardial ischemia either at rest or with minimal exertion. These symptoms and signs are similar to the chronic angina symptoms described above, consisting of substernal chest pain or discomfort that may radiate to the jaw, left shoulder or arm. Dyspnea, nausea, diaphoresis, or syncope may either accompany the chest discomfort or may be the only symptom of acute coronary syndrome. *About one-third of patients with MI have no chest pain per se*—these patients tend to be older, female, have diabetes, and be at higher risk for subsequent mortality. Patients with acute coronary syndromes have signs of heart failure in about 10% of cases, and this is also associated with higher risk of death.

Many hospitals have developed chest pain observation units to provide a systematic approach toward serial risk stratification to improve the triage process. In many cases, those who have not experienced new chest pain and have insignificant ECG changes and no cardiac biomarker elevation undergo treadmill exercise tests or imaging procedures to exclude ischemia at the end of an 8- to 24-hour period and are discharged directly from the emergency department if these tests are negative.

B. Laboratory Findings

Depending on the time from symptom onset to presentation, initial laboratory findings may be normal. The markers of cardiac myocyte necrosis (myoglobin, CK-MB and tropnin I and T) may all be used to identify acute MI. These markers have a well-described pattern of release over time in patients with MI (see Laboratory Findings, Acute Myocardial Infarction with ST-Segment Elevation, below). In patients with STEMI, these initial markers are often within normal limits as the patient is being rushed to immediate reperfusion. In patients without ST-segment elevation, it is the presence of abnormal CK-MB or troponin values that are associated with myocyte necrosis and the diagnosis of MI. High-sensitivity troponin assays allow rapid assessment of MI in emergency departments by using sex-based rule out algorithms. The universal definition of MI is a rise of cardiac biomarkers with at least one value above the 99th percentile of the upper reference limit together with evidence of myocardial ischemia with at least one of the following: symptoms of ischemia, ECG changes of new ischemia, new Q waves, or imaging evidence of new loss of viable myocardium or new wall motion abnormality.

Serum creatinine is an important determinant of risk, and estimated creatinine clearance is important to guide dosing of certain antithrombotics, including eptifibatide and enoxaparin.

C. ECG

Many patients with acute coronary syndromes will exhibit ECG changes during pain—either ST-segment elevation, ST-segment depression, or T-wave flattening or inversion. Dynamic ST-segment shift is the most specific for acute coronary syndrome. ST-segment elevation in lead AVR suggests left main or three-vessel disease.

▶ Treatment

A. General Measures

Treatment of acute coronary syndromes without ST elevation should be multifaceted. Patients who are at medium or high risk should be hospitalized, maintained at bed rest or at very limited activity for the first 24 hours, monitored, and given supplemental oxygen. Sedation with a benzodiazepine agent may help if anxiety is present.

B. Specific Measures

Figure 10–7 provides an algorithm for initial management of NSTEMI.

C. Antiplatelet and Anticoagulation Therapy

Patients should receive a combination of antiplatelet and anticoagulant agents on presentation. Fibrinolytic therapy should be *avoided* in patients without ST-segment elevation since they generally do not have an acute coronary occlusion, and the risk of such therapy appears to outweigh the benefit.

1. Antiplatelet therapy

A. ASPIRIN—Aspirin, 162–325 mg loading dose, then 81–325 mg daily, should be commenced immediately and continued for the first month. The 2012 ACC/AHA guidelines for longer-term aspirin treatment recommend aspirin 75–162 mg/day as preferable to higher doses with or without coronary stenting.

B. P2Y$_{12}$ INHIBITORS—ACC/AHA guidelines call for either a P2Y$_{12}$ inhibitor (clopidogrel, prasugrel [at the time of PCI], or ticagrelor) as a class I recommendation. The ESC guidelines provide a stronger recommendation for a P2Y$_{12}$ inhibitor up-front, as a class IA recommendation for all patients. Both sets of guidelines recommend postponing elective CABG surgery for at least 5 days after the last dose of clopidogrel or ticagrelor and at least 7 days after the last dose of prasugrel, due to risk of bleeding.

The Clopidogrel in Unstable Angina to Prevent Recurrent Events (CURE) trial demonstrated a 20% reduction in the composite end point of cardiovascular death, MI, and stroke with the addition of clopidogrel (300-mg loading dose, 75 mg/day for 9–12 months) to aspirin in patients with non–ST-segment elevation acute coronary syndromes. The large CURRENT trial showed that "double-dose" clopidogrel (600-mg initial oral loading dose, followed by 150 mg orally daily) for 7 days reduced stent thrombosis with a modest increase in major (but not fatal) bleeding and, therefore, it is an option for patients with acute coronary syndrome undergoing PCI.

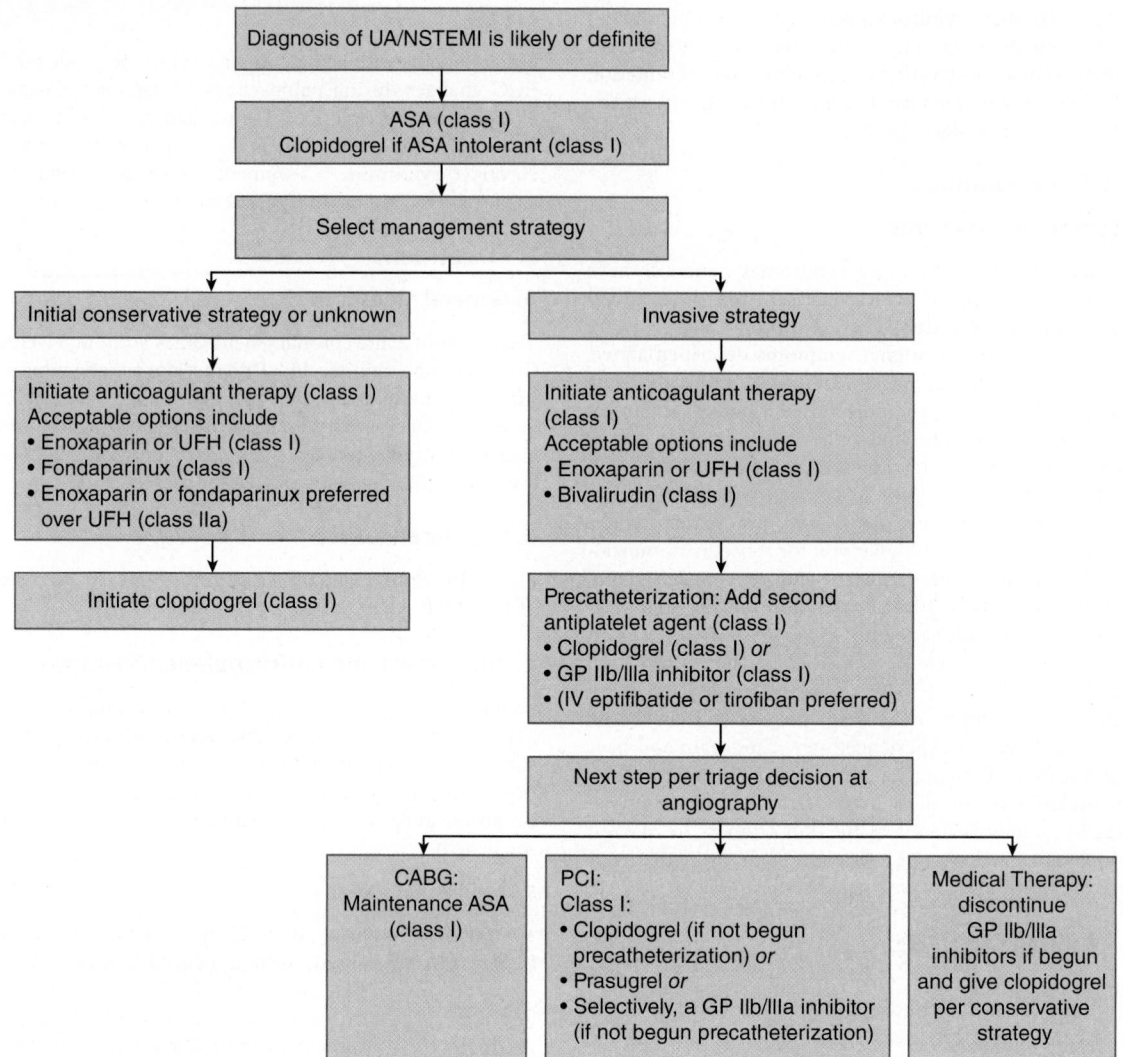

▲ **Figure 10–7.** Flowchart for class I and class IIa recommendations for initial management of unstable angina/non–ST-segment elevation myocardial infarction (UA/NSTEMI). ASA, aspirin; CABG, coronary artery bypass grafting; GP IIb/IIIa, glycoprotein IIb/IIIa; LOE, level of evidence; UFH, unfractionated heparin. (Reproduced, with permission, from Wright RS et al. 2011 ACCF/AHA Focused Update of the Guidelines for the Management of Patients With Unstable Angina/Non-ST-Elevation Myocardial Infarction (Updating the 2007 Guideline): a report of the American College of Cardiology Foundation/American Heart Association Task Force on Practice Guidelines. Circulation. 2011 May 10; 123(18):2022–60. Erratum in: Circulation. 2011 Sep 20;124(12):e337–40; Circulation. 2011 Jun 7;123(22):e625–6. © 2011 American Heart Association, Inc.)

The ESC guidelines recommend ticagrelor for all patients at moderate to high risk for acute coronary syndrome (class I recommendation). Prasugrel is recommended for patients who have not yet received another $P2Y_{12}$ inhibitor, for whom a PCI is planned, and who are not at high risk for life-threatening bleeding. Clopidogrel is reserved for patients who cannot receive either ticagrelor or prasugrel. Some studies have shown an association between assays of residual platelet function and thrombotic risk during $P2Y_{12}$ inhibitor therapy, and both the European and the US guidelines do not recommend routine platelet function testing to guide therapy (class IIb recommendation).

Prasugrel is both more potent and has a faster onset of action than clopidogrel. The TRITON trial compared prasugrel with clopidogrel in patients with STEMI or NSTEMI in whom PCI was planned; prasugrel resulted in a 19% relative reduction in death from cardiovascular causes, MI, or stroke, at the expense of an increase in serious bleeding (including fatal bleeding). Stent thrombosis was reduced by half. Because patients with prior stroke or TIA had higher risk of intracranial hemorrhage, prasugrel is contraindicated in such patients. Bleeding was also higher in patients with low body weight (less than 60 kg) and age 75 years or older, and caution should be used in these populations. For patients with STEMI treated with PCI, prasugrel appears to be especially effective (compared to clopidogrel) without a substantial increase in bleeding. For patients who will not receive revascularization, prasugrel, when compared to clopidogrel, had no overall benefit in the TRILOGY trial (the dose of prasugrel was lowered for older adults).

Ticagrelor has a faster onset of action than clopidogrel and a more consistent and potent effect. The PLATO trial showed that when ticagrelor was started at the time of presentation in acute coronary syndrome patients (UA/ NSTEMI and STEMI), it reduced cardiovascular death, MI, and stroke by 16% when compared with clopidogrel. In addition, there was a 22% relative risk reduction in mortality with ticagrelor. The overall rates of bleeding were similar between ticagrelor and clopidogrel, although non–CABG-related bleeding was modestly higher. The finding of a lesser treatment effect in the United States may have been related to use of higher-dose aspirin, and thus when using ticagrelor, low-dose aspirin (81 mg/day) is recommended.

c. Glycoprotein IIb/IIIa inhibitors—Small-molecule inhibitors of the platelet glycoprotein IIb/IIIa receptor are useful adjuncts in high-risk patients (usually defined by fluctuating ST-segment depression or positive biomarkers) with acute coronary syndromes, particularly when they are undergoing PCI. Tirofiban, 25 mcg/kg over 3 minutes, followed by 0.15 mcg/kg/min, and eptifibatide, 180 mcg/kg bolus followed by a continuous infusion of 2 mcg/kg/min, have both been shown to be effective. Downward dose adjustments of the infusions are required in patients with reduced kidney function. The bolus or loading dose remains unadjusted. For example, if the estimated creatinine clearance is below 50 mL/min, the eptifibatide infusion should be cut in half to 1 mcg/kg/min.

2. Anticoagulant therapy

a. Heparin—Several trials have shown that LMWH (enoxaparin 1 mg/kg subcutaneously every 12 hours) is somewhat more effective than unfractionated heparin in preventing recurrent ischemic events in the setting of acute coronary syndromes. However, the SYNERGY trial showed that unfractionated heparin and enoxaparin had similar rates of death or (re)infarction in the setting of frequent early coronary intervention.

b. Fondaparinux—Fondaparinux, a specific factor Xa inhibitor given in a dose of 2.5 mg subcutaneously once a day, was found in the OASIS-5 trial to be equally effective as enoxaparin among 20,000 patients at preventing early death, MI, and refractory ischemia, and resulted in a 50% reduction in major bleeding. This reduction in major bleeding translated into a significant reduction in mortality (and in death or MI) at 30 days. While catheter-related thrombosis was more common during coronary intervention procedures with fondaparinux, the FUTURA trial found that it can be controlled by adding unfractionated heparin (in a dose of 85 units/kg without glycoprotein IIb/IIIa inhibitors, and 60 units/kg with glycoprotein IIb/IIIa inhibitors) during the procedure. Guidelines recommend fondaparinux, describing it as especially favorable for patients who are initially treated medically and who are at high risk for bleeding, such as elderly individuals.

c. Direct thrombin inhibitors—The ACUITY trial showed that bivalirudin appears to be a reasonable alternative to heparin (unfractionated heparin or enoxaparin) plus a glycoprotein IIb/IIIa antagonist for many patients with acute coronary syndromes who are undergoing early coronary intervention. Bivalirudin (without routine glycoprotein IIb/IIIa inhibitor) is associated with substantially less bleeding than heparin plus glycoprotein IIb/IIIa inhibitor, although it may have numerically increased cardiovascular events. The ISAR REACT-4 trial showed that bivalirudin has similar efficacy compared to abciximab but better bleeding outcomes in NSTEMI patients. Bivalrudin does not currently have an FDA-approved indication for NSTEMI care.

D. Temporary Discontinuation of Antiplatelet Therapy for Procedures

Patients who have had recent coronary stents are at risk for thrombotic events, including stent thrombosis, if $P2Y_{12}$ inhibitors are discontinued for procedures (eg, dental procedures or colonoscopy). If possible, these procedures should be delayed until the end of the necessary treatment period with $P2Y_{12}$ inhibitors, which generally is at least 1 month with bare metal stents and 3–6 months with drug-eluting stents. With newer generation drug-eluting stents, elective stenting patients with bleeding risk may have $P2Y_{12}$ inhibitors stopped before 3 months. Before that time, if a procedure is necessary, risk and benefit of continuing the antiplatelet therapy through the time of the procedure should be assessed. Aspirin should generally be continued throughout the period of the procedure. Patients with polymer-free drug coated stents who are at high risk for bleeding and receiving a short course of dual antiplatelet therapy had fewer cardiovascular and bleeding events. A cardiologist should be consulted before temporary discontinuation of these agents.

E. Nitroglycerin

Nitrates are first-line therapy for patients with acute coronary syndromes presenting with chest pain. Nonparenteral therapy with sublingual or oral agents or nitroglycerin ointment is usually sufficient. If pain persists or recurs, intravenous nitroglycerin should be started. The usual initial dosage is 10 mcg/min. The dosage should be titrated upward by 10–20 mcg/min (to a maximum of 200 mcg/min) until angina disappears or mean arterial pressure drops by 10%. Careful—usually continuous—BP monitoring is required when intravenous nitroglycerin is used. Avoid hypotension (systolic BP less than 100 mm Hg). Tolerance to continuous nitrate infusion is common.

F. Beta-Blockers

Beta-blockers are an important part of the initial treatment of unstable angina unless otherwise contraindicated. The pharmacology of these agents is discussed in Chapter 11 and summarized in Table 11–9. Use of agents with intrinsic sympathomimetic activity should be avoided in this setting. Oral medication is adequate in most patients, but intravenous treatment with metoprolol, given as three 5-mg doses 5 minutes apart as tolerated and in the absence of heart failure, achieves a more rapid effect. Oral therapy should be titrated upward as BP permits.

G. Calcium Channel Blockers

Calcium channel blockers have not been shown to favorably affect outcome in unstable angina, and they should be used primarily as third-line therapy in patients with continuing angina who are taking nitrates and beta-blockers or those who are not candidates for these medications. In the presence of nitrates and without accompanying beta-blockers, diltiazem or verapamil is preferred, since nifedipine and the other dihydropyridines are more likely to cause reflex tachycardia or hypotension. The initial dosage should be low, but upward titration should proceed steadily (see Table 11–7).

H. Statins

The PROVE-IT trial provides evidence for starting a statin in the days immediately following an acute coronary syndrome. In this trial, more intensive therapy with atorvastatin 80 mg/day, regardless of total or LDL cholesterol level, improved outcome compared to pravastatin 40 mg/day, with the curves of death or major cardiovascular event separating as early as 3 months after starting therapy. **High-dose statins are recommended for all patients with acute coronary syndromes** (see Table 10–7).

▶ Indications for Coronary Angiography

For patients with acute coronary syndrome, including NSTEMI, risk stratification is important for determining intensity of care. Several therapies, including glycoprotein IIb/IIIa inhibitors, LMWH heparin, and early invasive catheterization, have been shown to have the greatest benefit in higher-risk patients with acute coronary syndrome. As outlined in the ACC/AHA guidelines, patients with any high-risk feature (Table 10–9) generally warrant an early invasive strategy with catheterization and revascularization. For patients without these high-risk features, either an invasive or noninvasive approach, using exercise (or pharmacologic stress for patients unable to exercise) stress testing to identify patients who have residual ischemia and/or high risk, can be used. Moreover, based on the ICTUS trial, a strategy based on selective coronary angiography and revascularization for instability or inducible ischemia, or both, even for patients with positive troponin, is acceptable (ACC/AHA class IIb recommendation).

Two risk-stratification tools are available that can be used at the bedside, the **GRACE Risk Score** (http://www.outcomes-umassmed.org/grace) and the **TIMI Risk Score** (http://www.timi.org). The GRACE Risk Score, which applies to patients with or without ST elevation, was developed in a more generalizable registry population and includes Killip class, BP, ST-segment deviation, cardiac arrest at presentation, serum creatinine, elevated creatine

Table 10–9. Indications for catheterization and percutaneous coronary intervention.[1]

Acute coronary syndromes (unstable angina and non-ST elevation MI)	
Class I	Early invasive strategy for any of the following high-risk indicators:
	Recurrent angina/ischemia at rest or with low-level activity
	Elevated troponin
	ST-segment depression
	Recurrent ischemia with evidence of HF
	High-risk stress test result
	EF < 40%
	Hemodynamic instability
	Sustained ventricular tachycardia
	PCI within 6 months
	Prior CABG
	In the absence of these findings, either an early conservative or early invasive strategy
Class IIa	Early invasive strategy for patients with repeated presentations for ACS despite therapy
Class III	Extensive comorbidities in patients in whom benefits of revascularization are not likely to outweigh the risks
	Acute chest pain with low likelihood of ACS
Acute MI after fibrinolytic therapy	
Class I	Cardiogenic shock or acute severe heart failure that develops after initial presentation
	Intermediate or high-risk findings on predischarge noninvasive ischemia testing
	Spontaneous or easily provoked myocardial ischemia
Class IIa	Failed reperfusion or reocclusion after fibrinolytic therapy
	Stable[2] patients after successful fibrinolysis, before discharge and ideally between 3 and 24 hours

[1]Class I indicates treatment is useful and effective, IIa indicates weight of evidence is in favor of usefulness/efficacy, class IIb indicates weight of evidence is less well established, and class III indicates intervention is not useful/effective and may be harmful. Level of evidence A recommendations are derived from large-scale randomized trials, and B recommendations are derived from smaller randomized trials or carefully conducted observational analyses.

[2]Although individual circumstances will vary, clinical stability is defined by the absence of low output, hypotension, persistent tachycardia, apparent shock, high-grade ventricular or symptomatic supraventricular tachyarrhythmias, and spontaneous recurrent ischemia.

ACCF/AHA, American College of Cardiology Foundation/American Heart Association; ACS, acute coronary syndrome; CABG, coronary artery bypass grafting; EF, ejection fraction; HF, heart failure; MI, myocardial infarction; PCI, percutaneous coronary intervention.

Data from O'Gara PT et al. 2013 ACCF/AHA guideline for the management of ST-elevation myocardial infarction: a report of the American College of Cardiology Foundation/American Heart Association Task Force on Practice Guidelines. Circulation. 2013;127. e362–e425.

kinase (CK)-MB or troponin, and heart rate. The TIMI Risk Score includes seven variables: age 65 years or older, three or more cardiac risk factors, prior coronary stenosis of 50% or more, ST-segment deviation, two anginal events in prior 24 hours, aspirin in prior 7 days, and elevated cardiac markers.

When to Refer

- All patients with acute MI should be referred to a cardiologist.
- Patients who are taking a $P2Y_{12}$ inhibitor following coronary stenting should consult a cardiologist before discontinuing treatment for nonemergency procedures.

Fanaroff AC et al. JAMA patient page. Acute coronary syndrome. JAMA. 2015 Nov 10;314(18):1990. [PMID: 26547478]

Hamm CW et al. ESC guidelines for the management of acute coronary syndromes in patients presenting without persistent ST-segment elevation: the Task Force for the Management of Acute Coronary Syndromes (ACS) in Patients Presenting Without Persistent ST-Segment Elevation of the European Society of Cardiology (ESC). Eur Heart J. 2011 Dec; 32(23):2999–3054. [PMID: 21873419]

Jneid H et al. 2012 ACCF/AHA focused update of the guideline for the management of patients with unstable angina/non–ST-elevation myocardial infarction (updating the 2007 guideline and replacing the 2011 focused update): a report of the American College of Cardiology Foundation/American Heart Association Task Force on Practice Guidelines. Circulation. 2012 Aug 14;126(7):875–910. [PMID: 22800849]

Levine GN et al. 2016 ACC/AHA Guideline focused update on duration of dual antiplatelet therapy in patients with coronary artery disease: a report of the American College of Cardiology/ American Heart Association Task Force on Clinical Practice Guidelines: An update of the 2011 ACCF/AHA/SCAI guideline for percutaneous coronary intervention, 2011 ACCF/ AHA guideline for coronary artery bypass graft surgery, 2012 ACC/AHA/ACP/AATS/PCNA/SCAI/STS guideline for the diagnosis and management of patients with stable ischemic heart disease, 2013 ACCF/AHA guideline for the management of ST-elevation myocardial infarction, 2014 AHA/ACC guideline for the management of patients with non–ST-elevation acute coronary syndromes, and 2014 ACC/AHA guideline on perioperative cardiovascular evaluation and management of patients undergoing noncardiac surgery. Circulation. 2016 Sep 6;134(10):e123–55. Erratum in: Circulation. 2016 Sep 6;134(10):e192–4. [PMID: 27026020]

Urban P et al; LEADERS FREE Investigators. Polymer-free drug-coated coronary stents in patients at high bleeding risk. N Engl J Med. 2015 Nov 19;373(21):2038–47. [PMID: 26466021]

ACUTE MYOCARDIAL INFARCTION WITH ST-SEGMENT ELEVATION

ESSENTIALS OF DIAGNOSIS

- ► Sudden but not instantaneous development of prolonged (more than 30 minutes) anterior chest discomfort (sometimes felt as "gas" or pressure).
- ► Sometimes painless, masquerading as acute heart failure, syncope, stroke, or shock.

- ► ECG: ST-segment elevation or left bundle branch block.
- ► Immediate reperfusion treatment is warranted.
- ► Primary PCI within 90 minutes of first medical contact is the goal and is superior to fibrinolytic therapy.
- ► Fibrinolytic therapy within 30 minutes of hospital presentation is the goal, and reduces mortality if given within 12 hours of onset of symptoms.

General Considerations

STEMI results, in most cases, from an occlusive coronary thrombus at the site of a preexisting (though not necessarily severe) atherosclerotic plaque. More rarely, infarction may result from prolonged vasospasm, inadequate myocardial blood flow (eg, hypotension), or excessive metabolic demand. Very rarely, MI may be caused by embolic occlusion, vasculitis, aortic root or coronary artery dissection, or aortitis. Cocaine, a cause of infarction, should be considered in young individuals without risk factors. A condition that may mimic STEMI is stress cardiomyopathy (also referred to as **tako-tsubo** or **apical ballooning syndrome**). ST elevation connotes an acute coronary occlusion and warrants *immediate* reperfusion therapy with activation of emergency services.

Clinical Findings

A. Symptoms

1. Premonitory pain—There is usually a worsening in the pattern of angina preceding the onset of symptoms of MI; classically the onset of angina occurs with minimal exertion or at rest.

2. Pain of infarction—Unlike anginal episodes, most infarctions occur *at rest*, and more commonly in the early morning. The pain is similar to angina in location and radiation but it may be more severe, and it builds up rapidly or in waves to maximum intensity over a few minutes or longer. Nitroglycerin has little effect; even opioids may not relieve the pain.

3. Associated symptoms—Patients may break out in a cold sweat, feel weak and apprehensive, and move about, seeking a position of comfort. They prefer not to lie quietly. Light-headedness, syncope, dyspnea, orthopnea, cough, wheezing, nausea and vomiting, or abdominal bloating may be present singly or in any combination.

4. Painless infarction—One-third of patients with acute MI present *without* chest pain, and these patients tend to be undertreated and have poor outcomes. Older patients, women, and patients with diabetes mellitus are more likely to present without chest pain. As many as 25% of infarctions are detected on routine ECG without any recallable acute episode.

5. Sudden death and early arrhythmias—Of all deaths from MI, about 50% occur before the patients arrive at the hospital, with death presumably caused by ventricular fibrillation.

B. Signs

1. General—Patients may appear anxious and sometimes are sweating profusely. The heart rate may range from marked bradycardia (most commonly in inferior infarction) to tachycardia, low cardiac output, or arrhythmia. The BP may be high, especially in former hypertensive patients, or low in patients with shock. Respiratory distress usually indicates heart failure. Fever, usually low grade, may appear after 12 hours and persist for several days.

2. Chest—The **Killip classification** is the standard way to classify heart failure in patients with acute MI and has powerful prognostic value. Killip class I is absence of rales and S_3, class II is rales that do not clear with coughing over one-third or less of the lung fields or presence of an S_3, class III is rales that do not clear with coughing over more than one-third of the lung fields, and class IV is cardiogenic shock (rales, hypotension, and signs of hypoperfusion).

3. Heart—The cardiac examination may be unimpressive or very abnormal. Jugular venous distention reflects RA hypertension, and a Kussmaul sign (failure of decrease of jugular venous pressure with inspiration) is suggestive of RV infarction. Soft heart sounds may indicate LV dysfunction. Atrial gallops (S_4) are the rule, whereas ventricular gallops (S_3) are less common and indicate significant LV dysfunction. Mitral regurgitation murmurs are not uncommon and may indicate papillary muscle dysfunction or, rarely, rupture. Pericardial friction rubs are uncommon in the first 24 hours but may appear later.

4. Extremities—Edema is usually not present. Cyanosis and cold temperature indicate low output. The peripheral pulses should be noted, since later shock or emboli may alter the examination.

C. Laboratory Findings

Cardiac-specific markers of myocardial damage include quantitative determinations of CK-MB, highly sensitive and conventional troponin I, and troponin T. Each of these tests may become positive as early as 4–6 hours after the onset of an MI and should be abnormal by 8–12 hours. Troponins are more sensitive and specific than CK-MB. "Highly sensitive" or "fourth-generation" troponin assays were approved in 2017 and are being used in the United States. They are the standard assays in most of Europe, with a 10- to 100-fold lower limit of detection, allowing MI to be detected earlier, using the change in value over 3 hours.

Circulating levels of troponins may remain elevated for 5–7 days or longer and therefore are generally not useful for evaluating suspected early reinfarction. Elevated CK-MB generally normalizes within 24 hours, thus being more helpful for evaluation of reinfarction. Low-level elevations of troponin in patients with severe chronic kidney disease may not be related to acute coronary disease but rather a function of the physiologic washout of the marker. While many conditions including chronic heart failure are associated with elevated levels of the high-sensitivity troponin assays, these assays may be especially useful when negative to exclude MI in patients reporting chest pain.

D. ECG

The extent of the ECG abnormalities, especially the sum of the total amount of ST-segment deviation, is a good indicator of the extent of acute infarction and risk of subsequent adverse events. The classic evolution of changes is from peaked ("hyperacute") T waves, to ST-segment elevation, to Q wave development, to T wave inversion. This may occur over a few hours to several days. The evolution of new Q waves (longer than 30 msec in duration and 25% of the R wave amplitude) is diagnostic, but Q waves do not occur in 30–50% of acute infarctions (**non-Q wave infarctions**). Left bundle branch block, especially when new (or not known to be old), in a patient with symptoms of an acute MI is considered to be a **"STEMI equivalent"**; reperfusion therapy is indicated for the affected patient. Concordant ST elevation (ie, ST elevation in leads with an overall positive QRS complex) with left bundle branch block is a specific finding indicating STEMI.

E. Chest Radiography

The chest radiograph may demonstrate signs of heart failure, but these changes often lag behind the clinical findings. Signs of aortic dissection, including mediastinal widening, should be sought as a possible alternative diagnosis.

F. Echocardiography

Echocardiography provides convenient bedside assessment of LV global and regional function. This can help with the diagnosis and management of infarction; echocardiography has been used successfully to make judgments about admission and management of patients with suspected infarction, including in patients with ST-segment elevation or left bundle branch block of uncertain significance, since normal wall motion makes an infarction unlikely. Doppler echocardiography is generally the most convenient procedure for diagnosing postinfarction mitral regurgitation or VSD.

G. Other Noninvasive Studies

Diagnosis of MI and extent of MI can be assessed by various imaging studies in addition to echocardiography. **MRI with gadolinium contrast enhancement** is the most sensitive test to detect and quantitate extent of infarction, with the ability to detect as little as 2 g of MI. **Technetium-99m pyrophosphate scintigraphy,** when injected at least 18 hours postinfarction, complexes with calcium in necrotic myocardium to provide a "hot spot" image of the infarction. This test is insensitive to small infarctions, and false-positive studies occur, so its use is limited to patients in whom the diagnosis by ECG and enzymes is not possible—principally those who present several days after the event or have intraoperative infarctions. **Scintigraphy with thallium-201** or **technetium-based perfusion tracers** will demonstrate "cold spots" in regions of diminished perfusion, which usually represent infarction when the radiotracer is administered at rest, but abnormalities do not distinguish recent from old damage. All of these tests may be considered after the patient has had revascularization.

H. Hemodynamic Measurements

These can be helpful in managing the patient with suspected cardiogenic shock. Use of PA catheters, however, has generally not been associated with better outcomes and should be limited to patients with severe hemodynamic compromise for whom the information would be anticipated to change management.

▶ Treatment

A. Aspirin, P2Y$_{12}$ Inhibitors (Prasugrel, Ticagrelor, and Clopidogrel)

All patients with definite or suspected acute MI should receive aspirin at a dose of 162 mg or 325 mg at once regardless of whether fibrinolytic therapy is being considered or the patient has been taking aspirin. Chewable aspirin provides more rapid blood levels. Patients with a definite aspirin allergy should be treated with a P2Y$_{12}$ inhibitor (clopidogrel, prasugrel, or ticagrelor).

P2Y$_{12}$ inhibitors, in combination with aspirin, have been shown to provide important benefits in patients with acute STEMI. Thus, guidelines call for a **P2Y$_{12}$ inhibitor to be added to aspirin for all patients with STEMI,** regardless of whether reperfusion is given, and continued for at least 14 days, and generally for 1 year. The preferred P2Y$_{12}$ inhibitors are prasugrel (60 mg orally on day 1, then 10 mg daily) or ticagrelor (180 mg orally on day 1, then 90 mg twice daily). Both of these medications demonstrated superior outcomes to clopidogrel in clinical studies of primary PCI. Clopidogrel should be administered as a loading dose of 300–600 mg orally for faster onset of action than the 75 mg maintenance dose. With fibrinolytic therapy, ticagrelor appears to be a reasonable alternative to clopidogrel, at least after an initial clopidogrel dose. Prasugrel is contraindicated in patients with history of stroke or who are older than 75 years.

B. Reperfusion Therapy

Patients with STEMI who seek medical attention within 12 hours of the onset of symptoms should be treated with reperfusion therapy, either primary PCI or fibrinolytic therapy. Patients without ST-segment elevation (previously labeled "non-Q wave" infarctions) do not benefit, and may derive harm, from thrombolysis.

1. Primary percutaneous coronary intervention— Immediate coronary angiography and primary PCI (including stenting) of the infarct-related artery have been shown to be *superior* to thrombolysis when done by experienced operators in high-volume centers with rapid time from first medical contact to intervention ("door-to-balloon"). US and European guidelines call for first medical contact or door-to-balloon times of 90 minutes or less. Several trials have shown that if efficient transfer systems are in place, transfer of patients with acute MI from hospitals without primary PCI capability to hospitals with primary PCI capability with first door-to-device times of 120 minutes or less can improve outcome compared with fibrinolytic therapy at the presenting hospital, although this requires sophisticated systems to ensure rapid identification, transfer, and expertise in PCI. Because PCI also carries a lower risk of hemorrhagic complications, including intracranial hemorrhage, it may be the preferred strategy in many older patients and others with contraindications to fibrinolytic therapy (see Table 10–10 for factors to consider in choosing fibrinolytic therapy or primary PCI).

A. STENTING—PCI with stenting is standard for patients with acute MI. Although randomized trials have shown a benefit with regard to fewer repeat interventions for restenosis with the use of drug-eluting stents in STEMI patients, and current generation drug-eluting stents have similar or lower rates of stent thrombosis than bare metal stents, bare metal stents may still be used for selected patients without the ability to obtain and comply with P2Y$_{12}$ inhibitor therapy. In the subgroup of patients with cardiogenic shock, early catheterization and percutaneous or surgical revascularization are the preferred management and have been shown to reduce mortality.

"Facilitated" PCI, whereby a combination of medications (full- or reduced-dose fibrinolytic agents, with or without glycoprotein IIb/IIIa inhibitors) is given followed by immediate PCI, is not recommended. Patients should be treated either with primary PCI or with fibrinolytic agents (and immediate rescue PCI for reperfusion failure), if it can be done promptly as outlined in the ACC/AHA and European guidelines. Timely access to most appropriate reperfusion, including primary PCI, can be expanded with development of regional systems of care, including emergency medical systems and networks of hospitals. Patients treated with fibrinolytic therapy appear to have improved outcomes if transferred for routine coronary angiography and PCI within 24 hours. The AHA has a program called "Mission: Lifeline" to support the development of regional systems of care (http://www.heart.org/missionlifeline).

B. ANTIPLATELET THERAPY AFTER DRUG-ELUTING OR BARE METAL STENTS—In patients with an acute coronary syndrome, **dual antiplatelet therapy** is indicated for 1 year in all patients (including those with medical therapy and those patients undergoing revascularization irrespective of stent type). For patients undergoing elective or stable PCI, the duration of dual antiplatelet therapy is recommended for at least 1 month for patients receiving bare metal stents. For patients receiving drug-eluting stents for acute coronary syndromes, dual antiplatelet therapy is recommended for at least 1 year by the ACC/AHA and European guidelines. These recommendations are based both on the durations of therapies during the studies evaluating the stents, and the pathophysiologic understanding of the timing of endothelialization following bare metal versus drug-eluting stent implantation. The DAPT (Dual Antiplatelet Therapy) study showed fewer death, MI, and stroke events with longer (up to 30 months) dual antiplatelet therapy for patients who had received drug-eluting stents, but it also showed more bleeding and a tendency for higher mortality. Treatment with clopidogrel for longer than 1 year after drug-eluting stents, therefore, should be individualized based on thrombotic and bleeding risks.

2. Fibrinolytic therapy

A. Benefit—Fibrinolytic therapy reduces mortality and limits infarct size in patients with STEMI (defined as 0.1 mV or more in two inferior or lateral leads or two contiguous precordial leads), or with left bundle branch block (not known to be old). The greatest benefit occurs if treatment is initiated within the first 3 hours after the onset of presentation, when up to a 50% reduction in mortality rate can be achieved. The magnitude of benefit declines rapidly thereafter, but a 10% relative mortality reduction can be achieved up to 12 hours after the onset of chest pain. The survival benefit is greatest in patients with large—usually anterior—infarctions. Primary PCI (including stenting) of the infarct-related artery, however, is superior to thrombolysis when done by experienced operators with rapid time from first medical contact to intervention ("door-to-balloon").

B. Contraindications—Major bleeding complications occur in 0.5–5% of patients, the most serious of which is intracranial hemorrhage. The major risk factors for intracranial bleeding are age 75 years or older, hypertension at presentation (especially over 180/110 mm Hg), low body weight (less than 70 kg), and the use of fibrin-specific fibrinolytic agents (alteplase, reteplase, tenecteplase). Although patients over age 75 years have a much higher mortality rate with acute MI and therefore may derive greater benefit, the risk of severe bleeding is also higher, particularly among patients with risk factors for intracranial hemorrhage, such as severe hypertension or recent stroke. Patients presenting more than 12 hours after the onset of chest pain may also derive a small benefit, particularly if pain and ST-segment elevation persist, but rarely does this benefit outweigh the attendant risk.

Absolute contraindications to fibrinolytic therapy include previous hemorrhagic stroke, other strokes or cerebrovascular events within 1 year, known intracranial neoplasm, recent head trauma (including minor trauma), active internal bleeding (excluding menstruation), or suspected aortic dissection. Relative contraindications are BP greater than 180/110 mm Hg at presentation, other intracerebral pathology not listed above as a contraindication, known bleeding diathesis, trauma within 2–4 weeks, major surgery within 3 weeks, prolonged (more than 10 minutes) or traumatic cardiopulmonary resuscitation, recent (within 2–4 weeks) internal bleeding, noncompressible vascular punctures, active diabetic retinopathy, pregnancy, active peptic ulcer disease, a history of severe hypertension, current use of anticoagulants (INR greater than 2.0–3.0), and (for streptokinase) prior allergic reaction or exposure to streptokinase or anistreplase within 2 years.

C. Fibrinolytic agents—The following fibrinolytic agents are available for acute MI and are characterized in Table 10–10.

Table 10–10. Fibrinolytic therapy for acute myocardial infarction.

	Alteplase; Tissue Plasminogen Activator (t-PA)	Reteplase	Tenecteplase (TNK-t-PA)	Streptokinase
Source	Recombinant DNA	Recombinant DNA	Recombinant DNA	Group C *Streptococcus*
Half-life	5 minutes	15 minutes	20 minutes	20 minutes
Usual dose	100 mg	20 units	40 mg	1.5 million units
Administration	Initial bolus of 15 mg, followed by 50 mg infused over the next 30 minutes and 35 mg over the following 60 minutes	10 units as a bolus over 2 minutes, repeated after 30 minutes	Single weight-adjusted bolus, 0.5 mg/kg	750,000 units over 20 minutes followed by 750,000 units over 40 minutes
Anticoagulation after infusion	Aspirin, 325 mg daily; heparin, 5000 units as bolus, followed by 1000 units per hour infusion, subsequently adjusted to maintain PTT 1.5–2 times control	Aspirin, 325 mg; heparin as with t-PA	Aspirin, 325 mg daily	Aspirin, 325 mg daily; there is no evidence that adjunctive heparin improves outcome following streptokinase
Clot selectivity	High	High	High	Low
Fibrinogenolysis	+	+	+	+++
Bleeding	+	+	+	+
Hypotension	+	+	+	+++
Allergic reactions	+	+	+	++
Reocclusion	10–30%	—	5–20%	5–20%
Approximate cost[1]	$10,560.43	$5964.98	$7034.24	Not available in the United States

[1]Average wholesale price (AWP, for AB-rated generic when available) for quantity listed.
PTT, partial thromboplastin time.
Source: IBM Micromedex, Red Book (electronic version). IBM Watson Health, Greenwood Village, CO, USA. Available at https://www.microdexsolutions.com (cited March 12, 2019). AWP may not accurately represent the actual pharmacy cost because wide contractual variations exist among institutions.

Alteplase (recombinant tissue plasminogen activator; t-PA) results in about a 50% reduction in circulating fibrinogen. In the first GUSTO trial, which compared a 90-minute dosing of t-PA (with unfractionated heparin) with streptokinase, the 30-day mortality rate with t-PA was one absolute percentage point lower (one additional life saved per 100 patients treated), though there was also a small increase in the rate of intracranial hemorrhage. An angiographic substudy confirmed a higher 90-minute patency rate and a higher rate of normal (TIMI grade 3) flow in patients.

Reteplase is a recombinant deletion mutant of t-PA that is slightly less fibrin specific. In comparative trials, it appeared to have efficacy similar to that of alteplase, but it has a longer duration of action and can be administered as two boluses 30 minutes apart.

Tenecteplase (TNK-t-PA) is a genetically engineered substitution mutant of native t-PA that has reduced plasma clearance, increased fibrin sensitivity, and increased resistance to plasminogen activator inhibitor-1. It can be given as a single weight-adjusted bolus. In the ASSENT 2 trial, this agent was equivalent to t-PA with regard to efficacy and resulted in significantly less noncerebral bleeding.

Streptokinase, commonly used outside of the United States, is somewhat less effective at opening occluded arteries and less effective at reducing mortality. It is non–fibrin-specific, causes depletion of circulating fibrinogen, and has a tendency to induce hypotension, particularly if infused rapidly. This can be managed by slowing or interrupting the infusion and administering fluids. There is controversy as to whether adjunctive heparin is beneficial in patients given streptokinase, unlike its administration with the more clot-specific agents. Allergic reactions, including anaphylaxis, occur in 1–2% of patients, and this agent should generally not be administered to patients with prior exposure.

(1) Selection of a fibrinolytic agent—In the United States, most patients are treated with alteplase, reteplase, or tenecteplase. The differences in efficacy between them are small compared with the potential benefit of treating a greater proportion of appropriate candidates in a more prompt manner. The principal objective should be to administer a thrombolytic agent within 30 minutes of presentation—or even during transport. The ability to administer tenecteplase as a single bolus is an attractive feature that may facilitate earlier treatment. The combination of a reduced-dose thrombolytic given with a platelet glycoprotein IIb/IIIa inhibitor does not reduce mortality but does cause a modest increase in bleeding complications.

(2) Postfibrinolytic management—After completion of the fibrinolytic infusion, aspirin (81–325 mg/day) and anticoagulation should be continued until revascularization or for the duration of the hospital stay (or up to 8 days). Anticoagulation with LMWH (enoxaparin or fondaparinux) is preferable to unfractionated heparin.

(A) Low-molecular-weight heparin—In the EXTRACT trial, enoxaparin significantly reduced death and MI at day 30 (compared with unfractionated heparin), at the expense of a modest increase in bleeding. In patients younger than age 75, enoxaparin was given as a 30-mg intravenous bolus and 1 mg/kg subcutaneously every 12 hours; in patients aged 75 years and older, it was given with no bolus and 0.75 mg/kg subcutaneously every 12 hours. This appeared to attenuate the risk of intracranial hemorrhage in older adults that had been seen with full-dose enoxaparin. Another antithrombotic option is fondaparinux, given at a dose of 2.5 mg subcutaneously once a day. There is no benefit of fondaparinux among patients undergoing primary PCI, and fondaparinux is not recommended as a sole anticoagulant during PCI due to risk of catheter thrombosis.

(B) Unfractionated heparin—Anticoagulation with intravenous heparin (initial dose of 60 units/kg bolus to a maximum of 4000 units, followed by an infusion of 12 units/kg/h to a maximum of 1000 units/hour, then adjusted to maintain an aPTT of 50–75 seconds beginning with an aPTT drawn 3 hours after thrombolytic) is continued for at least 48 hours after alteplase, reteplase, or tenecteplase, and with continuation of an anticoagulant until revascularization (if performed) or until hospital discharge (or day 8).

The VALIDATE trial found no benefit to bivalirudin compared to unfractionated heparin regarding the outcome of death, MI, or major bleeding.

(C) Prophylactic therapy against gastrointestinal bleeding—For all patients with STEMI treated with intensive antithrombotic therapy, prophylactic treatment with proton-pump inhibitors, or antacids and an H_2-blocker, is advisable, although certain proton-pump inhibitors, such as omeprazole and esomeprazole, decrease the effect of clopidogrel.

3. Assessment of myocardial reperfusion, recurrent ischemic pain, reinfarction—Myocardial reperfusion can be recognized clinically by the early cessation of pain and the resolution of ST-segment elevation. Although at least 50% resolution of ST-segment elevation by 90 minutes may occur without coronary reperfusion, ST resolution is a strong predictor of better outcome. Even with anticoagulation, 10–20% of reperfused vessels will reocclude during hospitalization, although reocclusion and reinfarction appear to be reduced following intervention. Reinfarction, indicated by recurrence of pain and ST-segment elevation, can be treated by readministration of a thrombolytic agent or immediate angiography and PCI.

C. General Measures

Cardiac care unit monitoring should be instituted as soon as possible. Patients without complications can be transferred to a telemetry unit after 24 hours. Activity should initially be limited to bed rest but can be advanced within 24 hours. Progressive ambulation should be started after 24–72 hours if tolerated. For patients without complications, discharge by day 4 appears to be appropriate. Low-flow oxygen therapy (2–4 L/min) should be given if oxygen saturation is reduced, but there is no value to routine use of oxygen.

D. Analgesia

An initial attempt should be made to relieve pain with sublingual nitroglycerin. However, if no response occurs after two or three tablets, intravenous opioids provide the most rapid and effective analgesia and may also reduce pulmonary congestion. Morphine sulfate, 4–8 mg, or meperidine, 50–75 mg, should be given. Subsequent small doses can be given every 15 minutes until pain abates.

Nonsteroidal anti-inflammatory agents, other than aspirin, should be avoided during hospitalization for STEMI due to increased risk of mortality, myocardial rupture, hypertension, heart failure, and kidney injury with their use.

E. Beta-Adrenergic Blocking Agents

Trials have shown modest short-term benefit from beta-blockers started during the first 24 hours after acute MI if there are no contraindications (metoprolol 25–50 mg orally twice daily). Aggressive beta-blockade can increase shock, with overall harm in patients with heart failure. Thus, early beta-blockade should be avoided in patients with any degree of heart failure, evidence of low output state, increased risk of cardiogenic shock, or other relative contraindications to beta-blockade. Carvedilol (beginning at 6.25 mg twice a day, titrated to 25 mg twice a day) was shown to be beneficial in the CAPRICORN trial following the acute phase of large MI.

F. Nitrates

Nitroglycerin is the agent of choice for continued or recurrent ischemic pain and is useful in lowering BP or relieving pulmonary congestion. However, routine nitrate administration is not recommended, since no improvement in outcome has been observed in the ISIS-4 or GISSI-3 trials. Nitrates should be avoided in patients who received phosphodiesterase inhibitors (sildenafil, vardenafil, and tadalafil) in the prior 24 hours.

G. Angiotensin-Converting Enzyme (ACE) Inhibitors

A series of trials (SAVE, AIRE, SMILE, TRACE, GISSI-III, and ISIS-4) have shown both short- and long-term improvement in survival with ACE inhibitor therapy. The benefits are greatest in patients with an EF of 40% or less, large infarctions, or clinical evidence of heart failure. Because substantial amounts of the survival benefit occur on the first day, ACE inhibitor treatment should be commenced early in patients without hypotension, especially patients with large or anterior MI. Given the benefits of ACE inhibitors for patients with vascular disease, it is reasonable to **use ACE inhibitors for *all* patients following STEMI who do not have contraindications.**

H. Angiotensin Receptor Blockers

Although there has been inconsistency in the effects of different ARBs on mortality for patients post-MI with heart failure and/or LV dysfunction, the VALIANT trial showed that valsartan 160 mg orally twice a day is equivalent to captopril in reducing mortality. Thus, valsartan should be used for all patients with ACE inhibitor intolerance, and is a reasonable, albeit more expensive, alternative to captopril. The combination of captopril and valsartan (at a reduced dose) was no better than either agent alone and resulted in more side effects.

I. Aldosterone Antagonists

The RALES trial showed that 25-mg spironolactone can reduce the mortality rate of patients with advanced heart failure, and the EPHESUS trial showed a 15% relative risk reduction in mortality with eplerenone 25 mg daily for patients post-MI with LV dysfunction (LVEF of 40% or less) and either clinical heart failure or diabetes. Kidney dysfunction or hyperkalemia are contraindications, and patients must be monitored carefully for development of hyperkalemia.

J. Calcium Channel Blockers

There are no studies to support the routine use of calcium channel blockers in most patients with acute MI—and indeed, they have the potential to exacerbate ischemia and cause death from reflex tachycardia or myocardial depression. Long-acting calcium channel blockers should generally be reserved for management of hypertension or ischemia as second- or third-line medications after beta-blockers and nitrates.

K. Long-Term Antithrombotic Therapy

Discharge on aspirin, 81–325 mg/day, since it is highly effective, inexpensive, and well tolerated, is a key quality indicator of MI care. Patients who received a coronary stent should also receive a $P2Y_{12}$ inhibitor (see Antiplatelet therapy after drug-eluting or bare metal stents, above).

Patients who have received a coronary stent and who require warfarin anticoagulation present a particular challenge, since **"triple therapy"** with aspirin, clopidogrel, and warfarin has a high risk of bleeding. Triple therapy should be (1) limited to patients with a clear indication for warfarin (such as $CHADS_2$ score of 2 or more or a mechanical prosthetic valve), (2) used for the shortest period of time (such as 1 month after placement of bare metal stent; drug-eluting stents that would require longer clopidogrel duration should be avoided if possible), (3) used with low-dose aspirin and with strategies to reduce risk of bleeding (eg, proton-pump inhibitors for patients with a history of gastrointestinal bleeding), and (4) used with consideration of a lower target anticoagulation intensity (INR 2.0–2.5, at least for the indication of atrial fibrillation) during the period of concomitant treatment with aspirin and $P2Y_{12}$ therapy. The PIONEER trial studied three treatment regimens for patients with atrial fibrillation who had coronary stent placement with a primary outcome of bleeding: (1) rivaroxaban 2.5 mg twice daily plus clopidogrel, (2) rivaroxaban 15 mg once daily plus clopidogrel, and (3) warfarin plus aspirin plus clopidogrel. There was less bleeding in the patients who received rivaroxaban plus clopidogrel than in those who received "triple therapy," although the trial was not powered to assess efficacy, and thus the low dose of rivaroxaban may be inadequate. Consensus statements recommend oral anticoagulation (with either warfarin or a DOAC) be combined with clopidogrel and with a relatively short duration of aspirin until hospital discharge up to 3 months for the typical patient with atrial fibrillation and coronary stents. Dabigatran, 110 mg and 150 mg, was also studied in patients with atrial fibrillation who underwent PCI.

Dual therapy with dabigatran and clopidogrel was shown to be beneficial for bleeding compared to triple therapy, with similar rates of thrombotic cardiovascular events. However, there were too few thrombotic events to be certain about efficacy of discontinuing the aspirin, and there was a suggestion that MI and stent thrombosis occurred more often with the 110-mg dose of dabigatran than with clopidogrel alone. Given the trial evidence to date, for a typical patient, it is reasonable to use a DOAC and clopidogrel and to discontinue aspirin at the time of hospital discharge.

L. Coronary Angiography

For patients who do not reperfuse based on lack of at least 50% resolution of ST elevation, rescue angioplasty should be performed and has been shown to reduce the composite risk of death, reinfarction, stroke, or severe heart failure. Patients treated with coronary angiography and PCI 3–24 hours after fibrinolytic therapy showed improved outcomes. Patients with recurrent ischemic pain prior to discharge should undergo catheterization and, if indicated, revascularization. PCI of a totally occluded infarct-related artery more than 24 hours after STEMI should generally not be performed in asymptomatic patients with one or two vessel disease without evidence of severe ischemia.

▶ When to Refer

All patients with acute MI should be referred to a cardiologist.

Cannon CP et al; RE-DUAL PCI Steering Committee and Investigators. Dual antithrombotic therapy with dabigatran after PCI in atrial fibrillation. N Engl J Med. 2017 Oct 19;377(16): 1513–24. [PMID: 28844193]
Erlinge D et al. Bivalirudin versus heparin monotherapy in myocardial infarction. N Engl J Med. 2017 Sep 21;377(12): 1132–42. [PMID: 28844201]

▶ Complications

A variety of complications can occur after MI even when treatment is initiated promptly.

A. Postinfarction Ischemia

In clinical trials of thrombolysis, recurrent ischemia occurred in about one-third of patients, was more common following NSTEMI than after STEMI, and had important short- and long-term prognostic implications. Vigorous medical therapy should be instituted, including nitrates and beta-blockers as well as aspirin 81–325 mg/day, anticoagulant therapy (unfractionated heparin, enoxaparin, or fondaparinux) and clopidogrel (75 mg orally daily). Most patients with postinfarction angina—and all who are refractory to medical therapy—should undergo early catheterization and revascularization by PCI or CABG.

B. Arrhythmias

Abnormalities of rhythm and conduction are common.

1. Sinus bradycardia—This is most common in inferior infarctions or may be precipitated by medications.

Observation or withdrawal of the offending agent is usually sufficient. If accompanied by signs of low cardiac output, atropine intravenously is usually effective. Temporary pacing is rarely required.

2. Supraventricular tachyarrhythmias—Sinus tachycardia is common and may reflect either increased adrenergic stimulation or hemodynamic compromise due to hypovolemia or pump failure. In the latter, beta-blockade is contraindicated. Supraventricular premature beats are common and may be premonitory for atrial fibrillation. Electrolyte abnormalities and hypoxia should be corrected and causative agents (especially aminophylline) stopped. Atrial fibrillation should be rapidly controlled or converted to sinus rhythm. Intravenous beta-blockers, such as metoprolol (2.5–5 mg intravenously every 2–5 minutes, maximum 15 mg over 10–minutes) or short-acting esmolol (50–200 mcg/kg/min), are the agents of choice if cardiac function is adequate. Intravenous diltiazem (5–15 mg/h) may be used if beta-blockers are contraindicated or ineffective. Electrical cardioversion (commencing with 100 J) may be necessary if atrial fibrillation is complicated by hypotension, heart failure, or ischemia, but the arrhythmia often recurs. Amiodarone (150 mg intravenous bolus and then 15–30 mg/h intravenously, or rapid oral loading dose for cardioversion of 400 mg three times daily) may be helpful to restore or maintain sinus rhythm.

3. Ventricular arrhythmias—Ventricular arrhythmias are most common in the first few hours after infarction and are a marker of high risk. Ventricular premature beats may be premonitory for ventricular tachycardia or fibrillation, but generally should *not* be treated in the absence of frequent or sustained ventricular tachycardia. Lidocaine is *not* recommended as a prophylactic measure.

Sustained ventricular tachycardia should be treated with a 1 mg/kg bolus of lidocaine if the patient is stable or by electrical cardioversion (100–200 J) if not. If the arrhythmia cannot be suppressed with lidocaine, procainamide (100 mg boluses over 1–2 minutes every 5 minutes to a cumulative dose of 750–1000 mg) or intravenous amiodarone (150 mg over 10 minutes, which may be repeated as needed, followed by 360 mg over 6 hours and then 540 mg over 18 hours) should be initiated, followed by an infusion of 0.5 mg/min (720 mg/24 hours). Ventricular fibrillation is treated electrically (300–400 J). All patients taking antiarrhythmics should be monitored with telemetry or ECGs during initiation. Unresponsive ventricular fibrillation should be treated with additional amiodarone and repeat cardioversion while cardiopulmonary resuscitation (CPR) is administered.

Accelerated idioventricular rhythm is a regular, wide-complex rhythm at a rate of 60–120/min. It may occur with or without reperfusion and should not be treated with antiarrhythmics, which could cause asystole.

4. Conduction disturbances—All degrees of AV block may occur in the course of acute MI. Block at the level of the AV node is more common than infranodal block and occurs in approximately 20% of inferior MIs. First-degree block is the most common and requires no treatment. Second-degree block is usually of the Mobitz type I form

(Wenckebach), is often transient, and requires treatment only if associated with a heart rate slow enough to cause symptoms. Complete AV block occurs in up to 5% of acute inferior infarctions, usually is preceded by Mobitz I second-degree block, and generally resolves spontaneously, though it may persist for hours to several weeks. The escape rhythm originates in the distal AV node or AV junction and hence has a narrow QRS complex and is reliable, albeit often slow (30–50 beats/min). Treatment is often necessary because of resulting hypotension and low cardiac output. Intravenous atropine (1 mg) usually restores AV conduction temporarily, but if the escape complex is wide or if repeated atropine treatments are needed, temporary ventricular pacing is indicated. The prognosis for these patients is only slightly worse than for patients in whom AV block does not develop.

In anterior infarctions, the site of block is distal, below the AV node, and usually a result of extensive damage of the His-Purkinje system and bundle branches. New first-degree block (prolongation of the PR interval) is unusual in anterior infarction; Mobitz type II AV block or complete heart block may be preceded by intraventricular conduction defects or may occur abruptly. The escape rhythm, if present, is an unreliable wide-complex idioventricular rhythm. Urgent ventricular pacing is mandatory, but even with successful pacing, morbidity and mortality are high because of the extensive myocardial damage. New conduction abnormalities, such as right or left bundle branch block or fascicular blocks, may presage progression, often sudden, to second- or third-degree AV block. Temporary ventricular pacing is recommended for new-onset alternating bilateral bundle branch block, bifascicular block, or bundle branch block with worsening first-degree AV block. Patients with anterior infarction who progress to second- or third-degree block even transiently should be considered for insertion of a prophylactic permanent ventricular pacemaker before discharge.

C. Myocardial Dysfunction

Persons with hypotension not responsive to fluid resuscitation or refractory heart failure or cardiogenic shock should be considered for urgent echocardiography to assess left and right ventricular function and for mechanical complications, right heart catheterization, and continuous measurements of arterial pressure. These measurements permit the accurate assessment of volume status and may facilitate decisions about volume resuscitation, selective use of pressors and inotropes, and mechanical support.

1. Acute LV failure—Dyspnea, diffuse rales, and arterial hypoxemia usually indicate LV failure. General measures include supplemental oxygen to increase arterial saturation to above 95% and elevation of the trunk. Diuretics are usually the initial therapy unless RV infarction is present. Intravenous furosemide (10–40 mg) or bumetanide (0.5–1 mg) is preferred because of the reliably rapid onset and short duration of action of these medications. Higher dosages can be given if an inadequate response occurs. Morphine sulfate (4 mg intravenously followed by increments of 2 mg) is valuable in acute pulmonary edema.

Diuretics are usually effective; however, because most patients with acute infarction are not volume overloaded, the hemodynamic response may be limited and may be associated with hypotension. In mild heart failure, sublingual isosorbide dinitrate (2.5–10 mg every 2 hours) or nitroglycerin ointment (6.25–25 mg every 4 hours) may be adequate to lower pulmonary capillary wedge pressure (PCWP). In more severe failure, especially if cardiac output is reduced and BP is normal or high, sodium nitroprusside may be the preferred agent. It should be initiated only with arterial pressure monitoring; the initial dosage should be low (0.25 mcg/kg/min) to avoid excessive hypotension, but the dosage can be increased by increments of 0.5 mcg/kg/min every 5–10 minutes up to 5–10 mcg/kg/min until the desired hemodynamic response is obtained. Excessive hypotension (mean BP less than 65–75 mm Hg) or tachycardia (greater than 10/min increase) should be avoided.

Intravenous nitroglycerin (starting at 10 mcg/min) also may be effective but may lower PCWP with less hypotension. Oral or transdermal vasodilator therapy with nitrates or ACE inhibitors is often necessary after the initial 24–48 hours.

Inotropic agents should be avoided if possible, because they often increase heart rate and myocardial oxygen requirements and worsen clinical outcomes. Dobutamine has the best hemodynamic profile, increasing cardiac output and modestly lowering PCWP, usually without excessive tachycardia, hypotension, or arrhythmias. The initial dosage is 2.5 mcg/kg/min, and it may be increased by similar increments up to 15–20 mcg/kg/min at intervals of 5–10 minutes. Dopamine is more useful in the presence of hypotension, since it produces peripheral vasoconstriction, but it has a less beneficial effect on PCWP. Digoxin has not been helpful in acute infarction except to control the ventricular response in atrial fibrillation, but it may be beneficial if chronic heart failure persists.

2. Hypotension and shock—Patients with hypotension (systolic BP less than 90 mm Hg, individualized depending on prior BP) and signs of diminished perfusion (low urinary output, confusion, cold extremities) that does not respond to fluid resuscitation should be presumed to have cardiogenic shock and should be considered for urgent catheterization and revascularization. Sparing use of **intra-aortic balloon pump (IABP)** support and hemodynamic monitoring with a PA catheter can be considered, although these later measures have not been shown to improve outcome. Up to 20% will have findings indicative of intravascular hypovolemia (due to diaphoresis, vomiting, decreased venous tone, medications—such as diuretics, nitrates, morphine, beta-blockers, calcium channel blockers, and thrombolytic agents—and lack of oral intake). These should be treated with successive boluses of 100 mL of normal saline until PCWP reaches 15–18 mm Hg to determine whether cardiac output and BP respond. Pericardial tamponade due to hemorrhagic pericarditis (especially after thrombolytic therapy or cardiopulmonary resuscitation) or ventricular rupture should be considered and excluded by echocardiography if clinically indicated. RV infarction, characterized by a normal PCWP but elevated RA pressure, can produce hypotension. This is discussed below.

Most patients with cardiogenic shock will have moderate to severe LV systolic dysfunction, with a mean EF of 30% in the SHOCK trial. If hypotension is only modest (systolic pressure higher than 90 mm Hg) and the PCWP is elevated, diuretics should be administered. If the BP falls, inotropic support will need to be added. A large randomized trial showed no benefit of IABP support in cardiogenic shock.

Norepinephrine (0.1–0.5 mcg/kg/min) is generally considered to be the most appropriate inotrope/vasopressor for cardiogenic shock based on limited randomized clinical trial evidence suggesting less arrhythmias and improved outcomes compared with dopamine. Dopamine is nonetheless also an option and can be initiated at a rate of 2–4 mcg/kg/min and increased at 5-minute intervals to the appropriate hemodynamic end point. At dosages lower than 5 mcg/kg/min, it improves renal blood flow; at intermediate dosages (2.5–10 mcg/kg/min), it stimulates myocardial contractility; at higher dosages (greater than 8 mcg/kg/min), it is a potent alpha-1-adrenergic agonist. In general, BP and cardiac index rise, but PCWP does not fall. Dopamine may be combined with nitroprusside or dobutamine (see above for dosing), or the latter may be used in its place if hypotension is not severe.

Patients with cardiogenic shock not due to hypovolemia have a poor prognosis, with 30-day mortality rates of 40–80%. The IABP-SHOCK II trial found that the use of an IABP does not offer a mortality benefit at 30 days or 1 year, compared with routine care with rapid revascularization, and is likely not helpful. Surgically implanted (or percutaneous) ventricular assist devices may be used in refractory cases. Emergent cardiac catheterization and coronary angiography followed by percutaneous or surgical revascularization offer the best chance of survival. Additionally, revascularization in shock should be aimed at the culprit artery only, avoiding multivessel PCI.

D. RV Infarction

RV infarction is present in one-third of patients with inferior wall infarction but is clinically significant in less than 50% of these. It presents as hypotension with relatively preserved LV function and should be considered whenever patients with inferior infarction exhibit low BP, raised venous pressure, and clear lungs. Hypotension is often exacerbated by medications that decrease intravascular volume or produce venodilation, such as diuretics, nitrates, and opioids. RA pressure and JVP are high, while PCWP is normal or low and the lungs are clear. The diagnosis is suggested by ST-segment elevation in right-sided anterior chest leads, particularly RV_4. The diagnosis can be confirmed by echocardiography or hemodynamic measurements. Treatment consists of fluid loading beginning with 500 mL of 0.9% saline over 2 hours to improve LV filling, and inotropic agents only if necessary.

E. Mechanical Defects

Partial or complete rupture of a papillary muscle or of the interventricular septum occurs in less than 1% of acute MIs and carries a poor prognosis. These complications occur in both anterior and inferior infarctions, usually 3–7 days after the acute event. They are detected by the appearance of a new systolic murmur and clinical deterioration, often with pulmonary edema. The two lesions are distinguished by the location of the murmur (apical versus parasternal) and by Doppler echocardiography. Hemodynamic monitoring is essential for appropriate management and demonstrates an increase in oxygen saturation between the RA and PA in VSD and, often, a large *v* wave with mitral regurgitation. Treatment by nitroprusside and, preferably, intra-aortic balloon counterpulsation (IABC) reduces the regurgitation or shunt, but surgical correction is mandatory. In patients remaining hemodynamically unstable or requiring continuous parenteral pharmacologic treatment or counterpulsation, early surgery is recommended, though mortality rates are high (15% to nearly 100%, depending on residual ventricular function and clinical status). Patients who are stabilized medically can have delayed surgery with lower risks (10–25%), although this may be due to the death of sicker patients, some of whom may have been saved by earlier surgery.

F. Myocardial Rupture

Complete rupture of the LV free wall occurs in less than 1% of patients and usually results in immediate death. It occurs 2–7 days postinfarction, usually involves the anterior wall, and is more frequent in older women. Incomplete or gradual rupture may be sealed off by the pericardium, creating a pseudoaneurysm. This may be recognized by echocardiography, radionuclide angiography, or LV angiography, often as an incidental finding. It demonstrates a narrow-neck connection to the LV. Early surgical repair is indicated, since delayed rupture is common.

G. LV Aneurysm

An LV aneurysm, a sharply delineated area of scar that bulges paradoxically during systole, develops in 10–20% of patients surviving an acute infarction. This usually follows anterior ST-elevation infarctions. Aneurysms are recognized by persistent ST-segment elevation (beyond 4–8 weeks), and a wide neck from the LV can be demonstrated by echocardiography, scintigraphy, or contrast angiography. They rarely rupture but may be associated with arterial emboli, ventricular arrhythmias, and heart failure. Surgical resection may be performed for these indications if other measures fail. The best results (mortality rates of 10–20%) are obtained when the residual myocardium contracts well and when significant coronary lesions supplying adjacent regions are bypassed.

H. Pericarditis

The pericardium is involved in approximately 50% of infarctions, but pericarditis is often not clinically significant. Twenty percent of patients with ST-elevation infarctions will have an audible friction rub if examined repetitively. Pericardial pain occurs in approximately the same proportion after 2–7 days and is recognized by its variation with respiration and position (improved by sitting). Often, no treatment is required, but aspirin (650 mg every 4–6 hours) will usually relieve the pain. Indomethacin and corticosteroids can cause impaired infarct healing and predispose to myocardial rupture, and therefore should generally be avoided in the early post-MI period. Likewise, anticoagulation should be used cautiously, since hemorrhagic pericarditis may result.

One week to 12 weeks after infarction, **Dressler syndrome** (post-MI syndrome) occurs in less than 5% of patients. This is an autoimmune phenomenon and presents as pericarditis with associated fever, leukocytosis, and, occasionally, pericardial or pleural effusion. It may recur over months. Treatment is the same as for other forms of pericarditis. A short course of nonsteroidal agents or corticosteroids may help relieve symptoms.

I. Mural Thrombus

Mural thrombi are common in large anterior infarctions but not in infarctions at other locations. Arterial emboli occur in approximately 2% of patients with known infarction, usually within 6 weeks. Anticoagulation with heparin followed by short-term (3-month) warfarin therapy (or DOAC therapy based on limited case report experience) results in clot resolution and prevents most emboli and should be considered in all patients with large anterior infarctions and evidence of LV thrombi. Mural thrombi can be detected by echocardiography or cardiac MRI.

Thiele H et al; CULPRIT-SHOCK Investigators. PCI strategies in patients with acute myocardial infarction and cardiogenic shock. N Engl J Med. 2017 Dec 21;377(25):2419–32. [PMID: 29083953]

► Postinfarction Management

After the first 24 hours, the focus of patient management is to prevent recurrent ischemia, improve infarct healing and prevent remodeling, and prevent recurrent vascular events. Patients with hemodynamic compromise, who are at high risk for death, need careful monitoring and management of volume status.

A. Risk Stratification

Risk stratification is important for the management of STEMI. GRACE and TIMI risk scores can be helpful tools. Patients with recurrent ischemia (spontaneous or provoked), hemodynamic instability, impaired LV function, heart failure, or serious ventricular arrhythmias should undergo cardiac catheterization (see Table 10–9). ACE inhibitor (or ARB) therapy is indicated in patients with clinical heart failure or LVEF of 40% or less. Aldosterone blockade is indicated for patients with an LVEF of 40% or less and either heart failure or diabetes mellitus.

For patients not undergoing cardiac catheterization, submaximal exercise (or pharmacologic stress testing for patients unable to exercise) before discharge or a maximal test after 3–6 weeks (the latter being more sensitive for ischemia) helps patients and clinicians plan the return to normal activity. Imaging in conjunction with stress testing adds additional sensitivity for ischemia and provides localizing information. Both exercise and pharmacologic stress imaging have successfully predicted subsequent outcome. One of these tests should be used prior to discharge in patients who have received thrombolytic therapy as a means of selecting appropriate candidates for coronary angiography.

B. Secondary Prevention

Postinfarction management should begin with identification and modification of risk factors. Treatment of hyperlipidemia and smoking cessation both prevent recurrent infarction and death. Statin therapy should be started before the patient is discharged from the hospital to reduce recurrent atherothrombotic events. BP control as well as cardiac rehabilitation and exercise are also recommended. They can be of considerable psychological benefit and appear to improve prognosis.

Beta-blockers improve survival rates, primarily by reducing the incidence of sudden death in high-risk subsets of patients, though their value may be less in patients without complications with small infarctions and normal exercise tests. While a variety of beta-blockers have been shown to be beneficial, for patients with LV dysfunction managed with contemporary treatment, carvedilol titrated to 25 mg orally twice a day has been shown to reduce mortality. Beta-blockers with intrinsic sympathomimetic activity have not proved beneficial in postinfarction patients.

Antiplatelet agents are beneficial; aspirin (81–325 mg daily, with 81 mg daily the preferred long-term dose) is recommended, and adding clopidogrel (75 mg daily) has been shown to provide additional short-term benefit after STEMI. Prasugrel provides further reduction in thrombotic outcomes compared with clopidogrel, at the cost of more bleeding. Likewise, ticagrelor provides benefit over clopidogrel but should be used with low-dose aspirin (81 mg/day). Warfarin anticoagulation for 3 months reduces the incidence of arterial emboli after large anterior infarctions and, according to the results of at least one study, it improves long-term prognosis; however, these studies were done before the routine use of aspirin and clopidogrel. An advantage to combining low-dose aspirin and warfarin has not been demonstrated, except perhaps in patients with atrial fibrillation.

Calcium channel blockers have *not* been shown to improve prognoses overall and should not be prescribed purely for secondary prevention. Antiarrhythmic therapy other than with beta-blockers has *not* been shown to be effective except in patients with symptomatic arrhythmias. Amiodarone has been studied in several trials of postinfarct patients with either LV dysfunction or frequent ventricular ectopy. Although survival was not improved, amiodarone was not harmful—unlike other agents in this setting. Therefore, it is the agent of choice for individuals with symptomatic postinfarction supraventricular arrhythmias. While implantable defibrillators improve survival for patients with postinfarction LV dysfunction and heart failure, the DINAMIT trial found no benefit to implantable defibrillators implanted in the 40 days following acute MI.

C. ACE Inhibitors and ARBs in Patients With LV Dysfunction

Patients who sustain substantial myocardial damage often experience subsequent progressive LV dilation and dysfunction, leading to clinical heart failure and reduced long-term survival. In patients with EFs less than 40%, long-term ACE inhibitor (or ARB) therapy prevents LV dilation and the onset of heart failure and prolongs survival. The HOPE trial, as well as an overview of trials of ACE inhibitors for secondary prevention, also demonstrated a reduction of approximately 20% in mortality rates and the occurrence of nonfatal MI and stroke with ramipril treatment of patients with coronary or peripheral vascular disease and without confirmed LV systolic dysfunction. Therefore, ACE inhibitor therapy should be strongly considered in this broader group of patients—and especially in patients with diabetes and those with even mild systolic hypertension, in whom the greatest benefit was observed (see Table 11–6).

D. Revascularization

Postinfarction patients not treated with primary PCI who appear likely to benefit from early revascularization with CABG if the anatomy is appropriate are (1) those who have undergone fibrinolytic therapy, especially if they have high-risk features (including systolic BP of less than 100 mm Hg, heart rate of greater than 100 beats/min, Killip class II or III, and ST-segment depression of 2 mm or more in the anterior leads); (2) patients with LV dysfunction (EF less than 30–40%); (3) patients with NSTEMI and high-risk features; and (4) patients with markedly positive exercise tests and multi-vessel disease. The value of revascularization in patients not treated with acute reperfusion therapy with preserved LV function who have mild ischemia and are not symptom limited is less clear. In general, patients without high-risk features who survive infarctions without complications, have preserved LV function (EF greater than 50%), and have no exercise-induced ischemia have an excellent prognosis and do not require invasive evaluation.

Smaller randomized trials have demonstrated that patients with noninfarct-related artery disease may benefit from revascularization strategies at the time of acute MI care, prior to hospital discharge.

O'Gara PT et al. 2013 ACCF/AHA guideline for the management of ST-elevation myocardial infarction: a report of the American College of Cardiology Foundation/American Heart Association Task Force on Practice Guidelines. Circulation. 2013 Jan 29;127(4):e362–425. Erratum in: Circulation. 2013 Dec 24;128(25):e481. [PMID: 23247304]

▼ DISORDERS OF RATE & RHYTHM

Abnormalities of cardiac rhythm and conduction can be symptomatic (syncope, near syncope, dizziness, fatigue, or palpitations) or asymptomatic. In addition, they can be lethal (sudden cardiac death) or dangerous to the extent that they reduce cardiac output, so that perfusion of the brain and myocardium is impaired. Stable supraventricular tachycardia (SVT) is generally well tolerated in patients without underlying heart disease but may lead to myocardial ischemia or heart failure in patients with coronary disease, valvular abnormalities, and systolic or diastolic myocardial dysfunction. Ventricular tachycardia, if prolonged, often results in hemodynamic compromise and may deteriorate into ventricular fibrillation if left untreated.

Whether slow heart rates produce symptoms at rest or with exertion depends on whether cerebral and peripheral perfusion can be maintained, which is generally a function of whether the patient is upright or supine and whether LV function is adequate to maintain stroke volume. If the heart rate abruptly slows, as with the onset of complete heart block or sinus arrest, syncope or convulsions (or both) may result. Unless a clear, reversible cause is found, most symptomatic patients require implantation of a permanent pacemaker.

The diagnosis of an abnormal tachyarrhythmia can generally be made via cardiac monitoring, including in-hospital and ambulatory ECG monitoring, event recorders (instruments that can be used for prolonged periods to record and transmit rhythm tracings when infrequent episodes occur), continuous mobile cardiac telemetry, or implantable loop recorders. More invasive testing, including catheter-based electrophysiologic studies (to assess sinus node function, AV conduction, and inducibility of arrhythmias), and tests of autonomic nervous system function (tilt-table testing) can also be performed.

Treatment of tachyarrhythmias varies and can include modalities such as antiarrhythmic medications and more invasive techniques such as catheter ablation.

▶ Antiarrhythmic Medications

Antiarrhythmic medications are frequently used to treat arrhythmias, but have variable efficacy and produce frequent side effects (Table 10–11). They are often divided into classes based on their electropharmacologic actions and many of these medications have multiple actions. The most frequently used classification scheme is the Vaughan-Williams, which consists of four classes.

Class I agents block membrane sodium channels. Three subclasses are further defined by the effect of the agents on the Purkinje fiber action potential. **Class Ia** medications (ie, quinidine, procainamide, disopyramide) slow the rate of rise of the action potential (V_{max}) and prolong its duration, thus slowing conduction and increasing refractoriness (moderate depression of phase 0 upstroke of the action potential). **Class Ib** agents (ie, lidocaine, mexiletine) shorten action potential duration; they do not affect conduction or refractoriness (minimal depression of phase 0 upstroke of the action potential). **Class Ic** agents (ie, flecainide, propafenone) prolong V_{max} and slow repolarization, thus slowing conduction and prolonging refractoriness, but more so than class Ia medications (maximal depression of phase 0 upstroke of the action potential).

Class II agents are the beta-blockers, which decrease automaticity, prolong AV conduction, and prolong refractoriness.

Class III agents (ie, amiodarone, dronedarone, sotalol, dofetilide, ibutilide) block potassium channels and prolong repolarization, widening the QRS and prolonging the QT

Table 10–11. Antiarrhythmic medications (listed in alphabetical order within class).

Agent	Intravenous Dosage	Oral Dosage	Therapeutic Plasma Level	Route of Elimination	Side Effects
Class Ia: Action: Sodium channel blockers: Depress phase 0 depolarization; slow conduction; prolong repolarization.					
Indications: Supraventricular tachycardia, ventricular tachycardia, symptomatic ventricular premature beats.					
Disopyramide		Immediate release: 100–200 mg every 6 h Sustained release: 200–400 mg every 12 h	2–8 mg/mL	Renal	Urinary retention, dry mouth, markedly ↓ LVF, QT prolongation
Procainamide	Loading: 10–17 mg/kg at 20–50 mg/min; Maintenance: 1–4 mg/min	50 mg/kg/day in divided doses every 4 h (short-acting)	4–10 mg/mL; NAPA (active metabolite), 10–20 mcg/mL	Renal	
Quinidine	6–10 mg/kg (intramuscularly or intravenously) over 20 min (rarely used parenterally)	324–648 mg every 8 h	2–5 mg/mL	Hepatic	GI, ↓ LVF, ↑ Dig
Class Ib: Action: Shorten repolarization.					
Indications: Ventricular tachycardia, prevention of ventricular fibrillation, symptomatic ventricular premature beats.					
Lidocaine	Loading: 1 mg/kg; Maintenance: 1–4 mg/min		1–5 mg/mL	Hepatic	CNS, GI, ↓ LVF
Mexiletine		100–300 mg every 8–12 h; maximum: 1200 mg/day	0.5–2 mg/mL	Hepatic	CNS, GI, leukopenia
Class Ic: Action: Depress phase 0 repolarization; slow conduction. (Propafenone is a weak calcium channel blocker and beta-blocker and prolongs action potential and refractoriness.)					
Indications: Ventricular tachycardia (in the absence of structural heart disease), refractory supraventricular tachycardia.					
Flecainide		50–150 mg twice daily	0.2–1 mg/mL	Hepatic	CNS, GI, AFL with 1:1 conduction, ventricular pro-arrhythmia
Propafenone		150–300 mg every 8–12 h	Note: Active metabolites	Hepatic	CNS, GI, AFL with 1:1 conduction, ventricular pro-arrhythmia
Class II: Action: Beta-blockers, slow AV conduction.					
Indications: Supraventricular tachycardia, ventricular tachycardia, symptomatic ventricular premature beats, long QT syndrome					
Esmolol	Loading: 500 mcg/kg over 1–2 min Maintenance: 50 mcg/kg/min	Other beta-blockers may be used concomitantly	Not established	Hepatic	↓ LVF, bradycardia, AV block
Metoprolol	5 mg every 5 min up to 3 doses	25–200 mg daily	Not established	Hepatic	↓ LVF, bradycardia, AV block, fatigue
Propranolol	1–3 mg every 5 min up to total of 5 mg	40–320 mg in 1–4 doses daily (depending on preparation)	Not established	Hepatic	↓ LVF, bradycardia, AV block, bronchospasm
Class III: Action: Prolong action potential.					
Indications: *Amiodarone:* refractory ventricular tachycardia, supraventricular tachycardia, prevention of ventricular tachycardia, atrial fibrillation, ventricular fibrillation; *Dofetilide:* atrial fibrillation and flutter; *Dronedarone:* atrial fibrillation (not persistent); *Ibutilide:* conversion of atrial fibrillation and flutter; *Sotalol:* ventricular tachycardia, atrial fibrillation.					
Amiodarone	150–300 mg infused rapidly, followed by 1 mg/min infusion for 6 h and then 0.5 mg/min for 18 h	800–1600 mg/day for 7–14 days; maintain at 100–400 mg/day	1–5 mg/mL	Hepatic	Pulmonary fibrosis, hypothyroidism, hyperthyroidism, photosensitivity, corneal and skin deposits, hepatitis, ↑ Dig, neurotoxicity, GI

(continued)

Table 10–11. Antiarrhythmic medications (listed in alphabetical order within class). (continued)

Agent	Intravenous Dosage	Oral Dosage	Therapeutic Plasma Level	Route of Elimination	Side Effects
Dofetilide		125–500 mcg every 12 h		Renal (dose must be reduced with kidney dysfunction)	Torsades de pointes in 3%; interaction with cytochrome P-450 inhibitors
Dronedarone		400 mg twice daily		Hepatic (contra-indicated in severe impairment)	QTc prolongation, HF. Contraindicated in HF (NYHA class IV or recent decompensa-tion), persistent AF
Ibutilide	1 mg over 10 min, followed by a second infusion of 0.5–1 mg over 10 min			Hepatic and renal	Torsades de pointes in up to 5% of patients within 3 h after administration; patients must be monitored with defi-brillator nearby
Sotalol	75 mg every 12 h	80–160 mg every 12 h (maximum 320 mg daily)		Renal (dosing interval should be extended if creatinine clearance is < 60 mL/min)	Early incidence of tors-ades de pointes, ↓ LVF, bradycardia, fatigue (and otherside effects associated with beta-blockers)

Class IV: Action: Slow calcium channel blockers.

Indications: Supraventricular tachycardia, ventricular tachycardia (outflow tract, idiopathic).

Agent	Intravenous Dosage	Oral Dosage	Therapeutic Plasma Level	Route of Elimination	Side Effects
Diltiazem	0.25 mg/kg over 2 min; second 0.35-mg/kg bolus after 15 min if response is inadequate; infusion rate, 5–15 mg/h	120–360 mg daily in 1–3 doses depending on preparation		Hepatic metabo-lism, renal excretion	Hypotension, ↓ LVF, bradycardia
Verapamil	2.5 mg bolus followed by additional boluses of 2.5–5 mg every 1–3 min; total 20 mg over 20 min; maintain at 5 mg/kg/min	80–120 mg every 6–8 h; 240–480 mg once daily with sustained-release preparation	0.1–0.15 mg/mL	Hepatic	Hypotension, ↓ LVF, constipation, ↑ Dig

Miscellaneous: Indications: Supraventricular tachycardia.

Agent	Intravenous Dosage	Oral Dosage	Therapeutic Plasma Level	Route of Elimination	Side Effects
Adenosine	6 mg rapidly followed by 12 mg after 1–2 min if needed; use half these doses if administered via central line			Adenosine receptor stimulation, metabolized in blood	Transient flushing, dyspnea, chest pain, AV block, sinus brady-cardia; effect ↓ by theophylline, ↑ by dipyridamole
Digoxin	0.5 mg over 20 min followed by increment of 0.25 or 0.125 mg to 1–1.5 mg over 24 h	1–1.5 mg over 24–36 h in 3 or 4 doses; maintenance, 0.125–0.5 mg/day	0.7–2 mg/mL	Renal	AV block, arrhythmias, GI, visual changes
Ivabradine		5–7.5 mg every 12 h		Renal and fecal	Bradycardia, phosphenes (visual brightness)

AF, atrial fibrillation; AV, atrioventricular; CNS, central nervous system; Dig, elevation of serum digoxin level; GI, gastrointestinal (nausea, vomiting, diarrhea); HF, heart failure; ↓LVF, reduced left ventricular function; NAPA, N-acetylprocainamide; NYHA, New York Heart Association; SLE, systemic lupus erythematosus.

interval. They decrease automaticity and conduction and prolong refractoriness.

Class IV agents are the calcium channel blockers, which decrease automaticity and AV conduction.

There are some antiarrhythmic agents that do not fall into one of these categories. The most frequently used are digoxin and adenosine. Digoxin inhibits the Na+, K+-ATPase pump. Digoxin prolongs AV nodal conduction and the AV nodal refractory period, but it shortens the action potential and decreases the refractoriness of the ventricular myocardium and Purkinje fibers. Adenosine can block AV nodal conduction and shortens atrial refractoriness.

Although the in vitro electrophysiologic effects of most of these agents have been defined, their use remains largely empiric. **All can exacerbate arrhythmias (proarrhythmic effect), and many depress LV function.**

The risk of antiarrhythmic agents has been highlighted by many studies, most notably the Coronary Arrhythmia Suppression Trial (CAST), in which two class Ic agents (flecainide, encainide) and a class Ia agent (moricizine) increased mortality rates in patients with asymptomatic ventricular ectopy after MI. Class Ic antiarrhythmic agents should therefore *not* be used in patients with prior myocardial infarction or structural heart disease.

The use of antiarrhythmic agents for specific arrhythmias is discussed below.

▶ Catheter Ablation for Cardiac Arrhythmias

Catheter ablation has become the primary modality of therapy for many symptomatic supraventricular arrhythmias, including AV nodal reentrant tachycardia, tachycardias involving accessory pathways, paroxysmal atrial tachycardia, and atrial flutter. Catheter ablation of atrial fibrillation is more complex and usually involves complete electrical isolation of the pulmonary veins (which are often the sites of initiation of atrial fibrillation) or placing linear lesions within the atria to prevent propagation throughout the atrial chamber. This technique is considered a reasonable therapy for symptomatic patients with medication-refractory atrial fibrillation or as an alternative to long-term antiarrhythmic medication treatment. Catheter ablation of ventricular arrhythmias has proved more difficult, but experienced centers have demonstrated reasonable success with all types of ventricular tachycardias including bundle-branch reentry, tachycardia originating in the ventricular outflow tract or papillary muscles, tachycardias originating in the specialized conduction system (fascicular ventricular tachycardia), and ventricular tachycardias occurring in patients with ischemic or dilated cardiomyopathy. Ablation of many of these arrhythmias can be performed from the endocardial surface via endovascular catheter placement or on the epicardial surface of the heart via a percutaneous subxiphoid approach.

Catheter ablation has also been successfully performed for the treatment of ventricular fibrillation when a uniform premature ventricular contraction (PVC) can be identified. In addition, patients with symptomatic PVCs or PVCs occurring at a high enough burden to result in a cardiomyopathy (usually more than 10,000/day) are often referred for catheter ablation as well.

Catheter ablation procedures are generally safe, with an overall major complication rate ranging from 1% to 5%. Major vascular damage during catheter insertion occurs in less than 2% of patients. There is a low incidence of perforation of the myocardial wall resulting in pericardial tamponade. Sufficient damage to the AV node to require permanent cardiac pacing occurs in less than 1% of patients. When transseptal access through the interatrial septum or retrograde LV catheterization is required, additional potential complications include damage to the heart valves, damage to a coronary artery, or systemic emboli. A rare but potentially fatal complication after catheter ablation of atrial fibrillation is the development of an atrio-esophageal fistula resulting from ablation on the posterior wall of the LA just overlying the esophagus, estimated to occur in less than 0.1% of procedures.

Calkins H et al. 2017 HRS/EHRA/ECAS/APHRS/SOLAECE expert consensus statement on catheter and surgical ablation of atrial fibrillation. Europace. 2018 Jan 1;20(1):e1–160. [PMID: 29016840]

SINUS ARRHYTHMIA, BRADYCARDIA, & TACHYCARDIA

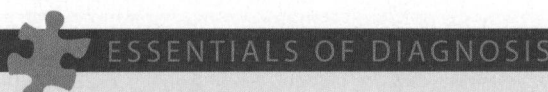

▶ ESSENTIALS OF DIAGNOSIS

▶ Wide variation in sinus rate is common in young, healthy individuals and generally not pathologic.

▶ Symptomatic bradycardia may require permanent pacemaker implantation, especially in the elderly or patients with underlying heart disease.

▶ Sinus tachycardia is usually secondary to another underlying process (ie, fever, pain, anemia, alcohol withdrawal).

▶ Sick sinus syndrome manifests as sinus bradycardia, pauses, or inadequate heart rate response to physiologic demands (chronotropic incompetence).

▶ General Considerations

Sinus arrhythmia is an irregularity of the normal heart rate defined as variation in the PP interval of more than 120 ms. This occurs commonly in young, healthy people due to changes in vagal influence on the sinus node during respiration (phasic) or independent of respiration (nonphasic). This is generally *not* a pathologic arrhythmia and requires no specific cardiac evaluation.

Sinus bradycardia is defined as a heart rate slower than 60 beats/min and may be due to increased vagal influence on the normal sinoatrial pacemaker or organic disease of the sinus node. In healthy individuals, and especially in patients who are in excellent physical condition, sinus bradycardia to rates of 50 beats/min or lower especially during sleep is a normal finding. However, in elderly patients and individuals with heart disease sinus bradycardia may be an indication of true sinus node pathology. When the sinus rate slows severely, the atrial-nodal junction or the nodal-His bundle junction may assume pacemaker activity for the heart, usually at a rate of 35–60 beats/min.

Sinus tachycardia is defined as a heart rate faster than 100 beats/min that is caused by rapid impulse formation from the sinoatrial node. It is a normal physiologic response to exercise or other conditions in which catecholamine release is increased. The rate infrequently exceeds 160 beats/min but may reach 180 beats/min in young persons. The onset and termination are usually gradual, in contrast to paroxysmal supraventricular tachycardia (PSVT) due to reentry. In rare instances, otherwise healthy individuals may present with "inappropriate" sinus tachycardia where persistently elevated basal heart rates are not in-line with physiologic demands. Long-term consequences of this disorder are few.

Sick sinus syndrome is a broad diagnosis applied to patients with sinus arrest, sinoatrial exit block (recognized by a pause equal to a multiple of the underlying PP interval or progressive shortening of the PP interval prior to a pause), or persistent sinus bradycardia. A common presentation in elderly patients is of recurrent SVTs (often atrial fibrillation) accompanied by bradyarrhythmias (**"tachy-brady syndrome"**). The long pauses that often follow the termination of tachycardia cause the associated symptoms. Sick sinus syndrome may also manifest as **chronotropic incompetence,** defined as an inappropriate heart rate response to the physiologic demands of exercise or stress, and is an underrecognized cause of poor exercise tolerance.

Clinical Findings

In most patients, sinus arrhythmia (bradycardia or tachycardia) does not cause symptoms in the absence of underlying cardiac disease or other comorbidities. When severe sinus bradycardia results in low cardiac output, however, patients may complain of weakness, confusion, or syncope if cerebral perfusion is impaired. Atrial, junctional and ventricular ectopic rhythms are more apt to occur with slow sinus rates. Sinus bradycardia is often exacerbated by medications (digitalis, calcium channel blockers, beta-blockers, sympatholytic agents, antiarrhythmics), and agents that may be responsible should be withdrawn prior to making the diagnosis.

Sinus tachycardia is most often a normal response to conditions that require an increase in cardiac output, including fever, pain, anxiety, anemia, heart failure, hypovolemia, or thyrotoxicosis. Alcohol and alcohol withdrawal are common causes of sinus tachycardia and other supraventricular arrhythmias. In patients with underlying cardiac disease, sinus tachycardia may cause dyspnea or chest pain due to increased myocardial oxygen demand or reduced coronary artery blood flow.

Symptoms from sinus node dysfunction are nonspecific and may be due to other causes. It is therefore essential that symptoms be demonstrated to coincide temporally with arrhythmias. This may require prolonged ambulatory monitoring or the use of an event recorder.

Treatment

Asymptomatic patients generally do not require treatment. For symptomatic patients with bradycardia or sick sinus syndrome, implantation of a permanent pacemaker is usually indicated. For patients with "tachy-brady syndrome," treatment of the associated tachyarrhythmia is often difficult without first instituting pacing, since beta-blockers, calcium channel blockers, and other antiarrhythmic agents may exacerbate the bradycardia. When a dual-chamber pacemaker is implanted for sinus node dysfunction with intact AV conduction, unnecessary ventricular pacing should be avoided because it may exacerbate heart failure, especially in patients with preexisting LV dysfunction. In most situations, sinus tachycardia will improve or resolve with treatment of the underlying cause. Inappropriate sinus tachycardia in the presence of symptoms (palpitations, dizziness, exertional intolerance) can be treated with a trial of beta-blockers or calcium channel blockers although treatment is often challenging. Ivabradine (5–7.5 mg twice daily), a selective inhibitor of the potassium funny channel (I_f) specific to the sinus node, appears to be an effective treatment option.

When to Refer

Patients with symptoms related to bradycardia or tachycardia when reversible etiologies have been excluded.

John RM et al. Sinus node and atrial arrhythmias. Circulation. 2016 May 10;133(19):1892–900. [PMID: 27166347]
Koruth JS et al. The clinical use of ivabradine. J Am Coll Cardiol. 2017 Oct 3;70(14):1777–84. [PMID: 28958335]

AV BLOCK

ESSENTIALS OF DIAGNOSIS

▶ Conduction disturbance between the atrium and ventricle that can be physiologic (due to enhanced vagal tone) or pathologic.

▶ Block occurs in the AV node (first-degree, second-degree Mobitz type I) or below the AV node (second-degree Mobitz type II, third-degree).

▶ Symptomatic AV block or block below the AV node in the absence of a reversible cause usually warrants permanent pacemaker implantation.

General Considerations

AV block can be physiologic (due to increased vagal tone) or pathologic (due to underlying heart disease such as ischemia, myocarditis, fibrosis of the conduction system, or after cardiac surgery). AV block is categorized as **first-degree** (PR interval greater than 200 msec with all atrial impulses conducted), **second-degree** (intermittent blocked beats), or **third-degree** (complete heart block, in which no atrial impulses are conducted to the ventricles).

Second-degree AV block is further subclassified into **Mobitz type I (Wenckebach),** in which the AV conduction time (PR interval) progressively lengthens before the blocked beat, and **Mobitz type II,** in which there are intermittently nonconducted atrial beats not preceded by lengthening AV conduction. When only 2:1 AV block is present on the ECG, the differentiation between Mobitz type I or Mobitz type II is more difficult. If the baseline PR interval is prolonged (greater than 200 msec) or the width of the QRS complex is narrow (less than 120 msec), the block is usually nodal (Mobitz type I); if the QRS complex is wide (greater than or equal to 120 msec), the block is more likely infranodal (Mobitz type II).

AV dissociation occurs when an intrinsic ventricular pacemaker is firing at a rate faster than or close to the sinus rate (accelerated idioventricular rhythm, ventricular premature beats, or ventricular tachycardia), such that atrial impulses arriving at the AV node when it is refractory may not be conducted. This phenomenon does not necessarily indicate AV block. No treatment is required aside from management of the causative arrhythmia.

► Clinical Findings

The clinical presentation of first-degree and Mobitz type I block is typically benign and rarely produces symptoms. Normal, physiologic block of this type occurs in response to increases in parasympathetic output. This is commonly seen during sleep, with carotid sinus massage, or in well-trained athletes. It may also occur as a medication effect (calcium channel blockers, beta-blockers, digitalis, or antiarrhythmics). Pathologic causes, including myocardial ischemia or infarction (discussed earlier), inflammatory processes (ie, Lyme disease), fibrosis, calcification, or infiltration (ie, amyloidosis or sarcoidosis), should be excluded.

Mobitz type II block and complete (third-degree) heart block are almost always due to pathologic disease involving the infranodal conduction system, and symptoms including fatigue, dyspnea, presyncope or syncope are common. With complete heart block, where no atrial impulses reach the ventricle, the ventricular escape rate is usually slow (less than 50 beats/min) and severity of symptoms may vary depending on the rate and stability of the escape rhythm. As for lesser degrees of AV block, pathologic causes should be explored.

Intraventricular conduction block is relatively common and may be transient (ie, related to increases in heart rate) or permanent. Right bundle branch block is often seen in patients with structurally normal hearts. The left bundle is composed of two components (anterior and posterior fascicles) and left bundle branch block is more often a marker of underlying cardiac disease, including ischemic heart disease, inflammatory or infiltrative disease, cardiomyopathy, and valvular heart disease. In asymptomatic patients with bifascicular block (block in two of three infranodal components—right bundle, left anterior, and left posterior fascicle), the incidence of occult complete heart block or progression to it is low.

► Treatment

Asymptomatic patients with first- or second-degree Mobitz type I AV block do not require any specific therapy. Patients should undergo treatment of any potentially reversible cause (ie, myocardial ischemia or medication effect). Symptomatic patients with any degree of heart block should be treated urgently with atropine (initial dose 0.5 mg given intravenously) or temporary pacing (transcutaneous or transvenous). The indications for permanent pacing are symptomatic bradyarrhythmias with any degree of AV block or asymptomatic high-degree AV block (second-degree Mobitz type II or third-degree heart block) with slow ventricular rates (less than 40 beats/min). Patients with presumed cardiac syncope with normal heart rates and rhythm but bifascicular or trifascicular block on ECG should also be considered for permanent pacing.

A standardized nomenclature for pacemaker generators is used, usually consisting of four letters. The first letter refers to the chamber that is paced (A, atrium; V, ventricle; D, dual [for both]). The second letter refers to the chamber that is sensed (also A, V, or D). An additional option (O) indicates absence of sensing. The third letter refers to how the pacemaker responds to a sensed event (I, inhibition by a sensed impulse; T, triggering by a sensed impulse; D, dual modes of response; O, no response to sensed impulse). The fourth letter refers to the programmability or rate modulation capacity (R, rate modulation), a function that can increase the pacing rate in response to motion or respiratory rate when the intrinsic heart rate is inappropriately low.

A dual-chamber pacemaker that senses and paces in both chambers is the most physiologic approach to pacing patients who remain in sinus rhythm. *AV synchrony* is particularly important in patients in whom atrial contraction produces a substantial increment in stroke volume and in those in whom sensing the atrial rate to provide rate-responsive ventricular pacing is useful. In patients with single-chamber ventricular pacemakers, the lack of an atrial kick may lead to the so-called **pacemaker syndrome**, in which the patient experiences signs of low cardiac output while upright. In patients with complete heart block with left ventricular systolic dysfunction, implantation of a pacemaker capable of direct capture of the native specialized conduction system (His bundle) or simultaneous left and right ventricular pacing (CRT-P) may be indicated. Complications from pacemaker implantation include infection, hematoma, cardiac perforation, pneumothorax, and lead dislodgement.

► When to Refer

Patients with symptomatic AV block (any degree) or asymptomatic high-degree (second-degree Mobitz type II or third-degree) AV block after reversible causes have been excluded.

Vijayaraman P et al. The continued search for physiological pacing: where are we now? J Am Coll Cardiol. 2017 Jun 27; 69(25):3099–114. [PMID: 28641799]

PAROXYSMAL SUPRAVENTRICULAR TACHYCARDIA (PSVT)

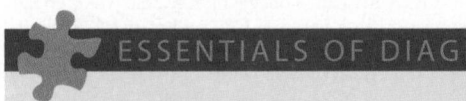

ESSENTIALS OF DIAGNOSIS

▶ Rapid, regular tachycardia most commonly seen in young adults and characterized by abrupt onset and offset.

▶ QRS duration narrow (less than 120 msec) except in the presence of bundle branch block or accessory pathway.

▶ Often responsive to vagal maneuvers, AV nodal blockers, or adenosine. Cardioversion rarely required.

▶ General Considerations

PSVT is an intermittent arrhythmia that is characterized by a sudden onset and offset and a regular ventricular response. Episodes may last from a few seconds to several hours or longer. PSVT often occurs in patients without structural heart disease. The most common mechanism for PSVT is reentry, which may be initiated or terminated by a fortuitously timed atrial or ventricular premature beat. The reentrant circuit usually involves dual pathways (a slow and a fast pathway) within the AV node; this is referred to as **AV nodal reentrant tachycardia (AVNRT)** and accounts for 60% of cases of PSVT. Less commonly (30% of cases), reentry is due to an accessory pathway between the atria and ventricles, referred to as **atrioventricular reciprocating tachycardia (AVRT)**. The pathophysiology and management of arrhythmias due to accessory pathways differ in important ways and are discussed separately below.

▶ Clinical Findings

A. Symptoms and Signs

Symptoms of PSVT can be quite variable depending on the degree of heart rate elevation, resultant hypotension or the presence of other comorbidities. Symptoms may include palpitations, diaphoresis, dyspnea, dizziness, and mild chest pain (even in the absence of associated CHD). Syncope is rare.

B. ECG

Obtaining a 12-lead ECG when feasible is important to help determine the tachycardia mechanism. The QRS duration will be narrow (less than 120 ms) except in cases of PSVT with aberrant conduction (left bundle branch block, right bundle branch block, or bystander accessory pathway). The heart rate is regular and is usually 160–220 beats/min but may be greater than 250 beats/min. The P wave usually differs in contour from sinus beats and is often simultaneous with or just after the QRS complex.

▶ Treatment

In the absence of structural heart disease, serious effects are rare, and most episodes resolve spontaneously. Particular effort should be made to terminate the episode quickly if cardiac failure, syncope, or anginal pain develops or if there is underlying cardiac or (particularly) coronary disease. Because reentry is the most common mechanism for PSVT, effective therapy requires that conduction be interrupted at some point in the reentry circuit and the vast majority of these circuits involve the AV node.

A. Mechanical Measures

A variety of maneuvers have been used to interrupt episodes, and patients may learn to perform these themselves. These maneuvers result in an acute increase in vagal tone and include the Valsalva maneuver, lowering the head between the knees, coughing, splashing cold water on the face, and breath holding. The **Valsalva maneuver** is performed with the patient semirecumbent (45 degrees), exerting around 40 mm Hg of intrathoracic pressure (by blowing through a 10 mL syringe) for at least 15 seconds. Moving the patient supine immediately following the strain maneuver and passively raising their legs for an additional 15 seconds may increase effectiveness of the maneuver. **Carotid sinus massage** is an additional technique often performed by clinicians but should be avoided if the patient has a carotid bruit. Firm but gentle pressure and massage are applied first over the right carotid sinus for 10–20 seconds and, if unsuccessful, then over the left carotid sinus. Pressure should not be exerted on both sides at the same time. **Facial contact with cold water** may cause transient bradycardia and termination of PSVT, a phenomenon known as the diving reflex. When performed properly, these maneuvers result in abrupt termination of the arrhythmia in 20–50% of cases.

B. Medication Therapy

If mechanical measures fail to terminate the arrhythmia, pharmacologic agents should be tried. **Intravenous adenosine** is recommended as the first-line agent due to its brief duration of action and minimal negative inotropic activity (Table 10–11). Because the half-life of adenosine is less than 10 seconds, the medication is given rapidly (in 1–2 seconds) as a 6 mg bolus followed by 20 mL of fluid. If this regimen is unsuccessful at terminating the arrhythmia, a second higher dose (12 mg) may be given. Adenosine causes block of electrical conduction through the AV node and results in termination of PSVT in approximately 90% of cases. Minor side effects are common and include transient flushing, chest discomfort, nausea, and headache. Adenosine may excite both atrial and ventricular tissue causing atrial fibrillation (in up to 12% of patients) or rarely ventricular arrhythmias and therefore administration should be performed with continuous cardiac monitoring and availability of an external defibrillator. Adenosine must also be used with caution in patients with reactive airways disease because it can promote bronchospasm.

When adenosine fails to terminate the arrhythmia or if a contraindication to its use is present, **intravenous calcium channel blockers**, including verapamil and diltiazem, may be used (Table 10–11). Verapamil in particular has been shown to be as effective at terminating PSVT in the acute setting (approximately 90%) as adenosine. Calcium channel blockers should be used with caution in patients with heart failure due to their negative inotropic effects. Their longer half-life compared to adenosine may result in prolonged hypotension despite restoration of normal rhythm.

Intravenous beta-blockers include esmolol (a very short-acting beta-blocker), propranolol, and metoprolol. While beta-blockers cause less myocardial depression than calcium channel blockers, the evidence of their effectiveness to terminate PSVT is limited. Although **intravenous amiodarone** is safe, it is usually not required and often ineffective for treatment of these arrhythmias.

C. Cardioversion

If the patient is hemodynamically unstable or if adenosine, beta-blockers, and calcium channel blockers are contraindicated or ineffective, synchronized electrical cardioversion (beginning at 100 J) should be performed.

▶ Prevention

A. Catheter Ablation

Because of concerns about the safety and the intolerability of antiarrhythmic medications, **radiofrequency ablation is the preferred approach to patients with recurrent symptomatic reentrant PSVT,** whether it is due to dual pathways within the AV node or to accessory pathways.

B. Medications

AV nodal blocking agents are the medications of choice as first-line medical therapy (Table 10–11). Beta-blockers or non-dihydropyridine calcium channel blockers, such as diltiazem and verapamil, are typically used first. Patients who do not respond to agents that increase refractoriness of the AV node may be treated with antiarrhythmics. The class Ic agents (flecainide, propafenone) can be used in patients without underlying structural heart disease. In patients with evidence of structural heart disease, class III agents, such as sotalol or amiodarone, should be used because of the lower incidence of ventricular proarrhythmia during long-term therapy.

▶ When to Refer

All patients with sustained or symptomatic PSVT should be referred to a cardiologist or cardiac electrophysiologist for long-term treatment options (including observation, pharmacotherapy, or ablation).

Appelboam A et al. Postural modification to the standard Valsalva manoeuvre for emergency treatment of supraventricular tachycardias (REVERT): a randomised controlled trial. Lancet. 2015 Oct 31;386(10005):1747–53. [PMID: 26314489]

Page RL et al. 2015 ACC/AHA/HRS guideline for the management of adult patients with supraventricular tachycardia: a report of the American College of Cardiology/American Heart Association Task Force on Clinical Practice Guidelines and the Heart Rhythm Society. J Am Coll Cardiol. 2016 Apr 5;67(13):e27–115. [PMID: 26409259]

PSVT DUE TO ACCESSORY AV PATHWAYS (Preexcitation Syndromes)

✦ ESSENTIALS OF DIAGNOSIS

▶ Two classic features of Wolff-Parkinson-White (WPW) pattern on ECG are short PR interval and wide, slurred QRS complex due to manifest preexcitation (delta wave).

▶ Most patients with WPW pattern do not have clinical history of arrhythmia but have a higher risk of sudden cardiac death due to rapidly conducted atrial fibrillation through the accessory pathway. Risk factors include age younger than 20, history of tachycardia, and rapid conduction properties at electrophysiologic testing.

▶ General Considerations

Accessory pathways or bypass tracts between the atrium and the ventricle bypass the compact AV node and can predispose to reentrant arrhythmias, such as AVRT and atrial fibrillation. When direct AV connections conduct antegrade (manifest preexcitation) they produce a classic **WPW pattern** on the baseline ECG consisting of a short PR interval and a wide, slurred QRS complex (**delta wave**) owing to early ventricular depolarization of the region adjacent to the pathway. Although the morphology and polarity of the delta wave can suggest the location of the pathway, mapping by intracardiac recordings is required for precise anatomic localization.

Accessory pathways occur in 0.1–0.3% of the population and facilitate reentrant arrhythmias owing to the disparity in refractory periods of the AV node and accessory pathway. **WPW syndrome** refers to a patient with baseline WPW pattern on ECG with associated SVT. Whether the tachycardia is associated with a narrow or wide QRS complex is frequently determined by whether antegrade conduction is through the node (narrow) or the bypass tract (wide). Some bypass tracts only conduct in a retrograde direction. In these cases, the bypass tract is termed "concealed" because it is not readily apparent on a baseline (sinus) ECG. **Orthodromic** reentrant tachycardia accounts for approximately 90% of AVRT episodes and is characterized by conduction antegrade down the AV node and retrograde up the accessory pathway, resulting in a narrow QRS complex (unless an underlying bundle branch block or interventricular conduction delay is present). **Antidromic** reentrant tachycardia conducts antegrade down the accessory pathway and retrograde through the AV node, resulting in a wide and often bizarre appearing QRS complex which may be mistaken for ventricular tachycardia. Accessory pathways often have shorter refractory periods than specialized conduction tissue and thus tachycardias involving accessory pathways have the potential to be more rapid.

Clinical Findings

Patients with WPW in whom arrhythmia develops often have palpitations, dizziness, or mild chest pain. Most patients that have a delta wave found incidentally on ECG (WPW pattern) do not have a clinical history of arrhythmia and are therefore asymptomatic. However, these patients are still at higher risk for sudden cardiac death than the general population. Atrial fibrillation with antegrade conduction down the accessory pathway and a rapid ventricular response will develop in up to 30% of patients with WPW. If this conduction is very rapid, it can potentially degenerate to ventricular fibrillation. The 10-year risk of sudden cardiac death in patients with WPW syndrome ranges from 0.15% to 0.24%. Risk factors include age younger than 20, a history of symptomatic tachycardia, and multiple accessory pathways.

Multiple risk stratification strategies have been proposed to identify asymptomatic patients with WPW pattern ECG who may be at higher risk for lethal cardiac arrhythmias. A sudden loss of preexcitation during exercise testing likely indicates an accessory pathway with poor conduction properties and therefore low risk for rapid anterograde conduction. In the absence of this finding or other signs of weak anterograde properties (intermittent preexcitation on resting or ambulatory ECG monitoring), patients may be referred for invasive electrophysiology testing. During the study, patients found to have the shortest preexcited R-R interval during atrial fibrillation of 250 msec or less or inducible SVT are at increased risk for sudden cardiac death and should undergo catheter ablation.

Treatment

A. Pharmacotherapy

Initial treatment of narrow-complex reentrant rhythms involving a bypass tract (orthodromic AVRT) is similar to other forms of PSVT and includes vagal maneuvers, intravenous adenosine, or verapamil. Treatment of wide-complex tachycardia in the presence of an accessory pathway, be it reentrant-type (antidromic AVRT) or atrial fibrillation with antegrade conduction down the bypass tract, must be managed differently. Agents such as calcium channel blockers and beta-blockers may increase the refractoriness of the AV node with minimal or no effect on the accessory pathway, often leading to faster ventricular rates and increasing the risk of ventricular fibrillation. Therefore, these agents should be avoided. Intravenous class Ia (procainamide) and class III (ibutilide) antiarrhythmic agents will increase the refractoriness of the bypass tract and are the medications of choice for wide-complex tachycardias involving accessory pathways. If hemodynamic compromise is present, electrical cardioversion is warranted.

B. Catheter Ablation

For long-term management, catheter ablation is the procedure of choice in patients with accessory pathways and recurrent symptoms or asymptomatic patients with WPW pattern on ECG and high-risk features at baseline or during electrophysiology study. Success rates for ablation of accessory pathways with radiofrequency catheters exceed 95% in appropriate patients. Major complications from catheter ablation are rare but include AV block, cardiac tamponade, and thromboembolic events. Minor complications, including hematoma at the catheter access site, occur in 1–2% of procedures. For patients not a candidate for catheter ablation, class Ic or class III antiarrhythmic medication may be considered.

When to Refer

- Asymptomatic patients with an incidental finding of WPW pattern on ECG with high-risk features.
- Symptomatic patients with recurrent or prolonged episodes despite treatment with AV nodal blocking agents.
- Patients with preexcitation and a history of atrial fibrillation or syncope.

Al-Khatib SM et al. Risk stratification for arrhythmic events in patients with asymptomatic pre-excitation: a systematic review for the 2015 ACC/AHA/HRS guideline for the management of adult patients with supraventricular tachycardia. Circulation. 2016 Apr 5;133(14):e575–86. [PMID: 26399661]

ATRIAL FIBRILLATION

ESSENTIALS OF DIAGNOSIS

- ► Presents as an irregularly irregular heart rhythm on examination and ECG.
- ► Prevention of stroke should be considered in all patients with risk factors for stroke (eg, heart failure, hypertension, age 65 or older, diabetes mellitus, prior history of stroke or TIA, and vascular disease).
- ► Heart rate control with beta-blocker or calcium channel blockers generally required. Restoration of sinus rhythm with cardioversion, antiarrhythmic medications, or catheter ablation in symptomatic patients.

General Considerations

Atrial fibrillation is the most common chronic arrhythmia, with an incidence and prevalence that rise with age, so that it affects approximately 9% of individuals over age 65 years. It occurs in rheumatic and other forms of valvular heart disease, dilated cardiomyopathy, ASD, hypertension, and CHD as well as in patients with no apparent cardiac disease; it may be the initial presenting sign in thyrotoxicosis, and this condition should be excluded with the initial episode.

Atrial fibrillation often appears in a **paroxysmal** fashion before becoming the established rhythm. Pericarditis, chest trauma, thoracic or cardiac surgery, thyroid disorders, obstructive sleep apnea, or pulmonary disease (pneumonia, pulmonary embolism) as well as medications such as theophylline and beta-adrenergic agonists may cause attacks in patients with normal hearts. Acute alcohol excess and alcohol withdrawal—and, in predisposed individuals, even consumption of small amounts of alcohol—may precipitate atrial fibrillation. This latter presentation, which is often termed **holiday heart,** is usually transient and self-limited. Short-term rate control usually suffices as treatment.

Atrial fibrillation, particularly when the ventricular rate is uncontrolled, can lead to LV dysfunction, heart failure, or myocardial ischemia (when underlying CAD is present). Perhaps the most serious consequence of atrial fibrillation is the propensity for thrombus formation due to stasis in the atria (particularly the left atrial appendage) and consequent embolization, most devastatingly to the cerebral circulation. Untreated, the rate of stroke is approximately 5% per year. However, patients with significant obstructive valvular disease, chronic heart failure or LV dysfunction, diabetes mellitus, hypertension, or age over 75 years and those with a history of prior stroke or other embolic events are at substantially higher risk (up to nearly 20% per year in patients with multiple risk factors) (Table 10–12). A substantial portion of the aging population with hypertension has **asymptomatic** or **"subclinical"** atrial fibrillation, which can be detected with monitoring devices and is also associated with increased risk of stroke, particularly if it lasts for 24 hours or longer. It is not clear whether, and for whom, oral anticoagulation should be used for subclinical atrial fibrillation, a question that is being addressed in ongoing clinical trials.

▶ Clinical Findings

A. Symptoms and Signs

Atrial fibrillation itself is rarely life-threatening; however, it can have serious consequences if the ventricular rate is sufficiently rapid to precipitate hypotension, myocardial ischemia, or tachycardia-induced myocardial dysfunction. Moreover, particularly in patients with risk factors, atrial fibrillation is a major preventable cause of stroke. Although many patients—particularly older or inactive individuals—have relatively few symptoms if the rate is controlled, some patients are aware of the irregular rhythm and may find it very uncomfortable. Most patients will complain of fatigue whether they experience other symptoms or not. The heart rate may range from quite slow to extremely rapid, but is uniformly irregular unless underlying complete heart block with junctional escape rhythm or a permanent ventricular pacemaker is in place. **Atrial fibrillation is the only common arrhythmia in which the ventricular rate is rapid and the rhythm very irregular.** Because of the varying stroke volumes resulting from fluctuating periods of diastolic filling, not all ventricular beats produce a palpable peripheral pulse. The difference between the apical rate and the pulse rate is the "pulse deficit"; this deficit is greater when the ventricular rate is high.

B. ECG

The surface ECG typically demonstrates erratic, disorganized atrial activity between discrete QRS complexes occurring in an irregular pattern. The atrial activity may be very fine and difficult to detect on the ECG, or quite coarse and often mistaken for atrial flutter.

C. Echocardiography

Echocardiography provides assessment of chamber volumes, left ventricular size and function, or the presence of concomitant valvular heart disease and should be performed in all patients with a new diagnosis of atrial fibrillation. TEE is the most sensitive imaging modality to identify thrombi in the left atrium or left atrial appendage prior to any attempt at chemical or electrical cardioversion.

▶ Treatment

A. Newly Diagnosed Atrial Fibrillation

1. Initial management

A. HEMODYNAMICALLY UNSTABLE PATIENT—If the patient is hemodynamically unstable—usually as a result of a rapid ventricular rate or associated cardiac or noncardiac conditions—hospitalization and immediate treatment of atrial fibrillation are required. Intravenous beta-blockers (esmolol, propranolol, and metoprolol) or calcium channel blockers (diltiazem and verapamil) are usually effective at

Table 10–12. CHADS$_2$ Risk Score for assessing risk of stroke and for selecting antithrombotic therapy for patients with atrial fibrillation.

	Condition	Points
C	Congestive heart failure	1
H	Hypertension (current or treated)	1
A	Age ≥ 75 years	1
D	Diabetes mellitus	1
S$_2$	Stroke or transient ischemic attack	2
CHADS$_2$ Score	Adjusted Stroke Rate, %/year (95% Confidence Interval)	Patients[1] (n = 1733)
0	1.9 (1.2 to 3.0)	120
1	2.8 (2.0 to 3.8)	463
2	4.0 (3.1 to 5.1)	523
3	5.9 (4.6 to 7.3)	337
4	8.5 (6.3 to 11)	220
5	12.5 (8.2 to 17.5)	65

[1]Validation performed in a population of Medicare beneficiaries aged 65 to 95 years who were not prescribed warfarin at hospital discharge.
Reproduced, with permission, from Gage BF et al. Validation of clinical classification schemes for predicting stroke: results from the National Registry of Atrial Fibrillation. JAMA. 2001;285(22):2864-70. Copyright © 2001 American Medical Association. All rights reserved.

rate control in the acute setting. Urgent electrical cardioversion is only indicated in patients with shock or severe hypotension, pulmonary edema, or ongoing MI or ischemia. There is a potential risk of thromboembolism in patients undergoing cardioversion who have not received anticoagulation therapy if atrial fibrillation has been present for more than 48 hours or is of unknown duration; however, in hemodynamically unstable patients the need for immediate rate control outweighs that risk. An initial shock with 100–200 J is administered in synchrony with the R wave. If sinus rhythm is not restored, an additional attempt with 360 J is indicated. If this fails, cardioversion may be successful after loading with intravenous ibutilide (1 mg over 10 minutes, repeated in 10 minutes if necessary).

B. Hemodynamically Stable Patient—If the patient has no symptoms, hemodynamic instability, or evidence of important precipitating conditions (such as silent MI or ischemia, decompensated heart failure, pulmonary embolism, or hemodynamically significant valvular disease), hospitalization is usually not necessary. In most of these cases, atrial fibrillation is an unrecognized chronic or paroxysmal condition and should be managed accordingly (see Subsequent Management, below). For new-onset atrial fibrillation, thyroid function tests and echocardiography to assess for occult valvular or myocardial disease should be performed.

In stable patients with atrial fibrillation, a strategy of **rate control** and **anticoagulation** is appropriate. This is true whether the conditions that precipitated atrial fibrillation are likely to persist (such as following cardiac or noncardiac surgery, with respiratory failure, or with pericarditis) or might resolve spontaneously over a period of hours to days (such as atrial fibrillation due to excessive alcohol intake, electrolyte imbalance or atrial fibrillation due to exposure to excessive theophylline or sympathomimetic agents). The choice of agent is guided by the hemodynamic status of the patient, associated conditions, and the urgency of achieving rate control. In the stable patient with atrial fibrillation, a beta-blocker or calcium channel blocker (orally or intravenously) is usually the first-line agent for ventricular rate control. In the setting of MI or ischemia, beta-blockers are the preferred agent. The most frequently used agents are either metoprolol (administered as a 5 mg intravenous bolus, repeated twice at intervals of 5 minutes and then given as needed by repeat boluses or orally at total daily doses of 25–200 mg) or, in unstable patients, esmolol (0.5 mg/kg intravenously, repeated once if necessary, followed by a titrated infusion of 0.05–0.2 mg/kg/min). If beta-blockers are contraindicated, calcium channel blockers are immediately effective. Diltiazem (10–20 mg bolus, repeated after 15 minutes if necessary, followed by a maintenance infusion of 5–15 mg/h) is the preferred calcium blocker if hypotension or LV dysfunction is present. Otherwise, verapamil (5–10 mg intravenously over 2–3 minutes, repeated after 30 minutes if necessary) may be used. Rate control using digoxin is slow (onset of action more than 1 hour with peak effect at 6 hours) and may be inadequate and is rarely indicated for use in the acute setting. Similarly, amiodarone, even when administered intravenously, has a relatively slow onset and is most useful as an adjunct

when rate control with the previously cited agents is incomplete or contraindicated or when cardioversion is planned in the near future. Care should be taken in patients with hypotension or heart failure because the rapid intravenous administration of amiodarone may worsen hemodynamics.

If the onset of atrial fibrillation was more than 48 hours prior to presentation (or unknown) and early cardioversion is considered necessary due to inability to adequately rate control, a transesophageal echocardiogram should be performed prior to cardioversion to exclude left atrial thrombus. If thrombus is present, the cardioversion is delayed until after a 4-week period of therapeutic anticoagulation. In any case, because atrial contractile activity may not recover for several weeks after restoration of sinus rhythm in patients who have been in atrial fibrillation for more than several days, cardioversion should be followed by anticoagulation *for at least 1 month* unless there is a strong contraindication.

2. Subsequent management—Up to two-thirds of patients experiencing a first episode of atrial fibrillation will spontaneously revert to sinus rhythm within 24 hours. In the absence of valvular heart disease, diabetes, hypertension or other risk factors for stroke, these patients may not require long-term anticoagulation beyond aspirin. If atrial fibrillation has been present for more than a week, spontaneous conversion is unlikely. In most cases immediate cardioversion is not required and management consists of rate control and anticoagulation whether or not the patient has been admitted to the hospital. Adequate rate control is usually achieved with beta-blockers or non-dihydropyridine calcium channel blockers. Long-term use of digoxin is associated with an increase in mortality in patients with chronic atrial fibrillation and is rarely indicated. Choice of the initial medication is best based on the presence of accompanying conditions: Hypertensive patients can be given beta-blockers or calcium blockers (see Tables 11–9 and 11–7). Patients with CHD or heart failure should receive a beta-blocker preferentially, whereas beta-blockers should be avoided in patients with severe chronic obstructive pulmonary disease (COPD) or asthma. In symptomatic patients, a resting heart rate of more than 80 beats/min is targeted. In asymptomatic patients without LV dysfunction, a more lenient resting heart rate of up to 100–110 beats/min is reasonable. Ambulatory monitoring to assess heart rate during exercise should be considered in all patients with a goal not to exceed maximum predicted heart rate (220 – age).

A. Anticoagulation—For patients with atrial fibrillation, even when it is paroxysmal or occurs rarely, the need for oral anticoagulation should be evaluated and treatment initiated for those without strong contraindication. Patients with **lone atrial fibrillation** (eg, no evidence of associated heart disease, hypertension, atherosclerotic vascular disease, diabetes mellitus, or history of stroke or TIA) under age 65 years need no antithrombotic treatment. Patients with **transient atrial fibrillation**, such as in the setting of acute MI or pneumonia, but no prior history of arrhythmia, are at high risk for future development of atrial fibrillation and appropriate anticoagulation should be initiated based on risk factors (Table 10–12). If the cause is reversible, such as after coronary artery bypass surgery or associated with hyperthyroidism, then long-term anticoagulation is not necessary.

In addition to the traditional five risk factors that comprise the **CHADS$_2$ score** (heart failure, hypertension, age 75 years or older, diabetes mellitus, and [2 points for] history of stroke or TIA), the European and American guidelines recommend that three additional factors included in the **CHA$_2$DS$_2$-VASc** score be considered: age 65–74 years, female sex, and presence of vascular disease (Table 10–13). The CHA$_2$DS$_2$-VASc score is especially relevant for patients who have a CHADS$_2$ score of 0 or 1; if the CHA$_2$DS$_2$-VASc score is greater than or equal to 2, oral anticoagulation is recommended, and if CHA$_2$DS$_2$-VASc score is 1, oral anticoagulation should be considered, taking into account risk, benefit, and patient preferences. (The use of warfarin is discussed in the section on Selecting Appropriate Anticoagulant Therapy in Chapter 14.) Unfortunately, studies show that *only about half* of patients with atrial fibrillation and an indication for oral anticoagulation are receiving it, and even when treated with warfarin, they are out of the target INR range nearly half the time. **One reason for undertreatment is the *misperception* that aspirin is useful for prevention of stroke due to atrial fibrillation.** In the 2016 European guidelines, aspirin is given a class III A recommendation, indicating that it should not be used because of harm (and with no good evidence of benefit). Cardioversion, if planned, should be performed after at least 3–4 weeks of anticoagulation at a therapeutic level (or after exclusion of left atrial appendage thrombus by transesophageal echocardiogram as discussed above). Anticoagulation clinics with systematic management of warfarin dosing and adjustment have been shown to result in better maintenance of target anticoagulation.

Four DOACs—dabigatran, rivaroxaban, apixaban, and edoxaban—have been shown to be at least as effective as warfarin for stroke prevention in patients with atrial fibrillation and have been approved by the FDA for this indication (Table 10–14). These medications have not been studied in patients with moderate or severe mitral stenosis, and they should not be used for patients with mechanical prosthetic valves. The term "nonvalvular atrial fibrillation" is no longer used in the European guidelines since most patients with other types of valvular heart disease have been included in trials of DOACs, which are equally effective in these patients.

Dabigatran (studied in the RE-LY trial) is superior to warfarin at preventing stroke at the 150 mg twice daily dose, and it is noninferior at the 110 mg twice daily dose, although this dose is not approved for treatment of atrial fibrillation in the United States. Both doses result in *less* intracranial hemorrhage than warfarin but also in *more* gastrointestinal bleeding than warfarin. Neither dabigatran nor any of the DOACs should be used in patients with mechanical prosthetic heart valves where the medications are less effective and riskier.

Rivaroxaban is noninferior to warfarin for stroke prevention in atrial fibrillation (in the ROCKET-AF trial). Rivaroxaban is dosed at 20 mg once daily, with a reduced

Table 10–13. CHA$_2$DS$_2$-VASc Risk Score for assessing risk of stroke and for selecting antithrombotic therapy for patients with atrial fibrillation.

CHA$_2$DS$_2$-VASc Risk Score	
Heart failure or LVEF ≤ 40%	1
Hypertension	1
Age ≥ 75 years	2
Diabetes mellitus	1
Stroke, transient ischemic attack, or thromboembolism	2
Vascular disease (previous myocardial infarction, peripheral artery disease, or aortic plaque)	1
Age 65–74 years	1
Female sex (but not a risk factor if female sex is the only factor)	1
Maximum score	9

Adjusted stroke rate according to CHA$_2$DS$_2$-VASc score

CHA$_2$DS$_2$-VASc Score	Patients (n = 7329)	Adjusted stroke rate (%/year)
0	1	0%
1	422	1.3%
2	1230	2.2%
3	1730	3.2%
4	1718	4.0%
5	1159	6.7%
6	679	9.8%
7	294	9.6%
8	82	6.7%
9	14	15.2%

CHA$_2$DS$_2$-VASc score = 0: recommend no antithrombotic therapy

CHA$_2$DS$_2$-VASc score = 1: recommend antithrombotic therapy with oral anticoagulation or antiplatelet therapy but preferably oral anticoagulation

CHA$_2$DS$_2$-VASc score = 2: recommend oral anticoagulation

CHA$_2$DS$_2$-VASc, Cardiac failure, Hypertension, Age ≥ 75 years (doubled), Diabetes, Stroke (doubled), Vascular disease, Age 65–74, and Sex category (female); LVEF, left ventricular ejection fraction. Data from Camm AJ et al. 2012 focused update of the ESC Guidelines for the management of atrial fibrillation: an update of the 2010 ESC Guidelines for the management of atrial fibrillation. Developed with the special contribution of the European Heart Rhythm Association. Eur Heart J. 2012 Nov;33(21) 2719–47.

dose (15 mg/day) for patients with creatinine clearances between 15 and 50 mL/min. It should be administered *with food*, since that results in a 40% higher drug absorption. Similar to dabigatran, there is substantially less intracranial hemorrhage with rivaroxaban than warfarin.

Apixaban is more effective than warfarin at stroke prevention while having a substantially lower risk of major

Table 10–14. Direct-acting oral anticoagulants for stroke prevention in patients with nonvalvular atrial fibrillation.

	Dabigatran	Rivaroxaban	Apixaban	Edoxaban
Class	Antithrombin	Factor Xa inhibitor	Factor Xa inhibitor	Factor Xa inhibitor
Bleeding risk compared to warfarin	Less intracranial bleeding Higher incidence of gastrointestinal bleeding	Less intracranial bleeding Higher incidence of gastrointestinal bleeding	Substantially lower risk of major bleeding Less intracranial bleeding	Lower risk of major bleeding Less intracranial bleeding
Dosage	110 mg twice daily 150 mg twice daily	20 mg once daily (give with food)	5 mg twice daily	60 mg once daily
Dosage adjustments	75 mg twice daily for creatinine clearance[1] 15–30 mL/min (approved in the United States but not tested in clinical trials)	15 mg once daily for creatinine clearance[1] < 50 mL/min	2.5 mg twice daily for patients with at least two of three risk factors: 1. Age ≥ 80 years 2. Body weight ≤ 60 kg 3. Serum creatinine ≥ 1.5 mg/dL	30 mg once daily for creatinine clearance[1] ≤ 50 mL/min FDA recommends not to use if creatinine clearance[1] > 95 mL/min

[1]Creatinine clearance calculated by Cockcroft-Gault equation.
Data from Nishimura RA et al. 2014 AHA/ACC Guideline for the Management of Patients With Valvular Heart Disease: A Report of the American College of Cardiology/American Heart Association Task Force on Practice Guidelines. Circulation. 2014 Jun 10;129(23):e521–643.

bleeding (in the ARISOTLE trial) and a lower risk of all-cause mortality. The apixaban dosage is 5 mg twice daily or 2.5 mg twice daily for patients with two of three high-risk criteria (age 80 years or older, body weight 60 kg or less, and serum creatinine of 1.5 mg/dL or more). Apixaban is associated with less intracranial hemorrhage and is well tolerated. Apixaban was also shown to be superior to aspirin (and better tolerated) in the AVERROES trial of patients deemed not suitable for warfarin.

Edoxaban, 60 mg once a day, is noninferior to warfarin for stroke prevention with lower rates of major bleeding and lower rates of hemorrhagic stroke (studied in the ENGAGE-AF trial). Edoxaban carries a boxed warning in FDA labelleling that it should not be used in patients whose creatinine clearance is more than 95 mL/min because it is less effective in this population. The dose is decreased to 30 mg/day for patients whose creatinine clearance is less than or equal to 50 mL/min.

These four DOACs have important advantages over warfarin, and therefore they are recommended preferentially over VKAs. In practice, these medications are often underdosed. They should be used at the doses shown to be effective in the clinical trials as shown in Table 10–14. Even though labeled for "nonvalvular" atrial fibrillation, the DOACs are safe and effective for patients with moderate or severe valvular abnormalities, with the exception of moderate or severe mitral stenosis. In part because of lower rates of intracerebral hemorrhage, DOACs have particular advantage over warfarin in the elderly and the frail, including patients with history of falls. For patients who fall, oral anticoagulation should generally be used, except for patients who are suffering head trauma with falls.

There are some patients with atrial fibrillation, however, who *should* be treated with VKAs. These patients include those who have mechanical prosthetic valves, advanced kidney disease (creatinine clearance less than 25 mL/min), or moderate or severe mitral stenosis, and those who cannot

afford the newer medications. Patients who have been stable while receiving warfarin for a long time, with a high time in target INR range, and who are at lower risk for intracranial hemorrhage will have relatively less benefit with a switch to a newer medication. It is important to note, however, that most patients who have intracranial hemorrhage while taking warfarin have had a recent INR below 3.0, so that good INR control does not ensure avoidance of intracranial bleeding. One way to reduce bleeding for patients taking oral anticoagulants is to avoid concurrent aspirin, unless the patient has a clear indication, like recent MI or coronary stent. Even then, use of oral anticoagulant plus clopidogrel without aspirin, or with only a brief period of "triple" therapy and then discontinuation of aspirin, may be a reasonable approach, as has been shown in clinical trials comparing rivaroxaban and dabigatran with warfarin.

There are some important practical issues with using the DOACs. It is important to monitor kidney function at baseline and at least once a year, or more often for those with impaired kidney function. Each of the medications interacts with other medications affecting the P-glycoprotein pathway, like oral ketoconazole, verapamil, dronederone, and phenytoin. Each of the medications has a half-life of about 10–12 hours for patients with normal kidney function. For elective procedures, stop the medications two to three half-lives (usually 24–48 hours) before procedures with low to moderate bleeding risk (ie, colonoscopy, dental extraction, cardiac catheterization), and five half-lives before procedures like major surgery. Discontinuation times should be extended in patients with impaired renal function, particularly with dabigatran. There are no practical tests to immediately measure the effect of the medications, although a normal aPTT suggests little effect with dabigatran, and a normal prothrombin suggests little effect with rivaroxaban. For rivaroxaban and apixaban, chromogenic Xa assays will measure the effect, but may not be readily available. For bleeding, standard measures (eg, diagnosing and controlling the source, stopping antithrombotic agents, and replacing blood products) should be taken. If the direct-acting medication was taken in the prior 2–4 hours, use activated oral charcoal to reduce absorption. If the patient is taking aspirin, consider platelet transfusion. Antidotes should be considered for life-threatening bleeding or for patients with need for immediate surgery, or both. For cardioversion, the DOACs appear to have similar rates of subsequent stroke as warfarin, as long as patients have been taking the medications and adherent for at least several weeks. Like with warfarin, there appears to be a 1.5- to 2-fold increased rate of bleeding associated with the use of aspirin in combination with the DOACs. Therefore, **aspirin should not be used with the DOACs unless there is a clear indication, such as acute coronary syndrome within the prior year.**

A patient with severe bleeding while taking dabigatran may be treated with the reversal agent **idarucizumab,** which is a humanized monoclonal antibody approved by the FDA for rapid reversal of the anticoagulation effects, for use in the event of severe bleeding or the need for an urgent procedure. This treatment is widely available in the United States. Andexanet alfa, an intravenous factor Xa decoy, is approved for reversal of factor Xa inhibitors. Four-factor prothrombin complex concentrate may partially reverse the effects of these agents. Due to the short half-life of the DOACs (10–12 hours with normal kidney function), supportive measures (local control, packed red blood cells, platelets) may suffice until the medication has cleared.

Each of the DOACs appears to be safe and effective around the time of electrical cardioversion. In each of these trials, and in one modest-sized prospective randomized trial of rivaroxaban that specifically addressed cardioversion, the rates of stroke were low (and similar to warfarin) with the DOACs when given for at least 3–4 weeks prior to cardioversion. An advantage of the DOACs is that when stable anticoagulation is desired before elective cardioversion, it is achieved faster than with warfarin.

Devices to exclude the left atrial appendage have been shown to protect against stroke, although they are not as effective as warfarin to prevent ischemic stroke; the most commonly used approved devices are the Watchman (United States and Europe) and Amulet (Europe), which are options for patients who are unsuitable for long-term anticoagulation.

B. Rate Control or Elective Cardioversion—Two large randomized controlled trials (the 4060-patient Atrial Fibrillation Follow-up Investigation of Rhythm Management, or AFFIRM trial; and the Rate Control Versus Electrical Cardioversion for Persistent Atrial Fibrillation, or RACE trial) compared strategies of rate control and rhythm control. In both, a strategy of rate control and long-term anticoagulation was associated with no higher rates of death or stroke—both, if anything, *favored rate control*—and only a modestly increased risk of hemorrhagic events over a strategy of restoring sinus rhythm and maintaining it with antiarrhythmic drug therapy. Of note is that exercise tolerance and quality of life were not significantly better in the rhythm control group. Nonetheless, the decision of

whether to attempt to restore sinus rhythm following the initial episode remains controversial. Elective cardioversion following an appropriate period of anticoagulation (minimum of 4 weeks) is generally recommended for the initial episode in patients in whom atrial fibrillation is thought to be of recent onset and when there is an identifiable precipitating factor. Similarly, cardioversion is appropriate in patients who remain symptomatic from the rhythm despite efforts to achieve rate control.

In cases in which elective cardioversion is required, it may be accomplished electrically or pharmacologically. A number of factors influence the success of electrical cardioversion. Biphasic energy waveform and anteroposterior electrode placement provide superior effectiveness. Pharmacologic cardioversion with **intravenous ibutilide** may be used (1 mg over 10 minutes, repeated in 10 minutes if necessary) in a setting in which the patient can undergo continuous ECG monitoring for at least 4–6 hours following administration. Pretreatment with intravenous magnesium (1–2 g) may prevent rare episodes of torsades de pointes associated with ibutilide administration. In patients in whom a decision has been made to continue antiarrhythmic therapy to maintain sinus rhythm (see next paragraph), cardioversion can be attempted with an agent that is being considered for long-term use. For instance, after therapeutic anticoagulation has been established, **amiodarone** can be initiated on an outpatient basis (400 mg twice daily for 2 weeks, followed by 200 mg twice daily for at least 2–4 weeks and then a maintenance dose of 200 mg daily). Because amiodarone increases the prothrombin time in patients taking warfarin and increases digoxin levels, careful monitoring of anticoagulation and medication levels is required.

Other agents that may be used for both cardioversion and maintenance therapy include dofetilide, propafenone, flecainide, and sotalol. **Dofetilide** (125–500 mcg twice daily orally) must be initiated in hospital due to the potential risk of torsades de pointes and the downward dose adjustment that is required for patients with renal impairment. **Propafenone** (150–300 mg orally every 8 hours) should be avoided in patients with structural heart disease (CAD, systolic dysfunction, or significant LVH). **Flecainide** (50–150 mg twice daily orally) should be used in conjunction with an AV nodal blocking medication, especially if there is a history of atrial flutter and should be avoided in patients with structural heart disease. **Sotalol** (80–160 mg orally twice daily) should be initiated in the hospital in patients with structural heart disease due to a risk of torsades de pointes; it is not very effective for converting atrial fibrillation but can be used to maintain sinus rhythm following cardioversion.

In patients treated long-term with an antiarrhythmic agent, sinus rhythm will persist in 30–50%. The most commonly used medications are amiodarone, dronedarone, sotalol, propafenone, flecainide, and dofetilide, but the latter four agents are associated with a clear risk of proarrhythmia in certain populations; dronedarone has less efficacy than amiodarone, and amiodarone frequently causes other adverse effects. Therefore, after an initial presentation of atrial fibrillation, it may be prudent to determine whether atrial fibrillation recurs during a period of

6 months without antiarrhythmic medications. If it does recur, the decision to restore sinus rhythm and initiate long-term antiarrhythmic therapy can be based on how well the patient tolerates atrial fibrillation. The decision to maintain long-term anticoagulation should be based on risk factors (CHADS$_2$ or CHA$_2$DS$_2$-VASc score, Tables 10–12 and 10–13) and not on the perceived presence or absence of atrial fibrillation as future episodes may be asymptomatic.

B. Recurrent and Refractory Atrial Fibrillation

1. Recurrent paroxysmal atrial fibrillation—Patients with recurrent paroxysmal atrial fibrillation are at similar stroke risk as those who are in atrial fibrillation chronically. Although these episodes may be apparent to the patient, many are not recognized and may be totally asymptomatic. Thus, extended continuous ambulatory monitoring or event recorders are indicated in those in whom paroxysmal atrial fibrillation is suspected. Long-term anticoagulation should be considered for all patients except in those who are under 65 years of age and have no additional stroke risk factors. Antiarrhythmic agents are first-line therapy for recurrent, symptomatic atrial fibrillation; however, they are not often successful in preventing all paroxysmal atrial fibrillation episodes.

2. Refractory atrial fibrillation—Atrial fibrillation should generally be considered refractory if it causes persistent symptoms or limits activity despite attempts at rate control. This is much more likely in younger individuals and those who are active or engage in strenuous exercise. Even in such individuals, combined use of a beta-blocker and a non-dihydropyridine calcium channel blocker can prevent excessive ventricular rates, though in some cases may cause excessive bradycardia during sedentary periods.

If antiarrhythmic or rate-control medications fail to improve the symptoms of atrial fibrillation, catheter ablation of foci in and around the pulmonary veins that initiate and maintain atrial fibrillation may be considered. **Pulmonary vein isolation** is a reasonable second-line therapy for individuals with symptomatic paroxysmal or persistent atrial fibrillation that is refractory to pharmacologic therapy and for select patients (older than 65 years or with concurrent heart failure) as first-line therapy. Ablation is successful about 50–70% of the time but more than one procedure may be required. The procedure is routinely performed in the electrophysiology laboratory using a catheter-based approach and can also be performed via a subxiphoid approach thorascopically, via thoracotomy, or via median sternotomy in the operating room by experienced surgeons. In symptomatic patients with poor rate-control and deemed inappropriate for pulmonary vein isolation, radiofrequency ablation of the AV node and permanent pacing ensure rate control and may facilitate a more physiologic rate response to activity, but this is used only as a last resort.

When to Refer

- Symptomatic atrial fibrillation with or without adequate rate control.

- Asymptomatic atrial fibrillation with poor rate control despite AV nodal blockers.
- Patients at risk for stroke who have not tolerated oral anticoagulants.

Kirchhof P et al. 2016 ESC Guidelines for the management of atrial fibrillation developed in collaboration with EACTS. Eur Heart J. 2016 Oct 7;37(38):2893–962. [PMID: 27567408]
Marrouche N et al; CASTLE-AF Investigators. Catheter ablation for atrial fibrillation with heart failure. N Engl J Med. 2018 Feb 1;378(5):417–27. [PMID: 29385358]
Piccini JP et al. Rhythm control in atrial fibrillation. Lancet. 2016 Aug 20;388(10046):829–40. [PMID: 27560278]
Van Gelder IC et al. Rate control in atrial fibrillation. Lancet. 2016 Aug 20;388(10046):818–28. [PMID: 27560277]

ATRIAL FLUTTER

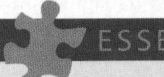 ESSENTIALS OF DIAGNOSIS

- ▶ Rapid, regular tachycardia presenting classically with 2 to 1 block in the AV node and ventricular heart rate of 150 beats/min. ECG shows "sawtooth" pattern of atrial activity (rate 300 beats/min).
- ▶ Stroke risk should be considered equivalent to that with atrial fibrillation.
- ▶ Catheter ablation is highly successful and is considered the definitive treatment for typical atrial flutter.

General Considerations

Atrial flutter is less common than fibrillation. It may occur in patients with structurally normal hearts but is more commonly seen in patients with COPD, valvular or structural heart disease, ASD, or surgically repaired congenital heart disease.

Clinical Findings

Patients typically present with complaints of palpitations, fatigue, or mild dizziness. In situations where the arrhythmia is unrecognized for a prolonged period of time, patients may present with symptoms and signs of heart failure (dyspnea, exertional intolerance, edema) due to tachycardia-induced cardiomyopathy. The ECG typically demonstrates a **"sawtooth"** pattern of atrial activity in the inferior leads (II, III, and AVF). The reentrant circuit generates atrial rates of 250–350 beats/min, usually with transmission of every second, third, or fourth impulse through the AV node to the ventricles.

Treatment

Ventricular rate control is accomplished using the same agents used in atrial fibrillation, but it is generally more difficult. Conversion of atrial flutter to sinus rhythm with class I antiarrhythmic agents is also difficult to achieve, and administration of these medications has been associated with slowing of the atrial flutter rate to the point at which 1:1 AV conduction can occur at rates in excess of 200 beats/min, with subsequent hemodynamic collapse. The intravenous class III antiarrhythmic agent ibutilide has been significantly more successful in converting atrial flutter (see Table 10–11). About 50–70% of patients return to sinus rhythm within 60–90 minutes following the infusion of 1–2 mg of this agent. Electrical cardioversion is also very effective for atrial flutter, with approximately 90% of patients converting following synchronized shocks of as little as 25–50 J.

Although the organization of atrial contractile function in this arrhythmia may provide some protection against thrombus formation, **the risk of thromboembolism should be considered equivalent to that with atrial fibrillation** due to the common coexistence of these arrhythmias. Precardioversion anticoagulation is not necessary for atrial flutter of less than 48 hours duration except in the setting of mitral valve disease. As with atrial fibrillation, anticoagulation should be continued for at least 4 weeks after electrical or chemical cardioversion and chronically in patients with risk factors for thromboembolism.

Catheter ablation is the treatment of choice for long-term management of atrial flutter owing to the high success rate and safety of the procedure. The anatomy of the typical circuit is well defined and catheter ablation within the right atrium results in immediate and permanent elimination of atrial flutter in more than 90% of patients. Due to the frequent coexistence of atrial flutter with atrial fibrillation, however, some patients may require catheter ablation of both arrhythmias. If pharmacologic therapy is chosen, class III antiarrhythmics (amiodarone or dofetilide) are generally preferred (see Table 10–11). Dofetilide is often given in conjunction with an AV nodal blocker (other than verapamil).

When to Refer

All patients with atrial flutter should be referred to a cardiologist or cardiac electrophysiologist for consideration of definitive treatment with catheter ablation.

ATRIAL TACHYCARDIA

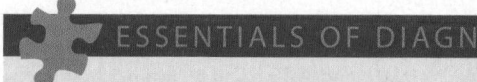

ESSENTIALS OF DIAGNOSIS

- ▶ Characterized by bursts of rapid, regular tachycardia.
- ▶ Multifocal atrial tachycardia commonly seen with severe COPD and presents with three or more distinct P wave morphologies on ECG, often confused for atrial fibrillation. Treatment of the underlying lung disease is most effective therapy.

General Considerations

Atrial tachycardia is an uncommon form of SVT characterized by paroxysms or bursts of rapid, regular arrhythmia due to focal atrial impulses originating outside of the normal sinus node. Common sites include the tricuspid annulus, the crista terminalis of the right atrium and the coronary sinus. **Multifocal atrial tachycardia** is a particular subtype seen in patients with severe COPD and characterized by varying P wave morphology (by definition, three or more foci) and markedly irregular PP intervals. The rate is usually between 100 beats/min and 140 beats/min, and it is often confused for atrial fibrillation. **Solitary atrial premature beats** are benign and generally not associated with underlying cardiac disease. They occur when an ectopic focus in the atria fires before the next sinus node impulse. The contour of the P wave usually differs from the patient's normal complex, unless the ectopic focus is near the sinus node. Acceleration of the heart rate by any means usually abolishes most premature beats.

Clinical Findings

Focal atrial tachycardias are usually intermittent and self-limiting although incessant forms do exist and may present with signs and symptoms of heart failure due to tachycardia-induced cardiomyopathy. Most patients report palpitations with an abrupt onset, similar to other forms of PSVT. Patients with underlying cardiac pathology (eg, CHD) can present with dyspnea or angina. Close inspection of the P wave on 12-lead ECG suggests a focus away from the sinus node, although certain locations (eg, high right atrial crista terminalis) may mimic sinus tachycardia. In this situation, the abrupt onset and offset of the arrhythmia is helpful in distinguishing atrial from sinus tachycardia, although electrophysiologic study is sometimes necessary.

Treatment

Initial management of atrial tachycardia is similar to other types of PSVT; however, vagal maneuvers and intravenous adenosine are generally less effective. Intravenous beta-blockers or calcium channel blockers can be given in the hemodynamically stable patient with a change to oral formulations for long-term managment. Antiarrhythmic medications or catheter ablation should be considered in patients who continue to have symptomatic episodes. Long-term anticoagulation is not indicated in the absence of coexistant atrial fibrillation or atrial flutter.

For patients with multifocal atrial tachycardia, treatment of the underlying condition (eg, COPD) is paramount; verapamil, 240–480 mg orally daily in divided doses may be effective in some patients.

When to Refer

All patients with atrial tachycardia in whom initial medical management fails should be referred to a cardiologist or cardiac electrophysiologist.

VENTRICULAR PREMATURE BEATS
(Ventricular Extrasystoles)

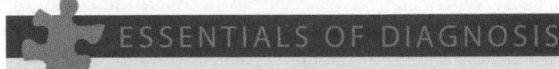

ESSENTIALS OF DIAGNOSIS

- ▶ Common but rarely symptomatic.
- ▶ Ambulatory ECG monitoring to quantify daily burden of PVCs. Asymptomatic patients with greater than 10% PVC burden should have periodic echocardiogram to exclude development of LV dysfunction.

General Considerations

Ventricular premature beats, or **PVCs,** are isolated beats typically originating from the outflow tract or His-Purkinje regions of ventricular tissue. In most patients, the presence of PVCs is a benign finding; however, they rarely may trigger ventricular tachycardia or ventricular fibrillation, especially in patients with underlying heart disease.

Clinical Findings

The patient may or may not sense the irregular beat, usually as a skipped beat. Exercise generally abolishes premature beats in normal hearts, and the rhythm becomes regular. Ventricular premature beats are characterized by wide QRS complexes that differ in morphology from the patient's normal beats. They are usually not preceded by a P wave, although retrograde ventriculoatrial conduction may occur. Bigeminy and trigeminy are arrhythmias in which every second or third beat is premature; these patterns confirm a reentry mechanism for the ectopic beat. Ambulatory ECG monitoring may reveal more frequent and complex ventricular premature beats than occur in a single routine ECG. An increased frequency of ventricular premature beats during exercise is associated with a higher risk of cardiovascular mortality and should be investigated further.

Treatment

If no associated cardiac disease is present and if the ectopic beats are asymptomatic, no therapy is indicated. Mild symptoms or anxiety from palpitations may be allayed with reassurance to the patient of the benign nature of this arrhythmia. If PVCs are frequent (bigeminal or trigeminal pattern), electrolyte abnormalities (especially hypokalemia or hyperkalemia and hypomagnesemia), hyperthyroidism, and occult heart disease should be excluded. In addition, an echocardiogram should be performed in patients in whom a burden of PVCs of greater than 10,000 per day has been documented by ambulatory ECG monitoring. Pharmacologic treatment is indicated only for patients who are symptomatic or who develop cardiomyopathy thought to be due to a high burden of PVCs (generally greater than 10% of daily heart beats). Beta-blockers or non-dihydropyridine calcium channel blockers are appropriate as first-line therapy. The class I and III antiarrhythmic agents (see Table 10–11) may be effective in reducing ventricular premature beats but are often poorly tolerated and can be proarrhythmic in up to 5% of patients. Catheter ablation is a well-established therapy for symptomatic individuals who do not respond to medication or for those patients whose burden of ectopic beats has resulted in a cardiomyopathy.

▶ When to Refer

Patients with symptomatic PVCs who do not respond to initial medical management or asymptomatic patients with daily PVC burden greater than 10% on ambulatory ECG monitoring should be referred to a cardiologist or cardiac electrophysiologist.

Tran CT et al. Premature ventricular contraction-induced cardiomyopathy: an emerging entity. Expert Rev Cardiovasc Ther. 2016 Nov;14(11):1227–34. [PMID: 27531417]

VENTRICULAR TACHYCARDIA

ESSENTIALS OF DIAGNOSIS

- ▶ Fast, wide QRS complex on ECG.
- ▶ Associated with ischemic heart disease, particularly in older patients.
- ▶ In the absence of reversible cause, implantable cardioverter defibrillator (ICD) is recommended if meaningful life expectancy is longer than 1 year.

General Considerations

Ventricular tachycardia is defined as three or more consecutive ventricular premature beats. It is classified as either **nonsustained** (lasting less than 30 seconds and terminating spontaneously) or **sustained** with a heart rate greater than 100 beats/min. In individuals without heart disease, nonsustained ventricular tachycardia is generally associated with a benign prognosis. In patients with structural heart disease, nonsustained ventricular tachycardia is associated with an increased risk of subsequent symptomatic ventricular tachycardia and sudden death, especially when seen more than 48 hours after MI.

Ventricular tachycardia is a frequent complication of acute MI and dilated cardiomyopathy but may occur in chronic coronary disease, hypertrophic cardiomyopathy, myocarditis, and in most other forms of myocardial disease. It can also be a consequence of atypical forms of cardiomyopathies, such as arrhythmogenic right ventricular cardiomyopathy. However, idiopathic ventricular tachycardia can also occur in patients with structurally normal hearts. **Accelerated idioventricular rhythm** is a regular wide complex rhythm with a rate of 60–120 beats/min, usually with a gradual onset. It occurs commonly in acute infarction and following reperfusion with thrombolytic medications. Treatment is not indicated unless there is hemodynamic compromise or more serious arrhythmias.

Torsades de pointes, a form of ventricular tachycardia in which QRS morphology twists around the baseline, may occur in the setting of severe hypokalemia, hypomagnesemia, or after administration of a medication that prolongs the QT interval. In nonacute settings, most patients with ventricular tachycardia have known or easily detectable cardiac disease, and the finding of ventricular tachycardia is an unfavorable prognostic sign.

► Clinical Findings

A. Symptoms and Signs

Patients commonly experience palpitations, dyspnea, or lightheadedness, but on rare occasion may be asymptomatic. Syncope or cardiac arrest can be presenting symptoms in patients with underlying cardiac disease or other severe comorbidities. Episodes may be triggered by exercise or emotional stress.

B. Diagnostic Studies

Comprehensive blood laboratory work should be performed because ventricular tachycardia can occur in the setting of hypokalemia and hypomagnesemia. Cardiac markers may be elevated when ventricular tachycardia presents in the setting of acute MI or as a consequence of underlying CAD and demand ischemia. In patients with sustained, hemodynamically tolerated ventricular tachycardia, a 12-lead ECG during tachycardia should be obtained. Cardiac evaluation with echocardiography or cardiac MRI, ambulatory ECG monitoring, and exercise testing may be warranted depending on the clinical situation. In survivors of cardiac arrest or those with life-threatening ventricular arrhythmia, invasive coronary angiography is recommended to establish or exclude the presence of significant CAD.

There is generally no role for invasive electrophysiologic study in patients with sustained ventricular tachycardia who otherwise meet criteria for ICD. In patients with structural heart disease and syncope of unknown cause, or in situations in which the mechanism of wide-complex tachycardia is uncertain, electrophysiologic study may provide important information.

C. Differentiation of Aberrantly Conducted Supraventricular Beats From Ventricular Beats

The distinction on 12-lead ECG of ventricular tachycardia from SVT with aberrant conduction may be difficult in patients with a wide-complex tachycardia; it is important because of the differing prognostic and therapeutic implications of each type. Findings favoring a **ventricular origin** include: (1) AV dissociation; (2) a QRS duration exceeding 0.14 second; (3) capture or fusion beats (infrequent); (4) left axis deviation with right bundle branch block morphology; (5) monophasic (R) or biphasic (qR, QR, or RS) complexes in V_1; and (6) a qR or QS complex in V_6. **Supraventricular origin** is favored by: (1) a triphasic QRS complex, especially if there was initial negativity in leads I and V_6; (2) ventricular rates exceeding 170 beats/min; (3) QRS duration longer than 0.12 second but not longer than 0.14 second; and (4) the presence of preexcitation syndrome. Patients with a wide-complex tachycardia, especially those with known cardiac disease, should be presumed to have ventricular tachycardia if the diagnosis is unclear.

► Treatment

A. Initial Management

The treatment of acute ventricular tachycardia is determined by the degree of hemodynamic compromise and the duration of the arrhythmia. In patients with structurally normal hearts, the prognosis is generally benign and syncope is uncommon. The etiology is often triggered activity from the right or left ventricular outflow tract and immediate treatment with a short-acting intravenous beta-blocker or verapamil may terminate the episode.

In the presence of known or suspected structural heart disease, assessment of hemodynamic stability determines the need for urgent direct current cardioversion. When ventricular tachycardia causes hypotension, heart failure, or myocardial ischemia, immediate synchronized direct current cardioversion with 100–360 J should be performed. If ventricular tachycardia recurs, intravenous amiodarone (150-mg bolus followed by 1 mg/min infusion for 6 hours and then 0.5 mg/min for 18 hours) should be administered to achieve a stable rhythm with further attempts at cardioversion as necessary. Significant hypotension can occur with rapid infusions of amiodarone. The management of ventricular tachycardia in the setting of acute MI is discussed in the Complications section of Acute Myocardial Infarction with ST-Segment Elevation.

In patients with sustained ventricular tachycardia who are hemodynamically stable, medical treatment with intravenous amiodarone, lidocaine or procainamide can be used; however direct current cardioversion should be performed if the ventricular tachycardia fails to terminate or symptoms worsen. Empiric magnesium replacement (1–2 g intravenously) may help especially for polymorphic ventricular tachycardia. If polymorphic ventricular tachycardia recurs, increasing the heart rate with isoproterenol infusion (up to 20 mcg/min) or atrial pacing with a temporary pacemaker (at 90–120 beats/min) will effectively shorten the QT interval to prevent further episodes.

B. Long-Term-Management

Patients with symptomatic or sustained ventricular tachycardia in the absence of a reversible precipitating cause (acute MI or ischemia, electrolyte imbalance, medication toxicity, etc) are at high risk for recurrence. In patients with structurally normal hearts and ventricular tachycardia with typical outflow tract (left bundle branch block with inferior axis) or left posterior fascicle (right bundle branch block with superior axis) appearance on ECG, suppressive treatment with beta-blocker or a non-dihydropyridine calcium channel blocker may be tried. Catheter ablation has a high success rate in these patients who fail initial medical treatment. In patients with significant LV dysfunction, subsequent sudden death is common and ICD implantation is recommended if meaningful survival is expected to be longer than 1 year. Beta-blockers are the mainstay for medical treatment of ventricular tachycardia in patients with structural heart disease. Antiarrhythmic medications have not been shown to lower mortality in these patients, but may decrease subsequent episodes and reduce the number of ICD shocks. Amiodarone is generally preferred in patients with structural heart disease but sotalol may be considered as well. Catheter ablation is an important treatment option for those patients with recurrent tachycardia who do not respond to or are intolerant of medical therapy; however, recurrence rates are high.

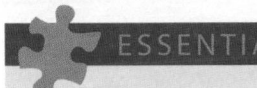 **When to Refer**

Any patient with sustained ventricular tachycardia or syncope of unknown cause in the presence of underlying structural cardiac disease.

Al-Khatib SM et al. 2017 AHA/ACC/HRS guideline for management of patients with ventricular arrhythmias and the prevention of sudden cardiac death: a report of the American College of Cardiology/American Heart Association Task Force on Clinical Practice Guidelines and the Heart Rhythm Society. J Am Coll Cardiol. 2017 Oct 25. pii: S0735-1097(17) 41306-4. [PMID: 29097296]

VENTRICULAR FIBRILLATION & SUDDEN DEATH

 ESSENTIALS OF DIAGNOSIS

► Most patients with sudden cardiac death have underlying CHD.

► In the absence of reversible cause, ICD is recommended.

General Considerations

Sudden cardiac death is defined as unexpected nontraumatic death in clinically well or stable patients who die within 1 hour after onset of symptoms. The causative rhythm in most cases is ventricular fibrillation. **Sudden cardiac arrest** is a term reserved for the successful resuscitation of ventricular fibrillation, either spontaneously or via intervention (defibrillation).

Clinical Findings

Approximately 70% of cases of sudden cardiac death are attributable to underlying CHD; in up to 40% of patients, sudden cardiac death may be the initial manifestation of CHD. Other forms of structural heart disease can predispose to sudden cardiac death including idiopathic cardiomyopathy, hypertrophic cardiomyopathy, valvular heart disease (aortic stenosis, pulmonic stenosis), congenital heart disease, arrhythmogenic right ventricular cardiomyopathy, and myocarditis. Five to 10% of cases of sudden cardiac death are primarily arrhythmic and occur in the absence of structural heart disease. Etiologies include long QT syndrome, Brugada syndrome, and catecholaminergic polymorphic ventricular tachycardia. Prompt evaluation to exclude reversible causes of sudden cardiac arrest should begin immediately following resuscitation. Laboratory testing should be performed to exclude severe electrolyte abnormalities (particularly hypokalemia and hypomagnesemia) and acidosis and to evaluate cardiac biomarkers. Caution should be taken in attributing cardiac arrest solely to an electrolyte disturbance,

however, because laboratory abnormalities may be secondary to resuscitation and not causative of the event. A 12-lead ECG should be performed to evaluate for ongoing ischemia or conduction system disease. Ventricular function should be evaluated with echocardiography. Coronary arteriography should be performed to exclude coronary disease as the underlying cause, since revascularization may prevent recurrence. In the absence of coronary disease, contrast-enhanced cardiac MRI may be used to evaluate for the presence of myocardial scar, which is a strong predictor of recurrent ventricular tachycardia/ventricular fibrillation in patients with nonischemic cardiomyopathy.

Treatment

Unless ventricular fibrillation occurs shortly after MI, is associated with ischemia, or is seen with a correctable process (such as an electrolyte abnormality or medication toxicity), surviving patients require intervention since recurrences are frequent. Survivors of cardiac arrest have improved long-term outcomes if a hypothermia protocol is rapidly initiated and continued for 24–36 hours after cardiac arrest.

Patients who survive sudden cardiac arrest have a high incidence of recurrence, so an ICD is generally indicated. Sudden cardiac arrest in the setting of acute ischemia or infarct should be managed with prompt coronary revascularization. However, implantation of a prophylactic ICD in patients immediately after MI is associated with a trend toward worse outcomes. These patients may be managed with a **wearable cardioverter defibrillator** until recovery of ventricular function can be assessed by echocardiogram at a later date (6–12 weeks following MI or coronary intervention).

When to Refer

All survivors of sudden cardiac arrest should be referred to a cardiologist or cardiac electrophysiologist.

Morin DP et al. Prediction and prevention of sudden cardiac death. Card Electrophysiol Clin. 2017 Dec;9(4):631–8. [PMID: 29173406]

INHERITED ARRHYTHMIA SYNDROMES

ESSENTIALS OF DIAGNOSIS

► Includes long QT syndrome, Brugada syndrome, and catecholaminergic polymorphic ventricular tachycardia.

► Genetic testing for patients with suspected congenital long QT syndrome based on family history, ECG or exercise testing, or severely prolonged QT interval (greater than 500 msec) on serial ECGs.

► Patients with long QT syndrome or catecholaminergic polymorphic ventricular tachycardia should be treated long term with an oral beta-blocker (nadolol or propranolol). ICD is indicated for patients with ventricular arrhythmia or syncope despite medical treatment.

General Considerations

Inherited arrhythmia syndromes may result in life-threatening ventricular arrhythmias due to gene mutations in cardiac channels resulting in abnormal electrolyte regulation across the cardiac cell membrane. **Congenital long QT syndrome** is an uncommon disease (1 in 2500 live births) that is characterized by a long QT interval (usually greater than 470 msec) and ventricular arrhythmia, typically polymorphic ventricular tachycardia. **Acquired long QT syndrome** is usually secondary to use of antiarrhythmic agents (sotalol, dofetilide), methadone, antidepressant medications, or certain antibiotics; electrolyte abnormalities; myocardial ischemia; or significant bradycardia. **Brugada syndrome** accounts for up to 20% of sudden cardiac death in the absence of structural heart disease and is most often due to a defect in a sodium channel gene. **Catecholaminergic polymorphic ventricular tachycardia** is a rare but important cause of sudden cardiac death associated with exercise.

Clinical Findings

Patients with an inherited arrhythmia syndrome have a variable clinical presentation; they may be asymptomatic or have palpitations, sustained tachyarrhythmia, syncope, or sudden cardiac arrest. In young patients, syncopal episodes may be misdiagnosed as a primary seizure disorder. Personal and family history should be thoroughly reviewed in all patients. A 12-lead ECG should be performed with careful attention to any abnormality in the ST segment, T wave, and QT interval. A corrected QT interval longer than 500 msec on serial ECGs in the absence of a secondary cause (medication or electrolyte abnormality) identifies a high-risk subset of patients with long QT syndrome. Ambulatory ECG monitoring may be used to evaluate for ventricular arrhythmias as well as dynamic changes to the QT interval or T wave. Exercise ECG testing may be performed in patients with suspected long QT syndrome to assess for lack of appropriate QT interval shortening with higher heart rates. Consultation with a genetic counselor and genetic testing are recommended for patients and family members with a high suspicion of an inherited arrhythmia syndrome.

Treatment

The management of acute polymorphic ventricular tachycardia (torsades de pointes) differs from that of other forms of ventricular tachycardia. Class Ia, Ic, or III antiarrhythmics, which prolong the QT interval, should be avoided—or withdrawn immediately if being used in patients with long QT syndrome. Intravenous beta-blockers may be effective in treating electrical storm due to long QT syndrome or catecholaminergic polymorphic ventricular tachycardia. Increasing the heart rate, whether by infusion of beta-agonist (dopamine or isoproterenol) or temporary atrial or ventricular pacing, is an effective approach that can both break and prevent the rhythm.

Long-term treatment of patients with inherited arrhythmia syndromes depends on the presence of high-risk features. Use of beta-blockers (particularly propranolol or nadolol) is the mainstay of treatment for patients with long

QT syndrome or catecholaminergic polymorphic ventricular tachycardia. Surgical cervicothoracic sympathectomy should be considered for patients who do not respond to or are intolerant of beta-blockers. There is no reliable medication therapy for Brugada syndrome and prevention of arrhythmias focuses on prompt treatment of exacerbating triggers, particularly fever. Antiarrhythmic medications should be avoided in patients with inherited arrhythmia syndromes except for specific identified genetic abnormalities under the direction of a specialist. ICD implantation is recommended for patients with an inherited arrhythmia syndrome in whom sudden cardiac arrest is the initial presentation. An ICD should be considered in patients with recurrent sustained ventricular arrhythmias or syncope despite medical therapy.

When to Refer

Any patient with known or suspected inherited arrhythmia syndrome or with severe corrected QT interval prolongation (greater than 500 msec on serial ECGs) should be referred to a cardiologist or cardiac electrophysiologist.

Tang PT et al. Ventricular arrhythmias and sudden cardiac death. Card Electrophysiol Clin. 2017 Dec;9(4):693–708. [PMID: 29173411]

SYNCOPE

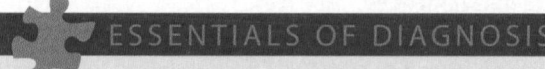

ESSENTIALS OF DIAGNOSIS

▶ Transient loss of consciousness and postural tone from vasodepressor or cardiogenic causes with prompt recovery without resuscitative measures.

▶ High-risk features include history of structural heart disease, abnormal ECG, and age older than 60 years.

General Considerations

Syncope is a symptom defined as a transient, self-limited loss of consciousness, usually leading to a fall. Thirty percent of the adult population will experience at least one episode of syncope. It accounts for approximately 3% of emergency department visits. A specific cause of syncope is identified in about 50% of cases during the initial evaluation. The prognosis is relatively favorable except when accompanying cardiac disease is present. In many patients with recurrent syncope or near syncope, arrhythmias are not the cause. This is particularly true when the patient has no evidence of associated heart disease by history, examination, standard ECG, or noninvasive testing. The history is the most important component of the evaluation to identify the cause of syncope.

Reflex (neurally mediated) syncope may be due to excessive vagal tone or impaired reflex control of the peripheral circulation. The most frequent type is **vasovagal syncope** or the "common faint," which is often initiated by a stressful, painful, or claustrophobic experience, especially in young women. Enhanced vagal tone with resulting hypotension is the cause of syncope in **carotid sinus hypersensitivity** and **postmicturition syncope;** vagal-induced sinus bradycardia, sinus arrest, and AV block are common accompaniments and may themselves be the cause of syncope.

Orthostatic (postural) hypotension is another common cause of vasodepressor syncope, especially in elderly patients; in diabetic patients or others with autonomic neuropathy; in patients with blood loss or hypovolemia; and in patients taking vasodilators, diuretics, and adrenergic-blocking medications. In addition, a syndrome of **chronic idiopathic orthostatic hypotension** exists primarily in older men. In most of these conditions, the normal vasoconstrictive response to assuming upright posture, which compensates for the abrupt decrease in venous return, is impaired.

Cardiogenic syncope can occur on a mechanical or arrhythmic basis. There is usually no prodrome; thus, injury secondary to falling is common. Mechanical problems that can cause syncope include aortic stenosis (where syncope may occur from autonomic reflex abnormalities or ventricular tachycardia), pulmonary stenosis, hypertrophic cardiomyopathy, congenital lesions associated with pulmonary hypertension or right-to-left shunting, and LA myxoma obstructing the mitral valve. Episodes are commonly exertional or postexertional. More commonly, cardiac syncope is due to disorders of automaticity (sick sinus syndrome), conduction disorders (AV block), or tachyarrhythmias (especially ventricular tachycardia and SVT with rapid ventricular rate).

Clinical Findings

A. Symptoms and Signs

Syncope is characteristically abrupt in onset, often resulting in injury, transient (lasting for seconds to a few minutes), and followed by prompt recovery of full consciousness.

Vasodepressor premonitory symptoms, such as nausea, diaphoresis, tachycardia, and pallor, are usual in the "common faint." Episodes can be aborted by lying down or removing the inciting stimulus. In orthostatic (postural) hypotension, a greater than normal decline (20 mm Hg) in BP immediately upon arising from the supine to the standing position is observed, with or without tachycardia depending on the status of autonomic (baroreceptor) function.

B. Diagnostic Tests

The evaluation for syncope depends on findings from the history and physical examination (especially orthostatic BP evaluation, auscultation of carotid arteries, and cardiac examination).

1. ECG—A resting ECG is recommended for all patients undergoing evaluation for syncope. High-risk findings on ECG include non-sinus rhythm, complete or partial left bundle branch block, and voltage criteria indicating left ventricular hypertrophy. Patients with a normal initial evaluation, including unremarkable history and physical, absence of cardiac disease or significant comorbidities and normal baseline ECG may not need further testing. When

initial evaluation suggests a possible cardiac arrhythmia, continuous ambulatory ECG monitoring, event recorder (for infrequent episodes), or an implantable cardiac monitor can be considered. Caution is required before attributing a patient's syncopal event to rhythm or conduction abnormalities observed during monitoring without concomitant symptoms. For instance, dizziness or syncope in older patients may be unrelated to incidentally observed bradycardia, sinus node abnormalities, or ventricular ectopy.

2. Autonomic testing—Tilt-table testing may be useful in patients with suspected vasovagal syncope where the diagnosis is unclear after initial evaluation, especially when syncope is recurrent. The hemodynamic response to tilting determines whether there is a cardioinhibitory, vasodepressor, or mixed response. The overall utility of the test is improved when there is a high pretest probability of neurally mediated syncope, since the sensitivity and specificity of the test in the general population is only moderate.

3. Electrophysiologic studies—Electrophysiologic study has limited role in the evaluation of syncope, particularly in patients without structural heart disease or when there is a low suspicion for arrhythmic etiology. In patients with ischemic heart disease, LV dysfunction, known conduction disease, or arrhythmia, electrophysiologic study may help elucidate the mechanism of syncope and guide treatment decisions. The diagnostic yield in patients with structural heart disease is approximately 50%.

Treatment

In patients with vasovagal syncope, treatment consists largely of education on the benign nature of the condition and counseling to avoid predisposing situations. Counterpressure maneuvers (squatting, leg-crossing, abdominal contraction) can be helpful in limiting or terminating episodes. Medical therapy is reserved for patients with symptoms despite these measures. Midodrine is an alpha-agonist that can increase the peripheral sympathetic neural outflow and decrease venous pooling during vasovagal episodes. Fludrocortisone and beta-blockers have also been used but generally provide minimal benefit. Selective serotonin reuptake inhibitors have shown some benefit in select patients. There is generally no indication for permanent pacemaker implantation in patients with vasovagal syncope unless prolonged, spontaneous episodes of syncope are recorded, especially in the absence of vasodepressor response on tilt-table testing.

If symptomatic bradyarrhythmias or supraventricular tachyarrhythmias are detected and felt to be the cause of syncope, therapy can usually be initiated without additional diagnostic studies. Permanent pacing is indicated in patients with syncope and documented severe pauses (greater than 3 seconds), bradycardia, or high-degree AV block (second-degree Mobitz type II or complete heart block) when symptoms are correlated to the arrhythmia.

An important consideration in patients who have experienced syncope, symptomatic ventricular tachycardia, or aborted sudden death is to provide recommendations concerning **automobile driving restrictions**. Patients with syncope thought to be due to temporary factors (acute MI, bradyarrhythmias subsequently treated with permanent pacing, medication effect, electrolyte imbalance) should be advised after recovery not to drive for at least 1 week. Other patients with symptomatic ventricular tachycardia or aborted sudden death, whether treated pharmacologically, with antitachycardia devices, or with ablation therapy, should not drive for at least 6 months. Longer restrictions are warranted in these patients if significant arrhythmias persist.

▶ When to Refer

- Patients with syncope and underlying structural heart disease, documented arrhythmia, or conduction disturbance.
- Unclear etiology of syncope with high-risk features (heart failure, abnormal ECG findings, advanced age, multiple unexplained episodes).

Shen WK et al. 2017 ACC/AHA/HRS guideline for the evaluation and management of patients with syncope: executive summary: a report of the American College of Cardiology/ American Heart Association Task Force on Clinical Practice Guidelines and the Heart Rhythm Society. J Am Coll Cardiol. 2017 Aug 1;70(5):620–63. [PMID: 28286222]

▼ HEART FAILURE

ESSENTIALS OF DIAGNOSIS

- ▶ LV failure: Either due to systolic or diastolic dysfunction. Predominant symptoms are those of low cardiac output and congestion, including dyspnea.

- ▶ RV failure: Symptoms of fluid overload predominate; usually RV failure is secondary to LV failure.

- ▶ Assessment of LV function is a crucial part of diagnosis and management.

- ▶ Optimal management of chronic heart failure includes combination medical therapies, such as ACE inhibitors, aldosterone antagonists, and beta-blockers.

▶ General Considerations

Heart failure is a common syndrome that is increasing in incidence and prevalence. Approximately 6.5 million patients in the United States have heart failure, and there are around 960,000 new cases each year, with 8 million or more patients projected to have heart failure by 2030. Each year in the United States, 900,000 patients are discharged from the hospital with a diagnosis of heart failure. It is primarily a disease of aging, with over 75% of existing and new cases occurring in individuals over 65 years of age. Seventy-five percent of heart failure patients have antecedent hypertension. The prevalence of heart failure rises from less than 1% in individuals below 60 years to nearly 10% in those over 80 years of age.

Heart failure may be right-sided or left-sided (or both). Patients with **left heart failure** may have symptoms of low cardiac output and elevated pulmonary venous pressure; dyspnea is the predominant feature. Signs of fluid retention predominate in **right heart failure**. Most patients exhibit symptoms or signs of both right- and left-sided failure, and LV dysfunction is the primary cause of RV failure. Approximately half of patients with heart failure have **preserved LV systolic function** and usually have some degree of diastolic dysfunction. Patients with reduced or preserved systolic function may have similar symptoms and it may be difficult to distinguish clinically between the two based on signs and symptoms. In developed countries, CAD with resulting MI and loss of functioning myocardium (**ischemic cardiomyopathy**) is the most common cause of systolic heart failure. Systemic hypertension remains an important cause of heart failure and, even more commonly in the United States, an exacerbating factor in patients with cardiac dysfunction due to other causes, such as CAD. Several processes may present with **dilated** or **congestive cardiomyopathy**, which is characterized by LV or biventricular dilation and generalized systolic dysfunction. These are discussed elsewhere in this chapter, but the most common are alcoholic cardiomyopathy, viral myocarditis (including infections by HIV), and dilated cardiomyopathies with no obvious underlying cause (idiopathic cardiomyopathy). Rare causes of dilated cardiomyopathy include infiltrative diseases (hemochromatosis, sarcoidosis, amyloidosis, etc), other infectious agents, metabolic disorders, cardiotoxins, and medication toxicity. Valvular heart diseases—particularly degenerative aortic stenosis and chronic aortic or mitral regurgitation—are not infrequent causes of heart failure. Persistent tachycardia, often related to atrial arrhythmias, can cause systolic dysfunction that may be reversible with controlling the rate. **Diastolic cardiac dysfunction** is associated with aging and related myocardial stiffening, as well as LVH, commonly resulting from hypertension. Conditions such as **hypertrophic** or **restrictive cardiomyopathy**, diabetes, and pericardial disease can produce the same clinical picture. Atrial fibrillation with or without rapid ventricular response may contribute to impaired left ventricular filling.

Heart failure is often preventable by early detection of patients at risk and by early intervention. The importance of these approaches is emphasized by US guidelines that have incorporated a classification of heart failure that includes four stages. **Stage A** includes patients at risk for developing heart failure (such as patients with hypertension). In the majority of these patients, development of heart failure can be prevented with interventions such as the aggressive treatment of hypertension, modification of coronary risk factors, and reduction of excessive alcohol intake. **Stage B** includes patients who have structural heart disease but no current or previously recognized symptoms of heart failure. Examples include patients with previous MI, other causes of reduced systolic function, LVH, or asymptomatic valvular disease. Both ACE inhibitors and beta-blockers prevent heart failure in the first two of these conditions, and more aggressive treatment of hypertension and early surgical intervention are effective in the latter two. **Stages C** and **D** include patients with clinical heart failure and the relatively small group of patients who have become refractory to the usual therapies, respectively.

► Clinical Findings

A. Symptoms

The most common symptom of patients with **left heart failure** is shortness of breath, chiefly exertional dyspnea at first and then progressing to orthopnea, paroxysmal nocturnal dyspnea, and rest dyspnea. Chronic nonproductive cough, which is often worse in the recumbent position, may occur. Nocturia due to excretion of fluid retained during the day and increased renal perfusion in the recumbent position is a common nonspecific symptom of heart failure, as is fatigue and exercise intolerance. These symptoms correlate poorly with the degree of cardiac dysfunction. Patients with **right heart failure** have predominate signs of fluid retention, with the patient exhibiting edema, hepatic congestion and, on occasion, loss of appetite and nausea due to edema of the gut or impaired gastrointestinal perfusion and ascites. Surprisingly, some individuals with severe LV dysfunction will display few signs of left heart failure and appear to have isolated right heart failure. Indeed, they may be clinically indistinguishable from patients with **cor pulmonale,** who have right heart failure secondary to pulmonary disease.

Patients with acute heart failure from MI, myocarditis, and acute valvular regurgitation due to endocarditis or other conditions usually present with pulmonary edema. Patients with episodic symptoms may be having LV dysfunction due to intermittent ischemia. Patients may also present with acute exacerbations of chronic, stable heart failure. Exacerbations may be caused by alterations in therapy (or patient noncompliance), excessive salt and fluid intake, arrhythmias, excessive activity, pulmonary emboli, intercurrent infection, or progression of the underlying disease.

Patients with heart failure are often categorized by the NYHA classification as **class I** (asymptomatic), **class II** (symptomatic with moderate activity), **class III** (symptomatic with mild activity), or **class IV** (symptomatic at rest). This classification is important since some of the treatments are indicated based on NYHA classification.

B. Signs

Many patients with heart failure, including some with severe symptoms, appear comfortable at rest. Others will be dyspneic during conversation or minor activity, and those with long-standing severe heart failure may appear cachectic or cyanotic. The vital signs may be normal, but tachycardia, hypotension, and reduced pulse pressure may be present. Patients often show signs of increased sympathetic nervous system activity, including cold extremities and diaphoresis. Important peripheral signs of heart failure can be detected by examination of the neck, the lungs, the abdomen, and the extremities. RA pressure may be estimated through the height of the pulsations in the jugular venous system. With the patient at 45 degrees, measure the height of the pulsation about the sternal angle, and add 5 cm to estimate the height above the left atrium, with a pressure greater than 8 cm being abnormal. In addition to the height of the venous pressure, abnormal pulsations, such as regurgitant *v* waves, should be sought. Examination of the carotid pulse may allow estimation of pulse pressure as well as detection of aortic stenosis. Thyroid examination may reveal occult hyperthyroidism or hypothyroidism, which are readily treatable causes of heart failure. Crackles at the lung bases reflect transudation of fluid into the alveoli. Pleural effusions may cause bibasilar dullness to percussion. Expiratory wheezing and rhonchi may be signs of heart failure. Patients with severe right heart failure may have hepatic enlargement—tender or nontender—due to passive congestion. Systolic pulsations may be felt in tricuspid regurgitation. Sustained moderate pressure on the liver may increase jugular venous pressure (a positive **hepatojugular reflux** is an increase of greater than 1 cm, which correlates with elevated pulmonary capillary wedge pressure). Ascites may also be present. Peripheral pitting edema is a common sign in patients with right heart failure and may extend into the thighs and abdominal wall.

Cardinal cardiac examination signs are a parasternal lift, indicating pulmonary hypertension; an enlarged and sustained LV impulse, indicating LV dilation and hypertrophy; a diminished first heart sound, suggesting impaired contractility; and an S_3 gallop originating in the LV and sometimes the RV. An S_4 is usually present in diastolic heart failure. Murmurs should be sought to exclude primary valvular disease; secondary mitral regurgitation and tricuspid regurgitation murmurs are common in patients with dilated ventricles. In chronic heart failure, many of the expected signs of heart failure may be absent despite markedly abnormal cardiac function and hemodynamic measurements.

C. Laboratory Findings

A blood count may reveal anemia and a high red-cell distribution width (RDW), both of which are associated with poor prognosis in chronic heart failure through poorly understood mechanisms. Kidney function tests can determine whether cardiac failure is associated with impaired kidney function that may reflect poor kidney perfusion. Chronic kidney disease is another poor prognostic factor in heart failure and may limit certain treatment options. Serum electrolytes may disclose hypokalemia, which increases the risk of arrhythmias; hyperkalemia, which may limit the use of inhibitors of the renin–angiotensin system; or hyponatremia, an indicator of marked activation of the renin–angiotensin system and a poor prognostic sign. Thyroid function should be assessed to detect occult thyrotoxicosis or myxedema, and iron studies should be checked to test for hemochromatosis. In unexplained cases, appropriate biopsies may lead to a diagnosis of amyloidosis. Myocardial biopsy may exclude specific causes of dilated cardiomyopathy but rarely reveals specific reversible diagnoses.

Serum BNP is a powerful prognostic marker that adds to clinical assessment in differentiating dyspnea due to heart failure from noncardiac causes. Two markers—**BNP** and **NT-proBNP**—provide similar diagnostic and prognostic information. BNP is expressed primarily in the ventricles and is elevated when ventricular filling pressures are high. It is quite sensitive in patients with symptomatic heart failure—whether due to systolic or to diastolic dysfunction—but less specific in older patients, women, and patients with COPD. Studies have shown that BNP can help in emergency department triage in the diagnosis of acute decompensated heart failure, such that an NT-proBNP less than 300 pg/mL or BNP less than 100 pg/mL, combined with a normal ECG, makes heart failure unlikely. BNP is less sensitive and specific to diagnose heart failure in the chronic setting. BNP may be helpful in guiding the intensity of diuretic and a more consistent use of disease-modifying therapies, such as ACE inhibitors and beta-blockers, for the management of chronic heart failure. BNP, but not NT-proBNP, is increased by neprilysin inhibitors, since neprilysin degrades BNP. Thus, while NT-proBNP is still reliable, BNP should *not* be used to monitor degree of heart failure when patients are treated with sacubitril/valsartan. Worsening breathlessness or weight associated with a rising BNP (or both) might prompt increasing the dose of diuretics. However, there is no proven value in using serial natriuretic peptide measurements to guide therapy, as shown in the GUIDE-IT trial. Elevation of serum troponin, and especially of high-sensitivity troponin, is common in both chronic and acute heart failure, and it is associated with higher risk of adverse outcomes.

D. ECG and Chest Radiography

ECG may indicate an underlying or secondary arrhythmia, MI, or nonspecific changes that often include low voltage, intraventricular conduction defects, LVH, and nonspecific repolarization changes. Chest radiographs provide information about the size and shape of the cardiac silhouette. Cardiomegaly is an important finding and is a poor prognostic sign. Evidence of pulmonary venous hypertension includes relative dilation of the upper lobe veins, perivascular edema (haziness of vessel outlines), interstitial edema, and alveolar fluid. In acute heart failure, these findings correlate moderately well with pulmonary venous pressure. However, patients with chronic heart failure may show relatively normal pulmonary vasculature despite markedly elevated pressures. Pleural effusions are common and tend to be bilateral or right-sided.

E. Additional Studies

Many studies have indicated that the clinical diagnosis of systolic myocardial dysfunction is often inaccurate. The primary confounding conditions are diastolic dysfunction of the heart with decreased relaxation and filling of the LV (particularly in hypertension and in hypertrophic states) and pulmonary disease.

The most useful test is the echocardiogram because it can differentiate heart failure with and without preserved LV systolic function. The echocardiogram can define the size and function of both ventricles and of the atria. LVEF is the most commonly used measurement to define systolic function. RV function is assessed by contractility and other measures, such as tricuspid annular plane systolic excursion. Echocardiography will also allow detection of pericardial effusion, valvular abnormalities, intracardiac shunts, and segmental wall motion abnormalities suggestive of old MI as opposed to more generalized forms of dilated cardiomyopathy.

Radionuclide angiography as well as cardiac MRI also measure LVEF and permit analysis of regional wall motion. These tests are especially useful when echocardiography is technically suboptimal, such as in patients with severe pulmonary disease. MRI can assess for presence of scar tissue and of infiltrative disease. When myocardial ischemia is suspected as a cause of LV dysfunction, as it should be unless there is another clear cause, stress testing or coronary angiography should be performed.

F. Cardiac Catheterization

In most patients with heart failure, clinical examination and noninvasive tests can determine LV size and function and valve function to support and refine the diagnosis. Left heart catheterization may be helpful to define the presence and extent of CAD, although CT angiography may also be appropriate, especially when the likelihood of coronary disease is low. Evaluation for coronary disease is particularly important when LV dysfunction may be partially reversible by revascularization. The combination of angina or noninvasive evidence of significant myocardial ischemia with symptomatic heart failure is often an indication for coronary angiography if the patient is a potential candidate for revascularization. Right heart catheterization may be useful to select and monitor therapy in patients refractory to standard therapy.

► Treatment: Heart Failure With Reduced LVEF

The treatment of heart failure is aimed at relieving symptoms, improving functional status, and preventing death and hospitalizations. Figure 10–8 outlines the role of the major pharmacologic and device therapies for heart failure with reduced LVEF (less than or equal to 40%). **The evidence of clinical benefit, including reducing death and hospitalization, as well as reducing sudden cardiac death, of most therapies is limited to patients with heart failure with reduced LVEF.** Treatment of heart failure with preserved LVEF is aimed at improving symptoms and treating comorbidities. Achieving target (or maximally tolerated up to target) dosing to obtain the benefits of these treatments that have been shown in clinical trials is important (Table 10–15).

A. Correction of Reversible Causes

The major reversible causes of heart failure with reduced EF, also called chronic systolic heart failure, include valvular lesions, myocardial ischemia, uncontrolled hypertension, arrhythmias (especially persistent tachycardias), alcohol- or drug-induced myocardial depression, hypothyroidism, intracardiac shunts, and high-output states. Calcium channel blockers with negative inotropy (specifically verapamil or diltiazem), antiarrhythmic medications, thiazolidinediones, and nonsteroidal anti-inflammatory agents may be important contributors to worsening heart failure. Some metabolic and infiltrative cardiomyopathies may be partially reversible, or their progression may be slowed; these include

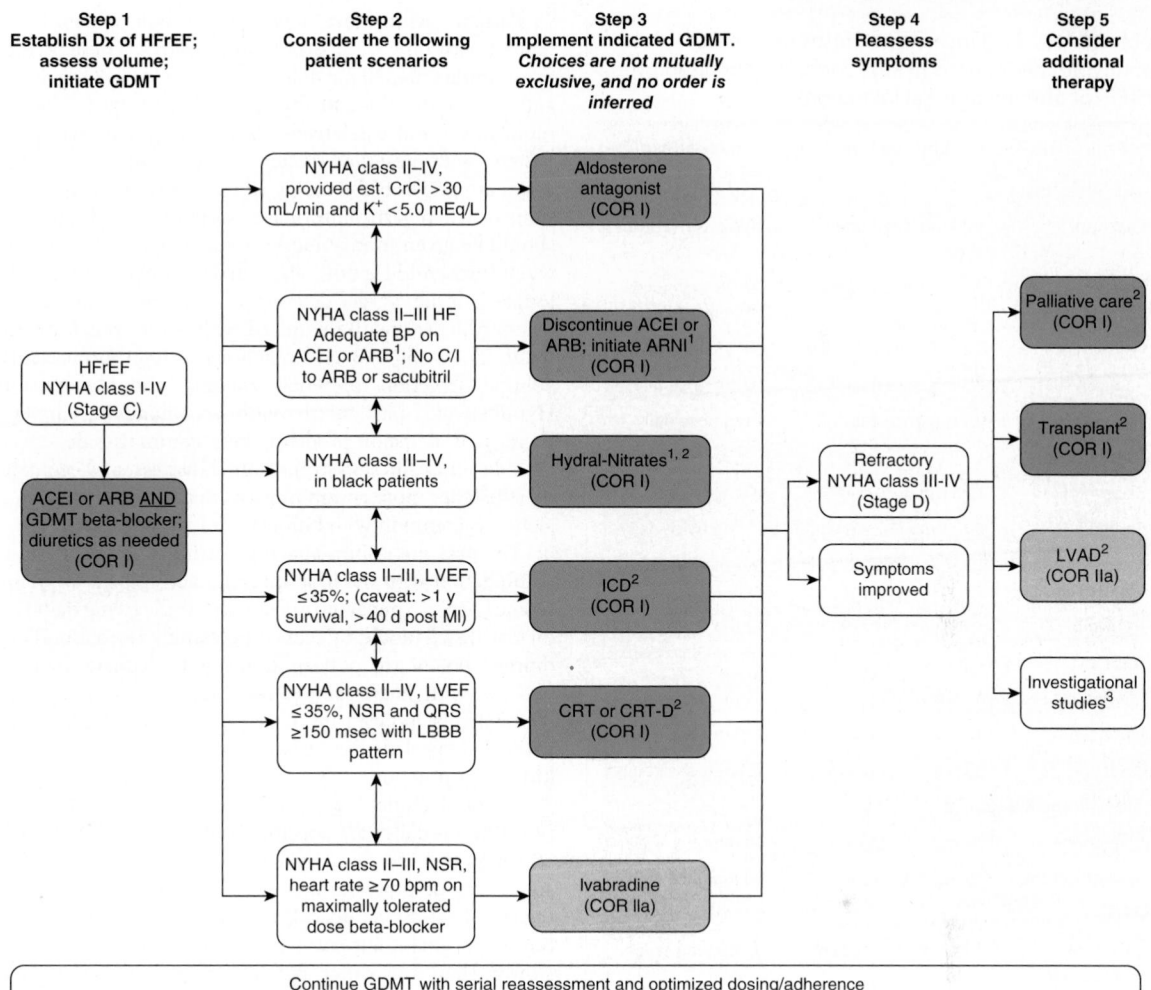

| Step 1
Establish Dx of HFrEF;
assess volume;
initiate GDMT | Step 2
Consider the following
patient scenarios | Step 3
Implement indicated GDMT.
*Choices are not mutually
exclusive, and no order is
inferred* | Step 4
Reassess
symptoms | Step 5
Consider
additional
therapy |

▲ Figure 10–8. Major pharmacologic and device therapies for heart failure with reduced left ventricular ejection fraction. For all medical therapies, dosing should be optimized and serial assessment exercised. ACEI, angiotensin-converting enzyme inhibitor; ARB, angiotensin receptor blocker; ARNI, angiotensin receptor-neprilysin inhibitor; BP, blood pressure; bpm, beats per minute; C/I, contraindication; COR, Class of Recommendation; CrCl, creatinine clearance; CRT-D, cardiac resynchronization therapy–device; Dx, diagnosis; GDMT, guideline-directed management and therapy; HF, heart failure; HFrEF, heart failure with reduced ejection fraction; ICD, implantable cardioverter-defibrillator; ISDN/HYD, isosorbide dinitrate hydral-nitrates; K+, potassium; LBBB, left bundle branch block; LVAD, left ventricular assist device; LVEF, left ventricular ejection fraction; MI, myocardial infarction; NSR, normal sinus rhythm; NYHA, New York Heart Association. (Figure reproduced, with permission, from Yancy CW et al. 2017 ACC/AHA/HFSA Focused Update of the 2013 ACCF/AHA Guideline for the Management of Heart Failure: A Report of the American College of Cardiology/American Heart Association Task Force on Clinical Practice Guidelines and the Heart Failure Society of America. Circulation. 2017 Aug 8;136(6):e137–e161. © 2017 American Heart Association, Inc.)

[1] The combination of ISDN/HYD with ARNI has not been robustly studied, BP response should be carefully monitored.

[2] See 2013 HF guidelines.

[3] Participation in investigational studies is also appropriate for stage C, NYHA class II and III HF.

hemochromatosis, sarcoidosis, and amyloidosis. Once possible reversible components are being addressed, the measures outlined below are appropriate.

B. Pharmacologic Treatment

See also the following section Acute Heart Failure & Pulmonary Edema.

1. Diuretic therapy—Diuretics are the most effective means of providing symptomatic relief to patients with moderate to severe heart failure with dyspnea and fluid overload, for heart failure with reduced and with preserved LVEF. Few patients with symptoms or signs of fluid retention can be optimally managed without a diuretic. However, excessive diuresis can lead to electrolyte imbalance and neurohormonal activation. A combination of a diuretic

Table 10–15. Evidence-based doses of disease-modifying medications in key randomized trials in HFrEF (or after myocardial infarction).

Medications	Starting Dose	Target Dose
ACE Inhibitors		
Captopril	6.25 mg three times daily	50 mg three times daily
Enalapril	2.5 mg twice daily	10–20 mg twice daily
Lisinopril	2.5–5.0 mg once daily	20–35 once daily
Ramipril	2.5 mg once daily	10 mg once daily
Trandolapril	0.5 mg once daily	4 mg once daily
Beta-Blockers		
Bisoprolol	1.25 mg once daily	10 mg once daily
Carvedilol	3.125 mg twice daily	25 mg twice daily
Metoprolol succinate (CR/XL)	12.5–25 mg once daily	200 mg once daily
Nebivolol	1.25 once daily	10 mg once daily
ARBs		
Candesartan	4–8 mg once daily	32 mg once daily
Valsartan	40 mg twice daily	160 mg twice daily
Losartan	50 mg once daily	150 mg once daily
Aldosterone Antagonist		
Eplerenone	25 mg once daily	50 mg once daily
Spironolactone	25 mg once daily	50 mg once daily
ARNI		
Sacubitril/valsartan	49/51 mg twice daily	97/103 mg twice daily
I$_f$ Channel Blocker		
Ivabradine	5 mg twice daily	7.5 mg twice daily

ACE, angiotensin-converting enzyme; ARBs, angiotensin receptor blockers; ARNI, angiotensin receptor-neprilysin inhibitor; HFrEF, heart failure with reduced ejection fraction.

and an ACE inhibitor should be the initial treatment in most symptomatic patients with heart failure and reduced LVEF, with the early addition of a beta-blocker.

When fluid retention is mild, **thiazide diuretics** or a similar type of agent (hydrochlorothiazide, 25–100 mg; metolazone, 2.5–5 mg; chlorthalidone, 25–50 mg; etc) may be sufficient. Thiazide or related diuretics often provide better control of hypertension than short-acting loop agents. The thiazides are generally *ineffective* when the glomerular filtration rate falls below 30–40 mL/min, a not infrequent occurrence in patients with severe heart failure. Metolazone maintains its efficacy down to a glomerular filtration rate of approximately 20–30 mL/min. Adverse reactions include hypokalemia and intravascular volume depletion with resulting prerenal azotemia, skin rashes, neutropenia and thrombocytopenia, hyperglycemia, hyperuricemia, and hepatic dysfunction.

Patients with more severe heart failure should be treated with one of the oral **loop diuretics.** These include furosemide (20–320 mg daily), bumetanide (1–8 mg daily), and torsemide (20–200 mg daily). These agents have a rapid onset and a relatively short duration of action. In patients with preserved kidney function, two or more daily doses are preferable to a single larger dose. In acute situations or when gastrointestinal absorption is in doubt, they should be given intravenously. Torsemide may be effective when furosemide is not, related to better absorption and a longer half life. Larger doses (up to 500 mg of furosemide or equivalent) may be required with severe renal impairment. The major adverse reactions include intravascular volume depletion, prerenal azotemia, and hypotension. Hypokalemia, particularly with accompanying digitalis therapy, is a major problem. Less common side effects include skin rashes, gastrointestinal distress, and ototoxicity (the latter more common with ethacrynic acid and possibly less common with bumetanide).

The **oral potassium-sparing agents** are often useful in combination with the loop diuretics and thiazides. Triamterene (37.5–75 mg daily) and amiloride (5–10 mg daily) act on the distal tubule to reduce potassium secretion. Their diuretic potency is only mild and not adequate for most patients with heart failure, but they may minimize the hypokalemia induced by more potent agents. Side effects include hyperkalemia, gastrointestinal symptoms, and kidney dysfunction.

Spironolactone (12.5–100 mg daily) and eplerenone (25–100 mg daily) are specific **inhibitors of aldosterone,** which is often increased in heart failure. These medications spare loss of potassium, they have some diuretic effect (especially at higher doses), and they also improve clinical outcomes, including survival. Their onsets of action are slower than the other potassium-sparing agents, and spironolactone's side effects include gynecomastia and hyperkalemia. Combinations of potassium supplements or ACE inhibitors and potassium-sparing medications can increase the risk of hyperkalemia but have been used with success in patients with persistent hypokalemia.

Patients with refractory edema may respond to combinations of a loop diuretic and thiazide-like agents. Metolazone, because of its maintained activity with chronic kidney disease, is the most useful agent for such a combination. Extreme caution must be observed with this approach, since massive diuresis and electrolyte imbalances often occur; 2.5 mg of metolazone orally should be added to the previous dosage of loop diuretic. In many cases this is necessary only once or twice a week, but dosages up to 10 mg daily have been used in some patients.

2. Inhibitors of the renin–angiotensin–aldosterone system—Inhibition of the renin–angiotensin–aldosterone system with ACE inhibitors should be part of the initial therapy of this syndrome based on their mortality benefits.

A. ACE INHIBITORS—At least seven ACE inhibitors have been shown to be effective for the treatment of heart failure or the related indication of postinfarction LV dysfunction (see Table 11–6). ACE inhibitors reduce mortality by approximately 20% in patients with symptomatic heart

Bronchospasm may occur in response to pulmonary edema and may itself exacerbate hypoxemia and dyspnea. Treatment with inhaled beta-adrenergic agonists or intravenous aminophylline may be helpful, but both may also provoke tachycardia and supraventricular arrhythmias.

In most cases, pulmonary edema responds rapidly to therapy. When the patient has improved, the cause or precipitating factor should be ascertained. In patients without prior heart failure, evaluation should include echocardiography and, in many cases, cardiac catheterization and coronary angiography. Patients with acute decompensation of chronic heart failure should be treated to achieve a euvolemic state and have their medical regimen optimized. Generally, an oral diuretic and an ACE inhibitor should be initiated, with efficacy and tolerability confirmed prior to discharge. In selected patients, early but careful initiation of beta-blockers in low doses should be considered.

MYOCARDITIS & THE CARDIOMYOPATHIES

INFECTIOUS MYOCARDITIS

ESSENTIALS OF DIAGNOSIS

▶ Often follows an upper respiratory infection.

▶ May present with chest pain (pleuritic or nonspecific) or signs of heart failure.

▶ Echocardiogram documents cardiomegaly and contractile dysfunction.

▶ Myocardial biopsy, though not sensitive, may reveal a characteristic inflammatory pattern. MRI has a role in diagnosis.

▶ General Considerations

Cardiac dysfunction due to primary myocarditis is presumedly caused by either an acute viral infection or a postviral immune response. Secondary myocarditis is the result of inflammation caused by nonviral pathogens, medications, chemicals, physical agents, or inflammatory diseases (such as systemic lupus erythematosus). The list of both infectious and noninfectious causes of myocarditis is extensive (Table 10–16).

Early-phase myocarditis is initiated by infection of cardiac tissue. The currently accepted definition of myocarditis is biopsy dependent and includes the observation of 14 or more lymphocytes/mcL including up to 4 monocytes/mcL with the presence of 7 or more CD3-positive T lymphocytes/mcL. Injury can be fulminant, subclinical, or chronic. Both cellular and humoral inflammatory processes contribute to the progression to chronic injury, and there are subgroups that appear to benefit from immunosuppression. The prevalence globally is about 22/100,000 patients annually.

Genetic predisposition is a likely factor in at least a few cases. Autoimmune myocarditis (eg, giant cell myocarditis) may occur with no identifiable viral infection.

Table 10–16. Causes of myocarditis.

1. INFECTIOUS CAUSES

RNA viruses: Picornaviruses (coxsackie A and B, echovirus, poliovirus, hepatitis virus), orthomyxovirus (influenza), paramyxoviruses (respiratory syncytial virus, mumps), togaviruses (rubella), flaviviruses (dengue fever, yellow fever)

DNA viruses: Adenovirus (A1, 2, 3, and 5), erythrovirus (Bi9V and 2), herpesviruses (human herpes virus 6 A and B, cytomegalovirus, Epstein-Barr virus, varicella-zoster), retrovirus (HIV)

Bacteria: Chlamydia (*Chlamydophila pneumoniae, C psittaci*), *Haemophilus influenzae, Legionella, Pneumophilia, Brucella, Clostridium, Francisella tularensis, Neisseria meningitis, Mycobacterium* (tuberculosis), *Salmonella, Staphylococcus, Streptococcus* A, *Streptococcus pneumoniae*, tularemia, tetanus, syphilis, *Vibrio cholera*

Spirocheta: *Borrelia recurrentis*, leptospira, *Treponema pallidum*

Rickettsia: *Coxiella burnetii, R rickettsii, R prowazekii*

Fungi: *Actinomyces, Aspergillus, Candida, Cryptococcus, Histoplasma, Nocardia*

Protozoa: *Entamoeba histolytica, Plasmodium falciparum, Trypanosoma cruzi, T burcei, T gondii, Leishmania*

Helminthic: *Ascaris, Echinococcus granulosus, Schistosoma, Trichenella spiralis, Wuchereria bancrofti*

2. NONINFECTIOUS CAUSES

Autoimmune diseases: Dermatomyositis, inflammatory bowel disease, rheumatoid arthritis, Sjögren syndrome, systemic lupus erythematosus, granulomatosis with polyangiitis, giant cell myocarditis

Medications: Aminophylline, amphetamine, anthracyclin, catecholamines, chloramphenicol, cocaine, cyclophosphamide, doxorubicin, 5-FU, mesylate, methysergide, phenytoin, trastuzumab, zidovudine

Hypersensitivity reactions due to medications: Azithromycin, benzodiazepines, clozapine, cephalosporins, dapsone, dobutamine, lithium, diuretics, thiazide, methyldopa, mexiletine, streptomycin, sulfonamides, nonsteroidal anti-inflammatory drugs, tetanus toxoid, tetracycline, tricyclic antidepressants

Hypersensitivity reactions due to venoms: Bee, wasp, black widow spider, scorpion, snake

Systemic diseases: Eosinophilic granulomatosis with polyangiitis (formerly known as Churg-Strauss syndrome), collagen diseases, sarcoidosis, Kawasaki disease, scleroderma

Other: Heat stroke, hypothermia, transplant rejection, radiation injury

▶ Clinical Findings

A. Symptoms and Signs

Patients may present several days to a few weeks after the onset of an acute febrile illness or a respiratory infection or they may present with heart failure without antecedent symptoms. The onset of heart failure may be gradual or may be abrupt and fulminant. In acute fulminant myocarditis, low output and shock may be present with severely depressed LV systolic function. A pericardial friction rub may be present. In the European Study of Epidemiology and Treatment of Inflammatory Heart Disease, 72% of participants had dyspnea, 32% had chest pain, and 18% had arrhythmias. Pulmonary and systemic emboli may occur. Pleural-pericardial chest pain is common. Examination reveals tachycardia, a gallop rhythm, and other evidence of heart failure or conduction defects. At times, the presentation may mimic an acute MI with ST changes, positive cardiac markers, and regional wall motion abnormalities despite normal coronaries. Microaneurysms may also occur and may be associated with serious ventricular arrhythmias. It has been estimated that approximately 10% of all dilated cardiomyopathy patients have viral myocarditis as the cause.

B. ECG and Chest Radiography

ECG may show sinus tachycardia, other arrhythmias, nonspecific repolarization changes, and intraventricular conduction abnormalities. The presence of Q waves or left bundle branch block portends a higher rate of death or cardiac transplantation. Ventricular ectopy may be the initial and only clinical finding. The chest radiograph is nonspecific, but cardiomegaly is frequent, though not universal. Evidence for pulmonary venous hypertension is common and frank pulmonary edema may be present.

C. Diagnostic Studies

There is no specific laboratory finding that is consistently present, though the white blood cell count is usually elevated and the sedimentation rate and CRP usually are increased. Troponin I or T levels are elevated in about one-third of patients, but CK-MB is elevated in only 10%. Other biomarkers, such as BNP and NT-proBNP, are usually elevated. Echocardiography provides the most convenient way of evaluating cardiac function and can exclude many other processes. MRI with gadolinium enhancement reveals spotty areas of injury throughout the myocardium, but both T2- and T1-weighted images are needed to achieve optimal results; correlation with endomyocardial biopsy results is poor.

D. Endomyocardial Biopsy

Confirmation of myocarditis still requires histologic evidence. The AHA/ACC/ESC class I recommendations for biopsy are (1) in patients with heart failure, a normal-sized or dilated LV less than 2 weeks after onset of symptoms, and hemodynamic compromise; or (2) in patients with a dilated LV 2 weeks to 3 months after onset of symptoms, new ventricular arrhythmias or AV nodal block (Mobitz II or complete heart block) or who do not respond to usual care after 1–2 weeks. In some cases, the identification of inflammation without viral genomes by polymerase chain reaction (PCR) suggests that immunosuppression might be useful. Because the cardiac involvement is often patchy, the diagnosis can be missed in up to one-half of cases.

▶ Treatment & Prognosis

Patients with fulminant myocarditis may present with acute cardiogenic shock. Acute myocarditis has been implicated as a cause of sudden death in 5–22% of such cases in athletes younger than 35 years. The ventricles are usually not dilated, but thickened (possibly due to myoedema). There is a high death rate, but if the patients recover, they are often left with no residual cardiomyopathy. Patients with subacute disease have a dilated cardiomyopathy and generally make an incomplete recovery. Those who present with chronic disease tend to have only mild dilation of the LV and eventually present with a more restrictive cardiomyopathy. Treatment is directed toward the clinical scenario with ACE inhibitors and beta-blockers if LVEF is less than 40%. Nonsteroidal anti-inflammatory medications should be used if myopericarditis-related chest pain occurs. Colchicine has been suggested if pericarditis predominates. Arrhythmias should be suppressed.

Specific antimicrobial therapy is indicated when an infecting agent is identified. Exercise should be limited during the recovery phase. Some experts believe digoxin should be avoided, and it likely has little value in this setting anyway. Controlled trials of immunosuppressive therapy with corticosteroids and intravenous immunoglobulin (IVIG) have not suggested a benefit, though some recommend IVIG given at 2 g/kg over 24 hours in proven cases. Uncontrolled trials suggest that interferon might have a supportive role. Similarly, antiviral medication (such as pleconaril for enteroviruses) has been tried empirically. Studies are lacking as to when to discontinue the chosen therapy if the patient improves. Patients with fulminant myocarditis require aggressive short-term support, including an IABP or an LV assist device. If severe pulmonary infiltrates accompany the fulminant myocarditis, extracorporeal membrane oxygenation (ECMO) support may be temporarily required and has had notable success.

▶ When to Refer

Patients in whom myocarditis is suspected should be seen by a cardiologist at a tertiary care center where facilities are available for diagnosis and therapies available should a fulminant course ensue. The facility should have ventricular support devices and transplantation options available.

Fung G et al. Myocarditis. Circ Res. 2016 Feb 5;118(3):496–514. [PMID: 26846643]

NONINFECTIOUS MYOCARDITIS

A variety of medications, illicit drugs, and toxic substances can produce acute or chronic myocardial injury; the clinical presentation varies widely. The phenothiazines, lithium, chloroquine, disopyramide, antimony-containing compounds, and arsenicals can also cause ECG changes, arrhythmias, or heart failure. Hypersensitivity reactions to sulfonamides, penicillins, and aminosalicylic acid as well as other medications can result in cardiac dysfunction. Radiation can cause an acute inflammatory reaction as well as a chronic fibrosis of heart muscle, usually in conjunction with pericarditis.

Cardiotoxicity from cocaine may occur from coronary artery spasm, MI, arrhythmias, and myocarditis. Because many of these processes are believed to be mediated by cocaine's inhibitory effect on norepinephrine reuptake by sympathetic nerves, beta-blockers have been used in patients with fixed stenosis. In documented coronary spasm, calcium channel blockers and nitrates may be effective. Usual therapy for heart failure or conduction system disease is warranted when symptoms occur. Other recreational drug use has been associated with myocarditis in various case reports.

Systemic disorders are also associated with myocarditis. These include giant cell myocarditis, eosinophilic myocarditis, celiac disease, granulomatosis with polyangiitis, and sarcoidosis. A benefit from immunosuppressive therapy, especially in giant cell myocarditis has been suggested in a number of observational studies, including those directed primarily at T cells (ie, using muromonab-CD3). Treatment of eosinophilic myocarditis includes the use of high-dose corticosteroids and removal of the offending medication or underlying trigger. Most studies suggest that HIV is only indirectly responsible for HIV cardiomyopathy, and other factors, gp 120 protein, adverse reaction to antiretroviral therapy, and opportunistic infections have been implicated more often. Epstein-Barr and herpex simplex viruses have been identified in some patients' myocardium.

The problem of cardiovascular side effects from cancer chemotherapy agents is an ever growing one. Anthracyclines (doxorubicin, daunorubicin, idarubicin, epirubicin, and mitoxantrone) remain the cornerstone of treatment of many malignancies. Heart failure can be expected in 5% of patients treated with a cumulative dose of $400-450 \text{ mg/m}^2$, and this rate is doubled if the patient is over age 65. While symptoms and evidence for myocardial dysfunction usually appear within 1 year of starting therapy, late onset manifestation of heart failure may appear up to a decade later. The major mechanism of cardiotoxicity is thought to be due to oxidative stress inducing both apoptosis and necrosis of myocytes. There is also disruption of the sarcomere. This pathologic understanding is the rationale behind the superoxide dismutase mimetic and iron-chelating agent, dexrazoxane, to protect from the injury. The use of trastuzumab in combination with anthracyclines increases the risk of cardiac dysfunction up to 28%; this has been an issue since combined use of these agents is particularly effective in *HER* 2–positive breast cancer. Other risk factors for patients receiving anthracyclines include the use of paxlitaxel, concurrent radiation, and preexisting cardiovascular disease (including hypertension, peripheral vascular disease, CAD, and diabetes).

In patients receiving chemotherapy, it is important to look for subtle signs of cardiovascular compromise. Echocardiography, cardiac MRI, and serial MUGA studies can provide concrete data regarding LV function. Biomarkers such as BNP or NT-proBNP may be of some value when serial measures are obtained. Other biomarkers may appear early in the course of myocardial injury (especially troponin and myeloperoxidase) and may allow for early detection of cardiotoxicity before other signs become evident. There is some evidence that beta-blocker therapy may reduce the negative effects on myocardial function. There are anecdotal data from animal models that nonsteroidal anti-inflammatory drugs may be harmful in patients with myocarditis. They should be avoided along with alcohol and strenuous physical exercise.

When to Refer

Many patients with myocardial injury from toxic agents can be monitored safely if ventricular function remains relatively preserved (EF greater than 40%) and no heart failure symptoms occur. Diastolic dysfunction may be subtle.

Once heart failure or a reduced LVEF becomes evident or significant conduction system disease becomes manifest, the patient should be evaluated and monitored by a cardiologist in case myocardial dysfunction worsens and further intervention becomes warranted.

Chaudhry MA et al. Modern day management of giant cell myocarditis. Int J Cardiol. 2015 Jan 15;178:82–4. [PMID: 25464225]
Rosa GM et al. Update on cardiotoxicity of anti-cancer treatments. Eur J Clin Invest. 2016 Mar;46(3):264–84. [PMID: 26728634]

DILATED CARDIOMYOPATHY

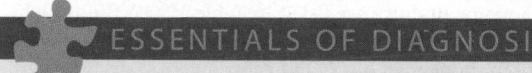

ESSENTIALS OF DIAGNOSIS

- ► Symptoms and signs of heart failure.
- ► Echocardiogram confirms LV dilation, thinning, and global dysfunction.
- ► Severity of RV dysfunction critical in long-term prognosis.

General Considerations

Heart failure definitions have changed over the years and patients with a dilated cardiomyopathy are generally placed into the category of heart failure with reduced ejection fraction where the LVEF is defined as less than or equal to 40%. In about half of the patients in this category there is LV enlargement and it is this group that defines dilated cardiomyopathy. This is a large group of heterogeneous myocardial disorders characterized by reduced myocardial contractility in the absence of abnormal loading conditions such as with hypertension or valvular disease. The prevalence averages 36 cases/100,000 in the United States and accounts for approximately 10,000 deaths annually. Blacks are afflicted three times as often as whites. The prognosis is poor with 50% mortality at 5 years once symptoms emerge.

The causes are multiple and diverse. Up to 20–35% have a familial etiology. A large proportion is idiopathic. Endocrine, inflammatory, and metabolic causes include obesity, diabetes, thyroid disease, celiac disease, systemic lupus erythematosus, acromegaly, and growth hormone deficiency. Toxic, drug-induced, and inflammatory causes are listed in the prior section. Nutritional diseases such as deficiency of thiamine, selenium, and carnitine have also been documented. Dilated cardiomyopathy may also be caused by prolonged tachycardia either from supraventricular arrhythmias, from very frequent PVCs (more than 15% of heart beats), or from frequent right ventricular pacing. Dilated cardiomyopathy is also associated with HIV, Chagas disease, rheumatologic disorders, iron overload, sleep apnea, amyloidosis, sarcoidosis, chronic alcohol usage, end-stage kidney disease, or cobalt exposure ("Quebec beer-drinkers cardiomyopathy"). Peripartum cardiomyopathy and stress-induced disease (tako-tsubo) are discussed separately.

► Clinical Findings

A. Symptoms and Signs

In most patients, symptoms of heart failure develop gradually. It is important to seek out a history of familial dilated cardiomyopathy and to identify behaviors that might predispose patients to the disease. The physical examination reveals rales, an elevated JVP, cardiomegaly, S_3 gallop rhythm, often the murmurs of functional mitral or tricuspid regurgitation, peripheral edema, or ascites. In severe heart failure, Cheyne-Stokes breathing, pulsus alternans, pallor, and cyanosis may be present.

B. ECG and Chest Radiography

The major findings are listed in Table 10–17. Sinus tachycardia is common. Other common abnormalities include left bundle branch block and ventricular or atrial arrhythmias. The chest radiograph reveals cardiomegaly, evidence for left and/or right heart failure, and pleural effusions (right more frequently than left).

C. Diagnostic Studies

In the 2017 AHA/ACCF heart failure guideline focused update, patients with dyspnea should have a BNP or NT-proBNP measured to help establish prognosis and disease severity (class I, level of evidence [LOE] A).

An echocardiogram is indicated to exclude unsuspected valvular or other lesions and confirm the presence of ventricular dilatation, reduced LV systolic function and associated RV systolic dysfunction, or pulmonary hypertension. Mitral Doppler inflow patterns also help in the diagnosis of concomitant diastolic dysfunction. Color flow Doppler can reveal tricuspid or mitral regurgitation, and continuous Doppler can estimate PA pressures. Intracavitary thrombosis is occasionally seen. Exercise or pharmacologic stress myocardial perfusion imaging may uncover underlying coronary disease. Radionuclide ventriculography provides a noninvasive measure of the EF and both RV and LV wall motion, though its use has been supplanted by cardiac MRI in most institutions. Cardiac MRI is particularly helpful in inflammatory or infiltrative processes, such as sarcoidosis or hemochromatosis, and is the diagnostic study of choice for RV dysplasia. MRI can also help define an ischemic etiology by noting gadolinium hyperenhancement consistent with myocardial scar from infarction or prior myocarditis. Cardiac catheterization is seldom of specific value unless myocardial ischemia is suspected, although right heart catheterization should be considered to help guide therapy when the clinical syndrome is not clear cut (class I indication, LOE C). Myocardial biopsy is rarely useful in establishing the diagnosis, although occasionally the underlying cause (eg, sarcoidosis, hemochromatosis) can be discerned. Its use is considered a

Table 10–17. Classification of the cardiomyopathies.

	Dilated	Hypertrophic	Restrictive
Frequent causes	Idiopathic, alcoholic, major catecholamine discharge, myocarditis, postpartum, doxorubicin, endocrinopathies, genetic diseases	Hereditary syndrome, possibly chronic hypertension in older adults	Amyloidosis, post-radiation, post–open heart surgery, diabetes, endomyocardial fibrosis
Symptoms	Left or biventricular heart failure	Dyspnea, chest pain, syncope	Dyspnea, fatigue, right heart failure > left heart failure
Physical examination	Cardiomegaly, S_3, elevated jugular venous pressure, rales	Sustained point of maximal impulse, S_4, variable systolic murmur, bisferiens carotid pulse	Elevated jugular venous pressure, Kussmaul sign
Electrocardiogram	ST–T changes, conduction abnormalities, ventricular ectopy	Left ventricular hypertrophy, exaggerated septal Q waves	ST–T changes, conduction abnormalities, low voltage
Chest radiograph	Enlarged heart, pulmonary congestion	Mild cardiomegaly	Mild to moderate cardiomegaly
Echocardiogram, nuclear studies, MRI	Left ventricular dilation and dysfunction	Left ventricular hypertrophy, asymmetric septal hypertrophy, small left ventricular size, normal or supranormal function, systolic anterior mitral motion, diastolic dysfunction	Small or normal left ventricular size, normal or mildly reduced left ventricular function. Gadolinium hyperenhancement on MRI
Cardiac catheterization	Left ventricular dilation and dysfunction, high diastolic pressures, low cardiac output. Coronary angiography important to exclude ischemic cause	Small, hypercontractile left ventricle, dynamic outflow gradient, diastolic dysfunction	High diastolic pressure, "square root" sign, normal or mildly reduced left ventricular function

class IIa indication with LOE of C. It should not be used routinely. Biopsy is most useful in transplant rejection.

Treatment

The management of heart failure is outlined in the section on heart failure in this chapter. Standard therapy includes control of BP and of contributing factors such as obesity, smoking, diabetes or potentially cardiotoxic agents. All patients with a remote history of MI or acute coronary syndrome and reduced LVEF should be given ACE inhibitors, ARBs, or sacubitril/valsartan. Beta-blockers should be included in this population as well. All patients with dilated cardiomyopathy regardless of etiology should be treated with beta-blockers and ACE inhibitors. If still symptomatic, aldosterone antagonsits should be added, and ARNI used instead of an ACE inhibitor or ARB. The use of the combination of all three of ACE inhibition, ARB, and aldosterone antagonists can create harm, though, and is discouraged due to concerns for hyperkalemia. Calcium channel blockers should be avoided except as necessary to control ventricular response in atrial fibrillation or flutter. If congestive symptoms are present, diuretics and an aldosterone antagonist should be added. In patients with class II–IV heart failure symptoms, an aldosterone receptor antagonist should be added when the LVEF is less than 35% (unless contraindicated). Care in the use of mineralocorticoid receptor antagonists is warranted when the glomerular filtration rate is less than 30 mL/min/1.73 m^2 or when the potassium is elevated. All patients with diabetes should be taking mineralocorticoid antagonists if the LVEF is less than or equal to 40%. Systemic BP control is extremely important. Use of the angiotensin receptor-neprilysin inhibitor, sacubitril/valsartan, has been approved for NYHA Heart Failure of Functional class II–IV. If the resting heart rate is greater than 70 beats per minute, the LVEF is less than 35% and the patient has chronic stable heart failure, the use of ivabradine to slow the heart rate has also been approved. Ivabradine should not replace other beta-blockers, however. Digoxin is a second-line medication but remains favored as an adjunct by some clinicians; digoxin may be beneficial to reduce recurrent hospitalizations and to control the ventricular response in atrial fibrillation in sedentary patients. Given the question of abnormal nitric oxide utilization in blacks, the use of hydralazine-nitrate combination therapy is recommended in this population. Sodium restriction is helpful, especially in acute heart failure. Continuous positive airway pressure can improve LV function in patients with sleep apnea.

When atrial fibrillation is present, heart rate control is important if sinus rhythm cannot be established or maintained. There are few data, however, to suggest an advantage of sinus rhythm over atrial fibrillation on long-term outcomes. Many patients may be candidates for cardiac synchronization therapy with biventricular pacing if there is significant mitral regurgitation and the QRS width is greater than 150 msec.

To help prevent sudden death, an ICD is reasonable (class IIa, LOE B) in asymptomatic ischemic cardiomyopathy patients with an LVEF of less than 30% on appropriate medical therapy (at least 40 days post-MI). Cardiac rehabilitation and exercise training have consistently been found to improve clinical status.

Few cases of cardiomyopathy are amenable to specific therapy for the underlying cause. Alcohol use should be discontinued, since there is often marked recovery of cardiac function following a period of abstinence in alcoholic cardiomyopathy. Endocrine causes (hyperthyroidism or hypothyroidism, acromegaly, and pheochromocytoma) should be treated. Immunosuppressive therapy is not indicated in chronic dilated cardiomyopathy. There are some patients who may benefit from implantable LV assist devices either as a bridge to transplantation or as a temporary measure until cardiac function returns. LV assist devices can be considered as *destination therapy* in patients who are not candidates for cardiac transplantation. Arterial and pulmonary emboli are more common in dilated cardiomyopathy than in ischemic cardiomyopathy and suitable candidates may benefit from long-term anticoagulation. All patients with atrial fibrillation should be so treated. DOACs are preferred over warfarin unless there is associated mitral stenosis. Either warfarin or a DOAC should be considered when a mobile LV thrombus is observed on the echocardiogram.

Prognosis

The prognosis of dilated cardiomyopathy without clinical heart failure is variable, with some patients remaining stable, some deteriorating gradually, and others declining rapidly. Once heart failure is manifest, the natural history is similar to that of other causes of heart failure, with an annual mortality rate of around 11–13%. The underlying cause of heart failure has prognostic value in patients with unexplained cardiomyopathy. Patients with peripartum cardiomyopathy or stress-induced cardiomyopathy appear to have a better prognosis than those with other forms of cardiomyopathy. Patients with cardiomyopathy due to infiltrative myocardial diseases, HIV infection, or doxorubicin therapy have an especially poor prognosis.

When to Refer

Patients with new or worsening symptoms of heart failure with dilated cardiomyopathy should be referred to a cardiologist. Patients with continued symptoms of heart failure and reduced LVEF (35% or less) should be referred for consideration of placement of an ICD or cardiac resynchronization therapy (if QRS duration is 150 msec or more, especially with a left bundle branch block pattern). Patients with advanced refractory symptoms should be referred for consideration of heart transplant or LV assist device therapy.

When to Admit

Patients with hypoxia, fluid overload, or pulmonary edema not readily resolved in an outpatient setting should be admitted.

Bozkurt B et al. Current diagnostic and treatment strategies for specific dilated cardiomyopathies: a scientific statement from the American Heart Association. Circulation. 2016 Dec 6;134(23):e579–646. [PMID: 27832612]

Japp AG et al. The diagnosis and evaluation of dilated cardiomy-opathy. J Am Coll Cardiol. 2016 Jun 28;67(25):2996–3010. [PMID: 27339497]

Witt CT et al. Adding the implantable cardioverter-defibrillator to cardiac resynchronization therapy is associated with improved long-term survival in ischaemic, but not in non-ischaemic cardiomyopathy. Europace. 2016 Mar;18(3):413–9. [PMID: 26378089]

Yancy CW et al. 2016 ACC/AHA/HFSA focused update on new pharmacological therapy for heart failure: an update of the 2013 ACCF/AHA guideline for the management of heart failure. J Am Coll Cardiol. 2016 Sep 27;68(13):1476–88. [PMID: 27216111]

Yancy CW et al. 2017 ACC/AHA/HFSA focused update of the 2013 ACCF/AHA guideline for the management of heart failure: a report of the American College of Cardiology/American Heart Association Task Force on Clinical Practice Guidelines and the Heart Failure Society of America. Circulation. 2017 Aug 8;136(6):e137–61. [PMID: 28455343]

STRESS CARDIOMYOPATHY

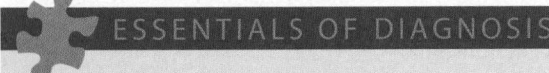

ESSENTIALS OF DIAGNOSIS

► Occurs after a major catecholamine discharge.

► Acute chest pain or shortness of breath.

► Predominately affects postmenopausal women.

► Presents as an acute anterior MI, but coronaries normal at cardiac catheterization.

► Imaging reveals apical left ventricular ballooning due to anteroapical stunning of the myocardium.

► Most patients recover completely, although there are complications similar to MI.

General Considerations

Stress cardiomyopathy (**tako-tsubo syndrome**) generally follows a high catecholamine surge. The resulting shape of the LV acutely suggests a rounded ampulla form similar to a Japanese octopus pot (tako-tsubo pot). Mid-ventricular ballooning has also been described. The key feature is that the myocardial stunning that occurs does not follow the pattern suggestive of coronary ischemia (even though about 15% of patients will have coexisting CAD, and some may have concomitant plaque rupture MI). Over two-thirds of patients report a prior stressful event, either emotional or physical, including hypoglycemia, lightning strikes, earth-quakes, postventricular tachycardia, during alcohol with-drawal, following surgery, during hyperthyroidism, after stroke, and following emotional stress ("broken-heart syndrome"). Virtually any event that triggers excess cate-cholamines has been implicated in a wide number of case reports. Pericarditis and even tamponade have been described in isolated cases. Recurrences have also been described. In Western countries it predominantly affects women (up to 90%), primarily postmenopausal. Among patients with stress cardiomyopathy, compared to patients with acute coronary syndrome, there are more neurologic

and psychiatric disorders. Patients with COPD, migraines, or affective disorders who take beta-agonists may have an increased risk of a poor outcome. The prognosis was ini-tially thought to be benign, but subsequent studies have demonstrated that both short-term mortality and long-term mortality are higher than thought. Indeed, mortality reported during the acute phase in hospitalized patients is approximately 4–5%, a figure comparable to that of STEMI in the era of primary percutaneous coronary interventions. Approximately 10% of patients will have cardiac and neuro-logic adverse outcomes over the next year.

The structures that mediate the stress response are in both the central and autonomic nervous systems. Acute stressors induce brain activation, increasing bioavailability of cortisol and catecholamine. Both circulating epineph-rine and norepinephrine released from adrenal medullary chromaffin cells and norepinephrine released locally from sympathetic nerve terminals are significantly increased. This catecholamine surge leads to myocardial damage through multiple mechanisms, including, direct catechol-amine toxicity, adrenoceptor-mediated damage, epicardial and microvascular coronary vasoconstriction and/or spasm, and increased cardiac workload. The relative pre-ponderance among postmenopausal women suggests that estrogen deprivation may be facilitating, possibly via endo-thelial dysfunction.

Clinical Findings

A. Symptoms and Signs

The symptoms are similar to any acute coronary syndrome. Typical angina and dyspnea are usually present. Syncope is rare, although arrhythmias are not uncommon.

B. ECG and Chest Radiography

The ECG reveals ST-segment elevation as well as deep anterior T-wave inversion. The chest radiograph is either normal or reveals pulmonary congestion. The dramatic T-wave inversions gradually resolve over time.

C. Diagnostic Studies

The echocardiogram reveals LV apical dyskinesia usually not consistent with any particular coronary distribution. The urgent cardiac catheterization reveals the LV apical ballooning in association with normal coronaries. Initial cardiac enzymes are positive but often taper quickly. In almost all cases, MRI hyperenhancement studies reveal no long-term scarring.

Treatment

Immediate therapy is similar to any acute MI. Initiation of long-term therapy depends on whether LV dysfunction persists. Most patients receive aspirin, beta-blockers, and ACE inhibitors until the LV fully recovers. Despite the presumed association with high catecholamines, the use of ACE inhibitors or ARBs, but not beta-blockers has been associated with improved long-term survival. See Treat-ment of Heart Failure with Reduced EF.

Prognosis

In a 2015 registry of 1759 patients, the rate of severe in-hospital complications, including shock and death, were similar between those with an acute coronary syndrome and tako-tsubo. Overall, prognosis is good unless there is a serious complication (such as mitral regurgitation, ventricular rupture, or ventricular tachycardia). Recovery of the LVEF is expected in most cases after a period of weeks to months. At times, the LV function recovers fully in a few days.

When to Refer

All patients with an acute coronary syndrome should be urgently seen by a cardiologist for further evaluation and monitored until resolution of the ventricular dysfunction.

Goica A et al. Novel developments in stress cardiomyopathy: from pathophysiology to prognosis. Int J Cardiol 2016;223:1053–58. [PMID: 27611570]

Templin C et al. Clinical features and outcome of takotsubo (stress) cardiomyopathy. N Engl J Med. 2015 Sep 3;373(10):929–38. [PMID: 26332547]

Tornvall P et al. A case-control study of the risk markers and mortality in Takotsubo stress cardiomyopathy. J Am Coll Cardiol. 2016 Apr 26;67(16):1931–6. [PMID: 27102508]

HYPERTROPHIC CARDIOMYOPATHY

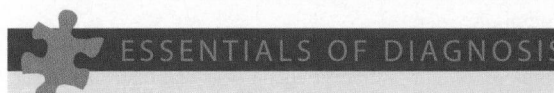

ESSENTIALS OF DIAGNOSIS

▶ May present with dyspnea, chest pain, syncope.

▶ Though LV outflow gradient is classic, symptoms are primarily related to diastolic dysfunction.

▶ Echocardiogram is diagnostic. Any area of LV wall thickness greater than 1.5 cm defines the disease.

▶ Increased risk of sudden death.

General Considerations

Hypertrophic cardiomyopathy is noted when there is LVH unrelated to any pressure or volume overload. The definition has evolved over time; while it traditionally has been defined by LV outflow obstruction due to septal hypertrophy, now it is considered present any time that **any LV wall is measured at more than 1.5 cm thick on an echocardiogram**. This allows for many forms to be considered that do not create LV outflow obstruction. The increased wall thickness reduces LV systolic stress, increases the EF, and can result in an "empty ventricle" at end-systole. The interventricular septum may be disproportionately involved (**asymmetric septal hypertrophy**), but in some cases the hypertrophy is localized to the mid-ventricle or to the apex. The LV outflow tract is usually narrowed during systole due to the hypertrophied septum and systolic anterior motion of the mitral valve occurs as the anterior mitral valve leaflet is pulled into the LV outflow. The obstruction is worsened by factors that increase myocardial contractility

(sympathetic stimulation, digoxin, and postextrasystolic beat) or that decrease LV filling (Valsalva maneuver, peripheral vasodilators). The amount of obstruction is preload and afterload dependent and can vary from day to day. The consequence of the hypertrophy is *elevated LV diastolic pressures* rather than systolic dysfunction. Rarely, systolic dysfunction develops late in the disease. The LV is usually more involved than the RV, and the atria are frequently significantly enlarged.

Hypertrophic cardiomyopathy is inherited as an autosomal-dominant trait with variable penetrance and is caused by mutations of one of a large number of genes, most of which code for myosin heavy chains or proteins regulating calcium handling. The prognosis is related to the specific gene mutation. Patients usually present in early adulthood. Elite athletes may demonstrate considerable hypertrophy that can be confused with hypertrophic cardiomyopathy, but generally diastolic dysfunction is not present in the athlete and this finding helps separate pathologic disease from **athletic hypertrophy**. The apical variety is particularly common in those of Asian descent. A hypertrophic cardiomyopathy in older adults (usually in association with hypertension) has also been defined as a distinct entity (often a sigmoid interventricular septum is noted with a knob of cardiac muscle below the aortic valve). Mitral annular calcification is often present. Mitral regurgitation is variable and often dynamic, depending on the degree of outflow tract obstruction.

Clinical Findings

A. Symptoms and Signs

The most frequent symptoms are dyspnea and chest pain (see Table 10–17). Syncope is also common and is typically postexertional, when diastolic filling diminishes due to fluid loss and tachycardia increasing LV outflow tract obstruction. Residual circulating catecholamines accentuate the changes. Arrhythmias are an important problem. Atrial fibrillation is a long-term consequence of chronically elevated LA pressures and is a poor prognostic sign. Ventricular arrhythmias are also common, and sudden death may occur, often after extraordinary exertion.

Features on physical examination include a bisferiens carotid pulse, triple apical impulse (due to the prominent atrial filling wave and early and late systolic impulses), and a loud S_4. The JVP may reveal a prominent *a* wave due to reduced RV compliance. In cases with LV outflow obstruction, a loud systolic murmur is present along the left sternal border that increases with upright posture or Valsalva maneuver and decreases with squatting. These maneuvers help differentiate the murmur of hypertrophic cardiomyopathy from that of aortic stenosis. In hypertrophic cardiomyopathy, reducing the LV volume *increases* the outflow obstruction and the murmur intensity; whereas in valvular aortic stenosis, reducing the stroke volume across the valve decreases the murmur. Mitral regurgitation is frequently present as well.

B. ECG and Chest Radiography

LVH is nearly universal in symptomatic patients, though entirely normal ECGs are present in up to 25%, usually in those with localized hypertrophy. Exaggerated septal Q waves inferolaterally may mimic MI. The chest radiograph is often unimpressive. Unlike with aortic stenosis, the ascending aorta is not dilated.

C. Diagnostic Studies

The echocardiogram is diagnostic, revealing LVH (involving the septum more commonly than the posterior walls), systolic anterior motion of the mitral valve, early closing followed by reopening of the aortic valve, a small and hypercontractile LV, and delayed relaxation and filling of the LV during diastole. The septum is usually 1.3–1.5 times the thickness of the posterior wall. Septal motion tends to be reduced. Doppler ultrasound reveals turbulent flow and a dynamic gradient in the LV outflow tract and, commonly, mitral regurgitation. Abnormalities in the diastolic filling pattern are present in 80% of patients.

Echocardiography can usually differentiate the disease from ventricular noncompaction, a congenital myocardial disease pattern with marked trabeculation that partially fills the LV cavity. Myocardial perfusion imaging may suggest septal ischemia in the presence of normal coronary arteries. Cardiac MRI confirms the hypertrophy and contrast enhancement frequently reveals evidence of scar at the junction of the RV attachment to the interventricular septum. Cardiac catheterization confirms the diagnosis and defines the presence or absence of CAD. Frequently, coronary arterial bridging (squeezing of the coronary in systole) occurs, especially in the septal arteries. Exercise studies are recommended to assess for ventricular arrhythmias and to document the BP response. Loop monitoring is recommended for determination of ventricular ectopy.

► Treatment

Beta-blockers should be the initial medication in symptomatic individuals, especially when dynamic outflow obstruction is noted on the echocardiogram. The resulting slower heart rates assist with diastolic filling of the stiff LV. Dyspnea, angina, and arrhythmias respond in about 50% of patients. Calcium channel blockers, especially verapamil, have also been effective in symptomatic patients. Verapamil is preferred due to its more potent effects on the myocardium. Their effect is due primarily to improved diastolic function; however, their vasodilating actions can also increase outflow obstruction and cause hypotension. Disopyramide is also effective because of its negative inotropic effects; it is usually used as an addition to the medical regimen rather than as primary therapy or to help control atrial arrhythmias. Diuretics are frequently necessary due to the high LV diastolic pressure and elevated LA pressures, but should be used with caution to avoid dehydration that would increase obstruction. Patients do best in sinus rhythm, and atrial fibrillation should be aggressively treated with antiarrhythmics or radiofrequency ablation. Dualchamber pacing may help prevent the progression of hypertrophy and obstruction. There appears to be an advantage to the use of short-AV delay biventricular pacing.

Patients with malignant ventricular arrhythmias and/or unexplained syncope in the presence of a positive family history for sudden death, with or without an abnormal BP response to exercise, are best managed with an implantable defibrillator. It is reasonable to consider an ICD for patients with hypertrophic cardiomyopathy (HCM) and maximum wall thickness of at least 30 mm, sudden cardiac death in a first-degree relative, and/or unexplained syncope in the last 6 months. Other factors include abnormal blood pressure response to exercise and gadolinium enhancement on MRI.

Excision of part of the outflow myocardial septum (myotomy–myomectomy) by experienced surgeons is successful in patients with severe symptoms unresponsive to medical therapy. A few surgeons advocate mitral valve replacement, since this results in resolution of the gradient and prevents associated mitral regurgitation. In some cases, myomectomy has been combined with an Alfieri stitch on the mitral valve (a stitch that binds the midportion of the anterior and posterior mitral valve leaflets together). Rare cases of progression to LV dilation or patients with intractable symptoms can be considered for cardiac transplantation. Nonsurgical septal ablation can be performed by injection of alcohol into septal branches of the left coronary artery to create a controlled myocardial infarct in the regions of greatest wall thickness. Figure 10–9 provides an algorithm for the treatment of hypertrophic cardiomyopathy as defined in the 2011 AHA/ACC guidelines.

Pregnancy results in an increased risk in patients with symptoms or outflow tract gradients of greater than 50 mm Hg. Genetic counseling is indicated before planned conception. In pregnant patients with hypertrophic cardiomyopathy, continuation of beta-blocker therapy is recommended.

► Prognosis

The natural history of hypertrophic cardiomyopathy is highly variable. Genetic testing is recommended if firstdegree relatives are available to participate. Some patients remain asymptomatic for many years or for life. Sudden death, especially during exercise, may be the initial event. The highest risk patients are those with (1) a personal history of serious ventricular arrhythmias or survival of a sudden death episode; (2) a family history of sudden death; (3) unexplained syncope; (4) documented nonsustained ventricular tachycardia, defined as three or more beats of ventricular tachycardia at 120 beats/min or more on ambulatory ECG monitoring; and (5) maximal LV wall thickness of 30 mm or more. In addition, patients in whom the systolic BP does not increase more than 20 mm Hg during treadmill stress testing are also at risk, as are those with double and compound genetic mutations and those with marked LV outflow tract obstruction. MRI data suggest that the extent of scarring on hyperenhancement may also be predictive of adverse events, and some studies suggest a substantial risk factor is defined if the amount of hyperenhancement scar exceeds 15% of the entire myocardium. Hypertrophic cardiomyopathy is the pathologic feature most frequently associated with sudden death in athletes.

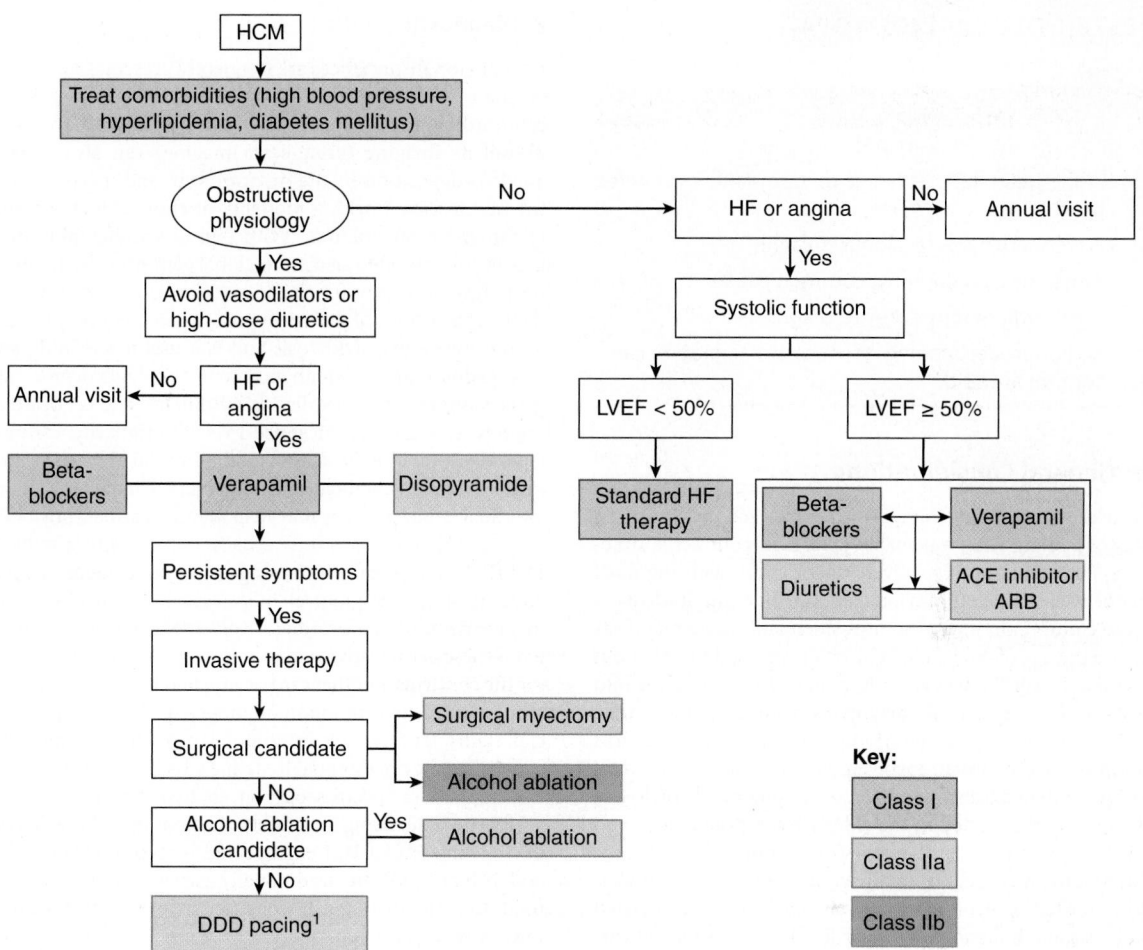

¹See section on AV Block in the text.

▲ **Figure 10–9.** Recommended therapeutic approach to the patient with hypertrophic cardiomyopathy (HCM). ACE, angiotensin-converting enzyme; ARB, angiotensin receptor blockers; HF, heart failure; LVEF, left ventricular ejection fraction. (Reproduced, with permission, from Gersh BJ et al. 2011 ACCF/AHA Guideline for the Diagnosis and Treatment of Hypertrophic Cardiomyopathy A Report of the American College of Cardiology Foundation/American Heart Association Task Force on Practice Guidelines Developed in Collaboration With the American Association for Thoracic Surgery, American Society of Echocardiography, American Society of Nuclear Cardiology, Heart Failure Society of America, Heart Rhythm Society, Society for Cardiovascular Angiography and Interventions, and Society of Thoracic Surgeons. J Am Coll Cardiol. 2011 Dec 13;58(25):e212–60. Copyright © Elsevier.)

Endocarditis prophylaxis is not indicated. A final stage may be a transition into a dilated cardiomyopathy in 5–10% of patients due to the long-term effects of LV remodeling; treatment at that stage is similar to that for dilated cardiomyopathy. An online calculator for risk of sudden cardiac death is available from the European Society of Cardiology (http://doc2do.com/hcm/webHCM.html).

► When to Refer

Patients should be referred to a cardiologist when symptoms are difficult to control, syncope has occurred, or there are any of the high-risk features present, which may denote the need for a prophylactic defibrillator.

Elliott PM et al. 2014 ESC guidelines on diagnosis and management of hypertrophic cardiomyopathy: the Task Force for the Diagnosis and Management of Hypertrophic Cardiomyopathy of the European Society of Cardiology (ESC). Eur Heart J. 2014 Oct 14;35(39):2733–79. [PMID: 25173338]

Gersh BJ et al. 2011 ACCF/AHA guideline for the treatment of hypertrophic cardiomyopathy. J Am Coll Cardiol. 2011 Dec 13;58(25):e212–60. [PMID: 22075469]

Maron BJ et al. How hypertrophic cardiomyopathy became a contemporary treatable genetic disease with low mortality shaped by 50 years of clinical research and practice. JAMA Cardiol. 2016 Apr 1;1(1):98–105. [PMID: 27437663]

Sen-Chowdry S et al. Update on hypertrophic cardiomyopathy and a guide to the guidelines. Nat Rev Cardiol. 2016 Nov;13(11):651–75. [PMID: 27681577]

RESTRICTIVE CARDIOMYOPATHY

ESSENTIALS OF DIAGNOSIS

► Right heart failure tends to dominate over left heart failure.

► Pulmonary hypertension is present.

► Amyloidosis is the most common cause.

► Echocardiography is key to diagnosis.

► Radionuclide imaging or myocardial biopsy can confirm amyloid.

► General Considerations

Restrictive cardiomyopathy is characterized by impaired diastolic filling with reasonably preserved contractile function. The condition is relatively uncommon, with the most frequent cause being amyloidosis. **Cardiac amyloidosis** is more common in men than in women and rarely manifests before the age of 40. While light-chain amyloid proteins can be toxic to cardiomyocytes, they may also internalize into many cell types and this may explain some of the cardiac dysfunction observed. The AL (light-chain) type is the most common, with cardiac involvement in 50%. Other forms include mutated transthyretin (ATTR) in familial amyloidosis (usually manifested in the elderly black population) and a wild-type transthyretin amyloidosis. Transthyretin is produced almost entirely in the liver. Secondary (AA) amyloidosis due to fragments of serum amyloid A protein associated with chronic inflammatory disorders is a rare cause of cardiac disease. An isolated atrial amyloid form is also recognized.

The differential diagnosis of a restrictive cardiomyopathy includes infiltrative disorders beside amyloidosis, such as sarcoidosis, Gaucher disease, and Hurler syndrome. Storage diseases such as hemochromatosis, Fabry disease, and glycogen storage diseases can also produce the picture. Noninfiltrative diseases, such as familial cardiomyopathy and pseudoxanthoma elasticum, can be implicated rarely, and other secondary causes include diabetes, scleroderma, radiation, chemotherapy, CAD, and longstanding hypertension.

► Clinical Findings

A. Symptoms and Signs

Restrictive cardiomyopathy must be distinguished from constrictive pericarditis (see Table 10–17). The key feature is that ventricular interaction is *accentuated* with respiration in constrictive pericarditis and that interaction is absent in restrictive cardiomyopathy. In addition, the pulmonary arterial pressure is invariably elevated in restrictive cardiomyopathy due to the high PCWP and is normal in uncomplicated constrictive pericarditis. Symptoms may include angina, syncope, stroke, and peripheral neuropathy. Periorbital purpura, a thickened tongue, or hepatomegaly are all suggestive physical findings of amyloidosis.

B. Diagnostic Studies

Conduction disturbances are frequently present. Low voltage on the ECG combined with ventricular hypertrophy on the echocardiogram is suggestive of disease. Technetium pyrophosphate imaging (bone scan imaging) can also identify amyloid deposition in the myocardium, and it has become the noninvasive imaging modality of choice for diagnosing transthyretin amyloidosis. With typical scintographic findings in patients without a monoclonal gammopathy, biopsy is no longer necessary for diagnosis. Cardiac MRI presents a distinctive pattern of diffuse hyperenhancement of the gadolinium image in amyloidosis and is a useful screening test. Late gadolinium hyperenhancement of a high degree suggests more extensive cardiac involvement. The echocardiogram reveals a small, thickened LV with bright myocardium (speckled), rapid early diastolic filling revealed by the mitral inflow Doppler, and biatrial enlargement. Characteristic longitudinal strain patterns may help identify cardiac amyloidosis. The LV chamber size is usually normal with a reduced LVEF. Atrial septal thickening may be evident. Rectal, abdominal fat, or gingival biopsies can confirm systemic involvement, but myocardial involvement may still be present if these are negative and requires endomyocardial biopsy for the confirmation that cardiac amyloid is present. Demonstration of tissue infiltration on biopsy specimens using special stains followed by immunohistochemical studies and genetic testing are essential to define which specific protein is involved. Mass spectroscopy on all tissue in question and TTR gene sequencing in patients in whom the TTR wild type or TTR mutant variant is suspected is recommended. BNP and NT-proBNP are traditionally elevated and have been used to help distinguish constrictive pericarditis from a restrictive cardiomyopathy.

► Treatment

In 2018, the medication tafamidis was shown to be effective in the Transthyretin Amyloidosis Cardiomyopathy Clinical Trial (ATTR-ACT). Tafamidis substantially improved survival, reduced hospitalization, and improved quality of life for patients with transthyretin amyloidosis cardiomyopathy. Tafamidis is approved in some countries, and has been given priority review status by the US FDA with a decision expected in 2019. Treatment for AL amyloidosis includes alkylator-based chemotherapy or high-dose melphalan followed by autologous stem cell transplantation. In immunoglobin light chain amyloidosis, standard- or high-dose chemotherapy with stem cell rescue is often pursued.

In acute cases, diuretics can help, but excessive diuresis can produce worsening kidney dysfunction. As with most patients with severe right heart failure, loop diuretics, thiazides, and aldosterone antagonists are all useful. Ultrafiltration devices may improve diuresis, although it is not clear if prognosis is improved. Atrial thrombi are not uncommon, although the role of anticoagulation in amyloidosis remains ill defined. Digoxin may precipitate arrhythmias and should not be used. Beta-blockers help slow heart rates and improve filling by increasing diastolic time. Verapamil presumably works by improving myocardial relaxation and increasing diastolic filling time. Slow heart rates are desired to allow for increased diastolic filling time. ACE inhibition or angiotensin II receptor blockade may improve diastolic filling at times and can be tried with caution if the systemic blood pressure is adequate. Corticosteroids may be helpful in sarcoidosis but they are more effective for conduction abnormalities than heart failure.

In amyloidosis, the therapeutic strategy depends on the characterization of the type of amyloid protein and extent of disease and may include chemotherapy or bone marrow transplantation. In familial amyloidosis (ATTR), tafamidis provides important benefits. In AL amyloidosis, chemotherapy and autologous stem cell transplantation have been tried with mixed success. Cardiac transplantation has also been used in patients with primary cardiac amyloidosis and no evidence of systemic involvement.

► When to Refer

All patients with the diagnosis of a restrictive cardiomyopathy should be referred to a cardiologist to decide etiology and plan appropriate treatment. Unexplained LVH with relatively preserved LVEF and symptoms of heart failure should raise the question of cardiac amyloid, particularly now that there is effective treatment available.

Gertz MA et al. Pathophysiology and treatment of cardiac amyloidosis. Nat Rev Cardiol. 2015 Feb;12(2):91–102. [PMID: 25311231]

Gillmore JD et al. Nonbiopsy diagnosis of cardiac transthyretin amyloidosis. Circulation. 2016 Jun 14;133(24):2404–12. [PMID: 27143678]

Maurer MS et al; ATTR-ACT Study Investigators. Tafamidis treatment for patients with transthyretin amyloid cardiomyopathy. N Engl J Med. 2018 Sep 13;379(11):1007–16. [PMID: 30145929]

Pereira NL et al. Spectrum of restrictive and infiltrative cardiomyopathies: part 1 of a 2-part series. J Am Coll Cardiol. 2018 Mar 13;71(10):1130–48. [PMID: 29519355]

Pereira NL et al. Spectrum of restrictive and infiltrative cardiomyopathies: part 2 of a 2-part series. J Am Coll Cardiol. 2018 Mar 13;71(10):1149–66. [PMID: 29519356]

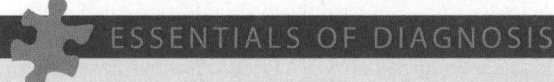

▼ RHEUMATIC FEVER

ESSENTIALS OF DIAGNOSIS

► More common in developing countries (100 cases/100,000 population) than in the United States (~2 cases/100,000 population).

► Peak incidence between ages 5 and 15 years.

► Revision of Jones criteria in 2015 includes echocardiographic findings.

► May involve mitral and other valves acutely, rarely leading to heart failure.

► General Considerations

Rheumatic fever is a systemic immune process that is a sequela of a beta-hemolytic streptococcal infection of the pharynx. It is a major scourge in developing countries and responsible for 250,000 deaths in young people worldwide each year. Over 15 million people have evidence for rheumatic heart disease. Signs of **acute rheumatic fever** usually commence 2–3 weeks after infection but may appear as early as 1 week or as late as 5 weeks. The disease has become quite uncommon in the United States, except in immigrants; however, there have been reports of new outbreaks in several regions of the United States. The peak incidence is between ages 5 and 15 years; rheumatic fever is rare before age 4 years or after age 40 years. Rheumatic carditis and valvulitis may be self-limited or may lead to slowly progressive valvular deformity. The characteristic lesion is a perivascular granulomatous reaction with valvulitis. The mitral valve is acutely attacked in 75–80% of cases, the aortic valve in 30% (but rarely as the sole valve involved), and the tricuspid and pulmonary valves in under 5% of cases.

The clinical profile of the infection includes carditis in 50–70% and arthritis in 35–66%, followed by chorea (10–30%, predominantly in girls) then subcutaneous nodules (0–10%) and erythema marginatum (in less than 6%). Echocardiography has been found to be superior to auscultation, and the 2015 guidelines introduced **subclinical carditis** to the Jones criteria to represent abnormal echocardiographic findings when auscultatory findings were either not present or not recognized.

Chronic rheumatic heart disease results from single or repeated attacks of rheumatic fever that produce rigidity and deformity of valve cusps, fusion of the commissures, or shortening and fusion of the chordae tendineae. Valvular stenosis or regurgitation results, and the two often coexist. In chronic rheumatic heart disease, the mitral valve alone is abnormal in 50–60% of cases; combined lesions of the aortic and mitral valves occur in 20%; pure aortic lesions are less common. Tricuspid involvement occurs in about 10% of cases, but only in association with mitral or aortic disease and is thought to be more common when recurrent infections have occurred. The pulmonary valve is rarely affected long term. A history of rheumatic fever is obtainable in only 60% of patients with rheumatic heart disease. A recent report estimated there were almost 320,000 deaths from rheumatic heart disease in 2015. It noted that from 1990 to 2015 this represented a 47.8% decline, but there were large regional differences. In 2015 alone, there were 33.4 million cases of rheumatic heart disease globally. These data emphasize that, while there has been progress against this disease, it remains a major cardiovascular problem in the poorest regions of the world.

► Clinical Findings

The presence of two major criteria—or one major and two minor criteria—establishes the diagnosis. While India, New Zealand, and Australia have all published revised guidelines since 2001, the 2015 recommendations have revised the Jones criteria (Table 10–18) in a scientific statement from the AHA where subclinical carditis is now recognized with the advent of echocardiography. The revised criteria also recognize that a lower threshold should be used to diagnosis acute rheumatic fever in high-risk populations.

Table 10–18. The 2015 revised Jones criteria.[1]

Population	Criteria	
	Major	Minor
Low risk	Carditis (clinical or subclinical)	Polyarthralgia
	Arthritis (polyarthritis only)	Fever (≥ 38.5°C)
	Chorea	ESR ≥ 60 mm/h or CRP ≥ 3.0 mg/dL (or both)
	Erythema marginatum	Prolonged PR interval (unless carditis is major criterion)
	Subcutaneous nodules	
Moderate and high risk	Carditis (clinical or subclinical)	Monoarthralgia
	Arthritis (monoarthritis, polyarthritis, polyarthalgia)	Fever (≥ 38°C)
	Chorea	ESR ≥ 30 mm/h or CRP ≥ 3.0 mg/dL (or both)
	Erythema marginatum	Prolonged PR interval (unless carditis is a major criterion)
	Subcutaneous nodules	

[1]For all patients with evidence of preceding group A streptococcal pharyngitis: initial acute rheumatic fever can be diagnosed when 2 major criteria or 1 major plus 2 minor criteria are met. Recurrent acute rheumatic fever can be diagnosed when 2 major or 1 major plus 2 minor or 3 minor criteria are met.

ESR, erythrocyte sedimentation rate; CRP, C-reactive protein.

Modified, with permission, from Gewitz, MH et al; American Heart Association Committee on Rheumatic Fever, Endocarditis, and Kawasaki Disease of the Council on Cardiovascular Disease in the Young. Revision of the Jones criteria for the diagnosis of acute rheumatic fever in the era of Doppler echocardiography. A scientific statement from the American Heart Association. Circulation. 2015 May 19;131(20):1806–18. © 2015 American Heart Association, Inc.

A. Major Criteria

1. Carditis—Carditis is most likely to be evident in children and adolescents. Any of the following suggests the presence of carditis: (1) pericarditis; (2) cardiomegaly, detected by physical signs, radiography, or echocardiography; (3) heart failure, right- or left-sided—the former perhaps more prominent in children, with painful liver engorgement due to tricuspid regurgitation; and (4) mitral or aortic regurgitation murmurs, indicative of dilation of a valve ring with or without associated valvulitis or morphologic findings on echocardiography of rheumatic valvulitis. The Carey–Coombs short mid-diastolic mitral murmur may be present due to inflammation of the mitral valve. It is a class I (LOE B) indication to perform echocardiography/Doppler studies on all cases of suspected or confirmed acute rheumatic fever.

2. Erythema marginatum and subcutaneous nodules—Erythema marginatum begins as rapidly enlarging macules that assume the shape of rings or crescents with clear centers. They may be raised, confluent, and either transient or persistent and usually on the trunk or proximal extremities. Subcutaneous nodules are uncommon except in children. They are small (2 cm or less in diameter), firm, and nontender and are attached to fascia or tendon sheaths over bony prominences. They persist for days or weeks, are recurrent, and are indistinguishable from rheumatoid nodules. Neither the rash nor nodules ever occur as the sole manifestation of acute rheumatic fever.

3. Sydenham chorea—This is the most definitive manifestation of acute rheumatic fever. Defined as involuntary choreoathetoid movements primarily of the face, tongue, and upper extremities, Sydenham chorea may be the sole manifestation of rheumatic fever. Girls are more frequently affected than boys, and occurrence in adults is rare.

4. Polyarthritis—This is a migratory polyarthritis that involves the large joints sequentially. In adults and in certain moderate- to high-risk populations, only a single joint may be affected. The arthritis lasts 1–5 weeks and subsides without residual deformity. Prompt response of arthritis to therapeutic doses of salicylates or nonsteroidal agents is characteristic.

B. Minor Criteria

These include fever, polyarthralgias, reversible prolongation of the PR interval, and an elevated erythrocyte sedimentation rate or CRP. A lower threshold is set for patients at high risk (Table 10–18). The 2015 guidelines stipulate that evidence for a preceding streptococcal infection can be defined by an increase or rising anti-streptolysin O titer or streptococcal antibodies (anti-DNAase B), a positive throat culture for group A beta-hemolytic streptococcal or a positive rapid group A streptococcal carbohydrate antigen test in a child with a high pretest probability of streptococcal pharyngitis.

▶ Treatment

A. General Measures

The patient should be kept at strict bed rest until the temperature returns to normal (without the use of antipyretic medications) and the sedimentation rate, plus the resting pulse rate, and the ECG have all returned to baseline.

B. Medical Measures

1. Salicylates—The salicylates markedly reduce fever and relieve joint pain and swelling. They have no effect on the natural course of the disease. Adults may require large doses of aspirin, 0.6–0.9 g every 4 hours; children are treated with lower doses.

2. Penicillin—Penicillin (benzathine penicillin, 1.2 million units intramuscularly once, or procaine penicillin, 600,000 units intramuscularly daily for 10 days) is used to eradicate streptococcal infection if present. Erythromycin may be substituted (40 mg/kg/day).

3. Corticosteroids—There is no proof that cardiac damage is prevented or minimized by corticosteroids. A short course of corticosteroids (prednisone, 40–60 mg orally daily, with tapering over 2 weeks) usually causes rapid improvement of the joint symptoms and is indicated when response to salicylates has been inadequate.

▶ Prevention of Recurrent Rheumatic Fever

Improvements in socioeconomic conditions and public health are critical to reducing bouts of rheumatic fever. The initial episode of rheumatic fever can usually be prevented by early treatment of streptococcal pharyngitis with penicillin (see Chapter 33). Prevention of recurrent episodes of rheumatic fever is critical. Recurrences of rheumatic fever are most common in patients who have had carditis during their initial episode and in children, 20% of whom will have a second episode within 5 years. The preferred method of prophylaxis is with benzathine penicillin G, 1.2 million units intramuscularly every 4 weeks. Oral penicillin (250 mg twice daily) is less reliable.

If the patient is allergic to penicillin, sulfadiazine (or sulfisoxazole), 1 g daily, or erythromycin, 250 mg orally twice daily, may be substituted. The macrolide azithromycin is similarly effective against group A streptococcal infection. If the patient has not had an immediate hypersensitivity (anaphylactic-type) reaction to penicillin, then cephalosporin may also be used.

Recurrences are uncommon after 5 years following the first episode and in patients over 21 years of age. Prophylaxis is usually discontinued after these times except in groups with a high risk of streptococcal infection—parents or teachers of young children, nurses, military recruits, etc. Secondary prevention of rheumatic fever depends on whether carditis has occurred. Current guidelines suggest that if there is no evidence for carditis, preventive therapy can be stopped at age 21 years. If carditis has occurred but there is no residual valvular disease, it can be stopped at 10 years after the acute rheumatic fever episode. If carditis has occurred with residual valvular involvement, it should be continued for 10 years after the last episode or until age 40 years if the patient is in a situation in which reexposure would be expected.

▶ Prognosis

Initial episodes of rheumatic fever may last months in children and weeks in adults. The immediate mortality rate is 1–2%. Persistent rheumatic carditis with cardiomegaly, heart failure, and pericarditis implies a poor prognosis; 30% of children thus affected die within 10 years after the initial attack. After 10 years, two-thirds of patients will have detectable valvular abnormalities (usually thickened valves with limited mobility), but significant symptomatic valvular heart disease or persistent cardiomyopathy occurs in less than 10% of patients with a single episode. In developing countries, acute rheumatic fever occurs earlier in life and recurs more frequently; thus the evolution to chronic valvular disease is both accelerated and more severe.

Gewitz MH et al; American Heart Association Committee on Rheumatic Fever, Endocarditis, and Kawasaki Disease of the Council on Cardiovascular Disease in the Young. Revision of the Jones criteria for the diagnosis of acute rheumatic fever in the era of Doppler echocardiography. A scientific statement from the American Heart Association. Circulation. 2015 May 19;131(20):1806–18. [PMID: 25908771]

Watkins DA et al. Global, regional, and national burden of rheumatic heart disease, 1990–2015. N Engl J Med. 2017 Aug 24;377(8):713–22. [PMID: 28834488]

Yacoub M et al. Eliminating acute rheumatic fever and rheumatic heart disease. Lancet. 2017 Jul 15;390(10091):212–3. [PMID: 28721865]

▼ DISEASES OF THE PERICARDIUM

ACUTE INFLAMMATORY PERICARDITIS

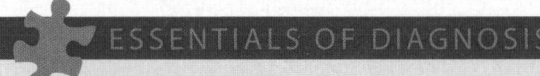
ESSENTIALS OF DIAGNOSIS

- ▶ Anterior pleuritic chest pain that is worse supine than upright.
- ▶ Pericardial rub.
- ▶ Fever common.
- ▶ Erythrocyte sedimentation rate or inflammatory CRP usually elevated.
- ▶ ECG reveals diffuse ST-segment elevation with associated PR depression.

▶ General Considerations

Acute (less than 2 weeks) inflammation of the pericardium may be infectious in origin or may be due to systemic diseases (autoimmune syndromes, uremia), neoplasm, radiation, drug toxicity, hemopericardium, postcardiac surgery, or contiguous inflammatory processes in the myocardium or lung. In many of these conditions, the pathologic process involves both the pericardium and the myocardium. Overall pericarditis accounts for 0.2% of hospital admissions and about 5% of patients with nonischemic chest pain seen in the emergency department. The ESC in 2015 proposed four definitions for pericarditis and elucidated diagnostic criteria for each (Table 10–19). **Viral infections** (especially infections with coxsackieviruses and echoviruses but also influenza, Epstein-Barr, varicella, hepatitis, mumps, and HIV viruses) are the most common cause of acute pericarditis and probably are responsible for many cases classified as idiopathic. Males—usually under age 50 years—are most commonly affected. The differential diagnosis primarily requires exclusion of acute MI. **Tuberculous pericarditis** is rare in developed countries but remains common in certain areas of the world. It results from direct lymphatic or hematogenous spread; clinical pulmonary involvement may

Table 10–19. Definitions and diagnostic criteria for pericarditis.

Pericarditis	Definition and Diagnosis
Acute	At least two of the following four listed findings: 1. Pericardial chest pain 2. Pericardial rub 3. New widespread ST-elevation or PR depression 4. Pericardial effusion (new or worsening)
	Additional supportive findings: 1. Elevated inflammatory markers (CRP, ESR, WBC) 2. Evidence for pericardial inflammation (CT or MRI)
Incessant	Pericarditis lasting longer than 4–6 weeks but less than 3 months without remission
Recurrent	Recurrence after a documented first espisode and a symptom-free interval of 4–6 weeks or longer
Chronic	Pericarditis lasting longer than 3 months

CRP, C-reactive protein; CT, computed tomography; ESR, erythrocyte sedimentation rate; MRI, magnetic resonance imaging; WBC, white blood cell count.
Modified, with permission, from Adler Y et al. 2015 ESC guidelines for the diagnosis and management of pericardial diseases: the Task Force for the Diagnosis and Management of Pericardial Diseases of the European Society of Cardiology (ESC) endorsed by: the European Association for Cardio-Thoracic Surgery (EACTS). Eur Heart J. 2015 Nov 7;36(42):2921–64. By permission of Oxford University Press and the European Society of Cardiology. © The European Society of Cardiology 2015. All rights reserved.

be absent or minor, although associated pleural effusions are common. **Bacterial pericarditis** is equally rare and usually results from direct extension from pulmonary infections. Pneumococci, though, can cause a primary pericardial infection. *Borrelia burgdorferi,* the organism responsible for Lyme disease, can also cause myopericarditis (and occasionally heart block). **Uremic pericarditis** is a common complication of chronic kidney disease. The pathogenesis is uncertain; it occurs both with untreated uremia and in otherwise stable dialysis patients. Spread of adjacent lung cancer as well as invasion by breast cancer, renal cell carcinoma, Hodgkin disease, and lymphomas are the most common **neoplastic processes** involving the pericardium and have become the most frequent causes of pericardial tamponade in many countries. Pericarditis may occur 2–5 days after infarction due to an inflammatory reaction to transmural myocardial necrosis (**post-MI** or **postcardiotomy pericarditis [Dressler syndrome]**). **Radiation** can initiate a fibrinous and fibrotic process in the pericardium, presenting as subacute pericarditis or constriction. Radiation pericarditis usually follows treatments of more than 4000 cGy delivered to ports including more than 30% of the heart.

Other causes of pericarditis include connective tissue diseases, such as lupus erythematosus and rheumatoid arthritis, drug-induced pericarditis (minoxidil, penicillins, clozapine), and myxedema. In addition, pericarditis may result from pericardial injury from invasive cardiac procedures (such as cardiac pacemaker and defibrillator perforation and intracardiac ablation, especially atrial fibrillation ablation), and the implantation of intracardiac devices (such as ASD occluder devices).

Pericarditis and myocarditis may coexist in 20–30% of patients. Myocarditis is often suspected when there is an elevation of serum troponins, although there are no data that suggest troponin elevations are associated with a poor prognosis.

▶ Clinical Findings

A. Symptoms and Signs

The presentation and course of inflammatory pericarditis depend on its cause, but most syndromes have associated chest pain, which is usually pleuritic and postural (relieved by sitting). The pain is substernal but may radiate to the neck, shoulders, back, or epigastrium. Dyspnea may also be present and the patient is often febrile. A pericardial **friction rub** is characteristic, with or without evidence of fluid accumulation or constriction. The presentation of tuberculous pericarditis tends to be subacute, but nonspecific symptoms (fever, night sweats, fatigue) may be present for days to months. Pericardial involvement develops in 1–8% of patients with pulmonary tuberculosis. Symptoms and signs of bacterial pericarditis are similar to those of other types of inflammatory pericarditides, but patients appear toxic and are often critically ill. Uremic pericarditis can present with or without symptoms; fever is absent. Often neoplastic pericarditis is painless, and the presenting symptoms relate to hemodynamic compromise or the primary disease. At times the pericardial effusion is very large, consistent with its chronic nature. Post-MI or postcardiotomy pericarditis (Dressler syndrome) usually presents as a recurrence of pain with pleural-pericardial features. A rub is often audible, and repolarization changes on the ECG may be confused with ischemia. Large effusions are uncommon, and spontaneous resolution usually occurs in a few days. Dressler syndrome occurs days to weeks to several months after MI or open heart surgery, may be recurrent, and probably represents an autoimmune syndrome. Patients present with typical pain, fever, malaise, and leukocytosis. Rarely, other symptoms of an autoimmune disorder, such as joint pain and fever, may occur. Tamponade is rare with Dressler syndrome after MI but not when it occurs postoperatively. The clinical onset of radiation pericarditis is usually within the first year but may be delayed for many years; often a full decade or more may pass before constriction becomes evident.

B. Laboratory Findings and Diagnostic Studies

The diagnosis of viral pericarditis is usually clinical, and leukocytosis is often present. Rising viral titers in paired sera may be obtained for confirmation but are rarely done. Cardiac enzymes may be slightly elevated, reflecting an epicardial myocarditis component. The echocardiogram is often normal or reveals only a trivial amount of extra fluid during the acute inflammatory process. The diagnosis of tuberculous pericarditis can be inferred if acid-fast bacilli are found elsewhere. The tuberculous pericardial effusions are usually small or moderate but may be large when chronic. The yield of mycobacterial organisms by pericardiocentesis is low; pericardial biopsy has a higher yield but may also be negative, and pericardiectomy may be required. If bacterial pericarditis is suspected on clinical grounds, diagnostic pericardiocentesis can be confirmatory. In uremic patients not on dialysis, the incidence of pericarditis correlates roughly with the level of blood urea nitrogen (BUN) and creatinine. The pericardium is characteristically "shaggy" in uremic pericarditis, and the effusion is hemorrhagic and exudative. The diagnosis of neoplastic pericarditis can occasionally be made by cytologic examination of the effusion or by pericardial biopsy, but it may be difficult to establish clinically if the patient has received mediastinal radiation within the previous year. Neoplastic pericardial effusions develop over a long period of time and may become quite huge (more than 2 L). The sedimentation rate is high in post-MI or post-cardiotomy pericarditis and can help confirm the diagnosis. Large pericardial effusions and accompanying pleural effusions are frequent. Myxedema pericardial effusions due to hypothyroidism usually are characterized by the presence of cholesterol crystals within the fluid.

C. Other Studies

The ECG usually shows generalized ST and T wave changes and may manifest a characteristic progression beginning with diffuse ST elevation, followed by a return to baseline and then to T-wave inversion. Atrial injury is often present and manifested by PR depression, especially in the limb leads. The chest radiograph is frequently normal but may show cardiac enlargement (if pericardial fluid is present), as well as signs of related pulmonary disease. Mass lesions and enlarged lymph nodes may suggest a neoplastic process. About 60% of patients have a pericardial effusion (usually mild) detectable by echocardiography. MRI and CT scan can visualize neighboring tumor in neoplastic pericarditis. A screening chest CT or MRI is often recommended to ensure there are no extracardiac diseases contiguous to the pericardium. A consensus statement from the American Society of Echocardiography proposes adding an elevated CRP and late gadolinium enhancement of the pericardium to confirmatory criteria for the diagnosis of pericarditis. There are data that the degree of quantitative delayed enhancement of the pericardium is associated with a higher rate of recurrent pericarditis. PET scanning can also be used to help define pericardial inflammation.

► Treatment

For acute pericarditis, experts suggest a restriction in activity until symptom resolution. For athletes, the duration of exercise restriction should be until resolution of symptoms and normalization of all laboratory tests (generally 3 months). The 2015 ESC guidelines recommend aspirin 750–1000 mg every 8 hours for 1–2 weeks with a taper by decreasing the dose 250–500 mg every 1–2 weeks or ibuprofen 600 mg every 8 hours for 1–2 weeks with a taper by decreasing the dose by 200–400 mg every 1–2 weeks. Gastroprotection should be included. Studies support initial treatment of the acute episode with colchicine to prevent recurrences. Colchicine should be added to the nonsteroidal anti-inflammatory medication at 0.5–0.6 mg once (for patients less than 70 kg) or twice (for patients more than 70 kg) daily and continued for at least 3 months.

Tapering of colchicine is not mandatory; however, in the last week of treatment, the dosage can be reduced every other day for patients less than 70 kg or once a day for those more than 70 kg. Aspirin and colchicine should be used instead of nonsteroidal anti-inflammatory medications in post-MI pericarditis (Dressler syndrome), since nonsteroidal anti-inflammatory medications and corticosteroids may have an adverse effect on myocardial healing. Aspirin in doses of 750–1000 mg three times daily for 1–2 weeks plus 3 months of colchicine is the recommended treatment for Dressler syndrome. Despite initial treatment, recurrence has been reported in about 30%.

Colchicine should be used for at least 6 months as therapy in all refractory cases and in recurrent pericarditis. At times a longer duration of therapy is required. The CRP is used to assess the effectiveness of treatment, and once it is normalized, tapering is initiated. Indomethacin in doses of 25–50 mg every 8 hours can also be considered in recurrent pericarditis in place of ibuprofen. Systemic corticosteroids can be added in patients with severe symptoms, in refractory cases, or in patients with immune-mediated etiologies, but such therapy may entail a higher risk of recurrence and may actually prolong the illness. Colchicine is recommended in addition to corticosteroids, again for at least 3 months, to help prevent recurrences. Prednisone in doses of 0.25–0.5 mg/kg/day orally is generally suggested with tapering over a 4–6 week period.

As a rule, symptoms subside in several days to weeks. The major early complication is tamponade, which occurs in less than 5% of patients. There may be recurrences in the first few weeks or months. Rarely, when colchicine therapy alone fails or cannot be tolerated (usually do to gastrointestinal symptoms), the pericarditis may require more significant immunosuppression, such as cyclophosphamide, azathioprine, intravenous human immunoglobulins, interleukin-1 receptor antagonists (anakinra), or methotrexate. If colchicine plus more significant immunosuppression fails, surgical pericardial stripping may be considered in recurrent cases even without clinical evidence for constrictive pericarditis.

Standard antituberculous medication therapy is usually successful for tuberculous pericarditis (see Chapter 9), but constrictive pericarditis can occur. Uremic pericarditis usually resolves with the institution of—or with more aggressive—dialysis. Tamponade is fairly common, and partial pericardiectomy (**pericardial window**) may be necessary. Whereas anti-inflammatory agents may relieve the pain and fever associated with uremic pericarditis, indomethacin and systemic corticosteroids do not affect its natural history. The prognosis with neoplastic effusion is poor, with only a small minority surviving 1 year. If it is compromising the clinical comfort of the patient, the effusion is initially drained percutaneously. Attempts at balloon pericardiotomy have been abandoned because outcomes were not more effective than simple drainage. A pericardial window, either by a subxiphoid approach or via video-assisted thoracic surgery, allows for partial pericardiectomy. Instillation of chemotherapeutic agents or tetracycline may be used to reduce the recurrence rate. Symptomatic therapy is the initial approach to radiation pericarditis, but recurrent effusions and constriction often require surgery.

When to Refer

Patients who do not respond initially to conservative management, who have recurrences, or who appear to be developing constrictive pericarditis should be referred to a cardiologist for further assessment.

Adler Y et al. 2015 ESC guidelines for the diagnosis and management of pericardial diseases: The Task Force for the Diagnosis and Management of Pericardial Diseases of the European Society of Cardiology (ESC) endorsed by: the European Association for Cardio-Thoracic Surgery (EACTS). Eur Heart J. 2015 Nov 7;36(42):2921–64. [PMID: 26320112]

Cremer PC et al. Complicated pericarditis: understanding risk factors and pathophysiology to inform imaging and treatment. J Am Coll Cardiol. 2016 Nov 29;68(21):2311–28. [PMID: 27884251]

Doctor NS et al. Acute pericarditis. Prog Cardiovasc Dis. 2017 Jan–Feb;59(4):349–59. [PMID: 27956197]

Imazio M et al. Acute and recurrent pericarditis. Cardiol Clin. 2017 Nov;35(4):505–13. [PMID: 29025542]

Imazio M et al. Evaluation and treatment of pericarditis. A systematic review. JAMA. 2015 Oct 13;314(14):1498–506. [PMID: 26461998]

Kumar A et al. Quantitative pericardial delayed hyperenhancement informs clinical course in recurrent pericarditis. JACC Cardiovasc Imaging. 2017 Nov;10(11):1337–46. [PMID: 28330665]

PERICARDIAL EFFUSION & TAMPONADE

ESSENTIALS OF DIAGNOSIS

Pericardial effusion

▶ Clinical impact determined by the speed of accumulation.

▶ May or may not cause pain.

Tamponade

▶ Tachycardia with an elevated JVP and either hypotension or a paradoxical pulse.

▶ Low voltage or electrical alternans on ECG.

▶ Echocardiography is diagnostic.

Pericardial effusion can develop during any of the acute pericarditis processes. Because the pericardium covers the ascending aorta and arch, aortic dissection and/or rupture can lead to tamponade as well. The *speed of accumulation* determines the physiologic importance of the effusion. Because of pericardial stretch, effusions larger than 1000 mL that develop slowly may produce no hemodynamic effects. Conversely, smaller effusions that appear rapidly can cause tamponade due to the curvilinear relationship between the volume of fluid and the intrapericardial pressure. Tamponade is characterized by elevated intrapericardial pressure (greater than 15 mm Hg), which restricts venous return and ventricular filling. As a result, the stroke volume and arterial pulse pressure fall, and the heart rate and venous pressure rise. Shock and death may result.

Clinical Findings

A. Symptoms and Signs

Pericardial effusions may be associated with pain if they occur as part of an acute inflammatory process or may be painless, as is often the case with neoplastic or uremic effusion. Dyspnea and cough are common, especially with tamponade. Cardiac tamponade can be a life-threatening syndrome evidenced by tachycardia, hypotension, pulsus paradoxicus, raised JVP, muffled heart sounds, and decreased ECG voltage or electrical alternans. Other symptoms may result from the primary disease. The prognosis is a function of the cause. Large idiopathic chronic effusions (over 3 months) have a 30–35% risk of progression to cardiac tamponade.

A pericardial friction rub may be present even with large effusions. In cardiac tamponade, tachycardia, tachypnea, a narrow pulse pressure, and a relatively preserved systolic pressure are characteristic. **Pulsus paradoxus** is defined as a decline of greater than 10 mm Hg in systolic pressure during inspiration. Since the RV and LV share the same pericardium, when there is significant pericardial effusion, as the RV enlarges with inspiratory filling, septal motion toward the LV chamber reduces LV filling and results in an accentuated drop in the stroke volume and systemic BP with inspiration (the paradoxical pulse). Central venous pressure is elevated and, since the intrapericardial, and thus intracardiac, pressures are high even at the initiation of diastole, there is no evident *y* descent in the RA, RV, or LV hemodynamic tracings because the pericardial pressure prevents early ventricular filling. This differs from constriction where most of the initial filling of the RV and LV occurs during early diastole (rapid *y* descent), and it is only in mid to late diastole that the ventricles can no longer fill. In tamponade, ventricular filling is inhibited throughout diastole. Edema or ascites are rarely present in tamponade; these signs favor a more chronic process.

B. Laboratory Findings

Laboratory tests tend to reflect the underlying processes (see causes of pericarditis under General Considerations above).

C. Diagnostic Studies

Chest radiograph can suggest chronic effusion by an enlarged cardiac silhouette with a globular configuration, but may appear normal in acute situations. The ECG often reveals nonspecific T wave changes and reduced QRS voltage. **Electrical alternans** is present only occasionally but is pathognomonic and is believed to be due to the heart swinging within the large effusion. Echocardiography is the primary method for demonstrating pericardial effusion and is quite sensitive. If tamponade is present, the high intrapericardial pressure may collapse lower pressure cardiac structures, such as the RA and RV. Cardiac CT and MRI also demonstrate pericardial fluid, pericardial thickening, and any associated contiguous lesions within the chest. Diagnostic pericardiocentesis or biopsy may be indicated for microbiologic and cytologic studies; a pericardial biopsy may be performed relatively simply through a small subxiphoid incision or by use of a video-assisted thoracoscopic surgical procedure. Unfortunately, the quality of the pericardial fluid itself rarely leads to a diagnosis, and any type of fluid (serous, serosanguinous, bloody, etc) can be seen in most diseases. Pericardial fluid analysis is most useful in excluding a bacterial cause and is occasionally helpful in malignancies. Effusions due to hypothyroidism or lymphatic obstruction may contain cholesterol or be chylous in nature, respectively.

Treatment

Small effusions can be followed clinically by careful observations of the JVP and by testing for a change in the paradoxical pulse. The most common cause of a paradoxical pulse is severe pulmonary disease, especially asthma, where marked changes in intrapleural pressures occur with inspiration and expiration. Serial echocardiograms are indicated if no intervention is immediately contemplated. Vasodilators and diuretics should be avoided. **When tamponade is present, urgent pericardiocentesis or cardiac surgery is required.** Because the pressure–volume relationship in the pericardial fluid is curvilinear and upsloping, removal of even a small amount of fluid often produces a dramatic fall in the intrapericardial pressure and immediate hemodynamic benefit; but complete drainage with a catheter is preferable. Continued or repeat drainage may be indicated, especially in malignant effusions. Pericardial windows via video-assisted thoracoscopy have been particularly effective in preventing recurrences when the underlying cause of the effusion continues to be present and are more effective than needle pericardiocentesis, subxiphoid surgical windows, or percutaneous balloon pericardiotomy. Effusions related to recurrent inflammatory pericarditis can be treated as noted above (see Acute Inflammatory Pericarditis). The presence of pericardial fluid in patients with pulmonary hypertension is a poor prognostic sign.

When to Refer

- Any unexplained pericardial effusion should be referred to a cardiologist.
- Trivial pericardial effusions are common, especially in heart failure, and need not be referred unless symptoms of pericarditis are evident.
- Hypotension or a paradoxical pulse suggesting the pericardial effusion is hemodynamically compromising the patient is a medical emergency and requires immediate drainage.
- Any echocardiographic signs of tamponade.

Adler Y et al. 2015 ESC guidelines for the diagnosis and management of pericardial diseases: the Task Force for the Diagnosis and Management of Pericardial Diseases of the European Society of Cardiology (ESC) endorsed by: the European Association for Cardio-Thoracic Surgery (EACTS). Eur Heart J. 2015 Nov 7;36(42):2921–64. [PMID: 26320112]

Azarbal A et al. Pericardial effusion. Cardiol Clin. 2017 Nov;35(4):515–24. [PMID: 29025543]

Cremer PC et al. Complicated pericarditis: understanding risk factors and pathophysiology to inform imaging and treatment. J Am Coll Cardiol. 2016 Nov 29;68(21):2311–28. [PMID: 27884251]

Horr SE et al. Comparison of outcomes of pericardiocentesis versus surgical pericardial window in patients requiring drainage of pericardial effusions. Am J Cardiol. 2017 Sep 1;120(5):883–90. [PMID: 28739031]

Langdon SE et al. Contemporary outcomes after pericardial window surgery: impact of operative technique. J Cardiothorac Surg. 2016 Apr 26;11(1):73. [PMID: 27118051]

CONSTRICTIVE PERICARDITIS

ESSENTIALS OF DIAGNOSIS

▶ Clinical evidence of right heart failure.

▶ No fall or an elevation of the JVP with inspiration (Kussmaul sign).

▶ Echocardiographic evidence for septal bounce and reduced mitral inflow velocities with inspiration.

▶ At times may be difficult to differentiate from restrictive cardiomyopathy.

▶ Cardiac catheterization may be necessary when clinical and echocardiographic features are equivocal.

General Considerations

Pericardial inflammation can lead to a thickened, fibrotic, adherent pericardium that restricts diastolic filling and produces chronically elevated venous pressures. In the past, tuberculosis was the most common cause of constrictive pericarditis, but while it remains so in underdeveloped countries, it is rare now in the rest of the world. Constrictive pericarditis rarely occurs following recurrent pericarditis. The risk of constrictive pericarditis due to viral or idiopathic pericarditis is less than 1%. Its occurrence increases following immune-mediated or neoplastic pericarditis (2–5%) and is highest after purulent bacterial pericarditis (20–30%). Other causes include post cardiac surgery, radiation therapy, and connective tissue disorders. A small number of cases are drug-induced or secondary to trauma, asbestosis, sarcoidosis, or uremia. At times, both pericardial tamponade and constrictive pericarditis may coexist, a condition referred to as **effusive-constrictive pericarditis**. The only definitive way to diagnose this condition is to reveal the underlying constrictive physiology once the pericardial fluid is drained. The differentiation of constrictive pericarditis from a restrictive cardiomyopathy may require cardiac catheterization and the utilization of all available noninvasive imaging methods.

Clinical Findings

A. Symptoms and Signs

The principal symptoms are slowly progressive dyspnea, fatigue, and weakness. Chronic edema, hepatic congestion, and ascites are usually present. Ascites often seems out of proportion to the degree of peripheral edema. The examination reveals these signs and a characteristically elevated jugular venous pressure with a rapid *y* descent. This can be detected at bedside by careful observation of the jugular pulse and noting an apparent increased pulse wave at the end of ventricular systole (due to the relative accentuation of the *v* wave by the rapid *y* descent). **Kussmaul sign**—a failure of the JVP to fall with inspiration—is also a frequent finding. The apex may actually retract with systole and a pericardial "knock" may be heard in early diastole. Pulsus paradoxus is unusual. Atrial fibrillation is common.

B. Diagnostic Studies

At times, constrictive pericarditis is extremely difficult to differentiate from restrictive cardiomyopathy and the two may coexist. When unclear, the use of both noninvasive testing and cardiac catheterization is required to sort out the difference.

1. Radiographic findings—The chest radiograph may show normal heart size or cardiomegaly. Pericardial calcification is best seen on the lateral view and is uncommon. It rarely involves the LV apex, and finding of calcification at the LV apex is more consistent with LV aneurysm.

2. Echocardiography—Echocardiography rarely demonstrates a thickened pericardium. A septal "bounce" reflecting the rapid early filling is common, though. RV/LV interaction may be demonstrated by an inspiratory reduction in the mitral inflow Doppler pattern of greater than 25%, much as in tamponade. Usually the initial mitral inflow into the LV is very rapid, and this can be demonstrated as well by the Doppler inflow (E wave) pattern. Other echocardiographic features can also help reveal constrictive physiology.

3. Cardiac CT and MRI—These imaging tests are only occasionally helpful. Pericardial thickening of more than 4 mm must be present to establish the diagnosis, but no pericardial thickening is demonstrable in 20–25% of patients with constrictive pericarditis. Some MRI techniques demonstrate the septal bounce and can provide further evidence for ventricular interaction.

4. Cardiac catheterization—This procedure is often confirmatory or can be diagnostic in difficult cases where the echocardiographic features are unclear or mixed. As a generality, the pulmonary pressure is low in constriction (as opposed to restrictive cardiomyopathy). In constrictive pericarditis, because of the need to demonstrate RV/LV interaction, cardiac catheterization should include simultaneous measurement of both the LV and RV pressure tracings with inspiration and expiration. This interaction can be demonstrated by cardiac MRI. Hemodynamically, patients with constriction have equalization of end-diastolic pressures throughout their cardiac chambers, there is rapid early filling then an abrupt increase in diastolic pressure ("square-root" sign), the RV end-diastolic pressure is more than one-third the systolic pressure, simultaneous measurements of RV and LV systolic pressure reveal a discordance with inspiration (the RV rises as the LV falls), and there is usually a Kussmaul sign (failure of the RA pressure to fall with inspiration). In restrictive cardiomyopathy, there is concordance of RV and LV systolic pressures with inspiration.

Treatment

Therapy should be aimed at the specific etiology initially. If there is laboratory evidence of ongoing inflammation, then anti-inflammatory medications may have a role. Once the hemodynamics are evident, the mainstay of treatment is diuresis. As in other disorders of right heart failure, the diuresis should be aggressive, using loop diuretics (oral torsemide or bumetanide if bowel edema is suspected or intravenous furosemide), thiazides, and aldosterone antagonists (especially in the presence of ascites and liver congestion). Surgical pericardiectomy should be recommended when diuretics are unable to control symptoms. Pericardiectomy removes only the pericardium between the phrenic nerve pathways, however, and most patients still require diuretics after the procedure, though symptoms are usually dramatically improved. Morbidity and mortality after pericardiectomy are high (up to 15%) and are greatest in those with the most disability prior to the procedure. Poor prognostic predictors include prior radiation, kidney dysfunction, higher pulmonary systolic pressures, abnormal LV systolic function, a lower serum sodium level, liver dysfunction, and older age. Pericardial calcium has no impact on survival. In a 2017 review by the Mayo Clinic of their 80-year experience with pericardial stripping, they noted the mortality from the procedure had dropped from 13.5% to 5.2% and the identified risk factors for mortality in their contemporary group included worsening heart failure, prior cardiac surgery, radiation, and the need for cardiopulmonary bypass.

▶ When to Refer

If the diagnosis of constrictive pericarditis is unclear or the symptoms of fluid retention resist medical therapy, then referral to a cardiologist is warranted to both establish the diagnosis and recommend therapy.

Adler Y et al. 2015 ESC guidelines for the diagnosis and management of pericardial diseases: the Task Force for the Diagnosis and Management of Pericardial Diseases of the European Society of Cardiology (ESC) endorsed by: the European Association for Cardio-Thoracic Surgery (EACTS). Eur Heart J. 2015 Nov 7;36(42):2921–64. [PMID: 26320112]

Cremer PC et al. Complicated pericarditis: understanding risk factors and pathophysiology to inform imaging and treatment. J Am Coll Cardiol. 2016 Nov 29;68(21):2311–28. [PMID: 27884251]

Geske JB et al. Differentiation of constriction and restriction: complex cardiovascular hemodynamics. J Am Coll Cardiol. 2016 Nov 29;68(21):2329–47. [PMID: 27884252]

Murashita T et al. Experience with pericardiectomy for constrictive pericarditis over eight decades. Ann Thorac Surg. 2017 Sep;104(3):742–50. [PMID: 28760468]

PULMONARY HYPERTENSION

ESSENTIALS OF DIAGNOSIS

▶ Mean PA pressure of 25 mm Hg or more.

▶ Dyspnea and often cyanosis.

▶ Enlarged pulmonary arteries on chest radiograph.

▶ Elevated JVP and RV heave.

▶ Echocardiography is often diagnostic.

General Considerations

The normal pulmonary bed offers about one-tenth as much resistance to blood flow as the systemic arterial system. Experts recommend that a diagnosis of idiopathic pulmonary hypertension should be firmly based on a **mean PA pressure of 25 mm Hg or more in association with a PCWP of less than 16 mm Hg at rest**.

The clinical classification of pulmonary hypertension by the Fourth World Symposium on Pulmonary Hypertension is outlined in Table 10–20. It is a complex disorder due to multiple causes.

Group I includes pulmonary arterial hypertension (PAH) related to an underlying pulmonary vasculopathy. It includes the former "primary" pulmonary hypertension

Table 10–20. Clinical classification of pulmonary hypertension.

I. Pulmonary arterial hypertension from pulmonary vasculopathy
Idiopathic pulmonary arterial hypertension
Heritable gene mutations
BMPR2 (bone morphogenic protein receptor type 2)
ALK1 (activin A receptor type II-like kinase-1), *endoglin* (with or without hereditary hemorrhagic telangiectasia)
Unknown
Drug and toxin-induced
Associated with
Connective tissue diseases
HIV infection
Portal hypertension
Congenital heart disease
Schistosomiasis
Chronic hemolytic anemia
Persistent pulmonary hypertension of the newborn
Pulmonary veno-occlusive disease and/or pulmonary capillary hemangiomatosis
II. Pulmonary hypertension due to left heart disease
Systolic dysfunction
Diastolic dysfunction
III. Pulmonary hypertension due to lung disease and/or hypoxia
Chronic obstructive pulmonary disease
Interstitial lung disease
Other pulmonary disease with mixed restrictive and obstructive pattern
IV. Chronic thromboembolic pulmonary hypertension
V. Pulmonary hypertension with unclear multifactorial mechanisms
Hematologic disorders: myeloproliferative disorders, splenectomy
Systemic disorders: sarcoidosis, pulmonary Langerhans cell histiocytosis: lymphangioleimyomatosis, neurofibromatosis, vasculitis
Metabolic disorders: glycogen storage disease, Gaucher disease, thyroid disorders
Others: tumoral obstruction, fibrosing mediastinitis, chronic renal failure on dialysis

Data from Simonneau G et al. Updated clinical classification of pulmonary hypertension. J Am Coll Cardiol. 2009 Jun 30;54(1 Suppl):S43–54.

under the term "idiopathic pulmonary hypertension" and is defined as pulmonary hypertension and elevated PVR in the absence of other disease of the lungs or heart. Its cause is unknown. About 6–10% have heritable PAH. Drug and toxic pulmonary hypertension have been described as associated with the use of anorexigenic agents that increase serotonin release and block its uptake. These include aminorex fumarate, fenfluramine, and dexfenfluramine. In some cases, there is epidemiologic linkage to ingestion of rapeseed oil or L-tryptophan and use of recreational drugs, such as amphetamines. Pulmonary hypertension associated with connective tissue disease includes cases associated with scleroderma—up to 8–12% of patients with scleroderma may be affected. Pulmonary hypertension has also been associated with HIV infection, portal hypertension, congenital heart disease (Eisenmenger syndrome), schistosomiasis, and chronic hemolytic anemia (eg, sickle cell anemia). In rare instances, obstruction of the pulmonary venous circulation may occur (pulmonary veno-occlusive disease and capillary hemangiomatosis).

Group II includes all cases related to left heart disease. **Group III** includes cases due to parenchymal lung disease, impaired control of breathing, or living at high altitude. This group encompasses those with idiopathic pulmonary fibrosis and COPD. **Group IV** represents patients with chronic thromboemboli. **Group V** includes multifactorial cases.

Clinical Findings

A. Symptoms and Signs

Common to all is exertional dyspnea, chest pain, fatigue, and lightheadedness as early symptoms; later symptoms include syncope, abdominal distention, ascites, and peripheral edema as RV function worsens. Chronic lung disease, especially sleep apnea, often is overlooked as a cause for pulmonary hypertension as is chronic thromboembolic disease. Patients with idiopathic pulmonary hypertension are characteristically young women who have evidence of right heart failure that is usually progressive, leading to death in 2–8 years without therapy. This is a decidedly different prognosis than patients with Eisenmenger physiology due to a left-to-right shunt; 40% of patients with Eisenmenger physiology are alive 25 years after the diagnosis has been made. Patients have manifestations of low cardiac output, with weakness and fatigue, as well as edema and ascites as right heart failure advances. Peripheral cyanosis is present, and syncope on effort may occur.

B. Diagnostic Studies

The European Society of Cardiology and European Respiratory Society updated guidelines for the diagnosis and treatment of pulmonary hypertension in 2015 (published in 2016). All patients with a high risk for PAH should undergo confirmatory right heart catheterization.

The laboratory evaluation of idiopathic pulmonary hypertension must exclude a secondary cause. A hypercoagulable state should be sought by measuring protein C and S levels, the presence of a lupus anticoagulant, the level of factor V Leiden, prothrombin gene mutations, and D-dimer. Chronic pulmonary emboli must be excluded (usually by ventilation-perfusion lung scan or contrast spiral CT); the ventilation-perfusion scan is the more sensitive test but not specific. If it is normal, then chronic thromboembolic pulmonary hypertension is very unlikely. The chest radiograph helps exclude a primary pulmonary etiology—evidence for patchy pulmonary edema may raise the suspicion of pulmonary veno-occlusive disease due to localized obstruction in pulmonary venous drainage. A sleep study may be warranted if sleep apnea is suspected. The ECG is generally consistent with RVH and RA enlargement. Echocardiography with Doppler helps exclude an intracardiac shunt and usually demonstrates an enlarged RV and RA—at times they may be huge and hypocontractile. Severe pulmonic or tricuspid valve regurgitation may be present. Interventricular septal flattening seen on the echocardiogram is consistent with pulmonary hypertension. Doppler interrogation of the tricuspid regurgitation jet provides an estimate of RV systolic pressure. Pulmonary function tests help exclude other disorders, though primary pulmonary hypertension may present with only a reduced carbon monoxide diffusing capacity of the lung (DL_{CO}) or severe desaturation (particularly if a PFO has been stretched open and a right-to-left shunt is present). A declining DL_{CO} in a scleroderma patient may precede the development of pulmonary hypertension. Chest CT demonstrates enlarged pulmonary arteries and excludes other causes (such as emphysema or interstitial lung disease). Pulmonary angiography (or magnetic resonance angiography or CT angiography) reveals loss of the smaller acinar pulmonary vessels and tapering of the larger ones. Catheterization allows measurement of pulmonary pressures and testing for vasoreactivity using a variety of agents, but nitric oxide is the preferred testing agent due to its ease of use and short half-life. A positive response is defined as one that decreases the pulmonary mean pressure by greater than 10 mm Hg, with the final mean PA pressure less than 40 mm Hg. Abdominal ultrasound is recommended to exclude portal hypertension. A lung biopsy is no longer suggested as relevant for the diagnosis.

Treatment & Prognosis

The treatment of PAH continues to evolve and depends on the etiology. For group I patients with a normal PCWP, treatment is related to the response to nitric oxide challenge with those responsive being initially treated with calcium channel blockers. The vast majority of patients, unfortunately, do not respond to the acute vasoreactivity testing. Specific PAH therapy is therefore recommended in this situation. This begins with monotherapy but expands to the use of sequential medication therapy when pulmonary pressures are not improved. In critically ill hypotensive patients inotropic support may be required and eventually lung transplantation considered. Balloon atrial septostomy is considered a IIb recommendation (on the notion that increased right to left shunting will improve cardiac output), but it is very rarely utilized.

Medication monotherapy varies in effectiveness depending on the etiologic classification. Only those in class I who respond to nitric oxide should get calcium channel blockers. The current medication therapies include endothelin-receptor blockers (ambrisentan, bosentan, macitentan),

phosphodiesterase type-5 inhibitors (sildenafil, tadalafil, and vardenafil), a guanylate cyclase stimulator (riociguat), prostanoids (epoprostenol, iloprost, treprostinil, and beraprost), and an IP-receptor agonist (selexipag). Various medication combinations have been approved and, when ineffective, sequential medication therapies may be used. Many medications interfere with HIV treatment, and this needs to be assessed if relevant. Due to inherent lung disease or left heart disease, there are no therapies that are specific to PAH. Bosentan, an endothelin receptor blocker, has received a class I indication for patients with Eisenmenger syndrome. Anticoagulation is often recommended and is required lifelong in chronic thromboembolic pulmonary hypertension; it should not be used if portal hypertension is present. There is an interest in the percutaneous treatment of inoperable chronic thromboembolic PAH with some data revealing the clinical feasibility of balloon pulmonary angioplasty. Riociguat remains the only approved medical therapy for chronic thromboembolic pulmonary hypertension patients deemed inoperable.

Counseling and patient education are also important. Aerobic exercise is recommended but no heavy physical exertion or isometric exercise. Routine immunizations are advised. Pregancy should be strongly discouraged and preventive measures taken to ensure it does not occur. Maternal mortality in severe PAH may be up to 50%.

Warfarin anticoagulation is recommended in all patients with idiopathic PAH and no contraindication. Diuretics are useful for the management of right-sided heart failure; clinical experience suggests loop diuretics (torsemide or butmetanide, which are absorbed even if bowel edema is present) plus spironolactone are preferable. Oxygen should be used to maintain oxygen saturation greater than 90%. Acute vasodilator testing (generally with nitric oxide) should be performed in all patients with idiopathic PAH who may be potential candidates for long-term therapy with calcium channel blockers. Patients with PAH caused by conditions other than idiopathic PAH respond poorly to oral calcium channel blockers, and there is little value of acute vasodilator testing in these patients.

When to Refer

All patients with suspected pulmonary hypertension should be referred to either a cardiologist or pulmonologist who specializes in pulmonary hypertension.

Galiè N et al. 2015 ESC/ERS guidelines for the diagnosis and treatment of pulmonary hypertension: the Joint Task Force for the Diagnosis and Treatment of Pulmonary Hypertension of the European Society of Cardiology (ESC) and the European Respiratory Society (ERS). Eur Heart J. 2016 Jan 1;37(1):67–119. [PMID: 26320113]

Liu HL et al. Efficacy and safety of pulmonary arterial hypertension-specific therapy in pulmonary arterial hypertension: a meta-analysis of randomized controlled trials. Chest. 2016 Aug;150(2):353–66. [PMID: 27048870]

Mahmud E et al. Chronic thromboembolic pulmonary hypertension: evolving therapeutic approaches for operable and inoperable disease. J Am Coll Cardiol. 2018 May 29; 71(21):2468–86. [PMID: 29793636]

Thenappan T et al. Pulmonary arterial hypertension: pathogenesis and clinical management. BMJ. 2018 Mar 14;360:j5492. [PMID: 29540357]

NEOPLASTIC DISEASES OF THE HEART

PRIMARY CARDIAC TUMORS

Primary cardiac tumors are rare and constitute only a small fraction of all tumors that involve the heart or pericardium. The most common primary tumor is **atrial myxoma**; it comprises about 50% of all tumors in adult case series. It is generally attached to the atrial septum and is more likely grow on the LA side of the septum rather than the RA. Patients with myxoma can rarely present with the characteristics of a systemic illness, with obstruction of blood flow at the mitral valve level or with signs of peripheral embolization. The syndrome includes fever, malaise, weight loss, leukocytosis, elevated sedimentation rate, and emboli (peripheral or pulmonary, depending on the location of the tumor). This is sometimes confused with infective endocarditis, lymphoma, other cancers, or autoimmune diseases. In other cases, the tumor may grow to considerable size and produce symptoms by simply obstructing mitral inflow. Episodic pulmonary edema (classically occurring when an upright posture is assumed) and signs of low output may result. Physical examination may reveal a diastolic sound related to motion of the tumor ("tumor plop") or a diastolic murmur similar to that of mitral stenosis. Right-sided myxomas may cause symptoms of right-sided failure. Familial myxomas occur as part of the Carney complex, which consists of myxomas, pigmented skin lesions, and endocrine neoplasia.

The diagnosis of atrial myxoma is established by echocardiography or by pathologic study of embolic material. Cardiac MRI is useful as an adjunct. Contrast angiography is frequently unnecessary, although it may demonstrate a "tumor blush" when the mass is vascular. Surgical excision is usually curative, though recurrences do occur and serial echocardiographic follow-up is recommended.

The second most common primary cardiac tumors are **valvular papillary fibroelastomas** and **atrial septal lipomas.** These tend to be benign and usually require no therapy, although large papillary fibroelastomas may embolize or cause valvular dysfunction and should be removed if large and mobile. Other primary cardiac tumors include rhabdomyomas (that often appear multiple in both the RV and LV), fibrous histiocytomas, hemangiomas, and a variety of unusual sarcomas. Some sarcomas may be of considerable size before discovery. Primary pericardial tumors, such as mesotheliomas related to asbestos exposure, may also occur. The diagnosis may be supported by an abnormal cardiac contour on radiograph. Echocardiography is usually helpful but may miss tumors infiltrating the ventricular wall. Cardiac MRI is the diagnostic procedure of choice along with gated CT imaging for all cardiac tumors.

SECONDARY CARDIAC TUMORS

Metastases from malignant tumors can also affect the heart. Most often this occurs in malignant melanoma, but other tumors that are known to metastasize to the heart include bronchogenic carcinoma; carcinoma of the breast; lymphoma; renal cell carcinoma; sarcomas; and, in patients with AIDS, Kaposi sarcoma. These are often clinically silent but may lead to pericardial tamponade, arrhythmias and conduction disturbances, heart failure, and peripheral emboli. The ECG may reveal regional Q waves. The diagnosis is often made by echocardiography, but cardiac MRI and CT scanning can often better delineate the extent of involvement. Metastatic tumors, especially lung or breast, may invade the pericardium and result in very large pericardial effusions as they result in slow accumulation of fluid. The prognosis is poor for all secondary cardiac tumors and treatment is generally palliative. On occasion, surgical resection for debulking or removal and chemotherapy may be effective in relieving symptoms.

▶ Treatment

Many primary tumors may be resectable. Atrial myxomas should be removed surgically due to the high incidence of embolization from these friable tumors. Recurrences require lifelong monitoring with echocardiography. Papillary fibroelastomas are usually benign but they should be removed if they appear mobile and are larger than 10 mm in size or if there is evidence of embolization at the time of discovery. Large pericardial effusions from metastatic tumors may be drained for comfort, but the fluid invariably recurs. Rhabdomyomas may be surgically cured if the tumor is accessible and can be removed while still leaving enough functioning myocardium intact.

▶ When to Refer

All patients with suspected cardiac tumors should be referred to a cardiologist or cardiac surgeon for evaluation and possible therapy.

Lichtenberger JP 3rd et al. MR imaging of cardiac masses. Top Magn Reson Imaging. 2018 Apr;27(2):103–11. [PMID: 29613965]
Taguchi S. Comprehensive review of the epidemiology and treatments for malignant adult cardiac tumors. Gen Thorac Cardiovasc Surg. 2018 May;66(5):257–62. [PMID: 29594875]
Wang Y et al. Surgical treatment of primary cardiac valve tumor: early and late results in eight patients. J Cardiothorac Surg. 2016 Feb 19;11:31. [PMID: 26891966]

TRAUMATIC HEART DISEASE

Trauma is the leading cause of death in patients aged 1–44 years; cardiac and vascular trauma is second only to neurologic injury as the reason for these deaths. Penetrating wounds to the heart are often lethal unless surgically repaired. In a 20-year review of penetrating trauma at a single institution, it was found that gunshot wounds were fatal 13 times more often than stab wounds and that factors such as hypotension, Glasgow Coma Score less than 8, Revised Trauma Score less than 7.84, associated injuries, and the more severe the injuries (Injury Severity Score greater than 25) all added to the mortality and morbidity risk.

Blunt trauma is a more frequent cause of cardiac injuries. This type of injury is common in motor vehicle accidents and may occur with any form of chest trauma, including CPR efforts. The most common injuries are myocardial contusions or hematomas. Other forms of nonischemic cardiac injury include metabolic injury due to burns, electrical current, or sepsis. These may be asymptomatic (particularly in the setting of more severe injuries) or may present with chest pain of a nonspecific nature or, not uncommonly, with a pericardial component. Elevations of cardiac enzymes are frequent but the levels do not correlate with prognosis. There are some data that the presence of certain other cardiac biomarkers, such as NT-proBNP, correlate better with significant myocardial injury. Echocardiography may reveal an akinetic segment or pericardial effusion. Cardiac MRI may also suggest acute injury. Coronary CT angiography or angiography can reveal a coronary dissection or acute occlusion if that is a concern. Pericardiocentesis is warranted if tamponade is evident. As noted above, tako-tsubo transient segmental myocardial dysfunction can occur due to the accompanying stress.

Severe trauma may also cause myocardial or valvular rupture. Cardiac rupture can involve any chamber, but survival is most likely if injury is to one of the atria or the RV. Hemopericardium or pericardial tamponade is the usual clinical presentation, and surgery is almost always necessary. Mitral and aortic valve rupture may occur during severe blunt trauma—the former presumably if the impact occurs during systole and the latter if during diastole. Patients reach the hospital in shock or severe heart failure. Immediate surgical repair is essential. The same types of injuries may result in transection of the aorta, either at the level of the arch or distal to the takeoff of the left subclavian artery at the ligmentum arteriosum. Transthoracic echocardiography and TEE are the most helpful and immediately available diagnostic techniques. CT and MRI may also be required to better define the injury before surgical intervention.

Blunt trauma may also result in damage to the coronary arteries. Acute or subacute coronary thrombosis is the most common presentation. The clinical syndrome is one of acute MI with attendant ECG, enzymatic, and contractile abnormalities. Emergent revascularization is sometimes feasible, either by the percutaneous route or by coronary artery bypass surgery. LV aneurysms are common outcomes of traumatic coronary occlusions, likely due to sudden occlusion with no collateral vascular support. Coronary artery dissection or rupture may also occur in the setting of blunt cardiac trauma.

As expected, patients with severe preexisting conditions fare the least well after cardiac trauma. Data from ReCONECT, a trauma consortium, reveal that mortality is linked to volume of cases seen at various centers, preexisting coronary disease or heart failure, intubation, age, and a severity scoring index.

Bellister SA et al. Blunt and penetrating cardiac trauma. Surg Clin North Am. 2017 Oct;97(5):1065–76. [PMID: 28958358]

Gosavi S et al. Cardiac trauma. Angiology. 2016;67(10):896–901. [PMID: 26802100]

Huis In't Veld MA et al. Blunt cardiac trauma review. Cardiol Clin. 2018 Feb;36(1):183–91. [PMID: 29173678]

Schellenberg M et al. Critical decisions in the management of thoracic trauma. Emerg Med Clin North Am. 2018 Feb;36(1):135–47. [PMID: 29132573]

Soto JR et al. Penetrating cardiac injuries at a Level II trauma center: a 15-year review. Am Surg. 2015 Mar;81(3):324–5. [PMID: 25760212]

HEART DISEASE & PREGNANCY

General principles to discuss with the patient include preconceptual counseling, pregnancy risk assessment, genetic risks, environmental risks, and pregnancy management. For some patients, it may also include a discussion regarding contraception, termination of a pregnancy, and a conversation about not only the delivery but what will happen post-pregnancy (including issues such as an eventual need for heart surgery or transplantation).

The **Cardiac Disease in Pregnancy Investigation (CARPREG I)** scoring system for risk from cardiac events for women with heart disease noted four major risk factors: (1) NYHA FC III or IV heart failure, (2) prior cardiac events, (3) mitral or aortic obstruction, and (4) LVEF less than 40%. One point is assigned to each. Patients with no points had a 5% risk, those with 1 point had a complication rate of 27%, while for those with 2 or more points, the risk was 74%. Other reviews have suggested that the major risk for adverse outcomes or death to either the mother or fetus include pulmonary hypertension (with pulmonary pressure greater than three-quarters of systemic pressure), maternal cyanosis, systemic ventricular dysfunction, poor maternal functional class, severe left-sided valvular obstruction, aortic coarctation, significantly dilated aortic root, significant unrepaired heart defects, and warfarin therapy in patients with mechanical valves. In 2018, this group reported the results from a follow-up study (CARPREG II). Cardiac complications occurred in 16% of pregnancies and were primarily related to arrhythmias and heart failure. Although the overall rates of cardiac complications during pregnancy did not change over the years, the frequency of pulmonary edema decreased (8% from 1994 to 2001 vs. 4% from 2001 to 2014). Ten predictors of maternal cardiac complications were identified: five general predictors (prior cardiac events or arrhythmias, poor functional class or cyanosis, high-risk valve disease/LV outflow tract obstruction, systemic ventricular dysfunction, no prior cardiac interventions); four lesion-specific predictors (mechanical valves, high-risk aortopathies, pulmonary hypertension, CAD); and one delivery of care predictor (late pregnancy assessment). These 10 predictors were incorporated into a new risk index **(CARPREG II)** shown in Figure 10–10.

In 2011, the World Health Organization outlined guidelines for the management of pregnancy in patients with congenital heart disease. This guideline also outlines risks to the fetus. Table 10–21 summarizes the observations and recommendations. Medication usage during pregnancy is always a difficult decision, since most have not been studied. ACE inhibitors and amiodarone are contraindicated. Beta-blockers (including labetalol, metoprolol, and sotalol), digoxin, and calcium channel blockers are generally well tolerated (especially nifedipine, amlodipine, or verapamil, although there is controversy with diltiazem). There are concerns about the use of atenolol and premature birth, and it should not be used. Labetalol has been found to be particularly useful for treating hypertension as has methyldopa. Diuretics can generally be given safely. Pregnancy is a hypercoagulant state; the use of warfarin is discussed above under valvular disease, but fundamentally the risk is

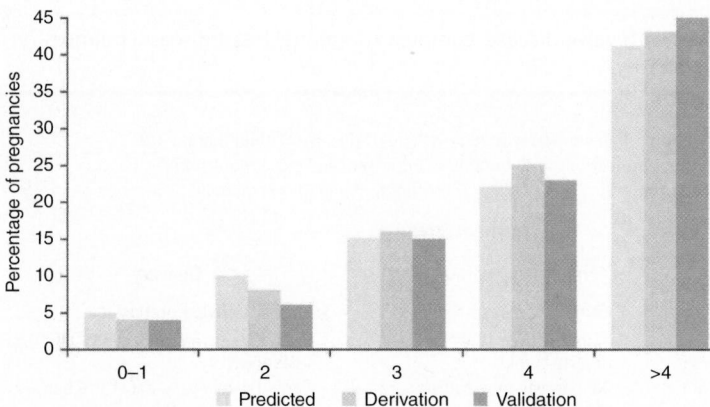

PREDICTOR	POINTS
Prior cardiac events or arrhythmias	3
Baseline NYHA III-IV or cyanosis	3
Mechanical valve	3
Ventricular dysfunction	2
High-risk left-sided valve disease/ left ventricular outflow tract obstruction	2
Pulmonary hypertension	2
Coronary artery disease	2
High-risk aortopathy	2
No prior cardiac intervention	1
Late pregnancy assessment	1

▲ **Figure 10–10.** Risk index for material cardiac complications in pregnancy (CARPREG II). The risk index is divided into five categories based on the sum of the points for a given pregnancy: 0 to 1 point; 2 points; 3 points; 4 points; and > 4 points. The predicted risks for primary cardiac events stratified according to point score were 0 to 1 point (5%), 2 points (10%), 3 points (15%), 4 points (22%), and > 4 points (41%). (Modified, with permission, from Silversides CK et al. Pregnancy outcomes in women with heart disease: the CARPREG II Study. J Am Coll Cardiol. 2018 May 29;71(21):2419–30. Copyright © 2018 by the American College of Cardiology Foundation. Published by Elsevier.)

dose related (not INR related) and can be used during the first trimester if the dose is 5 mg or less. For many patients, the most common potential complication is an atrial arrhythmia or systemic hypertension (systemic blood pressure greater than 140/90 mm Hg). Patients should be hospitalized if blood pressure exceeds 170/110 mm Hg.

Elkayam U et al. High-risk cardiac disease in pregnancy: part I. J Am Coll Cardiol. 2016 Jul 26;68(4):396–410. [PMID: 27443437]
Elkayam U et al. High-risk cardiac disease in pregnancy: part II. J Am Coll Cardiol. 2016 Aug 2;68(5):502–16. [PMID: 27443948]
Silversides CK et al. Pregnancy outcomes in women with heart disease: the CARPREG II study. J Am Coll Cardiol. 2018 May 29;71(21):2419–30. [PMID: 29793631]

CARDIOVASCULAR COMPLICATIONS OF PREGNANCY

Pregnancy-related hypertension (eclampsia and preeclampsia) is discussed in Chapter 19.

1. Cardiomyopathy of Pregnancy (Peripartum Cardiomyopathy)

In approximately 1 in 3000 to 4000 live births, dilated cardiomyopathy develops in the mother in the final month of pregnancy or within 6 months after delivery. Risk factors include preeclampsia, twin pregnancies, and African ethnicity. The cause is slowly being elucidated. A review from 2016 suggests a vasculo-hormonal hypothesis that requires two events. One is genetic, a reduction in a STAT3 transcription factor that results in cleavage of prolactin from the pituitary by cathepsin D. This results in a 16-kd fragment that increases microRNA 146a that results in myocardial apoptosis. The second is from the placenta, soluble tyrosine kinase that blocks VEGF (vascular endothelial growth factor). It appears both components may be necessary to effectively result in peripartum cardiomyopathy. The course of the disease is variable; most cases improve or resolve completely over several months, but others progress to refractory heart failure. About 60% of patients make a complete recovery. Serum BNP levels are routinely elevated in pregnancy, but serial values may be useful in predicting who may be at increased risk for a worse outcome. Beta-blockers have been administered judiciously to these patients, with at least anecdotal success. Diuretics, hydralazine, and nitrates help treat the heart failure with minimal risk to the fetus. Sotalol is acceptable for ventricular or atrial arrhythmias if other beta-blockers are ineffective. Some experts advocate anticoagulation because of an increased risk of thrombotic events, and both warfarin and heparin have their proponents. In severe cases, transient use of extracorporeal oxygenation (ECMO) has been lifesaving. Recurrence in subsequent pregnancies is common, particularly if cardiac function has not completely recovered, and subsequent pregnancies are to be discouraged if the EF remains less than 55%. The risk of recurrent heart failure in a subsequent pregnancy has been estimated to be about 1 in 5 (21%). Delivery of the baby is important, though the peak incidence of the problem is in the first week after delivery and a few cases appear up to 5 weeks after delivery. Since the anti-angiogenic cleaved prolactin fragment is considered causal for peripartum cardiomyopathy, bromocriptine (a prolactin release inhibitor) has been reported to be beneficial. A multicenter trial in Europe found LVEF improved to a greater extent in patients with peripartum cardiomyopathy who were given bromocriptine than those who were not given bromocriptine. In addition, bromocriptine treatment was associated with high rate of full LV recovery and low morbidity and mortality in peripartum cardiomyopathy patients compared with other peripartum cardiomyopathy cohorts not treated with bromocriptine. No significant differences were observed.

Arany Z et al. Peripartum cardiomyopathy. Circulation. 2016 Apr 5;133(14):1397–409. [PMID: 27045128]

Table 10–21. Management strategies for women with valve disease, complex congenital heart disease, pulmonary hypertension, aortopathy, and dilated cardiomyopathy.

High-Risk Heart Disease in Pregnancy
- Preconception counseling and pregnancy risk stratification for all women with high-risk heart disease of childbearing age
- In women considering pregnancy: Switch to safer cardiac medications and emphasize importance of close monitoring
- In women avoiding pregnancy: Discuss safe and effective contraception choices or termination in early pregnancy

Disease	Management Strategy		
	Pregnancy Not Advised	Pregnancy Management	Delivery
Valve disease	• Severe mitral and aortic valve disease • Mechanical prosthetic valves if effective anticoagulation not possible	• Close follow-up • Drug therapy for heart failure or arrhythmias • Balloon valvuloplasty or surgical valve replacement in refractory cases	• Vaginal delivery preferred • C-section in case of fetal or maternal instability • Early delivery for clinical and hemodynamic deterioration • Consider hemodynamic monitoring during labor and delivery
Complex congenital heart disease	• Significant ventricular dysfunction • Severe AV valve dysfunction • Falling Fontan circulation • Oxygen saturation < 85%	• Close follow-up	• Vaginal delivery preferred • C-section in case of fetal or maternal instability • Consider hemodynamic monitoring during labor and delivery
Pulmonary hypertension	• Established pulmonary arterial hypertension	• Close follow-up • Early institution of pulmonary vasodilators	• Vaginal delivery preferred • C-section in case of fetal or maternal instability • Timing of delivery depends on clinical and RV function • Early delivery advisable • Diuresis after delivery to prevent RV volume overload • Extended hospital stay after delivery

Aortopathy	*For some women—*
	• Marfan syndrome
	• Bicuspid aortic valve
	• Turner syndrome
	• Rapid growth of aortic diameter or family history of premature aortic dissection
		• Treat hypertension
		• Beta-blockers to reduce heart rate
		• Frequent echocardiographic assessment
		• Surgery during pregnancy or after C-section if large increase in aortic diameter
			• C-section in cases of significant aortic dilation
			  – Marfan syndrome > 40 mm
			  – Bicuspid aortic valve > 45 mm
			  – Turner syndrome: aortic size index > 20 mm/m²

Dilated cardiomyopathy	• LVEF < 40% • History of peripartum cardiomyopathy	• Close follow-up • Beta-blockers • Diuretic agents for volume overload • Vasodilators for hemodynamic and symptomatic improvement	• Vaginal delivery preferred • C-section in case of fetal or maternal instability • Consider hemodynamic monitoring during labor and delivery • Early delivery for clinical and hemodynamic deterioration

AV, atrioventricular; C-section, caesarean section; LV, left ventricular; LVEF, left ventricular ejection fraction; RV, right ventricular.

Modified, with permission, from Elkayam U et al. High-risk cardiac disease in pregnancy: Part I. J Am Coll Cardiol. 2016 Jul 26;68(4):396–410 © 2016 by the American College of Cardiology Foundation.

Hilfiker-Kleiner D et al. Bromocriptine for the treatment of peripartum cardiomyopathy: a multicentre randomized study. Eur Heart J. 2017 Sep 14;38(35):2671–9. [PMID: 28934837]

Sliwa K et al. Clinical characteristics of patients from the worldwide registry on peripartum cardiomyopathy (PPCM): EURObservational Research Programme in conjunction with the Heart Failure Association of the European Society of Cardiology Study Group on PPCM. Eur J Heart Fail. 2017 Sep;19(9):1131–41. [PMID: 28271625]

Sliwa K et al. Outcome of subsequent pregnancies in patients with a history of post-partum cardiomyopathy. Eur J Heart Fail. 2017;19:1131–41. [PMID: 28271625]

2. Coronary Artery & Aortic Vascular Abnormalities During Pregnancy

There have been a number of reports of MI during pregnancy. It is known that pregnancy predisposes to dissection of the aorta and other arteries, perhaps because of the accompanying connective tissue changes. The risk may be particularly high in patients with Marfan, Ehlers-Danlos, or Loeys-Dietz syndromes. In a review from 2015, the risk is highest in the third trimester, and coronary dissection, thrombosis, and atherosclerosis had about equal prevalence. The very highest cause was dissection overall, and it has a peak incidence in the early postpartum period. Paradoxical emboli through a PFO have been implicated in a few instances. Clinical management is essentially similar to that of other patients with acute infarction, unless there is a connective tissue disorder. If nonatherosclerotic dissection is present, coronary intervention may be risky, as further dissection can be aggravated. In most instances, conservative management is warranted. At times, extensive aortic dissection requires surgical intervention. The 2011 European guidelines suggest Marfan patients are particularly susceptible to further aortic expansion during pregnancy when the aortic diameter is more than 4.5 cm (greater or equal to 27 mm/m^2) and pregnancy be discouraged in these situations. Some data, however, suggest that there is an increased risk of dissection during pregnancy even when the aortic root is at 4.0 cm, since pregnancy appears to have a small, but significant, influence on aortic growth even at this size. The earlier 2010 ACC/AHA/AATS guidelines suggest elective repair is reasonable when the aortic root is greater than 4.0 cm in women with Marfan syndrome contemplating pregnancy; as the review notes, half of women with Marfan syndrome and this large of an aorta will need surgery since they are at risk for rupture or life-threatening aortic root growth during pregnancy.

Acute infarction during pregnancy is associated with an 8% maternal mortality and 56% incidence of premature delivery. If PCI is required, it is recommended that a bare metal stent be used to minimize antiplatelet usage. There are data that clopidogrel is safe, but ticagrelor, prasugrel, bivalirudin, and glycoprotein IIb/IIIa inhibitors should not be used. Statins are contraindicated in pregnancy.

Elkayam U et al. High-risk cardiac disease in pregnancy: part I. J Am Coll Cardiol. 2016 Jul 26;68(4):396–410. [PMID: 27443437]

Elkayam U et al. High-risk cardiac disease in pregnancy: part II. J Am Coll Cardiol. 2016 Aug 2;68(5):502–16. [PMID: 27443948]

Lameijer H et al. Ischaemic heart disease during pregnancy or post-partum: systematic review and case series. Neth Heart J. 2015 May;23(5):249–57. [PMID: 25911007]

Stout KK et al. 2018 AHA/ACC guideline for the management of adults with congenital heart disease: a report of the American College of Cardiology/American Heart Association Task Force on Clinical Practice Guidelines. J Am Coll Cardiol. 2019 Apr 2;73(12):e81–e192. [PMID: 30121239]

Tweet MS et al. Spontaneous coronary artery dissection associated with pregnancy. J Am Coll Cardiol. 2017 Jul 25;70(4): 426–35. [PMID: 28728686]

3. Management of Labor

Although vaginal delivery is usually well tolerated, unstable patients (including patients with severe hypertension and worsening heart failure) should have planned cesarean section. Spinal anesthesia results in a large drop in the systemic vascular resistant and can worsen right-to-left shunting. An increased risk of aortic rupture has been noted during delivery in patients with coarctation of the aorta and severe aortic root dilation with Marfan syndrome, and vaginal delivery should be avoided in these patients. For most patients, even those with complex congenital heart disease, vaginal delivery is the preferred method however.

Following delivery, there are numerous fluid shifts that occur with the initial blood-reducing preload accompanied by the loss of the afterload reduction provided by the placenta. Venous return increases as the uterus is no longer compressing the inferior vena cava and there is an infusion of fluid into the vascular system as the uterus quickly shrinks back toward its normal size. The sudden increase in preload and loss of afterload following delivery can result in heart failure during the first 48–72 hours after the delivery and that remains the high-risk time for susceptible patients.

CARDIOVASCULAR SCREENING OF ATHLETES

The sudden death of a competitive athlete inevitably becomes an occasion for local, if not national, publicity. On each occasion, the public and the medical community ask whether such events could be prevented by more careful or complete screening. Although each event is tragic, it must be appreciated that there are approximately 5 million competitive athletes at the high school level or above in any given year in the United States. The number of cardiac deaths occurring during athletic participation is unknown, but estimates at the high school level range from one in 100,000 to one in 300,000 participants. Death rates among more mature athletes increase as the prevalence of CAD rises. These numbers highlight the problem of how best to screen individual participants. Even an inexpensive test such as an ECG would generate an enormous cost if required of all athletes, and it is likely that only a few at-risk individuals would be detected. Echocardiography, either as a routine test or as a follow-up examination for abnormal ECGs, would be prohibitively expensive except for the elite professional athlete. Thus, the most feasible approach is that of a careful medical history and cardiac examination performed by personnel aware of the conditions responsible for most sudden deaths in competitive athletes.

It is important to point out that sudden death is much more common in the older than the younger athlete. Older athletes will generally seek advice regarding their fitness for participation. These individuals should recognize that strenuous exercise is associated with an increase in risk of sudden cardiac death and that appropriate training substantially reduces this risk. Prepartication screening for risk of sudden death in the older athlete is a complex issue and at present is largely focused on identifying inducible ischemia due to significant coronary disease.

In a series of 158 athletic deaths in the United States between 1985 and 1995, hypertrophic cardiomyopathy (36%) and coronary anomalies (19%) were by far the most frequent underlying conditions. LVH was present in another 10%, ruptured aorta (presumably due to Marfan syndrome or cystic medial necrosis) in 6%, myocarditis or dilated cardiomyopathy in 6%, aortic stenosis in 4%, and arrhythmogenic RV dysplasia in 3%. In addition, commotio cordis, or sudden death due to direct myocardial injury, may occur. More common in children, ventricular tachycardia or ventricular fibrillation may occur even after a minor direct blow to the heart; it is thought to be due to the precipitation of a PVC just prior to the peak of the T wave on ECG.

Table 10–22. 12-element AHA recommendations for preparticipation cardiovascular screening of competitive athletes.

Medical History
Personal History
1. Exertional chest pain/discomfort
2. Unexplained syncope/near-syncope
3. Excessive exertional and unexplained dyspnea/fatigue
4. Prior recognition of a heart murmur
5. Elevated systemic blood pressure
Family History
6. Premature death (sudden and unexpected, or otherwise) before age of 50 years due to heart disease in one or more relatives
7. Disability from heart disease in a close relative before age of 50 years
8. Specific knowledge of certain cardiac conditions in family members: hypertrophic cardiomyopathy, dilated cardiomyopathy, long QT syndrome or other ion channelopathies, Marfan syndrome, or other important arrhythmias
Physical Examination
9. Heart murmur
10. Diminished femoral pulse (to exclude coarctation)
11. Phenotype of Marfan syndrome
12. Brachial artery blood pressure (sitting position)

Reproduced, with permission, from Lawless CE et al. Protecting the heart of the American athlete: proceedings of the American College of Cardiology Sports and Exercise Cardiology Think Tank, October 18, 2012, Washington, DC. J Am Coll Cardiol. 2014 Nov 18–25;64(20):2146–71. Copyright © Elsevier.

A careful family and medical history and cardiovascular examination will identify most individuals at risk. An update in 2014 recommends that **all middle school and higher athletes undergo a medical screen questionnaire and examination.** The 12 elements in the examination are outlined in Table 10–22.

A family history of premature sudden death or cardiovascular disease, or of any of these predisposing conditions should mandate further workup, including an ECG and echocardiogram. Symptoms of unexplained fatigue or dyspnea, exertional chest pain, syncope, or near-syncope also warrant further evaluation. A Marfan-like appearance, significant elevation of BP, abnormalities of heart rate or rhythm, and pathologic heart murmurs or heart sounds should also be investigated before clearance for athletic participation is given. Such an evaluation is recommended before participation at the high school and college levels and every 2 years during athletic competition.

Stress-induced syncope or chest pressure may be the first clue to an anomalous origin of a coronary artery. Anatomically, this lesion occurs most often when the left anterior descending artery or left main coronary arises from the right coronary cusp and traverses between the aorta and pulmonary trunks. The "slit-like" orifice that results from the angulation at the vessel origin is thought to cause ischemia when the aorta and pulmonary arteries enlarge during rigorous exercise and tension is placed on the coronary.

The toughest distinction may be in sorting out the healthy athlete with LVH from the athlete with hypertrophic cardiomyopathy. In general, the healthy athlete's heart is *less* likely to have an unusual pattern of LVH (such as asymmetric septal hypertrophy), or to have LA enlargement, an abnormal ECG, an LV cavity less than 45 mm in diameter at end-diastole, an abnormal diastolic filling pattern, or a family history of hypertrophic cardiomyopathy. The athlete is more likely to be male than the individual with hypertrophic cardiomyopathy, where women are equally at risk. Increased risk is also evident in patients with the WPW syndrome, a prolonged QTc interval, or the Brugada syndrome on their ECG.

Selective use of routine ECG and stress testing is recommended in men above age 40 years and women above age 50 years who continue to participate in vigorous exercise and at earlier ages when there is a positive family history for premature CAD, hypertrophic cardiomyopathy, or multiple risk factors. Because at least some of the risk features (long QT, LVH, Brugada syndrome, WPW syndrome) may be evident on routine ECG screening, several cost-effectiveness studies have been done. Most suggest that preparticipation ECGs are of potential value, though what to do when the QTc is mildly increased is unclear. Many experts feel the high incidence of false-positive ECG studies make it very ineffective as a screening tool. With the low prevalence of cardiac anomalies in the general public, it has been estimated that 200,000 individual athletes would need to be screened to identify the single individual who would die suddenly. A report from Canada reviewing 74 sudden cardiac arrests during sports activity noted that the vast majority occurred during noncompetitive sports. The incidence during competitive sports was 0.76 per 100,000 athlete-years, and there was not a clear association with structural heart disease in most.

The issue of routine screening, therefore, remains controversial. A report from the United Kingdom in 2018, screening adolescent soccer players from 1996 to 2016 (that included ECG and echocardiography), identified diseases associated with sudden death in only 0.38% of the 11,168 athletes screened for a total of 118,351 person-years. The incidence of sudden death was about 7 per 100,000 athletes and most were related to cardiomyopathies that had not been detected on the screening procedures.

In 2017, a position paper from a number of European societies presented arguments regarding the use of a number of preparticipation screening options. The manuscript also provided input from a number of international sports organizations. They concluded that there were data to support obtaining the clinical history, performing a physical examination, and performing a 12-lead ECG on all participants. They did not recommend echocardiography as a screening tool.

In 2017, a consensus statement from the American Medical Society for Sports Medicine was published summarizing the current recommendations for the appropriate screening options in the various clinical scenarios. Once a high-risk individual has been identified, guidelines from the Bethesda conference and the ESC can be used to help determine whether the athlete may continue to participate in sporting events. Table 10–23 summarizes these recommendations.

Table 10–23. Recommendations for competitive sports participation among athletes with potential causes of SCD.

Condition	36th Bethesda Conference	European Society of Cardiology
Structural cardiac abnormalities		
HCM	Exclude athletes with a probable or definitive clinical diagnosis from all competitive sports. Genotype-positive/phenotype-negative athletes may still compete.	Exclude athletes with a probable or definitive clinical diagnosis from all competitive sports. Exclude genotype-positive/phenotype-negative individuals from competitive sports.
ARVC	Exclude athletes with a probable or definitive diagnosis from competitive sports.	Exclude athletes with a probable or definitive diagnosis from competitive sports.
CCAA	Exclude from competitive sports. Participation in all sports 3 months after successful surgery would be permitted for an athlete with ischemia, ventricular arrhythmia or tachyarrhythmia, or LV dysfunction during maximal exercise testing.	Not applicable.
Electrical cardiac abnormalities		
WPW	Athletes without structural heart disease, without a history of palpitations, or without tachycardia can participate in all competitive sports. In athletes with symptoms, electrophysiological study and ablation are recommended. Return to competitive sports is allowed after corrective ablation, provided that the ECG has normalized.	Athletes without structural heart disease, without a history of palpitations, or without tachycardia can participate in all competitive sports. In athletes with symptoms, electrophysiological study and ablation are recommended. Return to competitive sports is allowed after corrective ablation, provided that the ECG has normalized.
LQTS	Exclude any athlete with a previous cardiac arrest or syncopal episode from competitive sports. Asymptomatic patients restricted to competitive low-intensity sports. Genotype-positive/phenotype-negative athletes may still compete.	Exclude any athlete with a clinical or genotype diagnosis from competitive sports.
BrS	Exclude from all competitive sports except those of low intensity.	Exclude from all competitive sports.
CPVT	Exclude all patients with a clinical diagnosis from competitive sports. Genotype-positive/phenotype-negative patients may still compete in low-intensity sports.	Exclude all patients with a clinical diagnosis from competitive sports. Genotype-positive/phenotype-negative patients are also excluded.
Acquired cardiac abnormalities		
Commotio cordis	Eligibility for returning to competitive sport in survivors is a matter of individual clinical judgment. Survivors must undergo a thorough cardiovascular workup including 12-lead electrocardiography, ambulatory ECG monitoring, and echocardiography	Not applicable.
Myocarditis	Exclude from all competitive sports. Convalescent period of 6 months. Athletes may return to competition when test results normalize.	Exclude from all competitive sports. Convalescent period of 6 months. Athletes may return to competition when test results normalize.

ARVC, arrhythmogenic right ventricular cardiomyopathy; BrS, Brugada syndrome; CCAA, congenital coronary artery anomalies; CPVT, cathecholaminergic polymorphic ventricular tachycardia; ECG, electrocardiogram; HCM, hypertrophic cardiomyopathy; LQTS, long QT syndrome; LV, left ventricular; SCD, sudden cardiac death; WPW, Wolff-Parkinson-White syndrome.
Reproduced, with permission, from Chandra N et al. Sudden cardiac death in young athletes: practical challenges and diagnostic dilemmas. J Am Coll Cardiol. 2013 Mar 12;61(10):1027–40. Copyright © Elsevier.

Chugh SS et al. Sudden cardiac death in the older athlete. J Am Coll Cardiol. 2015 Feb 10;65(5):493–502. [PMID: 25660928]

Drezner JA et al. AMSSM position statement on cardiovascular preparticipation screening in athletes: current evidence, knowledge gaps, recommendations and future directions. Br J Sports Med. 2017 Feb; 51(3):153–67. [PMID: 27660369]

Landry CH et al; Rescu Investigators. Sudden cardiac arrest during participation in competitive sports. N Engl J Med. 2017 Nov 16;377(20):1943–53. [PMID: 29141175]

Malhotra A et al. Outcomes of cardiac screening in adolescent soccer players. N Engl J Med. 2018 Aug 9;379(6):524–34. [PMID: 30089062]

Mont L et al. Pre-participation cardiovascular evaluation for athletic participants to prevent sudden death: position paper from the EHRA and the EACPR, branches of the ESC. Endorsed by APHRS, HRS, and SOLAECE. Eur J Prev Cardiol. 2017 Jan;24(1):41–69. [PMID: 27815537]

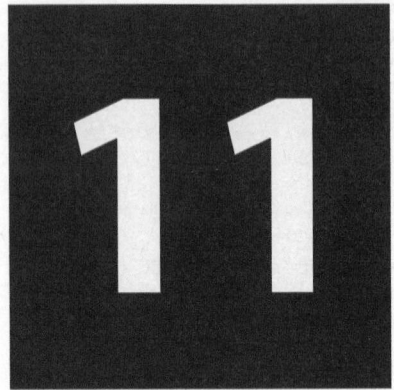

Systemic Hypertension

Michael Sutters, MD, MRCP (UK)

Based on data from the 2015–2016 NHANES survey, about one-third of adults in the United States are hypertensive. Hypertension is uncontrolled in almost half of affected individuals, and of those with uncontrolled hypertension, about 36% are unaware of the diagnosis. Even in patients in whom hypertension is diagnosed and treated, control is attained in only 60%. Cardiovascular morbidity and mortality increase as both systolic and diastolic blood pressures rise, but in individuals over age 50 years, the systolic pressure and pulse pressure are better predictors of complications than diastolic pressure. The prevalence of hypertension increases with age, and it is more common in blacks than in whites. Adequate blood pressure control reduces the incidence of acute coronary syndrome by 20–25%, stroke by 30–35%, and heart failure by 50%.

HOW IS BLOOD PRESSURE MEASURED & HYPERTENSION DIAGNOSED?

Blood pressure should be measured with a well-calibrated sphygmomanometer. The bladder width within the cuff should encircle at least 80% of the arm circumference. Readings should be taken after the patient has been resting comfortably, back supported in the sitting or supine position, for at least 5 minutes and at least 30 minutes after smoking or coffee ingestion. Automated office blood pressure readings, which are office-based devices that permit multiple automated measurements after a pre-programmed rest period, produce data that are independent of digit preference bias and the "white coat" phenomenon (where blood pressure is elevated in the clinic but normal at home). Blood pressure measurements taken outside the office environment, either by intermittent self-monitoring (home blood pressure) or with an automated device programmed to take measurements at regular intervals (ambulatory blood pressure) are more powerful predictors of outcomes and are advocated in clinical guidelines. Home measurements are also helpful in differentiating white coat hypertension from hypertension that is resistant to treatment, and in diagnosis of "masked hypertension" (where blood pressure is normal in the clinic but elevated at home). The cardiovascular risk associated with masked hypertension is similar to that observed in sustained hypertension.

A single elevated blood pressure reading is not sufficient to establish the diagnosis of hypertension. The major exceptions to this rule are hypertensive presentations with unequivocal evidence of life-threatening end-organ damage, as seen in hypertensive emergency, or in hypertensive urgency where blood pressure is greater than 220/125 mm Hg but life-threatening end-organ damage is absent. In less severe cases, the diagnosis of hypertension depends on a series of measurements of blood pressure, since readings can vary and tend to regress toward the mean with time. Patients whose initial blood pressure is in the hypertensive range exhibit the greatest fall toward the normal range between the first and second encounters. However, the concern for diagnostic precision needs to be balanced by an appreciation of the importance of establishing the diagnosis of hypertension as quickly as possible, since a 3-month delay in treatment of hypertension in high-risk patients is associated with a twofold increase in cardiovascular morbidity and mortality. Based on epidemiological data, the conventional 140/90 mm Hg threshold for the diagnosis of hypertension has been questioned. The 2017 guidelines from the American College of Cardiology and American Heart Association (ACC/AHA) suggest that, for conventional office-based measurement, **normal** be defined as less than 120/80 mm Hg, **elevated** as 120–129/less than 80 mm Hg, **stage 1** as 130–139/80–89 mm Hg and **stage 2** as greater than or equal to 140/90 mm Hg. As exemplified by Hypertension Canada's 2017 guidelines (Figure 11–1), automated and home blood pressure measurements are assuming greater prominence in the diagnostic algorithms published by many national hypertension workgroups. Equivalent blood pressure for these different modes of measurement are described in Table 11–1.

Ambulatory blood pressure readings are normally lowest at night and the loss of this nocturnal dip is a dominant predictor of cardiovascular risk, particularly risk of thrombotic stroke. An accentuation of the normal morning increase in blood pressure is associated with increased likelihood of cerebral hemorrhage. Furthermore, variability of systolic blood pressure predicts cardiovascular events independently of mean systolic blood pressure.

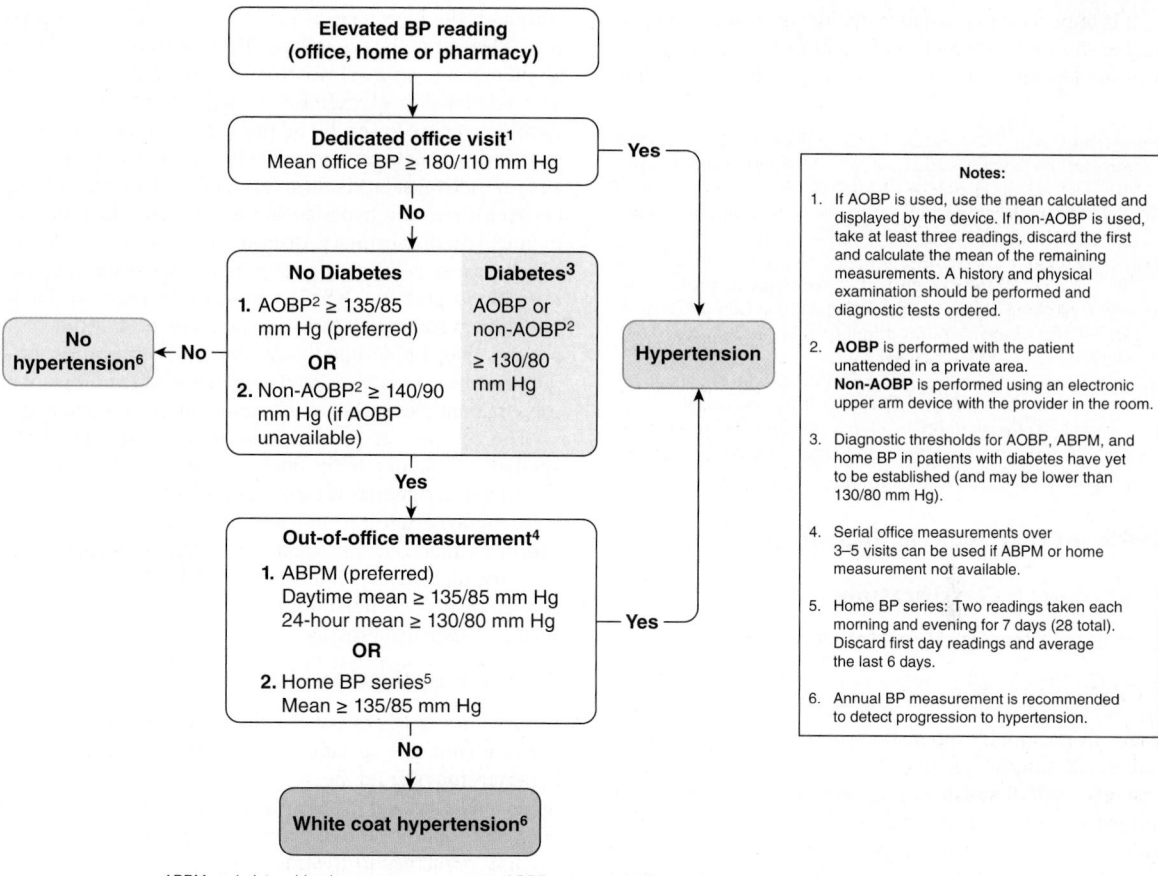

ABPM, ambulatory blood pressure measurement; AOBP, automated office blood pressure; BP, blood pressure.

▲ **Figure 11–1.** According to these recommendations, if AOBP measurements are not available, blood pressures recorded manually in the office may be substituted if taken as the mean of the last two readings of three consecutive readings. Note that the blood pressure threshold for diagnosing hypertension is higher if recorded manually in these guidelines. If home blood pressure monitoring is unavailable, office measurements recorded over three to five separate visits can be substituted. (Reproduced, with permission, from Leung AA et al; Hypertension Canada. Hypertension Canada's 2017 guidelines for diagnosis, risk assessment, prevention, and treatment of hypertension in adults. Can J Cardiol. 2017 May;33(5):557–76. Erratum in: Can J Cardiol. 2017 Dec;33(12):1733–4.)

Table 11–1. Corresponding blood pressure values across a range of blood pressure measurement methods.

Manual Measurement in Clinic[1]	Home Blood Pressure Measurement	Ambulatory Blood Pressure Measurement (Daytime)	Ambulatory Blood Pressure Measurement (Nighttime)	Ambulatory Blood Pressure Measurement (24-Hour)
120/80 mm Hg	120/80 mm Hg	120/80 mm Hg	100/65 mm Hg	115/75 mm Hg
130/80 mm Hg	130/80 mm Hg	130/80 mm Hg	110/65 mm Hg	125/75 mm Hg
140/90 mm Hg	135/85 mm Hg	135/85 mm Hg	120/70 mm Hg	130/80 mm Hg
160/100 mm Hg	145/90 mm Hg	145/90 mm Hg	140/85 mm Hg	145/90 mm Hg

[1]Clinic manual blood pressures are critically dependent on technique. The use of automated devices in an unattended setting typically result in systolic blood pressures 9–13 mm Hg lower than clinic manual pressures.
Data abstracted from Greenland P et al. The New 2017 ACC/AHA Guidelines "up the pressure" on diagnosis and treatment of hypertension. JAMA. 2017 Dec 5;318(21):2083–4.

It is important to recognize that the diagnosis of hypertension does not automatically entail drug treatment; this decision depends on the clinical setting, as discussed below.

Greenland P et al. The New 2017 ACC/AHA Guidelines "up the pressure" on diagnosis and treatment of hypertension. JAMA. 2017 Dec 5;318(21):2083–4. [PMID: 29159417]

Jin J. JAMA patient page. Checking blood pressure at home. JAMA. 2017 Jul 18;318(3):310. [PMID: 28719694]

Leung AA et al; Hypertension Canada. Hypertension Canada's 2017 guidelines for diagnosis, risk assessment, prevention, and treatment of hypertension in adults. Can J Cardiol. 2017 May;33(5):557–76. Erratum in: Can J Cardiol. 2017 Dec; 33(12):1733–4. [PMID: 28449828]

Melville S et al. Out-of-office blood pressure monitoring in 2018. JAMA. 2018 Nov 6;320(17):1805–6. [PMID: 30398589]

Myers MG. Automated office blood pressure—incorporating SPRINT into clinical practice. Am J Hypertens. 2017 Jan;30(1): 8–11. [PMID: 27551025]

APPROACH TO HYPERTENSION

▶ Etiology & Classification

A. Primary Essential Hypertension

"Essential hypertension" is the term applied to the 95% of hypertensive patients in which elevated blood pressure results from complex interactions between multiple genetic and environmental factors. The proportion regarded as "essential" will diminish with improved detection of clearly defined secondary causes and with better understanding of pathophysiology. Essential hypertension occurs in 10–15% of white adults and 20–30% of black adults in the United States. The onset is usually between ages 25 and 50 years; it is uncommon before age 20 years. The best understood pathways underlying hypertension include overactivation of the sympathetic nervous and renin-angiotensin-aldosterone systems (RAAS), blunting of the pressure-natriuresis relationship, variation in cardiovascular and renal development, and elevated intracellular sodium and calcium levels.

Exacerbating factors include obesity, sleep apnea, increased salt intake, excessive alcohol use, cigarette smoking, polycythemia, nonsteroidal anti-inflammatory drug (NSAID) therapy, and low potassium intake. Obesity is associated with an increase in intravascular volume, elevated cardiac output, activation of the renin-angiotensin system, and, probably, increased sympathetic outflow. Lifestyle-driven weight reduction lowers blood pressure modestly, but the dramatic weight reduction following bariatric surgery results in improved blood pressure in most patients, and actual remission of hypertension in 20–40% of cases. In patients with sleep apnea, treatment with continuous positive airway pressure (CPAP) has been associated with improvements in blood pressure. Increased salt intake probably elevates blood pressure in some individuals so dietary salt restriction is recommended in patients with hypertension. Excessive use of alcohol also raises blood pressure, perhaps by increasing plasma catecholamines. Hypertension can be difficult to control in patients who consume more than 40 g of ethanol (two drinks) daily or drink in "binges." Cigarette smoking raises blood pressure by increasing plasma norepinephrine.

Although the long-term effect of smoking on blood pressure is less clear, the synergistic effects of smoking and high blood pressure on cardiovascular risk are well documented. The relationship of exercise to hypertension is variable. Aerobic exercise lowers blood pressure in previously sedentary individuals, but increasingly strenuous exercise in already active subjects has less effect. The relationship between stress and hypertension is not established. Polycythemia, whether primary, drug-induced, or due to diminished plasma volume, increases blood viscosity and may raise blood pressure. NSAIDs produce increases in blood pressure averaging 5 mm Hg and are best avoided in patients with borderline or elevated blood pressures. Low potassium intake is associated with higher blood pressure in some patients; an intake of 90 mmol/day is recommended.

The complex of abnormalities termed the **"metabolic syndrome"** (upper body obesity, insulin resistance, and hypertriglyceridemia) is associated with both the development of hypertension and an increased risk of adverse cardiovascular outcomes. Affected patients usually also have low high-density lipoprotein (HDL) cholesterol levels and elevated catecholamines and inflammatory markers such as C-reactive protein.

B. Secondary Hypertension

Approximately 5% of patients have hypertension secondary to identifiable specific causes (Table 11–2). Secondary hypertension should be suspected in patients in whom hypertension develops at an early age or after the age of 50 years, and in those previously well controlled who become refractory to treatment. Hypertension resistant to three medications is another clue, although multiple medications are usually required to control hypertension in persons with diabetes. Secondary causes include genetic syndromes; kidney disease; renal vascular disease; primary hyperaldosteronism; Cushing syndrome; pheochromocytoma; coarctation of the aorta and hypertension associated with pregnancy, estrogen use, hypercalcemia, and medications.

1. Genetic causes—Hypertension can be caused by mutations in single genes, inherited on a Mendelian basis. Although rare, these conditions provide important insight into blood pressure regulation and possibly the genetic basis of essential hypertension. Glucocorticoid remediable aldosteronism is an autosomal dominant cause of early-onset

Table 11–2. Identifiable causes of hypertension.

Sleep apnea
Drug-induced or drug-related
Chronic kidney disease
Primary aldosteronism
Renovascular disease
Long-term corticosteroid therapy and Cushing syndrome
Pheochromocytoma
Coarctation of the aorta
Thyroid or parathyroid disease

Data from Chobanian AV et al. The Seventh Report of the Joint National Committee on Prevention, Detection, Evaluation, and Treatment of High Blood Pressure: the JNC 7 report. JAMA. 2003 May 21;289(19):2560–72.

hypertension with normal or high aldosterone and low renin levels. It is caused by the formation of a chimeric gene encoding both the enzyme responsible for the synthesis of aldosterone (transcriptionally regulated by angiotensin II) and an enzyme responsible for synthesis of cortisol (transcriptionally regulated by ACTH). As a consequence, aldosterone synthesis becomes driven by ACTH, which can be suppressed by exogenous cortisol. In the syndrome of apparent mineralocorticoid excess, early-onset hypertension with hypokalemic metabolic alkalosis is inherited on an autosomal recessive basis. Although plasma renin is low and plasma aldosterone level is very low in these patients, aldosterone antagonists are effective in controlling hypertension. This disease is caused by loss of function of the enzyme 11beta-hydroxysteroid dehydrogenase, which normally metabolizes cortisol and thus protects the otherwise "promiscuous" mineralocorticoid receptor in the distal nephron from inappropriate glucocorticoid activation. Similarly, glycyrrhetinic acid, found in licorice, causes increased blood pressure through inhibition of 11beta-hydroxysteroid dehydrogenase. The syndrome of hypertension exacerbated in pregnancy is inherited as an autosomal dominant trait. In these patients, a mutation in the mineralocorticoid receptor makes it abnormally responsive to progesterone and, paradoxically, to spironolactone. Liddle syndrome is an autosomal dominant condition characterized by early-onset hypertension, hypokalemic alkalosis, low renin, and low aldosterone levels. This is caused by a mutation that results in constitutive activation of the epithelial sodium channel of the distal nephron, with resultant unregulated sodium reabsorption and volume expansion. Gordon syndrome, or pseudohypoaldosteronism type II, presents with early-onset hypertension associated with hyperkalemia, metabolic acidosis and relative suppression of aldosterone. Inheritance is most often autosomal dominant. The underlying mutations occur in one of several genes encoding proteins that regulate the thiazide-sensitive NaCl co-transporter in the distal nephron, leading to constitutive activation of sodium and chloride reabsorption. The abnormalities in this syndrome are corrected by thiazide diuretics.

2. Kidney disease—Renal parenchymal disease is the most common cause of secondary hypertension, which results from increased intravascular volume and increased activity of the RAAS. Increased sympathetic nerve activity may also contribute.

3. Renal vascular hypertension—Renal artery stenosis is present in 1–2% of hypertensive patients. The most common cause is atherosclerosis, but fibromuscular dysplasia should be suspected in women under 50 years of age. Excessive renin release occurs due to reduction in renal perfusion pressure, while attenuation of pressure natriuresis contributes to hypertension in patients with a single kidney or bilateral lesions. Activation of the renal sympathetic nerves may also be important.

Renal vascular hypertension should be suspected in the following circumstances: (1) the documented onset is before age 20 or after age 50 years, (2) the hypertension is resistant to three or more drugs, (3) there are epigastric or renal artery bruits, (4) there is atherosclerotic disease of the aorta or peripheral arteries (15–25% of patients with symptomatic lower limb atherosclerotic vascular disease have renal artery

stenosis), (5) there is an abrupt increase (more than 25%) in the level of serum creatinine after administration of angiotensin-converting enzyme (ACE) inhibitors, or (6) episodes of pulmonary edema are associated with abrupt surges in blood pressure. (See Renal Artery Stenosis, Chapter 22.)

4. Primary hyperaldosteronism—Hyperaldosteronism should be considered in people with resistant hypertension, blood pressures consistently greater than 150/100 mm Hg, hypokalemia (although this is often absent), or adrenal incidentaloma, and in those with a family history of hyperaldosteronism. Hypersecretion of aldosterone is estimated to be present in 5–10% of hypertensive patients and, besides noncompliance, is the most common cause of resistant hypertension. The initial screening step is the simultaneous measurement of aldosterone and renin in blood in a morning sample collected after 30 minutes quietly seated. Hyperaldosteronism is suggested when the plasma aldosterone concentration is elevated (normal: 1–16 ng/dL) in association with suppression of plasma renin activity (normal: 1–2.5 ng/mL/h). However, the plasma aldosterone/renin ratio (normal less than 30) is not highly specific as a screening test. This is because "bottoming out" of renin assays leads to exponential increases in the plasma aldosterone/renin ratio even when aldosterone levels are normal. Hence, an elevated plasma aldosterone/renin ratio should probably not be taken as evidence of hyperaldosteronism unless the aldosterone level is actually supranormal.

During the workup for hyperaldosteronism, an initial plasma aldosterone/renin ratio can be measured while the patient continues taking usual medications. If under these circumstances the ratio proves negative or equivocal, medications that alter renin and aldosterone levels, including ACE inhibitors, angiotensin receptor blockers (ARBs), diuretics, beta-blockers, and clonidine, should be discontinued for 2 weeks before repeating the plasma aldosterone/renin ratio; spironolactone and eplerenone should be held for 4 weeks. Slow-release verapamil and alpha-receptor blockers can be used to control blood pressure during this drug washout period. Patients with a plasma aldosterone level greater than 16 ng/dL and an aldosterone/renin ratio of 30 or more might require further evaluation for primary hyperaldosteronism.

The lesion responsible for hyperaldosteronism is an adrenal adenoma or bilateral adrenal hyperplasia. Approximately 50% of aldosterone-secreting adenomas arise as a consequence of somatic mutations in genes encoding glomerulosa cell membrane ion transporters, with resultant elevation of intracellular calcium concentration.

5. Cushing syndrome—Hypertension occurs in about 80% of patients with spontaneous Cushing syndrome. Excess glucocorticoid may act through salt and water retention (via mineralocorticoid effects), increased angiotensinogen levels, or permissive effects in the regulation of vascular tone.

Diagnosis and treatment of Cushing syndrome are discussed in Chapter 26.

6. Pheochromocytoma—Pheochromocytomas are uncommon; they are probably found in less than 0.1% of all patients with hypertension and in approximately two individuals per million population. However, autopsy studies indicate that pheochromocytomas are very often undiagnosed in life. The blood pressure elevation caused by the catecholamine excess results mainly from alpha-receptor–mediated vasoconstriction of arterioles, with a contribution from beta-1-receptor–mediated increases in cardiac output and renin release. Chronic vasoconstriction of the arterial and venous beds leads to a reduction in plasma volume and predisposes to postural hypotension. Glucose intolerance develops in some patients. Hypertensive crisis in pheochromocytoma may be precipitated by a variety of drugs, including tricyclic antidepressants, antidopaminergic agents, metoclopramide, and naloxone. The diagnosis and treatment of pheochromocytoma are discussed in Chapter 26.

7. Coarctation of the aorta—This uncommon cause of hypertension is discussed in Chapter 10. Evidence of radial-femoral delay should be sought in all younger patients with hypertension.

8. Hypertension associated with pregnancy—Hypertension occurring de novo or worsening during pregnancy, including preeclampsia and eclampsia, is one of the most common causes of maternal and fetal morbidity and mortality (see Chapter 19). Autoantibodies with the potential to activate the angiotensin II type 1 receptor have been causally implicated in preeclampsia, in resistant hypertension, and in progressive systemic sclerosis.

9. Estrogen use—A small increase in blood pressure occurs in most women taking oral contraceptives. A more significant increase above 140/90 mm Hg is noted in about 5% of women, mostly in obese individuals older than age 35 who have been treated for more than 5 years. This is caused by increased hepatic synthesis of angiotensinogen. Postmenopausal estrogen does not generally cause hypertension but rather maintains endothelium-mediated vasodilation.

10. Other causes of secondary hypertension—Hypertension has been associated with hypercalcemia, acromegaly, hyperthyroidism, hypothyroidism, baroreceptor denervation, compression of the rostral ventrolateral medulla, and increased intracranial pressure. A number of medications may cause or exacerbate hypertension—most importantly cyclosporine, tacrolimus, angiogenesis inhibitors, and erythrocyte-stimulating agents (such as erythropoietin). Decongestants, NSAIDs, cocaine, and alcohol should also be considered. Over-the-counter products should not be overlooked, eg, a dietary supplement marketed to enhance libido was found to contain yohimbine, an alpha-2–antagonist, which can produce severe rebound hypertension in patients taking clonidine.

When to Refer

Referral to a hypertension specialist should be considered in cases of severe, resistant or early-/late-onset hypertension or when secondary hypertension is suggested by screening.

Byrd JB et al. Primary aldosteronism. Circulation. 2018 Aug 21; 138(8):823–35. [PMID: 30359120]

Owen JG et al. Bariatric surgery and hypertension. Am J Hypertens. 2017 Dec 8;31(1):11–7. [PMID: 28985287]

Raman G et al. Comparative effectiveness of management strategies for renal artery stenosis: an updated systematic review. Ann Intern Med. 2016 Nov 1;165(9):635–49. [PMID: 27536808]

Complications of Untreated Hypertension

Elevated blood pressure results in structural and functional changes in the vasculature and heart. Most of the adverse outcomes in hypertension are associated with thrombosis rather than bleeding, possibly because increased vascular shear stress converts the normally anticoagulant endothelium to a prothrombotic state. The excess morbidity and mortality related to hypertension approximately doubles for each 6 mm Hg increase in diastolic blood pressure. However, target-organ damage varies markedly between individuals with similar levels of office hypertension; home and ambulatory pressures are superior to office readings in the prediction of end-organ damage.

A. Hypertensive Cardiovascular Disease

Cardiac complications are the major causes of morbidity and mortality in primary (essential) hypertension. For any level of blood pressure, left ventricular hypertrophy is associated with incremental cardiovascular risk in association with heart failure (through systolic or diastolic dysfunction), ventricular arrhythmias, myocardial ischemia, and sudden death.

The occurrence of heart failure is reduced by 50% with antihypertensive therapy. Hypertensive left ventricular hypertrophy regresses with therapy and is most closely related to the degree of systolic blood pressure reduction. Diuretics have produced equal or greater reductions of left ventricular mass when compared with other drug classes. Conventional beta-blockers are less effective in reducing left ventricular hypertrophy but play a specific role in patients with established coronary artery disease or impaired left ventricular function.

B. Hypertensive Cerebrovascular Disease and Dementia

Hypertension is the major predisposing cause of hemorrhagic and ischemic stroke. Cerebrovascular complications are more closely correlated with systolic than diastolic blood pressure. The incidence of these complications is markedly reduced by antihypertensive therapy. Preceding hypertension is associated with a higher incidence of subsequent dementia of both vascular and Alzheimer types. Home and ambulatory blood pressure may be a better predictor of cognitive decline than office readings in older people. Effective blood pressure control may reduce the risk of development of cognitive dysfunction later in life, but once cerebral small-vessel disease is established, low blood pressure might exacerbate this problem.

C. Hypertensive Kidney Disease

Chronic hypertension is associated with injury to vascular, glomerular, and tubulointerstitial compartments within the kidney, accounting for about 25% of end-stage kidney disease. Nephrosclerosis is particularly prevalent in blacks, in whom susceptibility is linked to *APOL1* mutations and hypertension results from kidney disease rather than causing it.

D. Aortic Dissection

Hypertension is a contributing factor in many patients with dissection of the aorta. Its diagnosis and treatment are discussed in Chapter 12.

E. Atherosclerotic Complications

Most Americans with hypertension die of complications of atherosclerosis, but antihypertensive therapy seems to have a lesser impact on atherosclerotic complications compared with the other effects of treatment outlined above. Prevention of cardiovascular outcomes related to atherosclerosis probably requires control of multiple risk factors, of which hypertension is only one.

Seccia TM et al. Hypertensive nephropathy. Moving from classic to emerging pathogenetic mechanisms. J Hypertens. 2017 Feb; 35(2):205–12. [PMID: 27782909]

▶ Clinical Findings

The clinical and laboratory findings are mainly referable to involvement of the target organs: heart, brain, kidneys, eyes, and peripheral arteries.

A. Symptoms

Mild to moderate primary (essential) hypertension is largely asymptomatic for many years. The most frequent symptom, headache, is also very nonspecific. Accelerated hypertension is associated with somnolence, confusion, visual disturbances, and nausea and vomiting (hypertensive encephalopathy).

Hypertension in patients with pheochromocytomas that secrete predominantly norepinephrine is usually sustained but may be episodic. The typical attack lasts from minutes to hours and is associated with headache, anxiety, palpitation, profuse perspiration, pallor, tremor, and nausea and vomiting. Blood pressure is markedly elevated, and angina or acute pulmonary edema may occur. In primary aldosteronism, patients may have muscular weakness, polyuria, and nocturia due to hypokalemia; malignant hypertension is rare. Chronic hypertension often leads to left ventricular hypertrophy and diastolic dysfunction, which can present with exertional and paroxysmal nocturnal dyspnea. Cerebral involvement causes stroke due to thrombosis or hemorrhage from microaneurysms of small penetrating intracranial arteries. Hypertensive encephalopathy is probably caused by acute capillary congestion and exudation with cerebral edema, which is reversible.

B. Signs

Like symptoms, physical findings depend on the cause of hypertension, its duration and severity, and the degree of effect on target organs.

1. Blood pressure—Blood pressure is taken in both arms and, if lower extremity pulses are diminished or delayed, in the legs to exclude coarctation of the aorta. If blood pressure differs between right and left arms, the higher reading

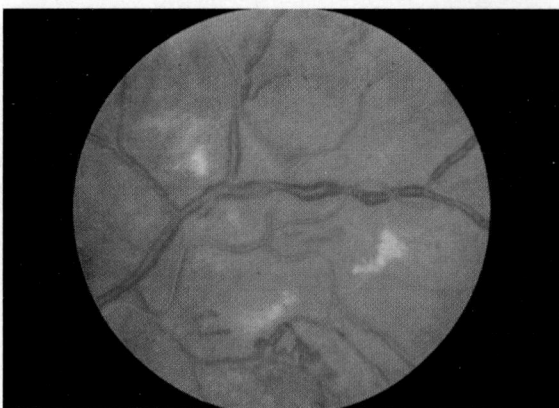

▲ **Figure 11–2.** Severe, chronic hypertensive retinopathy with hard exudates, increased vessel light reflexes, and sausage-shaped veins. (Used, with permission, from Richard E. Wyszynski, MD, in Knoop KJ, Stack LB, Storrow AB, Thurman RJ. *The Atlas of Emergency Medicine*, 4th ed. McGraw-Hill, 2016.)

should be recorded as the actual blood pressure and subclavian stenosis suspected in the other arm. An orthostatic drop of at least 20/10 mm Hg is often present in pheochromocytoma. Older patients may have falsely elevated readings by sphygmomanometry because of noncompressible vessels. This may be suspected in the presence of Osler sign—a palpable brachial or radial artery when the cuff is inflated above systolic pressure. Occasionally, it may be necessary to make direct measurements of intra-arterial pressure, especially in patients with apparent severe hypertension who do not tolerate therapy.

2. Retinas—Narrowing of arterial diameter to less than 50% of venous diameter, copper or silver wire appearance, exudates, hemorrhages, or hypertensive retinopathy are associated with a worse prognosis. the typical changes of severe hypertensive retinopathy are shown in Figure 11–2.

3. Heart—A left ventricular heave indicates severe hypertrophy. Aortic regurgitation may be auscultated in up to 5% of patients, and hemodynamically insignificant aortic regurgitation can be detected by Doppler echocardiography in 10–20%. A presystolic (S_4) gallop due to decreased compliance of the left ventricle is quite common in patients in sinus rhythm.

4. Pulses—Radial-femoral delay suggests coarctation of the aorta; loss of peripheral pulses occurs due to atherosclerosis, less commonly aortic dissection, and rarely Takayasu arteritis, all of which can involve the renal arteries.

C. Laboratory Findings

Recommended testing includes the following: hemoglobin; serum electrolytes and serum creatinine; fasting blood sugar level (hypertension is a risk factor for the development of diabetes, and hyperglycemia can be a presenting feature of pheochromocytoma); plasma lipids (necessary to calculate cardiovascular risk and as a modifiable risk factor); serum uric acid (hyperuricemia is a relative contraindication to diuretic therapy); and urinalysis.

D. Electrocardiography and Chest Radiographs

Electrocardiographic criteria are highly specific but not very sensitive for left ventricular hypertrophy. The "strain" pattern of ST–T wave changes is a sign of more advanced disease and is associated with a poor prognosis. A chest radiograph is not necessary in the workup for uncomplicated hypertension.

E. Echocardiography

The primary role of echocardiography should be to evaluate patients with clinical symptoms or signs of cardiac disease.

F. Diagnostic Studies

Additional diagnostic studies are indicated only if the clinical presentation or routine tests suggest secondary or complicated hypertension. These may include 24-hour urine free cortisol, urine or plasma metanephrines, and plasma aldosterone and renin concentrations to screen for endocrine causes of hypertension. Renal ultrasound will detect structural changes (such as polycystic kidneys, asymmetry, and hydronephrosis); echogenicity and reduced cortical volume are reliable indicators of advanced chronic kidney disease. Evaluation for renal artery stenosis should be undertaken in concert with subspecialist consultation.

G. Summary

Since most hypertension is essential or primary, few studies are necessary beyond those listed above. If conventional therapy is unsuccessful or if secondary hypertension is suspected, further studies and perhaps referral to a hypertension specialist are indicated.

Katsi V et al. Impact of arterial hypertension on the eye. Curr Hypertens Rep. 2012 Dec;14(6):581–90. [PMID: 22673879]

► Nonpharmacologic Therapy

Lifestyle modification may have an impact on morbidity and mortality and is recommended in all patients with elevated blood pressure. A diet rich in fruits, vegetables, and low-fat dairy foods and low in saturated and total fats (DASH diet) has been shown to lower blood pressure. Increased dietary fiber lowers blood pressure. For every 7 g of dietary fiber ingested, cardiovascular risk could be lowered by 9%. The effect of diet on blood pressure may be mediated by shifts in the microbial species in the gut, the intestinal microbiota. Additional lifestyle changes, listed in Table 11–3, can prevent or mitigate hypertension or its cardiovascular consequences.

Appel LJ. The effects of dietary factors on blood pressure. Cardiol Clin. 2017 May;35(2):197–212. [PMID: 28411894]
Marques FZ et al. Beyond gut feelings: how the gut microbiota regulates blood pressure. Nat Rev Cardiol. 2018 Jan;15(1):20–32. [PMID: 28836619]

► Who Should Be Treated With Medications?

Treatment should be offered to all persons in whom blood pressure reduction, irrespective of initial blood pressure levels, will reduce cardiovascular risk with an acceptably low rate of medication-associated adverse effects. The American College of Cardiology and the American Heart Association (ACC/AHA), Hypertension Canada (HC), and the European Society of Hypertension and European Society of Cardiology (ESH/ESC) have developed independent guidelines for the evaluation and management of hypertension. There is broad agreement that drug treatment is necessary in those with office-based blood pressures exceeding 160/100 mm Hg, irrespective of cardiac risk. Similarly, the American, Canadian, and European guidelines agree that treatment thresholds should be lower in the

Table 11–3. Lifestyle modifications to manage hypertension.[1]

Modification	Recommendation	Approximate Systolic BP Reduction, Range
Weight reduction	Maintain normal body weight (BMI, 18.5–24.9)	5–20 mm Hg/10 kg weight loss
Adopt DASH eating plan	Consume a diet rich in fruits, vegetables, and low-fat dairy products with a reduced content of saturated fat and total fat	8–14 mm Hg
Dietary sodium reduction	Reduce dietary sodium intake to no more than 100 mEq/day (2.4 g sodium or 6 g sodium chloride)	2–8 mm Hg
Physical activity	Engage in regular aerobic physical activity such as brisk walking (at least 30 minutes per day, most days of the week)	4–9 mm Hg
Moderation of alcohol consumption	Limit consumption to no more than two drinks per day (1 oz or 30 mL ethanol [eg, 24 oz beer, 10 oz wine, or 3 oz 80-proof whiskey]) in most men and no more than one drink per day in women and lighter-weight persons	2–4 mm Hg

[1]For overall cardiovascular risk reduction, stop smoking. The effects of implementing these modifications are dose- and time-dependent and could be higher for some individuals.

BMI, body mass index calculated as weight in kilograms divided by the square of height in meters; BP, blood pressure; DASH, Dietary Approaches to Stop Hypertension.

Data from Chobanian AV et al. The Seventh Report of the Joint National Committee on Prevention, Detection, Evaluation, and Treatment of High Blood Pressure: the JNC 7 report. JAMA. 2003 May 21;289(19):2560–72.

Table 11–4. Comparison of blood pressure treatment thresholds from the 2017 ACC/AHA guidelines, the 2018 Hypertension Canada guidelines, and the 2018 ESH/ESC guidelines.

Cardiovascular Risk	Guidelines[1]	Threshold for Pharmacotherapy (mm Hg)	Target (mm Hg)
Nonelevated	ACC/AHA	> 140/90	< 130/80 (reasonable)
	Hypertension Canada	> 160/100	< 140/90 (< 130/80 for diabetes)
	ESH/ESC	> 140/90[2]	All < 140/90, most < 130/80, not < 120
Elevated	ACC/AHA	< 130/80	< 130/80 (recommended)
	Hypertension Canada	> 140 systolic[3]	< 120 systolic
	ESH/ESC	> 130/80[3]	120–130/< 80
Elderly	ACC/AHA > 65 yr	> 130/80	< 130 systolic
	Hypertension Canada[4]	Not specified[4]	Not specified[4]
	ESH/ESC > 65 yr	> 140/90[5]	130–140/> 80[6]

[1]In all three sets of guidelines, blood pressure values are based upon nonautomated office blood pressure readings.
[2]Consider drug treatment if lifestyle changes fail to control blood pressure.
[3]Consider drug treatment if very high risk, eg, established cardiovascular disease, especially coronary disease.
Note: The > 130/80 mm Hg threshold for treatment of high-risk patients in the Canadian guidelines refers to automated blood pressure readings, which are lower than nonautomated readings.
[4]Recommendations for persons > 75 years are not explicitly stated in the Hypertension Canada guidelines. They removed separate goals for the elderly, but consider age > 75 years to be a risk signifier triggering an approach that many would view as overly aggressive in the extremely old.
[5]The European guidelines indicate a slightly more conservative treatment threshold of > 160/90 mm Hg for those > 80 years.
[6]This target range is also suggested in the European guidelines for patients > 80 years.
ACC, American College of Cardiology; AHA, American Heart Association; ESC, European Society of Cardiology; ESH, European Society of Hypertension.

presence of elevated cardiovascular risk. American guidelines stand apart in recommending initiation of antihypertensive pharmacotherapy in those with stage 1 hypertension (140–159/90–99 mm Hg) even if cardiovascular risk is not elevated. By contrast, the Canadian guidelines suggest lifestyle modifications in this low-cardiovascular-risk group, while the European guidelines recommend initiation of pharmacotherapy only if elevated pressure in this low-risk population persists after lifestyle modification. There is no outcomes evidence that mortality or risk of cardiovascular events can be reduced by treating mild hypertension (140/90–160/100 mm Hg) in low-risk individuals. Table 11–4 compares these three sets of guidelines. Since evaluation of total cardiovascular risk (Table 11–5) is important in deciding who to treat with antihypertensive medications, risk calculators are essential clinical tools. The ACC has developed an online toolkit relevant to primary prevention (https://tools.acc.org/ascvd-risk-estimator-plus/#!/calculate/estimate/), and an associated app called ASCVD Risk Estimator Plus (downloadable at https://www.acc.org/ASCVDApp).

▶ Goals of Treatment

Traditionally, the most widely accepted goal for blood pressure management has been less than 140/90 mm Hg. However, observational studies suggest that there does not seem to be a blood pressure level below which decrements in cardiovascular risk taper off, and a number of randomized

Table 11–5. Cardiovascular risk factors.

Major risk factors
Hypertension[1]
Cigarette smoking
Obesity (BMI ≥ 30)[1]
Physical inactivity
Dyslipidemia[1]
Diabetes mellitus[1]
Microalbuminuria or estimated GFR < 60 mL/min
Age (> 55 years for men, > 65 years for women)
Family history of premature cardiovascular disease (< 55 years for men, < 65 years for women)
Target-organ damage
Heart
Left ventricular hypertrophy
Angina or prior myocardial infarction
Prior coronary revascularization
Heart failure
Brain
Stroke or transient ischemic attack
Chronic kidney disease
Peripheral arterial disease
Retinopathy

[1]Components of the metabolic syndrome.
BMI indicates body mass index calculated as weight in kilograms divided by the square of height in meters; GFR, glomerular filtration rate.
Data from Chobanian AV et al. The Seventh Report of the Joint National Committee on Prevention, Detection, Evaluation, and Treatment of High Blood Pressure: the JNC 7 report. JAMA. 2003 May 21; 289(19):2560–72.

controlled trials have suggested that treatment to blood pressure targets considerably below 140 mm Hg may benefit certain patient groups.

The SPRINT study suggests that outcomes improve in nondiabetic patients with considerably elevated cardiovascular risk when treatment lowers systolic pressure to less than 120 mm Hg compared to less than 140 mm Hg. On the other hand, in the HOPE3 study of largely nondiabetic patients at somewhat lower risk than those in SPRINT, reducing blood pressure by an average of 6/3 mm Hg systolic from a baseline of 138/82 mm Hg provided no significant outcomes benefits. Therefore, it appears that blood pressure targets should be lower in people at greater estimated cardiovascular risk. In response to the SPRINT study, the 2018 Hypertension Canada guidelines urge prescribers to consider a blood pressure goal of less than 120/80 mm Hg in patients considered at elevated risk for cardiovascular events. The 2017 ACC/AHA guidelines take a different approach by defining a 130/80 mm Hg goal as "reasonable" in nonelevated risk patients, strengthening this to "recommended" in elevated risk hypertensive patients. The 2018 ESH/ESC guidelines specify a target of less than 140 mm Hg systolic for all, and less than 130 mm Hg for most if tolerated. There is a trend toward recommending similar treatment targets in the elderly; this topic is discussed in greater detail below. Some experts note that manual office measurements of around 130/80 mm Hg are likely to approximate the lower blood pressure targets specified in the SPRINT study, which used automated office blood pressure measuring devices that have been demonstrated to read 16/7 mm Hg lower than manual office readings. The 2018 Canadian guidelines acknowledge this disparity in measurement methods by specifying that automated office devices should be used in the monitoring of patients selected for the aggressive blood pressure goal of less than 120/80 mm Hg. Table 11–4 compares the treatment threshold and target recommendations laid out in the American, Canadian, and European guidelines.

Treatment to blood pressures less than 130 mm Hg systolic seems especially important in stroke prevention. The ACCORD study examined the effect of treatment of systolic pressures to below 130–135 mm Hg in patients with diabetes. Although the lower treatment goal significantly increased the risk of serious adverse effects (with no additional gain in terms of heart, kidney, or retinal disease), there was a significant additional reduction in the risk of stroke. Lower targets might be justified in diabetic patients at high risk for cerebrovascular events.

Similarly, in the SPS3 trial in patients who have had a lacunar stroke, treating the systolic blood pressure to less than 130 mm Hg (mean systolic blood pressure of 127 mm Hg among treated versus mean systolic blood pressure 138 mm Hg among untreated patients) probably reduced the risk of recurrent stroke (and with an acceptably low rate of adverse effects from treatment). Blood pressure management in acute stroke is discussed below.

▶ How Low To Go?

Although observational studies indicate that the blood pressure-risk relationship holds up at levels considerably below 120 mm Hg, there is uncertainty about whether this is true for treated blood pressure. This question was addressed in a secondary analysis of data from the ONTARGET and TRANSCEND studies in which participants with elevated cardiovascular risk but no history of stroke were treated with telmisartan (plus or minus ramipril), or placebo. The risk of the composite cardiovascular endpoint was lowest at a treated systolic blood pressure range between 120 mm Hg and 140 mm Hg. Increased risk was observed at blood pressures below and above this range. The risk of stroke was the only exception, with incremental benefit observed below a treated systolic of 120 mm Hg. With respect to diastolic blood pressure on treatment, composite risk began to increase at levels below 70 mm Hg. This suggests that the blood pressure–cardiovascular risk relationship evident in observational studies may not hold in the case of treated blood pressure and that there are grounds for a degree of caution in treating below a systolic pressure of 120 mm Hg.

In seeking to simplify decision making in the treatment of hypertension, some authors have suggested that a systolic blood pressure goal in the 120–130 mm Hg range would be safe and effective in high-risk patients, and a systolic blood pressure of around 130 mm Hg would be reasonable in lower-risk patients.

Data from multiple studies indicate that statins should be considered as part of the strategy to reduce overall cardiovascular risk. The HOPE3 study of persons at intermediate cardiovascular risk showed that 10 mg of rosuvastatin reduced average low-density lipoprotein (LDL) cholesterol from 130 mg/dL to 90 mg/dL (3.36–2.33 mmol/L), and significantly reduced the risk of multiple cardiovascular events, including myocardial infarction and coronary revascularization. Low-dose aspirin (81 mg/day) is likely to be beneficial in patients older than age 50 with either target-organ damage or elevated total cardiovascular risk (greater than 20–30%). Care should be taken to ensure that blood pressure is controlled to the recommended levels before starting aspirin to minimize the risk of intracranial hemorrhage.

ACCORD Study Group; Cushman WC et al. Effects of intensive blood-pressure control in type 2 diabetes mellitus. N Engl J Med. 2010 Apr 29;362(17):1575–85. [PMID: 20228401]

Böhm M et al. Achieved blood pressure and cardiovascular outcomes in high-risk patients: results from ONTARGET and TRANSCEND trials. Lancet. 2017 Jun 3;389(10085):2226–37. [PMID: 28390695]

Lonn EM et al; HOPE-3 Investigators. Blood-pressure lowering in intermediate-risk persons without cardiovascular disease. N Engl J Med. 2016 May 26;374(21):2009–20. [PMID: 27041480]

Sheppard JP et al. Benefits and harms of antihypertensive treatment in low-risk patients with mild hypertension. JAMA Intern Med. 2018 Dec ;178(12):1626–34. [PMID: 30383082]

SPRINT Research Group; Wright JT Jr et al. A randomized trial of intensive versus standard blood-pressure control. N Engl J Med. 2015 Nov 26;373(22):2103–16. [PMID: 26551272]

Williams B et al. 2018 Practice guidelines for the management of arterial hypertension of the European Society of Hypertension (ESH) and the European Society of Cardiology (ESC). Blood Press. 2018 Dec;27(6):314–40. [PMID: 30380928]

Yusuf S et al; HOPE-3 Investigators. Cholesterol lowering in intermediate-risk persons without cardiovascular disease. N Engl J Med. 2016 May 26;374(21):2021–31. [PMID: 27040132]

DRUG THERAPY: CURRENT ANTIHYPERTENSIVE AGENTS

There are many classes of antihypertensive drugs of which six (ACE inhibitors, ARBs, renin inhibitors, calcium channel blockers, diuretics, and beta-blockers) are suitable for initial therapy based on efficacy and tolerability. A number of considerations enter into the selection of the initial regimen for a given patient. These include the weight of evidence for beneficial effects on clinical outcomes, the safety and tolerability of the drug, its cost, demographic differences in response, concomitant medical conditions, and lifestyle issues. The specific classes of antihypertensive medications are discussed below, and guidelines for the choice of initial medications are offered.

A. Angiotensin-Converting Enzyme Inhibitors

ACE inhibitors are commonly used as the initial medication in mild to moderate hypertension (Table 11–6). Their primary mode of action is inhibition of the RAAS, but they also inhibit bradykinin degradation, stimulate the synthesis of vasodilating prostaglandins, and can reduce sympathetic nervous system activity. These latter actions may explain why they exhibit some effect even in patients with low plasma renin activity. ACE inhibitors appear to be more effective in younger white patients. They are relatively less effective in blacks and older persons and in predominantly systolic hypertension. Although as single therapy they achieve adequate antihypertensive control in only about 40–50% of patients, the combination of an ACE inhibitor and a diuretic or calcium channel blocker is potent.

ACE inhibitors are the agents of choice in persons with type 1 diabetes with frank proteinuria or evidence of kidney dysfunction because they delay the progression to end-stage renal disease. Many authorities have expanded this indication to include persons with type 1 and type 2 diabetes mellitus with microalbuminuria who do not meet the usual criteria for antihypertensive therapy. ACE inhibitors may also delay the progression of nondiabetic kidney disease. The Heart Outcomes Prevention Evaluation (HOPE) trial demonstrated that the ACE inhibitor ramipril reduced the number of cardiovascular deaths, nonfatal myocardial infarctions, and nonfatal strokes and also reduced the incidence of new-onset heart failure, kidney dysfunction, and new-onset diabetes in a population of patients at high risk for vascular events. Although this was not specifically a hypertensive population, the benefits were associated with a modest reduction in blood pressure, and the results inferentially support the use of ACE inhibitors in similar hypertensive patients. ACE inhibitors are a drug of choice (usually in conjunction with a diuretic and a beta-blocker) in patients with heart failure with reduced ejection fraction and are indicated also in asymptomatic patients with reduced ejection fraction. An advantage of the ACE inhibitors is their relative freedom from troublesome side effects. Severe hypotension can occur in patients with bilateral renal artery stenosis; sudden increases in creatinine may ensue but are usually reversible with the discontinuation of the ACE inhibitor. Hyperkalemia may develop in patients with kidney disease and type IV renal tubular acidosis (commonly seen in patients with diabetes) and in older adults. A baseline metabolic panel should be drawn prior to starting medications that interfere with the RAAS, repeated 1–2 weeks after initiation of therapy to evaluate changes in creatinine and potassium. Minor dose adjustments of these medications rarely trigger significant shifts in these values. A chronic dry cough is common, seen in 10% of patients or more, and may require stopping the drug. Skin rashes are observed with any ACE inhibitor. Angioedema is an uncommon but potentially dangerous side effect of all agents of this class because of their inhibition of kininase. Exposure of the fetus to ACE inhibitors during the second and third trimesters of pregnancy has been associated with a variety of defects due to hypotension and reduced renal blood flow.

B. Angiotensin II Receptor Blockers

ARBs can improve cardiovascular outcomes in patients with hypertension as well as in patients with related conditions, such as heart failure and type 2 diabetes with nephropathy. ARBs have not been compared with ACE inhibitors in randomized controlled trials in patients with hypertension, but two trials comparing losartan with captopril in heart failure and post–myocardial infarction left ventricular dysfunction showed trends toward worse outcomes in the losartan group. By contrast, valsartan seems as effective as ACE inhibitors in these settings. Within group heterogeneity of antihypertensive potency and duration of action might explain such observations. The Losartan Intervention for Endpoints (LIFE) trial in nearly 9000 hypertensive patients with electrocardiographic evidence of left ventricular hypertrophy—comparing losartan with the beta-blocker atenolol as initial therapy—demonstrated a significant reduction in stroke with losartan. Of note is that in diabetic patients, death and myocardial infarction were also reduced, and there was a lower occurrence of new-onset diabetes. In this trial, as in the Antihypertensive and Lipid-Lowering Treatment to Prevent Heart Attack Trial (ALLHAT), blacks treated with RAAS inhibitors exhibited less blood pressure reduction and less benefit with regard to clinical end points. In the treatment of hypertension, combination therapy with an ACE inhibitor and an ARB is not advised because it generally offers no advantage over monotherapy at maximum dose with addition of a complementary class where necessary.

Unlike ACE inhibitors, the ARBs rarely cause cough and are less likely to be associated with skin rashes or angioedema. However, as seen with ACE inhibitors, hyperkalemia can be a problem, and patients with bilateral renal artery stenosis may exhibit hypotension and worsened kidney function. Olmesartan has been linked to a sprue-like syndrome, presenting with abdominal pain, weight loss, and nausea, which subsides upon drug discontinuation. There is evidence from an observational study suggesting that ARBs and ACE inhibitors are less likely to be associated with depression than calcium channel blockers and beta-blockers.

C. Renin Inhibitors

Since renin cleavage of angiotensinogen is the rate-limiting step in the renin-angiotensin cascade, the most efficient inactivation of this system would be expected with renin inhibition.

Table 11–6. Antihypertensive drugs: renin and ACE inhibitors and angiotensin II receptor blockers.

Drug	Proprietary Name	Initial Oral Dosage	Dosage Range	Cost per Unit	Cost of 30 Days of Treatment (Average Dosage)[1]	Adverse Effects	Comments
Renin Inhibitors							
Aliskiren	Tekturna	150 mg once daily	150–300 mg once daily	$8.31/150 mg	$249.36	Angioedema, hypotension, hyperkalemia. Contraindicated in pregnancy.	Probably metabolized by CYP3A4. Absorption is inhibited by high-fat meal.
Aliskiren and HCTZ	Tekturna HCT	150 mg/12.5 mg once daily	150 mg/12.5 mg–300 mg/25 mg once daily	$8.31/150 mg/12.5 mg	$249.36		
ACE Inhibitors							
Benazepril	Lotensin	10 mg once daily	5–40 mg in 1 or 2 doses	$1.05/20 mg	$31.50	Cough, hypotension, dizziness, kidney dysfunction, hyperkalemia, angioedema; taste alteration and rash (may be more frequent with captopril); rarely, proteinuria, blood dyscrasia. Contraindicated in pregnancy.	More fosinopril is excreted by the liver in patients with kidney dysfunction (dose reduction may or may not be necessary). Captopril and lisinopril are active without metabolism. Captopril, enalapril, lisinopril, and quinapril are approved for heart failure.
Benazepril and HCTZ	Lotensin HCT	5 mg/6.25 mg once daily	5 mg/6.25 mg–20 mg/25 mg	$2.07/any dose	$62.10		
Benazepril and amlodipine	Lotrel	10 mg/2.5 mg once daily	10 mg/2.5 mg–40 mg/10 mg	$3.32/20 mg/10 mg	$99.60		
Captopril	Capoten	25 mg twice daily	50–450 mg in 2 or 3 doses	$1.36/25 mg	$81.60		
Captopril and HCTZ	Capozide	25 mg/15 mg twice daily	25 mg/15 mg–50 mg/25 mg	$2.85/25 mg/15 mg	$171.00		
Enalapril	Vasotec	5 mg once daily	5–40 mg in 1 or 2 doses	$1.00/20 mg	$30.00		
Enalapril and HCTZ	Vaseretic	5 mg/12.5 mg once daily	5 mg/12.5 mg–10 mg/25 mg	$1.19/10 mg/25 mg	$35.80		
Fosinopril	Monopril	10 mg once daily	10–80 mg in 1 or 2 doses	$1.19/20 mg	$35.70		
Fosinopril and HCTZ	Monopril-HCT	10 mg/12.5 mg once daily	10 mg/12.5 mg–20 mg/12.5 mg	$1.26/any dose	$37.80		
Lisinopril	Prinivil, Zestril	5–10 mg once daily	5–40 mg once daily	$0.08/20 mg	$2.45		
Lisinopril and HCTZ	Prinzide or Zestoretic	10 mg/12.5 mg once daily	10 mg/12.5 mg–20 mg/12.5 mg	$1.17/20 mg/12.5 mg	$35.10		
Moexipril	Univasc	7.5 mg once daily	7.5–30 mg in 1 or 2 doses	$1.39/7.5 mg	$41.70		
Moexipril and HCTZ	Uniretic	7.5 mg/12.5 mg once daily	7.5 mg/12.5 mg–15 mg/25 mg	$1.34/7.5 mg/12.5 mg	$40.20		

Drug	Proprietary Name	Initial Oral Dosage	Dosage Range	Cost per Unit	Cost of 30 Days Treatment	Adverse Effects	Comments
Perindopril	Aceon	4 mg once daily	4–16 mg in 1 or 2 doses	$2.80/8 mg	$84.00		
Perindopril and amlodipine	Prestalia	3.5 mg/2.5 mg once daily	14 mg/10 mg once daily	$5.87/7 mg/5 mg	$176.10		
Quinapril	Accupril	10 mg once daily	10–80 mg in 1 or 2 doses	$1.22/20 mg	$36.60		
Quinapril and HCTZ	Accuretic	10 mg/12.5 mg once daily	10 mg/12.5 mg–20 mg/25 mg	$1.22/20 mg/12.5 mg	$36.60		
Ramipril	Altace	2.5 mg once daily	2.5–20 mg in 1 or 2 doses	$1.62/5 mg	$48.60		
Trandolapril	Mavik	1 mg once daily	1–8 mg once daily	$1.21/4 mg	$36.30		
Trandolapril and verapamil	Tarka	2 mg/180 mg ER once daily	2 mg/180 mg ER–8 mg/480 mg ER	$5.29/any dose	$158.70		
Angiotensin II Receptor Blockers							
Azilsartan	Edarbi	40 mg once daily	40–80 mg once daily	$8.14/80 mg	$244.10	Hyperkalemia, kidney dysfunction, rare angioedema. Combinations have additional side effects. Contraindicated in pregnancy.	Losartan has a flat dose-response curve. Valsartan and irbesartan have wider dose-response ranges and longer durations of action. Addition of low-dose diuretic (separately or as combination pills) increases the response.
Azilsartan and chlorthalidone	Edarbychlor	40 mg/12.5 mg once daily	40 mg/12.5–40 mg/25 mg once daily	$7.68/any dose	$230.40		
Candesartan cilexitil	Atacand	16 mg once daily	8–32 mg once daily	$3.31/16 mg	$99.30		
Candesartan cilexitil and HCTZ	Atacand HCT	16 mg/12.5 mg once daily	32 mg/12.5 mg once daily	$4.72/16 mg/12.5 mg	$141.60		
Eprosartan	Teveten	600 mg once daily	400–800 mg in 1–2 doses	$3.43/600 mg	$102.90		
Irbesartan	Avapro	150 mg once daily	150–300 mg once daily	$3.07/150 mg	$92.10		
Irbesartan and HCTZ	Avalide	150 mg/12.5 mg once daily	150–300 mg irbesartan once daily	$3.72/150 mg/12.5 mg	$111.60		
Losartan and HCTZ	Hyzaar	50 mg/12.5 mg once daily	50 mg/12.5 mg–100 mg/25 mg tablets once daily	$0.28/50 mg/12.5 mg/tablet	$8.40		
Olmesartan	Benicar	20 mg once daily	20–40 mg once daily	$6.28/20 mg	$188.40		
Olmesartan and HCTZ	Benicar HCT	20 mg/12.5 mg once daily	20 mg/12.5 mg–40 mg/25 mg once daily	$6.28/20 mg/12.5 mg	$188.40		
Olmesartan and amlodipine	Azor	20 mg/5 mg once daily	20 mg/5 mg–40 mg/10 mg	$3.03/20 mg/5 mg	$90.90		

(continued)

Table 11–9. Antihypertensive drugs: beta-adrenergic blocking agents. (continued)

Drug	Proprietary Name	Initial Oral Dosage	Dosage Range	Cost per Unit	Cost of 30 Days of Treatment (Based on Average Dosage)[1]	Special Properties					Comments[5]
						Beta-1 Selectivity[2]	ISA[3]	MSA[4]	Lipid Solubility	Renal vs Hepatic Elimination	
Metoprolol and HCTZ	Lopressor HCT	50 mg/12.5 mg twice daily	50 mg/25 mg–200 mg/50 mg	$1.63/100 mg/25 mg	$48.90	+	0	+	+++	H	
Nadolol	Corgard	20 mg once daily	20–320 mg once daily	$3.97/40 mg	$119.10	0	0	0	0	R	
Nadolol and bendroflumethazide	Corzide	40 mg/5 mg once daily	40 mg/5 mg–80 mg/5 mg once daily	$4.66/40 mg/5 mg	$139.80						
Nebivolol	Bystolic	5 mg once daily	40 mg once daily	$5.73/5 mg	$171.90	+	0	0	++	H	Nitric oxide potentiating vasodilatory activity.
Pindolol	Visken	5 mg twice daily	10–60 mg in 2 doses	$1.10/5 mg	$66.00	0	++	+	+	H > R	In adults, 35% renal clearance.
Propranolol	Inderal / Inderal LA / InnoPran XL	20 mg twice daily / 80 mg ER once daily / 80 mg ER once nightly	40–640 mg in 2 doses / 120–640 mg ER once daily / 80–120 mg ER once nightly	$0.72/40 mg / $2.98/120 mg / $30.20/120 mg	$43.20 / $89.40 / $906.00	0	0	++	+++	H	Also indicated for angina and post-MI.
Propranolol and HCTZ	(generic)	40 mg/25 mg twice daily	80 mg/25 mg twice daily	$1.41/80 mg/25 mg	$84.60	0	0	++	+++	H	
Timolol	(generic)	5 mg twice daily	10–60 mg in 2 doses	$1.70/10 mg	$102.00	0	0	0	++	H > R	Also indicated for post-MI; 80% hepatic clearance.

[1]Average wholesale price (AWP, for AB-rated generic when available) for quantity listed. Source: IBM Micromedex Red Book (electronic version) IBM Watson Health. Greenwood Village, CO, USA. Available at https://www.micromedexsolutions.com, accessed March 12, 2019. AWP may not accurately represent the actual pharmacy cost because wide contractual variations exist among institutions.

[2]Agents with beta-1 selectivity are less likely to precipitate bronchospasm and decrease peripheral blood flow in low doses, but selectivity is only relative.

[3]Agents with ISA cause less resting bradycardia and lipid changes.

[4]MSA generally occurs at concentrations greater than those necessary for beta-adrenergic blockade. The clinical importance of MSA by beta-blockers has not been defined.

[5]Adverse effects of all beta-blockers: bronchospasm, fatigue, sleep disturbance and nightmares, bradycardia and atrioventricular block, worsening of heart failure, cold extremities, gastrointestinal disturbances, erectile dysfunction, ↑ triglycerides, ↓ high-density lipoprotein cholesterol, rare blood dyscrasias.

ANA, antinuclear antibody; ER, extended release; HCTZ, hydrochlorothiazide; ISA, intrinsic sympathomimetic activity; LE, lupus erythematosus; MI, myocardial infarction; MSA, membrane-stabilizing activity; SR, sustained release; 0, no effect; +, some effect; ++, moderate effect; +++, most effect.

Table 11–10. Alpha-adrenoceptor blocking agents, sympatholytics, and vasodilators.

Drug	Proprietary Names	Initial Dosage	Dosage Range	Cost per Unit	Cost of 30 Days of Treatment (Average Dosage)[1]	Adverse Effects	Comments
Alpha-Adrenoceptor Blockers							
Doxazosin	Cardura	1 mg at bedtime	1–16 mg once daily	$1.03/4 mg	$30.90 (4 mg once daily)	Syncope with first dose; postural hypotension, dizziness, palpitations, headache, weakness, drowsiness, sexual dysfunction, anticholinergic effects, urinary incontinence; first-dose effects may be less with doxazosin.	May ↑ HDL and ↓ LDL cholesterol. May provide short-term relief of obstructive prostatic symptoms. Less effective in preventing cardiovascular events than diuretics.
	Cardura XL	4 mg ER once daily	4–8 ER once daily	$6.42/4 mg ER	$192.60 (4 mg ER once daily)		
Prazosin	Minipress	1 mg at bedtime	2–20 mg in 2 or 3 doses	$2.18/5 mg	$130.80 (5 mg twice daily)		
Terazosin	Hytrin	1 mg at bedtime	1–20 mg in 1 or 2 doses	$1.60/1, 2, 5, 10 mg	$48.00 (5 mg once daily)		
Central Sympatholytics							
Clonidine	Catapres	0.1 mg twice daily	0.2–0.6 mg in 2 doses	$0.21/0.1 mg	$12.60 (0.1 mg twice daily)	Sedation, dry mouth, sexual dysfunction, headache, bradyarrhythmias; side effects may be less with guanfacine. Contact dermatitis with clonidine patch. Methyldopa also causes hepatitis, hemolytic anemia, fever.	"Rebound" hypertension may occur even after gradual withdrawal.
	Catapres TTS (transdermal patch)	0.1 mg/day patch weekly	0.1–0.3 mg/day patch weekly	$55.77/0.2 mg patch	$223.08 (0.2 mg weekly)		
Clonidine and chlorthalidone	Clorpres	0.1 mg/15 mg one to three times daily	0.1 mg/15 mg–0.3 mg/ 15 mg	$2.77/0.1 mg/ 15 mg	$166.20/0.1 mg/ 15 mg twice daily		
Guanfacine	Tenex	1 mg once daily	1–3 mg once daily	$0.87/1 mg	$26.10 (1 mg once daily)		
Methyldopa	Aldochlor	250 mg twice daily	500–2000 mg in 2 doses	$0.66/500 mg	$39.60 (500 mg twice daily)		Methyldopa should be avoided in favor of safer agents.

(continued)

Table 11–10. Alpha-adrenoceptor blocking agents, sympatholytics, and vasodilators. (continued)

Drug	Proprietary Names	Initial Dosage	Dosage Range	Cost per Unit	Cost of 30 Days of Treatment (Average Dosage)[1]	Adverse Effects	Comments
Peripheral Neuronal Antagonists							
Reserpine	(generic)	0.05 mg once daily	0.05–0.25 mg once daily	$1.19/0.1 mg	$35.70 (0.1 mg once daily)	Depression (less likely at low dosages, ie, < 0.25 mg), night terrors, nasal stuffiness, drowsiness, peptic disease, GI disturbances, bradycardia.	
Direct Vasodilators							
Hydralazine	Apresoline	25 mg twice daily	50–300 mg in 2–4 doses	$0.15/25 mg	$9.00 (25 mg twice daily)	GI disturbances, tachycardia, headache, nasal congestion, rash, LE-like syndrome.	May worsen or precipitate angina.
Minoxidil	(generic)	5 mg once daily	10–40 mg once daily	$1.29/10 mg	$38.70 (10 mg once daily)	Tachycardia, fluid retention, headache, hirsutism, pericardial effusion, thrombocytopenia.	Should be used in combination with beta-blocker and diuretic.

[1]Average wholesale price (AWP, for AB-rated generic when available) for quantity listed.
Source: IBM Micromedex Red Book (electronic version) IBM Watson Health. Greenwood Village, CO, USA. Available at https://www.micromedexsolutions.com, accessed March 12, 2019. AWP may not accurately represent the actual pharmacy cost because wide contractual variations exist among institutions.
ER, extended release; GI, gastrointestinal; LE, lupus erythematosus.

causes hepatitis and hemolytic anemia and should be restricted to individuals who have already tolerated long-term therapy. There is considerable experience with methyldopa in pregnant women, and it is still used for this population. Clonidine is available in patches, which may have particular value in noncompliant patients.

J. Peripheral Sympathetic Inhibitors

These agents are now used infrequently and usually in refractory hypertension. Reserpine remains a cost-effective antihypertensive agent (Table 11–10). Its reputation for inducing mental depression and its other side effects—sedation, nasal stuffiness, sleep disturbances, and peptic ulcers—has made it unpopular, though these problems are uncommon at low dosages. Guanethidine and guanadrel inhibit catecholamine release from peripheral neurons but frequently cause orthostatic hypotension (especially in the morning or after exercise), diarrhea, and fluid retention.

K. Arteriolar Dilators

Hydralazine and minoxidil (Table 11–10) relax vascular smooth muscle and produce peripheral vasodilation. When given alone, they stimulate reflex tachycardia, increase myocardial contractility, and cause headache, palpitations, and fluid retention. They are usually given in combination with diuretics and beta-blockers in resistant patients. Hydralazine produces frequent gastrointestinal disturbances and may induce a lupus-like syndrome. Minoxidil causes hirsutism and marked fluid retention; this very potent agent is reserved for the most refractory of cases.

▶ Antihypertensive Medications & the Risk of Cancer

A number of observational studies have examined the association between long-term exposure to antihypertensive medications and cancer. Weak associations have been suggested by some of these studies, but results have been very mixed. Examples of positive studies include an association between ACE inhibitors and lung cancer (hazard ratio 1.14) and between photosensitizing drugs and squamous skin cancer (the use of alpha-2-receptors blockers and diuretics was associated with a 17% increased risk of squamous cell cancer). The relationship between calcium channel blockers and breast cancer remains uncertain. In the absence of large-scale prospective studies with cancer as a prespecified outcome measure, the effect of antihypertensive drugs on the risk of cancer remains uncertain. By contrast, the beneficial effect of these drugs on cardiovascular outcomes has been clearly established. Concern about increased risk of cancer should not be minimized, but at present there are no compelling data to prompt a change in prescribing patterns.

Hicks BM et al. Angiotensin converting enzyme inhibitors and risk of lung cancer: population based cohort study. BMJ. 2018 Oct 24;363:k4209. [PMID: 30355745]
Su KA et al. Photosensitizing antihypertensive drug use and risk of cutaneous squamous cell carcinoma. Br J Dermatol. 2018 Nov;179(5):1088–94. [PMID: 29723931]

Wright CM et al. Calcium channel blockers and breast cancer incidence: an updated systematic review and meta-analysis of the evidence. Cancer Epidemiol. 2017 Oct;50(Pt A):113–24. [PMID: 28866282]

▶ Developing an Antihypertensive Regimen

Historically, data from large placebo-controlled trials supported the overall conclusion that antihypertensive therapy with diuretics and beta-blockers had a major beneficial effect on a broad spectrum of cardiovascular outcomes, reducing the incidence of stroke by 30–50% and of heart failure by 40–50%, and halting progression to accelerated hypertension syndromes. The decreases in fatal and nonfatal coronary heart disease and cardiovascular and total mortality were less dramatic, ranging from 10% to 15%. Similar placebo-controlled data pertaining to the newer agents are generally lacking, except for stroke reduction with the calcium channel blocker nitrendipine in the Systolic Hypertension in Europe trial. However, there is substantial evidence that ACE inhibitors, and to a lesser extent ARBs, reduce adverse cardiovascular outcomes in other related populations (eg, patients with diabetic nephropathy, heart failure, or postmyocardial infarction and individuals at high risk for cardiovascular events). Most large clinical trials that have compared outcomes in relatively unselected patients have failed to show a difference between newer agents—such as ACE inhibitors, calcium channel blockers, and ARBs—and the older diuretic-based regimens with regard to survival, myocardial infarction, and stroke. Where differences have been observed, they have mostly been attributable to subtle asymmetries in blood pressure control rather than to any inherent advantages of one agent over another. Recommendations for initial treatment identify ACE inhibitors, ARBs, and calcium channel blockers as valid choices. Because of their adverse metabolic profile, initial therapy with thiazides might best be restricted to older patients. Thiazides are acceptable as first-line therapy in blacks because of specific efficacy in this group.

As discussed above, beta-blockers are not ideal first-line drugs in the treatment of hypertension without compelling indications for their use (such as active coronary artery disease and heart failure). Vasodilator beta-blockers (such as carvedilol and nebivolol) may produce better outcomes than traditional beta-blockers; however, this possibility remains a theoretical consideration.

The American Diabetes Association has advocated evening dosing of one or more antihypertensive medications to restore nocturnal blood pressure dipping. Outcomes data to support this proposal are limited. The Spanish MAPEC study of such nocturnal antihypertensive dosing showed a significant reduction in a range of major cardiovascular events in 2156 participants over 5.6 years. However, there are concerns that ischemic optic neuropathy may be triggered by profound nocturnal hypotension. Thus, larger studies are necessary before this approach can be firmly recommended.

Drugs that interrupt the renin-angiotensin cascade are more effective in young, white persons, in whom renin tends to be higher. Calcium channel blockers and diuretics are more effective in older or black persons, in whom renin

Table 11–11. A step care approach to the initiation and titration of antihypertension medications.[1,2]

Step 1	ACE inhibitor/ARB **or**[3] Calcium channel blocker **or** Thiazide diuretic[4]
Step 2	ACE inhibitor/ARB **plus** Calcium channel blocker **or** thiazide diuretic[5]
Step 3	ACE inhibitor/ARB **plus** calcium channel blocker **plus** thiazide diuretic
Step 4	ACE inhibitor/ARB **plus** calcium channel blocker **plus** thiazide diuretic **plus** spironolactone[6]

[1]Allow 2 weeks to reach full effect of each drug. Proceed through steps until target blood pressure is attained.
[2]Beta-blockers can be used at any stage if specifically indicated, eg, heart failure or angina.
[3]The European guidelines recommend starting with low-dose combination of two antihypertensive drugs. American guidelines suggest initiation with dual therapy for stage 2 hypertension, > 160/100 mm Hg.
[4]Thiazide or calcium channel blocker is more effective initial therapy in older people and blacks.
[5]If required, add a calcium channel blocker rather than diuretic in younger patients to avoid long-term exposure to metabolic side effects of diuretics.
[6]Alternatives to spironolactone include eplerenone, amiloride, or triamterene. Watch for hyperkalemia, especially if also receiving ACE inhibitor/ARB. Avoid potassium-sparing diuretics in advanced CKD. If more than three drugs are required at maximum dose, consider specialist referral.
ACE, angiotensin-converting enzyme; ARB angiotensin receptor blocker; CKD chronic kidney disease.

levels are generally lower. Many patients require two or more medications and even then a substantial proportion fail to achieve the goal blood pressure. A stepped care approach to the drug treatment of hypertension is outlined in Table 11–11. In diabetic patients, three or four drugs are usually required to reduce systolic blood pressure to less than 140 mm Hg. In many patients, blood pressure cannot be adequately controlled with any combination. As a result, debating the appropriate first-line agent is less relevant than determining the most appropriate combinations of agents. The mnemonic ABCD can be used to remember four classes of antihypertensive medications. These four classes can be divided into two categories: AB and CD. AB refers to drugs that block the RAAS (**A**CE/ARB and **b**eta-blockers). CD refers to those that work in other pathways (**c**alcium channel blockers and **d**iuretics). As discussed above, beta-blockers are no longer considered first-line drugs in the absence of compelling indications. Combinations of drugs between the two categories are more potent than combinations from within a category. Many experts and practitioners recommend the use of fixed-dose combination antihypertensive agents as first-line therapy in patients with substantially elevated systolic pressures (greater than 160/100 mm Hg) or difficult-to-control hypertension (which is often associated with diabetes or kidney dysfunction). In light of unwanted metabolic effects, calcium channel blockers might be preferable to thiazides in the younger hypertensive patient requiring a second antihypertensive drug following initiation of therapy with an ACE inhibitor or ARB. Furthermore, based on the results from the ACCOMPLISH trial, a combination of ACE inhibitor and calcium channel blocker may also prove optimal for patients at high risk for cardiovascular events. The initial use of low-dose combinations allows faster blood pressure reduction without substantially higher intolerance rates and is likely to be better accepted by patients. Data from the ALTITUDE study (in patients with type 2 diabetes and chronic kidney disease or

cardiovascular disease or both) indicate that the addition of aliskiren to either ARB or ACE inhibitor was associated with worse outcomes and cannot be recommended, at least in this population. A suggested approach to treatment, tailored to patient demographics, is outlined in Table 11–12.

In sum, as a prelude to treatment, the patient should be informed of common side effects and the need for diligent compliance. In patients with mild or stage 1 hypertension (less than 160/90 mm Hg) in whom pharmacotherapy is indicated, treatment should start with a single agent or two-drug combination at a low dose. Follow-up visits should usually be at 4- to 6-week intervals to allow for full medication effects to be established (especially with diuretics) before further titration or adjustment. If, after titration to usual doses, the patient has shown a discernible but incomplete response and a good tolerance of the initial drug, another medication should be added. See Goals of Treatment, above. As a rule of thumb, a blood pressure reduction of 10 mm Hg can be expected for each antihypertensive agent added to the regimen and titrated to the optimum dose. In those with more severe hypertension (stage 2), or with comorbidities (such as diabetes) that are likely to render them resistant to treatment, initiation with combination therapy is advised and more frequent follow-up is indicated.

Patients who are compliant with their medications and who do not respond to conventional combination regimens should usually be evaluated for secondary hypertension before proceeding to more complex regimens.

▶ **Medication Nonadherence**

Adherence to antihypertensive treatment is alarmingly poor. In one European study of patients' antihypertensive medication compliance, there was a 40% discontinuation rate at 1 year after initiation. Only 39% of patients were found to be taking their medications continuously over a 10-year period. Collaborative care, utilizing physicians,

Table 11–12. Choice of antihypertensive agent based on demographic considerations.[1,2]

	Black, All Ages	All Others, Age < 55 Years	All Others, Age > 55 Years
First-line	CCB or diuretic	ACE inhibitor or ARB[3] or CCB or diuretic[4]	CCB or diuretic[5]
Second-line	ACE inhibitor or ARB[3] or vasodilating beta-blocker[6]	Vasodilating beta-blocker	ACE inhibitor or ARB[3] or vasodilating beta-blocker[6]
Resistant hypertension	Aldosterone receptor blocker	Aldosterone receptor blocker	Aldosterone receptor blocker
Additional options	Centrally acting alpha-agonist or peripheral alpha-antagonist[7]	Centrally acting alpha-agonist or peripheral alpha-antagonist[7]	Centrally acting alpha-agonist or peripheral alpha-antagonist[7]

[1]Compelling indications may alter the selection of an antihypertensive drug.
[2]Start with full dose of one agent, or lower doses of combination therapy. In stage 2 hypertension, consider initiating therapy with a fixed dose combination.
[3]Women of childbearing age should avoid ACE inhibitors and ARBs or discontinue as soon as pregnancy is diagnosed.
[4]The adverse metabolic effects of thiazide diuretics and beta-blockers should be considered in younger patients but may be less important in the older patient.
[5]For patients with significant kidney dysfunction, use loop diuretic instead of thiazide.
[6]There are theoretical advantages in the use of vasodilating beta-blockers such as carvedilol and nebivolol.
[7]Alpha-antagonists may precipitate or exacerbate orthostatic hypotension in older adults.
ACE, angiotensin-converting enzyme; ARB, angiotensin receptor blocker; CCB, calcium channel blocker.

pharmacists, social workers, and nurses to encourage compliance, has had a variable and often rather modest effect on blood pressure control. Adherence is enhanced by patient education and by use of home blood pressure measurement. The choice of antihypertensive medication is important. Better compliance has been reported for patients whose medications could be taken once daily or as combination pills. Adherence is best with ACE inhibitors and ARBs, and worse with beta-blockers and diuretics.

Consideration of Gender in Hypertension

Because of the preponderance of male recruitment into large-scale clinical trials, the impact of gender on the evaluation and management of hypertension remains uncertain. The limited data that exist suggest a steeper relationship in women between 24-hour ambulatory and night time systolic blood pressure and the risk of cardiovascular events. There are many gender-specific effects on the mechanisms and end organ impact of hypertension. In younger adults, men are more likely to be hypertensive than women, a relationship that reverses in later life. Regression of left ventricular hypertrophy in response to ACE inhibitors is less pronounced in women. Women are more likely to have isolated systolic hypertension, probably because they develop more active left ventricular systolic function and greater vascular stiffness than men. Fibromuscular dysplasia of the renal artery is much more common in women than men. As yet, however, there are no data to support a different blood pressure target in women.

Special Considerations in the Treatment of Diabetic Hypertensive Patients

Hypertensive patients with diabetes are at particularly high risk for cardiovascular events. Data from the ACCORD study of diabetic patients demonstrated that most of the benefits of blood pressure lowering were seen with a systolic target of less than 140 mm Hg. Although there was a reduction in stroke risk at a systolic target below 120/70 mm Hg, treatment to this lower target was associated with an *increased* risk of serious adverse effects. US and Canadian guidelines recommend a blood pressure goal of less than 130/80 mm Hg in diabetic patients. Because of the beneficial effects of ACE inhibitors in diabetic nephropathy, they should be part of the initial treatment regimen. ARBs or perhaps renin inhibitors may be substituted in those intolerant of ACE inhibitors. While the ONTARGET study showed that combinations of ACE inhibitors and ARBs in persons with atherosclerosis or type 2 diabetes with end-organ damage appeared to minimize proteinuria, this strategy slightly increased the risks of progression to dialysis and of death; thus, it is not recommended. Most diabetic patients require combinations of three to five agents to achieve target blood pressure, usually including a diuretic and a calcium channel blocker or beta-blocker. In addition to rigorous blood pressure control, treatment of persons with diabetes should include aggressive treatment of other risk factors.

Treatment of Hypertension in Chronic Kidney Disease

Hypertension is present in 40% of patients with a GFR of 60–90 mL/min, and 75% of patients with a GFR less than 30 mL/min. The rate of progression of chronic kidney disease is markedly slowed by treatment of hypertension. In the SPRINT trial, the reduction in cardiovascular risk associated with lower blood pressure targets was also observed in the subgroup with a GFR of less than 60 mL/min. However, an effect of *lower* blood pressure targets on the slowing of chronic kidney disease progression appears to be restricted to those with pronounced proteinuria. In the SPRINT trial, the lower blood pressure goal was associated with increased risk of acute kidney injury, but this was generally reversible and not associated with elevated biomarkers for ischemic injury. Most experts recommend a blood pressure target of less than 130/80 mm Hg in patients with chronic kidney disease, with consideration of more intensive lowering if proteinuria greater than 1 g per 24 hours is present. Medications that interrupt the renin-angiotensin cascade can slow the progression of kidney disease and are preferred for initial therapy, especially in those with albuminuria of greater than 300 mg/g creatinine. Transition from thiazide to loop diuretic is often necessary to control volume expansion as the eGFR falls below 30 mL/min. ACE inhibitors remain protective and safe in kidney disease associated with significant proteinuria and serum creatinine as high as 5 mg/dL (380 mcmol/L). However, the use of drugs blocking the RAAS cascade in patients with advanced chronic kidney disease should be supervised by a nephrologist. Kidney function and electrolytes should be measured 1 week after initiating treatment and subsequently monitored carefully in patients with kidney disease. An increase in creatinine of 20–30% is acceptable and expected; more exaggerated responses suggest the possibility of renal artery stenosis or volume contraction. Although lower blood pressure levels are associated with acute decreases in GFR, this appears not to translate into an increased risk of developing end-stage renal disease in the long term. Persistence with ACE inhibitor or ARB therapy in the face of hyperkalemia is probably not warranted, since other antihypertensive medications are renoprotective as long as goal blood pressures are maintained. However, diuretics can often be helpful in controlling mild hyperkalemia, and there are novel cation exchange polymers (such as patiromer) that sequester potassium in the gut and are more effective and better tolerated than sodium polystyrene sulfonate.

Hypertension Management in Blacks

Substantial evidence indicates that blacks are not only more likely to become hypertensive and more susceptible to the cardiovascular and renal complications of hypertension—they also respond differently to many antihypertensive medications. The REGARDS study illustrates these differences. At systolic blood pressures less than 120 mm Hg, black and white participants between 45 and 64 years of age had equal risk of stroke. For a 10 mm Hg increase in systolic blood pressure, the risk of stroke was threefold higher in black participants. At the level of stage 1 hypertension, the hazard ratio for stroke in black compared to white participants between 45 and 64 years of age was 2.35. This increased susceptibility may reflect genetic differences in the cause of hypertension or the subsequent responses to it, differences in occurrence of comorbid conditions such as diabetes or obesity, or environmental factors such as diet, activity, stress, or access to health care services. In any case, as in all persons with hypertension, a multifaceted program of education and lifestyle modification is warranted. Early introduction of combination therapy has been advocated, but there are no clinical trial data to support a lower than usual blood pressure goal (less than 140/90 mm Hg) in blacks. Because it appears that ACE inhibitors and ARBs—in the absence of concomitant diuretics—are less effective in blacks than in whites, initial therapy should generally be a diuretic or a diuretic in combination with a calcium channel blocker. However, inhibitors of the RAAS do lower blood pressure in black patients, are useful adjuncts to the recommended diuretic and calcium channel blockers, and should be used in patients with hypertension and compelling indications such as heart failure and kidney disease (especially in the presence of proteinuria) (Table 11–13). Black patients have an elevated risk of ACE inhibitor–associated angioedema and cough, so ARBs would be the preferred choice.

Treating Hypertension in Older Adults

Several studies in persons over 60 years of age have confirmed that antihypertensive therapy prevents fatal and nonfatal myocardial infarction and reduces overall cardiovascular mortality. In initiating therapy in older patients, pressure should be reduced more gradually with a safe intermediate systolic blood pressure goal of 160 mm Hg. The HYVET study indicated that a reasonable ultimate blood pressure goal would be 150/80 mm Hg. Updated guidelines suggest that blood pressure goals should not generally be influenced by age alone. An exploratory subgroup

Table 11–13. Recommended antihypertensive medications.

Indication	Antihypertensive Medication					
	Diuretic	Beta-Blocker	ACE Inhibitor	ARB	Calcium Channel Blocker	Aldosterone Antagonist
Heart failure	√	√	√	√		√
Following MI		√	√			√
High coronary disease risk	√	√	√		√	
Diabetes	√	√	√	√	√	
Chronic kidney disease			√	√		
Recurrent stroke prevention	√		√			

ACE, angiotensin-converting enzyme; ARB, angiotensin II receptor blocker; MI, myocardial infarction.

analysis of the SPRINT study found that people older than age 75 years showed benefit at the 120 mm Hg systolic treatment target. Importantly, these benefits were also evident in patients classified as frail. This more aggressive approach was, however, associated with greater risk of falls and worsening kidney function, indicating that close monitoring is required in elderly patients treated to lower blood pressure goals. In the SPRINT MIND study, the lower systolic blood pressure target of 120 mm Hg was associated with a 15% reduction in the incidence of mild cognitive impairment and probable all cause dementia compared to the 140 mm Hg in the target group. As discussed above, it is important to note that blood pressure measurements in the SPRINT study were made by automated devices, which are known to read lower than conventional office measurements. The same medications are used in older patients, but at 50% lower doses. As treatment is initiated, older patients should be carefully monitored for orthostasis, altered cognition and electrolyte disturbances. The elderly are especially susceptible to problems associated with polypharmacy, including drug interactions and dosing errors.

▶ Follow-Up of Patients Receiving Hypertension Therapy

Once blood pressure is controlled on a well-tolerated regimen, follow-up visits can be infrequent and laboratory testing limited to those appropriate for the patient and the medications used. Yearly monitoring of blood lipids is recommended, and an electrocardiogram could be repeated at 2- to 4-year intervals depending on whether initial abnormalities are present and on the presence of coronary risk factors. Patients who have had excellent blood pressure control for several years, especially if they have lost weight and initiated favorable lifestyle modifications, might be considered for a trial of reduced antihypertensive medications.

Boal AH et al. Monotherapy with major antihypertensive drug classes and risk of hospital admissions for mood disorders. Hypertension. 2016 Nov;68(5):1132–8. [PMID: 27733585]

Burnier M. Drug adherence in hypertension. Pharmacol Res. 2017 Nov;125(Pt B):142–9. [PMID: 28870498]

Carnethon MR et al; American Heart Association Council on Epidemiology and Prevention; Council on Cardiovascular Disease in the Young; Council on Cardiovascular and Stroke Nursing; Council on Clinical Cardiology; Council on Functional Genomics and Translational Biology; and Stroke Council. Cardiovascular health in African Americans: a scientific statement from the American Heart Association. Circulation. 2017 Nov 21;136(21):e393–423. [PMID: 29061565]

Chang AR et al. Blood pressure goals in patients with chronic kidney disease: a review of evidence and guidelines. Clin J Am Soc Nephrol. 2019 Jan 7;14(1):161–9. [PMID: 30455322]

Gudsoorkar PS et al. Changing concepts in hypertension management. J Hum Hypertens. 2017 Dec;31(12):763–7. [PMID: 28748919]

Kjeldsen SE et al. Intensive blood pressure lowering prevents mild cognitive impairment and possible dementia and slows development of white matter lesions in brain: the SPRINT Memory and Cognition IN Decreased Hypertension (SPRINT MIND) study. Blood Press. 2018 Oct;27(5):247–8. [PMID: 30175661]

Wenger NK et al. Hypertension across a woman's life cycle. J Am Coll Cardiol. 2018 Apr 24;71(16):1797–813. [PMID: 29673470]

RESISTANT HYPERTENSION

Resistant hypertension is defined as the failure to reach blood pressure control in patients who are adherent to full doses of an appropriate three-drug regimen (including a diuretic). Adherence is a major issue: the rate of partial or complete noncompliance probably approaches 50% in this group of patients; doxazosin, spironolactone, and hydrochlorothiazide were particularly unpopular in one Eastern European study based on drug assay. In the approach to resistant hypertension, the clinician should first confirm compliance and rule out "white coat hypertension," ideally using ambulatory or home-based measurement of blood pressure. Exacerbating factors should be considered (as outlined above). Finally, identifiable causes of resistant hypertension should be sought (Table 11–14). The clinician should pay particular attention to the type of diuretic being used in relation to the patient's kidney function. Aldosterone may play an important role in resistant hypertension and aldosterone receptor blockers can be very useful. If goal blood pressure cannot be achieved following completion of these steps, consultation with a hypertension specialist should be considered. Procedure-based approaches to resistant hypertension are being developed, but the Symplicity HTN 3 study failed to show that renal sympathetic ablation improved blood pressure compared to a sham-operated control group.

Wei FF et al. Diagnosis and management of resistant hypertension: state of the art. Nat Rev Nephrol. 2018 Jul;14(7):428–41. [PMID: 29700488]

Table 11–14. Causes of resistant hypertension.

Improper blood pressure measurement
Volume overload and pseudotolerance
Excess sodium intake
Volume retention from kidney disease
Inadequate diuretic therapy
Drug-induced or other causes
Nonadherence
Inadequate doses
Inappropriate combinations
Nonsteroidal anti-inflammatory drugs; cyclooxygenase-2 inhibitors
Cocaine, amphetamines, other illicit drugs
Sympathomimetics (decongestants, anorectics)
Oral contraceptives
Adrenal steroids
Cyclosporine and tacrolimus
Erythropoietin
Licorice (including some chewing tobacco)
Selected over-the-counter dietary supplements and medicines (eg, ephedra, ma huang, bitter orange)
Associated conditions
Obesity
Excess alcohol intake
Identifiable causes of hypertension (see Table 11–2)

Data from Chobanian AV et al. The Seventh Report of the Joint National Committee on Prevention, Detection, Evaluation, and Treatment of High Blood Pressure: the JNC 7 report. JAMA. 2003 May 21;289(19):2560–72.

HYPERTENSIVE URGENCIES & EMERGENCIES

Hypertensive emergencies have become less frequent in recent years but still require prompt recognition and aggressive but careful management. A spectrum of urgent presentations exists, and the appropriate therapeutic approach varies accordingly.

Hypertensive urgencies are situations in which blood pressure must be reduced within a few hours. These include patients with asymptomatic severe hypertension (systolic blood pressure greater than 220 mm Hg or diastolic pressure greater than 125 mm Hg that persists after a period of observation) and those with optic disk edema, progressive target-organ complications, and severe perioperative hypertension. Elevated blood pressure levels alone—in the absence of symptoms of new or progressive target-organ damage—rarely require emergency therapy. Parenteral drug therapy is not usually required, and partial reduction of blood pressure with relief of symptoms is the goal.

Hypertensive emergencies require substantial reduction of blood pressure within 1 hour to avoid the risk of serious morbidity or death. Although blood pressure is usually strikingly elevated (diastolic pressure greater than 130 mm Hg), the correlation between pressure and end-organ damage is often poor. *It is the presence of critical multiple end organ injury that determines the seriousness of the emergency and the approach to treatment.* Emergencies include hypertensive encephalopathy (headache, irritability, confusion, and altered mental status due to cerebrovascular spasm), hypertensive nephropathy (hematuria, proteinuria, and acute kidney injury due to arteriolar necrosis and intimal hyperplasia of the interlobular arteries), intracranial hemorrhage, aortic dissection, preeclampsia-eclampsia, pulmonary edema, unstable angina, or myocardial infarction. Encephalopathy or nephropathy accompanying hypertensive retinopathy has historically been termed **malignant hypertension**, but the therapeutic approach is identical to that used in other hypertensive emergencies.

Parenteral therapy is indicated in most hypertensive emergencies, especially if encephalopathy is present. The initial goal in hypertensive emergencies is to reduce the pressure by no more than 25% (within minutes to 1 or 2 hours) and then toward a level of 160/100 mm Hg within 2–6 hours. Excessive reductions in pressure may precipitate coronary, cerebral, or renal ischemia. To avoid such declines, the use of agents that have a predictable, dose-dependent, transient, and progressive antihypertensive effect is preferable (Table 11–15). In that regard, the use of sublingual or oral fast-acting nifedipine preparations is best avoided.

Acute ischemic stroke is often associated with marked elevation of blood pressure, which will usually fall spontaneously. In such cases, antihypertensives should only be used if the systolic blood pressure exceeds 180–200 mm Hg, and blood pressure should be reduced cautiously by 10–15% (Table 11–15). If thrombolytics are to be given, blood pressure should be maintained at less than 185/110 mm Hg during treatment and for 24 hours following treatment.

In intracerebral hemorrhage, the aim is to minimize bleeding by reducing the systolic blood pressure in most patients to 130–140 mm Hg within the first 6 hours. In acute subarachnoid hemorrhage, as long as the bleeding source remains uncorrected, a compromise must be struck between preventing further bleeding and maintaining cerebral perfusion in the face of cerebral vasospasm. In this situation, blood pressure goals depend on the patient's usual blood pressure. In previously normotensive patients, the target should be a systolic blood pressure of 110–120 mm Hg; in hypertensive patients, blood pressure should be treated to 20% below baseline pressure. In the treatment of hypertensive emergencies complicated by (or precipitated by) central nervous system injury, labetalol or nicardipine are good choices, since they are nonsedating and do not appear to cause significant increases in cerebral blood flow or intracranial pressure. Patients with subarachnoid hemorrhage should receive nimodipine for 3 weeks following presentation to minimize cerebral vasospasm. *In hypertensive emergencies arising from catecholaminergic mechanisms, such as pheochromocytoma or cocaine use, beta-blockers can worsen the hypertension because of unopposed peripheral vasoconstriction; nicardipine, clevidipine, or phentolamine is preferred.* Labetalol is useful in these patients if the heart rate must be controlled. Table 11–15 provides guidelines for the choice of antihypertensive agent based on the site of end-organ damage. ACE inhibitors are specifically indicated for hypertensive crisis from scleroderma.

► **Pharmacologic Management**

A. Parenteral Agents

Sodium nitroprusside is no longer the treatment of choice for acute hypertensive problems; in most situations, appropriate control of blood pressure is best achieved using combinations of nicardipine or clevidipine plus labetalol or esmolol. (Table 11–16 lists drugs, dosages, and adverse effects.)

1. Nicardipine—Intravenous nicardipine is the most potent and the longest acting of the parenteral calcium channel blockers. As a primarily arterial vasodilator, it has the potential to precipitate reflex tachycardia, and for that reason it should not be used without a beta-blocker in patients with coronary artery disease.

2. Clevidipine—Intravenous clevidipine is an L-type calcium channel blocker with a 1-minute half-life, which facilitates swift and tight control of severe hypertension. It acts on arterial resistance vessels and is devoid of venodilatory or cardiodepressant effects.

3. Labetalol—This combined beta- and alpha-blocking agent is the most potent adrenergic blocker for rapid blood pressure reduction. Other beta-blockers are far less potent. Excessive blood pressure drops are unusual. Experience with this agent in hypertensive syndromes associated with pregnancy has been favorable.

4. Esmolol—This rapidly acting beta-blocker is approved only for treatment of supraventricular tachycardia, but is often used for lowering blood pressure. It is less potent than labetalol and should be reserved for patients in whom there is particular concern about serious adverse events related to beta-blockers.

Table 11–15. Treatment of hypertensive emergency depending on primary site of end-organ damage. *See Table 11–16 for dosages.*

Type of Hypertensive Emergency	Recommended Drug Options and Combinations	Drugs to Avoid
Myocardial ischemia and infarction	Nicardipine plus esmolol[1] Nitroglycerin plus labetalol Nitroglycerin plus esmolol[1]	Hydralazine, diazoxide, minoxidil, nitroprusside
Acute kidney injury	Fenoldopam Nicardipine Clevidipine	
Aortic dissection	Esmolol plus nicardipine Esmolol plus clevidipine Labetalol Esmolol plus nitroprusside	Hydralazine, diazoxide, minoxidil
Acute pulmonary edema, LV systolic dysfunction	Nicardipine plus nitroglycerin[2] plus a loop diuretic Clevidipine plus nitroglycerin[2] plus a loop diuretic	Hydralazine, diazoxide, beta-blockers
Acute pulmonary edema, diastolic dysfunction	Esmolol plus low-dose nitroglycerin plus a loop diuretic Labetalol plus low-dose nitroglycerin plus a loop diuretic	
Ischemic stroke (systolic blood pressure > 180–200 mm Hg)	Nicardipine Clevidipine Labetalol	Nitroprusside, methyldopa, clonidine, nitroglycerin
Intracerebral hemorrhage (systolic blood pressure > 140–160 mm Hg)	Nicardipine Clevidipine Labetalol	Nitroprusside, methyldopa, clonidine, nitroglycerin
Hyperadrenergic states, including cocaine use	Nicardipine plus a benzodiazepine Clevidipine plus a benzodiazepine Phentolamine Labetalol	Beta-blockers
Preeclampsia, eclampsia	Labetalol Nicardipine	Diuretics, ACE inhibitors

[1]Avoid if LV systolic dysfunction.
[2]Drug of choice if LV systolic dysfunction is associated with ischemia.
ACE, angiotensin-converting enzyme; LV, left ventricular.

5. Fenoldopam—Fenoldopam is a peripheral dopamine-1 (DA_1) receptor agonist that causes a dose-dependent reduction in arterial pressure without evidence of tolerance, rebound, withdrawal, or deterioration of kidney function. In higher dosage ranges, tachycardia may occur. This drug is natriuretic, which may simplify volume management in acute kidney injury.

6. Enalaprilat—This is the active form of the oral ACE inhibitor enalapril. The onset of action is usually within 15 minutes, but the peak effect may be delayed for up to 6 hours. Thus, enalaprilat is used primarily as an adjunctive agent.

7. Diuretics—Intravenous loop diuretics can be very helpful when the patient has signs of heart failure or fluid retention, but the onset of their hypotensive response is slow, making them an adjunct rather than a primary agent for hypertensive emergencies. Low dosages should be used initially (furosemide, 20 mg, or bumetanide, 0.5 mg). They facilitate the response to vasodilators, which often stimulate fluid retention.

8. Hydralazine—Hydralazine can be given intravenously or intramuscularly, but its effect is less predictable than that of other drugs in this group. It produces reflex tachycardia and should not be given without beta-blockers in patients with possible coronary disease or aortic dissection. Hydralazine is used primarily in pregnancy and in children, but even in these situations, it is not a first-line drug.

9. Nitroglycerin, intravenous—This agent should be reserved for patients with accompanying acute coronary ischemic syndromes.

10. Nitroprusside sodium—This agent is given by controlled intravenous infusion gradually titrated to the desired effect. It lowers the blood pressure within seconds by direct arteriolar and venous dilation. Monitoring with

Table 11–16. Drugs for hypertensive emergencies and urgencies (in descending order of preference).

Agent	Action	Dosage	Onset	Duration	Adverse Effects	Comments
Hypertensive Emergencies						
Nicardipine (Cardene)	Calcium channel blocker	5 mg/h intravenously; may increase by 1–2.5 mg/h every 15 minutes to 15 mg/h	1–5 minutes	3–6 hours	Hypotension, tachycardia, headache.	May precipitate myocardial ischemia.
Clevidipine (Cleviprex)	Calcium channel blocker	1–2 mg/h intravenously initially; double rate every 90 seconds until near goal, then by smaller amounts every 5–10 minutes to a maximum of 32 mg/h	2–4 minutes	5–15 minutes	Headache, nausea, vomiting.	Lipid emulsion: contraindicated in patients with allergy to soy or egg.
Labetalol (Trandate)	Beta- and alpha-blocker	20–40 mg intravenously every 10 minutes to 300 mg; 2 mg/min infusion	5–10 minutes	3–6 hours	GI, hypotension, bronchospasm, bradycardia, heart block.	Avoid in acute LV systolic dysfunction, asthma. May be continued orally.
Esmolol (Brevibloc)	Beta-blocker	Loading dose 500 mcg/kg intravenously over 1 minute; maintenance, 25–200 mcg/kg/min	1–2 minutes	10–30 minutes	Bradycardia, nausea.	Avoid in acute LV systolic dysfunction, asthma. Weak antihypertensive.
Fenoldopam (Corlopam)	Dopamine receptor agonist	0.1–1.6 mcg/kg/min intravenously	4–5 minutes	< 10 minutes	Reflex tachycardia, hypotension, increased intraocular pressure.	May protect kidney function.
Enalaprilat (Vasotec)	ACE inhibitor	1.25 mg intravenously every 6 hours	15 minutes	6 hours or more	Excessive hypotension.	Additive with diuretics; may be continued orally.
Furosemide (Lasix)	Diuretic	10–80 mg orally or intravenously	15 minutes	4 hours	Hypokalemia, hypotension.	Adjunct to vasodilator.
Hydralazine (Apresoline)	Vasodilator	5–20 mg intravenously; may repeat after 20 minutes	10–30 minutes	2–6 hours	Tachycardia, headache, GI.	Avoid in coronary artery disease, dissection. Rarely used except in pregnancy.
Nitroglycerin	Vasodilator	0.25–5 mcg/kg/min intravenously	2–5 minutes	3–5 minutes	Headache, nausea, hypotension, bradycardia.	Tolerance may develop. Useful primarily with myocardial ischemia.
Nitroprusside (Nitropress)	Vasodilator	0.25–10 mcg/kg/min intravenously	Seconds	3–5 minutes	GI, CNS; thiocyanate and cyanide toxicity, especially with kidney and liver dysfunction; hypotension. Coronary steal, decreased cerebral blood flow, increased intracranial pressure.	No longer the first-line agent.
Hypertensive Urgencies						
Clonidine (Catapres)	Central sympatholytic	0.1–0.2 mg orally initially; then 0.1 mg every hour to 0.8 mg orally	30–60 minutes	6–8 hours	Sedation.	Rebound may occur.
Captopril (Capoten)	ACE inhibitor	12.5–25 mg orally	15–30 minutes	4–6 hours	Excessive hypotension.	
Nifedipine (Adalat, Procardia)	Calcium channel blocker	10 mg orally initially; may be repeated after 30 minutes	15 minutes	2–6 hours	Excessive hypotension, tachycardia, headache, angina, myocardial infarction, stroke.	Response unpredictable.

ACE, angiotensin-converting enzyme; CNS, central nervous system; GI, gastrointestinal; LV, left ventricular.

an intra-arterial line avoids hypotension. Nitroprusside—in combination with a beta-blocker—is useful in patients with aortic dissection.

B. Oral Agents

Patients with less severe acute hypertensive syndromes can often be treated with oral therapy. Suitable drugs will reduce the blood pressure over a period of hours. In those presenting as a consequence of noncompliance, it is usually sufficient to restore the patient's previously established oral regimen.

1. Clonidine—Clonidine, 0.2 mg orally initially, followed by 0.1 mg every hour to a total of 0.8 mg, will usually lower blood pressure over a period of several hours. Sedation is frequent, and rebound hypertension may occur if the drug is stopped.

2. Captopril—Captopril, 12.5–25 mg orally, will also lower blood pressure in 15–30 minutes. The response is variable and may be excessive. Captopril is the drug of choice in the management of scleroderma hypertensive crisis.

3. Nifedipine—The effect of fast-acting nifedipine capsules is unpredictable and may be excessive, resulting in hypotension and reflex tachycardia. Because myocardial infarction and stroke have been reported in this setting, the use of sublingual nifedipine is not advised. Nifedipine retard, 20 mg orally, appears to be safe and effective.

C. Subsequent Therapy

When the blood pressure has been brought under control, combinations of oral antihypertensive agents can be added as parenteral drugs are tapered off over a period of 2–3 days.

Cordonnier C et al. Intracerebral haemorrhage: current approaches to acute management. Lancet. 2018 Oct 6; 392(10154):1257–68. [PMID: 30319113]

Guiga H et al. Hospital and out-of-hospital mortality in 670 hypertensive emergencies and urgencies. J Clin Hypertens (Greenwich). 2017 Nov;19(11):1137–42. [PMID: 28866866]

Lawton MT et al. Subarachnoid hemorrhage. N Engl J Med. 2017 Jul 20;377(3):257–66. [PMID: 28723321]

Ipek E et al. Hypertensive crisis: an update on clinical approach and management. Curr Opin Cardiol. 2017 Jul;32(4):397–406. [PMID: 28306673]

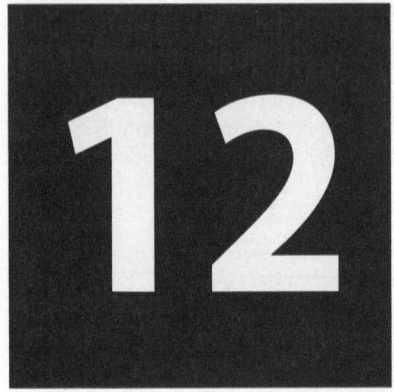

Blood Vessel & Lymphatic Disorders

Warren J. Gasper, MD
Joseph H. Rapp, MD
Meshell D. Johnson, MD

ATHEROSCLEROTIC PERIPHERAL VASCULAR DISEASE

OCCLUSIVE DISEASE: AORTA & ILIAC ARTERIES

ESSENTIALS OF DIAGNOSIS

► Claudication: cramping pain or tiredness in the calf, thigh, or hip while walking.
► Diminished femoral pulses.
► Tissue loss (ulceration, gangrene) or rest pain.

► General Considerations

Occlusive atherosclerotic lesions developing in the extremities, or peripheral artery disease (PAD), is evidence of a systemic atherosclerotic process. The prevalence of PAD is 30% in patients who are 50 years old, patients who have either diabetes mellitus or a history of tobacco use, or patients who are 70 years old without those risk factors. Pathologic changes of atherosclerosis may be diffuse, but flow-limiting stenoses occur segmentally. In the lower extremities, they classically occur in three anatomic segments: the aortoiliac segment, femoral-popliteal segment, and the infrapopliteal or tibial segment of the arterial tree. Lesions in the distal aorta and proximal common iliac arteries classically occur in white male smokers aged 50–60 years. Disease progression may lead to complete occlusion of one or both common iliac arteries, which can precipitate occlusion of the entire abdominal aorta to the level of the renal arteries.

► Clinical Findings

A. Symptoms and Signs

Approximately two-thirds of patients with PAD are either asymptomatic or do not have classic symptoms. Intermittent claudication, which is pain that occurs from insufficient blood flow when there is increased demand from exercise, is typically described as severe and cramping and primarily occurs in the calf muscles. The pain from aortoiliac lesions may extend into the thigh and buttocks and erectile dysfunction may occur from bilateral common iliac disease. Rarely, patients complain only of weakness in the legs when walking, or simply extreme limb fatigue. The symptoms are relieved with rest and are reproducible when the patient walks again. Femoral pulses are absent or very weak as are the distal pulses. Bruits may be heard over the aorta, iliac, and femoral arteries.

B. Doppler and Vascular Findings

The ratio of systolic blood pressure detected by Doppler examination at the ankle compared with the brachial artery (referred to as the ankle-brachial index [ABI]) is reduced to below 0.9 (normal ratio is 0.9–1.2); this difference is exaggerated by exercise. Both the dorsalis pedis and the posterior tibial arteries are measured and the higher of the two artery pressures is used for calculation. Segmental waveforms or pulse volume recordings obtained by strain gauge technology through blood pressure cuffs demonstrate blunting of the arterial inflow throughout the lower extremity.

C. Imaging

CT angiography (CTA) and magnetic resonance angiography (MRA) can identify the anatomic location of disease. Due to overlying bowel, duplex ultrasound has a limited role in imaging the aortoiliac segment. Imaging is required only when symptoms necessitate intervention, since a history and physical examination with vascular testing should appropriately identify the involved levels of the arterial tree.

► Treatment

A. Medical and Exercise Therapy

The cornerstones of PAD treatment are cardiovascular risk factor reduction and a structured exercise program. Essential elements include smoking cessation, antiplatelet therapy, lipid and blood pressure management, and weight loss. Nicotine replacement therapy, bupropion, and varenicline have established benefits in smoking cessation (see Chapter 1). Antiplatelet agents (such as aspirin, 81 mg orally daily) reduce overall cardiovascular morbidity and are recommended for all symptomatic patients. All patients with PAD should receive high-dose statin (eg, atorvastatin 80 mg daily if tolerated) to treat hypercholesterolemia and inflammation. A trial of cilostazol 100 mg orally twice a day, may improve walking distance in approximately two-thirds of patients.

Supervised exercise programs for PAD provide significant improvements in pain, walking distance, and quality of life and may be more effective than an endovascular treatment alone. A minimum training goal is a walking session of 30–45 minutes at least 3 days per week for a minimum of 12 weeks. Structured community or home-based exercise programs as well as alternative exercises (cycling, upper-body ergometry) may also be effective.

B. Endovascular Therapy

When the atherosclerotic lesions are focal, they can be effectively treated with angioplasty and stenting. This approach matches the results of surgery for single stenoses but both effectiveness and durability decrease with longer or multiple stenoses.

C. Surgical Intervention

A prosthetic aorto-femoral bypass graft that bypasses the diseased artery segments is a highly effective and durable treatment for this disease. Patients may be treated with a graft from the axillary artery to the femoral arteries (axillo-femoral bypass graft) or with a graft from the contralateral femoral artery (femoral-femoral bypass) when iliac disease is limited to one side. The operative risk of axillo-femoral and femoral-to-femoral bypass grafts is lower because the abdominal cavity is not entered and the aorta is not cross-clamped, but the grafts are less durable.

▶ Complications

The complications of the aorto-femoral bypass are those of any major abdominal surgery in a patient population with a high prevalence of cardiovascular disease. Mortality is low (2–3%), but morbidity is higher and includes a 5–10% rate of myocardial infarction. While endovascular approaches are safer and the complication rate is 1% to 3%, they are less durable with extensive disease.

▶ Prognosis

Patients with isolated aortoiliac disease may have a further reduction in walking distance without intervention, but symptoms rarely progress to rest pain or threatened limb loss. Life expectancy is limited by their attendant cardiovascular disease with a mortality rate of 25–40% at 5 years.

Symptomatic relief is generally excellent with supervised exercise or after intervention. After aorto-femoral bypass, a patency rate of 90% at 5 years is common. Endovascular patency rates and symptom relief for patients with short stenoses are also good with 80% symptom free at 3 years. Recurrence rates following endovascular treatment of extensive disease are 30–50%.

▶ When to Refer

Patients with progressive reduction in walking distance in spite of risk factor modification and supervised exercise programs and those with limitations that interfere with their activities of daily living should be referred for consultation to a vascular surgeon.

McDermott MM. Medical management of functional impairment in peripheral artery disease: a review. Prog Cardiovasc Dis. 2018 Mar–Apr;60(6):586–92. [PMID: 29727608]

Morcos R et al. The evolving treatment of peripheral arterial disease through guideline-directed recommendations. J Clin Med. 2018 Jan 9;7(1). [PMID: 29315259]

OCCLUSIVE DISEASE: FEMORAL & POPLITEAL ARTERIES

ESSENTIALS OF DIAGNOSIS

▶ Cramping pain or tiredness in the calf with exercise.

▶ Reduced popliteal and pedal pulses.

▶ Foot pain at rest, relieved by dependency.

▶ Foot gangrene or ischemic ulcers.

▶ General Considerations

The superficial femoral artery is the peripheral artery most commonly occluded by atherosclerosis. Atherosclerosis of the femoral-popliteal segment usually occurs about a decade after the development of aortoiliac disease, has an even gender distribution, and commonly affects black and Hispanic patients. The disease frequently occurs where the superficial femoral artery passes through the abductor magnus tendon in the distal thigh (Hunter canal). The common femoral artery and the popliteal artery are less commonly diseased but lesions in these vessels are debilitating, resulting in short-distance claudication.

▶ Clinical Findings

A. Symptoms and Signs

Symptoms of intermittent claudication caused by lesions of the common femoral artery, superficial femoral artery, and popliteal artery are confined to the calf. Occlusion or stenosis of the superficial femoral artery at the adductor canal when the patient has good collateral vessels from the profunda femoris will cause claudication at approximately 2–4 blocks. However, with concomitant disease of the profunda femoris or the popliteal artery, much shorter distances may trigger symptoms. With short-distance claudication, dependent rubor of the foot with blanching on elevation may be present. Chronic low blood flow states will also cause atrophic changes in the lower leg and foot with loss of hair, thinning of the skin and subcutaneous tissues, and disuse atrophy of the muscles. With segmental occlusive disease of the superficial femoral artery, the common femoral pulsation is normal, but the popliteal and pedal pulses are reduced.

B. Doppler and Vascular Findings

ABI values less than 0.9 are diagnostic of PAD and levels below 0.4 suggest critical limb ischemia. ABI readings depend on arterial compression. Since the vessels may be calcified in diabetes mellitus, chronic kidney disease, and in older adults, ABIs can be misleading. In such patients, the toe-brachial index is usually reliable with a value less than 0.7 considered diagnostic of PAD. Pulse volume recordings with cuffs placed at the high thigh, mid-thigh, calf, and ankle will delineate the levels of obstruction with reduced pressures and blunted waveforms.

C. Imaging

Duplex ultrasonography, CTA, or MRA all adequately show the anatomic location of the obstructive lesions and are done only if revascularization is planned.

► Treatment

A. Medical and Exercise Therapy

As with aortoiliac disease, risk factor reduction, medical optimization with a high-dose statin, and exercise treatment are the cornerstone of therapy. Cilostazol may improve intermittent claudication symptoms.

B. Surgical Intervention

Intervention is indicated if claudication is progressive, incapacitating, or interferes significantly with essential daily activities or employment. Intervention is mandatory if there is ischemic rest pain or ischemic ulcers threaten the foot.

1. Bypass surgery—The most effective and durable treatment for lesions of the superficial femoral artery is a femoral-popliteal bypass with autogenous saphenous vein. Synthetic material, usually polytetrafluoroethylene (PTFE), can be used, but these grafts do not have the durability of vein bypass.

2. Endovascular surgery—Endovascular techniques such as angioplasty and stenting, are often used for lesions of the superficial femoral artery. These techniques have lower morbidity than bypass surgery but also have lower rates of durability.

Endovascular therapy is most effective in patients undergoing aggressive risk factor modification in whom lesions measure less than 10 cm long. Paclitaxel-eluting stents or paclitaxel-coated balloons offer modest improvement over bare metal stents and noncoated balloons, but the success of local drug delivery in peripheral arteries is not as robust as in the coronary arteries. The 1-year patency rate is 50% for balloon angioplasty, 70% for drug-coated balloons, and 80% for stents. However, by 3 years the patency rates are significantly worse for all three techniques and reintervention for restenosis is common. In general, treating restenosis in stents is more difficult than in arteries that have undergone angioplasty.

3. Thromboendarterectomy—Removal of the atherosclerotic plaque is limited to the lesions of the common femoral and the profunda femoris arteries where bypass grafts and endovascular techniques have a more limited role.

► Complications

Open surgical procedures of the lower extremities, particularly long bypasses with vein harvest, have a risk of wound infection that is higher than in other areas of the body. Wound infection or seroma can occur in as many as 10–15% of cases. Myocardial infarction rates after open surgery are 5–10%, with a 1–4% mortality rate. Complication rates of endovascular surgery are 1–5%, making these therapies attractive despite their lower durability.

► Prognosis

The prognosis for motivated patients with isolated superficial femoral artery disease is excellent, and surgery is not recommended for mild or moderate claudication in these patients. However, when claudication significantly limits daily activity and undermines quality of life as well as overall cardiovascular health, intervention may be warranted. All interventions require close postprocedure follow-up with repeated ultrasound surveillance so that recurrent narrowing can be treated promptly to prevent complete occlusion. The reported patency rate of bypass grafts of the femoral artery, superficial femoral artery, and popliteal artery is 65–70% at 3 years, whereas the patency of angioplasty is less than 50% at 3 years.

Because of the extensive atherosclerotic disease, including associated coronary lesions, 5-year mortality among patients with lower extremity disease can be as high as 50%, particularly with involvement of the infrapopliteal vessels. However, with aggressive risk factor modification, substantial improvement in longevity has been reported.

► When to Refer

Patients with progressive symptoms, short-distance claudication, rest pain, or any ulceration should be referred to a peripheral vascular specialist.

Hiramoto JS et al. Interventions for lower extremity peripheral artery disease. Nat Rev Cardiol. 2018 Jun;15(6):332–50. [PMID: 29679023]
Rocha-Singh KJ et al; VIVA Physicians, Inc. Patient-level meta-analysis of 999 claudicants undergoing primary femoro-popliteal nitinol stent implantation. Catheter Cardiovasc Interv. 2017 Jun 1;89(7):1250–6. [PMID: 28303688]

OCCLUSIVE DISEASE: TIBIAL & PEDAL ARTERIES

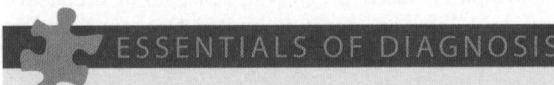

ESSENTIALS OF DIAGNOSIS

► Severe pain of the forefoot that is relieved by dependency.
► Pain or numbness of the foot with walking.
► Ulceration or gangrene of the foot or toes.
► Pallor when the foot is elevated.

General Considerations

Occlusive processes of the tibial arteries of the lower leg and pedal arteries in the foot occur primarily in patients with diabetes. There often is extensive calcification of the artery wall. While claudication is a common initial symptom of ischemia, it may not be present. The first manifestation of ischemia is frequently an ulcer or gangrene rather than claudication.

Clinical Findings

A. Symptoms and Signs

Unless there are concomitant lesions in the aortoiliac or femoral/superficial femoral artery segments, claudication may not occur. The gastrocnemius and soleus muscles may be supplied from collateral vessels from the popliteal artery; therefore, foot ischemia without attendant claudication may be the first sign of severe vascular insufficiency due to isolated tibial artery disease. The presence of ischemic rest pain or ulcers is termed **critical limb ischemia** and is associated with the highest rate of amputation. Classically, ischemic rest pain is confined to the dorsum of the foot and is relieved with dependency: the pain does not occur with standing, sitting or dangling the leg over the edge of the bed. It is severe and burning in character, and because it is present only when recumbent, it may awaken the patient from sleep. Because of the high incidence of neuropathy in these patients, it is important to differentiate rest pain from diabetic neuropathic dysesthesia. Leg night cramps, which are not a purely ischemic phenomenon, cause pain in the leg rather than the foot and should not be confused with ischemic rest pain.

On examination, depending on whether associated proximal disease is present, there may or may not be femoral and popliteal pulses, but the pedal pulses will be absent. Dependent rubor may be prominent with pallor on elevation. The skin of the foot is generally cool, atrophic, and hairless.

B. Doppler and Vascular Findings

The ABI may be quite low (in the range of 0.4 or lower). ABIs, however, may be falsely elevated when the medial layer of the arterial wall of the tibial arteries calcify (Mönckeberg medial calcific sclerosis) and are not compressible. Toe-brachial indexes should be used if noncompressible ankle arteries are encountered.

C. Imaging

Digital subtraction angiography is the gold standard method to delineate the anatomy of the tibial-popliteal segment. MRA or CTA is less helpful for detection of lesions in this location due to the small vasculature and other technical issues related to image resolution.

Treatment

Good foot care may prevent ulcers, and most diabetic patients will do well with a conservative regimen. However, if ulcerations appear and there is no significant healing within 2–3 weeks, blood flow studies (ankle-brachial index/toe-brachial index) are indicated. Poor blood flow and a foot ulcer or nightly ischemic rest pain requires revascularization to avoid a major amputation.

A. Bypass and Endovascular Techniques

Bypass with vein to the distal tibial or pedal arteries is an effective therapy to treat rest pain and heal ischemic ulcers of the foot. Because the foot often has relative sparing of vascular disease, these bypasses have had adequate patency rates (70% at 3 years). Fortunately, in nearly all series, limb preservation rates are much higher than patency rates.

Endovascular treatment with plain balloon angioplasty is effective for short segment lesions. The technical failure and reocclusion rates increase drastically with long segment disease in multiple tibial arteries. Drug-coated balloons or stents have not been successful in the tibial vessels.

B. Amputation

Patients with ischemic rest pain and ulcers are at high risk for amputation, particularly if revascularization cannot be done. Patients with diabetes and PAD have a 4-fold risk of critical limb ischemia compared with nondiabetic patients with PAD and have a risk of amputation up to 20-fold when compared to an age-matched population. Many patients who have below-the-knee or above-the-knee amputations due to vascular insufficiency never attain independent ambulatory status and often need assisted-living facilities. These factors combine to demand revascularization whenever possible to preserve the limb.

Complications

The complications of intervention are similar to those listed for superficial femoral artery disease with evidence that the overall cardiovascular risk of intervention increases with decreasing ABI. Patients with critical limb ischemia require aggressive risk factor modification. Wound infection rates after bypass are higher if there is an open wound in the foot.

Prognosis

Patients with tibial atherosclerosis have extensive atherosclerotic burden and a high prevalence of diabetes. Their prognosis without intervention is poor and complicated by the risk of amputation.

When to Refer

Patients with diabetes and foot ulcers should be referred for a formal vascular evaluation. Intervention may not be necessary but the severity of the disease will be quantified, which has implications for future symptom development. Any patient with an ulcer and a diabetic foot infection should be evaluated for an emergent operative incision and drainage. Broad-spectrum antibiotics should be given to cover gram-positive, gram-negative, and anaerobic organisms. Centers that have a multidisciplinary limb preservation center staffed with vascular surgeons, podiatrists, plastic and orthopedic surgeons, prosthetics and orthotic specialists, and diabetes specialists should be sought.

Mills JL. Lower limb ischaemia in patients with diabetic foot ulcers and gangrene: recognition, anatomic patterns and revascularization strategies. Diabetes Metab Res Rev. 2016 Jan; 32(Suppl 1):239–45. [PMID: 26455728]

Mills JL Sr et al. The Society for Vascular Surgery Lower Extremity Threatened Limb Classification System: risk stratification based on wound, ischemia, and foot infection (WIfI). J Vasc Surg. 2014 Jan;59(1):220–34.e1–2. [PMID: 24126108]

ACUTE ARTERIAL OCCLUSION OF A LIMB

ESSENTIALS OF DIAGNOSIS

- ▶ Sudden pain in an extremity with absent extremity pulses.
- ▶ Usually some neurologic dysfunction with numbness, weakness, or complete paralysis.
- ▶ Loss of light touch sensation requires revascularization within 3 hours for limb viability.

General Considerations

Acute occlusion may be due to an embolus or to thrombosis of a diseased atherosclerotic segment. Emboli large enough to occlude proximal arteries in the lower extremities are almost always from the heart. Over 50% of the emboli from the heart go to the lower extremities, 20% to the cerebrovascular circulation, and the remainder to the upper extremities and mesenteric and renal circulation. Atrial fibrillation is the most common cause of cardiac thrombus formation; other causes are valvular disease or thrombus formation on the ventricular surface of a large anterior myocardial infarct.

Emboli from arterial sources such as arterial ulcerations or calcified excrescences are usually small and go to the distal arterial tree (toes).

The typical patient with primary thrombosis has had a history of claudication and now has an acute occlusion. If the stenosis has developed over time, collateral blood vessels will develop, and the resulting occlusion may cause only minimal increase in symptoms.

Clinical Findings

A. Symptoms and Signs

The sudden onset of extremity pain, with loss or reduction in pulses, is diagnostic of acute arterial occlusion. This often will be accompanied by neurologic dysfunction, such as numbness or paralysis in extreme cases. With popliteal occlusion, symptoms may affect only the foot. With proximal occlusions, the whole leg may be affected. Signs of severe arterial ischemia include pallor, coolness of the extremity, and mottling. Impaired neurologic function progressing to anesthesia accompanied with paralysis suggests a poor prognosis.

B. Doppler and Laboratory Findings

There will be little or no flow found with Doppler examination of the distal vessels. Imaging, if done, may show an abrupt cutoff of contrast with embolic occlusion. Blood work may show myoglobin and metabolic acidosis.

C. Imaging

Whenever possible, imaging should be done in the operating room because obtaining angiography, MRA, or CTA may delay revascularization and jeopardize the viability of the extremity. However, in cases with only modest symptoms and where light touch of the extremity is maintained, imaging may be helpful in planning the revascularization procedure.

Treatment

Immediate revascularization is required in all cases of symptomatic acute arterial thrombosis. *Evidence of neurologic injury, including loss of light touch sensation, indicates that collateral flow is inadequate to maintain limb viability and revascularization should be accomplished within 3 hours.* Longer delays carry a significant risk of irreversible tissue damage. This risk approaches 100% at 6 hours.

A. Heparin

As soon as the diagnosis is made, unfractionated heparin should be administered (5000–10,000 units) intravenously, followed by a heparin infusion to maintain the activated partial thromboplastin time (aPTT) in the therapeutic range (60–85 seconds) (12–18 units/kg/h). This helps prevent clot propagation and may also help relieve associated vessel spasm. Anticoagulation may improve symptoms, but revascularization will still be required.

B. Endovascular Techniques

Catheter-directed chemical thrombolysis into the clot with tissue plasminogen activator (TPA) may be done but often requires 24 hours or longer to fully lyse the thrombus. This approach can be taken only in patients with an intact neurologic examination who do not have absolute contraindications such as bleeding diathesis, gastrointestinal bleeding, intracranial trauma, or neurosurgery within the past 3 months. A sheath is used to advance a TPA-infusing catheter through the clot. Heparin is administered systemically to prevent thrombus formation around the sheath. Frequent vascular and access site examinations are required during the thrombolytic procedure to assess for improved vascular perfusion and to guard against the development of a hematoma.

C. Surgical Intervention

General anesthesia is usually indicated; local anesthesia may be used in extremely high-risk patients if the exploration is to be limited to the common femoral artery. In extreme cases, it may be necessary to perform thromboembolectomy from the femoral, popliteal, and even the pedal vessels to revascularize the limb. The combined use of devices that pulverize and aspirate clot and intraoperative thrombolysis with TPA improves outcomes.

Complications

Complications of revascularization of an acutely ischemic limb can include severe metabolic acidosis, hyperkalemia, and cardiac arrest. In cases where several hours have elapsed but recovery of viable tissue may still be possible, significant levels of lactic acid, potassium, and other harmful agents may be released into the circulation during revascularization. Administering sodium bicarbonate (150 mEq NaHCO$_3$ in 1 liter of dextrose 5% in water) prior to reestablishing arterial flow is required. Surgery in the presence of thrombolytic agents and heparin carries a high risk of postoperative wound hematoma.

Prognosis

There is a 10–25% risk of amputation with an acute arterial embolic occlusion, and a 25% or higher in-hospital mortality rate. Prognosis for acute thrombotic occlusion of an atherosclerotic segment is generally better because the collateral flow can maintain extremity viability. The longer-term survival reflects the overall condition of the patient. In high-risk patients, an acute arterial occlusion is associated with a dismal prognosis.

OCCLUSIVE CEREBROVASCULAR DISEASE

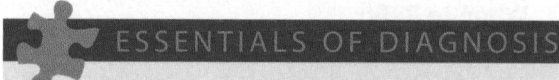

ESSENTIALS OF DIAGNOSIS

► Sudden onset of weakness and numbness of an extremity or the face, aphasia, dysarthria, or unilateral blindness (amaurosis fugax).
► Bruit heard loudest in the mid neck.

General Considerations

Unlike the other vascular territories, symptoms of ischemic cerebrovascular disease are predominantly due to emboli. The ischemia is reversible (transient ischemic attacks [TIAs]) when collateral flow reestablishes perfusion, but is a sign that the risk of additional emboli and a stroke is high. Most ischemic strokes are due to emboli from the heart. One-quarter of all ischemic strokes may be due to emboli from an arterial source; approximately 90% of these emboli originate from the proximal internal carotid artery, an area uniquely prone to the development of atherosclerosis. Intracranial atherosclerotic lesions are uncommon in western populations but are the most frequent location of cerebrovascular disease in Asian populations.

Clinical Findings

A. Symptoms and Signs

Generally, the symptoms of a TIA last only a few seconds to minutes (but may continue up to 24 hours) while

symptoms of a stroke persist beyond 24 hours. The most common lesions associated with carotid disease involve the anterior circulation in the cortex with both motor and sensory involvement. Emboli to the retinal artery cause unilateral blindness; when this blindness is transient, it is termed "amaurosis fugax." Posterior circulation symptoms referable to the brainstem, cerebellum, and visual regions of the brain may be due to atherosclerosis of the vertebral basilar systems and are much less common.

Signs of cerebrovascular disease may include carotid artery bruits. However, there is poor correlation between the degree of stenosis and the presence of the bruit. Furthermore, the presence of a bruit does not correlate with stroke risk. Nonfocal symptoms, such as dizziness and unsteadiness, seldom are related to cerebrovascular atherosclerosis.

B. Imaging

Duplex ultrasonography is the imaging modality of choice with high specificity and sensitivity for detecting and grading the degree of stenosis at the carotid bifurcation (see Chapter 24).

Excellent depiction of the full anatomy of the cerebrovascular circulation from aortic arch to cranium can be obtained with either MRA or CTA. Each of the modalities may have false-positive or false-negative findings. Since the decision to intervene in cases of carotid stenosis depends on an accurate assessment of the degree of stenosis, it is recommended that at least two modalities be used to confirm the degree of stenosis. Diagnostic cerebral angiography is reserved for cases where carotid artery stenting (CAS) is to be done.

Treatment

See Chapter 24 for a discussion of the medical management of occlusive cerebrovascular disease.

A. Asymptomatic Patients

Large studies have shown a 5-year reduction in stroke rate from 11.5% to 5.0% with surgical treatment of asymptomatic carotid stenosis that is greater than 60%. Patients with asymptomatic carotid stenosis may benefit from carotid intervention if their risk from intervention is low and their expected survival is longer than 5 years. Aggressive risk factor modification, including high potency statins, may be as valuable as intervention in these patients; the large NIH-sponsored CREST2 study is examining this issue.

Mild to moderate disease (30–50% stenosis) indicates the need for ongoing monitoring and aggressive risk factor modification. Patients with carotid stenosis that suddenly worsens are thought to have an unstable plaque and are at particularly high risk for embolic stroke.

B. Symptomatic Patients

Large randomized trials have shown that patients with TIAs or strokes from which they have completely or nearly completely recovered will benefit from carotid intervention if the ipsilateral carotid artery has a stenosis of more than 70% (Figure 12–1), and they are likely to benefit if the artery has a stenosis of 50–69%. In these situations, carotid

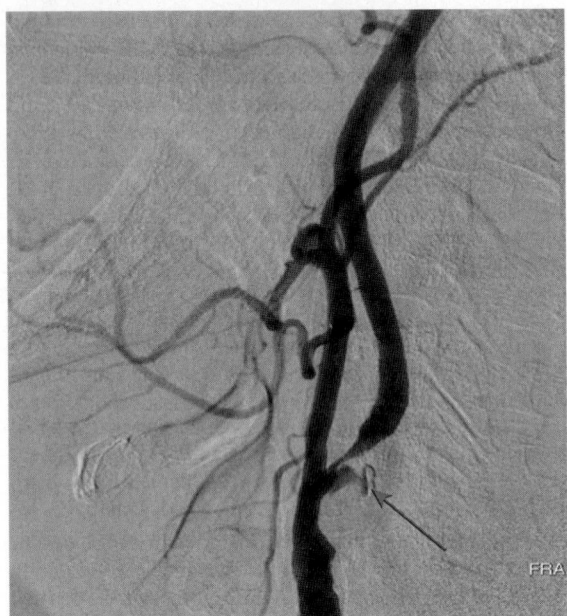

▲ **Figure 12–1.** Digital subtraction angiography of a high-grade (90%) stenosis of internal carotid artery, with ulceration (arrow). (Used, with permission, from Dean SM, Satiani B, Abraham WT. *Color Atlas and Synopsis of Vascular Diseases.* McGraw-Hill, 2014.)

endarterectomy (CEA) and, in selected cases, CAS have been shown to have a durable effect in preventing further events. In symptomatic patients, intervention should ideally be planned within 2 weeks since delays increase the risk of a second event.

▶ Complications

The most common complication from carotid intervention is cranial nerve injury, while the most dreaded complication is stroke from embolization or carotid occlusion. The American Heart Association's recommendations for upper limits of acceptable combined morbidity and mortality for these interventions is 3% for patients with asymptomatic carotid stenosis, 5% for those with TIAs, and 7% for patients with previous stroke. Higher rates of morbidity and mortality negate the therapeutic benefit of carotid intervention.

A. Carotid Endarterectomy

In the 2010 CREST study the stroke risk for CEA was 2.3%. CEA also carries a 1–2% risk of permanent cranial nerve injury (usually the vagus). There is also the risk of postoperative neck hematoma, which can cause acute airway compromise. Coronary artery disease is a comorbidity in most of these patients. Myocardial infarction rates after CEA are approximately 2–6%.

B. Angioplasty and Stenting

CAS had a stroke risk of 4.1% in the 2010 CREST study; patients over 70 years of age as well as women had higher stroke rates with CAS than with CEA. However, the risk of myocardial infarction was lower with CAS compared to CEA (1.1% vs 2.3%). CAS avoids both cranial nerve injury and neck hematoma. Nonetheless, emboli are more common during carotid angioplasty and stenting in spite of the use of embolic protection devices, especially when the carotid artery is tortuous and heavily calcified. In cases of restenosis after previous carotid intervention, CAS is an excellent choice since the risk of embolization is low and the risk of cranial nerve injury with surgery is high.

▶ Prognosis

Twenty-five percent of patients presenting with carotid stenosis and a TIA or small stroke will have further brain ischemia within 18 months with most of the events occurring within the first 6 months. Historically, patients with asymptomatic carotid stenosis are believed to have an annual stroke rate of just over 2% but this may be lower in the statin era. Prospective ultrasound screening at least annually is recommended in asymptomatic patients with known carotid stenosis to identify those who have evidence of plaque progression, which increases stroke risk. Concomitant coronary artery disease is common and is an important factor in these patients both for perioperative risk and long-term prognosis. Aggressive risk factor modification should be prescribed for patients with cerebrovascular disease regardless of planned intervention.

▶ When to Refer

Asymptomatic or symptomatic patients with a carotid stenosis of more than 70% and patients with carotid stenosis of less than 70% with symptoms of a TIA or stroke should be referred to a vascular specialist for consultation.

Brott TG et al; CREST Investigators. Long-term results of stenting versus endarterectomy for carotid-artery stenosis. N Engl J Med. 2016 Mar 17;374(11):1021–31. [PMID: 26890472]

Moresoli P et al. Carotid stenting versus endarterectomy for asymptomatic carotid artery stenosis: a systematic review and meta-analysis. Stroke. 2017 Aug;48(8):2150–7. [PMID: 28679848]

Zaidat OO et al; VISSIT Trial Investigators. Effect of a balloon-expandable intracranial stent vs medical therapy on risk of stroke in patients with symptomatic intracranial stenosis: the VISSIT randomized clinical trial. JAMA. 2015 Mar 24–31; 313(12):1240–8. [PMID: 25803346]

VISCERAL ARTERY INSUFFICIENCY (Intestinal Angina)

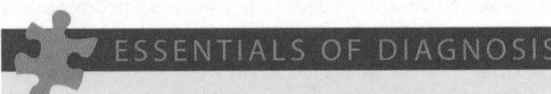

ESSENTIALS OF DIAGNOSIS

▶ Severe postprandial abdominal pain.

▶ Weight loss with a "fear of eating."

▶ **Acute mesenteric ischemia:** severe abdominal pain yet minimal findings on physical examination.

General Considerations

Acute visceral artery insufficiency results from either embolic occlusion or primary thrombosis of at least one major mesenteric vessel. Ischemia can also result from **non-occlusive mesenteric vascular insufficiency,** which is generally seen in patients with low flow states, such as heart failure, or hypotension. A **chronic syndrome** occurs when there is adequate perfusion for the viscera at rest but ischemia occurs with severe abdominal pain when flow demands increase with feeding. Because of the rich collateral network in the mesentery, generally at least two of the three major visceral vessels (celiac, superior mesenteric, inferior mesenteric arteries) are affected before symptoms develop. Ischemic colitis, a variant of mesenteric ischemia, usually occurs in the distribution of the inferior mesenteric artery. The intestinal mucosa is the most sensitive to ischemia and will slough if underperfused. The clinical presentation is similar to inflammatory bowel disease. Ischemic colitis can occur after aortic surgery, particularly aortic aneurysm resection or aortofemoral bypass for occlusive disease, when there is a sudden reduction in blood flow to the inferior mesenteric artery.

Clinical Findings

A. Symptoms and Signs

1. Acute intestinal ischemia—Patients with primary visceral arterial thrombosis often give an antecedent history consistent with chronic intestinal ischemia. The key finding with acute intestinal ischemia is severe, steady epigastric and periumbilical pain with minimal or no findings on physical examination of the abdomen because the visceral peritoneum is severely ischemic or infarcted and the parietal peritoneum is not involved. A high white cell count, lactic acidosis, hypotension, and abdominal distention may aid in the diagnosis.

2. Chronic intestinal ischemia—Patients are generally over 45 years of age and may have evidence of atherosclerosis in other vascular beds. Symptoms consist of epigastric or periumbilical postprandial pain lasting 1–3 hours. To avoid the pain, patients limit food intake and may develop a fear of eating. Weight loss is universal.

3. Ischemic colitis—Characteristic symptoms are left lower quadrant pain and tenderness, abdominal cramping, and mild diarrhea, which is often bloody.

B. Imaging and Colonoscopy

Contrast-enhanced CT is highly accurate at determining the presence of ischemic intestine. In patients with acute or chronic intestinal ischemia, a CTA or MRA can demonstrate narrowing of the proximal visceral vessels. In acute intestinal ischemia from a nonocclusive low flow state, angiography is needed to display the typical "pruned tree" appearance of the distal visceral vascular bed. Ultrasound scanning of the mesenteric vessels may show proximal obstructing lesions.

In patients with ischemic colitis, colonoscopy may reveal segmental ischemic changes, most often in the rectal sigmoid and splenic flexure where collateral circulation may be poor.

Treatment

A high suspicion of acute intestinal ischemia dictates immediate exploration to determine bowel viability. If the bowel remains viable, bypass using a prosthetic conduit can be done either from the supra-celiac aorta or common iliac artery to the celiac and the superior mesentery artery. In cases where bowel viability is questionable or bowel resection will be required, the bypass can be done with autologous vein to avoid the use of prosthetic conduits in a potentially contaminated field. Angioplasty and stenting of the arteries can be used but does not avoid a surgical evaluation of bowel viability.

In chronic intestinal ischemia, angioplasty and stenting of the proximal vessel may be beneficial depending on the anatomy of the stenosis. Should an endovascular solution not be available, an aorto-visceral artery bypass is the preferred management. The long-term results are highly durable. Visceral artery endarterectomy is reserved for cases with multiple lesions where bypass would be difficult.

The mainstay of treatment of **ischemic colitis** is maintenance of blood pressure and perfusion until collateral circulation becomes well established. The patient must be monitored closely for evidence of perforation, which will require resection.

Prognosis

The combined morbidity and mortality rates are 10–15% from surgical intervention in these debilitated patients. However, without intervention both acute and chronic intestinal ischemia are uniformly fatal. Adequate collateral circulation usually develops in those who have ischemic colitis, and the prognosis for this entity is better than chronic intestinal ischemia.

When to Refer

Any patient in whom there is a suspicion of intestinal ischemia should be urgently referred for imaging and possible intervention.

Alahdab F et al. A systematic review and meta-analysis of endovascular versus open surgical revascularization for chronic mesenteric ischemia. J Vasc Surg. 2018 May;67(5):1598–605. [PMID: 29571626]

Clair DG et al. Mesenteric ischemia. N Engl J Med. 2016 Mar 10; 374(10):959–68. [PMID: 26962730]

Eslami MH et al. Mortality of acute mesenteric ischemia remains unchanged despite significant increase in utilization of endovascular techniques. Vascular. 2016 Feb;24(1):44–52. [PMID: 25761854]

ACUTE MESENTERIC VEIN OCCLUSION

The hallmarks of acute mesenteric vein occlusion are postprandial pain and evidence of a hypercoagulable state. Acute mesenteric vein occlusion presents similarly to the arterial occlusive syndromes but is much less common. Patients at risk include those with paroxysmal nocturnal hemoglobinuria; protein C, protein S, or antithrombin deficiencies; or the *JAK2* mutation. These lesions are difficult to treat surgically, and thrombolysis is the mainstay of therapy. Aggressive long-term anticoagulation is required for these patients.

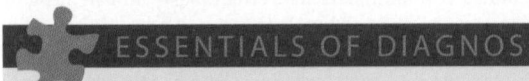

NONATHEROSCLEROTIC VASCULAR DISEASE

THROMBOANGIITIS OBLITERANS (Buerger Disease)

> **ESSENTIALS OF DIAGNOSIS**

> ▶ Typically occurs in male cigarette smokers.
> ▶ Distal extremities involved with severe ischemia, progressing to tissue loss.
> ▶ Thrombosis of the superficial veins may occur.
> ▶ Amputation will be necessary unless the patient stops smoking.

General Considerations

Buerger disease is a segmental, inflammatory, and thrombotic process of the distal-most arteries and occasionally veins of the extremities. Pathologic examination reveals arteritis in the affected vessels. The cause is not known but it is rarely seen in nonsmokers. Arteries most commonly affected are the plantar and digital vessels of the foot and lower leg. In advanced stages, the fingers and hands may become involved. The incidence of Buerger disease has decreased dramatically.

Clinical Findings

A. Symptoms and Signs

Buerger disease may be initially difficult to differentiate from routine peripheral vascular disease, but in most cases, the lesions are on the toes and the patient is younger than 40 years of age. The observation of superficial thrombophlebitis may aid the diagnosis. Because the distal vessels are usually affected, intermittent claudication is not common with Buerger disease, but rest pain, particularly pain in the distal most extremity (ie, toes), is frequent. This pain often progresses to tissue loss and amputation, unless the patient stops smoking. The progression of the disease seems to be intermittent with acute and dramatic episodes followed by some periods of remission.

B. Imaging

MRA or invasive angiography can demonstrate the obliteration of the distal arterial tree typical of Buerger disease.

Differential Diagnosis

In atherosclerotic peripheral vascular disease, the onset of tissue ischemia tends to be less dramatic than in Buerger disease, and symptoms of proximal arterial involvement, such as claudication, predominate.

Symptoms of Raynaud disease may be difficult to differentiate from Buerger disease. Repetitive atheroemboli may also mimic Buerger disease and may be difficult to differentiate. It may be necessary to image the proximal arterial tree to rule out sources of arterial microemboli.

Treatment

Smoking cessation is the mainstay of therapy and will halt the disease in most cases. As the distal arterial tree is occluded, revascularization is not possible. Sympathectomy is rarely effective.

Prognosis

If smoking cessation can be achieved, the outlook for Buerger disease may be better than in patients with premature peripheral vascular disease. If smoking cessation is not achieved, then the prognosis is generally poor, with amputation of both lower and upper extremities the eventual outcome.

Klein-Weigel P et al. Buerger's disease: providing integrated care. J Multidiscip Healthc. 2016 Oct 12;9:511–8. [PMID: 27785045]

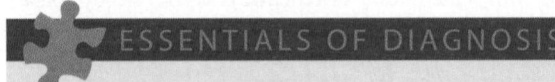

ARTERIAL ANEURYSMS

ABDOMINAL AORTIC ANEURYSM

> **ESSENTIALS OF DIAGNOSIS**

> ▶ Most aortic aneurysms are asymptomatic until rupture.
> ▶ Abdominal aortic aneurysms measuring 5 cm are palpable in 80% of patients.
> ▶ Back or abdominal pain with aneurysmal tenderness may precede rupture.
> ▶ Rupture is catastrophic; hypotension; excruciating abdominal pain that radiates to the back.

General Considerations

Dilatation of the infrarenal aorta is a normal part of aging. The aorta of a healthy young man measures approximately 2 cm. An aneurysm is considered present when the aortic diameter exceeds 3 cm, but aneurysms rarely rupture until their diameter exceeds 5 cm. Abdominal aortic aneurysms are found in 2% of men over 55 years of age; the male to female ratio is 4:1. Ninety percent of abdominal atherosclerotic aneurysms originate below the renal arteries. The aneurysms usually involve the aortic bifurcation and often involve the common iliac arteries.

Inflammatory aneurysms are an unusual variant. These have an inflammatory peel (similar to the inflammation seen with retroperitoneal fibrosis) that surrounds the aneurysm and encases adjacent retroperitoneal structures, such as the duodenum and, occasionally, the ureters.

► Clinical Findings

A. Symptoms and Signs

1. Asymptomatic—Although 80% of 5-cm infrarenal aneurysms are palpable on routine physical examination, most aneurysms are discovered on ultrasound or CT imaging as part of a screening program or during the evaluation of unrelated abdominal symptoms.

2. Symptomatic

A. Pain—Aneurysmal expansion may be accompanied by pain that is mild to severe midabdominal discomfort often radiating to the lower back. The pain may be constant or intermittent and is exacerbated by even gentle pressure on the aneurysm sack. Pain may also accompany inflammatory aneurysms. Most aneurysms have a thick layer of thrombus lining the aneurysmal sac, but embolization to the lower extremities is rarely seen.

B. Rupture—The sudden escape of blood into the retroperitoneal space causes severe pain, a palpable abdominal mass, and hypotension. Free rupture into the peritoneal cavity is a lethal event.

B. Laboratory Findings

In acute cases of a contained rupture, the hematocrit may be normal, since there has been no opportunity for hemodilution.

Patients with aneurysms may also have such cardiopulmonary diseases as coronary artery disease, carotid disease, kidney impairment, and emphysema, which are typically seen in elderly men who smoke. Preoperative testing may indicate the presence of these comorbid conditions, which increase the risk of intervention.

C. Imaging

Abdominal ultrasonography is the diagnostic study of choice for initial screening for the presence of an aneurysm. In approximately three-quarters of patients with aneurysms, curvilinear calcifications outlining portions of the aneurysm wall may be visible on plain films of the abdomen or back. CT scans provide a more reliable assessment of aneurysm diameter and should be done when the aneurysm nears the diameter threshold (5.5 cm) for treatment. Contrast-enhanced CT scans show the arteries above and below the aneurysm. The visualization of this vasculature is essential for planning repair.

Once an aneurysm is identified, routine follow-up with ultrasound will determine size and growth rate. The frequency of imaging depends on aneurysm size ranging from every 2 years for aneurysms smaller than 4 cm to every 6 months for aneurysms at or approaching 5 cm. When an aneurysm measures approximately 5 cm, a CTA with contrast should be done to more accurately assess the size of the aneurysm and define the anatomy.

► Screening

Data support the use of abdominal ultrasound to screen 65- to 75-year-old men, but not women, who are current or past smokers. Guidelines do not recommend repeated screening if the aorta shows no enlargement.

► Treatment

A. Elective Repair

In general, elective repair is indicated for aortic aneurysms larger than 5.5 cm in diameter or aneurysms that have undergone rapid expansion (more than 0.5 cm in 6 months). Symptoms such as pain or tenderness may indicate impending rupture and require urgent repair regardless of the aneurysm's diameter.

B. Aneurysmal Rupture

A ruptured aneurysm is a lethal event. Approximately half the patients exsanguinate prior to reaching a hospital. In the remainder, bleeding may be temporarily contained in the retroperitoneum (contained rupture), allowing the patient to undergo emergent surgery. However, only half of those patients will survive. Endovascular repair is available for ruptured aneurysm treatment in most major vascular centers, with the results offering some improvement over open repair for these critically ill patients.

C. Inflammatory Aneurysm

The presence of periaortic inflammation (inflammatory aneurysm) is not an indication for surgical treatment, unless there is associated compression of retroperitoneal structures, such as the ureter or pain upon palpation of the aneurysm. Interestingly, the inflammation that encases an inflammatory aneurysm recedes after either endovascular or open surgical aneurysm repair.

D. Assessment of Operative Risk

Aneurysms appear to be a variant of systemic atherosclerosis. Patients with aneurysms have a high rate of coronary disease. A 2004 trial demonstrated minimal value in addressing stable coronary artery disease prior to aneurysm resection. However, in patients with significant symptoms of coronary disease, the coronary disease should be treated first. Aneurysm resection should follow shortly thereafter because there is a slightly increased risk of aneurysm rupture after the coronary procedures.

E. Open Surgical Resection Versus Endovascular Repair

In open surgical aneurysm repair, a graft is sutured to the non-dilated vessels above and below the aneurysm. This involves an abdominal incision, extensive dissection, and interruption of aortic blood flow. The mortality rate is low (2–5%) in centers that have a high volume for this procedure and when it is performed in good-risk patients. Older, sicker patients may not tolerate the cardiopulmonary stresses of the operation. With endovascular repair, a stent-graft is used to line the aorta and exclude the aneurysm. The stent must be able to seal securely against the wall of the aorta above and below the aneurysm, thereby excluding blood from flowing into the aneurysm sac.

The anatomic requirements to securely achieve aneurysm exclusion vary according to the performance characteristics of the specific stent-graft device. Most studies have found that endovascular aneurysm repair offers patients reduced operative morbidity and mortality as well as shorter recovery periods. Long-term survival is equivalent between the two techniques. Patients who undergo endovascular repair, however, require more repeat interventions and need to be monitored postoperatively, since there is a 10–15% incidence of continued aneurysm growth post–endovascular repair.

F. Thrombus in an Aneurysm

The presence of thrombus within the aneurysm is not an indication for anticoagulation.

▶ Complications

Myocardial infarction, the most common complication, occurs in up to 10% of patients who undergo open aneurysm repair. The incidence of myocardial infarction is substantially lower with endovascular repair. For routine infrarenal aneurysms, renal injury is unusual; however, when it does occur, or if the baseline creatinine is elevated, it is a significant complicating factor in the postoperative period. Respiratory complications are similar to those seen in most major abdominal surgery. Gastrointestinal hemorrhage, even years after aortic surgeries, suggests the possibility of **graft enteric fistula,** most commonly between the aorta and the distal duodenum; the incidence of this complication is higher when the initial surgery is performed on an emergency basis.

▶ Prognosis

The mortality rate for an open elective surgical resection is 1–5%, and the mortality rate for endovascular therapy is 0.5–2%. Of those who survive surgery, approximately 60% are alive at 5 years; myocardial infarction is the leading cause of death. The endovascular approach is a consideration for high-risk patients because of the reduced perioperative morbidity and mortality.

Mortality rates of untreated aneurysms vary with aneurysm diameter. The mortality rate among patients with large aneurysms has been defined as follows: 12% annual risk of rupture with an aneurysm larger than 6 cm in diameter and a 25% annual risk of rupture in aneurysms of more than 7 cm diameter. In general, a patient with an aortic aneurysm larger than 5.5 cm has a threefold greater chance of dying of a consequence of rupture of the aneurysm than of dying of the surgical resection.

At present, endovascular aneurysm repair may be less definitive than open surgical repair and requires close follow up with an imaging procedure. Device migration, component separation, and graft limb thrombosis or kinking are common reasons for repeat intervention. With complete exclusion of blood from the aneurysm sac, the pressure is lowered, which causes the aneurysm to shrink. An "endoleak" from the top or bottom seal zones (type 1) or through a graft defect (type 3) is associated with a persistent risk of rupture. Indirect leakage of blood through lumbar and inferior mesenteric branches of the aneurysm (endoleak, type 2) produces an intermediate picture with somewhat reduced pressure in the sac, slow shrinkage, and low rupture risk. However, type 2 endoleak warrants close observation because aneurysm dilatation and rupture can occur.

▶ When to Refer

- Any patient with a 4.5-cm or larger aortic aneurysm should be referred for imaging and assessment by a vascular specialist.
- Urgent referrals should be made if the patient complains of pain and gentle palpation of the aneurysm confirms that it is the source, regardless of the aneurysmal size.

▶ When to Admit

Patients with a tender aneurysm to palpation or signs of aortic rupture require emergent hospital admission.

Brahmbhatt R et al. Improved trends in patient survival and decreased major complications after emergency ruptured abdominal aortic aneurysm repair. J Vasc Surg. 2016 Jan; 63(1):39–47. [PMID: 26506941]
Chaikof EL et al. The Society for Vascular Surgery practice guidelines on the care of patients with an abdominal aortic aneurysm. J Vasc Surg. 2018 Jan;67(1):2–77. [PMID: 29268916]
Patel RR et al. Endovascular versus open repair of abdominal aortic aneurysm in 15-years' follow-up of the UK endovascular aneurysm repair trial 1 (EVAR trial 1): a randomised controlled trial. Lancet. 2016 Nov 12;388(10058):2366–74. [PMID: 27743617]

THORACIC AORTIC ANEURYSMS

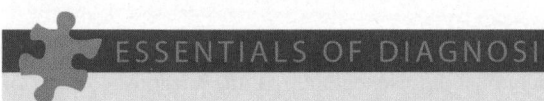

ESSENTIALS OF DIAGNOSIS

- ▶ Widened mediastinum on chest radiograph.
- ▶ With rupture, sudden onset of chest pain radiating to the back.

▶ General Considerations

Most thoracic aortic aneurysms are due to atherosclerosis; syphilis is a rare cause. Disorders of connective tissue and Ehlers-Danlos and Marfan syndromes also are rare causes but have important therapeutic implications. Traumatic, false aneurysms, caused by partial tearing of the aortic wall with deceleration injuries, may occur just beyond the origin of the left subclavian artery. Less than 10% of aortic aneurysms occur in the thoracic aorta.

▶ Clinical Findings

A. Symptoms and Signs

Most thoracic aneurysms are asymptomatic. When symptoms occur, they depend largely on the size and the position of the aneurysm and its rate of growth. Substernal back or neck pain may occur. Pressure on the trachea, esophagus, or superior vena cava can result in the following symptoms and signs: dyspnea, stridor, or brassy cough; dysphagia; and edema in the neck and arms as well as distended neck veins. Stretching of the left recurrent laryngeal nerve causes hoarseness. With aneurysms of the ascending aorta, aortic regurgitation may be present due to dilation of the aortic valve annulus. Rupture of a thoracic aneurysm is catastrophic because bleeding is rarely contained, allowing no time for emergent repair.

B. Imaging

The aneurysm may be diagnosed on chest radiograph by the calcified outline of the dilated aorta. CT scanning is the modality of choice to demonstrate the anatomy and size of the aneurysm and to exclude lesions that can mimic aneurysms, such as neoplasms or substernal goiter. MRI can also be useful. Cardiac catheterization and echocardiography may be required to describe the relationship of the coronary vessels to an aneurysm of the ascending aorta.

▶ Treatment

Indications for repair depend on the location of dilation, rate of growth, associated symptoms, and overall condition of the patient. Aneurysms measuring 6 cm or larger may be considered for repair. Aneurysms of the descending thoracic aorta are treated routinely by endovascular grafting. Repair of arch aneurysms should be undertaken only if there is a skilled surgical team with an acceptable record of outcomes for these complex procedures. The availability of thoracic aortic endograft technique for descending thoracic aneurysms or complex branched endovascular reconstructions for aneurysms involving the arch or visceral aorta (custom-made grafts with branches to the vessels involved in the aneurysm) does not change the indications for aneurysm repair. Aneurysms that involve the proximal aortic arch or ascending aorta represent particularly challenging problems. Open surgery is usually required; however, it carries substantial risk of morbidity (including stroke, diffuse neurologic injury, and intellectual impairment) because interruption of arch blood flow is required.

▶ Complications

With the exception of endovascular repair for discrete saccular aneurysms of the descending thoracic aorta, the morbidity and mortality of thoracic repair is higher than for infra-renal abdominal aortic aneurysm repair. Paraplegia remains a devastating complication. Most large series report approximately 4–10% rate of paraplegia following endovascular repair of thoracic aortic aneurysms. The spinal arterial supply is segmental through intercostal branches of the aorta with variable degrees of intersegmental connection. Therefore, the more extensive the aneurysm, the greater is the risk of paraplegia with repair. Prior infrarenal abdominal aortic surgery, subclavian or internal iliac artery occlusion, and hypotension all increase the paraplegia risk. Involvement of the aortic arch also increases the risk of stroke, even when the aneurysm does not directly affect the carotid artery.

▶ Prognosis

Generally, degenerative aneurysms of the thoracic aorta will enlarge and require repair to prevent death from rupture. Saccular aneurysms, particularly those distal to the left subclavian artery and the descending thoracic aorta, have good results with endovascular repair. Resection of aneurysms of the aortic arch requires a skilled surgical team for the major technical issues and should be attempted only in low-risk patients. Although available at specialty centers, branched or fenestrated endovascular grafting technology has demonstrated reduced morbidity and mortality.

▶ When to Refer

Patients with a 6-cm aneurysm who are deemed to have a reasonable surgical risk should be considered for repair, particularly if the aneurysm involves the descending thoracic aorta.

▶ When to Admit

Any patient with chest or back pain with a known or suspected thoracic aorta aneurysm must be brought to the hospital and undergo urgent imaging studies to rule out the aneurysm as a cause of the pain.

Gasper WJ et al. Assessing the anatomic applicability of the multibranched endovascular repair of thoracoabdominal aortic aneurysm technique. J Vasc Surg. 2013 Jun;57(6):1553–8. [PMID: 23395201]

Huang Q et al. Effect of left subclavian artery revascularisation in thoracic endovascular aortic repair: a systematic review and meta-analysis. Eur J Vasc Endovasc Surg. 2018 Nov; 56(5):644–51. [PMID: 30122331]

Patterson BO et al. Predicting mid-term all-cause mortality in patients undergoing elective endovascular repair of a descending thoracic aortic aneurysm. Ann Surg. 2016 Dec;264(6): 1162–7. [PMID: 26813915]

PERIPHERAL ARTERY ANEURYSMS

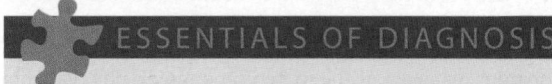

ESSENTIALS OF DIAGNOSIS

► Widened, prominent pulses.
► Acute leg or foot pain and paresthesias with loss of distal pulses.
► High association of popliteal aneurysms with abdominal aortic aneurysms.

▶ General Considerations

Like aortic aneurysms, peripheral artery aneurysms are silent until critically symptomatic. However, unlike aortic aneurysms, the presenting manifestations are due to peripheral embolization and thrombosis. Popliteal artery aneurysms account for 70% of peripheral arterial aneurysms. Popliteal aneurysms may embolize repetitively over time and occlude distal arteries. Due to the redundant parallel arterial supply to the foot, ischemia does not occur until a final embolus occludes flow.

Primary femoral artery aneurysms are much less common. However, pseudoaneurysms of the femoral artery following arterial punctures for arteriography and cardiac catheterization occur with an incidence ranging from 0.05% to 6% of arterial punctures.

Clinical Findings

A. Symptoms and Signs

The patient may be aware of a pulsatile mass when the aneurysm is in the groin, but popliteal aneurysms are often undetected by the patient and clinician. Rarely, peripheral aneurysms may produce symptoms by compressing the local vein or nerve. The first symptom may be due to ischemia of acute arterial occlusion. The symptoms range from sudden-onset pain and paralysis to short-distance claudication that slowly lessens as collateral circulation develops. Symptoms from recurrent embolization to the leg are often transient, if they occur at all. Sudden ischemia may appear in a toe or part of the foot, followed by slow resolution, and the true diagnosis may be elusive. The onset of recurrent episodes of pain in the foot, particularly if accompanied by cyanosis, suggests embolization and requires investigation of the heart and proximal arterial tree.

Because popliteal pulses are somewhat difficult to palpate even in normal individuals, a particularly prominent or easily felt pulse is suggestive of aneurysm and should be investigated by ultrasound. Since popliteal aneurysms are bilateral in 60% of cases, the diagnosis of thrombosis of a popliteal aneurysm is often aided by the palpation of a pulsatile aneurysm in the contralateral popliteal space. Approximately 50% of patients with popliteal aneurysms have an aneurysmal abdominal aorta.

B. Imaging Studies

Duplex color ultrasound is the most efficient investigation to confirm the diagnosis of peripheral aneurysm, measure its size and configuration, and demonstrate mural thrombus. MRA or CTA is required to define the aneurysm and local arterial anatomy for reconstruction. Arteriography is not recommended because mural thrombus reduces the apparent diameter of the lumen on angiography. Patients with popliteal aneurysms should undergo abdominal ultrasonography to determine whether an abdominal aortic aneurysm is also present.

Treatment

To prevent limb loss from thrombosis or embolization, surgery is indicated when an aneurysm is associated with any peripheral embolization, the aneurysm is larger than 2 cm, or a mural thrombus is present. Immediate or urgent surgery is indicated when acute embolization or thrombosis has caused acute ischemia. Bypass is generally performed. Endovascular exclusion of the aneurysm can be done but is reserved for high-risk patients. Intra-arterial thrombolysis may be done in the setting of acute ischemia, if examination (light touch) remains intact, suggesting that immediate surgery is not imperative. Acute pseudoaneurysms of the femoral artery due to arterial punctures can be successfully treated using ultrasound-guided compression. Open surgery

with prosthetic interposition grafting is preferred for primary aneurysms of the femoral artery.

Prognosis

Approximately one-third of untreated patients will require an amputation. The long-term patency of bypass grafts for femoral and popliteal aneurysms is generally excellent, but depends on the adequacy of the outflow tract. Late graft occlusion is less common than in similar surgeries for occlusive disease.

When to Refer

In addition to patients with symptoms of ischemia, any patient with a peripheral arterial aneurysm measuring 2 cm or with ultrasound evidence of thrombus within the aneurysm should be referred to prevent progression to limb-threatening ischemia.

Cervin A et al. Treatment of popliteal aneurysm by open and endovascular surgery: a contemporary study of 592 procedures in Sweden. Eur J Vasc Endovasc Surg. 2015 Sep;50(3):342–50. [PMID: 25911500]

AORTIC DISSECTION

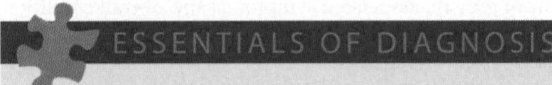

ESSENTIALS OF DIAGNOSIS

- ► Sudden searing chest pain with radiation to the back, abdomen, or neck in a hypertensive patient.
- ► Widened mediastinum on chest radiograph.
- ► Pulse discrepancy in the extremities.
- ► Acute aortic regurgitation may develop.

General Considerations

Aortic dissection occurs when a spontaneous intimal tear develops and blood dissects into the media of the aorta. The tear probably results from the repetitive torque applied to the ascending and proximal descending aorta during the cardiac cycle; hypertension is an important component of this disease process. **Type A dissection** involves the arch proximal to the left subclavian artery, and **type B dissection** occurs in the proximal descending thoracic aorta typically just beyond the left subclavian artery. Dissections may occur in the absence of hypertension but abnormalities of smooth muscle, elastic tissue, or collagen are more common in these patients. Pregnancy, bicuspid aortic valve, and coarctation also are associated with increased risk of dissection.

Blood entering the intimal tear may extend the dissection into the abdominal aorta, the lower extremities, the carotid arteries or, less commonly, the subclavian arteries. Both absolute pressure levels and the pulse pressure are important in propagation of dissection. *Aortic dissection is a true emergency and requires immediate control of blood pressure to limit the extent of the dissection.* With type A dissection, which has the worse prognosis, death may occur within hours due to rupture of the dissection into the pericardial sac or dissection into the coronary arteries, resulting in myocardial infarction. Rupture into the pleural cavity is also possible. The intimal/medial flap of the aortic wall created by the dissection may occlude major aortic branches, resulting in ischemia of the brain, intestines, kidney, or extremities.

► Clinical Findings

A. Symptoms and Signs

Severe persistent chest pain of sudden onset radiating down the back or possibly into the anterior chest is characteristic. Radiation of the pain into the neck may also occur. The patient is usually hypertensive. Syncope, hemiplegia, or paralysis of the lower extremities may occur. Intestinal ischemia or kidney injury may develop. Peripheral pulses may be diminished or unequal. A diastolic murmur may develop as a result of a dissection in the ascending aorta close to the aortic valve, causing valvular regurgitation, heart failure, and cardiac tamponade.

B. Electrocardiographic Findings

Left ventricular hypertrophy from long-standing hypertension is often present. Acute changes suggesting myocardial ischemia do not develop unless dissection involves the coronary artery ostium. Classically, inferior wall abnormalities predominate since dissection leads to compromise of the right rather than the left coronary artery. In some patients, the ECG may be completely normal.

C. Imaging

A multiplanar CT scan is the immediate diagnostic imaging modality of choice; clinicians should have a low threshold for obtaining a CT scan in any hypertensive patient with chest pain and equivocal findings on ECG.

The CT scan should include both the chest and abdomen to fully delineate the extent of the dissected aorta. MRI is an excellent imaging modality for chronic dissections, but in the acute situation, the longer imaging time and the difficulty of monitoring patients in the MRI scanner make the CT scan preferable. Chest radiographs may reveal an abnormal aortic contour or widened superior mediastinum. Although transesophageal echocardiography (TEE) is an excellent diagnostic imaging method, it is generally not readily available in the acute setting.

► Differential Diagnosis

Aortic dissection is most commonly misdiagnosed as myocardial infarction or other causes of chest pain such as pulmonary embolization. Dissections may occur with minimal pain; branch vessel occlusion of the lower extremity can mimic arterial embolus.

► Treatment

A. Medical

Aggressive measures to lower blood pressure should occur when an aortic dissection is suspected, even before the diagnostic studies have been completed. Treatment requires a simultaneous reduction of the systolic blood pressure to 100–120 mm Hg and pulse pressure. Beta-blockers have the

most desirable effect of reducing the left ventricular ejection force that continues to weaken the arterial wall and should be first-line therapy. Labetalol, both an alpha- and beta-blocker, lowers pulse pressure and achieves rapid blood pressure control. Give 20 mg over 2 minutes by intravenous injection. Additional doses of 40–80 mg intravenously can be given every 10 minutes (maximum dose 300 mg) until the desired blood pressure has been reached. Alternatively, 2 mg/min may be given by intravenous infusion, titrated to desired effect. In patients who have asthma, bradycardia, or other conditions that necessitate the patient's reaction to beta-blockers be tested, esmolol is a reasonable choice because of its short half-life. Give a loading dose of esmolol, 0.5 mg/kg intravenously over 1 minute, followed by an infusion of 0.0025–0.02 mg/kg/min. Titrate the infusion to a goal heart rate of 60–70 beats/min. If beta-blockade alone does not control the hypertension, nitroprusside may be added as follows: 50 mg of nitroprusside in 1000 mL of 5% dextrose and water, infused at a rate of 0.5 mL/min for a 70-kg person (0.3 mcg/kg/min); the infusion rate is increased by 0.5 mL every 5 minutes until adequate control of the pressure has been achieved. In patients with bronchial asthma, while there are no data supporting the use of the calcium channel antagonists, diltiazem and verapamil are potential alternatives to treatment with beta-blocking drugs. Morphine sulfate is the appropriate drug to use for pain relief. Long-term medical care of patients should include beta-blockers in their antihypertensive regimen.

B. Surgical Intervention

Urgent surgical intervention is required for all type A dissections. If a skilled cardiovascular team is not available, the patient should be transferred to an appropriate facility. The procedure involves grafting and replacing the diseased portion of the arch and brachiocephalic vessels as necessary. Replacement of the aortic valve may be required with reattachment of the coronary arteries.

Urgent surgery is required for **type B dissections** if there is aortic branch compromise resulting in malperfusion of the renal, visceral, or extremity vessels. The immediate goal of surgical therapy is to restore flow to the ischemic tissue, which is most commonly accomplished via a bypass. Endovascular stenting of the entry tear at the level of the subclavian artery may result in obliteration of the false lumen and restore flow into the branch vessel from the true lumen. The results, however, are unpredictable and should only be attempted by an experienced team. For acute type B dissections without malperfusion, evidence shows that long-term aortic-specific survival and late aneurysm formation rates are improved with early thoracic stent graft repair. Patients with uncomplicated type B dissections whose blood pressure is controlled and who survive the acute episode without complications may have long-term survival without surgical treatment.

► Prognosis & Follow-Up

The mortality rate for untreated type A dissections is approximately 1% per hour for 72 hours and over 90% at 3 months. Mortality is also extremely high for untreated type B dissections with malperfusion or rupture. The surgical and endovascular therapies for these patients are technically demanding and require an experienced team to achieve perioperative mortalities of less than 10%. Aneurysmal enlargement of the residual false lumen may develop despite adequate antihypertensive therapy. Yearly CT scans are required to monitor for aneurysm development. Indications for late aneurysm repair are determined by aneurysm size (6 cm or larger), similar to undissected thoracic aneurysms.

► When to Admit

All patients with an acute dissection should be hospitalized. Any dissection involving the aortic arch (type A) should be immediately repaired. Acute type B dissections require repair only when there is evidence of rupture or major branch occlusion.

Bossone E et al. Acute aortic syndromes: diagnosis and management, an update. Eur Heart J. 2018 Mar 1;39(9):739–49d. [PMID: 29106452]
Suzuki T et al. Medical management in type B aortic dissection. Ann Cardiothorac Surg. 2014 Jul;3(4):413–7. [PMID: 25133106]

▼ VENOUS DISEASES

VARICOSE VEINS

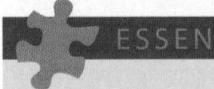

ESSENTIALS OF DIAGNOSIS

- ► Dilated, tortuous superficial veins in the legs.
- ► May be asymptomatic or associated with aching discomfort or pain.
- ► Often hereditary.
- ► Increased frequency after pregnancy.

► General Considerations

Varicose veins develop in the lower extremities. Periods of high venous pressure related to prolonged standing or heavy lifting are contributing factors, but the highest incidence occurs in women after pregnancy. Varicosities develop in over 20% of all adults.

The combination of progressive venous reflux and venous hypertension is the hallmark of chronic venous disease. The superficial veins are involved, typically the great saphenous vein and its tributaries, but the short saphenous vein (posterior lower leg) may also be affected. Distention of the vein prevents the valve leaflets from coapting, creating incompetence and reflux of blood toward the foot. Focal venous dilation and reflux leads to increased pressure and distention of the vein segment below that valve, which in turn causes progressive failure of the next lower valve. Perforating veins that connect the deep and superficial systems may become incompetent, allowing blood to reflux into the superficial veins from the deep system, increasing venous pressure and distention.

Secondary varicosities can develop as a result of obstructive changes and valve damage in the deep venous system following thrombophlebitis, or rarely as a result of proximal venous occlusion due to neoplasm or fibrosis. Congenital or acquired arteriovenous fistulas or venous malformations are also associated with varicosities and should be considered in young patients with varicosities.

► Clinical Findings

A. Symptoms and Signs

Symptom severity is not correlated with the number and size of the varicosities; extensive varicose veins may produce no subjective symptoms, whereas minimal varicosities may produce many symptoms. Dull, aching heaviness or a feeling of fatigue of the legs brought on by periods of standing is the most common complaint. Itching from venous eczema may occur either above the ankle or directly overlying large varicosities.

Dilated, tortuous veins of the thigh and calf are visible and palpable when the patient is standing. Longstanding varicose veins may progress to chronic venous insufficiency with associated ankle edema, brownish skin hyperpigmentation, and chronic skin induration or fibrosis. A bruit or thrill is never found with primary varicose veins and when found, alerts the clinician to the presence of an arteriovenous fistula or malformation.

B. Imaging

The identification of the source of venous reflux that feeds the symptomatic veins is necessary for effective surgical treatment. Duplex ultrasonography by a technician experienced in the diagnosis and localization of venous reflux is the test of choice for planning therapy. In most cases, reflux will arise from the greater saphenous vein.

► Differential Diagnosis

Varicose veins due to primary superficial venous reflux should be differentiated from those secondary to previous or ongoing obstruction of the deep veins (post-thrombotic syndrome). Pain or discomfort secondary to neuropathy should be distinguished from symptoms associated with coexistent varicose veins. Similarly, vein symptoms should be distinguished from pain due to intermittent claudication, which occurs after a predictable amount of exercise and resolves with rest. In adolescent patients with varicose veins, imaging of the deep venous system is obligatory to exclude a congenital malformation or atresia of the deep veins. Surgical treatment of varicose veins in these patients is contraindicated because the varicosities may play a significant role in venous drainage of the limb.

► Complications

Superficial thrombophlebitis of varicose veins is uncommon. The typical presentation is acute localized pain with tender, firm veins. The process is usually self-limiting, resolving within several weeks. The risk of deep venous thrombosis (DVT) or embolization is very low unless the thrombophlebitis extends into the great saphenous vein in the upper medial thigh. Predisposing conditions include pregnancy, local trauma, or prolonged periods of sitting.

In older patients, superficial varicosities may bleed with even minor trauma. The amount of bleeding can be alarming as the pressure in the varicosity is high.

Treatment

A. Nonsurgical Measures

Nonsurgical treatment is effective. Elastic graduated compression stockings (20–30 mm Hg pressure) reduce the venous pressure in the leg and may prevent the progression of disease. Good control of symptoms can be achieved when stockings are worn daily during waking hours and legs are elevated, especially at night. Compression stockings are well-suited for elderly patients or patients who do not want surgery.

B. Sclerotherapy

Direct injection of a sclerosing agent induces permanent fibrosis and obliteration of the target veins. Chemical irritants (eg, glycerin) or hypertonic saline are often used for small, less-than-4-mm reticular veins or telangiectasias. Foam sclerotherapy is used to treat the great saphenous vein, varicose veins larger than 4 mm, and perforating veins, often with local anesthesia alone. Injection of a cyanoacrylate adhesive is also available for treating the great saphenous vein. Foam sclerotherapy and cyanoacrylate adhesive therapy have similar clinical results as saphenous vein thermal ablation or stripping, although the long-term success rate may be lower and systemic embolization remains a concern. Complications such as phlebitis, tissue necrosis, or infection may occur with any sclerosing agent.

C. Surgical Measures

Treatment with endovenous thermal ablation (with either radiofrequency or laser) or, less commonly, with great saphenous vein stripping is effective for reflux arising from the great saphenous vein. Less common sources of reflux include the small saphenous vein (for varicosities in the posterior calf) and incompetent perforator veins arising directly from the deep venous system. Correction of reflux is performed at the same time as excision of the symptomatic varicose veins. Phlebectomy without correction of reflux results in a high rate of recurrent varicosities, as the uncorrected reflux progressively dilates adjacent veins. Concurrent reflux detected by ultrasonography in the deep system is not a contraindication to treatment of superficial reflux because the majority of deep vein dilatation is secondary to volume overload in this setting, which will resolve with correction of the superficial reflux.

Prognosis

Surgical treatment of superficial vein reflux and excision of varicose veins provide excellent results. The 5-year success rate (as defined as lack of pain and recurrent varicosities) is 85–90%. Simple excision (phlebectomy) or injection

sclerotherapy without correction of reflux is associated with higher rates of recurrence. Even after adequate treatment, secondary tissue changes may persist.

When to Refer

- Absolute indications for referral for saphenous ablation include thrombophlebitis and bleeding.
- Pain and cosmetic concerns are responsible for the majority of referrals for ablation.

Brittenden J et al. A randomized trial comparing treatments for varicose veins. N Engl J Med. 2014 Sep 25;371(13):1218–27. [PMID: 25251616]

DePopas E et al. Varicose veins and lower extremity venous insufficiency. Semin Intervent Radiol. 2018 Mar;35(1):56–61. [PMID: 29628617]

Hamann SAS et al. Editor's Choice—Five-year results of great saphenous vein treatment: a meta-analysis. Eur J Vasc Endovasc Surg. 2017 Dec;54(6):760–70. [PMID: 29033337]

SUPERFICIAL VENOUS THROMBOPHLEBITIS

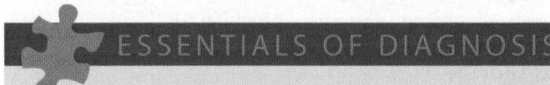
ESSENTIALS OF DIAGNOSIS

- ► Red, painful induration along a superficial vein, usually at the site of a recent intravenous line.
- ► Marked swelling of the extremity may not occur.

General Considerations

Short-term venous catheterization of superficial arm veins as well as the use of longer-term peripherally inserted central catheter (PICC) lines are the most common cause of superficial thrombophlebitis. Intravenous catheter sites should be observed daily for signs of local inflammation and should be removed if a local reaction develops in the vein. Serious thrombotic or septic complications can occur if this policy is not followed; *Staphylococcus aureus* is the most common pathogen. Other organisms, including fungi, may also be responsible.

Superficial thrombophlebitis may occur spontaneously, often in pregnant or postpartum women or in individuals with varicose veins, or it may be associated with trauma, as with a blow to the leg or following intravenous therapy with irritating solutions. It also may be a manifestation of systemic hypercoagulability secondary to abdominal cancer such as carcinoma of the pancreas and may be the earliest sign of these conditions. Superficial thrombophlebitis may be associated with occult DVT in about 20% of cases. Pulmonary emboli are exceedingly rare and occur from an associated DVT. (See Chapters 9 and 14 for discussion on deep venous thrombosis.)

Clinical Findings

In spontaneous superficial thrombophlebitis, the great saphenous vein is most often involved. The patient usually experiences a dull pain in the region of the involved vein.

Local findings consist of induration, redness, and tenderness along the course of a vein. The process may be localized, or it may involve most of the great saphenous vein and its tributaries. The inflammatory reaction generally subsides in 1–2 weeks; a firm cord may remain for a much longer period. Edema of the extremity is uncommon.

Localized redness and induration at the site of a recent intravenous line requires urgent attention. Proximal extension of the induration and pain with chills and high fever suggest septic phlebitis and requires urgent treatment.

► Differential Diagnosis

The linear rather than circular nature of the lesion and the distribution along the course of a superficial vein serve to differentiate superficial phlebitis from cellulitis, erythema nodosum, erythema induratum, panniculitis, and fibrositis. Lymphangitis and deep thrombophlebitis must also be considered.

► Treatment

For spontaneous thrombophlebitis if the process is well localized and not near the saphenofemoral junction, local heat and nonsteroidal anti-inflammatory medications are usually effective in limiting the process. If the induration is extensive or is progressing toward the saphenofemoral junction (leg) or cephalo-axillary junction (arm), ligation and division of the vein at the junction of the deep and superficial veins is indicated.

Anticoagulation therapy is usually not required for focal processes. Prophylactic dose low-molecular-weight heparin or fondaparinux is recommended for 5 cm or longer superficial thrombophlebitis of the lower limb veins (Table 14–14) and full anticoagulation is reserved for disease that is rapidly progressing or if there is concern for extension into the deep system (Table 14–16).

Septic superficial thrombophlebitis is an intravascular abscess and requires urgent treatment with heparin or fondaparinux (see Table 14–16) to limit additional thrombus formation as well as removal of the offending catheter in catheter-related infections (see Chapter 30). Treat with antibiotics (eg, vancomycin, 15 mg/kg intravenously every 12 hours, plus ceftriaxone, 1 g intravenously every 24 hours). If cultures are positive, therapy should be continued for 7–10 days or for 4–6 weeks if complicating endocarditis cannot be excluded. Surgical excision of the involved vein may also be necessary to control the infection.

► Prognosis

With spontaneous thrombophlebitis, the course is generally benign and brief. The prognosis depends on the underlying pathologic process. In patients with phlebitis secondary to varicose veins, recurrent episodes are likely unless correction of the underlying venous reflux and excision of varicosities is done. In contrast, the mortality from septic thrombophlebitis is 20% or higher and requires aggressive treatment. However, if the involvement is localized, the mortality is low and prognosis is excellent with early treatment.

Di Nisio M et al. Treatment for superficial thrombophlebitis of the leg. Cochrane Database Syst Rev. 2018 Feb 25;2:CD004982. [PMID: 29478266]

CHRONIC VENOUS INSUFFICIENCY

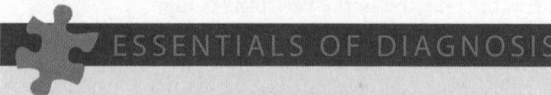

ESSENTIALS OF DIAGNOSIS

- ► History of prior DVT or leg injury.
- ► Edema, (brawny) skin hyperpigmentation, subcutaneous lipodermosclerosis in the lower leg.
- ► Large ulcerations at or above the medial ankle are common (venous ulcers).

► General Considerations

Chronic venous insufficiency is a severe manifestation of venous hypertension. One of the most common etiologies is prior deep venous thrombophlebitis (see Chapter 14), although about 25% of patients do not have a known history of DVT. In these cases, there may be a history of leg trauma or surgery; obesity is often a complicating factor. Progressive superficial venous reflux is also a common cause. Other causes include congenital or neoplastic obstruction of the pelvic veins or a congenital or acquired arteriovenous fistula.

The basic pathology is caused by valve leaflets that do not coapt because they are either thickened and scarred (post-thrombotic syndrome) or in a dilated vein and are therefore functionally inadequate. Proximal venous obstruction due to chronic thrombus or scarring compounds the problem. With the valves unable to stop venous blood from returning to the foot (venous reflux), the leg develops venous hypertension and an abnormally high hydrostatic force is transmitted to the subcutaneous veins and tissues of the lower leg. The resulting edema results in dramatic and deleterious secondary changes. The stigmata of chronic venous insufficiency include fibrosis of the subcutaneous tissue and skin, pigmentation of skin (hemosiderin taken up by the dermal macrophages), and, later, ulceration, which is extremely slow to heal. Itching may precipitate the formation of ulceration or local wound cellulitis. Dilation of the superficial veins may occur, leading to varicosities. Although surgical treatment for venous reflux can improve symptoms, controlling edema and the secondary skin changes usually require lifelong compression therapy.

► Clinical Findings

A. Symptoms and Signs

Progressive pitting edema of the leg (particularly the lower leg) is the primary presenting symptom. Secondary changes in the skin and subcutaneous tissues develop over time (Figure 12–2). The usual symptoms are itching, a dull discomfort made worse by periods of standing, and pain if an ulceration is present. The skin at the ankle is usually taut

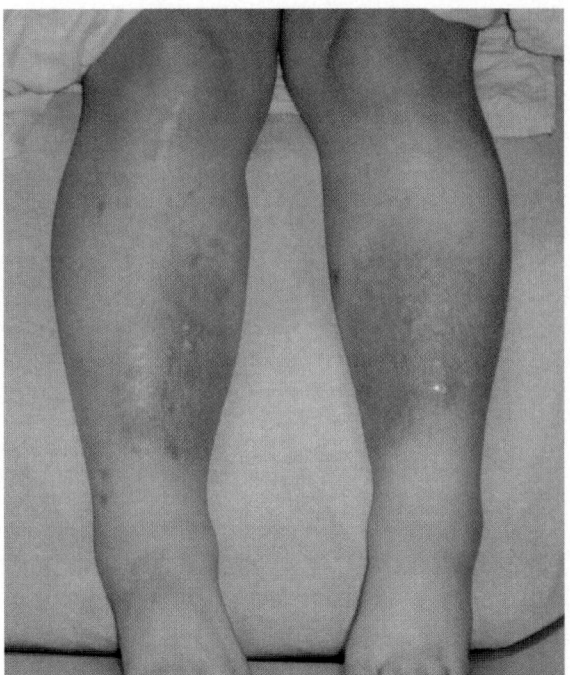

▲ **Figure 12–2.** Bilateral pretibial edema and erythema consistent with stasis dermatitis (sometimes mimicking cellulitis) in chronic venous insufficiency. (Used, with permission, from Dean SM, Satiani B, Abraham WT. *Color Atlas and Synopsis of Vascular Diseases.* McGraw-Hill, 2014.)

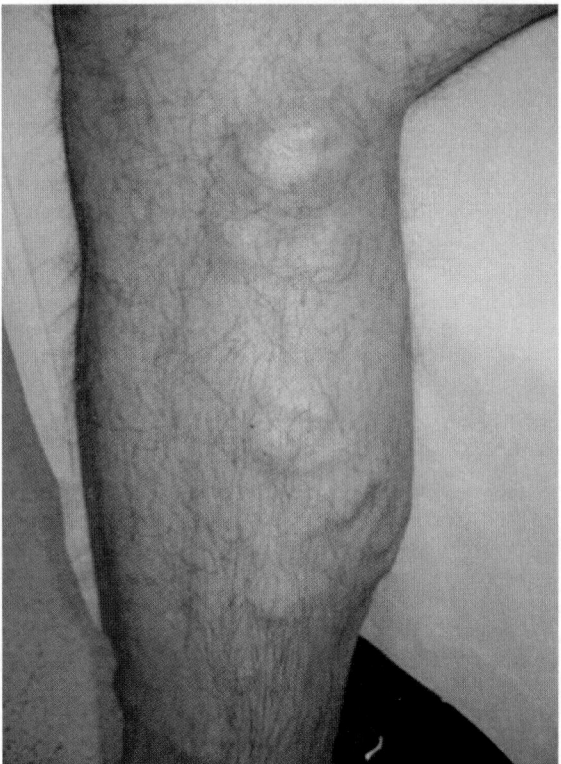

▲ **Figure 12–3.** Varicose veins, manifested as blue, subcutaneous, tortuous veins more than 3 mm in diameter. (Used, with permission, from Dean SM, Satiani B, Abraham WT. *Color Atlas and Synopsis of Vascular Diseases.* McGraw-Hill, 2014.)

from swelling, shiny, and a brownish pigmentation (hemosiderin) often develops. If the condition is longstanding, the subcutaneous tissues become thick and fibrous. Ulcerations may occur, usually just above the ankle, on the medial or anterior aspect of the leg. Healing results in a thin scar on a fibrotic base that often breaks down with minor trauma or further bouts of leg swelling. Varicosities may appear (Figure 12–3) that are associated with incompetent perforating veins. Cellulitis, which is often difficult to distinguish from the hemosiderin pigmentation, may be diagnosed by blanching erythema with pain.

B. Imaging

Patients with post-thrombotic syndrome or signs of chronic venous insufficiency should undergo duplex ultrasonography to determine whether superficial reflux is present and to evaluate the degree of deep reflux and obstruction.

▶ Differential Diagnosis

Patients with heart failure, chronic kidney disease, or decompensated liver disease may have bilateral edema of the lower extremities. Many medications can cause edema (eg, calcium channel blockers, nonsteroidal anti-inflammatory agents, thiazolidinediones). Swelling from lymphedema involves the feet and may be unilateral, but varicosities are absent. Edema from these causes pits easily and brawny discoloration is rare. Lipedema is a disorder of

adipose tissue that occurs almost exclusively in women, is bilateral and symmetric, and is characterized by stopping at a distinct line just above the ankles.

Primary varicose veins may be difficult to differentiate from the secondary varicosities of post-thrombotic syndrome or venous obstruction.

Other conditions associated with chronic ulcers of the leg include neuropathic ulcers usually from diabetes mellitus, arterial insufficiency (often very painful lateral ankle ulcers with absent pulses), autoimmune diseases (eg, Felty syndrome), sickle cell anemia, erythema induratum (bilateral and usually on the posterior aspect of the lower part of the leg), and fungal infections.

▶ Prevention

Irreversible tissue changes and associated complications in the lower legs can be reduced through early and aggressive anticoagulation of acute DVT to minimize the valve damages and by prescribing compression stockings if chronic edema develops after the DVT has resolved. Routine treatment of acute iliofemoral DVT with catheter-directed thrombolysis or mechanical thrombectomy does not reduce post-thrombotic syndrome and chronic venous insufficiency.

Treatment

A. General Measures

Fitted, graduated compression stockings (20–30 mm Hg pressure or higher) worn from the foot to just below the knee during the day and evening are the mainstays of treatment and are usually sufficient. When they are not, additional measures, such as avoidance of long periods of sitting or standing, intermittent elevations of the involved leg, and sleeping with the legs kept above the level of the heart, may be necessary to control the swelling. Pneumatic compression of the leg, which can pump the fluid out of the leg, is used in cases refractory to the above measures.

B. Ulceration

As the primary pathology is edema and venous hypertension, healing of the ulcer will not occur until the edema is controlled and compression is applied. Circumferential nonelastic bandages on the lower leg enhance the pumping action of the calf muscles on venous blood flow out of the calf. A lesion can often be treated on an ambulatory basis by means of a semi-rigid gauze boot made with Unna paste (Gelocast, Medicopaste) or a multi-layer compression dressing (eg, Profore). Initially, the ulcer needs to be debrided and the boot changed every 2–3 days to control ulcer drainage. As the edema and drainage subside, optimal healing is achieved when the boot is kept in place for 5–7 days. The ulcer, tendons, and bony prominences must be adequately padded. Alternatively, knee-high graduated compression stockings with an absorbent dressing may be used, if wound drainage is minimal. Home compression therapy with a pneumatic compression device is used in refractory cases, but many patients have severe pain with the "milking" action of the pump device. Some patients will require admission for complete bed rest and leg elevation to achieve ulcer healing. After the ulcer has healed, daily graduated compression stocking therapy is mandatory to prevent ulcer recurrence.

C. Vein Treatment (Reflux or Obstruction)

Treatment of superficial vein reflux (see Varicose Veins section, above) has been shown to decrease the recurrence rate of venous ulcers. Where there is substantial obstruction of the femoral and popliteal deep venous system, superficial varicosities supply the venous return and they should not be removed.

Using venous stents, treatment of chronic iliac deep vein stenosis or obstruction may improve venous ulcer healing and reduce the ulcer recurrence rate in severe cases.

Prognosis

Individuals with chronic venous insufficiency often have recurrent edema, particularly if they do not consistently wear support stockings that have at least 20–30 mm Hg compression.

When to Refer

- Patients with significant saphenous reflux should be evaluated for ablation.
- Patients with ulcers should be monitored by an interdisciplinary wound care team so that these challenging wounds receive aggressive care.

O'Donnell TF Jr et al. Management of venous leg ulcers: clinical practice guidelines of the Society for Vascular Surgery and the American Venous Forum. J Vasc Surg. 2014 Aug;60(2 Suppl): 3S–59S. [PMID: 24974070]

Raffetto JD. Pathophysiology of chronic venous disease and venous ulcers. Surg Clin North Am. 2018 Apr;98(2):337–47. [PMID: 29502775]

Seager MJ et al. Editor's Choice—A systematic review of endovenous stenting in chronic venous disease secondary to iliac vein obstruction. Eur J Vasc Endovasc Surg. 2016 Jan;51(1):100–20. [PMID: 26464055]

Vedantham S et al; ATTRACT Trial Investigators. Pharmacomechanical catheter-directed thrombolysis for deep-vein thrombosis. N Engl J Med. 2017 Dec 7;377(23):2240–52. [PMID: 29211671]

SUPERIOR VENA CAVAL OBSTRUCTION

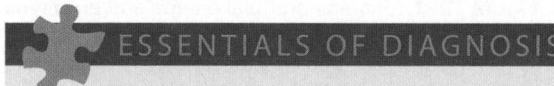

ESSENTIALS OF DIAGNOSIS

- ► Swelling of the neck, face, and upper extremities.
- ► Dilated veins over the upper chest and neck.

General Considerations

Partial or complete obstruction of the superior vena cava is a relatively rare condition that is usually secondary to neoplastic or inflammatory processes in the superior mediastinum. The most frequent causes are (1) neoplasms, such as lymphomas, primary malignant mediastinal tumors, or carcinoma of the lung with direct extension (over 80%); (2) chronic fibrotic mediastinitis, either of unknown origin or secondary to tuberculosis, histoplasmosis, pyogenic infections, or drugs, especially methysergide; (3) DVT, often by extension of the process from the axillary or subclavian vein into the innominate vein and vena cava associated with catheterization of these veins for dialysis or for hyperalimentation; (4) aneurysm of the aortic arch; and (5) constrictive pericarditis.

Clinical Findings

A. Symptoms and Signs

The onset of symptoms is acute or subacute. Symptoms include swelling of the neck and face and upper extremities. Symptoms are often perceived as congestion and present as headache, dizziness, visual disturbances, stupor, syncope, or cough. There is progressive obstruction of the venous drainage of the head, neck, and upper extremities. The cutaneous veins of the upper chest and lower neck become dilated, and flushing of the face and neck develops. Brawny edema of the face, neck, and arms occurs later, and cyanosis of these areas then appears. Cerebral and laryngeal edema ultimately result in impaired function of the brain as well as respiratory insufficiency. Bending over or lying down accentuates the symptoms; sitting quietly is generally preferred. The manifestations are more severe if the obstruction develops rapidly and if the azygos junction or the vena cava between that vein and the heart is obstructed.

B. Laboratory Findings

The venous pressure is elevated (often more than 20 cm of water) in the arm and is normal in the leg. Since lung cancer is a common cause, bronchoscopy is often performed; transbronchial biopsy, however, is relatively contraindicated because of venous hypertension and the risk of bleeding.

C. Imaging

Chest radiographs and a CT scan will define the location and often the nature of the obstructive process, and contrast venography or magnetic resonance venography (MRV) will map out the extent and degree of the venous obstruction and the collateral circulation. Brachial venography or radionuclide scanning following intravenous injection of technetium (Tc-99m) pertechnetate demonstrates a block to the flow of contrast material into the right heart and enlarged collateral veins. These techniques also allow estimation of blood flow around the occlusion as well as serial evaluation of the response to therapy.

Treatment

Conservative measures, such as elevation of the head of the bed and lifestyle modification to avoid bending over, are useful. Balloon angioplasty of the obstructed caval segment combined with stent placement provides prompt relief of symptoms and is the procedure of choice for all etiologies. Occasionally, anticoagulation is needed, while thrombolysis is rarely needed.

Urgent treatment for neoplasm consists of (1) cautious use of intravenous diuretics and (2) mediastinal irradiation, starting within 24 hours, with a treatment plan designed to give a high daily dose but a short total course of therapy to rapidly shrink the local tumor. Intensive combined therapy will palliate the process in up to 90% of patients. In patients with a subacute presentation, radiation therapy alone usually suffices. Chemotherapy is added if lymphoma or small-cell carcinoma is diagnosed.

Long-term outcome is complicated by risk of re-occlusion from either thrombosis or further growth of the neoplasm. Surgical procedures to bypass the obstruction are complicated by bleeding relating to high venous pressure. In cases where the thrombosis is secondary to an indwelling catheter, thrombolysis may be attempted. Clinical judgment is required since a long-standing clot may be fibrotic and the risk of bleeding will outweigh the potential benefit.

Prognosis

The prognosis depends on the nature and degree of obstruction and its speed of onset. Slowly developing forms secondary to fibrosis may be tolerated for years. A high degree of obstruction of rapid onset secondary to cancer is often fatal in a few days or weeks because of increased intracranial pressure and cerebral hemorrhage, but treatment of the tumor with radiation and chemotherapeutic drugs may result in significant palliation. Balloon angioplasty and stenting provide good relief, but may require re-treatment for recurrent symptoms secondary to thrombosis or restenosis.

When to Refer

Referral should occur with any patient with progressive head and neck swelling to rule out superior vena cava syndrome.

When to Admit

Any patient with acute edema of the head and neck or any patient in whom signs and symptoms of airway compromise, such as hoarseness or stridor, develop should be admitted.

Lepper PM et al. Superior vena cava syndrome in thoracic malignancies. Respir Care. 2011 May;56(5):653–66. [PMID: 21276318]

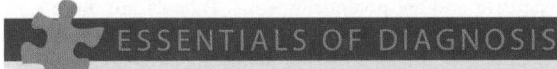

DISEASES OF THE LYMPHATIC CHANNELS

LYMPHANGITIS & LYMPHADENITIS

ESSENTIALS OF DIAGNOSIS

▶ Red streak from wound or area of cellulitis toward regional lymph nodes, which are usually enlarged and tender.

▶ Chills, fever, and malaise may be present.

General Considerations

Lymphangitis and lymphadenitis are common manifestations of a bacterial infection that is usually caused by hemolytic streptococci or *S aureus* (or by both organisms) and becomes invasive, generally from an infected wound. The wound may be very small or superficial, or an established abscess may be present, feeding bacteria into the lymphatics. The involvement of the lymphatics is often manifested by a red streak in the skin extending in the direction of the regional lymph nodes, which are, in turn, generally tender and engorged. Systemic manifestations include fever, chills, and malaise. The infection may progress rapidly, often in a matter of hours, and may lead to septicemia and even death.

Clinical Findings

A. Symptoms and Signs

Throbbing pain is usually present in the area of cellulitis at the site of bacterial invasion. Malaise, anorexia, sweating, chills, and fever of 38–40°C develop rapidly. The red streak, when present, may be definite or may be very faint and easily missed, especially in dark-skinned patients. It is usually tender or indurated in the area of cellulitis. The involved regional lymph nodes may be significantly enlarged and are usually quite tender. The pulse is often rapid.

B. Laboratory Findings

Leukocytosis with a left shift is usually present. Blood cultures may be positive, most often for staphylococcal or streptococcal species. Culture and sensitivity studies of the wound exudate or pus may be helpful in treatment of the more severe or refractory infections but are often difficult to interpret because of skin contaminants.

Differential Diagnosis

Lymphangitis may be confused with superficial thrombophlebitis, but the erythema and induration of thrombophlebitis is localized in and around the thrombosed vein. Venous thrombosis is not associated with lymphadenitis, and a wound of entrance with secondary cellulitis is generally absent.

Cat-scratch fever (*Bartonella henselae*) should be considered when lymphadenitis is present; the nodes, though often very large, are relatively nontender. Exposure to cats is common, but the patient may have forgotten about the scratch.

It is extremely important to differentiate cellulitis from acute streptococcal hemolytic gangrene or a necrotizing soft tissue infection. These are deeper infections that may be extensive and are potentially lethal. Patients are more seriously ill; there may be redness due to leakage of red cells, creating a non-blanching erythema; subcutaneous crepitus may be palpated or auscultated; and subcutaneous air may be present on radiography or CT scan. Immediate surgical consultation for wide debridement of all involved deep tissues should be pursued if a necrotizing infection is suspected.

Treatment

A. General Measures

Prompt treatment should include heat (hot, moist compresses or heating pad), elevation when feasible, and immobilization of the infected area. Analgesics may be prescribed for pain.

B. Specific Measures

Empiric antibiotic therapy for hemolytic streptococci or *S aureus* (or both organisms) should always be instituted. Cephalosporins or extended-spectrum penicillins are commonly used (eg, cephalexin, 0.5 g orally four times daily for 7–10 days; see Table 30–6). Trimethoprim-sulfamethoxazole (two double-strength tablets orally twice daily for 7–10 days) should be considered when there is concern

that the pathogen is methicillin-resistant *S aureus* (MRSA) (see Tables 30–4 and 30–6).

C. Wound Care

Any wound that is the initiating site of lymphangitis should be treated aggressively. Any necrotic tissue must be debrided and loculated pus drained.

Prognosis

With proper therapy including an antibiotic effective against the invading bacteria, control of the infection can usually be achieved in a few days. Delayed or inadequate therapy can lead to overwhelming infection with septicemia.

When to Admit

Infections causing lymphangitis should be treated in the hospital with intravenous antibiotics. Debridement may be required.

LYMPHEDEMA

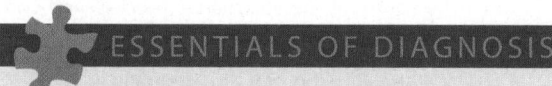

ESSENTIALS OF DIAGNOSIS

▶ Painless persistent edema of one or both lower extremities, primarily in young women.

▶ Pitting edema without ulceration, varicosities, or stasis pigmentation.

▶ There may be episodes of lymphangitis and cellulitis.

General Considerations

When lymphedema is due to congenital developmental abnormalities consisting of hypoplastic or hyperplastic involvement of the proximal or distal lymphatics, it is referred to as the **primary form**. The obstruction may be in the pelvic or lumbar lymph channels and nodes when the disease is extensive and progressive. The **secondary form** of lymphedema involves inflammatory or mechanical lymphatic obstruction from trauma, regional lymph node resection or irradiation, or extensive involvement of regional nodes by malignant disease or filariasis. Lymphedema may occur following surgical removal of the lymph nodes in the groin or axillae. Secondary dilation of the lymphatics that occurs in both forms leads to incompetence of the valve system, disrupts the orderly flow along the lymph vessels, and results in progressive stasis of a protein-rich fluid. Episodes of acute and chronic inflammation may be superimposed, with further stasis and secondary fibrosis.

Clinical Findings

Hypertrophy of the limb results, with markedly thickened and fibrotic skin and subcutaneous tissue (Figure 12–4) in very advanced cases.

Lymphangiography and radioactive isotope studies may identify focal defects in lymph flow but are of little value in

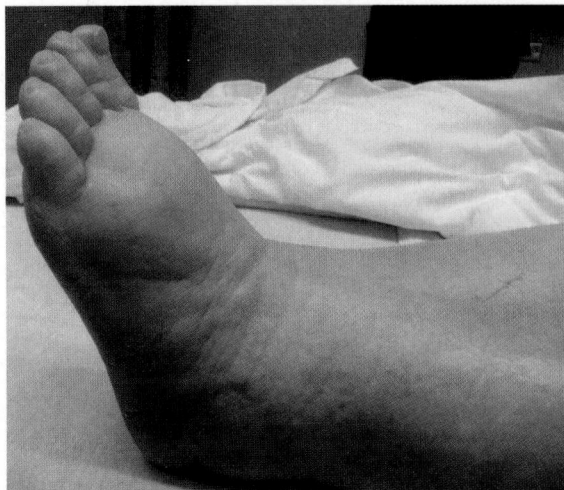

▲ **Figure 12–4.** Lymphedema with a dorsal pedal hump and exaggerated skin folds near the ankle. (Used, with permission, from Dean SM, Satiani B, Abraham WT. *Color Atlas and Synopsis of Vascular Diseases.* McGraw-Hill, 2014.)

planning therapy. T_2–weighted MRI has been used to identify lymphatics and proximal obstructing masses.

▶ Treatment

Since there is no effective cure for lymphedema, the treatment strategies are designed to control the problem and allow normal activity and function. Most patients can be treated with some of the following measures: (1) The flow of lymph out of the extremity can be aided through intermittent elevation of the extremity, especially during the sleeping hours (foot of bed elevated 15–20 degrees, achieved by placing pillows beneath the mattress); the constant use of graduated elastic compression stockings; and massage toward the trunk—either by hand or by means of pneumatic pressure devices designed to milk edema out of an extremity. Wound care centers specializing in the care of patients with lymphedema may be helpful. (2) Secondary cellulitis in the extremity should be avoided by means of good hygiene and treatment of any trichophytosis of the toes. Once an infection starts, it should be treated by periods of elevation and antibiotic therapy that covers *Staphylococcus* and *Streptococcus* organisms (see Table 30–6). Infections can be a serious and recurring problem and are often difficult to control. Prophylactic antibiotics have not been shown to be of benefit. (3) Intermittent courses of diuretic therapy, especially in those with premenstrual or seasonal exacerbations, are rarely helpful. (4) Amputation is used only for the rare complication of lymphangiosarcoma in the extremity.

▶ Prognosis

With aggressive treatment, including pneumatic compression devices, good relief of symptoms can be achieved. The long-term outlook is dictated by the associated conditions and avoidance of recurrent cellulitis.

Finnane A et al. Review of the evidence of lymphedema treatment effect. Am J Phys Med Rehabil. 2015 Jun;94(6):483–98. [PMID: 25741621]
Schaverien MV et al. New and emerging treatments for lymphedema. Semin Plast Surg. 2018 Feb;32(1):48–52. [PMID: 29636654]

▼ SHOCK

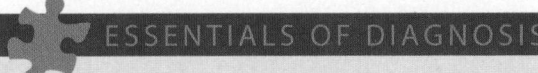

ESSENTIALS OF DIAGNOSIS

▶ Hypotension, tachycardia, oliguria, altered mental status.

▶ Peripheral hypoperfusion and impaired oxygen delivery.

▶ Four classifications: hypovolemic, cardiogenic, obstructive, or distributive.

▶ General Considerations

Shock occurs when the rate of arterial blood flow is inadequate to meet tissue metabolic needs. This results in regional hypoxia and subsequent lactic acidosis from anaerobic metabolism in peripheral tissues as well as eventual end-organ damage and failure.

▶ Classification

Table 12–1 outlines common causes and mechanisms associated with each type of shock.

A. Hypovolemic Shock

Hypovolemic shock results from decreased intravascular volume secondary to loss of blood or fluids and electrolytes. The etiology may be suggested by the clinical setting (eg, trauma) or by signs and symptoms of blood loss (eg, gastrointestinal bleeding) or dehydration (eg, vomiting or diarrhea). Compensatory vasoconstriction may transiently maintain the blood pressure but unreplaced losses of over 15% of the intravascular volume can result in hypotension and progressive tissue hypoxia.

B. Cardiogenic Shock

Cardiogenic shock results from cardiac failure with the resultant inability of the heart to maintain adequate tissue perfusion. The clinical definition of cardiogenic shock is evidence of tissue hypoxia due to decreased cardiac output (cardiac index less than 2.2 L/min/m²) in the presence of adequate intravascular volume. This is most often caused by myocardial infarction but can also be due to cardiomyopathy, myocardial contusion, valvular incompetence or stenosis, or arrhythmias. See Chapter 10.

C. Obstructive Shock

Cardiac tamponade, tension pneumothorax, and massive pulmonary embolism can cause an acute decrease in cardiac

Table 12–1. Classification of shock by mechanism and common causes.

Hypovolemic shock
Blood loss
Traumatic hemorrhage
Exsanguination
Hemothorax
Hemoperitoneum
Fracture (femur and pelvis)
Nontraumatic hemorrhage
Gastrointestinal bleed
AAA rupture
Ectopic pregnancy rupture
Volume loss
Burns
Skin integrity loss (toxic epidermal necrolysis)
Vomiting
Diarrhea
Hyperosmolar states (diabetic ketoacidosis)
Third spacing (eg, ascites, pancreatitis)
Decreased intake
Cardiogenic shock
Dysrhythmia
Bradycardias and blocks
Tachycardias
Myocardial disease
Left or right ventricular infarction
Dilated cardiomyopathy
Mechanical
Valvular
Aortic regurgitation from dissection
Papillary muscle rupture from ischemia
Acute valvular rupture from abscess
Ventricular aneurysm rupture
Ventricular septum rupture
Free wall ventricle rupture
Obstructive shock
Tension pneumothorax
Pericardial disease
Pericardial tamponade
Constrictive pericarditis
High-risk (massive) pulmonary embolism
Severe pulmonary hypertension
Auto PEEP from mechanical ventilation
Distributive shock
Anaphylactic shock
Septic shock
Neurogenic shock
Drug-induced vasodilation
Adrenal insufficiency

Modified, with permission, from Stone CK, Humphries RL (editors). *Current Emergency Diagnosis & Treatment*, 7th ed. McGraw-Hill, 2011. AAA, abdominal aortic aneurysm; PEEP, positive end expiratory pressure.

output resulting in shock. These are medical emergencies requiring prompt diagnosis and treatment.

D. Distributive Shock

Distributive or vasodilatory shock has many causes including sepsis, anaphylaxis, systemic inflammatory response syndrome (SIRS) produced by severe pancreatitis or burns, traumatic spinal cord injury, or acute adrenal insufficiency.

The reduction in systemic vascular resistance results in inadequate cardiac output and tissue hypoperfusion despite normal circulatory volume.

1. Septic shock—Sepsis is the most common cause of distributive shock and carries a mortality rate of 20–50%. The Society of Critical Care Medicine and the European Society of Intensive Care Medicine's 2016 definition for **sepsis** is life-threatening organ dysfunction caused by a dysregulated host response to infection. **Septic shock** is clinically defined as sepsis with fluid-unresponsive hypotension (systolic blood pressure less than 100 mm Hg), serum lactate level higher than 2 mmol/L, and a need for vasopressors to keep mean arterial pressure (MAP) above 65 mm Hg. The most common cause of septic shock in hospitalized patients is infection with gram-positive or gram-negative organisms, with a growing incidence of infection from multidrug-resistant organisms. Sepsis from fungal organisms is increasing, but remains less than that for bacterial infections. Risk factors for septic shock include bacteremia, extremes of age, diabetes, cancer, immunosuppression, and history of a recent invasive procedure.

The Third International Consensus Definitions for Sepsis and Septic Shock (SEPSIS-3) recommend using the Sequential Organ Failure Assessment (SOFA) score to define sepsis (https://en.wikipedia.org/wiki/SOFA_score); an increase of 2 or more SOFA score points in a patient with infection is diagnostic of sepsis with a predicted 10% mortality. The SEPSIS-3 group also introduced the quick SOFA (qSOFA) scoring system (https://en.wikipedia.org/wiki/SOFA_score); 1 point each is assigned for hypotension (systolic blood pressure below 100 mm Hg), altered mental status, or tachypnea (respiratory rate more than 22 breaths per minute). A qSOFA score of 2 or more in a patient with suspected infection suggests worsened clinical outcomes and may influence triage decisions for intensive care unit (ICU)-level care. Controversy remains over the utility of these definitions and scoring systems in the absence of strong evidence to advocate for universal adoption.

2. Systemic inflammatory response syndrome (SIRS)—Defined as a systemic response to a nonspecific infectious or noninfectious insult resulting in at least two of the following findings: (1) body temperature higher than 38°C (100.4°F) or lower than 36°C (96.8°F), (2) heart rate faster than 90 beats per minute, (3) respiratory rate more than 20 breaths per minute or hyperventilation with an arterial carbon dioxide tension ($Paco_2$) less than 32 mm Hg, or (4) abnormal white blood cell count (greater than 12,000/mcL or less than 4000/mcL or greater than 10% immature [band] forms). Vasodilatory shock from SIRS is often due to burns, pancreatitis, an autoimmune disorder, air or amniotic fluid embolus, ischemia, or trauma. A 2018 meta-analysis demonstrated that SIRS criteria have higher sensitivity than qSOFA, suggesting that SIRS may be a better screening tool for sepsis, while qSOFA may be better used as a predictor of ICU mortality.

3. Neurogenic shock—Neurogenic shock is caused by traumatic spinal cord injury or effects of an epidural or spinal anesthetic. This results in loss of sympathetic tone with a reduction in systemic vascular resistance and hypotension without a compensatory tachycardia. Reflex vagal parasympathetic stimulation evoked by pain, gastric dilation, or fright may simulate neurogenic shock, producing hypotension, bradycardia, and syncope.

4. Endocrine shock—Endocrine shock can arise from hyperthyroidism, hypothyroidism, or adrenal insufficiency. Adrenal insufficiency most often occurs with abrupt cessation of long-term corticosteroid use, but it can also be precipitated by infection, trauma, surgery, or pituitary injury (leading to secondary adrenal insufficiency). In addition to hypotension, symptoms include weakness, nausea, abdominal pain, and confusion. Hypothyroidism can lead to myxedema coma, presenting with vasodilation and depressed cardiac output. Shock from hyperthyroidism most often produces high-output cardiac failure.

▶ Clinical Findings

A. Symptoms and Signs

Hypotension is traditionally defined as a systolic blood pressure of 90 mm Hg or less or a MAP of less than 60–65 mm Hg but must be evaluated relative to the patient's normal blood pressure. A drop in systolic pressure of greater than 10–20 mm Hg or an increase in pulse of more than 15 beats per minute with positional change suggests depleted intravascular volume. However, blood pressure is often not the best indicator of end-organ perfusion because compensatory mechanisms, such as increased heart rate, increased cardiac contractility, and vasoconstriction can occur to prevent hypotension. Patients with hypotension often have cool or mottled extremities and weak or thready peripheral pulses. Splanchnic vasoconstriction may lead to oliguria, bowel ischemia, and hepatic dysfunction, which can ultimately result in multiorgan failure. Mentation may be normal or patients may become restless, agitated, confused, lethargic, or comatose as a result of inadequate perfusion of the brain.

Hypovolemic shock is evident when signs of hypoperfusion, such as oliguria, altered mental status, and cool extremities, are present. Jugular venous pressure is low, and there is a narrow pulse pressure indicative of reduced stroke volume. Rapid replacement of fluids can restore tissue perfusion. In **cardiogenic shock,** there are also signs of global hypoperfusion with oliguria, altered mental status, and cool extremities. Jugular venous pressure is elevated and there may be evidence of pulmonary edema with respiratory compromise in the setting of left-sided heart failure. A transthoracic echocardiogram (TTE) or a transesophageal echocardiogram (TEE) is an effective diagnostic tool to differentiate hypovolemic from cardiogenic shock. In hypovolemic shock, the left ventricle will be small because of decreased filling, but contractility is often preserved. In cardiogenic shock, there is a decrease in left ventricular contractility. The left ventricle may appear dilated and full because of the inability of the left ventricle to eject a sufficient stroke volume.

In **obstructive shock**, the central venous pressure may be elevated but the TTE or TEE may show reduced left ventricular filling, a pericardial effusion in the case of tamponade, or thickened pericardium in the case of pericarditis. Pericardiocentesis or pericardial window for pericardial tamponade, chest tube placement for tension pneumothorax, or catheter-directed thrombolytic therapy for massive pulmonary embolism can be life-saving in cases of obstructive shock.

In **distributive shock,** signs include hyperdynamic heart sounds, warm extremities initially, and a wide pulse pressure indicative of large stroke volume. The echocardiogram may show a hyperdynamic left ventricle. **Septic shock** is diagnosed when there is clinical evidence of infection in the setting of persistent hypotension and evidence of organ hypoperfusion, such as lactic acidosis, decreased urinary output, or altered mental status despite adequate volume resuscitation. **Neurogenic shock** is diagnosed when there is evidence of central nervous system injury and persistent hypotension despite adequate volume resuscitation. A history of long-term corticosteroid use or thyroid disease can increase the likelihood of **endocrine shock.**

B. Laboratory Findings and Imaging

Blood specimens should be evaluated for complete blood count, electrolytes, glucose, arterial blood gas determinations, coagulation parameters, lactate levels, typing and cross-matching, and bacterial cultures. An electrocardiogram and chest radiograph should also be part of the initial assessment. Point-of-care ultrasonography can rapidly assess global cardiac function, presence of pericardial effusion, and intravascular volume status via inferior vena cava inspection in cases of undifferentiated hypotension. A TTE can more formally assess right- and left-sided filling pressures and cardiac output.

▶ Treatment

A. General Measures

Treatment depends on prompt diagnosis and an accurate appraisal of inciting conditions. Initial management consists of basic life support with an assessment of the patient's circulation, airway, and breathing. This may entail airway intubation and mechanical ventilation. Ventilatory failure should be anticipated in patients with severe metabolic acidosis due to shock. Mechanical ventilation along with sedation can decrease respiratory muscle oxygen demand and allow improved oxygen delivery to hypoperfused tissues. Intravenous access and fluid resuscitation should be instituted along with cardiac monitoring and assessment of hemodynamic parameters such as blood pressure and heart rate. Cardiac monitoring can detect myocardial ischemia or malignant arrhythmias, which can be treated by standard advanced cardiac life support (ACLS) protocols.

Unresponsive or minimally responsive patients should have their glucose checked immediately, and if their glucose levels are low, 1 ampule of 50% dextrose intravenously should be given. An arterial line should be placed for continuous blood pressure measurement, and a Foley catheter should be inserted to monitor urinary output.

B. Hemodynamic Measurements

Early consideration is given to placement of a central venous catheter (CVC) for infusion of fluids and medications and for hemodynamic pressure measurements. A CVC can provide measurements of the central venous pressure (CVP) and the central venous oxygen saturation (ScvO$_2$), both of which can be used to manage septic and cardiogenic shock. Pulmonary artery catheters (PACs) allow measurement of the pulmonary artery pressure, left-sided filling pressure or the pulmonary capillary wedge pressure (PCWP), the mixed venous oxygen saturation (SvO$_2$), and cardiac output. Multiple studies suggest that PACs do not increase overall mortality or length of hospital stay but are associated with higher use of inotropes and intravenous vasodilators in select groups of critically ill patients. The attendant risks associated with PACs (infection, arrhythmias, vein thrombosis, and pulmonary artery rupture) can be as high as 4–9%; thus, the routine use of PACs cannot be recommended. However, in complex situations, PACs may be useful in distinguishing between cardiogenic and septic shock, so the value of the information they might provide must be carefully weighed in each patient. TTE is a noninvasive alternative to the PAC. TTE can provide information about the pulmonary artery pressure and current cardiac function, including cardiac output. The ScvO$_2$, which is obtained through the CVC, can be used as a surrogate for the SvO$_2$, which is obtained through the PAC. Pulse pressure variation, as determined by arterial waveform analysis, or stroke volume variation is much more sensitive than CVP as dynamic measures of fluid responsiveness in volume resuscitation, but these measurements have only been validated in patients who are mechanically ventilated with tidal volumes of 8 mL/kg, not triggering the ventilator, and in normal sinus rhythm. Point-of-care ultrasound measurements of the inferior vena cava (IVC) can suggest intravascular volume status and guide fluid replacement. If the patient is mechanically ventilated and the IVC dilates ~15–20% with respirations, they are likely to respond to intravenous fluids. If the patient is spontaneously breathing, they may be fluid-responsive if their IVC is less than 2 cm in diameter and collapses by more than 50% with each breath.

A CVP less than 5 mm Hg suggests hypovolemia, and a CVP greater than 18 mm Hg suggests volume overload, cardiac failure, tamponade, or pulmonary hypertension. A cardiac index lower than 2 L/min/m^2 indicates a need for inotropic support. A cardiac index higher than 4 L/min/m^2 in a hypotensive patient is consistent with early septic shock. The systemic vascular resistance is low (less than 800 dynes · s/cm^{-5}) in sepsis and neurogenic shock and high (greater than 1500 dynes · s/cm^{-5}) in hypovolemic and cardiogenic shock. Treatment is directed at maintaining a CVP of 8–12 mm Hg, a MAP of 65 mm Hg or higher, a cardiac index of 2–4 L/min/m^2, and a ScvO$_2$ greater than 70%.

C. Volume Replacement

Volume replacement is critical in the initial management of shock. **Hemorrhagic shock** is treated with immediate efforts to achieve hemostasis and rapid infusions of blood substitutes, such as type-specific or type O negative packed red blood cells (PRBCs) or whole blood, which provides extra volume and clotting factors. Each unit of PRBC or whole blood is expected to raise the hematocrit by 3%. **Hypovolemic shock** secondary to dehydration is managed with rapid boluses of isotonic crystalloid solutions, usually in 1-L increments. **Cardiogenic shock** in the absence of fluid overload requires smaller fluid challenges, usually in increments of 250 mL. **Septic shock** usually requires large volumes of fluid for resuscitation (usually more than 2 L) as the associated capillary leak releases fluid into the extravascular space. *Caution must be used with large-volume resuscitation with unwarmed fluids because this can produce hypothermia, which can lead to hypothermia-induced coagulopathy.* Warming of fluids before administration can avoid this complication.

Crystalloid solution is the resuscitation fluid of choice in most settings. Historically, 0.9% saline was the most widely used crystalloid solution in resuscitation. However, data suggests that balanced crystalloids, like lactated Ringer solution or Plasma-Lyte, are associated with less kidney injury, fewer instances of hyperchloremic metabolic acidosis, and decreased overall mortality. Comparisons of 0.9% saline and colloid (albumin) solutions in critically ill patients found no difference in outcome except in patients with traumatic brain injury, where albumin resuscitation led to higher mortality. Thus, the use of balanced crystalloid solutions for volume resuscitation in shock is favored.

D. Early Goal-Directed Therapy

Compensated shock can occur in the setting of normalized hemodynamic parameters with ongoing global tissue hypoxia. Traditional endpoints of resuscitation such as blood pressure, heart rate, urinary output, mental status, and skin perfusion can therefore be misleading. Following set protocols for the treatment of septic shock by adjusting the use of fluids, vasopressors, and inotropes as well as by using blood transfusions to meet hemodynamic targets (MAP 65 mm Hg or higher, CVP 8–12 mm Hg, ScvO$_2$ greater than 70%), termed **early goal-directed therapy (EGDT),** provided significant mortality benefits. Lactate clearance of more than 10% can be used as a substitute for ScvO$_2$ criteria if ScvO$_2$ monitoring is not available.

Two large randomized trials published in 2014 (ProCESS and ARISE) demonstrated no mortality benefit from the institution of EGDT, but this may have been due to earlier administration of antibiotics, components of EGDT becoming part of the "usual care" that clinicians deliver, and the effectiveness of education about detecting and treating sepsis in a timely fashion.

The Surviving Sepsis Campaign's recommendations for patients with sepsis or septic shock are to measure lactate level; obtain blood cultures prior to administration of broad-spectrum antibiotics, which should occur within 1 hour of sepsis diagnosis; and administer 30 mL/kg crystalloid for hypotension or lactate greater than 4 mmol/L within the first 3 hours of presentation. Vasopressors should be administered for hypotension not responsive to initial fluid resuscitation to maintain MAP 65 mm Hg or higher. Remeasure lactate if initial level was high, and reassess volume status and tissue perfusion frequently. A meta-analysis of hemodynamic optimization trials suggested that early treatment before the development of organ failure results in improved survival, and patients who respond well to initial efforts demonstrate a survival advantage over nonresponders.

E. Medications

1. Vasoactive therapy—Vasopressors and inotropic agents are administered only after adequate fluid resuscitation. Choice of vasoactive therapy depends on the presumed etiology of shock as well as cardiac output. If there is continued hypotension with evidence of high cardiac output after adequate volume resuscitation, then vasopressor support is needed to improve vasomotor tone. If there is evidence of low cardiac output with high filling pressures, inotropic support is needed to improve contractility.

For **vasodilatory shock** when increased vasoconstriction is required to maintain an adequate perfusion pressure, alpha-adrenergic catecholamine agonists (such as norepinephrine and phenylephrine) are generally used. Although norepinephrine is both an alpha-adrenergic and beta-adrenergic agonist, it preferentially increases MAP over cardiac output. The initial dose is 1–2 mcg/min as an intravenous infusion, titrated to maintain MAP at 65 mm Hg or higher. The usual maintenance dose is 2–4 mcg/min intravenously (maximum dose is 30 mcg/min). Patients with refractory shock may require dosages of 10–30 mcg/min intravenously. Epinephrine, also with both alpha-adrenergic and beta-adrenergic effects, may be used in severe shock and during acute resuscitation. It is the vasopressor of choice for **anaphylactic shock**. For severe shock, give 1 mcg/min as a continuous intravenous infusion initially and titrate to hemodynamic response; the usual dosage range is 1–10 mcg/min intravenously.

Dopamine has variable effects according to dosage. At low doses (2–5 mcg/kg/min intravenously), stimulation of dopaminergic and beta-adrenergic receptors produces increased glomerular filtration, heart rate, and contractility. At doses of 5–10 mcg/kg/min, beta-1-adrenergic effects predominate, resulting in an increase in heart rate and cardiac contractility. At higher doses (greater than 10 mcg/kg/min), alpha-adrenergic effects predominate, resulting in peripheral vasoconstriction. The maximum dose is typically 50 mcg/kg/min.

There is no evidence documenting a survival benefit from, or the superiority of, a particular vasopressor in **septic shock**. Norepinephrine is the initial vasopressor of choice in septic shock to maintain the MAP at 65 mm Hg or higher. Phenylephrine can be used for hyperdynamic septic shock if dysrhythmias or tachycardias prevent the use of agents with beta-adrenergic activity. In meta-analyses, the use of dopamine as a first-line vasopressor in septic shock resulted in an increase in 28-day mortality and a higher incidence of arrhythmic events. Dopamine should only be used as an alternative to norepinephrine in select patients with septic shock, including patients with significant bradycardia or low potential for tachyarrhythmias.

Vasopressin (antidiuretic hormone or ADH) is often used as an adjunctive therapy to catecholamine vasopressors in the treatment of **distributive** or **vasodilatory shock**. Vasopressin causes peripheral vasoconstriction via V1 receptors located on smooth muscle cells. Vasopressin also potentiates the effects of catecholamines on the vasculature and stimulates cortisol production. Intravenous infusion of vasopressin at a low dose (0.01–0.04 unit/min) as a second agent to norepinephrine may be safe and beneficial in septic patients with hypotension refractory to fluid resuscitation and conventional catecholamine vasopressors. Higher doses of vasopressin decrease cardiac output and may put patients at greater risk for splanchnic and coronary artery ischemia. Studies do not favor the use of vasopressin as first-line therapy.

Angiotensin II, a component of the renin-angiotensin-aldosterone system axis, is a potent direct vasoconstrictor that acts on the arteries and veins to increase blood pressure. Angiotensin II (marketed as Giapreza) can be considered as an *additional agent* in vasodilatory shock that is refractory to catecholamines and vasopressin. The recommended starting dose is 20 ng/kg/min via continuous intravenous infusion through a central venous line. It can be titrated every 5 minutes by increments of up to 15 ng/kg/min as needed to achieve MAP goals, but not to exceed 80 ng/kg/min during the first 3 hours of use. Maintenance doses should not exceed 40 ng/kg/min. Concurrent venous thromboembolism (VTE) prophylaxis is indicated as studies revealed a higher incidence of VTE with angiotensin II use.

There is insufficient evidence to recommend a specific vasopressor to use in **cardiogenic shock**, but expert opinion suggests that either norepinephrine or dopamine be used as a first-line agent. Dobutamine, a predominantly beta-adrenergic agonist, increases contractility and decreases afterload. It is used for patients with low cardiac output and high PCWP but who do not have hypotension. Dobutamine can be added to a vasopressor if there is reduced myocardial function (decreased cardiac output and elevated PCWP), or if there are signs of hypoperfusion despite adequate volume resuscitation and an adequate MAP. The initial dose is 0.1–0.5 mcg/kg/min intravenous infusion, which can be titrated every few minutes to hemodynamic effect; the usual dosage range is 2–20 mcg/kg/min intravenously. Tachyphylaxis can occur after 48 hours secondary to the down-regulation of beta-adrenergic receptors. Amrinone and milrinone are phosphodiesterase inhibitors that can be substituted for dobutamine. These drugs increase cyclic AMP levels and increase cardiac contractility, bypassing the beta-adrenergic receptor. Vasodilation is a side effect of both amrinone and milrinone.

2. Antibiotics—Definitive therapy for septic shock includes early initiation of empiric broad-spectrum antibiotics after appropriate cultures have been obtained and within 1 hour of recognition of septic shock. Imaging studies may prove useful to attempt localization of sources of infection. Surgical management may also be necessary if necrotic tissue or loculated infections are present in attempts to control the source of infection (see Table 30–5).

3. Corticosteroids—Corticosteroids are the treatment of choice in patients with shock secondary to adrenal insufficiency but studies do not support their use in patients with shock from sepsis or other etiologies. Trials where either high or low doses of corticosteroids were administered to patients in septic shock did not show improved survival; rather, some worse outcomes were observed from increased rates of secondary infections, even in patients who had relative adrenal insufficiency, defined by a cortisol response of 9 mcg/dL or less after one injection of 250 mcg of corticotropin.

F. Other Treatment Modalities

Cardiac failure may require use of transcutaneous or transvenous pacing or placement of an intra-arterial balloon pump or left ventricular assist device. Emergent revascularization by percutaneous angioplasty or coronary artery bypass surgery appears to improve long-term outcome with increased survival compared with initial medical stabilization for patients with myocardial ischemia leading to cardiogenic shock. Urgent hemodialysis or continuous venovenous hemofiltration may be indicated for maintenance of fluid and electrolyte balance during acute kidney injury resulting in shock from multiple modalities.

Fernando SM et al. Prognostic accuracy of the quick sequential organ failure assessment for mortality in patients with suspected infection: a systematic review and meta-analysis. Ann Intern Med. 2018 Feb 20;168(4):266–75. [PMID: 29404582]

Gamper G et al. Vasopressors for hypotensive shock. Cochrane Database Syst Rev. 2016 Feb 15;2:CD003709. [PMID: 26878401]

Khanna A et al; ATHOS-3 Investigators. Angiotensin II for the treatment of vasodilatory shock. N Engl J Med. 2017 Aug 3; 377(5):419–30. [PMID: 28528561]

Mouncey PR et al; ProMISe Trial Investigators. Trial of early, goal-directed resuscitation for septic shock. N Engl J Med. 2015 Apr 2;372(14):1301–11. [PMID: 25776532]

Peake SL et al; ARISE Investigators; ANZICS Clinical Trials Group. Goal-directed resuscitation for patients with early septic shock. N Engl J Med. 2014 Oct 16;371(16):1496–506. [PMID: 25272316]

Rhodes A et al. Surviving Sepsis Campaign: international guidelines for management of sepsis and septic shock: 2016. Crit Care Med. 2017 Mar;45(3):486–552. [PMID: 28098591]

Semler MW et al. Balanced crystalloids versus saline in critically ill adults. N Engl J Med. 2018 May 17;378(20):1951. [PMID: 29768150]

Seymour CW et al. Septic shock: advances in diagnosis and treatment. JAMA. 2015 Aug 18;314(7):708–17. [PMID: 26284722]

Singer M et al. The third international consensus definitions for sepsis and septic shock (Sepsis-3). JAMA. 2016 Feb 23; 315(8):801–10. [PMID: 26903338]

Yealy DM et al; ProCESS Investigators. A randomized trial of protocol-based care for early septic shock. N Engl J Med. 2014 May 1;370(18):1683–93. [PMID: 24635773]

Blood Disorders

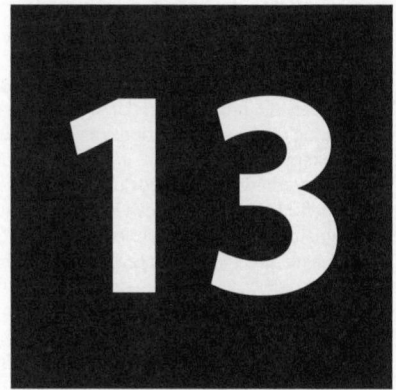

13

Lloyd E. Damon, MD
Charalambos Babis Andreadis, MD, MSCE

ANEMIAS

General Approach to Anemias

Anemia is present in adults if the hematocrit is below 41% (hemoglobin less than 13.6 g/dL [135 g/L]) in males or below 36% (hemoglobin less than 12 g/dL [120 g/L]) in females. Congenital anemia is suggested by the patient's personal and family history. The most common cause of anemia is iron deficiency. Poor diet may result in folic acid deficiency and contribute to iron deficiency, but bleeding is the most common cause of iron deficiency in adults. Physical examination demonstrates pallor. Attention to physical signs of primary hematologic diseases (lymphadenopathy; hepatosplenomegaly; or bone tenderness, especially in the sternum or anterior tibia) is important. Mucosal changes such as a smooth tongue suggest megaloblastic anemia.

Anemias are classified according to their pathophysiologic basis, ie, whether related to diminished production (relative or absolute reticulocytopenia) or to increased production due to accelerated loss of red blood cells (reticulocytosis) (Table 13–1), and according to red blood cell size (Table 13–2). A reticulocytosis occurs in one of three pathophysiologic states: acute blood loss, recent replacement of a missing erythropoietic nutrient, or reduced red blood cell survival (ie, hemolysis). A severely microcytic anemia (mean corpuscular volume [MCV] less than 70 fL) is due either to iron deficiency or thalassemia, while a severely macrocytic anemia (MCV greater than 120 fL) is almost always due to either megaloblastic anemia or to cold agglutinins in blood analyzed at room temperature. A bone marrow biopsy is generally needed to complete the evaluation of anemia when the blood laboratory evaluation fails to reveal an etiology, when there are additional cytopenias present, or when an underlying primary or secondary bone marrow process is suspected.

IRON DEFICIENCY ANEMIA

ESSENTIALS OF DIAGNOSIS

▸ Iron deficiency: serum ferritin is less than 12 ng/mL (27 pmol/L) or less than 30 ng/mL (67 pmol/L) if also anemic.

▸ Caused by bleeding unless proved otherwise.

▸ Responds to iron therapy.

General Considerations

Iron deficiency is the most common cause of anemia worldwide. The causes are listed in Table 13–3. Aside from circulating red blood cells, the major location of iron in the body is the storage pool as ferritin or as hemosiderin in macrophages.

The average American diet contains 10–15 mg of iron per day. About 10% of this amount is absorbed in the stomach, duodenum, and upper jejunum under acidic conditions. Dietary iron present as heme is efficiently absorbed (10–20%) but nonheme iron less so (1–5%), largely because of interference by phosphates, tannins, and other food constituents. The major iron transporter from the diet across the intestinal lumen is ferroportin, which also facilitates the transport of iron to apotransferrin in macrophages for delivery to erythroid progenitor cells prepared to synthesize hemoglobin. Hepcidin, which is increasingly produced during inflammation, negatively regulates iron transport by promoting the degradation of ferroportin. Small amounts of iron—approximately 1 mg/day—are normally lost through exfoliation of skin and mucosal cells.

Menstrual blood loss plays a major role in iron metabolism. The average monthly menstrual blood loss is approximately 50 mL but may be five times greater in some individuals. Women with heavy menstrual losses must absorb 3–4 mg of iron from the diet each day to maintain adequate iron stores, which is not commonly achieved. Women with menorrhagia of this degree will almost always become iron deficient without iron supplementation.

In general, iron metabolism is balanced between absorption of 1 mg/day and loss of 1 mg/day. Pregnancy and lactation upset the iron balance, since requirements increase to 2–5 mg of iron per day. Normal dietary iron cannot supply these requirements, and medicinal iron is needed during pregnancy and lactation. Decreased iron absorption can also cause iron deficiency, such as in people affected by celiac disease (gluten enteropathy), and it also commonly occurs after gastric resection or jejunal bypass surgery.

Table 13–1. Classification of anemia by red blood cell (RBC) pathophysiology.

Decreased RBC production (relative or absolute reticulocytopenia)
Hemoglobin synthesis lesion: iron deficiency, thalassemia, anemia of chronic disease, hypoerythropoietinemia
DNA synthesis lesion: megaloblastic anemia, folic acid deficiency, DNA synthesis inhibitor medications
Hematopoietic stem cell lesion: aplastic anemia, leukemia
Bone marrow infiltration: carcinoma, lymphoma, fibrosis, sarcoidosis, Gaucher disease, others
Immune-mediated inhibition: aplastic anemia, pure red cell aplasia
Increased RBC destruction or accelerated RBC loss (reticulocytosis)
Acute blood loss
Hemolysis (intrinsic)
Membrane lesion: hereditary spherocytosis, elliptocytosis
Hemoglobin lesion: sickle cell, unstable hemoglobin
Glycolysis lesion: pyruvate kinase deficiency
Oxidation lesion: glucose-6-phosphate dehydrogenase deficiency
Hemolysis (extrinsic)
Immune: warm antibody, cold antibody
Microangiopathic: thrombotic thrombocytopenic purpura, hemolytic-uremic syndrome, mechanical cardiac valve, paravalvular leak
Infection: *Clostridium perfringens*, malaria
Hypersplenism

The most important cause of iron deficiency anemia in adults is chronic blood loss, especially menstrual and gastrointestinal blood loss. Iron deficiency demands a search for a source of gastrointestinal bleeding if other sites of

Table 13–2. Classification of anemia by mean red blood cell volume (MCV).

Microcytic
Iron deficiency
Thalassemia
Anemia of chronic disease
Lead toxicity
Zinc deficiency
Macrocytic (Megaloblastic)
Vitamin B_{12} deficiency
Folate deficiency
DNA synthesis inhibitors
Macrocytic (Nonmegaloblastic)
Aplastic anemia
Myelodysplasia
Liver disease
Reticulocytosis
Hypothyroidism
Bone marrow failure state (eg, aplastic anemia, marrow infiltrative disorder, etc)
Copper deficiency
Normocytic
Kidney disease
Non-thyroid endocrine gland failure
Copper deficiency
Mild form of most acquired microcytic or macrocytic etiologies of anemia

Table 13–3. Causes of iron deficiency.

Deficient diet
Decreased absorption
Autoimmune gastritis
Celiac sprue
Helicobacter pylori gastritis
Hereditary iron-refractory iron deficiency anemia
Zinc deficiency
Increased requirements
Pregnancy
Lactation
Blood loss (chronic)
Gastrointestinal
Menstrual
Blood donation
Hemoglobinuria
Iron sequestration
Pulmonary hemosiderosis
Idiopathic

blood loss (menorrhagia, other uterine bleeding, and repeated blood donations) are excluded. Prolonged aspirin or nonsteroidal anti-inflammatory drug use may cause it even without a documented structural lesion. Celiac disease, even when asymptomatic, can cause iron deficiency through poor absorption in the gastrointestinal tract. Zinc deficiency is another cause of poor iron absorption. Chronic hemoglobinuria may lead to iron deficiency, but this is uncommon. Traumatic hemolysis due to a prosthetic cardiac valve and other causes of intravascular hemolysis (eg, paroxysmal nocturnal hemoglobinuria) should also be considered. The cause of iron deficiency is not found in up to 5% of cases.

Pure iron deficiency might prove refractory to oral iron replacement. Refractoriness is defined as a hemoglobin increment of less than 1 g/dL (10 g/L) after 4–6 weeks of 100 mg/day of elemental oral iron. The differential diagnosis in these cases (Table 13–3) includes malabsorption from autoimmune gastritis, *Helicobacter pylori* gastric infection, celiac disease, and hereditary iron-refractory iron deficiency anemia. Iron-refractory iron deficiency anemia is a rare autosomal recessive disorder due to mutations in the transmembrane serine protease 6 (*TMPRSS6*) gene, which normally down-regulates hepcidin. In iron-refractory iron deficiency anemia, hepcidin levels are normal to high and ferritin levels are high despite the iron deficiency.

► Clinical Findings

A. Symptoms and Signs

The primary symptoms of iron deficiency anemia are those of the anemia itself (easy fatigability, tachycardia, palpitations, and dyspnea on exertion). Severe deficiency causes skin and mucosal changes, including a smooth tongue, brittle nails, spooning of nails (koilonychia), and cheilosis. Dysphagia due to the formation of esophageal webs (Plummer-Vinson syndrome) may occur in severe iron deficiency. Many iron-deficient patients develop pica, craving for specific foods (ice chips, etc) often not rich in iron.

B. Laboratory Findings

Iron deficiency develops in stages. The first is depletion of iron stores without anemia followed by anemia with a normal red blood cell size (normal MCV) followed by anemia with reduced red blood cell size (low MCV). The reticulocyte count is low or inappropriately normal. Ferritin is a measure of total body iron stores. A ferritin value less than 12 ng/mL (27 pmol/L) (in the absence of scurvy) is a highly reliable indicator of reduced iron stores. Note that the lower limit of normal for ferritin generally is below 12 ng/mL (27 pmol/L) in women due to the fact that the normal ferritin range is generated by including healthy menstruating women who are iron deficient but not anemic. However, because serum ferritin levels may rise in response to inflammation or other stimuli, a normal or elevated ferritin level does not exclude a diagnosis of iron deficiency. A ferritin level less than 30 ng/mL (67 pmol/L) almost always indicates iron deficiency in anyone who is anemic. As iron deficiency progresses, serum iron values decline to less than 30 mcg/dL (67 pmol/L) and transferrin (the iron transport protein) levels rise to compensate, leading to transferrin saturations of less than 15%. Low transferrin saturation is also seen in anemia of inflammation, so caution in the interpretation of this test is warranted. Isolated iron deficiency anemia has a low hepcidin level, not yet a clinically available test. As the MCV falls (ie, microcytosis), the blood smear shows hypochromic microcytic cells. With further progression, anisocytosis (variations in red blood cell size) and poikilocytosis (variation in shape of red cells) develop. Severe iron deficiency will produce a bizarre peripheral blood smear, with severely hypochromic cells, target cells, and pencil-shaped or cigar-shaped cells. Bone marrow biopsy for evaluation of iron stores is rarely performed. If the biopsy is done, it shows the absence of iron in erythroid progenitor cells by Prussian blue staining. The platelet count is commonly increased, but it usually remains under 800,000/mcL (800 × 10^9/L).

► Differential Diagnosis

Other causes of microcytic anemia include anemia of chronic disease (specifically, anemia of inflammation), thalassemia, lead poisoning, and congenital X-linked sideroblastic anemia. Anemia of chronic disease is characterized by normal or increased iron stores in bone marrow macrophages and a normal or elevated ferritin level; the serum iron and transferrin saturation are low, often drastically so, and the total iron-binding capacity (TIBC) (the blood's capacity for iron to bind to transferrin) and transferrin are either normal or low. Thalassemia produces a greater degree of microcytosis for any given level of anemia than does iron deficiency and, unlike virtually every other cause of anemia, has a normal or elevated (rather than a low) red blood cell count as well as a reticulocytosis. In thalassemia, red blood cell morphology on the peripheral smear resembles severe iron deficiency.

► Treatment

The diagnosis of iron deficiency anemia can be made either by the laboratory demonstration of an iron-deficient state or by evaluating the response to a therapeutic trial of iron replacement. Since the anemia itself is rarely life-threatening, the most important part of management is identification of the cause—especially a source of occult blood loss.

A. Oral Iron

Ferrous sulfate, 325 mg once daily or every other day on an empty stomach, is a standard approach for replenishing iron stores. As oral iron stimulates hepcidin production, once daily or every other day dosing maximizes iron absorption compared to multiple doses per day, and with fewer side effects. Nausea and constipation limit compliance with ferrous sulfate. Extended-release ferrous sulfate with mucoprotease is a well-tolerated oral preparation. Taking ferrous sulfate with food reduces side effects but also its absorption. An appropriate response is a return of the hematocrit level halfway toward normal within 3 weeks with full return to baseline after 2 months. Iron therapy should continue for 3–6 months after restoration of normal hematologic values to replenish iron stores. Failure of response to iron therapy is usually due to noncompliance, although occasional patients may absorb iron poorly, particularly if the stomach is achlorhydric. Such patients may benefit from concomitant administration of oral ascorbic acid. Other reasons for failure to respond include incorrect diagnosis (anemia of chronic disease, thalassemia), celiac disease, and ongoing blood loss that exceeds the rate of new erythropoiesis. Treatment of *H pylori* infection, in appropriate cases, can improve oral iron absorption.

B. Parenteral Iron

The indications are intolerance of or refractoriness to oral iron (including those with iron-refractory iron deficiency anemia), gastrointestinal disease (usually inflammatory bowel disease) precluding the use of oral iron, and continued blood loss that cannot be corrected, such as chronic hemodialysis. Historical parenteral iron preparations, such as high-molecular-weight iron dextran, were problematic due to long infusion times (hours), polyarthralgia, and hypersensitivity reactions, including anaphylaxis. Current parenteral iron preparations coat the iron in protective carbohydrate shells or contain low-molecular-weight iron dextran, are safe, and can be administered over 15 minutes to 1 hour. Most iron deficient patients need 1–1.5 g of parenteral iron; this dose corrects for the iron deficit and replenishes iron stores for the future.

Ferric pyrophosphate citrate (Triferic) is an FDA-approved additive to the dialysate designed to replace the 5–7 mg of iron that patients with chronic kidney disease tend to lose during each hemodialysis treatment. Ferric pyrophosphate citrate delivers sufficient iron to the marrow to maintain hemoglobin and not increase iron stores; it may obviate the need for intravenous iron in hemodialysis patients.

► When to Refer

Patients should be referred to a hematologist if the suspected diagnosis is not confirmed or if they are not responsive to oral iron therapy.

Auerbach M et al. Single-dose intravenous iron for iron deficiency: a new paradigm. Hematology Am Soc Hematol Educ Program. 2016 Dec 2;2016(1):57–66. [PMID: 27913463]

Auerbach M et al. How we diagnose and treat iron deficiency anemia. Am J Hematol. 2016 Jan;91(1):31–8. [PMID: 26408108]

Camaschella C. Iron-deficiency anemia. N Engl J Med. 2015 May 7; 372(19):1832–43. [PMID: 25946282]

Hempel EV et al. The evidence-based evaluation of iron deficiency anemia. Med Clin North Am. 2016 Sep;100(5):1065–75. [PMID: 27542426]

ANEMIA OF CHRONIC DISEASE

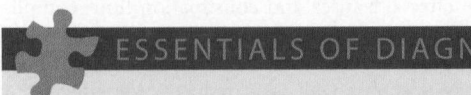

ESSENTIALS OF DIAGNOSIS

► Mild or moderate normocytic or microcytic anemia.

► Normal or increased ferritin and normal or reduced transferrin.

► Underlying chronic disease.

► General Considerations

Many chronic systemic diseases are associated with mild or moderate anemia. The anemias of chronic disease are characterized according to etiology and pathophysiology. First, the **anemia of inflammation** is associated with chronic inflammatory states (such as inflammatory bowel disease, rheumatoid arthritis, chronic infections, and malignancy) and is mediated through hepcidin (a negative regulator of ferroportin) primarily via elevated IL-6, resulting in reduced iron uptake in the gut and reduced iron transfer from macrophages to erythroid progenitor cells in the bone marrow. This is referred to as iron-restricted erythropoiesis since the patient is iron replete. There is also reduced responsiveness to erythropoietin, the elaboration of hemolysins that shorten red blood cell survival, and the production of inflammatory cytokines that dampen red cell production. The serum iron is low in the anemia of inflammation. Second, the **anemia of organ failure** can occur with kidney disease, liver failure, and endocrine gland failure. Erythropoietin is reduced and the red blood cell mass decreases in response to the diminished signal for red blood cell production; the serum iron is normal (except in chronic kidney disease where it is low due to the reduced hepcidin clearance and subsequent enhanced degradation of ferroportin). Third, the **anemia of older adults** is present in up to 20% of individuals over age 85 years in whom a thorough evaluation for an explanation of anemia is negative. The anemia is a consequence of (1) a relative resistance to red blood cell production in response to erythropoietin, (2) a decrease in erythropoietin production relative to the nephron mass, (3) a negative erythropoietic influence of higher levels of chronic inflammatory cytokines in older adults, and (4) the presence of various somatic mutations in myeloid genes typically associated with myeloid neoplasms. The latter condition is now referred to as **clonal cytopenias of undetermined significance,** which has a 1–1.5% per year rate of transformation to a myeloid neoplasm, such as a myelodysplastic syndrome. The serum iron is normal.

► Clinical Findings

A. Symptoms and Signs

The clinical features are those of the causative condition. The diagnosis should be suspected in patients with known chronic diseases. In cases of significant anemia, coexistent iron deficiency or folic acid deficiency should be suspected. Decreased dietary intake of iron or folic acid is common in chronically ill patients, many of whom will also have ongoing gastrointestinal blood losses. Patients undergoing hemodialysis regularly lose both iron and folic acid during dialysis.

B. Laboratory Findings

The hematocrit rarely falls below 60% of baseline (except in kidney failure). The MCV is usually normal or slightly reduced. Red blood cell morphology is usually normal, and the reticulocyte count is mildly decreased or normal.

1. Anemia of inflammation—In the anemia of inflammation, serum iron and transferrin values are low, and the transferrin saturation may be extremely low, leading to an erroneous diagnosis of iron deficiency. In contrast to iron deficiency, serum ferritin values should be normal or increased. A serum ferritin value less than 30 ng/mL (67 pmol/L) indicates coexistent iron deficiency. Anemia of inflammation has elevated hepcidin levels; however, no clinical test is yet available. A particular challenge is the diagnosis of iron deficiency in the setting of the anemia of inflammation, in which the serum ferritin can be as high as 200 ng/mL (450 pmol/L). The diagnosis is established by a bone marrow biopsy with iron stain. Absent iron staining indicates iron deficiency, whereas iron localized in marrow macrophages indicates pure anemia of inflammation. However, bone marrow biopsies are rarely done for this purpose. Two other tests all support iron deficiency in the setting of inflammation: a reticulocyte hemoglobin concentration of less than 28 pg or a soluble serum transferrin receptor (units: mg/L) to log ferritin (units: mcg/L) ratio of 1–8 (a ratio of less than 1 is virtually diagnostic of pure anemia of chronic disease). A functional test is hemoglobin response to oral or parenteral iron in the setting of inflammation when iron deficiency is suspected. A note of caution: certain circumstances of iron-restricted erythropoiesis (such as malignancy) will partially respond to parenteral iron infusion even when the iron stores are replete due to the immediate distribution of iron to erythropoietic progenitor cells after the infusion.

2. Other anemias of chronic disease—In the anemias of organ failure and of older adults, the iron studies are generally normal. The anemia of older persons is a diagnosis of exclusion. Clonal cytopenias of undetermined significance is diagnosed by sending a blood sample for myeloid gene sequencing.

► Treatment

In most cases, no treatment of the anemia is necessary and the primary management is to address the condition causing the anemia of chronic disease. When the anemia is severe or is adversely affecting the quality of life or functional status, then treatment involves either red blood cell transfusions or parenteral recombinant erythropoietin (epoetin alfa or darbepoetin). The FDA-approved indications for recombinant erythropoietin are hemoglobin less than 10 g/dL and anemia due to rheumatoid arthritis, inflammatory bowel disease, hepatitis C, zidovudine therapy in HIV-infected patients, myelosuppressive chemotherapy of solid malignancy (treated with palliative intent only), or chronic kidney disease (estimated glomerular filtration rate of less than 60 mL/min). The dosing and schedule of recombinant erythropoietin are individualized to maintain the hemoglobin between 10 g/dL (100 g/L) and 12 g/dL (120 g/L). The use of recombinant erythropoietin is associated with an increased risk of venothromboembolism and arterial thrombotic episodes, especially if the hemoglobin rises to greater than 12 g/dL (120 g/L). There is concern that recombinant erythropoietin is associated with reduced survival in patients with malignancy. For patients with end-stage renal disease receiving recombinant erythropoietin who are on hemodialysis, the anemia of chronic kidney disease can be more effectively corrected by adding soluble ferric pyrophosphate to their dialysate than by administering intravenous iron supplementation.

When to Refer

Referral to a hematologist is not usually necessary.

Cappellini MD et al. Iron deficiency across chronic inflammatory conditions: international expert opinion on definition, diagnosis, and management. Am J Hematol. 2017 Oct;92(10): 1068–78. [PMID: 28612425]

Fraenkel PG. Understanding anemia of chronic disease. Hematology Am Soc Hematol Educ Program. 2015;2015: 14–8. [PMID: 26637695]

Steensma DP. New challenges in evaluating anemia in older persons in the era of molecular testing. Hematology Am Soc Hematol Educ Program. 2016 Dec 2;2016(1):67–73. [PMID: 27913464]

THE THALASSEMIAS

ESSENTIALS OF DIAGNOSIS

- ▶ Microcytosis disproportionate to the degree of anemia.
- ▶ Positive family history.
- ▶ Lifelong personal history of microcytic anemia.
- ▶ Normal or elevated red blood cell count.
- ▶ Abnormal red blood cell morphology with microcytes, hypochromia, acanthocytes, and target cells.
- ▶ In beta-thalassemia, elevated levels of hemoglobin A_2 or F.

General Considerations

The thalassemias are hereditary disorders characterized by reduction in the synthesis of globin chains (alpha or beta).

Reduced globin chain synthesis causes reduced hemoglobin synthesis and a hypochromic microcytic anemia because of defective hemoglobinization of red blood cells. Thalassemias can be considered among the hyperproliferative hemolytic anemias, the anemias related to abnormal hemoglobin, and the hypoproliferative anemias, since all of these factors play a role in pathogenesis. The hallmark laboratory features are small (low MCV) and pale (low mean corpuscular hemoglobin [MCH]) red blood cells, anemia, and a normal to elevated red blood cell count (ie, a large number of the small and pale red blood cells are being produced). Although patients often exhibit an elevated reticulocyte count, generally the degree of reticulocyte output is inadequate to meet the degree of red blood cell destruction (hemolysis) occurring in the bone marrow and the patients remain anemic.

Normal adult hemoglobin is primarily hemoglobin A, which represents approximately 98% of circulating hemoglobin. Hemoglobin A is formed from a tetramer of two alpha chains and two beta globin chains—and is designated alpha2beta2. Two copies of the alpha-globin gene are located on each chromosome 16, and there is no substitute for alpha-globin in the formation of adult hemoglobin. One copy of the beta-globin gene resides on each chromosome 11 adjacent to genes encoding the beta-like globins delta and gamma (the so-called beta-globin gene cluster region). The tetramer of alpha2delta2 forms hemoglobin A_2, which normally comprises 1–3% of adult hemoglobin. The tetramer alpha2gamma2 forms hemoglobin F, which is the major hemoglobin of fetal life but which comprises less than 1% of normal adult hemoglobin.

The thalassemias are described as **thalassemia trait** when there are laboratory features without significant clinical impact, **thalassemia intermedia** when there is an occasional red blood cell transfusion requirement or other moderate clinical impact, and **thalassemia major** when the disorder is life-threatening and the patient is transfusion-dependent. Most patients with thalassemia major die of the consequences of iron overload from RBC transfusions.

Alpha-thalassemia is due primarily to gene deletions causing reduced alpha-globin chain synthesis (Table 13–4).

Table 13–4. Alpha-thalassemia syndromes.

Number of Alpha-Globin Genes Transcribed	Syndrome	Hematocrit	MCV
4	Normal	Normal	Normal
3	Silent carrier	Normal	Normal
2	Thalassemia minor (or trait)	28–40%	60–75 fL
1	Hemoglobin H disease	22–32%	60–70 fL
0	Hydrops fetalis[1]	< 18%	< 60 fL

[1]Die in utero.
MCV, mean corpuscular volume.

When to Refer

All patients with thalassemia intermedia or major should be referred to a hematologist. Any patient with an unexplained microcytic anemia should be referred to help establish a diagnosis. Patients with thalassemia minor or intermedia should be offered genetic counseling because offspring of thalassemic couples are at risk for inheriting thalassemia major.

Cappellini MD et al. New therapeutic targets in transfusion-dependent and -independent thalassemia. Hematology Am Soc Hematol Educ Program. 2017 Dec 8;2017(1):278–83. [PMID: 29222267]

Jagannath VA et al. Hematopoietic stem cell transplantation for people with B-thalassaemia major. Cochrane Database Syst Rev. 2016 Nov 30;11:CD008708. [PMID: 27900772]

Kwiatkowski JL. Current recommendations for chelation for transfusion-dependent thalassemia. Ann N Y Acad Sci. 2016 Mar;1368(1):107–14. [PMID: 27186943]

Srivastava A et al. Cure for thalassemia major—from allogeneic hematopoietic stem cell transplantation to gene therapy. Haematologica. 2017 Feb;102(2):214–23. [PMID: 27909215]

Taher AT et al. Thalassaemia. Lancet. 2018 Jan13;391(10116): 155–67. [PMID: 28774421]

Thompson AA et al. Gene therapy in patients with transfusion-dependent β-thalassemia. N Engl J Med. 2018 Apr 19;378(16): 1479–93. [PMID: 29669226]

VITAMIN B$_{12}$ DEFICIENCY

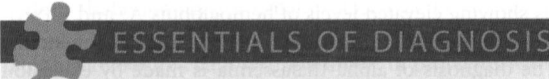

ESSENTIALS OF DIAGNOSIS

- ▶ Macrocytic anemia.
- ▶ Megaloblastic blood smear (macro-ovalocytes and hypersegmented neutrophils).
- ▶ Low serum vitamin B$_{12}$ level.

General Considerations

Vitamin B$_{12}$ belongs to the family of cobalamins and serves as a cofactor for two important reactions in humans. As methylcobalamin, it is a cofactor for methionine synthetase in the conversion of homocysteine to methionine, and as adenosylcobalamin for the conversion of methylmalonyl-coenzyme A (CoA) to succinyl-CoA. Vitamin B$_{12}$ comes from the diet and is present in all foods of animal origin. The daily absorption of vitamin B$_{12}$ is 5 mcg.

The liver contains 2–5 mg of stored vitamin B$_{12}$. Since daily utilization is 3–5 mcg, the body usually has sufficient stores of vitamin B$_{12}$ so that it takes more than 3 years for vitamin B$_{12}$ deficiency to occur if all intake or absorption immediately ceases.

Since vitamin B$_{12}$ is present in foods of animal origin, dietary vitamin B$_{12}$ deficiency is extremely rare but is seen in vegans—strict vegetarians who avoid all dairy products, meat, and fish (Table 13–6). Pernicious anemia is an autoimmune illness whereby autoantibodies destroy gastric parietal cells (that produce intrinsic factor) and cause atrophic gastritis or bind to and neutralize intrinsic factor, or both. Abdominal surgery may lead to vitamin B$_{12}$

Table 13–6. Causes of vitamin B$_{12}$ deficiency.

Dietary deficiency (rare)
Decreased production or absorption of intrinsic factor
Pernicious anemia (autoimmune)
Gastrectomy
Helicobacter pylori infection
Competition for vitamin B$_{12}$ in the gut
Blind loop syndrome
Fish tapeworm (rare)
Pancreatic insufficiency
Proton pump inhibitors
Decreased ileal absorption of vitamin B$_{12}$
Surgical resection
Crohn disease
Transcobalamin II deficiency (rare)

deficiency in several ways. Gastrectomy will eliminate the site of intrinsic factor production; blind loop syndrome will cause competition for vitamin B$_{12}$ by bacterial overgrowth in the lumen of the intestine; and surgical resection of the ileum will eliminate the site of vitamin B$_{12}$ absorption. Rare causes of vitamin B$_{12}$ deficiency include fish tapeworm (*Diphyllobothrium latum*) infection, in which the parasite uses luminal vitamin B$_{12}$; pancreatic insufficiency (with failure to inactivate competing cobalamin-binding proteins [R-factors]); severe Crohn disease, causing sufficient destruction of the ileum to impair vitamin B$_{12}$ absorption; and perhaps prolonged use of proton pump inhibitors.

Clinical Findings

A. Symptoms and Signs

Vitamin B$_{12}$ deficiency causes a moderate to severe anemia of slow onset; patients may have few symptoms relative to the degree of anemia. In advanced cases, the anemia may be severe, with hematocrits as low as 10–15%, and may be accompanied by leukopenia and thrombocytopenia. The deficiency also produces changes in mucosal cells, leading to glossitis, as well as other vague gastrointestinal disturbances such as anorexia and diarrhea. Vitamin B$_{12}$ deficiency also leads to a complex neurologic syndrome. Peripheral nerves are usually affected first, and patients complain initially of paresthesias. As the posterior columns of the spinal cord become impaired, patients complain of difficulty with balance or proprioception, or both. In more advanced cases, cerebral function may be altered as well, and on occasion dementia and other neuropsychiatric abnormalities may be present. It is critical to recognize that the nonhematologic manifestations of vitamin B$_{12}$ deficiency can be manifest despite a completely normal complete blood count.

Patients are usually pale and may be mildly icteric or sallow. Typically, later in the disease course, neurologic examination may reveal decreased vibration and position sense or memory disturbance (or both).

B. Laboratory Findings

The diagnosis of vitamin B$_{12}$ deficiency is made by finding a low serum vitamin B$_{12}$ (cobalamin) level. Whereas the normal vitamin B$_{12}$ level is greater than 210 pg/mL

(155 pmol/L), most patients with overt vitamin B_{12} deficiency have serum levels less than 170 pg/mL (126 pmol/L), with symptomatic patients usually having levels less than 100 pg/mL (74 pmol/L). The diagnosis of vitamin B_{12} deficiency in low or low-normal values (level of 170–210 pg/mL [126–155 pmol/L]) is best confirmed by finding an elevated level of serum methylmalonic acid (greater than 1000 nmol/L) or homocysteine. Of note, elevated levels of serum methylmalonic acid can be due to kidney disease.

The anemia of vitamin B_{12} deficiency is typically moderate to severe with the MCV quite elevated (110–140 fL). However, it is possible to have vitamin B_{12} deficiency with a normal MCV from coexistent thalassemia or iron deficiency; in other cases, the reason is obscure. Patients with neurologic symptoms and signs that suggest possible vitamin B_{12} deficiency should be evaluated for that deficiency despite a normal MCV or the absence of anemia. In typical cases, the peripheral blood smear is megaloblastic, defined as red blood cells that appear as macro-ovalocytes, (although other shape changes are usually present) and neutrophils that are hypersegmented (six [or greater]-lobed neutrophils or mean neutrophil lobe counts greater than four). The reticulocyte count is reduced. Because vitamin B_{12} deficiency can affect all hematopoietic cell lines, the white blood cell count and the platelet count are reduced in severe cases.

Other laboratory abnormalities include elevated serum lactate dehydrogenase (LD) and a modest increase in indirect bilirubin. These two findings reflect the intramedullary destruction of developing abnormal erythroid cells.

Bone marrow morphology is characteristically abnormal. Marked erythroid hyperplasia is present as a response to defective red blood cell production (ineffective erythropoiesis). Megaloblastic changes in the erythroid series include abnormally large cell size and asynchronous maturation of the nucleus and cytoplasm—ie, cytoplasmic maturation continues while impaired DNA synthesis causes retarded nuclear development. In the myeloid series, giant bands and meta-myelocytes are characteristically seen.

Differential Diagnosis

Vitamin B_{12} deficiency should be differentiated from folic acid deficiency, the other common cause of megaloblastic anemia, in which red blood cell folic acid is low while vitamin B_{12} levels are normal. The bone marrow findings of vitamin B_{12} deficiency are sometimes mistaken for a myelodysplastic syndrome (MDS) or even acute erythrocytic leukemia. The distinction between vitamin B_{12} deficiency and myelodysplasia is based on the characteristic morphology and the low vitamin B_{12} and elevated methylmalonic acid levels.

Treatment

Initially, patients with vitamin B_{12} deficiency are usually treated with parenteral therapy. Intramuscular or subcutaneous injections of 100–1000 mcg of vitamin B_{12} are adequate for each dose (with the higher dose recommended initially). Replacement is usually given daily for the first week, weekly for the next month, and then monthly for life.

The vitamin deficiency will recur if patients discontinue their therapy. Oral or sublingual methylcobalamin (1 mg/day) may be used instead of parenteral therapy once initial correction of the deficiency has occurred. Oral or sublingual replacement is effective, even in pernicious anemia, since approximately 1% of the dose is absorbed in the intestine via passive diffusion in the absence of active transport. It must be continued indefinitely and serum vitamin B_{12} levels must be monitored to ensure adequate replacement. For patients with neurologic symptoms caused by vitamin B_{12} deficiency, long-term parenteral vitamin B_{12} therapy is recommended, though its superiority over oral vitamin B_{12} therapy has not proven conclusively. Because some patients are concurrently folic acid deficient from intestinal mucosal atrophy, simultaneous folic acid replacement (1 mg daily) is advised for the first several months of vitamin B_{12} replacement.

Patients respond to therapy with an immediate improvement in their sense of well-being. Hypokalemia may complicate the first several days of therapy, particularly if the anemia is severe. A brisk reticulocytosis occurs in 5–7 days, and the hematologic picture normalizes in 2 months. Central nervous system symptoms and signs are potentially reversible if they have been present for less than 6 months. Red blood cell transfusions are rarely needed despite the severity of anemia, but when given, diuretics are also recommended to avoid heart failure because this anemia develops slowly and the plasma volume is increased at the time of diagnosis.

When to Refer

Referral to a hematologist is not usually necessary.

Green R. Vitamin B(12) deficiency from the perspective of a practicing hematologist. Blood. 2017 May 11;129(19):2603–11. [PMID: 28360040]

FOLIC ACID DEFICIENCY

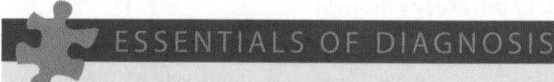

ESSENTIALS OF DIAGNOSIS

- ▶ Macrocytic anemia.
- ▶ Megaloblastic blood smear (macro-ovalocytes and hypersegmented neutrophils).
- ▶ Reduced folic acid levels in red blood cells or serum.
- ▶ Normal serum vitamin B_{12} level.

General Considerations

"Folic acid" is the term commonly used for pteroylmonoglutamic acid. Folic acid is present in most fruits and vegetables (especially citrus fruits and green leafy vegetables). Daily dietary requirements are 50–100 mcg. Total body stores of folic acid are approximately 5 mg, enough to supply requirements for 2–3 months.

Table 13–7. Causes of folic acid deficiency.

Dietary deficiency
Decreased absorption
Tropical sprue
Medications: phenytoin, sulfasalazine,
trimethoprim-sulfamethoxazole
Concurrent vitamin B_{12} deficiency
Increased requirement
Chronic hemolytic anemia
Pregnancy
Exfoliative skin disease
Excess loss: hemodialysis
Inhibition of reduction to active form
Methotrexate

The most common cause of folic acid deficiency is inadequate dietary intake (Table 13–7). Alcoholic or anorectic patients, persons who do not eat fresh fruits and vegetables, and those who overcook their food are candidates for folic acid deficiency. Reduced folic acid absorption is rarely seen, since absorption occurs from the entire gastrointestinal tract. However, medications such as phenytoin, trimethoprim-sulfamethoxazole, or sulfasalazine may interfere with its absorption. Folic acid absorption is poor in some patients with vitamin B_{12} deficiency due to gastrointestinal mucosal atrophy. Folic acid requirements are increased in pregnancy, hemolytic anemia, and exfoliative skin disease, and in these cases the increased requirements (5 to 10 times normal) may not be met by a normal diet.

Clinical Findings

A. Symptoms and Signs

The clinical features are similar to those of vitamin B_{12} deficiency. However, isolated folic acid deficiency does not result in the neurologic abnormalities of vitamin B_{12} deficiency.

B. Laboratory Findings

Megaloblastic anemia is identical to anemia resulting from vitamin B_{12} deficiency. A red blood cell folic acid level below 150 ng/mL (340 nmol/L) is diagnostic of folic acid deficiency. Whether to order a serum or a red blood cell folate level remains unsettled since there are few, if any, data to support one test over the other. Usually the serum vitamin B_{12} level is normal, and it should always be measured when folic acid deficiency is suspected. In some instances, folic acid deficiency is a consequence of the gastrointestinal mucosal megaloblastosis from vitamin B_{12} deficiency.

Differential Diagnosis

The megaloblastic anemia of folic acid deficiency should be differentiated from vitamin B_{12} deficiency by the finding of a normal vitamin B_{12} level and a reduced red blood cell (or serum) folic acid level. Alcoholic patients, who often have nutritional deficiency, may also have anemia of liver disease. Pure anemia of liver disease causes a macrocytic anemia but does not produce megaloblastic morphologic changes in the peripheral blood; rather, target cells are present. Hypothyroidism is associated with mild macrocytosis and also with pernicious anemia.

Treatment

Folic acid deficiency is treated with daily oral folic acid (1 mg). The response is similar to that seen in the treatment of vitamin B_{12} deficiency, with rapid improvement and a sense of well-being, reticulocytosis in 5–7 days, and total correction of hematologic abnormalities within 2 months. Large doses of folic acid may produce hematologic responses in cases of vitamin B_{12} deficiency, but permit neurologic damage to progress; hence, obtaining a serum vitamin B_{12} level in suspected folic acid deficiency is paramount.

When to Refer

Referral to a hematologist is not usually necessary.

Achebe MM et al. How I treat anemia in pregnancy: iron, cobalamin, and folate. Blood. 2017 Feb 23;129(8):940–9. [PMID: 28034892]

Green R et al. Megaloblastic anemias: nutritional and other causes. Med Clin North Am. 2017 Mar;101(2):297–317. [PMID: 28189172]

HEMOLYTIC ANEMIAS

The hemolytic anemias are a group of disorders in which red blood cell survival is reduced, either episodically or continuously. The bone marrow has the ability to increase erythroid production up to eightfold in response to reduced red cell survival, so anemia will be present only when the ability of the bone marrow to compensate is outstripped. This will occur when red cell survival is extremely short or when the ability of the bone marrow to compensate is impaired.

Hemolytic disorders are generally classified according to whether the defect is intrinsic to the red cell or due to some external factor (Table 13–8). Intrinsic defects have been described in all components of the red blood cell, including the membrane, enzyme systems, and hemoglobin; most of these disorders are hereditary. Hemolytic anemias due to external factors are immune and microangiopathic hemolytic anemias and infections of red blood cells.

Certain laboratory features are common to all hemolytic anemias. Haptoglobin, a normal plasma protein that binds and clears free hemoglobin released into plasma, may be depressed in hemolytic disorders. However, the haptoglobin level is influenced by many factors and is not always a reliable indicator of hemolysis, particularly in end-stage liver disease (its site of synthesis). When intravascular hemolysis occurs, transient hemoglobinemia ensues. Hemoglobin is filtered through the renal glomerulus and is usually reabsorbed by tubular cells. Hemoglobinuria will be present only when the capacity for reabsorption of hemoglobin by renal tubular cells is exceeded. In the

Table 13–8. Classification of hemolytic anemias.

Intrinsic
    Membrane defects: hereditary spherocytosis, hereditary
        elliptocytosis, paroxysmal nocturnal hemoglobinuria
    Glycolytic defects: pyruvate kinase deficiency, severe
        hypophosphatemia
    Oxidation vulnerability: glucose-6-phosphate dehydrogenase
        deficiency, methemoglobinemia
    Hemoglobinopathies: sickle cell syndromes, thalassemia,
        unstable hemoglobins, methemoglobinemia
Extrinsic
    Immune: autoimmune, lymphoproliferative disease,
        drug-induced
    Microangiopathic: thrombotic thrombocytopenic purpura,
        hemolytic-uremic syndrome, disseminated intravascular
        coagulation, valve hemolysis, metastatic adenocarcinoma,
        vasculitis, copper overload
    Infection: *Plasmodium, Clostridium, Borrelia*
    Hypersplenism
    Burns

absence of hemoglobinuria, evidence for prior intravascular hemolysis is the presence of hemosiderin in shed renal tubular cells (positive urine hemosiderin). With severe intravascular hemolysis, hemoglobinemia and methemalbuminemia may be present. Hemolysis increases the indirect bilirubin, and the total bilirubin may rise to 4 mg/dL (68 mcmol/L) or more. Bilirubin levels higher than this may indicate some degree of hepatic dysfunction. Serum LD levels are strikingly elevated in cases of microangiopathic hemolysis (thrombotic thrombocytopenic purpura, hemolytic-uremic syndrome) and may be elevated in other hemolytic anemias.

PAROXYSMAL NOCTURNAL HEMOGLOBINURIA

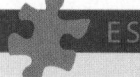
ESSENTIALS OF DIAGNOSIS

▸ Episodic hemoglobinuria.

▸ Thrombosis is common.

▸ Suspect in confusing cases of hemolytic anemia with or without pancytopenia.

▸ Flow cytometry demonstrates deficiencies of CD55 and CD59.

General Considerations

Paroxysmal nocturnal hemoglobinuria (PNH) is a rare acquired clonal hematopoietic stem cell disorder that results in abnormal sensitivity of the red blood cell membrane to lysis by complement and therefore hemolysis. Free hemoglobin is released into the blood that scavenges nitric oxide and promotes esophageal spasms, male erectile dysfunction, kidney damage, and thrombosis. Patients with significant PNH live about 10–15 years following diagnosis; thrombosis is the primary cause of death.

Clinical Findings

A. Symptoms and Signs

Classically, patients report episodic hemoglobinuria resulting in reddish-brown urine. Hemoglobinuria is most often noticed in the first morning urine due to the drop in blood pH while sleeping (hypoventilation) that facilitates this hemolysis. Besides anemia, these patients are prone to thrombosis, especially within mesenteric and hepatic veins, central nervous system veins (sagittal vein), and skin vessels (with formation of painful nodules). As this is a hematopoietic stem cell disorder, PNH may appear de novo or arise in the setting of aplastic anemia or myelodysplasia with possible progression to acute myeloid leukemia (AML). It is common that patients with idiopathic aplastic anemia have a small PNH clone (less than 2%) on blood or bone marrow analysis; this should not be considered true PNH per se, especially in the absence of a reticulocytosis or thrombosis.

B. Laboratory Findings

Anemia is of variable severity and frequency, so reticulocytosis may or may not be present at any given time. Abnormalities on the blood smear are nondiagnostic but may include macro-ovalocytes and polychromasia. Since the episodic hemolysis is mainly intravascular, urine hemosiderin is a useful test. Serum LD is characteristically elevated. Iron deficiency is commonly present, related to chronic iron loss from hemoglobinuria.

The white blood cell count and platelet count may be decreased and are always decreased in the setting of aplastic anemia. The best screening test is flow cytometry of blood erythrocytes, granulocytes, or monocytes to demonstrate deficiency of CD55 and CD59. The proportion of erythrocytes deficient in these proteins might be low due to the ongoing destruction of affected erythrocytes. The FLAER assay (fluorescein-labeled proaerolysin) by flow cytometry is more sensitive. Bone marrow morphology is variable and may show either generalized hypoplasia or erythroid hyperplasia or both. The bone marrow karyotype may be either normal or demonstrate a clonal abnormality.

Treatment

Many patients with PNH have mild disease not requiring intervention. In severe cases and in those occurring in the setting of myelodysplasia or previous aplastic anemia, allogeneic hematopoietic stem cell transplantation may prove curative. In patients with severe hemolysis (usually requiring red cell transfusions) or thrombosis (or both), treatment with eculizumab is warranted. Eculizumab is a humanized monoclonal antibody against complement protein C5. Binding of eculizumab to C5 prevents its cleavage so the membrane attack complex cannot assemble. Eculizumab improves quality of life and reduces hemolysis, transfusion requirements, fatigue, and thrombosis risk. Eculizumab is expensive and also increases the risk of *Neisseria meningitidis* infections; patients receiving the antibody should undergo meningococcal vaccination (including vaccines for serogroup B) and take oral penicillin (or equivalent) meningococcal prophylaxis. Iron replacement is indicated for treatment of iron deficiency when present, which may improve the anemia while also causing a transient increase in hemolysis. For unclear reasons, corticosteroids are effective in decreasing hemolysis.

When to Refer

Most patients with PNH should be under the care of a hematologist.

Brodsky RA. Complement in hemolytic anemia. Blood. 2015 Nov 26;126(22):2459–65. [PMID: 26582375]

Devalet B et al. Pathophysiology, diagnosis, and treatment of paroxysmal nocturnal hemoglobinuria: a review. Eur J Haematol. 2015 Sep;95(3):190–8. [PMID: 25753400]

Mohammed AA et al. Paroxysmal nocturnal hemoglobinuria: from bench to bed. Indian J Hematol Blood Transfus. 2016 Dec;32(4):383–91. [PMID: 27812245]

Parker CJ. Update on the diagnosis and management of paroxysmal nocturnal hemoglobinuria. Hematol Am Soc Hematol Educ Prog. 2016 Dec 2;2016(1):208–16. [PMID: 27913482]

GLUCOSE-6-PHOSPHATE DEHYDROGENASE DEFICIENCY

ESSENTIALS OF DIAGNOSIS

▶ X-linked recessive disorder seen commonly in American black men.

▶ Episodic hemolysis in response to oxidant drugs or infection.

▶ Bite cells and blister cells on the peripheral blood smear.

▶ Reduced levels of glucose-6-phosphate dehydrogenase between hemolytic episodes.

General Considerations

Glucose-6-phosphate dehydrogenase (G6PD) deficiency is a hereditary enzyme defect that causes episodic hemolytic anemia because of the decreased ability of red blood cells to deal with oxidative stresses. G6PD deficiency leads to excess oxidized glutathione (hence, inadequate levels of reduced glutathione) that forces hemoglobin to denature and form precipitants called Heinz bodies. Heinz bodies cause red blood cell membrane damage, which leads to premature removal of these red blood cells by reticuloendothelial cells within the spleen (ie, extravascular hemolysis).

Numerous G6PD isoenzymes have been described. The usual isoenzyme found in American blacks is designated G6PD-A and that found in whites is designated G6PD-B, both of which have normal function and stability and therefore no hemolytic anemia. Ten to 15 percent of American blacks have the variant G6PD isoenzyme designated A–, in which there is both a reduction in normal enzyme activity and a reduction in its stability. The A– isoenzyme activity declines rapidly as the red blood cell ages past 40 days, a fact that explains the clinical findings in this disorder. More than 150 G6PD isoenzyme variants have been described, including some Mediterranean, Ashkenazi Jewish, and Asian variants with very low enzyme activity, episodic hemolysis, and exacerbations due to oxidizing substances including fava beans. Patients with G6PD deficiency seem to be protected from malaria parasitic infection, have less coronary artery disease, and possibly have fewer cancers and greater longevity.

Clinical Findings

G6PD deficiency is an X-linked disorder affecting 10–15% of American hemizygous black males and rare female homozygotes. Female carriers are rarely affected—only when an unusually high percentage of cells producing the normal enzyme are X-inactivated.

A. Symptoms and Signs

Patients are usually healthy, without chronic hemolytic anemia or splenomegaly. Hemolysis occurs episodically as a result of oxidative stress on the red blood cells, generated either by infection or exposure to certain medications. Medications initiating hemolysis that should be avoided include dapsone, methylene blue, phenazopyridine, primaquine, rasburicase, toluidine blue, nitrofurantoin, trimethoprim/sulfamethoxazole, sulfadiazine, pegloticase, and quinolones. Other medications, such as chloroquine, quinine, high-dose aspirin, and isoniazid, have been implicated but are less certain as offenders since they are often given during infections. Even with continuous use of the offending medication, the hemolytic episode is self-limited because older red blood cells (with low enzyme activity) are removed and replaced with a population of young red blood cells (reticulocytes) with adequate functional levels of G6PD. Severe G6PD deficiency (as in Mediterranean variants) may produce a chronic hemolytic anemia.

B. Laboratory Findings

Between hemolytic episodes, the blood is normal. During episodes of hemolysis, the hemoglobin rarely falls below 8 g/dL (80 g/L), and there is reticulocytosis and increased serum indirect bilirubin. The peripheral blood cell smear often reveals a small number of "bite" cells—cells that appear to have had a bite taken out of their periphery, or "blister" cells. This indicates pitting of precipitated membrane hemoglobin aggregates (ie, Heinz bodies) by the splenic macrophages. Heinz bodies may be demonstrated by staining a peripheral blood smear with cresyl violet; they are not visible on the usual Wright-Giemsa–stained blood smear. Specific enzyme assays for G6PD reveal a low level but may be falsely normal if they are performed during or shortly after a hemolytic episode during the period of reticulocytosis. In these cases, the enzyme assays should be repeated weeks after hemolysis has resolved. In severe cases of G6PD deficiency, enzyme levels are always low.

Treatment

No treatment is necessary except to avoid known oxidant medications.

Belfield KD et al. Review and drug therapy implications of glucose-6-phosphate dehydrogenase deficiency. Am J Health Syst Pharm. 2018 Feb 1;75(3):97–104. [PMID: 29305344]

Luzzatto L et al. Glucose-6-phosphate dehydrogenase deficiency. Hematol Oncol Clin North Am. 2016 Apr;30(2):373–93. [PMID: 27040960]

SICKLE CELL ANEMIA & RELATED SYNDROMES

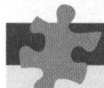 ESSENTIALS OF DIAGNOSIS

► Recurrent pain episodes.

► Positive family history and lifelong history of hemolytic anemia.

► Irreversibly sickled cells on peripheral blood smear.

► Hemoglobin S is the major hemoglobin seen on electrophoresis.

General Considerations

Sickle cell anemia is an autosomal recessive disorder in which an abnormal hemoglobin leads to chronic hemolytic anemia with numerous clinical consequences. A single DNA base change leads to an amino acid substitution of valine for glutamine in the sixth position on the beta-globin chain. The abnormal beta chain is designated beta^s and the tetramer of alpha-2beta^s-2 is designated hemoglobin S. Hemoglobin S is unstable and polymerizes in the setting of various stressors, including hypoxemia and acidosis, leading to the formation of sickled red blood cells. Sickled cells result in hemolysis and the release of ATP, which is converted to adenosine. Adenosine binds to its receptor (A2B), resulting in the production of 2,3-biphosphoglycerate and the induction of more sickling, and to its receptor (A2A) on natural killer cells, resulting in pulmonary inflammation. The free hemoglobin from hemolysis scavenges nitric oxide causing endothelial dysfunction, vascular injury, and pulmonary hypertension.

The rate of sickling is influenced by the intracellular concentration of hemoglobin S and by the presence of other hemoglobins within the cell. Hemoglobin F cannot participate in polymer formation, and its presence markedly retards sickling. Factors that increase sickling are red blood cell dehydration and factors that lead to formation of deoxyhemoglobin S (eg, acidosis and hypoxemia) either systemic or local in tissues. Hemolytic crises may be related to splenic sequestration of sickled cells (primarily in childhood before the spleen has been infarcted as a result of repeated sickling) or with coexistent disorders such as G6PD deficiency.

The beta^s gene is carried in 8% of American blacks, and 1 of 400 American black children will be born with sickle cell anemia; prenatal diagnosis is available when sickle cell anemia is suspected. Genetic counseling should be made available to patients.

Clinical Findings

A. Symptoms and Signs

The disorder has its onset during the first year of life, when hemoglobin F levels fall as a signal is sent to switch from production of gamma-globin to beta-globin. Chronic hemolytic anemia produces jaundice, pigment (calcium bilirubinate) gallstones, splenomegaly (early in life), and poorly healing ulcers over the lower tibia. Life-threatening severe anemia can occur during hemolytic or aplastic crises, the latter generally associated with viral or other infection or by folic acid deficiency causing reduced erythropoiesis, or infection caused by immunoincompetence from hyposplenism.

Acute painful episodes due to acute vaso-occlusion from clusters of sickled red cells may occur spontaneously or be provoked by infection, dehydration, or hypoxia. Common sites of acute painful episodes include the spine and long appendicular and thoracic bones. These episodes last hours to days and may produce low-grade fever. Acute vaso-occlusion may cause strokes due to sagittal sinus venous thrombosis or to bland or hemorrhagic central nervous system arterial ischemia and may also cause priapism. Vaso-occlusive episodes are not associated with increased hemolysis.

Repeated episodes of vascular occlusion especially affect the heart, lungs, and liver. The acute chest syndrome is characterized by acute chest pain, hypoxemia, and pulmonary infiltrates on a chest radiograph and must be distinguished from an infectious pneumonia. Ischemic necrosis of bones may occur, rendering the bone susceptible to osteomyelitis due to salmonellae and (somewhat less commonly) staphylococci. Infarction of the papillae of the renal medulla causes renal tubular concentrating defects and gross hematuria, more often encountered in sickle cell trait than in sickle cell anemia. Retinopathy similar to that noted in diabetes mellitus is often present and may lead to visual impairment. Pulmonary hypertension may develop and is associated with a poor prognosis. These patients are prone to delayed puberty. An increased incidence of infection is related to hyposplenism as well as to defects in the alternate complement pathway.

On examination, patients are often chronically ill and jaundiced. There is hepatomegaly, but the spleen is not palpable in adult life. The heart is enlarged with a hyperdynamic precordium and systolic murmurs and, in some cases, a pronounced increase in P2. Nonhealing ulcers of the lower leg and retinopathy may be present.

B. Laboratory Findings

Chronic hemolytic anemia is present. The hematocrit is usually 20–30%. The peripheral blood smear is characteristically abnormal, with irreversibly sickled cells comprising 5–50% of red cells. Other findings include reticulocytosis (10–25%), nucleated red blood cells, and hallmarks of hyposplenism such as Howell-Jolly bodies and target cells. The white blood cell count is characteristically elevated to 12,000–15,000/mcL, and reactive thrombocytosis may occur. Indirect bilirubin levels are high.

The diagnosis of sickle cell anemia is confirmed by hemoglobin electrophoresis (Table 13–9). Hemoglobin S

Table 13–9. Hemoglobin distribution in sickle cell syndromes.

Genotype	Clinical Diagnosis	Hb A	Hb S	Hb A$_2$	Hb F
AA	Normal	97–99%	0%	1–2%	< 1%
AS	Sickle trait	60%	40%	1–2%	< 1%
AS, alpha-thalassemia	Sickle trait, alpha-thalassemia	70–75%	25–30%	1–2%	< 1%
SS	Sickle cell anemia	0%	86–98%	1–3%	5–15%
SS, alpha-thalassemia (3 genes)	SS alpha-thalassemia, silent	0%	90%	3%	7–9%
SS, alpha-thalassemia (2 genes)	SS alpha-thalassemia, trait	0%	80%	3%	11–21%
S, beta^0-thalassemia	Sickle beta^0-thalassemia	0%	70–80%	3–5%	10–20%
S, beta$^+$-thalassemia	Sickle beta$^+$-thalassemia	10–20%	60–75%	3–5%	10–20%

Hb, hemoglobin; beta^0, no beta-globin produced; beta$^+$, some beta-globin produced.

will usually comprise 85–98% of hemoglobin. In homozygous S disease, no hemoglobin A will be present. Hemoglobin F levels are sometimes increased, and high hemoglobin F levels are associated with a more benign clinical course. Patients with S-beta$^+$-thalassemia and SS alpha-thalassemia also have a more benign clinical course than sickle cell anemia (SS) patients.

Treatment

When allogeneic hematopoietic stem cell transplantation is performed before the onset of significant end-organ damage, it can cure more than 80% of children with sickle cell anemia who have suitable HLA-matched donors. Transplantation remains investigational in adults. Other therapies modulate disease severity: cytotoxic agents, such as hydroxyurea, increase hemoglobin F levels epigenetically. Hydroxyurea (500–750 mg orally daily) reduces the frequency of painful crises in patients whose quality of life is disrupted by frequent pain crises (three or more per year). Long-term follow-up of patients taking hydroxyurea demonstrates it improves overall survival and quality of life with little evidence for secondary malignancy. The use of omega-3 (n-3) fatty acid supplementation may reduce vaso-occlusive episodes and reduce transfusion needs in patients with sickle cell anemia. L-glutamine has been shown to favorably modulate sickle pain crises and acute chest syndrome.

Supportive care is the mainstay of treatment for sickle cell anemia. Patients are maintained on folic acid supplementation (1 mg orally daily) and given transfusions for aplastic or hemolytic crises. When acute painful episodes occur, precipitating factors should be identified and infections treated if present. The patient should be kept well hydrated, given generous analgesics, and supplied oxygen if hypoxic. Pneumococcal vaccination reduces the incidence of infections with this pathogen while hydroxyurea and L-glutamine reduce hospitalizations for acute pain. Angiotensin-converting enzyme inhibitors are recommended in patients with microalbuminuria.

Exchange transfusions are indicated for the treatment of severe acute vaso-occlusive crises, intractable pain crises, acute chest syndrome, priapism, and stroke. Long-term transfusion therapy has been shown to be effective in reducing the risk of recurrent stroke in children. It has been recommended that children with SS who are aged 2–16 years have annual transcranial ultrasounds and, if the Doppler velocity is abnormal (200 cm/s or greater), the clinician should strongly consider beginning transfusions to prevent stroke. Iron chelation is needed for those on chronic transfusion therapy.

Prognosis

Sickle cell anemia becomes a chronic multisystem disease, leading to organ failure that may result in death. With improved supportive care, average life expectancy is now between 40 and 50 years of age.

When to Refer

Patients with sickle cell anemia should have their care coordinated with a hematologist and should be referred to a Comprehensive Sickle Cell Center, if one is available.

When to Admit

Patients should be admitted for management of acute chest crises, for aplastic crisis, or for painful episodes that do not respond to outpatient care.

Bauer DE et al. Curative approaches for sickle cell disease: a review of allogeneic and autologous strategies. Blood Cells Mol Dis. 2017 Sep;67:155–68. [PMID: 28893518]

Niihara Y et al. A phase 3 trial of l-glutamine in sickle cell disease. N Engl J Med. 2018 Jul 19;379(3):226–35. [PMID: 30021096]

Rees DC et al. How I manage red cell transfusions in patients with sickle cell disease. Br J Haematol. 2018 Feb;180(4):607–17. [PMID: 29377071]

SICKLE CELL TRAIT

People with the heterozygous hemoglobin genotype AS have **sickle cell trait.** These persons are hematologically normal, with no anemia and normal red blood cells on peripheral blood smear. Hemoglobin electrophoresis will reveal that approximately 40% of hemoglobin is hemoglobin S (Table 13–9). People with sickle cell trait experience more rhabdomyolysis during vigorous exercise but do not have increased mortality compared to the general population. They may be at increased risk for venous thromboembolism. Chronic sickling of red blood cells in the acidotic renal medulla results in microscopic and gross hematuria, hyposthenuria (poor urine concentrating ability), and possibly chronic kidney disease. No treatment is necessary but genetic counseling is recommended.

Naik RP et al. Sickle cell trait diagnosis: clinical and social implications. Hematology Am Soc Hematol Educ Program. 2015; 2015:160–7. [PMID: 26637716]

Nelson DA et al. Sickle cell trait, rhabdomyolysis, and mortality among U.S. Army soldiers. N Engl J Med. 2016 Aug 4;375(5): 435–42. [PMID: 27518662]

SICKLE THALASSEMIA

Patients with homozygous sickle cell anemia and alpha-thalassemia have less vigorous hemolysis and run higher hemoglobins than SS patients due to reduced red blood cell sickling related to a lower hemoglobin concentration within the red blood cell and higher hemoglobin F levels (Table 13–9). The MCV is low, and the red cells are hypochromic.

Patients who are compound heterozygotes for beta^s and beta-thalassemia are clinically affected with sickle cell syndromes. Sickle beta^0-thalassemia is clinically very similar to homozygous SS disease. Vaso-occlusive crises may be somewhat less severe, and the spleen is not always infarcted. The MCV is low, in contrast to the normal MCV of sickle cell anemia. Hemoglobin electrophoresis reveals no hemoglobin A but will show an increase in hemoglobins A$_2$ and F (Table 13–9).

Sickle beta$^+$-thalassemia is a milder disorder than homozygous SS disease, with fewer pain episodes but more acute chest syndrome than sickle beta^0-thalassemia. The spleen is usually palpable. The hemolytic anemia is less severe, and the hematocrit is usually 30–38%, with reticulocytes of 5–10%. Hemoglobin electrophoresis shows the presence of some hemoglobin A and elevated hemoglobins A$_2$ and F (Table 13–9). The MCV is low.

Benites BD et al. Sickle cell/β-thalassemia: comparison of Sβ(0) and Sβ(+) Brazilian patients followed at a single institution. Hematology. 2016 Dec;21(10):623–9. [PMID: 27237196]

Yu TT et al. Risk factors for venous thromboembolism in adults with hemoglobin SC or Sβ(+) thalassemia genotypes. Thromb Res. 2016 May;141:35–8. [PMID: 26962984]

AUTOIMMUNE HEMOLYTIC ANEMIA

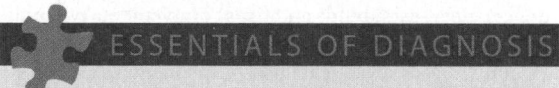

ESSENTIALS OF DIAGNOSIS

▶ Acquired hemolytic anemia caused by IgG autoantibody.

▶ Spherocytes and reticulocytosis on peripheral blood smear.

▶ Positive antiglobulin (Coombs) test.

▶ General Considerations

Autoimmune hemolytic anemia is an acquired disorder in which an IgG autoantibody is formed that binds to a red blood cell membrane protein and does so most avidly at body temperature (ie, a "warm" autoantibody). The antibody is most commonly directed against a basic component of the Rh system present on most human red blood cells. When IgG antibodies coat the red blood cell, the Fc portion of the antibody is recognized by macrophages present in the spleen and other portions of the reticuloendothelial system. The interaction between splenic macrophages and the antibody-coated red blood cell results in removal of red blood cell membrane and the formation of a spherocyte due to the decrease in surface-to-volume ratio of the surviving red blood cell. These spherocytic cells have decreased deformability and are unable to squeeze through the 2-mcm fenestrations of splenic sinusoids and become trapped in the red pulp of the spleen. When large amounts of IgG are present on red blood cells, complement may be fixed. Direct complement lysis of cells is rare, but the presence of C3b on the surface of red blood cells allows Kupffer cells in the liver to participate in the hemolytic process via C3b receptors. The destruction of red blood cells in the spleen and liver designates this as extravascular hemolysis.

Approximately one-half of all cases of autoimmune hemolytic anemia are idiopathic. The disorder may also be seen in association with systemic lupus erythematosus, other rheumatic disorders, chronic lymphocytic leukemia (CLL), or lymphomas. It must be distinguished from drug-induced hemolytic anemia. When penicillin (or other medications, especially cefotetan, ceftriaxone, and piperacillin) coats the red blood cell membrane, the autoantibody is directed against the membrane-drug complex. Fludarabine, an antineoplastic, causes autoimmune hemolytic anemia through its immunosuppression; there is defective self- versus non–self-immune surveillance permitting the escape of a B-cell clone, which produces the offending autoantibody.

▶ Clinical Findings

A. Symptoms and Signs

Autoimmune hemolytic anemia typically produces an anemia of rapid onset that may be life-threatening. Patients complain of fatigue and dyspnea and may present with angina pectoris or heart failure. On examination, jaundice and splenomegaly are usually present.

B. Laboratory Findings

The anemia is of variable degree but may be very severe, with hematocrit of less than 10%. Reticulocytosis is present, and spherocytes are seen on the peripheral blood smear. In cases of severe hemolysis, the stressed bone marrow may also release nucleated red blood cells. As with other hemolytic disorders, the serum indirect bilirubin is increased and the haptoglobin is low. Approximately 10% of patients with autoimmune hemolytic anemia have coincident immune thrombocytopenia (Evans syndrome).

The antiglobulin (Coombs) test forms the basis for diagnosis. The Coombs reagent is a rabbit IgM antibody raised against human IgG or human complement. The direct antiglobulin (Coombs) test (DAT) is performed by mixing the patient's red blood cells with the Coombs reagent and looking for agglutination, which indicates the presence of antibody or complement or both on the red blood cell surface. The indirect antiglobulin (Coombs) test is performed by mixing the patient's serum with a panel of type O red blood cells. After incubation of the test serum and panel red blood cells, the Coombs reagent is added. Agglutination in this system indicates the presence of free antibody (autoantibody or alloantibody) in the patient's serum.

The direct antiglobulin test is positive (for IgG, complement, or both) in about 90% of patients with autoimmune hemolytic anemia. The indirect antiglobulin test may or may not be positive. A positive indirect antiglobulin test indicates the presence of a large amount of autoantibody that has saturated binding sites on the red blood cell and consequently appears in the serum. Because the patient's serum usually contains the autoantibody, it may be difficult to obtain a "compatible" cross-match with homologous red blood cells for transfusions since the cross-match indicates the possible presence (true or false) of a red blood cell "alloantibody."

▶ Treatment

Initial treatment consists of prednisone, 1–2 mg/kg/day orally in divided doses. Patients with DAT-negative and DAT-positive autoimmune hemolysis respond equally well to corticosteroids. Transfused red blood cells will survive similarly to the patient's own red blood cells. Because of difficulty in performing the cross-match, possible "incompatible" blood may need to be given. Decisions regarding transfusions should be made in consultation with a hematologist and a blood bank specialist. Death from cardiovascular collapse can occur in the setting of rapid hemolysis. In patients with rapid hemolysis, therapeutic plasmapheresis should be performed early in management to remove autoantibodies. If prednisone is ineffective or if the disease recurs on tapering the dose, splenectomy should be considered, which may cure the disorder. Patients with autoimmune hemolytic anemia refractory to prednisone and splenectomy may also be treated with a variety of agents. Treatment with rituximab, a monoclonal antibody against the B cell antigen CD20, is effective in some cases. The suggested dose is 375 mg/m^2 intravenously weekly for 4 weeks. Rituximab is used in conjunction with corticosteroids as initial therapy in some patients with severe disease. Danazol, 400–800 mg/day orally, is less often effective than in immune thrombocytopenia but is well suited for long-term use because of its low toxicity profile. Immunosuppressive agents, including cyclophosphamide, vincristine, azathioprine, mycophenolate mofetil, alemtuzumab (an anti-CD52 antibody), or cyclosporine, may also be used. High-dose intravenous immune globulin (1 g/kg daily for 2 days) may be effective in controlling hemolysis. The benefit is short-lived (1–3 weeks), and the medication is very expensive. The long-term prognosis for patients with this disorder is good, especially if there is no other underlying autoimmune disorder or lymphoproliferative disorder. Treatment of an associated lymphoproliferative disorder will also treat the hemolytic anemia.

▶ When to Refer

Patients with autoimmune hemolytic anemia should be referred to a hematologist for confirmation of the diagnosis and subsequent care.

▶ When to Admit

Patients should be hospitalized for symptomatic anemia or rapidly falling hemoglobin levels.

Go RS et al. How I treat autoimmune hemolytic anemia. Blood. 2017 Jun 1;129(22):2971–9. [PMID: 28360039]

Hill A et al. Autoimmune hemolytic anemia. Hematology Am Soc Hematol Educ Program. 2018 Nov 30;2018(1):382–9. [PMID: 30504336]

Michel M et al. A randomized and double-blind controlled trial evaluating the safety and efficacy of rituximab for warm autoimmune hemolytic anemia in adults (the RIAHA study). Am J Hematol. 2017 Jan;91(1):23–7. [PMID: 27696475]

COLD AGGLUTININ DISEASE

ESSENTIALS OF DIAGNOSIS

- ▶ Increased reticulocytes on peripheral blood smear.
- ▶ Antiglobulin (Coombs) test positive only for complement.
- ▶ Positive cold agglutinin titer.

▶ General Considerations

Cold agglutinin disease is an acquired hemolytic anemia due to an IgM autoantibody (called a "cold agglutinin") usually directed against the I/i antigen on red blood cells. These IgM autoantibodies characteristically will react poorly with cells at 37°C but avidly at lower temperatures, usually at 0–4°C (ie, "cold" autoantibody). Since the blood temperature (even in the most peripheral parts of the body) rarely goes lower than 20°C, only cold autoantibodies reactive at relatively higher temperatures will produce clinical effects. Hemolysis results indirectly from attachment of IgM, which in the cooler parts of the circulation (fingers, nose, ears) binds and fixes complement. When the red blood cell returns to a warmer temperature, the IgM antibody dissociates, leaving complement on the cell. Complement lysis of red blood cells rarely occurs. Rather, C3b, present on the red blood cells, is recognized by Kupffer cells (which have receptors for C3b), and red blood cell sequestration and destruction in the liver ensues (extravascular hemolysis). In some cases, the complement membrane attack complex forms, lysing the red blood cells (intravascular hemolysis).

Most cases of chronic cold agglutinin disease are idiopathic. Others occur in association with Waldenström macroglobulinemia, lymphoma, or CLL, in which a monoclonal IgM paraprotein is produced. Acute postinfectious cold agglutinin disease occurs following mycoplasmal pneumonia or viral infection (infectious mononucleosis, measles, mumps, or cytomegalovirus [CMV] with autoantibody directed against antigen i rather than I).

► Clinical Findings

A. Symptoms and Signs

In chronic cold agglutinin disease, symptoms related to red blood cell agglutination occur on exposure to cold, and patients may complain of mottled or numb fingers or toes, acrocyanosis, episodic low back pain, and dark-colored urine. Hemolytic anemia is occasionally severe, but episodic hemoglobinuria may occur on exposure to cold. The hemolytic anemia in acute postinfectious syndromes is rarely severe.

B. Laboratory Findings

Mild anemia is present with reticulocytosis and rarely spherocytes. The blood smear made at room temperature shows agglutinated red blood cells (there is no agglutination on a blood smear made at body temperature). The direct antiglobulin (Coombs) test will be positive for complement only. Serum cold agglutinin titer will semi-quantitate the autoantibody. A monoclonal IgM is often found on serum protein electrophoresis and confirmed by serum immuno-electrophoresis. There is indirect hyperbilirubinemia and the haptoglobin is low during periods of hemolysis.

► Treatment

Treatment is largely symptomatic, based on avoiding exposure to cold. Splenectomy and prednisone are usually ineffective (except when associated with a lymphoproliferative disorder) since hemolysis takes place in the liver and blood stream. Rituximab is the treatment of choice. The dose is 375 mg/m² intravenously weekly for 4 weeks. Relapses may be effectively re-treated. High-dose intravenous immunoglobulin (2 g/kg) may be effective temporarily, but it is rarely used because of the high cost and short duration of benefit. Patients with severe disease may be treated with cytotoxic agents, such as bendamustine (plus rituximab), cyclophosphamide, fludarabine, or bortezomib, or with immunosuppressive agents, such as cyclosporine. As in warm IgG-mediated autoimmune hemolysis, it may be difficult to find compatible blood for transfusion. Red blood cells should be transfused through an in-line blood warmer.

Berentsen S et al. Bendamustine plus rituximab for chronic cold agglutinin disease: results of a Nordic prospective multicenter trial. Blood. 2017 Jul 27;130(4):537–41. [PMID: 28533306]

Berentsen S. Cold agglutinin disease. Hematology Am Soc Hematol Educ Program. 2016 Dec 2;2016(1):226–31. [PMID: 27913484]

Go RS et al. How I treat autoimmune hemolytic anemia. Blood. 2017 Jun 1;129(22):2971–9. [PMID: 28360039]

APLASTIC ANEMIA

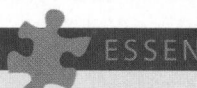

ESSENTIALS OF DIAGNOSIS

- ► Pancytopenia.
- ► No abnormal hematopoietic cells seen in blood or bone marrow.
- ► Hypocellular bone marrow.

► General Considerations

Aplastic anemia is a condition of bone marrow failure that arises from suppression of, or injury to, the hematopoietic stem cell. The bone marrow becomes hypoplastic, fails to produce mature blood cells, and pancytopenia develops.

There are a number of causes of aplastic anemia (Table 13–10). Direct hematopoietic stem cell injury may be caused by radiation, chemotherapy, toxins, or pharmacologic agents. Systemic lupus erythematosus may rarely cause suppression of the hematopoietic stem cell by an IgG autoantibody directed against it. However, the most common pathogenesis of aplastic anemia appears to be autoimmune suppression of hematopoiesis by a T-cell-mediated cellular mechanism, so called idiopathic aplastic anemia. In some cases of idiopathic aplastic anemia, defects in maintenance of the hematopoietic stem cell telomere length (dyskeratosis congenita) or in DNA repair pathways (Fanconi anemia) have been identified and are likely linked to both the initiation of bone marrow failure and the propensity to later progress to myelodysplasia, PNH, or AML. Complex detrimental immune responses to viruses can also cause aplastic anemia.

► Clinical Findings

A. Symptoms and Signs

Patients come to medical attention because of the consequences of bone marrow failure. Anemia leads to symptoms of weakness and fatigue, neutropenia causes vulnerability to bacterial or fungal infections, and thrombocytopenia results in mucosal and skin bleeding. Physical examination may reveal signs of pallor, purpura, and petechiae. Other abnormalities such as hepatosplenomegaly,

Table 13–10. Causes of aplastic anemia.

Autoimmune: idiopathic, systemic lupus erythematosus
Congenital: defects in telomere length maintenance or DNA repair
Chemotherapy, radiotherapy
Toxins: benzene, toluene, insecticides
Medications: chloramphenicol, gold salts, sulfonamides, phenytoin, carbamazepine, quinacrine, tolbutamide
Post-viral hepatitis (A, B, C, E, G, non-A through -G)
Non-hepatitis viruses (EBV, parvovirus, CMV, echovirus 3, others)
Pregnancy
Paroxysmal nocturnal hemoglobinuria

EBV, Epstein-Barr virus; CMV, cytomegalovirus.

lymphadenopathy, or bone tenderness should *not* be present, and their presence should lead to questioning the diagnosis.

B. Laboratory Findings

The hallmark of aplastic anemia is pancytopenia. However, early in the evolution of aplastic anemia, only one or two cell lines may be reduced.

Anemia may be severe and is always associated with reticulocytopenia. Red blood cell morphology is unremarkable, but there may be mild macrocytosis (increased MCV). Neutrophils and platelets are reduced in number, and no immature or abnormal forms are seen on the blood smear. The bone marrow aspirate and the bone marrow biopsy appear hypocellular, with only scant amounts of morphologically normal hematopoietic progenitors. The prior dictum that the bone marrow karyotype should be normal (or germline if normal variant) has evolved and some clonal abnormalities or other genetic aberrations may be present even in the setting of idiopathic aplastic anemia.

▶ Differential Diagnosis

Aplastic anemia must be differentiated from other causes of pancytopenia (Table 13–11). Hypocellular forms of myelodysplasia or acute leukemia may occasionally be confused with aplastic anemia. These are differentiated by the presence of cellular morphologic abnormalities, increased percentage of blasts, or abnormal karyotype in bone marrow cells typical of MDS or acute leukemia. Hairy cell leukemia has been misdiagnosed as aplastic anemia and should be recognized by the presence of splenomegaly and by abnormal "hairy" lymphoid cells in a hypocellular bone marrow biopsy. Pancytopenia with a normocellular bone marrow may be due to systemic lupus erythematosus, disseminated infection, hypersplenism, nutritional (eg, vitamin B$_{12}$ or folate) deficiency, or myelodysplasia. Isolated thrombocytopenia may occur early as aplastic anemia develops and may be confused with immune thrombocytopenia.

Table 13–11. Causes of pancytopenia.

Primary bone marrow disorders
Aplastic anemia
Myelodysplasia
Acute leukemia
Chronic idiopathic myelofibrosis
Infiltrative disease: lymphoma, myeloma, carcinoma, hairy cell leukemia, etc
Non–primary bone marrow disorders
Hypersplenism (with or without portal hypertension)
Systemic lupus erythematosus
Infection: tuberculosis, HIV, leishmaniasis, brucellosis, CMV, parvovirus B19
Nutritional deficiency (megaloblastic anemia)
Medications
Cytotoxic chemotherapy
Ionizing radiation

CMV, cytomegalovirus.

▶ Treatment

Mild cases of aplastic anemia may be treated with supportive care, including erythropoietic (epoetin or darbepoetin) or myeloid (filgrastim or sargramostim) growth factors, or both. Red blood cell transfusions and platelet transfusions are given as necessary, and antibiotics are used to treat infections.

Severe aplastic anemia is defined by a neutrophil count of less than 500/mcL, platelets less than 20,000/mcL, reticulocytes less than 1%, and bone marrow cellularity less than 20%. The treatment of choice for young adults (under age 40 years) who have an HLA-matched sibling is allogeneic bone marrow transplantation. Children or young adults may also benefit from allogeneic bone marrow transplantation using an unrelated donor. Because of the increased risks associated with unrelated donor allogeneic bone marrow transplantation compared to sibling donors, this treatment is usually reserved for patients who have not responded to immunosuppressive therapy.

For adults over age 40 years or those without HLA-matched hematopoietic stem cell donors, the treatment of choice for severe aplastic anemia is immunosuppression with equine antithymocyte globulin (ATG) plus cyclosporine. Equine ATG is given in the hospital in conjunction with transfusion and antibiotic support. A proven regimen is equine ATG 40 mg/kg/day intravenously for 4 days in combination with cyclosporine, 6 mg/kg orally twice daily. Equine ATG is superior to rabbit ATG, resulting in a higher response rate and better survival. Eltrombopag, a thrombopoietin mimetic, is now being added to ATG plus cyclosporine with tri-lineage hematologic responses as high as 90%. ATG should be used in combination with corticosteroids (prednisone or methylprednisolone 1–2 mg/kg/day orally for 1 week, followed by a taper over 2 weeks) to avoid ATG infusion reactions and serum sickness. Responses usually occur in 1–3 months and are usually only partial, but the blood counts rise high enough to give patients a safe and transfusion-free life. The full benefit of immunosuppression is generally assessed at 4 months post-equine ATG. Cyclosporine and eltrombopag are maintained at full doses for 6 months and then stopped in responding patients. Androgens (such as fluoxymesterone 10–20 mg/day orally in divided doses) have been widely used in the past, with a low response rate, and may be considered in mild cases.

▶ Course & Prognosis

Patients with severe aplastic anemia have a rapidly fatal illness if left untreated. Allogeneic bone marrow transplant from an HLA-matched sibling donor produces survival rates of over 80% in recipients under 20 years old and of about 65–70% in those 20 to 50 years old. Respective survival rates drop 10–15% when the donor is HLA-matched but unrelated. Equine ATG-cyclosporine immunosuppressive treatment leads to a response in approximately 70% of patients (including those with hepatitis virus–associated aplastic anemia) and in up to 90% of patients with the addition of eltrombopag. Up to one-third of patients will relapse with aplastic anemia after ATG-based therapy. Clonal hematologic disorders, such as PNH, AML, or myelodysplasia, may develop in one-quarter of patients treated with immuno-suppressive therapy after 10 years of follow-up. Factors that predict response to ATG-cyclosporine therapy are patient's age, reticulocyte count, lymphocyte count, and age-adjusted telomere length of leukocytes at the time of diagnosis.

▶ When to Refer

All patients should be referred to a hematologist.

▶ When to Admit

Admission is necessary for treatment of neutropenic infection, the administration of ATG, or allogeneic bone marrow transplantation.

Bacigalupo A. How I treat acquired aplastic anemia. Blood. 2017 Mar 16;129(11):1428–36. [PMID: 28096088]

Kumar R et al. Hematopoietic cell transplantation for aplastic anemia. Curr Opin Hematol. 2017 Nov;24(6):509–14. [PMID: 28877042]

Peslak SA et al. Diagnosis and treatment of aplastic anemia. Curr Treat Options Oncol. 2017 Nov 16;18(12):70. [PMID: 29143887]

Townsley DM et al. Eltrombopag added to standard immunosuppression for aplastic anemia. N Engl J Med. 2017 Apr 20; 376(16):1540–50. [PMID: 28423296]

NEUTROPENIA

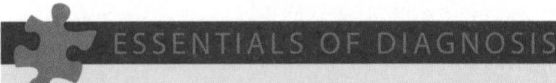

ESSENTIALS OF DIAGNOSIS

► Neutrophils less than 1800/mcL (1.8 × 10⁹/L).
► Severe neutropenia if neutrophils below 500/mcL (0.5 × 10⁹/L).

▶ General Considerations

Neutropenia is present when the absolute neutrophil count is less than 1800/mcL (1.8 × 10⁹/L), although blacks, Asians, and other specific ethnic groups may have normal neutrophil counts as low as 1200/mcL (1.2 × 10⁹/L). The neutropenic patient is increasingly vulnerable to infection by gram-positive and gram-negative bacteria and by fungi. The risk of infection is related to the severity of neutropenia. The risk of serious infection rises sharply with neutrophil counts below 500/mcL (0.5 × 10⁹/L), and a high risk of infection within days occurs with neutrophil counts below 100/mcL (0.1 × 10⁹/L) ("profound neutropenia"). The classification of neutropenic syndromes is unsatisfactory as the pathophysiology and natural history of different syndromes overlap. Patients with "chronic benign neutropenia" are free of infection despite very low stable neutrophil counts; they seem to physiologically respond adequately to infections and inflammatory stimuli with an appropriate neutrophil release from the bone marrow. In contrast, the neutrophil count of patients with cyclic neutropenia periodically oscillates (usually in 21-day cycles) between normal and low, with infections occurring during the nadirs. Congenital neutropenia is lifelong neutropenia punctuated with infection.

Table 13–12. Causes of neutropenia.

Bone marrow disorders
Congenital
Dyskeratosis congenita
Fanconi anemia
Cyclic neutropenia
Congenital neutropenia
Hairy cell leukemia
Large granular lymphoproliferative disorder
Myelodysplasia
Non–bone marrow disorders
Medications: antiretroviral medications, cephalosporins, chlorpromazine, chlorpropamide, cimetidine, methimazole, myelosuppressive cytotoxic chemotherapy, penicillin, phenytoin, procainamide, rituximab, sulfonamides
Aplastic anemia
Benign chronic neutropenia
Pure white cell aplasia
Hypersplenism
Sepsis
Other immune
Autoimmune (idiopathic)
Felty syndrome
Systemic lupus erythematosus
HIV infection

A variety of bone marrow disorders and nonmarrow conditions may cause neutropenia (Table 13–12). All of the causes of aplastic anemia (Table 13–10) and pancytopenia (Table 13–11) may cause neutropenia. The new onset of an isolated neutropenia is most often due to an idiosyncratic reaction to a medication, and agranulocytosis (complete absence of neutrophils in the peripheral blood) is almost always due to a drug reaction. In these cases, examination of the bone marrow shows an almost complete absence of granulocyte precursors with other cell lines undisturbed. Neutropenia in the presence of a normal bone marrow may be due to immunologic peripheral destruction (autoimmune neutropenia), sepsis, or hypersplenism. The presence in the serum of antineutrophil antibodies supports the diagnosis of autoimmune neutropenia but does not prove this as the pathophysiologic reason for neutropenia. **Felty syndrome** is an immune neutropenia associated with seropositive nodular rheumatoid arthritis and splenomegaly. Severe neutropenia may be associated with clonal disorders of T lymphocytes, often with the morphology of large granular lymphocytes, referred to as CD3-positive T-cell large granular lymphoproliferative disorder. Isolated neutropenia is an uncommon presentation of hairy cell leukemia or MDS. By its nature, myelosuppressive cytotoxic chemotherapy causes neutropenia in a predictable manner.

▶ Clinical Findings

Neutropenia results in stomatitis and in infections due to gram-positive or gram-negative aerobic bacteria or to fungi such as *Candida* or *Aspergillus*. The most common infectious syndromes are septicemia, cellulitis, pneumonia, and neutropenic fever of unknown origin. Fever in neutropenic patients should always be initially assumed to be of infectious origin until proven otherwise (Chapter 30).

Table 13–13. World Health Organization classification of myeloproliferative disorders (modified).

Myeloproliferative neoplasms
Chronic myeloid leukemia, *BCR-ABL1*–positive
Chronic neutrophilic leukemia
Polycythemia vera
Primary myelofibrosis (PMF)
Essential thrombocythemia
Chronic eosinophilic leukemia, not otherwise specified (NOS)
Myeloproliferative neoplasm, unclassifiable
Mastocytosis
Myelodysplastic/myeloproliferative neoplasms (MDS/MPN)
Myelodysplastic syndromes
Acute myeloid leukemia and related neoplasms
Acute myeloid leukemia with recurrent genetic abnormalities
Acute myeloid leukemia with myelodysplasia-related changes
Therapy-related myeloid neoplasms
Acute myeloid leukemia, NOS
Myeloid sarcoma
Myeloid proliferations related to Down syndrome
Acute leukemias of ambiguous lineage
B lymphoblastic leukemia/lymphoma
T lymphoblastic leukemia/lymphoma

Treatment

Treatment of neutropenia depends on its cause. Potential causative medications should be discontinued. Myeloid growth factors (filgrastim or sargramostim or biosimilar myeloid growth factors) help facilitate neutrophil recovery after offending medications are stopped. Chronic myeloid growth factor administration (daily or every other day) is effective at dampening the neutropenia seen in cyclic or congenital neutropenia. When Felty syndrome leads to repeated bacterial infections, splenectomy has been the treatment of choice, but sustained use of myeloid growth factors is effective and provides a nonsurgical alternative. Patients with autoimmune neutropenia often respond briefly to immunosuppression with corticosteroids and are best managed with intermittent doses of myeloid growth factors. The neutropenia associated with large granular lymphoproliferative disorder may respond to therapy with oral methotrexate, cyclophosphamide, or cyclosporine.

Fevers during neutropenia should be considered as infectious until proven otherwise. Febrile neutropenia is a life-threatening circumstance. Enteric gram-negative bacteria are of primary concern and often empirically treated with fluoroquinolones or third- or fourth-generation cephalosporins (see Infections in the Immunocompromised Patient, Chapter 30). For protracted neutropenia, fungal infections are problematic and empiric coverage with azoles (fluconazole for yeast and voriconazole, itraconazole, posaconazole, or isavuconazole for molds) or echinocandins is recommended. The neutropenia following myelosuppressive chemotherapy is predictable and is partially ameliorated by the use of myeloid growth factors. For patients with acute leukemia undergoing intense chemotherapy or patients with solid cancer undergoing high-dose chemotherapy, the prophylactic use of antimicrobial agents and myeloid growth factors is recommended.

When to Refer

Refer to a hematologist if neutrophils are persistently and unexplainably less than 1000/mcL (1.0×10^9/L).

When to Admit

Neutropenia by itself is not an indication for hospitalization. However, many patients with severe neutropenia have a serious underlying disease that may require inpatient treatment. Most patients with febrile neutropenia require hospitalization to treat infection.

Curtis BR. Non-chemotherapy drug-induced neutropenia: key points to manage the challenges. Hematology Am Soc Hematol Educ Program. 2017 Dec 8;2017(1):187–93. [PMID: 29222255]

Dale DC et al. An update on the diagnosis and treatment of chronic idiopathic neutropenia. Curr Opin Hematol. 2017 Jan; 24(1):46–53. [PMID: 27841775]

Newburger PE. Autoimmune and other acquired neutropenias. Hematology Am Soc Hematol Educ Program. 2016 Dec 2; 2016(1):38–42. [PMID: 27913460]

Palmblad J et al. How we diagnose and treat neutropenia in adults. Expert Rev Hematol. 2016 May;9(5):479–87. [PMID: 26778239]

LEUKEMIAS & OTHER MYELOPROLIFERATIVE NEOPLASMS

Myeloproliferative disorders are due to acquired clonal abnormalities of the hematopoietic stem cell. Since the stem cell gives rise to myeloid, erythroid, and platelet cells, qualitative and quantitative changes are seen in all of these cell lines. Classically, the myeloproliferative disorders produce characteristic syndromes with well-defined clinical and laboratory features (Tables 13–13 and 13–14). However, these disorders are grouped together because they may evolve from one into another and because hybrid disorders are commonly seen. All of the myeloproliferative disorders may progress to AML.

Table 13–14. Laboratory features of myeloproliferative neoplasms.

	White Count	Hematocrit	Platelet Count	Red Cell Morphology
Polycythemia vera	N or ↑	↑↑	N or ↑	N
Essential thrombocytosis	N or ↑	N	↑↑	N
Primary myelofibrosis	N or ↓ or ↑	↓	↓ or N or ↑	Abn
Chronic myeloid leukemia	↑↑	N or ↓	N or ↑ or ↓	N

Abn, abnormal; N, normal.

The Philadelphia chromosome seen in chronic myeloid leukemia (CML) was the first recurrent cytogenetic abnormality to be described in a human malignancy. Since that time, there has been tremendous progress in elucidating the genetic nature of these disorders, with identification of mutations in *JAK2, MPL, CALR, CSF3R,* and other genes.

Rumi E et al. Diagnosis, risk stratification, and response evaluation in classical myeloproliferative neoplasms. Blood. 2017 Feb 9; 129(6):680–92. [PMID: 28028026]

POLYCYTHEMIA VERA

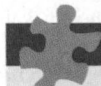

ESSENTIALS OF DIAGNOSIS

▶ *JAK2 (V617F)* mutation.
▶ Splenomegaly.
▶ Normal arterial oxygen saturation.
▶ Usually elevated white blood count and platelet count.

▶ General Considerations

Polycythemia vera is an acquired myeloproliferative disorder that causes overproduction of all three hematopoietic cell lines, most prominently the red blood cells. Erythroid production is independent of erythropoietin, and the serum erythropoietin level is low. A mutation in exon 14 of *JAK2 (V617F)*, a signaling molecule, has been demonstrated in 95% of cases. Additional *JAK2* mutations have been identified (exon 12) and suggest that *JAK2* is involved in the pathogenesis of this disease and is a potential therapeutic target.

True erythrocytosis, with an elevated red blood cell mass, should be distinguished from spurious erythrocytosis caused by a constricted plasma volume. Primary polycythemia (polycythemia vera) is a bone marrow disorder characterized by autonomous overproduction of erythroid cells.

▶ Clinical Findings

A. Symptoms and Signs

Headache, dizziness, tinnitus, blurred vision, and fatigue are common complaints related to expanded blood volume and increased blood viscosity. Generalized pruritus, especially following a warm shower or bath, is related to histamine release from the basophilia. Epistaxis is probably related to engorgement of mucosal blood vessels in combination with abnormal hemostasis. Sixty percent of patients are men, and the median age at presentation is 60 years. Polycythemia rarely occurs in persons under age 40 years.

Physical examination reveals plethora and engorged retinal veins. The spleen is palpable in 75% of cases but is nearly always enlarged when imaged. Thrombosis is the most common complication of polycythemia vera and the major cause of morbidity and death in this disorder. Thrombosis appears to be related both to increased blood viscosity and abnormal platelet function. Uncontrolled polycythemia leads to a very high incidence of thrombotic complications of surgery, and elective surgery should be deferred until the condition has been treated. Paradoxically, in addition to thrombosis, increased bleeding can also occur. There is a high incidence of peptic ulcer disease.

B. Laboratory Findings

According to the WHO 2016 criteria, the hallmark of polycythemia vera is a hematocrit (at sea level) that exceeds 49% in males or 48% in females. Red blood cell morphology is normal (Table 13–14). The white blood count is usually elevated to 10,000–20,000/mcL and the platelet count is variably increased, sometimes to counts exceeding 1,000,000/mcL. Platelet morphology is usually normal. White blood cells are usually normal, but basophilia and eosinophilia are frequently present. Erythropoietin levels are suppressed and are usually low. The diagnosis should be confirmed with *JAK2* mutation screening. The absence of a mutation in either exon 14 (most common) or 12 should lead the clinician to question the diagnosis.

The bone marrow is hypercellular, with panhyperplasia of all hematopoietic elements, but bone marrow examination is not necessary to establish the diagnosis. Iron stores are usually absent from the bone marrow, having been transferred to the increased circulating red blood cell mass. Iron deficiency may also result from chronic gastrointestinal blood loss. Bleeding may lower the hematocrit to the normal range (or lower), creating diagnostic confusion, and may lead to a situation with significant microcytosis with a normal hematocrit.

Vitamin B_{12} levels are strikingly elevated because of increased levels of transcobalamin III (secreted by white blood cells). Overproduction of uric acid may lead to hyperuricemia.

Although red blood cell morphology is usually normal at presentation, microcytosis, hypochromia, and poikilocytosis may result from iron deficiency following treatment by phlebotomy. Progressive hypersplenism may also lead to elliptocytosis.

▶ Differential Diagnosis

Spurious polycythemia, in which an elevated hematocrit is due to contracted plasma volume rather than increased red cell mass, may be related to diuretic use or may occur without obvious cause.

A secondary cause of polycythemia should be suspected if splenomegaly is absent and the high hematocrit is not accompanied by increases in other cell lines. Secondary causes of polycythemia include hypoxia and smoking; carboxyhemoglobin levels may be elevated in smokers (Table 13–15). A renal CT scan or sonogram may be considered to look for an erythropoietin-secreting cyst or tumor. A positive family history should lead to investigation for congenital high-oxygen-affinity hemoglobin. An absence of a mutation in *JAK2* suggests a different diagnosis. However, *JAK2* mutations are also commonly found in other myeloproliferative disorders, essential thrombocytosis, and myelofibrosis.

Polycythemia vera should be differentiated from other myeloproliferative disorders (Table 13–14). Marked elevation of the white blood count (above 30,000/mcL) suggests

Table 13–15. Causes of polycythemia.

Spurious polycythemia
Secondary polycythemia
Hypoxia: cardiac disease, pulmonary disease, high altitude
Carboxyhemoglobin: smoking
Erythropoietin-secreting tumors, eg, kidney lesions (rare)
Abnormal hemoglobins (rare)
Polycythemia vera

CML. Abnormal red blood cell morphology and nucleated red blood cells in the peripheral blood are seen in myelofibrosis. Essential thrombocytosis is suggested when the platelet count is strikingly elevated.

Treatment

The treatment of choice is phlebotomy. One unit of blood (approximately 500 mL) is removed weekly until the hematocrit is less than 45%; the hematocrit is maintained at less than 45% by repeated phlebotomy as necessary. Patients for whom phlebotomy is problematic (because of poor venous access or logistical reasons) may be managed primarily with hydroxyurea. Because repeated phlebotomy intentionally produces iron deficiency, the requirement for phlebotomy should gradually decrease. It is important to avoid medicinal iron supplementation, as this can thwart the goals of a phlebotomy program. A diet low in iron also is not necessary but will increase the intervals between phlebotomies. Maintaining the hematocrit at normal levels has been shown to decrease the incidence of thrombotic complications.

Occasionally, myelosuppressive therapy is indicated. Indications include a high phlebotomy requirement, thrombocytosis, and intractable pruritus. There is evidence that reduction of the platelet count to less than 600,000/mcL will reduce the risk of thrombotic complications. Hydroxyurea is widely used when myelosuppressive therapy is indicated. The usual dose is 500–1500 mg/day orally, adjusted to keep platelets less than 500,000/mcL without reducing the neutrophil count to less than 2000/mcL. The *JAK2* inhibitor ruxolitinib is FDA-approved for patients resistant or intolerant to hydroxyurea. In a randomized study comparing best available therapy with ruxolitinib, treatment with ruxolitinib was associated with greater benefit for both hematocrit control without phlebotomy (60%) and splenic volume reduction (38%). Symptom burden improved by greater than 50% in 49% of patients. Studies of pegylated alfa-2 interferon have demonstrated considerable efficacy, with hematologic responses in greater than 80%, as well as molecular responses in 20% (as measured by *JAK2* mutations). Patients in whom molecular responses were not achieved had a higher frequency of mutations outside the *JAK2* pathway and were more likely to acquire new mutations during therapy. Side effects were generally acceptable and much less significant than with nonpegylated forms of interferon. A randomized phase 3 trial comparing PEG-alpha-2 interferon to hydroxyurea demonstrated similar complete remission rates and modifications of disease features (spleen size, karyotype and histopathologic abnormalities) but with PEG-alpha-2 interferon causing more grade 3/4 adverse events. *Alkylating agents have been shown*

to increase the risk of conversion of this disease to acute leukemia and should be avoided.

Low-dose aspirin (75–81 mg/day orally) has been shown to reduce the risk of thrombosis without excessive bleeding, and should be part of therapy for all patients without contraindications to aspirin. Allopurinol 300 mg orally daily may be indicated for hyperuricemia. Antihistamine therapy with diphenhydramine or other H$_1$-blockers and, rarely, selective serotonin reuptake inhibitors are used to manage pruritus.

Prognosis

Polycythemia is an indolent disease with median survival of over 15 years. The major cause of morbidity and mortality is arterial thrombosis. Over time, polycythemia vera may convert to myelofibrosis or to CML. In approximately 5% of cases, the disorder progresses to AML, which is usually refractory to therapy.

When to Refer

Patients with polycythemia vera should be referred to a hematologist.

When to Admit

Inpatient care is rarely required.

Barbui T et al. The 2016 revision of WHO classification of myeloproliferative neoplasms: clinical and molecular advances. Blood Rev. 2016 Nov;30(6):453–9. [PMID: 27341755]

Mascarenhas J et al. Results of the myeloproliferative neoplasms — research consortium (MPN-RC) 112 randomized trial of pegylated interferon alfa-2a (PEG) versus hydroxyurea (HU) therapy for the treatment of high risk polycythemia vera (PV) and high risk essential thrombocythemia (ET). Blood. 2018 Dec 132:577.

Tefferi A et al. Polycythemia vera and essential thrombocythemia: 2019 update on diagnosis, risk-stratification and management. Am J Hematol. 2019;94:133–43. [PMID: 30281843]

ESSENTIAL THROMBOCYTOSIS

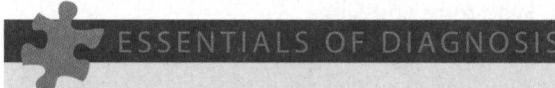

ESSENTIALS OF DIAGNOSIS

► Elevated platelet count in absence of other causes.
► Normal red blood cell mass.
► Absence of *bcr/abl* gene (Philadelphia chromosome).

General Considerations

Essential thrombocytosis is an uncommon myeloproliferative disorder of unknown cause in which marked proliferation of the megakaryocytes in the bone marrow leads to elevation of the platelet count. As with polycythemia vera, the finding of a high frequency of mutations of *JAK2* and others in these patients promises to advance the understanding of this disorder.

Clinical Findings

A. Symptoms and Signs

The median age at presentation is 50–60 years, and there is a slightly increased incidence in women. The disorder is often suspected when an elevated platelet count is found. Less frequently, the first sign is thrombosis, which is the most common clinical problem. The risk of thrombosis rises with age. Venous thromboses may occur in unusual sites such as the mesenteric, hepatic, or portal vein. Some patients experience erythromelalgia, painful burning of the hands accompanied by erythema; this symptom is reliably relieved by aspirin. Bleeding, typically mucosal, is less common and is related to a concomitant qualitative platelet defect. Splenomegaly is present in at least 25% of patients.

B. Laboratory Findings

An elevated platelet count is the hallmark of this disorder, and may be over 2,000,000/mcL (2000 × 10⁹/L) (Table 13–14). The white blood cell count is often mildly elevated, usually not above 30,000/mcL (30 × 10⁹/L), but with some immature myeloid forms. The hematocrit is normal. The peripheral blood smear reveals large platelets, but giant degranulated forms seen in myelofibrosis are not observed. Red blood cell morphology is normal.

The bone marrow shows increased numbers of megakaryocytes but no other morphologic abnormalities. The peripheral blood should be tested for the *bcr/abl* fusion gene (Philadelphia chromosome) since it can differentiate CML, where it is present, from essential thrombocytosis, where it is absent.

Differential Diagnosis

Essential thrombocytosis must be distinguished from secondary causes of an elevated platelet count. In reactive thrombocytosis, the platelet count seldom exceeds 1,000,000/mcL (1000 × 10⁹/L). Inflammatory disorders such as rheumatoid arthritis and ulcerative colitis cause significant elevations of the platelet count, as may chronic infection. The thrombocytosis of iron deficiency is observed only when anemia is significant. The platelet count is temporarily elevated after a splenectomy. *JAK2* mutations are found in over 50% of cases. *MPL* and *CALR* mutations frequently occur in patients with *JAK2*-negative essential thrombocytosis.

Regarding other myeloproliferative disorders, the lack of erythrocytosis distinguishes it from polycythemia vera. Unlike myelofibrosis, red blood cell morphology is normal, nucleated red blood cells are absent, and giant degranulated platelets are not seen. In CML, the Philadelphia chromosome (or *bcr/abl* by molecular testing) establishes the diagnosis.

Treatment

Patients are considered at high risk for thrombosis if they are older than 60 years, have a leukocyte count of 11,000/mcL (11 × 10⁹/L) or higher, or have a previous history of thrombosis. They also have a higher risk for bleeding. The risk of thrombosis can be reduced by control of the platelet count, which should be kept under 500,000/mcL (500 × 10⁹/L). The treatment of choice is oral hydroxyurea in a dose of 500–1000 mg/day. In rare cases in which hydroxyurea is not well tolerated because of anemia, low doses of anagrelide, 1–2 mg/day orally, may be added. Higher doses of anagrelide can be complicated by headache, peripheral edema, and heart failure. Pegylated interferon alfa-2 can induce significant hematologic responses and can potentially target the malignant clone in *CALR*-mutant cases. Strict control of coexistent cardiovascular risk factors is mandatory for all patients.

Vasomotor symptoms such as erythromelalgia and paresthesias respond rapidly to aspirin, and its long-term low-dose use (81 mg/day orally) may reduce the risk of thrombotic complications in low-risk patients. In the unusual event of severe bleeding, the platelet count can be lowered rapidly with plateletpheresis. In cases of marked thrombocytosis (greater than or equal to 1,000,000/mcL [1000 × 10⁹/L]) or of any evidence of bleeding, acquired von Willebrand syndrome must be excluded before starting low-dose aspirin.

Course & Prognosis

Essential thrombocytosis is an indolent disorder and allows long-term survival. Average survival is longer than 15 years from diagnosis, and the survival of patients younger than 50 years does not appear different from matched controls. The major source of morbidity—thrombosis—can be reduced by appropriate platelet control. Late in the course of the disease, the bone marrow may become fibrotic, and massive splenomegaly may occur, sometimes with splenic infarction. There is a 10–15% risk of progression to myelofibrosis after 15 years, and a 1–5% risk of transformation to acute leukemia over 20 years.

When to Refer

Patients with essential thrombocytosis should be referred to a hematologist.

Aruch D et al. Contemporary approach to essential thrombocythemia and polycythemia vera. Curr Opin Hematol. 2016 Mar; 23(2):150–60. [PMID: 26717193]
Rumi E et al. How I treat essential thrombocythemia. Blood. 2016 Nov 17;128(20):2403–14. [PMID: 27561316]

PRIMARY MYELOFIBROSIS

ESSENTIALS OF DIAGNOSIS

▶ Striking splenomegaly.

▶ Teardrop poikilocytosis on peripheral smear.

▶ Leukoerythroblastic blood picture; giant abnormal platelets.

▶ Initially hypercellular, then hypocellular bone marrow with reticulin or collagen fibrosis.

General Considerations

Primary myelofibrosis is a myeloproliferative disorder characterized by clonal hematopoiesis that is often but not always accompanied by *JAK2*, *CALR*, or *MPL* mutation; bone marrow fibrosis; anemia; splenomegaly; and a leukoerythroblastic peripheral blood picture with teardrop poikilocytosis. Myelofibrosis can also occur as a secondary process following the other myeloproliferative disorders (eg, polycythemia vera, essential thrombocytosis). It is believed that fibrosis occurs in response to increased secretion of platelet-derived growth factor (PDGF) and possibly other cytokines. In response to bone marrow fibrosis, extramedullary hematopoiesis takes place in the liver, spleen, and lymph nodes. In these sites, mesenchymal cells responsible for fetal hematopoiesis can be reactivated. According to the 2016 WHO classification, "prefibrotic" primary myelofibrosis is distinguished from "overtly fibrotic" primary myelofibrosis; the former might mimic essential thrombocytosis in its presentation and it is prognostically relevant to distinguish the two.

Clinical Findings

A. Symptoms and Signs

Primary myelofibrosis develops in adults over age 50 years and is usually insidious in onset. Patients most commonly present with fatigue due to anemia or abdominal fullness related to splenomegaly. Uncommon presentations include bleeding and bone pain. On examination, splenomegaly is almost invariably present and is commonly massive. The liver is enlarged in more than 50% of cases.

Later in the course of the disease, progressive bone marrow failure takes place as it becomes increasingly more fibrotic. Progressive thrombocytopenia leads to bleeding. The spleen continues to enlarge, which leads to early satiety. Painful episodes of splenic infarction may occur. The patient becomes cachectic and may experience severe bone pain, especially in the upper legs. Hematopoiesis in the liver leads to portal hypertension with ascites, esophageal varices, and occasionally transverse myelitis caused by myelopoiesis in the epidural space.

B. Laboratory Findings

Patients are almost invariably anemic at presentation. The white blood count is variable—either low, normal, or elevated—and may be increased to 50,000/mcL (50×10^9/L). The platelet count is variable. The peripheral blood smear is dramatic, with significant poikilocytosis and numerous teardrop forms in the red cell line. Nucleated red blood cells are present and the myeloid series is shifted, with immature forms including a small percentage of promyelocytes or myeloblasts. Platelet morphology may be bizarre, and giant degranulated platelet forms (megakaryocyte fragments) may be seen. The triad of teardrop poikilocytosis, leukoerythroblastic blood, and giant abnormal platelets is highly suggestive of myelofibrosis.

The bone marrow usually cannot be aspirated (dry tap), though early in the course of the disease it is hypercellular, with a marked increase in megakaryocytes. Fibrosis at this stage is detected by a silver stain demonstrating increased reticulin fibers. Later, biopsy reveals more severe fibrosis, with eventual replacement of hematopoietic precursors by collagen. There is no characteristic chromosomal abnormality. *JAK2* is mutated in ~65% of cases, and *MPL* and *CALR* are mutated in the majority of the remaining cases; 10% of cases are "triple-negative."

Differential Diagnosis

A leukoerythroblastic blood picture from other causes may be seen in response to severe infection, inflammation, or infiltrative bone marrow processes. However, teardrop poikilocytosis and giant abnormal platelet forms will not be present. Bone marrow fibrosis may be seen in metastatic carcinoma, Hodgkin lymphoma, and hairy cell leukemia. These disorders are diagnosed by characteristic morphology of involved tissues.

Of the other myeloproliferative disorders, CML is diagnosed when there is marked leukocytosis, normal red blood cell morphology, and the presence of the *bcr/abl* fusion gene. Polycythemia vera is characterized by an elevated hematocrit. Essential thrombocytosis shows predominant platelet count elevations.

Treatment

Observation with supportive care is a reasonable treatment strategy for asymptomatic patients with low or intermediate-1 Dynamic International Prognostic Scoring System (DIPSS)-plus risk disease, especially in the absence of high-risk mutations. Anemic patients are supported with transfusion. Anemia can also be controlled with androgens, prednisone, thalidomide, or lenalidomide. First-line therapy for myelofibrosis-associated splenomegaly is hydroxyurea 500–1000 mg/day orally, which is effective in reducing spleen size by half in approximately 40% of patients. Both thalidomide and lenalidomide may improve splenomegaly and thrombocytopenia in some patients. Splenectomy is not routinely performed but is indicated for medication-refractory splenic enlargement causing recurrent painful episodes, severe thrombocytopenia, or an unacceptable transfusion requirement. Perioperative complications can occur in 28% of patients and include infections, abdominal vein thrombosis, and bleeding. Radiation therapy has a role for painful sites of extramedullary hematopoiesis, pulmonary hypertension, or severe bone pain. Transjugular intrahepatic portosystemic shunt might also be considered to alleviate symptoms of portal hypertension.

Patients with DIPSS-plus high or intermediate-2 risk disease, or those patients harboring high-risk mutations such as *ASXL1* or *SRSF2*, should be considered for allogeneic stem cell transplant, which is currently the only potentially curative treatment modality in this disease. Nontransplant candidates may be treated with JAK2 inhibitors or immunomodulatory agents for symptom control. Ruxolitinib, the first JAK2 inhibitor to be FDA approved, results in reduction of spleen size and improvement of constitutional symptoms, but does not induce complete clinical or cytogenetic remissions or significantly affect *JAK2/CALR/MPL* mutant allele burden. Moreover, ruxolitinib can exacerbate cytopenias. The immunomodulatory medications lenalidomide and pomalidomide result in control of anemia in 25% and thrombocytopenia in ~58% of cases, without significant reduction in splenic size.

Course & Prognosis

The median survival from time of diagnosis is approximately 5 years. Therapies with biologic agents and the application of reduced-intensity allogeneic stem cell transplantation appear to offer the possibility of improving the outcome for many patients. End-stage myelofibrosis is characterized by generalized asthenia, liver failure, and bleeding from thrombocytopenia, with some cases terminating in AML. The DIPSS-plus incorporates clinical and genetic risk variables and is associated with overall survival. Most recently, DIPSS-plus-independent adverse prognostic relevance has been demonstrated for certain mutations including *ASXL1* and *SRSF2*, whereas patients with type 1/like *CALR* mutations, compared to their counterparts with other driver mutations, displayed significantly better survival.

When to Refer

Patients in whom myelofibrosis is suspected should be referred to a hematologist.

When to Admit

Admission is not usually necessary.

Bose P et al. Prognosis of primary myelofibrosis in the genomic era. Clin Lymphoma Myeloma Leuk. 2016 Aug;16(Suppl): S105–13. [PMID: 27521306]

Devlin R et al. Myelofibrosis: to transplant or not to transplant? Hematology Am Soc Hematol Educ Program. 2016 Dec 2; 2016(1):543–51. [PMID: 27913527]

Mesa RA et al. Ruxolitinib dose management as a key to long-term treatment success. Int J Hematol. 2016 Oct;104(4):420–9. [PMID: 27567907]

Tefferi A. Primary myelofibrosis: 2017 update on diagnosis, risk-stratification, and management. Am J Hematol. 2016 Dec; 91(12):1262–71. [PMID: 27870387]

CHRONIC MYELOID LEUKEMIA

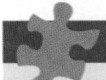

ESSENTIALS OF DIAGNOSIS

▶ Elevated white blood cell count.

▶ Markedly left-shifted myeloid series but with a low percentage of promyelocytes and blasts.

▶ Presence of *bcr/abl* gene (Philadelphia chromosome).

General Considerations

CML is a myeloproliferative disorder characterized by overproduction of myeloid cells. These myeloid cells continue to differentiate and circulate in increased numbers in the peripheral blood.

CML is characterized by a specific chromosomal abnormality and specific molecular abnormality. The **Philadelphia chromosome** is a reciprocal translocation between the long arms of chromosomes 9 and 22. The portion of 9q that is translocated contains *abl*, a protooncogene that is received at a specific site on 22q, the break point cluster (bcr). The fusion gene *bcr/abl* produces a novel protein that possesses tyrosine kinase activity. This disorder is the first recognized example of tyrosine kinase "addiction" by cancer cells.

Early CML ("chronic phase") does not behave like a malignant disease. Normal bone marrow function is retained, white blood cells differentiate and, despite some qualitative abnormalities, the neutrophils combat infection normally. However, untreated CML is inherently unstable, and without treatment the disease progresses to an accelerated and then acute blast phase, which is morphologically indistinguishable from acute leukemia. Remarkable advances in therapy have changed the natural history of the disease, and the relentless progression to more advanced stages of disease is at least greatly delayed, if not eliminated.

Clinical Findings

A. Symptoms and Signs

CML is a disorder of middle age (median age at presentation is 55 years). Patients usually complain of fatigue, night sweats, and low-grade fevers related to the hypermetabolic state caused by overproduction of white blood cells. Patients may also complain of abdominal fullness related to splenomegaly. In some cases, an elevated white blood count is discovered incidentally. Rarely, the patient will present with a clinical syndrome related to leukostasis with blurred vision, respiratory distress, or priapism. The white blood count in these cases is usually greater than 100,000/mcL (100×10^9/L) but less than 500,000/mcL (500×10^9/L). On examination, the spleen is enlarged (often markedly so), and sternal tenderness may be present as a sign of marrow overexpansion. In cases discovered during routine laboratory monitoring, these findings are often absent. Acceleration of the disease is often associated with fever (in the absence of infection), bone pain, and splenomegaly.

B. Laboratory Findings

CML is characterized by an elevated white blood cell count; the median white blood count at diagnosis is 150,000/mcL (150×10^9/L), although in some cases the white blood cell count is only modestly increased (Table 13–14). The peripheral blood is characteristic. The myeloid series is left shifted, with mature forms dominating and with cells usually present in proportion to their degree of maturation. Blasts are usually less than 5%. Basophilia and eosinophilia may be present. At presentation, the patient is usually not anemic. Red blood cell morphology is normal, and nucleated red blood cells are rarely seen. The platelet count may be normal or elevated (sometimes to strikingly high levels). A bone marrow biopsy is essential to ensure sufficient material for a complete karyotype and for morphologic evaluation to confirm the phase of disease. The bone marrow is hypercellular, with left-shifted myelopoiesis.

Myeloblasts compose less than 5% of marrow cells. The hallmark of the disease is the *bcr/abl* gene that is detected by the polymerase chain reaction (PCR) test in the peripheral blood and bone marrow.

With progression to the accelerated and blast phases, progressive anemia and thrombocytopenia occur, and the percentage of blasts in the blood and bone marrow increases. Blast-phase CML is diagnosed when blasts comprise more than 20% of bone marrow cells.

Differential Diagnosis

Early CML must be differentiated from the reactive leukocytosis associated with infection. In such cases, the white blood count is usually less than 50,000/mcL (50 × 10⁹/L), splenomegaly is absent, and the *bcr/abl* gene is not present.

CML must be distinguished from other myeloproliferative disease (Table 13–14). The hematocrit should not be elevated, the red blood cell morphology is normal, and nucleated red blood cells are rare or absent. Definitive diagnosis is made by finding the *bcr/abl* gene.

Treatment

Treatment is usually not emergent even with white blood counts over 200,000/mcL (200 × 10⁹/L), since the majority of circulating cells are mature myeloid cells that are smaller and more deformable than primitive leukemic blasts. In the rare instances in which symptoms result from extreme hyperleukocytosis (priapism, respiratory distress, visual blurring, altered mental status), emergent leukapheresis is performed in conjunction with myelosuppressive therapy.

In chronic-phase CML, the goal of therapy is normalization of the hematologic abnormalities and suppression of the malignant *bcr/abl*-expressing clone. The treatment of choice consists of a tyrosine kinase inhibitor (eg, imatinib, nilotinib, dasatinib) targeting the aberrantly active abl kinase. It is expected that a hematologic complete remission, with normalization of blood counts and splenomegaly will occur within 3 months of treatment initiation. Second, a major cytogenetic response should be achieved, ideally within 3 months but certainly within 6 months. A major cytogenetic response is identified when less than 35% of metaphases contain the Philadelphia chromosome. Lastly, a major molecular response is desired within 12 months and is defined as a 3-log reduction of the *bcr/abl* transcript as measured by quantitative PCR. This roughly corresponds to a *bcr/abl* ratio (compared to *abl*) of less than 0.01. Patients who achieve this level of molecular response have an excellent prognosis, with 100% of them remaining progression-free at 8 years. On the other hand, patients have a worse prognosis if these targets are not achieved, cytogenetic or molecular response is subsequently lost, or new mutations or cytogenetic abnormalities develop.

Imatinib mesylate was the first tyrosine kinase inhibitor to be approved and it results in nearly universal (98%) hematologic control of chronic-phase disease at a dose of 400 mg/day. The rate of a major molecular response with imatinib in chronic-phase disease is ~30% at 1 year. The second-generation tyrosine kinase inhibitors, nilotinib and dasatinib, are also used as front-line therapy and can significantly increase the rate of a major molecular response compared to imatinib (71% for nilotinib at 300–400 mg twice daily by 2 years, 64% for dasatinib at 100 mg/day by 2 years) and result in a lower rate of progression to advanced-stage disease. However, these agents can also salvage 90% of patients who do not respond to treatment with imatinib and may therefore be reserved for use in that setting. A dual *bcr/abl* tyrosine kinase inhibitor, bosutinib, is used for patients who are resistant or intolerant to the other tyrosine kinase inhibitors. The complete cytogenetic response rate to bosutinib is 25%, but it is not active against the *T315I* mutation.

Patients taking tyrosine kinase inhibitors should be monitored with a quantitative PCR assay. Those with a consistent increase in *bcr/abl* transcript or those with a suboptimal molecular response as defined above should undergo *abl* mutation testing and then be switched to an alternative tyrosine kinase inhibitor. The *T315I* mutation in *abl* is specifically resistant to therapy with imatinib, dasatinib, nilotinib, and bosutinib but appears to be sensitive to the third-generation agent ponatinib. However, ponatinib is associated with a high rate of vascular thrombotic complications. Lastly, omacetaxine—a non–tyrosine kinase inhibitor therapy approved for patients with CML who are resistant to at least two tyrosine kinase inhibitors—can produce major cytogenetic responses in 18% of patients. Patients in whom a good molecular response to any of these agents cannot be achieved or in whom diseases progresses despite therapy should be considered for allogeneic stem cell transplantation.

Patients with advanced-stage disease (accelerated phase or myeloid/lymphoid blast crisis) should be treated with a tyrosine kinase inhibitor alone or in combination with myelosuppressive chemotherapy. The doses of tyrosine kinase inhibitors in that setting are usually higher than those appropriate for chronic-phase disease. Since the duration of response to tyrosine kinase inhibitors in this setting is limited, patients who have accelerated or blast-phase disease should ultimately be considered for allogeneic stem cell transplantation.

Course & Prognosis

Since the introduction of imatinib therapy in 2001, and with the development of molecular-targeted agents, more than 80% of patients remain alive and without disease progression at 9 years. Patients with good molecular responses to tyrosine kinase inhibitor therapy have an excellent prognosis, with essentially 100% survival at 9 years, and it is likely that some fraction of these patients will be cured. Current studies suggest that tyrosine kinase inhibitor therapy may be safely discontinued after 2 years in patients who achieve a sustained major molecular response, with ~50–60% of patients remaining in molecular remission at least 1 year.

When to Refer

All patients with CML should be referred to a hematologist.

When to Admit

Hospitalization is rarely necessary and should be reserved for symptoms of leukostasis at diagnosis or for transformation to acute leukemia.

Barrett AJ et al. The role of stem cell transplantation for chronic myelogenous leukemia in the 21st century. Blood. 2015 May 21;125(21):3230–5. [PMID: 25852053]

Rosti G et al. Tyrosine kinase inhibitors in chronic myeloid leukaemia: which, when, for whom? Nat Rev Clin Oncol. 2017 Mar;14(3):141–54. [PMID: 27752053]

Steegmann JL et al. European LeukemiaNet recommendations for the management and avoidance of adverse events of treatment in chronic myeloid leukaemia. Leukemia. 2016 Aug; 30(8):1648–71. [PMID: 27121688]

MYELODYSPLASTIC SYNDROMES

ESSENTIALS OF DIAGNOSIS

► Cytopenias with a hypercellular bone marrow.
► Morphologic abnormalities in one or more hematopoietic cell lines.

General Considerations

The myelodysplastic syndromes are a group of acquired clonal disorders of the hematopoietic stem cell. They are characterized by the constellation of cytopenias, a usually hypercellular marrow, morphologic dysplasia, and genetic abnormalities. The disorders are usually idiopathic but may be caused by prior exposure to cytotoxic chemotherapy, radiation or both. In addition to cytogenetics, sequencing can detect genetic mutations in 80–90% of MDS patients. Importantly, acquired clonal mutations identical to those seen in MDS can occur in the hematopoietic cells of ~10% of apparently healthy older individuals, defining the disorder of **clonal hematopoiesis of indeterminate potential (CHIP).**

Myelodysplasia encompasses several heterogeneous syndromes. A key distinction is whether there is an increase in bone marrow blasts (greater than 5% of marrow elements). The category of MDS with excess blasts represents a more aggressive form of the disease, often leading to AML. Those without excess blasts are characterized by the degree of dysplasia, eg, MDS with single lineage dysplasia and MDS with multilineage dysplasia. The morphologic finding of **"ringed sideroblasts"** is retained in the 2016 WHO classification and is used to define a subcategory of the lower-risk MDS syndromes. Patients with **isolated 5q loss,** which is characterized by the cytogenetic finding of loss of part of the long arm of chromosome 5, comprise an important subgroup of patients with a different natural history. Lastly, patients with a proliferative syndrome including sustained peripheral blood monocytosis more than 1000/mcL (1.0×10^9/L) are termed **"chronic myelomonocytic leukemia" (CMML),** a disorder that shares features of myelodysplastic and myeloproliferative disorders. An

International Prognostic Scoring System (IPSS) classifies patients by risk status based on the percentage of bone marrow blasts, cytogenetics, and severity of cytopenias. The IPSS is associated with the rate of progression to AML and with overall survival, which can range from a median of 6 years for the low-risk group to 5 months for the high-risk patients.

Clinical Findings

A. Symptoms and Signs

Patients are usually over age 60 years. Many patients are asymptomatic when the diagnosis is made because of the finding of abnormal blood counts. Fatigue, infection, or bleeding related to bone marrow failure are usually the presenting symptoms and signs. The course may be indolent, and the disease may present as a wasting illness with fever, weight loss, and general debility. On examination, splenomegaly may be present in combination with pallor, bleeding, and various signs of infection. Myelodysplastic syndromes can also be accompanied by a variety of paraneoplastic syndromes prior to or following this diagnosis.

B. Laboratory Findings

Anemia may be marked with the MCV normal or increased, and transfusion support may be required. On the peripheral blood smear, macro-ovalocytes may be seen. The white blood cell count is usually normal or reduced, and neutropenia is common. The neutrophils may exhibit morphologic abnormalities, including deficient numbers of granules or deficient segmentation of the nucleus, especially a bilobed nucleus (Pelger-Huet abnormality). The myeloid series may be left shifted, and small numbers of promyelocytes or blasts may be seen. The platelet count is normal or reduced, and hypogranular platelets may be present.

The bone marrow is characteristically hypercellular but occasionally may be hypocellular. Erythroid hyperplasia is common, and signs of abnormal erythropoiesis include megaloblastic features, nuclear budding, or multinucleated erythroid precursors. The Prussian blue stain may demonstrate ringed sideroblasts. In the marrow, too, the myeloid series is often left shifted, with variable increases in blasts. Deficient or abnormal granules may be seen. A characteristic abnormality is the presence of dwarf megakaryocytes with a unilobed nucleus. Genetic abnormalities define MDS; there are frequent cytogenetic abnormalities involving the long arm of chromosome 5 as well as deletions of chromosomes 5 and 7. Some patients with an indolent form of the disease have an isolated partial deletion of chromosome 5 (MDS with isolated del[5q]). Aside from cytogenetic abnormalities, the most commonly mutated genes are *SF3B1, TET2, SRSF2, ASXL1, DNMT3A, RUNX1, U2AF1, TP53,* and *EZH2.*

Differential Diagnosis

Myelodysplastic syndromes should be distinguished from megaloblastic anemia, aplastic anemia, myelofibrosis, HIV-associated cytopenias, and acute or chronic drug effect. In subtle cases, cytogenetic evaluation of the bone marrow may help distinguish this clonal disorder from other causes of cytopenias. As the number of blasts increases in the bone marrow, myelodysplasia is arbitrarily separated from AML by the presence of less than 20% blasts.

Treatment

Myelodysplasia is a heterogeneous disease, and the appropriate treatment depends on a number of factors. For patients with anemia who have a low serum erythropoietin level (500 milliunits/mL or less), erythropoiesis-stimulating agents may raise the hematocrit and reduce the red cell transfusion requirement in 40%. Addition of intermittent granulocyte colony-stimulating factor (G-CSF) therapy may augment the erythroid response to epoetin. Unfortunately, the patients with the highest transfusion requirements are the least likely to respond. Patients who remain dependent on red blood cell transfusion and who do not have immediately life-threatening disease should receive iron chelation in order to prevent serious iron overload; the dose of oral agent deferasirox is 20 mg/kg/day. Patients affected primarily with severe neutropenia may benefit from the use of myeloid growth factors such as filgrastim. Oral thrombopoietin analogs, such as romiplostim and eltrombopag, that stimulate platelet production by binding the thrombopoietin receptor have shown effectiveness in raising the platelet count in myelodysplasia. Finally, occasional patients can benefit from immunosuppressive therapy including ATG. Predictors of response to ATG include age younger than 60 years, absence of 5q–, and presence of HLA DR15.

For patients who do not respond to these interventions, there are several therapeutic options available. Lenalidomide is approved for the treatment of transfusion-dependent anemia due to myelodysplasia. It is the treatment of choice in patients with MDS with isolated del(5q) with significant responses in 70% of patients, and responses typically lasting longer than 2 years. In addition, nearly half of these patients enter a cytogenetic remission with clearing of the abnormal 5q– clone. The recommended initial dose is 10 mg/day orally. The most common side effects are neutropenia and thrombocytopenia, but venous thrombosis occurs and warrants prophylaxis with aspirin, 325 mg/day orally. For patients with high-risk myelodysplasia, azacitidine is the treatment of choice. It can improve both symptoms and blood counts and prolong both overall survival and the time to conversion to acute leukemia. It is used at a dose of 75 mg/m^2 daily for 5–7 days every 28 days and up to six cycles of therapy may be required to achieve a response. Decitabine, a related hypomethylating agent, given at 20 mg/m^2 daily for 5 days every 28 days can produce similar hematologic responses but has not demonstrated a benefit in overall survival compared to supportive care alone. Combination therapy with azacitidine plus either lenalidomide or vorinostat, the histone deacetylase inhibitor, has shown preliminary promise in patients with high-risk disease and is being tested in a large prospective clinical trial. Allogeneic stem cell transplantation is the only curative therapy for myelodysplasia, but its role is limited by the advanced age of many patients and the indolent course of disease in some subsets of patients. The optimal use and timing of allogeneic transplantation are

controversial, but the use of reduced-intensity preparative regimens and alternative donor sources (cord blood, haplotype-matched) has expanded the role of this therapy. Agents targeting the emerging genetic mutations in MDS are in development.

Course & Prognosis

Myelodysplasia is an ultimately fatal disease, and allogeneic transplantation is the only curative therapy, with cure rates of 30–60% depending primarily on the risk status of the disease. Patients most commonly die of infections or bleeding. Patients with MDS with isolated del(5q) have a favorable prognosis, with 5-year survival over 90%. Other patients with low-risk disease (with absence of both excess blasts and adverse cytogenetics) may also do well, with similar survival. Those with excess blasts or CMML have a higher (30–50%) risk of developing acute leukemia, and short survival (less than 2 years) without allogeneic transplantation.

When to Refer

All patients with myelodysplasia should be referred to a hematologist.

When to Admit

Hospitalization is needed only for specific complications, such as severe infection.

Dao KT. Myelodysplastic syndromes: updates and nuances. Med Clin North Am. 2017 Mar;101(2):333–50. [PMID: 28189174]

de Witte T et al. Allogeneic hematopoietic stem cell transplantation for MDS and CMML: recommendations from an international expert panel. Blood. 2017 Mar 30;129(13):1753–62. [PMID: 28096091]

Kennedy JA et al. Clinical implications of genetic mutations in myelodysplastic syndrome. J Clin Oncol. 2017 Mar 20;35(9):968–74. [PMID: 28297619]

Sperling AS et al. The genetics of myelodysplastic syndrome: from clonal haematopoiesis to secondary leukaemia. Nat Rev Cancer. 2017 Jan;17(1):5–19. [PMID: 27834397]

ACUTE LEUKEMIA

ESSENTIALS OF DIAGNOSIS

▶ Short duration of symptoms, including fatigue, fever, and bleeding.

▶ Cytopenias or pancytopenia.

▶ Blasts in peripheral blood in 90% of patients.

▶ More than 20% blasts in the bone marrow.

General Considerations

Acute leukemia is a malignancy of the hematopoietic progenitor cell. These cells proliferate in an uncontrolled fashion and replace normal bone marrow elements. Most cases arise with no clear cause. However, radiation and some toxins (benzene) are leukemogenic. In addition, a number of chemotherapeutic agents (especially cyclophosphamide, melphalan, other alkylating agents, and etoposide) may cause leukemia. The leukemias seen after toxin or chemotherapy exposure often develop from a myelodysplastic prodrome and are often associated with abnormalities in chromosomes 5 and 7. Those related to etoposide may have abnormalities in chromosome 11q23 (MLL locus).

Most of the clinical findings in acute leukemia are due to replacement of normal bone marrow elements by the malignant cells. Less common manifestations result from organ infiltration (skin, gastrointestinal tract, meninges). Acute leukemia is potentially curable with combination chemotherapy.

The myeloblastic subtype, AML, is primarily an adult disease with a median age at presentation of 60 years and an increasing incidence with advanced age. Acute promyelocytic leukemia (APL) is characterized by the chromosomal translocation t(15;17), which produces the fusion gene *PML-RAR*-alpha, which interacts with the retinoic acid receptor to produce a block in differentiation that can be overcome with pharmacologic doses of retinoic acid. The lymphoblastic subtype of acute leukemia, ALL, comprises 80% of the acute leukemias of childhood. The peak incidence is between 3 and 7 years of age. It is also seen in adults, causing approximately 20% of adult acute leukemias.

Classification of the Leukemias

A. Acute Myeloid Leukemia (AML)

AML is primarily categorized based on recurrent structural chromosomal and molecular abnormalities. The cytogenetic abnormalities can be identified on traditional karyotyping or metaphase fluorescence in situ hybridization (FISH) and the molecular abnormalities are identified by either targeted or genome-wide sequencing of tumor DNA. Favorable cytogenetics such as t(8;21) producing a chimeric RUNX1/RUNX1T1 protein and inv(16)(p13;q22) are seen in 15% of cases and are termed the "core-binding factor" leukemias. These patients have a higher chance of achieving both short- and long-term disease control. Unfavorable cytogenetics confer a very poor prognosis. These consist of isolated monosomy 5 or 7, the presence of two or more other monosomies, or three or more separate cytogenetic abnormalities and account for 25% of the cases. The majority of cases of AML are of intermediate risk by traditional cytogenetics and have either a normal karyotype or chromosomal abnormalities that do not confer strong prognostic significance. However, there are several recurrent gene mutations with prognostic significance in this subgroup. On the one hand, internal tandem duplication in the gene *FLT3* occurs in ~30% of AML and is conditionally associated with a very poor prognosis in the setting of *NPM1* and *DNMT3A* mutation. Other mutations conferring a poor prognosis occur in *TET2, ASXL1, MLL-PTD, PHF6,* and *SRSF2*. On the other hand, a relatively favorable group of patients has been identified that lacks *FLT3-ITD* mutations and includes mutations of nucleophosmin 1 (*NPM1*) and *IDH1* or *IDH2* or carries *CEBPA* biallelic mutations.

B. Acute Promyelocytic Leukemia (APL)

In considering the various types of AML, APL is discussed separately because of its unique biologic features and response to non-chemotherapy treatments. APL is characterized by the cytogenetic finding of t(15;17) and the fusion gene *PML-RAR*-alpha. It is a highly curable form of leukemia (over 90%) with integration of all-trans-retinoic acid (ATRA) and arsenic trioxide (ATO) in induction, consolidation, and maintenance regimens.

C. Acute Lymphoblastic Leukemia (ALL)

ALL is most usefully classified by immunologic phenotype as follows: common, early B lineage, and T cell. Hyperdiploidy (with more than 50 chromosomes), especially of chromosomes 4, 10, and 17, and translocation t(12;21) (TEL-AML1), is associated with a better prognosis. Unfavorable cytogenetics are hypodiploidy (less than 44 chromosomes), the Philadelphia chromosome t(9;22), the t(4;11) translocation (which has fusion genes involving the *MLL* gene at 11q23), and a complex karyotype with more than five chromosomal abnormalities.

D. Mixed Phenotype Acute Leukemias

These leukemias consist of blasts that lack differentiation along the lymphoid or myeloid lineage or blasts that express both myeloid and lymphoid lineage-specific antigens. This group is considered very high risk and has a poor prognosis. The limited available data suggest that an "acute lymphoblastic leukemia–like" regimen followed by allogeneic stem cell transplant may be advisable; addition of a tyrosine kinase inhibitor in patients with t(9;22) translocation is recommended.

Clinical Findings

A. Symptoms and Signs

Most patients have been ill only for days or weeks. Bleeding (usually due to thrombocytopenia) occurs in the skin and mucosal surfaces, with gingival bleeding, epistaxis, or menorrhagia. Less commonly, widespread bleeding is seen in patients with disseminated intravascular coagulation (DIC) (in APL and monocytic leukemia). Infection is due to neutropenia, with the risk of infection rising as the neutrophil count falls below 500/mcL (0.5×10^9/L). Common presentations include cellulitis, pneumonia, and perirectal infections; death within a few hours may occur if treatment with appropriate antibiotics is delayed. Fungal infections are also commonly seen.

Patients may also seek medical attention because of gum hypertrophy and bone and joint pain. The most dramatic presentation is hyperleukocytosis, in which a markedly elevated circulating blast count (total white blood count greater than 100,000/mcL) leads to impaired circulation, presenting as headache, confusion, and dyspnea. Such patients require emergent chemotherapy with adjunctive leukapheresis since mortality approaches 40% in the first 48 hours.

On examination, patients appear pale and have purpura and petechiae; signs of infection may not be present. Stomatitis and gum hypertrophy may be seen in patients with monocytic leukemia, as may rectal fissures. There is variable enlargement of the liver, spleen, and lymph nodes. Bone tenderness may be present, particularly in the sternum, tibia, and femur.

B. Laboratory Findings

The hallmark of acute leukemia is the combination of pancytopenia with circulating blasts. However, blasts may be absent from the peripheral smear in as many as 10% of cases ("aleukemic leukemia"). The bone marrow is usually hypercellular and dominated by blasts. More than 20% blasts are required to make a diagnosis of acute leukemia.

Hyperuricemia may be seen. If DIC is present, the fibrinogen level will be reduced, the prothrombin time prolonged, and fibrin degradation products or fibrin D-dimers present. Patients with ALL (especially T cell) may have a mediastinal mass visible on chest radiograph. Meningeal leukemia will have blasts present in the spinal fluid, seen in approximately 5% of cases at diagnosis; it is more common in monocytic types of AML and can be seen with ALL.

The **Auer rod,** an eosinophilic needle-like inclusion in the cytoplasm, is pathognomonic of AML and, if seen, secures the diagnosis. The phenotype of leukemia cells is usually demonstrated by flow cytometry or immunohistochemistry. AML cells usually express myeloid antigens such as CD13 or CD33 and myeloperoxidase. ALL cells of B lineage will express CD19, and most cases will express CD10, formerly known as the "common ALL antigen." ALL cells of T lineage will usually not express mature T-cell markers, such as CD3, CD4, or CD8, but will express some combination of CD2, CD5, and CD7 and will not express surface immunoglobulin. Almost all ALL cells express terminal deoxynucleotidyl transferase (TdT).

▶ Differential Diagnosis

AML must be distinguished from other myeloproliferative disorders, CML, and myelodysplastic syndromes. Acute leukemia may also resemble a left-shifted bone marrow recovering from a previous toxic insult. If the diagnosis is in doubt, a bone marrow study should be repeated in several days to see if maturation has taken place. ALL must be separated from other lymphoproliferative disease such as CLL, lymphomas, and hairy cell leukemia. It may also be confused with the atypical lymphocytosis of mononucleosis and pertussis.

▶ Treatment

Most patients up to age 60 with acute leukemia are treated with the objective of cure. The first step in treatment is to obtain complete remission, defined as normal peripheral blood with resolution of cytopenias, normal bone marrow with no excess blasts, and normal clinical status. The type of initial chemotherapy depends on the subtype of leukemia.

1. AML—Most patients with AML are treated with a combination of an anthracycline (daunorubicin or idarubicin) plus cytarabine, either alone or in combination with other agents. This therapy will produce complete remissions in 80–90% of patients under age 60 years and in 50–60% of older patients (see Table 39–2). Older patients with AML who are not candidates for traditional chemotherapy may

be given 5-azacitidine, decitabine, or clofarabine initially with acceptable outcomes. Addition of the bcl2 inhibitor venetoclax to these agents shows higher complete remission rates in phase 2 studies.

Once a patient has entered remission, post-remission therapy should be given with curative intent whenever possible. Options include standard chemotherapy and allogeneic stem cell transplantation. The optimal treatment strategy depends on the patient's age and clinical status, and the genetic risk factor profile of the leukemia. Patients with a favorable genetic profile can be treated with chemotherapy alone or with autologous transplant with cure rates of 60–80%. Patients who do not enter remission (primary induction failure) or those with high-risk genetics have cure rates of less than 10% with chemotherapy alone and are referred for allogeneic stem cell transplantation. For intermediate-risk patients with AML, cure rates are 35–40% with chemotherapy and 40–60% with allogeneic transplantation. Addition of the FLT3 kinase inhibitor midostaurin to the induction, consolidation, and maintenance therapy of AML patients with *FLT3* mutation has been shown to prolong event-free and overall survival.

Patients over age 60 have had a poor prognosis, even in first remission, when treated with standard chemotherapy approaches, and only 10–20% become long-term survivors. The use of reduced-intensity allogeneic transplant has improved the outcome for such patients, with studies suggesting that up to 40% of selected patients may be cured.

Once leukemia has recurred after initial chemotherapy, the prognosis is poor. For patients in second remission, transplantation offers a 20–30% chance of cure. Targeted therapies directed at recurrent genetic mutations (*FLT3, IDH1/IDH2*) have shown promising activity in this setting, and the mutant isocitrate dehydrogenase 2 (IDH2) enzyme inhibitor enasidenib was approved by the FDA in 2017.

2. ALL—Adults with ALL are treated with combination chemotherapy, including daunorubicin, vincristine, prednisone, and asparaginase. This treatment produces complete remissions in 90% of patients. Those patients with Philadelphia chromosome-positive ALL (or *bcr-abl*-positive ALL) should have a tyrosine kinase inhibitor, such as dasatinib, added to their initial chemotherapy. Remission induction therapy for ALL is less myelosuppressive than treatment for AML and does not necessarily produce marrow aplasia. Patients should also receive central nervous system prophylaxis so that meningeal sequestration of leukemic cells does not develop.

After achieving complete remission, patients may be treated with either additional cycles of chemotherapy or high-dose chemotherapy and stem cell transplantation. Treatment decisions are made based on patient age and disease risk factors. Adults younger than 39 years have uniformly better outcomes when treated under pediatric protocols. Low-risk patients with ALL may be treated with chemotherapy alone with a 70% chance of cure. Intermediate-risk patients have a 30–50% chance of cure with chemotherapy, and high-risk patients are rarely cured with chemotherapy alone. High-risk patients with adverse cytogenetics or poor responses to chemotherapy are best treated with allogeneic transplantation. Minimal residual disease testing early on can also identify high-risk patients who will not be cured with chemotherapy alone. For patients with relapsed disease, the bispecific antibody blinatumomab has shown remarkable response rates as a bridge to transplantation and is considered superior to salvage chemotherapy options. Tisagenlecleucel is a therapy utilizing autologous T cells engineered to express an anti-CD-19 antigen receptor (CART-19) and is FDA-approved for the treatment of children and young adults with relapsed/refractory B-ALL.

Prognosis

Approximately 70–80% of adults with AML under age 60 years achieve complete remission and ~50% are cured using risk-adapted post-remission therapy. Older adults with AML achieve complete remission in up to 50% of instances. The cure rates for older patients with AML have been very low (approximately 10–20%) even if they achieve remission and are able to receive post-remission chemotherapy. Reduced-intensity allogeneic transplantation is increasingly being utilized in order to improve on these outcomes.

Patients younger than 39 years with ALL have excellent outcomes after undergoing chemotherapy followed by risk-adapted intensification and transplantation (cure rates of 60–80%). Patients with adverse cytogenetics, poor response to chemotherapy, or older age have a much lower chance of cure (cure rates of 20–40%).

When to Refer

All patients should be referred to a hematologist.

When to Admit

Most patients with acute leukemia will be admitted for treatment.

Döhner H et al. Diagnosis and management of AML in adults: 2017 ELN recommendations from an international expert panel. Blood. 2017 Jan 26;129(4):424–47. [PMID: 27895058]

Lo-Coco F et al. Current standard treatment of adult acute promyelocytic leukaemia. Br J Haematol. 2016 Mar;172(6): 841–54. [PMID: 26687281]

Marks DI et al. Management of adults with T-cell lymphoblastic leukemia. Blood. 2017 Mar 2;129(9):1134–42. Erratum in: Blood. 2017 Apr 13;129(15):2204. [PMID: 28115371]

Rytting ME et al. Acute lymphoblastic leukemia in adolescents and young adults. Cancer. 2017 Jul 1;123(13):2398–403. [PMID: 28328172]

Sanz MA et al. Emerging strategies for the treatment of older patients with acute myeloid leukemia. Ann Hematol. 2016 Oct; 95(10):1583–93. [PMID: 27118541]

CHRONIC LYMPHOCYTIC LEUKEMIA

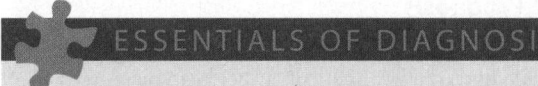

ESSENTIALS OF DIAGNOSIS

► B-cell lymphocytosis with CD19 expression greater than 5000/mcL.

► Coexpression of CD19, CD5 on lymphocytes.

General Considerations

CLL is a clonal malignancy of B lymphocytes. The disease is usually indolent, with slowly progressive accumulation of long-lived small lymphocytes. These cells are immune-incompetent and respond poorly to antigenic stimulation.

CLL is manifested clinically by immunosuppression, bone marrow failure, and organ infiltration with lymphocytes. Immunodeficiency is also related to inadequate antibody production by the abnormal B cells. With advanced disease, CLL may cause damage by direct tissue infiltration.

CLL usually pursues an indolent course, but some subtypes behave more aggressively; a variant, prolymphocytic leukemia, is more aggressive. The morphology of the latter is different, characterized by larger and more immature cells. In 5–10% of cases, CLL may be complicated by autoimmune hemolytic anemia or autoimmune thrombocytopenia. In approximately 5% of cases, while the systemic disease remains stable, an isolated lymph node transforms into an aggressive large-cell lymphoma (**Richter syndrome**).

Clinical Findings

A. Symptoms and Signs

CLL is a disease of older patients, with 90% of cases occurring after age 50 years and a median age at presentation of 70 years. Many patients will be incidentally discovered to have lymphocytosis. Others present with fatigue or lymphadenopathy. On examination, 80% of patients will have diffuse lymphadenopathy and 50% will have enlargement of the liver or spleen.

The long-standing Rai classification system remains prognostically useful: stage 0, lymphocytosis only; stage I, lymphocytosis plus lymphadenopathy; stage II, organomegaly (spleen, liver); stage III, anemia; stage IV, thrombocytopenia. These stages can be collapsed into low risk (stages 0–I), intermediate risk (stage II), and high risk (stages III–IV).

B. Laboratory Findings

The hallmark of CLL is isolated lymphocytosis. The white blood cell count is usually greater than 20,000/mcL (20 × 10^9/L) and may be markedly elevated to several hundred thousand. Usually 75–98% of the circulating cells are lymphocytes. Lymphocytes appear small and mature, with condensed nuclear chromatin, and are morphologically indistinguishable from normal small lymphocytes, but smaller numbers of larger and activated lymphocytes may be seen. The hematocrit and platelet count are usually normal at presentation. The bone marrow is variably infiltrated with small lymphocytes. The immunophenotype of CLL demonstrates coexpression of the B lymphocyte lineage marker CD19 with the T lymphocyte marker CD5; this finding is commonly observed only in CLL and mantle cell lymphoma. CLL is distinguished from mantle cell lymphoma by the expression of CD23, low expression of surface immunoglobulin and CD20, and the absence of a translocation or overexpression of cyclin D1. Patients whose CLL cells have mutated forms of the immunoglobulin gene

(IgVH somatic mutation) have a more indolent form of disease; these cells typically express low levels of the surface antigen CD38 and do not express the zeta-associated protein (ZAP-70). Conversely, patients whose cells have unmutated IgVH genes and high levels of ZAP-70 expression do less well and require treatment sooner. The assessment of genomic changes by FISH provides important prognostic information. The finding of deletion of chromosome 17p (TP53) confers the worst prognosis, while deletion of 11q (ATM) confers an inferior prognosis to the average genotype, and isolated deletion of 13q has a more favorable outcome.

Hypogammaglobulinemia is present in 50% of patients and becomes more common with advanced disease. In some, a small amount of IgM paraprotein is present in the serum.

Differential Diagnosis

Few syndromes can be confused with CLL. Viral infections producing lymphocytosis should be obvious from the presence of fever and other clinical findings; however, fever may occur in CLL from concomitant bacterial infection. Pertussis may cause a particularly high total lymphocyte count. Other lymphoproliferative diseases such as Waldenström macroglobulinemia, hairy cell leukemia, or lymphoma (especially mantle cell) in the leukemic phase are distinguished on the basis of the morphology and immunophenotype of circulating lymphocytes and bone marrow. Monoclonal B-cell lymphocytosis is a disorder characterized by fewer than 5000/mcL B cells and is considered a precursor to B-CLL.

Treatment

The treatment of CLL is evolving as several active targeted agents emerge. Most cases of early indolent CLL require no specific therapy, and the standard of care for early-stage disease has been observation. Indications for treatment include progressive fatigue, symptomatic lymphadenopathy, anemia, or thrombocytopenia. These patients have either symptomatic and progressive Rai stage II disease or stage III/IV disease. Initial treatment for patients younger than 70 years without significant comorbidities historically consisted of chemoimmunotherapy with either FCR (fludarabine with cyclophosphamide and rituximab) or BR (bendamustine with rituximab). The latter combination is better tolerated and associated with fewer adverse events but results in a shorter time to progression (see Table 39–3). The Bruton tyrosine kinase inhibitor ibrutinib is a well-tolerated, oral agent given at 420 mg daily; it has shown remarkable activity and duration of response in the front-line setting and is another option for patients who wish to avoid chemotherapy. Ibrutinib can be associated with hypertension, cardiac arrhythmias, rash, and increased infections. Caution should be exercised when this agent is used in conjunction with CYP3A inhibitors or inducers. In addition, there is a potential for serious bleeding when it is used in patients taking warfarin.

For older patients or young patients with significant comorbidities, chlorambucil, 0.6–1 mg/kg orally, every 2 or 3 weeks, had been the standard therapy. The monoclonal antibody obinutuzumab in combination with chlorambucil produces a significant number of responses (75%), including elimination of disease at the molecular level (in 17%), and offers another well-tolerated choice in this patient population. However, ibrutinib has become the standard of care in the United States for these patients, based on its tolerability profile.

For patients with relapsed or refractory disease, both idelalisib (a PI3 kinase delta inhibitor) and ibrutinib demonstrate significant activity, even for patients with high-risk genetics. Both of these agents can be associated with marked lymphocytosis due to release of tumor cells from the lymph nodes into the peripheral blood. This results in a significant early reduction in lymphadenopathy but a potentially misleading, more delayed clearance of peripheral blood and bone marrow. Idelalisib, 150 mg orally twice a day, is given in combination with rituximab. There are risks for colitis, liver injury, and fatal infectious complications in patients treated with idelalisib. Patients should be given antimicrobial prophylaxis and monitored closely while taking the drug. In patients with deletion of chromosome 17p, treatment with ibrutinib can result in a sustained duration of response (85% at 2 years), a breakthrough in this disease. The targeted oral bcl2 inhibitor venetoclax (slowly titrated up to 400 mg daily) is approved in the United States for this specific group of patients with similar response rates and a substantial number of minimal residual disease (MRD) negative responses. However, it can be associated with tumor lysis syndrome and neutropenia, and patients may require hospitalization for initial therapy.

Associated autoimmune hemolytic anemia or immune thrombocytopenia may require treatment with rituximab, prednisone, or splenectomy. Fludarabine should be avoided in patients with autoimmune hemolytic anemia since it may exacerbate it. Rituximab should be used with caution in patients with past hepatitis B virus (HBV) infection since HBV reactivation, fulminant hepatitis, and, rarely, death can occur without anti-HBV agent prophylaxis. Patients with recurrent bacterial infections and hypogammaglobulinemia benefit from prophylactic infusions of gamma globulin (0.4 g/kg/month), but this treatment is very expensive and can be justified only when these infections are severe. Patients undergoing therapy with a nucleoside analog (fludarabine, pentostatin) should receive anti-infective prophylaxis for *Pneumocystis jirovecii* pneumonia, herpes viruses, and invasive fungal infections until there is evidence of T-cell recovery.

Allogeneic transplantation offers potentially curative treatment for patients with CLL, but it should be used only in patients whose disease cannot be controlled by the available therapies. Nonmyeloablative allogeneic transplant can result in over 40% long-term disease control in CLL at the risk of moderate toxicity.

Prognosis

Therapies have changed the prognosis of CLL. In the past, median survival was approximately 6 years, and only 25% of patients lived more than 10 years. Patients with stage 0 or stage I disease have a median survival of 10–15 years, and these patients may be reassured that they can live a normal life for many years. Patients with stage III or stage IV disease had a median survival of less than 2 years in the past, but with current therapies, 2-year survival is now more than 90% and the long-term outlook appears to be substantially changed. For patients with high-risk and resistant forms of CLL, there is evidence that allogeneic transplantation can overcome risk factors and lead to long-term disease control.

When to Refer

All patients with CLL should be referred to a hematologist.

When to Admit

Hospitalization is rarely needed.

Fischer K et al. Optimizing frontline therapy of CLL based on clinical and biological factors. Hematology Am Soc Hematol Educ Program. 2017 Dec 8;2017(1):338–45. [PMID: 29222276]

Hallek M. Chronic lymphocytic leukemia: 2017 update on diagnosis, risk stratification, and treatment. Am J Hematol. 2017 Sep;92(9):946–65. [PMID: 28782884]

Jain N et al. Richter transformation of CLL. Expert Rev Hematol. 2016 Aug;9(8):793–801. [PMID: 27351634]

Kharfan-Dabaja MA et al. Clinical practice recommendations for use of allogeneic hematopoietic cell transplantation in chronic lymphocytic leukemia on behalf of the Guidelines Committee of the American Society for Blood and Marrow Transplantation. Biol Blood Marrow Transplant. 2016 Dec; 22(12):2117–25. [PMID: 27660167]

HAIRY CELL LEUKEMIA

ESSENTIALS OF DIAGNOSIS

- ► Pancytopenia.
- ► Splenomegaly, often massive.
- ► Hairy cells present on blood smear and especially in bone marrow biopsy.

General Considerations

Hairy cell leukemia is a rare malignancy of hematopoietic stem cells differentiated as mature B-lymphocytes with hairy cytoplasmic projections. The V600E mutation in the *BRAF* gene is recognized as the causal genetic event of hairy cell leukemia, since it is detectable in almost all cases at diagnosis and is present at relapse.

Clinical Findings

A. Symptoms and Signs

The disease characteristically presents in middle-aged men. The median age at presentation is 55 years, and there is a striking 5:1 male predominance. Most patients present with gradual onset of fatigue, others complain of symptoms related to markedly enlarged spleen, and some come to attention because of infection.

Splenomegaly is almost invariably present and may be massive. The liver is enlarged in 50% of cases; lymphadenopathy is uncommon.

Hairy cell leukemia is usually an indolent disorder whose course is dominated by pancytopenia and recurrent infections, including mycobacterial infections.

B. Laboratory Findings

The hallmark of hairy cell leukemia is pancytopenia. Anemia is nearly universal, and 75% of patients have thrombocytopenia and neutropenia. The "hairy cells" are usually present in small numbers on the peripheral blood smear and have a characteristic appearance with numerous cytoplasmic projections. The bone marrow is usually inaspirable (dry tap), and the diagnosis is made by characteristic morphology on bone marrow biopsy. The hairy cells have a characteristic histochemical staining pattern with tartrate-resistant acid phosphatase (TRAP). On immunophenotyping, the cells coexpress the antigens CD11c, CD20, CD22, CD25, CD103, and CD123. Pathologic examination of the spleen shows marked infiltration of the red pulp with hairy cells. This is in contrast to the usual predilection of lymphomas to involve the white pulp of the spleen.

Differential Diagnosis

Hairy cell leukemia should be distinguished from other lymphoproliferative diseases such as Waldenström macroglobulinemia and non-Hodgkin lymphomas. It also may be confused with other causes of pancytopenia, including hypersplenism due to any cause, aplastic anemia, and paroxysmal nocturnal hemoglobinuria.

Treatment

Treatment is indicated for symptomatic disease, ie, splenic discomfort, recurrent infections, or significant cytopenias. The treatment of choice is a nucleoside analog, specifically pentostatin or cladribine for a single course, producing a complete remission in 70–95% of patients. Treatment is associated with infectious complications, and patients should be closely monitored. The median duration of response is over 8 years and patients who relapse a year or more after initial therapy can be treated again with one of these agents. Rituximab can be used in the relapsed setting either as a single agent or in combination with a nucleoside analog. The BRAF inhibitor vemurafenib exhibits ~100% overall response rate in patients with refractory/relapsed hairy cell leukemia, with 35–40% complete remissions. The median relapse-free survival is ~19 months in patients who achieved complete remission and 6 months in those who obtained a partial response.

Course & Prognosis

More than 95% of patients with hairy cell leukemia live longer than 10 years.

Grever MR et al. Consensus guidelines for the diagnosis and management of patients with classic hairy cell leukemia. Blood. 2017 Feb 2;129(5):553–60. [PMID: 27903528]

Wierda WG et al. Hairy cell leukemia, version 2.2018, NCCN Clinical Practice Guidelines in Oncology. J Natl Compr Canc Netw. 2017 Nov;15(11):1414–27. [PMID: 29118233]

LYMPHOMAS

NON-HODGKIN LYMPHOMAS

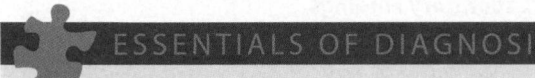

ESSENTIALS OF DIAGNOSIS

▶ Often present with painless lymphadenopathy.
▶ Diagnosis is made by tissue biopsy.

General Considerations

The non-Hodgkin lymphomas are a heterogeneous group of cancers of lymphocytes usually presenting as enlarged lymph nodes. The disorders vary in clinical presentation and course from indolent to rapidly progressive.

Molecular biology has provided clues to the pathogenesis of these disorders, often a matter of balanced chromosomal translocations whereby an oncogene becomes juxtaposed next to either an immunoglobulin gene (B-cell lymphoma) or the T-cell receptor gene or related gene (T-cell lymphoma). The net result is oncogene overexpression and development of lymphoma. The best-studied example is Burkitt lymphoma, in which a characteristic cytogenetic abnormality of translocation between the long arms of chromosomes 8 and 14 has been identified. The protooncogene c-*myc* is translocated from its normal position on chromosome 8 to the immunoglobulin heavy chain locus on chromosome 14. Overexpression of c-*myc* is related to malignant transformation through excess B-cell proliferation. In the follicular lymphomas, the t(14;18) translocation is characteristic and *bcl-2 is* overexpressed, resulting in protection against apoptosis, the usual mechanism of B-cell death.

Classification of the lymphomas is a dynamic area still undergoing evolution. The 2017 grouping (Table 13–16) separates diseases based on both clinical and pathologic features. Eighty-five percent of non-Hodgkin lymphomas are B-cell and 15% are T-cell or NK-cell in origin. Even though non-Hodgkin lymphomas represent a diverse group of diseases, they are historically divided in two categories based on clinical behavior and pathology: the indolent (low-grade) and the aggressive (intermediate- or high-grade).

Clinical Findings

A. Symptoms and Signs

Patients with non-Hodgkin lymphomas usually present with lymphadenopathy. Involved lymph nodes may be present peripherally or centrally (in the retroperitoneum, mesentery, and pelvis). The indolent lymphomas are usually disseminated at the time of diagnosis, and bone marrow involvement is frequent. Many patients with lymphoma have constitutional symptoms such as fever, drenching night sweats, and weight loss of greater than 10% of prior body weight (referred to as "B" symptoms).

On examination, lymphadenopathy may be isolated or diffuse, and extranodal sites of disease (such as the skin,

Table 13–16. World Health Organization classification of B-cell neoplasms (most common).

Precursor B-cell lymphoblastic lymphoma
Mature B-cell lymphomas
Chronic lymphocytic leukemia/small lymphocytic lymphoma
Monoclonal B-cell lymphocytosis
Hairy cell leukemia
Plasma cell myeloma
Diffuse large B-cell lymphoma
Primary diffuse large B-cell lymphoma of the CNS
High-grade B-cell lymphoma, with *MYC* and *BCL2* and/or *BCL6* rearrangements
Mediastinal large B-cell lymphoma
Follicular lymphoma
Small lymphocytic lymphoma
Lymphoplasmacytic lymphoma (Waldenström macroglobulinemia)
Mantle cell lymphoma
Burkitt lymphoma
Marginal zone lymphoma
MALT type
Nodal type
Splenic type
Mature T (and NK cell) lymphomas
Anaplastic large-cell lymphoma
Angioimmunoblastic T-cell lymphoma
Peripheral T-cell lymphoma, NOS
Cutaneous T-cell lymphoma (mycosis fungoides, Sézary syndrome)
Extranodal NK/T-cell lymphoma, nasal type
Adult T-cell leukemia/lymphoma
T-cell large granular lymphocytic leukemia
Hodgkin lymphoma
Nodular lymphocyte predominant Hodgkin lymphoma
Classic Hodgkin lymphoma
Posttransplant lymphoproliferative disorders
Histiocytic and dendritic cell neoplasms

CNS, central nervous system; MALT, mucosa-associated lymphoid tissue; NOS, not otherwise specified.

gastrointestinal tract, liver, and bone marrow) may be found. Patients with Burkitt lymphoma are noted to have abdominal pain or abdominal fullness because of the predilection of the disease for the abdomen.

Once a pathologic diagnosis is established, staging is done using a whole-body positron emission tomography (PET)/CT scan, a bone marrow biopsy, and, in patients with high-grade lymphoma or intermediate-grade lymphoma with high-risk features, a lumbar puncture.

B. Laboratory Findings

The peripheral blood is usually normal even with extensive bone marrow involvement by lymphoma. Circulating lymphoma cells in the blood are not commonly seen.

Bone marrow involvement is manifested as paratrabecular monoclonal lymphoid aggregates. In some high-grade lymphomas, the meninges are involved and malignant cells are found with cerebrospinal fluid cytology. The serum LD, a useful prognostic marker, is incorporated in risk stratification of treatment.

The diagnosis of lymphoma is made by tissue biopsy. Needle aspiration may yield evidence for non-Hodgkin lymphoma, but a lymph node biopsy (or biopsy of involved extranodal tissue) is required for accurate diagnosis and classification.

▶ Treatment

A. Indolent Lymphomas

The most common lymphomas in this group are follicular lymphoma, marginal zone lymphomas, and small lymphocytic lymphoma (SLL). The treatment of **indolent lymphomas** depends on the stage of disease and the clinical status of the patient. A small number of patients have limited disease with only one or two contiguous abnormal lymph node groups and may be treated with localized irradiation with curative intent. However, most patients (85%) with indolent lymphoma have disseminated disease at the time of diagnosis and are not considered curable. Historically, treatment of these patients has not affected overall survival; therefore, treatment is offered only when symptoms develop or for high tumor bulk. Following each treatment response, patients will experience a relapse at traditionally shorter intervals. Some patients will have temporary spontaneous remissions (8%). There are an increasing number of reasonable treatment options for indolent lymphomas, but no consensus exists on the best strategy. Treatment with rituximab (375 mg/m^2 intravenously weekly for 4 weeks) is commonly used either alone or in combination with chemotherapy and may be the only agent to affect overall survival in these disorders. Patients should be screened for hepatitis B because rare cases of fatal fulminant hepatitis have been described with the use of anti-CD20 monoclonal therapies without anti-HBV agent prophylaxis. Rituximab is added to chemotherapy regimens including bendamustine; cyclophosphamide, vincristine, and prednisone (R-CVP); and cyclophosphamide, doxorubicin, vincristine, and prednisone (R-CHOP) (see Table 39–3). Radioimmunoconjugates that fuse anti-B cell monoclonal antibodies with radioactive nuclides can produce higher response rates compared to antibody alone but are infrequently used. One such agent (yttrium-90 ibritumomab tiuxetan) is available in the United States. Some patients with clinically aggressive low-grade lymphomas may be appropriate candidates for allogeneic stem cell transplantation with curative intent. The role of autologous hematopoietic stem cell transplantation remains uncertain, but some patients with recurrent disease appear to have prolonged remissions without the expectation of cure.

Patients with mucosa-associated lymphoid tissue tumors of the stomach may be appropriately treated with combination antibiotics directed against *H pylori* and with acid blockade but require frequent endoscopic monitoring. Alternatively, mucosa-associated lymphoid tissue tumors confined to the stomach can also be cured with whole-stomach radiotherapy.

B. Aggressive Lymphomas

Patients with **diffuse large B-cell lymphoma** are treated with curative intent. Most patients are treated with six cycles of immunochemotherapy such as R-CHOP (see Table 39–3). Involved nodal radiotherapy (INRT) may be added for patients with bulky or extranodal disease. Patients with diffuse large B-cell lymphoma who relapse after initial chemotherapy can still be cured by autologous hematopoietic stem cell transplantation if their disease remains responsive to chemotherapy. For patients who do not respond to second-line chemotherapy, the FDA has approved the chimeric antigen receptor T-cell therapy axicabtagene ciloleucel, which has a durable complete response rate of ~40% but is associated with significant systemic cytokine release syndrome and neurotoxicity.

A subtype of diffuse large B-cell lymphoma with chromosomal translocations affecting *MYC*, such as t(8;14), and affecting *BCL2*, such as t(14;18), is called "double-hit lymphoma" and has a very aggressive course. Patients with this disease may do better with dose-adjusted R-EPOCH therapy. About 25% of patients with diffuse large B-cell lymphoma have been identified as "double-protein expressors" with overexpression of *MYC* and *BCL2* by immunohistochemistry. While the outcomes with R-CHOP are inferior, no definitive alternative treatment recommendations can be made at this time.

Mantle cell lymphoma is not effectively treated with standard immunochemotherapy regimens. Intensive initial immunochemotherapy including autologous hematopoietic stem cell transplantation has been shown to improve outcomes. Reduced-intensity allogeneic stem cell transplantation offers curative potential for selected patients. Ibrutinib and acalabrutinib are active in relapsed or refractory patients with mantle cell lymphoma. For **primary central nervous system lymphoma,** repetitive cycles of high-dose intravenous methotrexate with rituximab early in the treatment course produce better results than whole-brain radiotherapy and with less cognitive impairment.

Patients with **high-grade lymphomas** (Burkitt or lymphoblastic) require urgent, intense, cyclic chemotherapy in the hospital similar to that given for ALL, and they also require intrathecal chemotherapy as central nervous system prophylaxis.

Patients with **peripheral T-cell lymphomas** usually have advanced stage nodal and extranodal disease and typically have inferior response rates to therapy compared to patients with aggressive B-cell disease. Autologous stem cell transplantation is often incorporated in first-line therapy. The antibody-drug conjugate brentuximab vedotin has significant activity in patients with relapsed CD30 positive peripheral T-cell lymphomas, such as anaplastic large-cell lymphoma.

▶ Prognosis

The median survival of patients with indolent lymphomas is 10–15 years. These diseases ultimately become refractory to chemotherapy. This often occurs at the time of histologic progression of the disease to a more aggressive form of lymphoma.

The International Prognostic Index is widely used to categorize patients with aggressive lymphoma into risk groups. Factors that confer adverse prognosis are age over 60 years, elevated serum LD, stage III or stage IV disease, more than one extranodal site of disease, and poor performance status. Cure rates range from more than 80% for low-risk patients (zero risk factors) to less than 50% for high-risk patients (four or more risk factors).

For patients who relapse after initial chemotherapy, the prognosis depends on whether the lymphoma is still responsive to chemotherapy. If the lymphoma remains responsive to chemotherapy, autologous hematopoietic stem cell transplantation offers a 50% chance of long-term lymphoma-free survival.

The treatment of older patients with lymphoma has been difficult because of poorer tolerance of aggressive chemotherapy. The use of myeloid growth factors and prophylactic antibiotics to reduce neutropenic complications may improve outcomes.

Molecular profiling techniques using gene array technology and immunophenotyping have defined subsets of lymphomas with different biologic features and prognoses are being studied in clinical trials to determine choice of therapy.

▶ When to Refer

All patients with lymphoma should be referred to a hematologist or an oncologist.

▶ When to Admit

Admission is necessary only for specific complications of lymphoma or its treatment and for the treatment of all high-grade lymphomas.

Armitage JO. The aggressive peripheral T-cell lymphomas: 2017. Am J Hematol. 2017 Jul;92(7):706–15. [PMID: 28516671]

Campo E et al. Mantle cell lymphoma: evolving management strategies. Blood. 2015 Jan 1;125(1):48–55. [PMID: 25499451]

Chiappella A et al. Diffuse large B-cell lymphoma in the elderly: standard treatment and new perspectives. Expert Rev Hematol. 2017 Apr;10(4):289–97. [PMID: 28290728]

Kritharis A et al. Current therapeutic strategies and new treatment paradigms for follicular lymphoma. Cancer Treat Res. 2015;165:197–226. [PMID: 25655611]

Kubuschok B et al. Management of diffuse large B-cell lymphoma (DLBCL). Cancer Treat Res. 2015;165:271–88. [PMID: 25655614]

Paydas S. Primary central nervous system lymphoma: essential points in diagnosis and management. Med Oncol. 2017 Apr; 34(4):61. [PMID: 28315229]

HODGKIN LYMPHOMA

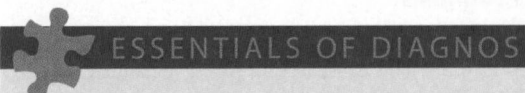

ESSENTIALS OF DIAGNOSIS

▶ Often painless lymphadenopathy.

▶ Constitutional symptoms may or may not be present.

▶ Pathologic diagnosis by lymph node biopsy.

▶ General Considerations

Hodgkin lymphoma is characterized by lymph node biopsy showing Reed-Sternberg cells in an appropriate reactive cellular background. The malignant cell is derived from B lymphocytes of germinal center origin.

▶ Clinical Findings

There is a bimodal age distribution, with one peak in the 20s and a second over age 50 years. Most patients seek medical attention because of a painless mass, commonly in the neck. Others may seek medical attention because of constitutional symptoms such as fever, weight loss, or drenching night sweats, or because of generalized pruritus. An unusual symptom of Hodgkin lymphoma is pain in an involved lymph node following alcohol ingestion.

An important feature of Hodgkin lymphoma is its tendency to arise within single lymph node areas and spread in an orderly fashion to contiguous areas of lymph nodes. Late in the course of the disease, vascular invasion leads to widespread hematogenous dissemination.

Hodgkin lymphoma is divided into two subtypes: classic Hodgkin (nodular sclerosis, mixed cellularity, lymphocyte rich, and lymphocyte depleted) and non-classic Hodgkin (nodular lymphocyte predominant). Hodgkin lymphoma should be distinguished pathologically from other malignant lymphomas and may occasionally be confused with reactive lymph nodes seen in infectious mononucleosis, cat-scratch disease, or drug reactions (eg, phenytoin).

Patients undergo a staging evaluation to determine the extent of disease, including serum chemistries, whole-body PET/CT scan, and bone marrow biopsy.

▶ Treatment

Chemotherapy is the mainstay of treatment for Hodgkin lymphoma and ABVD (doxorubicin, bleomycin, vinblastine, dacarbazine) remains the standard first-line regimen. Even though others such as Stanford V (cyclophosphamide, doxorubicin, vinblastine, vincristine, bleomycin, etoposide, prednisone) or escalated BEACOPP (bleomycin, etoposide, doxorubicin, cyclophosphamide, vincristine, procarbazine, prednisone) may improve response rates and reduce the need for consolidative radiotherapy, they are usually associated with increased toxicity and lack a definitive overall survival advantage. Low-risk patients are those with stage I or II disease without bulky lymphadenopathy or evidence of systemic inflammation. They traditionally receive a combination of short-course chemotherapy with INRT or a full course of chemotherapy alone (see Table 39–3). High-risk patients are those with stage III or IV disease or with stage II disease and a large mediastinal or other bulky mass. These patients are treated with a full course of ABVD for six cycles. Pulmonary toxicity can unfortunately occur following either chemotherapy (bleomycin) or radiation and should be treated aggressively in these patients, since it can lead to permanent fibrosis and death. A normal interim PET/CT scan after 2–4 cycles of chemotherapy can be used to identify patients with an excellent progression-free survival who can receive abbreviated chemotherapy or forego radiation altogether. Conversely, an abnormal interim PET/CT scan is associated with a worse prognosis and should prompt early intensification of treatment to achieve a complete response (CR).

Classic Hodgkin lymphoma relapsing after initial treatment is treatable with high-dose chemotherapy and autologous hematopoietic stem cell transplantation. This offers a 35–50% chance of cure when disease is still chemotherapy responsive. The antibody-drug conjugate brentuximab vedotin has shown impressive activity in patients relapsing after autologous stem cell transplantation (overall response rate [ORR] of 75%; CR of 34%) and is FDA-approved for this indication. It is being studied as front-line therapy, to replace the bleomycin in ABVD. Last, immune checkpoint inhibition by PD1 blockade with nivolumab or pembrolizumab has shown remarkable activity (ORR of 65%) in brentuximab failures.

▶ Prognosis

All patients should be treated with curative intent. Prognosis in advanced stage Hodgkin lymphoma is influenced by seven features: stage, age, gender, hemoglobin, albumin, white blood cell count, and lymphocyte count. The cure rate is 75% if zero to two risk features are present and 55% when three or more risk features are present. The prognosis of patients with stage IA or IIA disease is excellent, with 10-year survival rates in excess of 90%. Patients with advanced disease (stage III or IV) have 10-year survival rates of 50–60%. Poorer results are seen in patients who are older, those who have bulky disease, and those with lymphocyte depletion or mixed cellularity on histologic examination. Non-classic Hodgkin lymphoma (nodular lymphocyte predominant) is highly curable with radiotherapy alone for early-stage disease; however, for high-stage disease, it is characterized by long survival with repetitive relapses after chemotherapy.

▶ When to Refer

- All patients should be sent to an oncologist or hematologist.
- Secondary referral to a radiation oncologist might be appropriate.

▶ When to Admit

Patients should be admitted for complications of the disease or its treatment.

Bachanova V et al. Hodgkin lymphoma in the elderly, pregnant, and HIV-infected. Semin Hematol. 2016 Jul;53(3):203–8. [PMID: 27496312]

Connors JM. Risk assessment in the management of newly diagnosed classical Hodgkin lymphoma. Blood. 2015 Mar 12; 125(11):1693–702. [PMID: 25575542]

Donato EM et al. Immunotherapy for the treatment of Hodgkin lymphoma. Expert Rev Hematol. 2017 May;10(5):417–23. [PMID: 28359170]

PLASMA CELL MYELOMA

ESSENTIALS OF DIAGNOSIS

- ▶ Bone pain, often in the spine, ribs, or proximal long bones.
- ▶ Monoclonal immunoglobulin (ie, paraprotein) in the serum or urine.
- ▶ Clonal plasma cells in the bone marrow or in a tissue biopsy, or both.
- ▶ Organ damage due to plasma cells (eg, bones, kidneys, hypercalcemia, anemia) or other defined criteria.

▶ General Considerations

Plasma cell myeloma (previously called multiple myeloma) is a malignancy of hematopoietic stem cells terminally differentiated as plasma cells characterized by infiltration of the bone marrow, bone destruction, and paraprotein formation. The diagnosis is established when monoclonal plasma cells (either kappa or lambda light chain restricted) in the bone marrow (any percentage) or as a tumor (plasmacytoma), or both, are associated with end-organ damage (such as bone disease [lytic lesions seen on bone radiographs, magnetic resonance imaging {MRI}, or PET/CT scan], anemia [hemoglobin less than 10 g/dL {100 g/L}], hypercalcemia [calcium greater than 11.5 mg/dL {2.9 mmol/L}], or kidney injury [creatinine greater than 2 mg/dL {176.8 mcmol/L}]) with or without paraprotein elaboration. Sixty percent or more clonal plasma cells in the bone marrow, or a serum free kappa to lambda ratio of greater than 100 or less than 0.01 (both criteria regardless of end-organ damage), are also diagnostic of plasma cell myeloma. Smoldering myeloma is defined as 10–59% clonal plasma cells in the bone marrow, a serum paraprotein level of 3 g/dL (30 g/L) or higher, or both, without plasma cell–related end-organ damage.

Malignant plasma cells can form tumors (plasmacytomas) that may cause spinal cord compression or other soft-tissue–related problems. Bone disease is common and due to excessive osteoclast activation mediated largely by the interaction of the receptor activator of NF-kappa-B (RANK) with its ligand (RANKL). In plasma cell myeloma, osteoprotegerin (a decoy receptor for RANKL) is underproduced, thus promoting the binding of RANK with RANKL with consequent excessive bone resorption.

The paraproteins (monoclonal immunoglobulins) secreted by the malignant plasma cells may cause problems in their own right. Very high paraprotein levels (either IgG or IgA) may cause hyperviscosity, although this is more common with the IgM paraprotein in Waldenström macroglobulinemia. The light chain component of the immunoglobulin, when produced in excess, often leads to kidney injury (frequently aggravated by hypercalcemia or hyperuricemia, or both). Light chain components may be deposited in tissues as amyloid, resulting in kidney failure with albuminuria and a vast array of systemic symptoms.

Myeloma patients are prone to recurrent infections for a number of reasons, including neutropenia, the underproduction of normal immunoglobulins and the immunosuppressive effects of chemotherapy. Myeloma patients are especially prone to infections with encapsulated organisms such as *Streptococcus pneumoniae* and *Haemophilus influenzae*.

Clinical Findings

A. Symptoms and Signs

Myeloma is a disease of older adults (median age 65 years). The most common presenting complaints are those related to anemia, bone pain, kidney disease, and infection. Bone pain is most common in the back, hips, or ribs or may present as a pathologic fracture, especially of the femoral neck or vertebrae. Patients may also come to medical attention because of spinal cord compression from a plasmacytoma or the hyperviscosity syndrome (mucosal bleeding, vertigo, nausea, visual disturbances, alterations in mental status, hypoxia). Many patients are diagnosed because of laboratory findings of elevated total protein, hypercalcemia, proteinuria, elevated sedimentation rate, or abnormalities on serum protein electrophoresis obtained for symptoms or in routine screening studies. A few patients come to medical attention because of organ dysfunction due to amyloidosis.

Examination may reveal pallor, bone tenderness, or soft tissue masses. Patients may have neurologic signs related to neuropathy or spinal cord compression. Fever occurs mainly with infection. Acute oliguric or nonoliguric kidney injury may be present due to hypercalcemia, hyperuricemia, light chain cast injury, or primary amyloidosis.

B. Laboratory Findings

Anemia is nearly universal. Red blood cell morphology is normal, but rouleaux formation is common and may be marked. The absence of rouleaux formation, however, excludes neither plasma cell myeloma nor the presence of a serum paraprotein. The neutrophil and platelet counts are usually normal at presentation. Only rarely will plasma cells be visible on peripheral blood smear (plasma cell leukemia).

The hallmark of myeloma is the finding of a paraprotein on serum or urine protein electrophoresis (PEP) or immunofixation electrophoresis (IFE). The majority of patients will have a monoclonal spike visible in the gamma- or beta-globulin region of the PEP. The semi-quantification of the paraprotein on the PEP is referred to as the M-protein, and IFE will reveal this to be a monoclonal immunoglobulin. Approximately 15% of patients will have no demonstrable paraprotein in the serum on PEP because their myeloma cells produce only light chains and not intact immunoglobulin (but sometimes seen on serum IFE), and the light chains pass rapidly through the glomerulus into the urine. Urine PEP and IFE usually demonstrate the light chain paraprotein in this setting. The free light chain assay will sometimes demonstrate excess monoclonal light chains in serum and urine, and in a small proportion of patients, will be the only means to identify and quantify the paraprotein being produced. Overall, the paraprotein is IgG (60%), IgA (20%), or light chain only (15%) in plasma cell myeloma, with the remainder being rare cases of IgD, IgM, or biclonal gammopathy. In sporadic cases, no paraprotein is present ("nonsecretory myeloma"); these patients have particularly aggressive disease.

The bone marrow will be infiltrated by variable numbers of monoclonal plasma cells. The plasma cells may be morphologically abnormal often demonstrating multinucleation and vacuolization. The plasma cells will display marked skewing of the normal kappa-to-lambda light chain ratio, which will indicate their clonality. Many benign inflammatory processes can result in bone marrow plasmacytosis, but with the absence of clonality and morphologic atypia.

C. Imaging

Bone radiographs are important in establishing the diagnosis of myeloma. Lytic lesions are most commonly seen in the axial skeleton: skull, spine, proximal long bones, and ribs. At other times, only generalized osteoporosis is seen. The radionuclide bone scan is not useful in detecting bone lesions in myeloma, since there is usually no osteoblastic component. In the evaluation of patients with known or suspected plasma cell myeloma, MRI and PET scans are more sensitive to detect bone disease than plain radiographs and are preferred.

Differential Diagnosis

When a patient is discovered to have a paraprotein, the distinction between plasma cell myeloma or another lymphoproliferative malignancy with a paraprotein (CLL/SLL, Waldenström macroglobulinemia, non-Hodgkin lymphoma, primary amyloid, cryoglobulinemia) or monoclonal gammopathy of undetermined significance (MGUS) must be made. Plasma cell myeloma, smoldering plasma cell myeloma, and MGUS must be distinguished from reactive (benign) polyclonal hypergammaglobulinemia (which is commonly seen in cirrhosis or chronic inflammation).

Treatment

Patients with low-risk smoldering myeloma are observed. Those with high-risk smoldering disease may be treated with lenalidomide (an immunomodulatory agent) and dexamethasone since this therapy prolongs the time to symptomatic myeloma and may prolong survival compared to no treatment but at the expense of treatment-related side effects.

Most patients with plasma cell myeloma require treatment at diagnosis because of bone pain or other symptoms and complications related to the disease. The initial treatment generally involves triple therapy: an immunomodulatory agent, such as lenalidomide; a proteasome inhibitor, such as bortezomib or carfilzomib; and moderate- or high-dose dexamethasone. The major side effects of lenalidomide are neutropenia and thrombocytopenia, skin rash, venous thromboembolism, peripheral neuropathy, and possibly birth defects. Bortezomib and carfilzomib have the advantages of producing rapid responses and of being effective in poor-prognosis myeloma. The major side effect of bortezomib is neuropathy (both peripheral and autonomic), which is largely ameliorated when given subcutaneously rather than intravenously. Carfilzomib rarely causes neuropathy but sometimes causes pulmonary hypertension or cardiac systolic dysfunction that is usually reversible. In the setting of reduced kidney function, an alkylating agent (cyclophosphamide, orally or intravenously) is often incorporated into the induction therapy. An oral proteasome inhibitor, ixazomib, is available for relapsed disease. Pomalidomide, an immunomodulatory agent, is effective as salvage therapy after relapse. Other salvage agents include daratumumab (an anti-CD38 monoclonal antibody), elotuzumab (an anti-SLAMF7 monoclonal antibody), and panobinostat (a histone deacetylase inhibitor).

After initial therapy, many patients under age 80 years are consolidated with autologous hematopoietic stem cell transplantation following high-dose melphalan (an alkylating chemotherapeutic agent). Autologous stem cell transplantation prolongs both duration of remission and overall survival. Lenalidomide or thalidomide prolong remission and survival when given as posttransplant maintenance therapy but at the expense of an elevated rate of second malignancies. Proteasome inhibitors prolong remissions in high-risk patients after autologous stem cell transplantation.

Localized radiotherapy may be useful for palliation of bone pain or for eradicating tumor at the site of pathologic fracture. Vertebral collapse with its attendant pain and mechanical disturbance can be treated with vertebroplasty or kyphoplasty. Hypercalcemia and hyperuricemia should be treated aggressively and immobilization and dehydration avoided. The bisphosphonates (pamidronate 90 mg or zoledronic acid 4 mg intravenously monthly) reduce pathologic fractures in patients with bone disease and are an important adjunct in this subset of patients. The bisphosphonates are also used to treat myeloma-related hypercalcemia. However, long-term bisphosphonates have been associated with a risk of osteonecrosis of the jaw and other bony areas, so the use of bisphosphonates is limited to 1–2 years after definitive initial therapy. Myeloma patients with oliguric or anuric kidney disease at diagnosis should be treated aggressively with chemotherapy and considered for therapeutic plasma exchange (to reduce the paraprotein burden) because return of kidney function can commonly occur.

Prognosis

The outlook for patients with myeloma has been steadily improving for the past decade. The median survival of patients is more than 7 years. Patients with low-stage disease who lack high-risk genomic changes respond very well to treatment and derive significant benefit from autologous hematopoietic stem cell transplantation and have survivals approaching a decade. The International Staging System for myeloma relies on two factors: beta-2-microglobulin and albumin. Stage 1 patients have both beta-2-microglobulin less than 3.5 mg/L and albumin greater than 3.5 g/dL (survival more than 5 years). Stage 3

is established when beta-2-microglobulin is greater than 5.5 mg/L (survival less than 2 years). Stage 2 is established with values in between stage 1 and 3. Other adverse prognostic findings are an elevated serum LD or bone marrow genetic abnormalities established by FISH involving the immunoglobulin heavy chain locus at chromosome 14q32, multiple copies of the 1q21-23 locus, or 17p chromosome abnormalities (causing the loss or mutation of *TP53*).

When to Refer

All patients with plasma cell myeloma should be referred to a hematologist or an oncologist.

When to Admit

Hospitalization is indicated for treatment of acute kidney injury, hypercalcemia, or suspicion of spinal cord compression, for certain chemotherapy regimens, or for hematopoietic stem cell transplantation.

Dingli D et al. Therapy for relapsed multiple myeloma: guidelines from the Mayo stratification for myeloma and risk-adapted therapy. Mayo Clin Proc. 2017 Apr;92(4):578–98. [PMID: 28291589]

Gavriatopoulou M et al. Emerging treatment approaches for myeloma-related bone disease. Expert Rev Hematol. 2017 Mar; 10(3):217–28. [PMID: 28092987]

Jethava YS et al. Transplantation for multiple myeloma. Cancer Treat Res. 2016;169:227–50. [PMID: 27696266]

Laubach JP et al. Daratumumab, elotuzumab, and the development of therapeutic monoclonal antibodies in multiple myeloma. Clin Pharmacol Ther. 2017 Jan;101(1):81–8. [PMID: 27806428]

Richter J et al. Society of Hematologic Oncology state of the art update and next questions: multiple myeloma. Clin Lymphoma Myeloma Leuk. 2018 Nov;18(11):693–702. [PMID: 30287199]

Terpos E et al. The role of imaging in the treatment of patients with multiple myeloma in 2016. Am Soc Clin Oncol Educ Book. 2016;35:e407–17. [PMID: 27249748]

MONOCLONAL GAMMOPATHY OF UNDETERMINED SIGNIFICANCE

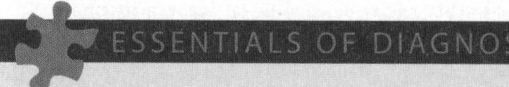

ESSENTIALS OF DIAGNOSIS

▶ Monoclonal immunoglobulin (ie, paraprotein) in the serum (less than 3 g/dL [less than 30 g/L]) or urine.

▶ Clonal plasma cells in the bone marrow less than 10% (if performed).

▶ No symptoms and no organ damage from the paraprotein.

General Considerations

MGUS is present in 1% of all adults (3% of those over age 50 years and more than 5% of those over age 70 years). Among all patients with paraproteins, MGUS is far more common than plasma cell myeloma. MGUS is defined as bone marrow monoclonal plasma cells less than 10% in the setting of a paraprotein (serum M-protein less than 3 g/dL [30 g/L]) and the absence of plasma cell–related end-organ damage. If an excess of serum free light chains (kappa or lambda) is established, the kappa to lambda ratio is 100 or less or 0.01 or greater. In approximately one-quarter of cases, MGUS progresses to overt malignant disease in a median of one decade. The transformation of MGUS to plasma cell myeloma is approximately 1% per year. Two adverse risk factors for progression of MGUS to a plasma cell or lymphoid disorder are an abnormal serum kappa to lambda free light chain ratio and a serum monoclonal protein (M-protein) level 1.5 g/dL or greater. Patients with MGUS have shortened survival (median 8.1 years vs 12.4 years for age- and sex-matched controls). In addition, 12% of patients with MGUS will convert to primary amyloidosis in a median of 9 years. Plasma cell myeloma, smoldering plasma cell myeloma, and MGUS must be distinguished from reactive (benign) polyclonal hypergammaglobulinemia (common in cirrhosis or chronic inflammation).

Laboratory Findings

To establish the diagnosis, serum and urine should be sent for PEP and IFE to search for a monoclonal protein; serum should be sent for free light chain analysis and quantitative immunoglobulins. Additional tests include a hemoglobin and serum albumin, calcium, and creatinine. If these additional tests are normal (or if abnormal is otherwise explained), then a bone marrow biopsy is usually deferred provided the serum M-protein is less than 3 g/dL (less than 30 g/L). In asymptomatic individuals, a skeletal survey (radiographs) is performed, but if there are some bone complaints or a question regarding bone disease, MRI or PET/CT imaging is preferred. MGUS is diagnosed if patients do not meet the criteria for smoldering plasma cell myeloma or plasma cell myeloma.

Treatment

Patients with MGUS are observed without treatment.

Kyle RA et al. Long-term follow up of monoclonal gammopathy of undetermined significance. N Engl J Med. 2018 Jan 18; 378(3):241–9. [PMID: 29342381]

Willrich MAV et al. Laboratory testing for monoclonal gammopathies: focus on monoclonal gammopathy of undetermined significance and smoldering multiple myeloma. Clin Biochem. 2018 Jan;51:38–47. [PMID: 28479151]

WALDENSTRÖM MACROGLOBULINEMIA

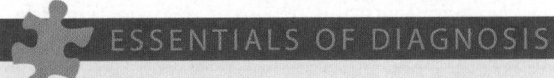

- ► Monoclonal IgM paraprotein.
- ► Infiltration of bone marrow by plasmacytic lymphocytes.
- ► Absence of lytic bone disease.

General Considerations

Waldenström macroglobulinemia is a syndrome of IgM hypergammaglobulinemia that occurs in the setting of a low-grade non-Hodgkin lymphoma characterized by B cells that are morphologically a hybrid of lymphocytes and plasma cells. These cells characteristically secrete the IgM paraprotein, and many clinical manifestations of the disease are related to this macroglobulin.

Clinical Findings

A. Symptoms and Signs

This disease characteristically develops insidiously in patients in their 60s or 70s. Patients usually present with fatigue related to anemia. Hyperviscosity of serum may be manifested in a number of ways. Mucosal and gastrointestinal bleeding is related to engorged blood vessels and platelet dysfunction. Other complaints include nausea, vertigo, and visual disturbances. Alterations in consciousness vary from mild lethargy to stupor and coma. The IgM paraprotein may also cause symptoms of cold agglutinin disease (hemolysis) or chronic demyelinating peripheral neuropathy.

On examination, there may be hepatosplenomegaly or lymphadenopathy. The retinal veins are engorged. Purpura may be present. There should be no bone tenderness.

B. Laboratory Findings

Anemia is nearly universal, and rouleaux formation is common, although the red blood cells are agglutinated when the blood smear is prepared at room temperature. The anemia is related in part to expansion of the plasma volume by 50–100% due to the presence of the paraprotein. Other blood counts are usually normal. The abnormal plasmacytic lymphocytes may appear in small numbers on the peripheral blood smear. The bone marrow is characteristically infiltrated by the plasmacytic lymphocytes.

The hallmark of macroglobulinemia is the presence of a monoclonal IgM spike seen on serum PEP in the beta-globulin region. The serum viscosity is usually increased above the normal of 1.4–1.8 times that of water. Symptoms of hyperviscosity usually develop when the serum viscosity is over four times that of water, and marked symptoms usually arise when the viscosity is over six times that of water. Because paraproteins vary in their physicochemical properties, there is no strict correlation between the concentration of paraprotein and serum viscosity.

The IgM paraprotein may cause a positive antiglobulin (Coombs) test for complement and have cold agglutinin or cryoglobulin properties. If macroglobulinemia is suspected but the serum PEP shows only hypogammaglobulinemia, the test should be repeated while taking special measures to maintain the blood at 37°C, since the paraprotein may precipitate out at room temperature. Bone radiographs are normal, and there is no evidence of kidney injury.

Differential Diagnosis

Waldenström macroglobulinemia is differentiated from MGUS by the finding of bone marrow infiltration with monoclonal malignant cells. It is distinguished from CLL by bone marrow morphology, the absence of CD5 expression, and the absence of lymphocytosis, and it is distinguished from plasma cell myeloma by bone marrow morphology, the finding of the characteristic IgM paraprotein, and the absence of lytic bone disease.

▶ Treatment

Patients with marked hyperviscosity syndrome (stupor, coma, pulmonary edema) should be treated on an emergency basis with plasmapheresis. On a chronic basis, some patients can be managed with periodic plasmapheresis alone. As with other indolent malignant lymphoid diseases, rituximab (375 mg/m² intravenously weekly for 4–8 weeks) has significant activity. However, a word of caution: the IgM often rises first after rituximab therapy before it falls. Combination therapy is recommended for advanced disease (see Table 39–3). *MYD88* is commonly mutated in Waldenström macroglobulinemia, and in patients with relapsed or refractory disease, the BTK inhibitor ibrutinib, at a dose of 420 mg daily, has shown significant activity with a 90% response rate and a 73% major response rate that can result in durable remissions. Bortezomib, lenalidomide, and bendamustine have also been shown to have activity in this disease. Autologous hematopoietic stem cell transplantation is reserved for relapsed or refractory patients.

▶ Prognosis

Waldenström macroglobulinemia is an indolent disease with a median survival rate of 5 years, and 10% of patients are alive at 15 years.

▶ When to Refer

All patients should be referred to a hematologist or an oncologist.

▶ When to Admit

Patients should be admitted for treatment of hyperviscosity syndrome.

Benevolo G et al. Current options to manage Waldenström's macroglobulinemia. Expert Rev Hematol. 2017 Jul;10(7):637–47. [PMID: 28592170]

Castillo JJ et al. Overall survival and competing risks of death in patients with Waldenström macroglobulinaemia: an analysis of the Surveillance, Epidemiology and End Results database. Br J Haematol. 2015 Apr;169(1):81–9. [PMID: 25521528]

Dimopoulos MA et al; INNOVATE Study Group and the European Consortium for Waldenström's Macroglobulinemia. Phase 3 trial of ibrutinib plus rituximab in Waldenström's macroglobulinemia. N Engl J Med. 2018 Jun 21;378(25):2399–410. [PMID: 29856685]

Oza A et al. Waldenström macroglobulinemia: prognosis and management. Blood Cancer J. 2015 Mar 27;5:e296. [PMID: 25815903]

Treon SP et al. Ibrutinib in previously treated Waldenström's macroglobulinemia. N Engl J Med. 2015 Apr 9;372(15):1430–40. [PMID: 25853747]

AMYLOIDOSIS

▶ ESSENTIALS OF DIAGNOSIS

▶ Congo red positive amyloid protein on tissue biopsy.
▶ Primary amyloid protein is kappa or lambda immunoglobulin light chain.
▶ Serum or urine (or both) light chain paraprotein.

▶ General Considerations

Amyloidosis is a rare condition whereby a protein abnormally deposits in tissue resulting in organ dysfunction. The propensity of a protein to be amyloidogenic is a consequence of disturbed translational or posttranslational protein folding and lack of consequential water solubility. The input of amyloid protein into tissues far exceeds its output, so amyloid build up inexorably proceeds to organ dysfunction and ultimately organ failure and premature death.

Amyloidosis is classified according to the type of amyloid protein deposited. The six main categories are **primary** (immunoglobulin light chain [AL]), **secondary** (serum protein A, produced in inflammatory conditions [AA]), **hereditary** (mutated transthyretin [TTR]; many others), **senile** (wild-type TTR; atrial natriuretic peptide; others), **dialysis-related** (beta-2-microglobulin, not filtered out by dialysis membranes [Abeta-2M]), and **LECT2** (associated with Latino patients). Amyloidosis is further classified as **localized** (amyloid deposits only in a single tissue type or organ) or, most common, **systemic** (widespread amyloid deposition).

▶ Clinical Findings

A. Symptoms and Signs

Patients with **localized amyloidosis** have symptoms and signs related to the affected single organ, such as hoarseness (vocal cords) or proptosis and visual disturbance (orbits). Patients with **systemic amyloidosis** have symptoms and signs of unexplained medical syndromes, including heart failure (infiltrative/restrictive cardiomyopathy), nephrotic syndrome, malabsorption and weight loss, hepatic dysfunction, autonomic insufficiency, carpal tunnel syndrome (often bilateral), and sensorimotor peripheral neuropathy. Other symptoms and signs include an enlarged tongue; waxy, rough plaques on skin; contusions (including the periorbital areas); cough or dyspnea; and disturbed deglutition. These symptoms and signs arise insidiously, and the diagnosis of amyloidosis is generally made late in the disease process.

B. Laboratory Findings

The diagnosis of amyloid protein requires a tissue biopsy that demonstrates deposition of a pink interstitial substance in the tissue with the hematoxylin and eosin stain. This protein stains red with Congo red and becomes an apple-green color when the light is polarized. Amyloid is a triple-stranded fibril composed of the amyloid protein, amyloid protein P, and glycosaminoglycan. The amyloid fibrils form beta-pleated sheets as demonstrated by electron microscopy. In primary amyloidosis, the amyloid protein is either the kappa or lambda immunoglobulin light chain.

When systemic amyloidosis is suspected, a blind aspiration of the abdominal fat pad will reveal amyloid two-thirds of the time. If the fat pad aspiration is unrevealing, then the affected organ needs biopsy. In 90% of patients with primary amyloidosis, analysis of the serum and urine will reveal a kappa or lambda light chain paraprotein by PEP, IFE, or free light chain assay; in the remainder, mass spectroscopy demonstrates light chain in the tissue biopsy. Lambda amyloid is more common than kappa amyloid, a relative proportion opposite from normal B-cell stoichiometry. Most patients with primary amyloidosis have a small excess of kappa- or lambda-restricted plasma cells in the bone marrow (but less than 10%). The bone marrow may or may not demonstrate interstitial amyloid deposition or amyloid in the blood vessels.

Patients with primary cardiac amyloidosis have an infiltrative cardiomyopathy with thick ventricular walls on echocardiogram that sometimes shows a specific speckling pattern. Paradoxically, QRS voltages are low on ECG. With renal amyloid, albuminuria is present, which can be in the nephrotic range. Late in renal involvement, kidney function decreases.

► Differential Diagnosis

Amyloidosis must be distinguished from MGUS and plasma cell myeloma or other malignant lymphoproliferative disorders with an associated paraprotein. Of note, 12% of patients with MGUS will convert to primary amyloidosis in a median of 9 years. One-fifth of patients who have primary amyloidosis will meet the diagnostic criteria for plasma cell myeloma; conversely, 5% of patients with plasma cell myeloma will have amyloid deposition of their paraprotein at diagnosis.

► Treatment

The treatment approach to primary amyloidosis closely resembles that of plasma cell myeloma. Prospective, randomized trials of plasma cell myeloma chemotherapy versus colchicine have demonstrated a survival benefit to chemotherapy. The goal is reduction of light chain production and deposition as a means to arrest progressive end-organ dysfunction. Active agents in primary amyloidosis include melphalan, cyclophosphamide, dexamethasone, lenalidomide, and bortezomib (see Table 39–3). The anti-CD38 monoclonal antibody daratumumab may have a role in treating this disorder. New antibodies are being developed that bind the deposited light chain and facilitate its breakage and dissolution. As in plasma cell myeloma, autologous hematopoietic stem cell transplantation after high-dose melphalan is used in patients with reasonable organ function and a good performance status. The treatment-related mortality, however, is higher in patients with primary amyloidosis than in plasma cell myeloma (6% vs 1%).

Some patients will demonstrate end-organ improvement after therapy. Agents are being developed that facilitate amyloid dissolution or correct protein folding abnormalities in the amyloid protein.

► Prognosis

Untreated primary amyloidosis is associated with progressive end-organ failure and premature death. There is no known cure for primary amyloidosis. Although virtually every tissue examined at autopsy will contain amyloid, patients with primary amyloidosis usually have one or two primary organs failing that clinically drive the presentation and prognosis. The cardiac biomarkers, B-type natriuretic peptide (BNP), N-terminal pro-BNP, and troponins T and I are prognostic in this disease regardless of overt clinical cardiac involvement. Historically, patients with predominantly cardiac or autonomic nerve presentations had survivals of 3–9 months, those with carpal tunnel syndrome or nephrosis had survivals of 1.5–3 years, and those with peripheral neuropathy had survivals of 5 years. These survivals are roughly doubled with plasma cell myeloma-like treatment. In those patients able to undergo autologous hematopoietic stem cell transplantation, the median survival approaches 5 years (and approaches 10 years for those achieving a complete hematologic remission).

► When to Refer

- All patients who have primary amyloidosis or in whom it is suspected should be referred to a hematologist or oncologist.
- All patients with hereditary amyloidosis should be referred to a hepatologist for consideration of liver transplantation.

► When to Admit

- Patients with systemic amyloidosis require hospitalization to treat exacerbations of end-organ failure, including heart, liver, or kidney.
- Patients with primary amyloidosis require hospitalization to undergo autologous hematopoietic stem cell transplantation.

Badar T et al. Recent advances in understanding and treating immunoglobulin light chain amyloidosis. F1000Res. 2018 Aug 29;7. [PMID: 30228867]

Gertz MA. Immunoglobulin light chain amyloidosis: 2016 update on diagnosis, prognosis, and treatment. Am J Hematol. 2016 Sep;91(9):447–56. [PMID: 27527836]

Zumbo G et al. New and developing therapies for AL amyloidosis. Expert Opin Pharmacother. 2017 Feb;18(2):139–49. [PMID: 28002971]

BLOOD TRANSFUSIONS

RED BLOOD CELL TRANSFUSIONS

Red blood cell transfusions are given to raise the hemoglobin levels in patients with anemia or to replace losses after acute bleeding episodes.

Preparations of Red Cells for Transfusion

Several types of preparations containing red blood cells are available.

A. Fresh Whole Blood

The advantage of whole blood for transfusion is the simultaneous presence of red blood cells, plasma, and fresh platelets. Fresh whole blood is not absolutely necessary, since all the above components are available separately. The major indications for use of whole blood are cardiac surgery or massive hemorrhage when more than 10 units of blood is required in a 24-hour period.

B. Packed Red Blood Cells

Packed red cells are the component most commonly used to raise the hemoglobin. Each unit has a volume of about 300 mL, of which approximately 200 mL consists of red blood cells. One unit of packed red cells will usually raise the hemoglobin by approximately 1 g/dL. Current guidelines recommend a transfusion "trigger" hemoglobin threshold of 7–8 g/dL (70–80 g/L) for hospitalized critically ill patients, those undergoing cardiothoracic surgery or repair of a hip fracture, those with upper gastrointestinal bleeding, and those with hematologic malignancy undergoing chemotherapy or hematopoietic cell transplant.

C. Leukocyte-Poor Blood

Most blood products are leukoreduced in-line during acquisition and are thus prospectively leukocyte-poor. Leukoreduced blood products reduce the incidence of leukoagglutination reactions, platelet alloimmunization, transfusion-related acute lung injury, and CMV exposure.

D. Autologous Packed Red Blood Cells

Patients scheduled for elective surgery may donate blood for autologous transfusion. These units may be stored for up to 35 days before freezing is necessary.

Compatibility Testing

Before transfusion, the recipient's and the donor's blood are typed and cross-matched to avoid hemolytic transfusion reactions. Although many antigen systems are present on red blood cells, only the ABO and Rh systems are specifically tested prior to all transfusions. The A and B antigens are the most important, because everyone who lacks one or both red cell antigens has IgM isoantibodies (called isoagglutinins) in his or her plasma against the missing antigen(s). The isoagglutinins activate complement and can cause rapid intravascular lysis of the incompatible red blood cells. In emergencies, type O/Rh-negative blood can be given to any recipient, but only packed cells should be given to minimize transfusion of donor plasma containing anti-A and anti-B antibodies.

The other important antigen routinely tested for is the D antigen of the Rh system. Approximately 15% of the population lacks this antigen. In patients lacking the antigen, anti-D antibodies are not naturally present, but the antigen

is highly immunogenic. A recipient whose red cells lack D and who receives D-positive blood may develop anti-D antibodies that can cause severe lysis of subsequent transfusions of D-positive red cells or reject a D-positive fetus.

Blood typing includes a cross-match assay of recipient serum for unusual alloantibodies directed against donor red blood cells by mixing recipient serum with panels of red blood cells representing commonly occurring minor red cell antigens. The screening is particularly important if the recipient has had previous transfusions or pregnancy.

Hemolytic Transfusion Reactions

The most severe hemolytic transfusion reactions are acute (temporally related to the transfusion), involving incompatible mismatches in the ABO system that are isoagglutinin-mediated. Most of these cases are due to clerical errors and mislabeled specimens. With current compatibility testing and double-check clerical systems, the risk of an acute hemolytic reaction is 1 in 76,000 transfused units of red blood cells. Death from acute hemolytic reaction occurs in 1 in 1.8 million transfused units. When hemolysis occurs, it is rapid and intravascular, releasing free hemoglobin into the plasma. The severity of these reactions depends on the dose of red blood cells given. The most severe reactions are those seen in surgical patients under anesthesia.

Delayed hemolytic transfusion reactions are caused by minor red blood cell antigen discrepancies and are typically less severe. The hemolysis usually takes place at a slower rate and is mediated by IgG alloantibodies causing extravascular red blood cell destruction. These transfusion reactions may be delayed for 5–10 days after transfusion. In such cases, the recipient has received red blood cells containing an immunogenic antigen, and in the time since transfusion, a new alloantibody has formed. The most common antigens involved in such reactions are Duffy, Kidd, Kell, and C and E loci of the Rh system. The current risk of a delayed hemolytic transfusion reaction is 1 in 6000 transfused units of red blood cells.

A. Symptoms and Signs

Major acute hemolytic transfusion reactions cause fever and chills, with backache and headache. In severe cases, there may be apprehension, dyspnea, hypotension, and cardiovascular collapse. Patients under general anesthesia will not manifest such symptoms, and the first indication may be tachycardia, generalized bleeding, or oliguria. *The transfusion must be stopped immediately.* In severe cases, acute DIC, acute kidney injury from tubular necrosis, or both can occur. Death occurs in 4% of acute hemolytic reactions due to ABO incompatibility. Delayed hemolytic transfusion reactions are usually without symptoms or signs.

B. Laboratory Findings

When an acute hemolytic transfusion episode is suspected, the identification of the recipient and of the transfusion product bag label should be rechecked. The transfusion product bag with its pilot tube must be returned to the blood bank, and a fresh sample of the recipient's blood must accompany the bag for retyping and re–cross-matching of donor and recipient blood samples. The hemoglobin will fail to rise by the expected amount. Coagulation studies may reveal evidence of acute kidney injury or acute DIC. The plasma-free hemoglobin in the recipient will be elevated resulting in hemoglobinuria.

In cases of delayed hemolytic reactions, there will be an unexpected drop in hemoglobin and an increase in the total and indirect bilirubins. The new offending alloantibody is easily detected in the patient's serum.

C. Treatment

If an acute hemolytic transfusion reaction is suspected, the transfusion should be stopped at once. The patient should be vigorously hydrated to prevent acute tubular necrosis. Forced diuresis with mannitol may help prevent or minimize acute kidney injury.

► Leukoagglutinin Reactions

Most transfusion reactions are not hemolytic but represent reactions to antigens present on transfused passenger leukocytes in patients who have been sensitized to leukocyte antigens through previous transfusions or pregnancy. Transfusion products relatively rich in leukocyte-rich plasma, especially platelets, are most likely to cause this. Moderate to severe leukoagglutinin reactions occur in 1% of red blood cell transfusions and 2% of platelet transfusions. Most commonly, fever and chills develop in patients within 12 hours after transfusion. In severe cases, cough and dyspnea may occur and the chest radiograph may show transient pulmonary infiltrates. Because no hemolysis is involved, the hemoglobin rises by the expected amount despite the reaction.

Leukoagglutinin reactions may respond to acetaminophen (500–650 mg orally) and diphenhydramine (25 mg orally or intravenously); corticosteroids, such as hydrocortisone (1 mg/kg intravenously), are also of value. Overall, leukoagglutination reactions are diminishing through the routine use of in-line leukotrapping during blood donation (ie, leukoreduced blood). Patients experiencing severe leukoagglutination episodes despite receiving leukoreduced blood transfusions should receive leukopoor or washed blood products.

► Hypersensitivity Reactions

Urticaria or bronchospasm may develop during or soon after a transfusion. These reactions are almost always due to exposure to allogeneic plasma proteins rather than to leukocytes. The risk is low enough that the routine use of antihistamine premedications has been eliminated before PRBC transfusions. However, a hypersensitivity reaction, including anaphylactic shock, may develop in patients who are IgA deficient because of antibodies to IgA in the patient's plasma directed against the IgA in the transfused blood product. Patients with such reactions may require transfusion of washed or even frozen red blood cells to avoid future severe reactions.

► Contaminated Blood

Blood products can be contaminated with bacteria. Platelets are especially prone to bacterial contamination because they cannot be refrigerated. Bacterial contamination occurs in 1 of every 30,000 red blood cell donations and 1 of every 5000 platelet donations. Receipt of a blood product contaminated with gram-positive bacteria will cause fever and bacteremia, but rarely causes a sepsis syndrome. Receipt of a blood product contaminated with gram-negative bacteria often causes septic shock, acute DIC, and acute kidney injury due to the transfused endotoxin and is usually fatal. Strategies to reduce bacterial contamination include enhanced venipuncture site skin cleansing, diverting of the first few milliliters of donated blood, use of single-donor blood products (as opposed to pooled-donor products), and point-of-care rapid bacterial screening in order to discard questionable units. Blood products infused with psoralen and then exposed to UVA light will have no living organisms in them, but add cost to acquisition of the blood product. The current risk of a septic transfusion reaction from a culture-negative unit of single-donor platelets (not psoralen treated) is 1 in 60,000. In any patient who may have received contaminated blood, the recipient and the donor blood bag should both be cultured, and antibiotics should be given immediately to the recipient.

► Infectious Diseases Transmitted Through Transfusion

Despite the use of only volunteer blood donors and the routine screening of blood, transfusion-associated viral diseases remain a problem. All blood products (red blood cells, platelets, plasma, cryoprecipitate) can transmit viral diseases. All blood donors are screened with questionnaires designed to detect (and therefore reject) donors at high risk for transmitting infectious diseases. All blood is screened for hepatitis B surface antigen, antibody to hepatitis B core antigen and syphilis, antibodies to HIV-1 and HIV-2 and NAT (nucleic acid amplification) for HIV, antibody to hepatitis C virus (HCV) and NAT for hepatitis C, antibody to human T-cell lymphotropic/leukemia virus (HTLV), and NAT for West Nile virus. Zika virus contamination is screened for by donor questionnaire but the routine use of an FDA-approved detection test has not been uniformly adopted to screen donated blood. It is recommended that blood donors get screened once for antibodies against *Trypanosoma cruzi*, the infectious agent that causes Chagas disease (and if negative, no further screening for additional blood donations).

With improved screening, the risk of posttransfusion hepatitis has steadily decreased after the receipt of screened "negative" blood products. The risk of acquiring hepatitis B is about 1 in 200,000 transfused units in the United States (vs about 1 in 21,000 to 1 in 600 transfused units in Asia). The risk of hepatitis C acquisition is 1 in 1.5 to 2 million transfused units in the United States. The risk of HIV acquisition is 1 in 2 million transfused units. Unscreened *but* leukoreduced blood products appear to be equivalent to CMV screened-negative blood products in terms of the risk of CMV transmission to a CMV-seronegative recipient.

Transfusion Graft-Versus-Host Disease

Allogeneic passenger lymphocytes within transfused blood products will engraft in some recipients and mount an alloimmune attack against tissues expressing discrepant HLA antigens causing graft-versus-host disease (GVHD). The symptoms and signs of transfusion-associated GVHD include fever, rash, diarrhea, hepatitis, lymphadenopathy, and severe pancytopenia. The outcome is usually fatal. Transfusion-associated GVHD occurs most often in recipients with immune defects, malignant lymphoproliferative disorders, solid tumors being treated with chemotherapy or immunotherapy, treatment with immunosuppressive medications (especially purine analogs such as fludarabine), or older patients undergoing cardiac surgery. HIV infection alone does not increase the risk. The use of leukoreduced blood products is inadequate to prevent transfusion-associated GVHD. This complication can be avoided by irradiating blood products (25 Gy or more) to prevent lymphocyte proliferation in blood products given to recipients at high risk for transfusion-associated GVHD.

Transfusion-Related Acute Lung Injury

Transfusion-related acute lung injury (TRALI) occurs in 1 in every 5000 transfused units of blood products. TRALI is clinically defined as noncardiogenic pulmonary edema after a blood product transfusion without other explanation. Transfused surgical and critically ill patients seem most susceptible. It has been associated with allogeneic antibodies in the donor plasma component that bind to recipient leukocyte antigens, including HLA antigens and other granulocyte- and monocyte-specific antigens (such as HNA-1a, -1b, -2a, and -3a). In 20% of cases, no antileukocyte antibodies are identified raising the concern that bioactive lipids or other substances that accumulate while the blood product is in storage can also mediate TRALI in susceptible recipients. Ten to 20% of female blood donors and 1–5% of male blood donors have antileukocyte antibodies in their serum. The risk of TRALI is reduced through the use of male-only plasma donors, when possible. There is no specific treatment for TRALI, only supportive care.

PLATELET TRANSFUSIONS

Platelet transfusions are indicated in cases of thrombocytopenia due to decreased platelet production. They are of some use in immune thrombocytopenia when active bleeding is evident, but the clearance of transfused platelets is rapid as they are exposed to the same pathophysiologic forces as the recipient's endogenous platelets. The risk of spontaneous bleeding rises when the platelet count falls to less than 80,000/mcL (80 × 10^9/L), and the risk of life-threatening spontaneous bleeding increases when the platelet count is less than 5000/mcL (5 × 10^9/L). Because of this, prophylactic platelet transfusions are often given at these very low levels, usually when less than 10,000/mcL (10 × 10^9/L). Platelet transfusions are also given prior to invasive procedures or surgery in thrombocytopenic patients, and the goal is often to raise the platelet count to 50,000/mcL (50 × 10^9/L) or more.

Platelets for transfusion are most commonly derived from single-donor apheresis collections (roughly the equivalent to the platelets recovered from six donations of whole blood). A single donor unit of platelets should raise the platelet count by 50,000 to 60,000 platelets per mcL (50–60 × 10^9/L) in a transfusion-naïve recipient without hypersplenism or ongoing platelet consumptive disorder. Transfused platelets typically last for 2 or 3 days. Platelet transfusion responses may be suboptimal with poor platelet increments and short platelet survival times. This may be due to one of several causes, including fever, sepsis, hypersplenism, DIC, large body habitus, low platelet dose in the transfusion, or platelet alloimmunization (from prior transfusions, prior pregnancy or prior organ transplantation). Many, but not all, alloantibodies causing platelet destruction are directed at HLA antigens. Patients requiring long periods of platelet transfusion support should be monitored to document adequate responses to transfusions so that the most appropriate product can be used. If random platelet transfusions prove inadequate, then the patient should be cross-matched with potential donors who might prove better able to provide adequate platelet-transfusion increments and platelet survival. Patients requiring ongoing platelet transfusions who become alloimmunized may benefit from HLA-matched platelets derived from either volunteer donors or family members.

TRANSFUSION OF PLASMA COMPONENTS

Fresh frozen plasma (FFP) is available in units of approximately 200 mL. FFP contains normal levels of all coagulation factors (about 1 unit/mL of each factor). FFP is used to correct coagulation factor deficiencies and to treat thrombotic thrombocytopenia purpura or other thrombotic microangiopathies. FFP is also used to correct or prevent coagulopathy in trauma patients receiving massive transfusion of PRBC. An FFP:PRBC ratio of 1:2 or more is associated with improved survival in trauma patients receiving massive transfusions, regardless of the presence of a coagulopathy.

Cryoprecipitate is made from fresh plasma by cooling the plasma to 4°C and collecting the precipitate. One unit of cryoprecipitate has a volume of approximately 15–20 mL and contains approximately 250 mg of fibrinogen and between 80 and 100 units of factor VIII and von Willebrand factor. Cryoprecipitate is most commonly used to supplement fibrinogen in cases of acquired hypofibrinogenemia (eg, DIC) or in rare instances of congenital hypofibrinogenemia. One unit of cryoprecipitate will raise the fibrinogen level by about 8 mg/dL (0.24 mcmol/L). Cryoprecipitate is sometimes used to temporarily correct the acquired qualitative platelet dysfunction associated with kidney disease.

Bryan AW Jr et al. Plasma transfusion demystified: a review of the key factors influencing the response to plasma transfusion. Lab Med. 2017 May 1;48(2):108–12. [PMID: 28444398]

Fasano RM et al. Platelet transfusion goals in oncology patients. Hematology Am Soc Hematol Educ Program. 2015;2015: 462–70. [PMID: 26637759]

Goodnough LT et al. Blood transfusion therapy. Med Clin North Am. 2017 Mar;101(2):431–47. [PMID: 28189180]

Hoeks MPA et al. Impact of red blood cell transfusion strategies in haemato-oncological patients: a systematic review and meta-analysis. Br J Haematol. 2017 Jul;178(1):137–51. [PMID: 28589623]

Kaufman RM et al. Platelet transfusion: a clinical practice guideline from the AABB. Ann Intern Med. 2015 Feb 3;162(3): 205–13. [PMID: 25383671]

Marfin AA et al. Granulocyte transfusion therapy. J Intensive Care Med. 2015 Feb;30(2):79–88. [PMID: 23920161]

Tariket S et al. Transfusion-related acute lung injury: transfusion, platelets and biological response modifiers. Expert Rev Hematol. 2016 May;9(5):497–508. [PMID: 26855042]

Disorders of Hemostasis, Thrombosis, & Antithrombotic Therapy

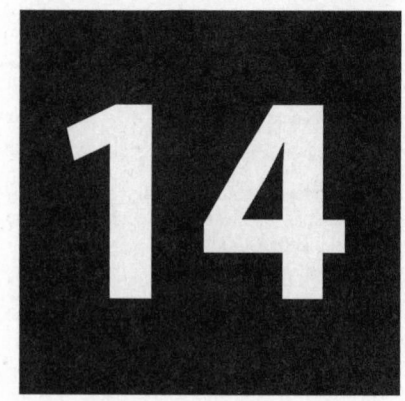

Andrew D. Leavitt, MD

Tracy Minichiello, MD

To evaluate patients for defects of hemostasis, the clinical context must be considered carefully (Table 14–1). Heritable defects are suggested by bleeding that begins in infancy or childhood, is recurrent, and occurs at multiple anatomic sites, although other patterns of presentation are possible. Acquired disorders of hemostasis typically are associated with bleeding that begins later in life and may relate to introduction of medications (eg, agents that affect platelet activity) or to onset of underlying medical conditions (such as kidney disease, liver disease, myelodysplasia, aortic stenosis, prosthetic aortic valve, myeloproliferative neoplasms), or may be idiopathic (acquired hemophilia A, acquired von Willebrand disease). Importantly, however, a sufficient hemostatic challenge (such as major trauma) may produce excessive bleeding even in individuals with normal hemostasis. A personal history of hemostatic challenges (eg, circumcision, trauma, injury during youth sports, tooth extractions, motor vehicle accidents, prior surgery, and pregnancy and delivery) and a family history of bleeding are critical when evaluating someone for a possible bleeding disorder.

PLATELET DISORDERS

THROMBOCYTOPENIA

Selected causes of thrombocytopenia are shown in Table 14–2. The age of the patient and presence of comorbid conditions can help direct the diagnostic workup.

The risk of clinically relevant spontaneous bleeding (including petechial hemorrhage and bruising) does not typically increase appreciably until the platelet count falls below 10,000–20,000/mcL, although patients with dysfunctional platelets or local vascular defects can bleed with higher platelet counts. Suggested platelet counts to prevent spontaneous bleeding or to provide adequate hemostasis around the time of invasive procedures are found in Table 14–3. However, most medical centers develop their own local guidelines to have a consistent approach to such complex situations.

DECREASED PLATELET PRODUCTION

1. Bone Marrow Failure

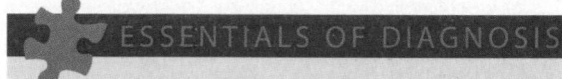

► Bone marrow failure states may be congenital or acquired.

► Most congenital marrow failure disorders present in childhood.

▶ General Considerations

Congenital conditions that cause thrombocytopenia include amegakaryocytic thrombocytopenia, the thrombocytopenia-absent radius syndrome, and Wiskott-Aldrich syndrome; these disorders usually feature isolated thrombocytopenia, whereas patients with Fanconi anemia and dyskeratosis congenita typically include cytopenias in other blood cell lineages. Mutations in genes (*FLI1, MYH9, GATA1, ETV6,* among others) that cause thrombocytopenia are being identified.

Acquired causes of bone marrow failure (see Chapter 13) leading to thrombocytopenia include, but are not limited to, acquired aplastic anemia, myelodysplastic syndrome (MDS), acquired amegakaryocytic thrombocytopenia (albeit a rare disorder), alcohol, and drugs. Unlike aplastic anemia, MDS is more common among older patients.

▶ Clinical Findings

See Chapter 13 for symptoms and signs of aplastic anemia. Acquired aplastic anemia typically presents with reductions in multiple blood cell lineages, and the CBC reveals pancytopenia (anemia, thrombocytopenia, and neutropenia). A bone marrow biopsy is required for diagnosis and reveals marked hypocellularity. MDS also presents as cytopenias and can have pancytopenia, but the marrow typically demonstrates hypercellularity. The presence of macrocytosis, ringed

Table 14–1. Evaluation of the bleeding patient.

Necessary Component of Evaluation	Diagnostic Correlate
Location	
Mucocutaneous (bruises, petechiae, gingivae, nosebleeds, GI, GU)	Suggests qualitative/quantitative platelet defects; vWD
Joints, soft tissue	Suggests disorders of coagulation factors
Onset	
Infancy/childhood	Suggests heritable condition
Adulthood	Suggests milder heritable condition or acquired defect of hemostasis (eg, ITP, medication, acquired factor VIII deficiency; acquired vWD)
Clinical Context	
Postsurgical	Anatomic/surgical defect must be ruled out
Pregnancy	vWD, HELLP syndrome, ITP, acquired factor VIII inhibitor
Sepsis	May indicate DIC
Exposure to anticoagulants	Rule out excessive anticoagulation
Personal History[1]	
Absent	Suggests acquired rather than congenital defect, or anatomic/surgical defect (if applicable)
Present	Suggests established acquired defect or congenital disorder
Family History	
Absent	Suggests acquired defect or no defect of hemostasis
Present	May signify hemophilia A or B, vWD, other heritable bleeding disorders

[1]Includes evaluation of prior spontaneous bleeding, as well as excessive bleeding with circumcision, menses, dental extractions, trauma, minor procedures (eg, endoscopy, biopsies), and major procedures (surgery).

DIC, disseminated intravascular coagulation; GI, gastrointestinal; GU, genitourinary; HELLP, hemolysis, elevated liver enzymes, low platelets; ITP, immune thrombocytopenia; vWD, von Willebrand disease.

sideroblasts on iron staining of the bone marrow aspirate, dysplasia of hematopoietic elements, or cytogenetic abnormalities (especially monosomy 5 or 7 and trisomy 8) is more suggestive of MDS.

▶ Differential Diagnosis

Adult patients with acquired amegakaryocytic thrombocytopenia (rare) have isolated thrombocytopenia and reduced or absent megakaryocytes in the bone marrow, which along with failure to respond to immunomodulatory

Table 14–2. Selected causes of thrombocytopenia.

> **Decreased production of platelets**
>   Congenital bone marrow failure (eg, Fanconi anemia, Wiskott-Aldrich syndrome; congenital amegakaryocytic thrombocytopenia)
>   Acquired bone marrow failure (eg, aplastic anemia, myelodysplasia, leukemia)
>   Exposure to chemotherapy, irradiation, medications (https://ouhsc.edu/platelets/ditp.html)
>   Marrow infiltration (neoplastic, infectious)
>   Nutritional (deficiency of vitamin B_{12}, folate)
>   Other: HIV infection, alcohol
> **Increased destruction of platelets**
>   Immune thrombocytopenia (primary)
>   Immune thrombocytopenia (secondary), including drug-induced or related to lymphoproliferative disorders (ie, CLL), hepatitis C virus, Epstein-Barr virus, or HIV
>   Heparin-induced thrombocytopenia
>   Thrombotic microangiopathy
>   Disseminated intravascular coagulation
>   Posttransfusion purpura
>   Neonatal alloimmune thrombocytopenia
>   Mechanical (aortic valvular dysfunction; extracorporeal bypass)
>   von Willebrand disease, type 2B
>   Hemophagocytosis
> **Increased sequestration of platelets**
>   Hypersplenism (eg, related to cirrhosis, myeloproliferative disorders, lymphoma)
> **Other conditions causing thrombocytopenia**
>   Gestational thrombocytopenia
>   Bernard-Soulier syndrome, gray platelet syndrome, May-Hegglin anomaly
>   Pseudothrombocytopenia

CLL, chronic lymphocytic leukemia.

regimens typically administered in immune thrombocytopenia (ITP), distinguishes them from patients with ITP.

▶ Treatment

A. Congenital Conditions

Treatment is varied but may include blood product support, blood cell growth factors, androgens and, in some cases, allogeneic hematopoietic stem cell transplantation.

Table 14–3. Desired platelet count ranges.

Clinical Scenario	Platelet Count (/mcL)
Prevention of spontaneous mucocutaneous bleeding	> 10,000–20,000
Insertion of central venous catheters	> 20,000–50,000[1]
Administration of therapeutic anticoagulation	> 30,000–50,000
Minor surgery and selected invasive procedures[2]	> 50,000–80,000
Major surgery	> 80,000–100,000

[1]A platelet target within the higher range of the reference is required for tunneled catheters.
[2]Such as endoscopy with biopsy.

B. Acquired Conditions

Patients with severe aplastic anemia are treated with immunosuppressive therapy or allogeneic hematopoietic stem cell transplantation (see Chapter 13).

Treatment of thrombocytopenia due to MDS, if clinically significant bleeding is present or if the risk of bleeding is high, is limited to chronic transfusion of platelets in most instances (Table 14–3). Additional treatment is discussed in Chapter 13.

Townsley DM et al. Eltrombopag added to standard immunosuppression for aplastic anemia. N Engl J Med. 2017 Apr 20; 376(16):1540–50. [PMID: 28423296]

2. Bone Marrow Infiltration

Replacement of the normal bone marrow elements by leukemic cells, myeloma, lymphoma, or other nonhematologic tumors, or by infections (such as mycobacterial disease or ehrlichiosis) may cause thrombocytopenia; however, abnormalities in other blood cell lines are usually present. These entities are easily diagnosed after examining the bone marrow biopsy and aspirate or determining the infecting organism from an aspirate specimen, and they often lead to a leukoerythroblastic peripheral blood smear (left-shifted myeloid lineage cells, nucleated red blood cells, and teardrop-shaped red blood cells). Treatment of thrombocytopenia is directed at eradication of the underlying infiltrative disorder, but platelet transfusion may be required if clinically significant bleeding is present.

3. Chemotherapy & Irradiation

Chemotherapeutic agents and irradiation may lead to thrombocytopenia by direct toxicity to megakaryocytes, hematopoietic progenitor cells, or both. The severity and duration of chemotherapy-induced depressions in the platelet count are determined by the specific regimen used, although the platelet count typically resolves more slowly following a chemotherapeutic insult than does neutropenia or anemia, especially if multiple cycles of treatment have been given. Until recovery occurs, patients may be supported with transfused platelets if bleeding is present or the risk of bleeding is high (Table 14–3). Initial studies suggest that that platelet growth factors, such as eltrombopag and romiplostim, may help prevent chemotherapy-induced thrombocytopenia and allow patients to receive their full chemotherapy doses on schedule.

Soff GA et al. Romiplostim for Chemotherapy-Induced Thrombocytopenia (CIT). Results of a phase 2 trial. Blood. 2017;130(Suppl 1):289.
Wang Z et al. Recombinant human thrombopoietin (rh-TPO) for the prevention of severe thrombocytopenia induced by high-dose cytarabine: a prospective, randomized, self-controlled study. Leuk Lymphoma. 2018 Dec;59(12):2821–8. [PMID: 29909708]

4. Nutritional Deficiencies

Thrombocytopenia, typically in concert with anemia, may be observed with a deficiency of folate (that may accompany alcoholism) or vitamin B_{12} (concomitant neurologic findings

may be manifest). In addition, thrombocytopenia can occur in very severe iron deficiency, albeit rarely, while thrombocytosis is far more common. Replacing the deficient vitamin or mineral results in improvement in the platelet count.

Briani C et al. Cobalamin deficiency: clinical picture and radiological findings. Nutrients. 2013 Nov 15;5(11):4521–39. [PMID: 24248213]

5. Cyclic Thrombocytopenia

Cyclic thrombocytopenia is a rare disorder that produces cyclic oscillations of the platelet count, usually with a periodicity of 3–6 weeks. The pathophysiologic mechanism responsible for the condition is unclear. Severe thrombocytopenia and bleeding typically occur at the platelet nadir. Oral contraceptive medications, androgens, azathioprine, and thrombopoietic growth factors have been used successfully in the management of cyclic thrombocytopenia.

INCREASED PLATELET DESTRUCTION

1. Immune Thrombocytopenia

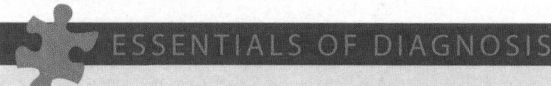

ESSENTIALS OF DIAGNOSIS

- ▶ Isolated thrombocytopenia (rule out pseudo-thrombocytopenia by review of peripheral smear).
- ▶ Assess for any new causative medications and HIV, hepatitis B, and hepatitis C infections.
- ▶ ITP is a diagnosis of exclusion.

▶ General Considerations

ITP is an autoimmune condition in which pathogenic antibodies bind platelets, accelerating their clearance from the circulation. Many patients with ITP also lack appropriate compensatory platelet production, thought, at least in part, to reflect the antibody's effect on megakaryocytopoiesis and thrombopoiesis. ITP is primary (idiopathic) in most adult patients, although it can be secondary, (ie, associated with connective tissue disease, such as systemic lupus erythematosus; lymphoproliferative disease, such as lymphoma; medications; and infections, such as hepatitis C virus and HIV infections). Antiplatelet antibody targets include glycoproteins IIb/IIIa and Ib/IX on the platelet membrane, although antibodies are demonstrable in only two-thirds of patients. In addition to production of antiplatelet antibodies, HIV and hepatitis C virus may lead to thrombocytopenia through additional mechanisms (for instance, by direct suppression of platelet production [HIV] and cirrhosis-related decreased TPO production and secondary splenomegaly [hepatitis C virus]).

▶ Clinical Findings

A. Symptoms and Signs

Mucocutaneous bleeding may be present, depending on the platelet count. Clinically relevant spontaneous bruising, epistaxis, gingival bleeding, or other types of hemorrhage generally do not occur until the platelet count has fallen below 10,000–20,000/mcL. Individuals with secondary ITP (such as due to collagen vascular disease, HIV or HCV infection, or lymphoproliferative malignancy) may have additional disease-specific findings.

B. Laboratory Findings

Typically, patients have isolated thrombocytopenia. If bleeding has occurred, anemia may also be present. Hepatitis B and C viruses and HIV infections should be excluded by serologic testing. Bone marrow should be examined in patients with unexplained cytopenias in two or more lineages, in patients older than 40 years with isolated thrombocytopenia, or in those who do not respond to primary ITP-specific therapy. A bone marrow biopsy is not necessary in all cases to make an ITP diagnosis in younger patients. Megakaryocyte morphologic abnormalities and hypocellularity or hypercellularity are not characteristic of ITP. ITP patients often have increased numbers of bone marrow megakaryocytes. If there are clinical findings suggestive of a lymphoproliferative

malignancy, a CT scan should be performed. In the absence of such findings, otherwise asymptomatic patients younger than 40 years with unexplained isolated thrombocytopenia of recent onset may be considered to have ITP. *Helicobacter pylori* infections can sometimes cause isolated thrombocytopenia.

▶ Treatment

Individuals with platelet counts less than 25,000–30,000/mcL or those with significant bleeding should be treated; the remainder may be monitored serially for progression, but that is a patient-specific decision. The mainstay of initial treatment of new-onset primary ITP is a short course of corticosteroids with or without intravenous immunoglobulin (IVIG) or anti-D (WinRho) (Figure 14–1). Response to corticosteroids is generally seen within 3–7 days of initiating treatment, with responses to IVIG typically seen in 24–36 hours. Platelet transfusions may be given concomitantly if active bleeding is present. Adding the anti-B cell monoclonal antibody rituximab to corticosteroids as first-line treatment may improve the initial response rate, but it is associated with increased toxicity and is not regarded as

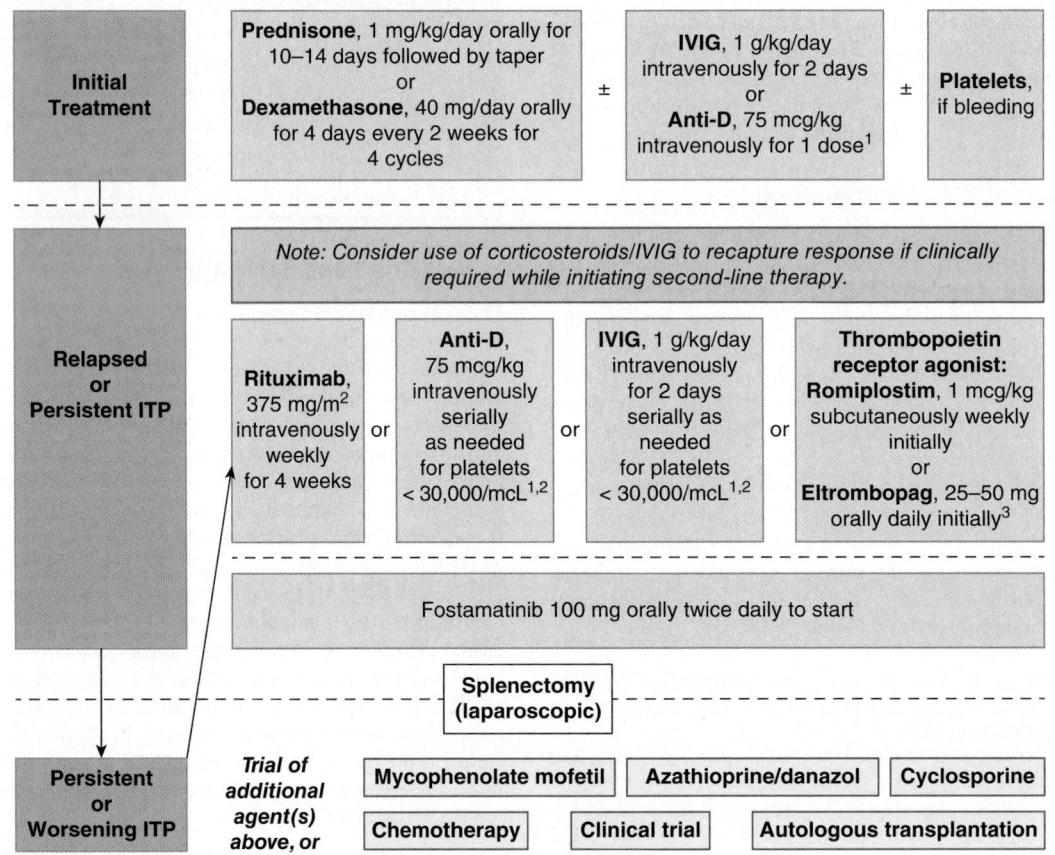

[1]Use in non-splenectomized, Rh blood type–positive, non-anemic patients only.
[2]May need to repeat infusion every 2–6 weeks to maintain platelet response.
[3]Recommended starting dose in Asians is 25 mg daily.

▲ **Figure 14–1.** Management of immune thrombocytopenia (ITP), a simplified overview. **Note:** All patients with ITP need to be managed by a hematologist because of the nuanced decision making required.

standard first-line therapy in most centers. Short course of high-dose dexamethasone is also an option for initial treatment.

Although over two-thirds of patients with ITP respond to initial treatment with oral corticosteroids, most relapse following reduction of the corticosteroid dose. Patients with a persistent platelet count less than 30,000/mcL or clinically significant bleeding are appropriate candidates for second-line treatments (Figure 14–1). These treatments are chosen empirically, bearing in mind potential toxicities and patient preference. IVIG or anti-D (WinRho) temporarily increases platelet counts (duration, up to 3 weeks, rarely longer), although serial IVIG or anti-D treatment (platelet counts less than 30,000/mcL) may allow adult patients to delay or avoid splenectomy. Rituximab leads to clinical responses in about 50% of adults with corticosteroid-refractory chronic ITP, which decreases to about 20% at 5 years. The TPO-mimetics romiplostim (administered subcutaneously weekly) and eltrombopag (taken orally daily) are approved for use in adult patients with chronic ITP who have not responded durably to corticosteroids, IVIG, or splenectomy and are typically taken indefinitely to maintain the platelet response, and they can be used as second-line therapy. Splenectomy has a durable response rate of over 50% and may be considered for cases of severe thrombocytopenia that fail to respond durably to initial treatment or are refractory to second-line agents; patients should receive pneumococcal, *Haemophilus influenzae* type b, and meningococcal vaccination at least 2 weeks before therapeutic splenectomy. If available, laparoscopic splenectomy is preferred. The Syk inhibitor fostamatinib represents a novel mechanism of action to treat ITP patients who do not respond to corticosteroids, TPO-mimetics, or rituximab. Additional treatments for ITP are found in Figure 14–1.

The goals of management of pregnancy-associated ITP are a platelet count of 10,000–30,000/mcL in the first trimester, greater than 30,000/mcL during the second or third trimester, and greater than 50,000/mcL prior to cesarean section or vaginal delivery. Moderate-dose oral prednisone or intermittent IVIG infusions are standard. Splenectomy is reserved for failure to respond to these therapies and may be performed in the first or second trimester. Management requires close interaction between obstetrician and hematologist.

For thrombocytopenia associated with HIV or hepatitis C virus, effective treatment of either infection leads to an amelioration of thrombocytopenia in most cases; refractory thrombocytopenia may be treated with infusion of IVIG or anti-D (HIV and hepatitis C virus), splenectomy (HIV), or interferon-alpha or eltrombopag (hepatitis C virus, including eradication). Treatment with corticosteroids is not recommended in hepatitis C virus infection. Occasionally, ITP treatment response is impaired due to *H pylori* infection, which should be ruled out in the appropriate situation.

► When to Refer

All patients with ITP should be referred to a hematologist for evaluation at the time of diagnosis.

► When to Admit

Patients with major hemorrhage or very severe thrombocytopenia associated with bleeding should be admitted and monitored in-hospital until the platelet count has stably risen to more than 20,000–30,000/mcL and hemodynamic stability has been achieved.

Bussel J et al. Fostamatinib for the treatment of adult persistent and chronic immune thrombocytopenia: results of two phase 3, randomized, placebo-controlled trials. Am J Hematol. 2018 Jul; 93(7):921–30. [PMID: 29696684]

Chaturvedi S et al. Splenectomy for immune thrombocytopenia: down but not out. Blood. 2018 Mar 15;131(11):1172–82. [PMID: 29295846]

Kuter DJ et al. TPO concentrations and response to romiplostim. Am J Hematol. 2014 Dec;89(12):1155–6. [PMID: 25132329]

Neunert C et al. Severe bleeding events in adults and children with primary immune thrombocytopenia: a systematic review. J Thromb Haemost. 2015 Mar;13(3):457–64. [PMID: 25495497]

Yang R et al. Therapeutic options for adult patients with previously treated immune thrombocytopenia—a systematic review and network meta-analysis. Hematology. 2019 Dec; 24(1):290–9. [PMID: 30661482]

2. Thrombotic Microangiopathy

ESSENTIALS OF DIAGNOSIS

► Microangiopathic hemolytic anemia and thrombocytopenia, without another plausible explanation, are sufficient for a presumptive diagnosis of thrombotic microangiopathy (TMA).

► Fever, neurologic abnormalities, and kidney disease may occur concurrently but are not required for diagnosis.

► Kidney dysfunction is more common and more severe in hemolytic-uremic syndrome (HUS).

► General Considerations

The TMAs include, but are not limited to, thrombotic thrombocytopenic purpura (TTP) and HUS. These disorders are characterized by thrombocytopenia due to the incorporation of platelets into fibrin thrombi in the microvasculature, and microangiopathic hemolytic anemia, which results from shearing of erythrocytes in fibrin networks in the microcirculation.

In idiopathic TTP, autoantibodies against ADAMTS-13 (a disintegrin and metalloproteinase with thrombospondin type 1 repeat, member 13), also known as the von Willebrand factor cleaving protease (vWFCP), lead to accumulation of ultra-large von Willebrand factor (vWF) multimers. The ultra-large multimers bridge and aggregate platelets in the absence of hemostatic triggers, which in turn leads to the vessel obstruction and various organ dysfunctions seen in TTP. In some cases of pregnancy-associated TMA, an antibody to ADAMTS-13 is present. In contrast, the activity of the ADAMTS-13 in congenital TTP is decreased due to a mutation in the gene encoding the molecule. Classic HUS, called Shiga toxin–mediated HUS, is thought to be secondary to toxin-mediated endothelial damage and is often contracted through the ingestion of undercooked ground beef contaminated with *Escherichia coli* (especially types O157:H7 or O145).

Complement-mediated HUS (formerly called atypical HUS) is not related to Shiga toxin. Patients with complement-mediated HUS often have genetic defects in proteins that regulate complement activity. Damage to endothelial cells—such as the damage that occurs in endemic HUS due to presence of toxins from *E coli* (especially type O157:H7 or O145) or in the setting of cancer, hematopoietic stem cell transplantation, or HIV infection—may also lead to TMA. Certain drugs (eg, cyclosporine, quinine, ticlopidine, clopidogrel, mitomycin C, and bleomycin) are associated with the development of TMA, possibly by promoting injury to endothelial cells, although inhibitory antibodies to ADAMTS-13 have been demonstrated in some cases.

▶ Clinical Findings

A. Symptoms and Signs

Microangiopathic hemolytic anemia and thrombocytopenia are presenting signs in all patients with TTP and most patients with HUS; in a subset of patients with HUS, the platelet count remains in the normal range. Only approximately 25% of patients with TMA manifest all components of the original pentad of findings (microangiopathic hemolytic anemia, thrombocytopenia, fever, kidney disease, and

neurologic system abnormalities) (Table 14–4). Most patients (especially children) with HUS have a recent or current diarrheal illness, often bloody. Neurologic manifestations, including headache, somnolence, delirium, seizures, paresis, and coma, may result from deposition of microthrombi in the cerebral vasculature.

B. Laboratory Findings

Laboratory features of TMA include those associated with microangiopathic hemolytic anemia (anemia, elevated lactate dehydrogenase [LD], elevated indirect bilirubin, decreased haptoglobin, reticulocytosis, schistocytes on the blood smear, and a negative direct antiglobulin test); thrombocytopenia; elevated creatinine; positive stool culture for *E coli* O157:H7 or stool assays for Shiga toxin; reductions in ADAMTS-13 activity with the presence (acquired TTP) or absence (inherited TTP) of ADAMTS-13 inhibitor; and mutations of genes encoding complement proteins (complement-mediated HUS; specialized laboratory assessment). Routine coagulation studies (prothrombin time [PT], activated partial thromboplastin time [aPTT], fibrinogen) are within the normal range in most patients with TTP or HUS.

▶ Treatment

Immediate administration of plasma exchange is essential in most cases because the TTP mortality rate is more than 95% without treatment. With the exception of children or adults with endemic diarrhea-associated HUS, who

Table 14–4. Presentation and management of thrombotic microangiopathies.

	TTP	Complement-Mediated HUS	Shiga Toxin–Mediated HUS
Patient population	Adults	Children (occasionally adults)	Usually children, often following bloody diarrhea
Pathogenesis	Acquired auto-antibody to ADAMTS-13	Some cases: heritable deficiency in function of complement regulatory proteins	Bacterial (such as enterotoxogenic *Escherichia coli*; Shiga toxin)
Thrombocytopenia	Typically severe, except in very early clinical course	Variable	May be mild/absent in a minority of patients
Fever	Typical	Variable	Atypical
Kidney disease	Typical, but may be mild	Typical	Typical
Neurologic impairment	Variable	Less than half of cases	Less than half of cases
Laboratory investigation	Decreased activity of ADAMTS-13; inhibitor usually identified	Defects in complement regulatory proteins	Typically normal ADAMTS-13 activity Positive stool culture for *E coli* 0157:H7 or detectable antibody to Shiga toxin
Management	TPE Hemodialysis for severe renal impairment Caplacizumab (selected patients) Platelet transfusions contraindicated unless TPE underway	Immediate TPE initially in most cases Eculizumab Supportive care Hemodialysis for severe renal impairment	Hemodialysis for severe kidney impairment Supportive care TPE rarely beneficial (exception: selected cases in adults)

ADAMTS-13, a disintegrin and metalloproteinase with a thrombospondin type 1 motif, member 13; HUS, hemolytic-uremic syndrome; TPE, therapeutic plasma exchange; TTP, thrombotic thrombocytopenic purpura.

generally recover with supportive care only, plasma exchange must be initiated as soon as the diagnosis of TMA is suspected and in all cases of TTP. Plasma exchange usually is administered once daily until the platelet count and LD have returned to normal for at least 2 days, after which the frequency of treatments may be tapered slowly while the platelet count and LD are monitored for relapse. In cases of insufficient response to once-daily plasma exchange, twice-daily treatments can be considered. Fresh frozen plasma (FFP) may be administered if immediate access to plasma exchange is not available or in cases of familial TMA. *Platelet transfusions are contraindicated* in the treatment of TMA due to reports of worsening TMA, possibly due to propagation of platelet-rich microthrombi. In cases of documented life-threatening bleeding, however, platelet transfusions may be given slowly and after plasma exchange is underway. Red blood cell transfusions may be administered in cases of clinically significant anemia. Hemodialysis should be considered for patients with significant kidney injury. Caplacizumab, an anti–von Willebrand factor (vWF) antibody that blocks the interaction between vWF and platelets, can reduce the time to platelet count normalization and thrombosis during treatment, and its role in TTP management is still being determined.

In cases of TTP relapse following initial treatment, plasma exchange should be reinstituted. If ineffective, or in cases of primary refractoriness, second-line treatments including rituximab (which has shown efficacy when administered preemptively in selected cases of relapsing TTP), corticosteroids, IVIG, vincristine, cyclophosphamide, and splenectomy should be used. Since idiopathic TTP is an autoimmune disorder (antibody inhibitor to ADAMTS-13), immunosuppression, often with rituximab, is often needed to prevent or reduce relapse events.

Cases of complement-mediated HUS may respond to plasma infusion initially; however, once this diagnosis is strongly suspected, apheresis is typically stopped and serial infusions of the anti-complement C5 antibody eculizumab are provided, which have produced sustained remissions in some patients. If irreversible kidney disease has occurred, hemodialysis or kidney transplantation may be necessary.

▶ When to Refer

Consultation by a hematologist or transfusion medicine specialist familiar with plasma exchange is required at the time of presentation. Patients with TMA require ongoing care by a hematologist.

▶ When to Admit

All patients with newly suspected or diagnosed TMA should be hospitalized immediately.

George JN et al. Syndromes of thrombotic microangiopathy associated with pregnancy. Hematology Am Soc Hematol Educ Program. 2015 Dec 5;2015(1):644–8. [PMID: 26637783]
Legendre CM et al. Terminal complement inhibitor eculizumab in atypical hemolytic-uremic syndrome. N Engl J Med. 2013 Jun 6;368(23):2169–81. [PMID: 23738544]

Sayani FA et al. How I treat refractory thrombotic thrombocytopenic purpura. Blood. 2015 Jun 18;125(25):3860–7. [PMID: 25784681]
Scully M et al; HERCULES Investigators. Caplacizumab treatment for acquired thrombotic thrombocytopenic purpura. N Engl J Med. 2019 Jan 24;380(4):335–46. [PMID: 30625070]
Scully M et al; International Working Group for Thrombotic Thrombocytopenic Purpura. Consensus on the standardization of terminology in thrombotic thrombocytopenic purpura and related thrombotic microangiopathies. J Thromb Haemost. 2017 Feb;15(2):312–22. [PMID: 27868334]

3. Heparin-Induced Thrombocytopenia

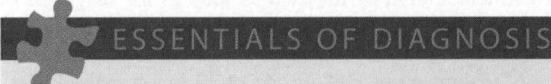
ESSENTIALS OF DIAGNOSIS

- ▶ Thrombocytopenia within 5–14 days of exposure to heparin.
- ▶ Decline in baseline platelet count of 50% or greater.
- ▶ Thrombosis occurs in up to 50% of cases; bleeding is uncommon.

▶ General Considerations

Heparin-induced thrombocytopenia (HIT) is an acquired disorder that affects approximately 3% of patients exposed to unfractionated heparin and 0.6% of patients exposed to low-molecular-weight heparin (LMWH). The condition results from formation of IgG antibodies to heparin-platelet factor 4 (PF4) complexes; the antibody:heparin-PF4 complex binds to and activates platelets independent of physiologic hemostasis, which leads to thrombocytopenia and thromboses.

▶ Clinical Findings

A. Symptoms and Signs

Patients are often asymptomatic, and due to the prothrombotic nature of HIT, bleeding usually does not occur. Thrombosis (at any venous or arterial site), however, may be detected in up to 50% of patients, up to 30 days post-diagnosis.

B. Laboratory Findings

A presumptive diagnosis of HIT is made when new-onset thrombocytopenia is detected in a patient (typically a hospitalized patient) within 5–14 days of exposure to heparin; other presentations (eg, rapid-onset HIT) are less common and reflect prior heparin exposure in the recent past. A decline of 50% or more from the baseline platelet count is typical. The 4T score (http://www.qxmd.com/calculate-online/hematology/hit-heparin-induced-thrombocytopenia-probability) is a clinical prediction rule for assessing pretest probability for HIT. Low 4T scores have been shown to be more predictive of excluding HIT, than are intermediate or high scores of predicting its presence. Once HIT is clinically suspected, the clinician must establish the diagnosis by performing a screening PF4-heparin antibody enzyme-linked immunosorbent assay (ELISA). If the PF4-heparin antibody ELISA is positive, the diagnosis must be confirmed using a functional assay (such as serotonin release assay). The magnitude of a positive ELISA result correlates with the clinical probability of HIT, but even high optical density values on the PF4 may be falsely positive. The confirmatory assay is essential.

▶ Treatment

Treatment should be initiated as soon as the diagnosis of HIT is suspected, before results of laboratory testing are available.

Management of HIT (Table 14–5) involves the immediate discontinuation of all forms of heparin. If thrombosis has not already been detected, duplex Doppler ultrasound of the lower extremities should be performed to rule out subclinical deep venous thrombosis (DVT). Despite thrombocytopenia, platelet transfusions are rarely necessary and should be avoided. Due to the substantial frequency of thrombosis among HIT patients, an alternative anticoagulant, typically a direct thrombin inhibitor (DTI) such as argatroban or bivalirudin, should be administered immediately while awaiting confirmatory testing. Fondaparinux is an option for some patients. For confirmed HIT, the DTI should be continued until the platelet count has recovered to at least 100,000/mcL, at which point treatment with a vitamin K antagonist (warfarin) may be initiated. The DTI should be continued until therapeutic anticoagulation with the vitamin K antagonist warfarin has been achieved (ie, international normalized ratio [INR] of 2.0–3.0); the infusion of argatroban must be temporarily discontinued before the INR is obtained so that it reflects the anticoagulant effect of warfarin alone. There is growing use of the subcutaneous indirect anti-Xa inhibitor fondaparinux for initial treatment of HIT. In all patients with HIT, some form of anticoagulation (warfarin or other) should be continued for at least 30 days, due to a persistent risk of thrombosis even after the platelet count has recovered, but in patients in whom thrombosis has been documented, anticoagulation should continue for 3–6 months.

Subsequent exposure to heparin should be avoided in all patients with a prior history of HIT, if possible. If its use is regarded as necessary for a procedure, it should be withheld until PF4-heparin antibodies are no longer detectable by ELISA (usually as of 100 days following an episode of HIT), and exposure should be limited to the shortest time period possible. A common example is a cardiac catheterization. The heparin is gone before the antibody returns, so HIT is avoided.

▶ When to Refer

Due to the tremendous thrombotic potential of the disorder and the complexity of use of the DTI, all patients with HIT should be evaluated by a hematologist.

▶ When to Admit

Most patients with HIT are hospitalized at the time of detection of thrombocytopenia. Typically, an outpatient in whom HIT is suspected should be admitted because the DTIs must be administered by continuous intravenous infusion. However, in selected cases, if they are a candidate for fondaparinux, admission is a clinical decision. Regardless, a hematologist needs to be involved as soon as the diagnosis is raised or treatment is indicated.

Table 14–5. Management of suspected or proven HIT.

I. Discontinue all forms of heparin. Send PF4-heparin ELISA (if indicated).
II. Begin treatment with direct thrombin inhibitor, or in some circumstances, fondaparinux.

Agent	Indication	Dosing
Argatroban	Prophylaxis or treatment of HIT	Continuous intravenous infusion of 0.5–1.2 mcg/kg/min, titrate to aPTT = 1.5 to 3 × the baseline value.[1] Max infusion rate ≤ 10 mcg/kg/min.
Bivalirudin	Percutaneous coronary intervention[2]	Bolus of 0.75 mg/kg intravenously followed by initial continuous intravenous infusion of 1.75 mg/kg/h. Manufacturer indicates monitoring should be by ACT.

III. Perform Doppler ultrasound of lower extremities to rule out subclinical thrombosis (if indicated).
IV. Follow platelet counts daily until recovery occurs.
V. When platelet count has recovered, transition anticoagulation to warfarin or fondaparinux; treat for 30 days (HIT) or 3–6 months (HITT).
VI. Document heparin allergy in medical record (confirmed cases).

[1]Hepatic insufficiency: initial infusion rate = 0.5 mcg/kg/min.
[2]Not approved for HIT/HITT.
ACT, activated clotting time; aPTT, activated partial thromboplastin time; ELISA, enzyme-linked immunosorbent assay; HIT, heparin-induced thrombocytopenia; HITT, heparin-induced thrombocytopenia and thrombosis; PF4, platelet factor 4.

Cuker A et al. American Society of Hematology 2018 guidelines for management of venous thromboembolism: heparin-induced thrombocytopenia. Blood Adv. 2018 Nov 27;2(22):3360–92. [PMID: 30482768]

Schindewolf M et al. Use of fondaparinux off-label or approved anticoagulants for management of heparin-induced thrombocytopenia. J Am Coll Cardiol. 2017 Nov 28;70(21):2636–48. [PMID: 29169470]

Warkentin TE et al. Serological investigation of patients with a previous history of heparin-induced thrombocytopenia who are reexposed to heparin. Blood. 2014 Apr 17;123(16):2485–93. [PMID: 24516044]

4. Disseminated Intravascular Coagulation

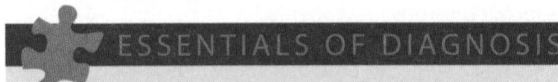

ESSENTIALS OF DIAGNOSIS

- ▶ A frequent cause of thrombocytopenia in hospitalized patients.
- ▶ Prolonged PT and aPTT, and low/declining fibrinogen.
- ▶ Thrombocytopenia.

General Considerations

Disseminated intravascular coagulation (DIC) is caused by uncontrolled local or systemic activation of coagulation, which leads to depletion of coagulation factors and fibrinogen and often results in thrombocytopenia as platelets are activated and consumed.

Numerous disorders are associated with DIC, including sepsis (in which coagulation is activated by presence of lipopolysaccharide), cancer, trauma, burns, and pregnancy-associated complications (in which tissue factor is released). Aortic aneurysm and cavernous hemangiomas may promote localized intravascular coagulation, and snake bites may result in DIC due to the introduction of exogenous toxins.

Clinical Findings

A. Symptoms and Signs

Bleeding in DIC usually occurs at multiple sites, such as intravenous catheters or incisions, and may be widespread (purpura fulminans). Malignancy-related DIC may manifest principally as thrombosis (Trousseau syndrome).

B. Laboratory Findings

In early DIC, the platelet count and fibrinogen levels may remain within the normal range, albeit reduced from baseline levels. There is progressive thrombocytopenia (rarely severe), prolongation of the PT, decrease in fibrinogen levels, and eventually elevation in the aPTT. D-dimer levels typically are elevated due to the activation of coagulation and diffuse cross-linking of fibrin followed by fibrinolysis. Schistocytes on the blood smear, due to shearing of red cells through the microvasculature, are present in 10–20% of patients. Laboratory abnormalities in the HELLP syndrome (hemolysis, elevated liver enzymes, low platelets), a severe form of DIC with a particularly high mortality rate that occurs in peripartum women, include elevated liver transaminases and kidney injury due to gross hemoglobinuria and pigment nephropathy. Malignancy-related DIC may feature normal platelet counts and coagulation studies, but clinicians often see a dropping platelet count and fibrinogen, with a rising INR, highlighting the importance of serial laboratory values to help make the diagnosis.

Treatment

The underlying causative disorder must be treated (eg, antimicrobials, chemotherapy, surgery, or delivery of conceptus). If clinically significant bleeding is present, hemostasis must be achieved (Table 14–6).

Blood products are administered if clinically significant hemorrhage has occurred or is thought likely to occur without intervention based on progressively rising PT, PTT, and dropping fibrinogen and platelets levels (Table 14–6). The goal of platelet therapy for most cases is greater than 20,000/mcL or greater than 50,000/mcL for serious bleeding, such as intracranial bleeding. FFP should be given only to patients with a prolonged aPTT and PT and significant bleeding. Cryoprecipitate may be given for bleeding or for fibrinogen levels less than 80–100 mg/dL. The clinician should correct the fibrinogen level with cryoprecipitate prior to giving FFP for prolonged PT and aPTT to see if the fibrinogen replacement alone corrects the PT and aPTT. The PT, aPTT, fibrinogen, and platelet count should be monitored at least every 6–8 hours in acutely ill patients with DIC.

In some cases of refractory bleeding despite replacement of blood products, administration of low doses of heparin can be considered. The clinician must remember that DIC is primarily a disorder of excessive clotting with secondary fibrinolysis, and that heparin can interfere with thrombin generation, which could then lead to a lessened consumption of coagulation proteins and platelets.

Table 14–6. Management of DIC.

I. Assess for underlying cause of DIC and treat.		
II. Establish baseline platelet count, PT, aPTT, D-dimer, fibrinogen.		
III. Transfuse blood products only if ongoing bleeding or high risk of bleeding.	**Platelets:** goal > 20,000/mcL (most patients) or > 50,000/mcL (severe bleeding, eg, intracranial hemorrhage)	
	Cryoprecipitate: goal fibrinogen level > 80–100 mg/dL	
	Fresh frozen plasma: goal PT and aPTT < 1.5 × normal	
	Packed red blood cells: goal hemoglobin > 8 g/dL or improvement in symptomatic anemia	
IV. Follow platelets, aPTT, PT, fibrinogen every 4–12 hours as clinically indicated.		
V. If persistent bleeding due to severe consumption or consumption that requires excessive blood product use, consider use of heparin[1] (initial infusion, 5 units/kg/h) and titrate to desired clinical goals; do not administer bolus.		
VI. Follow laboratory parameters every 4–12 hours as clinically indicated until DIC resolves		

[1]Contraindicated if platelets cannot be maintained at > 50,000/mcL, in cases of gastrointestinal or central nervous system bleeding, in conditions that may require surgical management, or placental abruption.
aPTT, activated partial thromboplastin time; DIC, disseminated intravascular coagulation; PT, prothrombin time.

An infusion of 5 units/kg/h (no bolus) may be used with appropriate clinical judgement, uptitrated as clinically appropriate. *Heparin, however, is contraindicated if the platelet count cannot be maintained at 50,000/mcL or more and in cases of central nervous system hemorrhage, gastrointestinal bleeding, placental abruption, and any other condition that is likely to require imminent surgery.* Fibrinolysis inhibitors may be considered in some patients with refractory DIC, but this can promote dangerous clotting and should be undertaken with great caution and only in consultation with a hematologist.

The treatment of HELLP syndrome must include evacuation of the uterus (eg, delivery of a term or near-term infant or removal of retained placental or fetal fragments). Patients with Trousseau syndrome require treatment of the underlying malignancy and administration of unfractionated heparin or subcutaneous therapeutic-dose LMWH as treatment of thrombosis, since warfarin typically is ineffective at secondary prevention of thromboembolism in the disorder. Typically, the heparin or LMWH treatment will gradually return the fibrinogen, PT (INR), aPTT, and platelet count back to normal, but it can take days. Oral anti-Xa agents or oral DTIs can be considered once stabilized with parenteral heparin or LMWH.

Immediate initiation of medical treatment (usually within 24 hours of diagnosis) is required for patients with acute promyelocytic leukemia (APL)–associated DIC, along with administration of blood products as clinically indicated.

▶ When to Refer

- Diffuse bleeding that is unresponsive to administration of blood products should be evaluated by a hematologist.
- All patients with DIC should be cared for by a hematologist prior to starting treatment with heparin or LMWH.

▶ When to Admit

Most patients with DIC are hospitalized when DIC is detected.

Feinstein DI. Disseminated intravascular coagulation in patients with solid tumors. Oncology (Williston Park). 2015 Feb; 29(2):96–102. [PMID: 25683828]

Iba T et al. Anticoagulant therapy for sepsis-associated disseminated intravascular coagulation: the view from Japan. J Thromb Haemost. 2014 Jul;12(7):1010–9. [PMID: 24801203]

Levi M. Diagnosis and treatment of disseminated intravascular coagulation. Int J Lab Hematol. 2014 Jun;36(3):228–36. [PMID: 24750668]

Wada H et al. Disseminated intravascular coagulation: testing and diagnosis. Clin Chim Acta. 2014 Sep 25;436:130–4. [PMID: 24792730]

OTHER CONDITIONS CAUSING THROMBOCYTOPENIA

1. Drug-Induced Thrombocytopenia

The mechanisms underlying drug-induced thrombocytopenia are thought in most cases to be immune, although exceptions exist (such as chemotherapy). Table 14–7 lists medications associated with thrombocytopenia. The typical presentation of drug-induced, antibody-mediated

Table 14–7. Selected medications causing drug-associated thrombocytopenia.[1]

Class	Examples
Chemotherapy	Most agents
Antiplatelet agents	Abciximab Anagrelide Eptifibatide Ticlopidine, tirofiban
Antimicrobial agents	Adefovir, indinavir, ritonavir Fluconazole Isoniazid Linezolid Penicillins Rifampin Sulfa drugs Vancomycin
Cardiovascular agents	Amiodarone Atorvastatin, simvastatin Captopril Digoxin Hydrochlorothiazide Procainamide
Gastrointestinal agents	Cimetidine, famotidine, ranitidine
Neuropsychiatric agents	Carbamazepine Haloperidol Methyldopa Phenytoin
Analgesic agents	Acetaminophen Diclofenac, ibuprofen, naproxen, sulindac
Anticoagulant agents	Heparin Low-molecular-weight heparin
Immunomodulator agents	Interferon-alpha Rituximab
Immunosuppressant agents	Mycophenolate mofetil Tacrolimus
Other agents	Immunizations Iodinated contrast dye

[1]See also https://www.ouhsc.edu/platelets/.

thrombocytopenia is severe thrombocytopenia and mucocutaneous bleeding 5–14 days after exposure to a new drug, although a range of presentations is possible. Discontinuation of the offending agent leads to resolution of thrombocytopenia within 3–7 days in most cases, but recovery kinetics depends on rate of drug clearance, which can be affected by liver and kidney function. Patients with severe thrombocytopenia should be given platelet transfusions with (immune cases only) or without IVIG. The University of Oklahoma Health Sciences center maintains a useful website for drug-induced thrombocytopenia (https://www.ouhsc.edu/platelets/).

2. Posttransfusion Purpura

Posttransfusion purpura (PTP) is a rare disorder that features sudden-onset thrombocytopenia in an individual who received transfusion of red cells, platelets, or plasma within

1 week prior to detection of thrombocytopenia. Antibodies against the human platelet antigen Pl[A1] are detected in most individuals with PTP. Patients with PTP often are either multiparous women or persons who have received transfusions previously. Severe thrombocytopenia and bleeding are typical. Initial treatment consists of administration of IVIG (1 g/kg/day for 2 days), which should be administered as soon as the diagnosis is suspected. Platelets are not indicated unless severe bleeding is present, but if they are to be administered, HLA-matched platelets are preferred. A second course or IVIG, plasma exchange, corticosteroids, TPO-mimetics, or splenectomy may be required in case of refractoriness. Pl[A1]-negative or washed blood products are preferred for subsequent transfusions, but data supporting various treatment options are limited.

3. von Willebrand Disease Type 2B

von Willebrand disease (vWD) type 2B leads to chronic, characteristically mild to moderate thrombocytopenia via an abnormal vWF molecule that binds platelets with increased affinity, resulting in aggregation and clearance.

4. Platelet Sequestration

One-third of the platelet mass is typically sequestered in the spleen. Splenomegaly, due to a variety of conditions, may lead to thrombocytopenia of variable severity. When possible, treatment of the underlying disorder should be pursued, but splenectomy, splenic embolization, or splenic irradiation may be considered in selected cases.

5. Pregnancy

Gestational thrombocytopenia is thought to result from progressive expansion of the blood volume that typically occurs during pregnancy, leading to hemodilution. Cytopenias result even though blood cell production is normal or increased. Platelet counts less than 100,000/mcL, however, are observed in less than 10% of pregnant women in the third trimester; decreases to less than 70,000/mcL should prompt consideration of pregnancy-related ITP as well as preeclampsia or a pregnancy-related thrombotic microangiopathy.

6. Infection or Sepsis

Both immune- and platelet production–mediated defects are possible, and there may be significant overlap with concomitant DIC. Regardless, the platelet count typically improves with effective antimicrobial treatment or after the infection has resolved. In some critically ill patients, a defect in immunomodulation may lead to bone marrow macrophages (histiocytes) engulfing cellular components of the marrow in a process also called hemophagocytosis. The phenomenon typically resolves with resolution of the infection, but with certain infections (Epstein-Barr virus) immunosuppression may be required. Hemophagocytosis also may arise in the setting of malignancy, in which case the disorder is usually unresponsive to treatment with immunosuppression. Sepsis-related thrombocytopenia may be due to increased hepatic clearance of platelets caused by loss of asialoglycoprotein moieties on the platelet surface.

7. Pseudothrombocytopenia

Pseudothrombocytopenia results from EDTA anticoagulant-induced platelet clumping; the phenomenon typically disappears when blood is collected in a tube containing citrate anticoagulant. Pseudothrombocytopenia diagnosis requires review of the peripheral blood smear.

Kasai J et al. Clinical features of gestational thrombocytopenia difficult to differentiate from immune thrombocytopenia diagnosed during pregnancy. J Obstet Gynaecol Res. 2015 Jan; 41(1):44–9. [PMID: 25163390]

Koyama K et al. Time course of immature platelet count and its relation to thrombocytopenia and mortality in patients with sepsis. PLoS One. 2018 Jan 30;13(1):e0192064. [PMID: 29381746]

Menis M et al. Posttransfusion purpura occurrence and potential risk factors among the inpatient US elderly, as recorded in large Medicare databases during 2011 through 2012. Transfusion. 2015 Feb;55(2):284–95. [PMID: 25065878]

QUALITATIVE PLATELET DISORDERS

CONGENITAL DISORDERS OF PLATELET FUNCTION

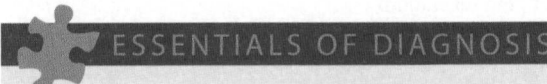

ESSENTIALS OF DIAGNOSIS

► Usually diagnosed in childhood.
► Family history usually is positive.
► May be diagnosed in adulthood when there is excessive bleeding.

► General Considerations

Heritable qualitative platelet disorders are far less common than acquired disorders of platelet function and lead to variably severe bleeding, often beginning in childhood. Occasionally, however, disorders of platelet function may go undetected until later in life when excessive bleeding occurs following a sufficient hemostatic challenge. Thus, the true incidence of hereditary qualitative platelet disorders is unknown.

Bernard-Soulier syndrome (BSS) is a rare, autosomal recessive bleeding disorder due to reduced or abnormal platelet membrane expression of glycoprotein Ib/IX (vWF receptor).

Glanzmann thrombasthenia results from a qualitative or quantitative abnormality in the platelet glycoprotein IIb/IIIa receptor on the platelet membrane and the fibrinogen receptor critical for linking platelets during initial platelet aggregation/platelet plug formation. Inheritance is autosomal recessive.

Under normal circumstances, activated platelets release the contents of platelet granules to reinforce the aggregatory response. Storage pool disease includes a spectrum of defects in release of alpha or dense (delta) platelet granules, or both (alpha-delta storage pool disease).

Clinical Findings

A. Symptoms and Signs

In patients with **Glanzmann thrombasthenia,** the onset of bleeding is usually in infancy or childhood. The degree of deficiency in IIb/IIIa may not correlate well with bleeding symptoms. Patients with **storage pool disease** are affected by variable bleeding, ranging from mild and trauma-related to spontaneous.

B. Laboratory Findings

In Bernard-Soulier syndrome, there are abnormally large platelets (approaching the size of red cells), moderate thrombocytopenia, and a prolonged bleeding time. Platelet aggregation studies show a marked defect in response to ristocetin, whereas aggregation in response to other agonists is normal; the addition of normal platelets corrects the abnormal aggregation. The diagnosis can be confirmed by platelet flow cytometry.

In Glanzmann thrombasthenia, platelet aggregation studies show marked impairment of aggregation in response to stimulation with various agonists, which reflects the critical role of the fibrinogen receptor in platelet plug formation.

Storage pool disease describes defects in the number, content, or function of platelet alpha or dense granules, or both. The gray platelet syndrome comprises abnormalities of platelet alpha granules, thrombocytopenia, and marrow fibrosis. The blood smear shows agranular platelets, and the diagnosis is confirmed with electron microscopy.

Albinism-associated storage pool disease involves defective dense granules in disorders of oculocutaneous albinism, such as the Hermansky-Pudlak and Chediak-Higashi syndromes. Electron microscopy confirms the diagnosis.

Non–albinism-associated storage pool disease results from quantitative or qualitative defects in dense granules and is seen in Ehlers-Danlos and Wiskott-Aldrich syndromes, among others.

The Quebec platelet disorder comprises mild thrombocytopenia, an abnormal platelet factor V molecule, and a prolonged bleeding time. Patients typically experience moderate bleeding. Interestingly, platelet transfusion does not ameliorate the bleeding. Patients have a prolonged bleeding time. Platelet aggregation studies characteristically show platelet dissociation following an initial aggregatory response, and electron microscopy confirms the diagnosis.

Treatment

The mainstay of treatment (including periprocedural prophylaxis) is transfusion of normal platelets, although desmopressin acetate (DDAVP), antifibrinolytic agents, and recombinant human activated factor VII each have a role in selected clinical situations.

Andrews RK et al. Bernard-Soulier syndrome: an update. Semin Thromb Hemost. 2013 Sep;39(6):656–62. [PMID: 23929303]
Orsini S et al; European Hematology Association-Scientific Working Group (EHA-SWG) on thrombocytopenias and platelet function disorders. Bleeding risk of surgery and its prevention in patients with inherited platelet disorders. Haematologica. 2017 Jul;102(7):1192–203. [PMID: 28385783]

ACQUIRED DISORDERS OF PLATELET FUNCTION

Platelet dysfunction is more commonly acquired than inherited; the widespread use of platelet-altering medications accounts for most of the cases of qualitative defects (Table 14–8). In cases where platelet function is irreversibly altered, platelet inhibition typically recovers within 7–9 days following discontinuation of the drug. In cases where platelet function is non-irreversibly affected, platelet inhibition recovers with clearance of the drug from the system. Transfusion of platelets may be required if clinically significant bleeding is present.

Zheng SL et al. Association of aspirin use for primary prevention with cardiovascular events and bleeding events: a systematic review and meta-analysis. JAMA. 2019 Jan 22;321(3):277-87. [PMID: 30667501]

DISORDERS OF COAGULATION

CONGENITAL DISORDERS OF COAGULATION

1. Hemophilia A & B

ESSENTIALS OF DIAGNOSIS

► **Hemophilia A:** congenital deficiency of coagulation factor VIII.
► **Hemophilia B:** congenital deficiency of coagulation factor IX.
► Recurrent hemarthroses and arthropathy.
► Risk of development of inhibitory antibodies to factor VIII or factor IX.
► In many older patients, infection with HIV or hepatitis C virus from receipt of contaminated blood products.

General Considerations

The frequency of hemophilia A is ~1 per 5000 live male births, whereas hemophilia B occurs in ~1 in 25,000 live male births. Inheritance is X-linked recessive, leading to affected males and carrier (affected) females with variable bleeding tendencies. Daughters of all affected males are obligate carriers. There is no race predilection. Factor activity testing is indicated for male infants with a hemophilic maternal pedigree who are asymptomatic or who experience excessive bleeding, for all daughters of affected males

Table 14–8. Causes of acquired platelet dysfunction.

Cause	Mechanism(s)	Treatment of Bleeding
Drug-Induced		
Salicylates (eg, aspirin)	Irreversible inhibition of platelet cyclooxygenase	Discontinuation of drug; platelet transfusion
NSAIDs (eg, ibuprofen)	Reversible inhibition of cyclooxygenase	
Glycoprotein IIb/IIIa inhibitors (eg, abciximab, tirofiban, eptifibatide)	↓ Binding of fibrinogen to PM IIb/IIIa receptor	
Thienopyridines (eg, clopidogrel, ticlopidine)	↓ ADP binding to PM receptor	
Dipyridamole	↓ Intracellular cAMP metabolism	
SSRIs (eg, paroxetine, fluoxetine)	↓ Serotonin in dense granules	
Omega-3 fatty acids (eg, DHA, EHA)	Disruption of PM phospholipid	
Antibiotics (eg, high-dose penicillin, nafcillin, ticarcillin, cephalothin, moxalactam)	Not fully elucidated; PM binding may interfere with receptor-ligand interactions	
Alcohol	↓ TXA2 release	
Disease-Related		
Uremia	↑ Nitric oxide; ↓ release of granules	DDAVP, high-dose estrogens; platelet transfusion, dialysis
Myeloproliferative disorder/myelodysplastic syndrome	Abnormal PM receptors, signal transduction, and/or granule release	Platelet transfusion; myelosuppressive treatment (myeloproliferative disorder)
Surgical Procedure-Related		
Cardiac bypass	Platelet activation in bypass circuit	Platelet transfusion

ADP, adenosine diphosphate; cAMP, cyclic adenosine monophosphate; DDAVP, desmopressin acetate; DHA, docosahexaenoic acid; EHA, eicosahexaenoic acid; NSAIDs, nonsteroidal anti-inflammatory drugs; PM, platelet membrane; SSRIs, selective serotonin release inhibitors; TXA2, thromboxane A2.

(100% chance of being affected) and carrier mothers (50% chance of being affected), and for an otherwise asymptomatic adolescent or adult who experiences unexpected excessive bleeding with trauma or invasive procedures.

Inhibitors to factor VIII will develop in approximately 20–25% of patients with severe hemophilia A, and inhibitors to factor IX will develop in less than 5% of patients with severe hemophilia B.

A substantial proportion of older patients with hemophilia acquired infection with HIV or HCV or both in the 1980s due to exposure to contaminated factor concentrates and blood products.

► **Clinical Findings**

A. Symptoms and Signs

Severe hemophilia (factor VIII activity less than 1%) presents in infant males or in early childhood with spontaneous bleeding into joints, soft tissues, or other locations. Spontaneous bleeding is rare in patients with mild hemophilia (factor VIII activity greater than 5%), but bleeding may occur with a significant hemostatic challenge (eg, surgery, trauma). Intermediate clinical symptoms are seen in patients with moderate hemophilia (factor VIII activity 1–5%). Female carriers of hemophilia can have a wide range of factor VIII activity and therefore have variable bleeding tendencies.

Significant hemophilic arthropathy is usually avoided in patients who have received long-term prophylaxis with factor concentrate starting in early childhood, whereas joint disease is common in adults who have experienced recurrent hemarthroses. Patients tend to have one or two "target" joints into which they bleed most often.

Inhibitor development to factor VIII or factor IX is characterized by bleeding episodes that are resistant to treatment with clotting factor VIII or IX concentrate, and by new or atypical bleeding.

B. Laboratory Findings

Hemophilia is diagnosed by demonstration of an isolated reproducibly low factor VIII or factor IX activity level, in the absence of other conditions. If the aPTT is prolonged, it typically corrects upon mixing with normal plasma. A variety of mutations, including inversions, large and small deletions, insertions, missense mutations, and nonsense mutations may be causative. Depending on the level of residual factor VIII or factor IX activity and the sensitivity of the thromboplastin used in the aPTT coagulation reaction, the aPTT may or may not be prolonged (although it typically is markedly prolonged in severe hemophilia). Hemophilia is classified according to the level of factor activity in the plasma. **Severe hemophilia** is characterized by less than 1% factor activity, **moderate hemophilia** features 1–5% factor activity and **mild hemophilia** features greater than 5% factor activity. Female carriers may become symptomatic if significant lyonization has occurred favoring the defective factor VIII or factor IX gene, leading to factor VIII or factor IX activity level markedly less than 50%. Typically, a clinical bleeding diathesis occurs once the factor activity is less than 20%, but bleeding can occur in trauma, surgery, and delivery if the factor activity is less than 50%.

In the presence of an inhibitor to factor VIII or factor IX, there is accelerated clearance of and suboptimal or absent rise in measured activity of infused factor, and the aPTT does not correct on mixing. The Bethesda assay measures the potency of the inhibitor.

► **Treatment**

Plasma-derived or recombinant factor VIII or IX products are the mainstay of treatment. The standard of care for most individuals with severe hemophilia is primary prophylaxis: by the age of 4 years, most children with severe hemophilia have begun twice- or thrice-weekly infusions of factor to prevent the recurrent joint bleeding that otherwise would characterize the disorder and lead to severe musculoskeletal morbidity. In selected cases of nonsevere

hemophilia, or as an adjunct to prophylaxis in severe hemophilia, treatment with factor products is given periprocedurally, prior to high-risk activities (such as sports), or as needed for bleeding episodes (Table 14–9). Recombinant factor VIII and factor IX molecules that are bioengineered to have an extended half-life may allow for extended dosing intervals in patients who are treated prophylactically. The decision to switch to a long-acting product is patient specific. The long-acting factor IX products have clear added value in reducing frequency of factor injections. This is not so clear with the long-acting factor VIII products. Patients with mild hemophilia A may respond to as-needed (on demand) intravenous or intranasal treatment with DDAVP. Antifibrinolytic agents may be useful in cases of mucosal bleeding and are commonly used adjunctively, such as following dental procedures. Gene therapy for hemophilia A and B is now a reality and is likely to change the treatment landscape over the next decade, transforming patient's lives and reducing or eliminating the need for prophylactic infusions of factor VIII or factor IX protein.

Factor inhibitors (antibodies that interfere with activity or half-life) are a major clinical problem for patients with hemophilia. It may be possible to overcome low-titer

Table 14–9. Treatment of bleeding in selected inherited disorders of hemostasis.

Disorder	Subtype	Treatment for Minor Bleeding	Treatment for Major Bleeding	Comment
Hemophilia A	Mild	DDAVP[1]	DDAVP[1] or factor VIII product	Treat for 3–10 days for major bleeding or following surgery, keeping factor activity level 50–80% initially. Adjunctive aminocaproic acid (EACA) may be useful for mucosal bleeding or procedures
	Moderate or severe	Factor VIII product	Factor VIII product	
Hemophilia B	Mild, moderate, or severe	Factor IX product	Factor IX product	
von Willebrand disease	Type 1	DDAVP	DDAVP, vWF product	
	Type 2	DDAVP,[1] vWF product	vWF product	
	Type 3	vWF product	vWF product	
Factor XI deficiency	—	FFP or EACA	FFP	Adjunctive EACA should be used for mucosal bleeding or procedures

[1]Mild hemophilia A and type 2A or 2B vWD patients: therapeutic trial must have previously confirmed an adequate response (ie, elevation of factor VIII or vWF activity level into the normal range) and (for type 2B) no exacerbation of thrombocytopenia. DDAVP is not typically effective for type 2M vWD. A vWF-containing factor VIII concentrate is preferred for treatment of type 2N vWD.

Notes:

DDAVP dose is 0.3 mcg/kg intravenously in 50 mL saline over 20 minutes, or nasal spray 300 mcg for weight > 50 kg or 150 mcg for < 50 kg, every 24 hours, maximum of three doses in a 72-hour period. If more than two doses are used in a 48-hour period, free water restriction and monitoring for hyponatremia is essential.

EACA dose is 50 mg/kg orally four times daily for 3–5 days; maximum 24 g/day, useful for mucosal bleeding/dental procedures.

Factor VIII product dose is 50 units/kg for severe hemophilia A intravenously initially followed by 25 units/kg every 8 hours followed by lesser doses at longer intervals once hemostasis has been established.

Factor IX product dose is 100 units/kg (120 units/kg if using Benefix) intravenously initially for severe hemophilia B followed by 50 units/kg (60 units/kg if using Benefix) every 8 hours followed by lesser doses at longer intervals once hemostasis has been established.

vWF-containing factor VIII product dose is 60–80 RCoF units/kg intravenously every 12 hours initially followed by lesser doses at longer intervals once hemostasis has been established.

FFP is typically administered in 4-unit boluses and may not need to be re-bolused after the initial administration due to the long half-life of factor XI.

DDAVP, desmopressin acetate; EACA, epsilon-aminocaproic acid; FFP, fresh frozen plasma; vWF, von Willebrand factor.

inhibitors (less than 5 Bethesda units [BU]) by giving larger doses of factor, whereas treatment of bleeding in the presence of a high-titer inhibitor (more than 5 BU) requires infusion of an activated prothrombin complex concentrate (such as FEIBA [factor eight inhibitor bypassing activity]) or recombinant activated factor VII. Recombinant porcine factor VIII is also an option but is reserved for selective circumstances because of its cost. Inhibitor tolerance induction, achieved by giving large doses (50–300 units/kg intravenously of factor VIII daily) for 6–18 months, succeeds in eradicating the inhibitor in 70% of patients with hemophilia A and in 30% of patients with hemophilia B. Patients with hemophilia B who receive inhibitor tolerance induction, however, are at risk for development of nephrotic syndrome and anaphylactic reactions, making eradication of their inhibitors less feasible. Additional immunomodulation may allow for eradication in selected inhibitor tolerance induction–refractory patients. Emicizumab is a novel bi-specific antibody that brings factors IX and X together, effectively replacing the cofactor function of factor VIII in the clotting cascade, offering new hope for patients with inhibitors. More recently, emicizumab has been demonstrated to be an effective option for patients without inhibitors.

Antiretroviral treatment should be administered to hemophilia patients with HIV infection. Patients with hepatitis C infection should be referred for treatment to eradicate the virus.

When to Refer

All patients with hemophilia should be seen regularly in a comprehensive hemophilia treatment center.

When to Admit

- Major invasive procedures because of the need for serial infusions of clotting factor concentrate.
- Bleeding that is unresponsive to outpatient treatment.

Aledort L et al. Factor VIII therapy for hemophilia A: current and future issues. Expert Rev Hematol. 2014 Jun;7(3):373–85. [PMID: 24717090]

George LA et al. Hemophilia B gene therapy with a high-specific-activity factor IX variant. N Engl J Med. 2017 Dec 7;377(23): 2215–27. [PMID: 29211678]

Mahlangu J et al. Emicizumab prophylaxis in patients who have hemophilia A without inhibitors. N Engl J Med. 2018 Aug 30; 379(9):811–22. [PMID: 30157389]

Manco-Johnson MJ et al; Joint Outcomes Committee of the Universal Data Collection, US Hemophilia Treatment Center Network. Prophylaxis usage, bleeding rates, and joint outcomes of hemophilia, 1999 to 2010: a surveillance project. Blood. 2017 Apr 27;129(17):2368–74. [PMID: 28183693]

Mazepa MA et al; US Hemophilia Treatment Center Network. Men with severe hemophilia in the United States: birth cohort analysis of a large national database. Blood. 2016 Jun 16; 127(24):3073–81. [PMID: 26983851]

Oldenburg J et al. Emicizumab prophylaxis in hemophilia A with inhibitors. N Engl J Med. 2017 Aug 31;377(9):809–18. [PMID: 28691557]

Rangarajan S et al. AAV5-factor VIII gene transfer in severe hemophilia A. N Engl J Med. 2017 Dec 28;377(26):2519–30. [PMID: 29224506]

2. von Willebrand Disease

ESSENTIALS OF DIAGNOSIS

▸ The most common inherited bleeding disorder.

▸ von Willebrand factor binds platelets to subendothelial surfaces, aggregates platelets, and prolongs the half-life of factor VIII.

General Considerations

vWF is an unusually large multimeric glycoprotein that binds to subendothelial collagen and its platelet receptor, glycoprotein Ib, bridging platelets to the subendothelial matrix at the site of vascular injury and contributing to linking them together in the platelet plug. vWF also has a binding site for factor VIII, prolonging factor VIII half-life in the circulation.

Between 75% and 80% of patients with vWD have type 1, a quantitative abnormality of the vWF molecule that usually does not feature an identifiable causal mutation in the vWF gene.

Type 2 vWD is seen in 15–20% of patients with vWD. In type 2A or 2B vWD, a qualitative defect in the vWF molecule is causative. Type 2N and 2M vWD are due to defects in vWF that decrease binding to factor VIII or to platelets, respectively. Importantly, type 2N vWD clinically resembles hemophilia A, with the exception of a family history that shows affected females. Factor VIII activity levels are decreased, and vWF activity and antigen (Ag) are normal. Type 2M vWD features a normal multimer pattern. Type 3 vWD is rare, and like type 1, is a quantitative defect, with mutational homozygosity or compound heterozygosity yielding very low levels of vWF and severe bleeding in infancy or childhood.

Clinical Findings

A. Symptoms and Signs

Patients with type 1 vWD usually have mild or moderate platelet-type bleeding (especially involving the integument and mucous membranes). Patients with type 2 vWD usually have moderate to severe bleeding that presents in childhood or adolescence. Patient with type 3 vWD demonstrate a severe bleeding phenotype.

B. Laboratory Findings

In type 1 vWD, the vWF activity (ristocetin co-factor assay) and the vWF Ag are mildly depressed, whereas the vWF multimer pattern is normal (Table 14–10). Laboratory testing of type 2A or 2B vWD typically shows a ratio of vWF Ag:vWF activity of approximately 2:1 and a multimer pattern that lacks the highest molecular weight multimers. Thrombocytopenia is common in type 2B vWD due to a gain-of-function mutation of the vWF molecule, which leads to increased binding to its receptor on platelets, resulting in platelet clearance; a ristocetin-induced platelet aggregation (RIPA) study shows an increase in platelet aggregation in response to low concentrations of

Table 14–10. Laboratory diagnosis of von Willebrand disease.

Type		vWF Activity	vWF Antigen	Factor VIII	RIPA	Multimer Analysis
1		↓	↓	Nl or ↓	↓	Normal pattern; uniform ↓ intensity of bands
2	A	↓↓	↓	↓	↓	Large and intermediate multimers decreased or absent
	B	↓↓	↓	↓	↑	Large multimers decreased or absent
	M	↓	↓	↓	↓	Normal pattern; uniform ↓ intensity of bands
	N	Nl	Nl	↓↓	Nl	Nl
3		↓↓↓	↓↓↓	↓↓↓	↓↓↓	Multimers absent

Nl, normal; RIPA, ristocetin-induced platelet aggregation; vWF, von Willebrand factor.

ristocetin. Except in the more severe forms of vWD that feature a significantly decreased factor VIII activity, aPTT and PT are most commonly normal in patients with vWD.

Treatment

The treatment of vWD is outlined in Table 14–9. DDAVP is useful in the treatment of mild bleeding in most cases of type 1 and some cases of type 2 vWD. DDAVP causes release of vWF and factor VIII from storage sites, leading to increases in vWF and factor VIII twofold to sevenfold that of baseline levels. A therapeutic trial to document sufficient vWF levels posttreatment is critical prior to depending on DDAVP as a treatment option. Due to tachyphylaxis and the risk of significant hyponatremia secondary to fluid retention, more than two doses should not be given in a 48-hour period. vWF-containing factor VIII concentrates or recombinant VWF products are used in all other clinical scenarios, and when bleeding is not controlled with DDAVP. Cryoprecipitate should not be given due to lack of viral inactivation. Antifibrinolytic agents (eg, aminocaproic acid or tranexamic acid) may be used adjunctively for mucosal bleeding or procedures. Pregnant patients with type I vWD usually do not require treatment at the time of delivery because of the natural physiologic increase in vWF levels (up to threefold that of baseline) that are observed by parturition. However, levels need to be confirmed in late pregnancy, and if they are low or if excessive bleeding is encountered, vWF products may be given. Moreover, patients are at risk for significant bleeding 1–2 weeks postpartum when vWF levels fall secondary to the fall in estrogen levels.

Abshire TC et al. Prophylaxis in severe forms of von Willebrand's disease: results from the von Willebrand Disease Prophylaxis Network (VWD PN). Haemophilia. 2013 Jan;19(1):76–81. [PMID: 22823000]

De Jong A et al. Developments in the diagnostic procedures for von Willebrand disease. J Thromb Haemost. 2016 Mar;14(3):449–60. [PMID: 26714181]

Kouides PA. Present day management of inherited bleeding disorders in pregnancy. Expert Rev Hematol. 2016 Oct;9(10):987–95. [PMID: 27459638]

Neff AT. Current controversies in the diagnosis and management of von Willebrand disease. Ther Adv Hematol. 2015 Aug;6(4):209–16. [PMID: 26288715]

Sharma R et al. Advances in the diagnosis and treatment of Von Willebrand disease. Blood. 2017 Nov 30;130(22):2386–91. [PMID: 29187375]

3. Factor XI Deficiency

Factor XI deficiency (also called hemophilia C) is inherited in an autosomal recessive manner (in contrast to X-linked inheritance for hemophilia A and B), leading to heterozygous or homozygous defects. It is most prevalent among individuals of Ashkenazi Jewish descent. Levels of factor XI, while variably reduced, do not correlate well with bleeding symptoms. Mild bleeding is most common, and diagnosis is often made after unexpected, excessive bleeding following surgery or trauma. Factor XI deficiency that can lead to provoked excessive bleeding does not always prolong the aPTT, which is important to remember. FFP is the mainstay of treatment in locales where the plasma-derived factor XI concentrate is not available. Administration of adjunctive aminocaproic acid or tranexamic acid is regarded as mandatory for procedures or bleeding episodes involving the mucosa (Table 14–9).

Bolton-Maggs PH. Factor XI deficiency—resolving the enigma? Hematology Am Soc Hematol Educ Program. 2009:97–105. [PMID: 20008187]

James P et al. Rare bleeding disorders—bleeding assessment tools, laboratory aspects and phenotype and therapy of FXI deficiency. Haemophilia. 2014 May;20(Suppl 4):71–5. [PMID: 24762279]

4. Less Common Heritable Disorders of Coagulation

Congenital deficiencies of clotting factors II, V, VII, and X are rare and typically are inherited in an autosomal recessive pattern. A prolongation in the PT (and aPTT for factor X, factor V, and factor II deficiency) that corrects upon mixing with normal plasma is typical. Definitive diagnosis requires testing for specific factor activity. The treatment of factor II deficiency is with a prothrombin complex concentrate; factor V deficiency is treated with infusions of FFP or platelets (which contain factor V in alpha granules); factor VII deficiency is treated with recombinant human activated factor VII at 15–30 mcg/kg every 4–6 hours. Factor X deficiency, previously treated with FFP, can now be treated with a FDA-approved plasma-derived factor X product (Coagadex).

Deficiency of factor XIII, a transglutamase that cross-links fibrin, characteristically leads to delayed bleeding that occurs hours to days after a hemostatic challenge (such as surgery or trauma). The condition is usually life-long, and spontaneous intracranial hemorrhages as well as recurrent pregnancy loss appear to occur with increased frequency in these patients compared with other congenital deficiencies. Cryoprecipitate or infusion of a plasma-derived factor XIII concentrate (appropriate for patients with A-subunit deficiency only) has been the mainstay of treatment for bleeding or surgical prophylaxis. Factor XIII has an A and B subunit. Recombinant factor XIII A-subunit (Tretten) can be used for patients deficient in the A subunit. Factor XIII deficiency does not cause a prolongation of the PT or aPTT.

de Moerloose P et al. Rare coagulation disorders: fibrinogen, factor VII and factor XIII. Haemophilia. 2016 Jul;22(Suppl 5): 61–5. [PMID: 27405678]
Peyvandi F et al. Treatment of rare factor deficiencies in 2016. Hematology Am Soc Hematol Educ Program. 2016 Dec 2; 2016(1):663–9. [PMID: 27913544]

ACQUIRED DISORDERS OF COAGULATION

1. Acquired Antibodies to Factor II

Patients with antiphospholipid antibodies occasionally have antibody specificity to coagulation factor II (prothrombin), leading typically to a severe hypoprothrombinemia and bleeding. Mixing studies may or may not reveal presence of an inhibitor, as the antibody typically binds a non-enzymatically active portion of the molecule that leads to accelerated clearance, but characteristically the PT is prolonged and levels of factor II are low. FFP should be administered for treatment of bleeding. Treatment is immunosuppressive.

2. Acquired Antibodies to Factor V

Products containing bovine factor V (such as topical thrombin or fibrin glue, frequently used in surgical procedures) can lead to formation of an anti–factor V antibody that cross-reacts with human factor V. Clinicopathologic manifestations range from a prolonged PT in an otherwise asymptomatic individual to severe bleeding. Mixing studies suggest the presence of an inhibitor, and the factor V activity level is low. In cases of serious or life-threatening bleeding, IVIG or platelet transfusions, or both, should be administered, and immunosuppression (as for acquired inhibitors to factor VIII) may be offered.

3. Acquired Antibodies to Factor VIII

Spontaneous antibodies to factor VIII (acquired hemophilia A) occasionally occur in adults without a prior history of hemophilia; older adults and patients with lymphoproliferative malignancy or connective tissue disease and those who are postpartum or postsurgical are at highest risk. The clinical presentation, which should be viewed as a medical emergency, typically includes extensive soft tissue ecchymoses, hematomas, and mucosal bleeding, as opposed to hemarthrosis characteristic of congenital hemophilia A. The aPTT is typically prolonged and does not correct upon mixing; factor VIII activity is found to be low and a Bethesda assay reveals the titer of the inhibitor. Inhibitors of low titer (less than 5 BU) may often

be overcome by infusion of high doses of factor VIII concentrates, whereas high-titer inhibitors (greater than 5 BU) must be treated with serial infusions of activated prothrombin complex concentrates, recombinant human activated factor VII, or recombinant porcine factor VIII (hemophilia A patients only). Along with establishment of hemostasis by one of these measures, immunosuppressive treatment with corticosteroids with or without oral cyclophosphamide or rituximab should be instituted; treatment with IVIG and plasmapheresis can be considered in refractory cases. Unlike in congenital factor VIII deficiency, the patient's bleeding does not correlate well with the factor VIII activity level, so the clinician must be concerned with any elevation of aPTT secondary to acquired factor VIII inhibitor. All such patients require immediate referral to a hematologist.

Astermark J. FVIII inhibitors: pathogenesis and avoidance. Blood. 2015 Mar 26;125(13):2045–51. [PMID: 25712994]
Gibson CJ et al. Clinical problem-solving. A Bruising Loss. N Engl J Med. 2016 Jul 7;375(1):76–81. [PMID: 27406351]
Tiede A et al. Prognostic factors for remission of and survival in acquired hemophilia A (AHA): results from the GTH-AH 01/2010 study. Blood. 2015 Feb 12;125(7):1091–7. [PMID: 25525118]
Zeng Y et al. Interventions for treating acute bleeding episodes in people with acquired hemophilia A. Cochrane Database Syst Rev. 2014 Aug 28;8:CD010761. [PMID: 25165992]

4. Vitamin K Deficiency

Vitamin K deficiency may occur as a result of deficient dietary intake of vitamin K (from green leafy vegetables, soybeans, and other sources), malabsorption, or decreased production by intestinal bacteria (due to treatment with chemotherapy or antibiotics). Vitamin K is required for normal function of vitamin K epoxide reductase that assists in posttranslational gamma-carboxylation of the coagulation factors II, VII, IX, and X, which is necessary for their activity. Thus, mild to moderate vitamin K deficiency typically features a prolonged PT (activity of the vitamin K–dependent factors is more reflected than in the aPTT; aPTT is prolonged if the deficiency is more severe) that corrects upon mixing; activity levels of individual clotting factors II, VII, IX, and X typically are low. Importantly, a concomitantly low factor V activity level is not indicative of isolated vitamin K deficiency, and may indicate an underlying defect in liver synthetic function. Hospitalized patients on broad-spectrum antibiotics who have poor or no oral intake are at high risk for vitamin K deficiency.

For treatment, vitamin K_1 (phytonadione) may be administered via intravenous or oral routes; the subcutaneous route is not recommended due to erratic absorption. The oral dose is 5–10 mg/day and absorption is typically excellent; at least partial improvement in the PT should be observed within 18–24 hours of administration. Intravenous administration results in faster normalization of a prolonged PT than oral administration; due to descriptions of anaphylaxis, parenteral doses should be administered at lower doses (1–5 mg/day) and slowly (eg, over 30 minutes) with concomitant monitoring. Overreplacement can make it difficult to resume warfarin when necessary.

5. Coagulopathy of Liver Disease

Impaired liver function due to cirrhosis or other causes leads to decreased synthesis of clotting factors, including factors II, V, VII, IX, X, and fibrinogen; whereas factor VIII levels, largely made in endothelial cells, may be elevated despite depressed levels of other coagulation factors. The PT (and with advanced disease, the aPTT) is typically prolonged and usually corrects on mixing with normal plasma. A normal factor V level, in spite of decreases in the activity of factors II, VII, IX, and X, however, suggests vitamin K deficiency rather than liver disease. Qualitative and quantitative deficiencies of fibrinogen also are prevalent among patients with advanced liver disease, typically leading to a prolonged PT, thrombin time, and reptilase time.

The coagulopathy of liver disease usually does not require hemostatic treatment unless bleeding occurs. Infusion of FFP may be considered if active bleeding is present and the aPTT and PT are prolonged; however, the effect is transient and concern for volume overload may limit infusions. Patients with bleeding and a fibrinogen level consistently below 80–100 mg/dL should receive cryoprecipitate. Liver transplantation, if feasible, results in production of coagulation factors at normal levels. The use of recombinant human activated factor VII in patients with bleeding varices is controversial, although some patient subgroups may experience benefit. The coagulopathy of liver disease can predispose to bleeding or thrombosis, so caution and experience are needed for optimal management.

Bianchini M et al. Coagulopathy in liver diseases: complication or therapy? Dig Dis. 2014;32(5):609–14. [PMID: 25034295]
Franchini M et al. Acquired factor V inhibitors: a systematic review. J Thromb Thrombolysis. 2011 May;31(4):449–57. [PMID: 21052780]
Tripodi A et al. The coagulopathy of chronic liver disease. N Engl J Med. 2011 Jul 14;365(2):147–56. [PMID: 21751907]

6. Warfarin Ingestion

See Antithrombotic Therapy section, below.

7. Disseminated Intravascular Coagulation

See above.

8. Heparin/Fondaparinux/Direct-Acting Oral Anticoagulant Use

See Classes of Anticoagulants, below.

9. Lupus Anticoagulants

Lupus anticoagulants prolong the aPTT by interfering with interactions between the clotting cascade and the phospholipid surface on which they function, but they do not lead to bleeding. In fact, they predispose to thrombosis. Lupus anticoagulants were so named because of their early identification in patients with connective tissue disease, although they also occur with increased frequency in individuals with underlying infection, inflammation, or malignancy, and they also can occur in asymptomatic individuals in the general population. A prolongation in the aPTT is observed that does not correct completely on mixing but that normalizes with excessive phospholipid. Specialized testing such as a positive hexagonal phase phospholipid neutralization assay, a prolonged dilute Russell viper venom time, and positive platelet neutralization assays can confirm the presence of a lupus anticoagulant. Rarely, the antibodies also interfere with factor II activity (see above), and that tiny subset of lupus anticoagulant patients are at risk for bleeding.

Adams M. Measurement of lupus anticoagulants: an update on quality in laboratory testing. Semin Thromb Hemost. 2013 Apr; 39(3):267–71. [PMID: 23424052]

OTHER CAUSES OF BLEEDING

Occasionally, abnormalities of the vasculature and integument may lead to bleeding despite normal hemostasis; congenital or acquired disorders may be causative. These abnormalities include Ehlers-Danlos syndrome, osteogenesis imperfecta, Osler-Weber-Rendu disease (hereditary hemorrhagic telangiectasia), and Marfan syndrome (heritable defects) and integumentary thinning due to prolonged corticosteroid administration or normal aging, amyloidosis, vasculitis, and scurvy (acquired defects). The bleeding time often is prolonged. If possible, treatment of the underlying condition should be pursued, but if this is not possible or feasible (ie, congenital syndromes), globally hemostatic agents such as DDAVP can be considered for treatment of bleeding.

Patients with hereditary hemorrhagic telangiectasia should be referred to a hereditary hemorrhagic telangiectasia center of excellence (https://curehht.org/understanding-hht/get-support/hht-treatment-centers/). Bevacizumab and tranexamic acid can be useful in the treatment of hereditary hemorrhagic telangiectasia.

Gaillard S et al; ATERO Study Group. Tranexamic acid for epistaxis in hereditary hemorrhagic telangiectasia patients: a European cross-over controlled trial in a rare disease. J Thromb Haemost. 2014 Sep;12(9):1494–502. [PMID: 25040799]
Iyer VN et al. Intravenous bevacizumab for refractory hereditary hemorrhagic telangiectasia-related epistaxis and gastrointestinal bleeding. Mayo Clin Proc. 2018 Feb;93(2):155–66. [PMID: 29395350]

ANTITHROMBOTIC THERAPY

The currently available anticoagulants include unfractionated heparin, LMWHs, fondaparinux, vitamin K antagonist (ie, warfarin), and DOACs (ie, dabigatran, rivaroxaban, apixaban, edoxaban). (For a discussion of the injectable DTIs, see section Heparin-Induced Thrombocytopenia above.)

▶ Classes of Anticoagulants

A. Unfractionated Heparin and LMWHs

Only about one-third of the molecules in a given preparation of unfractionated heparin contain the crucial pentasaccharide sequence that is necessary for binding of antithrombin and exerting its anticoagulant effect by converting thrombin from a slow inhibitor of coagulation factor activity to a rapid inhibitor. The degree of anticoagulation with unfractionated heparin is typically monitored by aPTT or anti-Xa level in patients who are receiving the drug in therapeutic doses, although the pharmacokinetics of unfractionated heparin are poorly predictable. Only a fraction of an infused dose of heparin is metabolized by the kidneys, however, making it safe to use in most patients with significant kidney disease. Heparin should be discontinued in patients who have bleeding, and in some cases, protamine sulfate should be administered; 1 mg of protamine neutralizes approximately 100 units of heparin sulfate, and the maximum dose is 50 mg intravenously.

Due to less protein and cellular binding, the pharmacokinetics of the LMWHs are much more predictable than those of unfractionated heparin, allowing for fixed weight-based dosing. All LMWHs are principally renally cleared and must be avoided or used with extreme caution in individuals with creatinine clearance less than 30 mL/min. A longer half-life permits once- or twice-daily subcutaneous dosing, allowing for greater convenience and outpatient therapy in selected cases. Most patients do not require monitoring, although monitoring using the anti-Xa activity level is appropriate for patients with moderate kidney disease, those with elevated body mass index or low weight, and selected pregnant patients. About 30% of the molecules in a dose of LMWH are long enough (ie, sufficiently negatively charged) to bind protamine sulfate, allowing for some neutralization of anticoagulant effect. LMWHs are associated with a lower frequency of HIT (approximately 0.6%) than unfractionated heparin.

B. Fondaparinux

Fondaparinux, which is chemically related to LMWHs, is a synthetic molecule consisting of the highly active pentasaccharide sequence. As such, it exerts almost no thrombin inhibition and works to indirectly inhibit factor Xa through binding to antithrombin. Fondaparinux, like the LMWHs, is almost exclusively metabolized by the kidneys, and should be avoided in patients with creatinine clearance less than 30 mL/min. Predictable pharmacokinetics allow for weight-based dosing. A particularly long half-life (17–21 hours) allows for once-daily subcutaneous dosing, but the absence of necessary charge characteristics leads to a lack of binding to protamine sulfate; therefore, unlike heparin, no effective neutralizing agent exists.

C. Vitamin K Antagonist (Warfarin)

The vitamin K antagonist warfarin inhibits the activity of the vitamin K–dependent carboxylase that is important for the posttranslational modification of coagulation factors II, VII, IX, and X. Although warfarin may be taken orally, leading to a significant advantage over the heparins and heparin derivatives, which must be given parenterally or subcutaneously, interindividual differences in response to the agent related to nutritional status, comorbid diseases, concomitant medications, and genetic polymorphisms lead to a poorly predictable anticoagulant response. Individuals taking warfarin must undergo periodic monitoring to verify the intensity of the anticoagulant effect. The intensity of

anticoagulant effect is reported as the INR, which corrects for differences in potency of commercially available thromboplastin used to perform the PT.[1]

D. Direct-Acting Oral Anticoagulants

Unlike warfarin, the DOACs (1) have a predictable dose effect and therefore do not require laboratory monitoring, (2) have anticoagulant activity independent of vitamin K with no need for dietary stasis, and (3) are renally metabolized to varying degrees so there are restrictions or dose reductions related to reduced kidney function (Table 14–11). While the DOACs have fewer drug interactions than warfarin, if DOACs are given with a potentially interacting medication, there is no reliable way to measure the impact on anticoagulant activity of the concomitant administration. There is no reliable way to measure adherence, either. There is a paucity of data on the use of DOACs in morbidly obese patients (more than 120 kg). There is a reversal agent available for dabigatran and for the anti-Xa inhibitors apixaban and rivaroxaban. The provider must carefully consider kidney function, weight, concomitant medications, indication for use, candidacy for lead-in parenteral therapy (as required for acute VTE treatment with edoxaban and dabigatran only) and anticipated patient adherence. Providers must be careful to dose each DOAC properly for the indication, kidney function, weight of patient, and for drug interactions. (See Table 14–11 for details.)

Routine monitoring is not recommended for patients taking DOACs. However, there are clinical scenarios where assessing anticoagulant activity may be helpful, including active bleeding, pending urgent surgery, suspected therapeutic failure, or concern for accumulation. There is no standardized laboratory assay to measure anticoagulant effect of the DOACs. They have varying effects on the PT and aPTT. A normal thrombin time excludes the presence of clinically relevant dabigatran levels; a normal aPTT likely excludes excess drug levels of dabigatran. A negative anti-Xa level likely excludes clinically relevant levels of rivaroxaban, apixaban, or edoxaban; a normal PT likely excludes excess drug levels of rivaroxaban but not apixaban or edoxaban. The INR is unreliable for the evaluation of factor Xa activity.

Connolly SJ et al; ANNEXA-4 Investigators. Andexanet alfa for acute major bleeding associated with factor Xa inhibitors. N Engl J Med. 2016 Sep 22;375(12):1131–41. [PMID: 27573206]

Rose AJ et al. Evidence-based best practices for outpatient management of warfarin. Ann Pharmacother. 2018 Oct;52(10):1042–6. [PMID: 29890846]

Streiff MB et al. Guidance for the treatment of deep vein thrombosis and pulmonary embolism. J Thromb Thrombolysis. 2016 Jan;41(1):32–67. Erratum in: J Thromb Thrombolysis. 2016 Apr;41(3):548. [PMID: 26780738]

Tomaselli GF et al. 2017 ACC Expert Consensus Decision Pathway on management of bleeding in patients on oral anticoagulants: a report of the American College of Cardiology Task Force on Expert Consensus Decision Pathways. J Am Coll Cardiol. 2017 Dec 19;70(24):3042–67. [PMID: 29203195]

---

[1]Importantly, because the INR is not standardized for abnormalities of factor V and fibrinogen, the INR should be used only in reference to anticoagulation in patients who are receiving warfarin.

Table 14–11. Direct-acting oral anticoagulants (DOACs) for VTE treatment and prevention.[1]

	Dabigatran	Rivaroxaban	Apixaban	Edoxaban	Betrixaban
Mechanism	Oral direct thrombin inhibitor	Oral direct factor Xa inhibitor	Oral direct factor Xa inhibitor	Oral direct factor Xa inhibitor	Oral direct factor Xa inhibitor
Approved uses	Atrial fibrillation VTE treatment and secondary prevention VTE replacement prophylaxis following hip replacement	Atrial fibrillation VTE treatment and secondary prevention VTE prophylaxis post-hip or knee replacement	Atrial fibrillation VTE treatment and secondary prevention VTE prophylaxis post-hip or knee replacement	Atrial fibrillation VTE treatment and secondary prevention	Prophylaxis of VTE in adults hospitalized for acute medical illness with moderate or severe restricted mobility and other risk factors for VTE
Frequency of dosing	Twice daily	Twice daily for first 21 days of acute VTE therapy, then daily Once daily for DVT prevention	Twice daily	Once daily	Once daily
Food	With or without food	With food (for 15- and 20-mg tablets)	With or without food	With or without food	With food
Crushable?	No	Can crush; do not administer via J tube	Can crush and administer orally or via NG tube	No data	
Renal clearance	80%	30–60%	25%	50%	15%
Kinetics	t½ = 12–17 hours; tmax = 2 hours	t½ = 5–9 hours; tmax = 3 hours	t½ = 12 hours; tmax = 3 hours	t½ = 10–14 hours; tmax = 2 hours	t½ = 19–27 hours; tmax = 3 hours
Influences INR?	↑ (or →)	↑↑ (or → at low concentrations)	↑ (or →)	↑	Unknown
Influences aPTT?	↑↑	↑	↑	↑	Unknown
Drug interactions (list not comprehensive)	**Avoid** rifampin, St John's wort, and possibly carbamazepine **Caution** with amiodarone, clarithromycin, dronedarone, ketoconazole, quinidine, verapamil. No dosage adjustment of dabigatran is recommended if CrCl > 50 mL/min **Reduce dose** to 75 mg orally twice daily if CrCl 30–50 mL/min and concurrent use of dronedarone or ketoconazole	**Avoid** carbamazepine, conivaptan, indinavir/ritonavir, itraconazole, ketoconazole, lopinavir/ritonavir, phenytoin, rifampin, ritonavir, St John's wort **Caution** with the concurrent use of combined P-gp inhibitors and/or weak or moderate inhibitors of CYP3A4 (eg, amiodarone, azithromycin, diltiazem, dronedarone, erythromycin, felodipine, quinidine, ranolazine, verapamil) with rivaroxaban, particularly in patients with impaired kidney function	**Avoid** carbamazepine, clarithromycin, phenytoin, rifampin, St John's wort, itraconazole, ketoconazole, and ritonavir in patients already taking apixaban even at a reduced dose of 2.5 mg twice daily **Caution** with clarithromycin, itraconazole, ketoconazole, and ritonavir	**Avoid** rifampin **Reduce dose** with certain P-gp inhibitors. Use has not been studied with many other P-gp inhibitors and inducers Some recommend avoiding concomitant use altogether	**Reduce dose** to 40 mg orally daily with concomitant use of P-gp inhibitors (eg, amiodarone, azithromycin, verapamil, ketoconazole, clarithromycin)

Switching from DOAC to warfarin (per AC Forum Clinical Guidance: either approach [ie, stop DOAC then start LMWH and warfarin; or overlap warfarin with DOAC] can be used for all DOAC to warfarin transitions. If overlapping warfarin and DOAC, measure INR just before next DOAC dose and stop DOAC when INR ≥ 2.0)	Start warfarin and overlap with dabigatran; CrCl C50 mL/min, overlap 3 days CrCl 30–50 mL/min, overlap 2 days CrCl 15–30 mL/min, overlap 1 day	Stop DOAC; start warfarin and LMWH at time of next scheduled DOAC dose and bridge until INR ≥ 2.0		For 60-mg dose, reduce dose to 30 mg and start warfarin concomitantly For 30-mg dose reduce dose to 15 mg and start warfarin concomitantly Stop edoxaban when INR ≥ 2.0	No data available
Warfarin to DOAC	Start when INR < 2.0	Start when INR < 3.0	Start when INR < 2.0	Start when INR ≤ 2.5	Start when INR < 2.5
Special considerations	Dyspepsia is common and starts within first 10 days GI bleeding risk higher with dabigatran vs warfarin	GI bleeding risk higher with rivaroxaban vs warfarin		Do not use if CrCl ≥ 95 mL/min	
Management of life-threatening bleeding	Idarucizumab 2 doses of 2.5 g intravenously no more than 15 min apart	Activated charcoal, supportive care, consider 4-component PCC Recombinant coagulation factor Xa (Andexxa) anticipated wide availability in 2019	Activated charcoal, supportive care, consider 4-component PCC Recombinant coagulation factor Xa (Andexxa) anticipated wide availability in 2019	Activated charcoal, supportive care, consider 4-component PCC	Activated charcoal, supportive care, consider 4-component PCC

[1]Previously called new (novel) oral anticoagulants and target-specific oral anticoagulants. Consult prescribing information for updated dosing.

aPTT, activated partial thromboplastin time; CrCl, creatinine clearance; DOAC, direct oral anticoagulant; GI, gastrointestinal; INR, international normalized ratio; LMWH, low-molecular-weight heparin; NG, nasogastric; PCC, prothrombin complex concentrate; P-gp, P-glycoprotein; VTE, venous thromboembolism.

Witt DM et al. American Society of Hematology 2018 guidelines
for management of venous thromboembolism: optimal management of anticoagulation therapy. Blood Adv. 2018 Nov 27;
2(22):3257–91. [PMID: 30482765]
Witt DM et al. Guidance for the practical management of warfarin
therapy in the treatment of venous thromboembolism.
J Thromb Thrombolysis. 2016 Jan;41(1):187–205. [PMID:
26780746]

Prevention of Venous Thromboembolic Disease

The frequency of venous thromboembolic disease (VTE) among hospitalized patients ranges widely; up to 20% of medical patients and 80% of critical care patients and high-risk surgical patients have been reported to experience this complication, which includes DVT and PE.

Avoidance of fatal PE, which occurs in up to 5% of high-risk inpatients as a consequence of hospitalization or surgery, is a major goal of pharmacologic prophylaxis. Tables 14–12 and 14–13 provide risk stratification for DVT/VTE among hospitalized surgical and medical inpatients. Standard pharmacologic prophylactic regimens are

Table 14–12. Risk stratification for DVT/VTE among surgical inpatients.

High risk
Recent major orthopedic surgery/arthroplasty/fracture
Abdominal/pelvic cancer undergoing surgery
Recent spinal cord injury or major trauma within 90 days
More than three of the intermediate risk factors (see below)
Intermediate risk
Not ambulating independently outside of room at least twice daily
Active infectious or inflammatory process
Active malignancy
Major surgery (nonorthopedic)
History of VTE
Stroke
Central venous access or PICC line
Inflammatory bowel disease
Prior immobilization (> 72 hours) preoperatively
Obesity (BMI > 30)
Patient age > 50 years
Hormone replacement or oral contraceptive therapy
Hypercoagulable state
Nephrotic syndrome
Burns
Cellulitis
Varicose veins
Paresis
HF (systolic dysfunction)
COPD exacerbation
Low risk
Minor procedure and age < 40 years with no additional risk factors
Ambulatory with expected length of stay of < 24 hours or minor surgery

BMI, body mass index; COPD, chronic obstructive pulmonary disease; DVT, deep venous thrombosis; HF, heart failure; PICC, peripherally inserted central catheter; VTE, venous thromboembolism.

Table 14–13. Padua Risk Assessment Model for VTE prophylaxis in hospitalized medical patients.

Condition	Points[1]
Active cancer, history of VTE, immobility, laboratory thrombophilia	3 points each
Recent (≤ 1 mo) trauma and/or surgery	2 points each
Age ≥ 70, acute MI or CVA, acute infection, rheumatologic disorder, BMI ≥ 30, hormonal therapy	1 point each

[1]A score ≥ 4 connotes high risk of VTE in the noncritically ill medical patients and pharmacologic prophylaxis is indicated, absent absolute contraindications.
BMI, body mass index; CVA, cerebrovascular accident; MI, myocardial infarction; VTE, venous thromboembolism.

listed in Table 14–14. Prophylactic strategies should be guided by individual risk stratification, with all moderate- and high-risk patients receiving pharmacologic prophylaxis, unless contraindicated. Contraindications to VTE prophylaxis for hospital inpatients at high risk for VTE are listed in Table 14–15. In patients at high risk for VTE with absolute contraindications to pharmacologic prophylaxis, mechanical devices such as intermittent pneumatic compression devices should be used, ideally portable devices with at least an 18-hour daily wear time.

It is recommended that VTE prophylaxis be used judiciously in hospitalized medical patients who are not critically ill since a comprehensive review of evidence suggested harm from bleeding in low-risk patients given low-dose heparin and skin necrosis in stroke patients given compression stockings. There are risk assessment models available to help the clinician identify patients who may benefit DVT prophylaxis (ie, Padua Risk Score and the IMPROVE risk score); however, neither is ideal and performance is limited (Table 14–13). The IMPROVE investigators also developed a bleeding risk model that may aid in identifying acutely ill medical inpatients at increased risk for bleeding. While one of the anti-Xa oral anticoagulants (betrixaban) has been approved for extended duration, out of hospital, DVT prophylaxis for hospitalized medical patients, how best to identify those who will have net clinical benefit from this practice is still unclear.

Certain high-risk surgical patients should be considered for extended-duration prophylaxis of approximately 1 month, including those undergoing total hip replacement, hip fracture repair, and abdominal and pelvic cancer surgery. If bleeding is present, if the risk of bleeding is high, or if the risk of VTE is high for the inpatient (Table 14–12) and therefore combined prophylactic strategies are needed, some measure of thromboprophylaxis may be provided through use of mechanical devices, including intermittent pneumatic compression devices, or graduated compression stockings.

Some ambulatory cancer patients undergoing chemotherapy who are at moderate to high risk of VTE (Khorona risk score ≥ 2) (https://www.mdcalc.com/khorana-risk-score-venous-thromboembolism-cancer-patients) may

Table 14–14. Pharmacologic prophylaxis of VTE in selected clinical scenarios.[1]

Anticoagulant	Dose	Frequency	Clinical Scenario	Comment
Enoxaparin	40 mg subcutaneously	Once daily	Most medical inpatients and critical care patients	—
			Surgical patients (moderate risk for VTE)	
			Abdominal/pelvic cancer surgery	Consider continuing for 4 weeks total duration after abdomino-pelvic cancer surgery
		Twice daily	Bariatric surgery	Higher doses may be required
	30 mg subcutaneously	Twice daily	Orthopedic surgery[2]	Give for at least 10 days. For THR, TKA, or HFS, consider continuing up to 1 month after surgery in high-risk patients
			Major trauma	Not applicable to patients with isolated lower extremity trauma
			Acute spinal cord injury	—
Dalteparin	2500 units subcutaneously	Once daily	Most medical inpatients	—
			Abdominal surgery (moderate risk for VTE)	Give for 5–10 days
	5000 units subcutaneously	Once daily	Orthopedic surgery[2]	First dose = 2500 units. Give for at least 10 days. For THR, TKA, or HFS, consider continuing up to 1 month after surgery in high-risk patients
			Abdominal surgery (higher risk for VTE)	Give for 5–10 days
			Medical inpatients	—
Fondaparinux	2.5 mg subcutaneously	Once daily	Orthopedic surgery[2]	Give for at least 10 days. For THR, TKA, or HFS, consider continuing up to 1 month after surgery in high-risk patients
Rivaroxaban	10 mg orally	Once daily	Orthopedic surgery: total hip and total knee replacement	Give for 12 days following total knee replacement; give for 35 days following total hip replacement
Apixaban	2.5 mg orally	Twice daily	Following hip or knee replacement surgery	Give for 12 days following total knee replacement; give for 35 days following total hip replacement
Dabigatran	110 mg orally first day, then 220 mg	Once daily	Following hip replacement surgery	For patients with CrCl > 30 mL/min
Betrixaban	Initial single dose of 160 mg, then 80 mg once daily with food Reduce dose for patients with severe renal impairment or taking P-gp inhibitors	Daily	Adult patients hospitalized for an acute medical illness with moderately to severely restricted mobility and other risk factors for VTE	Recommended duration of treatment is 35–42 days
Unfractionated heparin	5000 units subcutaneously	Three times daily	Higher VTE risk with low bleeding risk	Includes gynecologic surgery for malignancy and urologic surgery, medical patients with multiple risk factors for VTE
	5000 units subcutaneously	Twice daily	Hospitalized patients at intermediate risk for VTE	Includes gynecologic surgery (moderate risk)
			Patients with epidural catheters	LMWHs usually avoided due to risk of spinal hematoma
			Patients with severe kidney disease[3]	LMWHs contraindicated

(continued)

Table 14–14. Pharmacologic prophylaxis of VTE in selected clinical scenarios.[1] (continued)

Anticoagulant	Dose	Frequency	Clinical Scenario	Comment
Warfarin	(variable) oral	Once daily	Orthopedic surgery[2]	Titrate to goal INR = 2.5. Give for at least 10 days. For high-risk patients undergoing THR, TKA, or HFS, consider continuing up to 1 month after surgery
Aspirin	variable		Hip and knee replacement	

[1]All regimens administered subcutaneously, except for warfarin.
[2]Includes TKA, THR, and HFS.
[3]Defined as creatinine clearance < 30 mL/min.
CrCl, creatine clearance; HFS, hip fracture surgery; INR, international normalized ratio; LMWH, low-molecular-weight heparin; P-gp, P-glycoprotein; THR, total hip replacement; TKA, total knee arthroplasty; VTE, venous thromboembolic disease.

benefit from pharmacologic DVT prophylaxis, although bleeding risk is increased and caution should be taken, particularly in patients with gastrointestinal malignancy and other risk factors for anticoagulant-related bleeding (such as thrombocytopenia and kidney dysfunction).

Al Yami MS et al. Direct oral anticoagulants for extended thromboprophylaxis in medically ill patients: meta-analysis and risk/benefit assessment. J Blood Med. 2018 Feb 21;9:25–34. [PMID: 29503590]
Anderson DR et al. Aspirin or rivaroxaban for VTE prophylaxis after hip or knee arthroplasty. N Engl J Med. 2018 Feb 22; 378(8):699–707. [PMID: 29466159]

Table 14–15. Contraindications to VTE prophylaxis for medical or surgical hospital inpatients at high risk for VTE.

Absolute contraindications
Acute hemorrhage from wounds or drains or lesions
Intracranial hemorrhage within prior 24 hours
Heparin-induced thrombocytopenia (HIT): consider using fondaparinux
Severe trauma to head or spinal cord or extremities
Epidural anesthesia/spinal block within 12 hours of initiation of anticoagulation (concurrent use of an epidural catheter and anticoagulation other than low prophylactic doses of unfractionated heparin should require review and approval by service who performed the epidural or spinal procedure, eg, anesthesia/pain service, and in many cases, should be avoided entirely)
Currently receiving warfarin or heparin or LMWH or direct thrombin inhibitor for other indications
Relative contraindications
Coagulopathy (INR > 1.5)
Intracranial lesion or neoplasm
Severe thrombocytopenia (platelet count < 50,000/mcL)
Intracranial hemorrhage within past 6 months
Gastrointestinal or genitourinary hemorrhage within past 6 months

INR, international normalized ratio; LMWH, low-molecular-weight heparin; VTE, venous thromboembolic disease.
Adapted from guidelines used at the Veterans Affairs Medical Center, San Francisco, CA.

Schünemann HJ et al. American Society of Hematology 2018 guidelines for management of venous thromboembolism: prophylaxis for hospitalized and nonhospitalized medical patients. Blood Adv. 2018 Nov 27;2(22):3198–225. [PMID: 30482763]

Treatment of Venous Thromboembolic Disease

A. Anticoagulant Therapy

Treatment for VTE should be offered to patients with objectively confirmed DVT or PE, or to those in whom the clinical suspicion is high for the disorder but who have not yet undergone diagnostic testing (see Chapter 9). The management of VTE primarily involves administration of anticoagulants; the goal is to prevent recurrence, extension and embolization of thrombosis and to reduce the risk of postthrombotic syndrome. Suggested anticoagulation regimens are found in Table 14–16.

B. Selecting Appropriate Anticoagulant Therapy

Most patients with DVT alone may be treated as outpatients, provided that their risk of bleeding is low, and they have good follow-up. Table 14–17 outlines proposed selection criteria for outpatient treatment of DVT.

Among patients with PE, risk stratification should be done at time of diagnosis to direct treatment and triage. Patients with persistent hemodynamic instability are classified as high-risk patients (previously referred to as having "massive PE") and have an early PE-related mortality of more than 15%. These patients should be admitted to an intensive care unit and generally receive thrombolysis (both full-dose and half-dose regimens have been shown to be effective) and anticoagulation with intravenous heparin. Intermediate-risk patients (previously, "submassive PE") have a mortality rate of up to 15% and should be admitted to a higher level of inpatient care, with consideration of thrombolysis on a case-by-case basis. Catheter-directed techniques, if available, may be an option for patients who are poor candidates for systemic thrombolysis and/or in centers with expertise. Low-risk patients have a mortality rate less than 3% and are candidates for expedited discharge or outpatient therapy.

Table 14–16. Initial anticoagulation for VTE.[1]

Anticoagulant	Dose/Frequency	DVT, Lower Extremity	DVT, Upper Extremity	PE	VTE, With Concomitant Severe Kidney Disease[2]	VTE, Cancer-Related	Comment
Unfractionated Heparin							
Unfractionated heparin	80 units/kg intravenous bolus, then continuous intravenous infusion of 18 units/kg/h	×	×	×	×		Bolus may be omitted if risk of bleeding is perceived to be elevated. Maximum bolus, 10,000 units. Requires aPTT monitoring. Most patients: begin warfarin at time of initiation of heparin.
	330 units/kg subcutaneously × 1, then 250 units/kg subcutaneously every 12 hours	×					Fixed-dose; no aPTT monitoring required
LMWH and Fondaparinux							
Enoxaparin[3]	1 mg/kg subcutaneously every 12 hours	×	×	×			Most patients: begin warfarin at time of initiation of LMWH
Dalteparin[3]	200 units/kg subcutaneously once daily for first month, then 150 units/kg/day	×	×	×		×	Cancer: administer LMWH for ≥ 3–6 months; reduce dose to 150 units/kg after first month of treatment
Fondaparinux	5–10 mg subcutaneously once daily; use 7.5 mg for body weight 50–100 kg; 10 mg for body weight > 100 kg	×	×	×			
Direct-Acting Oral Anticoagulants (DOACs)							
Rivaroxaban	15 mg orally twice daily with food for 21 days then 20 mg orally daily with food	×	×	×			Contraindicated if CrCl < 30 mL/min
Apixaban	10 mg orally twice daily for first 7 days then 5 mg twice daily	×	×	×			Contraindicated if CrCl < 25 mL/min. Monotherapy without need for initial parenteral therapy
Dabigatran	5–10 days of parenteral anticoagulation, then 150 mg orally twice daily	×	×	×			Contraindicated if CrCl < 15 mL/min. Initial need for parenteral therapy
Edoxaban	5–10 days of parenteral anticoagulation, then 60 mg orally once daily; 30 mg once daily recommended if CrCl is between 15 and 50 mL/min, if weight ≤ 60 kg, or if certain P-gp inhibitors are present	×	×	×			Contraindicated if CrCl < 15 mL/min or > 95 mL/min. Initial need for parenteral therapy

[1]Obtain baseline hemoglobin, platelet count, aPTT, PT/INR, and creatinine prior to initiation of anticoagulation.
Anticoagulation is contraindicated in the setting of active bleeding.
[2]Defined as creatinine clearance < 30 mL/min.
[3]If body weight < 50 kg, reduce dose and monitor anti-Xa levels.
CrCl, creatinine clearance; DVT, deep venous thrombosis; PE, pulmonary embolism; P-gp, P-glycoprotein; VTE, venous thromboembolic disease (includes DVT and PE).
Note: An "×" denotes appropriate use of the anticoagulant.

Table 14–17. Patient selection for outpatient treatment of DVT.

Patients considered appropriate for outpatient treatment
  No clinical signs or symptoms of PE and pain controlled
  Motivated and capable of self-administration of injections
  Confirmed prescription insurance that covers injectable medication or patient can pay out-of-pocket for injectable agents
  Capable and willing to comply with frequent follow-up
  Initially, patients may need to be seen daily to weekly
Potential contraindications for outpatient treatment
  DVT involving inferior vena cava, iliac, common femoral, or upper extremity vein (these patients might benefit from vascular intervention)
  Comorbid conditions
  Active peptic ulcer disease, GI bleeding in past 14 days, liver synthetic dysfunction
  Brain metastases, current or recent CNS or spinal cord injury/surgery in the last 10 days, CVA ≤ 4–6 weeks
  Familial bleeding diathesis
  Active bleeding from source other than GI
  Thrombocytopenia
  Creatinine clearance < 30 mL/min
  Patient weighs < 55 kg (male) or < 45 kg (female)
  Recent surgery, spinal or epidural anesthesia in the past 3 days
  History of heparin-induced thrombocytopenia
  Inability to inject medication at home, reliably follow medication schedule, recognize changes in health status, understand or follow directions

DVT, deep vein thrombosis.

Because both intermediate- and low-risk patients are hemodynamically stable, additional assessment is necessary to differentiate the two. Echocardiography can be used to identify patients with right ventricular dysfunction, which connotes intermediate risk. An RV/LV ratio less than 1.0 on chest CT angiogram has been shown to have good negative predictive value for adverse outcome but suffers from inter-observer variability. Serum biomarkers such as B-type natriuretic peptide and troponin are most useful for their negative predictive value, and mainly in combination with other predictors. The Bova score, the PE severity index (PESI)/simplified PESI clinical risk scores (which do not require additional testing), accurately identify patients at low risk for 30-day PE-related mortality (Table 14–18) and thus potential candidates for expedited discharge or outpatient treatment. The PESI48 and sPESI48 scores identify a subgroup of patients hospitalized with intermediate-risk PE who are reclassified as low risk by 48 hours and may be appropriate for early discharge.

Selection of an initial anticoagulant should be determined by patient characteristics (kidney function, immediate bleeding risk, weight) and the clinical scenario (eg, whether thrombolysis is being considered, active cancer, thrombosis location).

1. Parenteral anticoagulants—

HEPARINS—In patients in whom parenteral anticoagulation is being considered, LMWHs are more effective than unfractionated heparin in the immediate treatment of DVT and PE and are preferred as initial treatment because

Table 14–18. Simplified Pulmonary Embolism Severity Index (PESI).

	Points
Age > 80 years old	1
Cancer	1
Chronic cardiopulmonary disease	1
Systolic blood pressure < 100 mm Hg	1
Oxygen saturation ≤ 90%	1

Severity Class	Points	30-Day Mortality
Low risk	0	1%
High risk	≥ 1	10%

Adapted, with permission, from Jiménez D et al; RIETE Investigators. Simplification of the pulmonary embolism severity index for prognostication in patients with acute symptomatic pulmonary embolism. Arch Intern Med. 2010 Aug 9;170(15):1383–9. Copyright © 2010 American Medical Association. All rights reserved.

of predictable pharmacokinetics, which allow for subcutaneous, once- or twice-daily dosing with no requirement for monitoring in most patients. Accumulation of LMWH and increased rates of bleeding have been observed among patients with severe kidney disease (creatinine clearance less than 30 mL/min), leading to a recommendation to use intravenous unfractionated heparin preferentially in these patients. *If concomitant thrombolysis is being considered, unfractionated heparin is indicated.* Patients with VTE and a perceived higher risk of bleeding (ie, post-surgery) may be better candidates for treatment with unfractionated heparin than LMWH given its shorter half-life and reversibility. Unfractionated heparin can be effectively neutralized with the positively charged protamine sulfate while protamine may only have partial reversal effect at best on LMWH. Use of unfractionated heparin leads to HIT in approximately 3% of patients, so most individuals require serial platelet count determinations during the initial 10–14 days of exposure.

Weight-based, fixed-dose daily subcutaneous fondaparinux (a synthetic factor Xa inhibitor) may also be used for the initial treatment of DVT and PE, with no increase in bleeding over that observed with LMWH. Its lack of reversibility, long half-life, and renal clearance limit its use in patients with an increased risk of bleeding or kidney disease.

2. Oral anticoagulants—

A. WARFARIN—If warfarin is chosen as the oral anticoagulant it will be initiated along with the parenteral anticoagulant, which is continued until INR is in therapeutic range. Most patients require 5 mg of warfarin daily for initial treatment, but lower doses (2.5 mg daily) should be considered for patients of Asian descent, older adults, and those with hyperthyroidism, heart failure, liver disease, recent major surgery, malnutrition, certain polymorphisms for the *CYP2C9* or the *VKORC1* genes or who are receiving

Table 14–19. Warfarin dosing adjustment guidelines for initiation of warfarin therapy.

Measurement Day	INR	Action
For Hospitalized Patients Newly Starting Therapy		
Day 1		5 mg (2.5 or 7.5 mg in select populations[1])
Day 2	< 1.5	Continue dose
	≥ 1.5	Decrease or hold dose[2]
Day 3	≤ 1.2	Increase dose[2]
	> 1.2 and < 1.7	Continue dose
	≥ 1.7	Decrease dose[2]
Day 4 until therapeutic	Daily increase < 0.2 units	Increase dose[2]
	Daily increase 0.2–0.3 units	Continue dose
	Daily increase 0.4–0.6 units	Decrease dose[2]
	Daily increase ≥ 0.7 units	Hold dose
For Outpatients Newly Starting Therapy		
Measure PT/INR on Day 1	Baseline	Start treatment with 2–7.5 mg
Measure PT/INR on Day 3–4	< 1.5	Increase weekly dose by 5–25%
	1.5–1.9	No dosage change
	2.0–2.5	Decrease weekly dose by 25–50%
	> 2.5	Decrease weekly dose by 50% or HOLD dose
Measure PT/INR on Day 5–7	< 1.5	Increase weekly dose by 10–25%
	1.5–1.9	Increase weekly dose by 0–20%
	2.0–3.0	No dosage change
	> 3.0	Decrease weekly dose by 10–25% or HOLD dose
Measure PT/INR on Day 8–10	< 1.5	Increase weekly dose by 15–35%
	1.5–1.9	Increase weekly dose by 5–20%
	2.0–3.0	No dosage change
	> 3.0	Decrease weekly dose by 10–25% or HOLD dose
Measure PT/INR on Day 11–14	< 1.6	Increase weekly dose by 15–35%
	1.6–1.9	Increase weekly dose by 5–20%
	2.0–3.0	No dosage change
	> 3.0	Decrease weekly dose by 5–20% or HOLD dose

[1]See text.
[2]In general, dosage adjustments should not exceed 2.5 mg or 50%.
Data from Kim YK et al. J Thromb Haemost 2010;8:101–6. From Center for Health Quality, Outcomes, and Economic Research, VA Medical Center, Bedford, MA.

concurrent medications that increase sensitivity to warfarin. Conversely, individuals of African descent, those with larger body mass index or hypothyroidism, and those who are receiving medications that increase warfarin metabolism may require higher initial doses (7.5 mg daily). Daily INR results should guide dosing adjustments in the hospitalized patient while at least biweekly INR results guide dosing in the outpatient (Table 14–19). Web-based warfarin dosing calculators that consider these clinical and genetic factors are available to help clinicians choose the appropriate starting dose (eg, see www.warfarindosing.org). Because an average of 5 days is required to achieve a steady-state reduction in the activity of vitamin K–dependent coagulation factors, the parenteral anticoagulant should be continued for at least 5 days and until the INR is more than 2.0. Meticulous follow-up should be arranged for all patients taking warfarin because of the bleeding risk that is associated with initiation of therapy. Once stabilized, the INR should be checked at an interval no longer than every 6 weeks and warfarin dosing should be adjusted by guidelines (Table 14–20) since this strategy has been shown to improve the time patients spend in the therapeutic range and their clinical outcomes. Supratherapeutic INRs should be managed according to evidence-based guidelines (Table 14–21).

Table 14–20. Warfarin-dosing adjustment guidelines for patients receiving long-term therapy, with target INR 2–3.

Patient INR	Weekly Dosing Change	
	Dose change	Follow-up INR
≤ 1.5	Increase by 10–15%	Within 1 week
1.51–1.79	If falling or low on two or more occasions, increase weekly dose by 5–10%.	7–14 days
1.80–2.29	Consider not changing the dose unless a consistent pattern has been observed.	7–14 days
2.3–3.0 (in range)	No change in dosage.	28 days (42 days if INR in range three times consecutively)
3.01–3.20	Consider not changing the dose unless a consistent pattern has been observed.	7–14 days
3.21–3.69	Do not hold warfarin. If rising or high on two or more occasions, decrease weekly dose by 5–10%.	7–14 days
3.70–4.99	Hold warfarin for 1 day and decrease weekly dose by 5–10%.	Within 1 week, sooner if clinically indicated
5.0–8.99	Hold warfarin. Clinical evaluation for bleeding. When INR is therapeutic, restart at lower dose (decrease weekly dose by 10–15%). Check INR at least weekly until stable.	Within 1 week, sooner if clinically indicated, then weekly until stabilized
≥ 9	See Table 14–21	

From Center for Health Quality, Outcomes, and Economic Research, VA Medical Center, Bedford, MA. Data from Kim YK et al. J Thromb Haemost 2010;8:101–6. See also Van Spall HE et al. Variation in warfarin dose adjustment practice is responsible for differences in the quality of anticoagulation control between centers and countries: an analysis of patients receiving warfarin in the randomized evaluation of long-term anticoagulation therapy (RE-LY) trial. Circulation. 2012 Nov 6;126(19):2309–16. [PMID: 23027801]

B. DIRECT-ACTING ORAL ANTICOAGULANTS—DOACs have a predictable dose effect, few drug-drug interactions, rapid onset of action, and freedom from laboratory monitoring (Table 14–11). Dabigatran, rivaroxaban, apixaban, and edoxaban are approved for treatment of acute DVT and PE. While rivaroxaban and apixaban can be used as monotherapy eliminating the need for parenteral therapy, patients who will be treated with dabigatran or edoxaban must first receive 5–10 days of parenteral anticoagulation and then be transitioned to the oral agent per prescribing information. Unlike warfarin, DOACs do not require an overlap or "bridge," since these agents are immediately active; the patient first receives a course of a parenteral agent, the agent is then stopped and the DOAC is started. Compared to warfarin and LMWH, the DOACs are all "noninferior" with respect to prevention of recurrent VTE; both rivaroxaban (in noncancer patients) and apixaban have a lower bleeding risk than warfarin and LMWH. Agent selection for acute treatment of VTE should be individualized and consider kidney function, concomitant medications, indication, ability to use LMWH bridge therapy, cost, and adherence.

LMWH is still endorsed as the preferred agent for treatment of cancer-related VTE according to American College of Chest Physicians and National Comprehensive Cancer Network guidelines. However, these guidelines were published prior to the Hokusai trial, which found the DOAC edoxaban to be noninferior to LMWH for treatment of cancer-associated VTE. While edoxaban resulted in reduced risk of recurrent DVT when compared to dalteparin, there was an increased risk of major bleeding, mostly in patients with gastrointestinal malignancies. In the SELECT D pilot study, rivaroxaban was found to be as effective as LMWH in preventing recurrent VTE in cancer patients; however, similar to the Hokusai trial, increased major bleeding rates were seen in patients taking a DOAC, particularly those with esophageal or gastroesophageal cancer. Based on these data, the Internal Society for Thrombosis and Haemostasis suggests use of specific DOACs for cancer patients with a diagnosis of acute VTE, no drug-drug interactions, and a low risk of bleeding but suggests use of LMWH for those with a high risk of bleeding, including patients with luminal gastrointestinal cancers with an intact primary tumor, and those at risk for bleeding from the genitourinary or gastrointestinal tract. Clinicians must be aware that many chemotherapeutic agents may interact with DOACs and their use should be avoided in cases of potential interactions because there is no easily accessible and reliable way to measure the anticoagulant effect of DOACs.

Evidence on using DOACs to manage antiphospholipid antibody syndrome is limited. Patients with high-risk antiphospholipid antibody syndrome were found to have a markedly increased risk of arterial events while taking rivaroxaban compared to warfarin. Warfarin is the preferred oral anticoagulant in these patients.

There is also limited data on use of DOACs in patients with splanchnic vein thrombosis as well as in patients in whom anticoagulation fails and thrombosis develops during treatment with LMWH or warfarin.

3. Duration of anticoagulation therapy—The clinical scenario in which the thrombosis occurred is the strongest predictor of recurrence and, in most cases, guides duration of anticoagulation (Table 14–22). In the first year after discontinuation of anticoagulation therapy, the frequency of recurrent VTE among individuals whose thrombosis occurred in the setting of a transient, major, reversible risk factor (such as surgery) is approximately 3% after completing 3 months of anticoagulation, compared with at least 8% for individuals whose thrombosis was

Table 14–21. American College of Chest Physicians Evidence-Based Clinical Practice Guidelines for the Management of Supratherapeutic INR.

Clinical Situation	INR	Recommendations
No significant bleed	Above therapeutic range but < 5.0	• Lower dose or omit dose • Monitor more frequently and resume at lower dose when INR falls within therapeutic range (if INR only slightly above range, may not be necessary to decrease dose)
	≥ 5.0 but < 9.0	• Hold next 1–2 doses • Monitor more frequently and resume therapy at lower dose when INR falls within therapeutic range • *Patients at high risk for bleeding*[1]: Hold warfarin and consider giving vitamin K$_1$ 1–2.5 mg orally; check INR in 24–48 h to ensure response to therapy
	≥ 9.0	• Hold warfarin • Vitamin K$_1$ 2.5–5 mg orally • Monitor frequently and resume therapy at lower dose when INR within therapeutic range
Serious/life-threatening bleed		• Hold warfarin and give 10 mg vitamin K by slow intravenous infusion supplemented by FFP, PCC, or recombinant factor VIIa (PCC preferred)

[1]Patients at higher risk for bleeding include elderly people, and conditions that increase the risk of bleeding include kidney disease, hypertension, falls, liver disease, and history of gastrointestinal or genitourinary bleeding.
FFP, fresh frozen plasma; INR, international normalized ratio; PCC, prothrombin complex concentrate.

unprovoked, and greater than 20% in patients with cancer. Patients with provoked VTE are generally treated with a minimum of 3 months of anticoagulation, whereas unprovoked VTE should prompt consideration of indefinite anticoagulation provided the patient is not at high risk for bleeding. Merely extending duration of anticoagulation beyond 3 months will not reduce risk of recurrence once anticoagulation is stopped; if anticoagulants are stopped after 3, 6, 12, or 18 months in a patient with unprovoked VTE, the risk of recurrence after cessation of therapy is similar. Individual risk stratification may help identify patients most likely to suffer recurrent disease and thus most likely to benefit from ongoing anticoagulation

therapy. Normal D-dimer levels 1 month after cessation of anticoagulation are associated with lower recurrence risk, although some would argue not low enough to consider stopping anticoagulant therapy, particularly in men. One risk scoring system uses body mass index, age, D-dimer, and post-phlebitic symptoms to identify women at lower risk for recurrence after unprovoked VTE. The Vienna Prediction Model, a simple scoring system based on age, sex, D-dimer, and location of thrombosis, can help estimate an individual's recurrence risk to guide duration of therapy decisions. The following facts are important to consider when determining duration of therapy: (1) men have a greater than twofold higher risk of recurrent VTE

Table 14–22. Duration of treatment of VTE.

Scenario	Suggested Duration of Therapy	Comments
Major transient risk factor (eg, major surgery, major trauma, major hospitalization)	3 months	VTE prophylaxis upon future exposure to transient risk factors
Cancer-related	≥ 3–6 months or as long as cancer active, whichever is longer	LMWH recommended for initial treatment (see Table 14–16)
Unprovoked	At least 3 months; consider indefinite if bleeding risk allows	May individually risk-stratify for recurrence with D-dimer, clinical risk scores, and clinical presentation
Recurrent unprovoked	Indefinite	
Underlying significant thrombophilia (eg, antiphospholipid antibody syndrome, antithrombin deficiency, protein C deficiency, protein S deficiency, ≥ two concomitant thrombophilic conditions)	Indefinite	To avoid false positives, consider delaying investigation for laboratory thrombophilia until 3 months after event

LMWH, low-molecular-weight heparin; VTE, venous thromboembolic disease.

Table 14–23. Candidates for thrombophilia workup if results will influence management.

Patients younger than 50 years
Strong family history of VTE
Clot in unusual locations
Recurrent thromboses
Women of childbearing age
Suspicion for APS

APS, antiphospholipid syndrome; VTE, venous thromboembolism.

compared to women, (2) recurrent PE is more likely to develop in patients with clinically apparent PE than in those with DVT alone and has a case fatality rate of nearly 10%, and (3) proximal DVT has a higher recurrence risk than distal DVT. Laboratory workup for thrombophilia is not recommended routinely for determining duration of therapy because clinical presentation is a much stronger predictor of recurrence risk. The workup may be pursued in patients younger than 50 years, with a strong family history, with a clot in unusual locations, or with recurrent thromboses (Table 14–23). In addition, a workup for thrombophilia may be considered in women of childbearing age in whom results may influence fertility and pregnancy outcomes and management or in those patients in whom results will influence duration of therapy. An important hypercoagulable state to identify is antiphospholipid syndrome because these patients have a marked increase in recurrence rates, are at risk for both arterial and venous disease, and in general receive bridge therapy during any interruption of anticoagulation. Due to effects of anticoagulants and acute thrombosis on many of the tests, the thrombophilia workup should be delayed in most cases until at least 3 months after the acute event, if it is indicated at all (Table 14–24). The benefit of anticoagulation must be weighed against the bleeding risks posed, and the benefit-risk ratio should be assessed at the initiation of therapy, at 3 months, and then at least annually in any patient receiving prolonged anticoagulant therapy. While bleeding risk scores have been developed to estimate risk of these complications, their performance may not offer any advantage over a clinician's subjective assessment, particularly in older individuals. Assessment of bleeding risk is of particular importance when identifying candidates for extended duration therapy for treatment of unprovoked VTE; it is recommended that patients with a high risk of bleeding receive a defined course of anticoagulation, rather than indefinite therapy, even if the VTE was unprovoked.

Secondary prevention (antithrombotic therapy offered after the initial 3–6 months of treatment) should be considered in patients with VTE that is not majorly provoked and is most compelling for those with unprovoked VTE. For patients who continue to take a DOAC to prevent recurrence, the dose can be reduced to prophylactic intensity after initial 6–12 months of therapy. Alternatively, low dose (81–100 mg) aspirin may be used; however, this will provide far less reduction in risk of recurrent VTE with similar bleeding risk.

Table 14–24. Laboratory evaluation of thrombophilia.

Hypercoagulable State	When to Suspect	Laboratory Workup	Influence of Anticoagulation and Acute Thrombosis
Antiphospholipid antibody syndrome	Unexplained DVT/PE CVA/TIA age < 50 Recurrent thrombosis (despite anticoagulation) Thrombosis at an unusual site Arterial and venous thrombosis Livedo reticularis, Raynaud phenomenon, thrombocytopenia, recurrent early pregnancy loss	Anti-cardiolipin IgG and/or IgM medium or high titer (ie, > 40 GPL or MPL, or > the 99th percentile)[1] Anti-beta-2 glycoprotein I IgG and/or IgM medium or high titer (> the 99th percentile)[1] Lupus anticoagulant[1]	Lupus anticoagulant can be falsely positive or falsely negative on anticoagulation
Protein C, S, antithrombin deficiencies	Thrombosis < 50 years of age with family history of VTE	Screen with protein C activity, free protein S, protein S activity, antithrombin activity	Acute thrombosis can result in decreased protein C, S and antithrombin activity. Warfarin can decrease protein C and S activity, heparin can cause decrease antithrombin activity. DOACs can increase protein C, S, and antithrombin activity
Factor V Leiden, prothrombin gene mutation	Thrombosis on OCPs, cerebral vein thrombosis, DVT/PE in white population	PCR for factor V Leiden or prothrombin gene mutation	No influence
Hyperhomocysteinemia		Fasting homocysteine	No influence

[1]Detected on two occasions not less than 12 weeks apart.
CVA/TIA, cerebrovascular accident/transient ischemic attack; DOACs, direct-acting oral anticoagulants; DVT/PE, deep venous thrombosis/pulmonary embolism; OCPs, oral contraceptives; PCR, polymerase chain reaction; VTE, venous thromboembolism.

Burnett AE et al. Guidance for the practical management of the direct oral anticoagulants (DOACs) in VTE treatment. J Thromb Thrombolysis. 2016 Jan;41(1):206–32. [PMID: 26780747]

Connors JM. Thrombophilia testing and venous thrombosis. N Engl J Med. 2017 Dec 7;377(23):2298. [PMID: 29211668]

Garcia D et al. Diagnosis and management of the antiphospholipid syndrome. N Engl J Med. 2018 May 24;378(21):2010–21. [PMID: 29791828]

Kearon C et al. Antithrombotic therapy for VTE disease: CHEST guideline and expert panel report. Chest. 2016 Feb;149(2):315–52. [PMID: 26867832]

Khorana AA et al. Role of direct oral anticoagulants in the treatment of cancer-associated venous thromboembolism: guidance from the SSC of the ISTH. J Thromb Haemost. 2018 Sep; 16(9):1891–4. [PMID: 30027649]

Konstantinides SV et al. Management of pulmonary embolism: an update. J Am Coll Cardiol. 2016 Mar 1;67(8):976–90. [PMID: 26916489]

MDCalc. Bova Score for pulmonary embolism complications. https://www.mdcalc.com/bova-score-pulmonary-embolism-complications

Raskob GE et al; Hokusai VTE Cancer Investigators. Edoxaban for the treatment of cancer-associated venous thromboembolism. N Engl J Med. 2018 Feb 15;378(7):615–24. [PMID: 29231094]

Young AM et al. Comparison of an oral factor Xa inhibitor with low molecular weight heparin in patients with cancer with venous thromboembolism: results of a randomized trial (SELECT-D). J Clin Oncol. 2018 Jul 10;36(20):2017-23. [PMID: 29746227]

C. Thrombolytic Therapy

Anticoagulation alone is appropriate treatment for most patients with PE; however, those with high-risk, massive PE, defined as PE with persistent hemodynamic instability, have an in-hospital mortality rate that approaches 30% and absent contraindications require immediate thrombolysis in combination with anticoagulation (Table 14–25). Systemic thrombolytic therapy has been used in selected patients with intermediate-risk, submassive PE, defined as PE without hemodynamic instability but with evidence of right ventricular compromise and myocardial injury. Thrombolysis in this cohort decreases risk of hemodynamic compromise but increases the risk of major hemorrhage and stroke. A lower dose of tPA (50% or less of the standard dose [100 mg] commonly used for the treatment of PE) has been evaluated in small trials but additional data are needed to routinely recommend its use. The use of thrombolysis in hemodynamically stable intermediate risk PE patients should be considered on a case-by-case basis. The use of catheter-directed therapy for acute PE may be considered for high-risk or intermediate-risk PE when systemic thrombolysis has failed or as an alternative to systemic thrombolytic therapy.

In patients with large proximal iliofemoral DVT, data from randomized controlled trials are conflicting on the benefit of catheter-directed thrombolysis in addition to treatment with anticoagulation; the CaVenT trial showed some reduction in risk of postthrombotic syndrome, but the larger ATTRACT trial failed to show reduction in postthrombotic syndrome but did find an increased risk of major bleeding.

Hennemeyer C et al. Outcomes of catheter-directed therapy plus anticoagulation versus anticoagulation alone for submassive and massive pulmonary embolism. Am J Med. 2019 Feb; 132(2):240–6. [PMID: 30367851]

Kiser TH et al. Half-dose versus full-dose alteplase for treatment of pulmonary embolism. Crit Care Med. 2018 Oct; 46(10):1617–25. [PMID: 29979222]

Konstantinides SV et al. Management of pulmonary embolism: an update. J Am Coll Cardiol. 2016 Mar 1;67(8):976–90. [PMID: 26916489]

Tapson VF et al. Systemic thrombolysis for pulmonary embolism: who and how. Tech Vasc Interv Radiol. 2017 Sep;20(3): 162–74. [PMID: 29029710]

Vedantham S et al; ATTRACT Trial Investigators. Pharmacomechanical catheter-directed thrombolysis for deep-vein thrombosis. N Engl J Med. 2017 Dec 7;377(23):2240–52. [PMID: 29211671]

Table 14–25. Thrombolytic therapies for pulmonary embolism.

Thrombolytic Agent	Dose	Frequency	Comment
High Risk (Massive Pulmonary Embolism)			
Alteplase	100 mg	Continuous intravenous infusion over 2 hours	Follow with continuous intravenous infusion of unfractionated heparin (see Table 14–16 for dosage)
	100 mg	Intravenous bolus × 1	Appropriate for acute management of cardiac arrest and suspected pulmonary embolism
Urokinase	4400 international units/kg	Intravenous bolus × 1 followed by 4400 international units/kg continuous intravenous infusion for 12 hours	Unfractionated heparin should be administered concurrently (see Table 14–16 for dosage)
Intermediate Risk (Submassive Pulmonary Embolism)			
rt-PA	50 mg/2 hours	Continuous infusion over 2 hours	
Tenecteplase	30–50 mg	Intravenous bolus × 1	
Alteplase	100 mg	(10-mg intravenous bolus, followed by a 90-mg intravenous infusion 2 hours)	

rt-PA, recombinant tissue plasminogen activator.

D. Nonpharmacologic Therapy

1. Graduated compression stockings—Graduated compressions stockings may provide symptomatic relief to selected patients with ongoing swelling but they do not reduce the risk of postthrombotic syndrome at 6 months. They are contraindicated in patients with peripheral vascular disease.

2. Inferior vena caval (IVC) filters—There is a paucity of data to support the use of IVC filters for the prevention of PE in any clinical scenario. There are two randomized, controlled trials of IVC filters for prevention of PE. In the first study, patients with documented DVT received full intensity, time-limited anticoagulation with or without placement of a permanent IVC filter. Patients with IVC filters had a lower rate of nonfatal asymptomatic PE at 12 days but an increased rate of DVT at 2 years. In the second study, patients with symptomatic PE and residual DVT plus at least one additional risk factor for severity received anticoagulation with or without a retrievable IVC filter. IVC filter use did not reduce the risk of symptomatic recurrent PE at 3 months. Most experts agree with placement of an IVC filter in patients with acute proximal DVT and an absolute contraindication to anticoagulation despite lack of evidence to support this practice. While IVC filters were once commonly used to prevent VTE recurrence in the setting of anticoagulation failure, many experts now recommend switching to an alternative agent or increasing the intensity of the current anticoagulant regimen instead. The remainder of the indications (submassive/intermediate-risk PE, free-floating iliofemoral DVT, perioperative risk reduction) are controversial. If the contraindication to anticoagulation is temporary (active bleeding with subsequent resolution), placement of a retrievable IVC filter may be considered so that the device can be removed once anticoagulation has been started and has been shown to be tolerated. Rates of IVC filter retrieval are very low, often due to a failure to arrange for its removal. Thus, if a device is placed, removal should be arranged at the time of device placement.

Complications of IVC filters include local thrombosis, tilting, migration, fracture, and inability to retrieve the device. When considering placement of an IVC filter, it is best to consider both short- and long-term complications, since devices intended for removal may become permanent. To improve patient safety, institutions should develop systems that guide appropriate patient selection for IVC filter placement, tracking, and removal.

Bikdeli B et al. Systematic review of efficacy and safety of retrievable inferior vena caval filters. Thromb Res. 2018 May;165: 79–82. [PMID: 29579576]

Kahn SR et al; SOX trial investigators. Compression stockings to prevent post-thrombotic syndrome: a randomised placebo-controlled trial. Lancet. 2014 Mar 8;383(9920):880–8. [PMID: 24315521]

Milovanovic L et al. Procedural and indwelling complications with inferior vena cava filters: frequency, etiology, and management. Semin Intervent Radiol. 2015 Mar;32(1):34–41. [PMID: 25762846]

Mismetti P et al; PREPIC2 Study Group. Effect of a retrievable inferior vena cava filter plus anticoagulation vs anticoagulation alone on risk of recurrent pulmonary embolism: a randomized clinical trial. JAMA. 2015 Apr 28;313(16):1627–35. [PMID: 25919526]

▶ When to Refer

- Presence of large iliofemoral VTE, IVC thrombosis, portal vein thrombosis, or Budd-Chiari syndrome for consideration of catheter-directed thrombolysis.
- High-risk PE for urgent embolectomy or catheter-directed therapies.
- Intermediate-risk PE if considering thrombolysis.
- History of HIT or prolonged PTT plus renal failure for alternative anticoagulation regimens.
- Consideration of IVC filter placement.
- Clots in unusual locations (eg, renal, hepatic, or cerebral vein), or simultaneous arterial and venous thrombosis, to assess possibility of a hypercoagulable state.
- Recurrent VTE while receiving therapeutic anticoagulation.

▶ When to Admit

- Documented or suspected intermediate- or high-risk PE and low-risk PE at high risk for bleeding or poor candidate for outpatient treatment.
- DVT with poorly controlled pain, high bleeding risk, or concerns about follow-up.
- Large iliofemoral DVT for consideration of thrombolysis.
- Acute DVT and absolute contraindication to anticoagulation for IVC filter placement.
- Venous thrombosis despite therapeutic anticoagulation.

Gastrointestinal Disorders

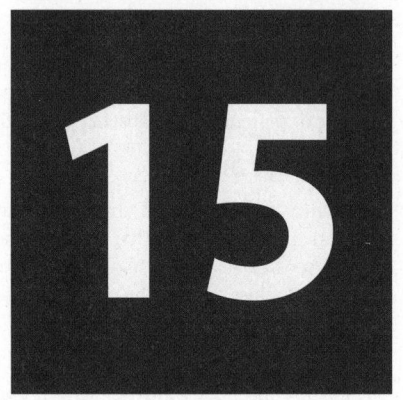

Kenneth R. McQuaid, MD

SYMPTOMS & SIGNS OF GASTROINTESTINAL DISEASE

DYSPEPSIA

ESSENTIALS OF DIAGNOSIS

- ▶ Predominant epigastric pain.
- ▶ May be associated epigastric fullness, nausea, heartburn, or vomiting.
- ▶ Endoscopy is warranted in all patients age 60 years or older and selected younger patients with alarm features.
- ▶ In all other patients, testing for *Helicobacter pylori* is recommended; if positive, antibacterial treatment is given.
- ▶ Patients who are *H pylori* negative or do not improve after *H pylori* eradication should be prescribed a trial of empiric proton pump inhibitor therapy.
- ▶ Patients with refractory symptoms should be offered a trial of tricyclic antidepressant, a prokinetic agent, or psychological therapy.

▶ General Considerations

Dyspepsia refers to acute, chronic, or recurrent pain or discomfort centered in the upper abdomen. A 2017 American College of Gastroenterology guideline has further defined clinically relevant dyspepsia as predominant epigastric pain for at least 1 month. The epigastric pain may be associated with other symptoms of heartburn, nausea, fullness, or vomiting. Heartburn (retrosternal burning) should be distinguished from dyspepsia. When heartburn is the dominant complaint, gastroesophageal reflux is nearly always present. Dyspepsia occurs in 10–20% of the adult population and accounts for 3% of general medical office visits.

▶ Etiology

A. Food or Drug Intolerance

Acute, self-limited "indigestion" may be caused by overeating, eating too quickly, eating high-fat foods, eating during stressful situations, or drinking too much alcohol or coffee. Many medications cause dyspepsia, including aspirin, nonsteroidal anti-inflammatory drugs (NSAIDs), antibiotics (metronidazole, macrolides), dabigatran, diabetes drugs (metformin, alpha-glucosidase inhibitors, amylin analogs, GLP-1 receptor antagonists), antihypertensive medications (angiotensin-converting enzyme [ACE] inhibitors, angiotensin-receptor blockers), cholesterol-lowering agents (niacin, fibrates), neuropsychiatric medications (cholinesterase inhibitors [donepezil, rivastigmine]), selective serotonin reuptake inhibitors (SSRIs) (fluoxetine, sertraline), serotonin-norepinephrine reuptake inhibitors (venlafaxine, duloxetine), Parkinson drugs (dopamine agonists, monoamine oxidase [MAO]-B inhibitors), corticosteroids, estrogens, digoxin, iron, and opioids.

B. Functional Dyspepsia

Functional dyspepsia refers to dyspepsia for which no organic etiology has been determined by endoscopy or other testing. This is the most common cause of *chronic* dyspepsia, accounting for the majority of patients. Symptoms may arise from a complex interaction of increased visceral afferent sensitivity, gastric delayed emptying or impaired accommodation to food or psychosocial stressors or may develop de novo following an enteric infection. Although benign, these symptoms may be chronic and difficult to treat.

C. Luminal Gastrointestinal Tract Dysfunction

Peptic ulcer disease is present in 5–15% of patients with dyspepsia. Gastroesophageal reflux disease (GERD) is present in up to 20% of patients with dyspepsia, even without significant heartburn. Gastric or esophageal cancer is identified in less than 1% but is extremely rare in persons under age 60 years with uncomplicated dyspepsia. Other causes include gastroparesis (especially in diabetes mellitus) and parasitic infection (*Giardia, Strongyloides, Anisakis*).

D. *Helicobacter pylori* Infection

Chronic gastric infection with *H pylori* is an important cause of peptic ulcer disease, and may cause dyspepsia in a small number of patients in the absence of peptic ulcer disease.

E. Pancreatic Disease

Pancreatic carcinoma and chronic pancreatitis may cause chronic epigastric pain that is more severe, sometimes radiates to the back, and usually is associated with anorexia, rapid weight loss, steatorrhea, or jaundice.

F. Biliary Tract Disease

The abrupt onset of epigastric or right upper quadrant pain due to cholelithiasis or choledocholithiasis should be readily distinguished from dyspepsia.

G. Other Conditions

Diabetes mellitus, thyroid disease, chronic kidney disease, myocardial ischemia, intra-abdominal malignancy, gastric volvulus or paraesophageal hernia, chronic gastric or intestinal ischemia, and pregnancy are sometimes accompanied by acute or chronic epigastric pain or discomfort.

▶ Clinical Findings

A. Symptoms and Signs

Given the nonspecific nature of dyspeptic symptoms, the history has limited diagnostic utility. It should clarify the chronicity, location, and quality of the epigastric pain, and its relationship to meals. The pain may be accompanied by one or more upper abdominal symptoms including postprandial fullness, heartburn, nausea, or vomiting. Concomitant weight loss, persistent vomiting, constant or severe pain, progressive dysphagia, hematemesis, or melena warrants endoscopy or abdominal CT imaging. Potentially offending medications and excessive alcohol use should be identified and discontinued if possible. The patient's reason for seeking care should be determined. Recent changes in employment, marital discord, physical and sexual abuse, anxiety, depression, and fear of serious disease may all contribute to the development and reporting of symptoms. Patients with functional dyspepsia often are younger, report a variety of abdominal and extragastrointestinal complaints, show signs of anxiety or depression, or have a history of use of psychotropic medications.

The symptom profile alone does not differentiate between functional dyspepsia and organic gastrointestinal disorders. Based on the clinical history alone, primary care clinicians misdiagnose nearly half of patients with peptic ulcers or gastroesophageal reflux.

The physical examination is rarely helpful. Signs of serious organic disease such as weight loss, organomegaly, abdominal mass, or fecal occult blood are to be further evaluated.

B. Laboratory Findings

In patients younger than age 60 with uncomplicated dyspepsia (in whom gastric cancer is rare), initial noninvasive strategies should be pursued. In patients older than age 60 years, initial laboratory work should include a blood count, electrolytes, liver enzymes, calcium, and thyroid function tests. The cost-effectiveness of routine laboratory studies is uncertain. In most patients younger than age 60, a noninvasive test for *H pylori* (urea breath test, fecal antigen test) should be performed first. Although serologic tests are inexpensive, performance characteristics are poor in low-prevalence populations, whereas breath and fecal antigen tests have 95% accuracy. If *H pylori* breath test or fecal antigen test results are negative in a patient not taking NSAIDs, peptic ulcer disease is virtually excluded.

C. Upper Endoscopy

Upper endoscopy is the study of choice to diagnose gastroduodenal ulcers, erosive esophagitis, and upper gastrointestinal malignancy. However, gastroduodenal ulcers and erosive esophagitis can be treated empirically with *H pylori* eradication or empiric proton pump inhibitor therapy or both. Therefore, upper endoscopy is mainly indicated to look for upper gastric or esophageal malignancy in patients over age 60 years with new-onset dyspepsia (in whom there is increased malignancy risk) and in selected younger patients with "alarm" features. In patients under age 60, the risk of malignancy is less than 1%—even among patients with reported "alarm" features. Recent guidelines therefore recommend against routine endoscopy for younger patients—even those with "alarm" features. However, endoscopy should be performed in patients with prominent "alarm" features, such as progressive weight loss, rapidly progressive dysphagia, severe vomiting, evidence of bleeding or anemia, or jaundice. It is also helpful for selected patients who are excessively concerned about serious underlying disease. For patients born in regions in which there is a higher incidence of gastric cancer, such as Central or South America, China and Southeast Asia, or Africa, an age threshold of 45 years may be more appropriate.

Endoscopic evaluation may also be warranted when symptoms fail to respond to initial empiric management strategies or when frequent symptom relapse occurs after discontinuation of empiric therapy.

D. Other Tests

In patients with refractory symptoms or progressive weight loss, antibodies for celiac disease or stool testing for ova and parasites or *Giardia* antigen, fat, or elastase may be considered. Abdominal imaging (ultrasonography or CT scanning) is performed only when pancreatic, biliary tract, vascular disease, or volvulus is suspected. Gastric emptying studies may be useful in patients with recurrent nausea and vomiting who have not responded to empiric therapies.

▶ Treatment

Initial empiric treatment is warranted for patients who are younger than age 60 years and who lack severe or worrisome "alarm" features. All other patients as well as patients whose symptoms do not to respond to or relapse after empiric treatment should undergo upper endoscopy with subsequent treatment directed at the specific disorder identified (eg, peptic ulcer, gastroesophageal reflux, cancer). When endoscopy is performed, gastric biopsies should be obtained to test for *H pylori* infection. If infection is present, antibacterial treatment should be given.

A. Empiric Therapy

H pylori–negative patients most likely have functional dyspepsia or atypical GERD and can be treated with an antisecretory agent (proton pump inhibitor) for 4 weeks. For patients who have symptom relapse after discontinuation of the proton pump inhibitor, intermittent or long-term proton pump inhibitor therapy may be considered. For patients in whom test results are positive for *H pylori*, antibiotic therapy proves definitive for patients with underlying peptic ulcers and may improve symptoms in a small subset (less than 10%) of infected patients with functional dyspepsia. Patients with persistent dyspepsia after *H pylori* eradication can be given a trial of proton pump inhibitor therapy.

B. Treatment of Functional Dyspepsia

Patients who have no significant findings on endoscopy as well as patients under age 60 who do not respond to *H pylori* eradication or empiric proton pump inhibitor therapy are presumed to have functional dyspepsia.

1. General measures—Most patients have mild, intermittent symptoms that respond to reassurance and lifestyle changes. Alcohol and caffeine should be reduced or discontinued. Patients with postprandial symptoms should be instructed to consume small, low-fat meals. A food diary, in which patients record their food intake, symptoms, and daily events, may reveal dietary or psychosocial precipitants of pain.

2. Anti–*H pylori* treatment—Meta-analyses have suggested that a small number of patients with functional dyspepsia (less than 10%) derive benefit from *H pylori* eradication therapy. Therefore, patients with functional dyspepsia should be tested and treated for *H pylori*.

3. Other pharmacologic agents—Drugs have demonstrated limited efficacy in the treatment of functional dyspepsia. One-third of patients derive relief from placebo. Antisecretory therapy for 4–8 weeks with proton pump inhibitors (omeprazole, esomeprazole, or rabeprazole 20 mg, dexlansoprazole or lansoprazole 30 mg, or pantoprazole 40 mg orally daily) may benefit up to 10% of patients. Low doses of antidepressants (eg, desipramine or nortriptyline, 25–50 mg orally at bedtime) benefit some patients, possibly by moderating visceral afferent sensitivity. Doses should be increased slowly to minimize side effects. Buspirone (10 mg three times daily 15 minutes before meals) is an antidepressant (serotonin 5-HT$_{1A}$ receptor agonist) that promotes accommodation of the gastric fundus and reduces postprandial bloating and fullness in some patients. Metoclopramide (5–10 mg three times daily) may improve symptoms but cannot be recommended for long-term use due to the risk of tardive dyskinesia. Other prokinetics have demonstrated modest efficacy in controlled trials but are not available in the United States.

4. Alternative therapies—Psychotherapy and hypnotherapy may be of benefit in selected motivated patients with functional dyspepsia. Herbal therapies (peppermint, caraway) may offer benefit with little risk of adverse effects.

Koduru P et al. Definition, pathogenesis, and management of that cursed dyspepsia. Clin Gastroenterol Hepatol. 2018 Apr; 16(4):467–79. [PMID: 28899670]

Moayyedi PM et al. ACG and CAG Clinical Guideline: management of dyspepsia. Am J Gastroenterol. 2017 Jul;112(7): 988–1013. [PMID: 28631728]

Pittayanon R et al. Prokinetics for functional dyspepsia: a systematic review and meta-analysis of randomized control trials. Am J Gastroenterol. 2019 Feb;114(2):233–43. [PMID: 30337705]

Vakil NB et al. White Paper AGA: functional dyspepsia. Clin Gastroenterol Hepatol. 2017 Aug;15(8):1191–4. [PMID: 28529164]

NAUSEA & VOMITING

Nausea is a vague, intensely disagreeable sensation of sickness or "queasiness" and is distinguished from anorexia. Vomiting often follows, as does retching (spasmodic respiratory and abdominal movements). Vomiting should be distinguished from regurgitation, the effortless reflux of liquid or food stomach contents; and from rumination, the chewing and swallowing of food that is regurgitated volitionally after meals.

The brainstem vomiting center is composed of a group of neuronal areas (area postrema, nucleus tractus solitarius, and central pattern generator) within the medulla that coordinate emesis. It may be stimulated by four different sources of afferent input: (1) Afferent vagal fibers from the gastrointestinal viscera are rich in serotonin 5-HT$_3$ receptors; these may be stimulated by biliary or gastrointestinal distention, mucosal or peritoneal irritation, or infections. (2) Fibers of the vestibular system, which have high concentrations of histamine H$_1$ and muscarinic cholinergic receptors. (3) Higher central nervous system centers (amygdala); here, certain sights, smells, or emotional experiences may induce vomiting. For example, patients receiving chemotherapy may start vomiting in anticipation of its administration. (4) The chemoreceptor trigger zone, located outside the blood-brain barrier in the area postrema of the medulla, which is rich in opioid, serotonin 5-HT$_3$, neurokinin 1 (NK$_1$), and dopamine D$_2$ receptors. This region may be stimulated by drugs and chemotherapeutic agents, toxins, hypoxia, uremia, acidosis, and radiation therapy. Although the causes of nausea and vomiting are many, a simplified list is provided in Table 15–1.

▶ Clinical Findings

A. Symptoms and Signs

Acute symptoms without abdominal pain are typically caused by food poisoning, infectious gastroenteritis, drugs, or systemic illness. Inquiry should be made into recent changes in medications, diet, other intestinal symptoms, or similar illnesses in family members. The acute onset of severe pain and vomiting suggests peritoneal irritation, acute gastric or intestinal obstruction, or pancreaticobiliary disease. Persistent vomiting suggests pregnancy, gastric outlet obstruction, gastroparesis, intestinal

Table 15–1. Causes of nausea and vomiting.

Visceral afferent stimulation	**Infections**
	Mechanical obstruction
	Gastric outlet obstruction: peptic ulcer disease, malignancy, gastric volvulus
	Small intestinal obstruction: adhesions, hernias, volvulus, Crohn disease, carcinomatosis
	Dysmotility
	Gastroparesis: diabetic, postviral, postvagotomy
	Small intestine: scleroderma, amyloidosis, chronic intestinal pseudo-obstruction, familial myoneuropathies
	Peritoneal irritation
	Peritonitis: perforated viscus, appendicitis, spontaneous bacterial peritonitis
	Viral gastroenteritis: Norwalk agent, rotavirus
	"Food poisoning": toxins from *Bacillus cereus, Staphylococcus aureus, Clostridium perfringens*
	Acute systemic infections
	Hepatobiliary or pancreatic disorders
	Hepatitis A or B
	Acute pancreatitis
	Cholecystitis or choledocholithiasis
	Topical gastrointestinal irritants
	Alcohol, NSAIDs, oral antibiotics
	Postoperative
	Other
	Cardiac disease: acute myocardial infarction, heart failure
	Urologic disease: stones, pyelonephritis
Vestibular disorders	**Vestibular disorders**
	Labyrinthitis, Ménière syndrome, motion sickness
CNS disorders	**Increased intracranial pressure**
	CNS tumors, subdural or subarachnoid hemorrhage
	Migraine
	Cyclical vomiting syndrome
	Infections
	Meningitis, encephalitis
	Psychogenic
	Anticipatory vomiting, anorexia nervosa and bulimia, psychiatric disorders
Irritation of chemoreceptor trigger zone	**Antitumor chemotherapy**
	Medications and drugs
	Opioids
	Marijuana
	Anticonvulsants
	Antiparkinsonism drugs
	Beta-blockers, antiarrhythmics, digoxin
	Oral contraceptives
	Cholinesterase inhibitors
	Diabetes medications (metformin, acarbose, pramlintide, exenatide)
	Radiation therapy
	Systemic disorders
	Diabetic ketoacidosis
	Uremia
	Adrenocortical crisis
	Parathyroid disease
	Hypothyroidism
	Pregnancy
	Paraneoplastic syndrome

CNS, central nervous system; NSAIDs, nonsteroidal anti-inflammatory drugs.

dysmotility, psychogenic disorders, and central nervous system or systemic disorders. Vomiting that occurs in the morning before breakfast is common with pregnancy, uremia, alcohol intake, and increased intracranial pressure. Inquiry should be made into use of cannabis products. Suspect cannabinoid hyperemesis syndrome in patients with prolonged use, especially in those who report compulsive showering or bathing. Vomiting immediately after meals strongly suggests bulimia or psychogenic causes. Vomiting of undigested food one to several hours after meals is characteristic of gastroparesis or a gastric outlet obstruction; physical examination may reveal a succussion splash. Patients with acute or chronic symptoms should be asked about neurologic symptoms (eg, headache, stiff neck, vertigo, and focal paresthesias or weakness) that suggest a central nervous system cause.

B. Special Examinations

With vomiting that is severe or protracted, serum electrolytes should be obtained to look for hypokalemia, azotemia, or metabolic alkalosis resulting from loss of gastric contents. Flat and upright abdominal radiographs or abdominal CT are obtained in patients with severe pain or suspicion of mechanical obstruction to look for free intraperitoneal air or dilated loops of small bowel. The cause of gastric outlet obstruction is best demonstrated by upper endoscopy, and the cause of small intestinal obstruction is best demonstrated with abdominal CT imaging. Gastroparesis is confirmed by nuclear scintigraphic studies or ^{13}C-octanoic acid breath tests, which show delayed gastric emptying and either upper endoscopy or barium upper gastrointestinal series showing no evidence of mechanical gastric outlet obstruction. Abnormal liver biochemical tests or elevated amylase or lipase suggest pancreaticobiliary disease, which may be investigated with an abdominal sonogram or CT scan. Central nervous system causes are best evaluated with either head CT or MRI.

▶ Complications

Complications include dehydration, hypokalemia, metabolic alkalosis, aspiration, rupture of the esophagus (Boerhaave syndrome), and bleeding secondary to a mucosal tear at the gastroesophageal junction (Mallory-Weiss syndrome).

▶ Treatment

A. General Measures

Most causes of acute vomiting are mild, self-limited, and require no specific treatment. Patients should ingest clear liquids (broths, tea, soups, carbonated beverages) and small quantities of dry foods (soda crackers). Ginger may be an effective nonpharmacologic treatment. For more severe acute vomiting, hospitalization may be required. Patients unable to eat and losing gastric fluids may become dehydrated, resulting in hypokalemia with metabolic alkalosis. Intravenous 0.45% saline solution with 20 mEq/L of potassium chloride is given in most cases to maintain hydration. A nasogastric suction tube for gastric or mechanical small bowel obstruction improves patient comfort and permits monitoring of fluid loss.

B. Antiemetic Medications

Medications may be given either to prevent or to control vomiting. Combinations of drugs from different classes may provide better control of symptoms with less toxicity in some patients. Table 15–2 outlines common antiemetic dosing regimens.

1. Serotonin 5-HT$_3$-receptor antagonists—Ondansetron, granisetron, dolasetron, and palonosetron are effective in preventing chemotherapy- and radiation-induced emesis when initiated prior to treatment. Due to its prolonged half-life and internalization of the 5-HT$_3$-receptor, palonosetron is superior to other 5-HT$_3$-receptor antagonists for the prevention of acute and delayed chemotherapy-induced emesis from moderately or highly emetogenic chemotherapeutic regimens. Although 5-HT$_3$-receptor antagonists are effective as single agents for the prevention of chemotherapy-induced nausea and vomiting, their efficacy is enhanced by combination therapy with a corticosteroid (dexamethasone) and an NK$_1$-receptor antagonist. Serotonin antagonists increasingly are used for the prevention of postoperative nausea and vomiting because of increased restrictions on the use of other antiemetic agents (such as droperidol).

2. Corticosteroids—Corticosteroids (eg, dexamethasone) have antiemetic properties, but the basis for these effects is unknown. These agents enhance the efficacy of serotonin receptor antagonists for preventing acute and delayed nausea and vomiting in patients receiving moderately to highly emetogenic chemotherapy regimens.

3. Neurokinin receptor antagonists—Aprepitant, fosaprepitant, and rolapitant are highly selective antagonists for NK$_1$-receptors in the area postrema. They are used in combination with corticosteroids and serotonin antagonists for the prevention of acute and delayed nausea and vomiting with highly emetogenic chemotherapy regimens. Netupitant is another oral NK$_1$-receptor antagonist that is administered in a fixed-dose combination with palonosetron. Combined therapy with a neurokinin-1 receptor antagonist prevents acute emesis in 80–90% and delayed emesis in more than 70% of patients treated with highly emetogenic regimens.

4. Dopamine antagonists—The phenothiazines, butyrophenones, and substituted benzamides (eg, prochlorperazine, promethazine) have antiemetic properties that are due to dopaminergic blockade as well as to their sedative effects. High doses of these agents are associated with antidopaminergic side effects, including extrapyramidal reactions and depression. With the advent of more effective and safer antiemetics, these agents are infrequently used, mainly in outpatients with minor, self-limited symptoms. The atypical antipsychotic agent olanzapine has potent antiemetic properties that may be mediated by blockade of both dopamine and serotonin neurotransmitters. It may be used in patients with poor control of chemotherapy-induced nausea and vomiting.

5. Antihistamines and anticholinergics—These drugs (eg, meclizine, dimenhydrinate, transdermal scopolamine) may be valuable in the prevention of vomiting arising from stimulation of the labyrinth, ie, motion sickness, vertigo, and migraines. They may induce drowsiness. A combination of oral vitamin B$_6$ and doxylamine is recommended by the American College of Obstetricians and Gynecologists as first-line therapy for nausea and vomiting during pregnancy.

6. Cannabinoids—Marijuana has been used widely as an appetite stimulant and antiemetic. Pure delta^9-tetrahydrocannabinol (THC) is the major active ingredient in marijuana and the most psychoactive and is available by prescription as dronabinol. In doses of 5–15 mg/m^2, oral dronabinol is effective in treating nausea associated with chemotherapy, but it is associated with central nervous system side effects in most patients. Some states allow the use of medical marijuana with a clinician's certification. Strains of medical marijuana with different proportions of

Table 15–2. Common antiemetic dosing regimens.

	Dosage	Route
Serotonin 5-HT$_3$ Antagonists		
Ondansetron	Doses vary: 4–8 mg twice daily for postoperative nausea and vomiting	Intravenously, orally
	8 mg twice daily for moderately or highly emetogenic chemotherapy	Intravenously, orally
Granisetron	1 mg once daily	Intravenously
	1–2 mg once daily	Orally
Dolasetron	12.5 mg postoperatively	Intravenously
	100 mg once daily	Orally
Palonosetron	0.25 mg once as a single dose 30 min before start of chemotherapy	Intravenously
	0.5 mg once as single dose	Orally
Corticosteroids		
Dexamethasone	4–12 mg once pre-induction for prevention of postoperative nausea and vomiting	Intravenously, orally
	8 mg once daily for chemotherapy	Intravenously, orally
Methylprednisolone	40–100 mg once daily	Intravenously, intramuscularly, orally
Dopamine Receptor Antagonists		
Metoclopramide	10–20 mg or 0.5 mg/kg every 6–8 hours	Intravenously
	10–20 mg every 6–8 hours	Orally
Prochlorperazine	5–10 mg every 4–6 hours	Intravenously, intramuscularly, orally
	25 mg suppository every 6 hours	Per rectum
Promethazine	12.5–25 mg every 6–8 hours	Intravenously, orally
	25 mg every 6–8 hours	Per rectum
Trimethobenzamide	200 mg every 6–8 hours	Orally
	250–300 mg every 6–8 hours	Intravenously, orally
Olanzapine	5–10 mg once daily on days 1–4 for chemotherapy	
Neurokinin Receptor Antagonists[1]		
Aprepitant	125 mg once before chemotherapy; then 80 mg on days 1 and 2 after chemotherapy	Orally
Fosaprepitant	150 mg once 30 minutes before chemotherapy	Intravenously
Rolapitant	180 mg once before chemotherapy	Orally
Netupitant/palonosetron	Netupitant 300 mg / palonosetron 0.50 mg once before chemotherapy	Orally

[1]Neurokinin receptor antagonists are used solely for highly emetogenic chemotherapy regimens in combination with 5-HT$_3$ antagonists or dexamethasone or both.

various naturally occurring cannabinoids (primarily THC and cannabidiol [CBD]) can be chosen to minimize its psychoactive effects.

Hesketh PJ et al. Antiemetics: American Society of Clinical Oncology clinical practice guideline update. J Clin Oncol. 2017 Oct;35(28):3240–61. [PMID: 28759346]

Lacy BE et al. Chronic nausea and vomiting: evaluation and treatment. Am J Gastroenterol. 2018 May;113(5):647–59. [PMID: 29545633]

Navari RM et al. Antiemetic prophylaxis for chemotherapy-induced nausea and vomiting. N Engl J Med. 2016 Apr 7; 374(14):1356–67. [PMID: 27050207]

Richards JR. Cannabinoid hyperemesis syndrome: pathophysiology and treatment in the emergency department. J Emerg Med. 2018 Mar;54(3):354–63. [PMID: 29310960]

Tageja N et al. Chemotherapy-induced nausea and vomiting: an overview and comparison of three consensus guidelines. Postgrad Med J. 2016 Jan;92(1083):34–40. [PMID: 26561590]

HICCUPS (Singultus)

Though usually a benign and self-limited annoyance, hiccups may be persistent and a sign of serious underlying illness. In patients on mechanical ventilation, hiccups can trigger a full respiratory cycle and result in respiratory alkalosis.

Causes of benign, self-limited hiccups include gastric distention (carbonated beverages, air swallowing, overeating), sudden temperature changes (hot then cold liquids, hot then cold shower), alcohol ingestion, and states of heightened emotion (excitement, stress, laughing). There are over 100 causes of recurrent or persistent hiccups due to gastrointestinal, central nervous system, cardiovascular, and thoracic disorders.

Clinical Findings

Evaluation of the patient with persistent hiccups should include a detailed neurologic examination, serum creatinine, liver chemistry tests, and a chest radiograph. When the cause remains unclear, CT or MRI of the head, chest, and abdomen, echocardiography, and upper endoscopy may help.

Treatment

A number of simple remedies may be helpful in patients with acute benign hiccups. (1) Irritation of the nasopharynx by tongue traction, lifting the uvula with a spoon, catheter stimulation of the nasopharynx, or eating 1 teaspoon (tsp) (7 g) of dry granulated sugar. (2) Interruption of the respiratory cycle by breath holding, Valsalva maneuver, sneezing, gasping (fright stimulus), or rebreathing into a bag. (3) Stimulation of the vagus by carotid massage. (4) Irritation of the diaphragm by holding knees to chest or by continuous positive airway pressure during mechanical ventilation. (5) Relief of gastric distention by belching or insertion of a nasogastric tube.

A number of drugs have been promoted as being useful in the treatment of hiccups. Chlorpromazine, 25–50 mg orally or intramuscularly, is most commonly used. Other agents reported to be effective include anticonvulsants (phenytoin, carbamazepine), benzodiazepines (lorazepam, diazepam), metoclopramide, baclofen, gabapentin, and occasionally general anesthesia.

Polito NB et al. Pharmacologic interventions for intractable and persistent hiccups: a systematic review. J Emerg Med. 2017 Oct;53(4):540–9. [PMID: 29079070]

Steger M et al. Systemic review: the pathogenesis and pharmacological treatment of hiccups. Aliment Pharmacol Ther. 2015 Nov;42(9):1037–50. [PMID: 26307025]

CONSTIPATION

Constipation occurs in 15% of adults and up to one-third of elderly adults and is a common reason for seeking medical attention. It is more common in women. Older individuals are predisposed due to comorbid medical conditions, medications, poor eating habits, decreased mobility, and in some cases, inability to sit on a toilet (bed-bound patients). The first step in evaluating the patient is to determine what is meant by "constipation." Patients may define constipation as infrequent stools (fewer than three in a week), hard stools, excessive straining, or a sense of incomplete evacuation. Table 15–3 summarizes the many causes of constipation, which are discussed below.

Etiology

A. Primary Constipation

Most patients have constipation that cannot be attributed to any structural abnormalities or systemic disease. Some of

Table 15–3. Causes of constipation in adults.

Most common
Inadequate fiber or fluid intake
Poor bowel habits
Systemic disease
Endocrine: hypothyroidism, hyperparathyroidism, diabetes mellitus
Metabolic: hypokalemia, hypercalcemia, uremia, porphyria
Neurologic: Parkinson disease, multiple sclerosis, sacral nerve damage (prior pelvic surgery, tumor), paraplegia, autonomic neuropathy
Medications
Opioids
Diuretics
Calcium channel blockers
Anticholinergics
Psychotropics
Calcium and iron supplements
NSAIDs
Clonidine
Cholestyramine
Structural abnormalities
Anorectal: rectal prolapse, rectocele, rectal intussusception, anorectal stricture, anal fissure, solitary rectal ulcer syndrome
Perineal descent
Colonic mass with obstruction: adenocarcinoma
Colonic stricture: radiation, ischemia, diverticulosis
Hirschsprung disease
Idiopathic megarectum
Slow colonic transit
Idiopathic: isolated to colon
Psychogenic
Eating disorders
Chronic intestinal pseudo-obstruction
Pelvic floor dyssynergia
Irritable bowel syndrome

NSAIDs, nonsteroidal anti-inflammatory drugs.

these patients have normal colonic transit time; however, a subset have slow colonic transit or defecatory disorders. Normal colonic transit time is approximately 35 hours; more than 72 hours is significantly abnormal. Slow colonic transit is commonly idiopathic but may be part of a generalized gastrointestinal dysmotility syndrome. Patients may complain of infrequent bowel movements and abdominal bloating. Slow transit is more common in women, some of whom have a history of psychosocial problems (depression, anxiety, eating disorder, childhood trauma) or sexual abuse. Normal defecation requires coordination between relaxation of the anal sphincter and pelvic floor musculature while abdominal pressure is increased. Patients with defecatory disorders (also known dyssynergic defecation)—women more often than men—have impaired relaxation or paradoxical contraction of the anal sphincter and/or pelvic floor muscles during attempted defecation that impedes the bowel movement. This problem may be acquired during childhood or adulthood. Patients may complain of excessive straining, sense of incomplete evacuation, or need for digital manipulation. Patients with primary complaints of abdominal pain or bloating with alterations in bowel habits (constipation, or alternating constipation and diarrhea) may have irritable bowel syndrome.

B. Secondary Constipation

Constipation may be caused by systemic disorders, medications, or obstructing colonic lesions. Systemic disorders can cause constipation because of neurologic gut dysfunction, myopathies, endocrine disorders, or electrolyte abnormalities (eg, hypercalcemia or hypokalemia); medication side effects are often responsible (eg, anticholinergics or opioids). Colonic lesions that obstruct fecal passage, such as neoplasms and strictures, are an uncommon cause but important in new-onset constipation. Such lesions should be excluded in patients older than age 50 years, in patients with "alarm" symptoms or signs (hematochezia, weight loss, anemia, or positive fecal occult blood tests [FOBT] or fecal immunochemical tests [FIT]), and in patients with a family history of colon cancer or inflammatory bowel disease. Defecatory difficulties also can be due to a variety of anorectal problems that impede or obstruct flow (perineal descent, rectal prolapse, rectocele), some of which may require surgery, and to Hirschsprung disease (usually suggested by lifelong constipation).

► Clinical Findings

A. Symptoms and Signs

All patients should undergo a history and physical examination to distinguish primary from secondary causes of constipation. Physical examination should include digital rectal examination with assessment for anatomic abnormalities, such as anal stricture, rectocele, rectal prolapse, or perineal descent during straining as well as assessment of pelvic floor motion during simulated defecation (ie, the patient's ability to "expel the examiner's finger"). Further diagnostic tests should be performed in patients with any of the following: age 50 years or older, severe constipation, signs of an organic disorders, alarm symptoms (hematochezia, weight loss, positive FOBT or FIT), or a family history of colon cancer or inflammatory bowel disease. These tests should include laboratory studies (complete blood count; serum electrolytes, calcium, glucose, and thyroid-stimulating hormone) and a colonoscopy or flexible sigmoidoscopy.

B. Special Examinations

Patients with refractory constipation not responding to routine medical management warrant further diagnostic studies. Anorectal manometry including a balloon expulsion test should be performed first to evaluate for defecatory disorders. Inability to expel a balloon (attached to a 16F Foley catheter) filled with 50 mL of warm water within 2 minutes while sitting on a toilet is strongly suggestive of pelvic floor dyssynergia. Defecography to further assess pelvic floor function may be considered in selected patients. Subsequent colon transit studies are recommended only after defecatory disorders have been excluded. Colon transit time may be assessed by radiopaque markers, scintigraphy, or wireless motility capsule.

► Treatment

A. Chronic Constipation

1. Dietary and lifestyle measures—Adverse psychosocial issues should be identified and addressed. Patients should be instructed on normal defecatory function and optimal toileting habits, including regular timing, proper positioning, and abdominal pressure. Adequate dietary fluid and fiber intake should be emphasized. A trial of fiber supplements is recommended (Table 15–4). Increased dietary fiber may cause distention or flatulence, which often diminishes over several days. Response to fiber therapy is not immediate, and increases in dosage should be made gradually over 7–10 days. Fiber is most likely to benefit patients with normal colonic transit, but it may not benefit patients with colonic inertia, defecatory disorders, opioid-induced constipation, or irritable bowel syndrome; it may even exacerbate symptoms in these patients. Regular exercise is associated with a decreased risk of constipation. When possible, discontinue medications that may be causing or contributing to constipation. Probiotics are widely promoted to patients in direct advertising for treatment of constipation. A 2014 meta-analysis of randomized controlled trials suggests probiotics improve stool frequency and consistency; however, more study is needed.

2. Laxatives—Laxatives may be given on an intermittent or chronic basis for constipation that does not respond to dietary and lifestyle changes (Table 15–4). There is no evidence that long-term use of these agents is harmful.

A. Osmotic laxatives—Treatment usually is initiated with regular (daily) use of an osmotic laxative. Nonabsorbable osmotic agents increase secretion of water into the intestinal lumen, thereby softening stools and promoting defecation. Magnesium hydroxide, nondigestible carbohydrates (sorbitol, lactulose), and polyethylene glycol are all efficacious and safe for treating acute and chronic cases. The dosages are adjusted to achieve soft to semi-liquid movements. Magnesium-containing saline laxatives should not be given to patients with chronic renal insufficiency. Nondigestible carbohydrates may induce bloating, cramps, and flatulence. Polyethylene glycol 3350 (Miralax) is a component of solutions traditionally used for colonic lavage prior to colonoscopy and does not cause flatulence. When used in conventional doses, the onset of action of these osmotic agents is generally within 24 hours. For more rapid treatment of acute constipation, purgative laxatives may be used, such as magnesium citrate. Magnesium citrate may cause hypermagnesemia.

B. Stimulant laxatives—For patients with incomplete response to osmotic agents, stimulant laxatives may be prescribed as needed as a "rescue" agent or on a regular basis three or four times a week. These agents stimulate fluid secretion and colonic contraction, resulting in a bowel movement within 6–12 hours after oral ingestion or 15–60 minutes after rectal administration. Oral agents are usually administered once daily at bedtime. Common preparations include bisacodyl, senna, and cascara (Table 15–4).

Table 15–4. Pharmacologic management of constipation.

Agent	Dosage	Onset of Action	Comments
Fiber Laxatives			
Bran powder	1–4 tbsp orally twice daily	Days	Inexpensive; may cause gas, flatulence
Psyllium	1 tsp once or twice daily	Days	(Metamucil; Perdiem)
Methylcellulose	1 tsp once or twice daily	Days	(Citrucel) Less gas, flatulence
Calcium polycarbophil	1 or 2 tablets once or twice daily	12–24 hours	(FiberCon) Does not cause gas; pill form
Guargum	1 tbsp once or twice daily	Days	(Benefiber) Non-gritty, tasteless, less gas
Stool Surfactants			
Docusate sodium	100 mg once or twice daily	12–72 hours	(Colace) Marginal benefit
Mineral oil	15–45 mL once or twice daily	6–8 hours	May cause lipoid pneumonia if aspirated
Osmotic Laxatives			
Magnesium hydroxide	15–30 mL orally once or twice daily	6–24 hours	(Milk of magnesia; Epsom salts) May cause hypermagnesemia if chronic kidney disease
Lactulose or 70% sorbitol	15–60 mL orally once daily to three times daily	6–48 hours	Cramps, bloating, flatulence
Polyethylene glycol (PEG 3350)	17 g in 8 oz liquid once or twice daily	6–24 hours	(Miralax) Less bloating than lactulose, sorbitol
Stimulant Laxatives			
Bisacodyl	5–20 mg orally as needed	6–8 hours	May cause cramps; avoid daily use if possible
Bisacodyl suppository	10 mg per rectum as needed	1 hour	
Cascara	4–8 mL or 2 tablets as needed	8–12 hours	(Nature's Remedy) May cause cramps; avoid daily use if possible
Senna	8.6–17.2 mg orally as needed	8–12 hours	(ExLax; Senekot) May cause cramps; avoid daily use if possible
Lubiprostone	24 mcg orally twice daily	12–48 hours	Expensive; may cause nausea. Contraindicated in pregnancy
Linaclotide	145 mcg orally once daily		Expensive; contraindicated in pediatric patients
Plecanatide	3 mg once daily		Expensive; contraindicated in pediatric patients
Enemas			
Tap water	500 mL per rectum	5–15 minutes	
Sodium phosphate enema	120 mL per rectum	5–15 minutes	Commonly used for acute constipation or to induce movement prior to medical procedures
Mineral oil enema	100–250 mL per rectum	5–15 minutes	To soften and lubricate fecal impaction
Agents Used for Acute Purgative or to Clean Bowel Prior to Medical Procedures			
Polyethylene glycol (PEG 3350)	4 L orally administered over 2–4 hours	< 4 hours	(GoLYTELY; CoLYTE; NuLYTE, MoviPrep) Used to cleanse bowel before colonoscopy
Magnesium citrate	10 oz orally	3–6 hours	Lemon-flavored

C. Chloride Secretory Agents—Several agents stimulate intestinal chloride secretion either through activation of chloride channels (lubiprostone) or guanylcyclase C (linaclotide and plecanatide), resulting in increased intestinal fluid and accelerated colonic transit. In multicenter controlled trials, patients treated with lubiprostone 24 mcg orally twice daily, linaclotide 145 mcg once daily, or plecanatide 3 mg once daily increased the number of bowel movements compared with patients treated with placebo.

Because these agents are expensive, they should be reserved for patients who have suboptimal response or side effects with less expensive agents.

D. Opioid-Receptor Antagonists—Long-term use of opioids can cause constipation by inhibiting peristalsis and increasing intestinal fluid absorption. Methylnaltrexone (450 mg orally once daily), naloxegol (25 mg orally once daily), and naldemedine (0.2 mg orally once daily) are mu-opioid receptor antagonists that block peripheral opioid receptors (including in the gastrointestinal tract) without affecting central analgesia. They are approved for the treatment of opioid-induced constipation in patients receiving opioids for chronic noncancer pain (see Chapter 5). A subcutaneous formulation of methylnaltrexone also is approved for treatment of patients receiving palliative care for advanced illness who have not responded to conventional laxative regimens.

B. Fecal Impaction

Severe impaction of stool in the rectal vault may result in obstruction to further fecal flow, leading to partial or complete large bowel obstruction. Predisposing factors include medications (eg, opioids), severe psychiatric disease, prolonged bed rest, neurogenic disorders of the colon, and spinal cord disorders. Clinical presentation includes decreased appetite, nausea and vomiting, and abdominal pain and distention. There may be paradoxical "diarrhea" as liquid stool leaks around the impacted feces. Firm feces are palpable on digital examination of the rectal vault. Initial treatment is directed at relieving the impaction with enemas (saline, mineral oil, or diatrizoate) or digital disruption of the impacted fecal material. Long-term care is directed at maintaining soft stools and regular bowel movements (as above).

▶ When to Refer

- Patients with refractory constipation for anorectal testing.
- Patients with defecatory disorders may benefit from biofeedback therapy.
- Patients with alarm symptoms or who are over age 50 should be referred for colonoscopy.
- Rarely, surgery (subtotal colectomy) is required for patients with severe colonic inertia.

Brenner DM et al. Chronic constipation. Gastroenterol Clin North Am. 2016 Jun;45(2):205–16. [PMID: 27261894]
Hale M et al. Naldemedine versus placebo for opioid-induced constipation (COMPOSE-1 and COMPOSE-2): two multicenter, phase 3, double-blind, randomized, parallel-group trials. Lancet Gastroenterol Hepatol. 2017 Aug;2(8):555–64. [PMID: 28576452]
Katakami N et al. Randomized phase III and extension studies of naldemedine in patients with opioid-induced constipation and cancer. J Clin Oncol 2017 Dec 1;35(34):3859–66. [PMID: 28968171]
Miner PB Jr et al. A randomized phase III clinical trial with plecanatide, a uroguanylin analog in patients with chronic idiopathic constipation. Am J Gastroenterol. 2017 Apr;112(4):613–21. [PMID: 28169285]
Murphy JA et al. Evidence based review of pharmacotherapy for opioid-induced constipation in noncancer pain. Ann Pharmacother. 2018 Apr;52(4):370–9. [PMID: 29092627]
Nee J et al. Efficacy of treatments for opioid-induced constipation: systematic review and meta-analysis. Clin Gastroenterol Hepatol. 2018 Oct;16(10):1569–84.e2. [PMID: 29374616]
Schoenfeld P et al. Low-dose linaclotide (72 μg) for chronic idiopathic constipation: a 12-week, randomized, double-blind, placebo-controlled trial. Am J Gastroenterol. 2018 Jan; 113(1):105–14. [PMID: 29091082]

GASTROINTESTINAL GAS

1. Belching

Belching (eructation) is the involuntary or voluntary release of gas from the stomach or esophagus. It occurs most frequently after meals, when gastric distention results in transient lower esophageal sphincter (LES) relaxation. Belching is a normal reflex and does not itself denote gastrointestinal dysfunction. Virtually all stomach gas comes from swallowed air. With each swallow, 2–5 mL of air is ingested, and excessive amounts may result in distention, flatulence, and abdominal pain. This may occur with rapid eating, gum chewing, smoking, and the ingestion of carbonated beverages. Evaluation should be restricted to patients with other complaints such as dysphagia, heartburn, early satiety, or vomiting.

Chronic excessive belching is almost always caused by supragastric belching (voluntary diaphragmatic contraction, followed by upper esophageal relaxation with air inflow to the esophagus) or true air swallowing (aerophagia), both of which are behavioral disorders that are more common in patients with anxiety or psychiatric disorders. These patients may benefit from referral to a behavioral or speech therapist.

Glasinovic E et al. Treatment of supragastric belching with cognitive behavioral therapy improves quality of life and reduces acid gastroesophageal reflux. Am J Gastroenterol. 2018 Apr;113(4):539–47. [PMID: 29460918]
Pauwels A et al. A randomized, double-blind, placebo-controlled, cross-over study using baclofen in the treatment of rumination syndrome. Am J Gastroenterol. 2018 (Jan);113(1):97–104. [PMID: 29206813]

2. Bloating & Flatus

Bloating is a complaint of increased abdominal pressure that may or may not be accompanied by visible distention. Organic causes of acute bloating with distention, vomiting, and/or pain include ascites, gastrointestinal obstruction (gastric fundoplication, gastric outlet obstruction, small intestine or colon obstruction, and constipation). Complaints of chronic abdominal distention or bloating are common. Some patients swallow excess air (aerophagia, poorly fitting dentures, sleep apnea, and rapid eating) or produce excess gas (excessive FODMAP [fermentable oligosaccharides, disaccharides, monosaccharides, and polyols] ingestion and malabsorption). Others have impaired gas propulsion or expulsion, increased bowel wall tension, enhanced visceral sensitivity, or altered viscerosomatic reflexes leading to abdominal protrusion. Many of these patients have an underlying functional gastrointestinal disorder such as irritable bowel syndrome or functional dyspepsia. Constipation should be treated, and exercise (which accelerates gas propulsion) is recommended. Medications that inhibit gastrointestinal motility should be avoided (opioids and calcium channel blockers).

Healthy adults pass **flatus** up to 20 times daily and excrete up to 750 mL. Flatus is derived from two sources: swallowed air (primarily nitrogen) and bacterial fermentation of undigested carbohydrate (which produces H_2, CO_2, and methane). A number of short-chain carbohydrates (FODMAPs) are incompletely absorbed in the small intestine and pass into the colon. These include lactose (dairy products); fructose (fruits, corn syrups, and some sweeteners); polyols (stone-fruits, mushrooms, and some sweeteners); and oligosaccharides (legumes, lentils, cruciferous vegetables, garlic, onion, pasta, and whole grains). Abnormal gas production may be caused by increased ingestion of these carbohydrates or, less commonly, by disorders of malabsorption. Foul odor may be caused by garlic, onion, eggplant, mushrooms, and certain herbs and spices.

Determining abnormal from normal amounts of flatus is difficult. Patients who report excess flatus may also complain of bloating, cramping, and altered stool habits (diarrhea or constipation). Patients with a long-standing history of flatulence and no other symptoms or signs of malabsorption disorders can be treated conservatively. Gum chewing and carbonated beverages should be avoided to reduce air swallowing. Lactose intolerance may be assessed by a 2-week trial of a lactose-free diet or by a hydrogen breath test. A list of foods containing FODMAPs should be provided and high FODMAP foods eliminated for 2–4 weeks. If symptoms improve, FODMAP groups may be sequentially introduced to identify triggers. Multiple low-FODMAP dietary guides are available; however, referral to a knowledgeable dietician may be helpful.

The nonprescription agent Beano (alpha-d-galactosidase enzyme) reduces gas caused by foods containing galacto-oligosaccharides (legumes, chickpeas, lentils) but not other FODMAPs. Activated charcoal may afford relief. Simethicone has no proven benefit.

Many patients report reduced flatus production with use of probiotics, although there has been limited controlled study of these agents for this purpose.

Kamboj AK et al. Workup and management of bloating. Clin Gastroenterol Hepatol. 2018 Jul;16(7):1030–3. [PMID: 29306037]
Malagelada JR et al. Bloating and abdominal distension: old misconceptions and current knowledge. Am J Gastroenterol. 2017 Aug;112(8):1221–31. [PMID: 28508867]
Omer A et al. Carbohydrate maldigestion and malabsorption. Clin Gastroenterol Hepatol. 2018 Aug;16(8):1197–9. [PMID: 29425782]

DIARRHEA

Diarrhea can range in severity from an acute self-limited episode to a severe, life-threatening illness. To properly evaluate the complaint, the clinician must determine the patient's normal bowel pattern and the nature of the current symptoms.

Approximately 10 L/d of fluid enter the duodenum of which all but 1.5 L/d are absorbed by the small intestine. The colon absorbs most of the remaining fluid, with less than 200 mL/d lost in the stool. Although diarrhea sometimes is defined as a stool weight of more than 200–300 g/24 h, quantification of stool weight is necessary only in some patients with chronic diarrhea. In most cases, the physician's working definition of diarrhea is increased stool frequency (more than three bowel movements per day) or liquidity of feces.

Table 15–5. Causes of acute infectious diarrhea.

Noninflammatory Diarrhea	Inflammatory Diarrhea
Viral Noroviruses, astrovirus, adenovirus, rotavirus, sapovirus	**Viral** Cytomegalovirus
Protozoal *Giardia lamblia* *Cryptosporidium* *Cyclospora*	**Protozoal** *Entamoeba histolytica*

Bacterial
1. Preformed enterotoxin production
  Staphylococcus aureus
  Bacillus cereus
  Clostridium perfringens
2. Enterotoxin production
  Enterotoxigenic
    Escherichia coli (ETEC)
  Vibrio cholera, Vibrio vulnificus
	Bacterial
	1. Cytotoxin production
	  Enterohemorrhagic
	    E coli O157:H5 and O157:H7 (EHEC)
	  Vibrio parahaemolyticus
	  Clostridioides difficile
	  Plesiomonas shigelloides
	2. Mucosal invasion
	  Shigella
	  Campylobacter jejuni
	  Salmonella
	  Enteroinvasive *E coli* (EIEC)
	  Aeromonas
	  Yersinia enterocolitica
	  Chlamydia
	  Neisseria gonorrhoeae
	  Listeria monocytogenes

The causes of diarrhea are myriad. In clinical practice, it is helpful to distinguish acute from chronic diarrhea, as the evaluation and treatment are entirely different (Tables 15–5 and 15–6).

1. Acute Diarrhea

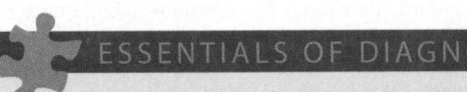

ESSENTIALS OF DIAGNOSIS

▶ Diarrhea of less than 2 weeks' duration is most commonly caused by invasive or noninvasive pathogens and their enterotoxins.

Acute noninflammatory diarrhea

▶ Watery, nonbloody.

▶ Usually mild, self-limited.

▶ Caused by a virus or noninvasive bacteria.

▶ Diagnostic evaluation is limited to patients with diarrhea that is severe or persists beyond 7 days.

Acute inflammatory diarrhea

▶ Blood or pus, fever.

▶ Usually caused by an invasive or toxin-producing bacterium.

▶ Diagnostic evaluation requires routine stool bacterial testing (including *E coli* O157:H5 and O157:H7) in all and testing as clinically indicated for *Clostridioides difficile* toxin, and ova and parasites.

Table 15–6. Causes of chronic diarrhea.

Osmotic diarrhea
CLUES: Stool volume decreases with fasting; increased stool osmotic gap
  1. Medications: antacids, lactulose, sorbitol
  2. Disaccharidase deficiency: lactose intolerance
  3. Factitious diarrhea: magnesium (antacids, laxatives)
Secretory diarrhea
CLUES: Large volume (> 1 L/day); little change with fasting; normal stool osmotic gap
  1. Hormonally mediated: VIPoma, carcinoid, medullary carcinoma of thyroid (calcitonin), Zollinger-Ellison syndrome (gastrin)
  2. Factitious diarrhea (laxative abuse); phenolphthalein, cascara, senna
  3. Villous adenoma
  4. Bile salt malabsorption (idiopathic, ileal resection; Crohn ileitis; postcholecystectomy)
  5. Medications
Inflammatory conditions
CLUES: Fever, hematochezia, abdominal pain
  1. Ulcerative colitis
  2. Crohn disease
  3. Microscopic colitis
  4. Malignancy: lymphoma, adenocarcinoma (with obstruction and pseudodiarrhea)
  5. Radiation enteritis
Medications
Common offenders: SSRIs, cholinesterase inhibitors, NSAIDs, proton pump inhibitors, angiotensin II receptor blockers, metformin, allopurinol
	Malabsorption syndromes
	CLUES: Weight loss, abnormal laboratory values; fecal fat > 10 g/24 h
	  1. Small bowel mucosal disorders: celiac disease, tropical sprue, Whipple disease, eosinophilic gastroenteritis, small bowel resection (short bowel syndrome), Crohn disease
	  2. Lymphatic obstruction: lymphoma, carcinoid, infectious (tuberculosis, MAI), Kaposi sarcoma, sarcoidosis, retroperitoneal fibrosis
	  3. Pancreatic disease: chronic pancreatitis, pancreatic carcinoma
	  4. Bacterial overgrowth: motility disorders (diabetes, vagotomy), scleroderma, fistulas, small intestinal diverticula
	Motility disorders
	CLUES: Systemic disease or prior abdominal surgery
	  1. Postsurgical: vagotomy, partial gastrectomy, blind loop with bacterial overgrowth
	  2. Systemic disorders: scleroderma, diabetes mellitus, hyperthyroidism
	  3. Irritable bowel syndrome
	Chronic infections
	  1. Parasites: *Giardia lamblia, Entamoeba histolytica, Strongyloides stercoralis, Capillaria philippinensis*
	  2. AIDS-related: Viral: Cytomegalovirus; Bacterial: *Clostridioides difficile, Mycobacterium avium* complex; Protozoal: Microsporidia (*Enterocytozoon bieneusi*), *Cryptosporidium, Cystoisospora belli* (formerly *Isospora belli*)
	Factitious
	See Osmotic and Secretory diarrhea above

MAI, *Mycobacterium avium-intracellulare;* NSAIDs, nonsteroidal anti-inflammatory drugs; SSRIs, selective serotonin reuptake inhibitors.

► **Etiology & Clinical Findings**

Diarrhea acute in onset and persisting for less than 2 weeks is most commonly caused by infectious agents, bacterial toxins (either preformed or produced in the gut), or medications. Community outbreaks (including nursing homes, schools, cruise ships) suggest a viral etiology or a common food source. Similar recent illnesses in family members suggest an infectious origin. Ingestion of improperly stored or prepared food implicates food poisoning. Pregnant women have an increased risk of developing listeriosis. Day care attendance or exposure to unpurified water (camping, swimming) may result in infection with *Giardia* or *Cryptosporidium.* Large *Cyclospora* outbreaks have been traced to contaminated produce. Recent travel abroad suggests "traveler's diarrhea" (see Chapter 30). Antibiotic administration within the preceding several weeks increases the likelihood of *C difficile* colitis. Finally, risk factors for HIV infection or sexually transmitted diseases should be determined. (AIDS-associated diarrhea is discussed in Chapter 31; infectious proctitis is discussed later in this chapter under Anorectal Infections.) Persons engaging in anal intercourse or oral-anal sexual activities are at risk for a variety of infections that cause proctitis, including gonorrhea, syphilis, lymphogranuloma venereum, and herpes simplex.

The nature of the diarrhea helps distinguish among different infectious causes (Table 15–5).

A. Noninflammatory Diarrhea

Watery, nonbloody diarrhea associated with periumbilical cramps, bloating, nausea, or vomiting suggests a small bowel source caused by either a virus (rotavirus, norovirus, adenovirus), a toxin-producing bacterium (enterotoxigenic *E coli* [ETEC], *Staphylococcus aureus, Bacillus cereus, Clostridium perfringens, Plesiomonas shigelloides*), or another agent (*Giardia*) that disrupts normal absorption and secretory process in the small intestine. Prominent vomiting suggests viral enteritis or *S aureus* food poisoning. Although typically mild, the diarrhea (which originates in the small intestine) can be voluminous and result in dehydration with hypokalemia and metabolic acidosis (eg, cholera). Because tissue invasion does not occur, fecal leukocytes are not present.

B. Inflammatory Diarrhea

The presence of fever and bloody diarrhea (dysentery) indicates colonic tissue damage caused by invasion (shigellosis, salmonellosis, *Campylobacter* or *Yersinia* infection, amebiasis) or a toxin (*C difficile, Aeromonas,* Shiga-toxin–producing *E coli* [STEC; also known as enterohemorrhagic *E coli*]). Because these organisms predominantly involve the colon, the diarrhea is small in volume (less than 1 L/day) and associated with left lower quadrant cramps, urgency, and tenesmus. Fecal leukocytes or lactoferrin usually are present in infections with invasive organisms. *E coli* O157:H7 is a Shiga-toxin–producing noninvasive organism most commonly acquired from contaminated meat that has resulted in several outbreaks of an acute, often severe hemorrhagic colitis. In 2011, an outbreak of severe gastroenteritis in Germany, caused by an unusual Shiga-toxin–producing strain, *E coli* O104:H4, was traced to contaminated sprouts. A major complication of STEC is hemolytic-uremic syndrome, which develops in 6–22% of cases. In immunocompromised and HIV-infected patients, cytomegalovirus (CMV) can cause intestinal ulceration with watery or bloody diarrhea.

Infectious dysentery must be distinguished from acute ulcerative colitis, which may also present acutely with fever, abdominal pain, and bloody diarrhea. Diarrhea that persists for more than 14 days is not attributable to bacterial pathogens (except for *C difficile*) and should be evaluated as chronic diarrhea.

► Evaluation

In over 90% of patients with acute noninflammatory diarrhea, the illness is mild and self-limited, responding within 5 days to simple rehydration therapy or antidiarrheal agents. The isolation rate of bacterial pathogens from stool cultures in patients with acute noninflammatory diarrhea is under 3%; therefore, diagnostic investigation is unnecessary

except in suspected outbreaks or in patients at high risk for spreading infection to others.

The goal of initial evaluation of acute diarrhea is to distinguish patients with mild disease from those with more serious illness. Prompt medical evaluation is indicated in the following situations (Figure 15–1): (1) signs of inflammatory diarrhea manifested by any of the following: fever (higher than 38.5°C), WBC 15,000/mcL or more, bloody diarrhea, or severe abdominal pain; (2) the passage of six or more unformed stools in 24 hours; (3) profuse watery diarrhea and dehydration; (4) frail older patients or nursing home residents; (5) immunocompromised patients (AIDS, posttransplantation); (6) exposure to antibiotics; (7) hospital-acquired diarrhea (onset following at least 3 days of hospitalization); or (8) systemic illness.

Physical examination pays note to the patient's level of hydration, mental status, and the presence of abdominal tenderness or peritonitis. Peritoneal findings may be present in infection with *C difficile* or STEC. Hospitalization is required in patients with severe dehydration, organ failure, marked abdominal pain, or altered mental status.

Stool should be sent for microbial assessment when patients have dysentery (bloody stools), severe illness, or persistent diarrhea beyond 7 days. In many centers, stool specimens are sent for microscopy (to assess for fecal white cells and protozoa) and bacterial cultures (requiring 48–72 hours). These traditional methods provide a positive

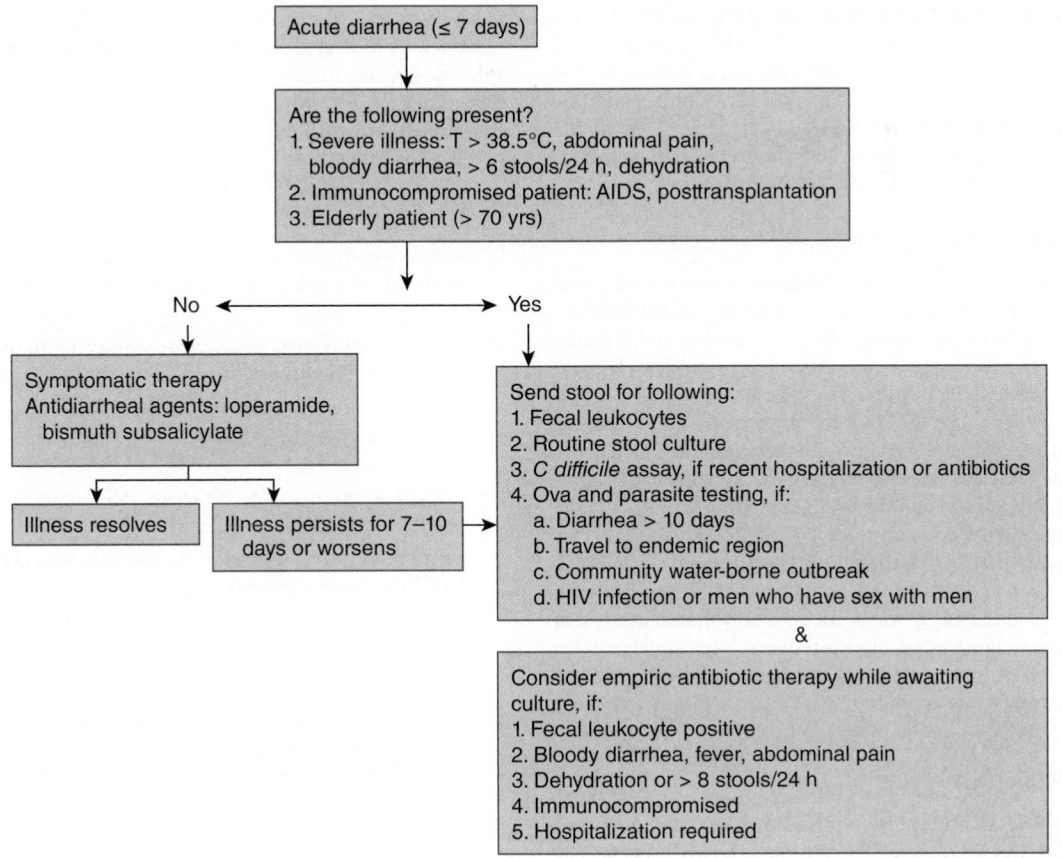

▲ **Figure 15–1.** Evaluation of acute diarrhea.

diagnosis in 60–75% of patients with dysenteric diarrhea but only in 6–20% with acute diarrhea. In patients who are hospitalized or who have a history of antibiotic exposure, a stool sample should be tested for *C difficile*. In lieu of conventional labor-intensive stool microscopy and culture, many centers perform microbial assessment using multiplex molecular techniques with nucleic acid amplification (eg, polymerase chain reaction [PCR] assays) that screen for a panel of pathogens, including viruses, protozoa, and bacteria and can detect potential pathogens in 35–54% of specimens within 1–4 hours.

▶ Treatment

A. Diet

Most mild diarrhea will not lead to dehydration provided the patient takes adequate oral fluids containing carbohydrates and electrolytes. Patients find it more comfortable to rest the bowel by avoiding high-fiber foods, fats, milk products, caffeine, and alcohol. Frequent feedings of tea, "flat" carbonated beverages, and soft, easily digested foods (eg, soups, crackers, bananas, applesauce, rice, toast) are encouraged.

B. Rehydration

In more severe diarrhea, dehydration can occur quickly, especially in children and frail older adults. Oral rehydration with fluids containing glucose, Na$^+$, K$^+$, Cl$^-$, and bicarbonate or citrate is preferred when feasible. A convenient mixture is ½ tsp salt (3.5 g), 1 tsp baking soda (2.5 g NaHCO$_3$), 8 tsp sugar (40 g), and 8 oz orange juice (1.5 g KCl), diluted to 1 L with water. Alternatively, oral electrolyte solutions (eg, Pedialyte, Gatorade) are readily available. Fluids should be given at rates of 50–200 mL/kg/24 h depending on the hydration status. Intravenous fluids (lactated Ringer injection) are preferred in patients with severe dehydration.

C. Antidiarrheal Agents

Antidiarrheal agents may be used safely in patients with mild to moderate diarrheal illnesses to improve patient comfort. Opioid agents help decrease the stool number and liquidity and control fecal urgency. However, they should not be used in patients with bloody diarrhea, high fever, or systemic toxicity and should be discontinued in patients whose diarrhea is worsening despite therapy. With these provisos, such drugs provide excellent symptomatic relief. Loperamide is preferred, in a dosage of 4 mg orally initially, followed by 2 mg after each loose stool (maximum: 8 mg/24 h).

Bismuth subsalicylate (Pepto-Bismol), two tablets or 30 mL orally four times daily, reduces symptoms in patients with traveler's diarrhea by virtue of its anti-inflammatory and antibacterial properties. It also reduces vomiting associated with viral enteritis. Anticholinergic agents (eg, diphenoxylate with atropine) are contraindicated in acute diarrhea because of the rare precipitation of toxic megacolon.

D. Antibiotic Therapy

1. Empiric treatment—Empiric antibiotic treatment of patients with acute, community-acquired diarrhea generally is not indicated. Even patients with inflammatory diarrhea caused by invasive pathogens usually have symptoms that will resolve within several days without antimicrobials. In centers in which stool microbial testing with rapid molecular assays is not available (yielding results within 5 hours), empiric treatment may be considered while the stool bacterial culture is incubating in certain patients: those with non–hospital-acquired diarrhea; those with moderate to severe fever, tenesmus, or bloody stools; and those with no suspicion of infection with STEC. It should also be considered in patients who are immunocompromised or who have significant dehydration. The oral drugs of choice for empiric treatment are the fluoroquinolones (eg, ciprofloxacin 500 mg, ofloxacin 400 mg, or levofloxacin 500 mg once daily) for 1–3 days. Alternatives include trimethoprim-sulfamethoxazole, 160/800 mg twice daily; or doxycycline, 100 mg twice daily. Macrolides and penicillins are no longer recommended because of widespread microbial resistance to these agents. Rifaximin (200 mg three times daily for 3 days) and azithromycin (1000 mg single dose or 500 mg daily for 3 days) are approved for empiric treatment of noninflammatory traveler's diarrhea (see Chapter 30).

2. Specific antimicrobial treatment—Antibiotics are not recommended in patients with nontyphoid *Salmonella*, *Campylobacter*, STEC, *Aeromonas*, or *Yersinia*, except in severe disease, because they do not hasten recovery or reduce the period of fecal bacterial excretion. The infectious bacterial diarrheas for which treatment is recommended are shigellosis, cholera, extraintestinal salmonellosis, listeriosis, and *C difficile*. The parasitic infections for which treatment is indicated are amebiasis, giardiasis, cryptosporidiosis, cyclosporiasis, and *Enterocytozoon bienusi* infection. Therapy for traveler's diarrhea, infectious (sexually transmitted) proctitis, and AIDS-related diarrhea is presented in Chapters 30 and 31.

▶ When to Admit

- Severe dehydration for intravenous fluids, especially if vomiting or unable to maintain sufficient oral fluid intake.

- Bloody diarrhea that is severe or worsening in order to distinguish infectious versus noninfectious cause.

- Severe abdominal pain, worrisome for toxic colitis, inflammatory bowel disease, intestinal ischemia, or surgical abdomen.

- Signs of severe infection or sepsis (temperature higher than 39.5°C, leukocytosis, rash).

- Severe or worsening diarrhea in patients who are older than 70 years or immunocompromised.

- Signs of hemolytic-uremic syndrome (acute kidney injury, thrombocytopenia, hemolytic anemia).

Acree M et al. Acute diarrheal infections in adults. JAMA. 2017 Sep 12;318(10):957–8. [PMID: 28898366]

Giddings SL et al. Traveler's diarrhea. Med Clin North Am. 2016 Mar;100(2):317–30. [PMID: 26900116]

Riddle MS et al. ACG Clinical Guideline: diagnosis, treatment, and prevention of acute diarrheal infections in adults. Am J Gastroenterol. 2016 May;111(5):602–22. [PMID: 27068718]

2. Chronic Diarrhea

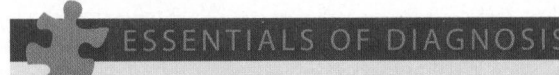

ESSENTIALS OF DIAGNOSIS

▶ Diarrhea present for longer than 4 weeks.

▶ Before embarking on extensive workup, common causes should be excluded, including medications, chronic infections, and irritable bowel syndrome.

▶ Etiology

The causes of chronic diarrhea may be grouped into the following major pathophysiologic categories: medications, osmotic diarrheas, secretory conditions, inflammatory conditions, malabsorptive conditions, motility disorders, chronic infections, and systemic disorders (Table 15–6).

A. Medications

Numerous medications can cause diarrhea. Common offenders include cholinesterase inhibitors, SSRIs, angiotensin II-receptor blockers, proton pump inhibitors, NSAIDs, metformin, allopurinol, and orlistat. All medications should be carefully reviewed, and discontinuation of potential culprits should be considered.

B. Osmotic Diarrheas

As stool leaves the colon, fecal osmolality is equal to the serum osmolality, ie, approximately 290 mOsm/kg. Under normal circumstances, the major osmoles are Na^+, K^+, Cl^-, and HCO_3^-. The stool osmolality may be estimated by multiplying the stool ($Na^+ + K^+$) × 2. The **osmotic gap** is the difference between the *measured* osmolality of the stool (or serum) and the *estimated* stool osmolality and is normally less than 50 mOsm/kg. An increased osmotic gap (greater than 75 mOsm/kg) implies that the diarrhea is caused by ingestion or malabsorption of an osmotically active substance. The most common causes are carbohydrate malabsorption (lactose, fructose, sorbitol), laxative abuse, and malabsorption syndromes. Osmotic diarrheas resolve during fasting. Those caused by malabsorbed carbohydrates are characterized by abdominal distention, bloating, and flatulence due to increased colonic gas production.

Carbohydrate malabsorption is common and should be considered in all patients with chronic, postprandial diarrhea. Patients should be asked about their intake of dairy products (lactose), fruits and artificial sweeteners (fructose and sorbitol), processed foods and soft drinks (high-fructose corn syrup), and alcohol. The diagnosis of carbohydrate malabsorption may be established by an elimination trial for 2–3 weeks or by hydrogen breath tests.

Ingestion of magnesium- or phosphate-containing compounds (laxatives, antacids) should be considered in enigmatic chronic diarrhea. The fat substitute olestra also causes diarrhea and cramps in occasional patients.

C. Secretory Conditions

Increased intestinal secretion or decreased absorption results in a high-volume watery diarrhea with a normal osmotic gap. There is little change in stool output during the fasting state, and dehydration and electrolyte imbalance may develop. Causes include endocrine tumors (stimulating intestinal or pancreatic secretion), bile salt malabsorption (stimulating colonic secretion), and microscopic colitis. Microscopic colitis is a common cause of chronic watery diarrhea in older adults (see Inflammatory Bowel Disease, below).

D. Inflammatory Conditions

Diarrhea is present in most patients with inflammatory bowel disease (ulcerative colitis, Crohn disease). A variety of other symptoms may be present, including abdominal pain, fever, weight loss, and hematochezia.

E. Malabsorptive Conditions

The major causes of malabsorption are small mucosal intestinal diseases, intestinal resections, lymphatic obstruction, small intestinal bacterial overgrowth, and pancreatic insufficiency. Its characteristics are weight loss, osmotic diarrhea, steatorrhea, and nutritional deficiencies. Significant diarrhea in the absence of weight loss is not likely to be due to malabsorption. The physical and laboratory abnormalities related to deficiencies of vitamins or minerals are discussed in Chapter 29.

F. Motility Disorders (Including Irritable Bowel Syndrome)

Irritable bowel syndrome is the most common cause of chronic diarrhea in young adults (see Irritable Bowel Syndrome, below). It should be considered in patients with lower abdominal pain and altered bowel habits who have no other evidence of serious organic disease (weight loss, nocturnal diarrhea, anemia, or gastrointestinal bleeding). Abnormal intestinal motility secondary to systemic disorders, radiation enteritis, or surgery may result in diarrhea due to rapid transit or to stasis of intestinal contents with bacterial overgrowth, resulting in malabsorption.

G. Chronic Infections

Chronic parasitic infections may cause diarrhea through a number of mechanisms. Pathogens most commonly associated with diarrhea include the protozoans *Giardia*, *Entamoeba histolytica*, and *Cyclospora* as well as the intestinal nematodes. Strongyloidiasis and capillariasis should be excluded in patients from endemic regions, especially in the presence of eosinophilia. Bacterial infections with *C difficile* and, uncommonly, *Aeromonas* and *Plesiomonas* may cause chronic diarrhea.

Immunocompromised patients are susceptible to infectious organisms that can cause acute or chronic diarrhea (see Chapter 31), including microsporidia, *Cryptosporidium*, CMV, *Cystoisospora belli* (formerly *Isospora belli*), *Cyclospora*, and *Mycobacterium avium* complex.

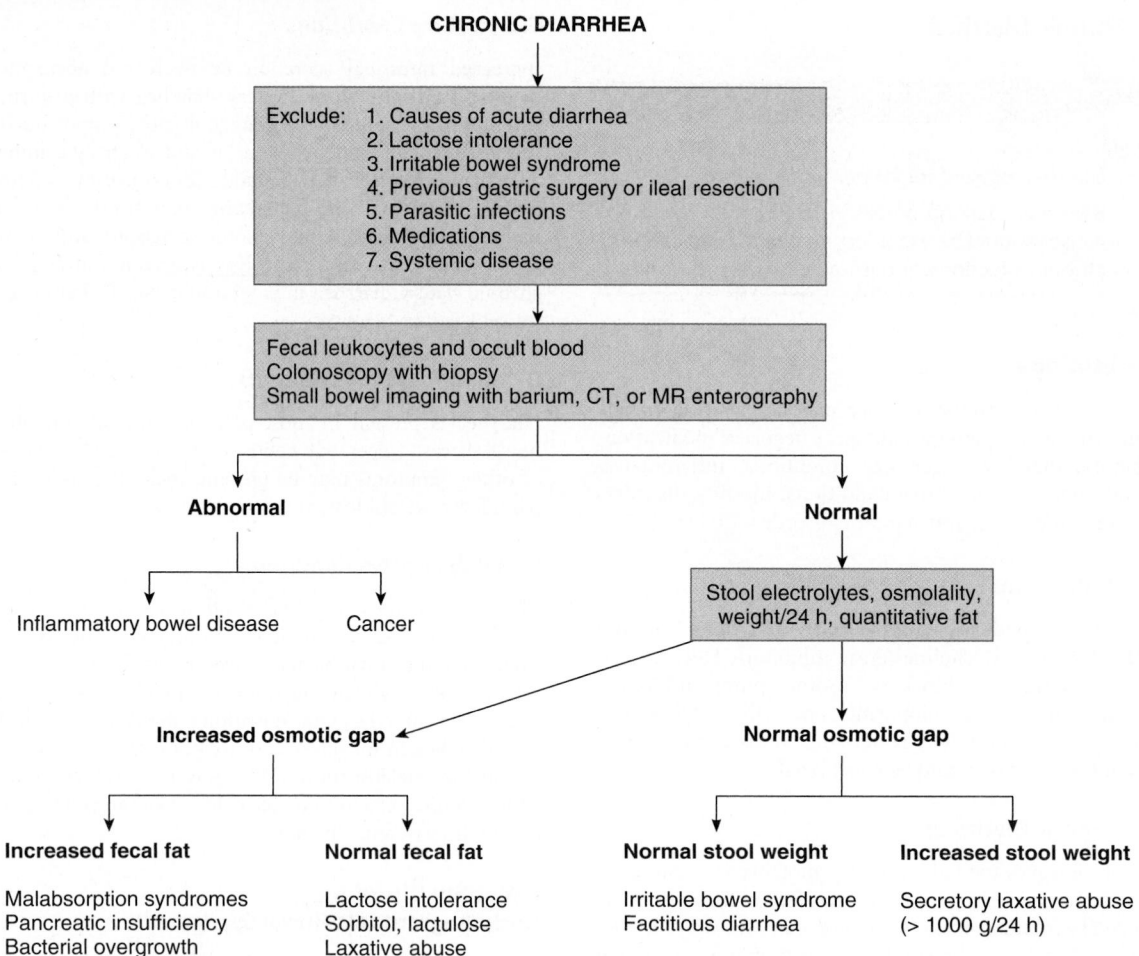

CHRONIC DIARRHEA

Exclude: 1. Causes of acute diarrhea
2. Lactose intolerance
3. Irritable bowel syndrome
4. Previous gastric surgery or ileal resection
5. Parasitic infections
6. Medications
7. Systemic disease

Fecal leukocytes and occult blood
Colonoscopy with biopsy
Small bowel imaging with barium, CT, or MR enterography

Abnormal　　　　　　　　　　　　　　　　　**Normal**

Inflammatory bowel disease　　　Cancer

Stool electrolytes, osmolality,
weight/24 h, quantitative fat

Increased osmotic gap　　　　　　　　　**Normal osmotic gap**

Increased fecal fat　　**Normal fecal fat**　　　**Normal stool weight**　　**Increased stool weight**

Malabsorption syndromes　Lactose intolerance　　Irritable bowel syndrome　Secretory laxative abuse
Pancreatic insufficiency　Sorbitol, lactulose　　Factitious diarrhea　　　(> 1000 g/24 h)
Bacterial overgrowth　　Laxative abuse

▲ **Figure 15–2.** Decision diagram for diagnosis of causes of chronic diarrhea.

H. Systemic Conditions

Chronic systemic conditions, such as thyroid disease, diabetes, and collagen vascular disorders, may cause diarrhea through alterations in motility or intestinal absorption.

▶ Clinical Findings

The history and physical examination commonly suggest the underlying pathophysiology that guides the subsequent diagnostic workup (Figure 15–2). The clinician should establish whether the diarrhea is continuous or intermittent, its relationship to meals, and whether it occurs at night or during fasting. The stool appearance may suggest a malabsorption disorder (greasy or malodorous), inflammatory disorder (containing blood or pus), or a secretory process (watery). The presence of abdominal pain suggests irritable bowel syndrome or inflammatory bowel disease. Medications, diet, and recent psychosocial stressors should be reviewed. Physical examination should assess for signs of malnutrition, dehydration, and inflammatory bowel disease.

Because chronic diarrhea is caused by so many conditions, the subsequent diagnostic approach is guided by the relative suspicion for the underlying cause, and no specific

algorithm can be followed in all patients. Prior to embarking on an extensive evaluation, the most common causes of chronic diarrhea should be considered, including medications, irritable bowel syndrome, and lactose intolerance. The presence of nocturnal diarrhea, weight loss, anemia, or positive results on FOBT are inconsistent with these disorders and warrant further evaluation. AIDS-associated diarrhea is discussed in Chapter 31.

A. Initial Diagnostic Tests

1. Routine laboratory tests—Complete blood count, serum electrolytes, liver chemistries, calcium, phosphorus, albumin, thyroid-stimulating hormone, vitamin A and D levels, international normalized ratio (INR), erythrocyte sedimentation rate, and C-reactive protein should be obtained in most patients. Serologic testing for celiac disease with an IgA tissue transglutaminase (tTG) test may be recommended in the evaluation of most patients with chronic diarrhea and all patients with signs of malabsorption. Anemia occurs in malabsorption syndromes (folate, iron deficiency, or vitamin B_{12}) as well as inflammatory conditions. Hypoalbuminemia is present in malabsorption, protein-losing

enteropathies, and inflammatory diseases. Hyponatremia and nonanion gap metabolic acidosis occur in secretory diarrheas. Increased erythrocyte sedimentation rate or C-reactive protein suggests inflammatory bowel disease.

2. Routine stool studies—Stool samples should be analyzed for ova and parasites, electrolytes (to calculate osmotic gap), qualitative staining for fat (Sudan stain), occult blood, and leukocytes or lactoferrin. Parasitic infections (*Giardia*, *E histolytica*, *Cryptosporidia*, and *Cyclospora*) may be diagnosed with stool antigen assays or microscopy with special stains. Alternatively, stool molecular diagnostic tests are available that screen for a panel of pathogens, providing results within 5 hours. As discussed previously, an increased osmotic gap suggests an osmotic diarrhea or disorder of malabsorption. A positive fecal fat stain suggests a disorder of malabsorption. The presence of fecal leukocytes or lactoferrin may suggest inflammatory bowel disease.

3. Endoscopic examination and mucosal biopsy—Most patients with chronic persistent diarrhea undergo colonoscopy with mucosal biopsy to exclude inflammatory bowel disease (including Crohn disease and ulcerative colitis), microscopic colitis, and colonic neoplasia. Upper endoscopy with small bowel biopsy is performed when a small intestinal malabsorptive disorder is suspected (celiac disease, Whipple disease) from abnormal laboratory studies or a positive fecal fat stain. It may also be done in patients with advanced AIDS to document *Cryptosporidium*, microsporidia, and *M avium-intracellulare* infection.

B. Further Studies

If the cause of diarrhea is still not apparent, further studies may be warranted.

1. 24-hour stool collection quantification of total weight and fat—A stool weight of less than 200–300 g/24 h excludes diarrhea and suggests a functional disorder such as irritable bowel syndrome. A weight greater than 1000–1500 g suggests a significant secretory process, including neuroendocrine tumors. A fecal fat determination in excess of 10 g/24 h confirms a malabsorptive disorder. Fecal elastase less than 100 mcg/g may be caused by pancreatic insufficiency. (See Celiac Disease and specific tests for malabsorption, below.)

2. Other imaging studies—Calcification on a plain abdominal radiograph confirms a diagnosis of chronic pancreatitis, although abdominal CT and endoscopic ultrasonography are more sensitive for the diagnosis of chronic pancreatitis as well as pancreatic cancer. Small intestinal imaging with CT or MRI enterography is helpful in the diagnosis of Crohn disease, small bowel lymphoma, carcinoid, and jejunal diverticula. Neuroendocrine tumors may be localized using somatostatin receptor scintigraphy. Retention of less than 11% at 7 days of intravenous 75Se-homotaurocholate on scintigraphy suggests bile salt malabsorption.

3. Laboratory tests—

A. SEROLOGIC TESTS FOR NEUROENDOCRINE TUMORS—Secretory diarrheas due to neuroendocrine tumors are rare but should be considered in patients with chronic, high-volume watery diarrhea (greater than 1 L/day) with a normal osmotic gap that persists during fasting. Measurements of the secretagogues of various neuroendocrine tumors may be assayed, including serum chromogranin A (pancreatic neuroendocrine tumors), vasoactive intestinal peptide (VIP) (VIPoma), calcitonin (medullary thyroid carcinoma), gastrin (Zollinger-Ellison syndrome), and urinary 5-hydroxyindoleacetic acid (5-HIAA) (carcinoid).

B. BREATH TEST—The diagnosis of small bowel bacterial overgrowth is suggested by a noninvasive breath tests (glucose or lactulose); however, a high rate of false-positive test results limits the utility of these tests. A definitive diagnosis of bacterial overgrowth is determined by aspirate of small intestinal contents for quantitative aerobic and anaerobic bacterial culture; however, this procedure is not available at most centers.

▶ Treatment

A number of antidiarrheal agents may be used in certain patients with chronic diarrheal conditions and are listed below. Opioids are safe in most patients with chronic, stable symptoms.

Loperamide: 4 mg orally initially, then 2 mg after each loose stool (maximum: 16 mg/day).

Diphenoxylate with atropine: One tablet orally three or four times daily as needed.

Codeine and **deodorized tincture of opium:** Because of potential habituation, these drugs are avoided except in cases of chronic, intractable diarrhea. Codeine may be given in a dosage of 15–60 mg orally every 4 hours; tincture of opium, 0.3–1.2 mL orally every 6 hours as needed.

Clonidine: Alpha-2-adrenergic agonists inhibit intestinal electrolyte secretion. Clonidine, 0.1–0.3 mg orally twice daily, or a clonidine patch, 0.1–0.2 mg/day, may help in some patients with secretory diarrheas, diabetic diarrhea, or cryptosporidiosis.

Octreotide: This somatostatin analog stimulates intestinal fluid and electrolyte absorption and inhibits intestinal fluid secretion and the release of gastrointestinal peptides. It is given for secretory diarrheas due to neuroendocrine tumors (VIPomas, carcinoid). Effective doses range from 50 mcg to 250 mcg subcutaneously three times daily.

Bile salt binders: Cholestyramine or colestipol (2–4 g once to three times daily) or colesevelam (625 mg, 1–3 tablets once or twice daily) may be useful in patients with bile salt-induced diarrhea, which may be idiopathic or secondary to intestinal resection or ileal disease.

Camilleri M et al. Pathophysiology, evaluation, and management of chronic watery diarrhea. Gastroenterology. 2017 Feb; 152(3):515–32. [PMID: 27773805]

DuPont HL. Persistent diarrhea: a clinical review. JAMA. 2016 Jun 28;315(24):2712–23. [PMID: 27357241]

Mohapatra S et al. Beyond O&P times three. Am J Gastroenterol. 2018 Jun;113(6):805–18. [PMID: 29867172]

Schiller LR et al. Chronic diarrhea: diagnosis and management. Clin Gastroenterol Hepatol. 2017 Feb;15(2):182–93. [PMID: 27496381]

GASTROINTESTINAL BLEEDING

1. Acute Upper Gastrointestinal Bleeding

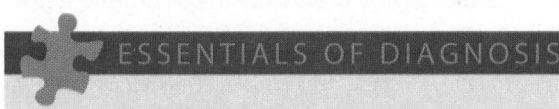

> ► Hematemesis (bright red blood or "coffee grounds").
> ► Melena in most cases; hematochezia in massive upper gastrointestinal bleeds.
> ► Volume status to determine severity of blood loss; hematocrit is a poor early indicator of blood loss.
> ► Endoscopy diagnostic and may be therapeutic.

► General Considerations

There are over 250,000 hospitalizations a year in the United States for acute upper gastrointestinal bleeding. In the United States, the mortality rate for nonvariceal upper gastrointestinal bleeding has declined steadily over the past 20 years to 2.1% in 2009. Mortality is higher in patients who are older than age 60 years and in patients in whom bleeding develops during hospitalization. Patients seldom die of exsanguination but rather of complications from an underlying disease.

The most common presentation of upper gastrointestinal bleeding is hematemesis or melena. Hematemesis may be either bright red blood or brown "coffee grounds" material. Melena develops after as little as 50–100 mL of blood loss in the upper gastrointestinal tract, whereas hematochezia requires a loss of more than 1000 mL. Although hematochezia generally suggests a lower bleeding source (eg, colonic), severe upper gastrointestinal bleeding may present with hematochezia in 10% of cases.

Upper gastrointestinal bleeding is self-limited in 80% of patients; urgent medical therapy and endoscopic evaluation are obligatory in the rest. Patients with bleeding more than 48 hours prior to presentation have a low risk of recurrent bleeding.

► Etiology

Acute upper gastrointestinal bleeding may originate from a number of sources. These are listed in order of their frequency and discussed in detail below.

A. Peptic Ulcer Disease

Peptic ulcers account for 40% of major upper gastrointestinal bleeding with an overall mortality rate of less than 5%. In North America, the incidence of bleeding from ulcers is declining due to eradication of *H pylori* and prophylaxis with proton pump inhibitors in high-risk patients.

B. Portal Hypertension

Portal hypertension accounts for 10–20% of upper gastrointestinal bleeding. Bleeding usually arises from esophageal varices and less commonly gastric or duodenal varices

or portal hypertensive gastropathy. Approximately 25% of patients with cirrhosis have medium to large esophageal varices, of whom 30% experience acute variceal bleeding within a 2-year period. Due to improved care, the hospital mortality rate has declined over the past 20 years from 40% to 15%. Nevertheless, a mortality rate of 60–80% is expected at 1–4 years due to recurrent bleeding or other complications of chronic liver disease.

C. Mallory-Weiss Tears

Lacerations of the gastroesophageal junction cause 5–10% of cases of upper gastrointestinal bleeding. Many patients report a history of heavy alcohol use or retching. Less than 10% have continued or recurrent bleeding.

D. Vascular Anomalies

Vascular anomalies are found throughout the gastrointestinal tract and may be the source of chronic or acute gastrointestinal bleeding. They account for 7% of cases of acute upper tract bleeding. The most common are **angioectasias** (angiodysplasias), which are 1–10 mm distorted, aberrant submucosal vessels caused by chronic, intermittent obstruction of submucosal veins. They have a bright red stellate appearance and occur throughout the gastrointestinal tract but most commonly in the right colon. **Telangiectasias** are small, cherry red lesions caused by dilation of venules that may be part of systemic conditions (hereditary hemorrhagic telangiectasia, CREST syndrome) or occur sporadically. The **Dieulafoy lesion** is an aberrant, large-caliber submucosal artery, most commonly in the proximal stomach that causes recurrent, intermittent bleeding.

E. Gastric Neoplasms

Gastric neoplasms result in 1% of upper gastrointestinal hemorrhages.

F. Erosive Gastritis

Because this process is superficial, it is a relatively unusual cause of severe gastrointestinal bleeding (less than 5% of cases) and more commonly results in chronic blood loss. Gastric mucosal erosions are due to NSAIDs, alcohol, or severe medical or surgical illness (stress-related mucosal disease).

G. Erosive Esophagitis

Severe erosive esophagitis due to chronic gastroesophageal reflux may rarely cause significant upper gastrointestinal bleeding, especially in patients who are bedbound long-term.

H. Others

An aortoenteric fistula complicates 2% of abdominal aortic grafts or, rarely, can occur as the initial presentation of a previously untreated aneurysm. Unusual causes of upper gastrointestinal bleeding include hemobilia (from hepatic tumor, angioma, penetrating trauma), pancreatic malignancy, and pseudoaneurysm (hemosuccus pancreaticus).

▶ Initial Evaluation & Treatment

A. Stabilization

The initial step is assessment of the hemodynamic status. A systolic blood pressure lower than 100 mm Hg identifies a high-risk patient with severe acute bleeding. A heart rate over 100 beats/min with a systolic blood pressure over 100 mm Hg signifies moderate acute blood loss. A normal systolic blood pressure and heart rate suggest relatively minor hemorrhage. Postural hypotension and tachycardia are useful when present but may be due to causes other than blood loss. Because the hematocrit may take 24–72 hours to equilibrate with the extravascular fluid, it is not a reliable indicator of the severity of acute bleeding.

In patients with significant bleeding, two 18-gauge or larger intravenous lines should be started prior to further diagnostic tests. Blood is sent for complete blood count, prothrombin time with INR, serum creatinine, liver enzymes, and blood typing and screening (in anticipation of the possible need for transfusion). In patients without hemodynamic compromise or overt active bleeding, aggressive fluid repletion can be delayed until the extent of the bleeding is further clarified. Patients with evidence of hemodynamic compromise are given 0.9% saline or lactated Ringer injection and cross-matched for 2–4 units of packed red blood cells. It is rarely necessary to administer type-specific or O-negative blood. Central venous pressure monitoring is desirable in some cases, but line placement should not interfere with rapid volume resuscitation.

Placement of a nasogastric tube is not routinely recommended in clinical guidelines but may be helpful in the initial assessment and triage of selected patients with suspected active upper tract bleeding. The aspiration of red blood or "coffee grounds" confirms an upper gastrointestinal source of bleeding, though up to 18% of patients with confirmed upper tract sources of bleeding have nonbloody aspirates—especially when bleeding originates in the duodenum. Erythromycin (250 mg) administered intravenously 30 minutes prior to upper endoscopy promotes gastric emptying and may improve the quality of endoscopic evaluation when substantial amounts of blood or clot in the stomach is suspected. Efforts to stop or slow bleeding by gastric lavage with large volumes of fluid are of no benefit and expose the patient to an increased risk of aspiration.

B. Blood Replacement

The amount of fluid and blood products required is based on assessment of vital signs, evidence of active bleeding from nasogastric aspirate, and laboratory tests. Sufficient packed red blood cells should be given to maintain a hemoglobin of no lower than 7–9 g/dL, based on the patient's hemodynamic status, comorbidities (especially cardiovascular disease), and presence of continued bleeding. In the absence of continued bleeding, the hemoglobin should rise approximately 1 g/dL for each unit of transfused packed red cells. Transfusion of blood should not be withheld from patients with massive active bleeding regardless of the hemoglobin value. In patients with severe gastrointestinal bleeding, it is desirable to transfuse blood before the hemoglobin reaches 7 g/dL to prevent decreases below that level occurring from hemodilution with fluid resuscitation. In actively bleeding patients, platelets are transfused if the platelet count is under 50,000/mcL and considered if there is impaired platelet function due to aspirin or clopidogrel use (regardless of the platelet count). Uremic patients (who also have dysfunctional platelets) with active bleeding are given three doses of desmopressin (DDAVP), 0.3 mcg/kg intravenously, at 12-hour intervals. Fresh frozen plasma is administered for actively bleeding patients with a coagulopathy and an INR greater than 1.8; however, endoscopy may be performed safely if the INR is less than 2.5. In the face of massive bleeding, administration of four factor prothrombin complex concentrates is preferred (rather than fresh frozen plasma) because it is more rapid and effective at correcting the INR and requires a smaller volume. Some patients with ongoing, serious gastrointestinal bleeding have taken the direct thrombin inhibitor, dabigatran, or factor Xa inhibitors. Although normal anticoagulation usually is restored within 24–48 hours in patients with normal kidney and liver function, reversal should be considered for ongoing severe or life-threatening bleeding. Idarucizumab (an intravenous monoclonal antibody) is approved for the reversal of dabigatran, and andexanet alfa (a modified factor Xa decoy protein) is approved for the reversal of apixaban and rivaroxaban.

C. Initial Triage

A preliminary assessment of risk based on several clinical factors aids in the resuscitation as well as the rational triage of the patient. Clinical predictors of increased risk of rebleeding and death include age over 60 years, comorbid illnesses, systolic blood pressure less than 100 mm Hg, pulse greater than 100 beats/min, and bright red blood in the nasogastric aspirate or on rectal examination.

1. High risk—Patients with active bleeding manifested by hematemesis or bright red blood on nasogastric aspirate, shock, persistent hemodynamic derangement despite fluid resuscitation, serious comorbid medical illness, or evidence of advanced liver disease require admission to an intensive care unit (ICU). After adequate resuscitation, endoscopy should be performed within 2–24 hours in most patients, but may be delayed in selected patients with serious comorbidities (eg, acute coronary syndrome) who do not have signs of continued bleeding.

2. Low to moderate risk—All other patients are admitted to a step-down unit or medical ward after appropriate stabilization for further evaluation and treatment. Patients without evidence of active bleeding undergo nonemergent endoscopy usually within 12–24 hours.

▶ Subsequent Evaluation & Treatment

Specific treatment of the various causes of upper gastrointestinal bleeding is discussed elsewhere in this chapter. The following general comments apply to most patients with bleeding.

The clinician's impression of the bleeding source is correct in only 40% of cases. Signs of chronic liver disease implicate bleeding due to portal hypertension, but a different lesion is identified in 25% of patients with cirrhosis. A history of dyspepsia, NSAID use, or peptic ulcer disease suggests peptic ulcer. Acute bleeding preceded by heavy alcohol ingestion or retching suggests a Mallory-Weiss tear, though most patients with Mallory-Weiss tears have neither.

A. Upper Endoscopy

Virtually all patients with upper tract bleeding should undergo upper endoscopy within 24 hours of arriving in the emergency department. The benefits of endoscopy in this setting are threefold.

1. To identify the source of bleeding—The appropriate acute and long-term medical therapy is determined by the cause of bleeding. Patients with portal hypertension will be treated differently from those with ulcer disease. If surgery or radiologic interventional therapy is required for uncontrolled bleeding, the source of bleeding identified at endoscopy will determine the approach.

2. To determine the risk of rebleeding and guide triage—Patients with a nonbleeding Mallory-Weiss tear, esophagitis, gastritis, and ulcers that have a clean, white base have a very low risk (less than 5%) of rebleeding. Patients with one of these findings who are younger than 60 years, without hemodynamic instability or transfusion requirement, without serious coexisting illness, and who have stable social support may be discharged from the emergency department or medical ward after endoscopy with outpatient follow-up. All others with one of these low-risk lesions should be observed on a medical ward for 24–48 hours. Patients with ulcers that are actively bleeding or have a visible vessel or adherent clot, or who have variceal bleeding usually require at least a 3-day hospitalization with closer initial observation in an ICU or step-down unit.

3. To render endoscopic therapy—Hemostasis can be achieved in actively bleeding lesions with endoscopic modalities such as cautery, injection, or endoclips. About 90% of bleeding or nonbleeding varices can be effectively treated immediately with injection of a sclerosant or application of rubber bands to the varices. Similarly, 90% of bleeding ulcers, angiomas, or Mallory-Weiss tears can be controlled with either injection of epinephrine, direct cauterization of the vessel by a heater probe or multipolar electrocautery probe, or application of an endoclip. Certain nonbleeding lesions such as ulcers with visible blood vessels, and angioectasias are also treated with these therapies. Specific endoscopic therapy of varices, peptic ulcers, and Mallory-Weiss tears is dealt with elsewhere in this chapter.

B. Acute Pharmacologic Therapies

1. Acid inhibitory therapy—Intravenous proton pump inhibitors (esomeprazole or pantoprazole, 80 mg bolus, followed by 8 mg/h continuous infusion for 72 hours) reduce the risk of rebleeding in patients with peptic ulcers with high-risk features (active bleeding, visible vessel, or adherent clot) after endoscopic treatment. **Oral proton pump inhibitors** (omeprazole, esomeprazole, or pantoprazole 40 mg; lansoprazole or dexlansoprazole 30–60 mg) once or twice daily are sufficient for lesions at low-risk for rebleeding (eg, esophagitis, gastritis, clean-based ulcers, and Mallory-Weiss tears).

Administration of continuous intravenous proton pump inhibitor *before* endoscopy results in a decreased number of ulcers with lesions that require endoscopic therapy. It therefore is standard clinical practice at many institutions to administer either an intravenous or a high-dose oral proton pump inhibitor prior to endoscopy in patients with significant upper gastrointestinal bleeding. Based on the findings during endoscopy, the intravenous proton pump inhibitor may be continued or discontinued.

2. Octreotide—Continuous intravenous infusion of octreotide (100 mcg bolus, followed by 50–100 mcg/h) reduces splanchnic blood flow and portal blood pressures and is effective in the initial control of bleeding related to portal hypertension. It is administered promptly to all patients with active upper gastrointestinal bleeding and evidence of liver disease or portal hypertension until the source of bleeding can be determined by endoscopy. In countries where it is available, terlipressin may be preferred to octreotide for the treatment of bleeding related to portal hypertension because of its sustained reduction of portal and variceal pressures and its proven reduction in mortality.

C. Other Treatment

1. Intra-arterial embolization—Angiographic treatment is used in patients with persistent bleeding from ulcers, angiomas, or Mallory-Weiss tears who have failed endoscopic therapy and are poor operative risks.

2. Transvenous intrahepatic portosystemic shunts (TIPS)—Placement of a wire stent from the hepatic vein through the liver to the portal vein provides effective decompression of the portal venous system and control of acute variceal bleeding. It is indicated in patients in whom endoscopic modalities have failed to control acute variceal bleeding.

Abougergi MS et al. Thirty-day readmission among patients with non-variceal upper gastrointestinal hemorrhage and effects on outcomes. Gastroenterology. 2018 Jul;155(1):38–46. [PMID: 29601829]

Kumar NL et al. Initial management and timing of endoscopy in nonvariceal upper GI bleeding. Gastrointest Endosc. 2016 Jul;84(1):10–17. [PMID: 26944336]

Laursen SB et al. Relationship between timing of endoscopy and mortality in patients with peptic ulcer bleeding: a nationwide cohort study. Gastrointest Endosc. 2017 May;85(5):936–44. [PMID: 27623102]

Nable JV et al. Gastrointestinal bleeding. Emerg Med Clin North Am. 2016 May;34(2):309–25. [PMID: 27133246]

Rogers KC et al. A new option for reversing the anticoagulant effect of Factor Xa inhibitors: andexanet alfa (ANDEXXA). Am J Med. 2019 Jan;132(1):38–41. [PMID: 30053385]

2. Acute Lower Gastrointestinal Bleeding

► Hematochezia usually present.

► Ten percent of cases of hematochezia due to upper gastrointestinal source.

► Evaluation with colonoscopy in stable patients.

► Massive active bleeding calls for evaluation with sigmoidoscopy, upper endoscopy, angiography, or nuclear bleeding scan.

General Considerations

Lower gastrointestinal bleeding is defined as that arising below the ligament of Treitz, ie, the small intestine or colon; however, up to 95% of cases arise from the colon. The severity of lower gastrointestinal bleeding ranges from mild anorectal bleeding to massive, large-volume hematochezia. Bright red blood that drips into the bowl after a bowel movement or is mixed with solid brown stool signifies mild bleeding, usually from an anorectosigmoid source, and can be evaluated in the outpatient setting. In patients hospitalized with gastrointestinal bleeding, lower tract bleeding is one-third as common as upper gastrointestinal hemorrhage and tends to have a more benign course. Patients hospitalized with lower gastrointestinal tract bleeding are less likely to present with shock or orthostasis (less than 20%) or to require transfusions (less than 40%). Spontaneous cessation of bleeding occurs in over 75% of cases, and hospital mortality is less than 4%.

Etiology

The cause of these lesions depends on both the age of the patient and the severity of the bleeding. In patients under 50 years of age, the most common causes are infectious colitis, anorectal disease, and inflammatory bowel disease. In older patients, significant hematochezia is most often seen with diverticulosis, angioectasias, malignancy, or ischemia. There is an increased risk of lower gastrointestinal bleeding in patients taking aspirin, nonaspirin antiplatelet agents, and NSAIDs.

A. Diverticulosis

Hemorrhage occurs in 3–5% of all patients with diverticulosis and is the most common cause of major lower tract bleeding, accounting for over 50% of cases. Diverticular bleeding usually presents as acute, painless, large-volume maroon or bright red hematochezia in patients over age 50 years. More than 95% of cases require less than 4 units of blood transfusion. Bleeding subsides spontaneously in 80% but may recur in up to 25% of patients.

B. Angioectasias

Angioectasias (angiodysplasias) occur throughout the upper and lower intestinal tracts and cause painless bleeding ranging from melena or hematochezia to occult blood loss. They are responsible for 5% of cases of lower gastrointestinal bleeding, where they are most often seen in the cecum and ascending colon. They are flat, red lesions (2–10 mm) with ectatic peripheral vessels radiating from a central vessel, and are most common in patients over age 70 years and in those with chronic renal failure. Bleeding in younger patients more commonly arises from the small intestine.

Ectasias can be identified in up to 6% of persons over age 60 years, so the mere presence of ectasias does not prove that the lesion is the source of bleeding, since active bleeding is seldom seen.

C. Neoplasms

Benign polyps and malignant carcinomas are associated with chronic occult blood loss or intermittent anorectal hematochezia. Furthermore, they may cause up to 7% of acute lower gastrointestinal hemorrhage.

After endoscopic removal of colonic polyps, important bleeding may occur up to 2 weeks later in 0.3% of patients. In general, prompt colonoscopy is recommended to treat postpolypectomy hemorrhage and minimize the need for transfusions.

D. Inflammatory Bowel Disease

Patients with inflammatory bowel disease (especially ulcerative colitis) often have diarrhea with variable amounts of hematochezia. Bleeding varies from occult blood loss to recurrent hematochezia mixed with stool. Symptoms of abdominal pain, tenesmus, and urgency are often present.

E. Anorectal Disease

Anorectal disease (hemorrhoids, fissures) usually results in small amounts of bright red blood noted on the toilet paper, streaking of the stool, or dripping into the toilet bowl; clinically significant blood loss can sometimes occur. Hemorrhoids are the source in 10% of patients admitted with lower bleeding. Rectal ulcers may account for up to 8% of lower bleeding, usually in elderly or debilitated patients with constipation.

F. Ischemic Colitis

This condition is seen commonly in older patients, most of whom have atherosclerotic disease. Most cases occur spontaneously due to transient episodes of nonocclusive ischemia. Ischemic colitis may also occur in 5% of patients after surgery for ileoaortic or abdominal aortic aneurysm. In younger patients, colonic ischemia may develop due to vasculitis, coagulation disorders, estrogen therapy, and long-distance running. Ischemic colitis results in hematochezia or bloody diarrhea associated with mild cramps. In most patients, the bleeding is mild and self-limited.

G. Others

Radiation-induced proctitis causes anorectal bleeding that may develop months to years after pelvic radiation. Endoscopy reveals multiple rectal telangiectasias. Acute infectious colitis (see Acute Diarrhea, above) commonly causes bloody diarrhea. Rare causes of lower tract bleeding include vasculitic ischemia, solitary rectal ulcer, NSAID-induced ulcers in the small bowel or right colon, small bowel diverticula, and colonic varices.

Clinical Findings

A. Symptoms and Signs

The color of the stool helps distinguish upper from lower gastrointestinal bleeding, especially when observed by the clinician. Brown stools mixed or streaked with blood predict a source in the rectosigmoid or anus. Large volumes of bright red blood suggest a colonic source; maroon stools imply a lesion in the right colon or small intestine; and black stools (melena) predict a source proximal to the ligament of Treitz. Although 10% of patients admitted with self-reported hematochezia have an upper gastrointestinal source of bleeding (eg, peptic ulcer), this almost always occurs in the setting of massive hemorrhage with hemodynamic instability. Painless large-volume bleeding usually suggests diverticular bleeding. Bloody diarrhea associated with cramping abdominal pain, urgency, or tenesmus is characteristic of inflammatory bowel disease, infectious colitis, or ischemic colitis.

B. Diagnostic Tests

Important considerations in management include exclusion of an upper tract source, anoscopy and sigmoidoscopy, colonoscopy, nuclear bleeding scans and angiography, and small intestine push enteroscopy or capsule imaging.

1. Exclusion of an upper tract source—A nasogastric tube with aspiration should be considered, especially in patients with hemodynamic compromise. Aspiration of red blood or dark brown ("coffee grounds") guaiac-positive material strongly implicates an upper gastrointestinal source of bleeding. Upper endoscopy should be performed in most patients presenting with hematochezia and hemodynamic instability to exclude an upper gastrointestinal source before proceeding with evaluation of the lower gastrointestinal tract.

2. Anoscopy and sigmoidoscopy—In otherwise healthy patients without anemia under age 45 years with small-volume bleeding, anoscopy and sigmoidoscopy are performed to look for evidence of anorectal disease, inflammatory bowel disease, or infectious colitis. If a lesion is found, no further evaluation is needed immediately unless the bleeding persists or is recurrent. In patients over age 45 years with small-volume hematochezia, the entire colon must be evaluated with colonoscopy to exclude tumor.

3. Colonoscopy—In patients with acute, large-volume bleeding requiring hospitalization, colonoscopy is the preferred initial study in most cases. The bowel first is purged rapidly by administration of a high-volume colonic lavage solution, given until the effluent is clear of blood and clots (4–8 L of GoLYTELY, CoLYTE, NuLYTE given orally or 1 L every 30 minutes over 2–5 hours by nasogastric tube). For patients with stable vital signs and whose lower

gastrointestinal bleeding appears to have stopped (more than 75% of patients), colonoscopy can be performed electively within 24 hours of admission after appropriate resuscitation and bowel cleansing. For patients who are resuscitated and hemodynamically stable but have signs of continued active bleeding during bowel preparation (less than 25% of patients), early colonoscopy (within 12–24 hours) should be performed. Preferably, this colonoscopy should be done within 1–2 hours of completing the bowel purgative when the bowel discharge is without clots. The probable site of bleeding can be identified in 70–85% of patients, and a high-risk lesion can be identified and treated in up to 25%. Early colonoscopy is associated with shorter hospitalizations.

4. Nuclear bleeding scans and angiography—In patients with massive lower gastrointestinal bleeding manifested by continued hemodynamic instability and hematochezia despite resuscitative efforts and in patients in whom colonoscopic hemostasis was unsuccessful, urgent radiographic imaging is warranted. Technetium-labeled red blood cell scanning can detect significant active bleeding and, in some cases, can localize the source to the small intestine, right colon, or left colon. Because most bleeding is slow or intermittent, less than half of nuclear studies are diagnostic and the accuracy of localization is poor. Increasingly, multidetector CT angiography is used instead of scintigraphy in an attempt to localize active bleeding. If scintigraphy or CT angiography demonstrates active bleeding, urgent angiography is performed in an attempt to localize the bleeding site and make embolization therapy possible. In patients with massive lower gastrointestinal bleeding and continued hemodynamic instability, urgent angiography may be performed without first attempting scintigraphy or CT angiography.

5. Small intestine push enteroscopy or capsule imaging—Up to 5% of acute episodes of lower gastrointestinal bleeding arise from the small intestine, eluding diagnostic evaluation with upper endoscopy and colonoscopy. Because of the difficulty of examining the small intestine and its relative rarity as a source of acute bleeding, evaluation of the small bowel is not usually pursued in patients during the initial episode of acute lower gastrointestinal bleeding. However, the small intestine is investigated in patients with unexplained recurrent hemorrhage of obscure origin.

Treatment

Initial stabilization, blood replacement, and triage are managed in the same manner as described above in Acute Upper Gastrointestinal Bleeding. In patients with ongoing bleeding, consideration should be given to discontinuation of antiplatelet agents and anticoagulants. Compared to persons who do not take long-term low-dose aspirin, the incidence of recurrent lower gastrointestinal bleeding within 5 years was higher in those who resumed low-dose aspirin postdischarge (18.9% vs 6.9%); however, these patients had a lower risk of serious cardiovascular events (22.8% vs 36.5%) and death (8.2% vs 26.7%).

A. Therapeutic Colonoscopy

High-risk lesions (eg, angioectasia or diverticulum, rectal ulcer with active bleeding, or a visible vessel) may be treated endoscopically with epinephrine injection, cautery (bipolar or heater probe), application of metallic endoclips or bands, or application of a hemostatic powder (TC-325). In diverticular hemorrhage with high-risk lesions identified at colonoscopy, rebleeding occurs in half of untreated patients compared with virtually no rebleeding in patients treated endoscopically. Radiation proctitis is effectively treated with applications of cautery therapy to the rectal telangiectasias, preferably with an argon plasma coagulator.

B. Intra-arterial Embolization

When a bleeding lesion is identified, angiography with selective embolization achieves immediate hemostasis in more than 95% of patients. Major complications occur in 5% (mainly ischemic colitis) and rebleeding occurs in up to 25%.

C. Surgical Treatment

Emergency surgery is required in less than 5% of patients with acute lower gastrointestinal bleeding due to the efficacy of colonoscopic and angiographic therapies. It is indicated in patients with ongoing bleeding that requires more than 6 units of blood within 24 hours or more than 10 total units in whom attempts at endoscopic or angiographic therapy failed. Most such hemorrhages are caused by a bleeding diverticulum or angioectasia.

Surgery may also be indicated in patients with two or more hospitalizations for diverticular hemorrhage depending on the severity of bleeding and the patient's other comorbid conditions.

Almadi MA et al. Patient presentation, risk stratification, and initial management in acute lower gastrointestinal bleeding. Gastrointest Endosc Clin N Am. 2018 Jul;28(3):363–77. [PMID: 29933781]

Becq A et al. Hemorrhagic angiodysplasia of the digestive tract: pathogenesis, diagnosis, and management. Gastrointest Endosc. 2017 Nov 86(5):792–806. [PMID: 28554655]

Gralnek IM et al. Acute lower gastrointestinal bleeding. N Engl J Med. 2017 Mar 16;376(11):1054–63. [PMID: 28296600]

Hookey L et al. Successful hemostasis of active lower GI bleeding using a hemostatic power as monotherapy, combination therapy, or rescue therapy. Gastrointest Endosc. 2019 Apr;89(4): 865–71. [PMID: 30612959]

Nagata N et al. Safety and effectiveness of early colonoscopy in management of acute lower gastrointestinal bleeding on the basis of propensity score matching analysis. Clin Gastroenterol Hepatol. 2016 Apr;14(4):558–64. [PMID: 26492844]

Soetikno R et al. The role of endoscopic hemostasis therapy in acute lower gastrointestinal hemorrhage. Gastrointest Endosc Clin N Am. 2018 Jul;28(3):391–408. [PMID: 29933783]

3. Small Bowel Bleeding

Bleeding from the small intestine can be overt or occult. *Overt* small bowel bleeding manifests as melena, maroon stools, or bright red blood per rectum. Up to 5–10% of patients admitted to hospitals with clinically overt gastrointestinal bleeding do not have a cause identified on upper endoscopy or colonoscopy and are presumed to have a small bowel source. In up to one-third of cases, however, a source of bleeding has been overlooked in the upper or lower tract on prior endoscopic studies. *Occult* small bowel bleeding refers to bleeding that is manifested by recurrent positive FOBTs or FITs or recurrent iron deficiency anemia, or both in the absence of visible blood loss. Occult small bowel bleeding is discussed in the next section.

The likely etiology of overt small bowel bleeding depends on the age of the patient. The most common causes of small intestinal bleeding in patients younger than 40 years are neoplasms (stromal tumors, lymphomas, adenocarcinomas, carcinoids), Crohn disease, celiac disease, and Meckel diverticulum. These disorders also occur in patients over age 40; however, angioectasias and NSAID-induced ulcers are far more common.

▶ Evaluation of Small Bowel Bleeding

The evaluation of overt small bowel bleeding depends on the age and overall health status of the patient, associated symptoms, and severity of the bleeding. Before pursuing evaluation of the small intestine, upper endoscopy and colonoscopy should be repeated to ascertain that a lesion in these regions has not been overlooked. Repeat upper endoscopy should be performed with a longer instrument (usually a colonoscope) to evaluate the distal duodenum. If these studies are unrevealing and the patient is hemodynamically stable, capsule endoscopy should be performed to evaluate the small intestine. Further management depends on the capsule endoscopic findings (most commonly, angioectasias (25%), ulcers (10–25%), and neoplasms (1–10%). Abdominal CT may be considered to exclude a hepatic or pancreatic source of bleeding. CT enterography may be considered if capsule endoscopy is unrevealing, since it is more sensitive for the detection of small bowel neoplasms. Laparotomy is warranted if a small bowel tumor is identified by capsule endoscopy or radiographic studies. Most other lesions identified by capsule imaging can be further evaluated with enteroscopes that use overtubes with balloons to advance the scope through most of the small intestine in a forward and retrograde direction (balloon-assisted enteroscopy). Neoplasms can be biopsied or resected, and angioectasias may be cauterized.

For massive or hemodynamically significant acute bleeding, urgent angiography is recommended (instead of capsule endoscopy) for localization and possible embolization of a bleeding vascular abnormality. For hemodynamically stable overt bleeding, CT angiography may be useful to localize bleeding and guide other interventions (enteroscopy or angiography with embolization). A nuclear scan for Meckel diverticulum should be obtained in patients under age 30. With the advent of capsule imaging and advanced endoscopic technologies for evaluating and treating bleeding lesions in the small intestine, intraoperative enteroscopy of the small bowel is seldom required.

4. Occult Gastrointestinal Bleeding

Occult gastrointestinal bleeding refers to bleeding that is not apparent to the patient. Chronic gastrointestinal blood loss of less than 100 mL/day may cause no appreciable change in stool appearance. Thus, occult bleeding in an adult is identified by a positive FOBT, FIT, or by iron deficiency anemia in the absence of visible blood loss. FOBT or

FIT may be performed in patients with gastrointestinal symptoms or as a screening test for colorectal neoplasia (see Chapter 39). From 2% to 6% of patients in screening programs have a positive FOBT or FIT.

In the United States, 2% of men and 5% of women have iron deficiency anemia (serum ferritin less than 30–45 mcg/L). In premenopausal women, iron deficiency anemia is most commonly attributable to menstrual and pregnancy-associated iron loss; however, a gastrointestinal source of chronic blood loss is present in 10%. Occult blood loss may arise from anywhere in the gastrointestinal tract. Among men and postmenopausal women, a potential gastrointestinal cause of blood loss can be identified in the colon in 15–30% and in the upper gastrointestinal tract in 35–55%; a malignancy is present in 10%. Iron deficiency on rare occasions is caused by malabsorption (especially celiac disease) or malnutrition. The most common causes of occult bleeding with iron deficiency are (1) neoplasms; (2) vascular abnormalities (angioectasias); (3) acid-peptic lesions (esophagitis, peptic ulcer disease, erosions in hiatal hernia); (4) infections (nematodes, especially hookworm; tuberculosis); (5) medications (especially NSAIDs or aspirin); and (6) other causes such as inflammatory bowel disease.

▶ Evaluation of Occult Bleeding

Asymptomatic adults with positive FOBTs or FITs that are performed for routine colorectal cancer screening should undergo colonoscopy (see Chapter 39). All symptomatic adults with positive FOBTs or FITs or iron deficiency anemia should undergo evaluation of the lower and upper gastrointestinal tract with colonoscopy and upper endoscopy, unless the anemia can be definitively ascribed to a nongastrointestinal source (eg, menstruation, blood donation, or recent surgery). Patients with iron deficiency anemia should be evaluated for possible celiac disease with either IgA anti-tissue transglutaminase or duodenal biopsy. After evaluation of the upper and lower gastrointestinal tract with upper endoscopy and colonoscopy, the origin of occult bleeding remains unexplained in 30–50% of patients. In many of these patients, a source for occult bleeding from a small intestine source is suspected.

In patients younger than 60 years with unexplained occult bleeding or iron deficiency after upper endoscopy and colonoscopy, it is recommended to pursue further evaluation of the small intestine for a source of obscure-occult bleeding in order to exclude a small intestinal neoplasm or inflammatory bowel disease. Patients over age 60 with obscure-occult bleeding who have a normal initial endoscopic evaluation and no other worrisome symptoms or signs (eg, abdominal pain, weight loss) most commonly have blood loss from small intestine angioectasias, which may be clinically unimportant. Therefore, it is reasonable to give an empiric trial of iron supplementation and observe the patient for evidence of clinically significant bleeding. For anemia that responds poorly to iron supplementation or recurrent or persistent chronic occult gastrointestinal blood loss, further evaluation is pursued for a source of obscure-occult bleeding with capsule endoscopy. If a small intestine source is identified, push enteroscopy, balloon-assisted enteroscopy, abdominal CT, angiography, or laparotomy is pursued, as indicated. When possible, antiplatelet agents (aspirin, NSAIDs, clopidogrel) should be discontinued. Patients with occult bleeding without a bleeding source identified after upper endoscopy, colonoscopy, and capsule endoscopy have a low risk of recurrent bleeding and usually can be managed with close observation.

ASGE Standards of Practice Committee; Gurudu SR et al. The role of endoscopy in the management of suspected small-bowel bleeding. Gastrointest Endosc. 2017 Jan;85(1):22–31. [PMID: 27374798]

Gerson LB et al. ACG clinical guideline: diagnosis and management of small bowel bleeding. Am J Gastroenterol. 2015 Sep;110(9):1265–87. [PMID: 26303132]

Holleran G et al. An overview of angiodysplasia: management and patient prospects. Expert Rev Gastroenterol Hepatol. 2018 Sep;12(9):863–72. [PMID: 30028221]

⏷ **DISEASES OF THE PERITONEUM**

ASSESSMENT OF THE PATIENT WITH ASCITES

▶ Etiology of Ascites

The term "ascites" denotes the pathologic accumulation of fluid in the peritoneal cavity. Healthy men have little or no intraperitoneal fluid, but women normally may have up to 20 mL depending on the phase of the menstrual cycle. The causes of ascites may be classified into two broad pathophysiologic categories: that which is associated with a normal peritoneum and that which occurs due to a diseased peritoneum (Table 15–7). The most common cause of ascites is portal hypertension secondary to chronic liver disease, which accounts for over 80% of patients with ascites. The management of portal hypertensive ascites is discussed in Chapter 16. The most common causes of nonportal hypertensive ascites include infections (tuberculous peritonitis), intra-abdominal malignancy, inflammatory disorders of the peritoneum, and ductal disruptions (chylous, pancreatic, biliary).

▶ Clinical Findings

A. Symptoms and Signs

The history usually is one of increasing abdominal girth, with the presence of abdominal pain depending on the cause. Because most ascites is secondary to chronic liver disease with portal hypertension, patients should be asked about risk factors for liver disease, especially alcohol consumption, transfusions, tattoos, injection drug use, a history of viral hepatitis or jaundice, and birth in an area endemic for hepatitis. A history of cancer or marked weight loss arouses suspicion of malignant ascites. Fevers may suggest infected peritoneal fluid, including bacterial peritonitis (spontaneous or secondary). Patients with chronic liver disease and ascites are at greatest risk for developing spontaneous bacterial peritonitis. In immigrants, immunocompromised hosts, or severely malnourished alcoholics, tuberculous peritonitis should be considered.

Physical examination should emphasize signs of portal hypertension and chronic liver disease. Elevated jugular

Table 15–7. Causes of ascites.

Normal Peritoneum

Portal hypertension (SAAG ≥ 1.1 g/dL)
1. Hepatic congestion[1]
   Heart failure
   Constrictive pericarditis
   Tricuspid insufficiency
   Budd-Chiari syndrome
   Veno-occlusive disease
2. Liver disease[2]
   Cirrhosis
   Alcoholic hepatitis
   Fulminant hepatic failure
   Massive hepatic metastases
   Hepatic fibrosis
   Acute fatty liver of pregnancy
3. Portal vein occlusion

Hypoalbuminemia (SAAG < 1.1 g/dL)
   Nephrotic syndrome
   Protein-losing enteropathy
   Severe malnutrition with anasarca

Miscellaneous conditions (SAAG < 1.1 g/dL)
   Chylous ascites
   Pancreatic ascites
   Bile ascites
   Nephrogenic ascites
   Urine ascites
   Myxedema (SAAG ≥ 1.1 g/dL)
   Ovarian disease

Diseased Peritoneum (SAAG < 1.1 g/dL)[2]

Infections
   Bacterial peritonitis
   Tuberculous peritonitis
   Fungal peritonitis
   HIV-associated peritonitis

Malignant conditions
   Peritoneal carcinomatosis
   Primary mesothelioma
   Pseudomyxoma peritonei
   Massive hepatic metastases
   Hepatocellular carcinoma

Other conditions
   Familial Mediterranean fever
   Vasculitis
   Granulomatous peritonitis
   Eosinophilic peritonitis

[1]Hepatic congestion is usually associated with SAAG ≥ 1.1 g/dL and ascitic fluid total protein > 2.5 g/dL.
[2]There may be cases of "mixed ascites" in which portal hypertensive ascites is complicated by a secondary process such as infection. In these cases, the SAAG is ≥ 1.1 g/dL.
SAAG, serum-ascites albumin gradient = serum albumin minus ascitic fluid albumin.

venous pressure may suggest right-sided heart failure or constrictive pericarditis. A large tender liver is characteristic of acute alcoholic hepatitis or Budd-Chiari syndrome (thrombosis of the hepatic veins). The presence of large abdominal wall veins with cephalad flow also suggests

portal hypertension; inferiorly directed flow implies hepatic vein obstruction. Signs of chronic liver disease include palmar erythema, cutaneous spider angiomas, gynecomastia, and muscle wasting. Asterixis secondary to hepatic encephalopathy may be present. Anasarca results from cardiac failure or nephrotic syndrome with hypoalbuminemia. Finally, firm lymph nodes in the left supraclavicular region or umbilicus may suggest intra-abdominal malignancy.

The physical examination is relatively insensitive for detecting ascitic fluid. In general, patients must have at least 1500 mL of fluid to be detected reliably by this method. Even the experienced clinician may find it difficult to distinguish between obesity and small-volume ascites. Abdominal ultrasound establishes the presence of fluid.

B. Laboratory Testing

1. Abdominal paracentesis—Abdominal paracentesis is performed as part of the diagnostic evaluation in all patients with new onset of ascites to help determine the cause. It also is recommended for patients admitted to the hospital with cirrhosis and ascites (in whom the prevalence of bacterial peritonitis is 10–20%) and when patients with known ascites deteriorate clinically (development of fever, abdominal pain, rapid worsening of kidney function, or worsened hepatic encephalopathy) to exclude bacterial peritonitis.

A. INSPECTION—Cloudy fluid suggests infection. Milky fluid is seen with chylous ascites due to high triglyceride levels. Bloody fluid is most commonly attributable to a traumatic paracentesis, but up to 20% of cases of malignant ascites are bloody.

B. ROUTINE STUDIES—

(1) Cell count—A white blood cell count with differential is the most important test. Normal ascitic fluid contains less than 500 leukocytes/mcL and less than 250 polymorphonuclear neutrophils (PMNs)/mcL. Any inflammatory condition can cause an elevated ascitic white blood cell count. A PMN count of greater than 250/mcL (neutrocytic ascites) with a PMN percentage of more than 75% of all white cells is highly suggestive of bacterial peritonitis, either spontaneous primary peritonitis or secondary peritonitis (ie, caused by an intra-abdominal source of infection, such as a perforated viscus or appendicitis). An elevated white count with a predominance of lymphocytes arouses suspicion of tuberculosis or peritoneal carcinomatosis.

(2) Albumin and total protein—The serum-ascites albumin gradient (SAAG) is the best single test for the classification of ascites into portal hypertensive and nonportal hypertensive causes (Table 15–7). Calculated by subtracting the ascitic fluid albumin from the serum albumin, the gradient correlates directly with the portal pressure. An SAAG of 1.1 g/dL or more suggests underlying portal hypertension, while gradients less than 1.1 g/dL implicate nonportal hypertensive causes.

The accuracy of the SAAG exceeds 95% in classifying ascites. It should be recognized, however, that approximately 4% of patients have "mixed ascites," ie, underlying cirrhosis with portal hypertension complicated by a second cause for ascites formation (such as malignancy or tuberculosis).

Thus, a high SAAG is indicative of portal hypertension but does not exclude concomitant malignancy.

The ascitic fluid total protein provides some additional clues to the cause. An elevated SAAG and a high protein level (greater than 2.5 g/dL) are seen in most cases of hepatic congestion secondary to cardiac disease or Budd-Chiari syndrome. However, an increased ascitic fluid protein is also found in up to 20% of cases of uncomplicated cirrhosis. Two-thirds of patients with malignant ascites have a total protein level more than 2.5 g/dL.

(3) Culture and Gram stain—The best technique consists of the inoculation of aerobic and anaerobic blood culture bottles with 5–10 mL of ascitic fluid at the patient's bedside, which increases the sensitivity for detecting bacterial peritonitis to over 85% in patients with neutrocytic ascites (greater than 250 PMNs/mcL), compared with approximately 50% sensitivity by conventional agar plate or broth cultures.

C. **OPTIONAL STUDIES**—Other laboratory tests are of utility in some specific clinical situations. Glucose and lactate dehydrogenase (LD) may be helpful in distinguishing spontaneous from secondary bacterial peritonitis. An elevated amylase may suggest pancreatic ascites or a perforation of the gastrointestinal tract with leakage of pancreatic secretions into the ascitic fluid. Perforation of the biliary tree is suspected with an ascitic bilirubin concentration that is greater than the serum bilirubin. An elevated ascitic creatinine suggests leakage of urine from the bladder or ureters. Ascitic fluid cytologic examination is ordered if peritoneal carcinomatosis is suspected. Adenosine deaminase may be useful for the diagnosis of tuberculous peritonitis.

C. Imaging

Abdominal ultrasound is useful in confirming the presence of ascites and in the guidance of paracentesis. Both ultrasound and CT imaging are useful in distinguishing between causes of portal and nonportal hypertensive ascites. Doppler ultrasound and CT can detect Budd-Chiari syndrome. In patients with nonportal hypertensive ascites, these studies are useful in detecting lymphadenopathy and masses of the mesentery and of solid organs such as the liver, ovaries, and pancreas. Furthermore, they permit directed percutaneous needle biopsies of these lesions. Ultrasound and CT are poor procedures for the detection of peritoneal carcinomatosis; the role of positron emission tomography (PET) imaging is unclear.

D. Laparoscopy

Laparoscopy is an important test in the evaluation of some patients with nonportal hypertensive ascites (low SAAG) or mixed ascites. It permits direct visualization and biopsy of the peritoneum, liver, and some intra-abdominal lymph nodes. Cases of suspected peritoneal tuberculosis or suspected malignancy with nondiagnostic CT imaging and ascitic fluid cytology are best evaluated by this method.

Gaetano JN et al. The benefit of paracentesis on hospitalized adults with cirrhosis and ascites. J Gastroenterol Hepatol. 2016 May;31(5):1025–30. [PMID: 26642977]

Pericleous M et al. The clinical management of abdominal ascites, spontaneous bacterial peritonitis and hepatorenal syndrome: a review of current guidelines and recommendations. Eur J Gastroenterol Hepatol. 2016 Mar;28(3):e10–8. [PMID: 26671516]
Solà E et al. Management of uninfected and infected ascites in cirrhosis. Liver Int. 2016 Jan;36(Suppl 1):109–15. [PMID: 26725907]

SPONTANEOUS BACTERIAL PERITONITIS

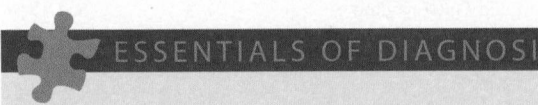
ESSENTIALS OF DIAGNOSIS

▶ A history of chronic liver disease and ascites.
▶ Fever and abdominal pain.
▶ Peritoneal signs uncommonly encountered on examination.
▶ Ascitic fluid neutrophil count greater than 250 white blood cells/mcL.

▶ General Considerations

"Spontaneous" bacterial infection of ascitic fluid occurs in the absence of an apparent intra-abdominal source of infection. It is seen with few exceptions in patients with ascites caused by chronic liver disease. Translocation of enteric bacteria across the gut wall or mesenteric lymphatics leads to seeding of the ascitic fluid, as may bacteremia from other sites. Approximately 20–30% of cirrhotic patients with ascites develop spontaneous peritonitis; however, the incidence is greater than 40% in patients with ascitic fluid total protein less than 1 g/dL, probably due to decreased ascitic fluid opsonic activity.

Virtually all cases of spontaneous bacterial peritonitis are caused by a monomicrobial infection. The most common pathogens are enteric gram-negative bacteria (*E coli, Klebsiella pneumoniae*) or gram-positive bacteria (*Streptococcus pneumoniae*, viridans streptococci, *Enterococcus* species). Anaerobic bacteria are not associated with spontaneous bacterial peritonitis.

▶ Clinical Findings

A. Symptoms and Signs

Eighty to 90 percent of patients with spontaneous bacterial peritonitis are symptomatic; in many cases the presentation is subtle. Spontaneous bacterial peritonitis may be present in 10–20% of patients hospitalized with chronic liver disease, sometimes in the absence of any suggestive symptoms or signs.

The most common symptoms are fever and abdominal pain, present in two-thirds of patients. Spontaneous bacterial peritonitis may also present with a change in mental status due to exacerbation or precipitation of hepatic encephalopathy, or sudden worsening of kidney function. Physical examination typically demonstrates signs of chronic liver disease with ascites. Abdominal tenderness is present in less than 50% of patients, and its presence suggests other processes.

B. Laboratory Findings

The most important diagnostic test is abdominal paracentesis. Ascitic fluid should be sent for cell count with differential, and blood culture bottles should be inoculated at the bedside; Gram stain and reagent strips are insensitive.

In the proper clinical setting, an ascitic fluid PMN count of greater than 250 cells/mcL (neutrocytic ascites) is presumptive evidence of bacterial peritonitis. The percentage of PMNs is greater than 50–70% of the ascitic fluid white blood cells and commonly approximates 100%. Patients with neutrocytic ascites are presumed to be infected and should be started—regardless of symptoms—on antibiotics. Although 10–30% of patients with neutrocytic ascites have negative ascitic bacterial cultures ("culture-negative neutrocytic ascites"), it is presumed that these patients have bacterial peritonitis and should be treated empirically. Occasionally, a positive blood culture identifies the organism when ascitic fluid is sterile.

Differential Diagnosis

Spontaneous bacterial peritonitis must be distinguished from secondary bacterial peritonitis, in which ascitic fluid has become secondarily infected by an intraabdominal infection. Even in the presence of perforation, clinical symptoms and signs of peritonitis may be lacking owing to the separation of the visceral and parietal peritoneum by the ascitic fluid. Causes of secondary bacterial peritonitis include appendicitis, diverticulitis, perforated peptic ulcer, and perforated gallbladder. Secondary bacterial infection accounts for 3% of cases of infected ascitic fluid.

Ascitic fluid total protein, LD, and glucose are useful in distinguishing spontaneous bacterial peritonitis from secondary infection. Up to two-thirds of patients with secondary bacterial peritonitis have at least two of the following: decreased glucose level (less than 50 mg/dL), an elevated LD level (greater than serum), and total protein greater than 1 g/dL. Ascitic neutrophil counts greater than 10,000/mcL also are suspicious; however, most patients with secondary peritonitis have neutrophil counts within the range of spontaneous peritonitis. The presence of multiple organisms on ascitic fluid Gram stain or culture is diagnostic of secondary peritonitis.

If secondary bacterial peritonitis is suspected, abdominal CT imaging of the upper and lower gastrointestinal tracts should be obtained to look for evidence of an intraabdominal source of infection. If these studies are negative and secondary peritonitis still is suspected, repeat paracentesis should be performed after 48 hours of antibiotic therapy to confirm that the PMN count is decreasing. Secondary bacterial peritonitis should be suspected in patients in whom the PMN count is not below the pretreatment value at 48 hours.

Neutrocytic ascites may also be seen in some patients with peritoneal carcinomatosis, pancreatic ascites, or tuberculous ascites. In these circumstances, however, PMNs account for less than 50% of the ascitic white blood cells.

Prevention

Up to 70% of patients who survive an episode of spontaneous bacterial peritonitis will have another episode within 1 year. Oral once-daily prophylactic therapy—with norfloxacin, 400 mg, ciprofloxacin, 250–500 mg, or trimethoprim-sulfamethoxazole, one double-strength tablet—has been shown to reduce the rate of recurrent infections to less than 20% and is recommended. Prophylaxis should be considered also in patients who have not had prior bacterial peritonitis but are at increased risk of infection due to low-protein ascites (total ascitic protein less than 1 g/dL). Although improvement in survival in cirrhotic patients with ascites treated with prophylactic antibiotics has not been shown, decision analytic modeling suggests that in patients with prior bacterial peritonitis or low ascitic fluid protein, the use of prophylactic antibiotics is a cost-effective strategy.

Treatment

Empiric therapy for spontaneous bacterial peritonitis should be initiated with a third-generation cephalosporin (such as cefotaxime, 2 g intravenously every 8–12 hours, or ceftriaxone, 1–2 g intravenously every 24 hours) or a combination beta-lactam/beta-lactamase agent (such as ampicillin/sulbactam, 2 g/1 g intravenously every 6 hours). Because of a high risk of nephrotoxicity in patients with chronic liver disease, aminoglycosides should not be used. Although the optimal duration of therapy is unknown, an empiric course of 5–10 days is recommended, or treatment until the ascites fluid PMN count decreases to less than 250 cells/mcL. For most infections, 5 days is sufficient; however, infections caused by more serious, virulent pathogens (S aureus, viridans streptococci, Pseudomonas, or Enterobacteriaceae) warrant 10 days of treatment. Patients without significant clinical improvement after 5 days should undergo repeat paracentesis to assess treatment efficacy. If the ascitic neutrophil count has not decreased by 25%, antibiotic coverage should be adjusted (guided by culture and sensitivity results, if available) and secondary causes of peritonitis excluded. If the ascitic PMN count has decreased but remains more than 250 cells/mcL, antibiotics should be continued for an additional 2–3 days before paracentesis is repeated. Patients with suspected secondary bacterial peritonitis should be given broad-spectrum coverage for enteric aerobic and anaerobic flora with a third-generation cephalosporin and metronidazole, pending identification and definitive (usually surgical) treatment of the cause.

Kidney injury develops in up to 40% of patients and is a major cause of death. Intravenous albumin increases effective arterial circulating volume and renal perfusion, decreasing both kidney injury and mortality. Intravenous albumin, 1.5 g/kg on day 1 and 1 g/kg on day 3, should be administered to patients at high risk for hepatorenal failure (ie, patients with baseline creatinine greater than 1 mg/dL, blood urea nitrogen [BUN] greater than 30 mg/dL, or bilirubin greater than 4 mg/dL). Nonselective beta-blockers increase the risk of hepatorenal syndrome in patients with bacterial peritonitis. They should be discontinued permanently due to their adverse impact on cardiac output and renal perfusion in advanced cirrhosis, both of which are associated with decreased long-term survival.

► Prognosis

The mortality rate of spontaneous bacterial peritonitis exceeds 30%. However, if the disease is recognized and treated early, the mortality rate is less than 10%. Since the majority of patients have underlying severe liver disease, many may die of liver failure, hepatorenal syndrome, or bleeding complications of portal hypertension. The most effective treatment for recurrent spontaneous bacterial peritonitis is liver transplantation.

Fiore M et al. Are third-generation cephalosporins still the empirical antibiotic treatment of community-acquired spontaneous bacterial peritonitis? A systematic review and meta-analysis. Eur J Gastroenterol Hepatol. 2018 Mar;30(3):329–36. [PMID: 29303883]

Fiore M et al. Current concepts and future strategies in the antimicrobial therapy of emerging Gram-positive spontaneous bacterial peritonitis. World J Hepatol. 2017 Oct 28;9(30):1166–75. [PMID: 29109849]

Jamtgaard L et al. Does albumin infusion reduce renal impairment and mortality in patients with spontaneous bacterial peritonitis? Ann Emerg Med. 2016 Apr;67(4):458–9. [PMID: 26234193]

Sidhu GS et al. Rifaximin versus norfloxacin for prevention of spontaneous bacterial peritonitis: a systematic review. BMJ Open Gastroenterol. 2017 Jul 17;4(1):e000154. [PMID: 28944070]

MALIGNANT ASCITES

Two-thirds of cases of malignant ascites are caused by peritoneal carcinomatosis. The most common tumors causing carcinomatosis are primary adenocarcinomas of the ovary, uterus, pancreas, stomach, colon, lung, or breast. The remaining one-third is due to lymphatic obstruction or portal hypertension due to hepatocellular carcinoma or diffuse hepatic metastases. Patients present with nonspecific abdominal discomfort and weight loss associated with increased abdominal girth. Nausea or vomiting may be caused by partial or complete intestinal obstruction. Abdominal CT may be useful to demonstrate the primary malignancy or hepatic metastases but seldom confirms the diagnosis of peritoneal carcinomatosis. In patients with carcinomatosis, paracentesis demonstrates a low serum ascites-albumin gradient (less than 1.1 mg/dL), an increased total protein (greater than 2.5 g/dL), and an elevated white cell count (often both neutrophils and mononuclear cells) but with a lymphocyte predominance. Cytology is positive in over 95%, but laparoscopy may be required in patients with negative cytology to confirm the diagnosis and to exclude tuberculous peritonitis, with which it may be confused. Malignant ascites attributable to portal hypertension usually is associated with an increased serum ascites-albumin gradient (greater than 1.1 g/dL), a variable total protein, and negative ascitic cytology. Ascites caused by peritoneal carcinomatosis does not respond to diuretics.

Patients may be treated with periodic large-volume paracentesis for symptomatic relief. Indwelling catheters can be left in place for patients approaching the end of life who require periodic paracentesis for symptomatic relief. Intraperitoneal chemotherapy is sometimes used to shrink the tumor, but the overall prognosis is extremely poor, with only 10% survival at 6 months. Ovarian cancers represent an exception to this rule. With newer treatments consisting of surgical debulking and intraperitoneal chemotherapy, long-term survival from ovarian cancer is possible.

Bohn KA et al. Repeat large-volume paracentesis versus tunneled peritoneal catheter placement for malignant ascites: a cost-minimization study. AJR Am J Roentgenol. 2015 Nov; 205(5):1126–34. [PMID: 26496562]

Chen BS et al. Permanent peritoneal ports for the management of recurrent malignant ascites: a retrospective review of safety and efficacy. Intern Med J. 2018 Dec;48(12):1524–8. [PMID: 30517990]

Ha T et al. Symptomatic fluid drainage: tunneled peritoneal and pleural catheters. Semin Intervent Radiol. 2017 Dec; 34(4):337–42. [PMID: 29249857]

Knight JA et al. Safety and effectiveness of palliative tunneled peritoneal drainage catheters in the management of refractory malignant and non-malignant ascites. Cardiovasc Intervent Radiol. 2018 May;41(5):753–61. [PMID: 29344716]

FAMILIAL MEDITERRANEAN FEVER

This is a rare autosomal recessive disorder of unknown pathogenesis that almost exclusively affects people of Mediterranean ancestry, especially Sephardic Jews, Armenians, Turks, and Arabs. Patients lack a protease in serosal fluids that normally inactivates interleukin-8 and the chemotactic complement factor 5A. Symptoms present in most patients before the age of 20 years. It is characterized by episodic bouts of acute peritonitis that may be associated with serositis involving the joints and pleura. Peritoneal attacks are marked by the sudden onset of fever, severe abdominal pain, and abdominal tenderness with guarding or rebound tenderness. If left untreated, attacks resolve within 24–48 hours. Because symptoms resemble those of surgical peritonitis, patients may undergo unnecessary exploratory laparotomy. Colchicine, 0.6 mg orally two or three times daily, has been shown to decrease the frequency and severity of attacks.

Özen S et al. Familial Mediterranean Fever: recent developments in pathogenesis and new recommendations for management. Front Immunol. 2017 Mar 23;8:253. [PMID: 28386255]

Papa R et al. Secondary, AA, amyloidosis. Rheum Dis Clin North Am. 2018 Nov;44(4):585–603. [PMID: 30274625]

MESOTHELIOMA

(See Chapter 39.)

DISEASES OF THE ESOPHAGUS

(See Chapter 39 for Esophageal Cancer.)

► Symptoms

Heartburn, dysphagia, and odynophagia almost always indicate a primary esophageal disorder.

A. Heartburn

Heartburn (pyrosis) is the feeling of substernal burning, often radiating to the neck. Caused by the reflux of acidic (or, rarely, alkaline) material into the esophagus, it is highly specific for GERD.

Table 15–8. Causes of oropharyngeal dysphagia.

Neurologic disorders
  Brainstem cerebrovascular accident, mass lesion
  Amyotrophic lateral sclerosis, multiple sclerosis, pseudobulbar palsy, post-polio syndrome, Guillain-Barré syndrome
  Parkinson disease, Huntington disease, dementia
  Tardive dyskinesia
Muscular and rheumatologic disorders
  Myopathies, polymyositis
  Oculopharyngeal dystrophy
  Sjögren syndrome
Metabolic disorders
  Thyrotoxicosis, amyloidosis, Cushing disease, Wilson disease
  Medication side effects: anticholinergics, phenothiazines
Infectious diseases
  Polio, diphtheria, botulism, Lyme disease, syphilis, mucositis (*Candida*, herpes)
Structural disorders
  Zenker diverticulum
  Cervical osteophytes, cricopharyngeal bar, proximal esophageal webs
  Oropharyngeal tumors
  Postsurgical or radiation changes
  Pill-induced injury
Motility disorders
  Upper esophageal sphincter dysfunction

Table 15–9. Causes of esophageal dysphagia.

Cause	Clues
Mechanical obstruction	**Solid foods worse than liquids**
Schatzki ring	Intermittent dysphagia; not progressive
Peptic stricture	Chronic heartburn; progressive dysphagia
Esophageal cancer	Progressive dysphagia; age over 50 years
Eosinophilic esophagitis	Young adults; small-caliber lumen, proximal stricture, corrugated rings, or white papules
Motility disorder	**Solid and liquid foods**
Achalasia	Progressive dysphagia
Diffuse esophageal spasm	Intermittent; not progressive; may have chest pain
Scleroderma	Chronic heartburn; Raynaud phenomenon
Ineffective esophageal motility	Intermittent; not progressive; commonly associated with GERD

B. Dysphagia

Difficulties in swallowing may arise from problems in transferring the food bolus from the oropharynx to the upper esophagus (oropharyngeal dysphagia) or from impaired transport of the bolus through the body of the esophagus (esophageal dysphagia). The history usually leads to the correct diagnosis.

1. Oropharyngeal dysphagia—The oropharyngeal phase of swallowing is a complex process requiring elevation of the tongue, closure of the nasopharynx, relaxation of the upper esophageal sphincter, closure of the airway, and pharyngeal peristalsis. A variety of mechanical and neuromuscular conditions can disrupt this process (Table 15–8). Problems with the oral phase of swallowing cause drooling or spillage of food from the mouth, inability to chew or initiate swallowing, or dry mouth. Pharyngeal dysphagia is characterized by an immediate sense of the bolus catching in the neck, the need to swallow repeatedly to clear food from the pharynx, or coughing or choking during meals. There may be associated dysphonia, dysarthria, or other neurologic symptoms.

2. Esophageal dysphagia—Esophageal dysphagia may be caused by **mechanical obstructions** of the esophagus or by **motility disorders** (Table 15–9). Patients with **mechanical obstruction** experience dysphagia, primarily for solids. This is recurrent, predictable, and, if the lesion progresses, will worsen as the lumen narrows. Patients with **motility disorders** have dysphagia for both solids and liquids. It is episodic, unpredictable, and can be progressive.

C. Odynophagia

Odynophagia is sharp substernal pain on swallowing that may limit oral intake. It usually reflects severe erosive disease. It is most commonly associated with infectious esophagitis due to *Candida*, herpesviruses, or CMV, especially in immunocompromised patients. It may also be caused by corrosive injury due to caustic ingestions and by pill-induced ulcers.

▶ Diagnostic Studies

A. Upper Endoscopy

Endoscopy is the study of choice for evaluating persistent heartburn, dysphagia, odynophagia, and structural abnormalities detected on barium esophagography. In addition to direct visualization, it allows biopsy of mucosal abnormalities and of normal mucosa (to evaluate for eosinophilic esophagitis) as well as dilation of strictures.

B. Videoesophagography

Oropharyngeal dysphagia is best evaluated with rapid-sequence videoesophagography.

C. Barium Esophagography

Patients with esophageal dysphagia often are evaluated first with a radiographic barium study to differentiate between mechanical lesions and motility disorders, providing important information about the latter in particular. In patients with esophageal dysphagia and a suspected motility disorder, barium esophagoscopy should be obtained first. In patients in whom there is a high suspicion of a mechanical lesion, many clinicians will proceed first to endoscopic evaluation because it better identifies mucosa lesions (eg, erosions) and permits mucosal biopsy and dilation. However, barium study is more sensitive for detecting subtle esophageal narrowing due to rings, achalasia, and proximal esophageal lesions.

D. Esophageal Manometry

Esophageal motility may be assessed using manometric techniques. High-resolution manometry with multiple, closely spaced sensors has replaced conventional manometry in most centers. Manometry is indicated (1) to determine the location of the LES to allow precise placement of a conventional electrode pH probe; (2) to establish the etiology of dysphagia in patients in whom a mechanical obstruction cannot be found, especially if a diagnosis of achalasia is suspected by endoscopy or barium study; and (3) for the preoperative assessment of patients being considered for antireflux surgery to exclude an alternative diagnosis (eg, achalasia) or possibly to assess peristaltic function in the esophageal body.

E. Esophageal pH Recording and Impedance Testing

The pH within the esophageal lumen may be monitored continuously for 24–48 hours. There are two kinds of systems in use: catheter-based and wireless. Traditional systems use a long transnasal catheter that is connected directly to the recording device. With wireless systems, a capsule is attached directly to the esophageal mucosa under endoscopic visualization and data are transmitted by radiotelemetry to the recording device. The recording provides information about the amount of esophageal acid reflux and the temporal correlations between symptoms and reflux.

Esophageal pH monitoring devices provide information about the amount of esophageal acid reflux but not nonacid reflux. Techniques using combined pH and multichannel intraluminal impedance allow assessment of acid and nonacid liquid reflux. They may be useful in evaluation of patients with atypical reflux symptoms or persistent symptoms despite therapy with proton pump inhibitors to diagnose hypersensitivity, functional symptoms, and symptoms caused by nonacid reflux.

Carlson DA et al. How to effectively use high-resolution esophageal manometry. Gastroenterology. 2016 Nov;151(5):789–92. [PMID: 27693348]

Dhawan I et al. Utility of esophageal high-resolution manometry in clinical practice: first, do HRM. Dig Dis Sci. 2018 Dec;63(12):3178–86. [PMID: 30276571]

Gyawali CP et al. Indications and interpretation of esophageal function testing. Ann N Y Acad Sci. 2018 Dec;1434(1):239–53. [PMID: 29754440]

Kahrilas PJ et al. Advances in management of esophageal motility disorders. Clin Gastroenterol Hepatol. 2018 Nov; 16(11):1692–700. [PMID: 29702296]

Roman S et al. High-resolution manometry improves the diagnosis of esophageal motility disorders in patients with dysphagia: a randomized multicenter study. Am J Gastroenterol. 2016 Mar;111(3):372–80. [PMID: 26832656]

Xiao Y et al. Tailored therapy for the refractory GERD patients by combined multichannel intraluminal impedance-pH monitoring. J Gastroenterol Hepatol. 2016 Feb;31(2):350–4. [PMID: 26202002]

GASTROESOPHAGEAL REFLUX DISEASE

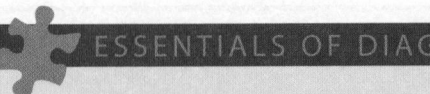

ESSENTIALS OF DIAGNOSIS

▶ Heartburn; may be exacerbated by meals, bending, or recumbency.

▶ Typical uncomplicated cases do not require diagnostic studies.

▶ Endoscopy demonstrates abnormalities in one-third of patients.

▶ General Considerations

GERD is a condition that develops when the reflux of stomach contents causes troublesome symptoms or complications. It affects 20% of adults. The two most common symptoms are heartburn and regurgitation. However, other symptoms of GERD include dyspepsia, dysphagia, belching, chest pain, cough, and hoarseness. Although most patients have mild disease, esophageal mucosal damage (reflux esophagitis) develops in up to one-third and more serious complications develop in a few others. Several factors may contribute to GERD.

A. Dysfunction of the Gastroesophageal Junction

The antireflux barrier at the gastroesophageal junction depends on LES pressure, the intra-abdominal location of the sphincter (resulting in a "flap valve" caused by angulation of the esophageal-gastric junction), and the extrinsic compression of the sphincter by the crural diaphragm. In most patients with GERD, baseline LES pressures are normal (10–35 mm Hg). Most reflux episodes occur during transient relaxations of the LES that are triggered by gastric distention by a vagovagal reflex. A subset of patients with GERD have an incompetent (less than 10 mm Hg) LES that results in increased acid reflux, especially when supine or when intra-abdominal pressures are increased by lifting or bending. A hypotensive sphincter is present in up to 50% of patients with severe erosive GERD.

Hiatal hernias are found in one-fourth of patients with nonerosive GERD, three-fourths of patients with severe erosive esophagitis, and over 90% of patients with Barrett esophagus. They are caused by movement of the LES above the diaphragm, resulting in dysfunction of the gastroesophageal junction reflux barrier. Hiatal hernias are common and may cause no symptoms; however, in patients with gastroesophageal reflux, they are associated with higher amounts of acid reflux and delayed esophageal acid clearance, leading to more severe esophagitis and Barrett esophagus. Increased reflux episodes occur during normal swallowing-induced relaxation, transient LES relaxations, and straining due to reflux of acid from the hiatal hernia sac into the esophagus.

Truncal obesity may contribute to GERD, presumably due to an increased intra-abdominal pressure, which contributes to dysfunction of the gastroesophageal junction and increased likelihood of hiatal hernia.

B. Irritant Effects of Refluxate

Esophageal mucosal damage is related to the potency of the refluxate and the amount of time it is in contact with the mucosa. Acidic gastric fluid (pH less than 4.0) is extremely caustic to the esophageal mucosa and is the major injurious agent in the majority of cases. In some patients, reflux of bile or alkaline pancreatic secretions may be contributory.

C. Abnormal Esophageal Clearance

Acid refluxate normally is cleared and neutralized by esophageal peristalsis and salivary bicarbonate. Patients with severe GERD may have diminished clearance due to hypotensive peristaltic contractions (less than 30 mm Hg) or intermittent failed peristalsis after swallowing. Certain medical conditions such as scleroderma are associated with diminished peristalsis. Sjögren syndrome, anticholinergic medications, and oral radiation therapy may exacerbate GERD due to impaired salivation.

D. Delayed Gastric Emptying

Impaired gastric emptying due to gastroparesis or partial gastric outlet obstruction potentiates GERD.

▶ Clinical Findings

A. Symptoms and Signs

The typical symptom is heartburn. This most often occurs 30–60 minutes after meals and upon reclining. Patients often report relief from taking antacids or baking soda. When this symptom is dominant, the diagnosis is established with a high degree of reliability. Many patients, however, have less specific dyspeptic symptoms with or without heartburn. Overall, a clinical diagnosis of gastroesophageal reflux has a sensitivity and specificity of only 65%. Severity is not correlated with the degree of tissue damage. In fact, some patients with severe esophagitis are only mildly symptomatic. Patients may complain of regurgitation—the spontaneous reflux of sour or bitter gastric contents into the mouth. Dysphagia occurs in one-third of patients and may be due to erosive esophagitis, abnormal esophageal peristalsis, or the development of an esophageal stricture.

"Atypical" or "extraesophageal" manifestations of gastroesophageal disease may occur, including asthma, chronic cough, chronic laryngitis, sore throat, noncardiac chest pain, and sleep disturbances. In the absence of heartburn or regurgitation, atypical symptoms are unlikely to be related to gastroesophageal reflux.

Physical examination and laboratory data are normal in uncomplicated disease.

B. Special Examinations

Initial diagnostic studies are not warranted for patients with typical GERD symptoms suggesting uncomplicated reflux disease. Patients with typical symptoms of heartburn and regurgitation should be treated empirically with a twice-daily H_2-receptor antagonist or a once-daily proton pump inhibitor for 4–8 weeks. Symptomatic response to empiric treatment (while clinically desirable) has only a 78% sensitivity and 54% specificity for GERD. Therefore, further investigation is required in patients with symptoms that persist despite empiric acid inhibitory therapy to identify complications of reflux disease and to diagnose other conditions, particularly in patients with "alarm features" (troublesome dysphagia, odynophagia, weight loss, iron deficiency anemia).

1. Upper endoscopy—Upper endoscopy is excellent for documenting the type and extent of tissue damage in gastroesophageal reflux; for detecting other gastroesophageal lesions that may mimic GERD; and for detecting GERD complications, including esophageal stricture, Barrett metaplasia, and esophageal adenocarcinoma. In the absence of prior antisecretory therapy, up to one-third of patients with GERD have visible mucosal damage (known as reflux esophagitis), characterized by single or multiple erosions or ulcers in the distal esophagus at the squamocolumnar junction. In patients treated with a proton pump inhibitor prior to endoscopy, preexisting reflux esophagitis may be partially or completely healed. The Los Angeles (LA) classification grades reflux esophagitis on a scale of A (one or more isolated mucosal breaks 5 mm or less that do not extend between the tops of two mucosal folds) to D (one or more mucosal breaks that involve at least 75% of the esophageal circumference).

2. Barium esophagography—This study should not be performed to diagnose GERD. In patients with severe dysphagia, it is sometimes obtained prior to endoscopy to identify a stricture.

3. Esophageal pH or combined esophageal pH-impedance testing—Esophageal pH monitoring measures the amount of esophageal acid reflux, whereas combined pH-impedance testing measures both acidic and nonacidic reflux. Both tests may also be useful to establish whether there is a temporal relationship between reflux events and symptoms. They are the most accurate studies for documenting gastroesophageal reflux but are unnecessary in most patients who have typical symptoms and satisfactory response to empiric antisecretory therapy. They are indicated in patients with typical symptoms who have unsatisfactory response to empiric therapy, patients with atypical or extraesophageal symptoms, and patients who are being considered for antireflux surgery.

▶ Differential Diagnosis

Symptoms of GERD may be similar to those of other diseases such as angina pectoris, eosinophilic esophagitis, esophageal motility disorders, dyspepsia, peptic ulcer, or functional disorders. Reflux erosive esophagitis may be confused with pill-induced damage, eosinophilic esophagitis, or infections (CMV, herpes, *Candida*).

▶ Complications

A. Barrett Esophagus

This is a condition in which the squamous epithelium of the esophagus is replaced by metaplastic columnar epithelium containing goblet and columnar cells (specialized intestinal metaplasia). Present in up to 15% of patients with chronic reflux, Barrett esophagus is believed to arise from chronic reflux-induced injury to the esophageal squamous epithelium; however, it is also increased in patients with truncal obesity independent of GERD. Barrett esophagus is suspected at endoscopy from the presence of orange, gastric type epithelium that extends upward more than 1 cm from the gastroesophageal junction into the distal tubular esophagus in a tongue-like or circumferential fashion. Biopsies obtained at endoscopy confirm the diagnosis. Three types of columnar epithelium may be identified: gastric cardiac, gastric fundic, and specialized intestinal metaplasia. There is agreement that the latter carries an increased risk of dysplasia; however, some authorities believe that gastric cardiac mucosa also raises risk.

Barrett esophagus does not provoke specific symptoms but gastroesophageal reflux does. Most patients have a long history of reflux symptoms, such as heartburn and regurgitation. Barrett esophagus should be treated with long-term proton pump inhibitors once or twice daily to control reflux symptoms. Although these medications do not appear to cause regression of Barrett esophagus, they may reduce the risk of cancer. Paradoxically, one-third of patients report minimal or no symptoms of GERD, suggesting decreased acid sensitivity of Barrett epithelium. Indeed, over 90% of individuals with Barrett esophagus in the general population do not seek medical attention.

The most serious complication of Barrett esophagus is esophageal adenocarcinoma. It is believed that most adenocarcinomas of the esophagus and many such tumors of the gastric cardia arise from dysplastic epithelium in Barrett esophagus. The incidence of adenocarcinoma in patients with Barrett esophagus has been estimated at 0.2–0.5% per year. Although this still is an 11-fold increased risk compared with patients without Barrett esophagus, adenocarcinoma of the esophagus remains a relatively uncommon malignancy in the United States (7000 cases/year). Given the large number of adults with chronic GERD relative to the small number in whom adenocarcinoma develops, a 2016 clinical guideline recommended against endoscopic screening for Barrett esophagus in adults with GERD except in men with two or more risk factors for adenocarcinoma (aged older than 50 years, truncal obesity, white race, current or prior history of smoking, family history of Barrett esophagus or esophageal adenocarcinoma) and in selected women with multiple risk factors.

In patients known to have nondysplastic Barrett esophagus, surveillance endoscopy every 3–5 years is recommended to look for low- or high-grade dysplasia or adenocarcinoma. However, given the relatively low risk of progression to cancer in patients with nondysplastic Barrett esophagus (0.2–0.5%/year), the risks and benefits of surveillance should be discussed with patients. During endoscopy, biopsies are obtained from nodular or irregular mucosa (which have an increased risk of high-grade dysplasia or cancer) as well as randomly from the esophagus every 1–2 cm. The finding of dysplasia should be confirmed by a second, expert pathologist. The risk of progression to adenocarcinoma is 0.7% per year for patients with low-grade dysplasia and 7% per year for

high-grade dysplasia. Approximately 13% of patients with high-grade dysplasia may harbor an unrecognized invasive esophageal cancer. Therefore, a repeat endoscopy by an endoscopist with expertise in advanced resection and ablation techniques is recommended.

On repeat endoscopy, all nodules should be removed with mucosal snare resection or dissection techniques to assess for the presence and depth of cancer; random biopsies should again be obtained. The subsequent management of patients with intramucosal cancer or high-grade dysplasia has rapidly evolved. Until recently, esophagectomy was recommended for patients deemed to have a low operative risk; however, this procedure is associated with high morbidity and mortality rates (40% and 1–5%, respectively). Therefore, endoscopic therapy is now standard care for all patients with low- or high-grade dysplasia and patients with well-differentiated intramucosal cancer (Tis and T1a) without lymphatic or vascular invasion. Of the patients who have cancer confined to the mucosa, less than 2% have recurrence of cancer or high-grade dysplasia after snare resection. Following resection, ablation of any remaining Barrett mucosa—including flat (nonnodular) high-grade dysplasia—is performed with radiofrequency wave electrocautery or cryotherapy. Current guidelines also recommend that patients with flat *low-grade* dysplasia (confirmed by a second expert pathologist) also be considered for ablation, reserving annual endoscopic surveillance to patients with increased comorbidities and reduced life-expectancy. The efficacy of endoscopic ablation therapies in patients with Barrett dysplasia is supported by several studies. When high-dose proton pump inhibitors are administered to normalize intraesophageal pH, radiofrequency wave ablation electrocautery eradication of Barrett columnar epithelium is followed by complete healing with normal squamous epithelium in greater than 78% of patients and elimination of dysplasia in 91%.

Endoscopic ablation techniques have a risk of complications (bleeding, perforation, strictures). Therefore, endoscopic eradication therapy currently is not recommended for patients with nondysplastic Barrett esophagus for whom the risk of developing esophageal cancer is low and treatment does not appear to be cost-effective.

B. Peptic Stricture

Stricture formation occurs in about 5% of patients with esophagitis. It is manifested by the gradual development of solid food dysphagia progressive over months to years. Often there is a reduction in heartburn because the stricture acts as a barrier to reflux. Most strictures are located at the gastroesophageal junction. Endoscopy with biopsy is mandatory in all cases to differentiate peptic stricture from stricture by esophageal carcinoma. Active erosive esophagitis is often present. Up to 90% of symptomatic patients are effectively treated with dilation with graduated polyvinyl catheters passed over a wire placed at the time of endoscopy or fluoroscopically, or balloons passed fluoroscopically or through an endoscope. Dilation is continued over one to several sessions. A luminal diameter of 13–17 mm is usually sufficient to relieve dysphagia. Long-term therapy with a proton pump inhibitor is required to decrease the likelihood of stricture recurrence. Some patients require intermittent dilation to maintain luminal patency, but operative management for strictures that do not respond to dilation is seldom required. Refractory strictures may benefit from endoscopic injection of triamcinolone into the stricture.

► Treatment

A. Medical Treatment

The goal of treatment is to provide symptomatic relief, to heal esophagitis (if present), and to prevent complications. In the majority of patients with uncomplicated disease, empiric treatment is initiated based on a compatible history without the need for further confirmatory studies. Patients not responding and those with suspected complications undergo further evaluation with upper endoscopy or esophageal manometry and pH recording.

1. Mild, intermittent symptoms—Patients with mild or intermittent symptoms that do not impact adversely on quality of life may benefit from lifestyle modifications with medical interventions taken as needed. Patients may find that eating smaller meals and elimination of acidic foods (citrus, tomatoes, coffee, spicy foods), foods that precipitate reflux (fatty foods, chocolate, peppermint, alcohol), and cigarettes may reduce symptoms. Weight loss should be recommended for patients who are overweight or have had recent weight gain. All patients should be advised to avoid lying down within 3 hours after meals (the period of greatest reflux). Patients with nocturnal symptoms should also elevate the head of the bed on 6-inch blocks or a foam wedge to reduce reflux and enhance esophageal clearance.

Patients with infrequent heartburn (less than once weekly) may be treated on demand with antacids or oral H_2-receptor antagonists. Antacids provide rapid relief of heartburn; however, their duration of action is less than 2 hours. Many are available over the counter. Those containing magnesium should not be used for patients with kidney disease, and patients with acute or chronic kidney disease should be cautioned appropriately.

The oral H_2-receptor antagonists come in a variety of strengths: cimetidine 200 mg; famotidine 10 mg and 20 mg; nizatidine 75 mg and 150 mg; and ranitidine 75 mg and 150 mg. Most of these drug strengths are now available over the counter without need for a prescription. When taken for active heartburn, these agents have a delay in onset of at least 30 minutes. However, once these agents take effect, they provide heartburn relief for up to 8 hours. When taken before meals known to provoke heartburn, these agents reduce the symptom.

2. Troublesome symptoms—

A. INITIAL THERAPY—Patients with troublesome reflux symptoms and patients with known complications of GERD (erosive esophagitis, Barrett esophagus, stricture) should be treated with a once-daily oral proton pump inhibitor (omeprazole or rabeprazole, 20 mg; omeprazole, 40 mg with sodium bicarbonate; lansoprazole, 30 mg; dexlansoprazole,

60 mg; esomeprazole or pantoprazole, 40 mg) taken 30 minutes before breakfast for 4–8 weeks. Because there appears to be little difference between these agents in efficacy or side effect profiles, the choice of agent is determined by cost. Oral omeprazole, 20 mg, and lansoprazole, 15 mg, are available as over-the-counter formulations. Once-daily proton pump inhibitors achieve adequate control of heartburn in 80–90% of patients, complete heartburn resolution in over 50%, and healing of erosive esophagitis (when present) in over 80%. Because of their superior efficacy and ease of use, proton pump inhibitors are preferred to H_2-receptor antagonists for the treatment of acute and chronic GERD. Approximately 10–20% of patients do not achieve symptom relief with a once-daily dose within 2–4 weeks and require a twice-daily proton pump inhibitor (taken 30 minutes before breakfast and dinner).

B. LONG-TERM THERAPY—In those who achieve good symptomatic relief with a course of empiric once-daily proton pump inhibitor, therapy may be discontinued after 8–12 weeks. Most patients (over 80%) will experience relapse of GERD symptoms, usually within 3 months. Patients whose symptoms relapse may be treated with either continuous proton pump inhibitor therapy, intermittent 2- to 4-week courses, or "on demand" therapy (ie, drug taken until symptoms abate) depending on symptom frequency and patient preference. Alternatively, twice daily H_2-receptor antagonists may be used to control symptoms in patients without erosive esophagitis. Patients who require twice-daily proton pump inhibitor therapy for initial symptom control and patients with complications of GERD, including severe erosive esophagitis, Barrett esophagus, or peptic stricture, should be maintained on long-term therapy with a once- or twice-daily proton pump inhibitor titrated to the lowest effective dose to achieve satisfactory symptom control.

Side effects of proton pump inhibitors are uncommon. Headache, diarrhea, and abdominal pain may occur with any of the agents but generally resolve when another formulation is tried. Potential risks of long-term use of proton pump inhibitors include an increased risk of infectious gastroenteritis (including *C difficile*), iron and vitamin B_{12} deficiency, hypomagnesemia, pneumonia, hip fractures (possibly due to impaired calcium absorption), and fundic gland polyps (which appear to be of no clinical significance). Recent observational studies report a slight increase in acute and chronic kidney disease (due to interstitial nephritis) and dementia; however, causality has not been established. Long-term proton pump inhibitor therapy should be prescribed to patients with appropriate indications and at the lowest effective dose.

3. Extraesophageal reflux manifestations—Establishing a causal relationship between gastroesophageal reflux and extraesophageal symptoms (eg, asthma, hoarseness, cough, sleep disturbances) is difficult. Gastroesophageal reflux seldom is the sole cause of extraesophageal disorders but may be a contributory factor. Although ambulatory esophageal pH testing can document the presence of increased acid esophageal reflux, it does not prove a causative connection. Current guidelines recommend that a trial of a twice-daily proton pump inhibitor be administered for 2–3 months in patients with suspected extraesophageal GERD syndromes who also have typical GERD symptoms. Improvement of extraesophageal symptoms suggests but does not prove that acid reflux is the causative factor. Esophageal impedance-pH testing or oropharyngeal pH testing may be performed in patients whose extraesophageal symptoms persist after 3 months of proton pump inhibitor therapy and may be considered before proton pump inhibitor therapy in patients without typical GERD symptoms in whom other causes of extraesophageal symptoms have been excluded.

4. Unresponsive disease—Approximately 5% do not respond to twice-daily proton pump inhibitors or a change to a different proton pump inhibitor. These patients should undergo endoscopy for detection of severe, inadequately treated reflux esophagitis and for other gastroesophageal lesions (including eosinophilic esophagitis) that may mimic GERD. Truly refractory esophagitis may be caused by gastrinoma with gastric acid hypersecretion (Zollinger-Ellison syndrome), pill-induced esophagitis, resistance to proton pump inhibitors, and medical noncompliance. Patients without endoscopically visible esophagitis should undergo ambulatory impedance-pH monitoring while taking a twice-daily proton pump inhibitor to determine whether the symptoms are correlated with acid or nonacid reflux episodes. The pH study is performed on therapy if the suspicion for GERD is high (to determine whether therapy has adequately suppressed acid esophageal reflux) and off therapy if the suspicion for GERD is low (to determine whether the patient has reflux disease). Combined esophageal pH monitoring with impedance monitoring is preferred over pH testing alone because of its ability to detect both acid and nonacid reflux events. Approximately 60% of patients with unresponsive symptoms do not have increased reflux and may be presumed to have a functional disorder. Treatment with a low-dose tricyclic antidepressant (eg, imipramine or nortriptyline 25 mg at bedtime) may be beneficial.

B. Surgical Treatment

Surgical fundoplication affords good to excellent relief of symptoms and healing of esophagitis in over 85% of properly selected patients and can be performed laparoscopically with low complication rates in most instances. Although patient satisfaction is high, typical reflux symptoms recur in 10–30% of patients. Furthermore, new symptoms of dysphagia, bloating, increased flatulence, dyspepsia, or diarrhea develop in over 30% of patients. In 2011, results from a randomized trial comparing laparoscopic fundoplication with prolonged medical therapy (esomeprazole 40 mg/day) for chronic GERD were reported. After 5 years, adequate GERD symptom control (symptom remission) was similar, occurring in 85–92% of patients; however, patients who had undergone fundoplication had increased dysphagia, bloating, and flatulence. A novel, minimally invasive magnetic artificial sphincter is FDA approved for the treatment of GERD in patients with hiatal hernias less than 3 cm in size. The device is made up of a flexible, elastic string of titanium beads (wrapped around a magnetic core)

that is placed laparoscopically below the diaphragm at the gastroesophageal junction. In clinical trials with over 1-year follow up, magnetic sphincter augmentation has demonstrated GERD symptom relief equivalent to laparoscopic fundoplication. The rate of laparoscopic device removal for persistent symptoms (mostly dysphagia) is 3–7%. Given the excellent safety and efficacy data demonstrated with this device to date, it may be considered as an alternative to fundoplication surgery for patients with GERD and hiatal hernias less than 3 cm in size, though outcomes of long-term follow up are awaited.

Surgical treatment is not recommended for patients who are well controlled with medical therapies but should be considered for (1) otherwise healthy, carefully selected patients with extraesophageal manifestations of reflux, as these symptoms often require high doses of proton pump inhibitors and may be more effectively controlled with antireflux surgery; (2) those with severe reflux disease who are unwilling to accept lifelong medical therapy due to its expense, inconvenience, or theoretical risks; and (3) patients with large hiatal hernias and persistent regurgitation despite proton pump inhibitor therapy. Gastric bypass (rather than fundoplication) should be considered for obese patients with GERD.

Several endoscopic procedures have been developed to treat GERD; however, none have found wide acceptance, largely due to limited long-term efficacy.

▶ When to Refer

- Patients with typical GERD whose symptoms do not resolve with empiric management with a twice-daily proton pump inhibitor.

- Patients with suspected extraesophageal GERD symptoms that do not resolve with 3 months of twice-daily proton pump inhibitor therapy.

- Patients with significant dysphagia or other alarm symptoms for upper endoscopy.

- Patients with Barrett esophagus for endoscopic surveillance.

- Patients who have Barrett esophagus with dysplasia or early mucosal cancer.

- Surgical fundoplication is considered.

Eluri S et al. Barrett's esophagus: diagnosis and management. Gastrointest Endosc. 2017 May;85(5):889–903. [PMID: 28109913]

Lee YY et al. Management of patients with functional heartburn. Gastroenterology. 2018 Jun;154(8):2018–21. [PMID: 29730025]

Patel A et al. Gastroesophageal reflux monitoring. JAMA. 2018 Mar 27;319(12):1271–2. [PMID: 29584823]

Richter JE et al. Efficacy of laparoscopic Nissen fundoplication vs transoral incisionless fundoplication or proton pump inhibitors in patients with gastroesophageal reflux disease: a systematic review and network meta-analysis. Gastroenterology. 2018 Apr;154(5):1298–308. [PMID: 29305934]

Standards of Practice Committee; Wani S et al. Endoscopic eradication therapy for patients with Barrett's esophagus-associated dysplasia and intramucosal cancer. Gastrointest Endosc. 2018 Apr;87(4):907–31.e9. [PMID: 29397943]

Tack J et al. Pathophysiology of gastroesophageal reflux disease. Gastroenterology. 2018 Jan;154(2):277–88. [PMID: 29037470]

Targownik L. Discontinuing long-term PPI therapy: why, with whom, and how? Am J Gastroenterol. 2018 Apr;113(4):519–28. [PMID: 29557943]

Vaezi MF et al. Extraesophageal symptoms and diseases attributed to GERD: where is the pendulum swinging now? Clin Gastroenterol Hepatol. 2018 Jul;16(7):1018–29. [PMID: 29427733]

Vaezi MF et al. White paper AGA: optimal strategies to define and diagnose gastroesophageal reflux disease. Clin Gastroenterol Hepatol. 2017 Aug;15(8):1162–72. [PMID: 28344064]

Yadlapati R et al. Complications of antireflux surgery. Am J Gastroenterol. 2018 Aug;113(8):1137–47. [PMID: 29899438]

Yadlapati R et al. Management options for patients with GERD and persistent symptoms on proton pump inhibitors: recommendations from an expert panel. Am J Gastroenterol. 2018 Jul;113(7):980–6. [PMID: 29686276]

INFECTIOUS ESOPHAGITIS

ESSENTIALS OF DIAGNOSIS

► Immunosuppressed patient.

► Odynophagia, dysphagia, and chest pain.

► Endoscopy with biopsy establishes diagnosis.

General Considerations

Infectious esophagitis occurs most commonly in immunosuppressed patients. Patients with AIDS, solid organ transplants, leukemia, lymphoma, and those receiving immunosuppressive drugs are at particular risk for opportunistic infections. *Candida albicans*, herpes simplex, and CMV are the most common pathogens. *Candida* infection may occur also in patients who have uncontrolled diabetes and those being treated with systemic corticosteroids, radiation therapy, or systemic antibiotic therapy. Herpes simplex can affect normal hosts, in which case the infection is generally self-limited.

Clinical Findings

A. Symptoms and Signs

The most common symptoms are odynophagia and dysphagia. Substernal chest pain occurs in some patients. Patients with candidal esophagitis are sometimes asymptomatic. Oral thrush is present in only 75% of patients with candidal esophagitis and 25–50% of patients with viral esophagitis and is therefore an unreliable indicator of the cause of esophageal infection. Patients with esophageal CMV infection may have infection at other sites such as the colon and retina. Oral ulcers (herpes labialis) are often associated with herpes simplex esophagitis.

B. Special Examinations

Treatment may be empiric. For diagnostic certainty, endoscopy with biopsy and brushings (for microbiologic and histopathologic analysis) is preferred because of its high diagnostic accuracy. The endoscopic signs of candidal esophagitis are diffuse, linear, yellow-white plaques adherent to the mucosa. CMV esophagitis is characterized by one to several large, shallow, superficial ulcerations. Herpes esophagitis results in multiple small, deep ulcerations.

Treatment

A. Candidal Esophagitis

Systemic therapy is required for esophageal candidiasis. An empiric trial of antifungal therapy is often administered without performing diagnostic endoscopy. Initial therapy is generally with fluconazole, 400 mg on day 1, then 200–400 mg/day orally for 14–21 days. Patients not responding to empiric therapy within 3–5 days should undergo endoscopy with brushings, biopsy, and culture to distinguish resistant fungal infection from other infections (eg, CMV, herpes). Esophageal candidiasis not responding to fluconazole therapy may be treated with itraconazole suspension (not capsules), 200 mg/day orally, or voriconazole, 200 mg orally twice daily. Refractory infection may be treated intravenously with caspofungin, 50 mg daily.

B. Cytomegalovirus Esophagitis

In patients with HIV infection, immune restoration with antiretroviral therapy is the most effective means of controlling CMV disease. Initial therapy is with ganciclovir, 5 mg/kg intravenously every 12 hours for 3–6 weeks. Neutropenia is a frequent dose-limiting side effect. Once resolution of symptoms occurs, it may be possible to complete the course of therapy with oral valganciclovir, 900 mg once daily. Patients who either do not respond to or cannot tolerate ganciclovir are treated acutely with foscarnet, 90 mg/kg intravenously every 12 hours for 3–6 weeks. The principal toxicities are acute kidney injury, hypocalcemia, and hypomagnesemia.

C. Herpetic Esophagitis

Immunocompetent patients may be treated symptomatically and generally do not require specific antiviral therapy. Immunosuppressed patients may be treated with oral acyclovir, 400 mg orally five times daily, or 250 mg/m^2 intravenously every 8–12 hours, usually for 14–21 days. Oral famciclovir, 500 mg orally three times daily, or valacyclovir, 1 g twice daily, are also effective but more expensive than generic acyclovir. Nonresponders require therapy with foscarnet, 40 mg/kg intravenously every 8 hours for 21 days.

Prognosis

Most patients with infectious esophagitis can be effectively treated with complete symptom resolution. Depending on the patient's underlying immunodeficiency, relapse of symptoms off therapy can raise difficulties. Long-term suppressive therapy is sometimes required.

Daniell HW. Acid suppressing therapy as a risk factor for *Candida* esophagitis. Dis Esophagus. 2016 Jul;29(5):479–83. [PMID: 25833302]

Grossi L et al. Esophagitis and its causes: who is "guilty" when acid is found "not guilty"? World J Gastroenterol. 2017 May 7; 23(17):3011–6. [PMID: 28533657]

Hoversten P et al. Infections of the esophagus: an update on risk factors, diagnosis, and management. Dis Esophagus. 2018 Dec 1;31(12). [PMID: 30295751]

PILL-INDUCED ESOPHAGITIS

A number of different medications may injure the esophagus, presumably through direct, prolonged mucosal contact or mechanisms that disrupt mucosal integrity. The most commonly implicated are the NSAIDs, potassium chloride pills, quinidine, zalcitabine, zidovudine, alendronate and risedronate, emepronium bromide, iron, vitamin C, and antibiotics (doxycycline, tetracycline, clindamycin, trimethoprim-sulfamethoxazole). Because injury is most likely to occur if pills are swallowed without water or while supine, hospitalized or bed-bound patients are at greater risk. Symptoms include severe retrosternal chest pain, odynophagia, and dysphagia, often beginning several hours after taking a pill. These may occur suddenly and persist for days. Some patients (especially older patients) have relatively little pain, presenting with dysphagia. Endoscopy may reveal one to several discrete ulcers that may be shallow or deep. Chronic injury may result in severe esophagitis with stricture, hemorrhage, or perforation. Healing occurs rapidly when the offending agent is eliminated. To prevent pill-induced damage, patients should take pills with 4 oz of water and remain upright for 30 minutes after ingestion. Known offending agents should not be given to patients with esophageal dysmotility, dysphagia, or strictures.

Grossi L et al. Esophagitis and its causes: who is "guilty" when acid is found "not guilty"? World J Gastroenterol. 2017 May 7; 23(17):3011–6. [PMID: 28533657]

BENIGN ESOPHAGEAL LESIONS

1. Mallory-Weiss Syndrome (Mucosal Laceration of Gastroesophageal Junction)

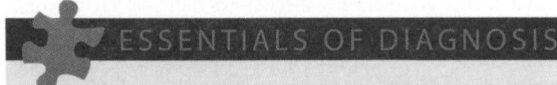

ESSENTIALS OF DIAGNOSIS

► Hematemesis; usually self-limited.
► Prior history of vomiting, retching in 50%.
► Endoscopy establishes diagnosis.

General Considerations

Mallory-Weiss syndrome is characterized by a nonpenetrating mucosal tear at the gastroesophageal junction that is hypothesized to arise from events that suddenly raise transabdominal pressure, such as lifting, retching, or vomiting. Alcoholism is a strong predisposing factor. Mallory-Weiss tears are responsible for approximately 5% of cases of upper gastrointestinal bleeding.

Clinical Findings

A. Symptoms and Signs

Patients usually present with hematemesis with or without melena. A history of retching, vomiting, or straining is obtained in about 50% of cases.

B. Special Examinations

As with other causes of upper gastrointestinal hemorrhage, upper endoscopy should be performed after the patient has been appropriately resuscitated. The diagnosis is established by identification of a 0.5- to 4-cm linear mucosal tear usually located either at the gastroesophageal junction or, more commonly, just below the junction in the gastric mucosa.

Differential Diagnosis

At endoscopy, other potential causes of upper gastrointestinal hemorrhage are found in over 35% of patients with Mallory-Weiss tears, including peptic ulcer disease, erosive gastritis, arteriovenous malformations, and esophageal varices. Patients with underlying portal hypertension are at higher risk for continued or recurrent bleeding.

Treatment

Patients are initially treated as needed with fluid resuscitation and blood transfusions. Most patients stop bleeding spontaneously and require no therapy. Endoscopic hemostatic therapy is employed in patients who have continuing active bleeding. Injection with epinephrine (1:10,000), cautery with a bipolar or heater probe coagulation device, or mechanical compression of the artery by application of an endoclip or band is effective in 90–95% of cases. Angiographic arterial embolization or operative intervention is required in patients who fail endoscopic therapy.

Corral JE et al. Mallory Weiss syndrome is not associated with hiatal hernia: a matched case-control study. Scand J Gastroenterol. 2017 Apr;52(4):462–4. [PMID: 28007004]

Nojkov B et al. Distinctive aspects of peptic ulcer disease, Dieulafoy's lesion, and Mallory-Weiss syndrome in patients with advanced alcoholic liver disease or cirrhosis. World J Gastroenterol. 2016 Jan 7;22(1):446–66. [PMID: 26755890]

2. Eosinophilic Esophagitis

General Considerations

Eosinophilia of the esophagus may be caused by eosinophilic esophagitis and GERD (and, rarely, celiac disease, Crohn disease, and pemphigus).

Eosinophilic esophagitis is a disorder in which food or environmental antigens are thought to stimulate an inflammatory response. Initially recognized in children, it is increasingly identified in young or middle-aged adults (estimated prevalence 43/100,000). A history of allergies or atopic conditions (asthma, eczema, hay fever) is present in over half of patients.

Clinical Findings

Most adults have a long history of dysphagia for solid-foods or an episode of food impaction. Heartburn or chest pain may be present. Children may have abdominal pain, vomiting, or failure to thrive. On laboratory tests, a few have eosinophilia or elevated IgE levels. Barium swallow studies may demonstrate a small-caliber esophagus; focal or long, tapered strictures; or multiple concentric rings. However, endoscopy with esophageal biopsy and histologic evaluation is required to establish the diagnosis. Endoscopic appearances include *e*dema, concentric *r*ings ("trachealization"), *e*xudates (white plaques), *f*urrows (vertical lines), and *s*trictures (EREFS); however, the esophagus is grossly normal in up to 5% of patients. Multiple biopsies (4–8) from the proximal and distal esophagus should be obtained to demonstrate multiple (greater than 15/high-powered field) eosinophils in the mucosa. Consideration should be given to the disorders that may cause increased esophageal eosinophils, including hypereosinophilic syndrome, eosinophilic gastroenteritis, achalasia, connective tissue disorders, drug hypersensitivity, and Crohn disease. Skin testing for food allergies may be helpful to identify causative factors.

Treatment

The goals of therapy are improvement of symptoms, reduction of inflammation, and prevention and treatment of esophageal strictures. Treatment options include proton pump inhibitors, topical corticosteroids, food elimination diets, and esophageal dilation. First-line therapy for most adults is a proton pump inhibitor orally twice daily for 2 months followed by repeat endoscopy and mucosal biopsy. Up to 50% of symptomatic patients with increased esophageal eosinophils have clinical and histologic improvement with proton pump inhibitor treatment. It is hypothesized that esophageal acid exposure may contribute to antigen-mediated eosinophilic inflammation. Proton pump inhibitor therapy should be discontinued in patients with persistent symptoms and inflammation.

In patients with continued symptoms, optimal treatment is uncertain. Referral to an allergist for evaluation of coexisting atopic disorders and for testing for food and environmental allergens may be considered, but studies suggest limited predictive value in adults. Empiric elimination of suspected dietary allergens leads to clinical, endoscopic and histologic improvement in 50–70% of adults. The most common allergenic foods are dairy, eggs, wheat, and soy followed by peanuts and shellfish. With progressive reintroduction of each food group, the trigger food group may be identified in up to 85% of patients. Topical corticosteroids lead to symptom resolution in 70% of adults. Either budesonide in sucralose suspension, 1 mg, or powdered fluticasone, 440–880 mcg (from foil-lined inhaler diskus), is administered twice daily for 2–4 weeks. Symptomatic relapse is common after discontinuation of therapy and may require maintenance therapy at reduced doses of 0.25 mg twice daily. Graduated dilation of strictures should be conducted in patients with dysphagia and strictures or narrow-caliber esophagus but should be performed cautiously because there is an increased risk of perforation and postprocedural chest pain.

Dellon ES et al. Epidemiology and natural history of eosinophilic esophagitis. Gastroenterology. 2018 Jan;154(2):319–32. [PMID: 28774845]

Dellon ES et al. Updated international consensus diagnostic criteria for eosinophilic esophagitis: proceedings of the AGREE Conference. Gastroenterology. 2018 Oct;155(4):1022–33. [PMID: 30009819]

Dougherty M et al. Esophageal dilation with either bougie or balloon technique as treatment for eosinophilic esophagitis: a systematic review. Gastrointest Endosc. 2017 Oct;86(4):581–91. [PMID: 28461094]

Greuter T et al. Long-term treatment of eosinophilic esophagitis with swallowed topical corticosteroids: development and evaluation of a therapeutic concept. Am J Gastroenterol. 2017 Oct;112(10):1527–35. [PMID: 28719593]

Straumann A et al. Diagnosis and treatment of eosinophilic esophagitis. Gastroenterology. 2018 Jan;154(2):346–59. [PMID: 28756235]

3. Esophageal Webs & Rings

Esophageal webs are thin, diaphragm-like membranes of squamous mucosa that typically occur in the mid or upper esophagus and may be multiple. They may be congenital but also occur with eosinophilic esophagitis, graft-versus-host disease, pemphigoid, epidermolysis bullosa, pemphigus vulgaris, and, rarely, in association with iron deficiency anemia (Plummer-Vinson syndrome). Esophageal "Schatzki" rings are smooth, circumferential, thin (less than 4 mm in thickness) mucosal structures located in the distal esophagus at the squamocolumnar junction. Their pathogenesis is controversial. They are associated in nearly all cases with a hiatal hernia, and reflux symptoms are common, suggesting that acid gastroesophageal reflux may be contributory in many cases. Most webs and rings are over 20 mm in diameter and are asymptomatic. Solid food dysphagia most often occurs with rings less than 13 mm in diameter. Characteristically, dysphagia is intermittent and not progressive. Large poorly chewed food boluses such as beefsteak are most likely to cause symptoms. Obstructing boluses may pass by drinking extra liquids or after regurgitation. In some cases, an impacted bolus must be extracted endoscopically. Esophageal webs and rings are best visualized using a barium esophagogram with full esophageal distention. Endoscopy is less sensitive than barium esophagography.

The majority of symptomatic patients with a single ring or web can be effectively treated with the passage of bougie dilators to disrupt the lesion or endoscopic electrosurgical incision of the ring. A single dilation may suffice, but repeat dilations are required in many patients. Patients who have heartburn or who require repeated dilation should receive long-term acid suppressive therapy with a proton pump inhibitor.

Jouhourian C et al. Abdominal compression during endoscopy (the Bolster technique) demonstrates hidden Schatzki rings (with videos). Gastrointest Endosc. 2016 May;83(5):1024–6. [PMID: 26548850]

4. Zenker Diverticulum

Zenker diverticulum is a protrusion of pharyngeal mucosa that develops at the pharyngoesophageal junction between the inferior pharyngeal constrictor and the cricopharyngeus. The cause is believed to be loss of elasticity of the upper esophageal sphincter, resulting in restricted opening during swallowing. Symptoms of dysphagia and regurgitation tend to develop insidiously over years in older, predominantly male patients. Initial symptoms include vague oropharyngeal dysphagia with coughing or throat discomfort. As the diverticulum enlarges and retains food, patients may note halitosis, spontaneous regurgitation of undigested food, nocturnal choking, gurgling in the throat, or a protrusion in the neck. Complications include aspiration pneumonia, bronchiectasis, and lung abscess. The diagnosis is best established by a videoesophagography.

Symptomatic patients require upper esophageal myotomy. Minimally invasive intraluminal approaches have been developed in which the septum between the esophagus and diverticulum is incised using a rigid or flexible endoscope or a diverticuloscope. Significant improvement occurs in over 90% of patients. Small asymptomatic diverticula may be observed.

Ishaq S et al. New and emerging techniques for endoscopic treatment of Zenker's diverticulum: state of the art review. Dig Endosc. 2018 Jul;30(4):449–60. [PMID: 29423955]

Le Mouel JP et al. Zenker diverticulum. N Engl J Med. 2017 Nov 30;377(22):e31. [PMID: 29171816]

Pang M et al. Comparison of flexible endoscopic cricopharyngeal myectomy and myotomy approaches for Zenker diverticulum repair. Gastrointest Endosc. 2019 Apr;89(4):880–6. [PMID: 30342027]

5. Esophageal Varices

ESSENTIALS OF DIAGNOSIS

► Develop secondary to portal hypertension.

► Found in 50% of patients with cirrhosis.

► One-third of patients with varices develop upper gastrointestinal bleeding.

► Diagnosis established by upper endoscopy.

► General Considerations

Esophageal varices are dilated submucosal veins that develop in patients with underlying portal hypertension and may result in serious upper gastrointestinal bleeding. The causes of portal hypertension are discussed in Chapter 16. Under normal circumstances, there is a 2–6 mm Hg pressure gradient between the portal vein and the inferior vena cava. When the gradient exceeds 10–12 mm Hg, significant portal hypertension exists. Esophageal varices are the most common cause of important gastrointestinal bleeding due to portal hypertension, though gastric varices and, rarely, intestinal varices may also bleed. Bleeding from esophageal varices most commonly occurs in the distal 5 cm of the esophagus.

The most common cause of portal hypertension is cirrhosis. Approximately 50% of patients with cirrhosis have esophageal varices. Bleeding from varices occurs in 30% of patients with esophageal varices. In the absence of any treatment, variceal bleeding spontaneously stops in about 50% of patients. Patients surviving this bleeding episode have a 60% chance of recurrent variceal bleeding, usually within the first 6 weeks. With current therapies, the in-hospital mortality rate associated with bleeding esophageal varices is 15%.

A number of factors have been identified that may portend an increased risk of bleeding from esophageal varices. The most important are (1) the size of the varices; (2) the presence at endoscopy of red wale markings (longitudinal dilated venules on the varix surface); (3) the severity of liver disease (as assessed by Child scoring); and (4) active alcohol abuse—patients with cirrhosis who continue to drink have an extremely high risk of bleeding.

► Clinical Findings

A. Symptoms and Signs

Patients with bleeding esophageal varices present with symptoms and signs of acute gastrointestinal hemorrhage. (See Acute Upper Gastrointestinal Bleeding, above.) In some cases, there may be preceding retching or dyspepsia attributable to alcoholic gastritis or withdrawal. Varices per se do not cause symptoms of dyspepsia, dysphagia, or retching. Variceal bleeding usually is severe, resulting in hypovolemia manifested by postural vital signs or shock. Twenty percent of patients with chronic liver disease in whom bleeding develops have a nonvariceal source of bleeding.

B. Laboratory Findings

These are identical to those listed above in the section on Acute Upper Gastrointestinal Bleeding.

► Initial Management

A. Acute Resuscitation

The initial management of patients with acute upper gastrointestinal bleeding is also discussed in the section on Acute Upper Gastrointestinal Bleeding. Variceal hemorrhage is life-threatening; rapid assessment and resuscitation with fluids or blood products are essential. Overtransfusion should be avoided as it leads to increased central and portal venous pressures, increasing the risk of rebleeding. Many patients with bleeding esophageal varices have coagulopathy due to underlying cirrhosis; fresh frozen plasma (20 mL/kg loading dose, then 10 mg/kg every 6 hours) or platelets should be administered to patients with INRs greater than 1.8–2.0 or with platelet counts less than 50,000/mcL in the presence of active bleeding. Recombinant factor VIIa has not demonstrated efficacy in controlled studies and is not recommended. The role of prothrombin complex concentrates requires further study. Patients with advanced liver disease are at high risk for poor outcome regardless of the bleeding source and should be transferred to an ICU.

B. Pharmacologic Therapy

1. Antibiotic prophylaxis—Cirrhotic patients admitted with upper gastrointestinal bleeding have a greater than 50% chance of developing a severe bacterial infection during hospitalization—such as bacterial peritonitis, pneumonia, or urinary tract infection. Most infections are caused by gram-negative organisms of gut origin. Prophylactic administration of oral or intravenous fluoroquinolones (eg, norfloxacin, 400 mg orally twice daily) or intravenous third-generation cephalosporins (eg, ceftriaxone, 1 g/day) for 5–7 days reduces the risk of serious infection to 10–20% as well as hospital mortality, especially in patients with Child-Pugh class C cirrhosis. Because of a rising incidence of infections caused by gram-positive organisms as well as fluoroquinolone-resistant organisms, intravenous third-generation cephalosporins may be preferred.

2. Vasoactive drugs—Octreotide and somatostatin infusions reduce portal pressures in ways that are poorly understood. Octreotide (50 mcg intravenous bolus followed by 50 mcg/h) or somatostatin (250 mcg/h)—not available in the United States—reduces splanchnic and hepatic blood flow and portal pressures in cirrhotic patients. Both agents appear to provide acute control of variceal bleeding in up to 80% of patients although neither has been shown to reduce mortality. Combined treatment with octreotide or somatostatin infusion and endoscopic therapy (band ligation or sclerotherapy) is superior to either modality alone in controlling acute bleeding and early rebleeding, and it may improve survival. In patients with advanced liver disease and upper gastrointestinal hemorrhage, it is reasonable to initiate therapy with octreotide or somatostatin on admission and continue for 3–5 days if varices are confirmed by endoscopy. If bleeding is determined by endoscopy not to be secondary to portal hypertension, the infusion can be discontinued.

Terlipressin, 1–2 mg intravenously every 4 hours (not available in the United States), is a synthetic vasopressin analog that causes a significant and sustained reduction in portal and variceal pressures while preserving renal perfusion. Where available, terlipressin may be preferred to somatostatin or octreotide. Terlipressin is contraindicated in patients with significant coronary, cerebral, or peripheral vascular disease.

3. Vitamin K—In cirrhotic patients with an abnormal prothrombin time, vitamin K (10 mg intravenously) should be administered.

4. Lactulose—Encephalopathy may complicate an episode of gastrointestinal bleeding in patients with severe liver disease. In patients with encephalopathy, lactulose should be administered in a dosage of 30 mL orally every 1–2 hours until evacuation occurs then reduced to 15–45 mL/h every 8–12 hours as needed to promote two or three bowel movements daily. (See Chapter 16.)

C. Emergent Endoscopy

Emergent endoscopy is performed after the patient's hemodynamic status has been appropriately stabilized (usually within 2–12 hours). In patients with active bleeding, endotracheal intubation is commonly performed to protect against aspiration during endoscopy. An endoscopic examination is performed to exclude other or associated causes of upper gastrointestinal bleeding such as Mallory-Weiss tears, peptic ulcer disease, and portal hypertensive gastropathy. In many patients, variceal bleeding has stopped spontaneously by the time of endoscopy, and the diagnosis of variceal bleeding is made presumptively. Immediate endoscopic treatment of the varices generally is performed with banding. In clinical practice, sclerotherapy seldom is used. These techniques arrest active bleeding in 80–90% of patients and reduce the chance of in-hospital recurrent bleeding to about 20%.

If banding is chosen, repeat sessions are scheduled at intervals of 2–4 weeks until the varices are obliterated or reduced to a small size. Banding achieves lower rates of rebleeding, complications, and death than sclerotherapy and should be considered the endoscopic treatment of choice. For patients with platelet counts less than 50,000/mcL, consideration should be given to preprocedure administration of avatrombopag, an oral thrombopoietin receptor agonist approved by the FDA in 2018. In phase III clinical trials at a dose of 40–60 mg/day for 5 consecutive days beginning 10–13 days prior to endoscopy, 68% of patients with baseline platelet counts less than 40,000/mcL and 88% with baseline counts 40,000–50,000/mcL achieved platelet counts greater than 50,000/mcL and avoided periprocedural platelet transfusions.

D. Balloon Tube Tamponade

Mechanical tamponade with specially designed nasogastric tubes containing large gastric and esophageal balloons (Minnesota or Sengstaken-Blakemore tubes) provides initial control of active variceal hemorrhage in 60–90% of patients; rebleeding occurs in 50%. Given its high rate of complications, mechanical tamponade is used as a temporizing measure only in patients with bleeding that cannot be controlled with pharmacologic or endoscopic techniques until more definitive decompressive therapy (eg, TIPS) can be provided.

E. Portal Decompressive Procedures

In the 10–20% of patients with variceal bleeding that cannot be controlled with pharmacologic or endoscopic therapy, emergency portal decompression may be considered.

1. Transvenous intrahepatic portosystemic shunts (TIPS)—Over a wire that is passed through a catheter inserted in the jugular vein, an expandable wire mesh stent (8–12 mm in diameter) is passed through the liver parenchyma, creating a portosystemic shunt from the portal vein to the hepatic vein. TIPS can control acute hemorrhage in over 90% of patients actively bleeding from gastric or esophageal varices. However, when TIPS is performed in the actively bleeding patient, the mortality approaches 40%, especially in patients requiring ventilatory support or blood pressure support and patients with renal insufficiency, bilirubin greater than 3 mg/dL, or encephalopathy. Therefore, TIPS should be considered in the 10–20% of patients with acute variceal bleeding that cannot be controlled with pharmacologic and endoscopic therapy, but it may not be warranted in patients with a particularly poor prognosis.

2. Emergency portosystemic shunt surgery—Emergency portosystemic shunt surgery is associated with a 40–60% mortality rate. At centers where TIPS is available, that procedure has instead become the preferred means of providing emergency portal decompression.

▶ Prevention of Rebleeding

Once the initial bleeding episode has been controlled, therapy is warranted to reduce the high risk (60%) of rebleeding.

A. Combination Beta-Blockers and Variceal Band Ligation

Nonselective beta-adrenergic blockers (propranolol, nadolol) reduce the risk of rebleeding from esophageal varices to about 40%. Likewise, long-term treatment with band ligation reduces the incidence of rebleeding to about 30%. In most patients, two to six treatment sessions (performed at 2- to 4-week intervals) are needed to eradicate the varices.

Meta-analyses of randomized controlled trials suggest that a *combination* of band ligation plus beta-blockers is superior to either variceal band ligation alone (RR 0.68) or beta-blockers alone (RR 0.71). Therefore, combination therapy is recommended for patients without contraindications to beta-blockers. Recommended starting doses of beta-blockers are propranolol (20 mg orally twice daily), long-acting propranolol (60 mg orally once daily), or nadolol (20–40 mg orally once daily), with gradual increases in the dosage every 1–2 weeks until the heart rate falls by 25% or reaches 55–60 beats/min, provided the systolic blood pressure remains above 90 mm Hg and the patient has no side effects. The average dosage of long-acting propranolol is 120 mg once daily and for nadolol, 80 mg once daily. One-third of patients with cirrhosis are intolerant of beta-blockers, experiencing fatigue or hypotension. Drug administration at bedtime may reduce the frequency and severity of side effects.

B. Transvenous Intrahepatic Portosystemic Shunt

TIPS has resulted in a significant reduction in recurrent bleeding compared with endoscopic sclerotherapy or band ligation—either alone or in combination with beta-blocker therapy. At 1 year, rebleeding rates in patients treated with TIPS versus various endoscopic therapies average 20% and 40%, respectively. However, TIPS was also associated with a higher incidence of encephalopathy (35% vs 15%) and did not result in a decrease in mortality. Another limitation of TIPS is that stenosis and thrombosis of the stents occur in the majority of patients over time with a consequent risk of rebleeding. Therefore, periodic monitoring with Doppler ultrasonography or hepatic venography is required. Stent patency usually can be maintained by balloon angioplasty or additional stent placement. Given these problems, TIPS should be reserved for patients who have recurrent (two or more) episodes of variceal bleeding that have failed endoscopic or pharmacologic therapies. TIPS is also useful in patients with recurrent bleeding from gastric varices or portal hypertensive gastropathy (for which endoscopic therapies cannot be used). TIPS is likewise considered in patients who are noncompliant with other therapies or who live in remote locations (without access to emergency care).

C. Surgical Portosystemic Shunts

Shunt surgery has a significantly lower rate of rebleeding compared with endoscopic therapy but also a higher incidence of encephalopathy. With the advent and widespread adoption of TIPS, surgical shunts are seldom performed.

D. Liver Transplantation

Candidacy for orthotopic liver transplantation should be assessed in all patients with chronic liver disease and bleeding due to portal hypertension. Transplant candidates should be treated with band ligation or TIPS to control bleeding pretransplant.

▶ Prevention of First Episodes of Variceal Bleeding

Among patients with varices that have not previously bled, bleeding occurs in 12% of patients each year, with a lifetime risk of 30%. Because of the high mortality rate associated with variceal hemorrhage, prevention of the initial bleeding episode is desirable. Therefore, patients with cirrhosis should undergo diagnostic endoscopy or capsule endoscopy to determine whether varices are present. Varices are present in 40% of patients with Child-Pugh class A cirrhosis and in 85% with Child-Pugh class C cirrhosis. In patients without varices on screening endoscopy, a repeat endoscopy is recommended in 3 years, since varices develop in 8% of patients per year. Patients with varices have a higher risk of bleeding if they have varices larger than 5 mm, varices with red wale markings, or Child-Pugh class B or C cirrhosis. The risk of bleeding in patients with varices smaller than 5 mm is 5% per year and with large varices is 15–20% per year. Patients with small varices without red wale marks and compensated (Child-Pugh class A) cirrhosis have a low-risk of bleeding; hence, prophylaxis is unnecessary, but endoscopy should be repeated in 1–2 years to reassess size.

Nonselective beta-adrenergic blockers are recommended to reduce the risk of first variceal hemorrhage in patients with medium/large varices and patients with small varices who either have variceal red wale marks or advanced cirrhosis (Child-Pugh class B or C). (See Combination Beta-Blockers and Variceal Band Ligation, above.) Band ligation is not recommended for small varices due to technical difficulties in band application. Prophylactic band ligation may be preferred over beta-blockers for patients at higher risk for bleeding, especially patients with medium/large varices with red wale markings or with advanced cirrhosis (Child-Pugh class B or C) as well as patients with contraindications to or intolerance of beta-blockers.

▶ When to Refer

- All patients with upper gastrointestinal bleeding and suspected varices should be evaluated by a physician skilled in therapeutic endoscopy.

- Patients being considered for TIPS procedures or liver transplantation.

- Patients with cirrhosis for endoscopic evaluation for varices.

When to Admit

All patients with acute upper gastrointestinal bleeding and suspected cirrhosis should be admitted to an ICU.

Albillos A et al; Baveno Cooperation. Stratifying risk in the prevention of recurrent variceal hemorrhage: results of an individual patient meta-analysis. Hepatology. 2017 Oct;66(4):1219–31. [PMID: 28543862]

Baiges A et al. Pharmacologic prevention of variceal bleeding and rebleeding. Hepatol Int. 2018 Feb;12(Suppl 1):68–80. [PMID: 29210030]

Brunner F et al. Prevention and treatment of variceal haemorrhage in 2017. Liver Int. 2017 Jan;37(Suppl 1):104–15. [PMID: 28052623]

Ibrahim M et al. New developments in managing variceal bleeding. Gastroenterology. 2018 May;154(7):1964–9. [PMID: 29481777]

Moon AM et al. Use of antibiotics among patients with cirrhosis and upper gastrointestinal bleeding is associated with reduced mortality. Clin Gastroenterol Hepatol. 2016 Nov;14(11):1629–37. [PMID: 27311621]

Terrault N et al. Avatrombopag before procedures reduces need for platelet transfusion in patients with chronic liver disease and thrombocytopenia. Gastroenterology. 2018 Sep;155(3):705–18. [PMID: 29778606]

ESOPHAGEAL MOTILITY DISORDERS

1. Achalasia

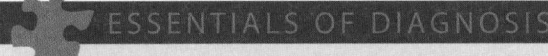

ESSENTIALS OF DIAGNOSIS

- ▶ Gradual, progressive dysphagia for solids and liquids.
- ▶ Regurgitation of undigested food.
- ▶ Barium esophagogram with "bird's beak" distal esophagus.
- ▶ Esophageal manometry confirms diagnosis.

General Considerations

Achalasia is an idiopathic motility disorder characterized by loss of peristalsis in the distal two-thirds (smooth muscle) of the esophagus and impaired relaxation of the LES. There appears to be denervation of the esophagus resulting primarily from loss of nitric oxide–producing inhibitory neurons in the myenteric plexus. The cause of the neuronal degeneration is unknown.

Clinical Findings

A. Symptoms and Signs

There is a steady increase in the incidence of achalasia with age; however, it can be seen in individuals as young as 25 years. Patients complain of the gradual onset of dysphagia for solid foods and, in the majority, of liquids also. Symptoms at presentation may have persisted for months to years. Substernal discomfort or fullness may be noted after eating. Many patients eat more slowly and adopt specific maneuvers such as lifting the neck or throwing the shoulders back to enhance esophageal emptying. Regurgitation of undigested food is common and may occur during meals or up to several hours later. Nocturnal regurgitation can provoke coughing or aspiration. Up to 50% of patients report substernal chest pain that is unrelated to meals or exercise and may last up to hours. Weight loss is common. Physical examination is unhelpful.

B. Imaging

Chest radiographs may show an air-fluid level in the enlarged, fluid-filled esophagus. Barium esophagography discloses characteristic findings, including esophageal dilation, loss of esophageal peristalsis, poor esophageal emptying, and a smooth, symmetric "bird's beak" tapering of the distal esophagus. Five minutes after ingestion of 8 oz of barium, a column height of more than 2 cm has a sensitivity and specificity of greater than 85% in differentiating achalasia from other causes of dysphagia. Without treatment, the esophagus may become markedly dilated ("sigmoid esophagus").

C. Special Examinations

After esophagography, endoscopy is always performed to evaluate the distal esophagus and gastroesophageal junction to exclude a distal stricture or a submucosal infiltrating carcinoma. The diagnosis is confirmed by esophageal manometry. The manometric features are complete absence of normal peristalsis and incomplete lower esophageal sphincteric relaxation with swallowing. Using high-resolution esophageal topographic tracings, three achalasia subtypes are recognized. Type III is a spastic variant with less favorable treatment outcomes (66%) than types I (81%) or II (96%).

Differential Diagnosis

Chagas disease is associated with esophageal dysfunction that is indistinguishable from idiopathic achalasia and should be considered in patients from endemic regions (Central and South America); it is becoming more common in the southern United States. Primary or metastatic tumors can invade the gastroesophageal junction, resulting in a picture resembling that of achalasia, called "pseudo-achalasia." Endoscopic ultrasonography and chest CT may be required to examine the distal esophagus in suspicious cases.

Treatment

A. Botulinum Toxin Injection

Endoscopically guided injection of botulinum toxin directly into the LES results in a marked reduction in LES pressure with initial improvement in symptoms in 65–85% of patients. However, symptom relapse occurs in over 50% of patients within 6–9 months and in all patients within 2 years. Because it is inferior to pneumatic dilation therapy and surgery in producing sustained symptomatic relief, this therapy is most appropriate for patients with comorbidities who are poor candidates for more invasive procedures.

B. Pneumatic Dilation

Up to 90% of patients derive good to excellent relief of dysphagia after one to three sessions of pneumatic dilation of the LES. Dilation is less effective in patients who are younger than age 45, have the type III variant, or have a dilated esophagus. Symptoms recur following pneumatic dilation in up to 35% within 10 years but usually respond to repeated dilation. Perforations occur in less than 3% of dilations and may require operative repair. The success of laparoscopic myotomy is not compromised by prior pneumatic dilation.

C. Surgery

A modified Heller cardiomyotomy of the LES and cardia results in good to excellent symptomatic improvement in over 90% of patients. Because gastroesophageal reflux develops in up to 20% of patients after myotomy, most surgeons also perform an antireflux procedure (fundoplication), and all patients are prescribed a once-daily proton pump inhibitor. Myotomy is performed with a laparoscopic approach and is preferred to the open surgical approach. Symptoms recur following cardiomyotomy in greater than 25% of cases within 10 years but usually respond to pneumatic dilation. A 2015 systematic review of nine randomized controlled trials reported treatment efficacy in 70–90% of patients treated with pneumatic dilation and 88–95% with laparoscopic myotomy. This was confirmed in a 2016 multicenter randomized trial, which found similar improvement with pneumatic dilation and Heller myotomy at 1 year. Thus, in experienced hands, the initial efficacies of pneumatic dilation and laparoscopic myotomy are nearly equivalent. Pneumatic dilation may be less effective in men younger than 45 years, so surgical myotomy may be preferred for them. Surgical myotomy may also be preferred for patients with the type III variant. Complete esophagectomy or percutaneous gastrostomy is required in 2–5% of patients in whom massive dilation of the esophagus (megaesophagus) develops despite dilation or myotomy. In megaesophagus, dysphagia, food retention, and regurgitation may decrease nutrition and quality of life and increase risk of aspiration.

D. Per Oral Endoscopic Myotomy (POEM)

Since 2011, selected, highly experienced centers in Southeast Asia and the United States have reported excellent results with a less invasive endoscopic procedure in which an endoscope is inserted into the patient's mouth and passed into the upper esophagus. After a small incision is made in the esophageal mucosa, the endoscope dissects through the submucosal space to the lower esophageal sphincter, where the circular muscle fibers of the cardia and distal esophagus are incised. In multiple uncontrolled studies involving thousands of patients, success rates of over 90% are reported, including patients with type III achalasia. Because a fundoplication is not performed, long-term antisecretory therapy for gastroesophageal reflux with a proton pump inhibitor is required in many patients. In expert centers, POEM may be the preferred treatment modality for type III achalasia (where a longer myotomy of

the distal esophagus is indicated) and an appropriate option in patients with type I and II achalasia who do not wish to have laparoscopic surgery.

Blonski W et al. Timed barium swallow: diagnostic role and predictive value in untreated achalasia, esophagogastric outflow obstruction, and non-achalasia dysphagia. Am J Gastroenterol. 2018 Feb;113(2):196–203. [PMID: 29257145]

Kahrilas PJ et al. Clinical practice update: the use of per-oral endoscopic myotomy in achalasia: expert review and best practice advice from the AGA Institute. Gastroenterology. 2017 Nov;153(5):1205–11. [PMID: 28989059]

Li QL et al. Outcomes of per-oral endoscopic myotomy for treatment of esophageal achalasia with a median follow-up of 49 months. Gastrointest Endosc. 2018 Jun;87(6):1405–12.e3. [PMID: 29108981]

Ngamruengphong S et al. Long-term outcomes of per-oral endoscopic myotomy in patients with achalasia with a minimum follow-up of 2 years: an international multicenter study. Gastrointest Endosc. 2017 May;85(5):927–33. [PMID: 27663714]

Pannala R et al. ASGE Technology Status Evaluation Report: Per-oral myotomy (with video). Gastrointest Endosc. 2016 Jun; 83(6):1051–60. [PMID: 27033144]

2. Other Primary Esophageal Motility Disorders

► Clinical Findings

A. Symptoms and Signs

Abnormalities in esophageal motility may cause dysphagia or chest pain. Dysphagia for liquids as well as solids tends to be intermittent and nonprogressive. Periods of normal swallowing may alternate with periods of dysphagia, which usually is mild though bothersome—rarely severe enough to result in significant alterations in lifestyle or weight loss. Dysphagia may be provoked by stress, large boluses of food, or hot or cold liquids. Some patients may experience anterior chest pain that may be confused with angina pectoris but usually is nonexertional. The pain generally is unrelated to eating. (See Chest Pain of Undetermined Origin, below.)

B. Diagnostic Tests

The evaluation of suspected esophageal motility disorders includes barium esophagography, upper endoscopy, and, in some cases, esophageal manometry. Barium esophagography is useful to exclude mechanical obstruction and to evaluate esophageal motility. The presence of simultaneous contractions (spasm), disordered peristalsis, or failed peristalsis supports a diagnosis of esophageal dysmotility. Upper endoscopy also is performed to exclude a mechanical obstruction (as a cause of dysphagia) and to look for evidence of erosive reflux esophagitis (a common cause of chest pain) or eosinophilic esophagitis (confirmed by esophageal biopsy). Manometry is not routinely used for mild to moderate symptoms because the findings seldom influence further medical management, but it may be useful in patients with persistent, disabling dysphagia to exclude achalasia and to look for other disorders of esophageal motility. These include diffuse esophageal spasm, hypercontractile ("jackhammer") esophagus, esophagogastric junction outflow obstruction, and findings of ineffective esophageal peristalsis (failed or weak esophageal peristalsis). The further evaluation of noncardiac chest pain is discussed below.

▶ Treatment

For patients with mild symptoms of dysphagia, therapy is directed at symptom reduction and reassurance. Patients should be instructed to eat more slowly and take smaller bites of food. In some cases, a warm liquid at the start of a meal may facilitate swallowing. Because unrecognized gastroesophageal reflux may cause dysphagia, a trial of a proton pump inhibitor (esomeprazole 40 mg, lansoprazole 30 mg) orally twice daily should be administered for 4–8 weeks. Treatment of patients with severe dysphagia is empiric. Suspected spastic disorders may be treated with (1) smooth muscle relaxants (isosorbide [10–20 mg four times daily] or nitroglycerin [0.4 mg sublingually as needed]); (2) calcium channel blockers (nifedipine [10 mg] or diltiazem [60–90 mg] 30–45 minutes before meals); (3) phosphodiesterase type 5 inhibitors (eg, sildenafil); (4) botulinum toxin injection into the lower esophagus; or (5) POEM. Esophageal dilation provides symptomatic relief in some cases.

Kahrilas PJ et al. Advances in management of esophageal motility disorders. Clin Gastroenterol Hepatol. 2018 Nov;16(11): 1692–700. [PMID: 29702296]

Khalaf M et al. Distal esophageal spasm: a review. Am J Med. 2018 Sep;131(9):1034–40. [PMID: 29605413]

Khan MA et al. Is POEM the answer for management of spastic esophageal disorders? A systematic review and meta-analysis. Dig Dis Sci. 2017 Jan;62(1):35–44. [PMID: 27858325]

Rohof WOA et al. Chicago Classification of esophageal motility disorders: lessons learned. Curr Gastroenterol Rep. 2017 Aug; 19(8):37. [PMID: 28730503]

CHEST PAIN OF UNDETERMINED ORIGIN

One-third of patients with chest pain undergo negative cardiac evaluation. Patients with recurrent noncardiac chest pain thus pose a difficult clinical problem. Because coronary artery disease is common and can present atypically, it must be excluded prior to evaluation for other causes.

Causes of noncardiac chest pain may include the following.

A. Chest Wall and Thoracic Spine Disease

These are easily diagnosed by history and physical examination.

B. Gastroesophageal Reflux

Up to 50% of patients have increased amounts of gastroesophageal acid reflux or a correlation between acid reflux episodes and chest pain demonstrated on esophageal pH testing. An empiric 4-week trial of acid-suppressive therapy with a high-dose proton pump inhibitor is recommended (eg, omeprazole or rabeprazole, 40 mg orally twice daily; lansoprazole, 30–60 mg orally twice daily; or esomeprazole or pantoprazole, 40 mg orally twice daily), especially in patients with reflux symptoms. In patients with

persistent symptoms, ambulatory esophageal pH or impedance and pH study may be useful to exclude definitively a relationship between acid and nonacid reflux episodes and chest pain events.

C. Esophageal Dysmotility

Esophageal motility abnormalities such as diffuse esophageal spasm or hypercontractile swallow ("jackhammer esophagus") are uncommon causes of noncardiac chest pain. In patients with chest pain and dysphagia, a barium swallow radiograph should be obtained to look for evidence of achalasia or diffuse esophageal spasm. Esophageal manometry is not routinely performed because of low specificity and the unlikelihood of finding a clinically significant disorder, but it may be recommended in patients with frequent symptoms.

D. Heightened Visceral Sensitivity

Some patients with noncardiac chest pain report pain in response to a variety of minor noxious stimuli such as physiologically normal amounts of acid reflux, inflation of balloons within the esophageal lumen, injection of intravenous edrophonium (a cholinergic stimulus), or intracardiac catheter manipulation. Low doses of oral antidepressants such as trazodone 50 mg or imipramine 10–50 mg reduce chest pain symptoms and are thought to reduce visceral afferent awareness. In a 2010 controlled crossover trial, over 50% of patients treated with venlafaxine, 75 mg once daily at bedtime, achieved symptomatic improvement compared with only 4% treated with placebo.

E. Psychological Disorders

A significant number of patients have underlying depression, anxiety, and panic disorder. Patients reporting dyspnea, sweating, tachycardia, suffocation, or fear of dying should be evaluated for panic disorder.

Viazis N et al. Proton pump inhibitor and selective serotonin reuptake inhibitor therapy for the management of noncardiac chest pain. Eur J Gastroenterol Hepatol. 2017 Sep;29(9):1054–8. [PMID: 28628496]

Yamasaki T et al. Noncardiac chest pain: diagnosis and management. Curr Opin Gastroenterol. 2017 Jul;33(4):293–300. [PMID: 28463855]

▼ DISEASES OF THE STOMACH & DUODENUM

(See Chapter 39 for Gastric Cancers.)

GASTRITIS & GASTROPATHY

The term "gastropathy" should be used to denote conditions in which there is epithelial or endothelial damage without inflammation, and "gastritis" should be used to denote conditions in which there is histologic evidence of inflammation. In clinical practice, the term "gastritis" is commonly applied to three categories: (1) erosive and hemorrhagic "gastritis" (gastropathy); (2) nonerosive, nonspecific (histologic) gastritis; and (3) specific types of gastritis, characterized by distinctive histologic and endoscopic features diagnostic of specific disorders.

1. Erosive & Hemorrhagic "Gastritis" (Gastropathy)

> ### ESSENTIALS OF DIAGNOSIS
>
> ▶ Most commonly seen in alcoholic or critically ill patients, or patients taking NSAIDs.
>
> ▶ Often asymptomatic; may cause epigastric pain, nausea, and vomiting.
>
> ▶ May cause hematemesis; usually insignificant bleeding.

General Considerations

The most common causes of erosive gastropathy are medications (especially NSAIDs), alcohol, stress due to severe medical or surgical illness, and portal hypertension ("portal gastropathy"). Major risk factors for stress gastritis include mechanical ventilation, coagulopathy, trauma, burns, shock, sepsis, central nervous system injury, liver failure, kidney disease, and multiorgan failure. The use of enteral nutrition reduces the risk of stress-related bleeding. Uncommon causes of erosive gastropathy include ischemia, caustic ingestion, and radiation. Erosive and hemorrhagic gastropathy typically are diagnosed at endoscopy, often being performed because of dyspepsia or upper gastrointestinal bleeding. Endoscopic findings include subepithelial hemorrhages, petechiae, and erosions. These lesions are superficial, vary in size and number, and may be focal or diffuse. There usually is no significant inflammation on histologic examination.

Clinical Findings

A. Symptoms and Signs

Erosive gastropathy is usually asymptomatic. Symptoms, when they occur, include anorexia, epigastric pain, nausea, and vomiting. There is poor correlation between symptoms and the number or severity of endoscopic abnormalities. The most common clinical manifestation of erosive gastritis is upper gastrointestinal bleeding, which presents as hematemesis, "coffee grounds" emesis, or bloody aspirate in a patient receiving nasogastric suction, or as melena. Because erosive gastritis is superficial, hemodynamically significant bleeding is rare.

B. Laboratory Findings

The laboratory findings are nonspecific. The hematocrit is low if significant bleeding has occurred; iron deficiency may be found.

C. Special Examinations

Upper endoscopy is the most sensitive method of diagnosis. Although bleeding from gastritis is usually insignificant, it cannot be distinguished on clinical grounds from more serious lesions such as peptic ulcers or esophageal varices. Hence, endoscopy is generally performed within 24 hours in patients with upper gastrointestinal bleeding to identify the source. An upper gastrointestinal series is sometimes obtained in lieu of endoscopy in patients with hemodynamically insignificant upper gastrointestinal bleeds to exclude serious (eg, mass) lesions but is insensitive for the detection of gastritis.

Differential Diagnosis

Epigastric pain may be due to peptic ulcer, gastroesophageal reflux, gastric cancer, biliary tract disease, food poisoning, viral gastroenteritis, and functional dyspepsia. With severe pain, one should consider a perforated or penetrating ulcer, pancreatic disease, esophageal rupture, ruptured aortic aneurysm, gastric volvulus, gastrointestinal ischemia, and myocardial ischemia. Causes of upper gastrointestinal bleeding include peptic ulcer disease, esophageal varices, Mallory-Weiss tear, and angioectasias.

Specific Causes & Treatment

A. Stress Gastritis

1. Prophylaxis—Stress-related mucosal erosions and subepithelial hemorrhages may develop within 72 hours in critically ill patients. Clinically overt bleeding occurs in 6% of ICU patients, but clinically important bleeding in less than 1.5%. Bleeding is associated with a higher mortality rate but is seldom the cause of death. Two of the most important risk factors for bleeding are coagulopathy (platelets less than 50,000/mcL or INR greater than 1.5) and respiratory failure with the need for mechanical ventilation for over 48 hours. When these two risk factors are absent, the risk of significant bleeding is only 0.1%. Other risk factors include traumatic brain injury, severe burns, sepsis, vasopressor therapy, corticosteroid therapy, and prior history of peptic ulcer disease and gastrointestinal bleeding. Early enteral tube feeding may decrease the risk of significant bleeding.

Prophylaxis should be routinely administered to critically ill patients with risk factors for significant bleeding upon admission. Prophylactic suppression of gastric acid with H_2-receptor antagonists (intravenous) or proton pump inhibitors (oral or intravenous) has been shown to reduce the incidence of clinically overt and significant bleeding but may increase the risk of nosocomial pneumonia. A 2016 meta-analysis of 19 randomized trials found that oral and intravenous proton pump inhibitors were superior to H_2-receptor antagonists in reducing the risk of overt bleeding (RR 0.48) and clinically important bleeding (RR 0.36) but did not affect the risk of pneumonia, length of ICU stay, or mortality. In a 2018 large randomized, placebo-controlled trial of ICU patients with increased risk of GI bleeding, patients who received intravenous pantoprazole, 40 mg/day, had a lower risk of clinically important GI bleeding (2.5%) compared with placebo (4.2%) but no difference in the incidence of pneumonia, *C difficile* infection, or myocardial infarction.

The optimal, cost-effective prophylactic regimen remains uncertain, hence clinical practices vary. For patients with nasoenteric tubes, immediate-release omeprazole (40 mg at 1 and 6 hours on day 1; then 40 mg once daily beginning on day 2) may be preferred because of lower cost and ease of administration. For patients requiring intravenous administration, continuous intravenous infusions of H_2-receptor antagonists provide adequate control of intragastric pH in most patients in the following doses over 24 hours: cimetidine (900–1200 mg), ranitidine (150 mg), or famotidine (20 mg). Alternatively, intravenous proton pump inhibitors, although more expensive, may be preferred due to superior efficacy. The optimal dosing of intravenous proton pump inhibitors is uncertain; however, in clinical trials pantoprazole doses ranging from 40 mg to 80 mg and administered every 8–24 hours appear equally effective.

2. Treatment—Once bleeding occurs, patients should receive continuous infusions of a proton pump inhibitor (esomeprazole or pantoprazole, 80 mg intravenous bolus, followed by 8 mg/h continuous infusion) as well as sucralfate suspension, 1 g orally every 4 to 6 hours. Endoscopy should be performed in patients with clinically significant bleeding to look for treatable causes, especially stress-related peptic ulcers with active bleeding or visible vessels. When bleeding arises from diffuse gastritis, endoscopic hemostasis techniques are not helpful.

B. NSAID Gastritis

Of patients receiving NSAIDs in clinical trials, 25–50% have gastritis and 10–20% have ulcers at endoscopy; however, symptoms of significant dyspepsia develop in about 5%. NSAIDs that are more selective for the cyclooxygenase (COX)-2 enzyme ("coxibs"), such as celecoxib, etodolac, and meloxicam, decrease the incidence of endoscopically visible ulcers by approximately 75% and significant ulcer complications by up to 50% compared with nonselective NSAIDs (nsNSAIDs). However, a twofold increase in the incidence in cardiovascular complications (myocardial infarction, cerebrovascular infarction, and death) in patients taking coxibs compared with placebo led to the withdrawal of two highly selective coxibs (rofecoxib and valdecoxib) from the market by the manufacturers. Celecoxib and all currently available nsNSAIDs (with notable exception of aspirin and possibly naproxen) are associated with increased risk of cardiovascular complications and therefore should be used with caution in patients with cardiovascular risk factors.

In population surveys, the rate of dyspepsia is increased 1.5- to 2-fold with nsNSAID and coxib use. However, dyspeptic symptoms correlate poorly with significant mucosal abnormalities or the development of adverse clinical events (ulcer bleeding or perforation). Given the frequency of dyspeptic symptoms in patients taking NSAIDs, it is neither feasible nor desirable to investigate all such cases. Patients with alarm symptoms or signs, such as severe pain, weight loss, vomiting, gastrointestinal bleeding, or anemia, should undergo diagnostic upper endoscopy. For other patients, symptoms may improve with discontinuation of the agent, reduction to the lowest effective dose, or administration with meals. Proton pump inhibitors have demonstrated efficacy in controlled trials for the treatment of NSAID-related dyspepsia and superiority to H_2-receptor antagonists for healing of NSAID-related ulcers even in the setting of continued NSAID use. Therefore, an empiric 2- to 4-week trial of an oral proton pump inhibitor (omeprazole, rabeprazole, or esomeprazole 20–40 mg/day; lansoprazole or dexlansoprazole, 30 mg/day; pantoprazole, 40 mg/day) is recommended for patients with NSAID-related dyspepsia, especially those in whom continued NSAID treatment is required. If symptoms do not improve, diagnostic upper endoscopy should be conducted.

C. Alcoholic Gastritis

Excessive alcohol consumption may lead to dyspepsia, nausea, emesis, and minor hematemesis—a condition sometimes labeled "alcoholic gastritis." However, it is not proven that alcohol alone actually causes significant erosive gastritis. Therapy with H_2-receptor antagonists, proton pump inhibitors, or sucralfate for 2–4 weeks often is empirically prescribed.

D. Portal Hypertensive Gastropathy

Portal hypertension commonly results in gastric mucosal and submucosal congestion of capillaries and venules, which is correlated with the severity of the portal hypertension and underlying liver disease. Usually asymptomatic, it may cause chronic gastrointestinal bleeding in 10% of patients and, less commonly, clinically significant bleeding with hematemesis. Treatment with propranolol or nadolol reduces the incidence of recurrent acute bleeding by lowering portal pressures. Patients who fail propranolol therapy may be successfully treated with portal decompressive procedures (see section above on treatment of esophageal varices).

Alshamsi F et al. Efficacy and safety of proton pump inhibitors for stress ulcer prophylaxis in critically ill patients: a systematic review and meta-analysis of randomized trials. Crit Care. 2016 May 4;20(1):120. [PMID: 27142116]
Krag M et al; SUP-ICU trial group. Pantoprazole in patients at risk for gastrointestinal bleeding in the ICU. N Engl J Med. 2018 Dec 6;379(23):2199–208. [PMID: 30354950]

2. Nonerosive, Nonspecific Gastritis

The diagnosis of nonerosive gastritis is based on histologic assessment of mucosal biopsies. Endoscopic findings are normal in many cases and do not reliably predict the presence of histologic inflammation. The main types of nonerosive gastritis are those due to *H pylori* infection, those associated with pernicious anemia, and eosinophilic gastritis. (See Specific Types of Gastritis below.)

A. *Helicobacter pylori* Gastritis

H pylori is a spiral gram-negative rod that resides beneath the gastric mucous layer adjacent to gastric epithelial cells. Although not invasive, it causes gastric mucosal inflammation with PMNs and lymphocytes.

In developed countries, the prevalence of *H pylori* is rapidly declining. In the United States, the prevalence rises from less than 10% in non-immigrants under age 30 years to over 50% in those over age 60 years. The prevalence is higher in non-whites and immigrants from developing countries and is correlated inversely with socioeconomic status. Transmission is from person to person, mainly during infancy and childhood; however, the mode of transmission is unknown.

Acute infection with *H pylori* may cause a transient clinical illness characterized by nausea and abdominal pain that may last for several days and is associated with acute histologic gastritis with PMNs. After these symptoms resolve, the majority progress to chronic infection with chronic, diffuse mucosal inflammation (gastritis) characterized by PMNs and lymphocytes. Although chronic *H pylori* infection with gastritis is present in 30–50% of the population, most persons are asymptomatic and suffer no sequelae. Three gastritis phenotypes occur which determine clinical outcomes. Most infected people have a mild, diffuse gastritis that does not disrupt acid secretion and seldom causes clinically important outcomes. About 15% of infected people have inflammation that predominates in the gastric antrum but spares the gastric body (where acid is secreted). People with this phenotype tend to have increased gastrin; increased acid production; and increased risk of developing peptic ulcers, especially duodenal ulcers. An even smaller subset of infected adults has inflammation that predominates in the gastric body. Over time, this may lead to destruction of acid-secreting glands with resultant mucosal atrophy, decreased acid secretion, and intestinal metaplasia. This phenotype is associated with an increased risk of gastric ulcers and gastric cancer. Long-term treatment with proton pump inhibitors can potentiate the development of *H pylori*–associated atrophic gastritis. Chronic *H pylori* gastritis leads to the development of duodenal or gastric ulcers in up to 10%, gastric cancer in 0.1–3%, and low-grade B cell gastric lymphoma (mucosa-associated lymphoid tissue lymphoma; MALToma) in less than 0.01%.

Eradication of *H pylori* may be achieved with antibiotics in over 85% of patients and leads to resolution of the chronic gastritis (see section on Peptic Ulcer Disease). Testing for *H pylori* is indicated for patients with either active or a past history of documented peptic ulcer disease, gastric MALToma, and a personal or family history of gastric carcinoma. Testing and empiric treatment are cost-effective in young patients (less than 60 years of age) with uncomplicated dyspepsia prior to further medical evaluation. Testing for and treating *H pylori* in patients with functional dyspepsia is generally recommended (see Dyspepsia, above). In addition, testing for (and, if positive, treating) *H pylori* infection is recommended in patients taking low-dose aspirin or NSAIDs long-term to reduce the risk of ulcer-related bleeding. Some groups recommend population-based screening of all asymptomatic persons in regions in which there is a high prevalence of *H pylori* and gastric cancer (such as Japan, Korea, and China) to reduce the incidence of gastric cancer. Population-based screening of asymptomatic individuals is not recommended in western countries, in which the incidence of gastric cancer is low, but should be considered in immigrants from high-prevalence regions.

1. Noninvasive testing for *H pylori*—Although serologic tests are easily obtained and widely available, clinical guidelines no longer endorse their use for testing for *H pylori* infection because they are less accurate than other noninvasive tests that measure active infection. Laboratory-based quantitative serologic ELISA tests have an overall accuracy of only 80%. In comparison, the fecal antigen immunoassay and [^{13}C] urea breath test have excellent sensitivity and specificity (greater than 95%) at a cost of less than $60. Although more expensive and cumbersome to perform, these tests of active infection are more cost-effective in most clinical settings because they reduce unnecessary treatment for patients without active infection.

Recent proton pump inhibitors or antibiotics significantly reduce the sensitivity of urea breath tests and fecal antigen assays (but not serologic tests). Prior to testing, proton pump inhibitors should be discontinued for 7–14 days and antibiotics for at least 28 days.

2. Endoscopic testing for *H pylori*—Endoscopy is not indicated to diagnose *H pylori* infection in most circumstances. However, when it is performed for another reason, gastric biopsy specimens can be obtained for detection of *H pylori* and tested for active infection by urease production. Histologic assessment of biopsies from the gastric antrum and body is more definitive but more expensive ($150–$250) than a rapid urease test. Histologic assessment is also indicated in patients with suspected MALTomas and, possibly, in patients with suspected infection whose rapid urease test is negative.

Chey WD et al. ACG Clinical Guideline: treatment of *Helicobacter pylori*. Am J Gastroenterol. 2017 Feb;112(2):212–39. [PMID: 28071659]
Sjomina O et al. Epidemiology of *Helicobacter pylori* infection. Helicobacter. 2018 Sep;23(Suppl 1):e12518. [PMID: 30203587]
Skrebinska S et al. Diagnosis of *Helicobacter pylori* infection. Helicobacter. 2018 Sep;23(Suppl 1):e12515. [PMID: 30203584]

B. Pernicious Anemia Gastritis

Pernicious anemia gastritis is a rare autoimmune disorder involving the fundic glands with resultant achlorhydria, decreased intrinsic factor secretion, and vitamin B_{12} malabsorption. Of patients with B_{12} deficiency, a small number have pernicious anemia. Most patients have malabsorption secondary to chronic *H pylori* infection that results in atrophic gastritis, small intestine bacterial overgrowth, or dietary insufficiency. Fundic histology in pernicious anemia is characterized by severe gland atrophy and intestinal metaplasia caused by autoimmune destruction of the gastric fundic mucosa. Anti-intrinsic factor antibodies are present in 70% of patients. Achlorhydria leads to pronounced hypergastrinemia (greater than 1000 pg/mL) due to loss of acid inhibition of gastrin G cells. Hypergastrinemia may induce hyperplasia of gastric enterochromaffin-like cells that may lead to the development of small, multicentric carcinoid tumors in 5% of patients. Metastatic spread is uncommon in lesions smaller than 2 cm. The risk of gastric adenocarcinoma is increased threefold, with a prevalence of 1–3%. Endoscopy with biopsy is indicated in patients with pernicious anemia at the time of diagnosis.

Patients with extensive atrophy and metaplasia involving the antrum and body, dysplasia or small carcinoids require periodic endoscopic surveillance. Pernicious anemia is discussed in detail in Chapter 13.

Minalyan A et al. Autoimmune atrophic gastritis: current perspectives. Clin Exp Gastroenterol. 2017 Feb 7;10:19–27. [PMID: 28223833]
Rusak E et al. Anti-parietal cell antibodies—diagnostic significance. Adv Med Sci. 2016 Jan 13;61(2):175–9. [PMID: 26918709]

3. Specific Types of Gastritis

▶ Infections

Acute bacterial infection of the gastric submucosa and muscularis with a variety of aerobic or anaerobic organisms produces a rare, rapidly progressive, life-threatening condition known as phlegmonous or necrotizing gastritis, which requires broad-spectrum antibiotic therapy and, in many cases, emergency gastric resection. Viral infection with CMV is seen in patients with AIDS and after bone marrow or solid organ transplantation. Endoscopic findings include thickened gastric folds and ulcerations. Fungal infection with mucormycosis and *Candida* may occur in immunocompromised and diabetic patients. Larvae of *Anisakis marina* ingested in raw fish or sushi may become embedded in the gastric mucosa, producing severe abdominal pain. Pain persists for several days until the larvae die. Endoscopic removal of the larvae provides rapid symptomatic relief.

PEPTIC ULCER DISEASE

🧩 ESSENTIALS OF DIAGNOSIS

- ▶ History of dyspepsia present in 80–90% of patients with variable relationship to meals.
- ▶ Ulcer symptoms characterized by rhythmicity and periodicity.
- ▶ Ulcer complications present without antecedent symptoms in 10–20% of patients.
- ▶ Most NSAID-induced ulcers are asymptomatic.
- ▶ Upper endoscopy with gastric biopsy for *H pylori* is the diagnostic procedure of choice in most patients.
- ▶ Gastric ulcer biopsy or documentation of complete healing necessary to exclude gastric malignancy.

▶ General Considerations

Peptic ulcer is a break in the gastric or duodenal mucosa that arises when the normal mucosal defensive factors are impaired or are overwhelmed by aggressive luminal factors such as acid and pepsin. By definition, ulcers extend through the muscularis mucosae and are usually over 5 mm in diameter. In the United States, there are about 500,000 new cases per year of peptic ulcer and 4 million ulcer recurrences; the lifetime prevalence of ulcers in the adult population is approximately 10%. Ulcers occur either in the duodenum, where over 95% are in the bulb or pyloric channel, or in the stomach, where benign ulcers are located most commonly in the antrum (60%) or at the junction of the antrum and body on the lesser curvature (25%).

Although ulcers can occur in any age group, duodenal ulcers most commonly occur in patients between the ages of 30 and 55 years, whereas gastric ulcers are more common in patients between the ages of 55 and 70 years. The incidence of duodenal ulcer disease has been declining dramatically for the past 30 years (due to the eradication of *H pylori*), but the incidence of gastric ulcers has not been declining (due to the widespread use of NSAIDs and low-dose aspirin).

▶ Etiology

There are two major causes of peptic ulcer disease: NSAIDs and chronic *H pylori* infection. Evidence of *H pylori* infection or NSAID ingestion should be sought in all patients with peptic ulcer. Alcohol, dietary factors, and stress do not appear to cause ulcer disease. Less than 5–10% of ulcers are caused by other conditions, including acid hypersecretory states (such as Zollinger-Ellison syndrome or systemic mastocytosis), CMV (especially in transplant recipients), Crohn disease, lymphoma, medications (eg, alendronate), or chronic medical illness (cirrhosis or chronic kidney disease), or are idiopathic. NSAID-induced and *H pylori*–associated ulcers will be presented in this section; Zollinger-Ellison syndrome will be discussed subsequently.

A. *H pylori*–Associated Ulcers

H pylori infection with associated gastritis and, in some cases, duodenitis appears to be a necessary cofactor for the majority of duodenal and gastric ulcers not associated with NSAIDs. Ulcer disease will develop in an estimated 10% of infected patients. The prevalence of *H pylori* infection in duodenal ulcer patients is 70–90%. The association with gastric ulcers is lower, but *H pylori* is found in most patients in whom NSAIDs cannot be implicated.

The natural history of *H pylori*–associated peptic ulcer disease is well defined. In the absence of specific antibiotic treatment to eradicate the organism, 85% of patients will have an endoscopically visible recurrence within 1 year. Half of these will be symptomatic. After successful eradication of *H pylori* with antibiotics, ulcer recurrence rates are reduced dramatically to 5–20% at 1 year. Most of these ulcer recurrences are due to NSAID use or, rarely, reinfection with *H pylori*.

B. NSAID-Induced Ulcers

There is a 10–20% prevalence of gastric ulcers and a 2–5% prevalence of duodenal ulcers in long-term NSAID users. Approximately 2–5%/year of long-term NSAID users will have an ulcer that causes clinically significant dyspepsia or a serious complication. The incidence of serious gastrointestinal complications (hospitalization, bleeding, perforation) is 0.2–1.9%/year. Meta-analyses of clinical trials detected an increased risk of upper gastrointestinal bleeding in patients taking low-dose aspirin (1 of 1000), coxibs (2 of 1000), and nsNSAIDs (4–6 of 1000). The risk of NSAID complications is greater within the first 3 months of therapy and in patients who are older than 60 years; who have a prior history of ulcer disease; or who take NSAIDs in combination with aspirin, corticosteroids, or anticoagulants.

Traditional nsNSAIDs inhibit prostaglandins through reversible inhibition of both COX-1 and COX-2 enzymes. Aspirin causes irreversible inhibition of COX-1 and COX-2 as well as of platelet aggregation. Coxibs (or selective NSAIDs) preferentially inhibit COX-2—the principal enzyme involved in prostaglandin production at sites of inflammation—while providing relative sparing of COX-1, the principal enzyme involved with mucosal cytoprotection in the stomach and duodenum. Celecoxib is the only coxib currently available in the United States, although other older NSAIDs (etodolac, meloxicam) may have similar COX-2/COX-1 selectivity.

Coxibs decrease the incidence of endoscopically visible ulcers by approximately 75% compared with nsNSAIDs. Of greater clinical importance, the risk of significant clinical events (obstruction, perforation, bleeding) is reduced by up to 50% in patients taking coxibs versus nsNSAIDs. However, a twofold increase in the incidence in cardiovascular complications (myocardial infarction, cerebrovascular infarction, and death) has been detected in patients taking coxibs compared with placebo, prompting the voluntary withdrawal of two highly selective coxibs (rofecoxib and valdecoxib) from the market by the manufacturers. A review by an FDA panel suggested that all NSAIDs (other than aspirin and, possibly, naproxen) may be associated with an increased risk of cardiovascular complications, but concluded that celecoxib, which has less COX-2 selectivity than rofecoxib and valdecoxib, does not have higher risk than other nsNSAIDs when used in currently recommended doses (200 mg/day). In 2016, a large, randomized, noninferiority trial comparing ibuprofen, naproxen, and celecoxib in arthritis patients with increased cardiovascular risk found no difference in cardiovascular safety between the three drugs over 3 years. However, celecoxib was associated with significantly fewer serious gastrointestinal events than both naproxen (hazard ratio 0.71) and ibuprofen (hazard ratio 0.65).

Use of even low-dose aspirin (81–325 mg/day) leads to a twofold increased risk of gastrointestinal bleeding complications. In randomized controlled trials, the absolute annual increase of gastrointestinal bleeding attributable to low-dose aspirin is only 0.12% higher than with placebo therapy. However, in population studies, gastrointestinal bleeding occurs in 1.2% of patients each year. Patients with a prior history of peptic ulcers or gastrointestinal bleeding have a markedly increased risk of complications on low-dose aspirin. It should be noted that low-dose aspirin in combination with NSAIDs or coxibs increases the risk of ulcer complications by up to tenfold compared with NSAIDs or low-dose aspirin alone. Dual antiplatelet therapy with aspirin and a thienopyridine (eg, clopidogrel) incurs a twofold to threefold increased risk of bleeding compared with aspirin alone.

H pylori infection increases the risk of ulcer disease and complications over threefold in patients taking NSAIDs or low-dose aspirin. It is hypothesized that NSAID initiation may potentiate or aggravate ulcer disease in susceptible infected individuals.

► **Clinical Findings**

A. Symptoms and Signs

Epigastric pain (dyspepsia), the hallmark of peptic ulcer disease, is present in 80–90% of patients. However, this complaint is not sensitive or specific enough to serve as a reliable diagnostic criterion for peptic ulcer disease. The clinical history cannot accurately distinguish duodenal from gastric ulcers. Less than 25% of patients with dyspepsia have ulcer disease at endoscopy. Twenty percent of patients with ulcer complications such as bleeding have no antecedent symptoms ("silent ulcers"). Nearly 60% of patients with NSAID-related ulcer complications do not have prior symptoms.

Pain is typically well localized to the epigastrium and not severe. It is described as gnawing, dull, aching, or "hunger-like." Approximately 50% of patients report relief of pain with food or antacids (especially those with duodenal ulcers) and a recurrence of pain 2–4 hours later. However, many patients deny any relationship to meals or report worsening of pain. Two-thirds of duodenal ulcers and one-third of gastric ulcers cause nocturnal pain that awakens the patient. A change from a patient's typical rhythmic discomfort to constant or radiating pain may reflect ulcer penetration or perforation. Most patients have symptomatic periods lasting up to several weeks with intervals of months to years in which they are pain free (periodicity).

Nausea and anorexia may occur with gastric ulcers. Significant vomiting and weight loss are unusual with uncomplicated ulcer disease and suggest gastric outlet obstruction or gastric malignancy.

The physical examination is often normal in uncomplicated peptic ulcer disease. Mild, localized epigastric tenderness to deep palpation may be present. FOBT or FIT is positive in one-third of patients.

B. Laboratory Findings

Laboratory tests are normal in uncomplicated peptic ulcer disease but are ordered to exclude ulcer complications or confounding disease entities. Anemia may occur with acute blood loss from a bleeding ulcer or less commonly from chronic blood loss. Leukocytosis suggests ulcer penetration or perforation. An elevated serum amylase in a patient with severe epigastric pain suggests ulcer penetration into the pancreas. A fasting serum gastrin level to screen for Zollinger-Ellison syndrome is obtained in some patients.

C. Endoscopy

Upper endoscopy is the procedure of choice for the diagnosis of duodenal and gastric ulcers. Duodenal ulcers are virtually never malignant and do not require biopsy. Three to 5 percent of benign-appearing gastric ulcers prove to be malignant. Hence, biopsies of the ulcer margin are almost always performed. Provided that the gastric ulcer appears benign to the endoscopist and adequate biopsy specimens reveal no evidence of cancer, dysplasia, or atypia, the patient may be monitored without further endoscopy. If these conditions are not fulfilled, follow-up endoscopy should be performed 12 weeks after the start of therapy to document complete healing; nonhealing ulcers are suspicious for malignancy.

D. Imaging

Barium upper gastrointestinal series is no longer recommended because it is less sensitive for detection of ulcers and less accurate for distinguishing benign from malignant ulcers than upper endoscopy. Abdominal CT imaging is obtained in patients with suspected complications of peptic ulcer disease (perforation, penetration, or obstruction).

E. Testing for *H pylori*

In patients in whom an ulcer is diagnosed by endoscopy, gastric mucosal biopsies should be obtained both for a rapid urease test and for histologic examination. The specimens for histology are discarded if the urease test is positive.

Noninvasive assessment for *H pylori* with fecal antigen assay or urea breath testing may be done in patients with a history of peptic ulcer disease to diagnose active infection or in patients following its treatment to confirm successful eradication. Both tests have a sensitivity and specificity of 95%. Proton pump inhibitors may cause false-negative urea breath tests and fecal antigen tests and should be withheld for at least 14 days before testing. Because of its lower sensitivity (85%) and specificity (79%), serologic testing should not be performed unless fecal antigen testing or urea breath testing is unavailable.

▶ Differential Diagnosis

Peptic ulcer disease must be distinguished from other causes of epigastric distress (dyspepsia). Over 50% of patients with dyspepsia have no obvious organic explanation for their symptoms and are classified as having functional dyspepsia (see sections above on Dyspepsia and Functional Dyspepsia). Atypical gastroesophageal reflux may be manifested by epigastric symptoms. Biliary tract disease is characterized by discrete, intermittent episodes of pain that should not be confused with other causes of dyspepsia. Severe epigastric pain is atypical for peptic ulcer disease unless complicated by a perforation or penetration. Other causes include acute pancreatitis, acute cholecystitis or choledocholithiasis, esophageal rupture, gastric volvulus, gastric or intestinal ischemia, and ruptured aortic aneurysm.

▶ Pharmacologic Agents

The pharmacology and use of several agents that enhance the healing of peptic ulcers are briefly discussed here. They may be divided into three categories: (1) acid-antisecretory agents, (2) mucosal protective agents, and (3) agents that promote healing through eradication of *H pylori*.

A. Acid-Antisecretory Agents

1. Proton pump inhibitors—Proton pump inhibitors covalently bind the acid-secreting enzyme H^+-K^+-ATPase, or "proton pump," permanently inactivating it. Restoration of acid secretion requires synthesis of new pumps, which have a half-life of 18 hours. Thus, although these agents have a serum half-life of less than 60 minutes, their duration of action exceeds 24 hours.

There are six oral proton pump inhibitors currently available: omeprazole, rabeprazole, esomeprazole, lansoprazole, dexlansoprazole, and pantoprazole. The available oral agents inhibit over 90% of 24-hour acid secretion, compared with under 65% for H_2-receptor antagonists in standard dosages. Despite minor differences in their pharmacology, they are equally efficacious in the treatment of peptic ulcer disease. Treatment with oral proton pump inhibitors results in over 90% healing of duodenal ulcers after 4 weeks and 90% of gastric ulcers after 8 weeks when given once daily (30 minutes before breakfast) at the following recommended doses: omeprazole, 20–40 mg; esomeprazole, 40 mg; rabeprazole, 20 mg; lansoprazole, 30 mg; dexlansoprazole, 30–60 mg; and pantoprazole, 40 mg. Compared with H_2-receptor antagonists, proton pump inhibitors provide faster pain relief and more rapid ulcer healing.

The proton pump inhibitors are remarkably safe for short-term therapy. Long-term use may lead to mild decreases in vitamin B_{12}, iron, magnesium, and calcium absorption. Observational studies suggest increased risks of enteric infections, including *C difficile* and bacterial gastroenteritis; pneumonia; and an increased risk of hip fracture (a 1.4-fold increase). Recent observational studies also report small increased risks of acute and chronic kidney disease (due to interstitial nephritis) and dementia; however, causality has not been demonstrated. Nonetheless, long-term proton pump inhibitor therapy should be prescribed only for patients with appropriate indications. Serum gastrin levels rise significantly in 3% of patients receiving long-term therapy but return to normal limits within 2 weeks after discontinuation.

2. H_2-receptor antagonists—Although H_2-receptor antagonists are effective in the treatment of peptic ulcer disease, proton pump inhibitors are now the preferred agents because of their ease of use and superior efficacy. Four H_2-receptor antagonists are available: cimetidine, ranitidine, famotidine, and nizatidine. For uncomplicated peptic ulcers, H_2-receptor antagonists may be administered once daily at bedtime as follows: ranitidine and nizatidine 300 mg, famotidine 40 mg, and cimetidine 800 mg. Duodenal and gastric ulcer healing rates of 85–90% are obtained within 6 weeks and 8 weeks, respectively.

B. Agents Enhancing Mucosal Defenses

Bismuth sucralfate, misoprostol, and antacids all have been shown to promote ulcer healing through the enhancement of mucosal defensive mechanisms. Given the greater efficacy and safety of antisecretory agents and better compliance of patients, these agents are no longer used as first-line therapy for active ulcers in most clinical settings.

C. *H pylori* Eradication Therapy

Eradication of *H pylori* has proved difficult. Combination regimens that use two or three antibiotics with a proton pump inhibitor or bismuth are required to achieve adequate rates of eradication and to reduce the number of failures due to antibiotic resistance. In the United States, up to 50% of strains are resistant to metronidazole and 10–20% are resistant to clarithromycin. Recommended regimens are listed in Table 15–10. Ideally, the optimal regimen would be determined by antibiotic susceptibility testing. However, this requires endoscopic biopsy, and few laboratories are equipped for *H pylori* cultures. Thus, in most clinical settings, therapy is chosen empirically. Until recently, in the United States a 14-day course of so-called triple therapy with a proton pump inhibitor, clarithromycin, and either amoxicillin or metronidazole (if penicillin allergic) was recommended as first-line therapy. However, a 2016 updated guideline from the Toronto Consensus group and 2017 guideline from the American College of Gastroenterology recommended that triple therapy no longer be used (due to increasing clarithromycin resistance) except in areas with known low-level clarithromycin

Table 15–10. Treatment options for peptic ulcer disease.

Active *Helicobacter pylori*–associated ulcer
1. Treat with anti–*H pylori* regimen for 14 days. Treatment options:

   Standard Bismuth Quadruple Therapy
   - Proton pump inhibitor orally twice daily[1,2]
   - Bismuth subsalicylate 262 mg two tablets orally four times daily or bismuth subcitrate 120–400 mg orally four times daily
   - Tetracycline 500 mg orally four times daily
   - Metronidazole 500 mg three times daily

   OR
   - Proton pump inhibitor orally twice daily[1]
   - Bismuth subcitrate potassium 140 mg/metronidazole 125 mg/tetracycline 125 mg (Pylera) three capsules orally four times daily for 10 days[3]

   Standard Nonbismuth Quadruple Therapy
   - Proton pump inhibitor orally twice daily
   - Amoxicillin 1000 mg twice daily
   - Metronidazole 500 mg twice daily
   - Clarithromycin 500 mg twice daily

   Standard Triple Therapy (No longer recommended except in locales where clarithromycin resistance is < 15%)
   - Proton pump inhibitor twice daily
   - Clarithromycin 500 mg twice daily
   - Amoxicillin 1 g orally twice daily (or, if penicillin allergic, metronidazole 500 mg orally twice daily)
2. After completion of course of *H pylori* eradication therapy, continue treatment with proton pump inhibitor[1] once daily for 4–6 weeks if ulcer is large (> 1 cm) or complicated.
3. Confirm successful eradication of *H pylori* with urea breath test, fecal antigen test, or endoscopy with biopsy at least 4 weeks after completion of antibiotic treatment and 1–2 weeks after completion of proton pump inhibitor treatment.

Active ulcer not attributable to *H pylori*
Consider other causes: NSAIDs, Zollinger-Ellison syndrome, gastric malignancy. Treatment options:
   - Proton pump inhibitors:[1]
       Uncomplicated duodenal ulcer: treat for 4 weeks
       Uncomplicated gastric ulcer: treat for 8 weeks
   - H$_2$-receptor antagonists:
       Uncomplicated duodenal ulcer: cimetidine 800 mg, ranitidine or nizatidine 300 mg, famotidine 40 mg, orally once daily at bedtime for 6 weeks
       Uncomplicated gastric ulcer: cimetidine 400 mg, ranitidine or nizatidine 150 mg, famotidine 20 mg, orally twice daily for 8 weeks
       Complicated ulcers: proton pump inhibitors[1] are the preferred drugs

Prevention of ulcer relapse
1. NSAID-induced ulcer: prophylactic therapy for high-risk patients (prior ulcer disease or ulcer complications, use of corticosteroids or anticoagulants, age > 60 years, serious comorbid illnesses). Treatment options:
   - Proton pump inhibitor once daily
   - Celecoxib (contraindicated in patients with increased risk of cardiovascular disease)
   - Misoprostol 200 mcg orally 4 times daily
2. Long-term "maintenance" therapy indicated in patients with recurrent ulcers who either are *H pylori*–negative or who have failed attempts at eradication therapy: once-daily oral proton pump inhibitor[1]

[1]Oral proton pump inhibitors: omeprazole 40 mg, rabeprazole 20 mg, lansoprazole 30 mg, dexlansoprazole 30–60 mg, pantoprazole 40 mg, esomeprazole 40 mg. Proton pump inhibitors are administered 30 minutes before meals.
[2]Preferred regimen in regions with high clarithromycin resistance or in patients who have previously received a macrolide antibiotic or are penicillin allergic. Effective against metronidazole-resistant organisms.
[3]Pylera is an FDA-approved formulation containing bismuth subcitrate 140 mg/tetracycline 125 mg/metronidazole 125 mg per capsule.
NSAIDs, nonsteroidal anti-inflammatory drugs.

resistance (less than 15%). In most settings, empiric treatment with a 14-day bismuth-based or a nonbismuth-based regimen of so-called quadruple therapy is now recommended as first-line therapy. Both achieve a greater than 85% eradication rate. The bismuth-based quadruple therapy regimen consists of bismuth, tetracycline, a proton pump inhibitor, and metronidazole or tinidazole (Table 15–10). It is effective even for metronidazole-resistant strains. Nonbismuth-based quadruple therapy consists of a proton pump inhibitor, amoxicillin, metronidazole, and clarithromycin; it is effective even for clarithromycin-resistant strains.

▶ Medical Treatment

Patients should be encouraged to eat balanced meals at regular intervals. There is no justification for bland or restrictive diets. Moderate alcohol intake is not harmful. Smoking retards the rate of ulcer healing and increases the frequency of recurrences and should be prohibited.

A. Treatment of *H pylori*–Associated Ulcers

1. Treatment of active ulcer—The goals of treatment of active *H pylori*–associated ulcers are to relieve dyspeptic symptoms, to promote ulcer healing, and to eradicate *H pylori* infection. Uncomplicated *H pylori*–associated ulcers should be treated for 14 days with one of the proton pump inhibitor–based *H pylori* eradication regimens listed in Table 15–10. At that point, no further antisecretory therapy is needed, provided the ulcer was small (less than 1 cm) and dyspeptic symptoms have resolved. For patients with large or complicated ulcers, an antisecretory agent should be continued for an additional 2–4 weeks (duodenal ulcer) or 4–6 weeks (gastric ulcer) after completion of the antibiotic regimen to ensure complete ulcer healing. A once-daily oral proton pump inhibitor (as listed in Table 15–10) is recommended. Confirmation of *H pylori* eradication is recommended for all patients more than 4 weeks after completion of antibiotic therapy and more than 2 weeks after discontinuation of the proton pump inhibitor either with noninvasive tests (urea breath test, fecal antigen test) or endoscopy with biopsy for histology.

2. Therapy to prevent recurrence—Successful eradication reduces ulcer recurrences to less than 20% after 1–2 years. The most common cause of recurrence after antibiotic therapy is failure to achieve successful eradication. Once cure has been achieved, reinfection rates are less than 0.5% per year. Although *H pylori* eradication has reduced the need for long-term maintenance antisecretory therapy to prevent ulcer recurrences, there remains a subset of patients who require long-term therapy with a proton pump inhibitor once daily. This subset includes patients with *H pylori*–positive ulcers who have not responded to repeated attempts at eradication therapy, patients with a history of *H pylori*–positive ulcers who have recurrent ulcers despite successful eradication, and patients with idiopathic ulcers (ie, *H pylori*–negative and not taking NSAIDs). In all patients with recurrent ulcers, NSAID usage (unintentional or surreptitious) and hypersecretory states (including gastrinoma) should be excluded.

B. Treatment of NSAID-Induced Ulcers

1. Treatment of active ulcers—In patients with NSAID-induced ulcers, the offending agent should be discontinued whenever possible. Both gastric and duodenal ulcers respond rapidly to therapy with H_2-receptor antagonists or proton pump inhibitors (Table 15–10) once NSAIDs are eliminated. All patients with NSAID-associated ulcers should undergo testing for *H pylori* infection. Antibiotic eradication therapy should be given if *H pylori* tests are positive.

2. Prevention of NSAID-induced ulcers—Clinicians should carefully weigh the benefits of NSAID therapy with the risks of cardiovascular and gastrointestinal complications. Both coxibs and nsNSAIDs may increase the risk of cardiovascular complications. Ulcer complications occur in up to 2% of all nsNSAID-treated patients per year, but in up to 10–20% per year of patients with multiple risk factors. These include age over 60 years, history of ulcer disease or complications, concurrent use of antiplatelet therapy (low-dose aspirin or clopidogrel, or both), concurrent therapy with anticoagulants or corticosteroids, and serious underlying medical illness. After considering the patient's risk of cardiovascular and gastrointestinal complications due to NSAID use, the clinician can decide what type of NSAID (nsNSAID vs coxib) is appropriate and what strategies should be used to reduce the risk of such complications. To minimize cardiovascular and gastrointestinal risks, all NSAIDs should be used at the lowest effective dose and for the shortest time necessary.

A. TEST FOR AND TREAT *H PYLORI* INFECTION—All patients with a known history of peptic ulcer disease who are treated with NSAIDs or antiplatelet agents (aspirin, clopidogrel) should be tested for *H pylori* infection and treated, if positive. Although *H pylori* eradication may decrease the risk of NSAID-related complications, co-therapy with a proton pump inhibitor is still required in high-risk patients.

B. PROTON PUMP INHIBITOR—Treatment with an oral proton pump inhibitor given once daily (rabeprazole 20 mg, omeprazole 20–40 mg, lansoprazole 30 mg, dexlansoprazole 30–60 mg, or pantoprazole or esomeprazole 40 mg) is effective in the prevention of NSAID-induced gastric and duodenal ulcers and is approved by the FDA for this indication. Among high-risk patients taking nsNSAIDs or coxibs, the incidence of endoscopically visible gastric and duodenal ulcers after 6 months of therapy in patients treated with esomeprazole 20–40 mg/day was 5%, compared with 17% who were given placebo. Nonetheless, proton pump inhibitors are not fully protective in high-risk patients in preventing NSAID-related complications. In prospective, controlled trials of patients with a prior history of NSAID-related ulcer complications, the incidence of recurrent bleeding was almost 5% after 6 months in patients taking nsNSAIDs and a proton pump inhibitor. In prospective, controlled trials of patients with a prior history of ulcer complications related to low-dose aspirin, the incidence of recurrent ulcer bleeding in patients taking low-dose aspirin alone was approximately 15% per year compared with 0–2% per year in patients taking low-dose aspirin and proton pump inhibitor and 9–14% per year in patients taking clopidogrel. Thus, proton pump inhibitors are highly effective in preventing complications related to low-dose aspirin, even in high-risk patients. Enteric coating of aspirin may reduce direct topical damage to the stomach but does not reduce complications.

C. Recommendations to reduce risk of ulcer complications from nsNSAIDs and coxibs—For patients with a low risk of cardiovascular disease who have no risk factors for gastrointestinal complications, an nsNSAID alone may be given. For patients with one or two gastrointestinal risk factors, a coxib alone or an nsNSAID with a proton pump inhibitor once daily should be given to reduce the risk of gastrointestinal complications. NSAIDs should be avoided if possible in patients with multiple risk factors; if required, however, combination therapy with a coxib or a partially COX-2 selective nsNSAID (etodolac, meloxicam) and a proton pump inhibitor once daily is recommended.

For patients with an increased risk of cardiovascular complications, it is preferable to avoid NSAIDs, if possible. Almost all patients with increased cardiovascular risk also will be taking antiplatelet therapy with low-dose aspirin or clopidogrel, or both. Because combination therapy with an nsNSAID and antiplatelet therapy increases the risks of gastrointestinal complications, these patients should all receive cotherapy with a proton pump inhibitor once daily or misoprostol.

D. Recommendations to reduce risk of ulcer complications with use of antiplatelet agents—The risk of significant gastrointestinal complications in persons taking low-dose aspirin (81–325 mg/day) or clopidogrel, or both, for cardiovascular prophylaxis is 0.5%/year. Aspirin, 81 mg/day, is recommended in most patients because it has a lower risk of gastrointestinal complications but equivalent cardiovascular protection compared with higher aspirin doses. Complications are increased with combinations of aspirin and clopidogrel or aspirin and anticoagulants. Clopidogrel does not cause gastrointestinal ulcers or erosions. However, its antiplatelet activity may promote bleeding from erosions or ulcers caused by low-dose aspirin or *H pylori*. Patients with dyspepsia or prior ulcer disease should be tested for *H pylori* infection and treated, if positive. Patients younger than 60–70 years who have no other risk factors for gastrointestinal complications may be treated with low-dose aspirin or dual antiplatelet therapy without a proton pump inhibitor. Virtually all other patients who require low-dose aspirin or aspirin plus anticoagulant therapy should receive a proton pump inhibitor once daily.

At the present time, the optimal management of patients who require dual antiplatelet therapy with clopidogrel and aspirin is uncertain. Clopidogrel is a prodrug that is activated by the cytochrome P450 CYP2C19 enzyme. All proton pump inhibitors inhibit CYP2C19 to varying degrees, with omeprazole having the highest and pantoprazole the least level of inhibition. In vitro and in vivo platelet aggregation studies demonstrate that proton pump inhibitors (especially omeprazole) may attenuate the antiplatelet effects of clopidogrel, although the clinical importance of this interaction is uncertain. The FDA has issued a warning that patients should avoid using clopidogrel with omeprazole and esomeprazole. A 2010 expert consensus panel concluded that once daily treatment with an oral proton pump inhibitor (pantoprazole 40 mg; rabeprazole 20 mg; lansoprazole or dexlansoprazole 30 mg) may be recommended for patients who have an increased risk of upper gastrointestinal bleeding (prior history of peptic ulcer disease or gastrointestinal bleeding; concomitant NSAIDs). For patients with a lower risk of gastrointestinal bleeding, the risks and benefits of proton pump inhibitors must be weighed. Pending further recommendations, an acceptable alternative is to treat with an oral H_2-receptor antagonist (famotidine 20 mg, ranitidine 150 mg, nizatidine 150 mg) twice daily; however, proton pump inhibitors are more effective in preventing upper gastrointestinal bleeding. Cimetidine is a CYP2C19 inhibitor and should not be used. An alternative strategy is ticagrelor, an antiplatelet agent approved for use with low-dose aspirin in the treatment of acute coronary syndrome. Like clopidogrel, ticagrelor blocks the platelet ADP p2y12 receptor; however, it does not require hepatic activation, it does not interact with the CYP2C19 enzyme, and its efficacy is not diminished by proton pump inhibitors.

C. Refractory Ulcers

Ulcers that are truly refractory to medical therapy are now uncommon. Less than 5% of ulcers are unhealed after 8 weeks of once daily therapy with proton pump inhibitors, and almost all benign ulcers heal with twice daily therapy. Thus, noncompliance is the most common cause of ulcer nonhealing. NSAID and aspirin use, sometimes surreptitious, are commonly implicated in refractory ulcers and must be stopped. *H pylori* infection should be sought and the infection treated, if present, in all refractory ulcer patients. Single or multiple linear gastric ulcers may occur in large hiatal hernias where the stomach slides back and forth through the diaphragmatic hiatus ("Cameron lesions"); this may be a cause of iron deficiency anemia. Other causes of nonhealing ulcers include acid hypersecretion (Zollinger-Ellison syndrome), unrecognized malignancy (adenocarcinoma or lymphoma), medications causing gastrointestinal ulceration (eg, iron or bisphosphonates), Crohn disease, and unusual infections (*H heilmanii*, CMV, mucormycosis). Fasting serum gastrin levels should be obtained to exclude gastrinoma with acid hypersecretion (Zollinger-Ellison syndrome). Repeat ulcer biopsies are mandatory after 2–3 months of therapy in all nonhealed ulcers to look for malignancy or infection. Patients with persistent nonhealing ulcers are referred for surgical therapy after exclusion of NSAID use and persistent *H pylori* infection.

Chey WD et al. ACG Clinical Guideline: treatment of *Helicobacter pylori* infection. Am J Gastroenterol. 2017 Feb;112(2):212–39. [PMID: 28071659]

Fallone CA et al. The Toronto Consensus for the treatment of *Helicobacter pylori* infection in adults. Gastroenterology. 2016 Jul;151(1):51–69. [PMID: 27102658]

Kavitt RT et al. Diagnosis and treatment of peptic ulcer disease. Am J Med. 2019 Apr;132(4):447–56. [PMID: 30611829]

Klatte DCF et al. Association between proton pump inhibitor use and risk of progression of chronic kidney disease. Gastroenterology. 2017 Sep;153(3):702–10. [PMID: 28583827]

Lanas A et al. Peptic ulcer disease. Lancet. 2017 Aug 5; 390(10094):613–24. [PMID: 28242110]
Vaezi MF et al. Complications of proton pump inhibitor therapy. Gastroenterology. 2017 Jul;153(1):35–48. [PMID: 28528705]

COMPLICATIONS OF PEPTIC ULCER DISEASE

1. Gastrointestinal Hemorrhage

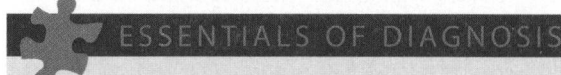

ESSENTIALS OF DIAGNOSIS

▶ "Coffee grounds" emesis, hematemesis, melena, or hematochezia.

▶ Emergent upper endoscopy is diagnostic and therapeutic.

▶ General Considerations

Approximately 50% of all episodes of upper gastrointestinal bleeding are due to peptic ulcer. Clinically significant bleeding occurs in 10% of ulcer patients. About 80% of patients stop bleeding spontaneously and generally have an uneventful recovery; the remaining 20% have more severe bleeding. The overall mortality rate for ulcer bleeding is 7%, but it is higher in older patients, in patients with comorbid medical problems, and in patients with hospital-associated bleeding. Mortality is also higher in patients who present with persistent hypotension or shock, bright red blood in the vomitus or nasogastric lavage fluid, or severe coagulopathy.

▶ Clinical Findings

A. Symptoms and Signs

Up to 20% of patients have no antecedent symptoms of pain; this is particularly true of patients receiving NSAIDs. Common presenting signs include melena and hematemesis. Massive upper gastrointestinal bleeding or rapid gastrointestinal transit may result in hematochezia rather than melena; this may be misinterpreted as signifying a lower tract bleeding source. Nasogastric lavage that demonstrates "coffee grounds" or bright red blood confirms an upper tract source. Recovered nasogastric lavage fluid that is negative for blood does not exclude active bleeding from a duodenal ulcer.

B. Laboratory Findings

The hematocrit may fall as a result of bleeding or expansion of the intravascular volume with intravenous fluids. The BUN may rise as a result of absorption of blood nitrogen from the small intestine and prerenal azotemia.

▶ Treatment

The assessment and initial management of upper gastrointestinal tract bleeding are discussed above. Specific issues pertaining to peptic ulcer bleeding are described below.

A. Medical Therapy

1. Antisecretory agents—Intravenous proton pump inhibitors should be administered for 3 days in patients with ulcers whose endoscopic appearance suggests a high risk of rebleeding after endoscopic therapy. Intravenous proton pump inhibitors have been associated with a reduction in rebleeding, transfusions, the need for further endoscopic therapy, and surgery in the subset of patients with high-risk ulcers, ie, an ulcer with active bleeding, visible vessel, or adherent clot. After initial successful endoscopic treatment of ulcer hemorrhage, intravenous esomeprazole, pantoprazole, or omeprazole (80 mg bolus injection, followed by 8 mg/h continuous infusion for 72 hours) reduces the rebleeding rate from approximately 20% to less than 10%; however, intravenous omeprazole is not available in the United States.

High-dose oral proton pump inhibitors (omeprazole 40 mg twice daily) also appear to be effective in reducing rebleeding but have not been compared with the intravenous regimen. Intravenous H_2-receptor antagonists have not been demonstrated to be of any benefit in the treatment of acute ulcer bleeding.

2. Long-term prevention of rebleeding—Recurrent ulcer bleeding develops within 3 years in one-third of patients if no specific therapy is given. In patients with bleeding ulcers who are *H pylori*–positive, successful eradication effectively prevents recurrent ulcer bleeding in almost all cases. It is therefore recommended that all patients with bleeding ulcers be tested for *H pylori* infection and treated if positive. Four to 8 weeks after completion of antibiotic therapy, a urea breath or fecal antigen test for *H pylori* should be administered or endoscopy performed with biopsy and histology for confirmation of successful eradication. In patients in whom *H pylori* persists or the small subset of patients whose ulcers are not associated with NSAIDs or *H pylori*, long-term acid suppression with a once-daily proton pump inhibitor should be prescribed to reduce the likelihood of recurrence of bleeding.

B. Endoscopy

Endoscopy is the preferred diagnostic procedure in almost all cases of upper gastrointestinal bleeding because of its high diagnostic accuracy, its ability to predict the likelihood of recurrent bleeding, and its availability for therapeutic intervention in high-risk lesions. Endoscopy should be performed within 24 hours in most cases. In cases of severe active bleeding, endoscopy is performed as soon as patients have been appropriately resuscitated and are hemodynamically stable.

On the basis of clinical and endoscopic criteria, it is possible to predict which patients are at a higher risk of rebleeding and therefore to make more rational use of hospital resources. Nonbleeding ulcers under 2 cm in size with a base that is clean have a less than 5% chance of rebleeding. Most young (under age 60 years), otherwise healthy patients with clean-based ulcers may be safely discharged from the emergency department or hospital after endoscopy. Ulcers that have a flat red or black spot have a less than 10% chance of significant rebleeding. Patients who are hemodynamically stable with these findings should be admitted to a hospital ward for 24–72 hours and may begin immediate oral feedings and antiulcer (or anti–*H pylori*) medication.

By contrast, the risk of rebleeding or continued bleeding in ulcers with a nonbleeding visible vessel is 50%, and with active bleeding, it is 80–90%. Endoscopic therapy with thermocoagulation (bipolar or heater probes) or application of endoscopic clips (akin to a staple) is the standard of care for such lesions because it reduces the risk of rebleeding, the number of transfusions, and the need for subsequent surgery. The optimal treatment of ulcers with a dense clot that adheres despite vigorous washing is controversial; removal of the clot followed by endoscopic treatment of an underlying vessel may be considered in selected high-risk patients. For actively bleeding ulcers, a combination of epinephrine injection followed by thermocoagulation or clip application commonly is used. These techniques achieve successful hemostasis of actively bleeding lesions in 90% of patients. After endoscopic therapy followed by an intravenous proton pump inhibitor, significant rebleeding occurs in less than 10%, of which over 70% can be managed successfully with repeat endoscopic treatment. After endoscopic treatment, patients should remain hospitalized for at least 72 hours, when the risk of rebleeding falls to below 3%.

C. Recurrent Bleeding

Less than 5% of patients have persistent or recurrent bleeding that cannot be controlled with endoscopic techniques. The availability of newer, larger over-the-scope clips ("bear claw") has further reduced the risk of persistent bleeding requiring other more aggressive interventions. In a randomized prospective study of patients with recurrent ulcer bleeding after conventional medical and endoscopic therapy, persistent bleeding occurred in 6% of patients treated with over-the-scope clips versus 42.4% treated with further conventional endoscopic modalities. For patients in whom endoscopic therapy is unsuccessful, percutaneous radiologic embolization or surgery should be considered. Overall surgical mortality for emergency ulcer bleeding is less than 6%. The prognosis is poorer for patients over age 60 years, those with serious underlying medical illnesses or chronic kidney disease, and those who require more than 10 units of blood transfusion.

2. Ulcer Perforation

Perforations develop in less than 5% of ulcer patients, usually from ulcers on the anterior wall of the stomach or duodenum. Perforation results in a chemical peritonitis that causes sudden, severe generalized abdominal pain that prompts most patients to seek immediate attention. Elderly or debilitated patients and those receiving long-term corticosteroid therapy may experience minimal initial symptoms, presenting late with bacterial peritonitis, sepsis, and shock. On physical examination, patients appear ill, with a rigid, quiet abdomen and rebound tenderness. Hypotension develops later after bacterial peritonitis has developed. If hypotension is present early with the onset of pain, other abdominal emergencies should be considered such as a ruptured aortic aneurysm, mesenteric infarction, or acute pancreatitis. Leukocytosis is almost always present. A mildly elevated serum amylase (less than twice normal) is sometimes seen with ulcer perforation. Abdominal CT usually establishes the diagnosis without need for further studies. The absence of free air may lead to a misdiagnosis of pancreatitis, cholecystitis, or appendicitis.

Laparoscopic perforation closure can be performed in many centers, significantly reducing operative morbidity compared with open laparotomy.

3. Gastric Outlet Obstruction

Gastric outlet obstruction occurs in less than 2% of patients with ulcer disease and is due to edema or cicatricial narrowing of the pylorus or duodenal bulb. With the advent of potent antisecretory therapy with proton pump inhibitors and the eradication of *H pylori*, obstruction now is less commonly caused by peptic ulcers than by gastric neoplasms or extrinsic duodenal obstruction by intra-abdominal neoplasms. The most common symptoms are early satiety, vomiting, and weight loss. Later, vomiting may develop that typically occurs one to several hours after eating and consists of partially digested food contents. Patients may develop dehydration, metabolic alkalosis, and hypokalemia. On physical examination, a succussion splash may be heard in the epigastrium. In most cases, nasogastric aspiration will result in evacuation of a large amount (greater than 200 mL) of foul-smelling fluid, which establishes the diagnosis. Patients are treated initially with intravenous isotonic saline and KCl to correct fluid and electrolyte disorders, an intravenous proton pump inhibitor, and nasogastric decompression of the stomach. Upper endoscopy is performed after 24–72 hours to define the nature of the obstruction and to exclude gastric neoplasm.

Abougergi MS et al. Thirty-day readmission among patients with non-variceal upper gastrointestinal hemorrhage and effects on outcomes. Gastroenterology. 2018 Jul;155(1):38–46. [PMID: 29601829]

Brandler J et al. Efficacy of over-the-scope clips in management of high-risk gastrointestinal bleeding. Clin Gastroenterol Hepatol. 2018 May;16(5):690–6. [PMID: 28756055]

Graham DY. Upper gastrointestinal bleeding due to a peptic ulcer. N Engl J Med. 2016 Sep 22;375(12):1197–8. [PMID: 27653583]

Kochhar R et al. Etiological spectrum and response to endoscopic balloon dilation in patients with benign gastric outlet obstruction. Gastrointest Endosc. 2018 Dec;88(6):899–908. [PMID: 30017869]

Nykänen T et al. Bleeding gastric and duodenal ulcers: case-control study comparing angioembolization and surgery. Scand J Gastroenterol. 2017 May;52(5):523–30. [PMID: 28270041]

Schmidt A et al. Over-the-scope clips are more effective than standard endoscopic therapy for patients with recurrent bleeding of peptic ulcers. Gastroenterology. 2018 Sep;155(3): 674–86.e6. [PMID: 29803838]

Shimomura A et al. New predictive model for acute gastrointestinal bleeding in patients taking oral anticoagulants: a cohort study. J Gastroenterol Hepatol. 2018 Jan;33(1):164–71. [PMID: 28544091]

ZOLLINGER-ELLISON SYNDROME (Gastrinoma)

 ESSENTIALS OF DIAGNOSIS

► Peptic ulcer disease; may be severe and atypical.

► Gastric acid hypersecretion.

► Diarrhea common, relieved by nasogastric suction.

► Most cases are sporadic; 25% with multiple endocrine neoplasia type 1 (MEN 1).

► General Considerations

Zollinger-Ellison syndrome is caused by gastrin-secreting gut neuroendocrine tumors (gastrinomas), which result in hypergastrinemia and acid hypersecretion. Less than 1% of peptic ulcer disease is caused by gastrinomas. Primary gastrinomas may arise in the pancreas (25%), duodenal wall (45%), or lymph nodes (5–15%), and in other locations including unknown primary sites (20%). Approximately 80% arise within the "gastrinoma triangle" bounded by the porta hepatis, the neck of the pancreas, and the third portion of the duodenum. Most gastrinomas are solitary or multifocal nodules that are potentially resectable. Approximately 25% of patients have small multicentric gastrinomas associated with MEN 1 that are more difficult to resect. Over two-thirds of gastrinomas are malignant, and one-third have already metastasized to the liver at initial presentation.

► Clinical Findings

A. Symptoms and Signs

Over 90% of patients with Zollinger-Ellison syndrome develop peptic ulcers. In most cases, the symptoms are indistinguishable from other causes of peptic ulcer disease, and therefore, the syndrome may go undetected for years. Ulcers usually are solitary and located in the duodenal bulb, but they may be multiple or occur more distally in the duodenum. Isolated gastric ulcers do not occur. Gastroesophageal reflux symptoms occur often. Diarrhea occurs in one-third of patients, in some cases in the absence of peptic symptoms. Gastric acid hypersecretion can cause direct intestinal mucosal injury and pancreatic enzyme inactivation, resulting in diarrhea, steatorrhea, and weight loss; nasogastric aspiration of stomach acid stops the diarrhea. Screening for Zollinger-Ellison syndrome with fasting gastrin levels should be done in patients with ulcers that are refractory to standard therapies, giant ulcers (larger than 2 cm), ulcers located distal to the duodenal bulb, multiple duodenal ulcers, frequent ulcer recurrences, ulcers associated with diarrhea, ulcers occurring after ulcer surgery, and ulcers with complications. Ulcer patients with hypercalcemia or family histories of ulcers (suggesting MEN 1) should also be screened. Finally, patients with peptic ulcers who are *H pylori* negative and who are not taking NSAIDs should be screened.

B. Laboratory Findings

The most sensitive and specific method for identifying Zollinger-Ellison syndrome is demonstration of an increased fasting serum gastrin concentration (greater than 150 pg/mL [150 ng/L]). If possible, levels should be obtained with patients not taking H_2-receptor antagonists for 24 hours or proton pump inhibitors for 6 days; however, withdrawal of the proton pump inhibitor may result in marked gastric hypersecretion with serious consequences and patients should be closely monitored. The median gastrin level is 500–700 pg/mL (500–700 ng/L), and 60% of patients have levels less than 1000 pg/mL (1000 ng/L). Hypochlorhydria with increased gastric pH is a much more common cause of hypergastrinemia than is gastrinoma. Therefore, a measurement of gastric pH (and, where available, a gastric secretory study) is performed in patients with fasting hypergastrinemia. Most patients have a basal acid output of over 15 mEq/h. A gastric pH of greater than 3.0 implies hypochlorhydria and excludes gastrinoma. In a patient with a serum gastrin level of greater than 1000 pg/mL (1000 ng/L) and acid hypersecretion, the diagnosis of Zollinger-Ellison syndrome is established. With lower gastrin levels (150–1000 pg/mL [150–1000 ng/L]) and acid secretion, a secretin stimulation test may be performed to distinguish Zollinger-Ellison syndrome from other causes of hypergastrinemia. Intravenous secretin (2 units/kg) produces a rise in serum gastrin of over 200 pg/mL (200 ng/L) within 2–30 minutes in 85% of patients with gastrinoma. An elevated serum calcium suggests hyperparathyroidism and MEN 1 syndrome. In all patients with Zollinger-Ellison syndrome, serum parathyroid hormone (PTH), prolactin, luteinizing hormone-follicle-stimulating hormone (LH-FSH), and growth hormone (GH) levels should be obtained to exclude MEN 1.

C. Imaging

Imaging studies are obtained in an attempt to determine whether there is metastatic disease and, if not, to identify the site of the primary tumor. CT and MRI scans are commonly obtained first to look for large hepatic metastases and primary lesions, but they have low sensitivity for small lesions. Gastrinomas express somatostatin receptors that bind radiolabeled octreotide. Somatostatin receptor scintigraphy (SRS) with single photon emission computed tomography (SPECT) allows total body imaging for detection of primary gastrinomas in the pancreas and lymph nodes, primary gastrinomas in unusual locations, and metastatic gastrinomas (liver and bone). The 80% sensitivity for tumor detection of SRS exceeds all other imaging studies combined. If SRS is positive for tumor localization, further imaging studies are not necessary. In patients with negative SRS, endoscopic ultrasonography (EUS) may be useful to detect small gastrinomas in the duodenal wall, pancreas, or peripancreatic lymph nodes. With a combination of SRS and EUS, more than 90% of primary gastrinomas can be localized preoperatively.

► Differential Diagnosis

Gastrinomas are one of several gut neuroendocrine tumors that have similar histopathologic features and arise either from the gut or pancreas. These include carcinoid, insulinoma, VIPoma, glucagonoma, and somatostatinoma. These tumors usually are differentiated by the gut peptides that they secrete; however, poorly differentiated neuroendocrine tumors may not secrete any hormones. Patients may present with symptoms caused by tumor metastases (jaundice, hepatomegaly) rather than functional symptoms. Once a diagnosis of a neuroendocrine tumor is established from the liver biopsy, the specific type of tumor can subsequently be determined. Both carcinoid and gastrinoma tumors may be detected incidentally during endoscopy after biopsy of a submucosal nodule and must be distinguished by subsequent studies.

Hypergastrinemia due to gastrinoma must be distinguished from other causes of hypergastrinemia. Atrophic gastritis with decreased acid secretion is detected by gastric secretory analysis. Other conditions associated with hypergastrinemia (eg, gastric outlet obstruction, vagotomy, chronic kidney disease) are associated with a negative secretin stimulation test.

▶ Treatment

A. Metastatic Disease

The most important predictor of survival is the presence of hepatic metastases. In patients with multiple hepatic metastases, initial therapy should be directed at controlling hypersecretion. Oral proton pump inhibitors (omeprazole, esomeprazole, rabeprazole, pantoprazole, or lansoprazole) are given at a dose of 40–120 mg/day, titrated to achieve a basal acid output of less than 10 mEq/h. At this level, there is complete symptomatic relief and ulcer healing. Owing to the slow growth of these tumors, 30% of patients with hepatic metastases have a survival of 10 years.

B. Localized Disease

Cure can be achieved only if the gastrinoma can be resected before hepatic metastatic spread has occurred. Lymph node metastases do not adversely affect prognosis. Laparotomy should be considered in all patients in whom preoperative studies fail to demonstrate hepatic or other distant metastases. A combination of preoperative studies, duodenotomy with careful duodenal inspection, and intraoperative palpation and sonography allows successful localization and resection in the majority of cases. The 15-year survival of patients who do not have liver metastases at initial presentation is over 95%. Surgery usually is not recommended in patients with MEN 1 due to the presence of multifocal tumors and long-term survival in the absence of surgery in most patients.

De Angelis C et al. Diagnosis and management of Zollinger-Ellison syndrome in 2017. Minerva Endocrinol. 2018 Jun; 43(2):212–20. [PMID: 28949124]

Norton JA et al. Gastrinomas: medical or surgical treatment. Endocrinol Metab Clin North Am. 2018 Sep;47(3):577–601. [PMID: 30098717]

Singh Ospina N et al. Assessing for multiple endocrine neoplasia type 1 in patients evaluated for Zollinger-Ellison Syndrome—clues to a safer diagnostic process. Am J Med. 2017 May; 130(5):603–5. [PMID: 28011308]

▶ DISEASES OF THE SMALL INTESTINE

MALABSORPTION

The term "malabsorption" denotes disorders in which there is a disruption of digestion and nutrient absorption. The clinical and laboratory manifestations of malabsorption are summarized in Table 15–11.

Table 15–11. Clinical manifestations and laboratory findings in malabsorption of various nutrients.

Manifestations	Laboratory Findings	Malabsorbed Nutrients
Steatorrhea (bulky, light-colored stools)	Increased fecal fat; decreased serum cholesterol; decreased serum carotene, vitamin A, vitamin D	Triglycerides, fatty acids, phospholipids, cholesterol. Fat-soluble vitamins: A, D, E, K
Diarrhea (increased fecal water)	Increased stool volume and weight; increased fecal fat; increased stool osmolality gap	Fats, carbohydrates
Weight loss; muscle wasting	Increased fecal fat; decreased carbohydrate (D-xylose) absorption	Fat, protein, carbohydrates
Microcytic anemia	Low serum iron	Iron
Macrocytic anemia	Decreased serum vitamin B_{12} or red blood cell folate	Vitamin B_{12} or folic acid
Paresthesia; tetany; positive Trousseau and Chvostek signs	Decreased serum calcium or magnesium	Calcium, vitamin D, magnesium
Bone pain; pathologic fractures; skeletal deformities	Osteopenia on radiograph; osteoporosis (adults); osteomalacia (children)	Calcium, vitamin D
Bleeding tendency (ecchymoses, epistaxis)	Prolonged prothrombin time or INR	Vitamin K
Edema	Decreased serum total protein and albumin; increased fecal loss of alpha-1-antitrypsin	Protein
Milk intolerance (cramps, bloating, diarrhea)	Abnormal lactose tolerance test	Lactose

INR, international normalized ratio.

Avitzur Y et al. Enteral approaches in malabsorption. Best Pract Res Clin Gastroenterol. 2016 Apr;30(2):295–307. [PMID: 27086892]
Wanten GJ. Parenteral approaches in malabsorption: home parenteral nutrition. Best Pract Res Clin Gastroenterol. 2016 Apr;30(2):309–18. [PMID: 27086893]

1. Celiac Disease

ESSENTIALS OF DIAGNOSIS

- ▶ *Typical symptoms*: weight loss, chronic diarrhea, abdominal distention, growth retardation.
- ▶ *Atypical symptoms*: dermatitis herpetiformis, iron deficiency anemia, osteoporosis.
- ▶ Abnormal serologic test results.
- ▶ Abnormal small bowel biopsy.
- ▶ Clinical improvement on gluten-free diet.

▶ General Considerations

Celiac disease (also called sprue, celiac sprue, and gluten enteropathy) is a permanent dietary disorder caused by an immunologic response to gluten, a storage protein found in certain grains, that results in diffuse damage to the proximal small intestinal mucosa with malabsorption of nutrients. Although symptoms may manifest between 6 months and 24 months of age after the introduction of weaning foods, the majority of cases present in childhood or adulthood. Population screening with serologic tests suggests that the global prevalence of this disease is 1.4%. In North America, the prevalence of biopsy-confirmed disease is 0.5%. Celiac disease develops only in people with the HLA-DQ2 (95%) or -DQ8 (5%) class II molecules, which are present in 40% of the population. Although the precise pathogenesis is unclear, celiac disease arises in a small subset of genetically susceptible (-DQ2 or -DQ8) individuals when dietary gluten stimulates an inappropriate immunologic response.

▶ Clinical Findings

The most important step in diagnosing celiac disease is to consider the diagnosis. Because of its protean manifestations, celiac disease is underdiagnosed in the adult population.

A. Symptoms and Signs

The gastrointestinal symptoms and signs of celiac disease depend on the length of small intestine involved and the patient's age when the disease presents. "Classic" symptoms of malabsorption, including diarrhea, steatorrhea, weight loss, abdominal distention, weakness, muscle wasting, or growth retardation, more commonly present in infants (younger than 2 years). Older children and adults are less likely to manifest signs of serious malabsorption. They may report chronic diarrhea, dyspepsia, or flatulence due to colonic bacterial digestion of malabsorbed nutrients, but the severity of weight loss is variable. Many adults have minimal or no gastrointestinal symptoms but present with extraintestinal "atypical"

manifestations, including fatigue, depression, iron deficiency anemia, osteoporosis, short stature, delayed puberty, amenorrhea, or reduced fertility. Approximately 40% of patients with positive serologic tests consistent with disease have no symptoms of disease; the natural history of these patients with "silent" disease is unclear.

Physical examination may be normal in mild cases or may reveal signs of malabsorption such as loss of muscle mass or subcutaneous fat, pallor due to anemia, easy bruising due to vitamin K deficiency, hyperkeratosis due to vitamin A deficiency, bone pain due to osteomalacia, or neurologic signs (peripheral neuropathy, ataxia) due to vitamin B_{12} or vitamin E deficiency (Table 15–11). Abdominal examination may reveal distention with hyperactive bowel sounds.

Dermatitis herpetiformis is regarded as a cutaneous variant of celiac disease. It is a characteristic skin rash consisting of pruritic papulovesicles over the extensor surfaces of the extremities and over the trunk, scalp, and neck. Dermatitis herpetiformis occurs in less than 10% of patients with celiac disease; however, almost all patients who present with dermatitis herpetiformis have evidence of celiac disease on intestinal mucosal biopsy, though it may not be clinically evident.

B. Laboratory Findings

1. Routine laboratory tests—Depending on the severity of illness and the extent of intestinal involvement, nonspecific laboratory abnormalities may be present that may raise the suspicion of malabsorption and celiac disease (Table 15–11). Limited proximal involvement may result only in microcytic anemia due to iron deficiency. Up to 3% of adults with iron deficiency not due to gastrointestinal blood loss have undiagnosed celiac disease. Megaloblastic anemia may be due to folate or vitamin B_{12} deficiency (due to terminal ileal involvement or associated autoimmune gastritis). Low serum calcium or elevated alkaline phosphatase may reflect impaired calcium or vitamin D absorption with osteomalacia or osteoporosis. Dual-energy x-ray densitometry scanning is recommended for all patients with sprue to screen for osteoporosis. Elevations of prothrombin time, or decreased vitamin A or D levels reflect impaired fat-soluble vitamin absorption. A low serum albumin may reflect small intestine protein loss or poor nutrition. Other deficiencies may include zinc and vitamin B_6. Mild elevations of aminotransferases are found in up to 40%.

2. Serologic tests—Serologic tests should be performed in all patients in whom there is a suspicion of celiac disease. The recommended test is the IgA tissue transglutaminase (IgA tTG) antibody, which has a 98% sensitivity and 98% specificity for the diagnosis of celiac disease. Antigliadin antibodies are not recommended because of their lower sensitivity and specificity. IgA antiendomysial antibodies are no longer recommended due to the lack of standardization among laboratories. An IgA level should be obtained in patients with a negative IgA tTG antibody when celiac disease is strongly suspected because up to 3% of patients with celiac disease have IgA deficiency. In patients with IgA deficiency, tests that measures IgG antibodies to tissue transglutaminase (IgG tTG) or to deamidated gliadin peptides (anti-DGP) have excellent sensitivity and specificity. Levels of all antibodies become undetectable after 3–24 months of dietary gluten withdrawal and may be used to monitor dietary compliance, especially in patients whose symptoms fail to resolve after institution of a gluten-free diet.

C. Mucosal Biopsy

Endoscopic mucosal biopsy of the proximal duodenum (bulb) and distal duodenum is the standard method for confirmation of the diagnosis in patients with a positive serologic test for celiac disease. Mucosal biopsy should also be pursued in patients with negative serologies when symptoms and laboratory studies are strongly suggestive of celiac disease. At endoscopy, atrophy or scalloping of the duodenal folds may be observed. Histology reveals abnormalities ranging from intraepithelial lymphocytosis alone to extensive infiltration of the lamina propria with lymphocytes and plasma cells, hypertrophy of the intestinal crypts, and blunting or complete loss of intestinal villi. An adequate normal biopsy excludes the diagnosis. Partial or complete reversion of these abnormalities occurs within 3–24 months after a patient is placed on a gluten-free diet, but symptom resolution remains incomplete in 30% of patients. If a patient with a compatible biopsy demonstrates prompt clinical improvement on a gluten-free diet and a decrease in serologic markers, a repeat biopsy is unnecessary.

► Differential Diagnosis

Many patients with chronic diarrhea or flatulence are erroneously diagnosed as having irritable bowel syndrome. Celiac disease must be distinguished from other causes of malabsorption, as outlined above. Severe panmalabsorption of multiple nutrients is almost always caused by mucosal disease. The histologic appearance of celiac disease may resemble other mucosal diseases such as tropical sprue, bacterial overgrowth, cow's milk intolerance, viral gastroenteritis, eosinophilic gastroenteritis, and mucosal damage caused by acid hypersecretion associated with gastrinoma. Documentation of clinical response to gluten withdrawal therefore is essential to the diagnosis.

Over the past decade, there has been a growing proportion (now 10%) of the population reporting symptoms after gluten ingestion who do not have serologic or histologic evidence of celiac disease. This has led to increases in gluten-free offerings from the restaurant and food industry. Foods with gluten often contain a number of other FODMAPs. A large 2013 study found that symptoms improved in gluten-sensitive patients when placed on a FODMAP-restricted diet and worsened to similar degrees when challenged in a double-blind crossover trial with gluten or whey proteins. A 2018 double-blind crossover trial in patients self-reporting gluten sensitivity reported significantly higher symptom scores during the fructan challenge than during the gluten or placebo challenges. These data suggest that self-reported wheat sensitivity may not be due to gluten intolerance and that the symptom improvement reported by patients with gluten restriction may be due to broader FODMAP elimination.

► Treatment

Removal of all gluten from the diet is essential to therapy—all wheat, rye, and barley must be eliminated. Although oats appear to be safe for many patients, commercial products may be contaminated with wheat or barley during processing. Because of the pervasive use of gluten products in manufactured foods and additives, in medications, and by restaurants, it is imperative that patients and their families confer with a knowledgeable dietitian to comply satisfactorily with this lifelong diet. Several excellent dietary guides and patient support groups are available. Most patients with celiac disease also have lactose intolerance either temporarily or permanently and should avoid dairy products until the intestinal symptoms have improved on the gluten-free diet. Dietary supplements (folate, iron, zinc, calcium, and vitamins A, B_6, B_{12}, D, and E) should be provided in the initial stages of therapy but usually are not required long-term with a gluten-free diet. Patients with confirmed osteoporosis may require long-term calcium, vitamin D, and bisphosphonate therapy.

Improvement in symptoms should be evident within a few weeks on the gluten-free diet. The most common reason for treatment failure is incomplete removal of gluten. Intentional or unintentional rechallenge with gluten may trigger acute severe diarrhea with dehydration and electrolyte imbalance, and may require TPN and intravenous or oral corticosteroids (prednisone 40 mg or budesonide 9 mg) for 2 or more weeks while a gluten-free diet is reinitiated.

► Prognosis & Complications

If appropriately diagnosed and treated, patients with celiac disease have an excellent prognosis. Celiac disease may be associated with other autoimmune disorders, including Addison disease, Graves disease, type 1 diabetes mellitus, myasthenia gravis, scleroderma, Sjögren syndrome, atrophic gastritis, and pancreatic insufficiency. In some patients, celiac disease may evolve and become refractory to the gluten-free diet. The most common cause is intentional or unintentional dietary noncompliance, which may be suggested by positive serologic tests. Celiac disease that is truly refractory to gluten withdrawal occurs in less than 5% and generally carries a poor prognosis. There are two types of refractory disease, which are distinguished by their intraepithelial lymphocyte phenotype. This diagnosis should be considered in patients previously responsive to the gluten-free diet in whom new weight loss, abdominal pain, and malabsorption develop.

Celiac Disease Foundation, 20350 Ventura Blvd, Suite #240, Woodland Hills, CA 91364. https://celiac.org

Leonard MM et al. Celiac disease and nonceliac gluten sensitivity: a review. JAMA. 2017 Aug 15;318(7):647–56. [PMID: 28810029]

Mahadev S et al. Prevalence of celiac disease in patients with iron deficiency anemia—a systematic review with meta-analysis. Gastroenterology. 2018 Aug;155(2):374–382. [PMID: 29689265]

Pearlman M et al. Who should be gluten-free? A review for the general practitioner. Med Clin North Am. 2019 Jan;103(1): 89–99. [PMID: 30466678]

Singh P et al. Global prevalence of celiac disease: systematic review and meta-analysis. Clin Gastroenterol Hepatol. 2018 Jun; 16(6):823–36. [PMID: 29551598]

Skodje GI et al. Fructan, rather than gluten, induces symptoms in patients with self-reported non-celiac gluten sensitivity. Gastroenterology. 2018 Feb;154(3):529–39. [PMID: 29102613]

Walker MM et al. Coeliac disease: review of diagnosis and management. Med J Aust. 2017 Aug 21;207(4):173–8. [PMID: 28814219]

2. Whipple Disease

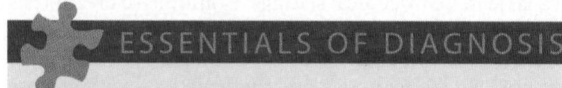

ESSENTIALS OF DIAGNOSIS

► Multisystem disease.

► Fever, lymphadenopathy, arthralgias.

► Weight loss, malabsorption, chronic diarrhea.

► Duodenal biopsy with periodic acid-Schiff (PAS)-positive macrophages with characteristic bacillus.

General Considerations

Whipple disease is a rare multisystem illness caused by infection with the bacillus *Tropheryma whipplei*. It may occur at any age but most commonly affects white men in the fourth to sixth decades. The source of infection is unknown, but no cases of human-to-human spread have been documented.

Clinical Findings

A. Symptoms and Signs

The clinical manifestations are protean; however, the most common are arthralgias, diarrhea, abdominal pain, and weight loss. Arthralgias or a migratory, nondeforming arthritis occurs in 80% and is typically the first symptom experienced. Gastrointestinal symptoms occur in approximately 75% of cases. They include abdominal pain, diarrhea, and some degree of malabsorption with distention, flatulence, and steatorrhea. Weight loss is the most common presenting symptom—seen in almost all patients. Loss of protein due to intestinal or lymphatic involvement may result in protein-losing enteropathy with hypoalbuminemia and edema. In the absence of gastrointestinal symptoms, the diagnosis often is delayed for several years. Intermittent low-grade fever occurs in over 50% of cases.

Physical examination may reveal hypotension (a late finding), low-grade fever, and evidence of malabsorption (see Table 15–11). Lymphadenopathy is present in 50%. Heart murmurs due to valvular involvement may be evident. Peripheral joints may be enlarged or warm, and peripheral edema may be present. Neurologic findings are cited above. Hyperpigmentation on sun-exposed areas is evident in up to 40%.

B. Laboratory Findings

If significant malabsorption is present, patients may have laboratory abnormalities as outlined in Table 15–11. There may be steatorrhea.

C. Histologic Evaluation

The diagnosis of Whipple disease is established in 90% of cases by endoscopic biopsy of the duodenum with histologic evaluation, which demonstrates infiltration of the lamina propria with PAS-positive macrophages that contain gram-positive bacilli (which are not acid-fast) and dilation of the lacteals. The remainder of cases are diagnosed by *T whipplei*–specific PCR or immunohistochemistry of duodenal biopsies or extraintestinal fluids (cerebrospinal, synovial) or tissue (lymph nodes, synovium, endocardium). The sensitivity of PCR is 97% and the specificity 100%. Because asymptomatic central nervous system infection occurs in 40% of patients, examination of the cerebrospinal fluid by PCR for *T whipplei* should be performed routinely.

Differential Diagnosis

Whipple disease should be considered in patients who present with signs of malabsorption, fever of unknown origin, lymphadenopathy, seronegative arthritis, culture-negative endocarditis, or multisystem disease. Small bowel biopsy readily distinguishes Whipple disease from other mucosal malabsorptive disorders, such as celiac disease.

Treatment

Antibiotic therapy results in a dramatic clinical improvement within several weeks, even in some patients with neurologic involvement. The optimal regimen is unknown. Complete clinical response usually is evident within 1–3 months; however, relapse may occur in up to one-third of patients after discontinuation of treatment. Therefore, prolonged treatment for at least 1 year is required. Drugs that cross the blood-brain barrier are preferred. A randomized controlled trial in 40 patients with 3–10 years' follow-up demonstrated 100% remission with either ceftriaxone 1 g intravenously twice daily or meropenem 1 g intravenously three times daily for 2 weeks, followed by trimethoprim-sulfamethoxazole 160/800 mg twice daily for 12 months. After treatment, repeat duodenal biopsies for histologic analysis and cerebrospinal fluid PCR should be obtained every 6 months for at least 1 year. The absence of PAS-positive material predicts a low likelihood of clinical relapse.

Prognosis

If untreated, the disease is fatal. Because some neurologic signs may be permanent, the goal of treatment is to prevent this progression. Patients must be followed closely after treatment for signs of symptom recurrence.

Biagi F et al. What is the best therapy for Whipple's disease? Our point of view. Scand J Gastroenterol. 2017 Apr;52(4):465–6. [PMID: 27924649]

Dolmans RA et al. Clinical manifestations, treatment, and diagnosis of *Tropheryma whipplei* infections. Clin Microbiol Rev. 2017 Apr;30(2):529–55. [PMID: 28298472]

Hujoel IA et al. *Tropheryma whipplei* infection (Whipple disease) in the USA. Dig Dis Sci. 2019 Jan;64(1):213–23. [PMID: 29572616]

3. Bacterial Overgrowth

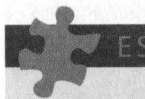

ESSENTIALS OF DIAGNOSIS

▶ Symptoms of distention, flatulence, diarrhea, and weight loss.

▶ Increased qualitative or quantitative fecal fat.

▶ Advanced cases associated with deficiencies of iron or vitamins A, D, and B_{12}.

▶ Diagnosis suggested by breath tests using glucose, lactulose, or ^{14}C-xylose as substrates.

▶ Diagnosis confirmed by jejunal aspiration with quantitative bacterial cultures.

▶ General Considerations

The small intestine normally contains a small number of bacteria. Bacterial overgrowth in the small intestine of whatever cause may result in malabsorption via a number of mechanisms. Bacterial deconjugation of bile salts may lead to inadequate micelle formation, resulting in decreased fat absorption with steatorrhea and malabsorption of fat-soluble vitamins (A, D). Microbial uptake of specific nutrients reduces absorption of vitamin B_{12} and carbohydrates. Bacterial proliferation also causes direct damage to intestinal epithelial cells and the brush border, further impairing absorption of proteins, carbohydrates, and minerals. Passage of the malabsorbed bile acids and carbohydrates into the colon leads to an osmotic and secretory diarrhea and increased flatulence.

Causes of bacterial overgrowth include (1) gastric achlorhydria (including proton pump inhibitor therapy); (2) anatomic abnormalities of the small intestine with stagnation (afferent limb of Billroth II gastrojejunostomy, resection of ileocecal valve, small intestine diverticula, obstruction, blind loop); (3) small intestine motility disorders (vagotomy, scleroderma, diabetic enteropathy, chronic intestinal pseudo-obstruction); (4) gastrocolic or coloenteric fistula (Crohn disease, malignancy, surgical resection); and (5) miscellaneous disorders. Bacterial overgrowth is an important cause of malabsorption in older patients, perhaps because of decreased gastric acidity or impaired intestinal motility. It may also be present in a subset of patients with irritable bowel syndrome.

▶ Clinical Findings

Many patients with bacterial overgrowth are asymptomatic. Symptoms are nonspecific and include flatulence, weight loss, abdominal pain, diarrhea, and sometimes steatorrhea. Severe cases may result in clinically significant vitamin and mineral deficiencies, including fat-soluble vitamins A or D, vitamin B_{12}, and iron (Table 15–11). Qualitative or quantitative fecal fat assessment typically is abnormal. Bacterial overgrowth should be considered in any patient with diarrhea, flatulence, weight loss, or macrocytic anemia, especially if the patient has a predisposing cause (such as prior gastrointestinal surgery). A stool collection should be obtained to corroborate the presence of steatorrhea. Vitamins A, D, B_{12}, and serum iron should be measured. A specific diagnosis can be established firmly only by an aspirate and culture of proximal jejunal secretion that demonstrates over 10^5 organisms/mL. However, this is an invasive and laborious test that requires careful collection and culturing techniques and therefore is not available in many clinical settings. Noninvasive breath tests are easier to perform and reported to have a sensitivity of 60–90% and a specificity of 85% compared with jejunal cultures. Breath hydrogen and methane tests with glucose or lactulose as substrates are commonly done because of their ease of use. A small bowel study (CT or MR enterography, barium radiography) may be obtained to look for mechanical factors predisposing to intestinal stasis.

Owing to the lack of an optimal test for bacterial overgrowth, many clinicians use an empiric antibiotic trial as a diagnostic and therapeutic maneuver in patients with predisposing conditions for bacterial overgrowth in whom unexplained diarrhea or steatorrhea develops.

▶ Treatment

Where possible, the anatomic defect that has potentiated bacterial overgrowth should be corrected. Otherwise, treatment as follows for 1–2 weeks with oral broad-spectrum antibiotics effective against enteric aerobes and anaerobes usually leads to dramatic improvement: twice-daily ciprofloxacin 500 mg, norfloxacin 400 mg, or amoxicillin clavulanate 875 mg, or a combination of metronidazole 250 mg three times daily plus either trimethoprim-sulfamethoxazole (one double-strength tablet) twice daily or cephalexin 250 mg four times daily. Rifaximin 400 mg three times daily is a nonabsorbable antibiotic that also appears to be effective but has fewer side effects than the other systemically absorbed antibiotics.

In patients in whom symptoms recur off antibiotics, cyclic therapy (eg, 1 week out of 4) may be sufficient. Continuous antibiotics should be avoided, if possible, to avoid development of bacterial antibiotic resistance.

Adike A et al. Small intestinal bacterial overgrowth: nutritional implications, diagnosis, and management. Gastroenterol Clin North Am. 2018 Mar;47(1):193–208. [PMID: 29413012]

Gatta L et al. Systematic review with meta-analysis: rifaximin is effective and safe for the treatment of small intestine bacterial overgrowth. Aliment Pharmacol Ther. 2017 Mar;45(5):604–16. [PMID: 28078798]

Krajicek EJ et al. Small intestinal bacterial overgrowth: a primary care review. Mayo Clin Proc. 2016 Dec;91(12):1828–33. [PMID: 27916156]

Rezaie A et al. Hydrogen and methane-based breath testing in gastrointestinal disorders: the North American consensus. Am J Gastroenterol. 2017 May;112(5):775–84. [PMID: 28323273]

4. Short Bowel Syndrome

Short bowel syndrome is the malabsorptive condition that arises secondary to removal of significant segments of the small intestine. The most common causes in adults are

Crohn disease, mesenteric infarction, radiation enteritis, volvulus, tumor resection, and trauma. The type and degree of malabsorption depend on the length and site of the resection and the degree of adaptation of the remaining bowel.

Terminal Ileal Resection

Resection of the terminal ileum results in malabsorption of bile salts and vitamin B_{12}, which are normally absorbed in this region. Patients with low serum vitamin B_{12} levels or resection of over 50 cm of ileum require monthly subcutaneous or intramuscular vitamin B_{12} injections. In patients with less than 100 cm of ileal resection, bile salt malabsorption stimulates fluid secretion from the colon, resulting in watery diarrhea. This may be treated with bile salt-binding resins (colestipol or cholestyramine, 2–4 g orally three times daily with meals or colesevelam, 625 mg, 1–3 tablets twice daily). Resection of over 100 cm of ileum leads to a reduction in the bile salt pool that results in steatorrhea and malabsorption of fat-soluble vitamins. Treatment is with a low-fat diet and vitamins supplemented with medium-chain triglycerides, which do not require micellar solubilization. Unabsorbed fatty acids bind with calcium, reducing its absorption and enhancing the absorption of oxalate. Oxalate kidney stones may develop. Calcium supplements should be administered to bind oxalate and increase serum calcium. Cholesterol gallstones due to decreased bile salts are common also. In patients with resection of the ileocolonic valve, bacterial overgrowth may occur in the small intestine, further complicating malabsorption (as outlined above).

Extensive Small Bowel Resection

Resection of up to 40–50% of the total length of small intestine usually is well tolerated. A more massive resection may result in "short bowel syndrome," characterized by weight loss and diarrhea due to nutrient, water, and electrolyte malabsorption. If the colon is preserved, 100 cm of proximal jejunum may be sufficient to maintain adequate oral nutrition with a low-fat, high–complex carbohydrate diet, though fluid and electrolyte losses may still be significant. In patients in whom the colon has been removed, at least 200 cm of proximal jejunum is typically required to maintain oral nutrition. Antidiarrheal agents (loperamide, 2–4 mg orally three times daily) slow transit and reduce diarrheal volume. Octreotide reduces intestinal transit time and fluid and electrolyte secretion. Gastric hypersecretion initially complicates intestinal resection and should be treated with proton pump inhibitors.

Patients with less than 100–200 cm of proximal jejunum remaining almost always require parenteral nutrition. Teduglutide (recombinant) is a glucagon-like peptide-2 analogue that stimulates small bowel growth and absorption and is FDA approved for the treatment of short bowel syndrome. In clinical trials, it resulted in a reduced need for parenteral nutrition. Small intestine transplantation has reported 5-year graft survival rates of 40%. Currently, it is performed chiefly in patients in whom serious problems develop due to parenteral nutrition.

Iyer KR et al. Independence from parenteral nutrition and intravenous fluid support during treatment with teduglutide among patients with intestinal failure associated with short bowel syndrome. JPEN J Parenter Enteral Nutr. 2017 Aug; 41(6):946–51. [PMID: 27875291]

Jeppesen PB et al. Factors associated with response to teduglutide in patients with short-bowel syndrome and intestinal failure. Gastroenterology. 2018 Mar;154(4):874–85. [PMID: 29174926]

Kochar B et al. Teduglutide for the treatment of short bowel syndrome—a safety evaluation. Expert Opin Drug Saf. 2018 Jul; 17(7):733–9. [PMID: 29848084]

Parrish CR et al. Managing the adult patient with short bowel syndrome. Gastroenterol Hepatol (N Y). 2017 Oct;13(10):600–8. [PMID: 29230136]

5. Lactase Deficiency

ESSENTIALS OF DIAGNOSIS

- ▶ Diarrhea, bloating, flatulence, and abdominal pain after ingestion of milk-containing products.
- ▶ Diagnosis supported by symptomatic improvement on lactose-free diet.
- ▶ Diagnosis confirmed by hydrogen breath test.

General Considerations

Lactase is a brush border enzyme that hydrolyzes the disaccharide lactose into glucose and galactose. The concentration of lactase enzyme levels is high at birth but declines steadily in most people of non-European ancestry during childhood and adolescence and into adulthood. As many as 90% of Asian Americans, 70% of African Americans, 95% of Native Americans, 50% of Mexican Americans, and 60% of Jewish Americans are lactose intolerant compared with less than 25% of white adults. Lactase deficiency may also arise secondary to other gastrointestinal disorders that affect the proximal small intestinal mucosa. These include Crohn disease, celiac disease, viral gastroenteritis, giardiasis, short bowel syndrome, and malnutrition. Malabsorbed lactose is fermented by intestinal bacteria, producing gas and organic acids. The nonmetabolized lactose and organic acids result in an increased stool osmotic load with an obligatory fluid loss.

Clinical Findings

A. Symptoms and Signs

Patients have great variability in clinical symptoms, depending both on the severity of lactase deficiency and the amount of lactose ingested. Because of the nonspecific nature of these symptoms, there is a tendency for both lactose-intolerant and lactose-tolerant individuals to mistakenly attribute a variety of abdominal symptoms to lactose intolerance. Most patients with lactose intolerance can drink at least one 8-oz serving of milk daily (12 g of lactose) without symptoms, though rare patients have almost complete intolerance. With mild to moderate amounts of lactose malabsorption, patients may experience bloating, abdominal cramps, and flatulence. With higher lactose ingestions, an osmotic diarrhea will result. Isolated lactase deficiency does not result in other signs of malabsorption or weight loss. If these findings are present, other gastrointestinal disorders should be pursued. Diarrheal specimens reveal an increased osmotic gap and a pH of less than 6.0.

B. Laboratory Findings

The most widely available test for the diagnosis of lactase deficiency is the hydrogen breath test. After ingestion of 50 g of lactose, a rise in breath hydrogen of more than 20 ppm within 90 minutes is a positive test, indicative of bacterial carbohydrate metabolism. In clinical practice, many clinicians prescribe an empiric trial of a lactose-free diet for 2 weeks. Resolution of symptoms (bloating, flatulence, diarrhea) is suggestive of lactase deficiency (though a placebo response cannot be excluded) and may be confirmed, if necessary, with a hydrogen breath test.

▶ Differential Diagnosis

The symptoms of late-onset lactose intolerance are nonspecific and may mimic a number of gastrointestinal disorders, such as inflammatory bowel disease, mucosal malabsorptive disorders, irritable bowel syndrome, and pancreatic insufficiency. Furthermore, lactase deficiency frequently develops secondary to other gastrointestinal disorders (as listed above). Concomitant lactase deficiency should always be considered in these gastrointestinal disorders.

▶ Treatment

The goal of treatment in patients with isolated lactase deficiency is achieving patient comfort. Patients usually find their "threshold" of intake at which symptoms will occur. Foods that are high in lactose include milk (12 g/cup), ice cream (9 g/cup), and cottage cheese (8 g/cup). Aged cheeses have a lower lactose content (0.5 g/oz). Unpasteurized yogurt contains bacteria that produce lactase and is generally well tolerated.

By spreading dairy product intake throughout the day in quantities of less than 12 g of lactose (one cup of milk), most patients can take dairy products without symptoms and do not require lactase supplements. Most food markets provide milk that has been pretreated with lactase, rendering it 70–100% lactose free. Lactase enzyme replacement is commercially available as nonprescription formulations (Lactaid, Lactrase, Dairy Ease). Caplets or drops of lactase may be taken with milk products, improving lactose absorption and eliminating symptoms. The number of caplets ingested depends on the degree of lactose intolerance. Patients who choose to restrict or eliminate milk products may have increased risk of osteoporosis. Calcium supplementation (calcium carbonate 500 mg orally two to three times daily) is recommended for susceptible patients.

Bayless TM et al. Lactase non-persistence and lactose intolerance. Curr Gastroenterol Rep. 2017 May;19(5):23. [PMID: 28421381]

Deng Y et al. Lactose intolerance in adults: biological mechanism and dietary management. Nutrients. 2015 Sep;7(9):8020–35. [PMID: 26393648]

INTESTINAL MOTILITY DISORDERS

1. Acute Paralytic Ileus

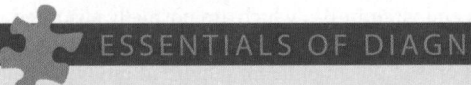

ESSENTIALS OF DIAGNOSIS

▶ Precipitating factors: surgery, peritonitis, electrolyte abnormalities, medications, severe medical illness.
▶ Nausea, vomiting, obstipation, distention.
▶ Minimal abdominal tenderness; decreased bowel sounds.
▶ Plain abdominal radiography with gas and fluid distention in small and large bowel.

▶ General Considerations

Ileus is a condition in which there is neurogenic failure or loss of peristalsis in the intestine in the absence of any mechanical obstruction. It is commonly seen in hospitalized patients as a result of (1) intra-abdominal processes such as recent gastrointestinal or abdominal surgery or peritoneal irritation (peritonitis, pancreatitis, ruptured viscus, hemorrhage); (2) severe medical illness such as pneumonia, respiratory failure requiring intubation, sepsis or severe infections, uremia, diabetic ketoacidosis, and electrolyte abnormalities (hypokalemia, hypercalcemia, hypomagnesemia, hypophosphatemia); and (3) medications that affect intestinal motility (opioids, anticholinergics, phenothiazines). Following surgery, small intestinal motility usually normalizes first (often within hours), followed by the stomach (24–48 hours), and the colon (48–72 hours). Postoperative ileus is reduced by the use of patient-controlled or epidural analgesia and avoidance of intravenous opioids as well as early ambulation, gum chewing, and initiation of a clear liquid diet.

▶ Clinical Findings

A. Symptoms and Signs

Patients who are conscious report mild diffuse, continuous abdominal discomfort with nausea and vomiting. Generalized abdominal distention is present with minimal abdominal tenderness but no signs of peritoneal irritation (unless due to the primary disease). Bowel sounds are diminished to absent.

B. Laboratory Findings

The laboratory abnormalities are attributable to the underlying condition. Serum electrolytes (sodium, potassium), magnesium, phosphorus, and calcium, should be obtained to exclude abnormalities as contributing factors.

C. Imaging

Plain film radiography of the abdomen demonstrates distended gas-filled loops of the small and large intestine. Air-fluid levels may be seen. Under some circumstances, it may be difficult to distinguish ileus from partial small bowel obstruction. A CT scan may be useful in such instances to exclude mechanical obstruction, especially in postoperative patients.

Differential Diagnosis

Ileus must be distinguished from mechanical obstruction of the small bowel or proximal colon. Pain from small bowel mechanical obstruction is usually intermittent, cramping, and associated initially with profuse vomiting. Acute gastroenteritis, acute appendicitis, and acute pancreatitis may all present with ileus.

Treatment

The primary medical or surgical illness that has precipitated adynamic ileus should be treated. Most cases of ileus respond to restriction of oral intake with gradual liberalization of diet as bowel function returns. Severe or prolonged ileus requires nasogastric suction and parenteral administration of fluids and electrolytes. Alvimopan is a peripherally acting mu-opioid receptor antagonist with limited absorption or systemic activity that reverses opioid-induced inhibition of intestinal motility. In five randomized controlled trials in postoperative patients, it reduced the time to first flatus, bowel movement, solid meal, and hospital discharge compared with placebo. Alvimopan, 12 mg orally twice daily (available only through a restricted program for short-term use—no more than 15 doses), may be considered in patients undergoing partial large or small bowel resection when postoperative opioid therapy is anticipated.

Güngördük K et al. Effects of coffee consumption on gut recovery after surgery of gynecological cancer patients: a randomized controlled trial. Am J Obstet Gynecol. 2017 Feb;216(2):145.e1–145. [PMID: 27780709]

Sultan S et al. Alvimopan for recovery of bowel function after radical cystectomy. Cochrane Database Syst Rev. 2017 May 2;5:CD012111. [PMID: 28462518]

2. Acute Colonic Pseudo-obstruction (Ogilvie Syndrome)

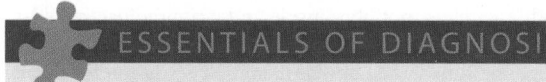

ESSENTIALS OF DIAGNOSIS

- Severe abdominal distention.
- Arises in postoperative state or with severe medical illness.
- May be precipitated by electrolyte imbalances, medications.
- Absent to mild abdominal pain; minimal tenderness.
- Massive dilation of cecum or right colon.

General Considerations

Spontaneous massive dilation of the cecum and proximal colon may occur in a number of different settings in hospitalized patients. Progressive cecal dilation may lead to spontaneous perforation with dire consequences. The risk of perforation correlates poorly with absolute cecal size and duration of colonic distention. Early detection and management are important to reduce morbidity and mortality. Colonic pseudo-obstruction is most commonly detected in postsurgical patients (mean 3–5 days), after trauma, and in medical patients with respiratory failure, metabolic imbalance, malignancy, myocardial infarction, heart failure, pancreatitis, or a recent neurologic event (stroke, subarachnoid hemorrhage, trauma). Liberal use of opioids or anticholinergic agents may precipitate colonic pseudo-obstruction in susceptible patients. It may also occur as a manifestation of colonic ischemia.

Clinical Findings

A. Symptoms and Signs

Many patients are on ventilatory support or are unable to report symptoms due to altered mental status. Abdominal distention is frequently noted by the clinician as the first sign, often leading to a plain film radiograph that demonstrates colonic dilation. Some patients are asymptomatic, although most report constant but mild abdominal pain. Nausea and vomiting may be present. Bowel movements may be absent, but up to 40% of patients continue to pass flatus or stool. Abdominal tenderness with some degree of guarding or rebound tenderness may be detected; however, signs of peritonitis are absent unless perforation has occurred. Bowel sounds may be normal or decreased.

B. Laboratory Findings

Laboratory findings reflect the underlying medical or surgical problems. Serum sodium, potassium, magnesium, phosphorus, and calcium should be obtained to exclude abnormalities as contributing factors. Significant fever or leukocytosis raises concern for colonic ischemia or perforation.

C. Imaging

Radiographs demonstrate colonic dilation, usually confined to the cecum and proximal colon. The upper limit of normal for cecal size is 9 cm. A cecal diameter greater than 10–12 cm is associated with an increased risk of colonic perforation. Varying amounts of small intestinal dilation and air-fluid levels due to adynamic ileus may be seen. Because the dilated appearance of the colon may raise concern that there is a distal colonic mechanical obstruction due to malignancy, volvulus, or fecal impaction, a CT scan or water-soluble (diatrizoate meglumine) enema may sometimes be performed.

Differential Diagnosis

Colonic pseudo-obstruction should be distinguished from distal colonic mechanical obstruction (as above) and toxic megacolon, which is acute dilation of the colon due to inflammation (inflammatory bowel disease) or infection (*C difficile*–associated colitis, CMV). Patients with toxic megacolon manifest fever; dehydration; significant abdominal pain; leukocytosis; and diarrhea, which is often bloody.

► Treatment

Conservative treatment is the appropriate first step for patients with no or minimal abdominal tenderness, no fever, no leukocytosis, and a cecal diameter smaller than 12 cm. The underlying illness is treated appropriately. A nasogastric tube and a rectal tube should be placed. Patients should be ambulated or periodically rolled from side to side and to the knee-chest position in an effort to promote expulsion of colonic gas. All drugs that reduce intestinal motility, such as opioids, anticholinergics, and calcium channel blockers, should be discontinued if possible. Enemas may be administered judiciously if large amounts of stool are evident on radiography. Oral laxatives are not helpful and may cause perforation, pain, or electrolyte abnormalities.

Conservative treatment is successful in over 80% of cases within 1–2 days. Patients must be watched for signs of worsening distention or abdominal tenderness. Cecal size should be assessed by abdominal radiographs every 12 hours. Intervention should be considered in patients with any of the following: (1) no improvement or clinical deterioration after 24–48 hours of conservative therapy; (2) cecal dilation greater than 10 cm for a prolonged period (more than 3–4 days); or (3) patients with cecal dilation greater than 12 cm. Neostigmine injection should be given unless contraindicated. A single dose (2 mg intravenously) results in rapid (within 30 minutes) colonic decompression in 75–90% of patients. Cardiac monitoring during neostigmine infusion is indicated for possible bradycardia that may require atropine administration. Colonoscopic decompression is indicated in patients who fail to respond to neostigmine. Colonic decompression with aspiration of air or placement of a decompression tube is successful in 70% of patients. However, the procedure is technically difficult in an unprepared bowel and has been associated with perforations in the distended colon. Dilation recurs in up to 50% of patients. In patients in whom colonoscopy is unsuccessful, a tube cecostomy can be created through a small laparotomy or with percutaneous radiologically guided placement.

► Prognosis

In most cases, the prognosis is related to the underlying illness. The risk of perforation or ischemia is increased with cecal diameter more than 12 cm and when distention has been present for more than 6 days. With aggressive therapy, the development of perforation is unusual.

Haj M et al. Ogilvie's syndrome: management and outcomes. Medicine (Baltimore). 2018 Jul;97(27):e11187. [PMID: 29979381]

Jayaram P et al. Postpartum acute colonic pseudo-obstruction (Ogilvie's syndrome): a systematic review of case reports and case series. Eur J Obstet Gynecol Reprod Biol. 2017 Jul;214: 145–9. [PMID: 28531835]

Wells CI et al. Acute colonic pseudo-obstruction: a systematic review of aetiology and mechanisms. World J Gastroenterol. 2017 Aug 14;23(30):5634–44. [PMID: 28852322]

3. Chronic Intestinal Pseudo-obstruction & Gastroparesis

Gastroparesis and chronic intestinal pseudo-obstruction are chronic conditions characterized by intermittent, waxing and waning symptoms and signs of gastric or intestinal obstruction in the absence of any mechanical lesions to account for the findings. They are caused by a heterogeneous group of endocrine disorders (diabetes mellitus, hypothyroidism, cortisol deficiency), postsurgical conditions (vagotomy, partial gastric resection, fundoplication, gastric bypass, Whipple procedure), neurologic conditions (Parkinson disease, muscular and myotonic dystrophy, autonomic dysfunction, multiple sclerosis, postpolio syndrome, porphyria), rheumatologic syndromes (progressive systemic sclerosis), infections (postviral, Chagas disease), amyloidosis, paraneoplastic syndromes, medications, and eating disorders (anorexia); a cause may not always be identified.

► Clinical Findings

A. Symptoms and Signs

Gastric involvement leads to chronic or intermittent symptoms of gastroparesis with postprandial fullness (early satiety), nausea, and vomiting (1–3 hours after meals). Patients with predominantly small bowel involvement may have abdominal distention, vomiting, diarrhea, and varying degrees of malnutrition. Abdominal pain is not common and should prompt investigation for structural causes of obstruction. Bacterial overgrowth in the stagnant intestine may result in malabsorption. Colonic involvement may result in constipation or alternating diarrhea and constipation.

B. Imaging

Plain film radiography may demonstrate dilation of the esophagus, stomach, small intestine, or colon resembling ileus or mechanical obstruction. Mechanical obstruction of the stomach, small intestine, or colon is much more common than gastroparesis or intestinal pseudo-obstruction and must be excluded with endoscopy or CT or barium enterography, especially in patients with prior surgery, recent onset of symptoms, or abdominal pain. In cases of unclear origin, studies based on the clinical picture are obtained to exclude underlying systemic disease. Gastric scintigraphy with a low-fat solid meal is the optimal means for assessing gastric emptying. Gastric retention of 60% after 2 hours or more than 10% after 4 hours is abnormal. Recently, the FDA approved both a wireless motility capsule and a nonradioactive, 13-C labeled blue-green algae (*Spirulina platensis*) to assess gastric emptying time. Small bowel manometry is useful for distinguishing visceral from myopathic disorders and for excluding cases of mechanical obstruction that are otherwise difficult to diagnose by endoscopy or radiographic studies.

► Treatment

There is no specific therapy for gastroparesis or pseudo-obstruction. Acute exacerbations are treated with nasogastric suction and intravenous fluids. Long-term treatment is directed at maintaining nutrition. Patients should eat small, frequent meals that are low in fiber, milk, gas-forming foods, and fat. Foods that are well tolerated include tea, ginger ale, soup, white rice, potatoes and sweet potatoes, fish, gluten-free foods, and applesauce. Some patients may require liquid enteral supplements. Agents that reduce gastrointestinal motility (opioids, anticholinergics) should be avoided. In diabetic patients, glucose levels should be maintained below 200 mg/dL, as hyperglycemia may slow gastric emptying even in the absence of diabetic neuropathy, and amylin and GLP-1 analogs (exenatide or pramlintide) should be discontinued. Metoclopramide (5–20 mg orally or 5–10 mg intravenously or subcutaneously four times daily) and erythromycin (50–125 mg orally three times daily) before meals are each of benefit in treatment of gastroparesis but not small bowel dysmotility. Since the use of metoclopramide for more than 3 months is associated with a less than 1% risk of tardive dyskinesia, patients are advised to discontinue the medication if neuromuscular side effects, particularly involuntary movements, develop. Older patients are at greatest risk. Gastric electrical stimulation with internally implanted neurostimulators has shown reduction in nausea and vomiting in small studies and one controlled trial in some patients with severe gastroparesis (especially those with diabetes mellitus); however, the mechanism of action is uncertain as improvement is not correlated with changes in gastric emptying. Many patients with gastroparesis have pylorospasm and antral hypomotility. Uncontrolled studies report symptom improvement with modalities that reduce intrapyloric pressure, including botulinum toxin injection, laparoscopic myotomy, and endoscopic myotomy. Bacterial overgrowth should be treated with intermittent antibiotics. Patients with predominant small bowel distention may require a venting gastrostomy to relieve distress. Some patients may require placement of a jejunostomy for long-term enteral nutrition. Patients unable to maintain adequate enteral nutrition require TPN or small bowel transplantation. Difficult cases should be referred to centers with expertise in this area.

Myint AS et al. Current and emerging therapeutic options for gastroparesis. Gastroenterol Hepatol (N Y). 2018 Nov;14(11):639–45. [PMID: 30538604]

Navas CM et al. Symptomatic management of gastroparesis. Gastrointest Endosc Clin N Am. 2019 Jan;29(1):55–70. [PMID: 30396528]

Shen S et al. Diabetic gastroparesis and nondiabetic gastroparesis. Gastrointest Endosc Clin N Am. 2019 Jan;29(1):15–25. [PMID: 30396524]

Zihni AM et al. Surgical management for gastroparesis. Gastrointest Endosc Clin N Am. 2019 Jan;29(1):85–95. [PMID: 30396530]

APPENDICITIS

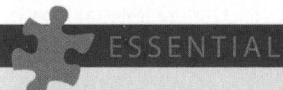

ESSENTIALS OF DIAGNOSIS

▶ *Early:* periumbilical pain; *later:* right lower quadrant pain and tenderness.

▶ Anorexia, nausea and vomiting, obstipation.

▶ Tenderness or localized rigidity at McBurney point.

▶ Low-grade fever and leukocytosis.

▶ General Considerations

Appendicitis is the most common abdominal surgical emergency, affecting approximately 10% of the population. It occurs most commonly between the ages of 10 and 30 years. It is initiated by obstruction of the appendix by a fecalith, inflammation, foreign body, or neoplasm. Obstruction leads to increased intraluminal pressure, venous congestion, infection, and thrombosis of intramural vessels. If untreated, gangrene and perforation develop within 36 hours.

▶ Clinical Findings

A. Symptoms and Signs

Appendicitis usually begins with vague, often colicky periumbilical or epigastric pain. Within 12 hours the pain shifts to the right lower quadrant, manifested as a steady ache that is worsened by walking or coughing. Almost all patients have nausea with one or two episodes of vomiting. Protracted vomiting or vomiting that begins before the onset of pain suggests another diagnosis. A sense of constipation is typical, and some patients administer cathartics in an effort to relieve their symptoms—though some report diarrhea. Low-grade fever (below 38°C) is typical; high fever or rigors suggest another diagnosis or appendiceal perforation.

On physical examination, localized tenderness with guarding in the right lower quadrant can be elicited with gentle palpation with one finger. When asked to cough, patients may be able to precisely localize the painful area, a sign of peritoneal irritation. Light percussion may also elicit pain. Although rebound tenderness is also present, it is unnecessary to elicit this finding if the above signs are present. The psoas sign (pain on passive extension of the right hip) and the obturator sign (pain with passive flexion and internal rotation of the right hip) are indicative of adjacent inflammation and strongly suggestive of appendicitis.

B. Atypical Presentations of Appendicitis

Owing to the variable location of the appendix, there are a number of "atypical" presentations. Because the retrocecal appendix does not touch the anterior abdominal wall, the pain remains less intense and poorly localized; abdominal tenderness is minimal and may be elicited in the right flank. The psoas sign may be positive. With pelvic appendicitis, there is pain in the lower abdomen, often on the left, with an urge to urinate or defecate. Abdominal tenderness is absent, but tenderness is evident on pelvic or rectal examination; the obturator sign may be present. In elderly patients, the diagnosis of appendicitis is often delayed because patients present with minimal, vague symptoms and mild abdominal tenderness. Appendicitis in pregnancy may present with pain in the right lower quadrant, periumbilical area, or right subcostal area owing to displacement of the appendix by the uterus.

C. Laboratory Findings

Moderate leukocytosis (10,000–20,000/mcL) with neutrophilia is common. Microscopic hematuria and pyuria are present in 25% of patients.

D. Imaging

Both abdominal ultrasound and CT scanning are useful in diagnosing appendicitis as well as excluding other diseases presenting with similar symptoms, including adnexal disease in younger women. However, CT scanning appears to be more accurate (sensitivity 94%, specificity 95%, positive likelihood ratio 13.3, negative likelihood ratio 0.09). Abdominal CT scanning is also useful in cases of suspected appendiceal perforation to diagnose a periappendiceal abscess. In patients in whom there is a clinically high suspicion of appendicitis, some surgeons feel that preoperative diagnostic imaging is unnecessary. However, studies suggest that even in this group, imaging studies suggest an alternative diagnosis in up to 15%.

Differential Diagnosis

Given its frequency and myriad presentations, appendicitis should be considered in the differential diagnosis of all patients with abdominal pain. It is difficult to reliably diagnose the disease in some cases. A several-hour period of close observation with reassessment usually clarifies the diagnosis. Absence of the classic migration of pain (from the epigastrium to the right lower abdomen), right lower quadrant pain, fever, or guarding makes appendicitis less likely. Ten to 20 percent of patients with suspected appendicitis have either a negative examination at laparotomy or an alternative surgical diagnosis. The widespread use of ultrasonography and CT has reduced the number of incorrect diagnoses to less than 2%. Still, in some cases diagnostic laparotomy or laparoscopy is required. The most common causes of diagnostic confusion are gastroenteritis and gynecologic disorders. Viral gastroenteritis presents with nausea, vomiting, low-grade fever, and diarrhea and can be difficult to distinguish from appendicitis. The onset of vomiting before pain makes appendicitis less likely. As a rule, the pain of gastroenteritis is more generalized and the tenderness less well localized. Acute salpingitis or tubo-ovarian abscess should be considered in young, sexually active women with fever and bilateral abdominal or pelvic tenderness. A twisted ovarian cyst may also cause sudden severe pain. The sudden onset of lower abdominal pain in the middle of the menstrual cycle suggests mittelschmerz. Sudden severe abdominal pain with diffuse pelvic tenderness and shock suggests a ruptured ectopic pregnancy. A positive pregnancy test and pelvic ultrasonography are diagnostic. Retrocecal or retroileal appendicitis (often associated with pyuria or hematuria) may be confused with ureteral colic or pyelonephritis. Other conditions that may resemble appendicitis are diverticulitis, Meckel diverticulitis, carcinoid of the appendix, perforated colonic cancer, Crohn ileitis, perforated peptic ulcer, cholecystitis, and mesenteric adenitis. It is virtually impossible to distinguish appendicitis from Meckel diverticulitis, but both require surgical treatment.

Complications

Perforation occurs in 20% of patients and should be suspected in patients with pain persisting for over 36 hours, high fever, diffuse abdominal tenderness or peritoneal findings, a palpable abdominal mass, or marked leukocytosis. Localized perforation results in a contained abscess, usually in the pelvis. A free perforation leads to suppurative peritonitis with toxicity. Septic thrombophlebitis (pylephlebitis) of the portal venous system is rare and suggested by high fever, chills, bacteremia, and jaundice.

Treatment

The treatment of early, uncomplicated appendicitis is surgical appendectomy in most patients. When possible, a laparoscopic approach is preferred to open laparotomy. Prior to surgery, patients should be given broad-spectrum antibiotics with gram-negative and anaerobic coverage to reduce the incidence of postoperative infections. Recommended preoperative intravenous regimens include cefoxitin or cefotetan 1–2 g every 8 hours; ampicillin-sulfabactam 3 g every 6 hours; or ertapenem 1 g as a single dose. Up to 80–90% of patients with uncomplicated appendicitis treated with antibiotics alone for 7 days have resolution of symptoms and signs. Therefore, conservative management with antibiotics alone may be considered in patients with a nonperforated appendicitis with surgical contraindications or with a strong preference to avoid surgery; however, appendectomy generally still is recommended in most patients to prevent recurrent appendicitis (20–35% within 1 year).

Emergency appendectomy is required in patients with perforated appendicitis with generalized peritonitis. The optimal treatment of stable patients with perforated appendicitis and a contained abscess is controversial. Surgery in this setting can be difficult. Many recommend percutaneous CT-guided drainage of the abscess with intravenous fluids and antibiotics to allow the inflammation to subside. An interval appendectomy may be performed after 6 weeks to prevent recurrent appendicitis.

Prognosis

The mortality rate from uncomplicated appendicitis is extremely low. Even with perforated appendicitis, the mortality rate in most groups is only 0.2%, though it approaches 15% in older adults.

Jaschinski T et al. Laparoscopic versus open surgery for suspected appendicitis. Cochrane Database Syst Rev. 2018 Nov 28;11: CD001546. [PMID: 30484855]

Nimmagadda N et al. Complicated appendicitis: immediate operation or trial of nonoperative management? Am J Surg. 2019 Apr;217(4):713–7. [PMID: 30635209]

Poprom N et al. The efficacy of antibiotic treatment versus surgical treatment of uncomplicated acute appendicitis: systematic review and network meta-analysis of randomized controlled trial. Am J Surg. 2018 Oct 9. [Epub ahead of print] [PMID: 30340760]

INTESTINAL TUBERCULOSIS

Intestinal tuberculosis is common in underdeveloped countries but rare in the United States except in immigrant groups or in patients with untreated AIDS. It is caused by both *Mycobacterium tuberculosis* and *M bovis*. Active pulmonary disease is present in less than 50% of patients.

The most frequent site of involvement is the ileocecal region; however, any region of the gastrointestinal tract may be involved. Patients may be without symptoms or complain of chronic abdominal pain, obstructive symptoms, weight loss, and diarrhea. An abdominal mass may be palpable. Complications include intestinal obstruction, hemorrhage, and fistula formation. The purified protein derivative (PPD) skin test may be negative, especially in patients with weight loss or AIDS. Abdominal CT may show thickening of the cecum and ileocecal valve and massive lymphadenopathy. Colonoscopy may demonstrate an ulcerated mass, multiple ulcers with steep edges and adjacent small sessile polyps, small ulcers or erosions, or small diverticula, most commonly in the ileocecal region. The differential diagnosis includes Crohn disease, carcinoma, lymphoma, and intestinal amebiasis. The diagnosis is established by either endoscopic or surgical biopsy revealing acid-fast bacilli, caseating granuloma, or positive cultures from the organism. Detection of tubercle bacilli in biopsy specimens by PCR is now the most sensitive means of diagnosis.

Treatment with standard antituberculous regimens (Tables 9–14 and 9–15) is effective.

Gan H et al. An analysis of the clinical, endoscopic, and pathologic features of intestinal tuberculosis. J Clin Gastroenterol. 2016 Jul;50(6):470–5. [PMID: 26974755]
Kentley J et al. Intestinal tuberculosis: a diagnostic challenge. Trop Med Int Health. 2017 Aug;22(8):994–9. [PMID: 28609809]

PROTEIN-LOSING ENTEROPATHY

Protein-losing enteropathy comprises a number of conditions that result in excessive loss of serum proteins into the gastrointestinal tract.

Hypoalbuminemia is the sine qua non of protein-losing enteropathy. However, a number of other serum proteins such as alpha-1-antitrypsin also are lost from the gut epithelium. In protein-losing enteropathy caused by lymphatic obstruction, loss of lymphatic fluid commonly results in lymphocytopenia (less than 1000/mcL), hypoglobulinemia, and hypocholesterolemia.

In most cases, protein-losing enteropathy is recognized as a sequela of a known gastrointestinal disorder. In patients in whom the cause is unclear, evaluation is indicated and is guided by the clinical suspicion. Protein-losing enteropathy must be distinguished from other causes of hypoalbuminemia, which include liver disease and nephrotic syndrome, and from heart failure. Protein-losing enteropathy is confirmed by determining the gut alpha-1-antitrypsin clearance (24-hour volume of feces × stool concentration of alpha-1-antitrypsin ÷ serum alpha-1-antitrypsin concentration). A clearance of more than 27 mL/24 h is abnormal.

Laboratory evaluation of protein-losing enteropathy includes serum protein electrophoresis, lymphocyte count, and serum cholesterol to look for evidence of lymphatic obstruction. Serum ANA and C3 levels are useful to screen for autoimmune disorders. Stool samples should be examined for ova and parasites. Evidence of malabsorption is evaluated by means of a stool qualitative fecal fat determination. Intestinal imaging is performed with small bowel enteroscopy biopsy, CT enterography, or wireless capsule endoscopy of the small intestine. Colonic diseases are excluded with colonoscopy. A CT scan of the abdomen is performed to look for evidence of neoplasms or lymphatic obstruction. Rarely, lymphangiography is helpful. In some situations, laparotomy with full-thickness intestinal biopsy is required to establish a diagnosis.

Treatment is directed at the underlying cause.

Levitt DG et al. Protein losing enteropathy: comprehensive review of the mechanistic association with clinical and subclinical disease states. Clin Exp Gastroenterol. 2017 Jul 17;10:147–68. [PMID: 28761367]

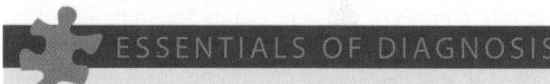

DISEASES OF THE COLON & RECTUM

(See Chapter 39 for Colorectal Cancer.)

IRRITABLE BOWEL SYNDROME

ESSENTIALS OF DIAGNOSIS

► Chronic functional disorder characterized by abdominal pain with alterations in bowel habits.

► Symptoms usually begin in late teens to early twenties.

► Limited evaluation to exclude organic causes of symptoms.

General Considerations

Irritable bowel syndrome can be defined as an idiopathic clinical entity characterized by chronic (more than 3 months) abdominal pain that occurs in association with altered bowel habits. These symptoms may be continuous or intermittent. The 2016 Rome IV consensus definition of irritable bowel syndrome is abdominal pain that has two of the following three features: (1) related to defecation, (2) associated with a change in frequency of stool, or (3) associated with a change in form (appearance) of stool. Symptoms of abdominal pain should be present on average at least 1 day per week. Other symptoms supporting the diagnosis include abnormal stool frequency; abnormal stool form (lumpy or hard; loose or watery); abnormal stool passage (straining, urgency, or feeling of incomplete evacuation); and abdominal bloating or a feeling of abdominal distention.

Patients may have other somatic or psychological complaints such as dyspepsia, heartburn, chest pain, headaches, fatigue, myalgias, urologic dysfunction, gynecologic symptoms, anxiety, or depression.

The disorder is a common problem presenting to both gastroenterologists and primary care physicians. Up to 10% of adults have symptoms compatible with the diagnosis, but most never seek medical attention. Approximately two-thirds of patients with irritable bowel syndrome are women.

Pathogenesis

A number of pathophysiologic mechanisms have been identified and may have varying importance in different individuals.

A. Abnormal Motility

A variety of abnormal myoelectrical and motor abnormalities have been identified in the colon and small intestine. In some cases, these are temporally correlated with episodes of abdominal pain or emotional stress. Differences between patients with constipation-predominant (slow intestinal transit) and diarrhea-predominant (rapid intestinal transit) syndromes are reported.

B. Visceral Hypersensitivity

Patients often have a lower visceral pain threshold, reporting abdominal pain at lower volumes of colonic gas insufflation or colonic balloon inflation than controls. Many patients complain of bloating and distention, which may be due to a number of different factors including increased visceral sensitivity, increased gas production, impaired gas transit through the intestine, or impaired rectal expulsion. Many patients report rectal urgency despite small rectal volumes of stool.

C. Intestinal Inflammation

The intestinal epithelium and immune system interact with the intra-intestinal microbiome, which is made up of an estimated 30,000 different microbial species. It is postulated that dietary factors, medications (antibiotics), or infections may increase intestinal permeability, leading to intestinal inflammation that may contribute to alterations in intestinal motility or visceral hypersensitivity. Increased inflammatory cells have been found in the mucosa, submucosa, and muscularis of some patients with irritable bowel syndrome, but their importance is unclear.

Symptoms compatible with irritable bowel syndrome develop within 1 year in over 10% of patients after an episode of bacterial gastroenteritis compared with less than 2% of controls. Women and patients with antibiotic exposure or psychological stress at the onset of gastroenteritis appear to be at increased risk for developing "postinfectious" irritable bowel syndrome.

Alterations in the intestinal microbiome composition may cause increased postprandial gas as well as bloating and distention due to degradation of undigested, fermentable carbohydrates in the small intestine or colon. An increase in breath hydrogen or methane excretion after lactulose ingestion has been reported in 65% of patients with irritable bowel syndrome, believed by some investigators to indicate small intestinal bacterial overgrowth. However, many investigators dispute these findings because overgrowth was confirmed in only 4% of patients using jejunal aspiration and bacterial culture.

D. Psychosocial Abnormalities

More than 50% of patients with irritable bowel who seek medical attention have underlying depression, anxiety, or somatization. Psychological abnormalities may influence how the patient perceives or reacts to illness and minor visceral sensations. Chronic stress may alter intestinal motility or modulate pathways that affect central and spinal processing of visceral afferent sensation.

Clinical Findings

A. Symptoms and Signs

Irritable bowel is a chronic condition. Symptoms usually begin in the late teens to twenties. The diagnosis is established in the presence of compatible symptoms and the judicious use of tests to exclude organic disease.

Abdominal pain usually is intermittent, crampy, and in the lower abdominal region. As previously stated, pain typically is associated with a change in stool frequency or form and may be improved or worsened by defecation. It does not usually occur at night or interfere with sleep. Patients with irritable bowel syndrome may be classified into one of four categories based on the predominant stool habits and stool form: irritable bowel syndrome with diarrhea, irritable bowel syndrome with constipation, irritable bowel syndrome with mixed constipation and diarrhea, or irritable bowel syndrome that is not subtyped. It is important to clarify what the patient means by these complaints. Patients with irritable bowel and constipation report infrequent bowel movements (less than three per week), hard or lumpy stools, or straining. Patients with irritable bowel syndrome with diarrhea refer to loose or watery stools, frequent stools (more than three per day), urgency, or fecal incontinence. Many patients report that they have a firm stool in the morning followed by progressively looser movements. Complaints of visible distention and bloating are common, though these are not always clinically evident.

The patient should be asked about "alarm symptoms" that suggest a diagnosis other than irritable bowel syndrome and warrant further investigation. The acute onset of symptoms raises the likelihood of organic disease, especially in patients older than 40–50 years. Nocturnal diarrhea, severe constipation or diarrhea, hematochezia, weight loss, and fever are incompatible with a diagnosis of irritable bowel syndrome and warrant investigation for underlying disease. Patients who have a family history of cancer, inflammatory bowel disease, or celiac disease should undergo additional evaluation.

A physical examination should be performed to look for evidence of organic disease and to allay the patient's anxieties. The physical examination usually is normal. Abdominal tenderness, especially in the lower abdomen, is common but not pronounced. A digital rectal examination should be performed in patients with constipation to screen for paradoxical anal squeezing during attempted straining that may suggest pelvic floor dyssynergia. A pelvic examination is recommended for postmenopausal women with recent onset constipation and lower abdominal pain to screen for gynecologic malignancy.

B. Laboratory Findings and Special Examinations

Although the vague nature of symptoms and patient anxiety may prompt clinicians to consider a variety of diagnostic studies, overtesting should be avoided, since the likelihood of serious organic disease is low. A 2013 study of primary care patients aged 30–50 years with suspected irritable bowel found that patients randomized to a strategy of extensive testing prior to diagnosis had higher health care costs but similar symptoms and satisfaction at 1 year as patients randomized to a strategy of minimal testing but a positive clinical diagnosis. A complete blood count should be obtained to screen for iron deficiency anemia. Serum C-reactive protein and fecal calprotectin level should be considered (especially in patients with diarrhea) to screen for inflammatory bowel disease and serologic testing for celiac disease (tissue transglutaminase [tTG] IgA) should be performed. Stool specimen examinations for ova and parasites should be obtained in patients with increased likelihood of infection (eg, day care workers, campers, foreign travelers). If these tests are negative, further testing is not necessary in most patients and education, reassurance, and initial empiric treatment is recommended. Routine sigmoidoscopy or colonoscopy is not recommended in young patients with symptoms of irritable bowel syndrome without alarm symptoms, but should be considered along with further laboratory testing in patients who do not improve with conservative management. In all patients aged 50 years or older who have not had a previous evaluation, colonoscopy should be obtained to exclude malignancy. When colonoscopy is performed, random mucosal biopsies should be obtained to look for evidence of microscopic colitis (which may have similar symptoms). Routine testing for bacterial overgrowth with hydrogen breath tests are not recommended.

▶ Differential Diagnosis

A number of disorders may present with similar symptoms. Examples include colonic neoplasia, inflammatory bowel disease (ulcerative colitis, Crohn disease, microscopic colitis), hyperthyroidism or hypothyroidism, parasites, malabsorption (especially celiac disease, bacterial overgrowth, lactase deficiency), causes of chronic secretory diarrhea (carcinoid), and gynecologic disorders (endometriosis, ovarian cancer). Psychiatric disorders such as depression, panic disorder, and anxiety must be considered as well. Women with refractory symptoms have an increased incidence of prior sexual and physical abuse. These diagnoses should be excluded in patients with presumed irritable bowel syndrome who do not improve within 2–4 weeks of empiric treatment or in whom subsequent alarm symptoms develop.

▶ Treatment

A. General Measures

As with other functional disorders, the most important interventions the clinician can offer are reassurance, education, and support. This includes identifying and responding to the patient's concerns, careful explanation of the pathophysiology and natural history of the disorder, setting realistic treatment goals, and involving the patient in the treatment process. Because irritable bowel symptoms are chronic, the patient's reasons for seeking consultation at this time should be determined. These may include major life events or recent psychosocial stressors, dietary or medication changes, concerns about serious underlying disease, or reduced quality of life and impairment of daily activities. In discussing with the patient the importance of the mind-gut interaction, it may be helpful to explain that alterations in visceral motility and sensitivity may be exacerbated by environmental, social, or psychological factors such as foods, medications, hormones, and stress. Symptoms such as pain, bloating, and altered bowel habits may lead to anxiety and distress, which in turn may further exacerbate bowel disturbances due to disordered communication between the gut and the central nervous system. Fears that the symptoms will progress, require surgery, or degenerate into serious illness should be allayed. The patient should understand that irritable bowel syndrome is a chronic disorder characterized by periods of exacerbation and quiescence. The emphasis should be shifted from finding the cause of the symptoms to finding a way to cope with them. Moderate exercise is beneficial. Clinicians must resist the temptation to chase chronic complaints with new or repeated diagnostic studies.

B. Dietary Therapy

Patients commonly report dietary intolerances. Proposed mechanisms for dietary intolerance include food allergy, hypersensitivity, effects of gut hormones, changes in bacterial flora, increased bacterial gas production (arising in the small or large intestine), and direct chemical irritation. Fatty foods, alcohol, caffeine, spicy foods, and grains are poorly tolerated by many patients with irritable bowel syndrome. In patients with diarrhea, bloating, and flatulence, lactose intolerance should be excluded with a hydrogen breath test or a trial of a lactose-free diet. A host of poorly absorbed, fermentable, monosaccharides and short-chain carbohydrates (FODMAPs) may exacerbate bloating, flatulence, and diarrhea in some patients. These include six food groups: fructose (corn syrups, apples, pears, honey, watermelon, raisins), lactose, fructans (garlic, onions, leeks, asparagus, artichokes), wheat-based products (breads, pasta, cereals, cakes), sorbitol (stone fruits), and raffinose (legumes, lentils, brussel sprouts, soybeans, cabbage). Dietary restriction of these fermentable carbohydrates for 2–4 weeks may improve symptoms (especially abdominal pain and bloating) in 50–65% of patients. Responders should gradually reintroduce different FODMAPs to identify food triggers. In a 2018 randomized placebo-controlled crossover trial, ingestion of alpha-galactosidase supplement ("Beano") with meals containing foods with high galactoside content (eg, beans, peas, lentils, soy) significantly improved bowel symptoms. Gluten has not been demonstrated to increase bowel symptoms independent of other FODMAPs, and a gluten-free diet is not recommended.

Poorly fermentable soluble fiber (psyllium, oatmeal) improves global symptoms in many patients and is recommended by the 2018 American College of Gastroenterology guideline. Fermentable or insoluble fiber (bran) may increase gas and bloating. The guideline does not recommend a gluten-free diet.

C. Pharmacologic Measures

More than two-thirds of patients with irritable bowel syndrome have mild symptoms that respond readily to education, reassurance, and dietary interventions. Drug therapy should be reserved for patients with moderate to severe symptoms that do not respond to conservative measures. These agents should be viewed as being adjunctive rather than curative. Given the wide spectrum of symptoms, no single agent is expected to provide relief in all or even most patients. Nevertheless, therapy targeted at the specific dominant symptom (pain, constipation, or diarrhea) may be beneficial.

1. Antispasmodic agents—Anticholinergic agents are used by some practitioners for treatment of acute episodes of pain or bloating despite a lack of well-designed trials demonstrating efficacy. Available agents include hyoscyamine, 0.125 mg orally (or sublingually as needed) or sustained-release, 0.037 mg or 0.75 mg orally twice daily; dicyclomine, 10–20 mg orally; or methscopolamine 2.5–5 mg orally before meals and at bedtime. Anticholinergic side effects are common, including urinary retention, constipation, tachycardia, and dry mouth. Hence, these agents should be used with caution in older patients and in patients with constipation. Peppermint oil formulations (which relax smooth muscle) may be helpful.

2. Antidiarrheal agents—Loperamide (2 mg orally three or four times daily) is effective for the treatment of patients with diarrhea, reducing stool frequency, liquidity, and urgency. It may best be used "prophylactically" in situations in which diarrhea is anticipated (such as stressful situations) or would be inconvenient (social engagements). Increased intracolonic bile acids due to alterations in enterohepatic circulation may contribute to diarrhea in a subset of patients with diarrhea. An empiric trial of bile salt-binding agents (cholestyramine 2–4 g with meals; colesevelam, 625 mg, 1–3 tablets twice daily) may be considered. Eluxadoline (75–100 mg twice daily) is an opioid antagonist that was approved by the FDA in 2016 for treatment of irritable bowel with diarrhea. In phase III trials, eluxadoline decreased abdominal pain and improved stool consistency in approximately 25% of patients versus 16–19% with placebo; however, sphincter of Oddi dysfunction and pancreatitis developed in a small percentage (0.5%) of patients. Given its minimal efficacy, adverse side effect profile, and unproven benefit versus loperamide, further study is needed before its use can be recommended.

3. Anticonstipation agents—Treatment with oral osmotic laxatives polyethylene glycol 3350 (Miralax, 17–34 g/day) may increase stool frequency, improve stool consistency, and reduce straining. Lactulose or sorbitol produces increased flatus and distention, which are poorly tolerated in patients with irritable bowel syndrome and should be avoided. Lubiprostone (8 mcg orally twice daily), linaclotide (290 mcg orally once daily), plecanatide (3 mg orally once daily), and tegaserod (6 mg orally twice daily) are newer agents approved for treatment of irritable bowel syndrome with constipation. Through different mechanisms, they stimulate increased intestinal chloride and fluid secretion, resulting in accelerated colonic transit. In clinical trials, lubiprostone led to global symptom improvement in 18% of patients compared with 10% of patients who received placebo. Trials of linaclotide included similar patient populations but measured different, FDA-defined primary end points. Higher combined response rates (defined as greater than 30% reduction in abdominal pain and more than three spontaneous bowel movements per week, including an increase of one or more from baseline) were found in 12.5% of linaclotide-treated patients compared with 4% of placebo-treated patients. Plecanatide was FDA approved in 2018 for the treatment of irritable bowel syndrome with constipation. Across two phase III trials, the proportion of patients with clinical response after 12 weeks of therapy (FDA-defined primary end points) with plecanatide (3 mg orally once daily) was 26% versus 16% with placebo. Tegaserod, a serotonin-4 (5-HT$_4$) receptor agonist, was originally approved by the FDA in 2002 for irritable bowel syndrome with constipation, but voluntarily withdrawn from the market in 2007 because of cardiovascular safety concerns. But in March 2019, it was reapproved by the FDA for women under age 65 after evaluation of clinical data from 29 placebo-controlled trials and newer treatment outcome data. Patients with intractable constipation should undergo further assessment for slow colonic transit and pelvic floor dysfunction (see Constipation, above).

4. Psychotropic agents—Patients with predominant symptoms of pain or bloating may benefit from low doses of tricyclic antidepressants, which are believed to have effects on motility, visceral sensitivity, and central pain perception that are independent of their psychotropic effects. Because of their anticholinergic effects, these agents may be more useful in patients with diarrhea-predominant than constipation-predominant symptoms. Oral nortriptyline, desipramine, or imipramine may be started at a low dosage of 10 mg at bedtime and increased gradually to 50–150 mg as tolerated. Response rates do not correlate with dosage, and many patients respond to doses of 50 mg or less daily. Side effects are common, and lack of efficacy with one agent does not preclude benefit from another. Agents with higher anticholinergic activity may improve diarrhea but worsen constipation. Improvement should be evident within 4 weeks. The oral serotonin reuptake inhibitors (sertraline, 25–100 mg daily; citalopram, 10–20 mg; paroxetine, 20–50 mg daily; or fluoxetine, 10–40 mg daily) may be used to treat irritable bowel symptoms as well as treat mood disorders. SSRIs may accelerate gastrointestinal transit and improve constipation. Anxiolytics should not be used chronically in irritable bowel syndrome because of their habituation potential. Patients with major depression or anxiety disorders should be identified and treated with therapeutic doses of appropriate agents.

5. Serotonin receptor antagonists—Serotonin is an important mediator of gastrointestinal motility and sensation. In patients with irritable bowel syndrome with diarrhea, 5-HT$_3$ antagonists may reduce diarrhea and improve overall symptoms through central and peripheral mechanisms. Alosetron is a 5-HT$_3$ antagonist that is FDA-approved for the treatment of women with severe irritable bowel syndrome with predominant diarrhea. Unfortunately, due to cases of severe constipation and a small (1:1000) but significant risk of ischemic colitis, alosetron is restricted to women with severe irritable bowel syndrome with diarrhea who have not responded to conventional therapies and who have been educated about the relative risks and benefits of the agent. It should not be used in patients with constipation. A randomized crossover trial of another 5-HT$_3$ antagonist, ondansetron 4–8 mg three times daily, showed overall superior symptom improvement, including stool frequency, consistency, and urgency. At this time, 5-HT$_3$ antagonists may be considered after careful discussion of the risks and benefits in carefully selected patients with severe diarrhea-predominant irritable bowel syndrome.

6. Nonabsorbable antibiotics—Rifaximin may be considered in patients with refractory symptoms, especially bloating. A 2012 meta-analysis identified a 9.9% greater improvement in bloating with rifaximin compared with placebo, a modest gain that is similar to other less expensive therapies. Symptom improvement may be attributable to suppression of bacteria in either the small intestine or colon, resulting in decreased bacterial carbohydrate fermentation, diarrhea, and bloating.

7. Probiotics—Meta-analyses of small controlled clinical trials of probiotics report improved symptoms of pain, bloating, and flatulence in some patients. It is hypothesized that alterations in gut flora may reduce symptoms through suppression of inflammation or reduction of bacterial gas production, resulting in reduced distention, flatus, and visceral sensitivity. Such therapy is attractive because it is safe, well tolerated, and inexpensive. Although promising, further study is needed to define the efficacy and optimal formulations of probiotic therapy. The 2018 American College of Gastroenterology guideline gave probiotics a weak recommendation.

D. Psychological Therapies

Cognitive-behavioral therapies, relaxation techniques, and hypnotherapy appear to be beneficial in some patients. Patients with underlying psychological abnormalities may benefit from evaluation by a psychiatrist or psychologist. Patients with severe disability should be referred to a pain treatment center.

Prognosis

The majority of patients with irritable bowel syndrome learn to cope with their symptoms and lead productive lives.

Brenner DM et al. Efficacy, safety, and tolerability of plecanatide in patients with irritable bowel syndrome with constipation: results of two phase 3 randomized clinical trials. Am J Gastroenterol. 2018 May;113(5):735–45. [PMID: 29545635]
Dionne J et al. A systematic review and meta-analysis evaluating the efficacy of a gluten-free diet and a low FODMAPS diet in treating symptoms of irritable bowel syndrome. Am J Gastroenterol. 2018 Sep;113(9):1290–300. [PMID: 30046155]
Eswaran S et al. A diet low in fermentable oligo-, di-, and monosaccharides and polyols improves quality of life and reduces activity impairment in patients with irritable bowel syndrome and diarrhea. Clin Gastroenterol Hepatol. 2017 Dec;15(12):1890–9. [PMID: 28668539]
Ford AC et al. American College of Gastroenterology monograph on management of irritable bowel syndrome. Am J Gastroenterol. 2018 Jun;113(Suppl 2):1–18. [PMID: 29950604]
Ford AC et al. Irritable bowel syndrome. N Engl J Med. 2017 Jun 29;376(26):2566–78. [PMID: 28657875]

Klem F et al. Prevalence, risk factors, and outcomes of irritable bowel syndrome after infectious enteritis: a systematic review and meta-analysis. Gastroenterology. 2017 Apr;152(5):1042–54. [PMID: 28069350]
Lackner JM et al. Improvement in gastrointestinal symptoms after cognitive behavior therapy for refractory irritable bowel syndrome. Gastroenterology. 2018 Jul;155(1):47–57. Erratum in: Gastroenterology. 2018 Oct;155(4):1281. [PMID: 29702118]
Staudacher HM et al. A diet low in FODMAPs reduces symptoms in patients with irritable bowel syndrome and a probiotic restores *Bifidobacterium* species: a randomized controlled trial. Gastroenterology. 2017 Oct;153(4):936–47. [PMID: 28625832]
Tuck CJ et al. Increasing symptoms in irritable bowel symptoms with ingestion of galacto-oligosaccharides are mitigated by α-galactosidase treatment. Am J Gastroenterol. 2018 Jan;113(1):124–34. [PMID: 28809383]

ANTIBIOTIC-ASSOCIATED COLITIS

ESSENTIALS OF DIAGNOSIS

► Most cases of antibiotic-associated diarrhea are not attributable to *C difficile* and are usually mild and self-limited.

► Symptoms of antibiotic-associated colitis vary from mild to fulminant; almost all colitis is attributable to *C difficile*.

► Diagnosis in most cases established by stool assay.

General Considerations

Antibiotic-associated diarrhea is a common clinical occurrence. Characteristically, the diarrhea occurs during the period of antibiotic exposure, is dose related, and resolves spontaneously after discontinuation of the antibiotic. In most cases, this diarrhea is mild, self-limited, and does not require any specific laboratory evaluation or treatment. Stool examination usually reveals no fecal leukocytes, and stool cultures reveal no pathogens. Although *C difficile* is identified in the stool of 15–25% of cases of antibiotic-associated diarrhea, it is also identified in 5–10% of patients treated with antibiotics who do not have diarrhea. Most cases of antibiotic-associated diarrhea are due to changes in colonic bacterial fermentation of carbohydrates and are not due to *C difficile*.

Antibiotic-associated colitis is a significant clinical problem almost always caused by *C difficile* infection that colonizes the colon and releases two toxins: TcdA and TcdB. This anaerobic bacterium is acquired by fecal-oral transmission of spores that colonize the colon of 3% of healthy adults and 8% of hospitalized patients. *C difficile* colitis is the major cause of diarrhea in patients hospitalized for more than 3 days, affecting up to 15 of every 1000 patients and increasing mean hospital stay costs as much as $30,000. In the United States, there are an estimated 453,000 cases per year with 29,000 associated deaths. Found throughout hospitals in patient rooms and bathrooms, *C difficile* is readily transmitted from patient to patient by hospital personnel. Fastidious hand washing and use of disposable gloves are helpful in minimizing transmission and reducing infections in hospitalized patients. In hospitalized patients, *C difficile* colitis occurs in approximately 20% of those who are colonized at admission and 3.5% of those not colonized. In both hospital-associated and community infections, most episodes of colitis occur in people who have received antibiotics that disrupt the normal bowel flora and thus allow the spores to germinate and the bacterium to flourish. Although almost all antibiotics have been implicated, colitis most commonly develops after use of ampicillin, clindamycin, third-generation cephalosporins, and fluoroquinolones. A 2017 meta-analysis of 19 clinical studies suggested that prophylactic administration of probiotics to hospitalized patients within 48 hours of antibiotic initiation reduces the risk of *C difficile* infection by more than 50%. Symptoms usually begin during or shortly after antibiotic therapy but may be delayed for up to 8 weeks. All patients with acute diarrhea should be asked about recent antibiotic exposure. Patients who are elderly; debilitated; immunocompromised; receiving multiple antibiotics or prolonged (more than 10 days) antibiotic therapy; receiving enteral tube feedings, proton pump inhibitors, or chemotherapy; or who have inflammatory bowel disease have a higher risk of acquiring *C difficile* and developing *C difficile*–associated diarrhea.

A more virulent strain of *C difficile* (NAP1) that contains an 18-base pair deletion of the TcdC inhibitory gene results in higher toxin A and B production. This hypervirulent strain is more prevalent among hospital-associated infections (31%) than community-acquired infections (19%) and has been associated with outbreaks of severe disease with up to 7% mortality.

▶ Clinical Findings

A. Symptoms and Signs

Most patients report mild to moderate greenish, foul-smelling watery diarrhea 5–15 times per day with lower abdominal cramps. Physical examination is normal or reveals mild left lower quadrant tenderness. The stools may have mucus but seldom gross blood. In most patients, colitis is most severe in the distal colon and rectum. Over half of hospitalized patients diagnosed with *C difficile* colitis have a white blood count greater than 15,000/mcL, and *C difficile* should be considered in all hospitalized patients with unexplained leukocytosis.

Severe or fulminant disease occurs in 10–15% of patients. It is characterized by fever; hemodynamic instability; and abdominal distention, pain, and tenderness. Most patients have profuse diarrhea (up to 30 stools/day); however, diarrhea may be absent or appear to be improving in patients with fulminant disease or ileus. Laboratory data suggestive of severe disease include a white blood count greater than 30,000/mcL, serum albumin less than 2.5 g/dL (due to protein-losing enteropathy), elevated serum lactate, or rising serum creatinine.

B. Special Examinations

1. Stool studies—Pathogenic strains of *C difficile* produce two toxins: toxin TcdA is an enterotoxin and toxin TcdB is a cytotoxin. Rapid enzyme immunoassays (EIAs) for toxins TcdA and TcdB have a 75–90% sensitivity with a single stool specimen; sensitivity increases to 90–95% with two specimens; however, these have now been supplanted in many laboratories by nucleic acid amplification tests (eg, PCR assays) that amplify the toxin TcdB gene. PCR assays are superior to EIA tests due to their high sensitivity (97%) as well as their ability to detect the NAP1 hypervirulent strain. Some laboratories first perform an assay for glutamate dehydrogenase (a common *C difficile* antigen), which has a high sensitivity and negative predictive value (greater than 95%). A negative glutamate dehydrogenase assay effectively excludes infection, while a positive assay requires confirmation with PCR or EIA to determine whether the strain that is present is toxin producing.

2. Flexible sigmoidoscopy—Flexible sigmoidoscopy is not needed in patients who have typical symptoms and a positive stool toxin assay. It may clarify the diagnosis in patients with positive *C difficile* toxin assays who have atypical symptoms or who have persistent diarrhea despite appropriate therapy. In patients with mild to moderate symptoms, there may be no abnormalities or only patchy or diffuse, nonspecific colitis indistinguishable from other causes. In patients with severe illness, true **pseudomembranous colitis** is seen.

3. Imaging studies—Abdominal radiographs or noncontrast abdominal CT scans are obtained in patients with severe or fulminant symptoms to look for evidence of colonic dilation and wall thickening. Abdominal CT also is useful in the evaluation of hospitalized patients with abdominal pain or ileus without significant diarrhea, in whom the presence of colonic wall thickening suggests unsuspected *C difficile* colitis. CT scanning is also useful in the detection of possible perforation.

▶ Differential Diagnosis

In the hospitalized patient in whom acute diarrhea develops after admission, the differential diagnosis includes simple antibiotic-associated diarrhea (not related to *C difficile*), enteral feedings, medications, and ischemic colitis. Other infectious causes are unusual in hospitalized patients in whom diarrhea develops more than 72 hours after admission, and it is not cost-effective to obtain stool cultures unless tests for *C difficile* are negative. Rarely, other organisms (staphylococci, *Clostridium perfringens*) have been associated with pseudomembranous colitis. *Klebsiella oxytoca* may cause a distinct form of antibiotic-associated hemorrhagic colitis that is segmental (usually in the right or transverse colon); spares the rectum; and is more common in younger, healthier outpatients.

▶ Complications

Severe colitis may progress quickly to fulminant disease, resulting in hemodynamic instability, respiratory failure, metabolic acidosis, megacolon (more than 7-cm diameter), perforation, and death. Chronic untreated colitis may result in weight loss and protein-losing enteropathy.

▶ Treatment

A. Immediate Treatment

If possible, antibiotic therapy should be discontinued and therapy with metronidazole, vancomycin, or fidaxomicin (a poorly absorbable macrolide antibiotic) should be initiated. For patients with mild disease, oral metronidazole (500 mg orally three times daily), vancomycin (125 mg orally four times daily), and fidaxomicin (200 mg orally two times daily) are equally effective for initial treatment. Vancomycin and fidaxomicin are significantly more expensive than metronidazole. At present, metronidazole remains the preferred first-line therapy in patients with mild disease, except in patients who are intolerant of metronidazole, patients with inflammatory bowel disease, pregnant women, and children, although vancomycin is increasingly used due to its superior efficacy against the NAP1 strain and the decreased cost of its generic version. The duration of initial therapy is usually 10–14 days. Symptomatic improvement occurs in most patients within 72 hours.

For patients with severe disease, characterized by a white blood cell count greater than 15,000/mcL, serum albumin less than 3 g/dL, or a rise in serum creatinine to more than 1.5 times baseline, vancomycin, 125 mg orally four times daily, is the preferred agent because it achieves significantly higher response rates (97%) than metronidazole (76%). In patients with severe, complicated disease, characterized by fever higher than 38.5°C, hypotension, mental status changes, ileus, megacolon, or WBC greater than 30,000/mcL, intravenous metronidazole, 500 mg every 6 hours, should be given—supplemented by vancomycin (500 mg four times daily administered by nasoenteric tube) and, in some cases, vancomycin enemas (500 mg in 100 mL every 6 hours). Intravenous vancomycin does not penetrate the bowel and should not be used. The efficacy of fidaxomicin for severe or fulminant disease requires further investigation. Early surgical consultation is recommended for all patients with severe or fulminant disease. Total abdominal colectomy or loop ileostomy with colonic lavage may be required in patients with toxic megacolon, perforation, sepsis, or hemorrhage.

B. Treatment of Relapse

Up to 25% of patients have a relapse of diarrhea from *C difficile* within 1 or 2 weeks after stopping initial therapy. This may be due to reinfection or failure to eradicate the organism. The optimal treatment regimen for recurrent relapses is evolving. The first episode of recurrent infection usually responds promptly to a second course of the same regimen used for the initial episode. Some patients, however, have further relapses that can be difficult to treat. For patients with two relapses, a 7-week tapering regimen of vancomycin is recommended: 125 mg orally four times daily for 14 days; twice daily for 7 days; once daily for 7 days; every other day for 7 days; and every third day for 2–8 weeks. Fidaxomicin may be appropriate for patients with recurrent *C difficile* infection or as initial therapy in patients believed to be at higher risk for recurrent disease. Patients treated with fidaxomicin have lower recurrence rates (15%)

of non-NAP1 *C difficile* strains than patients treated with vancomycin (25%).

For patients with three or more relapses, updated 2013 guidelines recommend consideration of an installation of a suspension of fecal bacteria from a healthy donor ("fecal microbiota transplant"). Until 2017, "fecal transplantation" was performed by installation into the terminal ileum or proximal colon (by colonoscopy) or into the duodenum and jejunum (by nasoenteric tube). Multiple case series reported disease remission after a single treatment in over 90% of patients with recurrent *C difficile* infection, and in a 2013 randomized study, duodenal infusion of donor feces led to resolution of *C difficile* diarrhea in 94%, which was dramatically higher than vancomycin treatment (31%). In 2017, a freeze-dried capsule fecal formulation became commercially available. In a multicenter, randomized controlled trial of 116 patients with recurrent *C difficile* infection, the proportion of patients without recurrent infection after 12 weeks was noninferior in patients treated with fecal transplantation administered by oral capsules versus colonoscopy-infusion (96.2% in both groups). Due to its efficacy and relative safety and ease of administration, fecal transplantation by oral capsule administration has become the preferred mode of fecal administration in most patients.

Kao D et al. Effect of oral capsule- vs colonoscopy-delivered fecal microbiota transplantation on recurrent *Clostridium difficile* infection: a randomized clinical trial. JAMA. 2017 Nov 28; 318(20):1985–93. [PMID: 29183074]

Krajicek E et al. Nuts and bolts of fecal microbiota transplantation. Clin Gastroenterol Hepatol. 2019 Jan;17(2):345–52. [PMID: 30268564]

Shen NT et al. Timely use of probiotics in hospitalized adults prevents *Clostridium difficile* infection: a systematic review with meta-regression analysis. Gastroenterology. 2017 Jun; 152(8):1889–900. [PMID: 28192108]

Vindigni SM et al. Managing *Clostridium difficile*: an old bug with new tricks. Am J Gastroenterol. 2018 Jul;113(7):932–5. [PMID: 29686272]

Wilcox MH et al; MODIFY I and MODIFY II Investigators. Bezlotoxumab for prevention of recurrent *Clostridium difficile* infection. N Engl J Med. 2017 Jan 26;376(4):305–17. [PMID: 28121498]

INFLAMMATORY BOWEL DISEASE

The term "inflammatory bowel disease" includes ulcerative colitis and Crohn disease. In the United States, there are approximately 1.6 million people with inflammatory bowel disease with adjusted annual incidences of 12.2 cases/100,000 and 10.7 cases/100,000 person-years for ulcerative colitis and Crohn disease, respectively. Ulcerative colitis is a chronic, recurrent disease characterized by diffuse mucosal inflammation involving only the colon. Ulcerative colitis invariably involves the rectum and may extend proximally in a continuous fashion to involve part or all of the colon. Crohn disease is a chronic, recurrent disease characterized by patchy transmural inflammation involving any segment of the gastrointestinal tract from the mouth to the anus.

Crohn disease and ulcerative colitis may be associated in 50% of patients with a number of extraintestinal manifestations, including oral ulcers, oligoarticular or polyarticular nondeforming peripheral arthritis, spondylitis or sacroiliitis, episcleritis or uveitis, erythema nodosum, pyoderma gangrenosum, hepatitis and sclerosing cholangitis, and thromboembolic events.

Pharmacologic Therapy

Although ulcerative colitis and Crohn disease appear to be distinct entities, several pharmacologic agents are used to treat both. Despite extensive research, there are still no specific therapies for these diseases. The mainstays of therapy are 5-aminosalicylic acid derivatives, corticosteroids, immunomodulating agents (such as mercaptopurine or azathioprine and methotrexate), and biologic agents.

A. 5-Aminosalicylic Acid (5-ASA)

5-ASA is a topically active agent that has a variety of antiinflammatory effects. It is used in the active treatment of ulcerative colitis and Crohn disease and during disease inactivity to maintain remission. It is readily absorbed from the small intestine but demonstrates minimal colonic absorption. A number of oral and topical compounds have been designed to target delivery of 5-ASA to the colon or small intestine while minimizing absorption. Commonly used formulations of 5-ASA are sulfasalazine, mesalamine, and azo compounds. Side effects of these compounds are uncommon but include nausea, rash, diarrhea, pancreatitis, and acute interstitial nephritis.

1. Oral mesalamine agents—These 5-ASA agents are coated in various pH-sensitive resins (Asacol, Apriso, and Lialda) or packaged in timed-release capsules (Pentasa). Pentasa releases 5-ASA slowly throughout the small intestine and colon. Asacol, Apriso, and Lialda tablets dissolve at pH 6.0–7.0, releasing 5-ASA in the terminal small bowel and proximal colon. Lialda has a multi-matrix system that gradually releases 5-ASA throughout the colon.

2. Azo compounds—Sulfasalazine, balsalazide, and olsalazine contain 5-ASA linked by an azo bond that requires cleavage by colonic bacterial azoreductases to release 5-ASA. Absorption of these drugs from the small intestine is negligible. After release within the colon, the 5-ASA works topically and is largely unabsorbed.

Sulfasalazine contains 5-ASA linked to a sulfapyridine moiety. It is unclear whether the sulfapyridine group has any anti-inflammatory effects. One gram of sulfasalazine contains 400 mg of 5-ASA. The sulfapyridine group, however, is absorbed and may cause side effects in 15–30% of patients—much higher than with other 5-ASA compounds. Dose-related side effects include nausea, headaches, leukopenia, oligospermia, and impaired folate metabolism. Allergic and idiosyncratic side effects are fever, rash, hemolytic anemia, neutropenia, worsened colitis, hepatitis, pancreatitis, and pneumonitis. Because of its side effects, sulfasalazine is less frequently used than other 5-ASA agents. It should always be administered in conjunction with folate. Eighty percent of patients intolerant of sulfasalazine can tolerate mesalamine.

3. Topical mesalamine—5-ASA is provided in the form of suppositories (Canasa; 1000 mg) and enemas (Rowasa;

4 g/60 mL). These formulations can deliver much higher concentrations of 5-ASA to the distal colon than oral compounds. Side effects are uncommon.

B. Corticosteroids

A variety of intravenous, oral, and topical corticosteroid formulations have been used in inflammatory bowel disease. They have utility in the short-term treatment of moderate to severe disease. However, long-term use is associated with serious, potentially irreversible side effects and is to be avoided. The agents, route of administration, duration of use, and tapering regimens used are based more on personal bias and experience than on data from rigorous clinical trials. The most commonly used intravenous formulations have been hydrocortisone or methylprednisolone, which are given by continuous infusion or every 6 hours. Oral formulations are prednisone or methylprednisolone. Adverse events commonly occur during short-term systemic corticosteroid therapy, including mood changes, insomnia, dyspepsia, weight gain, edema, elevated serum glucose levels, acne, and moon facies. Side effects of long-term use include osteoporosis, osteonecrosis of the femoral head, myopathy, cataracts, and susceptibility to infections. Calcium and vitamin D supplementation should be administered to all patients receiving long-term corticosteroid therapy. Bone densitometry should be considered in patients with inflammatory bowel disease with other risk factors for osteoporosis and in all patients with a lifetime use of corticosteroids for 3 months or more. Budesonide is an oral corticosteroid with high topical anti-inflammatory activity but low systemic activity due to high first-pass hepatic metabolism. An enteric-coated formulation is available (Entocort) that targets delivery to the terminal ileum and proximal colon. An enteric coated, multi-matrix, delayed-release formulation (budesonide MMX [Uceris]) is available that releases budesonide throughout the colon. Budesonide produces less suppression of the hypothalamic-pituitary-adrenal axis and fewer steroid-related side effects than hydrocortisone or prednisone. Topical preparations are provided as hydrocortisone suppositories (100 mg), foam (90 mg), and enemas (100 mg) and as budesonide foam (2 mg).

C. Immunomodulating Drugs and Other Small Molecules

1. Thiopurines (mercaptopurine and azathioprine)—These drugs are used in many patients with moderate to severe Crohn disease and ulcerative colitis either alone or in combination with anti-TNF agents. Thiopurines are used alone in patients who are corticosteroid-dependent in an attempt to reduce or withdraw corticosteroids and in patients in remission to reduce the risk of disease recurrence. Thiopurines are used in combination with biologic agents (especially anti-TNF agents) to reduce antibody formation against the biologic agent and to increase the likelihood of clinical remission through increased anti-TNF drug levels and possible synergistic effects. Azathioprine is converted in vivo to mercaptopurine. It is believed that the active metabolite of mercaptopurine is 6-thioguanine. Side effects of mercaptopurine and azathioprine, including allergic reactions (fever, rash, or arthralgias) and nonallergic reactions (nausea, vomiting, pancreatitis, hepatotoxicity, bone marrow suppression, infections), occur in 15% of patients. Thiopurines are associated with up to a 2.5-fold increased risk of non-Hodgkin lymphomas (0.5/1000 patient-years). The risk rises after 1–2 years of exposure and is higher in men younger than age 30 years and patients older than age 50 years. Thiopurines also are associated with a risk of human papillomavirus (HPV)–related cervical dysplasia and with an increased risk of nonmelanoma skin cancer. Younger patients also are at risk for severe primary Epstein-Barr virus (EBV) infection, if not previously exposed.

Three competing enzymes are involved in the metabolism of mercaptopurine to its active (6-thioguanine) and inactive but potentially toxic metabolites (6-MMP). About 1 person in 300 has a homozygous mutation of one of the enzymes that metabolizes thiopurine methyltransferase (TPMT), placing them at risk for profound immunosuppression; 1 person in 9 is heterozygous for TPMT, resulting in intermediate enzyme activity. Measurement of TPMT functional activity is recommended prior to initiation of therapy. Treatment should be withheld in patients with absent TPMT activity. The most effective dose of mercaptopurine is 1–1.5 mg/kg. For azathioprine, it is 2–3 mg/kg daily. For patients with normal TPMT activity, both drugs may be initiated at the weight-calculated dose. A complete blood count should be obtained weekly for 4 weeks, biweekly for 4 weeks, and then every 1–3 months for the duration of therapy. Liver biochemical tests should be measured periodically. Some clinicians prefer gradual dose escalation, especially for patients with intermediate TPMT activity or for whom TPMT measurement is not available; both drugs may be started at 25 mg/day and increased by 25 mg every 1–2 weeks while monitoring for myelosuppression until the target dose is reached. If the white blood count falls below 4000/mcL or the platelet count falls below 100,000/mcL, the medication should be held for at least 1 week before reducing the daily dose by 25–50 mg. Measurement of thiopurine metabolites (6-TG and 6-MMP) is of unproved value in most patients but is recommended in patients who have not responded to standard, weight-based dosing or in whom adverse effects develop.

2. Methotrexate—Low-dose oral methotrexate is used in combination with biologic agents to prevent immunogenicity. Methotrexate is an analog of dihydrofolic acid. Side effects of methotrexate include nausea, vomiting, stomatitis, infections, bone marrow suppression, hepatic fibrosis, and life-threatening pneumonitis. A complete blood count and liver chemistries should be monitored every 3 months. Folate supplementation (1 mg/day) should be administered. Because methotrexate is teratogenic, it should be discontinued in men and women at least 6 months before conception and during pregnancy.

3. Janus kinase inhibitors—Tofacitinib is a nonbiologic small-molecule inhibitor of Janus kinase (JAK 1/3), which is involved through the JAK-STAT pathway in modulation of multiple interleukins. It was approved by the FDA in 2018 for the treatment of moderate to severe ulcerative colitis (not Crohn disease). It has rapid oral absorption and lacks immunogenicity. When used as monotherapy, it has a low risk of adverse events (including infections) with the exception of herpes zoster (5% of patients). Vaccination with inactivated (not live) recombinant zoster (Shingrix) is recommended in all patients older than 50 years and in younger patients with other risk factors for reactivation. Elevations in both low-density lipoprotein (LDL) and high-density lipoprotein (HDL) are seen in 10–15% of patients within 4–8 weeks; however, the LDL/HDL ratio is unaltered and there has been no increase in cardiac events in long-term follow-up to 4 years. Prescribing guidelines recommend monitoring with a lipid panel within the first 8 weeks of treatment and with routine blood tests (liver tests, complete blood count) every 3 months.

D. Biologic Therapies

Although the etiology of inflammatory bowel disorders is uncertain, it appears that an abnormal response of the mucosal innate immune system to luminal bacteria may trigger inflammation, which is perpetuated by dysregulation of cellular immunity. A number of biologic therapies are available or in clinical testing that more narrowly target various components of the immune system. Biologic agents are highly effective for patients with moderate to severe disease and when administered early in the disease course may improve the natural history of disease. The potential benefits of these agents, however, must be carefully weighed with their high cost and risk of serious and potentially life-threatening side effects.

1. Anti-TNF therapies—TNF is one of the key proinflammatory cytokines in the T_H1 response. Four monoclonal antibodies to TNF currently are available for the treatment of inflammatory bowel disease: infliximab, adalimumab, golimumab, and certolizumab. All four agents bind and neutralize soluble as well as membrane-bound TNF on macrophages and activated T lymphocytes, thereby preventing TNF stimulation of effector cells.

Infliximab is a chimeric (75% human/25% mouse) IgG_1 antibody that is administered by intravenous infusion. A three-dose regimen of 5 mg/kg administered at 0, 2, and 6 weeks is recommended for acute induction, followed by infusions every 8 weeks for maintenance therapy. Acute infusion reactions occur in 5–10% of infusions but occur less commonly in patients receiving regularly scheduled infusions or concomitant immunomodulators (ie, azathioprine or methotrexate). Most reactions are mild or moderate (nausea; headache; dizziness; urticaria; diaphoresis; or mild cardiopulmonary symptoms that include chest tightness, dyspnea, or palpitations) and can be treated by slowing the infusion rate and administering acetaminophen and diphenhydramine. Severe reactions (hypotension, severe shortness of breath, rigors, severe chest discomfort) occur in less than 1% and may require oxygen, diphenhydramine, hydrocortisone, and epinephrine. Delayed serum sickness-like reactions occur in 1%. With repeated, intermittent intravenous injections, antibodies to infliximab develop in up to 40% of patients, which are associated with a shortened duration or loss of response and increased risk of acute or delayed infusion reactions. Giving infliximab in a regularly scheduled maintenance therapy (eg, every 8 weeks), concomitant use of infliximab with other immunomodulating agents (azathioprine, mercaptopurine, or methotrexate), or preinfusion treatment with corticosteroids (intravenous hydrocortisone 200 mg) significantly reduces the development of antibodies to less than 10%.

Adalimumab and golimumab are fully human IgG_1 antibodies that are administered by subcutaneous injection. For adalimumab, a dose of 160 mg at week 0 and 80 mg at week 2 is recommended for acute induction, followed by maintenance therapy with 40 mg subcutaneously every other week. For golimumab, a dose of 200 mg at week 0 and 100 mg at week 2 is recommended for acute induction, followed by maintenance therapy with 100 mg subcutaneously every 4 weeks.

Certolizumab is a fusion compound in which the Fab1 portion of a chimeric (95% human/5% mouse) TNF-antibody is bound to polyethylene glycol in order to prolong the drug half-life. However, certolizumab is infrequently used due to lower clinical efficacy.

Acute and delayed hypersensitivity reactions are rare with subcutaneous anti-TNF therapies. Antibodies to adalimumab or golimumab develop in 5% of patients and to certolizumab in 10%, which may lead to shortened duration or loss of response to the drug.

Serious infections with anti-TNF therapies may occur in 2–5% of patients, including sepsis, pneumonia, abscess, and cellulitis; however, controlled studies suggest the increased risk may be attributable to increased severity of disease and concomitant use of corticosteroids. Patients treated with anti-TNF therapies are at increased risk for the development of opportunistic infections with intracellular bacterial pathogens including tuberculosis, mycoses (candidiasis, histoplasmosis, coccidioidomycosis, nocardiosis), and listeriosis, and with reactivation of viral infections, including hepatitis B, herpes simplex, varicella zoster, and EBV. Prior to use of these agents, patients should be screened for latent tuberculosis with PPD testing and a chest radiograph. Antinuclear and anti-DNA antibodies occur in a large percentage of patients; however, the development of drug-induced lupus is rare. All agents may cause severe hepatic reactions leading to acute hepatic failure; liver biochemical tests should be monitored routinely during therapy. Anti-TNF therapies increase the risk of nonmelanoma skin cancer, hence annual dermatologic examinations are recommended. The risk of non-Hodgkin lymphoma is increased approximately 2.4-fold (0.4/1000 person-years) in patients taking anti-TNF monotherapy; however, the risk is much higher in patients receiving a combination of anti-TNF and a thiopurine (6.1-fold increase; 0.95/1000 person-years). Rare cases of optic neuritis and demyelinating diseases, including multiple sclerosis have been reported. Anti-TNF therapies may worsen heart failure in patients with cardiac disease.

In patients with active inflammatory bowel disease, monitoring of anti-TNF trough levels and any anti-drug antibodies can help guide therapy, especially in patients who have poor clinical response or who have lost clinical response. At present, recommended trough concentrations are greater than 3–7 mcg/mL for infliximab and greater than 7.5 mcg/mL for adalimumab. Patients with high titers of anti-drug antibodies should be switched to a different anti-TNF agent. Anti-TNF therapy is considered to have failed when patients have a poor response despite adequate anti-TNF trough concentrations; another class of drugs should be tried.

2. Anti-integrins—Anti-integrins decrease the trafficking of circulating leukocytes through the vasculature, reducing chronic inflammation. Vedolizumab is an anti-integrin that blocks the $alpha_4beta_7$ heterodimer, selectively blocking gut, but not brain, lymphocyte trafficking. Vedolizumab is FDA approved for patients with moderately active ulcerative colitis or Crohn disease who have an inadequate response to or intolerance of anti-TNF agents. Induction therapy is given as a 300-mg intravenous dose at weeks 0, 2, and 6. This is followed by maintenance therapy of 300 mg intravenously every 4–8 weeks based on clinical response or serum trough concentrations. Thus far, vedolizumab does not appear to be associated with an increased risk of serious infections or malignancy. Infusion reactions are uncommon. Antibodies develop in 5%, which may interfere with drug efficacy. Natalizumab is another anti-integrin compound that targets the $alpha_4$ integrin, thereby blocking trafficking to both the gut and brain. However, natalizumab may cause a reactivation of JC polyoma virus, leading to an increased incidence of progressive multifocal leukoencephalopathy (PML). To date, there are no cases of PML associated with vedolizumab, likely due to its greater selectivity for gut lymphocytes. With the advent of vedolizumab, natalizumab is now rarely used for inflammatory bowel disease.

3. Anti-IL-12/23 antibody—Ustekinumab is a human IgG_1 monoclonal antibody that binds the p40 subunit of IL-12 and IL-23, interfering with their receptor binding on T cells, NK cells, and antigen presenting cells. Ustekinumab was FDA approved in 2016 for the treatment of patients with moderate to severe Crohn disease (not ulcerative colitis) who have not responded to or are intolerant of conventional therapies. Induction therapy is given as a single, weight-based intravenous dose (approximately 5–7 mg/kg), followed by 90 mg every 8 weeks by subcutaneous injection. In extensive experience with its use in the treatment of psoriasis and clinical trial experience in treatment of Crohn disease, there has been no demonstrated increase in severe infections or malignancy, and other serious events are rare. Antibodies to ustekinumab develop in less than 5% of patients but their impact on treatment efficacy is uncertain.

Bonovas S et al. Biologic therapies and risk of infection and malignancy in patients with inflammatory bowel disease: a systematic review and network meta-analysis. Clin Gastroenterol Hepatol. 2016 Oct;14(10):1385–97. [PMID: 27189910]

Burke KE et al. Tofacitinib: a jak of all trades. Clin Gastroenterol Hepatol. 2019 Jan 5. [Epub ahead of print] [PMID: 30625401]

Cross RK et al. Is there a role for thiopurines in IBD? Am J Gastroenterol. 2018 Aug;113(8):1121–4. [PMID: 29946181]

Dreesen E et al. Evidence to support monitoring of vedolizumab trough concentrations in patients with inflammatory bowel diseases. Clin Gastroenterol Hepatol. 2018 Dec;16(12): 1937–46. [PMID: 29704680]

Farraye F et al. ACG Clinical Guideline: preventive care in inflammatory bowel disease. Am J Gastroenterol. 2017 Feb; 112(2):241–58. [PMID: 28071656]

Feuerstein JD et al. American Gastroenterological Association Institute guidelines on therapeutic drug monitoring in inflammatory bowel disease. Gastroenterology. 2017 Sep;153(3): 827–34. [PMID: 28780013]

Hanauer SB et al. Evolving considerations for thiopurine therapy for inflammatory bowel diseases—a clinical practice update: commentary. Gastroenterology. 2019 Jan;156(1):36–42. [PMID: 30195449]

Herfarth HH et al. Use of methotrexate in the treatment of inflammatory bowel diseases. Inflamm Bowel Dis. 2016 Jan; 22(1):224–33. [PMID: 26457382]

Kirchgesner J et al. Risk of serious and opportunistic infections associated with treatment of inflammatory bowel diseases. Gastroenterology. 2018 Aug;155(2):337–46. [PMID: 29655835]

Lemaitre M et al. Association between use of thiopurines or tumor necrosis factor antagonists alone or in combination and risk of lymphoma in patients with inflammatory bowel disease. JAMA. 2017 Nov 7;318(17):1679–86. [PMID: 29114832]

Papamichael K et al. Improved long-term outcomes of patients with inflammatory bowel disease receiving proactive compared with reactive monitoring of serum concentrations of infliximab. Clin Gastroenterol Hepatol. 2017 Oct;15(10):1580–8. [PMID: 28365486]

Willet N et al. Association between low trough levels of vedolizumab during induction therapy for inflammatory bowel diseases and need for additional doses within 6 months. Clin Gastroenterol Hepatol. 2017 Nov;15(11):1750–57. [PMID: 27890854]

▶ Social Support for Patients

Inflammatory bowel disease is a lifelong illness that can have profound emotional and social impacts on the individual. Patients should be encouraged to become involved in the Crohn's and Colitis Foundation of America (CCFA). National headquarters may be contacted at 733 Third Avenue, Suite 510, New York, NY 10017; phone 800-932-2423. Internet address: www.ccfa.org.

1. Crohn Disease

ESSENTIALS OF DIAGNOSIS

- ▶ Insidious onset.
- ▶ Intermittent bouts of low-grade fever, diarrhea, and right lower quadrant pain.
- ▶ Right lower quadrant mass and tenderness.
- ▶ Perianal disease with abscess, fistulas.
- ▶ Radiographic or endoscopic evidence of ulceration, stricturing, or fistulas of the small intestine or colon.

▶ General Considerations

One-third of cases of Crohn disease involve the small bowel only, most commonly the terminal ileum (ileitis). Half of all cases involve the small bowel and colon, most often the terminal ileum and adjacent proximal ascending colon (ileocolitis). In 20% of cases, the colon alone is affected. One-third of patients have associated perianal disease (fistulas, fissures, abscesses). Less than 5% of patients have symptomatic involvement of the upper intestinal tract. Unlike ulcerative colitis, Crohn disease is a transmural process that can result in mucosal inflammation and ulceration, stricturing, fistula development, and abscess formation. Cigarette smoking is strongly associated with the development of Crohn disease, resistance to medical therapy, and early disease relapse.

▶ Clinical Findings

A. Symptoms and Signs

Because of the variable location of involvement and severity of inflammation, Crohn disease may present with a variety of symptoms and signs. In eliciting the history, the clinician should take particular note of fevers, the patient's general sense of well-being, weight loss, the presence of abdominal pain, the number of liquid bowel movements per day, and prior surgical resections. Physical examination should focus on the patient's temperature, weight, and nutritional status, the presence of abdominal tenderness or mass, rectal examination, and extraintestinal manifestations. Approximately 20–30% of patients have an indolent, nonprogressive course. The majority will require specific therapies (often biologic agents) to reduce inflammation, improve quality of life, and reduce the risk of surgery and hospitalization. Most commonly, there is one or a combination of the following clinical constellations.

1. Chronic inflammatory disease—This is the most common presentation and is often seen in patients with ileitis or ileocolitis. Patients report malaise, weight loss, and loss of energy. In patients with ileitis or ileocolitis, there may be diarrhea, which is usually nonbloody and often intermittent. In patients with colitis involving the rectum or left colon, there may be bloody diarrhea and fecal urgency, which may mimic the symptoms of ulcerative colitis. Cramping or steady right lower quadrant or periumbilical pain is common. Physical examination reveals focal tenderness, usually in the right lower quadrant. A palpable, tender mass that represents thickened or matted loops of inflamed intestine may be present in the lower abdomen.

2. Intestinal obstruction—Narrowing of the small bowel may occur as a result of inflammation, spasm, or fibrotic stenosis. Patients report postprandial bloating, cramping pains, and loud borborygmi. This may occur in patients with active inflammatory symptoms (as above) or later in the disease from chronic fibrosis without other systemic symptoms or signs of inflammation.

3. Penetrating disease and fistulae—Sinus tracts that penetrate through the bowel, where they may be contained or form fistulas to adjacent structures, develop in a subset of patients. Penetration through the bowel can result in an intra-abdominal or retroperitoneal phlegmon or abscess manifested by fevers, chills, a tender abdominal mass, and leukocytosis. Fistulas between the small intestine and colon commonly are asymptomatic, but can result in diarrhea, weight loss, bacterial overgrowth, and malnutrition. Fistulas to the bladder produce recurrent infections. Fistulas to the vagina result in malodorous drainage and problems with personal hygiene. Fistulas to the skin usually occur at the site of surgical scars.

4. Perianal disease—One-third of patients with either large or small bowel involvement develop perianal disease manifested by large painful skin tags, anal fissures, perianal abscesses, and fistulas.

5. Extraintestinal manifestations—Extraintestinal manifestations may be seen with both Crohn disease and ulcerative colitis. These include arthralgias, arthritis, iritis or uveitis, pyoderma gangrenosum, or erythema nodosum. Oral aphthous lesions are common. There is an increased prevalence of gallstones due to malabsorption of bile salts from the terminal ileum. Nephrolithiasis with urate or calcium oxalate stones may occur.

B. Laboratory Findings

Laboratory values may reflect inflammatory activity or nutritional complications of disease. A complete blood count and serum albumin should be obtained in all patients. Anemia may reflect chronic inflammation, mucosal blood loss, iron deficiency, or vitamin B_{12} malabsorption secondary to terminal ileal inflammation or resection. Leukocytosis may reflect inflammation or abscess formation or may be secondary to corticosteroid therapy. Hypoalbuminemia may be due to intestinal protein loss, malabsorption, bacterial overgrowth, or chronic inflammation. The sedimentation rate or C-reactive protein level is elevated in many patients during active inflammation; however, one-third have a normal C-reactive protein level. Fecal calprotectin is an excellent noninvasive test. Elevated levels are correlated with active inflammation as demonstrated by ileocolonoscopy or radiologic CT or MR enterography. Stool specimens are sent for examination for routine pathogens and *C difficile* toxin by microscopy, culture, and toxin assay or by rapid multiplex PCR diagnostic assessment.

C. Special Diagnostic Studies

In most patients, the initial diagnosis of Crohn disease is based on a compatible clinical picture with supporting endoscopic, pathologic, and radiographic findings. Colonoscopy usually is performed first to evaluate the colon and terminal ileum and to obtain mucosal biopsies. Typical endoscopic findings include aphthoid, linear or stellate ulcers, strictures, and segmental involvement with areas of normal-appearing mucosa adjacent to inflamed mucosa. In 10% of cases, it may be difficult to distinguish ulcerative colitis from Crohn disease. Granulomas on biopsy are present in less than 25% of patients but are highly suggestive of Crohn disease. CT or MR enterography is obtained in patients with suspected small bowel involvement. Suggestive findings include ulcerations, strictures, and fistulas; in addition, CT or MR enterography may identify bowel wall thickening and vascularity, mucosal enhancement, and fat stranding. MR enterography, where available, may be preferred due its lack of radiation exposure. Capsule imaging

may help establish a diagnosis when clinical suspicion for small bowel involvement is high but radiographs are normal or nondiagnostic. Barium upper gastrointestinal series with small bowel follow through should no longer be performed except where CT or MR enterography is unavailable.

▶ Complications

A. Abscess

The presence of a tender abdominal mass with fever and leukocytosis suggests an abscess. Emergent CT of the abdomen is necessary to confirm the diagnosis. Patients should be given broad-spectrum antibiotics. Percutaneous drainage or surgery is usually required.

B. Obstruction

Small bowel obstruction may develop secondary to active inflammation or chronic fibrotic stricturing and is often acutely precipitated by dietary indiscretion. Patients should be given intravenous fluids with nasogastric suction. Systemic corticosteroids are indicated in patients with symptoms or signs of active inflammation but are unhelpful in patients with inactive, fixed disease. Patients unimproved on medical management require surgical resection of the stenotic area or stricturoplasty.

C. Abdominal and Rectovaginal Fistulas

Many fistulas are asymptomatic and require no specific therapy. Most symptomatic fistulas eventually require surgical therapy; however, medical therapy is effective in a subset of patients and is usually tried first in outpatients who otherwise are stable. Large abscesses associated with fistulas require percutaneous or surgical drainage. After percutaneous drainage, long-term antibiotics are administered in order to reduce recurrent infections until the fistula is closed or surgically resected. Anti-TNF agents may promote closure in up to 60% within 10 weeks; however, relapse occurs in over one-half of patients within 1 year despite continued therapy. Surgical therapy is required for symptomatic fistulas that do not respond to medical therapy. Fistulas that arise above (proximal to) areas of intestinal stricturing commonly require surgical treatment.

D. Perianal Disease

Patients with fissures, fistulas, and skin tags commonly have perianal discomfort. Successful treatment of active intestinal disease also may improve perianal disease. Specific treatment of perianal disease can be difficult and is best approached jointly with a surgeon with an expertise in colorectal disorders. Pelvic MRI is the best noninvasive study for evaluating perianal fistulas. Patients should be instructed on proper perianal skin care, including gentle wiping with a premoistened pad (baby wipes) followed by drying with a cool hair dryer, daily cleansing with sitz baths or a water wash, and use of perianal cotton balls or pads to absorb drainage. Oral antibiotics (metronidazole, 250 mg three times daily, or ciprofloxacin, 500 mg twice daily) may promote symptom improvement or healing in patients with fissures or uncomplicated fistulas; however, recurrent symptoms are common. Refractory fissures may benefit from mesalamine suppositories or topical 0.1% tacrolimus ointment. Immunomodulators or anti-TNF agents or both promote short-term symptomatic improvement from anal fistulas in two-thirds of patients and complete closure in up to one-half of patients; however, less than one-third maintain symptomatic remission during long-term maintenance treatment.

Anorectal abscesses should be suspected in patients with severe, constant perianal pain, or perianal pain in association with fever. Superficial abscesses are evident on perianal examination, but deep perirectal abscesses may be detected by digital examination or pelvic CT scan. Depending on the abscess location, surgical drainage may be achieved by incision, or catheter or seton placement. Surgery should be considered for patients with severe, refractory symptoms but is best approached after medical therapy of the Crohn disease has been optimized.

E. Carcinoma

Patients with colonic Crohn disease are at increased risk for developing colon carcinoma; hence, annual screening colonoscopy to detect dysplasia or cancer is recommended for patients with a history of 8 or more years of Crohn colitis. Patients with Crohn disease have an increased risk of lymphoma and of small bowel adenocarcinoma; however, both are rare.

F. Hemorrhage

Unlike ulcerative colitis, severe hemorrhage is unusual in Crohn disease.

G. Malabsorption

Malabsorption may arise after extensive surgical resections of the small intestine and from bacterial overgrowth in patients with enterocolonic fistulas, strictures, and stasis resulting in bacterial overgrowth. Serum levels of vitamins A, D, and B_{12} should be obtained at diagnosis and monitored periodically in patients with ileal inflammation or resection.

▶ Differential Diagnosis

Chronic cramping abdominal pain and diarrhea are typical of both irritable bowel syndrome and Crohn disease, but radiographic examinations are normal in the former. Celiac disease may cause diarrhea with malabsorption. Acute fever and right lower quadrant pain may resemble appendicitis or *Yersinia enterocolitica* enteritis. Intestinal lymphoma causes fever, pain, weight loss, and abnormal small bowel radiographs that may mimic Crohn disease. Patients with undiagnosed AIDS may present with fever and diarrhea. Segmental colitis may be caused by tuberculosis, *E histolytica, Chlamydia*, or ischemic colitis. *C difficile* or CMV infection may develop in patients with inflammatory bowel disease, mimicking disease recurrence. In patients from tuberculosis-endemic countries, it can be extremely difficult to distinguish active intestinal tuberculosis from Crohn disease, even with biopsies and PCR

analyses. Diverticulitis or appendicitis with abscess formation may be difficult to distinguish acutely from Crohn disease. NSAIDs may exacerbate inflammatory bowel disease and may also cause NSAID-induced colitis characterized by small bowel or colonic ulcers, erosion, or strictures that tend to be most severe in the terminal ileum and right colon.

▶ Treatment of Active Disease

Crohn disease is a chronic lifelong illness characterized by exacerbations and periods of remission. As no specific therapy exists, current treatment is directed toward symptomatic improvement and control of the disease process, in order to improve quality of life and reduce disease progression and complications. Although sustained clinical remission should be the therapeutic goal, this cannot be achieved in all patients. Choice of therapies depends on the disease location and severity, patient age and comorbidities, and patient preference. Early introduction of biologic therapy should be considered strongly in patients with risk factors for aggressive disease, including young age, perianal disease, stricturing disease, or need for corticosteroids. All patients with Crohn disease should be counseled to discontinue cigarettes.

A. Nutrition

1. Diet—Patients should eat a well-balanced diet with as few restrictions as possible. Eating smaller but more frequent meals may be helpful. Patients with diarrhea should be encouraged to drink fluids to avoid dehydration. Many patients report that certain foods worsen symptoms, especially fried or greasy foods. Because lactose intolerance is common, a trial off dairy products is warranted if flatulence or diarrhea is a prominent complaint. Patients with obstructive symptoms should be placed on a low-roughage diet, ie, no raw fruits or vegetables, popcorn, nuts, etc. Resection of more than 100 cm of terminal ileum results in fat malabsorption for which a low-fat diet is recommended. Parenteral vitamin B_{12} (1000 mcg subcutaneously per month) and oral vitamin D supplementation commonly is needed for patients with previous ileal resection or extensive terminal ileal disease.

2. Enteral therapy—Supplemental enteral therapy via nasogastric tube may be required for children and adolescents with poor intake and growth retardation.

3. Total parenteral nutrition—TPN is used short term in patients with active disease and progressive weight loss or those awaiting surgery who have malnutrition but cannot tolerate enteral feedings because of high-grade obstruction, high-output fistulas, severe diarrhea, or abdominal pain. It is required long term in a small subset of patients with extensive intestinal resections resulting in short bowel syndrome with malnutrition.

B. Symptomatic Medications

There are several potential mechanisms by which diarrhea may occur in Crohn disease in addition to active Crohn disease. A rational empiric treatment approach often yields therapeutic improvement that may obviate the need for corticosteroids or immunosuppressive agents. Involvement of the terminal ileum with Crohn disease or prior ileal resection may lead to reduced absorption of bile acids that may induce secretory diarrhea from the colon. This diarrhea commonly responds to cholestyramine 2–4 g, colestipol 5 g, or colesevelam 625 mg one to two times daily before meals to bind the malabsorbed bile salts. Patients with extensive ileal disease (requiring more than 100 cm of ileal resection) have such severe bile salt malabsorption that steatorrhea may arise. Such patients may benefit from a low-fat diet; bile salt-binding agents will exacerbate the diarrhea and should not be given. Patients with Crohn disease are at risk for the development of small intestinal bacterial overgrowth due to enteral fistulas, ileal resection, and impaired motility and may benefit from a course of broad-spectrum antibiotics (see Bacterial Overgrowth, above). Other causes of diarrhea include lactase deficiency and short bowel syndrome (described in other sections). Use of oral antidiarrheal agents may provide benefit in some patients. Loperamide (2–4 mg), diphenoxylate with atropine (one tablet), or tincture of opium (5–15 drops) may be given as needed up to four times daily. Because of the risk of toxic megacolon, these drugs should not be used in patients with active severe colitis.

C. Specific Drug Therapy

1. 5-Aminosalicylic acid agents—Mesalamine has long been used as initial therapy for the treatment of mild to moderately active colonic and ileocolonic Crohn disease. However, meta-analyses of published and unpublished trial data suggest that mesalamine is of no value in either the treatment of active Crohn disease or the maintenance of remission. Current treatment guidelines recommend against its use for Crohn disease.

2. Corticosteroids—Approximately one-half of patients with Crohn disease require corticosteroids at some time in their illness. Corticosteroids dramatically suppress the acute clinical symptoms or signs in most patients with both small and large bowel disease; however, they do not alter the underlying disease. An ileal-release budesonide preparation (Entocort), 9 mg once daily for 8–16 weeks, induces remission in 50–70% of patients with mild to moderate Crohn disease involving the terminal ileum or ascending colon. After initial treatment, budesonide is tapered over 2–4 weeks in 3 mg increments. In some patients, low-dose budesonide (6 mg/day) may be used for up to 1 year to maintain remission. Budesonide is superior to mesalamine but somewhat less effective than prednisone. However, because budesonide has markedly reduced acute and chronic steroid-related adverse effects, including smaller reductions of bone mineral density, it is preferred to other systemic corticosteroids for the treatment of mild to moderate Crohn disease involving the terminal ileum or ascending colon.

Prednisone or methylprednisolone, 40–60 mg/day, is generally administered to patients with Crohn disease that is severe, that involves the distal colon or proximal small intestine, or that has failed treatment with budesonide. Remission or significant improvement occurs in greater than 80%

of patients after 8–16 weeks of therapy. After improvement at 2 weeks, tapering proceeds at 5 mg/wk until a dosage of 20 mg/day is being given. Thereafter, slow tapering by 2.5 mg/wk is recommended. Approximately 20% of patients cannot be completely withdrawn from corticosteroids without experiencing a symptomatic flare-up. Furthermore, more than 50% of patients who achieve initial remission on corticosteroids will experience a relapse within 1 year. Use of long-term low corticosteroid doses (2.5–10 mg/day) should be avoided because of associated complications. Patients requiring long-term corticosteroid treatment should be given immunomodulatory drugs or biologic therapies or both in an effort to wean them from corticosteroids.

Patients with persisting symptoms despite oral corticosteroids or those with high fever, persistent vomiting, evidence of intestinal obstruction, severe weight loss, severe abdominal tenderness, or suspicion of an abscess should be hospitalized. In patients with a tender, palpable inflammatory abdominal mass, CT scan of the abdomen should be obtained prior to administering corticosteroids to rule out an abscess. If no abscess is identified, parenteral corticosteroids should be administered (as described for ulcerative colitis below).

3. Azathioprine, mercaptopurine, or methotrexate—The three main indications for immunomodulators in Crohn disease are (1) after induction therapy with corticosteroids to allow their withdrawal (particularly in patients who are corticosteroid-dependent) and to maintain remission; (2) for the induction of remission, in combination with anti-TNF therapy, in patients with moderate to severe active Crohn disease (discussed in next section); and (3) in combination with biologic agents to reduce the likelihood of neutralizing antibody formation. In the United States, mercaptopurine or azathioprine is more commonly used for induction of remission. Two randomized controlled trials in patients with newly diagnosed Crohn disease (treated with or without corticosteroids) found equivalent corticosteroid-free remissions rates in patients treated with thiopurines or placebo. Hence, guidelines recommend against the use of thiopurine monotherapy to induce remission.

4. Anti-TNF therapies—Infliximab, adalimumab, and certolizumab are used to induce and maintain remission in patients with moderate to severe Crohn disease, including fistulizing disease. These agents are also used to treat extraintestinal manifestations of Crohn disease (except optic neuritis).

A. ACUTE INDUCTION THERAPY—Anti-TNF therapies are recommended as the preferred first-line agents to induce remission in patients with moderate to severe Crohn disease, either as monotherapy or in combination with thiopurines. Up to two-thirds of patients have significant clinical improvement during acute induction therapy; dosing is described above. Currently, there are two major controversies about the use of anti-TNF agents: (1) whether anti-TNF agents should be reserved as second-line therapy in patients with moderate to severe Crohn disease who have not responded to prior therapy with corticosteroids and immunomodulators ("step-up" therapy) or whether they should be used early in the course of illness with the goal of inducing early remission and altering the natural history of the disease; and (2) whether an anti-TNF agent should be used alone or in combination with an immuno-modulator (azathioprine, mercaptopurine, or methotrexate) to enhance remission and reduce the development of antibodies to the anti-TNF agent. The best data support the use of anti-TNF agents early in the course of disease and suggest that "step-up therapy" (corticosteroids, followed by azathioprine, followed by infliximab) is obsolete, especially in patients with moderate to severe disease. Data in support of use of early combination therapy come from a large 2010 trial (SONIC) that compared three treatment arms: combination therapy with infliximab and azathioprine versus infliximab alone or azathioprine alone in patients with moderate to severe Crohn disease who had not previously been treated with immunomodulators or anti-TNF agents. After 6 months, clinical remission (57%) and mucosal healing (44%) was significantly higher with combination therapy than with either agent alone. However, post-hoc analyses of SONIC and other trials report that remission rates are similar between combination therapy and anti-TNF monotherapy when adjusted for the trough levels of infliximab. Low trough levels are associated with a decreased likelihood of remission and increased risk of developing anti-drug antibodies. Thus, if anti-TNF levels are measured during induction therapy to optimize long-term drug dosing, combination therapy may be unnecessary. Combination therapy with anti-TNF and azathioprine beyond 1 year may not be appropriate in men younger than 30 years of age in whom there is a higher risk of hepatosplenic T-cell lymphoma and in adults older than 50–60 years in whom there is a higher risk of lymphoma and infectious complications.

B. Maintenance therapy—After initial clinical response, symptom relapse occurs in more than 80% of patients within 1 year in the absence of further maintenance therapy. Therefore, scheduled maintenance therapy is usually recommended (eg, infliximab, 5 mg/kg infusion every 8 weeks; or adalimumab, 40 mg subcutaneous injection every 1–2 weeks). With long-term maintenance therapy, approximately two-thirds have continued clinical response and up to one-half have complete symptom remission. Loss of efficacy is due to low anti-TNF levels, the development of antibodies to the anti-TNF agent, or inflammation that is unresponsive to anti-TNF therapy. Serum anti-TNF trough levels and drug antibody levels may guide subsequent therapy in patients who have lost response. Patients with antibodies to the anti-TNF agent should be switched to another anti-TNF agent. Patients with low serum anti-TNF trough levels and absent drug antibodies should receive increased anti-TNF dosing (infliximab 10 mg/kg; adalimumab 80 mg) or decreased dosing intervals (infliximab every 6 weeks; adalimumab every week). Patients with inadequate response despite adequate anti-TNF trough levels should be changed to an alternative biologic agent, such as vedolizumab or ustekinumab. Concomitant therapy with anti-TNF agents and immunomodulating agents (azathioprine, mercaptopurine, or methotrexate) reduces the risk of development of antibodies to the anti-TNF agent but may increase the risk of complications (non-Hodgkin

lymphoma and opportunistic infections). For this reason, consideration should be given to stopping or reducing the dose of the immunomodulating agent after 6–12 months in patients who are in remission.

5. Anti-integrins—Anti-integrins may offer a therapeutic option for patients who do not respond to, or who lose response to, anti-TNF agents.

Vedolizumab is used primarily in patients with moderate to severe Crohn disease in whom anti-TNF therapy has failed or is not tolerated. The full clinical effects of vedolizumab may take 14 weeks to be apparent. A 2014 phase III trial studying patients with Crohn disease showed that when response was lost or side effects developed to one anti-TNF therapy, switching to vedolizumab (300 mg intravenously at weeks 0 and 2) resulted in clinical remission in 26.6% of patients at week 10 compared to 12.1% of patients treated with placebo. In another phase III trial, among patients demonstrating initial clinical improvement with vedolizumab induction therapy, 39% of patients treated with long-term vedolizumab (300 mg every 8 weeks) were in remission at 1 year compared with 21.6% of patients given placebo. Vedolizumab may be less effective than anti-TNF or ustekinumab in the treatment of fistulous disease.

6. Anti-IL-12/IL-23 antibody—Ustekinumab is approved by the FDA for treatment of patients with moderate to severe Crohn disease who have not responded to or are intolerant of conventional therapies. In a phase III trial involving 741 patients with Crohn disease in whom anti-TNF therapy failed, clinical response was seen in 34% of patients 6 weeks after a single-dose of intravenous ustekinumab compared to 21.5% with placebo. In a second phase III trial composed of patients in whom conventional therapy with immunomodulators or corticosteroids (but not anti-TNF) had failed, clinical improvement occurred in 55% compared to 28.7% with placebo. Among patients from both induction trials who were enrolled in a chronic maintenance trial (ustekinumab versus placebo subcutaneously every 8 weeks), 53% of those given ustekinumab were in clinical remission at week 44 versus 36% given the placebo.

▶ Indications for Surgery

Over 50% of patients will require at least one surgical procedure. The main indications for surgery are intractability to medical therapy, intra-abdominal abscess, massive bleeding, symptomatic refractory internal or perianal fistulas, and intestinal obstruction. Patients with chronic obstructive symptoms due to a short segment of ileal stenosis are best treated with resection or stricturoplasty (rather than long-term medical therapy), which promotes rapid return of well-being and elimination of corticosteroids. After surgery, endoscopic evidence of recurrence occurs in 60% within 1 year. Endoscopic recurrence precedes clinical recurrence by months to years; clinical recurrence occurs in 20% of patients within 1 year and 80% within 10–15 years. Therapy with metronidazole, 250 mg three times daily for 3 months, or long-term therapy with immunomodulators (mercaptopurine or azathioprine) has only been modestly effective in preventing clinical and endoscopic recurrence after ileocolic resection. In a 2016 controlled trial of 297 patients undergoing ileocolonic resection, endoscopic recurrence occurred in 30% of patients treated with infliximab every 8 weeks compared with 60% treated with placebo. It may be reasonable to initiate empiric infliximab postoperatively for patients at high risk for disease recurrence and to perform endoscopy in low-risk patients 6 months after surgery in order to identify patients with early endoscopic recurrence who may benefit from anti-TNF therapy.

▶ Prognosis

With proper medical and surgical treatment, the majority of patients are able to cope with this chronic disease and its complications and lead productive lives. Few patients die as a direct consequence of the disease.

▶ When to Refer

- For expertise in endoscopic procedures or capsule endoscopy.
- For follow-up of any patient requiring hospitalization.
- Patients with moderate to severe disease for whom therapy with immunomodulators or biologic agents is being considered.
- When surgery may be necessary.

▶ When to Admit

- An intestinal obstruction is suspected.
- An intra-abdominal or perirectal abscess is suspected.
- A serious infectious complication is suspected, especially in patients who are immunocompromised due to concomitant use of corticosteroids, immunomodulators, or anti-TNF agents.
- Patients with severe symptoms of diarrhea, dehydration, weight loss, or abdominal pain.
- Patients with severe or persisting symptoms despite treatment with corticosteroids.

Adedokun OJ et al. Pharmacokinetics and exposure response relationships of ustekinumab in patients with Crohn's disease. Gastroenterology. 2018 May;154(6):1660–71. [PMID: 29409871]

Bruining DH et al; Society of Abdominal Radiology Crohn's Disease-Focused Panel. Consensus recommendations for evaluation, interpretation, and utilization of computed tomography and magnetic resonance enterography in patients with small bowel Crohn's disease. Gastroenterology. 2018 Mar; 154(4):1172–94. [PMID: 29329905]

Cohen BL et al. Update on anti-tumor necrosis factor agents and other new drugs for inflammatory bowel disease. BMJ. 2017 Jun 19;357:j2505. [PMID: 28630047]

Danese S et al. Early intervention in Crohn's disease: towards disease modification trials. Gut. 2017 Dec;66(12):2179–87. [PMID: 28874419]

Feagan BG et al; UNITI–IM-UNITI Study Group. Ustekinumab as induction and maintenance therapy for Crohn's disease. N Engl J Med. 2016 Nov 17;375(20):1946–60. [PMID: 27959607]

Lee MJ et al. Efficacy of medical therapies for fistulizing Crohn's disease: systematic review and meta-analysis. Clin Gastroenterol Hepatol. 2018 Dec;16(12):1879–92. [PMID: 29374617]

Lichtenstein GR et al. ACG Clinical Guideline: management of Crohn's disease in adults. Am J Gastroenterol. 2018 Apr; 113(4):481–517. Erratum in: Am J Gastroenterol. 2018 Jul; 113(7):1101. [PMID: 29610508]

Rutgeerts P et al. Efficacy of ustekinumab for inducing endoscopic healing in patients with Crohn's disease. Gastroenterology. 2018 Oct;155(4):1045–58. [PMID: 29909019]

2. Ulcerative Colitis

ESSENTIALS OF DIAGNOSIS

- ▶ Bloody diarrhea.
- ▶ Lower abdominal cramps and fecal urgency.
- ▶ Anemia, low serum albumin.
- ▶ Negative stool cultures.
- ▶ Sigmoidoscopy is the key to diagnosis.

▶ General Considerations

Ulcerative colitis is an idiopathic inflammatory condition that involves the mucosal surface of the colon, resulting in diffuse friability and erosions with bleeding. Approximately one-fourth of patients have disease confined to the rectosigmoid region (proctosigmoiditis); one-half have disease that extends to the splenic flexure (left-sided colitis); and one-fourth have disease that extends more proximally (extensive colitis). In patients with distal colitis, the disease progresses with time to more extensive involvement in 25%. There is some correlation between disease extent and symptom severity. In most patients, the disease is characterized by periods of symptomatic flare-ups and remissions. Ulcerative colitis is more common in nonsmokers and former smokers. Disease severity may be lower in active smokers and may worsen in patients who stop smoking. Appendectomy before the age of 20 years for acute appendicitis is associated with a reduced risk of developing ulcerative colitis.

▶ Clinical Findings

A. Symptoms and Signs

The clinical profile in ulcerative colitis is highly variable. Bloody diarrhea is the hallmark. On the basis of several clinical and laboratory parameters, it is clinically useful to classify patients as having mild, moderate, or severe disease (Table 15–12). Patients should be asked about stool frequency, the presence and amount of rectal bleeding, cramps, abdominal pain, fecal urgency, tenesmus, and extraintestinal symptoms. Physical examination should focus on the patient's volume status as determined by orthostatic blood pressure and pulse measurements and by nutritional status. On abdominal examination, the clinician should look for tenderness and evidence of peritoneal inflammation. Red blood may be present on digital rectal examination.

1. Mild to moderate disease—Patients with mild to moderate disease have fewer than 4–6 bowel movements per day,

Table 15–12. Ulcerative colitis: assessment of disease activity.

	Mild	Moderate	Severe
Stool frequency (per day)	< 4	4–6	> 6 (mostly bloody)
Pulse (beats/min)	< 90	90–100	> 100
Hematocrit (%)	Normal	30–40	< 30
Weight loss (%)	None	1–10	> 10
Temperature (°F)	Normal	99–100	> 100
ESR (mm/h)	< 20	20–30	> 30
Albumin (g/dL)	Normal	3–3.5	< 3

ESR, erythrocyte sedimentation rate.

mild to moderate rectal bleeding, and no constitutional symptoms. Stools may be formed or loose in consistency. Because of rectal inflammation, there is fecal urgency and tenesmus. Left lower quadrant cramps relieved by defecation are common, but there is no significant abdominal pain or tenderness. There may be mild anemia and hypoalbuminemia.

2. Severe disease—Patients with severe disease have more than six bloody bowel movements per day, resulting in severe anemia, hypovolemia, and impaired nutrition with hypoalbuminemia. Abdominal pain and tenderness are present. "Fulminant colitis" is a subset of severe disease characterized by rapidly worsening symptoms with signs of toxicity.

B. Laboratory Findings

The degree of abnormality of the hematocrit, serum albumin, and inflammatory markers (erythrocyte sedimentation rate and C-reactive protein) reflects disease severity (Table 15–12).

C. Endoscopy

In acute colitis, the diagnosis is readily established by sigmoidoscopy. The mucosal appearance is characterized by edema, friability, mucopus, and erosions. Mild to moderate disease is characterized by erythema, friability, and erosions, and moderate to severe disease is characterized by deep ulceration and spontaneous bleeding. Colonoscopy should not be performed in patients with fulminant disease because of the risk of perforation. After patients have demonstrated improvement on therapy, colonoscopy is performed to determine the extent of disease.

D. Imaging

Abdominal imaging with plain radiographs or CT is obtained in patients with severe colitis to look for significant colonic dilation. Barium enemas are of little utility in the evaluation of acute ulcerative colitis and may precipitate toxic megacolon in patients with severe disease.

► Differential Diagnosis

The initial presentation of ulcerative colitis is indistinguishable from other causes of colitis, clinically as well as endoscopically. Thus, the diagnosis of idiopathic ulcerative colitis is reached after excluding other known causes of colitis. Infectious colitis should be excluded by sending stool specimens for routine testing to exclude *Salmonella, Shigella, Campylobacter, E coli* O157, *C difficile,* and amebiasis. Where available, microbial assessment using multiplex molecular techniques provides results within 1–4 hours with excellent sensitivity and is preferred to conventional labor-intensive stool microscopy, culture, and toxin testing. CMV colitis occurs in immunocompromised patients, including patients receiving prolonged corticosteroid therapy, and is diagnosed on mucosal biopsy. Gonorrhea, chlamydial infection, herpes, and syphilis are considerations in sexually active patients with proctitis. In elderly patients with cardiovascular disease, ischemic colitis may involve the rectosigmoid. A history of radiation to the pelvic region can result in proctitis months to years later. Crohn disease involving the colon but not the small intestine may be confused with ulcerative colitis. In 10% of patients, a distinction between Crohn disease and ulcerative colitis may not be possible.

► Treatment

There are two main treatment objectives: (1) to terminate the acute, symptomatic attack and (2) to prevent recurrence of attacks. The treatment of acute ulcerative colitis depends on the extent of colonic involvement and the severity of illness. Patients with systemic signs of inflammation (ie, anemia, low serum albumin, elevated C-reactive protein or erythrocyte sedimentation rate levels) and deep ulcerations with extensive disease on colonoscopy are at increased risk for hospitalization or surgery, and early aggressive therapy with corticosteroids, immunomodulators, or biologic agents is warranted.

A. Mild to Moderate Distal Colitis

Patients with disease confined to the rectum or rectosigmoid region generally have mild to moderate but distressing symptoms. Patients may be treated with topical mesalamine, topical corticosteroids, or oral aminosalicylates (5-ASA) according to patient preference and cost considerations. Topical mesalamine is the drug of choice and is superior to topical corticosteroids and oral 5-ASA. Mesalamine is administered as a suppository, 1000 mg once daily at bedtime for proctitis, and as an enema, 4 g at bedtime for proctosigmoiditis, for 4–8 weeks, with 75% of patients improving. Patients who either decline or are unable to manage topical therapy may be treated with oral 5-ASA, as discussed below. Although topical corticosteroids are a less expensive alternative to mesalamine, they are also less effective. Hydrocortisone enema or foam (80–100 mg) or budesonide foam are prescribed for proctitis or proctosigmoiditis. Systemic effects from short-term use are very slight. For patients with distal disease who do not improve with topical or oral mesalamine therapy, the following options may be considered: (1) a combination of a topical agent with an oral 5-ASA agent; (2) topical corticosteroid; or (3) addition of oral prednisone (as described below) or budesonide MMX 9 mg/day for 4–8 weeks to rectal and oral 5-ASA.

Most patients with proctitis or proctosigmoiditis who achieve complete remission with oral or rectal 5-ASA should continue indefinitely on the same therapy to reduce the likelihood of symptomatic relapse. Maintenance treatment with 5-ASA reduces the 12-month relapse rate from 75% to less than 40%. Some patients, however, may prefer intermittent therapy for symptomatic relapse. Topical corticosteroids are ineffective for maintaining remission of distal colitis.

B. Mild to Moderate Colitis

1. 5-ASA agents—Disease extending above the sigmoid colon is best treated with both an oral and rectal 5-ASA agent. For induction of remission, the optimal dose of oral 5-ASA (mesalamine or balsalazide) is 2–3 g once daily in combination with mesalamine 1 g suppository or 4 g enema at bedtime. Most patients improve within 4–8 weeks. Some patients may prefer to initiate therapy with an oral agent, adding topical therapy if initial response is inadequate. These agents achieve clinical improvement in 75% of patients and remission in 20–30%. Oral sulfasalazine (1.5–2 g twice daily) is uncommonly used due to its side effects but is sometimes prescribed in patients with significant arthritis. To minimize side effects, sulfasalazine is begun at a dosage of 500 mg twice daily and increased gradually over 1–2 weeks to 2 g twice daily. Folic acid, 1 mg/day orally, should be administered to all patients taking sulfasalazine.

2. Corticosteroids—Patients with mild to moderate disease who do not improve within 4–8 weeks of 5-ASA therapy should have an oral corticosteroid therapy added with budesonide MMX or prednisone. Budesonide MMX (Uceris) 9 mg/day orally for 4–8 weeks may be preferred in mild to moderate colitis due to its low incidence of corticosteroid-associated side effects, especially in those for whom other systemic corticosteroids are deemed high risk.

C. Moderate to Severe Colitis

1. Corticosteroids—An oral corticosteroid (prednisone or methylprednisolone) is recommended as the first-line agent for patients with moderate to severe disease or as second-line therapy in patients in whom initial 5-ASA therapy was ineffective. Depending on the severity of illness, the initial oral dose of prednisone is 40–60 mg daily. Rapid improvement is observed in most cases within 2 weeks. Thereafter, tapering of prednisone should proceed by 5–10 mg/wk. After tapering to 20 mg/day, slower tapering (2.5 mg/wk) is sometimes required. Complete tapering of prednisone without symptomatic flare-ups is possible in the majority of patients. Patients achieving remission should be maintained on oral mesalamine (2–4 g/day). Up to 30% of patients either do not respond to prednisone or have symptomatic flares during tapering that prevent its complete withdrawal. The addition of a thiopurine (azathioprine or mercaptopurine) is sometimes used in an effort to promote complete steroid withdrawal

and maintain long-term remission. However, therapy with biologic agents or tofacitinib is recommended for most patients with steroid dependency.

2. Anti-TNF agents—Infliximab, adalimumab, and golimumab are FDA approved in the United States for the treatment of patients with moderate to severe ulcerative colitis who have had an inadequate response to conventional therapies (oral corticosteroids, mercaptopurine or azathioprine, and mesalamine). Following a three-dose induction regimen of infliximab 5 mg/kg administered at 0, 2, and 6 weeks, clinical response occurs in 65%. During long-term maintenance treatment with infliximab 5–10 mg/kg every 4–8 weeks, clinical improvement or remission is achieved in approximately 50%. In two, large, controlled studies of patients with active moderate to severe colitis, initial induction therapy was followed by infliximab maintenance infusions (5 mg/kg) administered every 8 weeks for 30–54 weeks. At the end of the study (30 or 54 weeks), 35% were in clinical remission (and 21% were in corticosteroid-free remission), a modest but impressive response in patients with more refractory disease. Phase III trials of adalimumab and golimumab reported clinical response rates of 50–59% and remission rates of 16–21% after 8 weeks. Although the response and remission rates appear lower with adalimumab and golimumab than infliximab, differences in study design and patient populations limit comparisons. When initiating anti-TNF therapy, many clinicians add an immunomodulator (azathioprine, mercaptopurine, or methotrexate) for the first year. Combination therapy increases the likelihood of disease remission and reduces the development of antibodies that may result in secondary loss of response to anti-TNF therapies. After initiating anti-TNF therapy, serum trough levels and anti-drug antibody titers should be obtained at least once in order to optimize drug dosing.

3. Anti-integrin therapy—Vedolizumab, a monoclonal antibody directed against the $alpha_4 beta_7$ heterodimer, is FDA-approved for the treatment of moderate to severe ulcerative colitis in patients who have not responded to, lost response to, or been intolerant of other therapies. In a phase III clinical trial of patients with moderate to severe ulcerative colitis, vedolizumab induction (300 mg intravenously at 0, 2, and 6 weeks) led to clinical improvement in 47.1% of patients compared with 25.5% who were given placebo. Among patients who demonstrated initial clinical improvement, 41.8% of those given long-term maintenance treatment with vedolizumab (300 mg intravenously every 8 weeks) were in clinical remission at 1 year compared with 15.9% of those given placebo. At present, vedolizumab is recommended for treatment of acute cases and maintenance therapy in patients with moderate to severe ulcerative colitis who have not responded to or have lost response to anti-TNF therapy or immunomodulator therapy, or both.

4. Janus kinase Inhibitor—Tofacitinib, an oral, small-molecule JAK 1/3 inhibitor, was approved by the FDA in 2018 for the treatment of moderate to severe ulcerative colitis. In two phase III induction trials (OCTAVE 1 and 2), tofacitinib (10 mg orally twice daily) achieved remission after 8 weeks in 17.6% compared to 6% in those receiving a placebo. During long-term (1 year) follow-up, tofacitinib 10 mg/day maintained clinical response in 59.4% and remission in 41%. At present, tofacitinib may be preferred for patients who have not responded anti-TNF therapy. Although anti-TNF agents remain first-line therapy for most patients with moderate to severe colitis, tofacitinib is an increasingly attractive first-line agent due to its ease of administration (oral) and its safety profile.

5. Probiotics—Probiotics have not demonstrated significant benefit versus placebo in the treatment of mild to moderate ulcerative colitis in randomized, controlled trials. Nonetheless, various guidelines recommend that while they should not be used instead of other therapies with proven efficacy, they may be considered as adjunctive therapy for mild to moderate disease.

D. Severe and Fulminant Colitis

About 15% of patients with ulcerative colitis have a more severe course. Of these, a small subset has a fulminant course with rapid progression of symptoms over 1–2 weeks and signs of severe toxicity. These patients appear quite ill, with fever, prominent hypovolemia, hemorrhage requiring transfusion, and abdominal distention with tenderness. Toxic megacolon develops in less than 2% of cases of ulcerative colitis. It is characterized by colonic dilation of more than 6 cm on plain films with signs of toxicity.

1. General measures—Discontinue all oral intake for 24–48 hours or until the patient demonstrates clinical improvement. TPN is indicated only in patients with poor nutritional status or if feedings cannot be reinstituted within 7–10 days. All opioid or anticholinergic agents should be discontinued. Restore circulating volume with fluids, correct electrolyte abnormalities, and consider transfusion for significant anemia (hematocrit less than 25–28%). A plain abdominal radiograph or CT scan should be ordered on admission to look for evidence of colonic dilation. Send stools for assessment of bacterial pathogens, *C difficile* and parasites, either by conventional bacterial culture, *C difficile* toxin assay, and for ova and parasite examinations or by rapid, multiplex PCR assay. CMV superinfection should be considered in patients receiving long-term immunosuppressive therapy who are unresponsive to corticosteroid therapy. Due to a high risk of venous thromboembolic (VTE) disease, VTE prophylaxis should be administered to all hospitalized patients with inflammatory bowel disease. Surgical consultation should be sought for all patients with severe disease.

Patients with fulminant disease are at higher risk for perforation or toxic megacolon and must be monitored closely. Abdominal examinations should be repeated to look for evidence of worsening distention or pain. Broad-spectrum antibiotics should be administered to cover anaerobes and gram-negative bacteria. In addition to the therapies outlined above, nasogastric suction should be initiated. Patients should be instructed to roll from side to side and onto the abdomen in an effort to decompress the distended colon. Serial abdominal plain films should be obtained to look for worsening dilation or signs of ischemia. Patients with fulminant disease or toxic megacolon who worsen or do not improve within 48–72 hours should undergo surgery to prevent perforation. If the operation is performed before perforation, the mortality rate should be low.

2. Corticosteroid therapy—Methylprednisolone, 48–64 mg, or hydrocortisone, 300 mg, is administered intravenously in four divided doses or by continuous infusion over 24 hours. Higher or "pulse" doses are of no benefit. Hydrocortisone enemas (100 mg) may also be administered twice daily for treatment of urgency or tenesmus. Approximately 50–75% of patients achieve remission with systemic corticosteroids within 7–10 days. Once symptomatic improvement has occurred, oral fluids are reinstituted. If fluids are well tolerated, intravenous corticosteroids are discontinued and the patient is started on oral prednisone (as described for moderate disease). Patients without significant improvement within 3–5 days of intravenous corticosteroid therapy should be referred for surgery or considered for anti-TNF therapies or cyclosporine.

3. Anti-TNF therapies—Infusion of infliximab, 5–10 mg/kg, has been shown in uncontrolled and controlled studies to be effective in treating severe colitis in patients who did not improve within 4–7 days of intravenous corticosteroid therapy. In a controlled study of patients hospitalized for ulcerative colitis, colectomy was required within 3 months in 69% who received placebo therapy, compared with 47% who received infliximab. Thus, infliximab therapy should be considered in patients with severe ulcerative colitis who have not improved with intravenous corticosteroid therapy. Recent studies have demonstrated more rapid clearance of infliximab in patients with severe ulcerative colitis. Uncontrolled trials have found lower colectomy rates in patients administered higher doses of infliximab (three infusions of 5–10 mg/kg within 2–3 weeks) than with conventional dosing (5 mg/kg at 0, 2, and 6 weeks).

4. Cyclosporine—Intravenous cyclosporine (2–4 mg/kg/day as a continuous infusion) benefits 60–75% of patients with severe colitis who have not improved after 7–10 days of corticosteroids, but it is associated with significant toxicity (nephrotoxicity, seizures, infection, hypertension). Up to two-thirds of responders may be maintained in remission with a combination of oral cyclosporine for 3 months and long-term therapy with mercaptopurine or azathioprine. A 2011 randomized study of patients with severe colitis refractory to intravenous corticosteroids found similar response rates (85%) with cyclosporine and infliximab therapy.

5. Surgical therapy—Patients with severe disease who do not improve after corticosteroid, infliximab, or cyclosporine therapy are unlikely to respond to further medical therapy, and surgery is recommended.

▶ Risk of Colon Cancer

In patients with ulcerative colitis with disease proximal to the rectum and in patients with Crohn colitis, there is an increased risk of developing colon carcinoma. Although older meta-analyses from referral centers reported a high risk (8% after 20 years), more recent systematic reviews of population-based studies report a 2.4-fold increased risk (1.4% after a mean of 14 years of follow-up). Retrospective studies suggest that the risk of colon cancer may be reduced in patients treated with long-term 5-ASA therapy. Ingestion of folic acid, 1 mg/day, also is associated with a decreased risk of cancer development. Colonoscopies are recommended every 1–2 years in patients with colitis, beginning 8 years after diagnosis. Several prospective studies demonstrate that dye spraying with methylene blue or indigo carmine ("chromoendoscopy") enhances the detection of subtle mucosal lesions, thereby significantly increasing the detection of dysplasia compared with standard colonoscopy. At colonoscopy, all polypoid and nonpolypoid lesions should be resected, when possible, and biopsies obtained of endoscopically unresectable lesions.

Surgery in Ulcerative Colitis

Surgery is required in 25% of patients. Severe hemorrhage, perforation, and documented carcinoma are absolute indications for surgery. Surgery is indicated also in patients with fulminant colitis or toxic megacolon that does not improve within 48–72 hours, in patients with invisible flat dysplasia or non-endoscopically resectable dysplastic lesions on surveillance colonoscopy, and in patients with refractory disease requiring long-term corticosteroids to control symptoms.

Although total proctocolectomy (with placement of an ileostomy) provides complete cure of the disease, most patients seek to avoid it out of concern for the impact it may have on their bowel function, their self-image, and their social interactions. After complete colectomy, patients may have a standard ileostomy with an external appliance, a continent ileostomy, or an internal ileal pouch that is anastomosed to the anal canal (ileal pouch–anal anastomosis). The latter maintains intestinal continuity, thereby obviating an ostomy. Under optimal circumstances, patients have five to seven loose bowel movements per day without incontinence. Endoscopic or histologic inflammation in the ileal pouch ("pouchitis") develops in over 40% of patients, resulting in increased stool frequency, fecal urgency, cramping, and bleeding, but usually resolves with a 2-week course of oral metronidazole (250–500 mg three times daily) or ciprofloxacin (500 mg twice daily). Patients with frequently relapsing pouchitis may need continuous antibiotics. Probiotics containing nonpathogenic strains of lactobacilli, bifidobacteria, and streptococci (VSL#3) are effective in the maintenance of remission in patients with recurrent pouchitis.

Prognosis

Ulcerative colitis is a lifelong disease characterized by exacerbations and remissions. For most patients, the disease is readily controlled by medical therapy without need for surgery. The majority never require hospitalization. A subset of patients with more severe disease will require surgery, which results in complete cure of the disease. Properly managed, most patients with ulcerative colitis lead close to normal productive lives.

When to Refer

- Colonoscopy: for evaluation of activity and extent of active disease and for surveillance for neoplasia in patients with quiescent disease for more than 8–10 years.
- For follow-up of any patient requiring hospitalization.
- When surgical colectomy is indicated.

When to Admit

- Patients with severe disease manifested by frequent bloody stools, anemia, weight loss, and fever.
- Patients with fulminant disease manifested by rapid progression of symptoms, worsening abdominal pain, distention, high fever, and tachycardia.
- Patients with moderate to severe symptoms that do not respond to oral corticosteroids and require a trial of bowel rest and intravenous corticosteroids.

Bitton A et al; Canadian Association of Gastroenterology Severe Ulcerative Colitis Consensus Group. Treatment of hospitalized adult patients with severe ulcerative colitis: Toronto consensus statements. Am J Gastroenterol. 2012 Feb;107(2):179–94. [PMID: 22108451]

Brandse JF et al. Pharmacokinetic features and presence of antidrug antibodies associate with response to infliximab induction therapy in patients with moderate to severe ulcerative colitis. Clin Gastroenterol Hepatol. 2016 Feb;14(2):251–8. [PMID: 26545802]

Fumery M et al. Natural history of adult ulcerative colitis in population-based cohorts: a systematic review. Clin Gastroenterol Hepatol. 2018 Mar;16(3):343–56. [PMID: 28625817]

Hindryckx P et al. Review article: dose optimisation of infliximab for acute severe ulcerative colitis. Aliment Pharmacol Ther. 2017 Mar;45(5):617–30. [PMID: 28074618]

Kaltenbach T et al. Endoscopy in inflammatory bowel disease: advances in dysplasia detection and management. Gastrointest Endosc. 2017 Dec;86(6):962–71. [PMID: 28987547]

Ko CW et al; American Gastroenterological Association Institute Clinical Guidelines Committee. American Gastroenterological Association Institute guideline on the management of mild-to-moderate ulcerative colitis. Gastroenterology. 2019 Feb;156(3):748–64. [PMID: 30576644]

Laine L et al. SCENIC international consensus statement on surveillance and management of dysplasia in inflammatory bowel disease. Gastrointest Endosc. 2015 Mar;81(3):489–501. [PMID: 25708752]

Narula N et al. Vedolizumab for ulcerative colitis: treatment outcomes from the VICTORY Consortium. Am J Gastroenterol. 2018 Sep;113(9):1345–54. Erratum in: Am J Gastroenterol. 2018 Dec;113(12):1912. [PMID: 29946178]

Nguyen GC et al; IBD in Pregnancy Consensus Group; Canadian Association of Gastroenterology. The Toronto Consensus Statements for the management of inflammatory bowel disease in pregnancy. Gastroenterology. 2016 Mar;150(3):734–57. [PMID: 26688268]

Sandborn WJ et al. Safety of tofacitinib for treatment of ulcerative colitis, based on 4.4 years of data from global clinical trials. Clin Gastroenterol Hepatol. 2018 Nov 23. [Epub ahead of print] [PMID: 30476584]

Sandborn WJ et al. Tofacitinib as induction and maintenance therapy for ulcerative colitis. N Engl J Med. 2017 Aug 3;377(5):496–7. [PMID: 28767341]

Singh S et al. American Gastroenterological Association technical review on the management of mild-to-moderate ulcerative colitis. Gastroenterology. 2019 Feb;156(3):769–808.e29. [PMID: 30576642]

Singh S et al. Systematic review with network meta-analysis: first- and second-line pharmacotherapy for moderate-severe ulcerative colitis. Aliment Pharmacol Ther. 2018 Jan;47(2):162–75. [PMID: 29205406]

3. Microscopic Colitis

Microscopic colitis is an idiopathic condition that is found in up to 15% of patients who have chronic or intermittent watery diarrhea with normal-appearing mucosa at endoscopy. There are two major subtypes—lymphocytic colitis and collagenous colitis. In both, histologic evaluation of mucosal biopsies reveals chronic inflammation (lymphocytes, plasma cells) in the lamina propria and increased intraepithelial lymphocytes. **Collagenous colitis** is further characterized by the presence of a thickened band (greater than 10 mcm) of subepithelial collagen. Both forms occur more commonly in women, especially in the fifth to sixth decades. Symptoms tend to be chronic or recurrent but may remit in most patients after several years. A more severe illness characterized by abdominal pain, fatigue, dehydration, and weight loss may develop in a subset of patients. The cause of **microscopic colitis** usually is unknown. Several medications have been implicated as etiologic agents, including NSAIDs, proton pump inhibitors, low-dose aspirin, selective serotonin reuptake inhibitors, ACE inhibitors, and beta-blockers. Diarrhea usually abates within 30 days of stopping the offending medication. Celiac disease may be present in 2–9% of patients and should be excluded with serologic testing (anti-tissue transglutaminase IgA). Treatment is largely empiric since there are few well-designed, controlled treatment trials. Antidiarrheal therapy with loperamide is the first-line treatment, providing symptom improvement in up to 70%. For patients who do not respond to loperamide, bismuth subsalicylate (three 262-mg tablets three times daily) leads to complete response in up to 50% patients in some series. The next option is delayed-release budesonide (Entocort), 9 mg/day for 6–8 weeks. Budesonide has been shown in three prospective controlled studies to induce clinical remission in greater than 80% of patients; however, relapse occurs in most patients after stopping therapy. Remission is maintained in 75% of patients treated long-term with low doses of budesonide. In clinical practice, budesonide is tapered to the lowest effective dose for suppressing symptoms (3 mg every other day to 6 mg daily). For patients who do not respond to budesonide, uncontrolled studies report that treatment with bile-salt binding agents (cholestyramine, colestipol) or 5-ASAs (sulfasalazine, mesalamine) may be effective in some patients. Less than 3% of patients have refractory or severe symptoms, which may be treated with immunosuppressive agents (azathioprine or methotrexate) or anti-TNF agents (infliximab, adalimumab).

Cotter TG et al. Current approach to the evaluation and management of microscopic colitis. Curr Gastroenterol Rep. 2017 Feb; 19(2):8. [PMID: 28265892]
Gentile N et al. Prevalence, pathogenesis, diagnosis, and management of microscopic colitis. Gut Liver. 2018 May 15; 12(3):227–35. [PMID: 28669150]
Pardi DS. Diagnosis and management of microscopic colitis. Am J Gastroenterol. 2017 Jan;112(1):78–85. [PMID: 27897155]

DIVERTICULAR DISEASE OF THE COLON

Colonic diverticulosis increases with age, ranging from 5% in those under age 40, to 30% at age 60, to more than 50% over age 80 years in Western societies. Most are asymptomatic, discovered incidentally at endoscopy or on barium enema. Complications occur in less than 5%, including gastrointestinal bleeding and diverticulitis.

Colonic diverticula may vary in size from a few millimeters to several centimeters and in number from one to several dozen. Almost all patients with diverticulosis have involvement in the sigmoid and descending colon; however, only 15% have proximal colonic disease.

For over 40 years, it has been believed that diverticulosis arises after many years of a diet deficient in fiber. Recent epidemiologic studies challenge this theory, finding no association between the prevalence of asymptomatic diverticulosis and low dietary fiber intake or constipation. Thus, the etiology of diverticulosis is uncertain. The extent to which abnormal motility and hereditary factors contribute to diverticular disease is unknown. Patients with abnormal connective tissue are also disposed to development of diverticulosis, including Ehlers-Danlos syndrome, Marfan syndrome, and scleroderma.

1. Uncomplicated Diverticulosis

More than 90% of patients with diverticulosis have uncomplicated disease and no specific symptoms. In most, diverticulosis is an incidental finding detected during colonoscopic examination or barium enema examination. Some patients have nonspecific complaints of chronic constipation, abdominal pain, or fluctuating bowel habits. It is unclear whether these symptoms are due to alterations in the colonic motility, visceral hypersensitivity, gut microbiota, or low-grade inflammation. Physical examination is usually normal but may reveal mild left lower quadrant tenderness with a thickened, palpable sigmoid and descending colon. Screening laboratory studies should be normal in uncomplicated diverticulosis.

There is no reason to perform imaging studies for the purpose of diagnosing asymptomatic, uncomplicated disease. Diverticula are well seen on barium enema, colonoscopy, and CT imaging. Involved segments of colon may also be narrowed and deformed.

Patients in whom diverticulosis is discovered, especially patients with symptoms or a history of complicated disease should be treated with a high-fiber diet or fiber supplements (bran powder, 1–2 tbsp twice daily; psyllium or methylcellulose) (see section on constipation).

Cremon C et al. Diagnostic challenges of symptomatic uncomplicated diverticular disease. Minerva Gastroenterol Dietol. 2017 Jun;63(2):119–29. [PMID: 28079347]
Feuerstein JD et al. Diverticulosis and diverticulitis. Mayo Clin Proc. 2016 Aug;91(8):1094–104. [PMID: 27156370]
Scarpignato C et al. Management of colonic diverticular disease in the third millennium. Therap Adv Gastroenterol. 2018 May 20;11:1756284818771305. [PMID: 29844795]
Segev L et al. Natural history of bleeding risk in colonic diverticulosis. Minerva Gastroenterol Dietol. 2017 Jun;63(2):152–7. [PMID: 28240003]

2. Diverticulitis

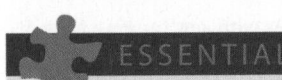

▶ Acute abdominal pain and fever.
▶ Left lower abdominal tenderness and mass.
▶ Leukocytosis.

▶ Clinical Findings

A. Symptoms and Signs

Diverticulitis is defined as macroscopic inflammation of a diverticulum that may reflect a spectrum from inflammation alone, to microperforation with localized paracolic inflammation, to macroperforation with either abscess or generalized peritonitis. Thus, there is a range from mild to severe disease. Most patients with localized inflammation or infection report mild to moderate aching abdominal pain, usually in the left lower quadrant. Constipation or loose stools may be present. Nausea and vomiting are frequent. In many cases, symptoms are so mild that the patient may not seek medical attention until several days after onset. Physical findings include a low-grade fever, left lower quadrant tenderness, and a palpable mass. Stool occult blood is common, but hematochezia is rare. Leukocytosis is mild to moderate. Patients with free perforation present with a more dramatic picture of generalized abdominal pain and peritoneal signs.

B. Imaging

In patients with mild symptoms and a presumptive diagnosis of diverticulitis, empiric medical therapy is started without further imaging in the acute phase. Patients who respond to acute medical management should undergo complete colonic evaluation with colonoscopy or radiologic imaging (CT colonography or barium enema) after resolution of clinical symptoms to corroborate the diagnosis or exclude other disorders such as colonic neoplasms. In patients who do not improve rapidly after 2–4 days of empiric therapy and in those with severe disease, CT scan of the abdomen is obtained to look for evidence of diverticulitis and determine its severity, and to exclude other disorders that may cause lower abdominal pain. The presence of colonic diverticula and wall thickening, pericolic fat infiltration, abscess formation, or extraluminal air or contrast suggests diverticulitis. Endoscopy and colonography are contraindicated during the initial stages of an acute attack because of the risk of free perforation.

▶ Differential Diagnosis

Diverticulitis must be distinguished from other causes of lower abdominal pain, including perforated colonic carcinoma, Crohn disease, appendicitis, ischemic colitis, *C difficile*-associated colitis, and gynecologic disorders (ectopic pregnancy, ovarian cyst or torsion), by abdominal CT scan,

pelvic ultrasonography, or radiographic studies of the distal colon that use water-soluble contrast enemas.

▶ Prevention

Two 2017 prospective cohort studies reported a lower risk of diverticulitis in men consuming diets high in fruits, vegetables, and whole grains than diets high in red meat and refined grains.

▶ Complications

Chronic inflammation or an untreated abscess may lead to fistula formation that may involve the bladder, ureter, vagina, uterus, bowel, and abdominal wall. Acute or chronic inflammation may result in stricturing of the colon with partial or complete obstruction.

▶ Treatment

A. Medical Management

Most patients can be managed with conservative measures. Patients with mild symptoms and no peritoneal signs may be managed initially as outpatients on a clear liquid diet. Although broad-spectrum oral antibiotics with anaerobic activity commonly are prescribed, large clinical trials confirm that antibiotics are not beneficial in uncomplicated disease. A 2015 American Gastroenterological Association guideline suggests that antibiotics should be used selectively for uncomplicated disease. Reasonable regimens include amoxicillin and clavulanate potassium (875 mg/125 mg) twice daily; or metronidazole, 500 mg three times daily; plus either ciprofloxacin, 500 mg twice daily, or trimethoprim-sulfamethoxazole, 160/800 mg twice daily orally, for 7–10 days or until the patient is afebrile for 3–5 days. Symptomatic improvement usually occurs within 3 days, at which time the diet may be advanced. Once the acute episode has resolved, a high-fiber diet is often recommended. Patients with increasing pain, fever, or inability to tolerate oral fluids require hospitalization. Patients with severe diverticulitis (high fevers, leukocytosis, or peritoneal signs) and patients who are elderly or immunosuppressed or who have serious comorbid disease require hospitalization acutely. Patients should be given nothing by mouth and should receive intravenous fluids. If ileus is present, a nasogastric tube should be placed. Intravenous antibiotics should be given to cover anaerobic and gram-negative bacteria. Single-agent therapy with either a second-generation cephalosporin (eg, cefoxitin), piperacillin-tazobactam, or ticarcillin clavulanate appears to be as effective as combination therapy (eg, metronidazole or clindamycin plus an aminoglycoside or third-generation cephalosporin [eg, ceftazidime, cefotaxime]). Symptomatic improvement should be evident within 2–3 days. Intravenous antibiotics should be continued for 5–7 days, before changing to oral antibiotics.

B. Surgical Management

Surgical consultation and repeat abdominal CT imaging should be obtained on all patients with severe disease or those who do not improve after 72 hours of medical management. Patients with a localized abdominal abscess 4 cm in size or larger are usually treated urgently with a percutaneous catheter drain placed by an interventional radiologist. This permits control of the infection and resolution of the immediate infectious inflammatory process. In this manner, a subsequent elective one-stage surgical operation can be performed (if deemed necessary) in which the diseased segment of colon is removed and primary colonic anastomosis performed. After recovery, the decision to perform elective surgery depends on the patient's age, comorbid disease, and frequency and severity of attacks. Patients with chronic disease resulting in fistulas or colonic obstruction will require elective surgical resection.

Indications for emergent surgical management include generalized peritonitis, large undrainable abscesses, and clinical deterioration despite medical management and percutaneous drainage. Surgery may be performed in one- or two-stage operations depending on the patient's nutritional status, severity of illness, and extent of intraabdominal peritonitis and abscess formation.

▶ Prognosis

Diverticulitis recurs in 15–30% of patients treated with medical management over 10–20 years. However, less than 5% have more than two recurrences. Recurrent mild attacks may warrant elective surgical resection in selected patients, especially those who have multiple attacks or those in whom chronic symptoms develop. Diverticulosis is not associated with an increased risk of colorectal cancer. Nonetheless, colorectal cancer may cause symptoms that may be confused with diverticulitis. Therefore, colonoscopy is recommended in patients over age 50 who have not undergone appropriate screening and should be considered in other high-risk patients, especially those with suspicious radiologic imaging, diverticulitis with complications or protracted symptoms, or family history of colorectal cancer.

▶ When to Refer

- Failure to improve within 72 hours of medical management.
- Presence of significant peridiverticular abscesses (4 cm or larger) requiring possible percutaneous or surgical drainage.
- Generalized peritonitis or sepsis.
- Recurrent attacks.
- Chronic complications, including colonic strictures or fistulas.

▶ When to Admit

- Severe pain or inability to tolerate oral intake.
- Signs of sepsis or peritonitis.
- CT scan showing signs of complicated disease (abscess, perforation, obstruction).
- Failure to improve with outpatient management.
- Immunocompromised or frail, elderly patient.

Ahmed AM et al. Surgical treatment of diverticulitis and its complications: a systematic review and meta-analysis of randomized control trials. Surgeon. 2018 Dec;16(6):372–83. [PMID: 30033140]

Gachabayov M et al. Laparoscopic approaches to complicated diverticulitis. Langenbecks Arch Surg. 2018 Feb;403(1):11–22. [PMID: 28875302]

Huston JM et al. Antibiotics versus no antibiotics for the treatment of acute uncomplicated diverticulitis: review of the evidence and future directions. Surg Infect (Larchmt). 2018 Oct;19(7):648–54. [PMID: 30204549]

Knott L et al. Medical management of diverticular disease. Clin Colon Rectal Surg. 2018 Jul;31(4):214–6. [PMID: 29942209]

Meara MP et al. Emergency presentations of diverticulitis. Surg Clin North Am. 2018 Oct;98(5):1025–46. [PMID: 30243445]

Shaban F et al. Perforated diverticulitis: to anastomose or not to anastomose? A systematic review and meta-analysis. Int J Surg. 2018 Oct;58:11–21. [PMID: 30165109]

Zoog E et al. An update on the current management of perforated diverticulitis. Am Surg. 2017 Dec 1;83(12):1321–8. [PMID: 29336748]

3. Diverticular Bleeding

Half of all cases of acute lower gastrointestinal bleeding are attributable to diverticulosis. For a full discussion, see the section on Acute Lower Gastrointestinal Bleeding, above.

POLYPS OF THE COLON

Polyps are discrete mass lesions that protrude into the intestinal lumen. Although most commonly sporadic, they may be inherited as part of a familial polyposis syndrome. Polyps may be divided into four major pathologic groups: mucosal adenomatous polyps (tubular, tubulovillous, and villous), mucosal serrated polyps (hyperplastic, sessile serrated polyps, and traditional serrated adenoma), mucosal nonneoplastic polyps (juvenile polyps, hamartomas, inflammatory polyps), and submucosal lesions (lipomas, lymphoid aggregates, carcinoids, pneumatosis cystoides intestinalis). Of polyps removed at colonoscopy, over 70% are adenomatous; most of the remainder are serrated. Adenomatous polyps and serrated polyps have significant clinical implications and will be considered further below.

NONFAMILIAL ADENOMATOUS & SERRATED POLYPS

Adenomas and serrated polyps may be non-polypoid (flat, slightly elevated, or depressed), sessile, or pedunculated (containing a stalk). They are present in 30% of adults over 50 years of age. Their significance is that over 95% of cases of adenocarcinoma of the colon are believed to arise from these lesions. It is proposed that there is a polyp → carcinoma sequence whereby nonfamilial colorectal cancer develops through a continuous process from normal mucosa to adenomatous or serrated polyp to carcinoma. The majority of cancers arise in adenomas after inactivation of the *APC* gene leads to chromosomal instability and inactivation or loss of other tumor suppressor genes. By contrast, cancers arising in the serrated pathway appear to have either *Kras* (traditional serrated adenomas) mutations or *BRAF* oncogene activation (sessile serrated adenomas) with methylation of CpG-rich promoter regions that leads to inactivation of tumor suppressor genes or mismatch repair genes (*MLH1*) with microsatellite instability.

Most adenomas are smaller than 1 cm and have a low risk of becoming malignant; less than 5% of these enlarge with time. Adenomas and serrated polyps are classified as "advanced" if they are 1 cm or larger or contain villous features or high-grade dysplasia. Advanced lesions are believed to have a higher risk of harboring or progressing to malignancy. It has been estimated from longitudinal studies that it takes an average of 5 years for a medium-sized polyp to develop from normal-appearing mucosa and 10 years for a gross cancer to arise. The prevalence of advanced adenomas is 6% and colorectal cancer 0.3%.

Most sessile serrated polyps and traditional serrated adenomas are believed to arise from hyperplastic polyps. It is believed that sessile serrated polyps and traditional serrated adenomas harbor an increased risk of colorectal cancer similar or greater to that of adenomas. Many pathologists cannot reliably distinguish between hyperplastic polyps and sessile serrated polyps. Hyperplastic polyps smaller than 5 mm located in the rectosigmoid region are of no consequence, except that they cannot reliably be distinguished from adenomatous lesions other than by biopsy. Hyperplastic polyps located in the proximal colon (ie, proximal to the splenic flexure) are associated with an increased risk of neoplasia, particularly those larger than 1 cm.

▶ Clinical Findings

A. Symptoms and Signs

Most patients with adenomatous and serrated polyps are completely asymptomatic. Chronic occult blood loss may lead to iron deficiency anemia. Large polyps may ulcerate, resulting in intermittent hematochezia.

B. Fecal Occult Blood or Multitarget DNA Tests

FOBT, FIT, and fecal DNA tests are available as part of colorectal cancer screening programs (see Chapter 39). FIT is a fecal immunochemical test for hemoglobin with a single specimen having a sensitivity of approximately 80% for colorectal cancer and 20–30% for advanced adenomas but a much lower sensitivity for serrated lesions. FIT is more sensitive than guaiac-based tests for the detection of colorectal cancer and advanced adenomas. In 2014, a test combining a fecal DNA test with a fecal immunochemical test for stool hemoglobin (under the proprietary name "Cologuard") was approved by the FDA. In a prospective comparative trial conducted in persons at average risk for colorectal cancer undergoing colonoscopy, the sensitivity for colorectal cancer for Cologuard was 92.3% compared to 73.8% for FIT and the sensitivity for large (greater than 1 cm) adenomas or serrated polyps for Cologuard was 42.4% compared to 23.8% for FIT.

C. Radiologic Tests

Polyps can be identified by means of barium enema examinations or CT colonography. Both studies require bowel cleansing with laxatives before the study and insertion of a rectal catheter for air insufflation during the study. CT colonography ("virtual colonoscopy") uses data from helical CT imaging with computer-enabled luminal image reconstruction to generate two-dimensional and three-dimensional images of the colon. Using optimal imaging software with multidetector helical CT scanners, several studies report a sensitivity of 90% or more for the detection of polyps larger than 10 mm in size. However, the accuracy for detection of polyps 5–9 mm in size is significantly lower (sensitivity 50%). A small proportion of these diminutive polyps harbor advanced histology (up to 1.2%) or carcinoma (less than 1%). Abdominal CT imaging also results in a radiation exposure that may lead to a small risk of cancer. Barium enema is no longer recommended due to its poor diagnostic accuracy.

D. Endoscopic Tests

Colonoscopy allows evaluation of the entire colon and is the best means of detecting and removing adenomatous and serrated polyps. It should be performed in all patients who have positive FOBT, FIT, or fecal DNA tests or iron deficiency anemia (see Occult Gastrointestinal Bleeding above), as the prevalence of colonic neoplasms is increased in these patients. Colonoscopy should also be performed in patients with polyps detected on radiologic imaging studies (CT colonography or barium enema) or adenomas detected on flexible sigmoidoscopy to remove these polyps and to fully evaluate the entire colon. The newest generation of capsule endoscopy of the colon has an 86% sensitivity and 88% specificity for detection of adenomas greater than 6 mm compared with colonoscopy, but only 29% sensitivity and 33% specificity for sessile serrated polyps. The bowel preparation required for the colon capsule study is more extensive than for colonoscopy and 10–30% of studies may be inadequate due to poor bowel preparation or failure to excrete the capsule. At this time, colonoscopy remains the best test in most patients to detect colorectal polyps. However, capsule endoscopy may be considered in patients who are unsuitable or unwilling to undergo colonoscopy or who have an incomplete colonoscopy.

▶ Treatment

A. Colonoscopic Polypectomy

Most adenomatous and serrated polyps are amenable to colonoscopic removal with biopsy forceps or snare cautery. Sessile polyps larger than 2–3 cm may be removed by snare cautery using a variety of techniques (eg, piecemeal or saline-lift assisted mucosal resection) or may require surgical resection. Patients with large sessile polyps removed in piecemeal fashion should undergo repeated colonoscopy in 2–6 months to verify complete polyp removal. Complications after colonoscopic polypectomy include perforation in 0.2% and clinically significant bleeding in 0.3–1% of patients.

B. Postpolypectomy Surveillance

Adenomas and serrated polyps can be found in 30–40% of patients when another colonoscopy is performed within 3–5 years after the initial examination and polyp removal. Periodic colonoscopic surveillance is therefore recommended to detect these "metachronous" lesions, which either may be new or may have been overlooked during the initial examination. Most of these polyps are small, without high-risk features, and of little immediate clinical significance. The probability of detecting advanced neoplasms at surveillance colonoscopy depends on the number, size, and histologic features of the polyps removed on initial (index) colonoscopy. Patients with 1–2 tubular adenomas smaller than 1 cm (without villous features or high-grade dysplasia) should have their next colonoscopy in 5–10 years. Patients with 3–10 adenomas, an adenoma larger than 1 cm, or an adenoma with villous features or high-grade dysplasia should have their next colonoscopy at 3 years. Patients with more than 10 adenomas should have a repeat colonoscopy at 1–2 years and may be considered for evaluation for a familial polyposis syndrome. Surveillance colonoscopy at 5 years is appropriate for patients with small (less than 1 cm) serrated polyps without cytologic dysplasia; surveillance colonoscopy at 3 years should be considered for serrated polyps larger than 1 cm and those with cytologic atypia. No surveillance is recommended for patients with small, typical hyperplastic polyps located in the distal colon and rectum.

Feagins LA. Colonoscopy, polypectomy, and the risk of bleeding. Med Clin North Am. 2019 Jan;103(1):125–35. [PMID: 30466669]

Mangas-Sanjuan C et al; Grupo de Cribado del Cáncer Colorrectal de la Sociedad Española de Epidemiología. Endoscopic surveillance after colonic polyps and colorectal cancer resection. 2018 update. Gastroenterol Hepatol. 2019 Mar;42(3): 188–201. [PMID: 30621911]

Robertson DJ et al. Recommendations on fecal immunochemical testing to screen for colorectal neoplasia: a consensus statement by the US Multi-Society Task Force on colorectal cancer. Gastrointest Endosc. 2017 Jan;85(1):2–21. [PMID: 27769516]

HEREDITARY COLORECTAL CANCER & POLYPOSIS SYNDROMES

Up to 4% of all colorectal cancers are caused by germline genetic mutations that impose on carriers a high lifetime risk of developing colorectal cancer (see Chapter 39). Because the diagnosis of these disorders has important implications for treatment of affected members and for screening of family members, it is important to consider these disorders in patients with a family history of colorectal cancer that has affected more than one family member, those with a personal or family history of colorectal cancer developing at an early age (50 years or younger), those with a personal or family history of multiple polyps (more than 20), and those with a personal or family history of multiple extracolonic malignancies.

1. Familial Adenomatous Polyposis

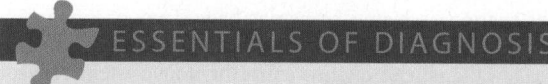

ESSENTIALS OF DIAGNOSIS

- ▶ Inherited condition characterized by early development of hundreds to thousands of colonic adenomatous polyps and even one or more adenocarcinoma(s).
- ▶ Variety of extracolonic manifestations, including duodenal adenomas, desmoid tumors, and osteomas.
- ▶ Attenuated variant with fewer than 500 (average 25) colonic adenomas.
- ▶ Genetic testing confirms mutation of *APC* gene (90%) or *MUTYH* gene (8%).
- ▶ Prophylactic colectomy recommended to prevent otherwise inevitable colorectal cancer (adenocarcinoma).

▶ General Considerations

Familial adenomatous polyposis (FAP) is a syndrome affecting 1:10,000 people and accounts for approximately 0.5% of colorectal cancer. The classic form of FAP is characterized by the development of hundreds to thousands of colonic adenomatous polyps and a variety of extracolonic manifestations. Of patients with classic FAP, approximately 90% have a mutation in the *APC* gene that is inherited in an autosomal dominant fashion and 8% have mutations in the *MUTYH* gene that are inherited in an autosomal recessive fashion. FAP arises de novo in 15% of patients in the absence of genetic mutations in the parents. An attenuated variant of FAP also has been recognized in which an average of only 25 polyps (range of 1–500) develop.

▶ Clinical Findings

A. Symptoms and Signs

Colorectal polyps develop by a mean age of 15 years and cancer at 40 years. Unless prophylactic colectomy is performed, colorectal cancer is inevitable by age 50 years. In attenuated FAP, the mean age for development of cancer is about 56 years.

Adenomatous polyps of the duodenum and periampullary area develop in over 90% of patients, resulting in a 5–8% lifetime risk of adenocarcinoma. Adenomas occur less frequently in the gastric antrum and small bowel and, in those locations, have a lower risk of malignant transformation. Gastric fundus gland polyps occur in over 50% but have an extremely low (0.6%) malignant potential.

A variety of other benign extraintestinal manifestations, including soft tissue tumors of the skin, desmoid tumors, osteomas, and congenital hypertrophy of the retinal pigment, develop in some patients with FAP. These extraintestinal manifestations vary among families, depending in part on the type or site of mutation in the

APC gene. Desmoid tumors are locally invasive fibromas, most commonly intra-abdominal, that may cause bowel obstruction, ischemia, or hemorrhage. They occur in 15% of patients and are the second leading cause of death in FAP. Malignancies of the central nervous system (Turcot syndrome) and tumors of the thyroid and liver (hepatoblastomas) may also develop in patients with FAP.

B. Genetic Testing

Genetic counseling and testing should be offered to patients found to have multiple adenomatous polyps at endoscopy and to first-degree family members of patients with FAP. Genetic testing is best performed by sequencing the *APC* gene to identify disease-associated mutations followed by *MUTYH* mutational assessment in patients with no detectable *APC* mutations. *APC* gene mutations are identified in 80% of patients with more than 1000, and 56% with 100–1000 polyps (ie, the classic phenotype of FAP). Recent guidelines also recommend that genetic testing be considered in individuals with as few as 10 adenomas to exclude a diagnosis of attenuated disease. *APC* or *MUTYH* mutations are found in 10% and 7%, respectively, of patients with 20–100 adenomas and 5% and 4%, respectively, of those with 10–19 adenomas.

► Treatment

Once the diagnosis has been established, complete proctocolectomy with ileoanal anastomosis or colectomy with ileorectal anastomosis is recommended, usually before age 20 years. Ileorectal anastomosis affords superior bowel function but has a 5% risk of development of rectal cancer, and for that reason frequent sigmoidoscopy with fulguration of polyps is required. Upper endoscopic evaluation of the stomach, duodenum, and periampullary area should be performed every 1–3 years to look for adenomas or carcinoma. Periampullary adenomas larger than 2 cm require surgical resection. Sulindac and celecoxib have been shown to decrease the number and size of polyps in the rectal stump but not the duodenum.

Boland PM et al. Recent progress in Lynch syndrome and other familial colorectal cancer syndromes. CA Cancer J Clin. 2018 May;68(3):217–31. [PMID: 29485237]

Byrne RM et al. Colorectal polyposis and inherited colorectal cancer syndromes. Ann Gastroenterol. 2018 Jan–Feb; 31(1):24–34. [PMID: 29333064]

Kanth P et al. Hereditary colorectal polyposis and cancer syndromes: a primer on diagnosis and management. Am J Gastroenterol. 2017 Oct;112(10):1509–25. [PMID: 28786406]

Lorans M et al. Update on hereditary colorectal cancer: improving the clinical utility of multigene panel testing. Clin Colorectal Cancer. 2018 Jun;17(2):e293–305. [PMID: 29454559]

2. Hamartomatous Polyposis Syndromes

Hamartomatous polyposis syndromes are rare and account for less than 0.1% of colorectal cancers.

Peutz-Jeghers syndrome is an autosomal dominant condition characterized by hamartomatous polyps throughout the gastrointestinal tract (most notably in the small intestine) as well as mucocutaneous pigmented macules on the lips, buccal mucosa, and skin. The hamartomas may become large, leading to bleeding, intussusception, or obstruction. Although hamartomas are not malignant, gastrointestinal malignancies (stomach, small bowel, and colon) develop in 40–60%, breast cancer in 30–50%, as well as a host of other malignancies of nonintestinal organs (gonads, pancreas). The defect has been localized to the serine threonine kinase 11 gene, and genetic testing is available.

Familial juvenile polyposis is also autosomal dominant and is characterized by multiple (more than ten) juvenile hamartomatous polyps located most commonly in the colon. There is an increased risk (up to 50%) of adenocarcinoma due to synchronous adenomatous polyps or mixed hamartomatous-adenomatous polyps. Genetic defects have been identified to loci on 18q and 10q (*MADH4* and *BMPR1A*). Genetic testing is available.

PTEN multiple hamartoma syndrome (Cowden disease) is characterized by hamartomatous polyps and lipomas throughout the gastrointestinal tract, trichilemmomas, and cerebellar lesions. An increased rate of malignancy is demonstrated in the thyroid, breast, and urogenital tract.

Byrne RM et al. Colorectal polyposis and inherited colorectal cancer syndromes. Ann Gastroenterol. 2018 Jan–Feb;31(1): 24–34. [PMID: 29333064]

Daniell J et al. An exploration of genotype-phenotype link between Peutz-Jeghers syndrome and *STK11*: a review. Fam Cancer. 2018 Jul;17(3):421–7. [PMID: 28900777]

Kanth P et al. Hereditary colorectal polyposis and cancer syndromes: a primer on diagnosis and management. Am J Gastroenterol. 2017 Oct;112(10):1509–25. [PMID: 28786406]

3. Lynch Syndrome

ESSENTIALS OF DIAGNOSIS

► Autosomal dominant inherited condition.

► Caused by mutations in a gene that detects and repairs DNA base-pair mismatches, resulting in DNA microsatellite instability and inactivation of tumor suppressor genes.

► Increased lifetime risk of colorectal cancer (22–75%), endometrial cancer (30–60%), and other cancers that may develop at young age.

► Evaluation warranted in patients with personal history of early-onset colorectal cancer or family history of colorectal, endometrial, or other Lynch syndrome–related cancers at young age or in multiple members.

► Diagnosis suspected by tumor tissue immunohistochemical staining for mismatch repair proteins or testing for microsatellite instability.

► Diagnosis confirmed by genetic testing.

► General Considerations

Lynch syndrome (also known as hereditary nonpolyposis colon cancer [HNPCC]) is an autosomal dominant condition in which there is a markedly increased risk of developing colorectal cancer as well as a host of other cancers, including endometrial, ovarian, renal or bladder, hepatobiliary, gastric, and small intestinal cancers. It is estimated to account for up to 3% of all colorectal cancers. Affected individuals have a 22–75% lifetime risk of developing colorectal carcinoma and a 30–60% lifetime risk of endometrial cancer, depending on the affected gene. Unlike individuals with familial adenomatous polyposis, patients with Lynch syndrome develop only a few adenomas, which may be flat and more often contain villous features or high-grade dysplasia. In contrast to the traditional polyp → cancer progression (which may take over 10 years), these polyps are believed to undergo rapid transformation over 1–2 years from normal tissue → adenoma → cancer. Colon and endometrial cancer tend to develop at an earlier age than sporadic, nonhereditary cancers (mean age 45–50 years). A germline mutation is identified in 20% of patients in whom colon cancer was diagnosed before age 50. Compared with patients with sporadic tumors of similar pathologic stage, those with Lynch syndrome tumors have improved survival. Synchronous or metachronous cancers occur within 10 years in up to 45% of patients.

Lynch syndrome is caused by a defect in one of several genes that are important in the detection and repair of DNA base-pair mismatches: *MLH1, MSH2, MSH6,* and *PMS2* or *EPCAM*, a promoter for *MSH2*. Germline mutations in *MLH1* and *MSH2* account for almost 90% of the known mutations in families with Lynch syndrome. Mutations in any of these mismatch repair genes result in a characteristic phenotypic DNA abnormality known as microsatellite instability.

Clinical Findings

A thorough family cancer history is essential to identify families that may be affected by the Lynch syndrome so that appropriate genetic and colonoscopic screening can be offered. The National Colorectal Cancer Roundtable recommends a simple three-question tool for identifying increased risk and meriting more detailed assessment: (1) Do you have a first-degree relative with colorectal cancer or another Lynch syndrome–related cancer diagnosed before age 50?; (2) Have you had colorectal cancer or polyps diagnosed before age 50?; and (3) Do you have three or more relatives with colorectal cancer? The PREMM5 probability model is available for calculating the likelihood of Lynch syndrome based on family and personal history (https://premm.dfci.harvard.edu/). Genetic evaluation is recommended for those with a personal or family history of colorectal cancer under age 50, a history of multiple family members with cancer, or a greater than 5% PREMM5 model-predicted chance of Lynch syndrome. Genetic testing can be performed with multigene panels that test for germline cancer genes (ie, Lynch, familial adenomatous polyposis, and hamartomatous syndromes) as well as others of uncertain significance for approximately $250. Referral to a genetic counselor therefore is recommended.

Personal and family history alone are insufficient to identify a significant proportion of patients with Lynch syndrome. For this reason, the National Comprehensive Cancer Network recommend that *all* colorectal cancers should undergo testing for Lynch syndrome with either immunohistochemistry or microsatellite instability. Universal testing has the greatest sensitivity for the diagnosis of Lynch syndrome and is cost-effective. Individuals whose tumors have normal immunohistochemical staining or do not have microsatellite instability are unlikely to have germline mutations in mismatch repair genes, do not require further genetic testing, and do not require intensive cancer surveillance. Up to 15% of sporadic (noninherited) tumors have microsatellite instability or absent *MLH1* staining due to somatic (noninherited) methylation of the *MLH1* gene promoter and somatic *BRAF* mutations, which must be excluded before further genetic testing is considered. Germline testing for gene mutations is positive in more than 90% of individuals whose tumors show absent histochemical staining of one of the mismatch repair genes or high level of microsatellite instability without a *BRAF* mutation.

Screening & Treatment

If a mutation is detected in a patient with cancer in one of the known mismatch genes, genetic testing of other first-degree family members is indicated. If genetic testing documents a Lynch syndrome gene mutation, affected relatives should be screened with colonoscopy every 1–2 years beginning at age 25 (or at age 5 years younger than the age at diagnosis of the youngest affected family member). If cancer is found, subtotal colectomy with ileorectal anastomosis (followed by annual surveillance of the rectal stump) should be performed. Women should undergo screening for endometrial and ovarian cancer beginning at age 30–35 years with pelvic examination, transvaginal ultrasound, and endometrial sampling. Prophylactic hysterectomy and oophorectomy are recommended to women at age 40 or once they have finished childbearing. Screening for gastric cancer with upper endoscopy should be considered every 2–3 years beginning at age 30–35 years.

Ballester V et al. How and when to consider genetic testing for colon cancer? Gastroenterology. 2018 Oct;155(4):955–9. [PMID: 30148981]

Idos G et al. When should patients undergo genetic testing for hereditary colon cancer syndromes? Clin Gastroenterol Hepatol. 2018 Feb;16(2):181–3. [PMID: 29133258]

Pearlman R et al; Ohio Colorectal Cancer Prevention Initiative Group. Prevalence and spectrum of germline cancer susceptibility gene mutations among patients with early-onset colorectal cancer. JAMA Oncol. 2017 Apr 1;3(4):464–71. [PMID: 27978560]

Samadder NJ et al. Cancer risk in families fulfilling the Amsterdam criteria for Lynch syndrome. JAMA Oncol. 2017 Dec 1; 3(12):1697–701. [PMID: 28772302]

Stoffel EM et al. Germline genetic features of young individuals with colorectal cancer. Gastroenterology. 2018 Mar;154(4): 897–905. [PMID: 29146522]

ANORECTAL DISEASES

(See Chapter 39 for Carcinoma of the Anus.)

HEMORRHOIDS

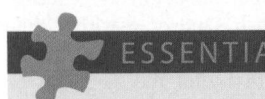

ESSENTIALS OF DIAGNOSIS

▶ Bright red blood per rectum.

▶ Protrusion, discomfort.

▶ Characteristic findings on external anal inspection and anoscopic examination.

General Considerations

Internal hemorrhoids are subepithelial vascular cushions consisting of connective tissue, smooth muscle fibers, and arteriovenous communications between terminal branches of the superior rectal artery and rectal veins. They are a normal anatomic entity, occurring in all adults, that contribute to normal anal pressures and ensure a water-tight closure of the anal canal. They commonly occur in three primary locations—right anterior, right posterior, and left lateral. External hemorrhoids arise from the inferior hemorrhoidal veins located below the dentate line and are covered with squamous epithelium of the anal canal or perianal region.

Hemorrhoids may become symptomatic as a result of activities that increase venous pressure, resulting in distention and engorgement. Straining at stool, constipation, prolonged sitting, pregnancy, obesity, and low-fiber diets all may contribute. With time, redundancy and enlargement of the venous cushions may develop and result in bleeding or protrusion.

Clinical Findings

A. Symptoms and Signs

Patients often attribute a variety of perianal complaints to "hemorrhoids." However, the principal problems attributable to internal hemorrhoids are bleeding, prolapse, and mucoid discharge. Bleeding is manifested by bright red blood that may range from streaks of blood visible on toilet paper or stool to bright red blood that drips into the toilet bowl after a bowel movement. Uncommonly, bleeding is severe and prolonged enough to result in anemia. Initially, internal hemorrhoids are confined to the anal canal (stage I). Over time, the internal hemorrhoids may gradually enlarge and protrude from the anal opening. At first, this mucosal prolapse occurs during straining and reduces spontaneously (stage II). With progression over time, the prolapsed hemorrhoids may require manual reduction after bowel movements (stage III) or may remain chronically protruding (stage IV). Chronically prolapsed hemorrhoids may result in a sense of fullness or discomfort and mucoid discharge, resulting in irritation of perianal skin and soiling of underclothes. Pain is unusual with internal hemorrhoids, occurring only when there is extensive inflammation and thrombosis of irreducible tissue or with thrombosis of an external hemorrhoid.

B. Examination

External hemorrhoids are readily visible on perianal inspection. Nonprolapsed internal hemorrhoids are not visible but may protrude through the anus with gentle straining while the clinician spreads the buttocks. Prolapsed hemorrhoids are visible as protuberant purple nodules covered by mucosa. The perianal region should also be examined for other signs of disease such as fistulas, fissures, skin tags, condyloma, anal cancer, or dermatitis. On digital examination, uncomplicated internal hemorrhoids are neither palpable nor painful. Anoscopic evaluation, best performed in the prone jackknife position, provides optimal visualization of internal hemorrhoids.

Differential Diagnosis

Small volume rectal bleeding may be caused by an anal fissure or fistula, neoplasms of the distal colon or rectum, ulcerative colitis or Crohn colitis, infectious proctitis, or rectal ulcers. Rectal prolapse, in which a full thickness of rectum protrudes concentrically from the anus, is readily distinguished from mucosal hemorrhoidal prolapse. Proctosigmoidoscopy or colonoscopy should be performed in all patients with hematochezia to exclude disease in the rectum or sigmoid colon that could be misinterpreted in the presence of hemorrhoidal bleeding.

Treatment

A. Conservative Measures

Most patients with early (stage I and stage II) disease can be managed with conservative treatment. To decrease straining with defecation, patients should be given instructions for a high-fiber diet and told to increase fluid intake with meals. Dietary fiber may be supplemented with bran powder (1–2 tbsp twice daily added to food or in 8 oz of liquid) or with commercial bulk laxatives (eg, Benefiber, Metamucil, Citrucel). Suppositories and rectal ointments have no demonstrated utility in the management of mild disease. Mucoid discharge may be treated effectively by the local application of a cotton ball tucked next to the anal opening after bowel movements.

B. Medical Treatment

Patients with stage I, stage II, and stage III hemorrhoids and recurrent bleeding despite conservative measures may be treated without anesthesia with injection sclerotherapy, rubber band ligation, or application of electrocoagulation (bipolar cautery or infrared photocoagulation). The choice of therapy is dictated by operator preference, but rubber band ligation is preferred due to its ease of use and high rate of efficacy. Major complications occur in less than 2%, including pelvic sepsis, pelvic abscess, urinary retention, and bleeding. Recurrence is common unless patients alter their dietary habits. Edematous, prolapsed (stage IV) internal hemorrhoids, may be treated acutely with topical creams, foams, or suppositories containing various combinations of emollients, topical anesthetics, (eg, pramoxine, dibucaine), vasoconstrictors (eg, phenylephrine), astringents (witch hazel), and corticosteroids. Common preparations include Preparation H (several formulations), Anusol HC, Proctofoam, Nupercainal, Tucks, and Doloproct (not available in the United States).

C. Surgical Treatment

Surgical excision (hemorrhoidectomy) is reserved for less than 5–10% of patients with chronic severe bleeding due to stage III or stage IV hemorrhoids or patients with acute thrombosed stage IV hemorrhoids with necrosis. Complications of surgical hemorrhoidectomy include postoperative pain (which may persist for 2–4 weeks) and impaired continence.

▶ Thrombosed External Hemorrhoid

Thrombosis of the external hemorrhoidal plexus results in a perianal hematoma. It most commonly occurs in otherwise healthy young adults and may be precipitated by coughing, heavy lifting, or straining at stool. The condition is characterized by the relatively acute onset of an exquisitely painful, tense and bluish perianal nodule covered with skin that may be up to several centimeters in size. Pain is most severe within the first few hours but gradually eases over 2–3 days as edema subsides. Symptoms may be relieved with warm sitz baths, analgesics, and ointments. If the patient is evaluated in the first 24–48 hours, removal of the clot may hasten symptomatic relief. With the patient in the lateral position, the skin around and over the lump is injected subcutaneously with 1% lidocaine using a tuberculin syringe with a 30-gauge needle. An ellipse of skin is then excised and the clot evacuated. A dry gauze dressing is applied for 12–24 hours, and daily sitz baths are then begun.

▶ When to Refer

- Stage I, II, or III: When conservative measures fail and expertise in medical procedures is needed (injection, banding, thermocoagulation).
- Stage IV: When surgical excision is required.

Jacobs DO. Hemorrhoids: what are the options in 2018? Curr Opin Gastroenterol. 2018 Jan;34(1):46–9. [PMID: 29076869]

Jamshidi R. Anorectal complaints: hemorrhoids, fissures, abscesses, fistulae. Clin Colon Rectal Surg. 2018 Mar;31(2):117–20. [PMID: 29487494]

Qureshi WA. Office management of hemorrhoids. Am J Gastroenterol. 2018 Jun;113(6):795–8. [PMID: 29487411]

Sandler RS et al. Rethinking what we know about hemorrhoids. Clin Gastroenterol Hepatol. 2019 Jan;17(1):8–15. [PMID: 29601902]

ANORECTAL INFECTIONS

A number of organisms can cause inflammation of the anal and rectal mucosa. Proctitis is characterized by anorectal discomfort, tenesmus, constipation, and mucus or bloody discharge. Most cases of proctitis are sexually transmitted, especially by anal-receptive intercourse. Infectious proctitis must be distinguished from noninfectious causes of anorectal symptoms, including anal fissures or fistulae, perirectal abscesses, anorectal carcinomas, and inflammatory bowel disease (ulcerative colitis or Crohn disease).

▶ Etiology & Management

Several organisms may cause infectious proctitis.

A. *Neisseria gonorrhoeae*

Gonorrhea may cause itching, burning, tenesmus, and a mucopurulent discharge, although many anorectal infections are asymptomatic. Rectal swab specimens should be taken during anoscopy for culture; Gram staining is unreliable. Cultures should also be taken from the pharynx and urethra in men and from the pharynx and cervix in women. Complications of untreated infections include strictures, fissures, fistulas, and perirectal abscesses. (For treatment, see Chapter 33.)

B. *Treponema pallidum*

Anal syphilis may be asymptomatic or may lead to perianal pain and discharge. With primary syphilis, the chancre may be at the anal margin or within the anal canal and may mimic a fissure, fistula, or ulcer. Proctitis or inguinal lymphadenopathy may be present. With secondary syphilis, condylomata lata (pale-brown, flat verrucous lesions) may be seen, with secretion of foul-smelling mucus. Although the diagnosis may be established with dark-field microscopy or fluorescent antibody testing of scrapings from the chancre or condylomas, this requires proper equipment and trained personnel. The VDRL or RPR test is positive in 75% of primary cases and in 99% of secondary cases. (For treatment, see Chapter 34.)

C. *Chlamydia trachomatis*

Chlamydial infection may cause proctitis similar to gonorrheal proctitis; however, some infections are asymptomatic. It also may cause lymphogranuloma venereum, characterized by proctocolitis with fever and bloody diarrhea, painful perianal ulcerations, anorectal strictures and fistulas, and inguinal adenopathy (buboes). Previously rare in developed countries, an increasing number of cases have been identified among men who have sex with men. The diagnosis is established by serology, culture, or PCR-based testing of rectal discharge or rectal biopsy. Recommended treatment is doxycycline 100 mg orally twice daily for 21 days.

D. Herpes simplex type 2

Herpes simplex type 2 virus is a common cause of anorectal infection. Symptoms occur 4–21 days after exposure and include severe pain, itching, constipation, tenesmus, urinary retention, and radicular pain from involvement of lumbar or sacral nerve roots. Small vesicles or ulcers may be seen in the perianal area or anal canal. Sigmoidoscopy is not usually necessary but may reveal vesicular or ulcerative lesions in the distal rectum. Diagnosis is established by viral culture, PCR, or antigen detection assays of vesicular fluid. Symptoms resolve within 2 weeks, but viral shedding may continue for several weeks. Patients may remain asymptomatic with or without viral shedding or may have recurrent mild relapses. Treatment of acute infection for 7–10 days with acyclovir, 400 mg, or famciclovir, 250 mg orally three times daily, or valacyclovir, 1 g twice daily, has been shown to reduce the duration of symptoms and viral shedding. Patients with AIDS and recurrent relapses may benefit from long-term suppressive therapy (see Chapter 31).

E. *Condylomata acuminata*

Condylomata acuminata (warts) are a significant cause of anorectal symptoms. Caused by the HPV, they may occur on the perianal area, in the anal canal, or on the genitals. Perianal or anal warts are seen in up to 25% of men who have sex with men. HIV-positive individuals with condylomas have a higher relapse rate after therapy and a higher rate of progression to high-grade dysplasia or anal cancer. The warts are located on the perianal skin and extend within the anal canal up to 2 cm above the dentate line. Patients may have no symptoms or may report itching, bleeding, and pain. The warts may be small and flat or verrucous, or may form a confluent mass that may obscure the anal opening. Warts must be distinguished from condyloma lata (secondary syphilis) or anal cancer. Biopsies should be obtained from large or suspicious lesions. Treatment can be difficult. Sexual partners should also be examined and treated. The treatment of anogenital warts is discussed in Chapter 30. The HPV vaccine, Gardasil-9 valent, has demonstrated efficacy in preventing anogenital warts and is now recommended for all persons aged 9-14 (2 or 3 doses) and persons aged 15-45 (3 doses), as well as all men of any age who have sex with men (see Chapters 1 and 30). HIV-positive individuals with condylomas who have detectable serum HIV RNA levels should have anoscopic surveillance for anal cancer every 3–6 months.

Davies D et al. Diagnosis and management of anorectal disorders in the primary care setting. Prim Care. 2017 Dec;44(4):709–20. [PMID: 29132530]

Diaz A et al. Lymphogranuloma venereum in Spain, 2005–2015: a literature review. Med Clin (Barc). 2018 Nov 21;151(10):412–7. [PMID: 30166126]

Workowski KA et al; Centers for Disease Control and Prevention (CDC). Sexually transmitted diseases treatment guidelines, 2015. MMWR Recomm Rep. 2015 Jun 5;64(RR-03):1–137. Erratum in: MMWR Recomm Rep. 2015 Aug 28;64(33):924. [PMID: 26042815]

FECAL INCONTINENCE

In a 2018 survey, 4.7% of US adults reported fecal incontinence within the prior 30 days. There are five general requirements for bowel continence: (1) solid or semisolid stool (even healthy young adults have difficulty maintaining continence with liquid rectal contents); (2) a distensible rectal reservoir (as sigmoid contents empty into the rectum, the vault must expand to accommodate); (3) a sensation of rectal fullness (if the patient cannot sense this, overflow may occur before the patient can take appropriate action); (4) intact pelvic nerves and muscles; and (5) the ability to reach a toilet in a timely fashion.

▶ Minor Incontinence

Many patients complain of inability to control flatus or slight soilage of undergarments that tends to occur after bowel movements or with straining or coughing. This may be due to local anal problems such as prolapsed hemorrhoids that make it difficult to form a tight anal seal or isolated weakness of the internal anal sphincter, especially if stools are somewhat loose. Patients should be treated with fiber supplements to provide greater stool bulk. Coffee and other caffeinated beverages should be eliminated. The perianal skin should be cleansed with moist, lanolin-coated tissue (baby wipes) to reduce excoriation and infection. After wiping, loose application of a cotton ball near the anal opening may absorb small amounts of fecal leakage. Prolapsing hemorrhoids may be treated with band ligation or surgical hemorrhoidectomy. Control of flatus and seepage may be improved by Kegel perineal exercises. Conditions such as ulcerative proctitis that cause tenesmus and urgency, chronic diarrheal conditions, and irritable bowel syndrome may result in difficulty in maintaining complete continence, especially if a toilet is not readily available. Loperamide may be helpful to reduce urge incontinence in patients with loose stools and may be taken in anticipation of situations in which a toilet may not be readily available. Older patients may require more time or assistance to reach a toilet, which may lead to incontinence. Scheduled toileting and the availability of a bedside commode are helpful. Elderly patients with chronic constipation may develop stool impaction leading to "overflow" incontinence.

▶ Major Incontinence

Complete uncontrolled loss of stool reflects a significant problem with central perception or neuromuscular function. Incontinence that occurs without awareness suggests a loss of central awareness (eg, dementia, cerebrovascular accident, multiple sclerosis) or peripheral nerve injury (eg, spinal cord injury, cauda equina syndrome, pudendal nerve damage due to obstetric trauma or pelvic floor prolapse, aging, or diabetes mellitus). Incontinence that occurs despite awareness and active efforts to retain stool suggests sphincteric damage, which may be caused by traumatic childbirth (especially forceps delivery), episiotomy, prolapse, prior anal surgery, and physical trauma.

Physical examination should include careful inspection of the perianal area for hemorrhoids, rectal prolapse, fissures, fistulas, and either gaping or a keyhole defect of the anal sphincter (indicating severe sphincteric injury or neurologic disorder). The perianal skin should be stimulated to confirm an intact anocutaneous reflex. Digital examination during relaxation gives valuable information about resting tone (due mainly to the internal sphincter) and contraction of the external sphincter and pelvic floor during squeezing. It also excludes fecal impaction. Anoscopy is required to evaluate for hemorrhoids, fissures, and fistulas. Proctosigmoidoscopy is useful to exclude rectal carcinoma or proctitis. Anal ultrasonography or pelvic MRI is the most reliable test for definition of anatomic defects in the external and internal anal sphincters. Anal manometry may also be useful to define the severity of weakness, to assess sensation, and to predict response to biofeedback training. In special circumstances, surface electromyography is useful to document sphincteric denervation and proctography to document perineal descent or rectal intussusception.

Patients who are incontinent only of loose or liquid stools are treated with bulking agents and antidiarrheal drugs (eg, loperamide, 2 mg before meals and prophylactically before social engagements, shopping trips, etc). Patients with incontinence of solid stool benefit from scheduled toilet use after glycerin suppositories or tap water enemas. Biofeedback training with anal sphincteric strengthening (Kegel) exercises (alternating 5-second squeeze and 10-second rest for 10 minutes twice daily) may be helpful in motivated patients to lower the threshold for awareness of rectal filling—or to improve anal sphincter squeeze function—or both. In 2012, the FDA approved two interventions for fecal incontinence. The first is a sterile gel (containing dextranomer and sodium hyaluronate) for submucosal injection into the proximal anal canal for the treatment of anal incontinence for patients who have not responded to conservative therapies, such as fiber supplements and antidiarrheal agents. This treatment is hypothesized to reduce incontinence episodes by bulking and narrowing the anal canal. In clinical trials, more than one-half of treated patients reported a greater than 50% reduction in the number of fecal incontinence episodes. The second is a sacral nerve stimulation device. In uncontrolled trials in selected patients, 83% of patients were improved with sacral stimulation. Inserts also are available that can be placed in the anus or vagina to enhance continence. Operative management is seldom needed, but should be considered in patients with major incontinence due to prior injury to the anal sphincter who have not responded to medical therapy.

When to Refer

- Conservative measures fail.
- Anorectal tests are deemed necessary (manometry, ultrasonography, electromyography).
- A surgically correctable lesion is suspected.

Forte ML et al. Systematic review of surgical treatments for fecal incontinence. Dis Colon Rectum. 2016 May;59(5):443–69. [PMID: 27050607]

Markland AD et al. Anal intercourse and fecal incontinence: evidence from the 2009–2010 National Health and Nutrition Examination Survey. Am J Gastroenterol. 2016 Feb;111(2):269–74. [PMID: 26753893]

Menees SB. My approach to fecal incontinence: it's all about consistency (stool, that is). Am J Gastroenterol. 2017 Jul;112(7):977–80. [PMID: 28631727]

Menees SB et al. Prevalence of and factors associated with fecal incontinence: results from a population-based survey. Gastroenterology. 2018 May;154(6):1672–81. [PMID: 29408460]

Rangan V et al. Risk factors for fecal urgency among individuals with and without diarrhea, based on data from the National Health and Nutrition Examination Survey. Clin Gastroenterol Hepatol. 2018 Sep;16(9):1450–8. [PMID: 29474972]

OTHER ANAL CONDITIONS

Anal Fissures

Anal fissures are linear or rocket-shaped ulcers that are usually less than 5 mm in length. Most fissures are believed to arise from trauma to the anal canal during defecation, perhaps caused by straining, constipation, or high internal sphincter tone. They occur most commonly in the posterior midline, but 10% occur anteriorly. Fissures that occur off the midline should raise suspicion for Crohn disease, HIV/AIDS, tuberculosis, syphilis, or anal carcinoma. Patients complain of severe, tearing pain during defecation followed by throbbing discomfort that may lead to constipation due to fear of recurrent pain. There may be mild associated hematochezia, with blood on the stool or toilet paper. Anal fissures are confirmed by visual inspection of the anal verge while gently separating the buttocks. Acute fissures look like cracks in the epithelium. Chronic fissures result in fibrosis and the development of a skin tag at the outermost edge (sentinel pile). Digital and anoscopic examinations may cause severe pain and may not be possible. Medical management is directed at promoting effortless, painless bowel movements. Fiber supplements and sitz baths should be prescribed. Topical anesthetics (5% lidocaine; 2.5% lidocaine plus 2.5% prilocaine) may provide temporary relief. Healing occurs within 2 months in up to 45% of patients with conservative management. Chronic fissures may be treated with topical 0.2–0.4% nitroglycerin, diltiazem 2% ointment, or nifedipine 0.5% (1 cm of ointment) applied twice daily just inside the anus with the tip of a finger for 4–8 weeks or injection of botulinum toxin (20 units) into the internal anal sphincter. All of these treatments result in healing in 50–80% of patients with chronic anal fissure, but headaches occur in up to 40% of patients treated with nitroglycerin. Botulinum toxin may cause transient anal incontinence. Fissures recur in up to 40% of patients after treatment. Chronic or recurrent fissures benefit from lateral internal sphincterotomy; however, minor incontinence may complicate this procedure.

Barnes TG et al. Fissurectomy combined with high-dose botulinum toxin is a safe and effective treatment for chronic anal fissure and a promising alternative to surgical sphincterotomy. Dis Colon Rectum. 2015 Oct;58(10):967–73. [PMID: 26347969]

Beaty JS et al. Anal fissure. Clin Colon Rectal Surg. 2016 Mar;29(1):30–7. [PMID: 26929749]

Jamshidi R. Anorectal complaints: hemorrhoids, fissures, abscesses, fistulae. Clin Colon Rectal Surg. 2018 Mar;31(2):117–20. [PMID: 29487494]

Lin JX et al. Optimal dosing of botulinum toxin for treatment of chronic anal fissure: a systematic review and meta-analysis. Dis Colon Rectum. 2016 Sep;59(9):886–94. [PMID: 27505118]

Sahebally SM et al. Botulinum toxin injection vs topical nitrates for chronic anal fissure: an updated systematic review and meta-analysis of randomized controlled trials. Colorectal Dis. 2018 Jan;20(1):6–15. [PMID: 29166553]

Perianal Abscess & Fistula

The anal glands located at the base of the anal crypts at the dentate line may become infected, leading to abscess formation. Other causes of abscess include anal fissure and Crohn disease. Abscesses may extend upward or downward through the intersphincteric plane. Symptoms of perianal abscess are throbbing, continuous perianal pain. Erythema, fluctuance, and swelling may be found in the perianal region on external examination or in the ischiorectal fossa on digital rectal examination. Perianal abscesses are treated with local incision and drainage, while ischiorectal abscesses require drainage in the operating room. After drainage of an abscess, most patients are found to have a fistula in ano.

Fistula in ano most often arises in an anal crypt and is usually preceded by an anal abscess. In patients with fistulas that connect to the rectum, other disorders such as Crohn disease, lymphogranuloma venereum, rectal tuberculosis, and cancer should be considered. Fistulas are associated with purulent discharge that may lead to itching, tenderness, and pain. The treatment of Crohn-related fistula is discussed elsewhere in this chapter. Treatment of simple idiopathic fistula in ano is by surgical incision or excision under anesthesia. Care must be taken to preserve the anal sphincters. Surgical fistulotomy for treatment of complex (high, transphincteric) anal fissures carries a high risk of incontinence. Techniques for healing the fistula while preserving the sphincter include an endoanal advancement flap over the internal opening and insertion of a bioprosthetic plug into the fistula opening.

Jamshidi R. Anorectal complaints: hemorrhoids, fissures, abscesses, fistulae. Clin Colon Rectal Surg. 2018 Mar;31(2): 117–20. [PMID: 29487494]

Schlichtemeier S et al. Treatment for complex anal fistula, are we any wiser? Colorectal Dis. 2018 Dec;20(12):1067–8. [PMID: 30506657]

Vogel JD et al. Clinical practice guideline for the management of anorectal abscess, fistula-in-ano, and rectovaginal fistula. Dis Colon Rectum. 2016 Dec;59(12):1117–33. [PMID: 27824697]

Williams G et al. The treatment of anal fistula: second ACPGBI Position Statement—2018. Colorectal Dis. 2018 Jul;20(Suppl 3): 5–31. [PMID: 30178915]

Perianal Pruritus

Perianal pruritus is characterized by perianal itching and discomfort. It may be caused by poor anal hygiene associated with fistulas, fissures, prolapsed hemorrhoids, skin tags, and minor incontinence. Conversely, overzealous cleansing with soaps may contribute to local irritation or contact dermatitis. Contact dermatitis, atopic dermatitis, bacterial infections (*Staphylococcus* or *Streptococcus*), parasites (pinworms, scabies), candidal infection (especially in diabetics), sexually transmitted disease (condylomata acuminata, herpes, syphilis, molluscum contagiosum), and other skin conditions (psoriasis, Paget disease, lichen sclerosis) must be excluded. In patients with idiopathic perianal pruritus, examination may reveal erythema, excoriations, or lichenified, eczematous skin. Education is vital to successful therapy. Spicy foods, coffee, chocolate, and tomatoes may cause irritation and should be eliminated. After bowel movements, the perianal area should be cleansed with nonscented wipes premoistened with lanolin followed by gentle drying. A piece of cotton ball should be tucked next to the anal opening to absorb perspiration or fecal seepage. Anal ointments and lotions may exacerbate the condition and should be avoided. A short course of high-potency topical corticosteroid may be tried, although efficacy has not been demonstrated. Diluted capsaicin cream (0.006%) led to symptomatic relief in 75% of patients in a double-blind crossover study.

Ansari P. Pruritus ani. Clin Colon Rectal Surg. 2016 Mar;29(1): 38–42. [PMID: 26929750]

Davies D et al. Diagnosis and management of anorectal disorders in the primary care setting. Prim Care. 2017 Dec;44(4):709–20. [PMID: 29132530]

Parés D et al. Management of common benign anorectal disease: what all physicians need to know. Am J Med. 2018 Jul; 131(7):745–51. [PMID: 29499172]

Liver, Biliary Tract, & Pancreas Disorders

Lawrence S. Friedman, MD

JAUNDICE & EVALUATION OF ABNORMAL LIVER BIOCHEMICAL TESTS

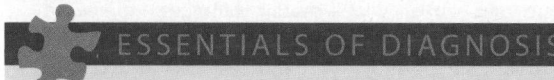

ESSENTIALS OF DIAGNOSIS

► Jaundice results from accumulation of bilirubin in body tissues; the cause may be hepatic or nonhepatic.

► Hyperbilirubinemia may be due to abnormalities in the formation, transport, metabolism, or excretion of bilirubin.

► Persistent mild elevations of the aminotransferase levels are common in clinical practice and caused most often by nonalcoholic fatty liver disease.

► Evaluation of obstructive jaundice begins with ultrasonography and is usually followed by cholangiography.

► General Considerations

Jaundice (icterus) results from the accumulation of bilirubin—a product of heme metabolism—in body tissues. Hyperbilirubinemia may be due to abnormalities in the formation, transport, metabolism, or excretion of bilirubin. Total serum bilirubin is normally 0.2–1.2 mg/dL (3.42–20.52 mcmol/L). Mean levels are higher in men than women, higher in whites and Hispanics than blacks, and correlate with an increased risk of symptomatic gallstone disease and inversely with the risk of stroke, respiratory disease, cardiovascular disease, and mortality, presumably because of an antioxidant effect. Jaundice may not be recognizable until serum bilirubin levels are about 3 mg/dL (51.3 mcmol/L).

Jaundice may be caused by predominantly unconjugated or conjugated bilirubin in the serum (Table 16–1). Unconjugated hyperbilirubinemia may result from overproduction of bilirubin because of hemolysis; impaired hepatic uptake of bilirubin due to certain drugs; or impaired conjugation of bilirubin by glucuronide, as in Gilbert

syndrome, due to mild decreases in uridine diphosphate (UDP) glucuronyl transferase, or Crigler-Najjar syndrome, caused by moderate decreases (type II) or absence (type I) of UDP glucuronyl transferase. Hemolysis alone rarely elevates the serum bilirubin level to more than 7 mg/dL (119.7 mcmol/L). Predominantly conjugated hyperbilirubinemia may result from impaired excretion of bilirubin from the liver due to hepatocellular disease, drugs, sepsis, or hereditary hepatocanalicular transport defects (such as Dubin-Johnson syndrome, progressive familial intrahepatic cholestasis syndromes, and intrahepatic cholestasis of pregnancy) or from extrahepatic biliary obstruction. Features of some hyperbilirubinemic syndromes are summarized in Table 16–2. The term "cholestasis" denotes retention of bile in the liver, and the term "cholestatic jaundice" is often used when conjugated hyperbilirubinemia results from impaired bile flow. Mediators of pruritus due to cholestasis have been identified to be lysophosphatidic acid and autotaxin, the enzyme that forms lysophosphatidic acid.

► Clinical Findings

A. Unconjugated Hyperbilirubinemia

Stool and urine color are normal, and there is mild jaundice and indirect (unconjugated) hyperbilirubinemia with no bilirubin in the urine. Splenomegaly occurs in all hemolytic disorders except in sickle cell disease.

B. Conjugated Hyperbilirubinemia

1. Hereditary cholestatic syndromes or intrahepatic cholestasis—The patient may be asymptomatic; cholestasis is often accompanied by pruritus, light-colored stools, and jaundice.

2. Hepatocellular disease—Malaise, anorexia, low-grade fever, and right upper quadrant discomfort are frequent. Dark urine, jaundice, and, in women, amenorrhea occur. An enlarged tender liver, spider telangiectasias, palmar erythema, ascites, gynecomastia, sparse body hair, fetor hepaticus, and asterixis may be present, depending on the cause, severity, and chronicity of liver dysfunction.

Table 16–1. Classification of jaundice.

Type of Hyperbilirubinemia	Location and Cause
Unconjugated hyperbilirubinemia (predominantly indirect bilirubin)	Increased bilirubin production (eg, hemolytic anemias, hemolytic reactions, hematoma, pulmonary infarction) Impaired bilirubin uptake and storage (eg, posthepatitis hyperbilirubinemia, Gilbert syndrome, Crigler-Najjar syndrome, drug reactions)
Conjugated hyperbilirubinemia (predominantly direct bilirubin)	**Hereditary Cholestatic Syndromes** (see also Table 16–2)
	Faulty excretion of bilirubin conjugates (eg, Dubin-Johnson syndrome, Rotor syndrome) or mutation in genes coding for bile salt transport proteins (eg, progressive familial intrahepatic cholestasis syndromes, benign recurrent intrahepatic cholestasis, and some cases of intrahepatic cholestasis of pregnancy)
	Hepatocellular Dysfunction
	Biliary epithelial and hepatocyte damage (eg, hepatitis, hepatic cirrhosis) Intrahepatic cholestasis (eg, certain drugs, biliary cirrhosis, sepsis, postoperative jaundice) Hepatocellular damage or intrahepatic cholestasis resulting from miscellaneous causes (eg, spirochetal infections, infectious mononucleosis, cholangitis, sarcoidosis, lymphomas, hyperthyroidism, industrial toxins)
	Biliary Obstruction
	Choledocholithiasis, biliary atresia, carcinoma of biliary duct, sclerosing cholangitis, IgG$_4$-related cholangitis, ischemic cholangiopathy, choledochal cyst, external pressure on bile duct, pancreatitis, pancreatic neoplasms

Ig, immunoglobulin.

C. Biliary Obstruction

There may be right upper quadrant pain, weight loss (suggesting carcinoma), jaundice, pruritus, dark urine, and light-colored stools. Symptoms and signs may be intermittent if caused by a stone, carcinoma of the ampulla, or cholangiocarcinoma. Pain may be absent early in pancreatic cancer. Occult blood in the stools suggests cancer of the ampulla. A palpable gallbladder (Courvoisier sign) is characteristic, but neither specific nor sensitive, of a pancreatic head tumor. Fever and chills are more common in benign obstruction with associated cholangitis.

▶ Diagnostic Studies

(See Tables 16–3 and 16–4.)

A. Laboratory Findings

Elevated serum alanine and aspartate aminotransferase (ALT and AST) levels reflect hepatocellular injury. Normal reference values for ALT and AST are lower than generally reported when persons with risk factors for fatty liver are excluded. The upper limit of normal for ALT is 29–33 units/L in men and 19–25 units/L in women. Levels decrease with age and correlate with body mass index and mortality from liver disease and inversely with caffeine consumption and physical activity. There is controversy about whether an elevated ALT level is associated with a low or high vitamin D level and with mortality from coronary artery disease, cancer, diabetes mellitus, and all causes. Truncal fat and early-onset paternal obesity are risk factors for increased ALT levels. Levels are mildly elevated in more than 25% of persons with untreated celiac disease and in type 1 diabetic patients with so-called glycogenic

hepatopathy and often rise transiently in healthy persons who begin taking 4 g of acetaminophen per day or experience rapid weight gain on a fast-food diet. Levels may rise strikingly but transiently in patients with acute biliary obstruction from choledocholithiasis. Nonalcoholic fatty liver disease is by far the most common cause of persistent mildly to moderately elevated aminotransferase levels. Elevated ALT and AST levels, often greater than 1000 units/L (20 mckat/L), are the hallmark of hepatocellular necrosis or inflammation. Elevated alkaline phosphatase levels are seen in cholestasis or infiltrative liver disease (such as tumor, granulomatous disease, or amyloidosis). Isolated alkaline phosphatase elevations of hepatic rather than bone, intestinal, or placental origin are confirmed by concomitant elevation of gamma-glutamyl transpeptidase or 5′-nucleotidase levels. Serum gamma-glutamyl transpeptidase levels appear to correlate with the risk of mortality and disability in the general population. The differential diagnosis of any liver test elevation always includes toxicity caused by drugs, herbal and dietary supplements, and toxins.

B. Imaging

Demonstration of dilated bile ducts by ultrasonography or CT indicates biliary obstruction (90–95% sensitivity). Ultrasonography, CT, and MRI may also demonstrate hepatomegaly, intrahepatic tumors, and portal hypertension. Use of color Doppler ultrasonography or contrast agents that produce microbubbles increases the sensitivity of transcutaneous ultrasonography for detecting small neoplasms. MRI is the most accurate technique for identifying isolated liver lesions such as hemangiomas, focal nodular hyperplasia, or focal fatty infiltration and for

Table 16–2. Hyperbilirubinemic disorders.

	Nature of Defect	Type of Hyperbilirubinemia	Clinical and Pathologic Characteristics
Gilbert syndrome[1]	Reduced activity of uridine diphosphate glucuronyl transferase	Unconjugated (indirect) bilirubin	Benign, asymptomatic hereditary jaundice. Hyperbilirubinemia increased by 24- to 36-hour fast. No treatment required. Associated with reduced mortality from cardiovascular disease.
Dubin-Johnson syndrome[2]	Reduced excretory function of hepatocytes	Conjugated (direct) bilirubin	Benign, asymptomatic hereditary jaundice. Gallbladder does not visualize on oral cholecystography. Liver darkly pigmented on gross examination. Biopsy shows centrilobular brown pigment. Prognosis excellent.
Rotor syndrome[3]	Reduced hepatic reuptake of bilirubin conjugates	Conjugated (direct) bilirubin	Similar to Dubin-Johnson syndrome, but liver is not pigmented and the gallbladder is visualized on oral cholecystography. Prognosis excellent.
Recurrent or progressive intrahepatic cholestasis[4]	Cholestasis, often on a familial basis	Predominantly conjugated (direct) bilirubin	Episodic attacks of or progressive jaundice, itching, and malaise. Onset in early life and may persist for a lifetime. Alkaline phosphatase increased. Cholestasis found on liver biopsy. (Biopsy may be normal during remission.) Prognosis is generally excellent for "benign" recurrent intrahepatic cholestasis but may not be for familial forms.
Intrahepatic cholestasis of pregnancy[5]	Cholestasis	Predominantly conjugated (direct) bilirubin	Benign cholestatic jaundice, usually occurring in the third trimester of pregnancy. Itching, gastrointestinal symptoms, and abnormal liver excretory function tests. Cholestasis noted on liver biopsy. Prognosis excellent, but recurrence with subsequent pregnancies or use of oral contraceptives is characteristic.

[1]Gilbert syndrome generally results from the addition of extra dinucleotide(s) TA sequences to the TATA promoter of the conjugating enzyme *UGT1A1*.
[2]Dubin-Johnson syndrome is caused by a mutation in the *ABCC2* gene coding for organic anion transporter multidrug resistance protein 2 in bile canaliculi on chromosome 10q24.
[3]Rotor syndrome is caused by mutations in the genes coding for organic anion transporting polypeptides OATP1B1 and OATP1B3 on chromosome 12p.
[4]Mutations in genes that control hepatocellular transport systems that are involved in the formation of bile and inherited as autosomal recessive traits are on chromosomes 18q21–22, 2q24, 7q21, and others in families with progressive familial intrahepatic cholestasis. Gene mutations on chromosome 18q21–22 alter a P-type ATPase expressed in the small intestine and liver and other tissues on chromosome 2q24 alter the bile acid export pump and also cause benign recurrent intrahepatic cholestasis. Less common causes of progressive familial intrahepatic cholestasis are mutations in genes that encode TJP2, FXR, and MYO5B.
[5]Mutations in genes (especially *ABCB4* and *ABCB11*) that encode biliary canalicular transporters account for many cases of intrahepatic cholestasis of pregnancy.

Table 16–3. Liver biochemical tests: normal values and changes in hepatocellular and obstructive jaundice.

Tests	Normal Values	Hepatocellular Jaundice	Obstructive Jaundice

Bilirubin[1]
  Direct
  Indirect
	
	0.1–0.3 mg/dL (1.71–5.13 mcmol/L)
	0.2–0.7 mg/dL (3.42–11.97 mcmol/L)
		
		Increased
		Increased
			
			Increased
			Increased

Urine bilirubin	None	Increased	Increased
Serum albumin	3.5–5.5 g/dL (35–55 g/L)	Decreased	Generally unchanged
Alkaline phosphatase	30–115 units/L (0.6–2.3 mkat/L)	Mildly increased (+)	Markedly increased (++++)
Prothrombin time	INR of 1.0–1.4. After vitamin K, 10% decrease in 24 hours	Prolonged if damage is severe; does not respond to parenteral vitamin K	Prolonged if obstruction is marked; generally responds to parenteral vitamin K
ALT, AST	ALT, ≤ 30 units/L (0.6 mkat/L) (men), ≤ 19 units/L (0.38 mkat/L) (women); AST, 5–40 units/L (0.1–0.8 mkat/L)	Increased, as in viral hepatitis	Minimally increased

[1]Measured by the van den Bergh reaction, which overestimates direct bilirubin in normal persons.
ALT, alanine aminotransferase; AST, aspartate aminotransferase; INR, international normalized ratio.

Table 16–4. Causes of serum aminotransferase elevations.[1]

Mild Elevations (< 5 × normal)	Severe Elevations (> 15 × normal)
Hepatic: ALT-predominant Chronic hepatitis B, C, and D Acute viral hepatitis (A–E, EBV, CMV) Steatosis/steatohepatitis Hemochromatosis Medications/toxins Autoimmune hepatitis Alpha-1-antitrypsin (alpha-1-antiprotease) deficiency Wilson disease Celiac disease Glycogenic hepatopathy **Hepatic: AST-predominant** Alcohol-related liver injury (AST:ALT > 2:1) Cirrhosis **Nonhepatic** Strenuous exercise Hemolysis Myopathy Thyroid disease Macro-AST	Acute viral hepatitis (A–E, herpes) Medications/toxins Ischemic hepatitis Autoimmune hepatitis Wilson disease Acute bile duct obstruction Acute Budd-Chiari syndrome Hepatic artery ligation

[1]Almost any liver disease can cause moderate aminotransferase elevations (5–15 × normal).

ALT, alanine aminotransferase; AST, aspartate aminotransferase; CMV, cytomegalovirus; EBV, Epstein-Barr virus.

Adapted, with permission, from Green RM et al. AGA technical review on the evaluation of liver chemistry tests. Gastroenterology. 2002 Oct;123(4):1367–84. Copyright © Elsevier.

detecting hepatic iron overload. The most sensitive techniques for detection of individual small hepatic metastases in patients eligible for resection are multiphasic helical or multislice CT; CT arterial portography, in which imaging follows intravenous contrast infusion via a catheter placed in the superior mesenteric artery; MRI with use of gadolinium or ferumoxides as contrast agents; and intraoperative ultrasonography. Dynamic gadolinium-enhanced MRI and MRI following administration of superparamagnetic iron oxide show promise in visualizing hepatic fibrosis. Because of its much lower cost, ultrasonography is preferable to CT (~six times more expensive) or MRI (~seven times more expensive) as a screening test. Positron emission tomography (PET) can be used to detect small pancreatic tumors and metastases. Ultrasonography can detect gallstones with a sensitivity of 95%.

Magnetic resonance cholangiopancreatography (MRCP) is a sensitive, noninvasive method of detecting bile duct stones, strictures, and dilatation; however, it is less reliable than endoscopic retrograde cholangiopancreatography (ERCP) for distinguishing malignant from benign strictures. ERCP requires a skilled endoscopist and may be used to demonstrate pancreatic or ampullary causes of jaundice, carry out sphincterotomy and stone extraction, insert a stent through an obstructing lesion, or facilitate

direct cholangiopancreatoscopy. Complications of ERCP include pancreatitis (5% or less) and, less commonly, cholangitis, bleeding, or duodenal perforation after sphincterotomy. Risk factors for post-ERCP pancreatitis include female sex, pregnancy, prior post-ERCP pancreatitis, suspected sphincter of Oddi dysfunction, and a difficult or failed cannulation. Percutaneous transhepatic cholangiography (PTC) is an alternative approach to evaluating the anatomy of the biliary tract. Serious complications of PTC occur in 3% and include fever, bacteremia, bile peritonitis, and intraperitoneal hemorrhage. Endoscopic ultrasonography (EUS) is the most sensitive test for detecting small lesions of the ampulla or pancreatic head and for detecting portal vein invasion by pancreatic cancer. It is also accurate for detecting or excluding bile duct stones.

C. Liver Biopsy

Percutaneous liver biopsy is considered the definitive study for determining the cause and histologic severity of hepatocellular dysfunction or infiltrative liver disease, although it is subject to sampling error and subjective interpretation. It is generally performed under ultrasound or, in some patients with suspected metastatic disease or a hepatic mass, CT guidance. A transjugular route can be used in patients with coagulopathy or ascites. The risk of bleeding after a percutaneous liver biopsy is approximately 0.6% and is increased in persons with a platelet count of 60,000/mcL (60×10^9/mcL) or less. The risk of death is up to 0.1%. Panels of blood tests (eg, FibroSure, nonalcoholic fatty liver disease [NAFLD] fibrosis score, enhanced liver fibrosis score) and elastography (vibration-controlled transient, shear wave, acoustic radiation force impulse, or magnetic resonance elastography) to measure liver stiffness are used for estimating the stage of liver fibrosis and degree of portal hypertension without the need for liver biopsy; they are most accurate for excluding advanced fibrosis.

▶ When to Refer

Patients with jaundice should be referred for diagnostic procedures.

▶ When to Admit

Patients with liver failure should be hospitalized.

Kwo PY et al. ACG Clinical Guideline: evaluation of abnormal liver chemistries. Am J Gastroenterol. 2017 Jan;112(1):18–35. [PMID: 27995906]

Lim JK et al. American Gastroenterological Association Institute guideline on the role of elastography in the evaluation of liver fibrosis. Gastroenterology. 2017 May;152(6):1536–43. [PMID: 28442119]

Newsome PN et al. Guidelines on the management of abnormal liver blood tests. Gut. 2018 Jan;67(1):6–19. [PMID: 29122851]

Tapper EB et al. Noninvasive imaging biomarker assessment of liver fibrosis by elastography in NAFLD. Nat Rev Gastroenterol Hepatol. 2018 May;15(5):274–82. [PMID: 29463906]

Tapper EB et al. Use of liver imaging and biopsy in clinical practice. N Engl J Med. 2017 Aug 24;377(8):756–68. [PMID: 28834467]

DISEASES OF THE LIVER

See Chapter 39 for Hepatocellular Carcinoma.

ACUTE HEPATITIS A

ESSENTIALS OF DIAGNOSIS

► Prodrome of anorexia, nausea, vomiting, malaise, aversion to smoking.

► Fever, enlarged and tender liver, jaundice.

► Normal to low white cell count; markedly elevated aminotransferases.

General Considerations

Hepatitis can be caused by viruses, including the five hepatotropic viruses—A, B, C, D, and E—and many drugs and toxic agents; the clinical manifestations may be similar regardless of cause. Hepatitis A virus (HAV) is a 27-nm RNA hepatovirus (in the picornavirus family) that causes epidemics or sporadic cases of hepatitis. HAV infection is hyperendemic in developing countries. Globally, 15 million people are infected with HAV annually. The virus is transmitted by the fecal-oral route by either person-to-person contact or ingestion of contaminated food or water, and its spread is favored by crowding and poor sanitation. Since introduction of the HAV vaccine in the United States in 1995, the incidence rate of HAV infection has declined from as much as 14 to 0.4 per 100,000 population, with a corresponding decline in the mortality rate from 0.1 to 0.02 death per 100,000 population and an increase in the mean age of infection and death. Common source outbreaks resulting from contaminated water or food, including inadequately cooked shellfish, continue to occur. In 2017, an outbreak in California and four other states affected a large number of homeless persons and resulted in many deaths. In addition, HAV infection has reemerged as a food-borne public health threat in Europe. Outbreaks among people who inject drugs or who are unvaccinated residents in institutions and cases among international adoptees and their contacts also occur. In the United States, international travel emerged as an important risk factor, accounting for over 40% of cases in the early 2000s.

The incubation period averages 30 days. HAV is excreted in feces for up to 2 weeks before clinical illness but rarely after the first week of illness. The mortality rate for hepatitis A is low, and acute liver failure due to hepatitis A is uncommon except for rare instances in which it occurs in a patient with concomitant chronic hepatitis C. There is no chronic carrier state. In the United States, about 30% of the population have serologic evidence of previous HAV infection.

Clinical Findings

A. Symptoms and Signs

Figure 16–1 shows the typical course of acute hepatitis A. Clinical illness is more severe in adults than in children, in

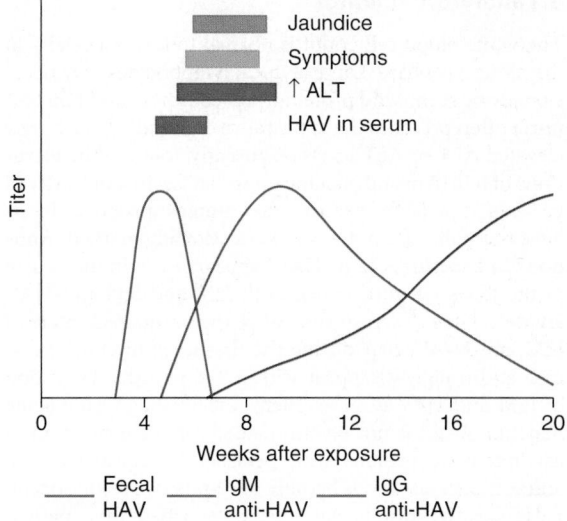

▲ **Figure 16–1.** The typical course of acute type A hepatitis. (HAV, hepatitis A virus; anti-HAV, antibody to hepatitis A virus; ALT, alanine aminotransferase.) (Reprinted, with permission, from Koff RS. Acute viral hepatitis. In: Friedman LS, Keeffe EB [editors]. *Handbook of Liver Disease*, 3rd ed. Philadelphia: Saunders Elsevier, 2012. Copyright © Elsevier.)

whom it is usually asymptomatic. The onset may be abrupt or insidious, with malaise, myalgia, arthralgia, easy fatigability, upper respiratory symptoms, and anorexia. A distaste for smoking, paralleling anorexia, may occur early. Nausea and vomiting are frequent, and diarrhea or constipation may occur. Fever is generally present but is low-grade except in occasional cases in which systemic toxicity may occur. Defervescence and a fall in pulse rate often coincide with the onset of jaundice.

Abdominal pain is usually mild and constant in the right upper quadrant or epigastrium, often aggravated by jarring or exertion, and rarely may be severe enough to simulate cholecystitis. Jaundice occurs after 5–10 days but may appear at the same time as the initial symptoms. In many patients, jaundice never develops. With the onset of jaundice, prodromal symptoms often worsen, followed by progressive clinical improvement. Stools may be acholic during this phase. Hepatomegaly—rarely marked—is present in over half of cases. Liver tenderness is usually present. Splenomegaly is reported in 15% of patients, and soft, enlarged lymph nodes—especially in the cervical or epitrochlear areas—may be noted.

The acute illness usually subsides over 2–3 weeks with complete clinical and laboratory recovery by 9 weeks. In some cases, clinical, biochemical, and serologic recovery may be followed by one or two relapses, but recovery is the rule. Acute cholecystitis occasionally complicates the course of acute hepatitis A. Other occasional extrahepatic complications include acute kidney injury, arthritis, vasculitis, acute pancreatitis, aplastic anemia, and a variety of neurologic manifestations.

B. Laboratory Findings

The white blood cell count is normal to low, especially in the preicteric phase. Large atypical lymphocytes may occasionally be seen. Mild proteinuria is common, and bilirubinuria often precedes the appearance of jaundice. Strikingly elevated ALT or AST levels occur early, followed by elevations of bilirubin and alkaline phosphatase; in a minority of patients, the latter persist after aminotransferase levels have normalized. Cholestasis is occasionally marked. Antibody to hepatitis A (anti-HAV) appears early in the course of the illness (Figure 16–1). Both IgM and IgG anti-HAV are detectable in serum soon after the onset. Peak titers of IgM anti-HAV occur during the first week of clinical disease and usually disappear within 3–6 months. Detection of IgM anti-HAV is an excellent test for diagnosing acute hepatitis A but is not recommended for the evaluation of asymptomatic persons with persistently elevated serum aminotransferase levels because false-positive results occur. False-negative results have been described in a patient receiving rituximab for rheumatoid arthritis. Titers of IgG anti-HAV rise after 1 month of the disease and may persist for years. IgG anti-HAV (in the absence of IgM anti-HAV) indicates previous exposure to HAV, noninfectivity, and immunity.

Differential Diagnosis

The differential diagnosis includes other viruses that cause hepatitis, particularly hepatitis B and C, and diseases such as infectious mononucleosis, cytomegalovirus infection, herpes simplex virus infection, Middle East respiratory syndrome, and infections caused by many other viruses, including influenza and Ebola virus; spirochetal diseases such as leptospirosis and secondary syphilis; brucellosis; rickettsial diseases such as Q fever; drug-induced liver injury; and ischemic hepatitis (shock liver). Occasionally, autoimmune hepatitis may have an acute onset mimicking acute viral hepatitis. Rarely, metastatic cancer of the liver, lymphoma, or leukemia may present as a hepatitis-like picture.

The prodromal phase of viral hepatitis must be distinguished from other infectious disease such as influenza, upper respiratory infections, and the prodromal stages of the exanthematous diseases. Cholestasis may mimic obstructive jaundice.

Prevention

Strict isolation of patients is not necessary, but hand washing after bowel movements is required. Unvaccinated persons who are exposed to HAV are advised to receive postexposure prophylaxis with a single dose of HAV vaccine or immune globulin (0.02 mL/kg) as soon as possible. The vaccine is preferred in healthy persons aged 1 year to 40 years, whereas immune globulin is preferred in those who are younger than 1 year or older than 40 years, are immunocompromised, or have chronic liver disease.

Vaccination with one of two effective inactivated hepatitis A vaccines available in the United States provides long-term immunity and is recommended for persons living in or traveling to endemic areas (including military personnel), patients with chronic liver disease upon diagnosis after prescreening for immunity (although the cost-effectiveness of vaccinating all patients with concomitant chronic hepatitis C has been questioned), persons with clotting-factor disorders who are treated with concentrates, men who have sex with men, animal handlers, illicit drug users, sewage workers, food handlers, close personal contacts of international adoptees, and children and caregivers in day-care centers and institutions. For healthy travelers, a single dose of vaccine at any time before departure can provide adequate protection. Routine vaccination is advised for all children in states with an incidence of hepatitis A at least twice the national average and has been approved by the Advisory Committee on Immunization Practices of the Centers for Disease Control and Prevention (CDC) for use in all children between ages 1 and 2 in the United States. HAV vaccine is also effective in the prevention of secondary spread to household contacts of primary cases. The recommended dose for adults is 1 mL (1440 ELISA units) of Havrix (GlaxoSmithKline) or 1 mL (50 units) of Vaqta (Merck) intramuscularly, followed by a booster dose at 6–18 months. A combined hepatitis A and B vaccine (Twinrix, GlaxoSmithKline) is available. HIV infection impairs the response to the HAV vaccine, especially in persons with a CD4 count less than 200/mcL.

Treatment

Bed rest is recommended only if symptoms are marked. If nausea and vomiting are pronounced or if oral intake is substantially decreased, intravenous 10% glucose is indicated.

Dietary management consists of palatable meals as tolerated, without overfeeding; breakfast is usually tolerated best. Strenuous physical exertion, alcohol, and hepatotoxic agents should be avoided. Small doses of oxazepam are safe because metabolism is not hepatic; morphine sulfate should be avoided.

Corticosteroids have no benefit in patients with viral hepatitis, including those with acute liver failure.

Prognosis

In most patients, clinical recovery is generally complete within 3 months. Laboratory evidence of liver dysfunction may persist for a longer period, but most patients recover completely. Hepatitis A does not cause chronic liver disease, although it may persist for up to 1 year, and clinical and biochemical relapses may occur before full recovery. The mortality rate is less than 1.0%, with a higher rate in older adults than in younger persons.

When to Admit

- Encephalopathy is present.
- International normalized ratio (INR) greater than 1.6.
- The patient is unable to maintain hydration.

Centers for Disease Control and Prevention (CDC). 2017—Outbreaks of hepatitis A in multiple states among people who are homeless and people who use drugs. https://www.cdc.gov/hepatitis/outbreaks/2017March-hepatitisA.htm

Lemon SM et al. Type A viral hepatitis: a summary and update on the molecular virology, epidemiology, pathogenesis and prevention. J Hepatol. 2018 Jan;68(1):167–84. [PMID: 28887164]

Linder KA et al. JAMA patient page. Hepatitis A. JAMA. 2017 Dec 19;318(23):2393. [PMID: 29094153]

ACUTE HEPATITIS B

ESSENTIALS OF DIAGNOSIS

▶ Prodrome of anorexia, nausea, vomiting, malaise, aversion to smoking.

▶ Fever, enlarged and tender liver, jaundice.

▶ Normal to low white blood cell count; markedly elevated aminotransferases early in the course.

▶ Liver biopsy shows hepatocellular necrosis and mononuclear infiltrate but is rarely indicated.

General Considerations

Hepatitis B virus (HBV) is a 42-nm hepadnavirus with a partially double-stranded DNA genome, inner core protein (hepatitis B core antigen, HBcAg), and outer surface coat (hepatitis B surface antigen, HBsAg). There are 10 different genotypes (A–J), which may influence the course of infection and responsiveness to antiviral therapy. HBV is usually transmitted by inoculation of infected blood or blood products or by sexual contact and is present in saliva, semen, and vaginal secretions. HBsAg-positive mothers may transmit HBV at delivery; the risk of chronic infection in the infant is as high as 90%.

Since 1990, the incidence of HBV infection in the United States has decreased from 8.5 to 1.5 cases per 100,000 population. The prevalence is 0.27% in persons aged 6 or older. Because of universal vaccination since 1992, exposure to HBV is now very low among persons aged 18 or younger. HBV is prevalent in men who have sex with men and in people who inject drugs (about 7% of HIV-infected persons are coinfected with HBV), but the greatest number of cases result from heterosexual transmission. Other groups at risk include patients and staff at hemodialysis centers, physicians, dentists, nurses, and personnel working in clinical and pathology laboratories and blood banks. Half of all patients with acute hepatitis B in the United States have previously been incarcerated or treated for a sexually transmitted disease. The risk of HBV infection from a blood transfusion in the United States is no higher than 1 in 350,000 units transfused. Screening for HBV infection is recommended for high-risk groups by the US Preventive Services Task Force.

The incubation period of hepatitis B is 6 weeks to 6 months (average 12–14 weeks). The onset of hepatitis B is more insidious, and the aminotransferase levels are higher on average than in HAV infection. Acute liver failure occurs in less than 1%, with a mortality rate of up to 60%. Following acute hepatitis B, HBV infection persists in

1–2% of immunocompetent adults, but in a higher percentage of children and immunocompromised adults. There are as many as 2.2 million persons (including an estimated 1.32 million foreign-born persons from endemic areas) with chronic hepatitis B in the United States and 248 million worldwide. Compared with the general population, the prevalence of chronic HBV infection is increased 2- to 3-fold in non-Hispanic blacks and 10-fold in Asians. Persons with chronic hepatitis B, particularly when HBV infection is acquired early in life and viral replication persists, are at substantial risk for cirrhosis and hepatocellular carcinoma (up to 25–40%); men are at greater risk than women.

▶ Clinical Findings

A. Symptoms and Signs

The clinical picture of viral hepatitis is extremely variable, ranging from asymptomatic infection without jaundice to acute liver failure and death in a few days to weeks. Figure 16–2 shows the typical course of acute HBV infection. The onset may be abrupt or insidious, and the clinical features are similar to those for acute hepatitis A. Serum sickness may be seen early in acute hepatitis B. Fever is generally present and is low-grade. Defervescence and a fall in pulse rate often coincide with the onset of jaundice. Infection caused by HBV may be associated with glomerulonephritis and polyarteritis nodosa.

The acute illness usually subsides over 2–3 weeks with complete clinical and laboratory recovery by 16 weeks. In 5–10% of cases, the course may be more protracted, but less than 1% will develop acute liver failure. Hepatitis B may become chronic.

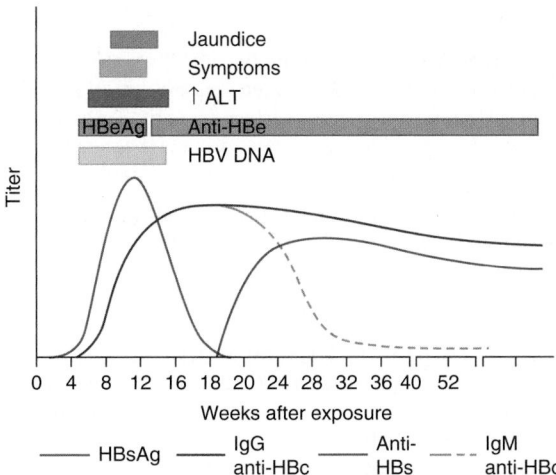

▲ **Figure 16–2.** The typical course of acute type B hepatitis. (anti-HBs, antibody to HBsAg; HBeAg, hepatitis Be antigen; HBsAg, hepatitis B surface antigen; anti-HBe, antibody to HBeAg; anti-HBc, antibody to hepatitis B core antigen; ALT, alanine aminotransferase.) (Reprinted, with permission, from Koff RS. Acute viral hepatitis. In: Friedman LS, Keeffe EB [editors]. *Handbook of Liver Disease*, 3rd ed. Philadelphia: Saunders Elsevier, 2012. Copyright © Elsevier.)

Table 16–5. Common serologic patterns in hepatitis B virus (HBV) infection and their interpretation.

HBsAg	Anti-HBs	Anti-HBc	HBeAg	Anti-HBe	Interpretation
+	–	IgM	+	–	Acute hepatitis B
+	–	IgG[1]	+	–	Chronic hepatitis B with active viral replication
+	–	IgG	–	+	Inactive HBV carrier state (low HBV DNA level) or HBeAg-negative chronic hepatitis B with active viral replication (high HBV DNA level)
+	+	IgG	+ or –	+ or –	Chronic hepatitis B with heterotypic anti-HBs (about 10% of cases)
–	–	IgM	+ or –	–	Acute hepatitis B
–	+	IgG	–	+ or –	Recovery from hepatitis B (immunity)
–	+	–	–	–	Vaccination (immunity)
–	–	IgG	–	–	False-positive; less commonly, infection in remote past

[1]Low levels of IgM anti-HBc may also be detected.

B. Laboratory Findings

The laboratory features are similar to those for acute hepatitis A, although serum aminotransferase levels are higher on average in acute hepatitis B, and marked cholestasis is not a feature. Marked prolongation of the prothrombin time in severe hepatitis correlates with increased mortality.

There are several antigens and antibodies as well as HBV DNA that relate to HBV infection and that are useful in diagnosis. Interpretation of common serologic patterns is shown in Table 16–5.

1. HBsAg—The appearance of HBsAg in serum is the first evidence of infection, appearing before biochemical evidence of liver disease, and persisting throughout the clinical illness. Persistence of HBsAg more than 6 months after the acute illness signifies chronic hepatitis B.

2. Anti-HBs—Specific antibody to HBsAg (anti-HBs) appears in most individuals after clearance of HBsAg and after successful vaccination against hepatitis B. Disappearance of HBsAg and the appearance of anti-HBs signal recovery from HBV infection, noninfectivity, and immunity.

3. Anti-HBc—IgM anti-HBc appears shortly after HBsAg is detected. In the setting of acute hepatitis, IgM anti-HBc indicates a diagnosis of acute hepatitis B, and it fills the serologic gap in rare patients who have cleared HBsAg but do not yet have detectable anti-HBs. IgM anti-HBc can persist for 3–6 months, and sometimes longer. IgM anti-HBc may also reappear during flares of previously inactive chronic hepatitis B. IgG anti-HBc also appears during acute hepatitis B but persists indefinitely, whether the patient recovers (with the appearance of anti-HBs in serum) or chronic hepatitis B develops (with persistence of HBsAg). In asymptomatic blood donors, an isolated anti-HBc with no other positive HBV serologic results may represent a falsely positive result or latent infection in which HBV DNA is detectable in serum only by polymerase chain reaction (PCR) testing.

4. HBeAg—HBeAg is a secretory form of HBcAg that appears in serum during the incubation period shortly after the detection of HBsAg. HBeAg indicates viral replication and infectivity. Persistence of HBeAg beyond 3 months indicates an increased likelihood of chronic hepatitis B. Its disappearance is often followed by the appearance of anti-HBe, generally signifying diminished viral replication and decreased infectivity.

5. HBV DNA—The presence of HBV DNA in serum generally parallels the presence of HBeAg, although HBV DNA is a more sensitive and precise marker of viral replication and infectivity. In some patients with chronic hepatitis B, HBV DNA is present at high levels without HBeAg in serum because of development of a mutation in the core promoter or precore region of the gene that codes HBcAg; these mutations prevent synthesis of HBeAg in infected hepatocytes. When additional mutations in the core gene are also present, the severity of HBV infection is enhanced and the risk of cirrhosis is increased.

▶ Differential Diagnosis

The differential diagnosis includes hepatitis A and the same disorders listed for the differential diagnosis of acute hepatitis A. In addition, coinfection with HDV must be considered.

▶ Prevention

Strict isolation of patients is not necessary. Thorough hand washing by medical staff who may contact contaminated utensils, bedding, or clothing is essential. Medical staff should handle disposable needles carefully and not recap them. Screening of donated blood for HBsAg, anti-HBc, and anti-HCV has reduced the risk of transfusion-associated hepatitis markedly. All pregnant women should undergo testing for HBsAg. HBV-infected persons should practice safe sex. Immunoprophylaxis of the neonate reduces the risk of perinatal transmission of HBV infection; when the mother's serum HBV DNA level is 200,000 international units/mL or higher (or the mother's serum HBsAg level is above 4–4.5 $\log_{10}$ international units/mL), antiviral treatment of the mother should also be initiated in the third trimester (see Chronic Hepatitis B & Chronic Hepatitis D). HBV-infected health care workers are not precluded from practicing medicine or dentistry if they follow CDC guidelines.

Hepatitis B immune globulin (HBIG) may be protective—or may attenuate the severity of illness—if given within 7 days after exposure (adult dose is 0.06 mL/kg body weight) followed by initiation of the HBV vaccine series. This approach is recommended for unvaccinated persons exposed to HBsAg-contaminated material via mucous membranes or through breaks in the skin and for individuals who have had sexual contact with a person with HBV infection (irrespective of the presence or absence of HBeAg in the source). HBIG is also indicated for newborn infants of HBsAg-positive mothers, with initiation of the vaccine series at the same time, both within 12 hours of birth (administered at different injection sites).

The CDC recommends HBV vaccination of all infants and children in the United States and all adults who are at risk for hepatitis B (including persons under age 60 with diabetes mellitus) or who request vaccination; the vaccine appears to be underutilized in adults for whom vaccination is recommended. Over 90% of recipients of the vaccine mount protective antibody to hepatitis B; immunocompromised persons, including patients receiving dialysis (especially those with diabetes mellitus), respond poorly (see Table 30–7). Reduced response to the vaccine may have a genetic basis in some cases and has also been associated with age over 40 years and celiac disease. The standard regimen for adults is 10–20 mcg (depending on the formulation) repeated again at 1 and 6 months, but alternative schedules have been approved, including accelerated schedules of 0, 1, 2, and 12 months and of 0, 7, and 21 days plus 12 months. For greatest reliability of absorption, the deltoid muscle is the preferred site of inoculation. Vaccine formulations free of the mercury-containing preservative thimerosal are given to infants under 6 months of age. A new vaccine, Heplisav-B, which uses a novel immune system–stimulating ingredient, was approved by the FDA for adults in 2017. Immunization requires only two injections, and Heplisav-B appears to be more effective than previous HBV vaccines. When documentation of seroconversion is considered desirable, postimmunization anti-HBs titers may be checked. Protection appears to be excellent even if the titer wanes—persisting for at least 20 years—and booster reimmunization is not routinely recommended but is advised for immunocompromised persons in whom anti-HBs titers fall below 10 milli-international units/mL. For vaccine nonresponders, three additional vaccine doses may elicit seroprotective anti-HBs levels in 30–50% of persons. Doubling of the standard dose may also be effective. Universal vaccination of neonates in countries endemic for HBV has reduced the incidence of hepatocellular carcinoma. Incomplete immunization is the most important predictor of liver disease among vaccinees.

Treatment

Treatment of acute hepatitis B is the same as that for acute hepatitis A. Encephalopathy or severe coagulopathy indicates acute liver failure, and hospitalization at a liver transplant center is mandatory. Antiviral therapy is generally unnecessary in patients with acute hepatitis B but is usually prescribed in cases of acute liver failure caused by HBV as well as in spontaneous reactivation of chronic hepatitis B presenting as acute-on-chronic liver failure (see Acute Liver Failure).

Prognosis

In most patients, clinical recovery is complete in 3–6 months. Laboratory evidence of liver dysfunction may persist for a longer period, but most patients recover completely. The mortality rate for acute hepatitis B is 0.1–1% but is higher with superimposed hepatitis D.

Chronic hepatitis, characterized by elevated aminotransferase levels for more than 3–6 months, develops in 1–2% of immunocompetent adults with acute hepatitis B, but in as many as 90% of infected neonates and infants and a substantial proportion of immunocompromised adults. Ultimately, cirrhosis develops in up to 40% of those with chronic hepatitis B; the risk of cirrhosis is even higher in HBV-infected patients coinfected with hepatitis C or HIV. Patients with cirrhosis are at risk for hepatocellular carcinoma at a rate of 3–5% per year. Even in the absence of cirrhosis, patients with chronic hepatitis B—particularly those with active viral replication—are at increased risk for hepatocellular carcinoma.

When to Refer

Refer patients with acute hepatitis who require liver biopsy for diagnosis.

When to Admit

- Encephalopathy is present.
- INR greater than 1.6.
- The patient is unable to maintain hydration.

Abara WE et al. Hepatitis B vaccination, screening, and linkage to care: best practice advice from the American College of Physicians and the Centers for Disease Control and Prevention. Ann Intern Med. 2017 Dec 5;167(11):794–804. [PMID: 29159414]

Anonymous. A two-dose hepatitis B vaccine for adults (Heplisav-B). Med Lett Drugs Ther. 2018 Jan 29;60(1539):17–8. [PMID: 29364196]

European Association for the Study of the Liver. EASL 2017 Clinical Practice Guidelines on the management of hepatitis B virus infection. J Hepatol. 2017 Aug;67(2):370–98. [PMID: 28427875]

Schillie S et al. Prevention of hepatitis B virus infection in the United States: recommendations of the Advisory Committee on Immunization Practices. MMWR Recomm Rep. 2018 Jan 12;67(1):1–31. [PMID: 29939980]

ACUTE HEPATITIS C & OTHER CAUSES OF ACUTE VIRAL HEPATITIS

Viruses other than HAV and HBV that can cause hepatitis are hepatitis C virus (HCV), hepatitis D virus (HDV) (delta agent), and hepatitis E virus (HEV) (an enterically transmitted hepatitis seen in epidemic form in Asia, the Middle East, and North Africa and sporadically in Western countries). Human pegivirus (formerly hepatitis G virus [HGV]) rarely, if ever, causes frank hepatitis. A related virus has been named human hepegivirus-1. A DNA virus designated the TT virus (TTV) has been identified in up to 7.5% of blood donors and found to be transmitted readily by blood transfusions, but an association between this virus and liver disease has not been established. A related virus known as SEN-V has been found in 2% of US blood donors, is transmitted by transfusion, and may account for some cases of transfusion-associated non-ABCDE hepatitis. In immunocompromised and rare immunocompetent persons, cytomegalovirus, Epstein-Barr virus, and herpes simplex virus should be considered in the differential diagnosis of hepatitis. Middle East respiratory syndrome (MERS), severe acute respiratory syndrome (SARS), Ebola virus infection, and influenza may be associated with marked serum aminotransferase elevations. Unidentified pathogens account for a small percentage of cases of acute viral hepatitis.

1. Hepatitis C

HCV is a single-stranded RNA virus (hepacivirus) with properties similar to those of flaviviruses. Seven major genotypes of HCV have been identified. In the past, HCV was responsible for over 90% of cases of posttransfusion hepatitis, yet only 4% of cases of hepatitis C were attributable to blood transfusions. Over 50% of cases are transmitted by injection drug use, and both reinfection and superinfection of HCV are common in people who actively inject drugs. Body piercing, tattoos, and hemodialysis are risk factors. The risk of sexual and maternal–neonatal transmission is low and may be greatest in a subset of patients with high circulating levels of HCV RNA. Having multiple sexual partners may increase the risk of HCV infection, and HIV coinfection, unprotected receptive anal intercourse with ejaculation, and sex while high on methamphetamine increase the risk of HCV transmission in men who have sex with men. Transmission via breastfeeding has not been documented. An outbreak of hepatitis C in patients with immune deficiencies has occurred in some recipients of intravenous immune globulin. Hospital- and outpatient facility–acquired transmission has occurred via multidose vials of saline used to flush Portacaths; through reuse of disposable syringes; through drug "diversion" and tampering with injectable opioids by an infected health care worker; through contamination of shared saline, radiopharmaceutical, and sclerosant vials; via inadequately disinfected endoscopy equipment; and between hospitalized patients on a liver unit. In the developing world, unsafe medical practices lead to a substantial number of cases of HCV infection. Covert transmission during bloody fisticuffs has even been reported, and incarceration in prison is a risk factor, with a frequency of 26% in the United States. In many patients, the source of infection is unknown. Coinfection with HCV is found in at least 30% of HIV-infected persons. HIV infection leads to an increased risk of acute liver failure and more rapid progression of chronic hepatitis C to cirrhosis; in addition, HCV increases the hepatotoxicity of antiretroviral therapy. The number of cases of chronic HCV infections in the United States is reported to have decreased from 3.2 million

in 2001 to 2.3 million in 2013, although estimates of at least 4.6 million exposed and 3.5 million currently infected have also been reported. The incidence of new cases of acute, symptomatic hepatitis C declined from 1992 to 2005, but an increase was observed in persons aged 15 to 24 after 2002, as a result of injection drug use. An increase has also been observed in women of reproductive age.

▶ Clinical Findings

A. Symptoms and Signs

Figure 16–3 shows the typical course of HCV infection. The incubation period for hepatitis C averages 6–7 weeks, and clinical illness is often mild, usually asymptomatic, and characterized by waxing and waning aminotransferase elevations and a high rate (greater than 80%) of chronic hepatitis. Spontaneous clearance of HCV following acute infection is more common (64%) in persons with the CC genotype of the *IFNL3* (*IL28B*) gene than in those with the CT or TT genotype (24% and 6%, respectively). In persons with the CC genotype, jaundice is more likely to develop during the course of acute hepatitis C. In pregnant patients with chronic hepatitis C, serum aminotransferase levels frequently normalize despite persistence of viremia, only to increase again after delivery.

B. Laboratory Findings

Diagnosis of hepatitis C is based on an enzyme immunoassay (EIA) that detects antibodies to HCV. Anti-HCV is not protective, and in patients with acute or chronic hepatitis, its presence in serum generally signifies that HCV is the cause. Limitations of the EIA include moderate sensitivity (false-negatives) for the diagnosis of acute hepatitis C early in the course and low specificity (false-positives) in some persons with elevated gamma-globulin levels. In these situations, a diagnosis of hepatitis C may be confirmed by using

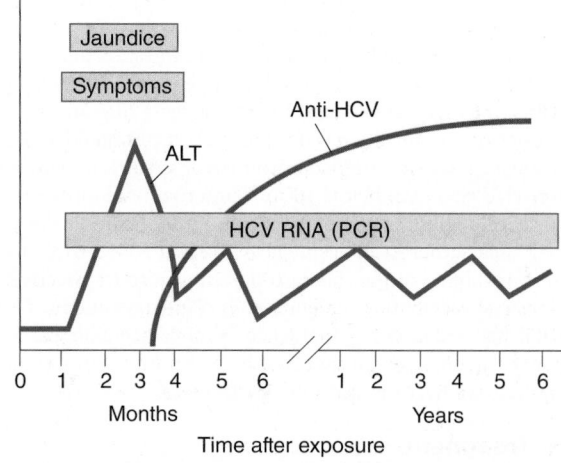

▲ **Figure 16–3.** The typical course of acute and chronic hepatitis C. (ALT, alanine aminotransferase; Anti-HCV, antibody to hepatitis C virus by enzyme immunoassay; HCV RNA [PCR], hepatitis C viral RNA by polymerase chain reaction.)

an assay for HCV RNA. Occasional persons are found to have anti-HCV without HCV RNA in the serum, suggesting recovery from HCV infection in the past.

Complications

HCV is a pathogenic factor in mixed cryoglobulinemia and membranoproliferative glomerulonephritis and may be related to lichen planus, autoimmune thyroiditis, lymphocytic sialadenitis, idiopathic pulmonary fibrosis, sporadic porphyria cutanea tarda, and monoclonal gammopathies. HCV infection confers a 20–30% or more increased risk of non-Hodgkin lymphoma, and chronic HCV infection (especially genotype 1) is associated with an increased risk of end-stage renal disease. Hepatic steatosis is a particular feature of infection with HCV genotype 3 and may also occur in patients infected with other HCV genotypes who have risk factors for fatty liver. On the other hand, chronic HCV infection is associated with a decrease in serum cholesterol and low-density lipoprotein levels.

Prevention

Testing donated blood for HCV has helped reduce the risk of transfusion-associated hepatitis C from 10% in 1990 to about 1 case per 2 million units in 2011. Birth cohort screening of persons born between 1945 and 1965 ("baby boomers") for HCV infection has been recommended by the CDC and the US Preventive Services Task Force; universal one-time testing has been suggested as an alternative approach. Screening of all pregnant women for HCV infection has been recommended by professional societies. HCV-infected persons should practice safe sex, but there is little evidence that HCV is spread easily by sexual contact or perinatally, and no specific preventive measures are recommended for persons in a monogamous relationship or for pregnant women. Because a majority of cases of HCV infection are acquired by injection drug use, public health officials have recommended avoidance of shared needles and access to needle exchange programs for injection drug users. As yet, there is no vaccine for HCV. Vaccination against HAV (after prescreening for prior immunity) and HBV is recommended for patients with chronic hepatitis C, just as vaccination against HAV is recommended for patients with chronic hepatitis B.

Treatment

In the past, treatment of patients with acute hepatitis C with a peginterferon-based regimen for 6–24 weeks was shown to appreciably decrease the risk of chronic hepatitis in patients in whom serum HCV RNA levels had failed to clear spontaneously after 3 months. Oral direct-acting agents have supplanted interferon-based therapy (see Chronic Viral Hepatitis), and a 6-week course of ledipasvir and sofosbuvir has been shown to prevent chronic hepatitis in patients with acute genotype-1 hepatitis C. Treatment of acute hepatitis C may be cost effective.

Prognosis

In most patients, clinical recovery is complete in 3–6 months. Laboratory evidence of liver dysfunction may persist for a longer period. The overall mortality rate is less than 1%, but the rate is reportedly higher in older people. Acute liver failure due to HCV is rare in the United States.

Chronic hepatitis, which progresses very slowly in many cases, develops in as many as 85% of all persons with acute hepatitis C. Ultimately, cirrhosis develops in up to 30% of those with chronic hepatitis C; the risk of cirrhosis and hepatic decompensation is higher in patients coinfected with both HCV and HBV or HIV. Patients with cirrhosis are at risk for hepatocellular carcinoma at a rate of 3–5% per year. Long-term morbidity and mortality in patients with chronic hepatitis C is lower in black than in white patients and lowest in those infected with HCV genotype 2 and highest in those with HCV genotype 3.

2. Hepatitis D (Delta Agent)

HDV is a defective RNA virus that causes hepatitis only in association with HBV infection and specifically only in the presence of HBsAg; it is cleared when the latter is cleared.

HDV may coinfect with HBV or may superinfect a person with chronic hepatitis B, usually by percutaneous exposure. When acute hepatitis D is coincident with acute HBV infection, the infection is generally similar in severity to acute hepatitis B alone. In chronic hepatitis B, superinfection by HDV appears to carry a worse short-term prognosis, often resulting in acute liver failure or severe chronic hepatitis that progresses rapidly to cirrhosis.

New cases of hepatitis D are now infrequent in the United States primarily because of the control of HBV infection (although rates of testing HBV carriers for HDV are inappropriately low), and cases seen today are usually from cohorts infected years ago who survived the initial impact of hepatitis D and now have cirrhosis. These patients are at risk for decompensation and have a threefold increased risk of hepatocellular carcinoma. New cases are seen primarily in immigrants from endemic areas, including Africa, central Asia, Eastern Europe, and the Amazon region of Brazil. More than 15 million people are infected worldwide. The diagnosis of hepatitis D is made by detection of antibody to hepatitis D antigen (anti-HDV) and, where available, hepatitis D antigen (HDAg) or HDV RNA in serum.

3. Hepatitis E

HEV is a 27- to 34-nm RNA hepevirus (in the Hepeviridae family) that is a major cause of acute hepatitis throughout Central and Southeast Asia, the Middle East, and North Africa, where it is responsible for waterborne hepatitis outbreaks. It is uncommon in the United States (although up to 16% of the population have antibodies to the virus) but should be considered in patients with acute hepatitis after a trip to an endemic area. In rare cases, hepatitis E can be mistaken for drug-induced liver injury. In industrialized countries, it may be spread by swine, and having a pet in the home and consuming undercooked organ meats or infected cow's milk are risk factors. The risk appears to be increased in patients undergoing hemodialysis. Illness generally is self-limited (no carrier state), but instances of chronic hepatitis with rapid progression to cirrhosis attributed to HEV have been reported in transplant recipients (particularly when tacrolimus rather than cyclosporine is used as the main immunosuppressant) and, rarely, in persons with HIV infection, preexisting liver disease, or cancer undergoing chemotherapy. The diagnosis of acute hepatitis E is made most readily by testing for IgM anti-HEV in serum, although available tests may not be reliable. Reported extrahepatic manifestations include arthritis; pancreatitis; monoclonal gammopathy; thrombocytopenia; a variety of neurologic complications, including Guillain-Barré syndrome and peripheral neuropathy; and hemophagocytic lymphohistiocytosis. In endemic regions, the mortality rate is high (15–25%) in pregnant women and correlates with high levels of HEV RNA in serum and gene mutations that lead to reduced expression of progesterone receptors. The risk of hepatic decompensation is increased in patients with underlying chronic liver disease. A 3-month course of treatment with oral ribavirin has been reported to induce sustained clearance of HEV RNA from the serum in 78% of patients with persistent HEV infection and may be considered in patients with severe acute hepatitis E. Improved public hygiene reduces the risk of HEV infection in endemic areas. Recombinant vaccines against HEV have shown promise in clinical trials, and one (Hecolin) is approved in China.

AASLD-IDSA HCV Guidance Panel. Hepatitis C Guidance 2018 Update: AASLD-IDSA recommendations for testing, managing, and treating hepatitis C virus infection. Clin Infect Dis. 2018 Oct 30;67(10):1477–92. [PMID: 30215672]

Bethea ED et al. Should we treat acute hepatitis C? A decision and cost-effectiveness analysis. Hepatology. 2018 Mar;67(3):837–46. [PMID: 29059461]

European Association for the Study of the Liver. EASL Clinical Practice Guidelines on hepatitis E virus infection. J Hepatol. 2018 Jun;68(6):1256–71. [PMID: 29609832]

Yartel AK et al. Hepatitis C virus testing for case identification in persons born during 1945–1965: results from three randomized controlled trials. Hepatology. 2018 Feb;67(2):524–33. [PMID: 28941361]

Zibbell JE et al. Increases in acute hepatitis C virus infection related to a growing opioid epidemic and associated injection drug use, United States, 2004 to 2014. Am J Public Health. 2018 Feb;108(2):175–81. [PMID: 29267061]

ACUTE LIVER FAILURE

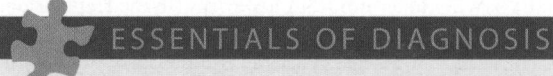

ESSENTIALS OF DIAGNOSIS

▶ May be fulminant or subfulminant; both forms carry a poor prognosis.

▶ Acetaminophen and idiosyncratic drug reactions are the most common causes.

▶ General Considerations

Acute liver failure may be fulminant or subfulminant. Fulminant hepatic failure is characterized by the development of hepatic encephalopathy within 8 weeks after the onset of acute liver injury. Coagulopathy (INR 1.5 or higher) is invariably present. Subfulminant hepatic failure occurs when these findings appear between 8 weeks and 6 months after the onset of acute liver injury and carries an equally poor prognosis. Acute-on-chronic liver failure refers to acute deterioration in liver function (often caused by infection) in a person with preexisting chronic liver disease.

An estimated 1600 cases of acute liver failure occur each year in the United States. Acetaminophen toxicity is the most common cause, accounting for at least 45% of cases. Suicide attempts account for 44% of cases of acetaminophen-induced hepatic failure, and unintentional overdoses ("therapeutic misadventures"), which are often a result of a decrease in the threshold toxic dose because of chronic alcohol use or fasting and have been reported after weight loss surgery, account for at least 48%. Other causes include idiosyncratic drug reactions (the second most common cause, with antituberculosis drugs, antiepileptics, and antibiotics implicated most commonly), viral hepatitis, poisonous mushrooms (*Amanita phalloides*), shock, hyperthermia, Budd-Chiari syndrome, malignancy (most commonly lymphomas), Wilson disease, Reye syndrome, fatty liver of pregnancy and other disorders of fatty acid oxidation, autoimmune hepatitis, parvovirus B19 infection and, rarely, grand mal seizures. The cause is indeterminate in approximately 5.5% of cases. The risk of acute liver failure is increased in patients with diabetes mellitus, and outcome is worsened by obesity. Herbal and dietary supplements are thought to be contributory to acute liver failure in a substantial portion of cases, regardless of cause, and may be associated with lower rates of transplant-free survival. Acute-on-chronic liver failure is often precipitated by a bacterial infection or an alcohol binge and alcoholic hepatitis.

Viral hepatitis now accounts for only 12% of all cases of acute liver failure. The decline of viral hepatitis as the principal cause of acute liver failure is due to universal vaccination of infants and children against hepatitis B and the availability of the hepatitis A vaccine. Acute liver failure may occur after reactivation of hepatitis B in carriers who receive immunosuppressive therapy. In endemic areas, hepatitis E is an important cause of acute liver failure, particularly in pregnant women. Hepatitis C is a rare cause of acute liver failure in the United States, but acute hepatitis A or B superimposed on chronic hepatitis C may cause acute liver failure.

▶ Clinical Findings

Gastrointestinal symptoms, systemic inflammatory response, and kidney dysfunction are common. Clinically significant bleeding is uncommon and reflects severe systemic inflammation rather than coagulopathy. Adrenal insufficiency and subclinical myocardial injury (manifesting as an elevated serum troponin I level) often complicate acute liver failure. Jaundice may be absent or minimal early in the course, but laboratory tests show severe hepatocellular damage. In acetaminophen toxicity, serum aminotransferase elevations are often towering (greater than 5000 units/L). In acute liver failure due to microvesicular steatosis (eg, fatty liver of pregnancy), serum aminotransferase elevations may be modest (less than 300 units/L). Over 10% of patients have an elevated serum amylase level at least three times the upper limit of normal, often as a result of renal dysfunction. The blood ammonia level is typically elevated and correlates (along with the Model for End-Stage Liver Disease [MELD] score) with the development of encephalopathy and intracranial hypertension. Intracranial hypertension rarely develops when the blood ammonia level is less than 75 mcmol/L and is invariable when it is greater than 200 mcmol/L. The severity of extrahepatic organ dysfunction (as assessed by the Sequential Organ Failure Assessment [SOFA]) also correlates with the likelihood of intracranial hypertension. Acute kidney injury frequently complicates acute-on-chronic liver failure.

▶ Treatment

The treatment of acute liver failure is directed toward achieving metabolic and hemodynamic stability. Intravascular volume should be preserved, but large-volume infusions of hypotonic fluids should be avoided. Norepinephrine is the preferred vasopressor. Hypoglycemia should be prevented. Intermittent renal replacement therapy may be required. To preserve muscle mass and immune function, enteral administration of protein, 1–1.5 g/kg/day, is advised, with careful monitoring of the ammonia level. Cerebral edema and sepsis are the leading causes of death. Prophylactic antibiotic therapy decreases the risk of infection, observed in up to 90%, but has no effect on survival and is not routinely recommended. Microbiological screening cultures should be obtained for patients admitted to hospital. For suspected sepsis, broad coverage is indicated. Despite a high rate of adrenal insufficiency, corticosteroids do not reduce mortality and may lower overall survival in patients with a high MELD score, although they may reduce vasopressor requirements. Stress gastropathy prophylaxis with an H_2-receptor blocker or proton pump inhibitor is recommended. Administration of acetylcysteine (140 mg/kg orally followed by 70 mg/kg orally every 4 hours for an additional 17 doses or 150 mg/kg in 5% dextrose intravenously over 15 minutes followed by 50 mg/kg over 4 hours and then 100 mg/kg over 16 hours) is indicated for acetaminophen toxicity up to 72 hours after ingestion. For massive acetaminophen overdoses, treatment with intravenous acetylcysteine may need to be extended in duration until the serum aminotransferase levels are declining and serum acetaminophen levels are undetectable. Treatment with acetylcysteine improves cerebral blood flow and oxygenation as well as transplant-free survival in patients with stage 1 or 2 encephalopathy due to fulminant hepatic failure of any cause. (Acetylcysteine treatment can prolong the prothrombin time, leading to the erroneous assumption that liver failure is worsening; it can also cause nausea, vomiting, and an anaphylactoid reaction [especially in persons with a history of asthma].) Penicillin G (300,000 to 1 million units/kg/day) or silibinin (silymarin or milk thistle), which is not licensed in the United States, is administered to patients with mushroom poisoning. Nucleoside analogs are recommended for patients with acute liver failure caused by HBV (see Chronic

Viral Hepatitis), and intravenous acyclovir has shown benefit in those with herpes simplex virus hepatitis. Plasmapheresis combined with D-penicillamine has been used in acute liver failure due to Wilson disease. Subclinical seizure activity is common in patients with acute liver failure, but the value of prophylactic phenytoin is uncertain.

Early transfer to a liver transplantation center is essential. The head of the patient's bed should be elevated to 30 degrees, and patients with stage 3 or 4 encephalopathy should be intubated. In some centers, extradural sensors are placed in patients at high risk for intracranial hypertension to monitor intracranial pressure for impending cerebral edema with the goal of maintaining the intracranial pressure below 20 mm Hg and the cerebral perfusion pressure above 70 mm Hg but may be associated with complications. Lactulose is generally avoided. Mannitol, 0.5 g/kg, or 100–200 mL of a 20% solution by intravenous infusion over 10 minutes, may decrease cerebral edema but should be used with caution in patients with advanced chronic kidney disease. Intravenously administered hypertonic saline to induce hypernatremia (serum sodium concentration of 145–155 mEq/L [145–155 mmol/L]) also may reduce intracranial hypertension. Hypothermia to a temperature of 32–34°C may reduce intracranial pressure when other measures have failed and may improve survival long enough to permit liver transplantation, although a controlled trial showed no benefit and some authorities recommend a target core temperature of 35–36°C. The value of hyperventilation is uncertain. A short-acting barbiturate, propofol, or intravenous boluses of indomethacin, 25 mg, is considered for refractory intracranial hypertension. Hemodialysis raises intracranial pressure and should be avoided, but plasma exchange may be used, if necessary, in patients with acute kidney injury.

▶ Prognosis

With earlier recognition of acute liver failure, the frequency of cerebral edema has declined, and overall survival has improved steadily since the 1970s and is now as high as 75%. However, the survival rate in acute liver failure with severe encephalopathy is as low as 20%, except for acetaminophen hepatotoxicity, in which the transplant-free survival is 65% and no more than 8% of patients undergo liver transplantation. For patients with acute liver failure of other causes, the outlook is poor in patients younger than 10 and older than 40 years of age and in those with an idiosyncratic drug reaction but appears to be improved when acetylcysteine is administered to patients with stage 1 or 2 encephalopathy. Spontaneous recovery is less likely for hepatitis B than for hepatitis A. Other adverse prognostic factors are a serum bilirubin level greater than 18 mg/dL (307.8 mcmol/L), INR higher than 6.5, onset of encephalopathy more than 7 days after the onset of jaundice, and a low factor V level (less than 20% of normal in patients younger than 30 years and 30% or less in those 30 years of age or older). For acetaminophen-induced acute liver failure, indicators of a poor outcome are acidosis (pH < 7.3), INR greater than 6.5, and azotemia (serum creatinine 3.4 mg/dL [283.22 mcmol/L] or higher), whereas a rising serum alpha-fetoprotein level predicts a favorable outcome. Other predictors of poor survival in patients with acute liver failure are an elevated blood lactate level (greater than 3.5 mEq/L [3.5 mmol/L]), elevated blood ammonia level (greater than 211 mcg/dL [124 mcmol/L]), and possibly hyperphosphatemia (greater than 3.7 mg/dL [1.2 mmol/L]). One study has shown that patients with persistent elevation of the arterial ammonia level (211 mcg/dL [122 mcmol/L] or higher) for 3 days have greater rates of complications and mortality than those with decreasing ammonia levels. The development of thrombocytopenia in the first week is associated with the development of multiorgan system failure and a poor outcome. A number of prognostic indices have been proposed: the "BiLE" score, based on the serum bilirubin, serum lactate, and etiology; the Acute Liver Failure Early Dynamic (ALFED) model, based on the arterial ammonia level, serum bilirubin, INR, and hepatic encephalopathy; and the Acute Liver Failure Study Group (ALFSG) index, based on coma grade, INR, serum bilirubin and phosphorous levels, and serum levels of M30, a cleavage product of cytokeratin-18 caspase. The likelihood of transplant-free survival on admission has been reported to be predicted by a regression model that incorporates the grade of hepatic encephalopathy, etiology, vasopressor use, and log transformations of the serum bilirubin and INR. For acetaminophen-induced acute liver failure, a model that incorporates hepatic encephalopathy grade equal to or greater than 3, Glasgow coma score, cardiovascular failure, mean arterial pressure, INR, serum bilirubin, serum AST, serum creatinine, arterial pH, and arterial lactate has shown good discrimination. In general, emergency liver transplantation is considered for patients with stage 2 to stage 3 encephalopathy or a MELD score of 30.5 or higher (see Cirrhosis) and is associated with a 70% survival rate at 5 years. For mushroom poisoning, liver transplantation should be considered when the interval between ingestion and the onset of diarrhea is less than 8 hours or the INR is 6.0 or higher, even in the absence of encephalopathy. Acute-on-chronic liver failure has a poor prognosis, particularly when associated with kidney dysfunction. Some patients may be candidates for liver transplantation.

▶ When to Admit

All patients with acute liver failure should be hospitalized.

Flamm SL et al. American Gastroenterological Association Institute guidelines for the diagnosis and management of acute liver failure. Gastroenterology. 2017 Feb;152(3):644–7. [PMID: 28056348]

Ganger DR et al; Acute Liver Failure Study Group. Acute liver failure of indeterminate etiology: a comprehensive systematic approach by an expert committee to establish causality. Am J Gastroenterol. 2018 Sep;113(9):1319–28. [PMID: 29946176]

Khan R et al. Modern management of acute liver failure. Gastroenterol Clin North Am. 2018 Jun;47(2):313–26. [PMID: 29735026]

Pyrsopoulos NT (guest editor). Acute liver failure. Clin Liver Dis. 2018;22:229–427. [Full issue]

Stravitz RT et al. Bleeding complications in acute liver failure. Hepatology. 2018 May;67(5):1931–42. [PMID: 29194678]

CHRONIC VIRAL HEPATITIS

> ### ESSENTIALS OF DIAGNOSIS

> ▶ Defined by chronic infection (HBV, HCV, HDV) for longer than 3–6 months.
> ▶ Diagnosis is usually made by antibody tests and viral nucleic acid in serum.

▶ General Considerations

Chronic hepatitis is defined as chronic necroinflammation of the liver of more than 3–6 months' duration, demonstrated by persistently elevated serum aminotransferase levels or characteristic histologic findings, often in the absence of symptoms. In many cases, the diagnosis of chronic hepatitis may be made on initial presentation. The causes of chronic hepatitis include HBV, HCV, and HDV as well as autoimmune hepatitis; alcoholic and nonalcoholic steatohepatitis; certain medications, such as isoniazid and nitrofurantoin; Wilson disease; alpha-1-antiprotease deficiency; and, rarely, celiac disease. Mortality from chronic HBV and HCV infection has been rising in the United States, and HCV has surpassed HIV as a cause of death. Chronic hepatitis is categorized on the basis of etiology; the grade of portal, periportal, and lobular inflammation (minimal, mild, moderate, or severe); and the stage of fibrosis (none, mild, moderate, severe, cirrhosis). In the absence of advanced cirrhosis, patients are often asymptomatic or have mild nonspecific symptoms.

1. Chronic Hepatitis B & Chronic Hepatitis D

▶ Clinical Findings & Diagnosis

Chronic hepatitis B afflicts 248 million people worldwide (2 billion overall have been infected; endemic areas include Asia and sub-Saharan Africa) and up to 2.2 million (predominantly males) in the United States. It may be noted as a continuum of acute hepatitis B or diagnosed because of repeated detection of HBsAg in serum, often with elevated aminotransferase levels.

Five phases of chronic HBV infection are recognized: immune tolerant phase, immune active (or immune clearance) phase, inactive HBsAg carrier state, reactivated chronic hepatitis B phase, and the HBsAg-negative phase. In the immune tolerant phase (**HBeAg-positive chronic HBV infection**), HBeAg and HBV DNA are present in serum and are indicative of active viral replication, and serum aminotransferase levels are normal, with little necroinflammation in the liver. This phase is common in infants and young children whose immature immune system fails to mount an immune response to HBV.

Persons in the immune tolerant phase and those who acquire HBV infection later in life may enter an immune active phase (**HBeAg-positive chronic hepatitis B**), in which aminotransferase levels are elevated and necroinflammation is present in the liver, with a risk of progression to cirrhosis (at a rate of 2–5.5% per year) and of hepatocellular carcinoma (at a rate of more than 2% per year in those with cirrhosis); low-level IgM anti-HBc is present in serum in about 70%.

Patients enter the inactive HBsAg carrier state (**HBeAg-negative chronic HBV infection**) when biochemical improvement follows immune clearance. This improvement coincides with disappearance of HBeAg and reduced HBV DNA levels (less than 10^5 copies/mL, or less than 20,000 international units/mL) in serum, appearance of anti-HBe, and integration of the HBV genome into the host genome in infected hepatocytes. Patients in this phase are at a low risk for cirrhosis (if it has not already developed) and hepatocellular carcinoma, and those with persistently normal serum aminotransferase levels infrequently have histologically significant liver disease, especially if the HBsAg level is low.

The reactivated chronic hepatitis B phase (**HBeAg-negative chronic hepatitis B**) may result from infection by a pre-core mutant of HBV or spontaneous mutation of the pre-core or core promoter region of the HBV genome during the course of chronic hepatitis caused by wild-type HBV. So-called HBeAg-negative chronic hepatitis B accounts for less than 10% of cases of chronic hepatitis B in the United States, up to 50% in southeast Asia, and up to 90% in Mediterranean countries, reflecting in part differences in the frequencies of HBV genotypes. In reactivated chronic hepatitis B, there is a rise in serum HBV DNA levels and possible progression to cirrhosis (at a rate of 8–10% per year), particularly when additional mutations in the core gene of HBV are present. Risk factors for reactivation include male sex and HBV genotype C as well as immunosuppression. Treatment of HCV infection with direct-acting antiviral agents has been reported to lead to instances of HBV reactivation. In patients with either HBeAg-positive or HBeAg-negative chronic hepatitis B, the risk of cirrhosis and of hepatocellular carcinoma correlates with the serum HBV DNA level. Other risk factors include advanced age, male sex, alcohol use, cigarette smoking, HBV genotype C, and coinfection with HCV or HDV. HIV coinfection is also associated with an increased frequency of cirrhosis when the CD4 count is low. Occasional patients reach the **HBsAg-negative phase,** in which anti-HBe remains the only serologic marker of HBV infection, serum ALT levels are normal, and HBV DNA is undetectable in serum but remains present in the liver.

Acute **hepatitis D** infection superimposed on chronic HBV infection may result in severe chronic hepatitis, which may progress rapidly to cirrhosis and may be fatal. Patients with long-standing chronic hepatitis D and B often have inactive cirrhosis and are at risk for decompensation and hepatocellular carcinoma. The diagnosis is confirmed by detection of anti-HDV or HDAg (or HDV RNA) in serum.

▶ Treatment

Patients with active viral replication (HBeAg and HBV DNA [10^5 copies/mL or more, or 20,000 international units/mL or more] in serum and elevated aminotransferase levels) may be treated with a nucleoside or nucleotide analog or with pegylated interferon. Nucleoside and nucleotide analogs are preferred because they are better tolerated and can be taken orally. For patients who are HBeAg-negative, the threshold for treatment is a serum HBV DNA level of 10^4 copies/mL or more, or 2000 international units/mL or more. If the threshold HBV DNA level for treatment is met but the serum ALT level is normal, treatment may still be considered in patients over age 35–40 if liver biopsy or a noninvasive assessment of liver fibrosis demonstrates a fibrosis stage of 2 of 4 (moderate) or higher. Therapy is aimed at reducing and maintaining the serum HBV DNA level to the lowest possible levels, thereby leading to normalization of the ALT level and histologic improvement. An additional goal in HBeAg-positive patients is seroconversion to anti-HBe, and some responders eventually clear HBsAg. Although nucleoside and nucleotide analogs generally have been discontinued 6–12 months after HBeAg-to-anti-HBe seroconversion, some patients (especially Asian patients) serorevert to HBeAg after discontinuation, have a rise in HBV DNA levels and recurrence of hepatitis activity, and require long-term therapy, which also is required when seroconversion does not occur and in patients with cirrhosis (at least until HBsAg clears and possibly indefinitely). HBeAg-negative patients with chronic hepatitis B also generally require long-term therapy because relapse is frequent when therapy is stopped.

The available nucleoside and nucleotide analogs—entecavir, tenofovir, lamivudine, adefovir, and telbivudine—differ in efficacy and rates of resistance; however, in HBeAg-positive patients, they all achieve an HBeAg-to-anti-HBe seroconversion rate of about 20% at 1 year, with higher rates after more prolonged therapy. The preferred first-line oral agents are entecavir and tenofovir. Entecavir is rarely associated with resistance unless a patient is already resistant to lamivudine. The daily dose is 0.5 mg orally for patients not resistant to lamivudine and 1 mg for patients who previously became resistant to lamivudine. Suppression of HBV DNA in serum occurs in nearly all treated patients, and histologic improvement is observed in 70% of patients. Entecavir has been reported to cause lactic acidosis when used in patients with decompensated cirrhosis. Tenofovir disoproxil fumarate, 300 mg orally daily, is equally effective and is used as a first-line agent or when resistance to a nucleoside analog has developed. Like entecavir, tenofovir has a low rate of resistance when used as initial therapy. Long-term use may lead to an elevated serum creatinine level and reduced serum phosphate level (Fanconi-like syndrome) that is reversible with discontinuation of the drug. Tenofovir alafenamide, 25 mg orally daily, is an alternative formulation of tenofovir that was approved by the FDA in 2016 and that may be associated with a lower rate of renal and bone toxicity than tenofovir disoproxil fumarate.

The first available nucleoside analog was lamivudine, 100 mg orally daily. No longer considered first-line therapy in the United States, it still may be used in countries in which cost is a deciding factor. Adefovir dipivoxil has activity against wild-type and lamivudine-resistant HBV but is the least potent of the oral antiviral agents for HBV and is now rarely if ever used. Telbivudine, given in a daily dose of 600 mg orally, is more potent than either lamivudine or adefovir but like them is associated with resistance. Elevated creatine kinase levels are common in patients treated with telbivudine.

Nucleoside and nucleotide analogs are well tolerated even in patients with decompensated cirrhosis (for whom the treatment threshold may be an HBV DNA level less than 10^4 copies/mL and therapy should be continued indefinitely) and may be effective in patients with rapidly progressive hepatitis B ("fibrosing cholestatic hepatitis") following organ transplantation. Combined use of a nucleoside and nucleotide analog or of peginterferon and a nucleoside or nucleotide analog has not been shown convincingly to have a substantial advantage over the use of one drug alone.

Nucleoside analogs are also recommended for inactive HBV carriers (and those positive only for anti-HBc) prior to the initiation of immunosuppressive therapy (including rituximab or anti-tumor necrosis factor antibody therapy) or cancer chemotherapy to prevent reactivation. In patients infected with both HBV and HIV, antiretroviral therapy, including two drugs active against both viruses (eg, tenofovir plus lamivudine or emtricitabine), has been recommended when treatment of HIV infection is indicated. Telbivudine and tenofovir are classified as pregnancy category B drugs, and lamivudine, a category C drug, has been shown to be safe in pregnant women with HIV infection. Antiviral therapy has been recommended, beginning in the third trimester, when the mother's serum HBV DNA level is 200,000 international units/mL or higher to reduce levels at the time of delivery.

Peginterferon alfa-2a is still an alternative to the oral agents in selected cases. A dose of 180 mcg subcutaneously once weekly for 48 weeks leads to sustained normalization of aminotransferase levels, disappearance of HBeAg and HBV DNA from serum, and appearance of anti-HBe in up to 40% of treated patients and results in improved survival. A response is most likely in patients with a low baseline HBV DNA level and high aminotransferase levels and is more likely in those who are infected with HBV genotype A than with other genotypes (especially genotype D). Moreover, many complete responders eventually clear HBsAg and develop anti-HBs in serum, and are thus cured. Relapses are uncommon in complete responders who seroconvert from HBeAg to anti-HBe. Peginterferon may be considered in order to avoid long-term therapy with an oral agent, as in young women who may want to become pregnant in the future. Patients with HBeAg-negative chronic hepatitis B have a response rate of 60% after 48 weeks of therapy with peginterferon, but the response may not be durable once peginterferon is stopped. The response to peginterferon is poor in patients with HIV coinfection.

In **chronic hepatitis D**, peginterferon alfa-2b (1.5 mcg/kg/wk for 48 weeks) may lead to normalization of serum aminotransferase levels, histologic improvement, and elimination of HDV RNA from serum in 20–50% of patients, but relapse may occur and tolerance is poor. Nucleoside and nucleotide analogs are generally not effective in treating chronic hepatitis D.

▶ Prognosis

The sequelae of chronic hepatitis secondary to hepatitis B include cirrhosis, liver failure, and hepatocellular carcinoma. The 5-year mortality rate is 0–2% in those without cirrhosis, 14–20% in those with compensated cirrhosis, and 70–86% following decompensation. The risk of cirrhosis and hepatocellular carcinoma correlates with serum HBV DNA levels, and a focus of therapy is to suppress HBV DNA levels below 300 copies/mL (60 international units/mL). In patients with cirrhosis, even low levels of HBV DNA in serum increase the risk of hepatocellular carcinoma compared with undetectable levels. HBV genotype C is associated with a higher risk of cirrhosis and hepatocellular carcinoma than other genotypes. Antiviral treatment improves the prognosis in responders, prevents (or leads to regression of) cirrhosis, and decreases the frequency of liver-related complications (although the risk of hepatocellular carcinoma does not become as low as that in inactive HBV carriers and hepatocellular carcinoma may even occur after clearance of HBsAg). A risk score (PAGE-B) based on a patient's age, sex, and platelet count has been reported to predict the 5-year risk of hepatocellular carcinoma in white patients taking entecavir or tenofovir.

2. Chronic Hepatitis C

▶ Clinical Findings & Diagnosis

Chronic hepatitis C develops in up to 85% of patients with acute hepatitis C. It is clinically indistinguishable from chronic hepatitis due to other causes and may be the most common. Worldwide, 170 million people are infected with HCV, with 1.8% of the US population infected. Peak prevalence in the United States (about 4%) is in persons born between 1945 and 1964. In approximately 40% of cases, serum aminotransferase levels are persistently normal. The diagnosis is confirmed by detection of anti-HCV by EIA. In rare cases of suspected chronic hepatitis C but a negative EIA, HCV RNA is detected by PCR testing. Progression to cirrhosis occurs in 20% of affected patients after 20 years, with an increased risk in men, those who drink more than 50 g of alcohol daily, and those who acquire HCV infection after age 40 years. The rate of fibrosis progression accelerates after age 50. African Americans have a higher rate of chronic hepatitis C but lower rates of fibrosis progression and response to therapy than whites. Immunosuppressed persons—including patients with hypogammaglobulinemia or HIV infection with a low CD4 count or those receiving immunosuppressants—appear to progress more rapidly to cirrhosis than immunocompetent persons with chronic hepatitis C. Tobacco and cannabis smoking and hepatic steatosis also appear to promote progression of fibrosis, but coffee consumption appears to slow progression. Persons with chronic hepatitis C and persistently normal serum aminotransferase levels usually have mild chronic hepatitis with slow or absent progression to cirrhosis; however, cirrhosis is present in 10% of these patients. Serum fibrosis testing (eg, FibroSure) or elastography may be used to identify the absence of fibrosis or presence of cirrhosis.

▶ Treatment

The introduction of direct-acting and host-targeting antiviral agents has rapidly expanded the therapeutic

Table 16–6. Direct-acting antiviral agents for HCV infection (in alphabetic order within class).[1]

Agent	Genotype(s)	Dose[2]	Comment
NS3/4A Protease Inhibitors			
Glecaprevir	1–6	300 mg orally once daily	Used in combination with pibrentasvir[3] with or without ribavirin
Grazoprevir	1 and 4	100 mg orally once daily	Used in combination with elbasvir[4]
Paritaprevir	1 and 4	150 mg orally once daily	Used in combination with ombitasvir and dasabuvir; ritonavir (100 mg) boosted;[5] for genotype 1b with cirrhosis and genotype 1a, used with ribavirin. Used in combination with ombitasvir, ritonavir boosting, and ribavirin for genotype 4[6]
Simeprevir	1 and 4	150 mg orally once daily	Used in combination with sofosbuvir
Voxilaprevir	1–6	100 mg orally once daily	Used in combination with sofosbuvir and velpatasvir[7]
NS5A Inhibitors			
Daclatasvir[8]	1–6	60 mg orally once daily	Used in combination with sofosbuvir (genotypes 1–6, with or without ribavirin depending on presence of cirrhosis) or with asunaprevir (not available in the United States)
Elbasvir	1–6	50 mg orally once daily	Used in combination with grazoprevir
Ledipasvir	1, 4–6	90 mg orally once daily	Used in combination with sofosbuvir[9]
Ombitasvir	1 and 4	25 mg orally once daily	Used in combination with paritaprevir (ritonavir boosted) with or without dasabuvir and with or without ribavirin as per paritaprevir above
Pibrentasvir	1–6	120 mg orally once daily	Used in combination with glecaprevir with or without ribavirin
Velpatasvir	1–6	100 mg orally once daily	Used in combination with sofosbuvir[10], may be used with sofosbuvir and voxilaprevir
NS5B Nucleos(t)ide Polymerase Inhibitor			
Sofosbuvir	1–6	400 mg orally once daily	Used in combination with ribavirin (genotypes 2 and 3) or with simeprevir (genotypes 1 and 4) or with daclatasvir (all genotypes) or with ledipasvir (genotypes 1, 3, and 4) or with velpatasvir (all genotypes) or with velpatasvir and voxilaprevir (all genotypes)
NS5B Non-Nucleos(t)ide Polymerase Inhibitor			
Dasabuvir	1 and 4	250 mg orally twice daily	Used in combination with paritaprevir (ritonavir boosted) and ombitasvir with or without ribavirin as per paritaprevir above

[1]Regimens approved by the FDA as of early 2019.

[2]The preferred regimen and duration of treatment may vary depending on HCV genotype, presence or absence of cirrhosis or chronic kidney disease, or nonresponse to prior therapy for HCV infection. In selected cases, testing for resistance-associated substitutions may be considered.

[3]Marketed as Mavyret (AbbVie).

[4]Marketed as Zepatier (Merck) for HCV genotypes 1 and 4 infection.

[5]Marketed as Viekira Pak and Viekira XR (AbbVie).

[6]Marketed as Technivie (AbbVie).

[7]Marketed as Vosevi (Gilead Sciences).

[8]Approved by the FDA for use with sofosbuvir in HCV genotypes 1 and 3 infection.

[9]Marketed as Harvoni (Gilead Sciences).

[10]Marketed as Epclusa (Gilead Sciences).

armamentarium against HCV (Table 16–6). Standard therapy for HCV infection from the late 1990s to the early 2010s was a combination of peginterferon plus ribavirin, and ribavirin continues to be used in some all-oral regimens. Sustained virologic response rates (negative HCV RNA in serum at 24 weeks after completion of therapy) for peginterferon plus ribavirin were 45% in patients with HCV genotype 1 infection and 70–80% in those with genotype 2 or 3 infection. Treatment with peginterferon-based

therapy is associated with frequent, often distressing, side effects, and discontinuation rates are as high as 15–30%.

After the introduction of all-oral regimens, the criterion for a sustained virologic response was shortened from 24 weeks to 12 weeks following the completion of treatment. The definition of clearance of HCV RNA requires use of a sensitive real-time reverse transcriptase-PCR assay to monitor HCV RNA during treatment (the lower limit of quantification should be 25 international units/mL or less, and the

Table 16–7. Recommended FDA-approved oral direct-acting antiviral (DAA) treatment regimens for HCV infection.[1]

Regimen	Indication
Sofosbuvir and ledipasvir	Genotypes 1 and 4
Grazoprevir and elbasvir	Genotypes 1 and 4
Sofosbuvir and daclatasvir	Alternative for genotypes 1–4
Sofosbuvir and velpatasvir	Genotypes 1–6
Sofosbuvir, velpatasvir, and voxilaprevir	DAA-experienced genotypes 1–6
Glecaprevir and pibrentasvir	Genotypes 1–6 and DAA-experienced genotype 1

[1]Based on the American Association for the Study of Liver Diseases/Infectious Diseases Society of America 2018 Guidance.

limit of detection should be 10–15 international units/mL). Several types of direct-acting antiviral agents have been developed (Tables 16–6 and 16–7). HCV protease inhibitors ("…previrs") generally have high antiviral potency but differ with respect to the development of resistance (although resistance-associated substitutions in the HCV genome tend not to persist after therapy with these agents is stopped). Some of the compounds show better response rates in HCV genotype 1b than in genotype 1a infection.

HCV polymerase inhibitors ("…buvirs") are categorized as nucleoside or nucleotide analog and non-nucleoside polymerase inhibitors. Nucleos(t)ide analogs are active against all HCV genotypes and have a high barrier to resistance. Non-nucleos(t)ide polymerase inhibitors are the weakest class of compounds against HCV because of a low barrier to resistance. Drugs in this class are generally more active against HCV genotype 1b than HCV genotype 1a. They have been developed to be used only in combination with the other direct-acting antiviral agents, mainly protease inhibitors and NS5A inhibitors. The first approved HCV NS5B nucleotide polymerase inhibitor was sofosbuvir in 2013.

Sofosbuvir was initially approved for use in combination with peginterferon and ribavirin in patients with HCV genotype 1 infection and with ribavirin alone in patients with HCV genotype 2 or 3 infection (see Table 16–6). Most patients with HCV genotype 2 or 3 infection, including those with HIV coinfection, are cured with 12 or 24 weeks of therapy, respectively. HCV genotype 2 responds much better to interferon-free sofosbuvir-based therapy than HCV genotype 3, but the sustained virologic response is 20–30% lower in patients with cirrhosis and the combination of sofosbuvir and ribavirin has been reported to cause lactic acidosis in some patients with advanced cirrhosis. Importantly, no sofosbuvir-resistant variants have been selected during therapy. The combination of sofosbuvir and simeprevir was found to be effective in HCV genotype 1 infection and has been approved by the FDA; the approval was thereafter extended to HCV genotypes 4, 5,

and 6. Sofosbuvir was also approved to be used in combination with ledipasvir.

The combination of paritaprevir (an NS3/4A protease inhibitor), boosted by ritonavir, plus ombitasvir (an NS5A inhibitor) and dasabuvir (an NS5B non-nucleoside polymerase inhibitor) is effective in HCV genotype-1 treatment-naive patients and prior nonresponders to interferon-based therapy, with or without cirrhosis, and has been approved by the FDA. The same combination without dasabuvir has also received FDA approval for HCV genotype 4 infection. Instances of hepatotoxicity have been reported with these regimens in patients with advanced cirrhosis. Daclatasvir in combination with sofosbuvir has proven effective in genotypes 1-, 2-, and 3-infected patients, including those coinfected with HIV, and was approved by the FDA in 2015 for HCV genotype 3 infection.

NS5A inhibitors ("…asvirs") are characterized by high antiviral potency at picomolar doses. The cross-genotype efficacy of these agents varies. Ledipasvir was the first NS5A inhibitor approved by the FDA in 2014 (see Table 16–6). Ledipasvir has potent activity against genotypes 1, 4, 5, and 6 HCV and has been formulated in combination with sofosbuvir. The combination is highly effective in both treatment-naive and treatment-experienced patients, even those with cirrhosis and is given in a fixed dose of ledipasvir 90 mg and sofosbuvir 400 mg once daily for 12 weeks in HCV genotype 1–infected treatment-naive patients and treatment-experienced patients without cirrhosis and for 24 weeks in treatment-experienced patients with cirrhosis. In treatment-naive patients without cirrhosis, the duration of treatment can be shortened to 8 weeks if the baseline HCV RNA level is less than 6 million international units/mL. Sustained virologic response rates are well above 90%, including in patients coinfected with HIV, and this regimen is a first-line therapy for HCV genotype 1. The combination of ledipasvir, sofosbuvir, and ribavirin achieves high rates of sustained virologic response in patients with HCV genotype 3 as well as in patients with HCV genotype 1 or 4 and advanced cirrhosis. Side effects are mild and include fatigue and headache. Concomitant use of a proton pump inhibitor, particularly twice-daily dosing in patients with cirrhosis, may reduce the effectiveness of the combination of ledipasvir and sofosbuvir. Re-treatment of occasional nonresponders or relapsers with resistance-associated substitutions that persist for years with an alternative regimen that may include sofosbuvir is often effective.

Over the past several years, the FDA has approved other highly effective combinations: 100 mg of grazoprevir (an NS3/4A protease inhibitor) plus 50 mg/day of elbasvir (an NS5A inhibitor) for HCV genotypes 1 and 4; 300 mg of glecaprevir (an NS3/4A protease inhibitor) plus 120 mg/day of pibrentasvir (an NS5A inhibitor) for genotypes 1–6 (pangenotypic); and another pangenotypic regimen, sofosbuvir and velpatasvir, with the addition of ribavirin in patients with cirrhosis and with the addition of voxilaprevir (an NS3A/N4 protease inhibitor) as "rescue" therapy in patients with nonresponse or relapse following initial treatment with an NS5A-containing regimen. The combination of glecaprevir and pibrentasvir is approved for 8 (rather than the usual 12) weeks in treatment-naïve, noncirrhotic patients, including those coinfected with HIV. It is also a pangenotypic option for patients with chronic kidney disease, including those receiving dialysis. Other "rescue" regimens are under study, including grazoprevir, ruzasvir (an NS5A inhibitor), and uprifosbuvir (an NS5B polymerase nucleotide inhibitor), with or without ribavirin, for patients who have not responded to NS5A-containing therapy. Where available, testing for resistance-associated substitutions may be helpful before re-treatment. Use of any regimen containing a protease inhibitor is contraindicated in patients with decompensated cirrhosis, and pretreatment testing for resistance-associated substitutions is recommended.

Overall treatment rates are still less than 20% and lowest among Hispanics and persons with Medicaid or indigent care insurance. The cost of direct-acting antiviral agents has been high (although declining), and lack of insurance coverage has often been a barrier to their use. Additional factors to consider in the selection of a regimen are the presence of cirrhosis or kidney dysfunction, prior treatment, potential drug interactions (of which there are many), and the likelihood that a patient may require liver transplantation in the future. For some regimens, an 8-week course of treatment may be effective in selected cases. Other agents that have been studied include NS3/4A protease inhibitors (eg, danoprevir, faldaprevir [now discontinued]); polymerase inhibitors (eg, mericitabine); virus entry, assembly, and secretion inhibitors; microRNA-122 antisense oligonucleotides (eg, miravirsen); cyclophilin A inhibitors (eg, alisporivir); interferon lambda-3; and therapeutic vaccines. HCV genotype 1 is now easy to cure with oral direct-acting agents, with expected sustained virologic response rates well above 90%, and virtually all HCV genotype 2 infection is curable with all-oral regimens. HCV genotype 3 infection, particularly in association with cirrhosis, has been the most challenging to treat, but the newest regimens have increased the likelihood of cure. Interferon is now rarely required, and the need for ribavirin is decreasing.

Antiviral therapy has been shown to be beneficial in the treatment of cryoglobulinemia associated with chronic hepatitis C; an acute flare of cryoglobulinemia may first require treatment with rituximab, cyclophosphamide plus methylprednisolone, or plasma exchange. As noted above, patients with HCV and HIV coinfection have been shown to respond well to treatment of HCV infection. Moreover, in persons coinfected with HCV and HIV, long-term liver disease–related mortality increases as HIV infection–related mortality is reduced by antiretroviral therapy. Occasional instances of reactivation of HBV infection, as well as herpesvirus, have occurred with direct-acting antiviral agents for HCV infection, and all candidates should be prescreened for HBV infection, with the initiation of antiviral prophylactic therapy in those who are HBsAg positive when treatment of HCV infection is begun.

Prognosis

Chronic hepatitis C is an indolent, often subclinical disease that may lead to cirrhosis and hepatocellular carcinoma after decades. The overall mortality rate in patients with transfusion-associated hepatitis C may be no different from that of an age-matched control population. Nevertheless, mortality or transplantation rates clearly rise to 5% per year once cirrhosis develops. A risk score combining age, sex, platelet count, and AST-to-ALT ratio has been proposed. There is some evidence that HCV genotype 1b is associated with a higher risk of hepatocellular carcinoma than other genotypes. Antiviral therapy has a beneficial effect on mortality and quality of life, is cost-effective, appears to retard and even reverse fibrosis, and reduces (but does not eliminate) the risk of decompensated cirrhosis and hepatocellular carcinoma in responders with advanced fibrosis. Even patients who achieve a sustained virologic response remain at an increased risk for mortality compared with the general population. An increased risk of death from extrahepatic cancers has been described in this group, as well as in patients who achieve suppression of HBV infection. Although mortality from cirrhosis and hepatocellular carcinoma due to hepatitis C is still substantial, the need for liver transplantation for chronic hepatitis C is now declining, and survival after transplantation is improving. The risk of mortality from drug addiction is higher than that for liver disease in patients with chronic hepatitis C. HCV infection appears to be associated with increased cardiovascular mortality, especially in persons with diabetes mellitus and hypertension. Statin use has been reported to be associated with improved virologic response to antiviral therapy and decreased progression of liver fibrosis and frequency of hepatocellular carcinoma.

▶ When to Refer

- For liver biopsy.
- For antiviral therapy.

▶ When to Admit

For complications of decompensated cirrhosis.

European Association for the Study of the Liver. EASL recommendations on treatment of hepatitis C 2018. J Hepatol. 2018 Aug;69(2):461–511. [PMID: 29650333]

Jacobson IM et al. American Gastroenterological Association Institute clinical practice update—expert review: care of patients who have achieved a sustained virologic response after antiviral therapy for chronic hepatitis C infection. Gastroenterology. 2017 May;152(6):1578–87. [PMID: 28344022]

Rizzetto M. Targeting hepatitis D. Semin Liver Dis. 2018 Feb;38(1):66–72. [PMID: 29471567]

Seto WK et al. Chronic hepatitis B virus infection. Lancet. 2018 Nov 24;392(10161):2313–24. [PMID: 30496122]

Tang LSY et al. Chronic hepatitis B infection: a review. JAMA. 2018 May 1;319(17):1802–13. [PMID: 29715359]

Terrault NA et al. Update on prevention, diagnosis, and treatment of chronic hepatitis B: AASLD 2018 hepatitis B guidance. Hepatology. 2018 Apr;67(4):1560–99. [PMID: 29405329]

Wong GL et al. Review article: long-term safety of oral anti-viral treatment for chronic hepatitis B. Aliment Pharmacol Ther. 2018 Mar;47(6):730–7. [PMID: 29359487]

Wong RJ et al. Race/ethnicity and insurance status disparities in access to direct acting antivirals for hepatitis C virus treatment. Am J Gastroenterol. 2018 Sep;113(9):1329–38. [PMID: 29523864]

AUTOIMMUNE HEPATITIS

ESSENTIALS OF DIAGNOSIS

► Usually young to middle-aged women.
► Chronic hepatitis with high serum globulins and characteristic liver histology.
► Positive antinuclear antibody (ANA) and/or smooth muscle antibody in most cases in the United States.
► Responds to corticosteroids.

General Considerations

Although autoimmune hepatitis is usually seen in young women, it can occur in either sex at any age. The incidence, which has been rising, and prevalence are estimated to be 8.5 and 107 per million population, respectively. The risk of autoimmune hepatitis is increased in first-degree relatives of affected patients.

Clinical Findings

A. Symptoms and Signs

The onset is usually insidious. About 20% of cases present with acute hepatitis (and occasionally acute liver failure), and some cases follow a viral illness (such as hepatitis A, Epstein-Barr infection, or measles) or exposure to a drug or toxin (such as nitrofurantoin, minocycline, hydralazine, methyldopa, or infliximab). Exacerbations may occur post-partum. Amenorrhea may be a presenting feature, and the frequency of depression appears to be increased. Thirty-four percent of patients, and particularly elderly patients, are asymptomatic. Examination may reveal a healthy-appearing young woman with multiple spider telangiectasias, cutaneous striae, acne, hirsutism, and hepatomegaly. Extrahepatic features include arthritis, Sjögren syndrome, thyroiditis, nephritis, ulcerative colitis, and Coombs-positive hemolytic anemia. Patients, especially elderly patients, with autoimmune hepatitis are at increased risk for cirrhosis, which, in turn, increases the risk of hepatocellular carcinoma (at a rate of about 1% per year).

B. Laboratory Findings

Serum aminotransferase levels may be greater than 1000 units/L, and the total bilirubin is usually increased. Autoimmune hepatitis has been classified as type I or type II, although the clinical features and response to treatment are similar between the two types. In type I (classic) autoimmune hepatitis, ANA or smooth muscle antibodies (either or both) are usually detected in serum. Serum gamma-globulin levels are typically elevated (up to 5–6 g/dL [0.05–0.06 g/L]); in such patients, the EIA for antibody to HCV may be falsely positive. Other antibodies, including atypical perinuclear antineutrophil cytoplasmic antibodies (pANCA) and antibodies to histones, F-actin, and alpha-actinin may be found. Antibodies to soluble liver antigen (anti-SLA)

characterize a variant of type I that is marked by severe disease, a high relapse rate after treatment, and absence of the usual antibodies (ANA and smooth muscle antibodies). Type II, seen more often in girls under age 14 in Europe, is characterized by circulating antibodies to liver-kidney microsome type 1 (anti-LKM1) without smooth muscle antibodies or ANA. In some cases, antibodies to liver cytosol type 1 are detected. Type II autoimmune hepatitis can be seen in patients with autoimmune polyglandular syndrome type 1. Concurrent primary biliary cholangitis (PBC) or primary sclerosing cholangitis ("overlap syndrome") has been recognized in 7–13% and 6–11% of patients with autoimmune hepatitis, respectively. Liver biopsy is indicated to help establish the diagnosis (interface hepatitis is the hallmark), evaluate disease severity and stage of fibrosis, and determine the need for treatment.

Simplified diagnostic criteria based on the detection of autoantibodies (1 point for a titer of > 1:40 or 2 points for a titer of > 1:80), elevated IgG levels (1 point for IgG level ≥ upper limit of normal or 2 points for level ≥ 1.1 times upper limit of normal), and characteristic histologic features (1 or 2 points depending on how typical the features are) and exclusion of viral hepatitis (2 points) can be useful for diagnosis; a score of 6 indicates probable and a score of 7 indicates definite autoimmune hepatitis with a high degree of specificity but moderate sensitivity. Diagnostic criteria for an overlap of autoimmune hepatitis and PBC ("Paris criteria") have been proposed.

Treatment

Prednisone with or without azathioprine improves symptoms; decreases the serum bilirubin, aminotransferase, and gamma-globulin levels; and reduces hepatic inflammation. Symptomatic patients with aminotransferase levels elevated 10-fold (or 5-fold if the serum globulins are elevated at least 2-fold) are optimal candidates for therapy, and asymptomatic patients with modest enzyme elevations may be considered for therapy depending on the clinical circumstances and histologic severity; however, asymptomatic patients usually remain asymptomatic, have either mild hepatitis or inactive cirrhosis on liver biopsy specimens, and have a good long-term prognosis without therapy.

Prednisone is given initially in a dose of 30 mg orally daily with azathioprine, 50 mg orally daily, which is generally well tolerated and permits the use of lower corticosteroid doses than a regimen beginning with prednisone 60 mg orally daily alone. Intravenous corticosteroids or prednisone, 60 mg orally daily, is recommended for patients with severe acute autoimmune hepatitis. Budesonide, 3 mg orally two or three times daily, may be at least as effective as prednisone as first-line treatment in patients with non-cirrhotic autoimmune hepatitis and associated with fewer side effects. Whether patients should undergo testing for the genotype or level of thiopurine methyltransferase prior to treatment with azathioprine to predict toxicity is debated. Blood counts are monitored weekly for the first 2 months of therapy and monthly thereafter because of the small risk of bone marrow suppression. The dose of prednisone is lowered from 30 mg/day after 1 week to 20 mg/day and again after 2 or 3 weeks to 15 mg/day. Treatment is response guided, and ultimately, a maintenance dose of 10 mg/day should be achieved. While symptomatic improvement is often prompt, biochemical improvement is more gradual, with normalization of serum aminotransferase levels after an average of 22 months. Histologic resolution of inflammation lags biochemical remission by 3–6 months, and repeat liver biopsy is recommended at least 3 months after the aminotransferase levels have normalized. Failure of aminotransferase levels to return to normal invariably predicts lack of histologic resolution.

The response rate to therapy with prednisone and azathioprine is 80%, with remission in 65% by 3 years. Older patients and those with HLA genotype *DRB1*04* are more likely to respond than younger patients and those with HLA *DRB1*03*, hyperbilirubinemia, or a high MELD score (12 or higher, see Cirrhosis). Fibrosis may reverse with therapy and rarely progresses after apparent biochemical and histologic remission. Once complete remission is achieved, therapy may be withdrawn, but the subsequent relapse rate is 90% by 3 years. Relapses may again be treated in the same manner as the initial episode, with the same remission rate. After successful treatment of a relapse, the patient may continue taking azathioprine (up to 2 mg/kg) or the lowest dose of prednisone with or without azathioprine (50 mg/day) needed to maintain aminotransferase levels as close to normal as possible; another attempt at withdrawing therapy may be considered in patients remaining in remission long term (eg, 4 years or longer). During pregnancy, flares can be treated with prednisone, and maintenance azathioprine does not have to be discontinued.

Nonresponders to corticosteroids and azathioprine (failure of serum aminotransferase levels to decrease by 50% after 6 months) may be considered for a trial of cyclosporine, tacrolimus, sirolimus, everolimus, methotrexate, rituximab, or infliximab. Mycophenolate mofetil, 1 g twice daily, is an effective alternative to azathioprine in patients who cannot tolerate it but is less effective in nonresponders to azathioprine and is a known teratogen that must be withdrawn prior to conception. It may be effective in up to 60% of patients refractory to or intolerant of corticosteroids. Occasionally, 6-mercaptopurine may be tolerated in patients who do not tolerate azathioprine. Bone density should be monitored—particularly in patients receiving maintenance corticosteroid therapy—and measures undertaken to prevent or treat osteoporosis (see Chapter 26). Liver transplantation may be required for treatment failures and patients with a severe acute presentation, but the outcome may be worse than that for PBC because of an increased rate of infectious complications. As immunosuppression is reduced, the disease has been recognized to recur in up to 70% of transplanted livers at 5 years (and rarely to develop de novo); sirolimus can be effective in such cases.

Overall long-term mortality of patients with autoimmune hepatitis appears to be twofold higher than that of the general population despite response to immunosuppressive therapy. Factors that predict the need for liver transplantation or that predict liver-related death include the following: (1) age 20 years or younger or age 60 years or older at presentation, (2) low serum albumin level at diagnosis, (3) cirrhosis at diagnosis, (4) the presence of anti-SLA, and (5) incomplete normalization of the serum ALT level after 6 months of treatment.

When to Refer

- For liver biopsy.
- For immunosuppressive therapy.

When to Admit

- Hepatic encephalopathy.
- INR greater than 1.6.

Grønbæk L et al. Family occurrence of autoimmune hepatitis: a Danish nationwide registry-based cohort study. J Hepatol. 2018 Oct;69(4):873–7. [PMID: 29885414]

Peiseler M et al. Efficacy and limitations of budesonide as a second-line treatment for patients with autoimmune hepatitis. Clin Gastroenterol Hepatol. 2018 Feb;16(2):260–7. [PMID: 28126427]

Roberts SK et al. Efficacy and safety of mycophenolate mofetil in patients with autoimmune hepatitis and suboptimal outcomes after standard therapy. Clin Gastroenterol Hepatol. 2018 Feb;16(2):268–77. [PMID: 29050991]

Schmeltzer PA et al. Clinical narrative: autoimmune hepatitis. Am J Gastroenterol. 2018 Jul;113(7):951–8. [PMID: 29755125]

ALCOHOLIC LIVER DISEASE

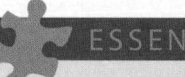

ESSENTIALS OF DIAGNOSIS

▶ Chronic alcohol intake usually exceeds 80 g/day in men and 30–40 g/day in women with alcoholic hepatitis or cirrhosis.

▶ Fatty liver is often asymptomatic.

▶ Fever, right upper quadrant pain, tender hepatomegaly, and jaundice characterize alcoholic hepatitis, but the patient may be asymptomatic.

▶ AST is usually elevated but usually not above 300 units/L (6 mckat/L); AST is greater than ALT, usually by a factor of 2 or more.

▶ Alcoholic hepatitis is often reversible, but it is the most common precursor of cirrhosis in the United States.

General Considerations

Excessive alcohol intake can lead to fatty liver, hepatitis, and cirrhosis. Validated tools, such as the Alcohol Use Disorders Inventory Test (AUDIT), can be used to identify persons with alcohol abuse and dependence (see Table 1–7). Alcoholic hepatitis is characterized by acute or chronic inflammation and parenchymal necrosis of the liver induced by alcohol. Alcoholic hepatitis is often a reversible disease but the most common precursor of cirrhosis in the United States. It is associated with four to five times the number of hospitalizations and deaths as hepatitis C.

The frequency of alcoholic cirrhosis is estimated to be 10–15% among persons who consume over 50 g of alcohol (4 oz of 100-proof whiskey, 15 oz of wine, or four 12-oz cans of beer) daily for over 10 years (although the risk of cirrhosis may be lower for wine than for a comparable intake of beer or spirits). The risk of cirrhosis is lower (5%) in the absence of other cofactors such as chronic viral hepatitis and obesity. Genetic factors may also account for differences in susceptibility to and severity of liver disease. Women appear to be more susceptible than men, in part because of lower gastric mucosal alcohol dehydrogenase levels, but young men who drink excessively are at increased risk for liver disease later in life when they are no longer drinking as much.

▶ Clinical Findings

A. Symptoms and Signs

The clinical presentation of alcoholic liver disease can vary from asymptomatic hepatomegaly to a rapidly fatal acute illness (acute-on-chronic liver failure) or end-stage cirrhosis. A recent period of heavy drinking, complaints of anorexia and nausea, and the demonstration of hepatomegaly and jaundice strongly suggest the diagnosis. Abdominal pain and tenderness, splenomegaly, ascites, fever, and encephalopathy may be present. Infection, including invasive aspergillosis, is common in patients with severe alcoholic hepatitis.

B. Laboratory Findings

In patients with steatosis, mild liver enzyme elevations may be the only laboratory abnormality. Anemia (usually macrocytic) may be present. Leukocytosis with a shift to the left is common in patients with severe alcoholic hepatitis. Leukopenia is occasionally seen and resolves after cessation of drinking. About 10% of patients have thrombocytopenia related to a direct toxic effect of alcohol on megakaryocyte production or to hypersplenism.

AST is usually elevated but infrequently above 300 units/L (6 mckat/L). AST is greater than ALT, usually by a factor of 2 or more. Serum alkaline phosphatase is generally elevated, but seldom more than three times the normal value. Serum bilirubin is increased in 60–90% of patients with alcoholic hepatitis.

Serum bilirubin levels greater than 10 mg/dL (171 mcmol/L) and marked prolongation of the prothrombin time (6 seconds or more above control) indicate severe alcoholic hepatitis with a mortality rate as high as 50%. The serum albumin is depressed, and the gamma-globulin level is elevated in 50–75% of individuals, even in the absence of cirrhosis. Increased transferrin saturation, hepatic iron stores, and sideroblastic anemia are found in many alcoholic patients. Folic acid deficiency may coexist.

C. Imaging

Imaging studies can detect moderate to severe hepatic steatosis reliably but not inflammation or fibrosis. Ultrasonography helps exclude biliary obstruction and identifies subclinical ascites. CT with intravenous contrast or MRI may be indicated in selected cases to evaluate patients for collateral vessels, space-occupying lesions of the liver, or concomitant disease of the pancreas.

D. Liver Biopsy

Liver biopsy, if done, demonstrates macrovesicular fat and, in patients with alcoholic hepatitis, polymorphonuclear infiltration with hepatic necrosis, Mallory (or Mallory-Denk) bodies (alcoholic hyaline), and perivenular and perisinusoidal fibrosis. Micronodular cirrhosis may be present as well. The findings are identical to those of nonalcoholic steatohepatitis.

▶ Differential Diagnosis

Alcoholic hepatitis may be closely mimicked by cholecystitis and cholelithiasis and by drug toxicity. Other causes of hepatitis or chronic liver disease may be excluded by serologic or biochemical testing, imaging studies, or liver biopsy. A formula based on the AST/ALT ratio, body mass index, mean corpuscular volume, and sex has been reported to reliably distinguish alcoholic liver disease from nonalcoholic fatty liver disease (NAFLD).

▶ Treatment

A. General Measures

Abstinence from alcohol is essential. Hospitalized patients should be monitored for alcohol withdrawal; the Clinical Institute Withdrawal Assessment for Alcohol (CIWA-Ar) is often used in practice (see Figure 25–3). Naltrexone, acamprosate, or baclofen may be considered in combination with counseling to reduce the likelihood of recidivism. Fatty liver is quickly reversible with abstinence. Every effort should be made to provide sufficient amounts of carbohydrates and calories in anorectic patients to reduce endogenous protein catabolism, promote gluconeogenesis, and prevent hypoglycemia. Nutritional support (30–40 [and no less than 21.5] kcal/kg with 1.0–1.5 g/kg as protein) improves liver disease, but not necessarily survival, in patients with malnutrition. Intensive enteral nutrition is difficult to implement, however. The administration of micronutrients, particularly folic acid, thiamine, and zinc, is indicated, especially when deficiencies are noted; glucose administration increases the thiamine requirement and can precipitate Wernicke-Korsakoff syndrome if thiamine is not coadministered. Nephrotoxic drugs should be avoided in patients with severe alcoholic hepatitis.

B. Pharmacologic Measures

Methylprednisolone, 32 mg/day orally, or the equivalent, for 1 month, may reduce short-term (1-month but not 6-month) mortality in patients with alcoholic hepatitis and encephalopathy or a Maddrey discriminant function index (defined by the patient's prothrombin time minus the control prothrombin time times 4.6 plus the total bilirubin in mg/dL) of 32 or more, or a MELD score of 20 or more (see Cirrhosis). Concomitant gastrointestinal bleeding or infection may not preclude treatment with corticosteroids if otherwise indicated, but treatment with prednisolone increases the risk of serious infections during and after treatment is completed. Prophylactic antibiotic therapy is under study. The combination of corticosteroids and N-acetylcysteine has been reported to further improve 1-month but not 6-month survival and reduce the risk of hepatorenal syndrome and infections; the combination may be superior to corticosteroids alone, but more data are needed.

Pentoxifylline, 400 mg orally three times daily for 4 weeks, decreases the risk of hepatorenal syndrome. It does not appear to reduce short-term mortality. Its use is not recommended in some guidelines, but it has been used when corticosteroids are contraindicated. The addition of pentoxifylline to prednisolone does not appear to improve survival but may reduce the frequency of hepatorenal syndrome compared with prednisolone alone. Other experimental therapies include propylthiouracil, oxandrolone, S-adenosyl-l-methionine, infliximab, antioxidants, granulocyte colony-stimulating factor, the combination of anakinra, zinc, and pentoxifylline, modulation of intestinal flora, and extracorporeal liver support. Colchicine does not reduce mortality in patients with alcoholic cirrhosis, and etanercept may increase mortality after 6 months.

▶ Prognosis

A. Short-Term

The overall mortality rate is 34% (20% within 1 month) without corticosteroid therapy. Individuals in whom the prothrombin time prohibits liver biopsy have a 42% mortality rate at 1 year. Other unfavorable prognostic factors are older age, a serum bilirubin greater than 10 mg/dL (171 mcmol/L), hepatic encephalopathy, coagulopathy, azotemia, leukocytosis, sepsis and other infections, systematic inflammatory response syndrome (which is associated with multiorgan failure), lack of response to corticosteroid therapy, and possibly a paucity of steatosis on a liver biopsy specimen and reversal of portal blood flow by Doppler ultrasonography. Concomitant gastrointestinal bleeding does not appear to worsen survival. Failure of the serum bilirubin level to decline after 7 days of treatment with corticosteroids predicts nonresponse and poor long-term survival, as does the Lille model (which includes age, serum creatinine, serum albumin, prothrombin time [or INR], serum bilirubin on admission, and serum bilirubin on day 7). The MELD score used for cirrhosis and the Glasgow alcoholic hepatitis score (based on age, white blood cell count, blood urea nitrogen, prothrombin time ratio, and bilirubin level) also correlate with mortality from alcoholic hepatitis and have higher specificities than the discriminant function and Lille score. A scoring system based on age, serum bilirubin, INR, and serum creatinine (ABIC) has been proposed, and at least one study has shown that the development of acute kidney injury is the most accurate predictor of 90-day mortality. Another scoring system based on hepatic encephalopathy, systemic inflammatory response syndrome, and MELD score has also been reported to predict acute kidney injury and mortality. The combination of the MELD score and Lille model

has also been reported to be the best predictor of short-term mortality among the scoring systems. Histologic features associated with 90-day mortality include the degree of fibrosis and neutrophil infiltration, presence of megamitochondria, and bilirubinostasis.

B. Long-Term

Overall mortality from alcoholic liver disease has declined slightly in the United States since 1980. Nevertheless, the 3-year mortality rate of persons who recover from acute alcoholic hepatitis is 10 times greater than that of control individuals of comparable age; the 5-year mortality rate is as high as 85%. Histologically severe disease is associated with continued excessive mortality rates after 3 years, whereas the death rate is not increased after the same period in those whose liver biopsy specimens show only mild alcoholic hepatitis. Complications of portal hypertension (ascites, variceal bleeding, hepatorenal syndrome), coagulopathy, and severe jaundice following recovery from acute alcoholic hepatitis also suggest a poor long-term prognosis.

The most important long-term prognostic factor is continued excessive drinking. The risk of alcoholic cirrhosis is greater in women than in men, associated with obesity, cigarette smoking, chronic hepatitis C, and low vitamin D levels; the risk is inversely associated with coffee drinking. Alcoholic cirrhosis is a risk factor for hepatocellular carcinoma, and the risk is highest in carriers of the *C282Y* mutation for hemochromatosis or those with increased hepatic iron. A 6-month period of abstinence is generally required before liver transplantation is considered, although this requirement has been questioned and early liver transplantation has been performed in selected patients with alcoholic hepatitis, with good outcomes. Optimal candidates have adequate social support, do not smoke, have no psychosis or personality disorder, are adherent to therapy, and have regular appointments with a psychiatrist or psychologist who specializes in addiction treatment. Patients with alcoholic liver disease are at higher risk for posttransplant malignancy than those with other types of liver disease because of alcohol and tobacco use.

▶ When to Refer

Refer patients with alcoholic hepatitis who require liver biopsy for diagnosis.

▶ When to Admit

- Hepatic encephalopathy.
- INR greater than 1.6.
- Total bilirubin 10 mg/dL or more.
- Inability to maintain hydration.

European Association for the Study of the Liver. EASL Clinical Practice Guidelines: management of alcohol-related liver disease. J Hepatol. 2018 Jul;69(1):154–81. [PMID: 29628280]
Fuster D et al. Alcohol use in patients with chronic liver disease. N Engl J Med. 2018 Sep 27;379(13):1251–61. [PMID: 30257164]

Lee BP et al. Outcomes of early liver transplantation for patients with severe alcoholic hepatitis. Gastroenterology. 2018 Aug; 155(2):422–30. [PMID: 29655837]

Louvet A et al. Corticosteroids reduce risk of death within 28 days for patients with severe alcoholic hepatitis, compared with pentoxifylline or placebo—a meta-analysis of individual data from controlled trials. Gastroenterology. 2018 Aug;155(2): 458–68. [PMID: 29738698]

Singal AK et al. ACG Clinical Guideline: alcoholic liver disease. Am J Gastroenterol. 2018 Feb;113(2):175–94. [PMID: 29336434]

DRUG- & TOXIN-INDUCED LIVER INJURY

ESSENTIALS OF DIAGNOSIS

► Drug-induced liver injury can mimic viral hepatitis, biliary tract obstruction, or other types of liver disease.

► Clinicians must inquire about the use of many widely used therapeutic agents, including over-the-counter "natural" and herbal and dietary supplements, in any patient with liver disease.

General Considerations

Many therapeutic agents may cause drug-induced liver injury, and up to 10% of patients with drug-induced liver injury die or undergo liver transplantation within 6 months of onset. In any patient with liver disease, the clinician must inquire carefully about the use of potentially hepatotoxic drugs or exposure to hepatotoxins, including over-the-counter herbal and dietary supplements. Khat chewing has been associated with an increased risk of chronic liver disease. The medications most commonly implicated are nonsteroidal anti-inflammatory drugs and antibiotics because of their widespread use. In some cases, coadministration of a second agent may increase the toxicity of the first (eg, isoniazid and rifampin, acetaminophen and alcohol). The diagnosis often depends on exclusion of other causes of liver disease. A relationship between increased serum ALT levels in premarketing clinical trials and postmarketing reports of hepatotoxicity has been identified. Except for drugs used to treat tuberculosis and HIV infection and possibly azithromycin, the risk of hepatotoxicity is not increased in patients with preexisting cirrhosis, but hepatotoxicity may be more severe and the outcome worse when it does occur. Older persons may be at higher risk for hepatotoxicity from certain agents, such as amoxicillin-clavulanic acid, isoniazid, and nitrofurantoin, and more likely to have persistent and cholestatic, rather than hepatocellular, injury compared with younger persons. Drug toxicity may be categorized on the basis of pathogenesis or predominant histologic appearance. Drug-induced liver injury can mimic viral hepatitis, biliary tract obstruction, or other types of liver disease. The development of jaundice in a patient with serum aminotransferase levels at least three times the upper limit of normal predicts a mortality rate of at least 10% ("Hy's Law"). A useful resource is the website https://livertox.nlm.nih.gov/.

Categorization by Pathogenesis

A. Direct Hepatotoxicity

Liver toxicity caused by this group of drugs is characterized by dose-related severity, a latent period following exposure, and susceptibility in all individuals. Examples include acetaminophen (whose toxicity is enhanced by fasting because of depletion of glutathione and by long-term alcohol use both because of depletion of glutathione and because of induction of cytochrome P450 2E1; and whose toxicity is possibly reduced by statins, fibrates, and nonsteroidal anti-inflammatory drugs, and acetylcysteine treatment). Other examples include alcohol, *Amanita phalloides* mushrooms, carbon tetrachloride, chloroform, heavy metals, mercaptopurine, niacin, plant alkaloids, phosphorus, pyrazinamide, tetracyclines, tipranavir, valproic acid, and vitamin A.

B. Idiosyncratic Reactions

Except for acetaminophen, most severe hepatotoxicity is idiosyncratic. Reactions of this type are (1) sporadic, (2) not related to dose above a general threshold of 100 mg/day, and (3) occasionally associated with features suggesting an allergic reaction, such as fever and eosinophilia (including drug rash with eosinophilia and systemic symptoms [DRESS] syndrome), which may be associated with a favorable outcome. In many instances, the drug is lipophilic, and toxicity results directly from a reactive metabolite that is produced only in certain individuals on a genetic basis. Illness tends to be more severe in blacks than in whites. Drug-induced liver injury may be observed only during post-marketing surveillance and not during preclinical trials. Examples include abacavir, amiodarone, aspirin, carbamazepine, chloramphenicol, dapsone, diclofenac, disulfiram, duloxetine, ezetimibe, flavocoxid (a "medical food"), fluoroquinolones (levofloxacin and moxifloxacin, in particular), flutamide, halothane, isoniazid, ketoconazole, lamotrigine, methyldopa, natalizumab, nevirapine, oxacillin, phenytoin, pyrazinamide, quinidine, rivaroxaban, streptomycin, temozolomide, thiazolidinediones, tolvaptan, and perhaps tacrine. Statins, like all cholesterol-lowering agents, may cause serum aminotransferase elevations but rarely cause true hepatitis, and even more rarely cause acute liver failure, and are no longer considered contraindicated in patients with liver disease. Most acute idiosyncratic drug-induced liver injury is reversible with discontinuation of the offending agent. Risk factors for chronicity (longer than 1 year) are older age, dyslipidemia, and severe acute injury.

Categorization by Histopathology

A. Cholestasis

1. Noninflammatory—Drug-induced cholestasis results from inhibition or genetic deficiency of various hepatobiliary transporter systems. The following drugs cause cholestasis: anabolic steroids containing an alkyl or ethinyl group at carbon 17, azathioprine, cetirizine, cyclosporine, diclofenac, estrogens, febuxostat, indinavir (increased risk of indirect hyperbilirubinemia in patients with Gilbert syndrome), mercaptopurine, methyltestosterone, tamoxifen, temozolomide, and ticlopidine.

2. Inflammatory—The following drugs cause inflammation of portal areas with bile duct injury (cholangitis [and, in some cases, bile duct loss]), often with allergic features such as eosinophilia: amoxicillin-clavulanic acid (among the most common causes of drug-induced liver injury), azathioprine, azithromycin, captopril, celecoxib, cephalosporins, chlorothiazide, chlorpromazine, chlorpropamide, erythromycin, mercaptopurine, penicillamine, prochlorperazine, semisynthetic penicillins (eg, cloxacillin), sulfadiazine, and temozolomide. Ketamine abuse may cause secondary biliary cirrhosis. Cholestatic and mixed cholestatic-hepatocellular toxicity is more likely than pure hepatocellular toxicity to lead to chronic liver disease.

B. Acute or Chronic Hepatitis

Medications that may result in acute or chronic hepatitis that is histologically and, in some cases, clinically similar to autoimmune hepatitis include minocycline and nitrofurantoin, most commonly, as well as aspirin, isoniazid (increased risk in HBV and HCV carriers), methyldopa, nonsteroidal anti-inflammatory drugs, propylthiouracil, terbinafine, tumor necrosis factor inhibitors, and varenicline. Histologic features that favor a drug cause include portal tract neutrophils and hepatocellular cholestasis. Hepatitis also can occur in patients taking cocaine, diclofenac, dimethyl fumarate, efavirenz, imatinib mesylate, ipilimumab, nivolumab, and other checkpoint inhibitors, methylenedioxymethamphetamine (MDMA; Ecstasy), nefazodone (has a black box warning for a potential to cause liver failure), nevirapine (like other protease inhibitors, increased risk in HBV and HCV carriers), pioglitazone, ritonavir (greater rate than other protease inhibitors), rosiglitazone, saquinavir, sulfonamides, telithromycin, and zafirlukast, as well as a variety of alternative remedies (eg, black cohosh, chaparral, germander, green tea extract, Herbalife products, Hydroxycut, jin bu huan, kava, saw palmetto, skullcap, and other traditional Chinese herbal preparations), in addition to dietary supplements (eg, 1, 3-dimethylamylamine in OxyELITE Pro, a weight-loss supplement withdrawn from the US market).

C. Other Reactions

1. Fatty liver

A. Macrovesicular—This type of liver injury may be produced by alcohol, amiodarone, corticosteroids, irinotecan, lomitapide, methotrexate, mipomersen, tamoxifen, vinyl chloride (in exposed workers), zalcitabine, and possibly oxaliplatin.

B. Microvesicular—Often resulting from mitochondrial injury, this condition is associated with didanosine, stavudine, tetracyclines, valproic acid, and zidovudine.

2. Granulomas—Allopurinol, hydralazine, pembrolizumab and other immune checkpoint inhibitors, phenytoin, pyrazinamide, quinidine, quinine, sulfasalazine, and vemurafenib can lead to granulomas and, in some cases, granulomatous hepatitis.

3. Fibrosis and cirrhosis—Methotrexate and vitamin A are associated with fibrosis and cirrhosis.

4. Sinusoidal obstruction syndrome (veno-occlusive disease)—This disorder may result from treatment with antineoplastic agents (eg, pre–bone marrow transplant, busulfan, gemtuzumab ozogamicin, oxaliplatin) and pyrrolizidine alkaloids (eg, comfrey).

5. Peliosis hepatis (blood-filled cavities)—Peliosis hepatis may be caused by anabolic steroids and oral contraceptive steroids as well as azathioprine and mercaptopurine, which may also cause nodular regenerative hyperplasia and other forms of liver injury.

6. Neoplasms—Neoplasms may result from therapy with oral contraceptive steroids, including estrogens (hepatic adenoma but not focal nodular hyperplasia) and vinyl chloride (angiosarcoma).

► When to Refer

Refer patients with drug- and toxin-induced hepatitis who require liver biopsy for diagnosis.

► When to Admit

Patients with liver failure should be hospitalized.

Andrade RJ et al. Hepatic damage by natural remedies. Semin Liver Dis. 2018 Feb;38(1):21–40. [PMID: 29471563]

De Martin E et al. Characterization of liver injury induced by cancer immunotherapy using immune checkpoint inhibitors. J Hepatol. 2018 Jun;68(6):1181–90. [PMID: 29427729]

Medina-Caliz I et al. Herbal and dietary supplement-induced liver injuries in the Spanish DILI Registry. Clin Gastroenterol Hepatol. 2018 Sep;16(9):1495–502. [PMID: 29307848]

Mukhinuthalapati PK et al. Celecoxib-induced liver injury: analysis of published case reports and cases reported to the Food and Drug Administration. J Clin Gastroenterol. 2018 Feb;52(2):114–22. [PMID: 28795997]

Navarro VJ et al. Liver injury from herbal and dietary supplements. Hepatology. 2017 Jan;65(1):363–73. [PMID: 27677775]

Reynolds K et al. Diagnosis and management of hepatitis in patients on checkpoint blockade. Oncologist. 2018 Sep;23(9):991–7. [PMID: 29853659]

NONALCOHOLIC FATTY LIVER DISEASE

ESSENTIALS OF DIAGNOSIS

► Often asymptomatic.

► Elevated aminotransferase levels, hepatomegaly, or steatosis on ultrasonography.

► Predominantly macrovesicular steatosis with or without inflammation and fibrosis on liver biopsy.

General Considerations

Nonalcoholic fatty liver disease (NAFLD) is estimated to affect 20–45% of the US population and has increased in incidence at least fivefold since the late 1990s. Even adolescents and young adults may be affected. The principal causes of NAFLD are obesity (present in 40% or more of affected patients), diabetes mellitus (in 20% or more), and hypertriglyceridemia (in 20% or more) in association with insulin resistance as part of the metabolic syndrome. The risk of NAFLD in persons with metabolic syndrome is 4 to 11 times higher than that of persons without insulin resistance. Nonobese persons (more frequently Asians) account for 3–30% of persons with NAFLD and have metabolic profiles characteristic of insulin resistance. Other causes of fatty liver include corticosteroids, amiodarone, diltiazem, tamoxifen, irinotecan, oxaliplatin, antiretroviral therapy, toxins (vinyl chloride, carbon tetrachloride, yellow phosphorus), endocrinopathies such as Cushing syndrome and hypopituitarism, polycystic ovary syndrome, hypothyroidism, hypobetalipoproteinemia and other metabolic disorders, obstructive sleep apnea (with chronic intermittent hypoxia), excessive dietary fructose consumption, starvation and refeeding syndrome, and total parenteral nutrition. NAFLD may be a predisposing factor in liver injury caused by some drugs. Gut dysbiosis and genetic factors play a role in NAFLD, and may account in part for an increased risk in Hispanics. The risk of NAFLD is increased in persons with psoriasis and appears to correlate with the activity of psoriasis. Soft drink consumption and cholecystectomy have been reported to be associated with NAFLD. Physical activity protects against the development of NAFLD.

In addition to macrovesicular steatosis, histologic features may include focal infiltration by polymorphonuclear neutrophils and Mallory hyalin, a picture indistinguishable from that of alcoholic hepatitis and referred to as nonalcoholic steatohepatitis (NASH), which affects 3–5% of the US population. In patients with NAFLD, older age, obesity, and diabetes mellitus are risk factors for advanced hepatic fibrosis and cirrhosis, whereas coffee consumption reduces the risk. In women, synthetic hormone use (oral contraceptives and hormone replacement therapy) increases the histologic severity of NASH. Cirrhosis caused by NASH appears to be uncommon in African Americans. Persons with NAFLD are at increased risk for cardiovascular disease, chronic kidney disease, and colorectal cancer.

Microvesicular steatosis is seen with Reye syndrome, didanosine or stavudine toxicity, valproic acid toxicity, high-dose tetracycline, or acute fatty liver of pregnancy and may result in acute liver failure. Women in whom fatty liver of pregnancy develops often have a defect in fatty acid oxidation due to reduced long-chain 3-hydroxyacyl-CoA dehydrogenase activity.

Clinical Findings

A. Symptoms and Signs

Most patients with NAFLD are asymptomatic or have mild right upper quadrant discomfort. Hepatomegaly is present in up to 75% of patients, but stigmata of chronic liver disease are uncommon. Rare instances of subacute liver failure caused by previously unrecognized NASH have been described. Signs of portal hypertension generally signify advanced liver fibrosis or cirrhosis, but occasionally occur in patients with mild or no fibrosis and severe steatosis.

B. Laboratory Findings

Laboratory studies may show mildly elevated aminotransferase and alkaline phosphatase levels; however, laboratory values may be normal in up to 80% of persons with hepatic steatosis. In contrast to alcoholic liver disease, the ratio of ALT to AST is almost always greater than 1 in NAFLD, but it decreases, often to less than 1, as advanced fibrosis and cirrhosis develop. Antinuclear or smooth muscle antibodies and an elevated serum ferritin level may each be detected in one-fourth of patients with NASH. Iron deficiency is also common and associated with female sex, obesity, increased waist circumference, diabetes mellitus, and black or Native American race.

C. Imaging

Macrovascular steatosis may be demonstrated on ultrasonography, CT, or MRI. However, imaging does not distinguish steatosis from steatohepatitis or detect fibrosis.

D. Liver Biopsy

Percutaneous liver biopsy is diagnostic and is the standard approach to assessing the degree of inflammation and fibrosis. The risks of the procedure must be balanced against the impact of the added information on management decisions and assessment of prognosis. Liver biopsy is generally not recommended in asymptomatic persons with unsuspected hepatic steatosis detected on imaging but normal liver biochemistry test results. The histologic spectrum of NAFLD includes fatty liver, isolated portal fibrosis, steatohepatitis, and cirrhosis. A risk score for predicting advanced fibrosis, known as BARD, is based on body mass index more than 28, AST/ALT ratio 0.8 or more, and diabetes mellitus; it has a high negative predictive value (ie, a low score reliably excludes advanced fibrosis). Another risk score for advanced fibrosis, the NAFLD Fibrosis Score (http://nafldscore.com) based on age, hyperglycemia, body mass index, platelet count, albumin, and AST/ALT ratio, has a positive predictive value of over 80% and identifies patients at increased risk for liver-related complications and death. Another index for predicting fibrosis that has also performed well is FIB-4, which is based on the platelet count, age, and serum AST and ALT levels. A clinical scoring system to predict the likelihood of NASH in morbidly obese persons includes six predictive factors: hypertension, type 2 diabetes mellitus, sleep apnea, AST greater than 27 units/L (0.54 mckat/L), ALT greater than 27 units/L (0.54 mckat/L), and non-black race.

Treatment

Treatment consists of lifestyle changes to remove or modify the offending factors. Weight loss, dietary fat restriction, and moderate exercise (through reduction of abdominal obesity) often lead to improvement in liver biochemical tests and steatosis in obese patients with NAFLD. A Mediterranean diet can reduce liver fat without weight loss and is often recommended. Loss of 3–5% of body weight appears necessary to improve steatosis, but loss of at least 10% may be needed to improve necroinflammation and fibrosis. Exercise may reduce liver fat with minimal or no weight loss and no reduction in ALT levels. Resistance training and aerobic exercise are equally effective in reducing hepatic fat content in patients with NAFLD and type 2 diabetes mellitus. Although avoidance of alcohol is recommended, modest wine consumption may not be detrimental. Various drugs for the treatment of NASH are under study. Vitamin E 800 international units/day (to reduce oxidative stress) appears to be of benefit in patients with NASH who do not have diabetes mellitus; there is controversy as to whether vitamin E increases the risk of prostate cancer in men. Thiazolidinediones reverse insulin resistance and, in most relevant studies, have improved both serum aminotransferase levels and histologic features of steatohepatitis but lead to weight gain. Metformin, which reduces insulin resistance, improves abnormal liver chemistries but may not reliably improve liver histology. Pentoxifylline improves liver biochemical test levels but is associated with a high rate of side effects, particularly nausea. Ursodeoxycholic acid, 12–15 mg/kg/day, has not consistently resulted in biochemical and histologic improvement in patients with NASH but may be effective when given in combination with vitamin E. Hepatic steatosis due to total parenteral nutrition may be ameliorated—and perhaps prevented—with supplemental choline. Obeticholic acid, a semisynthetic bile acid analog that has been approved for the treatment of primary biliary cholangitis, has been used. Statins are not contraindicated in persons with NAFLD and may protect against histologic progression in some patients. Bariatric surgery may be considered in patients with a body mass index greater than 35 and leads to histologic regression of NASH in most patients. Liver transplantation is indicated in appropriate candidates with advanced cirrhosis caused by NASH, now the third most common (and most rapidly increasing) indication for liver transplantation in the United States. Liver transplantation for NASH with advanced cirrhosis may be associated with increased mortality from cardiovascular disease and sepsis compared with liver transplantation for other indications.

Prognosis

Fatty liver often has a benign course and is readily reversible with discontinuation of alcohol (or no more than one glass of wine per day, which has been reported in some, but not other, studies to reduce the frequency of NASH in persons with NAFLD), or treatment of other underlying conditions; if untreated, fibrosis progresses at an average rate of 1 stage every 14 years, with 20% of patients progressing more rapidly. In patients with NAFLD, the likelihood of NASH is increased by the following factors: obesity, older age, non–African American ethnicity, female sex, diabetes mellitus, hypertension, higher ALT or AST level, higher AST/ALT ratio, low platelet count, elevated fasting C-peptide level, and a high ultrasound steatosis score. NASH may be associated with hepatic fibrosis in 40% of

cases with progression at a rate of 1 stage every 7 years; cirrhosis develops in 9–25%; and decompensated cirrhosis occurs in 30–50% of cirrhotic patients over 10 years. The course may be more aggressive in diabetic persons than in nondiabetic persons. Mortality is increased in patients with NAFLD, correlates with fibrosis stage, and is more likely to be the result of malignancy (including hepatocellular carcinoma, colorectal cancer, and breast cancer) and cardiovascular disease than liver disease. Risk factors for mortality are older age, male sex, white race, smoking, higher body mass index, hypertension, diabetes mellitus, and cirrhosis. Steatosis is a cofactor for the progression of fibrosis in patients with other causes of chronic liver disease, such as hepatitis C. Hepatocellular carcinoma is a complication of cirrhosis caused by NASH, as it is for other causes of cirrhosis, and has been reported even in the absence of cirrhosis. NASH accounts for a substantial percentage of cases labeled as cryptogenic cirrhosis and can recur following liver transplantation. Central obesity is an independent risk factor for death from cirrhosis of any cause.

When to Refer

Refer patients with NAFLD who require liver biopsy for diagnosis.

Chalasani N et al. The diagnosis and management of nonalcoholic fatty liver disease: practice guidance from the American Association for the Study of Liver Diseases. Hepatology. 2018 Jan;67(1):328–57. [PMID: 28714183]

Konerman MA et al. Pharmacotherapy for NASH: current and emerging. J Hepatol. 2018 Feb;68(2):362–75. [PMID: 29122694]

Loomba R. Role of imaging-based biomarkers in NAFLD: recent advances in clinical application and future research directions. J Hepatol. 2018 Feb;68(2):296–304. [PMID: 29203392]

Verhaegh P et al. Noninvasive tests do not accurately differentiate nonalcoholic steatohepatitis from simple steatosis: a systematic review and meta-analysis. Clin Gastroenterol Hepatol. 2018 Jun;16(6):837–61. [PMID: 28838784]

Younossi ZM et al. Current and future therapeutic regimens for nonalcoholic fatty liver disease and nonalcoholic steatohepatitis. Hepatology. 2018 Jul;68(1):361–71. [PMID: 29222911]

CIRRHOSIS

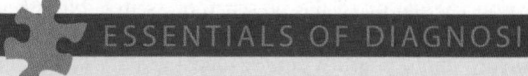

ESSENTIALS OF DIAGNOSIS

- ► End result of injury that leads to both fibrosis and regenerative nodules.
- ► May be reversible if cause is removed.
- ► The clinical features result from hepatic cell dysfunction, portosystemic shunting, and portal hypertension.

General Considerations

Cirrhosis, the eleventh leading cause of death globally and eighth leading cause of death in the United States with a prevalence rate of 0.27%, is the end result of hepatocellular injury that leads to both fibrosis and regenerative nodules throughout the liver. Hospitalization rates for cirrhosis and portal hypertension are rising in the United States, and patients with chronic liver disease have longer hospital stays, more readmissions, and less access to post-acute care than patients with other chronic diseases. Causes include chronic viral hepatitis; alcohol; drug toxicity; autoimmune and metabolic liver diseases, including NAFLD; and miscellaneous disorders. Celiac disease appears to be associated with an increased risk of cirrhosis. Many patients have more than one risk factor (eg, chronic hepatitis and alcohol use). Mexican Americans and African Americans have a higher frequency of cirrhosis than whites because of a higher rate of risk factors. In persons at increased risk for liver injury (eg, heavy alcohol use, obesity, iron overload), higher coffee and tea consumption and statin use reduce the risk of cirrhosis.

Clinically, cirrhosis is considered to progress through three stages that correlate with the thickness of fibrous septa: compensated, compensated with varices, and decompensated (ascites, variceal bleeding, encephalopathy, or jaundice). A diagnosis of acute-on-chronic liver failure should be made in a patient with cirrhosis and acute decompensation (new or worsening ascites, gastrointestinal hemorrhage, overt encephalopathy, worsening nonobstructive jaundice, or bacterial infection associated with other organ failure). Precipitating factors include infections, hemodynamic instability, heavy alcohol use, and drug hepatotoxicity.

► Clinical Findings

A. Symptoms and Signs

The clinical features of cirrhosis result from hepatocyte dysfunction, portosystemic shunting, and portal hypertension. Patients may have no symptoms for long periods. The onset of symptoms may be insidious or, less often, abrupt. Fatigue, disturbed sleep, muscle cramps, and weight loss are common. In advanced cirrhosis, anorexia is usually present and may be extreme, with associated nausea and occasional vomiting, as well as reduced muscle strength and exercise capacity. Abdominal pain may be present and is related either to hepatic enlargement and stretching of Glisson capsule or to the presence of ascites. Menstrual abnormalities (usually amenorrhea), erectile dysfunction, loss of libido, sterility, and gynecomastia may occur. Hematemesis is the presenting symptom in 15–25%. The risk of falls is increased in hospitalized patients with cirrhosis who are taking psychoactive medications.

Skin manifestations consist of spider telangiectasias (invariably on the upper half of the body), palmar erythema (mottled redness of the thenar and hypothenar eminences), and Dupuytren contractures. Evidence of vitamin deficiencies (glossitis and cheilosis) is common. Weight loss, wasting (due to sarcopenia), and the appearance of chronic illness are present. Jaundice—usually not an initial sign—is mild at first, increasing in severity during the later stages of the disease. In 70% of cases, the liver is enlarged, palpable, and firm if not hard and has a sharp or nodular edge; the left lobe may predominate. Splenomegaly is present in 35–50% of cases and is associated with an increased risk of complications of portal hypertension. The superficial veins of the abdomen and thorax are dilated, reflecting the intrahepatic obstruction to portal blood flow, as do rectal varices. The abdominal wall veins fill from below when compressed. Ascites, pleural effusions, peripheral edema, and ecchymoses are late findings. Encephalopathy, characterized by day-night reversal, asterixis, tremor, dysarthria, delirium, drowsiness and, ultimately coma also occurs late in the course except when precipitated by an acute hepatocellular insult or an episode of gastrointestinal bleeding or infection. Fever is present in up to 35% of patients and usually reflects associated alcoholic hepatitis, spontaneous bacterial peritonitis, or another intercurrent infection.

B. Laboratory Findings

Laboratory abnormalities are either absent or minimal in early or compensated cirrhosis. Anemia, a frequent finding, is often macrocytic; causes include suppression of erythropoiesis by alcohol as well as folate deficiency, hemolysis, hypersplenism, and occult or overt blood loss from the gastrointestinal tract. The white blood cell count may be low, reflecting hypersplenism, or high, suggesting infection. Thrombocytopenia, the most common cytopenia in cirrhotic patients, is secondary to alcoholic marrow suppression, sepsis, folate deficiency, or splenic sequestration. Prolongation of the prothrombin time may result from reduced levels of clotting factors (except factor VIII). However, bleeding risk correlates poorly with the prothrombin time because of concomitant abnormalities of fibrinolysis, and among hospitalized patients under age 45, cirrhosis is associated with an increased risk of venous thromboembolism.

Blood chemistries reflect hepatocellular injury and dysfunction, manifested by modest elevations of AST and alkaline phosphatase and progressive elevation of the bilirubin. Serum albumin decreases as the disease progresses; gammaglobulin levels are increased and may be as high as in autoimmune hepatitis. The risk of diabetes mellitus is increased in patients with cirrhosis, particularly when associated with HCV infection, alcoholism, hemochromatosis, or NAFLD. Vitamin D deficiency has been reported in as many as 91% of patients with cirrhosis. In cirrhosis of all causes, the following are common: (1) blunted cardiac inotropic and chronotropic responses to exercise, stress, and drugs, (2) prolongation of the QT interval in the setting of a hyperkinetic circulation, and (3) systolic and diastolic ventricular dysfunction in the absence of other known causes of cardiac disease ("cirrhotic cardiomyopathy"). Relative adrenal insufficiency appears to be common in patients with advanced cirrhosis, even in the absence of sepsis, and may relate in part to reduced synthesis of cholesterol and increased levels of proinflammatory cytokines.

C. Imaging

Ultrasonography is helpful for assessing liver size and detecting ascites or hepatic nodules, including small hepatocellular carcinomas. Together with a Doppler study, it may establish patency of the splenic, portal, and hepatic veins. Hepatic nodules are characterized further by contrast-enhanced CT or MRI. Nodules suspicious for malignancy may be biopsied under ultrasound or CT guidance.

D. Liver Biopsy

Liver biopsy may show inactive cirrhosis (fibrosis with regenerative nodules) with no specific features to suggest the underlying cause. Alternatively, there may be additional features of alcoholic liver disease, chronic hepatitis, NASH, or other specific causes of cirrhosis. Liver biopsy may be performed by laparoscopy or, in patients with coagulopathy and ascites, by a transjugular approach. Combinations of routine blood tests (eg, AST, platelet count), including the FibroSure test, serum markers of hepatic fibrosis (eg, hyaluronic acid, amino-terminal propeptide of type III collagen, tissue inhibitor of matrix metalloproteinase 1), ultrasound, or magnetic resonance elastography are potential alternatives to liver biopsy for the diagnosis or exclusion of cirrhosis. In persons with chronic hepatitis C, for example, a low FibroSure or elastography score reliably excludes advanced fibrosis, a high score reliably predicts advanced fibrosis, and intermediate scores are inconclusive.

E. Other Tests

Esophagogastroduodenoscopy confirms the presence of varices and detects specific causes of bleeding in the esophagus, stomach, and proximal duodenum. In selected cases, wedged hepatic vein pressure measurement may establish the presence and cause of portal hypertension.

▶ Differential Diagnosis

The most common causes of cirrhosis are alcohol, chronic hepatitis C infection, NAFLD, and hepatitis B infection. Hemochromatosis is the most commonly identified genetic disorder that causes cirrhosis. Other diseases associated with cirrhosis include Wilson disease, alpha-1-antitrypsin (alpha-1-antiprotease) deficiency, and celiac disease. PBC occurs more frequently in women than men. Secondary biliary cirrhosis may result from chronic biliary obstruction due to a stone, stricture, or neoplasm. Heart failure and constrictive pericarditis may lead to hepatic fibrosis ("cardiac cirrhosis") complicated by ascites. Hereditary hemorrhagic telangiectasia can lead to portal hypertension because of portosystemic shunting and nodular transformation of the liver as well as high-output heart failure. Many cases of cirrhosis are "cryptogenic," in which unrecognized NAFLD may play a role.

▶ Complications

Upper gastrointestinal tract bleeding may occur from varices, portal hypertensive gastropathy, or gastroduodenal ulcer (see Chapter 15). Varices may also result from portal vein thrombosis, which may complicate cirrhosis. Liver failure may be precipitated by alcoholism, surgery, and infection. Hepatic Kupffer cell (reticuloendothelial) dysfunction and decreased opsonic activity lead to an increased risk of systemic infection (which may be increased further by the use of proton pump inhibitors, which increase mortality fourfold). These infections include nosocomial infections, which may be classified as spontaneous bloodstream infections, urinary tract infections, pulmonary infections, spontaneous bacterial peritonitis, *Clostridioides difficile* infection, and intervention-related infections. These nosocomial infections are increasingly caused by multidrug-resistant bacteria. Osteoporosis occurs in 12–55% of patients with cirrhosis. The risk of hepatocellular carcinoma is increased greatly in persons with cirrhosis (see Chapter 39). Varices, ascites, and encephalopathy may arise when there is clinically significant portal hypertension (hepatic venous pressure gradient greater than 10 mm Hg).

▶ Treatment

A. General Measures

Most important is abstinence from alcohol. The diet should be palatable, with adequate calories (20–40 kcal/kg body weight per day depending on the patient's body mass index and the presence or absence of malnutrition) and protein (1–1.5 g/kg/day depending on the presence or absence of malnutrition) and, if there is fluid retention, sodium restriction. In the presence of hepatic encephalopathy, protein intake should be reduced to no less than 60–80 g/day. Vitamin supplementation is desirable. Muscle cramps may be helped by L-carnitine, 300 mg orally four times a day. Patients with cirrhosis should receive the HAV, HBV, and pneumococcal vaccines and a yearly influenza vaccine. Liver transplantation in appropriate candidates is curative. Care coordination and palliative care, when appropriate, have been shown to improve outcomes and reduce readmission rates.

B. Treatment of Complications

1. Ascites and edema—Diagnostic paracentesis is indicated for patients who have new ascites or who have been hospitalized for a complication of cirrhosis; it reduces mortality, especially if performed within 12 hours of admission. Serious complications of paracentesis, including bleeding, infection, or bowel perforation, occur in 1.6% of procedures and are associated with therapeutic (vs diagnostic) paracentesis and possibly with Child-Pugh class C, a platelet count less than 50,000/mcL (50×10^9/L), and alcoholic cirrhosis. In patients with coagulopathy, however, pre-paracentesis prophylactic transfusions do not appear to be necessary. In addition to a cell count and culture, the ascitic albumin level should be determined: a serum-ascites albumin gradient (serum albumin minus ascitic fluid albumin) greater than or equal to 1.1 suggests portal hypertension. An elevated ascitic adenosine deaminase level is suggestive of tuberculous peritonitis. Occasionally, cirrhotic ascites is chylous (rich in triglycerides); other causes of chylous ascites are malignancy, tuberculosis, and recent abdominal surgery or trauma.

In individuals with ascites, the urinary sodium concentration is often less than 10 mEq/L (10 mmol/L). Free water excretion is also impaired in cirrhosis, and hyponatremia may develop.

In all patients with cirrhotic ascites, dietary sodium intake may initially be restricted to 2000 mg/day; the intake of sodium may be liberalized slightly after diuresis ensues. Nonsteroidal anti-inflammatory drugs are contraindicated, and angiotensin-converting enzyme inhibitors and angiotensin II antagonists should be avoided. In some patients, ascites diminishes promptly with bed rest and dietary sodium restriction alone. Fluid intake is often restricted (to 800–1000 mL/day) in patients with hyponatremia. Treatment of severe hyponatremia (serum sodium less than 125 mEq/L [125 mmol/L]) with vasopressin receptor antagonists (eg, intravenous conivaptan, 20 mg daily) can be considered but such treatment is expensive, causes thirst, and does not improve survival; oral tolvaptan is contraindicated in patients with liver disease because of potential hepatotoxicity. Long-term intravenous administration of albumin has been reported to improve 18-month survival in patients with cirrhotic ascites.

A. DIURETICS—Spironolactone, generally in combination with furosemide, should be used in patients who do not respond to salt restriction alone. The dose of spironolactone is initially 100 mg orally daily and may be increased by 100 mg every 3–5 days (up to a maximal conventional daily dose of 400 mg/day, although higher doses have been used) until diuresis is achieved, typically preceded by a rise in the urinary sodium concentration. A "spot" urine sodium concentration that exceeds the potassium concentration correlates with a 24-hour sodium excretion greater than 78 mmol/day, which predicts diuresis in patients adherent to a salt-restricted diet. Monitoring for hyperkalemia is important. In patients who cannot tolerate spironolactone because of side effects, such as painful gynecomastia, amiloride (another potassium-sparing diuretic) may be used in a starting dose of 5–10 mg orally daily. Diuresis is augmented by the addition of a loop diuretic such as furosemide. This potent diuretic, however, will maintain its effect even with a falling glomerular filtration rate, with resulting prerenal azotemia. The dose of oral furosemide ranges from 40 mg/day to 160 mg/day, and blood pressure, urinary output, mental status, and serum electrolytes (especially potassium) should be monitored in patients taking the drug. The goal of weight loss in the ascitic patient without associated peripheral edema should be no more than 1–1.5 lb/day (0.5–0.7 kg/day).

B. LARGE-VOLUME PARACENTESIS—In patients with massive ascites and respiratory compromise, ascites refractory to diuretics ("diuretic resistant"), or intolerable diuretic side effects ("diuretic intractable"), large-volume paracentesis (more than 5 L) is effective. Intravenous albumin concomitantly at a dosage of 6–8 g/L of ascites fluid removed protects the intravascular volume and may prevent postparacentesis circulatory dysfunction, although the usefulness of this practice is debated and albumin is expensive. Large-volume paracentesis can be repeated daily until ascites is largely resolved and may decrease the need for hospitalization. If possible, diuretics should be continued in the hope of preventing recurrent ascites.

C. TRANSJUGULAR INTRAHEPATIC PORTOSYSTEMIC SHUNT (TIPS)—TIPS is an effective treatment of variceal bleeding refractory to standard therapy (eg, endoscopic band ligation) and has shown benefit in the treatment of severe refractory ascites. The technique involves insertion of an expandable metal stent between a branch of the hepatic vein and the portal vein over a catheter inserted via the internal jugular vein. Increased renal sodium excretion and control of ascites refractory to diuretics can be achieved in about 75% of selected cases. The success rate is lower in patients with underlying chronic kidney disease. TIPS appears to be the treatment of choice for refractory hepatic hydrothorax (translocation of ascites across the diaphragm to the pleural space); video-assisted thoracoscopy with pleurodesis using talc may be effective when TIPS is contraindicated. Complications of TIPS include hepatic encephalopathy in 20–30% of cases, infection, shunt stenosis in up to 60% of cases, and shunt occlusion in up to 30% of cases when bare stents are used; polytetrafluoroethylene-covered stents are associated with long-term patency rates of 80–90%. Long-term patency often requires periodic shunt revisions. In most cases, patency can be maintained by balloon dilation, local thrombolysis, or placement of an additional stent. TIPS is particularly useful in patients who require short-term control of variceal bleeding or ascites until liver transplantation can be performed. In patients with refractory ascites, TIPS results in lower rates of ascites recurrence and hepatorenal syndrome but a higher rate of hepatic encephalopathy than occurs with repeated large-volume paracentesis; a benefit in survival has been demonstrated in one study and a meta-analysis. Chronic kidney disease, diastolic cardiac dysfunction, refractory encephalopathy, and hyperbilirubinemia (greater than 5 mg/dL [85.5 mcmol/L]) are associated with mortality after TIPS.

2. Spontaneous bacterial peritonitis—Spontaneous bacterial peritonitis is heralded by abdominal pain, increasing ascites, fever, and progressive encephalopathy in a patient with cirrhotic ascites; symptoms are typically mild. (Analogously, spontaneous bacterial empyema may complicate hepatic hydrothorax and is managed similarly.) Risk factors in cirrhotic patients with ascites include gastroesophageal variceal bleeding and possibly use of a proton pump inhibitor. Paracentesis reveals an ascitic fluid with, most commonly, a total white cell count of up to 500 cells/mcL with a high polymorphonuclear (PMN) cell count (250/mcL or more) and a protein concentration of 1 g/dL (10 g/L) or less, corresponding to decreased ascitic opsonic activity. Cultures of ascites give the highest yield—80–90% positive—using specialized culture bottles inoculated at the bedside. Common isolates are *Escherichia coli* and *Streptococcus* spp. Gram-positive cocci are the most common isolates in patients who have undergone an invasive procedure such as central venous line placement, and the frequency of enterococcal isolates is increasing. Anaerobes are uncommon. Pending culture results, if there are 250 or more PMNs/mcL or symptoms or signs of infection, intravenous antibiotic therapy should be initiated with cefotaxime, 2 g every 8–12 hours for at least 5 days. Alternative choices include ceftriaxone, amoxicillin-clavulanic acid, and levofloxacin (in patients not receiving fluoroquinolone prophylaxis). Oral ofloxacin, 400 mg twice daily for 7 days, or, in a patient not already taking a fluoroquinolone for prophylaxis against bacterial peritonitis, a 2-day course of intravenous ciprofloxacin, 200 mg twice daily, followed by oral ciprofloxacin, 500 mg twice daily for 5 days, may be effective alternative regimens in selected patients. A carbapenem has been recommended for patients with hospital-acquired spontaneous bacterial peritonitis, which is increasingly caused by multidrug-resistant organisms. Supplemental administration of intravenous albumin, 1.5 g/kg at diagnosis and 1 g/kg on day 3, (which may have anti-inflammatory effects in addition to expanding plasma volume) prevents further renal impairment and reduces mortality, particularly in patients with a serum creatinine greater than 1 mg/dL (83.3 mcmol/L), blood urea nitrogen greater than 30 mg/dL (10.8 mmol/L), or total bilirubin greater than 4 mg/dL (68.4 mcmol/L). Response to therapy can be documented, if necessary, by a decrease in the PMN count of at least 50% on repeat paracentesis 48 hours after initiation of therapy. The overall mortality rate is high—up to 30% during hospitalization and up to 70% by 1 year. Mortality may be predicted by the 22/11 model: MELD score greater than 22 and peripheral white blood cell count higher than 11,000/mcL (11×10^9/L). Another model predictive of mortality includes the blood urea nitrogen, white blood cell count, Child-Pugh score, and mean arterial pressure. Patients with cirrhosis and septic shock have a high frequency of relative adrenal insufficiency, which if present requires administration of hydrocortisone.

In survivors of bacterial peritonitis, the risk of recurrent peritonitis may be decreased by long-term ciprofloxacin (eg, 500 mg orally once per day) or norfloxacin (400 mg orally daily; no longer available in the United States) or trimethoprim-sulfamethoxazole (eg, one double-strength tablet once per day). In cases of recurrent peritonitis, the causative organism is often resistant to fluoroquinolones and may become multidrug resistant in some cases. In high-risk cirrhotic patients without prior peritonitis (eg, those with an ascitic protein less than 1.5 g/dL and serum bilirubin greater than 3 mg/dL (51.3 mcmol/L), serum creatinine greater than 1.2 mg/dL (99.96 mcmol/L), blood urea nitrogen 25 mg/dL (9 mmol/L) or more, sodium 130 mEq/L (130 mmol/L or less), or Child-Pugh score of 9 or more, the risk of peritonitis, hepatorenal syndrome, and mortality for at least 1 year may be reduced by prophylactic trimethoprim-sulfamethoxazole, one double-strength tablet once per day, ciprofloxacin, 500 mg once per day, or norfloxacin, 400 mg orally once a day (though not in the United States). In patients hospitalized for acute variceal bleeding, intravenous ceftriaxone (1 g per day), followed by oral trimethoprim-sulfamethoxazole (one double-strength tablet once per day) or ciprofloxacin (500 mg every 12 hours), for a total of 7 days, reduces the risk of bacterial peritonitis. Nonantibiotic prophylactic strategies, including probiotics, bile acids, and statins, are under study.

3. Hepatorenal syndrome—Hepatorenal syndrome occurs in up to 10% of patients with advanced cirrhosis and ascites. It is characterized by (1) azotemia (increase in serum creatinine level of greater than 0.3 mg/dL [26.5 mcmol/L]) within 48 hours or increase by 50% or more from baseline within the previous 7 days in the absence of current or recent nephrotoxic drug use, (2) macroscopic signs of structural kidney injury, (3) shock, and (4) failure of kidney function to improve following 2 days of diuretic withdrawal and volume expansion with albumin, 1 g/kg up to a maximum of 100 g/day. Oliguria, hyponatremia, and a low urinary sodium concentration are typical features. Hepatorenal syndrome is diagnosed only when other causes of acute kidney injury (including prerenal azotemia and acute tubular necrosis) have been excluded. Acute kidney injury-hepatorenal syndrome (formerly type 1 hepatorenal syndrome) is typically associated with at least doubling of the serum creatinine to a level greater than 2.5 mg/dL (208.25 mcmol/L) or by halving of the creatinine clearance to less than 20 mL/min (0.34 mL/s/1.73 m^2 BSA) in less than 2 weeks. Chronic kidney disease-hepatorenal syndrome (formerly type 2 hepatorenal syndrome) is more slowly progressive and chronic. An acute decrease in cardiac output is often the precipitating event. In addition to discontinuation of diuretics, clinical improvement and an increase in short-term survival may follow intravenous infusion of albumin in combination with one of the following vasoconstrictor regimens for 7–14 days: oral midodrine plus octreotide, subcutaneously or intravenously; intravenous terlipressin (not yet available in the United States but the preferred agent where available); or intravenous norepinephrine. Oral midodrine, 7.5 mg three times daily, added to diuretics, increases the blood pressure and has also been reported to convert refractory ascites to diuretic-sensitive ascites. Prolongation of survival has been associated with use of MARS, a modified dialysis method that selectively removes albumin-bound substances. Improvement and sometimes normalization of kidney function may also follow placement of a TIPS; survival after 1 year is reported to be predicted by the combination of a serum bilirubin level less than 3 mg/dL (50 mcmol/L) and a platelet count greater than 75,000/mcL (75×10^9/L). Continuous venovenous hemofiltration and hemodialysis are of uncertain value in hepatorenal syndrome. Liver transplantation is the ultimate treatment of choice, but many patients die before a donor liver can be obtained. Mortality correlates with the MELD score and presence of a systemic inflammatory response. Acute kidney injury-hepatorenal syndrome is often irreversible in patients with a systemic infection. The 3-month probability of survival in cirrhotic patients with hepatorenal syndrome (15%) is lower than that for renal failure associated with infections (31%), hypovolemia (46%), and parenchymal kidney disease (73%).

4. Hepatic encephalopathy—Hepatic encephalopathy is a state of disordered central nervous system function resulting from failure of the liver to detoxify noxious agents of gut origin because of hepatocellular dysfunction and portosystemic shunting. The clinical spectrum ranges from day-night reversal and mild intellectual impairment to coma. Patients with covert (formerly minimal) hepatic encephalopathy have no recognizable clinical symptoms but demonstrate mild cognitive, psychomotor, and attention deficits on standardized psychometric tests and an increased rate of traffic accidents. The stages of overt encephalopathy are (1) mild confusion, (2) drowsiness, (3) stupor, and (4) coma. A revised staging system known as

SONIC (*spectrum of neurocognitive impairment in cirrhosis*) encompasses absent, covert, and stages 2 to 4 encephalopathy. Ammonia is the most readily identified and measurable toxin but is not solely responsible for the disturbed mental status. Bleeding into the intestinal tract may significantly increase the amount of protein in the bowel and precipitate encephalopathy. Other precipitants include constipation, alkalosis, and potassium deficiency induced by diuretics, opioids, hypnotics, and sedatives; medications containing ammonium or amino compounds; paracentesis with consequent hypovolemia; hepatic or systemic infection; and portosystemic shunts (including TIPS). In one study, risk factors for hepatic encephalopathy in patients with cirrhosis included a higher serum bilirubin level and use of a nonselective beta-blocker, whereas a higher serum albumin level and use of a statin were protective. The diagnosis is based primarily on detection of characteristic symptoms and signs, including asterixis. A smartphone app called EncephalApp using the "Stroop test" (asking the patient to name the color of a written word rather than the word itself, even when the word is the name of a different color) has proved useful for detecting covert hepatic encephalopathy. The role of neuroimaging studies (eg, cerebral PET, magnetic resonance spectroscopy) in the diagnosis of hepatic encephalopathy is evolving.

Protein is withheld during acute episodes if the patient cannot eat. When the patient resumes oral intake, protein intake should be 60–80 g/day as tolerated; vegetable protein is better tolerated than meat protein. Gastrointestinal bleeding should be controlled and blood purged from the gastrointestinal tract. This can be accomplished with 120 mL of magnesium citrate by mouth or nasogastric tube every 3–4 hours until the stool is free of gross blood or by administration of lactulose. The value of treating patients with covert hepatic encephalopathy is uncertain; probiotic agents may have some benefit.

Lactulose, a nonabsorbable synthetic disaccharide syrup, is digested by bacteria in the colon to short-chain fatty acids, resulting in acidification of colon contents. This acidification favors the formation of ammonium ion in the $NH_4^+ \leftrightarrow NH_3 + H^+$ equation; NH_4^+ is not absorbable, whereas NH_3 is absorbable and thought to be neurotoxic. Lactulose also leads to a change in bowel flora so that fewer ammonia-forming organisms are present. When given orally, the initial dose of lactulose for acute hepatic encephalopathy is 30 mL three or four times daily. The dose should then be titrated so that the patient produces 2–3 soft stools per day. When given rectally because the patient is unable to take medicines orally, the dose is 200 g/300 mL a solution of lactulose in saline or sorbitol as a retention enema for 30–60 minutes; it may be repeated every 4–6 hours. Bowel cleansing with a polyethylene glycol colonoscopy preparation is also effective in patients with acute overt hepatic encephalopathy and may be preferable. Continued use of lactulose after an episode of acute encephalopathy reduces the frequency of recurrences.

The ammonia-producing intestinal flora may also be controlled with an oral antibiotic. The nonabsorbable agent rifaximin, 550 mg orally twice daily, is preferred and has been shown as well to maintain remission of and reduce the risk of rehospitalization for hepatic encephalopathy over a 24-month period, with or without the concomitant use of lactulose. Metronidazole, 250 mg orally three times daily, has also shown benefit. Patients who do not respond to lactulose alone may improve with a course of an antibiotic added to treatment with lactulose.

Opioids and sedatives metabolized or excreted by the liver should be avoided. If agitation is marked, oxazepam, 10–30 mg, which is not metabolized by the liver, may be given cautiously by mouth or by nasogastric tube. Zinc deficiency should be corrected, if present, with oral zinc sulfate, 600 mg/day in divided doses. Sodium benzoate, 5 g orally twice daily, ornithine aspartate, 9 g orally three times daily, and L-acyl-carnitine (an essential factor in the mitochondrial transport of long-chain fatty acids), 4 g orally daily, may lower blood ammonia levels, but there is less experience with these drugs than with lactulose. Flumazenil is effective in about 30% of patients with severe hepatic encephalopathy, but the drug is short-acting and intravenous administration is required. Use of special dietary supplements enriched with branched-chain amino acids is usually unnecessary except in occasional patients who are intolerant of standard protein supplements.

5. Coagulopathy—Hypoprothrombinemia caused by malnutrition and vitamin K deficiency may be treated with vitamin K (eg, phytonadione, 5 mg orally or intravenously daily); however, this treatment is ineffective when synthesis of coagulation factors is impaired because of hepatic disease. In such cases, correcting the prolonged prothrombin time requires large volumes of fresh frozen plasma (see Chapter 14). Because the effect is transient, plasma infusions are not indicated except for active bleeding or before an invasive procedure, and even then, their value has been questioned because of concomitant alterations in antihemostatic factors and because bleeding risk does not correlate with the INR. Recombinant activated factor VIIa may be an alternative but is expensive and poses a 1–2% risk of thrombotic complications. In fact, bleeding risk in critically ill patients with cirrhosis has been shown to correlate with bleeding on hospital admission, a platelet count less than 30,000/mcL (30×10^9/L), a fibrinogen level less than 60 mg/dL (1.764 mcmol/L), and an activated partial thromboplastin time greater than 100 seconds. A thrombopoietin analog, eltrombopag, avatrombopag, or lusutrombopag, reduces the need for platelet transfusions in patients with cirrhosis and a platelet count less than 50,000/mcL (50×10^9/L) who undergo invasive procedures, but the first-generation agent, eltrombopag, is associated with an increased risk of portal vein thrombosis and arterial thromboembolism.

6. Hemorrhage from esophageal varices— See Chapter 15.

7. Hepatopulmonary syndrome and portopulmonary hypertension—Shortness of breath in patients with cirrhosis may result from pulmonary restriction and atelectasis caused by massive ascites or hepatic hydrothorax. The hepatopulmonary syndrome—the triad of chronic liver disease, an increased alveolar-arterial gradient while the patient is breathing room air, and intrapulmonary vascular dilatations or arteriovenous communications that result in a right-to-left intrapulmonary shunt—occurs in 5–32% of patients with cirrhosis. Patients often have greater dyspnea (platypnea) and arterial deoxygenation (orthodeoxia) in the upright than in the recumbent position. The diagnosis should be suspected in a cirrhotic patient with a pulse oximetry level of 96% or less.

Contrast-enhanced echocardiography is a sensitive screening test for detecting pulmonary vascular dilatations, whereas macroaggregated albumin lung perfusion scanning is more specific and may be used to confirm the diagnosis. High-resolution CT may be useful for detecting dilated pulmonary vessels that may be amenable to embolization in patients with severe hypoxemia (PO_2 less than 60 mm Hg [7.8 kPa]) who respond poorly to supplemental oxygen.

Medical therapy has been disappointing. Long-term oxygen therapy is recommended for severely hypoxemic patients. The syndrome may reverse with liver transplantation, although postoperative morbidity and mortality from severe hypoxemic respiratory failure are increased in patients with a preoperative arterial PO_2 less than 44 mm Hg (5.9 kPa) or with substantial intrapulmonary shunting. TIPS may provide palliation in patients with hepatopulmonary syndrome awaiting transplantation.

Portopulmonary hypertension occurs in 0.7% of patients with cirrhosis. Female sex and autoimmune hepatitis have been reported to be risk factors, and large spontaneous portosystemic shunts are present in many affected patients and are associated with a lack of response to treatment. In cases confirmed by right-sided heart catheterization, treatment with the prostaglandin epoprostenol, iloprost, or treprostinil (the latter two are easier to administer); the endothelin-receptor antagonist bosentan (no longer used because of potential hepatotoxicity), ambrisentan, or macitentan; the phosphodiesterase-5 inhibitor sildenafil, tadalafil, or vardenafil; the oral prostacyclin receptor agonist selexipag; or the direct cyclic GMP analog riociguat may reduce pulmonary hypertension and thereby facilitate liver transplantation; beta-blockers worsen exercise capacity and are contraindicated, and calcium channel blockers should be used with caution because they may worsen portal hypertension. Liver transplantation is contraindicated in patients with moderate to severe pulmonary hypertension (mean pulmonary pressure greater than 35 mm Hg).

C. Liver Transplantation

Liver transplantation is indicated in selected cases of irreversible, progressive chronic liver disease, acute liver failure, and certain metabolic diseases in which the metabolic defect is in the liver. Absolute contraindications include malignancy (except relatively small hepatocellular carcinomas in a cirrhotic liver—see Chapter 39), advanced cardiopulmonary disease (except hepatopulmonary syndrome), and sepsis. Relative contraindications include age over 70 years, morbid obesity, portal and mesenteric vein thrombosis, active alcohol or drug abuse, severe malnutrition, and lack of patient understanding. With the emergence of effective antiretroviral therapy for HIV disease, a major cause of mortality in these patients has shifted to liver disease caused by HCV and HBV infection; experience to date suggests

that the outcome of liver transplantation is comparable to that for non–HIV-infected liver transplant recipients. Patients with alcoholism should be abstinent for 6 months. Liver transplantation should be considered in patients with worsening functional status, rising bilirubin, decreasing albumin, worsening coagulopathy, refractory ascites, recurrent variceal bleeding, or worsening encephalopathy; prioritization is based on the MELD (or MELD-Na) score. Treatment of HCV infection should be deferred until after transplantation in patients in whom the MELD score is 21 or higher. Combined liver-kidney transplantation is indicated in patients with associated kidney failure presumed to be irreversible. The major impediment to more widespread use of liver transplantation is a shortage of donor organs. Adult living donor liver transplantation is an option for some patients, and extended-criteria donors are used. Five-year survival rates over 80% are now reported. Hepatocellular carcinoma, hepatitis B and C, and some cases of Budd-Chiari syndrome and autoimmune liver disease may recur in the transplanted liver. The incidence of recurrence of hepatitis B can be reduced by preoperative and postoperative treatment with a nucleoside or nucleotide analog and perioperative administration of HBIG, and hepatitis C can be treated with direct-acting antiviral agents. Immunosuppression is achieved with combinations of cyclosporine, tacrolimus, sirolimus, corticosteroids, azathioprine, and mycophenolate mofetil and may be complicated by infections, advanced chronic kidney disease, neurologic disorders, and drug toxicity, as well as graft rejection, vascular occlusion, or bile leaks. Patients taking these drugs are at risk for obesity, diabetes mellitus, and hyperlipidemia.

▶ Prognosis

The risk of death from compensated cirrhosis is 4.7 times that of the risk in the general population, and the risk from decompensated cirrhosis is 9.7 times higher. Use of statins appears to decrease the risk of decompensation in patients with compensated cirrhosis. Prognostic scoring systems for cirrhosis include the Child-Pugh score and MELD score (Table 16–8). The MELD (or MELD-Na) score, which incorporates the serum bilirubin, creatinine, and sodium levels and the INR, is also a measure of mortality risk in patients with end-stage liver disease and is particularly useful for predicting short- and intermediate-term survival and complications of cirrhosis (eg, bacterial peritonitis) as well as determining allocation priorities for donor livers. Additional (MELD-exception) points are given for patients with conditions such as hepatopulmonary syndrome and hepatocellular carcinoma that may benefit from liver transplantation. A MELD score of 17 or more is required for liver transplant listing. In patients with a relatively low MELD score (less than 21) and a low priority for liver transplantation, an elevated hepatic venous pressure gradient, persistent ascites, hepatic encephalopathy, and a low health-related quality of life are additional independent predictors of mortality, and further modifications of the MELD score are under consideration. Only 50% of patients with severe hepatic dysfunction (serum albumin less than 3 g/dL [30 g/L], bilirubin greater than

Table 16–8. Child-Pugh and Model for End-Stage Liver Disease (MELD) scoring systems for staging cirrhosis.

Child-Pugh Scoring System

Parameter	Numerical Score		
	1	2	3
Ascites	None	Slight	Moderate to severe
Encephalopathy	None	Slight to moderate	Moderate to severe
Bilirubin, mg/dL (mcmol/L)	< 2.0 (34.2)	2–3 (34.2–51.3)	> 3.0 (51.3)
Albumin, g/dL (g/L)	> 3.5 (35)	2.8–3.5 (28–35)	< 2.8 (28)
Prothrombin time (seconds increased)	1–3	4–6	> 6.0

Total Numerical Score and Corresponding Child-Pugh Class

Score	Class
5–6	A
7–9	B
10–15	C

MELD Scoring System

Original MELD = 11.2 $\log_e$ (INR) + 3.78 $\log_e$ (bilirubin [mg/dL]) + 9.57 $\log_e$ (creatinine [mg/dL]) + 6.43. (Range 6–40.)
The MELD-Na score was developed in 2016 by adding the serum sodium as a component: MELD-Na = MELD + (140 – Na) × (1 – 0.025 × MELD).

INR, international normalized ratio.

3 mg/dL [51.3 mcmol/L], ascites, encephalopathy, cachexia, and upper gastrointestinal bleeding) survive 6 months without transplantation. The risk of death in this subgroup of patients with advanced cirrhosis is associated with muscle wasting, age 65 years or older, mean arterial pressure 82 mm Hg or less, severe kidney dysfunction, cognitive dysfunction, ventilatory insufficiency, prothrombin time 16 seconds or longer, delayed and suboptimal treatment of sepsis, and second infections. For cirrhotic patients admitted to an intensive care unit, the Royal Free Hospital score, consisting of the serum bilirubin, INR, serum lactate, alveolar-arterial oxygen gradient, and blood urea nitrogen, has been reported to predict mortality. Severe kidney dysfunction increases mortality up to sevenfold in patients with cirrhosis. The ratio of neutrophils to lymphocytes in peripheral blood has been reported to correlate with mortality 1 year after a nonelective hospitalization in patients with cirrhosis. Obesity and diabetes mellitus appear to be risk factors for clinical deterioration and cirrhosis-related mortality, as is continued alcohol use in patients with alcoholic cirrhosis. The use of beta-blockers for portal hypertension is beneficial early in the course but becomes ineffective and may be associated with reduced survival in patients with refractory ascites, spontaneous bacterial peritonitis, sepsis, or severe alcoholic hepatitis because of their negative effect on cardiac compensatory reserve. In general, beta-blockers should be discontinued when the systolic blood pressure is less than 90 mm Hg, the serum sodium level is less than 130 mEq/L, or acute kidney injury has developed, although results of some studies have challenged these guidelines. Patients with cirrhosis are at risk for the development of hepatocellular carcinoma, with rates of 3–5% per year for alcoholic and viral hepatitis-related cirrhosis. Liver transplantation has markedly improved the outlook for patients with cirrhosis who are candidates and are referred for evaluation early in the course. Patients with compensated cirrhosis are given additional priority for liver transplantation if they are found to have a lesion larger than 2 cm in diameter consistent with hepatocellular carcinoma. In-hospital mortality from cirrhosis declined from 9.1% in 2002 to 5.4% in 2010 and that from variceal bleeding in patients with cirrhosis declined from over 40% in 1980 to 15% in 2000. Patients hospitalized with cirrhosis and an infection are at high risk for subsequent infections, particularly if they are older, taking a proton pump inhibitor, or receiving antibiotic prophylaxis for spontaneous bacterial peritonitis.

▶ When to Refer

- For liver biopsy.
- When the MELD score is 14 or higher.
- For upper endoscopy to screen for gastroesophageal varices.

▶ When to Admit

- Gastrointestinal bleeding.
- Stage 3–4 hepatic encephalopathy.
- Worsening kidney function.
- Severe hyponatremia.
- Serious infection.
- Profound hypoxia.

Asrani SK et al. Burden of liver diseases in the world. J Hepatol. 2019 Jan;70(1):151–71. [PMID: 30266282]

European Association for the Study of the Liver. EASL Clinical Practice Guidelines for the management of patients with decompensated cirrhosis. J Hepatol. 2018 Aug;69(2):406–60. [PMID: 29653741]

Mazzarelli C et al. Palliative care in end-stage liver disease: time to do better? Liver Transpl. 2018 Jul;24(7):961–8. [PMID: 29729119]

Mindikoglu AL et al. New developments in hepatorenal syndrome. Clin Gastroenterol Hepatol. 2018 Feb;16(2):162–77. [PMID: 28602971]

Northup P et al. Management of coagulation and anticoagulation in liver transplantation candidates. Liver Transpl. 2018 Aug;24(8):1119–32. [PMID: 30142249]

Speliotes EK et al. Treatment of dyslipidemia in common liver diseases. Clin Gastroenterol Hepatol. 2018 Aug;16(8):1189–96. [PMID: 29684459]

PRIMARY BILIARY CHOLANGITIS

- ▶ Occurs in middle-aged women.
- ▶ Often asymptomatic.
- ▶ Elevation of alkaline phosphatase, positive antimitochondrial antibodies, elevated IgM, increased cholesterol.
- ▶ Characteristic liver biopsy.
- ▶ In later stages, can present with fatigue, jaundice, features of cirrhosis, xanthelasma, xanthoma, steatorrhea.

General Considerations

Primary biliary cholangitis (PBC) is a chronic disease of the liver characterized by autoimmune destruction of small intrahepatic bile ducts and cholestasis. The designation "primary biliary cholangitis" has replaced "primary biliary cirrhosis" because many patients do not have cirrhosis. The disease is insidious in onset, occurs usually in women aged 40–60 years, and is often detected by the chance finding of elevated alkaline phosphatase levels. Estimated incidence and prevalence rates in the United States are 4.5 and 65.4 per 100,000, respectively, in women, and 0.7 and 12.1 per 100,000, respectively, in men. These rates may be increasing. The frequency of the disease among first-degree relatives of affected persons is 1.3–6%, the risk is increased in second- and third-degree relatives, and the concordance rate in identical twins is high. PBC is associated with HLA *DRB1*08* and *DQB1*. The disease may be associated with Sjögren syndrome, autoimmune thyroid disease, Raynaud syndrome, scleroderma, hypothyroidism, and celiac disease; all patients with PBC should be screened for these conditions. Infection with *Novosphingobium aromaticivorans* or *Chlamydophila pneumoniae* may trigger or cause PBC. A history of urinary tract infections (caused by *E coli* or *Lactobacillus delbrueckii*) and smoking, and possibly use of hormone replacement therapy and hair dye, are risk factors, and clustering of cases in time and space argues for a causative role of environmental agents.

Clinical Findings

A. Symptoms and Signs

Many patients are asymptomatic for years. The onset of clinical illness is insidious and is heralded by fatigue (excessive daytime somnolence) and pruritus. With progression, physical examination reveals hepatosplenomegaly. Xanthomatous lesions may occur in the skin and tendons and around the eyelids. Jaundice, steatorrhea, and signs of portal hypertension are late findings, although occasional patients have esophageal varices despite an early histologic stage. Autonomic dysfunction, including orthostatic hypotension and associated fatigue and cognitive dysfunction, appear to be common. The risk of low bone density, osteoporosis, and fractures is increased in patients with PBC (who tend to be older women) possibly due in part to polymorphisms of the vitamin D receptor.

B. Laboratory Findings

Blood counts are normal early in the disease. Liver biochemical tests reflect cholestasis with elevation of alkaline phosphatase, cholesterol (especially high-density lipoproteins), and, in later stages, bilirubin. Antimitochondrial antibodies are present in 95% of patients, and serum IgM levels are elevated.

Diagnosis

The diagnosis of PBC is based on the detection of cholestatic liver chemistries (often initially an isolated elevation of the alkaline phosphatase) and antimitochondrial antibodies in a titer greater than 1:40 in serum. Baseline ultrasonography should be obtained. Liver biopsy is not necessary for diagnosis unless antimitochondrial antibodies are absent but permits histologic staging: I, portal inflammation with granulomas; II, bile duct proliferation, periportal inflammation; III, interlobular fibrous septa; and IV, cirrhosis. Estimation of histologic stage by an "enhanced liver fibrosis (ELF) assay," which incorporates serum levels of hyaluronic acid, tissue inhibitor of metalloproteinase-1, and procollagen III aminopeptide, and by elastography has shown promise.

Differential Diagnosis

The disease must be differentiated from chronic biliary tract obstruction (stone or stricture), carcinoma of the bile ducts, primary sclerosing cholangitis, sarcoidosis, cholestatic drug toxicity (eg, chlorpromazine), and in some cases chronic hepatitis. Patients with a clinical and histologic picture of PBC but no antimitochondrial antibodies are said to have antimitochondrial antibody-negative PBC (previously termed "autoimmune cholangitis"), which has been associated with lower serum IgM levels and a greater frequency of smooth muscle antibodies and ANA. Many such patients are found to have antimitochondrial antibodies by immunoblot against recombinant proteins (rather than standard immunofluorescence). Some patients have overlapping features of PBC and autoimmune hepatitis.

Treatment

Cholestyramine (4 g) in water or juice three times daily may be beneficial for pruritus; colestipol and colesevelam may be better tolerated but have not been shown to reduce pruritus. Rifampin, 150–300 mg orally twice daily, is inconsistently beneficial. Opioid antagonists (eg, naloxone, 0.2 mcg/kg/min by intravenous infusion, or naltrexone, starting at 12.5 mg/day by mouth) show promise in the treatment of pruritus but may cause opioid withdrawal symptoms. The 5-hydroxytryptamine (5-HT$_3$) serotonin receptor antagonist ondansetron, 4 mg orally three times a day as needed, and the selective serotonin reuptake inhibitor sertraline, 75–100 mg/day orally, may also provide some benefit. For refractory pruritus, plasmapheresis or extracorporeal albumin dialysis may be needed. Modafinil, 100–200 mg/day orally, may improve daytime somnolence but is poorly tolerated. Deficiencies of vitamins A, D, and K may occur if steatorrhea is present and are aggravated when cholestyramine is administered.

Ursodeoxycholic acid (13–15 mg/kg/day in one or two doses) is the preferred medical treatment for PBC. It has been shown to slow the progression of disease (particularly in early-stage disease), stabilize histology, improve long-term survival, reduce the risk of developing esophageal varices, and delay (and possibly prevent) the need for liver transplantation, even in the absence of liver biochemical improvement. Complete normalization of liver biochemical tests occurs in 20% of treated patients within 2 years and 40% within 5 years, and survival is similar to that of healthy controls when the drug is given to patients with stage 1 or 2 PBC. Response rates have been reported to be lower in men than women (72% vs 80%) and higher in women diagnosed after age 70 than before age 30 (90% vs 50%). Ursodeoxycholic acid has also been reported to reduce the risk of recurrent colorectal adenomas in patients with PBC. Side effects include weight gain and rarely loose stools. The drug can be continued during pregnancy.

Obeticholic acid, a farnesoid-X receptor agonist, was approved by the FDA in 2016 for the treatment of PBC in patients with an incomplete response or intolerance to ursodeoxycholic acid. Obeticholic acid is begun in a dose of 5 mg orally daily and increased to 10 mg daily at 6 months if tolerated, based on the decline in serum alkaline phosphatase and bilirubin levels. In patients with Child-Pugh class B or C cirrhosis, the initial dose is 5 mg weekly. The principal side effect is pruritus. Given the expense of the drug, it may not be cost-effective.

Bezafibrate (not available in the United States) and fenofibrate, which activate peroxisome proliferator–activated receptors (PPARs) and inhibit bile acid synthesis, have shown promise as second-line agents and improve symptoms, liver biochemical test levels, and fibrosis. Colchicine (0.6 mg orally twice daily) and methotrexate (15 mg/wk orally) have had some reported benefit in improving symptoms and serum levels of alkaline phosphatase and bilirubin. Methotrexate may also improve liver histology in some patients, but overall response rates have been disappointing. For patients with advanced disease, liver transplantation is the treatment of choice.

▶ Prognosis

Without liver transplantation, survival averages 7–10 years once symptoms develop but has improved for younger women since the introduction of ursodeoxycholic acid. Progression to liver failure and portal hypertension may be accelerated by smoking. Patients with early-stage disease in whom the alkaline phosphatase and AST are less than 1.5 times normal and bilirubin is 1 mg/dL (17.1 mcmol/L) or less after 1 year of therapy with ursodeoxycholic acid (Paris II criteria) are at low long-term risk for cirrhosis and have a life expectancy similar to that of the healthy population. Pregnancy is well tolerated in younger patients. In advanced disease, an adverse prognosis is indicated by a high Mayo risk score that includes older age, high serum bilirubin, edema, low serum albumin, and prolonged prothrombin time as well as by variceal hemorrhage. Other prognostic models include the Globe index, which is based on age, serum bilirubin, serum albumin, serum alkaline phosphatase, and platelet count and, in treated patients, the UK-PBC score, which is based on the baseline serum albumin and platelet count and the serum bilirubin, aminotransferases, and alkaline phosphatase after 12 months of ursodeoxycholic acid. An increase in liver stiffness of more than 2.1 kilopascals per year indicates an adverse prognosis. A prediction tool for varices has been proposed based on the serum albumin, serum alkaline phosphatase, platelet count, and splenomegaly. Liver transplantation should be considered when the MELD-Na score is at least 15, total serum bilirubin at least 6, or Mayo risk score at least 7.8. Fatigue is associated with an increased risk of cardiac mortality and may not be reversed by liver transplantation. Among asymptomatic patients, at least one-third will become symptomatic within 15 years. The risk of hepatocellular carcinoma appears to be increased in patients with PBC; risk factors include older age, male sex, prior blood transfusions, advanced histologic stage, signs of cirrhosis or portal hypertension, and a biochemical nonresponse to ursodeoxycholic acid. Liver transplantation for advanced PBC is associated with a 1-year survival rate of 85–90%. The disease recurs in the graft in 20% of patients by 3 years, but this does not seem to affect survival.

▶ When to Refer

- For liver biopsy.
- For liver transplant evaluation.

▶ When to Admit

- Gastrointestinal bleeding.
- Stage 3–4 hepatic encephalopathy.
- Worsening kidney function.
- Severe hyponatremia.
- Profound hypoxia.

Carey EJ, Levy C (editors). Primary biliary cholangitis. Clin Liver Dis. 2018;22:429–624. [Full issue]

Corpechot C et al. A placebo-controlled trial of bezafibrate in primary biliary cholangitis. N Engl J Med. 2018 Jun 7;378(23):2171–81. [PMID: 29874528]

Hirschfield GM et al. The British Society of Gastroenterology/UK-PBC primary biliary cholangitis treatment and management guidelines. Gut. 2018 Sep;67(9):1568–94. [PMID: 29593060]

Kowdley KV et al. A randomized trial of obeticholic acid monotherapy in patients with primary biliary cholangitis. Hepatology. 2018 May;67(5):1890–902. [PMID: 29023915]

Levy C. Primary biliary cholangitis guidance update: implications for liver transplantation. Liver Transpl. 2018 Nov;24(11):1508–11. [PMID: 30091276]

Lu M et al. Increasing prevalence of primary biliary cholangitis and reduced mortality with treatment. Clin Gastroenterol Hepatol. 2018 Aug;16(8):1342–50. [PMID: 29277621]

HEMOCHROMATOSIS

ESSENTIALS OF DIAGNOSIS

▶ Usually suspected because of a family history or an elevated iron saturation or serum ferritin.

▶ Most patients are asymptomatic; the disease is rarely recognized clinically before the fifth decade.

▶ Hepatic abnormalities and cirrhosis, heart failure, hypogonadism, and arthritis.

▶ *HFE* gene mutation (usually *C282Y/C282Y*) is found in most cases.

▶ General Considerations

Hemochromatosis is an autosomal recessive disease caused in most cases by a mutation in the *HFE* gene on chromosome 6. The HFE protein is thought to play an important role in the process by which duodenal crypt cells sense body iron stores, and a mutation of the gene leads to increased iron absorption from the duodenum. A decrease in the synthesis or expression of hepcidin, the principal iron regulatory hormone, is thought to be a key pathogenic factor in all forms of hemochromatosis. About 85% of persons with well-established hemochromatosis are homozygous for the *C282Y* mutation (type 1a hemochromatosis). The frequency of *HFE* gene mutations averages 7% in Northern European and North American white populations, resulting in a 0.5% frequency of homozygotes (of whom 38–50% will develop biochemical evidence of iron overload but only 28% of men and 1% of women will develop clinical symptoms). The *HFE* gene mutation and hemochromatosis are uncommon in blacks and Asian American populations. A second genetic mutation (*H63D*) may contribute to the development of iron overload in a small percentage (1.5%) of persons who are compound heterozygotes for *C282Y* and *H63D* (type 1b); iron overload–related disease develops in few patients (particularly those who have a comorbidity such as diabetes mellitus and fatty liver). High serum ferritin levels are seen in hyperferritinemia cataract syndrome associated with mutations in the *FTL* (ferritin L-chain) gene. An uncommon juvenile-onset variant that is characterized by severe iron overload, cardiac dysfunction, hypogonadotropic hypogonadism, and a high mortality rate is usually linked to a mutation of a gene on chromosome 1q designated *HJV* that produces a protein called hemojuvelin (type 2a) or, rarely, to a mutation in the *HAMP* gene on chromosome 19 that encodes hepcidin (type 2b). Rare instances of hemochromatosis result from mutations in the genes that encode transferrin receptor 2 (*TFR2*) (type 3) and ferroportin (*SLC11A3*) (type 4).

Hemochromatosis is characterized by increased accumulation of iron as hemosiderin in the liver, pancreas, heart, adrenals, testes, pituitary, and kidneys. Cirrhosis is more likely to develop in affected persons who drink alcohol excessively or have obesity-related hepatic steatosis than in those who do not; other risk factors include age and diabetes mellitus. Eventually, hepatic and pancreatic insufficiency, heart failure, and hypogonadism may develop; overall mortality is increased slightly. Heterozygotes do not develop cirrhosis in the absence of associated disorders such as viral hepatitis or NAFLD.

▶ Clinical Findings

A. Symptoms and Signs

The onset of clinical disease is usually after age 50 years—earlier in men than in women; however, because of widespread liver biochemical testing and iron screening, the diagnosis is usually made long before symptoms develop. Early symptoms are nonspecific (eg, fatigue, arthralgia). Later clinical manifestations include arthropathy (and ultimately the need for joint replacement surgery in some cases), hepatomegaly and evidence of hepatic dysfunction, skin pigmentation (combination of slate-gray due to iron and brown due to melanin, sometimes resulting in a bronze color), cardiac enlargement with or without heart failure or conduction defects, diabetes mellitus with its complications, and erectile dysfunction in men. Population studies have shown an increased prevalence of liver disease but not of diabetes mellitus, arthritis, or heart disease in *C282Y* homozygotes. In patients in whom cirrhosis develops, bleeding from esophageal varices may occur, and there is a 15–20% frequency of hepatocellular carcinoma. Affected patients are at increased risk of infection with *Vibrio vulnificus*, *Listeria monocytogenes*, *Yersinia enterocolitica*, and other siderophilic organisms. The risk of porphyria cutanea tarda is increased in persons with the *C282Y* or *H63D* mutation, and *C282Y* homozygotes have twice the risk of colorectal and breast cancer than persons without the *C282Y* variant.

B. Laboratory Findings

Laboratory findings include mildly abnormal liver tests (AST, alkaline phosphatase), an elevated plasma iron with greater than 45% transferrin saturation, and an elevated serum ferritin (although a normal iron saturation or a normal ferritin does not exclude the diagnosis). Affected men are more likely than affected women to have an elevated ferritin level. Testing for *HFE* mutations is indicated in any patient with evidence of iron overload. Interestingly, in persons with an elevated serum ferritin, the likelihood of detecting *C282Y* homozygosity decreases with increasing ALT and AST levels, which are likely to reflect hepatic inflammation and secondary iron overload. In contrast to secondary iron overload, the serum ALT level is often normal.

C. Imaging

MRI and CT may show changes consistent with iron overload of the liver, and MRI-based techniques can quantitate hepatic iron stores and help assess the degree of hepatic fibrosis.

D. Liver Biopsy

In patients who are homozygous for *C282Y*, liver biopsy is often indicated to determine whether cirrhosis is present. Biopsy can be deferred, however, in patients in whom the serum ferritin level is less than 1000 mcg/L, serum AST level is normal, and hepatomegaly is absent; the likelihood of cirrhosis is low in these persons. Risk factors for advanced fibrosis include male sex, excess alcohol consumption, and diabetes mellitus. Liver biopsy is also indicated when iron overload is suspected even though the patient is neither homozygous for *C282Y* nor a *C282Y/H63D* compound heterozygote. In patients with hemochromatosis, the liver biopsy characteristically shows extensive iron deposition in hepatocytes and in bile ducts, and the hepatic iron index—hepatic iron content per gram of liver converted to micromoles and divided by the patient's age—is generally higher than 1.9 but no longer used for diagnosis. Only 5% of patients with hereditary hemochromatosis identified by screening in a primary care setting have cirrhosis.

Screening

Iron studies and *HFE* testing are recommended for all first-degree family members of a proband; children of an affected person (*C282Y* homozygote) need to be screened only if the patient's spouse carries the *C282Y* or *H63D* mutation. General population screening for hemochromatosis is not recommended because the clinical penetrance of *C282Y* homozygosity and morbidity and mortality from hemochromatosis are low. Patients with otherwise unexplained chronic liver disease, chondrocalcinosis, erectile dysfunction, and type 1 diabetes mellitus (especially late-onset) should be screened for iron overload.

Treatment

Affected persons are advised to avoid foods rich in iron (such as red meat), alcohol, vitamin C, raw shellfish, and supplemental iron. Weekly phlebotomies of 1 or 2 units (250–500 mL) of blood (each containing about 250 mg of iron) are indicated in all symptomatic patients, those with a serum ferritin level of at least 1000 mcg/L, and those with an increased fasting iron saturation and should be continued for up to 2–3 years to achieve depletion of iron stores. The hematocrit and serum iron values should be monitored. When iron store depletion is achieved (iron saturation less than 50% and serum ferritin level 50–100 mcg/L), phlebotomies (every 2–4 months) to maintain serum ferritin levels between 50 mcg/L and 100 mcg/L are continued, although compliance has been reported to decrease with time. Administration of a proton pump inhibitor, which reduces intestinal iron absorption, decreases the maintenance phlebotomy volume requirement. In *C282Y* homozygous women, a body mass index greater than 28 is associated with a lower phlebotomy requirement, possibly because hepcidin levels are increased by overweight. Complications of hemochromatosis—arthropathy, diabetes mellitus, heart disease, portal hypertension, and hypopituitarism—also require treatment.

The chelating agent deferoxamine is indicated for patients with hemochromatosis and anemia or in those with secondary iron overload due to thalassemia who cannot tolerate phlebotomies. The drug is administered intravenously or subcutaneously in a dose of 20–40 mg/kg/day infused over 24 hours and can mobilize 30 mg of iron per day; however, treatment is painful and time-consuming. Two oral chelators, deferasirox, 20 mg/kg once daily, and

deferiprone, 25 mg/kg three times daily, have been approved for treatment of iron overload due to blood transfusions and may be appropriate in persons with hemochromatosis who cannot tolerate phlebotomy; however, these agents have a number of side effects and drug-drug interactions.

The course of hemochromatosis is favorably altered by phlebotomy therapy, and there is some evidence that persons with hemochromatosis have better survival than that of the general population. With phlebotomy therapy, hepatic fibrosis may regress, and in precirrhotic patients, cirrhosis may be prevented. Cardiac conduction defects and insulin requirements improve with treatment. More severe joint symptoms are associated with persistent increases in the transferrin saturation, even if the serum ferritin level is maintained below 50 mcg/L. In patients with cirrhosis, varices may reverse, and the risk of variceal bleeding declines, although the risk of hepatocellular carcinoma persists. In those with an initial serum ferritin level greater than 1000 mcg/L (2247 pmol/L), the risk of death is fivefold greater than in those with a serum ferritin of 1000 mcg/L (2247 pmol/L) or less. In treated patients, only those with a serum ferritin greater than 2000 mcg/L (4494 pmol/L) have increased mortality, mainly related to liver disease. Since 1997, posttransplant survival rates have been excellent. Following liver transplantation, serum iron studies and hepcidin levels are normal, and phlebotomy is not required.

When to Refer

- For liver biopsy.
- For initiation of therapy.

Barton JC et al. Cirrhosis in hemochromatosis: independent risk factors in 368 HFE p.*C282Y* homozygotes. Ann Hepatol. 2018 Aug 24;17(5):871–9. [PMID: 30145563]

Brissot P et al. Pathophysiology and classification of iron overload diseases; update 2018. Transfus Clin Biol. 2019 Feb;26(1):80–8. [PMID: 30173950]

Radford-Smith DE et al. Haemochromatosis: a clinical update for the practising physician. Intern Med J. 2018 May;48(5):509–16. [PMID: 29722188]

Vanclooster A et al. Proton pump inhibitors decrease phlebotomy need in HFE hemochromatosis: double-blind randomized placebo-controlled trial. Gastroenterology. 2017 Sep; 153(3):678–80. [PMID: 28624580]

WILSON DISEASE

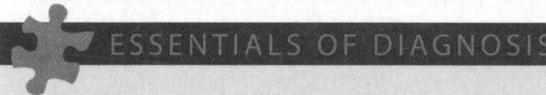

ESSENTIALS OF DIAGNOSIS

- ▶ Rare autosomal recessive disorder that usually occurs in persons under age 40.
- ▶ Excessive deposition of copper in the liver and brain.
- ▶ Serum ceruloplasmin, the plasma copper-carrying protein, is low.
- ▶ Urinary excretion of copper and hepatic copper concentration are high.

General Considerations

Wilson disease (hepatolenticular degeneration) is a rare autosomal recessive disorder that usually occurs in persons between 3 and 55 years of age. The worldwide prevalence is generally stated to be about 30 per million population, but the frequency of the allele appears to be greater than implied by this estimate. The condition is characterized by excessive deposition of copper in the liver and brain. The genetic defect, localized to chromosome 13 (*ATP7B*), has been shown to affect a copper-transporting adenosine triphosphatase in the liver and leads to copper accumulation in the liver and oxidative damage of hepatic mitochondria. Most patients are compound heterozygotes (ie, carry two different mutations). Over 600 mutations in the Wilson disease gene have been identified. The *H1069Q* mutation accounts for 37–63% of disease alleles in populations of Northern European descent. The major physiologic aberration in Wilson disease is excessive absorption of copper from the small intestine and decreased excretion of copper by the liver, resulting in increased tissue deposition, especially in the liver, brain, cornea, and kidney.

Clinical Findings

Wilson disease tends to present as liver disease in adolescents and neuropsychiatric disease in young adults, but there is great variability, and onset of symptoms after age 40 is more common than previously thought. The diagnosis should always be considered in any child or young adult with hepatitis, splenomegaly with hypersplenism, Coombs-negative hemolytic anemia, portal hypertension, and neurologic or psychiatric abnormalities. Wilson disease should also be considered in persons under 40 years of age with chronic or fulminant hepatitis.

Hepatic involvement may range from elevated liver biochemical tests (although the alkaline phosphatase may be low) to cirrhosis and portal hypertension. In patients with acute liver failure (seen much more often in females than males), the diagnosis of Wilson disease is suggested by an alkaline phosphatase (in units/L)-to-total bilirubin (in mg/dL) ratio less than 4 and an AST-to-ALT ratio greater than 2.2. The neurologic manifestations of Wilson disease are related to basal ganglia dysfunction and include an akinetic-rigid syndrome similar to parkinsonism, pseudosclerosis with tremor, ataxia, and a dystonic syndrome. Dysarthria, dysphagia, incoordination, and spasticity are common. Migraines, insomnia, and seizures have been reported. Psychiatric features include behavioral and personality changes and emotional lability and may precede characteristic neurologic features. The risk of depression is increased. The pathognomonic sign of the condition is the brownish or gray-green Kayser-Fleischer ring, which represents fine pigmented granular deposits in Descemet membrane in the cornea (Figure 16–4). The ring is usually most marked at the superior and inferior poles of the cornea. It is sometimes seen with the naked eye and is readily detected by slit-lamp examination. It may be absent in patients with hepatic manifestations only but is usually present in those with neuropsychiatric disease. Renal calculi, aminoaciduria, renal tubular acidosis,

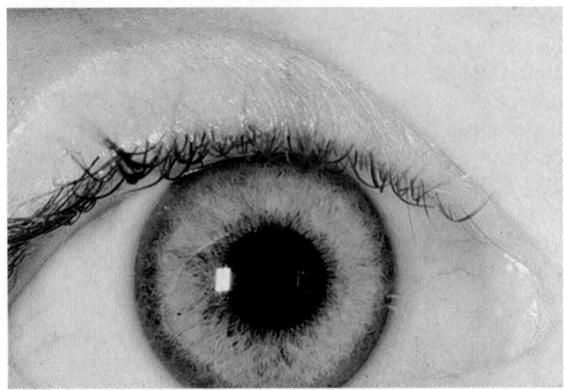

▲ **Figure 16–4.** Brownish Kayser-Fleischer ring at the rim of the cornea in a patient with Wilson disease. (Used, with permission, from Marc Solioz, University of Berne in Usatine RP, Smith MA, Chumley H, Mayeaux EJ Jr. *The Color Atlas of Family Medicine*, 2nd ed. New York, NY: McGraw-Hill, 2013.)

hypoparathyroidism, infertility, hemolytic anemia, and subcutaneous lipomas may occur.

Diagnosis

The diagnosis can be challenging, even with the use of scoring systems (eg, the Leipzig criteria), and is generally based on demonstration of increased urinary copper excretion (greater than 40 mcg/24 h and usually greater than 100 mcg/24 h) or low serum ceruloplasmin levels (less than 14 mg/dL [140 mg/L]; less than 10 mg/dL [100 mg/L] strongly suggests the diagnosis), and elevated hepatic copper concentration (greater than 250 mcg/g of dry liver) as well as Kayser-Fleischer rings, neurologic symptoms, and Coombs-negative hemolytic anemia. However, increased urinary copper (on three separate 24-hour collections) and a low serum ceruloplasmin level (by a standard immunologic assay) are useful but neither completely sensitive nor specific for Wilson disease, although an enzymatic assay for ceruloplasmin appears to be more accurate. The ratio of exchangeable copper to total copper in serum has been reported to improve diagnostic accuracy. In equivocal cases (when the serum ceruloplasmin level is normal), demonstration of a rise in urinary copper after a penicillamine challenge may be helpful, although the test has been validated only in children, lacks sensitivity, and is rarely used now. Liver biopsy may show acute or chronic hepatitis or cirrhosis. MRI of the brain may show evidence of increased basal ganglia, brainstem, and cerebellar copper even early in the course of the disease. If available, molecular analysis of *ATP7B* mutations can be diagnostic.

Treatment

Early treatment to remove excess copper before it can produce hepatic or neurologic damage is essential. Early in treatment, restriction of dietary copper (shellfish, organ foods, nuts, mushrooms, and chocolate) may be of value. Oral ᴅ-penicillamine (0.75–2 g/day in divided doses taken 1 h before or 2 h after food) has been the drug of choice and enhances urinary excretion of chelated copper. Oral pyridoxine, 50 mg per week, is added because D-penicillamine is an antimetabolite of this vitamin. If D-penicillamine treatment cannot be tolerated because of gastrointestinal intolerance, hypersensitivity, autoimmune reactions, nephrotoxicity, or bone marrow toxicity, consider the use of trientine, 250–500 mg three times a day, a chelating agent as effective as D-penicillamine but with a lower rate of adverse effects. Trientine is increasingly used as a first-line agent, although its cost has become exorbitant. Oral zinc acetate or zinc gluconate, 50 mg three times a day, interferes with intestinal absorption of copper, promotes fecal copper excretion, and has been used as first-line therapy in asymptomatic or pregnant patients and those with neurologic disease and as maintenance therapy after decoppering with a chelating agent, but adverse gastrointestinal effects often lead to discontinuation and its long-term efficacy and safety (including a risk of hepatotoxicity) have been questioned. Ammonium tetrathiomolybdate, which complexes copper in the intestinal tract, showed promise as initial therapy for neurologic Wilson disease, and a newer formulation, bis-choline tetrathiomolybdate, is more chemically stable and appears to be effective.

Treatment should continue indefinitely. The doses of penicillamine and trientine should be reduced during pregnancy. Supplemental vitamin E, an antioxidant, has been recommended but not rigorously studied. Once the serum nonceruloplasmin copper level is within the normal range (50–150 mcg/L), the dose of chelating agent can be reduced to the minimum necessary for maintaining that level. The prognosis is good in patients who are effectively treated before liver or brain damage has occurred, but long-term survival is reduced in patients with cirrhosis at diagnosis (84% after 20 years). Liver transplantation is indicated for acute liver failure (often after plasma exchange or dialysis with MARS as a stabilizing measure) and decompensated cirrhosis (with excellent outcomes). Liver transplantation is not generally recommended for intractable neurologic disease. All first-degree relatives, especially siblings, require screening with serum ceruloplasmin, liver biochemical tests, and slit-lamp examination or, if the causative mutation is known, with mutation analysis.

When to Refer

All patients with Wilson disease should be referred for diagnosis and treatment.

When to Admit

- Acute liver failure.
- Gastrointestinal bleeding.
- Stage 3–4 hepatic encephalopathy.
- Worsening kidney function.
- Severe hyponatremia.
- Profound hypoxia.

Pfeiffenberger J et al. Pregnancy in Wilson's disease: management and outcome. Hepatology. 2018 Apr;67(4):1261–9. [PMID: 28859232]

Poujois A et al. Answer to challenging issues in the management of Wilson's disease. Res Hepatol Gastroenterol. 2019 Feb; 43(1):e7–e8. [PMID: 30166252]

Schilsky ML. Wilson disease: diagnosis, treatment, and follow-up. Clin Liver Dis. 2017 Nov;21(4):755–67. [PMID: 28987261]

HEPATIC VENOUS OUTFLOW OBSTRUCTION (Budd-Chiari Syndrome)

ESSENTIALS OF DIAGNOSIS

- ▶ Right upper quadrant pain and tenderness.
- ▶ Ascites.
- ▶ Imaging studies show occlusion/absence of flow in the hepatic vein(s) or inferior vena cava.
- ▶ Clinical picture is similar in sinusoidal obstruction syndrome but major hepatic veins are patent.

General Considerations

Factors that predispose patients to hepatic venous outflow obstruction, or Budd-Chiari syndrome, including hereditary and acquired hypercoagulable states, can be identified in 75% of affected patients; multiple disorders are found in up to 45%. Up to 50% of cases are associated with polycythemia vera or other myeloproliferative neoplasms (which entail a 1% risk of Budd-Chiari syndrome). These cases are often associated with a specific mutation (*V617F*) in the gene that codes for JAK2 tyrosine kinase and may otherwise be subclinical. Other predispositions to thrombosis (eg, activated protein C resistance [factor V Leiden mutation] [25% of cases], protein C or S or antithrombin deficiency, hyperprothrombinemia [factor II *G20210A* mutation] [rarely], the methylenetetrahydrofolate reductase *TT677* mutation, antiphospholipid antibodies) may be identified in other cases. Hepatic vein obstruction may be associated with caval webs, right-sided heart failure or constrictive pericarditis, neoplasms that cause hepatic vein occlusion, paroxysmal nocturnal hemoglobinuria, Behçet syndrome, blunt abdominal trauma, use of oral contraceptives, and pregnancy. Some cytotoxic agents and pyrrolizidine alkaloids (comfrey or "bush teas") may cause sinusoidal obstruction syndrome (previously known as veno-occlusive disease because the terminal venules are often occluded), which mimics Budd-Chiari syndrome clinically. Sinusoidal obstruction syndrome may occur in patients who have undergone hematopoietic stem cell transplantation, particularly those with pretransplant serum aminotransferase elevations or fever during cytoreductive therapy with cyclophosphamide, azathioprine, carmustine, busulfan, etoposide, or gemtuzumab ozogamicin or those receiving high-dose cytoreductive therapy or high-dose total body irradiation. In India, China, and South Africa, Budd-Chiari syndrome is associated with a poor standard of living and often the result of occlusion of the hepatic portion of the inferior vena cava, presumably due to prior thrombosis. The clinical presentation is mild but the course is frequently complicated by hepatocellular carcinoma.

Clinical Findings

A. Symptoms and Signs

The presentation is most commonly subacute but may be fulminant, acute, or chronic. Clinical manifestations generally include tender, painful hepatic enlargement, jaundice, splenomegaly, and ascites. With chronic disease, bleeding varices and hepatic encephalopathy may be evident; hepatopulmonary syndrome may occur.

B. Imaging

Hepatic imaging studies may show a prominent caudate lobe, since its venous drainage may be occluded. The screening test of choice is contrast-enhanced, color, or pulsed-Doppler ultrasonography, which has a sensitivity of 85% for detecting evidence of hepatic venous or inferior vena caval thrombosis. MRI with spin-echo and gradient-echo sequences and intravenous gadolinium injection allows visualization of the obstructed veins and collateral vessels. Direct venography can delineate caval webs and occluded hepatic veins ("spider-web" pattern) most precisely.

C. Liver Biopsy

Percutaneous or transjugular liver biopsy in Budd-Chiari syndrome may be considered when the results of noninvasive imaging are inconclusive and frequently shows characteristic centrilobular congestion and fibrosis and often multiple large regenerative nodules. Liver biopsy is often contraindicated in sinusoidal obstruction syndrome because of thrombocytopenia, and the diagnosis is based on clinical findings.

Treatment

Ascites should be treated with salt and fluid restriction and diuretics. Treatable causes of Budd-Chiari syndrome should be sought. Prompt recognition and treatment of an underlying hematologic disorder may avoid the need for surgery; however, the optimal anticoagulation regimen is uncertain, and anticoagulation is associated with a high risk of bleeding, particularly in patients with portal hypertension and those undergoing invasive procedures. Low-molecular-weight heparins are preferred over unfractionated heparin because of a high rate of heparin-induced thrombocytopenia with the latter. Infusion of a thrombolytic agent into recently occluded veins has been attempted with success. Defibrotide, an adenosine receptor agonist that increases endogenous tissue plasminogen activator levels, has been approved by the FDA for the prevention and treatment of sinusoidal obstruction syndrome. The drug is given as an intravenous infusion every 6 hours for a minimum of 21 days. Serious adverse effects include hypotension and hemorrhage; the drug is expensive and has no benefit in severe sinusoidal obstruction syndrome. TIPS placement may be attempted in patients with Budd-Chiari syndrome

and persistent hepatic congestion or failed thrombolytic therapy and possibly in those with sinusoidal obstruction syndrome. Late TIPS dysfunction is less frequent with the use of polytetrafluoroethylene-covered stents than uncovered stents. TIPS is now preferred over surgical decompression (side-to-side portacaval, mesocaval, or mesoatrial shunt), which, in contrast to TIPS, has generally not been proven to improve long-term survival. Older age, a higher serum bilirubin level, and a greater INR predict a poor outcome with TIPS. Balloon angioplasty, in some cases with placement of an intravascular metallic stent, is preferred in patients with an inferior vena caval web and is being performed increasingly in patients with a short segment of thrombosis in the hepatic vein. Liver transplantation can be considered in patients with acute liver failure, cirrhosis with hepatocellular dysfunction, and failure of a portosystemic shunt, and outcomes have improved with the advent of patient selection based on the MELD score. Patients with Budd-Chiari syndrome often require lifelong anticoagulation and treatment of the underlying myeloproliferative disease; antiplatelet therapy with aspirin and hydroxyurea has been suggested as an alternative to warfarin in patients with a myeloproliferative disorder. For all patients with Budd-Chiari syndrome, a poor outcome has been reported to correlate with Child-Pugh class C and a lack of response to interventional therapy of any kind.

Prognosis

The overall 5-year survival rate is 50–90% with treatment (but less than 10% without intervention). Adverse prognostic factors in patients with Budd-Chiari syndrome are older age, high Child-Pugh score, ascites, encephalopathy, elevated total bilirubin, prolonged prothrombin time, elevated serum creatinine, concomitant portal vein thrombosis, and histologic features of acute liver disease superimposed on chronic liver injury. The 3-month mortality may be predicted by the Rotterdam score, which is based on encephalopathy, ascites, prothrombin time, and bilirubin. A serum ALT level at least fivefold above the upper limit of normal on presentation indicates hepatic ischemia and also predicts a poor outcome, particularly when the ALT level decreases slowly. The risk of hepatocellular carcinoma is increased; risk factors include cirrhosis, combined hepatic vein and inferior vena cava obstruction, and a long-segment inferior vena cava block.

When to Admit

All patients with hepatic vein obstruction should be hospitalized.

European Association for the Study of the Liver. EASL clinical practice guidelines: vascular diseases of the liver. J Hepatol. 2016 Jan;64(1):179–202. [PMID: 26516032]

Valla DC. Budd-Chiari syndrome/hepatic venous outflow tract obstruction. Hepatol Int. 2018 Feb;12(Suppl 1):168–80. [PMID: 28685257]

Van Wettere M et al. Diagnosis of Budd-Chiari syndrome. Abdom Radiol (NY). 2018 Aug;43(8):1896–907. [PMID: 29285598]

THE LIVER IN HEART FAILURE

Ischemic hepatitis, also called **ischemic hepatopathy, hypoxic hepatitis, shock liver**, or **acute cardiogenic liver injury** may affect 2.5 of every 100 patients admitted to an intensive care unit and results from an acute fall in cardiac output due to acute myocardial infarction, arrhythmia, or septic or hemorrhagic shock, usually in a patient with passive congestion of the liver. Clinical hypotension may be absent (or unwitnessed). In some cases, the precipitating event is arterial hypoxemia due to respiratory failure, sleep apnea, severe anemia, heat stroke, carbon monoxide poisoning, cocaine use, or bacterial endocarditis. More than one precipitant is common. Statin therapy prior to admission may protect against ischemic hepatitis.

The hallmark of ischemic hepatitis is a rapid and striking elevation of serum aminotransferase levels (often greater than 5000 units/L); an early rapid rise in the serum lactate dehydrogenase (LD) level (with an ALT-to-LD ratio less than 1.5) is also typical. Elevations of serum alkaline phosphatase and bilirubin are usually mild, but jaundice is associated with worse outcomes. The prothrombin time may be prolonged, and encephalopathy or hepatopulmonary syndrome may develop. The mortality rate due to the underlying disease is high (particularly in patients receiving vasopressor therapy or with septic shock, acute kidney disease, or coagulopathy), but in patients who recover, the aminotransferase levels return to normal quickly, usually within 1 week—in contrast to viral hepatitis.

In patients with **passive congestion of the liver** ("nutmeg liver") due to right-sided heart failure, the serum bilirubin level may be elevated, occasionally as high as 40 mg/dL (684 mcmol/L), due in part to hypoxia of perivenular hepatocytes, and its level is a predictor of mortality and morbidity. Serum alkaline phosphatase levels are normal or slightly elevated, and, in the absence of superimposed ischemia, aminotransferase levels are only mildly elevated. Hepatojugular reflux is present, and with tricuspid regurgitation the liver may be pulsatile. Ascites may be out of proportion to peripheral edema, with a high serum ascites-albumin gradient (greater than or equal to 1.1) and an ascitic fluid protein level of more than 2.5 g/dL (25 g/L). A markedly elevated serum N-terminal-proBNP or BNP level (greater than 364 pg/mL [364 ng/L]) has been reported to distinguish ascites due to heart failure from ascites due to cirrhosis in the absence of renal insufficiency. In severe cases, signs of encephalopathy may develop. Liver stiffness measurement by elastography is increased even in the absence of fibrosis. Mortality is generally attributable to the underlying heart disease but has also been reported to correlate with a noninvasive measure of liver stiffness. The MELD score excluding the INR (MELD-XI) predicts the clinical outcome.

Hilscher M et al. Congestive hepatopathy. Clin Liver Dis. 2016;8(3):68–71.

Lemmer A et al. Assessment of advanced liver fibrosis and the risk for hepatic decompensation in patients with congestive hepatopathy. Hepatology. 2018 Oct;68(4):1633–41. [PMID: 29672883]

Wells ML et al. Congestive hepatopathy. Abdom Radiol (NY). 2018 Aug;43(8):2037–51. [PMID: 29147765]

NONCIRRHOTIC PORTAL HYPERTENSION

 ESSENTIALS OF DIAGNOSIS

▶ Splenomegaly or upper gastrointestinal bleeding from esophageal or gastric varices in patients without liver disease.

▶ Portal vein thrombosis complicating cirrhosis.

▶ General Considerations

Causes of noncirrhotic portal hypertension include extrahepatic portal vein obstruction (portal vein thrombosis often with cavernous transformation [portal cavernoma]), splenic vein obstruction (presenting as gastric varices without esophageal varices), schistosomiasis, nodular regenerative hyperplasia, and arterial-portal vein fistula. Idiopathic noncirrhotic portal hypertension is common in India and has been attributed to chronic infections, exposure to medications or toxins, prothrombotic disorders, immunologic disorders, and genetic disorders that result in obliterative vascular lesions in the liver. It is rare in Western countries, where increased mortality is attributable to associated disorders and older age. Portal vein thrombosis may occur in 10–25% of patients with cirrhosis, is associated with the severity of the liver disease, and may be associated with hepatocellular carcinoma but not with increased mortality. Other risk factors are oral contraceptive use, pregnancy, chronic inflammatory diseases (including pancreatitis), injury to the portal venous system (including surgery), other malignancies, and treatment of thrombocytopenia with eltrombopag. Portal vein thrombosis may be classified as type 1, involving the main portal vein; type 2, involving one (2a) or both (2b) branches of the portal vein; or type 3, involving the trunk and branches of the portal vein. Additional descriptors are occlusive or nonocclusive; recent or chronic; extent (eg, into the mesenteric vein); and nature of any underlying liver disease. Splenic vein thrombosis may complicate pancreatitis or pancreatic cancer. Pylephlebitis (septic thrombophlebitis of the portal vein) may complicate intra-abdominal inflammatory disorders such as appendicitis or diverticulitis, particularly when anaerobic organisms (especially *Bacteroides* species) are involved. Nodular regenerative hyperplasia results from altered hepatic perfusion and can be associated with collagen vascular diseases; myeloproliferative disorders; and drugs, including azathioprine, 5-fluorouracil, and oxaliplatin. In patients infected with HIV, long-term use of didanosine and use of a combination of didanosine and stavudine have been reported to account for some cases of noncirrhotic portal hypertension often due to nodular regenerative hyperplasia; genetic factors may play a role. The term "obliterative portal venopathy" is used to describe primary occlusion of intrahepatic portal veins in the absence of cirrhosis, inflammation, or hepatic neoplasia.

Clinical Findings

A. Symptoms and Signs

Acute portal vein thrombosis usually causes abdominal pain. Aside from splenomegaly, the physical findings are not remarkable, although hepatic decompensation can follow severe gastrointestinal bleeding or a concurrent hepatic disorder, and intestinal infarction may occur when portal vein thrombosis is associated with mesenteric venous thrombosis. Ascites may occur in 25% of persons with noncirrhotic portal hypertension. Covert hepatic encephalopathy is reported to be common in patients with noncirrhotic portal vein thrombosis.

B. Laboratory Findings

Liver biochemical test levels are usually normal, but there may be findings of hypersplenism. An underlying hypercoagulable state is found in many patients with portal vein thrombosis; this includes myeloproliferative neoplasms (often associated with a specific mutation [V617F] in the gene coding for JAK2 tyrosine kinase, which is found in 24% of cases of portal vein thrombosis), mutation G20210A of prothrombin, factor V Leiden mutation, protein C and S deficiency, antiphospholipid syndrome, mutation TT677 of methylenetetrahydrofolate reductase, elevated factor VIII levels, hyperhomocysteinemia, and a mutation in the gene that codes for thrombin-activatable fibrinolysis inhibitor. It is possible, however, that in many cases evidence of hypercoagulability is a secondary phenomenon due to portosystemic shunting and reduced hepatic blood flow.

C. Imaging

Color Doppler ultrasonography and contrast-enhanced CT are usually the initial diagnostic tests for portal vein thrombosis. Magnetic resonance angiography (MRA) of the portal system is generally confirmatory. EUS may be helpful in some cases. In patients with jaundice, magnetic resonance cholangiography may demonstrate compression of the bile duct by a large portal cavernoma (portal biliopathy), a finding that may be more common in patients with an underlying hypercoagulable state than in those without one. In patients with pylephlebitis, CT may demonstrate an intra-abdominal source of infection, thrombosis or gas in the portal venous system, or a hepatic abscess.

D. Other Studies

Endoscopy shows esophageal or gastric varices. Needle biopsy of the liver may be indicated to diagnose schistosomiasis, nodular regenerative hyperplasia, and noncirrhotic portal fibrosis and may demonstrate sinusoidal dilatation. A low liver stiffness measurement by elastography may help distinguish noncirrhotic portal hypertension from cirrhosis.

Treatment

If splenic vein thrombosis is the cause of variceal bleeding, splenectomy is curative. For other causes of noncirrhotic portal hypertension, band ligation followed by beta-blockers to reduce portal pressure is initiated for variceal bleeding, and portosystemic shunting (including TIPS) is reserved for failures of endoscopic therapy; rarely, progressive liver dysfunction requires liver transplantation. Anticoagulation, particularly with low-molecular-weight heparin or thrombolytic therapy, may be indicated for isolated acute portal vein thrombosis (and leads to at least partial recanalization in up to 75% of cases when started within 6 months of thrombosis) and possibly for acute splenic vein thrombosis; an oral anticoagulant is continued long-term if a hypercoagulable disorder is identified or if an acute portal vein thrombosis extends into the mesenteric veins. There is a paucity of data on the use of direct-acting oral anticoagulants in patients with cirrhosis. The use of enoxaparin to prevent portal vein thrombosis and hepatic decompensation in patients with cirrhosis has shown promise.

When to Refer

All patients with noncirrhotic portal hypertension should be referred.

Hernández-Gea V et al. Idiopathic portal hypertension. Hepatology. 2018 Dec;68(6):2413–23. [PMID: 30066417]

Hoolwerf EW et al. Direct oral anticoagulants in patients with liver cirrhosis: a systematic review. Thromb Res. 2018 Oct; 170:102–8. [PMID: 30153564]

Loffredo L et al. Effects of anticoagulants in patients with cirrhosis and portal vein thrombosis: a systematic review and meta-analysis. Gastroenterology. 2017 Aug;153(2):480–7. [PMID: 28479379]

Loudin M et al. Portal vein thrombosis in cirrhosis. J Clin Gastroenterol. 2017 Aug;51(7):579–85. [PMID: 28489645]

Young K et al. Evaluation and management of acute and chronic portal vein thrombosis in patients with cirrhosis. Clin Liver Dis. 2017 Dec;10(6):152–6.

PYOGENIC HEPATIC ABSCESS

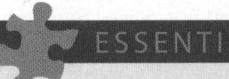

ESSENTIALS OF DIAGNOSIS

- ▶ Fever, right upper quadrant pain, jaundice.
- ▶ Often in setting of biliary disease, but up to 40% are "cryptogenic" in origin.
- ▶ Detected by imaging studies.

General Considerations

The incidence of liver abscess is 3.6 per 100,000 population in the United States and has increased since the 1990s. The liver can be invaded by bacteria via (1) the bile duct (acute "suppurative" [formerly ascending] cholangitis); (2) the portal vein (pylephlebitis); (3) the hepatic artery, secondary to bacteremia; (4) direct extension from an infectious process; and (5) traumatic implantation of bacteria through the abdominal wall. Risk factors for liver abscess include older age and male sex. Predisposing conditions and factors include presence of malignancy, diabetes mellitus, inflammatory bowel disease, and cirrhosis; necessity for liver transplantation; endoscopic sphincterotomy; and use of proton pump inhibitors. Statin use may reduce the risk of pyogenic liver abscess. Pyogenic liver abscess has been observed to be associated with a subsequent increased risk of gastrointestinal malignancy and hepatocellular carcinoma.

Acute cholangitis resulting from biliary obstruction due to a stone, stricture, or neoplasm is the most common identifiable cause of hepatic abscess in the United States. In 10% of cases, liver abscess is secondary to appendicitis or diverticulitis. At least 40% of abscesses have no demonstrable cause and are classified as cryptogenic; a dental source is identified in some cases. The most frequently encountered organisms are *E coli, Klebsiella pneumoniae, Proteus vulgaris, Enterobacter aerogenes*, and multiple microaerophilic and anaerobic species (eg, *Streptococcus anginosus* [also known as *S milleri*]). Liver abscess caused by virulent strains of *K pneumoniae* may be associated with thrombophlebitis of the portal or hepatic veins and hematogenously spread septic ocular or central nervous system complications; the abscess may be gas-forming, associated with diabetes mellitus, and result in a high mortality rate. *Staphylococcus aureus* is usually the causative organism in patients with chronic granulomatous disease. Uncommon causative organisms include *Salmonella, Haemophilus, Yersinia*, and *Listeria*. Hepatic candidiasis, tuberculosis, and actinomycosis are seen in immunocompromised patients and those with hematologic malignancies. Rarely, hepatocellular carcinoma can present as a pyogenic abscess because of tumor necrosis, biliary obstruction, and superimposed bacterial infection (see Chapter 39). The possibility of an amoebic liver abscess must always be considered (see Chapter 35).

Clinical Findings

A. Symptoms and Signs

The presentation is often insidious. Fever is almost always present and may antedate other symptoms or signs. Pain may be a prominent complaint and is localized to the right upper quadrant or epigastric area. Jaundice, tenderness in the right upper abdomen, and either steady or spiking fever are the chief physical findings. The risk of acute kidney injury is increased.

B. Laboratory Findings

Laboratory examination reveals leukocytosis with a shift to the left. Liver biochemical tests are nonspecifically abnormal. Blood cultures are positive in 50–100% of cases.

C. Imaging

Chest radiographs usually reveal elevation of the diaphragm if the abscess is in the right lobe of the liver. Ultrasonography, CT, or MRI may reveal the presence of intrahepatic lesions. On MRI, characteristic findings include high signal intensity on T2-weighted images and rim enhancement. The characteristic CT appearance of hepatic candidiasis, usually seen in the setting of systemic candidiasis, is that of multiple "bull's-eyes," but imaging studies may be negative in neutropenic patients.

Treatment

Treatment should consist of antimicrobial agents (generally a third-generation cephalosporin such as ceftriaxone 2 g intravenously every 24 hours and metronidazole 500 mg intravenously every 6 hours) that are effective against coliform organisms and anaerobes. Antibiotics are administered for 2–3 weeks, and sometimes up to 6 weeks. If the abscess is at least 5 cm in diameter or the response to antibiotic therapy is not rapid, intermittent needle aspiration, percutaneous or EUS-guided catheter drainage or stent placement or, if necessary, surgical (eg, laparoscopic) drainage should be done. Other suggested indications for abscess drainage are patient age of at least 55 years, symptom duration of at least 7 days, and involvement of two lobes of the liver. The underlying source (eg, biliary disease, dental infection) should be identified and treated. The mortality rate is still substantial (at least 5% in most studies) and is highest in patients with underlying biliary malignancy or severe multiorgan dysfunction. Other risk factors for mortality include older age, cirrhosis, chronic kidney disease, and other cancers. Hepatic candidiasis often responds to intravenous amphotericin B (total dose of 2–9 g). Fungal abscesses are associated with mortality rates of up to 50% and are treated with intravenous amphotericin B and drainage.

When to Admit

Nearly all patients with pyogenic hepatic abscess should be hospitalized.

Liao KF et al. Statin use correlates with reduced risk of pyogenic liver abscess: a population-based case-control study. Basic Clin Pharmacol Toxicol. 2017 Aug;121(2):144–49. [PMID: 28273396]

Peng YC et al. Risk of pyogenic liver abscess and endoscopic sphincterotomy: a population-based cohort study. BMJ Open. 2018 Mar 3;8(3):e018818. [PMID: 29502088]

Shi SH et al. Pyogenic liver abscess of biliary origin: the existing problems and their strategies. Semin Liver Dis. 2018 Aug;38(3):270–83. [PMID: 30041279]

Thng CB et al. Gas-forming pyogenic liver abscess: a world review. Ann Hepatobiliary Pancreat Surg. 2018 Feb;22(1):11–8. [PMID: 29536051]

BENIGN LIVER NEOPLASMS

Benign neoplasms of the liver must be distinguished from hepatocellular carcinoma, intrahepatic cholangiocarcinoma, and metastases (see Chapter 39). The most common benign neoplasm of the liver is the **cavernous hemangioma,** often an incidental finding on ultrasonography or CT. This lesion may enlarge in women who take hormonal therapy and must be differentiated from other space-occupying intrahepatic lesions, usually by contrast-enhanced MRI, CT, or ultrasonography. Rarely, fine-needle biopsy is necessary to differentiate these lesions and does not appear to carry an increased risk of bleeding. Surgical resection of cavernous hemangiomas is infrequently necessary but may be required for abdominal pain or rapid enlargement, to exclude malignancy, or to treat Kasabach-Merritt syndrome (consumptive coagulopathy complicating a hemangioendothelioma or rapidly growing hemangioma usually in infants).

In addition to rare instances of sinusoidal dilatation and peliosis hepatis, two distinct benign lesions with characteristic clinical, radiologic, and histopathologic features have been described in women taking oral contraceptives—focal nodular hyperplasia and hepatocellular adenoma. **Focal nodular hyperplasia** occurs at all ages and in both sexes and is probably not caused by the oral contraceptives. It is often asymptomatic and appears as a hypervascular mass, often with a central hypodense "stellate" scar on contrast-enhanced ultrasonography, CT, or MRI. Microscopically, focal nodular hyperplasia consists of hyperplastic units of hepatocytes that stain positively for glutamine synthetase with a central stellate scar containing proliferating bile ducts. It is not a true neoplasm but a proliferation of hepatocytes in response to altered blood flow. Focal nodular hyperplasia may also occur in patients with cirrhosis, with exposure to certain drugs such as azathioprine, and in antiphospholipid syndrome. The prevalence of hepatic hemangiomas is increased in patients with focal nodular hyperplasia.

Hepatocellular adenoma occurs most commonly in women in the third and fourth decades of life and is usually caused by oral contraceptives; acute abdominal pain may occur if the tumor undergoes necrosis or hemorrhage. The tumor may be associated with mutations in (1) the gene coding for hepatocyte nuclear factor 1 alpha (*HNF1alpha*) in 35% of cases (characterized by steatosis and a low risk of malignant transformation, although in men concomitant metabolic syndrome appears to increase the risk of malignant transformation); (2) the gene coding for beta-catenin (characterized by a high rate of malignant transformation) in 10–15% of cases; (3) genes resulting in activation of the IL6/JAK/STAT pathway, with the designation of inflammatory adenoma (previously termed "telangiectatic focal nodular hyperplasia"), which is associated with a high body mass index and serum biomarkers of inflammation (such as C-reactive protein and serum amyloid A) in 35–45% of cases; or (4) a sonic hedgehog-activated variant in 4–5%, which is associated with obesity. Unclassified adenomas account for up to 7% of tumors. Rare instances of multiple hepatocellular adenomas in association with maturity-onset diabetes of the young occur in families with a germline mutation in *HNF1alpha*. Hepatocellular adenomas (inflammatory or unclassified adenomas) also occur in patients with glycogen storage disease and familial adenomatous polyposis. The tumor is hypovascular. Grossly, the cut surface appears structureless. As seen microscopically, the hepatocellular adenoma consists of sheets of hepatocytes without portal tracts or central veins.

Cystic neoplasms of the liver, such as cystadenoma and cystadenocarcinoma, must be distinguished from simple and echinococcal cysts, von Meyenburg complexes (hamartomas), and polycystic liver disease.

► Clinical Findings

The only physical finding in focal nodular hyperplasia or hepatocellular adenoma is a palpable abdominal mass in a minority of cases. Liver function is usually normal. Contrast-enhanced ultrasonography, arterial phase helical CT, and especially multiphase dynamic MRI with contrast can distinguish an adenoma from focal nodular hyperplasia in 80–90% of cases and may suggest a specific subtype of adenoma (eg, homogeneous fat pattern in *HNF1alpha*-mutated adenomas and marked and persistent arterial enhancement in inflammatory adenomas).

► Treatment

Although oral contraceptives should not necessarily be discontinued in women who have focal nodular hyperplasia, affected women who continue taking oral contraceptives should undergo annual ultrasonography for 2–3 years to ensure that the lesion is not enlarging. The prognosis is excellent. Hepatocellular adenoma may undergo bleeding, necrosis, and rupture, often after hormone therapy, in the third trimester of pregnancy, or in men in whom the rate of malignant transformation is high. Resection is advised in all affected men and in women in whom the tumor causes symptoms or is 5 cm or greater in diameter, even in the absence of symptoms. If an adenoma is less than 5 cm in size, resection is also recommended if a beta-catenin gene mutation is present in a biopsy sample. In selected cases, laparoscopic resection or percutaneous radiofrequency ablation may be feasible. Rarely, liver transplantation is required. Regression of benign hepatic tumors may follow cessation of oral contraceptives. Transarterial embolization is the initial treatment for adenomas complicated by hemorrhage.

► When to Refer

- Diagnostic uncertainty.
- For surgery.

► When to Admit

- Severe pain.
- Rupture.

Garcia-Buitrago MT. Beta-catenin staining of hepatocellular adenomas. Gastroenterol Hepatol (N Y). 2017 Dec;13(12):740–3. [PMID: 29339950]

Nault JC et al. Molecular classification of hepatocellular adenoma in clinical practice. J Hepatol. 2017 Nov;67(5):1074–83. [PMID: 28733222]

van Aerts RMM et al. Clinical management of polycystic liver disease. J Hepatol. 2018 Apr;68(4):827–37. [PMID: 29175241]

van Rosmalen BV et al. Systematic review of transarterial embolization for hepatocellular adenomas. Br J Surg. 2017 Jun; 104(7):823–35. [PMID: 28518415]

Védie AL et al. Molecular classification of hepatocellular adenomas: impact on clinical practice. Hepat Oncol. 2018 Apr 9;5(1):HEP04. [PMID: 30302195]

DISEASES OF THE BILIARY TRACT

See Chapter 39 for Carcinoma of the Biliary Tract.

CHOLELITHIASIS (Gallstones)

ESSENTIALS OF DIAGNOSIS

▶ Often asymptomatic.

▶ Classic biliary pain ("episodic gallbladder pain") characterized by infrequent episodes of steady severe pain in epigastrium or right upper quadrant with radiation to right scapula.

▶ Detected on ultrasonography.

► General Considerations

Gallstones are more common in women than in men and increase in incidence in both sexes and all races with age. In the United States, the prevalence of gallstones is 8.6% in women and 5.5% in men. The highest rates are in persons over age 60, and rates are higher in Mexican Americans than in non-Hispanic whites and African Americans. Gallstone disease is associated with increased overall, cardiovascular, and cancer mortality. Although cholesterol gallstones are less common in black people, cholelithiasis attributable to hemolysis occurs in over a third of individuals with sickle cell disease. Native Americans of both the Northern and Southern Hemispheres have a high rate of cholesterol cholelithiasis, probably because of a predisposition resulting from "thrifty" (*LITH*) genes that promote efficient calorie utilization and fat storage. As many as 75% of Pima and other American Indian women over 25 years of age have cholelithiasis. Other genetic mutations that predispose persons to gallstones have been identified. Obesity is a risk factor for gallstones, especially in women. Rapid weight loss, as occurs after bariatric surgery, also increases the risk of symptomatic gallstone formation. Diabetes mellitus, glucose intolerance, and insulin resistance are risk factors for gallstones, and a high intake of carbohydrate and high dietary glycemic load increase the risk of cholecystectomy in women. Hypertriglyceridemia may promote gallstone formation by impairing gallbladder motility. The prevalence of gallbladder disease is increased in men (but not women) with cirrhosis and hepatitis C virus infection. Moreover, cholecystectomy has been reported to be associated with an increased risk of NAFLD and cirrhosis, possibly because gallstones and liver disease share risk factors.

The incidence of gallstones is high in individuals with Crohn disease; approximately one-third of those with inflammatory involvement of the terminal ileum have gallstones due to disruption of bile salt resorption that results in decreased solubility of the bile. Drugs such as clofibrate, octreotide, and ceftriaxone can cause gallstones. Prolonged fasting (over 5–10 days) can lead to formation of biliary "sludge" (microlithiasis), which usually resolves with refeeding but can lead to gallstones or biliary symptoms.

Pregnancy, particularly in obese women and those with insulin resistance, is associated with an increased risk of gallstones and of symptomatic gallbladder disease. Hormone replacement therapy appears to increase the risk of gallbladder disease and need for cholecystectomy; the risk is lower with transdermal than oral therapy. Gallstones detected by population screening have been reported to be associated with an increased risk of right-sided colon cancers. A low-carbohydrate diet and a Mediterranean diet as well as physical activity and cardiorespiratory fitness may help prevent gallstones. Consumption of caffeinated coffee appears to protect against gallstones in women, and a high intake of magnesium and of polyunsaturated and monounsaturated fats reduces the risk of gallstones in men. A diet high in fiber and rich in fruits and vegetables, and statin use reduce the risk of cholecystectomy, particularly in women. Aspirin and other nonsteroidal anti-inflammatory drugs may protect against gallstones.

Gallstones are classified according to their predominant chemical composition as cholesterol or calcium bilirubinate stones. The latter comprise less than 20% of the gallstones found in patients in the United States or Europe but 30–40% of gallstones found in patients in Japan.

► Clinical Findings

Table 16–9 lists the clinical and laboratory features of several diseases of the biliary tract as well as their treatment. Cholelithiasis is frequently asymptomatic and is discovered in the course of a routine radiographic study, surgery, or autopsy. Symptoms (biliary [or "episodic gallbladder"] pain) develop in 10–25% of patients (1–4% annually), and acute cholecystitis develops in 20% of these symptomatic persons over time. Risk factors for the development of symptoms or complications include female sex; young age; awareness of having gallstones; and large, multiple, and older stones. Occasionally, small intestinal obstruction due to "gallstone ileus" (or Bouveret syndrome when the obstructing stone is in the pylorus or duodenum) presents as the initial manifestation of cholelithiasis.

► Treatment

Nonsteroidal anti-inflammatory drugs (eg, diclofenac 50–75 mg intramuscularly) can be used to relieve biliary pain. Laparoscopic cholecystectomy is the treatment of choice for symptomatic gallbladder disease. Pain relief after cholecystectomy is most likely in patients with episodic pain (generally once a month or less), pain lasting 30 minutes to 24 hours, pain in the evening or at night, and the onset of symptoms 1 year or less before presentation. Patients may go home within 1 day of the procedure and return to work within days (instead of weeks for those undergoing open cholecystectomy). The procedure is often performed on an outpatient basis and is suitable for most patients, including those with acute cholecystitis. Conversion to a conventional open cholecystectomy may be necessary in 2–8% of cases (higher for acute cholecystitis than for uncomplicated cholelithiasis). Bile duct injuries occur in 0.1% of cases done by experienced surgeons, and the overall complication rate is 11% and correlates with the

Table 16–9. Diseases of the biliary tract.

	Clinical Features	Laboratory Features	Diagnosis	Treatment
Asymptomatic gallstones	Asymptomatic	Normal	Ultrasonography	None
Symptomatic gallstones	Biliary pain	Normal	Ultrasonography	Laparoscopic cholecystectomy
Cholesterolosis of gallbladder	Usually asymptomatic	Normal	Oral cholecystography	None
Adenomyomatosis	May cause biliary pain	Normal	Oral cholecystography	Laparoscopic cholecystectomy if symptomatic
Porcelain gallbladder	Usually asymptomatic, high risk of gallbladder cancer	Normal	Radiograph or CT	Laparoscopic cholecystectomy
Acute cholecystitis	Epigastric or right upper quadrant pain, nausea, vomiting, fever, Murphy sign	Leukocytosis	Ultrasonography, HIDA scan	Antibiotics, laparoscopic cholecystectomy
Chronic cholecystitis	Biliary pain, constant epigastric or right upper quadrant pain, nausea	Normal	Ultrasonography (stones), oral cholecystography (nonfunctioning gallbladder)	Laparoscopic cholecystectomy
Choledocholithiasis	Asymptomatic or biliary pain, jaundice, fever; gallstone pancreatitis	Cholestatic liver biochemical tests; leukocytosis and positive blood cultures in cholangitis; elevated amylase and lipase in pancreatitis	Ultrasonography (dilated ducts), EUS, MRCP, ERCP	Endoscopic sphincterotomy and stone extraction; antibiotics for cholangitis

ERCP, endoscopic retrograde cholangiopancreatography; EUS, endoscopic ultrasonography; HIDA, hepatic iminodiacetic acid; MRCP, magnetic resonance cholangiopancreatography.

patient's comorbidities, duration of surgery, and emergency admissions for gallbladder disease prior to cholecystectomy. There is generally no need for prophylactic cholecystectomy in an asymptomatic person unless the gallbladder is calcified, gallstones are 3 cm or greater in diameter, or the patient is a Native American or a candidate for bariatric surgery or cardiac transplantation. Cholecystectomy may increase the risk of esophageal, proximal small intestinal, and colonic adenocarcinomas as well as hepatocellular carcinoma because of increased duodenogastric reflux and changes in intestinal exposure to bile. In pregnant patients, a conservative approach to biliary pain is advised, but for patients with repeated attacks of biliary pain or acute cholecystitis, cholecystectomy can be performed—even by the laparoscopic route—preferably in the second trimester. Enterolithotomy alone is considered adequate treatment in most patients with gallstone ileus.

Ursodeoxycholic acid is a bile salt that when given orally for up to 2 years dissolves some cholesterol stones and may be considered in occasional, selected patients who refuse cholecystectomy. The dose is 8–13 mg/kg in divided doses daily. It is most effective in patients with a functioning gallbladder, as determined by gallbladder visualization on oral cholecystography, and multiple small "floating"

gallstones (representing not more than 15% of patients with gallstones). In half of patients, gallstones recur within 5 years after treatment is stopped. Ursodeoxycholic acid, 500–600 mg daily, and diets higher in fat reduce the risk of gallstone formation with rapid weight loss. Lithotripsy in combination with bile salt therapy for single radiolucent stones smaller than 20 mm in diameter was an option in the past but is no longer generally used in the United States.

▶ When to Refer

Patients should be referred when they require surgery.

Baiu I et al. JAMA patient page. Gallstones and biliary colic. JAMA. 2018 Oct 16;320(15):1612. [PMID: 30326127]

Ibrahim M et al. Gallstones: watch and wait, or intervene? Cleve Clin J Med. 2018 Apr;85(4):323–31. [PMID: 29634468]

Rebholz C et al. Genetics of gallstone disease. Eur J Clin Invest. 2018 Jul;48(7):e12935. [PMID: 29635711]

Shabanzadeh DM et al. Association between screen-detected gallstone disease and cancer in a cohort study. Gastroenterology. 2017 Jun;152(8):1965–74. [PMID: 28238770]

Wang Y et al. Gallstones and cholecystectomy in relation to risk of liver cancer. Eur J Cancer Prev. 2019 Mar;28(2):61–67. [PMID: 29738324]

ACUTE CHOLECYSTITIS

ESSENTIALS OF DIAGNOSIS

▶ Steady, severe pain and tenderness in the right hypochondrium or epigastrium.

▶ Nausea and vomiting.

▶ Fever and leukocytosis.

General Considerations

Cholecystitis is associated with gallstones in over 90% of cases. It occurs when a stone becomes impacted in the cystic duct and inflammation develops behind the obstruction. Acalculous cholecystitis should be considered when unexplained fever or right upper quadrant pain occurs within 2–4 weeks of major surgery or in a critically ill patient who has had no oral intake for a prolonged period; multiorgan failure is often present. Acute cholecystitis may be caused by infectious agents (eg, cytomegalovirus, cryptosporidiosis, microsporidiosis) in patients with AIDS or by vasculitis (eg, polyarteritis nodosa, Henoch-Schönlein purpura).

Clinical Findings

A. Symptoms and Signs

The acute attack is often precipitated by a large or fatty meal and is characterized by the sudden appearance of steady pain localized to the epigastrium or right hypochondrium, which may gradually subside over a period of 12–18 hours. Vomiting occurs in about 75% of patients and in half of instances affords variable relief. Fever is typical. Right upper quadrant abdominal tenderness (often with a Murphy sign, or inhibition of inspiration by pain on palpation of the right upper quadrant) is almost always present and is usually associated with muscle guarding and rebound tenderness (Table 16–9). A palpable gallbladder is present in about 15% of cases. Jaundice is present in about 25% of cases and, when persistent or severe, suggests the possibility of choledocholithiasis.

B. Laboratory Findings

The white blood cell count is usually high (12,000–15,000/mcL [12–15 ×10^9/L]). Total serum bilirubin values of 1–4 mg/dL (17.1–68.4 mcmol/L) may be seen even in the absence of bile duct obstruction. Serum aminotransferase and alkaline phosphatase levels are often elevated—the former as high as 300 units/mL, and even higher when associated with acute cholangitis. Serum amylase may also be moderately elevated.

C. Imaging

Plain films of the abdomen may show radiopaque gallstones in 15% of cases. ^{99m}Tc hepatobiliary imaging (using iminodiacetic acid compounds), also known as the hepatic iminodiacetic acid (HIDA) scan, is useful in demonstrating an obstructed cystic duct, which is the cause of acute cholecystitis in most patients. This test is reliable if the bilirubin is under 5 mg/dL (85.5 mcmol/L) (98% sensitivity and 81% specificity for acute cholecystitis). False-positive results can occur with prolonged fasting, liver disease, and chronic cholecystitis, and the specificity can be improved by intravenous administration of morphine, which induces spasm of the sphincter of Oddi. Right upper quadrant abdominal ultrasonography, which is often performed first, may show gallstones but is not as sensitive for acute cholecystitis (67% sensitivity, 82% specificity); findings suggestive of acute cholecystitis are gallbladder wall thickening, pericholecystic fluid, and a sonographic Murphy sign. CT may show complications of acute cholecystitis, such as perforation or gangrene.

Differential Diagnosis

The disorders most likely to be confused with acute cholecystitis are perforated peptic ulcer, acute pancreatitis, appendicitis in a high-lying appendix, perforated colonic carcinoma or diverticulum of the hepatic flexure, liver abscess, hepatitis, pneumonia with pleurisy on the right side, and myocardial ischemia. Definite localization of pain and tenderness in the right upper quadrant, with radiation around to the infrascapular area, strongly favors the diagnosis of acute cholecystitis. True cholecystitis without stones suggests acalculous cholecystitis.

Complications

A. Gangrene of the Gallbladder

Continuation or progression of right upper quadrant abdominal pain, tenderness, muscle guarding, fever, and leukocytosis after 24–48 hours suggests severe inflammation and possible gangrene of the gallbladder, resulting from ischemia due to splanchnic vasoconstriction and intravascular coagulation. Necrosis may occasionally develop without specific signs in the obese, diabetic, elderly, or immunosuppressed patient. Gangrene may lead to gallbladder perforation, usually with formation of a pericholecystic abscess, and rarely to generalized peritonitis. Other serious acute complications include emphysematous cholecystitis (secondary infection with a gas-forming organism) and empyema.

B. Chronic Cholecystitis and Other Complications

Chronic cholecystitis results from repeated episodes of acute cholecystitis or chronic irritation of the gallbladder wall by stones and is characterized pathologically by varying degrees of chronic inflammation of the gallbladder. Calculi are usually present. In about 4–5% of cases, the villi of the gallbladder undergo polypoid enlargement due to deposition of cholesterol that may be visible to the naked eye ("strawberry gallbladder," cholesterolosis). In other instances, hyperplasia of all or part of the gallbladder wall may be so marked as to give the appearance of a myoma (adenomyomatosis). Hydrops of the gallbladder results when acute cholecystitis subsides but cystic duct obstruction persists, producing distention of the gallbladder with a clear mucoid fluid. Occasionally, a stone in the neck of the gallbladder may compress the common hepatic duct and cause jaundice (Mirizzi syndrome). Xanthogranulomatous cholecystitis is a rare, aggressive variant of chronic cholecystitis characterized by grayish-yellow nodules or streaks, representing lipid-laden macrophages, in the wall of the gallbladder and often presents with acute jaundice.

Cholelithiasis with chronic cholecystitis may be associated with acute exacerbations of gallbladder inflammation, bile duct stone, fistulization to the bowel, pancreatitis and, rarely, carcinoma of the gallbladder. Calcified (porcelain) gallbladder is associated with gallbladder carcinoma and is generally an indication for cholecystectomy; the risk of gallbladder cancer may be higher when calcification is mucosal rather than intramural.

Treatment

Acute cholecystitis usually subsides on a conservative regimen, including withholding oral feedings, intravenous alimentation, analgesics, and intravenous antibiotics (generally a second- or third-generation cephalosporin such as ceftriaxone 1 g intravenously every 24 hours, with the addition of metronidazole, 500 mg intravenously every 6 hours), although the need for antibiotics has been questioned in patients undergoing immediate cholecystectomy. In severe cases, a fluoroquinolone such as ciprofloxacin, 400 mg intravenously every 12 hours, plus metronidazole may be given. Morphine or meperidine may be administered for pain. Because of the high risk of recurrent attacks (up to 10% by 1 month and over 20% by 1 year), cholecystectomy—generally laparoscopically—should be performed within 24 hours of admission to the hospital for acute cholecystitis. Compared with delayed surgery, surgery within 24 hours is associated with a shorter length of stay, lower costs, and greater patient satisfaction. If nonsurgical treatment has been elected, the patient (especially if diabetic or elderly) should be watched carefully for recurrent symptoms, evidence of gangrene of the gallbladder, or cholangitis. In high-risk patients, ultrasound-guided aspiration of the gallbladder, if feasible, percutaneous or EUS-guided cholecystostomy, or endoscopic insertion of a stent or nasobiliary drain into the gallbladder may postpone or even avoid the need for surgery. Immediate cholecystectomy is mandatory when there is evidence of gangrene or perforation.

Surgical treatment of chronic cholecystitis is the same as for acute cholecystitis. If indicated, cholangiography can be performed during laparoscopic cholecystectomy. Choledocholithiasis can also be excluded by either preoperative or postoperative MRCP or ERCP.

Prognosis

The overall mortality rate of cholecystectomy is less than 0.2%, but hepatobiliary tract surgery is a more formidable procedure in older patients, in whom mortality rates are higher; mortality rates are also higher in persons with diabetes mellitus and cirrhosis. A technically successful surgical procedure in an appropriately selected patient is generally followed by complete resolution of symptoms.

When to Admit

All patients with acute cholecystitis should be hospitalized.

Drachman DE et al. Case 27-2017. A 32-year-old man with acute chest pain. N Engl J Med. 2017 Aug 31;377(9):874–82. [PMID: 28854089]

Irani S et al. Similar efficacies of endoscopic ultrasound gallbladder drainage with a lumen-apposing metal stent versus percutaneous transhepatic gallbladder drainage for acute cholecystitis. Clin Gastroenterol Hepatol. 2017 May;15(5):738–45. [PMID: 28043931]

Khan MA et al. Efficacy and safety of endoscopic gallbladder drainage in acute cholecystitis: is it better than percutaneous gallbladder drainage? Gastrointest Endosc. 2017 Jan;85(1):76–87. [PMID: 27343412]

Portinari M et al. Do I need to operate on that in the middle of the night? Development of a nomogram for the diagnosis of severe acute cholecystitis. J Gastrointest Surg. 2018 Jun;22(6):1016–25. [PMID: 29464491]

PRE- & POSTCHOLECYSTECTOMY SYNDROMES

1. Precholecystectomy

In a small group of patients (mostly women) with biliary pain, conventional radiographic studies of the upper gastrointestinal tract and gallbladder—including cholangiography—are unremarkable. Emptying of the gallbladder may be markedly reduced on gallbladder scintigraphy following injection of cholecystokinin; cholecystectomy may be curative in such cases. Histologic examination of the resected gallbladder may show chronic cholecystitis or microlithiasis. An additional diagnostic consideration is sphincter of Oddi dysfunction.

2. Postcholecystectomy

Following cholecystectomy, some patients complain of continuing symptoms, ie, right upper quadrant pain, flatulence, and fatty food intolerance. The persistence of symptoms in this group of patients suggests the possibility of an incorrect diagnosis prior to cholecystectomy, eg, esophagitis, pancreatitis, radiculopathy, or functional bowel disease. Choledocholithiasis or bile duct stricture should be ruled out. Pain may also be associated with dilatation of the cystic duct remnant, neuroma formation in the ductal wall, foreign body granuloma, anterior cutaneous nerve entrapment syndrome, or traction on the bile duct by a long cystic duct.

The clinical presentation of right upper quadrant pain, chills, fever, or jaundice suggests biliary tract disease. EUS is recommended to demonstrate or exclude a stone or stricture. Biliary pain associated with elevated liver biochemical tests or a dilated bile duct in the absence of an obstructing lesion suggests sphincter of Oddi dysfunction. Biliary manometry may be useful for documenting elevated baseline sphincter of Oddi pressures typical of sphincter dysfunction when biliary pain is associated with elevated liver biochemical tests (twofold) or a dilated bile duct (greater than 10 mm) ("sphincter disorder," formerly type II sphincter of Oddi dysfunction), but is not necessary when both are present ("sphincter stenosis," formerly type I sphincter of Oddi dysfunction) and is associated with a high risk of pancreatitis. In the absence of either elevated liver biochemical tests or a dilated bile duct ("functional pain," formerly type III sphincter of Oddi dysfunction), a nonbiliary source of symptoms should be suspected, and biliary sphincterotomy does not benefit this group. (Analogous criteria have been developed for pancreatic sphincter dysfunction.) Biliary scintigraphy after intravenous administration of morphine and MRCP following intravenous administration of secretin have been studied as screening tests for sphincter dysfunction. Endoscopic sphincterotomy is most likely to relieve symptoms in patients with a sphincter disorder or stenosis, although many patients continue to have some pain. In some cases, treatment with a calcium channel blocker, long-acting nitrate, phosphodiesterase inhibitor (eg, vardenafil), duloxetine, or tricyclic antidepressants or possibly injection of the sphincter with botulinum toxin may be beneficial. The rate of psychosocial comorbidity with sphincter of Oddi dysfunction does not appear to differ from that of the general population. In refractory cases, surgical sphincteroplasty or removal of the cystic duct remnant may be considered.

When to Refer

Patients with sphincter of Oddi dysfunction should be referred for diagnostic procedures.

Cotton PB et al. The EPISOD study: long-term outcomes. Gastrointest Endosc. 2018 Jan;87(1):205–10. [PMID: 28455162]

Hyun JJ et al. Sphincter of Oddi dysfunction: sphincter of Oddi dysfunction or discordance? What is the state of the art in 2018? Curr Opin Gastroenterol. 2018 Sep;34(5):282–7. [PMID: 29916850]

Yang D et al. Cost effective therapy for sphincter of Oddi dysfunction. Clin Gastroenterol Hepatol. 2018 Mar;16(3): 328–30. [PMID: 28711688]

CHOLEDOCHOLITHIASIS & CHOLANGITIS

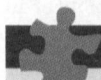

ESSENTIALS OF DIAGNOSIS

► Often a history of biliary pain, which may be accompanied by jaundice.

► Occasional patients present with painless jaundice.

► Nausea and vomiting.

► Cholangitis should be suspected with fever followed by hypothermia and gram-negative shock, jaundice, and leukocytosis.

► Stones in bile duct most reliably detected by ERCP or EUS.

General Considerations

About 15% of patients with gallstones have choledocholithiasis (bile duct stones). The percentage rises with age, and the frequency in elderly people with gallstones may be as high as 50%. Bile duct stones usually originate in the gallbladder but may also form spontaneously in the bile duct after cholecystectomy. The risk is increased twofold in persons with a juxtapapillary duodenal diverticulum. Symptoms and possible cholangitis result if there is obstruction.

Clinical Findings

A. Symptoms and Signs

A history of biliary pain or jaundice may be obtained. Biliary pain results from rapid increases in bile duct pressure due to obstructed bile flow. The features that suggest the presence of a bile duct stone are (1) frequently recurring attacks of right upper abdominal pain that is severe and persists for hours, (2) chills and fever associated with severe pain, and (3) a history of jaundice associated with episodes of abdominal pain (Table 16–9). The combination of pain, fever (and chills), and jaundice represents **Charcot triad** and denotes the classic picture of acute cholangitis. The addition of altered mental status and hypotension (**Reynolds pentad**) signifies acute suppurative cholangitis and is an endoscopic emergency. According to the Tokyo guidelines (2006), the diagnosis of acute cholangitis is established by the presence of either (1) the Charcot triad or (2) two elements of the Charcot triad plus laboratory evidence of an inflammatory response (eg, elevated white blood cell count, C-reactive protein), elevated liver biochemical test levels, and imaging evidence of biliary dilatation or a cause of obstruction.

Hepatomegaly may be present in calculous biliary obstruction, and tenderness is usually present in the right upper quadrant and epigastrium. Bile duct obstruction lasting more than 30 days results in liver damage leading to cirrhosis. Hepatic failure with portal hypertension occurs in untreated cases. In a population-based study from Denmark, acute cholangitis was reported to be a marker of occult gastrointestinal cancer.

B. Laboratory Findings

Acute obstruction of the bile duct typically produces a transient albeit striking increase in serum aminotransferase levels (often greater than 1000 units/L [20 mckat/L]). Bilirubinuria and elevation of the serum bilirubin are present if the bile duct remains obstructed; levels commonly fluctuate. Serum alkaline phosphatase levels rise more slowly. Not uncommonly, serum amylase elevations are present because of secondary pancreatitis. When extrahepatic obstruction persists for more than a few weeks, differentiation of obstruction from chronic cholestatic liver disease becomes more difficult. Leukocytosis is present in patients with acute cholangitis. Prolongation of the prothrombin time can result from the obstructed flow of bile to the intestine. In contrast to hepatocellular dysfunction, hypoprothrombinemia due to obstructive jaundice will respond to intravenous vitamin K, 10 mg, or water-soluble oral vitamin K (phytonadione, 5 mg) within 24–36 hours.

C. Imaging

Ultrasonography and CT may demonstrate dilated bile ducts, and radionuclide imaging may show impaired bile flow. EUS, helical CT, and magnetic resonance cholangiography are accurate in demonstrating bile duct stones and may be used in patients thought to be at intermediate risk for choledocholithiasis (age older than 55 years, cholecystitis, bile duct diameter greater than 6 mm on ultrasonography, serum bilirubin 1.8–4 mg/dL [30.78–68.4 mcmol/L], elevated serum liver enzymes, or pancreatitis). A decision analysis has suggested that magnetic resonance cholangiography is preferable when the risk of bile duct stones is low (less than 40%), and EUS is preferable when the risk is intermediate (40–91%). ERCP (occasionally with intraductal ultrasonography) or percutaneous transhepatic cholangiography (PTC) provides the most direct and accurate means of determining the cause, location, and extent of obstruction, but in patients at intermediate risk of choledocholithiasis, initial cholecystectomy with intraoperative cholangiography results in a shorter length of hospital stay, fewer bile duct investigations, and no increase in morbidity. If the likelihood that obstruction is caused by a stone is high (bile duct stone seen on ultrasonography, serum bilirubin greater than 4 mg/dL [68.4 mcmol/L], or acute cholangitis), ERCP with sphincterotomy and stone extraction or stent placement is the procedure of choice; meticulous technique is required to avoid causing acute cholangitis. Because the sensitivity of these criteria for choledocholithiasis is only 80%, it is not unreasonable for magnetic resonance cholangiography or EUS to be done before ERCP.

► Differential Diagnosis

The most common cause of obstructive jaundice is a bile duct stone. Next in frequency are neoplasms of the pancreas, ampulla of Vater, or bile duct or an obstructed stent placed previously for decompression of an obstructing tumor. Extrinsic compression of the bile duct may result from metastatic carcinoma (usually from the gastrointestinal tract or breast) involving porta hepatis lymph nodes or, rarely, from a large duodenal diverticulum. Gallbladder cancer extending into the bile duct often presents as obstructive jaundice. Chronic cholestatic liver diseases (PBC, sclerosing cholangitis, drug-induced) must be considered. Hepatocellular jaundice can usually be differentiated by the history, clinical findings, and liver biochemical tests, but liver biopsy is necessary on occasion. Recurrent pyogenic cholangitis should be considered in persons from Asia (and occasionally elsewhere) with intrahepatic biliary stones (particularly in the left ductal system) and recurrent cholangitis.

► Treatment

In general, bile duct stones, even small ones, should be removed, even in an asymptomatic patient. A bile duct stone in a patient with cholelithiasis or cholecystitis is usually treated by endoscopic sphincterotomy and stone extraction followed by laparoscopic cholecystectomy within 72 hours in patients with cholecystitis and within 2 weeks in those without cholecystitis. In select cases, laparoscopic cholecystectomy and ERCP can be performed in a single session.

An alternative approach, which is also associated with a shorter duration of hospitalization in patients at intermediate risk for choledocholithiasis, is laparoscopic cholecystectomy and bile duct exploration. For patients older than 70 years or poor-risk patients with cholelithiasis and choledocholithiasis, cholecystectomy may be deferred after endoscopic sphincterotomy because the risk of subsequent cholecystitis is low (although the risk of subsequent complications is lower when cholecystectomy is performed). ERCP with sphincterotomy, generally within 48 hours, should be performed before cholecystectomy in patients with gallstones and cholangitis, jaundice (serum total bilirubin greater than 4 mg/dL [68.4 mcmol/L]), a dilated bile duct (greater than 6 mm), or stones in the bile duct seen on ultrasonography or CT. (Stones may ultimately recur in up to 12% of patients, particularly in older patients, when the bile duct diameter is 15 mm or greater, or when brown pigment stones are found at the time of the initial sphincterotomy.) Endoscopic balloon dilation of the sphincter of Oddi is not associated with a higher rate of pancreatitis than endoscopic sphincterotomy if adequate dilation for more than 1 minute is carried out and it may be associated with a lower rate of stone recurrence. This procedure is generally reserved for patients with coagulopathy because the risk of bleeding is lower with balloon dilation than with sphincterotomy. EUS-guided biliary drainage and PTC with drainage are second-line approaches if ERCP fails or is not possible. In patients with biliary pancreatitis that resolves rapidly, the stone usually passes into the intestine, and ERCP prior to cholecystectomy is not necessary if intraoperative cholangiography is planned.

Choledocholithiasis discovered at laparoscopic cholecystectomy may be managed via laparoscopic or, if necessary, open bile duct exploration or by postoperative endoscopic sphincterotomy. Operative findings of choledocholithiasis are palpable stones in the bile duct, dilatation or thickening of the wall of the bile duct, or stones in the gallbladder small enough to pass through the cystic duct. Laparoscopic intraoperative cholangiography (or intraoperative ultrasonography) should be done at the time of cholecystectomy in patients with liver enzyme elevations but a bile duct diameter of less than 5 mm; if a ductal stone is found, the duct should be explored. In the post-cholecystectomy patient with choledocholithiasis, endoscopic sphincterotomy with stone extraction is preferable to transabdominal surgery. Lithotripsy (endoscopic or external), peroral cholangioscopy (choledoscopy), or biliary stenting may be a therapeutic consideration for large stones. For the patient with a T tube and bile duct stone, the stone may be extracted via the T tube.

Postoperative antibiotics are not administered routinely after biliary tract surgery. Cultures of the bile are always taken at operation. If biliary tract infection was present preoperatively or is apparent at operation, ampicillin-sulbactam (3 g intravenously every 6 hours) or piperacillin-tazobactam (3.375 or 4.5 g intravenously every 6 hours) or a third-generation cephalosporin (eg, ceftriaxone, 1 g intravenously every 24 hours) is administered postoperatively until the results of sensitivity tests on culture specimens are available. A T-tube cholangiogram should be done before the tube is removed, usually about 3 weeks after surgery.

A small amount of bile frequently leaks from the tube site for a few days.

Urgent ERCP with sphincterotomy and stone extraction (within 24–48 hours) is generally indicated for choledocholithiasis complicated by acute cholangitis and is preferred to surgery. Before ERCP, liver function should be evaluated thoroughly. The prothrombin time should be restored to normal by intravenous administration of vitamin K. For mild-to-moderately severe community-acquired acute cholangitis, ciprofloxacin (400 mg intravenously every 12 hours), penetrates well into bile and is effective treatment, with metronidazole (500 mg intravenously every 6–8 hours) for anaerobic coverage. An alternative regimen is ampicillin-sulbactam (3 g intravenously every 6 hours). Regimens for patients with severe or hospital-acquired acute cholangitis, and those potentially infected with an antibiotic-resistant pathogen, include intravenous piperacillin-tazobactam (3.375 or 4 g every 6 hours) or a carbopenem such as meropenem (1 g intravenously every 8 hours). Aminoglycosides (eg, gentamicin 5–7 mg/kg intravenously every 24 hours) may be added in cases of severe sepsis or septic shock but should not be given for more than a few days because the risk of aminoglycoside nephrotoxicity is increased in patients with cholestasis. Regimens that include drugs active against anaerobes are required when a biliary-enteric communication is present. Emergent decompression of the bile duct (within 12 hours), generally by ERCP, is required for patients who are septic or fail to improve on antibiotics within 12–24 hours. Medical therapy alone is most likely to fail in patients with tachycardia, a serum albumin less than 3 g/dL (30 g/L), marked hyperbilirubinemia, a high serum ALT level, a high white blood cell count, and a prothrombin time greater than 14 seconds on admission. If sphincterotomy cannot be performed, the bile duct can be decompressed by a biliary stent or nasobiliary catheter. Once decompression is achieved, antibiotics are generally continued for at least another 3 days. Elective cholecystectomy can be undertaken after resolution of cholangitis, unless the patient remains unfit for surgery. Mortality from acute cholangitis has been reported to correlate with a high total bilirubin level, prolonged partial thromboplastin time, presence of a liver abscess, and unsuccessful ERCP.

▶ When to Refer

All symptomatic patients with choledocholithiasis should be referred.

▶ When to Admit

All patients with acute cholangitis should be hospitalized.

Baiu I et al. JAMA patient page. Choledocholithiasis. JAMA. 2018 Oct 9;320(14):1506. [PMID: 30304429]

Park CH et al. Comparative efficacy of various endoscopic techniques for the treatment of common bile duct stones: a network meta-analysis. Gastrointest Endosc. 2018 Jan;87(1): 43–57. [PMID: 28756105]

Sharaiha RZ et al. Efficacy and safety of EUS-guided biliary drainage in comparison with percutaneous biliary drainage when ERCP fails: a systematic review and meta-analysis. Gastrointest Endosc. 2017 May;85(5):904–14. [PMID: 28063840]

Tan M et al. Association between early ERCP and mortality in patients with acute cholangitis. Gastrointest Endosc. 2018 Jan;87(1):185–92. [PMID: 28433613]

Williams E et al. Updated guideline on the management of common bile duct stones (CBDS). Gut. 2017 May;66(5):765–82. [PMID: 28122906]

Yang D et al. When does assessment for bile duct stones need to be performed prior to cholecystectomy for calculus gallbladder disease? Clin Gastroenterol Hepatol. 2018 Mar;16(3): 331–2. [PMID: 28669660]

BILIARY STRICTURE

Benign biliary strictures are the result of surgical (including liver transplantation) anastomosis or injury in about 95% of cases. The remainder of cases are caused by blunt external injury to the abdomen, pancreatitis, IgG_4-related disease, erosion of the duct by a gallstone, or prior endoscopic sphincterotomy.

Signs of injury to the duct may or may not be recognized in the immediate postoperative period. If complete occlusion has occurred, jaundice will develop rapidly; more often, however, a tear has been made accidentally in the duct, and the earliest manifestation of injury may be excessive or prolonged loss of bile from the surgical drains. Bile leakage resulting in a bile collection (biloma) may predispose to localized infection, which in turn accentuates scar formation and the ultimate development of a fibrous stricture.

Cholangitis is the most common complication of stricture. Typically, the patient experiences episodes of pain, fever, chills, and jaundice within a few weeks to months after cholecystectomy. Physical findings may include jaundice during an acute attack of cholangitis and right upper quadrant abdominal tenderness. Serum alkaline phosphatase is usually elevated. Hyperbilirubinemia is variable, fluctuating during exacerbations and usually remaining in the range of 5–10 mg/dL (85.5–171 mcmol/L). Blood cultures may be positive during an acute episode of cholangitis. Secondary biliary cirrhosis will inevitably develop if a stricture is not treated.

MRCP or multidetector CT is valuable in demonstrating the stricture and outlining the anatomy. ERCP is the first-line interventional approach and permits biopsy and cytologic specimens to exclude malignancy (in conjunction with EUS-guided fine-needle aspiration, an even more sensitive test for distal bile duct malignancy), sphincterotomy to allow a bile leak to close, and dilation (often repeated) and stent placement, thereby avoiding surgical repair in some cases. When ERCP is unsuccessful, dilation of a stricture may be accomplished by PTC or under EUS guidance. Placement of multiple plastic stents appears to be more effective than placement of a single stent. The use of covered metal stents, which are more easily removed endoscopically than uncovered metal stents, as well as bioabsorbable stents, is an alternative to use of plastic stents and requires fewer ERCPs to achieve stricture resolution. Uncovered metal stents, which often cannot be removed endoscopically, are generally avoided in benign strictures unless life expectancy is less than 2 years. Strictures related to chronic pancreatitis are more difficult than postsurgical strictures to treat endoscopically and may be best managed with a temporary covered metal stent. Following liver transplantation, endoscopic management is more successful for anastomotic than for nonanastomotic strictures. Results for nonanastomotic strictures may be improved with repeated dilations or the use of multiple plastic stents. Biliary strictures after live liver donor liver transplantation, particularly in patients with a late-onset (after 24 weeks) stricture or with intrahepatic biliary dilatation, are also challenging and require aggressive endoscopic therapy; in addition, the risk of post-ERCP pancreatitis appears to be increased. When malignancy cannot be excluded with certainty, additional endoscopic diagnostic approaches may be considered—if available—including intraductal ultrasonography, peroral cholangioscopy, confocal laser endomicroscopy, and fluorescence in situ hybridization. Differentiation from cholangiocarcinoma may ultimately require surgical exploration in 20% of cases. Operative treatment of a stricture frequently necessitates performance of an end-to-end ductal repair, choledochojejunostomy, or hepaticojejunostomy to reestablish bile flow into the intestine.

▶ When to Refer

All patients with biliary stricture should be referred.

▶ When to Admit

Patients with acute cholangitis should be hospitalized.

Hu B et al. Asia-Pacific consensus guidelines for endoscopic management of benign biliary strictures. Gastrointest Endosc. 2017 Jul;86(1):44–58. [PMID: 28283322]

Martins FP et al. Metal versus plastic stents for anastomotic biliary strictures after liver transplantation: a randomized controlled trial. Gastrointest Endosc. 2018 Jan;87(1):131–40. [PMID: 28455159]

Sun B et al. Review article: Asia-Pacific consensus recommendations on endoscopic tissue acquisition for biliary strictures. Aliment Pharmacol Ther. 2018 Jul;48(2):138–51. [PMID: 29876948]

PRIMARY SCLEROSING CHOLANGITIS

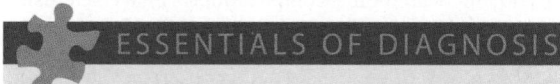

ESSENTIALS OF DIAGNOSIS

- ▶ Most common in men aged 20–50 years.
- ▶ Often associated with ulcerative colitis.
- ▶ Progressive jaundice, itching, and other features of cholestasis.
- ▶ Diagnosis based on characteristic cholangiographic findings.
- ▶ At least 10% risk of cholangiocarcinoma.

▶ General Considerations

Primary sclerosing cholangitis is an uncommon disease thought to result from an increased immune response to intestinal endotoxins and characterized by diffuse inflammation of the biliary tract leading to fibrosis and strictures of the biliary system. From 60% to 70% of affected persons are male, usually 20–50 years of age (median age 41). There is an incidence of nearly 3.3 per 100,000 in Asian Americans, 2.8 per 100,000 in Hispanic Americans, and 2.1 per 100,000 in African Americans, and an intermediate incidence in whites (and increasing) and a prevalence of 16.2 per 100,000 population (21 per 100,000 men and 6 per 100,000 women) in the United States. Primary sclerosing cholangitis is closely associated with inflammatory bowel disease (more commonly ulcerative colitis than Crohn colitis), which is present in approximately two-thirds of patients with primary sclerosing cholangitis; however, clinically significant sclerosing cholangitis develops in only 1–4% of patients with ulcerative colitis. Smoking is associated with a decreased risk of primary sclerosing cholangitis in patients who also have inflammatory bowel disease. Coffee consumption is also associated with a decreased risk of primary sclerosing cholangitis. Women with primary sclerosing cholangitis may be more likely to have recurrent urinary tract infections and less likely to use hormone replacement therapy than healthy controls. Associations with cardiovascular disease and diabetes mellitus have been reported. Primary sclerosing cholangitis is associated with the histocompatibility antigens HLA-B8 and -DR3 or -DR4, and first-degree relatives of patients with primary sclerosing cholangitis have a fourfold increased risk of primary sclerosing cholangitis and a threefold increased risk of ulcerative colitis. A subset of patients with primary sclerosing cholangitis have increased serum IgG_4 levels and distinct HLA associations (with a poorer prognosis) but do not meet criteria for IgG_4-related sclerosing cholangitis. The diagnosis of primary sclerosing cholangitis may be difficult to make after biliary surgery.

▶ Clinical Findings

A. Symptoms and Signs

Primary sclerosing cholangitis presents as progressive obstructive jaundice, frequently associated with fatigue, pruritus, anorexia, and indigestion. Patients may be diagnosed in the presymptomatic phase because of an elevated alkaline phosphatase level or a subclinical phase based on abnormalities on magnetic resonance cholangiography despite normal liver enzyme levels. Complications of chronic cholestasis, such as osteoporosis and malabsorption of fat-soluble vitamins, may occur late in the course. Risk factors for osteoporosis include older age, lower body mass index, and longer duration of inflammatory bowel disease. Esophageal varices on initial endoscopy are most likely in patients with a higher Mayo risk score based on age, bilirubin, albumin, and AST and a higher AST/ALT ratio, and new varices are likely to develop in those with a lower platelet count and higher bilirubin at 2 years. In patients with primary sclerosing cholangitis, ulcerative colitis is frequently characterized by rectal sparing and backwash ileitis.

B. Diagnostic Findings

The diagnosis of primary sclerosing cholangitis is generally made by MRCP, the sensitivity of which approaches that of ERCP. Characteristic cholangiographic findings are segmental fibrosis of bile ducts with saccular dilatations between strictures. Biliary obstruction by a stone or tumor should be excluded. Liver biopsy is not necessary for diagnosis when cholangiographic findings are characteristic. The disease may be confined to small intrahepatic bile ducts in about 15% of cases, in which case MRCP and ERCP are normal and the diagnosis is suggested by liver biopsy findings. These patients have a longer survival than patients with involvement of the large ducts and do not appear to be at increased risk for cholangiocarcinoma unless large-duct sclerosing cholangitis develops (which occurs in about 20% over 7–10 years). Liver biopsy may show characteristic periductal fibrosis ("onion-skinning") and allows staging, which is based on the degree of fibrosis and which correlates with liver stiffness as measured by elastography. Perinuclear ANCA as well as antinuclear, anticardiolipin, antithyroperoxidase, and anti-*Saccharomyces cerevisiae* antibodies and rheumatoid factor are frequently detected in serum. Occasional patients have clinical and histologic features of both sclerosing cholangitis and autoimmune hepatitis. Cholangitis in IgG_4-related disease may be difficult to distinguish from primary sclerosing cholangitis and even cholangiocarcinoma, is associated with autoimmune pancreatitis (see Chronic Pancreatitis), and is responsive to corticosteroids. A serum IgG_4 level more than four times the upper limit of normal or an IgG_4:IgG_1 ratio of more than 0.24 strongly suggests IgG_4-related sclerosing cholangitis, but in up to one-third of cases, the serum IgG_4 level is normal. Primary sclerosing cholangitis must also be distinguished from idiopathic adulthood ductopenia (a rare disorder that affects young to middle-aged adults who manifest cholestasis resulting from loss of interlobular and septal bile ducts yet who have a normal cholangiogram. It is caused in some cases by a mutation in the canalicular phospholipid transporter gene *ABCB4*). Primary sclerosing cholangitis must also be distinguished from other cholangiopathies (including PBC; cystic fibrosis; eosinophilic cholangitis; AIDS cholangiopathy; histiocytosis X; allograft rejection; graft-versus-host disease; ischemic cholangiopathy [often with biliary "casts," a rapid progression to cirrhosis, and a poor outcome] caused by hepatic artery thrombosis, shock, respiratory failure, or drugs; intra-arterial chemotherapy; and sarcoidosis).

► Complications

Cholangiocarcinoma may complicate the course of primary sclerosing cholangitis in up to 20% of cases (1.2% per year) and may be difficult to diagnose by cytologic examination or biopsy because of false-negative results. A serum CA 19-9 level above 100 units/mL is suggestive but not diagnostic of cholangiocarcinoma. Annual right-upper-quadrant ultrasonography or MRI with MRCP and serum CA 19-9 testing (a level of 20 is the threshold for further investigation) are recommended for surveillance, with ERCP and biliary cytology if the results are suggestive of malignancy. PET and peroral cholangioscopy may play roles in the early detection of cholangiocarcinoma. Patients with ulcerative colitis and primary sclerosing cholangitis are at high risk (tenfold higher than ulcerative colitis patients without primary sclerosing cholangitis) for colorectal neoplasia. The risks of gallstones, cholecystitis, gallbladder polyps, and gallbladder carcinoma appear to be increased in patients with primary sclerosing cholangitis.

► Treatment

Episodes of acute bacterial cholangitis may be treated with ciprofloxacin (750 mg twice daily orally or intravenously). Ursodeoxycholic acid in standard doses (10–15 mg/kg/day orally) may improve liver biochemical test results but does not appear to alter the natural history. However, withdrawal of ursodeoxycholic acid may result in worsening of liver biochemical test levels and increased pruritus, and ursodeoxycholic acid in intermediate doses (17–23 mg/kg/day) has been reported to be beneficial. Other approaches such as antibiotics (vancomycin, metronidazole, minocycline, azithromycin), obeticholic acid (a farnesoid-X receptor agonist), 24-norursodeoxycholic acid, budesonide, antitumor necrosis factor antibodies, simtuzumab (a monoclonal antibody to lysyl oxidase, an enzyme that functions as a profibrotic protein), cenicriviroc (a dual chemokine receptor [CCR] 5 and CCR2 antagonist), cyclosporine, tacrolimus, other antifibrotic agents, mitomycin C, and fecal microbial transplantation are under study. Careful endoscopic evaluation of the biliary tract may permit balloon dilation of localized strictures, and repeated dilation of a dominant stricture may improve survival, although such patients have reduced survival compared with patients who do not have a dominant stricture. Short-term (2–3 weeks) placement of a stent in a major stricture also may relieve symptoms and improve biochemical abnormalities, with sustained improvement after the stent is removed, but may not be superior to balloon dilation alone; long-term stenting may increase the rate of complications such as cholangitis and is not recommended. Cholecystectomy is indicated in patients with primary sclerosing cholangitis and a gallbladder polyp greater than 8 mm in diameter. In patients without cirrhosis, surgical resection of a dominant bile duct stricture may lead to longer survival than endoscopic therapy by decreasing the subsequent risk of cholangiocarcinoma. When feasible, extensive surgical resection of cholangiocarcinoma complicating primary sclerosing cholangitis may result in 5-year survival rates of greater than 50%. In patients with ulcerative colitis, primary sclerosing cholangitis is an independent risk factor for the development of colorectal dysplasia and cancer (especially in the right colon), and strict adherence to a colonoscopic surveillance program (yearly for those with ulcerative colitis and every 5 years for those without ulcerative colitis) is recommended. Whether treatment with ursodeoxycholic acid reduces the risk of colorectal dysplasia and carcinoma in patients with ulcerative colitis and primary sclerosing cholangitis is still uncertain. For patients with cirrhosis and clinical decompensation, liver transplantation is the treatment of choice; primary sclerosing cholangitis recurs in the graft in 30% of cases, with a possible reduction in the risk of recurrence when colectomy has been performed for ulcerative colitis before transplantation.

Prognosis

Survival of patients with primary sclerosing cholangitis averages 9–17 years, and up to 21 years in population-based studies. Adverse prognostic markers are older age, hepatosplenomegaly, higher serum bilirubin and AST levels, lower albumin levels, a history of variceal bleeding, a dominant bile duct stricture, and extrahepatic duct changes. Variceal bleeding is also a risk factor for cholangiocarcinoma. Patients in whom serum alkaline phosphatase levels decline by 40% or more (spontaneously, with ursodeoxycholic acid therapy, or after treatment of a dominant stricture) have longer transplant-free survival times than those in whom the alkaline phosphatase does not decline. Moreover, improvement in the serum alkaline phosphatase to less than 1.5 times the upper limit of normal is associated with a reduced risk of cholangiocarcinoma. The risk of progression can be predicted by three findings on MRI and MRCP: a cirrhotic appearance to the liver, portal hypertension, and enlarged perihepatic lymph nodes. The Amsterdam-Oxford model has been proposed to predict transplant-free survival and is based on disease subtype (large- vs. small-duct involvement), age at diagnosis, serum albumin, platelet count, serum AST, serum alkaline phosphatase, and serum bilirubin. Transplant-free survival can also be predicted by serum levels of markers of liver fibrosis—hyaluronic acid, tissue inhibitor of metalloproteinase-1, and propeptide of type III procollagen. Reduced quality of life is associated with older age, large-duct disease, and systemic symptoms. Although maternal primary sclerosing cholangitis is associated with preterm birth and cesarean section delivery, the risk of congenital malformations is not increased. Interestingly, patients with milder ulcerative colitis tend to have more severe primary cholangitis and a higher rate of liver transplantation. Actuarial survival rates with liver transplantation are as high as 72% at 5 years, but rates are much lower once cholangiocarcinoma has developed. Following transplantation, patients have an increased risk of non-anastomotic biliary strictures and—in those with ulcerative colitis—colon cancer, and the disease recurs in 25%. The retransplantation rate is higher than that for PBC. Those patients who are unable to undergo liver transplantation will ultimately require high-quality palliative care (see Chapter 5).

Alberts R et al. Genetic association analysis identifies variants associated with disease progression in primary sclerosing cholangitis. Gut. 2018 Aug;67(8):1517–24. [PMID: 28779025]

Ali AH et al. Surveillance for hepatobiliary cancers in patients with primary sclerosing cholangitis. Hepatology. 2018 Jun;67(6):2338–51. [PMID: 29244227]

de Vries EM et al. A novel prognostic model for transplant-free survival in primary sclerosing cholangitis. Gut. 2018 Oct;67(10):1864–9. [PMID: 28739581]

Dyson JK et al. Primary sclerosing cholangitis. Lancet. 2018 Jun 23;391(10139):2547–59. [PMID: 29452711]

Ponsioen CY et al. No superiority of stents vs balloon dilatation for dominant strictures in patients with primary sclerosing cholangitis. Gastroenterology. 2018 Sep;155(3):752–9. [PMID: 29803836]

DISEASES OF THE PANCREAS

See Chapter 39 for Carcinoma of the Pancreas and Periampullary Area.

ACUTE PANCREATITIS

ESSENTIALS OF DIAGNOSIS

▶ Abrupt onset of deep epigastric pain, often with radiation to the back.

▶ History of previous episodes, often related to alcohol intake.

▶ Nausea, vomiting, sweating, weakness.

▶ Abdominal tenderness and distention and fever.

▶ Leukocytosis, elevated serum amylase, elevated serum lipase.

General Considerations

The annual incidence of acute pancreatitis ranges from 13 to 45 per 100,000 population and has increased since 1990. Most cases of acute pancreatitis are related to biliary tract disease (a passed gallstone, usually 5 mm or less in diameter) or heavy alcohol intake. The exact pathogenesis is not known but may include edema or obstruction of the ampulla of Vater, reflux of bile into pancreatic ducts, and direct injury of pancreatic acinar cells by prematurely activated pancreatic enzymes. Among the numerous other causes or associations are hypercalcemia, hyperlipidemias (chylomicronemia, hypertriglyceridemia, or both), abdominal trauma (including surgery), drugs (including azathioprine, mercaptopurine, asparaginase, pentamidine, didanosine, valproic acid, tetracyclines, dapsone, isoniazid, metronidazole, estrogen and tamoxifen [by raising serum triglycerides], sulfonamides, mesalamine, celecoxib, sulindac, leflunomide, thiazides, simvastatin, fenofibrate, enalapril, methyldopa, procainamide, sitagliptin, exenatide, possibly corticosteroids, and others), vasculitis, infections (eg, mumps, cytomegalovirus, HEV, *M avium intracellulare* complex), peritoneal dialysis, cardiopulmonary bypass, single- or double-balloon enteroscopy, and ERCP. In patients with pancreas divisum, a congenital anomaly in which the dorsal and ventral pancreatic ducts fail to fuse, acute pancreatitis may result from stenosis of the minor papilla with obstruction to flow from the accessory pancreatic duct, although concomitant genetic mutations, particularly in the cystic fibrosis transmembrane conductance regulator (*CFTR*) gene, may actually account for acute pancreatitis in these patients. Acute pancreatitis may also result from the anomalous union of the pancreaticobiliary duct. Rarely, acute pancreatitis may be the presenting manifestation of a pancreatic or ampullary neoplasm. Celiac disease appears to be associated with an increased risk of acute and chronic pancreatitis. Apparently "idiopathic" acute pancreatitis is often caused by occult biliary microlithiasis but unlikely to be caused by sphincter of Oddi dysfunction involving the pancreatic duct. Between 15% and 25% of cases are truly idiopathic. Smoking, high dietary glycemic load, and abdominal adiposity increase the risk of pancreatitis, and older age and obesity increase the risk of a severe course; vegetable consumption, dietary fiber, and use of statins may reduce the risk of pancreatitis, and coffee drinking may reduce the risk of nonbiliary pancreatitis.

► Clinical Findings

A. Symptoms and Signs

Epigastric abdominal pain, generally abrupt in onset, is steady, boring, and severe and often made worse by walking and lying supine and better by sitting and leaning forward. The pain usually radiates into the back but may radiate to the right or left. Nausea and vomiting are usually present. Weakness, sweating, and anxiety are noted in severe attacks. There may be a history of alcohol intake or a heavy meal immediately preceding the attack or a history of milder similar episodes or biliary pain in the past.

The upper abdomen is tender, most often without guarding, rigidity, or rebound. The abdomen may be distended, and bowel sounds may be absent with associated ileus. Fever of 38.4–39°C, tachycardia, hypotension (even shock), pallor, and cool clammy skin are present in severe cases. Mild jaundice may be seen. Occasionally, an upper abdominal mass due to the inflamed pancreas or a pseudocyst may be palpated. Acute kidney injury (usually prerenal azotemia) may occur early in the course of acute pancreatitis.

B. Laboratory Findings

Serum amylase and lipase are elevated—usually more than three times the upper limit of normal—within 24 hours in 90% of cases; their return to normal is variable depending on the severity of disease. Lipase remains elevated longer than amylase and is slightly more accurate for the diagnosis of acute pancreatitis. Leukocytosis (10,000–30,000/mcL), proteinuria, granular casts, glycosuria (10–20% of cases), hyperglycemia, and elevated serum bilirubin may be present. Blood urea nitrogen and serum alkaline phosphatase may be elevated and coagulation tests abnormal. An elevated serum creatinine level (greater than 1.8 mg/dL [149.94 mcmol/L]) at 48 hours is associated with the development of pancreatic necrosis. In patients with clear evidence of acute pancreatitis, a serum ALT level of more than 150 units/L (3 mkat/L) suggests biliary pancreatitis. A decrease in serum calcium may reflect saponification and correlates with severity of the disease. Levels lower than 7 mg/dL (1.75 mmol/L) (when serum albumin is normal) are associated with tetany and an unfavorable prognosis. Patients with acute pancreatitis caused by hypertriglyceridemia generally have fasting triglyceride levels above 1000 mg/dL (10 mmol/L) and often have other risk factors for pancreatitis; in some cases, the serum amylase is not elevated substantially because of an inhibitor in the serum of patients with marked hypertriglyceridemia that interferes with measurement of serum amylase. An early rise in

the hematocrit value above 44% suggests hemoconcentration and predicts pancreatic necrosis. An elevated C-reactive protein concentration (greater than 150 mg/L [1500 mg/L]) at 48 hours suggests severe disease.

Other diagnostic tests that offer the possibility of simplicity, rapidity, ease of use, and low cost—including urinary trypsinogen-2, trypsinogen activation peptide, and carboxypeptidase B—are not widely available. In patients in whom ascites or a left pleural effusion develops, fluid amylase content is high. Electrocardiography may show ST–T wave changes.

C. Assessment of Severity

In addition to the individual laboratory parameters noted above, the severity of acute alcoholic pancreatitis can be assessed using several scoring systems (none of which has been shown to have high prognostic accuracy), including the **Ranson criteria** (Table 16–10). The **Sequential Organ Failure Assessment (SOFA)** score or **modified Marshall scoring system** can be used to assess injury to other organs, and the **Acute Physiology and Chronic Health Evaluation (APACHE II)** score is another tool for assessing severity. The severity of acute pancreatitis can also be predicted by the **Pancreatitis Activity Scoring System (PASS)** based on organ failure, intolerance to a solid diet, systemic inflammatory response syndrome, abdominal pain, and dose of intravenous morphine (or its equivalent). Another simple 5-point clinical scoring system (the **Bedside Index for Severity in Acute Pancreatitis,** or BISAP) based on blood urea nitrogen above 25 mg/dL (9 mmol/L), impaired mental status, systemic inflammatory response syndrome, age older than 60 years, and pleural effusion

Table 16–10. Ranson criteria for assessing the severity of acute pancreatitis.

Three or more of the following predict a severe course complicated by pancreatic necrosis with a sensitivity of 60–80%
Age over 55 years
White blood cell count > 16 × 10³/mcL (> 16 × 10⁹/L)
Blood glucose > 200 mg/dL (> 11 mmol/L)
Serum lactic dehydrogenase > 350 units/L (> 7 mkat/L)
Aspartate aminotransferase > 250 units/L (> 5 mkat/L)
Development of the following in the first 48 hours indicates a worsening prognosis
Hematocrit drop of more than 10 percentage points
Blood urea nitrogen rise > 5 mg/dL (> 1.8 mmol/L)
Arterial Po₂ of < 60 mm Hg (< 7.8 kPa)
Serum calcium of < 8 mg/dL (< 0.2 mmol/L)
Base deficit over 4 mEq/L
Estimated fluid sequestration of > 6 L
Mortality rates correlate with the number of criteria present

Number of Criteria	Mortality Rate
0–2	1%
3–4	16%
5–6	40%
7–8	100%

Table 16–11. Severity index for acute pancreatitis.

CT Grade	Points	Pancreatic Necrosis	Additional Points	Severity Index[1]	Mortality Rate[2]
A Normal pancreas	0	0%	0	0	0%
B Pancreatic enlargement	1	0%	0	1	0%
C Pancreatic inflammation and/or peripancreatic fat	2	< 30%	2	4	< 3%
D Single acute peripancreatic fluid collection	3	30–50%	4	7	6%
E Two or more acute peripancreatic fluid collections or retroperitoneal air	4	> 50%	6	10	> 17%

[1]Severity Index = CT Grade *Points* + Pancreatic Necrosis *Additional Points*.
[2]Based on the Severity Index.
Adapted with permission from Balthazar EJ. Acute pancreatitis: assessment of severity with clinical and CT evaluation. Radiology. 2002 Jun;223(3):603–13.

during the first 24 hours (before the onset of organ failure) identifies patients at increased risk for mortality. More simply, the presence of a systemic inflammatory response alone and an elevated blood urea nitrogen level on admission as well as a rise in blood urea nitrogen within the first 24 hours of hospitalization are independently associated with increased mortality; the greater the rise in blood urea nitrogen after admission, the greater the mortality rate. A model based on the change in serum amylase in the first 2 days after admission and the body mass index has been proposed. An early rise in serum levels of neutrophil gelatinase-associated lipocalin has also been proposed as a marker of severe acute pancreatitis. The absence of rebound abdominal tenderness or guarding, a normal hematocrit value, and a normal serum creatinine level (the "**harmless acute pancreatitis score**," or **HAPS**) predicts a nonsevere course with 98% accuracy. The **revised Atlanta classification** of the severity of acute pancreatitis uses the following three categories: (1) **mild** disease is the absence of organ failure and local ([peri]pancreatic necrosis or fluid collections) or systemic complications; (2) **moderate** disease is the presence of transient (under 48 hours) organ failure or local or systemic complications, or both; and (3) **severe** disease is the presence of persistent (48 hours or more) organ failure. A similar "**determinant-based**" classification also includes a category of **critical** acute pancreatitis characterized by both persistent organ failure and infected peripancreatic necrosis.

D. Imaging

Plain radiographs of the abdomen may show gallstones (if calcified), a "sentinel loop" (a segment of air-filled small intestine most commonly in the left upper quadrant), the "colon cutoff sign"—a gas-filled segment of transverse colon abruptly ending at the area of pancreatic inflammation—or focal linear atelectasis of the lower lobe of the lungs with or without pleural effusion. Ultrasonography is often not helpful in diagnosing acute pancreatitis because of intervening bowel gas but may identify gallstones in the gallbladder. Unenhanced CT is useful for demonstrating an enlarged pancreas when the diagnosis of pancreatitis is

uncertain, differentiating pancreatitis from other possible intra-abdominal catastrophes, and providing an initial assessment of prognosis but is often unnecessary early in the course (Table 16–11). Rapid-bolus intravenous contrast-enhanced CT following aggressive volume resuscitation is of particular value after the first 3 days of severe acute pancreatitis for identifying areas of necrotizing pancreatitis and assessing the degree of necrosis (although the use of intravenous contrast may increase the risk of complications of pancreatitis and of acute kidney injury and should be avoided when the serum creatinine level is above 1.5 mg/dL [124.95 mcmol/L].) MRI appears to be a suitable alternative to CT. Perfusion CT on day 3 demonstrating areas of ischemia in the pancreas has been reported to predict the development of pancreatic necrosis. The presence of a fluid collection in the pancreas correlates with an increased mortality rate. CT-guided needle aspiration of areas of necrotizing pancreatitis after the third day may disclose infection, usually by enteric organisms, which typically requires debridement. The presence of gas bubbles on CT implies infection by gas-forming organisms. EUS is useful in identifying occult biliary disease (eg, small stones, sludge, microlithiasis), which is present in a majority of patients with apparently idiopathic acute pancreatitis, and is indicated in persons over age 40 to exclude malignancy. ERCP is generally not indicated after a first attack of acute pancreatitis unless there is associated cholangitis or jaundice or a bile duct stone is known to be present, but EUS or MRCP should be considered, especially after repeated attacks of idiopathic acute pancreatitis. Following a single attack of idiopathic acute pancreatitis, a negative EUS examination predicts a low risk of relapse. In select cases, aspiration of bile for crystal analysis may confirm the suspicion of microlithiasis, and manometry of the pancreatic duct sphincter may detect sphincter of Oddi dysfunction as a cause of recurrent pancreatitis.

▶ Differential Diagnosis

Acute pancreatitis must be differentiated from an acutely perforated duodenal ulcer, acute cholecystitis, acute intestinal obstruction, leaking aortic aneurysm, renal colic, and acute mesenteric ischemia. Serum amylase may also be elevated in proximal intestinal obstruction, gastroenteritis, mumps not involving the pancreas (salivary amylase), and ectopic pregnancy and after administration of opioids and abdominal surgery. Serum lipase may also be elevated in many of these conditions.

Complications

Intravascular volume depletion secondary to leakage of fluids in the pancreatic bed and ileus with fluid-filled loops of bowel may result in prerenal azotemia and even acute tubular necrosis without overt shock. This sequence usually occurs within 24 hours of the onset of acute pancreatitis and lasts 8–9 days. Some patients require renal replacement therapy.

According to the revised Atlanta classification, fluid collections and necrosis may be acute (within the first 4 weeks) or chronic (after 4 weeks) and sterile or infected. Chronic collections, including pseudocysts and walled-off necrosis, are characterized by encapsulation. Sterile or infected necrotizing pancreatitis may complicate the course in 5–10% of cases and accounts for most of the deaths. The risk of infection does not correlate with the extent of necrosis. Pancreatic necrosis is often associated with fever, leukocytosis, and, in some cases, shock and is associated with organ failure (eg, gastrointestinal bleeding, respiratory failure, acute kidney injury) in 50% of cases. Because infected pancreatic necrosis is often an indication for debridement, fine-needle aspiration of necrotic tissue under CT guidance should be performed (if necessary, repeatedly) for Gram stain and culture.

A serious complication of acute pancreatitis is acute respiratory distress syndrome (ARDS); cardiac dysfunction may be superimposed. It usually occurs 3–7 days after the onset of pancreatitis in patients who have required large volumes of fluid and colloid to maintain blood pressure and urinary output. Most patients with ARDS require intubation, mechanical ventilation, and supplemental oxygen.

Pancreatic abscess (also referred to as infected or suppurative pseudocyst) is a suppurative process characterized by rising fever, leukocytosis, and localized tenderness and an epigastric mass usually 6 or more weeks into the course of acute pancreatitis. The abscess may be associated with a left-sided pleural effusion or an enlarging spleen secondary to splenic vein thrombosis. In contrast to infected necrosis, the mortality rate is low following drainage.

Pseudocysts, encapsulated fluid collections with high amylase content, commonly appear in pancreatitis when CT is used to monitor the evolution of an acute attack. Pseudocysts that are smaller than 6 cm in diameter often resolve spontaneously. They most commonly are within or adjacent to the pancreas but can present almost anywhere (eg, mediastinal, retrorectal) by extension along anatomic planes. Multiple pseudocysts are seen in 14% of cases. Pseudocysts may become secondarily infected, necessitating drainage as for an abscess. Pancreatic ascites may present after recovery from acute pancreatitis as a gradual increase in abdominal girth and persistent elevation of the serum amylase level in the absence of frank abdominal pain. Marked elevations in ascitic protein (greater than 3 g/dL)

and amylase (greater than 1000 units/L [20 mkat/L]) concentrations are typical. The condition results from disruption of the pancreatic duct or drainage of a pseudocyst into the peritoneal cavity.

Rare complications of acute pancreatitis include hemorrhage caused by erosion of a blood vessel to form a pseudoaneurysm and colonic necrosis. Portosplenomesenteric venous thrombosis frequently develops in patients with necrotizing acute pancreatitis but rarely leads to complications. Chronic pancreatitis develops in about 10% of cases. Permanent diabetes mellitus and exocrine pancreatic insufficiency occur uncommonly after a single acute episode.

Treatment

A. Treatment of Acute Disease

1. Mild disease—In most patients, acute pancreatitis is a mild disease ("nonsevere acute pancreatitis") that subsides spontaneously within several days. The pancreas is "rested" by a regimen of withholding food and liquids by mouth, bed rest, and, in patients with moderately severe pain or ileus and abdominal distention or vomiting, nasogastric suction. Goal-directed therapy with early fluid resuscitation (one-third of the total 72-hour fluid volume administered within 24 hours of presentation, 250–500 mL/h initially) may reduce the frequency of systemic inflammatory response syndrome and organ failure in this group of patients. Lactated Ringer solution may be preferable to normal saline; however, overly aggressive fluid resuscitation may lead to morbidity as well. Pain is controlled with meperidine, up to 100–150 mg intramuscularly every 3–4 hours as necessary. In those with severe liver or kidney dysfunction, the dose may need to be reduced. Morphine had been thought to cause sphincter of Oddi spasm but is now considered an acceptable alternative and, given the potential side effects of meperidine, may even be preferable. Oral intake of fluid and foods can be resumed when the patient is largely free of pain and has bowel sounds (even if the serum amylase is still elevated). Clear liquids are given first (this step may be skipped in patients with mild acute pancreatitis), followed by gradual advancement to a low-fat diet, guided by the patient's tolerance and by the absence of pain. Pain may recur on refeeding in 20% of patients. Following recovery from acute biliary pancreatitis, laparoscopic cholecystectomy is generally performed, preferably during the same hospital admission, and is associated with a reduced rate of recurrent gallstone-related complications compared with delayed cholecystectomy. In selected cases endoscopic sphincterotomy alone may be done. In patients with recurrent pancreatitis associated with pancreas divisum, insertion of a stent in the minor papilla (or minor papilla sphincterotomy) may reduce the frequency of subsequent attacks, although complications of such therapy are frequent. In patients with recurrent acute pancreatitis attributed to pancreatic sphincter of Oddi dysfunction, biliary sphincterotomy alone is as effective as combined biliary and pancreatic sphincterotomy in reducing the frequency of recurrent acute pancreatitis, but chronic pancreatitis may still develop in treated patients. Hypertriglyceridemia with acute pancreatitis has been treated with combinations of insulin, heparin, apheresis, and hemofiltration, but the benefit of these approaches has not been proven.

2. Severe disease—In more severe pancreatitis—particularly necrotizing pancreatitis—there may be considerable leakage of fluids, necessitating large amounts of intravenous fluids (eg, 500–1000 mL/h for several hours, then 250–300 mL/h) to maintain intravascular volume. Risk factors for high levels of fluid sequestration include younger age, alcohol etiology, higher hematocrit value, higher serum glucose, and systemic inflammatory response syndrome in the first 48 hours of hospital admission. Hemodynamic monitoring in an intensive care unit is required, and the importance of aggressive goal-directed intravenous hydration targeted to result in adequate urinary output, stabilization of blood pressure and heart rate, restoration of central venous pressure, and a modest decrease in hematocrit value cannot be overemphasized. Calcium gluconate must be given intravenously if there is evidence of hypocalcemia with tetany. Infusions of fresh frozen plasma or serum albumin may be necessary in patients with coagulopathy or hypoalbuminemia. With colloid solutions, the risk of ARDS may be increased. If shock persists after adequate volume replacement (including packed red cells), pressors may be required. For the patient requiring a large volume of parenteral fluids, central venous pressure and blood gases should be monitored at regular intervals. Enteral nutrition via a nasojejunal or possibly nasogastric feeding tube is preferable to parenteral nutrition in patients who will otherwise be without oral nutrition for at least 7–10 days and reduces the risk of multiorgan failure and mortality when started within 48 hours of admission, but may not be tolerated in some patients with an ileus and does not reduce the rates of infection and death compared with the introduction of an oral diet after 72 hours. Parenteral nutrition (including lipids) should be considered in patients who have severe pancreatitis and ileus; glutamine supplementation appears to reduce the risk of infectious complications and mortality. The routine use of antibiotics to prevent conversion of sterile necrotizing pancreatitis to infected necrosis is of no benefit and generally is not indicated in patients with less than 30% pancreatic necrosis. Imipenem (500 mg intravenously every 6 hours) and possibly cefuroxime (1.5 g intravenously three times daily, then 250 mg orally twice daily) administered for no more than 14 days to patients with sterile necrotizing pancreatitis has been reported in some studies to reduce the risk of pancreatic infection and mortality, but in general, prophylactic antibiotics are not recommended; meropenem and the combination of ciprofloxacin and metronidazole do not appear to reduce the frequency of infected necrosis, multiorgan failure, or mortality. When infected necrotizing pancreatitis is confirmed, imipenem or meropenem should be continued. Drug-resistant organisms are increasingly prevalent. In occasional cases, a fungal infection is found, and appropriate antifungal therapy should be prescribed. The role of intravenous somatostatin in severe acute pancreatitis is uncertain, and octreotide is thought to have no benefit. A small study has suggested benefit from pentoxifylline.

To date, probiotic agents have not been shown to reduce infectious complications of severe pancreatitis and may increase mortality. Nonsteroidal anti-inflammatory drugs (eg, indomethacin administered rectally) and aggressive hydration with lactated Ringer solution have been reported to reduce the frequency and severity of post-ERCP pancreatitis in persons at high risk, and rectal indomethacin is widely used, but studies of the benefit of indomethacin in unselected patients have yielded conflicting results. Placement of a stent across the pancreatic duct or orifice has been shown to reduce the risk of post-ERCP pancreatitis by 60–80% and is a common practice but has not been compared directly with rectal indomethacin.

B. Treatment of Complications and Follow-Up

A surgeon should be consulted in all cases of severe acute pancreatitis. If the diagnosis is in doubt and investigation indicates a strong possibility of a serious surgically correctable lesion (eg, perforated peptic ulcer), exploratory laparotomy is indicated. When acute pancreatitis is found unexpectedly, it is usually wise to close without intervention. If the pancreatitis appears mild and cholelithiasis or microlithiasis is present, cholecystectomy or cholecystostomy may be justified. When severe pancreatitis results from choledocholithiasis and jaundice (serum total bilirubin above 5 mg/dL [85.5 mcmol/L]) or cholangitis is present, ERCP with endoscopic sphincterotomy and stone extraction is indicated. MRCP may be useful in selecting patients for therapeutic ERCP. Endoscopic sphincterotomy does not appear to improve the outcome of severe pancreatitis in the absence of cholangitis or jaundice.

Necrosectomy may improve survival in patients with necrotizing pancreatitis and clinical deterioration with multiorgan failure or lack of resolution by 4 weeks and is often indicated for infected necrosis, although a select group of relatively stable patients with infected pancreatic necrosis may be managed with antibiotics alone. The goal is to debride necrotic pancreas and surrounding tissue and establish adequate drainage. Outcomes are best if necrosectomy is delayed until the necrosis has organized, usually about 4 weeks after disease onset. A "step-up" approach in which nonsurgical drainage of walled-off pancreatic necrosis under radiologic guidance with subsequent open surgical necrosectomy if necessary has been shown to reduce mortality and resource utilization in select patients with necrotizing pancreatitis and confirmed or suspected secondary infection. Endoscopic (transgastric or transduodenal) drainage combined with percutaneous drainage and, in some cases, laparoscopic guidance are additional options, depending on local expertise. Treatment is labor intensive, and multiple procedures are often required. Peritoneal lavage has not been shown to improve survival in severe acute pancreatitis, in part because the risk of late septic complications is not reduced.

The development of a pancreatic abscess is an indication for prompt percutaneous or surgical drainage. Chronic pseudocysts require endoscopic, percutaneous catheter, or surgical drainage when infected or associated with persisting pain, pancreatitis, or bile duct obstruction. For pancreatic infections, imipenem, 500 mg every 8 hours intravenously, is a good choice of antibiotic because it achieves bactericidal levels in pancreatic tissue for most causative organisms. Pancreatic duct leaks and fistulas may require endoscopic or surgical therapy.

Prognosis

Mortality rates for acute pancreatitis have declined from at least 10% to around 5% since the 1980s, but the mortality rate for severe acute pancreatitis (more than three Ranson criteria; see Table 16–10) remains at least 20%, with rates of 10% and 25% in those with sterile and infected necrosis, respectively. Severe acute pancreatitis is predicted by features of the systemic inflammatory response on admission; a persistent systemic inflammatory response is associated with a mortality rate of 25% and a transient response with a mortality rate of 8%. Half of the deaths occur within the first 2 weeks, usually from multiorgan failure. Multiorgan failure is associated with a mortality rate of at least 30%, and if it persists beyond the first 48 hours, the mortality rate is over 50%. Later deaths occur because of complications of infected necrosis. The risk of death doubles when both organ failure and infected necrosis are present. Moreover, hospital-acquired infections increase the mortality of acute pancreatitis, independent of severity. Readmission to the hospital for acute pancreatitis within 30 days may be predicted by a scoring system based on five factors during the index admission: eating less than a solid diet at discharge; nausea, vomiting, or diarrhea at discharge; pancreatic necrosis; use of antibiotics at discharge; and pain at discharge. Male sex, an alcohol etiology, and severe acute disease are risk factors. Recurrences are common (24%) in alcoholic pancreatitis, particularly in those who smoke (40%), but can be reduced by repeated, regularly scheduled interventions to eliminate alcohol consumption and smoking after discharge from the hospital. A severe initial attack also increases the risk of recurrence. The risk of chronic pancreatitis following an episode of acute alcoholic pancreatitis is 8% in 5 years, 13% in 10 years, and 16% in 20 years, and the risk of diabetes mellitus is increased more than twofold over 5 years. Overall, chronic pancreatitis develops in 36% of patients with recurrent acute pancreatitis; alcohol use and smoking are principal risk factors. An association between a diagnosis of acute pancreatitis and long-term risk of pancreatic cancer has been reported.

When to Admit

Nearly all patients with acute pancreatitis should be hospitalized.

Buxbaum J et al. The Pancreatitis Activity Scoring System predicts clinical outcomes in acute pancreatitis: findings from a prospective cohort study. Am J Gastroenterol. 2018 May; 113(5):755–64. [PMID: 29545634]

Crockett SD et al. American Gastroenterological Association Institute guideline on initial management of acute pancreatitis. Gastroenterology. 2018 Mar;154(4):1096–101. [PMID: 29409760]

James TW. Management of acute pancreatitis in the first 72 hours. Curr Opin Gastroenterol. 2018 Sep;34(5):330–5. [PMID: 29957661]

van Brunschot S et al. Minimally invasive and endoscopic versus open necrosectomy for necrotising pancreatitis: a pooled analysis of individual data for 1980 patients. Gut. 2018 Apr;67(4):697–706. [PMID: 28774886]

Vege SS et al. Initial medical treatment of acute pancreatitis: American Gastroenterological Association Institute technical review. Gastroenterology. 2018 Mar;154(4):1103–9. [PMID: 29421596]

CHRONIC PANCREATITIS

ESSENTIALS OF DIAGNOSIS

▶ Chronic or intermittent epigastric pain, steatorrhea, weight loss, abnormal pancreatic imaging.

▶ A mnemonic for the predisposing factors of chronic pancreatitis is TIGAR-O: toxic-metabolic, idiopathic, genetic, autoimmune, recurrent and severe acute pancreatitis, or obstructive.

General Considerations

Chronic pancreatitis occurs most often in patients with alcoholism (45–80% of all cases). The risk of chronic pancreatitis increases with the duration and amount of alcohol consumed, but pancreatitis develops in only 5–10% of heavy drinkers. Tobacco smoking is a risk factor for idiopathic chronic pancreatitis and has been reported to accelerate progression of alcoholic chronic pancreatitis. About 2% of patients with hyperparathyroidism develop pancreatitis. In tropical Africa and Asia, tropical pancreatitis, related in part to malnutrition, is the most common cause of chronic pancreatitis. A stricture, stone, or tumor obstructing the pancreas can lead to obstructive chronic pancreatitis. Autoimmune pancreatitis is associated with hypergammaglobulinemia (IgG_4 in particular), often with autoantibodies and other autoimmune diseases, and is responsive to corticosteroids. Affected persons are at increased risk for various cancers. Type 1 autoimmune pancreatitis (lymphoplasmacytic sclerosing pancreatitis, or simply autoimmune pancreatitis) is a multisystem disease, typically in a patient over age 60, characterized by lymphoplasmacytic infiltration and fibrosis on biopsy, associated bile duct strictures, retroperitoneal fibrosis, renal and salivary gland lesions, and a high rate of relapse after treatment. It is the pancreatic manifestation of IgG_4-related disease. Type 2 ("idiopathic duct-centric chronic pancreatitis") affects the pancreas alone, typically in a patient aged 40–50 years, and is characterized by intense duct-centric lymphoplasmacytic infiltration on biopsy, lack of systemic IgG_4 involvement, an association with inflammatory bowel disease in 25% of cases, often a tumor-like mass, and a low rate of relapse after treatment. Between 10% and 30% of cases of chronic pancreatitis are idiopathic, with either early onset (median age 23) or late onset (median age 62). Genetic factors may predispose to chronic pancreatitis in some of these cases and include mutations of the cystic fibrosis transmembrane conductance regulator (*CFTR*) gene, the pancreatic secretory trypsin inhibitory gene (*PSTI*, serine protease inhibitor, *SPINK1*), and possibly the gene for uridine 5′-diphosphate glucuronosyltransferase. Mutation of the cationic trypsinogen gene on chromosome 7 (serine protease 1, *PRSS1*) is associated with hereditary pancreatitis, transmitted as an autosomal dominant trait with variable penetrance. A useful mnemonic for the predisposing factors to chronic pancreatitis is TIGAR-O: toxic-metabolic, idiopathic, genetic, autoimmune, recurrent and severe acute pancreatitis, or obstructive.

The pathogenesis of chronic pancreatitis may be explained by the SAPE (*s*entinel *a*cute *p*ancreatitis *e*vent) hypothesis by which the first (sentinel) acute pancreatitis event initiates an inflammatory process that results in injury and later fibrosis ("necrosis-fibrosis"). In many cases, chronic pancreatitis is a self-perpetuating disease characterized by chronic pain or recurrent episodes of acute pancreatitis and ultimately by pancreatic exocrine or endocrine insufficiency (sooner in alcoholic pancreatitis than in other types). After many years, chronic pain may resolve spontaneously or as a result of surgery tailored to the cause of pain. Over 80% of adults develop diabetes mellitus within 25 years after the clinical onset of chronic pancreatitis.

▶ Clinical Findings

A. Symptoms and Signs

Persistent or recurrent episodes of epigastric and left upper quadrant pain are typical. The pain results in part from impaired inhibitory pain modulation by the central nervous system. Anorexia, nausea, vomiting, constipation, flatulence, and weight loss are common. During attacks, tenderness over the pancreas, mild muscle guarding, and ileus may be noted. Attacks may last only a few hours or as long as 2 weeks; pain may eventually be almost continuous. Steatorrhea (as indicated by bulky, foul, fatty stools) may occur late in the course.

B. Laboratory Findings

Serum amylase and lipase may be elevated during acute attacks; however, normal values do not exclude the diagnosis. Serum alkaline phosphatase and bilirubin may be elevated owing to compression of the bile duct. Glycosuria may be present. Excess fecal fat may be demonstrated on chemical analysis of the stool. Exocrine pancreatic insufficiency generally is confirmed by response to therapy with pancreatic enzyme supplements; the secretin stimulation test can be used if available (and has a high negative predictive factor for ruling out early acute chronic pancreatitis), as can detection of decreased fecal chymotrypsin or elastase levels, although the latter tests lack sensitivity and specificity. Vitamin B_{12} malabsorption is detectable in about 40% of patients, but clinical deficiency of vitamin B_{12} and fat-soluble vitamins is rare. Accurate diagnostic tests are available for the major trypsinogen gene mutations, but because of uncertainty about the mechanisms linking heterozygous *CFTR* and *PSTI* mutations with pancreatitis, genetic testing for mutations in these two genes is not currently recommended. Elevated IgG_4 levels, ANA, antibodies to lactoferrin

and carbonic anhydrase II, and other autoantibodies are often found in patients with autoimmune pancreatitis (especially type 1). Pancreatic biopsy, if necessary, shows a lymphoplasmacytic inflammatory infiltrate with characteristic IgG_4 immunostaining, which is also found in biopsy specimens of the major papilla, bile duct, and salivary glands, in type 1 autoimmune pancreatitis.

C. Imaging

Plain films show calcifications due to pancreaticolithiasis in 30% of affected patients. CT may show calcifications not seen on plain films as well as ductal dilatation and heterogeneity or atrophy of the gland. Occasionally, the findings raise suspicion of pancreatic cancer ("tumefactive chronic pancreatitis"). ERCP is the most sensitive imaging study for chronic pancreatitis and may show dilated ducts, intraductal stones, strictures, or pseudocyst but is infrequently used for diagnosis alone; moreover, the results may be normal in patients with so-called minimal change pancreatitis. MRCP (including secretin-enhanced MRCP) and EUS (with pancreatic tissue sampling) are less invasive alternatives to ERCP. Endoscopic ultrasonographic ("Rosemont") criteria for the diagnosis of chronic pancreatitis include hyperechoic foci with shadowing indicative of calculi in the main pancreatic duct and lobularity with honeycombing of the pancreatic parenchyma. Characteristic imaging features of autoimmune pancreatitis include diffuse enlargement of the pancreas, a peripheral rim of hypoattenuation, and irregular narrowing of the main pancreatic duct. In the United States, the diagnosis of autoimmune pancreatitis is based on the HISORt criteria: *h*istology, *i*maging, *s*erology, *o*ther *o*rgan involvement, and *r*esponse to corticosteroid *t*herapy.

▶ Complications

Opioid addiction is common. Other frequent complications include often brittle diabetes mellitus, pancreatic pseudocyst or abscess, cholestatic liver enzymes with or without jaundice, bile duct stricture, exocrine pancreatic insufficiency, malnutrition, osteoporosis, and peptic ulcer. Pancreatic cancer develops in 4% of patients after 20 years; the risk may relate to tobacco and alcohol use. In patients with hereditary pancreatitis, the risk of pancreatic cancer rises after age 50 years and reaches 19% by age 70 years (see Chapter 39).

▶ Treatment

A. Medical Measures

A low-fat diet should be prescribed. Alcohol is forbidden because it frequently precipitates attacks. Opioids should be avoided if possible. Preferred agents for pain are acetaminophen, nonsteroidal anti-inflammatory drugs, and tramadol, along with pain-modifying agents such as tricyclic antidepressants, selective serotonin reuptake inhibitors, and gabapentin or pregabalin. Exocrine pancreatic insufficiency is treated with pancreatic enzyme replacement therapy selected on the basis of high lipase activity (Table 16–12). A total dose of at least 40,000 units of lipase in capsules is given with each meal. Doses of 90,000 units or more of lipase per meal may be required in some cases. The tablets should be taken at the start of, during, and at the end of a meal. Concurrent administration of an H_2-receptor antagonist (eg, ranitidine, 150 mg orally twice daily), a proton pump inhibitor (eg, omeprazole, 20–60 mg orally daily), or sodium bicarbonate, 650 mg orally before and after meals, decreases the inactivation of lipase by acid and may thereby further decrease steatorrhea. In selected cases of alcoholic pancreatitis and in cystic fibrosis, enteric-coated microencapsulated preparations may offer an advantage; however, in patients with cystic fibrosis, high-dose pancreatic enzyme replacement therapy has been associated with strictures of the ascending colon. Pain secondary to idiopathic chronic pancreatitis may be alleviated in some cases by the use of pancreatic enzyme replacement therapy (not enteric-coated preparations) or octreotide, 200 mcg subcutaneously three times daily. Associated diabetes mellitus should be treated (see Chapter 27). Autoimmune pancreatitis is treated with prednisone 40 mg/day orally for 1–2 months, followed by a taper of 5 mg every 2–4 weeks. Nonresponse or relapse occurs in 45% of type 1 cases (particularly in those with concomitant IgG_4-associated cholangitis); rituximab is an effective induction and maintenance agent, and azathioprine or long-term low-dose corticosteroid use appears to reduce the risk of relapse.

B. Endoscopic and Surgical Treatment

Endoscopic therapy or surgery may be indicated in chronic pancreatitis to treat underlying biliary tract disease, ensure free flow of bile into the duodenum, drain persistent pseudocysts, treat other complications, eliminate obstruction of the pancreatic duct, attempt to relieve pain, or exclude pancreatic cancer. Liver fibrosis may regress after biliary drainage. Distal bile duct obstruction may be relieved by endoscopic placement of multiple bile duct stents. When obstruction of the duodenal end of the pancreatic duct can be demonstrated by ERCP, dilation of or placement of a stent in the duct and pancreatic duct stone lithotripsy or surgical resection of the tail of the pancreas with implantation of the distal end of the duct by pancreaticojejunostomy may be performed. Endoscopic therapy is successful in about 50% of cases. In patients who do not respond to endoscopic therapy, surgery is successful in about 50%. When the pancreatic duct is diffusely dilated, anastomosis between the duct after it is split longitudinally and a defunctionalized limb of jejunum (modified Puestow procedure), in some cases combined with resection of the head of the pancreas (Beger or Frey procedure), is associated with relief of pain in 80% of cases. In advanced cases, subtotal or total pancreatectomy may be considered as a last resort but has variable efficacy and causes pancreatic insufficiency and diabetes mellitus. Endoscopic or surgical (including laparoscopic) drainage is indicated for symptomatic pseudocysts and, in many cases, those over 6 cm in diameter. EUS may facilitate selection of an optimal site for endoscopic drainage. Pancreatic ascites or pancreaticopleural fistulas due to a disrupted pancreatic duct can be managed by endoscopic placement of a stent across the disrupted duct. Pancreatic sphincterotomy or fragmentation of stones in the pancreatic duct by lithotripsy and endoscopic removal of stones from the duct may relieve pain in selected patients. For patients with chronic pain and nondilated ducts, a percutaneous celiac plexus nerve block may be considered under either CT or EUS guidance, with pain relief (albeit often short-lived) in approximately 50% of patients. A single session of radiation therapy to the pancreas has been reported to relieve otherwise refractory pain.

► Prognosis

Chronic pancreatitis often leads to disability and reduced life expectancy; pancreatic cancer is the main cause

Table 16–12. FDA-approved pancreatic enzyme (pancrelipase) preparations.

Product	Enzyme Content/Unit Dose, USP Units		
	Lipase	Amylase	Protease
Immediate-Release Capsules			
Nonenteric-coated			
Viokace 10,440	10,440	39,150	39,150
Viokace 20,880	20,880	78,300	78,300
Delayed-Release Capsules			
Enteric-coated minimicrospheres			
Creon 3000	3000	15,000	9500
Creon 6000	6000	30,000	19,000
Creon 12,000	12,000	60,000	38,000
Creon 24,000	24,000	120,000	76,000
Creon 36,000	36,000	180,000	114,000
Enteric-coated minitablets			
Ultresa 13,800	13,800	27,600	27,600
Ultresa 20,700	20,700	46,000	41,400
Ultresa 23,000	23,000	46,000	41,400
Enteric-coated beads			
Zenpep 3000	3000	16,000	10,000
Zenpep 5000	5000	27,000	17,000
Zenpep 10,000	10,000	55,000	34,000
Zenpep 15,000	15,000	82,000	51,000
Zenpep 20,000	20,000	109,000	68,000
Zenpep 25,000	25,000	136,000	85,000
Enteric-coated microtablets			
Pancreaze 4200	4200	17,500	10,000
Pancreaze 10,500	10,500	43,750	25,000
Pancreaze 16,800	16,800	70,000	40,000
Pancreaze 21,000	21,000	61,000	37,000
Bicarbonate-buffered enteric-coated microspheres			
Peptyze 8000	8000	30,250	28,750
Peptyze 16,000	16,000	60,500	57,500

FDA, US Food and Drug Administration; USP, US Pharmacopeia.

of death. The prognosis is best in patients with recurrent acute pancreatitis caused by a remediable condition, such as cholelithiasis, choledocholithiasis, stenosis of the sphincter of Oddi, or hyperparathyroidism, and in those with autoimmune pancreatitis. Medical management of hyperlipidemia, if present, may also prevent recurrent attacks of pancreatitis. A chronic pancreatitis diagnosis score based on pain, hemoglobin A_{1c} level, C-reactive protein level, body mass index, and platelet count has been shown to correlate with hospital admissions and number of hospital days. In alcoholic pancreatitis, pain relief is most likely when a dilated pancreatic duct can be decompressed. In patients with disease not amenable to decompressive surgery, addiction to opioids is a frequent outcome of treatment. A poorer quality of life is associated with constant rather than intermittent pain, pain-related disability or unemployment, current smoking, and comorbidities.

When to Refer

All patients with chronic pancreatitis should be referred for diagnostic and therapeutic procedures.

When to Admit

- Severe pain.
- New jaundice.
- New fever.

Dominguez-Muñoz JE. Diagnosis and treatment of pancreatic exocrine insufficiency. Curr Opin Gastroenterol. 2018 Sep;34(5):349–54. [PMID: 29889111]

Lorenzo D et al; GETAID-AIP study group. Features of autoimmune pancreatitis associated with inflammatory bowel diseases. Clin Gastroenterol Hepatol. 2018 Jan;16(1):59–67. [PMID: 28782667]

Nagpal SJS et al. Autoimmune pancreatitis. Am J Gastroenterol. 2018 Sep;113(9):1301–9. [PMID: 29910463]

Vanga RR et al. Diagnostic performance of measurement of fecal elastase-1 in detection of exocrine pancreatic insufficiency: systematic review and meta-analysis. Clin Gastroenterol Hepatol. 2018 Aug;16(8):1220–8. [PMID: 29374614]

Yadav D et al. Managing chronic pancreatitis: the view from medical pancreatology. Am J Gastroenterol. 2018 Aug;113(8): 1108–10. [PMID: 29748562]

Breast Disorders

Armando E. Giuliano, MD, FACS, FRCSEd
Sara A. Hurvitz, MD, FACP

BENIGN BREAST DISORDERS

FIBROCYSTIC CONDITION

ESSENTIALS OF DIAGNOSIS

▶ Painful breast masses; often multiple and bilateral.

▶ Rapid fluctuation in mass size is common.

▶ Pain often worsens during premenstrual phase of cycle.

▶ Most common age is 30–50. Rare in postmenopausal women not receiving hormonal replacement.

▶ General Considerations

Fibrocystic condition is the most frequent lesion of the breast. Although commonly referred to as "fibrocystic disease," it does not, in fact, represent a pathologic or anatomic disorder. It is common in women 30–50 years of age but rare in postmenopausal women who are not taking hormonal replacement. Estrogen is considered a causative factor. There may be an increased risk in women who drink alcohol, especially women between 18 and 22 years of age.

The microscopic findings of fibrocystic condition include cysts (gross and microscopic), papillomatosis, adenosis, fibrosis, and ductal epithelial hyperplasia. Although fibrocystic condition has generally been considered to increase the risk of subsequent breast cancer, *only the variants with a component of epithelial proliferation (especially with atypia), papillomatosis, or increased breast density on mammogram represent true risk factors.*

▶ Clinical Findings

A. Symptoms and Signs

Fibrocystic condition may produce an asymptomatic mass in the breast that is discovered by accident, but pain or tenderness often calls attention to it. Discomfort often occurs or worsens during the premenstrual phase of the cycle, at which time the cysts tend to enlarge. Fluctuations in size

and rapid appearance or disappearance of a breast mass are common with this condition as are multiple or bilateral masses and serous nipple discharge. Patients will give a history of a transient lump in the breast or cyclic breast pain.

B. Diagnostic Tests

Mammography and ultrasonography should be used to evaluate a mass in a patient with fibrocystic condition. Ultrasonography alone may be used in women under 30 years of age. Because a mass due to fibrocystic condition is difficult to distinguish from carcinoma on the basis of clinical findings, *suspicious lesions should be biopsied.* Core needle biopsy, rather than fine-needle aspiration (FNA), is the preferable technique. Excisional biopsy is rarely necessary but should be done for lesions with atypia or where imaging and biopsy results are discordant. Surgery should be conservative, since the primary objective is to exclude cancer. Occasionally, FNA cytology will suffice. Simple mastectomy or extensive removal of breast tissue is rarely, if ever, indicated for fibrocystic condition.

▶ Differential Diagnosis

Pain, fluctuation in size, and multiplicity of lesions are the features most helpful in differentiating fibrocystic condition from carcinoma. If a dominant mass is present, the diagnosis of cancer should be assumed until disproven by biopsy. Mammography may be helpful, but the breast tissue in young women is usually too radiodense to permit a worthwhile study. Sonography is useful in differentiating a cystic mass from a solid mass, especially in women with dense breasts. Final diagnosis, however, depends on analysis of a biopsy specimen.

▶ Treatment

When the diagnosis of fibrocystic condition has been established by previous biopsy or is likely because the history is classic, aspiration of a discrete mass suggestive of a cyst is indicated to alleviate pain and, more importantly, to confirm the cystic nature of the mass. The patient is reexamined at intervals thereafter. If no fluid is obtained by aspiration, if fluid is bloody, if a mass persists after aspiration, or if at any time during follow-up a persistent or recurrent mass is noted, biopsy should be performed.

Breast pain associated with generalized fibrocystic condition is best treated by avoiding trauma and by wearing a good supportive brassiere during the night and day. Hormone therapy is not advisable because it does not cure the condition and has undesirable side effects. Danazol (100–200 mg orally twice daily), a synthetic androgen, is the only treatment approved by the US Food and Drug Administration (FDA) for patients with severe pain. This treatment suppresses pituitary gonadotropins, but androgenic effects (acne, edema, hirsutism) usually make this treatment intolerable; in practice, it is rarely used. Similarly, tamoxifen reduces some symptoms of fibrocystic condition, but because of its side effects, it is not useful for young women unless it is given to reduce the risk of cancer. Postmenopausal women receiving hormone replacement therapy may stop or change doses of hormones to reduce pain. Oil of evening primrose, a natural form of gamolenic acid, has been shown to decrease pain in 44–58% of users. The dosage of gamolenic acid is six capsules of 500 mg orally twice daily. Studies have also demonstrated a low-fat diet or decreasing dietary fat intake may reduce the painful symptoms associated with fibrocystic condition. Topical treatments such as nonsteroidal anti-inflammatory drugs are rarely of value.

The role of caffeine consumption in the development and treatment of fibrocystic condition is controversial. Some studies suggest that eliminating caffeine from the diet is associated with improvement while other studies refute the benefit entirely. Many patients are aware of these studies and report relief of symptoms after giving up coffee, tea, and chocolate. Similarly, many women find vitamin E (400 international units daily) helpful; however, these observations remain anecdotal.

▶ Prognosis

Exacerbations of pain, tenderness, and cyst formation may occur at any time until menopause, when symptoms usually subside, except in patients receiving hormonal replacement. The patient should be advised to examine her own breasts regularly just after menstruation and to inform her clinician if a mass appears. The risk of breast cancer developing in women with fibrocystic condition with a proliferative or atypical epithelial hyperplasia or papillomatosis is higher than that of the general population. These women should be monitored carefully with physical examinations and imaging studies.

Chetlen AL et al. Mastalgia: imaging work-up appropriateness. Acad Radiol. 2017 Mar;24:345–9. [PMID: 27916596]
Groen JW et al. Cyclic and non-cyclic breast pain: a systematic review on pain reduction, side effects, and quality of life for various treatments. Eur J Obstet Gynecol Reprod Biol. 2017 Dec;219:74–93. [PMID: 29059585]

FIBROADENOMA OF THE BREAST

This common benign neoplasm occurs most frequently in young women, usually within 20 years after puberty. It is somewhat more frequent and tends to occur at an earlier age in black women. Multiple tumors are found in 10–15% of patients.

The typical **fibroadenoma** is a round or ovoid, rubbery, discrete, relatively movable, nontender mass 1–5 cm in diameter. It is usually discovered accidentally. Clinical diagnosis in young patients is generally not difficult. In women over 30 years, fibrocystic condition of the breast and carcinoma of the breast must be considered. Cysts can be identified by aspiration or ultrasonography. Fibroadenoma does not normally occur after menopause but may occasionally develop after administration of hormones.

No treatment is usually necessary if the diagnosis can be made by core needle biopsy. Excision with pathologic examination of the specimen is performed if the diagnosis is uncertain or the lesion grows significantly. Cryoablation, or freezing of the fibroadenoma, appears to be a safe procedure if the lesion is a biopsy-proven fibroadenoma prior to ablation. Cryoablation is not appropriate for all fibroadenomas because some are too large to freeze or the diagnosis may not be certain. There is no obvious clinical advantage to cryoablation of a histologically proven fibroadenoma except that some patients may feel relief that a mass is gone. However, at times a mass of scar or fat necrosis replaces the mass of the fibroadenoma. Reassurance seems preferable. It is usually not possible to distinguish a large fibroadenoma from a phyllodes tumor on the basis of needle biopsy results or imaging alone and histology is usually required. Presumed fibroadenomas larger than 3–4 cm should be excised to rule out phyllodes tumors.

Phyllodes tumor is a fibroadenoma-like tumor with cellular stroma that grows rapidly. It may reach a large size and, if inadequately excised, will recur locally. The lesion can be benign or malignant. If benign, phyllodes tumor is treated by local excision. The treatment of malignant phyllodes tumor is more controversial, but complete removal of the tumor with a margin of normal tissue avoids recurrence. Because these tumors may be large, total mastectomy is sometimes necessary. Lymph node dissection is not performed, since the sarcomatous portion of the tumor metastasizes to the lungs and not the lymph nodes.

Co M et al. Mammary phyllodes tumour: a 15-year multicentre clinical review. J Clin Pathol. 2018 Jun;71(6):493–7. [PMID: 29146885]
Koh VCY et al. Size and heterologous elements predict metastases in malignant phyllodes tumours of the breast. Virchows Arch. 2018 Apr;472(4):615–21. [PMID: 29127495]
Krings G et al. Fibroepithelial lesions; the WHO spectrum. Semin Diagn Pathol. 2017 Sep;34(5):438–52. [PMID: 28688536]

NIPPLE DISCHARGE

In order of decreasing frequency, the following are the most common causes of nipple discharge in the nonlactating breast: duct ectasia, intraductal papilloma, and carcinoma. The important characteristics of the discharge and some other factors to be evaluated by history and physical examination are listed in Table 17–1.

Spontaneous, unilateral, serous or serosanguineous discharge from a single duct is usually caused by an ectatic duct or an intraductal papilloma or, rarely, by an

Table 17–1. Characteristics of nipple discharge in the nonpregnant, nonlactating woman.

Finding	Significance
Serous	Most likely benign FCC, ie, duct ectasia
Bloody	More likely neoplastic–papilloma, carcinoma
Associated mass	More likely neoplastic
Unilateral	Either neoplastic or non-neoplastic
Bilateral	Most likely non-neoplastic
Single duct	More likely neoplastic
Multiple ducts	More likely FCC
Milky	Endocrine disorders, medications
Spontaneous	Either neoplastic or non-neoplastic
Produced by pressure at single site	Either neoplastic or non-neoplastic
Persistent	Either neoplastic or non-neoplastic
Intermittent	Either neoplastic or non-neoplastic
Related to menses	More likely FCC
Premenopausal	More likely FCC
Taking hormones	More likely FCC

FCC, fibrocystic condition.

intraductal cancer. A mass may not be palpable. The involved duct may be identified by pressure at different sites around the nipple at the margin of the areola. Bloody discharge is suggestive of cancer but is more often caused by a benign papilloma in the duct. Cytologic examination may identify malignant cells, but negative findings do not rule out cancer, which is more likely in women over age 50 years. In any case, the involved bloody duct—and a mass if present—should be excised. A ductogram (a mammogram of a duct after radiopaque dye has been injected), like cytology, is of limited value since excision of the suspicious ductal system is indicated regardless of findings. Ductoscopy, evaluation of the ductal system with a small scope inserted through the nipple, has been attempted but is not effective management.

In premenopausal women, spontaneous multiple duct discharge, unilateral or bilateral, most noticeable just before menstruation, is often due to fibrocystic condition. Discharge may be green or brownish. Papillomatosis and ductal ectasia are usually detected only by biopsy. If a mass is present, it should be removed.

A milky discharge from multiple ducts in the nonlactating breast may occur from hyperprolactinemia. Serum prolactin levels should be obtained to search for a pituitary tumor. Thyroid-stimulating hormone (TSH) helps exclude causative hypothyroidism. Numerous antipsychotic medications and other medications may also cause a milky discharge that ceases on discontinuance of the medication.

Oral contraceptive agents or estrogen replacement therapy may cause clear, serous, or milky discharge from a single duct, but multiple duct discharge is more common.

In the premenopausal woman, the discharge is more evident just before menstruation and disappears on stopping the medication. If it does not stop, is from a single duct, and is copious, exploration should be performed since this may be a sign of cancer.

A purulent discharge may originate in a subareolar abscess and require removal of the abscess and the related lactiferous sinus.

When localization is not possible, no mass is palpable, and the discharge is nonbloody, the patient should be reexamined every 3 or 4 months for a year, and a mammogram and an ultrasound should be performed. Although most discharge is from a benign process, patients may find it annoying or disconcerting. To eliminate the discharge, proximal duct excision can be performed both for treatment and diagnosis.

Castellano I et al. The impact of malignant nipple discharge cytology (NDc) in surgical management of breast cancer patients. PLoS One. 2017 Aug 14;12(8):e0182073. [PMID: 28806416]

de Paula IB et al. Breast imaging in patients with nipple discharge. Radiol Bras. 2017 Nov–Dec;50(6):383–8. [PMID: 29307929]

Li GZ et al. Evaluating the risk of underlying malignancy in patients with pathologic nipple discharge. Breast J. 2018 Jul; 24(4):624–7. [PMID: 29520933]

FAT NECROSIS

Fat necrosis is a rare lesion of the breast but is of clinical importance because it produces a mass (often accompanied by skin or nipple retraction) that is usually indistinguishable from carcinoma even with imaging studies. In the past, most fat necrosis has been seen after trauma, but now fat necrosis is commonly seen after fat injections to augment breast size or fill defects after breast surgery. The resultant mass may be confused with cancer. If untreated, the mass gradually disappears. If imaging is not typical of fat necrosis, the safest course is to obtain a biopsy. Core needle biopsy is usually adequate. Fat necrosis is also common after segmental resection, radiation therapy, or flap reconstruction after mastectomy.

Nakada H et al. Fat necrosis after breast-conserving oncoplastic surgery. Breast Cancer. 2019 Jan;26(1):125–30. [PMID: 30151780]

BREAST ABSCESS

During nursing, an area of redness, tenderness, and induration may develop in the breast. The organism most commonly found in these abscesses is *Staphylococcus aureus* (see Puerperal Mastitis, Chapter 19).

Infection in the nonlactating breast is rare. A subareolar abscess may develop in young or middle-aged women who are not lactating. These infections tend to recur after incision and drainage unless the area is explored during a quiescent interval, with excision of the involved lactiferous duct or ducts at the base of the nipple. In the nonlactating breast, inflammatory carcinoma must always be considered. Thus, incision and biopsy of any indurated tissue with a small piece of erythematous skin is indicated when suspected abscess or cellulitis in the nonlactating breast does not resolve promptly with antibiotics. Often needle or catheter drainage is adequate to treat an abscess, but surgical incision and drainage may be necessary.

Barron AU et al. Do acute-care surgeons follow best practices for breast abscess management? A single-institution analysis of 325 consecutive cases. J Surg Res. 2017 Aug;216:169–71. [PMID: 28807202]

Saboo A et al. Trends in non-lactation breast abscesses in a tertiary hospital setting. ANZ J Surg. 2018 Jul–Aug;88(7–8): 739–44. [PMID: 29045009]

Taffurelli M et al. Recurrent periductal mastitis: surgical treatment. Surgery. 2016 Dec;160(6):1689–92. [PMID: 27616631]

DISORDERS OF THE AUGMENTED BREAST

At least 4 million American women have had breast implants. Breast augmentation is performed by placing implants under the pectoralis muscle or, less desirably, in the subcutaneous tissue of the breast. Most implants are made of an outer silicone shell filled with a silicone gel, saline, or some combination of the two. Capsule contraction or scarring around the implant develops in about 15–25% of patients, leading to a firmness and distortion of the breast that can be painful. Some require removal of the implant and surrounding capsule.

Implant rupture may occur in as many as 5–10% of women, and bleeding of gel through the capsule is noted even more commonly. Although silicone gel may be an immunologic stimulant, there is *no increase* in autoimmune disorders in patients with such implants. The FDA has advised symptomatic women with ruptured silicone implants to discuss possible surgical removal with their clinicians. However, women who are asymptomatic and have no evidence of rupture of a silicone gel prosthesis should probably not undergo removal of the implant. Women with symptoms of autoimmune illnesses often undergo removal, but no benefit has been shown.

Studies have failed to show any association between implants and an increased incidence of breast cancer. However, breast cancer may develop in a patient with an augmentation prosthesis, as it does in women without them. Detection in patients with implants may be more difficult because mammography is less able to detect early lesions. Mammography is better if the implant is subpectoral rather than subcutaneous. Prostheses should be placed retropectorally after mastectomy to facilitate detection of a local recurrence of cancer, which is usually cutaneous or subcutaneous and is easily detected by palpation. Rarely lymphoma of the breast with silicone implants has been reported.

If a cancer develops in a patient with implants, it should be treated in the same manner as in women without implants. Such women should be offered the option of mastectomy or breast-conserving therapy, which may require removal or replacement of the implant. Radiotherapy of the augmented breast often results in marked capsular contracture. Adjuvant treatments should be given for the same indications as for women who have no implants.

Clemens MW et al. NCCN consensus guidelines for the diagnosis and management of breast implant-associated anaplastic large cell lymphoma. Aesthet Surg J. 2017 Mar 1;37(3):285–9. [PMID: 28184418]

Doren EL et al. U.S. epidemiology of breast implant-associated anaplastic large cell lymphoma. Plast Reconstr Surg. 2017 May; 139(5):1042–50. [PMID: 28157769]

Elston JB et al. Complications and recurrence in implant-sparing oncologic breast surgery. Ann Plast Surg. 2017 Jun;78 (6S Suppl 5):S269–74. [PMID: 28328633]

CARCINOMA OF THE FEMALE BREAST

ESSENTIALS OF DIAGNOSIS

▶ Risk factors: Age, nulliparity, childbirth after age 30, family history of breast cancer or genetic mutations (*BRCA1*, *BRCA2*), and personal history of breast cancer or some types of proliferative conditions.

▶ **Early findings:** Single, nontender, firm to hard mass with ill-defined margins; mammographic abnormalities and no palpable mass.

▶ **Later findings:** Skin or nipple retraction; axillary lymphadenopathy; breast enlargement, erythema, edema, pain; fixation of mass to skin or chest wall.

▶ Incidence & Risk Factors

Breast cancer will develop in *one of eight* American women. Next to skin cancer, breast cancer is the most common cancer in women; it is second only to lung cancer as a cause of death. In 2018, there were approximately 268,670 new cases and 41,400 deaths from breast cancer in the United States. Worldwide, breast cancer is diagnosed in approximately 2.1 million women, and about 626,679 die of breast cancer each year, with the highest rates of diagnosis in Australia/New Zealand, Europe, and North America and lowest rates in Eastern/Middle Africa and South Central Asia. The highest rates of death are in black women in the United States and the lowest rates are in Korean women.

The most significant risk factor for the development of breast cancer is age. A woman's risk of breast cancer rises rapidly until her early 60s, peaks in her 70s, and then declines. A significant family history of breast or ovarian cancer may also indicate a high risk of developing breast cancer. Germline mutations in the *BRCA* family of tumor suppressor genes or other breast cancer susceptibility genes accounts for approximately 5–10% of breast cancer diagnoses and tend to cluster in certain ethnic groups, including women of Ashkenazi Jewish descent. Women with a mutation in the *BRCA1* gene, located on chromosome 17, have an estimated 85% chance of developing breast cancer in their lifetime. Other genes associated with an increased risk of breast and other cancers include *BRCA2* (associated with a gene on chromosome 13); ataxia-telangiectasia mutation (*ATM*), *BARD1*, *CHEK2*, *PALB2*, *RAD51D*; and mutation of the tumor suppressor gene *p53*. If a woman has a compelling family history (such as breast cancer diagnosed in two first-degree relatives, especially if diagnosed younger than age 50; ovarian cancer; male breast cancer; or a first-degree relative with bilateral breast cancer), genetic testing may be appropriate. In general, it is best for a woman who has a strong family history to meet with a genetics counselor to undergo a risk assessment and decide whether genetic testing is indicated.

Even when genetic testing fails to reveal a predisposing genetic mutation, women with a strong family history of breast cancer are at higher risk for development of breast cancer. Compared with a woman with no affected family members, a woman who has one first-degree relative with breast cancer has double the risk of developing breast cancer and a woman with two first-degree relatives with breast cancer has triple the risk of developing breast cancer. The risk is further increased for a woman whose affected family member was premenopausal at the time of diagnosis or had bilateral breast cancer. Lifestyle and reproductive factors also contribute to risk of breast cancer. Nulliparous women and women whose first full-term pregnancy occurred after the age of 30 have an elevated risk. Early menarche (under age 12) and late natural menopause (after age 55) are associated with an increase in risk, especially for hormone receptor–positive breast cancer. Combined oral contraceptive pills also appear to increase the risk of breast cancer, with longer use associated with higher risk. Several studies show that concomitant administration of progesterone and estrogen to postmenopausal women may increase the incidence of breast cancer, compared with the use of estrogen alone or with no hormone replacement treatment. Alcohol consumption, high dietary intake of fat, and lack of exercise may also increase the risk of breast cancer. Fibrocystic breast condition is also associated with an increased incidence of cancer when it is accompanied by proliferative changes, papillomatosis, atypical epithelial hyperplasia, and increased breast density on mammogram. A woman who had cancer in one breast is at increased risk for cancer developing in the other breast. In these women, a contralateral cancer develops at rate of 1% or 2% per year. Women with cancer of the uterine corpus have a risk of breast cancer significantly higher than that of the general population, and women with breast cancer have a comparably increased risk of endometrial cancer. Socioeconomic and racial factors have also been associated with breast cancer risk. Breast cancer tends to be diagnosed more frequently in women of higher socioeconomic status.

Women at greater than average risk for developing breast cancer (Table 17–2) should be identified by their clinicians and monitored carefully. Several risk assessment models have been validated (most extensively the Gail 2 model) to evaluate a woman's risk of developing cancer. Those with an exceptional family history should be counseled about the option of genetic testing. Some of these high-risk women may consider prophylactic mastectomy, oophorectomy, tamoxifen, or an aromatase inhibitor (AI).

Women with genetic mutations in whom breast cancer develops may be treated in the same way as women who do not have mutations (ie, lumpectomy), though there is an

Table 17–2. Factors associated with increased risk of breast cancer (listed in alphabetical order).

Age	Older
Family history	Breast cancer in parent, sibling, or child (especially bilateral or premenopausal)
Genetics	*BRCA1*, *BRCA2*, or other unknown mutations
Menstrual history	Early menarche (under age 12) Late menopause (after age 50)
Previous medical history	Endometrial cancer Proliferative forms of fibrocystic disease Cancer in other breast
Race	White
Reproductive history	Nulliparous or late first pregnancy

increased risk of ipsilateral and contralateral breast cancer after lumpectomy for these women. One study showed that of patients with a diagnosis of breast cancer who were found to be carriers of a *BRCA* mutation, approximately 50% chose to undergo bilateral mastectomy.

Bray F et al. Global cancer statistics 2018: GLOBOCAN estimates of incidence and mortality worldwide for 36 cancers in 185 countries. CA Cancer J Clin. 2018 Nov;68(6):394–424. [PMID: 30207593]

Couch FJ et al. Associations between cancer predisposition testing panel genes and breast cancer. JAMA Oncol. 2017 Sep 1;3(9):1190–6. [PMID: 28418444]

Frey MK et al. Prevalence of nonfounder *BRCA1/2* mutations in Ashkenazi Jewish patients presenting for genetic testing at a hereditary breast and ovarian cancer center. Cancer. 2019 Mar 1;125(5):690–7. [PMID: 30480775]

Ginsburg O et al. The global burden of women's cancers: a grand challenge in global health. Lancet. 2017 Feb 25;389(10071): 847–60. [PMID: 27814965]

Siegel RL et al. Cancer statistics, 2018. CA Cancer J Clin. 2018 Jan; 68(1):7–30. [PMID: 29313949]

▶ Prevention

Several clinical trials have evaluated the use of selective **estrogen receptor modulators (SERMs),** including tamoxifen and raloxifene, for prevention of breast cancer in women with no personal history of breast cancer but at high risk for developing the disease. A meta-analysis of nine of these studies including 83,399 women with a median follow-up of 65 months demonstrated a 38% reduction in breast cancer incidence (hazard ratio [HR], 0.62; 95% CI, 0.56, 0.69) with a 10-year cumulative incidence of 6.3% in control groups and 4.2% in SERM-treated groups. An increased risk of endometrial cancer, cataracts, and venous thromboembolic events but a reduced risk of vertebral fractures was seen in SERM groups. While SERMs have been shown to be effective at reducing the risk of breast cancer and saving costs, the use of this intervention by women has been relatively low, possibly due to the perceived risks and side effects of therapy.

Similar to SERMs, AIs, such as exemestane and anastrozole, have shown success in preventing breast cancer with a lower risk of uterine cancer and thromboembolic events, although bone loss is a significant side effect of this treatment.

Early Detection of Breast Cancer

A. Screening Programs

Screening detects breast cancer before it has spread to the lymph nodes in about 80% of the women evaluated. This increases the chance of survival to about 85% at 5 years.

Substantial evidence supports the use of **routine screening mammography;** however, recommendations relating to timing and frequency vary by different agencies and countries. About one-third of the abnormalities detected on screening mammograms will be found to be malignant when biopsy is performed. The probability of cancer on a screening mammogram is directly related to the Breast Imaging Reporting and Data System (BIRADS) assessment, and workup should be performed based on this classification. The sensitivity of mammography varies from approximately 60% to 90%. This sensitivity depends on several factors, including patient age, breast density, tumor size, tumor histology (lobular versus ductal), location, and mammographic appearance. In young women with dense breasts, mammography is less sensitive than in older women with fatty breasts, in whom mammography can detect at least 90% of malignancies. Smaller tumors, particularly those without calcifications, are more difficult to detect, especially in dense breasts. The lack of sensitivity and the low incidence of breast cancer in young women have led to questions concerning the value of mammography for screening in women 40–50 years of age. The specificity of mammography in women under 50 years varies from about 30% to 40% for nonpalpable mammographic abnormalities to 85% to 90% for clinically evident malignancies. Guidelines from at least six separate organizations exist in the United States and each differs slightly, making it somewhat complex for clinicians and patients to navigate. While the American College of Radiology, American Medical Association, and National Comprehensive Cancer Network (NCCN) recommend starting mammography screening at age 40, the US Preventive Services Task Force (USPSTF) recommends starting screening at age 50. Most guidelines recommend annual screening; however, the American Cancer Society recommends decreasing the frequency of screening to every 1–2 years starting at age 55 years and the USPSTF recommends routine mammography be done no more than every 2 years beginning at age 50 years. It is generally agreed that mammography should continue until life expectancy is shorter than 7–10 years, although the USPSTF recommends stopping screening after age 74 years regardless of life expectancy. Thus, clinicians should have an informed discussion with patients about screening mammography regarding its potential risks (eg, false positives, overdiagnosis, radiation exposure) and benefits (eg, early diagnosis), taking into consideration a patient's individual risk factors.

B. Imaging

1. Mammography—Mammography is the most reliable means of detecting breast cancer before a mass can be palpated. Most slowly growing cancers can be identified by mammography at least 2 years before reaching a size detectable by palpation.

Indications for mammography are as follows: (1) screening at regular intervals asymptomatic women at risk for developing breast cancer; (2) evaluating each breast when a diagnosis of potentially curable breast cancer has been made, and at regular intervals thereafter; (3) evaluating a questionable or ill-defined breast mass or other suspicious change in the breast; (4) searching for an occult breast cancer in women with metastatic disease in axillary nodes or elsewhere from an unknown primary; (5) screening women prior to cosmetic operations or prior to biopsy of a mass, to examine for an unsuspected cancer; (6) monitoring women with breast cancer who have been treated with breast-conserving surgery and radiation; and (7) monitoring the contralateral breast in women with breast cancer treated with mastectomy.

Film screen mammography has largely been replaced by digital mammography. Although full-field digital mammography provides an easier method to maintain and review mammograms and may improve image quality, it has not been proven to improve overall cancer detection and is less economical. It may offer screening benefits to women younger than age 50 years and to women with dense breasts. While computer-assisted detection may increase the sensitivity of mammography, it has not been shown to improve mortality rates. Tomosynthesis creates tomographic "slices" of the breast volume with a single acquisition. This technique may improve the sensitivity of mammogram especially in patients with dense breast tissue and reduces the number of callbacks but has not yet been shown in prospective studies to improve long-term patient outcomes.

Calcifications are the most easily recognized mammographic abnormality. The most common findings associated with carcinoma of the breast are clustered pleomorphic microcalcifications. Such calcifications are usually at least five to eight in number, aggregated in one part of the breast and differing from each other in size and shape, often including branched or V- or Y-shaped configurations. There may be an associated mammographic mass density or, at times, only a mass density with no calcifications. Such a density usually has irregular or ill-defined borders and may lead to architectural distortion within the breast, but may be subtle and difficult to detect.

Patients with a dominant or suspicious mass on examination must undergo biopsy despite mammographic findings. The mammogram should be obtained prior to biopsy so that other suspicious areas can be noted and the contralateral breast can be evaluated. *Mammography is never a substitute for biopsy* because it may not reveal clinical cancer, especially in a very dense breast.

Communication and documentation among the patient, the referring clinician, and the interpreting physician are critical for high-quality screening and diagnostic mammography. The patient should be told about *how* she will receive timely results of her mammogram; that mammography does not "rule out" cancer; and that she may receive a correlative examination such as ultrasound at the mammography facility if referred for a suspicious lesion. She should also be aware of the technique and need for breast compression and that this may be uncomfortable. The mammography facility should be informed in writing by the clinician of abnormal physical examination findings. The Agency for Health Care Policy and Research (AHCPR) Clinical Practice Guidelines strongly recommend that all mammography reports be communicated in writing to the patient and referring clinician. Legislation has been passed in a number of US states that requires imaging facilities to report to patients the density of their breasts. This may prompt women with dense breasts to discuss with their clinician whether or not additional screening options would be appropriate in addition to mammogram.

2. Other imaging—MRI and ultrasound may be useful screening modalities in women who are at high risk for breast cancer but not for the general population. The *sensitivity* of MRI is much higher than mammography; however, the *specificity* is significantly lower and this results in multiple unnecessary biopsies. The increased sensitivity despite decreased specificity may be considered a reasonable trade-off for those at increased risk for developing breast cancer but not for normal-risk population. The National Comprehensive Cancer Network guidelines recommend MRI in addition to screening mammography for high-risk women, including those with *BRCA1/2* mutations, those who have a lifetime risk of breast cancer of at least 20%, and those with a personal history of LCIS. Women who received radiation therapy to the chest in their teens or twenties are also known to be at high risk for developing breast cancer and screening MRI may be considered in addition to mammography.

C. Clinical Breast Examination and Self-Examination

Breast self-examination has *not* been shown to improve survival. Because of the lack of strong evidence demonstrating value, the American Cancer Society no longer recommends monthly breast self-examination. While breast self-examination is not a recommended practice, patients should recognize and report any breast changes to their clinicians as it remains an important facet of proactive care.

Welch HG et al. Breast-cancer tumor size, overdiagnosis, and mammography screening effectiveness. N Engl J Med. 2016 Oct 13;375(15):1438–47. [PMID: 27732805]

▶ Clinical Findings Associated With Early Detection of Breast Cancer

A. Symptoms and Signs

The presenting complaint in about 70% of patients with breast cancer is a lump (usually painless) in the breast. About 90% of these breast masses are discovered by the patient. Less frequent symptoms are breast pain; nipple discharge; erosion, retraction, enlargement, or itching of the nipple; and redness, generalized hardness,

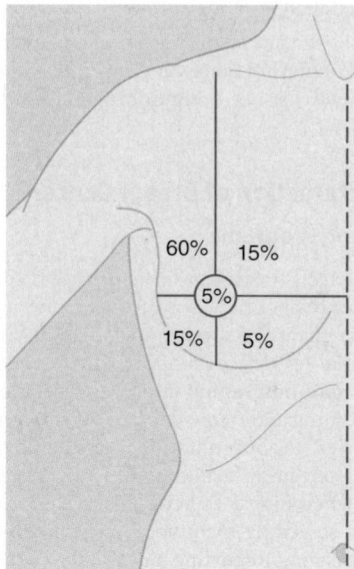

▲ **Figure 17–1.** Frequency of breast carcinoma at various anatomic sites.

enlargement, or shrinking of the breast. Rarely, an axillary mass or swelling of the arm may be the first symptom. Back or bone pain, jaundice, or weight loss may be the result of systemic metastases, but these symptoms are rarely seen on initial presentation.

The relative frequency of carcinoma in various anatomic sites in the breast is shown in Figure 17–1.

Inspection of the breast is the first step in physical examination and should be carried out with the patient sitting, arms at her sides and then overhead. Abnormal variations in breast size and contour, minimal nipple retraction, and slight edema, redness, or retraction of the skin can be identified (Figure 17–2). Asymmetry of the breasts and retraction or dimpling of the skin can often be accentuated by having the patient raise her arms overhead or press her hands on her hips to contract the pectoralis muscles. Axillary and supraclavicular areas should be thoroughly palpated for enlarged nodes with the patient

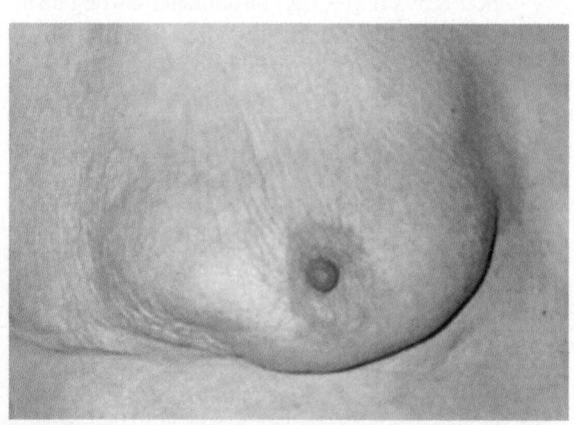

▲ **Figure 17–2.** Skin dimpling (Used, with permission, from Armando E. Giuliano, MD.)

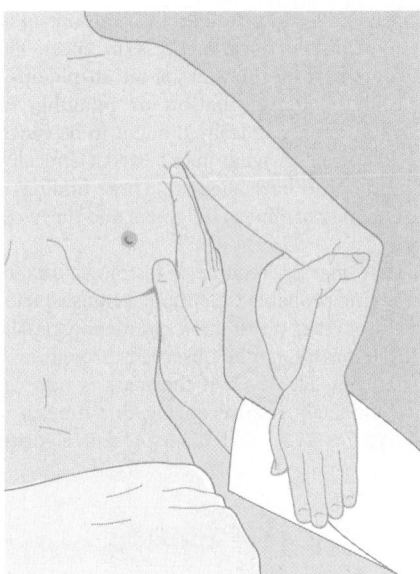

▲ **Figure 17–3.** Palpation of axillary region for enlarged lymph nodes.

sitting (Figure 17–3). Palpation of the breast for masses or other changes should be performed with the patient both seated and supine with the arm abducted. Palpation with a rotary motion of the examiner's fingers as well as a horizontal stripping motion has been recommended.

Breast cancer usually consists of a nontender, firm or hard mass with poorly delineated margins (caused by local infiltration). Very small (1–2 mm) erosions of the nipple epithelium may be the only manifestation of Paget disease of the breast (Figure 17–4). Watery, serous, or bloody discharge from the nipple is an occasional early sign but is more often associated with benign disease.

A lesion smaller than 1 cm in diameter may be difficult or impossible for the examiner to feel but may be discovered by the patient. She or he should always be asked to

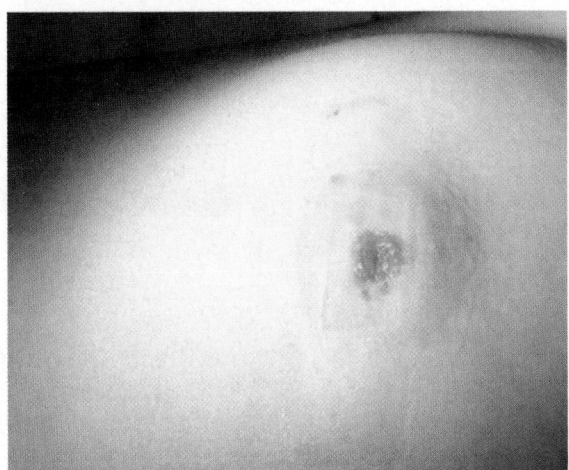

▲ **Figure 17–4.** Paget disease. (Used, with permission, from Armando E. Giuliano, MD.)

demonstrate the location of the mass; if the clinician fails to confirm the patient's suspicions and imaging studies are normal, the examination should be repeated in 2–3 months, preferably 1–2 weeks after the onset of menses. During the premenstrual phase of the cycle, increased innocuous nodularity may suggest neoplasm or may obscure an underlying lesion. If there is any question regarding the nature of an abnormality under these circumstances, the patient should be asked to return after her menses.

Metastases tend to involve regional lymph nodes, which may be palpable. One or two movable, nontender, not particularly firm axillary lymph nodes 5 mm or less in diameter are frequently present and are generally of no significance. Firm or hard nodes larger than 1 cm are typical of metastases. Axillary nodes that are matted or fixed to skin or deep structures indicate advanced disease (at least stage III). On the other hand, if the examiner thinks that the axillary nodes are involved, that impression will be borne out by histologic section in about 85% of cases. The incidence of positive axillary nodes increases with the size of the primary tumor. Noninvasive cancers (in situ) do not metastasize. Metastases are present in about 30% of patients with clinically negative nodes.

In most cases, no nodes are palpable in the supraclavicular fossa. Firm or hard nodes of any size in this location or just beneath the clavicle should be biopsied. Ipsilateral supraclavicular or infraclavicular nodes containing cancer indicate that the tumor is in an advanced stage (stage III or IV). Edema of the ipsilateral arm, commonly caused by metastatic infiltration of regional lymphatics, is also a sign of advanced cancer.

B. Laboratory Findings

Liver or bone metastases may be associated with elevation of serum alkaline phosphatase. Hypercalcemia is an occasional important finding in advanced cancer of the breast. Serum tumor markers such as carcinoembryonic antigen (CEA) and CA 15-3 or CA 27-29 are not recommended for diagnosis of early lesions or for routine surveillance for recurrence after a breast cancer diagnosis.

C. Imaging

1. For lesions felt only by the patient—Ultrasound is often valuable and mammography essential when an area is felt by the patient to be abnormal but the clinician feels no mass. MRI should not be used to rule out cancer because MRI has a false-negative rate of about 3–5%. Although lower than mammography, this false-negative rate cannot permit safe elimination of the possibility of cancer. False-negative results are more likely seen in infiltrating lobular carcinomas and DCIS than invasive ductal carcinoma.

2. For metastatic lesions—For patients with suspicious symptoms or signs (bone pain, abdominal symptoms, elevated liver biochemical tests) or locally advanced disease (clinically abnormal lymph nodes or large primary tumors), staging scans are indicated prior to surgery or systemic therapy. Chest imaging with CT or radiographs may be done to evaluate for pulmonary metastases. Abdominal imaging with CT or ultrasound may be obtained to evaluate for liver metastases. Bone scans using ^{99m}Tc-labeled phosphates or phosphonates are more sensitive than skeletal radiographs in detecting metastatic breast cancer. Bone scanning has not proved to be of clinical value as a routine preoperative test in the absence of symptoms, physical findings, or abnormal alkaline phosphatase or calcium levels. The frequency of abnormal findings on bone scan parallels the status of the axillary lymph nodes on pathologic examination. Positron emission tomography (PET) scanning alone or combined with CT (PET-CT) may also be used for detecting soft tissue or visceral metastases in patients with symptoms or signs of metastatic disease.

D. Diagnostic Tests

1. Biopsy—The diagnosis of breast cancer depends ultimately on examination of tissue or cells removed by biopsy.

Treatment should never be undertaken without an unequivocal histologic or cytologic diagnosis of cancer. **The safest course is biopsy examination of all suspicious lesions found on physical examination or imaging, or both.** About 60% of lesions clinically thought to be cancer prove on biopsy to be benign, while about 30% of clinically benign lesions are found to be malignant. These findings demonstrate the fallibility of clinical judgment and the necessity for biopsy.

All breast masses require a histologic diagnosis by biopsy with one probable exception: a nonsuspicious, presumably fibrocystic mass, in a premenopausal woman. Rather, these masses can be observed through one or two menstrual cycles. However, if the mass is not cystic and does not completely resolve during this time, it must be biopsied. Figures 17–5 and 17–6 present algorithms for

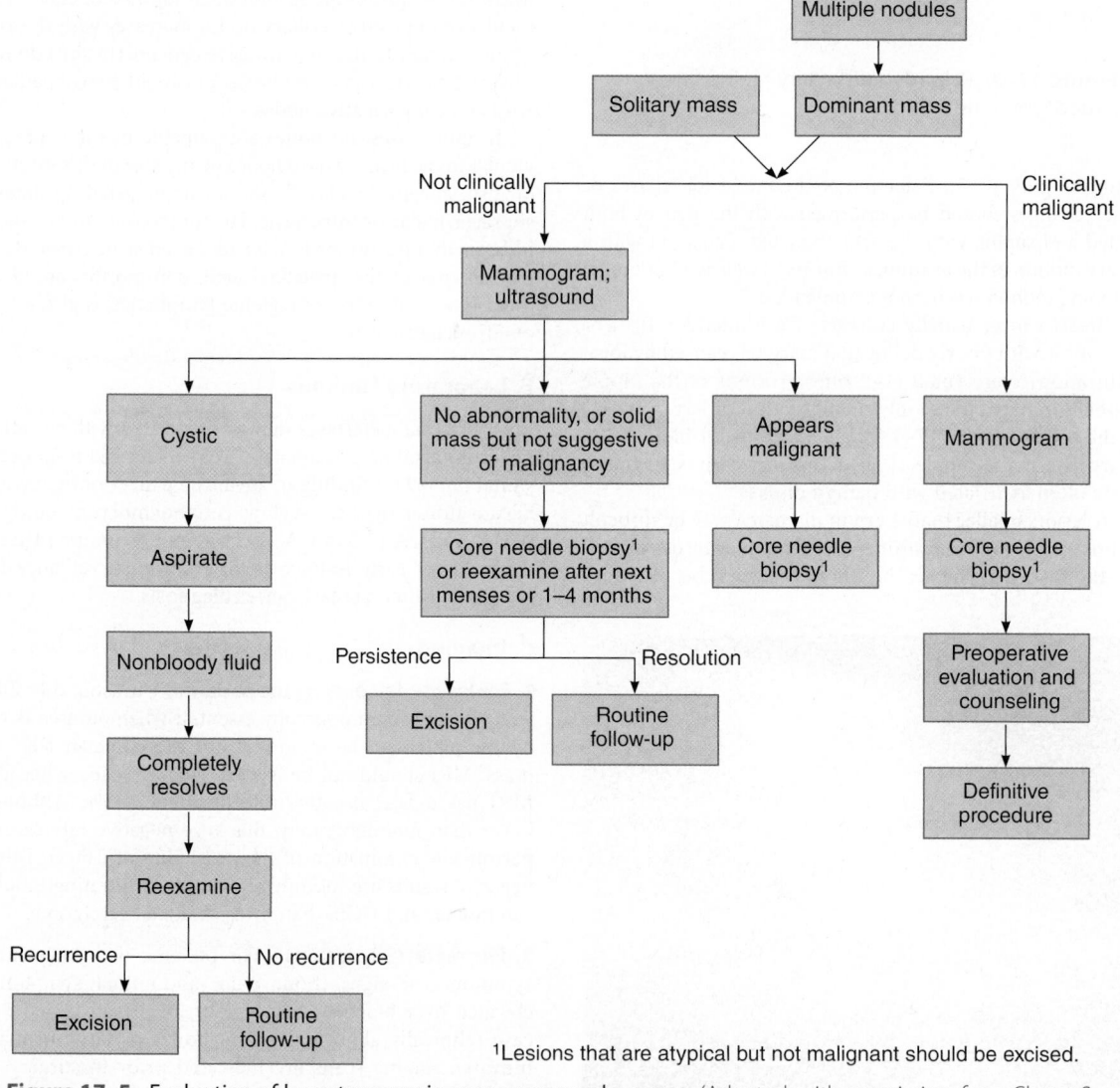

¹Lesions that are atypical but not malignant should be excised.

▲ **Figure 17–5.** Evaluation of breast masses in premenopausal women. (Adapted, with permission, from Chang S, Haigh PI, Giuliano AE. Breast disease. In: Berek JS, Hacker NF [editors], *Practical Gynecologic Oncology*, 4th ed, Philadelphia: Lippincott Williams & Wilkins, 2004.)

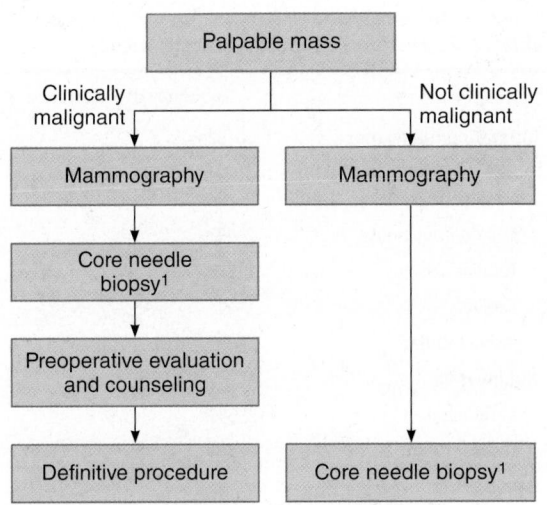

¹Lesions that are atypical but not malignant should be excised.

▲ **Figure 17–6.** Evaluation of breast masses in postmenopausal women. (Adapted, with permission, from Chang S, Haigh PI, Giuliano AE. Breast disease. In: Berek JS, Hacker NF [editors], *Practical Gynecologic Oncology*, 4th ed, Philadelphia: Lippincott Williams & Wilkins, 2004.)

management of breast masses in premenopausal and postmenopausal patients.

The simplest biopsy method is needle biopsy, either by aspiration of tumor cells (FNA cytology) or by obtaining a small core of tissue with a hollow needle (core needle biopsy).

Large-needle (core) biopsy removes a core of tissue with a large cutting needle and *is the diagnostic procedure of choice* for both palpable and image-detected abnormalities. Handheld biopsy devices make large-core needle (14-gauge) biopsy of a palpable mass easy and cost effective in the office with local anesthesia. As in the case of any needle biopsy, the main problem is sampling error due to improper positioning of the needle, giving rise to a false-negative test result. This is extremely unusual with image-guided biopsies. Core biopsy allows the tumor to be tested for the expression of biological markers, such as estrogen receptor (ER), progesterone receptor (PR) and *HER2*.

FNA cytology is a technique whereby cells are aspirated with a small needle and examined cytologically. This technique can be performed easily with virtually no morbidity and is much less expensive than excisional or open biopsy. The main disadvantages are that it requires a pathologist skilled in the cytologic diagnosis of breast cancer and it is subject to sampling problems. Furthermore, noninvasive cancers usually cannot be distinguished from invasive cancers and immunohistochemical tests to determine expression of hormone receptors and the amplification of the *HER2* oncogene cannot be reliably performed on FNA biopsies. The incidence of false-positive diagnoses is extremely low, perhaps 1–2%. The false-negative rate is as high as 10%. Most experienced clinicians would not leave a suspicious dominant mass in the breast even when FNA cytology is negative unless the clinical diagnosis, breast imaging studies, and cytologic studies were all in agreement, such as a fibrocystic lesion or fibroadenoma. Given the stated limitations, *FNA is not the modality of choice for sampling an abnormal breast mass and has been largely replaced by core needle biopsy.*

Open biopsy under local anesthesia as a separate procedure prior to deciding upon definitive treatment has become less common with the increased use of core needle biopsy. Needle biopsy, when positive, offers a more rapid approach with less expense and morbidity, but when nondiagnostic it must be followed by open biopsy. It generally consists of an excisional biopsy, which is done through an incision with the intent to remove the entire abnormality, not simply a sample. Intraoperative frozen section examination of a breast biopsy has generally been abandoned unless there is a high clinical suspicion of malignancy in a patient well prepared for the diagnosis of cancer and its treatment options.

In general, the two-step approach—outpatient large-needle core biopsy followed by definitive operation at a later date—is preferred in the diagnosis and treatment of breast cancer because patients can be given time to adjust to the diagnosis of cancer, can consider alternative forms of therapy, and can seek a second opinion if they wish. *There is no adverse effect on the cancer from the few weeks' delay of the two-step procedure.*

2. Biopsy with ultrasound guidance—Ultrasonography is performed primarily to differentiate cystic from solid lesions but may show signs suggestive of carcinoma. Ultrasonography may show an irregular mass within a cyst in the rare case of intracystic carcinoma. If a tumor is palpable and feels like a cyst, an 18-gauge needle can be used to aspirate the fluid and make the diagnosis of cyst. If a cyst is aspirated and the fluid is nonbloody, it does not have to be examined cytologically. If the mass does not recur, no further diagnostic test is necessary. Nonpalpable mammographic densities that appear benign should be investigated with ultrasound to determine whether the lesion is cystic or solid. These may even be needle biopsied with ultrasound guidance.

3. Biopsy with mammographic guidance ("stereotactic biopsy")—When a suspicious abnormality is identified by mammography alone and cannot be palpated by the clinician, the lesion should be biopsied under mammographic guidance. In the **computerized stereotactic guided core needle** technique, a biopsy needle is inserted into the lesion with mammographic guidance, and a core of tissue for histologic examination can then be examined. Vacuum assistance increases the amount of tissue obtained and improves diagnosis.

Mammographic localization biopsy is performed by obtaining a mammogram in two perpendicular views and placing a needle, hook-wire, or radioactive or radar-detectable seed localizer near the abnormality so that the surgeon can locate the lesion intraoperatively. After mammography confirms the position of the localizer in relation to the lesion, an incision is made and the localizer is identified. Often, the abnormality cannot even be palpated through the incision—as is the case with microcalcifications—and thus it is essential to obtain a mammogram of the specimen to document that the lesion was excised. At that time, a second marker needle can further localize the lesion for the pathologist. Image-guided core needle biopsies have proved equivalent to mammographic localization biopsies. Core biopsy is preferable to mammographic localization for accessible lesions since an operation can be avoided. A metal clip should be placed after any image-guided core biopsy to facilitate finding the site of the lesion if subsequent treatment is necessary.

4. Other imaging modalities—Other modalities of breast imaging have been investigated for diagnostic purposes. Automated breast ultrasonography is useful in distinguishing cystic from solid lesions but should be used only as a supplement to physical examination and mammography. MRI is highly sensitive but not specific and should not be used for screening except in highly selective cases. For example, MRI is useful in differentiating scar from recurrence postlumpectomy and may be valuable to screen high-risk women (eg, women with *BRCA* mutations). It may also be of value to examine for multicentricity when there is a known primary cancer; to examine the contralateral breast in women with cancer; to examine the extent of cancer, especially lobular carcinomas; or to determine the response to neoadjuvant chemotherapy. Moreover, MRI-detected suspicious findings that are not seen on mammogram or ultrasound may be biopsied under MRI guidance. PET scanning does not appear useful in evaluating the breast itself but is useful to examine for distant metastases.

5. Cytology—Cytologic examination of nipple discharge or cyst fluid may be helpful on rare occasions. As a rule, mammography (or ductography) and breast biopsy are required when nipple discharge or cyst fluid is bloody or cytologically questionable.

Differential Diagnosis

The lesions to be considered most often in the differential diagnosis of breast cancer are the following, in descending order of frequency: fibrocystic condition of the breast, fibroadenoma, intraductal papilloma, lipoma, and fat necrosis.

Staging

The American Joint Committee on Cancer and the International Union Against Cancer have a joint TNM (tumor, regional lymph nodes, distant metastases) staging system for breast cancer.

Pathologic Types

Numerous pathologic subtypes of breast cancer can be identified histologically (Table 17–3).

Except for the in situ cancers, the histologic subtypes have only a slight bearing on prognosis when outcomes are compared after accurate staging. The noninvasive cancers by definition are confined by the basement membrane of the ducts and lack the ability to spread. Histologic parameters for invasive cancers, including lymphovascular invasion and tumor grade, have been shown to be of prognostic value. Immunohistochemical analysis for expression of hormone

Table 17–3. Histologic types of breast cancer.

Type	Frequency of Occurrence
Infiltrating ductal (not otherwise specified)	80–90%
Medullary	5–8%
Colloid (mucinous)	2–4%
Tubular	1–2%
Papillary	1–2%
Invasive lobular	6–8%
Noninvasive	4–6%
Intraductal	2–3%
Lobular in situ	2–3%
Rare cancers	< 1%
Juvenile (secretory)	
Adenoid cystic	
Epidermoid	
Sudoriferous	

receptors and for overexpression of HER2 in the primary tumor offers prognostic and therapeutic information.

Special Clinical Forms of Breast Cancer

A. Paget Carcinoma

Paget carcinoma is not common (about 1% of all breast cancers). Over 85% of cases are associated with an underlying invasive or noninvasive cancer, usually a well differentiated infiltrating ductal carcinoma or a DCIS. The ducts of the nipple epithelium are infiltrated, but gross nipple changes are often minimal, and a tumor mass may not be palpable.

Because the nipple changes appear innocuous, the diagnosis is frequently missed. The first symptom is often itching or burning of the nipple, with superficial erosion or ulceration. These are often diagnosed and treated as dermatitis or bacterial infection, leading to delay or failure in detection. The diagnosis is established by biopsy of the area of erosion. When the lesion consists of nipple changes only, the incidence of axillary metastases is less than 5%, and the prognosis is excellent. When a breast mass is also present, the incidence of axillary metastases rises, with an associated marked decrease in prospects for cure by surgical or other treatment.

B. Inflammatory Carcinoma

This is the most malignant form of breast cancer and constitutes less than 3% of all cases. The clinical findings consist of a rapidly growing, sometimes painful mass that enlarges the breast. The overlying skin becomes erythematous, edematous, and warm. Often there is no distinct mass, since the tumor infiltrates the involved breast diffusely. The inflammatory changes, often mistaken for an infection, are caused by carcinomatous invasion of the subdermal lymphatics, with resulting edema and hyperemia. If the clinician suspects infection but the lesion does not respond rapidly (1–2 weeks) to antibiotics, biopsy should be performed. The diagnosis should be made when the redness involves more than one-third of the skin over the breast and biopsy shows infiltrating carcinoma with invasion of the subdermal lymphatics. Metastases tend to occur early and widely, and for this reason inflammatory carcinoma is rarely curable. Radiation, hormone therapy (if hormone receptor positive), anti-HER2 therapy (if HER2 overexpressing or amplified), and chemotherapy are the measures most likely to be of value initially rather than operation. Mastectomy is indicated when chemotherapy and radiation have resulted in clinical remission with no evidence of distant metastases. In these cases, residual disease in the breast may be eradicated.

Breast Cancer Occurring During Pregnancy or Lactation

Breast cancer complicates up to one in 3000 pregnancies. The diagnosis is frequently delayed, because physiologic changes in the breast may obscure the lesion and screening mammography is not done in young or pregnant women. Data are insufficient to determine whether interruption of pregnancy improves the prognosis of patients who are identified to have potentially curable breast cancer and who receive definitive treatment during pregnancy. Theoretically, the high levels of estrogen produced by the placenta as the pregnancy progresses could be detrimental to the patient with occult metastases of hormone-sensitive breast cancer. The decision whether or not to terminate the pregnancy must be made on an individual basis, taking into account the patient's clinical stage of the cancer and overall prognosis, the gestational age of the fetus, the potential for premature ovarian failure in the future with systemic therapy, and the patient's wishes.

It is important for primary care and reproductive specialists to aggressively work up any breast abnormality discovered in a pregnant woman. Pregnancy (or lactation) is not a contraindication to operation or treatment, and therapy should be based on the stage of the disease as in the nonpregnant (or nonlactating) woman. Women with early-stage gestational breast cancer who choose to continue their pregnancy should undergo surgery to remove the tumor and systemic therapy if indicated. Retrospective reviews of patients treated with anthracycline-containing regimens for gestational cancers (including leukemia and lymphomas) have established the relative safety of these regimens during pregnancy for both the patient and the fetus. Taxane-based and trastuzumab-based regimens have not been evaluated extensively, however. Radiation therapy should be delayed until after delivery. Overall survival rates have improved, since cancers are now diagnosed in pregnant women earlier than in the past and treatment has improved.

Bilateral Breast Cancer

Bilateral breast cancer occurs in less than 5% of cases, but there is as high as a 20–25% incidence of later occurrence of cancer in the second breast. Bilaterality occurs more often in familial breast cancer, in women under age 50 years, and when the tumor in the primary breast is lobular. The incidence of second breast cancers increases directly with the length of time the patient is alive after her first cancer—about 1–2% per year.

In patients with breast cancer, mammography should be performed before primary treatment and at regular intervals thereafter, to search for occult cancer in the opposite breast or conserved ipsilateral breast.

Noninvasive Cancer

Noninvasive cancer can occur within the ducts (**DCIS**) or lobules (**LCIS**). DCIS tends to be unilateral and most often progresses to invasive cancer if untreated. In approximately 40–60% of women who have DCIS treated with biopsy alone, invasive cancer develops within the same breast. LCIS is generally agreed to be a marker of an increased risk of breast cancer rather than a direct precursor of breast cancer itself. The probability of breast cancer (DCIS or invasive in either breast) in a woman in whom LCIS has been diagnosed is estimated to be 1% per year. If LCIS is detected on core needle biopsy, an excisional biopsy without lymph node sampling should be performed to rule out DCIS or invasive cancer since these are found in 10–20% of patients. The incidence of LCIS is rising, likely due to increased use of screening mammography. In addition, the rate of mastectomy after the diagnosis of LCIS is increasing in spite of the fact that mastectomy is only recommended in those patients who otherwise have an increased risk of breast cancer through family history, genetic mutation, or past exposure to thoracic radiation. Pleomorphic LCIS may behave more like DCIS and may be associated with invasive carcinoma. For this reason, pleomorphic LCIS should be surgically removed with clear margins.

The treatment of intraductal lesions is controversial. DCIS can be treated by wide excision with or without radiation therapy or with total mastectomy. Conservative management is advised in patients with small lesions amenable to lumpectomy. Patients in whom LCIS is diagnosed or who have received lumpectomy for DCIS may discuss chemoprevention (with hormonal blockade therapy) with their clinician, which is effective in reducing the risk of invasive breast cancer in DCIS that has been completely excised by breast-conserving surgery and in LCIS. Axillary metastases from in situ cancers should not occur unless there is an occult invasive cancer. Because one cannot perform a sentinel lymph node biopsy after mastectomy, one might consider performing a sentinel node biopsy in a patient undergoing mastectomy for DCIS in case an invasive component is discovered.

Hartman EK et al. The prognosis of women diagnosed with breast cancer before, during and after pregnancy: a meta-analysis. Breast Cancer Res Treat. 2016 Nov;160(2):347–60. [PMID: 27683280]

Vapiwala N et al. No impact of breast magnetic resonance imaging on 15-year outcomes in patients with ductal carcinoma in situ or early-stage invasive breast cancer managed with breast conservation therapy. Cancer. 2017 Apr 15;123(8):1324–32. [PMID: 27984658]

Biomarkers & Gene Expression Profiling

Determining the **ER, PR,** and **HER2** status of the tumor at the time of diagnosis of early breast cancer and, if possible, at the time of recurrence is critical, both to gauge a patient's prognosis and to determine the best treatment regimen. In addition to ER status and PR status, the rate at which tumor divides (assessed by an immunohistochemical stain for **Ki67**) and the grade and differentiation of the cells are also important prognostic factors. These markers may be obtained on core biopsy or surgical specimens, but not reliably on FNA cytology. Patients whose tumors are hormone receptor-positive tend to have a more indolent disease course than those whose tumors are receptor-negative. Moreover, treatment with an anti-hormonal agent is an essential component of therapy for hormone-receptor positive breast cancer at any stage. While up to 60% of patients with metastatic breast cancer will respond to hormonal manipulation if their tumors are ER-positive, less than 5% of patients with metastatic, ER-negative tumors will respond.

Another key element in determining treatment and prognosis is the amount of the *HER2* oncogene present in the cancer. HER2 overexpression (HER2-oncogene–positive breast cancer) is generally more aggressive than breast cancer with normal HER2 expression (HER2-negative breast cancer). Individually these biomarkers are predictive and thus provide insight to guide appropriate therapy. Moreover, when combined they provide useful information regarding risk of recurrence and prognosis. In general, tumors that lack expression of HER2, ER, and PR ("**triple negative**") have a higher risk of early recurrence and metastases and are associated with a worse survival compared with other types. Neither endocrine therapy nor HER2-targeted agents are useful for this type of breast cancer, leaving chemotherapy as the only treatment option. In contrast, patients with early stage, hormone receptor–positive breast cancer may not benefit from the addition of chemotherapy to hormonally targeted treatments. Several molecular tests have been developed to assess risk of recurrence and to predict which patients are most likely to benefit from chemotherapy. **Oncotype DX** (Genomic Health) evaluates the expression of 21 genes relating to ER, HER2, and proliferation in a tumor specimen and categorizes a patient's risk of recurrence (recurrence score) as high, intermediate, or low risk. This test is primarily indicated for ER-positive, lymph node-negative tumors but an ongoing study is addressing its predictive value in lymph node positive, ER positive breast cancer in a prospective manner. **MammaPrint** (Agendia) is an FDA-approved 70-gene signature assay that is available for evaluating prognosis. This test classifies patients into good and poor prognostic groups to predict clinical outcome and may be used on patients with hormone receptor positive or negative breast cancer. American Society of Clinical Oncology (ASCO) guidelines indicate this assay may be best used to help determine whether chemotherapy may be safely withheld in patients with hormone receptor–negative, HER2-negative, node-positive breast cancer at high clinical risk. ASCO does not recommend using this assay in hormone receptor–negative or HER2-positive breast cancer.

Ibraheem AF et al. Community clinical practice patterns and mortality in patients with intermediate Oncotype DX recurrence scores: who benefits from chemotherapy. Cancer. 2019 Jan 15;125(2):213–22. [PMID: 30387876]

Krop I et al. Use of biomarkers to guide decisions on adjuvant systemic therapy for women with early-stage invasive breast cancer: American Society of Clinical Oncology clinical practice guideline focused update. J Clin Oncol. 2017 Aug 20;35(24): 2838–47. [PMID: 28692382]

Mamounas EP et al. 21-gene recurrence score and locoregional recurrence in node-positive/ER-positive breast cancer treated with chemo-endocrine therapy. J Natl Cancer Inst. 2017 Jan 25;109(4):djw259. [PMID: 28122895]

Press MF et al. Assessment of ERBB2/HER2 status in HER2-equivocal breast cancers by FISH and 2013/2014 ASCO-CAP guidelines. JAMA Oncol. 2019 Mar 1;5(3):366–75. [PMID: 30520947]

Sparano JA et al. Adjuvant chemotherapy guided by a 21-gene expression assay in breast cancer. N Engl J Med. 2018 Jul 12; 379(2):111–21. [PMID: 29860917]

Wolff AC et al. Human epidermal growth factor receptor 2 testing in breast cancer: American Society of Clinical Oncology/ College of American Pathologists Clinical Practice Guideline Focused Update. Arch Pathol Lab Med. 2018 Nov;142(11): 1364–82. [PMID: 29846104]

Curative Treatment

Not all breast cancer is systemic at the time of diagnosis, and a pessimistic attitude concerning the management of breast cancer is unwarranted. Most patients with early breast cancer can be cured. Treatment with a curative intent is advised for clinical stage I, II, and III disease (see Table 39–2). Patients with locally advanced (T3, T4) and even inflammatory tumors may be cured with multimodality therapy, but metastatic disease will be diagnosed in most patients, and at that point, palliation becomes the goal of therapy. Treatment with palliative intent is appropriate for all patients with stage IV disease and for patients with unresectable local cancers.

A. Choice and Timing of Primary Therapy

The extent of disease and its biologic aggressiveness are the principal determinants of the outcome of primary therapy. Clinical and pathologic staging help in assessing extent of disease, but each is to some extent imprecise. Other factors such as tumor grade, hormone receptor assays, and *HER2* oncogene amplification are of prognostic value and are key to determining systemic therapy, but are not as relevant in determining the type of local therapy.

Controversy has surrounded the choice of primary therapy of stage I, II, and III breast carcinoma. Currently, the standard of care for stage I, stage II, and most stage III cancer is surgical resection followed by adjuvant radiation or systemic therapy, or both, when indicated. Neoadjuvant therapy has become popular since large tumors may be shrunk by chemotherapy prior to surgery, making some patients who require mastectomy candidates for lumpectomy. It is important for patients to understand all of the surgical options, including reconstructive options, prior to having surgery. Patients with large primary tumors, inflammatory cancer, or palpably enlarged lymph nodes should have staging scans performed to rule out distant metastatic disease prior to definitive surgery. In general, adjuvant systemic therapy is started when the breast has adequately healed, ideally within 4–8 weeks after surgery. While no prospective studies have defined the appropriate timing of adjuvant chemotherapy, a single institution study of over 6800 patients suggests that *systemic therapy should be started within 60 days of surgery*, especially in women with stage II or III breast cancer, triple-negative breast cancer or HER2-positive disease.

B. Surgical Resection

1. Breast-conserving therapy—Multiple, large, randomized studies including the Milan and NSABP trials show that disease-free and overall survival rates are similar for patients with stage I and stage II breast cancer treated with partial mastectomy (breast-conserving lumpectomy or "breast conservation") plus axillary dissection followed by radiation therapy and for those treated by modified radical mastectomy (total mastectomy plus axillary dissection).

Tumor size is a major consideration in determining the feasibility of breast conservation. The NSABP lumpectomy trial randomized patients with tumors as large as 4 cm. To achieve an acceptable cosmetic result, the patient must have a breast of sufficient size to enable excision of a 4-cm tumor without considerable deformity. Therefore, large tumor size is only a relative contraindication. Subareolar tumors, also difficult to excise without deformity, are not contraindications to breast conservation. Clinically detectable multifocality is a relative contraindication to breast-conserving surgery, as is fixation to the chest wall or skin or involvement of the nipple or overlying skin. The patient—not the surgeon—should be the judge of what is cosmetically acceptable. Given the relatively high risk of poor outcome after radiation, concomitant scleroderma is a contraindication to breast-conserving surgery. A history of prior therapeutic radiation to the ipsilateral breast or chest wall (or both) is also generally a contraindication for breast conservation.

Axillary dissection is primarily used to properly stage cancer and plan radiation and systemic therapy. Intraoperative lymphatic mapping and sentinel node biopsy identify lymph nodes most likely to harbor metastases if present (Figure 17–7). **Sentinel node biopsy** is a proven alternative to axillary dissection in patients without clinical

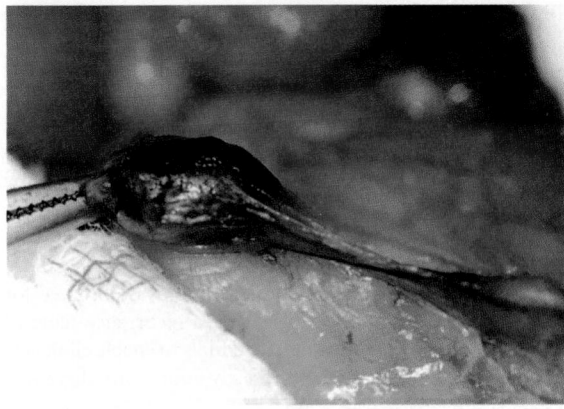

▲ **Figure 17–7.** Sentinel node. (Used, with permission, from Armando E. Giuliano, MD.)

evidence of axillary lymph node metastases. If sentinel node biopsy reveals no evidence of axillary metastases, it is highly likely that the remaining lymph nodes are free of disease and axillary dissection may be omitted. An important study from the American College of Surgeons Oncology Group randomized women with sentinel node metastases to undergo completion of axillary dissection or to receive no further axillary-specific treatment after lumpectomy; no difference in 10-year survival was found. *Omission of axillary dissection is acceptable for women with tumor-free sentinel nodes or those with involvement of one or two sentinel nodes who are treated with lumpectomy, whole breast irradiation, and adjuvant systemic therapy.*

Breast-conserving surgery with sentinel node biopsy and radiation is the preferred form of treatment for patients with early-stage breast cancer. Despite the numerous randomized trials showing no survival benefit of mastectomy over breast-conserving partial mastectomy with irradiation or of axillary dissection over sentinel node biopsy, these conservative procedures appear to be underutilized.

2. Mastectomy—Modified radical mastectomy was the standard therapy for most patients with early-stage breast cancer. This operation removes the entire breast, overlying skin, nipple, and areolar complex usually with underlying pectoralis fascia with the axillary lymph nodes in continuity. The major advantage of modified radical mastectomy is that radiation therapy may not be necessary, although radiation may be used when lymph nodes are involved with cancer or when the primary tumor is 5 cm or larger. The disadvantage of mastectomy is the cosmetic and psychological impact associated with breast loss. Radical mastectomy, which removes the underlying pectoralis muscle, should be performed rarely, if at all. Axillary node dissection is not indicated for noninvasive cancers because nodal metastases are rarely present. Skin-sparing and nipple-sparing mastectomy is available but is not appropriate for all patients. Breast reconstruction, immediate or delayed, should be discussed with patients who choose or require mastectomy. Patients should have an interview with a reconstructive plastic surgeon to discuss options prior to making a decision regarding reconstruction. Time is well spent preoperatively in educating the patient and family about these matters.

C. Radiotherapy

Radiotherapy after partial mastectomy consists of 5–7 weeks of five daily fractions to a total dose of 5000–6000 cGy. Most radiation oncologists use a boost dose to the cancer location. Shorter fractionation schedules may be reasonable for women over the age of 50 with early stage, lymph node–negative breast cancer. Accelerated partial breast irradiation, in which only the portion of the breast from which the tumor was resected is irradiated for 1–2 weeks, appears effective in achieving local control for selected patients; however, the prospective randomized NSABP B-39/RTOG 0413 trial failed to demonstrate noninferiority of partial breast irradiation compared to whole breast irradiation. With 4216 patients randomized and treated on this study, ipsilateral breast tumor recurrences at 10 years were slightly higher in the partial breast irradiation arm (4.8% vs 4.1%) and the 10-year relapse-free interval was significantly in favor of whole breast irradiation (93.4% vs 91.9%). Toxicity also tended to favor whole breast irradiation. In women over the age of 70 with small (less than 2 cm), lymph node–negative, hormone receptor–positive cancers, radiation therapy may be avoided. The recurrence rates after intra-operative radiation, while low, appear significantly higher than postoperative whole breast radiation therapy. However, in all of these situations, a balanced discussion with a radiation oncologist to weigh the risks and benefits of each approach is warranted.

Current studies suggest that radiotherapy after mastectomy may improve recurrence rates and survival in younger patients and those with tumors 5 cm or larger or positive lymph nodes.

Giuliano AE et al. Effect of axillary dissection vs no axillary dissection on 10-year overall survival among women with invasive breast cancer and sentinel node metastasis: The ACOSOG Z0011 (Alliance) Randomized Clinical Trial. JAMA. 2017 Sep 12;318(10):918–26. [PMID: 28898379]

Giuliano AE et al. Locoregional recurrence after sentinel lymph node dissection with or without axillary dissection in patients with sentinel lymph node metastases: long-term follow-up from the American College of Surgeons Oncology Group (Alliance) ACOSOG Z0011 Randomized Trial. Ann Surg. 2016 Sep;264(3):413–20. [PMID: 27513155]

Grover S et al. Survival after breast-conserving surgery with whole breast or partial breast irradiation in women with early stage breast cancer: a SEER data-base analysis. Breast J. 2017 May;23(3):292–8. [PMID: 27988987]

Lyman GH et al. Sentinel lymph node biopsy for patients with early-stage breast cancer: American Society of Clinical Oncology clinical practice guideline update. J Clin Oncol. 2017 Feb 10;35(5):561–4. [PMID: 27937089]

Poortmans PM et al; EORTC Radiation Oncology and Breast Cancer Groups. Internal mammary and medial supraclavicular irradiation in breast cancer. N Engl J Med. 2015 Jul 23; 373(4):317–27. [PMID: 26200978]

D. Adjuvant Systemic Therapy

The goal of systemic therapy, including hormone-modulating medications (endocrine therapy), cytotoxic chemotherapy, and HER2-targeted agents such as trastuzumab, is to kill cancer cells that have escaped the breast and axillary lymph nodes as *micro*metastases before they become *macro*metastases (ie, stage IV cancer). Systemic therapy improves survival and is advocated for most patients with curable breast cancer. In practice, most medical oncologists use adjuvant chemotherapy for patients with either node-positive or higher-risk (eg, hormone receptor–negative or HER2-positive) node-negative breast cancer and use endocrine therapy for all hormone receptor–positive invasive breast cancer unless contraindicated. Prognostic factors other than nodal status that are used to determine the patient's risks of recurrence are tumor size, ER and PR status, nuclear grade, histologic type, proliferative rate, oncogene expression (Table 17–4), and patient's age and menopausal status. In general, systemic chemotherapy decreases the chance of recurrence by about 30%, hormonal modulation

Table 17–4. Prognostic factors in node-negative breast cancer.

Prognostic Factors	Increased Recurrence	Decreased Recurrence
Size[1]	T3, T2	T1, T0
Hormone receptors (ER, PR)	Negative	Positive
Histologic grade	High	Low
S phase fraction	> 5%	< 5%
Lymphatic or vascular invasion	Present	Absent
HER2 oncogene amplification	High	Low
Epidermal growth factor receptor	High	Low
High Oncotype DX Recurrence Score or other genomic prognostic assays	High score	Low score

[1]See eTable 17–1 on *CMDT Online* for TNM staging for breast cancer.

decreases the relative risk of recurrence by 40–50% (for hormone receptor–positive cancer), and HER2-targeted therapy decreases the relative risk of recurrence by approximately 40% (for HER2-positive cancer). Systemic chemotherapy is usually given sequentially, rather than concurrently with radiation. In terms of sequencing, typically chemotherapy is given before radiation and endocrine therapy is started concurrent with or after radiation therapy.

The long-term advantage of systemic therapy is well established. All patients with invasive hormone receptor–positive tumors should consider the use of hormone-modulating therapy. Most patients with HER2-positive tumors should receive trastuzumab-containing chemotherapy regimens. In general, adjuvant systemic chemotherapy should not be given to women who have small node-negative breast cancers with favorable histologic findings and tumor biomarkers. The ability to predict more accurately which patients with HER2-negative, hormone receptor–positive, lymph node–negative tumors should receive chemotherapy is improving with the advent of prognostic tools, such as Oncotype DX and MammaPrint (see Biomarkers and Gene Expression Profiling above). In the MINDACT study, the 5-year distant metastasis–free survival improved by 1.5% in women with high clinical risk but low-risk gene expression as assessed by MammaPrint if they did *not* receive chemotherapy. In the TAILORx study, patients with an intermediate Oncotype DX recurrence score (11–25) were randomized to receive chemotherapy followed by endocrine therapy or endocrine therapy alone. This study demonstrated no significant benefit associated with adjuvant chemotherapy for patients with a recurrence score of less than 26, though some benefit was observed for women age 50 years or younger with a recurrence score of 16–25. These tests are thus validated tools to enable clinicians to better select patients who can safely omit chemotherapy.

1. Chemotherapy—The Early Breast Cancer Trialists' Collaborative Group (EBCTCG) meta-analysis involving over 28,000 women enrolled in 60 trials of adjuvant polychemotherapy versus no chemotherapy demonstrated a significant beneficial impact of chemotherapy on clinical outcome in non–stage IV breast cancer. This study showed that *adjuvant chemotherapy reduces the risk of recurrence and breast cancer–specific mortality in all women and also showed that women under the age of 50 derive the greatest benefit*.

A. Anthracycline- and cyclophosphamide-containing regimens—On the basis of the superiority of anthracycline-containing regimens in metastatic breast cancer, both doxorubicin and epirubicin have been studied extensively in the adjuvant setting. Studies comparing Adriamycin (doxorubicin) and cyclophosphamide (AC) or epirubicin and cyclophosphamide (EC) to cyclophospha-mide-methotrexate-5-fluorouracil (CMF) have shown that treatments with anthracycline-containing regimens are at least as effective as treatment with CMF. The EBCTCG analysis including over 14,000 patients enrolled in trials comparing anthracycline-based regimens to CMF, showed a small but statistically significant improved disease-free and overall survival with the use of anthracycline-based regimens. It should be noted, however, that most of these studies included a mixed population of patients with HER2-positive and HER2-negative breast cancer and were performed before the introduction of trastuzumab. Retro-spective analyses of a number of these studies suggest that anthracyclines may be primarily effective in tumors with HER2 overexpression or alteration in the expression of topoisomerase IIa (the target of anthracyclines and close to the *HER2* gene). Given this, for HER2-negative, node-negative breast cancer, four cycles of AC or six cycles of CMF are probably equally effective.

B. Taxanes—When taxanes (paclitaxel and docetaxel) emerged in the 1990s, multiple trials were conducted to evaluate their use in combination with anthracycline-based regimens. The majority of these trials showed an improvement in disease-free survival and at least one showed an improvement in overall survival with the taxane-based regimen. A meta-analysis of taxane versus non-taxane anthracycline-based regimen trials showed an improvement in disease-free and overall survival for the taxane-based regimens. Several regimens have been reported including AC followed by paclitaxel (AC-P) or docetaxel (Taxotere) (AC-T), docetaxel concurrent with AC (TAC), 5-fluorouracil-epirubicine-cyclophospha-mide (FEC)-docetaxel, and FEC-paclitaxel.

The US Oncology trial 9735 compared four cycles of AC with four cycles of docetaxel (Taxotere) and cyclophospha-mide (TC). With a median of 7 years' follow-up, this study showed a statistically significantly improved disease-free survival and overall survival in the patients who received TC. Subsequently, substudy results from the phase III MIN-DACT trial were presented in which 1301 patients with operable tumors were randomized 1:1 to standard anthra-cycline/cyclophosphamide-based therapy (with taxane in the 30% of patients with node-positive disease) or docetaxel plus capecitabine (DC). The 5-year disease-free survival was similar for the anthracycline arm (88.8%) and DC arm (90.7%) ($P = 0.263$) and 5-year overall survival was also similar (96.2% anthracycline vs 96.3% DC, $P = 0.722$).

The three Anthracyclines in early Breast Cancer (ABC) (USOR 06-090, NSABP B-46, NSABP B-49) trials (total N = 4242) each compared the TC regimen to anthracycline/taxane-based chemotherapy regimens (TaxAC) in HER2-negative early-stage breast cancer. An interim joint analysis showed that the invasive disease-free survival at 4 years was improved by 2.5% with the addition of an anthracycline ($P = 0.04$) but that the benefit of an anthracycline was primarily seen in triple-negative disease (HR 1.42, 95% CI 1.04, 1.94). No survival difference was observed at the time of interim reporting. In contrast, the West German Study Group phase III PlanB study compared six cycles of adjuvant TC to four cycles of EC followed by four cycles of docetaxel (EC-D) in 2449 patients with intermediate to high risk, HER2-negative breast cancer. Dose reductions were higher in the anthracycline arm (19.7% vs 6.6%, $P < 0.001$) and grade 3/4 toxicities were consistently and significantly higher in the anthracycline arm. TC demonstrated noninfe-riority to EC-D with a 5-year disease-free survival of 90% for each arm (HR TC vs. EC-D = 0.996; 95% CI [0.77–1.29]). In contrast to the ABC study, subset analysis indicated a similar disease-free survival in each treatment arm regardless of recurrence score, nodal status, Ki67 reactivity, grade, or tri-ple-negative subtype. A Danish phase III study was conducted to compare six cycles of TC to six cycles of EC-D in 2012 high-risk patients with *TOP2A* normal breast cancer. The 5-year disease-free survival was 87.9% for EC-D vs 88.3% for DC (HR, 1.00; $P = 1.00$). While it is generally agreed that *taxanes should be used for most patients receiving chemotherapy for early breast cancer, data relating to the benefits of anthracyclines are conflicting*; thus, a balanced discussion regarding the potential risks versus benefits of the addition of anthracyclines is warranted.

C. Duration and dose of chemotherapy—The ideal duration of adjuvant chemotherapy still remains uncertain. However, based on the meta-analysis performed in the Oxford Overview (EBCTCG), the current recommenda-tion is for 3–6 months of the commonly used regimens. Data suggest that the timing and sequencing of anthracy-cline-taxane–based chemotherapy may be important. Mul-tiple trials beginning in the 1980s sought to demonstrate whether dose-intensification of adjuvant chemotherapy by shortening the intervals between cycles ("dose-dense"), or by giving chemotherapy at full dose sequentially rather than concurrently at reduced doses is associated with bet-ter outcomes. The EBCTCG meta-analysis included 37,298 patients treated on 26 trials and showed a significant 3.4% absolute decrease and 14% relative risk reduction in breast cancer recurrences with dose-intensification. Moreover, the absolute 10-year breast cancer mortality was improved by 2.4%. While impressive, the benefit of dose-intensification appeared to be strongest in node-positive disease. Its benefit, if any, in HER2-positive disease in the era of HER2-targeted therapy has not been validated. Additionally, the use of dose-intensification in (non-anthracycline) taxane-based regimens has not been evaluated.

D. Chemotherapy side effects—Chemotherapy side effects, which are discussed in Chapter 39, are generally well controlled.

2. Targeted therapy—Targeted therapy refers to agents that are directed specifically against a protein or molecule expressed uniquely on tumor cells or in the tumor microenvironment.

A. HER2 OVEREXPRESSION—Approximately 20% of breast cancers are characterized by amplification of the *HER2* oncogene leading to overexpression of the HER2 oncoprotein. The poor prognosis associated with HER2 overexpression has been drastically improved with the development of HER2-targeted therapy. Trastuzumab (Herceptin [H]), a monoclonal antibody that binds to HER2, is effective in combination with chemotherapy in patients with HER2-overexpressing metastatic and early breast cancer. In the adjuvant setting, the first and most commonly studied chemotherapy backbone used with trastuzumab is AC-T. Subsequently, the BCIRG006 study showed similar efficacy for AC-TH and a nonanthracycline-containing regimen, TCH (docetaxel, carboplatin, trastuzumab). Both were significantly better than AC-T in terms of disease-free and overall survival and TCH had a lower risk of cardiac and bone marrow (leukemia/myelodysplasia) toxicity. Both AC-TH and TCH are FDA-approved for nonmetastatic, HER2-positive breast cancer. In these regimens, trastuzumab is given with chemotherapy and then continues beyond the course of chemotherapy with a goal, in general, to complete a full year. Neoadjuvant chemotherapy plus dual *HER2*-targeted therapy with trastuzumab and pertuzumab (also a HER2-targeted monoclonal antibody that prevents dimerization of HER2 with HER3 and has been shown to be synergistic in combination with trastuzumab) is a standard of care option available to patients with stage II/III HER2-positive breast cancer (see Neoadjuvant Therapy). The phase III randomized placebo-controlled adjuvant "APHINITY" study, reported in 2017, evaluated 1 year of adjuvant pertuzumab in combination with trastuzumab and showed a small but statistically significant reduction in recurrence of disease with pertuzumab (7.1% vs 8.7%, HR, 0.81; P = 0.045). The improved disease-free survival is most pronounced in patients with node-positive disease. Neratinib, an orally bioavailable dual HER1 (EGFR), HER2 tyrosine kinase inhibitor, is FDA-approved as adjuvant therapy. The phase III placebo-controlled EXTENET study demonstrated that neratinib improves invasive disease-free survival when given for 1 year after completion of a year of standard adjuvant trastuzumab-based therapy (median follow-up 5.2 years, stratified HR 0.73, 95% CI 0.57, 0.92, P = 0.0083). Neratinib is associated with gastrointestinal toxicity, most notably moderate to severe diarrhea in approximately 40% of patients who did not use antidiarrheal prophylaxis. Measures to mitigate this side effect are being evaluated in the CONTROL clinical trial (NCT02400476). Pending those final results, patients should be treated with upfront prophylaxis with loperamide.

Patients who undergo neoadjuvant trastuzumab-based chemotherapy and have residual disease remaining at the time of surgery have a comparatively poor outcome compared to those who achieve a pathologic complete response. In the phase III randomized KATHERINE trial, 1486 patients with residual disease after standard neoadjuvant trastuzumab/taxane-based therapy (18% of whom also received neoadjuvant pertuzumab) were randomized to receive the antibody-drug conjugate trastuzumab emtansine or standard trastuzumab for 14-cycles after surgery. Patients treated with trastuzumab emtansine had a statistically significantly improved 3-year invasive disease-free survival (88% vs 77%), associated with a 50% relative risk reduction. These data may lead to the FDA approval of trastuzumab emtansine in the adjuvant setting.

Retrospective studies have shown that even small (stage T1a,b) *HER2*-positive tumors have a worse prognosis compared with same-sized *HER2*-negative tumors and may thus be appropriate for trastuzumab-based regimens. The NSABP B43 study is ongoing to evaluate whether the addition of trastuzumab to radiation therapy is warranted for DCIS.

Cardiomyopathy develops in a small but significant percentage (0.4–4%) of patients who receive trastuzumab-based regimens. For this reason, anthracyclines and trastuzumab are rarely given concurrently and cardiac function is monitored periodically throughout therapy.

B. ENDOCRINE THERAPY—Adjuvant hormone modulation therapy is highly effective in decreasing relative risk of recurrence by 40–50% and mortality by 25% in women with hormone receptor–positive tumors regardless of menopausal status.

(1) Tamoxifen—The traditional regimen had been 5 years of the estrogen-receptor antagonist/agonist tamoxifen until the 2012 reporting of the Adjuvant Tamoxifen Longer Against Shorter (ATLAS) trial in which 5 versus 10 years of adjuvant tamoxifen were compared. In this study, disease-free and overall survival were significantly improved in women who received 10 years of tamoxifen, particularly after year 10. Though these results are impressive, the clinical application of long-term tamoxifen use must be discussed with patients individually, taking into consideration risks of tamoxifen (such as secondary uterine cancers, venous thromboembolic events, and side effects that impact quality of life). Ovarian suppression in addition to tamoxifen has been shown to significantly improve 8-year disease-free survival (83.2% vs 78.9%) and 8-year overall survival (93.3% vs 91.5%) compared to tamoxifen alone in the randomized Suppression of Ovarian Function Trial [SOFT] study, though the benefits appeared to be seen primarily in chemotherapy-treated patients with higher risk disease.

(2) Aromatase inhibitors—AIs, including anastrozole, letrozole, and exemestane, reduce estrogen production and are also effective in the adjuvant setting for postmenopausal women. AIs should not be used in a patient with functioning (premenopausal) ovaries since *they do not block ovarian production of estrogen*. At least seven large randomized trials enrolling more than 24,000 postmenopausal patients with hormone receptor–positive nonmetastatic breast cancer have compared the use of AIs with tamoxifen or placebo as adjuvant therapy. All of these studies have shown small but statistically significant improvements in disease-free survival (absolute benefits of 2–6%) with the use of AIs. In addition, AIs have been shown to reduce the risk of contralateral breast cancers and to have

fewer associated serious side effects (such as endometrial cancers and thromboembolic events) than tamoxifen. However, they are associated with accelerated bone loss and an increased risk of fractures as well as a musculoskeletal syndrome characterized by arthralgias or myalgias (or both) in the majority of patients. The American Society of Clinical Oncology and the NCCN have recommended that *postmenopausal* women with hormone receptor–positive breast cancer be offered an AI either initially or after tamoxifen therapy. HER2 status should not affect the use or choice of hormone therapy. A combined analysis of the SOFT and Tamoxifen and Exemestane Trial (TEXT) studies showed for the first time that exemestane plus ovarian suppression with triptorelin was associated with a reduced risk of relapse compared to tamoxifen, making this a viable adjuvant therapy option for *premenopausal* women with high-risk ER-positive breast cancers.

3. Bisphosphonates—Multiple randomized studies have evaluated the use of adjuvant bisphosphonates in addition to standard local and systemic therapy for early-stage breast cancer and have shown, in addition to improvement in bone density, a consistent reduction in the risk of metastatic recurrence in postmenopausal patients. A meta-analysis evaluating more than 18,000 women with early-stage breast cancer treated with bisphosphonates or placebo showed that bisphosphonates reduce the risk of cancer recurrence (especially in bone) and improve breast cancer–specific survival primarily in postmenopausal women. Side effects associated with bisphosphonate therapy include bone pain, fever, osteonecrosis of the jaw (rare, less than 1%), esophagitis or ulcers (for oral bisphosphonates), and kidney injury. Although the FDA has not yet approved the adjuvant use of bisphosphonates to reduce the risk of breast cancer recurrence, the 2017 jointly published guidelines of the Cancer Care Ontario and American Society of Clinical Oncology recommend that bisphosphonate use (zoledronic acid or clodronate) be considered in the adjuvant therapy plan for postmenopausal breast cancer patients. In addition, denosumab (another bone stabilizing medication), which is an antibody directed against receptor activator of nuclear factor kappa B ligand (RANK-L), was evaluated in the phase III adjuvant "D-CARE" study in which patients with early-stage breast cancer (all biologic subtypes) were randomized to receive denosumab or placebo. This study, reported by the American Society of Clinical Oncology in 2018, failed to demonstrate a reduction in breast cancer recurrences or deaths with RANK inhibition. It is speculated that one possible reason for this negative result may be due to the fact that premenopausal patients (who do not have a demonstrated metastatic recurrence benefit from bisphosphonates) were included in the study.

4. Adjuvant therapy in older women—Data relating to the optimal use of adjuvant systemic treatment for women over the age of 65 are limited. Results from the EBCTCG overview indicate that while adjuvant chemotherapy yields a smaller benefit for older women compared with younger women, it still improves clinical outcomes. Moreover, individual studies do show that older women with higher risk disease derive benefits from chemotherapy. One study compared the use of oral chemotherapy (capecitabine) to standard chemotherapy in older women and concluded that standard chemotherapy is preferred. Another study (USO TC vs AC) showed that women over the age of 65 derive similar benefits from the taxane-based regimen as women who are younger. The benefits of endocrine therapy for hormone receptor–positive disease appear to be independent of age. In general, decisions relating to the use of systemic therapy should take into account a patient's comorbidities and physiological age, more so than chronologic age.

E. Neoadjuvant Therapy

The use of systemic therapy prior to resection of the primary tumor (neoadjuvant) is a standard option that in many cases should be discussed with patients prior to surgery. This enables the assessment of in vivo sensitivity of the tumor to the selected systemic therapy. Patients with hormone receptor–negative, triple-negative, or HER2-positive breast cancer are more likely to have a pathologic complete response (meaning no residual invasive cancer at the time of surgery) to neoadjuvant chemotherapy than those with hormone receptor–positive breast cancer. A complete pathologic response at the time of surgery, especially in hormone receptor–negative tumors, is associated with improvement in event-free and overall survival. Neoadjuvant chemotherapy also increases the chance of breast conservation by shrinking the primary tumor in women who would otherwise need mastectomy for local control. Survival after neoadjuvant chemotherapy is similar to that seen with postoperative adjuvant chemotherapy.

1. HER2-positive breast cancer—Dual targeting of HER2 with two monoclonal antibodies, trastuzumab and pertuzumab, showed positive results in two clinical trials in the neoadjuvant setting, the TRYPHAENA and the NEO-SPHERE studies.

Based on these clinical trials, three regimens are FDA-approved in the *HER2*-positive neoadjuvant setting: docetaxel [T], cyclophosphamide [C], trastuzumab [H], and pertuzumab [P] (TCHP) for six cycles; 5-fluorouracil, epirubicin, cyclophosphamide [FEC] for 3 cycles followed by THP for 3 cycles; or THP for 4 cycles (followed by three cycles of postoperative FEC). After completing surgery, patients should resume trastuzumab to complete a full year.

2. Hormone receptor–positive, HER2-negative breast cancer—Patients with hormone receptor–positive breast cancer have a lower chance of achieving a pathologic complete response with neoadjuvant therapy than those patients with triple-negative or *HER2*-positive breast cancers. Studies indicate similar response rates with neoadjuvant endocrine therapy compared to neoadjuvant chemotherapy. Typically, responses are not appreciated unless 4–6 or more months of therapy are given. Outside of the clinical trial setting, the use of neoadjuvant hormonal therapy is generally restricted to postmenopausal patients who are unable or unwilling to tolerate chemotherapy.

3. Triple-negative breast cancer—No targeted therapy has been identified for patients with breast cancer that is lacking in *HER2* amplification or hormone receptor expression. Neoadjuvant chemotherapy leads to pathologic complete response in up to 40–50% of patients with triple-negative breast cancer. Patients who achieve a pathologic complete response seem to have a similar prognosis to other breast cancer subtypes with pathologic complete response. However, those patients with residual disease at the time of surgery have a poor prognosis. Based on the theory that triple-negative breast cancers may be more vulnerable to DNA-damaging agents, several studies have evaluated whether the addition of platinum salts to a neoadjuvant chemotherapy regimen is beneficial in this disease subtype, several of which have shown improved outcomes (pathologic complete response and disease-free survival) with platinum use. Other studies are ongoing to evaluate the pathologic complete response rates and long-term outcomes associated with incorporating platinums into standard chemotherapy regimens.

4. Timing of sentinel lymph node biopsy in neoadjuvant setting—There is considerable concern about the timing of sentinel lymph node biopsy, since the chemotherapy may affect cancer present in the lymph nodes. Several studies have shown that sentinel node biopsy can be done after neoadjuvant therapy. However, a large multicenter study, ACOSOG 1071, demonstrated a false-negative rate of 10.7%, well above the false-negative rate outside the neoadjuvant setting (less than 1–5%). If three nodes are removed and isotope and dye are used, the false-negative rate falls to an acceptable level. Some physicians recommend performing sentinel lymph node biopsy before administering the chemotherapy in order to avoid a false-negative result and to aid in planning subsequent radiation therapy. Others prefer to perform sentinel lymph node biopsy after neoadjuvant therapy to avoid a second operation and assess postchemotherapy nodal status. If a complete dissection is desired, this can be performed at the time of the definitive breast surgery. The SENTINA trial showed similarly poor results for sentinel node biopsy after neoadjuvant therapy. No study has evaluated the survival impact of no axillary treatment for node-positive patients who become node-negative after neoadjuvant therapy. Important questions remain to be answered involving the use of neoadjuvant therapy, including which neoadjuvant agents to use, duration of treatment, and additional postoperative therapy.

Early Breast Cancer Trialists' Collaborative Group (EBCTCG). Long-term outcomes for neoadjuvant versus adjuvant chemotherapy in early breast cancer: meta-analysis of individual patient data from ten randomised trials. Lancet Oncol. 2018 Jan;19(1):27–39. [PMID: 29242041]

▶ **Palliative Treatment**

Palliative treatments are aimed to manage symptoms, improve quality of life, and even prolong survival, without the expectation of achieving cure. In the United States, it is uncommon to have distant metastases at the time of diagnosis (de novo metastases). However, most patients who have a breast cancer recurrence after initial local and adjuvant therapy have metastatic rather than local (in breast) disease. Breast cancer most commonly metastasizes to the liver, lungs, and bone, causing symptoms such as fatigue, change in appetite, abdominal pain, cough, dyspnea, or bone pain. Headaches, imbalance, vision changes, vertigo, and other neurologic symptoms may be signs of brain metastases. Triple-negative (ER-, PR-, HER2-negative) and HER2-positive tumors have a higher rate of brain metastases than hormone receptor–positive, HER2-negative tumors.

A. Radiotherapy and Bisphosphonates

Palliative radiotherapy may be advised for primary treatment of locally advanced cancers with distant metastases to control ulceration, pain, and other manifestations in the breast and regional nodes. Irradiation of the breast and chest wall and the axillary, internal mammary, and supraclavicular nodes should be undertaken in an attempt to cure locally advanced and inoperable lesions when there is no evidence of distant metastases. A small number of patients in this group are cured in spite of extensive breast and regional node involvement.

Palliative irradiation is of value also in the treatment of certain bone or soft-tissue metastases to control pain or avoid fracture. Radiotherapy is especially useful in the treatment of isolated bony metastases, chest wall recurrences, brain metastases and sometimes, in lieu of the preferred option of orthopedic surgery for acute spinal cord compression.

In addition to radiotherapy, bisphosphonate therapy has shown excellent results in delaying and reducing skeletal events in women with bony metastases. Pamidronate and zoledronic acid are FDA-approved intravenous bisphosphonates given for bone metastases or hypercalcemia of malignancy from breast cancer. Denosumab, a fully human monoclonal antibody that targets RANK-ligand, is FDA-approved for the treatment of bone metastases from breast cancer, with data showing that it reduced the time to first skeletal-related event (eg, pathologic fracture) compared to zoledronic acid.

Caution should be exercised when combining radiation therapy with chemotherapy because toxicity of either or both may be augmented by their concurrent administration. In general, only one type of therapy should be given at a time unless it is necessary to irradiate a destructive lesion of weight-bearing bone while the patient is receiving chemotherapy. Systemic therapy should be changed only if the disease is clearly progressing. This is especially difficult to determine for patients with destructive bone metastases, since changes in the status of these lesions are difficult to determine radiographically.

B. Targeted Therapy

1. Hormonally based therapy for metastatic disease—The following therapies have all been shown to be effective in hormone receptor–positive metastatic breast cancer: administration of medications that block or downregulate estrogen receptors (such as tamoxifen or fulvestrant, respectively) or medications that block the synthesis of hormones (such as AIs);

Table 17–5. Hormonal agents commonly used for management of metastatic breast cancer (listed in alphabetical order).

Medications	Action	Dose, Route, Frequency	Major Side Effects
Anastrozole (Arimidex)	AI	1 mg orally daily	Hot flushes, skin rashes, nausea and vomiting, bone loss
Exemestane (Aromasin)	AI	25 mg orally daily	Hot flushes, increased arthralgia/arthritis, myalgia, bone loss
Fulvestrant (Faslodex)	Steroidal estrogen receptor antagonist	500 mg intramuscularly days 1, 15, 29 and then monthly	Gastrointestinal upset, headache, back pain, hot flushes, pharyngitis, injection site pain
Goserelin (Zoladex)	Synthetic luteinizing hormone releasing analog	3.6 mg subcutaneously monthly	Arthralgias, blood pressure changes, hot flushes, headaches, vaginal dryness, bone loss
Letrozole (Femara)	AI	2.5 mg orally daily	Hot flushes, arthralgia/arthritis, myalgia, bone loss
Leuprolid (Lupron)	Synthetic luteinizing hormone releasing analog	3.75 or 7.5 mg subcutaneously monthly	Arthralgias, blood pressure changes, hot flushes, headaches, vaginal dryness, bone loss
Megestrol acetate (Megace)	Progestin	40 mg orally four times daily	Fluid retention; venous thromboembolic events; rarely used except in very late stage, treatment-refractory disease
Tamoxifen citrate (Nolvadex)	SERM	20 mg orally daily	Hot flushes, uterine bleeding, thrombophlebitis, rash
Toremifene citrate (Fareston)	SERM	60 mg orally daily	Hot flushes, sweating, nausea, vaginal discharge, dry eyes, dizziness

AI, aromatase inhibitor; SERM, selective estrogen receptor modulator.

ablation of the ovaries, adrenals, or pituitary; and the administration of hormones (eg, estrogens, androgens, progestins); see Table 17–5. Because only 5–10% of women with ER-negative tumors respond, they should not receive endocrine therapy. Women within 1 year of their last menstrual period are arbitrarily considered to be premenopausal and should have surgical (bilateral oophorectomy) or chemical ovarian ablation (using a gonadotropin-releasing hormone [GnRH] analog such as leuprolide [Lupron], goserelin [Zoladex], or tritorelin). Premenopausal women who have had chemical or surgical ovarian ablation are then eligible to receive the same hormonally targeted therapies that are available to postmenopausal women. Current guidelines indicate that sequential hormonal therapy is the preferred treatment for hormone receptor–positive metastatic breast cancer except in the rare case when disease is immediately threatening visceral organs.

A. FIRST-LINE TREATMENT OPTIONS

(1) Hormonally targeted agents—Single-agent hormonally targeted therapy options include fulvestrant (500 mg intramuscularly days 1 and 15, then every month), tamoxifen (20 mg orally daily), or an AI (anastrozole, letrozole, or exemestane). The average time to progression associated with single agent first-line tamoxifen is 5–8 months and with AI is approximately 8–12 months. The side effect profile of AIs differs from tamoxifen. The main side effects of tamoxifen are nausea, skin rash, and hot flushes. Rarely, tamoxifen induces hypercalcemia in patients with bony metastases. Tamoxifen also increases the risk of venous thromboembolic events and uterine hyperplasia and cancer. The main side effects of AIs include hot flushes, vaginal dryness, and joint stiffness; however, osteoporosis and

bone fractures are significantly higher than with tamoxifen. Results from the phase III FALCON study (comparing first-line treatment with the pure estrogen antagonist fulvestrant to anastrozole) confirmed that the use of first-line fulvestrant improves progression-free survival by almost 3 months (HR 0.79, 95% CI 0.637, 0.999, $P = 0.0486$) with the largest treatment effect observed in patients without visceral disease. Overall survival data are needed.

(2) Hormonally targeted therapy plus cyclin dependent kinase inhibition—Hormonally driven breast cancer may be particularly sensitive to inhibition of cell cycle regulatory proteins, called cyclin dependent kinases (CDK). A phase III randomized, placebo-controlled study (PALOMA-2) of letrozole plus an oral CDK 4/6 inhibitor (palbociclib) for the first-line treatment of postmenopausal women with hormone receptor–positive advanced breast cancer demonstrated a striking and highly significant 10-month improvement in progression-free survival associated with the use of palbociclib. Two additional CDK4/6 inhibitors, ribociclib and abemaciclib, were also evaluated in placebo-controlled phase III trials (MONALEESA-2 and MONARCH-3, respectively) in the same disease setting and demonstrated a similar improvement in progression-free survival when added to an AI. These three studies all demonstrated a median progression-free survival of over 2 years; the longest median progression-free survival reported in metastatic ER-positive breast cancer to date, leading many to consider the use of a **CDK4/6 inhibitor plus AI the gold standard treatment in the first-line setting**. Importantly, these therapies yield objective response rates as good as or better than that seen with chemotherapy. All three agents are FDA-approved in the first-line setting in combination

with an AI. Overall survival results are not yet mature. Similar progression-free survival benefits were achieved with ribociclib in younger women in the phase III randomized trial (MONALEESA-7) that exclusively enrolled premenopausal women (treated with goserelin to suppress ovarian function in combination with endocrine therapy). In general, CDK4/6 inhibitors are well tolerated, though monitoring patients for grade 3/4 neutropenia (especially with ribociclib and palbociclib) and management of diarrhea (especially with abemaciclib) are necessary. Febrile neutropenia and infections are rare and use of growth factors is not required; however, palbociclib and ribociclib are given for 3 consecutive weeks, stopping for 1 week to allow white cell count to recover. Abemaciclib is given twice daily continuously (28-day cycles).

B. TREATMENT OPTIONS WHEN DISEASE PROGRESSES AFTER HORMONAL-BASED THERAPY

(1) Secondary or tertiary hormonal therapy—Patients who have disease progression following first-line hormonal therapy may be offered a different form of endocrine therapy. For example, if a patient has been treated with an AI as first-line therapy, fulvestrant or tamoxifen should be considered at the time of disease progression as second-line therapy.

(2) Fulvestrant plus CDK4/6 inhibitor—All three CDK4/6 inhibitors have also been evaluated in phase III trials (PALOMA-3, MONALEESA-3, MONARCH-2) in patients whose disease has progressed on prior endocrine therapy and all have shown a significant improvement in median progression-free survival with the addition of CDK4/6 inhibitor to fulvestrant compared to placebo plus fulvestrant. Palbociclib (125 mg orally daily) and abemaciclib (150 mg orally twice daily) are both FDA approved in combination with fulvestrant for this indication. Abemaciclib is also FDA-approved as a single agent (200 mg orally twice daily) for patients with advanced ER-positive breast cancer who have received prior endocrine therapy and chemotherapy. It should be noted that there is no evidence to date that use of a CDK4/6 inhibitor benefits patients whose disease has progressed despite therapy with a CDK4/6 inhibitor. Thus, at this time, use of any CDK4/6 inhibitor after disease progression on a CDK4/6 inhibitor is not appropriate outside of a clinical trial.

(3) Everolimus plus endocrine therapy—Everolimus (Afinitor) is an oral inhibitor of the mammalian target of rapamycin (MTOR)—a protein whose activation has been associated with the development of endocrine resistance. A phase III, placebo-controlled trial (BOLERO-2) evaluated the AI exemestane with or without everolimus in 724 patients with AI-resistant, hormone receptor–positive metastatic breast cancer and found that patients treated with everolimus had a significantly improved progression-free survival (7.8 months vs 3.2 months; HR, 0.45; 95% CI, 0.38–0.54; $P < 0.0001$) but no significant difference in overall survival. Everolimus has also been evaluated in combination with fulvestrant and shown to have similar improvements in progression-free survival compared to single agent fulvestrant. The main side effect of everolimus is stomatitis (mouth sores). This can be avoided, almost completely, by the prophylactic use of oral steroid mouthwash starting with cycle 1.

(4) Phosphatidylinositol-3-kinase (PI3K) inhibitors plus endocrine therapy—Approximately 40% of hormone receptor–positive breast cancers have activation of the PI3K-AKT-mTOR pathway, most commonly due to an activating mutation of PI3K on the *PIK3CA* gene. Taselisib and alpelisib are both oral alpha-isoform selective inhibitors of PI3K with clinical activity in *PIK3CA*-mutated breast cancer. Both were evaluated in randomized phase III clinical trials (fulvestrant with or without a PI3K inhibitor) in patients with hormone receptor–positive breast cancer who had been previously treated with an AI. In SANDPIPER, presented at the American Society of Clinical Oncology meeting in 2018, the addition of taselisib to fulvestrant was associated with a 2-month improvement (7.4 mos vs 5.4 mos) in *PIK3CA*-mutant tumors. The SOLAR-1 study presented at the European Society of Medical Oncology meeting in 2018 demonstrated over a 5-month improvement in median progression-free survival (11.0 mos vs 5.7 mos) associated with the addition of alpelisib to fulvestrant in patients with tumor *PIK3CA* mutations. Benefits with these PI3K inhibitors were not observed in wild-type tumors. Side effects of PI3K inhibitors include hyperglycemia, diarrhea, rash, and transaminitis.

2. HER2-targeted agents—For patients with *HER2*-positive tumors, trastuzumab plus chemotherapy significantly improves clinical outcomes, including survival compared to chemotherapy alone. **Pertuzumab** is an FDA-approved monoclonal antibody that targets the extracellular domain of *HER2* at a different epitope than targeted by trastuzumab and inhibits receptor dimerization. A phase III placebo-controlled randomized study (CLEOPATRA) showed that patients treated with the combination of pertuzumab, trastuzumab, and docetaxel had a significantly longer progression-free survival (18.5 months vs 12.4 months; HR, 0.62; 95% CI, 0.51–0.75; $P < 0.001$) compared with those treated with docetaxel and trastuzumab. Longer follow-up revealed a significant overall survival benefit associated with pertuzumab as well.

Lapatinib, an oral targeted medication that inhibits the intracellular tyrosine kinases of the epidermal growth factor and *HER2* receptors, is FDA-approved for the treatment of trastuzumab-resistant *HER2*-positive metastatic breast cancer in combination with capecitabine, thus, a completely oral regimen. The combination of trastuzumab plus lapatinib has been shown to be more effective than lapatinib alone for trastuzumab-resistant metastatic breast cancer. Moreover, several trials have shown a significant clinical benefit for continuing *HER2*-targeted agents beyond progression. T-DM1 ado-trastuzumab emtansine (Kadcyla) is an FDA-approved novel antibody-drug conjugate in which trastuzumab is stably linked to a derivative of maytansine, enabling targeted delivery of the cytotoxic chemotherapy to *HER2*-overexpressing cells. T-DM1 is associated with an improved progression-free and overall survival compared to lapatinib plus capecitabine in patients with *HER2*-positive, trastuzumab-pretreated advanced disease (EMILIA). Several other medications targeting *HER2* and its associated signaling pathways are in development, including neratinib, tucatinib (ONT-380), trastuzumab deruxtecan (DS-8201), margetuximab, pyrotinib, and *HER2*-targeted vaccines.

3. Targeting "triple-negative" breast cancer—Breast cancers lacking expression of the hormone receptors ER, PR, and *HER2* behave more aggressively and have traditionally been amenable only to therapy with cytotoxic chemotherapy, though emerging clinical trial data may lead to approval of new agents for this type of cancer. A phase II placebo-controlled randomized trial (LOTUS) demonstrated a significantly improved progression-free survival (6.2 mos vs 4.9 mos, stratified HR 0.60, $P = 0.037$) by adding the oral AKT inhibitor ipatasertib to first-line paclitaxel. These results need to be confirmed in a larger phase III study but are the first promising results of an AKT inhibitor for triple-negative breast cancer. Early phase clinical trials showed promise for immune checkpoint inhibitors (such as monoclonal antibodies that target PDL-1 or PD-1). Results from the first phase III randomized trial of immune therapy for triple-negative metastatic breast cancer (IMPASSION) were presented and published in 2018 and demonstrated that the anti-PD-L1 antibody atezolizumab added to nab-paclitaxel significantly improved the median progression-free survival in the intent to treat population (7.2 mos vs 5.5 mos) and in the population with PD-L-1 positive tumors (7.5 mos vs 5.0 mos) compared to nab-paclitaxel plus placebo. While median overall survival was not significantly improved in the intent to treat population, there was almost a 10-month improvement in overall survival in patients with PD-L-1 positive tumors (25.0 mos vs 15.5 mos). **These are the first results to demonstrate effectiveness of immune modulation therapy in breast cancer and will likely prove to be practice changing.** Another therapy garnering attention for triple-negative disease is sacituzumab govitecan, an antibody-drug conjugate that delivers SN-38 (active metabolite of the chemotherapy irinotecan) to Trop-2 overexpressing breast cancer cells. This antibody-drug conjugate has demonstrated significant clinical activity in heavily pretreated triple-negative breast cancer, leading to its priority review designation by the FDA. An ongoing phase III trial, ASCENT, is underway.

4. Targeting PARP in *BRCA1/2* mutation-associated breast cancer—Poly (adenosine diphosphate-ribose) polymerase (PARP) is an enzyme important in single-strand DNA repair. Patients who carry germline mutations in *BRCA1* or *BRCA2* have tumors with deficient double-strand DNA repair mechanisms. Experts have theorized that inhibiting PARP selectively kills *BRCA1/2* mutated cancers. A phase III clinical trial (OlympiAD) that compared olaparib (an oral PARP inhibitor) to treatment of physician's choice (single-agent chemotherapy) demonstrated a significantly improved progression-free survival (7.0 mos vs 4.2 mos, HR 0.58; $P < 0.001$), an improved response rate, and a lower rate of adverse events than standard therapy. Talazoparib, a second PARP inhibitor, has also been shown to improve outcomes similarly in the phase III EMBRACA study. Both olaparib and talazoparib are FDA-approved for *BRCA*-mutated metastatic breast cancer as single agents.

C. Palliative Chemotherapy

Cytotoxic medications should be considered for the treatment of metastatic breast cancer (1) if life- or organ-threatening visceral metastases are present (especially brain, liver, or lymphangitic pulmonary), (2) if hormonal treatment is unsuccessful or the disease has progressed after an initial response to hormonal manipulation (for hormone receptor–positive breast cancer), or (3) if the tumor is ER-negative or HER2-positive. Prior adjuvant chemotherapy does not seem to alter response rates in patients who relapse. A number of chemotherapy medications (including vinorelbine, paclitaxel, docetaxel, gemcitabine, ixabepilone, carboplatin, cisplatin, capecitabine, albumin-bound paclitaxel, eribulin, and liposomal doxorubicin) may be used as single agents with first-line objective response rates ranging from 30% to 50%.

Combination chemotherapy yields statistically significantly higher response rates and progression-free survival rates, but has not been conclusively shown to improve overall survival rates compared with sequential single-agent therapy. Combinations that have been tested in phase III studies and have proven efficacy compared with single-agent therapy include capecitabine/docetaxel, gemcitabine/paclitaxel, and capecitabine/ixabepilone (see Tables 39–3 and 39–13). Various other combinations of medications have been tested in phase II studies, and a number of clinical trials are ongoing to identify effective combinations. Patients should be encouraged to participate in clinical trials given the number of promising targeted therapies in development. It is generally appropriate to treat willing patients with multiple sequential lines of therapy as long as they tolerate the treatment and as long as their performance status is good (eg, at least ambulatory and able to care for self, up out of bed more than 50% of waking hours).

Bardia A. Efficacy and safety of anti-Trop-2 antibody drug conjugate sacituzumab govitecan (IMMU-132) in heavily pretreated patients with metastatic triple negative breast cancer. J Clin Oncol. 2017 Jul 1;35(19):2141–8. [PMID: 28291390]

Cameron D et al; Herceptin Adjuvant (HERA) Trial Study Team. 11 years' follow-up of trastuzumab after adjuvant chemotherapy in HER2-positive early breast cancer: final analysis of the HERceptin Adjuvant (HERA) trial. Lancet. 2017 Mar 25; 389(10075):1195–205. [PMID: 28215665]

Cardoso F et al; MINDACT Investigators. 70-Gene Signature as an aid to treatment decisions in early-stage breast cancer. N Engl J Med. 2016 Aug 25;375(8):717–29. [PMID: 27557300]

Cardoso F et al. Standard anthracycline-based vs. docetaxel-capecitabine in early breast cancer: results from the chemotherapy randomization (R-C) of EORTC 10041/BIG 3-04 MINDACT phase III trial. J Clin Oncol. 2017;35(suppl):abstr 516.

Dhesy-Thind S et al. Use of adjuvant bisphosphonates and other bone-modifying agents in breast cancer: a Cancer Care Ontario and American Society of Clinical Oncology clinical practice guideline. J Clin Oncol. 2017 Jun 20;35(18):2062–81. [PMID: 28618241]

Diéras V et al. Trastuzumab emtansine versus capecitabine plus lapatinib in patients with previously treated HER2-positive advanced breast cancer (EMILIA): a descriptive analysis of final overall survival results from a randomised, open-label, phase 3 trial. Lancet Oncol. 2017 Jun;18(6):732–42. [PMID: 28526536]

Early Breast Cancer Trialists' Collaborative Group (EBCTCG). Long-term outcomes for neoadjuvant versus adjuvant chemotherapy in early breast cancer: meta-analysis of individual patient data from ten randomised trials. Lancet Oncol. 2018 Jan;19(1):27–39. [PMID: 29242041]

Ejlertsen B et al. Adjuvant cyclophosphamide and docetaxel with or without epirubicin for early TOP2A-normal breast cancer: DBCG 07-READ, an open-label, phase III, randomized trial. J Clin Oncol. 2017 Aug 10;35(23):2639–46. [PMID: 28661759]

Finn RS et al. Palbociclib and letrozole in advanced breast cancer. N Engl J Med. 2016 Nov 17;375(20):1925–36. [PMID: 27959613]

Francis PA et al; SOFT and TEXT Investigators and the International Breast Cancer Study Group. Tailoring adjuvant endocrine therapy for premenopausal breast cancer. N Engl J Med. 2018 Jul 12;379(2):122–37. [PMID: 29863451]

Goetz MP et al. MONARCH 3: abemaciclib as initial therapy for advanced breast cancer. J Clin Oncol. 2017 Nov 10; 35(32):3638–46. [PMID: 28968163]

Harbeck N et al. Prospective WSG phase III PlanB trial: Final analysis of adjuvant 4xEC→4x doc vs. 6x docetaxel/cyclophosphamide in patients with high clinical risk and intermediate-to-high genomic risk HER2-negative, early breast cancer. J Clin Oncol. 2017;35(suppl):abstr 504.

Hortobagyi GN et al. Ribociclib as first-line therapy for HR-positive, advanced breast cancer. N Engl J Med. 2016 Nov 3;375(18): 1738–48. [PMID: 27717303]

Litton J et al. Talazoparib in patients with advanced breast cancer and a germline BRCA mutation. N Engl J Med. 2018 Aug 23; 379(8):753–63. [PMID: 30110579]

Martin M et al; ExteNET Study Group. Neratinib after trastuzumab-based adjuvant therapy in HER2-positive breast cancer (ExteNET): 5-year analysis of a randomised, double-blind, placebo-controlled, phase 3 trial. Lancet Oncol. 2017 Dec; 18(12):1688–1700. [PMID: 29146401]

National Comprehensive Cancer Network. NCCN guidelines: breast cancer. http://www.nccn.org/professionals/physician_gls/f_guidelines.asp

Robson M et al. Olaparib for metastatic breast cancer in patients with a germline BRCA mutation. N Engl J Med. 2017 Aug 10; 377(6):523–33. Erratum in: N Engl J Med. 2017 Oct 26; 377(17):1700. [PMID: 28578601]

Rugo HS et al. Prevention of everolimus-related stomatitis in women with hormone receptor-positive, HER2-negative metastatic breast cancer using dexamethasone mouthwash (SWISH): a single-arm, phase 2 trial. Lancet Oncol. 2017 May;18(5): 654–62. [PMID: 28314691]

Rugo HS et al. Endocrine therapy for hormone receptor-positive metastatic breast cancer: American Society of Clinical Oncology guideline. J Clin Oncol. 2016 Sep 1;34(25):3069–103. [PMID: 27217461]

Schmid P et al. Atezolizumab and nab-paclitaxel in advanced triple negative breast cancer. N Engl J Med. 2018 Nov 29; 379(22):2108–21. [PMID: 30345906]

Sledge GW Jr et al. MONARCH 2: abemaciclib in combination with fulvestrant in women with HR+/HER2- advanced breast cancer who had progressed while receiving endocrine therapy. J Clin Oncol. 2017 Sep 1;35(25):2875–84. [PMID: 28580882]

Tripathy D et al. Ribociclib plus endocrine therapy for premenopausal women with hormone-receptor-positive advanced breast cancer (MONALEESA-7): a randomised phase 3 trial. Lancet Oncol. 2018 Jul;19(7):904–15. [PMID: 29804902]

von Minckwitz G et al; APHINITY Steering Committee and Investigators. Adjuvant pertuzumab and trastuzumab in early HER2-positive breast cancer. N Engl J Med. 2017 Jul 13; 377(2):122–31. Erratum in: N Engl J Med. 2017 Aug 17; 377(7):702. [PMID: 28581356]

von Minckwitz G et al; KATHERINE Investigators. Trastuzumab emtansine for residual invasive HER2-positive breast cancer. N Engl J Med. 2019 Feb 14;380(7):617–28. [PMID: 30516102]

► Prognosis

Stage of breast cancer is the most reliable indicator of prognosis (Table 17–6). Axillary lymph node status is the best-analyzed prognostic factor and correlates with survival at all tumor sizes. When cancer is localized to the breast with no evidence of regional spread after pathologic

Table 17–6. Approximate survival of patients with breast cancer by TNM stage.

TNM Stage	5 Years	10 Years
0	95%	90%
I	85%	70%
IIA	70%	50%
IIB	60%	40%
IIIA	55%	30%
IIIB	30%	20%
IV	5–10%	2%
All	65%	30%

examination, the clinical cure rate with most accepted methods of therapy is 75% to more than 90%. In fact, patients with small mammographically detected biologically favorable tumors and no evidence of axillary spread have a 5-year survival rate greater than 95%. When the axillary lymph nodes are involved with tumor, the survival rate drops to 50–70% at 5 years and probably around 25–40% at 10 years. The use of biologic markers, such as ER, PR, grade, and HER2, helps identify high-risk tumor types as well as direct treatment used (see Biomarkers & Gene Expression Profiling). Gene analysis studies can predict disease-free survival for some subsets of patients. The American Joint Committee on Cancer (AJCC) Cancer Staging Manual 8th edition has incorporated these factors into staging.

Five-year statistics do not accurately reflect the final outcome of therapy. The mortality rate of breast cancer patients exceeds that of age-matched normal controls for nearly 20 years. Thereafter, the mortality rates are equal, though deaths that occur among breast cancer patients are often directly the result of tumor.

In general, breast cancer appears to be somewhat more aggressive and associated with worse outcomes in younger than in older women, and this may be related to the fact that fewer younger women have ER-positive tumors. Disparities in treatment outcome for different racial and ethnic backgrounds have been reported by several studies. These differences appear to be not only due to different socioeconomic factors (and a resulting difference in access to healthcare) but also due to differences in the subtype of breast cancer diagnosed.

For those patients whose disease progresses despite treatment, some studies suggest supportive group therapy may improve survival. As they approach the end of life, such patients will require meticulous palliative care (see Chapter 5).

DeSantis CE et al. Breast cancer statistics, 2017, racial disparity in mortality by state. CA Cancer J Clin. 2017 Nov;67(6):439–448. [PMID: 28972651]

Giuliano AE et al. Eighth edition of the AJCC Cancer Staging Manual: Breast Cancer. Ann Surg Oncol. 2018 Jul;25(7):1783–5. [PMID: 29671136]

Miller JW et al. Disparities in breast cancer survival in the United States (2001–2009): findings from the CONCORD-2 study. Cancer. 2017 Dec 15;(123 Suppl 24):5100–18. [PMID: 29205311]

Miller KD et al. Cancer statistics for hispanics/latinos, 2018. CA Cancer J Clin. 2018 Nov;68(6):425–45. [PMID: 30285281]

Pan H et al; EBCTCG. 20-year risks of breast-cancer recurrence after stopping endocrine therapy at 5 years. N Engl J Med. 2017 Nov 9;377(19):1836–46. [PMID: 29117498]

▶ Follow-Up Care

After primary therapy, patients with breast cancer should be monitored long term in order to detect recurrences and to observe the opposite breast for a second primary carcinoma. Local and distant recurrences occur most frequently within the first 2–5 years. During the first 2 years, most patients should be examined every 6 months, then annually thereafter. Special attention is paid to the contralateral breast because a new primary breast malignancy will develop in 20–25% of patients. In some cases, especially in hormone receptor–positive breast cancer, metastases are dormant for long periods and may appear 15 years or longer after removal of the primary tumor. Although studies have failed to show an adverse effect of hormonal replacement in disease-free patients, it is rarely used after breast cancer treatment, particularly if the tumor was hormone receptor–positive. Even pregnancy has not been associated with shortened survival of patients rendered disease free—yet many oncologists are reluctant to advise a young patient with breast cancer that it is safe to become pregnant. The use of estrogen replacement for conditions such as osteoporosis, vaginal dryness, and hot flushes may be considered for a woman with a history of breast cancer after discussion of the benefits and risks; however, it is not routinely recommended, especially given the availability of nonhormonal agents for these conditions (such as bisphosphonates and denosumab for osteoporosis).

A. Local Recurrence

The incidence of local recurrence correlates with tumor size, the presence and number of involved axillary nodes, the histologic type of tumor, the presence of skin edema or skin and fascia fixation with the primary tumor, and the type of definitive surgery and local irradiation. Local recurrence on the chest wall after total mastectomy and axillary dissection develops in as many as 8% of patients. When the axillary nodes are not involved, the local recurrence rate is less than 5%, but the rate is as high as 25% when they are heavily involved. A similar difference in local recurrence rate was noted between small and large tumors. Factors such as multifocal cancer, in situ tumors, lymphovascular invasion, positive resection margins, chemotherapy, and radiotherapy have an effect on local recurrence in patients treated with breast-conserving surgery. Adjuvant systemic therapy greatly decreases the rate of local recurrence.

Chest wall recurrences usually appear within the first several years but may occur as late as 15 or more years after mastectomy. All suspicious nodules and skin lesions should be biopsied. Local excision or localized radiotherapy may be feasible if an isolated nodule is present. If lesions are multiple or accompanied by evidence of regional involvement in the internal mammary or supraclavicular nodes, the disease is best managed by radiation treatment of the entire chest wall including the parasternal, supraclavicular, and axillary areas as well as systemic therapy.

Local recurrence after mastectomy usually signals the presence of widespread disease and is an indication for studies to search for metastases. Distant metastases will develop within a few years in most patients with locally recurrent tumor after mastectomy. When there is no evidence of metastases beyond the chest wall and regional nodes, irradiation for cure after complete local excision should be attempted. After partial mastectomy, local recurrence does not have as serious a prognostic significance as after mastectomy. However, those patients in whom a recurrence develops have a worse prognosis than those who do not. It is speculated that the ability of a cancer to recur locally after radiotherapy is a sign of aggressiveness and resistance to therapy. Completion of the mastectomy should be done for local recurrence after partial mastectomy; some of these patients will survive for prolonged periods, especially if the breast recurrence is DCIS or occurs more than 5 years after initial treatment. Systemic chemotherapy or hormonal treatment should be used for women in whom disseminated disease develops or those in whom local recurrence occurs.

B. Breast Cancer Survivorship Issues

Given that most women with non-metastatic breast cancer will be cured, a significant number of women face survivorship issues stemming from either the diagnosis or the treatment of the breast cancer, or both. These challenges include psychological struggles, upper extremity lymphedema, weight management problems, cardiovascular issues, bone loss, postmenopausal side effects, and fatigue. One randomized study reported that survivors who received psychological intervention from the time of diagnosis had a lower risk of recurrence and breast cancer–related mortality. A randomized study in older, overweight cancer survivors showed that diet and exercise reduced the rate of self-reported functional decline compared with no intervention. Cognitive dysfunction (also called "chemo brain") is a commonly reported symptom experienced by women who have undergone systemic treatment for early breast cancer.

1. Edema of the arm—Significant edema of the arm occurs in about 10–30% of patients after axillary dissection with or without mastectomy. It occurs more commonly in obese women, in women who had radiotherapy, and in women who had postoperative infection. Partial mastectomy with radiation to the axillary lymph nodes is followed by chronic edema of the arm in 10–20% of patients. Sentinel lymph node dissection has proved to be an accurate form of axillary staging without the side effects of edema or infection. Judicious use of radiotherapy, with treatment fields carefully planned to spare the axilla as much as possible, can greatly diminish the incidence of edema, which will occur in only 5% of patients if no radiotherapy is given to the axilla after a partial mastectomy and lymph node dissection.

Late or secondary edema of the arm may develop years after treatment, as a result of axillary recurrence or infection in the hand or arm, with obliteration of lymphatic channels. When edema develops, a careful examination of the axilla for recurrence or infection is performed. Infection in the arm or hand on the dissected side should be treated with antibiotics, rest, and elevation. If there is no sign of recurrence or infection, the swollen extremity should be treated with rest and elevation. A mild diuretic may be helpful. If there is no improvement, a compressor pump or manual compression decreases the swelling, and the patient is then fitted with an elastic glove or sleeve. Most patients are not bothered enough by mild edema to wear an uncomfortable glove or sleeve and will treat themselves with elevation or manual compression alone. Rarely, edema may be severe enough to interfere with use of the limb. A prospective randomized study has shown that twice weekly progressive weight lifting improves lymphedema symptoms and exacerbations and improves extremity strength.

2. Breast reconstruction—Breast reconstruction is usually feasible after total or modified radical mastectomy. Reconstruction should be discussed with patients prior to mastectomy, because it offers an important psychological focal point for recovery. Reconstruction is not an obstacle to the diagnosis of recurrent cancer. The most common breast reconstruction has been implantation of a silicone gel or saline prosthesis in the subpectoral plane between the pectoralis minor and pectoralis major muscles. Alternatively, autologous tissue can be used for reconstruction.

Autologous tissue flaps have the advantage of not feeling like a foreign body to the patient. The most popular autologous technique currently is reconstruction using abdominal tissue flaps. This includes the deep inferior epigastric perforator (**DIEP**) flap and the more traditional transrectus abdominis muscle (**TRAM**) flap. A latissimus dorsi flap can be swung from the back but offers less volume than the TRAM flap and thus often requires supplementation with an implant. Reconstruction may be performed immediately (at the time of initial mastectomy) or may be delayed until later, usually when the patient has completed adjuvant therapy. When considering reconstructive options, concomitant illnesses should be considered, since the ability of an autologous flap to survive depends on medical comorbidities. In addition, the need for radiotherapy may affect the choice of reconstruction as radiation may increase fibrosis around an implant or decrease the volume of a flap.

3. Risks of pregnancy—Clinicians are often asked to advise patients regarding the potential risk of future pregnancy after definitive treatment for early-stage breast cancer. **To date, no adverse effect of pregnancy on survival of women who have had breast cancer has been demonstrated.** When counseling patients, oncologists must take into consideration the patients' overall prognosis, age, comorbidities, and life goals.

In patients with inoperable or metastatic cancer (stage IV disease), induced abortion may be advisable because of the possible adverse effects of hormonal treatment, radiotherapy, or chemotherapy upon the fetus in addition to the expectant mother's poor prognosis.

Asdourian MS et al. Association between precautionary behaviors and breast cancer-related lymphedema in patients undergoing bilateral surgery. J Clin Oncol. 2017 Dec 10;35(35):3934–41. [PMID: 28976793]

Carroll JE et al. Cognitive performance in survivors of breast cancer and markers of biological aging. Cancer. 2019 Jan 15;125(2):298–306. [PMID: 30474160]

Dieli-Conwright CM et al. Hispanic ethnicity as a moderator of the effects of aerobic and resistance exercise in survivors of breast cancer. Cancer. 2019 Mar 15;125(6):910–20. [PMID: 30500981]

Gerstl B et al. Pregnancy outcomes after a breast cancer diagnosis: a systematic review and meta-analysis. Clin Breast Cancer. 2018 Feb;18(1):e79–88. [PMID: 28797766]

Hummel SB et al. Efficacy of internet-based cognitive behavioral therapy in improving sexual functioning of breast cancer survivors: results of a randomized controlled trial. J Clin Oncol. 2017 Apr 20;35(12):1328–40. [PMID: 28240966]

Janelsins MC et al. Cognitive complaints in survivors of breast cancer after chemotherapy compared with age-matched controls: an analysis from a nationwide, multicenter, prospective longitudinal study. J Clin Oncol. 2017 Feb 10;35(5):506–14. [PMID: 28029304]

Lambertini M et al. Long-term safety of pregnancy following breast cancer according to estrogen receptor status. J Natl Cancer Inst. 2018 Apr 1;110(4):426–9. [PMID: 29087485]

Mandelblatt JS et al. Cancer-related cognitive outcomes among older breast cancer survivors in the thinking and living with cancer study. J Clin Oncol. 2018 Oct 3. [Epub ahead of print] [PMID: 30281396]

Van Dyk K et al. The cognitive effects of endocrine therapy in survivors of breast cancer: a prospective longitudinal study up to 6 years after treatment. Cancer. 2019 Mar 1;125(5):681–9. [PMID: 30485399]

CARCINOMA OF THE MALE BREAST

ESSENTIALS OF DIAGNOSIS

► A painless lump beneath the areola in a man usually over 50 years of age.

► Nipple discharge, retraction, or ulceration may be present.

► Generally poorer prognosis than in women.

► General Considerations

Breast cancer in men is a rare disease; the incidence is only about 1% of all breast cancer diagnoses. The average age at occurrence is about 70 years, and there may be an increased incidence of breast cancer in men with prostate cancer. As in women, hormonal influences are probably related to the development of male breast cancer. There is a high incidence of both breast cancer and gynecomastia in Bantu men, theoretically owing to failure of estrogen inactivation by associated liver disease. It is important to note that first-degree relatives of men with breast cancer are considered to be at high risk. This risk should be taken into account when discussing options with the patient and family. In addition, *BRCA2* mutations are common in men with breast cancer. Men with breast cancer, especially with a history of prostate cancer, should receive genetic counseling. The prognosis, even in stage I cases, is worse in men than in women.

Clinical Findings

A painless lump, occasionally associated with nipple discharge, retraction, erosion, or ulceration, is the primary complaint. Examination usually shows a hard, ill-defined, nontender mass beneath the nipple or areola. Gynecomastia not uncommonly precedes or accompanies breast cancer in men. Nipple discharge is an uncommon presentation for breast cancer in men but is an ominous finding associated with carcinoma in nearly 75% of cases.

Breast cancer staging is the same in men as in women. Gynecomastia and metastatic cancer from another site (eg, prostate) must be considered in the differential diagnosis. Benign tumors are rare, and biopsy should be performed on all males with a defined breast mass.

Treatment

Treatment consists of modified radical mastectomy in operable patients, who should be chosen by the same criteria as women with the disease. Breast conserving therapy is rarely performed. Irradiation is the first step in treating localized metastases in the skin, lymph nodes, or skeleton that are causing symptoms. Examination of the cancer for hormone receptors and *HER2* overexpression is of value in determining adjuvant therapy. Over 95% of men have ER-positive tumors and less than 10% have overexpression of *HER2*. Androgen receptor is also commonly overexpressed in male breast cancer. Adjuvant systemic therapy and radiation are used for the same indications as in breast cancer in women.

Because breast cancer in men is frequently a disseminated disease, endocrine therapy is of considerable importance in its management. Tamoxifen is the main medication for management of advanced breast cancer in men. Tamoxifen (20 mg orally daily) should be the initial treatment. There is little data regarding the use of AIs in men. Castration in advanced breast cancer is a successful measure and more beneficial than the same procedure in women but is rarely used. Objective evidence of regression may be seen in 60–70% of men with endocrine therapy for metastatic disease—approximately twice the proportion in women. Bone is the most frequent site of metastases from breast cancer in men (as in women), and endocrine therapy relieves bone pain in most patients so treated. The longer the interval between mastectomy and recurrence, the longer the remission following treatment is likely. Corticosteroid therapy alone has been considered to be efficacious but probably has no value when compared with major endocrine ablation.

Chemotherapy should be administered for the same indications and using the same dosage schedules as for women with metastatic disease or for adjuvant treatment.

Prognosis

A large population-based, international study reported that after adjustment for prognostic features (age, stage, treatment), men have a significantly improved relative survival from breast cancer compared to women. For node-positive disease, 5-year survival is approximately 69%, and for node-negative disease, it is 88%. A practice-patterns database study reported that based on NCCN guidelines, only 59% of patients received the recommended chemotherapy, 82% received the recommended hormonal therapy, and 71% received the recommended post-mastectomy radiation, indicating a *relatively low adherence to NCCN guidelines for men*.

For those patients whose disease progresses despite treatment, meticulous efforts at palliative care are essential (see Chapter 5).

Giordano SH. Breast cancer in men. N Engl J Med. 2018 Jun 14; 378(24):2311–20. [PMID: 29897847]

Gynecologic Disorders

Jason Woo, MD, MPH, FACOG
Rachel K. Scott, MD, MPH, FACOG

PREMENOPAUSAL ABNORMAL UTERINE BLEEDING

 ESSENTIALS OF DIAGNOSIS

► Accurate diagnosis of abnormal uterine bleeding (AUB) depends on appropriate categorization and diagnostic tests.

► Pregnancy should always be ruled out as a cause of AUB in reproductive age women.

► The evaluation of AUB depends on the age and risk factors of the patient.

General Considerations

Normal menstrual bleeding lasts an average of 5 days (range, 2–7 days), with a mean blood loss of 40 mL per cycle. **Menorrhagia** is defined as blood loss of over 80 mL per cycle and frequently produces anemia. **Metrorrhagia** is defined as bleeding between periods. **Polymenorrhea** is defined as bleeding that occurs more often than every 21 days, and **oligomenorrhea** is defined as bleeding that occurs less frequently than every 35 days.

The International Federation of Gynecology and Obstetrics (FIGO) introduced the current classification system for abnormal uterine bleeding, and it was then endorsed by the American College of Obstetrics and Gynecology. The new classification system does not use the term "dysfunctional uterine bleeding." Instead, it uses the term **"abnormal uterine bleeding" (AUB)** and pairs it with descriptive terms denoting the bleeding pattern (ie, **heavy**, **light** and **menstrual**, **intermenstrual**) and etiology (the acronym **PALM-COEIN** standing for Polyp, Adenomyosis, Leiomyoma, Malignancy and hyperplasia, Coagulopathy, Ovulatory dysfunction, Endometrial, Iatrogenic, and Not yet classified). In adolescents, AUB often occurs as a result of persistent **anovulation** due to the immaturity of the hypothalamic-pituitary-ovarian axis and represents normal physiology. Once regular menses has been established during adolescence, **ovulatory dysfunction** AUB (AUB-O)

accounts for most cases. AUB in women aged 19–39 years is often a result of pregnancy, structural lesions, anovulatory cycles, use of hormonal contraception, or endometrial hyperplasia.

Clinical Findings

A. Symptoms and Signs

The diagnosis depends on the following: (1) a history of the duration and amount of flow, associated pain, and relationship to the last menstrual period (LMP), with the presence of blood clots or the degree of inconvenience caused by the bleeding serving as useful indicators; (2) a history of pertinent illnesses, such as recent systemic infections, other significant physical or emotional stressors, such as thyroid disease or weight change; (3) a history of medications (such as warfarin, heparin, or exogenous hormones); (4) a history of coagulation disorders in the patient or family members; (5) a complete physical examination to evaluate for excessive weight and signs of polycystic ovary syndrome (PCOS), thyroid disease, insulin resistance, or bleeding disorder; and (6) a pelvic examination to rule out vulvar, vaginal, or cervical lesions, pregnancy, uterine myomas, adnexal masses, adenomyosis, or infection.

B. Laboratory Studies

A complete blood count, pregnancy test, and thyroid tests should be done. For adolescents with heavy menstrual bleeding and adults with a positive screening history, coagulation studies should be considered, since up to 18% of women with severe menorrhagia have an underlying coagulopathy. Vaginal or urine samples should be obtained for polymerase chain reaction (PCR) or culture to rule out *Chlamydia* infection. If indicated, cervical cytology should also be obtained.

C. Imaging

Transvaginal ultrasound is useful to diagnose intrauterine or ectopic pregnancy or adnexal or uterine masses and to evaluate endometrial thickness. Sonohysterography or hysteroscopy may be used to diagnose endometrial polyps or subserous myomas. MRI is not a primary imaging modality for AUB but can more definitively diagnose submucous myomas and adenomyosis.

D. Cervical Biopsy and Endometrial Sampling

The purpose of endometrial sampling is to determine if hyperplasia or carcinoma is present. Sampling methods and other gynecologic diagnostic procedures are described in Table 18–1. Polyps, endometrial hyperplasia and, occasionally, submucous myomas are identified on endometrial biopsy. Endometrial sampling should be performed in patients with AUB who are older than 45 years, or in younger patients with a history of unopposed estrogen exposure or failed medical management and persistent

---

Table 18–1. Common gynecologic diagnostic procedures.

Colposcopy
Visualization of cervical, vaginal, or vulvar epithelium under 5–50 × magnification with and without dilute acetic acid to identify abnormal areas requiring biopsy. An office procedure.

Dilation & curettage (D&C)
Dilation of the cervix and curettage of the entire endometrial cavity, using a metal curette or suction cannula and often using forceps for the removal of endometrial polyps. Can usually be done in the office under local anesthesia or in the operating room under sedation or general anesthesia. D&C is often combined with hysteroscopy for improved sensitivity.

Endometrial biopsy
Blind sampling of the endometrium by means of a curette or small aspiration device without cervical dilation. Diagnostic accuracy similar to D&C. An office procedure performed with or without local anesthesia.

Endocervical curettage
Removal of endocervical epithelium with a small curette for diagnosis of cervical dysplasia and cancer. An office procedure performed with or without local anesthesia.

Hysterosalpingography
Injection of radiopaque dye through the cervix to visualize the uterine cavity and oviducts. Mainly used in investigation of infertility, to identify a space-occupying lesion, or to confirm fallopian tube inserts (Essure®) sterilization.

Hysteroscopy
Visual examination of the uterine cavity with a small fiberoptic endoscope passed through the cervix. Curettage, endometrial ablation, biopsies of lesions, and excision of myomas or polyps can be performed concurrently. Can be done in the office under local anesthesia or in the operating room under sedation or general anesthesia. Greater sensitivity for diagnosis of uterine pathology than D&C.

Laparoscopy
Visualization of the abdominal and pelvic cavity through a small fiberoptic endoscope passed through a subumbilical incision. Permits diagnosis, tubal sterilization, and treatment of many conditions previously requiring laparotomy. General anesthesia is used.

Saline infusion sonohysterography
Introduction of saline solution into endometrial cavity with a catheter to visualize submucous myomas or endometrial polyps by transvaginal ultrasound. May be performed in the office with oral or local analgesia, or both.

AUB. If the Papanicolaou smear abnormality requires it or a gross cervical lesion is seen, colposcopic-directed biopsies and endocervical curettage are usually indicated.

► Treatment

Treatment for premenopausal patients with AUB depends on the etiology of the bleeding, determined by history, physical examination, laboratory findings, imaging, and endometrial sampling. Patients with AUB secondary to submucosal myomas, infection, early abortion, thrombophilias, or pelvic neoplasms may require definitive therapy. A large proportion of premenopausal patients, however, have ovulatory dysfunction AUB (AUB-O).

AUB-O can be treated hormonally. Progestins, which limit and stabilize endometrial growth, are generally effective. For patients with irregular or light bleeding, medroxyprogesterone acetate, 10 mg/day orally, or norethindrone acetate, 5 mg/day orally, should be given for 10 days, following which withdrawal bleeding will occur. If successful, the treatment can be repeated for several cycles, starting medication on day 15 of subsequent cycles, or it can be reinstituted if amenorrhea or dysfunctional bleeding recurs. Nonsteroidal anti-inflammatory drugs (NSAIDs), such as naproxen or mefenamic acid, in the usual anti-inflammatory doses, will also often reduce blood loss in menorrhagia— even that associated with a copper intrauterine device (IUD). Women who are experiencing heavier bleeding can be given a taper of any of the combination oral contraceptives (with 30–35 mcg of estrogen estradiol) to control the bleeding. There are several commonly used contraceptive dosing regimens, including four times daily for 1 or 2 days followed by two pills daily through day 5 and then one pill daily through day 20; after withdrawal bleeding occurs, pills are taken in the usual dosage for three cycles. In cases of intractable heavy bleeding, a gonadotropin-releasing hormone (GnRH) agonist such as depot leuprolide, 3.75 mg intramuscularly monthly, can be used for up to 6 months to create a temporary cessation of menstruation by ovarian suppression. These therapies require 2–4 weeks to downregulate the pituitary and stop bleeding and will not stop bleeding acutely. In cases of heavy bleeding requiring hospitalization, intravenous conjugated estrogens, 25 mg every 4 hours for three or four doses, can be used, followed by oral conjugated estrogens, 2.5 mg daily, or ethinyl estradiol, 20 mcg orally daily, for 3 weeks, with the addition of medroxyprogesterone acetate, 10 mg orally daily for the last 10 days of treatment, or a combination oral contraceptive daily for 3 weeks. This will thicken the endometrium and control the bleeding.

If the abnormal bleeding is not controlled by hormonal treatment, hysteroscopy with tissue sampling or saline infusion sonohysterography is used to evaluate for structural lesions (such as polyps, submucous myomas) or neoplasms (such as endometrial cancer). In the absence of specific pathology, bleeding unresponsive to medical therapy may be treated with endometrial ablation, levonorgestrel-releasing IUD (LNG-IUD), or hysterectomy. While hysterectomy was used commonly in the past for bleeding unresponsive to medical therapy, the low risk of complications and the good short-term results of both endometrial ablation and LNG-IUD make them attractive alternatives to hysterectomy. Endometrial ablation may be performed through the hysteroscope with laser photocoagulation or electrocautery. Nonhysteroscopic techniques include balloon thermal ablation, cryoablation, free-fluid thermal ablation, impedance bipolar radiofrequency ablation, and microwave ablation. The latter methods are well-adapted to outpatient therapy under local anesthesia.

The LNG-IUD markedly reduces menstrual blood loss and may be a good alternative to other therapies. A risk-benefit review concluded the LNG-IUD is equally effective as surgical procedures in improving quality of life and is consistently a cost-effective option across a variety of countries and settings.

► When to Refer

- If bleeding is not controlled with first-line therapy.
- If expertise is needed for a surgical procedure.

► When to Admit

If bleeding is uncontrollable with first-line therapy or the patient is not hemodynamically stable.

Abbott JA. Adenomyosis and abnormal uterine bleeding (AUB-A)—pathogenesis, diagnosis, and management. Best Pract Res Clin Obstet Gynaecol. 2017 Apr;40:68–81. [PMID: 27810281]

Bacon JL. Abnormal uterine bleeding: current classification and clinical management. Obstet Gynecol Clin North Am. 2017 Jun; 44(2):179–93. [PMID: 28499529]

Bradley LD et al. The medical management of abnormal uterine bleeding in reproductive-aged women. Am J Obstet Gynecol. 2016 Jan;214(1):31–44. [PMID: 26254516]

Singh S et al. SOGC Clinical Practice Guideline No. 292. Abnormal uterine bleeding in pre-menopausal women. J Obstet Gynaecol Can. 2018 May;40(5):e391–415. [PMID: 29731212]

Wheeler KC et al. Transvaginal ultrasound for the diagnosis of abnormal uterine bleeding. Clin Obstet Gynecol. 2017 Mar; 60(1):11–7. [PMID: 28005589]

Whitaker L et al. Abnormal uterine bleeding. Best Pract Res Clin Obstet Gynaecol. 2016 Jul;34:54–65. [PMID: 26803558]

POSTMENOPAUSAL VAGINAL BLEEDING

ESSENTIALS OF DIAGNOSIS

- ► Vaginal bleeding that occurs 6 months or more following cessation of menstrual cycles.
- ► Postmenopausal bleeding of any amount always should be evaluated.
- ► Transvaginal ultrasound measurement of the endometrium is an important tool in evaluating the etiology of postmenopausal bleeding.

► General Considerations

The most common causes are endometrial atrophy, endometrial proliferation or hyperplasia, endometrial or cervical cancer, and administration of estrogens without or with added progestin. Other causes include atrophic vaginitis, trauma, endometrial polyps, friction ulcers of the cervix associated with prolapse of the uterus, and blood dyscrasias.

► Diagnosis

The vulva and vagina should be inspected for areas of bleeding, ulcers, or neoplasms. Cervical cytology should be obtained, if indicated. Transvaginal sonography should be used to measure endometrial thickness. An endometrial stripe measurement of 4 mm or less indicates a low likelihood of hyperplasia or endometrial cancer. If the endometrial thickness is greater than 4 mm or there is a heterogeneous appearance to the endometrium, endometrial sampling is indicated. Sonohysterography may be helpful in determining if the endometrial thickening is diffuse or focal. If the thickening is global, endometrial biopsy or D&C is appropriate. If focal, guided sampling with hysteroscopy should be done.

► Treatment

Simple endometrial hyperplasia calls for cyclic or continuous progestin therapy (medroxyprogesterone acetate, 10 mg/day orally, or norethindrone acetate, 5 mg/day orally) for 21 or 30 days of each month for 3 months. The use of a levonorgestrel intrauterine system is also a treatment option. Repeat sampling should be performed if symptoms recur. If endometrial hyperplasia with atypia or if carcinoma of the endometrium is found, hysterectomy is indicated.

► When to Refer

- Expertise in performing ultrasonography is required.
- Endometrial hyperplasia with atypia is present.
- Hysteroscopy is indicated.

Bar-On S et al. Is outpatient hysteroscopy accurate for the diagnosis of endometrial pathology among perimenopausal and postmenopausal women? Menopause. 2018 Feb;25(2):160–4. [PMID: 28763396]

Schramm A et al. Value of endometrial thickness assessed by transvaginal ultrasound for the prediction of endometrial cancer in patients with postmenopausal bleeding. Arch Gynecol Obstet. 2017 Aug;296(2):319–26. [PMID: 28634754]

Seckin B et al. Diagnostic value of sonography for detecting endometrial pathologies in postmenopausal women with and without bleeding. J Clin Ultrasound. 2016 Jul 8;44(6):339–46. [PMID: 26857098]

Turnbull HL et al. Investigating vaginal bleeding in postmenopausal women found to have an endometrial thickness of equal to or greater than 10 mm on ultrasonography. Arch Gynecol Obstet. 2017 Feb;295(2):445–50. [PMID: 27909879]

PREMENSTRUAL SYNDROME (Premenstrual Tension)

► General Considerations

The **premenstrual syndrome (PMS)** is a recurrent, variable cluster of troublesome physical and emotional symptoms that develop during the 5 days before the onset of menses and subside within 4 days after menstruation occurs. PMS intermittently affects about 40% of all premenopausal women, primarily those 25–40 years of age. In about 5–8% of affected women, the syndrome may be severe. Although not every woman experiences all the symptoms or signs at one time, many describe bloating, breast pain, ankle swelling, a sense of increased weight, skin disorders, irritability, aggressiveness, depression, inability to concentrate, libido change, lethargy, and food cravings. When emotional or mood symptoms predominate, along with physical symptoms, and there is a clear functional impairment with work or personal relationships, the term **"premenstrual dysphoric disorder" (PMDD)** may be applied. The pathogenesis of PMS/PMDD is still uncertain, and current treatment methods are mainly empiric. The clinician should provide support for both the patient's emotional and physical distress. This includes the following:

1. Careful evaluation of the patient, with understanding, explanation, and reassurance.
2. Advice to the patient to keep a daily diary of all symptoms for 2–3 months, such as the Daily Record of Severity of Problems, to evaluate the timing and characteristics of her symptoms. If her symptoms occur throughout the month rather than in the 2 weeks before menses, she may have depression or other mental health problems instead of or in addition to PMS.

▶ **Treatment**

For mild to moderate symptoms, a program of aerobic exercise; reduction of caffeine, salt, and alcohol intake; an increase in dietary calcium (to 1200 mg/day), vitamin D, or magnesium, and complex carbohydrates in the diet; and use of alternative therapies such as acupuncture and herbal treatments may be helpful, although these interventions remain unproven.

Medications that prevent ovulation, such as hormonal contraceptives, may lessen physical symptoms. These include continuous combined oral contraceptive pill or vaginal ring use; depot medroxyprogesterone acetate (DMPA), 150 mg intramuscularly every 3 months; etonogestrel subdermal (Nexplanon) progestin implant, every 3 years; high-dose progestin (eg, medroxyprogesterone acetate, 20–30 mg orally daily); or GnRH agonist with "add-back" therapy (eg, conjugated equine estrogen, 0.625 mg orally daily with medroxyprogesterone acetate, 2.5–5 mg orally daily).

When mood disorders predominate, several serotonin reuptake inhibitors have been shown to be effective in relieving tension, irritability, and dysphoria with few side effects. First-line medication therapy includes serotonergic antidepressants (citalopram, escitalopram, fluoxetine, sertraline, venlafaxine) either daily or only on symptom days. There are few data to support the use of calcium, vitamin D, and vitamin B_6 supplementation. There is insufficient evidence to support cognitive behavioral therapy.

Green-top Guideline No. 48. Management of premenstrual syndrome. BJOG. 2017 Feb;124(3):e73–105. [PMID: 27900828]

Naheed B et al. Non-contraceptive oestrogen-containing preparations for controlling symptoms of premenstrual syndrome. Cochrane Database Syst Rev. 2017 Mar 3;3:CD010503. [PMID: 28257559]

Yonkers KA et al. Premenstrual disorders. Am J Obstet Gynecol. 2018 Jan;218(1):68–74. [PMID: 28571724]

PELVIC PAIN

1. Primary Dysmenorrhea

Primary dysmenorrhea is menstrual pain associated with menstrual cycles in the absence of pathologic findings. Pain usually begins within 1–2 years after the menarche and may become progressively more severe. The frequency of cases increases up to age 20 and then decreases with both increasing age and parity. Fifty to 75% of women are affected by dysmenorrhea at some time and 5–6% have incapacitating pain.

▶ **Clinical Findings**

Primary dysmenorrhea is low, midline, wave-like, cramping pelvic pain often radiating to the back or inner thighs. Cramps may last for 1 or more days and may be associated with nausea, diarrhea, headache, and flushing. The pain is produced by uterine vasoconstriction, anoxia, and sustained contractions mediated by prostaglandins. The pelvic examination is normal between menses; examination during menses may produce discomfort, but there are no pathologic findings.

▶ **Treatment**

NSAIDs (ibuprofen, ketoprofen, mefenamic acid, naproxen) and the cyclooxygenase (COX)-2 inhibitor celecoxib are generally helpful. The medication should be started 1–2 days before expected menses. Symptoms can be suppressed with use of combined oral contraceptives, DMPA, etonogestrel subdermal (Nexplanon), or the LNG-IUD. Continuous use of oral contraceptives can be used to suppress menstruation completely and prevent dysmenorrhea. For women who do not wish to use hormonal contraception, other therapies that have shown at least some benefit include local heat; thiamine, 100 mg/day orally; vitamin E, 200 units/day orally from 2 days prior to and for the first 3 days of menses; and high-frequency transcutaneous electrical nerve stimulation.

2. Other Categories of Pelvic Pain

Unlike primary dysmenorrhea, other causes of pelvic pain may or may not be associated with the menstrual cycle but are more likely to be associated with pelvic pathology. Conditions such as endometriosis, adenomyosis, fibroids, pelvic inflammatory disease (PID), or other anatomic abnormalities of the pelvic organs, including the bowel or bladder, may present with symptoms during the menstrual cycle or with a more chronic nature.

▶ **Clinical Findings**

The history and physical examination may suggest endometriosis, adenomyosis, or fibroids. Other causes include

PID, submuchous myoma(s), IUD use, cervical stenosis with obstruction, or blind uterine horn (rare). Careful review of associated bowel or bladder symptoms should be done to exclude another pelvic organ source.

▶ Diagnosis

Pelvic imaging is useful for diagnosing the presence of uterine fibroids or other anomalies. Adenomyosis (the presence of islands of endometrial tissue in the myometrium) may be detected with ultrasound or MRI. Cervical stenosis may result from procedures done to the cervix, such as loop electrosurgical excision procedure (LEEP) or from an induced abortion. Such stenosis can create crampy pain at the time of expected menses with obstruction of blood flow. Laparoscopy may be used to diagnose endometriosis or other pelvic abnormalities not visualized by imaging.

▶ Treatment

A. Specific Measures

Combined estrogen and progestin and progestin-only hormonal contraceptives are first-line therapies in alleviating the symptoms of dysmenorrhea. Periodic use of analgesics, including the NSAIDs given for primary dysmenorrhea, may be beneficial, particularly in endometriosis. GnRH agonists are also an effective treatment of endometriosis, although their long-term use may be limited by cost or side effects. Adenomyosis may respond to the levonorgestrel-releasing intrauterine system, uterine artery embolization, or hormonal approaches used to treat endometriosis, but hysterectomy remains the definitive treatment of choice for women for whom childbearing is not a consideration. Cervical stenosis is easily cured by passing a sound into the uterine cavity after administering a paracervical block.

B. Surgical Measures

If disability is marked or prolonged, laparoscopy or exploratory laparotomy is usually warranted. Definitive surgery depends on the degree of disability and the findings at operation. Uterine fibroids may be removed or treated by uterine artery embolization. Hysterectomy may be done if other treatments have not worked but is usually a last resort.

▶ When to Refer

- Standard therapy fails to relieve pain.
- Suspicion of pelvic pathology, such as endometriosis, leiomyomas, or adenomyosis.

Ayorinde AA et al. Chronic pelvic pain in women of reproductive and post-reproductive age: a population-based study. Eur J Pain. 2017 Mar;21(3):445–55. [PMID: 27634190]

Bishop LA. Management of chronic pelvic pain. Clin Obstet Gynecol. 2017 Sep;60(3):524–30. [PMID: 28742584]

Brown J et al. Oral contraceptives for pain associated with endometriosis. Cochrane Database Syst Rev. 2018 May 22;5: CD001019. [PMID: 29786828]

Carey ET et al. Pharmacological management of chronic pelvic pain in women. Drugs. 2017 Mar;77(3):285–301. [PMID: 28074359]

Ferrero S et al. Current and emerging treatment options for endometriosis. Expert Opin Pharmacother. 2018 Jul;19(10): 1109–25. [PMID: 29975553]

Yosef A et al. Multifactorial contributors to the severity of chronic pelvic pain in women. Am J Obstet Gynecol. 2016 Dec; 215(6):760.e1–760. [PMID: 27443813]

VAGINITIS

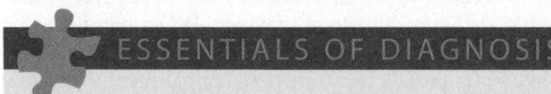

ESSENTIALS OF DIAGNOSIS

- ▶ Vaginal irritation.
- ▶ Pruritus.
- ▶ Abnormal or malodorous discharge.

▶ General Considerations

Inflammation and infection of the vagina are common gynecologic complaints, resulting from a variety of pathogens, allergic reactions to vaginal contraceptives or other products, vaginal atrophy, or friction during coitus. The normal vaginal pH is 4.5 or less, and *Lactobacillus* is the predominant organism. Normal secretions during the middle of the cycle, or during pregnancy, can be confused with vaginitis by concerned women.

▶ Clinical Findings

When the patient complains of vaginal irritation, pain, or unusual or malodorous discharge, a history should be taken, noting the onset of the LMP; recent sexual activity; use of contraceptives, tampons, or douches; recent changes in medications or use of antibiotics; and the presence of vaginal burning, pain, pruritus, or unusually profuse or malodorous discharge. The physical examination should include careful inspection of the vulva and speculum examination of the vagina and cervix. A vaginal, cervical, or urine sample can be obtained for detection of gonococcus and *Chlamydia,* if clinically indicated. A specimen of vaginal discharge is examined under the microscope in a drop of 0.9% saline solution to look for trichomonads or clue cells and in a drop of 10% potassium hydroxide to search for *Candida*. The vaginal pH should be tested; it is frequently greater than 4.5 in infections due to trichomonads and bacterial vaginosis. A bimanual examination to look for evidence of pelvic infection, namely cervical motion or adnexal tenderness, should follow. Point-of-care testing is available for all three main organisms that cause vaginitis and can be used if microscopy is not available or for confirmatory testing of microscopy.

A. Vulvovaginal Candidiasis

Pregnancy, diabetes, and use of broad-spectrum antibiotics or corticosteroids predispose patients to *Candida* infections. Heat, moisture, and occlusive clothing also contribute to the risk. Pruritus, vulvovaginal erythema, and a white curd-like discharge that is not malodorous are found (Figure 18–1). Microscopic examination with 10% potassium hydroxide

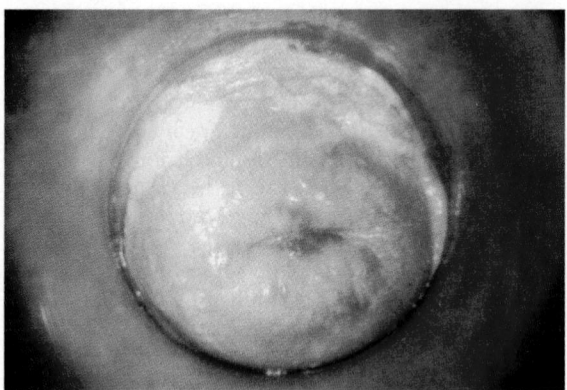

▲ Figure 18–1. Cervical candidiasis. (Public Health Image Library, CDC.)

reveals hyphae and spores. A swab for cultures with Nickerson medium or for PCR testing may be performed if *Candida* is suspected but not demonstrated.

B. *Trichomonas vaginalis* Vaginitis

This sexually transmitted protozoal flagellate infects the vagina, Skene ducts, and lower urinary tract in women and the lower genitourinary tract in men. Pruritus and a malodorous frothy, yellow-green discharge occur, along with diffuse vaginal erythema and red macular lesions on the cervix in severe cases ("**strawberry cervix**," Figure 18–2). Motile organisms with flagella are seen by microscopic examination of a wet mount with saline solution.

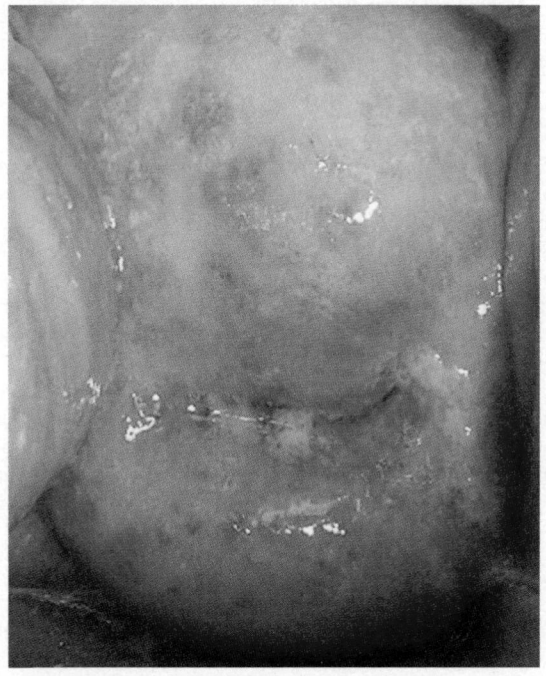

▲ Figure 18–2. Strawberry cervix in *Trichomonas vaginalis* infection, with inflammation and punctate hemorrhages. (Used, with permission, from Richard P. Usatine, MD.)

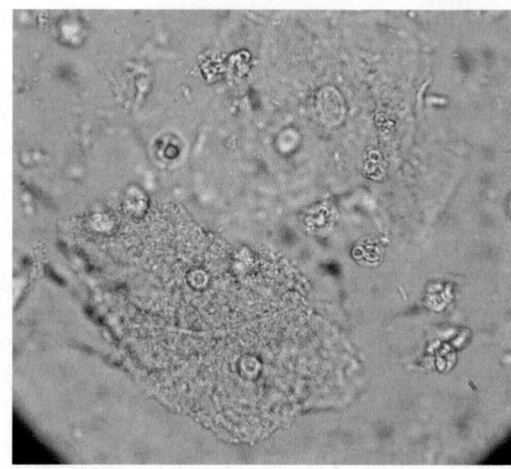

▲ Figure 18–3. Clue cells seen in bacterial vaginosis due to *Gardnerella vaginalis*. (Reproduced, with permission, from Richard P. Usatine, MD.)

C. Bacterial Vaginosis

This condition is a polymicrobial disease that is *not* sexually transmitted. An overgrowth of *Gardnerella* and other anaerobes is often associated with increased malodorous discharge without obvious vulvitis or vaginitis. The discharge is grayish and sometimes frothy, with a pH of 5.0–5.5. An amine-like ("fishy") odor is present if a drop of discharge is alkalinized with 10% potassium hydroxide. On wet mount in saline, epithelial cells are covered with bacteria to such an extent that cell borders are obscured (**clue cells**, Figure 18–3). Vaginal cultures are generally not useful in diagnosis; however, PCR testing is available.

▶ Treatment

A. Vulvovaginal Candidiasis

A variety of topical and oral regimens are available to treat vulvovaginal candidiasis. Women with uncomplicated vulvovaginal candidiasis will usually respond to a 1- to 3-day regimen of a topical azole or a one-time dose of oral fluconazole. Women with complicated infection (including four or more episodes in 1 year [*recurrent* vulvovaginal candidiasis], severe signs and symptoms, non-albicans species, uncontrolled diabetes, HIV infection, corticosteroid treatment, or pregnancy) should receive 7–14 days of a topical regimen or two doses of oral fluconazole 3 days apart. In recurrent non-albicans infections, 600 mg of boric acid in a gelatin capsule intravaginally once daily for 2 weeks is approximately 70% effective. If recurrence occurs, referral to a gynecologist or an infectious disease specialist is indicated.

1. Single-dose regimens—Effective single-dose regimens include miconazole (1200-mg vaginal suppository), tioconazole (6.5% cream, 5 g vaginally), sustained-release butoconazole (2% cream, 5 g vaginally), or fluconazole (150-mg oral tablet).

2. Three-day regimens—Effective 3-day regimens include butoconazole (2% cream, 5 g vaginally once daily), clotrimazole (2% cream, 5 g vaginally once daily), terconazole

(0.8% cream, 5 g, or 80-mg vaginal suppository once daily), or miconazole (200-mg vaginal suppository once daily).

3. Seven-day regimens—The following regimens are given once daily: clotrimazole (1% cream), miconazole (2% cream, 5 g, or 100-mg vaginal suppository), or terconazole (0.4% cream, 5 g).

4. Fourteen-day regimen—An effective 14-day regimen is nystatin (100,000-unit vaginal tablet once daily).

5. Recurrent vulvovaginal candidiasis (maintenance therapy)—Clotrimazole (500-mg vaginal suppository once weekly or 200 mg cream twice weekly) or fluconazole (100, 150, or 200 mg orally once weekly) are effective regimens for maintenance therapy for up to 6 months.

B. *Trichomonas vaginalis* Vaginitis

Treatment of both partners simultaneously is recommended; metronidazole or tinidazole, 2 g orally as a single dose or 500 mg orally twice a day for 7 days, is usually used.

In the case of treatment failure with metronidazole in the absence of reexposure, the patient should be re-treated with metronidazole, 500 mg orally twice a day for 7 days, or tinidazole, 2 g orally as a single dose. If treatment failure occurs again, give metronidazole or tinidazole, 2 g orally once daily for 5 days. If this is not effective in eradicating the organisms, metronidazole and tinidazole susceptibility testing can be arranged with the Centers for Disease Control and Prevention (CDC) at 404-718-4141 or at https://www.cdc.gov/std. Women infected with *T vaginalis* are at increased risk for concurrent infection with other sexually transmitted diseases (STDs) and should be offered comprehensive STD testing.

C. Bacterial Vaginosis

The recommended regimens are metronidazole (500 mg orally, twice daily for 7 days), clindamycin vaginal cream (2%, 5 g, once daily for 7 days), or metronidazole gel (0.75%, 5 g, twice daily for 5 days). Alternative regimens include clindamycin (300 mg orally twice daily for 7 days), clindamycin ovules (100 g intravaginally at bedtime for 3 days), tinidazole (2 g orally once daily for 3 days), or tinidazole (1 g orally once daily for 7 days). The National STD Curriculum offers a helpful training module to clinicians to review current recommendations for treatment of vaginitis (https://www.std.uw.edu/custom/self-study/vaginitis).

CONDYLOMA ACUMINATA

Warty growths on the vulva, perianal area, vaginal walls, or cervix are caused by various types of the human papillomavirus (HPV). Pregnancy and immunosuppression favor growth. Ninety percent of genital warts are caused by HPV 6 and 11. With increasing use of a quadrivalent HPV vaccine in the United States, the prevalence of HPV types 6, 11, 16 and 18 decreased from 11.5% in 2003–2006 to 4.3% in 2009–2012 among girls aged 14–19 years, and from 18.5% to 12.1% in women aged 20–24 years. Vulvar lesions may be obviously wart-like or may be diagnosed only after application of 4%

acetic acid (vinegar) and colposcopy, when they appear whitish, with prominent papillae. Vaginal lesions may show diffuse hypertrophy or a cobblestone appearance.

Recommended treatments for vulvar warts include podophyllum resin 10–25% in tincture of benzoin (do not use during pregnancy or on bleeding lesions) or 80–90% trichloroacetic or bichloroacetic acid, carefully applied to avoid the surrounding skin. The pain of bichloroacetic or trichloroacetic acid application can be lessened by a sodium bicarbonate paste applied immediately after treatment. Podophyllum resin must be washed off after 2–4 hours. Freezing with liquid nitrogen or a cryoprobe and electrocautery are also effective. Patient-applied regimens, useful when the entire lesion is accessible to the patient, include podofilox 0.5% solution or gel, imiquimod 5% cream, or sinecatechins 15% ointment. Vaginal warts may be treated with cryotherapy with liquid nitrogen or trichloroacetic acid. Extensive warts may require treatment with CO_2 laser, electrocautery, or excision under local or general anesthesia.

Grennan D. JAMA patient page. Genital warts. JAMA. 2018 Feb 5; 321(5):520. [PMID: 30721297]

Mills BB. Vaginitis: beyond the basics. Obstet Gynecol Clin North Am. 2017 Jun;44(2):159–77. [PMID: 28499528]

Sobel JD. Recurrent vulvovaginal candidiasis. Am J Obstet Gynecol. 2016 Jan;214(1):15–21. [PMID: 26164695]

Van Der Pol B. Clinical and laboratory testing for *Trichomonas vaginalis* infection. J Clin Microbiol. 2016 Jan;54(1):7–12. [PMID: 26491181]

Workowski KA et al; Centers for Disease Control and Prevention. Sexually transmitted diseases treatment guidelines, 2015. MMWR Recomm Rep. 2015 Jun 5;64(RR-03):1–137. Erratum: MMWR Recomm Rep. 2015 Aug 28;64(RR-03):924. [PMID: 26042815] https://www.cdc.gov/mmwr/preview/mmwrhtml/rr6403a1.htm

CERVICAL POLYPS

Cervical polyps commonly occur after menarche and are occasionally noted in postmenopausal women. The cause is not known, but inflammation may play an etiologic role. The principal symptoms are discharge and abnormal vaginal bleeding. However, abnormal bleeding should not be ascribed to a cervical polyp without sampling the endocervix and endometrium. The polyps are visible in the cervical os on speculum examination.

Cervical polyps must be differentiated from polypoid neoplastic disease of the endometrium, small submucous pedunculated myomas, large nabothian cysts, and endometrial polyps. Cervical polyps rarely contain dysplasia (0.5%) or malignant (0.5%) foci. Asymptomatic polyps in women under age 45 may be left untreated.

▶ Treatment

Cervical polyps can generally be removed in the office by avulsion with uterine packing forceps or ring forceps.

Levy RA et al. Cervical polyps: is histologic evaluation necessary? Pathol Res Pract. 2016 Sep;212(9):800–3. [PMID: 27465834]

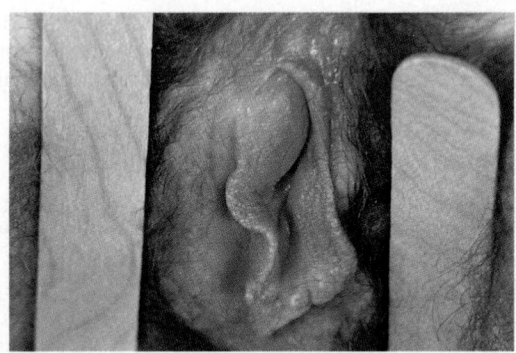

▲ **Figure 18–4.** Right-sided Bartholin cyst (abscess). The Bartholin gland is located in the lower two-thirds of the introitus. (From Susan Lindsley, Public Health Image Library, CDC.)

BARTHOLIN DUCT CYSTS & ABSCESSES

Trauma or infection may involve the Bartholin duct, causing obstruction of the gland. Drainage of secretions is prevented, leading to pain, swelling, and abscess formation (Figure 18–4). The infection usually resolves and pain disappears, but stenosis of the duct outlet with distention often persists. Reinfection causes recurrent tenderness and further enlargement of the duct.

The principal symptoms are periodic painful swelling on either side of the introitus and dyspareunia. A fluctuant swelling 1–4 cm in diameter lateral to either labium minus is a sign of occlusion of Bartholin duct. Tenderness is evidence of active infection.

Pus or secretions from the gland should be cultured for *Chlamydia* and other pathogens and treated accordingly (see Chapter 33); frequent warm soaks may be helpful. If an abscess develops, aspiration or incision and drainage are the simplest forms of therapy, but the problem may recur. Marsupialization (in the absence of an abscess), incision, and drainage with the insertion of an indwelling Word catheter, or laser treatment will establish a new duct opening. Antibiotics are unnecessary unless cellulitis is present. In women under 40 years of age, asymptomatic cysts do not require therapy; in women over age 40, biopsy or removal are recommended to rule out vulvar carcinoma.

► When to Refer

Surgical therapy (marsupialization) is indicated.

CERVICAL INTRAEPITHELIAL NEOPLASIA (CIN) (Dysplasia of the Cervix)

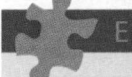 ESSENTIALS OF DIAGNOSIS

► The presumptive diagnosis is made by an abnormal Papanicolaou smear of an asymptomatic woman with no grossly visible cervical changes.

► Diagnose by colposcopically directed biopsy.

Table 18–2. Classification systems for Papanicolaou smears.

Numerical	Dysplasia	CIN	Bethesda System
1	Benign	Benign	Normal
2	Benign with inflammation	Benign with inflammation	Normal, ASC-US
3	Mild dysplasia	CIN I	Low-grade SIL
3	Moderate dysplasia	CIN II	High-grade SIL
3	Severe dysplasia	CIN III	
4	Carcinoma in situ		
5	Invasive cancer	Invasive cancer	Invasive cancer

ASC-US, atypical squamous cells of undetermined significance; CIN, cervical intraepithelial neoplasia; SIL, squamous intraepithelial lesion.

► General Considerations

The squamocolumnar junction of the cervix is an area of active squamous cell proliferation. In childhood, this junction is located on the exposed vaginal portion of the cervix. At puberty, because of hormonal influence and possibly because of changes in the vaginal pH, the squamous margin begins to encroach on the single-layered, mucus-secreting epithelium, creating an area of metaplasia (**transformation zone**). Infection with HPV (see Prevention, below) may lead to cellular abnormalities, which over a period of time develop into squamous cell dysplasia or cancer. There are varying degrees of dysplasia (Table 18–2), defined by the degree of cellular atypia; all atypia must be observed and treated if persistent or worsening.

► Clinical Findings

There are no specific symptoms or signs of CIN. The presumptive diagnosis is made by cytologic screening of an asymptomatic population with no grossly visible cervical changes. All visible abnormal cervical lesions should be biopsied (Figure 18–5).

► Screening & Diagnosis

A. Cytologic Examination (Papanicolaou Smear)

In immunocompetent women, cervical cancer screening should begin at age 21. The recommendation to start screening at age 21 years regardless of the age of onset of sexual intercourse is based on the very low incidence of cancer in younger women and the potential for adverse effects associated with treatment of young women with abnormal cytology screening results. In contrast to the high rate of infection with HPV in sexually active adolescents, invasive cervical cancer is very rare in women younger than age 21 years. The US Preventive Services

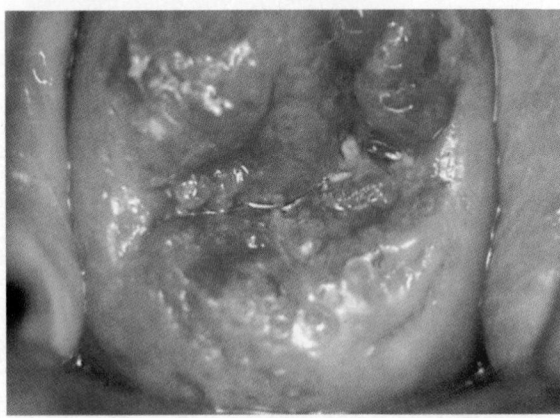

▲ **Figure 18–5.** Erosion of the cervix due to cervical intraepithelial neoplasia (CIN), a precursor lesion to cervical cancer. (Public Health Image Library, CDC.)

Task Force (USPSTF) 2018 statement recommends screening for cervical cancer in women aged 21 to 65 years as follows: for women aged 21 to 29 years, screening with cytology (conventional [Papanicolaou smear] or liquid based) alone every 3 years; and for women aged 30 to 65 years, screening with cytology alone every 3 years, with high-risk human papillomavirus (hrHPV) testing alone every 5 years, or with a combination of cytology and hrHPV testing (cotesting) every 5 years. These recommendations apply to women who have a cervix, regardless of their sexual history or HPV vaccination status. They do not apply to women who have previously been diagnosed with cervical cancer or a high-grade precancerous cervical lesion (ie, CIN grade II or III) or to women with immune compromise (eg, living with HIV) or with in utero exposure to diethylstilbestrol; such women may require more frequent screening.

The USPSTF recommends against screening for cervical cancer for women younger than age 21 years, for women older than age 65 years who have had adequate prior screening and are not otherwise at high risk for cervical cancer, and for women who have had a hysterectomy with removal of the cervix and who have no history of cervical cancer or a high-grade precancerous lesion.

The goal of screening is to identify high-grade precancerous cervical lesions to prevent their progression to cervical cancer. These high-grade cervical lesions may be treated with excisional and ablative therapies (see below). Early-stage cervical cancer may be treated with surgery (hysterectomy) or chemotherapy (see next section). Online guidelines are available for the management of abnormal screening test results at http://www.asccp.org/asccp-guidelines and https://www.uspreventiveservicestaskforce.org/Page/Document/RecommendationStatementFinal/cervical-cancer-screening2.

Cytologic reports from the laboratory may describe findings in one of several ways (see Table 18–2). The Bethesda System uses the terminology "atypical squamous cells of unknown significance" (**ASC-US**) and "squamous intraepithelial lesions," either low-grade (**LSIL**) or high-grade (**HSIL**). HPV DNA testing can be used as an adjunct in cervical cancer screening as a triage test to stratify risk in women age 21 years and older with a cytologic diagnosis of ASC-US and in postmenopausal women with a cytologic diagnosis of ASC-US or LSIL.

B. Colposcopy

Women with ASC-US and a negative HPV screening may be followed up in 1 year for a repeat Pap smear and HPV co-testing. If the HPV screen is positive, colposcopy is indicated. If HPV screening is unavailable, repeat cytology may be done at 12 months. All patients with SIL or atypical glandular cells should undergo colposcopy. Viewing the cervix with 10–20 × magnification allows for assessment of the size and margins of an abnormal transformation zone and determination of extension into the endocervical canal. The application of 3–5% acetic acid (vinegar) dissolves mucus, and the acid's desiccating action sharpens the contrast between normal and actively proliferating squamous epithelium. Abnormal changes include white patches and vascular atypia, which indicate areas of greatest cellular activity.

C. Biopsy

Colposcopically directed punch biopsy and endocervical curettage are office procedures. Data from both cervical biopsy and endocervical curettage are important in deciding on treatment.

▶ Prevention

Cervical infection with the HPV is associated with a high percentage of all cervical dysplasias and cancers. There are over 70 recognized HPV subtypes. Types 6 and 11 tend to cause genital warts and mild dysplasia and rarely progress to cervical cancer; types 16, 18, 31, and others cause higher-grade dysplasia. The HPV 9-valent (Gardasil-9) recombinant vaccine (9vHPV) is indicated for the prevention of cervical, vaginal, and vulvar cancers (in women) and anal cancers (in women and men) caused by HPV types 16, 18, 31, 33, 45, 52, and 58; genital warts (in women and men) caused by HPV types 6 and 11; and precancerous/dysplastic lesions of cervix, vagina, vulva (in women), and anus (in women and men) caused by HPV types 6, 11, 16, 18, 31, 33, 45, 52, and 58. Gardasil-9 is recommended for vaccination of females and males ages 9-45 years old. The earlier HPV 4-valent vaccine known as Gardasil that was indicated for prevention of diseases related to HPV types 6, 11, 16, and 18 has been discontinued in the United States. The use of HPV vaccination in the United States continues to increase. During 2016–2017, coverage increased for greater than or equal to 1 dose of HPV vaccine (from 60.4% to 65.5%). In 2017, 48.6% of adolescents were up to date with the three-dose HPV vaccine series compared with 43.4% in 2016.

Because complete coverage of all carcinogenic HPV types is not provided by either vaccine, all women need to have regular cervical cancer screening as outlined above. In addition to vaccination, preventive measures include limiting the number of sexual partners and thus exposure to HPV, using a diaphragm or condom for coitus, and smoking cessation and avoiding exposure to secondhand smoke.

Treatment

Treatment varies depending on the degree and extent of CIN. Biopsies should precede treatment, except in cases of HSIL where it may be appropriate to proceed directly to a LEEP.

A. Cryosurgery

The use of freezing (cryosurgery) is effective for noninvasive small lesions visible on the cervix without endocervical extension.

B. CO$_2$ Laser

This well-controlled method minimizes tissue destruction. It is colposcopically directed and requires special training. It may be used with large visible lesions. In current practice, it involves the vaporization of the transformation zone on the cervix and the distal 5–7 mm of endocervical canal.

C. Loop Excision

When the CIN is clearly visible in its entirety, a wire loop can be used for excisional biopsy. This office procedure, called **LEEP (loop electrosurgical excision procedure)**, done with local anesthesia is quick and uncomplicated. Cutting and hemostasis are achieved with a low-voltage electrosurgical machine.

D. Conization of the Cervix

Conization is surgical removal of the entire transformation zone and endocervical canal. It should be reserved for cases of severe dysplasia (CIN III) or carcinoma in situ, particularly those with endocervical extension. The procedure can be performed with scalpel, CO$_2$ laser, needle electrode, or large-loop excision.

Follow-Up

Because recurrence is possible—especially in the first 2 years after treatment—and because the false-negative rate of a single cervical cytologic test is 20%, close follow-up after colposcopy and biopsy is imperative. For CIN II or III, cytologic examination or cytology and colposcopy should be repeated at 12-month intervals for 2 years. If CIN II or III is identified at the margins of an endocervical curettage procedure, however, repeat cytology with endocervical curettage is instead recommended at 4–6 months. For CIN I, cytology should be performed at 12 months or HPV DNA testing can be done at 12 months. If testing is normal, routine cytologic screening can be resumed unless there is a discrepancy between the cytology and the endocervical curettage pathology (eg, HSIL on a Pap test and negative pathology on endocervical curettage), in which case cytology and HPV DNA co-testing at 12 and 14 months, an excisional diagnostic procedure, and a review of the cytology and pathology findings is indicated.

The American Society for Colposcopy and Cervical Pathology Guidelines for cervical cancer screening and management of abnormal Papanicolaou smears are available online (http://www.asccp.org/asccp-guidelines).

When to Refer

- Patients with CIN II/III should be referred to an experienced colposcopist.
- Patients requiring conization biopsy should be referred to a gynecologist.

Arbyn M et al. Prophylactic vaccination against human papillomaviruses to prevent cervical cancer and its precursors. Cochrane Database Syst Rev. 2018 May 9;5:CD009069. [PMID: 29740819]

Castle PE et al. Treatment of cervical intraepithelial lesions. Int J Gynaecol Obstet. 2017 Jul;138(Suppl 1):20–5. [PMID: 28691333]

Harper DM et al. HPV vaccines—a review of the first decade. Gynecol Oncol. 2017 Jul;146(1):196–204. [PMID: 28442134]

Melnikow J et al. Screening for cervical cancer with high-risk human papillomavirus testing: updated evidence report and systematic review for the US Preventive Services Task Force. JAMA. 2018 Aug 21;320(7):687–705. [PMID: 30140883]

Smith RA et al. Cancer screening in the United States, 2017: a review of current American Cancer Society guidelines and current issues in cancer screening. CA Cancer J Clin. 2017 Mar;67(2):100–21. [PMID: 28170086]

Ogilvie GS et al. Effect of screening with primary cervical HPV testing vs cytology testing on high-grade cervical intraepithelial neoplasia at 48 months: the HPV FOCAL randomized clinical trial. JAMA. 2018 Jul 3;320(1):43–52. [PMID: 29971397]

US Preventive Services Task Force; Curry SJ et al. Screening for cervical cancer: US Preventive Services Task Force Recommendation Statement. JAMA. 2018 Aug 21;320(7):674–86. [PMID: 30140884]

Vegunta S et al. Screening women at high risk for cervical cancer: special groups of women who require more frequent screening. Mayo Clin Proc. 2017 Aug;92(8):1272–7. [PMID: 28778260]

CARCINOMA OF THE CERVIX

ESSENTIALS OF DIAGNOSIS

- ► Increased risk in women who smoke and those with HIV or high-risk HPV types.
- ► Gross lesions should be evaluated by colposcopically directed biopsies and not cytology alone.

General Considerations

Cervical cancer is the third most common cancer in the world and the leading cause of cancer death among women in developing countries. It is considered a sexually transmitted disease as both squamous cell and adenocarcinoma of the cervix are secondary to infection with HPV, primarily types 16 and 18. Women infected with HIV are at an increased risk for high-risk HPV infection and CIN. Smoking and possibly dietary factors such as decreased circulating vitamin A appear to be cofactors. Squamous cell carcinoma (SCC) accounts for approximately 80% of cervical cancers, while adenocarcinoma accounts for 15% and adenosquamous carcinoma for 3–5%; neuroendocrine or small cell carcinomas are rare.

SCC appears first in the intraepithelial layers (the pre-invasive stage, or carcinoma in situ). Preinvasive cancer (CIN III) is a common diagnosis in women 25–40 years of age. Two to 10 years are required for carcinoma to penetrate the basement membrane and become invasive. While cervical cancer mortality has declined steadily in the United States due to high rates of screening and improved treatment, the rate of decline has slowed in recent years. In general, black women experienced much higher incidence and mortality than white women. The 5-year survival rate ranges from 63% for stage II cervical cancer to less than 20% for stage IV.

Clinical Findings

A. Symptoms and Signs

The most common signs are metrorrhagia, postcoital spotting, and cervical ulceration. Bladder and rectal dysfunction or fistulas and pain are late symptoms.

B. Cervical Biopsy and Endocervical Curettage or Conization

These procedures are necessary steps after a positive Papanicolaou smear to determine the extent and depth of invasion of the cancer. Even if the smear is positive, treatment with additional surgery or radiation is never justified until definitive diagnosis has been established through biopsy.

C. "Staging" or Estimate of Gross Spread of Cancer of the Cervix

Staging of invasive cervical cancer is achieved by clinical evaluation, usually conducted under anesthesia. Further examinations, such as ultrasonography, CT, MRI, lymphangiography, laparoscopy, and fine-needle aspiration, are valuable for treatment planning.

Complications

Metastases to regional lymph nodes occur with increasing frequency from stage I to stage IV. Paracervical extension occurs in all directions from the cervix. The ureters may become obstructed lateral to the cervix, causing hydroureter and hydronephrosis and consequently impaired kidney function. Almost two-thirds of patients with untreated carcinoma of the cervix die of uremia when ureteral obstruction is bilateral. Pain in the back, in the distribution of the lumbosacral plexus, is often indicative of neurologic involvement. Gross edema of the legs may be indicative of vascular and lymphatic stasis due to tumor. Vaginal fistulas to the rectum and urinary tract are severe late complications. Hemorrhage is the cause of death in 10–20% of patients with extensive invasive carcinoma.

Prevention

Vaccination with the recombinant 9-valent HPV vaccines (Gardasil-9) can prevent cervical cancer by targeting the HPV types that pose the greatest risk as well as protect against low-grade and precancerous lesions caused by other HPV types (see Cervical Intraepithelial Neoplasia).

Treatment

A. Emergency Measures

Vaginal hemorrhage originates from gross ulceration and cavitation in later stage cervical carcinoma. Ligation and suturing of the cervix are usually not feasible, but emergent vaginal packing, cautery, tranexamic acid, and irradiation are helpful to stop bleeding temporarily. Ligation, resection, or embolization of the uterine or hypogastric arteries may be lifesaving when other measures fail.

B. Specific Measures

1. Carcinoma in situ (stage 0)—In women for whom childbearing is not a consideration, total hysterectomy is the definitive treatment. In women who wish to retain the uterus, acceptable alternatives include cryosurgery, laser surgery, LEEP, or cervical conization. Close follow-up with Papanicolaou smears every 3 months for 1 year and every 6 months for another year is necessary after cryotherapy or laser.

2. Invasive carcinoma—Microinvasive carcinoma (stage IA1) is treated with simple, extrafascial hysterectomy. Stages IA2, IB1, and IIA cancers may be treated with either radical hysterectomy with concomitant radiation and chemotherapy or with radiation plus chemotherapy alone. Women with stage IB1 may be candidates for fertility-sparing surgery that includes radical trachelectomy and lymph node dissection with preservation of the uterus and ovaries. Stages IB2, IIB, III, and IV cancers are treated with radiation therapy plus concurrent chemotherapy.

Prognosis

The overall 5-year relative survival rate for carcinoma of the cervix is 68% in white women and 55% in black women in the United States. Survival rates are inversely proportionate to the stage of cancer: stage 0, 99–100%; stage IA, more than 95%; stage IB–IIA, 80–90%; stage IIB, 65%; stage III, 40%; and stage IV, less than 20%.

When to Refer

All patients with invasive cervical carcinoma (stage IA or higher) should be referred to a gynecologic oncologist.

American Cancer Society. Survival rates for cervical cancer, by stage, February 5, 2019. https://www.cancer.org/cancer/cervical-cancer/detection-diagnosis-staging/survival.html

Li H et al. Advances in diagnosis and treatment of metastatic cervical cancer. J Gynecol Oncol. 2016 Jul;27(4):e43. [PMID: 27171673]

Tsikouras P et al. Cervical cancer: screening, diagnosis and staging. J BUON. 2016 Mar–Apr;21(2):320–5. [PMID: 27273940]

US Preventive Services Task Force; Curry SJ et al. Screening for cervical cancer: US Preventive Services Task Force Recommendation Statement. JAMA. 2018 Aug 21;320(7):674–86. [PMID: 30140884]

Van Dyne EA et al. Trends in human papillomavirus-associated cancers—United States, 1999–2015. MMWR Morb Mortal Wkly Rep. 2018 Aug 24;67(33):918–24. [PMID: 30138307]

Verma J et al. New strategies for multimodality therapy in treating locally advanced cervix cancer. Semin Radiat Oncol. 2016 Oct;26(4):344–8. [PMID: 27619255]

LEIOMYOMA OF THE UTERUS
(Fibroid Tumor)

ESSENTIALS OF DIAGNOSIS

- ▶ Irregular enlargement of the uterus (may be asymptomatic).
- ▶ Heavy or irregular vaginal bleeding, dysmenorrhea.
- ▶ Pelvic pain and pressure.

▶ General Considerations

Uterine leiomyoma is the most common benign neoplasm of the female genital tract. It is a discrete, round, firm, often multiple uterine tumor composed of smooth muscle and connective tissue. The most convenient classification is by anatomic location: (1) intramural, (2) submucous, (3) subserous, (4) intraligamentous, (5) parasitic (ie, deriving its blood supply from an organ to which it becomes attached), and (6) cervical. Submucous myomas may become pedunculated and descend through the cervix into the vagina.

▶ Clinical Findings

A. Symptoms and Signs

In nonpregnant women, myomas are frequently asymptomatic. The two most common symptoms of uterine leiomyomas for which women seek treatment are AUB and pelvic pain or pressure. Occasionally, degeneration occurs, causing intense pain. The risk of miscarriage is increased if the myoma significantly distorts the uterine cavity and interferes with implantation. Fibroids rarely cause infertility by leading to bilateral tubal blockage; they more commonly cause miscarriage and pregnancy complications such as preterm labor, preterm delivery, and malpresentation.

B. Laboratory Findings

Iron deficiency anemia may result from blood loss.

C. Imaging

Ultrasonography will confirm the presence of uterine myomas and can be used sequentially to monitor growth. When multiple subserous or pedunculated myomas are being followed, ultrasonography is important to exclude ovarian masses. MRI can delineate intramural and submucous myomas accurately and is necessary prior to uterine artery embolization to assess blood flow to the fibroids. Hysterography or hysteroscopy can also confirm cervical or submucous myomas.

▶ Differential Diagnosis

Irregular myomatous enlargement of the uterus must be differentiated from the similar, but symmetric enlargement that may occur with pregnancy or adenomyosis. Subserous myomas must be distinguished from ovarian tumors.

Leiomyosarcoma is an unusual tumor occurring in 0.5% of women operated on for symptomatic myoma. It is very rare under the age of 40 and increases in incidence thereafter.

▶ Treatment

A. Emergency Measures

Emergency surgery may be required for acute torsion of a pedunculated myoma. If the patient is markedly anemic as a result of long, heavy menstrual periods, preoperative treatment with DMPA, 150 mg intramuscularly every 3 months, or use of a GnRH agonist, such as depot leuprolide, 3.75 mg intramuscularly monthly, will slow or stop bleeding, and medical treatment of anemia can be given prior to surgery. Levonorgestrel-containing IUDs have also been used to decrease the bleeding associated with fibroids; however, IUD placement can be more technically challenging in patients with fibroids.

B. Specific Measures

Women who have small asymptomatic myomas can be managed expectantly and evaluated annually. In patients wishing to defer surgical management, nonhormonal therapies (such as NSAIDs and tranexamic acid) have been shown to decrease menstrual blood loss. Hormonal therapies such as GnRH agonists and selective progesterone receptor modulators (SPRMs) such as low-dose mifepristone (5–10 mg/day) have been shown to reduce myoma volume, uterine size, and menstrual blood loss. Surgical intervention is based on the patient's symptoms and desire for future fertility. Uterine size alone is not an indication for surgery. Cervical myomas larger than 3–4 cm in diameter or pedunculated myomas that protrude through the cervix can cause bleeding, infection, degeneration, pain, or urinary retention and often require removal. Submucous myomas can be removed by hysteroscopic resection.

Because the risk of surgical complications increases with the increasing size of the myoma, preoperative reduction of myoma size is sometimes desirable prior to hysterectomy. GnRH analogs such as depot leuprolide, 3.75 mg intramuscularly monthly, can be used preoperatively for 3- to 4-month periods to induce reversible hypogonadism, to temporarily reduce the size of myomas, and reduce surrounding vascularity.

C. Surgical Measures

A variety of surgical measures are available for the treatment of myomas: myomectomy (hysteroscopic, laparoscopic, or abdominal) and hysterectomy (vaginal, laparoscopy-assisted vaginal, laparoscopic, abdominal, or robotic). Myomectomy is the treatment of choice for women who wish to preserve fertility. Uterine artery embolization is a minimally invasive treatment for uterine fibroids. In uterine artery embolization, the goal is to block the blood vessels supplying the fibroids, causing them to shrink. Magnetic resonance–guided high-intensity focused ultrasound, myolysis/radiofrequency ablation, and laparoscopic or vaginal occlusion of uterine vessels are newer interventions, with a smaller body of evidence.

Prognosis

Surgical therapy is curative. In women desiring future fertility, myomectomy can be offered, but patients should be counseled that recurrence is common, postoperative pelvic adhesions may impact fertility, and cesarean delivery may be necessary secondary to interruption of the myometrium.

When to Refer

Refer to a gynecologist for treatment of symptomatic leiomyomata.

When to Admit

For acute abdomen associated with an infarcted leiomyoma or hemorrhage not controlled by outpatient measures.

Donnez J et al. The current place of medical therapy in uterine fibroid management. Best Pract Res Clin Obstet Gynaecol. 2018 Jan;46:57–65. [PMID: 29169896]

Havryliuk Y et al. Symptomatic fibroid management: systematic review of the literature. JSLS. 2017 Jul–Sep;21(3). [PMID: 28951653]

Laughlin-Tommaso SK. Alternatives to hysterectomy: management of uterine fibroids. Obstet Gynecol Clin North Am. 2016 Sep;43(3):397–413. [PMID: 27521875]

Murji A et al. Selective progesterone receptor modulators (SPRMs) for uterine fibroids. Cochrane Database Syst Rev. 2017 Apr 26;4:CD010770. [PMID: 28444736]

CARCINOMA OF THE ENDOMETRIUM

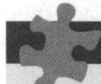

ESSENTIALS OF DIAGNOSIS

- ► Abnormal bleeding is the presenting sign in 90% of cases.
- ► Papanicolaou smear is frequently negative.
- ► After a negative pregnancy test, endometrial tissue is required to confirm the diagnosis.

General Considerations

Adenocarcinoma of the endometrium is the second most common cancer of the female genital tract. It occurs most often in women 50–70 years of age. Obesity, nulliparity, diabetes, polycystic ovaries with prolonged anovulation, unopposed estrogen therapy, and the extended use of tamoxifen for the treatment of breast cancer are also risk factors. Women with a family history of colon cancer (hereditary nonpolyposis colorectal cancer, Lynch syndrome) are at significantly increased risk, with a lifetime incidence as high as 30%.

Abnormal bleeding is the presenting sign in 90% of cases. Any postmenopausal bleeding requires investigation. Pain generally occurs late in the disease, with metastases or infection.

Papanicolaou smears of the cervix occasionally show atypical endometrial cells but are an insensitive diagnostic tool. Endocervical and endometrial sampling is the only reliable means of diagnosis. Simultaneous hysteroscopy can be a valuable addition in order to localize polyps or other lesions within the uterine cavity. Vaginal ultrasonography may be used to determine the thickness of the endometrium as an indication of hypertrophy and possible neoplastic change. The finding of a thin endometrial lining on ultrasound is clinically reassuring in cases where very little tissue is obtainable through endometrial biopsy.

Pathologic assessment is important in differentiating hyperplasias, which often can be treated with cyclic oral progestins.

Prevention

Prompt endometrial sampling for patients who report abnormal menstrual bleeding or postmenopausal uterine bleeding will reveal many incipient as well as clinical cases of endometrial cancer. Younger women with chronic anovulation are at risk for endometrial hyperplasia and subsequent endometrial cancer; they can significantly reduce the risk of hyperplasia with the use of oral contraceptives or cyclic progestin therapy.

Staging

Staging and prognosis are based on surgical and pathologic evaluation only. Examination under anesthesia, endometrial and endocervical sampling, chest radiography, intravenous urography, cystoscopy, sigmoidoscopy, transvaginal sonography, and MRI will help determine the extent of the disease and its appropriate treatment.

Treatment

Treatment consists of total hysterectomy and bilateral salpingo-oophorectomy. Peritoneal washings for cytologic examination are routinely taken and lymph node sampling may be done. If invasion deep into the myometrium has occurred or if sampled lymph nodes are positive for tumor, postoperative irradiation is indicated. Patients with stage III endometrial cancer are generally treated with surgery followed by chemotherapy and/or radiation therapy. A review by the Society of Gynecologic Oncology Clinical Practice Committee concluded "the use of adjuvant chemotherapy to treat stage I or II endometrial carcinoma is not supported by the available evidence." Palliation of advanced or metastatic endometrial adenocarcinoma may be accomplished with large doses of progestins, eg, medroxyprogesterone, 400 mg weekly intramuscularly, or megestrol acetate, 80–160 mg daily orally.

Prognosis

With early diagnosis and treatment, the overall 5-year survival is 80–85%. With stage I disease, the depth of myometrial invasion is the strongest predictor of survival, with a 98% 5-year survival with less than 66% depth of invasion and 78% survival with 66% or more invasion.

When to Refer

All patients with endometrial carcinoma should be referred to a gynecologic oncologist.

Bodurtha Smith AJ et al. Sentinel lymph node assessment in endometrial cancer: a systematic review and meta-analysis. Am J Obstet Gynecol. 2017 May;216(5):459–76. [PMID: 27871836]

Braun MM et al. Diagnosis and management of endometrial cancer. Am Fam Physician. 2016 Mar 15;93(6):468–74. [PMID: 26977831]

Morice P et al. Endometrial cancer. Lancet. 2016 Mar 12; 387(10023):1094–108. [PMID: 26354523]

Palisoul M et al. The clinical management of inoperable endometrial carcinoma. Expert Rev Anticancer Ther. 2016 May; 16(5):515–21. [PMID: 26999568]

Visser NCM et al. Accuracy of endometrial sampling in endometrial carcinoma: a systematic review and meta-analysis. Obstet Gynecol. 2017 Oct;130(4):803–13. [PMID: 28885397]

CARCINOMA OF THE VULVA

ESSENTIALS OF DIAGNOSIS

▶ History of genital warts.

▶ History of prolonged vulvar irritation, with pruritus, local discomfort, or slight bloody discharge.

▶ Early lesions may suggest or include non-neoplastic epithelial disorders.

▶ Late lesions appear as a mass, an exophytic growth, or a firm, ulcerated area in the vulva.

▶ Biopsy is necessary for diagnosis.

General Considerations

The majority of cancers of the vulva are squamous lesions that classically have occurred in women over 50 years of age. Several subtypes (particularly 16, 18, and 31) of HPV have been identified in some but not all vulvar cancers. About 70–90% of vulvar intraepithelial neoplasia (VIN) and 40–60% of vulvar cancers are HPV associated. As with squamous cell lesions of the cervix, a grading system of VIN from mild dysplasia to carcinoma in situ is used.

Differential Diagnosis

Benign vulvar disorders that must be excluded in the diagnosis of carcinoma of the vulva include chronic granulomatous lesions (eg, lymphogranuloma venereum, syphilis), condylomas, hidradenoma, or neurofibroma. Lichen sclerosus and other associated leukoplakic changes in the skin should be biopsied. The likelihood that a superimposed vulvar cancer will develop in a woman with a non-neoplastic epithelial disorder (vulvar dystrophy) is 1–5%.

Diagnosis

Biopsy is essential for the diagnosis of VIN and vulvar cancer and should be performed with any localized atypical vulvar lesion, including white patches. Multiple skin-punch specimens can be taken in the office under local anesthesia, with care to include tissue from the edges of each lesion sampled. Colposcopy of vulva, vagina, and cervix can help in identifying areas for biopsy and in planning further treatment.

Staging

Vulvar cancer generally spreads by direct extension into the vagina, urethra, perineum, and anus, with discontinuous spread into the inguinal and femoral lymph nodes. CT or MRI of the pelvis or abdomen is generally not required except in advanced cases for planning therapeutic options.

Treatment

A. General Measures

Early diagnosis and treatment of irritative or other predisposing causes, such as lichen sclerosis and VIN, should be pursued. A 7:3 combination of betamethasone and crotamiton is particularly effective for itching. After an initial response, fluorinated steroids should be replaced with hydrocortisone because of their skin atrophying effect. For lichen sclerosus, recommended treatment is clobetasol propionate cream 0.05% twice daily for 2–3 weeks, then once daily until symptoms resolve. Application one to three times a week can be used for long-term maintenance therapy.

B. Surgical Measures

High-grade VIN may be treated with a variety of approaches including topical chemotherapy, laser ablation, wide local excision, skinning vulvectomy, and simple vulvectomy. Small, invasive basal cell carcinoma of the vulva should be excised with a wide margin. If the VIN is extensive or multicentric, laser therapy or superficial surgical removal of vulvar skin may be required. In this way, the clitoris and uninvolved portions of the vulva may be spared.

Invasive carcinoma confined to the vulva without evidence of spread to adjacent organs or to the regional lymph nodes is treated with wide local excision and inguinal lymphadenectomy or wide local excision alone if invasion is less than 1 mm. To avoid the morbidity of inguinal lymphadenectomy, some guidelines recommend sentinel lymph node sampling for women with early-stage vulvar cancer. Patients with more advanced disease may receive preoperative radiation, chemotherapy, or both.

Prognosis

Basal cell vulvar carcinomas very seldom metastasize, and carcinoma in situ by definition has not metastasized. With adequate excision, the prognosis for both lesions is excellent. Patients with invasive vulvar SCC 2 cm in diameter or less, without inguinal lymph node metastases, have an 85–90% 5-year survival rate. If the lesion is larger than 2 cm and lymph node involvement is present, the likelihood of 5-year survival is approximately 40%.

When to Refer

All patients with invasive vulvar carcinoma should be referred to a gynecologic oncologist.

Allbritton JI. Vulvar neoplasms, benign and malignant. Obstet Gynecol Clin North Am. 2017 Sep;44(3):339–52. [PMID: 28778635]

American College of Obstetricians and Gynecologists. Committee Opinion No. 675 Summary: Management of vulvar intraepithelial neoplasia. Obstet Gynecol. 2016 Oct;128(4): 937–8. [PMID: 27661648]

Dellinger TH et al. Surgical management of vulvar cancer. J Natl Compr Canc Netw. 2017 Jan;15(1):121–8. [PMID: 28040722]

Koh WJ et al. Vulvar cancer, Version 1.2017, NCCN Clinical Practice Guidelines in Oncology. J Natl Compr Canc Netw. 2017 Jan;15(1):92–120. [PMID: 28040721]

Sznurkowski JJ. Vulvar cancer: initial management and systematic review of literature on currently applied treatment approaches. Eur J Cancer Care (Engl). 2016 Jul;25(4):638–46. [PMID: 26880231]

ENDOMETRIOSIS

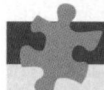

ESSENTIALS OF DIAGNOSIS

► Dysmenorrhea.

► Dyspareunia.

► Increased frequency among infertile women.

► Abnormal uterine bleeding.

General Considerations

Endometriosis is an aberrant growth of endometrium outside the uterus, particularly in the dependent parts of the pelvis and in the ovaries, whose principal manifestations are chronic pain and infertility. While retrograde menstruation is the most widely accepted cause, its pathogenesis and natural course are not fully understood. The overall prevalence in the United States is 6–10% and is four- to fivefold greater among infertile women. Endometriosis is associated with an increased risk of coronary heart disease.

Clinical Findings

The clinical manifestations of endometriosis are variable and unpredictable in both presentation and course. Dysmenorrhea, chronic pelvic pain, and dyspareunia, are among the well-recognized manifestations. A significant number of women with endometriosis, however, remain asymptomatic and most women with endometriosis have a normal pelvic examination. However, in some women, pelvic examination can disclose tender nodules in the cul-de-sac or rectovaginal septum, uterine retroversion with decreased uterine mobility, cervical motion tenderness, or an adnexal mass or tenderness.

Endometriosis must be distinguished from PID, ovarian neoplasms, and uterine myomas. Bowel invasion by endometrial tissue may produce blood in the stool that must be distinguished from bowel neoplasm.

Imaging is of limited value and is useful only in the presence of a pelvic or adnexal mass. Transvaginal ultrasonography is the imaging modality of choice to detect the presence of deeply penetrating endometriosis of the rectum or rectovaginal septum, while MRI should be reserved for equivocal cases of rectovaginal or bladder endometriosis. Ultimately, a definitive diagnosis of endometriosis is made only by histology of lesions removed at surgery.

► Treatment

A. Medical Treatment

Although there is no conclusive evidence that NSAIDs improve pain associated with endometriosis, these agents are reasonable options in appropriately selected patients. Medical treatment, using a variety of hormonal therapies, is effective in the amelioration of pain associated with endometriosis. However, there is no evidence that any of these agents increase the likelihood of pregnancy. Their preoperative use is of questionable value in reducing the difficulty of surgery. Most of these regimens are designed to inhibit ovulation over 4–9 months and lower hormone levels, thus preventing cyclic stimulation of endometriotic implants and inducing atrophy. The optimum duration of therapy is not clear, and the relative merits in terms of side effects and long-term risks and benefits show insignificant differences when compared with each other and, in mild cases, with placebo. Commonly used medical regimens include the following:

1. **Low-dose oral contraceptives** can be given cyclically or continuously; prolonged suppression of ovulation often inhibits further stimulation of residual endometriosis, especially if taken after one of the therapies mentioned here. Any of the combination oral contraceptives, the contraceptive patch, or vaginal ring may be used continuously for 6–12 months. Breakthrough bleeding can be treated with conjugated estrogens, 1.25 mg orally daily for 1 week, or estradiol, 2 mg daily orally for 1 week.

2. **Progestins,** specifically oral norethindrone acetate and subcutaneous DMPA, have been approved by the FDA for treatment of endometriosis-associated pain.

3. **Intrauterine progestin,** using the levonorgestrel intrauterine system, has also been shown to be effective in reducing endometriosis-associated pelvic pain, and it is recommended before surgery.

4. **GnRH agonists** are highly effective in reducing the pain syndromes associated with endometriosis. However, they are not superior to other methods such as combined oral contraceptives as first-line therapy. The GnRH analogs (such as long-acting injectable leuprolide acetate, 3.75 mg intramuscularly monthly, used for 6 months) suppresses ovulation. Side effects of vasomotor symptoms and bone demineralization may be relieved by "add-back" therapy, such as conjugated equine estrogen, 0.625 mg, or norethindrone, 5 mg orally daily.

5. **Danazol** is an androgenic medication that has been used for the treatment of endometriosis-associated pain. It should be used for 4–6 months in the lowest dose necessary to suppress menstruation, usually 200–400 mg orally twice daily. However, danazol has a high incidence of androgenic side effects that are more severe than other medications available, including decreased breast size, weight gain, acne, and hirsutism.

6. **Aromatase inhibitors** (such as anastrozole or letrozole) in combination with conventional therapy have been evaluated with positive results in premenopausal women with endometriosis-associated pain and pain recurrence.

B. Surgical Measures

Surgical treatment of endometriosis—particularly extensive disease—is effective both in reducing pain and in promoting fertility. Laparoscopic ablation of endometrial implants significantly reduces pain. Ablation of implants and, if necessary, removal of ovarian endometriomas enhance fertility, although subsequent pregnancy rates are inversely related to the severity of disease. Women with disabling pain for whom childbearing is not a consideration can be treated definitively with total abdominal hysterectomy and bilateral salpingo-oophorectomy. In premenopausal women, hormone replacement then may be used to relieve vasomotor symptoms. However, hormone replacement may lead to a recurrence of endometriosis and associated pain.

▶ Prognosis

There is little systematic research regarding either the progression of the disease or the prediction of clinical outcomes. The prognosis for reproductive function in early or moderately advanced endometriosis appears to be good with conservative therapy. Hysterectomy, with bilateral salpingo-oophorectomy, often is regarded as definitive therapy for the treatment of endometriosis associated with intractable pelvic pain, adnexal masses, or multiple previous ineffective conservative surgical procedures. However, symptoms may recur even after hysterectomy and oophorectomy.

▶ When to Refer

Refer to a gynecologist for laparoscopic diagnosis or treatment.

▶ When to Admit

Rarely necessary except for acute abdomen associated with ruptured or bleeding endometrioma.

Brown J et al. Nonsteroidal anti-inflammatory drugs for pain in women with endometriosis. Cochrane Database Syst Rev. 2017 Jan 23;1:CD004753. [PMID: 28114727]

Casper RF. Progestin-only pills may be a better first-line treatment for endometriosis than combined estrogen-progestin contraceptive pills. Fertil Steril. 2017 Mar;107(3):533–6. [PMID: 28162779]

Chaichian S et al. Comparing the efficacy of surgery and medical therapy for pain management in endometriosis: a systematic review and meta-analysis. Pain Physician. 2017 Mar; 20(3):185–95. [PMID: 28339429]

Flyckt R et al. Surgical management of endometriosis in patients with chronic pelvic pain. Semin Reprod Med. 2017 Jan; 35(1):54–64. [PMID: 28049215]

Fu J et al. Progesterone receptor modulators for endometriosis. Cochrane Database Syst Rev. 2017 Jul 25;7:CD009881. [PMID: 28742263]

Rafique S et al. Medical management of endometriosis. Clin Obstet Gynecol. 2017 Sep;60(3):485–96. [PMID: 28590310]

Singh SS et al. Surgery for endometriosis: beyond medical therapies. Fertil Steril. 2017 Mar;107(3):549–54. [PMID: 28189295]

Taylor HS et al. Treatment of endometriosis-associated pain with elagolix, an oral GnRH antagonist. N Engl J Med. 2017 Jul 6; 377(1):28–40. [PMID: 28525302]

PELVIC ORGAN PROLAPSE

▶ General Considerations

Cystocele, rectocele, and enterocele are vaginal hernias commonly seen in multiparous women. **Cystocele** is a hernia of the bladder wall into the vagina, causing a soft anterior fullness. Cystocele may be accompanied by **urethrocele,** which is not a hernia but a sagging of the urethra following its detachment from the pubic symphysis during childbirth. **Rectocele** is a herniation of the terminal rectum into the posterior vagina, causing a collapsible pouch-like fullness. **Enterocele** is a vaginal vault hernia containing small intestine, usually in the posterior vagina and resulting from a deepening of the pouch of Douglas. Two or all three types of hernia may occur in combination. Risk factors may include vaginal birth, genetic predisposition, advancing age, prior pelvic surgery, connective tissue disorders, and increased intra-abdominal pressure associated with obesity or straining associated with chronic constipation or coughing.

▶ Clinical Findings

Symptoms of pelvic organ prolapse may include sensation of a bulge or protrusion in the vagina, urinary or fecal incontinence, constipation, a sense of incomplete bladder emptying, and dyspareunia. The cause of pelvic organ prolapse, including prolapse of the uterus, vaginal apex, and anterior or posterior vaginal walls, is likely multifactorial.

▶ Treatment

The type of therapy depends on the extent of prolapse and the patient's age and her desire for menstruation, pregnancy, and coitus.

A. General Measures

Supportive measures include a high-fiber diet and laxatives to improve constipation. Weight reduction in obese patients and limitation of straining and lifting are helpful. Pelvic muscle training (Kegel exercises) is a simple, noninvasive intervention that may improve pelvic function and it has demonstrated clear benefit for women with urinary or fecal symptoms, especially incontinence. Pessaries may reduce cystocele, rectocele, or enterocele and are helpful in women who do not wish to undergo surgery or are poor surgical candidates.

B. Surgical Measures

The most common surgical procedure is vaginal or abdominal hysterectomy with additional attention to restoring apical support after the uterus is removed, including suspension either by vaginal uterosacral or sacrospinous fixation or by abdominal sacral colpopexy. Since stress incontinence is common after vault suspension procedures, an anti-incontinence procedure should be considered. However, in April 2019, the US FDA withdrew its previous (2016) class III (high risk) approval of surgical mesh intended for transvaginal repair of anterior compartment prolapse. Patients planning to have surgical repair of pelvic organ prolapse should discuss other treatment options than mesh with their clinician. If the patient desires pregnancy, the same procedures for vaginal suspension can be performed without hysterectomy, though limited data on pregnancy outcomes or prolapse outcomes are available. For elderly women who do not desire coitus, colpocleisis, the partial obliteration of the vagina, is surgically simple and effective. Uterine suspension with sacrospinous cervicocolpopexy may be an effective approach in older women who wish to avoid hysterectomy but preserve coital function. Women who have received transvaginal mesh for the surgical repair of pelvic organ prolapse but who are having no symptoms or complications related to it should continue with their annual check-ups and other routine follow-up care. They should let their clinician know that they have a surgical mesh implant, especially if they plan to have another pelvic surgery or related medical procedure. In addition, they should notify their clinician if they develop persistent vaginal bleeding or discharge, pelvic or groin pain, or dyspareunia.

When to Refer

- Refer to urogynecologist or gynecologist for incontinence evaluation.
- Refer if nonsurgical therapy is ineffective.

American College of Obstetricians and Gynecologists. Committee on Practice Bulletins—Gynecology and the American Urogynecologic Society. Practice Bulletin No. 176: Pelvic Organ Prolapse. Obstet Gynecol. 2017 Apr;129(4):e56–72. [PMID: 28333818]
American Urogynecologic Society (AUGS). Best Practice Statement: Evaluation and counseling of patients with pelvic organ prolapse. Female Pelvic Med Reconstr Surg. 2017 Sep/Oct; 23(5):281–7. [PMID: 28846554]
Coolen AWM et al. Primary treatment of pelvic organ prolapse: pessary use versus prolapse surgery. Int Urogynecol J. 2018 Jan; 29(1):99–107. [PMID: 28600758]
US FDA. Urogynecologic surgical mesh implants, April 16 2019. https://www.fda.gov/medical-devices/implants-and-prosthetics/urogynecologic-surgical-mesh-implant

PELVIC INFLAMMATORY DISEASE (Salpingitis, Endometritis)

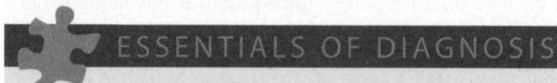

ESSENTIALS OF DIAGNOSIS

- ▸ Uterine, adnexal, or cervical motion tenderness.
- ▸ Abnormal discharge from the vagina or cervix.
- ▸ Absence of a competing diagnosis.

General Considerations

Pelvic inflammatory disease (PID) is a polymicrobial infection of the upper genital tract associated with the sexually transmitted organisms *Neisseria gonorrhoeae* and *Chlamydia trachomatis* as well as endogenous organisms, including anaerobes, *Haemophilus influenzae*, enteric gram-negative rods, and streptococci. It is most common in young, nulliparous, sexually active women with multiple partners and is a leading cause of infertility and ectopic pregnancy. The use of barrier methods of contraception may provide significant protection.

Clinical Findings

A. Symptoms and Signs

Patients with PID may have lower abdominal pain, chills and fever, menstrual disturbances, purulent cervical discharge, and cervical and adnexal tenderness. Right upper quadrant pain (**Fitz-Hugh and Curtis syndrome**) may indicate an associated perihepatitis. However, diagnosis of PID is complicated by the fact that many women may have subtle or mild symptoms that are not readily recognized as PID, such as postcoital bleeding, urinary frequency, or low back pain.

B. Minimum Diagnostic Criteria

Women with cervical motion, uterine, or adnexal tenderness should be considered to have PID and be treated with antibiotics unless there is a competing diagnosis such as ectopic pregnancy or appendicitis.

C. Additional Criteria

No single historical, physical, or laboratory finding is definitive for acute PID. The following criteria may be used to enhance the specificity of the diagnosis: (1) oral temperature higher than 38.3°C, (2) abnormal cervical or vaginal discharge with white cells on saline microscopy (greater than 1 leukocyte per epithelial cell), (3) elevated erythrocyte sedimentation rate, (4) elevated C-reactive protein, and (5) laboratory documentation of cervical infection with *N gonorrhoeae* or *C trachomatis*. Endocervical culture should be performed routinely, but treatment should not be delayed while awaiting results.

Differential Diagnosis

Appendicitis, ectopic pregnancy, septic abortion, hemorrhagic or ruptured ovarian cysts or tumors, torsion of an ovarian cyst, degeneration of a myoma, and acute enteritis must be considered. PID is more likely to occur when there is a history of PID, recent sexual contact, recent onset of menses, recent insertion of an IUD, or if the partner has a sexually transmitted disease. Acute PID is highly unlikely when recent (within 60 days) intercourse has not taken place. A sensitive serum pregnancy test should be obtained to rule out ectopic pregnancy. Pelvic and vaginal ultrasonography is helpful in the differential diagnosis of ectopic pregnancy of over 6 weeks and to rule out tubo-ovarian abscess. Laparoscopy is often used to diagnose PID, and it is imperative if the diagnosis is not certain or if the patient has not responded to antibiotic therapy after 48 hours. The appendix should be visualized at laparoscopy to rule out appendicitis. Cultures obtained at the time of laparoscopy are often specific and helpful.

Treatment

A. Antibiotics

Early treatment with appropriate antibiotics effective against *N gonorrhoeae, C trachomatis,* and the endogenous organisms listed above is essential to prevent long-term sequelae. The sexual partner should be examined and treated appropriately. Most women with mild to moderate disease can be treated successfully as an outpatient. The recommended outpatient regimen is a single dose of cefoxitin, 2 g intramuscularly, with probenecid, 1 g orally, plus doxycycline 100 mg orally twice a day for 14 days, or ceftriaxone 250 mg intramuscularly plus doxycycline, 100 mg orally twice daily, for 14 days. Metronidazole 500 mg orally twice daily for 14 days may also be added to either of these two regimens and will also treat bacterial vaginosis that is frequently associated with PID. For patients with severe disease or those who meet the other criteria for hospitalization, there are two recommended regimens. One regimen includes either cefotetan, 2 g intravenously every 12 hours, or cefoxitin, 2 g intravenously every 6 hours, plus doxycycline, 100 mg orally or intravenously every 12 hours. The other recommended regimen is clindamycin, 900 mg intravenously every 8 hours, plus gentamicin, a loading dose of 2 mg/kg intravenously or intramuscularly followed by a maintenance dose of 1.5 mg/kg every 8 hours (or as a single daily dose, 3–5 mg/kg). These regimens should be continued for a minimum of 24 hours after the patient shows significant clinical improvement. Then, an oral regimen should be given for a total course of antibiotics of 14 days with either doxycycline, 100 mg orally twice a day, or clindamycin, 450 mg orally four times a day. If a tubo-ovarian abscess is present, clindamycin or metronidazole should be used with doxycycline to complete the 14-day treatment for better anaerobic coverage.

B. Surgical Measures

Tubo-ovarian abscesses may require surgical excision or transcutaneous or transvaginal aspiration. Unless rupture is suspected, institute high-dose antibiotic therapy in the hospital, and monitor therapy with ultrasound. In 70% of cases, antibiotics are effective; in 30%, there is inadequate response in 48–72 hours, and surgical intervention is required. Unilateral adnexectomy is acceptable for unilateral abscess. Hysterectomy and bilateral salpingo-oophorectomy may be necessary for overwhelming infection or in cases of chronic disease with intractable pelvic pain.

Prognosis

In spite of treatment, long-term sequelae, including repeated episodes of infection, chronic pelvic pain, dyspareunia, ectopic pregnancy, or infertility, develop in one-fourth of women with acute disease. The risk of infertility increases with repeated episodes of salpingitis: it is estimated at 10% after the first episode, 25% after a second episode, and 50% after a third episode.

When to Admit

The following patients with acute PID should be admitted for intravenous antibiotic therapy:

- The patient has a tubo-ovarian abscess (direct inpatient observation for at least 24 hours before switching to outpatient parenteral therapy).
- The patient is pregnant.
- The patient is unable to follow or tolerate an outpatient regimen.
- The patient has not responded clinically to outpatient therapy within 72 hours.
- The patient has severe illness, nausea and vomiting, or high fever.
- Another surgical emergency, such as appendicitis, cannot be ruled out.

Bugg CW et al. Pelvic inflammatory disease: diagnosis and treatment in the emergency department. Emerg Med Pract. 2016 Dec;18(12):1–24. [PMID: 27879197]
Das BB et al. Pelvic inflammatory disease: improving awareness, prevention, and treatment. Infect Drug Resist. 2016 Aug 19; 9:191–7. [PMID: 27578991]
Ross J et al. 2017 European guideline for the management of pelvic inflammatory disease. Int J STD AIDS. 2018 Feb; 29(2):108–14. [PMID: 29198181]

OVARIAN CANCER & OVARIAN TUMORS

ESSENTIALS OF DIAGNOSIS

- ► Symptoms include vague gastrointestinal discomfort, pelvic pressure, or pain.
- ► Many cases of early-stage cancer are asymptomatic.
- ► Pelvic examination and ultrasound are mainstays of diagnosis.

General Considerations

Ovarian tumors are common. Most are benign, but malignant ovarian tumors are the leading cause of death from reproductive tract cancer. The wide range of types and patterns of ovarian tumors is due to the complexity of ovarian embryology and differences in tissues of origin.

In women with no family history of ovarian cancer, the lifetime risk is 1.6%, whereas a woman with one affected first-degree relative has a 5% lifetime risk. Ultrasound or tumor marker screening for women with one or no affected first-degree relatives have not been shown to reduce mortality from ovarian cancer, and the risks associated with unnecessary prophylactic surgical procedures outweigh the benefits in low-risk women. With two or more affected first-degree relatives, the risk is 7%. Approximately 3% of women with two or more affected first-degree relatives will have a **hereditary ovarian cancer syndrome** with a lifetime risk of 40%. Women with a *BRCA1* gene mutation have a 45% lifetime risk of ovarian cancer and those with a *BRCA2* mutation, a 25% risk. Consideration should be given to screening with transvaginal sonography and serum CA 125 testing, starting at age 30–35 years for women with *BRCA 1* or age 35–40 for women with *BRCA2* or 5–10 years earlier than the earliest age that ovarian cancer was first diagnosed in any family member. Of note, this screening regimen has not been shown to reduce mortality; thus, prophylactic oophorectomy should be considered at conclusion of childbearing.

Clinical Findings

A. Symptoms and Signs

Most women with both benign and malignant ovarian neoplasms are either asymptomatic or experience only mild nonspecific gastrointestinal symptoms or pelvic pressure. Women with advanced malignant disease may experience abdominal pain and bloating, and a palpable abdominal mass with ascites is often present.

B. Laboratory Findings

Serum CA 125 is elevated in 80% of women with epithelial ovarian cancer overall but in only 50% of women with early disease. CA 125 may be elevated in premenopausal women with benign disease (such as endometriosis), minimizing its usefulness in ovarian cancer screening. In premenopausal women with ovarian masses, other tumor markers (such as human chorionic gonadotropin [hCG], lactate dehydrogenase, or alpha-fetoprotein) may be indicators of the tumor type.

C. Imaging

Transvaginal sonography is useful for screening high-risk women but has inadequate sensitivity for screening low-risk women. Ultrasound is helpful in differentiating ovarian masses that are benign and likely to resolve spontaneously from those with malignant potential. Color Doppler imaging may further enhance the specificity of ultrasound diagnosis.

Differential Diagnosis

Once an ovarian mass has been detected, it must be categorized as functional, benign neoplastic, or potentially malignant. Predictive factors include age, size of the mass, ultrasound configuration, serum CA 125 level, the presence of symptoms, and whether the mass is unilateral or bilateral. Simple cysts up to 5 cm in diameter are almost universally benign in both premenopausal and postmenopausal patients. Most will resolve spontaneously and may be monitored without intervention. If the mass is larger or unchanged on repeat pelvic examination and transvaginal sonography, surgical evaluation is warranted.

Laparoscopic or robotic approaches may be used for oophorectomy and staging in early-stage ovarian cancer when the ovarian mass is small. In these cases, malignancy is often not diagnosed prior to the surgery. Data (retrospective) comparing open with laparoscopic approaches to ovarian cancer staging are limited. Laparotomy is generally preferred for staging and debulking if malignancy is suspected from findings on transvaginal ultrasound with morphologic scoring, color Doppler assessment of vascular quality, and CA 125 level.

Treatment

If a malignant ovarian mass is suspected, surgical evaluation should be performed by a gynecologic oncologist. For benign neoplasms, tumor removal or unilateral oophorectomy is usually performed. For ovarian cancer in an early stage, the standard therapy is complete surgical staging followed by hysterectomy and bilateral salpingo-oophorectomy with omentectomy and selective lymphadenectomy. With more advanced disease, in addition, aggressive removal of all visible tumor improves survival. Except for women with low-grade ovarian cancer in an early stage, postoperative chemotherapy is indicated (see Table 39–3). Several chemotherapy regimens are effective, such as the combination of cisplatin or carboplatin with paclitaxel, with clinical response rates of up to 60–70% (see Table 39–13).

Prognosis

Advanced disease is diagnosed in approximately 75% of women with ovarian cancer. The overall 5-year survival is approximately 17% with distant metastases, 36% with local spread, and 89% with early disease.

When to Refer

If a malignant mass is suspected, surgical evaluation should be performed by a gynecologic oncologist.

American College of Obstetricians and Gynecologists. Committee Opinion No. 716: The role of the obstetrician-gynecologist in the early detection of epithelial ovarian cancer in women at average risk. Obstet Gynecol. 2017 Sep;130(3):e146–9. [PMID: 28832487]

American College of Obstetricians and Gynecologists. Practice Bulletin No. 174: Evaluation and management of adnexal masses. Obstet Gynecol. 2016 Nov;128(5):e210–26. [PMID: 27776072]

American College of Obstetricians and Gynecologists. Practice Bulletin No. 182 Summary: Hereditary breast and ovarian cancer syndrome. Obstet Gynecol. 2017 Sep;130(3):657–9. [PMID: 28832475]

Biggs WS et al. Diagnosis and management of adnexal masses. Am Fam Physician. 2016 Apr 15;93(8):676–81. [PMID: 27175840]

Centers for Disease Control and Prevention (CDC). Ovarian cancer screening. 2018 Sept 12. https://www.cdc.gov/cancer/ovarian/basic_info/screening.htm

Doubeni CA et al. Diagnosis and management of ovarian cancer. Am Fam Physician. 2016 Jun 1;93(11):937–44. [PMID: 27281838]

US Preventive Services Task Force, Grossman DC et al. Screening for ovarian cancer: US Preventive Services Task Force Recommendation Statement. JAMA. 2018 Feb 13;319(6):588–94. [PMID: 29450531]

POLYCYSTIC OVARY SYNDROME

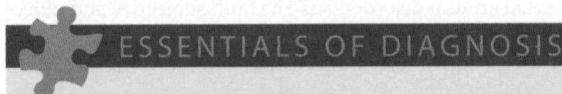

ESSENTIALS OF DIAGNOSIS

▶ Clinical or biochemical evidence of hyperandrogenism.

▶ Oligoovulation or anovulation.

▶ Polycystic ovaries on ultrasonography.

General Considerations

Polycystic ovary syndrome (PCOS) is a common endocrine disorder of unknown etiology affecting 5–10% of reproductive age women. PCOS is characterized by chronic anovulation, polycystic ovaries, and hyperandrogenism. It is associated with hirsutism and obesity as well as an increased risk of diabetes mellitus, cardiovascular disease, and metabolic syndrome. Unrecognized or untreated PCOS is a risk factor for cardiovascular disease. The Rotterdam Criteria identify **androgen production, ovulatory dysfunction,** and **polycystic ovaries** as the key diagnostic features of the disorder in adult women; the emerging consensus is that at least two of these features must be present for diagnosis. The classification system has been endorsed by the National Institutes of Health.

Clinical Findings

PCOS often presents as a menstrual disorder (ranging from amenorrhea to menorrhagia) and infertility. Skin disorders due to peripheral androgen excess, including hirsutism and acne, are common. Patients may also show signs of insulin resistance and hyperinsulinemia, and these women are at increased risk for early-onset type 2 diabetes and metabolic syndrome. Patients who do become pregnant are at increased risk for perinatal complications, such as gestational diabetes and preeclampsia. In addition, they have an increased long-term risk of endometrial cancer secondary to unopposed estrogen secretion.

Differential Diagnosis

Anovulation in the reproductive years may also be due to (1) premature ovarian failure (high follicle-stimulating hormone [FSH] and luteinizing hormone [LH] levels); (2) rapid weight loss, extreme physical exertion (normal FSH and LH levels for age), or obesity; (3) discontinuation of hormonal contraceptives (anovulation occurs for 6 months or more occasionally); (4) pituitary adenoma with elevated prolactin (galactorrhea may or may not be present); and (5) hyperthyroidism or hypothyroidism. To rule out other etiologies in women with suspected PCOS, serum FSH, LH, prolactin, and thyroid-stimulating hormone should be checked. Because of the high risk of insulin resistance and dyslipidemia, all women with suspected PCOS should have a hemoglobin A_{1C} and fasting glucose along with a lipid and lipoprotein profile. Women with clinical evidence of androgen excess should have total testosterone and sex hormone–binding globulin or free (bioavailable) testosterone and 17-hydroxyprogesterone measured. Women with stigmata of Cushing syndrome should have a 24-hour urinary free cortisol or a low-dose dexamethasone suppression test. Congenital adrenal hyperplasia and androgen-secreting adrenal tumors also tend to have high circulating androgen levels and anovulation with polycystic ovaries; these disorders must also be ruled out in women with presumed PCOS.

Treatment

In obese patients with PCOS, weight reduction and exercise are often effective in reversing the metabolic effects and in inducing ovulation. For those women who do not respond to weight loss and exercise, metformin therapy may be helpful. Metformin is beneficial for metabolic or glucose abnormalities, and it can improve menstrual function. Metformin has little or no benefit in the treatment of hirsutism, acne, or infertility. Contraceptive counseling should be offered to prevent unplanned pregnancy in case of a return of ovulatory cycles. For women who are seeking pregnancy and remain anovulatory, clomiphene or other medications can be used for ovarian stimulation (see section on Infertility below). Clomiphene is the first-line therapy for infertility. If induction of ovulation fails, treatment with gonadotropins, but at low dose to lower the risk of ovarian hyperstimulation syndrome, may be successful. Second-line therapies such as use of aromatase inhibitors or laparoscopic "ovarian drilling" are of unproved benefit. Women with PCOS are at greater risk than normal women for twin gestation with ovarian stimulation.

If the patient does not desire pregnancy and does not want or is not a candidate for contraception, then medroxyprogesterone acetate, 10 mg/day orally for the first 10 days of every 1–3 months, should be given to ensure regular shedding of the endometrium and thus avoid endometrial hyperplasia. If contraception is desired, combination contraceptives (pill, ring, or patch) can be used; this is also useful in controlling hirsutism, for which treatment must be continued for 6–12 months before results are seen. The levonorgestrel-containing IUD is another option to minimize uterine bleeding and protect against endometrial hyperplasia, but unlike the combined estrogen-progestin contraceptives, the IUD does not help control hirsutism.

Spironolactone is useful for hirsutism in doses of 25 mg three or four times daily. Flutamide, 125–250 mg orally daily, and finasteride, 5 mg orally daily, are also effective for treating hirsutism. Because these three agents are potentially teratogenic, they should be used only in conjunction with secure contraception. Topical eflornithine cream applied to affected facial areas twice daily for 6 months may be helpful in the majority of women. Hirsutism may also be managed with depilatory creams, electrolysis, and laser therapy. The combination of laser therapy and topical eflornithine may be particularly effective.

Weight loss, exercise, and treatment of unresolved metabolic derangements are important in preventing cardiovascular disease. Women with PCOS should be managed aggressively and should have regular monitoring of lipid profiles and glucose. In adolescent patients with

PCOS, hormonal contraceptives and metformin are treatment options.

When to Refer

- If expertise in diagnosis is needed.
- If patient is infertile.

Bednarska S et al. The pathogenesis and treatment of polycystic ovary syndrome: what's new? Adv Clin Exp Med. 2017 Mar–Apr; 26(2):359–67. [PMID: 28791858]

McCartney CR et al. Clinical practice: polycystic ovary syndrome. N Engl J Med. 2016 Jul 7;375(1):54–64. [PMID: 27406348]

Scoccia B. What is new in polycystic ovary syndrome? Best articles from the past year. Obstet Gynecol. 2016 Nov; 128(5):1174–6. [PMID: 27741186]

FEMALE SEXUAL DYSFUNCTION

General Considerations

Female sexual dysfunction is a common problem. Depending on the questions asked, surveys have shown that from 35% to 98% of women report sexual concerns. Questions related to sexual functioning should be asked as part of the routine medical history. Three helpful questions to broach the topic are "Are you currently involved in a sexual relationship?," "With men, women, or both?," and "Do you have any sexual concerns or any pain with sex?" If the woman is not involved in a sexual relationship, she should be asked if there are any concerns that are contributing to a lack of sexual behavior. If a history of sexual dysfunction is elicited, a complete history of factors that may affect sexual function should be taken. These factors include her reproductive history (including pregnancies and mode of delivery) as well as history of infertility, sexually transmitted diseases, rape or sexual violence, gynecologic or urologic disorders, endocrine abnormalities (such as diabetes mellitus or thyroid disease), neurologic problems, cardiovascular disease, psychiatric disease, and current prescription and over-the-counter medication use. A detailed history of the specific sexual dysfunction should be elicited, and a gynecologic examination should focus on findings that may contribute to sexual complaints.

Etiology

A. Disorders of Sexual Desire

Sexual desire in women is a complex and poorly understood phenomenon. Emotion is a key factor in sexual desire. Anger toward a partner, fear or anxiety related to previous sexual encounters, or history of sexual abuse violence may contribute to a lack of desire. Physical factors such as chronic illness, fatigue, depression, and specific medical disorders (such as diabetes mellitus, thyroid disease, or adrenal insufficiency) may also contribute. Menopause and attitudes toward aging may play a role. In addition, sexual desire may be influenced by other sexual dysfunction, such as arousal disorders, dyspareunia, or anorgasmia.

B. Sexual Arousal Disorders

Sexual arousal disorders may be both subjective and objective. Sexual stimulation normally leads to genital vasocongestion and lubrication. Some women may have a physiologic response to sexual stimuli, but may not subjectively feel aroused because of factors such as distractions; negative expectations; anxiety; fatigue; depression; or medications, such as selective serotonin reuptake inhibitors (SSRIs) or oral contraceptives. Other women with vaginal atrophy may lack both a subjective and physiologic response to sexual stimuli.

C. Orgasmic Disorders

In spite of subjective and physiologic arousal, women may experience a marked delay in orgasm, diminished sensation of an orgasm, or anorgasmia. The etiology is complex and typically multifactorial, but the disorder is usually amenable to treatment.

D. Sexual Pain Disorders

Dyspareunia and vaginismus are two subcategories of sexual pain disorders.

Dyspareunia is defined as recurrent or persistent genital pain associated with sexual intercourse that is not caused exclusively by lack of lubrication or by vaginismus and that causes marked distress or interpersonal difficulty. **Vulvodynia** is the most frequent cause of dyspareunia in premenopausal women. It is characterized by a sensation of burning along with other symptoms, including pain, itching, stinging, irritation, and rawness. The discomfort may be constant or intermittent, focal or diffuse, and experienced as either deep or superficial. There are generally no physical findings except minimal erythema that may be associated in a subset of patients with vulvodynia, those with vulvar vestibulitis. **Vulvar vestibulitis** is normally asymptomatic but pain is associated with touching or pressure on the vestibule, such as with vaginal entry or insertion of a tampon. Pain occurring with deep thrusting during coitus is usually due to acute or chronic infection of the cervix, uterus, or adnexa; endometriosis; adnexal tumors; or adhesions resulting from prior pelvic disease or operation.

Vaginismus is defined as recurrent or persistent involuntary spasm of the musculature of the outer third of the vagina that interferes with sexual intercourse, resulting from fear, pain, sexual violence, or a negative attitude toward sex, often learned in childhood, and causing marked distress or interpersonal difficulty. Other medical causes of sexual pain may include vulvovaginitis; vulvar disease, including lichen planus, lichen sclerosus, and lichen simplex chronicus; pelvic disease, such as endometriosis or chronic PID; or vaginal atrophy.

Treatment

A. Disorders of Sexual Desire

In the absence of specific medical disorders, arousal or orgasmic disorders or dyspareunia, the focus of therapy is psychological. Cognitive behavioral therapy, sexual therapy, and couples therapy may all play a role. Success with pharmacologic therapy, particularly the use of dopamine agonists or testosterone with estrogen, has been reported, but data from large long-term clinical trials are lacking.

B. Sexual Arousal Disorders

As with disorders of sexual desire, arousal disorders may respond to psychological therapy. The phosphodiesterase inhibitors used in men do not appear to benefit the majority of women with sexual arousal disorders. However, there is some evidence to suggest a role for sildenafil in women with sexual dysfunction due to multiple sclerosis, type 1 diabetes mellitus, spinal cord injury, and antidepressant medications if other established approaches fail. Flibanserin (Addyi), an antidepressant, was approved by the FDA in August 2015 as an effective treatment of hypoactive sexual desire disorder in premenopausal women; however, it must be used long term to be effective and has significant risks that require specific certifications of providers and pharmacies for dispensation to patients in the United States. While this medication remains available, it is not commonly prescribed.

C. Orgasmic Disorders

For many women, counseling or sex therapy may be adequate treatment. There is an FDA-approved vacuum device that increases clitoral blood flow and may improve the likelihood of orgasm.

D. Sexual Pain Disorders

Specific medical disorders, such as endometriosis, vulvovaginitis, or vaginal atrophy, should be treated as outlined in other sections of this chapter. Lichen planus and lichen simplex chronicus are addressed in Chapter 6. Lichen sclerosus, a thinning and whitening of the vulvar epithelium, is treated with clobetasol propionate 0.05% ointment, applied twice daily for 2–3 months.

Vaginismus may be treated initially with sexual counseling and education on anatomy and sexual functioning. The patient can be instructed in self-dilation, using a lubricated finger or dilators of graduated sizes. Before coitus (with adequate lubrication) is attempted, the patient—and then her partner—should be able to easily and painlessly introduce two fingers into the vagina. Penetration should never be forced, and the woman should always be the one to control the depth of insertion during dilation or intercourse. Injection of botulinum toxin has been used successfully in refractory cases.

Since the cause of vulvodynia is unknown, management is difficult. Few treatment approaches have been subjected to methodologically rigorous trials. A variety of topical agents have been tried, although only topical anesthetics (eg, estrogen cream and a compounded mixture of topical amitriptyline 2% and baclofen 2% in a water washable base) have been useful in relieving vulvodynia. Useful oral medications include tricyclic antidepressants, such as amitriptyline in gradually increasing doses from 10 mg/day to 75–100 mg/day; various SSRIs; and anticonvulsants, such

as gabapentin, starting at 300 mg three times daily and increasing to 1200 mg three times daily. Biofeedback and physical therapy, with a physical therapist experienced with the treatment of vulvar pain, have been shown to be helpful. Surgery—usually consisting of vestibulectomy—has been useful for women with introital dyspareunia. See also Chapter e6.

▶ When to Refer

- When symptoms or concerns persist despite first-line therapy.
- For expertise in surgical procedures.

American College of Obstetricians and Gynecologists. Committee Opinion No 706: Sexual health. Obstet Gynecol. 2017 Jul; 130(1):e42–7. [PMID: 28644338]

Clayton AH et al. Female sexual dysfunction. Psychiatr Clin North Am. 2017 Jun;40(2):267–84. [PMID: 28477652]

Dawson ML et al. The evaluation and management of female sexual dysfunction. J Fam Pract. 2017 Dec;66(12):722–8. [PMID: 29202143]

Goldstein I et al. Hypoactive sexual desire disorder: International Society for the Study of Women's Sexual Health (ISSWSH) Expert Consensus Panel Review. Mayo Clin Proc. 2017 Jan; 92(1):114–28. [PMID: 27916394]

Kingsberg SA et al. Female sexual dysfunction—medical and psychological treatments, Committee 14. J Sex Med. 2017 Dec; 14(12):1463–91. Erratum in: J Sex Med. 2018 Feb;15(2):270. [PMID: 29198504]

Stenson AL. Vulvodynia: diagnosis and management. Obstet Gynecol Clin North Am. 2017 Sep;44(3):493–508. [PMID: 28778645]

Zhou ES et al. Hormonal changes and sexual dysfunction. Med Clin North Am. 2017 Nov;101(6):1135–50. [PMID: 28992859]

INFERTILITY

A couple is said to be infertile if pregnancy does not result after 1 year of normal sexual activity without contraceptives. About 25% of couples experience infertility at some point in their reproductive lives; the incidence of infertility increases with age, with a decline in fertility beginning in the early 30s and accelerating in the late 30s. The male partner contributes to about 40% of cases of infertility, and a combination of factors is common. The most recent data from the CDC National Survey of Family Growth noted that 12% of women in the United States aged 15–44 have impaired fecundity.

A. Initial Testing

During the initial interview, the clinician can present an overview of infertility and discuss an evaluation and management plan. Private consultations with each partner separately are then conducted, allowing appraisal of psychosexual adjustment without embarrassment or criticism. Pertinent details (eg, sexually transmitted disease or prior pregnancies) must be obtained. The ill effects of cigarettes, alcohol, and other recreational drugs on male fertility should be discussed. Prescription medications that impair male potency and factors that may lead to scrotal hyperthermia, such as tight underwear or frequent use of saunas or hot tubs, should be discussed. The gynecologic history should include the menstrual pattern, the use and types of contraceptives, libido, sexual practices, frequency and success of coitus, and correlation of intercourse with time of ovulation. Family history includes repeated spontaneous abortions. The American Society for Reproductive Medicine provides patient information on the infertility evaluation and treatment (https://www.reproductivefacts.org/topics/topics-index/infertility/).

General physical and genital examinations are performed on the female partner. Basic laboratory studies include complete blood count, urinalysis, cervical culture for *Chlamydia,* rubella antibody determination, and thyroid function tests. If the woman has regular menses with minimal symptoms, the likelihood of ovulatory cycles is very high. A luteal phase serum progesterone above 3 ng/mL establishes ovulation. Couples should be advised that coitus resulting in conception occurs during the 6-day window around the day of ovulation. Ovulation predictor kits have largely replaced basal body temperatures for predicting ovulation, but temperature charting is a natural and inexpensive way to identify most fertile days. Basal body temperature charts cannot predict ovulation; they can only retrospectively confirm ovulation occurred.

A semen analysis should be completed to rule out a male factor for infertility. Men must abstain from sexual activity for at least 3 days before the semen is obtained. A clean, dry, wide-mouthed bottle for collection is preferred. Semen should be examined within 1–2 hours after collection. Semen is considered normal with the following minimum values: volume, 2.0 mL; concentration, 20 million sperm per milliliter; motility, 50% or more forward progression, 25% or more rapid progression; and normal forms, 30%. If the sperm count is abnormal, further evaluation includes physical examination of the male partner and a search for exposure to environmental and workplace toxins and alcohol or drug use.

B. Further Testing

1. Gross deficiencies of sperm (number, motility, or appearance) require a repeat confirmatory analysis. **Intracytoplasmic sperm injection (ICSI)** is the treatment option available for sperm deficiencies except for azoospermia (absence of sperm). ICSI requires the female partner to undergo **in vitro fertilization (IVF)**.

2. A screening pelvic ultrasound and hysterosalpingography to identify uterine cavity or tubal anomalies should be performed. Hysterosalpingography using an oil dye is performed within 3 days following the menstrual period if structural abnormalities are suspected. This radiographic study will demonstrate uterine abnormalities (septa, polyps, submucous myomas) and tubal obstruction. Oil-based (versus water-soluble) contrast media may improve pregnancy rates, but reports of complications using oil-based media resulted in a decrease in its usage. Women who have had prior pelvic inflammation should receive doxycycline, 100 mg orally twice daily, beginning immediately before and for 7 days after the radiographic study. IVF is recommended

as the primary treatment option for tubal disease. Surgery can be considered in women with mild tubal disease, but no rigorous research has evaluated surgical outcomes compared to IVF or expectant management.

3. Absent or infrequent ovulation requires additional laboratory evaluation. Elevated FSH and LH levels and low estradiol levels indicate ovarian insufficiency. Elevated LH levels in the presence of normal FSH levels may indicate the presence of polycystic ovaries. Elevation of blood prolactin (PRL) levels suggests a pituitary adenoma. In women over age 35, **ovarian reserve** should be assessed. A markedly elevated FSH (greater than 15–20 international units/L) on day 3 of the menstrual cycle suggests inadequate ovarian reserve. Although less widely used clinically, a Clomiphene Citrate Challenge Test, with measurement of FSH on day 10 after administration of clomiphene from days 5–9, can help confirm a diagnosis of diminished ovarian reserve. The number of antral follicles during the early follicular phase of the cycle can provide useful information about ovarian reserve and can confirm serum testing. Antimüllerian hormone can be used as part of the assessment of ovarian reserve. Unlike FSH, it can be measured at any time during the menstrual cycle and is less likely to be affected by hormones.

4. If all the above testing is normal, **unexplained infertility** is diagnosed. In approximately 25% of women whose basic evaluation is normal, the first-line therapy is usually controlled ovarian hyperstimulation (usually clomiphene citrate) and intrauterine insemination. IVF may be recommended as second-line therapy.

► Treatment

A. Medical Measures

Fertility may be restored by treatment of endocrine abnormalities, particularly hypothyroidism or hyperthyroidism. Women who are anovulatory as a result of low body weight or exercise may become ovulatory when they gain weight or decrease their exercise levels.

B. Surgical Measures

Excision of ovarian tumors or ovarian foci of endometriosis can improve fertility. Microsurgical relief of tubal obstruction due to salpingitis or tubal ligation will reestablish fertility in a significant number of cases, although with severe disease or proximal obstruction, IVF is preferable. Peritubal adhesions or endometriotic implants often can be treated via laparoscopy.

In a male with a varicocele, sperm characteristics may be improved following surgical treatment. For men who have sperm production but obstructive azoospermia, transepidermal sperm aspiration or microsurgical epidermal sperm aspiration has been successful.

C. Induction of Ovulation

1. Clomiphene citrate—Clomiphene citrate stimulates gonadotropin release, especially FSH. It acts as a selective estrogen receptor modulator, similar to tamoxifen and raloxifene, and binds to the estrogen receptor. The body perceives a low level of estrogen, decreasing the negative feedback on the hypothalamus, and there is an increased release of FSH and LH. When FSH and LH are present in the appropriate amounts and timing, ovulation occurs.

After a normal menstrual period or induction of withdrawal bleeding with progestin, 50 mg of clomiphene orally daily for 5 days, typically on days 3–7 of the cycle, should be given. If ovulation does not occur, the dosage is increased to 100 mg daily for 5 days. If ovulation still does not occur, the course is repeated with 150 mg daily and then 200 mg daily for 5 days. The maximum dosage is 200 mg. Ovulation and appropriate timing of intercourse can be facilitated with the addition of chorionic gonadotropin, 10,000 units intramuscularly. Monitoring of the follicles by transvaginal ultrasound usually is necessary to appropriately time the hCG injection. The rate of ovulation following this treatment is 90% in the absence of other infertility factors. The pregnancy rate is high. Twinning occurs in 5% of these patients, and three or more fetuses are found in rare instances (less than 0.5% of cases). Pregnancy is most likely to occur within the first three ovulatory cycles, and unlikely to occur after cycle six. In addition, several studies have suggested a twofold to threefold increased risk of ovarian cancer with the use of clomiphene for more than 1 year, so treatment with clomiphene is usually limited to a maximum of six cycles.

In the presence of increased androgen production (DHEA-S greater than 200 mcg/dL), the addition of dexamethasone, 0.5 mg orally, or prednisone, 5 mg orally, at bedtime, improves the response to clomiphene in selected patients. Dexamethasone should be discontinued after pregnancy is confirmed.

2. Letrozole—The aromatase inhibitor, letrozole, appears to be at least as effective as clomiphene for ovulation induction in women with PCOS. There is a reduced risk of multiple pregnancy, a lack of antiestrogenic effects, and a reduced need for ultrasound monitoring. The dose is 5–7.5 mg daily, starting on day 3 of the menstrual cycle. In women who have a history of estrogen dependent tumors, such as breast cancer, letrozole is preferred since the estrogen levels with this medication are much lower.

3. Cabergoline or bromocriptine—Cabergoline or bromocriptine is used only if PRL levels are elevated and there is no withdrawal bleeding following progesterone administration (otherwise, clomiphene is used). The initial dosage is 2.5 mg orally once daily, increased to 2.5 mg two or three times daily by 1.25 mg increments of cabergoline. The medication is discontinued once pregnancy occurs. Cabergoline causes fewer adverse effects than bromocriptine. However, it is much more expensive. Cabergoline is often used in patients who cannot tolerate the adverse effects of bromocriptine or who do not respond to bromocriptine.

4. Human menopausal gonadotropins (hMG) or recombinant FSH—hMG or recombinant FSH is indicated in cases of hypogonadotropism and most other types of anovulation resistant to clomiphene treatment. Because of the complexities, laboratory tests, and expense associated with this treatment, these patients should be referred to an infertility specialist.

D. Treatment of Endometriosis

See above.

E. Artificial Insemination in Azoospermia

If azoospermia is present, artificial insemination by a donor usually results in pregnancy, assuming female function is normal. The use of frozen sperm provides the opportunity for screening for sexually transmitted diseases, including HIV infection.

F. Assisted Reproductive Technology (ART)

Couples who have not responded to traditional infertility treatments, including those with tubal disease, severe endometriosis, oligospermia, and immunologic or unexplained infertility, may benefit from IVF. Gamete intrafallopian transfer and zygote intrafallopian transfer are rarely performed, although they may be an option in a few selected patients. These techniques are complex and require a highly organized team of specialists. All ART procedures involve ovarian stimulation to produce multiple oocytes, oocyte retrieval by transvaginal sonography–guided needle aspiration, and handling of the oocytes outside the body. With IVF, the eggs are fertilized in vitro and the embryos transferred to the uterus. ICSI allows fertilization with a single sperm. While originally intended for couples with male factor infertility, it is now used in two-thirds of all IVF procedures in the United States.

The chance of a multiple gestation pregnancy (ie, twins, triplets) is increased in all assisted reproductive procedures, increasing the risk of preterm delivery and other pregnancy complications. To minimize this risk, most infertility specialists recommend transferring only one embryo in appropriately selected patients with a favorable prognosis. In women with prior failed IVF cycles who are over the age of 40 who have poor embryo quality, up to 4 embryos may be transferred. In the event of a multiple gestation pregnancy, a couple may consider selective reduction to avoid the medical issues generally related to multiple births. This issue should be discussed with the couple *before* embryo transfer.

▶ Prognosis

The prognosis for conception and normal pregnancy is good if minor (even multiple) disorders can be identified and treated; it is poor if the causes of infertility are severe, untreatable, or of prolonged duration (over 3 years).

It is important to remember that in the absence of identifiable causes of infertility, 60% of couples will achieve a pregnancy within 3 years. Couples with unexplained infertility who do not achieve pregnancy within 3 years may be offered ovulation induction or assisted reproductive technology. Women over the age of 35 should be offered a more aggressive approach, with consideration of ART within 3–6 months of not achieving pregnancy with more conservative approaches. Also, offering appropriately timed information about adoption is considered part of a complete infertility regimen.

▶ When to Refer

Refer to reproductive endocrinologist if ART is indicated, or surgery is required.

Chua SJ et al. Surgery for tubal infertility. Cochrane Database Syst Rev. 2017 Jan 23;1:CD006415. [PMID: 28112384]

Gunn DD et al. Evidence-based approach to unexplained infertility: a systematic review. Fertil Steril. 2016 Jun;105(6):1566–74.e1. [PMID: 26902860]

Hanson B et al. Female infertility, infertility-associated diagnoses, and comorbidities: a review. J Assist Reprod Genet. 2017 Feb;34(2):167–77. [PMID: 27817040]

Jeelani R et al. Imaging and the infertility evaluation. Clin Obstet Gynecol. 2017 Mar;60(1):93–107. [PMID: 28106643]

CONTRACEPTION

Unintended pregnancies are a worldwide problem but disproportionately impact developing countries. Studies estimate that 40% of the 213 million pregnancies that occurred in 2012 were unintended. Globally, 50% ended in abortion, 13% ended in miscarriage, and 38% resulted in an unplanned birth. It is important for primary care providers to educate their patients about the benefits of contraception and to provide options that are appropriate and desirable for the patient.

1. Oral Contraceptives

A. Combined Oral Contraceptives

1. Efficacy and methods of use—Combined oral contraceptives have a perfect use failure rate of 0.3% and a typical use failure rate of 8%. Their primary mode of action is suppression of ovulation. The pills can be initially started on the first day of the menstrual cycle, the first Sunday after the onset of the cycle or on any day of the cycle. If started on any day other than the first day of the cycle, a backup method should be used. If an active pill is missed at any time, and no intercourse occurred in the past 5 days, two pills should be taken immediately and a backup method should be used for 7 days. If intercourse occurred in the previous 5 days, emergency contraception should be used immediately, and the pills restarted the following day. A backup method should be used for 5 days.

2. Benefits of oral contraceptives—Noncontraceptive benefits of oral contraceptives include lighter menses and improvement of dysmenorrhea symptoms, decreased risk of ovarian and endometrial cancer, and improvement in acne. Functional ovarian cysts are less likely with oral contraceptive use. The frequency of developing myomas is lower in patients who have taken oral contraceptives for longer than 4 years. There is also a beneficial effect on bone mass.

3. Selection of an oral contraceptive—Any of the combination oral contraceptives containing 35 mcg or less of ethinyl estradiol or 3 mg of estradiol valerate are suitable for most women. There is some variation in potency of the various progestins in the pills, but there are essentially no clinically significant differences for most women among the progestins in the low-dose pills. The available evidence is insufficient to determine whether triphasic oral contraceptives differ from monophasic oral contraceptives in effectiveness, bleeding patterns or discontinuation rates. Therefore, monophasic pills are recommended as a first choice for women starting oral contraceptive use. Women who have acne or hirsutism may benefit from treatment with desogestrel, drospirenone, or norgestimate, since they are the least androgenic. A combination regimen with 84 active and 7 inert pills that results in only four withdrawal bleeds per year is available. There is also a combination regimen that is taken continuously with withdrawal bleed. At the end of 1 years' use, 58% of the women had amenorrhea, and nearly 80% reported no bleeding requiring sanitary protection. Studies have not shown any significant risk from long-term amenorrhea in patients taking continuous oral contraceptives. The low-dose oral contraceptives commonly used in the United States are listed in Table 18–3.

4. Drug interactions—Several medications interact with oral contraceptives to decrease their efficacy by causing induction of microsomal enzymes in the liver, or by other mechanisms. Some commonly prescribed medications in this category are phenytoin, phenobarbital (and other barbiturates), primidone, topiramate, carbamazepine, and rifampin and St. John's Wort. Women taking these medications should use another means of contraception for maximum safety.

Antiretroviral medications, specifically ritonavir-boosted protease inhibitors, may significantly decrease the efficacy of combined oral contraceptives. Non-nucleoside reverse transcriptase inhibitors have smaller effects on oral contraceptive efficacy.

5. Contraindications and adverse effects—Oral contraceptives have been associated with many adverse effects; they are contraindicated with some conditions and should be used with caution in others (Table 18–4).

A. MYOCARDIAL INFARCTION—The risk of heart attack is higher with use of oral contraceptives, particularly with pills containing 50 mcg of estrogen or more. Cigarette smoking, obesity, hypertension, diabetes, or hypercholesterolemia increases the risk. Young nonsmoking women have minimal increased risk. Smokers over age 35 and women with other cardiovascular risk factors should use other non-estrogen–containing methods of birth control.

B. THROMBOEMBOLIC DISEASE—An increased rate of venous thromboembolism is found in oral contraceptive users, especially if the dose of estrogen is 50 mcg or more. While the overall risk is very low (5–6 per 100,000 woman-years compared to 50–300 per 100,000 pregnancies), several studies have reported a twofold increased risk in women using oral contraceptives containing the progestins gestodene (not available in the United States), drospirenone, or desogestrel compared with women using oral contraceptives with levonorgestrel and norethindrone. Women in whom thrombophlebitis develops should stop using this method, as should those at increased risk for thrombophlebitis because of surgery, fracture, serious injury, hypercoagulable condition, or immobilization. Women with a known thrombophilia should not use estrogen-containing contraceptives.

Table 18–3. Commonly used low-dose oral contraceptives (listed within each group in order of increasing estrogen dose).

Name	Progestin	Estrogen (Ethinyl Estradiol)	Cost per Month[1]
Combination			
Alesse[2,3]	0.1 mg levonorgestrel	20 mcg	$35.16
Loestrin 1/20[2]	1 mg norethindrone acetate	20 mcg	$28.65
Mircette[2]	0.15 mg desogestrel	20 mcg	$59.98
Yaz[2]	3 mg drospirenone	20 mcg	$70.84
Loestrin 21 1.5/30[2]	1.5 mg norethindrone acetate	30 mcg	$38.64
LoOvral[2]	0.3 mg norgestrel	30 mcg	$30.52
Levora[2]	0.15 mg levonorgestrel	30 mcg	$30.91
Desogen[2]	0.15 mg desogestrel	30 mcg	$35.28
Yasmin[2]	3 mg drospirenone	30 mcg	$76.72
Brevicon[2], Modicon[2]	0.5 mg norethindrone	35 mcg	$32.20
Demulen 1/35[2]	1 mg ethynodiol diacetate	35 mcg	$29.96
Ortho-Novum 1/35[2]	1 mg norethindrone	35 mcg	$29.49
Ortho-Cyclen[2]	0.25 mg norgestimate	35 mcg	$32.23
Gildagia[2]	0.4 mg norethindrone	35 mcg	$44.84
Combination: Extended-Cycle			
LoSeasonique (91-day cycle)[2]	0.10 mg levonorgestrel (days 1–84)/0 mg levonorgestrel (days 85–91)	20 mcg (84 days)/10 mcg (7 days)	$88.50
Amethyst (28-day pack)	90 mcg levonorgestrel	20 mcg	$63.60
Seasonique (91-day cycle)[2]	0.15 mg levonorgestrel (days 1–84)/0 mg levonorgestrel (days 85–91)	30 mcg (84 days)/10 mcg (7 days)	$88.50
Triphasic			
Estrostep[2]	1 mg norethindrone acetate (days 1–5) 1 mg norethindrone acetate (days 6–12) 1 mg norethindrone acetate (days 13–21)	20 mcg 30 mcg 35 mcg	$203.28
Cyclessa[2]	0.1 mg desogestrel (days 1–7) 0.125 mg desogestrel (days 8–14) 0.15 mg desogestrel (days 15–21)	25 mcg	$33.64
Ortho-Tri-Cyclen Lo	0.18 norgestimate (days 1–7) 0.215 norgestimate (days 8–14) 0.25 norgestimate (days 15–21)	25 mcg	$61.60
Trivora[2,3]	0.05 mg levonorgestrel (days 1–6) 0.075 mg levonorgestrel (days 7–11) 0.125 mg levonorgestrel (days 12–21)	30 mcg 40 mcg 30 mcg	$27.49
Ortho-Novum 7/7/7[2,3]	0.5 mg norethindrone (days 1–7) 0.75 mg norethindrone (days 8–14) 1 mg norethindrone (days 15–21)	35 mcg	$32.20
Ortho-Tri-Cyclen[2,3]	0.18 mg norgestimate (days 1–7) 0.215 mg norgestimate (days 8–14) 0.25 mg norgestimate (days 15–21)	35 mcg	$39.31
Tri-Norinyl[2,3]	0.5 mg norethindrone (days 1–7) 1 mg norethindrone (days 8–16) 0.5 mg norethindrone (days 17–21)	35 mcg	$39.35
Progestin-Only Minipill			
Ortho Micronor[2,3]	0.35 mg norethindrone to be taken continuously	None	$39.60

[1]Average wholesale price (AWP, for AB-rated generic when available) for quantity listed. Source: IBM Micromedex Redbook (electronic version), IBM Watson Health, Greenwood Village, CO, USA. Available at https://www.micromedexsolutions.com (cited April 25, 2019). AWP may not accurately represent the actual pharmacy cost because wide contractual variations exist among institutions.
[2]Generic equivalent available.
[3]Multiple other brands available.

Table 18–4. Contraindications to use of oral contraceptives.

Absolute contraindications
Pregnancy
Thrombophlebitis or thromboembolic disorders (past or present)
Stroke or coronary artery disease (past or present)
Cancer of the breast (known or suspected)
Undiagnosed abnormal vaginal bleeding
Estrogen-dependent cancer (known or suspected)
Hepatocellular adenoma (past or present)
Uncontrolled hypertension
Diabetes mellitus with vascular disease
Age over 35 and smoking > 15 cigarettes daily
Known thrombophilia
Migraine with aura
Active hepatitis
Surgery or orthopedic injury requiring prolonged immobilization
Relative contraindications
Migraine without aura
Hypertension
Heart or kidney disease
Diabetes mellitus
Gallbladder disease
Cholestasis during pregnancy
Sickle cell disease (S/S or S/C type)
Lactation

C. CEREBROVASCULAR DISEASE—Overall, a small increased risk of hemorrhagic stroke and subarachnoid hemorrhage and a somewhat greater increased risk of thrombotic stroke have been found; smoking, hypertension, and age over 35 years are associated with increased risk. Women should stop using estrogen-containing contraceptives if such warning symptoms as severe headache, blurred or lost vision, or other transient neurologic disorders develop.

D. CARCINOMA—There is no increased risk of breast cancer in women aged 35–64 who are current or former users of oral contraceptives. Women with a family history of breast cancer or women who started oral contraceptive use at a young age are not at increased risk. Combination oral contraceptives reduce the risk of endometrial carcinoma by 40% after 2 years of use and 60% after 4 or more years of use. The risk of ovarian cancer is reduced by 30% with pill use for less than 4 years, by 60% with use for 5–11 years, and by 80% after 12 or more years. Oral contraceptives have been associated with the development of benign hepatocellular adenomas and peliosis hepatis (blood-filled cavities) (but not focal nodular hyperplasia or hepatocellular carcinoma); hepatocellular adenomas may rarely cause rupture of the liver, hemorrhage, and death. The risk of hepatocellular adenoma increases with higher dosage, longer duration of use, and older age.

E. HYPERTENSION—Oral contraceptives may cause hypertension in some women; the risk is increased with longer duration of use and older age. Women in whom hypertension develops while using oral contraceptives should use other non-estrogen–containing contraceptive methods.

However, with regular blood pressure monitoring, non-smoking women with well-controlled mild hypertension may use oral contraceptives.

F. HEADACHE—Migraine or other vascular headaches may occur or worsen with pill use. If severe or frequent headaches develop while using this method, it should be discontinued. Women with migraine headaches *with an aura* should not use oral contraceptives.

G. LACTATION—Combined oral contraceptives can impair the quantity and quality of breast milk. While it is preferable to avoid the use of combination oral contraceptives during lactation, the effects on milk quality are small and are not associated with developmental abnormalities in infants. Combination oral contraceptives should be started no earlier than 6 weeks postpartum to allow for establishment of lactation. Progestin-only pills, levonorgestrel implants, and DMPA are alternatives with no adverse effects on milk quality.

H. OTHER DISORDERS—Depression may occur or be worsened with oral contraceptive use. Fluid retention may occur. Patients who had cholestatic jaundice during pregnancy may develop it while taking birth control pills.

I. OBESITY—Obese and overweight women have generally been excluded from oral contraceptive trials until recently, and some studies have suggested that oral contraceptives are less effective in overweight women. In addition, obesity is a risk factor for thromboembolic complications. It is important that obese women are not denied effective contraception as a result of concerns about complications or efficacy of oral contraceptives. Alternatives, including progestin only injections, implants, or intrauterine devices, should be considered as first options instead of oral contraceptives.

6. Minor side effects—Nausea and dizziness may occur in the first few months of pill use. A weight gain of 2–5 lb (0.9–2.25 kg) commonly occurs. Spotting or breakthrough bleeding between menstrual periods may occur, especially if a pill is skipped or taken late; this may be helped by switching to a pill of slightly greater potency (see section 3, above). Missed menstrual periods may occur, especially with low-dose pills. A pregnancy test should be performed if pills have been skipped or if two or more expected menstrual periods are missed. Fatigue and decreased libido can occur. Chloasma may occur, as in pregnancy, and is increased by exposure to sunlight.

B. Progestin Minipill

1. Efficacy and methods of use—A formulation containing 0.35 mg of norethindrone alone is available in the United States. The efficacy is similar to that of combined oral contraceptives but is highly dependent on consistent use (eg, taking the pill within the same 3-hour window every day). The minipill is believed to prevent conception by causing thickening of the cervical mucus to make it hostile to sperm, by causing alteration of ovum transport (which may account for the slightly higher rate of ectopic pregnancy with these pills), and by causing inhibition of implantation. Ovulation is inhibited inconsistently with this method. The minipill is begun on the first day of a menstrual cycle and then taken continuously for as long as contraception is desired; there is no "placebo week."

2. Advantages—The low dose of progestin and absence of estrogen make the minipill safe during lactation; it may increase the flow of milk. It is often tried by women who want minimal doses of hormones and by patients who are over age 35. The minipill lacks the cardiovascular side effects of combination pills. It can be safely used by women with sickle cell disease (S/S or S/C).

3. Complications and contraindications—Minipill users often have bleeding irregularities (eg, prolonged flow, spotting, or amenorrhea); such patients may need regular pregnancy tests. Ectopic pregnancies are more frequent, and complaints of abdominal pain should be investigated with this in mind. Many of the absolute contraindications and relative contraindications listed in Table 18–4 apply to the minipill; however, the contraceptive benefit of the minipill may outweigh the risks for patients who smoke, who are over age 35, or who have such conditions as superficial or deep venous thrombosis or known thromboembolic disorders or diabetes with vascular disease. Minor side effects of combination oral contraceptives such as weight gain and mild headache may also occur with the minipill.

Brown EJ et al. Contraception update: oral contraception. FP Essent. 2017 Nov;462:11–9. [PMID: 29172411]

Curtis KM et al. U.S. medical eligibility criteria for contraceptive use, 2016. MMWR Recomm Rep. 2016 Jul 29;65(3):1–103. [PMID: 27467196]

Curtis KM et al. U.S. selected practice recommendations for contraceptive use, 2016 MMWR Recomm Rep. 2016 Jul 29; 65(4):1–66. [PMID: 27467319]

Golobof A et al. The current status of oral contraceptives: progress and recent innovations. Semin Reprod Med. 2016 May; 34(3):145–51. [PMID: 26960906]

2. Contraceptive Injections & Implants (Long-Acting Progestins)

The injectable progestin **DMPA** is approved for contraceptive use in the United States. There has been extensive worldwide experience with this method over the past 3 decades. The medication is given as a deep intramuscular injection of 150 mg every 3 months and has a contraceptive efficacy of 99.7%. Common side effects include irregular bleeding, amenorrhea, weight gain, and headache. It is associated with bone mineral loss that is reversible after discontinuation of the method. Users commonly have irregular bleeding initially and subsequently develop amenorrhea. Ovulation may be delayed after the discontinuation. Contraindications are similar to those for the minipill.

A single-rod, subdermal progestin implant, etonogestrel subdermal (**Nexplanon**), is approved for use in the United States. Nexplanon is a 40-mm by 2-mm rod containing 68 mg of the progestin etonogestrel that is inserted in the inner aspect of the nondominant arm and remains effective for 3 years. Hormone levels drop rapidly after removal, and there is no delay in the return of fertility. In clinical trials, the pregnancy rate was 0.0% with 3 years of use. The side effect profile is similar to minipills, and DMPA. Irregular bleeding has been the most common reason for discontinuation. Both the American College of Obstetricians and Gynecologists and the American Academy of Pediatrics have recommended that adolescents should be encouraged to consider long-acting reversible contraception methods. In a large prospective study, a 75% reduction in unintended pregnancy was demonstrated with the use of long-acting reversible contraception.

American College of Obstetricians and Gynecologists. Committee Opinion No. 670: Immediate postpartum long-acting reversible contraception. Obstet Gynecol. 2016 Aug; 128(2):e32–7. [PMID: 27454734]

American College of Obstetricians and Gynecologists. Practice Bulletin No. 186: Long-acting reversible contraception: implants and intrauterine devices. Obstet Gynecol. 2017 Nov; 130(5):e251–69. [PMID: 29064972]

Deshmukh P et al. Contraception update: progestin-only implants and injections. FP Essent. 2017 Nov;462:25–9. [PMID: 29172413]

Dragoman MV et al. The safety of subcutaneously administered depot medroxyprogesterone acetate (104 mg/0.65 mL): a systematic review. Contraception. 2016 Sep;94(3):202–15. [PMID: 26874275]

Hubacher D et al. Long-acting reversible contraceptive acceptability and unintended pregnancy among women presenting for short-acting methods: a randomized patient preference trial. Am J Obstet Gynecol. 2017 Feb;216(2):101–9. [PMID: 27662799]

Sothornwit J et al. Immediate versus delayed postpartum insertion of contraceptive implant for contraception. Cochrane Database Syst Rev. 2017 Apr 22;4:CD011913. [PMID: 28432791]

Turok DK et al. New developments in long-acting reversible contraception: the promise of intrauterine devices and implants to improve family planning services. Fertil Steril. 2016 Nov;106(6):1273–81. [PMID: 27717553]

3. Other Hormonal Methods

A **transdermal contraceptive patch** containing norelgestromin (150 mcg) and ethinyl estradiol (20 mcg) and measuring 20 cm^2 is available. The patch is applied to the lower abdomen, upper torso, or buttock once a week for 3 consecutive weeks, followed by 1 week without the patch. It appears that the average steady-state concentration of ethinyl estradiol with the patch is approximately 60% higher than with a 35-mcg pill. However, there is currently no evidence for an increased incidence of estrogen-related side effects. The mechanism of action, side effects, and efficacy are similar to those associated with oral contraceptives, although compliance may be better. However, discontinuation for side effects is more frequent.

A **contraceptive vaginal ring** that releases 120 mcg of etonogestrel and 15 mcg of ethinyl estradiol daily is available. The ring is soft and flexible and is placed in the upper vagina for 3 weeks, removed, and replaced 1 week later, or can be removed and replaced after 4 weeks for continuous cycling, similar to oral contraceptives. The efficacy, mechanism of action, and systemic side effects are similar to those associated with oral contraceptives. Ring users may experience an increased incidence of vaginal discharge.

4. Intrauterine Devices

In the United States, the following devices are available: the levonorgestrel-releasing **Mirena, Liletta,** and **Skyla** IUDs and the copper-bearing **TCu380A.** The mechanism of action of the copper IUD is thought to involve either spermicidal or inhibitory effects on sperm capacitation and transport. The levonorgestrel-containing IUDs also cause thickening of cervical mucus, prevent endometrial thickening, and can inhibit ovulation. IUDs are not abortifacients.

Skyla and Liletta are FDA approved for 3 years, Mirena for 5 years, and the TCu380A for 10 years. The hormone-containing IUDs have the advantage of reducing cramping and menstrual flow.

The IUD is an excellent contraceptive method for most women. The devices are highly effective, with failure rates similar to those achieved with surgical sterilization. Nulliparity is not a contraindication to IUD use. Adolescents are also candidates for IUD use. Women who are not in mutually monogamous relationships should use condoms for protection from sexually transmitted diseases. Levonorgestrel-containing IUDs may have a protective effect against upper tract infection similar to that of the oral contraceptives.

A. Insertion

Insertion can be performed during or after the menses, at midcycle to prevent implantation, or later in the cycle if the patient has not become pregnant. There is growing evidence to suggest that IUDs can be safely inserted in the immediate postabortal and postpartum periods.

Both types of IUDs (levonorgestrel-releasing and copper bearing) may be inserted up to 48 hours after vaginal delivery, or prior to closure of the uterus at the time of cesarean section. Insertion immediately following abortion is acceptable if there is no sepsis and if follow-up insertion a month later will not be possible; otherwise, it is wise to wait until 4 weeks' postabortion. Misoprostol and NSAIDs given as premedications may help insertions in nulliparous patients or when insertion is not performed during menses.

B. Contraindications and Complications

Contraindications to use of IUDs are outlined in Table 18–5.

1. Pregnancy—A copper-containing IUD can be inserted within 5 days following a single episode of unprotected midcycle coitus as a **postcoital contraceptive**. An IUD should not be inserted into a pregnant uterus. If pregnancy occurs as an IUD failure, there is a greater chance of spontaneous abortion if the IUD is left in situ (50%) than if it is removed (25%). Spontaneous abortion with an IUD in place is associated with a high risk of severe sepsis, and death can occur rapidly. Women using an IUD who become pregnant should have the IUD removed if the string is visible. It can be removed at the time of abortion if that is desired. If the string is not visible and the patient wants to continue the pregnancy, she should be informed

Table 18–5. Contraindications to IUD use.

Absolute contraindications
Pregnancy
Acute or subacute pelvic inflammatory disease or purulent cervicitis
Significant anatomic abnormality of uterus
Unexplained uterine bleeding
Active liver disease (Mirena only)
Relative contraindications
History of pelvic inflammatory disease since the last pregnancy
Lack of available follow-up care
Menorrhagia or severe dysmenorrhea (copper IUD)
Cervical or uterine neoplasia

IUD, intrauterine device.

of the serious risk of sepsis and, occasionally, death with such pregnancies. She should be informed that any flu-like symptoms such as fever, myalgia, headache, or nausea warrant immediate medical attention for possible septic abortion.

Since the ratio of ectopic to intrauterine pregnancies is increased among IUD users, clinicians should search for adnexal masses in early pregnancy and should always check the products of conception for placental tissue following abortion.

2. Pelvic infection—There is an increased risk of pelvic infection during the first month following insertion; however, prophylactic antibiotics given at the time of insertion do not appear to decrease this risk. The subsequent risk of pelvic infection appears to be primarily related to the risk of acquiring sexually transmitted infections. Infertility rates do not appear to be increased among women who have previously used the currently available IUDs. At the time of insertion, women with an increased risk of sexually transmitted diseases should be screened for gonorrhea and *Chlamydia*. Women with a history of recent or recurrent pelvic infection are not good candidates for IUD use.

3. Menorrhagia or severe dysmenorrhea—The copper IUD can cause heavier menstrual periods, bleeding between periods, and more cramping, so it is generally not suitable for women who already suffer from these problems. Alternatively, the hormone-releasing IUD Mirena has been approved by the FDA to treat heavy menstrual bleeding. NSAIDs are also helpful in decreasing bleeding and pain in IUD users.

4. Complete or partial expulsion—Spontaneous expulsion of the IUD occurs in 10–20% of cases during the first year of use. Any IUD should be removed if the body of the device can be seen or felt in the cervical os.

5. Missing IUD strings—If the transcervical tail cannot be seen, this may signify unnoticed expulsion, perforation of the uterus with abdominal migration of the IUD, or simply retraction of the string into the cervical canal or uterus owing to movement of the IUD or uterine growth with pregnancy. Once pregnancy is ruled out, a cervical speculum may be used to visualize the IUD string in the cervical canal. If not visualized, one should probe for the IUD with a sterile sound or forceps designed for IUD removal after administering a paracervical block. If the IUD cannot be detected, pelvic ultrasound will demonstrate the IUD if it is in the uterus. Alternatively, obtain anteroposterior and lateral radiographs of the pelvis with another IUD or a sound in the uterus as a marker to confirm an extrauterine IUD. If the IUD is in the abdominal cavity, it should generally be removed by laparoscopy or laparotomy. Perforations of the uterus are less likely if insertion is performed slowly, with meticulous care taken to follow directions applicable to each type of IUD.

American College of Obstetricians and Gynecologists. Committee Opinion No. 670: Immediate postpartum long-acting reversible contraception. Obstet Gynecol. 2016 Aug;128(2): e32–7. [PMID: 27454734]

American College of Obstetricians and Gynecologists. Practice Bulletin No. 186: Long-acting reversible contraception: implants and intrauterine devices. Obstet Gynecol. 2017 Nov; 130(5):e251–69. [PMID: 29064972]

Lopez LM et al. Immediate postpartum insertion of intrauterine device for contraception. Cochrane Database Syst Rev. 2015 Jun 26;6:CD003036. [PMID: 26115018]

Moniz MH et al. Inpatient postpartum long-acting reversible contraception and sterilization in the United States, 2008–2013. Obstet Gynecol. 2017 Jun;129(6):1078–85. [PMID: 28486357]

5. Diaphragm & Cervical Cap

The **diaphragm (with contraceptive jelly)** is a safe and effective contraceptive method with features that make it acceptable to some women and not others. Failure rates range from 6% to 16%, depending on the motivation of the woman and the care with which the diaphragm is used. The advantages of this method are that it has no systemic side effects and gives significant protection against pelvic infection and cervical dysplasia as well as pregnancy. The disadvantages are that it must be inserted near the time of coitus and that pressure from the rim predisposes some women to cystitis after intercourse.

The **cervical cap (with contraceptive jelly)** is similar to the diaphragm but fits snugly over the cervix only (the diaphragm stretches from behind the cervix to behind the pubic symphysis). The cervical cap is more difficult to insert and remove than the diaphragm. The main advantages are that it can be used by women who cannot be fitted for a diaphragm because of a relaxed anterior vaginal wall or by women who have discomfort or develop repeated bladder infections with the diaphragm. However, failure rates are 9% (perfect use) and 16% (typical use) in nulliparous women and 26% (perfect use) and 32% (typical use) in parous women.

Because of the small risk of toxic shock syndrome, a cervical cap or diaphragm should not be left in the vagina for over 12–18 hours, nor should these devices be used during the menstrual period.

6. Contraceptive Foam, Cream, Film, Sponge, Jelly, & Suppository

These products are available without prescription, are easy to use, and have typical failure rates of 10–22%. All contain the spermicide nonoxynol-9, which also has some

virucidal and bactericidal activity. Nonoxynol-9 does not appear to adversely affect the vaginal colonization of hydrogen peroxide–producing lactobacilli. The FDA requires products containing nonoxynol-9 to include a warning that the products do not protect against HIV or other sexually transmitted diseases and that use of these products can irritate the vagina and rectum and may increase the risk of getting the AIDS virus from an infected partner. Low-risk women using a nonoxynol-9 product, with coital activity two to three times per week, are not at increased risk for epithelial disruption, compared with couples using condoms alone.

7. Condom

The male condom of latex, polyurethane or animal membrane affords protection against pregnancy—equivalent to that of a diaphragm and spermicidal jelly; latex and polyurethane (but not animal membrane) condoms also offer protection against many sexually transmitted diseases, including HIV. When a spermicide, such as vaginal foam, is used with the condom, the failure rate (approximately 2% with perfect use and 15% with typical use) approaches that of oral contraceptives. The disadvantages of condoms are dulling of sensation and spillage of semen due to tearing, slipping, or leakage with detumescence of the penis.

Two female condoms, one made of polyurethane and the other of synthetic nitrile, are available in the United States. The reported failure rates range from 5% to 21%; the efficacy is comparable to that of the diaphragm. These are the only female-controlled method that offers significant protection from both pregnancy and sexually transmitted diseases.

8. Contraception Based on Awareness of Fertile Periods

These methods are most effective when the couple restricts intercourse to the post-ovular phase of the cycle or uses a barrier method at other times. Well-instructed, motivated couples may be able to achieve low pregnancy rates with fertility awareness methods. However, properly done randomized clinical trials comparing the efficacy of most of these methods with other contraceptive methods do not exist.

9. Emergency Contraception

If unprotected intercourse occurs in midcycle and if the woman is certain she has not inadvertently become pregnant earlier in the cycle, the following regimens are effective in preventing implantation. These methods should be started as soon as possible and within 120 hours after unprotected coitus. (1) Levonorgestrel, 1.5 mg orally as a single dose (available in the United States prepackaged as Plan B and available over-the-counter for women aged 17 years and older), has a 1% failure rate when taken within 72 hours. It remains efficacious up to 120 hours after intercourse, though less so compared with earlier use. (2) If the levonorgestrel regimen is not available, a combination oral contraceptive containing ethinyl estradiol and levonorgestrel given twice in 12 hours may be used. At least 20 brands of pills may be used in this way. For specific dosages and instructions for each pill brand, consult "not-2-late" at http://ec.princeton.edu/. Used within 72 hours, the failure rate of these regimens is approximately 3%, but antinausea medication is often necessary. (3) Ulipristal, 30 mg orally as a single dose, has been shown to be more effective than levonorgestrel, especially when used between 72 and 120 hours, particularly among overweight women. It is available by prescription in the United States and Western Europe. (4) IUD insertion within 5 days after one episode of unprotected midcycle coitus will also prevent pregnancy; copperbearing IUDs have been tested and used for many years for this purpose. All victims of sexual violence should be offered emergency contraception.

Information on clinics or individual clinicians providing emergency contraception in the United States may be obtained by calling 1-888-668-2528.

American College of Obstetricians and Gynecologists. Committee Opinion No. 707: Access to emergency contraception. Obstet Gynecol. 2017 Jul;130(1):e48–52. [PMID: 28644339]

Batur P et al. Emergency contraception. Mayo Clin Proc. 2016 Jun; 91(6):802–7. [PMID: 27261868]

Fok WK et al. Update on emergency contraception. Curr Opin Obstet Gynecol. 2016 Dec;28(6):522–9. [PMID: 27676405]

Mittal S. Emergency contraception: which is the best? Minerva Ginecol. 2016 Dec;68(6):687–99. [PMID: 27082029]

Shen J et al. Interventions for emergency contraception. Cochrane Database Syst Rev. 2019 Jan 20;1:CD001324. [PMID: 30661244]

10. Abortion

Since the legalization of abortion in the United States in 1973, the related maternal mortality rate has fallen markedly, because illegal and self-induced abortions have been replaced by safer medical procedures. Abortions in the first trimester of pregnancy are performed by vacuum aspiration under local anesthesia or with medical regimens. Dilation and evacuation, a variation of vacuum aspiration is generally used in the second trimester. Techniques utilizing intra-amniotic instillation of hypertonic saline solution or various prostaglandins regimens, along with medical or osmotic dilators are occasionally used after 18 weeks. Several medical abortion regimens utilizing mifepristone and multiple doses of misoprostol have been reported as being effective in the second trimester. Overall, legal abortion in the United States has a mortality rate of less than 1:100,000. Rates of morbidity and mortality rise with length of gestation. In the United States, more than 60% of abortions are performed before 9 weeks, and more than 90% are performed before 13 weeks' gestation; only 1.2% are performed after 20 weeks. If abortion is chosen, every effort should be made to encourage the patient to seek an early procedure. In the United States, while numerous state laws limiting access to abortion and a federal law banning a rarely used variation of dilation and evacuation have been enacted, abortion remains legal and available until fetal viability, between 24 and 28 weeks' gestation, under *Roe v. Wade*.

Complications resulting from abortion include retained products of conception (often associated with infection and heavy bleeding), uterine perforation, and unrecognized ectopic pregnancy. Immediate analysis of the removed tissue for placenta can exclude or corroborate the diagnosis of ectopic pregnancy. Women who have fever, bleeding, or abdominal pain after abortion should be examined; use of broad-spectrum antibiotics and reaspiration of the uterus are frequently necessary. Hospitalization is advisable if acute salpingitis requires intravenous administration of antibiotics. Complications following illegal abortion often need emergency care for hemorrhage, septic shock, or uterine perforation.

Prophylactic antibiotics are indicated for surgical abortion; for example, a one-dose regimen of doxycycline, 200 mg orally can be given 1 hour before the procedure. Many clinics prescribe tetracycline, 500 mg orally four times daily for 5 days after the procedure, as presumptive treatment for *Chlamydia*. Rh immune globulin should be given to all Rh-negative women following abortion. Contraception should be thoroughly discussed and contraceptive supplies or pills provided at the time of abortion. There is growing evidence to support the safety and efficacy of immediate postabortal insertion of IUDs.

Mifepristone (RU 486) is approved by the FDA as an oral abortifacient at a dose of 600 mg on day 1, followed by 400 mcg orally of misoprostol on day 3. This combination is 95% successful in terminating pregnancies of up to 9 weeks' duration with minimum complications. A more commonly used, evidence-based regimen is mifepristone, 200 mg orally on day 1, followed by misoprostol, 800 mcg vaginally either immediately or within 6–8 hours. Although not approved by the FDA for this indication, a combination of intramuscular methotrexate, 50 mg/m^2 of body surface area, followed 3–7 days later by vaginal misoprostol, 800 mcg, is 98% successful in terminating pregnancy at 8 weeks or less. Minor side effects, such as nausea, vomiting, and diarrhea, are common with these regimens. There is a 5–10% incidence of hemorrhage or incomplete abortion requiring curettage. Medical abortion is generally considered as safe as surgical abortion in the first trimester but is associated with a lower success rate (requiring surgical abortion). Overall, the risk of uterine infection is lower with medical than with surgical abortion.

Bizjak I et al. Efficacy and safety of very early medical termination of pregnancy: a cohort study. BJOG. 2017 Dec;124(13): 1993–9. [PMID: 28856829]

Mark KS et al. Risk of complication during surgical abortion in obese women. Am J Obstet Gynecol. 2018 Feb;218(2):238. e1–5. [PMID: 29074080]

Nissi R et al. Mifepristone and misoprostol is safe and effective method in the second-trimester pregnancy termination. Arch Gynecol Obstet. 2016 Nov;294(6):1243–7. [PMID: 27522599]

Soon JA et al. Medications used in evidence-based regimens for medical abortion: an overview. J Obstet Gynaecol Can. 2016 Jul; 38(7):636–45. [PMID: 27591347]

11. Sterilization

In the United States, sterilization is the most popular method of birth control for couples who want no more children. Although sterilization is reversible in some instances, reversal surgery in both men and women is costly, complicated, and not always successful. Therefore, patients should be counseled carefully before sterilization and should view the procedure as permanent.

Male sterilization by vasectomy is a safe, simple procedure in which the vas deferens is severed and sealed through a scrotal incision under local anesthesia. Long-term follow-up studies on vasectomized men show no excess risk of cardiovascular disease. Despite past controversy, there is no definite association of vasectomy with prostate cancer.

Female sterilization procedures include laparoscopic bipolar electrocoagulation, salpingectomy, or plastic ring application on the uterine tubes, minilaparotomy with tubal resection, or hysteroscopic transcervical sterilization. The advantages of laparoscopy are minimal postoperative pain, small incisions, and rapid recovery. The advantages of minilaparotomy are that it can be performed with standard surgical instruments under local or general anesthesia. However, there is more postoperative pain and a longer recovery period. The cumulative 10-year failure rate for all methods combined is 1.85%, varying from 0.75% for postpartum partial salpingectomy and laparoscopic unipolar coagulation to 3.65% for spring clips; this fact should be discussed with women preoperatively. Some studies have found an increased risk of menstrual irregularities as a long-term complication of tubal ligation, but findings in different studies have been inconsistent. A method of transcervical sterilization, Essure®, can be performed as an outpatient procedure. Essure® involves the placement of an expanding microcoil of titanium into the proximal uterine tube under hysteroscopic guidance. The efficacy rate at 1 year is 99.8%. Tubal occlusion should be confirmed at 3 months with a hysterosalpingogram.

When to Refer

Refer to experienced clinicians for etonogestrel subdermal (Nexplanon) or other subcutaneous insertion, IUD insertion, tubal occlusion or ligation, vasectomy, or therapeutic abortion.

Antell K et al. Contraception update: sterilization. FP Essent. 2017 Nov;462:30–4. [PMID: 29172414]

Bhindi B et al. The association between vasectomy and prostate cancer: a systematic review and meta-analysis. JAMA Intern Med. 2017 Sep 1;177(9):1273–86. [PMID: 28715534]

Danis RB et al. Postpartum permanent sterilization: could bilateral salpingectomy replace bilateral tubal ligation? J Minim Invasive Gynecol. 2016 Sep–Oct;23(6):928–32. [PMID: 27234430]

SEXUAL VIOLENCE

ESSENTIALS OF DIAGNOSIS

▶ The legal definition of rape varies by state and geographic location. The term "sexual violence" is used by the CDC and will be used in this discussion. It can be committed by a stranger, but more commonly by an assailant known to the victim, including a current or former partner or spouse (a form of intimate partner violence [IPV]).

▶ All victims of sexual violence should be offered emergency contraception, and counseled that this method does not induce abortion.

▶ The large number of individuals affected, the enormous health care costs, and the need for a multidisciplinary approach make sexual violence and IPV important health care issues.

▶ Knowledge of state laws and collection of evidence requirements are essential for clinicians evaluating possible victims of sexual violence, including IPV.

General Considerations

Rape, or sexual assault, is legally defined in different ways in various jurisdictions. Clinicians and emergency department personnel who deal with victims of sexual violence should be familiar with the laws pertaining to sexual assault in their own state. From a medical and psychological viewpoint, it is essential that persons treating victims of sexual violence recognize the nonconsensual and violent nature of the crime. About 95% of reported victims of sexual violence are women. Each year in the United States, 4.8 million incidents of physical or sexual assault are reported by women. Penetration may be vaginal, anal, or oral and may be by the penis, hand, or a foreign object. The absence of genital injury does not imply consent by the victim. The assailant may be unknown to the victim or, more frequently, may be an acquaintance or even the spouse.

"Unlawful sexual intercourse," or statutory rape, is intercourse with a female before the age of majority even with her consent.

Health care providers can have a significant impact in increasing the reporting of sexual violence and in identifying resources for the victims. The International Rescue Committee has developed a multimedia training tool to encourage competent, compassionate, and confidential clinical care for sexual violence survivors in low-resource settings. They studied this intervention in over 100 healthcare providers, and found knowledge and confidence in clinical care for sexual violence survivors increased from 49% to 62% ($P < 0.001$) and 58% to 73% ($P < 0.001$), respectively, following training. There was also a documented increase in eligible survivors receiving emergency contraception from 50% to 82% ($P < 0.01$), HIV postexposure prophylaxis from 42% to 92% ($P < 0.001$), and sexually transmitted infection prophylaxis and treatment from 45% to 96% ($P < 0.01$). This training encourages providers to offer care in the areas of pregnancy and sexually transmitted infection prevention as well as assistance for psychological trauma.

Because sexual violence is a personal crisis, each patient will react differently, but anxiety disorders and posttraumatic stress disorder (PTSD) are common sequelae. The **rape trauma syndrome** comprises two principal phases. (1) Immediate or acute: Shaking, sobbing, and restless activity may last from a few days to a few weeks. The patient may experience anger, guilt, or shame or may repress these emotions. Reactions vary depending on the victim's personality and the circumstances of the attack. (2) Late or chronic:

Problems related to the attack may develop weeks or months later. The lifestyle and work patterns of the individual may change. Sleep disorders or phobias often develop. Loss of self-esteem can lead to suicide, albeit rarely.

Clinicians and emergency department personnel who deal with victims of sexual violence should work with community rape crisis centers or other sources of ongoing psychological support and counseling.

► General Office Procedures

The clinician who first sees the alleged victim of sexual violence should be empathetic and prepared with appropriate evidence collection and treatment materials. Standardized information and training, such as the program created by the International Rescue Committee, can be a helpful resource to the providers caring for these patients. Many emergency departments have a protocol for sexual violence victims and personnel who are trained in interviewing and examining victims of sexual violence.

► Treatment

1. Give analgesics or sedatives if indicated. Administer tetanus toxoid if deep lacerations contain soil or dirt particles.

2. Give ceftriaxone, 125 mg intramuscularly, to prevent gonorrhea. In addition, give metronidazole, 2 g as a single dose, and azithromycin 1 g orally or doxycycline 100 mg orally twice daily for 7 days to prevent chlamydial infection. Incubating syphilis will probably be prevented by these medications, but the VDRL test should be repeated 6 weeks after the assault.

3. Prevent pregnancy by using one of the methods discussed under Emergency Contraception.

4. Vaccinate against hepatitis B.

5. Offer HIV prophylaxis (see Chapter 31).

6. Because women who are sexually assaulted are at increased risk for long-term psychological sequelae, such as PTSD and anxiety disorders, it is critical that the patient and her family and friends have a source of ongoing counseling and psychological support.

► When to Refer

All women who seek care for sexual assault should be referred to a facility that has expertise in the management of victims of sexual violence and is capable of performing expert forensic examination, if requested.

American College of Obstetricians and Gynecologists. The role of obstetrician-gynecologists in supporting survivors of sexual assault, November, 2018. https://www.acog.org/-/media/Statements-of-Policy/Public/96Survivors-of-Sexual-Assault-Oct17-2018.pdf

Crawford-Jakubiak JE et al; Committee on Child Abuse and Neglect; Committee on Adolescence. Care of the adolescent after an acute sexual assault. Pediatrics. 2017 Mar;139(3). Erratum in: Pediatrics. 2017 Jun;139(6). [PMID: 28242861]

Vrees RA. Evaluation and management of female victims of sexual assault. Obstet Gynecol Surv. 2017 Jan;72(1):39–53. [PMID: 28134394]

MENOPAUSAL SYNDROME

ESSENTIALS OF DIAGNOSIS

► Menopause is a retrospective diagnosis after 12 months of amenorrhea.

► Approximately 80% of women will experience hot flushes and night sweats.

► Elevated FSH and low estradiol can help confirm the diagnosis.

► General Considerations

The term "menopause" denotes the final cessation of menstruation, either as a normal part of aging or as the result of surgical removal of both ovaries. In a broader sense, as the term is commonly used, it denotes a 1- to 3-year period during which a woman adjusts to a diminishing and then absent menstrual flow and the physiologic changes that may be associated with lowered estrogen levels—hot flushes, night sweats, and vaginal dryness.

The average age at menopause in Western societies is 51 years. Premature menopause is defined as ovarian failure and menstrual cessation before age 40; this often has a genetic or autoimmune basis. Surgical menopause due to bilateral oophorectomy is common and can cause more severe symptoms owing to the sudden rapid drop in sex hormone levels.

There is no objective evidence that cessation of ovarian function is associated with severe emotional disturbance or personality changes. However, mood changes toward depression and anxiety can occur at this time. Disruption of sleep patterns associated with the menopause can affect mood and concentration and cause fatigue. Furthermore, the time of menopause often coincides with other major life changes, such as departure of children from the home, a midlife identity crisis, or divorce.

► Clinical Findings

A. Symptoms and Signs

1. Cessation of menstruation—Menstrual cycles generally become irregular as menopause approaches. Anovular cycles occur more often, with irregular cycle length and occasional menorrhagia. Menstrual flow usually diminishes in amount owing to decreased estrogen secretion, resulting in less abundant endometrial growth. Finally, cycles become longer, with missed periods or episodes of spotting only. When no bleeding has occurred for 1 year, the menopausal transition can be said to have occurred. Any bleeding after 6 months of the cessation of menses warrants investigation by endometrial curettage or aspiration to rule out endometrial cancer.

2. Hot flushes—Hot flushes (feelings of intense heat over the trunk and face, with flushing of the skin and sweating) occur in over 80% of women as a result of the decrease in ovarian hormones. Hot flushes can begin before the cessation of menses. Menopausal vasomotor symptoms last longer than previously thought, and there are ethnic differences in the duration of symptoms. Vasomotor symptoms were found to last more than 7 years in more than 50% of the women. African-American women reported the longest duration of vasomotor symptoms. The etiology of hot flushes is unknown. Occurring at night, they often cause sweating and insomnia and result in fatigue on the following day.

3. Vaginal atrophy—With decreased estrogen secretion, thinning of the vaginal mucosa and decreased vaginal lubrication occur and may lead to dyspareunia. The introitus decreases in diameter. Pelvic examination reveals pale, smooth vaginal mucosa and a small cervix and uterus. The ovaries are not normally palpable after the menopause. Continued sexual activity will help prevent vaginal atrophy.

4. Osteoporosis—Osteoporosis may occur as a late sequela of menopause. The US Preventive Services Task Force recommends screening for osteoporosis beginning at age 65. The most recent June 2018 USPSTF recommendation summary can be found at https://www.uspreventiveservicestaskforce .org/Page/Document/UpdateSummaryFinal/osteoporosis-screening1.

B. Laboratory Findings

Serum FSH, LH, and estradiol levels are of little diagnostic value because of unpredictable variability during the menopausal transition but can provide confirmation if the FSH is elevated and the estradiol is low. Vaginal cytologic examination will show a low estrogen effect with predominantly parabasal cells, indicating lack of epithelial maturation due to hypoestrogenism.

▶ Treatment

A. Natural Menopause

Education and support from health providers, midlife discussion groups, and reading material will help most women having difficulty adjusting to the menopause. Physiologic symptoms can be treated with both hormonal or nonhormonal therapies. Hormonal replacement therapy has been shown to be effective in treating perimenopausal and menopausal symptoms but is not effective in prevention of chronic conditions such as coronary heart disease.

1. Vasomotor symptoms—For women with mild symptoms, lifestyle modification, such as increased hydration, decreased caffeine consumption, tobacco cessation, and dressing in layers are first-line therapies to be undertaken before consideration of other nonhormonal or hormonal medical treatments. For women with moderate to severe vasomotor symptoms, hormone replacement estrogen or estrogen/progestin regimens are the most effective approach to symptom relief. Conjugated estrogens, 0.3 mg, 0.45 mg, or 0.625 mg; 17-beta-estradiol, 0.5 or 1 mg; or estrone sulfate, 0.625 mg can be given once daily orally; or estradiol can be given transdermally as skin patches that are changed

once or twice weekly and secrete 0.05–0.1 mg of hormone daily. Unless the patient has undergone hysterectomy, a combination regimen of an estrogen with a progestin such as medroxyprogesterone, 1.5 or 2.5 mg, or norethindrone, 0.1, 0.25, or 0.5 mg, should be used to prevent endometrial hyperplasia or cancer. There is also a patch available containing estradiol and the progestin levonorgestrel. Oral hormones can be given in several differing regimens. Give estrogen on days 1–25 of each calendar month, with 5–10 mg of oral medroxyprogesterone acetate added on days 14–25. Withhold hormones from day 26 until the end of the month, when the endometrium will be shed, producing a light, generally painless monthly period. Alternatively, give the estrogen along with a progestin daily, without stopping. This regimen causes some initial bleeding or spotting, but within a few months it produces an atrophic endometrium that will not bleed. If the patient has had a hysterectomy, a progestin need not be used.

Postmenopausal women generally should not use combination progestin-estrogen therapy for more than 3 or 4 years (see discussion below). Women who cannot find relief with alternative approaches may wish to consider continuing use of combination therapy after a thorough discussion of the risks and benefits. Alternatives to hormone therapy for vasomotor symptoms include SSRIs such as paroxetine, 12.5 mg or 25 mg/day orally, or venlafaxine, 75 mg/day orally. Gabapentin, an antiseizure medication, is also effective at 900 mg/day orally. Clonidine given orally or transdermally, 100–150 mcg daily, may also reduce the frequency of hot flushes, but its use is limited by side effects, including dry mouth, drowsiness, and hypotension. There is some evidence that soy isoflavones may be effective in treating menopausal symptoms. Other compounds including red clover and black cohosh have not been shown to be effective. Because little is known about adverse effects, particularly with long-term use, dietary supplements should be used with caution.

2. Vaginal atrophy—A vaginal ring containing 2 mg of estradiol can be left in place for 3 months and is suitable for long-term use. Although serum estrogen level increases associated with vaginal rings are lower than other routes of administration, it is recommended that the ring be used with caution. ACOG suggests that vaginal estrogen is an option for urogenital symptoms even in breast cancer survivors. Short-term use of estrogen vaginal cream will relieve symptoms of atrophy, but because of variable absorption, therapy with either the vaginal ring or systemic hormone replacement is preferable. A low-dose estradiol tablet (10 mcg) is available and is inserted in the vagina daily for 2 weeks and then twice a week for long-term use. Testosterone propionate 1–2%, 0.5–1 g, in a vanishing cream base used in the same manner is also effective if estrogen is contraindicated. A bland lubricant such as unscented cold cream or water-soluble gel can be helpful at the time of coitus.

3. Osteoporosis—(See also discussion in Chapter 26.) Women should ingest at least 800 mg of calcium daily throughout life. Nonfat or low-fat milk products, calcium-fortified orange juice, green leafy vegetables, corn tortillas, and canned sardines or salmon consumed with the bones are good dietary sources. Vitamin D, at least 800 international units/day from food, sunlight, or supplements, is necessary to enhance calcium absorption and maintain bone mass. A daily program of energetic walking and exercise to strengthen the arms and upper body helps maintain bone mass. Screening bone densitometry is recommended for women beginning at age 65 (see Chapter 1). Women most at risk for osteoporotic fractures should consider bisphosphonates, raloxifene, or hormone replacement therapy. This includes white and Asian women, especially if they have a family history of osteoporosis, are thin, short, cigarette smokers, have a history of hyperthyroidism, use corticosteroid medications long term, or are physically inactive.

B. Risks of Hormone Therapy

Double-blind, randomized, controlled trials have shown no overall cardiovascular benefit with estrogen-progestin replacement therapy in a group of postmenopausal women with or without established coronary disease. Both in the Women's Health Initiative (WHI) trial and the Heart and Estrogen/Progestin Replacement Study (HERS), the overall health risks (increased risk of coronary heart events; strokes; thromboembolic disease; gallstones; and breast cancer, including an increased risk of mortality from breast cancer) exceeded the benefits from the long-term use of combination estrogen and progesterone. An ancillary study of the WHI study showed that not only did estrogen-progestin hormone replacement therapy not benefit cognitive function, but there was a small increased risk of cognitive decline in that group compared with women in the placebo group. The unopposed estrogen arm of the WHI trial demonstrated a decrease in the risk of hip fracture, a small but not significant decrease in breast cancer, but an increased risk of stroke and no evidence of protection from coronary heart disease. The study also showed a small increase in the combined risk of mild cognitive impairment and dementia with estrogen use compared with placebo, similar to the estrogen-progestin arm. Women who have been receiving long-term estrogen-progestin hormone replacement therapy, even in the absence of complications, should be encouraged to stop, especially if they do not have menopausal symptoms. However, the risks appear to be lower in women starting therapy at the time of menopause and higher in previously untreated women starting therapy long after menopause. Therapy should be individualized as the risk-benefit profile varies with age and individual risk factors. (See also discussions of estrogen and progestin replacement therapy in Chapter 26.)

C. Surgical Menopause

The abrupt hormonal decrease resulting from oophorectomy generally results in severe vasomotor symptoms and rapid onset of dyspareunia and osteoporosis unless treated. If not contraindicated, estrogen replacement is generally started immediately after surgery. Conjugated estrogens 1.25 mg orally, estrone sulfate 1.25 mg orally, or estradiol 2 mg orally is given for 25 days of each month. After age 45–50 years, this dose can be tapered to 0.625 mg of conjugated estrogens or equivalent.

Del Carmen MG et al. Management of menopausal symptoms in women with gynecologic cancers. Gynecol Oncol. 2017 Aug; 146(2):427–35. [PMID: 28625396]

Gartlehner G et al. Hormone therapy for the primary prevention of chronic conditions in postmenopausal women: evidence report and systematic review for the US Preventive Services Task Force. JAMA. 2017 Dec 12;318(22):2234–49. [PMID: 29234813]

Lipold LD et al. Is there a time limit for systemic menopausal hormone therapy? Cleve Clin J Med. 2016 Aug;83(8):605–12. [PMID: 27505882]

Lumsden MA et al. Diagnosis and management of menopause: The National Institute of Health Care and Excellence (NICE) guideline. JAMA Intern Med. 2016 Aug 1;176(8):1205–6. [PMID: 27322881]

The NAMS 2017 Hormone Therapy Position Statement Advisory Panel. The 2017 hormone therapy position statement of The North American Menopause Society. Menopause. 2017 Jul;24(7):728–53. [PMID: 28650869]

Obstetrics & Obstetric Disorders

Vanessa L. Rogers, MD

Scott W. Roberts, MD

DIAGNOSIS OF PREGNANCY

It is advantageous to diagnose pregnancy as promptly as possible when a sexually active woman misses a menstrual period or has symptoms suggestive of pregnancy. Prenatal care can begin early for a desired pregnancy, and potentially harmful medications and activities such as drug and alcohol use, smoking, and occupational chemical exposure can be eliminated. In the event of an unwanted pregnancy, counseling about adoption or termination of the pregnancy can be provided at an early stage.

Pregnancy Tests

All urine or blood pregnancy tests rely on the detection of human chorionic gonadotropin (hCG) produced by the placenta. Levels increase shortly after implantation, approximately double every 48 hours (this rise can range from 30% to 100% in normal pregnancies), reach a peak at 50–75 days, and fall to lower levels in the second and third trimesters. Pregnancy tests are performed on serum or urine and are accurate at the time of the missed period or shortly after it.

Compared with intrauterine pregnancies, **ectopic pregnancies** may show lower levels of hCG that plateau or fall in serial determinations. Quantitative assays of hCG repeated at 48-hour intervals are used in the diagnosis of ectopic pregnancy as well as in cases of molar pregnancy, threatened abortion, and missed abortion. Comparison of hCG levels between laboratories may be misleading in a given patient because different international standards may produce results that vary by as much as twofold. hCG levels can also be problematic because they require a series of measurements. Progesterone levels, however, remain relatively stable in the first trimester. A single measurement of progesterone is the best indicator of whether a pregnancy is viable, although there is a broad indeterminate zone. A value less than 10 nmol/L predicts pregnancy failure while a value greater than 25 ng/mL (80 nmol/L) indicates a pregnancy will be successful. There is uncertainty when the value is between these two points. Combining several serum biomarkers (beta hCG and progesterone) may provide a better prediction of pregnancy viability. **Pregnancy of unknown location** is a term used to describe a situation where a woman has a positive pregnancy test, but the location and viability of the pregnancy are not known because it is not seen on transvaginal ultrasound.

Manifestations of Pregnancy

The following symptoms and signs are usually due to pregnancy, but none are diagnostic. A record of the time and frequency of coitus is helpful for diagnosing and dating a pregnancy.

A. Symptoms

Amenorrhea, nausea and vomiting, breast tenderness and tingling, urinary frequency and urgency, "quickening" (perception of first movement noted at about the 18th week), weight gain.

B. Signs (in Weeks From Last Menstrual Period)

Breast changes (enlargement, vascular engorgement, colostrum) start to occur very early in pregnancy and continue until the postpartum period. Cyanosis of the vagina and cervical portio and softening of the cervix occur in about the 7th week. Softening of the cervicouterine junction takes place in the 8th week, and generalized enlargement and diffuse softening of the corpus occurs after the 8th week. When a woman's abdomen will start to enlarge depends on her body habitus but typically starts in the 16th week.

The uterine fundus is palpable above the pubic symphysis by 12–15 weeks from the last menstrual period and reaches the umbilicus by 20–22 weeks. Fetal heart tones can be heard by Doppler at 10–12 weeks of gestation.

Differential Diagnosis

The nonpregnant uterus enlarged by myomas can be confused with the gravid uterus, but it is usually very firm and irregular. An ovarian tumor may be found midline, displacing the nonpregnant uterus to the side or posteriorly. Ultrasonography and a pregnancy test will provide accurate diagnosis in these circumstances.

ESSENTIALS OF PRENATAL CARE

The first prenatal visit should occur as early as possible after the diagnosis of pregnancy and should include the following: history, physical examination, advice to the patient, and appropriate tests and procedures.

► History

The patient's age, ethnic background, and occupation should be obtained. The onset of the last menstrual period and its normality, possible conception dates, bleeding after the last menstruation, medical history, all prior pregnancies (duration, outcome, and complications), and symptoms of present pregnancy should be documented. The patient's nutritional habits should be discussed with her, as well as any use of caffeine, tobacco, alcohol, or drugs (Table 19–1). Whether there is any family history of congenital anomalies and heritable diseases, a personal history of childhood varicella, prior sexually transmitted diseases (STDs), or risk factors for HIV infection should be determined. The woman should be screened for domestic violence. She should also be asked about recent travel to determine the possibility of exposure to the Zika virus.

► Physical Examination

Height, weight, and blood pressure should be measured, and a general physical examination should be done, including a breast examination. Abdominal and pelvic examination should include the following: (1) estimate of uterine size or measure of fundal height; (2) evaluation of bony pelvis for symmetry and adequacy; (3) evaluation of cervix for structural anatomy, infection, effacement, dilation; (4) detection of fetal heart tones by Doppler device after 10 weeks.

Table 19–1. Common drugs that are teratogenic or fetotoxic.[1]

ACE inhibitors	Lithium
Alcohol	Methotrexate
Androgens	Misoprostol
Angiotensin-II receptor blockers	NSAIDs (third trimester)
Antiepileptics (phenytoin, valproic acid, carbamazepine)	Opioids (prolonged use)
	Radioiodine (antithyroid)
Benzodiazepines	Reserpine
Cyclophosphamide	Ribavirin
Diazoxide	Sulfonamides (second and
Diethylstilbestrol	third trimesters)
Disulfiram	Tetracycline (third trimester)
Ergotamine	Thalidomide
Estrogens	Tobacco smoking
Griseofulvin	Warfarin and other coumarin
Isotretinoin	anticoagulants

[1]Many other drugs are also contraindicated during pregnancy. Evaluate any drug for its need versus its potential adverse effects. Further information can be obtained from the manufacturer or from any of several teratogenic registries around the country.
Go to https://www.fda.gov/ScienceResearch/SpecialTopics/Womens HealthResearch/ucm134848.htm for more information.
ACE, angiotensin-converting enzyme; NSAIDs, nonsteroidal anti-inflammatory drugs.

► Laboratory Tests

See Tests & Procedures, below.

► Advice to Patients

A. Prenatal Visits

Prenatal care should begin early and maintain a schedule of regular prenatal visits: 4–28 weeks, every 4 weeks; 28–36 weeks, every 2 weeks; 36 weeks on, weekly.

B. Diet

The patient should be counseled to eat a balanced diet containing the major food groups. See Nutrition in Pregnancy, below.

1. Prenatal vitamins with 30–60 mg of elemental iron and 0.4 mg of folic acid should be prescribed. Supplements that are not specified for pregnant women should be avoided as they may contain dangerous amounts of certain vitamins.

2. Caffeine intake should be decreased to 0–1 cup of coffee, tea, or caffeinated cola daily.

3. The patient should be advised to avoid eating raw or rare meat as well as fish known to contain elevated levels of mercury.

4. Patients should be encouraged to eat fresh fruits and vegetables (washed before eating).

C. Medications

Only medications prescribed or authorized by the obstetric provider should be taken.

D. Alcohol and Other Drugs

Patients should be encouraged to abstain from alcohol, tobacco, and all recreational ("street") drugs. No safe level of alcohol intake has been established for pregnancy. Fetal effects are manifest in the **fetal alcohol syndrome**, which includes growth restriction; facial, skeletal, and cardiac abnormalities; and serious central nervous system dysfunction. These effects are thought to result from direct toxicity of ethanol as well as of its metabolites such as acetaldehyde.

Cigarette smoking results in fetal exposure to carbon monoxide and nicotine, and this is thought to eventuate in a number of adverse pregnancy outcomes. An increased risk of placental abruption (abruptio placentae), placenta previa, and premature rupture of the membranes is documented among women who smoke. Preterm delivery, low birth weight, and ectopic pregnancy are also more likely among smokers. Women who smoke should quit smoking or at least reduce the number of cigarettes smoked per day to as few as possible. Clinicians should ask all pregnant women about their smoking history and offer smoking cessation counseling during pregnancy, since women are more motivated to change at this time. Pregnant women should also avoid exposure to environmental smoke ("passive smoking"), smokeless tobacco, and e-cigarettes (see Tables 1–4, 1–5). Pharmacotherapy for smoking cessation has been used with mixed results. Studies of buproprion and nicotine replacement systems are inadequate to properly weigh risks and benefits, and prolonged cessation from smoking has not been proven.

Sometimes compounding the above effects on pregnancy outcome are the independent adverse effects of illicit drugs. Cocaine use in pregnancy is associated with an increased risk of premature rupture of membranes, preterm delivery, placental abruption, intrauterine growth restriction, neurobehavioral deficits, and sudden infant death syndrome. Similar adverse effects on pregnancy are associated with amphetamine use, perhaps reflecting the vasoconstrictive properties of both amphetamines and cocaine. Adverse effects associated with opioid use include intrauterine growth restriction, prematurity, and fetal death.

E. Radiographs and Noxious Exposures

Radiographs should be avoided unless essential and approved by a clinician. Abdominal shielding should be used whenever possible. The patient should be told to inform her other health care providers that she is pregnant. Chemical or radiation hazards should be avoided as should excessive heat in hot tubs or saunas. Patients should be told to avoid handling cat feces or cat litter and to wear gloves when gardening to avoid infection with toxoplasmosis.

F. Rest and Activity

The patient should be encouraged to obtain adequate rest each day. She should abstain from strenuous physical work or activities, particularly when heavy lifting or weight bearing is required. Regular exercise can be continued at a mild to moderate level; however, exhausting or hazardous exercises or new athletic training programs should be avoided during pregnancy. Exercises that require a great deal of balance should also be done with caution.

G. Birth Classes

The patient should be encouraged to enroll in a childbirth preparation class with a family member, if possible, well before her due date.

▶ **Tests & Procedures**

A. Each Visit

Weight, blood pressure, fundal height, and fetal heart rate are measured, and a urine specimen is obtained and tested for protein and glucose. Any concerns the patient may have about pregnancy, health, and nutrition should be addressed.

B. 6–12 Weeks

Confirm uterine size and growth by pelvic examination. Document fetal heart tones (audible at 10–12 weeks of gestation by Doppler). Urinalysis; culture of a clean-voided midstream urine sample; random blood glucose; complete blood count (CBC) with red cell indices; serologic test for syphilis, rubella antibody titer; varicella immunity; blood group; Rh type; and antibody screening for anti-Rh$_o$(D), hepatitis B surface antigen (HBsAg), and HIV

should be performed. Women at increased risk for infection should be tested for *Chlamydia trachomatis* and *Neisseria gonorrhoeae*. Women who are at least 21 years old should undergo cervical cancer screening. All women of African origin should have sickle cell screening. Women of African, Asian, or Mediterranean ancestry with anemia or low mean corpuscular volume (MCV) values should have hemoglobin electrophoresis performed to identify abnormal hemoglobins (Hb S, C, F, alpha-thalassemia, beta-thalassemia). Tuberculosis testing is indicated for high-risk populations. Blood screening for Tay-Sachs, Canavan disease, and familial dysautonomia is offered to couples who are of Eastern and Central European Jewish (Ashkenazi) descent. Couples of French Canadian or Cajun ancestry should also be screened as possible Tay-Sachs carriers. Screening for cystic fibrosis and spinal muscular atrophy is offered to all pregnant women. Hepatitis C antibody screening should be offered to pregnant women who are at high risk for infection. Fetal aneuploidy screening is available in the first and second trimester and should be offered to all women, ideally before 20 weeks' gestation. Noninvasive first trimester screening for Down syndrome includes ultrasonographic nuchal translucency and serum levels of PAPP-A (pregnancy-associated plasma protein A) and the free beta subunit of hCG. For pregnancies at high risk for aneuploidy, noninvasive testing with cell free fetal DNA from maternal plasma has a higher detection rate for Down syndrome than other noninvasive tests, but it has a lower detection rate for trisomy 13 and 18, and it does not screen for neural tube defects. Screening for other conditions may be available upon request at certain laboratories. If indicated and requested by the patient, chorionic villus sampling can be performed during this period (11–13 weeks).

C. 16–20 Weeks

The maternal serum "quad screen" for aneuploidy and spina bifida (alpha-fetoprotein, hCG, estradiol, and inhibin A) and amniocentesis are performed as indicated and requested by the patient during this time. First- and second-trimester serum screening tests have similar detection rates. When first and second trimester screening tests for Down syndrome are combined (integrated screening), the detection rates are even higher. Fetal ultrasound examination to determine pregnancy dating and evaluate fetal anatomy is also done. An earlier examination provides the most accurate dating, and a later examination demonstrates fetal anatomy in greatest detail. The best compromise is at 18–20 weeks of gestation. Cervical length measurement (greater than 2.5 cm is normal) is not performed universally in all practices, but is used by some clinicians to identify women at risk for preterm birth.

D. 24 Weeks to Delivery

The patient should be instructed about the symptoms and signs of preterm labor and rupture of membranes. Ultrasound examination is performed as indicated. Typically, fetal size and growth are evaluated when fundal height is 3 cm less than or more than expected for gestational age. In multi-fetal pregnancies, ultrasound should be performed every 2–6 weeks to evaluate for discordant growth.

E. 24–28 Weeks

Screening for gestational diabetes is performed using a 50-g glucose load (Glucola) and a 1-hour post-Glucola blood glucose determination. Abnormal values (greater than or equal to 140 mg/dL or 7.8 mmol/L) should be followed up with a 3-hour glucose tolerance test (see Table 19–4).

F. 28 Weeks

If initial antibody screen for anti-$Rh_o(D)$ is negative, repeat antibody testing for Rh-negative patients is performed, but the result is not required before $Rh_o(D)$ immune globulin is administered.

G. 28–32 Weeks

A CBC is done to evaluate for anemia of pregnancy. Screening for syphilis and HIV is also performed at this time. Providers should familiarize themselves with the laws in their state since testing requirements vary.

H. 28 Weeks to Delivery

Fetal position and presentation are determined. The patient is asked about symptoms or signs of preterm labor or rupture of membranes at each visit. Maternal perception of fetal movement should be assessed at each visit. Antepartum fetal testing in the form of nonstress tests and biophysical profiles can be performed as medically indicated.

I. 36 Weeks to Delivery

Repeat syphilis and HIV testing (depending on state laws) and tests for *N gonorrhoeae* and *C trachomatis* should be performed in at-risk patients. The indicators of onset of labor, admission to the hospital, management of labor and delivery, and options for analgesia and anesthesia should be discussed with the patient. Weekly cervical examinations are not necessary unless indicated to assess a specific clinical situation. Patients should not be delivered prior to 39 completed weeks without a clinical indication.

The CDC recommends universal prenatal culture-based screening for group B streptococcal colonization in pregnancy. A single standard culture of the distal vagina and anorectum is collected at 35–37 weeks. No prophylaxis is needed if the screening culture is negative. Patients whose cultures are positive receive intrapartum penicillin prophylaxis during labor. Except when group B streptococci are found in urine, asymptomatic colonization is not to be treated before labor. Patients who have had a previous infant with invasive group B streptococcal disease or who have group B streptococcal bacteriuria during this pregnancy should receive intrapartum prophylaxis regardless, so rectovaginal cultures are not needed. Patients whose cultures at 35–37 weeks were not done or whose results are not known should receive prophylaxis if they have a risk factor for early-onset neonatal disease, including intrapartum temperature 38°C or higher, membrane rupture more than 18 hours, or delivery before 37 weeks' gestation.

The routine recommended regimen for prophylaxis for group B streptococcal colonization is penicillin G, 5 million units intravenously as a loading dose and then 2.5–3 million units intravenously every 4 hours until delivery. In penicillin-allergic patients not at high risk for anaphylaxis, 2 g of cefazolin can be given intravenously as an initial dose and then 1 g intravenously every 8 hours until delivery. In patients at high risk for anaphylaxis, vancomycin 1 g intravenously every 12 hours until delivery is used or, after confirmed susceptibility testing of group B streptococcal isolate to both clindamycin and erythromycin, clindamycin 900 mg intravenously every 8 hours until delivery.

J. 41 Weeks

The patient should have a cervical examination to determine the probability of successful induction of labor. Induction is undertaken if the cervix is favorable (generally, cervix 2 cm or more dilated, 50% or more effaced, vertex at –1 station, soft cervix, and midposition); if unfavorable, antepartum fetal testing is begun. Induction is performed at 42 weeks' gestation regardless of the cervical examination findings; some providers elect induction at 41 weeks regardless of the cervical examination findings.

NUTRITION IN PREGNANCY

Nutrition in pregnancy can affect maternal health and infant size and well-being. Pregnant women should have nutrition counseling early in prenatal care and access to supplementary food programs if necessary. Counseling should stress abstention from alcohol, smoking, and recreational drugs. Caffeine and artificial sweeteners should be used only in small amounts.

Recommendations regarding weight gain in pregnancy should be based on maternal body mass index (BMI) preconceptionally or at the first prenatal visit. According to the National Academy of Medicine guidelines, total weight gain should be 25–35 lbs (11.3–15.9 kg) for normal weight women (BMI of 18.5–24.9) and 15–25 lbs (6.8–11.3 kg) for overweight women. For obese women (BMI of 30 or greater), weight gain should be limited to 11–20 lbs (5.0–9.1 kg). Excessive maternal weight gain has been associated with increased birth weight as well as postpartum retention of weight. Not gaining weight in pregnancy, conversely, has been associated with low birth weight. Nutrition counseling must be tailored to the individual patient.

The increased calcium needs of pregnancy (1200 mg/day) can be met with milk, milk products, green vegetables, soybean products, corn tortillas, and calcium carbonate supplements.

The increased need for iron and folic acid should be met with foods as well as vitamin and mineral supplements. (See Anemia section.) Megavitamins should not be taken in pregnancy, as they may result in fetal malformation or disturbed metabolism. However, a balanced prenatal supplement containing 30–60 mg of elemental iron, 0.4 mg of folate, and the recommended daily allowances of various vitamins and minerals is widely used in the United States and is probably beneficial to many women with marginal diets. There is evidence that periconceptional folic acid supplements can decrease the risk of neural tube defects in the fetus. For this reason, the United States Public Health Service recommends the consumption of

0.4 mg of folic acid per day for all pregnant and reproductive age women. Women with a prior pregnancy complicated by neural tube defect may require higher supplemental doses as determined by their providers.

American College of Obstetricians and Gynecologists. ACOG Committee Opinion No. 548: Weight gain during pregnancy. Obstet Gynecol. 2013 Jan;121(1):210–2. [Reaffirmed 2018] [PMID: 23262962]

Haider BA et al. Multiple-micronutrient supplementation for women during pregnancy. Cochrane Database Syst Rev. 2015 Nov 1;(11):CD004905. [PMID: 26522344]

PREVENTION OF RHESUS ALLOIMMUNIZATION

The antibody anti-$Rh_o(D)$ causes severe hemolytic disease of the newborn. About 15% of whites and much lower proportions of blacks and Asians are $Rh_o(D)$–negative. If an $Rh_o(D)$–negative woman carries an $Rh_o(D)$–positive fetus, antibodies against $Rh_o(D)$ may develop in the mother when fetal red cells enter her circulation during small feto-maternal bleeding episodes in the early third trimester or during delivery, abortion, ectopic pregnancy, placental abruption, or other instances of antepartum bleeding. This antibody, once produced, remains in the woman's circulation and poses the threat of hemolytic disease for subsequent Rh-positive fetuses.

Passive immunization against hemolytic disease of the newborn is achieved with $Rh_o(D)$ immune globulin, a purified concentrate of antibodies against $Rh_o(D)$ antigen. The $Rh_o(D)$ immune globulin (one vial of 300 mcg intramuscularly) is given to the mother within 72 hours after delivery (or spontaneous or induced abortion or ectopic pregnancy). The antibodies in the immune globulin destroy fetal Rh-positive cells so that the mother will not produce anti-$Rh_o(D)$. During her next Rh-positive gestation, erythroblastosis will be prevented. An additional safety measure is the routine administration of the immune globulin at the 28th week of pregnancy. The passive antibody titer that results is too low to significantly affect an Rh-positive fetus. The maternal clearance of the globulin is slow enough that protection will continue for 12 weeks. Once a woman is alloimmunized, $Rh_o(D)$ immune globulin is no longer helpful and should not be given.

LACTATION

Breastfeeding should be encouraged by education throughout pregnancy and the puerperium. Mothers should be told the benefits of breastfeeding, including infant immunity, emotional satisfaction, mother-infant bonding, and economic savings. The period of amenorrhea associated with frequent and consistent breastfeeding provides some (although not reliable) birth control until menstruation begins at 6–12 months postpartum or the intensity of breastfeeding diminishes. Even a brief period of nursing is beneficial. Transfer of immunoglobulins, macrophages, and lymphocytes in colostrum and breast milk immunoprotects the infant against many systemic and enteric infections. The intestinal flora of breastfed infants inhibit the growth of pathogens. Breastfed infants have fewer bacterial and viral infections, fewer gastrointestinal tract infections, and fewer allergy problems than bottle-fed infants. Furthermore, they are less apt to be obese as children and adults.

Frequent breastfeeding on an infant-demand schedule enhances milk flow and successful breastfeeding. Mothers breastfeeding for the first time need help and encouragement from providers, nurses, and other nursing mothers. Milk supply can be increased by increased suckling and increased rest.

Nursing mothers should have a fluid intake of over 3 L/day. The United States RDA calls for 21 g of extra protein (over the 44 g/day baseline for an adult woman) and 550 extra kcal/day in the first 6 months of nursing. Calcium intake should be 1200 mg/day. Continuation of a prenatal vitamin and mineral supplement is wise. Strict vegetarians who avoid both milk and eggs should always take vitamin B_{12} supplements during pregnancy and lactation.

1. Effects of Drugs in a Nursing Mother

Drugs taken by a nursing mother may accumulate in milk and be transmitted to the infant (Table 19–2). The amount of drug entering the milk depends on the drug's lipid solubility, mechanism of transport, and degree of ionization.

2. Suppression of Lactation

The simplest and safest method of suppressing lactation after it has started is to gradually transfer the baby to a bottle or a cup over a 3-week period. Milk supply will decrease with decreased demand, and minimal discomfort ensues. If nursing must be stopped abruptly, the mother should avoid nipple stimulation, refrain from expressing milk, and use a snug brassiere. Ice packs and analgesics can be helpful. This same technique can be used in cases where suppression is desired before nursing has begun. Engorgement will gradually recede over a 2- to 3-day period. Hormonal suppression of lactation is no longer practiced.

Martin CR et al. Review of infant feeding: key features of breast milk and infant formula. Nutrients. 2016 May 11;8(5):E279. [PMID: 27187450]

TRAVEL & IMMUNIZATIONS DURING PREGNANCY

During an otherwise normal low-risk pregnancy, travel can be planned most safely up to the 32nd week. Commercial flying in pressurized cabins does not pose a threat to the fetus. An aisle seat will allow frequent walks. Adequate fluids should be taken during the flight. Travelling to endemic areas of yellow fever (Africa or Latin America) or of Zika virus (Latin America) is not advisable; since Zika virus can be sexually transmitted, partner travel should also be discussed (see Chapter 32). Similarly, it is inadvisable to travel to areas of Africa or Asia where chloroquine-resistant falciparum malaria is a hazard, since complications of malaria are more common in pregnancy.

Ideally, all immunizations should precede pregnancy. *Live virus products are contraindicated during pregnancy*

Table 19–2. Drugs and substances that require a careful assessment of risk before they are prescribed for breastfeeding women.[1]

Drugs	Concern
Atenolol	Has been associated with hypotension and bradycardia in the infant. Metoprolol and propranolol are preferred.
Ciprofloxacin	Association with adverse effects on fetal cartilage and bone. Must weigh risks versus benefits.
Codeine, oxycodone	Cause CNS depression. Unpredictable metabolism.
Cyclophosphamide	Neonatal neutropenia. No breastfeeding.
Diphenhydramine	Present in very small quantities in milk; sources are conflicting with regard to its safety.
Fluoxetine	Present in breast milk in higher levels than other SSRIs. Watch for adverse effects like an infant's fussiness and crying.
Lisinopril	Unknown effects. Captopril or enalapril is preferred if an ACE inhibitor is needed.
Lithium	Circulating levels in the neonate are variable. Follow infant's serum creatinine and blood urea nitrogen levels and thyroid function tests.
Tetracyclines	Concern for bone growth and dental staining.
Valproic acid	Long-term effects are unknown. Although levels in milk are low, it is teratogenic, so it should be avoided if possible.

[1]The above list is not all-inclusive. For additional information, see the below reference from which this information is adapted or the online drug and lactation database, Lactmed, at http://toxnet.nlm.nih.gov/newtoxnet/lactmed.htm.
ACE, angiotensin-converting enzyme; CNS, central nervous system; SSRIs, selective serotonin reuptake inhibitors.
Data from Rowe H et al. Maternal medication, drug use, and breastfeeding. Pediatr Clin North Am. 2013 Feb;60(1):275–94.

(measles, rubella, yellow fever, and smallpox). Inactivated polio vaccine should be given subcutaneously instead of the oral live-attenuated vaccine. The varicella vaccine should be given 1–3 months before becoming pregnant. Vaccines against pneumococcal pneumonia, meningococcal meningitis, and hepatitis A can be used as indicated. Pregnant women who are considered to be at high-risk for hepatitis B and who have not been previously vaccinated should be vaccinated during pregnancy. The HPV vaccine is not recommended for pregnant women. However, adverse outcomes have not been described when used during pregnancy.

The CDC lists pregnant women as a high-risk group for influenza. Annual influenza vaccination is indicated in all women who are pregnant or will be pregnant during the "flu season." It can be given in the first trimester. The CDC also recommends that every pregnant woman receive a dose of Tdap during each pregnancy irrespective of her prior vaccination history. The optimal timing for such Tdap administration is between 27 and 36 weeks of gestation, in order to maximize the antibody response of the pregnant woman against pertussis and the passive antibody transfer to the infant. For any woman who was not previously vaccinated with Tdap and for whom the vaccine was not given during her pregnancy, Tdap should be administered immediately postpartum. Further, any teenagers or adults not previously vaccinated who will have close contact with the infant should also receive it, ideally 2 weeks before exposure to the child. This vaccination strategy is referred to as "cocooning," and its purpose is to protect the infant aged younger than 12 months who is at particularly high risk for lethal pertussis.

Hepatitis A vaccine contains formalin-inactivated virus and can be given in pregnancy when needed. Pooled immune globulin to prevent hepatitis A is safe and does not carry risk of HIV transmission. Chloroquine can be used for malaria prophylaxis in pregnancy, and proguanil is also safe.

Water should be purified by boiling, since iodine purification may provide more iodine than is safe during pregnancy.

Prophylactic antibiotics or bismuth subsalicylate should not be used during pregnancy to prevent diarrhea. Oral rehydration and treatment of bacterial diarrhea with erythromycin or ampicillin if necessary is preferred.

American College of Obstetricians and Gynecologists. ACOG Committee Opinion No. 741: Maternal immunization. Obstet Gynecol. 2018 Jun;131(6):e214–7. [PMID: 29794683]

OBSTETRIC COMPLICATIONS OF THE FIRST & SECOND TRIMESTERS

VOMITING OF PREGNANCY & HYPEREMESIS GRAVIDARUM

 ESSENTIALS OF DIAGNOSIS

► Morning or evening nausea and vomiting.
► Persistent vomiting severe enough to result in weight loss, dehydration, starvation ketosis, hypochloremic alkalosis, hypokalemia.
► May have transient elevation of liver enzymes.
► Appears related to high or rising serum hCG.
► More common with multi-fetal pregnancies or hydatidiform mole.

► General Considerations

Nausea and vomiting begin soon after the first missed period and cease by the fifth month of gestation. Up to three-fourths of women complain of nausea and vomiting during early pregnancy, with the vast majority noting nausea throughout the day. This problem exerts no adverse effects on the pregnancy and does not presage other complications.

Persistent, severe vomiting during pregnancy—hyperemesis gravidarum—can be disabling and require hospitalization. Hyperthyroidism can be associated with hyperemesis gravidarum, so it is advisable to determine thyroid-stimulating hormone (TSH) and free thyroxine (FT_4) values in these patients. Of note, these patients will not have a goiter.

Treatment

A. Mild Nausea and Vomiting of Pregnancy

In most instances, only reassurance and dietary advice are required. Because of possible teratogenicity, drugs used during the first half of pregnancy should be restricted to those of major importance to life and health. Vitamin B_6 (pyridoxine), 50–100 mg/day orally, is nontoxic and may be helpful in some patients. Pyridoxine alone or in combination with doxylamine (10 mg doxylamine succinate and 10 mg pyridoxine hydrochloride, two tablets at bedtime) is first-line pharmacotherapy. Antiemetics, antihistamines, and antispasmodics are generally unnecessary to treat nausea of pregnancy.

B. Hyperemesis Gravidarum

With more severe nausea and vomiting, it may become necessary to hospitalize the patient. In this case, a private room with limited activity is preferred. It is recommended to give nothing by mouth until the patient is improving, and maintain hydration and electrolyte balance by giving appropriate parenteral fluids and vitamin supplements as indicated. Antiemetics such as promethazine (12.5–25 mg orally, rectally, or intravenously every 4–6 hours), metoclopramide (5–10 mg orally or intravenously every 6 hours), or ondansetron (4–8 mg orally or intravenously every 8 hours) should be started. Ondansetron has been associated in some studies with congenital anomalies. Data are limited, but the risks and benefits of treatment should be addressed with the patient. Antiemetics will likely need to be given intravenously initially. Rarely, total parenteral nutrition may become necessary but only if enteral feedings cannot be done. As soon as possible, the patient should be placed on a dry diet consisting of six small feedings daily. Antiemetics may be continued orally as needed. After in-patient stabilization, the patient can be maintained at home even if she requires intravenous fluids in addition to her oral intake. There are conflicting studies regarding the use of corticosteroids for the control of hyperemesis gravidarum, and it has also been associated with fetal anomalies. Therefore, this treatment should be withheld before 10 weeks' gestation and until more accepted treatments have been exhausted.

When to Refer

- Patient does not respond to first-line outpatient management.
- There is concern for other pathology (ie, hydatidiform mole).

When to Admit

- Patient is unable to tolerate any food or water.
- Condition precludes the patient from ingesting necessary medications.
- Weight loss.
- Presence of a hydatidiform mole.

American College of Obstetricians and Gynecologists. ACOG Practice Bulletin No. 189: Nausea and vomiting of pregnancy. Obstet Gynecol. 2018 Jan;131(1):e15–30. [PMID: 29266076]

SPONTANEOUS ABORTION

ESSENTIALS OF DIAGNOSIS

- ▶ Intrauterine pregnancy at less than 20 weeks.
- ▶ Low or falling levels of hCG.
- ▶ Bleeding, midline cramping pain.
- ▶ Open cervical os.
- ▶ Complete or partial expulsion of products of conception.

General Considerations

About three-fourths of spontaneous abortions occur before the 16th week; of these, three-fourths occur before the 8th week. Almost 20% of all clinically recognized pregnancies terminate in spontaneous abortion.

More than 60% of spontaneous abortions result from chromosomal defects due to maternal or paternal factors; about 15% appear to be associated with maternal trauma, infections, dietary deficiencies, diabetes mellitus, hypothyroidism, the lupus anticoagulant-anticardiolipin-antiphospholipid antibody syndrome, or anatomic malformations. There is no reliable evidence that abortion may be induced by psychic stimuli such as severe fright, grief, anger, or anxiety. In about one-fourth of cases, the cause of abortion cannot be determined. There is no evidence that video display terminals or associated electromagnetic fields are related to an increased risk of spontaneous abortion.

It is important to distinguish women with a history of incompetent cervix from those with more typical early abortion. Characteristically, incompetent cervix presents as "silent" cervical dilation (ie, with minimal uterine contractions) in the second trimester. When the cervix reaches 4 cm or more, active uterine contractions or rupture of the membranes may occur secondary to the degree of cervical dilation. This does not change the primary diagnosis. Factors that predispose to incompetent cervix are a history of incompetent cervix with a previous pregnancy, cervical conization or surgery, cervical injury, diethylstilbestrol (DES) exposure, and anatomic abnormalities of the cervix. Prior to pregnancy or during the first trimester, there are no methods for determining whether the cervix will eventually be incompetent. After 14–16 weeks, ultrasound may be used to evaluate the internal anatomy of the lower uterine segment and cervix for the funneling and shortening abnormalities consistent with cervical incompetence.

Clinical Findings

A. Symptoms and Signs

1. Threatened abortion—Bleeding or cramping occurs, but the pregnancy continues. The cervix is not dilated.

2. Inevitable abortion—The cervix is dilated and the membranes may be ruptured, but passage of the products of conception has not yet occurred. Bleeding and cramping persist, and passage of the products of conception is considered inevitable.

3. Complete abortion—Products of conception are completely expelled. Pain ceases, but spotting may persist. Cervical os is closed.

4. Incomplete abortion—The cervix is dilated. Some portion of the products of conception remains in the uterus. Only mild cramps are reported, but bleeding is persistent and often excessive.

5. Missed abortion—The pregnancy has ceased to develop, but the conceptus has not been expelled. Symptoms of pregnancy disappear. There may be a brownish vaginal discharge but no active bleeding. Pain does not develop. The cervix is semifirm and slightly patulous; the uterus becomes smaller and irregularly softened; the adnexa are normal.

B. Laboratory Findings

Pregnancy tests show low or falling levels of hCG. A CBC should be obtained if bleeding is heavy. Determine Rh type, and give $Rh_o(D)$ immune globulin if Rh-negative. All tissue recovered should be assessed by a pathologist and may be sent for genetic analysis in selected cases.

C. Ultrasonographic Findings

The gestational sac can be identified at 5–6 weeks from the last menstruation, a fetal pole at 6 weeks, and fetal cardiac activity at 6–7 weeks by transvaginal ultrasound. Serial observations are often required to evaluate changes in size of the embryo. Diagnostic criteria of early pregnancy loss are a crown-rump length of 7 mm or more and no heartbeat or a mean sac diameter of 25 mm or more and no embryo.

Differential Diagnosis

The bleeding that occurs in abortion of a uterine pregnancy must be differentiated from the abnormal bleeding of an ectopic pregnancy and anovulatory bleeding in a nonpregnant woman. The passage of hydropic villi in the bloody discharge is diagnostic of hydatidiform mole.

Treatment

A. General Measures

1. Threatened abortion—Bed rest for 24–48 hours followed by gradual resumption of usual activities has been offered in

the past. Studies do not support that this strategy is beneficial. Abstinence from sexual activity has also been suggested without proven benefit. Data are lacking to support the administration of progestins to all women with a threatened abortion. If during the patient's evaluation, an infection is diagnosed (ie, urinary tract infection), it should be treated.

2. Missed abortion—This calls for counseling regarding the fate of the pregnancy and planning for its elective termination at a time chosen by the patient and clinician. Management can be medical or surgical. Each has risks and benefits. Medically induced first-trimester termination with prostaglandins (ie, misoprostol given vaginally or orally in a dose of 200–800 mcg) is safe, effective, less invasive, and more private than surgical intervention; however, if it is unsuccessful or if there is excessive bleeding, a surgical procedure (dilation and curettage) may still be needed. Patients must be counseled about the different therapeutic options.

B. Surgical Measures

1. Incomplete or inevitable abortion—Prompt removal of any products of conception remaining within the uterus is required to stop bleeding and prevent infection. Analgesia and a paracervical block are useful, followed by uterine exploration with ovum forceps or uterine aspiration. Regional anesthesia may be required.

2. Cerclage and restriction of activities—A cerclage is the treatment of choice for incompetent cervix, but a viable intrauterine pregnancy should be confirmed prior to placement of the cerclage.

A variety of suture materials including a 5-mm Mersilene tape or No. 2 nonabsorbable monofilament suture can be used to create a purse-string type of stitch around the cervix, using either the McDonald or Shirodkar method. Cerclage should be undertaken with caution when there is advanced cervical dilation or when the membranes are prolapsed into the vagina. *Rupture of the membranes and infection are specific contraindications to cerclage.* Cervical cultures for *N gonorrhoeae, C trachomatis*, and group B streptococci should be obtained before elective placement of a cerclage. *N gonorrhoeae* and *C trachomatis* should be treated before placement.

When to Refer

- Patient with history of two second-trimester losses.
- Vaginal bleeding in a pregnant patient that resembles menstruation in a nonpregnant woman.
- Patient with an open cervical os.
- No signs of uterine growth in serial examinations of a pregnant patient.
- Leakage of amniotic fluid.

When to Admit

- Open cervical os.
- Heavy vaginal bleeding.
- Leakage of amniotic fluid.

American College of Obstetricians and Gynecologists. ACOG Practice Bulletin No. 142: Cerclage for the management of cervical insufficiency. Obstet Gynecol. 2014 Feb; 123(2 Pt 1): 372–9. [Reaffirmed 2016] [PMID: 24451674]

American College of Obstetricians and Gynecologists. ACOG Practice Bulletin No. 150: Early pregnancy loss. Obstet Gynecol. 2015 May;125(5):1258–67. [Reaffirmed 2017] [PMID: 25932865]

RECURRENT ABORTION

According to the American Society of Reproductive Medicine, recurrent pregnancy loss is defined as the loss of two or more previable (less than 24 weeks' gestation or 500 g) pregnancies in succession. Recurrent abortion affects about 1–5% of couples. Abnormalities related to recurrent abortion can be identified in approximately 50% of these couples. If a woman has lost three previous pregnancies without identifiable cause, she still has at least a 55% chance of carrying a fetus to viability.

Recurrent abortion is a clinical rather than pathologic diagnosis. The clinical findings are similar to those observed in other types of abortion. It is appropriate to begin a medical evaluation in a woman who has had two first-trimester losses.

Treatment

A. Preconception Therapy

Preconception therapy is aimed at detection of maternal or paternal defects that may contribute to abortion. A thorough history and examination is essential. A random blood glucose test and thyroid function studies (including thyroid antibodies) can be done if history indicates a possible predisposition to diabetes mellitus or thyroid disease. Detection of lupus anticoagulant and other hemostatic abnormalities (proteins S and C and antithrombin deficiency, hyperhomocysteinemia, anticardiolipin antibody, factor V Leiden mutations) and an antinuclear antibody test may be indicated. Hysteroscopy, saline infusion sonogram, or hysterography can be used to exclude submucosal myomas and congenital anomalies of the uterus. In women with recurrent losses, resection of a uterine septum, if present, has been recommended. Chromosomal (karyotype) analysis of both partners can be done to rule out balanced translocations (found in 3–4% of infertile couples), but karyotyping is expensive and may not be helpful.

Many therapies have been tried to prevent recurrent pregnancy loss from immunologic causes. Low-molecular-weight heparin (LMWH), aspirin, intravenous immunoglobulin, and corticosteroids have all been used but the definitive treatment has not yet been determined (see Antiphospholipid Syndrome, below). Prophylactic dose heparin and low-dose aspirin have been recommended for women with antiphospholipid antibodies and recurrent pregnancy loss.

B. Postconception Therapy

The patient should be provided early prenatal care and scheduled frequent office visits. Empiric sex steroid

hormone therapy is complicated and should be done by an expert if undertaken.

Prognosis

The prognosis is excellent if the cause of abortion can be corrected or treated.

Homer HA. Modern management of recurrent miscarriage. Aust N Z J Obstet Gynaecol. 2019 Feb;59(1):36–44. [PMID: 30393965]

ECTOPIC PREGNANCY

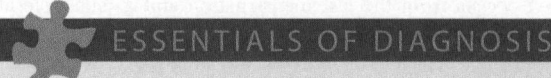

ESSENTIALS OF DIAGNOSIS

► Amenorrhea or irregular bleeding and spotting.
► Pelvic pain, usually adnexal.
► Adnexal mass by clinical examination or ultrasound.
► Failure of serum beta-hCG to double every 48 hours.
► No intrauterine pregnancy on transvaginal ultrasound with serum beta-hCG greater than 2000 milli-units/mL.

General Considerations

Ectopic implantation occurs in approximately 2% of first trimester pregnancies. About 98% of ectopic pregnancies are tubal. Other sites of ectopic implantation are the peritoneum or abdominal viscera, the ovary, and the cervix. Any condition that prevents or retards migration of the fertilized ovum to the uterus can predispose to an ectopic pregnancy, including a history of infertility, pelvic inflammatory disease, ruptured appendix, and prior tubal surgery. Combined intrauterine and extrauterine pregnancy (heterotopic) may occur rarely. In the United States, undiagnosed or undetected ectopic pregnancy is one of the most common causes of maternal death during the first trimester.

Clinical Findings

A. Symptoms and Signs

Severe lower quadrant pain occurs in almost every case. It is sudden in onset, stabbing, intermittent, and does not radiate. Backache may be present during attacks. Shock occurs in about 10%, often after pelvic examination. At least two-thirds of patients give a history of abnormal menstruation; many have been infertile.

Blood may leak from the tubal ampulla over a period of days, and considerable blood may accumulate in the peritoneum. Slight but persistent vaginal spotting is usually reported, and a pelvic mass may be palpated. Abdominal distention and mild paralytic ileus are often present.

B. Laboratory Findings

The CBC may show anemia and slight leukocytosis. Quantitative serum pregnancy tests will show levels generally lower than expected for normal pregnancies of the same duration. If beta-hCG levels are followed over a few days, there may be a slow rise or a plateau rather than the near doubling every 2 days associated with normal early intrauterine pregnancy or the falling levels that occur with spontaneous abortion. A progesterone level can also be measured to assess the viability of the pregnancy.

C. Imaging

Ultrasonography can reliably demonstrate a gestational sac 5–6 weeks from the last menstruation and a fetal pole at 6 weeks if located in the uterus. An empty uterine cavity raises a strong suspicion of extrauterine pregnancy, which can occasionally be revealed by transvaginal ultrasound. Specified levels of serum beta-hCG have been reliably correlated with ultrasound findings of an intrauterine pregnancy. For example, a beta-hCG level of 6500 milli-units/mL with an empty uterine cavity by transabdominal ultrasound is highly suspicious for an ectopic pregnancy. Similarly, a beta-hCG value of 2000 milli-units/mL or more can be indicative of an ectopic pregnancy if no products of conception are detected within the uterine cavity by transvaginal ultrasound. Serum beta-hCG values can vary by laboratory.

D. Special Examinations

Laparoscopy is the surgical procedure of choice both to confirm an ectopic pregnancy and in most cases to permit removal of the ectopic pregnancy without the need for exploratory laparotomy.

Ectopic pregnancy should be suspected when postabortal tissue examination fails to reveal chorionic villi. Steps must be taken for immediate diagnosis, including prompt microscopic tissue examination, ultrasonography, and serial beta-hCG titers every 48 hours.

▶ Differential Diagnosis

Clinical and laboratory findings suggestive or diagnostic of pregnancy will distinguish ectopic pregnancy from many acute abdominal illnesses such as acute appendicitis, acute pelvic inflammatory disease, ruptured corpus luteum cyst or ovarian follicle, and urinary calculi. Uterine enlargement with clinical findings similar to those found in ectopic pregnancy is also characteristic of an aborting uterine pregnancy or hydatidiform mole.

▶ Treatment

Patients must be warned about the complications of an ectopic pregnancy and monitored closely. In a stable patient with normal liver and renal function tests, methotrexate (50 mg/m^2) intramuscularly—given as single or multiple doses—is acceptable medical therapy for early ectopic pregnancy. Favorable criteria are that the pregnancy should be less than 3.5 cm in largest dimension and unruptured, with no active bleeding and no fetal heart tones. Several small studies have not found an increased risk of fetal malformations or pregnancy losses in women who conceive within 6 months of methotrexate therapy.

When a patient with an ectopic pregnancy is unstable or when surgical therapy is planned, the patient is hospitalized. Blood is typed and cross-matched. The goal is to diagnose and operate before there is frank rupture of the tube and intra-abdominal hemorrhage. *The use of methotrexate in an unstable patient is absolutely contraindicated.*

Surgical treatment is definitive. In most patients, diagnostic laparoscopy is the initial surgical procedure performed. Depending on the size of the ectopic pregnancy and whether or not it has ruptured, salpingostomy with removal of the ectopic pregnancy or a partial or complete salpingectomy can usually be performed. Clinical conditions permitting, patency of the contralateral tube can be established by injection of indigo carmine into the uterine cavity and flow through the contralateral tube confirmed visually by the surgeon; iron therapy for anemia may be necessary during convalescence. Rh$_o$(D) immune globulin (300 mcg) should be given to Rh-negative patients.

▶ Prognosis

Repeat tubal pregnancy occurs in about 10% of cases. This should not be regarded as a contraindication to future pregnancy, but the patient requires careful observation and early ultrasound confirmation of an intrauterine pregnancy.

▶ When to Refer

- Severe abdominal pain.
- Palpation of an adnexal mass on pelvic examination.
- Abdominal pain and vaginal bleeding in a pregnant patient.

▶ When to Admit

Presence of symptoms or signs of a ruptured ectopic pregnancy.

Brady PC. New evidence to guide ectopic pregnancy diagnosis and management. Obstet Gynecol Surv. 2017 Oct;72(10): 618–25. [PMID: 29059454]

GESTATIONAL TROPHOBLASTIC DISEASE (Hydatidiform Mole & Choriocarcinoma)

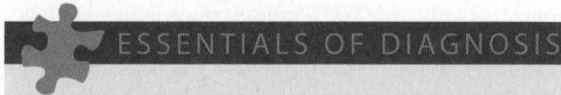

ESSENTIALS OF DIAGNOSIS

Hydatidiform mole

- ▶ Amenorrhea.
- ▶ Irregular uterine bleeding.
- ▶ Serum beta-hCG greater than 40,000 milli-units/mL.
- ▶ Passage of grapelike clusters of enlarged edematous villi per vagina.

► Uterine ultrasound shows characteristic heterogeneous echogenic image and no fetus or placenta.

► Cytogenetic composition is 46,XX (85%), of paternal origin.

Choriocarcinoma

► Persistence of detectable beta-hCG after mole evacuation.

General Considerations

Gestational trophoblastic disease is a spectrum of disorders that includes hydatidiform mole (partial and complete), invasive mole (local extension into the uterus or vagina), choriocarcinoma (malignancy often complicated by distant metastases), and placental site trophoblastic tumor. Complete moles show no evidence of a fetus on ultrasonography. The majority are 46,XX, with all chromosomes of paternal origin. Partial moles generally show evidence of an embryo or gestational sac; are triploid, slower-growing, and less symptomatic; and often present clinically as a missed abortion. Partial moles tend to follow a benign course, while complete moles have a greater tendency to become choriocarcinoma.

In North America, the frequency of gestational trophoblastic disease is 1:1500 pregnancies. The highest rates occur in Asians. Risk factors include prior spontaneous abortion, a history of mole, and age younger than 21 or older than 35. Approximately 10% of women require further treatment after evacuation of the mole; choriocarcinoma develops in 2–3% of women.

Clinical Findings

A. Symptoms and Signs

Uterine bleeding, beginning at 6–16 weeks, is observed in most instances. In some cases, the uterus is larger than would be expected in a normal pregnancy of the same duration. Excessive nausea and vomiting may occur. Bilaterally enlarged cystic ovaries are sometimes palpable. They are the result of ovarian hyperstimulation due to excess beta-hCG.

Preeclampsia-eclampsia may develop during the second trimester of an untreated molar pregnancy, but this is unusual because most are diagnosed early.

Choriocarcinoma may be manifested by continued or recurrent uterine bleeding after evacuation of a mole or following delivery, abortion, or ectopic pregnancy. The presence of an ulcerative vaginal tumor, pelvic mass, or distant metastases may be the presenting manifestation.

B. Laboratory Findings

Hydatidiform moles are generally characterized by high serum beta-hCG values, which can range from high normal to the millions. Levels are higher with complete moles than with partial moles. Serum beta-hCG values, if extremely high, can assist in making the diagnosis, but they are more helpful in managing response to treatment. Hematocrit, creatinine, blood type, liver biochemical tests,

and thyroid function tests should also be measured. High beta-hCG levels can cause the release of thyroid hormone, and rarely, symptoms of hyperthyroidism. Patients with hyperthyroidism may require beta-blocker therapy until the mole has been evacuated.

C. Imaging

The preoperative diagnosis of hydatidiform mole is confirmed by ultrasound. Placental vesicles can be easily seen on transvaginal ultrasound. A preoperative chest film is indicated to rule out pulmonary metastases of the trophoblast.

Treatment

A. Specific (Surgical) Measures

The uterus should be emptied as soon as the diagnosis of hydatidiform mole is established, preferably by suction curettage. Ovarian cysts should not be resected nor ovaries removed; spontaneous regression of theca lutein cysts will occur with elimination of the mole. The products of conception removed from the uterus should be sent to a pathologist for review. In patients who have completed their childbearing, hysterectomy is an acceptable alternative. Hysterectomy does not preclude the need for follow-up of beta-hCG levels.

B. Follow-Up Measures

Weekly quantitative beta-hCG level measurements are initially required. Following successful surgical evacuation, moles show a progressive decline in beta-hCG. After three negative weekly tests (less than 5 milli-units/mL), the interval may be increased to every 1 month for an additional 6 months. The purpose of this follow-up is to identify persistent nonmetastatic and metastatic disease, including choriocarcinoma, which is more likely to occur if the initial beta-hCG is high and the uterus is large. If levels plateau or begin to rise, the patient should be evaluated by repeat laboratory tests, chest film, and dilatation and curettage (D&C) before the initiation of chemotherapy. Effective contraception (preferably birth control pills) should be prescribed to avoid the hazard and confusion of elevated beta-hCG from a new pregnancy. The beta-hCG levels should be negative for 6 months before pregnancy is attempted again. Because the risk of recurrence of a molar pregnancy is 1–2%, an ultrasound should be performed in the first trimester of the pregnancy following a mole to ensure that the pregnancy is normal. In addition, a beta-hCG level should then be checked 6 weeks' postpartum (after the subsequent normal pregnancy) to ensure there is no persistent trophoblastic tissue, and the placenta should be examined by a pathologist.

C. Antitumor Chemotherapy

If malignant tissue is discovered at surgery or during the follow-up examination, chemotherapy is indicated. For low-risk patients with a good prognosis, methotrexate is considered first-line therapy followed by dactinomycin (see Table 39–3). Patients with high-risk disease should be referred to a cancer center, where multiple-agent chemotherapy probably will be given.

Prognosis

Five-year survival after courses of chemotherapy, even when metastases have been demonstrated, can be expected in at least 85% of cases of choriocarcinoma.

When to Refer

- Uterine size exceeds that anticipated for gestational age.
- Vaginal bleeding similar to menstruation.
- Pregnant patient with a history of a molar pregnancy.

When to Admit

- Confirmed molar pregnancy by ultrasound and laboratory studies.
- Heavy vaginal bleeding in a pregnant patient under evaluation.

Brown J et al. 15 years of progress in gestational trophoblastic disease: scoring, standardization, and salvage. Gynecol Oncol. 2017 Jan;144(1):200–7. [PMID: 27743739]

OBSTETRIC COMPLICATIONS OF THE SECOND & THIRD TRIMESTERS

PREECLAMPSIA-ECLAMPSIA

ESSENTIALS OF DIAGNOSIS

Preeclampsia

▶ Blood pressure of 140 mm Hg or higher systolic or 90 mm Hg or higher diastolic after 20 weeks of gestation.

▶ Proteinuria of 0.3 g or more in 24 hours.

▶ When hypertension is present with severe features of preeclampsia, seizure prophylaxis could be beneficial.

Preeclampsia with severe features

▶ Blood pressure of 160 mm Hg or higher systolic or 110 mm Hg or higher diastolic.

▶ Progressive kidney injury.

▶ Thrombocytopenia.

▶ Hemolysis, elevated liver enzymes, low platelets (HELLP).

▶ Pulmonary edema.

▶ Vision changes or headache.

Eclampsia

▶ Seizures in a patient with evidence of preeclampsia.

General Considerations

Preeclampsia is defined as the presence of newly elevated blood pressure and proteinuria during pregnancy. Eclampsia is diagnosed when seizures develop in a patient with evidence of preeclampsia. Historically, the presence of three elements was required for the diagnosis of preeclampsia: hypertension, proteinuria, and edema. Edema was difficult to objectively quantify and is no longer a required element. In addition, proteinuria may not always be present.

Preeclampsia-eclampsia can occur any time after 20 weeks of gestation and up to 6 weeks' postpartum. It is a disease unique to pregnancy, with the only cure being delivery of the fetus and placenta. Preeclampsia develops in approximately 7% of pregnant women in the United States; of those, eclampsia will develop in 5% (0.04% of pregnant women). Primiparas are most frequently affected; however, the incidence of preeclampsia-eclampsia is increased with multi-fetal pregnancies, chronic hypertension, diabetes mellitus, kidney disease, collagen-vascular and autoimmune disorders, and gestational trophoblastic disease. Uncontrolled eclampsia is a significant cause of maternal death.

Clinical Findings

Clinically, the severity of preeclampsia-eclampsia can be measured with reference to the six major sites in which it exerts its effects: the central nervous system, the kidneys, the liver, the hematologic system, the vascular system, and the fetal-placental unit. By evaluating each of these areas for the presence of mild to severe preeclampsia, the degree of involvement can be assessed, and an appropriate management plan can be formulated that balances the severity of disease and gestational age (Table 19–3).

A. Preeclampsia

1. Without severe features—Patients usually have few complaints, and the diastolic blood pressure is less than 110 mm Hg. Edema may be present. The platelet count is over 100,000/mcL, antepartum fetal testing is reassuring (see Tests & Procedures, above), central nervous system irritability is minimal, epigastric pain is not present, and liver enzymes are not elevated.

2. With severe features—Symptoms are more dramatic and persistent. Patients may complain of headache and changes in vision. The blood pressure is often above 160/110 mm Hg. Thrombocytopenia (platelet count less than 100,000/mcL) may be present and progress to disseminated intravascular coagulation. Severe epigastric pain may be present from hepatic subcapsular hemorrhage with significant stretch or rupture of the liver capsule. HELLP syndrome (hemolysis, elevated liver enzymes, low platelets) is an advanced form of severe preeclampsia.

B. Eclampsia

The occurrence of seizures defines eclampsia. It is a manifestation of severe central nervous system involvement. Other findings of preeclampsia are observed.

Table 19–3. Indicators of mild to moderate versus severe preeclampsia-eclampsia.

Site	Indicator	Mild to Moderate	Severe
Central nervous system	Symptoms and signs	Hyperreflexia	Seizures Blurred vision Scotomas Headache Clonus Irritability
Kidney	Proteinuria Urinary output	0.3–5 g/24 h > 30 mL/h	> 5 g/24 h or catheterized urine with 4+ protein < 30 mL/h
Liver	AST, ALT, LD	Normal liver enzymes	Elevated liver enzymes Epigastric pain Ruptured liver
Hematologic	Platelets Hemoglobin	Normal	< 100,000/mcL Low, normal, or elevated
Vascular	Blood pressure Retina	< 160/110 mm Hg Arteriolar spasm	> 160/110 mm Hg Retinal hemorrhages
Fetal-placental unit	Growth restriction Oligohydramnios Fetal distress	Absent Absent Absent	Present Present Present

ALT, alanine aminotransferase; AST, aspartate aminotransferase; LD, lactate dehydrogenase.

▶ Differential Diagnosis

Preeclampsia-eclampsia can mimic and be confused with many other diseases, including chronic hypertension, chronic kidney disease, primary seizure disorders, gallbladder and pancreatic disease, immune thrombocytopenia, thrombotic thrombocytopenic purpura, and hemolytic-uremic syndrome. It must always be considered in any pregnant woman beyond 20 weeks of gestation with consistent signs and symptoms. Although it is most common in the third trimester, it can occur earlier, especially in women with comorbid conditions like hypertension, kidney disease, and systemic lupus erythematosus. It is particularly difficult to diagnose when a preexisting disease such as hypertension is present.

▶ Treatment

Based on evidence and expert consensus, the American College of Obstetricians and Gynecologists (ACOG) supports considering the use of low-dose aspirin (81 mg orally daily) initiated between 12 weeks' and 28 weeks' gestation for women at increased risk for preeclampsia; risk factors include a history of preeclampsia, multifetal gestation, chronic hypertension, diabetes mellitus, kidney disease, or autoimmune diseases (such as systemic lupus erythematosus or antiphospholipid syndrome). In clinical studies, diuretics, dietary restriction or enhancement, sodium restriction, and vitamin-mineral supplements (eg, calcium or vitamin C and E) have not been confirmed to be useful. The only cure is delivery of the fetus at a time as favorable as possible for its survival.

A. Preeclampsia

Early recognition is the key to treatment. This requires careful attention to the details of prenatal care—especially subtle changes in blood pressure and weight. The objectives are to prolong pregnancy if possible to allow fetal lung maturity while preventing progression to severe disease and eclampsia. The critical factors are the gestational age of the fetus, fetal pulmonary maturity, and the severity of maternal disease. Preeclampsia-eclampsia at term is managed by delivery. Prior to term, severe preeclampsia-eclampsia requires delivery with very few exceptions. Epigastric pain, seizures, severe range blood pressures, thrombocytopenia, and visual disturbances are strong indications for delivery of the fetus. Marked proteinuria alone can be managed more conservatively.

1. Home management—Home management may be attempted for patients with preeclampsia without severe features and a stable home situation. This requires assistance at home, rapid access to the hospital, a reliable patient, and the ability to obtain frequent blood pressure readings. A home health nurse can often provide frequent home visits and assessments.

2. Hospital care—Hospitalization is required for women with preeclampsia with severe features or those with unreliable home situations. Regular assessments of blood pressure, urine protein, and fetal heart tones and activity are required. A CBC with platelet count, electrolyte panel, and liver enzymes should be checked regularly, with frequency dependent on severity. A 24-hour urine collection for total protein and creatinine clearance should be obtained on admission and repeated as indicated. Magnesium sulfate is not used until the diagnosis of severe preeclampsia is made and delivery planned (see Eclampsia, below).

Fetal evaluation should be obtained as part of the workup. If the patient is being admitted to the hospital, fetal testing should be performed on the same day to assess fetal well-being. This may be done by fetal heart rate testing with nonstress testing or by biophysical profile. A regular schedule of fetal surveillance must then be followed. Daily fetal kick counts can be recorded by the patient herself. If the fetus is less than 34 weeks' gestation, corticosteroids (betamethasone 12 mg intramuscularly every 24 h for two doses, or dexamethasone 6 mg intramuscularly every 12 h for four doses) can be administered to the mother. *However, when a woman is clearly suffering from unstable severe preeclampsia, delivery should not be delayed for fetal lung maturation or administration of corticosteroids.*

The method of delivery is determined by the maternal and fetal status. A vaginal delivery is preferred because it has less blood loss than a cesarean section and requires less coagulation factors. Cesarean section is reserved for the usual fetal indications. For mild preeclampsia, delivery should take place at term.

B. Eclampsia

1. Emergency care—If the patient is convulsing, she is turned on her side to prevent aspiration and to improve blood flow to the placenta. The seizure may be stopped by giving an intravenous bolus of either magnesium sulfate, 4–6 g, or lorazepam, 2–4 mg over 4 minutes or until the seizure stops. Magnesium sulfate is the preferred agent, and alternatives should be used only if magnesium sulfate is unavailable. A continuous intravenous infusion of magnesium sulfate is then started at a rate of 2–3 g/h unless the patient is known to have significantly reduced kidney function. Magnesium blood levels are then checked every 4–6 hours and the infusion rate adjusted to maintain a therapeutic blood level (4–7 mEq/L). Urinary output is checked hourly and the patient assessed for signs of possible magnesium toxicity such as loss of deep tendon reflexes or decrease in respiratory rate and depth, which can be reversed with calcium gluconate, 1 g intravenously over 2 minutes.

2. General care—In patients who have preeclampsia with severe features, magnesium sulfate should be given intravenously, 4- to 6-g load over 15–20 minutes followed by 2–3 g/h maintenance, for seizure prophylaxis. The occurrence of eclampsia necessitates delivery once the patient is stabilized. It is important, however, that assessment of the status of the patient and fetus take place first. Continuous fetal monitoring must be performed and maternal blood typed and crossmatched quickly. A urinary catheter is inserted to monitor urinary output, and a CBC with platelets, electrolytes, creatinine, and liver enzymes are obtained. If hypertension is present with systolic values of 160 mm Hg or higher or diastolic values 110 mm Hg or higher, antihypertensive medications should be administered to reduce the blood pressure to 140–150/90–100 mm Hg. Lower blood pressures than this may induce placental insufficiency through reduced perfusion. Hydralazine given in 5- to 10-mg increments intravenously every 20 minutes is frequently used to lower blood pressure. Labetalol, 10–20 mg intravenously, every 20 minutes as needed, can also be used. The 2017 ACOG guidelines for treatment of emergency hypertension include the use of immediate-release oral nifedipine (not sublingual), particularly for patients who do not have intravenous access. Nifedipine should not be used in conjunction with magnesium sulfate for seizure prophylaxis.

3. Delivery—Delivery is mandated once eclampsia has occurred. Vaginal delivery is preferred. The rapidity with which delivery must be achieved depends on the fetal and maternal status following the seizure and the availability of laboratory data on the patient. Oxytocin, given intravenously and titrated to a dose that results in adequate contractions, may be used to induce or augment labor. Oxytocin should only be administered by a clinician specifically trained in its use. Regional analgesia or general anesthesia is acceptable. Cesarean section is used for the usual obstetric indications.

4. Postpartum—Magnesium sulfate infusion (2–3 g/h) should be continued for 24 hours postpartum. Late-onset preeclampsia-eclampsia can occur during the postpartum period. It is usually manifested by either hypertension or seizures. Treatment is the same as prior to delivery—ie, with hydralazine and magnesium sulfate.

▶ When to Refer

- New onset of hypertension and proteinuria in a pregnant patient more than 20 weeks' gestation.
- New onset of seizure activity in a pregnant patient.

▶ When to Admit

- Symptoms of preeclampsia with severe features in a pregnant patient with elevated blood pressure above baseline.
- Evaluation for preeclampsia when severe features of the disease are suspected.
- Evaluation for preeclampsia in a patient with an unstable home environment.
- Evidence of eclampsia.

American College of Obstetrics and Gynecologists. Committee Opinion No. 692: Emergent therapy for acute-onset, severe hypertension during pregnancy and the postpartum period. Obstet Gynecol. 2017 Apr;129(4):e90–5. [PMID: 28333820]

American College of Obstetricians and Gynecologists. Hypertension in pregnancy. Report of the American College of Obstetricians and Gynecologists' Task Force on Hypertension in Pregnancy. Obstet Gynecol. 2013 Nov;122(5):1122–31. [PMID: 24150027]

American College of Obstetricians and Gynecologists. Practice Advisory on low-dose aspirin and prevention of preeclampsia, 2016. https://www.acog.org/Clinical-Guidance-and-Publications/Practice-Advisories/Practice-Advisory-Low-Dose-Aspirin-and-Prevention-of-Preeclampsia-Updated-Recommendations

Mol BW et al. Pre-eclampsia. Lancet. 2016 Mar 5;387(10022): 999–1011. [PMID: 26342729]

PRETERM LABOR

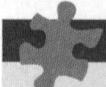

ESSENTIALS OF DIAGNOSIS

- ▶ Preterm regular uterine contractions approximately 5 minutes apart.
- ▶ Cervical dilatation, effacement, or both.

General Considerations

Preterm birth is defined as delivery prior to 37 weeks' gestation, and spontaneous preterm labor with or without premature rupture of the fetal membranes is responsible for at least two-thirds of all preterm births. Prematurity is the largest single contributor to infant mortality, and survivors are at risk for a myriad of short- and long-term complications. Rates of infant death and long-term neurologic impairment are inversely related to gestational age at birth. The cusp of viability in contemporary practice is 23–25 weeks' gestation, and infants born prior to 23 weeks rarely survive. About two-thirds of the preterm births occur between 34 weeks and 36 weeks and 6 days (termed "late preterm birth"), and good outcomes are expected at these gestational ages. Importantly, however, even these late preterm infants are at significantly increased risk for both morbidity and mortality when compared to those infants born at term.

Major risk factors for spontaneous preterm labor include a past history of preterm birth and a short cervical length as measured by transvaginal ultrasound. Patients with one or both of these risk factors have largely been the focus of recent intervention trials aiming to prevent preterm birth. Other known risk factors are many but include black race, multi-fetal pregnancies, intrauterine infection, substance abuse, smoking, periodontal disease, and socioeconomic deprivation.

Clinical Findings

In women with regular uterine contractions and cervical change, the diagnosis of preterm labor is straightforward. However, symptoms such as pelvic pressure, cramping, or vaginal discharge may be the first complaints in high-risk patients who later develop preterm labor. Because these complaints may be vague and irregular uterine contractions are common, distinguishing which patients merit further evaluation can be problematic. In some cases, this distinction can be facilitated by the use of fetal fibronectin measurement in cervicovaginal specimens. This test is most useful when it is negative (less than 50 ng/mL), since the negative predictive value for delivery within 7–14 days is 93–97%. A negative test, therefore, usually means the patient can be reassured and discharged home. Because of its low sensitivity, however, fetal fibronectin is not recommended as a screening test in asymptomatic women.

Treatment

A. General Measures

Patients must be educated to identify symptoms associated with preterm labor to avoid unnecessary delay in their evaluation. In patients who are believed to be at increased risk for preterm delivery, conventional recommendations are for limited activity and bed rest. Randomized trials, however, have failed to demonstrate improved outcomes in women placed on activity restriction. Paradoxically, such recommendations may place a woman at an *increased* risk to deliver preterm. Women with preterm labor at the threshold of viability present unique ethical and obstetric challenges and are best managed in consultation with maternal-fetal medicine and neonatology specialists. The families in such situations should be actively and continually engaged about decisions regarding the aggressiveness of resuscitative efforts.

B. Corticosteroids

In pregnancies between 23 and 34 weeks' gestation where preterm birth is anticipated, a single short course of corticosteroids should be administered to promote fetal lung maturity. Such therapy has been demonstrated to reduce the frequency of respiratory distress syndrome, intracranial hemorrhage, and even death in preterm infants. Betamethasone, 12 mg intramuscularly repeated once 24 hours later, or dexamethasone, 6 mg intramuscularly repeated every 12 hours for four doses, both cross the placenta and are the preferred treatments in this setting. A single repeat course of antenatal corticosteroids should be considered in women who are at risk for preterm delivery within the next 7 days, and whose prior dose of antenatal corticosteroids was administered more than 14 days previously. Rescue course corticosteroids could be provided as early as 7 days from the prior dose, if indicated by the clinical scenario. Administration of betamethasone may be considered in pregnant women between 34 0/7 and 36 6/7 weeks of gestation at imminent risk for preterm birth within 7 days, and who have not received a previous course of antenatal corticosteroids.

Although antibiotics have not been proven to forestall delivery, women in preterm labor should receive antimicrobial prophylaxis against group B *Streptococcus*.

C. Tocolytic Agents

Numerous tocolytic pharmacologic agents have been given in an attempt to forestall preterm birth, although none are completely effective, and there is no evidence that such therapy directly improves neonatal outcomes. Administering tocolytic agents, however, remains a reasonable approach to the initial management of preterm labor and may provide sufficient prolongation of pregnancy to administer a course of corticosteroids and (if appropriate) transport the patient to a facility better equipped to care for premature infants. Maintenance therapy (continuation of treatment beyond 48 hours) is not effective at preventing preterm birth and is not recommended. Likewise, despite the finding that preterm labor is associated with intrauterine infection in certain cases, there is no evidence that antibiotics forestall delivery in women with preterm labor and intact membranes.

Magnesium sulfate is commonly used (but no longer recommended as a first-line agent) for tocolysis, and there is evidence that it may also be protective against cerebral palsy in infants from 24 weeks' to 32 weeks' gestation when given at time of birth. It may also be used for women in labor at the prescribed gestational ages for neuroprotection in preterm infants. Magnesium sulfate is given intravenously as a 4- to 6-g bolus followed by a continuous infusion of 2 g/h. Magnesium levels are not typically checked but should be monitored if there is any concern for toxicity.

Magnesium sulfate is entirely cleared by the kidney and must, therefore, be used with caution in women with any degree of kidney disease.

Beta-adrenergic drugs such as **terbutaline** can be given as an intravenous infusion starting at 2.5 mcg/min or as a subcutaneous injection starting at 250 mcg given every 30 minutes. Oral terbutaline is not recommended because of the lack of proven efficacy and concerns about maternal safety. Serious maternal side effects have been reported with the use of terbutaline and include tachycardia, pulmonary edema, arrhythmias, metabolic derangements (such as hyperglycemia and hypokalemia), and even death. Pulmonary edema occurs with increased frequency with concomitant administration of corticosteroids, large volume intravenous fluid infusion, maternal sepsis, or prolonged tocolysis. Because of these safety concerns, the US Food and Drug Administration warns that terbutaline be administered exclusively in a hospital setting and discontinued after 48–72 hours of treatment.

Nifedipine, 20 mg orally every 6 hours, and **indomethacin**, 50 mg orally once then 25 mg orally every 6 hours up to 48 hours, have also been used with limited success. Nifedipine should not be given in conjunction with magnesium sulfate. Overall, evidence supports the use of first-line tocolytic treatment with beta-adrenergic receptor agonists, calcium channel blockers, or indomethacin for short-term prolongation of pregnancy (up to 48 hours) to allow for the administration of antenatal steroids.

Before attempts are made to prevent preterm delivery with tocolytic agents, the patient should be assessed for conditions in which delivery would be indicated. Severe preeclampsia, lethal fetal anomalies, placental abruption, and intrauterine infection are all examples of indications for preterm delivery. In such cases, attempts to forestall delivery would be inappropriate.

▶ Preterm Birth Prevention

Strategies aimed at preventing preterm birth in high-risk women—principally those with a history of preterm birth or a shortened cervix (or both)—have focused on the administration of progesterone or progesterone compounds and the use of cervical cerclage. Prospective randomized controlled trials have demonstrated reductions in rates of preterm birth in high-risk women with singleton pregnancies who received progesterone supplementation, although the optimal preparation, dose, and route of administration (intramuscular injection versus vaginal suppository) are unclear. Although the issue has not been settled, there is also some evidence that progesterone therapy may decrease rates of preterm birth in nulliparous women who are found to have a shortened cervix as measured by transvaginal ultrasound. ACOG does not recommend universal transvaginal cervical length screening but acknowledges that this strategy may be considered.

There is also evidence that women with a previous spontaneous preterm birth and a shortened cervix (less than 25 mm before 24 weeks' gestation) may benefit from placement of a cervical cerclage. Incidentally detected short cervical length in the second trimester in the absence of a prior singleton preterm birth is not diagnostic of

cervical insufficiency, and cerclage is not indicated in this setting. In twin and triplet gestations, however, neither progesterone administration nor cervical cerclage placement has been effective at prolonging pregnancy, and these therapies are not recommended in women with multi-fetal pregnancies.

▶ When to Refer

- Symptoms of increased pelvic pressure or cramping in high-risk patients.
- Regular uterine contractions.
- Rupture of membranes.
- Vaginal bleeding.

▶ When to Admit

- Cervical dilation of 2 cm or more prior to 34 weeks' gestation.
- Contractions that cause cervical change.
- Rupture of membranes.

American College of Obstetricians and Gynecologists. ACOG Practice Bulletin No. 130: Prediction and prevention of preterm birth. Obstet Gynecol. 2012 Oct;120(4):964–73. [Reaffirmed 2018] [PMID: 22996126]

American College of Obstetricians and Gynecologists. ACOG Practice Bulletin No. 142: Cerclage for the management of cervical insufficiency. Obstet Gynecol. 2014 Feb;123(2 Pt 1): 372–9. [Reaffirmed 2016] [PMID: 24451674]

American College of Obstetricians and Gynecologists. ACOG Practice Bulletin No. 171: Management of preterm labor. Obstet Gynecol. 2016 Oct;128:e155–64. [PMID: 27661654]

American College of Obstetricians and Gynecologists. Committee Opinion No. 713: Antenatal corticosteroid therapy for fetal maturation. Obstet Gynecol. 2017 Aug;130(2):e102–9. [PMID: 28742678]

THIRD-TRIMESTER BLEEDING

Five to 10 percent of women have vaginal bleeding in late pregnancy. The clinician must distinguish between placental causes (placenta previa, placental abruption, vasa previa) and nonplacental causes (labor, infection, disorders of the lower genital tract, systemic disease). The approach to bleeding in late pregnancy depends on the underlying cause, the gestational age at presentation, the degree of blood loss, and the overall status of the mother and her fetus. The cause of antepartum bleeding after midpregnancy is unknown in one-third of cases.

▶ Treatment

A. General Measures

The patient should initially be observed closely with continuous fetal monitoring to assess for fetal distress. A complete blood count with platelets and a prothrombin time (INR) should be obtained and repeated serially if the bleeding continues. If hemorrhage is significant or if there is evidence of acute hypovolemia, the need for transfusion should be anticipated and an appropriate volume of red cells prepared with cross-matching. Ultrasound examination should be performed to determine placental location. Digital pelvic examinations are done only after ultrasound examination has ruled out placenta previa. Administration of anti-D immune globulin may be required for women who are Rh negative.

B. Placenta Previa

Placenta previa occurs when the placenta implants over the internal cervical os. Risk factors for this condition include previous cesarean delivery, increasing maternal age, multiparity, and smoking. If the diagnosis is initially made in the first or second trimester, the ultrasound should be repeated in the third trimester. Persistence of placenta previa at this point is an indication for cesarean as the route of delivery. Painless vaginal bleeding is the characteristic symptom in placenta previa and can range from light spotting to profuse hemorrhage. Hospitalization for extended evaluation is the appropriate initial management approach. For pregnancies that have reached 37 weeks' gestation or beyond with continued bleeding, cesarean delivery is generally indicated. Pregnancies at 36 weeks or earlier are candidates for expectant management provided the bleeding is not prodigious, and a subset of these women can be discharged if the bleeding and contractions completely subside.

C. Morbidly Adherent Placenta

Morbidly adherent placenta is a general term describing an abnormally adherent placenta that has invaded into the uterus. The condition can be further classified depending on whether the depth of invasion is limited to the endometrium (*accreta*), extends into the myometrium (*increta*), or invades beyond the uterine serosa (*percreta*). The most important risk factor for a morbidly adherent placenta is a prior uterine scar—typically from one or more prior cesarean deliveries. The focus of invasion usually involves the scar itself, and *placenta previa* is commonly associated with morbid adherence. Of serious concern for the field of obstetrics, the incidence of these syndromes has increased dramatically over the last 50 years commensurate with the increasing cesarean delivery rate.

After delivery of the infant, almost always in a repeat cesarean section, the morbidly adherent placenta does not separate normally, and the bleeding that results can be torrential. Emergency hysterectomy is usually required to stop the hemorrhage, and transfusion requirements are often massive. Because of the considerable increase in both maternal morbidity and mortality associated with this condition, careful preoperative planning is imperative when the diagnosis is suspected antenatally. Ultrasound findings such as intraplacental lacunae, bridging vessels into the bladder, and loss of the retroplacental clear space suggest placental invasion in women who have placenta previa. *Importantly, however, even if ultrasound findings are subtle, an abnormally adherent placenta should be suspected in any patient with one or more prior cesarean deliveries and an anterior placenta previa.* Ideally, delivery planning should involve a multidisciplinary team, and the surgery should take place at an institution with appropriate personnel and a blood bank equipped to handle patients requiring massive transfusion. It has been demonstrated that a systematic approach to management with a multidisciplinary team improves patient outcomes. Evidence-based recommendations regarding delivery timing are lacking, but the goal is to have a planned, late-preterm cesarean delivery. As such, delivery at 34–36 weeks in a stable patient seems a reasonable approach.

D. Placental Abruption

Placental abruption is the premature separation of the placenta from its implantation site before delivery. Hypertension is a known risk factor for abruption. Other risk factors include multiparity, cocaine use, smoking, previous abruption, and thrombophilias. Classic symptoms are vaginal bleeding, uterine tenderness, and frequent contractions, but the clinical presentation is highly variable. There is often concealed hemorrhage when the placenta abrupts, which causes increased pressure in the intervillous space. Excess amounts of thromboplastin escape into the maternal circulation and defibrination occurs. Profound coagulopathy and acute hypovolemia from blood loss can occur and are more likely with an abruption severe enough to kill the fetus. Ultrasound may be helpful to exclude placenta previa, but failure to identify a retroplacental clot does not exclude abruption. In most cases, abruption is an indication for immediate cesarean delivery because of the high risk of fetal death.

American College of Obstetricians and Gynecologists. Committee Opinion No. 529: Placenta accreta. Obstet Gynecol. 2012 Jul; 120(1):207–11. [Reaffirmed 2017] [PMID: 22914422]

American College of Obstetricians and Gynecologists. Practice Bulletin No. 183: Postpartum hemorrhage. Obstet Gynecol. 2017 Oct;130(4):e168–86. [PMID: 28937571]

Bartels HC et al. Association of implementing a multidisciplinary team approach in the management of morbidly adherent placenta with maternal morbidity and mortality. Obstet Gynecol. 2018 Nov;132(5):1167–76. [PMID: 30234729]

Shamshirsaz AA et al. Outcomes of planned compared with urgent deliveries using a multidisciplinary team approach for morbidly adherent placenta. Obstet Gynecol. 2018 Feb; 131(2):234–41. [PMID: 29324609]

OBSTETRIC COMPLICATIONS OF THE PERIPARTUM PERIOD

PUERPERAL MASTITIS

Postpartum mastitis occurs sporadically in nursing mothers, usually with symptom onset after discharge from the hospital. *Staphylococcus aureus* is usually the causative agent. Women nursing for the first time and those with difficulty breastfeeding appear to be at greatest risk. Rarely, inflammatory carcinoma of the breast can be mistaken for puerperal mastitis (see also Chapter 17). Unfortunately, strategies aimed at preventing mastitis in breastfeeding women have been unsuccessful.

Mastitis frequently begins within 3 months after delivery and may start with an engorged breast and a sore or fissured nipple. Cellulitis is typically unilateral with the affected area of breast being red, tender, and warm. Fever and chills are common complaints as well. Treatment consists of antibiotics effective against penicillin-resistant staphylococci (dicloxacillin 500 mg orally every 6 hours or a cephalosporin for 10–14 days) and regular emptying of the breast by nursing or by using a mechanical suction device. Although nursing of the infected breast is safe for the infant, local inflammation of the nipple may complicate latching. Failure to respond to usual antibiotics within 3 days may represent an organizing abscess or infection with a resistant organism. When the causative organism is methicillin-resistant *S aureus* (MRSA), the risk for abscess formation is increased when compared with infection caused by nonresistant staphylococcal species. If an abscess is suspected, ultrasound of the breast can help confirm the diagnosis. In these cases, aspiration or surgical evacuation is usually required. Changing antibiotics based on culture sensitivity (to vancomycin or trimethoprim-sulfamethoxazole, for example) is useful, especially if the clinical course is not improving appropriately.

Fernández L et al. Prevention of infectious mastitis by oral administration of *Lactobacillus salivarius* PS2 during late pregnancy. Clin Infect Dis. 2016 Mar 1;62(5):568–73. [PMID: 26611780]

Mediano P et al. Microbial diversity in milk of women with mastitis: potential role of coagulase-negative staphylococci, viridans group streptococci, and corynebacteria. J Hum Lact. 2017 May;33(2):309–18. [PMID: 28418794]

Yu Z et al. High-risk factors for suppurative mastitis in lactating women. Med Sci Monit. 2018 Jun 19;24:4192–7. [PMID: 29916453]

CHORIOAMNIONITIS & METRITIS

> ### ESSENTIALS OF DIAGNOSIS
>
> ▶ Fever not attributable to another source.
> ▶ Uterine tenderness.
> ▶ Tachycardia in the mother, fetus, or both.

General Considerations

Pelvic infections are relatively common problems encountered during the peripartum period. Chorioamnionitis is an infection of the amnion and chorion (fetal parts), usually occurring during labor. Uterine infection after delivery is often called endometritis or endomyometritis, but the term "metritis" is probably most accurate to emphasize that the infection extends throughout the uterine tissue. These infections are polymicrobial and are most commonly attributed to urogenital pathogens. The single most important risk factor for puerperal infection is cesarean delivery, which increases the risk from 5- to 20-fold. Other recognized risk factors include prolonged labor, use of internal monitors, nulliparity, multiple pelvic examinations, prolonged rupture of membranes, and lower genital tract infections. Although maternal complications such as

dysfunctional labor and postpartum hemorrhage are increased with clinical chorioamnionitis, the principal reason to initiate treatment is to prevent morbidity in the offspring. Neonatal complications such as sepsis, pneumonia, intraventricular hemorrhage, and cerebral palsy are increased in the setting of chorioamnionitis. Intrapartum initiation of antibiotics, however, significantly reduces neonatal morbidity.

Clinical Findings

Puerperal infections are diagnosed principally by the presence of fever (38°C or higher) in the absence of any other source and one or more of the following signs: maternal or fetal tachycardia (or both), and uterine tenderness. Foul-smelling lochia may be present, but is an insensitive marker of infection as many women without infection also experience an unpleasant odor. Likewise, some life-threatening infections such as necrotizing fasciitis are typically odorless. Cultures are typically not done because of the polymicrobial nature of the infection.

Treatment

Treatment is empiric with broad-spectrum antibiotics that will cover gram-positive and gram-negative organisms if still pregnant and gram-negative organisms and anaerobes if postpartum. A common regimen for chorioamnionitis is ampicillin, 2 g intravenously every 6 hours, and gentamicin, 2 mg/kg intravenous load then 1.5 mg/kg intravenously every 8 hours. A common regimen for metritis is gentamicin, 2 mg/kg intravenous load then 1.5 mg/kg intravenously every 8 hours, and clindamycin, 900 mg intravenously every 8 hours. Antibiotics are stopped in the mother when she has been afebrile (and asymptomatic) for 24 hours. No oral antibiotics are subsequently needed. Patients with metritis who do not respond in the first 24–48 hours may have an enterococcal component of metritis and require additional gram-positive coverage (such as ampicillin) to the regimen.

Higgins RD et al; Chorioamnionitis Workshop Participants. Evaluation and management of women and newborns with a maternal diagnosis of chorioamnionitis: summary of a workshop. Obstet Gynecol. 2016 Mar;127(3):426–36. [PMID: 26855098]

Mackeen AD et al. Antibiotic regimens for postpartum endometritis. Cochrane Database Syst Rev. 2015 Feb 2;(2):CD001067. [PMID: 25922861]

MEDICAL CONDITIONS COMPLICATING PREGNANCY

ANEMIA

Normal pregnancy is characterized by an increase in maternal plasma volume of about 50% and an increase in red cell volume of about 25%. Because of these changes, the mean hemoglobin and hematocrit values are lower than in the nonpregnant state. Anemia in pregnancy is considered when the hemoglobin measurement is below 11 g/dL. By far, the most common causes are iron deficiency and acute blood loss anemia, the latter usually occurring in the peripartum period. Symptoms such as fatigue and dyspnea that would otherwise suggest the presence of anemia in non-pregnant women are common in pregnant women; therefore, periodic measurement of hematocrits in pregnancy is essential so that anemia can be identified and treated. In addition to its impact on maternal health, untoward pregnancy outcomes such as low birthweight and preterm delivery have been associated with second- and third-trimester anemia.

A. Iron Deficiency Anemia

The increased requirement for iron over the course of pregnancy is appreciable in order to support fetal growth and expansion of maternal blood volume. Dietary intake of iron is generally insufficient to meet this demand, and it is recommended that all pregnant women receive about 30 mg of elemental iron per day in the second and third trimesters. Oral iron therapy is commonly associated with gastrointestinal side effects, such as nausea and constipation, and these symptoms often contribute to noncompliance. If supplementation is inadequate, however, anemia often becomes evident by the third trimester of pregnancy. Because iron deficiency is by far the most common cause of anemia in pregnancy, treatment is usually empiric and consists of 60–100 mg of elemental iron per day and a diet containing iron-rich foods. Iron studies can confirm the diagnosis if necessary (see Chapter 13), and further evaluation should be considered in patients who do not respond to oral iron. Intermittent iron supplementation (eg, every other day) has been associated with fewer side effects and may be reasonable for women who cannot tolerate daily therapy.

B. Folic Acid Deficiency Anemia

Megaloblastic anemia in pregnancy is almost always caused by folic acid deficiency, since vitamin B_{12} deficiency is extremely uncommon in the childbearing years. Folate deficiency is usually caused by inadequate dietary intake of fresh leafy vegetables, legumes, and animal proteins.

The diagnosis is made by finding macrocytic red cells and hypersegmented neutrophils on a blood smear (see Chapter 13). However, blood smears in pregnancy may be difficult to interpret, since they frequently show iron deficiency changes as well. With established folate deficiency, a supplemental dose of 1 mg/day and a diet with increased folic acid is generally sufficient to correct the anemia.

C. Sickle Cell Anemia

Women with sickle cell anemia are subject to serious complications in pregnancy. The anemia becomes more severe, and acute pain crises often occur more frequently. When compared with women who do not have hemoglobinopathies, women with hemoglobin SS are at increased risk for infections (especially pulmonary and urinary tract), thromboembolic events, pregnancy-related hypertension, transfusion, cesarean delivery, preterm birth, and fetal growth restriction. There also continues to be an increased rate of maternal mortality, despite an increased recognition

of the high-risk nature of these pregnancies. Intensive medical treatment may improve the outcomes for both mother and fetus. Prophylactically transfusing packed red cells to lower the level of hemoglobin S and elevate the level of hemoglobin A is a controversial practice without clear benefit. Most women with sickle cell disease will not require iron supplementation, but folate requirements can be appreciable due to red cell turnover from hemolysis.

D. Other Anemias

Although many of the inherited or acquired causes of anemia are relatively rare in women of childbearing age, they can be encountered in pregnancy. The implications for the mother and her offspring vary widely depending on the etiology of anemia. For example, mild microcytic anemia may be caused by iron deficiency, but it could also represent anemia of chronic disease as a result of previously undiagnosed malignancy. As such, women who have anemia caused by a disorder besides a nutritional deficiency are best managed in conjunction with a maternal fetal medicine specialist and a hematologist. Additionally, women who have an inherited form of anemia (hemoglobinopathies and thalassemia syndromes, for example) should be offered genetic counseling; prenatal diagnosis, if available, should be discussed if the parents wish to know whether the fetus is affected.

American College of Obstetricians and Gynecologists. ACOG Practice Bulletin No. 95: Anemia in pregnancy. Obstet Gynecol. 2008 Jul;112(1):201–7. [Reaffirmed 2017] [PMID: 18591330]

American College of Obstetricians and Gynecologists. ACOG Practice Bulletin No. 78: Hemoglobinopathies in pregnancy. Obstet Gynecol 2007 Jan;109(1):229–37. [Reaffirmed 2018] [PMID: 17197616]

Hathaway AR. Sickle cell disease in pregnancy. South Med J. 2016 Sep;109(9):554–6. [PMID: 27598360]

ANTIPHOSPHOLIPID SYNDROME

The antiphospholipid syndrome (APS) is characterized by the presence of specific autoantibodies in association with certain clinical conditions, most notably arterial and venous thrombosis and adverse pregnancy outcomes. Clinically, the diagnosis can be suspected after any of the following outcomes: an episode of thrombosis, three or more unexplained consecutive spontaneous abortions prior to 10 weeks' gestation, one or more unexplained deaths of a morphologically normal fetus after 10 weeks' gestation, or a preterm delivery at less than 34 weeks due to preeclampsia or placental insufficiency. In addition to these clinical features, laboratory criteria include the identification of at least one of the following three antiphospholipid antibodies: (1) anticardiolipin antibodies, (2) anti-beta-2-glycoprotein I antibodies, or (3) the lupus anticoagulant (see Chapter 20).

The optimal treatment for APS in pregnancy is unclear but generally involves administration of a heparin compound (unfractionated or LMWH) in prophylactic amounts (5000–10,000 units subcutaneously twice per day for the former) and low-dose aspirin (81 mg). Although anticoagulation is particularly prudent in women with a history of thrombosis, there is also evidence that this management reduces the risk for spontaneous abortion in women with recurrent pregnancy loss from APS. It is not clear whether continuation of therapy beyond the first trimester decreases the risk for stillbirth or placental dysfunction; however, treatment is typically continued through pregnancy and the early postpartum period for thromboprophylaxis. LMWH is also commonly used for this indication (30–40 mg subcutaneously once per day); however, it is not clear that LMWH has the same effect on reducing the risk of recurrent abortion as unfractionated heparin. Either prophylactic or therapeutic dosing strategies may be appropriate depending on the patient's history and clinical risk factors. The use of corticosteroids and intravenous immunoglobulin is of unclear benefit in these patients, and neither treatment is recommended.

American College of Obstetricians and Gynecologists. No. 132: Antiphospholipid syndrome. Obstet Gynecol. 2012 Dec; 120(6):1514–21. [Reaffirmed 2017] [PMID: 23168789]

Santos TDS et al. Antiphospholipid syndrome and recurrent miscarriage: a systematic review and meta-analysis. J Reprod Immunol. 2017 Sep;123:78–87. [PMID: 28985591]

THYROID DISEASE

See Chapter 26.

Thyroid disease is relatively common in pregnancy, and in their overt states, both hypothyroidism and hyperthyroidism have been consistently associated with adverse pregnancy outcomes. Fortunately, these risks are mitigated by adequate treatment. It is essential to understand the gestational age-specific effects that pregnancy has on thyroid function tests, since these biochemical markers are required to make the diagnosis of thyroid dysfunction. Failure to recognize these physiologic alterations can result in misclassification or misdiagnosis. Women who have a history of a thyroid disorder or symptoms that suggest thyroid dysfunction should be screened with thyroid function tests. Screening asymptomatic pregnant women, however, is of unproven benefit and is not currently recommended.

Overt hypothyroidism is defined by an elevated serum TSH level with a depressed FT_4 level. The condition in pregnancy has consistently been associated with an increase in complications such as spontaneous abortion, preterm birth, preeclampsia, placental abruption, and impaired neuropsychological development in the offspring. The most common etiology is Hashimoto (autoimmune) thyroiditis. Many of the symptoms of hypothyroidism mimic those of normal pregnancy, making its clinical identification difficult. Initial treatment is empiric with oral levothyroxine started at 75–100 mcg/day. Thyroid function tests can be repeated at 4–6 weeks and the dose adjusted as necessary with the goal of normalizing the TSH level (preferably to a trimester-specific gestational reference range). An increase in the dose of levothyroxine may be required in the second and third trimesters.

Subclinical hypothyroidism is defined as an increased serum TSH with a normal FT_4 level. Although some studies have found associations with untoward pregnancy outcomes such as miscarriage, preterm birth, and preeclampsia, others have failed to confirm these findings. There is currently no evidence, however, that identification and treatment of subclinical hypothyroidism will prevent any of these outcomes. Data from an NIH-sponsored Maternal-Fetal Medicine Units Network randomized, controlled trial demonstrated no improvement in cognitive function of 5-year-olds born to women screened and treated for subclinical hypothyroidism. For these reasons, the American College of Obstetricians and Gynecologists and the American Association of Clinical Endocrinologists recommend against universal screening for thyroid disease in pregnancy.

Overt hyperthyroidism, defined as excessive production of thyroxine with a depressed (usually undetectable) serum TSH level, is also associated with increased risks in pregnancy. Spontaneous abortion, preterm birth, preeclampsia, and maternal heart failure occur with increased frequency with untreated thyrotoxicosis. Thyroid storm, although rare, can be a life-threatening complication. Medical treatment of thyrotoxicosis is usually accomplished with the antithyroid drugs propylthiouracil or methimazole. Although teratogenicity has not been clearly established, in utero exposure to methimazole has been associated with aplasia cutis and choanal and esophageal atresia in the offspring of pregnancies so treated. Propylthiouracil is not believed to be teratogenic, but it has been associated with the rare complications of hepatotoxicity and agranulocytosis. Recommendations by the American Thyroid Association are to treat with propylthiouracil in the first trimester and convert to methimazole for the remainder of the pregnancy. The therapeutic target for the FT_4 level is the upper limit of the normal reference range. The TSH levels generally stay suppressed even with adequate treatment. A beta-blocker can be used for such symptoms as palpitations or tremors. Fetal hypothyroidism or hyperthyroidism is uncommon but can occur with maternal Graves disease, which is the most common cause of hyperthyroidism in pregnancy. *Radioiodine ablation is absolutely contraindicated in pregnancy because it may destroy the fetal thyroid as well.*

Transient autoimmune thyroiditis can occur in the postpartum period and is evident within the first year after delivery. The first phase, occurring up to 4 months postpartum, is a hyperthyroid state. Over the next few months, there is a transition to a hypothyroid state, which may require treatment with levothyroxine. Spontaneous resolution to a euthyroid state within the first year is the expected course; however, some women remain hypothyroid beyond this time (see Chapter 26).

American College of Obstetricians and Gynecologists. Practice Bulletin No. 148: Thyroid disease in pregnancy. Obstet Gynecol. 2015 Apr;125(4):996–1005. [Reaffirmed 2017] [PMID: 25798985]

Casey BM et al; Eunice Kennedy Shriver National Institute of Child Health and Human Development Maternal–Fetal Medicine Units Network. Treatment of subclinical hypothyroidism or hypothyroxinemia in pregnancy. N Engl J Med. 2017 Mar 2; 376(9):815–25. [PMID: 28249134]

DIABETES MELLITUS

Normal pregnancy can be characterized as a state of increased insulin resistance that helps ensure a steady stream of glucose delivery to the developing fetus. Thus, both mild fasting hypoglycemia and postprandial hyperglycemia are physiologic. These metabolic changes are felt to be hormonally mediated with likely contributions from human placental lactogen, estrogen, and progesterone.

A. Gestational Diabetes Mellitus

Gestational diabetes mellitus is abnormal glucose tolerance in pregnancy and is generally believed to be an exaggeration of the pregnancy-induced physiologic changes in carbohydrate metabolism. Alternatively, pregnancy may unmask an underlying propensity for glucose intolerance, which will be evident in the nonpregnant state at some future time if not in the immediate postpartum period. Indeed, at least 50% of women with gestational diabetes are diagnosed with overt diabetes at some point in their lifetime. During the pregnancy, the principal concern in women identified to have gestational diabetes is excessive fetal growth, which can result in increased maternal and perinatal morbidity. Shoulder dystocia occurs more frequently in infants of diabetic mothers because of fetal overgrowth and increased fat deposition on the shoulders. Cesarean delivery and preeclampsia are also significantly increased in women with diabetes, both gestational and overt.

All asymptomatic pregnant women should undergo laboratory screening for gestational diabetes after 24 weeks' gestation. The diagnostic thresholds for glucose tolerance tests in pregnancy are not universally agreed upon, and importantly, adverse pregnancy outcomes appear to occur along a continuum of glucose intolerance even if the diagnosis of gestational diabetes is not formally assigned. A two-stage testing strategy is recommended by the American College of Obstetricians and Gynecologists, starting with a 50-g screening test offered to all pregnant women at 24–28 weeks' gestation. If this test is abnormal, the diagnostic test is a 100-g oral glucose tolerance test (Table 19–4).

Women in whom gestational diabetes is diagnosed should undergo nutrition counseling, and medications are typically initiated for those with persistent fasting hyperglycemia. Insulin has historically been considered the standard medication used to achieve glycemic control. Oral hypoglycemic agents, principally glyburide and metformin, have been evaluated in short-term clinical trials and appear to achieve similar degrees of glycemic control to insulin without increasing maternal or neonatal morbidity. These medications, however, have not been approved by the US Food and Drug Administration for this indication, and the long-term safety of oral agents has not been adequately studied in the women so treated or in their offspring. The current standard of care, nonetheless, is that either insulin or oral agents are appropriate first-line therapy. Insulin regimens commonly include multiple daily injections of a split dose mix of intermediate-acting and short-acting agents. Regular and NPH insulins, as well as insulin lispro and aspart, do not cross the placenta. Once therapy is initiated, blood glucose surveillance is important

Table 19–4. Screening and diagnostic criteria for gestational diabetes mellitus.

Screening for gestational diabetes mellitus
1. 50-g oral glucose load, administered between 24 and 28 weeks, without regard to time of day or time of last meal.
2. Venous plasma glucose measured 1 hour later.
3. Value of 140 mg/dL (7.8 mmol/L) or above in venous plasma indicates the need for a diagnostic glucose tolerance test.

Diagnosis of gestational diabetes mellitus
1. 100-g oral glucose load, administered in the morning after overnight fast lasting at least 8 hours but not more than 14 hours, and following at least 3 days of unrestricted diet (> 150 g carbohydrate) and physical activity.
2. Venous plasma glucose is measured fasting and at 1, 2, and 3 hours. Patient should remain seated and should not smoke throughout the test.
3. The diagnosis of gestational diabetes is made when two or more of the following venous plasma concentrations are met or exceeded: fasting, 95 mg/dL (5.3 mmol/L); 1 hour, 180 mg/dL (10 mmol/L); 2 hours, 155 mg/dL (8.6 mmol/L); 3 hours, 140 mg/dL (7.8 mmol/L).

to assess for adequacy of glycemic control. Capillary blood glucose levels should be checked four times per day, once fasting and three times after meals. Euglycemia is considered to be 60–90 mg/dL (3.3–5.0 mmol/L) while fasting and less than 120 mg/dL (6.7 mmol/L) 2 hours postprandially. Intensive therapy with dietary modifications or insulin therapy, or both, has been demonstrated to decrease rates of macrosomia, shoulder dystocia, and preeclampsia. Because of the increased prevalence of overt diabetes in women identified to have gestational diabetes, they should be screened at 6–12 weeks' postpartum with a fasting plasma glucose test or a 2-hour oral glucose tolerance test (75-g glucose load).

B. Overt Diabetes Mellitus

Overt diabetes is diabetes mellitus that antedates the pregnancy. As in gestational diabetes, fetal overgrowth from inadequately controlled hyperglycemia remains a significant concern because of the increased maternal and perinatal morbidity that accompany macrosomia. Women with overt diabetes are subject to a number of other complications as well. Spontaneous abortions and third-trimester stillbirths occur with increased frequency in these women. There is also at least a twofold to threefold increased risk for fetal malformations, as hyperglycemia during organogenesis is teratogenic. The most common malformations in offspring of diabetic women are cardiac, skeletal, and neural tube defects. For the mother, the likelihood of infections and pregnancy-related hypertension is increased.

Preconception counseling and evaluation in a diabetic woman is ideal to maximize the pregnancy outcomes. This provides an opportunity to optimize glycemic control and evaluate for evidence of end-organ damage. The initial evaluation of diabetic women should include a complete chemistry panel, HbA_{1c} determination, 24-hour urine collection for total protein and creatinine clearance, funduscopic examination, and an ECG. Hypertension is common and may require treatment. Optimally, euglycemia should be established before conception and maintained during pregnancy with daily home glucose monitoring by the patient. There is an inverse relationship between glycemic control and the occurrence of fetal malformations, and women whose periconceptional glycosylated hemoglobin levels are at or near normal levels have rates of malformations that approach baseline. A well-planned dietary program is a key component, with an intake of 1800–2200 kcal/day divided into three meals and three snacks. Insulin is given subcutaneously in a split-dose regimen as described above for women with gestational diabetes. The use of continuous insulin pump therapy may be helpful for some patients.

Throughout the pregnancy, diabetic women should be seen every 2–3 weeks and more frequently depending on the clinical condition. Adjustments in the insulin regimen may be necessary as the pregnancy progresses to maintain optimal glycemic control. A specialized ultrasound is often performed around 20 weeks to screen for fetal malformations. Symptoms and signs of infections should be evaluated and promptly treated. In the third trimester, fetal surveillance is indicated, and women with diabetes should receive serial antenatal testing (usually in the form of a nonstress test or biophysical profile). The timing of delivery is dictated by the quality of diabetic control, the presence or absence of medical complications, and fetal status. The goal is to reach 39 weeks (38 completed weeks) and then proceed with delivery. Confirmation of lung maturity may be appropriate if preterm delivery is contemplated.

American College of Obstetricians and Gynecologists. Practice Bulletin No. 60. Pregestational diabetes mellitus. Obstet Gynecol. 2005 Mar;105(3):675–85. [Reaffirmed 2016] [PMID: 15738045]

American College of Obstetricians and Gynecologists. Practice Bulletin No. 180: Gestational diabetes mellitus. Obstet Gynecol. 2017 Jul;130(1):e17–37. [PMID: 28644336]

Bryant SN et al. Diabetic ketoacidosis complicating pregnancy. J Neonatal Perinatal Med. 2017;10(1):17–23. [PMID: 28304323]

Melamed N et al. Induction of labor before 40 weeks is associated with lower rate of cesarean delivery in women with gestational diabetes mellitus. Am J Obstet Gynecol. 2016 Mar; 214(3):364.e1–8. [PMID: 26928149]

Moyer VA et al. Screening for gestational diabetes mellitus: U.S. Preventive Services Task Force recommendation statement. Ann Intern Med. 2014 Mar 18;160(6):414–20. [PMID: 24424622]

CHRONIC HYPERTENSION

Chronic hypertension is estimated to complicate up to 5% of pregnancies. To establish this diagnosis, hypertension should antedate the pregnancy or be evident before 20 weeks' gestation to differentiate it from pregnancy-related hypertension. This distinction can be problematic when the initial presentation is after 20 weeks, but chronic hypertension is confirmed if the blood pressure remains elevated beyond 12 weeks' postpartum. Risk factors for chronic hypertension include older maternal age, African-American race, and obesity. While essential hypertension is by far the most common cause, secondary causes should be sought when clinically indicated.

Women with chronic hypertension are at increased risk for adverse maternal and perinatal outcomes. Superimposed preeclampsia develops in up to 20% of women with mild hypertension, but the risk increases up to 50% when there is severe baseline hypertension (160/110 mm Hg or higher) and may be even higher when there is evidence of end-organ damage. When preeclampsia is superimposed on chronic hypertension, there is a tendency for it to occur at an earlier gestational age, be more severe, and impair fetal growth. Women with chronic hypertension are also at increased risk for placental abruption, cesarean delivery, preterm birth, and perinatal mortality.

Ideally, women with chronic hypertension should undergo a preconceptional evaluation to detect end-organ damage, assess the need for antihypertensive therapy, and discontinue teratogenic medications. The specific tests ordered may vary depending on the severity of the hypertensive disorder, but an evaluation of kidney and cardiac function (eg, 24-hour urine protein and maternal echocardiogram if mother takes medications) is appropriate.

If the woman is not known to have chronic hypertension, then initiation of antihypertensive therapy in pregnant women is indicated only if the blood pressure is sustained at or above 160/105 mm Hg or if there is evidence of end-organ damage. Treatment of hypertension has not been demonstrated to improve pregnancy outcomes, but it is indicated in women with significant hypertension for long-term maternal cardiovascular health. Although methyldopa has the longest record of safety in pregnancy, nifedipine and labetalol are also acceptable, and these three agents are recommended above all others when initiating therapy in pregnancy. Care must be taken not to excessively reduce the blood pressure, as this may decrease uteroplacental perfusion. The goal is a modest reduction in blood pressure and avoidance of severe hypertension.

If a woman with mild chronic hypertension is stable on a medical regimen when she becomes pregnant, it is usually appropriate to continue this therapy, although the benefits of doing so are not well established. *Angiotensin-converting enzyme (ACE) inhibitors and angiotensin receptor blockers, however, are contraindicated in all trimesters of pregnancy.* These medications are teratogenic in the first trimester and cause fetal hypocalvaria and acute kidney injury in the second and third trimesters.

When there is sustained severe hypertension despite multiple medications or significant end-organ damage from hypertensive disease, pregnancy is not likely to be tolerated well. In these situations, therapeutic abortion may be appropriate. If the pregnancy is continued, the woman must be counseled that the maternal and perinatal risks are appreciable, and complications such as superimposed preeclampsia and fetal growth restriction should be anticipated.

American College of Obstetricians and Gynecologists; Task Force on Hypertension in Pregnancy. Hypertension in pregnancy. Obstet Gynecol. 2013 Nov;122(5):1122–31. [PMID: 24150027]

Morgan JL et al. Blood pressure profiles across pregnancy in women with chronic hypertension. Am J Perinatol. 2016 Oct; 33(12):1128–32. [PMID: 27322664]

Moussa HN et al. Pregnancy outcomes in women with pre-eclampsia superimposed on chronic hypertension with and without severe features. Am J Perinatol. 2017 Mar;34(4): 403–8. [PMID: 27606778]

HEART DISEASE

Normal pregnancy physiology is characterized by cardiovascular adaptations in the mother. Cardiac output increases markedly as a result of both augmented stroke volume and an increase in the resting heart rate, and the maternal blood volume expands by up to 50%. These changes may not be tolerated well in women with functional or structural abnormalities of the heart. Thus, although only a small number of pregnancies are complicated by cardiac disease, these contribute disproportionately to overall rates of maternal morbidity and mortality. Most cardiac disease in women of childbearing age in the United States is caused by congenital heart disease. Ischemic heart disease, however, is being seen more commonly in pregnant women due to increasing rates of comorbid conditions, such as diabetes mellitus, hypertension, and obesity.

For practical purposes, the best single measurement of cardiopulmonary status is defined by the New York Heart Association Functional Classification. Most pregnant women with cardiac disease have class I or II functional disability, and although good outcomes are generally anticipated in this group, complications such as preeclampsia, preterm birth, and low birth weight appear to occur with increased frequency. Women with more severe disability (class III or IV) are rare in contemporary obstetrics; however, the maternal mortality is markedly increased in this setting and is usually the result of heart failure. Because of these risks, therapeutic abortion for maternal health should be considered in women who are severely disabled from cardiac disease. Specific conditions that have been associated with a particularly high risk for maternal death include Eisenmenger syndrome, primary pulmonary hypertension, Marfan syndrome with aortic root dilatation, and severe aortic or mitral stenosis. In general, these conditions should be considered contraindications to pregnancy.

The importance of preconceptional counseling for women with heart disease cannot be overstated. A thorough evaluation prior to pregnancy provides an opportunity for comprehensive risk assessment and detailed planning. Once pregnant, women with cardiac disease are best treated by a team of practitioners with experience in caring for such patients. Heart failure and arrhythmias are the most common cardiovascular complications associated with heart disease in pregnancy, and adverse maternal and fetal outcomes are increased when they occur. Symptoms of volume overload should therefore be evaluated and treated promptly. Labor management depends on the underlying cardiac lesion and the degree of disability. Women with a history of arrhythmia should have continuous cardiac monitoring throughout labor, delivery, and the immediate postpartum period. Cesarean delivery is generally reserved for obstetric indications but may be appropriate for women in whom Valsalva maneuvers are contraindicated. The early postpartum period is a critical time for fluid management. Patients who are predisposed to heart failure should be monitored closely during the puerperium.

Infective endocarditis prophylaxis is not recommended for a vaginal or cesarean delivery in the absence of infection, except in the very small subset of patients at highest risk for adverse outcomes from endocarditis. The women at highest risk include those with cyanotic heart disease, prosthetic valves, or both. If infection is present, such as chorioamnionitis, the underlying infection should be treated with the usual regimen and additional agents are not needed specifically for endocarditis prophylaxis. Prophylaxis, if required, should be given intravenously (see Table 33–5).

American College of Obstetricians and Gynecologists. Practice Bulletin No. 199: Use of prophylactic antibiotics in labor and delivery. Obstet Gynecol. 2018 Sep;132(3):e103–19. [PMID: 30134425]
Canobbio MM et al. Management of pregnancy in patients with complex congenital heart disease: a scientific statement for healthcare professionals from the American Heart Association. 2017 Feb 21;135(8):e50–87. [PMID: 28082385]

ASTHMA

(See also Chapter 9.)

Asthma is one of the most common medical conditions encountered in pregnancy. Women with mild to moderate asthma can generally expect excellent pregnancy outcomes, but severe or poorly controlled asthma has been associated with a number of pregnancy complications, including preterm birth, small-for-gestational-age infants, and preeclampsia. The effects of pregnancy on asthma are likely minimal as asthma severity in the pregnancy has been reported to be similar to its severity during the year preceding the pregnancy. Strategies for treatment are similar to those in nonpregnant women. Patients should be educated about symptom management and avoidance of asthma triggers. Baseline pulmonary function tests can provide an objective assessment of lung function and may help the patient with self-monitoring of her asthma severity using a peak flow meter. As in nonpregnant women, treatment algorithms generally follow a stepwise approach, and commonly used medications, particularly those for mild to moderate asthma symptoms, are generally considered safe in pregnancy. Concerns about teratogenicity and medication effects on the fetus should be thoroughly discussed with the patient to decrease noncompliance rates. Inhaled beta-2-agonists are indicated for all asthma patients, and low to moderate dose inhaled corticosteroids are added for persistent symptoms when a rescue inhaler alone is inadequate. Systemic corticosteroid administration is reserved for severe exacerbations but should not be withheld, if indicated, irrespective of gestational age. Cromolyn, leukotriene receptor antagonists, and theophylline are appropriate alternative therapies if first-line management is ineffective. The primary goals of management in pregnancy include minimizing symptoms and avoiding hypoxic episodes to the fetus. Prostaglandin F2a and ergonovine—medications frequently used to treat postpartum uterine atony—should be avoided because they can precipitate bronchospasm in women with asthma.

Ali Z et al. Exacerbations of asthma during pregnancy: impact on pregnancy complications and outcome. J Obstet Gynaecol. 2016 May;36(4):455–61. [PMID: 26467747]

American College of Obstetricians and Gynecologists. Practice Bulletin No. 90: Asthma in pregnancy. Obstet Gynecol. 2008 Feb;111 (2 Pt 1):457–64. [Reaffirmed 2016] [PMID: 18238988]

SEIZURE DISORDERS

Epilepsy is one of the most common serious neurologic disorders in pregnant women. Many of the commonly used antiepileptic drugs are known human teratogens. Therefore, the principal objectives in managing pregnancy in epileptic women are achieving adequate control of seizures while minimizing exposure to medications that can cause congenital malformations. Certain women who are contemplating pregnancy and have been seizure-free for 2–5 years may be considered candidates for discontinuation of antiseizure medication prior to pregnancy. For those who continue to require treatment, however, therapy with one medication is preferred. Selecting a regimen should be based on the type of seizure disorder and the risks associated with each medication. Valproic acid should not be considered first-line therapy because it has consistently been associated with higher rates of fetal malformations than most other commonly used antiepileptic drugs, and it may be associated with impaired neurocognitive development in the offspring. Phenytoin and carbamazepine both have established patterns of associated fetal malformations. Concerns about teratogenicity have prompted increasing use of the newer antiepileptic drugs such as lamotrigine, topiramate, oxcarbazepine, and levetiracetam. Although the safety of these medications in pregnancy continues to be evaluated, experiences from ongoing registries and large, population-based studies suggest that in utero exposure to the newer antiepileptic drugs in the first trimester of pregnancy carries a lower risk of major malformations than older medications. Some studies, however, suggest that topiramate is associated with a slightly increased risk of oral clefts, and one birth registry found an increase in oral clefts among women taking lamotrigine. Several small studies have found an association between levetiracetam and low birth weight. Lamotrigine and levetiracetam are considered the least teratogenic. Although it is recommended that pregnant women with epilepsy be given supplemental folic acid, it is unclear if supplemental folate decreases rates of fetal malformations in women taking anticonvulsant therapy. Antiepileptic medications may be affected by volume of distribution changes in pregnancy, and serum levels should be followed when appropriate.

Harden C et al. Epilepsy in pregnancy. Neurol Clin. 2019 Feb; 37(1):53–62. [PMID: 30470275]

Patel SI et al. Management of epilepsy during pregnancy: an update. Ther Adv Neurol Disord. 2016 Mar;9(2):118–29. [PMID: 27006699]

INFECTIOUS CONDITIONS COMPLICATING PREGNANCY

URINARY TRACT INFECTION

The urinary tract is especially vulnerable to infections during pregnancy because the altered secretions of steroid sex hormones and the pressure exerted by the gravid uterus on the ureters and bladder cause hypotonia and congestion and predispose to urinary stasis. Labor and delivery and urinary retention postpartum also may initiate or aggravate infection. *Escherichia coli* is the offending organism in over two-thirds of cases.

From 2% to 15% of pregnant women have asymptomatic bacteriuria, which some believe to be associated with an increased risk of preterm birth. It is estimated that pyelonephritis will develop in 20–40% of these women if untreated.

An evaluation for asymptomatic bacteriuria at the first prenatal visit is recommended for all pregnant women. If a urine culture is positive, treatment should be initiated. Nitrofurantoin (100 mg orally twice daily), ampicillin (250 mg orally four times daily), and cephalexin (250 mg orally four times daily) are acceptable medications for 4–7 days. Sulfonamides should be avoided in the third trimester because they may interfere with bilirubin binding and thus impose a risk of neonatal hyperbilirubinemia and kernicterus. Fluoroquinolones are also contraindicated because of their potential teratogenic effects on fetal cartilage and bone. Patients with recurrent bacteriuria should receive suppressive medication (once daily dosing of an appropriate antibiotic) for the remainder of the pregnancy. Acute pyelonephritis requires hospitalization for intravenous administration of antibiotics and crystalloids until the patient is afebrile; this is followed by a full course of oral antibiotics.

Glaser AP et al. Urinary tract infection and bacteriuria in pregnancy. Urol Clin North Am. 2015 Nov;42(4):547–60. [PMID: 26475951]

Kalinderi K et al. Urinary tract infection during pregnancy: current concepts on a common multifaceted problem. J Obstet Gynaecol. 2018 May;38(4):448–53. [PMID: 29402148]

GROUP B STREPTOCOCCAL INFECTION

Group B streptococci frequently colonize the lower female genital tract, with an asymptomatic carriage rate in pregnancy of 10–30%. This rate depends on maternal age, gravidity, and geographic variation. Vaginal carriage is asymptomatic and intermittent, with spontaneous clearing in approximately 30% and recolonization in about 10% of women. Adverse perinatal outcomes associated with group B streptococcal colonization include urinary tract infection, intrauterine infection, premature rupture of membranes, preterm delivery, and postpartum metritis.

Women with postpartum metritis due to infection with group B streptococci, especially after cesarean section, develop fever, tachycardia, and abdominal pain, usually within 24 hours after delivery. Approximately 35% of these women are bacteremic.

Group B streptococcal infection is a common cause of neonatal sepsis. Transmission rates are high, yet the rate of neonatal sepsis is surprisingly low at less than 1:1000 live births. Unfortunately, the mortality rate associated with early-onset disease can be as high as 20–30% in premature infants. In contrast, it is approximately 2–3% in those at term. Moreover, these infections can contribute markedly to chronic morbidity, including mental retardation and neurologic disabilities. Late-onset disease develops through contact with hospital nursery personnel. Up to 45% of these health care workers can carry the bacteria on their skin and transmit the infection to newborns.

CDC recommendations for screening and prophylaxis for group B streptococcal colonization are set forth above (see Essentials of Prenatal Care: Tests and Procedures).

Le Doare K et al; GBS Intrapartum Antibiotic Investigator Group. Intrapartum antibiotic chemoprophylaxis policies for the prevention of Group B streptococcal disease worldwide: systematic review. Clin Infect Dis. 2017 Nov 6;65(Suppl 2): S143–51. [PMID: 29117324]

VARICELLA

Commonly known as chickenpox, varicella-zoster virus (VZV) infection has a fairly benign course when incurred during childhood but may result in serious illness in adults, particularly during pregnancy. Infection results in lifelong immunity. Approximately 95% of women born in the United States have VZV antibodies by the time they reach reproductive age. The incidence of VZV infection during pregnancy has been reported as up to 7:10,000.

▶ Clinical Findings

A. Symptoms and Signs

The incubation period for this infection is 10–20 days. A primary infection follows and is characterized by a flu-like syndrome with malaise, fever, and development of a pruritic maculopapular rash on the trunk, which becomes vesicular and then crusts. Pregnant women are prone to the development of VZV pneumonia, often a fulminant infection sometimes requiring respiratory support. After primary infection, the virus becomes latent, ascending to dorsal root ganglia. Subsequent reactivation can occur as zoster, often under circumstances of immunocompromise, although this is rare during pregnancy.

Two types of fetal infection have been documented. The first is congenital VZV syndrome, which typically occurs in 0.4–2% of fetuses exposed to primary VZV infection during the first trimester. Anomalies include limb and digit abnormalities, microphthalmos, and microcephaly.

Infection during the second and third trimesters is less threatening. Maternal IgG crosses the placenta, protecting the fetus. The only infants at risk for severe infection are those born after maternal viremia but before development of maternal protective antibody. Maternal infection manifesting 5 days before or up to 2 days after delivery is the time period believed to be most hazardous for transmission to the fetus.

B. Laboratory Findings

Diagnosis is commonly made on clinical grounds. Laboratory verification is made by enzyme-linked immunosorbent assay (ELISA), fluorescent antibody, and hemagglutination inhibition antibody techniques. Serum obtained by cordocentesis may be tested for VZV IgM to document fetal infection. Vesicular fluid can be sent for qualitative varicella polymerase chain reaction (PCR) assay.

▶ Treatment

Varicella-zoster immune globulin (VZIG) has been shown to prevent or modify the symptoms of infection in exposed persons. Treatment success depends on identification of susceptible women at or just following exposure. Exposed women with a questionable or negative history of chickenpox should be checked for antibody, since the overwhelming majority will have been previously exposed. If the antibody is negative, VZIG (625 units intramuscularly) should ideally be given within 96 hours of exposure for greatest efficacy, but the CDC reports it can be given for up to 10 days. There are no known adverse effects of VZIG administration during pregnancy, although the incubation period for disease can be lengthened. Infants born to women in whom symptoms develop in the period from 5 days before delivery to 2 days after delivery should also receive VZIG (125 units).

Pregnant women with varicella may benefit from treatment with oral acyclovir, 800 mg orally four times daily for 5 days, if started within 24 hours of rash onset. Treatment has been shown to improve maternal symptoms but does not prevent congenital varicella. Infected pregnant women should be closely observed and hospitalized at the earliest signs of pulmonary involvement. Intravenous acyclovir (10 mg/kg intravenously every 8 hours) is recommended in the treatment of VZV pneumonia.

American College of Obstetricians and Gynecologists. ACOG Practice Bulletin No. 151: Cytomegalovirus, parvovirus B19, varicella zoster, and toxoplasmosis in pregnancy. Obstet Gynecol. 2015 Jun;125(6):1510–25. [Reaffirmed 2017] [PMID: 26000539]

Centers for Disease Control and Prevention (CDC). Updated recommendations for use of VariZIG—United States, 2013. MMWR Morb Mortal Wkly Rep. 2013 July 19;62(28):574–6. [PMID: 23863705]

TUBERCULOSIS

The diagnosis of tuberculosis in pregnancy is made by history taking, physical examination, and testing, with special attention to women in high-risk groups. Women at high risk include those who are from endemic areas, those infected with HIV, drug users, health care workers, and close contacts of people with tuberculosis. Chest radiographs should not be obtained as a routine screening measure in pregnancy but should be used only in patients with a positive test or with suggestive findings in the history and physical examination. Abdominal shielding must be used if a chest radiograph is obtained. Both tuberculin skin testing and interferon gamma release assays are acceptable tests in pregnancy.

Decisions on treatment depend on whether the patient has active disease or is at high risk for progression to active disease. Pregnant women with latent disease not at high risk for disease progression can receive treatment postpartum, which does not preclude breastfeeding. The concentration of medication in breast milk is neither toxic nor adequate for treatment of the newborn. Treatment is with isoniazid and ethambutol or isoniazid and rifampin (see Chapters 9 and 33). Because isoniazid therapy may result in vitamin B_6 deficiency, a supplement of 50 mg/day of vitamin B_6 should be given simultaneously. There is concern that isoniazid, particularly in pregnant women, can cause hepatitis. Liver biochemical tests should be performed regularly in pregnant women who receive treatment. Streptomycin, ethionamide, and most other antituberculous drugs should be avoided in pregnancy. If adequately treated, tuberculosis in pregnancy has an excellent prognosis.

Nahid P et al. Official American Thoracic Society/Centers for Disease Control and Prevention/Infectious Diseases Society of America Clinical Practice Guidelines: treatment of drug-susceptible tuberculosis. Clin Infect Dis. 2016 Oct 1; 63(7):e147–95. [PMID: 27516382]

HIV/AIDS DURING PREGNANCY

Asymptomatic HIV infection is associated with a normal pregnancy rate and no increased risk of adverse pregnancy outcomes. There is no evidence that pregnancy causes AIDS progression.

Previously, two-thirds of HIV-positive neonates acquired their infection close to, or during, the time of delivery. Routine HIV screening in pregnancy, including the use of rapid HIV tests in Labor and Delivery units, and the use of antiretroviral drugs has markedly reduced this transmission risk to approximately 2%. In an HIV-positive pregnant woman, a CD4 count, plasma RNA level, and resistance testing (if virus is detectable, and the patient has not already had this) should be obtained at the first prenatal visit. Treatment should not be delayed while waiting for the results of resistance testing. Prior or current antiretroviral use should be reviewed. A woman already taking and tolerating an acceptable antiretroviral regimen does not have to discontinue it in the first trimester. Patients should also be tested for hepatitis C, tuberculosis, toxoplasmosis, and cytomegalovirus.

Women not taking medication should be offered combination antiretroviral therapy (commonly a dual nucleoside reverse transcriptase inhibitor combination and a ritonavir-boosted protease inhibitor) after counseling regarding the potential impact of therapy on both mother and fetus (see Chapter 31). Antiretroviral therapy should be offered regardless of viral load and CD4 count. Whether to start in the first or second trimester should be determined on a case-by-case basis, but it should be started as early as reasonably possible. It can be started in the first trimester after explanation of risks and benefits, provided the mother is not experiencing nausea and vomiting. The majority of drugs used to treat HIV/AIDS have thus far proven to be safe in pregnancy with an acceptable risk/benefit ratio. Efavirenz has been linked with a small increase in anomalies (myelomeningocele) and should not be used in the first trimester of pregnancy. However, efavirenz does not need to be discontinued if a virologically suppressed patient becomes pregnant while taking it. Standard of care also includes administration of intravenous zidovudine (2 mg/kg intravenously over 1 hour followed by 1 mg/kg/h intravenously) begun 3 hours before cesarean delivery and continued through the surgery until cord clamping in women whose viral load near delivery is greater than or equal to 1000 copies/mL or unknown. Antiretroviral therapy on the patient's usual schedule should be continued in labor. Intravenous zidovudine is not required for antiretroviral therapy-compliant women with a suppressed viral load.

The use of prophylactic elective cesarean section at 38 weeks (before the onset of labor or rupture of the membranes) to prevent vertical transmission of HIV infection from mother to fetus has been shown to further reduce the transmission rate. In patients with a viral load of less than 1000 copies/mL, there may be no additional benefit of cesarean delivery, and those women can be offered a vaginal delivery. Amniotomy should not be performed in the setting of viremia unless there is a clear obstetric indication. Amniotomy has not been associated with an increased risk of perinatal transmission when the mother is receiving antiretroviral therapy and virologically suppressed. Internal monitors, particularly the fetal scalp electrode, should be avoided. Methergine (used for postpartum hemorrhage) should be avoided in patients receiving certain regimens. HIV-infected women should be advised not to breastfeed their infants.

The Public Health Task Force provides guidelines for the management of HIV/AIDS in pregnancy that are regularly updated and available at http://www.aidsinfo.nih.gov. In addition, there is the National Perinatal HIV Hotline, which provides free consultation regarding perinatal HIV care (1-888-448-8765).

Panel on Treatment of HIV-Infected Pregnant Women and Prevention of Perinatal Transmission. Recommendations for use of antiretroviral drugs in pregnant HIV-1 infected women for maternal health and interventions to reduce perinatal HIV transmission in the United States. 2018 Oct 26. https://aidsinfo.nih.gov/ContentFiles/lvguidelines/PerinatalGL.pdf

MATERNAL HEPATITIS B & C CARRIER STATE

There are an estimated 350 million chronic carriers of **hepatitis B virus** worldwide (see also Chapter 1). In the United States, 1.4 million people are infected, with the highest rate among Asian Americans. All pregnant women should be screened for HBsAg. Transmission of the virus to the baby after delivery is likely if both surface antigen and e antigen are positive. Vertical transmission can be blocked by the immediate postdelivery administration to the newborn of hepatitis B immunoglobulin and hepatitis B vaccine intramuscularly. The vaccine dose is repeated at 1 and

6 months of age. Third trimester administration of tenofovir disoproxil fumarate, 300 mg orally once per day starting at 28–32 weeks and continuing through delivery (first line), lamivudine, or telbivudine to women with a viral load of greater than 10^6–10^8 copies/mL has been shown to reduce vertical transmission particularly if the viral load is less than 10^6 copies/mL at delivery. This therapy appears safe in pregnancy although long-term follow-up data are lacking. Pregnant women with chronic hepatitis B should have liver biochemical tests and viral load testing during the pregnancy. Hepatitis B infection is not a contraindication to breastfeeding, and antiviral therapy if given does not need to be continued postpartum.

Hepatitis C virus infection is the most common chronic blood-borne infection in the United States. The average rate of hepatitis C virus (HCV) infection among infants born to HCV-positive, HIV-negative women is 5–6%. However, the average infection rate increases to 10–11% when mothers are coinfected with HCV and HIV. The principal factor associated with transmission is the presence of HCV RNA in the mother at the time of birth. Treatment is not recommended in pregnancy. Interferon and ribavirin have been considered contraindicated. Ledipasvir/sofosbuvir (Harvoni) has been shown to be safe in animal studies, but there are no human studies on safety or efficacy at reducing vertical transmission.

Pan CQ et al; China Study Group for the Mother-to-Child Transmission of Hepatitis B. Tenofovir to prevent hepatitis B transmission in mothers with high viral load. N Engl J Med. 2016 Jun 16;374(24):2324–34. [PMID: 27305192]

Society for Maternal-Fetal Medicine (SMFM). Hepatitis C in pregnancy: screening, treatment, and management. Am J Obstet Gynecol. 2017 Nov;217(5):B2–12. [PMID: 28782502]

HERPES GENITALIS

Infection of the lower genital tract by herpes simplex virus type 2 (HSV-2) (see also Chapter 6) is a common STD with potentially serious consequences to pregnant women and their newborn infants. Although up to 25% of women in an obstetric practice may have antibodies to HSV-2, a history of the infection is unreliable and the incidence of neonatal infection is low (10–60/100,000 live births). Most infected neonates are born to women with no history, symptoms, or signs of infection.

Women who have had *primary* herpes infection late in pregnancy are at high risk for shedding virus at delivery. Some experts suggest use of prophylactic acyclovir, 400 mg orally three times daily, to decrease the likelihood of active lesions at the time of labor and delivery.

Women with a history of *recurrent* genital herpes have a lower neonatal attack rate than women infected during the pregnancy, but they should still be monitored with clinical observation and culture of any suspicious lesions. Since asymptomatic viral shedding is not predictable by antepartum cultures, current recommendations do not include routine cultures in individuals with a history of herpes without active disease. However, when labor begins, vulvar and cervical inspection should be performed.

Cesarean delivery is indicated at the time of labor if there are prodromal symptoms or active genital lesions.

For treatment, see Chapter 32. The use of acyclovir in pregnancy is acceptable, and prophylaxis starting at 36 weeks' gestation has been shown to decrease the number of cesarean sections performed for active disease.

American College of Obstetricians and Gynecologists. ACOG Practice Bulletin No. 82: Management of herpes in pregnancy. Obstet Gynecol. 2007 Jun;109(6):1489–98. [Reaffirmed 2018] [PMID: 17569194]

SYPHILIS, GONORRHEA, & *CHLAMYDIA TRACHOMATIS* INFECTION

These STDs have significant consequences for mother and child (see also Chapters 33 and 34). Untreated syphilis in pregnancy can cause late abortion, stillbirth, transplacental infection, and congenital syphilis. Gonorrhea can produce large-joint arthritis by hematogenous spread as well as ophthalmia neonatorum. Maternal chlamydial infections are largely asymptomatic but are manifested in the newborn by inclusion conjunctivitis and, at age 2–4 months, by pneumonia. The diagnosis of each can be reliably made by appropriate laboratory tests. All women should be tested for syphilis and *C trachomatis* as part of their routine prenatal care. Repeat testing is dependent on risk factors, prevalence, and state laws. A pregnant patient treated for *C trachomatis* should have a test of cure 3–4 weeks later and then 3 months after that because of high reinfection rates. Women at risk should be tested for gonorrhea. The sexual partners of women with STDs should be identified and treated also if possible; the local health department can assist with this process.

Workowski KA et al; Centers for Disease Control and Prevention (CDC). Sexually transmitted diseases treatment guidelines, 2015. MMWR Recomm Rep. 2015 Jun 5;64(RR-03):1–137. [PMID: 26042815]

GASTROINTESTINAL, HEPATIC, & BILIARY DISORDERS OF PREGNANCY

Complications involving the gastrointestinal tract, liver, and gallbladder are common in pregnancy. Nausea and vomiting in the first trimester affect the majority of pregnant women to some degree (see Obstetric Complications of the First & Second Trimesters). Nausea and vomiting in the last half of pregnancy, however, are never normal; a thorough evaluation of such complaints is mandatory. Some of these conditions are incidental to pregnancy (eg, appendicitis), while others are related to the gravid state and tend to resolve with delivery (eg, acute fatty liver of pregnancy). Importantly, the myriad anatomic and physiologic changes associated with normal pregnancy must be considered when assessing for a disease state. Likewise, interpretation of laboratory studies must take into account the pregnancy-associated changes in hepatic protein production.

For conditions in which surgery is clinically indicated, operative intervention should never be withheld based solely on the fact that a woman is pregnant. While purely elective surgery is avoided during pregnancy, women who undergo surgical procedures for an urgent or emergent indication during pregnancy do not appear to be at increased risk for adverse outcomes. Obstetric complications, when they occur, are more likely to be associated with the underlying maternal illness. Recommendations have held that the optimal time for semi-elective surgery is the second trimester to avoid exposure to anesthesia in the first trimester and the enlarged uterus in the third. Importantly, however, there is no convincing evidence that general anesthesia induces malformations or increases the risk for abortion.

CHOLELITHIASIS & CHOLECYSTITIS

Cholelithiasis is common in pregnancy as physiologic changes such as increased cholesterol production and incomplete gallbladder emptying predispose to gallstone formation. The diagnosis is usually suspected based on classic symptoms of nausea, vomiting, and right upper quadrant pain, usually after meals, and is confirmed with right upper quadrant ultrasound. Symptomatic cholelithiasis without cholecystitis is usually managed conservatively, but recurrent symptoms are common. Cholecystitis results from obstruction of the cystic duct and often is accompanied by bacterial infection. Medical management with antibiotics is reasonable in selected cases, but definitive treatment with cholecystectomy will help prevent complications such as gallbladder perforation and pancreatitis. Cholecystectomy has successfully been performed in all trimesters of pregnancy and should not be withheld based on the stage of pregnancy if clinically indicated. Laparoscopy is preferred in the first half of pregnancy, but becomes more technically challenging in the last trimester due to the enlarged uterus and cephalad displacement of abdominal contents.

Obstruction of the common bile duct, which can lead to cholangitis, is an indication for surgical removal of gallstones and establishment of biliary drainage. Endoscopic retrograde cholangiopancreatography (ERCP) with or without sphincterotomy is a nonsurgical alternative. Pregnant women can safely undergo ERCP provided that precautions are taken to minimize fetal exposure to radiation. There does, however, appear to be a slightly higher rate of post-procedure pancreatitis in pregnant women who undergo ERCP. Magnetic resonance cholangiopancreatography (MRCP) can also be of use in patients with suspected common bile duct obstruction. This study is particularly useful for those women in whom the etiology of common duct dilatation is unclear on ultrasound. MRCP can provide detailed evaluation of the entire biliary system and the pancreas while avoiding ionizing radiation.

Athwal R et al. Surgery for gallstone disease during pregnancy does not increase fetal or maternal mortality: a meta-analysis. Hepatobiliary Surg Nutr. 2016 Feb;5(1):53–7. [PMID: 26904557]

Cappell MS et al. Systematic review of safety and efficacy of therapeutic endoscopic-retrograde-cholangiopancreatography during pregnancy including studies of radiation-free therapeutic endoscopic-retrograde-cholangiopancreatography. World J Gastrointest Endosc. 2018 Oct 16;10(10):308–21. [PMID: 30364767]

ACUTE FATTY LIVER OF PREGNANCY

Acute fatty liver of pregnancy, a disorder limited to the gravid state, occurs in the third trimester of pregnancy and causes acute hepatic failure. With improved recognition and immediate delivery, the maternal mortality rate in contemporary reports is about 4%. The disorder is usually seen after the 35th week of gestation and is more common in primigravidas and those with twins. The incidence is about 1:10,000 deliveries.

The etiology of acute fatty liver of pregnancy is likely poor placental mitochondrial function. Many cases may be due to a homozygous fetal deficiency of long-chain acyl coenzyme A dehydrogenase (LCHAD).

▶ Clinical Findings

Pathologic findings are unique to the disorder, with fatty engorgement of hepatocytes. Clinical onset is gradual, with nausea and vomiting being the most common presenting symptoms. Varying degrees of flu-like symptoms are also typical. Eventually, symptoms progress to those of fulminant hepatic failure: jaundice, encephalopathy, disseminated intravascular coagulation, and death. On examination, the patient shows signs of hepatic failure.

Laboratory findings include marked elevation of alkaline phosphatase but only moderate elevations of alanine aminotransferase (ALT) and aspartate aminotransferase (AST). Hypocholesterolemia and hypofibrinogenemia are typical, and hypoglycemia can be extreme. Coagulopathy is also frequently seen with depressed procoagulant protein production. Kidney function should be assessed for hepatorenal syndrome. The white blood cell count is elevated, and the platelet count is depressed.

▶ Differential Diagnosis

The differential diagnosis is that of fulminant hepatitis. Liver aminotransferases for fulminant hepatitis are higher (greater than 1000 units/mL) than those for acute fatty liver of pregnancy (usually 500–1000 units/mL). Preeclampsia may involve the liver but typically does not cause jaundice; the elevations in liver biochemical tests in patients with preeclampsia usually do not reach the levels seen in patients with acute fatty liver of pregnancy.

▶ Treatment

Diagnosis of acute fatty liver of pregnancy mandates immediate delivery. Intensive supportive care with ICU-level observation is essential and typically includes administration of blood products and glucose as well as correction of acidemia. Vaginal delivery is preferred. Resolution of encephalopathy and laboratory derangements occurs over days with supportive care, and recovery is usually complete. Rare cases of liver transplantation have been reported.

Zhang YP et al. Acute fatty liver of pregnancy: a retrospective analysis of 56 cases. Chin Med J (Engl). 2016 May 20; 129(10):1208–14. [PMID: 27174330]

INTRAHEPATIC CHOLESTASIS OF PREGNANCY

Intrahepatic cholestasis of pregnancy is characterized by incomplete clearance of bile acids in genetically susceptible women. The principal symptom is pruritus, which can be generalized but tends to have a predilection for the palms and soles. Presentation is typically in the third trimester, and women with multi-fetal pregnancies are at increased risk. The finding of an elevated serum bile acid level, ideally performed in the fasting state, confirms the diagnosis. Associated laboratory derangements include modest elevations in hepatic transaminase levels and mild hyperbilirubinemia. Although rare, the bilirubin level may be sufficiently elevated to result in clinical jaundice. The symptoms and laboratory abnormalities resolve quickly after delivery but can recur in subsequent pregnancies or with exposure to combination oral contraceptives.

Ursodeoxycholic acid (8–10 mg/kg/day) is the treatment of choice and results in decreased pruritus in most women.

Adverse fetal outcomes, particularly preterm birth, non-reassuring fetal status, meconium-stained amniotic fluid, and stillbirth, have consistently been reported in women with cholestasis of pregnancy. The risk for adverse perinatal outcomes appears to correlate with disease severity as measured by the degree of bile acid elevation, and women with fasting bile acids greater than 40 mcmol/L have been reported to be at greatest risk. Because of the risks associated with cholestasis of pregnancy, many clinicians recommend antenatal testing in the third trimester and elective early delivery in attempt to avoid stillbirth. Evidence-based recommendations regarding such management practices, however, are not currently available.

Bicocca MJ et al. Intrahepatic cholestasis of pregnancy: review of six national and regional guidelines. Eur J Obstet Gynecol Reprod Biol. 2018 Dec;231:180–7. [PMID: 30396107]

APPENDICITIS

Appendicitis occurs in about 1 of 1500 pregnancies. The diagnosis is more difficult to make clinically in pregnant women where the appendix is displaced cephalad from McBurney point. Furthermore, nausea, vomiting, and mild leukocytosis occur in normal pregnancy, so with or without these findings, any complaint of right-sided pain should raise suspicion. Imaging can help confirm the diagnosis if clinical findings are equivocal. Abdominal sonography is a reasonable initial imaging choice, but nonvisualization of the appendix is common in pregnancy. CT scanning is more sensitive than ultrasound, and with proper shielding, the radiation exposure to the fetus is minimized. MRI is also used to evaluate for appendicitis in pregnant women and is a reasonable alternative to CT scanning. Unfortunately, the diagnosis of appendicitis is not made until the appendix has ruptured in at least 20% of obstetric patients. Peritonitis in these cases can lead to preterm labor or abortion. With early diagnosis and appendectomy, the prognosis is good for mother and baby.

Prodromidou A et al. Outcomes after open and laparoscopic appendectomy during pregnancy: a meta-analysis. Eur J Obstet Gynecol Reprod Biol. 2018 Jun;225:40–50. [PMID: 29656140]

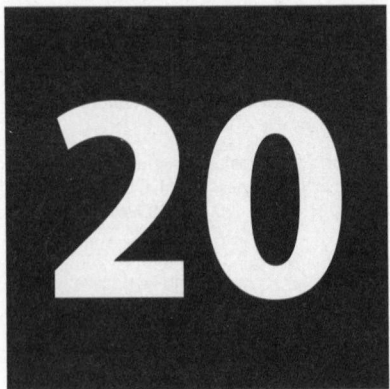

Rheumatologic, Immunologic, & Allergic Disorders

David B. Hellmann, MD, MACP

John B. Imboden Jr., MD

▶ Diagnosis & Evaluation

A. Examination of the Patient

Two helpful clinical clues for diagnosing arthritis are the joint pattern and the presence or absence of extra-articular manifestations. The joint pattern is defined by the answers to three questions: (1) Is inflammation present? (2) How many joints are involved? and (3) What joints are affected? Joint inflammation manifests as warmth, swelling, and morning stiffness of at least 30 minutes' duration. Overlying erythema occurs with the intense inflammation of crystal-induced and septic arthritis. Both the number of affected joints and the specific sites of involvement affect the differential diagnosis (Table 20–1). Some diseases—gout, for example—are characteristically monarticular, whereas other diseases, such as rheumatoid arthritis, are usually polyarticular. The location of joint involvement can also be distinctive. Only two diseases frequently cause prominent involvement of the distal interphalangeal (DIP) joint: osteoarthritis and psoriatic arthritis. Extra-articular manifestations such as fever (eg, gout, Still disease, endocarditis), rash (eg, systemic lupus erythematosus [SLE], psoriatic arthritis, Still disease), nodules (eg, rheumatoid arthritis, gout), or neuropathy (eg, polyarteritis nodosa, granulomatosis with polyangiitis) narrow the differential diagnosis further.

B. Arthrocentesis and Examination of Joint Fluid

If the diagnosis is uncertain, synovial fluid should be examined whenever possible (Table 20–2). Most large joints are easily aspirated, and contraindications to arthrocentesis are few. The aspirating needle should never be passed through an overlying cellulitis or psoriatic plaque because of the risk of introducing infection. For patients who are receiving direct-acting oral anticoagulants or long-term anticoagulation therapy with warfarin, joints can be aspirated with a small-gauge needle (eg, 22F); the international normalized ratio (INR) should be less than 3.0 for patients taking warfarin.

1. Types of studies

A. Gross examination—Clarity is an approximate guide to the degree of inflammation. Noninflammatory fluid is transparent, mild inflammation produces translucent fluid, and purulent effusions are opaque. Bleeding disorders, trauma, and traumatic taps are the most common causes of bloody effusions.

B. Cell count—The synovial fluid white cell count discriminates between noninflammatory (less than 2000 white cells/mcL [2.0×10^9/L]), inflammatory (2000–75,000 white cells/mcL [2.0×10^9/L–75.0 $\times 10^9$/L]), and purulent (greater than 100,000 white cells/mcL [100×10^9/L]) joint effusions. Synovial fluid glucose and protein levels add little information and should not be ordered.

C. Microscopic examination—Compensated polarized light microscopy identifies and distinguishes monosodium urate (gout, negatively birefringent) and calcium pyrophosphate (pseudogout, positive birefringent) crystals. Gram stain has specificity but limited sensitivity (50%) for septic arthritis.

D. Culture—Bacterial cultures as well as special studies for gonococci, tubercle bacilli, or fungi are ordered as appropriate.

2. Interpretation

Synovial fluid analysis is diagnostic in infectious or microcrystalline arthritis. Although the severity of inflammation in synovial fluid can overlap among various conditions, the synovial fluid white cell count is a helpful guide to diagnosis (Table 20–3).

DEGENERATIVE JOINT DISEASE (Osteoarthritis)

 ESSENTIALS OF DIAGNOSIS

▶ A degenerative disorder with minimal articular inflammation.

▶ No systemic symptoms.

▶ Pain relieved by rest; morning stiffness brief.

▶ Radiographic findings: narrowed joint space, osteophytes, increased subchondral bone density, bony cysts.

Table 20–1. Diagnostic value of the joint pattern.

Characteristic	Status	Representative Disease
Inflammation	Present	Rheumatoid arthritis, SLE, gout
	Absent	Osteoarthritis
Number of involved joints	Monarticular	Gout, trauma, septic arthritis, Lyme disease, osteoarthritis
	Oligoarticular (2–4 joints)	Reactive arthritis, psoriatic arthritis, inflammatory bowel disease
	Polyarticular (≥ 5 joints)	Rheumatoid arthritis, SLE
Site of joint involvement	Distal interphalangeal	Osteoarthritis, psoriatic arthritis (not rheumatoid arthritis)
	Metacarpophalangeal, wrists	Rheumatoid arthritis, SLE, calcium pyrophosphate deposition disease (not osteoarthritis)
	First metatarsal phalangeal	Gout, osteoarthritis

SLE, systemic lupus erythematosus.

General Considerations

Osteoarthritis, the most common form of joint disease, is chiefly a disease of aging. Ninety percent of all people have radiographic features of osteoarthritis in weight-bearing joints by age 40. Symptomatic disease also increases with age. Sex is also a risk factor; osteoarthritis develops in women more frequently than in men.

This arthropathy is characterized by degeneration of cartilage and by hypertrophy of bone at the articular margins. Inflammation is usually minimal. Hereditary and mechanical factors may be involved in the pathogenesis.

Obesity is a risk factor for osteoarthritis of the knee, hand, and probably of the hip. Recreational running does not increase the incidence of osteoarthritis, but participation in competitive contact sports does. Jobs requiring frequent bending and carrying increase the risk of knee osteoarthritis (see Chapter 41).

Clinical Findings

A. Symptoms and Signs

Degenerative joint disease is divided into two types: (1) primary, which most commonly affects some or all of the following: the DIP and the proximal interphalangeal (PIP) joints of the fingers, the carpometacarpal joint of the thumb, the hip, the knee, the metatarsophalangeal (MTP) joint of the big toe, and the cervical and lumbar spine; and (2) secondary, which may occur in any joint as a sequela to articular injury. The injury may be acute, as in a fracture; or chronic, as that due to occupational overuse of a joint or metabolic disease (eg, hyperparathyroidism, hemochromatosis, ochronosis) or joint inflammation (eg, rheumatoid arthritis).

The onset is insidious. Initially, there is articular stiffness, seldom lasting more than 15 minutes; this develops later into pain on motion of the affected joint and is made worse by activity or weight bearing and relieved by rest. Flexion contracture or varus deformity of the knee is not unusual, and bony enlargements of the DIP (Heberden nodes) and PIP (Bouchard nodes) are occasionally prominent (Figure 20–1). There is no ankylosis, but limitation of motion of the affected joint or joints is common. Crepitus may often be felt over the knee. Joint effusion and other articular signs of inflammation are mild. There are no systemic manifestations.

B. Laboratory Findings

Osteoarthritis does not cause elevation of the erythrocyte sedimentation rate (ESR) or other laboratory signs of inflammation. Synovial fluid is noninflammatory.

C. Imaging

Radiographs may reveal narrowing of the joint space; osteophyte formation and lipping of marginal bone; and thickened, dense subchondral bone. Bone cysts may also be present.

Table 20–2. Examination of joint fluid.

Measure	(Normal)	Group I (Noninflammatory)	Group II (Inflammatory)	Group III (Purulent)
Volume (mL) (knee)	< 3.5	Often > 3.5	Often > 3.5	Often > 3.5
Clarity	Transparent	Transparent	Translucent to opaque	Opaque
Color	Clear	Yellow	Yellow to opalescent	Yellow to green
WBC (per mcL)	< 200	< 2000	2000–75,000[1]	> 100,000[2]
Polymorphonuclear leukocytes	< 25%	< 25%	50% or more	75% or more
Culture	Negative	Negative	Negative	Usually positive[2]

[1]Gout, rheumatoid arthritis, and other inflammatory conditions occasionally have synovial fluid WBC counts > 75,000/mcL but rarely > 100,000/mcL.
[2]Most purulent effusions are due to septic arthritis. Septic arthritis, however, can present with group II synovial fluid, particularly if infection is caused by organisms of low virulence (eg, *Neisseria gonorrhoeae*) or if antibiotic therapy has been started.
WBC, white blood cell count.

Table 20–3. Differential diagnosis by joint fluid groups.

Noninflammatory (< 2000 white cells/mcL)	Inflammatory (2000–75,000 white cells/mcL)	Purulent (> 100,000 white cells/mcL)	Hemorrhagic
Osteoarthritis Traumatic arthritis Osteonecrosis Charcot arthropathy	Rheumatoid arthritis Systemic lupus erythematosus Polydermatomyositis Scleraderma Systemic necrotizing vasculitides Polychondritis Gout Calcium pyrophosphate deposition disease Hydroxyapatite deposition disease Juvenile rheumatoid arthritis Ankalosing spondylitis Psoriatic arthritis Reactive arthritis Chronic inflammatory bowel disease Hypogammaglobulinemia Sarcoidosis Rheumatic fever Indolent/low virulence infections (viral, mycobacterial, fungal, Whipple disease, Lyme disease)	Septic arthritis (bacterial)	Trauma Pigmented villonodular synovitis Tuberculosis Neoplasia Coagulopathy Charcot arthropathy

Reproduced, with permission, from Klippel JH et al (eds). *Primer on the Rheumatic Diseases*, 13th ed. Springer, 2008.

Differential Diagnosis

Because articular inflammation is minimal and systemic manifestations are absent, degenerative joint disease should seldom be confused with other arthritides. The distribution of joint involvement in the hands also helps distinguish osteoarthritis from rheumatoid arthritis. Osteoarthritis chiefly affects the DIP and PIP joints and spares the wrist and metacarpophalangeal (MCP) joints; rheumatoid arthritis involves the wrists and MCP joints and spares the DIP joints. Furthermore, the joint enlargement is bony-hard and cool in osteoarthritis but spongy and warm in rheumatoid arthritis. Skeletal symptoms due to degenerative changes in joints—especially in the spine—may cause coexistent metastatic neoplasia, osteoporosis, plasma cell myeloma, or other bone disease to be overlooked.

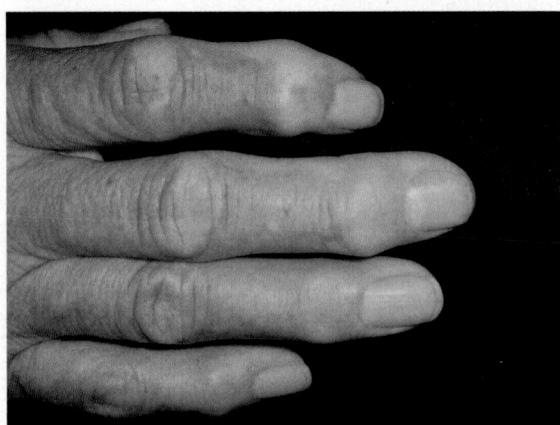

▲ **Figure 20–1.** Osteoarthritis in an older woman with Heberden nodes at the distal interphalangeal joints. There is some swelling beginning at the proximal interphalangeal joints creating Bouchard nodes. (Used, with permission, from Richard P. Usatine, MD.)

Prevention

Weight reduction reduces the risk of developing symptomatic knee osteoarthritis. Correcting leg length discrepancy of greater than 1 cm with shoe modification may prevent knee osteoarthritis from developing in the shorter leg. Maintaining normal vitamin D levels may reduce the occurrence and progression of osteoarthritis, in addition to being important for bone health.

Treatment

A. General Measures

Patients with osteoarthritis of the hand may benefit from assistive devices and instruction on techniques for joint protection; splinting is beneficial for those with symptomatic osteoarthritis of the first carpometacarpal joint. Patients with mild to moderate osteoarthritis of the knee or hip should participate in a regular exercise program (eg, a supervised walking program, hydrotherapy classes) and, if overweight, should lose weight. The use of assistive devices (eg, a cane on the contralateral side) can improve functional status.

B. Medical Management

1. Oral nonsteroidal anti-inflammatory drugs (NSAIDs)— NSAIDs (see Table 5–7) are more effective than acetaminophen for osteoarthritis but have greater toxicity. NSAIDs inhibit cyclooxygenase (COX), the enzyme that converts arachidonic acid to prostaglandins. Prostaglandins play important roles in promoting inflammation, but they also help maintain homeostasis in several organs—especially the stomach, where prostaglandin E serves as a local hormone responsible for gastric mucosal cytoprotection. COX exists in two isomers—COX-1, which is expressed continuously in many cells and is responsible for the homeostatic effects of prostaglandins, and COX-2, which is induced by cytokines and expressed in inflammatory tissues. Most NSAIDs inhibit both isomers. Celecoxib is the only selective COX-2 inhibitor currently available in the United States.

Gastrointestinal toxicity, such as gastric ulceration, perforation, and gastrointestinal hemorrhage, are the most common serious side effects of NSAIDs. The overall rate of bleeding with NSAID use in the general population is low (1:6000 users or less) but is increased by the risk factors of long-term use, higher NSAID dose, concomitant corticosteroids or anticoagulants, the presence of rheumatoid arthritis, history of peptic ulcer disease or alcoholism, and age over 70. *Proton pump inhibitors (eg, omeprazole 20 mg orally daily) reduce the incidence of serious gastrointestinal toxicity and should be used for patients with risk factors for NSAID-induced gastrointestinal toxicity.* Patients who have recently recovered from an NSAID-induced bleeding gastric ulcer appear to be at high risk for rebleeding (about 5% in 6 months) when an NSAID is reintroduced, even if prophylactic measures (such as proton pump inhibitors) are used. Compared with nonselective NSAIDs, celecoxib is less likely in some circumstances to cause upper gastrointestinal tract adverse events.

All of the NSAIDs, including aspirin and celecoxib, can produce renal toxicity, including interstitial nephritis, nephrotic syndrome, prerenal azotemia, and aggravation of hypertension. Hyperkalemia due to hyporeninemic hypoaldosteronism is seen rarely. The risk of renal toxicity is low but is increased by the following risk factors: age older than 60 years, history of kidney disease, heart failure, ascites, and diuretic use.

All NSAIDs, except the nonacetylated salicylates and the COX-2 inhibitor celecoxib, interfere with platelet function and prolong bleeding time. Aspirin irreversibly inhibits platelet function, so the bleeding time effect resolves only as new platelets are made. In contrast, the effect of nonselective NSAIDs on platelet function is reversible and resolves as the drug is cleared. Concomitant administration of a nonselective NSAID can interfere with the ability of aspirin to acetylate platelets and thus may interfere with the cardioprotective effects of low-dose aspirin. *The US Food and Drug Administration (FDA) has warned that all NSAIDs can increase the risk of myocardial infarction and stroke in patients with or without risk factors for heart disease or known heart disease.* While the cardiovascular risk is related to the dose and duration of treatment, stroke and myocardial infarction can occur within the first week of treatment. Cardiovascular risks associated with naproxen, ibuprofen, and moderate dose celecoxib (200 mg orally daily) are comparable.

Chondroitin sulfate and glucosamine, alone or in combination, are no better than placebo in reducing pain in patients with knee or hip osteoarthritis.

2. Topical therapies—Topical NSAIDs (eg, 4 g of diclofenac gel 1% applied to the affected joint four times daily) appear more effective than placebo for knee and hand osteoarthritis and have lower rates of systemic side effects than with oral NSAIDs. Few studies have compared the efficacy of oral and topical NSAIDs. Because of their attractive safety profile, topical NSAIDs should be considered early in the treatment of patients with mild osteoarthritis affecting a few joints, especially of the hand or knee.

Topical capsaicin may be of benefit for osteoarthritis of the hand or the knee.

3. Acetaminophen—Patients with mild osteoarthritis may benefit from acetaminophen (2.6–4 g/day orally). Growing awareness of the danger of hepatotoxicity from high doses of acetaminophen and clearer appreciation that its impact on pain is frequently neglible, acetaminophen is no longer recommended as first-line treatment for osteoarthritis of the hip or knee.

4. Intra-articular injections—Many patients with moderately severe osteoarthritis of the knee who do not respond to NSAIDs receive intra-articular injections of corticosteroids, hyaluronate, or platelet-rich plasma. Although each of these can temporarily reduce pain, none has convincingly produced long-term benefits in reducing pain or preserving function. For example, a 2-year controlled trial demonstrated that injecting the knee with triamcinolone every 6 months was no more effective than injecting saline in reducing knee pain. The American College of Rheumatology does not recommend corticosteroid injections for osteoarthritis of the hand.

C. Surgical Measures

Total hip and knee replacements provide excellent symptomatic and functional improvement when involvement of that joint severely restricts walking or causes pain at rest, particularly at night. Arthroscopic surgery for knee osteoarthritis is ineffective.

► Prognosis

Symptoms may be quite severe and limit activity considerably (especially with involvement of the hips, knees, and cervical spine).

► When to Refer

Refer patients to an orthopedic surgeon when recalcitrant symptoms or functional impairment, or both, warrant consideration of joint replacement surgery of the hip or knee.

Jones IA et al. Intra-articular treatment options for knee osteoarthritis. Nat Rev Rheumatol. 2019 Feb;15(2):77–90. [PMID: 30498258]

O'Neill TW et al. Update on the epidemiology, risk factors and disease outcomes of osteoarthritis. Best Pract Res Clin Rheumatol. 2018 Apr;32(2):312–26. [PMID: 30527434]

CRYSTAL DEPOSITION ARTHRITIS

1. Gouty Arthritis

ESSENTIALS OF DIAGNOSIS

► Acute, monarticular arthritis, often of the first MTP joint; recurrence is common.

► Polyarticular involvement more common in patients with longstanding disease.

► Identification of urate crystals in joint fluid or tophi is diagnostic.

► Dramatic therapeutic response to NSAIDs.

► With chronicity, urate deposits in subcutaneous tissue, bone, cartilage, joints, and other tissues.

components of the interleukin-1 receptor) have efficacy for the management of acute gout, but these drugs have not been approved by the FDA for this indication.

C. Management Between Attacks

Treatment during symptom-free periods is intended to minimize urate deposition in tissues, which causes chronic tophaceous arthritis, and to reduce the frequency and severity of recurrences. Potentially reversible causes of hyperuricemia are a high-purine diet, obesity, alcohol consumption, and use of certain medications. Patients with a single episode of gout who have normal kidney function and are willing to lose weight and stop drinking alcohol are at low risk for another attack and may not require long-term medical therapy. In contrast, individuals with mild chronic kidney disease or with a history of multiple attacks of gout are likely to benefit from pharmacologic treatment. In general, the higher the uric acid level and the more frequent the attacks, the more likely that long-term medical therapy will be beneficial. All patients with tophaceous gout should receive urate-lowering therapy.

1. Diet—Excessive alcohol consumption can precipitate attacks and should be avoided. Beer consumption appears to confer a higher risk of gout than does whiskey or wine. Although dietary purines usually contribute only 1 mg/dL to the serum uric acid level, moderation in eating foods with high purine content is advisable (Table 20–5). Patients should avoid organ meats and beverages sweetened with

Table 20–5. The purine content of foods.[1]

Low-purine foods
Refined cereals and cereal products, cornflakes, white bread, pasta, flour, arrowroot, sago, tapioca, cakes
Milk, milk products, and eggs
Sugar, sweets, and gelatin
Butter, polyunsaturated margarine, and all other fats
Fruit, nuts, and peanut butter
Lettuce, tomatoes, and green vegetables (except those listed below)
Cream soups made with low-purine vegetables but without meat or meat stock
Water, fruit juice, cordials, and carbonated drinks
High-purine foods
All meats, including organ meats, and seafood
Meat extracts and gravies
Yeast and yeast extracts, beer, and other alcoholic beverages
Beans, peas, lentils, oatmeal, spinach, asparagus, cauliflower, and mushrooms

[1]The purine content of a food reflects its nucleoprotein content and turnover. Foods containing many nuclei (eg, liver) have many purines, as do rapidly growing foods such as asparagus. The consumption of large amounts of a food containing a small concentration of purines may provide a greater purine load than consumption of a small amount of a food containing a large concentration of purines.
Reproduced, with permission, from Emmerson BT. The management of gout. N Engl J Med. 1996 Feb 15;334(7):445–51. Copyright © 1996 Massachusetts Medical Society. Reprinted with permission from Massachusetts Medical Society.

high fructose corn syrup. A high liquid intake and, more importantly, a daily urinary output of 2 L or more will aid urate excretion and minimize urate precipitation in the urinary tract.

2. Avoidance of hyperuricemic medications—Thiazide and loop diuretics inhibit renal excretion of uric acid and, if possible, should be avoided in patients with gout. Similarly, niacin can raise serum uric acid levels and should be discontinued if there are therapeutic alternatives. Low doses of aspirin also aggravate hyperuricemia.

3. Colchicine prophylaxis—There are two indications for daily colchicine administration. First, colchicine can be used to prevent future attacks for the individual who has mild hyperuricemia and only occasional attacks of gouty arthritis. Second, colchicine can be used when urate-lowering therapy is started to suppress attacks precipitated by abrupt changes in the serum uric acid level. For either indication, the usual dose is 0.6 mg orally either once or twice a day. Colchicine is renally cleared. Patients who have coexisting moderate chronic kidney disease should take colchicine only once a day or once every other day in order to avoid peripheral neuromyopathy and other complications of colchicine toxicity.

4. Reduction of serum uric acid—Indications for a urate-lowering therapy in a person with gout include frequent acute arthritis (two or more episodes per year), tophaceous deposits, or chronic kidney disease (stage 2 or worse). The American College of Rheumatology guidelines recommend a treat-to-target approach for urate-lowering therapy. The minimum goal of urate-lowering therapy is a serum uric acid at or below 6 mg/dL or 357 mcmol/L (ie, below the level at which serum is supersaturated with uric acid, thereby allowing urate crystals to solubilize); in some cases, control of gout may require lowering serum uric acid to less than 5 mg/dL or 297.4 mcmol/L. Lowering serum uric acid levels is not of benefit for the treatment of an acute gout flare.

Three classes of agents may be used to lower the serum uric acid—xanthine oxidase inhibitors (allopurinol or febuxostat), uricosuric agents, and uricase (pegloticase).

A. Xanthine oxidase inhibitors—Allopurinol and febuxostat are the preferred first-line agents for lowering urate. They reduce plasma uric acid levels by blocking the final enzymatic steps in the production of uric acid. Allopurinol and febuxostat should not be used together, but they can be tried sequentially if the initial agent fails to lower serum uric acid to the target level or if it is not tolerated. The most frequent adverse effect with either medication is the precipitation of an acute gouty attack; thus, patients generally should be receiving prophylactic doses of colchicine.

Hypersensitivity to allopurinol occurs in 2% of cases, usually within the first few months of therapy, and it can be life-threatening. The most common initial sign of hypersensitivity is a pruritic rash that may progress to toxic epidermal necrolysis, particularly if allopurinol is continued; vasculitis and hepatitis are other manifestations. Patients should be instructed to stop allopurinol immediately if a rash develops. Chronic kidney disease and concomitant thiazide therapy are risk factors. There is a strong association between allopurinol hypersensitivity and HLA-B*5801, which is a prevalent allele in certain East Asian populations. Current recommendations are to screen for HLA-B*5801 prior to initiating allopurinol in Koreans with stage 3 or worse chronic kidney disease, and in all persons of Han Chinese and Thai descent.

The initial daily dose of allopurinol is 100 mg/day orally (50 mg/day for those with stage 4 or worse chronic kidney disease); the dose of allopurinol should be titrated upward every 2–5 weeks to achieve the target serum uric acid level (either less than or equal to 6.0 mg/dL [357 mcmol/L] for men or less than or equal to 5.0 mg/dL [297.4 mcmol/L] for women). Successful treatment usually requires a dose of at least 300 mg of allopurinol daily. The maximum daily dose is 800 mg.

Allopurinol interacts with other drugs. The combined use of allopurinol and ampicillin causes a drug rash in 20% of patients. Allopurinol can increase the half-life of probenecid, while probenecid increases the excretion of allopurinol. Thus, a patient taking both drugs may need to use slightly higher than usual doses of allopurinol and lower doses of probenecid.

Febuxostat does not cause the hypersensitivity reactions seen with allopurinol and can be given without dose adjustment to patients with mild to moderate kidney disease. However, abnormal liver tests may develop in 2–3% of patients taking febuxostat. In addition, one clinical study showed that febuxostat was associated with a slightly higher rate of fatal and nonfatal cardiovascular events than allopurinol (0.97 vs 0.58 per 100 patient-years). The initial dose of febuxostat is 40 mg/day orally. If the target serum uric acid is not reached, the dose of febuxostat can be increased to 80 mg/day and then to the maximum dose of 120 mg/day.

B. Uricosuric drugs—Uricosuric drugs lower serum uric acid levels by blocking the tubular reabsorption of filtered urate, thereby increasing uric acid excretion by the kidney. Probenecid (0.5 g/day orally) and lesinurad (200 mg/day orally) are the uricosurics of choice in the United States, and are typically reserved for patients who cannot achieve a serum uric acid of less than or equal to 6.0 mg/dL with allopurinol or febuxostat alone. Lesinurad carries an FDA black box warning that acute kidney injury can occur with treatment, especially when lesinurad is used as monotherapy; it is contraindicated in patients with a creatinine clearance of less than 45 mL/min. Probenecid can be added to a xanthine oxidase inhibitor or used as monotherapy. Probenecid should not be used in patients with a creatinine clearance of less than 50 mL/min due to limited efficacy; contraindications include a history of nephrolithiasis (uric acid or calcium stones) and evidence of overproduction of uric acid (ie, greater than 800 mg of uric acid in a 24-hour urine collection). To reduce the development of uric acid stones (which occur in up to 11%), patients should be advised to increase their fluid intake and clinicians should consider prescribing an alkalinizing agent (eg, potassium citrate, 30–80 mEq/day orally) to maintain a urinary pH > 6.0.

C. Uricase—Pegloticase, a recombinant uricase that must be administered intravenously (8 mg every 2 weeks), is indicated for the rare patient with refractory chronic tophaceous gout. Pegloticase carries an FDA black box warning, which advises administering the drug only in health care settings and by health care professionals prepared to manage anaphylactic and other serious infusion reactions.

D. Chronic Tophaceous Arthritis

With rigorous medical compliance, allopurinol, febuxostat, or pegloticase shrinks tophi and in time can lead to their disappearance. Resorption of extensive tophi requires maintaining a serum uric acid below 6 mg/dL. Surgical excision of large tophi offers mechanical improvement in selected deformities.

E. Gout in the Transplant Patient

Hyperuricemia and gout commonly develop in many transplant patients because they have decreased kidney function and require drugs that inhibit uric acid excretion (especially cyclosporine and diuretics). Treating acute gout in these patients is challenging. Often the best approach for monarticular gout—after excluding infection—is injecting corticosteroids into the joint. For polyarticular gout, increasing the dose of systemic corticosteroid may be the only alternative. Since transplant patients often have multiple attacks of gout, long-term relief requires lowering the serum uric acid with allopurinol or febuxostat. (Kidney dysfunction seen in many transplant patients makes uricosuric agents ineffective.) Both allopurinol and febuxostat inhibit the metabolism of azathioprine and should be avoided in patients who must take azathioprine.

▶ Prognosis

Without treatment, the acute attack may last from a few days to several weeks. The intervals between acute attacks vary up to years, but the asymptomatic periods often become shorter if the disease progresses. Chronic gouty arthritis occurs after repeated attacks of acute gout, but only after inadequate treatment. The younger the patient at the onset of disease, the greater the tendency to a progressive course. Destructive arthropathy is rarely seen in patients whose first attack is after age 50.

Bardin T et al. The role of febuxostat in gout. Curr Opin Rheumatol. 2019 Mar;31(2):152–8. [PMID: 30601228]

Janssen CA et al. Anakinra for the treatment of acute gout flares: a randomized, double-blind, placebo-controlled, active-comparator, non-inferiority trial. Rheumatology (Oxford). 2019 Jan 2. [Epub ahead of print] [PMID: 30602035]

2. Calcium Pyrophosphate Deposition

Calcium pyrophosphate deposition (CPPD) in fibrocartilage and hyaline cartilage (chondrocalcinosis) can cause an acute crystal-induced arthritis ("pseudogout"), a degenerative arthropathy, and a chronic inflammatory polyarthritis ("pseudorheumatoid arthritis"). CPPD also can be an asymptomatic condition detected as incidental chondrocalcinosis on radiographs. The prevalence of CPPD increases with age. Hyperparathyroidism, familial hypocalcuric hypercalcemia, hemochromatosis, and hypomagnesemia confer risk of CPPD, but most cases have no associated condition.

Pseudogout is most often seen in persons aged 60 or older, is characterized by acute, recurrent and rarely chronic arthritis involving large joints (most commonly the knees and the wrists) and is almost always accompanied by radiographic chondrocalcinosis of the affected joints. The crowned dens syndrome, caused by pseudogout of the atlantoaxial junction associated with "crown-like" calcifications around the dens, manifests with severe neck pain, rigidity, and high fever that can mimic meningitis or polymyalgia rheumatica. Pseudogout, like gout, frequently develops 24–48 hours after major surgery. Identification of calcium pyrophosphate crystals in joint aspirates is diagnostic. NSAIDs are helpful in the treatment of acute episodes. Colchicine, 0.6 mg orally once or twice daily, is more effective for prophylaxis than for acute attacks. Aspiration of the inflamed joint and intra-articular injection of triamcinolone, 10–40 mg, depending on the size of the joint, are also of value in resistant cases.

The degenerative arthropathy associated with CPPD can involve joints not usually affected by osteoarthritis (eg, glenohumeral joint, wrist, patellofemoral compartment of the knee). The "pseudorheumatoid arthritis" of CPPD affects the metacarpophalangeal joints and wrists. In both conditions, radiographs demonstrate chondrocalcinosis and degenerative changes such as asymmetric joint space narrowing and osteophyte formation.

Lee JS et al. Clinical features and risk of recurrence of acute calcium pyrophosphate crystal arthritis. Clin Exp Rheumatol. 2019 Mar–Apr;37(2):254–9. [PMID: 30148438]

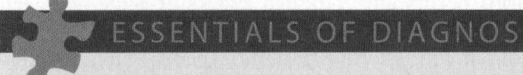

AUTOIMMUNE DISEASES

RHEUMATOID ARTHRITIS

ESSENTIALS OF DIAGNOSIS

► Usually insidious onset with morning stiffness and joint pain.

► Symmetric polyarthritis with predilection for small joints of the hands and feet; deformities common with progressive disease.

► **Radiographic findings:** juxta-articular osteoporosis, joint erosions, and joint space narrowing.

► Rheumatoid factor and antibodies to cyclic citrullinated peptides (anti-CCP) are present in 70–80%.

► **Extra-articular manifestations:** subcutaneous nodules, interstitial lung disease, pleural effusion, pericarditis, splenomegaly with leukopenia, and vasculitis.

► General Considerations

Rheumatoid arthritis is a chronic systemic inflammatory disease whose major manifestation is synovitis of multiple joints. It has a prevalence of 1% and is more common in women than men (female:male ratio of 3:1). Rheumatoid arthritis can begin at any age, but the peak onset is in the fourth or fifth decade for women and the sixth to eighth decades for men. The cause is not known. Susceptibility to rheumatoid arthritis is genetically determined with multiple genes contributing. Inheritance of HLA-DRB1 alleles encoding a distinctive five-amino-acid sequence known as the "shared epitope" is the best characterized genetic risk factor. Untreated, rheumatoid arthritis causes joint destruction with consequent disability and shortens life expectancy. Early, aggressive treatment is the standard of care.

The pathologic findings in the joint include chronic synovitis with formation of a pannus, which erodes cartilage, bone, ligaments, and tendons. Effusion and other manifestations of inflammation are common.

► Clinical Findings

A. Symptoms and Signs

1. Joint symptoms—The clinical manifestations of rheumatoid disease are highly variable, but joint symptoms usually predominate. Although acute presentations may occur, the onset of articular signs of inflammation is usually insidious, with prodromal symptoms of vague periarticular pain or stiffness. Symmetric swelling of multiple joints with tenderness and pain is characteristic. Monarticular disease is occasionally seen initially. Stiffness persisting for longer than 30 minutes (and usually many hours) is prominent in the morning. Stiffness may recur after daytime inactivity and be much more severe after strenuous activity. Although any diarthrodial joint may be affected, PIP joints of the fingers, MCP joints (Figure 20–3),

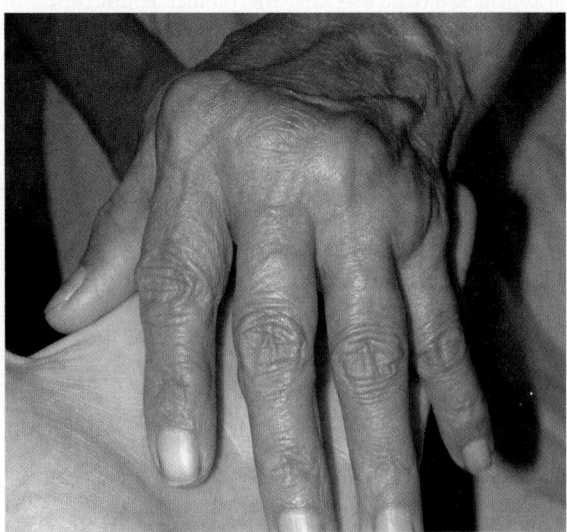

▲ **Figure 20–3.** Rheumatoid arthritis with ulnar deviation at the metacarpophalangeal (MCP) joints. (Used, with permission, from Richard P. Usatine, MD.)

wrists, knees, ankles, and MTP joints are most often involved. Synovial cysts and rupture of tendons may occur. Entrapment syndromes are common—particularly of the median nerve at the carpal tunnel of the wrist. Rheumatoid arthritis can affect the neck but spares the other components of the spine and does not involve the sacroiliac joints. In advanced disease, atlantoaxial (C1–C2) subluxation can lead to myelopathy.

2. Rheumatoid nodules—Twenty percent of patients have subcutaneous rheumatoid nodules, most commonly situated over bony prominences but also observed in the bursae and tendon sheaths (Figure 20–4). Nodules are occasionally seen in the lungs, the sclerae, and other tissues. Nodules correlate with the presence of rheumatoid factor in serum ("seropositivity"), as do most other extra-articular manifestations.

3. Ocular symptoms—Dryness of the eyes, mouth, and other mucous membranes is found especially in advanced disease (see Sjögren syndrome). Other ocular manifestations include episcleritis, scleritis, scleromalacia due to scleral nodules, and peripheral ulcerative keratitis.

4. Other symptoms—Interstitial lung disease is not uncommon (estimates of prevalence vary widely according to method of detection) and manifests clinically as cough and progressive dyspnea. Pericarditis and pleural disease, when present, are usually silent clinically. Patients with active joint disease often have palmar erythema. Occasionally, a small vessel vasculitis develops and manifests as tiny hemorrhagic infarcts in the nail folds or finger pulps. Necrotizing arteritis is well reported but rare. A small subset of patients with rheumatoid arthritis have Felty syndrome, the occurrence of splenomegaly and neutropenia, usually in the setting of severe, destructive arthritis. Felty syndrome must be distinguished from large granular lymphoproliferative disorder, with which it shares many features.

B. Laboratory Findings

Anti-CCP antibodies and rheumatoid factor, an IgM antibody directed against the Fc region of IgG, are present in 70–80% of patients with established rheumatoid arthritis. Rheumatoid factor has a sensitivity of only 50% in early disease. Anti-CCP antibodies are the most specific blood test for rheumatoid arthritis (specificity ~95%). Rheumatoid factor can occur in other autoimmune disease and in chronic infections, including hepatitis C, syphilis, subacute bacterial endocarditis, and tuberculosis. The prevalence of rheumatoid factor positivity also rises with age in healthy individuals. Approximately 20% of rheumatoid patients have antinuclear antibodies.

The ESR and levels of C-reactive protein (CRP) are typically elevated in proportion to disease activity. Anemia of chronic disease is common. The white cell count is normal or slightly elevated, but leukopenia may occur, often in the presence of splenomegaly (eg, Felty syndrome). The platelet count is often elevated, roughly in proportion to the severity of overall joint inflammation. Initial joint fluid examination confirms the inflammatory nature of the arthritis (see Table 20–2).

Arthrocentesis is needed to diagnose superimposed septic arthritis, which is a common complication of rheumatoid arthritis and should be considered whenever a patient with rheumatoid arthritis has one joint inflamed out of proportion to the rest.

C. Imaging

Of all the laboratory tests, radiographic changes are the most specific for rheumatoid arthritis. Radiographs obtained during the first 6 months of symptoms, however, are usually normal. The earliest changes occur in the hands or feet and consist of soft tissue swelling and juxta-articular demineralization. Later, diagnostic changes of uniform joint space narrowing and erosions develop. The erosions are often first evident at the ulnar styloid and at the juxta-articular margin, where the bony surface is not protected by cartilage. Characteristic changes also occur in the cervical spine, with C1–2 subluxation, but these changes usually take many years to develop. Although both MRI and ultrasonography are more sensitive than radiographs in detecting bony and soft tissue changes in rheumatoid arthritis, their value in early diagnosis relative to that of plain radiographs has not been established.

► Differential Diagnosis

The differentiation of rheumatoid arthritis from other joint conditions and immune-mediated disorders can be difficult. In contrast to rheumatoid arthritis, osteoarthritis spares the wrist and the MCP joints. Osteoarthritis is not associated with constitutional manifestations, and the joint pain is characteristically relieved by rest, unlike the morning stiffness of rheumatoid arthritis. Signs of articular inflammation, prominent

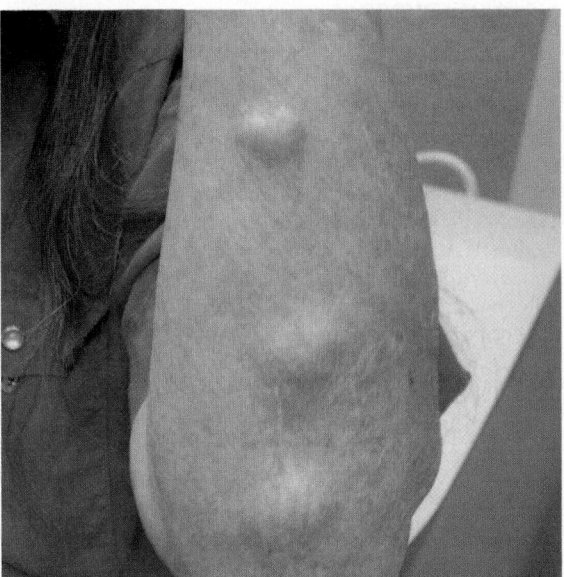

▲ **Figure 20–4.** Rheumatoid nodules over the extensor surface of the forearm. (Used, with permission, from Richard P. Usatine, MD, in Usatine RP, Smith MA, Mayeaux EJ Jr, Chumley H. *The Color Atlas of Family Medicine,* 2nd ed. McGraw-Hill, 2013.)

in rheumatoid arthritis, are usually minimal in degenerative joint disease. CPPD disease can cause a degenerative arthropathy of the MCPs and wrists; radiographs are usually diagnostic. Although gouty arthritis is almost always intermittent and monarticular in the early years, it may evolve with time into a chronic polyarticular process that mimics rheumatoid arthritis. Gouty tophi can resemble rheumatoid nodules but are not associated with rheumatoid factor, whose sensitivity for rheumatoid nodules approaches 100%. The early history of intermittent monoarthritis and the presence of synovial urate crystals are distinctive features of gout. Spondyloarthropathies, particularly earlier in their course, can be a source of diagnostic uncertainty; predilection for lower extremities and involvement of the spine and sacroiliac joints point to the correct diagnosis. Chronic Lyme arthritis typically involves only one joint, most commonly the knee, and is associated with positive serologic tests (see Chapter 34). Acute viral infections, most notably with Chikungunya virus and parvovirus B19, can cause a polyarthritis that mimics early-onset rheumatoid arthritis. However, fever is common, the arthritis usually resolves within weeks, and serologic studies confirm recent infection. Chronic infection with hepatitis C can cause a chronic nonerosive polyarthritis associated with rheumatoid factor; tests for anti-CCP antibodies are negative.

Malar rash, photosensitivity, discoid skin lesions, alopecia, high titer antibodies to double-stranded DNA, glomerulonephritis, and central nervous system abnormalities point to the diagnosis of SLE. Polymyalgia rheumatica occasionally causes polyarthralgias in patients over age 50, but these patients remain rheumatoid factor–negative and have chiefly proximal muscle pain and stiffness, centered on the shoulder and hip girdles. Joint pain that can be confused with rheumatoid arthritis presents in a substantial minority of patients with granulomatosis with polyangiitis. This diagnostic error can be avoided by recognizing that, in contrast to rheumatoid arthritis, the arthritis of granulomatosis with polyangiitis preferentially involves large joints (eg, hips, ankles, wrists) and usually spares the small joints of the hand. Rheumatic fever is characterized by the migratory nature of the arthritis, an elevated antistreptolysin titer, and a more dramatic and prompt response to aspirin; carditis and erythema marginatum may occur in adults, but chorea and subcutaneous nodules virtually never do. Finally, a variety of cancers produce paraneoplastic syndromes, including polyarthritis. One form is hypertrophic pulmonary osteoarthropathy most often produced by lung and gastrointestinal carcinomas, characterized by a rheumatoid-like arthritis associated with clubbing, periosteal new bone formation, and a negative rheumatoid factor. Diffuse swelling of the hands with palmar fasciitis occurs in a variety of cancers, especially ovarian carcinoma.

▶ Treatment

The primary objectives in treating rheumatoid arthritis are reduction of inflammation and pain, preservation of function, and prevention of deformity. Success requires early, effective pharmacologic intervention. Disease-modifying antirheumatic drugs (DMARDs) should be started as soon as the diagnosis of rheumatoid disease is certain and then adjusted with the aim of suppressing disease activity. NSAIDs provide some symptomatic relief in rheumatoid arthritis but do not prevent erosions or alter disease progression. They are not appropriate for monotherapy and should only be used in conjunction with DMARDs, if at all. The American College of Rheumatology recommends using standardized assessments, such as the Disease Activity Score 28 Joints (www.das-score.nl/das28/en/) or the Clinical Disease Activity Index, to gauge therapeutic responses, with the target of mild disease activity or remission by these measures.

A. Corticosteroids

Low-dose corticosteroids (eg, oral prednisone 5–10 mg daily) produce a prompt anti-inflammatory effect and slow the rate of articular erosion. These often are used as a "bridge" to reduce disease activity until the slower acting DMARDs take effect or as adjunctive therapy for active disease that persists despite treatment with DMARDs. No more than 10 mg of prednisone or equivalent per day is appropriate for articular disease. Many patients do reasonably well on 5–7.5 mg daily. (The use of 1-mg tablets, to facilitate doses of less than 5 mg/day, is encouraged.) Higher doses are used to manage serious extra-articular manifestations (eg, pericarditis, necrotizing scleritis). When the corticosteroids are to be discontinued, they should be tapered gradually on a planned schedule appropriate to the duration of treatment. All patients receiving long-term corticosteroid therapy should take measures to prevent osteoporosis (Table 26–16).

Intra-articular corticosteroids may be helpful if one or two joints are the chief source of difficulty. Intra-articular triamcinolone, 10–40 mg depending on the size of the joint to be injected, may be given for symptomatic relief but not more than four times a year.

B. DMARDs

1. Synthetic DMARDs—

A. METHOTREXATE—Methotrexate is usually the initial synthetic DMARD of choice for patients with rheumatoid arthritis. It is generally well tolerated and often produces a beneficial effect in 2–6 weeks. The usual initial dose is 7.5 or 10 mg of methotrexate orally once weekly. If the patient has tolerated methotrexate but has not responded in 1 month, the dose can be increased to 15 mg orally once per week. The maximal dose is usually 20–25 mg/wk. The most frequent side effects are gastric irritation and stomatitis. Cytopenia, most commonly leukopenia or thrombocytopenia but rarely pancytopenia, due to bone marrow suppression, is another important potential problem. The risk of developing pancytopenia is much higher in patients whose serum creatinine is greater than 2 mg/dL (176.8 mcmol/L). Hepatotoxicity with fibrosis and cirrhosis is an important toxic effect that correlates with cumulative dose and is uncommon with appropriate monitoring of liver biochemical tests. Methotrexate is contraindicated in a patient with any form of chronic hepatitis, in pregnant women, and in any patient with significant kidney dysfunction (estimated glomerular filtration rate less than 30 mL/min). Heavy alcohol use increases the hepatotoxicity, so patients should be advised to drink alcohol in extreme moderation, if at all. Diabetes mellitus, obesity, and kidney disease also increase the risk of hepatotoxicity. Liver biochemical tests should be monitored at least every 12 weeks, along with a complete blood count. The dose of methotrexate should be reduced if aminotransferase levels are elevated, and the drug should be discontinued if abnormalities persist despite dosage reduction. Gastric irritation, stomatitis, cytopenias, and hepatotoxicity are reduced by prescribing either daily folate (1 mg orally) or weekly leucovorin calcium (2.5–5 mg taken orally 24 hours after the dose of methotrexate). Hypersensitivity to methotrexate can cause an acute or subacute interstitial pneumonitis that can be life-threatening but which usually responds to cessation of the drug and institution of corticosteroids. Because methotrexate is teratogenic, women of childbearing age as well as men must use effective contraception while taking the medication. Methotrexate is associated with an increased risk of B-cell lymphomas, some of which resolve following the discontinuation of the medication. The combination of methotrexate and other folate antagonists, such as trimethoprim-sulfamethoxazole, should be used cautiously since pancytopenia can result. Amoxicillin can decrease renal clearance of methotrexate, leading to toxicity. Probenecid also increases methotrexate drug levels and toxicity and should be avoided.

B. Sulfasalazine—This drug is a second-line agent for rheumatoid arthritis. It is usually introduced at a dosage of 0.5 g orally twice daily and then increased each week by 0.5 g until the patient improves or the daily dose reaches 3 g. Side effects, particularly neutropenia and thrombocytopenia, occur in 10–25% and are serious in 2–5%. Sulfasalazine also causes hemolysis in patients with glucose-6-phosphate dehydrogenase (G6PD) deficiency, so a G6PD level should be checked before initiating sulfasalazine. Patients with aspirin sensitivity should not be given sulfasalazine. Patients taking sulfasalazine should have complete blood counts monitored every 2–4 weeks for the first 3 months, then every 3 months.

C. Leflunomide—Leflunomide, a pyrimidine synthesis inhibitor, is FDA-approved for treatment of rheumatoid arthritis and is administered as a single oral daily dose of 20 mg. The most frequent side effects are diarrhea, rash, reversible alopecia, and hepatotoxicity. Some patients experience dramatic unexplained weight loss. The drug is teratogenic and has a half-life of 2 weeks. Thus, it is contraindicated in premenopausal women who wish to bear children or in men who wish to father children.

D. Antimalarials—Hydroxychloroquine sulfate is the antimalarial agent most often used against rheumatoid arthritis. Monotherapy with hydroxychloroquine should be reserved for patients with mild disease because only a small percentage will respond and in some of those cases only after 3–6 months of therapy. Hydroxychloroquine is often used in combination with other conventional DMARDs, particularly methotrexate and sulfasalazine. The advantage of hydroxychloroquine is its comparatively low toxicity, especially at a dosage of 200–400 mg/day orally (not to exceed 5 mg/kg/day). The prevalence of the most important reaction, pigmentary retinitis that can lead to visual loss, is a function of duration of therapy, occurring in less than 2% of patients (dosed properly) during the first 10 years of use but rising to 20% after 20 years of treatment. Ophthalmologic examinations every 12 months are

required. Other reactions include neuropathies and myopathies of both skeletal and cardiac muscle, which usually improve when the drug is withdrawn.

E. Janus kinase inhibitors—Tofacitinib, an inhibitor of Janus kinase 3, is used to manage severe rheumatoid arthritis that is refractory to methotrexate. Baricitinib, an inhibitor of Janus kinases 1 and 2, is approved for disease that has failed to respond to inhibitors of tumor necrosis factor. Janus kinase inhibitors are oral agents that can be used either as monotherapy or in combination with methotrexate. Tofacitinib is administered in a dose of 5 mg or 10 mg twice daily; the dose of baricitinib is 2 mg daily. Patients should be screened and treated for latent tuberculosis prior to receiving these drugs.

2. Biologic DMARDs—

A. Tumor necrosis factor inhibitors—Inhibitors of tumor necrosis factor (TNF)—a pro-inflammatory cytokine—are frequently added to the treatment of patients who have not responded adequately to methotrexate and are increasingly used as initial therapy in combination with methotrexate for patients with poor prognostic factors.

Five inhibitors are in use: etanercept, infliximab, adalimumab, golimumab, and certolizumab pegol. Etanercept, a soluble recombinant TNF receptor:Fc fusion protein, is usually administered at a dosage of 50 mg subcutaneously once per week. Infliximab, a chimeric monoclonal antibody, is administered at a dosage of 3–10 mg/kg intravenously; infusions are repeated after 2, 6, 10, and 14 weeks and then are administered every 8 weeks. Adalimumab, a human monoclonal antibody that binds to TNF, is given at a dosage of 40 mg subcutaneously every other week. The dose for golimumab, a human anti-TNF monoclonal antibody, is 50 mg subcutaneously once monthly. Certolizumab pegol is a PEGylated Fab fragment of an anti-TNF monoclonal antibody; the dose is 200–400 mg subcutaneously every 2 to 4 weeks. Each drug produces substantial improvement in more than 60% of patients. Each is usually very well tolerated. Minor irritation at injection sites is the most common side effect of etanercept and adalimumab. Rarely, nonrecurrent leukopenia develops in patients. TNF plays a physiologic role in combating many types of infection; TNF inhibitors have been associated with a several-fold increased risk of serious bacterial infections and a striking increase in granulomatous infections, particularly reactivation of tuberculosis. Screening for latent tuberculosis (see Chapter 9) is mandatory before the initiation of TNF blockers. It is prudent to suspend TNF blockers when a fever or other manifestations of a clinically important infection develops in a patient. Demyelinating neurologic complications that resemble multiple sclerosis have been reported rarely in patients taking etanercept, but the true magnitude of this risk—likely quite small—has not been determined with precision. While there are conflicting data with respect to increased risk of malignancy, there is an FDA safety alert about case reports of malignancies, including leukemias, in patients treated with TNF inhibitors. Infliximab was associated with increased morbidity in a heart failure trial, therefore, TNF inhibitors should be used with extreme caution in patients with heart failure. Infliximab can rarely cause anaphylaxis and induce anti-DNA antibodies (but rarely clinically evident SLE).

B. ABATACEPT—Abatacept, a recombinant protein made by fusing a fragment of the Fc domain of human IgG with the extracellular domain of a T-cell inhibitory receptor (CTLA4), blocks T-cell costimulation and produces clinically meaningful responses in approximately 50% of individuals whose disease did not respond to the combination of methotrexate and a TNF inhibitor.

C. RITUXIMAB—Rituximab, a humanized mouse monoclonal antibody that depletes B cells, can be used in combination with methotrexate for patients whose disease has been refractory to treatment with a TNF inhibitor.

D. TOCILIZUMAB—Tocilizumab is a monoclonal antibody that blocks the receptor for IL-6, an inflammatory cytokine involved in the pathogenesis of rheumatoid arthritis. It is used most often in combination with methotrexate for patients whose disease has been refractory to treatment with a TNF inhibitor.

3. Combination DMARDs—As a general rule, DMARDs have greater efficacy when administered in combination than when used individually. The most commonly used combination is methotrexate with one of the TNF inhibitors, which is more effective than methotrexate alone. Still, most patients who require DMARD therapy are given methotrexate monotherapy initially because methotrexate alone usually works and is less expensive and less toxic than combination therapy. The combination of methotrexate, sulfasalazine, and hydroxychloroquine is also effective and is not inferior to the combination of methotrexate plus etanercept for those who have not responded to methotrexate monotherapy. Biologic DMARDs should not be used in combination.

▶ **Course & Prognosis**

After months or years, deformities may occur; the most common are ulnar deviation of the fingers, boutonnière deformity (hyperextension of the DIP joint with flexion of the PIP joint), "swan-neck" deformity (flexion of the DIP joint with extension of the PIP joint), valgus deformity of the knee, and volar subluxation of the MTP joints. The excess mortality associated with rheumatoid arthritis is largely due to cardiovascular disease that appears to be a result of deleterious effects of chronic systemic inflammation on the vascular system.

▶ **When to Refer**

Early referral to a rheumatologist is essential for diagnosis and the timely introduction of effective therapy.

Aletaha D et al. Diagnosis and management of rheumatoid arthritis: a review. JAMA. 2018 Oct 2;320(13):1360–72. [PMID: 30285183]

Boleto G et al. Safety of combination therapy with two bDMARDs in patients with rheumatoid arthritis: a systematic review and meta-analysis. Semin Arthritis Rheum. 2018 Dec 18. [Epub ahead of print] [PMID: 30638975]

van der Woude D et al. Update on the epidemiology, risk factors, and disease outcomes of rheumatoid arthritis. Best Pract Res Clin Rheumatol. 2018 Apr;32(2):174–87. [PMID: 30527425]

ADULT STILL DISEASE

Still disease is a systemic form of juvenile chronic arthritis in which high spiking fevers are much more prominent, especially at the outset, than arthritis. This syndrome also occurs in adults. Most adults are in their 20s or 30s; onset after age 60 is rare. The fever is dramatic, often with daily spikes to 40°C, associated with sweats and chills, and then plunging to normal or several degrees below normal in the absence of antipyretics. Many patients initially complain of sore throat. An evanescent salmon-colored nonpruritic rash, chiefly on the chest and abdomen, is a characteristic feature. The rash can easily be missed since it often appears only with the fever spike. Many patients also have lymphadenopathy and pericardial effusions. Joint symptoms are mild or absent in the beginning, but a destructive arthritis, especially of the wrists, may develop months later. Anemia and leukocytosis, with white blood counts sometimes exceeding 40,000/mcL, are the rule. Serum ferritin levels are often strikingly elevated (greater than 3000 mg/mL or 6741 pmol/L). The diagnosis of adult Still disease is strongly suggested by the quotidian fever pattern, sore throat, and the classic rash but requires exclusion of other causes of fever. About half of the patients respond to NSAIDs, and half require prednisone, sometimes in doses greater than 60 mg/day orally. Targeting IL-1 with anakinra or canakinumab or IL-6 with tocilizumab can be effective for patients with refractory disease. The course of adult Still disease can be monophasic, intermittent, or chronic. Macrophage activation syndrome is a life-threatening complication of adult Still disease and manifests as fever; splenomegaly; cytopenias; hypertriglyceridemia; hypofibrinogenemia; marked elevation of serum ferritin; elevated soluble CD25; depressed natural killer cell activity; and hemophagocytosis in bone marrow, spleen, and lymph nodes.

Kim MJ et al. Association between fever pattern and clinical manifestations of adult-onset Still's disease: unbiased analysis using hierarchical clustering. Clin Exp Rheumatol. 2018 Nov–Dec;36(6 Suppl 115):74–9. [PMID: 30582502]

SYSTEMIC LUPUS ERYTHEMATOSUS

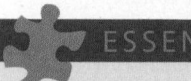

ESSENTIALS OF DIAGNOSIS

▶ Occurs mainly in young women.

▶ Rash over areas exposed to sunlight.

▶ Joint symptoms in 90% of patients.

▶ Anemia, leukopenia, thrombocytopenia.

▶ Glomerulonephritis, central nervous system disease, and complications of antiphospholipid antibodies are major sources of disease morbidity.

▶ **Serologic findings:** antinuclear antibodies (100%), anti–double-stranded DNA antibodies (approximately two-thirds), and low serum complement levels (particularly during disease flares).

► General Considerations

SLE is an inflammatory autoimmune disorder characterized by autoantibodies to nuclear antigens. It can affect multiple organ systems. Many of its clinical manifestations are secondary to the trapping of antigen-antibody complexes in capillaries of visceral structures or to autoantibody-mediated destruction of host cells (eg, thrombocytopenia). The clinical course is marked by spontaneous remission and relapses. The severity may vary from a mild episodic disorder to a rapidly fulminant, life-threatening illness.

The incidence of SLE is influenced by many factors, including sex, race, and genetic inheritance. About 85% of patients are women. Sex hormones play a role; most cases develop after menarche and before menopause. Among older individuals, the sex distribution is more equal. Race is also a factor, as SLE occurs in 1:1000 white women but in 1:250 black women. Familial occurrence of SLE has been repeatedly documented, and the disorder is concordant in 25–70% of identical twins. If a mother has SLE, her daughters' risks of developing the disease are 1:40 and her sons' risks are 1:250. Aggregation of serologic abnormalities (positive antinuclear antibody) is seen in asymptomatic family members, and the prevalence of other rheumatic diseases is increased among close relatives of patients. The importance of specific genes in SLE is emphasized by the high frequency of certain HLA haplotypes, especially DR2 and DR3, and null complement alleles.

The diagnosis of SLE should be suspected in patients having a multisystem disease with a positive test for antinuclear antibodies. It is imperative to ascertain that the condition has not been induced by a drug (see Drug-Induced Lupus below).

The diagnosis of SLE can be made with reasonable probability if 4 of the 11 criteria set forth in Table 20–6 are met. These criteria, developed as guidelines for the inclusion of patients in research studies, do not supplant clinical judgment in the diagnosis of SLE.

► Clinical Findings

A. Symptoms and Signs

The systemic features include fever, anorexia, malaise, and weight loss. Most patients have skin lesions at some time; the characteristic "butterfly" (malar) rash affects less than half of patients. Other cutaneous manifestations are panniculitis (lupus profundus), discoid lupus, typical fingertip lesions, periungual erythema, nail fold infarcts, and splinter hemorrhages. Alopecia is common. Mucous membrane lesions tend to occur during periods of exacerbation. Raynaud phenomenon, present in about 20% of patients, often antedates other features of the disease.

Joint symptoms, with or without active synovitis, occur in over 90% of patients and are often the earliest manifestation. The arthritis can lead to reversible swan-neck deformities, but radiographic erosions and subcutaneous nodules are rare.

Ocular manifestations include conjunctivitis, photophobia, transient or permanent monocular blindness, and blurring of vision. Cotton-wool spots on the retina (cytoid

Table 20–6. Criteria for the classification of SLE. (A patient is classified as having SLE if any 4 or more of 11 criteria are met.)

1. Malar rash
2. Discoid rash
3. Photosensitivity
4. Oral ulcers
5. Arthritis
6. Serositis
7. Kidney disease
a. > 0.5 g/day proteinuria, or
b. ≥ 3+ dipstick proteinuria, or
c. Cellular casts
8. Neurologic disease
a. Seizures, or
b. Psychosis (without other cause)
9. Hematologic disorders
a. Hemolytic anemia, or Leukopenia (< 4000/mcL), or
b. Lymphopenia (< 1500/mcL), or
c. Thrombocytopenia (< 100,000/mcL)
10. Immunologic abnormalities
a. Antibody to native DNA, or
b. Antibody to Sm, or
c. Antibodies to antiphospholipid antibodies based on (1) IgG or IgM anticardiolipin antibodies, (2) lupus anticoagulant, or (3) false-positive serologic test for syphilis
11. Positive ANA

ANA, antinuclear antibody; SLE, systemic lupus erythematosus. Modified and reproduced, with permission, from Tan EM et al. The 1982 revised criteria for the classification of systemic lupus erythematosus. Arthritis Rheum. 1982 Nov;25(11):1271-7, and data from Hochberg MC. Updating the American College of Rheumatology revised criteria for the classification of systemic lupus erythematosus. Arthritis Rheum. 1997 Sep;40(9):1725.

bodies) represent degeneration of nerve fibers due to occlusion of retinal blood vessels.

Pleurisy, pleural effusion, bronchopneumonia, and pneumonitis are frequent. Restrictive lung disease can develop. Alveolar hemorrhage is uncommon but life-threatening. Interstitial lung disease is rare.

The pericardium is affected in the majority of patients. Heart failure may result from myocarditis and hypertension. Cardiac arrhythmias are common. Atypical verrucous endocarditis of Libman-Sacks is usually clinically silent but occasionally can produce acute or chronic valvular regurgitation—most commonly mitral regurgitation.

Mesenteric vasculitis occasionally occurs in SLE and may closely resemble polyarteritis nodosa, including the presence of aneurysms in medium-sized blood vessels. Abdominal pain (particularly postprandial), ileus, peritonitis, and perforation may result.

Neurologic complications of SLE include psychosis, cognitive impairment, seizures, peripheral and cranial neuropathies, transverse myelitis, and strokes. Severe depression and psychosis are sometimes exacerbated by the administration of large doses of corticosteroids.

Several forms of glomerulonephritis may occur, including mesangial, focal proliferative, diffuse proliferative, and membranous (see Chapter 22). Some patients may also have interstitial nephritis. With appropriate therapy, the survival rate even for patients with serious chronic kidney disease (proliferative glomerulonephritis) is favorable, albeit a substantial portion of patients with severe lupus nephritis still eventually require renal replacement therapy.

Hematologic manifestations include leukopenia, autoimmune hemolytic anemia, immune thrombocytopenia, and thrombotic thrombocytopenic purpura.

B. Laboratory Findings

(Tables 20–7 and 20–8.) SLE is characterized by the production of many different autoantibodies. Antinuclear antibody tests based on immunofluorescence assays using HEp-2 cells (a human cell line) as a source of nuclei are nearly 100% sensitive for SLE but not specific—ie, they are positive in low titer in up to 20% of healthy adults and also in many patients with nonlupus conditions such as rheumatoid arthritis, autoimmune thyroid disease, scleroderma, and Sjögren syndrome. False-negative results can occur with tests for antinuclear antibodies based on multiplex assays that use specific nuclear antigens rather than cell lines. Therefore, SLE should not be excluded on the basis of a negative multiplex assay for antinuclear antibodies. Antibodies to double-stranded DNA and to Sm are specific for SLE but not sensitive, since they are present in only 60% and 30% of patients, respectively. Depressed serum complement—a finding suggestive of disease activity—often returns toward normal in remission. Anti–double-stranded DNA antibody levels also correlate with disease activity in some patients; anti-Sm levels do not. Other autoantibodies commonly seen in SLE include antibodies to SS-A/Ro, SS-B/La, ribonucleoprotein (RNP), and phospholipid. Antibodies to SS-A/Ro are associated with subacute cutaneous lupus; during pregnancy these autoantibodies can cross the placenta and damage the developing fetal conduction system, producing congenital heart block.

Table 20–8. Frequency (%) of laboratory abnormalities in systemic lupus erythematosus.

Anemia	60%
Leukopenia	45%
Thrombocytopenia	30%
Antiphospholipid antibodies	
Anti-cardiolipin antibody	25%
Lupus anticoagulant	7%
Anti-beta-2-glycoprotein 1	25%
Direct Coombs-positive	30%
Proteinuria	30%
Hematuria	30%
Hypocomplementemia	60%
ANA	95–100%
Anti-native DNA	50%
Anti-Sm	20%

ANA, antinuclear antibody; Anti-Sm, anti-Smith antibody.
Modified and reproduced, with permission, from Hochberg MC et al. Systemic lupus erythematosus: a review of clinicolaboratory features and immunologic matches in 150 patients with emphasis on demographic subsets. Medicine (Baltimore). 1985 Sep; 64(5): 285–95.

During disease flares, elevations in the ESR are common, but the serum CRP is usually normal unless there is serositis or arthritis. Abnormality of urinary sediment is almost always found in association with kidney lesions. Showers of red blood cells, with or without casts, and proteinuria (varying from mild to nephrotic range) are frequent during exacerbation of the disease.

Table 20–7. Frequency (%) of autoantibodies in rheumatic diseases.[1]

	ANA	Anti-Native DNA	Rheumatoid Factor	Anti-Sm	Anti-SS-A	Anti-SS-B	Anti-SCL-70	Anti-Centromere	Anti-Jo-1	ANCA
Rheumatoid arthritis	30–60	0–5	70	0	0–5	0–2	0	0	0	0
Systemic lupus erythematosus	95–100	60	20	10–25	15–20	5–20	0	0	0	0–1
Sjögren syndrome	95	0	75	0	65	65	0	0	0	0
Diffuse scleroderma	>95	0	30	0	0	0	33	1	0	0
Limited scleroderma (CREST syndrome)	>95	0	30	0	0	0	20	50	0	0
Polymyositis/dermatomyositis	80	0	33	0	0	0	0	0	20–30	0
Granulomatosis with polyangiitis	0–15	0	50	0	0	0	0	0	0	93–96[1]

[1]Frequency for generalized, active disease.
ANA, antinuclear antibodies; Anti-Sm, anti-Smith antibody; anti-SCL-70, anti-scleroderma antibody; ANCA, antineutrophil cytoplasmic antibody; CREST, calcinosis cutis, Raynaud phenomenon, esophageal motility disorder, sclerodactyly, and telangiectasia.

Differential Diagnosis

Differential diagnosis includes drug-induced lupus, rheumatoid arthritis, systemic vasculitis, scleroderma, primary antiphospholipid syndrome, inflammatory myopathies, viral hepatitis, sarcoidosis, and acute drug reactions.

Treatment

Since the various manifestations of SLE affect prognosis differently and since SLE activity often waxes and wanes, drug therapy—both the choice of agents and the intensity of their use—must be tailored to match disease severity. Patients should be cautioned against sun exposure and should apply a protective lotion to the skin while out of doors. Skin lesions often respond to the local administration of corticosteroids. Minor joint symptoms can usually be alleviated by rest and NSAIDs.

Antimalarials (hydroxychloroquine) may be helpful in treating lupus rashes or joint symptoms and appear to reduce the incidence of severe disease flares. The dose of hydroxychloroquine is 200 or 400 mg/day orally and should not exceed 5 mg/kg/day; annual monitoring for retinal changes is recommended. Drug-induced neuropathy and myopathy may be erroneously ascribed to the underlying disease.

Corticosteroids are required for the control of certain complications. (Systemic corticosteroids are not usually given for minor arthritis, skin rash, leukopenia, or the anemia associated with chronic disease.) Glomerulonephritis, hemolytic anemia, pericarditis or myocarditis, alveolar hemorrhage, central nervous system involvement, and thrombotic thrombocytopenic purpura all require corticosteroid treatment and often other interventions as well. Forty to 60 mg of oral prednisone is often needed initially; however, the lowest dose of corticosteroid that controls the condition should be used (Table 26–16). Central nervous system lupus may require higher doses of corticosteroids than are usually given; however, corticosteroid psychosis may mimic lupus cerebritis, in which case reduced doses are appropriate. Immunosuppressive agents such as cyclophosphamide, mycophenolate mofetil, and azathioprine are used in cases resistant to corticosteroids. Treatment of severe lupus nephritis includes an induction phase and a maintenance phase. Cyclophosphamide, which improves renal survival but not patient survival, has been used for many years as the standard treatment for both phases of lupus nephritis. Cyclophosphamide can be administered according to the National Institutes of Health regimen (3–6 monthly intravenous pulses [0.5–1 g/m^2] for induction followed by maintenance infusions every 3 months) or the Euro-Lupus regimen (500 mg intravenously every 2 weeks for 6 doses followed by maintenance with azathioprine). Mycophenolate mofetil appears to be an equally effective alternative treatment to cyclophosphamide for many patients with lupus nephritis. Very close follow-up is needed to watch for potential side effects when immunosuppressants are given; these agents should be administered by clinicians experienced in their use. When cyclophosphamide is required, gonadotropin-releasing hormone analogs can be given to protect a woman against the risk of premature ovarian failure. Belimumab, a monoclonal antibody that inhibits the activity of a B-cell growth factor, is FDA approved for treating antibody-positive SLE patients with active disease who have not responded to standard therapies (eg, NSAIDs, antimalarials, or immunosuppressive therapies); it is not recommended for lupus nephritis or for use in conjunction with cyclophosphamide. Rituximab is usually reserved for life-threatening or organ-threatening manifestations that have failed conventional therapies.

Course & Prognosis

Ten-year survival rates exceeding 85% are routine. In most patients, the illness pursues a relapsing and remitting course. Prednisone, often needed in doses of 40 mg/day orally or more during severe flares, can usually be tapered to low doses (5–10 mg/day) when the disease is inactive. However, there are some in whom the disease pursues a virulent course, leading to serious impairment of vital structures such as lungs, heart, brain, or kidneys, and the disease may lead to death. With improved control of lupus activity and with increasing use of corticosteroids and immunosuppressive drugs, the mortality and morbidity patterns in lupus have changed. Mortality in SLE shows a bimodal pattern. In the early years after diagnosis, infections—especially with opportunistic organisms—are the leading cause of death, followed by active SLE, chiefly due to kidney or central nervous system disease. In later years, accelerated atherosclerosis, linked to chronic inflammation, becomes a major cause of death. Indeed, the incidence of myocardial infarction is five times higher in persons with SLE than in the general population. Therefore, it is especially important for SLE patients to avoid smoking and to minimize other conventional risk factors for atherosclerosis (eg, hypercholesterolemia, hypertension, obesity, and inactivity). Patients with SLE should receive influenza vaccination every year and pneumococcal vaccination every 5 years. Since SLE patients have a higher risk of developing malignancy (especially lymphoma, lung cancer, and cervical cancer), preventive cancer screening recommendations should be followed assiduously. With more patients living longer, it has become evident that avascular necrosis of bone, affecting most commonly the hips and knees, is responsible for substantial morbidity. Nonetheless, the outlook for most patients with SLE is increasingly favorable.

When to Refer

- Appropriate diagnosis and management of SLE requires the active participation of a rheumatologist.
- The severity of organ involvement dictates referral to other subspecialists, such as nephrologists and pulmonologists.

When to Admit

- Rapidly progressive glomerulonephritis, pulmonary hemorrhage, transverse myelitis, and other severe organ-threatening manifestations of lupus usually require in-patient assessment and management.
- Severe infections, particularly in the setting of immunosuppressant therapy, should prompt admission.

Fava A et al. Systemic lupus erythematosus: diagnosis and clinical management. J Autoimmun. 2019 Jan;96:113. [PMID: 30448290]

Gatto M et al. New therapeutic strategies in systemic lupus erythematosus management. Nat Rev Rheumatol. 2019 Jan; 15(1):30–48. [PMID: 30538302]

Ospina FE et al. Distinguishing infections vs flares in patients with systemic lupus erythematosus. Rheumatology (Oxford). 2017 Apr 1;56(Suppl 1):i46–54. [PMID: 27744359]

DRUG-INDUCED LUPUS

Drug-induced lupus shares several clinical and serologic features with SLE but is due to ongoing exposure to a drug and resolves when the offending drug is discontinued. In contrast to SLE, the sex ratio is nearly equal. As a general rule, drug-induced lupus presents with fever, arthralgia, myalgia, and serositis but not renal involvement, neurologic symptoms, or other features of SLE. Serologic testing reveals elevated titers of antinuclear antibodies in all patients, but antibodies to DNA, Sm, RNP, SS-A, and SS-B are rare. Antibodies to histones are common but also are seen in SLE and thus do not distinguish drug-induced lupus from SLE. Complement levels are usually normal. There are definite associations between the development of drug-induced lupus and the use of hydralazine, isoniazid, and minocycline as well as several medications no longer commonly prescribed (procainamide, quinidine, methyldopa, chlorpromazine). The list of drugs implicated as possible causes of drug-induced lupus in observational studies and case reports is extensive. The incidence of drug-induced lupus in patients taking hydralazine for a year or longer is as high as 5–8%; for most other medications, the risk is considerably lower (less than 1%). TNF inhibitors can induce antibodies to DNA, but the incidence of lupus-like syndromes on these medications is low (0.5–1%).

Pérez-De-Lis M et al. Autoimmune diseases induced by biological agents. A review of 12,731 cases (BIOGEAS Registry). Expert Opin Drug Saf. 2017 Nov;16(11):1255–71. [PMID: 28854831]

ANTIPHOSPHOLIPID SYNDROME

ESSENTIALS OF DIAGNOSIS

▶ Hypercoagulability; recurrent arterial or venous thromboses.

▶ Thrombocytopenia is common.

▶ Recurrent fetal loss.

▶ Recurrent events are common; lifetime anticoagulation with warfarin is recommended.

General Considerations

Primary antiphospholipid syndrome (APS) is diagnosed in patients who have venous or arterial occlusions or pregnancy complications (ie, three or more first-trimester miscarriages, unexplained fetal death, and premature birth before 34 weeks of gestation attributable to severe preeclampsia, eclampsia, or placental insufficiency) with persistent (12 weeks or longer), high-titer, diagnostic antiphospholipid antibodies but no other features of SLE (see Chapter 19). Diagnostic antiphospholipid antibodies are IgG or IgM anticardiolipin, or IgG or IgM antibodies to beta-2-glycoprotein 1, and lupus anticoagulant. In less than 1% of patients with antiphospholipid antibodies, a potentially devastating syndrome known as the "catastrophic antiphospholipid syndrome" occurs, leading to diffuse thromboses, thrombotic microangiopathy, and multi-organ system failure.

▶ Clinical Findings

A. Symptoms and Signs

Patients are often asymptomatic until suffering a thrombotic complication of this syndrome or a pregnancy loss. Thrombotic events may occur in either the arterial or venous circulations. Thus, deep venous thromboses, pulmonary emboli, and cerebrovascular accidents are typical clinical events among patients with the APS. In case-control studies, 3.1% of patients in the general population who experienced a venous thrombotic event (in the absence of cancer) tested positive for the lupus anticoagulant (versus 0.9% of controls, yielding an odds ratio of 3.6). For women younger than 50 years in whom stroke developed, the odds ratio for having the lupus anticoagulant is 43.1. Budd-Chiari syndrome, cerebral sinus vein thrombosis, myocardial or digital infarctions, hemorrhagic infarction of the adrenal glands (due to adrenal vein thrombosis), and other thrombotic events also occur. A variety of other symptoms and signs are often attributed to the APS, including thrombocytopenia, mental status changes, livedo reticularis, skin ulcers, microangiopathic nephropathy, and cardiac valvular dysfunction—typically mitral regurgitation due to Libman-Sacks endocarditis. Livedo racemosa is strongly associated with the subset of patients with APS in whom arterial ischemic events develop. Pregnancy losses that are associated with APS include unexplained fetal death after the first trimester, one or more premature births before 34 weeks because of eclampsia or preeclampsia, or three or more unexplained miscarriages during the first trimester.

B. Laboratory Findings

As noted in the discussion of SLE, three types of antiphospholipid antibody are associated with this syndrome: (1) anti-cardiolipin antibodies, (2) antibodies to beta-2 glycoprotein, and (3) a "lupus anticoagulant" that prolongs certain phospholipid-dependent coagulation tests (see below). Antibodies to cardiolipin and to beta-2 glycoprotein are typically measured with enzyme immunoassays. Anti-cardiolipin antibodies can produce a biologic false-positive test for syphilis (ie, a positive rapid plasma reagin but negative specific anti-treponemal assay). In general, IgG anti-cardiolipin antibodies are believed to be more pathologic than IgM. Presence of the lupus anticoagulant is a stronger risk factor for thrombosis or pregnancy loss than is the presence of antibodies to either beta-2-glycoprotein I or anticardiolipin. A clue to the presence of a lupus anticoagulant, which may occur in individuals who do not have SLE, may be

detected by a prolongation of the partial thromboplastin time (which, paradoxically, is associated with a thrombotic tendency rather than a bleeding risk). Testing for the lupus anticoagulant involves phospholipid-dependent functional assays of coagulation, such as the Russell viper venom time (RVVT). In the presence of a lupus anticoagulant, the RVVT is prolonged and does not correct with mixing studies but does with the addition of excess phospholipid.

Differential Diagnosis

The exclusion of other autoimmune disorders, particularly those in the SLE spectrum, is essential because such disorders may be associated with additional complications requiring alternative treatments. Other genetic or acquired conditions associated with hypercoagulability such as protein C, protein S, or antithrombin deficiency and factor V Leiden should be excluded. Catastrophic APS has a broad differential, including sepsis, pulmonary-renal syndromes, systemic vasculitis, disseminated intravascular coagulation, and thrombotic thrombocytopenic purpura.

Treatment

Patients should be given warfarin to maintain an INR of 2.0–3.0. The efficacy and safety of direct-acting oral anticoagulants for the antiphospholipid syndrome have not been established. Patients who have recurrent thrombotic events on this level of anticoagulation may require higher INRs (greater than 3.0), but the bleeding risk increases substantially with this degree of anticoagulation. Guidelines indicate that patients with APS should be treated with anticoagulation for life. Because of the teratogenic effects of warfarin, subcutaneous heparin and low-dose aspirin (81 mg) is the usual approach to prevent pregnancy complications in women with APS (see Chapter 19). In patients with catastrophic APS, a three-pronged approach is taken in the acute setting: intravenous heparin, high doses of corticosteroids, and either intravenous immune globulin or plasmapheresis.

Sciascia S et al. Diagnosing antiphospholipid syndrome: 'extra-criteria' manifestations and technical advances. Nat Rev Rheumatol. 2017 Sep;13(9):548–60. [PMID: 28769114]

Zuo Y et al. Primary thrombosis prophylaxis in persistently antiphospholipid antibody-positive individuals: where do we stand in 2018? Curr Rheumatol Rep. 2018 Sep 10;20(11):66. [PMID: 30203272]

RAYNAUD PHENOMENON

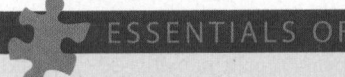

ESSENTIALS OF DIAGNOSIS

▶ Paroxysmal bilateral digital pallor and cyanosis followed by rubor.

▶ Precipitated by cold or emotional stress; relieved by warmth.

▶ **Primary form:** benign course; usually affects young women.

▶ **Secondary form:** can cause digital ulceration or gangrene.

General Considerations

Raynaud phenomenon (RP) is a syndrome of paroxysmal digital ischemia, most commonly caused by an exaggerated response of digital arterioles to cold or emotional stress. The initial phase of RP, mediated by excessive vasoconstriction, consists of well-demarcated digital pallor or cyanosis; the subsequent (recovery) phase of RP, caused by vasodilation, leads to intense hyperemia and rubor. Although RP chiefly affects fingers, it can also affect toes and other acral areas such as the nose and ears. RP is classified as primary (idiopathic or Raynaud disease) or secondary. Nearly one-third of the population reports being "sensitive to the cold" but does not experience the paroxysms of digital pallor, cyanosis, and erythema characteristic of RP. Primary RP occurs in 2–6% of adults, is especially common in young women, and poses more of a nuisance than a threat to good health. In contrast, secondary RP is less common, is chiefly associated with rheumatic diseases (especially scleroderma), and is frequently severe enough to cause digital ulceration or gangrene.

Clinical Findings

In early attacks of RP, only one or two fingertips may be affected; as it progresses, all fingers down to the distal palm may be involved. The thumbs are rarely affected. During recovery there may be intense rubor, throbbing, paresthesia, pain, and slight swelling. Attacks usually terminate spontaneously or upon returning to a warm room or putting the extremity in warm water. The patient is usually asymptomatic between attacks. Sensory changes that often accompany vasomotor manifestations include numbness, stiffness, diminished sensation, and aching pain.

Primary RP appears first between ages 15 and 30, almost always in women. It tends to be mildly progressive and, unlike secondary RP (which may be unilateral and may involve only one or two fingers), symmetric involvement of the fingers of both hands is the rule. Spasm becomes more frequent and prolonged. Unlike secondary RP, primary RP does not cause digital pitting, ulceration, or gangrene.

Nailfold capillary abnormalities are among the earliest clues that a person has secondary rather than primary RP. The nailfold capillary pattern can be visualized by placing a drop of grade B immersion oil at the patient's cuticle and then viewing the area with an ophthalmoscope set to 20–40 diopters. Dropout of capillaries and dilation of the remaining capillary loops indicate the patient has a secondary form of RP, most commonly scleroderma (Table 20–9). While highly specific for secondary RP, nailfold capillary changes have a low sensitivity. Digital pitting or ulceration or other abnormal physical findings (eg, skin tightening, loss of extremity pulse, rash, swollen joints) can also provide evidence of secondary RP.

Primary RP must be differentiated from the numerous causes of secondary RP (Table 20–9). The history and examination may suggest the diagnosis of scleroderma, SLE, and mixed connective tissue disease; RP is often the first manifestation of limited scleroderma (CREST syndrome). The diagnosis of many of these rheumatic diseases can be confirmed with specific serologic tests (see Table 20–7).

Table 20–9. Causes of secondary Raynaud phenomenon.

Rheumatic diseases
  Scleroderma
  Systemic lupus erythematosus
  Dermatomyositis/polymyositis
  Sjögren syndrome
  Vasculitis (polyarteritis nodosa, Takayasu disease, Buerger disease)
Neurovascular compression and occupational
  Carpal tunnel syndrome
  Thoracic outlet obstruction
  Vibration injury
Medications
  Serotonin agonists (sumatriptan)
  Sympathomimetic drugs (decongestants)
  Chemotherapy (bleomycin, vinblastine)
  Ergotamine
  Caffeine
  Nicotine
Hematologic disorders
  Cryoglobulinemia
  Polycythemia vera
  Paraproteinemia
  Cold agglutinins
Endocrine disorders
  Hypothyroidism
  Pheochromocytoma
Miscellaneous
  Atherosclerosis
  Embolic disease
  Migraine
  Exposure to epoxy resins
  Sequela of frostbite

RP may occur in patients with the thoracic outlet syndromes. In these disorders, involvement is generally unilateral, and symptoms referable to brachial plexus compression tend to dominate the clinical picture. Carpal tunnel syndrome should also be considered, and nerve conduction tests are appropriate in selected cases.

▶ Differential Diagnosis

The differentiation from Buerger disease (thromboangiitis obliterans) is usually not difficult, since thromboangiitis obliterans is generally a disease of men, particularly smokers; peripheral pulses are often diminished or absent; and, when RP occurs in association with thromboangiitis obliterans, it is usually in only one or two digits.

In acrocyanosis, cyanosis of the hands is permanent and diffuse; the sharp and paroxysmal line of demarcation with pallor does not occur with acrocyanosis. Frostbite may lead to chronic RP.

Erythromelalgia can mimic the rubor phase of RP; exacerbation by heat and relief with cold readily distinguish erythromelalgia from RP.

▶ Treatment

A. General Measures

Patients should wear gloves or mittens whenever outside in temperatures that precipitate attacks. Keeping the body warm is also a cornerstone of initial therapy. Wearing warm shirts, coats, and hats will help prevent the exaggerated vasospasm that causes RP and that is not prevented by warming only the hands. The hands should be protected from injury at all times; wounds heal slowly, and infections are consequently hard to control. Softening and lubricating lotion to control the fissured dry skin should be applied to the hands frequently. Smoking should be stopped and sympathomimetic drugs (eg, decongestants, diet pills, and amphetamines) should be avoided. For most patients with primary RP, general measures alone are sufficient to control symptoms. Medical or surgical therapy should be considered in patients who have severe symptoms or are experiencing tissue injury from digital ischemia.

B. Medications

Calcium channel blockers are first-line therapy for RP. Calcium channel blockers produce a modest benefit and are more effective in primary RP than secondary RP. Slow release nifedipine (30–180 mg/day orally), amlodipine (5–20 mg/day orally), felodipine, isradipine, or nisoldipine are popular and more effective than verapamil, nicardipine, and diltiazem. Other medications that are sometimes effective in treating RP include angiotensin-converting enzyme inhibitors, sympatholytic agents (eg, prazosin), topical nitrates, phosphodiesterase inhibitors (eg, sildenafil, tadalafil, and vardenafil), selective serotonin reuptake inhibitors (fluoxetine), endothelin-receptor inhibitors (ie, bosentan), statins, parenteral prostaglandins (prostaglandin E_1), and oral prostaglandins (misoprostol).

C. Surgical Measures

Sympathectomy may be indicated when attacks have become frequent and severe, when they interfere with work and well-being, and particularly when trophic changes have developed and medical measures have failed. Digital sympathectomy may improve secondary RP.

▶ Prognosis

Primary RP is benign and largely a nuisance for affected individuals who are exposed to cold winters or excessive air conditioning. The prognosis of secondary RP depends on the severity of the underlying disease. Unfortunately, severe pain from ulceration and gangrene is not rare with scleroderma, especially the CREST variant.

▶ When to Refer

Appropriate management of patients with secondary RP often requires consultation with a rheumatologist.

▶ When to Admit

Patients with severe digital ischemia as evidenced by demarcation should be admitted for intensive therapy.

Roustit M et al. On-demand sildenafil as a treatment for Raynaud Phenomenon: a series of n-of-1 trials. Ann Intern Med. 2018 Nov 20;169(10):694–703. [PMID: 30383134]

SCLERODERMA (Systemic Sclerosis)

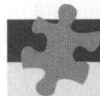
General Considerations

Scleroderma (systemic sclerosis) is a rare chronic disorder characterized by diffuse fibrosis of the skin and internal organs. Symptoms usually appear in the third to fifth decades, and women are affected two to three times as frequently as men.

Two forms of scleroderma are generally recognized: limited (80% of patients) and diffuse (20%). In limited scleroderma, which is also known as the CREST syndrome (representing calcinosis cutis, Raynaud phenomenon, esophageal motility disorder, sclerodactyly, and telangiectasia), the hardening of the skin (scleroderma) is limited to the face and hands. In contrast, in diffuse scleroderma, the skin changes also involve the trunk and proximal extremities. Tendon friction rubs over the forearms and shins occur uniquely (but not universally) in diffuse scleroderma. In general, patients with limited scleroderma have better outcomes than those with diffuse disease, largely because kidney disease or interstitial lung disease rarely develops in patients with limited disease. Cardiac disease is also more characteristic of diffuse scleroderma. Patients with limited disease, however, are more susceptible to digital ischemia, leading to finger loss, and to life-threatening pulmonary hypertension. Small and large bowel hypomotility, which may occur in either form of scleroderma, can cause constipation alternating with diarrhea, malabsorption due to bacterial overgrowth, pseudoobstruction, and severe bowel distention with rupture.

Clinical Findings

A. Symptoms and Signs

Raynaud phenomenon is usually the initial manifestation and can precede other signs and symptoms by years in cases of limited scleroderma. Polyarthralgia, weight loss, and malaise are common early features of diffuse scleroderma but are infrequent in limited scleroderma. Cutaneous disease usually, but not always, develops before visceral involvement and can manifest initially as non-pitting subcutaneous edema associated with pruritus. With time the skin becomes thickened and hidebound, with loss of normal folds. Telangiectasia, pigmentation, and depigmentation are characteristic. Ulceration about the fingertips and subcutaneous calcification are seen. Dysphagia and symptoms of reflux due to esophageal dysfunction are common and result from abnormalities in motility and later from fibrosis. Fibrosis and atrophy of the gastrointestinal tract cause hypomotility. Large-mouthed diverticuli occur in the jejunum, ileum, and colon. Diffuse pulmonary fibrosis and pulmonary vascular disease are reflected in restrictive lung physiology and low diffusing capacities. Cardiac abnormalities include pericarditis, heart block, myocardial fibrosis, and right heart failure secondary to pulmonary hypertension. Scleroderma renal crisis, resulting from intimal proliferation of smaller renal arteries and usually associated with hypertension, is a marker for a poor outcome even though many cases can be treated effectively with angiotensin-converting enzyme inhibitors.

B. Laboratory Findings

Mild anemia is often present. In scleroderma renal crisis, the peripheral blood smear shows findings consistent with a microangiopathic hemolytic anemia (due to mechanical damage to red cells from diseased small vessels). Elevation of the ESR is unusual. Proteinuria appears in association with renal involvement. Antinuclear antibody tests are nearly always positive, frequently in high titers (Table 20–7). The scleroderma antibody (anti-SCL-70), directed against topoisomerase III, is found in one-third of patients with diffuse systemic sclerosis and in 20% of those with CREST syndrome. Although present in only a small number of patients with diffuse scleroderma, anti-SCL-70 antibodies may portend a poor prognosis, with a high likelihood of serious internal organ involvement (eg, interstitial lung disease). Anticentromere antibodies are seen in 50% of those with CREST syndrome and in 1% of individuals with diffuse scleroderma (Table 20–7). Anticentromere antibodies are highly specific for limited scleroderma, but they also occur occasionally in overlap syndromes. Anti-RNA polymerase III antibodies develop in 10–20% of scleroderma patients overall and correlate with the development of diffuse skin disease and renal hypertensive crisis.

Differential Diagnosis

Early in its course, scleroderma can cause diagnostic confusion with other causes of Raynaud phenomenon, particularly SLE, mixed connective tissue disease, and the inflammatory myopathies. Eosinophilic fasciitis is a rare disorder presenting with skin hardening that resemble diffuse scleroderma. The inflammatory abnormalities, however, are limited to the fascia rather than the dermis and epidermis. Moreover, patients with eosinophilic fasciitis are distinguished from those with scleroderma by the presence of peripheral blood eosinophilia, the absence of Raynaud phenomenon, the good response to prednisone, and an association (in some cases) with paraproteinemias. Diffuse skin thickening and visceral involvement are features of scleromyxedema; the presence of a paraprotein, the absence of Raynaud phenomenon, and distinct skin histology point to scleromyxedema. Diabetic cheiropathy typically develops in longstanding, poorly controlled diabetes mellitus and can mimic sclerodactyly. Morphea and linear scleroderma cause sclerodermatous changes limited to circumscribed areas of the skin and usually have excellent outcomes.

► Treatment

Treatment of scleroderma is symptomatic and supportive and focuses on the organ systems involved. There is no effective therapy for the underlying disease process. However, interventions for management of specific organ manifestations of this disease have improved substantially. First-line therapy for moderately severe Raynaud syndrome is a calcium channel blocker, eg, long-acting nifedipine, 30–120 mg/day orally. Poor responders can be treated with a PDE-5 inhibitor, eg, sildenafil 50 mg orally twice daily. Severe Raynaud syndrome can be treated with intravenous iloprost. Patients with esophageal disease should take medications in liquid or crushed form. Esophageal reflux can be reduced and the risk of scarring diminished by avoidance of late-night meals and by the use of proton pump inhibitors (eg, omeprazole, 20–40 mg/day orally), which achieve near-complete inhibition of gastric acid production and are remarkably effective for refractory esophagitis. Patients with delayed gastric emptying maintain their weight better if they eat small, frequent meals and remain upright for at least 2 hours after eating. Malabsorption due to bacterial overgrowth responds to antibiotics, eg, tetracycline, 500 mg four times orally daily, often prescribed cyclically. The hypertensive crises associated with scleroderma renal crisis must be treated early and aggressively (in the hospital) with angiotensin-converting enzyme inhibitors, eg, captopril, initiated at 25 mg orally every 6 hours and titrated up as tolerated to a maximum of 100 mg every 6 hours. Apart from the patient with myositis, prednisone has little or no role in the treatment of scleroderma; doses higher than 15 mg/day may precipitate scleroderma renal crisis. In patients with early diffuse scleroderma, methotrexate has been used in the treatment of skin disease, arthritis, and myositis. The usual initial dose is 7.5 mg of methotrexate orally once weekly. If the patient has tolerated methotrexate but has not responded in 1 month, the dose can be increased to 15 mg orally once per week. The maximal dose is usually 20–25 mg/wk. Cyclophosphamide improves dyspnea and pulmonary function tests modestly in patients with severe interstitial lung disease; this highly toxic drug should only be administered by physicians familiar with its use. Mycophenolate mofetil, 1 g twice daily, stabilized lung function in small, uncontrolled studies of patients with interstitial lung disease. Bosentan, an endothelin receptor antagonist, improves exercise capacity and cardiopulmonary hemodynamics in patients with pulmonary hypertension and helps prevent digital ulceration. Sildenafil, prostaglandins (delivered by continuous intravenous infusion or intermittent inhalation), or riociguat may also be useful in treating pulmonary hypertension. For patients with severe, diffuse scleroderma, myeloablation followed by autologous stem cell transplantation is superior to immunosuppression with cyclophosphamide but has greater toxicity.

The 9-year survival rate in scleroderma averages approximately 40%. The prognosis tends to be worse in those with diffuse scleroderma, in blacks, in men, and in older patients. Lung disease—in the form of pulmonary fibrosis or pulmonary arterial hypertension—is the number one cause of mortality. Death from advanced heart failure or chronic kidney disease is also common. Those persons in whom severe internal organ involvement does not develop in the first 3 years have a substantially better prognosis, with 72% surviving at least 9 years. Breast and lung cancer may be more common in patients with scleroderma. Studies conducted in a small number of patients with simultaneous onset of cancer and scleroderma have demonstrated that the scleroderma developed as a consequence of an immune response directed at the cancer.

► When to Refer

- Appropriate management of scleroderma requires frequent consultations with a rheumatologist.
- Severity of organ involvement dictates referral to pulmonologists, gastroenterologists, or nephrologists.

Goldin JG et al. Longitudinal changes in quantitative interstitial lung disease on computed tomography after immunosuppression in the Scleroderma Lung Study II. Ann Am Thorac Soc. 2018 Nov;15(11):1286–95. [PMID: 30265153]

Kowal-Bielecka O et al; EUSTAR Coauthors. Update of EULAR recommendations for the treatment of systemic sclerosis. Ann Rheum Dis. 2017 Aug;76(8):1327–39. [PMID: 27941129]

Sullivan KM et al; SCOT Study Investigators. Myeloablative autologous stem-cell transplantation for severe scleroderma. N Engl J Med. 2018 Jan 4;378(1):35–47. [PMID: 29298160]

IDIOPATHIC INFLAMMATORY MYOPATHIES (Polymyositis & Dermatomyositis)

ESSENTIALS OF DIAGNOSIS

- ► Bilateral proximal muscle weakness.
- ► **Dermatomyositis:** characteristic cutaneous manifestations (Gottron papules, heliotrope rash); increased risk of malignancy.
- ► Elevated creatine kinase, myositis-specific antibodies, diagnostic muscle biopsy.
- ► Mimics include inclusion body myositis and statin-induced immune-mediated necrotizing myopathy.

► General Considerations

Polymyositis and dermatomyositis are systemic disorders of unknown cause whose principal manifestation is muscle weakness. Although their clinical presentations (aside from the presence of certain skin findings in dermatomyositis, some of which are pathognomonic) and treatments are similar, the two diseases are pathologically quite distinct. They affect persons of any age group, but the peak incidence is in the fifth and sixth decades of life. Women are affected twice as commonly as men, and the diseases (particularly polymyositis) also occur more often among blacks than whites. There is an increased risk of malignancy in adult patients with dermatomyositis. Indeed, up to one patient in four with dermatomyositis has an occult malignancy. Malignancies may be evident at the time of presentation with the muscle disease but may not be detected until months afterward in some cases. The malignancies most commonly associated with dermatomyositis in descending order of frequency are ovarian, lung, pancreatic, stomach, colorectal, and non-Hodgkin lymphoma. Patients may have skin disease without overt muscle involvement, a condition termed dermatomyositis sine myositis; these patients can have aggressive interstitial lung disease. Myositis may also be associated with other connective tissue diseases, especially scleroderma, systemic lupus erythematosus, mixed connective tissue disease, and Sjögren syndrome.

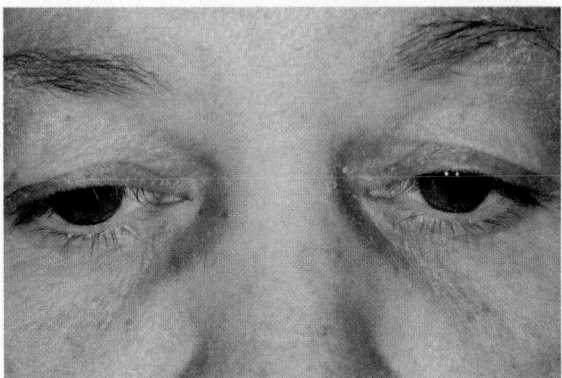

▲ **Figure 20–5.** Bilateral heliotrope rash, which is a pathognomonic sign of dermatomyositis. (Used, with permission, from Richard P. Usatine, MD, in Usatine RP, Smith MA, Mayeaux EJ Jr, Chumley H. *The Color Atlas of Family Medicine*, 2nd ed. McGraw-Hill, 2013.)

▶ Clinical Findings

A. Symptoms and Signs

Polymyositis may begin abruptly, but the usual presentation is one of progressive muscle weakness over weeks to months. The weakness chiefly involves proximal muscle groups of the upper and lower extremities as well as the neck. Leg weakness (eg, difficulty in rising from a chair or climbing stairs) typically precedes arm symptoms. In contrast to myasthenia gravis, polymyositis and dermatomyositis do not cause facial or ocular muscle weakness. Pain and tenderness of affected muscles occur in one-fourth of cases, but these are rarely the chief complaints. About one-fourth of patients have dysphagia. In contrast to scleroderma, which affects the smooth muscle of the lower esophagus and can cause a "sticking" sensation below the sternum, polymyositis or dermatomyositis involves the striated muscles of the upper pharynx and can make initiation of swallowing difficult. Muscle atrophy and contractures occur as late complications of advanced disease. Clinically significant myocarditis is uncommon even though there is often creatine kinase-MB elevation. Patients who are bed-bound from myositis should be screened for respiratory muscle weakness that can be severe enough to cause CO_2 retention and can progress to require mechanical ventilation.

The characteristic rash of **dermatomyositis** is dusky red and may appear in a malar distribution mimicking the classic rash of SLE. Facial erythema beyond the malar distribution is also characteristic of dermatomyositis. Erythema also occurs over other areas of the face, neck, shoulders, and upper chest and back ("shawl sign"). Periorbital edema and a purplish (heliotrope) suffusion over the eyelids are typical signs (Figure 20–5). Coloration of the heliotrope and other rashes of dermatomyositis can be affected by skin tone. In blacks, the rashes may appear more hyperpigmented than erythematous or violaceous. Periungual erythema, dilations of nailfold capillaries, Gottron papules (raised violaceous lesions overlying the dorsa of DIP, PIP, and MCP joints), and Gottron sign (erythematous rash on the extensors surfaces

of the fingers, elbows, and knees) are highly suggestive. Scalp involvement by dermatomyositis may mimic psoriasis. Infrequently, the cutaneous findings of this disease precede the muscle inflammation by weeks or months. Diagnosing polymyositis in patients over age 70 years can be difficult because weakness may be overlooked or attributed erroneously to idiopathic frailty. A subset of patients with polymyositis and dermatomyositis have the **"antisynthetase syndrome,"** a group of findings including inflammatory nonerosive arthritis, fever, Raynaud phenomenon, "mechanic's hands" (hyperkeratosis along the radial and palmar aspects of the fingers), interstitial lung disease, and often severe muscle disease associated with certain autoantibodies (eg, anti-Jo-1 antibodies).

B. Laboratory Findings

Measurement of serum levels of muscle enzymes, especially creatine kinase and aldolase, is most useful in diagnosis and in assessment of disease activity. Polymyositis can be misdiagnosed as hepatitis because of elevations in serum levels of muscle-derived alanine aminotransferase (ALT) and aspartate aminotransferase (AST) levels. Anemia is uncommon. The ESR and CRP are often normal and are not reliable indicators of disease activity. Rheumatoid factor is found in a minority of patients. Antinuclear antibodies can be present, especially when there is an associated connective tissue disease. A number of autoantibodies are seen exclusively in patients with myositis and are associated with distinctive clinical features (Table 20–10). These myositis-specific antibodies include (1) anti-Jo-1 antibody (seen in the subset of patients who have antisynthetase syndrome), (2) anti-Mi-2 (associated with dermatomyositis), (3) anti-SRP (anti-signal recognition particle, associated with rapidly progressive, severe polymyositis, and dysphagia), (4) anti-155/140 (strongly associated with dermatomyositis with malignancy), and (5) anti-MDA5 (melanocyte differentiation-associated protein 5, linked to dermatomyositis with cutaneous ulcerations and rapidly progressive interstitial lung disease). Chest radiographs are

Table 20–10. Myositis-specific antibodies.

Antibody	Clinical Association
Anti-Jo-1 and other antisynthetase antibodies	Polymyositis or dermatomyositis with interstitial lung disease, arthritis, mechanic's hands
Anti-Mi-2	Dermatomyositis with rash more than myositis
Anti-MDA5 (anti-CADM 140)	Dermatomyositis with rapidly progressive lung disease, cutaneous ulcers
Anti-155/140	Cancer-associated myositis
Anti-140	Juvenile dermatomyositis
Anti-SAE	Cancer-associated dermatomyositis, dermatomyositis with rapidly progressive lung disease
Anti-signal recognition particle	Severe, acute necrotizing myopathy
Anti-HMG CoA reductase	Necrotizing myopathy related to statin use

Adapted, with permission, from Imboden JB, Hellmann DB, Stone JH (editors): *Current Diagnosis & Treatment Rheumatology*, 3rd ed. McGraw-Hill, 2013.

usually normal unless there is associated interstitial lung disease. Electromyographic abnormalities can point toward a myopathic, rather than a neurogenic, cause of weakness. MRI can detect early and patchy muscle involvement, can guide biopsies, and often is more useful than electromyography. The search for an occult malignancy should begin with a history and physical examination, supplemented with a complete blood count, comprehensive biochemical panel, serum protein electrophoresis, and urinalysis, and should include age- and risk-appropriate cancer screening tests. Given the especially strong association of ovarian carcinoma and dermatomyositis, transvaginal ultrasonography, CT scanning, and CA-125 levels may be useful in women. No matter how extensive the initial screening, some malignancies will not become evident for months after the initial presentation.

C. Muscle Biopsy

Biopsy of clinically involved muscle is the only specific diagnostic test. The pathology findings in polymyositis and dermatomyositis are distinct. Although both include lymphoid inflammatory infiltrates, the findings in dermatomyositis are localized to perivascular regions and there is evidence of humoral and complement-mediated destruction of microvasculature associated with the muscle. In addition to its vascular orientation, the inflammatory infiltrate in dermatomyositis centers on the interfascicular septa and is located around, rather than in, muscle fascicles. A pathologic hallmark of dermatomyositis is perifascicular atrophy. In contrast, the pathology of polymyositis

characteristically includes endomysial infiltration of the inflammatory infiltrate. However, false-negative biopsies sometimes occur in both disorders because of the sometimes patchy distribution of pathologic abnormalities.

▶ Differential Diagnosis

Muscle inflammation may occur as a component of SLE, scleroderma, Sjögren syndrome, and overlap syndromes. In those cases, associated findings usually permit the precise diagnosis of the primary condition.

Inclusion body myositis, because of its tendency to mimic polymyositis, is a common cause of "treatment-resistant polymyositis." In contrast to the epidemiologic features of polymyositis, however, the typical inclusion body myositis patient is white, male, and over the age of 50. The onset of inclusion body myositis is more insidious than that of polymyositis or dermatomyositis (eg, occurring over years rather than months), and asymmetric distal motor weakness is common in inclusion body myositis. Creatine kinase levels in inclusion body myositis are often minimally elevated and are normal in 25%. Electromyography may show a mixed picture of myopathic and neurogenic abnormalities. Muscle biopsy shows characteristic intracellular vacuoles by light microscopy and either tubular or filamentous inclusions in the nucleus or cytoplasm by electron microscopy. Inclusion body myositis is less likely to respond to therapy.

Hypothyroidism is a common cause of proximal muscle weakness associated with elevations of serum creatine kinase. Hyperthyroidism and Cushing disease may both be associated with proximal muscle weakness with normal levels of creatine kinase. Patients with polymyalgia rheumatica are over the age of 50 and—in contrast to patients with polymyositis—have pain but no objective weakness; creatine kinase levels are normal. Disorders of the peripheral and central nervous systems (eg, chronic inflammatory polyneuropathy, multiple sclerosis, myasthenia gravis, Lambert-Eaton disease, and amyotrophic lateral sclerosis) can produce weakness but are distinguished by characteristic symptoms and neurologic signs and often by distinctive electromyographic abnormalities. A number of systemic vasculitides (polyarteritis nodosa, microscopic polyangiitis, eosinophilic granulomatosis with polyangiitis [formerly called Churg-Strauss syndrome], granulomatosis with polyangiitis, and mixed cryoglobulinemia) can produce profound weakness through vasculitic neuropathy. The muscle weakness associated with these disorders, however, is typically distal and asymmetric, at least in the early stages.

Limb-girdle muscular dystrophy can present in early adulthood with a clinical picture that mimics polymyositis: proximal muscle weakness, elevations in serum levels of creatine kinase, and inflammatory changes on muscle biopsy. Failure to respond to treatment for polymyositis or the presence of atypical clinical features such as scapular winging or weakness of ankle plantar flexors should prompt genetic testing for limb-girdle muscular dystrophy.

Many drugs, including corticosteroids, alcohol, clofibrate, penicillamine, tryptophan, and hydroxychloroquine, can produce proximal muscle weakness. Long-term use of colchicine at doses as low as 0.6 mg twice a day in patients with moderate chronic kidney disease can produce a mixed neuropathy-myopathy that mimics polymyositis. The weakness and muscle enzyme elevation reverse with cessation of the drug. Polymyositis can occur as a complication of HIV or HTLV-1 infection and with zidovudine therapy as well.

HMG-CoA reductase inhibitors can cause myopathy and rhabdomyolysis. Although only about 0.1% of patients taking a statin drug alone develop myopathy, concomitant administration of other drugs (especially gemfibrozil, cyclosporine, niacin, macrolide antibiotics, azole antifungals, and protease inhibitors) increases the risk. Statin use has also been linked to the development of an immune-mediated necrotizing myositis, which persists after the statin has been discontinued and is associated with autoantibodies to HMG-CoA reductase.

The use of immune check point inhibitors to treat cancer can cause rheumatic and musculoskeletal symptoms, including myalgia.

► Treatment

Most patients respond to corticosteroids. Often a daily dose of 40–60 mg or more of oral prednisone is required initially. The dose is then adjusted downward while monitoring muscle strength and serum levels of muscle enzymes. Long-term use of corticosteroids is often needed, and the disease may recur or reemerge when they are withdrawn. Patients with an associated neoplasm have a poor prognosis, although remission may follow treatment of the tumor; corticosteroids may or may not be effective in these patients. In patients resistant or intolerant to corticosteroids, therapy with methotrexate or azathioprine may be helpful. Intravenous immune globulin is effective for dermatomyositis resistant to prednisone. Mycophenolate mofetil (1–1.5 g orally twice daily) may be useful as a steroid-sparing agent. Rituximab is effective in some patients with inflammatory myositis unresponsive to prednisone. Since the rash of dermatomyositis is often photosensitive, patients should limit sun exposure. Hydroxychloroquine (200–400 mg/day orally not to exceed 5 mg/kg) can also help ameliorate the skin disease.

► When to Refer

- All patients with myositis should be referred to a rheumatologist or neurologist.
- Severe lung disease may require consultation with a pulmonologist.

► When to Admit

- Signs of rhabdomyolysis.
- New onset of dysphagia.
- Respiratory insufficiency with hypoxia or carbon dioxide retention.

Cappelli LC et al. Rheumatic and musculoskeletal immune-related adverse events due to immune checkpoint inhibitors: a systematic review of the literature. Arthritis Care Res (Hoboken). 2017 Nov;69(11):1751–63. [PMID: 27998041]

Milone M. Diagnosis and management of immune-mediated myopathies. Mayo Clin Proc. 2017 May;92(5):826–37. [PMID: 28473041]

Wolstencroft PW et al. Dermatomyositis clinical and pathological phenotypes associated with myositis-specific autoantibodies. Curr Rheumatol Rep. 2018 Apr 10;20(5):28. [PMID: 29637414]

MIXED CONNECTIVE TISSUE DISEASE & OVERLAP SYNDROMES

Many patients with symptoms and signs compatible with a connective tissue disease have features consistent with more than one type of rheumatic disease. Special attention has been drawn to antinuclear antibody–positive patients who have overlapping features of SLE, scleroderma, and inflammatory myopathy together with autoantibodies to RNP. Some consider these patients to have a distinct entity ("mixed connective tissue disease"), and others view this as a subset of SLE characterized by a higher prevalence of Raynaud phenomenon, polyarthritis, myositis, and pulmonary hypertension and a lower incidence of renal involvement. Other patients have features of more than one connective tissue disease (eg, rheumatoid arthritis and SLE, SLE and scleroderma) in the absence of anti-RNP antibodies and are referred to as having an "overlap syndrome." Treatments are guided more by the distribution and severity of patients' organ system involvement than by therapies specific to these overlap syndromes.

Reiseter S et al. Progression and mortality of interstitial lung disease in mixed connective tissue disease: a long-term observational nationwide cohort study. Rheumatology (Oxford). 2018 Feb 1;57(2):255–62. [PMID: 28379478]

SJÖGREN SYNDROME

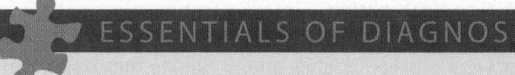

ESSENTIALS OF DIAGNOSIS

- ► Women (average age 50 years) compose 90% of patients.
- ► Dryness of eyes and dry mouth (sicca components) are the most common features; they occur alone or with rheumatoid arthritis or other connective tissue disease.
- ► Rheumatoid factor and antinuclear antibodies are common.
- ► Increased incidence of lymphoma.

► General Considerations

Sjögren syndrome is a systemic autoimmune disorder whose clinical presentation is usually dominated by dryness of the eyes and mouth due to immune-mediated dysfunction of the lacrimal and salivary glands. The disorder is predominantly seen in women, with a ratio of 9:1; most cases develop between the ages of 40 and 60 years. Sjögren syndrome can occur in isolation ("primary" Sjögren syndrome) or in association with another rheumatic disease.

Sjögren syndrome is most frequently associated with rheumatoid arthritis but also occurs with SLE, primary biliary cholangitis, scleroderma, polymyositis, Hashimoto thyroiditis, polyarteritis, and interstitial pulmonary fibrosis.

▶ Clinical Findings

A. Symptoms and Signs

Keratoconjunctivitis sicca results from inadequate tear production caused by lymphocyte and plasma cell infiltration of the lacrimal glands. Ocular symptoms are usually mild. Burning, itching, and the sensation of having a foreign body or a grain of sand in the eye occur commonly. For some patients, the initial manifestation is the inability to tolerate wearing contact lenses. Many patients with more severe ocular dryness notice ropy secretions across their eyes, especially in the morning. Photophobia may signal corneal ulceration resulting from severe dryness. For most patients, symptoms of dryness of the mouth (xerostomia) dominate those of dry eyes. Patients frequently complain of a "cotton mouth" sensation and difficulty swallowing foods, especially dry foods like crackers, unless they are washed down with liquids. The persistent oral dryness causes most patients to carry water bottles or other liquid dispensers from which they sip constantly. A few patients have such severe xerostomia that they have difficulty speaking. Persistent xerostomia results often in rampant dental caries; caries at the gum line strongly suggest Sjögren syndrome. Some patients are most troubled by loss of taste and smell. Parotid enlargement, which may be chronic or relapsing, develops in one-third of patients. Dryness may involve the nose, throat, larynx, bronchi, vagina, and skin.

Systemic manifestations include dysphagia, small vessel vasculitis, pleuritis, obstructive airways disease and interstitial lung disease (in the absence of smoking), neuropsychiatric dysfunction (most commonly peripheral neuropathies), and pancreatitis; they may be related to the associated diseases noted above. Renal tubular acidosis (type I, distal) occurs in 20% of patients. Chronic interstitial nephritis, which may result in impaired kidney function, may be seen.

B. Laboratory Findings

Laboratory findings include mild anemia, leukopenia, and eosinophilia. Polyclonal hypergammaglobulinemia, rheumatoid factor positivity (70%), and antinuclear antibodies (95%) are all common findings. Antibodies against SS-A and SS-B (also called Ro and La, respectively) are often present in primary Sjögren syndrome and tend to correlate with the presence of extra-glandular manifestations (Table 20–7). Thyroid-associated autoimmunity is a common finding among patients with Sjögren syndrome.

Useful ocular diagnostic tests include the Schirmer test, which measures the quantity of tears secreted. Lip biopsy, a simple procedure, reveals characteristic lymphoid foci in accessory salivary glands. Biopsy of the parotid gland should be reserved for patients with atypical presentations such as unilateral gland enlargement that suggest a neoplastic process.

▶ Differential Diagnosis

Isolated complaints of dry mouth are most commonly due to medication side effects. Chronic hepatitis C can cause sicca symptoms and rheumatoid factor positivity. Minor salivary gland biopsies reveal lymphocytic infiltrates but not to the extent of Sjögren syndrome, and tests for anti-SS-A and anti-SS-B are negative. Involvement of the lacrimal or salivary glands, or both in sarcoidosis can mimic Sjögren syndrome; biopsies reveal noncaseating granulomas. Rarely, amyloid deposits in the lacrimal and salivary glands produce sicca symptoms. IgG_4-related systemic disease (characterized by high serum IgG_4 levels and infiltration of tissues with IgG_4^+ plasma cells) can result in lacrimal and salivary gland enlargement that mimics Sjögren syndrome.

▶ Treatment & Prognosis

Treatment of sicca symptoms is symptomatic and supportive. Artificial tears applied frequently will relieve ocular symptoms and avert further desiccation. Topical ocular 0.05% cyclosporine also improves ocular symptoms and signs of dryness. The mouth should be kept well lubricated. Sipping water frequently or using sugar-free gums and hard candies usually relieves dry mouth symptoms. Pilocarpine (5 mg orally four times daily) and the acetylcholine derivative cevimeline (30 mg orally three times daily) may improve xerostomia symptoms. Atropinic drugs and decongestants decrease salivary secretions and should be avoided. A program of oral hygiene, including fluoride treatment, is essential in order to preserve dentition. If there is an associated rheumatic disease, its systemic treatment is not altered by the presence of Sjögren syndrome.

Although Sjögren syndrome may compromise patients' quality of life significantly, the disease is usually consistent with a normal life span. Poor prognoses are influenced mainly by the presence of systemic features associated with underlying disorders, the development in some patients of lymphocytic vasculitis, the occurrence of a painful peripheral neuropathy, and the complication (in a minority of patients) of lymphoma. Severe systemic inflammatory manifestations are treated with prednisone or various immunosuppressive medications. The patients at greatest risk for developing lymphoma are those with severe exocrine dysfunction, marked parotid gland enlargement, splenomegaly, vasculitis, peripheral neuropathy, anemia, and mixed monoclonal cryoglobulinemia (3–10% of the total Sjögren population).

▶ When to Refer

- Presence of systemic symptoms or signs.
- Ocular dryness not responsive to artificial tears.

▶ When to Admit

Presence of severe systemic signs such as vasculitis unresponsive to outpatient management.

Mariette X et al. Primary Sjögren's syndrome. N Engl J Med. 2018 Mar 8;378(10):931–9. [PMID: 29514034]

IgG$_4$-RELATED DISEASE

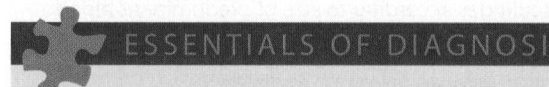

ESSENTIALS OF DIAGNOSIS

► Predominantly affects men (75% of patients); average age older than 50 years.

► Protean manifestations caused by lymphoplasmacytic infiltrates in any organ or tissue, especially the pancreas, lacrimal glands, biliary tract, and retroperitoneum.

► Subacute onset; fever, constitutional symptoms rare.

► Diagnostic histopathology.

General Considerations

IgG$_4$-related disease is a systemic disorder of unknown cause marked by highly characteristic fibroinflammatory changes that can affect virtually any organ. Elevations of serum IgG$_4$ levels occur often but are not diagnostic. The disorder chiefly affects men over the age of 50 years.

Clinical Findings

A. Symptoms and Signs

IgG$_4$-related disease can affect any organ of the body, can be localized or generalized, demonstrates the same distinctive histopathology at all sites of involvement, produces protean manifestations depending on location and extent of involvement, and causes disease that ranges in severity from asymptomatic to organ- or life-threatening. The inflammatory infiltration in IgG$_4$-related disease frequently produces tumefactive masses that can be found during physical examination or on imaging. Some of the common presenting manifestations include enlargement of submandibular glands, proptosis from periorbital infiltration, retroperitoneal fibrosis, mediastinal fibrosis, inflammatory aortic aneurysm, and pancreatic mass with autoimmune pancreatitis. IgG$_4$-related disease can also affect the thyroid (formerly Reidel thyroiditis), kidney, meninges, pituitary, sinuses, lung, prostate, breast, and bone. Most symptomatic patients with IgG$_4$-related disease present subacutely; fever and constitutional symptoms are usually absent. Nearly half of the patients with IgG$_4$-related disease also have allergic disorders such as sinusitis or asthma.

B. Laboratory Findings

The infiltrating lesions in IgG$_4$-related disease often produce tumors or fibrotic changes that are evident on CT or MRI imaging. However, the cornerstone of diagnosis is the histopathology. The key pathological findings are a dense lymphoplasmacytic infiltrate rich in IgG$_4$ plasma cells, storiform (matted and irregularly whorled) fibrosis, and obliterative phlebitis. Serum IgG$_4$ levels are usually, but not invariably, elevated so this finding cannot be used as the sole diagnostic criterion.

Differential Diagnosis

IgG$_4$-related disease can mimic many disorders including sarcoidosis, Sjögren syndrome (lacrimal gland enlargement), pancreatic cancer (pancreatic mass), and granulomatosis with polyangiitis (proptosis). Some cases of retroperitoneal fibrosis and mediastinal fibrosis are caused by IgG$_4$-related disease. Lymphoma can mimic some of the histopathologic features of IgG$_4$-related disease.

Treatment & Prognosis

Patients who are asymptomatic and have no organ-threatening disease can be monitored carefully. Spontaneous resolution can occur. The optimal therapy for symptomatic patients has not been defined, but initial therapy is usually oral prednisone 0.6 mg/kg/day, tapered over weeks or months depending on response. Patients who do not respond to prednisone or respond only to sustained high doses of prednisone can be treated with rituximab, mycophenolate mofetil, or azathioprine. The degree of fibrosis in affected organs determines the patient's responsiveness to treatment.

When to Refer

• Presence of systemic symptoms or signs.

• Symptoms or signs not responsive to prednisone.

When to Admit

Presence of severe systemic signs unresponsive to outpatient management.

AbdelRazek MA et al. IgG4-related disease of the central and peripheral nervous systems. Lancet Neurol. 2018 Feb; 17(2):183–92. [PMID: 29413316]

Wallwork R et al. Rituximab for idiopathic and IgG4-related retroperitoneal fibrosis. Medicine (Baltimore). 2018 Oct; 97(42):e12631. [PMID: 30334947]

RHABDOMYOLYSIS

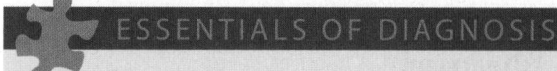

ESSENTIALS OF DIAGNOSIS

► Associated with crush injuries to muscle, immobility, drug toxicities, and hypothermia.

► Usually markedly elevated muscle enzymes.

General Considerations

Rhabdomyolysis is a syndrome of acute necrosis of skeletal muscle associated with myoglobinuria and markedly elevated creatine kinase levels. Acute tubular necrosis is a common complication of rhabdomyolysis and is due to the toxic effects of filtering excessive quantities of myoglobin in the setting of hypovolemia (see Acute Tubular Necrosis in Chapter 22). Many patients in whom rhabdomyolysis develops are volume-contracted and, therefore, oliguric renal failure is encountered routinely. Compartment syndrome, disseminated intravascular coagulation, and cardiac arrhythmias are serious but less common complications of rhabdomyolysis.

Rhabdomyolysis is a common complication of severe crush injuries to muscle. Cocaine use and alcohol intoxication, particularly in the setting of prolonged immobility and exposure hypothermia, are leading causes of hospital admissions for rhabdomyolysis. Use of statins is another important cause of rhabdomyolysis. The presence of compromised kidney and liver function, diabetes mellitus, and hypothyroidism as well as concomitant use of other medications increase the risk of rhabdomyolysis in patients taking statins. The cytochrome P450 liver enzymes metabolize all statins except for pravastatin and rosuvastatin. Drugs that block the action of cytochrome P450 include protease inhibitors, erythromycin, itraconazole, clarithromycin, diltiazem, and verapamil. Use of these drugs concomitantly with the statins (but not pravastatin or rosuvastatin) can increase the risk of development of rhabdomyolysis. The likelihood of rhabdomyolysis also increases when statins are used with niacin and fibric acids (gemfibrozil, clofibrate, and fenofibrate). Rhabdomyolysis is an uncommon complication of polymyositis, dermatomyositis, and the myopathy of hypothyroidism, despite the high levels of creatine kinase often seen in these conditions.

Often there is little evidence for muscle injury on clinical assessment of the patients with rhabdomyolysis—specifically, myalgias and weakness are usually absent. The first clue to muscle necrosis in such individuals may be a urinary dipstick testing positive for "blood" (actually myoglobin) in the absence of red cells in the sediment. This myoglobinuria results in a false-positive reading for hemoglobin. Urine tests for myoglobin are insensitive, however, and are positive in only 25% of patients with rhabdomyolysis. Such an abnormality should prompt determination of the serum creatine kinase level, which invariably is elevated (usually markedly so). Other commonly encountered laboratory abnormalities in rhabdomyolysis include elevated serum levels of AST, ALT, and lactate dehydrogenase (due to release of these enzymes from skeletal muscle), hyperkalemia, and hypocalcemia. The massive acute elevations of muscle enzymes peak quickly and usually resolve within days once the inciting injury has been removed.

▶ Treatment

Vigorous fluid resuscitation (eg, 4–6 L/day but often more in the setting of severe crush injuries) is indicated. Urine alkalinization (to minimize precipitation of myoglobin within tubules) has been recommended to reduce kidney injury, but definitive evidence for the efficacy of this measure is lacking. Myopathic complications of statins usually resolve within several weeks of discontinuing the drug.

Cervellin G et al. Non-traumatic rhabdomyolysis: background, laboratory features, and acute clinical management. Clin Biochem. 2017 Aug;50(12):656–62. [PMID: 28235546]

Panzio N et al. Molecular mechanisms and novel therapeutic approaches to rhabdomyolysis-induced acute kidney injury. Kidney Blood Press Res. 2015;40(5):520–32. [PMID: 26512883]

Table 20–11. Classification scheme of primary vasculitides according to size of predominant blood vessels involved.

Predominantly large-vessel vasculitides
Takayasu arteritis
Giant cell arteritis (temporal arteritis)
Behçet disease[1]
Predominantly medium-vessel vasculitides
Polyarteritis nodosa
Buerger disease
Primary angiitis of the central nervous system
Predominantly small-vessel vasculitides
Cutaneous leukocytoclastic angiitis ("hypersensitivity vasculitis")
Immune-complex mediated
Henoch-Schönlein purpura
Essential cryoglobulinemia[2]
"ANCA-associated" disorders[3]
Granulomatosis with polyangiitis[2]
Microscopic polyangiitis[2]
Eosinophilic granulomatosis with polyangiitis[2]

[1]May involve small-, medium-, and large-sized blood vessels.
[2]Frequent overlap of small- and medium-sized blood vessel involvement.
[3]Not all forms of these disorders are always associated with ANCA.
ANCA, antineutrophil cytoplasmic antibodies.

▼ VASCULITIS SYNDROMES

"Vasculitis" is a heterogeneous group of disorders characterized by inflammation within the walls of affected blood vessels. The major forms of primary systemic vasculitis are listed in Table 20–11. The first consideration in classifying cases of vasculitis is the size of the major vessels involved: large, medium, or small. The presence of the clinical signs and symptoms shown in Table 20–12 helps distinguish among these three groups. After determining the size of

Table 20–12. Typical clinical manifestations of large-, medium-, and small-vessel involvement by vasculitis.

Large	Medium	Small
Constitutional symptoms: fever, weight loss, malaise, arthralgias/arthritis		
Limb claudication	Cutaneous nodules	Purpura
Asymmetric blood pressures	Ulcers	Vesiculobullous lesions
Absence of pulses	Livedo reticularis	Urticaria
Bruits	Digital gangrene	Glomerulonephritis
Aortic dilation	Mononeuritis multiplex	Alveolar hemorrhage
	Microaneurysms	Cutaneous extravascular necrotizing granulomas
		Splinter hemorrhages
		Uveitis
		Episcleritis
		Scleritis

the major vessels involved, other issues that contribute to the classification include the following:

- Does the process involve arteries, veins, or both?
- What are the patient's demographic characteristics (age, sex, ethnicity, smoking status)?
- Which organs are involved?
- Is there hypocomplementemia or other evidence of immune complex deposition?
- Is there granulomatous inflammation on tissue biopsy?
- Are antineutrophil cytoplasmic antibodies (ANCA) present?

In addition to the disorders considered to be primary vasculitides, there are also multiple forms of vasculitis that are associated with other known underlying conditions. These "secondary" forms of vasculitis occur in the setting of chronic infections (eg, hepatitis B or C, subacute bacterial endocarditis), connective tissue disorders, inflammatory bowel disease, malignancies, and reactions to medications. Only the major primary forms of vasculitis are discussed here.

Elefante E et al. One year in review 2018: systemic vasculitis. Clin Exp Rheumatol. 2018 Mar–Apr;36 Suppl 111(2):12–32. [PMID: 29799395]
Grau RG. Drug-induced vasculitis: new insights and a changing lineup of suspects. Curr Rheumatol Rep. 2015 Dec;17(12):71. [PMID: 26503355]

POLYMYALGIA RHEUMATICA & GIANT CELL ARTERITIS

ESSENTIALS OF DIAGNOSIS

▶ Age over 50 years.

▶ Markedly elevated ESR and CRP.

▶ **Polymyalgia rheumatica:** pain and stiffness in shoulders and hips lasting for several weeks without other explanation.

▶ **Giant cell arteritis:** headache, jaw claudication, polymyalgia rheumatica, visual abnormalities.

General Considerations

Polymyalgia rheumatica and giant cell arteritis probably represent a spectrum of one disease. Both affect the same population (patients over the age of 50), and the incidence of the disease increases with each decade of life. Both show preference for the same HLA haplotypes, and show similar patterns of cytokines in blood and arteries. Giant cell arteritis is a systemic panarteritis affecting medium-sized and large vessels. Giant cell arteritis is also called temporal arteritis because the temporal artery is frequently involved, as are other extracranial branches of the carotid artery. Polymyalgia rheumatica and giant cell arteritis also frequently coexist. The important differences between the two

conditions are that polymyalgia rheumatica alone does not cause blindness and responds to low-dose (10–20 mg/day orally) prednisone therapy, whereas giant cell arteritis can cause blindness and large artery complications and requires high-dose (40–60 mg/day) prednisone.

Clinical Findings

A. Polymyalgia Rheumatica

Polymyalgia rheumatica is a clinical diagnosis based on pain and stiffness of the shoulder and pelvic girdle areas, frequently in association with fever, malaise, and weight loss. In approximately two-thirds of cases, polymyalgia occurs in the absence of giant cell arteritis. Because of the stiffness and pain in the shoulders, hips, and lower back, patients have trouble combing their hair, putting on a coat, or rising from a chair. In contrast to polymyositis and polyarteritis nodosa, polymyalgia rheumatica does not cause muscular weakness either through primary muscle inflammation or secondary to nerve infarction. A few patients have joint swelling, particularly of the knees, wrists, and sternoclavicular joints.

B. Giant Cell Arteritis

The mean age at onset is approximately 79 years. About 50% of patients with giant cell arteritis also have polymyalgia rheumatica. The classic symptoms suggesting that a patient has arteritis are headache, scalp tenderness, visual symptoms (particularly amaurosis fugax or diplopia), jaw claudication, or throat pain. Of these symptoms, jaw claudication has the highest positive predictive value. The temporal artery is usually normal on physical examination but may be nodular, enlarged, tender, or pulseless. Blindness usually results from the syndrome of anterior ischemic optic neuropathy, caused by occlusive arteritis of the posterior ciliary branch of the ophthalmic artery. The ischemic optic neuropathy of giant cell arteritis may produce no funduscopic findings for the first 24–48 hours after the onset of blindness.

Asymmetry of pulses in the arms, a murmur of aortic regurgitation, or bruits heard near the clavicle resulting from subclavian artery stenoses identify patients in whom giant cell arteritis has affected the aorta or its major branches. Clinically evident large vessel involvement—characterized chiefly by aneurysm of the thoracic aorta or stenosis of the subclavian, vertebral, carotid, and basilar arteries—occurs in approximately 25% of patients with giant cell arteritis, sometimes years after the diagnosis. Subclinical large artery disease is the rule: positron emission tomography scans reveal inflammation in the aorta and its major branches in nearly 85% of untreated patients. Forty percent of patients with giant cell arteritis have nonclassical symptoms at presentation, including large artery involvement causing chiefly aortic regurgitation or arm claudication, respiratory tract problems (most frequently dry cough), mononeuritis multiplex (most frequently with painful paralysis of a shoulder), or fever of unknown origin. Giant cell arteritis accounts for 15% of all cases of fever of unknown origin in patients over the age of 65. The fever can be as high as 40°C and is frequently associated with rigors and sweats. In contrast to patients with infection, patients with giant cell arteritis and fever usually have normal white blood cell counts (before prednisone is started). Thus, in an older patient with fever of unknown origin, marked elevations of acute-phase reactants, and a normal white blood count, giant cell arteritis must be considered even in the absence of specific features such as headache or jaw claudication. In some cases, instead of having the well-known symptom of jaw claudication, patients complain of vague pain affecting other locations, including the tongue, nose, or ears. Indeed, unexplained head or neck pain in an older patient may signal the presence of giant cell arteritis.

C. Laboratory Findings

1. Polymyalgia rheumatica—Anemia and elevated acute-phase reactants (often markedly elevated ESRs, for example) are present in the most cases, but cases of polymyalgia rheumatica occurring with normal acute-phase reactants are well documented.

2. Giant cell arteritis—Nearly 90% of patients with giant cell arteritis have ESRs higher than 50 mm/h. The ESR in this disorder is often more than 100 mm/h, but cases in which the ESR is lower or even normal do occur. In one series, 5% of patients with biopsy-proven giant cell arteritis had ESRs below 40 mm/h. Although the CRP is slightly more sensitive, patients with biopsy-proven giant cell arteritis with normal CRP have also been described. Most patients also have a mild normochromic, normocytic anemia and thrombocytosis. The alkaline phosphatase (liver source) is elevated in 20% of patients with giant cell arteritis.

► Differential Diagnosis

The differential diagnosis of malaise, anemia, and striking acute-phase reactant elevations includes rheumatic diseases (such as rheumatoid arthritis, other systemic vasculitides, plasma cell myeloma, and other malignant disorders) and chronic infections (such as bacterial endocarditis and osteomyelitis).

► Treatment

A. Polymyalgia Rheumatica

Patients with isolated polymyalgia rheumatica (ie, those not having "above the neck" symptoms of headache, jaw claudication, scalp tenderness, or visual symptoms) are treated with prednisone, 10–20 mg/day orally. If the patient does not experience a dramatic improvement within 72 hours, the diagnosis should be revisited. Usually after 2–4 weeks of treatment, slow tapering of the prednisone can be attempted. Most patients require some dose of prednisone for a minimum of approximately 1 year; 6 months is too short in most cases. Disease flares are common (50% or more) as prednisone is tapered. The addition of weekly methotrexate may increase the chance of successfully tapering prednisone in some patients.

B. Giant Cell Arteritis

The urgency of early diagnosis and treatment in giant cell arteritis relates to the prevention of blindness. Once blindness develops, it is usually permanent. Therefore, when a patient has symptoms and findings suggestive of temporal arteritis, therapy with prednisone (60 mg/day orally) should be initiated immediately and a temporal artery biopsy performed promptly thereafter. For patients who seek medical attention for visual loss, intravenous pulse methylprednisolone (eg, 1 g daily for 3 days) has been advocated; unfortunately, few patients recover vision no matter what the initial treatment. Retrospective studies suggest that low-dose aspirin (~81 mg/day orally) may reduce the chance of visual loss or stroke in patients with giant cell arteritis and should be added to prednisone in the initial treatment. Although it is prudent to obtain a temporal artery biopsy as soon as possible after instituting treatment, diagnostic findings of giant cell arteritis may still be present 2 weeks (or even considerably longer) after starting corticosteroids. Typically, a positive biopsy shows inflammatory infiltrate in the media and adventitia with lymphocytes, histiocytes, plasma cells, and giant cells. An adequate biopsy specimen is essential (at least 2 cm in length is ideal), because the disease may be segmental. Unilateral temporal artery biopsies are positive in approximately 80–85% of patients, but bilateral biopsies add incrementally to the yield (10–15% in some studies, less in others). Imaging of the temporal artery with ultrasonography, MRI, or CT angiography can sometimes obviate the need for biopsy. Temporal artery biopsy is abnormal in only 50% of patients with large artery disease (eg, arm claudication and unequal upper extremity blood pressures). In these patients, magnetic resonance angiography or CT angiography will establish the diagnosis by demonstrating long stretches of narrowing of the subclavian and axillary arteries. Prednisone should be continued in a dosage of 60 mg/day orally for about 1 month before tapering. When only the symptoms of polymyalgia rheumatica are present, temporal artery biopsy is not necessary.

After 1 month of high-dose prednisone, almost all patients will have a normal ESR. When tapering and adjusting the dosage of prednisone, the ESR (or CRP) is a useful but not absolute guide to disease activity. A common error is treating the ESR rather than the patient. The ESR often rises slightly as the prednisone is tapered, even as the disease remains quiescent. Because elderly individuals often have baseline ESRs that are above the normal range, mild ESR elevations should not be an occasion for renewed treatment with prednisone in patients who are asymptomatic. Tocilizumab, an inhibitor of the IL-6 receptor, is FDA approved for giant cell arteritis that can reduce the prolonged use of prednisone and its side effects, including weight gain, osteoporosis, diabetes, hypertension, and proximal muscle weakness. Clinical trials demonstrate that patients treated initially with both tocilizumab and prednisone can taper off of prednisone more rapidly and successfully than patients treated with prednisone alone. After 1 year of treatment, tocilizumab achieves corticosteroid-free remission in approximately 50% of patients. Longer follow-up is needed to determine the recommended role of tocilizumab treating giant cell arteritis. Methotrexate has been less promising; it was modestly effective in one double-blind, placebo-controlled treatment trial but ineffective in another. Anti-TNF therapies do not work in giant cell arteritis. Thoracic aortic aneurysms occur 17 times more frequently in patients with giant cell arteritis than in normal individuals and can result in aortic regurgitation, dissection, or rupture. The aneurysms can develop at any time but typically occur 7 years after the diagnosis of giant cell arteritis is made.

Buttgereit F et al. Polymyalgia rheumatica and giant cell arteritis: a systematic review. JAMA. 2016 Jun 14;315(22):2442–58. [PMID: 27299619]

Dejaco C et al. Giant cell arteritis and polymyalgia rheumatica: current challenges and opportunities. Nat Rev Rheumatol. 2017 Oct;13(10):578–92. [PMID: 28905861]

Stone JH et al. Trial of tocilizumab in giant-cell arteritis. N Engl J Med. 2017 Jul 27;377(4):317–28. [PMID: 28745999]

TAKAYASU ARTERITIS

Takayasu arteritis is a granulomatous vasculitis of the aorta and its major branches. Rare in North America but more prevalent in the Far East, it primarily affects women and typically has its onset in early adulthood. Takayasu arteritis can present with nonspecific constitutional symptoms of malaise, fever, and weight loss or with manifestations of vascular inflammation and damage: diminished pulses, unequal blood pressures in the arms, carotidynia (tenderness over the carotid arteries), bruits over carotids and subclavian arteries, retinopathy, limb claudication, and hypertension. There are no specific laboratory abnormalities; the ESR and the CRP level are elevated in most cases. The diagnosis is established by imaging studies, usually MRI, which can detect inflammatory thickening of the walls of affected vessels, or CT angiography, which can provide images of the stenoses, occlusions, and dilations characteristic of arteritis. Corticosteroids (eg, oral prednisone, 1 mg/kg for 1 month, followed by a taper over several months to 10 mg daily) are the mainstays of treatment. The addition of methotrexate, azathioprine, or mycophenolate mofetil to prednisone may be more effective than the prednisone alone. Case series suggest that biologic therapy with either inhibitors of TNF (eg, infliximab) or the IL-6 receptor (tocilizumab) may be effective for patients refractory to prednisone. Takayasu arteritis has a chronic relapsing and remitting course that requires ongoing monitoring and adjustment of therapy.

Comarmond C et al; French Takayasu Network. Long-term outcomes and prognostic factors of complications in Takayasu arteritis: a multicenter study of 318 patients. Circulation. 2017 Sep 19;136(12):1114–22. [PMID: 28701469]

Gudbrandsson B et al. TNF inhibitors appear to inhibit disease progression and improve outcome in Takayasu arteritis; an observational, population-based time trend study. Arthritis Res Ther. 2017 May 18;19(1):99. [PMID: 28521841]

Langford CA et al; Vasculitis Clinical Research Consortium. A randomized, double-blind trial of abatacept (CTLA-4Ig) for the treatment of Takayasu arteritis. Arthritis Rheumatol. 2017 Apr;69(4):846–53. [PMID: 28133931]

Mekinian A et al; French Takayasu Network. Efficacy of biological-targeted treatments in Takayasu arteritis: multicenter, retrospective study of 49 patients. Circulation. 2015 Nov 3; 132(18):1693–700. [PMID: 26354797]

POLYARTERITIS NODOSA

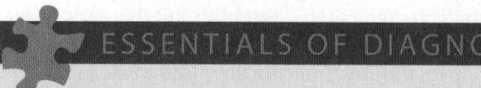

ESSENTIALS OF DIAGNOSIS

► Medium-sized arteries are affected.

► Clinical findings depend on the arteries involved; lungs are spared.

► Common features include fever, abdominal pain, extremity pain, livedo reticularis, mononeuritis multiplex.

► Kidney involvement causes renin-mediated hypertension.

► Anemia and elevated acute-phase reactants (ESR or CRP or both).

► Associated with hepatitis B (10% of cases).

► General Considerations

Polyarteritis nodosa is a necrotizing arteritis of medium-sized vessels that has a predilection for involving the skin, peripheral nerves, mesenteric vessels (including renal arteries), heart, and brain but spares the lungs. Polyarteritis nodosa is relatively rare, with a prevalence of about 30 per 1 million people. Approximately 10% of cases of polyarteritis nodosa are caused by hepatitis B. Most cases of hepatitis B–associated disease occur within 6 months of hepatitis B infection. Mutations in the gene for adenosine deaminase 2 have been identified in early-onset familial polyarteritis.

► Clinical Findings

A. Symptoms and Signs

The clinical onset is usually insidious, with fever, malaise, weight loss, and other symptoms developing over weeks to months. Pain in the extremities is often a prominent early feature caused by arthralgia, myalgia (particularly affecting the calves), or neuropathy. The combination of mononeuritis multiplex (with the most common finding being foot-drop) and features of a systemic illness is one of the earliest specific clues to the presence of an underlying vasculitis. Polyarteritis nodosa is among the forms of vasculitis most commonly associated with vasculitic neuropathy.

In polyarteritis nodosa, the typical skin findings—livedo reticularis, subcutaneous nodules, and skin ulcers—reflect the involvement of deeper, medium-sized blood vessels. Digital gangrene is not an unusual occurrence. The most common cutaneous presentation is lower extremity ulcerations, usually occurring near the malleoli. Involvement of the renal arteries leads to a renin-mediated hypertension (much less characteristic of vasculitides involving smaller blood vessels). For unclear reasons, classic polyarteritis nodosa seldom (if ever) involves the lung, with the occasional exception of the bronchial arteries.

Abdominal pain—particularly diffuse periumbilical pain precipitated by eating—is common but often difficult to attribute to mesenteric vasculitis in the early stages. Nausea and vomiting are common symptoms. Infarction compromises the function of major viscera and may lead to acalculous cholecystitis or appendicitis. Some patients present dramatically with an acute abdomen caused by mesenteric vasculitis and gut perforation or with hypotension resulting from rupture of a microaneurysm in the liver, kidney, or bowel.

Newly acquired hypertension from renin-mediated kidney disease frequently occurs. Subclinical cardiac involvement is common in polyarteritis nodosa, and overt cardiac dysfunction occasionally occurs (eg, myocardial infarction secondary to coronary vasculitis, or myocarditis).

B. Laboratory Findings

Most patients with polyarteritis nodosa have a slight anemia, and leukocytosis is common. Acute-phase reactants are often (but not always) strikingly elevated. A major challenge in making the diagnosis of polyarteritis nodosa, however, is the absence of a disease-specific serologic test (eg, an autoantibody). Patients with classic polyarteritis nodosa are ANCA-negative but may have low titers of rheumatoid factor or antinuclear antibodies, both of which are nonspecific findings. Appropriate tests for active hepatitis B infection (HBsAg, HBeAg, hepatitis B viral load) should be performed. Patients with childhood onset of polyarteritis nodosa should undergo genetic evaluation for mutations in the genes for adenosine deaminase 2.

C. Biopsy and Angiography

The diagnosis of polyarteritis nodosa requires confirmation with either a tissue biopsy or an angiogram. Biopsies of symptomatic sites such as skin (from the edge of an ulcer or the center of a nodule), nerve, or muscle have sensitivities of approximately 70%. The least invasive tests should usually be obtained first, but biopsy of an involved organ is essential. If performed by experienced clinicians, tissue biopsies normally have high benefit-risk ratios because of the importance of establishing the diagnosis. Patients in whom polyarteritis nodosa is suspected—eg, on the basis of mesenteric ischemia or new-onset hypertension occurring in the setting of a systemic illness—may be diagnosed by the angiographic finding of aneurysmal dilations in the renal, mesenteric, or hepatic arteries. Angiography must be performed cautiously in patients with baseline kidney disease.

▶ Treatment

For polyarteritis nodosa, corticosteroids in high doses (up to 60 mg of oral prednisone daily) may control fever and constitutional symptoms and heal vascular lesions. Pulse methylprednisolone (eg, 1 g intravenously daily for 3 days) may be necessary for patients who are critically ill at presentation. The addition of cyclophosphamide lowers the risk of disease-related death and morbidity among patients who have severe disease. Methotrexate or azathioprine are used

to maintain remissions induced by cyclophosphamide. For patients with polyarteritis nodosa associated with hepatitis B, the preferred treatment regimen is a short course of prednisone accompanied by anti-HBV therapy and plasmapheresis (three times a week for up to 6 weeks). Inhibitors of TNF are first-line therapy for the polyarteritis associated with deficiency of adenosine deaminase 2.

▶ Prognosis

Without treatment, the 5-year survival rate in this disorder is poor—on the order of 10%. With appropriate therapy, remissions are possible in many cases and the 5-year survival rate has improved to 60–90%. Poor prognostic factors are chronic kidney disease with serum creatinine greater than 1.6 mg/dL (141 mcmol/L), proteinuria greater than 1 g/day, gastrointestinal ischemia, central nervous system disease, and cardiac involvement. In the absence of any of these five factors, 5-year survival is nearly 90%. Survival at 5 years drops to 75% with one poor prognostic factor present and to about 50% with two or more factors. Substantial morbidity and even death may result from adverse effects of cyclophosphamide and corticosteroids (Table 26–16). Consequently, these therapies require careful monitoring and expert management. In contrast to many other forms of systemic vasculitis, disease relapses in polyarteritis following the successful induction of remission are the exception rather than the rule, occurring in only about 20% of cases.

Hashem H et al. Deficiency of adenosine deaminase 2 (DADA2), an inherited cause of polyarteritis nodosa and a mimic of other systemic rheumatologic disorders. Curr Rheumatol Rep. 2017 Oct 5;19(11):70. [PMID: 28983775]

Puéchal X et al; French Vasculitis Study Group. Adding azathioprine to remission-induction glucocorticoids for eosinophilic granulomatosis with polyangiitis (Churg-Strauss), microscopic polyangiitis, or polyarteritis nodosa without poor prognosis factors: a randomized, controlled trial. Arthritis Rheumatol. 2017 Nov;69(11):2175–86. [PMID: 28678392]

Ozen S. The changing face of polyarteritis nodosa and necrotizing vasculitis. Nat Rev Rheumatol. 2017 Jun;13(6):381–6. [PMID: 28490787]

GRANULOMATOSIS WITH POLYANGIITIS

ESSENTIALS OF DIAGNOSIS

- ▶ Classic triad of upper and lower respiratory tract disease and glomerulonephritis.
- ▶ Suspect if upper respiratory tract symptoms (eg, nasal congestion, sinusitis) are refractory to usual treatment.
- ▶ Kidney disease often rapidly progressive.
- ▶ Venous thromboembolism commonly occurs.
- ▶ ANCAs (90% of patients), usually directed against proteinase-3 (less commonly against myeloperoxidase present in severe, active disease).
- ▶ Tissue biopsy usually necessary for diagnosis.

General Considerations

Granulomatosis with polyangiitis, which has an estimated incidence of approximately 12 cases per million individuals per year, is the prototype of diseases associated with anti-neutrophil cytoplasmic antibodies (ANCA). Other "ANCA-associated vasculitides" include microscopic polyangiitis and eosinophilic granulomatosis with polyangiitis. Granulomatosis with polyangiitis is characterized in its full expression by vasculitis of small arteries, arterioles, and capillaries, necrotizing granulomatous lesions of both upper and lower respiratory tract, glomerulonephritis, and other organ manifestations. Without treatment, generalized disease is invariably fatal, with most patients surviving less than 1 year after diagnosis. It occurs most commonly in the fourth and fifth decades of life and affects men and women with equal frequency.

Clinical Findings

A. Symptoms and Signs

The disorder usually develops over 4–12 months. Upper respiratory tract symptoms develop in 90% of patients and lower respiratory tract symptoms develop in 60% of patients; some patients may have both upper and lower respiratory tract symptoms. Upper respiratory tract symptoms can include nasal congestion, sinusitis, otitis media, mastoiditis, inflammation of the gums, or stridor due to subglottic stenosis. Since many of these symptoms are common, the underlying disease is not often suspected until the patient develops systemic symptoms or the original problem is refractory to treatment. The lungs are affected initially in 40% and eventually in 80%, with symptoms including cough, dyspnea, and hemoptysis. Other early symptoms can include a migratory oligoarthritis with a predilection for large joints; a variety of symptoms related to ocular disease (unilateral proptosis from orbital pseudotumor; red eye from scleritis [Figure 20–6], episcleritis, anterior uveitis, or peripheral ulcerative keratitis); purpura or other skin lesions; and dysesthesia due to neuropathy. Renal involvement, which develops in three-fourths of the cases, may be subclinical until kidney disease is advanced. Fever, malaise, and weight loss are common.

Physical examination can be remarkable for congestion, crusting, ulceration, bleeding, and even perforation of the nasal septum. Destruction of the nasal cartilage with "saddle nose" deformity occurs late. Otitis media, proptosis, scleritis, episcleritis, and conjunctivitis are other common findings. Newly acquired hypertension, a frequent feature of polyarteritis nodosa, is rare in granulomatosis with polyangiitis. Venous thrombotic events (eg, deep venous thrombosis and pulmonary embolism) are a common occurrence in granulomatosis with polyangiitis, at least in part because of the tendency of the disease to involve veins as well as arteries. Although limited forms of granulomatosis with polyangiitis have been described in which the kidney is spared initially, kidney disease will develop in the majority of untreated patients.

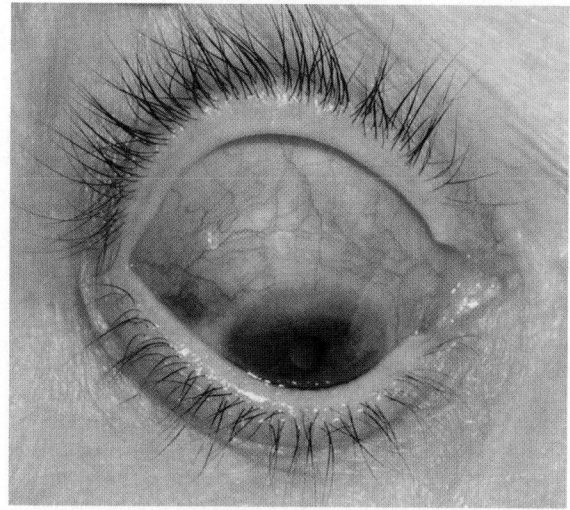

▲ **Figure 20–6.** Scleritis in a patient with granulomatosis with polyangiitis. (Used, with permission, from Everett Allen, MD, in Usatine RP, Smith MA, Mayeaux EJ Jr, Chumley H. *The Color Atlas of Family Medicine*, 2nd ed. McGraw-Hill, 2013.)

B. Laboratory Findings

1. Serum tests and urinalysis—Most patients have slight anemia, mild leukocytosis, and elevated acute-phase reactants. If there is kidney involvement, there is proteinuria and the urinary sediment contains red cells, with or without white cells, and often has red cell casts.

Serum tests for ANCA help in the diagnosis of granulomatosis with polyangiitis and related forms of vasculitis (Table 20–7). Several different types of ANCA are recognized, but the two subtypes relevant to systemic vasculitis are those directed against proteinase-3 (PR3) and myeloperoxidase (MPO). Antibodies to these two antigens are termed "PR3-ANCA" and "MPO-ANCA," respectively. The cytoplasmic pattern of immunofluorescence (c-ANCA) caused by PR3-ANCA has a high specificity (more than 90%) for either granulomatosis with polyangiitis or a closely related disease, microscopic polyangiitis (or, less commonly, eosinophilic granulomatosis with polyangiitis). In the setting of active disease, particularly cases in which the disease is severe and generalized to multiple organ systems, the sensitivity of PR3-ANCA is greater than 95%. A substantial percentage of patients with "limited" granulomatosis with polyangiitis—disease that does not pose an immediate threat to life and is often confined to the respiratory tract—are ANCA-negative. Furthermore, ANCA levels correlate erratically with disease activity, and changes in titer should not dictate changes in therapy in the absence of supporting clinical data. The perinuclear (p-ANCA) pattern, caused by MPO-ANCA, is more likely to occur in microscopic polyangiitis or eosinophilic granulomatosis with polyangiitis but may also be found in granulomatosis with polyangiitis. Approximately 10–25% of patients with classic granulomatosis with polyangiitis have MPO-ANCA. All positive immunofluorescence assays for ANCA should be confirmed by enzyme immunoassays for the specific autoantibodies directed against PR3 or MPO.

2. Histologic findings—Although ANCA testing may be helpful when used properly, there remains the need in most cases for confirmation of the diagnosis by tissue biopsy. Histologic features of granulomatosis with polyangiitis include vasculitis, granulomatous inflammation, geographic necrosis, and acute and chronic inflammation. The full range of pathologic changes is usually evident only on thoracoscopic lung biopsy; granulomas, observed only rarely in kidney biopsy specimens, are found much more commonly on lung biopsy specimens. Nasal biopsies often do not show vasculitis but may show chronic inflammation and other changes which, interpreted by an experienced pathologist, can serve as convincing evidence of the diagnosis. Kidney biopsy discloses a segmental necrotizing glomerulonephritis with multiple crescents; this is characteristic but not diagnostic. Pathologists characterize the kidney lesion of granulomatosis with polyangiitis (and other forms of "ANCA-associated vasculitis") as a pauci-immune glomerulonephritis because of the relative absence (compared with immune complex–mediated disorders) of IgG, IgM, IgA, and complement proteins within glomeruli.

C. Imaging

Chest CT is more sensitive than chest radiography; lesions include infiltrates, nodules, masses, and cavities. Pleural effusions are uncommon. Often the radiographs prompt concern about lung cancer. Hilar adenopathy large enough to be evident on chest film is unusual in granulomatosis with polyangiitis; if present, sarcoidosis, tumor, or infection is more likely. Other common radiographic abnormalities include extensive sinusitis and even bony sinus erosions.

▶ Differential Diagnosis

In most patients with granulomatosis with polyangiitis, refractory sinusitis or otitis media is initially suspected. When upper respiratory tract inflammation persists and is accompanied by additional systemic inflammatory signs (eg, red eye from scleritis, joint pain, and swelling), the diagnosis of granulomatosis with polyangiitis should be considered. Initial complaints of joint pain can lead to a misdiagnosis of rheumatoid arthritis. Arriving at the correct diagnosis is aided by awareness that rheumatoid arthritis typically involves small joints of the hand, whereas granulomatosis with polyangiitis favors large joints, such as the hip, knee, elbow, and shoulder. Lung cancer may be the first diagnostic consideration for some middle-aged patients in whom cough, hemoptysis, and lung masses are presenting symptoms and signs; typically, evidence of glomerulonephritis, a positive ANCA or, ultimately, the lung biopsy findings will point to the proper diagnosis. Granulomatosis with polyangiitis shares with SLE, anti–glomerular basement membrane disease, and microscopic polyangiitis the ability to cause an acute pulmonary-renal syndrome. Approximately 10–25% of patients with classic granulomatosis with polyangiitis have MPO-ANCA. Owing to involvement of the same types of blood vessels, similar patterns of organ involvement, and the possibility of failing to identify granulomatous pathology on tissue biopsies because of sampling error, granulomatosis with polyangiitis is often difficult to differentiate from microscopic polyangiitis. The crucial distinctions between the two disorders are the tendencies for granulomatosis with polyangiitis to involve the upper respiratory tract (including the ears) and to cause granulomatous inflammation. Cocaine use can cause destruction of midline tissues—the nose and palate—that mimics granulomatosis with polyangiitis. Indeed, distinguishing between the two conditions can be challenging because patients with cocaine-mediated midline destructive disease frequently have positive tests for PR-3-ANCA and lesional biopsies that demonstrate vasculitis. In contrast to granulomatosis with polyangiitis, cocaine-mediated midline destructive disease does not cause pulmonary or renal disease. IgG$_4$-related disease may mimic some of the manifestations of granulomatosis with polyangiitis.

▶ Treatment

Early treatment is crucial in preventing the devastating end-organ complications of this disease, and often in preserving life. While granulomatosis with polyangiitis may involve the sinuses or lung for months, once proteinuria or hematuria develops, progression to advanced chronic kidney disease can be rapid (over several weeks). Current practice divides treatment into two phases: induction of remission and maintenance of remission. Choice of induction therapy is dictated by whether the patient has mild disease (ie, no significant kidney dysfunction or immediately life-threatening disease) or severe disease (ie, life- or organ-threatening disease such as rapidly progressive glomerulonephritis or pulmonary hemorrhage).

A. Induction of Remission

For patients with severe disease, the treatment options for inducing remission are corticosteroids and either rituximab or cyclophosphamide.

1. Rituximab plus prednisone—Rituximab, a B-cell depleting antibody, is FDA approved in combination with corticosteroids (prednisone 1 mg/kg orally daily) for the treatment of granulomatosis with polyangiitis and microscopic polyangiitis. Studies demonstrate that rituximab is not less effective than cyclophosphamide for remission induction in these conditions. Indeed, post-hoc analysis of one clinical trial demonstrated that rituximab is more effective than cyclophosphamide for treating relapses of granulomatosis with polyangiitis and microscopic polyangiitis.

2. Cyclophosphamide and prednisone—Remissions can be induced in more than 90% of patients treated with prednisone (1 mg/kg daily) plus cyclophosphamide (2 mg/kg/day orally with adjustments required for acute or chronic kidney disease and patients over age 70). Cyclophosphamide is best given daily by mouth; intermittent high-dose intravenous cyclophosphamide is less effective. To minimize toxicity, patients are treated with cyclophosphamide for only 3–6 months; once remission is achieved, the patient is switched to a maintenance regimen more likely to be tolerated well.

Both rituximab and cyclophosphamide increase the risk of developing life-threatening opportunistic infections (including progressive multifocal leukoencephalopathy [PML]). *Whenever cyclophosphamide or rituximab is used,* Pneumocystis jirovecii *prophylaxis with single-strength oral trimethoprim-sulfamethoxazole daily is essential.*

B. Maintenance of Remission

There are three options for maintaining remission in patients with normal or near normal kidney function after rituximab or cyclophosphamide induction: azathioprine (up to 2 mg/kg/day orally), methotrexate (20–25 mg/wk administered either orally or intramuscularly), or rituximab (500 mg administered intravenously when remission is achieved, repeated in 14 days, then repeated every 6 months three more times). Methotrexate should not be used in patients with kidney dysfunction. One randomized, controlled trial comparing rituximab and azathioprine for maintenance of remission showed that the risk of relapse over 28 months was 5% with rituximab and 29% with azathioprine. Before the institution of azathioprine, patients should be tested (through a commercially available blood test) for deficiencies in the level of thiopurine methyltransferase, an enzyme essential to the metabolism of azathioprine.

Because of its superior side-effect profile, methotrexate is viewed as an appropriate substitute for cyclophosphamide or rituximab for initial and maintenance treatment in patients who have mild disease and normal kidney function.

Maritati F et al. Methotrexate versus cyclophosphamide for remission maintenance in ANCA-associated vasculitis: a randomised trial. PLoS One. 2017 Oct 10;12(10):e0185880. [PMID: 29016646]

Puéchal X et al; French Vasculitis Study Group. Long-term outcomes among participants in the wegent trial of remission-maintenance therapy for granulomatosis with polyangiitis (Wegener's) or microscopic polyangiitis. Arthritis Rheumatol. 2016 Mar;68(3):690–701. [PMID: 26473755]

Singer O et al. Update on maintenance therapy for granulomatosis with polyangiitis and microscopic polyangiitis. Curr Opin Rheumatol. 2017 May;29(3):248–53. [PMID: 28306595]

Unizony S et al; RAVE-ITN Research Group. Clinical outcomes of treatment of anti-neutrophil cytoplasmic antibody (ANCA)-associated vasculitis based on ANCA type. Ann Rheum Dis. 2016 Jun;75(6):1166–9. [PMID: 26621483]

MICROSCOPIC POLYANGIITIS

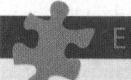

ESSENTIALS OF DIAGNOSIS

▶ Necrotizing vasculitis of small- and medium-sized arteries and veins.

▶ Most common cause of pulmonary-renal syndrome: diffuse alveolar hemorrhage and glomerulonephritis.

▶ ANCA in 75% of cases.

▶ General Considerations

Microscopic polyangiitis is a pauci-immune nongranulomatous necrotizing vasculitis that (1) affects small blood vessels (capillaries, venules, or arterioles), (2) often causes glomerulonephritis and pulmonary capillaritis, and (3) is often associated with ANCA on immunofluorescence testing (directed against MPO, a constituent of neutrophil granules). Because microscopic polyangiitis may involve medium-sized as well as small blood vessels and because it tends to affect capillaries within the lungs and kidneys, its spectrum overlaps those of both polyarteritis nodosa and granulomatosis with polyangiitis.

In rare instances, medications, particularly propylthiouracil, hydralazine, allopurinol, penicillamine, minocycline, and sulfasalazine, induce a systemic vasculitis associated with high titers of p-ANCA and features of microscopic polyangiitis.

▶ Clinical Findings

A. Symptoms and Signs

A wide variety of findings suggesting vasculitis of small blood vessels may develop in microscopic polyangiitis. These include "palpable" (or "raised") purpura and other signs of cutaneous vasculitis (ulcers, splinter hemorrhages, vesiculobullous lesions).

Microscopic polyangiitis is the most common cause of pulmonary-renal syndromes, being several times more common than anti–glomerular basement membrane disease. Interstitial lung fibrosis that mimics usual interstitial pneumonitis is the presenting condition. Pulmonary hemorrhage may occur. The pathologic findings in the lung are typically those of capillaritis.

Vasculitic neuropathy (mononeuritis multiplex) is also common in microscopic polyangiitis.

B. Laboratory Findings

Three-fourths of patients with microscopic polyangiitis are ANCA-positive, usually anti-myeloperoxidase antibodies (MPO-ANCA) that cause a p-ANCA pattern on immunofluorescence testing. ANCA directed against proteinase-3 (PR3-ANCA) can also be observed.

Elevated acute-phase reactants are also typical of active disease. Microscopic hematuria, proteinuria, and red blood cell casts in the urine may occur. The kidney lesion is a segmental, necrotizing glomerulonephritis, often with localized intravascular coagulation and the observation of intraglomerular thrombi upon renal biopsy.

▶ Differential Diagnosis

Distinguishing this disease from granulomatosis with polyangiitis may be challenging in some cases. Microscopic polyangiitis is not associated with the chronic destructive upper respiratory tract disease often found in granulomatosis with polyangiitis. Moreover, as noted, a critical difference between the two diseases is the absence of granulomatous inflammation in microscopic polyangiitis.

Because their treatments may differ, microscopic polyangiitis must also be differentiated from polyarteritis nodosa.

Treatment

Microscopic polyangiitis is usually treated in the same way as granulomatosis with polyangiitis: patients with severe disease, typically involving pulmonary hemorrhage and glomerulonephritis, require urgent induction treatment with corticosteroids and either cyclophosphamide or rituximab. If cyclophosphamide is chosen, it may be administered either in an oral daily regimen or via intermittent (usually monthly) intravenous pulses; following induction of remission, cyclophosphamide may be replaced with azathioprine, rituximab, or methotrexate (provided the patient has normal kidney function). In cases of drug-induced MPO-ANCA–associated vasculitis, the offending medication should be discontinued; significant organ involvement (eg, pulmonary hemorrhage, glomerulonephritis) requires immunosuppressive therapy.

Prognosis

The key to effecting good outcomes is early diagnosis. Compared with patients who have granulomatosis with polyangiitis, those who have microscopic polyangiitis are more likely to have significant fibrosis on renal biopsy because of later diagnosis. The likelihood of disease recurrence following remission in microscopic polyangiitis is about 33%.

Bossuyt X et al. Position paper: Revised 2017 international consensus on testing of ANCAs in granulomatosis with polyangiitis and microscopic polyangiitis. Nat Rev Rheumatol. 2017 Nov;13(11):683–92. [PMID: 28905856]

BuBui VL et al. Clinical significance of a positive antineutrophil cytoplasmic antibody (ANCA) test. JAMA. 2016 Sep 6;316 (9):984–5. [PMID: 27599333]

Imboden JB. Involvement of the peripheral nervous system in polyarteritis nodosa and antineutrophil cytoplasmic antibodies-associated vasculitis. Rheum Dis Clin North Am. 2017 Nov; 43(4):633–9. [PMID: 29061248]

Maritati F et al. Methotrexate versus cyclophosphamide for remission maintenance in ANCA-associated vasculitis: a randomised trial. PLoS One. 2017 Oct 10;12(10):e0185880. [PMID: 29016646]

Wechsler ME et al; EGPA Mepolizumab Study Team. Mepolizumab or placebo for eosinophilic granulomatosis with polyangiitis. N Engl J Med. 2017 May 18;376(20):1921–32. [PMID: 28514601]

LEVAMISOLE-ASSOCIATED PURPURA

Exposure to levamisole, a prevalent adulterant of illicit cocaine in North America, can induce a distinctive clinical syndrome of retiform purpura and cutaneous necrosis affecting the extremities, ears, and skin overlying the zygomatic arch. Biopsies reveal widespread thrombosis of small cutaneous vessels with varying degrees of vasculitis. The syndrome is associated with the lupus anticoagulant, IgM antibodies to cardiolipin, and very high titers of p-ANCAs (due to autoantibodies to elastase, lactoferrin, cathepsin-G, and other neutrophil components rather than to myeloperoxidase alone). There is no consensus on treatment of levamisole-induced purpura, but early lesions can resolve with abstinence. Use of levamisole-adulterated cocaine also has been linked to neutropenia, agranulocytosis, and pauci-immune glomerulonephritis.

Cascio MJ et al. Cocaine/levamisole-associated autoimmune syndrome: a disease of neutrophil-mediated autoimmunity. Curr Opin Hematol. 2018 Jan;25(1):29–36. [PMID: 29211697]

CRYOGLOBULINEMIA

Cryoglobulinemia can be associated with an immune-complex mediated, small-vessel vasculitis. Chronic infection with hepatitis C is the most common underlying condition; cryoglobulinemic vasculitis also can occur with other chronic infections (such as subacute bacterial endocarditis, osteomyelitis, HIV, and hepatitis B), with connective tissues diseases (especially Sjögren syndrome), and with lympho-proliferative disorders. The cryoglobulins associated with vasculitis are cold-precipitable immune complexes consisting of rheumatoid factor and IgG (rheumatoid factor is an autoantibody to the constant region of IgG). The rheumatoid factor component can be monoclonal (type II cryoglobulins) or polyclonal (type III cryoglobulins). (Type I cryoglobulins are cryoprecipitable monoclonal proteins that lack rheumatoid factor activity; these cause cold-induced hyperviscosity syndromes, not vasculitis, and are associated with B-cell lymphoproliferative diseases.)

Clinical Findings

Cryoglobulinemic vasculitis typically manifests as recurrent palpable purpura (predominantly on the lower extremities) and peripheral neuropathy. A proliferative glomerulonephritis can develop and can manifest as rapidly progressive glomerulonephritis. Abnormal liver biochemical tests, abdominal pain, digital gangrene, and pulmonary disease may also occur. The diagnosis is based on a compatible clinical picture and a positive serum test for cryoglobulins. The presence of a disproportionately low C4 level can be a diagnostic clue to the presence of cryoglobulinemia.

Treatment

Antiviral regimens that do not include interferon are first-line therapy for hepatitis C–associated cryoglobulinemic vasculitis that is neither life- nor organ-threatening. Patients with severe cryoglobulinemic vasculitis (eg, extensive digital gangrene, extensive neuropathy, and rapidly progressive glomerulonephritis) and hepatitis C should receive immunosuppressive therapy with corticosteroids and either rituximab or cyclophosphamide as well as interferon-free antiviral therapy; plasma exchange may provide additional benefit in selected cases. Relapse of vasculitis with cryoglobulinemia following clearing of hepatitis C infection has been reported in a small percentage of patients.

Bonacci MB et al. Long-term outcomes of patients with HCV-associated cryoglobulinemic vasculitis after virologic cure. Gastroenterology. 2018 Aug;155(2):311–5. [PMID: 29705529]

Desbois AC et al. Cryoglobulinemia vasculitis: how to handle. Curr Opin Rheumatol. 2017 Jul;29(4):343–7. [PMID: 28368978]

HENOCH-SCHÖNLEIN PURPURA

Henoch-Schönlein purpura, the most common systemic vasculitis in children, occurs in adults as well. Typical features are palpable purpura, arthritis, and hematuria. Abdominal pain occurs less frequently in adults than in children. Pathologic features include leukocytoclastic vasculitis with IgA deposition. The cause is not known.

The purpuric skin lesions are typically located on the lower extremities but may also be seen on the hands, arms, trunk, and buttocks. Joint symptoms are present in the majority of patients, the knees and ankles being most commonly involved. Abdominal pain secondary to vasculitis of the intestinal tract is often associated with gastrointestinal bleeding. Hematuria signals the presence of a renal lesion that is usually reversible, although it occasionally may progress to chronic kidney disease. Children tend to have more frequent and more serious gastrointestinal vasculitis, whereas adults more often suffer from chronic kidney disease. Biopsy of the kidney reveals segmental glomerulonephritis with crescents and mesangial deposition of IgA.

Chronic courses with persistent or intermittent skin disease are more likely to occur in adults than in children. The value of corticosteroids has been controversial. In children, prednisone (1–2 mg/kg/day orally) does not decrease the frequency of proteinuria 1 year after onset of disease. Severe disease is often treated with aggressive immunosuppressive agents, such as mycophenolate mofetil, but there is no consensus as to the efficacy of this approach or the optimal therapeutic regimen.

Audemard-Verger A et al; French Vasculitis Study Group. Characteristics and management of IgA vasculitis (Henoch-Schönlein) in adults: data from 260 patients included in a French multicenter retrospective survey. Arthritis Rheumatol. 2017 Sep;69(9):1862–70. [PMID: 28605168]

Heineke MH et al. New insights in the pathogenesis of immunoglobulin A vasculitis (Henoch-Schönlein purpura). Autoimmun Rev. 2017 Dec;16(12):1246–53. [PMID: 29037908]

Hong S et al. Late-onset IgA vasculitis in adult patients exhibits distinct clinical characteristics and outcomes. Clin Exp Rheumatol. 2016 May–Jun;34(3 Suppl 97):S77–83. [PMID: 26842218]

Milani GP et al. Prevalence and characteristics of nonblanching, palpable skin lesions with a linear pattern in children with Henoch-Schönlein syndrome. JAMA Dermatol. 2017 Nov 1; 153(11):1170–3. [PMID: 28678983]

RELAPSING POLYCHONDRITIS

This disease is characterized by inflammatory destructive lesions of cartilaginous structures, principally the ears, nose, trachea, and larynx. Nearly 40% of cases are associated with another disease, especially either other immunologic disorders (such as SLE, rheumatoid arthritis, or Hashimoto thyroiditis) or cancers (such as plasma cell myeloma) or hematologic disorders (such as myelodysplastic syndrome). The disease, which is usually episodic, affects males and females equally. The cartilage is painful, swollen, and tender during an attack and subsequently becomes atrophic, resulting in permanent deformity. Biopsy of the involved cartilage shows inflammation and chondrolysis.

Laryngotracheal and bronchial chondritis can lead to life-threatening airway narrowing and collapse. Noncartilaginous manifestations of the disease include fever, episcleritis, uveitis, deafness, aortic regurgitation, and rarely glomerulonephritis. In 85% of patients, a migratory, asymmetric, and seronegative arthropathy occurs, affecting both large and small joints and the costochondral junctions. Diagnosing this uncommon disease is especially difficult since the signs of cartilage inflammation (such as red ears or nasal pain) may be more subtle than the fever, arthritis, rash, or other systemic manifestations.

Prednisone, 0.5–1 mg/kg/day orally, is often effective. Dapsone (100–200 mg/day orally) or methotrexate (7.5–20 mg orally per week) may also have efficacy, sparing the need for long-term high-dose corticosteroid treatment. Involvement of the tracheobronchial tree may respond to inhibitors of TNF.

Kingdon J et al. Relapsing polychondritis: a clinical review for rheumatologists. Rheumatology (Oxford). 2018 Sep 1;57(9): 1525–32. [PMID: 29126262]

BEHÇET SYNDROME

ESSENTIALS OF DIAGNOSIS

▶ Recurrent, painful oral and genital aphthous ulcers.

▶ Erythema nodosum–like lesions; follicular rash; and the pathergy phenomenon.

▶ Anterior or posterior uveitis. Posterior uveitis may be asymptomatic until significant damage to the retina has occurred.

▶ Neurologic lesions can mimic multiple sclerosis.

General Considerations

Named after the Turkish dermatologist who first described it, Behçet disease is of unknown cause and most commonly occurs in persons of Asian, Turkish, or Middle Eastern background. The protean manifestations are believed to result from vasculitis that may involve all types of blood vessels: small, medium, and large, on both the arterial and venous side of the circulation.

Clinical Findings

A. Symptoms and Signs

The hallmark of Behçet disease is painful aphthous ulcerations in the mouth. These lesions, which usually are multiple, may be found on the tongue, gums, and inner surfaces of the oral cavity. Genital lesions, similar in appearance, are also common but do not occur in all patients. Other cutaneous lesions of Behçet disease include tender, erythematous, papular lesions that resemble erythema nodosum. (On biopsy, however, many of these lesions are shown to be secondary to vasculitis rather than septal panniculitis.) These erythema nodosum–like lesions have a tendency to ulcerate, a major difference between the lesions of Behçet disease and the erythema nodosum seen in cases of sarcoidosis and inflammatory bowel disease. An erythematous follicular rash that occurs frequently on the upper extremities may be a subtle feature of the disease. The **pathergy phenomenon** is frequently underappreciated (unless the patient is asked); in this phenomenon, sterile pustules develop at sites where needles have been inserted into the skin (eg, for phlebotomy) in some patients.

A nonerosive arthritis occurs in about two-thirds of patients, most commonly affecting the knees and ankles. Eye involvement may be one of the most devastating complications of Behçet disease. Posterior uveitis, in essence a retinal venulitis, may lead to the insidious destruction of large areas of the retina before the patient becomes aware of visual problems. Anterior uveitis, associated with the triad of photophobia, blurred vision, and a red eye, is intensely symptomatic. This complication may lead to a hypopyon, the accumulation of pus in the anterior chamber. If not treated properly with mydriatic agents to dilate the pupil and corticosteroid eyedrops to diminish inflammation, the anterior uveitis may lead to synechial formation between the iris and lens, resulting in permanent pupillary distortion.

Central nervous system involvement is another cause of major potential morbidity. The central nervous system lesions may mimic multiple sclerosis radiologically. Findings include sterile meningitis (recurrent meningeal headaches associated with a lymphocytic pleocytosis), cranial nerve palsies, seizures, encephalitis, mental disturbances, and spinal cord lesions. Aphthous ulcerations of the ileum and cecum and other forms of gastrointestinal involvement develop in approximately a quarter of patients. Large vessel vasculitis can lead to pulmonary artery aneurysms and life-threatening pulmonary hemorrhage. Finally, patients have a hypercoagulable tendency that may lead to complicated venous thrombotic events, particularly multiple deep venous thrombosis, pulmonary emboli, cerebral sinus thrombosis, and other problems associated with clotting.

The clinical course may be chronic but is often characterized by remissions and exacerbations.

B. Laboratory Findings

There are no pathognomonic laboratory features of Behçet disease. Although acute-phase reactants are often elevated, there is no autoantibody or other assay that is distinctive. No markers of hypercoagulability specific to Behçet have been identified.

▶ Treatment

Both colchicine (0.6 mg once to three times daily orally) and thalidomide (100 mg/day orally) help ameliorate the mucocutaneous findings. Apremilast, a selective phosphodiesterase-4 inhibitor, is effective for the treatment of the oral ulcers. Corticosteroids (1 mg/kg/day of oral prednisone) are a mainstay of initial therapy for severe disease

manifestations. Azathioprine (2 mg/kg/day orally) may be an effective steroid-sparing agent. Infliximab, cyclosporine, or cyclophosphamide is indicated for severe ocular and central nervous system complications of Behçet disease.

Bulur I et al. Behçet disease: new aspects. Clin Dermatol. 2017 Sep–Oct;35(5):421–34. [PMID: 28916023]
Greco A et al. Behçet's disease: new insights into pathophysiology, clinical features and treatment options. Autoimmun Rev. 2018 Jun;17(6):567–75. [PMID: 29631062]
Hatemi I et al. Gastrointestinal involvement in Behçet Disease. Rheum Dis Clin North Am. 2018 Feb;44(1):45–64. [PMID: 29149927]

PRIMARY ANGIITIS OF THE CENTRAL NERVOUS SYSTEM

Primary angiitis of the central nervous system is a syndrome with several possible causes that produces small- and medium-sized vasculitis limited to the brain and spinal cord. Biopsy-proved cases have predominated in men who have a history of weeks to months of headaches, encephalopathy, and multifocal strokes. Systemic symptoms and signs are absent, and routine laboratory tests, including ESR and CRP, are usually normal. MRI of the brain is almost always abnormal, and the spinal fluid often reveals a mild lymphocytosis and a modest increase in protein level. Angiograms classically reveal a "string of beads" pattern produced by alternating segments of arterial narrowing and dilation. However, neither the MRI nor the angiogram appearance is specific for vasculitis. Indeed, in one study, none of the patients who had biopsy-proved central nervous system vasculitis had an angiogram showing "the string of beads," and none of the patients with the classic angiographic findings had a positive brain biopsy for vasculitis. Review of many studies suggests that the sensitivity of angiography varies greatly (from 40% to 90%) and the specificity is only approximately 30%. Many conditions, including vasospasm, can produce the same angiographic pattern as vasculitis. Definitive diagnosis requires a compatible clinical picture; exclusion of infection (including subacute bacterial endocarditis), neoplasm (especially intravascular lymphoma), or metabolic disorder or drug exposure (eg, cocaine) that can mimic primary angiitis of the central nervous system; and a positive brain biopsy. In contrast to biopsy-proved cases, patients with angiographically defined central nervous system vasculopathy are chiefly women who have had an abrupt onset of headaches and stroke (often in the absence of encephalopathy) with normal spinal fluid findings. Many patients who fit this clinical profile may have reversible cerebral vasoconstriction rather than true vasculitis. Such cases may best be treated with calcium channel blockers (such as nimodipine or verapamil) and possibly a short course of corticosteroids. Biopsy-proved cases usually improve with prednisone therapy and often require cyclophosphamide. Treatment response correlates with the size of arteries involved: vasculitis of small cortical and leptomeningeal vessels is associated with a better response and outcome than vasculitis of larger arteries. Cases of central nervous system vasculitis associated with cerebral amyloid angiopathy often respond well to corticosteroids, albeit the long-term natural history remains poorly defined.

Mandal J et al. Primary angiitis of the central nervous system. Rheum Dis Clin North Am. 2017 Nov;43(4):503–18. [PMID: 29061238]

Salvarani C et al. Management of primary and secondary central nervous system vasculitis. Curr Opin Rheumatol. 2016 Jan; 28(1):21–8. [PMID: 26599380]

Schuster S et al. Subtypes of primary angiitis of the CNS identified by MRI patterns reflect the size of affected vessels. J Neurol Neurosurg Psychiatry. 2017 Sep;88(9):749–55. [PMID: 28705900]

LIVEDO RETICULARIS & LIVEDO RACEMOSA

Livedo reticularis produces a mottled, purplish discoloration of the skin with reticulated cyanotic areas surrounding paler central cores. This distinctive "fishnet" pattern is caused by spasm or obstruction of perpendicular arterioles, combined with pooling of blood in surrounding venous plexuses. Idiopathic livedo reticularis is a benign condition that worsens with cold exposure, improves with warming, and primarily affects the extremities. Apart from cosmetic concerns, it is usually asymptomatic. Systemic symptoms or the development of cutaneous ulcerations point to the presence of an underlying disease.

Secondary livedo reticularis, now more properly known as livedo racemosa, occurs in association with diseases that cause vascular obstruction or inflammation. Livedo racemosa resembles idiopathic livedo reticularis but has a wider distribution (often found on trunk and buttocks as well as extremities) and its lesions are more irregular, broken, and circular. Of particular importance is the link with antiphospholipid antibody syndrome. Livedo racemosa is the presenting manifestation of 25% of patients with antiphospholipid antibody syndrome and is strongly associated with the subgroup that has arterial thromboses, including those with Sneddon syndrome (livedo reticularis and cerebrovascular events). Other underlying causes of livedo racemosa include the vasculitides (particularly polyarteritis nodosa), cholesterol emboli syndrome, thrombocythemia, cryoglobulinemia, cold agglutinin disease, primary hyperoxaluria (due to vascular deposits of calcium oxalate), and disseminated intravascular coagulation.

Franco Marques G et al. The management of livedoid vasculopathy focused on direct oral anticoagulants (DOACs): four case reports successfully treated with rivaroxaban. Int J Dermatol. 2018 Jun;57(6):732–41. [PMID: 29663354]

Sajjan VV et al. Livedo reticularis: a review of the literature. Indian Dermatol Online J. 2015 Sep–Oct;6(5):315–21. [PMID: 26500860]

SERONEGATIVE SPONDYLOARTHROPATHIES

The seronegative spondyloarthropathies are ankylosing spondylitis, psoriatic arthritis, reactive arthritis, the arthritis associated with inflammatory bowel disease, and undifferentiated spondyloarthropathy. These disorders are noted for male predominance, onset usually before age 40, inflammatory arthritis of the spine and sacroiliac joints, asymmetric oligoarthritis of large peripheral joints, enthesopathy (inflammation of where ligaments, tendons, and joint capsule insert into bone), uveitis in a significant minority, the absence of autoantibodies in the serum, and a striking association with HLA-B27. HLA-B27 is positive in up to 90% of patients with ankylosing spondylitis and 75% with reactive arthritis. HLA-B27 also occurs in 50% of the psoriatic and inflammatory bowel disease patients who have sacroiliitis. Patients with only peripheral arthritis in these latter two syndromes do not show an increase in HLA-B27.

ANKYLOSING SPONDYLITIS

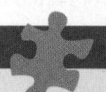

ESSENTIALS OF DIAGNOSIS

► Chronic low backache in young adults, generally worst in the morning.

► Progressive limitation of back motion and of chest expansion.

► Transient (50%) or persistent (25%) peripheral arthritis.

► Anterior uveitis in 20–25%.

► Diagnostic radiographic changes in sacroiliac joints.

► Negative serologic tests for rheumatoid factor and anti-CCP antibodies.

► HLA-B27 testing is most helpful when there is an intermediate probability of disease.

► General Considerations

Ankylosing spondylitis is a chronic inflammatory disease of the joints of the axial skeleton, manifested clinically by pain and progressive stiffening of the spine. The age at onset is usually in the late teens or early 20s. The incidence is greater in males than in females, and symptoms are more prominent in men, with ascending involvement of the spine more likely to occur.

► Clinical Findings

A. Symptoms and Signs

The onset is usually gradual, with intermittent bouts of back pain that may radiate into the buttocks. The back pain is worse in the morning and usually associated with stiffness that lasts hours. The pain and stiffness improve with activity, in contrast to back pain due to mechanical causes and degenerative disease, which improves with rest and worsens with activity. As the disease advances, symptoms progress in a cephalad direction, and back motion becomes limited, with the normal lumbar curve flattened and the thoracic curvature exaggerated. Chest expansion is often limited as a consequence of costovertebral joint involvement. In advanced cases, the entire spine becomes fused, allowing no motion in any direction. Transient acute arthritis of the peripheral joints occurs in about 50% of cases, and permanent changes in the peripheral joints—most commonly the hips, shoulders, and knees—are seen in about 25%. Enthesopathy, a hallmark of the spondyloarthropathies, can manifest as swelling of the Achilles tendon at its insertion, plantar fasciitis (producing heel pain), or "sausage" swelling of a finger or toe (less common in ankylosing spondylitis than in psoriatic arthritis).

Anterior uveitis is associated in as many as 25% of cases and may be a presenting feature. Spondylitic heart disease, characterized chiefly by atrioventricular conduction defects and aortic regurgitation occurs in 3–5% of patients with longstanding severe disease. Constitutional symptoms similar to those of rheumatoid arthritis are absent in most patients.

B. Laboratory Findings

The ESR is elevated in 85% of cases, but serologic tests for rheumatoid factor and anti-CCP antibodies are negative. Anemia of chronic disease may be present but is often mild. HLA-B27 is found in 90% of white patients and 50% of black patients with ankylosing spondylitis. Because this antigen occurs in 8% of the healthy white population and 2% of healthy blacks, it is not a specific diagnostic test but is most useful when there is intermediate probability of disease.

C. Imaging

The earliest radiographic changes are usually in the sacroiliac joints. In the first 2 years of the disease process, the sacroiliac changes may be detectable only by MRI. Indeed, patients who have symptoms and findings of ankylosing spondylitis and sacroiliitis evident by MRI but not by conventional radiographs are classified as having nonradiographic axial spondyloarthritis. Later, erosion and sclerosis of these joints often become evident on plain radiographs; the sacroiliitis of ankylosing spondylitis is bilateral and symmetric. Inflammation where the annulus fibrosus attaches to the vertebral bodies initially causes sclerosis ("the shiny corner sign") and then characteristic squaring of the vertebral bodies. The term "bamboo spine" describes the late radiographic appearance of the spinal column in which the vertebral bodies are fused by vertically oriented, bridging syndesmophytes formed by the ossification of the annulus fibrosus and calcification of the anterior and lateral spinal ligaments. Fusion of the posterior facet joints of the spine is also common.

Additional radiographic findings include periosteal new bone formation on the iliac crest, ischial tuberosities and calcanei, and alterations of the pubic symphysis and sternomanubrial joint similar to those of the sacroiliacs. Radiologic changes in peripheral joints, when present, tend to be asymmetric and lack the demineralization and erosions seen in rheumatoid arthritis.

▶ Differential Diagnosis

Low back pain due to mechanical causes, disk disease, and degenerative arthritis is very common. Onset of back pain prior to age 30 and an "inflammatory" quality of the back pain (ie, morning stiffness and pain that improve with activity) should raise the possibility of ankylosing spondylitis. In contrast to ankylosing spondylitis, rheumatoid arthritis predominantly affects multiple, small, peripheral joints of the hands and feet. Rheumatoid arthritis spares the sacroiliac joints and only affects the cervical component of the spine. Bilateral sacroiliitis indistinguishable from ankylosing spondylitis is seen with the spondylitis associated with inflammatory bowel disease. Sacroiliitis associated with reactive arthritis and psoriasis, on the other hand, is often asymmetric or even unilateral. Osteitis condensans ilii (sclerosis on the iliac side of the sacroiliac joint) is an asymptomatic, postpartum radiographic finding that is occasionally mistaken for sacroiliitis. Diffuse idiopathic skeletal hyperostosis (DISH) causes exuberant osteophytes ("enthesophytes") of the spine that occasionally are difficult to distinguish from the syndesmophytes of ankylosing spondylitis. The enthesophytes of DISH are thicker and more anterior than the syndesmophytes of ankylosing spondylitis, and the sacroiliac joints are normal in DISH.

▶ Treatment

NSAIDs remain first-line treatment of ankylosing spondylitis and may slow radiographic progression of spinal disease. TNF inhibitors have established efficacy for NSAID-resistant axial disease; responses are often substantial and durable. Etanercept (50 mg subcutaneously once a week), adalimumab (40 mg subcutaneously every other week), infliximab (5 mg/kg every other month by intravenous infusion), golimumab (50 mg subcutaneously once a month), or certolizumab (200 mg subcutaneously every other week) is reasonable for patients whose symptoms are refractory to NSAIDs. Secukinumab, an inhibitor of the proinflammatory cytokine IL-17A, is also highly effective in the treatment of ankylosing spondylitis. Corticosteroids have minimal impact on the arthritis—particularly the spondylitis—of ankylosing spondylitis and can worsen osteopenia. All patients should be referred to a physical therapist for instruction in postural exercises.

▶ Prognosis

Almost all patients have persistent symptoms over decades; rare individuals experience long-term remissions. The severity of disease varies greatly, with about 10% of patients having work disability after 10 years. Developing hip disease within the first 2 years of disease onset presages a worse prognosis. TNF inhibitors provide symptomatic relief and improve quality of life for many patients with ankylosing spondylitis.

Landewé R et al. Efficacy and safety of continuing versus withdrawing adalimumab therapy in maintaining remission in patients with non-radiographic axial spondyloarthritis (ABILITY-3): a multicentre, randomised, double-blind study. Lancet. 2018 Jul 14;392(10142):134–44. [PMID: 29961640]

Marzo-Ortega H et al; Measure 2 Study Group. Secukinumab and sustained improvement in signs and symptoms of patients with active ankylosing spondylitis through two years: results from a phase III study. Arthritis Care Res (Hoboken). 2017 Jul; 69(7):1020–9. [PMID: 28235249]

Taurog JD et al. Ankylosing spondylitis and axial spondyloarthritis. N Engl J Med. 2016 Jun 30;374(26):2563–74. [PMID: 27355535]

Ward MM et al. American College of Rheumatology/Spondylitis Association of America/Spondyloarthritis Research and Treatment Network 2015 recommendations for the treatment of ankylosing spondylitis and nonradiographic axial spondyloarthritis. Arthritis Rheumatol. 2016 Feb;68(2):282–98. [PMID: 26401991]

PSORIATIC ARTHRITIS

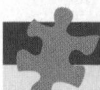

ESSENTIALS OF DIAGNOSIS

► Psoriasis precedes arthritis in 80% of cases.
► **Arthritis:** usually asymmetric, with "sausage" appearance of fingers and toes; polyarthritis that resembles rheumatoid arthritis also occurs.
► Sacroiliac joint involvement common.
► **Radiographic findings:** osteolysis; pencil-in-cup deformity; relative lack of osteoporosis; bony ankylosis; asymmetric sacroiliitis and atypical syndesmophytes.

► General Considerations

Although psoriasis usually precedes the onset of arthritis, arthritis precedes (by up to 2 years) or occurs simultaneously with the skin disease in approximately 20% of cases.

► Clinical Findings

A. Symptoms and Signs

The patterns or subsets of psoriatic arthritis include the following:

1. A symmetric polyarthritis that resembles rheumatoid arthritis. Usually, fewer joints are involved than in rheumatoid arthritis.

2. An oligoarticular form that may lead to considerable destruction of the affected joints.

3. A pattern of disease in which the DIP joints are primarily affected. Early, this may be monarticular, and often the joint involvement is asymmetric. Pitting of the nails and onycholysis frequently accompany DIP involvement.

4. A severe deforming arthritis (arthritis mutilans) in which osteolysis is marked.

5. A spondylitic form in which sacroiliitis and spinal involvement predominate; 50% of these patients are HLA-B27-positive.

Arthritis is at least five times more common in patients with severe psoriatic skin disease than in those with only mild skin findings. Occasionally, however, patients may have a single patch of psoriasis (typically hidden in the scalp, gluteal cleft, or umbilicus) and are unaware of its presence. Thus, a detailed search for cutaneous lesions is essential in patients with arthritis of new onset. Also, the psoriatic lesions may have cleared when arthritis appears—in such cases, the history is most useful in diagnosing previously unexplained cases of monoarthritis or oligoarthritis. Nail pitting is sometimes a clue. "Sausage" swelling of one or more digits is a common manifestation of enthesopathy in psoriatic arthritis.

B. Laboratory Findings

Laboratory studies show an elevation of the ESR; rheumatoid factor and anti-CCP antibodies are not present. Uric acid levels may be high, reflecting the active turnover of skin affected by psoriasis. There is a correlation between the extent of psoriatic involvement and the level of uric acid, but gout is no more common than in patients without psoriasis. Desquamation of the skin may also reduce iron stores.

C. Imaging

Radiographic findings are most helpful in distinguishing the disease from other forms of arthritis. There are marginal erosions of bone and irregular destruction of joint and bone, which, in the phalanx, may give the appearance of a sharpened pencil. Fluffy periosteal new bone may be marked, especially at the insertion of muscles and ligaments into bone. Such changes will also be seen along the shafts of metacarpals, metatarsals, and phalanges. Psoriatic spondylitis causes asymmetric sacroiliitis and syndesmophytes, which are coarser than those seen in ankylosing spondylitis. In psoriatic arthritis as in ankylosing spondylitis, MRI is more sensitive in detecting axial abnormalities than plain radiographs, especially in the first few years of disease onset. Ultrasonography and MRI are more sensitive than conventional radiographs in detecting peripheral arthritis, enthesitis, and dactylitis.

► Treatment

NSAIDs are usually sufficient for mild cases. For patients with peripheral arthritis, methotrexate (7.5–20 mg orally once a week) is generally considered the drug of choice for patients who have not responded to NSAIDs; methotrexate is not effective for axial arthritis. Methotrexate can improve both the cutaneous and arthritic manifestations. For patients with axial disease or peripheral arthritis that is refractory to methotrexate, treatment with a TNF inhibitor (at doses similar to the treatment of ankylosing spondylitis) is usually effective for both arthritis and psoriatic skin disease. Patients who do not respond to TNF inhibitors can be treated with ustekinumab, a monoclonal antibody that inhibits IL-12 and IL-23, or either secukinumab or ixekizumab, which inhibit IL-17. Apremilast, an oral phosphodiesterase-4 inhibitor, is an option for patients who cannot use, or choose not to use, biologic agents. Corticosteroids are less effective in psoriatic arthritis than in other forms of inflammatory arthritis and may precipitate pustular psoriasis during tapers. Successful treatment directed at the skin lesions alone (eg, by PUVA therapy) occasionally is accompanied by an improvement in peripheral articular symptoms.

Gladman D et al. Tofacitinib for psoriatic arthritis in patients with an inadequate response to TNF inhibitors. N Engl J Med. 2017 Oct 19;377(16):1525–36. [PMID: 29045207]

Naik GS et al. Th17 inhibitors in active psoriatic arthritis: a systematic review and meta-analysis of randomized controlled clinical trials. Dermatology. 2017;233(5):366–77. [PMID: 29258093]

Schemoul J et al. Treatment strategies for psoriatic arthritis. Joint Bone Spine. 2018 Oct;85(5):537–44. [PMID: 29155104]

Van den Bosch F et al. Clinical management of psoriatic arthritis. Lancet. 2018 Jun 2;391(10136):2285–94. [PMID: 29893227]

REACTIVE ARTHRITIS

ESSENTIALS OF DIAGNOSIS

▶ Oligoarthritis, conjunctivitis, urethritis, and mouth ulcers most common features.

▶ Usually follows dysentery or a sexually transmitted infection.

▶ HLA-B27–positive in 50–80% of patients.

► General Considerations

Reactive arthritis is precipitated by antecedent gastrointestinal and genitourinary infections and manifests as an asymmetric sterile oligoarthritis, typically of the lower extremities. It is frequently associated with enthesitis. Extra-articular manifestations are common and include urethritis, conjunctivitis, uveitis, and mucocutaneous lesions. Reactive arthritis occurs most commonly in young men and is associated with HLA-B27 in 80% of white patients and 50–60% of blacks.

► Clinical Findings

A. Symptoms and Signs

Most cases of reactive arthritis develop within 1–4 weeks after either a gastrointestinal infection (usually with *Shigella*, *Salmonella*, *Yersinia*, or *Campylobacter*) or a sexually transmitted infection (with *Chlamydia trachomatis* or perhaps *Ureaplasma urealyticum*). Whether the inciting infection is sexually transmitted or dysenteric does not affect the subsequent manifestations but does influence the gender ratio: The ratio is 1:1 after enteric infections but 9:1 with male predominance after sexually transmitted infections. Synovial fluid from affected joints is culture-negative. A clinically indistinguishable syndrome can occur without an apparent antecedent infection, suggesting that subclinical

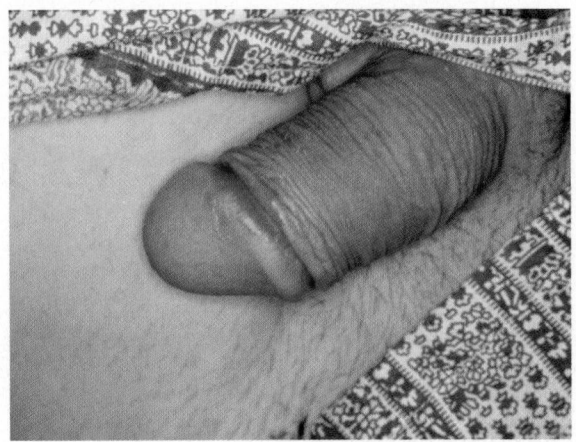

▲ **Figure 20–7.** Circinate balanitis due to reactive arthritis. (From Susan Lindsley, Dr. M. F. Rein, Public Health Image Library, CDC.)

infection can precipitate reactive arthritis or that there are other, as yet unrecognized, triggers.

The arthritis is most commonly asymmetric and frequently involves the large weight-bearing joints (chiefly the knee and ankle); sacroiliitis or ankylosing spondylitis is observed in at least 20% of patients, especially after frequent recurrences. Systemic symptoms including fever and weight loss are common at the onset of disease. The mucocutaneous lesions may include balanitis (Figure 20–7), stomatitis, and keratoderma blennorrhagicum, indistinguishable from pustular psoriasis. Involvement of the fingernails in reactive arthritis also mimics psoriatic changes. When present, conjunctivitis is mild and occurs early in the disease course. Anterior uveitis, which can develop at any time in HLA-B27-positive patients, is a more clinically significant ocular complication. Carditis and aortic regurgitation may occur. While most signs of the disease disappear within days or weeks, the arthritis may persist for several months or become chronic. Recurrences involving any combination of the clinical manifestations are common and are sometimes followed by permanent sequelae, especially in the joints (eg, articular destruction).

B. Imaging

Radiographic signs of permanent or progressive joint disease may be seen in the sacroiliac as well as the peripheral joints.

► Differential Diagnosis

Gonococcal arthritis can initially mimic reactive arthritis, but the marked improvement after 24–48 hours of antibiotic administration in gonococcal arthritis and the culture results distinguish the two disorders. Rheumatoid arthritis, ankylosing spondylitis, and psoriatic arthritis must also be considered. By causing similar oral, ocular, and joint lesions, Behçet disease may also mimic reactive arthritis. The oral lesions of reactive arthritis, however, are typically painless, in contrast to those of Behçet disease.

HIV is not more common in sexually active men with reactive arthritis.

Treatment

NSAIDs have been the mainstay of therapy. Antibiotics given at the time of a nongonococcal sexually transmitted infection reduce the chance that the individual will develop this disorder. For chronic reactive arthritis associated with chlamydial infection, combination antibiotics taken for 6 months are more effective than placebo. Patients who do not respond to NSAIDs may respond to sulfasalazine, 1000 mg orally twice daily, or to methotrexate, 7.5–20 mg orally per week. For those patients with recent-onset disease that is refractory to NSAIDs and these DMARDs, anti-TNF agents, which are effective in the other spondyloarthropathies, may be effective.

Courcoul A et al. A bicentre retrospective study of features and outcomes of patients with reactive arthritis. Joint Bone Spine. 2018 Mar;85(2):201–5. [PMID: 28238883]
García-Kutzbach A et al. Reactive arthritis: update 2018. Clin Rheumatol. 2018 Apr;37(4):869–74. [PMID: 29455267]

ARTHRITIS & INFLAMMATORY INTESTINAL DISEASES

One-fifth of patients with **inflammatory bowel disease** have arthritis, which complicates Crohn disease somewhat more frequently than it does ulcerative colitis. In both diseases, two distinct forms of arthritis occur. The first is peripheral arthritis—usually a nondeforming asymmetric oligoarthritis of large joints—in which the activity of the joint disease parallels that of the bowel disease. The arthritis usually begins months to years after the bowel disease, but occasionally the joint symptoms develop earlier and may be prominent enough to cause the patient to overlook intestinal symptoms. The second form of arthritis is a spondylitis that is indistinguishable by symptoms or radiographs from ankylosing spondylitis and follows a course independent of the bowel disease. About 50% of these patients are HLA-B27 positive.

Controlling the intestinal inflammation usually eliminates the peripheral arthritis. NSAIDs can be effective when the arthritis is mild but must be used cautiously since they can exacerbate inflammatory bowel disease. TNF inhibitors are attractive therapies because they are effective both for the bowel and for the joints. Range-of-motion exercises as prescribed for ankylosing spondylitis can be helpful.

About two-thirds of patients with **Whipple disease** experience arthralgia or arthritis, most often an episodic, large-joint polyarthritis. The arthritis usually precedes the gastrointestinal manifestations by years and often resolves as the diarrhea develops. Thus, Whipple disease should be considered in the differential diagnosis of unexplained episodic arthritis.

Malaty HM et al. Characterization and prevalence of spondyloarthritis and peripheral arthritis among patients with inflammatory bowel disease. Clin Exp Gastroenterol. 2017 Sep 27;10:259–63. [PMID: 29026327]

INFECTIOUS ARTHRITIS

NONGONOCOCCAL ACUTE BACTERIAL (Septic) ARTHRITIS

ESSENTIALS OF DIAGNOSIS

► Acute onset of inflammatory monarticular arthritis, most often in large weight-bearing joints and wrists.
► Common risk factors include previous joint damage and injection drug use.
► Infection with causative organism commonly found elsewhere in body.
► Joint effusions are usually large, with white blood cell counts commonly over 50,000/mcL.

General Considerations

Lyme disease is discussed in Chapter 34.

Nongonococcal acute bacterial arthritis is most often due to hematogenous seeding of the joint; direct inoculation from penetrating trauma is rare. The key risk factors are bacteremia (eg, injection drug use, endocarditis, infection at other sites), damaged joints (eg, rheumatoid arthritis), prosthetic joints, compromised immunity (eg, advanced age, diabetes mellitus, advanced chronic kidney disease, alcoholism, cirrhosis, and immunosuppressive therapy), and loss of skin integrity (eg, cutaneous ulcer or psoriasis). *Staphylococcus aureus* is the most common cause of nongonococcal septic arthritis, accounting for about 50% of all cases. Methicillin-resistant *S aureus* (MRSA) and group B *Streptococcus* have become increasing frequent and important causes of septic arthritis. Gram-negative septic arthritis causes about 10% of cases and is especially common in injection drug users and in immunocompromised persons. *Escherichia coli* and *Pseudomonas aeruginosa* are the most common gram-negative isolates in adults. Pathologic changes include varying degrees of acute inflammation, with synovitis, effusion, abscess formation in synovial or subchondral tissues, and, if treatment is not adequate, articular destruction.

Clinical Findings

A. Symptoms and Signs

The onset is usually acute, with pain, swelling, and heat of the affected joint worsening over hours. The knee is most frequently involved; other commonly affected sites are the hip, wrist, shoulder, and ankle. Unusual sites, such as the sternoclavicular or sacroiliac joint, can be involved in injection drug users. Chills and fever are common but are absent in up to 20% of patients. Infection of the hip usually does not produce apparent swelling but results in groin pain greatly aggravated by walking. More than one joint is involved in 15% of cases of septic arthritis; risk factors for multiple joint involvement include rheumatoid arthritis, associated endocarditis, and infection with group B streptococci.

B. Laboratory Findings

Synovial fluid analysis is critical for diagnosis. The leukocyte count of the synovial fluid is always inflammatory (greater than 2000/mcL), usually exceeds 50,000/mcL, and often is more than 100,000/mcL, with 90% or more polymorphonuclear cells (Table 20–2). Gram stain of the synovial fluid is positive in 75% of staphylococcal infections and in 50% of gram-negative infections. Synovial fluid cultures are positive in 70–90% of cases; administration of antibiotics prior to arthrocentesis reduces the likelihood of a positive culture result. Blood cultures are positive in approximately 50% of patients.

C. Imaging

Imaging tests generally add little to the diagnosis of septic arthritis. Indeed, other than demonstrating joint effusion, radiographs are usually normal early in the disease; however, evidence of demineralization may develop within days of onset. MRI and CT are more sensitive in detecting fluid in joints that are not accessible to physical examination (eg, the hip). Bony erosions and narrowing of the joint space followed by osteomyelitis and periostitis may be seen within 2 weeks.

D. Prosthetic Joint Infection

The clinical and laboratory manifestations of prosthetic joint infection is influenced by whether the infection is early (less than 3 months after surgery), delayed (3–12 months after surgery), or late (more than 12 months after surgery). Early infections present with acute redness and swelling and are usually caused by *S aureus* and gram-negative organisms. Delayed infections often present with subtle manifestations: pain is common but only 50% of patients will have fever. Less virulent organisms, such as coagulase-negative *Staphylococcus*, *Propionibacterium acnes*, and enterococci, are most common causes of delayed infections. Late infections present with acute pain, swelling, and fever and are often caused by hematogenous seeding of *S aureus*, gram-negative bacilli, and hemolytic streptococci.

▶ Differential Diagnosis

Gout and pseudogout can cause acute, very inflammatory monarticular arthritis and high-grade fever; the failure to find crystals on synovial fluid analysis excludes these diagnoses. A well-recognized but uncommon initial presentation of rheumatoid arthritis is an acute inflammatory monoarthritis ("pseudoseptic"). The most common articular manifestation of chronic Lyme disease is inflammatory monoarthritis of the knee, which yields synovial fluid that is Gram stain and culture negative. Acute rheumatic fever commonly involves several joints; Still disease may mimic septic arthritis, but laboratory evidence of infection is absent. Pyogenic arthritis may be superimposed on other types of joint disease, notably rheumatoid arthritis. Indeed, septic arthritis must be excluded by joint fluid examination in any patient with rheumatoid arthritis who has a joint strikingly more inflamed than the other joints.

▶ Prevention

There is no evidence that patients with prosthetic joints undergoing procedures should receive antibiotic prophylaxis to prevent joint infection unless the patient has a prosthetic heart valve or the procedure requires antibiotics to prevent a surgical site infection. However, the topic remains controversial. The American Academy of Orthopedic Surgeons advocates prescribing antibiotic prophylaxis for any patient with a prosthetic joint replacement undergoing a procedure that can cause bacteremia.

▶ Treatment

The effective treatment of septic arthritis requires appropriate antibiotic therapy together with drainage of the infected joint. Hospitalization is always necessary. If the likely causative organism cannot be determined clinically or from the synovial fluid Gram stain, treatment should be started with broad-spectrum antibiotic coverage effective against staphylococci, streptococci, and gram-negative organisms. The recommendation for initial treatment is to give vancomycin (1 g intravenously every 12 hours, adjusted for age, weight, and renal function) plus a third-generation cephalosporin: ceftriaxone, 1–2 g intravenously daily (or every 12 hours if concomitant meningitis or endocarditis is suspected); or cefotaxime, 1–2 g intravenously every 8 hours; or ceftazidime, 1–2 g intravenously every 8 hours. Antibiotic therapy should be adjusted when culture results become available; the duration of antibiotic therapy is usually 4–6 weeks.

Early orthopedic consultation is essential. Effective drainage is usually achieved through early arthroscopic lavage and debridement together with drain placement. Open surgical drainage should be performed when conservative treatment fails, when there is concomitant osteomyelitis requiring debridement, or when the involved joint (eg, hip, shoulder, sacroiliac joint) cannot be drained by more conservative means. Immobilization with a splint and elevation are used at the onset of treatment. Early active motion exercises within the limits of tolerance will hasten recovery. Options for treating prosthetic joint infections depend, in part, on the timing of the infection and include chronic suppression, debridement without removal of the prosthesis, or one- or two-stage exchange of the prosthesis.

▶ Prognosis

The outcome of septic arthritis depends largely on the antecedent health of the patient, the causative organism (eg, *S aureus* bacterial arthritis is associated with a poor functional outcome in about 40% of cases), and the promptness of treatment. Five to 10 percent of patients with an infected joint die of respiratory complications of sepsis. The mortality rate is 30% for patients with polyarticular sepsis.

Bony ankylosis and articular destruction commonly also occur if treatment is delayed or inadequate.

Butler BA et al. Early diagnosis of septic arthritis in immuno-compromised patients. J Orthop Sci. 2018 May;23(3):542–5. [PMID: 29519562]

Kapadia BH et al. Periprosthetic joint infection. Lancet. 2016 Jan 23;387(10016):386–94. [PMID: 26135702]

Nair R et al. Septic arthritis and prosthetic joint infections in older adults. Infect Dis Clin North Am. 2017 Dec;31(4):715–29. [PMID: 29079156]

GONOCOCCAL ARTHRITIS

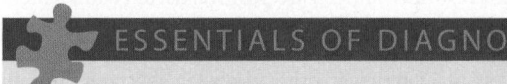
ESSENTIALS OF DIAGNOSIS

- ▶ Prodromal migratory polyarthralgias.
- ▶ Tenosynovitis is the most common sign.
- ▶ Purulent monoarthritis in 50%.
- ▶ Characteristic skin lesions.
- ▶ Most common in young women during menses or pregnancy.
- ▶ Symptoms of urethritis frequently absent.
- ▶ Dramatic response to antibiotics.

▶ General Considerations

In contrast to nongonococcal bacterial arthritis, gonococcal arthritis usually occurs in otherwise healthy individuals. Host factors, however, influence the expression of the disease: gonococcal arthritis is two to three times more common in women than in men, is especially common during menses and pregnancy, and is rare after age 40. Gonococcal arthritis is also common in men who have sex with men, whose high incidence of asymptomatic gonococcal pharyngitis and proctitis predisposes them to disseminated gonococcal infection. Recurrent disseminated gonococcal infection should prompt testing of the patient's CH50 level to evaluate for a congenital deficiency of a terminal complement component (C5, C6, C7, or C8).

▶ Clinical Findings

A. Symptoms and Signs

One to 4 days of migratory polyarthralgias involving the wrist, knee, ankle, or elbow are common at the outset. Thereafter, two patterns emerge. The first pattern is characterized by tenosynovitis that most often affects wrists, fingers, ankles, or toes and is seen in 60% of patients. The second pattern is purulent monoarthritis that most frequently involves the knee, wrist, ankle, or elbow and is seen in 40% of patients. Less than half of patients have fever, and less than one-fourth have any genitourinary symptoms. Most patients will have asymptomatic but highly characteristic skin lesions that usually consist of 2 to 10 small necrotic pustules distributed over the extremities, especially the palms and soles.

B. Laboratory Findings

The peripheral blood leukocyte count averages about 10,000 cells/mcL and is elevated in less than one-third of patients. The synovial fluid white blood cell count usually ranges from 30,000 to 60,000 cells/mcL. The synovial fluid Gram stain is positive in one-fourth of cases and culture in less than half. Positive blood cultures are uncommon. Urethral, throat, cervical, and rectal cultures should be done in all patients, since they are often positive in the absence of local symptoms. Urinary nucleic acid amplification tests have excellent sensitivity and specificity for the detection of *Neisseria gonorrhoeae* in genitourinary sites.

C. Imaging

Radiographs are usually normal or show only soft tissue swelling.

▶ Differential Diagnosis

Reactive arthritis can produce acute monoarthritis, urethritis, and fever in a young person but is distinguished by negative cultures and failure to respond to antibiotics. Lyme disease involving the knee is less acute, does not show positive cultures, and may be preceded by known tick exposure and characteristic rash. The synovial fluid analysis will exclude gout, pseudogout, and nongonococcal bacterial arthritis. Rheumatic fever and sarcoidosis can produce migratory tenosynovitis but have other distinguishing features. Infective endocarditis with septic arthritis can mimic disseminated gonococcal infection. Meningococcemia occasionally presents with a clinical picture that resembles disseminated gonococcal infection; blood cultures establish the correct diagnosis. Early hepatitis B infection is associated with circulating immune complexes that can cause a rash and polyarthralgias. In contrast to disseminated gonococcal infection, the rash in hepatitis B is urticarial.

▶ Treatment

In most cases, patients in whom gonococcal arthritis is suspected should be admitted to the hospital to confirm the diagnosis, to exclude endocarditis, and to start treatment. The recommended initial treatment is azithromycin (1 g orally as a single dose) and a third-generation cephalosporin: ceftriaxone, 1 g intravenously daily (or every 12 hours if concomitant meningitis or endocarditis is suspected); or cefotaxime, 1 g intravenously every 8 hours; or ceftizoxime, 1 g intravenously every 8 hours. Azithromycin enhances eradication of gonorrhea and covers potential coinfection with *Chlamydia*. Because of the increasing prevalence of resistant strains of gonococci, step-down treatment from parenteral to oral antibiotics is no longer recommended in the absence of culture results documenting sensitivity to the antibiotic being selected. Otherwise, once improvement has been achieved for 24–48 hours, patients must receive ceftriaxone 250 mg intramuscularly every 24 hours to complete a 7- to 14-day course.

▶ Prognosis

Generally, gonococcal arthritis responds dramatically in 24–48 hours after initiation of antibiotics, and drainage of the infected joint(s) is required infrequently. Complete recovery is the rule.

Sena Corrales G et al. Gonococcal arthritis in human immuno-deficiency virus-infected patients. Review of the literature. Reumatol Clin. 2017 Jan–Feb;13(1):39–41. [PMID: 26826910]

RHEUMATIC MANIFESTATIONS OF HIV INFECTION

Infection with HIV has been associated with various rheumatic disorders, most commonly arthralgias and arthritis. HIV painful articular syndrome causes severe arthralgias in an oligoarticular, asymmetric pattern that resolve within 24 hours; the joint examination is normal. HIV-associated arthritis is an asymmetric oligoarticular process with objective findings of arthritis and a self-limited course that ranges from weeks to months. Psoriatic arthritis and reactive arthritis occur in HIV-infected individuals and can be severe. These spondyloarthropathies can respond to NSAIDs, though many cases are unresponsive. Along with antiretroviral therapies, immunosuppressive medications can be used if necessary in HIV-infected patients, though with caution. Muscle weakness associated with an elevated creatine kinase can be due to nucleoside reverse transcriptase inhibitor-associated myopathy or HIV-associated myopathy; the clinical presentations of each resemble idiopathic polymyositis but the muscle biopsies show minimal inflammation. Less commonly, an inflammatory myositis indistinguishable from idiopathic polymyositis occurs. Other rheumatic manifestations of HIV include diffuse infiltrative lymphocytosis syndrome (with parotid gland enlargement) and various forms of vasculitis. The use of antiretroviral therapy has been associated with a marked decreased frequency of painful articular syndromes, psoriatic arthritis, spondyloarthropathy, and diffuse infiltrative lymphocytosis syndrome, and an increased frequency of the immune reconstitution inflammatory syndrome (IRIS) and osteoporosis.

Adizie T et al. Inflammatory arthritis in HIV positive patients: a practical guide. BMC Infect Dis. 2016 Mar 1;16:100. [PMID: 26932524]
Mehsen-Cêtre N et al. Osteoarticular manifestations associated with HIV infection. Joint Bone Spine. 2017 Jan;84(1):29–33. [PMID: 27238195]

VIRAL ARTHRITIS

Arthralgias occur frequently in the course of acute infections with many viruses, but frank arthritis is uncommon with the notable exceptions of acute parvovirus B19 infection and Chikungunya fever. Parvovirus B19 causes an acute polyarthritis in 50–60% of adult cases (infected children develop the febrile exanthem known as "slapped cheek fever"). The arthritis can mimic rheumatoid arthritis but is almost always self-limited and resolves within several weeks. The diagnosis is established by the presence of IgM antibodies specific for parvovirus B19. Chikungunya fever is an arthropod-borne viral infection that is endemic to West Africa but has spread to multiple locations including the Indian Ocean islands, the Caribbean and Central and Latin America. Clinical manifestations include high fever, rash, and incapacitating bone pain. Acute polyarthralgia and polyarthritis are common and can persist for months or years.

Self-limited polyarthritis is common in acute hepatitis B infection and typically occurs before the onset of jaundice. Urticaria or other types of skin rash may be present. Indeed, the clinical picture resembles that of serum sickness. Serum transaminase levels are elevated, and tests for hepatitis B surface antigen are positive. Serum complement levels are often low during active arthritis and become normal after remission of arthritis. The incidence of hepatitis B–associated polyarthritis has fallen substantially with the introduction of hepatitis B vaccination. Effective vaccination programs in the United States have eliminated acute rubella infections, formerly a common cause of virally induced polyarthritis. Changes in the rubella vaccine (an attenuated live vaccine) have greatly reduced the incidence of rubella vaccine–induced polyarthritis as well.

Chronic infection with hepatitis C is associated with chronic polyarthralgia in up to 20% of cases and with chronic polyarthritis in 3–5%. Both can mimic rheumatoid arthritis, and the presence of rheumatoid factor in most hepatitis C–infected individuals leads to further diagnostic confusion. Indeed, hepatitis C–associated arthritis is frequently misdiagnosed as rheumatoid arthritis. Distinguishing hepatitis C–associated arthritis/arthralgias from the co-occurrence of hepatitis C and rheumatoid arthritis can be difficult. Rheumatoid arthritis always causes objective arthritis (not just arthralgias) and can be erosive (hepatitis C–associated arthritis is nonerosive). The presence of anti-CCP antibodies points to the diagnosis of rheumatoid arthritis.

Hua C et al. Chikungunya virus-associated disease. Curr Rheumatol Rep. 2017 Oct 5;19(11):69. [PMID: 28983760]
Runowska M et al. Chikungunya virus: a rheumatologist's perspective. Clin Exp Rheumatol. 2018 May–Jun;36(3):494–501. [PMID: 29533749]

INFECTIONS OF BONES

ACUTE PYOGENIC OSTEOMYELITIS

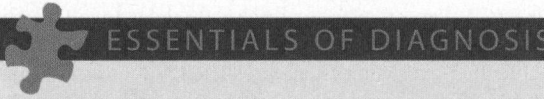

ESSENTIALS OF DIAGNOSIS

▶ Fever associated with pain and tenderness of involved bone.

▶ Diagnosis usually requires culture of bone biopsy.

▶ Elevated ESR and CRP.

▶ Radiographs early in the course are typically negative.

General Considerations

Osteomyelitis is a serious infection that is often difficult to diagnose and treat. Infection of bone occurs as a consequence of (1) hematogenous dissemination of bacteria, (2) invasion from a contiguous focus of infection, and (3) skin breakdown in the setting of vascular insufficiency.

Clinical Findings

A. Symptoms and Signs

1. Hematogenous osteomyelitis—Osteomyelitis resulting from bacteremia is a disease associated with sickle cell disease, injection drug users, diabetes mellitus, or older adults. Patients with this form of osteomyelitis often present with sudden onset of high fever, chills, and pain and tenderness of the involved bone. The site of osteomyelitis and the causative organism depend on the host. Among patients with hemoglobinopathies such as sickle cell anemia, osteomyelitis is caused most often by salmonellae; *S aureus* is the second most common cause. Osteomyelitis in injection drug users develops most commonly in the spine. Although in this setting *S aureus* is most common, gram-negative infections, especially *P aeruginosa* and *Serratia* species, are also frequent pathogens. Rapid progression to epidural abscess causing fever, pain, and sensory and motor loss is not uncommon. In older patients with hematogenous osteomyelitis, the most common sites are the thoracic and lumbar vertebral bodies. Risk factors for these patients include diabetes, intravenous catheters, and indwelling urinary catheters. These patients often have more subtle presentations, with low-grade fever and gradually increasing bone pain.

2. Osteomyelitis from a contiguous focus of infection—Prosthetic joint replacement, pressure injury (formerly called pressure ulcer), neurosurgery, and trauma most frequently cause soft tissue infections that can spread to bone. *S aureus* and *Staphylococcus epidermidis* are the most common organisms. Polymicrobial infections, rare in hematogenously spread osteomyelitis, are more common in osteomyelitis due to contiguous spread. Localized signs of inflammation are usually evident, but high fever and other signs of toxicity are usually absent. Septic arthritis and cellulitis can also spread to contiguous bone.

3. Osteomyelitis associated with vascular insufficiency—Patients with diabetes mellitus and vascular insufficiency are susceptible to developing a very challenging form of osteomyelitis. The foot and ankle are the most commonly affected sites. Infection originates from an ulcer or other break in the skin that is usually still present when the patient presents but may appear disarmingly unimpressive. Bone pain is often absent or muted by the associated neuropathy. Fever is also commonly absent. Two of the best bedside clues that the patient has osteomyelitis are the ability to easily advance a sterile probe through a skin ulcer to bone and an ulcer area larger than 2 cm^2.

B. Imaging and Laboratory Findings

The ESR and serum CRP are almost always elevated and can be useful parameters to follow during the course of therapy.

The plain film is the most readily available imaging procedure to establish the diagnosis of osteomyelitis, but it can be falsely negative initially. Early radiographic findings may include soft tissue swelling, loss of tissue planes, and periarticular demineralization of bone. About 2 weeks after onset of symptoms, erosion of bone and alteration of cancellous bone appear, followed by periostitis.

MRI, CT, and nuclear medicine bone scanning are more sensitive than conventional radiography. MRI is the most sensitive and is particularly helpful in demonstrating the extent of soft tissue involvement. Radionuclide bone scanning is most valuable when osteomyelitis is suspected but no site is obvious. Nuclear medicine studies may also detect multifocal sites of infection. Ultrasound is useful in diagnosing the presence of effusions within joints and extra-articular soft tissue fluid collections but not in detecting bone infections.

Identifying the offending organism is a crucial step in selection of antibiotic therapy. Bone biopsy for culture is required except in those with hematogenous osteomyelitis, who have positive blood cultures. Cultures from overlying ulcers, wounds, or fistulas are unreliable.

Differential Diagnosis

Acute hematogenous osteomyelitis should be distinguished from suppurative arthritis, rheumatic fever, and cellulitis. More subacute forms must be differentiated from tuberculosis or mycotic infections of bone and Ewing sarcoma or, in the case of vertebral osteomyelitis, from metastatic cancer. When osteomyelitis involves the vertebrae, it commonly traverses the disk—a finding not observed in cancer. Charcot arthropathy of the foot or ankle can mimic osteomyelitis, particularly in patients with diabetes but does not cause an elevated ESR or serum CRP.

Complications

Inadequate treatment of bone infections results in chronicity of infection, and this possibility is increased by delaying diagnosis and treatment. Extension to adjacent bone or joints may complicate acute osteomyelitis. Recurrence of bone infections often results in anemia of chronic disease, a markedly elevated ESR, weight loss, weakness and, rarely, amyloidosis or nephrotic syndrome. Pseudoepitheliomatous hyperplasia, squamous cell carcinoma, or fibrosarcoma may occasionally arise in persistently infected tissues.

Treatment

Most patients require both debridement of necrotic bone and prolonged administration of antibiotics. Patients with vertebral body osteomyelitis and epidural abscess may require urgent neurosurgical decompression. Depending on the site and extent of debridement, surgical procedures to stabilize, fill in, cover, or revascularize may be needed.

Oral therapy with quinolones (eg, ciprofloxacin, 750 mg twice daily) for 6–8 weeks has been shown to be as effective as standard parenteral antibiotic therapy for chronic osteomyelitis with susceptible organisms. When treating osteomyelitis caused by *S aureus*, quinolones are usually combined with rifampin, 300 mg orally twice daily.

Prognosis

If sterility of the lesion is achieved within 2–4 days, a good result can be expected in most cases if there is no compromise of the patient's immune system. However, progression of the disease to a chronic form may occur. It is especially common in the lower extremities and in patients in whom circulation is impaired (eg, diabetics).

Courjon J et al; DTS (Duration of Treatment for Spondylodiscitis) Study Group. Pyogenic vertebral osteomyelitis of the elderly: Characteristics and outcomes. PLoS One. 2017 Dec 5; 12(12):e0188470. [PMID: 29206837]

Peters EJ et al; International Working Group on the Diabetic Foot. Interventions in the management of infection in the foot in diabetes: a systematic review. Diabetes Metab Res Rev. 2016 Jan;32(Suppl 1):145–53. [PMID: 26344844]

TUBERCULOSIS OF BONES & JOINTS

SPINAL TUBERCULOSIS (Pott Disease)

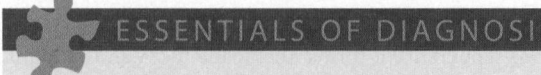

ESSENTIALS OF DIAGNOSIS

► Seen primarily in immigrants from developing countries or immunocompromised patients.

► Back pain and gibbus deformity.

► Radiographic evidence of vertebral involvement.

► Evidence of *Mycobacterium tuberculosis* in aspirate or biopsies of spinal lesions.

General Considerations

In the developing world, children primarily bear the burden of musculoskeletal tuberculosis. In the United States, however, musculoskeletal infection is more often seen in adult immigrants from countries where tuberculosis is prevalent, or it develops in the setting of immunosuppression (eg, HIV infection, therapy with TNF inhibitors). Spinal tuberculosis (Pott disease) accounts for about 50% of musculoskeletal infection due to *M tuberculosis* (see Chapter 9). Seeding of the vertebrae may occur through hematogenous spread from the respiratory tract at the time of primary infection, with clinical disease developing years later as a consequence of reactivation, or through lymphatics from infected foci in the pleura or kidneys. The thoracic and lumbar vertebrae are the most common sites of spinal involvement; vertebral infection is associated with paravertebral cold abscesses in 75% of cases.

Clinical Findings

A. Symptoms and Signs

Patients complain of back pain, often present for months and sometimes associated with radicular pain and lower extremity weakness. Constitutional symptoms are usually absent, and less than 20% have active pulmonary disease. Destruction of the anterior aspect of the vertebral body can produce the characteristic gibbus deformity.

B. Laboratory Findings

Most patients have a positive reaction to purified protein derivative (PPD) or a positive interferon-gamma release assay. Cultures of paravertebral abscesses and biopsies of vertebral lesions are positive in up to 70–90%. Biopsies reveal characteristic caseating granulomas in most cases. Isolation of *M tuberculosis* from an extraspinal site is sufficient to establish the diagnosis in the proper clinical setting.

C. Imaging

Radiographs can reveal lytic and sclerotic lesions and bony destruction of vertebrae but are normal early in the disease course. CT scanning can demonstrate paraspinal soft tissue extensions of the infection; MRI is the imaging technique of choice to detect compression of the spinal cord or cauda equina.

Differential Diagnosis

Spinal tuberculosis must be differentiated from subacute and chronic spinal infections due to pyogenic organisms, *Brucella*, and fungi as well as from malignancy.

Complications

Paraplegia due to compression of the spinal cord or cauda equina is the most serious complication of spinal tuberculosis.

Treatment

Antimicrobial therapy should be administered for 6–9 months, usually in the form of isoniazid, rifampin, pyrazinamide, and ethambutol for 2 months followed by isoniazid and rifampin for an additional 4–7 months (see also Chapter 9). Medical management alone is often sufficient. Surgical intervention, however, may be indicated when there is neurologic compromise or severe spinal instability.

Dunn RN et al. Spinal tuberculosis. Bone Joint J. 2018 Apr 1; 100-B(4):425–31. [PMID: 29629596]

Hu HT et al. Vertebral column decortication for the management of sharp angular spinal deformity in Pott disease: case report. Medicine (Baltimore). 2017 Nov;96(45):e8592. [PMID: 29137084]

TUBERCULOUS ARTHRITIS

Infection of peripheral joints by *M tuberculosis* usually presents as a monoarticular arthritis lasting for weeks to months (or longer), but less often, it can have an acute presentation that mimics septic arthritis. Any joint can be involved; the hip and knee are most commonly affected. Constitutional symptoms and fever are present in only a small number of cases. Tuberculosis also can cause a chronic tenosynovitis of the hand and wrist. Joint destruction occurs far more slowly than in septic arthritis due to pyogenic organisms. Synovial fluid is inflammatory but not to the degree seen in pyogenic infections, with synovial white cell counts in the range of 10,000–20,000 cells/mcL. Smears of synovial fluid are positive for acid-fast bacilli in a minority of cases; synovial fluid cultures, however, are positive in 80% of cases. Because culture results may take weeks, the diagnostic procedure of choice usually is synovial biopsy, which yields characteristic pathologic findings and positive cultures in greater than 90%. Antimicrobial therapy is the mainstay of treatment. Rarely, a reactive, sterile polyarthritis associated with erythema nodosum (Poncet disease) develops in patients with active pulmonary or extrapulmonary tuberculosis.

ARTHRITIS IN SARCOIDOSIS

The frequency of arthritis among patients with sarcoidosis is variously reported between 10% and 35%. It is usually acute in onset, but articular symptoms may appear insidiously and often antedate other manifestations of the disease. Knees and ankles are most commonly involved, but any joint may be affected. Distribution of joint involvement is usually polyarticular and symmetric. The arthritis is commonly self-limited, resolving after several weeks or months and rarely resulting in chronic arthritis, joint destruction, or significant deformity. Sarcoid arthropathy is often associated with erythema nodosum, but the diagnosis is contingent on the demonstration of other extra-articular manifestations of sarcoidosis and, notably, biopsy evidence of noncaseating granulomas. Despite the clinical appearance of an inflammatory arthritis, synovial fluid often is noninflammatory (ie, less than 2000 leukocytes/mcL). In chronic arthritis, radiographs show typical changes in the bones of the extremities with intact cortex and cystic changes.

Treatment of arthritis in sarcoidosis is usually symptomatic and supportive. Colchicine may be of value. Patients with severe and progressive joint disease may respond to corticosteroids or to TNF inhibitors.

Ungprasert P et al. Clinical characteristics of sarcoid arthropathy: a population-based study. Arthritis Care Res (Hoboken). 2016 May;68(5):695–9. [PMID: 26415117]

Zhou Y et al. Clinical characteristics of patients with bone sarcoidosis. Semin Arthritis Rheum. 2017 Aug;47(1):143–48. [PMID: 28274482]

MISCELLANEOUS RHEUMATOLOGIC DISORDERS

THORACIC OUTLET SYNDROMES

Thoracic outlet syndromes result from compression of the neurovascular structures supplying the upper extremity. Symptoms and signs arise from intermittent or continuous pressure on elements of the brachial plexus (more than 90% of cases) or the subclavian or axillary vessels (veins or arteries) by a variety of anatomic structures of the shoulder girdle region. The neurovascular bundle can be compressed between the anterior or middle scalene muscles and a normal first thoracic rib or a cervical rib. Most commonly thoracic outlet syndromes are caused by scarred scalene neck muscle secondary to neck trauma or sagging of the shoulder girdle resulting from aging, obesity, or pendulous breasts. Faulty posture, occupation, or thoracic muscle hypertrophy from physical activity (eg, weight-lifting, baseball pitching) may be other predisposing factors.

Thoracic outlet syndromes present in most patients with some combination of four symptoms involving the upper extremity: pain, numbness, weakness, and swelling. The predominant symptoms depend on whether the compression chiefly affects neural or vascular structures. The onset of symptoms is usually gradual but can be sudden. Some patients spontaneously notice aggravation of symptoms with specific positioning of the arm. Pain radiates from the point of compression to the base of the neck, the axilla, the shoulder girdle region, arm, forearm, and hand. Paresthesias are common and distributed to the volar aspect of the fourth and fifth digits. Sensory symptoms may be aggravated at night or by prolonged use of the extremities. Weakness and muscle atrophy are the principal motor abnormalities. Vascular symptoms consist of arterial ischemia characterized by pallor of the fingers on elevation of the extremity, sensitivity to cold and, rarely, gangrene of the digits or venous obstruction marked by edema, cyanosis, and engorgement.

The symptoms of thoracic outlet syndromes can be provoked within 60 seconds over 90% of the time by having a patient elevate the arms in a "stick-em-up" position (ie, abducted 90 degrees in external rotation). Reflexes are usually not altered. Obliteration of the radial pulse with certain maneuvers of the arm or neck, once considered a highly sensitive sign of thoracic outlet obstruction, does not occur in most cases.

Chest radiography will identify patients with cervical rib (although most patients with cervical ribs are asymptomatic). MRI with the arms held in different positions is useful in identifying sites of impaired blood flow. Intra-arterial or venous obstruction is confirmed by angiography. Determination of conduction velocities of the ulnar and other peripheral nerves of the upper extremity may help localize the site of their compression.

Thoracic outlet syndrome must be differentiated from osteoarthritis of the cervical spine, tumors of the superior pulmonary sulcus, cervical spinal cord, or nerve roots, and periarthritis of the shoulder.

Treatment is directed toward relief of compression of the neurovascular bundle. Greater than 95% of patients can be treated successfully with conservative therapy consisting of physical therapy and avoiding postures or activities that compress the neurovascular bundle. Some women will benefit from a support bra. Operative treatment, required by less than 5% of patients, is more likely to relieve the neurologic rather than the vascular component that causes symptoms.

Buller LT et al. Thoracic outlet syndrome: current concepts, imaging features, and therapeutic strategies. Am J Orthop (Belle Mead NJ). 2015 Aug;44(8):376–82. [PMID: 26251937]

Matos JM et al. Outcomes following operative management of thoracic outlet syndrome in the pediatric patients. Vascular. 2018 Aug;26(4):410–7. [PMID: 29301465]

FIBROMYALGIA

ESSENTIALS OF DIAGNOSIS

▶ Most frequent in women aged 20–50.

▶ Chronic widespread musculoskeletal pain syndrome with multiple tender points.

▶ Fatigue, headaches, numbness common.

▶ Objective signs of inflammation absent; laboratory studies normal.

▶ General Considerations

Fibromyalgia is a common syndrome, affecting 3–10% of the general population. It shares many features with the chronic fatigue syndrome, namely, an increased frequency among women aged 20–50, absence of objective findings, and absence of diagnostic laboratory test results. While many of the clinical features of the two conditions overlap, musculoskeletal pain predominates in fibromyalgia whereas lassitude dominates the chronic fatigue syndrome.

The cause is unknown, but aberrant perception of painful stimuli, sleep disorders, depression, and viral infections have all been proposed. Fibromyalgia can be a complication of hypothyroidism, rheumatoid arthritis or, in men, sleep apnea.

▶ Clinical Findings

The patient complains of chronic aching pain and stiffness, frequently involving the entire body but with prominence of pain around the neck, shoulders, low back, and hips. Fatigue, sleep disorders, subjective numbness, chronic headaches, and irritable bowel symptoms are common. Even minor exertion aggravates pain and increases fatigue. Physical examination is normal except for "trigger points" of pain produced by palpation of various areas such as the trapezius, the medial fat pad of the knee, and the lateral epicondyle of the elbow.

▶ Differential Diagnosis

Fibromyalgia is a diagnosis of exclusion. A detailed history and repeated physical examination can obviate the need for extensive laboratory testing. Rheumatoid arthritis and SLE present with objective physical findings or abnormalities on routine testing. Thyroid function tests are useful, since hypothyroidism can produce a secondary fibromyalgia syndrome. Polymyositis produces weakness rather than pain. The diagnosis of fibromyalgia probably should be made hesitantly in a patient over age 50 and should never be invoked to explain fever, weight loss, or any other objective signs. Polymyalgia rheumatica produces shoulder and pelvic girdle pain, is associated with anemia and an elevated ESR, and occurs after age 50. Hypophosphatemic states, such as oncogenic osteomalacia, can cause musculoskeletal pain unassociated with physical findings. In contrast to fibromyalgia, oncogenic osteomalacia usually produces pain in only a few areas and is associated with a low serum phosphate level.

▶ Treatment

A multidisciplinary approach is most effective. Patient education is essential. Patients can be comforted that they have a diagnosable syndrome treatable by specific though imperfect therapies and that the course is not progressive. Cognitive behavioral therapy, including programs that emphasize mindfulness meditation, is often helpful. The following medications have shown modest efficacy: amitriptyline, fluoxetine, duloxetine, milnacipran, chlorpromazine, cyclobenzaprine, pregabalin, or gabapentin. Amitriptyline is initiated at a dosage of 10 mg orally at bedtime and gradually increased to 40–50 mg depending on efficacy and toxicity. Less than 50% of the patients experience a sustained improvement. Exercise programs are also beneficial. NSAIDs are generally ineffective. Tramadol and acetaminophen combinations have ameliorated symptoms modestly in short-term trials. Opioids and corticosteroids are ineffective and should not be used to treat fibromyalgia. Acupuncture is also ineffective.

▶ Prognosis

All patients have chronic symptoms. With treatment, however, many do eventually resume increased activities. Progressive or objective findings do not develop.

Clauw DJ. Fibromyalgia and related conditions. Mayo Clin Proc. 2015 May;90(5):680–92. [PMID: 25939940]

Lichtenstein A et al. The complexities of fibromyalgia and its comorbidities. Curr Opin Rheumatol. 2018 Jan;30(1):94–100. [PMID: 29040155]

Welsch P et al. Serotonin and noradrenaline reuptake inhibitors (SNRIs) for fibromyalgia. Cochrane Database Syst Rev. 2018 Feb 28;2:CD010292. [PMID: 29489029]

COMPLEX REGIONAL PAIN SYNDROME

Complex regional pain syndrome (formerly called reflex sympathetic dystrophy) is a rare disorder of the extremities characterized by autonomic and vasomotor instability.

The cardinal symptoms and signs are pain localized to an arm or leg, swelling of the involved extremity, disturbances of color and temperature in the affected limb, dystrophic changes in the overlying skin and nails, and limited range of motion. Strikingly, the findings are not limited to the distribution of a single peripheral nerve. Most cases are preceded by surgery or direct physical trauma, often of a relatively minor nature, to the soft tissues, bone, or nerve. Early mobilization after injury or surgery reduces the likelihood of developing the syndrome. Any extremity can be involved, but the syndrome most commonly occurs in the hand and is associated with ipsilateral restriction of shoulder motion ("shoulder-hand" syndrome). This syndrome proceeds through phases: pain, swelling, and skin color and temperature changes develop early and, if untreated, lead to atrophy and dystrophy. The swelling in complex regional pain syndrome is diffuse ("catcher's mitt hand") and not restricted to joints. Pain is often burning in quality, intense, and often greatly worsened by minimal stimuli such as light touch. The shoulder-hand variant of this disorder sometimes complicates myocardial infarction or injuries to the neck or shoulder. Complex regional pain syndrome may occur after a knee injury or after arthroscopic knee surgery. There are no systemic symptoms. In the early phases of the syndrome, bone scans are sensitive, showing diffuse increased uptake in the affected extremity; radiographs eventually reveal severe generalized osteopenia. In the posttraumatic variant, this is known as Sudeck atrophy. Symptoms and findings are bilateral in some. This syndrome should be differentiated from other cervicobrachial pain syndromes, rheumatoid arthritis, thoracic outlet obstruction, and scleroderma, among others.

Early treatment offers the best prognosis for recovery. For mild cases, NSAIDs (eg, naproxen 250–500 mg twice daily orally) can be effective. For more severe cases associated with edema, prednisone, 30–60 mg/day orally for 2 weeks and then tapered over 2 weeks, can be effective. Pain management is important and facilitates physical therapy, which plays a critical role in efforts to restore function. Some patients will also benefit from antidepressant agents (eg, nortriptyline initiated at a dosage of 10 mg orally at bedtime and gradually increased to 40–75 mg at bedtime) or from anticonvulsants (eg, gabapentin 300 mg three times daily orally). Bisphosphonates, calcitonin, regional nerve blocks, and dorsal-column stimulation have also been reported to be helpful. Patients who have restricted shoulder motion may benefit from the treatment described for scapulohumeral periarthritis. The prognosis partly depends on the stage in which the lesions are encountered and the extent and severity of associated organic disease.

Petersen PB et al. Risk factors for post-treatment complex regional pain syndrome (CRPS): an analysis of 647 cases of CRPS from the Danish Patient Compensation Association. Pain Pract. 2018 Mar;18(3):341–9. [PMID: 28691184]

Tajerian M et al. New concepts in complex regional pain syndrome. Hand Clin. 2016 Feb;32(1):41–9. [PMID: 26611388]

Urits I et al. Complex regional pain syndrome, current concepts and treatment options. Curr Pain Headache Rep. 2018 Feb 5;22(2):10. [PMID: 29404787]

RHEUMATOLOGIC MANIFESTATIONS OF CANCER

Rheumatologic syndromes may be the presenting manifestations for a variety of cancers. Dermatomyositis in adults, for example, is often associated with cancer. Hypertrophic pulmonary osteoarthropathy, which is characterized by the triad of polyarthritis, new onset of clubbing, and periosteal new bone formation, is associated with both malignant diseases (eg, lung and intrathoracic cancers) and nonmalignant ones (eg, cyanotic heart disease, cirrhosis, and lung abscess). Cancer-associated polyarthritis is rare, has both oligoarticular and polyarticular forms, and should be considered when "seronegative rheumatoid arthritis" develops abruptly in an elderly patient. Palmar fasciitis manifests as bilateral palmar swelling with finger contractures and may be the first indication of cancer, particularly ovarian carcinoma. Remitting seronegative synovitis with non-pitting edema ("RS3PE") presents with a symmetric small-joint polyarthritis associated with non-pitting edema of the hands; it can be idiopathic or associated with malignancy. Palpable purpura due to leukocytoclastic vasculitis may be the presenting complaint in myeloproliferative disorders. Hairy cell leukemia can be associated with medium-sized vessel vasculitis such as polyarteritis nodosa. Acute leukemia can produce joint pains that are disproportionately severe in comparison to the minimal swelling and heat that are present. Leukemic arthritis complicates approximately 5% of cases. Rheumatic manifestations of myelodysplastic syndromes include cutaneous vasculitis, lupus-like syndromes, neuropathy, and episodic intense arthritis. Erythromelalgia, a painful warmth and redness of the extremities that (unlike Raynaud) improves with cold exposure or with elevation of the extremity, is often associated with myeloproliferative diseases, particularly essential thrombocythemia. The discovery that the immune response to various neoplasms can cause scleroderma, at least in a few patients, suggests the possibility that many autoimmune disorders may be caused by cancer immune surveillance. Cancer therapies, especially selective estrogen receptor modulators, aromatase inhibitors, and immune checkpoint inhibitors, can cause myalgia, arthralgia, arthritis, and autoimmune disorders.

Durieux V et al. Autoimmune paraneoplastic syndromes associated to lung cancer: a systematic review of the literature. Lung Cancer. 2017 Apr;106:102–9. [PMID: 28285683]

NEUROGENIC ARTHROPATHY (Charcot Joint)

Neurogenic arthropathy is joint destruction resulting from loss or diminution of proprioception, pain, and temperature perception. Although initially described in the knees of patients with tabes dorsalis, it is more frequently seen in association with diabetic neuropathy (foot and ankle) or syringomyelia (shoulder). As normal muscle tone and protective reflexes are lost, secondary degenerative joint disease ensues, resulting in an enlarged, boggy, relatively painless joint with extensive cartilage erosion, osteophyte formation, and multiple loose joint bodies. Radiographs can reveal striking osteolysis that mimics osteomyelitis or dramatic destruction of the joint with subluxation, fragmentation of bone, and bony sclerosis.

Treatment is directed toward the primary disease; mechanical devices are used to assist in weight bearing and prevention of further trauma. In some instances, amputation becomes unavoidable.

Shazadeh Safavi P et al. A systematic review of current surgical interventions for Charcot neuroarthropathy of the midfoot. J Foot Ankle Surg. 2017 Nov–Dec;56(6):1249–52. [PMID: 28778632]

PALINDROMIC RHEUMATISM

Palindromic rheumatism is a disease of unknown cause characterized by frequent recurring attacks (at irregular intervals) of acutely inflamed joints. Periarticular pain with swelling and transient subcutaneous nodules may also occur. The attacks cease within several hours to several days. The knee and finger joints are most commonly affected, but any peripheral joint may be involved. Systemic manifestations other than fever do not occur. Although hundreds of attacks may take place over a period of years, there is no permanent articular damage. Laboratory findings are usually normal. Palindromic rheumatism must be distinguished from acute gouty arthritis and an atypical acute onset of rheumatoid arthritis. In some patients, palindromic rheumatism is a prodrome of rheumatoid arthritis.

Symptomatic treatment with NSAIDs is usually all that is required during the attacks. Hydroxychloroquine may be of value in preventing recurrences.

OSTEONECROSIS
(Avascular Necrosis of Bone)

Osteonecrosis is a complication of corticosteroid use, alcoholism, trauma, SLE, pancreatitis, gout, sickle cell disease, dysbaric syndromes (eg, "the bends"), knee meniscectomy, and infiltrative diseases (eg, Gaucher disease). The most commonly affected sites are the proximal and distal femoral heads, leading to hip or knee pain. Other commonly affected sites include the ankle, shoulder, and elbow. Osteonecrosis of the jaw has been associated with use of bisphosphonate therapy, usually when the bisphosphonate is used for treating metastatic cancer or plasma cell myeloma rather than osteoporosis. Initially, radiographs are often normal; MRI, CT scan, and bone scan are all more sensitive techniques. Treatment involves avoidance of weight bearing on the affected joint for at least several weeks. The value of surgical core decompression is controversial. For osteonecrosis of the hip, a variety of procedures designed to preserve the femoral head have been developed for early disease, including vascularized and nonvascularized bone grafting procedures. These procedures are most effective in avoiding or forestalling the need for total hip arthroplasty in young patients who do not have advanced disease. Without a successful intervention of this nature, the natural history of avascular necrosis is usually progression of the bony infarction to cortical collapse, resulting in significant joint dysfunction. Total hip replacement is the usual outcome for all patients who are candidates for that procedure.

Chughtai M et al. An evidence-based guide to the treatment of osteonecrosis of the femoral head. Bone Joint J. 2017 Oct; 99-B(10):1267–79. [PMID: 28963146]

Hao YQ et al. Core decompression, lesion clearance and bone graft in combination with Tongluo Shenggu decoction for the treatment of osteonecrosis of the femoral head: a retrospective cohort study. Medicine (Baltimore). 2018 Oct;97(41): e12674. [PMID: 30313059]

Ruggiero SL. Diagnosis and staging of medication-related osteonecrosis of the jaw. Oral Maxillofac Surg Clin North Am. 2015 Nov;27(4):479–87. [PMID: 26293329]

ALLERGIC & IMMUNOLOGIC DISORDERS

Antoine Azar, MD

N. Franklin Adkinson Jr., MD

Allergy is an immunologically mediated hypersensitivity reaction to a foreign antigen manifested by tissue inflammation and organ dysfunction. The clinical expression of allergic disease depends on prior immunologic responsiveness, antigen exposure, and genetically influenced host factors such as atopy. Atopic patients have a genetically aggregated predisposition to a limited number of disorders: allergic rhinitis (Chapter 8), allergic asthma (Chapter 9), atopic dermatitis (Chapter 6), and IgE-mediated food allergies. Although these disorders tend to aggregate in families designated as "atopic," each of these disorders can occur in individuals without personal or familial history of an atopic diathesis. In addition, many mast cell and IgE-dependent disorders (eg, many drug and chemical sensitivities, eosinophilic disorders, mast cell stability syndromes, chronic urticaria) occur equally frequently in atopic and nonatopic persons.

The timing of the onset of clinical allergic syndromes after exposure to a suspected allergen serves as a useful clinical marker on which to base diagnosis and treatment. Reactions will usually be either *immediate* (generally occurring within 60 minutes after initial exposure), or *delayed*, appearing after many hours to days or weeks of antigen exposure.

IMMEDIATE HYPERSENSITIVITY

IgE antibodies occupy receptor sites on mast cells. Within minutes after exposure to the allergen, a multivalent antigen links adjacent IgE molecules, activating and degranulating mast cells. Clinical manifestations can be explained by the effects of released mediators on target end organs. Both preformed and newly generated mediators cause vasodilation and permeability changes, visceral smooth muscle contraction, mucous secretory gland stimulation, vascular permeability, and tissue inflammation. Arachidonic acid metabolites, cytokines, and other mediators (such as chemoattractants) induce a late-phase inflammatory response that appears several hours later in affected tissues when antigen exposure is continuous (eg, pollen) or chronic.

1. Anaphylaxis

General Considerations

Anaphylaxis is the most serious and potentially life-threatening manifestation of mast cell and basophil mediator release. Anaphylaxis is defined clinically under the following circumstances: (1) an allergen exposure followed by the acute onset of illness involving skin or mucosal tissue and either respiratory compromise or hypotension (systolic blood pressure less than 90 mm Hg or 30% less than known baseline); (2) a likely allergen exposure followed by the acute onset of two or more of the following conditions: skin or mucosal tissue involvement, respiratory compromise, hypotension, and persistent gastrointestinal symptoms; or (3) a known allergen exposure followed by hypotension.

IgE-dependent anaphylaxis is usually an acute syndrome initiated by a new allergen exposure after a prior silent exposure has sensitized the patient with IgE antibodies. Thus, anaphylaxis (or systemic allergic reactions which do not meet the definition of anaphylaxis) cannot occur on first-time exposure to allergens like drugs, insect venoms, latex, and foods. In contrast, other syndromes of anaphylaxis (sometimes called "anaphylactoid"), such as reactions to radiocontrast media and most NSAID and opioid reactions, is pseudoallergic without known immunologic mechanisms and can occur with first-time exposure.

Clinical Findings

A. Symptoms and Signs

Symptoms and signs typically occur within 30 minutes of initial exposure but may appear up to several hours later. These include (in order of frequency) (1) skin manifestations, typically urticaria but also flushing, blotchy rashes, and pruritus; (2) respiratory distress, including wheezing, stridor, bronchospasm, and airway angioedema; (3) gastrointestinal symptoms, including cramping, emesis, and diarrhea (especially in food allergy); and (4) hypotension, often manifested as lightheadedness, dizziness, or syncope. The condition is potentially fatal, especially if untreated, and can affect both nonatopic and atopic persons.

B. Laboratory Findings

Identification of anaphylaxis is clinical as the need for treatment is urgent. Elevated serum levels of mast cell mediators, such as tryptase and histamine, may be detected shortly after a reaction providing support to the diagnosis. Referral to an allergy specialist is standard because of concern for a future reaction and need for appropriate interventions and education. Specific IgE serum or skin testing may be performed to suspected allergens. Skin testing, which is usually more sensitive, optimally occurs 4–6 weeks after a severe reaction to avoid falsely negative testing during a post-reaction "refractory" period. The positive predictive value of these tests is highly dependent on a suggestive temporal relationship to putative allergen exposure.

Treatment

Early administration of intramuscular epinephrine at the onset of suspected anaphylaxis is the cornerstone of therapy. Supportive measures, such as oxygen, intravenous fluids and, if required, airway management are also appropriate. Adjunctive pharmacologic therapies include antihistamines, bronchodilators, and corticosteroids. Self-administered epinephrine at the earliest signs of recurrence can be life-sparing, whereas antihistamines and corticosteroids have limited value in reversing anaphylactic syndromes.

When to Refer

Patients with new or unexplained onset of anaphylaxis should be evaluated by an allergist.

Lieberman P et al. Anaphylaxis—a practice parameter update 2015. Ann Allergy Asthma Immunol. 2015 Nov;115(5): 341–84. [PMID: 26505932]
Muraro A et al; EAACI Food Allergy and Anaphylaxis Guidelines Group. Anaphylaxis: guidelines from the European Academy of Allergy and Clinical Immunology. Allergy. 2014 Aug;69(8):1026–45. [PMID: 24909803]
Williams KW et al. Anaphylaxis and urticaria. Immunol Allergy Clin North Am. 2015 Feb;35(1):199–219. [PMID: 25459585]

2. Food Allergy

Immediate allergic reactions within 2 hours of ingestion of foods are much less common among adults than children. Most acute systemic food allergy is caused by proteins in milk, egg, wheat, soy, fish, shellfish, peanuts, and tree nuts. Milk and egg allergies in atopic children are often outgrown by adulthood. Shellfish, peanuts, and tree nuts are the most common causes of food anaphylaxis in adults. Diagnosis of food allergy relies on a combination of history, skin tests, and serum specific IgE tests. There is no role for specific IgG testing for evaluating food hypersensitivity. Because of frequent false-positive IgE tests, especially among atopic patients, oral food challenge remains the gold standard for diagnosis. However, this procedure should only be conducted by an experienced provider in a well-equipped setting. Management involves strict avoidance of the culprit food and guaranteed access to self-administered epinephrine.

Other IgE-mediated food reactions include oral allergy syndrome and hypersensitivity to alpha-gal (galactose-alpha-1,3-galactose). Oral allergy syndrome, also known as pollen-associated food allergy syndrome, is the result of cross-reactivity between food and pollen proteins. Affected individuals have known seasonal pollen allergies (most commonly tree pollens) and experience itching of the oral mucosa upon ingestion of certain raw fruits and vegetables. In contrast to systemic food allergy, symptoms are limited to the oropharynx and usually do not involve other organ systems or progress to anaphylaxis.

Alpha-gal (galactose-alpha-1,3-galactose) is a carbohydrate found in red mammalian meats, including beef, pork and lamb but not in human tissues. Sensitization to this epitope has been linked to tick bites, so nonatopic individuals are at risk. In contrast to conventional systemic food allergy, the reaction to red meat typically occurs 4–6 hours after ingestion.

Kattan JD et al. Optimizing the diagnosis of food allergy. Immunol Allergy Clin North Am. 2015 Feb;35(1):61–76. [PMID: 25459577]

Muraro A et al. EAACI food allergy and anaphylaxis guidelines: diagnosis and management of food allergy. Allergy. 2014 Aug;69(8):1008–25. [PMID: 24909706]

3. Drug Allergy

Skin testing for immediate allergy to drugs is reliable for high molecular weight proteins (eg, cytokines, antisera, enzymes) but often not as reliable for low-molecular-weight compounds (eg, most drugs), which must bind to larger proteins (as haptens) to become immunogenic. With the exception of beta-lactam antibiotics like penicillins and some intraoperative drugs, in vivo skin testing for low-molecular-weight drugs is largely unvalidated, and interpretable only if the test is positive at a nonirritating concentration. Testing for IgE-mediated allergy to penicillin is available because the immunochemistry has been delineated and appropriate skin testing reagents are available. Skin testing with the major and minor metabolic determinants of penicillin has a very high (more than 98%) negative predictive value. Referral of individuals who relate histories of acute penicillin reactions to an allergist for skin testing is worthwhile because more than 90% have negative testing, indicating loss of allergic sensitization. Such patients may then safely receive penicillins and related antibiotics.

Chiriac AM et al. Drug allergy diagnosis. Immunol Allergy Clin North Am. 2014 Aug;34(3):461–7. [PMID: 25017672]

Kelso JM. Drug and vaccine allergy. Immunol Allergy Clin North Am. 2015 Feb;35(1):221–30. [PMID: 25459586]

Mirakian R et al; Standards of Care Committee of the British Society for Allergy and Clinical Immunology. Management of allergy to penicillins and other beta-lactams. Clin Exp Allergy. 2015 Feb;45(2):300–27. [PMID: 25623506]

4. Venom Allergy

The most common insects causing systemic allergic reactions include honeybees, vespids (yellow jackets, hornets, wasps), and fire ants. Systemic reactions often occur after several unremarkable stinging events and can develop at any age. Patients at highest risk for a severe reaction are those who have had a history of recent and severe reactions. The risk of a systemic reaction appears to decline over time since the last sting. If a systemic allergy is suspected, referral to an allergist for testing and, if appropriate, initiation of venom immunotherapy, is recommended. In the interim, making self-administrated epinephrine available is indicated for those with continuing exposure.

5. Pseudoallergic Reactions

Pseudoallergic (anaphylactoid) reactions (Table 20–13) resemble immediate hypersensitivity reactions but are not mediated by allergen-IgE interaction. Examples include radiocontrast reactions, opioid reactions (direct mast cell activation), and "red man syndrome" from rapid infusion of vancomycin. In contrast to IgE-mediated reactions, these can often be prevented by prophylactic medical regimens.

▶ Radiocontrast Media Reactions

Reactions to radiocontrast media are not IgE antibody–mediated, yet they are clinically similar to anaphylaxis and can be life-threatening. If a patient has had an anaphylactoid reaction to conventional radiocontrast media, the risk for a second reaction upon reexposure may be as high as 30%. Patients with a history of atopy are at increased risk.

Management includes use of low-osmolality contrast preparations and prophylactic administration of prednisone (50 mg orally every 6 hours beginning 13 hours before the procedure) and diphenhydramine (25–50 mg orally, intramuscularly or intravenously 60 minutes before the procedure). The use of lower-osmolality radiocontrast media in combination with the pretreatment regimen decreases the incidence of recurrent reactions to less than 1%.

Red Man Syndrome

Like radiocontrast media reactions, the "red man syndrome" (Table 20–13) results in anaphylactoid symptoms, especially flushing, pruritus, and erythema of the upper body. First described as a vancomycin infusion reaction, it is related to the rate of drug administration resulting in direct activation of mast cells. Management includes administration of an antihistamine such as diphenhydramine, 25–50 mg intravenously or intramuscularly, and reinitiation of the vancomycin infusion at no more than half the former rate. In patients who have previously experienced a vancomycin infusion reaction, premedication with an H_1-antagonist (eg, diphenhydramine) and H_2-antagonist (eg, cimetidine) is recommended 1 hour prior to the infusion. Although rare, IgE sensitization to vancomycin does occur and should be suspected in patients who have received multiple courses of the drug. Skin testing is helpful because vancomycin, as a "complete allergen," can elicit positive skin tests. Desensitization to vancomycin is possible for patients with positive skin tests and no acceptable alternative antibiotic.

Davis PL. Anaphylactoid reactions to the nonvascular administration of water-soluble iodinated contrast media. AJR Am J Roentgenol. 2015 Jun;204(6):1140–5. [PMID: 26001221]

6. Aspirin (NSAID) Exacerbated Respiratory Disease

Although aspirin (NSAID) hypersensitivity is a feature of this condition, the reaction is a result of aberrant arachidonic acid metabolism, rather than a product of an IgE-activated process. The inhibition of cyclooxygenase-1 (COX-1) by these anti-inflammatory drugs results in the overproduction of cysteinyl leukotrienes and increased expression of leukotriene receptors, leading to increased airway responsiveness, bronchospasm, rhinorrhea, and nasal congestion. Reactions outside of the respiratory system can also occur, including ocular, cutaneous, and gastric symptoms.

Table 20–13. Uncommon allergic and pseudoallergic conditions.

Disease	Pathogenesis	Symptoms and Signs	Diagnostic Findings[1]	Treatment
Allergic bronchopulmonary aspergillosis	Immunologic response to pulmonary fungal colonization	Often underlying moderate to severe allergic asthma and/or cystic fibrosis, with wheezing, cough productive of thick brown sputum, fever, weight loss, fatigue	**Elevated serum total IgE (> 1000 ng/mL); skin test positive to *Aspergillus*; positive *Aspergillus* precipitins,** eosinophilia (off corticosteroids) (total eosinophils > 1000 cells/mcL), pulmonary infiltrates, central bronchiectasis	Oral corticosteroids, antifungal (azole) agent
Hereditary angioedema	Quantitative or functional C1 esterase inhibitor deficiency, resulting in increased serum bradykinin levels	Unpredictable swelling of face, lips, tongue, hands, feet; no urticaria; gastrointestinal tract swelling causing severe abdominal pain	**Decreased C1 esterase inhibitor serum level and/or function,** decreased serum C4 level	Prophylactic treatment: Danazol, tranexamic acid Acute treatment: C1 esterase inhibitor product, kallikrein inhibitor, bradykinin receptor antagonist
Hypereosinophilic syndromes	Leukoproliferative disorder characterized by overproduction of eosinophils	Symptoms related to eosinophilic infiltration of organs: angioedema, urticaria, pruritic papules, chronic cough, splenomegaly, heart failure	**Eosinophilia (eosinophils > 1500 cells/mcL),** elevated serum vitamin B_{12} level, elevated serum tryptase level, anemia, PDGFRA gene mutation	Corticosteroids, tyrosine kinase inhibitors
Mastocytosis	Mast cell hyperplasia	Pruritus, flushing, nausea, vomiting, diarrhea, abdominal pain, hypotension	**Dense bone marrow mast cell infiltrate (≥ 15/hpf) on biopsy, elevated serum tryptase level (> 20 ng/mL),** atypical mast cell morphology, *cKIT* mutation	Antihistamine, cromolyn, epinephrine, chemotherapy directed at underlying mast cell hyperplasia
"Red man syndrome" (acute infusion reaction)	Direct activation of mast cells by vancomycin (opioids and other drugs)	Flushing, pruritus, and erythema, especially of the upper body, during intravenous infusion of drug	Clinical history and physical examination, no role for laboratory testing	Antihistamine pretreatment 1 hour prior to subsequent vancomycin (or opioid and other causative drug) infusions, decreased rate of infusion
Serum sickness (and serum sickness-like syndromes)	Mediated by circulating immune complexes	Fever, pruritic urticarial or maculopapular rash, lymphadenopathy, arthralgias, arthritis, nephritis	**Increased ESR, leukocytosis,** possible low serum C3 and C4 levels	Self-limited illness: NSAIDs, antihistamines Severe illness: Corticosteroids, plasma exchange

[1]Key diagnostic findings in bold.

cKIT, stem cell factor receptor or CD117; ESR, erythrocyte sedimentation rate; NSAID, nonsteroidal anti-inflammatory drug; PDGFRA, platelet-derived growth factor receptor alpha.

In addition to aspirin or NSAID sensitivity, patients with aspirin exacerbated respiratory disease typically have chronic rhinosinusitis with nasal polyps and asthma, a syndrome referred to as "Samter triad" or "triad asthma." Diagnosis is largely based on history and clinical findings. If required, a positive aspirin challenge can demonstrate the NSAID hypersensitivity, the presence of which may suggest increased responsiveness to treatments such as nasal polypectomy and aspirin desensitization. Patients who require daily aspirin or NSAID treatment can be desensitized to permit such treatment. Desensitization and long-term aspirin therapy have also been shown to reduce the need for nasal polypectomy and asthma therapy. Referral to an allergy specialist is appropriate for consideration of such desensitization.

Saff RR et al. Management of patients with nonaspirin-exacerbated respiratory disease aspirin hypersensitivity reactions. Allergy Asthma Proc. 2015 Jan–Feb;36(1):34–9. [PMID: 25562554]
Simon RA et al. Update on aspirin desensitization for chronic rhinosinusitis with polyps in aspirin-exacerbated respiratory disease (AERD). Curr Allergy Asthma Rep. 2015 Mar; 15(3):508. [PMID: 25663486]

ALLERGY TESTING

To maximize the positive predictive value of allergy testing, a positive test result must be correlated with the history. Patients selected for testing include those with moderate to severe disease, those who are potential candidates for allergen immunotherapy, and those with strong predisposing factors for atopic diatheses, eg, a strong family history of atopy or ongoing exposure to potential sources of allergen. Since the development of rhinitis precedes the presentation of asthma in over half of cases, early intervention may decrease the risk of more severe clinical illness. The type of immune response must be consistent with the nature of the disease. For example, IgE antibody causes allergic rhinitis but not allergic contact dermatitis. IgE antibodies are detected by in vivo (skin tests) or in vitro methods.

Adkinson NF Jr et al. Clinical history-driven diagnosis of allergic diseases: utilizing in vitro IgE testing. J Allergy Clin Immunol Pract. 2015 Nov–Dec;3(6):871–6. [PMID: 26553614]

DELAYED HYPERSENSITIVITY

According to the Gell and Coombs classification, type IV delayed hypersensitivity is mediated by activated T cells, which accumulate in areas of antigen deposition. A common example is allergic contact dermatitis, which develops when a low-molecular-weight sensitizing substance serves as a hapten for dermal proteins, becoming a complete antigen. Sensitized T cells release cytokines, activating macrophages and promoting subsequent dermal inflammation; this typically occurs 48–72 hours after contact. Another common expression of delayed hypersensitivity is drug allergy that occurs after a similar process and that often results in maculopapular or morbilliform exanthems. T-cell–mediated hypersensitivity is now understood to involve both Th1 and Th2 cells. In addition, subsequent inflammation and tissue damage occur via various effector cell types, including monocytes, eosinophils, and neutrophils.

1. Drug Exanthems

The clinical manifestation of these reactions is vast (Chapter 6), ranging from the commonly observed morbilliform rash to skin sloughing observed in Stevens-Johnson syndrome and toxic epidermal necrolysis. Given the range of cutaneous findings, the differential diagnosis is broad and includes miliaria, lichen planus, folliculitis, pityriasis rosea, tinea corporis, and mycosis fungoides. Physical examination of rash characteristics, dermatologic consultation, and biopsy findings can help narrow the differential. While a whole spectrum of drugs can result in exanthems, there are no commercially available laboratory or other diagnostic tests to reliably identify the culprit drug.

Management consists mainly of immediate cessation of suspected medications and monitoring for symptom resolution. Systemic corticosteroids may be indicated for extensive dermatitis or other organ involvement.

Martin SF. New concepts in cutaneous allergy. Contact Dermatitis. 2015 Jan;72(1):2–10. [PMID: 25348820]
Naisbitt DJ et al. In vitro diagnosis of delayed-type drug hypersensitivity: mechanistic aspects and unmet needs. Immunol Allergy Clin North Am. 2014 Aug;34(3):691–705. [PMID: 25017686]
Pavlos R et al. T cell-mediated hypersensitivity reactions to drugs. Annu Rev Med. 2015;66:439–54. [PMID: 25386935]

2. Drug-Induced Hypersensitivity Syndrome (Drug Reaction With Eosinophilia & Systemic Symptoms)

▶ General Considerations

Potentially life-threatening, systemic drug-induced hypersensitivity reactions most commonly occur with exposure to anticonvulsants and sulfonamides, although many other classes of drugs, including other antimicrobials and antidepressants, have been implicated. The onset of symptoms typically occurs 2–6 weeks after drug initiation. As suggested by its alternative name, drug reaction with eosinophilia and systemic symptoms (DRESS), it typically includes eosinophilia and/or lymphocytosis and systemic symptoms such as fever and lymph node enlargement, along with the rash. The exact pathogenesis of DRESS is not well elucidated but may include deficient drug metabolism due to genetic mutations in specific detoxification enzymes; reactivation of herpesviruses including HHV-6, HHV-7, cytomegalovirus, and Epstein-Barr virus; and a genetic predisposition based on the presence of specific HLA haplotypes.

HLA Haplotypes & Risk of Delayed-Onset Drug Hypersensitivity Syndromes

Activated cytotoxic CD8 T lymphocytes play a key role in the pathogenesis of serious, drug-induced adverse cutaneous reactions, such as toxic epidermal necrolysis. There are striking, medication-specific associations between inheritance of particular HLA-B alleles and risk of these hypersensitivity reactions in defined populations. Most notably, B*57:01 confers risk for reactions to abacavir; B*15:02, for carbamazepine; B*58:01, for allopurinol; and B*13:01, for dapsone. The most likely mechanism is a direct interaction between the drug and the antigen-binding cleft of the HLA-B molecule, such that many "self" antigens subsequently bound by the HLA-B molecule are perceived as "foreign," eliciting massive CD8 T-cell activation. Current FDA recommendations call for testing for the relevant HLA-B allele prior to initiating therapy with abacavir in all patients and with carbamazepine in Asian patients. The American College of Rheumatology recommends such testing before starting allopurinol therapy in patients of Korean descent, especially those with kidney disease, and Han Chinese and individuals of Thai extraction. Pretreatment HLA testing for other drugs or in other populations may not be useful at the present time due to low prevalence of the implicated isotypes.

Clinical Findings

A. Symptoms and Signs

Drug-induced hypersensitivity syndrome often begins with pruritus and fever, but cutaneous manifestations generally follow soon thereafter, most commonly an erythematous morbilliform rash. Although the entire skin surface can be involved, the face, trunk, and upper and lower extremities are commonly affected. The most common systemic findings involve the lymphatic (lymphadenopathy), hematologic and hepatic systems, although renal, pulmonary and cardiac involvement is also documented.

B. Laboratory Findings

Laboratory abnormalities include leukocytosis with eosinophilia (greater than 1.5×10^9/L) and atypical lymphocytosis; elevated hepatic transaminases (more than 2 times upper limits of normal) and alkaline phosphatase, and increased serum creatinine, pyuria, and proteinuria, which may indicate the development of interstitial nephritis. The most common skin biopsy findings are a dense, perivascular lymphocytic infiltrate in the papillary dermis with eosinophils and dermal edema.

Treatment

Management consists of cessation of the causative medication and initiation of systemic corticosteroids. A dose of 1.0 mg/kg of oral prednisone is recommended as a starting dose, followed by a gradual taper occurring over 3–6 months after laboratory normalization and stabilization. Additional supportive therapies may include antipyretics for fever, topical steroids for skin lesions, or fluid and electrolyte replacement in the case of more severe exfoliative dermatitis.

Cheng CY et al. HLA associations and clinical implications in T-cell mediated drug hypersensitivity reactions: an updated review. J Immunol Res. 2014;2014:565320. [PMID: 24901010]

Husain Z et al. DRESS syndrome: Part I. Clinical perspectives. J Am Acad Dermatol. 2013 May;68(5):693.e1–14. [PMID: 23602182]

Husain Z et al. DRESS syndrome: Part II. Management and therapeutics. J Am Acad Dermatol. 2013 May;68(5):709.e1–9. [PMID: 23602183]

Schwartz RA et al. Toxic epidermal necrolysis. Part I. Introduction, history, classification, clinical diagnosis, systemic manifestations, etiology, and immunopathogenesis. J Am Acad Dermatol. 2013 Aug;69(2):173.e1–13. [PMID: 23866878]

PRIMARY IMMUNODEFICIENCY DISORDERS IN ADULTS

Primary immunologic deficiency diseases are estimated to affect 1 in 4000 individuals; many are genetically determined and present in childhood. Nonetheless, several important immunodeficiency disorders present in adulthood, most notably the antibody deficiency syndromes: selective IgA deficiency, common variable immunodeficiency, and specific (functional) antibody deficiency (Table 20–14). Antibody deficiency predisposes patients to recurrent infections, particularly of the respiratory tract, including refractory chronic rhinosinusitis, bronchitis, pneumonia, and bronchiectasis. Patients are most susceptible to infections with encapsulated bacteria (eg, *Haemophilus influenzae*, *Streptococcus pneumoniae*, *Neisseria meningitides*). However, any part of the innate or adaptive immune system can be defective and results in infections with different spectra of organisms.

1. Selective Immunoglobulin A Deficiency

Selective IgA deficiency is the most common primary immunodeficiency disorder and is characterized by undetectable serum IgA levels (lower than 7 mg/dL) with normal levels of IgG and IgM; its prevalence is about 1 in 500 individuals (Table 20–14). Most affected individuals are asymptomatic. A minority of patients have recurrent infections such as sinusitis, otitis, and bronchitis. Selective IgA deficiency can be associated with atopic diseases and autoimmune disorders, including Graves disease, SLE, juvenile rheumatoid arthritis, type 1 diabetes mellitus, and celiac disease.

Some individuals with undetectable levels of serum IgA may have high titers of anti-IgA antibodies and are at risk for anaphylactic reactions to IgA following exposure to it through infusions of plasma (or blood transfusions). Treatment with commercial immune globulin is not indicated and may very rarely result in anaphylactic reactions.

When to Refer

• Refer patients with anaphylaxis following infusions of plasma (or blood transfusions) to an immunologist for further evaluation of possible IgA deficiency.

Table 20–14. Selected immunodeficiency syndromes.

Disease	Clinical Presentation	Diagnosis[1]	Treatment
Common variable immunodeficiency	Most common symptomatic primary immunodeficiency disorder Recurrent sinopulmonary infections, parasitic (especially *Giardia lamblia*) gastrointestinal infections, autoimmune diseases, and increased risk of malignancy	**Low serum IgG,** low serum IgA and/or IgM; **poor antibody response to immunizations;** exclusion of secondary causes of hypogammaglobulinemia	Subcutaneous or intravenous immunoglobulins Prophylactic antibiotics
Selective IgA deficiency	Most prevalent primary immunodeficiency; most cases asymptomatic; recurrent sinopulmonary infections; atopic disorders, rheumatoid arthritis and systemic lupus erythematosus common; rarely, anaphylaxis to transfusion of blood or blood products	**Undetectable serum IgA** levels (< 7 mg/dL), normal serum IgG and IgM levels	Early use of antibiotics for bacterial infections Prophylactic antibiotics for symptomatic patients with recurrent infections
Adult T-cell deficiencies	Opportunistic infections (similar to HIV); eg, CMV, EBV, other herpes viruses, mycobacteria, and fungi (*Candida, Cryptococcus, Pneumocystis*)	Exclude HIV infection; obtain CD4 and CD8 T-cell counts, and in vitro T-cell function	Antibiotics; some patients are candidates for bone marrow transplantation
Complement disorders	"Early" complement component deficiencies: autoimmune diseases "Late" complement component (C5–C8) deficiencies: recurrent meningococcal or gonococcal infections	Screen with CH50 and AH50. Obtain individual serum complement levels if abnormal	Prompt administration of antibiotics
Granulocyte disorders	Recurrent invasive skin and soft tissue infections, abscesses requiring incision and drainage Common organisms are *S aureus*, gram-negative bacilli, *Nocardia, Aspergillus*	CBC with differential to evaluate neutrophil count Dihydrorhodamine assay to evaluate neutrophil oxidative burst	Antimicrobial prophylaxis; interferon in patients with chronic granulomatous disease

[1]Key diagnostic findings in bold.
CMV, cytomegalovirus; EBV, Epstein-Barr virus.
Modified, with permission, from Ashar B, Miller R, Sisson S (editors): *Johns Hopkins Internal Medicine Board Review Certification and Recertification*, 5th ed. © Elsevier, 2015.

- Refer patients with undetectable serum IgA and recurrent sinopulmonary infections, celiac disease, giardiasis, or a family history of immunodeficiency to an immunologist.

Bonilla FA et al. Practice parameter for the diagnosis and management of primary immunodeficiency. J Allergy Clin Immunol. 2015 Nov;136(5):1186–205. [PMID: 26371839]
Singh K et al. IgA deficiency and autoimmunity. Autoimmun Rev. 2014 Feb;13(2):163–77. [PMID: 24157629]

2. Common Variable Immunodeficiency

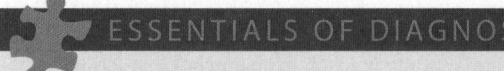

ESSENTIALS OF DIAGNOSIS

▶ Frequent sinopulmonary infections secondary to humoral immune deficiency.

▶ Low serum immunoglobulin levels and deficient functional antibody responses.

▶ Primary defect may be with B cells or T cells.

▶ General Considerations

The most common symptomatic primary immunodeficiency disorder is common variable immunodeficiency, a heterogeneous immunodeficiency disorder clinically characterized by an increased incidence of recurrent infections, autoimmune phenomena, and neoplastic diseases. The onset is generally in early adulthood but it can occur at any age. The prevalence of common variable immunodeficiency is about 1 in 25,000 in the United States. Most cases are sporadic; about 10–20% are familial.

▶ Clinical Findings

A. Symptoms and Signs

Increased susceptibility to infections, especially with encapsulated organisms, is the hallmark of the disease. Virtually all patients suffer from recurrent sinusitis; bronchitis, otitis, pharyngitis, and pneumonia are common infections. Infections may be prolonged or associated with unusual complications such as meningitis or sepsis.

Gastrointestinal infections and dysfunction are commonly associated with common variable immunodeficiency, and a sprue-like syndrome, with diarrhea, steatorrhea, malabsorption, protein-losing enteropathy, and hepatosplenomegaly, may develop in patients. Paradoxically, there is an increased incidence of autoimmune disease (20%), although patients may not display the usual serologic markers. Autoimmune cytopenias are most common, but autoimmune endocrinopathies, seronegative rheumatic disease, and gastrointestinal disorders are also commonly seen. Lymph nodes may be enlarged in these patients, yet biopsies show marked reduction in plasma cells. Noncaseating granulomas are frequently found in the spleen, liver, lungs, or skin. There is an increased propensity for the development of B-cell neoplasms (50- to 400-fold increased risk of lymphoma), and gastric carcinomas. Chronic lung disease is one of the most common complications of common variable immunodeficiency.

B. Laboratory Findings

Assess serum quantitative immunoglobulin levels. All patients with common variable immunodeficiency have a reduced serum IgG level, either serum IgM or IgA or both are reduced as well. Demonstration of functional or quantitative defects in antibody production is essential and is typically performed by checking antibody response to polysaccharide (Pneumovax) and protein antigens (such as tetanus and diphtheria). The diagnosis is made in patients who have reduced serum immunoglobulins and poor antibody response to vaccines, after exclusion of secondary causes (eg, proteinuria, protein-losing enteropathy, drug effects such as rituximab, antiepileptics, chronic lymphocytic leukemia, lymphoma, and plasma cell myeloma).

The absolute B-cell count in the peripheral blood in most patients, despite the underlying cellular defect, is normal. A subset of these patients has concomitant T-cell immunodeficiency with increased numbers of activated CD8 cells, splenomegaly, and decreased delayed-type hypersensitivity.

▶ Treatment

Patients with common variable immunodeficiency should be treated aggressively with antibiotics at the first sign of infection. Since antibody deficiency predisposes patients to high-risk pyogenic infections, antibiotic coverage should be sure to cover encapsulated bacteria. Infections with other microorganisms also can develop, including viruses, parasites, and extracellular gram-positive or gram-negative bacteria (such as *S aureus* or *P aeruginosa*). Mainstay of preventive therapy is with subcutaneous or intravenous immunoglobulin replacement therapy, typically provided every 1–4 weeks, with a typical monthly dose of 300–600 mg/kg. Subcutaneous injections of IgG offer the convenience of self-administration at home and lower incidence of adverse effects. Adjustment of the dosage or infusion interval is made primarily on the basis of clinical responses, in addition to serum IgG levels. Such therapy is essential for decreasing the incidence of potentially life-threatening infections, increasing quality of life, and reducing the progression of lung disease.

▶ When to Refer

- Refer patients with low serum immunoglobulins and history of recurrent or unusual infections, autoimmune disease, or family history of immunodeficiency.

- The presence of bronchiectasis without a known underlying cause such as cystic fibrosis should raise the suspicion of a primary immunodeficiency; even when serum immunoglobulins are normal, the patient can have a specific antibody deficiency that would warrant further evaluation.

3. Specific (Functional) Antibody Deficiency

Specific antibody deficiency is characterized by decreased or absent IgG antibody response to vaccines in the setting of normal or mildly decreased serum immunoglobulin levels. The clinical spectrum can range from mild to severe with features very similar to common variable immunodeficiency.

Bonilla FA et al; Joint Task Force on Practice Parameters, representing the American Academy of Allergy, Asthma & Immunology; the American College of Allergy, Asthma & Immunology; and the Joint Council of Allergy, Asthma & Immunology. Practice parameter for the diagnosis and management of primary immunodeficiency. J Allergy Clin Immunol. 2015 Nov;136(5):1186–205.e1–78. [PMID: 26371839]

Gathmann B et al; European Society for Immunodeficiencies Registry Working Party. Clinical picture and treatment of 2212 patients with common variable immunodeficiency. J Allergy Clin Immunol. 2014 Jul;134(1):116–26. [PMID: 24582312]

Kashani S et al. Clinical characteristics of adults with chronic rhinosinusitis and specific antibody deficiency. J Allergy Clin Immunol Pract. 2015 Mar–Apr;3(2):236–42. [PMID: 25609325]

Wall LA et al. Specific antibody deficiencies. Immunol Allergy Clin North Am. 2015 Nov;35(4):659–70. [PMID: 26454312]

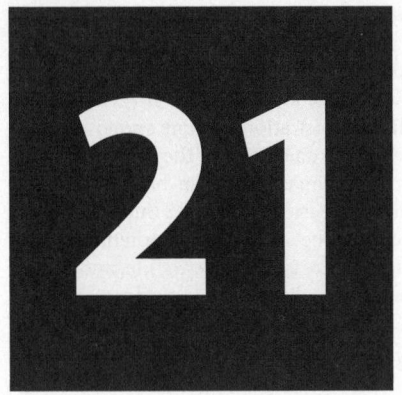

21

Electrolyte & Acid-Base Disorders

Naomi B. Anker, MD

Kerry C. Cho, MD

ASSESSMENT OF THE PATIENT

The diagnosis and treatment of fluid and electrolyte disorders are based on (1) careful history, (2) physical examination and assessment of total body water and its distribution, (3) serum osmolality and electrolyte concentrations, and (4) urine osmolality and electrolyte concentrations.

A. Body Water and Fluid Distribution

Total body water is different in men than in women, and it decreases with age (Table 21–1). Among adults, approximately 40–60% of body weight is water. Fat has a lower water content than muscle; individuals with more fat have a lower ratio of total body water to body weight. Two-thirds of total body water is intracellular, while one-third is extracellular. Only one-fourth of extracellular fluid (ECF) (or approximately 5% of body weight) is intravascular. Total body water content fluctuates and acute changes can be evaluated clinically by measuring changes in body weight.

B. Serum Electrolytes

The cause of electrolyte disorders may be determined by reviewing the history, underlying diseases, and medications, though further diagnostic tests, most often blood or urine laboratory tests, are often required.

C. Evaluation of Urine

The urine concentration of an electrolyte can be helpful in determining whether the kidney is appropriately (or inappropriately) excreting or retaining an electrolyte in response to high or low serum levels. A 24-hour urine collection for daily electrolyte excretion is the gold standard

Table 21–1. Approximate total body water (as percentage of body weight) in relation to age and sex.

Age	Male	Female
Young and middle aged adults	60%	50%
Older adults	50%	45%

for renal electrolyte handling, but it is slow and can be challenging to perform correctly. A more convenient method is the fractional excretion (Fe) of an electrolyte X (Fe_x) calculated from a spot urine sample:

$$FE_x\ (\%) = [(Ux/Sx)/(UCr/SCr)] \times 100$$
$$= [(Ux \times SCr)/(Sx \times UCr)] \times 100$$

A low fractional excretion indicates renal reabsorption (high avidity or electrolyte retention), while a high fractional excretion indicates renal wasting (low avidity or electrolyte excretion). Thus, the fractional excretion can often help the clinician determine whether the kidney's response is appropriate for a specific electrolyte disorder.

D. Serum Osmolality

Solute concentration is measured by osmolality in millimoles per kilogram. Osmolarity is measured in millimoles of solute per liter of solution. At physiologic solute concentrations (normally 285–295 mmol/kg), the two measurements are clinically interchangeable. Tonicity refers to osmolytes that are impermeable to cell membranes. Differences in tonicity across cell membranes lead to osmosis (shift of water across the cell membrane from an area of higher tonicity to one of lower tonicity). Substances that easily permeate cell membranes (eg, urea and ethanol) do not contribute to tonicity and thus do not cause water shifts across fluid compartments. These substances are sometimes called "ineffective osmoles."

Serum osmolality (Osm) can be estimated using the following formula:

$$Osm = 2(Na^+\ mEq/L) + \frac{Glucose\ mg/dL}{18} + \frac{BUN\ mg/dL}{2.8}$$

(1 mOsm/L of glucose equals 180 mg/L or 18 mg/dL and 1 mOsm/L of urea nitrogen equals 28 mg/L or 2.8 mg/dL).

Sodium is the major extracellular cation; doubling the serum sodium in the formula for estimated osmolality accounts for counterbalancing anions. A discrepancy between measured and estimated osmolality of more than 10 mmol/kg is referred to as an osmolal gap. An osmolal gap suggests the presence of unmeasured osmoles such as ethanol, methanol, ethylene glycol, mannitol, propylene glycol, and isopropanol.

DISORDERS OF SODIUM CONCENTRATION

HYPONATREMIA

 ESSENTIALS OF DIAGNOSIS

► Thorough history and volume status examination are essential to determine etiology.

► Hyponatremia reflects excess water relative to sodium; total body sodium may be appropriate, low, or high.

► Hypotonic fluids commonly contribute to hyponatremia in hospitalized patients.

► General Considerations

Defined as a serum sodium concentration less than 135 mEq/L (135 mmol/L), hyponatremia is the most common electrolyte abnormality in hospitalized patients. Hyponatremia can be subclassified as mild (130–134 mEq/L), moderate (125–129 mEq/L), or severe (below 125 mEq/L).

A common misconception is that the sodium concentration is a reflection of total body sodium. In fact, total body sodium can be low, normal, or high in hyponatremia since the kidney independently regulates sodium and water homeostasis. Hyponatremia reflects water imbalance relative to sodium, which frequently, but not always, is secondary to elevated levels of antidiuretic hormone (ADH), causing the kidney to retain water. A diagnostic algorithm using serum osmolality and volume status separates the causes of hyponatremia into therapeutically useful categories (Figure 21–1).

► Etiology

A. Isotonic and Hypertonic Hyponatremia

Serum osmolality identifies isotonic and hypertonic hyponatremia, although these cases can often be identified by careful history or previous laboratory tests.

Isotonic hyponatremia, also called pseudohyponatremia, is a laboratory artifact that can cause the sodium concentration to be underestimated in the setting of an abnormally elevated percentage of serum that is solid rather than liquid, such as with hyperlipidemia or hyperproteinemia. Pseudohyponatremia does not occur if the serum sodium is measured with an ion-specific electrode in a direct assay of an undiluted serum specimen.

Hypertonic hyponatremia, also called translocational hyponatremia, occurs when a large amount of a substance that cannot easily cross the cell membrane is added to the ECF compartment. This change in tonicity "pulls" intracellular water into the ECF and dilutes the sodium concentration. Classic examples of this phenomenon are hyperglycemia and iatrogenic mannitol. Hypertonic hyponatremia is not a disorder of sodium or water; rather, it is water redistributing in response to a change in tonicity. When the offending substance is cleared (for example when the hyperglycemia is treated), the ECF tonicity decreases and water shifts back into the intracellular space. Occasionally, hyponatremia is misidentified as hypertonic hyponatremia because the serum osmolality is elevated. However, the substance raising the serum osmolality is an ineffective osmole. For example, in kidney disease, the calculated osmolality may be elevated because of high urea levels. The urea, however, moves freely in and out of cells, and it does not contribute to tonicity or cause translocational hyponatremia.

For hypertonic hyponatremia from hyperglycemia, it is useful to estimate what the sodium concentration would be if the hyperglycemia resolved in order to evaluate the underlying sodium and water balance. Some experts recommend a single correction factor, wherein the serum sodium concentration decreases by 1.6 mEq/L (or 1.6 mmol/L) for every 100 mg/dL (5.56 mmol/L) rise in plasma glucose above normal. Other experts advocate correction factors as high as 2.4 mEq/L per 100 mg/dL.

B. Hypotonic Hyponatremia

Most cases of hyponatremia are hypotonic, highlighting sodium's role as the predominant extracellular osmole. Many causes of hypotonic hyponatremia relate to either appropriate or inappropriate ADH secretion. Normally, the pituitary gland secretes ADH when the osmolality increases or there is substantially low effective arterial blood volume. ADH promotes water reabsorption in the distal nephron, thus minimizing urinary water losses. Clinically, volume status is a useful way to categorize hypotonic hyponatremia (Figure 21–1).

1. Hypovolemic hypotonic hyponatremia—Hypovolemic hyponatremia occurs with renal or extrarenal volume loss and hypotonic fluid replacement. Total body sodium and total body water are decreased. To maintain intravascular volume, the pituitary increases ADH secretion, causing free water retention from the hypotonic fluid replacement. The body sacrifices serum osmolality to preserve intravascular volume. In short, losses of water and salt are replaced, at least in part, by water alone. Urine sodium can be a clue as to whether volume losses are more likely renal (U_{Na} greater than 20 mEq/L) or extrarenal (U_{Na} below 10 mEq/L), though urinary sodium excretion also depends on sodium and fluid intake.

Cerebral salt wasting has been described as a distinct and rare subset of hypovolemic hyponatremia seen in patients with intracranial disease (eg, hemorrhage, infections, cerebrovascular accidents, tumors, and neurosurgery). Presenting features include hypotonic hyponatremia with hypovolemia and renal salt wasting. Clinically, it can be challenging to differentiate from syndrome of inappropriate ADH (SIADH) (discussed below), which is much more common among those with neurologic injury and hyponatremia.

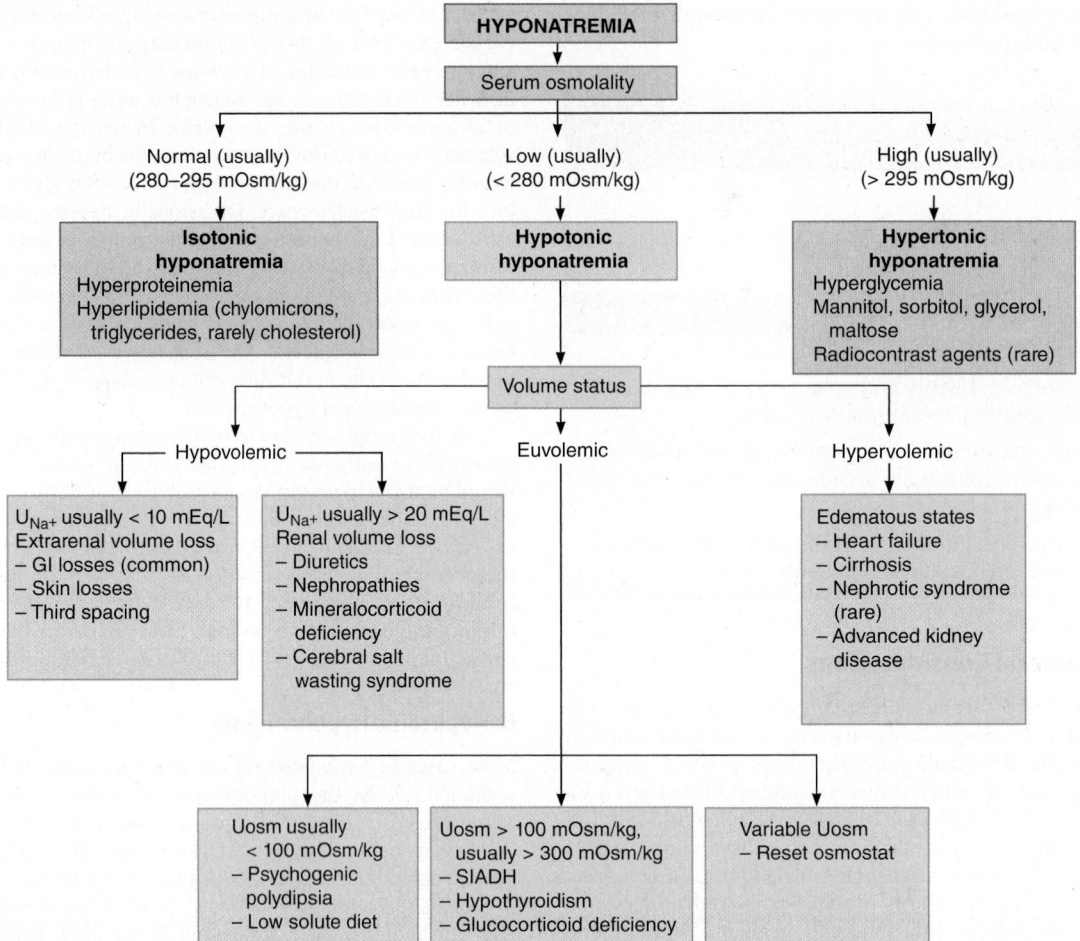

▲ **Figure 21–1.** Evaluation of hyponatremia using serum osmolality and extracellular fluid volume status. GI, gastrointestinal; SIADH, syndrome of inappropriate antidiuretic hormone; Uosm, urine osmolality. (Modified, with permission, from Narins RG et al. Diagnostic strategies in disorders of fluid, electrolyte and acid-base homeostasis. Am J Med. 1982 Mar;72(3):496–520. Copyright © Elsevier.)

2. Euvolemic hypotonic hyponatremia—Euvolemic hyponatremia has the broadest differential diagnosis. Diseases in this category are often divided into those with a high urine osmolality and those with a low urine osmolality. Reset osmostat is a relatively uncommon cause of (generally mild) euvolemic hypotonic hyponatremia and has variable urine osmolality.

A. Syndrome of inappropriate antidiuretic hormone secretion—SIADH is a common cause of euvolemic hypotonic hyponatremia, particularly among hospitalized patients. ADH is generally secreted in response to hyperosmolality or very low effective arterial blood volume, but many conditions and medications can lead to ADH secretion in the absence of these physiologic stimuli (ie, ADH secretion is inappropriate). In SIADH, there is a nonphysiologic ADH secretion, which means that water is inappropriately retained leading to relatively concentrated urine (urine osmolality is usually greater than 300 mOsm/kg). Urinary solute handling remains preserved; thus, urine sodium

is generally not low (U_{Na} greater than 20 mEq/L), although it will depend on dietary ingestion of sodium. Conditions associated with SIADH (Table 21–2) include CNS disorders, pulmonary disorders, and malignancies. Some common symptoms, such as pain and nausea, stimulate ADH release.

B. Hormonal abnormalities—Severe hypothyroidism and glucocorticoid insufficiency can cause hyponatremia that cannot be differentiated from SIADH by urine or serum electrolytes alone. These disorders can generally be identified by testing hormone levels.

C. Psychogenic polydipsia and low solute diet—Water balance in euvolemic people depends on water intake, solute intake, and renal diluting capacity. Marked free water intake relative to solute intake produces hyponatremia. Among euvolemic people who have normal serum osmolality, solute and water excretion approximate solute and water intake. The maximal urine dilution in healthy adults is about 50 mOsm/kg. Because even maximally dilute

Table 21–2. Common causes of syndrome of inappropriate ADH secretion (SIADH).

Central nervous system disorders
  Brain tumor
  Encephalitis
  Guillain-Barré syndrome
  Head trauma
  Hydrocephalus
  Meningitis
  Psychosis, acute
  Stroke
  Subarachnoid hemorrhage
Pulmonary lesions
  Pneumonia, including fungal and mycobacterial
  Other intrathoracic infections
  Neoplasms
  Respiratory failure or positive pressure ventilation or both
Malignancies
  Small cell carcinoma of the lung
  Other small cell carcinomas
  Pituitary tumors, craniopharyngioma
  Squamous cell cancers of the head and neck
  Most other malignancies have been reported to cause SIADH
    but are uncommon
Drugs
  Antidepressants: tricyclics, SSRIs, monoamine oxidase inhibitors
  Antineoplastics: cyclophosphamide, vincristine, vinblastine
  Carbamazepine, oxcarbamazepine
  Clofibrate
  Desmopressin (DDAVP), vasopressin (ADH)
  Methylenedioxymethamphetamine (MDMA; Ecstasy)
  Antipsychotics, typicals more often than atypicals
  Amiodarone
  Chlorpropamide, tolbutamide
  NSAIDs (rare without another concomitant etiology)
Others
  Acute intermittent porphyria
  AIDS
  Hereditary
  Nausea
  Pain
  Postoperative
  Stress

ADH, antidiuretic hormone; NSAIDs, nonsteroidal anti-inflammatory drugs; SSRIs, selective serotonin reuptake inhibitors.

urine has an obligate solute concentration, there is a maximal amount of water a healthy person can drink before becoming hyponatremic, even if ADH is appropriately suppressed. This maximal amount of water depends on the solute intake (the more solute that is taken in, the more water that can be ingested and excreted successfully). In psychogenic polydipsia, patients generally ingest a normal amount of solute and have normal kidney function. However, when water intake exceeds 10–15 L/day, even normally functioning kidneys with a normal amount of solute to excrete begin to retain water because the kidney cannot excrete pure free water. Patients with low solute intake or those who cannot dilute their urine osmolality to 50 mOsm/kg become hyponatremic with less water intake.

With a low solute diet (sometimes called "beer potomania" or "tea and toast diet"), a patient's daily water intake may be

less than 10 L. However, the maximal amount of free water these patients can ingest before becoming hyponatremic is lower because the kidney cannot excrete water that is devoid of solute.

Patients with significant chronic kidney disease (CKD) may not be able to dilute their urine to 50 mOsm/kg. Rather, their maximally dilute urine may be as high as 100–250 mOsm/kg even if ADH is maximally suppressed. Therefore, a relatively modest increase in water intake or decrease in solute intake can result in hyponatremia when there is impaired ability to dilute urine.

D. Reset osmostat—Reset osmostat is a rare cause of hyponatremia characterized by appropriate ADH regulation in response to water deprivation and fluid challenges. Patients with reset osmostat regulate serum sodium and serum osmolality around a lower set point, concentrating or diluting urine in response to hyperosmolality and hypoosmolality. The mild hypoosmolality of pregnancy is a form of reset osmostat.

E. Thiazide diuretics—Thiazides can induce severe hyponatremia in a small percentage of patients who clinically appear hypovolemic or euvolemic. The mechanism is likely more complex than volume contraction leading to ADH secretion, since thiazides generally do not produce substantial volume losses. Loop diuretics do not cause hyponatremia as frequently likely because loop diuretics impair urinary concentrating ability by reducing the medullary concentrating gradient.

F. Exercise-associated hyponatremia—Hyponatremia after exercise, especially endurance events such as triathlons and marathons, is generally thought to be a combination of excessive hypotonic fluid intake and inappropriate ADH secretion. Endurance athletes should drink water according to thirst rather than according to specified hourly rates of fluid intake. Specific universal recommendations for fluid replacement rates are not possible given the variability of sweat production, renal water excretion, and environmental conditions. Electrolyte-containing sport drinks do not protect against hyponatremia since they are markedly hypotonic relative to serum.

G. Other causes—Use of 3,4-methylenedioxymethamphetamine (MDMA, also known as Ecstasy) can lead to hyponatremia and severe neurologic symptoms, including seizures, cerebral edema, and brainstem herniation. MDMA and its metabolites increase ADH release from the hypothalamus. Primary polydipsia may contribute to hyponatremia since MDMA users typically increase fluid intake while intoxicated.

3. Hypervolemic hypotonic hyponatremia—Hypervolemic hyponatremia occurs in cirrhosis, heart failure, nephrotic syndrome, and advanced kidney disease (Figure 21–1). In cirrhosis and heart failure, effective arterial blood volume is decreased due to peripheral vasodilation or decreased cardiac output. Increased ADH secretion, secondary to low effective arterial blood volume, results in water retention. Note the pathophysiologic similarity to hypovolemic hyponatremia: The body sacrifices osmolality in an attempt to restore effective arterial blood volume.

Clinical Findings

A. Symptoms and Signs

Whether hypotonic hyponatremia is symptomatic depends on its severity and acuity. The symptoms of hypotonicity are mainly neurologic and relate to brain edema. Chronic hyponatremia can be severe yet remarkably asymptomatic because the brain has adapted by decreasing its tonicity over weeks to months. Acute disease that has developed over hours to days can be severely symptomatic with relatively modest hyponatremia. Mild hyponatremia (sodium concentrations of 130–135 mEq/L) is usually asymptomatic, though it has been linked to gait disturbances, falls, and fractures. Mild symptoms of nausea and malaise progress to headache, lethargy, and disorientation as the sodium concentration drops. The most serious symptoms are seizure and, very rarely, coma, brainstem herniation, and death.

Evaluation starts with a careful history for new medications and changes in fluid and solute intake (polydipsia, anorexia, intravenous fluid rates and composition) and fluid output (vomiting, diarrhea, ostomy output, polyuria, oliguria, insensible losses). The physical examination should help categorize the patient's volume status into hypovolemia, euvolemia, or hypervolemia.

B. Laboratory Findings

Laboratory assessment should include serum electrolytes, creatinine, and osmolality as well as urine sodium, potassium, and osmolality. The etiology of most cases of hyponatremia will be apparent from the history, physical, and basic laboratory tests. Additional tests of thyroid and adrenal function will occasionally be necessary.

SIADH is a clinical diagnosis. Classically, it is characterized by (1) hypotonic hyponatremia; (2) absence of heart, kidney, or liver disease; (3) normal thyroid and adrenal function (see Chapter 26); and (4) urine sodium usually over 20 mEq/L. In clinical practice, ADH levels are not measured. Patients with SIADH may or may not have low blood urea nitrogen (BUN) (less than 5–10 mg/dL) and hypouricemia (less than 4 mg/dL), which are thought to result from increased urea and uric acid clearance. Elevated BUN may reflect volume contraction, which if present, would need to be corrected before an additional etiology of hyponatremia (eg, SIADH) could be diagnosed.

Complications

Overly rapid correction of hypotonic hyponatremia, particularly severe chronic hypotonic hyponatremia, can cause cerebral osmotic demyelination syndrome. Osmotic demyelination syndrome symptoms generally present several days after the rapid sodium correction. While a variety of neurologic symptoms can occur, the classic presentation altered mental status, quadriparesis, and pseudobulbar symptoms that develop within a few days of rapid sodium correction. Risk factors for osmotic demyelination syndrome include serum sodium less than 120 mEq/L, malnourishment, and liver disease. Symptoms may be reversible or permanent. Diagnosis can be confirmed with MRI, though MRI findings may occasionally be delayed so

a normal MRI in the acute setting does not entirely exclude osmotic demyelination syndrome.

Treatment

Pseudohyponatremia from hypertriglyceridemia or hyperproteinemia requires no therapy directed toward the hyponatremia except confirmation with the clinical laboratory. **Translocational hyponatremia** from glucose or mannitol can be managed with hyperglycemia treatment or mannitol discontinuation. Rapid reduction in serum osmolality associated with correction of substantial hyperglycemia may cause cerebral edema and many authors recommend that this potential complication be considered when selecting fluids for treatment of severe hyperglycemia.

Mild to moderate **hypotonic hyponatremia** is generally treated according to the presumed etiology. Regardless of etiology, experts generally recommend correction rates for chronic hypotonic hyponatremia of 4–6 mEq/L/24 h and no more than 6–8 mEq/L/24 h. Slow correction in chronic hyponatremia is intended to avoid rapid shifts that may lead to osmotic demyelination syndrome. **Acute hyponatremia,** for example postoperative hyponatremia, can be corrected quickly. Symptomatic and severe hypotonic hyponatremia are discussed separately below.

Hypovolemic hyponatremic patients require adequate fluid resuscitation, usually with isotonic fluid, to suppress the hypovolemic stimulus for ADH release. Diuretics should be withheld in hypovolemic patients and the underlying etiology of volume depletion addressed. Patients believed to have cerebral salt wasting may benefit from hypertonic saline (with close monitoring) since this obviates the need to distinguish between cerebral salt wasting and SIADH when neurologic catastrophe have occurred and when obtaining and maintaining stable osmolality and sodium levels are critically important.

Hypotonic hypervolemic hyponatremic patients generally require loop diuretics to correct increased total body water and sodium; patients with hypotonic hypervolemic hyponatremia and severe acute or chronic kidney injury generally require dialysis. V_2 receptor antagonists (such as tolvaptan) may be helpful for severe hypervolemic hyponatremia from heart failure but are contraindicated in cirrhosis. V_2 receptor antagonists can only be safely initiated in the hospital, with careful attention to urinary output and serum sodium to avoid rapid overcorrection.

Hypotonic euvolemic hyponatremia should be treated based on the underlying etiology and acuity. Acute hyponatremia can and generally should be corrected quickly. Psychogenic polydipsia can correct quickly with water restriction alone; if hyponatremia is moderate to severe, patients need close monitoring during treatment to avoid overcorrection. It is imperative to monitor serum sodium carefully (every 2–8 hours depending on the severity of the hyponatremia) as well as hourly urinary output. High urinary output strongly suggests that serum sodium will rise rapidly unless oral intake is also relatively high. If there is concern for overcorrection, a stat serum sodium should be checked and the fluid restriction should be temporarily liberalized or lifted entirely. In the case of clinician uncertainty, overcorrection, or severe hyponatremia thought secondary to psychogenic polydipsia, subspecialist consultation should be obtained. In general, low solute diet can be treated with increased oral solute intake as well as fluid restriction with monitoring for overcorrection, except with severe hyponatremia when more aggressive therapies with close monitoring would be indicated. Patients with psychogenic polydipsia or low solute diet who have an impaired ability to maximally clear free water because of CKD will require a higher solute intake and/or lower fluid intake than individuals with these disorders who are able to maximally dilute their urine.

Mild to moderate **hypotonic euvolemic hyponatremia** secondary to SIADH will often respond to restricting fluid intake, withholding offending medications, or treating pain and nausea. Increased solute intake (such as salt tablets or urea) and loop diuretics can also be used to increase water clearance in refractory cases that are not severe. Among inpatients, 2 g of sodium chloride two or three times daily is often a reasonable dose in these cases, though the expected rate of sodium rises in SIADH in response to salt tablets depends on urinary electrolyte losses and nephrology consultation can best recommend the proper dose and monitoring frequency for an individual patient. Oral urea is an evidence-based therapy for SIADH but is an infrequent choice in the United States because it is challenging to obtain. Loop diuretics can be added in patients with SIADH who have substantially concentrated urine and who are assuredly not hypovolemic. Loop diuretics prevent maximal urinary concentration by diluting the medullary concentrating gradient in the kidney. Starting dose should be on the low end (eg, furosemide, 10–20 mg orally twice daily). All these therapies require close monitoring of serum sodium and volume status. Demeclocycline, which induces diabetes insipidus (DI), is a second- or third-line choice. Overly rapid correction of chronic hyponatremia should be avoided, particularly when the underlying etiology of SIADH is treated. At times, SIADH can be so severe that the patient's maximally dilute urine is hypertonic compared with saline. In those cases, normal saline infusion will cause worsening hyponatremia because patients will excrete the sodium chloride from the saline but will be unable to excrete all the water in which the sodium chloride was dissolved. Hyponatremia secondary to severe SIADH, particularly those cases in which the sum of the spot urine potassium and sodium is greater than the serum sodium ($U_K + U_{Na}$ greater than S_{Na}), may be challenging to correct with fluid restriction and salt tablets alone, in which case 3% saline or a V_2 antagonist can be considered (see below) in consultation with a nephrologist. The hyponatremia associated with adrenal insufficiency or hypothyroidism can usually be treated with fluid restriction to achieve a slow and steady rise in serum sodium as well as addressing the underlying cause.

Patients with **symptomatic** or **severe hyponatremia** (or both) generally require hospitalization for careful monitoring of fluid balance and weight, treatment, and frequent sodium checks. Inciting medications should be discontinued if possible. In acute symptomatic hyponatremia and chronic hyponatremia with severe symptoms (such as seizure), patients can be given 100 mL of 3% hypertonic saline infused over 10 minutes (repeated twice as necessary) aiming to immediately reverse symptoms. Generally, the 24-hour correction goal rate of 4–6 mEq/L (for chronic hyponatremia) is still recommended, so after a brief period of rapid correction, no further correction may be needed until the next day. Chronic hyponatremic patients at high risk for demyelination who are corrected too rapidly are candidates for treatment with a combination of desmopressin (DDAVP) and intravenous dextrose 5% to re-lower the serum sodium in consultation with nephrology. Acute hypernatremia can be corrected more quickly because there is much less concern for osmotic demyelination syndrome.

In severe chronic euvolemic hypotonic hyponatremia that is symptomatic or not responsive to fluid restriction, but without seizure or other immediately life-threatening symptoms, the clinician can deliver 3% hypertonic saline at a slow rate, adjusting in real time, to achieve a correction rate of 4–6 mEq/L/24 h. This approach is generally used for SIADH, since the other etiologies of hypovolemic and euvolemic hypotonic hyponatremia are usually responsive to treatments directed at the underlying etiology. Hypertonic saline is generally avoided in hypervolemic hyponatremia in the absence of critical symptomatic hyponatremia out of concern for worsening volume overload. The amount of 3% hypertonic saline that should be given to treat severe hyponatremia and non-critical symptoms is an area of active debate. In the past, complex equations such as

$$\text{Goal } S_{Na} \text{ (mEq/L)} = [S_{Na} \text{ (mEq/L)} \times \text{total body water (L)}] \\ + [513 \text{ mEq/L} \times \text{amount of 3\% saline (L)}] \\ /[\text{total body water (L)} \\ + \text{amount of 3\% saline (L)}]$$

have been used to choose an initial 3% hypertonic saline infusion rate, but limitations to this approach include the potential for mathematical error and possible inaccuracy of the equations, particularly if they do not account for urinary losses. The most recent United States hyponatremia treatment guidelines from 2013 recommend that 3% hypertonic saline be given at an initial rate of 0.5–2 mL/kg/h without further calculation of an infusion rate. There should then be frequent monitoring of serum sodium to avoid overcorrection, which is less likely to occur if the initial rate of infusion is with the lower end of the recommended range. Regardless of the strategy used, close monitoring of serum sodium (initially every 1–2 hours) and urine output is strongly recommended with titration of the 3% hypertonic saline infusion rate to achieve the goal correction rate. A high urinary output may be the first sign that ADH secretion has stopped and the patient is at even higher risk of overcorrection. Some experts add DDAVP to reduce the risk of overcorrection (see below). Nephrology consultation is indicated for all patients with severe hyponatremia, since there are several approaches to treatment, minimal data to support therapy, and a high risk of overcorrection.

Vasopressin 2 (V_2) receptors mediate the diuretic effect of ADH, and the use of V_2 receptor antagonists can be considered for patients with euvolemic hyponatremia, generally secondary to SIADH or hypervolemic hyponatremia from heart failure. V_2 receptor antagonists can also be considered for patients with a sodium level below 125 mEq/L or milder hyponatremia that is symptomatic and resistant to fluid restriction. The starting dose of tolvaptan is 15 mg orally daily; it can be increased to 30 mg daily and 60 mg daily at 24-hour intervals if hyponatremia persists or if the increase in sodium concentration is less than 4–6 mEq/L over the preceding 24 hours. Conivaptan is given as an intravenous loading dose of 20 mg delivered over 30 minutes, then as 20 mg continuously over 24 hours. Subsequent infusions may be administered for an additional 1–3 days at 20–40 mg/day by continuous infusion. Tolvaptan is approved for up to 30 days and conivaptan for up to 4 days. V_2 receptor antagonists are contraindicated in patients with liver disease, including cirrhosis. The standard free water restriction for hyponatremic patients should be lifted for patients receiving V_2 receptor antagonists since the aquaresis can result in excessive sodium correction in a fluid-restricted patient. Similarly, V_2 receptor antagonists should not be used concomitantly with 3% hypertonic saline. V_2 receptor antagonists must be initiated in the hospital because meticulous monitoring of the urinary output and serum sodium is necessary. Often, high hourly urinary output is the first sign that a patient's water diuresis is excessive (with attendant risk of over-correction) when taking these medications.

When to Refer

- Nephrology or endocrinology consultation should be obtained in severe, symptomatic, refractory, or complicated cases of hyponatremia.
- Aggressive therapies with hypertonic saline, V_2 antagonists, or dialysis mandate specialist consultation as do cases where saline overcorrects or the patient does not respond as predicted to initial therapy.
- Consultation may be necessary with severe liver or heart disease.

When to Admit

- Symptomatic or severe hyponatremia.
- Patient requires aggressive therapies that need close monitoring and frequent laboratory testing.

Henry DA. In the clinic: hyponatremia. Ann Intern Med. 2015 Aug 4;163(3):ITC1–19. [PMID: 26237763]

Hoorn EJ et al. Diagnosis and treatment of hyponatremia: compilation of the guidelines. J Am Soc Nephrol. 2017 May; 28(5):1340–9. [PMID: 28174217]

Peri A. Management of hyponatremia: causes, clinical aspects, differential diagnosis and treatment. Expert Rev Endocrinol Metab. 2018 Dec 11:1–9. [PMID: 30596344]

Sterns RH. Treatment of severe hyponatremia. Clin J Am Soc Nephrol. 2018 Apr 6;13(4):641–9. [PMID: 29295830]

HYPERNATREMIA

ESSENTIALS OF DIAGNOSIS

- ▶ Increased thirst and water intake are the main defense against hypernatremia.
- ▶ Urine osmolality helps differentiate renal from nonrenal water loss.

General Considerations

Hypernatremia is defined as a sodium concentration greater than 145 mEq/L. All patients with hypernatremia have hyperosmolality, unlike hyponatremic patients who can have a low, normal, or high serum osmolality. The hypernatremic patient is typically hypovolemic due to hypotonic fluid losses, or, less often, hypodipsia or adipsia. Hypotonic fluid losses can be renal (such as with DI or inappropriately dilute urine from diuretics) or nonrenal (such as with gastrointestinal [GI] losses or burns). Hypervolemic hypernatremia is less common but can be an iatrogenic complication in hospitalized patients who receive substantial amounts of intravenous sodium salts, and rarely in other settings as well (such as with sea water ingestion). Hypernatremia in primary aldosteronism is mild and usually does not cause symptoms.

Normally, the hypothalamus senses minimal changes in serum osmolality. High osmolality triggers two responses: the first is to secrete ADH, which acts on the kidney to minimize urinary water losses, and the second is to stimulate thirst. These two mechanisms are complimentary. For example, in DI, where the kidney is inappropriately losing free water either because of impaired ADH secretion or inability of the kidney to sense ADH appropriately, the thirst mechanism is generally sufficient to avoid hypernatremia. Thus, whatever the underlying disorder, excess water loss generally only causes hypernatremia when either the thirst mechanism is not intact or adequate water intake is not possible.

Clinical Findings

A. Symptoms and Signs

When the patient is dehydrated, orthostatic hypotension and oliguria are typical findings. Because water shifts from the cells to the intravascular space to protect volume status, these symptoms may be delayed. Lethargy, irritability, and weakness are early signs. Hyperthermia, delirium, seizures, and coma may be seen with severe hypernatremia (ie, sodium greater than 158 mEq/L). In acute hyperosmolality, somnolence and confusion can appear when the osmolality exceeds 320–330 mOsm/kg (320–330 mmol/kg); coma, respiratory arrest, and death can result when osmolality exceeds 340–350 mOsm/kg (340–350 mmol/kg). Symptoms in older adults may not be specific; a recent change in consciousness is associated with a poor prognosis. Osmotic cerebral demyelination is an uncommon but reported consequence of acute severe hypernatremia.

B. Laboratory Findings

1. Urine osmolality greater than 400 mOsm/kg—Renal water-conserving ability is functioning.

A. NONRENAL LOSSES—Hypernatremia will develop if water intake falls behind hypotonic fluid losses from excessive sweating, the respiratory tract, or bowel movements. Lactulose causes an osmotic diarrhea with loss of free water.

B. RENAL LOSSES—While severe hyperglycemia can cause translocational hyponatremia, progressive volume depletion from glucosuria can result in hypernatremia. Osmotic diuresis can occur with the use of mannitol or urea.

2. Urine osmolality less than 250 mOsm/kg—Hypernatremia with a dilute urine (osmolality less than 250 mOsm/kg) is characteristic of DI. Central DI results from inadequate ADH release. Nephrogenic DI results from renal insensitivity to ADH; common causes include lithium, demeclocycline, relief of urinary obstruction, interstitial nephritis, hypercalcemia, and hypokalemia.

▶ Treatment

Treatment of hypernatremia includes correcting the cause of the fluid loss, replacing water, and replacing electrolytes (as needed). In response to increases in plasma osmolality, brain cells synthesize idiogenic osmoles, which are solutes that cause intracellular fluid shifts. Osmole production begins 4–6 hours after dehydration and takes several days to reach steady state. If hypernatremia is rapidly corrected, the osmotic imbalance may cause cerebral edema and potentially severe neurologic impairment. There is no consensus about the optimal rates of sodium correction in chronic hypernatremia among adults. Based primarily on data out of the pediatrics literature, many experts advocate a maximum sodium correction rate per day of 10 mEq/L in chronic hypernatremia out of concern for cerebral edema. However, acute hypernatremia should be corrected more quickly to avoid osmotic cerebral demyelination. Expert consultation should be requested in cases where the optimal rate of correction is unclear.

A. Choice of Type of Fluid for Replacement

1. Hypernatremia with hypovolemia—Hypovolemic patients can receive isotonic fluid to restore euvolemia and to treat hyperosmolality. Even 0.9% normal saline (308 mOsm/kg or 308 mmol/kg), which has the highest osmolality of the usual isotonic fluids, is hypoosmolar compared with substantially hyperosmolar plasma. After adequate volume resuscitation, hypotonic fluid should be used to replace any remaining free water deficit (Table 21–3). If the patient is euvolemic, 0.45% saline and 5% dextrose are common choices. Oral water is an excellent option in patients who are able to drink water safely.

Table 21–3. Electrolyte concentrations in common isotonic crystalloids.

	Plasma-Lyte A (mmol/L)	Lactated Ringer (mmol/L)	Saline (mmol/L)
Sodium	140	130	154
Potassium	5	4	
Magnesium	1.5		
Calcium		1.5	
Chloride	98	109	154
Acetate	27		
Gluconate	23		
Lactate		28	

2. Hypernatremia with euvolemia—Water ingestion or intravenous 5% dextrose will result in the excretion of excess sodium in the urine. If the glomerular filtration rate (GFR) is decreased, diuretics will increase urinary sodium excretion but may impair renal concentrating ability, increasing the quantity of water that needs to be replaced.

3. Hypernatremia with hypervolemia—Treatment includes 5% dextrose solution to reduce hyperosmolality. Loop diuretics may be necessary to promote natriuresis and lower total body sodium. In severe rare cases with kidney disease, hemodialysis may be necessary to correct the excess total body sodium and water.

B. Calculation of Water Deficit

Fluid replacement should include the free water deficit (equation below) and additional maintenance fluid to replace ongoing and anticipated fluid losses. Ongoing losses may be substantial, particularly in the setting of DI. Chronic hypernatremia should be corrected slowly to avoid cerebral edema.

1. Acute hypernatremia—In acute dehydration without much solute loss, free water loss is similar to the weight loss. Initially, a 5% dextrose solution may be used if losses are primarily free water. As correction of water deficit progresses, therapy should continue with 0.45% saline with dextrose.

2. Chronic hypernatremia—The water deficit is calculated to restore normal sodium concentration, typically 140 mEq/L. Conservatively, though, the maximum sodium correction rate per day should not exceed 10 mEq/L in chronic hypernatremia. High ongoing water losses should be added to the water deficit that needs to be repleted over 24 hours. Serum sodium should be measured every 2–8 hours depending on cerebral edema risk, water dose, and route (more frequent monitoring should occur with higher doses of water and with the intravenous route as opposed to the oral route). Oral water replacement is generally preferred, when clinically possible. If the water replacement route must be intravenous, the free water replacement should be as dextrose 5% in water rather than sterile water (which can cause hemolysis).

Total body water (TBW) (Table 21–1) correlates with muscle mass and therefore decreases with advancing age, cachexia, and dehydration and is lower in women than in men. Current TBW equals 40–60% current body weight.

$$\text{Free water deficit (in L)} = \text{Current TBW} \times \frac{[S_{Na}] - 140}{140}$$

▶ When to Refer

Patients with refractory or unexplained hypernatremia should be referred for subspecialist consultation.

▶ When to Admit

- Patients with symptomatic hypernatremia require hospitalization for evaluation and treatment.

- Significant comorbidities or concomitant acute illnesses, especially if contributing to hypernatremia, may necessitate hospitalization.

Liamis G et al. Evaluation and treatment of hypernatremia: a practical guide for physicians. Postgrad Med. 2016;128(3):299–306. [PMID: 26813151]

Morley JE. Dehydration, hypernatremia, and hyponatremia. Clin Geriatr Med. 2015 Aug;31(3):389–99. [PMID: 26195098]

Muhsin SA et al. Diagnosis and treatment of hypernatremia. Best Pract Res Clin Endocrinol Metab. 2016 Mar;30(2):189–203. [PMID: 27156758]

Tsipotis E et al. Hospital-associated hypernatremia spectrum and clinical outcomes in an unselected cohort. Am J Med. 2018 Jan;131(1):72–82. [PMID: 28860033]

DISORDERS OF POTASSIUM CONCENTRATION

HYPOKALEMIA

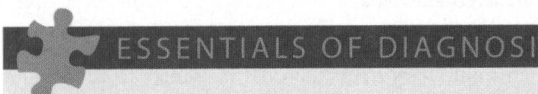

ESSENTIALS OF DIAGNOSIS

▶ Serum potassium level less than 3.5 mEq/L (3.5 mmol/L).

▶ Severe hypokalemia may induce arrhythmias and rhabdomyolysis.

▶ Transtubular potassium concentration gradient (TTKG) can distinguish renal from nonrenal loss of potassium.

General Considerations

Hypokalemia can result from insufficient dietary potassium intake, intracellular shifting of potassium from the extracellular space, extrarenal potassium loss, or renal potassium loss (Table 21–4). Cellular uptake of potassium is increased by insulin and beta-adrenergic stimulation and blocked by alpha-adrenergic stimulation. Aldosterone is an important regulator of total body potassium, increasing potassium secretion in the distal renal tubule. The most common cause of hypokalemia, especially in developing countries, is gastrointestinal loss from infectious diarrhea. The potassium concentration in intestinal secretion is ten times higher (80 mEq/L) than in gastric secretions. Hypokalemia in the presence of acidosis suggests profound potassium depletion and requires urgent treatment. Self-limited hypokalemia occurs in 50–60% of trauma patients, perhaps related to enhanced release of epinephrine.

Hypokalemia induced by beta-2-adrenergic agonists and diuretics may substantially increase the risk of arrhythmias. Hypokalemia increases the likelihood of digitalis toxicity. Numerous genetic mutations affect fluid and electrolyte metabolism, including disorders of potassium metabolism (Table 21–5).

Magnesium is an important cofactor for potassium uptake and maintenance of intracellular potassium levels.

Table 21–4. Causes of hypokalemia.

Decreased potassium intake
Potassium shift into the cell
Alkalosis
Barium intoxication
Beta-adrenergic agonists
Increased postprandial secretion of insulin
Periodic paralysis (hypokalemic)
Trauma (via beta-adrenergic stimulation)
Renal potassium loss
Increased aldosterone (mineralocorticoid) effects
Primary hyperaldosteronism
Secondary aldosteronism (dehydration, heart failure)
Bartter syndrome, Gitelman syndrome
Cushing syndrome, ectopic ACTH-producing tumor
Congenital abnormality of steroid metabolism (eg, adrenogenital syndrome, 17-alpha-hydroxylase defect, apparent mineralocorticoid excess, 11-beta-hydroxylase deficiency)
Licorice (European)
Renin-producing tumor
Renovascular hypertension, malignant hypertension
Increased flow to distal nephron
Diuretics (furosemide, thiazides)
Salt-losing nephropathy, polyuria
Hypomagnesemia
Unreabsorbable anion
Bicarbonaturia
Carbenicillin, penicillin
Hippurate from toluene use or glue sniffing
Renal tubular acidosis (type I or II)
Liddle syndrome
Extrarenal potassium loss
Vomiting, diarrhea, laxative abuse
Villous adenoma, Zollinger-Ellison syndrome

Loop diuretics (eg, furosemide) cause substantial renal potassium and magnesium losses. Magnesium depletion should be considered in refractory hypokalemia.

Clinical Findings

A. Symptoms and Signs

Muscular weakness, fatigue, and muscle cramps are frequent complaints in mild to moderate hypokalemia. Gastrointestinal smooth muscle involvement may result in constipation or ileus. Flaccid paralysis, hyporeflexia, hypercapnia, tetany, and rhabdomyolysis may be seen with severe hypokalemia (less than 2.5 mEq/L). The presence of hypertension may be a clue to the diagnosis of hypokalemia from aldosterone or mineralocorticoid excess (Table 21–5). Renal manifestations include nephrogenic DI and interstitial nephritis.

B. Laboratory Findings

Urinary potassium concentration is low (less than 20 mEq/L) as a result of extrarenal loss (eg, diarrhea, vomiting) and inappropriately high (greater than 40 mEq/L) with renal loss (eg, mineralocorticoid excess, Bartter syndrome, Liddle syndrome) (Table 21–4).

Table 21–5. Genetic disorders associated with electrolyte metabolism disturbances.

Disease	Site of Mutation
Potassium	
Hypokalemia	
Hypokalemic periodic paralysis	Dihydropyridine-sensitive skeletal muscle voltage-gated calcium channel
Bartter syndrome	Na^+-K^+-$2Cl^-$ cotransporter, K^+ channel (ROMK), or Cl^- channel of thick ascending limb of Henle (hypofunction), barttin
Gitelman syndrome	Thiazide-sensitive Na^+-Cl^- cotransporter
Liddle syndrome	Beta or gamma subunit of amiloride-sensitive Na^+ channel (hyperfunction)
Apparent mineralocorticoid excess	11-beta-hydroxysteroid dehydrogenase (failure to inactivate cortisol)
Glucocorticoid-remediable hyperaldosteronism	Regulatory sequence of 11-beta-hydroxysteroid controls aldosterone synthase inappropriately
Hyperkalemia	
Hyperkalemic periodic paralysis	Alpha subunit of calcium channel
Pseudohypoaldosteronism type I	Beta or gamma subunit of amiloride-sensitive Na^+ channel (hypofunction)
Pseudohypoaldosteronism type II (Gordon syndrome)	WNK2, WNK4
Calcium	
Familial hypocalciuric hypercalcemia	Ca^{2+}-sensing protein (hypofunction)
Familial hypocalcemia	Ca^{2+}-sensing protein (hyperfunction)
Phosphate	
Hypophosphatemic rickets	*PEX* gene, FGF23
Magnesium	
Hypomagnesemia-hypercalciuria syndrome	Paracellin-1
Water	
Nephrogenic diabetes insipidus	V_2 receptor (Type 1), aquaporin-2
Acid-base	
Proximal RTA	Na^+ HCO_3^- cotransporter
Distal RTA	Cl^- HCO_3^- exchanger, H^+-ATPase
Proximal and distal RTA	Carbonic anhydrase II

FGF23, fibroblast growth factor 23; RTA, renal tubular acidosis; V_2, vasopressin.

The transtubular $[K^+]$ gradient (TTKG) is a simple and rapid evaluation of net potassium secretion. TTKG is calculated as follows:

$$TTKG = \frac{Urine\ K^+ / Plasma\ K^+}{Urine\ Osm / Plasma\ Osm}$$

Hypokalemia with a TTKG more than 4 suggests renal potassium loss with increased distal K^+ secretion. In such cases, plasma renin and aldosterone levels are helpful in differential diagnosis. The presence of nonabsorbed anions, such as bicarbonate, increases the TTKG.

C. Electrocardiogram

The electrocardiogram (ECG) may show decreased amplitude and broadening of T waves, prominent U waves, premature ventricular contractions, and depressed ST segments.

► Treatment

Oral potassium supplementation is the safest and easiest treatment for mild to moderate deficiency. Dietary potassium is almost entirely coupled to phosphate—rather than chloride—and is therefore less effective in correcting potassium loss associated with chloride depletion from diuretics or vomiting.

Intravenous potassium is indicated for patients with severe hypokalemia and for those who cannot take oral supplementation. For severe deficiency, potassium may be given through a peripheral intravenous line in a concentration up to 40 mEq/L and at rates up to 10 mEq/h. Concentrations of up to 20 mEq/h may be given through a central venous catheter. Continuous ECG monitoring is indicated, and the serum potassium level should be checked every 3–6 hours. Avoid glucose-containing fluid to prevent further shifts of potassium into the cells. Magnesium deficiency should be corrected, particularly in refractory hypokalemia.

► When to Refer

Patients with unexplained hypokalemia, refractory hypokalemia, or suggestive alternative diagnoses (eg, aldosteronism or hypokalemic periodic paralysis) should be referred for endocrinology or nephrology consultation.

► When to Admit

Patients with symptomatic or severe hypokalemia, especially with cardiac manifestations, require cardiac monitoring, potassium supplementation, and frequent laboratory testing.

Gumz ML et al. An integrated view of potassium homeostasis. N Engl J Med. 2015 Jul 2;373(1):60–72. Erratum in: N Engl J Med. 2015 Sep 24;373(13):1281. [PMID: 26132942]

Palmer BF et al. Physiology and pathophysiology of potassium homeostasis. Adv Physiol Educ. 2016 Dec;40(4):480–90. [PMID: 27756725]

Wu KL et al. Identification of the causes for chronic hypokalemia: importance of urinary sodium and chloride excretion. Am J Med. 2017 Jul;130(7):846–55. [PMID: 28213045]

HYPERKALEMIA

ESSENTIALS OF DIAGNOSIS

▶ Serum potassium level greater than 5.0 mEq/L (5.0 mmol/L).

▶ Hyperkalemia may develop in patients taking angiotensin-converting enzyme (ACE) inhibitors, angiotensin-receptor blockers, potassium-sparing diuretics, or their combination, even with no or only mild kidney dysfunction.

▶ The ECG may be normal despite life-threatening hyperkalemia.

▶ Measurement of plasma potassium level differentiates potassium leak from blood cells from truly elevated serum potassium.

▶ Rule out extracellular potassium shift from the cells in acidosis and assess renal potassium excretion.

General Considerations

Hyperkalemia usually occurs in patients with advanced kidney disease but can also develop with normal kidney function (Table 21–6). Acidosis causes intracellular potassium to shift extracellularly. Serum potassium concentration rises about 0.7 mEq/L for every decrease of 0.1 pH unit during acidosis. Fist clenching during venipuncture may raise the potassium concentration by 1–2 mEq/L by causing acidosis and potassium shift from cells. In the absence of acidosis, serum potassium concentration rises about 1 mEq/L when there is a total body potassium excess of 1–4 mEq/kg. However, the higher the serum potassium concentration, the smaller the excess necessary to raise the potassium levels further.

Mineralocorticoid deficiency from Addison disease or CKD is another cause of hyperkalemia with decreased renal excretion of potassium. Mineralocorticoid resistance due to genetic disorders, interstitial kidney disease, or urinary tract obstruction also leads to hyperkalemia.

ACE inhibitors or angiotensin-receptor blockers (ARBs) may cause hyperkalemia. The concomitant use of spironolactone, eplerenone, or beta-blockers further increases the risk of hyperkalemia. Thiazide or loop diuretics and sodium bicarbonate may minimize hyperkalemia. Persistent mild hyperkalemia in the absence of ACE inhibitor or ARB therapy is usually due to type IV renal tubular acidosis (RTA). Heparin inhibits aldosterone production in the adrenal glands, causing hyperkalemia.

Trimethoprim is structurally similar to amiloride and triamterene, and all three drugs inhibit renal potassium excretion through suppression of sodium channels in the distal nephron.

Cyclosporine and tacrolimus can induce hyperkalemia in organ transplant recipients, especially kidney transplant patients, partly due to suppression of the basolateral Na^+–K^+-ATPase in principal cells. Hyperkalemia is

Table 21–6. Causes of hyperkalemia.

Spurious/Pseudohyperkalemia
Leakage from erythrocytes when separation of serum from clot is delayed (plasma K^+ normal)
Marked thrombocytosis or leukocytosis with release of intracellular K^+ (plasma K^+ normal)
Repeated fist clenching during phlebotomy, with release of K^+ from forearm muscles
Specimen drawn from arm with intravenous K^+ infusion
Decreased K^+ excretion
Kidney disease, acute and chronic
Renal secretory defects (may or may not have reduced kidney function): kidney transplant, interstitial nephritis, systemic lupus erythematosus, sickle cell disease, amyloidosis, obstructive nephropathy
Hypoaldosteronism
Addison disease
Type IV renal tubular acidosis
Heparin
Drugs that inhibit potassium excretion: spironolactone, eplerenone, drospirenone, NSAIDs, ACE inhibitors, angiotensin II receptor blockers, triamterene, amiloride, trimethoprim, pentamidine, cyclosporine, tacrolimus
Shift of K^+ from within the cell
Massive release of intracellular K^+ in burns, rhabdomyolysis, hemolysis, severe infection, internal bleeding, vigorous exercise
Metabolic acidosis (in the case of organic acid accumulation—eg, lactic acidosis—a shift of K^+ does not occur since organic acid can easily move across the cell membrane)
Hypertonicity (solvent drag)
Insulin deficiency (metabolic acidosis may not be apparent)
Hyperkalemic periodic paralysis
Drugs: succinylcholine, arginine, digitalis toxicity, beta-adrenergic antagonists
Alpha-adrenergic stimulation?
Excessive intake of K^+
Especially in patients taking medications that decrease potassium secretion (see above)

ACE, angiotensin-converting enzyme; NSAIDs, nonsteroidal anti-inflammatory drugs.

commonly seen in HIV patients and has been attributed to impaired renal excretion of potassium due to pentamidine or trimethoprim-sulfamethoxazole or to hyporeninemic hypoaldosteronism.

Clinical Findings

Hyperkalemia impairs neuromuscular transmission, causing muscle weakness, flaccid paralysis, and ileus. Electrocardiography is not a sensitive method for detecting hyperkalemia, since nearly half of patients with a serum potassium level greater than 6.5 mEq/L will not manifest ECG changes. ECG changes in hyperkalemia include bradycardia, PR interval prolongation, peaked T waves, QRS widening, and biphasic QRS–T complexes. Conduction disturbances, such as bundle branch block and atrioventricular block, may occur. Ventricular fibrillation and cardiac arrest are terminal events.

Prevention

Inhibitors of the renin-angiotensin-aldosterone axis (ie, ACE inhibitors, ARBs, and spironolactone) and potassium-sparing diuretics (eplerenone, triamterene) should be used cautiously in patients with heart failure, liver failure, and kidney disease. Laboratory monitoring should be performed within 1 week of drug initiation or dosage increase.

Treatment

The diagnosis should be confirmed by repeat laboratory testing to rule out spurious hyperkalemia, especially in the absence of medications that cause hyperkalemia or in patients without kidney disease or a previous history of hyperkalemia. Plasma potassium concentration can be measured to avoid spurious hyperkalemia due to potassium leakage out of red cells, white cells, and platelets. Kidney dysfunction should be ruled out at the initial assessment.

Treatment consists of withholding exogenous potassium, identifying the cause, reviewing the patient's medications and dietary potassium intake, and correcting the hyperkalemia. Emergent treatment is indicated when cardiac toxicity, muscle paralysis, or severe hyperkalemia (potassium greater than 6.5 mEq/L) is present, even in the absence of ECG changes. Insulin, bicarbonate, and beta-agonists shift potassium intracellularly within minutes of administration (Table 21–7). Intravenous calcium may be given to antagonize the cell membrane effects of potassium, but its use should be restricted to life-threatening hyperkalemia in patients taking digitalis because hypercalcemia may cause digitalis toxicity. Hemodialysis may be required to remove potassium in patients with acute or chronic kidney injury. Patiromer binds potassium in the intestine and is FDA-approved for the treatment of chronic hyperkalemia in patients with CKD who take at least one drug that inhibits the renin-angiotensin-aldosterone system. Patiromer may decrease the absorption of orally administered drugs. Another potassium binder sodium zirconium cyclosilicate is FDA approved for hyperkalemia treatment. Little is known about these agents as treatment in end-stage renal disease. Sodium polystyrene has been widely used for decades although its efficacy and safety have been questioned. It may not increase potassium excretion above laxatives alone and has been associated with colonic necrosis, both with and without sorbitol coadministration. The FDA has recommended that sodium polystyrene should not be administered in sorbitol, but the mixture remains commonly available. Its use should be restricted to patients with life-threatening hyperkalemia when dialysis is not available and other therapies (eg, diuretics) have failed. Sodium polystyrene is contraindicated in patients with risk factors for colonic necrosis, such as bowel obstruction, ileus, and postoperative state.

When to Refer

Patients with hyperkalemia from kidney disease and reduced renal potassium excretion should see a nephrologist.

When to Admit

Patients with severe hyperkalemia greater than 5.5–6 mEq/L, any degree of hyperkalemia associated with ECG changes, or concomitant illness (eg, tumor lysis, rhabdomyolysis, metabolic acidosis, acute kidney injury) should be sent to the emergency department for immediate treatment. The appropriate triage of patients with milder hyperkalemia and without any of the concerning features mentioned above will depend on provider and patient comfort, presumed etiology of hyperkalemia, and the ability to monitor closely in outpatient setting.

Kovesdy CP et al. Potassium homeostasis in health and disease: a scientific workshop cosponsored by the National Kidney Foundation and the American Society of Hypertension. J Am Soc Hypertens. 2017 Dec;11(12):783–800. [PMID: 29030153]

Kovesdy CP. Updates in hyperkalemia: outcomes and therapeutic strategies. Rev Endocr Metab Disord. 2017 Mar;18(1):41–7. [PMID: 27600582]

Montford JR et al. How dangerous is hyperkalemia? J Am Soc Nephrol. 2017 Nov;28(11):3155–65. [PMID: 28778861]

DISORDERS OF CALCIUM CONCENTRATION

The normal total plasma (or serum) calcium concentration is 8.5–10.5 mg/dL (or 2.1–2.6 mmol/L). Ionized calcium (normal: 4.6–5.3 mg/dL [or 1.15–1.32 mmol/L]) is physiologically active and necessary for muscle contraction and nerve function.

The calcium-sensing receptor, a transmembrane protein that detects the extracellular calcium concentration, is in the parathyroid gland and the kidney. Functional defects in this protein are associated with diseases of abnormal calcium metabolism such as familial hypocalcemia and familial hypocalciuric hypercalcemia (Table 21–5).

HYPOCALCEMIA

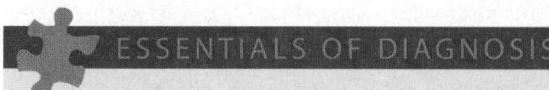

ESSENTIALS OF DIAGNOSIS

► Often mistaken as a neurologic disorder.

► Decreased serum parathyroid hormone (PTH), vitamin D, or magnesium levels.

► Despite a low total serum calcium, calcium metabolism is likely normal if ionized calcium level is normal.

General Considerations

The most common cause of low total serum calcium is hypoalbuminemia. When serum albumin concentration is lower than 4 g/dL (40 g/L), serum Ca^{2+} concentration is reduced by 0.8–1 mg/dL (0.20–0.25 mmol/L) for every 1 g/dL (10 g/L) of albumin.

The most accurate measurement of serum calcium is the ionized calcium concentration. True hypocalcemia

Table 21–7. Treatment of hyperkalemia.

Rapid					
Modality	**Mechanism of Action**	**Onset**	**Duration**	**Prescription**	**K$^+$ Removed From Body?**
Calcium	Antagonizes cardiac conduction abnormalities	0–5 minutes	1 hour	Calcium gluconate 10%, 5–30 mL intravenously; or calcium chloride 5%, 5–30 mL intravenously	No
Bicarbonate	Distributes K$^+$ into cells	15–30 minutes	1–2 hours	NaHCO$_3$, 50–100 mEq intravenously **Note:** Sodium bicarbonate may not be effective in end-stage kidney disease patients; dialysis is more expedient and effective. Some patients may not tolerate the additional sodium load of bicarbonate therapy.	No, does shift potassium into cells slightly
Insulin	Distributes K$^+$ into cells	15–60 minutes	4–6 hours	Regular insulin, 5–10 units intravenously, plus glucose 50%, 25 g intravenously. Must check glucose very frequently afterward.	No, does shift potassium into cells
Albuterol	Distributes K$^+$ into cells	15–30 minutes	2–4 hours	Nebulized albuterol, 10–20 mg in 4 mL normal saline, inhaled over 10 minutes **Note:** Much higher doses are necessary for hyperkalemia therapy (10–20 mg) than for airway disease (2.5 mg).	No, does shift potassium into cells slightly

Slower (should only be used in conjunction with above therapies in hyperkalemic emergency)				
Modality	**Mechanism of Action**	**Onset of Action**	**Prescription**	**K$^+$ Removed From Body?**
Loop diuretic	Renal K$^+$ excretion	0.5–2 hours	Furosemide, 40–160 mg intravenously **Note:** Diuretics may not be effective in patients with acute and chronic kidney diseases.	Yes
Cation exchangers (eg, kayexalate, patiromer, sodium zirconium cyclosilicate)	Ion-exchange resin binds K$^+$	1–3 hours	Depends on the agent chosen. Patiromer and sodium zirconium cyclosilicate have not been specifically studied in hyperkalemic emergency but some experts advocate their use over kayexalate based on better adverse effect profile.	Yes
Hemodialysis[1]	Extracorporeal K$^+$ removal	1–8 hours	Dialysate [K$^+$] 1–2 mEq/L **Note:** A fast and effective therapy for hyperkalemia, hemodialysis can be delayed by vascular access placement and equipment and/or staffing availability. Serum K can be rapidly corrected within minutes, but post-dialysis rebound can occur.	Yes
Peritoneal dialysis	Peritoneal K$^+$ removal	1–4 hours	Frequent exchanges **Note:** Strategy generally limited to those receiving peritoneal dialysis already.	Yes

[1]Can be both acute immediate and urgent treatment of hyperkalemia.
Modified and reproduced, with permission, from Cogan MG. *Fluid and Electrolytes: Physiology and Pathophysiology.* McGraw-Hill, 1991.

Table 21–8. Causes of hypocalcemia.

Decreased intake or absorption
Malabsorption
Small bowel bypass, short bowel
Vitamin D deficit (decreased absorption, decreased production of 25-hydroxyvitamin D or 1,25-dihydroxyvitamin D)
Increased loss
Alcoholism
Chronic kidney disease
Diuretic therapy
Endocrine disease
Hypoparathyroidism (genetic, acquired; including hypomagnesemia and hypermagnesemia)
Post-parathyroidectomy (hungry bone syndrome)
Pseudohypoparathyroidism
Calcitonin secretion with medullary carcinoma of the thyroid
Familial hypocalcemia
Associated diseases
Pancreatitis
Rhabdomyolysis
Septic shock
Physiologic causes
Decreased serum albumin[1]
Decreased end-organ response to vitamin D
Hyperphosphatemia
Aminoglycoside antibiotics, plicamycin, loop diuretics, foscarnet

[1]Ionized calcium concentration is normal.

(decreased ionized calcium) implies insufficient action of PTH or active vitamin D. Important causes of hypocalcemia are listed in Table 21–8.

The most common cause of hypocalcemia is advanced CKD, in which decreased production of active vitamin D_3 (1,25 dihydroxyvitamin D_3) and hyperphosphatemia both play a role (see Chapter 22). Some cases of primary hypoparathyroidism are due to mutations of the calcium-sensing receptor in which inappropriate suppression of PTH release leads to hypocalcemia (see Chapter 26). Magnesium depletion reduces both PTH release and tissue responsiveness to PTH, causing hypocalcemia. Hypocalcemia in pancreatitis is a marker of severe disease. Elderly hospitalized patients with hypocalcemia and hypophosphatemia, with or without an elevated PTH level, are likely vitamin D deficient.

► Clinical Findings

A. Symptoms and Signs

Hypocalcemia increases excitation of nerve and muscle cells, primarily affecting the neuromuscular and cardiovascular systems. Spasm of skeletal muscle causes cramps and tetany. Laryngospasm with stridor can obstruct the airway. Convulsions, perioral and peripheral paresthesias, and abdominal pain can develop. Classic physical findings include Chvostek sign (contraction of the facial muscle in response to tapping the facial nerve) and Trousseau sign (carpal spasm occurring with occlusion of the brachial artery by a blood pressure cuff). QT prolongation predisposes to ventricular arrhythmias. In chronic hypoparathyroidism, cataracts and calcification of basal ganglia may appear (see Chapter 26).

B. Laboratory Findings

Serum calcium concentration is low (less than 8.5 mg/dL [2.1 mmol/L]). In true hypocalcemia, the ionized serum calcium concentration is also low (less than 4.6 mg/dL [1.15 mmol/L]). Serum phosphate is usually elevated in hypoparathyroidism or in advanced CKD, whereas it is suppressed in early CKD or vitamin D deficiency.

Serum magnesium concentration is commonly low. In respiratory alkalosis, total serum calcium is normal but ionized calcium is low. The ECG shows a prolonged QT interval.

► Treatment[1]

A. Severe, Symptomatic Hypocalcemia

In the presence of tetany, arrhythmias, or seizures, intravenous calcium gluconate is indicated.[1] Because of the short duration of action, continuous calcium infusion is usually required. Ten to 15 milligrams of calcium per kilogram body weight, or six to eight 10-mL vials of 10% calcium gluconate (558–744 mg of calcium), are added to 1 L of D_5W and infused over 4–6 hours. By monitoring the serum calcium level frequently (every 4–6 hours), the infusion rate is adjusted to maintain the serum calcium level at 7–8.5 mg/dL.

B. Asymptomatic Hypocalcemia

Oral calcium (1–2 g) and vitamin D preparations, including active vitamin D sterols, are used. Calcium carbonate is well tolerated and less expensive than many other calcium tablets. A check of urinary calcium excretion is recommended after the initiation of therapy because hypercalciuria (urine calcium excretion greater than 300 mg or 7.5 mmol per day) or urine calcium:creatinine ratio greater than 0.3 may impair kidney function in these patients. The low serum calcium associated with hypoalbuminemia does not require replacement therapy. If serum Mg^{2+} is low, therapy must include magnesium replacement, which by itself will usually correct hypocalcemia.

► When to Refer

Patients with complicated hypocalcemia from hypoparathyroidism, familial hypocalcemia, or CKD require referral to an endocrinologist or nephrologist, as do those requiring intravenous calcium repletion.

► When to Admit

Patients with tetany, arrhythmias, seizures, as well as those with severe hypocalcemia, require immediate therapy and immediate consultation with a nephrologist or an endocrinologist.

Aberegg SK. Ionized calcium in the ICU: should it be measured and corrected? Chest. 2016 Mar;149(3):846–55. [PMID: 26836894]

Rosner MH. Hypocalcemia in a patient with cancer. Clin J Am Soc Nephrol. 2017 Apr 3;12(4):696–9. [PMID: 28274993]

Schafer AL et al. Hypocalcemia: diagnosis and treatment. In: De Groot LJ et al, editors. Endotext. 2016 Jan 3. [PMID: 25905251]

[1]See also Chapter 26 for discussion of the treatment of hypoparathyroidism.

HYPERCALCEMIA

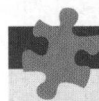

► Most common causes: primary hyperparathyroidism and malignancy-associated hypercalcemia.

► Hypercalciuria usually precedes hypercalcemia.

► Asymptomatic, mild hypercalcemia (above 10.5 mg/dL [2.6 mmol/L]) is usually due to primary hyperparathyroidism; symptomatic, severe hypercalcemia (above 14 mg/dL [3.5 mmol/L]) is usually due to hypercalcemia of malignancy.

General Considerations

Important causes of hypercalcemia are listed in Table 21–9. Primary hyperparathyroidism and malignancy account for 90% of cases. Primary hyperparathyroidism is the most common cause of hypercalcemia (usually mild) in ambulatory patients. Chronic hypercalcemia (over 6 months) or some manifestation such as nephrolithiasis also suggests a benign cause. Tumor production of PTH-related proteins (PTHrP) is the most common paraneoplastic endocrine syndrome, accounting for most cases of hypercalcemia in inpatients. The neoplasm is clinically apparent in nearly all cases when the hypercalcemia is detected, and the prognosis is poor. Granulomatous diseases, such as sarcoidosis and

Table 21–9. Causes of hypercalcemia.

Increased intake or absorption
Milk-alkali syndrome
Vitamin D or vitamin A excess
Endocrine disorders
Primary hyperparathyroidism
Secondary or tertiary hyperparathyroidism (usually associated with hypocalcemia)
Acromegaly
Adrenal insufficiency
Pheochromocytoma
Thyrotoxicosis
Neoplastic diseases
Tumors producing PTH-related proteins (ovary, kidney, lung)
Plasma cell myeloma (elaboration of osteoclast-activating factor)
Lymphoma (occasionally from production of calcitriol)
Miscellaneous causes
Thiazide diuretics
Granulomatous diseases (production of calcitriol)
Paget disease of bone
Hypophosphatasia
Immobilization
Familial hypocalciuric hypercalcemia
Complications of kidney transplantation
Lithium intake

PTH, parathyroid hormone.

tuberculosis, cause hypercalcemia via overproduction of active vitamin D_3 (1,25 dihydroxyvitamin D_3).

Milk-alkali syndrome has had a resurgence due to calcium ingestion for prevention of osteoporosis. Heavy calcium carbonate intake causes hypercalcemic acute kidney injury, likely from renal vasoconstriction. The decreased GFR impairs bicarbonate excretion, while hypercalcemia stimulates proton secretion and bicarbonate reabsorption. Metabolic alkalosis decreases calcium excretion, maintaining hypercalcemia.

Hypercalcemia causes nephrogenic DI through activation of calcium-sensing receptors in collecting ducts, which reduces ADH-induced water permeability. Volume depletion further worsens hypercalcemia.

Clinical Findings

A. Symptoms and Signs

The history and physical examination should focus on the duration of hypercalcemia and evidence for a neoplasm. Hypercalcemia may affect gastrointestinal, kidney, and neurologic function. Mild hypercalcemia is often asymptomatic. Symptoms usually occur if the serum calcium is higher than 12 mg/dL (3 mmol/L) and tend to be more severe if hypercalcemia develops acutely. Symptoms include constipation and polyuria, except in hypocalciuric hypercalcemia, in which polyuria is absent. Other symptoms include nausea, vomiting, anorexia, peptic ulcer disease, renal colic, and hematuria from nephrolithiasis. Polyuria from hypercalciuria-induced nephrogenic DI can result in volume depletion and acute kidney injury. Neurologic manifestations range from mild drowsiness to weakness, depression, lethargy, stupor, and coma in severe hypercalcemia. Ventricular ectopy and idioventricular rhythm occur and can be accentuated by digitalis.

B. Laboratory Findings

The ionized calcium exceeds 1.32 mmol/L. A high serum chloride concentration and a low serum phosphate concentration in a ratio greater than 33:1 (or greater than 102 if SI units are utilized) suggests primary hyperparathyroidism where PTH decreases proximal tubular phosphate reabsorption. A low serum chloride concentration with a high serum bicarbonate concentration, along with elevated BUN and creatinine, suggests milk-alkali syndrome. Severe hypercalcemia (greater than 14 mg/dL [3.5 mmol/L]) generally occurs in malignancy. More than 300 mg (7.5 mmol) per day of urinary calcium excretion suggests hypercalciuria; less than 100 mg (2.5 mmol) per day suggests hypocalciuria. Hypercalciuric patients—such as those with malignancy or those receiving oral active vitamin D therapy—may easily develop hypercalcemia in case of volume depletion. Serum phosphate may or may not be low, depending on the cause. Hypocalciuric hypercalcemia occurs in milk-alkali syndrome, thiazide diuretic use, and familial hypocalciuric hypercalcemia.

The chest radiograph may reveal malignancy or granulomatous disease. The ECG can show a shortened QT interval.

Measurements of PTH and PTHrP help distinguish between hyperparathyroidism (elevated PTH) and malignancy-associated hypercalcemia (suppressed PTH, elevated PTHrP).

► Treatment

Until the primary cause can be identified and treated, renal excretion of calcium is promoted through aggressive hydration and forced calciuresis. The tendency in hypercalcemia is hypovolemia from nephrogenic DI. In volume-depleted patients with normal cardiac and kidney function, 0.9% saline can initially be given rapidly (250–500 mL/h). A meta-analysis questioned the efficacy and safety profile of intravenous furosemide for hypercalcemia. Thiazides can worsen hypercalcemia.

Bisphosphonates are the treatment of choice for hypercalcemia of malignancy. Although they are safe, effective, and normalize calcium in more than 70% of patients, bisphosphonates may require up to 48–72 hours before reaching full therapeutic effect. Calcitonin may be helpful in the short-term until bisphosphonates reach therapeutic levels. In emergency cases, dialysis with low calcium dialysate may be needed. Denosumab, a monoclonal antibody against RANKL inhibits osteoclasts, reducing bone resorption and serum calcium levels; this medication is FDA-approved for malignancy-associated hypercalcemia refractory to bisphosphonate therapy. The calcimimetic agent cinacalcet suppresses PTH secretion and decreases serum calcium concentration; it has been recommended for use in patients with symptomatic or severe primary hyperparathyroidism who are unable to undergo parathyroidectomy and patients with inoperable parathyroid carcinoma. (See Chapters 26 and 39.)

► When to Refer

- Patients may require referral to an oncologist or endocrinologist depending on the cause of hypercalcemia.
- Patients with granulomatous diseases (eg, tuberculosis and other chronic infections, granulomatosis with polyangiitis, sarcoidosis) may require assistance from infectious disease specialists, rheumatologists, or pulmonologists.

► When to Admit

- Patients with symptomatic or severe hypercalcemia require immediate treatment.
- Unexplained hypercalcemia with associated conditions, such as acute kidney injury or suspected malignancy, may require urgent treatment and expedited evaluation.

Ahmad S et al. Hypercalcemic crisis: a clinical review. Am J Med. 2015 Mar;128(3):239–45. [PMID: 25447624]

Bazari H et al. Case records of the Massachusetts General Hospital. Case 24-2016. A 66-year-old man with malaise, weakness, and hypercalcemia. N Engl J Med. 2016 Aug 11;375(6):567–74. [PMID: 27509105]

Minisola S et al. The diagnosis and management of hypercalcemia. BMJ. 2015 Jun 2;350:h2723. [PMID: 26037642]

Tebben PJ et al. Vitamin D-mediated hypercalcemia: mechanisms, diagnosis, and treatment. Endocr Rev. 2016 Oct;37(5):521–47. [PMID: 27588937]

Thosani S et al. Denosumab: a new agent in the management of hypercalcemia of malignancy. Future Oncol. 2015;11(21):2865–71. [PMID: 26403973]

DISORDERS OF PHOSPHORUS CONCENTRATION

Plasma phosphorus is mainly inorganic phosphate and represents a small fraction (less than 0.2%) of total body phosphate. Important determinants of plasma inorganic phosphate are renal excretion, intestinal absorption, and shift between the intracellular and extracellular spaces. The kidney is the most important regulator of the serum phosphate level. PTH decreases reabsorption of phosphate in the proximal tubule while 1,25-dihydroxyvitamin D_3 increases reabsorption. Renal proximal tubular reabsorption of phosphate is decreased by volume expansion, corticosteroids, and proximal tubular dysfunction (as in Fanconi syndrome). Fibroblast growth factor 23 (FGF23) is a potent phosphaturic hormone. Intestinal absorption of phosphate is facilitated by active vitamin D. PTH stimulates phosphate release from bone and renal phosphate excretion; primary hyperparathyroidism can lead to hypophosphatemia and depletion of bone phosphate stores. By contrast, growth hormone augments proximal tubular reabsorption of phosphate. Cellular phosphate uptake is stimulated by various factors and conditions, including alkalemia, insulin, epinephrine, feeding, hungry bone syndrome, and accelerated cell proliferation.

Phosphorus metabolism and homeostasis are intimately related to calcium metabolism. See sections on metabolic bone disease in Chapter 26.

HYPOPHOSPHATEMIA

ESSENTIALS OF DIAGNOSIS

- ► Severe hypophosphatemia may cause tissue hypoxia and rhabdomyolysis.
- ► Renal loss of phosphate can be diagnosed by calculating the fractional excretion of phosphate ($F_E PO_4$).
- ► PTH and FGF23 are the major factors that increase urine phosphate.

► General Considerations

The leading causes of hypophosphatemia are listed in Table 21–10. Hypophosphatemia may occur in the presence of normal phosphate stores. Serious depletion of body phosphate stores may exist with low, normal, or high serum phosphate concentrations.

Serum phosphate levels decrease transiently after food intake; thus, fasting samples are recommended for

Table 21–10. Causes of hypophosphatemia.

Diminished supply or absorption
Starvation
Parenteral alimentation with inadequate phosphate content
Malabsorption syndrome, small bowel bypass
Absorption blocked by oral antacids with aluminum or magnesium
Vitamin D–deficient and vitamin D–resistant osteomalacia
Increased loss
Phosphaturic drugs: theophylline, diuretics, bronchodilators, corticosteroids
Hyperparathyroidism (primary or secondary)
Hyperthyroidism
Renal tubular defects with excessive phosphaturia (congenital, Fanconi syndrome induced by monoclonal gammopathy, heavy metal poisoning), alcoholism
Hypokalemic nephropathy
Inadequately controlled diabetes mellitus
Hypophosphatemic rickets
Phosphatonins of oncogenic osteomalacia (eg, FGF23 production)
Intracellular shift of phosphorus
Administration of glucose
Anabolic steroids, estrogen, oral contraceptives, beta-adrenergic agonists, xanthine derivatives
Hungry bone syndrome
Respiratory alkalosis
Salicylate poisoning
Electrolyte abnormalities
Hypercalcemia
Hypomagnesemia
Metabolic alkalosis
Abnormal losses followed by inadequate repletion
Diabetes mellitus with acidosis, particularly during aggressive therapy
Recovery from starvation or prolonged catabolic state
Chronic alcoholism, particularly during restoration of nutrition; associated with hypomagnesemia
Recovery from severe burns

FGF23, fibroblast growth factor 23.

accuracy. **Moderate hypophosphatemia** (1.0–2.4 mg/dL [0.32–0.79 mmol/L]) occurs commonly in hospitalized patients and may not reflect decreased phosphate stores.

In **severe hypophosphatemia** (less than 1 mg/dL [0.32 mmol/L]), the affinity of hemoglobin for oxygen increases through a decrease in the erythrocyte 2,3-biphosphoglycerate concentration, impairing tissue oxygenation and cell metabolism and resulting in muscle weakness or even rhabdomyolysis. Severe hypophosphatemia is common and multifactorial in alcoholic patients. In acute alcohol withdrawal, increased plasma insulin and epinephrine along with respiratory alkalosis promote intracellular shift of phosphate. Vomiting, diarrhea, and poor dietary intake contribute to hypophosphatemia. Chronic alcohol use results in a decrease in the renal threshold of phosphate excretion. This renal tubular dysfunction reverses after a month of abstinence. Patients with chronic obstructive pulmonary disease and asthma commonly have hypophosphatemia, attributed to xanthine derivatives causing shifts of phosphate intracellularly and the phosphaturic effects of beta-adrenergic agonists, loop diuretics, xanthine derivatives, and corticosteroids. Refeeding or glucose administration to phosphate-depleted patients may cause fatal hypophosphatemia.

▶ **Clinical Findings**

A. Symptoms and Signs

Acute, severe hypophosphatemia (less than 1.0 mg/dL [0.32 mmol/L]) can lead to rhabdomyolysis, paresthesias, and encephalopathy (irritability, confusion, dysarthria, seizures, and coma). Respiratory failure or failure to wean from mechanical ventilation may occur as a result of diaphragmatic weakness. Arrhythmias and heart failure are uncommon but serious manifestations. Hematologic manifestations include acute hemolytic anemia from erythrocyte fragility, platelet dysfunction with petechial hemorrhages, and impaired chemotaxis of leukocytes (leading to increased susceptibility to gram-negative sepsis).

Chronic severe depletion may cause anorexia, pain in muscles and bones, and fractures.

B. Laboratory Findings

Urine phosphate excretion is a useful clue in the evaluation of hypophosphatemia. The normal renal response to hypophosphatemia is decreased urinary phosphate excretion to less than 100 mg/day, and a fractional excretion of phosphate ($F_E PO_4$) less than 5%. The main factors regulating $F_E PO_4$ are PTH and phosphate intake. Increased PTH or phosphate intake decreases $F_E PO_4$ (ie, more phosphate is excreted into the urine).

Measurement of plasma PTH or PTHrP levels may be helpful. The clinical utility of serum FGF levels is undetermined except in uncommon diseases.

Other clinical features may be suggestive of hypophosphatemia, such as hemolytic anemia and rhabdomyolysis. Fanconi syndrome may present with any combination of uricosuria, aminoaciduria, normoglycemic glucosuria, normal anion gap metabolic acidosis, and phosphaturia. In chronic hypophosphatemia, radiographs and bone biopsies show changes resembling osteomalacia.

▶ **Treatment**

Hypophosphatemia can be prevented by including phosphate in repletion and maintenance fluids. A rapid decline in calcium levels can occur with parenteral administration of phosphate; oral replacement of phosphate is preferable. Moderate hypophosphatemia (1.0–2.5 mg/dL [or 0.32–0.79 mmol/L]) is usually asymptomatic and does not require treatment. The hypophosphatemia in patients with diabetic ketoacidosis (DKA) will usually correct with normal dietary intake. Chronic hypophosphatemia can be treated with oral phosphate repletion. Mixtures of sodium and potassium phosphate salts may be given to provide 0.5–1 g (16–32 mmol) of phosphate per day. For severe, symptomatic hypophosphatemia (less than 1 mg/dL [0.32 mmol/L]), an infusion should provide 279–310 mg/12 h (or 9–10 mmol/12 h) until the serum phosphorus exceeds 1 mg/dL and the patient can be switched to oral therapy.

The infusion rate should be decreased if hypotension occurs. Monitoring of plasma phosphate, calcium, and potassium every 6 hours is necessary because the response to phosphate supplementation is not predictable. Magnesium deficiency often coexists and should be treated.

Contraindications to phosphate replacement include hypoparathyroidism, advanced CKD, tissue damage and necrosis, and hypercalcemia. When an associated hyperglycemia is treated, phosphate accompanies glucose into cells, and hypophosphatemia may ensue.

When to Refer

- Patients with refractory hypophosphatemia with increased urinary phosphate excretion may require evaluation by an endocrinologist (eg, for hyperparathyroidism and vitamin D disorders) or a nephrologist (eg, for renal tubular defects).

- Patients with decreased gastrointestinal absorption may require referral to a gastroenterologist.

When to Admit

Patients with severe or refractory hypophosphatemia will require intravenous phosphate.

Kraft MD. Phosphorus and calcium: a review for the adult nutrition support clinician. Nutr Clin Pract. 2015 Feb;30(1):21–33. Erratum in: Nutr Clin Pract. 2015 Jun;30(3):450. [PMID: 25550328]

Manghat P et al. Phosphate homeostasis and disorders. Ann Clin Biochem. 2014 Nov;51(Pt 6):631–56. [PMID: 24585932]

HYPERPHOSPHATEMIA

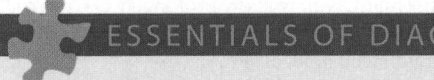

ESSENTIALS OF DIAGNOSIS

- ▶ Advanced CKD is the most common cause.
- ▶ Hyperphosphatemia in the presence of hypercalcemia imposes a high risk of metastatic calcification.

General Considerations

Advanced CKD with decreased urinary excretion of phosphate is the most common cause of hyperphosphatemia. Other causes are listed in Table 21–11.

Clinical Findings

A. Symptoms and Signs

The clinical manifestations are those of the underlying disorder or associated condition.

B. Laboratory Findings

In addition to elevated phosphate, blood chemistry abnormalities are those of the underlying disease.

Table 21–11. Causes of hyperphosphatemia.

Massive load of phosphate into the extracellular fluid
Exogenous sources
Hypervitaminosis D
Laxatives or enemas containing phosphate
Intravenous phosphate supplement
Endogenous sources
Rhabdomyolysis (especially if chronic kidney disease coexists)
Cell lysis by chemotherapy of malignancy, particularly lymphoproliferative diseases
Metabolic acidosis (lactic acidosis, ketoacidosis)
Respiratory acidosis (phosphate incorporation into cells is disturbed)
Decreased excretion into urine
Chronic kidney disease
Acute kidney injury
Hypoparathyroidism
Pseudohypoparathyroidism
Acromegaly
Pseudohyperphosphatemia
Plasma cell myeloma
Hyperbilirubinemia
Hypertriglyceridemia
Hemolysis in vitro

Treatment

Treatment is directed at the underlying cause. Exogenous sources of phosphate, including enteral or parenteral nutrition and medications, should be reduced or eliminated. Dietary phosphate absorption can be reduced by oral phosphate binders, such as calcium carbonate, calcium acetate, sevelamer carbonate, lanthanum carbonate, and aluminum hydroxide. Sevelamer, lanthanum, and aluminum may be used in patients with hypercalcemia, although aluminum use should be limited to a few days because of the risk of aluminum accumulation and neurotoxicity. In acute kidney injury and advanced CKD, dialysis will reduce serum phosphate.

When to Admit

Patients with acute severe hyperphosphatemia require hospitalization for emergent therapy, possibly including dialysis. Concomitant illnesses, such as acute kidney injury or cell lysis, may necessitate admission.

Criscuolo M et al. Tumor lysis syndrome: review of pathogenesis, risk factors and management of a medical emergency. Expert Rev Hematol. 2016;9(2):197–208. [PMID: 26629730]

Felsenfeld AJ et al. Pathophysiology of calcium, phosphorus, and magnesium dysregulation in chronic kidney disease. Semin Dial. 2015 Nov–Dec;28(6):564–77. [PMID: 26303319]

Ketteler M et al. Treating hyperphosphatemia—current and advancing drugs. Expert Opin Pharmacother. 2016 Oct; 17(14):1873–9. [PMID: 27643443]

Leaf DE et al. A physiologic-based approach to the evaluation of a patient with hyperphosphatemia. Am J Kidney Dis. 2013 Feb; 61(2):330–6. [PMID: 22938849]

DISORDERS OF MAGNESIUM CONCENTRATION

Normal plasma magnesium concentration is 1.8–3.0 mg/dL (or 0.75–1.25 mmol/L), with about one-third bound to protein and two-thirds existing as free cation. Magnesium excretion is via the kidney. Magnesium's physiologic effects on the nervous system resemble those of calcium.

Altered magnesium concentration usually provokes an associated alteration of Ca^{2+}. Both hypomagnesemia and hypermagnesemia can decrease PTH secretion or action. Severe hypermagnesemia (greater than 5 mg/dL [2.1 mmol/L]) suppresses PTH secretion with consequent hypocalcemia; this disorder is typically seen only in patients receiving magnesium therapy for preeclampsia. Severe hypomagnesemia causes PTH resistance in end organs and eventually decreased PTH secretion in severe cases.

HYPOMAGNESEMIA

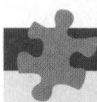

ESSENTIALS OF DIAGNOSIS

▶ Serum concentration of magnesium may be normal even in the presence of magnesium depletion. Check urinary magnesium excretion if renal magnesium wasting is suspected.

▶ Causes neurologic symptoms and arrhythmias.

▶ Impairs release of PTH.

▶ General Considerations

Causes of hypomagnesemia are listed in Table 21–12. Normomagnesemia does not exclude magnesium depletion because only 1% of total body magnesium is in the ECF. Hypomagnesemia and hypokalemia share many etiologies, including diuretics, diarrhea, alcoholism, aminoglycosides, and amphotericin. Renal potassium wasting also occurs from hypomagnesemia, and is refractory to potassium replacement until magnesium is repleted. Hypomagnesemia also suppresses PTH release and causes end-organ resistance to PTH and low 1,25-dihydroxyvitamin D_3 levels. The resultant hypocalcemia is refractory to calcium replacement until the magnesium is normalized. Molecular mechanisms of magnesium wasting have been revealed in some hereditary disorders. There is an FDA warning about hypomagnesemia for patients taking proton pump inhibitors. The presumed mechanism is decreased intestinal magnesium absorption, but it is not clear why this complication develops in only a small fraction of patients taking these medications.

▶ Clinical Findings

A. Symptoms and Signs

Common symptoms are those of hypokalemia and hypocalcemia, with weakness and muscle cramps. Marked neuromuscular and central nervous system hyperirritability may

Table 21–12. Causes of hypomagnesemia.

Diminished absorption or intake
Malabsorption, chronic diarrhea, laxative abuse
Proton pump inhibitors
Prolonged gastrointestinal suction
Small bowel bypass
Malnutrition
Alcoholism
Total parenteral alimentation with inadequate Mg^{2+} content
Increased renal loss
Diuretic therapy (loop diuretics, thiazide diuretics)
Hyperaldosteronism, Gitelman syndrome
Hyperparathyroidism, hyperthyroidism
Hypercalcemia
Volume expansion
Tubulointerstitial diseases
Transplant kidney
Drugs (aminoglycoside, cetuximab, cisplatin, amphotericin B, pentamidine)
Others
Diabetes mellitus
Post-parathyroidectomy (hungry bone syndrome)
Respiratory alkalosis
Pregnancy

produce tremors, athetoid movements, jerking, nystagmus, Babinski response, confusion, and disorientation. Cardiovascular manifestations include hypertension, tachycardia, and ventricular arrhythmias.

B. Laboratory Findings

Urinary excretion of magnesium exceeding 10–30 mg/day or a fractional excretion greater than 2% indicates renal magnesium wasting. Hypocalcemia and hypokalemia are often present. The ECG may show prolonged QT interval, due to lengthening of the ST segment. PTH secretion is often suppressed (see Hypocalcemia).

▶ Treatment

Magnesium oxide, 250–500 mg orally once or twice daily, is useful for treating chronic hypomagnesemia. Symptomatic hypomagnesemia requires intravenous magnesium sulfate 1–2 g over 5–60 minutes mixed in either dextrose 5% or 0.9% normal saline. Torsades de pointes in the setting of hypomagnesemia can be treated with 1–2 g of magnesium sulfate in 10 mL of dextrose 5% solution pushed intravenously over 15 minutes. Severe, non–life-threatening deficiency can be treated at a rate to 1–2 g/h over 3–6 hours. Magnesium sulfate may also be given intramuscularly in a dosage of 200–800 mg/day (8–33 mmol/day) in four divided doses. Serum levels must be monitored daily and dosage adjusted to keep the concentration from rising above 3 mg/dL (1.23 mmol/L). Tendon reflexes may be checked for hyporeflexia of hypermagnesemia. K^+ and Ca^{2+} replacement may be required, but patients with hypokalemia and hypocalcemia of hypomagnesemia do not recover without magnesium supplementation.

Patients with normal kidney function can excrete excess magnesium; hypermagnesemia should not develop with replacement dosages. In patients with CKD, magnesium replacement should be done cautiously to avoid hypermagnesemia. Reduced doses (50–75% dose reduction) and more frequent monitoring (at least twice daily) are indicated.

Cheungpasitporn W et al. Dysmagnesemia in hospitalized patients: prevalence and prognostic importance. Mayo Clin Proc. 2015 Aug;90(8):1001–10. [PMID: 26250725]
Gommers LM et al. Hypomagnesemia in type 2 diabetes: a vicious circle? Diabetes. 2016 Jan;65(1):3–13. [PMID: 26696633]

HYPERMAGNESEMIA

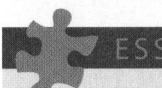

ESSENTIALS OF DIAGNOSIS

► Often associated with advanced CKD and chronic intake of magnesium-containing drugs.

General Considerations

Hypermagnesemia is almost always the result of advanced CKD and impaired magnesium excretion. Antacids and laxatives are underrecognized sources of magnesium. Pregnant patients may have severe hypermagnesemia from intravenous magnesium for preeclampsia and eclampsia. Magnesium replacement should be done cautiously in patients with CKD; dose reductions up to 75% may be necessary to avoid hypermagnesemia.

Clinical Findings

A. Symptoms and Signs

Muscle weakness, decreased deep tendon reflexes, mental obtundation, and confusion are characteristic manifestations. Weakness, flaccid paralysis, ileus, urinary retention, and hypotension are noted. Serious findings include respiratory muscle paralysis and cardiac arrest.

B. Laboratory Findings

Serum Mg^{2+} is elevated. In the common setting of CKD, BUN, creatinine, potassium, phosphate, and uric acid may all be elevated. Serum Ca^{2+} is often low. The ECG may show increased PR interval, broadened QRS complexes, and peaked T waves, probably related to associated hyperkalemia.

Treatment

Exogenous sources of magnesium should be discontinued. Calcium antagonizes Mg^{2+} and may be given intravenously as calcium chloride, 500 mg or more at a rate of 100 mg (4.1 mmol) per minute. Hemodialysis or peritoneal dialysis may be necessary to remove magnesium, particularly with severe kidney disease.

Long-term use of magnesium hydroxide and magnesium sulfate should be avoided in patients with advanced stages of CKD.

Broman M et al. Analysis of hypo- and hypermagnesemia in an intensive care unit cohort. Acta Anaesthesiol Scand. 2018 May; 62(5):648–57. [PMID: 29341068]
Chang WT et al. Calcium, magnesium, and phosphate abnormalities in the emergency department. Emerg Med Clin North Am. 2014 May;32(2):349–66. [PMID: 24766937]
Haider DG et al. Hypermagnesemia is a strong independent risk factor for mortality in critically ill patients: results from a cross-sectional study. Eur J Intern Med. 2015 Sep;26(7):504–7. [PMID: 26049918]

ACID–BASE DISORDERS

Assessment of a patient's acid-base status requires measurement of arterial pH, P_{CO_2}, and plasma bicarbonate (HCO_3^-). Blood gas analyzers directly measure pH and P_{CO_2}. The HCO_3^- value is calculated from the Henderson–Hasselbalch equation:

$$pH = 6.1 + \log \frac{HCO_3^-}{0.03 \times PCO_2}$$

The total venous CO_2 measurement is a more direct determination of HCO_3^-. Because of the dissociation characteristics of carbonic acid (H_2CO_3) at body pH, dissolved CO_2 is almost exclusively in the form of HCO_3^-, and for clinical purposes the total carbon dioxide content is equivalent (± 3 mEq/L) to the HCO_3^- concentration:

$$H^+ + HCO_3^- \leftrightarrow H_2CO_3 \leftrightarrow CO_2 + H_2O$$

Venous blood gases can provide useful information for acid-base assessment since the arteriovenous differences in pH and P_{CO_2} are small and relatively constant. Venous blood pH is usually 0.03–0.04 units lower than arterial blood pH, and venous blood P_{CO_2} is 7 or 8 mm Hg higher than arterial blood P_{CO_2}. Calculated HCO_3^- concentration in venous blood is at most 2 mEq/L higher than arterial blood HCO_3^-. Arterial and venous blood gases will not be equivalent during a cardiopulmonary arrest; arterial samples should be obtained for the most accurate measurements of pH and P_{CO_2}.

TYPES OF ACID–BASE DISORDERS

There are two types of acid-base disorders: acidosis and alkalosis. These disorders can be either metabolic (decreased or increased HCO_3^-) or respiratory (decreased or increased P_{CO_2}). Primary respiratory disorders affect blood acidity by changes in P_{CO_2}, and primary metabolic disorders are disturbances in HCO_3^- concentration. A primary disturbance is usually accompanied by a compensatory response, but the compensation does not fully correct the pH disturbance of the primary disorder. If the pH is < 7.40, the primary process is acidosis, either respiratory (P_{CO_2} greater than 40 mm Hg) or metabolic (HCO_3^- less than 24 mEq/L). If the pH is > 7.40, the primary process is alkalosis, either respiratory (P_{CO_2} less than 40 mm Hg) or metabolic (HCO_3^- greater than 24 mEq/L). One respiratory or metabolic disorder with its

Table 21–13. Primary acid-base disorders and expected compensation.

Disorder	Primary Defect	Compensatory Response	Magnitude of Compensation
Respiratory acidosis			
Acute	↑ PCO_2	↑ HCO_3^-	↑ HCO_3^- 1 mEq/L per 10 mm Hg ↑ PCO_2
Chronic	↑ PCO_2	↑ HCO_3^-	↑ HCO_3^- 3.5 mEq/L per 10 mm Hg ↑ PCO_2
Respiratory alkalosis			
Acute	↓ PCO_2	↓ HCO_3^-	↓ HCO_3^- 2 mEq/L per 10 mm Hg ↓ PCO_2
Chronic	↓ PCO_2	↓ HCO_3^-	↓ HCO_3^- 5 mEq/L per 10 mm Hg ↓ PCO_2
Metabolic acidosis	↓ HCO_3^-	↓ PCO_2	↓ PCO_2 1.3 mm Hg per 1 mEq/L ↓ HCO_3^-
Metabolic alkalosis	↑ HCO_3^-	↑ PCO_2	↑ PCO_2 0.7 mm Hg per 1 mEq/L ↑ HCO_3^-

appropriate compensatory response is a simple acid-base disorder.

MIXED ACID-BASE DISORDERS

Two or three simultaneous disorders can be present in a mixed acid-base disorder, but there can never be two primary respiratory disorders. Uncovering a mixed acid-base disorder is clinically important, and requires a methodical approach to acid-base analysis (see box Step-by-Step Analysis of Acid-Base Status). Once the primary disturbance has been determined, the clinician should assess whether the compensatory response is appropriate (Table 21–13). An inadequate or an exaggerated response indicates the presence of another primary acid-base disturbance.

STEP-BY-STEP ANALYSIS OF ACID-BASE STATUS

Step 1: Determine the primary (or main) disorder—whether it is metabolic or respiratory—from blood pH, HCO_3^-, and PCO_2 values.

Step 2: Determine the presence of mixed acid-base disorders by calculating the range of compensatory responses (see Table 21–13).

Step 3: Calculate the anion gap (see Table 21–14).

Step 4: Calculate the corrected HCO_3^- concentration if the anion gap is increased (see above).

Step 5: Examine the patient to determine whether the clinical signs are compatible with the acid-base analysis.

The anion gap should always be calculated for two reasons. First, it is possible to have an abnormal anion gap even if the sodium, chloride, and bicarbonate concentrations are normal. Second, an anion gap larger than 20 mEq/L suggests a primary metabolic acid-base disturbance regardless of the pH or serum bicarbonate level because a markedly abnormal anion gap is never a compensatory response to a respiratory disorder. In patients

with an increased anion gap metabolic acidosis, clinicians should calculate the corrected bicarbonate. In increased anion gap acidoses, there should be a mole for mole decrease in HCO_3^- as the anion gap increases. A corrected HCO_3^- value higher or lower than normal (24 mEq/L) indicates the concomitant presence of metabolic alkalosis or normal anion gap metabolic acidosis, respectively.

Filippatos T et al. Acid-base and electrolyte disorders associated with the use of antidiabetic drugs. Expert Opin Drug Saf. 2017 Oct;16(10):1121–32. [PMID: 28748724]

Gomez H et al. Understanding acid base disorders. Crit Care Clin. 2015 Oct;31(4):849–60. [PMID: 26410149]

Hamm LL et al. Acid-base homeostasis. Clin J Am Soc Nephrol. 2015 Dec 7;10(12):2232–42. [PMID: 26597304]

Scheiner B et al. Acid-base disorders in liver disease. J Hepatol. 2017 Nov;67(5):1062–73. [PMID: 28684104]

Seifter JL. Integration of acid-base and electrolyte disorders. N Engl J Med. 2014 Nov 6;371(19):1821–31. [PMID: 25372090]

Wiener SW. Toxicologic acid-base disorders. Emerg Med Clin North Am. 2014 Feb;32(1):149–65. [PMID: 24275173]

METABOLIC ACIDOSIS

 ESSENTIALS OF DIAGNOSIS

▶ Decreased HCO_3^- with acidemia.

▶ Classified into increased anion gap acidosis and normal anion gap acidosis.

▶ Lactic acidosis, ketoacidosis, and toxins produce metabolic acidoses with the largest anion gaps.

▶ Normal anion gap acidosis is mainly caused by gastrointestinal HCO_3^- loss or RTA. Urinary anion gap may help distinguish between these causes.

▶ General Considerations

The hallmark of metabolic acidosis is decreased HCO_3^-. Metabolic acidoses are classified by the anion gap, usually normal or increased (Table 21–14). The anion gap is the difference between readily measured anions and cations.

Table 21–14. Anion gap in metabolic acidosis.[1]

Decreased (< 6 mEq)
  Hypoalbuminemia (decreased unmeasured anion)
  Plasma cell dyscrasias
    Monoclonal protein (cationic paraprotein accompanied by
      chloride and bicarbonate)
  Bromide intoxication
Increased (> 12 mEq)
  Metabolic anion
    Diabetic ketoacidosis
    Alcoholic ketoacidosis
    Lactic acidosis
    Chronic kidney disease (advanced stages) (PO_4^{3-}, SO_4^{2-})
    Starvation
    Metabolic alkalosis (increased number of negative charges
      on protein)
    5-Oxoproline acidosis from acetaminophen toxicity
  Drug or chemical anion
    Salicylate intoxication
    Sodium carbenicillin therapy
    Methanol (formic acid)
    Ethylene glycol (oxalic acid)
Normal (6–12 mEq)
  Loss of HCO_3
    Diarrhea
    Recovery from diabetic ketoacidosis
    Pancreatic fluid loss, ileostomy (unadapted)
    Carbonic anhydrase inhibitors
  Chloride retention
    Renal tubular acidosis
    Ileal loop bladder
  Administration of HCl equivalent or NH_4Cl
    Arginine and lysine in parenteral nutrition

[1]Reference ranges for anion gap may vary based on differing laboratory methods.

In plasma,

$$[Na^+] + \begin{matrix} \text{Unmeasured} \\ \text{cations} \end{matrix} = (HCO_3^- + Cl^-) + \begin{matrix} \text{Unmeasured} \\ \text{anions} \end{matrix}$$

$$\text{Anion gap} = Na^+ - (HCO_3^- + Cl^-)$$

Major unmeasured cations are calcium (2 mEq/L), magnesium (2 mEq/L), gamma-globulins, and potassium (4 mEq/L). Major unmeasured anions are albumin (2 mEq/L per g/dL), phosphate (2 mEq/L), sulfate (1 mEq/L), lactate (1–2 mEq/L), and other organic anions (3–4 mEq/L). Traditionally, the normal anion gap has been 12 ± 4 mEq/L. With current auto-analyzers, the reference range may be lower (6 ± 1 mEq/L), primarily from an increase in Cl⁻ values. Despite its usefulness, the anion gap can be misleading. Non–acid-base disorders may cause errors in anion gap interpretation; these disorders include hypoalbuminemia, hypernatremia, or hyponatremia; antibiotics (eg, carbenicillin is an unmeasured anion; polymyxin is an unmeasured cation) may also cause errors in anion gap interpretation. Although not usually associated with metabolic acidosis, a decreased anion gap can occur because of a reduction in unmeasured anions or an increase in unmeasured cations. In hypoalbuminemia, a 2 mEq/L decrease in anion gap will occur for every 1 g/dL decline in serum albumin.

INCREASED ANION GAP ACIDOSIS (Increased Unmeasured Anions)

Normochloremic metabolic acidosis generally results from addition of organic acids such as lactate, acetoacetate, beta-hydroxybutyrate, and exogenous toxins. Other anions such as isocitrate, alpha-ketoglutarate, malate, and D-lactate may contribute to the anion gap of lactic acidosis, DKA, and acidosis of unknown etiology. Uremia causes an increased anion gap metabolic acidosis from unexcreted organic acids and anions.

A. Lactic Acidosis

Lactic acidosis is a common cause of metabolic acidosis, producing an elevated anion gap and decreased serum pH when present without other acid-base disturbances. Lactate is formed from pyruvate in anaerobic glycolysis. Normally, lactate levels remain low (1 mEq/L) because of metabolism of lactate principally by the liver through gluconeogenesis or oxidation via the Krebs cycle.

In lactic acidosis, lactate levels are at least 4–5 mEq/L but commonly 10–30 mEq/L. There are two basic types of lactic acidosis.

Type A (hypoxic) lactic acidosis is more common, resulting from decreased tissue perfusion; cardiogenic, septic, or hemorrhagic shock; and carbon monoxide or cyanide poisoning. These conditions increase peripheral lactic acid production and decrease hepatic metabolism of lactate as liver perfusion declines.

Type B lactic acidosis may be due to metabolic causes (eg, diabetes, ketoacidosis, liver disease, kidney disease, infection, leukemia, or lymphoma) or toxins (eg, ethanol, methanol, salicylates, isoniazid, or metformin). Propylene glycol can cause lactic acidosis from decreased liver metabolism; it is used as a vehicle for intravenous drugs, such as nitroglycerin, etomidate, and diazepam. Parenteral nutrition without thiamine causes severe refractory lactic acidosis from deranged pyruvate metabolism. Patients with short bowel syndrome may develop d-lactic acidosis with encephalopathy due to carbohydrate malabsorption and subsequent fermentation by colonic bacteria. Nucleoside analog reverse transcriptase inhibitors can cause type B lactic acidosis due to mitochondrial toxicity.

Idiopathic lactic acidosis, usually in debilitated patients, has an extremely high mortality rate. (For treatment of lactic acidosis, see below and Chapter 27.)

B. Diabetic Ketoacidosis (DKA)

DKA is characterized by hyperglycemia and metabolic acidosis with an increased anion gap:

$$H^+ + B^- + NaHCO_3 \leftrightarrow CO_2 + NaB + H_2O$$

where B⁻ is beta-hydroxybutyrate or acetoacetate, the ketones responsible for the increased anion gap. The anion gap should be calculated from the measured serum electrolytes; correction of the serum sodium for the dilutional effect of hyperglycemia will exaggerate the anion gap. Diabetics with ketoacidosis may have lactic acidosis from tissue hypoperfusion and increased anaerobic metabolism.

During the recovery phase of DKA, a hyperchloremic non-anion gap acidosis can develop because saline resuscitation results in chloride retention, restoration of GFR, and ketoaciduria. Ketone salts (NaB) are formed as bicarbonate is consumed:

$$HB + NaHCO_3 \rightarrow NaB + H_2CO_3$$

The kidney reabsorbs ketone anions poorly but can compensate for the loss of anions by increasing the reabsorption of Cl^-.

Patients with DKA and normal kidney function may have marked ketonuria and severe metabolic acidosis but only a mildly increased anion gap. Thus, the size of the anion gap correlates poorly with the severity of the DKA; the urinary loss of Na^+ or K^+ salts of beta-hydroxybutyrate will lower the anion gap without altering the H^+ excretion or the severity of the acidosis. Urine dipsticks for ketones test primarily for acetoacetate and, to a lesser degree, acetone but not the predominant ketoacid, beta-hydroxybutyrate. Dipstick tests for ketones may become more positive even as the patient improves due to the metabolism of beta-hydroxybutyrate. Thus, the patient's clinical status and pH are better markers of improvement than the anion gap or ketone levels.

C. Alcoholic Ketoacidosis

Chronically malnourished patients who consume large quantities of alcohol daily may develop alcoholic ketoacidosis. Most of these patients have mixed acid-base disorders (10% have a triple acid-base disorder). Although decreased HCO_3^- is usual, 50% of the patients may have normal or alkalemic pH. Three types of metabolic acidosis are seen in alcoholic ketoacidosis: (1) Ketoacidosis is due to beta-hydroxybutyrate and acetoacetate excess. (2) Lactic acidosis: Alcohol metabolism increases the NADH:NAD ratio, causing increased production and decreased utilization of lactate. Accompanying thiamine deficiency, which inhibits pyruvate carboxylase, further enhances lactic acid production in many cases. Moderate to severe elevations of lactate (greater than 6 mmol/L) are seen with concomitant disorders such as sepsis, pancreatitis, or hypoglycemia. (3) Hyperchloremic acidosis from bicarbonate loss in the urine is associated with ketonuria (see above). Metabolic alkalosis occurs from volume contraction and vomiting. Respiratory alkalosis results from alcohol withdrawal, pain, or associated disorders such as sepsis or liver disease. Half of the patients have hypoglycemia or hyperglycemia. When serum glucose levels are greater than 250 mg/dL (13.88 mmol/L), the distinction from DKA is difficult. The absence of a diabetic history and normoglycemia after initial therapy support the diagnosis of alcoholic ketoacidosis.

D. Toxins

(See also Chapter 38.) Multiple toxins and drugs increase the anion gap by increasing endogenous acid production. Common examples include methanol (metabolized to formic acid), ethylene glycol (glycolic and oxalic acid), and salicylates (salicylic acid and lactic acid). The latter can cause a mixed disorder of metabolic acidosis with respiratory alkalosis. In toluene poisoning, the metabolite hippurate is rapidly excreted by the kidney and may present as a normal anion gap acidosis. Isopropanol, which is metabolized to acetone, increases the osmolar gap, but not the anion gap. If there is a concern for toxin ingestion, the Poison Control Center should be contacted immediately; in the United States, the center is available 24 hours at 1-800-222-1222.

E. Uremic Acidosis

As the GFR drops below 15–30 mL/min, the kidneys are increasingly unable to synthesize NH_3. The reduced excretion of H^+ and organic acids (eg, phosphate and sulfate) as NH_4Cl results in an increased anion gap metabolic acidosis.

NORMAL ANION GAP ACIDOSIS

The two major causes are gastrointestinal HCO_3^- loss and defects in renal acidification (renal tubular acidosis) (Table 21–15). The urinary anion gap can differentiate between these causes.

A. Gastrointestinal HCO_3^- Loss

The gastrointestinal tract secretes bicarbonate at multiple sites. Small bowel and pancreatic secretions contain large amounts of HCO_3^-; massive diarrhea or pancreatic drainage can result in HCO_3^- loss. Hyperchloremia occurs because the ileum and colon secrete HCO_3^- in exchange for Cl^- by countertransport. The resultant volume contraction causes increased Cl^- retention by the kidney in the setting of decreased HCO_3^-. Patients with ureterosigmoidostomies can develop hyperchloremic metabolic acidosis because the colon secretes HCO_3^- in the urine in exchange for Cl^-.

B. Renal Tubular Acidosis (RTA)

Hyperchloremic acidosis with a normal anion gap and normal (or near normal) GFR, and in the absence of diarrhea, defines RTA. The defect is either inability to excrete H^+ (inadequate generation of new HCO_3^-) or inadequate reabsorption of HCO_3^-. Three major types can be differentiated by the clinical setting, urinary pH, urinary anion gap, and serum K^+ level. The pathophysiologic mechanisms of RTA have been elucidated by identifying the responsible molecules and gene mutations.

1. Classic distal RTA (type I)—This disorder is characterized by selective deficiency in H^+ secretion in alpha intercalated cells in the collecting tubule. Despite acidosis, urinary pH cannot be acidified and is above 5.5, which retards the binding of H^+ to phosphate ($H^+ + HPO_4^{2-} \rightarrow H_2PO_4$) and inhibits titratable acid excretion. Furthermore, urinary excretion of $NH_4^+Cl^-$ is decreased, and the urinary anion gap is positive. Enhanced K^+ excretion occurs probably because there is less competition from H^+ in the distal nephron transport system. Furthermore, hyperaldosteronism occurs in response to renal salt wasting, which will increase potassium excretion. Nephrocalcinosis and nephrolithiasis are often seen in patients with distal RTA since chronic acidosis decreases tubular calcium reabsorption.

Table 21–15. Hyperchloremic, normal anion gap metabolic acidoses.

	Renal Defect	Serum [K⁺]	Distal H⁺ Secretion		Urinary Anion Gap	Treatment
			Urine pH	Titratable Acid		
Gastrointestinal HCO₃⁻ loss	None	↓	< 5.5	↑↑	Negative	Na⁺, K⁺, and HCO₃⁻ as required
Renal tubular acidosis						
I. Classic distal	Distal H⁺ secretion	↓	> 5.5	↓	Positive	NaHCO₃ (1–3 mEq/kg/day)
II. Proximal	Proximal HCO₃⁻ reabsorption	↓	Variable	Normal	Positive	NaHCO₃ or KHCO₃ (10–15 mEq/kg/day), thiazide
IV. Hyporeninemic hypoaldosteronism	Distal Na⁺ reabsorption, K⁺ secretion, and H⁺ secretion	↑	Variable	↓	Positive	Fludrocortisone (0.1–0.5 mg/day), dietary K⁺ restriction, furosemide (40–160 mg/day), NaHCO₃ (1–3 mEq/kg/day)

Modified and reproduced, with permission, from Cogan MG. *Fluid and Electrolytes: Physiology and Pathophysiology.* McGraw-Hill, 1991.

Hypercalciuria, alkaline urine, and lowered level of urinary citrate cause calcium phosphate stones and nephrocalcinosis. Distal RTA develops as a consequence of paraproteinemias, autoimmune disease, and drugs and toxins such as amphotericin.

2. Proximal RTA (type II)—Proximal RTA is due to a selective defect in the proximal tubule's ability to reabsorb filtered HCO₃⁻. Carbonic anhydrase inhibitors (acetazolamide) can cause proximal RTA. About 90% of filtered HCO₃⁻ is absorbed by the proximal tubule. A proximal defect in HCO₃⁻ reabsorption will overwhelm the distal tubule's limited capacity to reabsorb HCO₃⁻, resulting in bicarbonaturia and metabolic acidosis. Distal delivery of HCO₃⁻ declines as the plasma HCO₃⁻ level decreases. When the plasma HCO₃⁻ level drops to 15–18 mEq/L, the distal nephron can reabsorb the diminished filtered load of HCO₃⁻. Bicarbonaturia resolves, and the urinary pH can be acidic. Thiazide-induced volume contraction can be used to enhance proximal HCO₃⁻ reabsorption, leading to the decrease in distal HCO₃⁻ delivery and improvement of bicarbonaturia and renal acidification. The increased delivery of HCO₃⁻ to the distal nephron increases K⁺ secretion, and hypokalemia results if a patient is loaded with excess HCO₃⁻ and K⁺ is not adequately supplemented. Proximal RTA can exist with other proximal reabsorption defects, such as Fanconi syndrome, resulting in glucosuria, aminoaciduria, phosphaturia, and uricosuria. Causes include plasma cell myeloma (formerly called multiple myeloma) and nephrotoxic drugs.

3. Hyporeninemic hypoaldosteronemic RTA (type IV)—Type IV is the most common RTA in clinical practice. The defect is aldosterone deficiency or antagonism, which impairs distal nephron Na⁺ reabsorption and K⁺ and H⁺ excretion. Renal salt wasting and hyperkalemia are frequently present. Common causes are diabetic nephropathy, tubulointerstitial renal diseases, hypertensive nephrosclerosis, and AIDS. In patients with these disorders, drugs,

such as ACE inhibitors, ARBs, spironolactone, and NSAIDs, can exacerbate the hyperkalemia.

C. Dilutional Acidosis

Rapid dilution of plasma volume by 0.9% NaCl may cause hyperchloremic acidosis.

D. Recovery from DKA

See Increased Anion Gap Acidosis (Increased Unmeasured Anions).

E. Posthypocapnia

In prolonged respiratory alkalosis, HCO₃⁻ decreases and Cl⁻ increases from decreased renal NH₄⁺Cl⁻ excretion. If the respiratory alkalosis is corrected quickly, HCO₃⁻ will remain low until the kidneys can generate new HCO₃⁻, which generally takes several days. In the meantime, the increased Pco₂ with low HCO₃⁻ causes metabolic acidosis.

F. Hyperalimentation

Hyperalimentation fluids may contain amino acid solutions that acidify when metabolized, such as arginine hydrochloride and lysine hydrochloride.

► Assessment of Hyperchloremic Metabolic Acidosis by Urinary Anion Gap

Increased renal NH₄⁺Cl⁻ excretion to enhance H⁺ removal is the normal physiologic response to metabolic acidosis. The daily urinary excretion of NH₄Cl can be increased from 30 mEq to 200 mEq in response to acidosis.

The urinary anion gap (Na⁺ + K⁺ – Cl⁻) reflects the ability of the kidney to excrete NH₄Cl. The urinary anion gap differentiates between gastrointestinal and renal causes of hyperchloremic acidosis. If the cause is gastrointestinal

HCO_3^- loss (diarrhea), renal acidification remains normal and NH_4Cl excretion increases, and the urinary anion gap is negative. If the cause is distal RTA, the urinary anion gap is positive, since the basic lesion in the disorder is the inability of the kidney to excrete H^+ as NH_4Cl. In proximal (type II) RTA, the kidney has defective HCO_3^- reabsorption, leading to increased HCO_3^- excretion rather than decreased NH_4Cl excretion; the urinary anion gap is often negative.

Urinary pH may not readily differentiate between the two causes. Despite acidosis, if volume depletion from diarrhea causes inadequate Na^+ delivery to the distal nephron and therefore decreased exchange with H^+, urinary pH may not be lower than 5.3. In the presence of this relatively high urinary pH, however, H^+ excretion continues due to buffering of NH_3 to NH_4^+, since the pK of this reaction is as high as 9.1. Potassium depletion, which can accompany diarrhea (and surreptitious laxative abuse), may also impair renal acidification. Thus, when volume depletion is present, the urinary anion gap is a better measure of ability to acidify the urine than urinary pH.

When large amounts of other anions are present in the urine, the urinary anion gap may not be reliable. In such a situation, NH_4^+ excretion can be estimated using the urinary osmolar gap where urine concentrations and osmolality are in mmol/L.

NH_4^+ excretion (mmol/L) = 0.5 × Urinary osmolar gap
= 0.5 [U Osm − 2(U Na^+ + U K^+) + U urea + U glucose]

► Clinical Findings

A. Symptoms and Signs

Symptoms of metabolic acidosis are mainly those of the underlying disorder. Compensatory hyperventilation is an important clinical sign and may be misinterpreted as a primary respiratory disorder; Kussmaul breathing (deep, regular, sighing respirations) may be seen with severe metabolic acidosis.

B. Laboratory Findings

Blood pH, serum HCO_3^-, and P_{CO_2} are decreased. Anion gap may be normal (hyperchloremic) or increased (normochloremic). Hyperkalemia may be seen.

► Treatment

A. Increased Anion Gap Acidosis

Treatment is aimed at the underlying disorder, such as insulin and fluid therapy for diabetes and appropriate volume resuscitation to restore tissue perfusion. The metabolism of lactate will produce HCO_3^- and increase pH. Supplemental HCO_3^- is indicated for treatment of hyperkalemia (see Table 21–7) and some forms of normal anion gap acidosis but has been controversial for treatment of increased anion gap metabolic acidosis with respect to efficacy and safety. Large amounts of HCO_3^- may have deleterious effects, including hypernatremia, hyperosmolality, volume overload, and worsening of intracellular acidosis.

In addition, alkali administration stimulates phosphofructokinase activity, thus exacerbating lactic acidosis via enhanced lactate production. Ketogenesis is also augmented by alkali therapy.

In salicylate intoxication, alkali therapy must be started to decrease central nervous system damage unless blood pH is already alkalinized by respiratory alkalosis, since an increased pH converts salicylate to more impermeable salicylic acid. In alcoholic ketoacidosis, thiamine should be given with glucose to avoid Wernicke encephalopathy. The bicarbonate deficit can be calculated as follows:

HCO_3^- deficit = 0.5 × body weight in kg × (24 − HCO_3^-)

Half of the calculated deficit should be administered within the first 3–4 hours to avoid overcorrection and volume overload. In methanol intoxication, inhibition of alcohol dehydrogenase by fomepizole is standard care. Ethanol had previously been used as a competitive substrate for alcohol dehydrogenase, which metabolizes to formaldehyde.

B. Normal Anion Gap Acidosis

Treatment of RTA is mainly achieved by administration of alkali (either as bicarbonate or citrate) to correct metabolic abnormalities and prevent nephrocalcinosis and CKD.

Large amounts of oral alkali (10–15 mEq/kg/day) (Table 21–15) may be required to treat proximal RTA because most of the alkali is excreted into the urine, which exacerbates hypokalemia. Thus, a mixture of sodium and potassium salts is preferred. Thiazides may reduce the amount of alkali required, but hypokalemia may develop. Treatment of type 1 distal RTA requires less alkali (1–3 mEq/kg/day) than proximal RTA. Potassium supplementation may be necessary.

For type IV RTA, dietary potassium restriction may be necessary and potassium-retaining drugs should be withdrawn. Fludrocortisone may be effective in cases with hypoaldosteronism, but should be used with care, preferably in combination with loop diuretics. In some cases, oral alkali supplementation (1–3 mEq/kg/day) may be required.

► When to Refer

Most clinicians will refer patients with renal tubular acidoses to a nephrologist for evaluation and possible alkali therapy.

► When to Admit

Patients will require emergency department evaluation or hospital admission depending on the severity of the acidosis and underlying conditions.

Fayfman M et al. Management of hyperglycemic crises: diabetic ketoacidosis and hyperglycemic hyperosmolar state. Med Clin North Am. 2017 May;101(3):587–606. [PMID: 28372715]

Lalau JD et al. Metformin-associated lactic acidosis (MALA): moving towards a new paradigm. Diabetes Obes Metab. 2017 Nov;19(11):1502–12. [PMID: 28417525]

Palmer BF et al. Electrolyte and acid-base disturbances in patients with diabetes mellitus. N Engl J Med. 2015 Aug 6; 373(6):548–59. [PMID: 26244308]

Seheult J et al. Lactic acidosis: an update. Clin Chem Lab Med. 2017 Mar 1;55(3):322–33. [PMID: 27522622]

Sharma S et al. Comprehensive clinical approach to renal tubular acidosis. Clin Exp Nephrol. 2015 Aug;19(4):556–61. [PMID: 25951806]

Suetrong B et al. Lactic acidosis in sepsis: it's not all anaerobic: implications for diagnosis and management. Chest. 2016 Jan; 149(1):252–61. [PMID: 26378980]

METABOLIC ALKALOSIS

ESSENTIALS OF DIAGNOSIS

▶ High HCO_3^- with alkalemia.

▶ Evaluate effective circulating volume by physical examination.

▶ Urinary chloride concentration differentiates saline-responsive alkalosis from saline-unresponsive alkalosis.

▶ Classification

Metabolic alkalosis is characterized by high HCO_3^-. Abnormalities that generate HCO_3^- are called "initiation factors," whereas abnormalities that promote renal conservation of HCO_3^- are called "maintenance factors." Thus, metabolic alkalosis may remain even after the initiation factors have resolved.

The causes of metabolic alkalosis are classified into two groups based on "saline responsiveness" using the urine Cl^- as a marker for volume status (Table 21–16). Saline-responsive metabolic alkalosis is a sign of extracellular volume contraction, and saline-unresponsive alkalosis implies excessive total body bicarbonate with either euvolemia or hypervolemia. The compensatory increase in Pco_2 rarely exceeds 55 mm Hg; higher Pco_2 values imply a superimposed primary respiratory acidosis.

A. Saline-Responsive Metabolic Alkalosis

Much more common than saline-unresponsive alkalosis, saline-responsive alkalosis is characterized by normotensive extracellular volume contraction and hypokalemia. Hypotension and orthostasis may be seen. In vomiting or nasogastric suction, loss of acid (HCl) initiates the alkalosis, but volume contraction from Cl^- loss maintains the alkalosis because the kidney avidly reabsorbs Na^+ to restore the ECF. Increased sodium reabsorption necessitates increased HCO_3^- reabsorption proximally, and the urinary pH remains acidic despite alkalemia (paradoxical aciduria). Renal Cl^- reabsorption is high, and urine Cl^- is low (less than 20 mEq/L). In alkalosis, bicarbonaturia may force Na^+ excretion as the accompanying cation even if volume depletion is present. Therefore, urine Cl^- is preferred to urine Na^+ as a measure of extracellular volume. Diuretics may limit the utility of urine chloride by increasing urine chloride and sodium excretion, even in the setting of volume contraction.

Metabolic alkalosis is generally associated with hypokalemia due to the direct effect of alkalosis on renal potassium excretion and secondary hyperaldosteronism from volume depletion. Hypokalemia exacerbates the metabolic alkalosis by increasing bicarbonate reabsorption in the proximal tubule and hydrogen ion secretion in the distal tubule. Administration of KCl will correct the disorder.

1. Contraction alkalosis—Diuretics decrease extracellular volume from urinary loss of NaCl and water. The plasma HCO_3^- concentration increases because the ECF volume contracts around a stable total body bicarbonate. Contraction alkalosis is the opposite of dilutional acidosis.

Table 21–16. Metabolic alkalosis.

Saline-Responsive (U_{Cl} < 20 mEq/L)	Saline-Unresponsive (U_{Cl} > 40 mEq/L)
Excessive body bicarbonate content	**Excessive body bicarbonate content**
Renal alkalosis	Renal alkalosis
Diuretic therapy	Normotensive
Poorly reabsorbable anion therapy: carbenicillin, penicillin, sulfate, phosphate	Bartter syndrome (renal salt wasting and secondary hyperaldosteronism)
Posthypercapnia	Severe potassium depletion
Gastrointestinal alkalosis	Refeeding alkalosis
Loss of HCl from vomiting or nasogastric suction	Hypercalcemia and hypoparathyroidism
Intestinal alkalosis: chloride diarrhea	Hypertensive
$NaHCO_3$ (baking soda)	Endogenous mineralocorticoids
Sodium citrate, lactate, gluconate, acetate	Primary aldosteronism
Transfusions	Hyperreninism
Antacids	Adrenal enzyme (11-beta-hydroxylase and 17-alpha-hydroxylase) deficiency
Normal body bicarbonate content	Liddle syndrome
"Contraction alkalosis"	Exogenous alkali
	Exogenous mineralocorticoids
	Licorice

2. Posthypercapnia alkalosis—In chronic respiratory acidosis, the kidney decreases bicarbonate excretion, increasing plasma HCO_3^- concentration (see Table 21–13). Hypercapnia directly affects the proximal tubule to decrease NaCl reabsorption, which can cause extracellular volume depletion. If PCO_2 is rapidly corrected, metabolic alkalosis will exist until the kidney excretes the retained bicarbonate. Many patients with chronic respiratory acidosis receive diuretics, which further exacerbates the metabolic alkalosis.

B. Saline-Unresponsive Alkalosis

1. Hyperaldosteronism—Primary hyperaldosteronism causes extracellular volume expansion and hypertension by increasing distal sodium reabsorption. Aldosterone increases H^+ and K^+ excretion, producing metabolic alkalosis and hypokalemia. In an attempt to decrease extracellular volume, high levels of NaCl are excreted resulting in a high urine Cl^- (greater than 20 mEq/L). Therapy with NaCl will only increase volume expansion and hypertension and will not treat the underlying problem of mineralocorticoid excess.

2. Alkali administration with decreased GFR—The normal kidney has a substantial capacity for bicarbonate excretion, protecting against metabolic alkalosis even with large HCO_3^- intake. However, urinary excretion of bicarbonate is inadequate in CKD. If large amounts of HCO_3^- are consumed, as with intensive antacid therapy, metabolic alkalosis will occur. Lactate, citrate, and gluconate can also cause metabolic alkalosis because they are metabolized to bicarbonate. In milk-alkali syndrome, sustained heavy ingestion of absorbable antacids and milk causes hypercalcemic kidney injury and metabolic alkalosis. Volume contraction from renal hypercalcemic effects exacerbates the alkalosis.

▶ Clinical Findings

A. Symptoms and Signs

There are no characteristic symptoms or signs. Orthostatic hypotension may be encountered. Concomitant hypokalemia may cause weakness and hyporeflexia. Tetany and neuromuscular irritability occur rarely.

B. Laboratory Findings

The arterial blood pH and bicarbonate are elevated. With respiratory compensation, the arterial PCO_2 is increased. Serum potassium and chloride are decreased. There may be an increased anion gap. The urine chloride can differentiate between saline-responsive (less than 25 mEq/L) and unresponsive (greater than 40 mEq/L) causes.

▶ Treatment

Mild alkalosis is generally well tolerated. Severe or symptomatic alkalosis (pH > 7.60) requires urgent treatment.

A. Saline-Responsive Metabolic Alkalosis

Therapy for saline-responsive metabolic alkalosis is correction of the extracellular volume deficit with isotonic saline.

Diuretics should be discontinued. H_2-blockers or proton pump inhibitors may be helpful in patients with alkalosis from nasogastric suctioning. If pulmonary or cardiovascular disease prohibits adequate resuscitation, acetazolamide will increase renal bicarbonate excretion. Hypokalemia may develop because bicarbonate excretion may induce kaliuresis. Severe cases, especially those with reduced kidney function, may require dialysis with low-bicarbonate dialysate.

B. Saline-Unresponsive Metabolic Alkalosis

Therapy for saline-unresponsive metabolic alkalosis includes surgical removal of a mineralocorticoid-producing tumor and blockage of aldosterone effect with an ACE inhibitor or with spironolactone (see Chapter 26). Metabolic alkalosis in primary aldosteronism can be treated only with potassium repletion.

Feldman M et al. Respiratory compensation to a primary metabolic alkalosis in humans. Clin Nephrol. 2012 Nov;78(5):365–9. [PMID: 22854166]

Peixoto AJ et al. Treatment of severe metabolic alkalosis in a patient with congestive heart failure. Am J Kidney Dis. 2013 May;61(5):822–7. [PMID: 23481366]

Soifer JT et al. Approach to metabolic alkalosis. Emerg Med Clin North Am. 2014 May;32(2):453–63. [PMID: 24766943]

Yi JH et al. Metabolic alkalosis from unsuspected ingestion: use of urine pH and anion gap. Am J Kidney Dis. 2012 Apr; 59(4):577–81. [PMID: 22265393]

RESPIRATORY ACIDOSIS (Hypercapnia)

Respiratory acidosis results from hypoventilation and subsequent hypercapnia. Pulmonary and extrapulmonary disorders can cause hypoventilation.

Acute respiratory failure is associated with severe acidosis and only a small increase in the plasma bicarbonate. After 6–12 hours, the primary increase in PCO_2 evokes a renal compensation to excrete more acid and to generate more HCO_3^-; complete metabolic compensation by the kidney takes several days.

Chronic respiratory acidosis is generally seen in patients with underlying lung disease, such as chronic obstructive pulmonary disease. Renal excretion of acid as NH_4Cl results in hypochloremia. When chronic respiratory acidosis is corrected suddenly, posthypercapnic metabolic alkalosis ensues until the kidneys excrete the excess bicarbonate over 2–3 days.

▶ Clinical Findings

A. Symptoms and Signs

With acute onset, somnolence, confusion, mental status changes, asterixis, and myoclonus may develop. Severe hypercapnia increases cerebral blood flow, cerebrospinal fluid pressure, and intracranial pressure; papilledema and pseudotumor cerebri may be seen.

B. Laboratory Findings

Arterial pH is low and PCO_2 is increased. Serum HCO_3^- is elevated but does not fully correct the pH. If the disorder is chronic, hypochloremia is seen. Respiratory etiologies of respiratory acidosis usually have a wide A-a gradient; a relatively normal A-a gradient suggests a nonpulmonary (eg, central) etiology.

Treatment

If opioid overdose is a possible diagnosis or there is no other obvious cause for hypoventilation, the clinician should consider a diagnostic and therapeutic trial of intravenous naloxone (see Chapter 38). In all forms of respiratory acidosis, treatment is directed at the underlying disorder to improve ventilation.

Bruno CM et al. Acid-base disorders in patients with chronic obstructive pulmonary disease: a pathophysiological review. J Biomed Biotechnol. 2012;2012:915150. [PMID: 22500110]
Chebbo A et al. Hypoventilation syndromes. Med Clin North Am. 2011 Nov;95(6):1189–202. [PMID: 22032434]
Schwartzstein RM et al. Rising PaCO$_2$ in the ICU: using a physiologic approach to avoid cognitive biases. Chest. 2011 Dec;140(6):1638–42. [PMID: 22147823]

RESPIRATORY ALKALOSIS

Respiratory alkalosis occurs when hyperventilation reduces the PCO_2, increasing serum pH. The most common cause of respiratory alkalosis is hyperventilation syndrome (Table 21–17), but bacterial septicemia and cirrhosis are other common causes. In pregnancy, progesterone stimulates the respiratory center, producing an average PCO_2 of 30 mm Hg and respiratory alkalosis. Symptoms of acute respiratory alkalosis are related to decreased cerebral blood flow induced by the disorder.

Determination of appropriate metabolic compensation may reveal an associated metabolic disorder (see Mixed Acid-Base Disorders).

As in respiratory acidosis, the metabolic compensation is greater if the respiratory alkalosis is chronic (see Table 21–13). Although serum HCO_3^- is frequently less than 15 mEq/L in metabolic acidosis, such a low level in respiratory alkalosis is unusual and may represent a concomitant primary metabolic acidosis.

Clinical Findings

A. Symptoms and Signs

In acute cases (hyperventilation), there is light-headedness, anxiety, perioral numbness, and paresthesias. Tetany occurs from a low ionized calcium, since severe alkalosis increases calcium binding to albumin.

B. Laboratory Findings

Arterial blood pH is elevated, and PCO_2 is low. Serum bicarbonate is decreased in chronic respiratory alkalosis.

Treatment

Treatment is directed toward the underlying cause. In acute hyperventilation syndrome from anxiety, the traditional treatment of breathing into a paper bag should be

Table 21–17. Causes of respiratory alkalosis.

Hypoxia
Decreased inspired oxygen tension
High altitude
Ventilation/perfusion inequality
Hypotension
Severe anemia
CNS-mediated disorders
Voluntary hyperventilation
Anxiety-hyperventilation syndrome
Neurologic disease
Cerebrovascular accident (infarction, hemorrhage)
Infection
Trauma
Tumor
Pharmacologic and hormonal stimulation
Salicylates
Nicotine
Xanthines
Pregnancy (progesterone)
Hepatic failure
Gram-negative septicemia
Recovery from metabolic acidosis
Heat exposure
Pulmonary disease
Interstitial lung disease
Pneumonia
Pulmonary embolism
Pulmonary edema
Mechanical overventilation

Adapted, with permission, from Gennari FJ. Respiratory acidosis and alkalosis. In: *Maxwell and Kleeman's Clinical Disorders of Fluid and Electrolyte Metabolism*, 5th ed. Narins RG (editor). McGraw-Hill, 1994.

discouraged because it does not correct PCO_2 and may decrease PO_2. Reassurance may be sufficient for the anxious patient, but sedation may be necessary if the process persists. Hyperventilation is usually self-limited since muscle weakness caused by the respiratory alkalemia will suppress ventilation. Rapid correction of chronic respiratory alkalosis may result in metabolic acidosis as PCO_2 is increased with a previous compensatory decrease in HCO_3^-. The severity of hypocapnia in critically ill patients has been associated with adverse outcomes.

Batlle D et al. Metabolic acidosis or respiratory alkalosis? Evaluation of a low plasma bicarbonate using the urine anion gap. Am J Kidney Dis. 2017 Sep;70(3):440–4. [PMID: 28599903]
Palmer BF. Evaluation and treatment of respiratory alkalosis. Am J Kidney Dis. 2012 Nov;60(5):834–8. [PMID: 22871240]

FLUID MANAGEMENT

Intravenous fluids for the hospitalized patient can be divided into two categories: resuscitation fluid and maintenance fluid. Resuscitation fluid is for hypovolemic patients to correct volume loss (see Chapter 12). Maintenance fluid is for a euvolemic patient who is unable to ingest enough electrolytes and water to keep up with ongoing losses.

Historically 0.45% saline with or without potassium supplementation has been used as a maintenance fluid. Hypotonic fluid replacement, however, has been strongly associated with the development of hyponatremia in hospitalized patients. Isotonic fluids may be acceptable, or even preferable, in most patients requiring maintenance fluids. The choice of fluid replacement should be individualized based on serum electrolytes and the rate and type of ongoing fluid losses, which can vary between patients. Obtaining electrolyte studies on the fluid losses can help predict appropriate repletion (Table 21–18). Adjustments to intravenous fluid replacement should be made based on frequent electrolyte and volume assessments. If intravenous fluids are the only source of water, electrolytes, and calories for longer than approximately 1 week, parenteral nutrition containing amino acids, lipids, trace metals, and vitamins may be indicated (see Chapter 29).

Moritz ML et al. Maintenance intravenous fluids in acutely ill patients. N Engl J Med. 2015 Oct;373(14):1350–60. [PMID: 26422725]

Table 21–18. Approximate electrolyte concentration of common gastrointestinal losses.

	Approximate Electrolyte Composition			
	Na^+ (mEq/L)	K^+ (mEq/L)	Cl^- (mEq/L)	HCO_3^- (mEq/L)
Gastric	20–80	5–20	100–150	
Pancreatic	120–140	5–15	40–60	70–110
Biliary	120–140	5–15	80–120	30–50
Small bowel	100–140	5–15	80	6–130
Colon	30–140	30–70	15	20–80

Myburgh JA et al. Resuscitation fluids. N Engl J Med. 2013 Sep 26;369(13):1243–51. [PMID: 24066745]

Semler MW et al; SMART Investigators and the Pragmatic Critical Care Research Group. Balanced crystalloids versus saline in critically ill adults. N Engl J Med. 2018 Mar 1;378(9):829–39. [PMID: 29485925]

Kidney Disease

Tonja C. Dirkx, MD
Tyler Woodell, MD, MCR

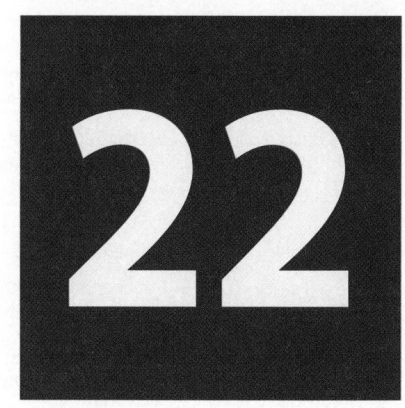

Although some patients with kidney disease experience hypertension, edema, nausea, or hematuria that may lead to its discovery, kidney disease is often discovered incidentally during a routine medical evaluation. The initial approach to kidney disease is to assess the cause and severity of renal abnormalities. In all cases, this evaluation includes (1) estimation of disease duration, (2) careful examination of the urine, and (3) assessment of the glomerular filtration rate (GFR). The history and physical examination, though equally important, are variable among renal syndromes—thus, specific symptoms and signs are discussed under each disease entity.

ASSESSMENT OF KIDNEY DISEASE

Kidneys may be damaged by a variety of injuries; data helpful in the evaluation of kidney disease include estimation of disease duration, examination of the urine and quantification of urinary protein excretion, and estimation of the glomerular filtration rate (eGFR). Additionally, renal imaging (most often ultrasonography) can be helpful. Kidney biopsy may be performed in select cases as noted below and particularly when glomerulonephritis is suspected.

Disease Duration

Kidney disease can be acute or chronic. Acute kidney injury (AKI) is worsening of kidney function over hours to days, resulting in retention of waste products (such as urea nitrogen) and creatinine in the blood. Retention of these substances is called azotemia. Chronic kidney disease (CKD) is the abnormal loss of kidney function over months to years. Differentiating between AKI and CKD is important for diagnosis and treatment, and certain clues may help distinguish the two. For instance, oliguria is only observed in AKI, whereas anemia (from low kidney erythropoietin production) suggests CKD. Additionally, small kidney size on ultrasound or other imaging is more consistent with CKD, whereas normal to large kidney size can be seen with both acute and chronic disease.

Urinalysis

Examination of the urine can provide important clues to underlying kidney disease. A urine specimen should be collected in midstream or by bladder catheterization and examined within 1 hour after collection to avoid destruction of formed elements. Urinalysis includes a dipstick examination followed by microscopy if the dipstick has positive findings. The dipstick examination measures urinary pH, specific gravity, protein, hemoglobin, glucose, ketones, bilirubin, nitrites, and leukocyte esterase. Microscopy of centrifuged urinary sediment permits examination of formed elements—crystals, cells, casts, and infectious organisms. A bland (normal) sediment is common, especially in CKD and acute nonparenchymal disorders, such as limited effective blood flow to the kidney or urinary obstruction. Urinary casts form when urine flow is slow, leading to precipitation of Tamm-Horsfall mucoprotein in the renal tubule; if there are many red or white blood cells in the urine, cellular casts may form. The presence of protein on dipstick examination strongly suggests underlying glomerular disease. If the glomerular basement membrane (GBM) is damaged (eg, by inflammation), red blood cells may leak into the urinary space and appear dysmorphic (also called acanthocytes). Thus, proteinuria, hematuria with acanthocytes, and red blood cells casts are highly suggestive of glomerulonephritis. Heavy proteinuria and lipiduria are consistent with nephrotic syndrome. Pigmented granular casts (also termed "muddy brown casts") and renal tubular epithelial cells alone or in casts are hallmarks of acute tubular necrosis (ATN). White blood cells (including neutrophils and eosinophils), white blood cell casts (Table 22–1), and proteinuria of varying degree can be seen with pyelonephritis and interstitial nephritis; Wright and Hansel stains can detect eosinophiluria. Pyuria alone can indicate a urinary tract infection. Proteinuria and hematuria are discussed more thoroughly below.

A. Proteinuria

Proteinuria is defined as excessive protein excretion in the urine, generally greater than 150 mg/24 h in adults. Proteinuria more than 1–2 g/day is usually a sign of

Table 22–1. Significance of specific urinary casts.

Type	Significance
Hyaline casts	Concentrated urine, febrile disease, after strenuous exercise, during diuretic therapy (not indicative of kidney disease)
Red cell casts	Glomerulonephritis
White cell casts	Pyelonephritis, interstitial nephritis (indicative of infection or inflammation)
Renal tubular cell casts	Acute tubular necrosis, interstitial nephritis
Coarse, granular casts	Nonspecific; can represent acute tubular necrosis
Broad, waxy casts	Chronic kidney disease (indicative of stasis in enlarged collecting tubules)

underlying glomerular kidney disease, whereas proteinuria less than 1 g/day can be due to multiple causes along the nephron segment, as listed below. Proteinuria can be accompanied by other clinical abnormalities—elevated blood urea nitrogen (BUN) and serum creatinine levels, abnormal urine sediment, or evidence of systemic illness (eg, fever, rash, vasculitis).

There are several reasons proteinuria may develop: (1) **Functional proteinuria** is a benign process stemming from stressors such as acute illness, exercise, and "orthostatic proteinuria." The latter condition, generally found in people under 30 years of age, usually causes protein excretion less than 1 g/day. The orthostatic nature of the proteinuria is confirmed by measuring an 8-hour overnight supine urinary protein excretion, which should be less than 50 mg. (2) **Overload proteinuria** can result from overproduction of circulating, filterable plasma proteins (monoclonal gammopathies), such as Bence Jones proteins associated with plasma cell myeloma (formerly multiple myeloma). Protein electrophoresis from the serum or urine will exhibit a discrete, monoclonal protein spike. Other examples of overload proteinuria include myoglobinuria in rhabdomyolysis and hemoglobinuria in hemolysis. (3) **Glomerular proteinuria** results from effacement of epithelial cell foot processes and altered glomerular permeability with an increased filtration fraction of normal plasma proteins, as in diabetic nephropathy. Protein electrophoresis will have a pattern exhibiting a large albumin spike indicative of the increased permeability of albumin across the damaged GBM. (4) **Tubular proteinuria** occurs as a result of faulty reabsorption of normally filtered proteins in the proximal tubule, such as beta-2-microglobulin and immunoglobulin light chains. Causes may include ATN, toxic injury (lead, aminoglycosides, and certain antiretrovirals), drug-induced interstitial nephritis, and hereditary metabolic disorders (Wilson disease and Fanconi syndrome).

Evaluation of proteinuria by urinary dipstick does not actually measure protein but instead detects the negative electrochemical charge that characterizes albumin. As a result, positively charged Bence Jones proteins are often missed with dipstick analysis. Bence Jones proteins can be detected by the addition of sulfosalicylic acid to the urine specimen or by directly measuring urine protein (discussed below).

While urinary dipstick is commonly used as a screening test for proteinuria, formal investigation typically requires direct evaluation of daily urinary protein excretion, which can be estimated with a random urine sample or measured from a timed urine collection (typically over 24 hours). Collection of a random urine sample is far simpler, and the ratio of urinary protein-to-creatinine concentration ($[U_{protein}]/[U_{creatinine}]$) correlates with a 24-hour urinary protein collection (less than 0.2 is normal and corresponds to excretion of less than 200 mg/24 h). In a 24-hour urine collection, proteinuria more than 150 mg is abnormal and greater than 3.5 g is consistent with nephrotic range proteinuria. One benefit of a random urinary protein-to-creatinine ratio is the minimization of error from overcollection or undercollection of urine in the 24-hour specimen. A kidney biopsy may be indicated to determine the cause of abnormal proteinuria, if present, particularly if accompanied by AKI. The clinical sequelae of proteinuria are discussed in the section on Nephrotic Spectrum Glomerular Diseases.

B. Hematuria

Hematuria is clinically significant if there are more than three red cells per high-power field on at least two occasions. It is usually detected incidentally by the urine dipstick examination or clinically following an episode of macroscopic hematuria. The diagnosis must be confirmed via microscopic examination, as false-positive dipstick tests can be caused by myoglobin, oxidizing agents, beets and rhubarb, hydrochloric acid, and bacteria. Transient hematuria is common, but it is less often of clinical significance in patients younger than 40 years due to lower concern for malignancy.

Hematuria may be due to renal or extrarenal causes. Most worrisome are urologic malignancies (see Chapter 39). Extrarenal causes are addressed in Chapter 23. Renal causes account for approximately 10% of cases and are best considered anatomically as glomerular or extraglomerular. Glomerular causes include immunoglobulin A (IgA) nephropathy, thin GBM disease, membranoproliferative glomerulonephritis (MPGN), other hereditary glomerular diseases (eg, Alport syndrome), and systemic nephritic syndromes. The most common extraglomerular sources include cysts; calculi; interstitial nephritis; and genitourinary neoplasms from the kidney, prostate, or bladder. Currently, due to insufficient evidence, the United States Preventive Services Task Force gives no recommendation to screen for hematuria to test for bladder cancer in asymptomatic adults.

▶ Glomerular Filtration Rate (GFR)

The GFR provides a useful measure of kidney function at the level of the glomerulus and can either be measured directly using biomarkers (most commonly creatinine) or estimated using validated formulae. The GFR measures the amount of plasma ultrafiltered across the glomerular capillaries and reflects the ability of the kidneys to filter fluids and various substances, including medications; it is often used to determine drug dosing. Daily GFR in normal individuals is variable, with a range of 150–250 L/24 h or 100–120 mL/min/1.73 m^2 of body surface area. Patients with kidney disease can have decreased GFR from any process that causes loss of nephron (and thus glomerular) mass. However, they can also have normal or increased GFR, either from hyperfiltration at the glomerulus or disease at a different segment of the nephron, interstitium, or vascular supply.

GFR can be measured by determining the renal clearance of plasma substances that are not bound to plasma proteins, are freely filterable across the glomerulus and are neither secreted nor reabsorbed along the renal tubules. The renal clearance of a substance is defined as:

$$C = \frac{U \times \dot{V}}{P}$$

where C is the clearance, U and P are the respective urine and plasma concentrations of the substance (mg/dL), and $\dot{V}$ is the urine flow rate (mL/min). In clinical practice, the clearance rate of endogenous creatinine (termed **creatinine clearance**) is the primary way to measure GFR. Creatinine is a product of muscle metabolism produced at a relatively constant rate and cleared by renal excretion. It is freely filtered by the glomerulus and not reabsorbed by the renal tubules. With stable kidney function, creatinine production and excretion are equal; thus, plasma creatinine concentrations remain constant. However, creatinine is not a perfect indicator of GFR for the following reasons: (1) a small amount is normally eliminated by tubular secretion, and the fraction secreted progressively increases as GFR declines (thus overestimating GFR); (2) with severe kidney failure, gut microorganisms degrade creatinine; (3) dietary meat intake and muscle mass affect plasma creatinine levels; (4) commonly used drugs such as aspirin, dolutegravir, probenecid, and trimethoprim reduce tubular secretion of creatinine, increasing the plasma creatinine concentration and falsely suggesting kidney dysfunction; and (5) the accuracy of the measurement necessitates a stable plasma creatinine concentration over a 24-hour period, so when values are changing during the development of and recovery from AKI, the creatinine clearance is unhelpful.

One way to measure creatinine clearance is to perform a timed urine collection and determine the plasma creatinine level midway through the collection. An incomplete or prolonged urine collection is a common source of error. A method of estimating the completeness of the collection is to calculate a 24-hour creatinine excretion; the amount should be constant:

$$U_{cr} \times \dot{V} = 15 - 20 \text{ mg/kg for healthy young women}$$

$$U_{cr} \times \dot{V} = 20 - 25 \text{ mg/kg for healthy young men}$$

The creatinine clearance (C_{cr}) is approximately 100 mL/min/1.73 m^2 in healthy young women and 120 mL/min/ 1.73 m^2 in healthy young men. The creatinine clearance declines by an average of 0.8 mL/min/yr after age 40 years as part of the aging process, but this is variable, with 35% of subjects in one study having no decline in kidney function over 10 years.

Given the tedious nature of timed urine collections for measuring GFR, GFR is far more commonly estimated using formulae that have been validated using patient characteristics (such as age, weight, race, and sex) and plasma creatinine levels. In fact, the Kidney Disease Improving Global Outcomes workgroup recommends estimated GFR (eGFR) formulae as the primary method for evaluating GFR. They recommend using the 2009 CKD-Epidemiology (EPI) Collaboration creatinine equation (https://www.kidney.org/content/ckd-epi-creatinine-equation-2009). An alternative creatinine-based GFR estimating equation is acceptable if it improves accuracy over the CKD-EPI equation. Several web-based calculators will calculate the eGFR (eg, http://touchcalc.com/e_gfr). Creatinine clearance can also be estimated using the Modification of Diet in Renal Disease (MDRD) Study equation, but multiple studies across many populations show that the CKD-EPI equation is more accurate. It is important to note that another formula, the Cockcroft-Gault formula, is still commonly used to determine drug dosing, but it was developed before the standardization of creatinine assays currently in use today and, thus, its use is not recommended. **Cystatin C** is another endogenous marker of GFR that is filtered freely at the glomerulus, produced at a relatively constant rate, and less dependent on muscle mass. It is reabsorbed and partially metabolized in the renal tubular epithelial cells. Adding the measurement of cystatin C to serum creatinine can improve the accuracy of the eGFR. A large meta-analysis showed that cystatin C alone or in combination with serum creatinine is a stronger predictor of important clinical events, such as end-stage renal disease (ESRD) or death, than serum creatinine alone. Use of cystatin C improves classification of kidney disease and prediction of outcomes among at-risk individuals.

BUN is another index used in assessing kidney function. It is synthesized mainly in the liver and is the end product of protein catabolism. Urea is freely filtered by the glomerulus, but about 30–70% is reabsorbed in the renal tubules. Unlike creatinine clearance, which overestimates GFR, urea clearance underestimates GFR. Urea reabsorption in the kidney decreases in volume replete patients and increases (in conjunction with increased sodium reabsorption) in hypovolemic patients (who, therefore, have an increased BUN). A normal BUN:creatinine ratio is approximately 10:1, although this can vary between individuals. With volume depletion, the ratio can increase to 20:1 or higher. Other causes of increased BUN include increased catabolism (gastrointestinal [GI] bleeding, cell lysis, and corticosteroid usage), increased dietary protein, and decreased renal perfusion prompting increased sodium (and therefore BUN) reabsorption (eg, heart failure, renal artery stenosis) (Table 22–2). Reduced BUN levels are seen in liver disease and in the syndrome of inappropriate antidiuretic hormone (SIADH).

Table 22–2. Conditions affecting BUN independently of GFR.

Increased BUN
Reduced effective circulating blood volume (prerenal azotemia)
Catabolic states (gastrointestinal bleeding, corticosteroid use)
High-protein diets
Tetracycline
Decreased BUN
Liver disease
Malnutrition
Sickle cell anemia
SIADH

BUN, blood urea nitrogen; GFR, glomerular filtration rate; SIADH, syndrome of inappropriate antidiuretic hormone.

As patients approach ESRD, a more accurate measure of GFR than creatinine clearance is the average of the creatinine and urea clearances. The creatinine clearance overestimates GFR, as mentioned above, while the urea clearance underestimates GFR. Therefore, an average of the two more accurately approximates the true GFR.

KIDNEY BIOPSY

Indications for percutaneous needle biopsy include (1) unexplained AKI or CKD; (2) unexplained proteinuria and hematuria; (3) previously identified and treated lesions to guide future therapy; (4) systemic diseases associated with kidney dysfunction, such as systemic lupus erythematosus (SLE), anti-GBM disease (Goodpasture syndrome), and granulomatosis with polyangiitis, to confirm the extent of renal involvement and to guide management; and (5) kidney transplant dysfunction, to evaluate for transplant rejection or other causes of AKI. Importantly, kidney biopsies typically should be performed only if the results will influence the treatment plan or facilitate discussion about prognosis; patients unwilling to accept therapy based on biopsy findings should not undergo kidney biopsy. Relative contraindications include a solitary or ectopic kidney (exception: transplant allografts), horseshoe kidney, ESRD, congenital anomalies, and multiple cysts. Absolute contraindications include an uncorrected bleeding disorder; severe uncontrolled hypertension; renal infection; renal neoplasm; hydronephrosis; or uncooperative patients, including those who are unable to lie flat for the procedure.

Prior to a kidney biopsy, patients should not use medications that prolong clotting times, and blood pressure should be less than 160/90 mm Hg. Blood work should include hemoglobin concentration, platelet count, prothrombin time, and partial thromboplastin time. After biopsy, hematuria occurs in nearly all patients, although less than 10% will have macroscopic hematuria. Patients should remain supine for 4–6 hours postbiopsy and should be closely monitored when the hemoglobin is more than 1 g/dL lower than baseline by 6 hours postbiopsy.

Percutaneous kidney biopsies are generally safe. The major risk is bleeding, which may occur up to 72 hours post biopsy. More than half of patients will have at least a small hematoma; approximately 1% of patients will experience significant bleeding requiring a blood transfusion. Anticoagulation therapy should be held for 5–7 days postbiopsy if possible. The risks of nephrectomy and mortality are about 0.06–0.08%. When a percutaneous needle biopsy is technically not feasible and kidney tissue is deemed clinically essential, a closed biopsy via interventional radiologic techniques or open biopsy under general anesthesia can be performed.

Cavanaugh C et al. Urine sediment examination in the diagnosis and management of kidney disease: Core Curriculum 2019. Am J Kidney Dis. 2019 Feb;73(2):258–72. [PMID: 30249419]

Hogan JJ et al. The native kidney biopsy: update and evidence for best practice. Clin J Am Soc Nephrol. 2016 Feb;11:354–62. [PMID: 26339068]

Levey AS et al. Assessment of glomerular filtration rate in health and disease: a state of the art review. Clin Pharmacol Ther. 2017 Sep;102(3):405–19. [PMID: 28474735]

O'Neill WC. Renal relevant radiology: use of ultrasound in kidney disease and nephrology procedures. Clin J Am Soc Nephrol. 2014 Feb;9(2):373–81. [PMID: 24458082]

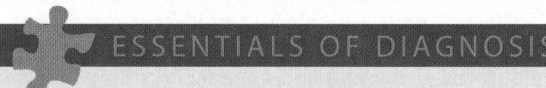

ACUTE KIDNEY INJURY

ESSENTIALS OF DIAGNOSIS

▶ Rapid increase in serum creatinine.

▶ Oliguria may be present.

▶ Symptoms and signs depend on cause.

▶ General Considerations

AKI is defined as an absolute increase in serum creatinine by 0.3 mg/dL or more within 48 hours or a relative increase of greater than or equal to 1.5 times baseline that is known or presumed to have occurred within 7 days. AKI is characterized as oliguric if urine production is less than 400–500 mL/day or less than 20 mL/h. Clinically, AKI is characterized by an inability to maintain acid-base, fluid, and electrolyte balance and to excrete nitrogenous wastes. The three stages of AKI defined by the 2012 Kidney Disease Improving Global Outcomes Clinical Practice Guidelines for Acute Kidney Injury are based on the elevation in serum creatinine or decline in urinary output, both of which correlate with prognosis. **Stage 1** is a 1.0- to 1.5-fold increase in serum creatinine or a decline in urinary output to less than 0.5 mL/kg/h over 6–12 hours; **stage 2** is a 2.0- to 2.9-fold increase in serum creatinine or decline in urinary output to less than 0.5 mL/kg/h over 12 hours or longer; **stage 3** is a 3-fold or greater increase in serum creatinine, an increase in serum creatinine to greater than or equal to 4 mg/dL, a decline in urinary output to less than 0.3 mL/kg/h for 24 hours or longer, anuria for 12 hours or longer, or initiation of renal replacement therapy. In the absence of functioning kidneys, serum creatinine concentration will typically increase by 1–1.5 mg/dL daily, although with certain conditions, such as rhabdomyolysis, serum creatinine can increase more rapidly. On average, 5% of hospital admissions and 30% of intensive care unit (ICU) admissions carry a diagnosis of AKI, and AKI will develop in 25% of hospitalized patients. Patients with AKI of any type are at higher risk for all-cause mortality according to prospective cohort studies, even if renal recovery is substantial. The rates of AKI in the hospital setting have increased steadily since the 1980s and are continuing to rise.

Clinical Findings

A. Symptoms and Signs

Although many patients will not experience any symptoms or exhibit any signs of AKI, the buildup of waste products can sometimes cause nonspecific symptoms and signs collectively termed **uremia.** Uremia can cause nausea, vomiting, malaise, and altered sensorium. Additionally, patients may experience symptoms and signs of the underlying disease process causing their AKI (eg, SLE). Hypertension can occur, and fluid homeostasis is often impaired. Hypovolemia can cause states of low blood flow to the kidneys, sometimes termed **prerenal azotemia,** whereas hypervolemia can result from intrinsic or postrenal disease. Pericardial effusions can occur with uremia and may result in cardiac tamponade; a pericardial friction rub can be present, signaling pericarditis. Arrhythmias can occur, especially with hyperkalemia. The lung examination may reveal rales in the presence of hypervolemia. AKI can cause nonspecific diffuse abdominal pain and ileus as well as platelet dysfunction; bleeding and clotting disorders are more common in affected patients. The neurologic examination sometimes reveals encephalopathic changes with asterixis and confusion; seizures may ensue in significant AKI.

B. Laboratory Findings

By definition, elevated serum creatinine (and often BUN) levels are present, though these elevations do not distinguish AKI from CKD. Metabolic acidosis (due to decreased clearance of organic and nonorganic acids) is often noted. Hyperkalemia can occur from impaired renal potassium excretion or from extracellular shifting of potassium into the blood as a result of metabolic acidosis. With hyperkalemia, ECG can reveal peaked T waves, PR prolongation, and QRS widening. A long QT segment can occur with hypocalcemia. Hyperphosphatemia occurs when phosphorus cannot be secreted by damaged tubules either with or without increased cell catabolism. Anemia can occur as a result of decreased erythropoietin production over weeks, and associated platelet dysfunction is typical.

Classification & Etiology

AKI is commonly divided into three categories: prerenal causes (kidney hypoperfusion leading to lower GFR), intrinsic kidney disease, and postrenal causes (any obstruction to urinary outflow). Identifying the cause is the first step toward treatment (Table 22–3).

A. Prerenal Causes

Prerenal causes are the most common etiology of AKI, accounting for 40–80% of cases depending on the population studied. Prerenal azotemia is due to renal hypoperfusion, which is an appropriate physiologic change. If reversed quickly with restoration of renal blood flow

Table 22–3. Classification and differential diagnosis of acute kidney injury.

| | Prerenal Azotemia | Postrenal Azotemia | Intrinsic Renal Disease | | |
			Acute Tubular Necrosis	Acute Glomerulonephritis	Acute Interstitial Nephritis
Etiology	Poor renal perfusion	Obstruction of the urinary tract	Ischemia, nephrotoxins	Immune complex-mediated, pauci-immune, anti-GBM related, monoclonal immunoglobulin–mediated, C3 glomerulopathy	Allergic reaction; drug reaction; infection, collagen vascular disease
Serum BUN:Cr ratio	> 20:1	> 20:1	< 20:1	> 20:1	< 20:1
U_{Na} (mEq/L)	< 20	Variable	> 20	< 20	Variable
FE_{Na} (%)	< 1	Variable	> 1 (when oliguric)	< 1	< 1; > 1
Urine osmolality (mOsm/kg)	> 500	< 400	250–300	Variable	Variable
Urinary sediment	Benign or hyaline casts	Normal or red cells, white cells, or crystals	Granular (muddy brown) casts, renal tubular casts	Red cells, dysmorphic red cells, and red cell casts	White cells, white cell casts, with or without eosinophils

BUN:Cr, blood urea nitrogen:creatinine ratio; FE_{Na}, fractional excretion of sodium; GBM, glomerular basement membrane; U_{Na}, urinary concentration of sodium.

(eg, fluid resuscitation), renal parenchymal damage often does not occur. If hypoperfusion persists, ischemia can lead to intrinsic kidney injury.

Decreased renal perfusion can occur in several ways, such as a decrease in intravascular volume, a change in vascular resistance, or low cardiac output. Causes of volume depletion include hemorrhage (eg, from trauma), GI losses, excessive diuresis, and extravascular space sequestration (eg, pancreatitis, burns, and peritonitis).

Changes in vascular resistance can occur systemically with sepsis, anaphylaxis, anesthesia, and afterload-reducing drugs. Blockade of the renin-angiotensin-aldosterone system, such as with angiotensin-converting enzyme (ACE) inhibitors, limits efferent renal arteriolar constriction out of proportion to afferent arteriolar constriction; GFR will decrease with these medications. Nonsteroidal anti-inflammatory drugs (NSAIDs) minimize afferent arteriolar vasodilation by inhibiting prostaglandin-mediated signals. Thus, in cirrhosis and heart failure, when prostaglandins are recruited to increase renal blood flow, NSAIDs will have particularly deleterious effects. Epinephrine, norepinephrine, high-dose dopamine, anesthetic agents, and calcineurin inhibitors also can cause renal vasoconstriction. Renal artery stenosis causes increased resistance and decreased renal perfusion.

Low cardiac output is a state of low effective renal arterial blood flow. This occurs in states of cardiogenic shock, heart failure, pulmonary embolism, and pericardial tamponade. Arrhythmias and valvular disorders can also reduce cardiac output. In the intensive care setting, positive pressure ventilation will decrease venous return and, in effect, cardiac output.

When GFR falls acutely, it is important to determine whether AKI is due to prerenal or intrinsic causes. The history and physical examination are important, and laboratory data may be helpful in distinguishing between these causes. In prerenal AKI, the BUN:creatinine ratio often exceeds 20:1 due to increased urea reabsorption. In an oliguric patient, another useful index is the fractional excretion of sodium (FE_{Na}). With decreased GFR, the kidney reabsorbs salt and water avidly if there is no intrinsic tubular dysfunction. Thus, oliguric patients with prerenal AKI should have a low fractional excretion of sodium (less than 1%). Oliguric patients with intrinsic kidney dysfunction typically have a high fractional excretion of sodium (greater than 1–2%). The FE_{Na} is calculated as follows: FE_{Na} = clearance of Na^+/GFR = clearance of Na^+/C_{cr}:

$$FE_{Na} = \frac{Urine_{Na} / Serum_{Na}}{Urine_{cr} / Serum_{cr}} \times 100\%$$

The equation was specifically created and validated to assess the difference between *oliguric* ATN and prerenal states; its utility in nonoliguric patients is limited. Further, because diuretics act by increasing sodium excretion, if the FE_{Na} is high within 12–24 hours after diuretic administration, the cause of AKI cannot be accurately assessed. In contrast, a low FE_{Na} *despite* receiving diuretics offers strong evidence of prerenal states in oliguric patients. Given the limitations of FE_{Na} calculations, urine microscopy is typically a more valuable tool for determining cause of AKI. Patients with prerenal azotemia typically have bland urine sediments, though may sometimes have hyaline casts. In contrast, patients with ATN often have renal tubular epithelial cells or muddy brown casts visible on urine microscopy. Additionally, urinary biomarkers other than creatinine have emerged as promising tools to distinguish between prerenal azotemia and ATN.

Treatment of prerenal AKI depends entirely on the causes, but achievement of euvolemia, attention to serum electrolytes, and avoidance of nephrotoxic drugs are benchmarks of therapy. This involves careful assessment of volume status, cardiac function, diet, and drug usage.

B. Postrenal Causes

Postrenal causes of AKI are the least common, accounting for approximately 5–10% of cases, but are important to detect because of their reversibility. Postrenal azotemia occurs when urinary flow from both kidneys, or a single functioning kidney, is obstructed. Occasionally, postrenal uropathies can occur when a single kidney is obstructed if the contralateral kidney cannot compensate for the loss in function, (eg, in a patient with advanced CKD). Obstruction leads to elevated intraluminal pressure and resultant kidney parenchymal damage, with marked effects on renal blood flow and tubular function and a decrease in GFR.

Postrenal causes of AKI include urethral obstruction, bladder dysfunction or obstruction, and obstruction of both ureters or renal pelvises. In men, benign prostatic hyperplasia is the most common cause. Patients taking anticholinergic drugs are at risk for urinary retention. Obstruction can also be caused by bladder, prostate, and cervical cancers; retroperitoneal fibrosis; and neurogenic bladder (eg, from diabetes mellitus). Less common causes are blood clots, bilateral ureteral stones, urethral stones or strictures, and bilateral papillary necrosis.

Patients may be anuric or polyuric and may experience lower abdominal or back pain. Polyuria can occur in the setting of partial obstruction with resultant tubular dysfunction and an inability to appropriately reabsorb salt and water loads. Obstruction can be constant or intermittent and partial or complete. On examination, the patient may have an enlarged prostate, distended bladder, or mass detected on pelvic examination.

Laboratory examination may initially reveal high urine osmolality, low urine sodium, high BUN:creatinine ratio, and low FE_{Na} (as tubular function may not be compromised initially). These indices are similar to a prerenal picture because extensive intrinsic renal damage has not yet occurred. After several days, however, the urine sodium increases as the kidneys fail and are unable to concentrate the urine—thus, isosthenuria is present. The urine sediment is generally bland.

Patients with AKI and suspected postrenal insults should undergo bladder catheterization and ultrasonography to assess for hydroureter, hydronephrosis, or large bladder volume despite the inability or lack of sensation to void. After reversal of the underlying process, patients often undergo a postobstructive diuresis, and care should be taken to avoid volume depletion or electrolyte derangements. Rarely, obstruction is not diagnosed by ultrasonography. For example, patients with retroperitoneal fibrosis from tumor or radiation may not show dilation of the urinary tract. If suspicion persists, a CT scan or MRI (without gadolinium, which can cause nephrogenic systemic fibrosis if given to patients with eGFR less than 30 mL/min/1.73 m^2) can establish the diagnosis. Prompt treatment of obstruction within days by catheters, stents, or other surgical procedures can result in partial or complete reversal of AKI.

C. Intrinsic Acute Kidney Injury

Intrinsic renal disorders account for up to 50% of all cases of AKI referred to a nephrologist. Intrinsic dysfunction is considered after prerenal and postrenal causes have been excluded. The potential sites of injury are the tubules, interstitium, vasculature, and glomeruli.

▶ When to Refer

- If a patient has signs of AKI that have not reversed over 1–2 weeks without uremia, the patient can usually be referred to a nephrologist rather than admitted.
- If a patient has signs of persistent urinary tract obstruction, the patient should be referred to a urologist.

▶ When to Admit

The patient should be admitted if there is sudden loss of kidney function resulting in abnormalities that cannot be handled expeditiously in an outpatient setting (eg, hyperkalemia, volume overload, uremia) or other requirements for acute intervention, such as emergent urologic procedures or dialysis.

Malhotra R et al. Biomarkers for the early detection and prognosis of acute kidney injury. Clin J Am Soc Nephrol. 2017 Jan 6; 12(1):149–73. [PMID: 27827308]

Okusa MD et al. Reading between the (guide)lines—the KDIGO practice guideline on acute kidney injury in the individual patient. Kidney Int. 2014 Jan;85(1):39–48. [PMID: 24067436]

Ostermann M et al. Acute kidney injury 2016: diagnosis and diagnostic workup. Crit Care. 2016 Sep 27;20(1):299–312. [PMID: 27670788]

Thomas ME et al. The definition of acute kidney injury and its use in practice. Kidney Int. 2015 Jan;87(1):62–73. [PMID: 25317932]

ACUTE TUBULAR NECROSIS

ESSENTIALS OF DIAGNOSIS

- ▶ AKI.
- ▶ Ischemic or toxic insult or underlying sepsis.
- ▶ Urine sediment with pigmented granular casts and renal tubular epithelial cells is pathognomonic but not essential.

▶ General Considerations

AKI due to tubular damage is termed "acute tubular necrosis (ATN)" and accounts for approximately 85% of intrinsic AKI. The two major causes of ATN are ischemia and nephrotoxin exposure. Ischemic ATN is characterized not only by inadequate GFR but also by renal blood flow that is inadequate to maintain parenchymal cellular perfusion. Renal tubular damage with low effective arterial blood flow to kidneys can result in tubular necrosis and apoptosis. This occurs in the setting of prolonged hypotension or hypoxemia, such as volume depletion or shock. Underlying sepsis is also an independent risk factor for ATN. Major surgical procedures can involve prolonged periods of hypoperfusion, which are exacerbated by vasodilating anesthetic agents.

A. Exogenous Nephrotoxins

Aminoglycosides cause some degree of ATN in up to 25% of hospitalized patients receiving therapeutic levels of the drugs. Nonoliguric kidney injury typically occurs after 5–10 days of exposure. Predisposing factors include underlying kidney damage, volume depletion, and advanced age. Aminoglycosides can remain in renal tissue for up to a month, so renal recovery may be delayed after stopping the medication. Monitoring drug levels is important, and trough levels are particularly helpful in predicting renal toxicity. Gentamicin and tobramycin are equally nephrotoxic; streptomycin is the least nephrotoxic of the aminoglycosides, likely due to the number of cationic amino side chains present on each molecule.

Amphotericin B is typically nephrotoxic after a dose of 2–3 g. This causes a type 1 (distal) renal tubular acidosis with severe vasoconstriction and tubular damage, which can lead to hypokalemia and nephrogenic diabetes insipidus. **Vancomycin**, intravenous **acyclovir**, and several **cephalosporins** have also been known to cause or be associated with ATN.

Radiographic contrast media may be directly nephrotoxic. Contrast nephropathy is the third leading cause of incident AKI in hospitalized patients and is thought to result from the synergistic combination of direct renal tubular epithelial cell toxicity and renal medullary ischemia. Predisposing factors include advanced age; CKD with serum creatinine greater than 2 mg/dL; volume depletion; diabetic nephropathy; heart failure; plasma cell myeloma; repeated doses of contrast; and recent exposure to other nephrotoxic agents, including NSAIDs and ACE inhibitors. The combination of preexisting diabetes mellitus and CKD are associated with the greatest risk (15–50%) for contrast nephropathy. Lower volumes of contrast with lower osmolality are recommended in high-risk patients. Toxicity usually occurs within 24–48 hours after the radiocontrast study. Nonionic contrast media may be less toxic, but this has not been well proven. Prevention of contrast nephropathy is the goal when using these agents. The mainstay of therapy is 500–1000 mL of intravenous 0.9% (normal) saline over 10–12 hours both before and after the contrast administration—cautiously in patients with preexisting cardiac dysfunction; oral intake of fluids is an acceptable alternative for outpatient studies. Isotonic intravenous volume repletion is superior to hypotonic intravenous solutions, and both are superior to oral solutions in small studies. Other nephrotoxic agents should be avoided during the day before and after dye administration. Neither mannitol nor furosemide offers benefit over 0.9% (normal) saline administration. In fact, furosemide may lead to increased rates of kidney dysfunction in this setting. *N*-acetylcysteine and sodium bicarbonate can no longer be recommended as preventive therapies for contrast nephropathy based on lack of efficacy.

Cyclosporine toxicity is usually dose dependent. It causes distal tubular dysfunction (a type 4 renal tubular acidosis) and severe vasoconstriction. Regular blood level monitoring is important to prevent both acute and chronic nephrotoxicity. In patients who are taking cyclosporine to prevent kidney allograft rejection, kidney biopsy is often necessary to distinguish transplant rejection from cyclosporine toxicity. Kidney function usually improves after reducing the dose or stopping the drug.

Other exogenous nephrotoxins include antineoplastics, such as cisplatin and organic solvents, and heavy metals such as mercury, cadmium, and arsenic. Herbal medicines are also increasingly recognized as potentially nephrotoxic. Exogenous nephrotoxins more commonly cause damage than endogenous nephrotoxins.

B. Endogenous Nephrotoxins

Endogenous nephrotoxins include heme-containing products, uric acid, and paraproteins. **Myoglobinuria** from rhabdomyolysis leads to ATN. Necrotic muscle releases large amounts of myoglobin, which is freely filtered across the glomerulus. The myoglobin is reabsorbed by the renal tubules, and direct damage occurs. Distal tubular obstruction from pigmented casts and intrarenal vasoconstriction can also cause damage. This type of kidney injury occurs in the setting of crush injury, or muscle necrosis from prolonged unconsciousness, seizures, cocaine, and alcohol abuse. Dehydration and acidosis predispose to the development of myoglobinuric AKI. Patients may report muscle pain and often have signs of muscle injury. Rhabdomyolysis of clinical importance commonly occurs with a serum creatine kinase (CK) greater than 20,000–50,000 international units/L; one study showed that 58% of patients with AKI from rhabdomyolysis had CK levels greater than 16,000 international units/L, while only 11% of patients without kidney injury had CK values greater than 16,000 international units/L. The globin moiety of myoglobin will cause the urine dipstick to read falsely positive for hemoglobin: the urine appears dark brown, but no red cells are present. With lysis of muscle cells, patients also become hyperkalemic, hyperphosphatemic, and hyperuricemic. Hypocalcemia may ensue due to phosphorus and calcium precipitation. The mainstay of treatment is volume repletion with normal saline. Adjunctive treatments with mannitol and alkalinization of the urine have not been proven to change outcomes in human trials. As patients recover, calcium can move back from tissues to plasma, so early exogenous calcium administration for hypocalcemia is not recommended unless the patient is symptomatic or the level becomes exceedingly low in an unconscious patient; calcium repletion can result in hypercalcemia later in the course of the illness.

Hemoglobin can cause a similar form of ATN. Massive intravascular hemolysis is seen in transfusion reactions and in certain hemolytic anemias. Reversal of the underlying disorder and hydration are the mainstays of treatment.

Hyperuricemia can occur in the setting of rapid cell turnover and lysis. Chemotherapy for germ cell neoplasms and leukemia and lymphoma are the primary causes. Spontaneous tumor lysis syndrome is a less common cause. AKI occurs with intratubular deposition of uric acid crystals; serum uric acid levels are often greater than 15–20 mg/dL and urine uric acid levels are typically greater than 600 mg/24 h. A urine uric acid to urine creatinine ratio greater than 1.0 identifies individuals at risk for AKI. Allopurinol or rasburicase can be used prophylactically, and rasburicase with or without dialysis is often used for treatment in diagnosed cases.

Bence Jones proteinuria seen in conjunction with plasma cell myeloma can cause direct tubular toxicity and tubular obstruction. Other renal complications from plasma cell myeloma include hypercalcemia and renal tubular dysfunction, including proximal renal tubular acidosis (see Plasma Cell Myeloma below).

▶ Clinical Findings

A. Symptoms and Signs

See Acute Kidney Injury.

B. Laboratory Findings

Hyperkalemia and hyperphosphatemia are commonly present. The BUN:creatinine ratio is usually less than 20:1 because tubular function is not intact, as described in the general section on AKI (Table 22–3). Urinary output can be oliguric or nonoliguric, with oliguria portending a worse prognosis. Urine sodium concentration and the FE_{Na} are typically elevated, indicative of tubular dysfunction. Urine microscopy may show evidence of acute tubular damage; the presence of two or more muddy brown casts or renal tubular epithelial cells are strongly predictive of ATN but have a low negative predictive value (see Table 22–1). In some instances, kidney biopsy is necessary.

▶ Treatment

Treatment of ATN is aimed at hastening recovery and avoiding complications. Preventive measures should be taken to avoid volume overload and hyperkalemia. A prospective randomized controlled trial did not show a benefit from loop diuretics on either recovery from AKI or death. Widespread use of diuretics in critically ill patients with AKI should be used only when otherwise clinically indicated (eg, in states of volume overload), although unresponsiveness to high-dose diuretics has been shown to predict future need for acute dialysis in this population (termed "furosemide stress test"). Disabling side effects of supranormal diuretic dosing include hearing loss and cerebellar dysfunction. This is mainly due to peak furosemide levels and can be minimized by the use of a continuous furosemide infusion. A starting dose of 0.1–0.3 mg/kg/h is appropriate, increasing to a maximum of 0.5–1 mg/kg/h, as needed; a bolus of 1–1.5 mg/kg should be administered with each dose escalation. Thiazide diuretics can be used to augment urinary output; metolazone (2.5–5 mg orally every 12–24 hours) or chlorothiazide (250–500 mg intravenously every 8–12 hours) are reasonable choices. Metolazone is less expensive than intravenous chlorothiazide and has reasonable bioavailability. Short-term effects of loop diuretics include activation of the renin-angiotensin system. A 2012 randomized controlled trial did not show a benefit on mortality from plasma ultrafiltration compared to intravenous diuretics in patients with decompensated heart failure. Thus, ultrafiltration should generally be reserved for ICU patients with AKI in need of volume removal who are nonresponsive to diuretics, with the recognition that this has not ultimately improved survival in this patient population. Nutritional support should meet daily needs while preventing excessive catabolism. Dietary protein restriction of 0.6 g/kg/day helps prevent metabolic acidosis. Hypocalcemia and hyperphosphatemia can be improved with dietary modification and phosphate-binding agents taken with meals three times daily; examples include aluminum hydroxide (500 mg orally) over the short term, and calcium carbonate (500–1500 mg orally), calcium acetate (667 mg, two or three tablets), sevelamer carbonate (800–1600 mg orally), and lanthanum carbonate (1000 mg orally) over longer periods. Hypocalcemia should not be treated in patients with rhabdomyolysis unless they are symptomatic. Hypermagnesemia can occur because of reduced magnesium excretion by the renal tubules, so magnesium-containing antacids and laxatives should be avoided in these patients. Dosages of all medications must be adjusted for drugs eliminated by the kidney.

Indications for dialysis in AKI from ATN or other intrinsic disorders include life-threatening electrolyte disturbances (such as hyperkalemia), volume overload unresponsive to diuresis, refractory acidosis, and uremic complications (eg, encephalopathy, pericarditis, and seizures). In gravely ill patients, less severe but worsening abnormalities may also be indications for dialytic support. There is growing evidence that neither more intensive nor earlier initiation of renal replacement therapy for patients with AKI confers any survival benefit.

Course & Prognosis

The clinical course of ATN is often divided into three phases: initial injury, maintenance, and recovery. The maintenance phase is expressed as either oliguric (urinary output less than 500 mL/day) or nonoliguric. Nonoliguric ATN is associated with better outcomes than oliguric ATN, though conversion from oliguric to nonoliguric states with the use of diuretics has not been shown to alter prognosis. While dopamine has sometimes been used for this purpose, numerous studies have shown that its use in this setting is not beneficial. Average duration of the maintenance phase is 1–3 weeks, but some cases may last several months. Cellular repair and removal of tubular debris occur during this period. The recovery phase can be heralded by diuresis. This can be due to inability of recovering renal tubules to reabsorb salt and water appropriately, and a solute diuresis from elevated BUN levels. GFR begins to rise; BUN and serum creatinine fall.

The mortality rate associated with AKI is 20–50% in hospitalized settings, and up to 70% for those in the ICU requiring dialysis with additional comorbid illnesses, both of which are actually slightly improved according to retrospective cohort studies conducted within the past decade. Increased mortality is associated with advanced age, severe underlying disease, and multisystem organ failure. Leading causes of death are infections, fluid and electrolyte disturbances, and worsening of underlying disease.

▶ When to Refer

- When uncertainty exists as to the cause of or treatment for AKI.
- For fluid, electrolyte, and acid-base abnormalities that are recalcitrant to interventions.
- Nephrology referral improves outcomes in AKI.

▶ When to Admit

A patient with symptoms or signs of AKI that require immediate intervention, such as administration of intravenous fluids or dialytic therapy, or that require a team approach that cannot be coordinated as an outpatient.

Barbar SD et al; IDEAL-ICU Trial Investigators and the CRICS TRIGGERSEP Network. Timing of renal-replacement therapy in patients with acute kidney injury and sepsis. N Engl J Med. 2018 Oct 11;379(15):1431–42. [PMID: 30304656]

Gaudry S et al; AKIKI Study Group. Initiation strategies for renal-replacement therapy in the intensive care unit. N Engl J Med. 2016 Jul 14;375(2):122–33. [PMID: 27181456]

Koyner JL et al. Furosemide stress test and biomarkers for the prediction of AKI severity. J Am Soc Nephrol. 2015 Aug;26(8):2023–31. [PMID: 25655065]

Weisbord SD et al; PRESERVE Trial Group. Outcomes after angiography with sodium bicarbonate and acetylcysteine. N Engl J Med. 2018 Feb 15;378(7):603–14. [PMID: 29130810]

Yang B et al. Nephrotoxicity and Chinese herbal medicine. Clin J Am Soc Nephrol. 2018 Oct 8;13(10):1605–11. [PMID: 29615394]

INTERSTITIAL NEPHRITIS

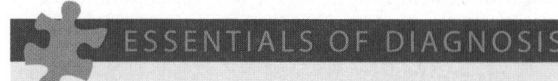
ESSENTIALS OF DIAGNOSIS

- ▶ Fever.
- ▶ Transient maculopapular rash.
- ▶ Acute or chronic kidney injury.
- ▶ Pyuria (including eosinophiluria), white blood cell casts, and hematuria.

▶ General Considerations

Acute interstitial nephritis accounts for 10–15% of cases of intrinsic renal failure. An interstitial inflammatory response with edema and possible tubular cell damage is the typical pathologic finding.

Although drugs account for over 70% of cases, acute interstitial nephritis also occurs in infectious diseases, immunologic disorders, or as idiopathic conditions. The most common drugs implicated are penicillins and cephalosporins, sulfonamides and sulfonamide-containing diuretics, NSAIDs, proton pump inhibitors, rifampin, phenytoin, and allopurinol. Infectious causes include streptococcal infections, leptospirosis, cytomegalovirus, histoplasmosis, and Rocky Mountain spotted fever. SLE, Sjögren syndrome, sarcoidosis, and cryoglobulinemia can also cause interstitial nephritis, though they are more classically associated with glomerulonephritis.

Clinical Findings

Clinical features can include fever (more than 80% of cases), rash (25–50%), arthralgias, and peripheral blood eosinophilia (80%). The classic triad of fever, rash, and arthralgias is present in only 10–15% of cases. The urine often contains white cells (95%), red cells, and white cell casts. Proteinuria can be a feature, particularly in NSAID-induced interstitial nephritis, but is usually modest (less than 2 g/24 h). Eosinophiluria is neither very sensitive nor specific for interstitial nephritis but can be detected by Wright or Hansel stain. Although the clinical history and laboratory data can often give clues to the diagnosis, kidney biopsy is sometimes needed for confirmation.

Treatment & Prognosis

Acute interstitial nephritis often carries a good prognosis, with recovery occurring over weeks to months. Urgent dialytic therapy may be necessary in up to one-third of all referred patients before resolution but patients rarely progress to ESRD. Those with prolonged oliguria and advanced age have a worse prognosis. Treatment consists of supportive measures and removal of the inciting agent. If kidney injury persists after these steps, a short course of corticosteroids can be considered, although the data to support use of corticosteroids are not substantial and their efficacy may depend on the time that has elapsed between onset of AKI and their initiation. Short-term, high-dose methylprednisolone (0.5–1 g/day intravenously for 1–4 days) or prednisone (60 mg/day orally for 1–2 weeks) followed by a prednisone taper can be used in these more severe cases of drug-induced interstitial nephritis.

GLOMERULONEPHRITIS

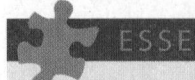

ESSENTIALS OF DIAGNOSIS

- ► Hematuria, mild proteinuria.
- ► Non-dysmorphic or dysmorphic red cells.
- ► Red cell casts pathognomonic but not required for diagnosis.
- ► Dependent edema and hypertension.
- ► AKI.

General Considerations

Acute glomerulonephritis is a relatively uncommon cause of AKI, accounting for about 5% of cases. Pathologically, inflammatory glomerular lesions are seen. These include mesangioproliferative, focal and diffuse proliferative, and crescentic lesions. The larger the percentage of glomeruli involved and the more severe the lesion, the more likely it is that the patient will have a poor clinical outcome.

Acute glomerulonephritis is classified according to the pathophysiologic process, which can be aided by serologic analysis. Markers include anti-GBM antibodies, antineutrophil cytoplasmic antibodies (ANCAs), and other immune markers of disease.

Immune complex deposition usually occurs when moderate antigen excess over antibody production occurs. Complexes formed with marked antigen excess tend to remain in the circulation. Antibody excess with large antigen–antibody aggregates usually results in phagocytosis and clearance of the precipitates by the mononuclear phagocytic system in the liver and spleen. Causes include IgA nephropathy, infection-related glomerulonephritis, lupus nephritis, and cryoglobulinemic glomerulonephritis (often associated with hepatitis C virus [HCV]).

Anti-GBM–associated acute glomerulonephritis is either confined to the kidney or associated with pulmonary hemorrhage. The latter is termed "Goodpasture syndrome." Injury is related to autoantibodies against type IV collagen in the GBM rather than to immune complex deposition.

Pauci-immune acute glomerulonephritis is a form of small-vessel vasculitis associated with ANCAs, causing kidney diseases without direct immune complex deposition or antibody binding. Tissue injury is believed to be due to cell-mediated immune processes. An example is granulomatosis with polyangiitis, a systemic necrotizing vasculitis of small arteries and veins associated with intravascular and extravascular granuloma formation. In addition to glomerulonephritis, these patients can have upper airway, pulmonary, and skin manifestations of disease. Cytoplasmic ANCA (c-ANCA) is the common pattern. Microscopic polyangiitis is another pauci-immune vasculitis causing acute glomerulonephritis, which is more commonly associated with perinuclear staining (p-ANCA). ANCA-associated and anti-GBM–associated acute glomerulonephritides can evolve to crescentic glomerulonephritis and often have poor outcomes unless treatment is started early.

Other vascular causes of acute glomerulonephritis include hypertensive emergencies and the thrombotic microangiopathies such as hemolytic-uremic syndrome and thrombotic thrombocytopenic purpura (see Chapter 14).

Clinical Findings

A. Symptoms and Signs

Patients with acute glomerulonephritis are often hypertensive and edematous with an abnormal urinary sediment. The edema is found first in body parts with low tissue tension, such as the periorbital and scrotal regions.

B. Laboratory Findings

Serum creatinine can rise over days to months, depending on the rapidity of the underlying process. The BUN:creatinine ratio is not a reliable marker of kidney function and is more reflective of the patient's underlying volume status. Dipstick and microscopic evaluation will reveal evidence of hematuria and typically mild proteinuria (usually less than 3 g/day); there may be cellular elements such as dysmorphic red cells, red cell casts, and white cells. Red cell casts are specific for glomerulonephritis, and a detailed search is warranted. Either spot urinary protein-creatinine ratios or 24-hour urine collections can quantify protein excretion; the latter can quantify creatinine clearance when renal function is stable. However, in cases of rapidly changing serum creatinine values, the urinary creatinine clearance is an unreliable marker of GFR. The FE_{Na} is usually low unless the renal tubulointerstitial space is affected, and renal dysfunction is marked (see Table 22–3).

Additional tests include serum complement levels (C3, C4, CH50) that may be low in immune complex glomerulonephritis aside from IgA nephropathy or C3 glomerulopathy and normal in pauci-immune, anti-GBM–related, and monoclonal immunoglobulin–mediated glomerulonephritides. Other tests include ASO titers, anti-GBM antibody levels, ANCAs, antinuclear antibody titers, cryoglobulins, hepatitis serologies, serum protein electrophoresis and serum free light chains, blood cultures, and renal ultrasound. With few exceptions, however, a kidney biopsy is ultimately necessary to confirm the diagnosis, irrespective of laboratory data.

Treatment

Depending on the nature and severity of disease, treatment might include high-dose corticosteroids, rituximab, and cytotoxic agents (such as cyclophosphamide). Plasma exchange can be used in Goodpasture syndrome and pauci-immune glomerulonephritis as a temporizing measure until chemotherapy can take effect. Treatment and prognosis for specific diseases are discussed more fully below.

Moledina DG et al. Drug-induced acute interstitial nephritis. Clin J Am Soc Nephrol. 2017 Dec 7;12(12):2046–9. [PMID: 28893923]
Moledina DG et al. Treatment of drug-induced acute tubulointerstitial nephritis: the search for better evidence. Clin J Am Soc Nephrol. 2018 Dec 7;13(12):1785–7. [PMID: 30397028]
Sethi S et al. Mayo Clinic/Renal Pathology Society consensus report on pathologic classification, diagnosis, and reporting of GN. J Am Soc Nephrol. 2016 May;27(5):1278–87. [PMID: 26567243]

CARDIORENAL SYNDROME

ESSENTIALS OF DIAGNOSIS

▶ **Cardiac dysfunction:** acute or chronic heart failure, ischemic injury, or arrhythmias.

▶ **Kidney disease:** acute or chronic, depending on the type of cardiorenal syndrome.

General Considerations

Cardiorenal syndrome is a pathophysiologic disorder of the heart and kidneys wherein the acute or chronic deterioration of one organ results in the acute or chronic deterioration of the other. This syndrome is classified into five types as a matter of convention, though achieving euvolemia is the overarching therapeutic goal regardless of type.

Type 1 consists of AKI stemming from acute cardiac disease. Type 2 is CKD due to chronic cardiac disease. Type 3 is acute cardiac disease as a result of AKI. Type 4 is chronic cardiac decompensation from CKD. Type 5 consists of heart and kidney dysfunction due to other acute or chronic systemic disorders (such as sepsis). Identifying and defining this common syndrome may assist in the future with treatments to improve its morbidity and mortality. Although novel agents are being examined for future therapies, the mainstay of treatment is to address the primary underlying cardiac or renal dysfunction.

Ronco C et al. Cardiorenal syndrome in western countries: epidemiology, diagnosis and management approaches. Kidney Dis (Basel). 2017 Jan;2(4):151–63. [PMID: 28232932]

CHRONIC KIDNEY DISEASE

ESSENTIALS OF DIAGNOSIS

▶ Decline in the GFR over months to years.

▶ Persistent proteinuria or abnormal renal morphology may be present.

▶ Hypertension in most cases.

▶ Symptoms and signs of uremia when nearing end-stage disease.

▶ Bilateral small or echogenic kidneys on ultrasound in advanced disease.

General Considerations

CKD affects at least 10% of Americans. Many may be unaware of the condition because they remain asymptomatic until the disease is near end stage. The National Kidney Foundation's staging system helps clinicians formulate practice plans (Table 22–4). Over 70% of cases of late-stage CKD (stage 5 CKD and ESRD) in the United States are due to diabetes mellitus or hypertension/vascular disease. Glomerulonephritis, cystic diseases, chronic tubulointerstitial diseases, and other urologic diseases account for the remainder (Table 22–5). Genetic polymorphisms of the *APOL-1* gene have been shown to be associated with an increased risk of the development of CKD in persons of African descent.

CKD usually leads to a progressive decline in kidney function even if the inciting cause can be identified and treated or removed. Destruction of nephrons leads to compensatory hypertrophy and supranormal GFR of the

Table 22–4. Stages of chronic kidney disease: a clinical action plan.[1,2]

Stage[3]	Description	GFR (mL/min/1.73 m^2)	Action
1	Kidney damage with normal or ↑↑ GFR	≥90	Diagnosis and treatment of underlying etiology if possible. Treatment of comorbid conditions. Estimate progression, work to slow progression. Cardiovascular disease risk reduction.
2	Kidney damage with mildly ↓ GFR	60–89	
3a	Mildly-moderately ↓ GFR	45–59	As above, and evaluating and treating complications.
3b	Moderately-severely ↓ GFR	30–44	
4	Severely ↓ GFR	15–29	Preparation for end-stage renal disease.
5	End-stage renal disease	<15 (or dialysis)	Dialysis, transplant, or palliative care.

[1]Based on National Kidney Foundation, KDOQI, and KDIGO Chronic Kidney Disease Guidelines.
[2]Chronic kidney disease is defined as either kidney damage or GFR < 60 mL/min/1.73 m^2 for 3 or more months. Kidney damage is defined as pathologic abnormalities or markers of damage, including abnormalities in blood or urine tests or imaging studies.
[3]At all stages, persistent albuminuria confers added risk for chronic kidney disease progression and cardiovascular disease in the following gradations: <30 mg/day = lowest added risk, 30–300 mg/day = mildly increased risk, > 300–1000 mg/day moderately increased risk, > 1000 mg/day = severely increased risk.
GFR, glomerular filtration rate.
Modified and reproduced, with permission, from Kidney Disease: Improving Global Outcomes (KDIGO) CKD Work Group. KDIGO 2012 Clinical Practice Guideline for the Evaluation and Management of Chronic Kidney Disease. Kidney Int. 2013 Jan;3(1) (Suppl):1–150. Copyright © 2013 International Society of Nephrology. Published by Elsevier Inc. All rights reserved.

Table 22–5. Major causes of chronic kidney disease.

Glomerular Diseases

Primary glomerular diseases
  Focal segmental glomerulosclerosis
  Membranoproliferative glomerulonephritis
  IgA nephropathy
  Membranous nephropathy
  Alport syndrome (hereditary nephritis)
Secondary glomerular diseases
  Diabetic nephropathy
  Renal amyloidosis
  Postinfectious glomerulonephritis
  HIV-associated nephropathy
  Collagen-vascular diseases (eg, SLE)
  HCV-associated membranoproliferative glomerulonephritis

Tubulointerstitial Nephritis

  Drug hypersensitivity
  Heavy metals
  Analgesic nephropathy
  Reflux/chronic pyelonephritis
  Sickle cell nephropathy
  Idiopathic

Cystic Diseases

  Polycystic kidney disease
  Medullary cystic disease

Obstructive Nephropathies

  Prostatic disease
  Nephrolithiasis
  Retroperitoneal fibrosis/tumor
  Congenital

Vascular Diseases

  Hypertensive nephrosclerosis
  Renal artery stenosis

HCV, hepatitis C virus; SLE, systemic lupus erythematosus.

remaining nephrons in order to maintain overall homeostasis. As a result, the serum creatinine may remain relatively normal even in the face of significant loss of renal mass and is, therefore, a relatively insensitive marker for renal damage and scarring. In addition, compensatory hyperfiltration leads to overwork injury in the remaining nephrons, which in turn causes progressive glomerular sclerosis and interstitial fibrosis. Angiotensin receptor blockers (ARBs) and ACE inhibitors can help reduce hyperfiltration injury and are particularly helpful in slowing the progression of proteinuric CKD.

While CKD is an independent risk factor for cardiovascular disease (CVD), proteinuric CKD confers the highest risk. Most patients with stage 3 CKD die of underlying CVD prior to progression to ESRD.

▶ Clinical Findings

A. Symptoms and Signs

In the early stages, CKD is asymptomatic. Symptoms develop slowly with the progressive decline in GFR, are nonspecific, and do not manifest until kidney disease is far advanced (GFR less than 5–10 mL/min/1.73 m^2). At this point, the accumulation of metabolic waste products, or uremic toxins, results in the uremic syndrome. General symptoms of uremia may include fatigue, anorexia, nausea, and a metallic taste in the mouth. Neurologic symptoms such as irritability, memory impairment, insomnia, restless legs, paresthesias, and twitching may be due to uremia. Generalized pruritus (without rash) may occur, as may decreased libido and menstrual irregularities. Pericarditis, a rare complication of CKD, may present with pleuritic chest pain. Medications that are cleared by the kidneys will accumulate as kidney function worsens and toxicity may ensue; an important example is insulin and an increasing risk of significant hypoglycemia if doses are not appropri-ately reduced as GFR declines.

The most common physical finding in CKD is hyper-tension; this is due in part to impaired sodium excretion. It is often present in early stages of CKD and tends to worsen with CKD progression. In later stages of CKD, sodium retention may lead to typical physical signs of volume over-load. Uremic signs are seen with a profound decrease in GFR (less than 5–10 mL/min/1.73 m^2) and may include a generally sallow and ill appearance, halitosis (uremic fetor), and the uremic encepholopathic signs of decreased mental status, asterixis, myoclonus, and possibly seizures.

Symptoms and signs of uremia warrant immediate hos-pital admission and nephrology consultation for initiation of dialysis. The uremic syndrome is ameliorated with dia-lytic therapy.

In any patient with kidney disease, it is important to identify and correct all possibly reversible insults or exac-erbating factors (Table 22–6). Urinary tract infections, obstruction, hypovolemia, hypotension, nephrotoxins (such as NSAIDs, aminoglycosides, or proton pump inhib-itors), severe or emergent hypertension, and heart failure should be excluded.

B. Laboratory Findings

CKD is usually defined by an abnormal GFR persisting for at least 3 months. Persistent proteinuria or abnormalities on renal imaging (eg, polycystic kidneys) are also diagnos-tic of CKD, even when eGFR is normal. It is helpful to plot the inverse of serum creatinine ($1/S_{Cr}$) or eGFR (if reported by the laboratory) versus time. If three or more prior mea-surements are available, the time to ESRD can be roughly estimated (Figure 22–1). If the slope of the line acutely declines, new and potentially reversible renal insults should be excluded as outlined above. Anemia, hyperphosphate-mia, hypocalcemia, hyperkalemia, and metabolic acidosis are common complications of advanced CKD. The urinary

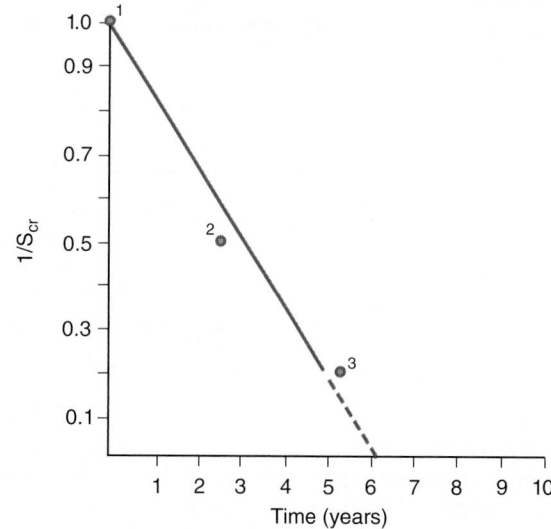

^{1} Value of serum creatinine level = 1.0 mg/dL
^{2} Value of serum creatinine level = 2.0 mg/dL
^{3} Value of serum creatinine level = 5.0 mg/dL

▲ **Figure 22–1.** Decline in kidney function (expressed as the reciprocal of serum creatinine as shown here, or as estimated glomerular filtration rate [eGFR]) plotted against time to end-stage renal disease (ESRD). The solid line indicates the linear decline in kidney function over time. The dotted line indicates the approximate time to ESRD.

sediment may show broad waxy casts as a result of dilated, hypertrophic nephrons. Proteinuria may be present. If so, it should be quantified as described above. Quantification of urinary protein is important for several reasons. First, it helps narrow the differential diagnosis of the etiology of the CKD (Table 22–5); for example, glomerular diseases tend to present with protein excretion of more than 1 g/day. Second, the presence of proteinuria is associated with more rapid progression of CKD and with increased risk of cardiovascular mortality.

C. Imaging

The finding of small, echogenic kidneys bilaterally (less than 9–10 cm) by ultrasonography suggests the chronic parenchymal scarring of advanced CKD. Large kidneys can be seen with adult polycystic kidney disease, diabetic nephropathy, HIV-associated nephropathy, plasma cell myeloma, amyloidosis, and obstructive uropathy.

▶ Complications

The complications of CKD tend to occur at relatively pre-dictable stages of disease as noted in Figure 22–2.

A. Cardiovascular Complications

Patients with CKD experience greater morbidity and mor-tality from CVD in comparison to the general population. Roughly 80% of patients with CKD die, primarily of CVD,

Table 22–6. Reversible causes of kidney injury.

Reversible Factors	Diagnostic Clues
Infection	Urine culture and sensitivity tests
Obstruction	Bladder catheterization, then renal ultrasound
Extracellular fluid volume depletion or significant hypotension relative to baseline	Blood pressure and pulse, including orthostatic pulse
Hypokalemia, hypercalcemia, and hyperuricemia (usually >15 mg/dL)	Serum electrolytes, calcium, phosphate, uric acid
Nephrotoxic agents	Drug history
Severe/urgent hypertension	Blood pressure, chest radiograph
Heart failure	Physical examination, chest radiograph

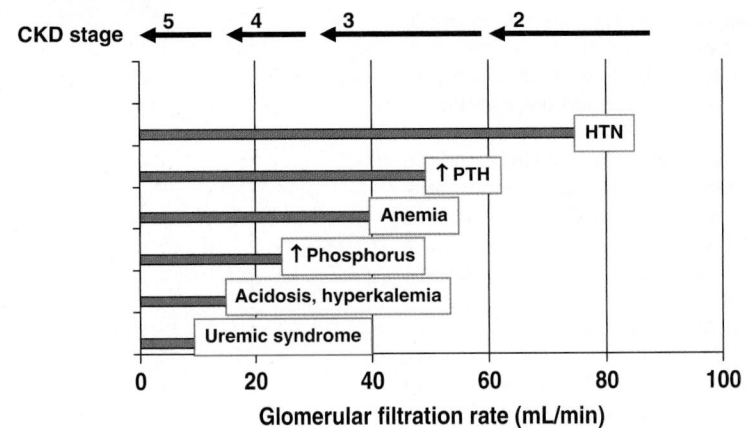

▲ **Figure 22–2.** Complications of chronic kidney disease (CKD) by stage and glomerular filtration rate (GFR). Complications arising from CKD tend to occur at the stages depicted, although there is considerable variability noted in clinical practice. HTN, hypertension; PTH, parathyroid hormone. (Adapted, with permission, from William Bennett, MD.)

before reaching the need for dialysis. Of those undergoing dialysis, 45% will die of a cardiovascular cause. The mechanisms for enhanced cardiovascular mortality in CKD are complex and include abnormal phosphorus and calcium homeostasis, increased burden of oxidative stress, increased vascular reactivity, increased left ventricular hypertrophy, and underlying coexistent comorbidities such as hypertension and diabetes mellitus.

1. Hypertension—Hypertension is the most common complication of CKD; it tends to be progressive and salt-sensitive. Hyperreninemic states and exogenous erythropoietin administration can also exacerbate hypertension.

As with other patient populations, control of hypertension should focus on both nonpharmacologic therapy (eg, diet, exercise, weight loss, treatment of obstructive sleep apnea) and pharmacologic therapy. CKD results in disturbed sodium homeostasis such that the ability of the kidney to adjust to variations in sodium and water intake becomes limited as GFR declines. A low salt diet (2 g/day) is often essential to control blood pressure and help avoid overt volume overload. Diuretics are nearly always needed to help control hypertension (see Table 11–8); thiazides work well in early CKD, but in those with a GFR less than 30 mL/min/1.73 m², loop diuretics are more effective. However, volume contraction as a result of very low sodium intake (especially with intercurrent illness) or over-diuresis in the presence of impaired sodium homeostasis can result in AKI. Initial drug therapy for proteinuric patients should include ACE inhibitors or ARBs (see Table 11–6). When an ACE inhibitor or an ARB is initiated or uptitrated, patients must have serum creatinine and potassium checked within 7–14 days. Hyperkalemia or a rise in serum creatinine greater than 30% from baseline mandates reduction or cessation of the drug. An ACE inhibitor and ARB should not be used in combination. CKD is a common cause of refractory hypertension and additional agents from other classes are often needed. Current guidelines differ with respect to blood pressure goals in CKD; those from the Joint National Commission suggest a blood pressure goal of less than 140/90 mm Hg, while the American Heart Association advocates for less than 130/80 mm Hg. Additionally, patients with CKD may be at risk for renal hypoperfusion and AKI with overtreatment of hypertension. Thus, many experts agree that more studies are needed in this patient population, and that it is prudent to continue with an individualized approach to blood pressure control.

2. Coronary artery disease—Patients with CKD are at higher risk for death from CVD than the general population. Traditional modifiable risk factors for CVD, such as hypertension, tobacco use, and hyperlipidemia, should be aggressively treated in patients with CKD. Uremic vascular calcification involving disordered phosphorus homeostasis and other mediators may also be a cardiovascular risk factor in these patients.

3. Heart failure—The complications of CKD result in increased cardiac workload due to hypertension, volume overload, and anemia. Patients with CKD may also have accelerated rates of atherosclerosis and vascular calcification resulting in vessel stiffness. All of these factors contribute to left ventricular hypertrophy and heart failure with preserved ejection fraction, which is common in CKD. Over time, heart failure with decreased ejection fraction may also develop. Diuretic therapy, in addition to prudent fluid and salt restriction, is usually necessary. Thiazides may be adequate therapy for most patients through CKD stage 3, but loop diuretics are usually needed when the GFR is less than 30 mL/min/1.73 m²; higher doses may be needed as kidney function declines. Digoxin is excreted by the kidney, and its toxicity is exacerbated in the presence of electrolyte disturbances, which are common in CKD. ACE inhibitors and ARBs can be used for patients with advanced CKD with close monitoring of blood pressure as well as for hyperkalemia and worsening kidney function.

4. Pericarditis—Pericarditis rarely develops in uremic patients; typical findings include pleuritic chest pain and a friction rub. Development of a significant effusion may result in pulsus paradoxus, an enlarged cardiac silhouette on chest radiograph, and low QRS voltage and electrical alternans on ECG. The effusion is generally hemorrhagic, and anticoagulants should be avoided if this diagnosis is suspected. Cardiac tamponade can occur; therefore, uremic pericarditis is a mandatory indication for hospitalization and initiation of hemodialysis.

B. Disorders of Mineral Metabolism

The metabolic bone disease of CKD refers to the complex disturbances of calcium and phosphorus metabolism, parathyroid hormone (PTH), active vitamin D, and fibroblast growth factor-23 (FGF-23) homeostasis (see Chapter 21 and Figure 22–3). A typical pattern seen as early as CKD stage 3 is hyperphosphatemia, hypocalcemia, and hypovitaminosis D, resulting in secondary hyperparathyroidism. These abnormalities can contribute to vascular calcification and may be responsible in part for the accelerated CVD and excess mortality seen in the CKD population. Epidemiologic studies in humans show an association between elevated phosphorus levels and increased risk of cardiovascular mortality in early CKD through ESRD. As yet, there are no intervention trials suggesting the best course of treatment in these patients; control of mineral and PTH levels per current guidelines is discussed below.

Bone disease, or **renal osteodystrophy,** in advanced CKD is common and there are several types of lesions. Renal osteodystrophy can be diagnosed only by bone biopsy, which is rarely done. The most common bone disease, **osteitis fibrosa cystica,** is a result of secondary hyperparathyroidism and the osteoclast-stimulating effects of PTH. This is a high-turnover disease with bone resorption and subperiosteal lesions; it can result in bone pain and proximal muscle weakness. **Adynamic bone disease,** or low-bone turnover, is becoming more common; it may result iatrogenically from suppression of PTH or via spontaneously low PTH production. **Osteomalacia** is characterized by lack of bone mineralization. In the past, osteomalacia was associated with aluminum toxicity—either as a result of

chronic ingestion of prescribed aluminum-containing phosphorus binders or from high levels of aluminum in impure dialysate water. Currently, osteomalacia is more likely to result from hypovitaminosis D; there is also theoretical risk of osteomalacia associated with use of bisphosphonates in advanced CKD.

All of the above entities increase the risk of fractures. Aluminum exposure should be avoided. In addition, treatment may involve correction of calcium, phosphorus, and 25-OH vitamin D levels toward normal values, and mitigation of hyperparathyroidism. Understanding the interplay between these abnormalities can help target therapy (Figure 22–3). Declining GFR leads to phosphorus retention. This results in hypocalcemia as phosphorus complexes with calcium, deposits in soft tissues, and stimulates PTH. Loss of renal mass and low 25-OH vitamin D levels often seen in CKD patients result in low 1,25(OH) vitamin D production by the kidney. Because 1,25(OH) vitamin D is a suppressor of PTH production, hypovitaminosis D also leads to secondary hyperparathyroidism.

The first step in treatment of metabolic bone disease is control of hyperphosphatemia. This involves dietary phosphorus restriction initially (see section on dietary management), followed by the administration of oral phosphorus binders if targets are not achieved. Oral phosphorus binders block absorption of dietary phosphorus in the gut and are given thrice daily with meals. These should be titrated to a near-normal serum phosphorus level. Calcium-containing binders (calcium carbonate, 650 mg/tablet, or calcium acetate, 667 mg/capsule, used at doses of one to three pills per meal) are relatively inexpensive but may contribute to positive calcium balance and vascular calcification; overt hypercalcemia may also occur. Thus, current guidelines suggest limiting their use in favor of the non-calcium–containing binders sevelamer carbonate (800–3200 mg/meal) and lanthanum carbonate (500–1000 mg/meal). Aluminum hydroxide is a highly effective phosphorus binder but can cause osteomalacia and neurologic complications when used long-term. It can be used in the acute setting for severe hyperphosphatemia or for short periods (eg, 3 weeks) in CKD patients.

Once serum phosphorus levels are controlled, active vitamin D (1,25[OH] vitamin D, or calcitriol) or active vitamin D analogs are recommended to treat secondary hyperparathyroidism in advanced CKD and ESRD. Serum 25-OH vitamin D levels should be measured and brought to normal (see Chapter 26) prior to considering administration of active vitamin D. Active vitamin D (calcitriol) increases serum calcium and phosphorus levels; both need to be monitored closely during calcitriol therapy, and its dose should be decreased if hypercalcemia or hyperphosphatemia occurs. Typical calcitriol dosing is 0.25 or 0.5 mcg orally daily or every other day. Cinacalcet targets the calcium-sensing receptors of the parathyroid gland and suppresses PTH production. Cinacalcet, 30–90 mg orally once a day, can be used if elevated serum phosphorus or calcium levels prohibit the use of vitamin D analogs; cinacalcet can cause serious hypocalcemia, and patients should be closely monitored for this complication. Optimal PTH levels in CKD are not known, but because skeletal resistance to PTH

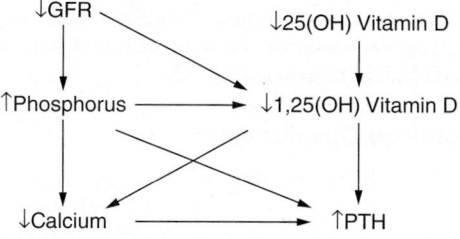

▲ **Figure 22–3.** Mineral abnormalities of chronic kidney disease (CKD). Decline in glomerular filtration rate (GFR) and loss of renal mass lead directly to increased serum phosphorus and hypovitaminosis D. Both of these abnormalities result in hypocalcemia and hyperparathyroidism. Many CKD patients also have nutritional 25(OH) vitamin D deficiency. PTH, parathyroid hormone.

develops with uremia, relatively high levels are targeted in advanced CKD to avoid adynamic bone disease. Expert guidelines generally suggest goal PTH levels near or just above the upper limit of normal for moderate CKD, and at least twofold and up to ninefold the upper limit of normal for ESRD.

C. Hematologic Complications

1. Anemia—The anemia of CKD is primarily due to decreased erythropoietin production, which often becomes clinically significant during stage 3 CKD. CKD is also associated with high hepcidin levels, which blocks GI iron absorption and mobilization of iron from body stores; this results in a functional iron deficiency—the so-called "anemia of chronic disease." The approach to a patient with CKD and anemia begins with ensuring that the bone marrow has tools with which to respond to erythropoietin. Thus, thyroid function tests, serum vitamin B_{12} levels, and iron stores should be checked. Serum ferritin and iron saturation are measured in patients with CKD but are targeted to higher goals due to a functional blockade of iron utilization in this population. In CKD, a serum ferritin below 100–200 ng/mL or iron saturation less than 20% is suggestive of iron deficiency. Iron stores may be repleted with oral or parenteral iron; iron therapy should probably be withheld if the serum ferritin is greater than 500–800 ng/mL, even if the iron saturation is less than 20%. Oral therapy with ferrous sulfate, gluconate, or fumarate, 325 mg once to three times daily, is the initial therapy in pre-ESRD CKD. For those who do not respond due to poor GI absorption or lack of tolerance, intravenous iron (eg, iron sucrose or iron gluconate) may be necessary.

Erythropoiesis-stimulating agents (ESAs, eg, recombinant erythropoietin [epoetin alfa or beta] and darbepoetin) are used to treat the anemia of CKD if other treatable causes are excluded. There is likely no benefit of starting an ESA before hemoglobin (Hgb) values are less than 9 g/dL. The starting dose of epoetin alfa is 50 units/kg (3000–4000 units/dose) once or twice a week, and darbepoetin is started at 0.45 mcg/kg and administered every 2–4 weeks; epoetin beta is given every 2–4 weeks. These agents can be given intravenously (eg, to the hemodialysis patient) or subcutaneously (to both the predialysis or dialysis patient); subcutaneous dosing of epoetin alfa is roughly 30% more effective than intravenous dosing. ESAs should be titrated to an Hgb of 10–11 g/dL for optimal safety; studies show that targeting a higher Hgb increases the risk of stroke and possibly other cardiovascular events. When titrating doses, Hgb levels should rise no more than 1 g/dL every 3–4 weeks. Hypertension is a common complication of treatment with ESAs.

2. Coagulopathy—The bleeding diathesis that may occur in stage 4–5 CKD is mainly due to platelet dysfunction, but severe anemia may also contribute.

Treatment is required only in patients who are symptomatic. Raising the Hgb to 9–10 g/dL in anemic patients can reduce risk of bleeding via improved clot formation. Desmopressin (25 mcg intravenously every 8–12 hours for two doses) is a short-lived but effective treatment for platelet dysfunction and it is often used in preparation for surgery or kidney biopsy. Conjugated estrogens, 2.5–5 mg orally for 5–7 days, may have an effect for several weeks but are seldom used. Dialysis improves the bleeding time.

D. Hyperkalemia

Potassium balance generally remains intact in CKD until stages 4–5. However, hyperkalemia may occur at earlier stages when certain conditions are present, such as type 4 renal tubular acidosis (seen in patients with diabetes mellitus), high potassium diets, or medications that decrease renal potassium secretion (amiloride, triamterene, spironolactone, eplerenone, NSAIDs, ACE inhibitors, ARBs) or block cellular potassium uptake (beta-blockers). Other causes include acidemic states and any type of cellular destruction causing release of intracellular contents, such as hemolysis and rhabdomyolysis.

Treatment of acute hyperkalemia is discussed in Chapter 21 (see Table 21–6). Cardiac monitoring is indicated for any ECG changes seen with hyperkalemia or a serum potassium level greater than 6.0–6.5 mEq/L or mmol/L. Chronic hyperkalemia is best treated with dietary potassium restriction (2 g/day) and minimization or elimination of any medications that may impair renal potassium excretion, as noted above. Loop diuretics may also be administered for their kaliuretic effect as long as the patient is not volume-depleted.

E. Acid-Base Disorders

Damaged kidneys are unable to excrete the 1 mEq/kg/day of acid generated by metabolism of dietary animal proteins in the typical Western diet. The resultant metabolic acidosis is primarily due to decreased GFR; proximal or distal tubular defects may contribute to or worsen the acidosis. Excess hydrogen ions are buffered by bone; the consequent leaching of calcium and phosphorus from the bone contributes to the metabolic bone disease described above. Chronic acidosis can also result in muscle protein catabolism as well as growth retardation in children with CKD and may accelerate progression of CKD. The serum bicarbonate level should be normalized. Reduction in the intake of dietary animal protein and the administration of oral sodium bicarbonate (in doses of 0.5–1.0 mEq/kg/day divided twice daily and titrated as needed) may achieve this goal. Citrate salts increase the absorption of dietary aluminum and should be avoided in CKD.

F. Neurologic Complications

Uremic encephalopathy, resulting from the aggregation of uremic toxins, does not occur until GFR falls below 5–10 mL/min/1.73 m^2. Symptoms begin with difficulty in concentrating and can progress to lethargy, confusion, seizure, and coma. Physical findings may include altered mental status, weakness, and asterixis. These findings improve with dialysis.

Other neurologic complications that can manifest with advanced CKD include peripheral neuropathies (stocking-glove or isolated mononeuropathies), erectile dysfunction, autonomic dysfunction, and restless leg syndrome. These may not improve with dialysis therapy.

G. Endocrine Disorders

There is risk of hypoglycemia in treated diabetic patients with advanced CKD due to decreased renal elimination of insulin. Doses of oral hypoglycemics and insulin may need reduction. The risk of lactic acidosis with metformin is due to both dose and eGFR; it should be discontinued when eGFR is less than 30 mL/min/1.73 m^2. Whether to discontinue metformin when the eGFR is between 30 mL/min and 60 mL/min is controversial.

Decreased libido and erectile dysfunction are common in advanced CKD. Men have decreased testosterone levels; women are often anovulatory. Women with serum creatinine less than 1.4 mg/dL are not at increased risk for poor outcomes in pregnancy; however, those with serum creatinine greater than 1.4 mg/dL may experience faster progression of CKD with pregnancy. Fetal survival is not compromised, however, unless CKD is advanced. Despite a high degree of infertility in patients with ESRD, pregnancy can occur in this setting; however, fetal mortality approaches 50%, and babies who survive are often premature. In female patients with ESRD, renal transplantation with a well-functioning allograft affords the best chances for a successful pregnancy.

▶ Treatment

A. Slowing Progression

Treatment of the underlying cause of CKD is vital. Control of diabetes should be aggressive in early CKD; risk of hypoglycemia increases in advanced CKD, and glycemic targets may need to be relaxed to avoid this dangerous complication. Blood pressure control is vital to slow progression of all forms of CKD; agents that block the renin-angiotensin-aldosterone system are particularly important in proteinuric disease (see section on hypertension regarding blood pressure goals). Several small studies suggest a possible benefit of oral bicarbonate therapy in slowing CKD progression when acidemia is present; treating hyperuricemia, if present, may also retard progression and lower blood pressure, but strong clinical evidence for this is lacking. Obese patients should be encouraged to lose weight. Management of traditional cardiovascular risk factors should also be emphasized.

B. Dietary Management

Patients with CKD should be evaluated by a renal nutritionist. Patient-specific recommendations should be made concerning protein, salt, water, potassium, and phosphorus intake to help manage CKD progression and complications.

1. Protein restriction—Reduced intake of animal protein to 0.6-0.8 g/kg/day may retard CKD progression and is likely not harmful in the otherwise well-nourished patient; it is not advisable in those with cachexia or low serum albumin in the absence of the nephrotic syndrome.

2. Salt and water restriction—In advanced CKD, the kidney is unable to adapt to large changes in sodium intake. Intake of greater than 3–4 g/day can lead to hypertension and hypervolemia, whereas intake of less than 1 g/day can lead to volume depletion and hypotension. A goal of 2 g/day of sodium is reasonable for most patients. Daily fluid restriction to 2 L may be needed if volume overload is present.

3. Potassium restriction—Restriction is needed once the GFR has fallen below 10–20 mL/min/1.73 m^2, or earlier if the patient is hyperkalemic. Patients should receive detailed lists describing potassium content of foods and should limit their intake to less than 50–60 mEq/day (2 g/day). An aggressive bowel regimen should be instituted for patients with hyperkalemia (more than two bowel movements daily), since a higher percentage of potassium is excreted through the gastrointestinal tract as GFR declines.

4. Phosphorus restriction—Guidelines suggest lowering elevated serum phosphorus levels toward normal in all stages of CKD. Dietary phosphate restriction to 800–1000 mg/day is the first step. Processed foods and cola beverages are often preserved with highly bioavailable phosphorus and should be avoided. Foods rich in phosphorus such as eggs, dairy products, nuts, beans, and meat may also need to be limited, although care must be taken to avoid protein malnutrition. When GFR is less than 20–30 mL/min/1.73 m^2, dietary restriction is rarely sufficient to reach target levels, and phosphorus binders are usually required.

C. Medication Management

Many drugs are excreted by the kidney; dosages should be adjusted for GFR. Insulin doses may need to be decreased as noted above. Magnesium-containing medications, such as laxatives or antacids, and phosphorus-containing medicines, (eg, cathartics) should be avoided. Active morphine metabolites can accumulate in advanced CKD; this problem is not encountered with other opioid agents. Drugs with potential nephrotoxicity (NSAIDs, intravenous contrast, as well as others noted in the Acute Kidney Injury section) should be avoided.

D. Treatment of ESRD

When GFR declines to 5–10 mL/min/1.73 m^2, renal replacement therapy (hemodialysis, peritoneal dialysis, or kidney transplantation) is required to sustain life. Patient education is important in understanding which mode of therapy is most suitable, as is timely preparation for treatment; therefore, referral to a nephrologist should take place in late stage 3 CKD, or when the GFR is declining rapidly. Such referral has been shown to improve mortality. Preparation for ESRD treatment requires a team approach with the involvement of dieticians, social workers, primary care clinicians, and nephrologists. For very elderly patients, or those with multiple debilitating or life-limiting comorbidities, dialysis therapy may not meaningfully prolong life, and the option of palliative care should be discussed with the patient and family. Conversely, for patients who are otherwise relatively healthy, evaluation for possible kidney transplantation should be considered prior to initiation of dialysis.

1. Dialysis—Dialysis initiation should be considered when GFR is 10 mL/min/1.73 m². Studies suggest that the well-selected patient without overt uremic symptoms may wait to initiate dialysis until GFR is closer to 7 mL/min/1.73 m². Other indications for dialysis, which may occur when GFR is 10–15 mL/min/1.73 m², include (1) uremic symptoms, (2) fluid overload unresponsive to diuresis, and (3) refractory hyperkalemia.

A. HEMODIALYSIS—Vascular access for hemodialysis can be accomplished by an arteriovenous fistula (the preferred method) or prosthetic graft; creation of dialysis access should be considered well before dialysis initiation. An indwelling catheter is used when there is no useable vascular access. Because catheters confer a high risk of bloodstream infection, they should be considered a temporary measure. Native fistulas typically last longer than prosthetic grafts but require a longer time after surgical construction for maturation (6–8 weeks for a fistula versus 2 weeks for a graft). Infection, thrombosis, and aneurysm formation are complications seen more often in grafts than fistulas. *Staphylococcus* species are the most common cause of soft tissue infections and bacteremia.

Treatment at a hemodialysis center occurs three times a week. Sessions last 3–5 hours depending on patient size and type of dialysis access. Home hemodialysis is often performed more frequently (3–6 days per week for shorter sessions) and requires a trained helper. Results of trials comparing quotidian modalities (nocturnal and frequent home hemodialysis) to conventional in-center dialysis have not thus far shown significant mortality differences, but there may be improvements in blood pressure control, mineral metabolism, and quality of life.

B. PERITONEAL DIALYSIS—With peritoneal dialysis, the peritoneal membrane is the "dialyzer." Dialysate is instilled into the peritoneal cavity through an indwelling catheter; water and solutes move across the capillary bed that lies between the visceral and parietal layers of the membrane into the dialysate during a "dwell." After equilibration, the dialysate is drained, and fresh dialysate is instilled—this is an "exchange."

The most common complication of peritoneal dialysis is peritonitis. Peritonitis may present with nausea and vomiting, abdominal pain, diarrhea or constipation, and fever. The normally clear dialysate becomes cloudy; and a diagnostic peritoneal fluid cell count greater than 100 white blood cells/mcL with a differential of greater than 50% polymorphonuclear neutrophils is present. *Staphylococcus aureus* is the most common infecting organism, but streptococci and gram-negative species may also be causative. Empiric intraperitoneal administration of either vancomycin or a first-generation cephalosporin (cefazolin) plus a third-generation cephalosporin (ceftazidime) should be instituted with the first signs of peritonitis and subsequently tailored based on culture results.

2. Kidney transplantation—Many patients with ESRD are otherwise healthy enough to be suitable for transplantation, although standard criteria for recipient selection are lacking between transplant centers. Two-thirds of kidney allografts come from deceased donors, with the remainder from living related or unrelated donors. Over 100,000 patients are on the waiting list for a deceased donor transplant in the United States; the average wait is 2–6 years, depending on geographic location and recipient blood type.

3. Medical management of ESRD—As noted above, some patients are not candidates for kidney transplantation and may not benefit from dialysis. Very elderly persons may die soon after dialysis initiation; those who do not may nonetheless rapidly lose functional status in the first year of treatment. The decision to initiate dialysis in patients with limited life expectancy should be weighed against possible deterioration in quality of life. For patients with ESRD who elect not to undergo dialysis or who withdraw from dialysis, progressive uremia with gradual suppression of sensorium results in a painless death within days to months. Hyperkalemia may intervene with a fatal cardiac dysrhythmia. Diuretics, volume restriction, and opioids, as described in Chapter 5, may help decrease the symptoms of volume overload. Involvement of a palliative care team is essential.

▶ Prognosis in ESRD

Compared with kidney transplant recipients and age-matched controls, mortality is higher for patients undergoing dialysis. There is likely little difference in survival for well-matched peritoneal versus hemodialysis patients.

Survival rates on dialysis depend on the underlying disease process. Five-year Kaplan-Meier survival rates vary from 37% for patients with diabetes to 54% for patients with glomerulonephritis. Overall 5-year survival is currently estimated at 40%. Patients undergoing dialysis have an average life-expectancy of 3–5 years, but survival for as long as 25 years may be achieved depending on comorbidities. The most common cause of death is cardiac disease (more than 50%). Other causes include infection, cerebrovascular disease, and malignancy. Diabetes, advanced age, a low serum albumin, lower socioeconomic status, and inadequate dialysis are all significant predictors of mortality; high fibroblast growth factor (FGF)-23 levels are a novel marker for mortality in ESRD.

▶ When to Refer

- A patient with stage 3–5 CKD should be referred to a nephrologist for management in conjunction with the primary care provider.
- A patient with other forms of CKD such as those with proteinuria greater than 1 g/day or polycystic kidney disease should be referred to a nephrologist at earlier stages.

▶ When to Admit

- Admission should be considered for patients with decompensation of problems related to CKD, such as worsening of acid-base status, electrolyte abnormalities, and volume overload, that cannot be appropriately treated in the outpatient setting.
- Admission is appropriate when a patient needs to start dialysis and is not stable for its outpatient initiation.

Grill AK et al. Approach to the detection and management of chronic kidney disease: what primary care providers need to know. Can Fam Physician. 2018 Oct;64(10):728–35. [PMID: 30315015]

Kalantar-Zadeh K et al. Nutritional management of chronic kidney disease. N Engl J Med. 2017 Nov 2;377(18):1765–76. [PMID: 29091561]

Palmer BF et al. Renal considerations in the treatment of hypertension. Am J Hypertens. 2018 Mar 10;31(4):394–401. [PMID: 29373638]

Whelton PK et al. 2017 ACC/AHA/AAPA/ABC/ACPM/AGS/APhA/ASH/ASPC/NMA/PCNA Guideline for the prevention, detection, evaluation, and management of high blood pressure in adults: executive summary: a report of the American College of Cardiology/American Heart Association Task Force on Clinical Practice Guidelines. Hypertension. 2018 Jun;71(6):1269–324. [PMID: 29133354]

Whittaker CF et al. Medication safety principles and practice in CKD. Clin J Am Soc Nephrol. 2018 Nov 7;13(11):1738–46. [PMID: 29915131]

Zoccali C et al; European Renal and Cardiovascular Medicine (EURECA-m) Working Group of the European Renal Association—European Dialysis Transplantation Association (ERA-EDTA). The systemic nature of CKD. Nat Rev Nephrol. 2017 Jun;13(6):344–58. [PMID: 28435157]

RENAL ARTERY STENOSIS

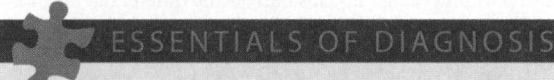

ESSENTIALS OF DIAGNOSIS

► Produced by atherosclerotic occlusive disease (80–90% of patients) or fibromuscular dysplasia (10–15%).

► Hypertension.

► AKI in patients starting ACE inhibitor therapy if stenosis is bilateral.

General Considerations

Atherosclerotic ischemic renal disease accounts for most cases of renal artery stenosis. Fibromuscular dysplasia is a less common cause of renal artery stenosis. Approximately 5% of Americans with hypertension suffer from renal artery stenosis. It occurs most commonly in those over 45 years of age with a history of atherosclerotic disease. Other risk factors include CKD, diabetes mellitus, tobacco use, and hypertension.

Clinical Findings

A. Symptoms and Signs

Patients with atherosclerotic ischemic renal disease may have refractory hypertension, new-onset hypertension (in an older patient), pulmonary edema with poorly controlled blood pressure, and AKI upon starting an ACE inhibitor. In addition to hypertension, physical examination may reveal an audible abdominal bruit on the affected side. Fibromuscular dysplasia primarily affects young women. Unexplained hypertension in a woman younger than 40 years is a reason to screen for this disorder.

B. Laboratory Findings

BUN and serum creatinine may be elevated if there is significant renal ischemia. Patients with bilateral renal artery stenosis may have hypokalemia, a finding that reflects activation of the renin-angiotensin-aldosterone system in response to reduced blood flow (a "prerenal" state).

C. Imaging

Abdominal ultrasound can reveal either asymmetric kidney size if one renal artery is affected more than the other or small hyperechoic kidneys if both are affected.

Three prevailing methods used for screening are Doppler ultrasonography, CT angiography, and magnetic resonance angiography (MRA). According to the American College of Cardiology/American Heart Association guidelines, one of these should be undertaken if a corrective procedure would be performed when a positive test result is found. **Doppler ultrasonography** is highly sensitive and specific (85% and 92% respectively in a meta-analysis of 88 studies) and relatively inexpensive. However, this method is extremely operator and patient dependent.

CT angiography consists of intravenous digital subtraction angiography with arteriography. A noninvasive procedure, it uses a spiral (helical) CT scan with intravenous contrast injection. The sensitivities from various studies range from 77% to 98%, with specificities in the range of 90–94%.

MRA is an excellent but expensive way to screen for renal artery stenosis, particularly in those with atherosclerotic disease. Sensitivity is 77–100%, although one flawed study showed a sensitivity of only 62%. Specificity ranges from 71% to 96%. Turbulent blood flow can cause false-positive results. The imaging agent for MRA (gadolinium) has been associated with nephrogenic systemic fibrosis, which occurs primarily in patients with a GFR of less than 15 mL/min/1.73 m^2, and rarely in patients with a GFR of 15–29 mL/min/1.73 m^2. This fibrosis has also occurred in those with AKI and kidney transplants.

Renal angiography is the gold standard for diagnosis but it is more invasive than the three screening tests discussed above. Thus, it is performed after a positive screening test. CO_2 subtraction angiography can be used in place of dye when the risk of dye nephropathy exists—eg, in diabetic patients with kidney injury. Lesions are most commonly found in the proximal third or ostial region of the renal artery. The risk of atheroembolic phenomena after angiography ranges from 5% to 10%. Fibromuscular dysplasia has a characteristic "beads-on-a-string" appearance on angiography.

Treatment

Treatment of atherosclerotic ischemic renal disease is controversial. Options include medical management, angioplasty with or without stenting, and surgical bypass. Two large randomized trials showed that vascular intervention is no better than optimal medical management in typical patients with renal artery stenosis. Angioplasty might reduce the number of antihypertensive medications but does not significantly change the progression of kidney dysfunction in comparison to patients medically managed. Stenting produces significantly better results than angioplasty.

However, with medical management blood pressure and serum creatinine are similar at 6 months compared with both angioplasty and stents. Angioplasty is equally as effective as, and safer than, surgical revision.

Treatment of fibromuscular dysplasia with percutaneous transluminal angioplasty is often curative, which is in stark contrast to treatments for atherosclerotic disease.

Cooper CJ et al; CORAL Investigators. Stenting and medical therapy for atherosclerotic renal-artery stenosis. N Engl J Med. 2014 Jan 2;370(1):13–22. [PMID: 24245566]

Gupta R et al. Renal artery stenosis: new findings from the CORAL trial. Curr Cardiol Rep. 2017 Sep;19(9):75. [PMID: 28752274]

GLOMERULAR DISEASES

Glomerular diseases can be challenging to understand clinically because the glomerulus is a histologically complex structure (consisting of the epithelial cells [podocytes], basement membrane, capillary endothelium, and mesangium). The following are examples of injuries that can affect any or all of the constituents of the glomerulus: (1) overwork injury, as in CKD; (2) an inflammatory process, such as SLE; (3) a podocyte protein mutation, as in hereditary focal segmental glomerulosclerosis (FSGS); or (4) a deposition disease, as in diabetes or amyloidosis.

When a glomerular disease is suspected, a kidney biopsy may be needed to clarify the etiology.

▶ Classification

Clinically, a glomerular disease can be classified as being in one of two clinical spectra—either in the nephritic spectrum or the nephrotic spectrum (Figure 22–4). At the "least severe" end of the **nephritic spectrum**, the findings of asymptomatic glomerular hematuria (ie, dysmorphic red blood cells with or without some proteinuria [<1 g/day]) are characteristic. The nephritic *syndrome*, comprising glomerular hematuria, subnephrotic proteinuria (less than 3 g/day), edema, and elevated creatinine, falls in the mid-portion of the spectrum. The rapidly progressive glomerulonephridities (RPGNs), with systemic symptoms, are at the "most severe" and clinically urgent end of the nephritic spectrum. The **nephrotic spectrum** is comprised of diseases that present primarily with proteinuria of at least 0.5–1 g/day and a bland urine sediment (no cells or cellular casts). At the more severe end of the nephrotic spectrum is the nephrotic *syndrome*, consisting of nephrotic-range proteinuria (>3 g/day), hypoalbuminemia, edema, hyperlipidemia, and urinary oval fat bodies. Differentiating between a clinical presentation within the nephritic spectrum versus the nephrotic spectrum is important because it helps narrow the differential diagnosis of the underlying glomerular disease (Tables 22–7 and 22–8).

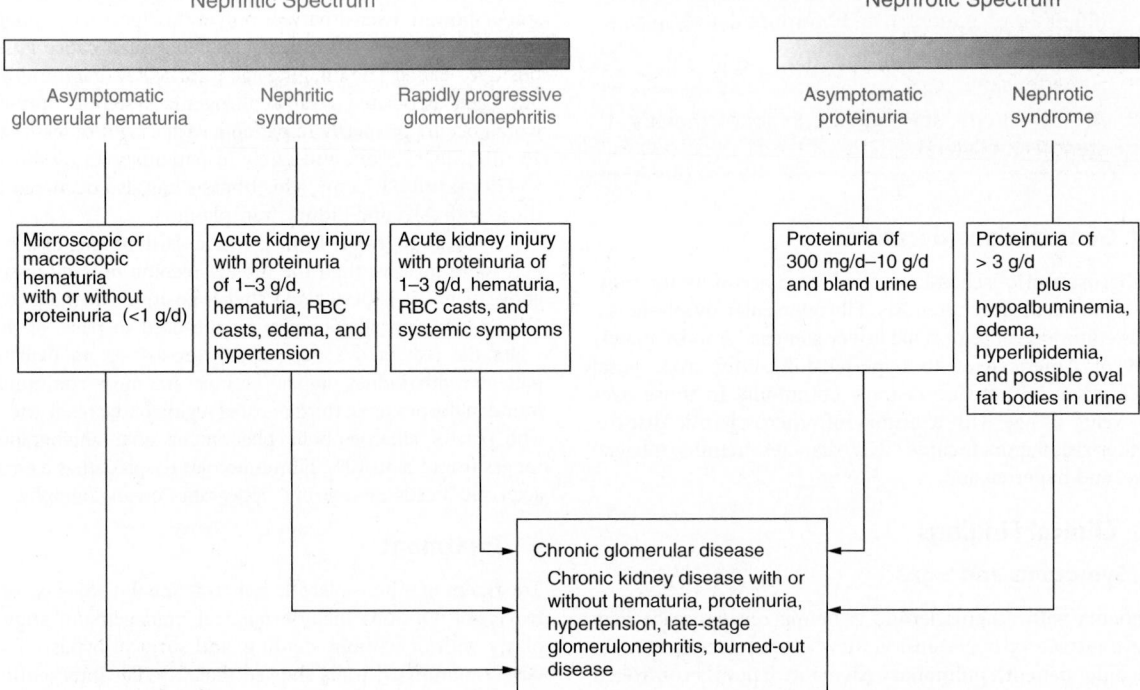

▲ **Figure 22–4.** Glomerular diseases present within one of the clinical spectra shown; the exact presentation is determined by the severity of the underlying disease and the pattern of injury. Nephritic diseases are characterized by the presence of an active urine sediment with glomerular hematuria and often with proteinuria. Nephrotic spectrum diseases are proteinuric with bland urine sediments (no cells or cellular casts). All glomerular diseases may progress to a chronic, scarred state. (Adapted, with permission, from Megan Troxell, MD, PhD.)

Table 22–7. Classification and findings in glomerulonephritis: nephritic spectrum presentations.

	Typical Presentation	Association/Notes	Serology
Postinfectious glomerulonephritis	Children: abrupt onset of nephritic syndrome and acute kidney injury but can present anywhere in nephritic spectrum	Streptococci, other bacterial infections (eg, staphylococci, endocarditis, shunt infections)	Rising ASO titers, low complement levels
IgA nephropathy (Berger disease) and Henoch-Schönlein purpura, systemic IgA vasculitis	Classically: gross hematuria with respiratory tract infection; can present anywhere in nephritic spectrum; Henoch-Schönlein purpura with vasculitic rash and gastrointestinal hemorrhage	Abnormal IgA glycosylation in both primary (familial predisposition) and secondary disease (associated with cirrhosis, HIV, celiac disease) Henoch-Schönlein purpura in children after an inciting infection	No serologic tests helpful; complement levels are normal
Pauci-immune (granulomatosis with polyangiitis, eosinophilic granulomatosis with polyangiitis, polyarteritis, idiopathic crescentic glomerulonephritis)	Classically as crescentic or RPGN, but can present anywhere in nephritic spectrum; may have respiratory tract/sinus symptoms in granulomatosis with polyangiitis	See Figure 22–5	ANCAs: MPO or PR3 titers high; complement levels normal
Anti-GBM glomerulonephritis; Goodpasture syndrome	Classically as crescentic or RPGN, but can present anywhere in nephritic spectrum; with pulmonary hemorrhage in Goodpasture syndrome	May develop as a result of respiratory irritant exposure (chemicals or tobacco use)	Anti-GBM antibody titers high; complement levels normal
Cryoglobulin-associated glomerulonephritis	Often acute nephritic syndrome; often with systemic vasculitis including rash and arthritis	Most commonly associated with chronic hepatitis C; may occur with other chronic infections or some connective tissue diseases	Cryoglobulins positive; rheumatoid factor may be elevated; complement levels low
MPGN	Classically presents with acute nephritic syndrome, but can see nephrotic syndrome features in addition	Most patients are < 30 years old Type I/immune complex most common Type II (dense deposit disease) and C3 glomerulonephritis	Low complement levels, may have findings of underlying infection or paraproteinemia
Hepatitis C infection	Anywhere in nephritic spectrum	Can cause MPGN pattern of injury or cryoglobulinemic glomerulonephritis; membranous nephropathy pattern of injury uncommon	Low complement levels; positive hepatitis C serology; rheumatoid factor may be elevated
Systemic lupus erythematosus	Anywhere in nephritic spectrum, depending on pattern/severity of injury	Treatment depends on clinical course and International Society of Nephrology and Renal Pathology Society (ISN/RPS) classification on biopsy	High ANA and anti-double-stranded DNA titers; low complement levels

ANA, antinuclear antibodies; ANCAs: antineutrophil cytoplasmic antibodies; GBM, glomerular basement membrane; MPGN, membranoproliferative glomerulonephritis; MPO, myeloperoxidase; PR3, proteinase 3; RPGN, rapidly progressive glomerulonephritis.

Glomerular diseases can also be classified according to whether they cause only renal abnormalities (primary renal disease) or whether the renal abnormalities result from a systemic disease (secondary renal disease).

Further evaluation prior to kidney biopsy may include serologic testing for systemic diseases that can result in glomerular damage (Figure 22–5).

Cavanaugh C et al. Urine sediment examination in the diagnosis and management of kidney disease: Core Curriculum 2019. Am J Kidney Dis. 2019 Feb;73(2):258–72. [PMID: 30249419]

Couser WG et al. The etiology of glomerulonephritis: roles of infection and autoimmunity. Kidney Int. 2014 Nov;86(5):905–14. [PMID: 24621918]

Floege J et al. Primary glomerulonephritides. Lancet. 2016 May 14;387(10032):2036–48. [PMID: 26921911]

Leung N et al. Dysproteinemias and glomerular Disease. Clin J Am Soc Nephrol. 2018 Jan 6;13(1):128–39. [PMID: 29114004]

Long JD et al. Autoimmune kidney diseases associated with chronic viral infections. Rheum Dis Clin North Am. 2018 Nov;44(4):675–98. [PMID: 30274630]

Ponticelli C et al. Glucocorticoids in the treatment of glomerular diseases: pitfalls and pearls. Clin J Am Soc Nephrol. 2018 May 7;13(5):815–22. [PMID: 29475991]

Table 22–8. Classification and findings in glomerulonephritis: nephrotic spectrum presentations.

Disease	Typical Presentation	Association/Notes
Minimal change disease (nil disease; lipoid nephrosis)	Child with sudden onset of full nephrotic syndrome	Children: associated with allergy or viral infection Adults: associated with Hodgkin disease, NSAIDs
Membranous nephropathy	Anywhere in nephrotic spectrum, but nephrotic syndrome not uncommon; particular predisposition to hypercoagulable state	Primary (idiopathic) may be associated with antibodies to PLA$_2$R Secondary may be associated with non-Hodgkin lymphoma, carcinoma (gastrointestinal, renal, bronchogenic, thyroid), gold therapy, penicillamine, SLE, chronic hepatitis B or C infection
Focal and segmental glomerulosclerosis	Anywhere in nephrotic spectrum; children with congenital disease have nephrotic syndrome	Children: congenital disease with podocyte gene mutation, or in spectrum of disease with minimal change disease Adults: associated with heroin abuse, HIV infection, reflux nephropathy, obesity, pamidronate, podocyte protein mutations, *APOL1* mutations
Amyloidosis	Anywhere in nephrotic spectrum	AL: plasma cell dyscrasia with Ig light chain overproduction and deposition; check SPEP and UPEP AA: serum amyloid protein A overproduction and deposition in response to chronic inflammatory disease (rheumatoid arthritis, inflammatory bowel disease, chronic infection)
Diabetic nephropathy	High GFR (hyperfiltration) → microalbuminuria → frank proteinuria → decline in GFR	Diabetes diagnosis precedes diagnosis of nephropathy by years
HIV-associated nephropathy	Heavy proteinuria, often nephrotic syndrome, progresses to ESRD relatively quickly	Usually seen in antiviral treatment-naïve patients (rare in antiretroviral therapy era), predilection for those of African descent (*APOL1* mutations)
Membranoproliferative glomerulonephropathy	Classically presents with acute nephritic syndrome, some may also exhibit nephrotic features	Immune complex–MPGN are idiopathic or secondary to infections, paraproteinemia, or systemic autoimmune disease; C3 glomerulopathies are due to alternative complement pathway dysregulation

ESRD, end-stage renal disease; GFR, glomerular filtration rate; NSAIDs, nonsteroidal anti-inflammatory drugs; PLA$_2$R, phospholipase A$_2$ receptor; SLE, systemic lupus erythematosus; SPEP/UPEP, serum and urine protein electrophoresis.

NEPHRITIC SPECTRUM GLOMERULAR DISEASES

ESSENTIALS OF DIAGNOSIS

▶ **Asymptomatic glomerular hematuria**
 –Hematuria with dysmorphic RBCs
 –Proteinuria < 1 g/day
▶ **Nephritic syndrome** in more severe cases
 –Glomerular hematuria (and RBC casts if glomerular bleeding is heavy)
 –Proteinuria of 1–3 g/day
 –Hypertension
 –Edema
 –Rising creatinine over days to months
▶ **Rapidly progressive glomerulonephritis** in most severe cases
 –AKI with rising creatinine over days to months
 –Glomerular hematuria (and RBC casts)
 –Proteinuria of 1–3 g/day
 –Systemic symptoms
 –Hypertension and edema uncommon

▶ General Considerations

"Glomerulonephritis" is a term given to those diseases that present in the nephritic spectrum and usually signifies an inflammatory process causing renal dysfunction. It can be acute, developing over days to weeks, with or without resolution, or may be more chronic and indolent with progressive scarring. As noted above, diseases that cause a nephritic spectrum presentation may present with glomerular hematuria and proteinuria, with nephritic syndrome, or with RPGN (Figure 22–4). The presentation depends on the severity of the underlying inflammation and the pattern of injury caused by the disease process.

▶ Clinical Findings

A. Symptoms and Signs

If the nephritic syndrome is present, the acute decrease in GFR leads to sodium retention. This is clinically manifested by edema, first seen in regions of low tissue pressure such as the periorbital and scrotal areas, and by hypertension. Heavy glomerular bleeding from inflammation may result in gross hematuria (smoky or cola-colored urine).

B. Laboratory Findings

1. Serologic testing—Serologic tests, including complement levels, antinuclear antibodies, cryoglobulins,

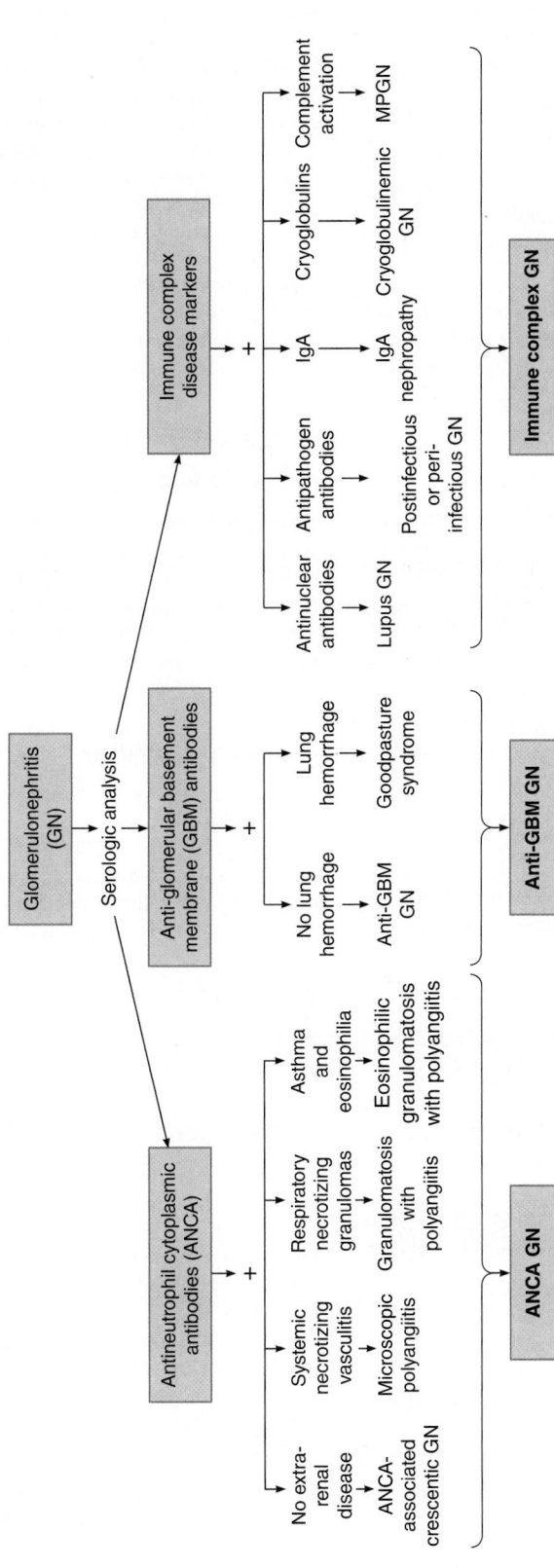

▲ **Figure 22–5.** Serologic analysis of patients with glomerulonephritis. MPGN, membranoproliferative glomerulonephritis. (Modified, with permission, from Greenberg A et al. *Primer on Kidney Diseases.* Academic Press, 1994; and Jennette JC, Falk RJ. Diagnosis and management of glomerulonephritis and vasculitis presenting as acute renal failure. Med Clin North Am. 1990;74(4):893–908. © Elsevier.)

hepatitis serologies, ANCAs, anti-GBM antibodies, and antistreptolysin O (ASO) titers (Figure 22–5) based on the history and physical examination help narrow the differential diagnosis of the nephritic spectrum disorder.

2. Urinalysis—The urine dipstick is positive for protein and blood. Urinary microscopy reveals red blood cells that are misshapen or dysmorphic from traversing a damaged glomerular filtration barrier. Red blood cell casts are seen with heavy glomerular bleeding and tubular stasis. When quantified, proteinuria is usually subnephrotic (less than 3 g/day).

3. Biopsy—Kidney biopsy should be considered if there are no contraindications (eg, bleeding disorders, thrombocytopenia, uncontrolled hypertension). Important morphologic information is gleaned from light, electron, and immunofluorescent microscopy.

▶ Treatment

General measures for all include treatment of hypertension and of fluid overload if present. Antiproteinuric therapy with an ACE inhibitor or ARB should be considered for those without AKI. For those with profound AKI, dialysis may be needed. The inflammatory glomerular injury may require immunosuppressive agents (see specific diseases discussed below).

▶ When to Refer

Any patient in whom a glomerulonephritis is suspected should be referred to a nephrologist.

▶ When to Admit

Any suspicion of acute nephritic syndrome or RPGN warrants consideration of immediate hospitalization.

Kazi SN et al. Work-up of hematuria. Prim Care. 2014 Dec; 41(4):737–48. [PMID: 25439531]
Tan Y et al. Complement in glomerular diseases. Nephrology (Carlton). 2018 Oct;23(Suppl 4):11–5. [PMID: 30298653]

1. Infection-Related & Postinfectious Glomerulonephritis

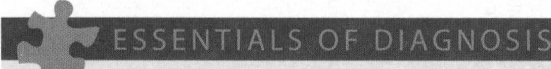

ESSENTIALS OF DIAGNOSIS

- ▶ Proteinuria.
- ▶ Glomerular hematuria.
- ▶ Symptoms 1–3 weeks after some infections (often pharyngitis or impetigo) or during course of other infections (eg, pneumonia or endocarditis).

▶ General Considerations

Postinfectious glomerulonephritis is most often due to infection with nephritogenic group A beta-hemolytic

streptococcal infections (pharyngitis or impetigo). It can occur sporadically or in clusters and during epidemics. with onset up to 1–3 weeks after infection (average 7–10 days).

Other infections have been associated with glomerulonephritis including bacteremic states (especially with *S aureus*), bacterial pneumonias, deep-seated abscesses, gram-negative infections, infective endocarditis, and shunt infections; viral, fungal, and parasitic causes of glomerulonephritis include hepatitis B or C, HIV, cytomegalovirus infection, infectious mononucleosis, coccidioidomycosis, malaria, mycobacteria, syphilis, and toxoplasmosis. These entities result in glomerular injury during active infection, and are better termed "infection-related glomerulonephritis" rather than "postinfectious glomerulonephritis."

▶ Clinical Findings

A. Symptoms and Signs

Disease presentation can vary widely across the nephritic spectrum from asymptomatic glomerular hematuria (especially in epidemic cases) with minimal change in kidney function, to nephritic syndrome with hypertension, edema, and perhaps gross glomerular hematuria (smokey-colored urine); the most severe cases may result in oliguric AKI requiring dialysis.

B. Laboratory Findings

Serum complement levels are low; in postinfectious glomerulonephritis due to group A streptococcal infection, anti-streptolysin O (ASO) titers can be high unless the immune response has been blunted with previous antibiotic treatment. Glomerular hematuria and subnephrotic proteinuria are present. Kidney biopsy shows a diffuse proliferative pattern of injury on light microscopy. Immunofluorescence demonstrates granular deposition of IgG and C3 in the mesangium and along the capillary basement membrane. Electron microscopy shows large, dense subepithelial deposits or "humps."

▶ Treatment

The underlying infection should be identified and treated appropriately; otherwise, treatment for postinfectious glomerulonephritis is supportive. Antihypertensives, salt restriction, and diuretics should be used if needed. Corticosteroids have not been shown to improve outcomes but have been tried in severe cases. Prognosis depends on the severity of the glomerular injury and age of the patient. Children are more likely to fully recover; adults are more prone to the development of severe disease (RPGN with crescent formation) and CKD.

Hunt EAK et al. Infection-related glomerulonephritis. Pediatr Clin North Am. 2019 Feb;66(1):59–72. [PMID: 30454751]
Maness DL et al. Poststreptococcal illness: recognition and management. Am Fam Physician. 2018 Apr 15;97(8):517–22. [PMID: 29671499]

2. IgA Nephropathy

ESSENTIALS OF DIAGNOSIS

▸ Proteinuria: minimal to nephrotic range.

▸ Glomerular hematuria: microscopic is common; macroscopic (gross) after infection.

▸ Positive IgA staining on kidney biopsy.

General Considerations

IgA nephropathy (Berger disease) is a primary renal disease of IgA deposition in the glomerular mesangium. The inciting cause is unknown but is likely due to deficient O-linked glycosylation of IgA subclass 1 molecules. IgA nephropathy can be a primary (renal-limited) disease, or it can be secondary to hepatic cirrhosis, celiac disease, and infections such as HIV and cytomegalovirus. Susceptibility to IgA nephropathy is inheritable.

IgA nephropathy is the most common primary glomerular disease worldwide, particularly in Asia. It is most commonly seen in children and young adults, with males affected two to three times more commonly than females.

Clinical Findings

The classical presentation of IgA nephropathy is an episode of gross hematuria associated with a mucosal viral infection, often of the upper respiratory tract. The urine becomes red or smokey-colored 1–2 days after illness onset—a so-called synpharyngitic presentation in contradistinction to the latent period seen in postinfectious glomerulonephritis. However, IgA nephropathy can also present anywhere along the nephritic spectrum from asymptomatic microscopic hematuria to RPGN (Figure 22–4). Rarely, nephrotic syndrome can be present as well.

There are no serologic tests that aid in this diagnosis; serum IgA subclass 1 testing may be a possibility in the future. Serum complements are normal. The typical pattern of injury seen on kidney biopsy is a focal glomerulonephritis with mesangial proliferation; immunofluorescence demonstrates diffuse mesangial IgA and C3 deposits.

Treatment

The disease course of primary IgA nephropathy varies widely among patients; treatment approach needs to be tailored to risk for progression. Patients with low risk for progression (no hypertension, normal GFR, minimal proteinuria) can be monitored annually. Patients at higher risk (proteinuria greater than 1.0 g/day, decreased GFR, or hypertension or any combination of these three conditions) should be treated with an ACE inhibitor or ARB. Therapy should be titrated to reduce proteinuria to less than 1 g/day and to control blood pressure in the range of 125/75 mm Hg to 130/80 mm Hg. Addition of corticosteroids (eg, methylprednisolone, 1 g/day intravenously for 3 days during months 1, 3, and 5, plus prednisone in a dosage of 0.5 mg/kg orally every other day for 6 months) in patients with GFR greater than 50 mL/min/1.73 m² and persistent proteinuria greater than 1 g/day has been shown to reduce proteinuria, but there seems to be little durable effect, and risk of infection and hyperglycemia is significant. Azathioprine and mycophenolate mofetil have also been used in patients at high risk for progression, but studies with these agents are small and their use is not routinely recommended. For the rare patient with IgA neuropathy and a rapidly progressive clinical course with crescent formation on biopsy, cyclophosphamide and corticosteroid therapy should be considered (see section on ANCA-associated vasculitis below). Kidney transplantation is an excellent option for patients with ESRD, but recurrent disease has been documented in 30% of patients 5–10 years posttransplant. Fortunately, recurrent disease rarely leads to failure of the allograft.

Prognosis

Approximately one-third of patients experience spontaneous clinical remission. Progression to ESRD occurs in 20–40% of patients. The remaining patients have chronic microscopic hematuria and a stable serum creatinine. The most unfavorable prognostic indicator is proteinuria greater than 1 g/day; other unfavorable prognostic indicators include hypertension, tubulointerstitial fibrosis, glomerulosclerosis, or glomerular crescents on biopsy, and abnormal GFR on presentation.

Barratt J et al. Treatment of IgA nephropathy: evolution over half a century. Semin Nephrol. 2018 Sep;38(5):531–40. [PMID: 30177025]

Rodrigues JC et al. IgA nephropathy. Clin J Am Soc Nephrol. 2017 Apr 3;12(4):677–86. [PMID: 28159829]

Saha MK et al. Secondary IgA nephropathy. Kidney Int. 2018 Oct;94(4):674–81. [PMID: 29804660]

3. Henoch-Schönlein Purpura

Henoch-Schönlein purpura is a systemic small-vessel leukocytoclastic vasculitis associated with IgA subclass 1 deposition in vessel walls. It is most common in children and is often associated with an inciting infection, such as group A streptococcus or other exposure. There is a male predominance. It classically presents with palpable purpura in the lower extremities and buttock area; arthralgias; and abdominal symptoms, such as nausea, colic, and melena. A decrease in GFR is common with a nephritic presentation. The renal lesions can be identical to those found in IgA nephropathy, and the underlying pathophysiology appears to be similar. Most patients with microscopic hematuria and minimal proteinuria recover fully over several weeks. Progressive CKD and possibly ESRD are more likely to develop in those with the nephrotic syndrome and the presence of both nephritic and nephrotic syndrome features poses the worst renal prognosis. Histologic classification of the lesions in children may also provide prognostic information. Although several treatment regimens of various immunosuppressive agents have been clinically tested, none have been definitively proven to alter the course of severe Henoch-Schönlein purpura nephritis.

Rituximab treatment and plasma exchange have been successful for severe disease according to several case reports, but clinical trials are lacking. Rapidly progressive disease with crescent formation on biopsy may be treated as in ANCA-associated vasculitis (see section below).

Further details about Henoch-Schönlein purpura are provided in Chapter 20.

Fenoglio R et al. Rituximab therapy for IgA-vasculitis with nephritis: a case series and review of the literature. Immunol Res. 2017 Feb;65(1):186–192. [PMID: 27449502]
González-Gay MA et al. IgA vasculitis: genetics and clinical and therapeutic management. Curr Rheumatol Rep. 2018 Apr 2; 20(5):24. [PMID: 29611051]

4. Pauci-Immune Glomerulonephritis (ANCA-Associated)

Pauci-immune necrotizing glomerulonephritis is caused by the following systemic ANCA-associated small-vessel vasculitides: granulomatosis with polyangiitis, microscopic polyangiitis, and eosinophilic granulomatosis with polyangiitis (formerly Churg-Strauss disease; see Chapter 20). ANCA-associated glomerulonephritis can also present as a primary renal lesion without systemic involvement; this is termed "idiopathic crescentic glomerulonephritis." The pathogenesis of these entities appears to involve cytokine-primed neutrophils presenting cytoplasmic antigens on their surfaces (proteinase 3 and myeloperoxidase). Circulating ANCAs then bind to these antigens and activate a neutrophil respiratory burst with consequent vascular damage; primed neutrophils also appear to activate the alternative complement pathway. Putative environmental exposures that may incite the initial response include *S aureus* and silica. Immunofluorescence of kidney biopsy specimens demonstrates lack of immunoglobulin or complement deposition, hence the term "pauci-immune." Renal involvement classically presents as an RPGN, but more indolent presentations can be seen as well.

▶ Clinical Findings

A. Symptoms and Signs

Symptoms of a systemic inflammatory disease, including fever, malaise, and weight loss may be present and usually precede initial presentation by several months. In addition to hematuria and proteinuria from glomerular inflammation, some patients exhibit purpura from dermal capillary involvement and mononeuritis multiplex from nerve arteriolar involvement. Ninety percent of patients with granulomatosis with polyangiitis have upper (especially sinus) or lower respiratory tract symptoms with nodular lesions that can cavitate and bleed. Hemoptysis is a concerning sign and usually warrants hospitalization and aggressive immunosuppression.

B. Laboratory Findings

Serologically, ANCA subtype analysis is done to determine whether antiproteinase-3 antibodies (PR3-ANCA) or antimyeloperoxidase antibodies (MPO-ANCA) are present. Most patients with granulomatosis with polyangiitis are PR3 positive; the remainder are MPO positive or, more rarely, do not demonstrate circulating ANCA. Microscopic angiitis is generally associated with MPO ANCA. Renal biopsy demonstrates necrotizing lesions and crescents on light microscopy; immunofluorescence is negative for immune complex deposition.

▶ Treatment

Treatment should be instituted early if aggressive disease is present. Induction therapy of high-dose corticosteroids (methylprednisolone, 1–2 g/day intravenously for 3 days, followed by prednisone, 1 mg/kg orally for 1 month, with a slow taper over the next 6 months) and cytotoxic agents (cyclophosphamide, 0.5–1 g/m² intravenously per month or 1.5–2 mg/kg orally for 3–6 months) is followed by long-term azathioprine or mycophenolate mofetil. Rituximab has been shown to be noninferior to cyclophosphamide for induction and is also used in refractory or relapsing cases and as an alternative to azathioprine for maintenance of remission. Plasma exchange has been used in conjunction with induction therapy in particularly severe cases; however, its efficacy is not supported by a large trial. Patients receiving cyclophosphamide should receive prophylaxis for *Pneumocystis jirovecii*, such as trimethoprim-sulfamethoxazole double-strength orally 3 days per week.

▶ Prognosis

Without treatment, prognosis is extremely poor. However, with aggressive treatment, complete remission can be achieved in about 75% of patients. Prognosis depends on the extent of renal involvement before treatment is started and may be worse in those with PR3-associated disease. ANCA titers may be monitored to follow treatment efficacy; rising titers may herald relapse.

Chen M et al. Complement in ANCA-associated vasculitis: mechanisms and implications for management. Nat Rev Nephrol. 2017 Jun;13(6):359–67. [PMID: 28316335]
Salvadori M et al. Antineutrophil cytoplasmic antibody associated vasculitides with renal involvement: Open challenges in the remission induction therapy. World J Nephrol. 2018 May 6; 7(3):71–83. [PMID: 29736379]
Yates M et al. EULAR/ERA-EDTA recommendations for the management of ANCA-associated vasculitis. Ann Rheum Dis. 2016 Sep;75(9):1583–94. [PMID: 27338776]
Zonozi R et al. Renal involvement in antineutrophil cytoplasmic antibody-associated vasculitis. Rheum Dis Clin North Am. 2018 Nov;44(4):525–43. [PMID: 30274621]

5. Anti-Glomerular Basement Membrane Glomerulonephritis & Goodpasture Syndrome

Autoantibodies to epitopes of the GBM cause a glomerulonephritis (anti-GBM disease); concomitant immune attack on alveolar basement membranes results in pulmonary hemorrhage as well (Goodpasture syndrome) (Figure 22–5). Anti-GBM–associated glomerulonephritis accounts for 10–20% of patients with acute RPGN. The incidence peaks in the third decade of life during which time males are predominantly affected and lung involvement is more common, and again in the sixth and seventh decades with less gender specificity and pulmonary involvement. Goodpasture syndrome has been associated with pulmonary infection, tobacco use, and exposure to hydrocarbon solvents or alemtuzumab; HLA-DR2 and -B7 antigens may predispose as well.

► Clinical Findings

A. Symptoms and Signs

The onset of disease may be preceded by an upper respiratory tract infection; hemoptysis, dyspnea, and possible respiratory failure may ensue. Other findings are consistent with an RPGN, although rare cases may present with much milder forms of the nephritic spectrum of disease (eg, glomerular hematuria and proteinuria with minimal kidney dysfunction).

B. Laboratory Findings

Chest radiographs may demonstrate pulmonary infiltrates if pulmonary hemorrhage is present. Serum complement levels are normal. Circulating anti-GBM antibodies are present in over 90% of patients. A small percentage of patients also have elevated ANCA titers; these patients should be treated with plasma exchange as for anti-GBM disease. Kidney biopsy typically shows crescent formation with light microscopy, with linear IgG staining along the GBM with immunofluorescence.

► Treatment

Patients with pulmonary hemorrhage and strong clinical suspicion of Goodpasture syndrome should be treated emergently—possibly prior to confirming the diagnosis with serology and kidney biopsy. Treatment is a combination of plasma exchange therapy daily for up to 2 weeks to remove circulating antibodies, and administration of corticosteroids and cyclophosphamide to prevent formation of new antibodies and control the inflammatory response. Rituximab has been used in a small number of patients with refractory disease. Patients with oliguric AKI or who require dialysis upon presentation have a poor prognosis. Anti-GBM antibody titers should decrease as the clinical course improves.

Henderson SR et al. Diagnostic and management challenges in Goodpasture's (anti-glomerular basement membrane) disease. Nephrol Dial Transplant. 2018 Feb 1;33(2):196–202 [PMID: 28459999]

Segelmark M et al. Anti-glomerular basement membrane disease: an update on subgroups, pathogenesis and therapies. Nephrol Dial Transplant. 2018 Oct 29. [Epub ahead of print] [PMID: 30371823]

van Daalen EE et al. Predicting outcome in patients with anti-GBM glomerulonephritis. Clin J Am Soc Nephrol. 2018 Jan 6; 13(1):63–72. [PMID: 29162595]

6. Cryoglobulin-Associated Glomerulonephritis

Essential (mixed) cryoglobulinemia is a vasculitis caused by cold-precipitable immunoglobulins (cryoglobulins). The most common underlying etiology is HCV infection; in these cases, there is clonal expansion of B lymphocytes, which produce IgM rheumatoid factor. Rheumatoid factor, HCV antigen and polyclonal anti-HCV IgG form complexes that deposit in vessels and incite inflammation. Other overt or occult infections (eg, viral, bacterial, and fungal) as well as some connective tissue diseases can also be cause cryoglobulinemic vasculitis.

Patients exhibit purpuric and necrotizing skin lesions in dependent areas, arthralgias, fever, and hepatosplenomegaly. Serum complement levels are low and rheumatoid factor is often elevated. Kidney biopsy may show several different patterns of injury; there may be crescent formation, glomerular capillary thrombi, or MPGN (see below). Treatment consists of aggressively targeting the causative infection. Pulse corticosteroids, plasma exchange, rituximab, and cytotoxic agents have been used when there is little risk of exacerbating the underlying infection or when no infection is present. See also Hepatitis C Virus–Associated Renal Disease.

Montero N et al. Treatment for hepatitis C virus-associated mixed cryoglobulinaemia. Cochrane Database Syst Rev. 2018 May 7;5:CD011403. [PMID: 29734473]

Zaidan M et al; CryoVas Study Group. Spectrum and prognosis of noninfectious renal mixed cryoglobulinemic GN. J Am Soc Nephrol. 2016 Apr;27(4):1213–24. [PMID: 26260165]

7. Membranoproliferative Glomerulonephritis & C3 Glomerulopathies

MPGN is a relatively rare pattern of glomerular injury that can present anywhere along the nephritic spectrum from asymptomatic glomerular hematuria to acute nephritic syndrome with bouts of gross hematuria to RPGN; nephrotic syndrome can also be seen. MPGN is currently classified pathologically into immune-complex and C3-related disease. Etiologies of immune complex–mediated MPGN include chronic infection (most commonly HCV, but bacterial and parasitic infections may also be causative), a paraproteinemia, or an underlying autoimmune disease (such as lupus); it can also be idiopathic (especially in children and young adults). In these cases, the pathogenesis is likely a chronic antigenemia leading to classical complement pathway activation with immune complex deposition; however, it is now recognized that some cases may result from alternative complement pathway dysregulation. C3-related MPGN is caused by several inherited or acquired abnormalities in the alternative complement pathway. Both types result in low circulating C3 complement; C4 is low in immune complex disease. Light microscopy of both types shows varying degrees of mesangial hypercellularity, endocapillary proliferation and capillary wall remodeling resulting in double contours of the GBM ("tram track" appearance). Immunofluorescence and electron microscopy provide distinguishing information. Immune complex–mediated MPGN reveals C3 and IgG or IgM staining (or both) on immunofluorescence; electron microscopy demonstrates mesangial and subepithelial deposits. C3 glomerulonephritis is distinguished by lack of immunoglobulin staining on immunofluorescence, but can appear similar to immune complex disease with respect to light and electron microscopy. An additional but rare type of C3 glomerular injury is "dense deposit disease" based on thick ribbon-like deposits seen on electron microscopy. Together, dense deposit disease and C3 glomerulonephritis are now termed "C3 glomerulopathies."

Treatment of immune complex MPGN should be directed at any identifiable underlying cause. Treatment of idiopathic immune complex disease is controversial and controlled trial data are lacking. For those with mild disease, ACE inhibitors and ARBs should be used. For severe disease, a combination of oral cyclophosphamide or mycophenolate mofetil plus corticosteroids could be considered; rituximab is also sometimes used. Those with RPGN and crescents on biopsy may be treated the same as those with ANCA-associated disease provided secondary causes have been ruled out. Despite therapy, most will progress to ESRD. Treatment for the C3 glomerulopathies is in evolution as novel therapies to target the dysregulated alternative complement cascade are being explored; small, uncontrolled series suggest a possible benefit of eculizumab. Less favorable prognostic findings include dense deposit disease, early decline in GFR, hypertension, and persistent nephrotic syndrome. All types of MPGN recur with high frequency after kidney transplantation; however, dense deposit disease recurs more commonly. Plasma exchange has been used with mixed results to treat posttransplant recurrence of MPGN.

Lionaki S et al. Understanding the complement-mediated glomerular diseases: focus on membranoproliferative glomerulonephritis and C3 glomerulopathies. APMIS. 2016 Sep; 124(9):725–35. [PMID: 27356907]

Noris M et al. Autoimmune abnormalities of the alternative complement pathway in membranoproliferative glomerulonephritis and C3 glomerulopathy. Pediatr Nephrol. 2018 Jun 9. [Epub ahead of print] [PMID: 29948306]

8. Hepatitis C Virus–Associated Kidney Disease

Kidney disease can occur in the setting of HCV infection. The three patterns of kidney injury associated with HCV are secondary MPGN (most common), cryoglobulinemic glomerulonephritis, and membranous nephropathy. The clinical presentation is dictated by the underlying pattern of injury. Many patients have elevated serum transaminases and an elevated rheumatoid factor. Hypocomplementemia is very common, with C4 typically more reduced than C3; complement levels and rheumatoid factor tend to be normal if there is a membranous pattern of injury.

▶ Treatment

Viral suppression or eradication is the cornerstone of treatment of HCV–associated kidney disease (see Chapter 16). Use of most direct-acting antiviral agents appears to be safe in those with reduced GFR, with the exception of sofosbuvir. Therapy with rituximab and possibly corticosteroids and plasmapheresis should be initiated in patients with severe vasculitis prior to the initiation of antiviral therapy.

Fabrizi F et al. Treatment choices for hepatitis C in patients with kidney disease. Clin J Am Soc Nephrol. 2018 May 7;13(5): 793–5. [PMID: 29523677]

Jadoul M et al. Executive summary of the 2018 KDIGO Hepatitis C in CKD Guideline: welcoming advances in evaluation and management. Kidney Int. 2018 Oct;94(4):663–73. [PMID: 30243313]

Pol S et al. Hepatitis C virus and the kidney. Nat Rev Nephrol. 2019 Feb;15(2):73–86. [PMID: 30455426]

9. Systemic Lupus Erythematosus

Renal involvement in SLE is very common; estimates range from 35% to 90%, with higher estimates encompassing subclinical disease. Rates of lupus nephritis are highest in nonwhites. The pathogenesis may be dysregulated cellular apoptosis resulting in autoantibodies against nucleosomes; antibody/nucleosome complexes then bind to components of the glomerulus to form immune complex glomerular disease. See Chapter 20 for further discussion of SLE.

The term "lupus nephritis" encompasses many possible patterns of renal injury—most cases present within the nephritic spectrum (class I–IV). Nonglomerular syndromes include tubulointerstitial nephritis and vasculitis. All patients with SLE should have routine urinalyses to monitor for the appearance of hematuria or proteinuria. If urinary abnormalities are detected, kidney biopsy is often performed. The 2003 International Society of Nephrology and Renal Pathology Society (ISN/RPS) classification of renal glomerular lesions is class I, minimal mesangial nephritis; class II, mesangial proliferative nephritis; class III, focal (less than 50% of glomeruli affected with capillary involvement) proliferative nephritis; class IV, diffuse (greater than 50% of glomeruli affected with capillary involvement) proliferative nephritis; class V, membranous nephropathy; and class VI, advanced sclerosis without residual disease activity. Classes III and IV, the most severe forms of lupus nephritis, are further classified as active or chronic, and global or segmental, which confers additional prognostic value.

▶ Treatment

Individuals with **class I** and **class II lesions** generally require no treatment; corticosteroids or calcineurin inhibitors should be considered for those with class II lesions with nephrotic-range proteinuria. Transformation of these types to a more active lesion may occur and is usually accompanied by an increase in lupus serologic activity (eg, rising titers of anti–double-stranded DNA antibodies and falling C3 and C4 levels) and increasing proteinuria or falling GFR. Repeat biopsy in such patients is recommended. Some experts recommend hydroxychloroquine treatment in all patients with lupus nephritis, regardless of histological class. Patients with extensive **class III lesions** and all **class IV lesions** should receive aggressive immunosuppressive therapy. The features signifying the poorest prognosis in patients with class III or IV lesions include elevated serum creatinine, lower complement levels, male sex, presence of antiphospholipid antibodies, nephrotic-range proteinuria, African descent (possibly in association with *APOL1* risk alleles), and poor response to therapy. Immunosuppressive therapy for class V lupus nephritis is indicated if superimposed proliferative lesions exist. Class VI lesions should not be treated.

Treatment of **class III** or **IV lupus nephritis** consists of induction therapy, followed by maintenance treatment. All induction therapy includes corticosteroids (eg, methylprednisolone 1 g intravenously daily for 3 days followed by prednisone, 1 mg/kg orally daily with subsequent taper over 6–12 months) in combination with either cyclophosphamide or mycophenolate mofetil. Data suggest that blacks and Hispanics respond more favorably to mycophenolate mofetil rather than cyclophosphamide; in addition, mycophenolate mofetil has a more favorable side-effect profile than cyclophosphamide and should be favored when preservation of fertility is a consideration. Mycophenolate mofetil induction is typically given at 2–3 g/day, then tapered to 1–2 g/day for maintenance. Cyclophosphamide induction regimens vary but usually involve monthly intravenous pulse doses (500–1000 mg/m^2) for 6 months. Induction is followed by daily oral mycophenolate mofetil or azathioprine maintenance therapy; mycophenolate mofetil may be superior to azathioprine maintenance and causes few adverse effects. Maintenance with calcineurin inhibitors may also be considered, but the relapse rate is high upon discontinuation of these agents. With standard therapy, remission rates with induction vary from 80% for partial remission to 50–60% for full remission; it may take more than 6 months to see these effects. Relapse is common and rates of disease flare are higher in those who do not experience complete remission; similarly, progression to ESRD is more common in those who relapse more frequently, or in whom no remission has been achieved. Studies to assess safety and efficacy of newer biologic immunomodulatory drugs for lupus nephritis are ongoing.

The normalization of various laboratory tests (double-stranded DNA antibodies, serum C3, C4, CH50 levels) can be useful in monitoring treatment. Urinary protein levels and sediment activity are also helpful markers. Patients with SLE who undergo dialysis have a favorable prospect for long-term survival; interestingly, systemic lupus symptoms may become quiescent with the development of ESRD. Patients with SLE undergoing kidney transplants can have recurrent renal disease, although rates are relatively low.

Almaani S et al. Update on lupus nephritis. Clin J Am Soc Nephrol. 2017 May 8;12(5):825–35. [PMID: 27821390]

Bomback AS. Nonproliferative forms of lupus nephritis: an overview. Rheum Dis Clin North Am. 2018 Nov;44(4):561–9. [PMID: 30274623]

McClure M et al. Update on lupus nephritis for GPs. Lupus. 2018 Oct;27(1 Suppl):11–4. [PMID: 30452323]

Meliambro K et al. Therapy for proliferative lupus nephritis. Rheum Dis Clin North Am. 2018 Nov;44(4):545–60. [PMID: 30274622]

Pinheiro SVB et al. Pediatric lupus nephritis. J Bras Nefrol. 2018 Nov 14. [Epub ahead of print] [PMID: 30465590]

Tunnicliffe DJ et al. Immunosuppressive treatment for proliferative lupus nephritis. Cochrane Database Syst Rev. 2018 Jun 29; 6:CD002922. [PMID: 29957821]

NEPHROTIC SPECTRUM GLOMERULAR DISEASES

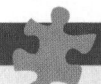

ESSENTIALS OF DIAGNOSIS

► Bland urine sediment (few if any cells or cellular casts).

► Nephrotic syndrome is characterized by the following:

–Heavy proteinuria (urine protein excretion greater than 3 g per 24 hours).

–Hypoalbuminemia (albumin less than 3 g/dL).

–Peripheral edema.

–Hyperlipidemia.

–Oval fat bodies may be seen in the urine.

► General Considerations

In American adults, the most common cause of nephrotic spectrum glomerular disease is diabetes mellitus. Other causes of this presentation include minimal change disease, FSGS, membranous nephropathy, and amyloidosis. Any of these entities can present on the less severe end of the spectrum with a bland urinalysis and proteinuria, or with the most severe presentation of the nephrotic syndrome. Serum creatinine may or may not be abnormal at the time of presentation, depending on the severity and acuity of the disease.

► Clinical Findings

A. Symptoms and Signs

Patients with subnephrotic range proteinuria do not manifest symptoms of the kidney disease. In those with the nephrotic syndrome, peripheral edema is present and is most likely due to sodium retention and, at albumin levels less than 2 g/dL (20 g/L), arterial underfilling from low plasma oncotic pressure. Edema may present in dependent regions, such as the lower extremities, or it may become generalized and include periorbital edema. Dyspnea due to pulmonary edema, pleural effusions, and diaphragmatic compromise with ascites can occur.

B. Laboratory Findings

1. Urinalysis—Proteinuria occurs as a result of effacement of podocytes (foot processes) and an alteration of the negative charge of the GBM. The urinary dipstick is a good screening test for proteinuria; however, it detects only albumin. The addition of sulfosalicylic acid to the urine causes total protein to precipitate, allowing for the possible discovery of paraproteins (and albumin). A spot urine protein to urine creatinine ratio gives a reasonable approximation of grams of protein excreted per day; a 24-hour urine sample for protein excretion is rarely needed.

Microscopically, the urinary sediment has relatively few cellular elements or casts. However, if marked hyperlipidemia is present, urinary oval fat bodies may be seen. They appear as "grape clusters" under light microscopy and "Maltese crosses" under polarized light.

2. Blood chemistries—The nephrotic syndrome results in hypoalbuminemia (less than 3 g/dL [30 g/L]) and hypoproteinemia (less than 6 g/dL [60 g/L]). Hyperlipidemia occurs in over 50% of patients with early nephrotic syndrome, and becomes more frequent and worsens in degree as the severity of the nephrotic syndrome increases. A fall in oncotic pressure triggers increased hepatic production of lipids (cholesterol and apolipoprotein B). There is also decreased clearance of very low-density lipoproteins, causing hypertriglyceridemia. Patients may also have an elevated erythrocyte sedimentation rate as a result of alterations in some plasma components such as increased levels of fibrinogen. Patients may become deficient in vitamin D, zinc, and copper from loss of binding proteins in the urine.

Laboratory testing to determine the underlying cause may include complement levels, serum and urine protein electrophoresis, antinuclear antibodies, and serologic tests for viral hepatitides.

3. Kidney biopsy—Kidney biopsy is often performed in adults with new-onset idiopathic nephrotic syndrome if a primary renal disease that may require immunosuppressive therapy is suspected. Chronically and significantly decreased GFR indicates irreversible kidney disease mitigating the usefulness of kidney biopsy. In the setting of long-standing diabetes mellitus type 1 or 2, proteinuric renal disease is rarely biopsied unless atypical features (such as significant glomerular hematuria or cellular casts) are also present, or if there is other reason to suspect an additional renal lesion.

▶ Treatment

A. Protein Loss

In those with subnephrotic proteinuria or mild nephrotic syndrome, dietary protein restriction may be helpful in slowing progression of renal disease (see CKD section). In those with proteinuria greater than 10 g/day, protein malnutrition may occur and daily protein intake should replace daily urinary protein losses.

In both diabetic and nondiabetic patients, therapy that is aimed at reducing proteinuria may also reduce progression of renal disease. ACE inhibitors and ARBs lower urine protein excretion by reducing glomerular capillary pressure; they also have antifibrotic effects. These agents can be used in patients with reduced GFR as long as significant hyperkalemia (potassium greater than 5.2–5.5 mEq/L or mmol/L) does not occur and serum creatinine rises less than 30%; patients should be monitored closely to avoid AKI and hyperkalemia. Combination therapy of an ARB and an ACE inhibitor is not recommended because of the risk of AKI and hyperkalemia.

B. Edema

Dietary salt restriction is essential for managing edema; most patients also require diuretic therapy. Both thiazide and loop diuretics are highly protein bound; therefore, with hypoalbuminemia and decreased GFR, diuretic delivery to the kidney is reduced, and patients often require larger doses. A combination of loop and thiazide diuretics can potentiate the diuretic effect and may be needed for patients with refractory fluid retention.

C. Hyperlipidemia

Hypercholesterolemia and hypertriglyceridemia occur as noted above. Dietary modification and exercise should be advocated; however, effective lipid-lowering usually also requires pharmacologic treatment (see Chapter 28). There is significant risk of rhabdomyolysis in patients with CKD who take gemfibrozil in combination with statins; combining fenofibrate or niacin with a statin may be safer.

D. Hypercoagulable State

Patients with serum albumin less than 2 g/dL (20 g/L) can become hypercoagulable. Nephrotic patients have urinary losses of antithrombin, protein C, and protein S and increased platelet activation. Patients are prone to renal vein thrombosis, pulmonary embolus, and other venous thromboemboli, particularly with membranous nephropathy. Anticoagulation therapy with warfarin is warranted for at least 3–6 months in patients with evidence of thrombosis in any location. Patients with renal vein thrombosis, pulmonary embolus, or recurrent thromboemboli require indefinite anticoagulation. After an initial clotting event, ongoing nephrotic syndrome poses a risk of thrombosis recurrence, and continued anticoagulation should be considered until resolution of the nephrotic syndrome.

▶ When to Refer

Any patient with the nephrotic syndrome should be referred immediately to a nephrologist for volume and blood pressure management, assessment for kidney biopsy, and treatment of the underlying disease. Proteinuria of more than 1 g/day without the nephrotic syndrome also merits nephrology referral, though with less urgency.

▶ When to Admit

Patients with edema refractory to outpatient therapy or rapidly worsening kidney function that may require inpatient interventions should be admitted.

Agrawal S et al. Dyslipidaemia in nephrotic syndrome: mechanisms and treatment. Nat Rev Nephrol. 2018 Jan;14(1):57–70. [PMID: 29176657]

Bierzynska A et al. Recent advances in understanding and treating nephrotic syndrome. F1000Res. 2017 Feb 9;6:121. [PMID: 28232870]

Fried LF et al; VA NEPHRON-D Investigators. Combined angiotensin inhibition for the treatment of diabetic nephropathy. N Engl J Med. 2013 Nov 14;369(20):892–903. [PMID: 24206457]

McCloskey O et al. Diagnosis and management of nephrotic syndrome. Practitioner. 2017 Feb;261(1801):11–5. [PMID: 29020719]

Sexton DJ et al. Direct-acting oral anticoagulants as prophylaxis against thromboembolism in the nephrotic syndrome. Kidney Int Rep. 2018 Mar 3;3(4):784–93. [PMID: 29989039]

Snyder S et al. Workup for proteinuria. Prim Care. 2014 Dec; 41(4):719–35. [PMID: 25439530]

NEPHROTIC SPECTRUM DISEASE IN PRIMARY RENAL DISORDERS

MINIMAL CHANGE DISEASE

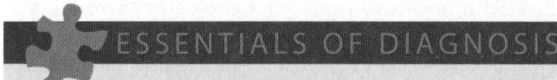

ESSENTIALS OF DIAGNOSIS

► Nephrotic-range proteinuria.

► Kidney biopsy shows no changes on light microscopy.

► Characteristic foot-process effacement on electron microscopy.

General Considerations

Minimal change disease is the most common cause of proteinuric renal disease in children, accounting for about 80% of cases. It often remits upon treatment with a course of corticosteroids. Indeed, children with nephrotic syndrome are often treated for minimal change disease empirically without a biopsy diagnosis. Biopsy should be considered for children with nephrotic syndrome who exhibit unusual features (such as signs of other systemic illness), or who are steroid-resistant or relapse upon withdrawal of corticosteroid therapy; the latter two conditions may indicate an underlying focal and segmental glomerulosclerosis (discussed below) rather than minimal change disease. Minimal change disease is less common in adults, accounting for 20–25% of cases of primary nephrotic syndrome in those over age 40 years. This entity can be idiopathic but also occurs following viral upper respiratory infections (especially in children), in association with neoplasms such as Hodgkin disease, with drugs (lithium), and with hypersensitivity reactions (especially to NSAIDs and bee stings).

Clinical Findings

A. Symptoms and Signs

Patients present with nephrotic syndrome, which confers susceptibility to infection, tendency toward thromboembolic events, severe hyperlipidemia, and possibly protein malnutrition. Minimal change disease can cause AKI due to renal tubular damage and interstitial edema.

B. Laboratory and Histologic Findings

There is no helpful serologic testing. When kidney biopsy is performed (see considerations above), glomeruli appear normal on light microscopy and immunofluorescence. On electron microscopy, there is a characteristic effacement of podocyte foot processes. Mesangial cell proliferation may be seen in a subgroup of patients; this finding is associated with more hematuria and hypertension and poor response to standard corticosteroid treatment.

Treatment

Treatment is with prednisone, 60 mg/m²/day orally; remission in steroid-responsive minimal change disease generally occurs within 4–8 weeks. Adults often require longer courses of therapy than children, requiring up to 16 weeks to achieve a response. Treatment should be continued for several weeks after complete remission of proteinuria, and dosing tapers should be individualized. A significant number of patients will relapse and require repeated corticosteroid treatment. Patients with frequent relapses or corticosteroid resistance may require cyclophosphamide, a calcineurin inhibitor (tacrolimus, cyclosporine), or rituximab to induce subsequent remissions. Progression to ESRD is rare. Complications most often arise from prolonged corticosteroid use.

Noone DG et al. Idiopathic nephrotic syndrome in children. Lancet. 2018 Jul 7;392(10141):61–74. Erratum in: Lancet. 2018 Jul 28;392(10144):282. [PMID: 29910038]

FOCAL SEGMENTAL GLOMERULOSCLEROSIS

General Considerations

This relatively common renal pattern of injury results from damage to podocytes; such damage may be a primary/renal-limited disorder or may be secondary to another underlying disease state. Primary causes fall into three categories: (1) heritable abnormalities in any one of several podocyte proteins, or to underlying type 4 collagen mutations; (2) polymorphisms in the *APOL1* gene in those of African descent; or (3) increased levels of a circulating permeability factor. Secondary causes include renal overwork injury, obesity, hypertension, chronic urinary reflux, HIV infection, or analgesic or bisphosphonate exposure. Genetic testing in primary cases is becoming more common, especially in the pediatric population.

Clinical Findings

Proteinuria is present in patients with FSGS. In FSGS caused by a primary renal disease, 80% of children and 50% of adults have overt nephrotic syndrome; however, when it develops due to a secondary cause, frank nephrotic syndrome is uncommon. Decreased GFR is present in 25–50% of those with FSGS at time of diagnosis.

Diagnosis requires kidney biopsy; there is no helpful serologic test. Light microscopy shows sclerosis of segments of some, but not all, glomeruli. On immunofluorescence, IgM and C3 are seen in the sclerotic lesions, although it is presumed that these immune components are simply trapped in the sclerotic glomeruli and not pathogenetic. As in minimal change disease, electron microscopy shows fusion of epithelial foot processes.

Treatment

Treatment for all forms of FSGS should include diuretics for edema, ACE inhibitors or ARBs to control proteinuria and hypertension, and statins or niacin for hyperlipidemia. Immunosuppression therapy (oral prednisone, 1 mg/kg/day for 4–16 weeks followed by a slow taper) is reserved for nephrotic primary FSGS cases presumed to be due to a circulating permeability factor; in those with steroid-resistance or intolerance, calcineurin inhibitors and mycophenolate mofetil can be considered. Kidney transplantation in this subgroup of FSGS patients is complicated by a relatively high relapse rate and risk of graft loss. Plasma exchange therapy, and possibly rituximab, just prior to the transplant surgery and with early signs of relapse, appear to be beneficial. Those with *APOL1*-associated and nonhereditary primary renal disease may not benefit from immunosuppression, although robust clinical trials are lacking. Patients with secondary FSGS do not benefit from immunosuppressive therapy; treatment should be directed at the inciting cause.

De Vriese AS et al. Differentiating primary, genetic, and secondary FSGS in adults: a clinicopathologic approach. J Am Soc Nephrol. 2018 Mar;29(3):759–74. [PMID: 29321142]

Freedman BI et al. *APOL1*-associated nephropathy: a key contributor to racial disparities in CKD. Am J Kidney Dis. 2018 Nov;72(5S1):S8–16. [PMID: 30343724]

Sharif B et al. Advances in molecular diagnosis and therapeutics in nephrotic syndrome and focal and segmental glomerulosclerosis. Curr Opin Nephrol Hypertens. 2018 May;27(3):194–200. [PMID: 29465426]

MEMBRANOUS NEPHROPATHY

ESSENTIALS OF DIAGNOSIS

- ▶ Varying degrees of proteinuria, may have nephrotic syndrome.
- ▶ Associated with coagulopathy, eg, renal vein thrombosis, if nephrotic syndrome present.
- ▶ "Spike and dome" pattern on kidney biopsy from subepithelial deposits.
- ▶ Secondary causes notably include hepatitis B virus and carcinomas.

▶ General Considerations

Membranous nephropathy is the most common cause of primary nephrotic syndrome in adults, most often presenting in the fifth and sixth decades. It is an immune-mediated disease characterized by immune complex deposition in the subepithelial portion of glomerular capillary walls. The antigen in the primary form of the disease appears to be a phospholipase A_2 receptor (PLA_2R) on the podocyte in 70–80% of patients. Secondary disease is associated with underlying carcinomas (some of these cases may involve autoimmunity to podocyte-expressed thrombospondin type-1 domain-containing 7A [THSD7A]); infections, such as hepatitis B and C, endocarditis, and syphilis; autoimmune disease, such as SLE, mixed connective tissue disease, and thyroiditis; and certain drugs, such as NSAIDs and captopril. The course of disease is variable, with about 50% of patients progressing to ESRD over 3–10 years.

Poorer outcome is associated with concomitant tubulointerstitial fibrosis, male sex, elevated serum creatinine, hypertension, and proteinuria greater than 10 g/day.

Patients with membranous nephropathy and nephrotic syndrome have a higher risk of hypercoagulable state than those with nephrosis from other etiologies; there is a particular predisposition to renal vein thrombosis in these patients.

▶ Clinical Findings

A. Symptoms and Signs

Patients may be asymptomatic or may have edema or frothy urine. Venous thrombosis, such as an unprovoked deep venous thrombosis, may be an initial sign. There may be symptoms or signs of an underlying infection or neoplasm (especially lung, stomach, breast, and colon cancers) in secondary membranous nephropathy.

B. Laboratory Findings

Hypoalbuminemia and hyperlipidemia are characteristic laboratory findings in the nephrotic syndrome. Evaluation for secondary causes including serologic testing for SLE, syphilis, and viral hepatitides, and age- and risk-appropriate cancer screening should be performed. Serum evaluation for circulating PLA_2R antibodies to assess for idiopathic membranous nephropathy is possible; additionally, titers can be followed during treatment. Renal biopsy is indicated for all glomerular diseases except for classical presentations of diabetic nephropathy and minimal change disease. Biopsy findings in membranous nephropathy include increased capillary wall thickness without inflammatory changes or cellular proliferation; when stained with silver methenamine, a "spike and dome" pattern results from projections of excess GBM between the subepithelial deposits. Immunofluorescence shows IgG and C3 staining along capillary loops. Electron microscopy shows a discontinuous pattern of dense deposits along the subepithelial surface of the basement membrane.

▶ Treatment

Underlying causes must be excluded prior to consideration of treatment. Idiopathic/primary disease treatment depends on the risk of renal disease progression. Roughly 30% of patients present with subnephrotic proteinuria (less than 3 g/day) and most have a good prognosis with conservative management, including antiproteinuric therapy with ACE inhibitor or ARB if blood pressure is greater than 125/75 mm Hg. Spontaneous remission may develop even in those with heavy proteinuria (about 30% of cases). Thus, use of immunosuppressive agents should be limited to those at highest risk for progression and with salvageable renal function. Patients with nephrotic syndrome despite 6 months of conservative management and serum creatinine less than 3.0 mg/dL (265 mcmol/L) may elect therapy with rituximab or with corticosteroids and cyclophosphamide for 6 months. Calcineurin inhibitors with or without corticosteroids may be considered as well. Remission may take up to 6 months. Patients with primary membranous nephropathy are excellent candidates for transplant.

Angioi A et al. Treatment of primary membranous nephropathy: where are we now? J Nephrol. 2018 Aug;31(4):489–502. [PMID: 28875476]

Hofstra JM et al. Should aspirin be used for primary prevention of thrombotic events in patients with membranous nephropathy? Kidney Int. 2016 May;89(5):981–3. [PMID: 27083274]

NEPHROTIC SPECTRUM DISEASE FROM SYSTEMIC DISORDERS

DIABETIC NEPHROPATHY

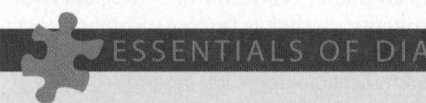

ESSENTIALS OF DIAGNOSIS

▸ Evidence of diabetes mellitus, typically over 10 years.

▸ Albuminuria usually precedes decline in GFR.

▸ Other end-organ damage, such as retinopathy, is common.

▸ General Considerations

Diabetic nephropathy is the most common cause of ESRD in the United States. The incidence is approximately 30% in both type 1 and type 2 diabetes mellitus. ESRD is much more likely to develop in persons with type 1 diabetes mellitus, in part due to fewer comorbidities and deaths before ESRD ensues. With the current epidemic of obesity and type 2 diabetes mellitus, rates of diabetic nephropathy are projected to continue to increase. Patients at higher risk include males, African Americans, Native Americans, and those with a family history of kidney disease. Mortality rates are higher for diabetics with kidney disease compared to those without CKD.

▸ Clinical Findings

Diabetic nephropathy develops about 10 years after the onset of diabetes mellitus. It may be present at the time type 2 diabetes mellitus is diagnosed. The first stage of classic diabetic nephropathy is hyperfiltration with an increase in GFR, followed by the development of microalbuminuria (30–300 mg/day). With progression, albuminuria increases to greater than 300 mg/day and can be detected on a urine dipstick as overt proteinuria; the GFR subsequently declines over time. Yearly screening for microalbuminuria is recommended for all diabetic patients to detect disease at its earliest stage; however, diabetic nephropathy can, less commonly present as nonproteinuric CKD.

The most common lesion in diabetic nephropathy is diffuse glomerulosclerosis, but nodular glomerulosclerosis (Kimmelstiel-Wilson nodules) is pathognomonic. The kidneys are usually enlarged. Kidney biopsy is not required in most patients, though, unless atypical findings are present, such as sudden onset of proteinuria, nephritic spectrum features (see above), massive proteinuria (greater than 10 g/day), urinary cellular casts, or rapid decline in GFR.

Patients with diabetes are prone to other renal diseases. These include papillary necrosis, chronic interstitial nephritis, and type 4 (hyporeninemic hypoaldosteronemic) renal tubular acidosis. Patients are more susceptible to AKI from many insults, including intravenous contrast material and concomitant use of an ACE inhibitor or ARB with NSAID.

▸ Treatment

With the onset of microalbuminuria, aggressive treatment is necessary. Strict glycemic control should be emphasized early in diabetic nephropathy, with recognition of risk of hypoglycemia as CKD becomes advanced (see CKD section). Recommended blood pressure goals should be tailored to the individual patient: based on the ACCORD trial, those with microalbuminuria (30–300 mg/day) and preserved GFR and those with significant CVD likely derive little benefit from blood pressure lowering much below 140/90 mm Hg, although the 2017 guidelines from the American Heart Association advocate treatment to 130/80 mm Hg or less. Those with overt proteinuria (especially when more than 1 g/day) benefit from a goal of less than 130/80 mm Hg. ACE inhibitors and ARBs in those with microalbuminuria lower the rate of progression to overt proteinuria and slow progression to ESRD by reducing intraglomerular pressure and via antifibrotic effects; these agents are not absolutely indicated in diabetics without albuminuria. Diabetic patients, especially with advanced CKD, are at relatively high risk for AKI and hyperkalemia with inhibition of the renin-angiotensin system, so monitoring for hyperkalemia or a decline in GFR more than 30% within ~2 weeks of the initiation or uptitration of this therapy is prudent, with dose reduction or discontinuation of therapy if these complications are encountered. Combination ARB and ACE inhibitor therapy is not recommended due to lack of efficacy and increased adverse events of hyperkalemia and AKI. Newer antidiabetic agents, including canagliflozin and empagliflozin (SGLT inhibitors), linagliptin (DPP-4 inhibitor), and liraglutide (GLP-1 receptor antagonist), show early promise in slowing the progression of early diabetic nephropathy, but more experience with these agents is needed; the SGLT inhibitors should not be used in advanced CKD. Treatment of other cardiovascular risk factors and obesity is crucial. Many with diabetes have multiple comorbid conditions; therefore, in patients undergoing dialysis who progress to ESRD, mortality over the first 5 years is high. Patients who are relatively healthy, however, benefit from renal transplantation.

Lo C et al. Insulin and glucose-lowering agents for treating people with diabetes and chronic kidney disease. Cochrane Database Syst Rev. 2018 Sep 24;9:CD011798. [PMID: 30246878]

Ruospo M et al. Glucose targets for preventing diabetic kidney disease and its progression. Cochrane Database Syst Rev. 2017 Jun 8;6:CD010137. [PMID: 28594069]

Umanath K et al. Update on diabetic nephropathy: Core Curriculum 2018. Am J Kidney Dis. 2018 Jun;71(6):884–95. [PMID: 29398179]

Zelniker TA et al. SGLT2 inhibitors for primary and secondary prevention of cardiovascular and renal outcomes in type 2 diabetes: a systematic review and meta-analysis of cardiovascular outcome trials. Lancet. 2019 Jan 5;393(10166):31–9. [PMID: 30424892]

HIV-ASSOCIATED NEPHROPATHY

HIV-associated nephropathy usually presents with nephrotic syndrome and declining GFR in patients with active HIV infection. Most patients are of African descent, likely due to the association of *APOL1* polymorphisms with increased risk for HIV-associated nephropathy. HIV-associated nephropathy is usually associated with low CD4 counts and AIDS, but it can also be the initial presentation of HIV disease. Patients with HIV are at risk for kidney disease other than HIV-associated nephropathy, such as toxicity from antiretroviral medications such as tenofovir, vascular disease, and diabetes, or an immune complex–mediated glomerular disease (HIV-immune complex disease).

Classic HIV-associated nephropathy results in an FSGS pattern of injury with glomerular collapse; severe tubulointerstitial damage may also be present.

HIV-associated nephropathy is becoming less common in the era of HIV screening and more effective antiretroviral therapy. Small, uncontrolled studies have shown that antiretroviral therapy slows progression of disease. ACE inhibitors or ARBs can be used to control blood pressure and proteinuria. Kidney biopsy is necessary for diagnosis and to rule out other causes of kidney dysfunction. Corticosteroid treatment may be considered for those with significant inflammation on biopsy; caution should be exercised when administering these drugs to immunocompromised individuals. Patients who progress to ESRD and are otherwise healthy are good candidates for kidney transplantation.

Ekrikpo UE et al. Chronic kidney disease in the global adult HIV-infected population: a systematic review and meta-analysis. PLoS One. 2018 Apr 16;13(4):e0195443. [PMID: 29659605]
Hou J et al. Changing concepts of HIV infection and renal disease. Curr Opin Nephrol Hypertens. 2018 May;27(3):144–52. [PMID: 29337702]

RENAL AMYLOIDOSIS

Amyloidosis is caused by tissue deposition of an abnormally folded protein (amyloid). Several different proteins can form amyloid fibrils. Primary amyloidosis, or AL amyloidosis, is the most common form and is due to a plasma cell dyscrasia causing overproduction and deposition of monoclonal Ig light chains (see Chapter 13). Secondary amyloidosis, or AA amyloidosis, results from a chronic inflammatory disease such as rheumatoid arthritis, inflammatory bowel disease, or chronic infection; in these cases, there is deposition of an acute phase reactant, serum amyloid A protein. Other less common forms of amyloidosis may be encountered.

Proteinuria, decreased GFR, and nephrotic syndrome are presenting symptoms and signs of renal involvement in amyloidosis; evidence of other organ involvement, such as the heart, is common. Serum and urine protein electrophoresis should be done as screening tests; if a monoclonal spike is found on either, serum free light chains should be quantified. Amyloid-affected kidneys are often larger than 10 cm. Pathologically, glomeruli are filled with amorphous deposits that show green birefringence with Congo red staining.

AL amyloidosis progresses to ESRD in an average of 2–3 years. Five-year overall survival is less than 20%, with death occurring from ESRD and heart disease. Standard treatment is a combination of melphalan, corticosteroids, and the proteosome inhibitor bortezomib. A greater than 90% reduction in the level of serum free light chains correlates with improved renal outcomes. Melphalan and stem cell transplantation are associated with a high (45%) mortality rate, but can induce remission in 80% of survivors; however, few patients are eligible for this treatment. In AA amyloidosis, remission can occur if the underlying disease is treated. Renal transplantation is an option.

Gertz MA. Immunoglobulin light chain amyloidosis: 2018 update on diagnosis, prognosis, and treatment. Am J Hematol. 2018 Sep;93(9):1169–80. [PMID: 30040145]
Ryšavá R. AL amyloidosis: advances in diagnostics and treatment. Nephrol Dial Transplant. 2018 Oct 8. [Epub ahead of print] [PMID: 30299492]

TUBULOINTERSTITIAL DISEASES

Tubulointerstitial disease may be acute or chronic. Acute disease is most commonly associated with medications, infectious agents, and systemic rheumatologic disorders. Interstitial edema, infiltration with polymorphonuclear neutrophils, and tubular cell necrosis can be seen. (See Acute Kidney Injury, above, and Table 22–9.) Chronic disease is associated with insults from an acute factor or progressive insults without any obvious acute cause. Interstitial fibrosis and tubular atrophy are present, with a mononuclear cell predominance. The chronic disorders are described below.

CHRONIC TUBULOINTERSTITIAL DISEASES

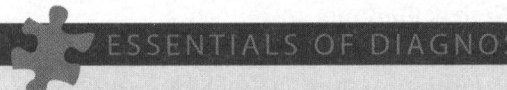

ESSENTIALS OF DIAGNOSIS

▶ Kidney size is small and contracted.

▶ Decreased urinary concentrating ability.

▶ Hyperchloremic metabolic acidosis.

▶ Reduced GFR.

▶ General Considerations

The most common cause of *chronic* tubulointerstitial disease is **obstructive uropathy**, which may result from prolonged or recurrent obstruction. The major causes are prostate disease in men; ureteral calculus in a single functioning kidney; bilateral ureteral calculi; carcinoma of the cervix, colon, or bladder; and retroperitoneal tumors or fibrosis.

Reflux nephropathy from **vesicoureteral reflux** is primarily a disorder of childhood and occurs when urine passes retrograde from the bladder to the kidneys during

Table 22–9. Causes of acute tubulointerstitial nephritis (abbreviated list).

Drug Reactions
Antibiotics
Beta-lactam antibiotics: methicillin, penicillin, ampicillin, cephalosporins
Ciprofloxacin
Erythromycin
Sulfonamides
Tetracycline
Vancomycin
Trimethoprim-sulfamethoxazole
Ethambutol
Rifampin
Nonsteroidal anti-inflammatory drugs
Diuretics
Thiazides
Furosemide
Miscellaneous
Allopurinol
Cimetidine
Phenytoin
Proton pump inhibitors
Systemic Infections
Bacteria
Streptococcus
Corynebacterium diphtheriae
Legionella
Viruses
Epstein-Barr
Others
Mycoplasma
Rickettsia rickettsii
Leptospira icterohaemorrhagiae
Toxoplasma
Idiopathic
Tubulointerstitial nephritis-uveitis

voiding. It is the second most common cause of chronic tubulointerstitial disease. It occurs as a result of an incompetent vesicoureteral sphincter. Urine can extravasate into the interstitium, triggering an inflammatory response that leads to fibrosis over time. The inflammatory response is due to either bacteria or normal urinary components.

Analgesic nephropathy is most commonly seen in patients who ingest large quantities of pain medication. The drugs of concern are phenacetin, paracetamol, aspirin, and other NSAIDs; acetaminophen is a possible but less certain culprit. Ingestion of at least 1 g/day for 3 years of these analgesics is considered necessary for kidney dysfunction to develop, and most patients grossly underestimate their analgesic use. This disorder occurs most frequently in individuals who are using analgesics for chronic headaches, muscular pains, and arthritis; female sex, older age, and malnutrition are risk factors for analgesic nephropathy. Tubulointerstitial inflammation and papillary necrosis are seen on pathologic examination. Papillary tip and inner medullary concentrations of some analgesics are tenfold higher than in the renal cortex. Phenacetin—once a

common cause of this disorder and now rarely available—is metabolized in the papillae by the prostaglandin hydroperoxidase pathway to reactive intermediates that bind covalently to interstitial cell macromolecules, causing necrosis. Aspirin and other NSAIDs can cause damage by their metabolism to active intermediates, which can result in cell necrosis. These drugs also decrease medullary blood flow (via inhibition of prostaglandin synthesis) and decrease glutathione levels, which are necessary for detoxification.

Environmental exposure to **heavy metals**—such as lead, cadmium, mercury, and bismuth—is seen infrequently now in the United States but can cause tubulointerstitial disease. Individuals at risk for lead-induced tubulointerstitial disease are those with occupational exposure (eg, welders who work with lead-based paint) and drinkers of alcohol distilled in automobile radiators ("moonshine" whiskey users). Lead is filtered by the glomerulus and is transported across the proximal convoluted tubules, where it accumulates and causes cell damage. Fibrosed arterioles and cortical scarring also lead to damaged kidneys. The proximal tubular dysfunction from cadmium exposure can cause hypercalciuria and nephrolithiasis.

A form of chronic tubulointerstitial disease disproportionately affecting male agricultural workers in Central America is an important cause of ESRD. While the exact pathophysiology is still unknown, the term **Mesoamerican nephropathy** is applied to reflect the geographic region in which this disease occurs. Affected individuals tend to be 30–50 years of age without diabetes, hypertension, or other causes of kidney disease who work under hot conditions, particularly in sugar cane or cotton fields, and thus are susceptible to dehydration.

► Clinical Findings

A. General Findings

Polyuria is common because tubular damage leads to inability to concentrate the urine. Volume depletion can also occur as a result of a salt-wasting defect in some individuals.

Patients can become hyperkalemic both because the GFR is lower and the distal tubules become aldosterone resistant. A hyperchloremic renal tubular acidosis is characteristic from a type 1 or type 4 renal tubular acidosis. Less commonly, a proximal (type 2) renal tubular acidosis is seen due to direct proximal tubular damage. The cause of the renal tubular acidosis is threefold: (1) reduced ammonia production, (2) inability to acidify the distal tubules, and (3) proximal tubular bicarbonate wasting. The urinalysis is nonspecific, as opposed to that seen in acute interstitial nephritis; a few cells may be seen, and broad waxy casts are often present. Proteinuria is typically less than 2 g/day (owing to inability of the proximal tubule to reabsorb freely filterable proteins).

B. Specific Findings

1. Obstructive uropathy—In partial obstruction, patients can exhibit polyuria (possibly due to vasopressin insensitivity and poor ability to concentrate the urine) or oliguria (due to decreased GFR). Azotemia and hypertension (due to increased renin-angiotensin production) are usually present. Abdominal, rectal, and genitourinary examinations may be helpful. Urinalysis can show hematuria, pyuria, and bacteriuria but is often bland. Abdominal ultrasound may detect mass lesions, hydroureter, and hydronephrosis. CT scanning and MRI provide more detailed information and can be considered if clinical suspicion remains despite a normal ultrasound.

2. Vesicoureteral reflux—Vesicoureteral reflux is typically diagnosed in young children with a history of recurrent urinary tract infections; it can also develop after kidney transplantation. This entity can be detected before birth via screening fetal ultrasonography or after birth via voiding cystourethrography. Less commonly, this entity is not diagnosed until adolescence or young adulthood when patients present with hypertension and substantial proteinuria, unusual in most tubular diseases. At this point, renal ultrasound or IVP can show renal scarring and hydronephrosis. IVP is relatively contraindicated in patients with kidney dysfunction who are at higher risk for contrast nephropathy. Although not usually necessary, kidney biopsies of patients with vesicoureteral reflux typically show nonspecific scarring of the tubulointerstitium and glomeruli. Although most damage occurs before age 5 years, progressive renal deterioration to ESRD continues as a result of early insults.

3. Analgesics—Patients can exhibit hematuria, mild proteinuria, polyuria (from tubular damage), anemia (from GI bleeding or erythropoietin deficiency), and sterile pyuria. Sloughed papillae can be found in the urine when papillary necrosis occurs. An IVP may be helpful for detecting these—contrast will fill the area of the sloughed papillae, leaving a "ring shadow" sign at the papillary tip. However, IVP is rarely used in patients with significant kidney dysfunction, given the need for dye and associated AKI risk.

4. Heavy metals—Proximal tubular damage from lead exposure can cause decreased secretion of uric acid, resulting in hyperuricemia and saturnine gout. Patients commonly are hypertensive. Diagnosis is most reliably performed with a calcium disodium edetate (EDTA) chelation test. Urine excretion of greater than 600 mg of lead in 24 hours following 1 g of EDTA indicates excessive lead exposure. The proximal tubular dysfunction from cadmium can cause hypercalciuria and nephrolithiasis.

5. Mesoamerican nephropathy—In addition to low-grade proteinuria, hyperuricemia and hypokalemia are consistently (but not universally) identified among affected individuals. On kidney biopsy, chronic tubulointerstitial injury may be accompanied by areas of glomerular ischemia despite very mild vascular changes.

▶ Treatment

Treatment depends first on identifying the disorder responsible for kidney dysfunction. The degree of interstitial fibrosis that has developed can help predict recovery of kidney function. Once there is evidence of parenchymal loss (small shrunken kidneys or interstitial fibrosis on biopsy), little can prevent the progression to ESRD. Treatment is then directed at medical management. Tubular dysfunction may require potassium and phosphorus restriction and sodium, calcium, or bicarbonate supplements.

If hydronephrosis is present, the obstruction should be promptly relieved. Prolonged obstruction leads to further tubular damage—particularly in the distal nephron—which may be irreversible despite relief of obstruction. Neither surgical correction of reflux nor medical therapy with antibiotics can prevent deterioration toward ESRD once renal scarring has occurred.

Patients in whom lead nephropathy is suspected should continue chelation therapy with EDTA if there is no evidence of irreversible renal damage (eg, renal scarring or small kidneys). Continued exposure should be avoided.

Treatment of analgesic nephropathy requires withdrawal of all analgesics. Stabilization or improvement of renal function may occur if significant interstitial fibrosis is not present. Ensuring volume repletion during exposure to analgesics may also have some beneficial effects.

Patients with Mesoamerican nephropathy should be counseled to remain adequately hydrated and, if possible, minimize heat exposure. NSAIDs should be avoided due to their hemodynamic effects (reduced renal blood flow and glomerular filtration), which may exacerbate renal injury in states of volume depletion and hot climates.

▶ When to Refer

- Patients with stage 3–5 CKD should be referred to a nephrologist when tubulointerstitial diseases are suspected. Other select cases of stage 1–2 CKD should also be referred.
- Patients with urologic abnormalities should be referred to a urologist.

Madero M et al. Pathophysiologic insight into MesoAmerican nephropathy. Curr Opin Nephrol Hypertens. 2017 Jul; 26(4):296–302. [PMID: 28426518]
Perazella MA. Clinical approach to diagnosing acute and chronic tubulointerstitial disease. Adv Chronic Kidney Dis. 2017 Mar; 24(2):57–63. [PMID: 28284380]

CYSTIC DISEASES OF THE KIDNEY

Renal cysts are epithelium-lined cavities filled with fluid or semisolid material that develop primarily from renal tubular elements. One or more simple cysts are found in 50% of individuals over the age of 50 years. They are rarely symptomatic and have little clinical significance. In contrast, generalized cystic diseases are associated with cysts scattered throughout the cortex and medulla of both kidneys and can progress to ESRD (Table 22–10).

SIMPLE OR SOLITARY CYSTS

Simple cysts account for 65–70% of all renal masses. They are generally found at the outer cortex and contain fluid that is consistent with an ultrafiltrate of plasma. Most are found incidentally on ultrasonographic examination. Simple cysts are typically asymptomatic but can become infected.

The major diagnostic objective with simple cysts is to differentiate them from malignancy, abscess, or polycystic kidney disease. Renal cystic disease can develop in dialysis

Table 22–10. Clinical features of renal cystic disease.

	Simple Renal Cysts	Acquired Renal Cysts	Autosomal Dominant Polycystic Kidney Disease	Medullary Sponge Kidney	Medullary Cystic Kidney
Prevalence	Common	Dialysis patients	1:1000	1:5000	Rare
Inheritance	None	None	Autosomal dominant	None	Autosomal dominant
Age at onset	...	...	20–40	40–60	Adulthood
Kidney size	Normal	Small	Large	Normal	Small
Cyst location	Cortex and medulla	Cortex and medulla	Cortex and medulla	Collecting ducts	Corticomedullary junction
Hematuria	Occasional	Occasional	Common	Rare	Rare
Hypertension	None	Variable	Common	None	None
Associated complications	None	Adenocarcinoma in cysts	Urinary tract infections, renal calculi, cerebral aneurysms 10–15%, hepatic cysts 40–60%	Renal calculi, urinary tract infections	Polyuria, salt wasting
Kidney failure	Never	Always	Frequently	Never	Always

patients and has the potential to progress to malignancy. Ultrasound and CT scanning are the recommended procedures for evaluating these masses. Simple cysts must meet three sonographic criteria to be considered benign: (1) echo free, (2) sharply demarcated mass with smooth walls, and (3) an enhanced back wall (indicating good transmission through the cyst). Complex cysts can have thick walls, calcifications, solid components, and mixed echogenicity. On CT scan, simple cysts should have smooth thin walls that are sharply demarcated and should not enhance with contrast media. A renal cell carcinoma will enhance but typically is of lower density than the rest of the parenchyma. Arteriography can also be used to evaluate a mass preoperatively. A renal cell carcinoma is hypervascular in 80%, hypovascular in 15%, and avascular in 5% of cases.

If a cyst is benign, periodic reevaluation is the standard of care. If the lesion is not consistent with a simple cyst, urologic consultation and possible surgical exploration is recommended.

Cramer MT et al. Cystic kidney disease: a primer. Adv Chronic Kidney Dis. 2015 Jul;22(4):297–305. [PMID: 26088074]

AUTOSOMAL DOMINANT POLYCYSTIC KIDNEY DISEASE

 ESSENTIALS OF DIAGNOSIS

▶ Multiple cysts in both kidneys; total number of cysts depends on patient age.

▶ Combination of hypertension and abdominal mass suggestive of disease.

▶ Autosomal dominant chromosomal abnormalities present in some patients.

▶ Family history and large, palpable kidneys are compelling but not necessary.

General Considerations

Polycystic kidney disease is among the most common hereditary diseases in the United States, affecting 500,000 individuals, or 1 in 800 live births. ESRD develops by age 60 years in up to 50% of patients. The disease has variable penetrance but accounts for 10% of dialysis patients in the United States. At least two genes account for this disorder: *ADPKD1* on the short arm of chromosome 16 (85–90% of patients) and *ADPKD2* on chromosome 4 (10–15%). Patients with the *PKD2* mutation have slower progression of disease and longer life expectancy than those with *PKD1*. Other sporadic cases without these mutations are also recognized.

Clinical Findings

Abdominal or flank pain and microscopic or gross hematuria are present in most patients. A history of urinary tract infections and nephrolithiasis is common. A family history is present in 75% of cases, and more than 50% of patients have hypertension that may precede clinical manifestations of the disease. Patients have large kidneys that may be palpable on abdominal examination. The combination of hypertension and an abdominal mass should suggest the disease. Forty to 50 percent have concurrent hepatic cysts; pancreatic and splenic cysts may occur. Hemoglobin tends to be maintained as a result of erythropoietin production by the cysts. The urinalysis may show hematuria and mild proteinuria. In patients with a confirmed family history of *PKD1*, ultrasonography confirms the diagnosis—two or more cysts in patients under age 30 years (sensitivity of 88.5%), two or more cysts in each kidney in patients aged 30–59 years (sensitivity of 100%), and four or more cysts in each kidney in patients aged 60 years or older are diagnostic for autosomal dominant polycystic kidney disease. Importantly, these criteria do *not* apply to individuals without a known family history; patients without a known family history of polycystic kidney disease require additional diagnostic evaluation including CT scanning, which reveals innumerable cysts in cases of polycystic kidney disease

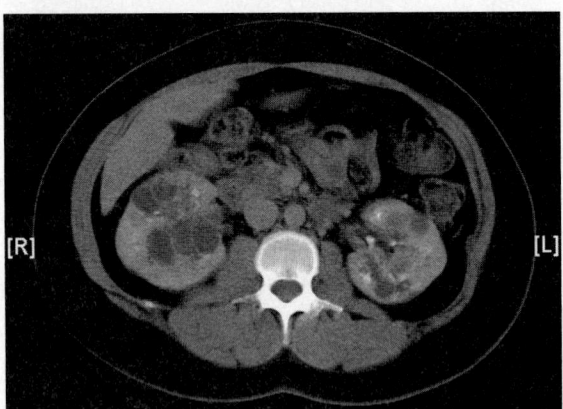

▲ **Figure 22–6.** Polycystic kidney disease. CT scan showing bilateral polycystic kidneys in a 43-year-old woman who presented with newly diagnosed hypertension and microscopic hematuria. (Used, with permission, from Michael Freckleton, MD, in Usatine RP, Smith MA, Mayeaux EJ Jr, Chumley H. *The Color Atlas of Family Medicine,* 2nd ed. McGraw-Hill, 2013.)

(Figure 22–6); the presence of multiple hepatic cysts can aid in establishing the diagnosis. In some cases, genetic testing for *ADPKD1* and *ADPKD2* mutations may be required.

▶ Complications & Treatment

A. Pain

Abdominal or flank pain is caused by infection, bleeding into cysts, and nephrolithiasis. Bed rest and analgesics are recommended. Cyst decompression can help with chronic pain.

B. Hematuria

Gross hematuria is most commonly due to rupture of a cyst into the renal pelvis, but it can also be caused by a kidney stone or urinary tract infection. Hematuria typically resolves within 7 days with bed rest and hydration. Recurrent bleeding should suggest the possibility of underlying renal cell carcinoma, particularly in men over age 50 years.

C. Renal Infection

An infected renal cyst should be suspected in patients who have flank pain, fever, and leukocytosis. Blood cultures may be positive, and urinalysis may be normal if the cyst does not communicate directly with the urinary tract. CT scans can be helpful because an infected cyst may have increased wall thickness. Bacterial cyst infections are difficult to treat. Antibiotics with cystic penetration (eg, fluoroquinolones or trimethoprim-sulfamethoxazole) should be used. Treatment may require 2 weeks of parenteral therapy followed by long-term oral therapy.

D. Nephrolithiasis

Up to 20% of patients have kidney stones, primarily calcium oxalate. Hydration (2–3 L/day) is recommended in order to prevent precipitation of stones.

E. Hypertension

Fifty percent of patients have hypertension at time of presentation, and it will develop in most patients during the course of the disease. Cyst-induced ischemia appears to cause activation of the renin-angiotensin system, and cyst decompression can lower blood pressure temporarily. Hypertension should be treated with an ACE inhibitor or an ARB as the preferred drug if tolerated; a randomized controlled trial comparing aggressive control (blood pressures 95–110/60–75 mm Hg) to usual care (blood pressures 120–130/70–80 mm Hg) showed that aggressive control slowed the increase of kidney volume but not the decline in GFR.

F. Cerebral Aneurysms

About 10–15% of these patients have arterial aneurysms in the circle of Willis. Screening arteriography is not recommended unless the patient has a family history of aneurysms, is employed in a high-risk profession (such as airline pilot), or is undergoing elective surgery with a high risk of developing moderate to severe perioperative hypertension.

G. Other Complications

Vascular problems include mitral valve prolapse in up to 25% of patients, aortic aneurysms, and aortic valve abnormalities. Colonic diverticula are more common in patients with polycystic kidneys.

▶ Prognosis

Cyst growth in polycystic kidney disease is thought to be sensitive to cyclic AMP production, which is stimulated by the hormone vasopressin. Indeed, vasopressin receptor antagonists decrease the rate of change in total kidney volume and eGFR decline, and one such medication (tolvaptan) is FDA approved for the treatment of autosomal dominant polycystic kidney disease. It should be noted that liberal ingestion of water will have the same physiologic effect on vasopressin, and patients should be encouraged to drink at least 2 L of water daily. Other agents such as octreotide, sirolimus, and tyrosine kinase inhibitors decrease the rate of cyst growth but not the decline in kidney function. Avoidance of caffeine may prevent cyst formation due to effects on G-coupled proteins. Treatment of hypertension and a low-protein diet may slow the progression of disease, although this is not well proven.

Chebib FT et al. Autosomal dominant polycystic kidney disease: Core Curriculum 2016. Am J Kidney Dis. 2016 May;67(5): 792–810. [PMID: 26530876]

Chebib FT et al. Recent advances in the management of autosomal dominant polycystic kidney disease. Clin J Am Soc Nephrol. 2018 Nov 7;13(11):1765–76. [PMID: 30049849]

MEDULLARY SPONGE KIDNEY

This disease is a relatively common and benign disorder that is present at birth and not usually diagnosed until the fourth or fifth decade. It can be caused by autosomal dominant mutations in the *MCKD1* or *MCKD2* genes on chromosomes 1 and 16, respectively. Kidneys have a marked irregular enlargement of the medullary and interpapillary collecting ducts. This is associated with medullary cysts that are diffuse, giving a "Swiss cheese" appearance in these regions.

▶ Clinical Findings

Medullary sponge kidney presents with gross or microscopic hematuria, recurrent urinary tract infections, or nephrolithiasis. Common abnormalities are a decreased urinary concentrating ability and nephrocalcinosis; less common is incomplete type 1 distal renal tubular acidosis. The diagnosis can be made by CT, which shows cystic dilatation of the distal collecting tubules, a striated appearance in this area, and calcifications in the renal collecting system.

▶ Treatment

There is no known therapy. Adequate fluid intake (2 L/day) helps prevent stone formation. If hypercalciuria is present, thiazide diuretics are recommended because they decrease calcium excretion. Alkali therapy is recommended if renal tubular acidosis is present.

▶ Prognosis

Renal function is well maintained unless there are complications from recurrent urinary tract infections and nephrolithiasis.

Meola M et al. Clinical scenarios in chronic kidney disease: cystic renal diseases. Contrib Nephrol. 2016;188:120–30. [PMID: 27169740]

Sun H et al. Safety and efficacy of minimally invasive percutaneous nephrolithotomy in the treatment of patients with medullary sponge kidney. Urolithiasis. 2016 Oct;44(5):421–6. [PMID: 26671346]

MULTISYSTEM DISEASES WITH VARIABLE KIDNEY INVOLVEMENT

PLASMA CELL MYELOMA

Plasma cell myeloma is a malignancy of plasma cells (see Chapter 13) that can cause a variety of renal disorders. "Myeloma kidney" (formally called cast nephropathy) is the most common kidney disease in plasma cell myeloma and occurs when light chain immunoglobulins (Bence Jones protein) in the urine cause renal toxicity and tubular obstruction by precipitating in the distal tubules. Plasma cell myeloma may also cause Fanconi syndrome, a type 2 proximal renal tubular acidosis characterized by hypophosphatemia and inappropriate glycosuria. Proteinuria in myeloma kidney is exclusively tubular; hence, urine dipstick findings are minimal since glomerular proteinuria and hematuria are not present. Hypercalcemia and hyperuricemia are frequently seen. Glomerular amyloidosis can develop in patients with plasma cell myeloma; in these patients, dipstick protein tests are positive due to glomerular epithelial cell foot process effacement and albumin "spilling" into the Bowman capsule with resultant albuminuria; hematuria

may or may not be present. Other conditions resulting in kidney dysfunction include plasma cell infiltration of the renal parenchyma and hyperviscosity syndrome compromising renal blood flow. The presence of myeloma-related kidney disease does not itself preclude use of contrast dye for imaging studies; standard precautions for the use of intravenous contrast and gadolinium in patients with reduced GFR apply to patients with myeloma-related kidney disease. Therapy for AKI attributed to plasma cell myeloma includes correction of hypercalcemia, volume repletion, and chemotherapy for the underlying malignancy. Plasmapheresis has been proposed to reduce the burden of circulating monoclonal proteins, but results have been equivocal and its use is controversial.

Dimopoulos MA et al. International Myeloma Working Group recommendations for the diagnosis and management of myeloma-related renal impairment. J Clin Oncol. 2016 May1;34(13):1544–57. [PMID: 26976420]

Rosner MH et al. Paraprotein-related kidney disease: diagnosing and treating monoclonal gammopathy of renal significance. Clin J Am Soc Nephrol. 2016 Dec 7;11(12):2280–7. [PMID: 27526705]

Sethi S et al. The complexity and heterogeneity of monoclonal immunoglobulin-associated renal diseases. J Am Soc Nephrol. 2018 Jul;29(7):1810–23. [PMID: 29703839]

SICKLE CELL DISEASE

Kidney dysfunction associated with sickle cell disease is most commonly due to sickling of red blood cells in the renal medulla because of low oxygen tension and hypertonicity. Congestion and stasis lead to hemorrhage, interstitial inflammation, and papillary infarcts with resultant necrosis. Clinically, hematuria is common. Damage to renal capillaries also leads to diminished concentrating ability. Isosthenuria (urine osmolality equal to that of serum) is routine, and patients can easily become dehydrated. These abnormalities are also encountered in patients with sickle cell trait. Sickle cell glomerulopathy is less common but will inexorably progress to ESRD. Its primary clinical manifestation is proteinuria. Optimal treatment requires adequate hydration and control of the sickle cell disease.

Naik RP et al. Sickle cell trait and the risk of ESRD in blacks. J Am Soc Nephrol. 2017 Jul;28(7):2180–7. [PMID: 28280138]

Naik RP et al. The spectrum of sickle hemoglobin-related nephropathy: from sickle cell disease to sickle trait. Expert Rev Hematol. 2017 Dec;10(12):1087–94. [PMID: 29048948]

Nath KA et al. Sickle cell disease: renal manifestations and mechanisms. Nat Rev Nephrol. 2015 Mar;11(3):161–71. [PMID: 25668001]

TUBERCULOSIS

The classic renal manifestation of tuberculosis is the presence of microscopic pyuria with a sterile urine culture—or "sterile pyuria." More often, other bacteria are also present. Microscopic hematuria is often present with pyuria. Urine cultures are the gold standard for diagnosis. Three to six first morning midstream specimens should be performed to improve sensitivity. Papillary necrosis and cavitation of the renal parenchyma occur less frequently, as do ureteral strictures and calcifications. Adequate drug therapy can result in resolution of renal involvement.

Figueiredo AA et al. Urogenital tuberculosis. Microbiol Spectr. 2017 Jan;5(1). [PMID: 28087922]

GOUT & THE KIDNEY

The kidney is the primary organ for excretion of uric acid. Patients with proximal tubular dysfunction have decreased excretion of uric acid and are more prone to gouty arthritis attacks. Depending on the pH and uric acid concentration, deposition can occur in the tubules, the interstitium, or the urinary tract. The more alkaline pH of the interstitium causes urate salt deposition, whereas the acidic environment of the tubules and urinary tract causes uric acid crystal deposition at high concentrations.

Three disorders are commonly seen: (1) uric acid nephrolithiasis, (2) acute uric acid nephropathy, and (3) chronic urate nephropathy. Kidney dysfunction with uric acid nephrolithiasis stems from obstructive physiology. Acute uric acid nephropathy presents similarly to acute tubulointerstitial nephritis with direct toxicity from uric acid crystals. Chronic urate nephropathy is caused by deposition of urate crystals in the alkaline medium of the interstitium; this can lead to fibrosis and atrophy. Epidemiologically, hyperuricemia and gout have been associated with worse cardiovascular outcomes.

Treatment between gouty attacks involves avoidance of food and drugs causing hyperuricemia (see Chapter 20), aggressive hydration, and pharmacotherapy aimed at reducing serum uric acid levels (such as with allopurinol and febuxostat). The three disorders mentioned above are seen in both "overproducers" and "underexcretors" of uric acid. The latter situation may seem counterintuitive; however, these patients have hyperacidic urine, which explains the deposition of relatively insoluble uric acid crystals. For those with uric acid nephrolithiasis, fluid intake should exceed 3 L/day, and use of a urinary alkalinizing agent can be considered.

Mallat SG et al. Hyperuricemia, hypertension, and chronic kidney disease: an emerging association. Curr Hypertens Rep. 2016 Oct;18(10):74. [PMID: 27696189]

Singh JA et al. Comparative effectiveness of allopurinol versus febuxostat for preventing incident renal disease in older adults: an analysis of Medicare claims data. Ann Rheum Dis. 2017 Oct;76(10):1669–78. [PMID: 28584186]

NEPHROGENIC SYSTEMIC FIBROSIS

Nephrogenic systemic fibrosis is a multisystem disorder seen only in patients with CKD (primarily with an eGFR less than 15 mL/min/1.73 m^2, but rarely with a GFR of 15–29 mL/min/1.73 m^2), AKI, and after kidney transplantation. Histopathologically, there is an increase in dermal spindle cells positive for CD34 and procollagen I. Collagen bundles with mucin and elastic fibers are also noted.

Nephrogenic systemic fibrosis was first recognized in hemodialysis patients in 1997 and has been strongly linked to use of contrast agents containing gadolinium. Incidence is projected to be 1–4% in the highest risk (ESRD) population that has received gadolinium, and lower in patients with less severe kidney dysfunction. Reassuringly, the incidence has decreased over time and is thought to result from modified preparations of gadolinium as well as carefully identifying individuals who should avoid exposure altogether. There is an FDA warning regarding avoidance of exposure to this agent for patients with an eGFR less than 30 mL/min/1.73 m^2.

▶ Clinical Findings

Nephrogenic systemic fibrosis affects several organ systems, including the skin, muscles, lungs, and cardiovascular system. The most common manifestation is a debilitating fibrosing skin disorder that can range from skin-colored to erythematous papules, which coalesce to brawny patches. The skin can be thick and woody in areas and is painful out of proportion to findings on examination.

▶ Treatment

Several case reports and series describe benefit after treatment with corticosteroids, photopheresis, plasmapheresis, and sodium thiosulfate, but their true efficacy is unknown. Patients already on dialysis who absolutely require gadolinium typically receive prolonged hemodialysis on 3 consecutive days, but this is based on expert opinion rather than high-quality evidence.

Bruce R et al. Incidence of nephrogenic systemic fibrosis using gadobenate dimeglumine in 1423 patients with renal insufficiency compared with gadodiamide. Invest Radiol. 2016 Nov;51(11):701–5. [PMID: 26885631]

Todd DJ et al. Gadolinium-induced fibrosis. Annu Rev Med. 2016;67:273–91. [PMID: 26768242]

Urologic Disorders

Mathew Sorensen, MD, MS, FACS

Thomas J. Walsh, MD, MS

Kevin A. Ostrowski, MD

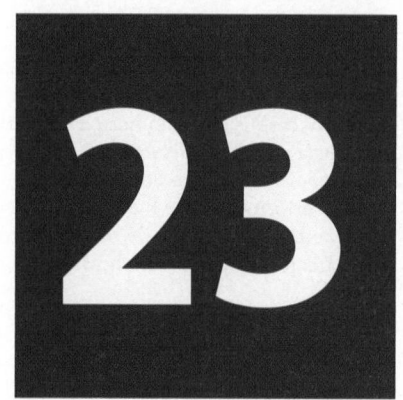

HEMATURIA

ESSENTIALS OF DIAGNOSIS

▶ Both gross and microscopic hematuria require evaluation.

▶ The upper urinary tract should be imaged, and cystoscopy should be performed if there is hematuria in the absence of an identifiable benign cause.

▶ General Considerations

An **upper tract source** (kidneys and ureters) can be identified in 10% of patients with gross or microscopic hematuria. For upper tract sources, stone disease accounts for 40%, medical kidney disease (medullary sponge kidney, glomerulonephritis, papillary necrosis) for 20%, renal cell carcinoma for 10%, and urothelial cell carcinoma of the ureter or renal pelvis for 5%. Medication ingestion and associated medical problems may provide diagnostic clues. Analgesic use (papillary necrosis), cyclophosphamide (chemical cystitis), antibiotics (interstitial nephritis), diabetes mellitus, sickle cell trait or disease (papillary necrosis), a history of stone disease, or malignancy should all be investigated. The **lower tract source** of gross hematuria (in the absence of infection) is most commonly from urothelial carcinoma of the bladder. Microscopic hematuria in the male is most commonly from benign prostatic hyperplasia (13%), kidney stones (6%), or urethral stricture (1.4%). The presence of hematuria in patients receiving antiplatelet or anticoagulation therapy cannot be presumed to be due to the medication; a complete evaluation is warranted consisting of upper tract imaging, cystoscopy, and urine cytology (see Chapter 39 for Bladder Cancer, Cancers of the Ureter & Renal Pelvis, Renal Cell Carcinoma, and Other Primary Tumors of the Kidney).

▶ Clinical Findings

A. Symptoms and Signs

If gross hematuria occurs, a description of the timing (initial, terminal, total) may provide a clue to the localization of disease. Associated symptoms (ie, renal colic, irritative voiding symptoms, constitutional symptoms) should be investigated. Physical examination should emphasize signs of systemic disease (fever, rash, lymphadenopathy, abdominal or pelvic masses) as well as signs of medical kidney disease (hypertension, volume overload). Urologic evaluation may demonstrate an enlarged prostate, flank mass, or urethral disease.

B. Laboratory Findings

Initial laboratory investigations include a urinalysis and urine culture. Microhematuria is defined as three or more red blood cells per high-power field on a microscopic evaluation of the urine. A positive dipstick reading for heme merits microscopic examination to confirm or refute the diagnosis of hematuria. If hematuria is present, proteinuria, dysmorphic red blood cells, and urinary casts suggest renal origin. Irritative voiding symptoms, bacteriuria, and a positive urine culture suggest urinary tract infection, but followup urinalysis is important after treatment to ensure resolution of the hematuria. An estimate of kidney function should be obtained, since intrinsic kidney disease has implications for further evaluation and management of patients with hematuria. Urine cytology and other urinary-based markers are not routinely recommended in the evaluation of asymptomatic microscopic hematuria.

C. Imaging

The upper tract should be imaged using a CT-intravenous pyelogram (CT-IVP), which is an abdominal and pelvic CT scan without contrast, with contrast, and with excretory delayed imaging to identify neoplasms of the kidney or ureter as well as benign conditions such as urolithiasis, obstructive uropathy, papillary necrosis, medullary sponge kidney, or polycystic kidney disease. For patients with relative or absolute contraindications that preclude a CT-IVP (such as kidney dysfunction, intravenous contrast allergy, or pregnancy), a magnetic resonance urogram without and with contrast can be performed. The role of ultrasonographic evaluation of the urinary tract for hematuria is unclear. Although it may provide adequate information for the kidney, its sensitivity in detecting ureteral disease is lower.

D. Cystoscopy

Cystoscopy is necessary to assess for bladder or urethral neoplasm, benign prostatic enlargement, and radiation or chemical cystitis; it is indicated for patients with gross hematuria and those over age 35 years with asymptomatic microscopic hematuria. For gross hematuria, cystoscopy is ideally performed while the patient is actively bleeding to allow better localization (ie, lateralize to one side of the upper tracts, bladder, or urethra).

▶ Follow-Up

In patients with negative evaluations, repeat evaluations may be warranted to avoid a missed malignancy; however, the ideal frequency of such evaluations is not defined. Urinary cytology can be obtained after initial negative evaluation or in persons with risk factors (irritative voiding symptoms, tobacco use, chemical exposures), and cystoscopy and upper tract imaging may be repeated 1 year after an initial negative evaluation.

▶ When to Refer

In the absence of a clear benign etiology (such as an infection, menstruation, vigorous exercise, medical renal disease, viral illness, trauma, or recent urologic procedure), hematuria (either gross or microscopic) requires evaluation.

Davis R et al. Diagnosis, evaluation and follow-up of asymptomatic microhematuria (AMH) in adults: AUA guideline. J Urol. 2012 Dec;188(6 Suppl):2473–81. [PMID: 23098784]

Halpern JA et al. Cost-effectiveness of common diagnostic approaches for evaluation of asymptomatic microscopic hematuria. JAMA Intern Med. 2017 Jun 1;177(6):800–7. [PMID: 28418451]

Kaag MG et al. Clinical guidelines: clearing murky water—a guideline-based approach to haematuria. Nat Rev Urol. 2016 May;13(5):243–4. [PMID: 27071454]

Kiragu D et al. Evaluation of patients with asymptomatic microhematuria. JAMA. 2015 Nov 3;314(17):1865–6. [PMID: 26529165]

Nielsen M et al. Hematuria as a marker of occult urinary tract cancer: advice for high-value care from the American College of Physicians. Ann Intern Med. 2016 Apr 5;164(7):488–97. [PMID: 26810935]

Sountoulides P et al. Non-visible asymptomatic haematuria: a review of the guidelines from the urologist's perspective. Expert Rev Anticancer Ther. 2017 Mar;17(3):203–16. [PMID: 28116915]

GENITOURINARY TRACT INFECTIONS

Urinary tract infections are among the most common entities encountered in medical practice. In acute infections, a single pathogen is usually found, whereas two or more pathogens are often seen in chronic infections. Coliform bacteria are responsible for most non-nosocomial, uncomplicated urinary tract infections, with *Escherichia coli* being the most common. Such infections typically are sensitive to a wide variety of orally administered antibiotics and respond quickly. Nosocomial infections often are due to more resistant pathogens and may require parenteral antibiotics. Renal infections are of particular concern because if they are inadequately treated, loss of kidney function

may result. A urine culture is recommended for patients with suspected urinary tract infection and ideally should be obtained prior to the initiation of antibiotic therapy. Previously, a colony count greater than 10^5/mL was considered the criterion for urinary tract infection. However, it is now recognized that up to 50% of women with symptomatic infections have lower counts. In addition, the presence of pyuria correlates poorly with the diagnosis of urinary tract infection, and thus urinalysis alone is not adequate for diagnosis. With respect to treatment, soft tissue infections (pyelonephritis, prostatitis) require therapy for 1–2 weeks, while mucosal infections (cystitis) require only 1–3 days of therapy.

1. Acute Cystitis

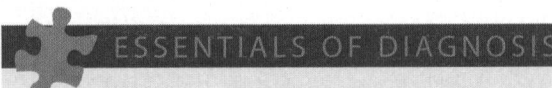

ESSENTIALS OF DIAGNOSIS

▶ Irritative voiding symptoms.

▶ Patient usually afebrile.

▶ Positive urine culture; blood cultures may also be positive.

▶ General Considerations

Acute cystitis is an infection of the bladder most commonly due to the coliform bacteria (especially *E coli*) and occasionally gram-positive bacteria (enterococci). The route of infection is typically ascending from the urethra. Viral cystitis due to adenovirus is sometimes seen in children but is rare in adults. Uncomplicated cystitis in men is rare and implies a pathologic process such as infected stones, prostatitis, or chronic urinary retention requiring further investigation.

▶ Clinical Findings

A. Symptoms and Signs

Irritative voiding symptoms (frequency, urgency, dysuria) and suprapubic discomfort are common. Women may experience gross hematuria, and symptoms may often appear following sexual intercourse. Physical examination may elicit suprapubic tenderness, but examination is often unremarkable. Systemic toxicity is absent.

B. Laboratory Findings

Urinalysis shows pyuria, bacteriuria, and varying degrees of hematuria. The degree of pyuria and bacteriuria does not necessarily correlate with the severity of symptoms. Urine culture is positive for the offending organism, but colony counts exceeding 10^5/mL are not required for the diagnosis. Patients with long-term urinary catheters (indwelling urinary [Foley] or suprapubic catheter) or urostomy urinary diversions are expected to be colonized with bacteria, and thus, urinalysis and urine culture are most helpful in directing therapy rather than determining whether symptomatic infection exists.

C. Imaging

Because uncomplicated cystitis is rare in men, elucidation of the underlying problem with appropriate investigations, such as abdominal ultrasonography, postvoid residual testing, and cystoscopy, is warranted. Follow-up imaging using CT scanning is warranted if pyelonephritis, recurrent infections, or anatomic abnormalities are suspected.

▶ Differential Diagnosis

In women, infectious processes such as vulvovaginitis and pelvic inflammatory disease can usually be distinguished by pelvic examination and urinalysis. In men, urethritis and prostatitis may be distinguished by physical examination (urethral discharge or prostatic tenderness).

Noninfectious causes of cystitis-like symptoms include pelvic irradiation, chemotherapy (cyclophosphamide), bladder carcinoma, interstitial cystitis, voiding dysfunction disorders, and psychosomatic disorders.

▶ Prevention

The risk of developing a urinary tract infection can be reduced by drinking plenty of fluid and emptying the bladder frequently and completely. Women in whom urinary tract infections tend to develop after intercourse should be advised to void before, and especially after intercourse, and may benefit from a postcoital single dose of antibiotic. Postmenopausal women with recurrent urinary tract infections (three or more episodes per year) may benefit from a topical estrogen cream. Daily cranberry tablets may reduce the risk of cystitis, though the data are conflicting. Women with recurrent episodes of cystitis (three or more episodes per year) may also benefit, after treatment of the urinary tract infection, from prophylactic antibiotic therapy to prevent recurrences. Prior to institution of antibiotic prophylaxis, a thorough urologic evaluation is warranted to exclude any anatomic abnormality (eg, stones, reflux, fistula). An initial course of 6- to 12-months of prophylactic antibiotics can be offered. The benefits of prophylactic antibiotics should be weighed against the risks of developing bacterial resistance.

The risk of acquiring a catheter-associated urinary tract infection in hospitalized patients can be minimized by using indwelling catheters only when necessary, implementing systems to ensure removal of catheters when no longer needed, using antimicrobial catheters in high-risk patients, using external collection devices in select men, identifying significant postvoid residuals by ultrasound, maintaining proper insertion techniques, and utilizing alternatives such as intermittent catheterization.

▶ Treatment

Uncomplicated cystitis in women can be treated with short-term antimicrobial therapy, which consists of single-dose therapy or 1–7 days of therapy. Fosfomycin, nitrofurantoin, and trimethoprim-sulfamethoxazole are the medications of choice for uncomplicated cystitis (Table 23–1). The US Food and Drug Administration (FDA) advises restricting fluoroquinolone use for uncomplicated infections, including

Table 23–1. Empiric therapy for urinary tract infections.

Diagnosis	Antibiotic	Route	Duration	Cost per Duration Noted[1]
Acute cystitis[a]				
	First-line:			
	Trimethoprim-sulfamethoxazole, 160/800 mg, (one DS tablet) every 12 hours[2]	Oral	3 days	$2.25
	Nitrofurantoin (macrocrystals), 100 mg every 12 hours	Oral	5 days	$33.76
	Fosfomycin, 3 g packet once	Oral	1 day	$104.30
	Second-line:			
	Ciprofloxacin, 250 mg every 12 hours[3]	Oral	3 days	$27.21
	Levofloxacin, 250–500 mg daily[3]	Oral	3 days	$50.46
	Alternative agents:			
	Cephalexin, 500 mg every 6–12 hours	Oral	7 days	$38.53
	Amoxicillin/clavulanate, 500/125 mg every 12 hours	Oral	3 days	$22.00
	Cefpodoxime, 100 mg every 12 hours	Oral	3 days	$40.44
Acute pyelonephritis[a]				
	Hospitalized:			
	Ampicillin, 1 g every 6 hours, plus gentamicin, 1 mg/kg every 8 hours	Intravenous	14 days	$291.14, not including intravenous supplies
	Ceftriaxone, 1 g daily	Intravenous	14 days	$25.20
	Ciprofloxacin, 400 mg every 12 hours	Intravenous	14 days	$787.50

(continued)

Table 23–1. Empiric therapy for urinary tract infections. (Continued)

Diagnosis	Antibiotic	Route	Duration	Cost per Duration Noted[1]
Acute pyelonephritis[a] (cont.)	**Non-hospitalized:**			
	Initial intravenous dose:[4]			
	Ceftriaxone, 1 g	Intravenous	Once	$1.80
	Ciprofloxacin, 400 mg	Intravenous	Once	$28.12
	Gentamicin, 5 mg/kg	Intravenous	Once	$21.80
	Followed by one of these oral regimens:			
	Ciprofloxacin, 500 mg every 12 hours[2]	Oral	7 days	$69.00
	Levofloxacin, 750 mg daily	Oral	5 days	$146.05
	Trimethoprim-sulfamethoxazole, 160/800 mg (one DS tablet) every 12 hours[5]	Oral	14 days	$10.44
Acute bacterial prostatitis[b]	**Hospitalized:**			
	Ampicillin, 2 g every 6 hours, plus gentamicin, 1.5 mg/kg every 8 hours	Intravenous	Until afebrile	$20.80/day, not including intravenous supplies
	Followed by one of these outpatient oral regimens:			
	Trimethoprim-sulfamethoxazole, 160/800 mg (one DS tablet) every 12 hours[5]	Oral	3 weeks	$15.75/3 weeks
	Ciprofloxacin, 250–500 mg every 12 hours	Oral	3 weeks	$207.00/3 weeks
Chronic bacterial prostatitis[b]	**First-line:**			
	Ciprofloxacin, 500 mg every 12 hours	Oral	1–3 months	$295.80/month
	Levofloxacin, 750 mg daily	Oral	28 days	$689.08
	Second-line:			
	Doxycycline, 100 mg twice daily	Oral	4–12 weeks	$196.80/month
	Azithromycin, 500 mg daily	Oral	4–12 weeks	$467.10/month
	Clarithromycin, 500 mg daily	Oral	4–12 weeks	$135.60/month
Acute epididymitis[c]				
Sexually transmitted (under age 35)	Ceftriaxone, 250 mg as single dose, **plus** Doxycycline, 100 mg every 12 hours	Intramuscular Oral	Once 10 days	$0.90/250 mg $98.90 (10 days)
Sexual transmitted in men who practice insertive anal sex	Ceftriaxone, 250 mg as single dose **plus** Levofloxacin, 500 mg daily **or** Ofloxacin, 300 mg every 12 hours	Intramuscular Oral Oral	Once 10 days 10 days	$0.90/250 mg $168.20 (10 days) $113.80 (10 days)
Non–sexually transmitted, usually enteric organisms (over age 35)	Levofloxacin, 500 mg daily Ofloxacin, 300 mg every 12 hours	Oral Oral	10 days 10 days	$168.20 (10 days) $113.80 (10 days)

[1]Average wholesale price (AWP, for AB-rated generic when available) for quantity listed. Source: IBM Micromedex Red Book (electronic version) IBM Watson Health, Greenwood Village, CO, USA. Available at https://www.micromedexsolutions.com (cited April 25, 2019). AWP may not accurately represent the actual pharmacy cost because wide contractual variations exist among institutions.

[2]Increasing resistance noted.

[3]FDA advises restricting fluoroquinolone use for some uncomplicated infections, including uncomplicated urinary tract infections.

[4]Infectious Diseases Society of America (IDSA) recommends an initial 24-hour intravenous dose of antibiotic when local resistance of the selected oral regimen exceeds 10%. Please refer to local antibiograms.

[5]Increasing resistance noted (up to 20%).

Sources:

[a]Treatment regimens based upon Gupta K et al. Treatment of acute uncomplicated cystitis and pyelonephritis in women: a 2010 update by the Infectious Diseases Society of America and European Society for Microbiology and Infectious Diseases. Clin Infect Dis. 2011;52(5):e103-e120.

[b]Treatment regimens based upon Sharp VJ et al. Prostatitis: diagnosis and treatment. Am Fam Physician. 2010 Aug 15;82(4):397-406.

[c]Treatment regimens based upon Workowski KA et al; Centers for Disease Control and Prevention. Sexually transmitted diseases treatment guidelines, 2015. MMWR Recomm Rep. 2015 Jun 5;64(RR-03):1-137. Erratum in: MMWR Recomm Rep. 2015 Aug 28;64(33):924.

uncomplicated urinary tract infections. Local patterns of bacterial resistance should be consulted to identify best treatment options. Some antibiotics may be ineffective because of the emergence of resistant organisms. A review of the literature proposed that acute uncomplicated cystitis in women can be diagnosed without office evaluation or urine culture, and that appropriate first-line therapies include trimethoprim-sulfamethoxazole (160/800 mg twice daily for 3 days), nitrofurantoin (100 mg twice daily for 5–7 days), and fosfomycin trometamol (3 g single dose). In men, uncomplicated urinary tract infection is rare; thus, the duration of antibiotic therapy depends on the underlying etiology. Hot sitz baths or urinary analgesics (phenazopyridine, 200 mg orally three times daily) may provide symptomatic relief. Postmenopausal women with recurrent cystitis can be treated with vaginal estrogen cream 0.5 g nightly for 2 weeks and then twice weekly thereafter.

► Prognosis

Infections typically respond rapidly to therapy, and failure to respond suggests resistance to the selected medication or anatomic abnormalities requiring further investigation.

► When to Refer

- Suspicion or radiographic evidence of anatomic abnormality.
- Evidence of urolithiasis.
- Recurrent cystitis due to bacterial persistence.

Arnold JJ et al. Common questions about recurrent urinary tract infections in women. Am Fam Physician. 2016 Apr 1; 93(7):560–9. [PMID: 27035041]

Bader MS et al. An update on the management of urinary tract infections in the era of antimicrobial resistance. Postgrad Med. 2017 Mar;129(2):242–58. [PMID: 27712137]

Datta R et al. Nitrofurantoin vs fosfomycin: rendering a verdict in a trial of acute uncomplicated cystitis. JAMA. 2018 May 1; 319(17):1771–2. [PMID: 29710273]

Grigoryan L et al. Diagnosis and management of urinary tract infection in the outpatient setting: a review. JAMA. 2014 Oct 22–29;312(16):1677–84. [PMID: 25335150]

Huttner A et al. Effect of 5-day nitrofurantoin vs single-dose fosfomycin on clinical resolution of uncomplicated lower urinary tract infection in women: a randomized clinical trial. JAMA. 2018 May 1;319(17):1781–9. [PMID: 29710295]

US Food & Drug Administration. FDA Drug Safety Communication: FDA updates warnings for oral and injectable fluoroquinolone antibiotics due to disabling side effects. 2016 Jul 26. http://www.fda.gov/Drugs/DrugSafety/ucm511530.htm

2. Acute Pyelonephritis

ESSENTIALS OF DIAGNOSIS

- ► Fever.
- ► Flank pain.
- ► Irritative voiding symptoms.
- ► Positive urine culture.

► General Considerations

Acute pyelonephritis is an infectious inflammatory disease involving the kidney parenchyma and renal pelvis. Gram-negative bacteria are the most common causative agents including *E coli, Proteus, Klebsiella, Enterobacter,* and *Pseudomonas.* Gram-positive bacteria are less commonly seen but include *Enterococcus faecalis* and *Staphylococcus aureus.* The infection usually ascends from the lower urinary tract—with the exception of *S aureus,* which usually is spread by a hematogenous route.

► Clinical Findings

A. Symptoms and Signs

Symptoms include fever, flank pain, shaking chills, and irritative voiding symptoms (urgency, frequency, dysuria). Associated nausea and vomiting and diarrhea are common. Signs include fever and tachycardia. Costovertebral angle tenderness is usually pronounced.

B. Laboratory Findings

Complete blood cell count shows leukocytosis and a left shift. Urinalysis shows pyuria, bacteriuria, and varying degrees of hematuria. White cell casts may be seen. Urine culture demonstrates heavy growth of the offending organism, and blood culture may also be positive.

C. Imaging

In complicated pyelonephritis, renal ultrasound may show hydronephrosis from a stone or other source of obstruction. CT scan may demonstrate decreased perfusion of the kidney or focal areas within the kidney and nonspecific perinephric fat stranding.

► Differential Diagnosis

The differential diagnosis includes acute cystitis or a lower urinary source. Acute intra-abdominal disease such as appendicitis, cholecystitis, pancreatitis, or diverticulitis must be distinguished from pyelonephritis. A normal urinalysis is usually seen in gastrointestinal disorders; however, on occasion, inflammation from adjacent bowel (appendicitis or diverticulitis) may result in hematuria or sterile pyuria. Abnormal liver biochemical tests or elevated amylase levels may assist in the differentiation. Lower-lobe pneumonia is distinguishable by the abnormal chest radiograph.

In males, the main differential diagnosis for acute pyelonephritis also includes acute epididymitis and acute prostatitis. Physical examination and the location of the pain should permit this distinction.

► Complications

Sepsis with shock can occur with acute pyelonephritis. In diabetic patients, emphysematous pyelonephritis resulting from gas-producing organisms may be life-threatening if not adequately treated. Healthy adults usually recover complete kidney function, yet if coexistent kidney disease is present, scarring or chronic pyelonephritis may result. Inadequate therapy could result in abscess formation.

Treatment

Urine and blood cultures are obtained to identify the causative agent and to determine antimicrobial sensitivity. In the inpatient setting, intravenous ampicillin and an aminoglycoside are initiated prior to obtaining sensitivity results (Table 23–1). In the outpatient setting, empiric therapy may be initiated (Table 23–1). Antibiotics are adjusted according to sensitivities. If local antibiograms demonstrate local resistance rates for the oral regimen exceed 10%, an initial 24-hour intravenous dose of antibiotic is required. Fevers may persist for up to 72 hours even with appropriate antibiotics; failure to respond within 48 hours warrants imaging (CT or ultrasound) to exclude complicating factors that may require intervention. Catheter drainage may be necessary in the face of urinary retention and nephrostomy drainage if there is ureteral obstruction. In inpatients, intravenous antibiotics are continued for 24 hours after the fever resolves, and oral antibiotics are then given to complete a 14-day course of therapy.

Prognosis

With prompt diagnosis and appropriate treatment, acute pyelonephritis carries a good prognosis. Complicating factors, underlying kidney disease, and increasing patient age may lead to a less favorable outcome.

When to Refer

- Evidence of complicating factors (urolithiasis, obstruction).
- Failure of clinical improvement in 48 hours.

When to Admit

- Severe infections or complicating factors, evidence of sepsis, or need for parenteral antibiotics.
- Need for radiographic imaging or drainage of urinary tract obstruction.

Bader MS et al. An update on the management of urinary tract infections in the era of antimicrobial resistance. Postgrad Med. 2017 Mar;129(2):242–58. [PMID: 27712137]

Dawson-Hahn EE et al. Short-course versus long-course oral antibiotic treatment for infections treated in outpatient settings: a review of systematic reviews. Fam Pract. 2017 Sept 1;34(5):511–9. [PMID: 28486675]

Gupta K et al. International clinical practice guidelines for the treatment of acute uncomplicated cystitis and pyelonephritis in women: a 2010 update by the Infectious Disease Society of America and the European Society for Microbiology and Infectious Diseases. Clin Infect Dis. 2011 Mar 1;52(5):e103–20. [PMID: 21292654]

Talan DA et al; EMERGEncy ID Net Study Group. Fluoroquinolone-resistant and extended-spectrum β-lactamase-producing *Escherichia coli* infections in patients with pyelonephritis, United States. Emerg Infect Dis. 2016 Sep;22(9). [PMID: 27532362]

Wagenlehner FM et al. Ceftolozane-tazobactam compared with levofloxacin in the treatment of complicated urinary-tract infections, including pyelonephritis: a randomised, double-blind, phase 3 trial (ASPECT-cUTI). Lancet. 2015 May 16; 385(9981):1949–56. [PMID: 25931244]

Yoon YK et al. Role of piperacillin/tazobactam as a carbapenem-sparing antibiotic for treatment of acute pyelonephritis due to extended-spectrum β-lactamase-producing *Escherichia coli*. Int J Antimicrob Agents. 2017 Apr;49(4):410–15. [PMID: 28263710]

3. Acute Bacterial Prostatitis

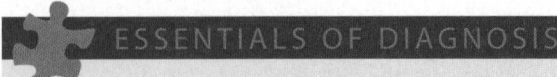

ESSENTIALS OF DIAGNOSIS

- ► Fever.
- ► Irritative voiding symptoms.
- ► Perineal or suprapubic pain; exquisite tenderness common on rectal examination.
- ► Positive urine culture.

General Considerations

Acute bacterial prostatitis is usually caused by gram-negative rods, especially *E coli* and *Pseudomonas* species, and less commonly by gram-positive organisms (eg, enterococci). The most likely routes of infection include ascent up the urethra and reflux of infected urine into the prostatic ducts. Lymphatic and hematogenous routes are probably rare.

Clinical Findings

A. Symptoms and Signs

Perineal, sacral, or suprapubic pain, fever, and irritative voiding complaints are common. Varying degrees of obstructive symptoms may occur as the acutely inflamed prostate swells, which may lead to urinary retention. High fevers and a warm and often exquisitely tender prostate are detected on examination. Care should be taken to perform a gentle rectal examination, since vigorous manipulations may result in septicemia. Prostatic massage is contraindicated.

B. Laboratory Findings

Complete blood count shows leukocytosis and a left shift. Urinalysis shows pyuria, bacteriuria, and varying degrees of hematuria. Urine cultures will demonstrate the offending pathogen (Table 23–2).

C. Imaging

Acute prostatitis can progress to prostatic abscess and a pelvic CT or transrectal ultrasound is indicated in patients who do not respond to antibiotics in 24–48 hours.

Differential Diagnosis

Acute pyelonephritis or acute epididymitis should be distinguishable by the location of pain as well as by physical examination. Acute diverticulitis is occasionally confused with acute prostatitis; however, the history and urinalysis should permit clear distinction. Urinary retention from benign or malignant prostatic enlargement is distinguishable by initial or follow-up rectal examination and postvoid residual bladder scan.

Table 23–2. Clinical characteristics of prostatitis and chronic pelvic pain syndrome.

Findings	Acute Bacterial Prostatitis	Chronic Bacterial Prostatitis	Chronic Nonbacterial Prostatitis	Chronic Pelvic Pain Syndrome
Fever	+	–	–	–
Urinalysis	+	–	–	–
Expressed prostate secretions	Contraindicated	+ WBC + Culture	+ WBC – Culture	– WBC – Culture
Postprostatic massage urine specimen	Contraindicated	+ Culture	– Culture	– Culture

WBC, white blood cell.

Treatment

Hospitalization may be required, and parenteral antibiotics (ampicillin and aminoglycoside) should be initiated until organism sensitivities are available (Table 23–1). After the patient is afebrile for 24–48 hours, oral antibiotics (eg, quinolones if organism is sensitive) are used to complete 4–6 weeks of therapy. If urinary retention develops, an in-and-out catheterization to relieve the initial obstruction or short-term (12 hours) small indwelling urinary catheter is appropriate.

Prognosis

Acute bacterial prostatitis is relatively simple to treat, since bacteria are eradicated with appropriate antibiotic therapy. Progression to chronic bacterial prostatitis is rare.

When to Refer

- Evidence of urinary retention.
- Evidence of chronic prostatitis.

When to Admit

- Signs of sepsis.
- Need for surgical drainage of bladder or prostatic abscess.

Coker TJ et al. Acute bacterial prostatitis: diagnosis and management. Am Fam Physician. 2016 Jan;93(2):114–20. [PMID: 26926407]

Gill BC. Bacterial prostatitis. Curr Opin Infect Dis. 2016 Feb; 29 (1):86–91. [PMID: 26555038]

Khan FU et al. Comprehensive overview of prostatitis. Biomed Pharmacother. 2017 Oct;94:1064–76. [PMID: 28813783]

Schaeffer AJ et al. Clinical Practice. Urinary tract infections in older men. N Engl J Med. 2016 Feb 11;374(6):562–71. [PMID: 26863357]

4. Chronic Bacterial Prostatitis

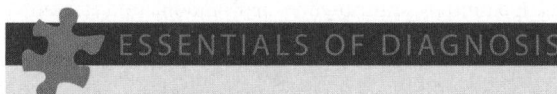
ESSENTIALS OF DIAGNOSIS

- ▶ Irritative voiding symptoms.
- ▶ Perineal or suprapubic discomfort, often dull and poorly localized.
- ▶ Positive expressed prostatic secretions and culture.

General Considerations

Although chronic bacterial prostatitis may evolve from acute bacterial prostatitis or recurrent urinary tract infection, over half of affected men have no history of acute infection. Gram-negative rods are the most common etiologic agents, but only one gram-positive organism (*Enterococcus*) is associated with chronic infection. Routes of infection are the same as discussed for acute infection.

Clinical Findings

A. Symptoms and Signs

Clinical manifestations are variable. Most patients have varying degrees of irritative voiding symptoms, urethral pain, and obstructive urinary symptoms. Low back and perineal pain are common. Many patients (25–43%) report a history of urinary tract infections. Physical examination is often unremarkable, although the prostate may feel normal, boggy, or indurated. A postvoid residual urine volume should be measured to evaluate for urinary retention.

B. Laboratory Findings

Urinalysis is normal unless a secondary cystitis is present. Expressed prostatic secretions or a postprostatic massage voided urine or both demonstrate increased numbers of leukocytes (greater than 5–10 per high-power field) and bacterial growth when cultured (Table 23–2). Culture of the secretions and the postprostatic massage urine specimen is necessary to make the diagnosis. Leukocyte and bacterial counts from expressed prostatic secretions do not correlate with severity of symptoms. If no organisms are identified on culture, then nonbacterial prostatitis, chronic pelvic pain, or interstitial cystitis should be suspected.

C. Imaging

Imaging tests are typically not necessary.

Differential Diagnosis

Chronic urethritis may mimic chronic prostatitis, though cultures of the fractionated urine may localize the source of infection to the initial specimen, which would come from the urethra. Cystitis may be secondary to prostatitis, but urine samples after prostatic massage may localize the infection to the prostate. Other chronic prostatic conditions, such as nonbacterial prostatitis, chronic pelvic pain, or interstitial cystitis, are distinguished from chronic bacterial prostatitis by examination and culture of prostatic secretions and postprostatic massage urine sample. Anal disease may share some of the symptoms of prostatitis, but physical examination should distinguish between the two.

Treatment

As in acute prostatitis, if patients are febrile or systemically ill, they may require admission and initial intravenous therapy with broad-spectrum antibiotics, such as ampicillin plus gentamicin, a third-generation cephalosporin, or a fluoroquinolone (Table 23–1). Therapy would then continue with oral trimethoprim-sulfamethoxazole, fluoroquinolones, or an extended-spectrum beta-lactamase antibiotic based on culture and sensitivities of expressed prostatic secretion or postprostatic massage urine. The optimal duration of therapy remains controversial, ranging from 4 to 6 weeks. Symptomatic relief may be provided by anti-inflammatory agents (indomethacin, ibuprofen), hot sitz baths, and alphablockers (tamsulosin, alfuzosin, silodosin).

Prognosis

Chronic bacterial prostatitis may be recurrent, can be difficult to cure, and often requires repeated courses of therapeutic antibiotics.

When to Refer

- Persistent symptoms.
- Consideration of enrollment in clinical trials.

Holt JD et al. Common questions about chronic prostatitis. Am Fam Physician. 2016 Feb 15;93(4):290–6. [PMID: 26926816]

Khan FU et al. Comprehensive overview of prostatitis. Biomed Pharmacother. 2017 Oct;94:1064–76. [PMID: 28813783]

Schaeffer AJ et al. Clinical Practice. Urinary tract infections in older men. N Engl J Med. 2016 Feb 11;374(6):562–71. [PMID: 26863357]

Zaidi N et al. Management of chronic prostatitis. Curr Urol Rep. 2018 Aug 31;19(11):88. [PMID: 30167899]

5. Nonbacterial Chronic Prostatitis/Chronic Pelvic Pain Syndrome

ESSENTIALS OF DIAGNOSIS

- ▶ Irritative voiding symptoms.
- ▶ Perineal or suprapubic discomfort, similar to that of chronic bacterial prostatitis.
- ▶ Presence of white blood cells in expressed prostatic secretions but negative culture.

General Considerations

Nonbacterial chronic prostatitis and chronic pelvic pain syndromes are caused by an interrelated cascade of inflammatory, immunologic, endocrine, muscular, neuropathic, and psychologic mechanisms. There are a variety of subtypes based on the most pronounced symptoms. Chronic perineal, suprapubic, or pelvic pain is the most common presenting symptom, though men may complain of pain in the testes, groin, and low back. Pain during or after ejaculation is one of the most prominent and bothersome symptoms in many patients. Psychosocial factors (depression, anxiety, catastrophizing, poor social support, stress) also likely play an important role in the exacerbation of chronic pelvic pain symptoms. Because the cause of nonbacterial prostatitis remains unknown, the diagnosis is usually one of exclusion, and treatment may require multimodal therapy. Quality of life is greatly decreased for many patients with chronic nonbacterial prostatitis and chronic pelvic pain syndrome.

Clinical Findings

A. Symptoms and Signs

The clinical presentation is identical to that of chronic bacterial prostatitis; however, no history of urinary tract infections is typically present. The National Institutes of Health Chronic Prostatitis Symptom Index (NIH-CPSI) (www.prostatitisclinic.com/graphics/questionnaire2.pdf) has been validated to quantify symptoms of chronic nonbacterial prostatitis or chronic pelvic pain syndrome.

B. Laboratory Findings

Increased numbers of leukocytes are typically seen in expressed prostatic secretions, but cultures of both expressed prostatic secretions and postprostatic urine specimens are negative.

Differential Diagnosis

The major distinction is from chronic bacterial prostatitis. The absence of positive cultures makes the distinction (Table 23–2). In older men with irritative voiding symptoms and negative cultures, bladder cancer must be excluded. Urinary cytologic examination and cystoscopy are warranted.

Treatment

Multimodal therapy is recommended according to the various phenotypes of patient presentation. Patients with voiding symptoms are treated with an alpha-blocker (tamsulosin, alfuzosin, silodosin). Antibiotics are used to treat newly diagnosed, antimicrobial-naive patients. Psychosocial disorders are treated with cognitive behavioral therapy, antidepressants, anxiolytics, and, if necessary, referral to mental health specialists. Neuropathic pain is treated with gabapentinoids, amitriptyline, neuromodulation, acupuncture, or, if necessary, referral to a pain management specialist. Pelvic floor muscle dysfunction may respond to diazepam, biofeedback techniques, pelvic floor physical therapy (eg, kegel exercises), pelvic shock wave lithotripsy, and heat therapy. Sexual dysfunction with pain symptoms is treated with sexual therapy and phosphodiesterase-5 inhibitors (eg, sildenafil, tadalafil, vardenafil). Surgery is not recommended for chronic prostatitis.

Prognosis

Annoying, recurrent symptoms are common, but serious sequelae have not been identified.

Franco JV et al. Non-pharmacological interventions for treating chronic prostatitis/chronic pelvic pain syndrome. Cochrane Database Syst Rev. 2018 Jan 26;1:CD012551. Update in: Cochrane Database Syst Rev 2018 May 12;5:CD012551. [PMID: 29372565]

Holt JD et al. Common questions about chronic prostatitis. Am Fam Physician. 2016 Feb;93(4):290–6. [PMID: 26926816]

Kaplan SA, McVary KT (editors). *Male Lower Urinary Tract Symptoms and Benign Prostatic Hyperplasia,* 1st ed. Wiley-Blackwell; Hoboken, NJ, 2014.

Magistro G et al. Contemporary management of chronic prostatitis/chronic pelvic pain syndrome. Eur Urol. 2016 Feb;69(2):286–97. [PMID: 26411805]

Polackwich AS et al. Chronic prostatitis/chronic pelvic pain syndrome: a review of evaluation and therapy. Prostate Cancer Prostatic Dis. 2016 Jun;19(2):132–8. [PMID: 26951713]

Sandhu J et al. Recent advances in managing chronic prostatitis/chronic pelvic pain syndrome. F1000Res. 2017 Sep 25;6. [PMID: 29034074]

6. Acute Epididymitis

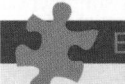

ESSENTIALS OF DIAGNOSIS

- ► Fever.
- ► Irritative voiding symptoms.
- ► Painful enlargement of epididymis.

General Considerations

Most cases of acute epididymitis are infectious and can be divided into one of two categories that have different age distributions and etiologic agents. **Sexually transmitted forms** typically occur in men under age 35 years, are associated with urethritis, and result from *Chlamydia trachomatis* or *Neisseria gonorrhoeae.* **Men who practice insertive anal intercourse** may have acute epididymitis from sexually transmitted and enteric organisms. **Non–sexually transmitted forms** typically occur in men age 35 years and older, are associated with urinary tract infections and prostatitis, and are caused by enteric gram-negative rods. The route of infection is probably via the urethra to the ejaculatory duct and then down the vas deferens to the epididymis. Amiodarone has been associated with self-limited epididymitis, which is a dose-dependent phenomenon.

Clinical Findings

A. Symptoms and Signs

Symptoms may follow chronic dysfunctional voiding, urinary retention, sexual activity, or trauma. Associated symptoms of urethritis (pain at the tip of the penis and urethral discharge) or cystitis (irritative voiding symptoms) may occur. Pain develops in the scrotum and may radiate along the spermatic cord or to the flank. Scrotal swelling and tenderness are usually apparent. Severe cases may develop systemic symptoms such as fever. Early in the course, the epididymis may be distinguishable from the testis; however, later the two may appear as one enlarged, tender mass. A reactive hydrocele may develop. The prostate may be tender on rectal examination.

B. Laboratory Findings

A complete blood count shows leukocytosis and a left shift. In the sexually transmitted variety, Gram staining of a smear of urethral discharge may be diagnostic of gram-negative intracellular diplococci *(N gonorrhoeae).* White cells without visible organisms on urethral smear represent nongonococcal urethritis, and *C trachomatis* is the most likely pathogen. In the non-sexually transmitted variety, urinalysis shows pyuria, bacteriuria, and varying degrees of hematuria. Urine cultures will demonstrate the offending pathogen.

C. Imaging

Scrotal ultrasound may aid in the diagnosis if examination is difficult because of the presence of a large hydrocele or because questions exist regarding the diagnosis.

Differential Diagnosis

Tumors generally cause painless enlargement of the testis. Urinalysis is negative, and examination reveals a normal epididymis. Scrotal ultrasound is helpful to define the pathology. Testicular torsion usually occurs in prepubertal males but is occasionally seen in young adults. Acute onset of symptoms and a negative urinalysis favor testicular torsion or torsion of one of the testicular or epididymal appendages. Prehn sign (elevation of the scrotum improves pain from epididymitis) may be helpful but is not reliable. A distal ureteral stone often presents with referred pain into the ipsilateral groin and scrotum, but the scrotum is not tender to palpation and a scrotal ultrasound is normal.

Treatment

Bed rest, ice, and scrotal elevation are important in the acute phase. Treatment is directed toward the identified pathogen (Table 23–1). The sexually transmitted variety in patients under age 35 is treated with an intramuscular injection of ceftriaxone 250 mg plus 10 days of oral doxycycline 100 mg four times daily; any sexual partners from the preceding 60 days must be evaluated and treated as well. Men who practice insertive anal intercourse receive an intramuscular injection of ceftriaxone 250 mg and 10 days of an oral fluoroquinolone (eg, ciprofloxacin 500 mg twice daily) to cover sexually transmitted and enteric organisms. Non–sexually transmitted forms are treated for 10 days with a fluoroquinolone, at which time evaluation of the urinary tract is warranted to identify underlying disease. Symptoms and signs of epididymitis that do not subside within 3 days require re-evaluation of the diagnosis and therapy.

Prognosis

Prompt treatment usually results in a favorable outcome. If significant scrotal swelling has developed, this may take 4 weeks to resolve. Delayed or inadequate treatment may result in epididymo-orchitis, decreased fertility, or abscess formation.

When to Refer

- Persistent symptoms and infection despite antibiotic therapy.
- Signs of sepsis or abscess formation.

Centers for Disease Control and Prevention. 2015 Sexually Transmitted Disease Treatment Guidelines: Epididymitis. 2015 Jun 4. https://www.cdc.gov/std/tg2015/epididymitis.htm

McConaghy JR et al. Epididymitis: an overview. Am Fam Physician. 2016 Nov 1;94(9):723–6. [PMID: 27929243]

Srinath H. Acute scrotal pain. Aust Fam Physician. 2013 Nov; 42(11):790–2. [PMID: 24217099]

INTERSTITIAL CYSTITIS

ESSENTIALS OF DIAGNOSIS

- ► Pain with bladder filling; urinary urgency and frequency.
- ► Submucosal petechiae or ulcers on cystoscopic examination.
- ► Diagnosis of exclusion.

General Considerations

Interstitial cystitis (painful bladder syndrome) is characterized by pain with bladder filling that is relieved by emptying and is often associated with urgency and frequency with a dramatic exaggeration of normal sensations. This is a diagnosis of exclusion, and patients must have a negative urine culture and cytology and no other obvious cause such as radiation cystitis, chemical cystitis (cyclophosphamide), vaginitis, urethral diverticulum, or genital herpes. Up to 40% of patients referred to urologists for interstitial cystitis may actually be found to have a different diagnosis after careful evaluation. What was once considered a bladder disorder is now considered a chronic pain syndrome.

Population-based studies have demonstrated a prevalence of between 18 and 40 per 100,000 people. Both sexes are involved, but most patients are women, with a mean age of 40 years at onset. Patients with interstitial cystitis are more likely to report bladder problems in childhood, and there appears to be a higher prevalence of these in women. Up to 50% of patients may experience spontaneous remission of symptoms, with a mean duration of 8 months without treatment.

The etiology of interstitial cystitis is unknown, and it is most likely not a single disease but rather several diseases with similar symptoms. Associated diseases include severe allergies, irritable bowel syndrome, or inflammatory bowel disease. Theories regarding the cause of interstitial cystitis include increased epithelial permeability, neurogenic causes (sensory nervous system abnormalities), and autoimmunity.

Clinical Findings

A. Symptoms and Signs

Pain, pressure, or discomfort with bladder filling that is relieved with urination, and urgency, frequency, and nocturia are the most common symptoms. Patients should be asked about exposure to pelvic radiation or treatment with cyclophosphamide. Examination should exclude genital herpes, vaginitis, or a urethral diverticulum.

B. Laboratory Findings

Urinalysis, urine culture, and urinary cytologies are obtained to examine for infectious causes and bladder malignancy; in interstitial cystitis, they are all normal. Urodynamic testing can be done to assess bladder sensation and compliance and to exclude detrusor instability.

C. Cystoscopy

The bladder is distended with fluid (hydrodistention) to detect glomerulations (submucosal hemorrhage), which may or may not be present. Biopsy should be performed to exclude other causes such as carcinoma, eosinophilic cystitis, and tuberculous cystitis. The presence of submucosal mast cells is *not* needed to make the diagnosis of interstitial cystitis.

Differential Diagnosis

Exposures to radiation or cyclophosphamide are discovered by the history. Bacterial cystitis, genital herpes, or vaginitis can be excluded by urinalysis, culture, and physical examination. A urethral diverticulum may be suspected if palpation of the urethra demonstrates an indurated mass that results in the expression of pus from the urethral meatus. Urethral carcinoma presents as a firm mass on palpation.

Treatment

There is no cure for interstitial cystitis, but most patients achieve symptomatic relief from one of several approaches, including hydrodistention, which is usually done as part of the diagnostic evaluation. Approximately 20–30% of patients notice symptomatic improvement following this maneuver. Also of importance is the measurement of bladder capacity during hydrodistention, since patients with very small bladder capacities (less than 200 mL) are unlikely to respond to medical therapy.

Amitriptyline (10–75 mg/day orally) is often used as first-line medical therapy in patients with interstitial cystitis. Both central and peripheral mechanisms may contribute to its activity. Nifedipine (30–60 mg/day orally) and other calcium channel blockers have also demonstrated some activity in patients with interstitial cystitis. Pentosan polysulfate sodium (Elmiron) is an oral synthetic sulfated polysaccharide that helps restore integrity to the epithelium of the bladder in a subset of patients and has been evaluated in a placebo-controlled trial. Other options include intravesical instillation of dimethyl sulfoxide

(DMSO) and heparin. Intravesical bacillus Calmette-Guérin (BCG) is not beneficial.

Further treatment modalities include transcutaneous electric nerve stimulation (TENS), acupuncture, stress reduction, exercise, biofeedback, massage, and pelvic floor relaxation. Surgical therapy for interstitial cystitis should be considered only as a last resort and may require cysto-urethrectomy with urinary diversion.

► When to Refer

Persistent and bothersome symptoms in the absence of identifiable cause.

Cox A et al. CUA guideline: diagnosis and treatment of intersti-tial cystitis/bladder pain syndrome. Can Urol Assoc J. 2016 May–Jun;10(5-6):E136–55. [PMID: 27790294]

Giusto LL et al. An evaluation of the pharmacotherapy for inter-stitial cystitis. Expert Opin Pharmacother. 2018 Jul;19(10):1097–108. [PMID: 29972328]

Hanno PM et al; American Urological Association. Diagnosis and treatment of interstitial cystitis/bladder pain syndrome: AUA guideline amendment. J Urol. 2015 May;193(5):1545–53. [PMID: 25623737]

Patanaik SS et al. Etiology, pathophysiology and biomarkers of interstitial cystitis/painful bladder syndrome. Arch Gynecol Obstet. 2017 Jun;295(6):1341–59. [PMID: 28391486]

Rawls WF et al. Dimethyl sulfoxide (DMSO) as intravesical therapy for interstitial cystitis/bladder pain syndrome: a review. Neurourol Urodyn. 2017 Sep;36(7):1677–84. [PMID: 28220525]

Zhang W et al. Intravesical treatment of interstitial cystitis/painful bladder syndrome: a network meta-analysis. Int Urogynecol J. 2017 Apr;28(4):515–25. [PMID: 27614759]

URINARY STONE DISEASE

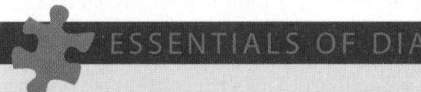

ESSENTIALS OF DIAGNOSIS

► Severe flank pain.

► Nausea and vomiting.

► Identification on noncontrast CT or ultrasonography.

► General Considerations

Urinary stone disease is exceeded in frequency as a uri-nary tract disorder only by infections and prostatic dis-ease. It is estimated to afflict 240,000–720,000 Americans per year. The prevalence of kidney stones has increased to 8.8%, or 1 in 11 Americans, representing a 70% increase over the last 15 years. While men are more frequently affected by urolithiasis than women, with a ratio of 1.5:1, the prevalence of stones in women is increasing. Initial presentation usually occurs in the third through fifth decades, and more than 50% of patients will become recurrent stone formers.

Urinary calculi are polycrystalline aggregates composed of varying amounts of crystalloid and a small amount of organic matrix. Stone formation requires saturated urine that is dependent on solute concentration, ionic strength,

pH, and complexation. There are five major types of uri-nary stones: **calcium oxalate**, **calcium phosphate**, **struvite** (magnesium ammonium phosphate), **uric acid**, and **cystine.** The most common types are those composed of calcium oxalate or phosphate (85%), and for that reason most uri-nary stones are radiopaque on plain abdominal radio-graphs. Although pure uric acid stones are radiolucent, uric acid stones are frequently composed of a combination of uric acid and calcium oxalate and thus may be radio-paque. Cystine stones frequently have a smooth-edged ground-glass appearance and are radiolucent.

Geographic factors contribute to the development of stones. High humidity and elevated temperatures appear to be contributing factors, and the incidence of symptomatic ureteral stones is greatest in such areas during hot summer months. Higher incidence rates of stones have also been associated with sedentary lifestyle, obesity, hypertension, insulin resistance and poor glycemic control, carotid calci-fication, and cardiovascular disease.

Many commonly prescribed medications increase the risk of formation of kidney stones, including carbonic anhydrase inhibitors (topiramate, zonisamide, acetazol-amide), systemic corticosteroids (prednisone), antiretrovi-ral protease inhibitors (indinavir), gout medications (probenecid), diuretics (furosemide, bumetanide, torse-mide, triamterene), decongestants (guaifenesin, ephed-rine), and laxatives (if abused for weight loss). The risk of stones from calcium supplementation is controversial. Thus, if calcium supplementation is medically necessary, it is recommended that the calcium supplement be taken with meals, and restricted to no more than 2000 mg of total calcium intake daily (including dietary sources).

Inadequate hydration is another very important dietary factor in the development of urinary stones. Finally, high protein and salt intake as well as restricted dietary calcium intake are other important risk factors.

Genetic factors may contribute to urinary stone forma-tion. While approximately 50% of calcium-based stones are thought to have a heritable component, other stone types are better characterized genetically. For example, cystinuria is an autosomal recessive disorder. Homozygous individuals have markedly increased excretion of cystine and frequently have numerous recurrent episodes of urinary stones. Distal renal tubular acidosis may be transmitted as a hereditary trait, and urolithiasis occurs in up to 75% of affected patients.

► Clinical Findings

A. Symptoms and Signs

Obstructing urinary stones usually present with acute, unremitting, and severe colic. Pain most often occurs sud-denly and may awaken patients from sleep. It is typically localized to the flank and may be associated with nausea and vomiting. In sharp contrast to patients with an acute abdomen, patients with kidney stones are constantly mov-ing trying to find a comfortable position. The pain may occur episodically and may radiate anteriorly over the abdomen. As the stone progresses down the ureter, the pain may be referred into the ipsilateral groin. If the stone becomes lodged at the uretero-vesicular junction, patients may complain of marked urinary urgency and frequency and in men, pain may radiate to the tip of the penis. After the stone passes into the bladder, there typically is minimal pain with passage through the urethra. Stone size does not correlate with the severity of the symptoms. If the stone fails to pass and obstruction persists, patients will often have a marked decrease in discomfort. As many as 25% of patients with resolution of pain will have a persistent stone and thus follow-up imaging is recommended in all patients if the stone has not been witnessed to pass.

B. Laboratory Findings

Regardless of symptom severity, urinalysis usually reveals microscopic or gross hematuria (~90%). However, the absence of microhematuria does not exclude urinary stones. Urinary pH may provide a valuable clue to the possible stone type. Normal urinary pH is 5.8–6.2, and persistent urinary pH < 5.5 is suggestive of uric acid stones. In contrast, a persistent urinary pH > 7.2 is suggestive of a struvite (infection-related) stone and pH > 7.5, a calcium phosphate stone. Patients with calcium oxalate–based stones typically have a normal urinary pH.

C. Metabolic Evaluation

Stone analysis on recovered stones can facilitate counseling for prevention of recurrence. Patients with uncomplicated first-time stones should undergo dietary counseling as outlined below and can be offered an optional complete metabolic evaluation.

General dietary counseling includes encouraging patients to augment their fluid intake to increase their urine volume (goal urinary output = 2.5 L/day). This typically requires a fluid intake of 3 L/day or more. Stone formers should reduce their sodium intake (goal less than or equal to 3500 mg/day), and reduce their animal protein intake (eggs, fish, chicken, pork, and beef). Detailed medical and dietary history, serum chemistries, and urinalysis should be obtained for all patients with newly diagnosed nephrolithiasis. A 24-hour urine collection to determine urinary volume, creatinine, pH, calcium, uric acid, oxalate, phosphate, sodium, and citrate excretion is recommended for interested patients with their first stone, for all patients who have recurrent stones, and for patients at high risk for recurrence. Results are used to personalize medical management to individual patient risk factors. In addition, a serum parathyroid hormone level should be checked when hyperparathyroidism is suspected and a serum uric acid should be obtained to exclude severe hyperuricemia, which can lead to crystal deposition in the kidneys or heart.

D. Imaging

A plain abdominal radiograph (kidney, ureter, and bladder [KUB]) and renal ultrasound examination will diagnose up to 80% of stones. Since more than 60% of patients with acute renal colic will have a stone in the distal 4 cm of the ureter, attention should be directed to that region when examining radiographs and ultrasonographic studies. Noncontrast CT is the most accurate imaging modality for evaluating flank pain given its increased sensitivity and specificity over other tests; however, ultrasonography

(which is devoid of ionizing radiation) is a safe and effective alternative for initial evaluation of renal colic and one that can be used in the emergency department with good accuracy. If CT scan is used, it should be obtained in the prone position to help differentiate distal ureterovesicular stones from those that have already passed into the urinary bladder. A "low-dose" imaging protocol should be used when available and repeated CT scans should be minimized due to the substantial cumulative radiation exposure that patients with recurrent stones can face. Stone density can be estimated with Hounsfield units (HU) on CT scans to help determine stone type. All stones, whether radiopaque or radiolucent on plain abdominal radiographs, will be visible on noncontrast CT except the rare protease inhibitor calculus (with indinavir). Pain from a kidney stone is due to the dilatation of the ureter and kidney from the obstruction, and thus small nonobstructing kidney stones are typically not associated with pain.

▶ Medical Treatment & Prevention

To reduce the recurrence rate of urinary stones, dietary modification is important. Metabolic evaluation often identifies a modifiable risk factor that can further reduce stone recurrence rates. If no medical treatment is provided, stones will generally recur in 50% of patients within 5 years. Some stone types (eg, uric acid, cystine) are more prone to rapid recurrence than others. An increased fluid intake is of greatest importance in reducing stone recurrence. Increasing fluid intake to ensure a voided volume of 2.5 L/day is recommended (normal average voided volume is 1.6 L/day). Urine should be clear or light yellow at each void. Medical therapy should be tailored to the patient's metabolic workup and the activity of their stone disease. Routine follow-up every 6–8 months and annual imaging (preferably with ultrasonography) will help encourage medical compliance, assess for interval stone formation or growth, and permit adjustments in medical therapy based on repeat metabolic studies.

A. General Dietary Recommendations

A 24-hour urinary sodium level of greater than 150 mmol/day indicates excessive sodium intake. **Sodium intake** should be limited to less than 3500 mg daily. Excessive sodium intake will increase renal sodium and calcium excretion, increase urinary monosodium urates (that can act as a nidus for stone growth), increase the relative saturation of calcium phosphate, and decrease urinary citrate excretion. All of these factors encourage stone growth.

A urinary sulfate level of greater than 20 mEq/day indicates excessive animal protein intake. **Animal protein intake** should be spread out through the day, not all consumed during any individual meal, and is best limited to 1 g/kg/day. An increased protein load during an individual meal can lead to acidic urine and also increases calcium, oxalate, and uric acid excretion and decrease urinary citrate excretion.

Dietary calcium intake should not be restricted in an effort to decrease stone formation because it may paradoxically lead to increased stone formation due to increased oxalate absorption and consequent hyperoxaluria.

B. Calcium Nephrolithiasis

1. Hypercalciuria—Elevated urinary calcium levels (greater than 4 mg/kg/day or greater than 250 mg/day for males and greater than 200 mg/day for females) lead to hypercalciuric calcium nephrolithiasis. Hypercalciuria can be caused by absorptive, resorptive, and renal disorders. The categorization system provided below was proposed in the 1970s and provides a simplified explanation of the causes of hypercalciuria; however, it is not routinely used in clinical practice. Thiazide diuretics decrease renal calcium excretion; after primary hyperparathyroidism has been excluded, thiazide diuretics should be offered to patients with high urinary calcium and recurrent calcium stones. Chlorthalidone and indapamide are first-line agents since they can be administered once a day, while hydrochlorothiazide for hypercalciuria should be administered twice a day. All patients respond to thiazide diuretics with decreases in urinary calcium unless they have primary hyperparathyroidism or are nonadherent with taking the medication. Clinicians should periodically test patients taking thiazide diuretics for hypokalemia, since they may require potassium supplementation.

Absorptive hypercalciuria is secondary to increased absorption of calcium at the level of the small bowel, predominantly in the jejunum, and can be further subdivided into types I, II, and III.

Type I absorptive hypercalciuria is independent of calcium intake. There is increased urinary calcium on a regular or even a calcium-restricted diet. Historic studies have reported that thiazides may have limited long-term utility (less than 5 years) in this subgroup.

Type II absorptive hypercalciuria is diet-dependent and fortunately rare. Decreasing calcium intake by 50% (approximately 400 mg/day) will decrease the hypercalciuria to normal values (150–200 mg/24 h). There is no specific medical therapy. In the past, type I and type II absorptive hypercalciuria were distinguished by using an oral calcium load test; however, this is no longer routinely performed in clinical practice.

Type III absorptive hypercalciuria is secondary to a renal phosphate leak. This results in increased vitamin D synthesis and secondarily increased small bowel absorption of calcium. This can be readily reversed by orthophosphates (250 mg orally three to four times per day), presently available without need for a prescription. Orthophosphates do not change intestinal absorption but rather inhibit vitamin D synthesis.

Resorptive hypercalciuria is secondary to hyperparathyroidism. Hypercalcemia, hypophosphatemia, elevated serum parathyroid hormone, and urinary hypercalciuria are present. Appropriate surgical resection of the parathyroid adenoma is curative in 75% of patients with kidney stones and primary hyperparathyroidism. Medical management is typically reserved for patients who are elderly or frail.

Renal hypercalciuria is the most common form of hypercalciuria and occurs when the renal tubules are unable to efficiently reabsorb filtered calcium. Spilling calcium in the urine may result in secondary hyperparathyroidism with normal serum calcium. A thiazide diuretic is an effective long-term therapy in patients with this disorder because it corrects the urinary calcium losses and is associated with an increase in bone mineral density of approximately 1% per year while receiving therapy.

2. Hyperuricosuria—Hyperuricosuric calcium nephrolithiasis is defined by elevated urinary uric acid levels (greater than 800 mg/day for males and greater than 750 mg/day for females). It is usually secondary to dietary purine excess or endogenous uric acid metabolic defects. Excess uric acid in the urine can lead to uric acid stones if the urine pH is low, or to calcium stones at higher urine pH due to formation of a monosodium urate crystal that then calcifies in a process known as heterogenous nucleation. Dietary purine restriction can reduce hyperuricosuria in 85% of cases. Patients with hyperuricosuria, normocalciuria, and recurrent calcium oxalate stones can be successfully treated with allopurinol.

3. Hyperoxaluria—Hyperoxaluric calcium nephrolithiasis (greater than 40 mg/day of urinary oxalate) is usually due to either an intestinal malabsorption disorder or a mismatch in dietary calcium and oxalate intake. When dietary calcium and oxalate intake are consumed concurrently, they are unable to be absorbed systemically as they are bound together in the intestinal tract. If dietary calcium is restricted, or dietary oxalate is excessive, free oxalate is rapidly absorbed and excreted in the urine. Treatment includes adhering to a diet containing moderate calcium intake (1000–1200 mg daily) and avoiding high-oxalate-containing foods. Low-dose calcium carbonate (250 mg) can be consumed with meals if dietary calcium increases do not successfully reach 1000 mg daily. Patients with a history of chronic diarrhea, inflammatory bowel disease, malabsorption, supplement use, or gastric bypass surgery are also at risk for hyperoxaluria. In these situations, increased intestinal fat or bile (or both) combine with calcium to form a soap-like product. Calcium is therefore unavailable to bind to oxalate, leading to free oxalate absorption. A small increase in oxalate absorption significantly increases stone formation. If the diarrhea or steatorrhea cannot be effectively curtailed, oral calcium should be increased with meals, either by ingesting dairy products or taking low-dose calcium carbonate supplements (250 mg). Excess ascorbic acid (greater than 2000 mg/day) will substantially increase urinary oxalate levels. Rare enzymatic liver defects can lead to primary hyperoxaluria that is routinely fatal without a combined liver and kidney transplantation.

4. Hypocitraturia—Urinary citrate is the most important inhibitor of stone formation, and citrate levels less than 450 mg/day increase the risk of stones. Urinary citrate binds to calcium in solution, thereby decreasing available calcium for precipitation and subsequent stone formation. **Hypocitraturic calcium nephrolithiasis** is usually idiopathic. Urinary citrate excretion is influenced by systemic acid-base balance and serum potassium levels, and thus, hypocitraturia occurs secondary to any metabolic acidemia (chronic diarrhea, distal renal tubular acidosis), or with systemic potassium losses (long-term treatment with thiazide or loop diuretics). Metabolic acidosis enhances citrate transport into the proximal tubular cells where it is consumed by the citric acid cycle in their mitochondria. Potassium citrate supplements (eg, Urocit-K™) are usually effective treatment in these situations; a typical dose is 40–60 mEq total daily intake, divided either into two or three daily doses. Alternatively, oral lemonade has been shown to increase urinary citrate by about 150 mg/24 h.

C. Uric Acid Calculi

Urinary pH is the most important contributor to uric acid stone formation, and thus efforts should focus on alkalinizing the urine as first-line therapy (oral potassium citrate or sodium bicarbonate), while efforts to decrease urinary uric acid (allopurinol) should be reserved for patients continuing to form stones despite adequate urinary alkalinization. Urine pH is consistently less than 5.5 in patients who form pure uric acid stones. Increasing the urinary pH dramatically increases uric acid solubility, leading to prevention of stone formation (urine pH over 6.0) and even stone dissolution (urine pH over 6.5). Nitrazine pH test strips are often useful to some patients in reinforcing adherence to urinary alkalinization efforts. Less common contributors to uric acid stone formation include hyperuricemia, myeloproliferative disorders, chemotherapy for malignancies with rapid cell turnover or cell death, abrupt and dramatic weight loss, and uricosuric medications (probenecid). If hyperuricemia is present or the patient has a history of recurrent gout, in addition to hyperuricosuria, allopurinol (300 mg/day orally) may be given for stone prevention.

D. Struvite Calculi

Struvite stones are composed of magnesium-ammonium-phosphate and are typically visible on plain radiographs. They are most common in women with recurrent urinary tract infections with urease-producing organisms, including *Proteus, Pseudomonas, Providencia,* and, less commonly, *Klebsiella, Staphylococcus,* and *Mycoplasma* (but not *E coli*). They rarely present as a first symptomatic ureteral stone. Frequently, a struvite stone is discovered as a large staghorn calculus forming a cast of the renal collecting system. Urinary pH is high, routinely above 7.2. Struvite stones are relatively soft and amenable to percutaneous removal. Appropriate perioperative antibiotics are required. They can recur rapidly, and efforts should be taken to render the patient stone-free.

E. Cystine Calculi

Cystine stones are caused by a genetic metabolic defect resulting in abnormal excretion of cystine. These stones are exceptionally challenging to manage medically. Prevention is centered around marked increased fluid intake during the day and night to achieve a urinary volume of 3–4 L/day, decrease in sodium and dietary cystine intake, and urinary alkalinization (typically with high-dose potassium citrate) with a goal urinary pH greater than 7.0. Refractory stone formers may be treated with disulfide inhibitors such as tiopronin (alpha-mercaptoproprionylglycine) or penicillamine. There are no known inhibitors of cystine calculi.

▶ Medical Expulsion & Surgical Treatment

In the acute setting, forced intravenous fluids will not push stones down the ureter. Forced diuresis can be counterproductive and exacerbate pain; instead, a euvolemic state should be achieved. Signs of infection, including associated fever, tachycardia, hypotension, and elevated white blood cell count, may indicate a urinary tract infection behind the obstructing stone. Any obstructing stone with associated infection is a **medical emergency** requiring urology consultation and prompt drainage of the kidney with a ureteral stent or a percutaneous nephrostomy tube. Antibiotics alone are inadequate and only used as an adjunct to urinary drainage behind the obstruction.

A. Ureteral Stones

Impediment to urine flow by ureteral stones usually occurs at three sites: the ureteropelvic junction, the crossing of the ureter over the iliac artery, or the ureterovesicular junction. Stones smaller than 5–6 mm in diameter on a plain abdominal radiograph usually pass spontaneously. Medical expulsive therapy with alpha-blockers (such as tamsulosin, 0.4 mg orally once daily) in combination with an anti-inflammatory agent (such as ibuprofen 600 mg orally three times per day), with or without a short course of a low-dose oral corticosteroid (such as prednisone 10 mg orally daily for 5–10 days), may increase the rate of spontaneous stone passage and appears to be most effective for distal stones. Medical expulsive therapy with appropriate pain medications and imaging follow-up is appropriate for a few weeks. If the stone fails to pass within 4 weeks, the patient has fever, intolerable pain, or persistent nausea or vomiting, or the patient must return to work or anticipates travel, then surgical intervention is indicated.

Stones in the mid and distal ureter that require surgical removal are best managed with ureteroscopic stone extraction, though extracorporeal shock wave lithotripsy (SWL) can be offered as second-line therapy. Ureteroscopic stone extraction involves placement of a small endoscope through the urethra, bladder, and into the ureter. Under direct vision, basket extraction or laser fragmentation followed by fragment extraction is performed. A ureteral stent is often placed temporarily to allow drainage of the kidney while the swelling and inflammation from the stone and procedure resolve.

SWL utilizes an external energy source focused on the stone with the aid of fluoroscopy or ultrasonography. SWL is typically performed under anesthesia as an outpatient procedure with the goal of stone fragmentation. Most stone fragments then pass uneventfully within 2 weeks. Occasionally, stone fragments will obstruct the ureter after SWL. Conservative management will usually result in spontaneous resolution with eventual passage of the stone fragments. Fragments that have not passed within 6 weeks are unlikely to do so without intervention.

Proximal ureteral stones—those above the superior margin of the sacroiliac joint—as well as intrarenal stones can be treated with SWL or ureteroscopy. SWL is less successful with larger stones and those that are very dense. After cases of SWL failure, ureteroscopic extraction will be required.

B. Renal Calculi

Patients with asymptomatic, nonobstructing renal calculi, urinary tract infection, or obstruction may not warrant surgical treatment. If surveillance is elected, they should be monitored with serial abdominal radiographs or renal ultrasonographic examinations every 3–12 months. If calculi are growing or become symptomatic, intervention should be undertaken. SWL is most effective for stones less than 1 cm in the lower pole of the kidney or less than 2 cm elsewhere in the kidney. SWL is less effective for stones that are very hard (cystine stones, calcium oxalate stones greater than 1000–1200 Hounsfield units on CT scan) and for obese patients (skin-to-stone distance greater than 10–12 cm). Ureteroscopy and laser lithotripsy is effective for multiple stones and larger stones, though very large stones may require multiple treatment sessions. Stones larger than 15–20 mm and staghorn stones (large branched stones occupying at least two renal calices) are best treated via percutaneous nephrolithotomy. Percutaneous nephrolithotomy is performed by inserting a needle into the appropriate renal calyx and dilating a tract large enough to allow a nephroscope to pass directly into the kidney. In this fashion, larger and more complex renal stones can be inspected, fragmented, and removed. In unusual cases, laparoscopic, robotic-assisted, or open stone removal may be considered. Perioperative antibiotic coverage should be given for any stone procedure, ideally based on preoperative urine culture.

When to Refer

- Evidence of urinary obstruction.
- Urinary stone with associated flank pain.
- Anatomic abnormalities, solitary kidney, or chronic kidney disease.
- Concomitant pyelonephritis or recurrent infection.

When to Admit

- Intractable nausea and vomiting or pain.
- Obstructing stone with fever or other signs of infection.

Assimos D et al. Surgical management of stones: American Urological Association/Endourological Society Guideline, Part I. J Urol. 2016 Oct;196(4):1153–60. [PMID: 27238616]

Gambaro G et al. Metabolic diagnosis and medical prevention of calcium nephrolithiasis and its systemic manifestations: a consensus statement. J Nephrol. 2016 Dec;29(6):715–34. [PMID: 27456839]

Hernandez N et al. Cessation of ureteric colic does not necessarily mean that a ureteral stone has been expelled. J Urol. 2018 Apr;199(4):1011–4. [PMID: 29107030]

Pearle MS et al. Medical management of kidney stones: AUA guideline. J Urol. 2014 Aug;192(2):316–24. [PMID: 24857648]

Pickard R et al. Medical expulsive therapy in adults with ureteric colic: a multicentre, randomised, placebo-controlled trial. Lancet. 2015 Jul 25;386(9991):341–9. [PMID: 25998582]

Rodgers AL. Physicochemical mechanisms of stone formation. Urolithiasis. 2017 Feb;45(1):27–32. [PMID: 27928586]

Scales CD Jr et al; NIDDK Urologic Diseases in America Project. Quality of acute care for patients with urinary stones in the United States. Urology. 2015 Nov;86(5):914–21. [PMID: 26335495]

Smith-Bindman R et al. Ultrasonography versus computed tomography for suspected nephrolithiasis. N Engl J Med. 2014 Sep 18;371(12):1100–10. [PMID: 25229916]

Song L et al. 24-hour urine calcium in the evaluation and management of nephrolithiasis. JAMA. 2017 Aug 1;318(5):474–5. [PMID: 28763529]

Taguchi K et al. Genetic risk factors for idiopathic urolithiasis: a systemic review of the literature and causal network analysis. Eur Urol Focus. 2017 Feb;3(1):72–81. [PMID: 28720371]

MALE ERECTILE DYSFUNCTION & SEXUAL DYSFUNCTION

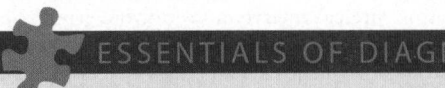

ESSENTIALS OF DIAGNOSIS

- ► Erectile dysfunction can have organic and psychogenic etiologies, and the two frequently overlap.
- ► Organic erectile dysfunction may be an early sign of cardiovascular disease and requires evaluation.
- ► Peyronie disease is a common, benign fibrotic disorder of the penis that causes pain, penile deformity, and sexual dysfunction.

General Considerations

Erectile dysfunction is the consistent inability to attain or maintain a sufficiently rigid penile erection for sexual intercourse. More than half of men aged 40–70 years have erectile dysfunction and its incidence increases with age. Normal male erection is a neurovascular event relying on an intact autonomic and somatic nerve supply to the penis, arterial blood flow supplied by the paired cavernosal arteries, and smooth and striated musculature of the corpora cavernosa and pelvic floor. Erection is initiated by nerve impulses in the pelvic plexus leading to an increase in arterial flow, active relaxation of the smooth muscle within the sinusoids of the corpora cavernosa, and an increase in venous resistance. Contraction of the ischiocavernosus muscle causes further rigidity of the penis with intracavernosal pressures exceeding systolic blood pressure. Nitric oxide is the key neurotransmitter that initiates and sustains erections.

Male sexual dysfunction is manifested in a variety of ways, and patient history is critical to the proper classification and treatment. A **loss of libido** may indicate androgen deficiency. **Loss of erections** may result from neurogenic, arterial, venous, hormonal, or psychogenic causes. Concurrent medical problems may damage one or more of the mechanisms. The most common cause of erectile dysfunction is a decrease in arterial flow resultant from progressive vascular disease. Endothelial dysfunction results from the decreased bioavailability of nitric oxide with subsequent impairment of arterial vasodilation. Erectile dysfunction may be an early manifestation of endothelial dysfunction, which precedes more severe atherosclerotic cardiovascular disease. Many medications, especially antihypertensive, antidepressant, and opioid agents, are associated with erectile dysfunction.

Peyronie disease is a fibrotic disorder of the tunica albuginea of the penis resulting in varying degrees of penile pain, curvature, or deformity. Peyronie disease develops in approximately 5–10% of men and is more common with increased age. While 10% of men improve spontaneously, 50% will stabilize and the remainder will progress if left untreated. Penile deformity can impair normal sexual function and impact self-esteem.

Priapism is the occurrence of penile erection lasting longer than 4 hours resulting in ischemic injury of the corpora cavernosa from venous congestion and cessation of arterial inflow (low flow or "ischemic" priapism). Ischemic priapism is a medical emergency requiring immediate medical or surgical intervention to avoid irreversible penile damage. Ischemic priapism may be caused by red blood cell dyscrasias, drug use, and any of the treatments for erectile dysfunction.

Anejaculation is the loss of seminal emission and may result from androgen deficiency by decreasing prostate and seminal vesicle secretions, or by sympathetic denervation as a result of spinal cord injury, diabetes mellitus or pelvic or retroperitoneal surgery or radiation. **Retrograde ejaculation** may occur as a result of mechanical disruption of the bladder neck, due to congenital abnormalities, transurethral prostate surgery, pelvic radiation, sympathetic denervation, or treatment with alpha-blockers. **Premature ejaculation** is the distressful, recurrent ejaculation with minimal stimulation before a person desires. Primary premature ejaculation may be treated with behavioral modification, sexual health counseling, local anesthetic agents, and systemic medications. Secondary premature ejaculation is due to erectile dysfunction and responds to treatment of the underlying disorder.

▶ Clinical Findings

A. Symptoms and Signs

Erectile dysfunction should be distinguished from problems with penile deformity, libido, orgasm, and ejaculation. The severity, intermittency, and timing of erectile dysfunction should be noted. The history should include inquiries about dyslipidemia, hypertension, depression, neurologic disease, diabetes mellitus, kidney disease, endocrine disorders, and cardiac or peripheral vascular disease. Pelvic trauma, surgery, or irradiation increases a man's likelihood of erectile dysfunction. Histories of prostate cancer treatment or Peyronie disease should be elicited. The ability to attain but not maintain an erection may be the first sign of endothelial dysfunction and further cardiovascular risk stratification should be considered. Medication use should be reviewed. Special attention should be given to the use of nitrate-containing medications. Alcohol, tobacco, marijuana, and other recreational drug use are associated with an increased risk of sexual dysfunction. The use of pornography to maintain sexual arousal should be elicited.

During the physical examination, vital signs, body habitus (obesity), and secondary sexual characteristics should be assessed. Basic cardiovascular and neurologic examinations should be performed. The genitalia should be examined, noting the stretched length of the penis, the presence of Peyronie disease and any abnormalities in size or consistency of either testicle.

B. Laboratory Findings

Laboratory evaluation should be performed in select cases based on patient history and examination. Possible testing includes a lipid profile, glucose, and testosterone. Patients with abnormalities of testosterone may require further evaluation with measurement of free testosterone and luteinizing hormone (LH) to distinguish hypothalamic-pituitary dysfunction from primary testicular failure.

▶ Treatment

Treatment of men suffering from sexual dysfunction should be patient centered and goal oriented. Lifestyle modification and reduction of cardiovascular risk factors are important components of treatment and should include smoking cessation; reduction of alcohol intake; diet; exercise; and treatment of diabetes, dyslipidemia, and hypertension. Men who have a psychogenic component to their erectile dysfunction or who are experiencing emotional distress will benefit from sexual health therapy or counseling.

A. Hormonal Replacement

In men with hypogonadism who have undergone complete endocrinologic evaluation, restoration of normal testosterone levels may improve sexual quality of life (see Male Hypogonadism in Chapter 26.)

B. Vasoactive Therapy

1. Oral agents—Sildenafil, vardenafil, tadalafil, and avanafil inhibit phosphodiesterase type 5 (PDE-5), preventing the degradation of cGMP and increasing blood flow into the penis. These medications are similar but have variable effectiveness in different patients. The medications have variable durations of onset, activity, and side effects. Each medication should be initiated at the lowest dose and titrated to achieve the desired effect. There is no impact on libido and priapism is exceedingly rare. These medications are contraindicated in patients taking nitroglycerin or nitrates, since there may be exaggerated cardiac preload reduction causing hypotension and syncope. All patients being evaluated for acute chest pain should be asked about the use of PDE-5 inhibitors before administering nitroglycerin and close monitoring of blood pressure is warranted if there is concern regarding medication overlap.

The combination of PDE-5 inhibitors and alpha-receptor blockers (prescribed for lower urinary tract symptoms) may cause a larger reduction in systemic blood pressure than when PDE-5 inhibitors are used alone. However, these two classes of medication may be safely used in combination if they are initiated and titrated in a stepwise fashion.

2. Injectable or suppository medications—Injection of prostaglandin E_2 into the corpora cavernosa is an acceptable form of treatment for many men with erectile dysfunction. Injections are performed using a tuberculin-type syringe or a metered-dose injection device. The base and lateral aspect of the penis is used as the injection site to avoid injury to the superficial blood and nerve supply located dorsally. Complications are rare and include priapism, penile pain, bruising, fibrosis, and infection. Prostaglandin E$_2$ (alprostadil urethral) can also be delivered via an intraurethral suppository. Prostaglandin E$_2$ is often compounded with papaverine, phentolamine, or atropine in order to increase effectiveness. Patients using such compounded agents should be cautioned about the increased risk of priapism and variability of drug effect due to differences in compounding.

C. Vacuum Erection Device

The vacuum erection device creates negative pressure around the penis, drawing blood into the corpora cavernosa. Once tumescence is achieved, an elastic constriction band is placed around the penile base to prevent loss of erection. Such devices are effective but may cause penile discomfort leading to a high rate of disuse. Serious complications are rare.

D. Penile Prosthetic Surgery

Penile prostheses are implanted directly into the paired corpora cavernosa and may be semi-rigid (malleable) or inflatable (self-contained hydraulic device). Inflatable devices are most commonly used and result in a natural appearance and function because they emulate the tumescence and detumescence of the normal erection. Complications of surgery are rare but include mechanical failure, infection, and injury to adjacent anatomic structures. For men who elect this treatment, personal and partner satisfaction rates are very high due to enhanced spontaneity and reliability of erections.

E. Medical and Surgical Therapy for Peyronie Disease

Oral medications for Peyronie disease have not been approved by the FDA; however, off-label use of multiple vasodilatory, anti-inflammatory, and antioxidant medications is common. Injectable collagenase *Clostridium histolyticum* is the only FDA-approved medication for the treatment of Peyronie disease. Collagenase enzymatically severs disordered collagen fibers after injection into the central portion of the penile plaque. Surgical treatment is an alternative for men with compromised sexual function due to severe curvature, lesions causing penile instability, or with inadequate results from collagenase. The choice of corrective procedure should be tailored to each patient after a detailed evaluation of disease severity and sexual function.

▶ When to Refer

- Patients with inadequate response to oral medications, who are unable to tolerate side effects or who are dissatisfied with their current treatment.
- Patients with Peyronie disease or other penile deformity.
- Patients with a history of pelvic or perineal trauma, surgery, or radiation.

- Ischemic priapism is a medical emergency and requires immediate referral to a urologist or the emergency department for intervention to allow restoration of penile blood perfusion.

Bennett N Jr. Sexual dysfunction: behavioral, medical, and surgical treatment. Med Clin North Am. 2018 Mar;102(2):349–60. [PMID: 29406063]

Gabrielson AT et al. Collagenase *Clostridium histolyticum* in the treatment of urologic disease: current and future impact. Sex Med Rev. 2018 Jan;6(1):143–56. [PMID: 28454897]

Mobley DF et al. Recent advances in the treatment of erectile dysfunction. Postgrad Med J. 2017 Nov;93(1105):679–85. [PMID: 28751439]

Razdan S et al. Effect of prescription medications on erectile dysfunction. Postgrad Med J. 2018 Mar;94(1109):171–8. [PMID: 29103015]

MALE INFERTILITY

ESSENTIALS OF DIAGNOSIS

- ▶ Male infertility is common, contributing to 50% of infertility cases.
- ▶ Causes include decreased or absent sperm production or function, or obstruction of the male genital tract.
- ▶ Abnormal semen quality may indicate poor health or increased risk of certain health conditions.

▶ General Considerations

Infertility is the inability of a couple to conceive a child after 1 year of sexual intercourse without contraceptive use. It affects 15–20% of US couples and 50% of cases result from male factors. The evaluation of both partners is critical for treatment success. Following a detailed history and physical examination, a semen analysis should be performed at least twice, on two separate occasions (Figure 23–1). Because spermatogenesis requires approximately 75 days, it is important to review health events and gonadotoxic exposures from the preceding 3 months. Male infertility is associated with a higher risk of testicular germ cell cancer and with a higher rate of medical comorbidity. These men should be counseled and screened appropriately and taught testicular self-examination.

▶ Clinical Findings

A. Symptoms and Signs

The history should include prior testicular insults (torsion, cryptorchidism, trauma), infections (mumps orchitis, epididymitis, sexually transmitted infections), environmental factors (excessive heat, radiation, chemotherapy, prolonged pesticide exposure), medications (testosterone, finasteride, cimetidine, selective serotonin reuptake inhibitors, and spironolactone may affect spermatogenesis; phenytoin may lower FSH; sulfasalazine and

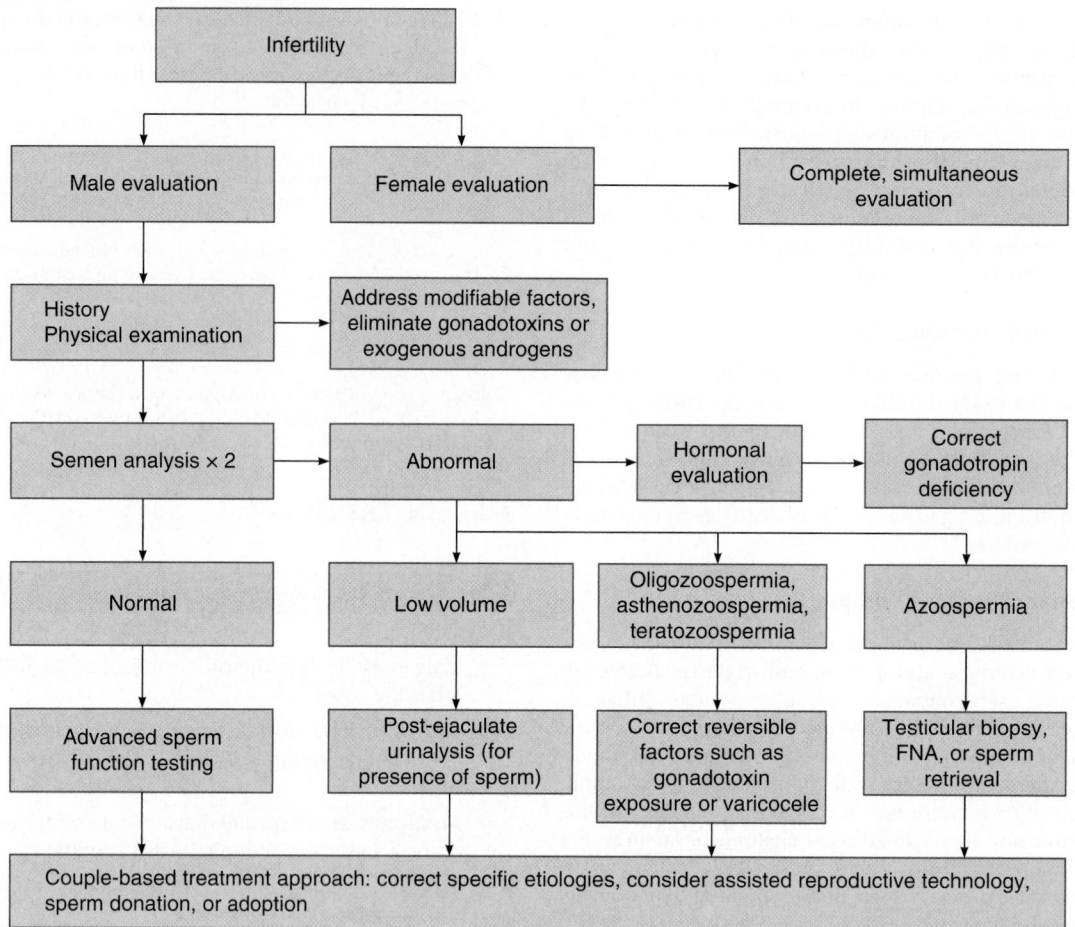

▲ **Figure 23–1.** Couple-based approach to evaluation and treatment of male factor infertility. FNA, fine-needle aspiration.

nitrofurantoin affect sperm motility; tamsulosin causes retrograde ejaculation), and other drugs (alcohol, tobacco, marijuana). Sexual function, frequency and timing of intercourse, use of lubricants, and each partner's previous fertility are important. The past medical or surgical history may reveal chronic disease, including, obesity, cardiovascular, thyroid, or liver disease (decreased spermatogenesis); diabetes mellitus (decreased spermatogenesis, retrograde or anejaculation); or radical pelvic or retroperitoneal surgery (absent seminal emission secondary to sympathetic nerve injury).

Physical examination should assess features of hypogonadism: underdeveloped sexual characteristics, diminished male pattern hair distribution (axillary, body, facial, pubic), body habitus, gynecomastia, and obesity. Testicular size should be noted (normal size approximately 4.5 × 2.5 cm, volume 18 mL). **Varicoceles** are abnormally dilated and refluxing veins of the pampiniform plexus that can be identified in the standing position by gentle palpation of the spermatic cord and, on occasion, may only be appreciated with the Valsalva maneuver. The vasa deferentia, epididymides, and prostate should be palpated (absence of all or part of one or both of the vasa deferentia may indicate the presence of a cystic fibrosis variant, congenital bilateral or unilateral absence of the vasa deferentia).

B. Laboratory Findings

Semen analysis should be performed after 3–5 days of ejaculatory abstinence. The specimen should be analyzed within 1 hour after collection. Abnormal sperm concentrations are less than 15 million/mL (**oligozoospermia** is the presence of less than 15 million sperm/mL in the ejaculate; **azoospermia** is the complete absence of sperm). Normal semen volume should be equal to or greater than 1.5 mL (lesser volumes may be due to retrograde ejaculation, ejaculatory duct obstruction, congenital bilateral absence of the vasa deferentia, or hypogonadism). Normal sperm motility and morphology demonstrate greater than 39% motile cells and greater than 3% normal morphology. Abnormal motility (asthenozoospermia) may result from varicocele, antisperm antibodies, infection, abnormalities of the sperm flagella, or ejaculatory duct obstruction. Abnormal morphology may result from a varicocele, infection, or exposure to gonadotoxins (eg, tobacco, marijuana).

Endocrine evaluation is warranted if sperm concentration is below 10 million sperm/mL or if the history and physical examination suggest an endocrinologic origin. Initial testing should include serum testosterone and FSH. Specific abnormalities in these hormones should prompt additional testing, including serum LH and prolactin. Elevated FSH and LH levels and low testosterone levels (**hypergonadotropic** or **primary hypogonadism**) are associated with primary testicular failure. Low FSH and LH associated with low testosterone (**hypogonadotropic** or **secondary hypogonadism**) may be of hypothalamic or pituitary origin. Elevation of serum prolactin may indicate the presence of prolactinoma.

C. Genetic Testing

Men with sperm concentrations less than 10 million/mL should consider testing for Y chromosome microdeletions and karyotypic abnormalities. Gene deletions from the long arm of the Y chromosome may cause azoospermia or oligozoospermia with age-related decline in spermatogenesis that is transmissible to male offspring. Karyotyping may reveal Klinefelter syndrome. Partial or complete absence of the vasa deferentia should prompt testing for gene mutations associated with cystic fibrosis.

D. Imaging

Scrotal ultrasound can aid in characterizing the testes and may detect a testicular mass or a subclinical varicocele. Men with low ejaculate volume and no evidence of retrograde ejaculation should undergo transrectal ultrasound to evaluate the prostate and seminal vesicles. MRI of the sella turcica should be performed in men with elevated prolactin or hypogonadotropic hypogonadism to evaluate the anterior pituitary gland. MRI of the pelvis and scrotum should be considered in men for whom the testes cannot be identified in the scrotum by physical examination or ultrasound. Men with unilateral absence of the vas deferens should have abdominal ultrasound or CT to exclude absence of the ipsilateral kidney.

▶ Treatment

A. General Measures

Education about intercourse timing in relation to the woman's ovulatory cycle as well as the avoidance of spermicidal lubricants should be discussed. In cases of gonadotoxic exposure or medication-related factors, the offending agent should be removed whenever feasible. Patients with active genitourinary tract infections should be treated with appropriate antibiotics. Healthy lifestyle habits, including diet, exercise, and avoidance of gonadotoxins (tobacco, excessive alcohol, and marijuana), should be reinforced.

B. Varicocele

Varicocelectomy is performed to stop retrograde blood flow in abnormal spermatic cord veins. Surgical ligation, which is accomplished via a subinguinal incision with the aid of a surgical microscope and Doppler ultrasound, is the gold standard approach given its high success and low complication rates. Percutaneous venographic embolization of varicoceles is feasible but incurs both radiation and intravenous contrast exposure.

C. Endocrine Therapy

Hypogonadotropic hypogonadism may be treated with human chorionic gonadotropin (2000 international units intramuscularly three times a week) once primary pituitary disease has been excluded or treated. If sperm concentration fails to rise after 12 months, recombinant FSH therapy should be initiated (150 international units subcutaneously three times a week).

D. Ejaculatory Dysfunction Therapy

Patients with retrograde ejaculation may benefit from alpha-adrenergic agonists (pseudoephedrine, 60 mg orally three times a day) or imipramine (25 mg orally three times a day). Medical failures may require the collection of post-ejaculation urine for intrauterine insemination. Anejaculation can be treated with vibratory stimulation or electroejaculation in select cases.

E. Ductal Obstruction

Obstruction of the vas deferens after vasectomy may be managed by microsurgical vasectomy reversal or by surgical sperm retrieval in combination with in vitro fertilization.

F. Assisted Reproductive Techniques

Intrauterine insemination and in vitro fertilization (with or without intracytoplasmic sperm injection) are alternatives for patients in whom other means of treating reduced sperm concentration, motility, or functionality have failed. Intrauterine insemination should be performed only when adequate numbers of motile sperm are noted in an ejaculate sample. With the use of intracytoplasmic sperm injection, some men with azoospermia may still initiate a pregnancy by surgical retrieval of sperm from the testicle, epididymis, or vas deferens.

▶ When to Refer

- Couples with infertility or who are concerned about their fertility potential.
- Men with known genital insults, genetic diagnoses, or syndromes that preclude natural fertility.
- Reproductive-aged men with newly diagnosed cancer or other disease that may require cytotoxic therapies with interest in fertility preservation.

Avellino G et al. Common urologic diseases in older men and their treatment: how they impact fertility. Fertil Steril. 2017 Feb;107(2):305–11. [PMID: 28073432]

Duthie EA et al. A conceptual framework for patient-centered fertility treatment. Reprod Health. 2017 Sep 7;14(1):114. [PMID: 28882134]

Gundersen TD et al. Association between use of marijuana and male reproductive hormones and semen quality: a study among 1,215 healthy young men. Am J Epidemiol. 2015 Sep 15; 182(6):473–81. [PMID: 26283092]

Jensen CFS et al. Varicocele and male infertility. Nat Rev Urol. 2017 Sep;14(9):523–33. [PMID: 28675168]

Kashanian JA et al. JAMA patient page. Male infertility. JAMA. 2015 May 5;313(17):1770. [PMID: 25942742]

Krausz C et al. Genetics of male infertility. Nat Rev Urol. 2018 Jun;15(6):369–84. [PMID: 29622783]

Lotti F et al. Sexual dysfunction and male infertility. Nat Rev Urol. 2018 May;15(5):287–307. [PMID: 29532805]

BENIGN PROSTATIC HYPERPLASIA

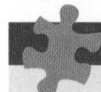

ESSENTIALS OF DIAGNOSIS

▶ Obstructive or irritative voiding symptoms.

▶ May have enlarged prostate on rectal examination.

▶ Absence of urinary tract infection, neurologic disorder, stricture disease, prostatic or bladder malignancy.

▶ General Considerations

Benign prostatic hyperplasia is the most common benign tumor in men, and its incidence is age related. The prevalence of histologic benign prostatic hyperplasia in autopsy studies rises from approximately 20% in men aged 41–50 years, to 50% in men aged 51–60, and to over 90% in men over 80 years of age. Although clinical evidence of disease occurs less commonly, symptoms of prostatic obstruction are also age related. At age 55 years, approximately 25% of men report obstructive voiding symptoms. At age 75 years, 50% of men report a decrease in the force and caliber of the urinary stream.

Risk factors for the development of benign prostatic hyperplasia are poorly understood. Some studies have suggested a genetic predisposition and some have noted racial differences. Approximately 50% of men under age 60 years who undergo surgery for benign prostatic hyperplasia may have a heritable form of the disease. This form is most likely an autosomal dominant trait, and first-degree male relatives of such patients carry an increased relative risk of approximately fourfold.

▶ Clinical Findings

A. Symptoms

The symptoms of benign prostatic hyperplasia can be divided into obstructive and irritative complaints. **Obstructive symptoms** include hesitancy, decreased force and caliber of the stream, sensation of incomplete bladder emptying, double voiding (urinating a second time within 2 hours), straining to urinate, and postvoid dribbling. **Irritative symptoms** include urgency, frequency, and nocturia.

The American Urological Association (AUA) symptom index (Table 23–3) is perhaps the single most important tool used in the evaluation of patients with this disorder and should be calculated for all patients before starting therapy. The answers to seven questions quantitate the severity of obstructive or irritative complaints on a scale of 0–5. Thus, the score can range from 0 to 35, in increasing severity of symptoms.

A detailed history focusing on the urinary tract should be obtained to exclude other possible causes of symptoms such as prostate cancer or disorders unrelated to the prostate such as urinary tract infection, neurogenic bladder, or urethral stricture.

Table 23–3. American Urological Association symptom index for benign prostatic hyperplasia.[1]

Questions to Be Answered	Not at All	Less Than One Time in Five	Less Than Half the Time	About Half the Time	More Than Half the Time	Almost Always
1. Over the past month, how often have you had a sensation of not emptying your bladder completely after you finish urinating?	0	1	2	3	4	5
2. Over the past month, how often have you had to urinate again less than 2 hours after you finished urinating?	0	1	2	3	4	5
3. Over the past month, how often have you found you stopped and started again several times when you urinated?	0	1	2	3	4	5
4. Over the past month, how often have you found it difficult to postpone urination?	0	1	2	3	4	5
5. Over the past month, how often have you had a weak urinary stream?	0	1	2	3	4	5
6. Over the past month, how often have you had to push or strain to begin urination?	0	1	2	3	4	5
7. Over the past month, how many times did you most typically get up to urinate from the time you went to bed at night until the time you got up in the morning?	0	1	2	3	4	5

[1]Sum of seven circled numbers equals the symptom score. See text for explanation.

Reproduced, with permission, from Barry MJ et al; Measurement Committee of the American Urological Association. The American Urological Association symptom index for benign prostatic hyperplasia. J Urol. 2017 Feb;197(2S):S189–97.

B. Signs

A physical examination, digital rectal examination (DRE), and a focused neurologic examination should be performed on all patients. The size and consistency of the prostate should be noted, but prostate size does not correlate with the severity of symptoms or the degree of obstruction. Benign prostatic hyperplasia usually results in a smooth, firm, elastic enlargement of the prostate. Induration, if detected, must alert the clinician to the possibility of cancer, and further evaluation is needed (ie, prostate-specific antigen [PSA] testing, transrectal ultrasound, and biopsy). Examination of the lower abdomen should be performed to assess for a distended bladder.

C. Laboratory Findings

Urinalysis should be performed to exclude infection or hematuria. Clinicians should consider obtaining a serum PSA test, particularly in patients whose life expectancy is longer than 10 years. PSA certainly increases the ability to detect prostate cancer over DRE alone; however, because there is much overlap between levels seen in benign prostatic hyperplasia and prostate cancer, its use remains controversial (see Chapter 39).

D. Imaging

Upper tract imaging (CT or renal ultrasound) is recommended only in the presence of concomitant urinary tract disease or complications from benign prostatic hyperplasia (ie, hematuria, urinary tract infection, chronic kidney disease, history of stone disease). As included in the Choosing Wisely (ABIM Foundation) initiative, neither creatinine nor imaging should be routinely ordered for patients with benign prostatic hyperplasia.

E. Cystoscopy

Cystoscopy is not recommended to determine the need for treatment but may assist in determining the surgical approach in patients opting for invasive therapy.

F. Additional Tests

Cystometrograms and urodynamic profiles should be reserved for patients with suspected neurologic disease or those who have failed prostate surgery. Flow rates, postvoid residual urine determination, and pressure-flow studies are considered optional.

▶ Differential Diagnosis

A history of prior urethral instrumentation, urethritis, or trauma should be elucidated to exclude urethral stricture or bladder neck contracture. Hematuria and pain are commonly associated with bladder stones. Carcinoma of the prostate may be detected by abnormalities on the DRE or an elevated PSA (see Chapter 39). A urinary tract infection can mimic the irritative symptoms of benign prostatic hyperplasia and can be readily identified by urinalysis and culture; however, a urinary tract infection can also be a complication of benign prostatic hyperplasia. Carcinoma of the bladder, especially carcinoma in situ, may also present with irritative voiding complaints; however, urinalysis usually shows evidence of hematuria (see Chapter 39). Patients with a neurogenic bladder may also have many of the same symptoms and signs as those with benign prostatic hyperplasia; however, a history of neurologic disease, stroke, diabetes mellitus, or back injury may be obtained, and diminished perineal or lower extremity sensation or alterations in rectal sphincter tone or the bulbocavernosus reflex might be observed on examination. Simultaneous alterations in bowel function (constipation) might also suggest the possibility of a neurologic disorder.

▶ Treatment

Clinical practice guidelines exist for the evaluation and treatment of patients with benign prostatic hyperplasia (Figure 23–2). Following evaluation as outlined above, patients should be offered various forms of therapy for benign prostatic hyperplasia. Patients are advised to consult with their primary care clinicians and make an educated decision on the basis of the relative efficacy and side effects of the treatment options (Table 23–4).

Patients with mild symptoms (AUA scores 0–7) should be managed by watchful waiting only. Medical therapy is appropriate for many others. Absolute surgical indications include refractory urinary retention (failing at least one attempt at catheter removal), large bladder diverticula, or any of the following sequelae of benign prostatic hyperplasia: recurrent urinary tract infection, recurrent gross hematuria, bladder stones, or chronic kidney disease.

A. Watchful Waiting

The risk of progression or complications is uncertain. However, in men with symptomatic disease, it is clear that progression is not inevitable and that some men undergo spontaneous improvement or resolution of their symptoms.

Retrospective studies on the natural history of benign prostatic hyperplasia are inherently subject to bias, relating in part to patient selection and also to the type and extent of follow-up. Very few prospective studies addressing the natural history have been reported. One small series demonstrated that approximately 10% of symptomatic men may progress to urinary retention while 50% of patients demonstrate marked improvement or resolution of symptoms. A large randomized study compared finasteride with placebo in men with moderate to severely symptomatic disease and enlarged prostates on DRE. Patients in the placebo arm demonstrated a 7% risk of developing urinary retention over 4 years.

Men with moderate or severe symptoms can also be observed if they so choose. The optimal interval for follow-up is not defined, nor are the specific end points for intervention.

B. Medical Therapy

1. Alpha-blockers—Alpha-blockers can be classified according to their receptor selectivity as well as their half-life (Table 23–5).

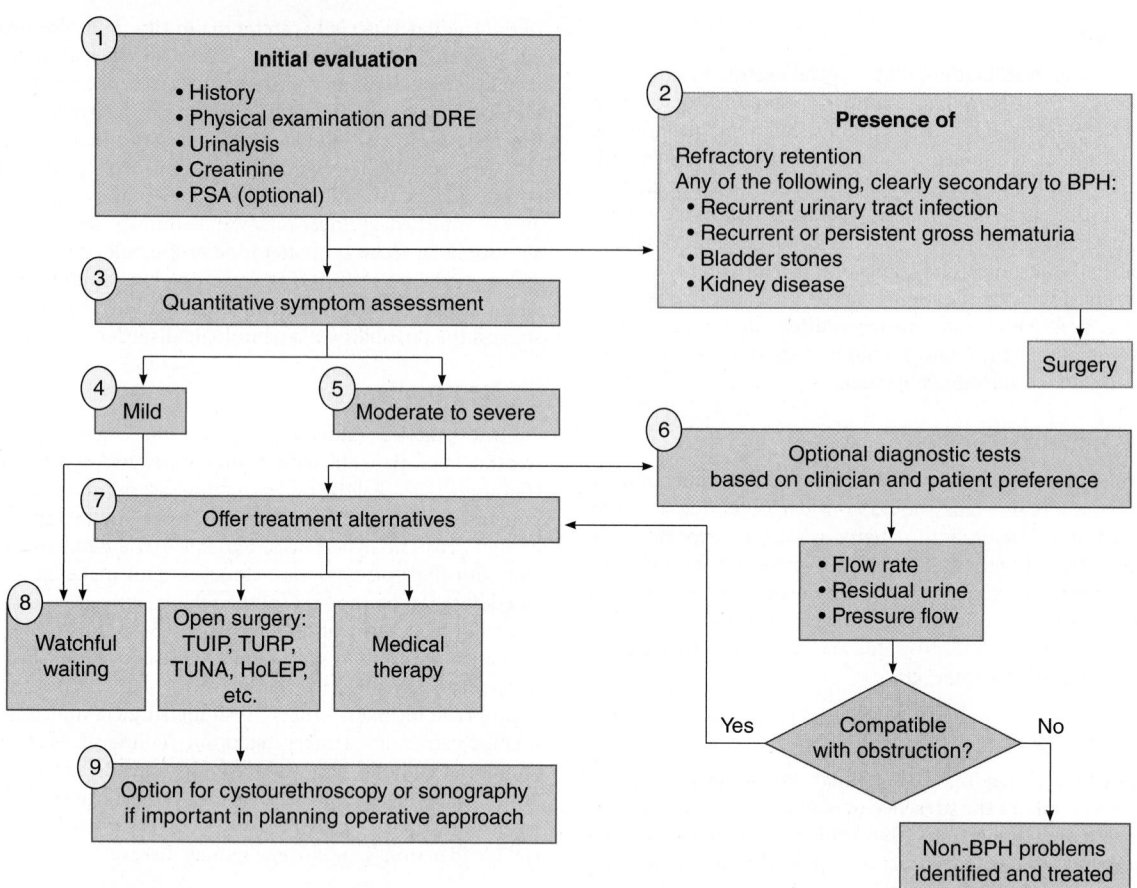

▲ **Figure 23–2.** Benign prostatic hyperplasia decision diagram. BPH, benign prostatic hyperplasia; DRE, digital rectal examination; HoLEP, Holmium laser enucleation of the prostate; PSA, prostate-specific antigen; TUIP, transurethral incision of the prostate; TUNA, transurethral needle ablation; TURP, transurethral resection of the prostate.

Table 23–4. Summary of benign prostatic hyperplasia treatment outcomes.[1]

Outcome	TUIP	Open Surgery	TURP	Watchful Waiting	Alpha-Blockers	Finasteride[2]
Chance for improvement[1]	78–83%	94–99.8%	75–96%	31–55%	59–86%	54–78%
Degree of symptom improvement (% reduction in symptom score)	73%	79%	85%	Unknown	51%	31%
Morbidity and complications[1]	2.2–33.3%	7–42.7%	5.2–30.7%	1–5%	2.9–43.3%	13.6–8.8%
Death within 30–90 days[1]	0.2–1.5%	1–4.6%	0.5–3.3%	0.8%	0.8%	0.8%
Total incontinence[1]	0.1–1.1%	0.3–0.7%	0.7–1.4%	2%	2%	2%
Need for operative treatment for surgical complications[1]	1.3–2.7%	0.6–14.1%	0.7–10.1%	0	0	0
Erectile dysfunction[1]	3.9–24.5%	4.7–39.2%	3.3–34.8%	3%	3%	2.5–5.3%
Retrograde ejaculation	6–55%	36–95%	25–99%	0	4–11%	0
Loss of work in days	7–21	21–28	7–21	1	3.5	1.5
Hospital stay in days	1–3	5–10	3–5	0	0	0

[1]90% confidence interval.
[2]Most of the data reviewed for finasteride are derived from three trials that have required an enlarged prostate for entry. The chance of improvement in men with symptoms yet minimally enlarged prostates may be much less, as noted from the VA Cooperative Trial.
TUIP, transurethral incision of the prostate; TURP, transurethral resection of the prostate.

Table 23–5. Alpha-blockade for benign prostatic hyperplasia.

Agent	Action	Oral Dose
Alfuzosin	Alpha-1a-blockade	10 mg daily
Doxazosin	Alpha-1-blockade	1–8 mg daily
Prazosin	Alpha-1-blockade	1–5 mg twice daily
Terazosin	Alpha-1-blockade	1–10 mg daily
Silodosin	Alpha-1a-blockade	4 or 8 mg daily
Tamsulosin	Alpha-1a-blockade	0.4 or 0.8 mg daily
Tadalafil	Phosphodiesterase type 5 inhibitor	5 mg daily

Prazosin is an effective short-acting, nonselective alpha-blocker; however, it requires dose titration and twice daily dosing. Typical side effects include orthostatic hypotension, dizziness, tiredness, retrograde ejaculation, rhinitis, and headache.

Long-acting, nonselective alpha-blockers allow for once-a-day dosing, but dose titration is still necessary because side effects similar to those seen with prazosin may occur. Terazosin improves symptoms and in numerous studies is superior to placebo or finasteride. Terazosin is started at a dosage of 1 mg orally daily for 3 days, increased to 2 mg orally daily for 11 days, then 5 mg orally daily. Additional dose escalation to 10 mg orally daily can be performed if necessary. Doxazosin is started at a dosage of 1 mg orally daily for 7 days, increased to 2 mg orally daily for 7 days, then 4 mg orally daily. Additional dose escalation to 8 mg orally daily can be performed if necessary.

Alpha-1a-receptors are localized to the prostate and bladder neck. Selective blockade of these receptors results in fewer systemic side effects than alpha-blocker therapy (orthostatic hypotension, dizziness, tiredness, rhinitis, and headache), thus obviating the need for dose titration. The typical dose of tamsulosin is 0.4 mg orally daily taken 30 minutes after a meal. Alfuzosin is a long-acting alpha-1a-blocker; its dose is 10 mg orally once daily with food and does not require titration. Several randomized, double-blind, placebo-controlled trials have been performed comparing terazosin, doxazosin, tamsulosin, and alfuzosin with placebo. All agents have demonstrated safety and efficacy. Floppy iris syndrome, a complication of cataract surgery, can occur in patients taking alpha-blockers and alpha-1a-blockers.

2. 5-alpha-reductase inhibitors—Finasteride and dutasteride block the conversion of testosterone to dihydrotestosterone. These medications impact the epithelial component of the prostate, resulting in reduction in size of the gland and improvement in symptoms. Six months of therapy is required for maximum effects on prostate size (20% reduction) and symptomatic improvement.

Several randomized, double-blind, placebo-controlled trials have been performed comparing finasteride with placebo. Efficacy, safety, and durability are well established. However, symptomatic improvement is seen only in men with enlarged prostates (greater than 40 mL by ultrasonographic examination). Side effects include decreased libido, decrease in volume of ejaculate, and erectile dysfunction. Serum PSA is reduced by approximately 50% in patients receiving finasteride therapy, but the % free PSA is unchanged. Therefore, in order to compare with pre-finasteride PSA levels, the serum PSA of a patient taking finasteride should be doubled.

A report suggests that finasteride therapy may decrease the incidence of urinary retention and the need for operative treatment in men with enlarged prostates and moderate to severe symptoms. The larger the prostate over 40 mL, the greater the relative-risk reduction. However, optimal identification of appropriate patients for prophylactic therapy remains to be determined. Dutasteride is a dual 5-alpha-reductase inhibitor that appears to be similar to finasteride in its effectiveness; its dose is 0.5 mg orally daily.

Both finasteride and dutasteride have been shown to be effective chemopreventive agents for prostate cancer in large, randomized clinical trials. A 25% risk reduction was observed in men with both low and high risk for prostate cancer. However, despite the strength of the evidence for 5-alpha-reductase inhibitors in reducing the risk of prostate cancer, an FDA advisory committee recommended against labeling these agents for prostate cancer chemoprevention, citing the potential increased risk of high-grade tumors in these studies (1.8% vs 1.0% for finasteride and 1% vs 0.5% for dutasteride), isolated risk reduction in low-grade tumors, and inability to apply the findings to the general population. Moreover, the FDA has included the increased risk of being diagnosed with high-grade prostate cancer in the labels of all 5-alpha-reductase inhibitors.

3. Phosphodiesterase-5 inhibitor—Tadalafil is approved by the FDA to treat the signs and symptoms of benign prostatic hyperplasia; it is also approved for use in men with both urinary symptoms and erectile dysfunction. The data from two randomized, double-blind, placebo-controlled trials demonstrated significant improvements in standardized measurements of urinary function between 2 and 4 weeks after initiating treatment at 5 mg once daily, with minimal adverse effects.

4. Combination therapy—The Medical Therapy of Prostatic Symptoms (MTOPS) trial was a large, randomized, placebo-controlled trial comparing finasteride, doxazosin, the combination of the two, and placebo in 3047 men observed for a mean of 4.5 years. Long-term combination therapy with doxazosin and finasteride was safe and reduced the risk of overall clinical progression of benign prostatic hyperplasia significantly more than did treatment with either medication alone. Combination therapy and finasteride alone reduced the long-term risk of acute urinary retention and the need for invasive therapy. Combination therapy had the risks of additional side effects and the cost of two medications.

5. Phytotherapy—Phytotherapy is the use of plants or plant extracts for medicinal purposes. Several plant extracts have been popularized, including the saw palmetto berry, the bark of *Pygeum africanum*, the roots of *Echinacea purpurea* and *Hypoxis rooperi*, pollen extract, and the leaves of the trembling poplar. However, a prospective, randomized, double-blind, placebo-controlled trial revealed no improvement in symptoms, urinary flow rate, or quality of life for men with benign prostatic hyperplasia with saw palmetto treatment compared with placebo.

C. Conventional Surgical Therapy

1. Transurethral resection of the prostate (TURP)—Over 95% of prostate surgeries can be performed endoscopically (through the urethra). TURP is the gold standard treatment for surgical treatment of benign prostatic hyperplasia, and it often requires a 1- to 2-day hospital stay. While there are only a few head-to-head surgical studies comparing TURP to minimally invasive therapies, most studies show symptom scores and flow rate improvements are superior following TURP compared to any minimally invasive therapy. The risks of TURP include retrograde ejaculation (75%), erectile dysfunction (less than 5%), and urinary incontinence (less than 1%). Potential complications include (1) bleeding; (2) urethral stricture or bladder neck contracture; (3) perforation of the prostate capsule with extravasation; and (4) transurethral resection syndrome, a hypervolemic, hyponatremic state resulting from absorption of the hypotonic irrigating solution. This syndrome was much more prevalent when TURPs were most often performed with monopolar electrocautery but, with the increased use of bipolar TURPs (using saline irrigation), it is now very rare. Clinical manifestations of the syndrome include nausea, vomiting, confusion, hypertension, bradycardia, and visual disturbances. The risk of transurethral resection syndrome increases with monopolar resection times over 90 minutes. Treatment includes diuresis and, in severe cases, hypertonic saline administration (see Hyponatremia, Chapter 21).

2. Transurethral incision of the prostate (TUIP)—Men with moderate to severe symptoms and small prostates often have posterior commissure hyperplasia or an "elevated bladder neck." These patients will often benefit from incision of the prostate. The procedure is more rapid and less morbid than TURP. Outcomes in well-selected patients are comparable, though a lower rate of retrograde ejaculation has been reported (25%).

3. Simple prostatectomy (Open/Robotic)—When the prostate is very large, open or robotic enucleation is necessary. What size is "too large" depends upon the surgeon's experience with TURP. Glands over 100 g are usually considered for enucleation. In addition to size, other relative indications for open prostatectomy include concomitant bladder diverticulum or bladder stone and whether dorsal lithotomy positioning is or is not possible.

Simple prostatectomies can be performed with either a suprapubic or retropubic approach. Simple suprapubic prostatectomy is performed transvesically and is the operation of choice if there is concomitant bladder pathology. After the prostatic adenoma is removed, both a urethral and a suprapubic catheter are inserted prior to closure. In simple retropubic prostatectomy, the bladder is not entered but rather a transverse incision is made in the surgical capsule of the prostate and the adenoma is enucleated as described above; only a urethral catheter is needed at the end of the case. These operations can also be performed via robotic-assisted laparoscopic techniques with shorter hospital stays, less blood loss, and decreased need for a suprapubic catheter.

D. Minimally Invasive Therapy

1. Laser therapy—Several coagulation necrosis techniques have been utilized. Transurethral laser-induced prostatectomy (TULIP) is performed under transrectal ultrasound guidance. The instrument is placed in the urethra and transrectal ultrasound is used to direct the device as it is slowly pulled from the bladder neck to the apex. The depth of treatment is monitored with ultrasound.

Most urologists prefer to use visually directed laser techniques. Visual coagulative necrosis is performed under cystoscopic control, and the laser fiber is pulled through the prostate at several designated areas depending on the size and configuration of the gland. Coagulative techniques do not create an immediate visual defect in the prostatic urethra—tissue is sloughed over the course of several weeks up to 3 months following the procedure.

Visual contact ablative techniques take longer in the operating room because the laser fiber is placed in direct contact with the prostate tissue, which is vaporized. Photovaporization of the prostate (PVP), an alternative laser technique, uses a high-power KTP laser. An immediate defect is obtained in the prostatic urethra, similar to that seen during TURP.

Interstitial laser therapy places laser fibers directly into the prostate, usually under cystoscopic control. Irritative voiding symptoms may be less in these patients as the urethral mucosa is spared and prostate tissue is resorbed by the body rather than sloughed.

Holmium laser enucleation of the prostate (HoLEP) is a technique of enucleating the adenomatous lobes intact and morcellating the tissue within the bladder. Advantages of HoLEP compared with other methods include ability to treat all prostate sizes, low re-treatment rates, few complications, and shorter duration of catheterization.

Advantages to laser surgery include minimal blood loss, rarity of transurethral resection syndrome, ability to treat patients during anticoagulant therapy, and outpatient surgery. Disadvantages are the lack of tissue for pathologic examination, longer postoperative catheterization time, variable effectiveness, more frequent irritative voiding complaints, and expense of laser fibers and generators.

Large multicenter, randomized studies with long-term follow-up are needed to compare laser prostate surgery with TURP and other forms of minimally invasive surgery.

2. Transurethral needle ablation of the prostate (TUNA)—This procedure uses a specially designed urethral catheter that is passed into the urethra. Interstitial radiofrequency needles are then deployed from the tip of the catheter, piercing the mucosa of the prostatic urethra. Radiofrequencies are then used to heat the tissue, resulting in coagulative necrosis. Subjective and objective improvement in voiding occurs. In randomized trials comparing TUNA to TURP, similar improvement was seen when comparing life scores, peak urinary flow rates, and

postvoid residual urine. Bladder neck and median lobe enlargement are not well treated by TUNA. A technique was approved by the FDA in 2015 that delivers the radiofrequency energy through water vapor.

3. Transurethral electrovaporization of the prostate— This technique uses the standard resectoscope. High current densities result in heat vaporization of tissue, creating a cavity in the prostatic urethra. This procedure usually takes longer than a standard TURP. Long-term comparative data are needed.

4. Hyperthermia—Microwave hyperthermia is most commonly delivered with a transurethral catheter. Some devices cool the urethral mucosa to decrease the risk of injury. However, if temperatures do not go above 45°C, cooling is unnecessary. Symptom score and flow rate improvement are obtained, but (as with laser surgery) large randomized studies with long-term follow-up are needed to assess durability and cost-effectiveness.

5. Implant to open prostatic urethra (UroLift)—A minimally invasive, FDA-approved implant can be used to retract the enlarged lobes of the prostate in symptomatic men age 50 years and older with an enlarged prostate (less than 80 g). This implant staples the prostatic lobes to open the prostatic urethral lumen. This is done in the clinic setting with local analgesia. Short-term data show improved symptoms and voiding flows with minimal impact on erectile or ejaculatory function. Long-term comparative data are needed.

6. Water vapor thermal therapy (Rezum)—This minimally invasive, FDA-approved technique uses a transurethral device to deliver steam into the prostatic tissue and thermally destroy it. This procedure is done in the clinic or ambulatory surgery setting with 3-year data showing improvement in symptoms and voiding flows with minimal impact on erectile or ejaculatory function compared with medical therapy.

▶ When to Refer

- Progression to urinary retention.
- Patient dissatisfaction with medical therapy.
- Need for surgical intervention or further evaluation (cystoscopy).

Barry MJ et al; Measurement Committee of the American Urological Association. The American Urological Association symptom index for benign prostatic hyperplasia. J Urol. 2017 Feb; 197(2S):S189–97. [PMID: 28012747]

Hecht SL et al. Diagnostic work-up of lower urinary tract symptoms. Urol Clin North Am. 2016 Aug;43(3):299–309. [PMID: 27476123]

Kim EH et al. Management of benign prostatic hyperplasia. Annu Rev Med. 2016;67:137–51. [PMID: 26331999]

McVary KT et al. Three-year outcomes of the prospective, randomized controlled Rezüm System study: convective radiofrequency thermal therapy for treatment of lower urinary tract symptoms due to benign prostatic hyperplasia. Urology. 2018 Jan;111:1–9. [PMID: 29122620]

Pattanaik S et al. Phosphodiesterase inhibitors for lower urinary tract symptoms consistent with benign prostatic hyperplasia. Cochrane Database Syst Rev. 2018 Nov 16;11:CD010060. [PMID: 30480763]

Rukstalis D et al. Prostatic Urethral Lift (PUL) for obstructive median lobes: 12 month results of the MedLift Study. Prostate Cancer Prostatic Dis. 2018 Dec 12. [Epub ahead of print] [PMID: 30542055]

Sun F et al. Transurethral procedures in the treatment of benign prostatic hyperplasia: a systematic review and meta-analysis of effectiveness and complications. Medicine (Baltimore). 2018 Dec;97(51):e13360. [PMID: 30572440]

Thomas D et al. Emerging drugs for the treatment of benign prostatic hyperplasia. Expert Opin Emerg Drugs. 2017 Sep; 22(3):201–12. [PMID: 28829208]

Villa L et al. Silodosin: an update on efficacy, safety and clinical indications in urology. Adv Ther. 2019 Jan;36(1):1–18. [PMID: 30523608]

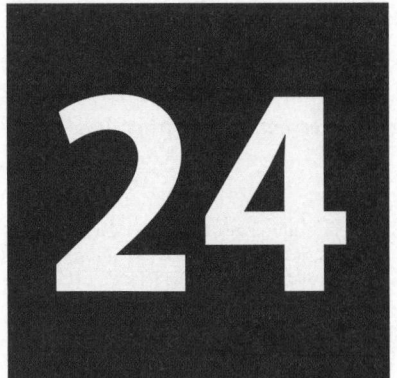

Nervous System Disorders

24

Vanja C. Douglas, MD
Michael J. Aminoff, MD, DSc, FRCP

HEADACHE

Headache is such a common complaint and can occur for so many different reasons that its proper evaluation may be difficult. New, severe, or acute headaches are more likely than chronic headaches to relate to an intracranial disorder; the approach to such headaches is discussed in Chapter 2. **Chronic headaches** may be primary or secondary to another disorder. Common **primary** headache syndromes include migraine, tension-type headache, and cluster headache. Important **secondary** causes to consider include intracranial lesions, head injury, cervical spondylosis, dental or ocular disease, temporomandibular joint dysfunction, sinusitis, hypertension, depression, and a wide variety of general medical disorders. Although underlying structural lesions are not present in most patients presenting with headache, it is nevertheless important to bear this possibility in mind. About one-third of patients with brain tumors, for example, present with a primary complaint of headache.

1. Migraine

ESSENTIALS OF DIAGNOSIS

- ► Headache, usually pulsatile, lasting 4–72 hours.
- ► Pain is typically, but not always, unilateral.
- ► Nausea, vomiting, photophobia, and phonophobia are common accompaniments.
- ► Pain is aggravated with routine physical activity.
- ► An aura of transient neurologic symptoms (commonly visual) may precede head pain.
- ► Commonly, head pain occurs with no aura.

► General Considerations

The pathophysiology of migraine probably relates to neuronal dysfunction in the trigeminal system resulting in release of vasoactive neuropeptides such as calcitonin gene-related peptide leading to neurogenic inflammation, sensitization, and headache. Migraine aura is hypothesized to result from cortical spreading depression, a wave of neuronal and glial depolarization that moves slowly across the cerebral cortex corresponding to the clinical symptoms (ie, occipital cortex and visual aura). Migraine often exhibits a complex, polygenic pattern of inheritance. Sometimes, an autosomal dominant inheritance pattern is apparent, as in **familial hemiplegic migraine (FHM),** in which attacks of lateralized weakness represent the aura.

► Clinical Findings

Typical migrainous headache is a lateralized throbbing headache that occurs episodically following its onset in adolescence or early adult life. In many cases, the headaches do not conform to this pattern, although their associated features and response to antimigrainous preparations nevertheless suggest a similar basis. In this broader sense, migrainous headaches may be lateralized or generalized, may be dull or throbbing, and are sometimes associated with anorexia, nausea, vomiting, photophobia, phonophobia, osmophobia, cognitive impairment, and blurring of vision. They usually build up gradually and last several hours or longer. Focal disturbances of neurologic function (**migraine aura**) may precede or accompany the headaches. Visual disturbances occur commonly and may consist of field defects (**scotoma**); of luminous visual hallucinations such as stars, sparks, unformed light flashes (**photopsia**), geometric patterns, or zigzags of light; or of some combination of field defects and luminous hallucinations (**scintillating scotomas**). Other focal disturbances such as aphasia or numbness, paresthesias, clumsiness, dysarthria, dysequilibrium, or weakness in a circumscribed distribution may also occur.

In rare instances, the neurologic or somatic disturbance accompanying typical migrainous headaches becomes the sole manifestation of an attack ("**migraine equivalent**"). Very rarely, the patient may be left with a permanent neurologic deficit following a migrainous attack, and migraine with aura may be a risk factor for stroke.

Patients often give a family history of migraine. Attacks may be triggered by emotional or physical stress, lack or excess of sleep, missed meals, specific foods (eg, chocolate), alcoholic beverages, bright lights, loud noise, menstruation, or use of oral contraceptives.

An uncommon variant is **basilar artery migraine,** in which blindness or visual disturbances throughout both visual fields are accompanied or followed by dysarthria, dysequilibrium, tinnitus, and perioral and distal paresthesias and are sometimes followed by transient loss or impairment of consciousness or by a confusional state. This, in turn, is followed by a throbbing (usually occipital) headache, often with nausea and vomiting.

In **ophthalmoplegic migraine,** lateralized pain—often about the eye—is accompanied by nausea, vomiting, and diplopia due to transient external ophthalmoplegia. The ophthalmoplegia is due to third nerve palsy, sometimes with accompanying sixth nerve involvement, and may outlast the orbital pain by several days or even weeks. The ophthalmic division of the fifth nerve has also been affected in some patients. Ophthalmoplegic migraine is rare and a diagnosis of exclusion; more common causes of a painful ophthalmoplegia are internal carotid artery aneurysms and diabetes.

▶ **Treatment**

Management of migraine consists of avoidance of any precipitating factors, together with prophylactic or symptomatic pharmacologic treatment if necessary.

A. Symptomatic Therapy

During acute attacks, rest in a quiet, darkened room may be helpful until symptoms subside. A simple analgesic (eg, aspirin, acetaminophen, ibuprofen, or naproxen) taken immediately often provides relief, but prescription medication is sometimes necessary. *To prevent medication overuse, use of simple analgesics should be limited to 15 days or less per month, and combination analgesics should be limited to no more than 10 days per month.*

1. Ergotamines—Cafergot, a combination of ergotamine tartrate (1 mg) and caffeine (100 mg), is often particularly helpful; one or two tablets are taken at the onset of headache or warning symptoms, followed by one tablet every 30 minutes, if necessary, up to six tablets per attack and no more than 10 days per month. Cafergot given rectally (one-half to one suppository containing 2 mg of ergotamine) or dihydroergotamine mesylate (0.5–1 mg intravenously or 1–2 mg subcutaneously or intramuscularly) may be useful when vomiting precludes use of oral medications. Ergotamine-containing preparations should be avoided during pregnancy, in patients with cardiovascular disease or its risk factors, and in patients taking potent CYP 3A4 inhibitors.

2. Triptans—The triptans are 5-HT$_1$ receptor agonists that inhibit release of vasoactive neuropeptides. Sumatriptan is a rapidly effective agent for aborting attacks when given subcutaneously by an autoinjection device (4–6 mg once subcutaneously, may repeat once after 2 hours if needed; maximum dose 12 mg/24 h). Nasal and oral preparations are available but may be less effective due to slower absorption. Zolmitriptan is available in oral and nasal formulations.

The dose is 5 mg orally or in one nostril once; this may be repeated once after 2 hours. The maximum dose for both formulations is 10 mg/24 h. Other triptans are available, including rizatriptan (5–10 mg orally at onset, may repeat every 2 hours twice [maximum dose 30 mg/24 h]); naratriptan (1–2.5 mg orally at onset, may repeat once after 4 hours [maximum dose 5 mg/24 h]); almotriptan (6.25–12.5 mg orally at onset, may repeat dose once after 2 hours [maximum dose 25 mg/24 h]); frovatriptan (2.5 mg orally at onset, may repeat after 2 hours once [maximum dose 7.5 mg/24]); and eletriptan (20–40 mg orally at onset; may repeat after 2 hours once [maximum dose 80 mg/24 h]). Eletriptan is useful for immediate therapy and frovatriptan, which has a longer half-life, may be worthwhile for patients with prolonged attacks or attacks provoked by menstrual periods. Patients often experience greater benefit when the triptan is combined with naproxen (500 mg orally).

Triptans may cause nausea and vomiting. They should probably be avoided in women who are pregnant, and in patients with hemiplegic or basilar migraine, a history of stroke or transient ischemic attack (TIA), or uncontrolled hypertension. In patients whose hypertension is controlled, triptans are commonly used safely, although caution is advised. Triptans are contraindicated in patients with coronary or peripheral vascular disease and Prinzmetal angina.

3. Other agents—Prochlorperazine is effective and may be administered rectally (25 mg suppository), intravenously or intramuscularly (5–10 mg), or orally (5–10 mg). Intravenous metoclopramide (10–20 mg) or chlorpromazine (25–50 mg) is also particularly useful in the emergency department setting. Various butalbital-containing combination oral analgesics risk overuse and dependence and should only be used as a last resort. Opioid analgesics should be avoided because of high rates of rebound headache and the tendency to develop medication overuse headache.

4. Neuromodulation—Single-pulse transcranial magnetic stimulation was effective in aborting migraine with aura, and noninvasive vagus nerve stimulation was effective in aborting migraine with or without aura in separate sham-controlled trials. Both are approved in the United States and the former in Europe. Transcranial magnetic stimulation is contraindicated in patients with epilepsy.

B. Preventive Therapy

Preventive treatment may be necessary if migraine headaches occur more frequently than *two or three times a month* or significant disability is associated with attacks. Avoidance of triggers and maintenance of homeostasis with regular sleep, meals, and hydration should not be neglected; a headache diary may be useful to identify triggers. Some more common agents used for prophylaxis are listed in Table 24–1. The medication chosen first will vary with the individual patient, depending on factors such as comorbid obesity, depression, anxiety, hypertension, and patient preference. Several medications may have to be tried in turn before headaches are brought under control. Once a medication has been found to help, it should be continued for several months. If the patient remains headache-free, the dose may be tapered and the medication

Table 24–1. Pharmacologic prophylaxis of migraine (listed in alphabetical order within classes).

Medication	Usual Adult Oral Daily Dose	Selected Side Effects and Comments
Antiepileptic[1]		
Topiramate	100 mg (divided twice daily)	Somnolence, nausea, dyspepsia, irritability, dizziness, ataxia, nystagmus, diplopia, glaucoma, renal calculi, weight loss, hypohidrosis, hyperthermia.
Valproic acid[2,3]	500–1000 mg (divided twice daily)	Nausea, vomiting, diarrhea, drowsiness, alopecia, weight gain, hepatotoxicity, thrombocytopenia, tremor, pancreatitis.
Cardiovascular		
Candesartan[3]	8–32 mg once daily	Dizziness, cough, diarrhea, fatigue.
Guanfacine	1 mg once daily	Dry mouth, somnolence, dizziness, constipation, erectile dysfunction.
Propranolol[4]	80–240 mg (divided twice to four times daily)	Fatigue, dizziness, hypotension, bradycardia, depression, insomnia, nausea, vomiting, constipation.
Verapamil[5]	120–240 mg (divided three times daily)	Headache, hypotension, flushing, edema, constipation. May aggravate atrioventricular nodal heart block and heart failure.
Antidepressant[6]		
Amitriptyline[7]	10–150 mg at bedtime	Sedation, dry mouth, constipation, weight gain, blurred vision, edema, hypotension, urinary retention.
Venlafaxine	37.5–150 mg extended release once daily	Nausea, somnolence, dry mouth, dizziness, diaphoresis, sexual dysfunction, anxiety, weight loss.
Monoclonal antibodies against calcitonin gene–related peptide		
Erenumab	70–140 mg subcutaneously once monthly	Injection site reactions, constipation, muscle cramps, antibody development.
Fremanezumab	225 mg subcutaneously once monthly	Injection site reactions, antibody development.
Galcanezumab	120 mg subcutaneously daily × 2 doses, followed by 120 mg monthly	Injection site reactions, antibody development.
Other		
Acupuncture		More rapid pain relief and fewer side effects than pharmacologic treatment.
Botulinum toxin A	Intramuscular injection	Injection site reaction, hypersensitivity, muscle weakness.
Riboflavin	400 mg once daily	Yellow-orange discoloration of urine

[1]Gabapentin and possibly other antiepileptics have also been used successfully.
[2]Avoid during pregnancy.
[3]Not FDA-approved for this indication.
[4]Other beta-adrenergic antagonists such as atenolol, metoprolol, nadolol, and timolol are similarly effective.
[5]Other calcium channel antagonists (eg, nimodipine, nicardipine, and diltiazem) may also help.
[6]Depression is commonly comorbid with migraine disorder and may warrant separate treatment.
[7]Other tricyclic antidepressants (eg, nortriptyline and imipramine) may help similarly.

eventually withdrawn. Transcutaneous supraorbital neurostimulation reduced the number of migraine days per month in a sham-controlled randomized trial and is approved in the United States. In **chronic migraine** (at least 15 days per month with headaches lasting 4 hours per day or longer), acupuncture is as effective as prophylactic pharmacologic treatment, and botulinum toxin type A reduces headache frequency. Monoclonal antibodies that block the calcitonin gene-related peptide receptor also reduce headache frequency in chronic migraine. Some other neurostimulation techniques look promising, including single-pulse transcranial magnetic stimulation, vagus nerve stimulators, and implantable occipital nerve stimulation, but critical appraisal is necessary.

2. Tension-Type Headache

This is the most common type of primary headache disorder. Patients frequently complain of pericranial tenderness, poor concentration, and other nonspecific symptoms, in addition to constant daily headaches that are often vise-like or tight in quality but not pulsatile. Headaches may be exacerbated by emotional stress, fatigue, noise, or glare. The headaches are usually generalized, may be most intense about the neck or back of the head, and are not associated with focal neurologic symptoms. There is diagnostic overlap with migraine.

The therapeutic approach is similar to that in migraine, except that triptans and ergotamines are not indicated.

Treatment of comorbid anxiety or depression is important. Behavioral therapies that may be effective include biofeedback and relaxation training.

3. Cluster Headache

Cluster headache affects predominantly middle-aged men. The pathophysiology is unclear but may relate to activation of cells in the ipsilateral hypothalamus, triggering the trigeminal autonomic vascular system. There is often no family history of headache or migraine. Episodes of severe unilateral periorbital pain occur daily for several weeks and are often accompanied by one or more of the following: ipsilateral nasal congestion, rhinorrhea, lacrimation, redness of the eye, and Horner syndrome (ptosis, pupillary meiosis, and facial anhidrosis or hypohidrosis). During attacks, patients are often restless and agitated. Episodes typically occur at night, awaken the patient, and last between 15 minutes and 3 hours. Spontaneous remission then occurs, and the patient remains well for weeks or months before another bout of closely spaced attacks. Bouts may last for 4 to 8 weeks and may occur up to several times per year. During a bout, many patients report alcohol triggers an attack; others report that stress, glare, or ingestion of specific foods occasionally precipitates attacks. In occasional patients, remission does not occur. This variant has been referred to as **chronic cluster headache**. In longstanding cases, Horner syndrome may persist between attacks.

Cluster headache is one of the **trigeminal autonomic cephalgias**, which include hemicrania continua, paroxysmal hemicrania, and short-lasting neuralgiform headache attacks with conjunctival injection and tearing. Similar to cluster headache, the other trigeminal autonomic cephalgias consist of unilateral periorbital pain associated with ipsilateral autonomic symptoms; they are distinguished from cluster headache by different attack duration and frequency and their exquisite responsiveness to indomethacin.

Treatment of an individual attack with oral medications is generally unsatisfactory, but subcutaneous (6 mg) or intranasal (20 mg/spray) sumatriptan or inhalation of 100% oxygen (12–15 L/min for 15 minutes via a non-rebreather mask) may be effective. Zolmitriptan (5- and 10-mg nasal spray) is also effective. Dihydroergotamine (0.5–1 mg intramuscularly or intravenously) or viscous lidocaine (1 mg of 4–6% solution intranasally) is sometimes effective.

Various prophylactic agents include oral medications such as lithium carbonate (start at 300 mg daily, titrating according to serum levels and treatment response up to a typical total daily dose of 900–1200 mg, divided three or four times), verapamil (start at 240 mg daily, increase by 80 mg every 2 weeks to 960 mg daily, with routine ECG to monitor the PR interval), topiramate (100–400 mg daily), and civamide (not available in the United States). As there is often a delay before these medications are effective, transitional therapy is often used. Prednisone (60 mg daily for 5 days followed by gradual withdrawal over 7–10 days) is effective in 70–80% of patients, and suboccipital corticosteroid injection about the greater occipital nerve is effective in 75%. Ergotamine tartrate can be given as rectal suppositories (0.5–1 mg at night or twice daily), by mouth (2 mg daily), or by subcutaneous injection (0.25 mg three times daily for 5 days per week). Electrical stimulation of the vagus nerve at headache onset successfully aborts pain in 30–50% of attacks, and twice daily prophylactic stimulation reduces attack number in chronic cluster headache; this treatment is approved in the United States. In Europe, sphenopalatine ganglion stimulation is approved for treatment of cluster headache based on efficacy in one randomized sham-controlled study. Limited evidence suggests that electrical stimulation of the occipital nerve by an implantable device may be helpful, especially in chronic cluster headache.

4. Posttraumatic Headache

A variety of nonspecific symptoms may follow closed head injury, regardless of whether consciousness is lost (see Head Injury). Headache is often a conspicuous feature. It usually appears within a day or so following injury, may worsen over the ensuing weeks, and then gradually subsides. It is usually a constant dull ache, with superimposed throbbing that may be localized, lateralized, or generalized. Headaches are sometimes accompanied by nausea, vomiting, or scintillating scotomas and often respond to simple analgesics; severe headaches may necessitate preventive treatment as outlined for migraine.

5. Primary Cough Headache

Severe head pain may be produced by coughing (and by straining, sneezing, and laughing) but, fortunately, usually lasts for only a few minutes or less. Intracranial lesions, usually in the posterior fossa (eg, Arnold-Chiari malformation), are present in about 10% of cases, and brain tumors or other space-occupying lesions may present in this way. Accordingly, *CT scanning or MRI should be undertaken in all patients.*

The disorder is usually self-limited, although it may persist for several years. For unknown reasons, symptoms sometimes clear completely after lumbar puncture. Indomethacin (75–150 mg daily orally) may provide relief. Similar activity-triggered headache syndromes include primary exertional headache and primary headache associated with sexual activity.

6. Headache Due to Giant Cell (Temporal or Cranial) Arteritis

This topic is discussed in Chapter 20.

7. Headache Due to Intracranial Mass Lesion

Intracranial mass lesions of all types may cause headache owing to displacement of vascular structures and other pain-sensitive tissues. While pain and location are nonspecific, headache may be worse upon lying down, awaken the patient at night, or peak in the morning after overnight recumbency. *The key feature prompting brain imaging is a new or worsening headache in middle or later life.* Other features suggesting an intracranial lesion include signs or symptoms of infection or malignancy such as fever, night sweats, and weight loss; immunocompromise; or history of malignancy. Signs of focal or diffuse cerebral dysfunction or of increased intracranial pressure (eg, papilledema) also necessitate investigation.

8. Medication Overuse (Analgesic Rebound) Headache

In approximately half of all patients with **chronic daily headaches,** medication overuse is responsible. Patients have chronic pain or severe headache unresponsive to medication (typically defined as no effect after having been used regularly for more than 3 months). Ergotamines, triptans, medications containing butalbital, and opioids cause medication overuse headache when taken on more than 10 days per month; acetaminophen, acetylsalicylic acid, and nonsteroidal anti-inflammatory drugs may also be offenders if taken on more than 15 days per month. Early initiation of a migraine preventive therapy permits withdrawal of analgesics and eventual relief of headache.

9. Headache Due to Other Neurologic Causes

Cerebrovascular disease may be associated with headache, but the mechanism is unclear. Headache may occur with internal carotid artery occlusion or carotid dissection and after carotid endarterectomy. Acute severe headache (**"thunderclap"**) accompanies subarachnoid hemorrhage, carotid or vertebral artery dissection, cerebral venous thrombosis, ischemic or hemorrhagic stroke, reversible cerebral vasoconstriction syndrome, hypertensive crisis, posterior reversible leukoencephalopathy syndrome, pituitary apoplexy, spontaneous intracranial hypotension, vasculitis, and meningeal infections; accompanying focal neurologic signs, impairment of consciousness, and signs of meningeal irritation indicate the need for further investigations. Headaches are also a feature of pseudotumor cerebri (idiopathic intracranial hypertension).

Dull or throbbing headache is a frequent sequela of lumbar puncture and may last for several days. It is aggravated by the erect posture and alleviated by recumbency. The mechanism is unclear, but the headache is commonly attributed to leakage of cerebrospinal fluid through the dural puncture site. Its incidence may be reduced if an atraumatic needle (instead of a beveled, cutting needle) is used for the lumbar puncture.

► When to Refer

- Thunderclap onset.
- Increasing headache unresponsive to simple measures.
- History of trauma, hypertension, fever, visual changes.
- Presence of neurologic signs or of scalp tenderness.

► When to Admit

Suspected subarachnoid hemorrhage or other structural intracranial lesion.

Chiang CC et al. Treatment of medication-overuse headache: a systematic review. Cephalalgia. 2016 Apr;36(4):371–86. [PMID: 26122645]

Puledda F et al. An update on migraine: current understanding and future directions. J Neurol. 2017 Sep;264(9):2031–9. [PMID: 28321564]

Vukovic-Cvetkovic V et al. Neurostimulation for the treatment of chronic migraine and cluster headache. Acta Neurol Scand. 2019 Jan;139(1):4–17. [PMID: 30291633]

FACIAL PAIN

1. Trigeminal Neuralgia

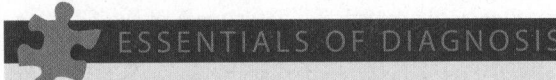
ESSENTIALS OF DIAGNOSIS

- ► Brief episodes of stabbing facial pain.
- ► Pain is in the territory of the second and third division of the trigeminal nerve.
- ► Pain exacerbated by touch.

► General Considerations

Trigeminal neuralgia ("tic douloureux") is most common in middle and later life. It affects women more frequently than men. Pain may be due to an anomalous artery or vein impinging on the trigeminal nerve.

► Clinical Findings

Momentary episodes of sudden lancinating facial pain commonly arise near one side of the mouth and shoot toward the ipsilateral ear, eye, or nostril. The pain may be triggered by such factors as touch, movement, drafts, and eating. In order to lessen the likelihood of triggering further attacks, many patients try to hold the face still while talking. Spontaneous remissions for several months or longer may occur. As the disorder progresses, however, the episodes of pain become more frequent, remissions become shorter and less common, and a dull ache may persist between the episodes of stabbing pain. Symptoms remain confined to the distribution of the trigeminal nerve (usually the second or third division) on one side only.

► Differential Diagnosis

The characteristic features of the pain in trigeminal neuralgia usually distinguish it from other causes of facial pain. Neurologic examination shows no abnormality except in a few patients in whom trigeminal neuralgia is symptomatic of some underlying lesion, such as multiple sclerosis or a brainstem neoplasm, in which case the finding will depend on the nature and site of the lesion. Multiple sclerosis must be suspected in a patient younger than 40 years in whom trigeminal neuralgia is the presenting symptom, even if there are no other neurologic signs. Bilateral symptoms should also prompt further investigation. Brain MRI need only be obtained when a secondary cause is suspected; it is usually normal in classic trigeminal neuralgia.

Treatment

The medications most helpful for treatment are oxcarbazepine (although not approved by the FDA for this indication) or carbamazepine, with monitoring by serial blood counts and liver biochemical tests. If these medications are ineffective or cannot be tolerated, phenytoin should be tried. (Doses and side effects of these medications are shown in Table 24–2.) Baclofen (10–20 mg orally three or four times daily), topiramate (50 mg orally twice daily), or lamotrigine (400 mg orally daily) may also be helpful, either alone or in combination with one of these other agents. Gabapentin may also relieve pain, especially in patients who do not respond to conventional medical therapy and those with multiple sclerosis. Depending on response and tolerance, up to 3600 mg daily orally is given in divided doses.

For neuralgia refractory to medical treatment, several surgical treatment options are available that provide initial pain relief in at least 80% of patients. Microvascular surgical decompression with separation of the anomalous vessel (usually not visible on CT scans, MRI, or arteriograms) from the nerve root produces long-term relief of symptoms in roughly 75% of patients. Three less invasive techniques are based on destruction of nociceptive trigeminal nerve fibers, which causes sensory loss in addition to symptom relief in half of patients: (1) radiofrequency rhizotomy produces long-term pain relief in 60% of patients, (2) percutaneous balloon compression of the trigeminal ganglion in 67%, and (3) stereotactic radiosurgery to the trigeminal nerve root in 45%. In elderly patients with a limited life expectancy, radiofrequency rhizotomy and stereotactic radiosurgery are sometimes preferred because both can be performed without general anesthesia and have few complications. Surgical exploration is inappropriate in patients with trigeminal neuralgia due to multiple sclerosis, but the less invasive techniques are sometimes helpful.

Table 24–2. Medication treatment for seizures in adults (in alphabetical order within classes).

Medication	Usual Adult Daily Oral Dose	Minimum No. of Daily Doses	Time to Steady-State Medication Levels	Optimal Medication Level and Laboratory Monitoring[1]	Selected Side Effects and Idiosyncratic Reactions
Generalized or Focal Seizures					
Brivaracetam[2,3]	50–100 mg	2	1–2 days	CBC, liver biochemical tests	Somnolence, fatigue, ataxia, vertigo, psychosis, leukopenia, hypersensitivity (bronchospasm and angioedema).
Cannabidiol[4]	5–20 mg/kg	2	11–13 days	Liver biochemical tests at baseline, 1, 3, and 6 months	Somnolence, fatigue, anorexia, weight loss, anemia, diarrhea, rash, sleep disorder, infections. Elevation in liver enzymes may occur; reduce dose in hepatic impairment.
Carbamazepine[2]	400–1600 mg (immediate or extended release)	2	3–4 days	4–8 mcg/mL CBC, liver biochemical tests, BUN/Cr	Nystagmus, dysarthria, diplopia, ataxia, drowsiness, nausea, blood dyscrasias, hepatotoxicity, hyponatremia, Stevens-Johnson syndrome.[5] **May exacerbate myoclonic seizures.**
Clobazam[6]	10–40 mg	2	7–10 days		Lethargy and somnolence, ataxia, insomnia, dysarthria, aggression, constipation, fever, Stevens-Johnson syndrome.
Clorazepate[3]	22.5–90 mg	2	10 days		Sedation, dizziness, confusion, ataxia, depression, dependency/abuse.
Eslicarbazepine[2,3]	400–1200 mg	1	4 days	Serum sodium and chloride; liver biochemical tests	As for carbamazepine.
Ezogabine[3]	300–1200 mg	3	2–3 days	ECG to assess QT interval	Dizziness, somnolence, confusion, vertigo, nausea, ataxia, psychiatric disturbances, prolonged QT interval, retinal abnormalities.[7]
Felbamate[2,3,6,8]	1200–3600 mg	3	4–5 days	CBC and reticulocytes, liver biochemical tests	Anorexia, nausea, vomiting, headache, insomnia, weight loss, dizziness, hepatotoxicity, fatal aplastic anemia. Reserved for refractory epilepsy.

(continued)

Table 24–2. Medication treatment for seizures in adults (in alphabetical order within classes). (continued)

Medication	Usual Adult Daily Oral Dose	Minimum No. of Daily Doses	Time to Steady-State Medication Levels	Optimal Medication Level and Laboratory Monitoring[1]	Selected Side Effects and Idiosyncratic Reactions
Gabapentin[3]	900–3600 mg	3	1 day		Sedation, fatigue, ataxia, nystagmus, weight loss.
Lacosamide[2,3]	100–400 mg	2	3 days	ECG if known cardiac conduction problems or severe cardiac disease	Vertigo, diplopia, nausea, headache, fatigue, ataxia, tremor, anaphylactoid reactions, PR prolongation, cardiac dysrhythmia, suicidality.
Lamotrigine[3,6,9,10]	100–500 mg	2	4–5 days		Sedation, skin rash, visual disturbances, dyspepsia, ataxia.
Levetiracetam[3,9,11]	1000–3000 mg	2	2 days		Somnolence, ataxia, headache, behavioral changes.
Oxcarbazepine[2,3]	900–1800 mg	2	2–3 days	Serum sodium	As for carbamazepine.
Perampanel[2,3,9]	4–12 mg	1	3 weeks		Dizziness, somnolence, irritability, weight gain, falls, ataxia, dysarthria, blurred vision.
Phenobarbital[2,12]	100–200 mg	1	14–21 days	10–40 mcg/mL CBC, liver biochemical tests, BUN/Cr	Drowsiness, nystagmus, ataxia, skin rashes, learning difficulties, hyperactivity.
Phenytoin[2,12]	200–400 mg	1	5–10 days	10–20 mcg/mL CBC, liver biochemical tests, folate	Nystagmus, ataxia, dysarthria, sedation, confusion, gingival hyperplasia, hirsutism, megaloblastic anemia, blood dyscrasias, skin rashes, fever, systemic lupus erythematosus, lymphadenopathy, peripheral neuropathy, dyskinesias. **May exacerbate myoclonic seizures.**
Pregabalin[3]	150–300 mg	2	2–4 days		Somnolence, dizziness, poor concentration, weight gain, thrombocytopenia, skin rashes, anaphylactoid reactions.
Primidone[2,12]	750–1500 mg	3	4–7 days	5–12 mcg/mL CBC	Sedation, nystagmus, ataxia, vertigo, nausea, skin rashes, megaloblastic anemia, irritability.
Rufinamide[6]	800–3200 mg	2	2 days		Somnolence, headache, dizziness, suicidality, Stevens-Johnson syndrome, leukopenia, shortened QT interval, nausea, vomiting.
Tiagabine[3]	32–56 mg	2	2 days		Somnolence, anxiety, dizziness, poor concentration, tremor, diarrhea.
Topiramate[2,3,6,9,12]	200–400 mg	2	4 days	Serum bicarbonate, BUN/Cr in elderly patients	Somnolence, nausea, dyspepsia, irritability, dizziness, ataxia, nystagmus, diplopia, glaucoma, renal calculi, weight loss, hypohidrosis, hyperthermia.
Valproic acid[2,3,13,14]	1500–2000 mg	2–3	2–4 days	50–100 mcg/mL CBC, liver biochemical tests	Nausea, vomiting, diarrhea, drowsiness, alopecia, weight gain, hepatotoxicity, thrombocytopenia, tremor, pancreatitis. **Teratogenic; avoid in women of childbearing age.**

(continued)

Table 24–2. Medication treatment for seizures in adults (in alphabetical order within classes). (continued)

Medication	Usual Adult Daily Oral Dose	Minimum No. of Daily Doses	Time to Steady-State Medication Levels	Optimal Medication Level and Laboratory Monitoring[1]	Selected Side Effects and Idiosyncratic Reactions
Vigabatrin[3,15]	3000 mg	2	2 days		Somnolence, anorexia, nausea, vomiting, agitation, hostility, confusion, suicidality, neutropenia, Stevens-Johnson syndrome, permanent visual field loss.[7]
Zonisamide[3]	200–600 mg	1	14 days	BUN/Cr, serum bicarbonate	Somnolence, ataxia, anorexia, nausea, vomiting, rash, confusion, renal calculi. Do not use in patients with sulfonamide allergy.
Absence Seizures					
Clonazepam[6,11,13,16,17]	0.04–0.2 mg/kg	2	7–10 days	20–80 ng/mL CBC, liver biochemical tests	Drowsiness, ataxia, irritability, behavioral changes, exacerbation of tonic-clonic seizures.
Ethosuximide[13]	500–1500 mg	2	5–10 days	40–100 mcg/mL CBC, liver biochemical tests, urinalysis	Nausea, vomiting, anorexia, headache, lethargy, unsteadiness, blood dyscrasias, systemic lupus erythematosus, urticaria, pruritus.
Valproic acid[2,3,13,14]	1500–2000 mg	2–3	2–4 days	See above	Nausea, vomiting, diarrhea, drowsiness, alopecia, weight gain, hepatotoxicity, thrombocytopenia, tremor, pancreatitis.
Myoclonic Seizures					
Clonazepam[6,11,13,16,17]	0.04–0.2 mg/kg	2	7–10 days	See above	Drowsiness, ataxia, irritability, behavioral changes, exacerbation of tonic-clonic seizures.
Valproic acid[2,3,13,14]	1500–2000 mg	2–3	2–4 days	See above	Nausea, vomiting, diarrhea, drowsiness, alopecia, weight gain, hepatotoxicity, thrombocytopenia, tremor, pancreatitis.
Levetiracetam[3,9,11]	1000–3000 mg	2	2 days		Somnolence, ataxia, headache, behavioral changes.

BUN, blood urea nitrogen; CBC, complete blood count; Cr, creatinine; ECG, electrocardiogram. Note that many factors influence optimal dose of these drugs including age, tolerance, and concomitant medication.

[1]Patients starting treatment with any antiepileptic drug should be monitored for new or worsening depression or suicidal thoughts, especially during the first weeks of therapy. Baseline measurement of creatinine clearance is advisable in renally metabolized drugs.
[2]Approved as monotherapy for focal-onset seizures.
[3]Approved as adjunctive therapy for focal-onset seizures.
[4]Approved for treatment of seizures in Lennox-Gastaut and Dravet syndrome in patients 2 years and older.
[5]Carriers of the HLA-B*1502 allele are at higher risk for Stevens-Johnson syndrome. Patients of Asian ancestry should be tested for this allele prior to initiation of therapy.
[6]Approved as adjunctive therapy for Lennox-Gastaut syndrome.
[7]Regular ophthalmologic examination is recommended.
[8]Not to be used as a first-line drug; when used, blood counts should be performed regularly (every 2–4 weeks). Should be used only in selected patients because of risk of aplastic anemia and hepatic failure. It is advisable to obtain written informed consent before use.
[9]Approved as adjunctive therapy for primary generalized tonic-clonic seizures.
[10]Approved as monotherapy (after conversion from another drug) in focal-onset seizures.
[11]Approved as adjunctive therapy for myoclonic seizures.
[12]Approved as initial monotherapy for primary generalized tonic-clonic seizures.
[13]Approved as monotherapy and adjunctive therapy for absence seizures.
[14]Approved as adjunctive therapy for patients with multiple seizure types including absence seizures.
[15]Approved as monotherapy for infantile spasms.
[16]Approved as monotherapy for Lennox-Gastaut syndrome.
[17]Approved as monotherapy for myoclonic seizures.

2. Atypical Facial Pain

Facial pain without the typical features of trigeminal neuralgia is generally a constant, often burning pain that may have a restricted distribution at its onset but soon spreads to the rest of the face on the affected side and sometimes involves the other side, the neck, or the back of the head as well. The disorder is especially common in middle-aged women, many of them depressed, but it is not clear whether depression is the cause of or a reaction to the pain. Simple analgesics should be given a trial, as should tricyclic antidepressants, carbamazepine, oxcarbazepine, and phenytoin; the response is often disappointing. Opioid analgesics pose a danger of addiction. Attempts at surgical treatment are not indicated.

3. Glossopharyngeal Neuralgia

Glossopharyngeal neuralgia is an uncommon disorder in which pain similar in quality to that in trigeminal neuralgia occurs in the throat, about the tonsillar fossa, and sometimes deep in the ear and at the back of the tongue. The pain may be precipitated by swallowing, chewing, talking, or yawning and is sometimes accompanied by syncope. In most instances, no underlying structural abnormality is present; multiple sclerosis is sometimes responsible. Oxcarbazepine and carbamazepine are the treatments of choice and should be tried before any surgical procedures are considered. Microvascular decompression is often effective and is generally preferred over destructive surgical procedures such as partial rhizotomy in medically refractory cases.

4. Postherpetic Neuralgia

Postherpetic neuralgia develops in about 15% of patients who have herpes zoster (shingles). This complication seems especially likely to occur in elderly or immunocompromised persons, when the rash is severe, and when the first division of the trigeminal nerve is affected. It also relates to the duration of the rash before medical consultation. A history of shingles and the presence of cutaneous scarring resulting from shingles aid in the diagnosis. Severe pain with shingles correlates with the intensity of postherpetic symptoms.

Acyclovir (800 mg five times daily) or valacyclovir (1000 mg three times daily), when given within 72 hours of rash onset, reduces the incidence of postherpetic neuralgia by almost half; systemic corticosteroids do *not* help prevent postherpetic neuralgia (see Chapter 6). Management of the established complication is with simple analgesics. If they fail to help, a trial of a tricyclic antidepressant (eg, amitriptyline or nortriptyline, up to 100–150 mg daily orally) is often effective. Other patients respond to gabapentin (up to 3600 mg daily orally) or pregabalin (up to 600 mg/daily orally). Subcutaneous injection of botulinum toxin A into the affected region produced sustained pain relief in 87% of patients in a small placebo-controlled trial. Topical application of capsaicin cream (eg, Zostrix, 0.025%) may be helpful, as may topical lidocaine (5%). The administration of **recombinant zoster vaccine** to patients over the age of 50 years is important in reducing the likelihood of herpes zoster and reducing the severity of postherpetic neuralgia should a reactivation occur.

5. Facial Pain Due to Other Causes

Facial pain may be caused by temporomandibular joint dysfunction in patients with malocclusion, abnormal bite, or faulty dentures. There may be tenderness of the masticatory muscles, and sometimes pain begins at the onset of chewing. This pattern differs from that of jaw (masticatory) claudication, a symptom of giant cell arteritis, in which pain develops progressively with mastication. Treatment of the underlying joint dysfunction relieves symptoms.

A relationship of facial pain to chewing or temperature changes may suggest a dental disturbance. The cause is sometimes not obvious, and diagnosis requires careful dental examination and radiographs. Sinusitis and ear infections causing facial pain are usually recognized by a history of respiratory tract infection, fever, and, in some instances, nasal or aural discharge. There may be localized tenderness. Radiologic evidence of sinus infection or mastoiditis is confirmatory.

Glaucoma is an important ocular cause of facial pain, usually localized to the periorbital region.

On occasion, pain in the jaw may be the principal manifestation of angina pectoris. Precipitation by exertion and radiation to more typical areas suggests a cardiac origin.

▶ When to Refer

- Worsening pain unresponsive to simple measures.
- Continuing pain of uncertain cause.
- For consideration of surgical treatment (trigeminal or glossopharyngeal neuralgia).

Donnet A et al. French guidelines for diagnosis and treatment of classical trigeminal neuralgia (French Headache Society and French Neurosurgical Society). Rev Neurol (Paris). 2017 Mar; 173(3):131–51. [PMID: 28314515]

EPILEPSY

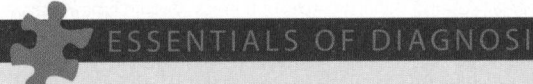

ESSENTIALS OF DIAGNOSIS

▶ Recurrent unprovoked seizures.

▶ Characteristic electroencephalographic changes accompany seizures.

▶ Mental status abnormalities or focal neurologic symptoms may persist for hours postictally.

▶ General Considerations

The term "epilepsy" denotes any disorder characterized by recurrent *unprovoked* seizures. A seizure is a transient disturbance of cerebral function due to an abnormal paroxysmal neuronal discharge in the brain. Epilepsy is relatively common, affecting approximately 0.5% of the population in the United States.

Patients with recurrent seizures provoked by a readily reversible cause, such as withdrawal from alcohol or drugs, hypoglycemia, hyperglycemia, or uremia, are not considered to have epilepsy.

▶ Classification of Epilepsy

According to the International League Against Epilepsy classification system, recurrent seizures should be classified first by seizure type, second by epilepsy type, and third, if possible, by epilepsy syndrome. The etiology of recurrent seizures should be sought at each stage of classification (see Etiology of Epilepsy).

A. Seizure Types

The International League Against Epilepsy distinguishes seizures affecting only part of the brain (focal seizures) from those that are generalized.

1. Focal onset seizures—The initial clinical and electroencephalographic manifestations of focal (partial) seizures indicate that only a restricted part of one cerebral hemisphere has been activated. The ictal manifestations depend on the area of the brain involved. Focal seizures are classified by motor or nonmotor onset as well as by whether awareness is impaired.

A. MOTOR VERSUS NONMOTOR ONSET—Seizures with motor onset may be **clonic, tonic, atonic, myoclonic,** or **hyperkinetic,** or may manifest as **automatisms** or **epileptic spasms.** The most commonly observed focal motor seizures consist of clonic jerking or automatisms. Nonmotor seizures may be manifested by sensory symptoms (eg, paresthesias or tingling, gustatory, olfactory, visual or auditory sensations), behavior arrest, cognitive symptoms (eg, speech arrest, déjà vu, jamais vu), emotional symptoms (eg, fear), or autonomic symptoms or signs (eg, abnormal epigastric sensations, sweating, flushing, pupillary dilation). Focal sensory and motor seizures may spread (or "march") to different parts of the limb or body depending on their cortical representation and were previously called "simple partial" seizures.

B. AWARE VERSUS IMPAIRED AWARENESS—Awareness is defined as knowledge of self and environment and of events occurring during a seizure. Impaired awareness may be preceded, accompanied, or followed by the various motor and nonmotor symptoms mentioned above. Such seizures were previously called "complex partial" seizures.

C. FOCAL TO BILATERAL TONIC-CLONIC—Focal seizures sometimes involve loss of awareness and evolve to bilateral tonic-clonic seizures, in a process previously called "secondary generalization."

2. Generalized onset seizures—Generalized seizures are thought to originate in or rapidly spread to involve bilateral cortical networks. In some cases, the distinction between focal and generalized onset can only be made by electroencephalogram (EEG). Generalized seizures are classified into those with motor or nonmotor features. Awareness is typically lost with generalized seizures but may be retained partially in the briefest absence attacks and some myoclonic seizures.

A. NONMOTOR (ABSENCE) SEIZURES—These are characterized by impairment of consciousness, sometimes with mild clonic, tonic, myoclonic, or atonic components (ie, reduction or loss of postural tone), autonomic components (eg, enuresis), or accompanying automatisms. Onset and termination of attacks are abrupt. If attacks occur during conversation, the patient may miss a few words or may break off in midsentence for a few seconds. The impairment of external awareness is so brief that the patient is unaware of it. **Absence ("petit mal") seizures** almost always begin in childhood and frequently cease by the age of 20 years or are then replaced by other forms of generalized seizure. Electroencephalographically, such attacks are associated with bursts of bilaterally synchronous and symmetric 3-Hz spike-wave activity. A normal background in the electroencephalogram and normal or above-normal intelligence imply a good prognosis for the ultimate cessation of these seizures. **Atypical absence seizures** may demonstrate more marked changes in tone, or attacks may have a more gradual onset and termination than in typical absence seizures. They commonly occur in patients with multiple seizure types, may be accompanied by developmental delay or mental retardation, and are associated with slower spike-wave discharges than those in typical absence attacks.

B. MOTOR SEIZURES—Types of generalized motor seizures include **tonic-clonic, clonic, tonic, myoclonic, myoclonic-tonic-clonic, myoclonic-atonic, atonic,** and **epileptic spasms.** During tonic-clonic seizures there is sudden loss of consciousness, the patient becomes rigid and falls to the ground, and respiration is arrested. This tonic phase, which usually lasts for under 1 minute, is followed by a clonic phase in which there is jerking of the body musculature that may last for 2 or 3 minutes and is then followed by a stage of flaccid coma. During the seizure, the tongue or lips may be bitten, urinary or fecal incontinence may occur, and the patient may be injured. Immediately after the seizure, the patient may recover consciousness, drift into sleep, have a further convulsion without recovery of consciousness between the attacks (**status epilepticus),** or after recovering consciousness have a further convulsion (**serial seizures).** In other cases, patients may behave in an abnormal fashion in the immediate postictal period, without subsequent awareness or memory of events (**postepileptic automatism).** Headache, disorientation, confusion, drowsiness, nausea, soreness of the muscles, or some combination of these symptoms commonly occurs postictally. Myoclonic seizures consist of single or multiple myoclonic jerks. Atonic seizures consist of very brief (less than 2 seconds) loss of muscle tone and often result in falls (**epileptic drop attacks). Epileptic spasms** are sudden flexion or extension of truncal muscles; these seizures usually manifest during infancy.

3. Unknown onset seizures—In some circumstances, seizures cannot be classified because of incomplete information or because they do not fit into any category. Generally, with additional information from the history or from video-EEG telemetry, the seizure onset can be correctly classified.

B. Epilepsy Types

The International League Against Epilepsy classifies epilepsy by the seizure type. Thus, epilepsy may be **focal**, **generalized,** or **combined generalized and focal.** The EEG may be helpful in facilitating classification.

C. Epilepsy Syndromes

Epilepsy syndromes are defined by constellations of seizure types, EEG findings, and imaging features, and often also depend on age at onset and comorbidities. Not every patient with epilepsy can be given a syndromic diagnosis. Several well-known epilepsy syndromes exist but are beyond the scope of this chapter.

► Etiology of Epilepsy

In parallel to classifying the seizure type, epilepsy type, and epilepsy syndrome (if applicable), the cause of the patient's seizures should be sought. The International League Against Epilepsy lists six broad etiologic categories; sometimes a patient's seizures have more than one etiology.

A. Structural Etiology

1. Pediatric age groups—Congenital abnormalities and perinatal injuries may result in seizures presenting in infancy or childhood.

2. Mesial temporal sclerosis—Hippocampal sclerosis is a recognized cause of focal and secondarily generalized seizures of uncertain etiology.

3. Trauma—Trauma is an important cause of seizures at any age, but especially in young adults. Posttraumatic epilepsy is more likely to develop if the dura mater was penetrated and generally becomes manifest within 2 years following the injury. Seizures developing in the first week after head injury do not necessarily imply that future attacks will occur. There is no evidence that prophylactic anticonvulsant medication treatment reduces the incidence of posttraumatic epilepsy.

4. Tumors and other space-occupying lesions—Neoplasms may lead to seizures at any age, but they are an especially important cause of seizures in middle and later life, when the incidence of neoplastic disease increases. Seizures are commonly the initial symptoms of the tumor and often are focal in character. They are most likely to occur with structural lesions involving the frontal, parietal, or temporal regions. *Tumors must be excluded by imaging studies (MRI preferred over CT) in all patients with onset of seizures after 20 years of age, focal seizures or signs, or a progressive seizure disorder.*

5. Vascular diseases—Stroke and other vascular diseases become increasingly frequent causes of seizures with advancing age and are the most common cause of seizures with onset at age 60 years or older.

6. Degenerative disorders—Alzheimer disease and other degenerative disorders are a cause of seizures in later life.

B. Genetic Etiology

This category encompasses a broad range of disorders, for which the age at onset ranges from the neonatal period to adolescence or even later in life. Monogenic disorders tend to exhibit an autosomal dominant pattern of inheritance, and where the mutation is known, the responsible gene often encodes a neuronal ion channel. A genetic etiology may also underpin certain epilepsies with a metabolic or structural basis.

C. Infectious Etiology

Infectious diseases must be considered in all age groups as potentially reversible causes of seizures. Seizures may occur with an acute infective or inflammatory illness, such as bacterial meningitis or herpes encephalitis, or in patients with more longstanding or chronic disorders, such as neurosyphilis or cerebral cysticercosis. In patients with AIDS, seizures may result from central nervous system toxoplasmosis, cryptococcal meningitis, secondary viral encephalitis, or other infective complications. Seizures are a common sequela of supratentorial brain abscess, developing most frequently in the first year after treatment.

D. Metabolic Etiology

Inborn errors of metabolism and other inherited conditions may cause epilepsy as one of their manifestations (eg, pyridoxine deficiency, mitochondrial disease); these disorders typically present during childhood.

E. Immune Etiology

Autoimmune diseases such as systemic lupus erythematosus and autoimmune limbic encephalitis may cause epilepsy; often the epilepsy can be cured with immunotherapy and lifelong antiepileptic medication treatment is not necessary.

F. Unknown Etiology

In many cases, the cause of epilepsy cannot be determined.

► Clinical Findings

A. Symptoms and Signs

Nonspecific changes such as headache, mood alterations, lethargy, and myoclonic jerking alert some patients to an impending seizure hours before it occurs. These prodromal symptoms are distinct from the aura; the aura that may precede a generalized seizure by a few seconds or minutes is itself a part of the seizure indicating focal onset from a restricted part of the brain.

In most patients, seizures occur unpredictably at any time and without any relationship to posture or ongoing activities. Occasionally, however, they occur at a particular time (eg, during sleep) or in relation to external precipitants such as lack of sleep, missed meals, emotional stress, menstruation, alcohol ingestion (or alcohol withdrawal), or use of certain recreational drugs. Fever and nonspecific infections may also precipitate seizures in epileptic patients. In a few patients, seizures are provoked by specific stimuli such as flashing lights or a flickering television set (**photosensitive epilepsy**), music, or reading.

Clinical examination between seizures shows no abnormality in patients with idiopathic epilepsy, but in the immediate postictal period, extensor plantar responses may be seen. The presence of lateralized or focal signs postictally suggests that seizures may have a focal origin. In patients with symptomatic epilepsy, the findings on examination will reflect the underlying cause.

B. Laboratory and Other Studies

Initial investigations after a first seizure should include complete blood count, serum glucose, electrolytes, creatinine, calcium, magnesium, and liver biochemical tests to exclude various causes of provoked seizures and to provide a baseline for subsequent monitoring of long-term effects of treatment. Routine laboratory investigations are not usually necessary after recurrent seizures in patients with known epilepsy. A lumbar puncture may be necessary when any sign of infection is present or in the evaluation of new-onset seizures in the acute setting.

C. Imaging

MRI is indicated for patients with focal neurologic symptoms or signs, focal seizures, or electroencephalographic findings of a focal disturbance. It should also be performed in patients with clinical evidence of a progressive disorder and in those with new onset of seizures after the age of 20 years because of the possibility of an underlying neoplasm. CT is generally less sensitive than MRI in detecting small structural brain abnormalities but may be used when MRI is contraindicated or unavailable.

Electroencephalography may support the clinical diagnosis of epilepsy (by demonstrating paroxysmal abnormalities containing spikes or sharp waves), provide a guide to prognosis, and help classify the seizure disorder. Classification of the disorder is important for determining the most appropriate anticonvulsant medication with which to start treatment. For example, absence and focal seizures with impaired awareness may be difficult to distinguish clinically, but the electroencephalographic findings and treatment of choice differ in these two conditions. Finally, by localizing the epileptogenic source, the electroencephalographic findings are important in evaluating candidates for surgical treatment.

▶ Differential Diagnosis

The distinction between the various disorders likely to be confused with generalized seizures is usually made on the basis of the history. The importance of obtaining an eyewitness account of the attacks cannot be overemphasized.

A. Differential Diagnosis of Focal Seizures

1. TIAs—These are distinguished from seizures by their longer duration, lack of spread, and negative (eg, weakness or numbness) rather than positive (eg, convulsive jerking or paresthesias) symptoms. Level of consciousness, which is unaltered, does not distinguish them.

2. Migraine aura—Migraine aura may produce positive or negative symptoms, tends to spread slowly from one part of the body to another (over minutes rather than seconds), and is usually longer in duration (minutes to hours). It is usually, but not always, followed by a typical migraine headache.

3. Panic attacks—These may be hard to distinguish from focal seizures unless there is evidence of an anxiety disorder between attacks and the attacks have a clear relationship to external circumstances.

4. Rage attacks—These are situational and lead to goal-directed aggressive behavior.

B. Differential Diagnosis of Generalized Seizures

1. Syncope—Syncopal episodes usually occur in relation to postural change, emotional stress, instrumentation, pain, or straining. They are typically preceded by pallor, sweating, nausea, and malaise and lead to loss of consciousness accompanied by flaccidity; recovery occurs rapidly with recumbency, and there is no postictal headache or confusion. In some instances, however, motor accompaniments and urinary incontinence may simulate a seizure.

2. Cardiac disease—Cerebral hypoperfusion due to a disturbance of cardiac rhythm should be suspected in patients with known cardiac or vascular disease or in elderly patients who present with episodic loss of consciousness. Prodromal symptoms are typically absent. Cardiac rhythm monitoring may be necessary to establish the diagnosis; external event recorders or implantable loop recorders may be valuable if the disturbances of consciousness are rare. A relationship of attacks to physical activity and the finding of a systolic murmur are suggestive of aortic stenosis.

3. Brainstem ischemia—Loss of consciousness is preceded or accompanied by other brainstem signs. Basilar artery migraine and vertebrobasilar vascular disease are discussed elsewhere in this chapter.

4. Psychogenic nonepileptic seizure (PNES)—Simulating an epileptic seizure, a PNES may occur due to a conversion disorder or malingering. Many patients also have epileptic seizures or a family history of epilepsy. A history of childhood physical or sexual abuse is common. Although a PNES tends to occur at times of emotional stress, this may also be the case with epileptic seizures.

Clinically, the attacks superficially resemble tonic-clonic seizures, but there may be obvious preparation before a PNES. Moreover, there is usually no tonic phase; instead, there may be an asynchronous thrashing of the limbs and the attack rarely leads to injury. Eyes are often forcibly closed during PNES, unlike epileptic seizures, in which they are typically open. Consciousness may be normal or "lost," but in the latter context the occurrence of goal-directed behavior or of shouting, swearing, etc, indicates that it is feigned. Postictally, there are no changes in behavior or neurologic findings.

Often, clinical observation is insufficient to discriminate epileptic from nonepileptic seizures and **video electroencephalographic monitoring** is required. Elevation of serum prolactin level to at least twice the upper limit of normal can be seen between 10 and 20 minutes after a seizure or syncopal event but not after a PNES. However, prolactin measurement has limited clinical utility because levels are normal after an epileptic seizure in roughly half of patients and a baseline prolactin must be drawn 6 hours after the attack.

► Treatment

A. General Measures

For patients with epilepsy, medication is prescribed with the goal of preventing further attacks and is usually continued until there have been no seizures for at least 2 years. Epileptic patients should be advised to avoid situations that could be dangerous or life-threatening if further seizures should occur. Legislation may require clinicians to report to the state authorities any patients with seizures or other episodic disturbances of consciousness; *driving cessation* for 6 months or as legislated is appropriate following an unprovoked seizure.

1. Choice of medication—Medication selection depends on seizure type (Table 24–2). The dose of the selected anticonvulsant is gradually increased until seizures are controlled or side effects prevent further increases. If seizures continue despite treatment at the maximal tolerated dose, a second medication is added and the dose increased depending on tolerance; the first medication is then gradually withdrawn. In most patients with seizures of a single type, satisfactory control can be achieved with a single anticonvulsant. Treatment with two medications may further reduce seizure frequency or severity but usually only at the cost of greater toxicity. Treatment with more than two medications is almost always unhelpful unless the patient is having seizures of different types. Other factors to consider in selecting an anticonvulsant include likely side effects, teratogenicity, interactions with other medications and oral contraceptives, and route of metabolism.

All antiepileptics are potentially teratogenic, although the teratogenicity of the newer antiseizure medications is less clear. Nevertheless, antiepileptic medication must be given to pregnant women with epilepsy to prevent seizures, which can pose serious risk to the fetus from trauma, hypoxia, or other factors.

2. Monitoring—Individual differences in drug metabolism cause a given dose of a medication to produce different blood concentrations in different patients, and this will affect the therapeutic response. In general, *the dose of an antiepileptic agent is increased to achieve the desired clinical response regardless of the serum drug level.* When a dose is reached that either controls seizures or is the maximum tolerated, then a steady-state trough drug level may be obtained for future reference; rechecking this level may be appropriate during pregnancy, if a breakthrough seizure occurs, a dose change occurs, or another (potentially interacting) medication is added to the regimen. A laboratory's therapeutic range for a medication is only a guide; many patients achieve good seizure control with no adverse effect at serum levels that exceed the stipulated range, and in these cases no dose adjustment is needed. The most common cause of a lower concentration of medication than

expected for the prescribed dose is suboptimal patient adherence. Adherence can be improved by limiting to a minimum the number of daily doses. Recurrent seizures or status epilepticus may result if medications are taken erratically, and in some circumstances nonadherent patients may be better off without any medication. All anticonvulsants have side effects, and many require baseline and regular laboratory monitoring (Table 24–2).

3. Discontinuance of medication—Only when adult patients have been seizure-free for 2 years should withdrawal of medication be considered. Unfortunately, there is no way of predicting which patients can be managed successfully without treatment, although seizure recurrence is more likely in patients who initially did not respond to therapy, those with seizures having focal features or of multiple types, and those with continuing electroencephalographic abnormalities. Dose reduction should be gradual (over weeks or months), and medications should be withdrawn one at a time. If seizures recur, treatment is reinstituted with the previously effective regimen.

4. Surgical treatment—Patients with seizures refractory to two or more medications may be candidates for operative treatment. Surgical resection is most efficacious when there is a single well-defined seizure focus, particularly in the temporal lobe. Among well-chosen patients, up to 70% remain seizure-free after extended follow-up. Deep brain or cortical stimulation for medically refractory focal-onset seizures may be of benefit.

5. Vagal nerve stimulation—Treatment by chronic vagal nerve stimulation for adults and adolescents with medically refractory focal seizures is approved in the United States and provides an alternative approach for patients who are not optimal candidates for surgical treatment. The mechanism of therapeutic action is unknown. Adverse effects consist mainly of transient hoarseness during stimulus delivery.

B. Special Circumstances

1. Solitary seizures—In patients who have had only one seizure or a flurry of seizures over a brief period of several hours, investigation as outlined earlier should exclude an underlying cause requiring specific treatment. An electroencephalogram should be obtained, preferably within 24 hours after the seizure. Prophylactic anticonvulsant treatment is generally not required unless further attacks occur or investigations reveal underlying pathology. The risk of seizure recurrence varies in different series between about 30% and 70%, with higher risk of recurrence in patients with structural brain lesions or abnormalities on electroencephalogram. Epilepsy should *not* be diagnosed on the basis of a solitary seizure. If seizures occur in the context of transient, nonrecurrent systemic disorders such as hyponatremia or hypoglycemia, the diagnosis of epilepsy is inaccurate, and long-term prophylactic anticonvulsant treatment is unnecessary.

2. Alcohol withdrawal seizures—The characteristic alcohol withdrawal seizure pattern is one or more generalized tonic-clonic seizures that may occur within 48 hours or so of withdrawal from alcohol after a period of high or prolonged intake. If the seizures have consistently focal features, the possibility of an associated structural abnormality, often traumatic in origin, must be considered. Treatment with anticonvulsants is generally not required for alcohol withdrawal seizures, since they are self-limited. Benzodiazepines are effective and safe for preventing further seizures (see Chapter 25). Status epilepticus may complicate alcohol withdrawal and is managed along conventional lines. Further attacks will not occur if the patient abstains from alcohol.

3. Tonic-clonic status epilepticus—Poor adherence to the anticonvulsant regimen is the most common cause; however, any disorder that can cause a single seizure may be responsible. The mortality rate may be as high as 20%, and among survivors the incidence of neurologic and cognitive sequelae is high. The prognosis relates to the underlying cause as well as the length of time between onset of status epilepticus and the start of effective treatment.

Status epilepticus is a medical emergency. Initial management includes maintenance of the airway and 50% dextrose (25–50 mL) intravenously in case hypoglycemia is responsible. If seizures continue, an intravenous bolus of lorazepam, 4 mg, is given at a rate of 2 mg/min and repeated once after 10 minutes if necessary; alternatively, 10 mg of midazolam is given intramuscularly, and again after 10 minutes if necessary. Diazepam can also be given rectally as a gel (0.2 mg/kg). These measures are usually effective in halting seizures for a brief period. Respiratory depression and hypotension may complicate the treatment and are treated as in other circumstances, including intubation and mechanical ventilation and admission to an intensive care unit.

Regardless of the response to lorazepam or midazolam, fosphenytoin or phenytoin should be administered intravenously to initiate long-term seizure control. Fosphenytoin (18–20 mg phenytoin equivalents [PE]/kg) is rapidly and completely converted to phenytoin following intravenous administration and is preferred because it is less likely to cause reactions at the infusion site, can be given with all common intravenous solutions, and may be administered at a faster rate (150 mg PE/min). When fosphenytoin is not available, phenytoin (18–20 mg/kg) is given intravenously at a rate of 50 mg/min. Phenytoin is best injected directly but can also be given in saline; it precipitates, however, if injected into glucose-containing solutions. Because arrhythmias may develop during rapid administration of fosphenytoin or phenytoin, electrocardiographic monitoring is prudent. Hypotension may occur, especially if diazepam has also been given.

If seizures continue, phenobarbital is then given in a loading dose of 10–20 mg/kg intravenously by slow or intermittent injection (50 mg/min). Respiratory depression and hypotension are especially common with this therapy. Alternatively or additionally, intravenous valproate is used for status epilepticus (loading dose 20–40 mg/kg over 15 min); although valproate is not approved by the FDA for this indication, it has been used with success.

If these measures fail, general anesthesia with ventilatory assistance may be required; some experts recommend proceeding directly to general anesthesia if convulsions do not cease after the initial 18–20 PE/kg fosphenytoin load. Intravenous midazolam may provide control of refractory status epilepticus; the suggested loading dose is 0.2 mg/kg, followed by 0.05–0.2 mg/kg/h. Propofol (1–2 mg/kg as an intravenous bolus, followed by infusion at 2–15 mg/kg/h depending on response) may also be used, as may pentobarbital (15 mg/kg intravenously, followed by 0.5–4 mg/kg/h).

After status epilepticus is controlled, an oral medication program for the long-term management of seizures is started, and investigations into the cause of the disorder are pursued.

4. Nonconvulsive status epilepticus—In some cases, status epilepticus presents not with convulsions, but with a fluctuating abnormal mental status, confusion, impaired responsiveness, and automatism. Electroencephalography establishes the diagnosis. The treatment approach outlined above applies to any type of status epilepticus, although intravenous anesthesia is usually not necessary. The prognosis is a reflection of the underlying cause rather than of continuing seizures.

▶ **When to Refer**

- Behavioral episodes of uncertain nature.
- Seizures are difficult to control with monotherapy.
- There is a progressive neurologic disorder.

▶ **When to Admit**

- Status epilepticus.
- Frequent seizures requiring rapid medication titration and electroencephalographic monitoring.
- For inpatient monitoring when PNES is suspected.

Betjemann JP et al. Status epilepticus in adults. Lancet Neurol. 2015 Jun;14(6):615–24. [PMID: 25908090]

Fisher RS et al. Operational classification of seizure types by the International League Against Epilepsy: position paper of the ILAE commission for classification and terminology. Epilepsia. 2017 Apr;58(4):522–30. [PMID: 28276060]

Gavvala JR et al. JAMA patient page. Epilepsy. JAMA. 2016 Dec 27;316(24):2686. [PMID: 28027369]

Kanner AM et al. Practice guideline update summary: efficacy and tolerability of the new antiepileptic drugs I: Treatment of new-onset epilepsy. Epilepsy Curr. 2018 Jul–Aug;18(4):260–8. [PMID: 30254527]

Scheffer IE et al. ILAE classification of the epilepsies: position paper of the ILAE commission for classification and terminology. Epilepsia. 2017 Apr;58(4):512–21. [PMID: 28276062]

DYSAUTONOMIA

ESSENTIALS OF DIAGNOSIS

▶ Postural hypotension or abnormal heart rate regulation.

▶ Abnormalities of sweating, intestinal motility, sexual function, or sphincter control.

▶ Syncope may occur.

▶ Symptoms occur in isolation or any combination.

General Considerations

Dysautonomia may occur as a result of pathological processes in the central or peripheral nervous system. It is manifested by a variety of symptoms related to abnormalities of blood pressure regulation, thermoregulatory sweating, gastrointestinal function, sphincter control, sexual function, respiration, and ocular function. The differential diagnosis depends on the time course of autonomic dysfunction and whether dysautonomia is an isolated symptom or associated with central or peripheral neurologic symptoms and signs.

A. Causes in the Central Nervous System

Disease at certain sites, regardless of its nature, may lead to dysautonomic symptoms. Postural hypotension, which is usually the most troublesome and disabling symptom, may result from spinal cord transection and other myelopathies (eg, due to tumor or syringomyelia) above the T6 level or from brainstem lesions such as syringobulbia and posterior fossa tumors. Sphincter or sexual disturbances may result from cord lesions at any level. Certain primary degenerative disorders are responsible for dysautonomia occurring in isolation (**pure autonomic failure**) or in association with more widespread abnormalities (**multisystem atrophy**) that may include parkinsonism, pyramidal symptoms, and cerebellar deficits. Postural hypotension is also a prominent symptom of idiopathic Parkinson disease and dementia with Lewy bodies.

B. Causes in the Peripheral Nervous System

A pure autonomic neuropathy may occur acutely or subacutely after a viral infection or as a paraneoplastic disorder related usually to small cell lung cancer, particularly in association with certain antibodies, such as anti-Hu or those directed at neuronal nicotinic ganglionic acetylcholine receptors. Dysautonomia is often conspicuous in patients with Guillain-Barré syndrome, manifesting with marked hypotension or hypertension or cardiac arrhythmias that may have a fatal outcome. It may also occur with diabetic, uremic, amyloidotic, and various other metabolic or toxic neuropathies; in association with leprosy or Chagas disease; and as a feature of certain hereditary neuropathies with autosomal dominant or recessive inheritance or an X-linked pattern. Autonomic symptoms are prominent in the crises of hepatic porphyria. Patients with botulism or the Lambert-Eaton myasthenic syndrome may have constipation, urinary retention, and a sicca syndrome as a result of impaired cholinergic function.

Clinical Findings

A. Symptoms and Signs

Dysautonomic symptoms include syncope, postural hypotension, paroxysmal hypertension, persistent tachycardia without other cause, facial flushing, hypohidrosis or hyperhidrosis, vomiting, constipation, diarrhea, dysphagia, abdominal distention, disturbances of micturition or defecation, erectile dysfunction, apneic episodes, and declining night vision. In syncope, prodromal malaise, nausea, headache, diaphoresis, pallor, visual disturbance, loss of postural tone, and a sense of weakness and impending loss of consciousness are followed by actual loss of consciousness. It is usually accompanied by hypotension and bradycardia and may occur in response to emotional stress, postural hypotension, vigorous exercise in a hot environment, obstructed venous return to the heart, acute pain or its anticipation, fluid loss, and a variety of other circumstances. Although the patient is usually flaccid, some motor activity is not uncommon, and urinary (and rarely fecal) incontinence may also occur, thereby simulating a seizure. Recovery is rapid once the patient becomes recumbent, but headache, nausea, and fatigue commonly persist.

B. Evaluation of the Patient

The extent and severity of autonomic dysfunction should be determined, and the presence of associated neurologic symptoms and signs ascertained. Bedside testing of autonomic function includes examination of pupillary reactivity, examination of the skin for areas of excessive or reduced sweating and of the hands and feet for color or temperature changes, as well as assessment of blood pressure and heart rate in the supine position and 2 minutes after standing. With dysautonomia, postural hypotension is not accompanied by a compensatory rise in heart rate. Specialized tests include the cardiovascular response to the Valsalva maneuver and deep respiration, tilt-table testing, the thermoregulatory sweat test, the quantitative sudomotor axon reflex test, and the quantitative direct and indirect axon reflex test. Tests of gastrointestinal motility and urodynamics may be helpful when symptoms of dysmotility, incontinence, or urinary retention are present.

The neurologic examination should focus on detecting signs of parkinsonism, cerebellar dysfunction, disorders of neuromuscular transmission, and peripheral neuropathy. All patients should be tested for vitamin B_{12} deficiency and diabetes. Patients with acute or subacute isolated dysautonomia should undergo testing for ganglionic acetylcholine receptor, anti-Hu, voltage-gated potassium channel complex, and voltage-gated calcium channel antibodies. For those with evidence of peripheral neuropathy, nerve conduction studies; electromyography; and testing for HIV, amyloidosis, Sjögren syndrome, and Fabry disease are indicated. If there is evidence of central pathology, imaging studies will exclude a treatable structural cause. If the neurologic examination is normal, reversible, nonneurologic causes of symptoms must be considered. Isolated postural hypotension and syncope may relate to a reduced cardiac output, paroxysmal cardiac dysrhythmias, volume depletion, various medications, and endocrine and metabolic disorders such as Addison disease, hypothyroidism or hyperthyroidism, pheochromocytoma, and carcinoid syndrome.

Treatment

The most disabling symptoms are usually postural hypotension and syncope. Abrupt postural change, prolonged recumbency, heavy meals, and other precipitants should be avoided. Medications associated with postural hypotension should be discontinued or reduced in dose. Treatment may include wearing waist-high elastic hosiery, salt supplementation, sleeping in a semierect position (which minimizes the natriuresis and diuresis that occur during recumbency), ingestion of 500 mL water 30 minutes before arising, and fludrocortisone (0.1–0.5 mg orally daily). Vasoconstrictor agents may be helpful and include midodrine (2.5–10 mg orally three times daily), droxidopa (100–600 mg orally three times daily), and ephedrine (15–30 mg orally three times daily). Other agents that have been used occasionally or experimentally are dihydroergotamine, yohimbine, pyridostigmine, and clonidine; refractory cases may respond to erythropoietin (epoetin alfa) or desmopressin. Patients must be monitored for recumbent hypertension. Postprandial hypotension is helped by caffeine. There is no satisfactory treatment for disturbances of sweating, but an air-conditioned environment is helpful in avoiding extreme swings in body temperature.

► When to Refer

- When the diagnosis is uncertain.
- When symptoms persist despite conventional treatment.

Palma JA. Epidemiology, diagnosis, and management of neurogenic orthostatic hypotension. Mov Disord Clin Pract. 2017 May–Jun;4(3):298–308. [PMID: 28713844]

TRANSIENT ISCHEMIC ATTACKS

ESSENTIALS OF DIAGNOSIS

- ► Focal neurologic deficit of acute onset.
- ► Clinical deficit resolves completely within 24 hours.
- ► Risk factors for vascular disease often present.

► General Considerations

Transient ischemic attacks (TIAs) are characterized by focal ischemic cerebral neurologic deficits that last for *less than 24 hours* (usually less than 1–2 hours). About 30% of patients with stroke have a history of TIAs and 5–10% of patients with TIAs will have a stroke within 90 days. The natural history of attacks is variable. Some patients will have a major stroke after only a few attacks, whereas others may have frequent attacks for weeks or months without having a stroke. The risk of stroke is high in the first 3 months after an attack, particularly in the first month and especially within the first 48 hours. The stroke risk is greater in patients older than 60 years, in patients with diabetes, or after TIAs that last longer than 10 minutes and with symptoms or signs of weakness, speech impairment, or gait disturbance. In general, carotid ischemic attacks are more liable than vertebrobasilar ischemic attacks to be followed by stroke.

Urgent intervention in TIA patients reduces rates of subsequent stroke, and **the condition should be treated with a similar sense of urgency as unstable angina.**

► Etiology

An important cause of transient cerebral ischemia is embolization. In many patients with these attacks, a source is readily apparent in the heart or a major extracranial artery to the head, and emboli sometimes are visible in the retinal arteries. An embolic phenomenon explains why separate attacks may affect different parts of the territory supplied by the same major vessel. Cardiac causes of embolic ischemic attacks include atrial fibrillation, heart failure, infective and nonbacterial thrombotic endocarditis, atrial myxoma, and mural thrombi complicating myocardial infarction. Atrial septal defects and patent foramen ovale may permit venous thromboemboli to reach the brain (**paradoxical emboli**). An ulcerated plaque on a major artery to the brain may serve as a source of emboli. In the anterior circulation, atherosclerotic changes occur most commonly in the region of the carotid bifurcation extracranially; these changes may cause a bruit. Atherosclerosis also affects the vertebrobasilar system and the major intracranial vessels including the middle and anterior cerebral arteries.

Less common abnormalities of blood vessels that may cause TIAs include fibromuscular dysplasia, which affects particularly the cervical internal carotid artery; atherosclerosis of the aortic arch; inflammatory arterial disorders such as giant cell arteritis, polyarteritis, and granulomatous angiitis; and meningovascular syphilis. Critical stenosis of a major extracranial or intracranial artery may cause TIA, especially in the setting of hypotension.

Hematologic causes of TIA include polycythemia, sickle cell disease, hyperviscosity syndromes, and the antiphospholipid antibody syndrome. Severe anemia may also lead to transient focal neurologic deficits in patients with preexisting cerebral arterial disease.

The **subclavian steal syndrome** may lead to transient vertebrobasilar ischemia. Symptoms develop when there is localized stenosis or occlusion of one subclavian artery proximal to the source of the vertebral artery, so that blood is "stolen" from the vertebral artery to supply the arm. A bruit in the supraclavicular fossa, unequal radial pulses, and a difference of 20 mm Hg or more between the systolic blood pressures in the arms should suggest the diagnosis in patients with vertebrobasilar TIAs.

► Clinical Findings

A. Symptoms and Signs

The symptoms of TIAs vary markedly among patients; however, the symptoms in a given individual tend to be constant in type. Onset is abrupt and without warning, and recovery usually occurs rapidly, often within a few minutes. The specific symptoms depend on the arterial distribution affected, as outlined in the subsequent section on stroke. Of note, TIA *rarely* causes of loss of consciousness or acute confusion but is often erroneously blamed for such symptoms.

B. Imaging

CT or MRI scan is indicated within 24 hours of symptom onset, in part to exclude the possibility of a small cerebral hemorrhage or a cerebral tumor masquerading as a TIA. MRI with diffusion-weighted sequences is particularly sensitive for revealing acute or subacute infarction, which is seen in up to one-third of cases despite resolution of clinical symptoms and indicates a high risk of subsequent stroke. Noninvasive imaging of the cervical vasculature should also be performed; carotid duplex ultrasonography is useful for detecting significant stenosis of the internal carotid artery, and MR or CT angiography permits broader visualization of cervical and intracranial vasculature.

C. Laboratory and Other Studies

Clinical and laboratory evaluation must include assessment for hypertension, heart disease, hematologic disorders, diabetes mellitus, hyperlipidemia, and peripheral vascular disease. It should include complete blood count, fasting blood glucose and serum cholesterol determinations, and may include serologic tests for syphilis and HIV infection. An ECG should be obtained. Echocardiography with agitated saline contrast is performed if a cardioembolic source is likely, and blood cultures are obtained if endocarditis is suspected. Ambulatory ECG monitoring is indicated to detect paroxysmal atrial fibrillation and, if the cause of the TIA remains elusive, extended monitoring may detect paroxysmal atrial fibrillation in up to 20% of patients.

▶ Differential Diagnosis

Focal seizures usually cause abnormal motor or sensory phenomena such as clonic limb movements, paresthesias, or tingling, rather than weakness or loss of feeling. Symptoms generally spread ("march") up the limb and may lead to a generalized tonic-clonic seizure.

Classic migraine is easily recognized by the visual premonitory symptoms, followed by nausea, headache, and photophobia, but less typical cases may be hard to distinguish. Patients with migraine are typically younger, commonly have a history of episodes since adolescence and report that other family members have a similar disorder.

Focal neurologic deficits may occur during periods of hypoglycemia in diabetic patients receiving insulin or oral hypoglycemic agent therapy.

▶ Treatment

A. Medical Measures

Medical treatment is aimed at preventing further attacks and stroke. Treat diabetes mellitus, hematologic disorders, and hypertension, preferably with an angiotensin-converting enzyme inhibitor or angiotensin receptor blocker. A statin should be started regardless of the current low-density lipoprotein level (LDL), although this practice is only supported by randomized trial data in patients with an LDL greater than 100 mg/dL. Cigarette smoking should be stopped, and cardiac sources of embolization should be treated appropriately. Weight reduction and regular physical activity should be encouraged when appropriate. An antiplatelet or anticoagulant should be started as soon as imaging has established the absence of hemorrhage.

1. Hospitalization—Hospitalization should be considered for patients seen within a week of the attack, when they are at increased risk for early recurrence. One commonly used method to assess recurrence risk is the **ABCD²score;** points are assigned for each of the following criteria: age 60 years or older (1 point), blood pressure 140/90 mm Hg or higher (1 point), clinical symptoms of focal weakness (2 points) or speech impairment without weakness (1 point), duration of 60 minutes or longer (2 points) or 10–59 minutes (1 point), or diabetes mellitus (1 point). An ABCD² score of 4 or more points has been suggested as a threshold for hospital admission. The **ABCD²I** (with an additional 3 points for any abnormal diffusion-weighted MRI finding or any infarct [new or old] on noncontrast CT) has been proposed as a better predictor of subsequent stroke risk. Admission is also advisable for patients with crescendo attacks, symptomatic carotid stenosis, or a known cardiac source of emboli or hypercoagulable state; such hospitalization facilitates early intervention for any recurrence and rapid institution of secondary prevention measures.

2. Anticoagulation—*The chief indication for anticoagulation after TIA is atrial fibrillation.* Patients with metal heart valves, left ventricular thrombus, and the antiphospholipid antibody syndrome should also receive anticoagulation therapy. Treatment is with warfarin (target INR 2.0–3.0); bridging warfarin with heparin is not necessary, but some experts advocate treatment with aspirin until the INR becomes therapeutic. For long-term anticoagulation in the setting of atrial fibrillation, apixaban (2.5–5 mg orally twice daily), dabigatran (150 mg orally twice daily), edoxaban (60 mg orally daily), and rivaroxaban (20 mg orally daily) are options. Combination antiplatelet-anticoagulation therapy is only indicated in patients with mechanical heart valves or those with a separate indication for antiplatelet therapy such as a cardiac stent. In patients with cardiomyopathy and an ejection fraction under 35% without atrial fibrillation, warfarin (target INR 2.0–3.0) reduces ischemic stroke risk compared to aspirin but results in a roughly equivalent increase in the risk of major hemorrhage; treatment in this population should therefore be individualized.

3. Antiplatelet therapy—*All patients in whom anticoagulation is not indicated should be treated with short-term dual antiplatelet therapy and long-term monotherapy to reduce the frequency of TIAs and the incidence of stroke.* Treatment should be initiated within 12 hours after the TIA or minor stroke (defined by an National Institutes of Health Stroke Scale of 3 or less) with an oral loading dose of clopidogrel (300–600 mg) followed by 75 mg/day orally plus aspirin (50–325 mg daily orally) for 21–90 days, followed by monotherapy with aspirin (81 mg daily orally), aspirin combined with extended-release dipyridamole (200 mg twice daily orally), or clopidogrel (75 mg daily orally). Cilostazol (100 mg twice daily) had similar efficacy as aspirin at long-term stroke prevention in an Asian population with less risk of hemorrhage. Combining clopidogrel with aspirin beyond 90 days increases the risk of hemorrhagic complications and is not recommended.

B. Surgical or Endovascular Measures

1. Carotid revascularization—When arteriography reveals a surgically accessible high-grade stenosis (70–99% in luminal diameter) on the side appropriate to carotid ischemic attacks, operative treatment (**carotid endarterectomy**) or **endovascular intervention** reduces the risk of ipsilateral carotid stroke, especially when TIAs are of recent onset (less than 1 month) and when the perioperative morbidity and mortality risk is estimated to be less than 6%. Endovascular therapy carries a slightly higher procedural stroke risk than endarterectomy in patients older than 70 years and is generally reserved for younger patients whose neck anatomy is unfavorable for surgery. Patients with symptomatic carotid stenosis of 50–69% derive moderate benefit from intervention, but surgery is not indicated for mild stenosis (less than 50%).

2. Closure of patent foramen ovale—Carefully selected patients with patent foramen ovale (PFO) and right-to-left shunt benefit from PFO closure and antiplatelet therapy. Patients should be considered for PFO closure if they are between 18 and 60 years old; have had a cryptogenic stroke or TIA; and do not have uncontrolled diabetes, hypertension, or a specific indication for long-term anticoagulation. A cryptogenic stroke does not have an identified mechanism, such as large artery atherosclerosis (greater than or equal to 30–50% stenosis of the intracranial or cervical arteries or a plaque greater than or equal to 4mm thick in the aortic arch), known cardioembolic source (eg, atrial fibrillation), small vessel arteriolosclerosis (eg, lacunar stroke smaller than 1.5 cm in diameter), hypercoagulable state, or dissection. Patients with moderate to large interatrial shunts or associated atrial septal aneurysms appear to benefit most from PFO closure. See also Chapter 10.

▶ When to Refer

All patients should be referred for urgent investigation and *treatment to prevent stroke.*

▶ When to Admit

If seen within a week of a TIA, patients should be considered for admission when they have an ABCD^2 score of 4 points or more, when outpatient evaluation is impractical, or when there are multiple attacks, carotid stenosis of greater than 70%, or other concern for early recurrence or stroke.

Johnston SC et al; Clinical Research Collaboration, Neurological Emergencies Treatment Trials Network, and the POINT Investigators. Clopidogrel and aspirin in acute ischemic stroke and high-risk TIA. N Engl J Med. 2018 Jul 19;379(3): 215–25. [PMID: 29766750]

Sposato LA et al. Diagnosis of atrial fibrillation after stroke and transient ischaemic attack: a systematic review and meta-analysis. Lancet Neurol. 2015 Apr;14(4):377–87. [PMID: 25748102]

STROKE

ESSENTIALS OF DIAGNOSIS

▶ Sudden onset of neurologic deficit of cerebrovascular origin.

▶ Patient often has hypertension, diabetes mellitus, tobacco use, atrial fibrillation, or atherosclerosis.

▶ Distinctive neurologic signs reflect the region of the brain involved.

▶ General Considerations

In the United States, stroke is the fifth leading cause of death and a leading cause of disability. Risk factors for stroke include hypertension, diabetes mellitus, hyperlipidemia, cigarette smoking, cardiac disease, HIV infection, trigeminal herpes zoster, recreational drug abuse, heavy alcohol consumption, and a family history of stroke.

Strokes are subdivided pathologically into infarcts and hemorrhages. The distinction may be difficult clinically; CT scanning is essential to clarify the pathologic basis (Table 24–3).

1. Lacunar Infarction

Lacunar infarcts are small lesions (usually less than 1.5 cm in diameter) that occur in the distribution of short penetrating arterioles in the basal ganglia, pons, cerebellum, internal capsule, thalamus and, less commonly, the deep cerebral white matter (Table 24–3). Lacunar infarcts are associated with poorly controlled hypertension or diabetes and have been found in several clinical syndromes, including contralateral pure motor hemiparesis or pure hemisensory deficit, ipsilateral ataxia with hemiparesis, and dysarthria with clumsiness of the hand. The neurologic deficit may progress over 24–36 hours before stabilizing.

Early mortality and risk of stroke recurrence is higher for patients with nonlacunar than lacunar infarcts. The prognosis for recovery from the deficit produced by a lacunar infarct is usually good, with partial or complete resolution occurring over the following 4–6 weeks in many instances. Treatment is as described for TIA and cerebral infarction.

2. Cerebral Infarction

Thrombotic or embolic occlusion of a major vessel leads to cerebral infarction. Causes are identical to the disorders predisposing to TIAs. The resulting deficit depends on the

Table 24–3. Features of the major stroke subtypes.

Stroke Type and Subtype	Clinical Features	Diagnosis	Treatment
Ischemic Stroke			
Lacunar infarct	Small (< 1.5 cm) lesions in the basal ganglia, pons, cerebellum, or internal capsule; less often in deep cerebral white matter; prognosis generally good; clinical features depend on location, but may worsen over first 24–36 hours.	MRI with diffusion-weighted sequences usually defines the area of infarction; CT is insensitive acutely but can be used to exclude hemorrhage.	Antiplatelet; control risk factors (hypertension, tobacco use, hypercholesterolemia, and diabetes mellitus).
Carotid circulation obstruction	See text—signs vary depending on occluded vessel.	Noncontrast CT to exclude hemorrhage but findings may be normal during first 6–24 hours of an ischemic stroke; diffusion-weighted MRI is gold standard for identifying acute stroke; electrocardiography, carotid duplex studies, echocardiography, blood glucose, complete blood count, and tests for hyperlipidemia are indicated; ambulatory ECG monitoring, including extended monitoring in selected instances; CTA, MRA, or conventional angiography in selected cases; tests for hypercoagulable states in selected cases.	0–3 hours in United States: intravenous thrombolytics (approved in Europe for up to 4.5 hours). 0–6 hours: endovascular mechanical embolectomy. 6–24 hours: endovascular mechanical embolectomy in select cases. Secondary prevention: antiplatelet agent is first-line therapy; anticoagulation without heparin bridge for cardioembolic strokes due to atrial fibrillation and other select cases when no contraindications exist; control risk factors as above.
Vertebrobasilar occlusion	See text—signs vary based on location of occluded vessel.	As for carotid circulation obstruction.	As for carotid circulation obstruction.
Hemorrhagic Stroke			
Spontaneous intracerebral hemorrhage	Commonly associated with hypertension; also with bleeding disorders, amyloid angiopathy. Hypertensive hemorrhage is located commonly in the basal ganglia, pons, thalamus, cerebellum, and less commonly the cerebral white matter.	Noncontrast CT is superior to MRI for detecting bleeds of < 48 hours duration; laboratory tests to identify bleeding disorder: angiography may be indicated to exclude aneurysm or AVM in younger patients without hypertension. Do *not* perform lumbar puncture.	Lower systolic blood pressure to 140 mm Hg; cerebellar bleeds or hematomas with gross mass effect may require urgent surgical evacuation. AVM: surgical resection indicated to prevent further bleeding; other modalities to treat nonoperable AVMs available at specialized centers.
Subarachnoid hemorrhage	Present with sudden onset of worst headache of life, may lead rapidly to loss of consciousness; signs of meningeal irritation often present; etiology usually aneurysm or AVM, but 20% have no source identified.	CT to confirm diagnosis, but may be normal in rare instances; if CT negative and suspicion high, perform lumbar puncture to look for red blood cells or xanthochromia; angiography to determine source of bleed in candidates for treatment.	Lower systolic blood pressure to < 140 mm Hg immediately. Aneurysm: prevent further bleeding by clipping aneurysm or coil embolization; nimodipine helps prevent vasospasm; once aneurysm has been obliterated intravenous fluids and induced hypertension to prevent vasospasm; angioplasty may also reverse symptomatic vasospasm. AVM: as above.

AVMs, arteriovenous malformations; CTA, computed tomography angiography; MRA, magnetic resonance angiography.

particular vessel involved and the extent of any collateral circulation. Cerebral ischemia leads to release of excitatory and other neuropeptides that may augment calcium flux into neurons, thereby leading to cell death and increasing the neurologic deficit.

▶ Clinical Findings

A. Symptoms and Signs

Onset is usually abrupt, and there may then be very little progression except that due to brain swelling. Clinical evaluation should always include examination of the heart for murmurs and rhythm irregularities. Auscultating over the carotid or subclavian vessels may reveal a bruit but is not sensitive enough to substitute for vascular imaging.

1. Obstruction of carotid circulation—Occlusion of the **anterior cerebral artery** distal to its junction with the anterior communicating artery causes weakness and cortical sensory loss in the contralateral leg and sometimes mild weakness of the arm, especially proximally. There may be a contralateral grasp reflex, paratonic rigidity, abulia (lack of initiative), or frank confusion. Urinary incontinence is not uncommon, particularly if behavioral disturbances are conspicuous. Bilateral anterior cerebral infarction is especially likely to cause marked behavioral changes and memory disturbances. Unilateral anterior cerebral artery occlusion proximal to the junction with the anterior communicating artery is generally well tolerated because of the collateral supply from the other side.

Middle cerebral artery occlusion leads to contralateral hemiplegia, hemisensory loss, and homonymous hemianopia (ie, bilaterally symmetric loss of vision in half of the visual fields), with the eyes deviated to the side of the lesion. If the dominant hemisphere is involved, global aphasia is also present. It may be impossible to distinguish this clinically from occlusion of the internal carotid artery. With occlusion of either of these arteries, there may also be considerable swelling of the hemisphere during the first 72 hours. For example, an infarct involving one cerebral hemisphere may lead to such swelling that the function of the other hemisphere or the rostral brainstem is disturbed and coma results. Occlusions of different branches of the middle cerebral artery cause more limited findings. For example, involvement of the superior division in the dominant hemisphere leads to a predominantly expressive (**Broca**) aphasia and to contralateral paralysis and loss of sensations in the arm, the face and, to a lesser extent, the leg. Inferior branch occlusion in the dominant hemisphere produces a receptive (**Wernicke**) aphasia and a homonymous visual field defect. With involvement of the nondominant hemisphere, speech and comprehension are preserved, but there may be a left hemispatial neglect syndrome or constructional and visuospatial deficits.

Occlusion of the **ophthalmic or central retinal artery** leads to sudden painless visual loss with retinal pallor and a macular cherry red spot on fundoscopic examination. Sudden, transient vision loss in one eye (**amaurosis fugax**) is a TIA in this arterial territory. Patients with a **cilioretinal artery** (approximately 25%) may have macular sparing due to collateral blood supply.

2. Obstruction of vertebrobasilar circulation—Occlusion of the **posterior cerebral artery** may lead to a thalamic syndrome in which contralateral hemisensory disturbance occurs, followed by the development of spontaneous pain and hyperpathia. There is often a macular-sparing homonymous hemianopia and sometimes a mild, usually temporary, hemiparesis. Depending on the site of the lesion and the collateral circulation, the severity of these deficits varies and other deficits may also occur, including involuntary movements and alexia. Occlusion of the main artery beyond the origin of its penetrating branches may lead solely to a macular-sparing hemianopia.

Vertebral artery occlusion below the origin of the anterior spinal and posterior inferior cerebellar arteries may be clinically silent because the circulation is maintained by the other vertebral artery. If the remaining vertebral artery is congenitally small or severely atherosclerotic, however, a deficit similar to that of basilar artery occlusion is seen unless there is good collateral circulation from the anterior circulation through the circle of Willis. An obstruction of the **posterior inferior cerebellar artery** or an obstruction of the vertebral artery just before it branches to this vessel leads to the lateral medullary syndrome, characterized by vertigo and nystagmus (vestibular nucleus), ipsilateral spinothalamic sensory loss involving the face (trigeminal nucleus and tract), dysphagia (nucleus ambiguus), limb ataxia (inferior cerebellar peduncle), and Horner syndrome (descending sympathetic fibers), combined with contralateral spinothalamic sensory loss involving the limbs.

Occlusion of both **vertebral arteries** or the **basilar artery** leads to coma with pinpoint pupils, flaccid quadriplegia and sensory loss, and variable cranial nerve abnormalities. With partial basilar artery occlusion, there may be diplopia, visual loss, vertigo, dysarthria, ataxia, weakness or sensory disturbances in some or all of the limbs, and discrete cranial nerve palsies. In patients with hemiplegia of pontine origin, the eyes are often deviated to the paralyzed side, whereas in patients with a hemispheric lesion, the eyes commonly deviate from the hemiplegic side. When the small paramedian arteries arising from the basilar artery are occluded, contralateral hemiplegia and sensory deficit occur in association with an ipsilateral cranial nerve palsy at the level of the lesion.

Occlusion of any of the major **cerebellar arteries** produces vertigo, nausea, vomiting, nystagmus, and ipsilateral limb ataxia. Contralateral spinothalamic sensory loss in the limbs may also be present. Deafness due to cochlear infarction may follow occlusion of the anterior inferior cerebellar artery, which may also cause ipsilateral facial spinothalamic sensory loss and weakness. Massive cerebellar infarction may lead to obstructive hydrocephalus, coma, tonsillar herniation, and death.

B. Imaging

A CT scan of the head (without contrast) should be performed immediately, before the administration of aspirin or other antithrombotic agents, to *exclude cerebral hemorrhage* (Table 24–3). CT is relatively insensitive to acute ischemic stroke within the first 6–12 hours, and subsequent MRI with diffusion-weighted sequences helps define the distribution and extent of infarction as well as exclude tumor or other differential considerations. CT angiography of the head and neck should be performed to identify large vessel occlusions amenable to endovascular therapy in patients presenting within 6 hours of stroke onset and should be considered in those presenting between 6 and 24 hours, together with CT perfusion studies. Regardless of timing of presentation, imaging of the cervical vasculature is indicated as part of a search to identify the source of the stroke. In patients with a PFO and otherwise cryptogenic stroke, the intracranial vasculature must be imaged to rule out large vessel atherosclerosis before PFO closure can be considered.

C. Laboratory and Other Studies

Investigations should include a complete blood count, blood glucose determination, and fasting lipid panel. Serologic tests for syphilis and HIV infection may be included depending on the circumstances. Screening for antiphospholipid antibodies (lupus anticoagulants, anticardiolipin, and anti-beta2-glycoprotein antibodies); the factor V Leiden mutation; abnormalities of protein C, protein S, or antithrombin; or a prothrombin gene mutation is indicated only if a hypercoagulable disorder is suspected (eg, a young patient without apparent risk factors for stroke) or needs to be ruled out if PFO closure is under consideration. While elevated serum homocysteine is a risk factor for stroke, lowering homocysteine levels with vitamin supplementation has not been shown to decrease stroke risk, and therefore, routinely checking homocysteine is *not* recommended. Electrocardiography or continuous cardiac monitoring for at least 24 hours will help exclude a recent myocardial infarction or a cardiac arrhythmia that might be a source of embolization. While atrial fibrillation will be discovered in approximately 10% of patients with ischemic stroke during their hospitalization, it is estimated that an arrhythmia will be found in an additional 10% with prolonged ambulatory ECG monitoring after discharge; this testing is indicated in cases where atrial fibrillation is suspected (eg, nonlacunar stroke and left atrial enlargement on echocardiography or lack of intracranial or carotid atherosclerosis) but has not been demonstrated. Echocardiography (with agitated saline contrast) should be performed in cases of nonlacunar stroke to exclude valvular disease, right-to-left shunting, and cardiac thrombus. Blood cultures should be performed if endocarditis is suspected but are not required routinely. Examination of the cerebrospinal fluid is not always necessary but may be helpful if cerebral vasculitis or another inflammatory or infectious cause of stroke is suspected, but it should be delayed until after CT or MRI to exclude any risk for herniation due to mass effect.

▶ Treatment

Management is divided into acute and chronic phases: the first is aimed at minimizing disability and the second at preventing recurrent stroke. A combination of thrombolysis and endovascular therapies is available to patients who present within 24 hours of stroke onset, determined by when the patient was last normal.

Intravenous thrombolytic therapy with recombinant tissue plasminogen activator (rtPA; 0.9 mg/kg to a maximum of 90 mg, with 10% given as a bolus over 1 minute and the remainder over 1 hour) improves the chance of recovery without significant disability at 90 days from 26% to 39% if given within 3 hours from stroke onset; it is still effective up to 4.5 hours from stroke onset. Treatment should be initiated as soon as possible; outcome is directly related to the time from stroke onset to treatment. Intravenous thrombolysis is approved in Europe for use up to 4.5 hours from stroke onset but only for up to 3 hours in the United States, although off-label use during the 3- to 4.5-hour window is standard. In patients with systolic pressure greater than 185 mm Hg or diastolic pressure greater than 110 mm Hg, the blood pressure should be lowered to less than 185/110 mm Hg with intravenous labetalol or nicardipine to enable rtPA administration. Due to the risk of hemorrhage, rtPA should not be used beyond 4.5 hours, or in other situations where it is medically contraindicated.

Several randomized trials have demonstrated an increased likelihood of achieving functional independence after **endovascular mechanical embolectomy** by stent retrievers as an adjunct to intravenous rtPA. Patients with large vessel occlusion (about 20% of patients with acute ischemic stroke) in whom treatment can be initiated within 6 hours of stroke onset are eligible for embolectomy, as are patients who present between 6 hours and 24 hours and also have a large ischemic penumbra identified by perfusion CT, perfusion MRI, or diffusion-weighted MRI. A subset of patients who awaken with stroke symptoms, were last normal at bedtime, and do not have a large vessel occlusion may benefit from rtPA based on MRI features that show early ischemia likely under 4.5 hours in duration.

Early management of a completed stroke otherwise requires **general supportive measures.** Management in a stroke care unit has been shown to improve outcomes, likely due to early rehabilitation and prevention of medical complications. During the acute stage, there may be marked brain swelling and edema, with symptoms and signs of increasing intracranial pressure, an increasing neurologic deficit, or herniation syndrome. Elevated intracranial pressure is managed by head elevation and osmotic agents such as mannitol. Maintenance of an adequate cerebral perfusion pressure helps prevent further ischemia. Early decompressive hemicraniectomy (within 48 hours of stroke onset) for malignant middle cerebral artery infarctions reduces mortality and improves functional outcome. Attempts to lower the blood pressure of hypertensive patients during the acute phase (ie, within 72 hours) of a stroke should generally be *avoided* unless the purpose is to enable the safe administration of rtPA, as there is loss of cerebral autoregulation, and lowering the blood pressure may further compromise ischemic areas. However, if the systolic pressure exceeds 220 mm Hg, it can be lowered using intravenous labetalol or nicardipine with continuous monitoring to 170–200 mm Hg, and then after 72 hours, it can be reduced further to less than 140/90 mm Hg. Blood pressure augmentation is usually not necessary in patients with relative hypotension but maintenance of intravenous hydration is important.

Prophylactic and medical measures are discussed in the section on TIAs and should guide management. Once hemorrhage has been excluded by CT, aspirin (325 mg orally daily) is started immediately unless the patient received thrombolysis, in which case aspirin is initiated after a follow-up CT has ruled out thrombolytic-associated hemorrhage at 24 hours. Dual antiplatelet therapy should be used temporarily for patients with minor stroke (National Institutes of Health Stroke Scale of 3 or less). Anticoagulant medications are started when indicated, as discussed in the section on TIAs. *There is generally no advantage in delay*, and the common fear of causing hemorrhage into a previously infarcted area is misplaced, since there is a far greater risk of further embolism to the cerebral circulation if treatment is withheld.

Physical therapy has an important role in the management of patients with impaired motor function. Passive movements at an early stage will help prevent contractures. As cooperation increases and some recovery begins, active movements will improve strength and coordination. In all cases, early mobilization and active rehabilitation are important. Occupational therapy may improve morale and motor skills, while speech therapy may help expressive aphasia or dysarthria. Because of the risk for dysphagia following stroke, access to food and drink is typically restricted until an appropriate swallowing evaluation; the head of the bed should be kept elevated to prevent aspiration. Urinary catheters should not be placed and, if placed, removed within 24–48 hours.

Prognosis

The prognosis for survival after cerebral infarction is better than after cerebral or subarachnoid hemorrhage. Patients receiving treatment with rtPA are at least 30% more likely to have minimal or no disability at 3 months than those not treated by this means. Those treated with mechanical embolectomy are also at least 30% more likely to achieve functional independence. Loss of consciousness after a cerebral infarct implies a poorer prognosis than otherwise. The extent of the infarct governs the potential for rehabilitation. Patients who have had a cerebral infarct are at risk for additional strokes and for myocardial infarcts. The prophylactic measures discussed earlier reduce this risk. Antiplatelet therapy reduces the recurrence rate by 30% among patients without a cardiac cause for the stroke who are not candidates for carotid endarterectomy. Nevertheless, the cumulative risk of recurrence of noncardioembolic stroke is still 3–7% annually.

When to Refer

All patients should be referred.

When to Admit

All patients should be hospitalized, preferably in a stroke care unit.

Albers GW et al; DEFUSE 3 Investigators. Thrombectomy for stroke at 6 to 16 hours with selection by perfusion imaging. N Engl J Med. 2018 Feb 2;378(8):708–18. [PMID: 29364767]
Muth CC. JAMA patient page. Recovery after stroke. JAMA. 2016 Dec13;316(22):2440. [PMID: 27959997]
Nogueira RG et al; DAWN Trial Investigators. Thrombectomy 6 to 24 hours after stroke with a mismatch between deficit and infarct. N Engl J Med. 2018 Jan 4;378(1):11–21. [PMID: 29129157]
Powers WJ et al. 2018 Guidelines for the early management of patients with acute ischemic stroke: a guideline for healthcare professionals from the American Heart Association/American Stroke Association. Stroke. 2018 Mar;49(3):e46–110. [PMID: 29367334]

3. Intracerebral Hemorrhage

Spontaneous, nontraumatic intracerebral hemorrhage in patients with no angiographic evidence of an associated vascular anomaly (eg, aneurysm or angioma) is usually due to hypertension. The pathologic basis for hemorrhage is probably the presence of microaneurysms that develop on perforating vessels in hypertensive patients. Hypertensive intracerebral hemorrhage occurs most frequently in the basal ganglia, pons, thalamus, cerebellum and less commonly in the cerebral white matter. Hemorrhage may extend into the ventricular system or subarachnoid space, and signs of meningeal irritation are then found. In older adults, cerebral amyloid angiopathy is another important and frequent cause of hemorrhage, which is usually lobar in distribution, sometimes recurrent, and associated with a better immediate prognosis than hypertensive hemorrhage. Arteriovenous malformations are an important cause of intracerebral hemorrhage in younger patients.

Other causes of nontraumatic intracerebral hemorrhage include hematologic and bleeding disorders (eg, leukemia, thrombocytopenia, hemophilia, or disseminated intravascular coagulation), anticoagulant therapy, liver disease, high alcohol intake, cocaine and methamphetamine abuse, herpes simplex encephalitis, vasculitis, moyamoya disease, reversible cerebral vasoconstriction syndrome, and primary or secondary brain tumors. There is also an association with advancing age and male sex. Bleeding is primarily into the subarachnoid space when it occurs from an intracranial aneurysm, but it may be partly intraparenchymal as well. Hemorrhage can also occur into arterial and venous cerebral infarcts.

Clinical Findings

A. Symptoms and Signs

With hemorrhage into the cerebral hemisphere, consciousness is initially lost or impaired in about one-half of patients. Vomiting occurs very frequently at the onset of bleeding, and headache is sometimes present. Focal symptoms and signs then develop, depending on the site of the hemorrhage. With hypertensive hemorrhage, there is generally a rapidly evolving neurologic deficit with hemiplegia or hemiparesis. A hemisensory disturbance is also present with more deeply placed lesions. With lesions of the putamen, loss of conjugate lateral gaze may be conspicuous. With thalamic hemorrhage, there may be a loss of upward gaze, downward or skew deviation of the eyes, lateral gaze palsies, and pupillary inequalities.

Cerebellar hemorrhage may present with sudden onset of nausea and vomiting, dysequilibrium, ataxia of gait, limbs, or trunk; headache; and loss of consciousness that may terminate fatally within 48 hours. Pontine hemorrhage causes some combination of lateral conjugate gaze palsies to the side of the lesion; small reactive pupils; contralateral hemiplegia; peripheral facial weakness; and periodic respiration. These signs may be bilateral with larger pontine hemorrhage, and the patient may become locked in, with quadriplegia and preserved consciousness.

B. Imaging

CT scanning (without contrast) is important not only in confirming that hemorrhage has occurred but also in determining the size and site of the hematoma. MRI is equally sensitive when magnetic susceptibility weighted sequences (eg, gradient echo) are used. If the patient's condition permits further intervention, CT angiography, MR angiography, or cerebral angiography may be undertaken to determine whether an aneurysm or arteriovenous malformation is present. In patients under age 55 with lobar hemorrhage and no history of hypertension, a contrast-enhanced MRI may indicate a nonhypertensive cause such as an underlying neoplasm.

C. Laboratory and Other Studies

A complete blood count, platelet count, prothrombin and partial thromboplastin times, liver biochemical tests, and kidney function tests may reveal a predisposing cause for the hemorrhage. *Lumbar puncture is contraindicated* because it may precipitate a herniation syndrome in patients with a large hematoma, and CT scanning is superior in detecting intracerebral hemorrhage.

▶ Treatment

Patients should be admitted to an intensive care unit for observation and supportive care. The systolic blood pressure should be lowered to 140 mm Hg with intravenous labetalol or nicardipine, although randomized trials targeting systolic blood pressures of less than 140 mm Hg and less than 180 mm Hg have not shown a difference in outcomes. Thrombocytopenia should be treated with platelet transfusion; the specific threshold for treatment and the goal platelet count after transfusion vary with patient characteristics and provider experience. Coagulopathies should be reversed using fresh frozen plasma, prothrombin complex concentrates, vitamin K, or specific reversal agents (eg, protamine for heparin; idarucizumab for dabigatran; and andexanet alfa for apixaban, betrixaban, edoxaban, and rivaroxaban). Hemostatic therapy with recombinant activated factor VII in patients without underlying coagulopathy has not improved survival or functional outcome. Intracranial pressure may require monitoring and osmotic therapy. Ventricular drainage may be required in patients with intraventricular hemorrhage and acute hydrocephalus. Decompression may be helpful when a superficial hematoma in cerebral white matter is exerting a mass effect and causing incipient herniation. In patients with cerebellar hemorrhage who are deteriorating neurologically or who have brainstem compression or hydrocephalus, prompt surgical evacuation of the hematoma is appropriate because spontaneous unpredictable deterioration may otherwise lead to a fatal outcome and because operative treatment may lead to complete resolution of the clinical deficit. The treatment of underlying structural lesions or bleeding disorders depends on their nature. There is no specific treatment for cerebral amyloid angiopathy.

▶ When to Refer

All patients should be referred.

▶ When to Admit

All patients should be hospitalized.

Hemphill JC III et al. Guidelines for the management of spontaneous intracerebral hemorrhage: a guideline for healthcare professionals from the American Heart Association/American Stroke Association. Stroke. 2015 Jul;46(7):2032–60. [PMID: 26022637]

Qureshi AI et al; ATACH-2 Trial Investigators and the Neurological Emergency Treatment Trials Network. Intensive blood-pressure lowering in patients with acute cerebral hemorrhage. N Engl J Med. 2016 Sep 15;375(11):1033–43. [PMID: 27276234]

4. Spontaneous Subarachnoid Hemorrhage

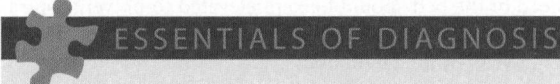
ESSENTIALS OF DIAGNOSIS

▶ Sudden ("thunderclap") severe headache.
▶ Signs of meningeal irritation usually present.
▶ Obtundation is common.
▶ Focal deficits frequently absent.

▶ General Considerations

Between 5% and 10% of strokes are due to subarachnoid hemorrhage. Trauma is the most common cause of subarachnoid hemorrhage, the prognosis of which depends on the severity of the head injury. Spontaneous (nontraumatic) subarachnoid hemorrhage frequently results from the rupture of an arterial saccular ("berry") aneurysm or from an arteriovenous malformation.

▶ Clinical Findings

A. Symptoms and Signs

Subarachnoid hemorrhage has a characteristic clinical picture. Its onset is with sudden ("thunderclap") headache of a severity never experienced previously by the patient. This may be followed by nausea and vomiting and by a loss or impairment of consciousness that can either be transient or progress inexorably to deepening coma and death. If consciousness is regained, the patient is often confused and irritable and may show other symptoms of an altered mental status. Neurologic examination generally reveals nuchal rigidity and other signs of meningeal irritation, except in deeply comatose patients.

Most aneurysms are asymptomatic until they rupture, but they may cause a focal neurologic deficit by compressing adjacent structures. Occasional patients with aneurysms have headaches, sometimes accompanied by nausea and neck stiffness, a few hours or days before massive subarachnoid hemorrhage occurs. This has been attributed to "warning leaks" of a small amount of blood from the aneurysm.

A higher risk of subarachnoid hemorrhage is associated with older age, female sex, nonwhite ethnicity, hypertension, tobacco smoking, high alcohol consumption (exceeding 150 g per week), previous symptoms, posterior circulation aneurysms, and larger aneurysms. Focal neurologic signs are usually absent but, when present, may relate either to a focal intracerebral hematoma (from arteriovenous malformations) or to ischemia in the territory of the vessel with a ruptured aneurysm.

B. Imaging

A CT scan (preferably with CT angiography) should be performed immediately to confirm that hemorrhage has occurred and to search for clues regarding its source. It is preferable to MRI because it is faster and more sensitive in detecting hemorrhage in the first 24 hours. CT findings sometimes are normal in patients with suspected hemorrhage, and the cerebrospinal fluid must then be examined for the presence of blood or xanthochromia before the possibility of subarachnoid hemorrhage is discounted.

Cerebral arteriography is undertaken to determine the source of bleeding. In general, bilateral carotid and vertebral arteriography are necessary because aneurysms are often multiple, while arteriovenous malformations may be supplied from several sources. The procedure allows an interventional radiologist to treat an underlying aneurysm or arteriovenous malformation by various techniques. If arteriograms show no abnormality, the examination should be repeated after 2 weeks because vasospasm or thrombus may have prevented detection of an aneurysm or other vascular anomaly during the initial study. CT or MR angiography may also be revealing but is less sensitive than conventional arteriography.

C. Laboratory and Other Studies

The cerebrospinal fluid demonstrates an elevated red blood cell count. Subarachnoid hemorrhage can be differentiated from a traumatic lumbar puncture by the lack of clearing of red blood cells from the first and fourth tube of cerebrospinal fluid or by the presence of xanthochromia, which occurs due to lysis of red blood cells and takes at least 2 hours to develop. The absolute red blood cell count is also helpful: in the absence of xanthochromia, a red blood cell count of less than 2000×10^6/L is very unlikely to be due to subarachnoid hemorrhage. Electrocardiographic evidence of arrhythmias or myocardial ischemia has been well described and probably relates to excessive sympathetic activity. Peripheral leukocytosis and transient glycosuria are also common findings.

▶ Treatment

All patients should be hospitalized and seen by a neurologist. The measures outlined below in the section on stupor and coma are applied to comatose patients. Conscious patients are confined to bed, advised against any exertion or straining, treated symptomatically for headache and anxiety, and given laxatives or stool softeners. The systolic blood pressure should be lowered to 140 mm Hg until the aneurysm is treated definitively. Seizure prophylaxis is not necessary unless a convulsion has occurred (see Table 24–2).

Patients are generally hospitalized for at least 14 days to monitor, prevent, and treat vasospasm.

The major aim of treatment is to prevent further hemorrhage. The risk of further hemorrhage from a ruptured aneurysm is greatest within a few days of the first hemorrhage; approximately 20% of patients will have further bleeding within 2 weeks and 40% within 6 months. Definitive treatment, ideally within 2 days of the hemorrhage, requires surgical clipping of the aneurysm or endovascular treatment by coil embolization; the latter is sometimes feasible even for inoperable aneurysms and has a lower morbidity than surgery.

▶ Complications

Spontaneous subarachnoid hemorrhage may result in severe complications, so monitoring is necessary, usually in an intensive care unit. Hemiplegia or other focal deficit sometimes may follow aneurysmal bleeding after a delay of 2–14 days due to focal arterial spasm. The etiology of **vasospasm** is uncertain and likely multifactorial, and it sometimes leads to significant cerebral ischemia or infarction and may further aggravate any existing increase in intracranial pressure. Transcranial Doppler ultrasound may be used to screen noninvasively for vasospasm, but conventional arteriography is required to document and treat vasospasm when the clinical suspicion is high. *Nimodipine has been shown to reduce the incidence of ischemic deficits from arterial spasm;* a dose of 60 mg every 4 hours orally for 21 days is given prophylactically to all patients. After surgical obliteration of all aneurysms, symptomatic vasospasm may also be treated by intravascular volume expansion and induced hypertension; transluminal balloon angioplasty of involved intracranial vessels is also helpful.

Acute hydrocephalus, which sometimes occurs due to cerebrospinal fluid outflow disruption by the subarachnoid blood, should be suspected if the patient deteriorates clinically; a repeat CT scan should be obtained. Acute hydrocephalus frequently causes intracranial hypertension severe enough to require temporary, and less commonly prolonged or permanent, intraventricular cerebrospinal fluid shunting. **Renal salt-wasting** is another complication of subarachnoid hemorrhage that may develop abruptly during the first several days of hospitalization. The resulting hyponatremia and cerebral edema may exacerbate intracranial hypertension and may require carefully titrated treatment with oral sodium chloride or intravenous hyperosmotic sodium solution. Daily measurement of the serum sodium level allows for the early detection of this complication. **Hypopituitarism** may occur as a late complication of subarachnoid hemorrhage.

Blok KM et al. CT within 6 hours of headache onset to rule out subarachnoid hemorrhage in nonacademic hospitals. Neurology. 2015 May 12;84(19):1927–32. [PMID: 25862794]

Perry JJ et al. Differentiation between traumatic tap and aneurysmal subarachnoid hemorrhage: prospective cohort study. BMJ. 2015 Feb 18;350:h568. [PMID: 25694274]

Perry JJ et al. Validation of the Ottowa subarachnoid hemorrhage rule in patients with acute headache. CMAJ. 2017 Nov 13; 189(45):E1379–85. [PMID: 29133539]

5. Intracranial Aneurysm

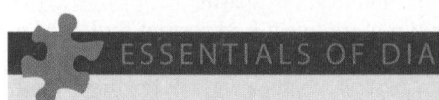

- ► Subarachnoid hemorrhage or focal deficit.
- ► Abnormal imaging studies.

General Considerations

Saccular aneurysms (**"berry" aneurysms**) tend to occur at arterial bifurcations, are frequently multiple (20% of cases), and are usually asymptomatic. They are associated with polycystic kidney disease, moyamoya disease, familial aldosteronism type 1, and coarctation of the aorta. Risk factors for aneurysm formation include cigarette smoking, hypertension, and female sex. Most aneurysms are located on the anterior part of the circle of Willis—particularly on the anterior or posterior communicating arteries, at the bifurcation of the middle cerebral artery, and at the bifurcation of the internal carotid artery. Mycotic aneurysms resulting from septic embolism occur in more distal vessels and often at the cortical surface. The most significant complication of intracranial aneurysms is a subarachnoid hemorrhage, which is discussed in the preceding section.

Clinical Findings

A. Symptoms and Signs

Aneurysms may cause a focal neurologic deficit by compressing adjacent structures. However, most are asymptomatic or produce only nonspecific symptoms until they rupture, at which time subarachnoid hemorrhage results. Its manifestations, complications, and management were outlined in the preceding section.

B. Imaging

Definitive evaluation is by digital subtraction angiography (bilateral carotid and vertebral studies), which generally indicates the size and site of the lesion, sometimes reveals multiple aneurysms, and may show arterial spasm if rupture has occurred. Visualization by CT or MR angiography is not usually adequate if operative treatment is under consideration because lesions may be multiple and small lesions are sometimes missed, but these modalities can be used to screen patients who have two or more first-degree relatives with intracranial aneurysms.

Treatment

The major aim of treatment is to prevent hemorrhage. Management of ruptured aneurysms was described in the section on subarachnoid hemorrhage. Symptomatic but unruptured aneurysms merit prompt treatment, either surgically or by endovascular techniques. The decision to treat or monitor asymptomatic aneurysms discovered incidentally is complicated and depends on aneurysm size, location, risk factors for rupture, and treatment-related morbidity; risk scores to guide decision-making are available.

When to Refer

All patients should be referred.

When to Admit

- All patients with a subarachnoid hemorrhage.
- All patients for detailed imaging.
- All patients undergoing surgical or endovascular treatment.

Etminan N et al. The unruptured intracranial aneurysm treatment score: a multidisciplinary consensus. Neurology. 2015 Sep 8;85(10):881–9. [PMID: 26276380]

6. Arteriovenous Malformations

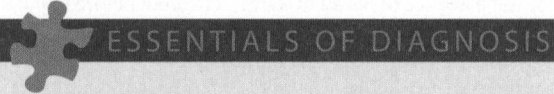

- ► Sudden onset of subarachnoid and intracerebral hemorrhage.
- ► Distinctive neurologic signs reflect the region of the brain involved.
- ► Signs of meningeal irritation in patients presenting with subarachnoid hemorrhage.
- ► Seizures or focal deficits may occur.

General Considerations

Arteriovenous malformations are congenital vascular malformations that result from a localized maldevelopment of part of the primitive vascular plexus and consist of abnormal arteriovenous communications without intervening capillaries. They vary in size, ranging from massive lesions that are fed by multiple vessels and involve a large part of the brain to lesions so small that they are hard to identify at arteriography, surgery, or autopsy. In approximately 10% of cases, there is an associated arterial aneurysm, while 1–2% of patients presenting with aneurysms have associated arteriovenous malformations. Clinical presentation may relate to hemorrhage from the malformation or an associated aneurysm or may relate to cerebral ischemia due to diversion of blood by the anomalous arteriovenous shunt or due to venous stagnation. Regional maldevelopment of the brain, compression or distortion of adjacent cerebral tissue by enlarged anomalous vessels, and progressive gliosis due to mechanical and ischemic factors may also be contributory.

Clinical Findings

Most cerebral arteriovenous malformations are supratentorial, usually lying in the territory of the middle cerebral artery. Up to 70% bleed at some point in their natural history, most commonly before the patient reaches the age of 40 years. Arteriovenous malformations that have bled once are more likely to bleed again, at an approximate rate of 4.5% annually. A higher risk of bleeding is also observed if there is an associated aneurysm, deep venous drainage, or deep brain location; size of the malformation and sex are not associated with risk of hemorrhage.

A. Symptoms and Signs

Initial symptoms consist of hemorrhage in 30–60% of cases, recurrent seizures in 20–40%, headache in 5–25%, and miscellaneous complaints (including focal deficits) in 10–15%. Hemorrhage is commonly intracerebral as well as into the subarachnoid space and is fatal in about 10% of cases. Seizures are more likely with frontal or parietal arteriovenous malformations. Headaches are especially likely when the external carotid arteries are involved in the malformation. These sometimes simulate migraine, but more commonly are nonspecific in character, with nothing about them to suggest an underlying structural lesion. Brainstem and cerebellar arteriovenous malformations may cause obstructive hydrocephalus.

In patients presenting with subarachnoid hemorrhage, examination may reveal an abnormal mental status and signs of meningeal irritation. Additional findings may help localize the lesion and sometimes indicate that intracranial pressure is increased. A **cranial bruit** always suggests the possibility of a cerebral arteriovenous malformation, but bruits may also be found with aneurysms, meningiomas, acquired arteriovenous fistulas, and arteriovenous malformations involving the scalp, calvarium, or orbit. Bruits are best heard over the ipsilateral eye or mastoid region and are of some help in lateralization but of no help in localization. Absence of a bruit does not exclude the possibility of arteriovenous malformation.

B. Imaging

In patients with suspected hemorrhage, CT scanning indicates whether subarachnoid or intracerebral bleeding has recently occurred, helps localize its source, and may reveal the arteriovenous malformation. When intracranial hemorrhage is confirmed but the source of hemorrhage is not evident on the CT scan, arteriography is necessary to exclude aneurysm or arteriovenous malformation. MR and CT angiography are not sensitive enough for this purpose. Even if the findings on CT scan suggest arteriovenous malformation, arteriography is required to establish the nature of the lesion with certainty and to determine its anatomic features so that treatment can be planned. The examination must generally include bilateral opacification of the internal and external carotid arteries and the vertebral arteries.

In patients presenting without hemorrhage, CT scan or MRI usually reveals the underlying abnormality, and MRI frequently also shows evidence of old or recent hemorrhage that may have been asymptomatic. The nature and detailed anatomy of any focal lesion identified by these means are delineated by angiography, especially if operative treatment is under consideration.

▶ Treatment

Surgical treatment to prevent further hemorrhage is justified in patients with arteriovenous malformations that have bled, provided that the lesion is accessible and the patient has a reasonable life expectancy. Surgical treatment is also appropriate if intracranial pressure is increased and to prevent further progression of a focal neurologic deficit. In patients presenting solely with seizures, anticonvulsant treatment is usually sufficient (Table 24–2), and operative treatment is unnecessary unless seizures cannot be controlled medically.

Definitive operative treatment consists of excision of the arteriovenous malformation if it is surgically accessible. Stereotactic radiosurgery is used to treat inoperable cerebral arteriovenous malformations. Arteriovenous malformations that are inoperable because of their location are sometimes treated solely by embolization; although the risk of hemorrhage is not reduced, neurologic deficits may be stabilized or even reversed by this procedure. Embolization is more commonly performed as an adjunct to surgery or radiosurgery; it is also used to treat intranidal aneurysms.

▶ When to Refer

All patients should be referred.

▶ When to Admit

- All patients with a subarachnoid or cerebral hemorrhage.
- All patients for detailed imaging.
- All patients undergoing surgical or endovascular treatment.

Osbun JW et al. Arteriovenous malformations: epidemiology, clinical presentation, and diagnostic evaluation. Handb Clin Neurol. 2017;143:25–9. [PMID: 28552148]

7. Intracranial Venous Thrombosis

Intracranial venous thrombosis may occur in association with intracranial or maxillofacial infections, hypercoagulable states, polycythemia, sickle cell disease, cyanotic congenital heart disease and in pregnancy or during the puerperium. Genetic factors are also important. The disorder is characterized by headache, focal or generalized convulsions, drowsiness, confusion, increased intracranial pressure, and focal neurologic deficits—and sometimes by evidence of meningeal irritation. The diagnosis is confirmed by CT or MR venography or angiography.

Treatment includes anticonvulsants if seizures have occurred (Table 24–2) and—if necessary—measures to reduce intracranial pressure. Anticoagulation with dose-adjusted intravenous heparin or weight-adjusted subcutaneous low-molecular-weight heparin, followed by oral warfarin anticoagulation for 6 months reduces morbidity and mortality of venous sinus thrombosis. Concomitant intracranial hemorrhage related to the venous thrombosis does not contraindicate heparin therapy. In cases refractory to heparin, endovascular techniques including catheter-directed thrombolytic therapy (urokinase) and thrombectomy are sometimes helpful but may increase the risk for major hemorrhage.

When to Refer

All patients should be referred.

When to Admit

All patients should be hospitalized.

8. Spinal Cord Vascular Diseases

ESSENTIALS OF DIAGNOSIS

▸ Sudden onset of back or limb pain and neurologic deficit in limbs.

▸ Motor, sensory, or reflex changes in limbs depending on level of lesion.

▸ Imaging studies distinguish between infarct and hematoma.

Infarction of the Spinal Cord

Infarction of the spinal cord is rare. It typically occurs in the territory of the anterior spinal artery because this vessel, which supplies the anterior two-thirds of the cord, is itself supplied by only a limited number of feeders. Infarction usually results from interrupted flow in one or more of these feeders, eg, with aortic dissection, aortic aneurysm, aortography, polyarteritis, severe hypotension, or after surgical repair of the thoracic or abdominal aorta. The paired posterior spinal arteries, by contrast, are supplied by numerous arteries at different levels of the cord. Spinal cord hypoperfusion may lead to a central cord syndrome with distal weakness of lower motor neuron type and loss of pain and temperature appreciation, with preserved posterior column function.

Since the anterior spinal artery receives numerous feeders in the cervical region, infarcts almost always occur caudally. Clinical presentation is characterized by acute onset of flaccid, areflexive paraplegia that evolves after a few days or weeks into a spastic paraplegia with extensor plantar responses. There is an accompanying dissociated sensory loss, with impairment of appreciation of pain and temperature but preservation of sensations of vibration and joint position.

The risk of spinal cord infarction in the setting of abdominal aortic surgery and thoracic endovascular repair may be reduced by intraoperative cerebrospinal fluid drainage through a catheter placed in the lumbar subarachnoid space to reduce intraspinal pressure. If signs of infarction are noted after surgery, blood pressure augmentation for 24–48 hours in addition to lumbar drainage has been noted anecdotally to improve outcomes. Treatment is otherwise symptomatic.

Epidural or Subdural Hemorrhage

Epidural or subdural hemorrhage may lead to sudden severe back pain followed by an acute compressive myelopathy necessitating urgent spinal MRI or myelography and surgical evacuation. It may occur in patients with bleeding disorders or those who are taking anticoagulants, sometimes following trauma or lumbar puncture. Epidural hemorrhage may also be related to a vascular malformation or tumor deposit.

Spinal Dural Arteriovenous Fistulae

Spinal dural arteriovenous fistulae are congenital lesions that present with spinal subarachnoid hemorrhage or myeloradiculopathy. Since most of these malformations are located in the thoracolumbar region, they lead to motor and sensory disturbances in the legs and to sphincter disorders. Pain in the legs or back is often severe. Examination reveals an upper, lower, or mixed motor deficit in the legs; sensory deficits are also present and are usually extensive, although occasionally they are confined to a radicular distribution. Cervical spinal dural arteriovenous fistulae lead also to symptoms and signs in the arms. Spinal MRI may not detect the spinal dural arteriovenous fistula, although most cases show either T2 hyperintensity in the cord or perimedullary flow voids. Myelography (performed with the patient prone and supine) may detect serpiginous filling defects due to enlarged vessels. Selective spinal arteriography is required to confirm the diagnosis and plan treatment. Most lesions are extramedullary, are posterior to the cord (lying either intradurally or extradurally), and can easily be treated by ligation of feeding vessels and excision of the fistulous anomaly or by embolization procedures. Delay in treatment may lead to increased and irreversible disability or to death from recurrent subarachnoid hemorrhage.

When to Refer

All patients should be referred.

When to Admit

All patients should be hospitalized.

Rabinstein AA. Vascular myelopathies. Continuum (Minneap Minn). 2015 Feb;21(1 Spinal Cord Disorders):67–83. [PMID: 25651218]

INTRACRANIAL & SPINAL MASS LESIONS

1. Primary Intracranial Tumors

ESSENTIALS OF DIAGNOSIS

▸ Generalized or focal disturbance of cerebral function, or both.

▸ Increased intracranial pressure in some patients.

▸ Neuroradiologic evidence of space-occupying lesion.

General Considerations

Roughly one-third of all primary intracranial neoplasms (Table 24–4) are meningiomas, one-quarter are gliomas,

Table 24–4. Primary intracranial tumors (listed by major histology grouping and by incidence within each group).

Tumor	Clinical Features	Treatment and Prognosis
Tumors of Meninges		
Meningioma	Originates from the dura mater or arachnoid; compresses rather than invades adjacent neural structures. Increasingly common with advancing age. Tumor size varies greatly. Symptoms vary with tumor site—eg, unilateral proptosis (sphenoidal ridge); anosmia and optic nerve compression (olfactory groove). Tumor is usually benign and readily detected by CT scanning; may lead to calcification and bone erosion visible on plain radiographs of skull.	Treatment is surgical. Tumor may recur if removal is incomplete.
Tumors of Neuroepithelial Origin		
Glioblastoma multiforme	Presents commonly with nonspecific complaints and increased intracranial pressure. As it grows, focal deficits develop. O^6-methylguanine-DNA methyltransferase promoter methylation positivity (seen in 40% of cases) and isocitrate dehydrogenase 1/2 mutations (seen in 10% of cases) carry better prognosis.	Course is rapidly progressive, with poor prognosis (< 20% survival at 2 years). Total surgical removal is usually not possible. Radiation therapy and temozolamide may prolong survival. Tumor treatment fields added to temozolamide after completion of radiation therapy prolong survival.
Astrocytoma	Presentation similar to glioblastoma multiforme but course more protracted, often over several years. Cerebellar astrocytoma may have a more benign course. Isocitrate dehydrogenase 1/2 mutations (seen in a majority of cases) carry better prognosis in grade II and III tumors.	Prognosis is variable. By the time of diagnosis, total excision is usually impossible; tumor may be radiosensitive and temozolamide is also helpful in grade II and III tumors. In cerebellar astrocytoma, total surgical removal is often possible.
Ependymoma	Glioma arising from the ependyma of a ventricle, especially the fourth ventricle; leads to early signs of increased intracranial pressure. Arises also from central canal of cord.	Tumor is best treated surgically if possible. Radiation therapy may be used for residual tumor.
Oligodendroglioma	Slow-growing. Usually arises in cerebral hemisphere in adults. Calcification may be visible on skull radiograph. Co-deletion of 1p/19q and isocitrate dehydrogenase 1/2 mutation required for diagnosis.	Treatment is surgical and usually successful. Radiation and chemotherapy (temozolamide or procarbazine, lomustine, and vincristine) are used in grade II and III tumors.
Brainstem glioma	Presents during childhood with cranial nerve palsies and then with long tract signs in the limbs. Signs of increased intracranial pressure occur late.	Tumor is inoperable; treatment is by irradiation and shunt for increased intracranial pressure.
Neuronal and mixed neuronal-glial tumors	Slow-growing; usually arise in cerebral hemispheres; often associated with seizures. Some are benign (eg, dysembryoblastic neuroepithelial tumors) and some have malignant potential (eg, ganglioglioma).	Resection is not always necessary for benign tumors unless seizures are medically refractory, but is indicated for those with malignant potential.
Medulloblastoma	Seen most frequently in children. Generally arises from roof of fourth ventricle and leads to increased intracranial pressure accompanied by brainstem and cerebellar signs. May seed subarachnoid space. Wingless activated tumors carry best prognosis (> 90% 5-year survival).	Treatment consists of surgery combined with radiation therapy and chemotherapy; 5-year survival exceeds 70%. Wingless activated tumors may require less aggressive treatment.
Pineal tumor	Presents with increased intracranial pressure, sometimes associated with impaired upward gaze (Parinaud syndrome) and other deficits indicative of midbrain lesion.	Ventricular decompression by shunting is followed by surgical approach to tumor; irradiation is indicated if tumor is malignant. Prognosis depends on histopathologic findings and extent of tumor.
Tumors of the Sellar Region		
Pituitary adenoma	Functioning adenomas present with symptoms of hormone secretion; nonfunctioning adenomas present with symptoms of local mass effect (eg, bitemporal hemianopsia, hypopituitarism) or are found incidentally.	Prolactin-secreting adenomas are treated with bromocriptine or cabergoline. Others are surgically resected. Pituitary hormone replacement may be required.
Craniopharyngioma	Originates from remnants of Rathke pouch above the sella, depressing the optic chiasm. May present at any age but usually in childhood, with endocrine dysfunction and bitemporal visual field defects.	Treatment is surgical, but total removal may not be possible. Radiation may be used for residual tumor.

(continued)

Table 24–4. Primary intracranial tumors (listed by major histology grouping and by incidence within each group). (continued)

Tumor	Clinical Features	Treatment and Prognosis
Tumors of Cranial and Spinal Nerves		
Acoustic neurinoma (also referred to as acoustic neuroma)	Ipsilateral hearing loss is most common initial symptom. Subsequent symptoms may include tinnitus, headache, vertigo, facial weakness or numbness, and long tract signs. (May be familial and bilateral when related to neurofibromatosis.) Most sensitive screening tests are MRI and brainstem auditory evoked potential.	Treatment is excision by translabyrinthine surgery, craniectomy, or a combined approach. Outcome is usually good.
Lymphomas		
Primary cerebral lymphoma	Associated with AIDS and other immunodeficient states. Presentation may be with focal deficits or with disturbances of cognition and consciousness. May be indistinguishable from cerebral toxoplasmosis.	Treatment is high-dose methotrexate and corticosteroids followed by radiation therapy. Prognosis depends on CD4 count at diagnosis.
Unclassified		
Cerebellar hemangioblastoma	Presents with dysequilibrium, ataxia of trunk or limbs, and signs of increased intracranial pressure. Sometimes familial. May be associated with retinal and spinal vascular lesions, polycythemia, and renal cell carcinoma.	Treatment is surgical. Radiation is used for residual tumor.

and the remainder are pituitary adenomas (see Chapter 26), neurofibromas, and other tumors. Certain tumors, especially neurofibromas, hemangioblastomas, and retinoblastomas, may have a familial basis, and congenital factors bear on the development of craniopharyngiomas. Tumors may occur at any age, but certain gliomas show particular age predilections.

Clinical Findings

A. Symptoms and Signs

Intracranial tumors typically present with headache, seizures, or focal neurologic deficits. New headaches or symptoms of elevated intracranial pressure, such as headaches awaking a patient from sleep or worsening with Valsalva maneuver, cough, or recumbency, are suggestive of brain tumor. Intracranial tumors may also lead to a generalized disturbance of cerebral function with personality changes, intellectual decline, emotional lability, nausea, and malaise.

1. Frontal lobe lesions—Tumors of the frontal lobe often lead to progressive intellectual decline, slowing of mental activity, personality changes, and contralateral grasp reflexes. They may lead to expressive aphasia if the posterior part of the left inferior frontal gyrus is involved. Anosmia may also occur as a consequence of pressure on the olfactory nerve. Precentral lesions may cause focal motor seizures or contralateral pyramidal deficits.

2. Temporal lobe lesions—Tumors of the uncinate region may be manifested by seizures with olfactory or gustatory hallucinations, motor phenomena such as licking or smacking of the lips, and some impairment of external awareness without actual loss of consciousness. Temporal lobe lesions also lead to depersonalization, emotional changes, behavioral disturbances, sensations of déjà vu or jamais vu, micropsia or macropsia (objects appear smaller or larger than they are), visual field defects (crossed upper quadrantanopia), and auditory illusions or hallucinations. Left-sided lesions may lead to dysnomia and receptive aphasia, while right-sided involvement sometimes disturbs the perception of musical notes and melodies.

3. Parietal lobe lesions—Tumors in this location characteristically cause contralateral disturbances of sensation and may cause sensory seizures, sensory loss or inattention, or some combination of these symptoms. The sensory loss is cortical in type and involves postural sensibility and tactile discrimination, so that the appreciation of shape, size, weight, and texture is impaired. Objects placed in the hand may not be recognized (astereognosis). Extensive parietal lobe lesions may produce contralateral hyperpathia and spontaneous pain (thalamic syndrome). Involvement of the optic radiation leads to a contralateral homonymous field defect that sometimes consists solely of lower quadrantanopia. Lesions of the left angular gyrus cause Gerstmann syndrome (a combination of alexia, agraphia, acalculia, right-left confusion, and finger agnosia), whereas involvement of the left submarginal gyrus causes ideational apraxia. Anosognosia (the denial, neglect, or rejection of a paralyzed limb) is seen in patients with lesions of the nondominant (right) hemisphere. Constructional apraxia and dressing apraxia may also occur with right-sided lesions.

4. Occipital lobe lesions—Tumors of the occipital lobe characteristically produce contralateral homonymous hemianopia or a partial field defect. With left-sided or bilateral lesions, there may be visual agnosia both for objects and for colors, while irritative lesions on either side can cause unformed visual hallucinations. Bilateral occipital lobe involvement causes cortical blindness in which there is preservation of pupillary responses to light and lack of awareness of the defect by the patient. There may also be loss of color perception, prosopagnosia (inability to identify a familiar face), simultagnosia (inability to integrate and interpret a composite scene as opposed to its individual elements), and Balint syndrome (failure to turn the eyes to a particular point in space, despite preservation of spontaneous and reflex eye movements). The denial of blindness or a field defect constitutes Anton syndrome.

5. Brainstem and cerebellar lesions—Brainstem lesions lead to cranial nerve palsies, ataxia, incoordination, nystagmus, and pyramidal and sensory deficits in the limbs on one or both sides. Intrinsic brainstem tumors, such as gliomas, tend to produce an increase in intracranial pressure only late in their course. Cerebellar tumors produce marked ataxia of the trunk if the vermis cerebelli is involved and ipsilateral appendicular deficits (ataxia, incoordination and hypotonia of the limbs) if the cerebellar hemispheres are affected.

6. Herniation syndromes—If the pressure is increased in a particular cranial compartment, brain tissue may herniate into a compartment with lower pressure. The most familiar syndrome is herniation of the temporal lobe uncus through the tentorial hiatus, which causes compression of the third cranial nerve, midbrain, and posterior cerebral artery. The earliest sign of this is ipsilateral pupillary dilation, followed by stupor, coma, decerebrate posturing, and respiratory arrest. Another important herniation syndrome consists of displacement of the cerebellar tonsils through the foramen magnum, which causes medullary compression leading to apnea, circulatory collapse, and death.

7. False localizing signs—Tumors may lead to neurologic signs other than by direct compression or infiltration, thereby leading to errors of clinical localization. These false localizing signs include third or sixth nerve palsy and bilateral extensor plantar responses produced by herniation syndromes, and an extensor plantar response occurring ipsilateral to a hemispheric tumor as a result of compression of the opposite cerebral peduncle against the tentorium.

B. Imaging

MRI with gadolinium enhancement is the preferred method to detect the lesion and to define its location, shape, and size; the extent to which normal anatomy is distorted; and the degree of any associated cerebral edema or mass effect. CT scanning with radiocontrast enhancement could be performed; however, it is less helpful than MRI for small lesions or tumors in the posterior fossa. The characteristic appearance of meningiomas on MRI or CT scanning is virtually diagnostic, ie, a lesion in a typical site (parasagittal and sylvian regions, olfactory groove, sphenoidal ridge, tuberculum sellae) that appears as a homogeneous area of increased density in noncontrast scans and enhances uniformly with contrast. Additional MRI sequences that may be helpful in differentiating gliomas from other intracranial pathology include perfusion imaging, magnetic resonance spectroscopy, and diffusion-weighted imaging,

although none are specific enough to obviate the need for tissue sampling. Arteriography is largely reserved for presurgical embolization of highly vascular tumors. In patients with normal hormone levels and an intrasellar mass, angiography is sometimes necessary to distinguish with confidence between a pituitary adenoma and an arterial aneurysm.

C. Laboratory and Other Studies

When glial neoplasms are suspected, biopsy is necessary for definitive histologic diagnosis and molecular analysis. The World Health Organization classifies glial tumors by both histology and genetic characteristics. Lumbar puncture is rarely necessary; the findings are seldom diagnostic, and the procedure carries the risk of causing a herniation syndrome.

▶ Treatment

Treatment depends on the type and site of the tumor (Table 24–4) and the condition of the patient. Some benign tumors, especially meningiomas discovered incidentally during brain imaging for another purpose, may be monitored with serial annual imaging. For symptomatic tumors, complete surgical removal may be possible if the tumor is extra-axial (eg, meningioma, acoustic neuroma) or is not in a critical or inaccessible region of the brain (eg, cerebellar hemangioblastoma). Surgery also permits the diagnosis to be verified and may be beneficial in reducing intracranial pressure and relieving symptoms even if the neoplasm cannot be completely removed. Clinical deficits are sometimes due in part to obstructive hydrocephalus, in which case simple surgical shunting procedures often produce dramatic benefit. In patients with malignant gliomas, survival correlates to the extent of initial resection.

Radiation therapy increases median survival rates regardless of any preceding surgery, and its combination with chemotherapy provides additional benefit. Indications for irradiation in the treatment of patients with other primary intracranial neoplasms depend on tumor type and accessibility and the feasibility of complete surgical removal. Long-term neurocognitive deficits may complicate radiation therapy. Temozolomide is a commonly used oral and intravenous chemotherapeutic for gliomas, and the use of monoclonal antibodies like bevacizumab as a component of therapy may be helpful (see Table 39–2). The addition of low-intensity, 200 kHz frequency alternating electric fields (**tumor treatment fields**) delivered extracranially at least 18 hours daily, improves progression-free survival by 2.7 months and median survival by 4.9 months compared to temozolomide alone. Combination therapy with procarbazine, lomustine, and vincristine in patients with oligodendroglioma and p1/19q co-deletion is under investigation, and treatment of glioblastoma multiforme with a recombinant nonpathogenic polio-rhinovirus chimera showed promise in a phase I clinical trial.

Corticosteroids help reduce cerebral edema and are usually started before surgery. Herniation is treated with intravenous dexamethasone (10–20 mg as a bolus, followed by 4 mg every 6 hours) and intravenous mannitol (20% solution given in a dose of 1.5 g/kg over about 30 minutes).

Anticonvulsants are also commonly administered in standard doses (see Table 24–2), but are not indicated for prophylaxis in patients who have no history of seizures. For those patients with difficult to treat symptoms or those needing help with advance care planning, specialty palliative care consultation is appropriate (see Chapter 5).

When to Refer

All patients should be referred.

When to Admit

- All patients with increased intracranial pressure.
- All patients requiring biopsy, surgical treatment, or shunting procedures.

Louis DN et al. The 2016 World Health Organization classification of tumors of the central nervous system: a summary. Acta Neuropathol. 2016 Jun;131(6):803–20. [PMID: 27157931]

Oberheim Bush NA et al. Treatment strategies for low-grade glioma in adults. J Oncol Pract. 2016 Dec;12(12):1235–41. [PMID: 27943684]

Stupp R et al. Effect of tumor-treating fields plus maintenance temozolomide vs maintenance temozolomide alone on survival in patients with glioblastoma: a randomized clinical trial. JAMA. 2017 Dec 19;318(23):2306–16. Erratum in: JAMA. 2018 May 1;319(17):1824. [PMID: 29260225]

van den Bent MJ et al. Diffuse infiltrating oligodendroglioma and astrocytoma. J Clin Oncol. 2017 Jul 20;35(21):2394–401. [PMID: 28640702]

2. Metastatic Intracranial Tumors

A. Cerebral Metastases

Metastatic brain tumors present in the same way as other cerebral neoplasms, ie, with increased intracranial pressure, with focal or diffuse disturbance of cerebral function, or with both of these manifestations. Indeed, in patients with a single cerebral lesion, the metastatic nature of the lesion may become evident only on histopathologic examination. In other patients, there is evidence of widespread metastatic disease, or an isolated cerebral metastasis develops during treatment of the primary neoplasm.

The most common source of intracranial metastasis is carcinoma of the lung; other primary sites are the breast, kidney, skin (melanoma), and gastrointestinal tract. Most cerebral metastases are located supratentorially. Laboratory and radiologic studies used to evaluate patients with metastases are those described for primary neoplasms. They include MRI and CT scanning performed both with and without contrast. Lumbar puncture is necessary only in patients with suspected carcinomatous meningitis. In patients with verified cerebral metastasis from an unknown primary, investigation is guided by symptoms and signs. In women, mammography is indicated; in men under 50, germ cell origin is sought.

In patients with only a single, surgically accessible cerebral metastasis who are otherwise well (ie, a high level of functioning and little or no evidence of extracranial disease), it may be possible to remove the lesion and then treat with irradiation; the latter may also be selected as the sole treatment. In patients with multiple metastases or widespread systemic disease, the prognosis is poor; stereotactic radiosurgery, whole-brain radiotherapy, or both may help in some instances, but in others, treatment is palliative only.

Ba JL et al. Current and emerging treatments for brain metastases. Oncology (Williston Park). 2015 Apr;29(4):250–7. [PMID: 25952487]

B. Leptomeningeal Metastases (Carcinomatous Meningitis)

The neoplasms metastasizing most commonly to the leptomeninges are carcinoma of the breast and lung, lymphomas, and leukemia (see Chapter 39). Leptomeningeal metastases lead to multifocal neurologic deficits, which may be associated with infiltration of cranial and spinal nerve roots, direct invasion of the brain or spinal cord, obstructive or communicating hydrocephalus, or some combination of these factors.

The diagnosis is confirmed by examination of the cerebrospinal fluid. Findings may include elevated cerebrospinal fluid pressure, pleocytosis, increased protein concentration, and decreased glucose concentration. Cytologic studies may indicate that malignant cells are present; if not, lumbar puncture should be repeated at least twice to obtain further samples for analysis.

CT scans showing contrast enhancement in the basal cisterns or showing hydrocephalus without any evidence of a mass lesion support the diagnosis. Gadolinium-enhanced MRI is more sensitive and frequently shows enhancing foci in the leptomeninges. Myelography may show deposits on multiple nerve roots.

Treatment is by irradiation to symptomatic areas, combined with intrathecal chemotherapy in select patients. The long-term prognosis is poor—only about 10% of patients survive for 1 year—and palliative care is therefore important (see Chapter 5).

Passarin MG et al. Leptomeningeal metastasis from solid tumors: a diagnostic and therapeutic challenge. Neurol Sci. 2015 Jan; 36(1):117–23. [PMID: 25022241]

3. Intracranial Mass Lesions in AIDS Patients

Primary cerebral lymphoma is a common complication in patients with AIDS. This leads to disturbances in cognition or consciousness, focal motor or sensory deficits, aphasia, seizures, and cranial neuropathies. Similar clinical disturbances may result from **cerebral toxoplasmosis**, which is also a common complication in patients with AIDS (see Chapters 31 and 35). Neither CT nor MRI findings distinguish these two disorders, serologic tests for toxoplasmosis are unreliable in AIDS patients, and although the finding of Epstein-Barr virus DNA in the spinal fluid by polymerase chain reaction suggests lymphoma, it is not specific enough to initiate treatment. Accordingly, for neurologically stable patients, a *trial of treatment for toxoplasmosis* with pyrimethamine and sulfadiazine is recommended for 3 weeks; the imaging studies are then repeated, and if any lesion has improved, the regimen is continued indefinitely. If any lesion does not improve, cerebral biopsy is necessary (see also Chapter 31). Primary cerebral lymphoma in AIDS patients is treated with corticosteroids, high-dose methotrexate, and antiretroviral therapy. Rituximab may be used in some patients. Whole-brain irradiation may not be necessary.

Cryptococcal meningitis is a common opportunistic infection in AIDS patients. Clinically, it may resemble cerebral toxoplasmosis or lymphoma, but cranial CT scans are usually normal (see Chapter 36).

4. Primary & Metastatic Spinal Tumors

Approximately 10% of spinal tumors are intramedullary. Ependymoma is the most common type of intramedullary tumor; the remainder are other types of glioma. Extramedullary tumors may be extradural or intradural in location. Among the primary extramedullary tumors, neurofibromas and meningiomas are relatively common, benign, and may be intradural or extradural. Carcinomatous metastases, lymphomatous or leukemic deposits, and myeloma are usually extradural; in the case of metastases, the prostate, breast, lung, and kidney are common primary sites.

Tumors may lead to spinal cord dysfunction by direct compression, by ischemia secondary to arterial or venous obstruction and, in the case of intramedullary lesions, by invasive infiltration.

▶ Clinical Findings

A. Symptoms and Signs

Symptoms usually develop insidiously. Pain is often conspicuous with extradural lesions; is characteristically aggravated by coughing or straining; may be radicular, localized to the back, or felt diffusely in an extremity; and may be accompanied by motor deficits, paresthesias, or numbness, especially in the legs. Bladder, bowel, and sexual dysfunction may occur. When sphincter disturbances occur, they are usually particularly disabling. Pain, however, often precedes specific neurologic symptoms from epidural metastases.

Examination may reveal localized spinal tenderness. A segmental lower motor neuron deficit or dermatomal sensory changes (or both) are sometimes found at the level of the lesion, while an upper motor neuron deficit and sensory disturbance are found below it.

B. Imaging

MRI with contrast or CT myelography is used to identify and localize the lesion. The combination of known tumor elsewhere in the body, back pain, and either abnormal plain films of the spine or neurologic signs of cord compression is an indication to perform this on an *urgent* basis.

C. Laboratory Findings

The cerebrospinal fluid is often xanthochromic and contains a greatly increased protein concentration with normal cell content and glucose concentration.

▶ Treatment

Intramedullary tumors are treated by decompression and surgical excision (when feasible) and by irradiation. The prognosis depends on the cause and severity of cord compression before it is relieved.

Treatment of epidural spinal metastases consists of surgical decompression, radiation, or both. Dexamethasone is also given in a high dosage (eg, 10–96 mg once intravenously, followed by 4–25 mg four times daily for 3 days orally or intravenously, followed by rapid tapering of the dosage, depending on initial dose and response) to reduce cord swelling and relieve pain. Radiation alone is often all that is required in patients with radiosensitive tumors. Surgical decompression is reserved for patients with tumors that are unresponsive to irradiation or who have previously been irradiated, for those with spinal instability, and for patients in whom there is some uncertainty about the diagnosis. The long-term outlook is poor, but treatment may at least delay the onset of major disability.

Chamberlain MC. Neoplastic myelopathies. Continuum (Minneap Minn). 2015 Feb;21(1 Spinal Cord Disorders):132–45. [PMID: 25651222]

5. Brain Abscess

ESSENTIALS OF DIAGNOSIS

▶ Signs of expanding intracranial mass.
▶ Signs of primary infection or congenital heart disease are sometimes present.
▶ Fever may be absent.

▶ General Considerations

Brain abscess presents as an intracranial space-occupying lesion and arises as a sequela of disease of the ear or nose, may be a complication of infection elsewhere in the body, or may result from infection introduced intracranially by trauma or surgical procedures. The most common infective organisms are streptococci, staphylococci, and anaerobes; mixed infections also occur.

▶ Clinical Findings

A. Symptoms and Signs

Headache, drowsiness, inattention, confusion, and seizures are early symptoms, followed by signs of increasing intracranial pressure and then a focal neurologic deficit. There may be little or no systemic evidence of infection.

B. Imaging and Other Investigations

A CT scan of the head characteristically shows an area of contrast enhancement surrounding a low-density core. Similar abnormalities may be found in patients with metastatic neoplasms. MRI findings often permit earlier recognition of focal cerebritis or an abscess. Stereotactic needle aspiration may enable a specific etiologic organism to be identified. Examination of the cerebrospinal fluid does not help in diagnosis and may precipitate a herniation syndrome. Peripheral leukocytosis is sometimes present.

▶ Treatment

Treatment consists of intravenous antibiotics combined with surgical drainage (aspiration or excision), if necessary, to reduce the mass effect or sometimes to establish the diagnosis. Abscesses smaller than 2 cm can often be cured medically. Broad-spectrum antibiotics, selected based on risk factors and likely organisms, are used if the infecting organism is unknown (see Chapter 33). An initial empiric multi-antibiotic regimen typically includes ceftriaxone (2 g intravenously every 12 hours), metronidazole (15 mg/kg intravenous loading dose, followed by 7.5 mg/kg intravenously every 6 hours), and vancomycin (1 g intravenously every 12 hours). The regimen is altered once culture and sensitivity data are available. Antimicrobial treatment is usually continued parenterally for 6–8 weeks and is followed by oral treatment for certain infections, such as nocardiosis, actinomycosis, fungal infections, and tuberculosis. The patient should be monitored by serial CT scans or MRI every 2 weeks and at deterioration. Dexamethasone (4–25 mg four times daily intravenously or orally, depending on severity, followed by tapering of dose, depending on response) may reduce any associated edema, but intravenous mannitol is sometimes required.

Chow F. Brain and spinal epidural abscess. Continuum (Minneap Minn). 2018 Oct;24(5):1327–48. [PMID: 30273242]

NONMETASTATIC NEUROLOGIC COMPLICATIONS OF MALIGNANT DISEASE

A variety of nonmetastatic neurologic complications of malignant disease can be recognized. **Metabolic encephalopathy** due to electrolyte abnormalities, infections, drug overdose, or the failure of some vital organ may be reflected by drowsiness, lethargy, restlessness, insomnia, agitation, confusion, stupor, or coma. The mental changes are usually associated with tremor, asterixis, and multifocal myoclonus. The electroencephalogram is generally diffusely slowed. Laboratory studies are necessary to detect the cause of the encephalopathy, which must then be treated appropriately.

Immune suppression resulting from either the malignant disease or its treatment (eg, by chemotherapy) predisposes patients to brain abscess, progressive multifocal leukoencephalopathy, meningitis, herpes zoster infection, and other opportunistic infectious diseases. Moreover, an overt or occult cerebrospinal fluid fistula, as occurs with some tumors, may also increase the risk of infection. MRI or CT scanning aids in the early recognition of a brain abscess, but metastatic brain tumors may have a similar appearance. Examination of the cerebrospinal fluid is essential in the evaluation of patients with meningitis and encephalitis but is of no help in the diagnosis of brain abscess.

Cerebrovascular disorders that cause neurologic complications in patients with systemic cancer include nonbacterial thrombotic endocarditis and septic embolization. Cerebral, subarachnoid, or subdural hemorrhages may occur in patients with myelogenous leukemia and may be found in association with metastatic tumors, especially melanoma. Spinal subdural hemorrhage sometimes occurs after lumbar puncture in patients with marked thrombocytopenia.

Disseminated intravascular coagulation occurs most commonly in patients with acute promyelocytic leukemia or with some adenocarcinomas and is characterized by a fluctuating encephalopathy, often with associated seizures, that frequently progresses to coma or death. There may be few accompanying neurologic signs. **Venous sinus thrombosis,** which usually presents with convulsions and headaches, may also occur in patients with leukemia or lymphoma. Examination commonly reveals papilledema and focal or diffuse neurologic signs. Anticonvulsants, anticoagulants, and medications to lower the intracranial pressure may be of value.

Autoimmune paraneoplastic disorders occur when the immune system reacts against neuronal antigens expressed by tumor cells. The clinical manifestations depend on the autoantibody. Symptoms may precede those due to the neoplasm itself. Several distinct syndromes are common, including paraneoplastic cerebellar degeneration, limbic encephalitis, encephalomyelitis, anti-NMDA receptor-associated encephalitis, opsoclonus/myoclonus, sensory neuronopathy, retinopathy, and dermatomyositis.

Paraneoplastic cerebellar degeneration occurs most commonly in association with carcinoma of the lung, but also in breast and gynecologic cancers and Hodgkin lymphoma. Typically, there is a pancerebellar syndrome causing dysarthria, nystagmus, and ataxia of the trunk and limbs. The disorder is associated with anti-Yo, -Tr, -voltage-gated calcium channel (VGCC), and Zic antibodies. Treatment is of the underlying malignant disease. **Limbic encephalitis**, characterized by impaired recent memory, disturbed affect, hallucinations, and seizures, occurs in some patients with tumors of the lungs, breast, thymus, and germ cells. Associated antibodies include anti-Hu, -Ma2, -CV2/CRMP5, -voltage-gated potassium channel (VGKC), -leucine rich glioma inactivated 1 (LGI1), -contactin associated protein-like 2 (Caspr2), -dipeptidyl-peptidase-like protein-6 (DPPX), -AMPA receptor, -GABA$_A$ receptor, and -GABA$_B$ receptor. **Anti-DPPX encephalitis** is typically preceded by a severe and prolonged diarrheal prodrome. A more generalized **encephalomyelitis** occurs with anti-Hu, -CV2/CRMP5, -Ma2, and -amphiphysin antibodies in the context of a similar spectrum of tumors. **Anti-NMDA receptor-associated encephalitis** causes a characteristic syndrome of severe psychiatric symptoms, dyskinesias, dysautonomia, and hypoventilation, and is frequently associated with ovarian teratoma. **Opsoclonus/myoclonus**, a syndrome of involuntary, erratic, and conjugate saccadic eye movements and myoclonic movements of the limbs, occurs in patients with lung, breast, and gynecologic tumors, often without an identifiable antibody. **Sensory neuronopathy**, typically caused by anti-Hu antibodies in small cell lung cancer or other carcinomas, manifests itself with asymmetric, multifocal sensory nerve root deficits leading to pain, numbness, sensory ataxia, and sometimes hearing loss. Both a **sensorimotor** and a **purely sensory polyneuropathy** have been associated with circulating anti-MAG or anti-Hu antibodies. The sensorimotor polyneuropathy may be mild and occur in the course of known malignant disease, or it may have an acute or subacute onset, lead to severe disability, and occur before there is any clinical evidence of the cancer, occasionally following a remitting course. An **autonomic neuropathy** may also occur as a paraneoplastic disorder related to the presence of anti-Hu antibodies or to antibodies against ganglionic acetylcholine receptors (anti-nAChR). Paraneoplastic **retinopathy** occurs due to antirecoverin or antibipolar cell antibodies associated with small cell lung cancer or melanoma. **Dermatomyositis** (see Chapter 20) or the **Lambert-Eaton myasthenic syndrome** may be seen in patients with underlying carcinoma. Identification of an antibody is not always possible in a suspected autoimmune paraneoplastic condition, and a search for an underlying neoplasm should be undertaken. Treatment of the neoplasm offers the best hope for stabilization or improvement of the neurologic symptoms, which often are not completely reversible. Specific treatment of the antibody-mediated symptoms by intravenous immunoglobulin (IVIG) administration, plasmapheresis, corticosteroids, or other immunosuppressive regimens is frequently attempted despite limited evidence of efficacy. Encephalitides involving antibodies directed against neuronal cell surface antigens, such as VGKC, LGI1, Caspr2, AMPA, NMDA, $GABA_{B\ and\ A}$ receptors, and DPPX, can occur either as paraneoplastic phenomena or in isolation, and typically respond well to immunotherapy.

Höftberger R et al. Update on neurological paraneoplastic syndromes. Curr Opin Oncol. 2015 Nov;27(6):489–95. [PMID: 26335665]

Linnoila J et al. Autoantibody-associated central nervous system neurologic disorders. Semin Neurol. 2016 Aug;36(4):382–96. [PMID: 27643908]

PSEUDOTUMOR CEREBRI (Idiopathic Intracranial Hypertension)

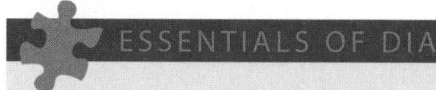

ESSENTIALS OF DIAGNOSIS

► Headache, worse on straining.
► Visual obscurations or diplopia may occur.
► Examination reveals papilledema.
► Abducens palsy is commonly present.

General Considerations

There are many causes of pseudotumor cerebri. Thrombosis of the transverse venous sinus as a complication of otitis media or chronic mastoiditis is one cause, and sagittal sinus thrombosis may lead to a clinically similar picture. Other causes include chronic pulmonary disease, systemic lupus erythematosus, uremia, endocrine disturbances such as hypoparathyroidism, hypothyroidism, or Addison disease, vitamin A toxicity, and the use of tetracycline or oral contraceptives. Cases have also followed withdrawal of corticosteroids after long-term use. In most instances, however, no specific cause can be found, and the disorder remits spontaneously after several months. This idiopathic variety—known as idiopathic intracranial hypertension—occurs most commonly among overweight women aged 20–44. In all cases, screening for a space-occupying lesion of the brain is important.

Clinical Findings

A. Symptoms and Signs

Symptoms consist of headache, diplopia, and other visual disturbances due to papilledema and abducens nerve dysfunction. Pulse-synchronous tinnitus may also occur. Examination reveals papilledema and some enlargement of the blind spots, but patients otherwise look well.

B. Imaging

Investigations reveal no evidence of a space-occupying lesion. CT or MRI shows small or normal ventricles and an empty sella turcica. MR venography is important in screening for thrombosis of the intracranial venous sinuses. In some cases, stenosis of one or more of the venous sinuses will be observed.

C. Laboratory Findings

Lumbar puncture confirms the presence of intracranial hypertension, but the cerebrospinal fluid is normal. Laboratory studies help exclude some of the other causes mentioned earlier.

Treatment

Untreated intracranial hypertension sometimes leads to secondary optic atrophy and permanent visual loss. Acetazolamide (250–500 mg orally three times daily, increasing slowly to a maintenance dose of up to 4000 mg daily, divided two to four times daily) reduces formation of cerebrospinal fluid. Like acetazolamide, the antiepileptic medication topiramate (Table 24–2) is a carbonic anhydrase inhibitor and was shown to be similarly effective in an open label study; topiramate has the added benefit of causing weight loss. Furosemide (20–40 mg daily) may be helpful as adjunct therapy. Corticosteroids (eg, prednisone 60–80 mg daily) are sometimes prescribed, but side effects and the risk of relapse on withdrawal have discouraged their use. Obese patients should be advised to lose weight. Repeated lumbar puncture to lower the intracranial pressure by removal of cerebrospinal fluid is effective as a temporizing measure, but pharmacologic approaches to treatment provide better long-term relief. Treatment is monitored by checking visual acuity and visual fields, funduscopic appearance, and pressure of the cerebrospinal fluid. The disorder may worsen after a period of stability, indicating the need for long-term follow-up.

If medical treatment fails to control the intracranial pressure, surgical placement of a lumboperitoneal or ventriculoperitoneal shunt or optic nerve sheath fenestration should be undertaken to preserve vision. Venous sinus stenting is under study as a therapy for dural venous sinus stenosis.

In addition to the above measures, any specific cause of intracranial hypertension requires appropriate treatment. Thus, hormone therapy should be initiated if there is an underlying endocrine disturbance. Discontinuing the use of tetracycline, oral contraceptives, or vitamin A will allow for resolution of intracranial hypertension due to these agents. If corticosteroid withdrawal is responsible, the medication should be reintroduced and then tapered more gradually.

When to Refer

All patients should be referred.

When to Admit

All patients with worsening vision requiring shunt placement or optic nerve sheath fenestration should be hospitalized.

Madriz Peralta G et al. An update of idiopathic intracranial hypertension. Curr Opin Ophthalmol. 2018 Nov;29(6): 495–502. [PMID: 30169466]

SELECTED NEUROCUTANEOUS DISEASES

Because the nervous system develops from the epithelial layer of the embryo, a number of congenital diseases include both neurologic and cutaneous manifestations. Among these disorders, three are discussed below, and von Hippel-Lindau disease is discussed in Chapter 26.

1. Tuberous Sclerosis

Tuberous sclerosis may occur sporadically or on a familial basis with autosomal dominant inheritance. Neurologic presentation is with seizures and progressive psychomotor retardation beginning in early childhood. The cutaneous abnormality **adenoma sebaceum** becomes manifest usually between 5 and 10 years of age and typically consists of reddened nodules on the face (cheeks, nasolabial folds, sides of the nose, and chin) and sometimes on the forehead and neck. Other typical cutaneous lesions include subungual fibromas, shagreen patches (leathery plaques of subepidermal fibrosis, situated usually on the trunk), and leaf-shaped hypopigmented spots. Associated abnormalities include retinal lesions and tumors, benign rhabdomyomas of the heart, lung cysts, benign tumors in the viscera, and bone cysts.

The disease is slowly progressive and leads to increasing mental deterioration. There is no specific treatment, but anticonvulsants may help in controlling seizures.

2. Neurofibromatosis

Neurofibromatosis may occur either sporadically or on a familial basis with autosomal dominant inheritance. Two distinct forms are recognized: **Type 1 (Recklinghausen disease)** is characterized by multiple hyperpigmented macules, Lisch nodules, and neurofibromas, and results from mutations in the *NF1* gene on chromosome 17. **Type 2** is characterized by bilateral eighth nerve tumors, often accompanied by other intracranial or intraspinal tumors, and is associated with mutations in the *NF2* (merlin) gene on chromosome 22.

Neurologic presentation is usually with symptoms and signs of tumor. Multiple neurofibromas characteristically are present and may involve spinal or cranial nerves, especially the eighth nerve. Examination of the superficial cutaneous nerves usually reveals palpable mobile nodules. In some cases, there is marked overgrowth of subcutaneous tissues (plexiform neuromas), sometimes with an underlying bony abnormality. Associated cutaneous lesions include axillary freckling and patches of cutaneous pigmentation (café au lait spots). Malignant degeneration of neurofibromas occasionally occurs and may lead to peripheral sarcomas. Meningiomas, gliomas (especially optic nerve gliomas), bone cysts, pheochromocytomas, scoliosis, and obstructive hydrocephalus may also occur.

3. Sturge-Weber Syndrome

Sturge-Weber syndrome consists of a congenital, usually unilateral, cutaneous capillary angioma involving the upper face, leptomeningeal angiomatosis, and, in many patients, choroidal angioma. It has no sex predilection and usually occurs sporadically. The cutaneous angioma sometimes has a more extensive distribution over the head and neck and is often quite disfiguring, especially if there is associated overgrowth of connective tissue. Focal or generalized seizures are the usual neurologic presentation and may commence at any age. There may be contralateral homonymous hemianopia, hemiparesis and hemisensory disturbance, ipsilateral glaucoma, and mental subnormality. Skull radiographs taken after the first 2 years of life usually reveal gyriform ("tramline") intracranial calcification, especially in the parieto-occipital region, due to mineral deposition in the cortex beneath the intracranial angioma.

Treatment is aimed at controlling seizures pharmacologically (Table 24–2), but surgical treatment may be necessary. Ophthalmologic advice should be sought concerning the management of choroidal angioma and of increased intraocular pressure.

MOVEMENT DISORDERS

1. Essential (Familial) Tremor

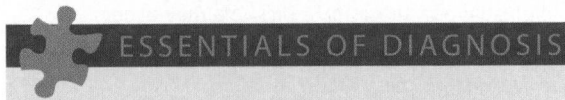

ESSENTIALS OF DIAGNOSIS

► Postural tremor of hands, head, or voice.
► Family history common.
► May improve temporarily with alcohol.
► No abnormal findings other than tremor.

General Considerations

The cause of essential tremor is uncertain, but it is sometimes inherited in an autosomal dominant manner.

Clinical Findings

Tremor may begin at any age and is enhanced by emotional stress. The tremor usually involves one or both hands, the head, or the hands and head, while the legs tend to be spared. The tremor is not present at rest, but emerges with action. Examination reveals no other abnormalities. Ingestion of a small quantity of alcohol commonly provides remarkable but short-lived relief by an unknown mechanism.

Although the tremor may become more conspicuous with time, it generally leads to little disability. Occasionally, it interferes with manual skills and leads to impairment of handwriting. Speech may also be affected if the laryngeal muscles are involved.

Treatment

Treatment is often unnecessary. When it is required because of disability, propranolol (60–240 mg daily orally) may be helpful. Long-term therapy is typical; however, intermittent therapy is sometimes useful in patients whose tremor becomes exacerbated in specific predictable situations. Primidone may be helpful when propranolol is ineffective, but patients with essential tremor are often very sensitive to it. Therefore, the starting dose is 50 mg daily orally, and the daily dose is increased by 50 mg every 2 weeks depending on the patient's response; a maintenance dose of 125 mg three times daily orally is commonly effective. Occasional patients do not respond to these measures but are helped by alprazolam (up to 3 mg daily orally in divided doses), topiramate (titrated up to a dose of 400 mg daily orally in divided doses over about 8 weeks), or gabapentin (1800 mg daily orally in divided doses). Botulinum toxin A may reduce tremor, but adverse effects include dose-dependent weakness of the injected muscles.

Disabling tremor unresponsive to medical treatment may be helped by high-frequency thalamic stimulation ("deep brain stimulation") on one or both sides, according to the laterality of symptoms. Focused transcranial ultrasound thalamotomy using MRI guidance is also effective, as is stereotactic radiosurgery for upper extremity tremor.

When to Refer

- When refractory to first-line treatment with propranolol or primidone.
- When additional neurologic signs are present (ie, parkinsonism).

When to Admit

Patients requiring surgical treatment (deep brain stimulator placement) should be hospitalized.

Elias WJ et al. A randomized trial of focused ultrasound thalamotomy for essential tremor. N Engl J Med. 2016 Aug 25; 375(8):730–9. [PMID: 27557301]

Schneider SA et al. Medical and surgical treatment of tremors. Neurol Clin. 2015 Feb;33(1):57–75. [PMID: 25432723]

2. Parkinson Disease

ESSENTIALS OF DIAGNOSIS

- ▶ Any combination of tremor, rigidity, bradykinesia, and progressive postural instability ("parkinsonism").
- ▶ Cognitive impairment is sometimes prominent.

General Considerations

Parkinsonism is a relatively common disorder that occurs in all ethnic groups, with an approximately equal sex distribution. The most common variety, idiopathic Parkinson disease, begins most often between 45 and 65 years of age and is a progressive disease.

Etiology

Parkinsonism may rarely occur on a familial basis, and the parkinsonian phenotype may result from mutations of several different genes. Postencephalitic parkinsonism is becoming increasingly rare. Exposure to certain toxins (eg, manganese dust, carbon disulfide) and severe carbon monoxide poisoning may lead to parkinsonism. Reversible parkinsonism may develop in patients receiving neuroleptic medications (see Chapter 25), reserpine, or metoclopramide. Only rarely is hemiparkinsonism the presenting feature of a progressive space-occupying lesion.

In idiopathic Parkinson disease, dopamine depletion due to degeneration of the dopaminergic nigrostriatal system leads to an imbalance of dopamine and acetylcholine, which are neurotransmitters normally present in the corpus striatum. Treatment of the motor disturbance is directed at redressing this imbalance by blocking the effect of acetylcholine with anticholinergic medications or by the administration of levodopa, the precursor of dopamine. Prior use of ibuprofen is associated with a *decreased* risk of developing Parkinson disease; age, family history, male sex, ongoing herbicide/pesticide exposure, and significant prior head trauma are risk factors.

Clinical Findings

Tremor, rigidity, bradykinesia, and postural instability are the cardinal motor features of parkinsonism and may be present in any combination. **Nonmotor manifestations** include affective disorders (depression, anxiety, and apathy), psychosis, cognitive changes, fatigue, sleep disorders, anosmia, autonomic disturbances, sensory complaints or pain, and seborrheic dermatitis. Dementia or mild cognitive impairment will eventually develop in many patients.

The tremor of about four to six cycles per second is most conspicuous at rest, is enhanced by emotional stress, and is often less severe during voluntary activity. Although it may ultimately be present in all limbs, the tremor is commonly confined to one limb or to the limbs on one side for months or years before it becomes more generalized. In some patients, tremor is absent.

Rigidity (an increase in resistance to passive movement) is responsible for the characteristically flexed posture seen in many patients, but the most disabling symptoms of parkinsonism are due to bradykinesia, manifested as a slowness of voluntary movement and a reduction in automatic movements such as swinging of the arms while walking. Curiously, however, effective voluntary activity may briefly be regained during an emergency (eg, the patient is able to leap aside to avoid an oncoming motor vehicle).

Clinical diagnosis of the well-developed syndrome is usually simple. The patient has a relatively immobile face with widened palpebral fissures, infrequent blinking, and a fixity of facial expression. Seborrhea of the scalp and face is common. There is often mild blepharoclonus, and a tremor may be present about the mouth and lips. Repetitive tapping (about twice per second) over the bridge of the nose produces a sustained blink response (Myerson sign). Other findings may include saliva drooling from the mouth, perhaps due to impairment of swallowing; soft and poorly modulated voice; a variable rest tremor and rigidity in some or all of the limbs; slowness of voluntary movements; impairment of fine or rapidly alternating movements; and micrographia. There is typically no muscle weakness (provided that sufficient time is allowed for power to be developed) and no alteration in the tendon reflexes or plantar responses. It is difficult for the patient to arise from a sitting position and begin walking. The gait itself is characterized by small shuffling steps and a loss of the normal automatic arm swing; there may be unsteadiness on turning, difficulty in stopping, and a tendency to fall.

▶ Differential Diagnosis

Diagnostic problems may occur in mild cases, especially if tremor is minimal or absent. For example, mild hypokinesia or slight tremor is commonly attributed to old age. **Depression,** with its associated expressionless face, poorly modulated voice, and reduction in voluntary activity, can be difficult to distinguish from mild parkinsonism, especially since the two disorders may coexist. The family history, the character of the tremor, and lack of other neurologic signs should distinguish essential tremor from parkinsonism. **Wilson disease** can be distinguished by its early age at onset, the presence of other abnormal movements, Kayser-Fleischer rings, and chronic hepatitis, and by increased concentrations of copper in the tissues. **Huntington disease** presenting with rigidity and bradykinesia may be mistaken for parkinsonism unless the family history and accompanying dementia are recognized. In **multisystem atrophy** (previously called the **Shy-Drager syndrome**), autonomic insufficiency (leading to postural hypotension, anhidrosis, disturbances of sphincter control, erectile dysfunction, etc) may be accompanied by parkinsonism, pyramidal deficits, lower motor neuron signs, or cerebellar dysfunction. In **progressive supranuclear palsy,**

bradykinesia and rigidity are accompanied by a supranuclear disorder of eye movements, pseudobulbar palsy, pseudo-emotional lability (pseudobulbar affect), and axial dystonia. **Creutzfeldt-Jakob disease** may be accompanied by features of parkinsonism, but progression is rapid, dementia is usual, myoclonic jerking is common, ataxia and pyramidal signs may be conspicuous, and the MRI and electroencephalographic findings are usually characteristic. In **corticobasal degeneration**, asymmetric parkinsonism is accompanied by conspicuous signs of cortical dysfunction (eg, apraxia, sensory inattention, dementia, aphasia). **Diffuse Lewy body disease** is characterized by prominent visual hallucinations and cognitive impairment that begin before or within 1 year of onset of the motor features of parkinsonism.

▶ Treatment

Treatment is symptomatic. There is great interest in developing disease-modifying therapies, but trials of several putative neuroprotective agents have shown no benefit. Trials of various gene therapies have shown limited or no benefit.

A. Medical Measures

Medication is not required early in the course of Parkinson disease, but the nature of the disorder and the availability of medical treatment for use when necessary should be discussed with the patient.

1. Amantadine—Patients with mild symptoms but no disability may be helped by amantadine. This medication improves all of the clinical features of parkinsonism, but its mode of action is unclear. Side effects include restlessness, confusion, depression, skin rashes, edema, nausea, constipation, anorexia, postural hypotension, and disturbances of cardiac rhythm. However, these are relatively uncommon with the usual dose. It also ameliorates dyskinesias resulting from chronic levodopa therapy. Amantadine is available in immediate-release (100 mg orally two or three times daily) and extended-release once-daily formulations.

2. Levodopa—Levodopa, which is converted in the body to dopamine, improves all of the major features of parkinsonism, including bradykinesia, but does *not* stop progression of the disorder. The most common early side effects of levodopa are nausea, vomiting, and hypotension, but cardiac arrhythmias may also occur. Dyskinesias, restlessness, confusion, and other behavioral changes tend to occur somewhat later and become more common with time. **Levodopa-induced dyskinesias** may take any conceivable form, including chorea, athetosis, dystonia, tremor, tics, and myoclonus. An even later complication is the **wearing off effect** or the **on-off phenomenon,** in which abrupt but transient fluctuations in the severity of parkinsonism occur unpredictably but frequently during the day. The "off" period of marked bradykinesia has been shown to relate in some instances to falling plasma levels of levodopa. During the "on" phase, dyskinesias are often conspicuous but mobility is increased. However, such response fluctuations may relate to advancing disease rather than to levodopa therapy itself.

Carbidopa, which inhibits the enzyme responsible for the breakdown of levodopa to dopamine, does not cross the blood-brain barrier. When levodopa is given in combination with carbidopa, the extracerebral breakdown of levodopa is diminished. This reduces the amount of levodopa required daily for beneficial effects, and it lowers the incidence of nausea, vomiting, hypotension, and cardiac irregularities. Such a combination does not prevent the development of response fluctuations and the incidence of other side effects (dyskinesias or psychiatric complications) may actually be increased.

Sinemet, a commercially available preparation that contains carbidopa and levodopa in a fixed ratio (1:10 or 1:4), is generally used. Treatment is started with a small dose—eg, one tablet of Sinemet 25/100 (containing 25 mg of carbidopa and 100 mg of levodopa) three times daily—and gradually increased depending on the response. Sinemet CR is a controlled-release formulation (containing 25 or 50 mg of carbidopa and 100 or 200 mg of levodopa). It is mainly useful when taken at bedtime to lessen motor disability upon awakening. A formulation of carbidopa/levodopa (Rytary) containing both immediate- and delayed-release beads provides a smoother response in patients with fluctuations. The commercially available combination of levodopa with both carbidopa and entacapone (Stalevo) may also be helpful in this context and is discussed in the following section on COMT inhibitors. Response fluctuations are also reduced by keeping the daily intake of *protein* at the recommended minimum and taking the main protein meal as the last meal of the day. A continuous infusion of a carbidopa-levodopa enteral suspension through a percutaneous gastrojejunostomy tube by a portable infusion pump reduces "off" time in patients with advanced Parkinson disease.

The dyskinesias and behavioral side effects of levodopa are dose-related, but reduction in dose may eliminate any therapeutic benefit. Levodopa-induced dyskinesias may also respond to amantadine.

Levodopa therapy is contraindicated in patients with psychotic illness or narrow-angle glaucoma. It should not be given to patients taking monoamine oxidase A inhibitors or within 2 weeks of their withdrawal, because hypertensive crises may result. Sudden discontinuation of levodopa can precipitate neuroleptic malignant syndrome and should be avoided.

3. Dopamine agonists—Dopamine agonists, such as pramipexole and ropinirole, act directly on dopamine receptors, and their use in parkinsonism is associated with a lower incidence of the response fluctuations and dyskinesias that occur with long-term levodopa therapy. They are effective in both early and advanced stages of Parkinson disease. They are often given either before the introduction of levodopa or with a low dose of Sinemet 25/100 (carbidopa 25 mg and levodopa 100 mg, one tablet three times daily) when dopaminergic therapy is first introduced; the dose of Sinemet is kept constant, while the dose of the agonist is gradually increased.

Pramipexole is started at a dosage of 0.125 mg three times daily orally, and the dose is built up gradually to between 0.5 and 1.5 mg three times daily. Ropinirole is begun at 0.25 mg three times daily orally and gradually increased; most patients require between 2 and 8 mg three times daily for benefit. Extended-release, once-daily formulations of pramipexole and ropinirole have similar efficacy and tolerability as the immediate release versions. Rotigotine is a dopamine agonist absorbed transdermally from a skin patch; it is started at 2 mg once daily and increased weekly by 2 mg daily until achieving an optimal response, up to a maximum of 8 mg daily. Adverse effects of these various agonists include fatigue, somnolence, nausea, peripheral edema, dyskinesias, confusion, and postural hypotension. Less commonly, an irresistible urge to sleep may occur, sometimes in inappropriate and hazardous circumstances. Impulse control disorders involving gambling, shopping, or sexual activity also occur. Local skin reactions may occur with the rotigotine patch. The **dopamine agonist withdrawal syndrome** develops occasionally in patients in whom a dopamine agonist is tapered. It consists of a combination of distressing physical and psychological symptoms that are refractory to levodopa and other dopaminergic medications and may persist for months or longer. There is no effective treatment. The dopamine agonist should be reintroduced and tapered more gradually if possible.

4. Selective monoamine oxidase inhibitors—Rasagiline, a selective monoamine oxidase B inhibitor, has a clear symptomatic benefit in some patients at a daily oral dose of 1 mg, taken in the morning; it may also be used for adjunctive therapy in patients with response fluctuations to levodopa. Selegiline (5 mg orally with breakfast and lunch) or safinamide (50 mg orally daily, increased to 100 mg daily after 14 days) are also approved as adjunctive treatments. By inhibiting the metabolic breakdown of dopamine, these medications may improve fluctuations or declining response to levodopa.

Studies have suggested (but failed to show conclusively) that rasagiline may slow the progression of Parkinson disease, and it appears to delay the need for other symptomatic therapies. For these reasons, rasagiline is often started early, particularly for patients who are young or have mild disease. However, the FDA has rejected an expansion of rasagiline's indication to include disease modification.

5. COMT inhibitors—Catecholamine-*O*-methyltransferase (COMT) inhibitors reduce the metabolism of levodopa to 3-*O*-methyldopa and thereby alter the plasma pharmacokinetics of levodopa, leading to more sustained plasma levels and more constant dopaminergic stimulation of the brain. Treatment with entacapone or tolcapone results in reduced response fluctuations, with a greater period of responsiveness to administered levodopa. **Tolcapone** is given in a dosage of 100 mg or 200 mg three times daily orally, and **entacapone** is given as 200 mg with each dose of Sinemet. **Opicapone,** a long-acting, peripherally selective COMT inhibitor, taken once daily (50 mg) at bedtime, is available in Europe but not yet in the United States. The dose of Sinemet taken concurrently may have to be reduced by up to one-third to avoid side effects. Diarrhea is sometimes troublesome. Because rare cases of fulminant hepatic failure have followed its use, tolcapone should be avoided in patients with preexisting liver disease. Serial liver biochemical tests should be performed at 2-week intervals for the first year and at longer intervals thereafter in patients receiving the medication—as recommended by the manufacturer. Serious hepatotoxicity has not been reported with entacapone or opicapone.

Stalevo is the commercial preparation of levodopa combined with both carbidopa and entacapone. It is best used in patients already stabilized on equivalent doses of carbidopa/levodopa and entacapone. It is priced at or below the price of the individual ingredients (ie, carbidopa/levodopa and entacapone) and has the added convenience of requiring fewer tablets to be taken daily. It is available in three strengths: Stalevo 50 (12.5 mg of carbidopa, 50 mg of levodopa, and 200 mg of entacapone), Stalevo 100 (25 mg of carbidopa, 100 mg of levodopa, and 200 mg of entacapone), and Stalevo 150 (37.5 mg of carbidopa, 150 mg of levodopa, and 200 mg of entacapone).

6. Anticholinergic medications—Anticholinergics are more helpful in alleviating tremor and rigidity than bradykinesia. Treatment is started with a small dose and gradually increased until benefit occurs or side effects limit further increments. If treatment is ineffective, the medication is gradually withdrawn and another preparation then tried. However, these medications are often poorly tolerated, especially in older adults.

7. Antipsychotics—Confusion and psychotic symptoms may occur as a side effect of dopaminergic therapy or as a part of the underlying illness. They often respond to the atypical antipsychotic agents clozapine and quetiapine, which have few extrapyramidal side effects and do not block the effects of dopaminergic medication. Clozapine may rarely cause marrow suppression, and weekly blood counts are therefore necessary for patients taking it. The patient is started on 6.25 mg at bedtime and the dosage increased to 25–100 mg/day as needed. In low doses, it may also improve iatrogenic dyskinesias. Typical antipsychotic agents and the second-generation antipsychotic agents risperidone and olanzapine may cause *worsening* of motor symptoms and should be avoided. Pimavanserin (34 mg once daily), a serotonin(2A) agonist, is also effective in treating the psychosis of Parkinson disease.

B. General Measures

Physical therapy or speech therapy helps many patients. Cognitive impairment and psychiatric symptoms may be helped by a cholinesterase inhibitor, such as rivastigmine (3–12 mg orally daily or 4.6 or 9.5 mg/24 hours transdermally daily). The quality of life can often be improved by the provision of simple aids to daily living, eg, rails or banisters placed strategically about the home, special table cutlery with large handles, nonslip rubber table mats, and devices to amplify the voice.

C. Stimulation and Ablative Treatments

High-frequency stimulation of the subthalamic nuclei or globus pallidus internus may benefit many of the motor features of the disease but does not affect its natural history. Electrical stimulation of the brain has the advantage over ablative thalamotomy and pallidotomy procedures of being reversible and of causing minimal or no damage to the brain, and is therefore the preferred surgical approach to treatment. It is reserved for patients without cognitive impairment or psychiatric disorder who have a good response to levodopa, but in whom dyskinesias or response fluctuations are problematic. It frequently takes 3–6 months after surgery to adjust stimulator programming and to achieve optimal results. Side effects include depression, apathy, impulsivity, executive dysfunction, and decreased verbal fluency in a subset of patients. Focused ultrasound thalamotomy may help patients with medically refractory tremor-predominant parkinsonism who are reluctant to undergo surgery.

D. Gene Therapy

Injections of adeno-associated viruses encoding various human genes have been made into the subthalamic nucleus or putamen in various clinical trials. These approaches may be useful in the future but remain experimental.

▶ When to Refer

All patients should be referred.

▶ When to Admit

Patients requiring surgical treatment should be admitted.

National Institute for Health and Care Excellence (2017) Parkinson's disease in adults. NICE Guideline (NG71). 2017 July. https://www.nice.org.uk/guidance/ng71

Rughani A et al. Congress of Neurological Surgeons systematic review and evidence-based guideline on subthalamic nucleus and globus pallidus internus deep brain stimulation for the treatment of patients with Parkinson's disease: executive summary. Neurosurgery. 2018 Jun 1;82(6):753–6. [PMID: 29538685]

3. Huntington Disease

ESSENTIALS OF DIAGNOSIS

▶ Gradual onset and progression of chorea and dementia or behavioral change.

▶ Family history of the disorder.

▶ Responsible gene identified on chromosome 4.

▶ General Considerations

Huntington disease is characterized by chorea and dementia. It is inherited in an autosomal dominant manner and occurs throughout the world, in all ethnic groups, with a prevalence rate of about 5 per 100,000. There is an expanded and unstable CAG trinucleotide repeat in the huntingtin gene at 4p16.3; longer repeat lengths correspond to an earlier age of onset and faster disease progression.

Clinical Findings

A. Symptoms and Signs

Clinical onset is usually between 30 and 50 years of age. The disease is progressive and usually leads to a fatal outcome within 15–20 years. The initial symptoms may consist of either abnormal movements or intellectual changes, but ultimately both occur. The earliest mental changes are often behavioral, with irritability, moodiness, antisocial behavior, or a psychiatric disturbance, but a more obvious dementia subsequently develops. The dyskinesia may initially be no more than an apparent fidgetiness or restlessness, but eventually choreiform movements and some dystonic posturing occur. A parkinsonian syndrome with progressive rigidity and akinesia (rather than chorea) sometimes occurs in association with dementia, especially in cases with childhood onset. The diagnosis is established with a widely available genetic test, although such testing should be pursued under the guidance of a licensed genetic counselor.

B. Imaging

CT scanning or MRI usually demonstrates cerebral atrophy and atrophy of the caudate nucleus in established cases. Positron emission tomography (PET) has shown reduced striatal metabolic rate.

Differential Diagnosis

Chorea developing with no family history of choreoathetosis should not be attributed to Huntington disease, at least not until other causes of chorea have been excluded clinically and by appropriate laboratory studies. Nongenetic causes of chorea include stroke, systemic lupus erythematosus and antiphospholipid antibody syndrome, paraneoplastic syndromes, infection with HIV, and various medications. In younger patients, self-limiting Sydenham chorea develops after group A streptococcal infections on rare occasions. If a patient presents solely with progressive intellectual failure, it may not be possible to distinguish Huntington disease from other causes of dementia unless there is a characteristic family history or a dyskinesia develops.

Huntington disease–like (HDL) disorders resemble Huntington disease but are caused by other genetic mutations. A clinically similar autosomal dominant disorder **(dentatorubral-pallidoluysian atrophy),** manifested by chorea, dementia, ataxia, and myoclonic epilepsy, is uncommon except in persons of Japanese ancestry. Treatment is as for Huntington disease.

Treatment

There is no cure for Huntington disease; progression cannot be halted; and treatment is purely symptomatic. The reported biochemical changes suggest a relative underactivity of neurons containing GABA and acetylcholine or a relative overactivity of dopaminergic neurons. Tetrabenazine, a medication that interferes with the vesicular storage of biogenic amines, is widely used to treat the dyskinesia. The starting dose is 12.5 mg twice or three times daily orally, increasing by 12.5 mg every 5 days depending on response

and tolerance; the usual maintenance dose is 25 mg three times daily. Side effects include depression, postural hypotension, drowsiness, and parkinsonian features; tetrabenazine should not be given within 14 days of taking monoamine oxidase inhibitors and is not indicated for the treatment of levodopa-induced dyskinesias. Reserpine is similar in depleting central monoamines but has more peripheral effects and a worse side-effect profile, making its use problematic in Huntington disease; if utilized, the dose is built up gradually to between 2 mg and 5 mg orally daily, depending on the response. Deutetrabenazine is also effective in reducing chorea in Huntington disease and may have fewer side effects than tetrabenazine but direct comparisons are lacking. The starting dose is 6 mg once daily orally, increased to 6 mg twice daily after 1 week and by 6-mg increments weekly thereafter, to a maximum of 24 mg twice daily. Treatment with medications blocking dopamine receptors, such as phenothiazines or haloperidol, may control the dyskinesia and any behavioral disturbances. Haloperidol treatment is usually begun with a dose of 1 mg once or twice daily orally, which is then increased every 3 or 4 days depending on the response; alternatively, atypical antipsychotic agents such as quetiapine (increasing from 25 mg daily orally up to 100 mg twice daily orally as tolerated) may be tried. Amantadine in a dose of 200 mg to 400 mg daily orally is sometimes helpful for chorea. Deep brain stimulation has been used successfully to treat chorea in a small number of patients. Behavioral disturbances may respond to clozapine. Attempts to compensate for the relative GABA deficiency by enhancing central GABA activity or to compensate for the relative cholinergic underactivity by giving choline chloride have not been therapeutically helpful.

Offspring should be offered *genetic counseling.* Genetic testing permits presymptomatic detection and definitive diagnosis of the disease.

When to Refer

All patients should be referred.

Huntington Study Group. Effect of deutetrabenazine on chorea among patients with Huntington disease: a randomized clinical trial. JAMA. 2016 Jul 5;316(1):40–50. [PMID: 27380342]

4. Idiopathic Torsion Dystonia

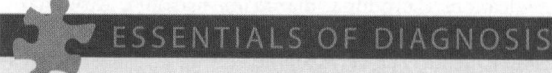

ESSENTIALS OF DIAGNOSIS

▶ Dystonic movements and postures.
▶ Normal birth and developmental history. No other neurologic signs.
▶ Investigations (including CT scan or MRI) reveal no cause of dystonia.

General Considerations

Idiopathic torsion dystonia may occur sporadically or on a hereditary basis, with autosomal dominant, autosomal recessive, and X-linked recessive modes of transmission. Symptoms may begin in childhood or later and persist throughout life.

Clinical Findings

The disorder is characterized by the onset of abnormal movements and postures in a patient with a normal birth and developmental history, no relevant past medical illness, and no other neurologic signs. Investigations (including CT scan) reveal no cause for the abnormal movements. Dystonic movements of the head and neck may take the form of torticollis, blepharospasm, facial grimacing, or forced opening or closing of the mouth. The limbs may also adopt abnormal but characteristic postures. The age at onset influences both the clinical findings and the prognosis. With onset in childhood, there is usually a family history of the disorder, symptoms commonly commence in the legs, and progression is likely until there is severe disability from generalized dystonia. In contrast, when onset is later, a positive family history is unlikely, initial symptoms are often in the arms or axial structures, and severe disability does not usually occur, although generalized dystonia may ultimately develop in some patients. If all cases are considered together, about one-third of patients eventually become so severely disabled that they are confined to chair or bed, while another one-third are affected only mildly.

Differential Diagnosis

Perinatal anoxia, birth trauma, and kernicterus are common causes of dystonia, but abnormal movements usually then develop before the age of 5, the early development of the patient is usually abnormal, and a history of seizures is not unusual. Moreover, examination may reveal signs of mental retardation or pyramidal deficit in addition to the movement disorder. Dystonic posturing may also occur in Wilson disease, Huntington disease, or parkinsonism; as a sequela of encephalitis lethargica or previous neuroleptic medication therapy; and in certain other disorders. In these cases, diagnosis is based on the history and accompanying clinical manifestations.

Treatment

Idiopathic torsion dystonia usually responds poorly to medications. Levodopa, diazepam, baclofen, carbamazepine, amantadine, or anticholinergic medication such as trihexyphenidyl or benztropine (in high dosage) is occasionally helpful; if not, a trial of treatment with tetrabenazine, phenothiazines, or haloperidol may be worthwhile. In each case, the dose has to be individualized, depending on response and tolerance. However, the doses of these latter medications that are required for benefit lead usually to mild parkinsonism. Pallidal deep brain stimulation is helpful for medically refractory dystonia and has a lower morbidity than stereotactic thalamotomy, which is sometimes helpful in patients with predominantly unilateral limb dystonia. Potential adverse events of deep brain stimulation include cerebral infection or hemorrhage, broken leads, affective changes, and dysarthria.

A distinct variety of dominantly inherited dystonia, caused by a mutation in the gene for GTP cyclohydrolase I on chromosome 14q, is remarkably responsive to levodopa; therefore, a levodopa trial is warranted in all patients.

When to Refer

All patients should be referred.

When to Admit

Patients requiring surgical treatment should be admitted.

Fox MD et al. Brain stimulation for torsion dystonia. JAMA Neurol. 2015 Jun;72(6):713–9. [PMID: 25894231]

5. Focal Torsion Dystonia

A number of the dystonic manifestations that occur in idiopathic torsion dystonia may also occur as isolated phenomena. They are best regarded as focal dystonias that either occur as formes frustes of idiopathic torsion dystonia in patients with a positive family history or represent a focal manifestation of the adult-onset form of that disorder when there is no family history. Medical treatment is generally unsatisfactory. A trial of the medications used in idiopathic torsion dystonia is worthwhile, however, since a few patients do show some response. In addition, with restricted dystonias such as blepharospasm or torticollis, local injection of botulinum A toxin into the overactive muscles may produce worthwhile benefit for several weeks or months and can be repeated as needed.

Both blepharospasm and oromandibular dystonia may occur as an isolated focal dystonia. The former is characterized by spontaneous involuntary forced closure of the eyelids for a variable interval. Oromandibular dystonia is manifested by involuntary contraction of the muscles about the mouth causing, for example, involuntary opening or closing of the mouth, roving or protruding tongue movements, and retraction of the platysma. Cervical dystonia (spasmodic torticollis), usually with onset between 25 and 50 years of age, is characterized by a tendency for the neck to twist to one side. This initially occurs episodically, but eventually the neck is held to the side. Some patients have a sensory trick ("geste antagoniste") that lessens the dystonic posture, eg, touching the side of the face. Spontaneous resolution may occur in the first year or so. The disorder is otherwise usually lifelong. Local injection of botulinum A toxin provides benefit in most cases. Deep brain stimulation of the globus pallidus interna is an option if medical treatment and botulinum toxin injection are unsuccessful.

Writer's cramp is characterized by dystonic posturing of the hand and forearm when the hand is used for writing and sometimes when it is used for other tasks, eg, playing the piano or using a screwdriver or eating utensils. Medication treatment is usually unrewarding, and patients are often best advised to learn to use the other hand for activities requiring manual dexterity. Injections of botulinum A toxin are helpful in some instances.

Fox MD et al. Brain stimulation for torsion dystonia. JAMA Neurol. 2015 Jun;72(6):713–9. [PMID: 25894231]

6. Myoclonus

Occasional myoclonic jerks may occur in anyone, especially when drifting into sleep. **General or multifocal myoclonus** is common in patients with idiopathic epilepsy and is especially prominent in certain hereditary disorders characterized by seizures and progressive intellectual decline, such as the lipid storage diseases. It is also a feature of subacute sclerosing panencephalitis and Creutzfeldt-Jakob disease. Generalized myoclonic jerking may accompany uremic and other metabolic encephalopathies, result from therapy with levodopa or tricyclic antidepressants, occur in alcohol or drug withdrawal states, or follow anoxic brain damage. It also occurs on a hereditary or sporadic basis as an isolated phenomenon in otherwise healthy subjects.

Segmental myoclonus is a rare manifestation of a focal spinal cord lesion. It may also be the clinical expression of **epilepsia partialis continua**, a disorder in which a repetitive focal epileptic discharge arises in the contralateral sensorimotor cortex, sometimes from an underlying structural lesion. An electroencephalogram is often helpful in clarifying the epileptic nature of the disorder, and CT or MRI scan may reveal the causal lesion.

Myoclonus may respond to certain anticonvulsant medications, especially valproic acid or levetiracetam, or to one of the benzodiazepines, particularly clonazepam (see Table 24–2). It may also respond to piracetam (up to 16.8 g daily; not available in the United States). Myoclonus following anoxic brain damage is often responsive to oxitriptan (5-hydroxytryptophan), the precursor of serotonin, and sometimes to clonazepam. Oxitriptan is given in gradually increasing doses up to 1–1.5 mg daily. In patients with segmental myoclonus, a localized lesion should be searched for and treated appropriately.

7. Wilson Disease

In this metabolic disorder, abnormal movement and posture may occur with or without coexisting signs of liver involvement. Psychiatric and neuropsychological manifestations are common. Wilson disease is discussed in Chapter 16.

8. Drug-Induced Abnormal Movements

Phenothiazines, butyrophenones, and metoclopramide may produce a wide variety of abnormal movements, including parkinsonism, akathisia (ie, motor restlessness), acute dystonia, chorea, and tardive dyskinesias or dystonia; several of these are also produced by aripiprazole. These complications are discussed in Chapter 25. Chorea may also develop in patients receiving levodopa, bromocriptine, anticholinergic medications, phenytoin, carbamazepine, lithium, amphetamines, or oral contraceptives, and it resolves with withdrawal of the offending substance. Similarly, dystonia may be produced by levodopa, bromocriptine, lithium, or carbamazepine; and parkinsonism by reserpine and tetrabenazine. Postural tremor may occur with a variety of medications, including epinephrine, isoproterenol, amiodarone, theophylline, caffeine, lithium, thyroid hormone, tricyclic antidepressants, and valproic acid.

9. Restless Legs Syndrome

This common disorder, affecting 1–5% of people, may occur as a primary (idiopathic) disorder or in relation to Parkinson disease, pregnancy, iron deficiency anemia, or peripheral neuropathy (especially uremic or diabetic). It may have a hereditary basis, and several genetic loci have been associated with the disorder. Restlessness and curious sensory disturbances lead to an irresistible urge to move the limbs, especially during periods of relaxation; movement of the limbs provides relief. The urge occurs exclusively in the evening and at night or is worse at night than during the day. Most patients also have periodic limb movements of sleep and one-third have periodic limb movements during relaxed wakefulness; both consist of brief involuntary flexion at the ankle, knee, and hip. Disturbed nocturnal sleep and excessive daytime somnolence may result. *Ferritin levels should always be measured;* treatment with oral iron sulfate in patients with levels less than or equal to 75 mcg/L (13.4 mcmol/L) should be attempted prior to initiation of other pharmacotherapies. Therapy is with nonergot dopamine agonists, such as pramipexole (0.125–0.5 mg orally once daily), ropinirole (0.25–4 mg orally once daily 2 to 3 hours before bedtime), or rotigotine (1–3 mg/24 h transdermal patch once daily) or with gabapentin enacarbil (300–1200 mg orally each evening). Gabapentin (starting with 300 mg orally daily, increasing to approximately 1800 mg daily depending on response and tolerance) and pregabalin (150–300 mg orally divided twice to three times daily) are related medications that improve symptoms. Levodopa is helpful but may lead to an augmentation of symptoms, so that its use is generally reserved for those who do not respond to other measures. Extended-release oxycodone-naloxone (2.5–5 mg to 5–10 mg orally twice daily) is useful in patients with severe symptoms or those who are refractory to first-line therapies.

Winkelman JW et al. Practice guideline summary: treatment of restless legs syndrome in adults: report of the Guideline Development, Dissemination, and Implementation Subcommittee of the American Academy of Neurology. Neurology. 2016 Dec 13;87(24):2585–93. [PMID: 27856776]

10. Gilles de la Tourette Syndrome

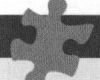 ESSENTIALS OF DIAGNOSIS

► Multiple motor and phonic tics.

► Symptoms begin before age 18 years.

► Tics occur frequently for at least 1 year.

► Tics vary in number, frequency, and nature over time.

Clinical Findings

Simple tics occur transiently in up to 25% of children, remit within weeks to months, and do not require treatment. Tourette syndrome is a more complex disorder. Motor tics are the initial manifestation in 80% of cases and most commonly involve the face, whereas in the remaining 20%, the initial symptoms are phonic tics; ultimately a combination of different motor and phonic tics develop in all patients. Tics are preceded by an urge that is relieved upon performance of the movement or vocalization; they can be temporarily suppressed but eventually the urge becomes overwhelming. These are noted first in childhood, generally between the ages of 2 and 15. Motor tics occur especially about the face, head, and shoulders (eg, sniffing, blinking, frowning, shoulder shrugging, head thrusting, etc). Phonic tics commonly consist of grunts, barks, hisses, throat-clearing, coughs, etc, but sometimes also of verbal utterances including coprolalia (obscene speech). There may also be echolalia (repetition of the speech of others), echopraxia (imitation of others' movements), and palilalia (repetition of words or phrases). Some tics may be self-mutilating in nature, such as nail-biting, hair-pulling, or biting of the lips or tongue. The disorder is chronic, but the course may be punctuated by relapses and remissions. *Obsessive-compulsive disorder (OCD) and attention deficit hyperactivity disorder (ADHD) are commonly associated* and may be more disabling than the tics themselves. A family history is sometimes obtained.

Examination usually reveals no abnormalities other than the tics. In addition to OCD, psychiatric disturbances may occur because of the associated cosmetic and social embarrassment. The diagnosis of the disorder is often delayed for years, the tics being interpreted as psychiatric illness or some other form of abnormal movement. Patients are thus often subjected to unnecessary treatment before the disorder is recognized. The tic-like character of the abnormal movements and the absence of other neurologic signs should differentiate this disorder from other movement disorders presenting in childhood. Wilson disease, however, can simulate the condition and should be excluded.

Treatment

Treatment is symptomatic and may need to be continued indefinitely. Habit reversal training or other forms of behavioral therapy can be effective alone or in combination with pharmacotherapy. Alpha-adrenergic agonists, such as clonidine (start 0.05 mg orally at bedtime, titrating to 0.3–0.4 mg orally daily, divided three to four times per day) or guanfacine (start 0.5 mg orally at bedtime, titrating to a maximum of 3–4 mg orally daily, divided twice daily) are first-line therapies because of a favorable side-effect profile compared with typical antipsychotics, which are the only FDA-approved therapies for the disorder. They also have the advantage of improving the symptoms of concomitant ADHD. Many specialists favor the use of tetrabenazine. The atypical antipsychotic risperidone (1–6 mg daily orally) is more effective than placebo in controlling tics and more effective than pimozide in improving symptoms of comorbid OCD and may be tried before the typical antipsychotic agents. When a typical antipsychotic is required in cases of

severe tics, haloperidol is generally regarded as the medication of choice. It is started in a low dose (0.25 mg daily orally) that is gradually increased (by 0.25 mg every 4 or 5 days) until there is maximum benefit with a minimum of side effects or until side effects limit further increments. A total daily oral dose of between 2 mg and 8 mg is usually optimal, but higher doses are sometimes necessary. Fluphenazine (1–15 mg orally daily) and pimozide (1–10 mg orally daily) are alternatives. Typical antipsychotics can cause significant weight gain and carry a risk of tardive dyskinesias and other long-term, potentially irreversible motor side effects. Small randomized trials or observational studies have reported benefit from topiramate, nicotine, tetrahydrocannabinol, baclofen, and clonazepam. A number of other medications, including deutetrabenazine, valbenazine, and ecopipam, are being studied for the treatment of tics.

Injection of botulinum toxin type A at the site of the most distressing tics is sometimes worthwhile and has fewer side effects than systemic antipsychotic therapy. Bilateral high-frequency deep brain stimulation at various sites has been helpful in some, otherwise intractable, cases.

When to Refer

All patients should be referred.

When to Admit

Patients undergoing surgical (deep brain stimulation) treatment should be admitted.

Martinez-Ramirez D et al. Efficacy and safety of deep brain stimulation in Tourette syndrome: the International Tourette Syndrome Deep Brain Stimulation Public Database and Registry. JAMA Neurol. 2018 Mar 1;75(3):353–9. [PMID: 29340590]
Serajee FJ et al. Advances in Tourette syndrome: diagnoses and treatment. Pediatr Clin North Am. 2015 Jun;62(3):687–701. [PMID: 26022170]

DEMENTIA

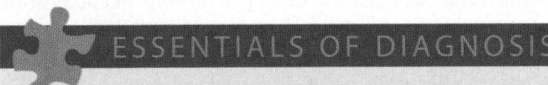

ESSENTIALS OF DIAGNOSIS

▶ Progressive intellectual decline.

▶ Not due to delirium or psychiatric disease.

▶ Age is the main risk factor, followed by family history and vascular disease risk factors.

General Considerations

Dementia is a progressive decline in intellectual function that is *severe enough to compromise social or occupational functioning*. **Mild cognitive impairment** describes a decline that has not resulted in a change in the level of function. Although a few patients identify a precipitating event, most experience an insidious onset and gradual progression of symptoms.

Dementia typically begins after age 60, and the prevalence doubles approximately every 5 years thereafter; in persons aged 85 and older, around half have dementia. The prevalence of Alzheimer dementia is predicted to be 15 million by 2060 in the United States. In most cases, the cause of dementia is acquired, either as a sporadic primary neurodegenerative disease or as the result of another disorder, such as stroke (Table 24–5). Other risk factors for dementia include family history, diabetes mellitus, cigarette smoking, hypertension, obesity, a history of significant head injury, and hearing loss. Vitamin D deficiency and chronic sleep deprivation may also increase the risk of dementia. Dementia is more prevalent among women, but this may be accounted for by their longer life expectancy. Physical activity seems to be protective; education, ongoing intellectual stimulation, and social engagement may also be protective, perhaps by promoting **cognitive reserve**, an improved capacity to compensate for insidious neurodegeneration.

Dementia is distinct from delirium and psychiatric disease. **Delirium** is an acute confusional state that often occurs in response to an identifiable trigger, such as drug or alcohol intoxication or withdrawal (eg, Wernicke encephalopathy, described below), medication side effects (especially medications with anticholinergic properties, antihistamines, benzodiazepines, sleeping aids, opioids, neuroleptics, corticosteroids, and other sedative or psychotropic agents), infection (consider occult urinary tract infection or pneumonia in elderly patients), metabolic disturbance (including an electrolyte abnormality; hypoglycemia or hyperglycemia; or a nutritional, endocrine, renal, or hepatic disorder), sleep deprivation, or other neurologic disease (seizure, including a postictal state, or stroke). Delirium typically involves *fluctuating* levels of arousal, including drowsiness or agitation, and it improves after removal or treatment of the precipitating factor. Patients with dementia are especially susceptible to episodes of delirium, but recognition of dementia is not possible until delirium lifts. For this reason, dementia is typically diagnosed in outpatients who are otherwise medically stable, rather than in acutely ill patients in the hospital.

Table 24–5. Common causes of age-related dementia.

Disorder	Pathology	Clinical Features
Alzheimer disease	Plaques containing beta-amyloid peptide, and neurofibrillary tangles containing tau protein, occur throughout the neocortex.	• Most common age-related neurodegenerative disease; incidence doubles every 5 years after age 60. • Short-term memory impairment is early and prominent in most cases. • Variable deficits of executive function, visuospatial function, and language.
Vascular dementia	Multifocal ischemic change.	• Stepwise or progressive accumulation of cognitive deficits in association with repeated strokes. • Symptoms depend on localization of strokes.
Dementia with Lewy bodies	Histologically indistinguishable from Parkinson disease: alpha-synuclein-containing Lewy bodies occur in the brainstem, midbrain, olfactory bulb, and neocortex. Alzheimer pathology may coexist.	• Cognitive dysfunction, with prominent visuospatial and executive deficits. • Psychiatric disturbance, with anxiety, visual hallucinations, and fluctuating delirium. • Parkinsonian motor deficits with or after other features. • Cholinesterase inhibitors lessen delirium; poor tolerance of neuroleptics and dopaminergics.
Frontotemporal dementia (FTD)	Neuropathology is variable and defined by the protein found in intraneuronal aggregates. Tau protein, TAR DNA-binding protein 43 (TDP-43), or fused-in-sarcoma (FUS) protein account for most cases.	• Peak incidence in the sixth decade; approximately equal to Alzheimer disease as a cause of dementia in patients under 60 years old. • Familial cases result from mutations in genes for tau, progranulin, or others. **Behavioral variant FTD** • Deficits in empathy, social comportment, insight, abstract thought, and executive function. • Behavior is disinhibited, impulsive, and ritualistic, with prominent apathy and increased interest in sex or sweet/fatty foods. • Relative preservation of memory. • Focal right frontal atrophy. • Association with amyotrophic lateral sclerosis. **Semantic variant primary progressive aphasia** • Deficits in word-finding, single-word comprehension, object and category knowledge, and face recognition. • Behaviors may be similar to behavioral variant FTD. • Focal, asymmetric temporal pole atrophy. **Nonfluent/agrammatic variant primary progressive aphasia** • Speech is effortful with dysarthria, phonemic errors, sound distortions, and poor grammar. • Focal extrapyramidal signs and apraxia of the right arm and leg are common; overlaps with corticobasal degeneration. • Focal left frontal atrophy.

Psychiatric disease sometimes leads to complaints of impaired cognition (**pseudodementia**). Impaired attention is usually to blame, and in some patients with depression or anxiety, poor focus and concentration may even be a primary complaint. The symptoms should improve with appropriate psychiatric treatment. Mood disorders are commonly seen in patients with neurodegenerative disease and in some cases are an early symptom. There is some evidence that a persistent, untreated mood disorder may predispose to the development of an age-related dementia, and psychiatric symptoms can clearly exacerbate cognitive impairment in patients who already have dementia; therefore, *suspicion of dementia should not distract from appropriate screening for and treatment of depression or anxiety.*

▶ Clinical Findings

A. Symptoms and Signs

Symptoms and signs of the common causes of dementia are detailed in Table 24–5. Clinicians should be aware that a patient's insight into a cognitive change may be vague or absent, and collateral history is essential to a proper evaluation. As patients age, primary care clinicians should inquire periodically about the presence of any cognitive symptoms.

Symptoms depend on the area of the brain affected. **Short-term memory loss**, involving the repeating of questions or stories and a diminished ability to recall the details of recent conversations or events, frequently results from pathologic changes in the hippocampus. **Word-finding difficulty** often involves difficulty recalling the names of people, places, or objects, with low-frequency words affected first, eventually resulting in speech laden with pronouns and circumlocutions. This problem is thought to arise from pathology at the temporoparietal junction of the left hemisphere. Problems with articulation, fluency, comprehension, or word meaning are anatomically distinct and less common. **Visuospatial dysfunction** may result in poor navigation and getting lost in familiar places, impaired recognition of previously familiar faces and buildings, or trouble discerning an object against a background. The right parietal lobe is one of the brain areas implicated in such symptoms. **Executive dysfunction** may manifest by easy distractibility, impulsivity, mental inflexibility, concrete thought, slowed processing speed, poor planning and organization, or impaired judgment. Localization may vary and could include the frontal lobes or subcortical areas like the basal ganglia or cerebral white matter. **Apathy** or indifference, separate from depression, is common and may have a similar anatomy as executive dysfunction. **Apraxia**, or the loss of learned motor behaviors, may result from dysfunction of the frontal or parietal lobes, especially the left parietal lobe.

The time of symptom onset must be established, but subtle, early symptoms are often apparent only in retrospect. Another event, such as an illness or hospitalization, may lead to new recognition of existing symptoms. Symptoms often accumulate over time, and the nature of the earliest symptom is most helpful in forming the differential diagnosis. The history should establish risk factors for dementia, including family history, other chronic illnesses, and vascular disease risk factors. Finally, it is important to document the patient's current capacity to perform basic and instrumental activities of daily living (see Chapter 4) and to note the extent of decline from the premorbid level of function. Indeed, *it is this functional assessment that defines the presence and severity of dementia.*

The physical examination is important to identify any occult medical illness. In addition, eye movement abnormalities, parkinsonism, or other motor abnormalities may help identify an underlying neurologic condition. The workup should prioritize the exclusion of conditions that are reversible or require separate therapy. Screening for depression is necessary, along with imaging and laboratory workup, as indicated below.

B. Neuropsychological Assessment

Brief quantification of cognitive impairment is indicated in a patient complaining of cognitive symptoms or if caregivers raise similar concerns. The Folstein Mini Mental State Exam (MMSE), Montreal Cognitive Assessment (MoCA), Mini-Cog, and other similar tests are brief, objective, and widely used but have important limitations: they are insensitive to mild cognitive impairment, they may be biased negatively by the presence of language or attention problems, and they do not correlate with functional capacity.

A neuropsychiatric evaluation by a trained neuropsychologist or psychometrician may be appropriate. The goal of such testing is to enhance localization by defining the cognitive domains that are impaired as well as to quantify the degree of impairment. There is no standard battery of tests, but a variety of metrics is commonly used to assess the symptom types highlighted above. Assessments are most accurate when a patient is well rested, comfortable, and otherwise medically stable.

C. Imaging

Brain imaging with MRI or CT without contrast is indicated in any patient with a new, progressive cognitive complaint. The goal is to exclude occult cerebrovascular disease, tumor, or other identifiable structural abnormality, rather than to provide positive evidence of a neurodegenerative disease. Global or focal brain atrophy may be worse than expected for age and could suggest a particular neurodegenerative process, but such findings are rarely specific.

Positron-emission tomography (PET) with fluorodeoxyglucose (FDG) does not confirm or exclude any specific cause of dementia but may be useful as an element of the workup in specific clinical circumstances, such as discriminating between Alzheimer disease and frontotemporal dementia in a patient with some symptoms of each. PET imaging with a radiolabeled ligand for beta-amyloid, one of the pathologic proteins in Alzheimer disease, is highly sensitive to amyloid pathology and may provide positive evidence for Alzheimer disease in a patient with cognitive decline. However, after age 60 or 70, amyloid plaques can accumulate in the absence of cognitive impairment; thus, the specificity of a positive amyloid scan diminishes with age. Single photon-emission computed tomography offers similar information as FDG-PET but is less sensitive. PET imaging with radiolabeled ligands for tau, a pathogenic protein in Alzheimer disease, progressive supranuclear palsy, and some forms of frontotemporal dementia, also may help refine premortem diagnostic accuracy.

D. Laboratory Findings

Serum levels of vitamin B_{12}, free T_4, and thyroid-stimulating hormone should be measured for any patient with cognitive symptoms. A serum rapid plasma reagin (RPR) and testing for HIV should be considered. Other testing should be driven by clinical suspicion, and often includes a complete blood count, serum electrolytes, glucose, and lipid profile.

Although the presence of one or two ApoE epsilon-4 alleles indicates an increased risk of Alzheimer disease and ApoE genotyping is clinically available, it is of limited clinical utility. Finding an ApoE epsilon-4 allele in a young patient with dementia might raise the index of suspicion for Alzheimer disease, but obtaining a genotype in an elderly patient is unlikely to be helpful, and doing so in an asymptomatic patient as a marker of risk for Alzheimer disease is inappropriate until a preventive therapy becomes available. Spinal fluid protein measurements are also available; levels of beta-amyloid decrease and tau protein increase in Alzheimer disease, but this testing shares some of the same concerns as amyloid PET imaging.

► Differential Diagnosis

In elderly patients with gradually progressive cognitive symptoms and no other complaint or sign, a neurodegenerative disease is likely (Table 24–5). Decline beginning before age 60, rapid progression, fluctuating course, unintended weight loss, systemic complaints, or other unexplained symptoms or signs raise suspicion for a process other than a neurodegenerative disease. In this case, the differential is broad and includes infection or inflammatory disease (consider a lumbar puncture to screen for cells or antibodies in the spinal fluid), neoplasm or a paraneoplastic condition, endocrine or metabolic disease, drugs or toxins, or other conditions. **Normal pressure hydrocephalus** is a difficult diagnosis to establish. Symptoms include gait apraxia (sometimes described as a "magnetic" gait, as if the feet are stuck to the floor), urinary incontinence, and dementia. CT scanning or MRI of the brain reveals ventricles that are enlarged in obvious disproportion to sulcal widening and overall brain atrophy.

► Treatment

A. Nonpharmacologic Approaches

Aerobic exercise (45 minutes most days of the week) and **frequent mental stimulation** may reduce the rate of functional decline and decrease the demented patient's caregiving needs, and these interventions may reduce the risk of dementia in normal individuals. The most efficacious manner of mental stimulation is a matter of debate: maintaining as active a role in the family and community as practically possible is most likely to be of benefit, emphasizing activities at which the patient feels confident.

Patients with neurodegenerative diseases have a limited capacity to regain lost skills; for instance, memory drills in a patient with Alzheimer disease are more likely to lead to frustration than benefit and studies show that computerized cognitive training does *not* improve cognition or function in demented patients. Vitamin E (1000 international units twice daily) appears to reduce the rate of functional decline in patients with Alzheimer disease, but does not affect cognition or prevent the development of Alzheimer disease in patients with mild cognitive impairment.

B. Cognitive Symptoms

Cholinesterase inhibitors are first-line therapy for Alzheimer disease and dementia with Lewy bodies (Table 24–5). They provide modest, symptomatic treatment for cognitive dysfunction and may prolong the capacity for independence but do not prevent disease progression. Commonly used medications include donepezil (start at 5 mg orally daily for 4 weeks, then increase to 10 mg daily; a 23 mg daily dose is approved for moderate to severe Alzheimer disease, although its very modest additional efficacy over the 10 mg dose is overshadowed by an increased risk of side effects); rivastigmine (start at 1.5 mg orally twice daily, then increasing every 2 weeks by 1.5 mg twice daily to a goal of 3–6 mg twice daily; or 4.6, 9.5, or 13.3 mg/24 hours transdermally daily); and galantamine (start at 4 mg orally twice daily, then increasing every 4 weeks by 4 mg twice daily to a goal of 8–12 mg twice daily; a once-daily extended-release formulation is also available). Cholinesterase inhibitors are *not* given for frontotemporal dementia because they may worsen behavioral symptoms. Nausea and diarrhea are common side effects; syncope and cardiac dysrhythmia are uncommon but more serious. An ECG is often obtained before and after starting therapy, particularly in a patient with cardiac disease or a history of syncope.

Memantine (start at 5 mg orally daily, then increase by 5 mg per week up to a target of 10 mg twice daily) is approved for the treatment of moderate to severe Alzheimer disease. In frontotemporal dementia, memantine is ineffective and may worsen cognition. There is some evidence that memantine may improve cognition and behavior among patients with dementia with Lewy bodies.

Disease-modifying medications are not yet available for Alzheimer disease. Aducanumab, an antibody directed against aggregated beta-amyloid, showed promise in a phase II trial; phase III trials are ongoing.

C. Mood and Behavioral Disturbances

Selective serotonin reuptake inhibitors are generally safe and well tolerated in elderly, cognitively impaired patients, and they may be efficacious for the treatment of depression, anxiety, or agitation. There is evidence to support the use of citalopram (10–30 mg orally daily) for agitation; side effects include QTc prolongation and worsened cognition at the highest dose. Paroxetine should be avoided because it has anticholinergic effects; avoid all tricyclic antidepressants for the same reason. Other antidepressant agents, such as buproprion or venlafaxine, may be tried.

Insomnia is common, and trazodone (25–50 mg orally at bedtime as needed) can be safe and effective. Over-the-counter antihistamine hypnotics must be avoided, along with benzodiazepines, because of their tendency to worsen cognition and precipitate delirium. Other prescription hypnotics such as zolpidem may result in similar adverse reactions.

For agitation, impulsivity, and other behaviors that interfere with safe caregiving, causes of delirium (detailed above) should first be considered. When no reversible trigger is identified, treatment should be approached in a staged manner. Behavioral interventions, such as reorientation and distraction from anxiety-provoking stimuli, are first-line. Ensure that the patient is kept active during the day with both physical exercise and mentally stimulating activities, and that there is adequate sleep at night. Reassess the level of caregiving, and consider increasing the time spent directly with an attendant. Next, ensure that appropriate pharmacologic treatment of cognition and mood is optimized. Finally, as a last resort, when other measures prove insufficient and the patient's behaviors raise safety concerns, consider pharmacologic therapy. Citalopram or low doses of an atypical antipsychotic medication such as quetiapine (start 25 mg orally daily as needed, increasing to two to three times daily as needed) can be tried; even though atypical agents cause extrapyramidal side effects less frequently than typical antipsychotics, they should be used with particular caution in a patient at risk for falls, especially if parkinsonian signs are already present. Regularly scheduled dosing of antipsychotics is not recommended, and if implemented should be reassessed on a frequent basis (eg, weekly), with attempts to taper off as tolerated. There is an FDA black box warning against the use of all antipsychotic medications in elderly demented patients because of an *increased risk of death;* the reason for the increased mortality is unclear. The combination of dextromethorphan and quinidine (up to 30/10 mg orally twice daily) has shown promise in early clinical trials.

▶ Special Circumstances

A. Rapidly Progressive Dementia

When dementia develops quickly, with obvious decline over a few weeks to a few months, the syndrome may be classified as a **rapidly progressive dementia.** The differential diagnosis for typical dementias is still relevant, but additional etiologies must be considered, including prion disease; infections; toxins; neoplasms; and autoimmune and inflammatory diseases, including corticosteroid-responsive (Hashimoto) encephalopathy and antibody-mediated paraneoplastic syndromes. Workup should begin with brain MRI with contrast and diffusion-weighted imaging, routine laboratory studies (serum vitamin B_{12}, free T_4, and thyroid-stimulating hormone levels), serum RPR, HIV antibody, Lyme serology, rheumatologic tests (erythrocyte sedimentation rate, C-reactive protein, and antinuclear antibody), anti-thyroglobulin and anti-thyroperoxidase antibody levels, paraneoplastic autoimmune antibodies (see Nonmetastatic Neurologic Complications of Malignant Disease, above),

and cerebrospinal fluid studies (cell count and differential; protein and glucose levels; protein electrophoresis for oligoclonal bands; IgG index [spinal-fluid-to-serum-gamma-globulin level] ratio; and VDRL). Depending on the clinical context, it may be necessary to exclude Wilson disease (24-hour urine copper level), heavy metal intoxication (24-hour urine heavy metal panel), and infectious encephalitis (cerebrospinal fluid polymerase chain reaction for Whipple disease, herpes simplex virus, cytomegalovirus, varicella-zoster virus, and other viruses).

Creutzfeldt-Jakob disease is a relatively common cause of rapidly progressive dementia (see Chapter 32). Family history is important since mutations in *PRNP*, the gene for the prion protein, account for around 15% of cases. Diffusion-weighted MRI is the most helpful diagnostic tool, classically revealing cortical ribboning (a gyral pattern of hyperintensity) as well as restricted diffusion in the caudate and anterior putamen. An electroencephalogram often shows periodic complexes. Real time quaking induced conversion (RT-QuIC), in which patient cerebrospinal fluid is mixed with recombinant prion protein and aggregation of prion protein is detected, is a sensitive and specific diagnostic test. Reflecting the high rate of neuronal death, cerebrospinal fluid levels of the intraneuronal proteins tau, 14-3-3, and neuron-specific enolase are often elevated, although this finding is neither sensitive nor specific.

B. Driving and Dementia

It is recommended that any patient with mild dementia or worse should discontinue driving. Most states have laws regulating driving among cognitively impaired individuals, and many require the clinician to report the patient's diagnosis to the public health department or department of motor vehicles. There is *no* evidence that driving classes help patients with neurodegenerative diseases.

▶ When to Refer

All patients with new, unexplained cognitive decline should be referred.

▶ When to Admit

Admission to the hospital should be avoided in patients with dementia due to increased risk of developing hospital-acquired delirium.

Apostolova LG. Alzheimer disease. Continuum (Minneap Minn). 2016 Apr;22(2 Dementia):419–34. [PMID: 27042902]

Brookmeyer R et al. Forecasting the prevalence of preclinical and clinical Alzheimer's disease in the United States. Alzheimers Dement. 2018 Feb;14(2):121–9. [PMID: 29233480]

Farina N et al. Vitamin E for Alzheimer's dementia and mild cognitive impairment. Cochrane Database Syst Rev. 2017 Apr 18;4:CD002854. [PMID: 28418065]

Geschwind MD. Rapidly progressive dementia. Continuum (Minneap Minn). 2016 Apr;22(2 Dementia):510–37. [PMID: 27042906]

Guure CB et al. Impact of physical activity on cognitive decline, dementia, and its subtypes: meta-analysis of prospective studies. Biomed Res Int. 2017;2017:9016924. [PMID: 28271072]

Livingston G et al. Dementia prevention, intervention, and care. Lancet. 2017 Dec 16;390(10113):2673–734. [PMID: 28735855]

Sevigny J et al. The antibody aducanumab reduces Aβ plaques in Alzheimer's disease. Nature. 2016 Sep 1;537(7618):50–6. [PMID: 27582220]

MULTIPLE SCLEROSIS

 ESSENTIALS OF DIAGNOSIS

▶ Episodic neurologic symptoms.

▶ Patient usually under 55 years of age at onset.

▶ Single pathologic lesion cannot explain clinical findings.

▶ Multiple foci best visualized by MRI.

▶ General Considerations

This common neurologic disorder, which probably has an autoimmune basis, has its greatest incidence in young adults. Epidemiologic studies indicate that multiple sclerosis is much more common in persons of western European lineage who live in temperate zones. No population with a high risk for multiple sclerosis exists between latitudes 40° N and 40° S. A genetic susceptibility to the disease is present. Pathologically, focal—often perivenular—areas of demyelination with reactive gliosis are found scattered in the white matter of the brain and spinal cord and in the optic nerves. Axonal damage also occurs.

▶ Clinical Findings

A. Symptoms and Signs

The common initial presentation is weakness, numbness, tingling, or unsteadiness in a limb; spastic paraparesis; retrobulbar optic neuritis; diplopia; dysequilibrium; or a sphincter disturbance such as urinary urgency or hesitancy. Symptoms may disappear after a few days or weeks, although examination often reveals a residual deficit.

Several forms of the disease are recognized. In most patients, there is an interval of months or years after the initial episode before new symptoms develop or the original ones recur (**relapsing-remitting disease**). Eventually, however, relapses and usually incomplete remissions lead to increasing disability, with weakness, spasticity, and ataxia of the limbs, impaired vision, and urinary incontinence. The findings on examination at this stage commonly include optic atrophy; nystagmus; dysarthria; and pyramidal, sensory, or cerebellar deficits in some or all of the limbs. In some of these patients, the clinical course changes so that a steady deterioration occurs, unrelated to acute relapses (**secondary progressive disease**). Less commonly, symptoms are steadily progressive from their onset, and disability develops at a relatively early stage (**primary progressive disease**). The diagnosis cannot be made with confidence unless the total clinical picture indicates involvement of *different parts of the central nervous system at different times*. Fatigue is common in all forms of the disease.

A number of factors (eg, infection) may precipitate or trigger exacerbations. Relapses are reduced in pregnancy but are more likely during the 2 or 3 months following pregnancy, possibly because of the increased demands and stresses that occur in the postpartum period.

B. Imaging

MRI of the brain and cervical cord has a major role in excluding other causes of neurologic dysfunction and in demonstrating the presence of multiple lesions. In T1-weighted images, hypointense "black holes" probably represent areas of permanent axonal damage. Gadolinium-enhanced T1-weighted images may highlight areas of active inflammation with breakdown of the blood-brain barrier, which helps identify newer lesions. T2-weighted images provide information about disease burden or total number of lesions, which typically appear as areas of high signal intensity. CT scans are less helpful than MRI.

In patients with myelopathy alone and no clinical or laboratory evidence of more widespread disease, MRI or myelography is necessary to exclude a congenital or acquired surgically treatable lesion. In patients with mixed pyramidal and cerebellar deficits in the limbs, the foramen magnum region must be visualized to exclude the possibility of Arnold-Chiari malformation, in which parts of the cerebellum and lower brainstem are displaced into the cervical canal.

C. Laboratory and Other Studies

A definitive diagnosis can never be based solely on the laboratory findings. If there is clinical evidence of only a single lesion in the central nervous system, multiple sclerosis cannot properly be diagnosed unless it can be shown that other regions are affected subclinically. Visual, brainstem auditory, and somatosensory evoked potentials are helpful in this regard, but other disorders may also be characterized by multifocal electrophysiologic abnormalities reflecting disease of central white matter. Certain infections (eg, HIV, Lyme disease, syphilis), connective tissue diseases (eg, systemic lupus erythematosus, Sjögren syndrome), sarcoidosis, metabolic disorders (eg, vitamin B_{12} deficiency), and lymphoma may therefore require exclusion.

There may be mild lymphocytosis or a slightly increased protein concentration in the cerebrospinal fluid, especially soon after an acute relapse. Elevated IgG in cerebrospinal fluid and discrete bands of IgG (oligoclonal bands) are present in many patients. The presence of such bands is not specific, however, since they have been found in a variety of inflammatory neurologic disorders and occasionally in patients with vascular or neoplastic disorders of the nervous system.

Vitamin D deficiency may be associated with an increased risk of developing multiple sclerosis; whether supplementation prevents the disease or disease progression is under study.

D. Diagnosis

Multiple sclerosis should not be diagnosed unless there is evidence that two or more different regions of the central white matter (*dissemination in space*) have been affected at different times (*dissemination in time*); the most widely used diagnostic algorithm is the 2017 revision to the McDonald criteria. The diagnosis may be made in a patient with two or more typical attacks and objective evidence on clinical examination of two lesions (eg, optic disk atrophy and pyramidal weakness), or objective evidence of one lesion with clear-cut historical evidence the other attack was typical of multiple sclerosis and in a distinct neuroanatomic location. To fulfill the criterion of dissemination in space in a patient with two clinical attacks but objective clinical evidence of only one lesion, MRI should demonstrate at least one lesion in at least two of four typical sites (periventricular, cortical or juxtacortical, infratentorial, or spinal); alternatively, an additional attack localized to a different site suffices. The criterion of dissemination in time in a patient with only one attack can be fulfilled by the simultaneous presence of gadolinium-enhancing and non-enhancing lesions at any time (including at initial examination); the presence of oligoclonal bands unique to the cerebrospinal fluid; a new lesion on follow-up MRI; or a second attack. Lesions in the optic nerve on MRI in patients with optic neuritis cannot be used to fulfill the McDonald criteria for dissemination in space or time. Primary progressive disease requires at least a year of progression, plus two of three of the following: at least one typical brain lesion, at least two spinal lesions, or oligoclonal banding in the cerebrospinal fluid.

In patients with a single clinical event who do not satisfy criteria for multiple sclerosis, a diagnosis of a **clinically isolated syndrome (CIS)** is made. Such patients are at risk for developing multiple sclerosis and are sometimes offered beta-interferon or glatiramer acetate therapy, which may delay progression to clinically definite disease. Follow-up MRI should be considered 6–12 months later to assess for the presence of any new lesion.

Treatment

At least partial recovery from acute exacerbations can reasonably be expected, but further relapses may occur without warning. Some disability is likely to result eventually, but about half of all patients are without significant disability even 10 years after onset of symptoms. Current treatments are chiefly aimed at preventing relapses, thereby reducing disability.

Recovery from acute relapses may be hastened by treatment with corticosteroids, but the extent of recovery is unchanged. Intravenous therapy is often given first—typically methylprednisolone 1 g daily for 3 days—followed by oral prednisone at 60–80 mg daily for 1 week with a taper over the ensuing 2–3 weeks, but randomized trials show similar efficacy whether the initial high dose is given orally or intravenously. Long-term treatment with corticosteroids provides no benefit and does not prevent further relapses. Transient exacerbation of symptoms relating to intercurrent infection or heat requires no added treatment.

In patients with relapsing disease, numerous medications have well-established efficacy at *reducing the frequency of attacks* (Table 24–6). The initial agent is chosen after considering medication tolerance and risks, patient preference, and disease severity. Glatiramer acetate or an interferon is often used initially due to favorable side effect profiles and availability, although the efficacy of early treatment with higher intensity therapy is being explored. In general, the medications most effective in reducing relapses have stronger immunomodulatory effects and more, albeit rare, serious adverse effects. Prescription of these agents should be managed by a specialist.

Ocrelizumab is the only medication effective in slowing disability progression in primary progressive multiple sclerosis and is approved for this indication by the FDA.

For patients with severe or secondary progressive disease, limited evidence supports immunosuppressive therapy with rituximab, cyclophosphamide, azathioprine, methotrexate, or mitoxantrone. Plasmapheresis is sometimes helpful in patients with severe relapses unresponsive to corticosteroids.

Symptomatic therapy for spasticity, neurogenic bladder, or fatigue may be required. Fatigue is especially common in multiple sclerosis, and modafinil (200 mg orally every morning) is an effective and FDA-approved therapy for this indication. Dalfampridine (an extended-release formulation of 4-aminopyridine administered as 10 mg orally twice daily) is efficacious at improving timed gait in multiple sclerosis. Depression and even suicidality can occur in multiple sclerosis and may worsen with interferon beta-1a therapy; screening and conventional treatment of such symptoms are appropriate.

▶ When to Refer

All patients, but especially those with progressive disease despite standard therapy, should be referred.

▶ When to Admit

- Patients requiring plasma exchange for severe relapses unresponsive to corticosteroids.
- During severe relapses.
- Patients unable to manage at home.

Hauser SL et al; OPERA I and OPERA II Clinical Investigators. Ocrelizumab versus interferon beta-1a in relapsing multiple sclerosis. N Engl J Med. 2017 Jan 19;376(3):221–34. [PMID: 28002679]

Montalban X et al; ORATORIO Clinical Investigators. Ocrelizumab versus placebo in primary progressive multiple sclerosis. N Engl J Med. 2017 Jan 19;376(3):209–20. [PMID: 28002688]

Rae-Grant A et al. Practice guideline recommendations summary: disease-modifying therapies for adults with multiple sclerosis: report of the Guideline Development, Dissemination, and Implementation Subcommittee of the American Academy of Neurology. Neurology. 2018 Apr 24;90(17): 777–88. [PMID: 29686116]

Thompson AJ et al. Diagnosis of multiple sclerosis: 2017 revisions of the McDonald criteria. Lancet Neurol. 2018 Feb; 17(2):162–73. [PMID: 29275977]

Table 24–6. Treatment of multiple sclerosis (in alphabetical order within categories).[1]

Medication	Dose
Acute Episode, Including Relapse[2]	
Dexamethasone	160 mg orally daily for 3–5 days
Methylprednisolone	1 g intravenously or orally daily for 3–5 days
Relapse Prevention, First-Line Treatment	
Cladribine (Mavenclad)	1.75 mg/kg orally divided between weeks 1 and 5, repeated once in 1 year
Dimethyl fumarate (Tecfidera)	240 mg orally twice daily
Fingolimod (Gilenya)	0.5 mg orally daily
Glatiramer acetate (Copaxone)	20 mg subcutaneously daily
Interferon β-1a (Rebif)	44 mcg subcutaneously three times per week
Interferon β-1a (Avonex)	30 mcg intramuscularly once per week
Interferon β-1b (Betaseron, Extavia)	0.25 mg subcutaneously on alternate days
Ocrelizumab (Ocrevus)	300 mg intravenously on day 1 and day 15, followed by 600 mg every 6 months
Teriflunomide (Aubagio)	14 mg orally daily
Relapse Prevention for Disease Activity Despite Use of First-Line Treatment	
Alemtuzumab (Lemtrada)	12 mg intravenously daily for 5 days; 3-day course given 1 year later
Cladribine (Mavenclad)	1.75 mg/kg orally divided between weeks 1 and 5, repeated once in 1 year
Dimethyl fumarate (Tecfidera)	240 mg orally twice daily
Fingolimod (Gilenya)	0.5 mg orally daily
Mitoxantrone	12 mg/m^2 intravenously every 3 months; maximum lifetime dose, 140 mg/m^2
Natalizumab (Tysabri)	300 mg intravenously monthly
Ocrelizumab (Ocrevus)	300 mg intravenously on day 1 and day 15, followed by 600 mg every 6 months
High Disease Activity (Typically with Multiple Gadolinium-Enhancing Lesions on MRI)	
Alemtuzumab (Lemtrada)	12 mg intravenously daily for 5 days; 3-day course given 1 year later
Fingolimod (Gilenya)	0.5 mg orally daily
Natalizumab (Tysabri)	300 mg intravenously monthly
Ocrelizumab (Ocrevus)	300 mg intravenously on day 1 and day 15, followed by 600 mg every 6 months

[1]Several of these agents require special monitoring or pretreatment; some should be avoided during pregnancy. Readers should refer to the manufacturer's guidelines.
[2]For corticosteroid-refractory relapses, plasmapheresis may be used.
Reproduced, with permission, from Aminoff MJ et al. *Clinical Neurology*, 9th ed, McGraw-Hill Education, 2015.

NEUROMYELITIS OPTICA

This disorder is characterized by optic neuritis and acute myelitis with MRI changes that extend over at least three segments of the spinal cord. An isolated myelitis or optic neuritis may also occur. Previously known as **Devic disease** and once regarded as a variant of multiple sclerosis, neuromyelitis optica is associated with a specific antibody marker (NMO-IgG) targeting the water channel aquaporin-4 in 80% of cases, and with antibodies to myelin oligodendrocyte glycoprotein (MOG-IgG) in approximately 33% of NMO-IgG seronegative patients. MRI of the brain typically does not show widespread white matter involvement, but such changes do not exclude the diagnosis. Treatment is by long-term immunosuppression. First-line therapy is with rituximab (two 1 g intravenous infusions spaced by 2 weeks, or four weekly infusions of 375 mg/m^2; re-dosing may occur every 6 months or when CD19/20-positive or CD27-positive lymphocytes become detectable), mycophenolate mofetil (500–1500 mg orally twice daily, titrated until the absolute lymphocyte count falls below 1500/mcL), or azathioprine (2.5–3 mg/kg orally). Acute relapses are treated with corticosteroids at doses similar to those outlined for multiple sclerosis and with plasma exchange for severe relapses unresponsive to corticosteroids.

Nikoo Z et al. Comparison of the efficacy of azathioprine and rituximab in neuromyelitis optica spectrum disorder: a randomized clinical trial. J Neurol. 2017 Sep;264(9):2003–9. [PMID: 28831548]

Wingerchuk DM et al; International Panel for NMO Diagnosis. International consensus diagnostic criteria for neuromyelitis optica spectrum disorders. Neurology. 2015 Jul 14;85(2): 177–89. [PMID: 26092914]

VITAMIN E DEFICIENCY

Vitamin E deficiency may produce a disorder somewhat similar to Friedreich ataxia. There is spinocerebellar degeneration involving particularly the posterior columns of the spinal cord and leading to limb ataxia, sensory loss, absent tendon reflexes, slurring of speech and, in some cases, pigmentary retinal degeneration. The disorder may occur as a consequence of malabsorption or on a hereditary basis (eg, abetalipoproteinemia).

SPASTICITY

The term "spasticity" is commonly used for an upper motor neuron deficit, but it properly refers to a velocity-dependent increase in resistance to passive movement that affects different muscles to a different extent, is not uniform in degree throughout the range of a particular movement, and is commonly associated with other features of pyramidal deficit. It is often a major complication of stroke, cerebral or spinal injury, static perinatal encephalopathy, and multiple sclerosis.

Physical therapy with appropriate stretching programs is important during rehabilitation after the development of an upper motor neuron lesion and in subsequent management of the patient. The aim is to prevent joint and muscle *contractures* and perhaps to modulate spasticity.

Medication management is important also, but treatment may increase functional disability when increased extensor tone is providing additional support for patients with weak legs. Dantrolene weakens muscle contraction by interfering with the role of calcium. It is best avoided in patients with poor respiratory function or severe myocardial disease. Treatment is begun with 25 mg once daily, increased by 25 mg every 3 days, depending on tolerance, to a maximum of 100 mg four times daily. Side effects include diarrhea, nausea, weakness, hepatic dysfunction (that may rarely be fatal, especially in women older than 35), drowsiness, light-headedness, and hallucinations.

Baclofen is an effective medication for treating spasticity of spinal origin and painful flexor (or extensor) spasms. The maximum recommended daily oral dose is 80 mg; treatment is started with a dose of 5 or 10 mg twice daily orally and then built up gradually. Side effects include gastrointestinal disturbances, lassitude, fatigue, sedation, unsteadiness, confusion, and hallucinations. Diazepam may modify spasticity by its action on spinal interneurons and perhaps also by influencing supraspinal centers, but effective doses often cause intolerable drowsiness and vary with different patients. Tizanidine, a centrally acting alpha-2-adrenergic agonist, is as effective as these other agents and is probably better tolerated. The daily dose is built up gradually, usually to 8 mg taken three times daily. Side effects include sedation, lassitude, hypotension, and dryness of the mouth. Cannabinoids are also effective in reducing spasticity, but are associated with side effects, including dizziness, drowsiness, and fatigue.

Intramuscular injection of botulinum toxin has been used to relax targeted muscles.

In patients with severe spasticity that is unresponsive to other therapies and is associated with marked disability, intrathecal injection of phenol or alcohol may be helpful. Surgical options include implantation of an intrathecal baclofen pump, rhizotomy, or neurectomy. Severe contractures may be treated by surgical tendon release.

Spasticity may be exacerbated by decubitus ulcers, urinary or other infections, and nociceptive stimuli.

MYELOPATHIES IN AIDS

A variety of myelopathies may occur in patients with AIDS. These are discussed in Chapter 31.

MYELOPATHY OF HUMAN T-CELL LEUKEMIA VIRUS INFECTION

Human T-cell leukemia virus (HTLV-1), a human retrovirus, is transmitted by breastfeeding, sexual contact, blood transfusion, and contaminated needles. Most patients are asymptomatic, but after a variable latent period (which may be as long as several years), a myelopathy develops in some instances. The MRI, electrophysiologic, and cerebrospinal fluid findings are similar to those of multiple sclerosis, but HTLV-1 antibodies are present in serum and spinal fluid. There is no specific treatment, but intravenous or oral corticosteroids may help in the initial inflammatory phase of the disease. Prophylactic measures are important. Needles or syringes should not be shared; infected patients should not breastfeed their infants or donate blood, semen, or other tissue. Infected patients should use condoms to prevent sexual transmission.

SUBACUTE COMBINED DEGENERATION OF THE SPINAL CORD

Subacute combined degeneration of the spinal cord is due to **vitamin B$_{12}$ deficiency**, such as occurs in pernicious anemia. It is characterized by myelopathy with spasticity, weakness, proprioceptive loss, and numbness due to degeneration of the corticospinal tracts and posterior columns. Polyneuropathy, mental changes, or optic neuropathy also develop in some patients. Megaloblastic anemia may also occur, but this does not parallel the neurologic disorder, and the former may be obscured if folic acid supplements have been taken. Treatment is with vitamin B$_{12}$. For pernicious anemia, a convenient therapeutic regimen is 1000 mcg cyanocobalamin intramuscularly daily for 1 week, then weekly for 1 month, and then monthly for the remainder of the patient's life. Oral cyanocobalamin replacement is not advised for pernicious anemia when neurologic symptoms are present. A similar syndrome is caused by recreational abuse of inhaled nitrous oxide due to its interference with vitamin B$_{12}$ metabolism. Copper deficiency, caused by malabsorption or excess zinc ingestion, may also be responsible.

WERNICKE ENCEPHALOPATHY & KORSAKOFF SYNDROME

Wernicke encephalopathy is characterized by confusion, ataxia, and nystagmus leading to ophthalmoplegia (lateral rectus muscle weakness, conjugate gaze palsies); peripheral neuropathy may also be present. It is due to thiamine deficiency and in the United States occurs most commonly in patients with alcoholism. It may also occur in patients with AIDS or hyperemesis gravidarum, and after bariatric surgery. In suspected cases, thiamine (100 mg) is given intravenously immediately and then intramuscularly on a daily basis until a satisfactory diet can be ensured after which the same dose is given orally. Some guidelines recommend initial doses of 200–500 mg intravenously three times daily for the first 5–7 days of treatment. Intravenous glucose given *before* thiamine may precipitate the syndrome or worsen the symptoms. The diagnosis is confirmed by the response in 1 or 2 days to treatment, which must not be delayed while awaiting laboratory confirmation of thiamine deficiency from a blood sample obtained prior to thiamine administration. **Korsakoff syndrome** occurs in more severe cases; it includes anterograde and retrograde amnesia and sometimes confabulation, and may not be recognized until after the initial delirium has lifted.

STUPOR & COMA

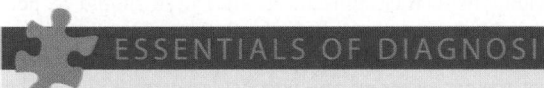

ESSENTIALS OF DIAGNOSIS

- ▶ Level of consciousness is depressed.
- ▶ Stuporous patients respond only to repeated vigorous stimuli.
- ▶ Comatose patients are unarousable and unresponsive.

▶ General Considerations

The patient who is stuporous is unresponsive except when subjected to repeated vigorous stimuli, while the comatose patient is unarousable and unable to respond to external events or inner needs, although reflex movements and posturing may be present.

Coma is a major complication of serious central nervous system disorders. It can result from seizures, hypothermia, metabolic disturbances, or structural lesions causing bilateral cerebral hemispheric dysfunction or a disturbance of the brainstem reticular activating system. A mass lesion involving one cerebral hemisphere may cause coma by compression of the brainstem.

▶ Assessment & Emergency Measures

The diagnostic workup of the comatose patient must proceed concomitantly with management. Supportive therapy for respiration or blood pressure is initiated; in hypothermia, all vital signs may be absent and all such patients should be rewarmed before the prognosis is assessed.

The patient can be positioned on one side with the neck partly extended, dentures removed, and secretions cleared by suction; if necessary, the patency of the airways is maintained with an oropharyngeal airway. Blood is drawn for serum glucose, electrolyte, and calcium levels; arterial blood gases; liver biochemical and kidney function tests; and toxicologic studies as indicated. Thiamine (100 mg), dextrose 50% (25 g), and naloxone (0.4–1.2 mg) are given intravenously without delay.

Further details are then obtained from attendants of the patient's medical history, the circumstances surrounding the onset of coma, and the time course of subsequent events. Abrupt onset of coma suggests subarachnoid hemorrhage, brainstem stroke, or intracerebral hemorrhage, whereas a slower onset and progression occur with other structural or mass lesions. Urgent noncontrast CT scanning of the head is appropriate if it can be obtained directly from the emergency department, in order to identify intracranial hemorrhage, brain herniation, or other structural lesion that may require immediate neurosurgical intervention. A metabolic cause is likely with a preceding intoxicated state or agitated delirium. On examination, attention is paid to the behavioral response to painful stimuli, the pupils and their response to light, the response to touching the cornea with a wisp of sterile gauze, position of the eyes and their movement in response to passive movement of the head and ice-water caloric stimulation, and the respiratory pattern.

A. Response to Painful Stimuli

Purposeful limb withdrawal from painful stimuli implies that sensory pathways from and motor pathways to the stimulated limb are functionally intact. Unilateral absence of responses despite application of stimuli to both sides of the body in turn implies a corticospinal lesion; bilateral absence of responsiveness suggests brainstem involvement, bilateral pyramidal tract lesions, or psychogenic unresponsiveness. Decorticate (flexor) posturing may occur with lesions of the internal capsule and rostral cerebral peduncle and decerebrate (extensor) posturing with dysfunction or destruction of the midbrain and rostral pons. Decerebrate posturing occurs in the arms accompanied by flaccidity or slight flexor responses in the legs in patients with extensive brainstem damage extending down to the pons at the trigeminal level.

B. Ocular Findings

1. Pupils—Hypothalamic disease processes may lead to unilateral Horner syndrome, while bilateral diencephalic involvement or destructive pontine lesions may lead to small but reactive pupils. Ipsilateral pupillary dilation with no direct or consensual response to light occurs with compression of the third cranial nerve, eg, with uncal herniation. The pupils are slightly smaller than normal but responsive to light in many metabolic encephalopathies; however, they may be fixed and dilated following overdosage with atropine or scopolamine, and pinpoint (but responsive) with opioids.

2. Corneal reflex—Touching the cornea with a wisp of sterile gauze or cotton should elicit a blink reflex. The afferent limb of the arc is mediated by the fifth cranial nerve; the efferent limb by the seventh nerve. A unilateral absent corneal reflex implies damage to the ipsilateral pons or a trigeminal deficit. Bilateral loss can be seen with large pontine lesions or in deep pharmacologic coma.

3. Eye movements—Conjugate deviation of the eyes to the side suggests the presence of an ipsilateral hemispheric lesion, a contralateral pontine lesion, or ongoing seizures from the contralateral hemisphere. A mesencephalic lesion leads to downward conjugate deviation. Dysconjugate ocular deviation in coma implies a structural brainstem lesion unless there was preexisting strabismus.

The oculomotor responses to passive head turning and to caloric stimulation relate to each other and provide complementary information. In response to brisk rotation of the head from side to side and to flexion and extension of the head, normally conscious patients with open eyes do not exhibit contraversive conjugate eye deviation (**oculocephalic reflex**) unless there is voluntary visual fixation or bilateral frontal pathology. With cortical depression in lightly comatose patients, a brisk oculocephalic reflex is seen. With brainstem lesions, this oculocephalic reflex becomes impaired or lost, depending on the site of the lesion.

The **oculovestibular reflex** is tested by caloric stimulation using irrigation with ice water. In normal subjects, jerk nystagmus is elicited for about 2 or 3 minutes, with the slow component toward the irrigated ear. In unconscious patients with an intact brainstem, the fast component of the nystagmus disappears, so that the eyes tonically deviate toward the irrigated side for 2–3 minutes before returning to their original position. With impairment of brainstem function, the response becomes abnormal and finally disappears. In metabolic coma, oculocephalic and oculovestibular reflex responses are preserved, at least initially.

C. Respiratory Patterns

Diseases causing coma may lead to respiratory abnormalities. **Cheyne-Stokes respiration** (in which episodes of deep breathing alternate with periods of apnea) may occur with bihemispheric or diencephalic disease or in metabolic disorders. **Central neurogenic hyperventilation** occurs with lesions of the brainstem tegmentum; **apneustic breathing** (in which there are prominent end-inspiratory pauses) suggests damage at the pontine level (eg, due to basilar artery occlusion); and **atactic breathing** (a completely irregular pattern of breathing with deep and shallow breaths occurring randomly) is associated with lesions of the lower pontine tegmentum and medulla.

1. Stupor & Coma Due to Structural Lesions

Supratentorial mass lesions tend to affect brain function in a systematic way. There may initially be signs of hemispheric dysfunction, such as hemiparesis. As coma develops and deepens, cerebral function becomes progressively disturbed, producing a predictable progression of neurologic signs that suggest rostrocaudal deterioration.

Thus, as a supratentorial mass lesion begins to impair the diencephalon, the patient becomes drowsy, then stuporous, and finally comatose. There may be Cheyne-Stokes respiration; small but reactive pupils or an ipsilateral third nerve palsy due to uncal herniation; normal oculocephalic responses with side-to-side head movements but sometimes an impairment of reflex upward gaze with brisk flexion of the head; tonic ipsilateral deviation of the eyes in response to vestibular stimulation with cold water; and initially a positive response to pain but subsequently only decorticate posturing. With further progression, midbrain failure occurs. Motor dysfunction progresses from decorticate to bilateral decerebrate posturing in response to painful stimuli; Cheyne-Stokes respiration is gradually replaced by sustained central hyperventilation; the pupils become middle-sized and fixed; and the oculocephalic and oculovestibular reflex responses become impaired, abnormal, or lost. As the pons and then the medulla fail, the pupils remain unresponsive; oculovestibular responses are unobtainable; respiration is rapid and shallow; and painful stimuli may lead only to flexor responses in the legs. Finally, respiration becomes irregular and stops, the pupils often then dilating widely.

In contrast, a **subtentorial (ie, brainstem) lesion** may lead to an early, sometimes abrupt disturbance of consciousness without any orderly rostrocaudal progression of neurologic signs. Compressive lesions of the brainstem, especially cerebellar hemorrhage, may be clinically indistinguishable from intraparenchymal processes.

A structural lesion is suspected if the findings suggest focality. In such circumstances, a CT scan should be performed before, or instead of, a lumbar puncture in order to avoid any risk of cerebral herniation. Further management is of the causal lesion and is considered separately under the individual disorders.

2. Stupor & Coma Due to Metabolic Disturbances

Patients with a metabolic cause of coma generally have signs of patchy, diffuse, and symmetric neurologic involvement that cannot be explained by loss of function at any single level or in a sequential manner, although focal or lateralized deficits may occur in hypoglycemia. Pupillary reactivity is usually preserved. Comatose patients with meningitis, encephalitis, or subarachnoid hemorrhage may also exhibit little in the way of focal neurologic signs, however, and clinical evidence of meningeal irritation is sometimes very subtle in comatose patients. Examination of the cerebrospinal fluid in such patients is essential to establish the correct diagnosis.

In patients with coma due to cerebral ischemia and hypoxia, the absence of pupillary light reflexes 24 hours after return of spontaneous circulation indicates that there is little chance of regaining independence; absent corneal reflexes or absent or extensor motor responses at 72 hours also indicate a grim prognosis. Physical findings are less reliable predictors of outcome among those treated with therapeutic hypothermia, although absent corneal or pupillary light reflexes at 72 hours likely indicate a poor prognosis, as do bilaterally absent cortical somatosensory evoked potentials in response to median nerve stimulation after the patient has returned to normothermia.

Treatment of metabolic encephalopathy is of the underlying disturbance and is considered in other chapters. If the cause of the encephalopathy is obscure, all medications except essential ones may have to be withdrawn in case they are responsible for the altered mental status.

3. Brain Death

Brain death occurs when there is complete and irreversible cessation of all brain function; although the organs can be maintained with mechanical ventilation for the purposes of donation, in most countries the diagnosis of brain death is equivalent to a declaration of death. To diagnose brain death, the cause of coma must be established, compatible with a known cause of brain death, and irreversible. Reversible coma simulating brain death may be seen with hypothermia (temperature lower than 32°C) and overdosage with central nervous system depressant drugs, and these conditions must be excluded by warming the patient and allowing enough time for all sedating medications to be metabolized (ie, at least five half-lives) or by measuring serum levels. Severe blood pressure, electrolyte, acid-base, and endocrine derangements cannot be present.

Finally, a neurologic examination must demonstrate that the patient is comatose (ie, no eye opening and no response to central or peripheral pain); has lost all brainstem reflex responses, including the pupillary, corneal, oculovestibular, oculocephalic, oropharyngeal, and cough reflexes; and has no respiratory drive. The response to pain should be absent or only consist of spinal reflex movements; decerebrate or decorticate posturing is not consistent with brain death. Absence of respiratory drive is demonstrated with an **apnea test** (absence of spontaneous respiratory activity at a $PACO_2$ of at least 60 mm Hg or after a rise of 20 mm Hg from baseline).

Certain ancillary tests may assist the determination of brain death if an apnea test cannot be performed but are not essential. These include an isoelectric electroencephalogram, when the recording is made according to the recommendations of the American Clinical Neurophysiology Society, and demonstration of an absent cerebral circulation by intravenous radioisotope cerebral angiography or by four-vessel contrast cerebral angiography.

4. Persistent Vegetative State

Patients with severe bilateral hemispheric disease may show some improvement from an initially comatose state, so that, after a variable interval, they appear to be awake but lie motionless and without evidence of awareness or higher mental activity. This is called a "persistent" vegetative state once it has lasted over 4 weeks and has also been variously referred to as akinetic mutism, apallic state, or coma vigil. Patients in a vegetative state from a medical cause (eg, anoxic brain injury) for more than 3 months and from a traumatic brain injury for more than 12 months are said to be in a "chronic" vegetative state, from which a few patients may regain consciousness but remain severely disabled.

5. Minimally Conscious State

In this state, patients exhibit inconsistent evidence of consciousness. There is some degree of functional recovery of

behaviors suggesting self- or environmental awareness, such as basic verbalization or context-appropriate gestures, emotional responses (eg, smiling) to emotional but not neutral stimuli, or purposive responses to environmental stimuli (eg, a finger movement or eye blink apparently to command). Further improvement is manifest by the restoration of communication with the patient. The minimally conscious state may be temporary or permanent. Little information is available about its natural history or long-term outlook, which reflects the underlying cause. The likelihood of useful functional recovery diminishes with time; after 12 months, patients are likely to remain severely disabled and without a reliable means of communication. Prognostication is difficult. Amantadine (100–200 mg orally daily) may hasten recovery when given to patients in a vegetative or minimally conscious state 4–16 weeks after traumatic brain injury.

6. Locked-In Syndrome (De-efferented State)

Acute destructive lesions (eg, infarction, hemorrhage, demyelination, encephalitis) involving the ventral pons and sparing the tegmentum may lead to a mute, quadriparetic but conscious state in which the patient is capable of blinking and voluntary eye movement in the vertical plane, with preserved pupillary responses to light. Such a patient can mistakenly be regarded as comatose. Clinicians should recognize that "locked-in" individuals are fully aware of their surroundings. The prognosis is usually poor, but recovery has occasionally been reported in some cases, including resumption of independent daily life. A similar condition may occur with severe Guillain-Barré syndrome and has a better prognosis.

Citerio G et al. Brain death: the European perspective. Semin Neurol. 2015 Apr;35(2):139–44. [PMID: 25839722]

Giacino JT et al. Practice guideline update recommendations summary: disorders of consciousness: report of the Guideline Development, Dissemination, and Implementation Subcommittee of the American Academy of Neurology; the American Congress of Rehabilitation Medicine; and the National Institute on Disability, Independent Living, and Rehabilitation Research. Neurology. 2018 Sep 4;91(10):450–60. [PMID: 30089618]

Wijdicks EF. Determining brain death. Continuum (Minneap Minn). 2015 Oct;21(5 Neurocritical Care):1411–24. [PMID: 26426238]

HEAD INJURY

Trauma is the most common cause of death in young people, and head injury accounts for almost half of these trauma-related deaths. Head injury severity ranges from **concussion** to **severe traumatic brain injury (TBI).** Concussion is broadly defined as an *alteration in mental status caused by trauma with or without loss of consciousness.* The term concussion is often used synonymously with mild TBI. Grades of TBI are traditionally defined by the Glasgow Coma Scale (GCS) measured 30 minutes after injury (Table 24–7).

Head trauma may cause cerebral injury through a variety of mechanisms (Table 24–8). Central to management is determination of which patients need head imaging and

Table 24–7. Glasgow Coma Scale.[1]

Points	Eye Opening	Verbal Response	Motor Response
1	None	None	None
2	To pain	Vocal but not verbal	Extension
3	To voice	Verbal but not conversational	Flexion
4	Spontaneous	Conversational but disoriented	Withdraws from pain
5	Spontaneous	Oriented	Localizes pain
6	Spontaneous	Oriented	Obeys commands

[1]GCS score indicating severity of traumatic brain injury (TBI): **mild**, 13–15; **moderate**, 9–12; **severe**, ≤ 8.
Reproduced, with permission, from Aminoff MJ et al. *Clinical Neurology*, 9th ed, McGraw-Hill Education, 2015; Data from Teasdale G, Jennett B. Assessment of coma and impaired consciousness. A practical scale. *Lancet*. 1974;304:81–4.

observation. Of particular concern is identification of patients with epidural and subdural hematoma, who may present with normal neurologic findings shortly after injury (lucid interval) but rapidly deteriorate thereafter, and in whom surgical intervention is life-saving.

► **Clinical Findings**

A. Symptoms and Signs

Common symptoms of concussion that develop acutely include headache, nausea, vomiting, confusion, disorientation, dizziness, and imbalance. A period of amnesia encompassing the traumatic event and a variable period of time leading up to the trauma is typical. Loss of consciousness may occur. Additional symptoms of photophobia, phonophobia, difficulty concentrating, irritability, and sleep and mood disturbances may develop over the following hours to days. Examination is usually normal, although orientation and attention, short-term memory, and reaction time may be impaired. Persistent or progressive decline in the level of consciousness after the initial injury, or focal neurologic findings, suggests the need for urgent imaging and neurosurgical consultation.

Patients should also be examined for signs of scalp lacerations, facial and skull fracture, and neck injury. The clinical signs of basilar skull fracture include bruising about the orbit (raccoon sign), blood in the external auditory meatus (Battle sign), and leakage of cerebrospinal fluid (which can be identified by its glucose or beta-2-transferrin content) from the ear or nose. Cranial nerve palsies (involving especially the first, second, third, fourth, fifth, seventh, and eighth nerves in any combination) may also occur. The head and neck should be immobilized until imaging can be performed.

Table 24–8. Acute cerebral sequelae of head injury.

Sequelae	Clinical Features	Pathology
Concussion	A transient, trauma-induced alteration in mental status that may or may not involve loss of consciousness. Symptoms and signs include headache, nausea, disorientation, irritability, amnesia, clumsiness, visual disturbances, and focal neurologic deficit.	Unknown; likely mild diffuse axonal injury and excitotoxic neuronal injury. Cerebral contusion may occur.
Cerebral contusion or laceration	Loss of consciousness longer than with concussion. Focal neurologic deficits are often present. May lead to death or severe residual neurologic deficit.	Bruising on side of impact (coup injury) or contralaterally (contrecoup injury). Vasogenic edema, multiple petechial hemorrhages, and mass effect. May have subarachnoid bleeding. Herniation may occur in severe cases. Cerebral laceration specifically involves tearing of the cerebral tissue and pia-arachnoid overlying a contusion.
Acute epidural hemorrhage	Headache, confusion, somnolence, seizures, and focal deficits occur several hours after injury (lucid interval) and lead to coma, respiratory depression, and death unless treated by surgical evacuation.	Tear in meningeal artery, vein, or dural sinus, leading to hematoma visible on CT scan.
Acute subdural hemorrhage	Similar to epidural hemorrhage, but interval before onset of symptoms is longer. Neurosurgical consultation for consideration of evacuation.	Hematoma from tear in veins from cortex to superior sagittal sinus or from cerebral laceration, visible on CT scan.
Cerebral hemorrhage	Generally develops immediately after injury. Clinically resembles hypertensive hemorrhage. Surgery to relieve mass effect is sometimes necessary.	Hematoma, visible on CT scan.
Diffuse axonal injury	Persistent loss of consciousness, coma, or persistent vegetative state resulting from severe rotational shearing forces or deceleration.	Imaging may be normal or may show tiny, scattered white matter hemorrhages. Histology reveals torn axons.

B. Imaging and Other Investigations

Current recommendations are that head CT be performed in patients with concussion and any of the following: GCS score less than 15; focal neurologic deficit; seizure; coagulopathy; aged 65 or older; skull fracture; persistent headache or vomiting; retrograde amnesia exceeding 30 minutes; intoxication; or soft tissue injury of the head or neck. Otherwise, patients can be sent home as long as a responsible caregiver can *check the patient at hourly intervals* for the next 24 hours. Patients requiring imaging should be admitted unless the head CT is normal, the GCS score is 15, there have been no seizures, there is no predisposition to bleeding, and they can be monitored by a caregiver at home.

Because injury to the spine may have accompanied head trauma, cervical spine radiographs (three views) or CT should always be obtained in comatose patients and in patients with severe neck pain or a deficit possibly related to cord compression.

▶ Treatment

Head injury can often be prevented by helmets, seatbelts, and other protective equipment.

After intracranial bleeding has been excluded clinically or by head CT, treatment of mild TBI is aimed at promoting resolution of postconcussive symptoms and *preventing recurrent injury,* which increases the risk of chronic neurobehavioral impairment and delays recovery. Rarely, a recurrent concussion while a patient is still symptomatic from a first concussion may lead to fatal cerebral edema (**second impact syndrome**). These observations form the basis of the recommendation that patients at risk for recurrent concussion (eg, athletes) be held out of the risky activity until their concussive symptoms have fully resolved.

In patients hospitalized with moderate or severe TBI, management often requires a multidisciplinary approach due to multiple concomitant injuries. Elevated intracranial pressure can result from diffuse axonal injury or a hematoma requiring surgical evacuation, or from a variety of medical causes. Decompressive craniectomy may reduce otherwise refractory intracranial hypertension but does not improve neurologic outcome. Hypothermia is associated with worsened functional outcomes.

Because bridging veins between the brain and venous sinuses become more vulnerable to shear injury as the brain atrophies, a **subdural hematoma** may develop days or weeks following head injury in elderly patients or even occur spontaneously. Clinical presentation can be subtle, often with mental changes such as slowness, drowsiness, headache, confusion, or memory disturbance. Focal neurologic deficits such as hemiparesis or hemisensory disturbance are less common. Surgical intervention is indicated if the hematoma is 10 mm or more in thickness or there is a midline shift of 5 mm or more; if there is a decline in GCS score of 2 or more from injury to hospital admission; or if one or both pupils are fixed and dilated.

Scalp lacerations and depressed skull fractures should be treated surgically as appropriate. Simple skull fractures require no specific treatment. If there is any leakage of cerebrospinal fluid, conservative treatment, with elevation of the head, restriction of fluids, and administration of acetazolamide (250 mg orally four times daily), is often helpful; if the leak continues for more than a few days, lumbar subarachnoid drainage may be necessary. Antibiotics are given if infection occurs, based on culture and sensitivity studies; vaccination against pneumococcus is recommended (see Table 30–7). Only very occasional patients require intracranial repair of the dural defect because of persistence of the leak or recurrent meningitis.

▶ Prognosis

Moderate and severe TBI may result in permanent cognitive and motor impairment depending on the severity and location of the initial injury. Initial GCS and head CT findings have prognostic value. Among patients with a GCS score of 8 or less at presentation, mortality approaches 30% and only one-third of survivors regain functional independence. Cognitive impairment tends to affect frontal and temporal lobe function, causing deficits in attention, memory, judgment, and executive function. Behavioral dysregulation, depression, and disinhibition can impair social functioning. Anosmia, presumably due to shearing of fibers from the nasal epithelium, is common.

Epilepsy can develop after TBI, especially with more severe injury. Among patients with severe TBI (typically loss of consciousness for at least 12–24 hours, intracranial hematoma, depressed skull fracture, or cerebral contusion), phenytoin or levetiracetam is typically given for 7 days to reduce the incidence of early posttraumatic seizures; this is done exclusively to minimize acute complications resulting from such seizures and does not prevent the development of posttraumatic epilepsy.

Among patients with mild TBI, symptoms of concussion resolve in most patients by 1 month and in the vast majority by 3 months. Prolonged postconcussive symptoms are uncommon, persisting at 1 year in 10–15% of patients. Risk factors for prolonged postconcussive symptoms included active litigation regarding the injury; repeated concussions; and GCS score of 13 or less at presentation. Headaches often have migrainous features and may respond to tricyclic antidepressants or beta-blockers (Table 24–1). Opioids should be avoided to minimize the risk of medication overuse headache. Mood symptoms may respond to antidepressants, anxiolytics, and cognitive behavioral therapy.

There appears to be an association between head trauma and the later development of neurodegenerative disease, such as Alzheimer disease, Parkinson disease, or amyotrophic lateral sclerosis (ALS). Normal pressure hydrocephalus may also occur. Repetitive, mild head injury, such as that which occurs in athletes or military personnel, can lead to **chronic traumatic encephalopathy**, a distinct pathologic entity associated with mood and cognitive changes and characterized by the abnormal aggregation of tau or other proteins either focally or globally in the cerebral cortex. Whether chronic traumatic encephalopathy is a static response to recurrent head injury or a progressive neurodegenerative disease is not known, but the severity of neuropathology appears to correlate to lifetime exposure to repetitive head injury.

When to Refer

- Patients with focal neurologic deficits, altered consciousness, or skull fracture.
- Patients with late complications of head injury, eg, posttraumatic seizure disorder or normal pressure hydrocephalus.

When to Admit

- Patients with concussion and GCS score less than 15, predisposition to bleeding, seizure, or no responsible caregiver at home.
- Patients with abnormal head CT.

Levin HS et al. Diagnosis, prognosis, and clinical management of mild traumatic brain injury. Lancet Neurol. 2015 May;14(5):506–17. [PMID: 25801547]
Mez J et al. Clinicopathological evaluation of chronic traumatic encephalopathy in players of American football. JAMA. 2017 Jul 25;318(4):360–70. [PMID: 28742910]
Thompson K et al. Pharmacological treatment for preventing epilepsy following traumatic brain injury. Cochrane Database Syst Rev. 2015 Aug 10;(8):CD009900. [PMID: 26259048]

SPINAL TRAUMA

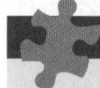

ESSENTIALS OF DIAGNOSIS

- ► History of preceding trauma.
- ► Development of acute neurologic deficit.
- ► Signs of myelopathy on examination.

General Considerations

While spinal cord damage may result from whiplash injury, severe injury usually relates to fracture-dislocation causing compression or angular deformity of the cord either cervically or in the lower thoracic and upper lumbar regions. Extreme hypotension following injury may also lead to cord infarction.

Clinical Findings

Total cord transection results in immediate flaccid paralysis and loss of sensation below the level of the lesion. Reflex activity is lost for a variable period, and there is urinary and fecal retention. As reflex function returns over the following days and weeks, spastic paraplegia or quadriplegia develops, with hyperreflexia and extensor plantar responses, but a flaccid atrophic (lower motor neuron) paralysis may be found depending on the segments of the cord that are affected. The bladder and bowels also regain some reflex function, permitting urine and feces to be expelled at intervals. As spasticity increases, flexor or extensor spasms (or both) of the legs become troublesome, especially if the patient develops bed sores or a urinary tract infection. Paraplegia with the legs in flexion or extension may eventually result.

With lesser degrees of injury, patients may be left with mild limb weakness, distal sensory disturbance, or both. Sphincter function may also be impaired, urinary urgency and urge incontinence being especially common. More particularly, a unilateral cord lesion leads to an ipsilateral motor disturbance with accompanying impairment of proprioception and contralateral loss of pain and temperature appreciation below the lesion (**Brown-Séquard syndrome**). A central cord syndrome may lead to a lower motor neuron deficit at the level of the lesion and loss of pain and temperature appreciation below it, with sparing of posterior column functions. With more extensive involvement, posterior column sensation may also be impaired and pyramidal weakness develops. A radicular deficit may occur at the level of the injury—or, if the cauda equina is involved, there may be evidence of disturbed function in several lumbosacral roots.

Treatment

Treatment of the injury consists of immobilization and—if there is cord compression—early decompressive laminectomy and fusion (within 24 hours). Early treatment with high doses of corticosteroids (eg, methylprednisolone, 30 mg/kg by intravenous bolus, followed by 5.4 mg/kg/h for 23 hours) may improve neurologic recovery if commenced within 8 hours after injury, although the evidence is limited and some neurosurgical guidelines do not recommend their use. Anatomic realignment of the spinal cord by traction and other orthopedic procedures is important. Subsequent care of the residual neurologic deficit—paraplegia or quadriplegia—requires treatment of spasticity and care of the skin, bladder, and bowels.

When to Refer

All patients with focal neurologic deficits should be referred.

When to Admit

- Patients with neurologic deficits.
- Patients with spinal cord injury, compression, or acute epidural or subdural hematoma.
- Patients with vertebral fracture-dislocation likely to compress the cord.

Stein DM et al. Management of acute spinal cord injury. Continuum (Minneap Minn). 2015 Feb;21(1 Spinal Cord Disorders):159–87. [PMID: 25651224]

SYRINGOMYELIA

Destruction or degeneration of gray and white matter adjacent to the central canal of the cervical spinal cord leads to cavitation and accumulation of fluid within the spinal cord. The precise pathogenesis is unclear, but many cases are associated with **Arnold-Chiari malformation**, in which there is displacement of the cerebellar tonsils, medulla, and fourth ventricle into the spinal canal, sometimes with accompanying meningomyelocele. In such circumstances, the cord cavity connects with and may merely represent a dilated central canal. In other cases, the cause of cavitation is less clear. There is a characteristic clinical picture, with segmental atrophy, areflexia, and loss of pain and temperature appreciation in a "cape" distribution, owing to the destruction of fibers crossing in front of the central canal in the mid-cervical spinal cord. Thoracic kyphoscoliosis is usually present. With progression, involvement of the long motor and sensory tracts occurs as well, so that a pyramidal and sensory deficit develops in the legs. Upward extension of the cavitation (syringobulbia) leads to dysfunction of the lower brainstem and thus to bulbar palsy, nystagmus, and sensory impairment over one or both sides of the face.

Syringomyelia, ie, cord cavitation, may also occur in association with an intramedullary tumor or following severe cord injury, and the cavity then does not communicate with the central canal.

In patients with Arnold-Chiari malformation, CT scans reveal a small posterior fossa and enlargement of the foramen magnum, along with other associated skeletal abnormalities at the base of the skull and upper cervical spine. MRI reveals the syrinx as well as the characteristic findings of the Arnold-Chiari malformation, including the caudal displacement of the fourth ventricle and herniation of the cerebellar tonsils through the foramen magnum. Focal cord enlargement is found at myelography or by MRI in patients with cavitation related to past injury or intramedullary neoplasms.

Treatment of Arnold-Chiari malformation with associated syringomyelia is by suboccipital craniectomy and upper cervical laminectomy, with the aim of decompressing the malformation at the foramen magnum. The cord cavity should be drained and, if necessary, an outlet for the fourth ventricle can be made. In cavitation associated with intramedullary tumor, treatment is surgical, but radiation therapy may be necessary if complete removal is not possible. Posttraumatic syringomyelia is also treated surgically if it leads to increasing neurologic deficits or to intolerable pain.

DEGENERATIVE MOTOR NEURON DISEASES

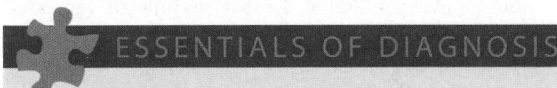

ESSENTIALS OF DIAGNOSIS

- ► Weakness.
- ► No sensory loss or sphincter disturbance.
- ► Progressive course.
- ► No identifiable underlying cause other than genetic basis in familial cases.

General Considerations

This group of degenerative disorders is characterized clinically by weakness and variable wasting of affected muscles, without accompanying sensory changes.

Motor neuron disease in adults generally commences between 30 and 60 years of age. There is degeneration of the anterior horn cells in the spinal cord, the motor nuclei of the lower cranial nerves, and the corticospinal and corticobulbar pathways. The disorder is usually sporadic, but familial cases may occur and several genetic mutations or loci have been identified. Cigarette smoking may be one risk factor.

Classification

Five varieties have been distinguished on clinical grounds.

A. Progressive Bulbar Palsy

Bulbar involvement predominates owing to disease processes affecting primarily the motor nuclei of the cranial nerves.

B. Pseudobulbar Palsy

Bulbar involvement predominates in this variety also, but it is due to bilateral corticobulbar disease and thus reflects upper motor neuron dysfunction. There may be a "pseudobulbar affect," with uncontrollable episodes of laughing or crying to stimuli that would not normally have elicited such marked reactions.

C. Progressive Spinal Muscular Atrophy

This is characterized primarily by a lower motor neuron deficit in the limbs due to degeneration of the anterior horn cells in the spinal cord.

D. Primary Lateral Sclerosis

There is a purely upper motor neuron deficit in the limbs.

E. Amyotrophic Lateral Sclerosis (ALS)

A mixed upper and lower motor neuron deficit is found in the limbs. This disorder is sometimes associated with cognitive decline (in a pattern consistent with frontotemporal dementia), a pseudobulbar affect, or parkinsonism. Approximately 10% of ALS cases are familial and have been associated with mutations at several different genetic loci, including a hexanucleotide repeat on chromosome 9 that also associates with frontotemporal dementia.

Differential Diagnosis

The spinal muscular atrophies (SMAs) are inherited syndromes caused most often by mutations of the survival motor neuron 1 (*SMN1*) gene on chromosome 5. Different mutations result in more or less severe disruptions of the protein, resulting in an age of onset that ranges from infancy (SMA type I; Werdnig-Hoffmann disease), to early (type II) or late childhood (type III; Kugelberg-Welander syndrome), to adulthood (type IV). X-linked bulbospinal neuronopathy (Kennedy syndrome) is associated with an expanded trinucleotide repeat sequence on the androgen receptor gene and carries a more benign prognosis than other forms of motor neuron disease.

There are reports of juvenile SMA due to hexosaminidase deficiency. Pure motor syndromes resembling motor neuron disease may also occur in association with monoclonal gammopathy or multifocal motor neuropathies with conduction block. A motor neuronopathy may also develop in Hodgkin disease and has a relatively benign prognosis. Infective anterior horn cell diseases (polio virus or West Nile virus infection) can generally be distinguished by the acute onset and monophasic course of the illness, as discussed in Chapter 32.

Clinical Findings

A. Symptoms and Signs

Difficulty in swallowing, chewing, coughing, breathing, and talking (dysarthria) occurs with bulbar involvement. In progressive bulbar palsy, there is drooping of the palate; a depressed gag reflex; pooling of saliva in the pharynx; a weak cough; and a wasted, fasciculating tongue. In pseudobulbar palsy, the tongue is contracted and spastic and cannot be moved rapidly from side to side. Limb involvement is characterized by motor disturbances (weakness, stiffness, wasting, fasciculations) reflecting lower or upper motor neuron dysfunction; there are no objective changes on sensory examination, although there may be vague sensory complaints. The sphincters are generally spared. Cognitive changes or pseudobulbar affect may be present. The disorder is progressive, and ALS is usually fatal within 3–5 years; death usually results from pulmonary infections. Patients with bulbar involvement generally have the poorest prognosis, while patients with primary lateral sclerosis often have a longer survival despite profound quadriparesis and spasticity.

B. Laboratory and Other Studies

Electromyography may show signs of acute and chronic partial denervation with reinnervation. In patients with suspected ALS, the diagnosis should not be made with confidence unless such changes are found in at least three spinal regions (cervical, thoracic, lumbosacral) or two spinal regions and the bulbar musculature. Motor conduction velocity is usually normal but may be slightly reduced, and sensory conduction studies are also normal. Biopsy of a wasted muscle shows the histologic changes of denervation but is not necessary for diagnosis. The serum creatine kinase may be slightly elevated but never reaches the extremely high values seen in some of the muscular dystrophies. The cerebrospinal fluid is normal. To diagnose SMA, molecular genetic testing for pathogenic variants of SMN1 is available. There are abnormal findings on rectal biopsy and reduced hexosaminidase A in serum and leukocytes in patients with juvenile SMA due to hexosaminidase deficiency.

Treatment

Riluzole, 50 mg orally twice daily, which reduces the presynaptic release of glutamate, increased short-term survival in ALS in randomized trials. Edaravone, a free radical scavenger, slows disease progression in patients with mild disease. It is administered in monthly cycles as a 60 mg intravenous infusion on days 1–14 in the first month and days 1–10 in the subsequent months.

Noninvasive ventilation at least 4 hours per day in patients with a maximal inspiratory pressure less than 60 cm H_2O may prolong survival in ALS. Symptomatic and supportive measures to treat spasticity (discussed earlier), drooling, and dysphagia, prevent contractures, and preserve mobility are important. Drooling is treated with over-the-counter decongestants, anticholinergic medications (such as trihexyphenidyl, amitriptyline, or atropine), botulinum toxin injections into the salivary glands, or use of a portable suction machine. Physical and occupational therapy are helpful throughout the disease course. Combination dextromethorphan/quinidine (20 mg/10 mg, one tablet orally once or twice daily) may relieve symptoms of pseudobulbar affect. A semiliquid diet or gastrostomy tube feeding may be needed if dysphagia is severe; it is advisable to perform the procedure before the forced vital capacity falls below 50% of predicted to minimize the risk of complications. Tracheostomy is sometimes performed if respiratory muscles are severely affected; however, in the terminal stages of these disorders, realistic expectations and advance care planning should be discussed. Information on palliative care is provided in Chapter 5.

Treatment of spinal muscular atrophy takes advantage of the fact that the SMN protein is also encoded by a second gene, SMN2, that usually does not translate functional protein due to aberrant splicing. Nusinersen is an antisense oligonucleotide that modulates premessenger RNA splicing of the SMN2 gene and results in increased production of the full length protein. Intrathecal administration resulted in achievement of motor milestones and prolonged survival in infants with type 1 SMA and improved motor function in children with later-onset disease. Gene therapy with intravenous delivery of an intact SMN1 gene using a viral vector also shows promise.

When to Refer

All patients (to exclude other treatable causes of symptoms and signs) should be referred.

When to Admit

Patients may need to be admitted for initiation or titration of noninvasive ventilation, or for periods of increased requirement of noninvasive ventilator support during pulmonary infections.

Edaravone (MCI-186) ALS 19 Study Group. Safety and efficacy of edaravone in well defined patients with amyotrophic lateral sclerosis: a randomized, double-blind, placebo-controlled trial. Lancet Neurol. 2017 Jul;16(7):505–12. [PMID: 28522181]

Finkel RS et al; ENDEAR Study Group. Nusinersen versus sham control in infantile-onset spinal muscular atrophy. N Engl J Med. 2017 Nov 2;377(18):1723–32. [PMID: 29091570]

Mendell JR et al. Single-dose gene-replacement therapy for spinal muscular atrophy. N Engl J Med. 2017 Nov 2;377(18):1713–22. [PMID: 29091557]

Mercuri E et al; CHERISH Study Group. Nusinersen versus sham control in later-onset spinal muscular atrophy. N Engl J Med. 2018 Feb 15;378(7):625–35. [PMID: 29443664]

PERIPHERAL NEUROPATHIES

Peripheral neuropathies can be categorized on the basis of the structure primarily affected. The predominant pathologic feature may be **axonal degeneration (axonal or neuronal neuropathies)** or **paranodal or segmental demyelination.** The distinction may be possible on the basis of neurophysiologic findings. Motor and sensory conduction velocity can be measured in accessible segments of peripheral nerves. In axonal neuropathies, conduction velocity is normal or reduced only mildly and needle electromyography provides evidence of denervation in affected muscles. In demyelinating neuropathies, conduction may be slowed considerably in affected fibers, and in more severe cases, conduction is blocked completely, without accompanying electromyographic signs of denervation.

POLYNEUROPATHIES & MONONEURITIS MULTIPLEX

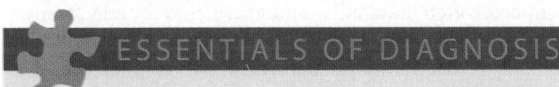

ESSENTIALS OF DIAGNOSIS

- Weakness, sensory disturbances, or both in the extremities.
- Pain is common.
- Depressed or absent tendon reflexes.
- May be family history of neuropathy.
- May be history of systemic illness or toxic exposure.

General Considerations

Diffuse **polyneuropathies** lead to a symmetric sensory, motor, or mixed deficit, often most marked distally. They include the hereditary, metabolic, and toxic disorders; idiopathic inflammatory polyneuropathy (**Guillain-Barré syndrome**); and the peripheral neuropathies that may occur as a nonmetastatic complication of malignant diseases. Involvement of motor fibers leads to flaccid weakness that is most marked distally; dysfunction of sensory fibers causes impaired sensory perception. Tendon reflexes are depressed or absent. Paresthesias, pain, and muscle tenderness may also occur. Multiple mononeuropathies (**mononeuropathy multiplex**) suggest a patchy multifocal disease process such as vasculopathy (eg, diabetes, arteritis), an infiltrative process (eg, leprosy, sarcoidosis), radiation damage, or an immunologic disorder (eg, brachial plexopathy).

Clinical Findings

The cause of polyneuropathy or mononeuritis multiplex is suggested by the history, mode of onset, and predominant clinical manifestations. Laboratory workup includes a complete blood count, serum protein electrophoresis with reflex to immunofixation or immunotyping, determination of plasma urea and electrolytes, liver biochemical tests,

thyroid function tests, vitamin B_{12} level, tests for rheumatoid factor and antinuclear antibody, HBsAg determination, a serologic test for syphilis, fasting blood glucose level and hemoglobin A_{1c}, urinary heavy metal levels, cerebrospinal fluid examination, and chest radiography. These tests should be ordered selectively, as guided by symptoms and signs. Measurement of nerve conduction velocity can confirm the peripheral nerve origin of symptoms and provides a means of following clinical changes, as well as indicate the likely disease process (ie, axonal or demyelinating neuropathy). Cutaneous nerve biopsy may help establish a precise diagnosis (eg, polyarteritis, amyloidosis). In about half of cases, no specific cause can be established; of these, slightly less than half are subsequently found to be familial.

Treatment

Treatment is of the underlying cause, when feasible, and is discussed below under the individual disorders. Physical therapy helps prevent contractures, and splints can maintain a weak extremity in a position of useful function. Anesthetic extremities must be protected from injury. To guard against burns, patients should check the temperature of water and hot surfaces with a portion of skin having normal sensation, measure water temperature with a thermometer, and use cold water for washing or lower the temperature setting of their hot-water heaters. Shoes should be examined frequently during the day for grit or foreign objects in order to prevent pressure lesions.

Patients with polyneuropathies or mononeuritis multiplex are subject to additional nerve injury at pressure points and should therefore avoid such behavior as leaning on elbows or sitting with crossed legs for lengthy periods.

Neuropathic, burning pain may respond to simple analgesics, such as aspirin or nonsteroidal anti-inflammatory agents, and to gabapentin (300 mg orally three times daily, titrated up to a maximum of 1200 mg orally three times daily as necessary) or pregabalin (50–100 mg orally three times daily). Duloxetine (60 mg orally once or twice daily), venlafaxine (start 37.5 mg orally twice daily, and titrate up to 75 mg orally two to three times daily), or tricyclic antidepressants (eg, amitriptyline 10–150 mg orally at bedtime daily) may be helpful, especially in painful diabetic neuropathy. Medical cannabis may provide some relief, but long-term safety data are lacking. The use of a frame or cradle to reduce contact with bedclothes may be helpful. Many patients experience episodic stabbing pains, which may respond to gabapentin, pregabalin, carbamazepine (start 100 mg orally twice daily, and titrate up to 400 mg orally twice daily), or tricyclic antidepressants. Opioids may be necessary for severe hyperpathia or pain induced by minimal stimuli, but their use generally should be avoided.

Symptoms of **autonomic dysfunction** are occasionally troublesome. Treatment of postural hypotension is discussed earlier in this chapter. Erectile dysfunction can be treated with phosphodiesterase inhibitors; a flaccid neuropathic bladder may respond to parasympathomimetic medications such as bethanechol chloride, 10–50 mg three or four times daily.

Callaghan BC et al. Distal symmetric polyneuropathy: a review. JAMA. 2015 Nov 24;314(20):2172–81. [PMID: 26599185]

Watson JC et al. Peripheral neuropathy: a practical approach to diagnosis and symptom management. Mayo Clin Proc. 2015 Jul; 90(7):940–51. [PMID: 26141332]

1. Inherited Neuropathies

A. Charcot-Marie-Tooth Disease (HMSN Type I, II)

There are several distinct varieties of Charcot-Marie-Tooth disease, usually with an autosomal dominant mode of inheritance, but occasional cases occur on a sporadic, recessive, or X-linked basis. Clinical presentation may be with foot deformities or gait disturbances in childhood or early adult life. Slow progression leads to the typical features of polyneuropathy, with distal weakness and wasting that begin in the legs, a variable amount of distal sensory loss, and depressed or absent tendon reflexes. Tremor is a conspicuous feature in some instances. Hereditary motor and sensory neuropathy (HMSN) type I is characterized by demyelination on electrodiagnostic studies and is usually caused by mutations in the peripheral myelin protein 22 or myelin protein zero gene. In HMSN type II, electrodiagnostic studies show axonal loss rather than demyelination; one-third of cases are due to mutations in the gene mitofusin 2.

A similar disorder may occur in patients with progressive distal spinal muscular atrophies, but there is no sensory loss; electrophysiologic investigation reveals that motor conduction velocity is normal or only slightly reduced, and nerve action potentials are normal.

B. Dejerine-Sottas Disease (HMSN Type III)

The disorder may occur on a sporadic, autosomal dominant or, less commonly, autosomal recessive basis. Onset in infancy or childhood leads to a progressive motor and sensory polyneuropathy with weakness, ataxia, sensory loss, and depressed or absent tendon reflexes. The peripheral nerves may be palpably enlarged and are characterized pathologically by segmental demyelination, Schwann cell hyperplasia, and thin myelin sheaths. Electrophysiologically, there is a slowing of conduction, and sensory action potentials may be unrecordable.

C. Friedreich Ataxia

This disorder, the only known autosomal recessive trinucleotide repeat disease, is caused by expansion of a poly-GAA locus in the gene for frataxin on chromosome 9, leading to symptoms in childhood or early adult life. The gait becomes ataxic, the hands become clumsy, and other signs of cerebellar dysfunction develop accompanied by weakness of the legs and extensor plantar responses. Involvement of peripheral sensory fibers leads to sensory disturbances in the limbs and depressed tendon reflexes. There is bilateral pes cavus. Pathologically, there is a marked loss of cells in the posterior root ganglia and degeneration of peripheral sensory fibers. In the central nervous system, changes are conspicuous in the posterior and lateral columns of the cord. Electrophysiologically,

conduction velocity in motor fibers is normal or only mildly reduced, but sensory action potentials are small or absent. Cardiac disease is the most common cause of death.

In the differential diagnosis for Friedreich ataxia are other spinocerebellar ataxias, a growing group of at least 30 inherited disorders, each involving a different identified gene. These heterogeneous disorders, which frequently (but not exclusively) exhibit an autosomal dominant inheritance pattern and poly-CAG expansion of the affected gene, typically cause cerebellar ataxia and varying combinations of other symptoms (such as peripheral neuropathy, ophthalmoparesis, dysarthria, and pyramidal and extrapyramidal signs).

D. Refsum Disease (HMSN Type IV)

This autosomal recessive disorder is due to a disturbance in phytanic acid metabolism. Pigmentary retinal degeneration is accompanied by progressive sensorimotor polyneuropathy and cerebellar signs. Auditory dysfunction, cardiomyopathy, and cutaneous manifestations may also occur. Motor and sensory conduction velocities are reduced, often markedly, and there may be electromyographic evidence of denervation in affected muscles. Dietary restriction of phytanic acid and its precursors may be helpful therapeutically. Plasmapheresis to reduce stored phytanic acid may help at the initiation of treatment.

E. Porphyria

Peripheral nerve involvement may occur during acute attacks in both **variegate porphyria** and **acute intermittent porphyria.** Motor symptoms usually occur first, and weakness is often most marked proximally and in the upper limbs rather than the lower. Sensory symptoms and signs may be proximal or distal in distribution. Autonomic involvement is sometimes pronounced. The electrophysiologic findings are in keeping with the results of neuropathologic studies suggesting that the neuropathy is axonal in type (see Chapter 40).

F. Familial Amyloid Polyneuropathy

Sensory and autonomic symptoms are especially conspicuous, whereas distal wasting and weakness occur later. The polyneuropathy is axonal and likely results from amyloid deposition within the peripheral nerves due to mutations in the genes encoding transthyretin, apolipoprotein A1, or gelsolin. Transthyretin amyloidosis is the most common; is associated with cardiomyopathy, nephropathy, leptomeningeal involvement, and vitreous opacity; and is treatable with liver transplantation, the small interfering ribonucleic acid patisiran (0.3 mg/kg up to 30 mg intravenously once every 3 weeks), or the antisense oligonucleotide inotersen (284 mg subcutaneously weekly).

2. Neuropathies Associated with Systemic & Metabolic Disorders

A. Diabetes Mellitus

In this disorder, involvement of the peripheral nervous system may lead to symmetric sensory or mixed polyneuropathy, asymmetric motor radiculoneuropathy or plexopathy (diabetic amyotrophy), thoracoabdominal radiculopathy, autonomic neuropathy, or isolated lesions of individual nerves. These may occur singly or in any combination and are discussed in Chapter 27.

B. Uremia

Uremia may lead to a symmetric sensorimotor polyneuropathy that tends to affect the lower limbs more than the upper limbs and is more marked distally than proximally (see Chapter 22). The diagnosis can be confirmed electrophysiologically because motor and sensory conduction velocity is moderately reduced. The neuropathy improves both clinically and electrophysiologically with kidney transplantation and to a lesser extent with chronic dialysis.

C. Alcoholism and Nutritional Deficiency

Many patients with alcoholism have an axonal distal sensorimotor polyneuropathy that is frequently accompanied by painful cramps, muscle tenderness, and painful paresthesias and is often more marked in the legs than in the arms. Symptoms of autonomic dysfunction may also be conspicuous. Motor and sensory conduction velocity may be slightly reduced, even in subclinical cases, but gross slowing of conduction is uncommon. Treatment is similar to diabetic polyneuropathy but also includes abstinence from alcohol. A similar distal sensorimotor polyneuropathy is a well-recognized feature of beriberi (thiamine deficiency). In vitamin B_{12} deficiency, distal sensory polyneuropathy may develop but is usually overshadowed by central nervous system manifestations (eg, myelopathy, optic neuropathy, or intellectual changes).

D. Paraproteinemias

A symmetric sensorimotor polyneuropathy that is gradual in onset, progressive in course, and often accompanied by pain and dysesthesias in the limbs may occur in patients (especially men) with **plasma cell myeloma** (formerly multiple myeloma). The neuropathy is of the axonal type in classic lytic myeloma, but segmental demyelination (primary or secondary) and axonal loss may occur in sclerotic myeloma and lead to predominantly motor clinical manifestations. Both demyelinating and axonal neuropathies are also observed in patients with paraproteinemias without myeloma. A small fraction will develop myeloma if serially followed. The demyelinating neuropathy in these patients may be due to the monoclonal proteins reacting to a component of the nerve myelin. The neuropathy of classic plasma cell myeloma is poorly responsive to therapy. The polyneuropathy of benign monoclonal gammopathy may respond to immunosuppressant medications and plasmapheresis.

Polyneuropathy may also occur in association with monoclonal gammopathy of unknown significance, macroglobulinemia, and cryoglobulinemia and sometimes responds to plasmapheresis. Many patients with an IgM M-protein will have antibodies to myelin-associated glycoprotein (MAG); these patients may respond to treatment with rituximab. Entrapment neuropathy, such as carpal tunnel syndrome, is more common than polyneuropathy in patients with (nonhereditary) generalized amyloidosis.

3. Neuropathies Associated with Infectious & Inflammatory Diseases

A. Leprosy

Leprosy is an important cause of peripheral neuropathy in certain parts of the world. Sensory disturbances are mainly due to involvement of intracutaneous nerves. In tuberculoid leprosy, they develop at the same time and in the same distribution as the nerve; trunks lying beneath the lesion are also involved. In lepromatous leprosy, there is more extensive sensory loss, and this develops earlier and to a greater extent in the coolest regions of the body, such as the dorsal surfaces of the hands and feet, where the bacilli proliferate most actively. Motor deficits result from involvement of superficial nerves where their temperature is lowest, eg, the ulnar nerve in the region proximal to the olecranon groove, the median nerve as it emerges from beneath the forearm flexor muscle to run toward the carpal tunnel, the peroneal nerve at the head of the fibula, and the posterior tibial nerve in the lower part of the leg; patchy facial muscular weakness may also occur owing to involvement of the superficial branches of the seventh cranial nerve.

Motor disturbances in leprosy are suggestive of multiple mononeuropathy, whereas sensory changes resemble those of distal polyneuropathy. Examination, however, relates the distribution of sensory deficits to the temperature of the tissues; in the legs, for example, sparing frequently occurs between the toes and in the popliteal fossae, where the temperature is higher. Treatment is with antileprotic agents (see Chapter 33).

B. AIDS

A variety of neuropathies occur in HIV-infected patients (see Chapter 31).

C. Lyme Borreliosis

The neurologic manifestations of Lyme disease include meningitis, meningoencephalitis, polyradiculoneuropathy, mononeuropathy multiplex, and cranial neuropathy. Serologic tests establish the underlying disorder. Lyme disease and its treatment are discussed in depth in Chapter 34.

D. Sarcoidosis

Cranial nerve palsies (especially facial palsy), multiple mononeuropathy and, less commonly, symmetric polyneuropathy may all occur, the latter sometimes preferentially affecting either motor or sensory fibers. Improvement may occur with use of corticosteroids.

E. Polyarteritis

Involvement of the vasa nervorum by the vasculitic process may result in infarction of the nerve. Clinically, one encounters an asymmetric sensorimotor polyneuropathy (mononeuritis multiplex) that pursues a waxing and waning course. Corticosteroids and cytotoxic agents— especially cyclophosphamide—may be of benefit in severe cases (Chapter 20).

F. Rheumatoid Arthritis

Compressive or entrapment neuropathies, ischemic neuropathies, mild distal sensory polyneuropathy, and severe progressive sensorimotor polyneuropathy can occur in rheumatoid arthritis.

4. Neuropathy Associated with Critical Illness

Patients in intensive care units with sepsis and multiorgan failure sometimes develop polyneuropathies. This may be manifested initially by unexpected difficulty in weaning patients from a mechanical ventilator and in more advanced cases by wasting and weakness of the extremities and loss of tendon reflexes. Sensory abnormalities are relatively inconspicuous. The neuropathy is axonal in type. Its pathogenesis is obscure, and treatment is supportive. The prognosis is good provided patients recover from the underlying critical illness.

5. Toxic Neuropathies

Axonal polyneuropathy may follow exposure to industrial agents or pesticides such as acrylamide, organophosphorus compounds, hexacarbon solvents, methyl bromide, and carbon disulfide; metals such as arsenic, thallium, mercury, and lead; and medications such as phenytoin, amiodarone, perhexiline, isoniazid, nitrofurantoin, vincristine, and pyridoxine in high doses. Detailed occupational, environmental, and medical histories and recognition of clusters of cases are important in suggesting the diagnosis. Treatment is by preventing further exposure to the causal agent. Isoniazid neuropathy is prevented by pyridoxine supplementation.

Diphtheritic neuropathy results from a neurotoxin released by the causative organism and is common in many areas. Palatal weakness may develop 2–4 weeks after infection of the throat, and infection of the skin may similarly be followed by focal weakness of neighboring muscles. Disturbances of accommodation may occur about 4–5 weeks after infection and distal sensorimotor demyelinating polyneuropathy after 1–3 months.

6. Neuropathies Associated with Malignant Diseases

A variety of neuropathies have been associated with nonmetastatic complications of malignancy and were discussed earlier.

7. Acute Idiopathic Polyneuropathy (Guillain-Barré Syndrome)

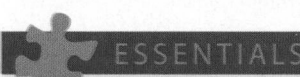

> ► Acute or subacute progressive polyradiculoneuropathy.
> ► Weakness is more severe than sensory disturbances.
> ► Acute dysautonomia may be life-threatening.

► General Considerations

This acute or subacute polyradiculoneuropathy sometimes follows infective illness, inoculations, or surgical procedures. There is an association with preceding *Campylobacter jejuni* enteritis. The disorder probably has an immunologic basis, but the precise mechanism is unclear.

► Clinical Findings

A. Symptoms and Signs

The main complaint is of weakness that varies widely in severity in different patients and often has a proximal emphasis and symmetric distribution. It usually begins in the legs, spreading to a variable extent but frequently involving the arms and often one or both sides of the face. The muscles of respiration or deglutition may also be affected. Sensory symptoms are usually less conspicuous than motor ones, but distal paresthesias and dysesthesias are common, and neuropathic or radicular pain is present in many patients. Autonomic disturbances are also common, may be severe, and are sometimes life-threatening; they include tachycardia, cardiac irregularities, hypotension or hypertension, facial flushing, abnormalities of sweating, pulmonary dysfunction, and impaired sphincter control. The axonal subtypes of the syndrome (**acute motor axonal neuropathy [AMAN]** and **acute motor and sensory axonal neuropathy [AMSAN]**) are caused by antibodies to gangliosides on the axon membrane. The **Miller Fisher syndrome,** another subtype, is characterized by the clinical triad of ophthalmoplegia, ataxia, and areflexia, and is associated with anti-GQ1b antibodies.

B. Laboratory Findings

The cerebrospinal fluid characteristically contains a high protein concentration with a normal cell count, but these changes may take up to 2 weeks to develop; white blood cell counts greater than 50 cells/mcL should prompt consideration of alternative diagnoses. Electrophysiologic studies may reveal marked abnormalities, which do not necessarily parallel the clinical disorder in their temporal course.

► Differential Diagnosis

When the diagnosis is made, the history and appropriate laboratory studies should exclude the possibility of porphyric, diphtheritic, or toxic (heavy metal, hexacarbon, organophosphate) neuropathies, and of HIV infection. The temporal course excludes other peripheral neuropathies. Poliomyelitis, botulism, and tick paralysis must also be considered as they cause weakness of acute onset. The presence of pyramidal signs, a markedly asymmetric motor deficit, a sharp sensory level, or early sphincter involvement should suggest a focal cord lesion.

► Treatment

Treatment with prednisone is ineffective and may prolong recovery time. Plasmapheresis is of value; it is best performed within the first few days of illness and is particularly useful for clinically severe or rapidly progressive cases or those with ventilatory impairment. IVIG (400 mg/kg/day for 5 days) is equally helpful. Patients should be admitted to intensive care units if their forced vital capacity is declining, and intubation is considered if the forced vital capacity reaches 15 mL/kg, the maximum inspiratory pressure reaches –30 mm Hg, or dyspnea becomes evident. Declining oxygen saturation is a late indicator of neuromuscular respiratory failure. Respiratory toilet and chest physical therapy help prevent atelectasis. Marked hypotension may respond to volume replacement or pressor agents. Thromboprophylaxis is important.

Prognosis

Most patients eventually make a good recovery, but this may take many months, and about 20% of patients are left with persisting disability. Approximately 3% of patients with acute idiopathic polyneuropathy have one or more clinically similar relapses, sometimes several years after the initial illness.

When to Refer

All patients should be referred.

When to Admit

All patients should be hospitalized until their condition is stable and there is no respiratory compromise.

Willison HJ et al. Guillain-Barré syndrome. Lancet. 2016 Aug 13; 388(10045):717–27. [PMID: 26948435]

8. Chronic Inflammatory Polyneuropathy

Chronic inflammatory demyelinating polyneuropathy, an acquired immunologically mediated disorder, is clinically similar to Guillain-Barré syndrome except that it has a relapsing or steadily progressive course over months or years and that autonomic dysfunction is generally less common. It may present as an exclusively motor disorder or with a mixed sensorimotor disturbance. In the relapsing form, partial recovery may occur after some relapses, but in other instances there is no recovery between exacerbations. Although remission may occur spontaneously with time, the disorder frequently follows a progressive downhill course leading to severe functional disability.

Electrodiagnostic studies show marked slowing of motor and sensory conduction, and focal conduction block. Signs of partial denervation may also be present owing to secondary axonal degeneration. Nerve biopsy may show chronic perivascular inflammatory infiltrates in the endoneurium and epineurium, without accompanying evidence of vasculitis. However, a normal nerve biopsy result or the presence of nonspecific abnormalities does not exclude the diagnosis.

Corticosteroids may arrest or reverse the downhill course. Treatment is usually begun with prednisone, 60–80 mg orally daily, continued for 2–3 months or until a definite response has occurred. If no response has occurred despite 3 months of treatment, a higher dose may be tried. In responsive cases, the dose is gradually tapered, but most patients become corticosteroid-dependent, often requiring prednisone, 20 mg daily on alternate days, on a long-term basis. IVIG can be used in place of, or in addition to corticosteroids, and is best used as the initial treatment in pure motor syndromes; a weekly regimen of 0.2–0.4 g/kg of a 20% subcutaneous immunoglobulin solution is an effective alternative but has not been compared directly to corticosteroids or IVIG. When both IVIG and corticosteroids are ineffective, plasma exchange may be worthwhile. Consistent with the notion that the condition is antibody mediated, rituximab has shown promise. Immunosuppressant or immunomodulatory medications (such as azathioprine) may be added when the response to other measures is unsatisfactory or to enable maintenance doses of corticosteroids to be lowered. Symptomatic treatment is also important.

Mahdi-Rogers M et al. Immunomodulatory treatment other than corticosteroids, immunoglobulin and plasma exchange for chronic inflammatory demyelinating polyneuropathy. Cochrane Database Syst Rev. 2017 May 8;5:CD003280. [PMID: 28481421]

MONONEUROPATHIES

ESSENTIALS OF DIAGNOSIS

► Focal motor or sensory deficit.
► Deficit is in territory of an individual peripheral nerve.

An individual nerve may be injured along its course or may be compressed, angulated, or stretched by neighboring anatomic structures, especially at a point where it passes through a narrow space (**entrapment neuropathy**). The relative contributions of mechanical factors and ischemia to the local damage are not clear. With involvement of a sensory or mixed nerve, pain is commonly felt distal to the lesion. Symptoms never develop with some entrapment neuropathies, resolve rapidly and spontaneously in others, and become progressively more disabling and distressing in yet other cases. The precise neurologic deficit depends on the nerve involved. Percussion of the nerve at the site of the lesion may lead to paresthesias in its distal distribution.

Entrapment neuropathy may be the sole manifestation of subclinical polyneuropathy, and this must be borne in mind and excluded by nerve conduction studies. Such studies are also indispensable for the localization of the focal lesion.

In patients with acute compression neuropathy such as may occur in intoxicated individuals (**Saturday night palsy**), no treatment is necessary. Complete recovery generally occurs, usually within 2 months, presumably because the underlying pathology is demyelination. However, axonal degeneration can occur in severe cases, and recovery then takes longer and may never be complete.

In chronic compressive or entrapment neuropathies, avoidance of aggravating factors and correction of any underlying systemic conditions are important. Local infiltration of the region about the nerve with corticosteroids may be of value; in addition, surgical decompression may help if there is a progressively increasing neurologic deficit or if electrodiagnostic studies show evidence of partial denervation in weak muscles.

Peripheral nerve tumors are uncommon, except in neurofibromatosis type 1, but also give rise to mononeuropathy. This may be distinguishable from entrapment neuropathy only by noting the presence of a mass along the course of the nerve and by demonstrating the precise site of the lesion with appropriate electrophysiologic studies. Treatment of symptomatic lesions is by surgical removal if possible.

1. Carpal Tunnel Syndrome

See Chapter 41.

2. Pronator Teres or Anterior Interosseous Syndrome

The median nerve gives off its motor branch, the anterior interosseous nerve, below the elbow as it descends between the two heads of the pronator teres muscle. A lesion of either nerve may occur in this region, sometimes after trauma or owing to compression from, for example, a fibrous band. With anterior interosseous nerve involvement, there is no sensory loss, and weakness is confined to the pronator quadratus, flexor pollicis longus, and the flexor digitorum profundus to the second and third digits. Weakness is more widespread and sensory changes occur in an appropriate distribution when the median nerve itself is affected. The prognosis is variable. If improvement does not occur spontaneously, decompressive surgery may be helpful.

3. Ulnar Nerve Lesions

Ulnar nerve lesions are likely to occur in the elbow region as the nerve runs behind the medial epicondyle and descends into the cubital tunnel. In the condylar groove, the ulnar nerve is exposed to pressure or trauma. Moreover, any increase in the carrying angle of the elbow, whether congenital, degenerative, or traumatic, may cause excessive stretching of the nerve when the elbow is flexed. Ulnar nerve lesions may also result from thickening or distortion of the anatomic structures forming the cubital tunnel, and the resulting symptoms may also be aggravated by flexion of the elbow, because the tunnel is then narrowed by tightening of its roof or inward bulging of its floor. A severe lesion at either site causes sensory changes in the fifth and medial half of the fourth digits and along the medial border of the hand. There is weakness of the ulnar-innervated muscles in the forearm and hand. With a cubital tunnel lesion, however, there may be relative sparing of the flexor carpi ulnaris muscle. Electrophysiologic evaluation using nerve stimulation techniques allows more precise localization of the lesion.

Initial treatment consists of avoiding pressure on the medial elbow (eg, avoid resting the elbows on arm rests; pad the elbow during sleep) and preventing prolonged elbow flexion, especially at night. Splints are available to keep the elbow from flexing beyond 45 to 90 degrees. If conservative measures are unsuccessful in relieving symptoms and preventing further progression, surgical treatment may be necessary. This consists of nerve transposition if the lesion is in the condylar groove, or a release procedure if it is in the cubital tunnel.

Ulnar nerve lesions may also develop at the wrist or in the palm of the hand, usually owing to repetitive trauma or to compression from ganglia or benign tumors. They can be subdivided depending on their presumed site. Compressive lesions are treated surgically. If repetitive mechanical trauma is responsible, this is avoided by occupational adjustment or job retraining.

4. Radial Nerve Lesions

The radial nerve is particularly liable to compression or injury in the axilla (eg, by crutches or by pressure when the arm hangs over the back of a chair). This leads to weakness or paralysis of all the muscles supplied by the nerve, including the triceps. Sensory changes may also occur but are often surprisingly inconspicuous, being marked only in a small area on the back of the hand between the thumb and index finger. Injuries to the radial nerve in the spiral groove occur characteristically during deep sleep, as in intoxicated individuals, and there is then sparing of the triceps muscle, which is supplied more proximally. The nerve may also be injured at or above the elbow; its purely motor posterior interosseous branch, supplying the extensors of the wrist and fingers, may be involved immediately below the elbow, but then there is sparing of the extensor carpi radialis longus, so that the wrist can still be extended. The superficial radial nerve may be compressed by handcuffs or a tight watch strap.

5. Femoral Neuropathy

The clinical features of femoral nerve palsy consist of weakness and wasting of the quadriceps muscle, with sensory impairment over the anteromedian aspect of the thigh and sometimes also of the leg to the medial malleolus, and a depressed or absent knee jerk. Isolated femoral neuropathy may occur in patients with diabetes or from compression by retroperitoneal neoplasms or hematomas (eg, expanding aortic aneurysm). Femoral neuropathy may also result from pressure from the inguinal ligament when the thighs are markedly flexed and abducted, as in the lithotomy position.

6. Meralgia Paresthetica

The lateral femoral cutaneous nerve, a sensory nerve arising from the L2 and L3 roots, may be compressed or stretched in obese or diabetic patients and during pregnancy. The nerve usually runs under the outer portion of the inguinal ligament to reach the thigh, but the ligament sometimes splits to enclose it. Hyperextension of the hip or increased lumbar lordosis—such as occurs during pregnancy—leads to nerve compression by the posterior fascicle of the ligament. However, entrapment of the nerve at any point along its course may cause similar symptoms, and several other anatomic variations predispose the nerve to damage when it is stretched. Pain, paresthesia, or numbness occurs about the outer aspect of the thigh, usually unilaterally, and is sometimes relieved by sitting. The pain stops at the knee, unlike the pain from lower lumbar sciatica that radiates to the foot. Examination shows no abnormalities except in severe cases when cutaneous sensation is impaired in the affected area. Symptoms are usually mild and commonly settle spontaneously. Hydrocortisone injections medial to the anterosuperior iliac spine often relieve symptoms temporarily, while nerve decompression by transposition may provide more lasting relief.

7. Sciatic & Common Peroneal (Fibular) Nerve Palsies

Misplaced deep intramuscular injections are probably still the most common cause of sciatic nerve palsy. Trauma to the buttock, hip, or thigh may also be responsible. The resulting clinical deficit depends on whether the whole nerve has been affected or only certain fibers. In general, the peroneal (fibular) fibers of the sciatic nerve are more susceptible to damage than those destined for the tibial nerve. A sciatic nerve lesion may therefore be difficult to distinguish from peroneal (fibular) neuropathy unless there is electromyographic evidence of involvement of the short head of the biceps femoris muscle. The common peroneal (fibular) nerve itself may be compressed or injured in the region of the head and neck of the fibula, eg, by sitting with crossed legs or wearing high boots. There is weakness of dorsiflexion and eversion of the foot, accompanied by numbness or blunted sensation of the anterolateral aspect of the calf and dorsum of the foot.

8. Tarsal Tunnel Syndrome

The tibial nerve, the other branch of the sciatic, supplies several muscles in the lower extremity, gives origin to the sural nerve, and then continues as the posterior tibial nerve to supply the plantar flexors of the foot and toes. It passes through the tarsal tunnel behind and below the medial malleolus, giving off calcaneal branches and the medial and lateral plantar nerves that supply small muscles of the foot and the skin on the plantar aspect of the foot and toes. Compression of the posterior tibial nerve or its branches between the bony floor and ligamentous roof of the tarsal tunnel leads to pain, paresthesias, and numbness over the bottom of the foot, especially at night, with sparing of the heel. Muscle weakness may be hard to recognize clinically. Compressive lesions of the individual plantar nerves may also occur more distally, with clinical features similar to those of the tarsal tunnel syndrome. Treatment is surgical decompression.

When to Refer

- If there is uncertainty about the diagnosis.
- Symptoms or signs are progressing despite treatment.

BELL PALSY

ESSENTIALS OF DIAGNOSIS

▸ Sudden onset of lower motor neuron facial palsy.
▸ Hyperacusis or impaired taste may occur.
▸ No other neurologic abnormalities.

General Considerations

Bell palsy is an idiopathic facial paresis of lower motor neuron type that has been attributed to an inflammatory reaction involving the facial nerve near the stylomastoid foramen or in the bony facial canal. In some instances, this may be due to reactivation of herpes simplex or varicella zoster virus infection in the geniculate ganglion. The disorder is more common in pregnant women and in persons with diabetes mellitus.

Clinical Findings

The facial paresis (Figure 24–1) generally comes on abruptly, but it may worsen over the following day or so. Pain about

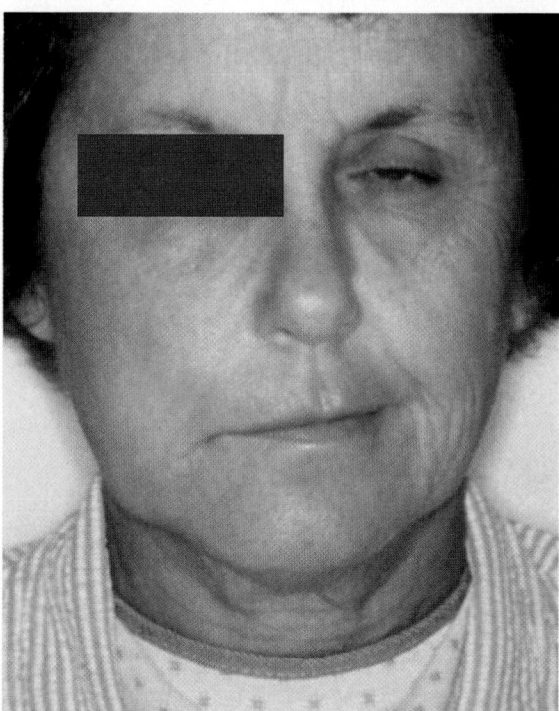

▲ **Figure 24–1.** Facial palsy caused by an infection with *Borrelia burgdorferi* (Lyme disease). (Public Health Image Library, CDC.)

the ear precedes or accompanies the weakness in many cases but usually lasts for only a few days. The face itself feels stiff and pulled to one side. There may be ipsilateral restriction of eye closure and difficulty with eating and fine facial movements. A disturbance of taste is common, owing to involvement of chorda tympani fibers, and hyperacusis due to involvement of fibers to the stapedius occurs occasionally. In cases due to herpes zoster infection, vesicles may be observed in the external ear canal.

Differential Diagnosis

Lower motor neuron facial palsy can be differentiated from stroke by clinical examination. A stroke or other central lesion will not cause hyperacusis or disturbance of taste, generally spares the forehead, and is accompanied by other focal deficits. An isolated facial palsy may occur in patients with HIV seropositivity, sarcoidosis, Lyme disease (Figure 24–1; also see Chapter 34), or any process causing an inflammatory reaction in the subarachnoid space, such as meningitis. Whenever facial palsies occur bilaterally, or a facial palsy occurs in conjunction with other neurologic deficits, MRI brain imaging should be undertaken and other investigations considered.

Treatment

Approximately 60% of cases of Bell palsy recover completely without treatment, presumably because the lesion is so mild that it leads merely to conduction block. Treatment with corticosteroids (prednisone 60 mg orally daily for 5 days followed by a 5-day taper, or prednisolone 25 mg orally twice daily for 10 days) increases the chance of a complete recovery at 9–12 months by 12–15%. Treatment with acyclovir or valacyclovir is only indicated when there is evidence of herpetic vesicles in the external ear canal. It is helpful to protect the eye with lubricating drops (or lubricating ointment at night) and a patch if eye closure is not possible. There is no evidence that surgical procedures to decompress the facial nerve are of benefit. Physical therapy may improve facial function.

Madhok VB et al. Corticosteroids for Bell's palsy (idiopathic facial paralysis). Cochrane Database Syst Rev. 2016 Jul 18; 7:CD001942. [PMID: 27428352]

DISCOGENIC NECK PAIN

ESSENTIALS OF DIAGNOSIS

▶ Neck pain, sometimes radiating to arms.

▶ Restricted neck movements.

▶ Motor, sensory, or reflex changes in arms with root involvement.

▶ Neurologic deficit in legs, gait disorder, or sphincter disturbance with cord involvement.

General Considerations

A variety of congenital abnormalities may involve the cervical spine and lead to neck pain; these include hemivertebrae, fused vertebrae, basilar impression, and instability of the atlantoaxial joint. Traumatic, degenerative, infective, and neoplastic disorders may also lead to pain in the neck. When rheumatoid arthritis involves the spine, it tends to affect especially the cervical region, leading to pain, stiffness, and reduced mobility; displacement of vertebrae or atlantoaxial subluxation may lead to cord compression that can be life-threatening if not treated by fixation. Further details are given in Chapter 41 and discussion here is restricted to disk disease.

1. Acute Cervical Disk Protrusion

Acute cervical disk protrusion leads to pain in the neck and radicular pain in the arm, exacerbated by head movement. With lateral herniation of the disk, motor, sensory, or reflex changes may be found in a radicular (usually C6 or C7) distribution on the affected side (Figure 24–2); with more centrally directed herniations, the spinal cord may also be involved, leading to spastic paraparesis and sensory disturbances in the legs, sometimes accompanied by impaired sphincter function. The diagnosis is confirmed by MRI or CT myelography. In mild cases, the prognosis is good and complete recovery occurs in a majority of patients with conservative therapy. Evidence does not support any specific intervention, and some combination of bed rest, activity restriction, immobilization of the neck in a collar for several weeks, and physical therapy is generally prescribed. If these measures are unsuccessful or the patient has a significant neurologic deficit, surgical removal of the protruding disk may be necessary.

2. Cervical Spondylosis

Cervical spondylosis results from chronic cervical disk degeneration, with herniation of disk material, secondary calcification, and associated osteophytic outgrowths. One or more of the cervical nerve roots may be compressed, stretched, or angulated; and myelopathy may also develop as a result of compression, vascular insufficiency, or recurrent minor trauma to the cord. Patients present with neck pain and restricted head movement, occipital headaches, radicular pain and other sensory disturbances in the arms, weakness of the arms or legs, or some combination of these symptoms. Examination generally reveals that lateral flexion and rotation of the neck are limited. A segmental pattern of weakness or dermatomal sensory loss (or both) may be found unilaterally or bilaterally in the upper limbs, and tendon reflexes mediated by the affected root or roots are depressed. The C5 and C6 nerve roots are most commonly involved, and examination frequently then reveals weakness of muscles supplied by these roots (eg, deltoids, supraspinatus and infraspinatus, biceps, brachioradialis), pain or sensory loss about the shoulder and outer border of the arm and forearm, and depressed biceps and brachioradialis reflexes. Spastic paraparesis may also be present if there is an associated myelopathy, sometimes accompanied by urinary urgency, incontinence, or posterior column or spinothalamic sensory deficits in the legs.

Plain radiographs of the cervical spine show osteophyte formation, narrowing of disk spaces, and encroachment on the intervertebral foramina, but such changes are common in middle-aged persons and may be unrelated to

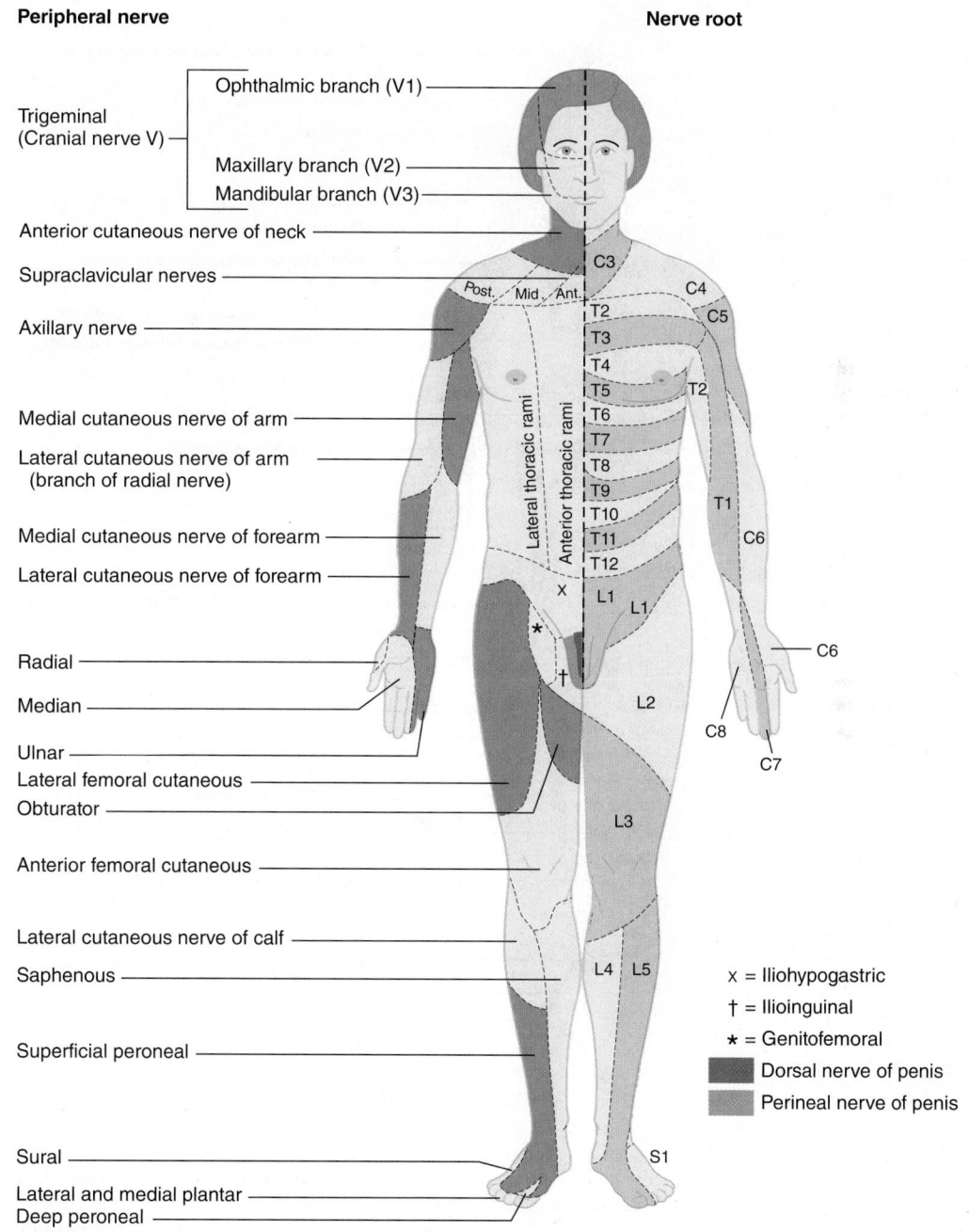

Peripheral nerve   **Nerve root**

Ophthalmic branch (V1)
Trigeminal (Cranial nerve V)
Maxillary branch (V2)
Mandibular branch (V3)
Anterior cutaneous nerve of neck
Supraclavicular nerves
Axillary nerve
Medial cutaneous nerve of arm
Lateral cutaneous nerve of arm (branch of radial nerve)
Medial cutaneous nerve of forearm
Lateral cutaneous nerve of forearm
Radial
Median
Ulnar
Lateral femoral cutaneous
Obturator
Anterior femoral cutaneous
Lateral cutaneous nerve of calf
Saphenous
Superficial peroneal
Sural
Lateral and medial plantar
Deep peroneal

x = Iliohypogastric
† = Ilioinguinal
★ = Genitofemoral
Dorsal nerve of penis
Perineal nerve of penis

▲ **Figure 24–2.** Cutaneous innervation. The segmental or radicular (root) distribution is shown on the left side of the body and the peripheral nerve distribution on the right side. Segmental maps show differences depending on how they were constructed (single root stimulation or section; local anesthetic injection into single dorsal root ganglia). (Adapted, with permission, from Aminoff MJ, Greenberg DA, Simon RP. *Clinical Neurology*, 9th ed. McGraw-Hill Education, 2015.)

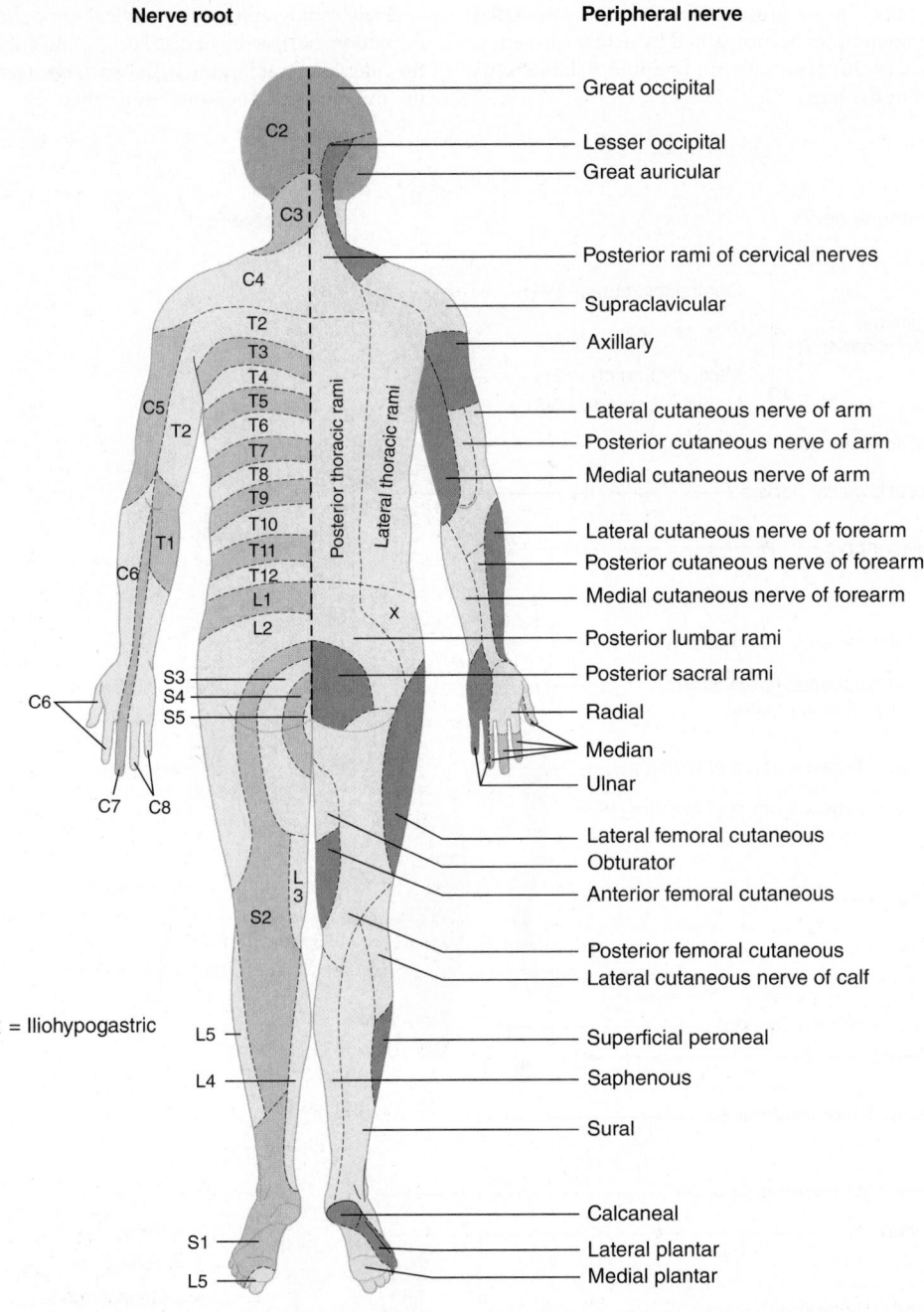

Nerve root

Peripheral nerve

- Great occipital
- Lesser occipital
- Great auricular
- Posterior rami of cervical nerves
- Supraclavicular
- Axillary
- Lateral cutaneous nerve of arm
- Posterior cutaneous nerve of arm
- Medial cutaneous nerve of arm
- Lateral cutaneous nerve of forearm
- Posterior cutaneous nerve of forearm
- Medial cutaneous nerve of forearm
- Posterior lumbar rami
- Posterior sacral rami
- Radial
- Median
- Ulnar
- Lateral femoral cutaneous
- Obturator
- Anterior femoral cutaneous
- Posterior femoral cutaneous
- Lateral cutaneous nerve of calf
- Superficial peroneal
- Saphenous
- Sural
- Calcaneal
- Lateral plantar
- Medial plantar

x = Iliohypogastric

▲ **Figure 24–2.** (continued)

the presenting complaint. CT or MRI helps confirm the diagnosis and exclude other structural causes of the myelopathy.

Restriction of neck movements by a cervical collar may relieve pain. Local injection of anesthetics or corticosteroids, for instance by a pain management specialist, may be of benefit. Operative treatment may be necessary to prevent further progression if there is a significant neurologic deficit; bowel or bladder symptoms; or if root pain is severe, persistent, and unresponsive to conservative measures.

▶ **When to Refer**

- Pain unresponsive to simple measures.
- Patients with neurologic deficits.
- Patients in whom surgical treatment is under consideration.

When to Admit

- Patients with progressive or significant neurologic deficit.
- Patients with sphincter involvement (from cord compression).
- Patients requiring surgical treatment.

Iyer S et al. Cervical radiculopathy. Curr Rev Musculoskelet Med. 2016 Sep;9(3):272–80. [PMID: 27250042]

BRACHIAL & LUMBAR PLEXUS LESIONS

1. Brachial Plexus Neuropathy

Brachial plexus neuropathy may be idiopathic, sometimes occurring in relationship to a number of different nonspecific illnesses or factors. In other instances, brachial plexus lesions follow trauma or result from congenital anomalies, neoplastic involvement, or injury by various physical agents. In rare instances, the disorder occurs on a familial basis.

Idiopathic brachial plexus neuropathy (**neuralgic amyotrophy**) characteristically begins with severe pain about the shoulder, followed within a few days by weakness, reflex changes, and sensory disturbances involving especially the C5 and C6 segments but affecting any nerve in the brachial plexus. Symptoms and signs are usually unilateral but may be bilateral. Wasting of affected muscles is sometimes profound. The disorder relates to disturbed function of cervical roots or part of the brachial plexus, but its precise cause is unknown. Recovery occurs over the ensuing months but may be incomplete. Treatment is purely symptomatic.

2. Cervical Rib Syndrome

Compression of the C8 and T1 roots or the lower trunk of the brachial plexus by a cervical rib or band arising from the seventh cervical vertebra leads to weakness and wasting of intrinsic hand muscles, especially those in the thenar eminence, accompanied by pain and numbness in the medial two fingers and the ulnar border of the hand and forearm. Electromyography, nerve conduction studies, and somatosensory evoked potential studies may help confirm the diagnosis. MRI may be especially helpful in revealing the underlying compressive structure. Plain radiographs or CT scanning sometimes shows the cervical rib or a large transverse process of the seventh cervical vertebra, but normal findings do not exclude the possibility of a cervical band. Treatment of the disorder is by surgical excision of the rib or band.

3. Lumbosacral Plexus Lesions

A lumbosacral plexus lesion may develop in association with diseases such as diabetes, cancer, or bleeding disorders or in relation to injury. It occasionally occurs as an isolated phenomenon similar to idiopathic brachial plexopathy, and pain and weakness then tend to be more conspicuous than sensory symptoms. The distribution of symptoms and signs depends on the level and pattern of neurologic involvement.

Van Eijk JJ et al. Neuralgic amyotrophy: an update on diagnosis, pathophysiology, and treatment. Muscle Nerve. 2016 Mar; 53(3):337–50. [PMID: 26662794]

DISORDERS OF NEUROMUSCULAR TRANSMISSION

1. Myasthenia Gravis

ESSENTIALS OF DIAGNOSIS

- ► Fluctuating weakness of commonly used voluntary muscles, producing symptoms such as diplopia, ptosis, and difficulty in swallowing.
- ► Activity increases weakness of affected muscles.
- ► Short-acting anticholinesterases transiently improve the weakness.

General Considerations

Myasthenia gravis occurs at all ages, sometimes in association with a thymic tumor or thyrotoxicosis, as well as in rheumatoid arthritis and lupus erythematosus. It is most common in young women with HLA-DR3; if thymoma is associated, older men are more commonly affected. Onset is usually insidious, but the disorder is sometimes unmasked by a coincidental infection that leads to exacerbation of symptoms. Exacerbations may also occur before the menstrual period and during or shortly after pregnancy. Symptoms are due to a variable degree of block of neuromuscular transmission caused by autoantibodies binding to acetylcholine receptors; these are found in most patients with the disease and have a primary role in reducing the number of functioning acetylcholine receptors. Additionally, cellular immune activity against the receptor is found.

Clinical Findings

A. Symptoms and Signs

Patients present with ptosis, diplopia, difficulty in chewing or swallowing, respiratory difficulties, limb weakness, or some combination of these problems. Weakness may remain localized to a few muscle groups or may become generalized. The external ocular muscles and certain other cranial muscles, including the masticatory, facial, and pharyngeal muscles, are especially likely to be affected, and the respiratory and limb muscles may also be involved. Symptoms often fluctuate in intensity during the day, and this diurnal variation is superimposed on a tendency to longer-term spontaneous relapses and remissions that may last for weeks. Nevertheless, the disorder follows a slowly progressive course and may have a fatal outcome owing to respiratory complications such as aspiration pneumonia.

Clinical examination confirms the weakness and fatigability of affected muscles. In most cases, the extraocular muscles are involved, and this leads to ocular palsies and ptosis, which are commonly asymmetric. Pupillary responses are normal. The bulbar and limb muscles are often weak, but the pattern of involvement is variable. Sustained activity of affected muscles increases the weakness, which improves after a brief rest. Sensation is normal, and there are usually no reflex changes.

Life-threatening exacerbations of myasthenia (so-called **myasthenic crisis**) may lead to respiratory weakness requiring immediate admission to the intensive care unit, where respiratory function can be monitored and ventilator support is readily available.

B. Laboratory and Other Studies

Assay of serum for elevated levels of circulating acetylcholine receptor antibodies is useful because it has a sensitivity of 80–90% for the diagnosis of myasthenia gravis. Certain patients without antibodies to acetylcholine receptors have serum antibodies to muscle-specific tyrosine kinase (MuSK), which should therefore be determined; these patients are more likely to have facial, respiratory, and proximal muscle weakness than those with antibodies to acetylcholine receptors. Other antibodies associated with myasthenia gravis include low-density lipoprotein receptor-related protein 4 (LRP4) and agrin, but tests for these antibodies are not widely commercially available.

Electrophysiologic demonstration of a decrementing muscle response to repetitive 2- or 3-Hz stimulation of motor nerves indicates a disturbance of neuromuscular transmission. Such an abnormality may even be detected in clinically strong muscles with certain provocative procedures. Needle electromyography of affected muscles shows a marked variation in configuration and size of individual motor unit potentials, and single-fiber electromyography reveals an increased jitter, or variability, in the time interval between two muscle fiber action potentials from the same motor unit.

C. Imaging

A CT scan of the chest with and without contrast should be obtained to demonstrate a coexisting thymoma.

▶ Treatment

Anticholinesterase medications provide symptomatic benefit without influencing the course of the disease. Neostigmine, pyridostigmine, or both can be used, the dose being determined on an individual basis. The usual dose of neostigmine is 7.5–30 mg (average, 15 mg) orally taken four times daily; of pyridostigmine, 30–180 mg (average, 60 mg) orally four times daily. Overmedication may temporarily increase weakness. A wide range of medications (eg, aminoglycosides) may exacerbate myasthenia gravis and should be avoided.

Thymectomy should be performed when a thymoma is present. A multicenter randomized trial demonstrated the benefit of thymectomy even in the absence of a radiologically identifiable thymoma, with improved strength, lower immunosuppression requirements, and fewer hospitalizations in the surgically treated group. Thus, *thymectomy should be considered in all patients younger than age 65* unless weakness is restricted to the extraocular muscles. If the disease is of recent onset and only slowly progressive, operation is sometimes delayed for a year or so, in the hope that spontaneous remission will occur.

Treatment with corticosteroids is indicated for patients who have responded poorly to anticholinesterase medications. Some patients experience transient exacerbation of weakness and even develop respiratory failure within the first 1–2 weeks if corticosteroids are initiated at high doses (eg, prednisone 1 mg/kg/day). Therefore, in stable patients, corticosteroids are introduced gradually in the outpatient setting. Prednisone can be started at 20 mg orally daily and increased by 10 mg increments weekly to a target of 1 mg/kg/day (maximum daily dose 100 mg). For patients hospitalized with severe myasthenia and treated with intravenous immunoglobulin or plasmapheresis, the higher dose can be given initially because the more rapid onset of action of the former two therapies mitigates the initial dip in strength due to corticosteroids. Corticosteroids can be prescribed as alternate-day or daily treatment, with alternate-day therapy potentially mitigating side effects. Once the patient has stabilized at the initial high dose, corticosteroids can gradually be tapered to a relatively low maintenance level (eg, 10 mg prednisone orally daily) as improvement occurs; total withdrawal is difficult, however. Treatment with azathioprine may be effective in allowing a lower dose of corticosteroids. The usual dose is 2–3 mg/kg orally daily after a lower initial dose. Other immunosuppressive agents that are used in myasthenia gravis to reduce the corticosteroid dose include mycophenolate mofetil, rituximab, cyclosporine, methotrexate, and tacrolimus.

In patients with major disability, plasmapheresis or IVIG therapy may be beneficial and have similar efficacy. It is also useful for stabilizing patients before thymectomy and for managing acute crisis.

▶ When to Refer

All patients should be referred.

▶ When to Admit

- Patients with acute exacerbation or respiratory involvement.
- Patients requiring plasmapheresis.
- For thymectomy.

Sanders DB et al. International consensus guidance for management of myasthenia gravis: executive summary. Neurology. 2016 Jul 26;87(4):419–25. [PMID: 27358333]

Wolfe GI et al; MGTX Study Group. Randomized trial of thymectomy in myasthenia gravis. N Engl J Med. 2016 Aug 11; 375(6):511–22. [PMID: 27509100]

2. Myasthenic Syndrome (Lambert-Eaton Myasthenic Syndrome)

ESSENTIALS OF DIAGNOSIS

- ▶ Variable weakness, typically improving with activity.
- ▶ Dysautonomic symptoms may also be present.
- ▶ A history of malignant disease may be obtained.

Clinical Findings

Myasthenic syndrome may be associated with small cell carcinoma, sometimes developing before the tumor is diagnosed, and occasionally occurs with certain autoimmune diseases. There is defective release of acetylcholine in response to a nerve impulse, caused by P/Q-type voltage-gated calcium channel antibodies, and this leads to weakness, especially of the proximal muscles of the limbs. Unlike myasthenia gravis, however, power steadily *increases* with sustained contraction. The diagnosis can be confirmed electrophysiologically, because the muscle response to stimulation of its motor nerve increases remarkably after exercise or if the nerve is stimulated repetitively at high rates (50 Hz), even in muscles that are not clinically weak.

Treatment

Treatment with intravenous immunoglobulin, plasmapheresis, and immunosuppressive medication therapy (prednisone and azathioprine) may lead to clinical and electrophysiologic improvement, in addition to therapy aimed at tumor when present. Prednisone is usually initiated in a daily dose of 60–80 mg orally and azathioprine in a daily dose of 2 mg/kg orally. Symptomatic therapy includes the use of potassium channel antagonists; of these, 3,4-diaminopyridine (60–80 mg/day orally in three divided doses) has been best studied and appears efficacious. Guanidine hydrochloride (25–50 mg/kg/day orally in divided doses) is an alternative and is occasionally helpful in seriously disabled patients, but adverse effects of the medication include marrow suppression. The response to treatment with anticholinesterase medications such as pyridostigmine or neostigmine is usually disappointing.

3. Botulism

The toxin of *Clostridium botulinum* prevents the release of acetylcholine at neuromuscular junctions and autonomic synapses. Botulism occurs most commonly following the ingestion of contaminated home-canned food; outbreaks have also occurred among drug abusers due to wound infection after injection of contaminated heroin. The diagnosis should be suggested by the development of sudden, fluctuating, severe weakness with preserved sensation in a previously healthy person. Symptoms begin within 72 hours following ingestion of the toxin and may progress for several days. Typically, there is diplopia, ptosis, facial weakness, dysphagia, and nasal speech, followed by respiratory difficulty and finally by weakness that appears last in the limbs. Blurring of vision (with unreactive dilated pupils) is characteristic, and there may be dryness of the mouth, constipation (paralytic ileus), and postural hypotension. The tendon reflexes are not affected unless the involved muscles are very weak. If the diagnosis is suspected, the local health authority should be notified and a sample of serum and contaminated food (if available) sent to be assayed for toxin. Support for the diagnosis may be obtained by electrophysiologic studies; with repetitive stimulation of motor nerves at fast rates, the muscle response increases in size progressively.

Patients should be hospitalized in case respiratory assistance becomes necessary. Treatment is with heptavalent antitoxin, in patients without known allergy to horse serum. Potassium channel antagonists may provide symptomatic relief as they do in Lambert-Eaton myasthenic syndrome. Anticholinesterase medications are of no value. Respiratory assistance and other supportive measures should be provided as necessary. Further details are provided in Chapter 33.

4. Disorders Associated with Use of Aminoglycosides

Aminoglycoside antibiotics, eg, gentamicin, may produce a clinical disturbance similar to botulism by preventing the release of acetylcholine from nerve endings, but symptoms subside rapidly as the responsible medication is eliminated from the body. These antibiotics are particularly dangerous in patients with preexisting disturbances of neuromuscular transmission and are therefore best avoided in patients with myasthenia gravis.

MYOPATHIC DISORDERS

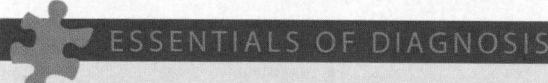

ESSENTIALS OF DIAGNOSIS

▸ Muscle weakness without sensory loss, often in a characteristic distribution.

▸ Serum creatine kinase elevated in most cases.

▸ Age at onset, time course, and inheritance pattern may suggest underlying disorder.

General Considerations

Myopathies can be inherited or acquired. Acquired myopathies often present acutely or subacutely while inherited myopathies are typically insidious in onset. Patients typically complain of weakness affecting proximal muscles, such as difficulty climbing stairs, arising from a chair, or reaching overhead, or of head drop. Sensory symptoms are absent. A detailed family history is required.

Examination shows weakness of proximal muscles. In some cases, there is a more specific pattern of weakness (eg, quadriceps and finger flexor weakness in inclusion body myositis). Extraocular muscle involvement is rarely seen, except in certain mitochondrial disorders, oculopharyngeal muscular dystrophy, and hyperthyroidism; when present, it should suggest the possibility of a neuromuscular junction disorder. Reflexes are normal or diminished in proportion to the degree of weakness. Sensation is normal.

Initial testing should include serum creatine kinase determination. Consider testing thyroid-stimulating hormone, cortisol, vitamin D, and calcium. Antibodies specific to certain inflammatory myopathies and connective tissue disease can be checked when these conditions are suspected (see Chapter 20). Electromyography will reveal small motor units and early recruitment; it is helpful in confirming the localization of weakness to the muscle and suggesting a suitable site for biopsy, as does MRI. The electromyographic findings may be normal in corticosteroid and mitochondrial myopathies. Muscle biopsy establishes the diagnosis when inflammatory, mitochondrial, metabolic, or certain inherited myopathies are suspected. In cases where the family history or pattern of weakness suggests a specific genetic disorder, genetic testing can be pursued directly and biopsy may not be needed. Selected common and treatable myopathies are discussed below.

1. Muscular Dystrophies

These inherited myopathic disorders are subdivided by mode of inheritance, age at onset, and clinical features, as shown in Table 24–9. In the **Duchenne** type, pseudohypertrophy of muscles frequently occurs at some stage; intellectual disability is common; and there may be skeletal deformities, muscle contractures, and cardiac involvement. A genetic defect on the short arm of the X chromosome has been identified in Duchenne dystrophy. The affected gene codes for the protein dystrophin, which is markedly reduced or absent from the muscle of patients with the disease. Dystrophin levels are generally normal in the **Becker** variety, but the protein is qualitatively altered. The diagnosis is usually made with genetic testing; muscle biopsy is needed occasionally. Duchenne muscular dystrophy can be recognized early in pregnancy in about 95% of women by genetic studies; in late pregnancy, DNA probes can be used on fetal tissue obtained for this purpose by amniocentesis. The genes causing some of the other muscular dystrophies are listed in Table 24–9.

In 2016, the FDA provisionally approved the medication eteplirsen for Duchenne muscular dystrophy, an antisense oligonucleotide that may benefit the 13% of patients with this disorder who have a dystrophin mutation that benefits from exon 51 skipping. Patients treated with eteplirsen had more functional dystrophin on muscle biopsy than controls and a slower rate of disease progression than matched historical controls. Prednisone (0.75 mg/kg orally daily or

Table 24–9. Selected muscular dystrophies.[1]

Disorder	Inheritance	Age at Onset (years)	Distribution	Prognosis	Genetic Association
Duchenne type	X-linked recessive	1–5	Pelvic, then shoulder girdle; later, limb and respiratory muscles.	Rapid progression. Death within about 15 years after onset.	Xp21; Dystrophin (loss of functional expression).
Becker	X-linked recessive	5–25	Pelvic, then shoulder girdle.	Slow progression. May have normal life span.	Xp21; Dystrophin (reduced functional expression).
Limb-girdle (Erb)	Autosomal recessive, dominant, or sporadic	10–30	Pelvic or shoulder girdle initially, with later spread to the other.	Variable severity and rate of progression. Possible severe disability in middle life.	Multiple.
Facioscapulohumeral	Autosomal dominant	Any age	Face and shoulder girdle initially; later, pelvic girdle and legs.	Slow progression. Minor disability. Usually normal life span.	4q35.2; Double homeobox protein 4. 18p11.32; Structural maintenance of chromosome's flexible hinge domain-containing protein 1.
Emery-Dreifuss	X-linked recessive or autosomal dominant	5–10	Humeroperoneal or scapuloperoneal.	Variable.	Multiple.
Distal	Autosomal dominant or recessive	40–60	Onset distally in extremities; proximal involvement later.	Slow progression.	Multiple.
Oculopharyngeal	Autosomal dominant	Any age	Ptosis, external ophthalmoplegia, and dysphagia.	Slow progression	14q11.2–q13; Poly (A)-binding protein-2.
Myotonic dystrophy	Autosomal dominant	Any age (usually 20–40)	Face, neck, distal limbs.	Slow progression.	19q13.32; Myotonin-protein kinase. 3q21.3; Cellular nucleic acid-binding protein.

[1]Not all possible genetic loci are shown.

10 mg/kg orally given weekly over 2 days) or deflazacort (0.9 mg/kg orally daily) improves muscle strength and function in boys with Duchenne dystrophy, but side effects need to be monitored. Although both corticosteroid preparations cause similar side effects, weight gain at 1 year is less with deflazacort. Prolonged bed rest must be avoided, as inactivity often leads to worsening of the underlying muscle disease. Physical therapy and orthopedic procedures may help counteract deformities or contractures.

2. Myotonic Dystrophy

Myotonic dystrophy, a slowly progressive, dominantly inherited disorder, usually manifests itself in the third or fourth decade but occasionally appears early in childhood. Two types, with a different genetic basis, have been recognized. Myotonia leads to complaints of muscle stiffness and is evidenced by the marked delay that occurs before affected muscles can relax after a contraction. This can often be demonstrated clinically by delayed relaxation of the hand after sustained grip or by percussion of the belly of a muscle. In addition, there is weakness and wasting of the facial, sternocleidomastoid, and distal limb muscles. Associated clinical features include cataracts, frontal baldness, testicular atrophy, diabetes mellitus, cardiac abnormalities, and intellectual changes. Electromyographic sampling of affected muscles reveals myotonic discharges in addition to changes suggestive of myopathy.

It is difficult to determine whether medication therapy for myotonia is safe or effective. When myotonia is disabling, treatment with a sodium channel blocker—such as phenytoin (100 mg orally three times daily), procainamide (0.5–1 g orally four times daily), or mexiletine (150–200 mg orally three times daily)—may be helpful, but the associated side effects, particularly for antiarrhythmic medications, are often limiting. Neither the weakness nor the course of the disorder is influenced by treatment. Cardiac function should be monitored, and pacemaker placement may be considered if there is evidence of heart block.

3. Myotonia Congenita

Myotonia congenita is commonly inherited as a dominant trait. Generalized myotonia without weakness is usually present from birth, but symptoms may not appear until early childhood. Patients complain of muscle stiffness that is enhanced by cold and inactivity and relieved by exercise. Muscle hypertrophy, at times pronounced, is also a feature. A recessive form with later onset is associated with slight weakness and atrophy of distal muscles. Treatment with procainamide, tocainide, mexiletine, or phenytoin may help the myotonia, as in myotonic dystrophy.

4. Mitochondrial Myopathies

The mitochondrial myopathies are a clinically diverse group of disorders that on pathologic examination of skeletal muscle with the modified Gomori stain show characteristic "ragged red fibers" containing accumulations of abnormal mitochondria. Patients may present with progressive external ophthalmoplegia or with limb weakness that is exacerbated or induced by activity. Other patients present with central neurologic dysfunction, eg, myoclonic epilepsy (**myoclonic epilepsy, ragged red fiber syndrome, or MERRF**), or the combination of myopathy, encephalopathy, lactic acidosis, and stroke-like episodes (**MELAS**). Migraine is a common symptom. Systemic features include but are not limited to diabetes mellitus, hearing loss, retinopathy, cardiomyopathy, gastric dysmotility, and short stature. The serum creatine kinase is usually normal. Mitochondrial myopathies result from separate abnormalities of mitochondrial DNA. Treatment is symptomatic and palliative, but various experimental approaches are being explored.

5. Acid Maltase Deficiency (Pompe disease)

This is a glycogen storage disease due to mutations in the gene encoding acid alpha-1,4-glucosidase. Age at presentation ranges from infancy to the late fifties and depends on the degree of residual enzyme activity. The juvenile and adult-onset forms present with slowly progressive proximal weakness that includes respiratory failure. Cardiomyopathy is less common in the adult form. Serum creatine kinase is mildly elevated. Muscle biopsy shows glycogen containing lysosomal vacuoles, but the diagnosis is suggested by detecting reduced acid-1,4-alpha-glucosidase activity on a dried blood spot, and confirmed by genetic testing. Treatment with recombinant alpha-glucosidase (20 mg/kg intravenously every 2 weeks) stabilizes disease progression and results in improvement in respiratory function.

6. Dermatomyositis, Anti-Synthetase Syndromes, Immune-mediated Necrotizing Myopathies, & Polymyositis

See Chapter 20.

7. Inclusion Body Myositis

This disorder, of unknown cause, begins insidiously, usually after middle age, with progressive proximal weakness of first the lower and then the upper extremities, and affecting facial and pharyngeal muscles. Weakness often begins in the quadriceps femoris in the lower limbs and the forearm flexors in the upper limbs. Distal weakness is usually mild. Serum creatine kinase levels may be normal or increased. The diagnosis is confirmed by muscle biopsy. Anticytosolic 5'-nucleotidase 1A antibodies are detected in one-third of cases and may be associated with a more severe phenotype. Corticosteroid and immunosuppressive therapy is sometimes offered but is usually ineffective, and IVIG therapy is not recommended.

8. Endocrine Myopathies

Myopathy is observed with hypothyroidism, hyperthyroidism, Cushing syndrome and disease, Addison disease, vitamin D deficiency, and both hyperparathyroidism and hypoparathyroidism (the latter mediated by calcium derangements). In hypothyroidism, there may be associated entrapment neuropathies, and examination may show delayed relaxation of tendon reflexes, muscle enlargement, or myoedema. Hyperthyroidism can cause both distal and proximal weakness and rarely a bulbar myopathy. Serum creatine kinase is normal except in hypothyroid myopathy, which can also be painful. Treatment is of the underlying endocrinopathy.

9. Critical Illness Myopathy

Myopathy may occur in association with critical illness, typically in patients who received neuromuscular blocking agents and corticosteroids. It is frequently discovered when patients unexpectedly require prolonged ventilatory support. There can be an associated sensorimotor polyneuropathy. Serum creatine kinase may be elevated initially but has frequently returned to normal or is below normal by the time the condition is suspected. Treatment is supportive.

10. Toxic Myopathies

Myopathy can occur in patients taking aminocaproic acid, amiodarone, chloroquine, colchicine, corticosteroids, cyclosporine, daptomycin, emetine, fibrates, gemcitabine, nucleoside reverse transcriptase inhibitors, or statin medications. Myopathy also occurs with chronic alcoholism, whereas acute reversible muscle necrosis may occur shortly after acute alcohol, cocaine, or methamphetamine intoxication, and with propofol infusion. Inflammatory myopathy may occur in patients taking penicillamine and can by induced by programmed death-1 inhibitors; myotonia may be induced by clofibrate, and preexisting myotonia may be exacerbated or unmasked by depolarizing muscle relaxants (eg, suxamethonium), beta-blockers (eg, propranolol), fenoterol, ritodrine and, possibly, certain diuretics. Valproic acid can precipitate or worsen myopathy in patients with mitochondrial disorders or carnitine palmitoyltransferase II deficiency.

▶ When to Refer

All patients should be referred to establish the diagnosis and underlying cause.

▶ When to Admit

- For respiratory assistance.
- For rhabdomyolysis.

Feingold B et al. Management of cardiac involvement associated with neuromuscular diseases: a scientific statement from the American Heart Association. Circulation. 2017 Sep 26; 136(13):e200–31. [PMID: 28838934]

Gloss D et al. Practice guideline update summary: corticosteroid treatment of Duchenne muscular dystrophy: report of the guideline development subcommittee of the American Academy of Neurology. Neurology. 2016 Feb 2;86(5):465–72. [PMID: 26833937]

Mendell JR et al. Longitudinal effect of eteplirsen versus historical control on ambulation in Duchenne muscular dystrophy. Ann Neurol. 2016 Feb;79(2):257–71. [PMID: 26573217]

PERIODIC PARALYSIS SYNDROMES

Periodic paralysis may have a familial (dominant inheritance) basis. The syndromes to be described are *channelopathies* that manifest as abnormal, often potassium-sensitive, muscle-membrane excitability and lead clinically to episodes of flaccid weakness or paralysis, sometimes in association with abnormalities of the plasma potassium level. Strength is initially normal between attacks, but progressive myopathic weakness may develop in up to one-third of patients as they age. **Hypokalemic periodic paralysis** is characterized by attacks that tend to occur on awakening, after exercise, or after a heavy meal and may last for several days. Patients should avoid excessive exertion. A low-carbohydrate and low-salt diet may help prevent attacks. An ongoing attack may be aborted by potassium chloride given orally or by intravenous drip, provided the ECG can be monitored and kidney function is satisfactory. In young Asian men, it is commonly associated with hyperthyroidism; treatment of the endocrine disorder prevents recurrences. A nonselective beta-adrenergic blocker may prevent attacks until the endocrine abnormality has been treated. In **hyperkalemic periodic paralysis,** attacks also tend to occur after exercise but usually last for less than 1 hour. They may be terminated by intravenous calcium gluconate (1–2 g) or by intravenous diuretics (furosemide, 20–40 mg), glucose, or glucose and insulin. **Normokalemic periodic paralysis** is similar clinically to the hyperkalemic variety, but the plasma potassium level remains normal during attacks. Several randomized trials support the use of dichlorphenamide (50–100 mg orally twice daily) for prevention of attacks in both hyperkalemic and hypokalemic periodic paralysis; acetazolamide (250–750 mg orally daily) is also effective. Chlorothiazide may also be used to prevent attacks in hyperkalemic periodic paralysis.

▶ When to Refer

All patients should be referred.

Sansone VA et al; Muscle Study Group. Randomized, placebo-controlled trials of dichlorphenamide in periodic paralysis. Neurology. 2016 Apr 12;86(15):1408–16. [PMID: 26865514]

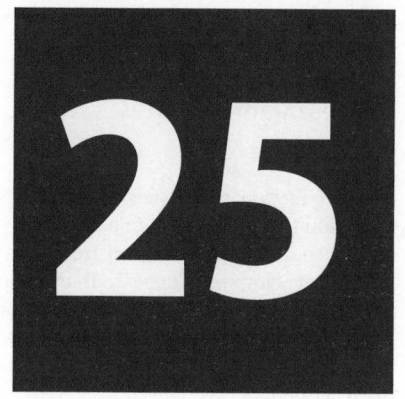

Psychiatric Disorders

Kristin S. Raj, MD
Nolan Williams, MD
Charles DeBattista, DMH, MD

The fifth edition of the American Psychiatric Association's *Diagnostic and Statistical Manual (DSM-5)* is the common language that clinicians use for psychiatric conditions. It utilizes specific criteria with which to objectively assess symptoms for use in clinical diagnosis and communication.

COMMON PSYCHIATRIC DISORDERS

ADJUSTMENT DISORDERS

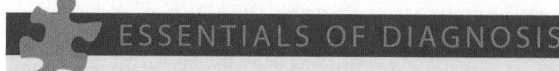

ESSENTIALS OF DIAGNOSIS

▶ Anxiety or depression in reaction to an identifiable stress, though out of proportion to the severity of the stressor.

▶ Symptoms are not at the severity of a major depressive episode or with the chronicity of generalized anxiety disorder (GAD).

▶ General Considerations

An individual experiences stress when adaptive capacity is overwhelmed by events. The event may be an insignificant one when objectively considered, and even favorable changes (eg, promotion and transfer) requiring adaptive behavior can produce stress. For everyone, stress is subjectively defined, and the response to stress is a function of each person's personality and physiologic endowment.

Opinion differs about what events are most apt to produce stress reactions. The causes of stress are different at different ages—eg, in young adulthood, the sources of stress are found in the marriage or parent-child relationship, the employment relationship, and the struggle to achieve financial stability; in the middle years, the focus shifts to changing spousal relationships, problems with aging parents, and problems associated with having young adult offspring who themselves are encountering stressful situations; in old age, the principal concerns are apt to be retirement, loss of physical and mental capacity, major personal losses, and thoughts of death.

▶ Clinical Findings

An individual may react to stress by becoming anxious or depressed, by developing a physical symptom, by running away, drinking alcohol, overeating, starting an affair, or in limitless other ways. Common subjective responses are anxiety, sadness, fear, rage, guilt, and shame. Acute and reactivated stress may be manifested by restlessness, irritability, fatigue, increased startle reaction, and a feeling of tension. Inability to concentrate, sleep disturbances (insomnia, bad dreams), and somatic preoccupations often lead to self-medication, most commonly with alcohol or other central nervous system depressants. Emotional and behavioral distressing symptomatology in response to stress is called **adjustment disorder**, with the major symptom specified (eg, "adjustment disorder with depressed mood"). *Even with an identifiable stressor, if the patient meets syndromal criteria for another disorder such as major depression, then the convention would be to diagnose a major depression and not an adjustment disorder with depressed mood.*

▶ Differential Diagnosis

Adjustment disorders are distinguished from anxiety disorders, mood disorders, bereavement, other stress disorders such as posttraumatic stress disorder (PTSD), and personality disorders exacerbated by stress and from somatic disorders with psychic overlay. Unlike many other psychiatric disorders, such as bipolar disorder or schizophrenia, adjustment disorders are *wholly situational* and usually resolve when the stressor resolves or the individual effectively adapts to the situation. Adjustment disorders may have symptoms that overlap with other disorders, such as anxiety symptoms, but they occur in reaction to an identifiable life stressor such as a difficult work situation or romantic breakup. An adjustment disorder that persists and worsens can potentially evolve into another psychiatric disorder such as major depression or GAD. However, that is not the case for most patients. Patients with adjustment disorders have marked distress after a stressor and significant impairment in social or occupational functioning but not to the degree experienced by patients with a more severe disorder such as major depressive disorder or PTSD.

By definition, an adjustment disorder occurs within 3 months of an identifiable stressor.

Treatment

A. Behavioral

Stress reduction techniques include immediate symptom reduction (eg, rebreathing in a bag for hyperventilation) or early recognition and removal from a stress source before full-blown symptoms appear. It is often helpful for the patient to keep a daily log of stress precipitators, responses, and alleviators. Relaxation, mindfulness-based stress reduction, and exercise techniques are also helpful in improving the reaction to stressful events.

B. Social

The stress reactions of life crisis problems are a function of psychosocial upheaval. While it is not easy for the patient to make necessary changes (or they would have been made long ago), it is important for the clinician to establish the framework of the problem, since the patient's denial system may obscure the issues. Clarifying the problem in the patient's psychosocial context allows the patient to begin viewing it within the proper frame and facilitates the difficult decisions the patient eventually must make (eg, change of job).

C. Psychological

Prolonged in-depth psychotherapy is seldom necessary in cases of isolated stress response or adjustment disorder. Supportive psychotherapy (see above) with an emphasis on strengthening of existing coping mechanisms is a helpful approach so that time and the patient's own resiliency can restore the previous level of function. In addition, cognitive behavioral therapy has long been established to treat acute stress and facilitate recovery in patients with an adjustment disorder.

D. Pharmacologic

Judicious use of sedatives (eg, lorazepam, 0.5–1 mg two or three times daily orally) for a limited time and as part of an overall treatment plan can provide relief from acute anxiety symptoms. Problems arise when the situation becomes chronic through inappropriate treatment or when the treatment approach supports the development of chronicity. There are occasions where the short-term use of selective serotonin reuptake inhibitors (SSRIs) targeting dysphoria and anxiety may be useful.

Prognosis

Return to satisfactory function after a short period is part of the clinical picture of this syndrome. Resolution may be delayed if others' responses to the patient's difficulties are thoughtlessly harmful or if the secondary gains outweigh the advantages of recovery. The longer the symptoms persist, the worse the prognosis. There is also evidence that stress-related disorders are associated with increased risk of autoimmune disease, although this mechanism has yet to be elucidated.

Song H et al. Association of stress-related disorders with subsequent autoimmune disease. JAMA. 2018 Jun 19;319(23): 2388–400. [PMID: 29922828]

TRAUMA & STRESSOR-RELATED DISORDERS

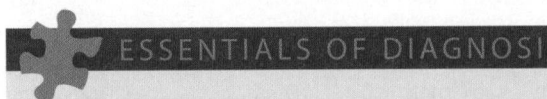

ESSENTIALS OF DIAGNOSIS

► Exposure to a traumatic or life-threatening event.
► Flashbacks, intrusive images, and nightmares, often represent reexperiencing the event.
► Avoidance symptoms, including numbing, social withdrawal, and avoidance of stimuli associated with the event.
► Increased vigilance, such as startle reactions and difficulty falling asleep.
► Symptoms impair functioning.

General Considerations

Posttraumatic stress disorder (PTSD) has been reclassified from an anxiety disorder to a trauma and stressor-related disorder in the *DSM-5*. PTSD is a syndrome characterized by "reexperiencing" a traumatic event (eg, sexual assault, severe burns, military combat) and decreased responsiveness and avoidance of current events associated with the trauma. The 2005 National Comorbidity Survey Report estimated the lifetime prevalence of PTSD among adult Americans at 6.8% with a point prevalence of 3.6% and with women having rates twice as high as men. Many individuals with PTSD (20–40%) have experienced other associated problems, including divorce, parenting problems, difficulties with the law, and substance abuse.

Clinical Findings

The key to establishing the diagnosis of PTSD lies in the *history of exposure to a perceived or actual life-threatening event, serious injury, or sexual violence.* This can include serious medical illnesses, and the prevalence of PTSD is higher in people who have experienced serious illnesses such as cancer. The symptoms of PTSD include intrusive thoughts (eg, flashbacks, nightmares), avoidance (eg, withdrawal), negative thoughts and feelings, and increased reactivity. Patients with PTSD can experience physiologic hyperarousal, including startle reactions, illusions, overgeneralized associations, sleep problems, nightmares, dreams about the precipitating event, impulsivity, difficulties in concentration, and hyperalertness. The symptoms may be precipitated or exacerbated by events that are a reminder of the original traumatic event. Symptoms frequently arise after a long latency period (eg, child abuse can result in later-onset PTSD). *DSM-5* includes the requirement that the symptoms persist for at least 1 month. In some individuals, the symptoms fade over months or years, and in others they may persist for a lifetime.

▶ Differential Diagnosis

In 75% of cases, PTSD occurs with comorbid depression or panic disorder, and there is considerable overlap in the symptom complexes of all three conditions. **Acute stress disorder** has many of the same symptoms as PTSD, but symptoms persist for only 3 days to a month after the trauma. The other major comorbidity is alcohol and substance abuse. The Primary Care-PTSD Screen and the PTSD Checklist are two useful screening instruments in primary care clinics or community settings with populations at risk for trauma exposure.

▶ Treatment

A. Psychotherapy

Psychotherapy should be initiated *as soon as possible* after the traumatic event, and it should be brief (typically 8–12 sessions), once the individual is in a safe environment. Cognitive processing therapy, prolonged exposure therapy, and eye-movement desensitization reprocessing have been effective in significantly reducing the duration of symptoms. In these approaches, the individual confronts the traumatic situation and learns to view it with less reactivity. Psychological debriefing in a single session, once a mainstay in prevention of PTSD, is now considered to be *ineffective and possibly harmful*. Posttraumatic stress syndromes respond to interventions that help patients integrate the event in an adaptive way with some sense of mastery in having survived the trauma. Partner relationship problems are a major area of concern, and it is important that the clinician have available a dependable referral source when marriage counseling is indicated.

Treatment of any comorbid substance abuse is an essential part of the recovery process for patients with PTSD. In patients with comorbid substance use disorders, there is evidence for better outcomes when substance abuse treatment is delivered alongside trauma-focused psychotherapy. Support groups and 12-step programs such as Alcoholic Anonymous are often very helpful.

Video telepsychiatry for psychotherapy or medication management allows for access to these resources that some patients, such as those in rural settings, may not otherwise have. There is similar efficacy in reduction of PTSD symptoms in women veterans with video teletherapy as with in-person therapy, and the practice of telepsychiatry is expanding.

B. Pharmacotherapy

SSRIs are helpful in ameliorating depression, panic attacks, sleep disruption, and startle responses in PTSD. Sertraline and paroxetine are approved by the US Food and Drug Administration (FDA) for this purpose, and the SSRIs are the only class of medications approved for the treatment of PTSD. They are, therefore, considered the pharmacotherapy of choice for PTSD. Early treatment of anxious arousal with beta-blockers (eg, propranolol, 80–160 mg orally daily) may lessen the peripheral symptoms of anxiety (eg, tremors, palpitations) but has not been shown to help prevent development of PTSD. Similarly, noradrenergic agents such as clonidine (titrated from 0.1 mg orally at bedtime to 0.2 mg three times a day) have been shown to help with the hyperarousal symptoms of PTSD. The alpha-adrenergic blocking agent prazosin (2–10 mg orally at bedtime) has mixed evidence for decreasing nightmares and improving quality of sleep in PTSD. Benzodiazepines, such as clonazepam, are generally thought to be *contraindicated* in the treatment of PTSD. The risks of benzodiazepines, including addiction and disinhibition, are thought to outweigh the anxiolytic and sleep benefits in most patients. Trazodone (25–100 mg orally at bedtime) is commonly prescribed as a non–habit forming hypnotic agent. Second-generation antipsychotics have not demonstrated significant utility in the treatment of PTSD, but agents such as quetiapine 50–300 mg/day may have a limited role in treating agitation and sleep disturbance in PTSD patients. Work with novel agents such as MDMA (methylenedioxymethamphetamine; also called Ecstasy) have shown early promise in the treatment of PTSD and are in phase III trials as of 2019.

▶ Prognosis

The sooner therapy is initiated after the trauma, the better the prognosis. A study published in 2018 comparing sertraline and prolonged exposure therapy for patients with PTSD demonstrated that patients who received their preferred treatment were more likely to be adherent, respond to treatment, and have lower self-reported PTSD, depression, and anxiety symptoms. Approximately half of patients with PTSD experience chronic symptoms. Prognosis is best in those with good premorbid psychiatric functioning. Individuals experiencing an acute stress disorder typically do better long-term than those experiencing a delayed posttraumatic disorder. Individuals who experience trauma resulting from a natural disaster (eg, earthquake or hurricane) tend to do better than those who experience a traumatic interpersonal encounter (eg, rape or combat).

Hoskins M et al. Pharmacotherapy for post-traumatic stress disorder: systematic review and meta-analysis. Br J Psychiatry. 2015 Feb;206(2):93–100. [PMID: 25644881]

Roberts NP et al. Psychological therapies for post-traumatic stress disorder and comorbid substance use disorder. Cochrane Database Syst Rev. 2016 Apr 4;4:CD010204. [PMID: 27040448]

Spoont MR et al. Does this patient have posttraumatic stress disorder? Rational clinical examination systematic review. JAMA. 2015 Aug 4;314(5):501–10. Erratum in: JAMA. 2016 Jan 5;315(1):90. [PMID: 26241601]

Zoellner LA et al. Doubly randomized preference trial of prolonged exposure versus sertraline for treatment of PTSD. Am J Psychiatry. 2019 Apr 1;176(4):287–96. [PMID: 30336702]

ANXIETY DISORDERS

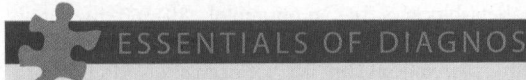

ESSENTIALS OF DIAGNOSIS

▶ Persistent excessive anxiety or chronic fear and associated behavioral disturbances.

▶ Somatic symptoms referable to the autonomic nervous system or to a specific organ system (eg, dyspnea, palpitations, paresthesias).

▶ Not limited to an adjustment disorder.

▶ Not a result of physical disorders, other psychiatric conditions (eg, schizophrenia), or drug abuse (eg, cocaine).

▶ General Considerations

Stress, fear, and anxiety all tend to be interactive. The principal components of anxiety are **psychological** (tension, fears, difficulty in concentration, apprehension) and **somatic** (tachycardia, hyperventilation, shortness of breath, palpitations, tremor, sweating). Sympathomimetic symptoms of anxiety are both a response to a central nervous system state and a reinforcement of further anxiety. Anxiety can become *self-generating,* since the symptoms reinforce the reaction, causing it to spiral. Additionally, avoidance of triggers of anxiety leads to reinforcement of the anxiety. The person continues to associate the trigger with anxiety and never relearns through experience that the trigger need not always result in fear, or that anxiety will naturally improve with prolonged exposure to an objectively neutral stressor.

Anxiety may be free-floating, resulting in acute anxiety attacks, occasionally becoming chronic. Lack of structure is frequently a contributing factor, as noted in those people who have "Sunday neuroses." They do well during the week with a planned work schedule but cannot tolerate the unstructured weekend. Planned-time activities tend to bind anxiety, and many people have increased difficulties when this is lost, as in retirement.

▶ Clinical Findings

A. Generalized Anxiety Disorder

Anxiety disorders are the most prevalent psychiatric disorders. About 7% of women and 4% of men will meet criteria for GAD over a lifetime. GAD becomes chronic in many patients with over half of patients having the disorder for longer than 2 years. Anxiety disorder in the elderly is twice as common as dementia and four to six times more common than major depression, and it is associated with poorer quality of life and contributes to the onset of disability. The anxiety symptoms of apprehension, worry, irritability, difficulty in concentrating, insomnia, or somatic complaints are present more days than not for at least 6 months. Manifestations can include cardiac (eg, tachycardia, increased blood pressure), gastrointestinal (eg, increased acidity, nausea, epigastric pain), and neurologic

(eg, headache, near-syncope) systems. The focus of the anxiety may be a number of everyday activities.

B. Panic Disorder

Panic attacks are recurrent, unpredictable episodes of intense surges of anxiety accompanied by marked physiologic manifestations. **Agoraphobia,** fear of being in places where escape is difficult, such as open spaces or public places where one cannot easily hide, may be present and may lead the individual to confine his or her life to home. Distressing symptoms and signs such as dyspnea, tachycardia, palpitations, dizziness, paresthesias, choking, smothering feelings, and nausea are associated with feelings of impending doom (alarm response). Although these symptoms may lead to overlap with some of the same bodily complaints found in the somatic symptom disorders, the key to the diagnosis of panic disorder is the psychic pain and suffering the individual expresses. **Panic disorder** is diagnosed when panic attacks are accompanied by a chronic fear of the recurrence of an attack or a maladaptive change in behavior to try to avoid potential triggers of the panic attack. Recurrent **sleep panic attacks** (not nightmares) occur in about 30% of panic disorders. **Anticipatory anxiety** develops in all these patients and further constricts their daily lives. Panic disorder tends to be familial, with onset usually under age 25; it affects 3–5% of the population, and the female-to-male ratio is 2:1. The premenstrual period is one of heightened vulnerability. Patients frequently undergo evaluations for emergent medical conditions (eg, heart attack or hypoglycemia), which are then ruled out before the correct diagnosis is made. Gastrointestinal symptoms (eg, stomach pain, heartburn, diarrhea, constipation, nausea and vomiting) are common, occurring in about one-third of cases. Myocardial infarction, pheochromocytoma, hyperthyroidism, and various recreational drug reactions can mimic panic disorder and should be considered in the differential diagnosis. Patients who have panic disorder can become demoralized, hypochondriacal, agoraphobic, and depressed. These individuals are at increased risk for major depression and suicide. Alcohol abuse (in about 20%) results from self-treatment and is frequently combined with dependence on sedatives. Some patients have atypical panic attacks associated with seizure-like symptoms that often include psychosensory phenomena (a history of stimulant abuse often emerges). About 25% of panic disorder patients also have obsessive-compulsive disorder (OCD).

C. Phobic Disorders

Phobias are fears of a specific object or situation (eg, spiders, height) that are out of proportion to the danger posed, and they tend to be chronic. **Social phobias** are global or specific; in the former, all social situations are poorly tolerated, while the latter group includes performance anxiety (eg, fear of public speaking). While patients with **simple phobias** such as fear of heights may function as long as they do not have to be in tall buildings or airplanes, a patient with agoraphobia may not be able to function vocationally or interpersonally.

▶ Treatment

In all cases, underlying medical disorders must be ruled out (eg, cardiovascular, endocrine, respiratory, and neurologic disorders and substance-related syndromes, both intoxication and withdrawal states).

A. Pharmacologic

1. Generalized anxiety disorder—Antidepressants including the SSRIs and serotonin norepinephrine reuptake inhibitors (SNRIs) are first-line treatment and safe and effective in the long-term management of GAD. Some patients may find more noradrenergic SNRIs such as levomilnacipran too activating to tolerate. The antidepressants appear to be as effective as the benzodiazepines without the risks of tolerance or dependence. However, benzodiazepines take effect more quickly if not immediately, which can be beneficial in brief acute management (Table 25–1).

Antidepressants are the first-line medications for sustained treatment of GAD, having the advantage of not causing physiologic dependency problems. *Antidepressants can themselves be anxiogenic when first started*—thus, at the initiation of treatment, patient education and at times concomitant short-term treatment with a benzodiazepine is indicated. SSRIs, such as escitalopram and paroxetine, are FDA-approved. The SNRIs venlafaxine and duloxetine are FDA-approved for the treatment of GAD in usual antidepressant doses. Initial daily dosing should start low

Table 25–1. Commonly used antianxiety and hypnotic agents (listed in alphabetical order within classes).

Medication	Usual Daily Oral Doses	Usual Daily Maximum Doses	Cost for 30 Days of Treatment Based on Maximum Dosage[1]
Benzodiazepines (used for anxiety)			
Alprazolam (Xanax)[2]	0.5 mg	4 mg	$101.40
Chlordiazepoxide (Librium)[3]	10–20 mg	100 mg	$36.72
Clonazepam (Klonopin)[3]	1–2 mg	10 mg	$152.25
Clorazepate (Tranxene)[3]	15–30 mg	60 mg	$260.40
Diazepam (Valium)[3]	5–15 mg	30 mg	$27.00
Lorazepam (Ativan)[2]	2–4 mg	4 mg	$75.60
Oxazepam (Serax)[2]	10–30 mg	60 mg	$95.40
Benzodiazepines (used for sleep)			
Estazolam (Prosom)[2]	1 mg	2 mg	$29.70
Flurazepam (Dalmane)[3]	15 mg	30 mg	$26.40
Midazolam (Versed)[4]	5 mg		$1.24/dose
Quazepam (Doral)[3]	7.5 mg	15 mg	$675.00
Temazepam (Restoril)[2]	15 mg	30 mg	$24.30
Triazolam (Halcion)[5]	0.125 mg	0.25 mg	$110.00
Miscellaneous (used for anxiety)			
Buspirone (Buspar)[2]	10–30 mg	60 mg	$238.80
Phenobarbital[3]	15–30 mg	90 mg	$35.70
Miscellaneous (used for sleep)			
Eszopiclone (Lunesta)[5]	2–3 mg	3 mg	$349.80
Hydroxyzine (Vistaril)[2]	50 mg	100 mg	$67.20
Ramelteon (Rozerem)	8 mg	8 mg	$466.80
Suvorexant (Belsomra)	5–10 mg	20 mg	$417.90
Zaleplon (Sonata)[6]	5–10 mg	10 mg	$113.70
Zolpidem (Ambien)[5]	5–10 mg	10 mg	$138.60

[1]Average wholesale price (AWP, for AB-rated generic when available) for quantity listed. Source: IBM Micromedex Red Book (electronic version) IBM Watson Health, Greenwood, CO, USA. Available at https://www.micromedexsolutions.com (cited April 25, 2019). AWP may not accurately represent the actual pharmacy cost because wide contractual variations exist among institutions.
[2]Intermediate physical half-life (10–20 hours).
[3]Long physical half-life (> 20 hours).
[4]Intravenously for procedures.
[5]Short physical half-life (1–6 hours).
[6]Short physical half-life (about 1 hour).

(37.5–75 mg for venlafaxine and 30 mg for duloxetine) and be titrated upward as needed. While most antidepressants including tricyclic antidepressants (TCAs) and mono-amine oxidase (MAO) inhibitors are often effective in the treatment of anxiety disorders, their side effects and drug interactions make them second- or third-line agents. Bus-pirone, sometimes used as an augmenting agent in the treatment of depression and compulsive behaviors, is also effective for generalized anxiety. Buspirone is usually given in a total dose of 30–60 mg/day in divided doses. Higher doses are sometimes associated with side effects of gastro-intestinal symptoms and dizziness. Bupropion may be the most anxiogenic antidepressant and does *not* have evi-dence in treatment of anxiety disorders. There is a 2- to 4-week delay before antidepressants and buspirone take effect, and *patients require education regarding this lag.* Sleep is sometimes negatively affected. Gabapentin (titrated to doses of 900–1800 mg orally daily) appears effective and lacks the habit-forming potential of the benzodiazepines. Unfortunately, like buspirone, many patients find gabapen-tin less effective than benzodiazepines in the management of acute anxiety. Beta-blockers, such as propranolol, may help reduce peripheral somatic symptoms. Alcohol is the most frequently self-administered drug and should be strongly discouraged.

2. Panic disorder—Antidepressants are the first-line phar-macotherapy for panic disorder. Several SSRIs, including fluoxetine, paroxetine, and sertraline, are approved for the treatment of panic disorder. The SNRI venlafaxine is FDA approved for treatment of panic disorder. As with GAD, panic disorder is often a chronic condition; the long-term use of benzodiazepines can result in tolerance or even ben-zodiazepine dependence. While panic disorder often responds to high-potency benzodiazepines such as clonaz-epam and alprazolam, the best use of these agents is gener-ally early in the course of treatment concurrently with an antidepressant. Once the antidepressant has begun working after 4 or more weeks, the benzodiazepine may be tapered.

Whether the indications for benzodiazepines are anxi-ety or insomnia, the medications should be used judi-ciously. The longer-acting benzodiazepines are used for the treatment of alcohol withdrawal and anxiety symptoms; the intermediate medications are useful as sedatives for insomnia (eg, lorazepam), while short-acting agents (eg, midazolam) are used for medical procedures such as endoscopy. Benzodiazepines may be given orally, and sev-eral are available in intramuscular or parenteral formula-tions. In psychiatric disorders, the benzodiazepines are usually given orally; in controlled medical environments (eg, the intensive care unit [ICU]), where the rapid onset of respiratory depression can be assessed, they often are given intravenously. Lorazepam does not produce active metabo-lites and has a half-life of 10–20 hours; these characteristics are useful in treating elderly patients or those with liver dysfunction. Ultra–short-acting agents, such as triazolam, have half-lives of 1–3 hours and may lead to rebound with-drawal anxiety. Longer-acting benzodiazepines, such as flurazepam, diazepam, and clonazepam, produce active metabolites, have half-lives of 20–120 hours, and should be avoided in the elderly; however, some clinicians prefer

clonazepam because of its long half-life and thus ease of dosing to once or twice a day. Since people vary widely in their response and since the medications are long lasting, the dosage must be individualized. Once this is established, an adequate and scheduled dose early in the course of symptom development will obviate the need for "pill pop-ping," which can contribute to dependency problems.

The side effects of all the benzodiazepine antianxiety agents are patient and dose dependent. As the dosage exceeds the levels necessary for sedation, the side effects include disinhibition, ataxia, dysarthria, nystagmus, and delirium. (The patient should be told not to operate machinery and drive with caution until he or she is well stabilized without side effects.)

Paradoxical agitation, anxiety, psychosis, confusion, mood lability, and anterograde amnesia have been reported, particularly with the shorter-acting benzodiazepines. These agents produce cumulative clinical effects with repeated dosage (especially if the patient has not had time to metabo-lize the previous dose), additive effects when given with other classes of sedatives or alcohol, and residual effects after termination of treatment (particularly in the case of medications that undergo slow biotransformation).

Overdosage results in respiratory depression, hypoten-sion, shock syndrome, coma, and death. Flumazenil, a benzodiazepine antagonist, is effective in overdosage. Overdosage (see Chapter 38) and withdrawal states are *medical emergencies.* Serious side effects of chronic exces-sive dosage are development of tolerance, resulting in increasing dose requirements, and physiologic depen-dence, resulting in withdrawal symptoms similar in appear-ance to alcohol and barbiturate withdrawal (withdrawal effects must be distinguished from reemergent anxiety). Abrupt withdrawal of sedative medications may cause seri-ous and even fatal convulsive seizures. Psychosis, delirium, and autonomic dysfunction have also been described. Both duration of action and duration of exposure are major fac-tors related to likelihood of withdrawal.

Common withdrawal symptoms after low to moderate daily use of benzodiazepines are classified as somatic (dis-turbed sleep, tremor, nausea, muscle aches), psychological (anxiety, poor concentration, irritability, mild depression), or perceptual (poor coordination, mild paranoia, mild con-fusion). The presentation of symptoms will vary depending on the half-life of the medication. Benzodiazepine interac-tions with other medications are listed in Table 25–2.

Antidepressants have been used in conjunction with beta-blockers in resistant cases. Propranolol (40–160 mg/day orally) can mute the peripheral symptoms of anxiety with-out significantly affecting motor and cognitive perfor-mance. They block symptoms mediated by sympathetic stimulation (eg, palpitations, tremulousness) but not non-adrenergic symptoms (eg, diarrhea, muscle tension). Con-trary to common belief, *they usually do not cause depression as a side effect* and can be used cautiously in patients with depression.

3. Phobic disorders—Social phobias and agoraphobia may be treated with SSRIs, such as paroxetine, sertraline, and fluvoxamine. In addition, phobic disorders often respond to SNRIs such as venlafaxine. Gabapentin, an antiseizure

Table 25–2. Benzodiazepine interactions with other medications (listed in alphabetical order).

Medication	Effects
Antacids	Decreased absorption of benzodiazepines
Cimetidine	Increased half-life of diazepam and triazolam
Contraceptives	Increased levels of diazepam and triazolam
Digoxin	Alprazolam and diazepam raise digoxin level
Disulfiram	Increased duration of action of sedatives
Isoniazid	Increased plasma diazepam
Levodopa	Inhibition of antiparkinsonism effect
Propoxyphene	Impaired clearance of diazepam
Rifampin	Decreased plasma diazepam
Warfarin	Decreased prothrombin time

medication with anxiolytic properties, is an alternative to antidepressants in the treatment of social phobia in a dosage of 300–3600 mg/day, depending on response versus sedation. Specific phobias such as performance or test anxiety may respond to moderate doses of beta-blockers, such as propranolol, 20–40 mg 1 hour prior to exposure. Specific phobias tend to respond to behavioral therapies such as systematic desensitization, which is when the patient is gradually exposed to the feared object or situation in a controlled setting.

B. Behavioral

Behavioral approaches are widely used in various anxiety disorders, often in conjunction with medication. Any of the behavioral techniques can be used beneficially in altering the contingencies (precipitating factors or rewards) supporting any anxiety-provoking behavior. Relaxation techniques can sometimes be helpful in reducing anxiety. Desensitization, by exposing the patient to graded doses of a phobic object or situation, is an effective technique and one that the patient can practice outside the therapy session. Emotive imagery, wherein the patient imagines the anxiety-provoking situation while at the same time learning to relax, helps decrease the anxiety when the patient faces the real-life situation. Physiologic symptoms in panic attacks respond well to relaxation training. Both GAD and panic disorder appear to respond as well to cognitive behavioral therapy as they do to medications.

C. Psychological

Cognitive behavioral therapy is the first-line psychotherapy in treatment of panic disorder, GAD, and phobias. These approaches share a common cognitive component of examining the thoughts associated with the fear and behavioral technique of exposing the individual to the feared object or situation. *The combination of medication and cognitive behavioral therapy is more effective than either alone.* Mindfulness meditation can also be effective in decreasing symptoms of anxiety. Group therapy is the treatment of choice when the anxiety is clearly a function of the patient's difficulties in dealing with social settings. Acceptance and commitment therapy have been used with some success in anxiety disorders. It encourages individuals to keep focused on life goals while they "accept" the presence of anxiety in their lives.

D. Social

Peer support groups for panic disorder and agoraphobia have been particularly helpful. Social modification may require measures such as family counseling to aid acceptance of the patient's symptoms and avoid counterproductive behavior in behavioral training. Any help in maintaining the social structure is anxiety-alleviating, and work, school, and social activities should be maintained. School and vocational counseling may be provided by professionals, who often need help from the clinician in defining the patient's limitations.

▶ Prognosis

Anxiety disorders are usually long-standing and may be difficult to treat. All can be relieved to varying degrees with medications and behavioral techniques. The prognosis is better if the commonly observed anxiety-panic-phobia-depression cycle can be broken with a combination of the therapeutic interventions discussed above.

Craske MG et al. Anxiety. Lancet. 2016 Dec 17;388(10063): 3048–59. [PMID: 27349358]

Koychev I et al. Anxiety in older adults often goes undiagnosed. Practitioner. 2016 Jan;260(1789):17–20. [PMID: 27180498]

Pompoli A et al. Psychological therapies for panic disorder with or without agoraphobia in adults: a network meta-analysis. Cochrane Database Syst Rev. 2016 Apr 13;4:CD011004. [PMID: 27071857]

Porter E et al. A systematic review of predictors and moderators of improvement in cognitive-behavioral therapy for panic disorder and agoraphobia. Clin Psychol Rev. 2015 Dec;42: 179–92. [PMID: 26443228]

OBSESSIVE-COMPULSIVE DISORDER & RELATED DISORDERS

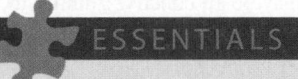
ESSENTIALS OF DIAGNOSIS

▶ Preoccupations or rituals (repetitive psychologically triggered behaviors) that are distressing to the individual.

▶ Symptoms are excessive or persistent beyond potentially developmentally normal periods.

▶ General Considerations

Obsessive-compulsive disorder (OCD), classified as an anxiety disorder in the *DSM-IV,* now is part of a separate category of Obsessive-Compulsive Disorder and Related Disorders in *DSM-5.* In OCD, the irrational idea or impulse repeatedly and unwantedly intrudes into awareness. **Obsessions** (recurring distressing thoughts, such as fears of exposure to germs) and **compulsions** (repetitive actions such as washing one's hands many times or cognitions such as counting rituals) are usually recognized by the individual as unwanted or unwarranted and are resisted, but anxiety often is alleviated only by ritualistic performance of the compulsion or by deliberate contemplation of the intruding idea or emotion. Some patients with OCD only experience obsessions, while some experience both obsessions and compulsions. Many patients do not volunteer the symptoms and must be asked about them. There is an overlapping of OCD with some features in other disorders ("**OCD spectrum**"), including tics, trichotillomania (hair pulling), excoriation disorder (skin picking), hoarding, and body dysmorphic disorder. The incidence of OCD in the general population is 2–3% and there is a high comorbidity with major depression: major depression will develop in two-thirds of OCD patients during their lifetime. Male-to-female ratios are similar, with the highest rates occurring in the young, divorced, separated, and unemployed (all high-stress categories). Neurologic abnormalities of fine motor coordination and involuntary movements are common. Under extreme stress, these patients sometimes exhibit paranoid and delusional behaviors, often associated with depression, and can mimic schizophrenia.

▶ Treatment

A. Pharmacologic

OCD responds to serotonergic antidepressants including SSRIs and clomipramine in about 60% of cases and usually requires a longer time to response than depression (up to 12 weeks). Clomipramine has proved effective in doses equivalent to those used for depression. Fluoxetine has been widely used in this disorder but in doses higher than those used in depression (up to 60–80 mg orally daily). The other SSRI medications, such as sertraline, paroxetine, and fluvoxamine, are used with comparable efficacy each with its own side-effect profile. There is some evidence that antipsychotics and topiramate may be helpful as adjuncts to the SSRIs in treatment-resistant cases. Alternatively, low-dose clomipramine may be an effective adjunct to an SSRI in some patients, though caution should be used when prescribing multiple serotonergic agents given the risk of serotonin syndrome. Plasma levels of clomipramine and its metabolite should be checked 2–3 weeks after a dosing of 50 mg/day has been achieved, with levels being kept under 500 ng/mL to avoid toxicity.

B. Behavioral

OCD may respond to a variety of behavioral techniques. One common strategy is exposure and response prevention. As in the treatment of simple phobias, exposure and response prevention involves gradually exposing the OCD spectrum patient to situations that the patient fears, such as perceived germs or situations that a hoarder must part with things they are hoarding. By gradually exposing patients to

increasingly stressful situations and helping them manage their anxiety without performing the unwanted behavior, OCD spectrum patients are often able to develop some mastery over the behaviors.

C. Psychological

In addition to behavioral techniques, OCD may respond to psychological therapies including cognitive behavioral therapy in which the patient learns to identify maladaptive cognitions associated with obsessive thoughts and challenge those cognitions. For example, an OCD patient may fear that if he does not wash his hands 50 times after shaking hands, he or someone close to him might develop a serious disease. These cognitions can be identified and gradually replaced with more rational thoughts. A technique used to help quell obsessive thoughts is "thought stopping." In this technique, the patient is taught to identify an obsessive thought and then to derail it. For example, the patient may be taught to say "STOP" any time an obsessive thought is present. In time, thought stopping can mitigate some of the obsessive thoughts.

D. Social

OCD can have devastating effects on the ability of a patient to lead a normal life. Educating both the patient and family about the course of illness and treatment options is extremely useful in setting appropriate expectations. Severe OCD is commonly associated with vocational disability, and the clinician may sometimes need to facilitate a leave of absence from work or encourage vocational rehabilitation to get the patient back to work.

E. Procedures

Transcranial magnetic stimulation also is FDA-approved for OCD. Psychosurgery has a limited place in selected cases of severe unremitting OCD. Experimental work has suggested a role for deep brain stimulation in OCD, and it is FDA approved on a humanitarian device exemption basis for refractory OCD patients.

▶ Prognosis

OCD is usually a chronic disorder with a waxing and waning course. As many as 40% of patients in whom OCD problems develop in childhood will experience remission as adults. However, it is less common for OCD to remit without treatment when it develops during adulthood.

Hirschtritt ME et al. Obsessive-compulsive disorder: advances in diagnosis and treatment. JAMA. 2017 Apr 4;317(13):1358–67. [PMID: 28384832]

Trevizol AP et al. Transcranial magnetic stimulation for obsessive-compulsive disorder: an updated systematic review and meta-analysis. J ECT. 2016 Dec;32(4):262–6. [PMID: 27327557]

FEEDING & EATING DISORDERS

See Chapter 29.

SOMATIC SYMPTOM DISORDERS
(Abnormal Illness Behaviors)

ESSENTIALS OF DIAGNOSIS

► Prominent physical symptoms may involve one or more organ systems and are associated with distress, impairment, or both.

► Sometimes able to correlate symptom development with psychosocial stresses.

► Combination of biogenetic and developmental patterns.

General Considerations

Any organ system can be affected in somatic symptom disorders. In *DSM-5*, somatic symptom disorders encompass disorders that were listed under somatic disorders in *DSM-IV*, including conversion disorder, hypochondriasis, somatization disorder, and pain disorder secondary to psychological factors. Vulnerability in one or more organ systems and exposure to family members with somatization problems plays a major role in the development of particular symptoms, and the "functional" versus "organic" dichotomy is a hindrance to good treatment. Clinicians should suspect psychiatric disorders in a number of conditions. For example, 45% of patients describing palpitations had lifetime psychiatric diagnoses including generalized anxiety, depression, panic, and somatic symptom disorders. Similarly, 33–44% of patients who undergo coronary angiography for chest pain but have negative results have been found to have panic disorder.

In any patient presenting with a condition judged to be somatic symptom disorder, depression must be considered in the diagnosis.

Clinical Findings

A. Conversion Disorder (Functional Neurologic Symptom Disorder)

"Conversion" of psychic conflict into physical neurologic symptoms in parts of the body innervated by the sensorimotor system (eg, paralysis, aphonic) is a disorder that commonly occurs concomitantly with panic disorder or depression. The somatic manifestation that takes the place of anxiety is often paralysis, and in some instances the dysfunction may have symbolic meaning (eg, arm paralysis in marked anger so the individual cannot use the arm to strike someone). Nonepileptic seizures can be difficult to differentiate from intoxication states or panic attacks and can occur in patients who also have epileptic seizures. Lack of postictal confusion, closed eyes during the seizure, ictal crying, and a fluctuating course can suggest nonepileptic seizures; some symptoms such as asynchronous movements or pelvic thrusting can occur in both nonepileptic seizures and frontal lobe seizures. Electroencephalography, particularly in a video-electroencephalography assessment unit, during the attack is the most helpful diagnostic aid in

excluding epileptic seizures. A serum prolactin levels rise more than twice baseline abruptly in the postictal state is more likely to be associated with an epileptic seizure. La belle indifférence (an unconcerned affect) is not a significant identifying characteristic, as commonly believed, since individuals even with genuine medical illness may exhibit a high level of denial. It is important to identify physical disorders with unusual presentations (eg, multiple sclerosis, systemic lupus erythematosus).

B. Somatic Symptom Disorder

Somatic symptom disorder is characterized by one or more somatic symptoms that are associated with significant distress or disability. The somatic symptoms are associated with disproportionate and persistent thoughts about the seriousness of the symptoms, a high level of anxiety about health, or excessive time and energy devoted to these symptoms. The patient's focus on somatic symptoms is usually chronic. Panic, anxiety, and depression are often present, and major depression is an important consideration in the differential diagnosis. There is a significant relationship (20%) to a lifetime history of panic-agoraphobia-depression. It usually occurs before age 30 and is ten times more common in women. Preoccupation with medical and surgical therapy becomes a lifestyle that may exclude other activities. Patients most often first present to primary care physicians and experience reassurance regarding their physical condition as only briefly helpful or dismissive. Patients' complaints of symptoms should always be first carefully medically evaluated.

C. Factitious Disorders

These disorders, in which symptom production is *intentional*, are not somatic symptom conditions in that symptoms are produced consciously, in contrast to the unconscious process of the other somatic symptom disorders. They are characterized by self-induced or described symptoms or false physical and laboratory findings for the purpose of deceiving clinicians or other health care personnel. The deceptions may involve self-mutilation, fever, hemorrhage, hypoglycemia, seizures, and an almost endless variety of manifestations—often presented in an exaggerated and dramatic fashion (**Munchausen syndrome**). Factitious disorder imposed on another, previously termed **Munchausen by proxy**, is diagnosed when someone (often a parent) creates an illness in another person (often a child) for perceived psychological benefit of the first person, such as sympathy or a relationship with clinicians. The duplicity may be either simple or extremely complex and difficult to recognize. The patients are frequently connected in some way with the health professions and there is no apparent external motivation other than achieving the patient role. A poor clinician-patient relationship and "doctor shopping" tend to exacerbate the problem.

Complications

Sedative and analgesic dependency is the most common iatrogenic complication. Patients may pursue medical or surgical treatments that induce iatrogenic problems. Thus, identifying patients with a potential somatic symptom disorder and attempting to limit tests, procedures, and medications that may lead to harm are quite important.

Treatment

A. Medical

Medical support with careful attention to **building a therapeutic clinician-patient relationship is the mainstay of treatment.** It must be accepted that the patient's distress is real. *Every problem not found to have an organic basis is not necessarily a mental disease.* Diligent attempts should be made to relate symptoms to adverse developments in the patient's life. It may be useful to have the patient keep a meticulous diary, paying particular attention to various pertinent factors evident in the history. Regular, frequent, short appointments that are not symptom-contingent may be helpful. Medications (frequently abused) should not be prescribed to replace appointments. One person should be the primary clinician, and consultants should be used mainly for evaluation. An empathic, realistic, optimistic approach must be maintained in the face of the expected ups and downs. Ongoing reevaluation is necessary, since somatization can coexist with a concurrent physical illness.

B. Psychological

The primary clinician can use psychological approaches when it is clear that the patient is ready to make some changes in lifestyle in order to achieve symptomatic relief. This is often best approached with orientation toward pragmatic current changes rather than an exploration of early experiences that the patient frequently fails to relate to current distress. Group therapy with other individuals who have similar problems is sometimes of value to improve coping, allow ventilation, and focus on interpersonal adjustment. Hypnosis used early can be helpful in resolving conversion disorders. If the primary clinician has been working with the patient on psychological problems related to the physical illness, the groundwork is often laid for successful psychiatric referral.

For patients who have been identified as having a factitious disorder, early psychiatric consultation is indicated. There are two main treatment strategies for these patients. One consists of a conjoint confrontation of the patient by both the primary clinician and the psychiatrist. The patient's disorder is portrayed as a cry for help, and psychiatric treatment is recommended. The second approach avoids direct confrontation and attempts to provide a face-saving way to relinquish the symptom without overt disclosure of the disorder's origin. Techniques such as biofeedback and self-hypnosis may foster recovery using this strategy.

C. Behavioral

Behavioral therapy is probably best exemplified by **biofeedback** techniques. In biofeedback, the particular abnormality (eg, increased peristalsis) must be recognized and monitored by the patient and therapist (eg, by an electronic stethoscope to amplify the sounds). This is immediate feedback, and after learning to recognize it, the patient can

then learn to identify any change thus produced (eg, a decrease in bowel sounds) and so become a conscious originator of the feedback instead of a passive recipient. Relief of the symptom operantly conditions the patient to utilize the maneuver that relieves symptoms (eg, relaxation causing a decrease in bowel sounds). With emphasis on this type of learning, the patient is able to identify symptoms early and initiate the countermaneuvers, thus decreasing the symptomatic problem. Migraine and tension headaches have been particularly responsive to biofeedback methods.

D. Social

Social endeavors include family, work, and other interpersonal activity. Family members should come for some appointments with the patient so they can learn how best to live with the patient. This is particularly important in treatment of somatic and pain disorders. Peer support groups provide a climate for encouraging the patient to accept and live with the problem. Ongoing communication with the employer may be necessary to encourage long-term continued interest in the employee. Employers can become just as discouraged as clinicians in dealing with employees who have chronic problems.

Prognosis

The prognosis is better if the primary clinician is able to intervene early before the situation has deteriorated. After the problem has crystallized into chronicity, it is more difficult to effect change.

Katz J et al. Chronic pain, psychopathology, and DSM-5 somatic symptom disorder. Can J Psychiatry. 2015 Apr;60(4):160–7. [PMID: 26174215]

Tavel ME. Somatic symptom disorders without known physical causes: one disease with many names? Am J Med. 2015 Oct;128(10):1054–8. [PMID: 26031885]

CHRONIC PAIN DISORDERS

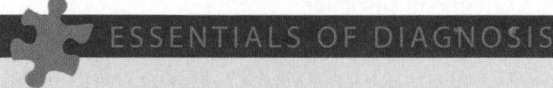
ESSENTIALS OF DIAGNOSIS

► Chronic complaints of pain.
► Symptoms frequently exceed signs.
► Minimal relief with standard treatment.
► History of having seen many clinicians.
► Frequent use of several nonspecific medications.

General Considerations

A problem in the management of pain is the lack of distinction between acute and chronic pain syndromes. Most clinicians are adept at dealing with acute pain problems but face greater challenges in treating a patient with a chronic pain disorder. Patients with chronic pain can frequently take many medications, stay in bed a great deal, have seen many clinicians, have lost skills, and experience little joy in either work or play. All relationships suffer (including those with clinicians), and life becomes a constant search for relief. The search results in complex clinician-patient relationships that usually include many medication trials, particularly sedatives, with adverse consequences (eg, irritability, depressed mood) related to long-term use. Treatment failures provoke angry responses and depression from both the patient and the clinician, and the pain syndrome is exacerbated. When frustration becomes too great, a new clinician is found, and the cycle is repeated. The longer the existence of the pain disorder, the more important become the psychological factors of anxiety and depression. As with all other conditions, it is counterproductive to speculate about whether the pain is "real." *It is real to the patient,* and acceptance of the problem must precede a mutual endeavor to alleviate the disturbance.

► Clinical Findings

Components of the chronic pain syndrome consist of anatomic changes, chronic anxiety and depression, anger, and changed lifestyle. Usually, the anatomic problem is

irreversible, since it has already been subjected to many interventions with increasingly unsatisfactory results. An algorithm for assessing chronic pain and differentiating it from other psychiatric conditions is illustrated in Figure 25–1.

Chronic anxiety and depression produce heightened irritability and overreaction to stimuli. A marked decrease in pain threshold is apparent. This pattern develops into a preoccupation with the body and a constant need for reassurance. Patients may have started avoiding usual behaviors when they first developed pain, and then chronic avoidance of usual physical functioning can lead to the development of chronic pain. The pressure on the clinician becomes wearing and often leads to covert rejection of the patient, such as not being available or making referrals to other clinicians.

This is perceived by the patient, who then intensifies the effort to find help, and the typical cycle is repeated. Anxiety and depression are seldom discussed, almost as if there is a tacit agreement not to deal with these issues.

Changes in lifestyle involve some of the pain behaviors. These usually take the form of a *family script* in which the

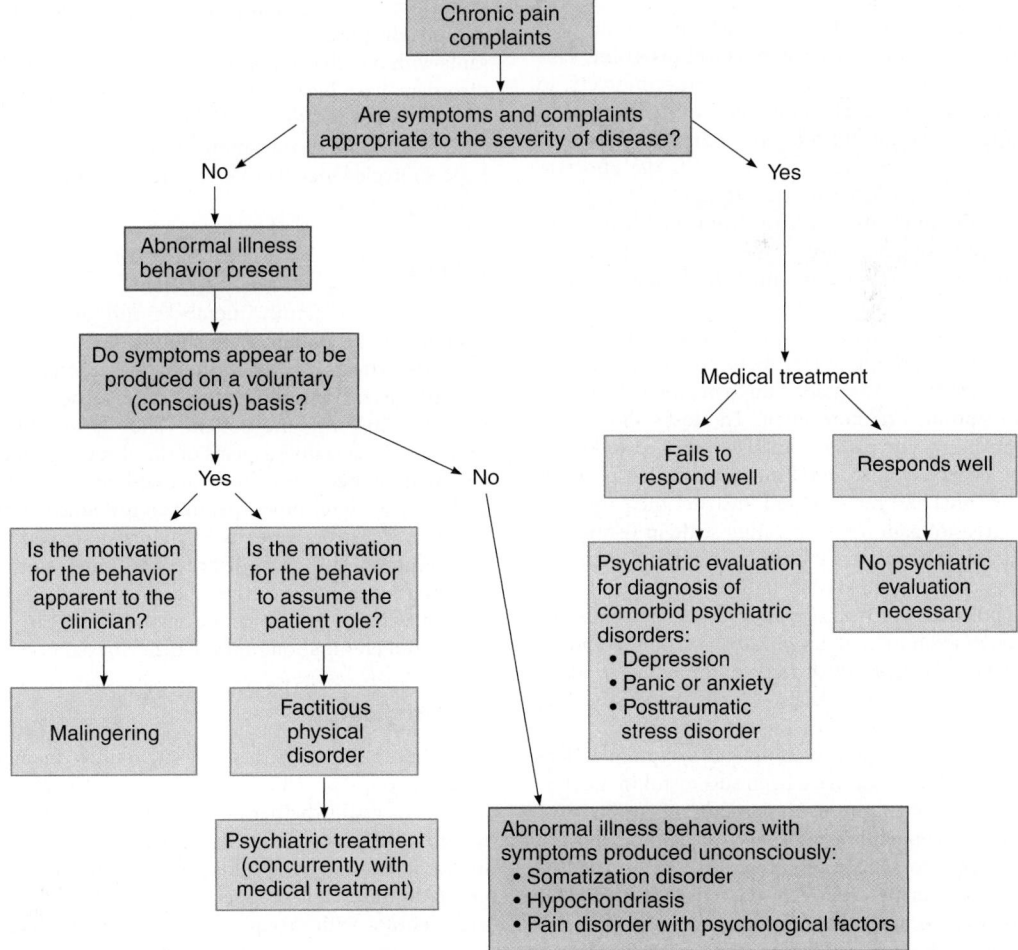

▲ **Figure 25–1.** Algorithm for assessing psychiatric component of chronic pain. (Adapted and reproduced, with permission, from Eisendrath SJ. Psychiatric aspects of chronic pain. Neurology. 1995 Dec;45(12 Suppl 9):S26–34.)

patient accepts the role of being sick, and this role then becomes the focus of most family interactions and may become important in maintaining the family, so that neither the patient nor the family wants the patient's role to change. Cultural factors frequently play a role in the behavior of the patient and how the significant people around the patient cope with the problem. Some cultures encourage demonstrative behavior, while others value the stoic role.

Another secondary gain that can maintain the patient in the sick role is financial compensation or other benefits. Frequently, such systems are structured so that they reinforce the maintenance of sickness and discourage any attempts to give up the role. Clinicians unwittingly reinforce this role because of the very nature of the practice of medicine, which is to respond to complaints of illness. Helpful suggestions from the clinician are often met with responses like, "Yes, but…." Medications then become the principal approach, and drug dependency problems may develop.

▶ Treatment

A. Behavioral

The cornerstone of a unified approach to chronic pain syndromes is a **comprehensive behavioral program.** This is necessary to identify and eliminate pain reinforcers, to decrease medication use, and to use effectively those positive reinforcers that shift the focus from the pain. It is critical that the patient be made a partner in the effort to manage and function better in the setting of ongoing pain symptoms. The clinician must shift from the idea of biomedical cure to ongoing care of the patient. The patient should agree to discuss the pain only with the clinician and not with family members; this tends to stabilize the patient's personal life, since the family is usually tired of the subject. At the beginning of treatment, the patient should be assigned self-help tasks graded up to maximal activity as a means of positive reinforcement. The tasks should not exceed capability. The patient can also be asked to keep a self-rating chart to log accomplishments, so that progress can be measured and remembered. Instruct the patient to record degrees of pain on a self-rating scale in relation to various situations and mental attitudes so that similar circumstances can be avoided or modified.

Avoid positive reinforcers for pain such as marked sympathy and attention to pain. Emphasize a positive response to productive activities, which remove the focus of attention from the pain. Activity is also desensitizing, since the patient learns to tolerate increasing activity levels.

Biofeedback techniques (see Somatic Symptom Disorders, above) and hypnosis have been successful in ameliorating some pain syndromes. Hypnosis tends to be most effective in patients with a high level of denial, who are more responsive to suggestion. Hypnosis can be used to lessen anxiety, alter perception of the length of time that pain is experienced, and encourage relaxation. Mindfulness-based stress reduction programs have been useful in helping individuals develop an enhanced capacity to live a higher quality life with persistent pain.

B. Medical

A *single clinician in charge* of the comprehensive treatment approach is the highest priority. Consultations as indicated and technical procedures done by others are appropriate, but the care of the patient should remain in the hands of the primary clinician. Referrals should not be allowed to raise the patient's hopes unrealistically or to become a way for the clinician to reject the case. The attitude of the clinician should be one of honesty, interest, and hopefulness—not for a cure but for control of pain and improved function. If the patient manifests opioid addiction, detoxification may be an early treatment goal.

Medical management of chronic pain is addressed in Chapter 5. *The harms of opioids generally outweigh the benefits in chronic pain management.* A fixed schedule lessens the conditioning effects of these medications. SNRIs (eg, venlafaxine, milnacipran, and duloxetine) and TCAs (eg, nortriptyline) in doses up to those used in depression may be helpful, particularly in neuropathic pain syndromes. Both duloxetine and milnacipran are approved for the treatment of fibromyalgia; duloxetine is also indicated in chronic pain conditions. In general, the SNRIs tend to be safer in overdose than the TCAs; suicidality is often an important consideration in treating patients with chronic pain syndromes. Gabapentin and pregabalin, anticonvulsants with possible applications in the treatment of anxiety disorders, have been shown to be useful in somatic symptom disorders and fibromyalgia.

In addition to medications, a variety of nonpharmacologic strategies may be offered, including physical therapy and acupuncture.

C. Social

Involvement of family members and other significant persons in the patient's life should be an early priority. The best efforts of both patient and therapists can be unwittingly sabotaged by other persons who may feel that they are "helping" the patient. They frequently tend to reinforce the negative aspects of the chronic pain disorder. The patient becomes more dependent and less active, and the pain syndrome becomes an immutable way of life. The more destructive pain behaviors described by many experts in chronic pain disorders are the results of well-meaning but misguided efforts of family members. Ongoing therapy with the family can be helpful in the early identification and elimination of these behavior patterns.

D. Psychological

In addition to group therapy with family members and others, groups of patients can be helpful if properly led. The major goal, whether of individual or group therapy, is to gain patient involvement. A group can be a powerful instrument for achieving this goal, with the development of group loyalties and cooperation. People will frequently make efforts with group encouragement that they would never make alone. Individual therapy should be directed toward strengthening existing coping mechanisms and improving self-esteem. For example, teaching patients to challenge expectations induced by chronic pain may lead to improved functioning. As an illustration, many chronic pain patients, making assumptions more derived from acute injuries, *incorrectly believe they will damage themselves by attempting to function.* The rapport between patient and clinician, as in all psychotherapeutic efforts, is the major factor in therapeutic success.

Beal BR et al. An overview of pharmacologic management of chronic pain. Med Clin North Am. 2016 Jan;100(1):65–79. [PMID: 26614720]

Dale R et al. Multimodal treatment of chronic pain. Med Clin North Am. 2016 Jan;100(1):55–64. [PMID: 26614719]

Markozannes G et al. An umbrella review of the literature on the effectiveness of psychological interventions for pain reduction. BMC Psychol. 2017 Aug 31;5(1):31. [PMID: 28859685]

Mills S et al. Identification and management of chronic pain in primary care: a review. Curr Psychiatry Rep. 2016 Feb;18(2):22. [PMID: 26820898]

PSYCHOSEXUAL DISORDERS

The stages of sexual activity include **excitement** (arousal), **orgasm,** and **resolution.** The precipitating excitement or arousal is psychologically determined. Arousal response leading to orgasm is a physiologic and psychological phenomenon of vasocongestion, a parasympathetic reaction causing erection in men and labial-clitoral congestion in women. The orgasmic response includes emission in men and clonic contractions of the analogous striated perineal muscles of both men and women. Resolution is a gradual return to normal physiologic status.

While the arousal stimuli—vasocongestive and orgasmic responses—constitute a single response in a well-adjusted person, they can be considered as separate stages that can produce different syndromes responding to different treatment procedures.

▶ Clinical Findings

There are three major groups of sexual disorders.

A. Paraphilias

In these conditions, formerly called "deviations" or "variations," the excitement stage of sexual activity is associated with sexual objects or orientations different from those usually associated with adult sexual stimulation. The stimulus may be a woman's shoe, a child, animals, instruments of torture, or incidents of aggression. The pattern of sexual stimulation is usually one that has early psychological roots. When paraphilias are associated with distress, impairment, or risk of harm, they become paraphilic disorders. Some paraphilias or paraphilic disorders include exhibitionism, transvestism, voyeurism, pedophilia, incest, sexual sadism, and sexual masochism.

B. Gender Dysphoria

Gender dysphoria is distress associated with the incongruence between one's experienced or expressed gender and one's assigned gender. As a disorder, it is defined by significant distress or impairment; those experiencing this incongruence but without the distress would *not* meet criteria for having gender dysphoria. Screening should be done for conditions related to the oppression and stigmatization that transgender people face, including a high risk of suicide.

C. Sexual Dysfunctions

This category includes a large group of vasocongestive and orgasmic disorders. Often, they involve problems of sexual adaptation, education, and technique that are often initially discussed with, diagnosed by, and treated by the primary care provider.

There are two conditions common in men: erectile dysfunction and ejaculation disturbances.

Erectile dysfunction is inability to achieve or maintain an erection firm enough for satisfactory intercourse; patients sometimes use the term incorrectly to mean premature ejaculation. Decreased nocturnal penile tumescence occurs in some depressed patients. Psychological erectile dysfunction is caused by interpersonal or intrapsychic factors (eg, partner disharmony, depression). Organic factors are discussed in Chapter 23.

Ejaculation disturbances include premature ejaculation, inability to ejaculate, and retrograde ejaculation. (Ejaculation is possible in patients with erectile dysfunction.) Ejaculation is usually connected with orgasm, and ejaculatory control is an acquired behavior that is minimal in adolescence and increases with experience. Pathogenic factors are those that interfere with learning control, most frequently sexual ignorance. Intrapsychic factors (anxiety, guilt, depression) and interpersonal maladaptation (partner problems, unresponsiveness of mate, power struggles) are also common. Organic causes include interference with sympathetic nerve distribution (often due to surgery or radiation) and the effects of pharmacologic agents (eg, SSRIs or sympatholytics).

In women, the most common forms of sexual dysfunction are orgasmic disorder and hyposexual desire disorder (see Chapter 18).

Orgasmic disorder is a complex condition in which there is a general lack of sexual responsiveness. The woman has difficulty in experiencing erotic sensation and does not have the vasocongestive response. Sexual activity varies from active avoidance of sex to an occasional orgasm. **Orgasmic dysfunction**—in which a woman has a vasocongestive response but varying degrees of difficulty in reaching orgasm—is sometimes differentiated from **anorgasmia.** Causes for the dysfunctions include poor sexual techniques, early traumatic sexual experiences, interpersonal disharmony (partner struggles, use of sex as a means of control), and intrapsychic problems (anxiety, fear, guilt). Organic causes include any conditions that might cause pain in intercourse, pelvic pathology, mechanical obstruction, and neurologic deficits.

Hyposexual desire disorder consists of diminished or absent libido in either sex and may be a function of organic or psychological difficulties (eg, anxiety, phobic avoidance). Any chronic illness can reduce desire as can aging. Hormonal disorders, including hypogonadism or use of antiandrogen compounds such as cyproterone acetate, and chronic kidney disease contribute to deterioration in sexual desire. Although menopause may lead to diminution of sexual desire in some women, the relationship between menopause and libido is complicated and may be influenced by sociocultural factors. Alcohol, sedatives, opioids, marijuana, and some medications may affect sexual drive and performance.

▶ Treatment

A. Paraphilias

1. Psychological—Paraphilias, particularly those of a more superficial nature (eg, voyeurism) and those of recent onset, are responsive to psychotherapy in some cases. The prognosis is much better if the motivation comes from the individual rather than the legal system; unfortunately, judicial intervention is frequently the only stimulus to treatment because the condition persists and is reinforced until conflict with the law occurs. Therapies frequently focus on barriers to normal arousal response; the expectation is that the variant behavior will decrease as normal behavior increases.

2. Behavioral—In some cases, paraphilic disorders improve with modeling, role-playing, and conditioning procedures.

3. Social—Although they do not produce a change in sexual arousal patterns or gender role, self-help groups have facilitated adjustment to an often hostile society. Attention to the family is particularly important in helping people in such groups to accept their situation and alleviate their guilt about the role they think they had in creating the problem.

4. Pharmacologic—Medroxyprogesterone acetate, a suppressor of libidinal drive, can be used to mute disruptive sexual behavior in men. Onset of action is usually within 3 weeks, and the effects are generally reversible. Fluoxetine or other SSRIs at depression doses may reduce some of the compulsive sexual behaviors including the paraphilias. A focus of study in the treatment of severe paraphilia has been agonists of luteinizing hormone–releasing hormone (LHRH). Case reports and open label studies suggest that LHRH-agonists may play a role in preventing relapse in some patients with paraphilia.

B. Gender Dysphoria

1. Psychological—Individuals with gender dysphoria often find benefit from psychotherapy, providing them with a safe place to explore and understand their thoughts and feelings, and to identify their own specific needs and desires and adjust to a changing life.

2. Social—Peer support groups, parent psychoeducation and support, and community empowerment are important social components of treatment.

3. Medical—Some individuals with gender dysphoria choose to pursue surgery or hormone therapy or both. Most recommendations prior to surgery include that the individual spends significant time prior living as their desired gender. Rates of suicide fall significantly after surgery but still remain much higher than the general population.

C. Sexual Dysfunction

1. Psychological—The use of psychotherapy by itself is best suited for those cases in which interpersonal difficulties or intrapsychic problems predominate. Anxiety and guilt about parental injunctions against sex may contribute to sexual dysfunction. Even in these cases, however, a combined behavioral-psychological approach usually produces results most quickly.

2. Behavioral—Syndromes resulting from conditioned responses have been treated by conditioning techniques, with excellent results. Masters and Johnson have used behavioral approaches in all of the sexual dysfunctions, with concomitant supportive psychotherapy and with improvement of the communication patterns of the couple.

3. Social—The proximity of other people (eg, a mother-in-law) in a household is frequently an inhibiting factor in sexual relationships. In such cases, some social engineering may alleviate the problem.

4. Medical—Even if the condition is not reversible, identification of the specific cause helps the patient to accept the condition. Partner disharmony, with its exacerbating effects, may thus be avoided. Of all the sexual dysfunctions, erectile dysfunction is the condition most likely to have an organic basis. Sildenafil, tadalafil, and vardenafil are phosphodiesterase type 5 inhibitors that are effective oral agents for the treatment of penile erectile dysfunction (eg, sildenafil 25–100 mg orally 1 hour prior to intercourse). These agents are effective for SSRI-induced erectile dysfunction in men and in some cases for SSRI-associated sexual dysfunction in women. Use of the medications in conjunction with any nitrates can have significant hypotensive effects leading to death in rare cases. Because of their common effect in delaying ejaculation, the SSRIs have been effective in premature ejaculation.

Flibanserin is a $5-HT_{1A}$-agonist/$5-HT_2$-antagonist that is FDA approved for the treatment of female hyposexual desire disorder. This is the first medication marketed to improve sexual desire in women. Women treated with flibanserin have a marginally higher number of sexual events. The medication interacts with alcohol, causing hypotensive events, so patients need to be educated about this risk. Flibanserin is taken 100 mg orally at bedtime to circumvent the side effects of dizzinesss, sleepiness, and nausea.

Holoyda BJ et al. The biological treatment of paraphilic disorders: an updated review. Curr Psychiatry Rep. 2016 Feb;18(2):19. [PMID: 26800994]

Jaspers L et al. Efficacy and safety of flibanserin for the treatment of hypoactive sexual desire disorder in women: a systematic review and meta-analysis. JAMA Intern Med. 2016. Apr; 176(4):453–62. [PMID: 26927498]

Wylie K et al. Serving transgender people: clinical care considerations and service delivery models in transgender health. Lancet. 2016 Jul 23;388(10042):401–11. [PMID: 27323926]

PERSONALITY DISORDERS

> ### ESSENTIALS OF DIAGNOSIS

> ► Long history dating back to childhood.
> ► Recurrent maladaptive behavior.
> ► Difficulties with interpersonal relationships or society.
> ► Depression with anxiety when maladaptive behavior fails.

General Considerations

An individual's personality structure, or character, is an integral part of self-image. It reflects genetics, interpersonal influences, and recurring patterns of behavior adopted in order to cope with the environment. The classification of subtypes of personality disorders depends on the predominant symptoms and their severity. The most severe disorders—those that bring the patient into greatest conflict with society—tend to be antisocial (psychopathic) or borderline.

Classification & Clinical Findings

See Table 25–3.

Differential Diagnosis

Patients with personality disorders tend to experience anxiety and depression when pathologic coping mechanisms fail and may first seek treatment when this occurs. Occasionally, the more severe cases may decompensate into psychosis under stress and mimic other psychotic disorders.

Treatment

A. Social

Social and therapeutic environments such as day hospitals, halfway houses, and self-help communities utilize peer "pressure" to modify the self-destructive behavior. The patient with a personality disorder often has failed to profit from experience, and difficulties with authority can impair the learning experience. The use of peer relationships and the repetition possible in a structured setting of a helpful community enhance the behavioral treatment opportunities and increase learning. When problems are detected early, both the school and the home can serve as foci of intensified social pressure to change the behavior, particularly with the use of behavioral techniques.

B. Behavioral

The behavioral techniques used are principally **operant conditioning** and **aversive conditioning.** The former simply emphasizes the recognition of acceptable behavior and its reinforcement with praise or other tangible rewards. Aversive responses usually mean punishment, although this can range from a mild rebuke to some specific punitive responses such as deprivation of privileges. Extinction plays a role in that an attempt is made not to respond to inappropriate behavior, and the lack of response eventually causes the person to abandon that type of behavior. Pouting and tantrums, for example, diminish quickly when such behavior elicits no reaction. These traits are less likely to develop in children at risk for development of antisocial tendencies due to a genetic predisposition when they are given positive reinforcement for positive behaviors. **Dialectical behavioral therapy** is a program of individual and group therapy specifically designed for patients with chronic suicidality and borderline personality disorder. It blends mindfulness and a cognitive-behavioral model to address self-awareness, interpersonal functioning, affective

Table 25–3. Personality disorders: Classification and clinical findings (listed in alphabetical order).

Personality Disorder	Clinical Findings
Antisocial	Selfish, callous, promiscuous, impulsive, unable to learn from experience, often has legal problems.
Avoidant	Fears rejection, hyperreacts to rejection and failure, with poor social endeavors and low self-esteem.
Borderline	Impulsive; has unstable and intense interpersonal relationships; is suffused with anger, fear, and guilt; lacks self-control and self-fulfillment; has identity problems and affective instability; is suicidal (a serious problem—up to 80% of hospitalized borderline patients make an attempt at some time during treatment, and the incidence of completed suicide is as high as 5%); aggressive behavior, feelings of emptiness, and occasional psychotic decompensation.
Dependent	Passive, overaccepting, unable to make decisions, lacks confidence, with poor self-esteem.
Histrionic (hysterical)	Dependent, immature, seductive, egocentric, vain, emotionally labile.
Narcissistic	Exhibitionist, grandiose, preoccupied with power, lacks interest in others, with excessive demands for attention.
Obsessive compulsive	Perfectionist, egocentric, indecisive, with rigid thought patterns and need for control.
Paranoid	Defensive, oversensitive, secretive, suspicious, hyperalert, with limited emotional response.
Schizoid	Shy, introverted, withdrawn, avoids close relationships.
Schizotypal	Superstitious, socially isolated, suspicious, with limited interpersonal ability, eccentric behaviors, and odd speech.

lability, and reactions to stress. There is also evidence that mindfulness alone is effective for borderline personality disorder.

C. Psychological

Psychological interventions can be conducted in group and individual settings. Group therapy is helpful when specific interpersonal behavior needs to be improved. This mode of treatment also has a place with so-called "acting-out" patients, ie, those who frequently act in an impulsive and inappropriate way. The peer pressure in the group tends to impose restraints on rash behavior. The group also quickly identifies the patient's types of behavior and helps improve the validity of the patient's self-assessment, so that the antecedents of the unacceptable behavior can be effectively handled, thus decreasing its frequency. Individual therapy should initially be supportive, ie, helping the patient to restabilize and mobilize coping mechanisms. If the individual has the ability to observe his or her own behavior, a longer-term and more introspective therapy may be warranted. The therapist must be able to handle countertransference feelings (which are frequently negative), maintain appropriate boundaries in the relationship, and refrain from premature confrontations and interpretations.

D. Pharmacologic

Hospitalization is indicated in the case of serious suicidal or homicidal danger. In most cases, treatment can be accomplished in the day treatment center or self-help community. Pharmacotherapy should be directed to specific symptom clusters. Antidepressants have improved anxiety, depression, and sensitivity to rejection in some patients with borderline personality disorder. SSRIs also have a role in reducing aggressive behavior in impulsive aggressive patients (eg, fluoxetine 20–60 mg orally daily or sertraline 50–200 mg orally daily). Antipsychotics may be helpful in targeting hostility, agitation, and as adjuncts to antidepressant therapy (eg, olanzapine [2.5–10 mg/day orally], risperidone [0.5–2 mg/day orally], or haloperidol [0.5–2 mg/day orally, split into two doses]). In some cases, these medications are required only for several days and can be discontinued after the patient has regained a previously established level of adjustment; they can also provide ongoing support. Anticonvulsants, including carbamazepine, 400–800 mg orally daily in divided doses, lamotrigine, 50–200 mg/day and valproate 500–2000 mg/day, have been shown to decrease the severity of behavioral dyscontrol in some personality disorder patients. Patients with a schizotypal personality often improve with antipsychotics, while those with avoidant personality may benefit from strategies that reduce anxiety, including the use of SSRIs and benzodiazepines.

Prognosis

Antisocial and borderline categories generally have a guarded prognosis. Those patients with a history of parental abuse and a family history of mood disorder tend to have the most challenging treatments.

Moukaddam N et al. Difficult patients in the emergency department: personality disorders and beyond. Psychiatr Clin North Am. 2017 Sep;40(3):379–95. [PMID: 28800796]

Sng AA et al. Mindfulness for personality disorders. Curr Opin Psychiatry. 2016 Jan;29(1):70–6. [PMID: 26651010]

Stoffers JM et al. Pharmacotherapy for borderline personality disorder—current evidence and recent trends. Curr Psychiatry Rep. 2015 Jan;17(1):534. [PMID: 25413640]

SCHIZOPHRENIA SPECTRUM DISORDERS

ESSENTIALS OF DIAGNOSIS

▶ Social withdrawal, usually slowly progressive, with decrease in emotional expression or motivation or both.

▶ Deterioration in personal care with disorganized behaviors or decreased reactivity to the environment or both.

▶ Disorganized thinking, often inferred from speech that switches topics oddly or is incoherent.

▶ Auditory hallucinations, often of a derogatory nature.

▶ Delusions, fixed false beliefs despite conflicting evidence, frequently of a persecutory nature.

General Considerations

Schizophrenia is manifested by a massive disruption of thinking, mood, and overall behavior as well as poor filtering of stimuli. The cause of schizophrenia is believed to be multifactorial, with genetic, environmental, and neurotransmitter pathophysiologic components. At present, there is no laboratory method for confirming the diagnosis of schizophrenia. There may or may not be a history of a major disruption in the individual's life (failure, loss, physical illness) before gross psychotic deterioration is evident.

Other psychotic disorders on this spectrum are conditions that are similar to schizophrenia in their acute symptoms, but have a less pervasive influence over the long term. The patient usually attains higher levels of functioning. The acute psychotic episodes tend to be less disruptive of the person's lifestyle, with a fairly quick return to previous levels of functioning.

Classification

A. Schizophrenia

Schizophrenia is the most common of the psychotic disorders that are all characterized by a loss of contact with reality. The term psychosis is broad and most often refers to having paranoia, auditory hallucinations, delusions, or all of these symptoms. One percent of the population suffers from schizophrenia. Schizophrenia is a chronic disorder that is characterized by increasing social and vocational disability that begins in late adolescence or early adulthood and tends to continue through life. The average age of onset for men is 18 years and for women is 25 years.

Symptoms have been classified into positive and negative categories. **Positive symptoms** include hallucinations, delusions, and disorganized speech; these symptoms appear to be related to increased dopaminergic (D_2) activity in the mesolimbic region, and all patients have at least one or two of these symptoms to meet criteria for diagnosis. There is often a component of paranoia involved. They may also have disorganized behavior, lack of emotional/cognitive responsiveness, or both. **Negative symptoms** include diminished sociability, restricted affect, and poverty of speech; these symptoms appear to be related to decreased D_2 activity in the mesocortical system. Level of functioning is markedly below that before the onset of symptoms, which must last at least 6 months in some form.

B. Delusional Disorder

Delusional disorders are psychoses in which the predominant symptoms are persistent delusions (ie, beliefs that are false yet fixed despite being shown evidence that they are unfounded) with minimal impairment of daily functioning. Intellectual and occupational activities are little affected, whereas social and partner functioning tends to be markedly involved. Hallucinations are not usually present. Common delusional themes include paranoid delusions of persecution, delusions of being related to or loved by a well-known person, and delusions that one's partner is unfaithful.

C. Schizoaffective Disorder

Schizoaffective disorders are those cases that fail to fit comfortably either in the schizophrenia or in the affective categories. They are usually cases with affective symptoms (either a major depressive episode, manic episode, or hypomanic episode) that precede or develop concurrently with psychotic manifestations, and the psychotic symptoms occur in the absence of any mood symptoms. The psychotic symptoms begin before the mood episode begins and can continue to linger for some time after resolution of the mood episode but do not remain permanently. Because of this, the long-term prognosis is better than for schizophrenia.

D. Schizophreniform Disorders

Schizophreniform disorders are similar in their symptoms to schizophrenic disorders except that the duration of prodromal, acute, and residual symptoms is longer than 1 month but less than 6 months.

E. Brief Psychotic Disorders

Brief psychotic disorders are defined as psychotic symptoms lasting less than 1 month. They are the result of psychological stress. The shorter duration is significant and correlates with a more acute onset and resolution as well as a much better prognosis.

▶ Clinical Findings

A. Symptoms and Signs

The symptoms and signs of schizophrenia *vary markedly among individuals as well as in the same person at different times.* The patient's appearance may be bizarre, although the usual finding is mildly to moderately unkempt. Motor activity is generally reduced, although extremes ranging from catatonic stupor to frenzied excitement occur. Social behavior is characterized by marked withdrawal coupled with disturbed interpersonal relationships and a reduced ability to experience pleasure. Dependency and a poor self-image are common. Verbal utterances are variable, the language being concrete yet symbolic, with unassociated rambling statements (at times interspersed with mutism) during an acute episode. Neologisms (made-up words or phrases), echolalia (repetition of words spoken by others), and verbigeration (repetition of senseless words or phrases) are occasionally present. Affect is usually flattened, with occasional inappropriateness. *Depression is present in almost all cases* but may be less apparent during the acute psychotic episode and more obvious during recovery. Depression is sometimes confused with akinetic side effects of antipsychotic medications. It is also related to boredom, which increases symptoms and decreases the response to treatment. Work is generally unavailable and time unfilled, providing opportunities for counterproductive activities such as drug abuse, withdrawal, and increased psychotic symptoms.

Thought content may vary from a paucity of ideas to a rich complex of delusional fantasy with archaic thinking. One frequently notes after a period of conversation that little if any information has actually been conveyed. Incoming stimuli produce varied responses. In some cases, a simple question may trigger explosive outbursts, whereas at other times there may be no overt response whatsoever (catatonia). When paranoid ideation is present, the patient is often irritable and less cooperative. Delusions (false beliefs) are characteristic of paranoid thinking, and they usually take the form of a preoccupation with the supposedly threatening behavior exhibited by other individuals. This ideation may cause the patient to adopt active countermeasures such as locking doors and windows, taking up weapons, covering the ceiling with aluminum foil to counteract radar waves, and other bizarre efforts. Somatic delusions revolve around issues of bodily decay or infestation. Perceptual distortions usually include auditory hallucinations—visual hallucinations are more commonly associated with organic mental states—and may include illusions (distortions of reality) such as figures changing in size or lights varying in intensity. Cenesthetic hallucinations (eg, a burning sensation in the brain, feeling blood flowing in blood vessels) occasionally occur. Lack of humor, feelings of dread, depersonalization (a feeling of being apart from the self), and fears of annihilation may be present. Any of the above symptoms generate higher anxiety levels, with heightened arousal and occasional panic and suicidal ideation, as the individual fails to cope.

The development of the acute episode in schizophrenia frequently is the end product of a gradual decompensation. Frustration and anxiety appear early, followed by depression and alienation, along with progressive ineffectiveness in day-to-day coping. This often leads to feelings of panic and increasing disorganization, with loss of the ability to test and evaluate the reality of perceptions.

The stage of so-called **psychotic resolution** includes delusions, autistic preoccupations, and psychotic insight, with acceptance of the decompensated state. The process is frequently complicated by the use of caffeine, alcohol, and other recreational drugs. Life expectancy of patients with schizophrenia is as much as 20% shorter than that of cohorts in the general population and is often associated with comorbid conditions such as the metabolic syndrome, which may be induced or exacerbated by the atypical antipsychotic agents.

Polydipsia may produce water intoxication with hyponatremia—characterized by symptoms of confusion, lethargy, psychosis, seizures, and occasionally death—in any psychiatric disorder, but most commonly in schizophrenia. These problems exacerbate the schizophrenic symptoms and can be confused with them. Possible pathogenetic factors in polydipsia include a hypothalamic defect, inappropriate antidiuretic hormone (ADH) secretion, antipsychotic medications (anticholinergic effects, stimulation of hypothalamic thirst center, effect on ADH), smoking (nicotine and syndrome of inappropriate antidiuretic hormone [SIADH]), psychotic thought processes (delusions), and other medications (eg, diuretics, antidepressants, lithium, alcohol) (see Chapter 21).

B. Imaging

Ventricular enlargement and cortical atrophy, as seen on CT scan, have been correlated with chronic course, severe cognitive impairment, and nonresponsiveness to antipsychotic medications. Decreased frontal lobe activity seen on PET scan has been associated with negative symptoms.

▶ Differential Diagnosis

The diagnosis of schizophrenia is best made over time because repeated observations increase the reliability of the diagnosis. One should not hesitate to reconsider the diagnosis of schizophrenia in any person who has received that diagnosis in the past, particularly when the clinical course has been atypical. A number of these patients have been found to actually have bipolar disorder, which has responded well to lithium. Manic episodes often mimic schizophrenia. However, schizophrenia is less likely to be associated with the decreased need for sleep, increase in goal-directed activity, and overconfidence, symptoms that are typical of mania. However, thought disorder, auditory hallucinations, and delusions are commonly seen in manic psychosis.

Psychotic depressions, brief reactive psychosis, delusional disorder, and any illness with psychotic ideation tend to be confused with schizophrenia, partly because of the regrettable tendency to use the terms interchangeably.

Medical disorders such as thyroid dysfunction, adrenal and pituitary disorders, reactions to toxic materials (eg, mercury, PCBs), and almost all of the organic mental states in the early stages must be ruled out. Postpartum psychosis is discussed under Mood Disorders. Complex partial seizures, especially when psychosensory phenomena are present, are an important differential consideration. Toxic drug states arising from prescription, over-the-counter, herbal and street drugs may mimic all of the psychotic disorders. The chronic use of amphetamines, cocaine, and other stimulants frequently produces a psychosis that is almost identical to the acute paranoid schizophrenic episode. Drug-induced psychoses can have all the positive symptoms of schizophrenia but less commonly have the negative symptoms. The presence of formication (sensation of insects crawling on or under the skin) and stereotypy suggests the possibility of stimulant abuse. Phencyclidine, a common street drug, may cause a reaction that is difficult to distinguish from other psychotic disorders. Cerebellar signs, excessive salivation, dilated pupils, and increased deep tendon reflexes should alert the clinician to the possibility of a toxic psychosis. Industrial chemical toxicity (both organic and metallic), degenerative disorders, and metabolic deficiencies must be considered in the differential diagnosis.

Catatonia, a psychomotor disturbance that may involve decreased motor activity, decreased interaction, or excessive and odd motor activity, is frequently assumed to exist solely as a component of schizophrenic disorders. However, it can actually be the end product of a number of illnesses, including a number of organic conditions as well as other psychiatric disorders such as bipolar disorder. Neoplasms, viral and bacterial encephalopathies, central nervous system hemorrhage, metabolic derangements such as diabetic ketoacidosis, sedative withdrawal, and liver and kidney malfunction have all been implicated. It is particularly important to realize that drug toxicity (eg, overdoses of antipsychotic medications such as fluphenazine or haloperidol) can cause catatonic syndrome, which may be misdiagnosed as a catatonic schizophrenia and inappropriately treated with more antipsychotic medication. Catatonia is also seen in other major psychiatric disorders, including bipolar disorder and major depression.

▶ Treatment

A. Pharmacologic (see Side Effects, below)

Hospitalization is sometimes necessary, particularly when the patient's behavior shows gross disorganization. The presence of competent family members or social support lessens the need for hospitalization, and each case should be judged individually. The major considerations are to prevent self-inflicted harm or harm to others and to provide the patient's basic needs. A full medical evaluation and CT scan or MRI of the brain should be considered in first episodes of psychosis.

Antipsychotic medications are the treatment of choice. The relapse rate can be reduced by 50% with proper maintenance antipsychotic therapy. Long-acting, injectable antipsychotics are used in nonadherent patients or nonresponders to oral medication or patients who choose the ease of not taking a daily pill.

Antipsychotic medications include the **"typical or first-generation"** antipsychotics (phenothiazines, thioxanthenes, butyrophenones, dihydroindolones, dibenzoxazepines, and benzisoxazoles) and the newer **"atypical**

Table 25–4. Commonly used antipsychotic medications (listed in alphabetical order).

Medication	Usual Daily Oral Dose	Usual Daily Maximum Dose[1]	Cost per Unit	Cost for 30 Days of Treatment Based on Maximum Dosage[2]
Aripiprazole (Abilify)	10–15 mg	30 mg	$45.35/30 mg	$1360.50
Asenapine (Saphris)	10–20 mg	20 mg	$24.02/10 mg	$1441.20
Cariprazine (Vraylar)	1.5–6 mg	6 mg	$48.03/6 mg	$1440.90
Chlorpromazine (Thorazine; others)	100–400 mg	1 g	$17.86/200 mg	$2679.00
Clozapine (Clozaril)	300–450 mg	900 mg	$2.73/100 mg	$737.10
Fluphenazine (Permitil, Prolixin)[3]	2–10 mg	60 mg	$1.15/10 mg	$207.00
Haloperidol (Haldol)	2–5 mg	60 mg	$2.76/20 mg	$248.40
Iloperidone (Fanapt)	12–24 mg	24 mg	$46.39/12 mg	$2783.40
Loxapine (Loxitane)	20–60 mg	200 mg	$2.57/50 mg	$308.40
Lurasidone (Latuda)	40–80 mg	80 mg	$48.94/80 mg	$1468.20
Olanzapine (Zyprexa)	5–10 mg	20 mg	$39.79/20 mg	$1193.70
Paliperidone (Invega)	6–12 mg	12 mg	$30.53/6 mg	$1831.80
Perphenazine (Trilafon)[3]	16–32 mg	64 mg	$3.90/16 mg	$468.00
Quetiapine (Seroquel)	200–400 mg	800 mg	$19.93/400 mg	$1195.80
Risperidone (Risperdal)[4]	2–6 mg	10 mg	$7.06/2 mg	$1059.00
Thiothixene (Navane)[3]	5–10 mg	80 mg	$3.36/10 mg	$806.40
Trifluoperazine (Stelazine)	5–15 mg	60 mg	$2.45/10 mg	$441.00
Ziprasidone (Geodon)	40–160 mg	160 mg	$10.76/80 mg	$645.60

[1]Can be higher in some cases.
[2]Average wholesale price (AWP, for AB-rated generic when available) for quantity listed. Source: IBM Micromedex Red Book (electronic version) IBM Watson Health, Greenwood, CO, USA. Available at https://www.micromedexsolutions.com (cited April 25, 2019). AWP may not accurately represent the actual pharmacy cost because wide contractual variations exist among institutions.
[3]Indicates piperazine structure.
[4]For risperidone, daily doses above 6 mg increase the risk of extrapyramidal syndrome. Risperidone 6 mg is approximately equivalent to haloperidol 20 mg.

or second-generation" antipsychotics (clozapine, risperidone, olanzapine, quetiapine, aripiprazole, ziprasidone, paliperidone, asenapine, iloperidone, lurasidone, and cariprazine) (Tables 25–4 and 25–5). Generally, increasing milligram potency of the typical antipsychotics is associated with decreasing anticholinergic and adrenergic side effects and increasing extrapyramidal symptoms. Data suggest similar antipsychotic efficacy for first- and second-generation antipsychotics, but a tendency for the second-generation antipsychotics to be better tolerated leading to enhanced compliance.

The phenothiazines comprise the bulk of the currently used "typical" or first-generation antipsychotic medications. The only butyrophenone commonly used in psychiatry is haloperidol, which is different in structure but similar in action and side effects to the piperazine phenothiazines such as fluphenazine, perphenazine, and trifluoperazine. These medications and haloperidol (dopamine [D_2] receptor blockers) have high potency and a paucity of autonomic side effects and act to markedly lower arousal levels.

Clozapine, the first "atypical" (novel) antipsychotic medication developed, has dopamine (D_4) receptor-blocking activity as well as central serotonergic, histaminergic, and alpha-noradrenergic receptor-blocking activity. It is effective in the treatment of about 30% of psychoses resistant to other antipsychotic medications, and it may have specific efficacy in decreasing suicidality in patients with schizophrenia. Risperidone is an antipsychotic that blocks some serotonin receptors (5-HT_2) and dopamine receptors (D_2). Risperidone causes fewer extrapyramidal side effects than the typical antipsychotics at doses less than 6 mg. It appears to be as effective as haloperidol and possibly as effective as clozapine in treatment-resistant patients without necessitating weekly white cell counts, as required with clozapine therapy. Risperidone is available in a long-acting injectable preparation.

Olanzapine is a potent blocker of 5-HT_2 and dopamine D_1, D_2, and D_4 receptors. High doses of olanzapine (10–20 mg daily) appear to be more effective than lower doses. The medication is somewhat more effective than haloperidol in the treatment of negative symptoms, such as withdrawal, psychomotor retardation, and poor interpersonal relationships. It is available in an orally disintegrating form for patients who are unable to tolerate standard oral dosing

Table 25–5. Relative potency and side effects of antipsychotic medications (listed in alphabetical order).

Medication	Chlorpromazine:Drug Potency Ratio	Anticholinergic Effects[1]	Extrapyramidal Effect[1]
Aripiprazole	1:20	1	1
Chlorpromazine	1:1	4	1
Clozapine	1:1	4	—
Fluphenazine	1:50	1	4
Haloperidol	1:50	1	4
Iloperidone	1:25	1	1
Loxapine	1:10	2	3
Lurasidone	1:5	1	2
Olanzapine	1:20	1	1
Perphenazine	1:10	2	3
Quetiapine	1:1	1	1
Risperidone	1:50	1	3
Thiothixene	1:20	1	4
Trifluoperazine	1:20	1	4
Ziprasidone	1:1	1	1

[1]1, weak effect; 4, strong effect.

and in an injectable form for the management of acute agitation associated with schizophrenia and bipolar disorder. Olanzapine is available in a long-term injectable preparation, but this formulation tends to be used less commonly than other depot formulations because some patients experience severe sedation and delirium, which occurs in about 0.5–1% of patients.

Quetiapine is an antipsychotic with greater 5-HT$_2$ relative to D$_2$ receptor blockade as well as a relatively high affinity for alpha-1- and alpha-2-adrenergic receptors. It appears to be as efficacious as haloperidol in treating positive and negative symptoms of schizophrenia, with fewer extrapyramidal side effects even at high doses.

Ziprasidone has both anti-dopamine receptor and anti-serotonin receptor effects, with good efficacy for both positive and negative symptoms of schizophrenia. Aripiprazole is a partial agonist at the dopamine D$_2$ and serotonin 5-HT$_1$ receptors and an antagonist at 5-HT$_2$ receptors, and it is effective against positive and negative symptoms of schizophrenia. It functions as an antagonist or agonist, depending on the dopaminergic activity at the dopamine receptors. This may help decrease side effects. Aripiprazole is approved as an augmentation agent for treatment-resistant depression, even when psychosis is not present, and as a maintenance treatment for bipolar disorder. Aripiprazole is available as an acute injectable preparation as well as a long-term injectable preparation that is given once monthly in patients who are not able to adhere to daily oral dosing. Asenapine, approved for the treatment of schizophrenia and bipolar disorder (mixed or manic state), appears to be particularly helpful in treating negative symptoms of schizophrenia. Paliperidone, the active metabolite of risperidone, is available as a capsule and a monthly injection. Lurasidone is FDA-approved and has been shown to be effective in treating acute decompensation in patients with chronic schizophrenia. Cariprazine is a partial agonist of the D$_2$ and D$_3$ receptor and is approved by the FDA for the treatment of schizophrenia and bipolar disorder. Akathisia, weight gain, and insomnia are among the more commonly reported side effects with cariprazine. Because cariprazine is not a potent D$_2$-antagonist, it is less likely to increase prolactin levels than most antipsychotics.

1. Clinical indications—The antipsychotics are used to treat all forms of the schizophrenias as well as drug-induced psychoses, psychotic depression, augmentation of unipolar depression, acute mania, and the prevention of mood cycles in bipolar disorder. They are also effective in Tourette syndrome and behavioral dyscontrol in autistic patients. While frequently used to treat agitation in dementia patients, no antipsychotic has been shown to be reliably effective in this population and may *increase the risk of early mortality in elderly dementia patients.* Antipsychotics quickly lower the arousal (activity) level and, perhaps indirectly, gradually improve socialization and thinking. The improvement rate for treating positive symptoms is about 80%. Patients whose behavioral symptoms worsen with use of antipsychotic medications may have an undiagnosed organic condition such as anticholinergic toxicity.

Symptoms that are ameliorated by these medications include hyperactivity, hostility, aggression, delusions, hallucinations, irritability, and poor sleep. Individuals with acute psychosis and good premorbid function respond quite well. The most common cause of failure in the treatment of acute psychosis is inadequate dosage, and the most common cause of relapse is noncompliance.

Although first-generation antipsychotics are efficacious in the treatment of positive symptoms of schizophrenia, such as hallucinations and delusions, second-generation antipsychotics are thought to have efficacy in reducing positive symptoms and some efficacy in treating negative symptoms. Antidepressant medications may be used in conjunction with antipsychotics if significant depression is present. Resistant cases may require concomitant use of lithium, carbamazepine, or valproic acid. The addition of a benzodiazepine medication to the antipsychotic regimen may prove helpful in treating the agitated or catatonic psychotic patient who has not responded to antipsychotics alone—lorazepam, 1–2 mg orally, can produce a rapid resolution of catatonic symptoms and may allow maintenance with a lower antipsychotic dose. Electroconvulsive therapy (ECT) has also been effective in treating catatonia and in treating schizophrenia when used in combination with medications.

2. Dosage forms and patterns—The dosage range is quite broad (Table 25–4). For example, risperidone, 0.25–1 mg orally at bedtime, may be sufficient for the elderly person with mild dementia with psychosis (especially in view of the increased risk of stroke and death in the elderly), whereas up to 6 mg/day may be used in a young patient with acute schizophrenia. For quick response, an atypical antipsychotic may be started in combination with a benzodiazepine (eg, risperidone oral solution, 2 mg, or olanzapine, 10 mg orally, and lorazepam, 2 mg orally, every 2–4 hours as needed). In an acutely distressed, psychotic patient one might use haloperidol, 10 mg intramuscularly, which is absorbed rapidly and achieves an initial tenfold plasma level advantage over equal oral doses. Psychomotor agitation, racing thoughts, and general arousal are quickly reduced. The dose can be repeated every 3–4 hours; when the patient is less symptomatic, oral doses can replace parenteral administration in most cases. In the elderly, both atypical (eg, risperidone 0.25 mg–0.5 mg daily or olanzapine 1.25 mg daily) and typical (eg, haloperidol 0.5 mg daily or perphenazine 2 mg daily) antipsychotics, often used effectively in small doses for behavioral control, have been linked to premature death in some cases.

Absorption of oral medications may be increased or decreased by concomitant administration of other medications (eg, antacids tend to decrease the absorption of antidepressants). Previous gastrointestinal surgery may alter pH, motility, and surface areas available for drug absorption. There are racial genetic-based enzyme differences in metabolizing the antipsychotic medications—eg, many Asians require only about half the usual dosage. Bioavailability is influenced by other factors such as smoking or hepatic microsomal enzyme stimulation with alcohol or barbiturates and enzyme-altering medications such as carbamazepine or methylphenidate. Antipsychotic plasma drug level determinations are not currently of major clinical assistance.

Divided daily doses are not necessary after a maintenance dose has been established, and most patients can then be maintained on a single daily dose, usually taken at bedtime. This is particularly appropriate in a case where the sedative effect of the medication is desired for nighttime sleep, and undesirable sedative effects can be avoided during the day. First-episode patients especially should be tapered off medications after about 6 months of stability and carefully monitored; their rate of relapse is lower than that of multiple-episode patients.

Psychiatric patients—particularly paranoid individuals—often neglect to take their medication. In these cases and in nonresponders to oral medication, the enanthate and decanoate (the latter is slightly longer-lasting and has fewer extrapyramidal side effects) forms of fluphenazine or the decanoate form of haloperidol may be given by deep subcutaneous injection or intramuscularly to achieve an effect that will usually last 7–28 days. A patient who cannot be depended on to take oral medication (or who overdoses on minimal provocation) will generally agree to come to the clinician's office for a "shot." The usual dose of the fluphenazine long-acting preparations is 25 mg every 2 weeks. Dosage and frequency of administration vary from about 12.5 mg monthly to 100 mg weekly. Use the smallest effective amount as infrequently as possible. A monthly injection of 25 mg of fluphenazine decanoate is equivalent to about 15–20 mg of oral fluphenazine daily. Risperidone was the first atypical antipsychotic available in a long-acting injectable form (25–50 mg intramuscularly every 2 weeks). Concomitant use of a benzodiazepine (eg, lorazepam, 2 mg orally twice daily) may permit reduction of the required dosage of oral or parenteral antipsychotic medication. Long-acting injectables are now available for risperidone, paliperidone, aripiprazole, and olanzapine.

Intravenous haloperidol, the antipsychotic most commonly used by this route, is often used in critical care units in the management of agitated, delirious patients. Intravenous haloperidol should be given no faster than 1 mg/min to reduce cardiovascular side effects, such as torsades de pointes. Current practice indicates that ECG monitoring should be used whenever haloperidol is being administered intravenously.

Some antipsychotic agents are available for intranasal administration. The intranasal form of loxapine has a more rapid onset of action for the treatment of agitation (about 10 minutes) than either intramuscular or oral antipsychotic agents. Also, intranasal administration tends to be less traumatic to patients than getting an injection. However, intranasal loxapine requires the cooperation of the patient and is more expensive than generic antipsychotic injectable preparations.

There have been investigations for novel compounds involving other therapeutics targets such as the glutamate system as well as the inflammatory cascade.

3. Side effects—For both typical and atypical antipsychotic agents, a range of side effects has been reported. The most common anticholinergic side effects include **dry mouth** (which can lead to ingestion of caloric liquids and weight gain or hyponatremia), **blurred near vision, urinary retention** (particularly in elderly men with enlarged prostates), **delayed gastric emptying, esophageal reflux, ileus, delirium,** and precipitation of **acute glaucoma** in patients with narrow anterior chamber angles. Other autonomic effects include **orthostatic hypotension** and **sexual dysfunction**—problems in achieving erection, ejaculation (including retrograde ejaculation), and orgasm in men (approximately 50% of cases) and women (approximately 30%). Delay in achieving orgasm is often a factor in medication noncompliance. **Electrocardiographic changes** occur frequently, but clinically significant arrhythmias are much less common. Elderly patients and those with pre-existing cardiac disease are at greater risk. The most frequently seen electrocardiographic changes include diminution of the T wave amplitude, appearance of prominent U waves, depression of the ST segment, and prolongation of the QT interval (Table 25–6). Ziprasidone can produce QTc prolongation. A pretreatment ECG is indicated for patients at risk for cardiac sequelae (including patients taking other medications that might prolong the QTc interval). In some critical care patients, torsades de pointes has been associated with the use of high-dose intravenous haloperidol (usually greater than 30 mg/24 h).

Associations have been suggested between the atypical antipsychotics and new-onset **diabetes, hyperlipidemia, and weight gain** (Table 25–6). The FDA has particularly noted the risk of hyperglycemia and new-onset diabetes in this class of medication that is *not* related to weight gain. The risk of diabetes mellitus is increased in patients taking clozapine and olanzapine. Monitoring of weight, fasting blood sugar, and lipids prior to initiation of treatment and at regular intervals thereafter is an important part of medication monitoring. The addition of metformin to olanzapine may improve drug-induced weight gain in patients with drug-naïve, first-episode schizophrenia. Antipsychotic medications in general may have **metabolic and endocrine effects,** including weight gain, hyperglycemia, impaired temperature regulation in hot weather, and water intoxication, which may be due to inappropriate ADH secretion. **Lactation and menstrual irregularities** are common (antipsychotic medications should be avoided, if possible, in breast cancer patients because of potential trophic effects of elevated prolactin levels on the breast). Both antipsychotic and antidepressant medications **inhibit sperm motility. Bone marrow depression** and **cholestatic**

jaundice occur rarely; these are hypersensitivity reactions, and they usually appear in the first 2 months of treatment. They subside on discontinuance of the medication. There is cross-sensitivity among all of the phenothiazines, and a medication from a different group should be used when allergic reactions occur.

Clozapine is associated with a 1.6% risk of **agranulocytosis** (higher in persons of Ashkenazi Jewish ancestry), and its use must be strictly monitored with weekly blood counts during the first 6 months of treatment, with monitoring every other week thereafter. The risk of developing agranulocytosis is approximately 2.5 times higher in patients with a polymorphism for *HLADQB1* gene. Thus, this genetic test may be worthwhile to perform before initiating clozapine. Discontinuation of the medication requires weekly monitoring of the white blood cell count for 1 month. Clozapine has been associated with fatal myocarditis and is contraindicated in patients with severe heart disease. In addition, clozapine lowers the seizure threshold and has many side effects, including sedation, hypotension, increased liver biochemical levels, hypersalivation, respiratory arrest, weight gain, and changes in both the ECG and the electroencephalogram. Notably, adynamic ileus is a rare side effect of clozapine that can be fatal, and patients should be closely monitored and treated quickly and preemptively for constipation.

Photosensitivity, retinopathy, and **hyperpigmentation** are associated with use of fairly high dosages of chlorpromazine. The appearance of particulate melanin deposits in the lens of the eye is related to the total dose given, and patients on long-term medication should have periodic eye examinations. Teratogenicity has not been causally related to these medications, but prudence is indicated particularly in the first trimester of pregnancy. The seizure threshold is lowered, but it is safe to use these medications in epileptics who take anticonvulsants.

The **neuroleptic malignant syndrome (NMS)** is a catatonia-like state manifested by extrapyramidal signs, blood pressure changes, altered consciousness, and

Table 25–6. Adverse factors associated with atypical antipsychotic medications (listed in alphabetical order).

Medication	Weight Gain	Hyperlipidemia	New-Onset Diabetes Mellitus	QTc Prolongation[1]
Aripiprazole	+/–	–	–	++
Asenapine	+/–	+/–	+/–	+++
Clozapine	+++	+++	+++	+/–
Lurasidone	–	–	–	–
Olanzapine	+++	+++	+++	+/–
Paliperidone	+	+/–	+/–	+++
Quetiapine	++	++	++	+++
Risperidone	++	++	++	+
Ziprasidone	+/–	–	–	+++

[1]QTc prolongation is a side effect of many medications and suggests a possible risk for arrhythmia. Prescriber's Letter 2011;18(12):271207.

hyperpyrexia; it is an uncommon but serious complication of antipsychotic treatment. Muscle rigidity, involuntary movements, confusion, dysarthria, and dysphagia are accompanied by pallor, cardiovascular instability, fever, pulmonary congestion, and diaphoresis and may result in stupor, coma, and death. The cause may be related to a number of factors, including poor dosage control of antipsychotic medication, affective illness, decreased serum iron, dehydration, and increased sensitivity of dopamine receptor sites. Lithium in combination with an antipsychotic medication may increase vulnerability, which is already increased in patients with an affective disorder. In most cases, the symptoms develop within the first 2 weeks of antipsychotic drug treatment. The syndrome may occur with small doses of the medications. Intramuscular administration is a risk factor. Elevated creatine kinase and leukocytosis with a shift to the left are present early in about half of cases. Treatment includes controlling fever and providing fluid support. Dopamine agonists such as bromocriptine, 2.5–10 mg orally three times a day, and amantadine, 100–200 mg orally twice a day, have also been useful. Dantrolene, 50 mg intravenously as needed, is used to alleviate rigidity (do not exceed 10 mg/kg/day due to hepatotoxicity risk). There is ongoing controversy about the efficacy of these three agents as well as the use of calcium channel blockers and benzodiazepines. ECT has been used effectively in resistant cases. Clozapine has been used with relative safety and fair success as an antipsychotic medication for patients who have had NMS.

Akathisia is the most common (about 20%) extrapyramidal symptom. It usually occurs early in treatment (but may persist after antipsychotics are discontinued) and is frequently mistaken for anxiety or exacerbation of psychosis. It is characterized by a subjective desire to be in constant motion followed by an inability to sit or stand still and consequent pacing. It may induce suicidality or feelings of fright, rage, terror, or sexual torment. Insomnia is often present. It is crucial to educate patients in advance about these potential side effects so that the patients do not misinterpret them as signs of increased illness. In all cases, reevaluate the dosage requirement or the type of antipsychotic medication. One should inquire also about cigarette smoking, which in women has been associated with an increased incidence of akathisia. Antiparkinsonism medications (such as trihexyphenidyl, 2–5 mg orally three times daily) may be helpful, but first-line treatment often includes a benzodiazepine (such as clonazepam 0.5–1 mg orally three times daily). In resistant cases, symptoms may be alleviated by propranolol, 30–80 mg/day orally, diazepam, 5 mg orally three times daily, or amantadine, 100 mg orally three times daily.

Acute dystonias usually occur early, although a late (tardive) occurrence is reported in patients (mostly men after several years of therapy) who previously had early severe dystonic reactions and a mood disorder. Younger patients are at higher risk for acute dystonias. The most common signs are bizarre muscle spasms of the head, neck, and tongue. Frequently present are torticollis, oculogyric crises, swallowing or chewing difficulties, and masseter spasms. Laryngospasm is particularly dangerous. Back,

arm, or leg muscle spasms are occasionally reported. Diphenhydramine, 50 mg intramuscularly, is effective for the acute crisis; one should then give benztropine mesylate, 2 mg orally twice daily, for several weeks, and then discontinue gradually, since few of the extrapyramidal symptoms require long-term use of the antiparkinsonism medications (all of which are about equally efficacious—though trihexyphenidyl tends to be mildly stimulating and benztropine mildly sedating).

Drug-induced parkinsonism is indistinguishable from idiopathic parkinsonism, but it is reversible, occurs later in treatment than the preceding extrapyramidal symptoms, and in some cases appears after antipsychotic withdrawal. The condition includes the typical signs of apathy and reduction of facial and arm movements (akinesia, which can mimic depression), festinating gait, rigidity, loss of postural reflexes, and pill-rolling tremor. Patients with AIDS seem particularly vulnerable to extrapyramidal side effects. High-potency antipsychotics often require antiparkinsonism medications (see Table 24–6). The antipsychotic dosage should be reduced, and immediate relief can be achieved with antiparkinsonism medications in the same dosages as above. After 4–6 weeks, these antiparkinsonism medications can often be discontinued with no recurrent symptoms. In any of the extrapyramidal symptoms, amantadine, 100–400 mg orally daily, may be used instead of the antiparkinsonism medications. Antipsychotic-induced catatonia is similar to catatonic stupor with rigidity, drooling, urinary incontinence, and cogwheeling. It usually responds slowly to withdrawal of the offending medication and use of antiparkinsonism agents.

Tardive dyskinesia is a syndrome of abnormal involuntary stereotyped movements of the face, mouth, tongue, trunk, and limbs that may occur after months or (usually) years of treatment with antipsychotic agents. The syndrome affects 20–35% of patients who have undergone long-term antipsychotic therapy. Predisposing factors include older age, many years of treatment, cigarette smoking, and diabetes mellitus. Pineal calcification is higher in this condition by a margin of 3:1. There are no clear-cut differences among the antipsychotic medications in the development of tardive dyskinesia. (Although the atypical antipsychotics appear to offer a lower risk of tardive dyskinesia, long-term effects have not been investigated.) However, clozapine is unique in that it has been found to treat antipsychotic-induced tardive dyskinesia. Early manifestations of tardive dyskinesia include fine worm-like movements of the tongue at rest, difficulty in sticking out the tongue, facial tics, increased blink frequency, or jaw movements of recent onset. Later manifestations may include bucco-linguo-masticatory movements, lip smacking, chewing motions, mouth opening and closing, disturbed gag reflex, puffing of the cheeks, disrupted speech, respiratory distress, or choreoathetoid movements of the extremities (the last being more prevalent in younger patients). The symptoms do not necessarily worsen and in rare cases may lessen even though antipsychotic medications are continued. The dyskinesias do not occur during sleep and can be voluntarily suppressed for short periods. Stress and movements in other parts of the body will often aggravate the condition.

Early signs of dyskinesia must be differentiated from those reversible signs produced by ill-fitting dentures or nonantipsychotic medications such as levodopa, TCAs, antiparkinsonism agents, anticonvulsants, and antihistamines. Other neurologic conditions such as Huntington chorea can be differentiated by history and examination.

The emphasis should be on prevention of side effects. Use the least amount of antipsychotic medication necessary to mute the psychotic symptoms. Detect early manifestations of dyskinesias. When these occur, stop anticholinergic medications and gradually discontinue antipsychotic medications, if clinically feasible. Weight loss and cachexia sometimes appear on withdrawal of antipsychotics. In an indeterminate number of cases, the dyskinesias will remit. Keep the patient off the medications until reemergent psychotic symptoms dictate their resumption, at which point they are restarted in low doses and gradually increased until there is clinical improvement. If antipsychotic medications are restarted, clozapine and olanzapine appear to offer less risk of recurrence. The use of adjunctive agents such as benzodiazepines or lithium may help directly or indirectly by allowing control of psychotic symptoms with a low dosage of antipsychotics. If the dyskinesic syndrome recurs and it is necessary to continue antipsychotic medications to control psychotic symptoms, informed consent should be obtained. Benzodiazepines, buspirone (in doses of 15–60 mg/day orally), phosphatidylcholine, clonidine, calcium channel blockers, vitamin E, omega-3 fatty acids, and propranolol all have had limited usefulness in treating the dyskinetic side effects.

B. Social

Environmental considerations are most important in the individual with a chronic illness, who usually has a history of repeated hospitalizations, a continued low level of functioning, and symptoms that never completely remit. Family rejection and work failure are common. In these cases, board and care homes staffed by personnel experienced in caring for psychiatric patients are most important. There is frequently an inverse relationship between stability of the living situation and the amounts of required antipsychotic medications, since the most salutary environment is one that reduces stimuli. Nonresidential self-help groups such as Recovery, Inc., should be utilized whenever possible. They provide a setting for sharing, learning, and mutual support and are frequently the only social involvement with which this type of patient is comfortable. Vocational rehabilitation and work agencies (eg, Goodwill Industries, Inc.) provide assessment, training, and job opportunities at a level commensurate with the person's clinical condition.

C. Psychological

The need for psychotherapy varies markedly depending on the patient's current status and history. In a person with a single psychotic episode and a previously good level of adjustment, supportive psychotherapy may help the patient reintegrate the experience, gain some insight into antecedent problems, and become a more self-observant individual who can recognize early signs of stress. Research suggests that cognitive behavioral therapy—in conjunction with medication management—has efficacy in the treatment of symptoms of schizophrenia. Cognitive behavioral therapy for schizophrenia involves helping the individual challenge psychotic thinking and alters response to hallucinations. Similarly, a form of psychotherapy called acceptance and commitment therapy has shown value in helping prevent hospitalizations in schizophrenia. Cognitive remediation therapy is another approach to treatment that may help patients with schizophrenia become better able to focus their disorganized thinking. Family therapy may also help alleviate the patient's stress and to assist relatives in coping with the patient.

D. Behavioral

Behavioral techniques (see above) are most frequently used in therapeutic settings such as day treatment centers, but they can also be incorporated into family situations or any therapeutic setting. Many behavioral techniques (eg, positive reinforcement—whether it be a word of praise or an approving nod—after some positive behavior) can be a powerful instrument for helping a person learn behaviors that will facilitate social acceptance. Music from portable digital players or smartphones with earphones is one of many ways to divert the patient's attention from auditory hallucinations.

▶ Prognosis

For most patients with any psychosis, the prognosis is good for alleviation of positive symptoms such as hallucinations or delusions treated with medication. Negative symptoms such as diminished affect and sociability are much more difficult to treat but appear mildly responsive to atypical antipsychotics. Cognitive deficits, such as the executive dysfunction that is common to schizophrenia, also do not appear as responsive to antipsychotics as do positive symptoms. Unfortunately, both negative symptoms and cognitive deficits appear to contribute more to long-term disability than do positive symptoms. Unavailability of structured work situations and lack of family therapy or access to other social support are two other reasons why the prognosis is so guarded in such a large percentage of patients.

Buckley PF et al. Schizophrenia research: a progress report. Psychiatr Clin North Am. 2015 Sep;38(3):373–7. [PMID: 26300028]

Owen MJ et al. Schizophrenia. Lancet. 2016 Jul 2;388(10039): 86–97. [PMID: 26777917]

Tseng PT et al. Significant effect of valproate augmentation therapy in patients with schizophrenia: a meta-analysis study. Medicine (Baltimore). 2016 Jan;95(4):e2475. [PMID: 26825886]

Yang AC et al. New targets for schizophrenia treatment beyond the dopamine hypothesis. Int J Mol Sci. 2017 Aug 3;18(8):E1689. [PMID: 28771182]

MOOD DISORDERS (Depression & Mania)

ESSENTIALS OF DIAGNOSIS

Present in most depressions

▶ Mood varies from mild sadness to intense despondency and feelings of guilt, worthlessness, and hopelessness.

▶ Difficulty in thinking, including inability to concentrate, ruminations, and lack of decisiveness.

▶ Loss of interest, with diminished involvement in work and recreation.

▶ Somatic complaints such as disrupted, lessened, or excessive sleep; loss of energy; change in appetite; decreased sexual drive.

Present in some severe depressions

▶ Psychomotor retardation or agitation.

▶ Delusions of a somatic or persecutory nature.

▶ Withdrawal from activities.

▶ Physical symptoms of major severity, eg, anorexia, insomnia, reduced sexual drive, weight loss, and various somatic complaints.

▶ Suicidal ideation.

Possible symptoms in mania

▶ Mood ranging from euphoria to irritability.

▶ Sleep disruption.

▶ Hyperactivity.

▶ Racing thoughts.

▶ Grandiosity or extreme overconfidence.

▶ Variable psychotic symptoms.

▶ General Considerations

Depression is extremely common, with up to 30% of primary care patients having depressive symptoms. Depression may be the final expression of (1) genetic factors (neurotransmitter dysfunction), (2) developmental problems (personality problems, childhood events), or (3) psychosocial stresses (divorce, unemployment). It frequently presents in the form of somatic complaints with negative medical workups. *Although sadness and grief are normal responses to loss, depression is not.* Patients experiencing normal grief tend to produce sympathy and sadness in the clinician caregiver; depression often produces frustration and irritation in the clinician. Grief is usually accompanied by intact self-esteem, whereas depression is marked by a sense of guilt and worthlessness.

Mania is often combined with depression and may occur alone, together with depression in a mixed episode, or in cyclic fashion with depression.

▶ Clinical Findings

In general, there are four major types of depression, with similar symptoms in each group.

A. Adjustment Disorder with Depressed Mood

Depression may occur in reaction to some identifiable stressor or adverse life situation, usually loss of a person by death (grief reaction), divorce, etc; financial reversal (crisis); or loss of an established role, such as being needed. Anger is frequently associated with the loss, and this in turn often produces a feeling of guilt. The disorder occurs within 3 months of the stressor and causes significant impairment in social or occupational functioning. The symptoms range from mild sadness, anxiety, irritability, worry, and lack of concentration, discouragement, and somatic complaints to the more severe symptoms of frank depression. *When the full criteria for major depressive disorder are present, however, then that diagnosis should be made and treatment instituted even when there is a known stressor.* The presence of a stressor is not the determining diagnostic driver, it is the resultant syndromal complex. One should not neglect treatment for major depression simply because it may appear to be an understandable reaction to a particular stress or difficulty.

B. Depressive Disorders

The subclassifications include major depressive disorder and dysthymia.

1. Major depressive disorder—A major depressive disorder consists of a syndrome of mood, physical and cognitive symptoms that occurs at any time of life. Many consider a physiologic or metabolic aberration to be causative. Complaints vary widely but most frequently include a loss of interest and pleasure (anhedonia), withdrawal from activities, and feelings of guilt. Also included are inability to concentrate, some cognitive dysfunction, anxiety, chronic fatigue, feelings of worthlessness, somatic complaints (unexplained somatic complaints frequently indicate depression), loss of sexual drive, and thoughts of death. Unemployment has been associated with increase in depression risk. Diurnal variation with improvement as the day progresses is common. Vegetative signs that frequently occur are insomnia, anorexia with weight loss, and constipation. Occasionally, severe agitation and psychotic ideation are present. **Psychotic major depression** occurs up to 14% of all patients with major depression and 25% of patients who are hospitalized with depression. Psychotic symptoms (delusions, paranoia) are more common in depressed persons who are older than 50 years. Paranoid symptoms may range from general suspiciousness to ideas of reference with delusions. The somatic delusions frequently revolve around feelings of impending annihilation or somatic concerns (eg, that the body is rotting away with cancer). Hallucinations are less common than unusual beliefs and tend not to occur independent of delusions.

In addition to psychotic major depression, other subcategories include **major depression with atypical features** that is characterized by hypersomnia, overeating, lethargy, and mood reactivity in which the mood brightens in response to positive events or news. **Melancholic major depression** is characterized by a lack of mood reactivity seen in atypical depression, the presence of a prominent anhedonia, and more severe vegetative symptoms. **Major depression with a seasonal onset (seasonal affective disorder)** is a dysfunction of circadian rhythms that occurs more commonly in the fall and winter months and is believed to be due to decreased exposure to full-spectrum light. Common symptoms include carbohydrate craving, lethargy, hyperphagia, and hypersomnia. **Major depression with peripartum onset** occurs during pregnancy or starts up to 4 weeks after delivery.

Half of depressions associated with the peripartum period start during pregnancy. Most women (up to 80%) experience some mild letdown of mood in the postpartum period. For some of these (10–15%), the symptoms are more severe and similar to those usually seen in serious depression, with an increased emphasis on concerns related to the baby (obsessive thoughts about harming it or inability to care for it). When psychotic symptoms occur, there is frequently associated sleep deprivation, volatility of behavior, and manic-like symptoms. Postpartum psychosis is much less common (less than 2%), often occurs within the first 2 weeks, and requires early and aggressive management. Biologic vulnerability with hormonal changes and psychosocial stressors all play a role. The chances of a second episode are about 25% and may be reduced with prophylactic treatment.

2. Persistent depressive disorder (dysthymia)—
Dysthymia is a chronic depressive disturbance. Sadness, loss of interest, and withdrawal from activities over a period of 2 or more years with a relatively persistent course are necessary for this diagnosis. Generally, the symptoms are milder but longer-lasting than those in a major depressive episode.

3. Premenstrual dysphoric disorder—Depressive symptoms occur during the late luteal phase (last 2 weeks) of the menstrual cycle. (See also Chapter 18.)

C. Bipolar Disorder

Bipolar disorder consists of episodic mood shifts into mania, major depression, hypomania, and mixed mood states. The ability of bipolar disorder to mimic aspects of many other coincident major mental health disorders and a high comorbidity with substance abuse can make the initial diagnosis of bipolar disorder difficult. **Bipolar I** is diagnosed when an individual has manic episodes. For individuals who experience hypomanic episodes without frank mania, the diagnosis is **bipolar II**.

1. Mania—A manic episode is a mood state characterized by elation with hyperactivity, overinvolvement in life activities, increased irritability, flight of ideas, easy distractibility, and little need for sleep. The overenthusiastic quality of the mood and the expansive behavior initially attract others, but the irritability, mood lability with swings into depression, aggressive behavior, and grandiosity usually lead to marked interpersonal difficulties. Activities may occur that are later regretted, eg, excessive spending, resignation from a job, a hasty marriage, sexual acting out, and exhibitionistic behavior, with alienation of friends and family. Atypical manic episodes can include gross delusions, paranoid ideation of severe proportions, and auditory hallucinations usually related to some grandiose perception. The episodes begin abruptly (sometimes precipitated by life stresses) and may last from several days to months. Generally, the manic episodes are of shorter duration than the depressive episodes. *In almost all cases, the manic episode is part of a broader bipolar disorder.* Patients with four or more discrete episodes of a mood disturbance in 1 year have "rapid cycling." (Substance abuse, particularly cocaine, can mimic rapid cycling.) These patients have a higher incidence of hypothyroidism. Patients with mania differ from patients with schizophrenia in that the former use more effective interpersonal maneuvers, are more sensitive to the social maneuvers of others, and are more able to utilize weakness and vulnerability in others to their own advantage. Creativity has been positively correlated with mood disorders, but the best work done is between episodes of mania and depression.

2. Cyclothymic disorder—This is a chronic mood disturbance with episodes of subsyndromal depression and hypomania. The symptoms must have at least a 2-year duration and are milder than those that occur in depressive or manic episodes. Occasionally, the symptoms will escalate into a full-blown manic or depressive episode, in which case reclassification as bipolar I or II would be warranted.

D. Mood Disorders Secondary to Illness and Medications

Any illness, severe or mild, can cause significant depression. Conditions such as rheumatoid arthritis, multiple sclerosis, stroke, and chronic heart disease are particularly likely to be associated with depression, as are other chronic illnesses. Depression is common in cancer, as well, with a particularly high degree of comorbidity in pancreatic cancer. Hormonal variations clearly play a role in some depressions. Varying degrees of depression occur at various times in schizophrenic disorders, central nervous system disease, and organic mental states. Alcohol dependency frequently coexists with serious depression.

The classic model of **drug-induced depression** occurred with the use of reserpine, both in clinical settings and as a pharmacologic probe in research settings. Corticosteroids and oral contraceptives are commonly associated with mood changes such as depression and hypomania. Antihypertensive medications such as methyldopa, guanethidine, and clonidine have been associated with the development of depressive syndromes, as have digitalis and antiparkinsonism medications (eg, levodopa). Interferon is strongly associated with depressed mood and fatigue as a side effect; consultation with a psychiatrist prior to prescribing these agents is indicated in cases where there is a history of depression. It is unusual for beta-blockers to produce depression when given for short periods, such as in the treatment of performance anxiety. Sustained use of beta-blockers for medical conditions such as hypertension may be associated with depression in some patients, although most individuals do not suffer this adverse effect. One study associated the use of beta-blockers with a significant reduction in risk of depressive symptoms 1 year after a percutaneous coronary intervention. Infrequently, disulfiram and anticholinesterase medications may be associated with symptoms of depression. All stimulant use results in a depressive syndrome when the drug is withdrawn. Alcohol, sedatives, opioids, and most of the psychedelic drugs are depressants and, paradoxically, are often used in self-treatment of depression. Corticosteroids may be associated with hypomania.

Differential Diagnosis

Since depression may be a part of any illness—either reactively or as a secondary symptom—careful attention must be given to personal life adjustment problems and the role of medications (eg, reserpine, corticosteroids, levodopa). Schizophrenia, partial complex seizures, organic brain syndromes, panic disorders, and anxiety disorders must be differentiated. Thyroid dysfunction and other endocrinopathies should be ruled out. Malignancies, including central and gastrointestinal tumors are sometimes associated with depressive symptoms and may antecede the diagnosis of tumor. Strokes, particularly dominant hemisphere lesions, can occasionally present with a syndrome that looks like major depression. Medication-induced depressive symptoms are also quite common.

Complications

The most important complication is **suicide**, which often includes some elements of aggression. Suicide rates in the general population vary from 9 per 100,000 in Spain to 14 per 100,000 in the United States to 58 per 100,000 in Hungary. In individuals hospitalized for depression, the lifetime risk rises to 10–15%. In patients with bipolar I disorder, the risk is higher, with up to 20% of individuals dying of suicide. Men over the age of 50 are more likely to *complete* a suicide because of their tendency to attempt suicide with more violent means, particularly guns. On the other hand, women make more *attempts* but are less likely to complete a suicide. An increased suicide rate is being observed in the younger population, aged 15–35. Patients with cancer, respiratory illnesses, AIDS, and those being maintained on hemodialysis have higher suicide rates. Alcohol use is a significant factor in many suicide attempts.

There are several groups of people who make suicide attempts. One group includes those individuals with acute situational problems. These individuals may be acutely distressed by a recent breakup in a relationship or another type of disappointment. This group also includes those who may not be diagnosed as having depression, but who are overwhelmed by a stressful situation often with an aspect of public humiliation (eg, victims of cyber-bullying). A suicide attempt in such cases may be an impulsive or aggressive act not associated with significant depression.

Another high-risk group includes individuals with severe depression. Severe depression may be due to conditions such as medical illness (eg, AIDS, whose victims have a suicide rate over 20 times that of the general population) or comorbid psychiatric disorders (eg, panic disorders). Anxiety, panic, and fear are major findings in suicidal behavior. A patient may seem to make a dramatic improvement, but the lifting of depression may be due to the patient's decision to commit suicide. Another high-risk group are individuals with psychotic illness who tend not to verbalize their concerns and are often successful in their suicide attempt, although they make up only a small percentage of the total.

Suicide is 10 times more prevalent in patients with schizophrenia than in the general population, and jumping from bridges is a more common means of attempted suicide by patients with schizophrenia than by others. In one study of 100 people who jumped from bridges, 47% had schizophrenia.

The immediate goal of psychiatric evaluation is to assess the current suicidal risk and the need for hospitalization versus outpatient management. *Perhaps the one most useful question is to ask the person how many hours per day he or she thinks about suicide.* If it is more than 1 hour, the individual is at high risk. Further assessing the risk by inquiring about intent, plans, means, and suicide-inhibiting factors (eg, strong ties to children or the church) is essential. Alcohol, hopelessness, delusional thoughts, and complete or nearly complete loss of interest in life or ability to experience pleasure are all positively correlated with suicide attempts. Other risk factors are previous attempts, a family history of suicide, medical or psychiatric illness (eg, anxiety, depression, psychosis), male sex, older age, contemplation of violent methods, a humiliating social stressor, and drug use (including long-term sedative or alcohol use), which contributes to impulsiveness or mood swings. Successful treatment of the patient at risk for suicide cannot be achieved if the patient continues to abuse drugs. An attempt is less likely to be suicidal, for example, if small amounts of poison or medication were ingested or scratching of wrists was superficial, if the act was performed in the vicinity of others or with early notification of others, or if the attempt was arranged so that early detection would be anticipated.

The patient's current mood status is best evaluated by direct evaluation of plans and concerns about the future, personal reactions to the attempt, and thoughts about the reactions of others. Measurement of mood is often facilitated by using a standardized instrument such as the Hamilton or Montgomery-Asberg clinician-administered rating scales or the self-administered Patient Health Questionnaire-9. Scales allow for initial assessment as well as ongoing treatment tracking. Suicide risk can be specifically assessed using an instrument such as the Columbia-Suicide Severity Risk Scale. The patient's immediate resources should also be assessed—people who can be significantly involved (most important), family support, job situation, financial resources, etc.

If hospitalization is not indicated after a suicide attempt, the clinician must formulate and institute a treatment plan or make an adequate referral. (The National Suicide Prevention Lifeline, 1-800-273-8255, may be of assistance.) Medication should be dispensed in small amounts to at-risk patients. Although TCAs and SSRIs are associated with an equal incidence of suicide attempts, the risk of a completed suicide is much higher with TCA overdose. Guns and medications should be removed from the patient's household. Driving should be interdicted until the patient improves. The problem is often worsened by the long-term complications of the suicide attempt, eg, brain damage due to hypoxia, peripheral neuropathies caused by staying for long periods in one position causing nerve compressions, and medical or surgical problems such as esophageal strictures and tendon dysfunctions.

▶ Treatment of Depression

A. Medical

Milder forms of depression usually do not require medication therapy and can be managed by psychotherapy and the passage of time. In severe cases—particularly when vegetative signs are significant and symptoms have persisted for more than a few weeks—antidepressant medication therapy is often effective. Medication therapy is also suggested by a family history of major depression in first-degree relatives or a past history of prior episodes.

The antidepressant medications may be classified into four groups: (1) the newer antidepressants, including the SSRIs, SNRIs, and bupropion, vilazodone, vortioxetine, and mirtazapine, (2) the TCAs and clinically similar medications, (3) the MAO inhibitors (Table 25–7), and (4) stimulants. ECT and repetitive transcranial magnetic stimulation are procedural treatments for depression. These modalities are described in greater detail below.

Hospitalization is necessary if suicide is a major consideration or if complex treatment modalities are required.

Medication selection is influenced by the history of previous response or lack thereof if that information is available. A positive family history of response to a particular medication suggests that the patient may respond similarly. If no background information is available, a medication such as sertraline, 25 mg orally daily and increasing gradually up to 200 mg, or venlafaxine at 37.5 mg/day and titrated gradually to a maximum dose of 225 mg/day can be selected and a *full trial* instituted. The medication trial should be monitored for worsening mood or suicidal ideation with patient assessments every 1–2 weeks until week 6. The STAR*D trial suggests that if the response to the first medication is inadequate, the best alternatives are to switch to a second agent that may be from the same or different class of antidepressant; another option is to try augmenting the first agent with bupropion (150–450 mg/day), lithium (eg, 300–900 mg/day orally), thyroid medication (eg, liothyronine, 25–50 mcg/day orally), or a second-generation antipsychotic (eg, aripiprazole [5–15 mg/day] or olanzapine [5–15 mg/day]). The latter course is often taken when there has been at least a partial response to the initial medication. The Agency for Health Care Policy and Research has produced clinical practice guidelines that outline one algorithm of treatment decisions (Figure 25–2).

Psychotic depression should be treated with a combination of an antipsychotic such as olanzapine and an antidepressant such as an SSRI at their usual doses. Mifepristone may have specific and early activity against psychotic depression. ECT is generally regarded as the single most effective treatment for psychotic depression.

Major depression with atypical features or seasonal onset can be treated with bupropion or an SSRI with good results. MAO inhibitors appear more effective than TCAs, and a MAO inhibitor may be used if more benign antidepressant strategies prove unsuccessful.

Melancholic depression may respond to ECT, TCAs, and SNRIs, which are preferable to SSRIs. However, SSRIs are often used in the treatment of melancholic depression and are effective in many cases.

Caution: Depressed patients often have suicidal thoughts, and the amount of medication dispensed should be appropriately controlled particularly if prescribing a MAO inhibitor, TCA, and to a lesser extent, venlafaxine. At the same time, *adults with untreated depression are at higher risk for suicide than those who are treated sufficiently to reduce symptoms.* It has been thought that in children and adolescent populations, antidepressants may be associated with some slightly increased risk of suicidality. One meta-analysis indicates that suicidality persists even after symptoms of depression are treated, suggesting other causes such as increased impulsivity among younger patients. After age 25, antidepressants may have neutral or possibly protective effects until age 65 years or older. The older TCAs have a narrow therapeutic index. One advantage of the newer medications is their wider margin of safety. Nonetheless, even with newer agents, because of the possibility of suicidality early in antidepressant treatment, close follow-up is indicated. In all cases of pharmacologic management of depressed states, caution is indicated until the risk of suicide is considered minimal.

1. SSRIs, SNRIs, and atypical antidepressants—The SSRIs include fluoxetine, sertraline, paroxetine, fluvoxamine, citalopram and its enantiomer escitalopram (Table 25–7). The chief advantages of these agents are that they are generally well tolerated, the starting dose is typically a therapeutic dose for most patients, and they have much lower lethality in overdose compared to TCAs or MAO inhibitors. (Notably, citalopram carries a warning regarding QT prolongation in doses above 40 mg, and 20 mg is considered the maximum dose for patients older than 60 years. There is no similar FDA warning for escitalopram.) The SNRIs include venlafaxine, desvenlafaxine, duloxetine, milnacipran, and levomilnacipran. In addition to possessing the strong serotonin reuptake blocking properties of the SSRIs, the SNRIs are also norepinephrine reuptake blockers. The combined serotonergic-noradrenergic properties of these medications may provide benefits in pain conditions such as neuropathy and fibromyalgia as well as conditions such as stress incontinence. The atypical antidepressants are bupropion, nefazodone, trazodone, vilazodone, vortioxetine, and mirtazapine (Table 25–7). All of these antidepressants are effective in the treatment of depression, both typical and atypical. The SSRI medications have been effective in the treatment of panic disorder, bulimia, GAD, OCD, and PTSD.

Table 25–7. Commonly used antidepressant medications (listed in alphabetical order within classes).

Medication	Usual Daily Oral Dose (mg)	Usual Daily Maximum Dose (mg)	Sedative Effects[1]	Anticholinergic Effects[1]	Cost per Unit	Cost for 30 Days of Treatment Based on Maximum Dosage[2]
SSRIs						
Citalopram (Celexa)	20	40	< 1	1	$2.53/40 mg	$75.90
Escitalopram (Lexapro)	10	20	< 1	1	$4.51/20 mg	$135.30
Fluoxetine (Prozac, Sarafem)	5–40	80	< 1	< 1	$2.48/20 mg	$297.60
Fluvoxamine (Luvox)	100–300	300	1	< 1	$2.64/100 mg	$237.60
Paroxetine (Paxil)	20–30	50	1	1	$2.64/20 mg	$161.10
Sertraline (Zoloft)	50–150	200	< 1	< 1	$2.71/100 mg	$162.60
SNRIs						
Desvenlafaxine (Pristiq)	50	100	1	< 1	$11.47/100 mg	$344.10
Duloxetine (Cymbalta)	40	60	2	3	$7.85/60 mg	$235.50
Levomilnacipran (Fetzima)	40	120	1	1	$15.71/80 mg	$471.36
Milnacipran (Savella)	100	200	1	1	$7.64/100 mg	$458.32
Venlafaxine XR (Effexor)	150–225	225	1	< 1	$4.67/75 mg	$420.30
Tricyclic and Clinically Similar Compounds						
Amitriptyline (Elavil)	150–250	300	4	4	$2.14/150 mg	$128.40
Amoxapine (Asendin)	150–200	400	2	2	$1.98/100 mg	$237.60
Clomipramine (Anafranil)	100	250	3	3	$11.24/75 mg	$1348.80
Desipramine (Norpramin)	100–250	300	1	1	$5.74/100 mg	$498.60
Doxepin (Sinequan)	150–200	300	4	3	$1.97/100 mg	$177.30
Imipramine (Tofranil)	150–200	300	3	3	$1.16/50 mg	$219.60
Maprotiline (Ludiomil)	100–200	300	4	2	$2.34/75 mg	$280.80
Nortriptyline (Aventyl, Pamelor)	100–150	150	2	2	$4.22/75 mg	$253.20
Protriptyline (Vivactil)	15–40	60	1	3	$3.30/10 mg	$594.00
Trimipramine (Surmontil)	75–200	200	4	4	$9.44/100 mg	$566.40
Monoamine Oxidase Inhibitors						
Phenelzine (Nardil)	45–60	90	…	…	$0.84/15 mg	$151.20
Selegiline transdermal (Emsam)	6 (skin patch)	12	…	…	$65.98/6 mg patch	$1979.50
Tranylcypromine (Parnate)	20–30	50	…	…	$3.60/10 mg	$540.00
Other Compounds						
Bupropion SR (Wellbutrin SR)	300	400[3]	< 1	< 1	$3.51/200 mg	$210.60
Bupropion XL (Wellbutrin XL)	300[4]	450[4]	< 1	< 1	$4.77/300 mg	$286.20
Mirtazapine (Remeron)	15–45	45	4	2	$2.43/30 mg	$77.70
Nefazodone (Serzone)	150–600	600	3	1	$4.98/200 mg	$448.20
Trazodone (Desyrel)	100–300	400	4	< 1	$1.10/100 mg	$132.00
Vilazodone (Viibryd)	10–40	40	1	1	$10.89/40 mg	$326.70
Vortioxetine (Brintellix)	10	20	<1	< 1	$15.35/20 mg	$460.50

[1]1, weak effect; 4, strong effect.
[2]Average wholesale price (AWP, for AB-rated generic when available) for quantity listed. Source: IBM Micromedex Red Book (electronic version) IBM Watson Health, Greenwood, CO, USA. Available at https://www.micromedexsolutions.com (cited April 25, 2019). AWP may not accurately represent the actual pharmacy cost because wide contractual variations exist among institutions.
[3]200 mg twice daily.
[4]Wellbutrin XL is a once-daily form of bupropion. Bupropion is still available as immediate release, and, if used, no single dose should exceed 150 mg.
SNRIs, serotonin norepinephrine reuptake inhibitors; SSRIs, selective serotonin reuptake inhibitors.

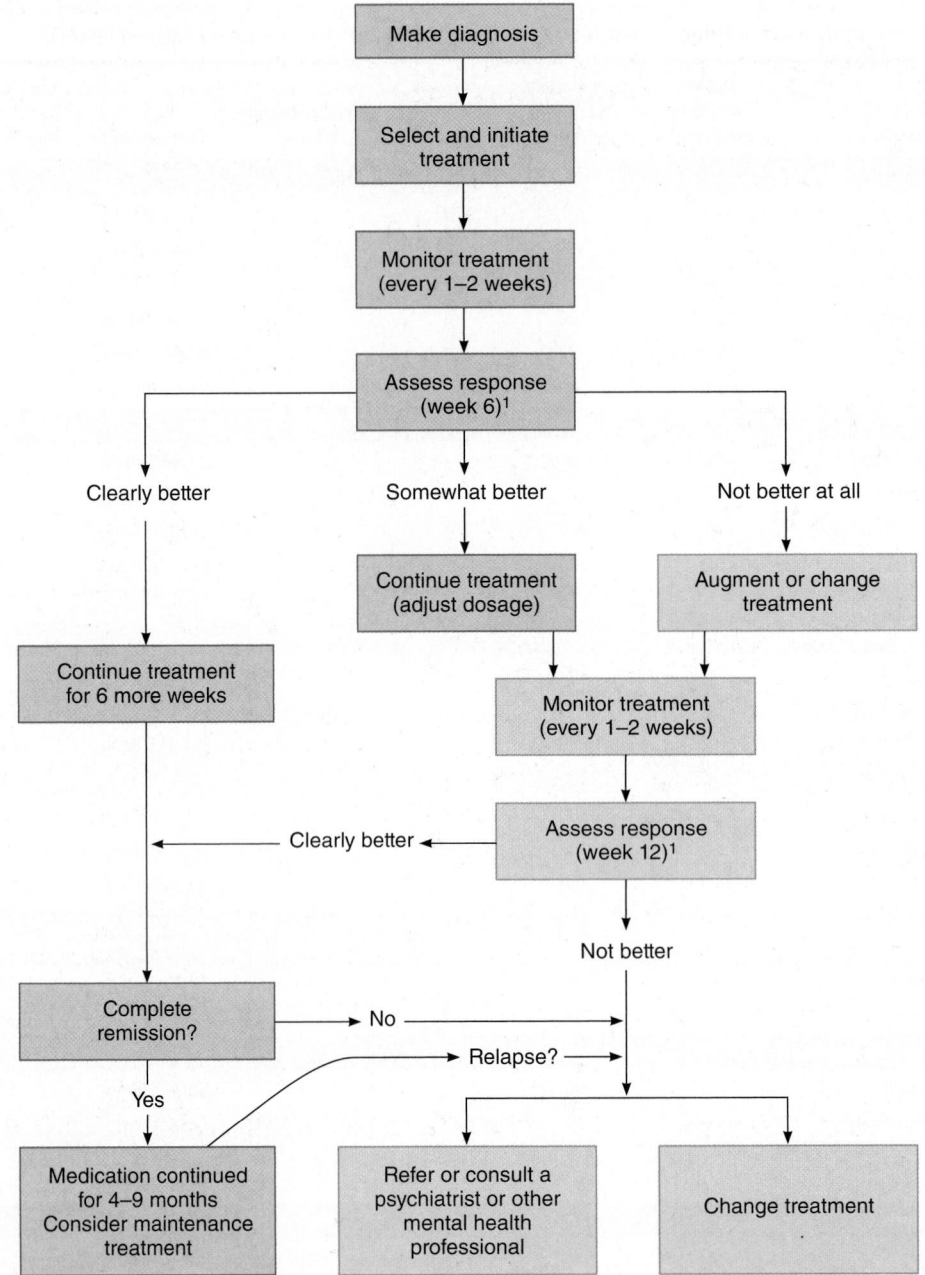

Figure 25–2. Overview of treatment for depression. (Reproduced from Agency for Health Care Policy and Research: Depression in Primary Care. Vol. 2: Treatment of Major Depression. United States Department of Health and Human Services, 1993.)

[1]Times of assessment (weeks 6 and 12) rest on very modest data. It may be necessary to revise the treatment plan earlier for patients not responding at all.

Most of the medications in this group tend to be activating and are given in the morning so as not to interfere with sleep. Some patients, however, may have sedation, requiring that the medication be given at bedtime. This reaction occurs most commonly with paroxetine, fluvoxamine, and mirtazapine. The SSRIs can be given in once-daily dosage. Nefazodone and trazodone are usually given twice daily. Bupropion and venlafaxine are available in extended-release formulations and can be given once daily. There is usually some delay in response; fluoxetine, for example, requires 2–6 weeks to act in depression, 4–8 weeks to be effective in panic disorder, and 6–12 weeks in treatment of OCD. The starting dose (10 mg) is given for 1 week before increasing to the average daily oral dose of 20 mg for depression, while OCD may require up to 80 mg daily. Some patients, particularly the elderly, may tolerate and benefit from as little as 10 mg/day or every other day. The other SSRIs have shorter half-lives and a lesser effect on hepatic enzymes, which reduces their impact on the metabolism of other medications (thus not increasing significantly the serum concentrations of other medications as much as fluoxetine). The shorter half-lives also allow for more rapid clearing if adverse side effects appear. Venlafaxine appears to be more effective with doses greater than 200 mg/day orally, although some individuals respond to doses as low as 75 mg/day.

The side effects common to all of these medications are headache, nausea, tinnitus, insomnia, and nervousness. Akathisia has been common with the SSRIs; other extrapyramidal symptoms (eg, dystonias) have occurred infrequently but particularly in withdrawal states. Because SSRIs affect platelet serotonin levels, abnormal bleeding can occur. Sertraline and citalopram appear to be the safest agents in this class when used with warfarin. Sexual side effects of erectile dysfunction, retrograde ejaculation, and dysorgasmia are very common with the SSRIs. Oral phosphodiesterase-5 inhibitors (such as sildenafil, 25–50 mg; tadalafil, 5-20 mg; or vardenafil, 10–20 mg taken 1 hour prior to sexual activity) can improve erectile dysfunction in some patients and have been shown to improve other SSRI-induced sexual dysfunction in both men and women. Adjunctive bupropion (75–150 mg orally daily) may also enhance sexual arousal. Cyproheptadine, 4 mg orally prior to sexual activity, may be helpful in countering drug-induced anorgasmia but also is quite sedating and may counter the therapeutic benefits of SSRIs as well. Taking a "drug holiday," ie, skipping a day of medication periodically when sexual activity is anticipated, can also decrease sexual side effects. The SSRIs are strong serotonin uptake blockers and may in high dosage or in combination with MAO inhibitors, including the antiparkinsonian drug selegiline, cause a **"serotonin syndrome."** This syndrome is manifested by rigidity, hyperthermia, autonomic instability, myoclonus, confusion, delirium, and coma. This syndrome can be a particularly troublesome problem in the elderly. Research indicates that SSRIs are safer agents to use than TCAs in patients with cardiac disease; the SSRI sertraline is a safe and effective antidepressant treatment in patients with acute myocardial infarction or unstable angina.

Withdrawal symptoms, including dizziness, paresthesias, dysphoric mood, agitation, and a flu-like state, have been reported for the shorter-acting SSRIs and SNRIs but may occur with other classes including the TCAs and MAO inhibitors. These medications should be discontinued gradually over a period of weeks or months to reduce the risk of withdrawal phenomena.

Fluoxetine, fluvoxamine, sertraline, venlafaxine, and citalopram in customary antidepressant doses may increase the risk of major fetal malformation when used during pregnancy; however, the absolute risk of congenital defects is considered low. Maternal major mood disorder in pregnancy by itself carries its own risks to the mother and fetus and has been linked to low birth weight and preterm delivery. Postpartum effects of prenatal depression have not been studied. The decision to use SSRIs and other psychotropic agents during pregnancy and postpartum must be a collaborative decision based on a thorough risk-benefit analysis for each individual.

Venlafaxine lacks significant anticholinergic side effects. Nausea, nervousness, and profuse sweating appear to be the major side effects. Venlafaxine appears to have few drug-drug interactions. It does require monitoring of blood pressure because dose-related hypertension may develop in some individuals. Venlafaxine prescribing in the United Kingdom has been restricted to psychiatrists. Venlafaxine appears to carry a greater risk of lethal arrhythmias in instances of overdose relative to the SSRIs, but less risk than with the TCAs. Desvenlafaxine, a newer form of the medication, is started at its target dose of 50 mg/day orally and does not require upward titration although higher doses have been well studied and some patients benefit from 100 mg/day. Duloxetine may also result in small increases in blood pressure. Common side effects include dry mouth, dizziness, and fatigue. Inhibitors of 1A2 and 2D6 may increase duloxetine levels with a risk of toxicity. Milnacipran, approved for the treatment of fibromyalgia, and levomilnacipran, approved for the treatment of major depression, carry many of the side effects common to other SNRIs including a mild tachycardia, hypertension, sexual side effects, mydriasis, urinary constriction, and occasional abnormal bleeding. Levomilnacipran is started at 20 mg/day orally then increased to 40 mg/day after 2–3 days. The target dose is 40–120 mg given once daily. Milnacipran is typically started at 12.5 mg/day orally, titrated to 12.5 mg twice daily after 2 days, and then to 25 mg twice daily after 7 days. The target dose is typically 100–200 mg/day given in in two divided doses. While not approved for the treatment of major depression, the evidence suggests that milnacipran, like levomilnacipran, is an effective antidepressant agent.

Nefazodone appears to lack the anticholinergic effects of the TCAs and the agitation sometimes induced by SSRIs. Nefazodone should not be given with terfenadine, astemizole, or cisapride, which are not commercially available in the United States. Because nefazodone inhibits the liver's cytochrome P450 3A4 isoenzymes, concurrent use of these medications can lead to serious QT prolongation, ventricular tachycardia, or death. Through the same mechanism of enzyme inhibition, nefazodone can elevate cyclosporine levels sixfold to tenfold. Nefazodone carries an FDA warning given its association with liver failure in rare cases. Pretreatment and ongoing monitoring of liver biochemical enzymes are indicated.

Mirtazapine is thought to enhance central noradrenergic and serotonergic activity with minimal sexual side effects compared with the SSRIs. Its action as a potent antagonist of histaminergic receptors may make it a useful agent for patients with depression and insomnia. It is also an effective antiemetic due to its antagonism of the 5-HT$_3$ receptor. Its most common adverse side effects include somnolence, increased appetite, weight gain, lipid abnormalities, and dizziness. The labeling for mirtazapine indicated that agranulocytosis was seen in 2 of 2796 patients in premarketing studies. An association of agranulocytosis or a clinically significant neutropenia with the medication appears to be modest. Although it is metabolized by P450 isoenzymes, it is not an inhibitor of this system. It is given in a single oral dose at bedtime starting at 15 mg and increasing in 15-mg increments every week or every other week up to 45 mg.

Vortioxetine is an antidepressant that blocks serotonin reuptake, is a partial agonist of the 5-HT$_{1A}$ receptor, and effects a variety of other serotonin receptor sites. The side effects attributed to its serotonergic effects include gastrointestinal upset and sexual dysfunction. Vortioxetine has demonstrated efficacy in improving cognitive symptoms of depression and received regulatory approval for this indication in Europe. Vortioxetine is typically dosed at 10 mg/day orally and may be increased to 20 mg/day.

2. Tricyclic antidepressants (TCAs) and clinically similar medications—TCAs were the mainstay of medication therapy for depression for many years. They have also been effective in panic disorder, pain syndromes, and anxiety states. Specific ones have been studied and found to be effective in OCD (clomipramine), enuresis (imipramine), psychotic depression (amoxapine), and reduction of craving in cocaine withdrawal (desipramine).

TCAs are characterized more by their similarities than by their differences. They tend to affect both serotonin and norepinephrine reuptake; some medications act mainly on the former and others principally on the latter neurotransmitter system. Individuals receiving the same dosages vary markedly in therapeutic drug levels achieved (elderly patients require smaller doses), and determination of plasma drug levels is helpful when clinical response has been disappointing. Nortriptyline is usually effective when plasma levels are between 50 and 150 ng/mL; imipramine at plasma levels of 200–250 ng/mL; and desipramine at plasma levels of 100–250 ng/mL. High blood levels are not more effective than moderate levels and may be counterproductive (eg, delirium, seizures). Patients with gastrointestinal side effects benefit from plasma level monitoring to assess absorption of the drug. Most TCAs can be given in a single dose at bedtime, starting at fairly low doses (eg, nortriptyline 25 mg orally) and increasing by 25 mg every several days as tolerated until the therapeutic response is achieved (eg, nortriptyline, 100–150 mg) or to maximum dose if necessary (eg, nortriptyline, 150 mg). *The most common cause of treatment failure is an inadequate trial.* A full trial consists of giving a therapeutic daily dosage for at least 6 weeks. Because of marked anticholinergic and sedating side effects, clomipramine is started at a low dose (25 mg/day orally) and increased slowly in divided doses up to 100 mg/day, held at that level for several days, and then gradually increased as necessary up to 250 mg/day. The TCAs have anticholinergic side effects to varying degrees (amitriptyline 100 mg is equivalent to atropine 5 mg). One must be particularly wary of the effect in elderly men with prostatic hyperplasia. The anticholinergic effects also predispose to other medical problems such as constipation, confusion, heat stroke, or dental problems from xerostomia. Orthostatic hypotension is fairly common, is not dose-dependent, and may not remit with time on medication; this may predispose to falls and hip fractures in the elderly.

Cardiac effects of the TCAs are functions of the anticholinergic effect, direct myocardial depression, quinidine-like effect, and interference with adrenergic neurons. These factors may produce altered rate, rhythm, and contractility, particularly in patients with preexisting cardiac disease, such as bundle-branch or bifascicular block. Even relatively small overdoses (eg, 1500 mg of imipramine) have resulted in lethal arrhythmias. Electrocardiographic changes range from benign ST segment and T wave changes and sinus tachycardia to a variety of complex and serious arrhythmias, the latter requiring a change in medication. Because TCAs have class I antiarrhythmic effects, they should be used with caution in patients with ischemic heart disease, arrhythmias, or conduction disturbances. SSRIs or the atypical antidepressants are better initial choices for this population.

TCAs lower the seizure threshold so this is of particular concern in patients with a propensity for seizures. Loss of libido and erectile, ejaculatory, and orgasmic dysfunction are fairly common and can compromise compliance. Trazodone rarely causes priapism (1 in 9000), but when it occurs, it requires treatment within 12 hours (epinephrine 1:1000 injected into the corpus cavernosum). Delirium, agitation, and mania are infrequent complications of the TCAs but can occur. Sudden discontinuation of some of these medications can produce "cholinergic rebound," manifested by headaches and nausea with abdominal cramps. Overdoses of TCAs are often serious because of the narrow therapeutic index and quinidine-like effects (see Chapter 38).

3. Monoamine oxidase inhibitors—The MAO inhibitors are generally used as third-line medications for depression (after a failure of SSRIs, SNRIs, TCAs, or the atypical antidepressants) because of the dietary and other restrictions required (Table 25–8). They should be considered third-line medications for refractory panic disorder as well as depression; however, this hierarchy has become more flexible since MAO inhibitor skin patches (selegiline) have become available. They deliver the MAO inhibitor to the bloodstream bypassing the gastrointestinal tract so that dietary restrictions are not necessary in the lowest dosage strength (6 mg/24 h).

The MAO inhibitors commonly cause symptoms of orthostatic hypotension (which may persist) and sympathomimetic effects of tachycardia, sweating, and tremor. Nausea, insomnia (often associated with intense afternoon drowsiness), and sexual dysfunction are common. Zolpidem 5–10 mg orally at bedtime can ameliorate MAO-induced insomnia. Central nervous system effects include

Table 25–8. Principal dietary restrictions in MAOI use.

1. Cheese, except cream cheese and cottage cheese and fresh yogurt
2. Fermented or aged meats such as bologna, salami
3. Broad bean pods such as Chinese bean pods
4. Liver of all types
5. Meat and yeast extracts
6. Red wine, sherry, vermouth, cognac, beer, ale
7. Soy sauce, shrimp paste, sauerkraut

MAOI, monoamine oxidase inhibitor.

agitation and toxic psychoses. Dietary limitations (see Table 25–8) and abstinence from medication products containing phenylpropanolamine, phenylephrine, meperidine, dextromethorphan, and pseudoephedrine are mandatory for MAO-A type inhibitors (those marketed for treatment of depression), since the reduction of available MAO leaves the patient vulnerable to exogenous amines (eg, tyramine in foodstuffs).

4. Stimulants and other medications under investigation— Dextroamphetamine (5–30 mg/day orally) and methylphenidate (10–45 mg/day orally) may be effective for the short-term treatment of some depressive symptoms in medically ill and geriatric patients. The stimulants are notable for rapid onset of action (hours) and a paucity of side effects (tachycardia, agitation) in most patients. They are usually given in two divided doses early in the day (eg, 7 am and noon) so as to avoid interfering with sleep. These agents may also be useful as adjunctive agents in refractory depression. Intravenous infusion of the dissociative anesthetic ketamine has been shown to lead to a rapid improvement in depressive symptoms in 50–70% of patients with depression. The effects of a single treatment are short-lived (about 3–7 days). Ketamine acts both through the glutamate system as well as the opioid system. Other NMDA antagonists and opioid system agents continue to be evaluated in the treatment of resistant depression. Esketamine has been designated by the FDA as a potential breakthrough medication and has been approved, with significant restrictions, for the treatment of depression for patients who have been inadequately treated by two other antidepressant medications. However, there are ongoing concerns about long-term use of esketamine or ketamine, including the risk of abuse, psychotomimetic side effects, and the risk of uropathy.

5. Switching and combination therapy— If the therapeutic response has been poor after an adequate trial with the chosen medication, the diagnosis should be reassessed. Assuming that the trial has been adequate and the diagnosis is correct, a trial with a second medication is appropriate. In switching from one group to another, an adequate "washout time" must be allowed. This is critical in certain situations—eg, in switching from a MAO inhibitor to a TCA, allow 2–3 weeks between stopping one medication and starting another; in switching from an SSRI to a MAO inhibitor, allow 4–5 weeks for fluoxetine and at least 2 weeks for other SSRIs. In switching within groups—eg, from one TCA to another (amitriptyline to desipramine, etc)—no washout time is needed, and one can rapidly decrease the dosage of one medication while increasing the other. In clinical practice, adjunctive treatment with lithium, buspirone, or thyroid hormone may be helpful in depression. The adjunctive use of low-dose atypical antipsychotics such as aripiprazole, olanzapine, and quetiapine in the treatment of patients with refractory depression is supported by research. The side effect risk is the same as when treating psychosis. Adding an atypical agent requires monitoring body mass index, lipids, and glucose. Combining two antidepressants, or adding an antipsychotic to an antidepressant, requires caution and is usually reserved for

clinicians who feel comfortable managing this or after psychiatric consultation.

6. Maintenance and tapering— When clinical relief of symptoms is obtained, medication is continued for 12 months in the effective maintenance dosage, which is the dosage required in the acute stage. The full dosage should be continued indefinitely when the individual has a first episode before age 20 or after age 50, is over age 40 with two episodes, has at least one episode after age 50, or has had three episodes at any age. *Major depression generally should be considered a chronic/intermittent disease with most patients having relapses in time and some patients never fully recovering from a depressive episode.* If the medication is being tapered, it should be done gradually over several months, monitoring closely for relapse.

7. Drug interactions— Interactions with other medications are listed in Table 25–9.

8. Electroconvulsive therapy— ECT causes a generalized central nervous system seizure (peripheral convulsion is not necessary) by means of electric current. The key objective is to exceed the seizure threshold, which can be accomplished by a variety of means. The mechanism of action is not known, but it is thought to involve major neurotransmitter responses at the cell membrane.

ECT is the most effective (about 70–85%) treatment of severe depression. In treatment-resistant depression, remission rates from ECT are lower (around 48%). It is particularly effective for the delusions and agitation commonly seen with depression in the elderly. It is indicated when medical conditions preclude the use of antidepressants, nonresponsiveness to these medications, and extreme suicidality. Comparative controlled studies of ECT in severe depression show that it is more effective than pharmacotherapy. It is also effective in the treatment of mania and psychoses during pregnancy (when medications may be contraindicated). It has also been shown to be helpful in chronic schizophrenic disorders when clozapine alone is not fully effective.

The most common side effects of ECT are memory disturbance and headache. Memory loss or confusion is usually related to the number and frequency of ECT treatments and proper oxygenation during treatment. Unilateral ECT is associated with less memory loss than bilateral ECT. Both anterograde and retrograde memory loss may occur, but short term-retrograde memory loss is more common. While some memory deficits may persist, memory loss tends to improve in a few weeks after the last ECT treatment. There have been reports that lithium administration concurrent with ECT resulted in greater memory loss.

Increased intracranial pressure is a relative contraindication. Other problems such as cardiac disorders, aortic aneurysms, bronchopulmonary disease, and venous thrombosis must be evaluated in light of the severity of the medical problem versus the need for ECT. Serious complications arising from ECT occur in less than 1 in 1000 cases. Most of these problems are cardiovascular or respiratory in nature (eg, aspiration of gastric contents, arrhythmias, myocardial infarction). Poor patient understanding and lack of acceptance of the technique by the public are the biggest obstacles to the use of ECT.

Table 25–9. Antidepressant drug interactions with other medications (listed in alphabetical order within classes).

Medication	Effects
Tricyclic and Other Non-MAOI Antidepressants	
Antacids	Decreased absorption of antidepressants
Anticoagulants	Increased hypoprothrombinemic effect
Cimetidine	Increased antidepressant blood levels and psychosis
Clonidine	Decreased antihypertensive effect
Digitalis	Increased incidence of heart block
Disulfiram	Increased antidepressant blood levels
Haloperidol	Increased antidepressant levels
Insulin	Decreased blood sugar
Lithium	Increased lithium levels with fluoxetine
Methyldopa	Decreased antihypertensive effect
Other anticholinergic medications	Marked anticholinergic responses
Phenytoin	Increased blood levels
Procainamide	Decreased ventricular conduction
Procarbazine	Hypertensive crisis
Propranolol	Increased hypotension
Quinidine	Decreased ventricular conduction
Rauwolfia derivatives	Increased stimulation
Sedatives	Increased sedation
Sympathomimetic medications	Increased vasopressor effect
Terfenadine,[1] astemizole,[1] cisapride[1]	Torsades de pointes
MAOIs	
Antihistamines	Increased sedation
Belladonna-like medications	Increased blood pressure
Dextromethorphan	Same as meperidine
Guanethidine	Decreased blood pressure
Insulin	Decreased blood sugar
Levodopa	Increased blood pressure
Meperidine	Increased agitation, serotonin syndrome, death
Methyldopa	Decreased blood pressure
Pseudoephedrine	Hypertensive crisis (increased blood pressure)
Reserpine	Increased blood pressure/ hypertensive crisis
Succinylcholine	Increased neuromuscular blockade
Sulfonylureas	Decreased blood sugar
Sympathomimetic medications	Increased blood pressure/hypertensive crisis
SSRIs, SNRIs, triptans	Serotonin syndrome, death

[1]Terfenadine, astemizole, and cisapride are not commercially available in the United States.

MAOIs, monoamine oxidase inhibitors; SNRIs, serotonin norepinephrine reuptake inhibitors; SSRIs, selective serotonin reuptake inhibitors.

9. Phototherapy—Phototherapy is used in major depression with seasonal onset. It consists of indirect eye exposure to a light source of greater than 2500 lux for 2 hours daily or 10,000 lux for 20 minutes daily to increase the photoperiod of the day. Light visors are an adaptation that provides greater mobility and an adjustable light intensity but may not be as effective. The dosage varies, with some patients requiring morning and night exposure. One effect is alteration of biorhythm through melatonin mechanisms.

10. Repetitive transcranial magnetic stimulation—Repetitive transcranial magnetic stimulation (rTMS) is used to treat nonpsychotic treatment-resistant depression and involves the application of electromagnetic pulses to the dorsolateral prefrontal cortex. Its use in depression is approved by the FDA for individuals who have not tolerated or responded to at least one or more standard antidepressant medications. It is usually delivered in a course of 20–30 sessions over 4–6 weeks. rTMS neither requires general anesthesia nor is it associated with cognitive side effects. Several meta-analyses have demonstrated that in nonpsychotic depression, rTMS is noninferior to ECT. There is a small risk of seizure (1:30,000 in post market research), and this is due primarily to operator error. The most common side effects are scalp sensitivity under the coil and transient headache.

11. Other treatments—Vagus nerve stimulation has shown promise in about one-third of extremely refractory cases and is approved by the FDA but has not been approved by insurers. Data have demonstrated that the effects plateau around 18 months to 2 years and are durable at 5 years. Deep brain stimulation continues to be explored for the treatment of refractory depression but two multisite randomized controlled studies in two separate targets (subgenual cingulate and ventral capsule/ventral striatum) have not shown success to date. There has been one successful trial but the study methodology was a derivation of the traditional randomized controlled trial. This is still considered an experimental approach, and the appropriate target and methodology are unknown.

B. Psychological

It is often challenging to engage an individual in penetrating psychotherapeutic endeavors during the acute stage of a severe depression. While medications may be taking effect, a supportive and behavioral approach to strengthen existing coping mechanisms and appropriate consideration of the patient's continuing need to function at work, to engage in recreational activities, etc, are necessary as the severity of the depression lessens. Therapy during or just after the acute stage may focus on coping techniques, with some practice of alternative choices. If the patient is not seriously depressed, it is often appropriate to initiate intensive psychotherapeutic efforts, since flux periods are a good time to effect change. A catharsis of repressed anger and guilt may be beneficial. Depression-specific psychotherapies help improve self-esteem, increase assertiveness, and lessen dependency. Interpersonal psychotherapy for depression has shown efficacy in the treatment of acute depression, helping patients master interpersonal stresses and develop new coping strategies. Cognitive behavioral therapy for depression addresses patients' patterns of negative thoughts, called cognitive distortions, which lead to feelings of depression and anxiety. Treatment usually includes homework assignments such as keeping a journal of cognitive distortions and of positive responses to them. *The combination of medication therapy plus interpersonal psychotherapy or cognitive behavioral therapy is generally more effective than either modality alone.* It is usually helpful to involve the spouse or other significant family members early in treatment. Mindfulness-based cognitive therapy has reduced relapse rates in several randomized controlled trials. In two studies, it was as effective as maintenance medication in preventing relapse. This therapy incorporates meditation and teaches patients to distance themselves from depressive thinking. It may be a preferable alternative for individuals who wish to have an alternative to long-term medications to stay free of depressive episodes.

C. Social

Flexible use of appropriate social services can be of major importance in the treatment of depression. Since alcohol abuse is often associated with depression, early involvement in alcohol treatment programs such as Alcoholics Anonymous can be important to future success (see Alcohol Use Disorder [Alcoholism]). The structuring of daily activities during severe depression is often quite difficult for the patient, and loneliness is often a major factor. The help of family, employer, or friends is often necessary to mobilize the patient who experiences no joy in daily activities and tends to remain uninvolved and to deteriorate. Insistence on sharing activities will help involve the patient in simple but important daily functions. In some severe cases, the use of day treatment centers or support groups of a specific type (eg, mastectomy groups) is indicated. It is not unusual for a patient to have multiple legal, financial, and vocational problems requiring legal and vocational assistance.

D. Behavioral

When depression is a function of self-defeating coping techniques such as passivity, the role-playing approach can be useful. Behavioral techniques, including desensitization, may be used in problems such as phobias where depression is a by-product. When depression is a regularly used interpersonal style, behavioral counseling to family members or others can help in extinguishing the behavior in the patient. Behavioral activation, a technique of motivating depressed patients to begin engaging in pleasurable activities, has been shown to be a useful depression-specific psychotherapy. Exercise, especially aerobic and supervised by exercise professionals, has evidence in improving depressive symptoms.

▶ Treatment of Bipolar Disorder, Manic & Depressive Episodes

Acute manic or hypomanic symptoms will respond to the mood stabilizers lithium or valproic acid after several days of treatment, but it is increasingly common to use second-generation antipsychotics as first-line agents.

The antipsychotics do not require serum level monitoring. High-potency benzodiazepines (eg, clonazepam) may also be useful adjuncts in managing the agitation and sleep disturbance that are features of manic and hypomanic episodes.

A. Antipsychotics

Acute manic symptoms may be treated initially with a second-generation antipsychotic such as olanzapine, (eg, 5–20 mg orally), risperidone (2–3 mg orally), or aripiprazole (15–30 mg) in conjunction with a benzodiazepine if indicated. All of the available oral second-generation antipsychotics and many of the first-generation agents appear to be more rapidly effective in the management of acute mania than are mood stabilizers such as lithium or valproate. Alternatively, when behavioral control is immediately necessary, olanzapine in an injectable form (2.5–10 mg intramuscularly) or haloperidol, 5–10 mg orally or intramuscularly repeated as needed until symptoms subside, may be used. The dosage of the antipsychotic may be gradually reduced after lithium or another mood stabilizer is started. Olanzapine, quetiapine, ziprasidone, aripiprazole, and the long-acting injectable risperidone are approved as maintenance treatments for bipolar disorder to prevent subsequent cycles of both mania and depression.

B. Valproic Acid

Valproic acid (divalproex) is a first-line treatment for mania because it has a broader index of safety than lithium. This issue is particularly important in AIDS or other medically ill patients prone to dehydration or malabsorption with wide swings in serum lithium levels. Valproic acid has also been used effectively in panic disorder and migraine headache. Treatment is often started at a dose of 750 mg/day orally in divided doses, and dosage is then titrated to achieve therapeutic serum levels. Oral loading in acutely manic bipolar patients in an inpatient setting (initiated at a dosage of 20 mg/kg/day) can safely achieve serum therapeutic levels in 2–3 days. Concomitant use of aspirin may increase valproate levels, carbamazepine or phenytoin may decrease valproate levels, while warfarin levels may be elevated by valproate. Gastrointestinal symptoms and weight gain are the main side effects. Liver enzyme biochemical tests, complete blood counts, glucose levels, and weight should be monitored at 2 weeks, 4 weeks, and 3 months initially and annually or more frequently thereafter based on clinical judgment. Significant teratogenic effects are a concern so pregnancy should be ruled out prior to initiation. In utero exposure to valproate has been associated with adversely affecting intellectual development in the fetus and there is an FDA warning to that effect. Thus, alternatives to valproate should be considered in women of childbearing years who might become pregnant.

C. Lithium

Lithium significantly decreases the frequency and severity of both manic and depressive attacks in about 50–70% of patients, and is FDA approved for maintenance and manic episodes. Lithium appears to work best in patients with classic bipolar I disorder. Antipsychotics, valproate, lamotrigine, and carbamazepine may be more effective than lithium in the management of rapid cycling and mixed episodes. A positive response to lithium is more predictable if the patient has a low frequency of episodes (no more than two per year with intervals free of psychopathology). A positive response occurs more frequently in individuals who have blood relatives with a diagnosis of manic or hypomanic episodes.

In addition to its use in bipolar disorder, lithium is sometimes useful in the prophylaxis of recurrent unipolar depressions (perhaps undiagnosed bipolar disorder) and in lowering the risk of suicide. Lithium may ameliorate nonspecific aggressive behaviors and dyscontrol syndromes. *Most patients with bipolar disease can be managed longterm with lithium alone,* although some will require continued or intermittent use of an antipsychotic, antidepressant, or carbamazepine. An excellent resource for information is the Lithium Information Center, https://www.uwhealth.org/health/topic/multum/lithium/d00061a1.html.

Before treatment, the clinical workup should include a medical history and physical examination; complete blood count; T_4, thyroid-stimulating hormone, blood urea nitrogen (BUN), serum creatinine, and serum electrolyte determinations; urinalysis; and electrocardiography (in patients over age 45 or with a history of cardiac disease). Compliance with lithium therapy is adversely affected by the loss of some hypomanic experiences valued by the patient. These include social extroversion and a sense of heightened enjoyment in many activities such as sex and business dealings, often with increased productivity in the latter.

1. Dosage—The common starting dosage of lithium carbonate is 300 mg orally two or three times daily, with trough blood levels measured after 5 days of treatment. In a small minority of patients, a slow release form or units of different dosage may be required. Lithium citrate is available as a syrup. The dosage is that required to maintain blood levels in the therapeutic range. For acute attacks, this ranges from 1 to 1.5 mEq/L. Although there is controversy about the optimal long-term maintenance dose, many clinicians reduce the acute level to 0.6–1 mEq/L in order to reduce side effects. The dose required to meet this need will vary in different individuals. For acute mania, doses of 1200–1800 mg/day are generally recommended. Augmentation of antidepressants is usually achieved with half of these doses. Once-a-day dosage is acceptable, but most patients have less nausea when they take the medication in divided doses with meals.

Lithium is readily absorbed, with peak serum levels occurring within 1–3 hours and complete absorption in 8 hours. Half of the total body lithium is excreted in 18–24 hours (95% in the urine). Blood for lithium levels should be drawn 12 hours after the last dose. Serum levels should be measured 5–7 days after initiation of treatment and changes in dose. For maintenance treatment, lithium levels should be monitored initially every 1–2 months but may be measured every 6–12 months in stable, long-term patients. Levels should be monitored more closely when there is any condition that causes volume depletion (eg, diarrhea, dehydration, use of diuretics).

2. Side effects—**Early side effects,** including mild gastrointestinal symptoms (take lithium with food and in divided doses), fine tremors (treat with propranolol, 20–60 mg/day orally, only if persistent), slight muscle weakness, and some degree of somnolence, can occur and are usually transient. Moderate polyuria (reduced renal responsiveness to ADH) and polydipsia (associated with increased plasma renin concentration) are often present. Potassium administration can blunt this effect, as may once-daily dosing of lithium. Weight gain (often a result of calories in fluids taken for polydipsia) and leukocytosis not due to infection are fairly common.

Thyroid side effects include goiter (3%; often euthyroid) and hypothyroidism (10%; concomitant administration of lithium and iodide or lithium and carbamazepine enhances the hypothyroid and goitrogenic effect of either medication). Most clinicians treat lithium-induced hypothyroidism (more common in women) with thyroid hormone while continuing lithium therapy. Changes in the glucose tolerance test toward a diabetes-like curve, nephrogenic diabetes insipidus (usually resolving about 8 weeks after cessation of lithium therapy), nephrotic syndrome, edema, folate deficiency, and pseudotumor cerebri (ophthalmoscopy is indicated if there are complaints of headache or blurred vision) can occur. Thyroid and kidney function should be checked at 4- to 6-month intervals. Hypercalcemia and elevated parathyroid hormone levels occur in some patients. Electrocardiographic abnormalities (principally T wave flattening or inversion) may occur during lithium administration but are not of major clinical significance. Sinoatrial block may occur, particularly in the elderly. Other medications that prolong intraventricular conduction, such as TCAs, must be used cautiously in conjunction with lithium. Lithium impairs ventilatory function in patients with airway obstruction. Lithium alone does not have a significant effect on sexual function, but when combined with benzodiazepines (clonazepam in most symptomatic patients), it causes sexual dysfunction in about 50% of men. Lithium may precipitate or exacerbate psoriasis in some patients and can also cause acne. Most of these side effects subside when lithium is discontinued; when residual side effects exist, they are usually not serious.

Side effects from long-term lithium therapy include the development of cogwheel rigidity and, occasionally, other extrapyramidal signs. Lithium potentiates the parkinsonian effects of haloperidol. Long-term lithium therapy has also been associated with a relative lowering of the level of memory and perceptual processing (affecting compliance in some cases). Some impairment of attention and emotional reactivity has also been noted. Lithium-induced delirium with therapeutic lithium levels is an infrequent complication usually occurring in the elderly and may persist for several days after serum levels have become negligible. Encephalopathy has occurred in patients receiving combined lithium and antipsychotic therapy and in those who have cerebrovascular disease, thus requiring careful evaluation of patients who develop neurotoxic signs at subtoxic blood levels.

Some reports have suggested that the long-term use of lithium may have adverse effects on kidney function (with interstitial fibrosis, tubular atrophy, or nephrogenic diabetes insipidus). Persistent polyuria should require an investigation of the kidney's ability to concentrate urine. A rise in serum creatinine levels is an indication for in-depth evaluation of kidney function and consideration of alternative treatments if the individual can tolerate a change. Incontinence has been reported in women, apparently related to changes in bladder cholinergic-adrenergic balance.

Prospective studies suggest that the overall risk imposed by lithium in pregnancy may be overemphasized. However, lithium exposure in early pregnancy does minimally increase the frequency of congenital anomalies, notably Ebstein and other major cardiovascular anomalies. For women who take psychotropic medications who become pregnant, the decision to make a change in medication is complex and requires informed consent regarding the relative risks to the patient and fetus. Indeed, the risk of untreated bipolar disorder carries its own risks for pregnancy. Mothers who take lithium should use formula to feed their newborn, since concentration in breast milk is one-third to half that in serum.

Frank toxicity usually occurs at blood lithium levels greater than 2 mEq/L. Because sodium and lithium are reabsorbed at the same loci in the proximal renal tubules, any sodium loss (diarrhea, use of diuretics, or excessive perspiration) increases lithium levels. Symptoms and signs include vomiting and diarrhea, the latter exacerbating the problem since more sodium is lost and more lithium is absorbed. Other symptoms and signs, some of which may not be reversible, include tremors, marked muscle weakness, confusion, dysarthria, vertigo, choreoathetosis, ataxia, hyperreflexia, rigidity, lack of coordination, myoclonus, seizures, opisthotonos, and coma. Toxicity is more severe in the elderly, who should be maintained on slightly lower serum levels. Lithium overdosage may be accidental or intentional or may occur as a result of poor monitoring. Significant overdoses of lithium are typically managed with hemodialysis since the medication is excreted completely by the kidneys.

See Chapter 38 for the treatment of patients with massive ingestions of lithium or blood lithium levels greater than 2.5 mEq/L.

3. Drug interactions—Patients receiving lithium should use diuretics with caution and only under close medical supervision. The thiazide diuretics cause increased lithium reabsorption from the proximal renal tubules, resulting in increased serum lithium levels (Table 25–10), and adjustment of lithium intake must be made to compensate for this. Reduce lithium dosage by 25–40% when the patient is receiving 50 mg of hydrochlorothiazide daily. Potassium-sparing diuretics (spironolactone, amiloride, triamterene) may also increase serum lithium levels and require careful monitoring of lithium levels. Loop diuretics (furosemide, ethacrynic acid, bumetanide) do not appear to alter serum lithium levels. Concurrent use of lithium and angiotensin-converting enzyme inhibitors requires a 50–75% reduction in lithium intake, as does prolonged concurrent use of nonsteroidal anti-inflammatory medication.

Table 25–10. Lithium interactions with other medications (listed in alphabetical order).

Medication	Effects
ACE inhibitors	↑ Lithium levels
Celecoxib	↑ Lithium levels
Fluoxetine	↑ Lithium levels
Ibuprofen	↑ Lithium levels
Indomethacin	↑ Lithium levels
Methyldopa	Rigidity, mutism, fascicular twitching
Osmotic diuretics (urea, mannitol)	↑ Lithium excretion
Phenylbutazone	↑ Lithium levels
Potassium-sparing diuretics (spironolactone, amiloride, triamterene)	↑ Lithium levels
Sodium bicarbonate	↑ Lithium excretion
Succinylcholine	↑ Duration of action of succinylcholine
Theophylline, aminophylline	↑ Lithium excretion
Thiazide diuretics	↑ Lithium levels
Valproic acid	↓ Lithium levels

ACE, angiotensin-converting enzyme.

D. Carbamazepine

Carbamazepine is used in the treatment of bipolar patients who cannot be satisfactorily treated with lithium (nonresponsive, excessive side effects, or rapid cycling). It is often effective at 800–1600 mg/day orally. It has also been used in the treatment of trigeminal neuralgias and alcohol withdrawal as well as in patients with behavioral dyscontrol. It has been used to treat residual symptoms in previous stimulant abusers (eg, PTSD with impulse control problems). Dose-related side effects include sedation and ataxia. Dosages start at 400–600 mg orally daily and are increased slowly to therapeutic levels. Skin rashes and a mild reduction in white count are common. SIADH occurs rarely. Nonsteroidal anti-inflammatory medications (except aspirin), the antibiotics erythromycin and isoniazid, the calcium channel blockers verapamil and diltiazem (but not nifedipine), fluoxetine, propoxyphene, and cimetidine all increase carbamazepine levels. Carbamazepine can be effective in conjunction with lithium, although there have been reports of reversible neurotoxicity with the combination. Carbamazepine stimulates hepatic microsomal enzymes and so tends to decrease levels of haloperidol and oral contraceptives. It also lowers T_4, free T_4, and T_3 levels. Cases of fetal malformation (particularly spina bifida) have been reported along with growth deficiency and developmental delay. Liver biochemical tests and complete blood counts should be monitored in patients taking carbamazepine. Genetic studies suggest that screening for the

HLA-B1502 allele in the Han Chinese population and the HLA-A3101 allele in northern Europeans may help target individuals more susceptible to a serious rash. Oxcarbazepine, a derivative of carbamazepine, does not appear to induce its own metabolism, and is associated with fewer drug interactions, although it may impose a higher risk of hyponatremia. FDA-approved for partial seizures, oxcarbazepine may have efficacy in acute mania. It appears to be a safer alternative to carbamazepine due to its lower risk of hepatotoxicity.

E. Lamotrigine

Lamotrigine is thought to inhibit neuronal sodium channels and the release of the excitatory amino acids, glutamate and aspartate. It is FDA-approved for the maintenance treatment of bipolar disorder. Two double-blind studies support its efficacy in the treatment of acute bipolar depression as adjunctive therapy or as monotherapy, but several other controlled studies failed to demonstrate benefit. Likewise, lamotrigine has not proven effective in the management of acute mania. Its metabolism is inhibited by coadministration of valproic acid—doubling its half-life—and accelerated by hepatic enzyme-inducing agents such as carbamazepine. More frequent mild side effects include headache, dizziness, nausea, and diplopia. Rash occurring in 10% of patients may be an indication for immediate cessation of dosing, since lamotrigine has been associated with Stevens-Johnson syndrome (1:1000) and, rarely, toxic epidermal necrolysis. The medication should be stopped for a rash associated with systemic symptoms including fever, lymphadenopathy, and oral mucosa ulcerations, and the patient sent to an emergency department. Any new rash associated with lamotrigine use should be evaluated by a dermatologist. Dosing starts at 25–50 mg/day orally and is titrated upward slowly to decrease the likelihood of rash. Slower titration and a lower total dose are indicated for patients taking valproic acid.

▶ Prognosis

Most depressive episodes are usually time-limited, and the prognosis with treatment is good if a pathologic pattern of adjustment does not intervene. Major affective disorders frequently respond well to a full trial of medication treatment. However, at least 20% of patients will have a more chronic illness lasting 2 or more years. Many patients do not sustain a complete remission of symptoms and most depressive episodes recur. *At least 80% of patients who have a single major depressive episode will have one or more recurrences within 15 years of the index episode.* Many patients, therefore, require long-term maintenance therapy with antidepressants.

Mania has a good prognosis with adequate treatment, although patient adherence to treatment is often quite challenging. Few effective treatments exist for bipolar depression, which include quetiapine, lurasidone, and the combination of fluoxetine and olanzapine. Most patients with bipolar disorder require treatment with two or more medications such as lithium, antipsychotics, and sleeping agents. Breakthrough manic or depressive episodes are common, even

with adherence to maintenance treatments, although maintenance therapy lessens the risk of recurrent episodes.

Bergfeld IO et al. Deep brain stimulation of the ventral anterior limb of the internal capsule for treatment-resistant depression: a randomized clinical trial. JAMA Psychiatry. 2016 May 1;73(5):456–64. [PMID: 27049915]

Beyer JL et al. Suicide behaviors in bipolar disorder: a review and update for the clinician. Psychiatr Clin North Am. 2016 Mar;39(1):111–23. [PMID: 26876322]

Bobo WV. The diagnosis and management of bipolar I and II disorders: clinical practice update. Mayo Clin Proc. 2017 Oct;92(10):1532–51. [PMID: 28888714]

Fountoulakis KN et al. The International College of Neuro-Psychopharmacology (CINP) treatment guidelines for bipolar disorder in adults (CINP-BD-2017), part 3: the clinical guidelines. Int J Neuropsychopharmacol. 2017 Feb 1; 20(2):180–95. [PMID: 27941079]

Fountoulakis KN et al. The International College of Neuropsychopharmacology (CINP) treatment guidelines for bipolar disorder in adults (CINP-BD-2017), part 4: unmet needs in the treatment of bipolar disorder and recommendations for future research. Int J Neuropsychopharmacol. 2017 Feb 1;20(2):196–205. [PMID: 27677983]

Malhi GS et al. Depression. Lancet. 2018 Nov 24;392(10161): 2299–312. [PMID: 30396512]

Orsolini L et al. Serotonin reuptake inhibitors and breastfeeding: a systematic review. Hum Psychopharmacol. 2015 Jan;30(1): 4–20. [PMID: 25572308]

Robinson GE. Controversies about the use of antidepressants in pregnancy. J Nerv Ment Dis. 2015 Mar;203(3):159–63. [PMID: 25714252]

Schuch FB et al. Exercise as a treatment for depression: a meta-analysis adjusting for publication bias. J Psychiatr Res. 2016 Jun;77:42–51. [PMID: 26978184]

Viktorin A et al. Association of antidepressant medication use during pregnancy with intellectual disability in offspring. JAMA Psychiatry. 2017 Oct 1;74(10):1031–8. [PMID: 28700807]

Williams NR et al. Attenuation of antidepressant effects of ketamine by opioid receptor antagonism. Am J Psychiatry. 2018 Dec 1;175(12):1205–15. [PMID: 30153752]

Williams NR et al. NMDA antagonist treatment of depression. Curr Opin Neurobiol. 2016 Feb;36:112–7. [PMID: 26687375]

ATTENTION-DEFICIT/HYPERACTIVITY DISORDER

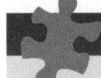
ESSENTIALS OF DIAGNOSIS

▶ Persistent patterns of inability to sustain attention, excessive motor activity/restlessness/impulsivity, or both.

▶ Symptoms interfere with daily functioning.

▶ Symptoms began prior to age 12 and in at least two settings (ie, school/work, home, with friends/family).

▶ Clinical Findings

While attention-deficit/hyperactivity disorder (ADHD) begins in childhood, symptoms persist into adulthood in approximately two-thirds of patients, with half of those still requiring medication to aid in their functioning. The prevalence of ADHD in adults is estimated to be 4–5%. ADHD is never diagnosed in some patients during childhood because they may not have presented for assessment at that time or were able to compensate for symptoms at the time. The specific presenting symptoms in adulthood tend to be inattention, restlessness, and impulsivity, whereas hyperactivity has often improved. At least five inattention symptoms (such as making careless mistakes, being easily sidetracked, trouble keeping deadlines or with organization, losing belongings, being forgetful in daily chores/tasks) are required to meet criteria for this subtype of ADHD, or five hyperactivity/impulsivity symptoms (such as feeling restless and leaving a seat though expected to remain, feeling "driven by a motor," interrupting others, cannot wait his or her turn) for this subtype. It is often useful to have patients provide questionnaires to other adult observers, including those who knew them during childhood, such as parents. This collateral data can help prevent diagnosing ADHD in someone who is seeking stimulants but without symptomatology as well as aid in making the diagnosis, since evidence shows that many adults who do have ADHD often underreport symptoms.

► Treatment

A. Pharmacologic

Stimulants such as methylphenidate and amphetamine are the most effective treatment, with some of the largest effect sizes for medication treatment in psychiatric disorders. These come in both short-acting and long-acting formulations. Caution should be used to assess for potential substance abuse or diversion as well as for comorbid mood disorders that may not respond well to a stimulant prior to prescribing these medications. Atomoxetine, a nonstimulant, is a second-line agent that is FDA-approved for ADHD; it affects norepinephrine and dopamine transport and makes more of these neurotransmitters available in the brain. Bupropion has evidence of efficacy as well and may be considered in patients in whom a stimulant is contraindicated or in those who also suffer from major depression. Desipramine, a tricyclic antidepressant, also can be effective for ADHD and may be considered in patients who have additional needs, such as a concomitant depression or neuropathic pain. Guanfacine and clonidine are two additional nonstimulant medications used primarily to treat blood pressure but with some efficacy in ADHD as well.

B. Behavioral and Other Treatments

Psychoeducation regarding ADHD should be given to all patients. Many patients are able to implement behavioral changes that either improve their functioning, such as creating calendars and organizational schemes or doing tasks in multiple timed short spurts, or can help them avoid tasks that are challenging for them in favor of complementary tasks they are more suited to (ie, selecting jobs that value more activity rather than sustained focus, or sharing in the chores at home that do not require attention to detail). Cognitive behavioral therapy has some evidence for helping residual symptoms after medication management has been optimized.

Clemow DB et al. Atomoxetine in patients with ADHD: a clinical and pharmacological review of the onset, trajectory, duration of response and implications for patients. J Psychopharmacol. 2015 Dec;29(12):1221–30. [PMID: 26349559]

Epstein T et al. Immediate-release methylphenidate for attention deficit hyperactivity disorder (ADHD) in adults. Cochrane Database Syst Rev. 2014 Sep 18;(9):CD005041. Update in: Cochrane Database Syst Rev. 2016;(5):CD005041. [PMID: 25230710]

Fredriksen M et al. Long-term pharmacotherapy of adults with attention deficit hyperactivity disorder: a literature review and clinical study. Basic Clin Pharmacol Toxicol. 2016 Jan;118(1):23–31. [PMID: 26404187]

Jensen CM et al. Cognitive behavioural therapy for ADHD in adults: systematic review and meta-analyses. Atten Defic Hyperact Disord. 2016 Mar;8(1):3–11. [PMID: 26801998]

Simon N et al. Methylphenidate in adults with attention deficit hyperactivity disorder and substance use disorders. Curr Pharm Des. 2015;21(23):3359–66. [PMID: 26088112]

Torgersen T et al. Optimal management of ADHD in older adults. Neuropsychiatr Dis Treat. 2016 Jan 8;12:79–87. [PMID: 26811680]

AUTISM SPECTRUM DISORDERS

ESSENTIALS OF DIAGNOSIS

► Persistent issues with social communication and interactions.

► Repetitive behaviors, interests, or activities.

► Symptoms interfere with functioning.

► May or may not have accompanying language or intellectual impairment.

► Clinical Findings

Autism spectrum disorder is a neurodevelopmental disorder in which patients suffer from pervasive difficulties with social communication and have repetitive, restricted interests and behaviors. Autism spectrum disorder affects about 1% of the adult population with an estimated heritability of about 90%. Approximately 20–30% of individuals in whom autism is diagnosed also have a substance use problem as well as a higher risk of ADHD, mood, or obsessive-compulsive disorders. The National Institute of Health and Care Excellence (NICE) guidelines recommend that assessment of autism spectrum disorder should be a comprehensive and multidisciplinary approach that includes asking about core autism spectrum disorder difficulties, early development, medical and family history, behavior, education, employment, needs assessment, risks, physical examination with potential laboratory testing, and feedback to the individual.

► Treatment

No treatments for the core symptoms of autism spectrum disorder in adults have been validated. There is some evidence for therapy to address social cognitions and behaviors. Use of repetitive transcranial magnetic stimulation for the treatment of autism spectrum disorder is under investigation.

Jin J. JAMA patient page. Screening for autism spectrum disorder. JAMA. 2016 Feb 16;315(7):718. [PMID: 26881385]
Murphy CM et al. Autism spectrum disorder in adults: diagnosis, management, and health services development. Neuropsychiatr Dis Treat. 2016 Jul 7;12:1669–86. [PMID: 27462160]

SLEEP-WAKE DISORDERS

Sleep consists of two distinct states as shown by electroencephalographic studies: (1) REM (rapid eye movement) sleep, also called dream sleep, D state sleep, or paradoxic sleep, and (2) NREM (non-REM) sleep, also called S stage sleep, which is divided into stages 1, 2, 3, and 4 and is recognizable by different electroencephalographic patterns. Stages 3 and 4 are "delta" sleep. Dreaming occurs mostly in REM and to a lesser extent in NREM sleep.

Sleep is a cyclic phenomenon, with four or five REM periods during the night accounting for about one-fourth of the total night's sleep (1.5–2 hours). The first REM period occurs about 80–120 minutes after onset of sleep and lasts about 10 minutes. Later REM periods are longer (15–40 minutes) and occur mostly in the last several hours of sleep. Most stage 4 (deepest) sleep occurs in the first several hours.

Age-related changes in normal sleep include an unchanging percentage of REM sleep and a marked decrease in stage 3 and stage 4 sleep, with an increase in wakeful periods during the night. These normal changes, early bedtimes, and daytime naps play a role in the increased complaints of insomnia in older people. Variations in sleep patterns may be due to circumstances (eg, "jet lag") or to idiosyncratic patterns ("night owls") in persons who perhaps because of different "biologic rhythms" habitually go to bed late and sleep late in the morning. Creativity and rapidity of response to unfamiliar situations are impaired by loss of sleep. There are also rare individuals who have chronic difficulty in adapting to a 24-hour sleep-wake cycle (**desynchronization sleep disorder**), which can be resynchronized by altering exposure to light.

The three major sleep disorders are discussed below. Any persistent sleep disorder that is not attributable to another condition should be evaluated by a sleep specialist.

1. Insomnia

▶ Classification & Clinical Findings

Patients may complain of difficulty getting to sleep or staying asleep, intermittent wakefulness during the night, early morning awakening, or combinations of any of these. Transient episodes are usually of little significance. Stress, caffeine, physical discomfort, daytime napping, and early bedtimes are common factors.

Psychiatric disorders are often associated with persistent insomnia. Depression is usually associated with fragmented sleep, decreased total sleep time, earlier onset of REM sleep, a shift of REM activity to the first half of the night, and a loss of slow wave sleep—all of which are nonspecific findings. In manic disorders, a reduced total sleep time and a decreased need for sleep are cardinal features and important early sign of impending mania. In addition to a decreased amount of sleep, manic episodes are characterized by a shortened REM latency and increased REM activity. Sleep-related panic attacks occur in the transition from stage 2 to stage 3 sleep in some patients with a longer REM latency in the sleep pattern preceding the attacks.

Abuse of alcohol may cause or be secondary to the sleep disturbance. *There is a tendency to use alcohol as a means of getting to sleep without realizing that it disrupts the normal sleep cycle.* Acute alcohol intake produces a decreased sleep latency with reduced REM sleep during the first half of the night. REM sleep is increased in the second half of the night, with an increase in total amount of slow wave sleep (stages 3 and 4). Vivid dreams and frequent awakenings are common. Chronic alcohol abuse increases stage 1 and decreases REM sleep (most medications delay or block REM sleep), with symptoms persisting for many months after the individual has stopped drinking. Acute alcohol or other sedative withdrawal causes delayed onset of sleep and REM rebound with intermittent awakening during the night.

Heavy smoking (more than a pack a day) causes difficulty falling asleep—apparently independently of the often associated increase in coffee drinking. Excess intake near bedtime of caffeine, cocaine, and other stimulants (eg, over-the-counter cold remedies) causes decreased total sleep time—mostly NREM sleep—with some increased sleep latency.

Sedative-hypnotics—specifically, the benzodiazepines, which are the most commonly prescribed medications to promote sleep—tend to increase total sleep time, decrease sleep latency, and decrease nocturnal awakening, with variable effects on NREM sleep. Nonbenzodiazepine hypnotics have similar effects on sleep as do the benzodiazepines, though some evidence shows improved slow wave sleep and less residual next-morning somnolence with non-benzodiazepines, such as zolpidem. Withdrawal causes just the opposite effects and results in continued use of the drug for the purpose of preventing withdrawal symptoms. Antidepressants decrease REM sleep (with marked rebound on withdrawal in the form of nightmares) and have varying effects on NREM sleep. The effect on REM sleep correlates with reports that REM sleep deprivation produces improvement in some depressions.

Persistent insomnias are also related to a wide variety of medical conditions, particularly delirium, pain, respiratory distress syndromes, uremia, asthma, thyroid disorders, and nocturia due to benign prostatic hyperplasia. Sleep apnea and restless leg movement are described below. Adequate analgesia and proper treatment of medical disorders will reduce symptoms and decrease the need for sedatives.

▶ Treatment

In general, there are two broad classes of treatment for insomnia, and the two may be combined: psychological (cognitive-behavioral) and pharmacologic. In situations of acute distress, such as a grief reaction, pharmacologic measures may be most appropriate. *With primary insomnia, however, initial efforts should be psychologically based.* This is particularly true in the elderly to avoid the potential adverse reactions of medications. The elderly population is at risk for complaints of insomnia because sleep becomes lighter and more easily disrupted with aging. Medical disorders that become more common with age may also predispose to insomnia.

A. Psychological

Psychological strategies should include educating the patient regarding good **sleep hygiene:** (1) Go to bed only when sleepy. (2) Use the bed and bedroom only for sleeping and sex. (3) If still awake after 20 minutes, leave the bedroom, pursue a restful activity (such as a bath or meditation), and only return when sleepy. (4) Get up at the same time every morning regardless of the amount of sleep during the night. (5) Discontinue caffeine and nicotine, at least in the evening if not completely. (6) Establish a daily exercise regimen. (7) Avoid alcohol as it may disrupt continuity of sleep. (8) Limit fluids in the evening. (9) Learn and practice relaxation techniques. (10) Establish a bedtime ritual and a routine time for going to sleep. Research suggests that cognitive behavioral therapy for insomnia is as effective as zolpidem with benefits sustained 1 year after treatment.

B. Pharmacologic

When the above measures are insufficient, medications may be useful. Lorazepam (0.5 mg orally nightly), temazepam (7.5–15 mg orally nightly), and the nonbenzodiazepine hypnotics zolpidem (5–10 mg orally nightly, with a limit of 5 mg indicated for women) and zaleplon (5–10 mg orally nightly) are often effective for the elderly population and can be given in larger doses—twice what is prescribed for the elderly—in younger patients. Zolpidem is also available as a sublingual tablet to treat insomnia characterized by middle-of-the-night awakening with difficulty falling back to sleep. The dose is 1.75 mg for women and 3.5 mg for men, taken once per night. Eszopiclone (2–3 mg orally) is similar in action to zolpidem and zaleplon and, like oral zolpidem, is approved for long-term use. A lower dose of 1 mg is indicated in the elderly or those with hepatic impairment. It is important to note that short-acting agents like triazolam or zolpidem may lead to amnestic episodes if used on a daily ongoing basis. Longer-acting agents such as flurazepam (half-life of more than 48 hours) may accumulate in the elderly and lead to cognitive slowing, ataxia, falls, and somnolence. In general, it is appropriate to use medications for short courses of 1–2 weeks. The medications described above have largely replaced barbiturates as hypnotic agents because of their greater safety in overdose and their lesser hepatic enzyme induction effects. Antihistamines such as diphenhydramine (25 mg orally nightly) or hydroxyzine (25 mg orally nightly) may also be useful for sleep, as they produce no pharmacologic dependency; their anticholinergic effects may, however, produce confusion or urinary symptoms in the elderly. Trazodone, an atypical antidepressant, is a non–habit-forming, effective sleep medication in lower than antidepressant doses (25–150 mg orally at bedtime). Priapism is a rare side effect requiring emergent treatment. Ramelteon, 8 mg orally at bedtime, is a melatonin receptor agonist that helps with sleep onset and does not appear to have abuse potential. It appears to be safe for ongoing use without the development of tolerance.

The dual orexin receptor antagonists (DORAs) class of hypnotics are approved to help initiate and maintain sleep. DORAs such as suvorexant may be more effective than other hypnotics for some patients. However, the role of suvorexant has not been established relative to other hypnotics and is more expensive since it is not generically available. DORAs have shown a significant increase in depressive symptoms in a subset of patients, so other hypnotics may be a better choice in depressed patients. The dose of suvorexant is 10–20 mg orally given about 30 minutes before bedtime.

2. Hypersomnias (Disorders of Excessive Sleepiness)

▶ Classification & Clinical Findings

A. Breathing-Related Sleep Disorders

Obstructive sleep apnea is by far the most common of the breathing-related sleep disorders that include **central sleep apnea** and **sleep-related hypoventilation**. Obstructive sleep apnea hypopnea is characterized by snoring, gasping, or breathing pauses during sleep and five or more apneas or hypopneas per hour or evidence by polysomnography. (See Chapter 9.)

B. Narcolepsy Hypocretin Deficiency Syndrome

Narcolepsy consists of a tetrad of symptoms: (1) sudden, brief (about 15 minutes) sleep attacks that may occur during any type of activity; (2) cataplexy—sudden loss of muscle tone involving specific small muscle groups or generalized muscle weakness that may cause the person to slump to the floor, unable to move, often associated with emotional reactions and sometimes confused with seizure disorder; (3) sleep paralysis—a generalized flaccidity of muscles with full consciousness in the transition zone between sleep and waking; and (4) hypnagogic hallucinations, visual or auditory, which may precede sleep or occur during the sleep attack. The attacks are characterized by an abrupt transition into REM sleep—a necessary criterion for diagnosis. The disorder begins in early adult life, affects both sexes equally, and usually levels off in severity at about 30 years of age.

REM sleep behavior disorder, characterized by motor dyscontrol and often violent dreams during REM sleep, may be related to narcolepsy.

C. Kleine-Levin Syndrome

This syndrome, which occurs mostly in young men, is characterized by hypersomnic attacks three or four times a year lasting up to 2 days, with hyperphagia, hypersexuality, irritability, and confusion on awakening. It has often been associated with antecedent neurologic insults. It usually remits after age 40.

D. Periodic Limb Movement Disorder

Periodic lower leg movements occur only during sleep with subsequent daytime sleepiness, anxiety, depression, and cognitive impairment. Restless leg syndrome includes movements while awake as well.

E. Shift Work Sleep Disorder

Shift work sleep disorder occurs when there is excessive fatigue as a consequence of work occurring during the normal sleep period.

▶ Treatment

Narcolepsy can be managed by daily administration of a stimulant such as dextroamphetamine sulfate, 10 mg orally in the morning, with increased dosage as necessary. Modafinil and its enantiomer armodafinil are schedule IV medications FDA-approved for treating the excessive daytime fatigue of narcolepsy, sleepiness associated with obstructive sleep apnea, as well as for shift work sleep disorder. Usual dosing is 200–400 mg orally each morning for modafinil and 150–250 mg orally in the morning for armodafinil. The mechanism of action of modafinil and armodafil is unknown, yet they are thought to be less of an abuse risk than stimulants that are primarily dopaminergic. Common side effects include headache and anxiety; however, modafinil appears to be generally well tolerated. Modafinil may reduce the efficacy of cyclosporine, oral contraceptives, and other medications by inducing their hepatic metabolism. Imipramine, 75–100 mg orally daily, has been effective in treatment of cataplexy but not narcolepsy.

Periodic limb movement disorder and REM sleep behavior disorder can be treated with clonazepam with variable results. There is no treatment for Kleine-Levin syndrome, although lithium can prevent recurrences in some.

Treatment of sleep apnea is discussed in Chapter 9.

3. Parasomnias (Abnormal Behaviors during Sleep)

These disorders (sleep terror, nightmares, sleepwalking, and enuresis) are fairly common in children but less so in adults.

Abbott SM et al. Circadian rhythm sleep-wake disorders. Psychiatr Clin North Am. 2015 Dec;38(4):805–23. [PMID: 26600110]

Khoury J et al. Primary sleep disorders. Psychiatr Clin North Am. 2015 Dec;38(4):683–704. [PMID: 26600103]

Reid KJ et al. Jet lag and shift work disorder. Sleep Med Clin. 2015 Dec;10(4):523–35. [PMID: 26568127]

Rhyne DN et al. Suvorexant in insomnia: efficacy, safety and place in therapy. Ther Adv Drug Saf. 2015 Oct;6(5):189–95. [PMID: 26478806]

Trauer JM et al. Cognitive behavioral therapy for chronic insomnia: a systematic review and meta-analysis. Ann Intern Med. 2015 Aug 4;163(3):191–204. [PMID: 26054060]

Winkelman JW. Clinical practice. Insomnia disorder. N Engl J Med. 2015 Oct 8;373(15):1437–44. [PMID: 26444730]

DISORDERS OF AGGRESSION

Aggression and violence are symptoms rather than diseases, and most frequently they are not necessarily associated with an underlying medical condition. Clinicians are unable to predict dangerous behavior with greater than chance accuracy. Depression, schizophrenia, personality disorders, mania, paranoia, temporal lobe dysfunction, and organic mental states may be associated with acts of aggression. Impulse control disorders are characterized by physical abuse (usually of the aggressor's domestic partner or children), by pathologic intoxication, by impulsive sexual activities, and by reckless driving. Anabolic steroid usage by athletes has been associated with increased tendencies toward violent behavior.

In the United States, a significant proportion of all violent deaths are alcohol related. The ingestion of even small amounts of alcohol can result in pathologic intoxication that resembles an acute organic mental condition. Amphetamines, crack cocaine, and other stimulants are frequently associated with aggressive behavior. Phencyclidine is a drug commonly associated with violent behavior that is occasionally of a bizarre nature, partly due to lowering of the pain threshold. Domestic violence and rape are much more widespread than previously recognized. Awareness of the problem is to some degree due to increasing recognition of the rights of women and the understanding by women that they do not have to accept abuse. Acceptance of this kind of aggressive behavior inevitably leads to more, with the ultimate aggression being murder—20–50% of murders in the United States occur within the family. Police are called more for domestic disputes than all other criminal incidents combined. Children living in such family situations frequently become victims of abuse.

Features of individuals who have been subjected to long-term physical or sexual abuse are as follows: trouble expressing anger, staying angry longer, general passivity in relationships, feeling "marked for life" with an accompanying feeling of deserving to be victimized, lack of trust, and dissociation of affect from experiences. They are prone to express their psychological distress with somatization symptoms, often pain complaints. They may also have symptoms related to posttraumatic stress, as discussed above. The clinician should be suspicious about the origin of any injuries not fully explained, particularly if such incidents recur.

▶ Treatment

A. Psychological

Management of any acutely potentially violent individual includes appropriate psychological maneuvers. Move slowly, talk slowly with clarity and reassurance, and evaluate the situation. Strive to create a setting that is minimally disturbing, and eliminate people or things threatening to the violent individual. Do not threaten and do not touch or crowd the person. Allow no weapons in the area (an increasing problem in hospital emergency departments). Proximity to a door is comforting to both the patient and the examiner. Use a negotiator who the violent person can relate to comfortably. Food and drink are helpful in defusing the situation (as are cigarettes for those who smoke). Honesty is important. Make no false promises, bolster the patient's self-esteem, and continue to engage the subject verbally until the situation is under control. This type of individual does better with strong external controls to replace the lack of inner controls over the long term. Close probationary supervision and judicially mandated restrictions can be most helpful. There should be a major effort to help the individual avoid drug use (eg, Alcoholics Anonymous). Victims of abuse are essentially treated as any victim of trauma and, not infrequently, have evidence of PTSD.

B. Pharmacologic

Pharmacologic means are often necessary whether or not psychological approaches have been successful. This is particularly true in the agitated or psychotic patient. The medications of choice in seriously violent or psychotic aggressive states are antipsychotics, given intramuscularly if necessary, every 1–2 hours until symptoms are alleviated. A number of second-generation intramuscular antipsychotics are FDA approved in the management of acute agitation, and include aripiprazole (9.75 mg/1.3 mL), ziprasidone (10-mg/0.5 mL), and olanzapine (10 mg/2 mL). The second-generation antipsychotics appear less likely than first-generation medications like haloperidol (2.5–5 mg) to cause acute extrapyramidal symptoms. However, the second-generation medications appear no more effective than first-generation medications and generally are more expensive. Benzodiazepine sedatives (eg, diazepam, 5 mg orally or intravenously every several hours) can be used for mild to moderate agitation, but are sometimes associated with a disinhibition of aggressive impulses similar to alcohol. Chronic aggressive states, particularly in intellectual disabilities and brain damage (rule out causative organic conditions and medications such as anticholinergic medications in amounts sufficient to cause confusion), have been ameliorated with risperidone, 0.5–2 mg/day orally, propranolol, 40–240 mg/day orally, or pindolol, 5 mg twice daily orally (pindolol causes less bradycardia and hypotension than propranolol). Carbamazepine and valproic acid are effective in the treatment of aggression and explosive disorders, particularly when associated with known or suspected brain lesions. Lithium and SSRIs are also effective for some intermittent explosive outbursts. Buspirone (10–45 mg/day orally) is helpful for aggression, particularly in patients with intellectual disabilities.

C. Physical

Physical management is necessary if psychological and pharmacologic means are not sufficient. It requires the active and visible presence of an adequate number of personnel (five or six) to reinforce the idea that the situation is under control despite the patient's lack of inner controls. Such an approach often precludes the need for actual physical restraint. Seclusion rooms and restraints should be used only when necessary (ambulatory restraints are an alternative), and the patient must then be observed at frequent intervals. Narrow corridors, small spaces, and crowded areas exacerbate the potential for violence in an anxious patient.

D. Other Interventions

The treatment of victims (eg, battered women) is challenging and often complicated by their reluctance to leave the situation. Reasons for staying vary, but common themes include the fear of more violence because of leaving, the hope that the situation may ameliorate (in spite of steady worsening), and the financial aspects of the situation, which are seldom to the woman's advantage. Concerns for the children often finally compel the woman to seek help. An early step is to get the woman into a therapeutic situation that provides the support of others in similar straits. Al-Anon is frequently a valuable asset when alcohol is a factor. The group can support the victim while she gathers strength to consider alternatives without being paralyzed by fear. Many cities offer temporary emergency centers and counseling. Use the available resources, attend to any medical or psychiatric problems, and maintain a compassionate interest. Some states require clinicians to report injuries caused by abuse or suspected abuse to police authorities. See Chapter e6 for detailed discussion.

Nash RP et al. Acute pharmacological management of behavioral and emotional dysregulation following a traumatic brain injury: a systematic review of the literature. Psychosomatics. 2019 Mar–Apr;60(2):139–52. [PMID: 30665668]

SUBSTANCE USE DISORDERS

The term "dependency" was previously used to describe a severe form of substance abuse and drug addiction characterized by the triad of: (1) a **psychological dependence or craving** and the behavior involved in procurement of the drug; (2) **physiologic dependence,** with withdrawal symptoms on discontinuance of the drug; and (3) **tolerance,** ie, the need to increase the dose to obtain the desired effects. The terms "dependency" and "abuse" were dropped in *DSM-5* in favor of the single term "substance use disorder," ranging from mild to severe. Many patients could have a severe and life-threatening abuse problem without ever being dependent on a drug.

There is accumulating evidence that an impairment syndrome exists in many former (and current) drug users. It is believed that drug use produces damaged neurotransmitter receptor sites and that the consequent imbalance produces symptoms that may mimic other psychiatric illnesses. "Kindling"—repeated stimulation of the brain—renders the individual more susceptible to focal brain activity with minimal stimulation. Stimulants and depressants can produce kindling, leading to relatively spontaneous effects no longer dependent on the original stimulus. These effects may be manifested as mood swings, panic, psychosis, and occasionally overt seizure activity. The imbalance also results in frequent job changes, partner problems, and generally erratic behavior. Patients with PTSD frequently have treated themselves with a variety of drugs. Chronic abusers of a wide variety of drugs exhibit cerebral atrophy on CT scans, a finding that may relate to the above symptoms. Early recognition is important, mainly to establish realistic treatment programs that are chiefly symptom-directed.

The clinician faces three problems with substance use disorders: (1) the prescribing of substances such as sedatives, stimulants, or opioids that might produce dependency; (2) the treatment of individuals who have already abused drugs, most commonly alcohol; and (3) the detection of illicit drug use in patients presenting with psychiatric symptoms. The usefulness of **urinalysis for detection of drugs** varies markedly with different drugs and under different circumstances (pharmacokinetics is a major factor). Water-soluble drugs (eg, alcohol, stimulants, opioids) are eliminated in a day or so. Lipophilic substances (eg, barbiturates, tetrahydrocannabinol) appear in the urine over longer periods of time: several days in most cases, 1–2 months in chronic marijuana users. Sedative drug determinations are quite variable, amount of drug and duration of use being important determinants. False-positives can be a problem related to ingestion of some legitimate medications (eg, phenytoin for barbiturates, phenylpropanolamine for amphetamines, chlorpromazine for opioids) and some foods (eg, poppy seeds for opioids, coca leaf tea for cocaine). Manipulations can alter the legitimacy of the testing. Dilution, either in vivo or in vitro, can be detected by checking urine-specific gravity. Addition of ammonia, vinegar, or salt may invalidate the test, but odor and pH determinations are simple. Hair analysis can determine drug use over longer periods, particularly sequential drug-taking patterns. The sensitivity and reliability of such tests are considered good, and the method may be complementary to urinalysis.

ALCOHOL USE DISORDER (Alcoholism)

Meshell D. Johnson, MD

ESSENTIALS OF DIAGNOSIS

► Physiologic dependence as manifested by evidence of withdrawal when intake is interrupted.

► Tolerance to the effects of alcohol.

► Evidence of alcohol-associated illnesses, such as alcoholic liver disease, cerebellar degeneration.

► Continued drinking despite strong medical and social contraindications and life disruptions.

► Impairment in social and occupational functioning.

► Depression.

► Blackouts.

General Considerations

Alcohol use disorder is a syndrome consisting of two phases: **at-risk drinking** and moderate to severe **alcohol misuse.** At-risk drinking is the repetitive use of alcohol, often to alleviate anxiety or solve other emotional problems. A moderate to severe alcohol use disorder is similar to that which occurs following the repeated use of other sedative-hypnotics and is characterized by recurrent use of alcohol despite disruption in social roles (family and work), alcohol-related legal problems, and taking safety risks by oneself and with others. The National Institute on Alcohol Abuse and Alcoholism formally defines at-risk drinking as *more than 4 drinks per day or 14 drinks per week for men or more than 3 drinks per day or 7 drinks per week for women.* A drink is defined by the Centers for

Disease Control and Prevention (CDC) as 12 oz of beer, 8 oz of malt liquor, 5 oz of wine, or 1.3 oz or a "shot" of 80-proof distilled spirits of liquor. Individuals with at-risk drinking are at an increased risk for developing or are developing an alcohol use disorder. Alcohol and other drug abuse patients have a much higher prevalence of lifetime psychiatric disorders. While male-to-female ratios in alcoholic treatment agencies remain at 4:1, there is evidence that the rates are converging. Women delay seeking help, and when they do, they tend to seek it in medical or mental health settings. Adoption and twin studies indicate some genetic influence. Ethnic distinctions are important—eg, 40% of Japanese have aldehyde dehydrogenase deficiency and are more susceptible to the effects of alcohol. Depression is often present and should be evaluated carefully. The majority of suicides and intrafamily homicides involve alcohol. Alcohol is a major factor in rapes and other assaults.

There are several screening instruments that may help identify an alcohol use disorder. One of the most useful is the **Alcohol Use Disorder Identification Test (AUDIT)** (see Table 1–7).

McNeely J et al. A brief patient self-administered substance use screening tool for primary care: two-site validation study of the Substance Use Brief Screen (SUBS). Am J Med. 2015 Jul;128(7):784.e9–19. [PMID: 25770031]

McNeely J et al. Performance of the Tobacco, Alcohol, Prescription Medication, and Other Substance Use (TAPS) tool for substance use screening in primary care patients. Ann Intern Med. 2016 Nov 15;165(10):690–9. [PMID: 27595276]

► Clinical Findings

A. Acute Intoxication

The signs of alcoholic intoxication are the same as those of overdosage with any other central nervous system depressant: drowsiness, errors of commission, psychomotor dysfunction, disinhibition, dysarthria, ataxia, and nystagmus. For a 70-kg person, an ounce of whiskey, a 4- to 6-oz glass of wine, or a 12-oz bottle of beer (roughly 15, 11, and 13 grams of alcohol, respectively) may raise the level of alcohol in the blood by 25 mg/dL. For a 50-kg person, the blood alcohol level would rise even higher (35 mg/dL) with the same consumption. Blood alcohol levels below 50 mg/dL rarely cause significant motor dysfunction (the legal limit for driving under the influence is commonly 80 mg/dL). Intoxication as manifested by ataxia, dysarthria, and nausea and vomiting indicates a blood level greater than 150 mg/dL, and lethal blood levels range from 350 mg/dL to 900 mg/dL. In severe cases, overdosage is marked by respiratory depression, stupor, seizures, shock syndrome, coma, and death. Serious overdoses are frequently due to a combination of alcohol with other sedatives.

B. Withdrawal

There is a wide spectrum of manifestations of alcohol withdrawal, ranging from anxiety, decreased cognition, and tremulousness, through increasing irritability and hyperreactivity to full-blown delirium tremens (DTs). **Alcohol** withdrawal syndrome can be categorized as mild, moderate, or severe withdrawal, withdrawal seizures, and DTs. Symptoms of mild withdrawal, including tremor, anxiety, tachycardia, nausea, vomiting, and insomnia, begin within 6 hours after the last drink, often before the blood alcohol levels drop to zero, and usually have passed by day 2. Severe or major withdrawal occurs 48–96 hours after the last drink and is usually preceded by prolonged heavy alcohol use. Symptoms include disorientation, agitation, diaphoresis, whole body tremor, vomiting, hypertension, and hallucinations (visual > tactile > auditory). Moderate withdrawal symptoms and signs fall between those of minor and major withdrawal. Withdrawal seizures can occur as early as 8 hours after the last drink but usually do not manifest more than 48 hours after alcohol cessation. Seizures are more prevalent in persons who have a history of withdrawal syndromes. These seizures are generalized tonic-clonic seizures, are brief in duration, and resolve spontaneously. If withdrawal is untreated, these seizures can recur in about 60% of patients. DTs will develop in approximately half of these patients. If seizures are focal, associated with trauma or fever, or have an onset more than 48 hours after the last drink, another etiology for seizures must be considered. DT is the most severe form of alcohol withdrawal. It is an acute organic psychosis that usually manifests 48–72 hours after the last drink, but may occur up to 7–10 days later. It is characterized by extreme mental confusion, agitation, tremor, diaphoresis, sensory hyperacuity, visual hallucinations (often of snakes, bugs, etc), and autonomic hyperactivity (tachycardia and hypertension). Complications of DTs include (1) dehydration, (2) electrolyte disturbances (hypokalemia, hypomagnesemia), (3) arrhythmias and seizures, and (4) cardiovascular collapse and death. *The acute withdrawal syndrome is often unexpected,* occurring when the patient has been hospitalized for an unrelated problem, thus presenting as a diagnostic dilemma. Suspect alcohol withdrawal in every unexplained delirium. The mortality rate from DTs, which was upward of 35%, has steadily decreased with early diagnosis and improved treatment.

In addition to the immediate withdrawal symptoms, there is evidence of persistent longer-term ones, including sleep disturbances, anxiety, depression, excitability, fatigue, and emotional volatility. These symptoms may persist for 3–12 months, and in some cases they become chronic.

C. Alcoholic (Organic) Hallucinosis

This syndrome occurs either during heavy drinking or on withdrawal and is characterized by a paranoid psychosis without the tremulousness, confusion, and clouded sensorium seen in withdrawal syndromes. The patient appears normal except for the auditory hallucinations, which are frequently persecutory and may cause the patient to behave aggressively and in a paranoid fashion.

D. Chronic Alcoholic Brain Syndromes

These encephalopathies are characterized by increasing erratic behavior, memory and recall problems, and emotional instability—the usual signs of organic brain injury due to any cause. Wernicke-Korsakoff syndrome due to thiamine deficiency may develop with a series of episodes. Wernicke encephalopathy consists of the triad of confusion, ataxia, and ophthalmoplegia (typically sixth nerve palsy). Early recognition and treatment with thiamine can minimize damage. One of the possible sequelae is Korsakoff psychosis, characterized by both anterograde and retrograde amnesia, with confabulation early in the course. Early recognition and treatment with intravenous thiamine and B complex vitamins can minimize damage. Excessive alcohol consumption in men has been associated with faster cognitive decline compared with light to moderate alcohol consumption.

E. Laboratory Findings

Ethanol may contribute to the presence of an otherwise unexplained osmolar gap. There may also be increased serum liver biochemical tests, uric acid, and triglycerides and decreased serum potassium and magnesium. The most definitive biologic marker for chronic alcoholism is carbohydrate deficient transferrin, which can detect heavy use (60 mg/day over 7–10 days) with high specificity. Other useful tests for diagnosing alcohol use disorder are gamma-glutamyl transpeptidase (GGT) measurement (levels greater than 30 units/L are suggestive of heavy drinking) and mean corpuscular volume (MCV) (more than 95 fL in men and more than 100 fL in women). If both are elevated, a serious alcohol problem is likely. Use of other recreational drugs with alcohol skews and negates the significance of these tests. Concomitant elevations of high-density lipoprotein (HDL) cholesterol and gamma-glutamyl transpeptidase concentrations also can help identify heavy drinkers.

▶ Differential Diagnosis

The differential diagnosis of alcoholism is essentially between primary alcohol use disorder (when no other major psychiatric diagnosis exists) and secondary alcohol use disorder (when alcohol is used as self-medication for major underlying psychiatric problems such as schizophrenia or affective disorder). The differentiation is important, since the latter group requires treatment for the specific psychiatric problem. In primary and secondary alcoholism, at-risk drinking can be distinguished from alcohol addiction by taking a careful psychiatric history and evaluating the degree to which recurrent drinking impacts the social role functioning and physical safety of the individual.

The differential diagnosis of alcohol withdrawal includes other sedative withdrawals and other causes of delirium. Acute alcoholic hallucinosis must be differentiated from other acute paranoid states such as amphetamine psychosis or paranoid schizophrenia. The form of the brain syndrome is of little help—eg, chronic brain syndromes from systemic lupus erythematosus may be associated with confabulation similar to that resulting from longstanding alcoholism.

▶ Complications

The medical, economic, and psychosocial problems of alcoholism are staggering. The central and peripheral nervous system complications include chronic brain syndromes, cerebellar degeneration, cardiomyopathy, and peripheral neuropathies. Direct effects on the liver include cirrhosis, esophageal varices, and eventual hepatic failure. Indirect effects include protein abnormalities, coagulation defects, hormone deficiencies, and an increased incidence of liver neoplasms.

Fetal alcohol syndrome includes one or more of the following developmental defects in the offspring of alcoholic women: (1) low birth weight and small size with failure to catch up in size or weight, (2) mental retardation, with an average IQ in the 60s, and (3) a variety of birth defects, with a large percentage of facial and cardiac abnormalities. The risk is appreciably higher with the more alcohol ingested by the mother each day.

◢ Treatment of At-Risk Drinking

A. Psychological

The most important consideration for the clinician is to suspect the problem early and take a nonjudgmental attitude, although this does not mean a passive one. The problem of denial must be faced, preferably with significant family members at the first meeting. This means dealing from the beginning with any *enabling behavior* of the spouse or other significant people. Enabling behavior allows the patient with an alcohol use disorder to avoid facing the consequences of his or her behavior.

There must be an emphasis on the things that can be done. This approach emphasizes the fact that the clinician cares and strikes a positive and hopeful note early in treatment. Valuable time should not be wasted trying to find out why the patient drinks; come to grips early with the immediate problem of how to stop the drinking. Although total abstinence should be the ultimate goal, a **harm reduction model** indicates that gradual progress toward abstinence can be a useful treatment strategy.

Motivational interviewing, a model of counseling that addresses both the patient's ambivalence and motivation for change, may contribute to reduced consumption over time.

B. Social

Encourage the patient to attend **Alcoholics Anonymous** meetings and the spouse to attend **Al-Anon** meetings. Success is usually proportionate to the utilization of Alcoholics Anonymous, religious counseling, and other resources. The patient should be seen frequently for short periods.

Do not underestimate the importance of religion, particularly since the patient with alcohol use disorder is often a dependent person who needs a great deal of support. Early enlistment of the help of a concerned religious adviser can often provide the turning point for a personal conversion to sobriety.

One of the most important considerations is the patient's job—*fear of losing a job is one of the most powerful motivations for giving up alcohol.* The business community is aware of the problem; about 70% of the Fortune 500 companies offer programs to their employees to help with the problem of alcoholism. Some specific recommendations that can be offered to employers include (1) avoid placement in jobs where the alcoholic patient must be

alone, eg, as a traveling buyer or sales executive, (2) use supervision but not surveillance, (3) keep competition with others to a minimum, and (4) avoid positions that require quick decision making on important matters (high-stress situations). In general, commitment to abstinence and avoidance of situations that might be conducive to drinking are most predictive of a good outcome.

C. Medical

Hospitalization is not usually necessary. It is sometimes used to dramatize a situation and force the patient to face the problem of alcoholism, but generally it should be used for medical indications. Alcohol is responsible for about 88,000 deaths in the United States each year.

Because of the many medical complications of alcoholism, a complete physical examination with appropriate laboratory tests is mandatory, with special attention to the liver and nervous system. Use of sedatives as a replacement for alcohol is not desirable. The usual result is concomitant use of sedatives and alcohol and worsening of the problem. Lithium is not helpful in the treatment of alcoholism.

Disulfiram (250–500 mg/day orally) has been used for many years as an aversive medication to discourage alcohol use. Disulfiram inhibits aldehyde dehydrogenase, causing toxic reactions when alcohol is consumed. The results have generally been of limited effectiveness and depend on the motivation of the individual to be compliant.

Naltrexone, an opiate antagonist, in a dosage of 50 mg orally daily, lowers relapse rates over the 3–6 months after cessation of drinking, apparently by lessening the pleasurable effects of alcohol. One study suggests that naltrexone is most effective when given during periods of drinking in combination with therapy that supports abstinence but accepts the fact that relapses occur. Naltrexone is FDA approved for maintenance therapy. Studies indicate that it reduces alcohol craving when used as part of a comprehensive treatment program. Acamprosate (333–666 mg orally three times daily) helps reduce craving and maintain abstinence and can be continued even during periods of relapse. Both acamprosate and oral naltrexone have been associated with reduction in return to drinking.

D. Behavioral

Conditioning approaches historically have been used in some settings in the treatment of alcoholism, most commonly as a type of aversion therapy. For example, the patient is given a drink of whiskey and then a shot of apomorphine, and proceeds to vomit. In this way a strong association is built up between the drinking and vomiting. Although this kind of treatment has been successful in some cases, after appropriate informed consent, many people do not sustain the learned aversive response.

◢ Treatment of Hallucinosis & Withdrawal

A. Hallucinosis

Alcoholic hallucinosis, which can occur either during or on cessation of a prolonged drinking period, is not a typical withdrawal syndrome and is handled differently. Since the symptoms are primarily those of a psychosis in the presence of a clear sensorium, they are handled like any other psychosis: hospitalization (when indicated) and adequate amounts of antipsychotic medications. Haloperidol, 5 mg orally twice a day for the first day or so, usually ameliorates symptoms quickly, and the medication can be decreased and discontinued over several days as the patient improves. It then becomes necessary to deal with the chronic alcohol abuse, which has been discussed.

B. Withdrawal

The onset of withdrawal symptoms is usually 6–36 hours, and the peak intensity of symptoms is 48–72 hours after alcohol consumption is stopped. Providing adequate central nervous system depressants (eg, benzodiazepines) is important to counteract the excitability resulting from sudden cessation of alcohol intake. The choice of a specific sedative is less important than using adequate doses to bring the patient to a level of moderate sedation, and this will vary from person to person.

All patients should be evaluated for their risk of alcohol withdrawal. Mild dependency requires "drying out." For outpatients, in some instances, a short course of tapering long-acting benzodiazepines—eg, diazepam, 20 mg/day orally initially, decreasing by 5 mg daily—may be a useful adjunct. When the history or presentation suggests that patients are actively in withdrawal or at significant risk for withdrawal, they should be hospitalized. Risk factors include a recent drinking history, frequent alcohol consumption, a past history of withdrawal, seizures, hallucinosis, or DTs, a past history of needing medication for detoxification, or a history of benzodiazepine or barbiturate use, abuse, or dependency.

For all hospitalized patients, general management includes ensuring adequate hydration, correction of electrolyte imbalances (particularly magnesium, calcium, and potassium), and administering the vitamins thiamine (100 mg intravenously daily for 3 days then orally daily), folic acid (1 mg orally daily), and a multivitamin orally daily. Thiamine should be given *prior* to any glucose-containing solutions to decrease the risk of precipitating Wernicke encephalopathy or Korsakoff syndrome. Alcohol withdrawal is treated with benzodiazepines. Continual assessment is recommended to determine the severity of withdrawal, and **symptom-driven medication regimens**, which have been shown to prevent undersedation as well as oversedation and to reduce total benzodiazepine usage over fixed-dose schedules, should be used. The severity of withdrawal will determine a patient's level of care. For those at risk for withdrawal and with mild withdrawal symptoms, admission to a medical unit is adequate. For those with moderate withdrawal, a higher acuity hospital environment is recommended. Those with severe withdrawal should be admitted to the ICU.

1. Assessing alcohol withdrawal symptom severity—The **Clinical Institute Withdrawal Assessment for Alcohol, Revised (CIWA-Ar)** is a validated tool that is widely used to determine severity of alcohol withdrawal. This survey assesses symptoms in 10 areas and can be administered

relatively quickly (Figure 25–3). One caveat is that the patient must be able to communicate his or her symptoms to the provider. The maximum attainable score is 67. Clinical judgment should be used to determine final dosing of medications to patients who are in alcohol withdrawal because dosing will vary between patients and degrees of withdrawal.

2. Treating alcohol withdrawal symptoms based on CIWA-Ar score—

A. MINIMAL WITHDRAWAL SYMPTOMS (CIWA-AR SCORE LESS THAN 8)—Patients who have a history suggestive of alcohol withdrawal risk with minimal withdrawal symptoms are suitable for withdrawal prophylaxis. The recommended benzodiazepine options include chlordiazepoxide or lorazepam orally, tapered over 3 days. The protocol calls for nursing assessment of sedation and withdrawal symptoms (CIWA-Ar) every 6 hours. If prophylactic medication is indicated, a sample tapering regimen may include lorazepam, 1 mg orally every 6 hours for 1 day, then 1 mg orally every 8 hours for 1 day, then 1 mg orally every 12 hours for 1 day, then discontinue; or chlordiazepoxide, 50 mg orally every 6 hours for 1 day, 25 mg orally every 6 hours for 2 days, then discontinue. Avoid chlordiazepoxide in the elderly or in patients with liver disease. Lorazepam is preferred in patients with liver disease. Sedation is assessed 30–60 minutes after each medication dose. The benzodiazepine dose is held for oversedation or if the respiratory rate is less than 10 breaths per minute. For CIWA-Ar score greater than 8, the provider must be notified, because this is suggestive of active withdrawal, and escalation of treatment must occur.

B. MILD WITHDRAWAL SYMPTOMS (CIWA-AR SCORE 8–15)—For patients in mild withdrawal, either chlordiazepoxide orally or lorazepam orally or intravenously can be used. Initially, chlordiazepoxide 50 mg orally or lorazepam 1 or 2 mg orally or intravenously is given hourly for 2 hours. Patients must be assessed for level of sedation and withdrawal symptoms (CIWA-Ar) every 4 hours. Dosing is adjusted as necessary to control symptoms without excessive sedation. After the first 2 hours, chlordiazepoxide or lorazepam is given every 4 hours and as needed. Typical dosing may include chlordiazepoxide 25–50 mg orally or lorazepam 0.5–1 mg orally or intravenously every 4 hours as needed. Additional doses of benzodiazepines should be given if the CIWA-Ar score remains between 8 and 15.

C. MODERATE WITHDRAWAL (CIWA-AR SCORE 16–20)—For patients in moderate withdrawal, chlordiazepoxide 100 mg orally or lorazepam 3 or 4 mg orally or intravenously is given every hour for the first 2 hours. CIWA-Ar monitoring should occur every 2 hours. Dosing is adjusted to control symptoms without excessive sedation. After initial dosing, continued treatment could include chlordiazepoxide 50 mg orally or lorazepam 1–2 mg orally or intravenously every 2 hours as needed for CIWA-Ar score between 16 and 20, and chlordiazepoxide 25 mg orally or lorazepam 0.5–1 mg orally or intravenously every 2 hours for CIWA-Ar score between 8 and 15. The maximum dose

Patient: _____ **Date:** _____ **Time:** _____ (24 hour clock, midnight = 00:00)

Pulse or heart rate, taken for 1 minute: _____ **Blood pressure:** _____

NAUSEA AND VOMITING — Ask "Do you feel sick to your stomach? Have you vomited?" Observation.

0   no nausea and no vomiting
1   mild nausea with no vomiting
2
3
4   intermittent nausea with dry heaves
5
6
7   constant nausea, frequent dry heaves and vomiting

TREMOR — Arms extended and fingers spread apart. Observation.

0   no tremor
1   not visible, but can be felt fingertip to fingertip
2
3
4   moderate, with patient's arms extended
5
6
7   severe, even with arms not extended

PAROXYSMAL SWEATS — Observation.

0   no sweat visible
1   barely perceptible sweating, palms moist
2
3
4   beads of sweat obvious on forehead
5
6
7   drenching sweats

ANXIETY — Ask "Do you feel nervous?" Observation.

0   no anxiety, at ease
1   mildly anxious
2
3
4   moderately anxious, or guarded, so anxiety is inferred
5
6
7   severely anxious, equivalent…

TACTILE DISTURBANCES — Ask "Have you any itching, pins and needles sensations, any burning, any numbness, or do you feel bugs crawling on or under your skin?" Observation.

0   none
1   very mild itching, pins and needles, burning, or numbness
2   mild itching, pins and needles, burning, or numbness
3   moderate itching, pins and needles, burning, or numbness
4   moderately severe hallucinations (formications)
5   severe hallucinations
6   extremely severe hallucinations
7   continuous hallucinations

AUDITORY DISTURBANCES — Ask "Are you more aware of sounds around you? Are they harsh? Do they frighten you? Are you hearing anything that is disturbing to you? Are you hearing things you know are not there?" Observation.

0   not present
1   very mild harshness or ability to frighten
2   mild harshness or ability to frighten
3   moderate harshness or ability to frighten
4   moderately severe auditory hallucinations
5   severe hallucinations
6   extremely severe hallucinations
7   continuous hallucinations

VISUAL DISTURBANCES — Ask "Does the light appear to be too bright? Is its color different? Does it hurt your eyes? Are you seeing anything that is disturbing to you? Are you seeing things you know are not there?" Observation.

0   not present
1   very mild photosensitivity
2   mild sensitivity
3   moderate sensitivity
4   moderately severe visual hallucinations
5   severe hallucinations
6   extremely severe hallucinations
7   continuous hallucinations

HEADACHE, FULLNESS IN HEAD — Ask "Does your head feel different? Does it feel like there is a band around your head?" Do not rate for dizziness or lightheadedness. Otherwise, rate severity.

0   not present
1   very mild
2   mild
3   moderate
4   moderately severe
5   severe
6   very severe
7   extremely severe

▲ **Figure 25–3.** Alcohol withdrawal assessment. (Reproduced from Sullivan JT et al. Assessment of alcohol withdrawal: The revised clinical institute withdrawal assessment for alcohol scale [CIWA-Ar]. *Br J Addict* 1989;84:1353. This scale is not copyrighted and may be used freely.)

AGITATION — Observation.

0 normal activity
1 somewhat more than normal activity
2
3
4 moderately fidgety and restless
5
6
7 paces back and forth during most of the interview, or constantly thrashes about

ORIENTATION AND CLOUDING OF SENSORIUM — Ask "What is today's date?... Who am I?". Serial additions: "Please count up by 5's — 0, 5, 10…"

0 oriented and can do serial additions
1 cannot do serial additions or is uncertain about date
2 disoriented for date by no more than 2 calendar days
3 disoriented for date by more than 2 calendar days
4 disoriented for date and place or person

Total **CIWA-Ar** Score _____

Rater's Initials _____

Maximum Possible Score 67

This assessment for monitoring withdrawal symptoms requires approximately 5 minutes to administer. The maximum score is 67 (see instrument). Patients scoring less than 8 (or 10, according to some experts) do not usually need additional medication for withdrawal.

▲ **Figure 25–3.** (*continued*)

of chlordiazepoxide is 600 mg in 24 hours. Continuous pulse oximetry and cardiac monitoring should be considered. The degree of sedation should be monitored 30–60 minutes after each oral dose of medication and for 15 minutes after each parenteral dose.

D. Severe withdrawal (CIWA-Ar score greater than 20)—Patients with severe withdrawal are at risk for the development of DTs and should be transferred or admitted to the ICU. Intravenous lorazepam is the medication of choice for treating severe withdrawal. Lorazepam 1–2 mg intravenously every 15 minutes can be given until patient is calm and sedated but awake. Initial CIWA-Ar monitoring should occur every 30 minutes. The patient can then receive lorazepam 2 mg orally or intravenously every hour as needed when the CIWA-Ar score is between 16 and 20, and lorazepam 1–2 mg orally or intravenously every hour as needed when the CIWA-Ar score is between 8 and 15. If the patient requires more than 8 mg/h of lorazepam as an initial dose or continues to demonstrate observable agitation, tremors, tachycardia, or hypertension despite high doses of lorazepam, consider adding dexmedetomidine. Dexmedetomidine, an alpha-2-agonist, produces sedation with minimal effect on respiratory drive. It is not recommended as a sole agent for the treatment of alcohol withdrawal but as adjunctive therapy along with benzodiazepines to decrease the hyperadrenergic output in patients with severe alcohol withdrawal not controlled by benzodiazepines or in patients at risk for respiratory depression from high-dose benzodiazepine administration. The recommended dosing of dexmedetomidine is 0.2–0.7 mcg/kg/h, with lorazepam 1–2 mg intravenously every 8 hours plus lorazepam 1–2 mg intravenously every hour as needed for agitation. In limited cases of severe withdrawal requiring frequent lorazepam boluses for at least 6 hours, continuous intravenous lorazepam infusion can be considered, but the patient must be monitored extremely carefully for signs of respiratory depression. Continuous pulse oximetry and close observance of the patient's respiratory status is required. Sedation is assessed 15 minutes after each intravenous dose. If withdrawal symptoms are

refractory to escalating benzodiazepine usage, despite the addition of dexmedetomidine, escalation to propofol should be considered. Patients receiving large doses of benzodiazepines often require intubation for airway protection, at which time initiation of propofol infusion for sedation, in addition to treatment of refractory alcohol withdrawal, is recommended. Phenobarbital monotherapy for alcohol withdrawal is used at some institutions, but randomized controlled trials comparing the efficacy of phenobarbital to benzodiazepines are lacking.

In all cases, benzodiazepines should be held if the patient is too sedated or has a respiratory rate less than 10 breaths per minute. Do not bolus lorazepam in doses greater than 4 mg intravenously. Mixing benzodiazepines, eg, chlordiazepoxide orally every 8 hours with lorazepam, is not recommended. Instead, select a single agent and titrate as needed. Once a patient has been stable for 24 hours, the benzodiazepine dose can be reduced by 20% daily until withdrawal is complete.

3. Managing other withdrawal-associated conditions—Meticulous examination for other medical problems is necessary. Alcoholic hypoglycemia can occur with low blood alcohol levels (see Chapter 27). Patients with severe alcohol use disorder commonly have liver disease with associated clotting disorders and are also prone to injury—and the combination all too frequently leads to undiagnosed subdural hematoma.

Phenytoin does *not* appear to be useful in managing alcohol withdrawal seizures per se. Sedating doses of benzodiazepines are effective in treating alcohol withdrawal seizures. Thus, other anticonvulsants are not usually needed unless there is a preexisting seizure disorder.

Chronic brain syndromes secondary to a long history of alcohol intake are not clearly responsive to thiamine and vitamin replenishment. Attention to the social and environmental care of this type of patient is paramount.

4. Initiating psychological and social measures—The psychological and behavioral treatment methods outlined under Treatment of At-Risk Drinking become the primary considerations after successful treatment of alcoholic hallucinosis or withdrawal. Psychological and social measures should be initiated in the hospital prior to discharge. This increases the possibility of continued posthospitalization treatment.

Mehta AJ. Alcoholism and critical illness: a review. World J Crit Care Med. 2016 Feb 4;5(1):27–35. [PMID: 26855891]

Oks M et al. The safety and utility of phenobarbital use for the treatment of severe alcohol withdrawal syndrome in the medical intensive care unit. J Intensive Care Med. 2018 Jan 1. [Epub ahead of print] [PMID: 29925291]

Schmidt KJ et al. Treatment of severe alcohol withdrawal. Ann Pharmacother. 2016 May;50(5):389–401. [PMID: 26861990]

Sullivan SM et al. Comparison of phenobarbital-adjunct versus benzodiazepine-only approach for alcohol withdrawal syndrome in the emergency department. Am J Emerg Med. 2018 Oct 11. [Epub ahead of print] [PMID: 30414743]

Soyka M et al; WFSBP Task Force on Treatment Guidelines for Substance Use Disorders. Guidelines for biological treatment of substance use and related disorders, part 1: Alcoholism, first revision. World J Biol Psychiatry. 2017 Mar;18(2): 86–119. [PMID: 28006997]

OTHER DRUG & SUBSTANCE USE DISORDERS

1. Opioids

While the terms "opioids" and "narcotics" both refer to a group of drugs with actions that mimic those of morphine, the term "opioids" is used when discussing medications prescribed in a controlled manner by a clinician, and the term "narcotics" is used to connote illicit drug use. All of the opioid analgesics can be reversed by the opioid antagonist naloxone.

The clinical symptoms and signs of mild narcotic intoxication include changes in mood, with feelings of euphoria; drowsiness; nausea with occasional emesis; needle tracks; and miosis. The incidence of snorting and inhaling ("smoking") heroin is increasing, particularly among cocaine users. This coincides with a decrease in the availability of methaqualone (no longer marketed) and other sedatives used to temper the cocaine "high" (see discussion of cocaine under Stimulants, below). Overdosage causes respiratory depression, peripheral vasodilation, pinpoint pupils, pulmonary edema, coma, and death.

Tolerance and withdrawal are major concerns when continued use of opioids occurs, although withdrawal causes only moderate morbidity (similar in severity to a bout of "flu"). Addicted patients sometimes consider themselves more addicted than they really are and may not require a withdrawal program. Grades of withdrawal are categorized from 0 to 4: **grade 0** includes craving and anxiety; **grade 1,** yawning, lacrimation, rhinorrhea, and perspiration; **grade 2,** previous symptoms plus mydriasis, piloerection, anorexia, tremors, and hot and cold flashes with generalized aching; **grades 3 and 4,** increased intensity of previous symptoms and signs, with increased temperature, blood pressure, pulse, and respiratory rate and depth. In withdrawal from the most severe addiction, vomiting, diarrhea, weight loss, hemoconcentration, and spontaneous ejaculation or orgasm commonly occur.

Treatment for overdosage (or suspected overdosage) is discussed in Chapter 38.

Treatment for withdrawal begins if grade 2 signs develop. If a withdrawal program is necessary, use methadone, 10 mg orally (use parenteral administration if the patient is vomiting), and observe. If signs (piloerection, mydriasis, cardiovascular changes) persist for more than 4–6 hours, give another 10 mg; continue to administer methadone at 4- to 6-hour intervals until signs are not present (rarely greater than 40 mg of methadone in 24 hours). Divide the total amount of medication required over the first 24-hour period by 2 and give that amount every 12 hours. Each day, reduce the total 24-hour dose by 5–10 mg. Thus, a moderately addicted patient initially requiring 30–40 mg of methadone could be withdrawn over a 4- to 8-day period. Clonidine, 0.1 mg orally several times daily over a 10- to 14-day period, is both an alternative and an adjunct to methadone detoxification; it is not necessary to taper the dose. Clonidine is helpful in alleviating cardiovascular symptoms but does not significantly relieve anxiety, insomnia, or generalized aching. There is a protracted abstinence syndrome of metabolic, respiratory, and blood pressure changes over a period of 3–6 months. Alternative strategies for the treatment of opioid withdrawal have included rapid and ultrarapid detoxification techniques. However, data do not support the use of either method.

Opioid antagonists (eg, naltrexone) can also be used successfully for treatment of the patient who has been free of opioids for 7–10 days. Naltrexone blocks the narcotic "high" of heroin when 50 mg is given orally every 24 hours initially for several days and then 100 mg is given every 48–72 hours. A monthly injectable form of naltrexone is available and may enhance compliance. Liver disorders are a major contraindication. Buprenorphine, a partial agonist, is a mainstay of office-based treatment of opiate dependency. Its use requires certified training along with a special license from the Drug Enforcement Agency. Buprenorphine is a mu partial agonist and kappa antagonist. Unlike conventional opioids, buprenorphine may have a role in the treatment of major depression.

Methadone maintenance programs are of some value in chronic recidivism. Under carefully controlled supervision, the narcotic addict is maintained on fairly high doses of methadone (40–120 mg/day) that satisfy craving and block the effects of heroin to a great degree.

2. Sedatives (Anxiolytics)

See Anxiety Disorders, this chapter.

3. Psychedelics

All of the common psychedelics (LSD, mescaline, psilocybin, dimethyltryptamine, and other derivatives of phenylalanine and tryptophan) can produce similar behavioral and physiologic effects. An initial feeling of tension is followed by emotional release such as crying or laughing (1–2 hours). Later and at higher doses, perceptual distortions occur, with visual illusions and hallucinations, and occasionally there is fear of ego disintegration (2–3 hours). Major changes in time sense and mood lability then occur

(3–4 hours). A feeling of detachment and a sense of destiny and control occur (4–6 hours). Of course, reactions vary among individuals, and some of the drugs produce markedly different time frames. Occasionally, the acute episode is terrifying (a "bad trip"), which may include panic, depression, confusion, or psychotic symptoms. Preexisting emotional problems, the attitude of the user, and the setting where the drug is used affect the experience.

Treatment of the acute episode primarily involves protection of the individual from erratic behavior that may lead to injury or death. A structured environment is usually sufficient until the drug is metabolized. In severe cases, antipsychotic medications with minimal side effects (eg, haloperidol, 5 mg intramuscularly) may be given every several hours until the individual has regained control. In cases where "flashbacks" occur (mental imagery from a "bad trip" that is later triggered by mild stimuli such as marijuana, alcohol, or psychic trauma), a short course of an antipsychotic medication—eg, olanzapine, 5–10 mg/day orally, or risperidone, 2 mg/day orally, initially, and up to 20 mg/day and 6 mg/day, respectively—is usually sufficient. Lorazepam or clonazepam, 1–2 mg orally every 2 hours as needed for acute agitation, may be a useful adjunct. An occasional patient may have "flashbacks" for much longer periods and may require small doses of antipsychotic medications over the longer term.

4. Phencyclidine

Phencyclidine (PCP, angel dust, peace pill, hog) is simple to produce and mimics to some degree the traditional psychedelic drugs. PCP is a common deceptive substitute for LSD, tetrahydrocannabinol, and mescaline. It is available in crystals, capsules, and tablets to be inhaled, injected, swallowed, or smoked (it is commonly sprinkled on marijuana).

Absorption after smoking is rapid, with onset of symptoms in several minutes and peak symptoms in 15–30 minutes. Mild intoxication produces euphoria accompanied by a feeling of numbness. Moderate intoxication (5–10 mg) results in disorientation, detachment from surroundings, distortion of body image, combativeness, unusual feats of strength (partly due to its anesthetic activity), and loss of ability to integrate sensory input, especially touch and proprioception. Physical symptoms include dizziness, ataxia, dysarthria, nystagmus, retracted upper eyelid with blank stare, hyperreflexia, and tachycardia. There are increases in blood pressure, respiration, muscle tone, and urine production. Usage in the first trimester of pregnancy is associated with an increase in spontaneous abortion and congenital defects. Severe intoxication (20 mg or more) produces an increase in degree of moderate symptoms, with the addition of seizures, deepening coma, hypertensive crisis, and severe psychotic ideation. The drug is particularly long-lasting (several days to several weeks) owing to high lipid solubility, gastroenteric recycling, and the production of active metabolites. Overdosage may be fatal, with the major causes of death being hypertensive crisis, respiratory arrest, and convulsions. Acute rhabdomyolysis has been reported and can result in myoglobinuric kidney failure.

Differential diagnosis involves the whole spectrum of street drugs, since in some ways phencyclidine mimics sedatives, psychedelics, and marijuana in its effects. Blood and urine testing can detect the acute problem.

Treatment is discussed in Chapter 38.

5. Marijuana

Cannabis sativa, a hemp plant, is the source of marijuana. Mercury may be a contaminant in marijuana grown in volcanic soil. The drug is usually inhaled by smoking but vaporizing is increasingly popular. Effects occur in 10–20 minutes and last 2–3 hours. "Joints" of good quality contain about 500 mg of marijuana (which contains approximately 5–15 mg of tetrahydrocannabinol with a half-life of 7 days).

With moderate dosage, recreational marijuana (higher in the THC versus CBD component) produces two phases: mild euphoria followed by sleepiness. In the acute state, the user has an altered time perception, less inhibited emotions, psychomotor problems, impaired immediate memory, and conjunctival injection. High doses produce transient psychotomimetic effects. No specific treatment is necessary except in the case of the occasional "bad trip," in which case the person is treated in the same way as for psychedelic usage. Marijuana frequently aggravates existing mental illness and adversely affects motor performance.

Studies of long-term effects have conclusively shown abnormalities in the pulmonary tree. Laryngitis and rhinitis are related to prolonged use, along with chronic obstructive pulmonary disease. Electrocardiographic abnormalities are common, but no chronic cardiac disease has been linked to marijuana use. Long-term usage has resulted in depression of plasma testosterone levels and reduced sperm counts. Abnormal menstruation and failure to ovulate have occurred in some women. Cognitive impairments are common. Health care utilization for a variety of health problems is increased in long-term marijuana smokers. Sudden withdrawal produces insomnia, nausea, myalgia, and irritability. Psychological effects of long-term marijuana usage are still unclear. Urine testing is reliable if samples are carefully collected and tested. Detection periods span 4–6 days in short-term users and 20–50 days in long-term users.

6. Stimulants: Amphetamines & Cocaine

Stimulant abuse is quite common, either alone or in combination with abuse of other drugs. The stimulants include illicit drugs such as methamphetamine ("speed")—one variant is a smokable form called "ice," which gives an intense and fairly long-lasting high—and methylphenidate and dextroamphetamine, which are under prescription control. Street availability of amphetamines remains high. Moderate usage of any of the stimulants produces hyperactivity, a sense of enhanced physical and mental capacity, and sympathomimetic effects. The clinical picture of acute stimulant intoxication includes sweating, tachycardia, elevated blood pressure, mydriasis, hyperactivity, and an acute brain syndrome with confusion and disorientation. Tolerance develops quickly, and, as the dosage is increased, hypervigilance, paranoid ideation (with delusions of parasitosis), stereotypy, bruxism, tactile hallucinations of insect infestation, and full-blown psychoses occur, often with persecutory ideation and aggressive responses. Stimulant withdrawal is characterized by depression with symptoms of hyperphagia and hypersomnia.

People who have used stimulants chronically (eg, anorexigenics) occasionally become sensitized ("kindling") to future use of stimulants. In these individuals, even small amounts of mild stimulants such as caffeine can cause symptoms of paranoia and auditory hallucinations.

Cocaine is a stimulant. It is a product of the coca plant. The derivatives include seeds, leaves, coca paste, cocaine hydrochloride, and the free base of cocaine. Cocaine hydrochloride is the salt and the most commonly used form. Freebase, a purer (and stronger) derivative called "crack," is prepared by simple extraction from cocaine hydrochloride.

There are various modes of use. Coca leaf chewing involves toasting the leaves and chewing with alkaline material (eg, the ash of other burned leaves) to enhance buccal absorption. One achieves a mild high, with onset in 5–10 minutes and lasting for about an hour. Intranasal use is simply snorting cocaine through a straw. Absorption is slowed somewhat by vasoconstriction (which may eventually cause tissue necrosis and septal perforation); the onset of action is in 2–3 minutes, with a moderate high (euphoria, excitement, increased energy) lasting about 30 minutes. The purity of the cocaine is a major determinant of the high. Intravenous use of cocaine hydrochloride or "freebase" is effective in 30 seconds and produces a short-lasting, fairly intense high of about 15 minutes' duration. The combined use of cocaine and ethanol results in the metabolic production of cocaethylene by the liver. This substance produces more intense and long-lasting cocaine-like effects. Smoking freebase (volatilized cocaine because of the lower boiling point) acts in seconds and results in an intense high lasting several minutes. The intensity of the reaction is related to the marked lipid solubility of the freebase form and produces by far the most severe medical and psychiatric symptoms.

Cardiovascular collapse, arrhythmias, myocardial infarction, and transient ischemic attacks have been reported. Seizures, strokes, migraine symptoms, hyperthermia, and lung damage may occur, and there are several obstetric complications, including spontaneous abortion, abruptio placentae, teratogenic effects, delayed fetal growth, and prematurity. Cocaine can cause anxiety, mood swings, and delirium, and chronic use can cause the same problems as other stimulants.

Clinicians should be alert to cocaine use in patients presenting with unexplained nasal bleeding or septal perforations, headaches, fatigue, insomnia, anxiety, depression, and chronic hoarseness. Sudden withdrawal of the drug is not life-threatening but usually produces craving, sleep disturbances, hyperphagia, lassitude, and severe depression (sometimes with suicidal ideation) lasting days to weeks.

Treatment is imprecise and difficult. Since the high is related to blockage of dopamine reuptake, the dopamine agonist bromocriptine, 1.5 mg orally three times a day, alleviates some of the symptoms of craving associated with

acute cocaine withdrawal. Treatment of psychosis is the same as that of any psychosis: antipsychotic medications in dosages sufficient to alleviate the symptoms. Any medical symptoms (eg, hyperthermia, seizures, hypertension) are treated specifically. These approaches should be used in conjunction with a structured program, most often based on the Alcoholics Anonymous model. Hospitalization may be required if self-harm or violence toward others is a perceived threat (usually indicated by paranoid delusions).

7. Caffeine

Caffeine, along with nicotine and alcohol, is one of the most commonly used drugs worldwide. Tea, cocoa, and cola drinks also contribute to an intake of caffeine that is often astoundingly high in a large number of people. Low to moderate doses (30–200 mg/day) tend to improve some aspects of performance (eg, vigilance). The approximate content of caffeine in a (180-mL) cup of beverage is as follows: brewed coffee, 80–140 mg; instant coffee, 60–100 mg; decaffeinated coffee, 1–6 mg; black leaf tea, 30–80 mg; tea bags, 25–75 mg; instant tea, 30–60 mg; cocoa, 10–50 mg; and 12-oz cola drinks, 30–65 mg. A 2-oz chocolate candy bar has about 20 mg. Some herbal teas (eg, "morning thunder") contain caffeine. Caffeine-containing analgesics usually contain approximately 30 mg per unit. Symptoms of caffeinism (usually associated with ingestion of over 500 mg/day) include anxiety, agitation, restlessness, insomnia, a feeling of being "wired," and somatic symptoms referable to the heart and gastrointestinal tract. It is common for a case of caffeinism to present as an anxiety disorder. It is also common for caffeine and other stimulants to precipitate severe symptoms in compensated schizophrenic and manic-depressive patients. Chronically depressed patients often use caffeine drinks as self-medication. This diagnostic clue may help distinguish some major affective disorders. Discontinuation of caffeine (greater than 250 mg/day) can produce withdrawal symptoms, such as headaches, irritability, lethargy, and occasional nausea.

8. Miscellaneous Drugs & Solvents

The principal over-the-counter drugs of concern are an assortment of antihistaminic agents, frequently in combination with a mild analgesic promoted as cold remedies.

Antihistamines usually produce some central nervous system depression—thus their use as over-the-counter sedatives. Practically all of the so-called sleep aids are antihistamines. The mixture of antihistamines with alcohol usually exacerbates the central nervous system effects. Scopolamine and bromides generally have been removed from over-the-counter products.

The abuse of laxatives sometimes can lead to electrolyte disturbances that may contribute to the manifestations of a delirium. The greatest use of laxatives tends to be in the elderly and in those with eating disorders, both of whom are the most vulnerable to physiologic changes.

Anabolic steroids are abused by people who wish to increase muscle mass for cosmetic reasons or for greater strength. In addition to the medical problems, the practice is associated with significant mood swings, aggressiveness, and paranoid delusions. Alcohol and stimulant use are higher in these individuals. Withdrawal symptoms of steroid dependency include fatigue, depressed mood, restlessness, and insomnia.

Amyl nitrite is used as an "orgasm expander." The changes in time perception, "rush," and mild euphoria caused by the drug prompted its nonmedical use. Subjective effects last from 5 seconds to 15 minutes. Tolerance develops readily, but there are no known withdrawal symptoms. Abstinence for several days reestablishes the previous level of responsiveness. Long-term effects may include damage to the immune system and respiratory difficulties.

Sniffing of solvents and inhaling of gases (including aerosols) produce a form of inebriation similar to that of the volatile anesthetics. Agents include gasoline, toluene, petroleum ether, lighter fluids, cleaning fluids, paint thinners, and solvents that are present in many household products (eg, nail polish). Typical intoxication states include euphoria, slurred speech, hallucinations, and confusion, and with high doses, acute manifestations are unconsciousness and cardiorespiratory depression or failure; chronic exposure produces a variety of symptoms related to the liver, kidney, bone marrow, or heart. Lead encephalopathy can be associated with sniffing leaded gasoline. In addition, studies of workers chronically exposed to jet fuel showed significant increases in neurasthenic symptoms, including fatigue, anxiety, mood changes, memory difficulties, and somatic complaints. These same problems have been noted in long-term solvent abuse.

The so-called designer drugs are synthetic substitutes for commonly used recreational drugs. Common designer drugs include methyl analogues of fentanyl used as heroin substitutes. MDMA is also a designer drug with high abuse potential and purported neurotoxicity. Often not detected by standard toxicology screens, these substances can present a vexing problem for clinicians faced with symptoms from a totally unknown cause.

Bohnert ASB et al. Understanding links among opioid use, overdose, and suicide. N Engl J Med. 2019 Jan 3;380(1):71–9. [PMID: 30601750]

Manhapra A et al. Pain and addiction: an integrative therapeutic approach. Med Clin North Am. 2018 Jul;102(4):745–63. [PMID: 29933827]

Mirijello A et al. Identification and management of alcohol withdrawal syndrome. Drugs. 2015 Mar;75(4):353–65. [PMID: 25666543]

NEUROCOGNITIVE DISORDERS

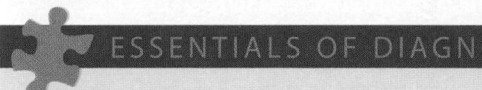

ESSENTIALS OF DIAGNOSIS

► Transient or permanent brain dysfunction with alterations in awareness or attention.

► Cognitive impairment to varying degrees.

► Impaired recall and recent memory, inability to focus attention and problems in perceptual processing, often with psychotic ideation.

► Random psychomotor activity such as stereotypy.

► Emotional disorders frequently present: depression, anxiety, irritability.

► Behavioral disturbances: impulse control, sexual acting-out, attention deficits, aggression, and exhibitionism.

► **General Considerations**

The organic problem may be a primary brain disorder or a secondary manifestation of some general disorder. All of the cognitive disorders show *some degree of impaired thinking* depending on the site of involvement, the rate of onset and progression, and the duration of the underlying brain lesion. Emotional disturbances (eg, depression) are often present as significant comorbidities. The behavioral disturbances tend to be more common with chronicity, more directly related to the underlying personality or central nervous system vulnerability to drug side effects, and not necessarily correlated with cognitive dysfunction.

The causes of cognitive disorders are listed in Table 25–11.

► **Clinical Findings**

The many manifestations include problems with orientation, short or fluctuating attention span, loss of recent memory and recall, impaired judgment, emotional lability, lack of initiative, impaired impulse control, inability to reason through problems, depression (worse in mild to moderate types), confabulation (not limited to alcohol organic brain syndrome), constriction of intellectual functions, visual and auditory hallucinations, and delusions. Physical findings will vary according to the cause. The electroencephalogram usually shows generalized slowing in delirium.

A. Delirium

Delirium (acute confusional state) is a transient global disorder of attention, with clouding of consciousness, usually a result of systemic problems (eg, medications, hypoxemia). See Chapters 4 and 24. Onset is usually rapid. The mental status fluctuates (impairment is usually least in the morning), with varying inability to concentrate, maintain attention, and sustain purposeful behavior. There is a marked deficit of short-term memory and recall. Anxiety and irritability are common. Orientation problems follow the inability to retain information. Perceptual disturbances (often visual hallucinations) and psychomotor restlessness with insomnia are common. **"Sundowning"**—mild to moderate delirium at night—is more common in patients with preexisting dementia and may be precipitated by hospitalization, medications, and sensory deprivation.

B. Dementia

Dementia is characterized by chronicity and deterioration of selective mental functions. See Chapters 4 and 24.

In all types of dementia, loss of impulse control (sexual and language) is common. **Pseudodementia** is a term previously applied to depressed patients who appear to be demented. These patients are often identifiable by their

Table 25–11. Etiology of delirium and other cognitive disorders.

Disorder	Possible Causes
Intoxication	Alcohol, sedatives, bromides, analgesics (eg, pentazocine), psychedelic drugs, stimulants, and household solvents.
Medication withdrawal	Withdrawal from alcohol, sedative-hypnotics, corticosteroids.
Long-term effects of alcohol	Wernicke-Korsakoff syndrome.
Infections	Septicemia; meningitis and encephalitis due to bacterial, viral, fungal, parasitic, or tuberculous organisms or to central nervous system syphilis; acute and chronic infections due to the entire range of microbiologic pathogens.
Endocrine disorders	Thyrotoxicosis, hypothyroidism, adrenocortical dysfunction (including Addison disease and Cushing syndrome), pheochromocytoma, insulinoma, hypoglycemia, hyperparathyroidism, hypoparathyroidism, panhypopituitarism, diabetic ketoacidosis.
Respiratory disorders	Hypoxia, hypercapnia.
Metabolic disturbances	Fluid and electrolyte disturbances (especially hyponatremia, hypomagnesemia, and hypercalcemia), acid-base disorders, hepatic disease (hepatic encephalopathy), kidney failure, porphyria.
Nutritional deficiencies	Deficiency of vitamin B_1 (beriberi), vitamin B_{12} (pernicious anemia), folic acid, nicotinic acid (pellagra); protein-calorie malnutrition.
Trauma	Subdural hematoma, subarachnoid hemorrhage, intracerebral bleeding, concussion syndrome.
Cardiovascular disorders	Myocardial infarctions, cardiac arrhythmias, cerebrovascular spasms, hypertensive encephalopathy, hemorrhages, embolisms, and occlusions indirectly cause decreased cognitive function.
Neoplasms	Primary or metastatic lesions of the central nervous system, cancer-induced hypercalcemia.
Seizure disorders	Ictal, interictal, and postictal dysfunction.
Collagen-vascular and immunologic disorders	Autoimmune disorders, including systemic lupus erythematosus, Sjögren syndrome, and AIDS.
Degenerative diseases	Alzheimer disease, Pick disease, multiple sclerosis, parkinsonism, Huntington chorea, normal pressure hydrocephalus.
Medications	Anticholinergic medications, antidepressants, H_2-blocking agents, digoxin, salicylates (long-term use), and a wide variety of other over-the-counter and prescribed medications.

tendency to complain about memory problems vociferously rather than try to cover them up. They usually say they cannot complete cognitive tasks but with encouragement can often do so. They can be considered to have depression-induced reversible dementia that improves when the depression resolves. In many geriatric patients, however, the depression appears to be an insult that often unmasks a progressive dementia.

C. Amnestic Syndrome

This is a memory disturbance without delirium or dementia. It is usually associated with thiamine deficiency and chronic alcohol use (eg, Korsakoff syndrome). There is an impairment in the ability to learn new information or recall previously learned information.

D. Substance-Induced Hallucinosis

This condition is characterized by persistent or recurrent hallucinations (usually auditory) without the other symptoms usually found in delirium or dementia. Alcohol or hallucinogens are often the cause. There does not have to be any other mental disorder, and there may be complete spontaneous resolution.

► Treatment

See Chapters 4 and 24 for detailed discussion.

Deardorff WJ et al. The use of cholinesterase inhibitors across all stages of Alzheimer's disease. Drugs Aging. 2015 Jul;32(7): 537–47. [PMID: 26033268]

Wong N et al. Managing delirium in the emergency department: tools for targeting underlying etiology. Emerg Med Pract. 2015 Oct;17(10):1–20. [PMID: 26367083]

PSYCHIATRIC PROBLEMS ASSOCIATED WITH HOSPITALIZATION & ILLNESS

► Diagnostic Categories

A. Acute Problems

1. Delirium with psychotic features secondary to the medical or surgical problem, or compounded by effect of treatment.

2. Acute anxiety, often related to ignorance and fear of the immediate problem as well as uncertainty about the future.

3. Anxiety as an intrinsic aspect of the medical problem (eg, hyperthyroidism).

4. Denial of illness, which may present during acute or intermediate phases of illness.

B. Intermediate Problems

1. Depression as a function of the illness or acceptance of the illness, often associated with realistic or fantasied hopelessness about the future.

2. Behavioral problems, often related to denial of illness and, in extreme cases, causing the patient to leave the hospital against medical advice.

C. Recuperative Problems

1. Decreasing cooperation as the patient sees that improvement and compliance are not compelled.

2. Readjustment problems with family, job, and society.

► General Considerations

A. Acute Problems

1. "Intensive care unit psychosis"—The ICU environment may contribute to the etiology of delirium. Critical care unit factors include sleep deprivation, increased arousal, mechanical ventilation, and social isolation. Other causes include those common to delirium and require vigorous investigation (see Delirium).

2. Presurgical and postsurgical anxiety states—Anxiety before or after surgery is common and commonly ignored. **Presurgical anxiety** is very common and is principally a fear of death (many surgical patients make out their wills). Patients may be fearful of anesthesia (improved by the preoperative anesthesia interview), the mysterious operating room, and the disease processes that might be uncovered by the surgeon. Such fears frequently cause people to delay examinations that might result in earlier surgery and a greater chance of cure.

The opposite of this is **surgery proneness,** the quest for surgery to escape from overwhelming life stresses. Some polysurgery patients may be classified as having factitious disorders. Dynamic motivations include the need to get medical care as a way of getting dependency needs met, the desire to outwit authority figures, unconscious guilt, or a masochistic need to suffer. Frequent surgery may also be related to a somatic symptom disorder, particularly body dysmorphic disorder (an obsession that a body part is disfigured). More apparent reasons may include an attempt to get relief from pain and a lifestyle that has become almost exclusively medically oriented, with all of the risks entailed in such an endeavor.

Postsurgical anxiety states are usually related to pain, procedures, and loss of body image. Acute pain problems are quite different from chronic pain disorders (see Chronic Pain Disorders, this chapter); the former are readily handled with adequate analgesic medication (see Chapter 5). Alterations in body image, as with amputations, ostomies, and mastectomies, often raise concerns about relationships with others.

3. Iatrogenic problems—These usually pertain to medications, complications of diagnostic and treatment procedures, and impersonal and unsympathetic staff behavior. Polypharmacy is often a factor. Patients with unsolved diagnostic problems are at higher risk. They are desirous of relief, and the quest engenders more diagnostic procedures with a higher incidence of complications. The upset patient and family may be very demanding. Excessive demands usually result from anxiety. Such behavior is best handled with calm and measured responses.

B. Intermediate Problems

1. Prolonged hospitalization—Prolonged hospitalization presents unique problems in certain hospital services, eg, burn units or orthopedic services. The acute problems of the severely burned patient are discussed in Chapter 37. The problems often are behavioral difficulties related to length of hospitalization and necessary procedures. For example, in burn units, pain is a major problem in addition to anxiety about procedures. Disputes with staff are common and often concern pain medication or ward privileges. Some patients regress to infantile behavior and dependency. Staff members must agree about their approach to the patient in order to ensure the smooth functioning of the unit.

Denial of illness may present in some patients. Intervention by an authority figure (eg, immediate work supervisor) may help the patient accept treatment and eventually abandon the coping mechanism of denial.

2. Depression—Mood disorders ranging from mild adjustment disorder to major depressive disorder frequently occur during prolonged hospitalizations. A key to the diagnosis of depression in the medical setting is the individual's loss of self-esteem; they often think of themselves as worthless and are guilt ridden. Therapeutic medications (eg, corticosteroids) may be a factor. Depression can contribute to irritability and overt anger. Severe depression can lead to anorexia, which further complicates healing and metabolic balance. It is during this period that the issue of disfigurement arises—relief at survival gives way to concern about future function and appearance.

C. Recuperative Problems

1. Anxiety—Anxiety about return to the posthospital environment can cause regression to a dependent position. Complications increase, and staff forbearance again is tested. Anxiety occurring at this stage usually is handled more easily than previous behavior problems.

2. Posthospital adjustment—Adjustment difficulties after discharge are related to the severity of the deficits and the use of outpatient facilities (eg, physical therapy, rehabilitation programs, psychiatric outpatient treatment). Some patients may experience posttraumatic stress symptoms (eg, from traumatic injuries or even from necessary medical treatments). Lack of appropriate follow-up can contribute to depression in the patient, who may feel that he or she is making poor progress and may have thoughts of "giving up." Reintegration into work, educational, and social endeavors may be slow.

Clinical Findings

The symptoms that occur in these patients are similar to those discussed in previous sections of this chapter, eg, delirium, stress and adjustment disorders, anxiety, and depression. Behavior problems may include lack of cooperation, increased complaints, demands for medication, sexual approaches to nurses, threats to leave the hospital, and actual signing out against medical recommendations. The stress of hospitalization often brings out these more primitive defense mechanisms than the patient displays in daily life.

Complications

Prolongation of hospitalization causes increased expense, deterioration of patient-staff relationships, and increased probabilities of iatrogenic and legal problems. The possibility of increasing posthospital treatment problems is enhanced.

Treatment

A. Medical

The most important consideration by far is to have one clinician in charge, a clinician whom the patient trusts and who is able to oversee multiple treatment approaches (see Somatic Symptom Disorders, above). In acute problems, attention must be paid to metabolic imbalance, alcohol withdrawal, and previous drug use—prescribed, recreational, or over-the-counter. Adequate sleep and analgesia are important in enhancing a patient's coping abilities.

Many clinicians are attuned to the early detection of the surgery-prone patient. Plastic and orthopedic surgeons are at particular risk. Appropriate consultations may help detect some problems and mitigate future ones.

Postsurgical anxiety states can be alleviated by personal attention from the surgeon. Anxiety is not so effectively lessened by ancillary medical personnel, whom the patient perceives as lesser authorities, until after the clinician has reassured the patient. "Patient-controlled analgesia" can improve pain control, decrease anxiety, and minimize side effects.

Depression should be recognized early. If severe, it may be treated by antidepressant medications (see Antidepressant Medications, above). High levels of anxiety can be lowered with judicious use of anxiolytic agents. Unnecessary medications tend to reinforce the patient's impression that there must be a serious illness or medication would not be required.

B. Psychological

Prepare the patient and family for what is to come. This includes the types of units where the patient will be quartered, the procedures that will be performed, and any disfigurements that will result from surgery. Repetition improves understanding. The nursing staff can be helpful, since patients frequently confide a lack of understanding to a nurse but are reluctant to do so to the physician.

Denial of illness is frequently a block to acceptance of treatment. This too should be handled with family members present (to help the patient face the reality of the situation) in a series of short interviews (for reinforcement). Dependency problems resulting from long hospitalization are best handled by focusing on the changes to come as the patient makes the transition to the outside world. Key figures are teachers, vocational counselors, and physical therapists. Challenges should be realistic and practical and handled in small steps.

Depression is usually related to the loss of familiar hospital supports, and the outpatient therapists and counselors help to lessen the impact of the loss. Some of the impact can be alleviated by anticipating, with the patient and family, the signal features of the common depression to help prevent the patient from assuming a permanent sick role.

Suicide is always a concern when a patient is faced with despair. An honest, compassionate, and supportive approach will help sustain the patient during this trying period.

C. Behavioral

Prior desensitization can significantly allay anxiety about medical procedures. A "dry run" can be done to reinforce the oral description. Cooperation during acute problem periods can be enhanced by the use of appropriate reinforcers such as a favorite nurse or helpful family member. People who are positive reinforcers are even more helpful during the intermediate phases when the patient becomes resistant to the seemingly endless procedures (eg, debridement of burned areas).

Specific situations (eg, psychological dependency on the respirator) can be corrected by weaning with appropriate reinforcers (eg, watching a favorite movie on a DVD player or laptop when disconnected from the ventilator). Behavioral approaches should be used in a positive and optimistic way for maximal reinforcement.

Relaxation techniques, hypnosis, and attentional distraction can be used to block side effects of a necessary treatment (eg, nausea in cancer chemotherapy).

D. Social

A change in environment requires adaptation. Because of the illness, admission and hospitalization may be more easily handled than discharge. A predischarge evaluation must be made to determine whether the family will be able to cope with the physical or mental changes in the patient. Working with the family while the patient is in the acute stage may presage a successful transition later on.

Development of a new social life can be facilitated by various self-help organizations (eg, the stoma club). Sharing problems with others in similar circumstances eases the return to a social life, which may be quite different from that prior to the illness.

Prognosis

The prognosis is good in all patients who have reversible medical and surgical conditions. It is guarded when there is serious functional loss that impairs vocational, educational, or societal possibilities—especially in the case of progressive and ultimately life-threatening illness.

Hshieh TT et al. Delirium in the elderly. Psychiatr Clin North Am. 2018 Mar;41(1):1–17. [PMID: 29412839]

Endocrine Disorders

Paul A. Fitzgerald, MD

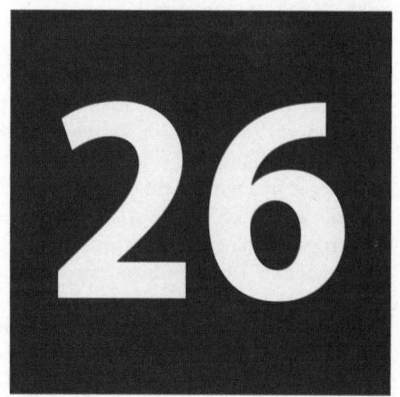

ANTERIOR HYPOPITUITARISM

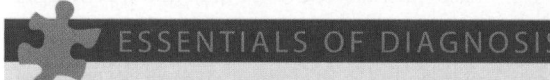

ESSENTIALS OF DIAGNOSIS

► **Adrenocorticotropic hormone (ACTH) deficiency:** reduced adrenal secretion of cortisol and epinephrine; aldosterone secretion remains intact.

► **Growth hormone (GH) deficiency:** short stature in children; asthenia, obesity, and increased cardiovascular risk in adults.

► **Prolactin (PRL) deficiency:** postpartum lactation failure.

► **Thyroid-stimulating hormone (TSH) deficiency:** secondary hypothyroidism.

► **Luteinizing hormone (LH)** and **follicle-stimulating hormone (FSH) deficiency:** hypogonadism and infertility in men and women.

► General Considerations

The anterior pituitary hormones are GH, PRL, ACTH, TSH, LH, and FSH. The posterior pituitary hormones are oxytocin and arginine vasopressin (AVP), also known as antidiuretic hormone (ADH).

1. Hypopituitarism with mass lesions—Pituitary adenomas can cause anterior hypopituitarism, particularly when they are large macroadenomas (1 cm or more in diameter). Nonfunctioning pituitary adenomas are more likely than functioning pituitary adenomas to grow large enough to cause anterior hypopituitarism; they rarely cause diabetes insipidus. Other mass lesions include craniopharyngioma, meningioma, germinoma, glioma, chordoma, metastatic lesions, and cysts (Rathke cleft, dermoid, arachnoid). Vascular lesions include pituitary tumor apoplexy, acute Sheehan syndrome, intrasellar carotid aneurysm, and subarachnoid hemorrhage. Inflammatory/infiltrative lesions include granulomatosis with polyangiitis, xanthomatosis, giant cell granuloma, Langerhans cell histiocytosis, sarcoidosis, syphilis, and tuberculosis. Infectious lesions can be bacterial, fungal, or parasitic.

Lymphocytic hypophysitis is an autoimmune disorder affecting the pituitary gland. Spontaneous lymphocytic hypophysitis is more common in women (71%) and most frequently presents during pregnancy or postpartum. The condition is often associated with other autoimmune conditions, such as systemic lupus erythematosus (SLE) or Hashimoto thyroiditis. Immune checkpoint inhibitor hypophysitis can be caused by several immunity-enhancing drugs, particularly the anti-CTLA-4 agents ipilimumab and tremelimumab (10–15%), as well as with the anti-PD-1 agents pembrolizumab and nivolumab. Symptoms of hypophysitis develop on average 9 weeks after beginning the medication and as late as 19 months after commencing therapy.

2. Hypopituitarism without mass lesions—Congenital combined hypopituitarism occurs in syndromes such as septo-optic dysplasia and in patients with various gene mutations that cause a progressive loss of anterior pituitary function in childhood. Congenital hypogonadotropic hypogonadism can be caused by mutations in any of the many genes that control the production or release of gonadotropin-releasing hormone (GnRH), LH, or FSH. Prader-Willi syndrome is a genetic disorder where genes on the paternal chromosome 15 are deleted or unexpressed. Kallmann syndrome is caused by various gene mutations that impair the development or migration of GnRH-synthesizing neurons from the olfactory bulb to the hypothalamus. Congenital GH deficiency occurs as an isolated pituitary hormone deficiency in about one-third of cases.

Acquired hypopituitarism without a visible mass lesion on MRI can result from cranial radiation therapy, pituitary surgery, encephalitis, cerebral malaria, hemochromatosis, autoimmunity, or coronary artery bypass grafting (CABG). Bexarotene chemotherapy causes a high rate of pituitary insufficiency with central hypothyroidism. At least one pituitary hormone deficiency develops in about 25–30% of survivors of moderate to severe traumatic brain injury and in about 55% of survivors of aneurysmal subarachnoid hemorrhage. Some degree of hypopituitarism, most commonly GH deficiency and hypogonadotropic hypogonadism, occurs in one-third of ischemic stroke patients. Other cases of acquired hypopituitarism can be idiopathic or associated with an empty sella on MRI.

In functional hypopituitarism, GH deficiency can occur with malnutrition, chronic kidney disease, opioid therapy, and normal aging. LH and FSH deficiency with hypogonadotropic hypogonadism occurs in serious illness, malnutrition, anorexia nervosa, alcoholism, opioid therapy, Cushing syndrome (spontaneous or iatrogenic), and hyperprolactinemia (drug-induced or spontaneous). Therapy with GnRH agonists (eg, leuprolide) also causes hypogonadotropic hypogonadism that can persist after therapy is stopped. Partial hypogonadotropic hypogonadism commonly develops in men with normal aging or obesity, since they have serum free testosterone levels that are low or near the lower end of normal reference ranges while serum FSH and LH levels remain normal. Hypothalamic amenorrhea frequently develops in women during periods of severe emotional or physical stress, intense exercise programs, severe caloric restriction, or eating disorders. ACTH suppression with functional isolated secondary adrenal insufficiency occurs in patients receiving megesterol acetate, patients on high-dose opioid therapy (15%), and in patients exposed to excess endogenous or exogenous corticosteroids (parenteral, oral, inhaled, or topical). TSH deficiency can be caused by mitotane or bexarotene, resulting in secondary hypothyroidism.

Sheehan syndrome refers to hypopituitarism caused by postpartum pituitary necrosis, usually following severe postpartum uterine hemorrhage. It is usually characterized by postpartum amenorrhea and inability to lactate. *Hypopituitarism can occur acutely, usually with severe secondary adrenal insufficiency that may be fatal unless recognized and treated.* Acute hypopituitarism may also be associated with diabetes insipidus. However, hypopituitarism in Sheehan syndrome usually occurs gradually over 10–20 years; the diagnosis is typically delayed an average of 9 years. Manifestations in affected women are typically hyponatremia, hypoglycemia, or anemia. In acute Sheehan syndrome, MRI shows an enlarged pituitary with only a thin rim of enhancement with gadolinium. After 1 year, MRI shows atrophy of the pituitary and a partially empty sella.

▶ Clinical Findings

When hypopituitarism is caused by a mass lesion or hypophysitis, patients may have headaches or visual field defects. Nonspecific symptoms, such as fatigue, dizziness and hypotension, confusion, cognitive dysfunction, sexual dysfunction, polydipsia, or cold intolerance, can develop.

A. Symptoms and Signs

1. GH (somatropin) deficiency—Congenital GH deficiency can present in newborns with hypoglycemia, jaundice, and a small penis and later with short stature in childhood.

GH deficiency in adults is often undiagnosed, since maximum height has already been reached and other manifestations are nonspecific. Symptoms vary in severity from mild to severe, resulting in a variable spectrum of nonspecific symptoms that include mild to moderate central obesity, reduced physical and mental energy, impaired concentration and memory, and depression. Patients may also have variably reduced muscle and bone mass, increased low-density lipoprotein (LDL) cholesterol, and reduced cardiac output with exercise. When other more recognizable pituitary hormone deficits are present, there is a high likelihood of concurrent GH deficiency.

2. Gonadotropin deficiency (hypogonadotropic hypogonadism)—In gonadotropin deficiency, insufficiencies of LH and FSH cause hypogonadism and infertility.

Congenital gonadotropin deficiency is characterized by partial or complete lack of pubertal development. The sense of olfaction (smell) is entirely normal in 58% (normosmic isolated hypogonadotropic hypogonadism), or hyposmic or anosmic in 42% (Kallmann syndrome). Patients frequently have abnormal genitalia (25%), kidney anomalies (28%), midline craniofacial defects (50%), neurologic deficits (42%), and musculoskeletal malformations. Some affected women have menarche followed by secondary amenorrhea. Some affected males also have congenital adrenal hypoplasia with X-linked inheritance; affected boys who survive childhood can present with failure to enter puberty.

Prader-Willi syndrome presents with cryptorchidism, mental retardation, short stature, hyperflexibility, autonomic dysregulation, cognitive impairment, hyperphagia with obesity, hypogonadotropic hypogonadism, or primary hypogonadism.

Acquired gonadotropin deficiency is characterized by the gradual loss of facial, axillary, pubic, and body hair. Men may note diminished libido, erectile dysfunction, muscle atrophy, infertility, and osteopenia. Women have amenorrhea, infertility, and osteoporosis.

3. TSH deficiency—TSH deficiency causes hypothyroidism (see Hypothyroidism, below).

4. ACTH deficiency—Central adrenal insufficiency is caused by ACTH deficiency. There is functional atrophy of the adrenal cortex within 2 weeks of pituitary damage, which results in diminished cortisol. Adrenal mineralocorticoid secretion continues, so manifestations of adrenal insufficiency in hypopituitarism are usually less striking than in bilateral adrenal gland destruction (see Primary Adrenal Insufficiency [Addison disease], below). Patients with partial ACTH deficiency have some cortisol secretion and may not have symptoms until stressed by illness or surgery.

5. PRL deficiency—This presents in women with failure to lactate in the puerperium.

6. Panhypopituitarism—This condition refers to a deficiency of several or all pituitary hormones. Hypopituitarism typically presents with difficulty breastfeeding and amenorrhea due to hypogonadotropic hypogonadism (62%), diabetes insipidus (54%), headache (50%), hypothyroidism (48%), ACTH deficiency (47%), GH deficiency (37%), and hyperprolactinemia (36%), which clinicians may mistake for a prolactinoma.

7. Hypothalamic damage—This can cause obesity and cognitive impairment. Hypopituitarism occurs but usually along with increased serum levels of PRL. Local tumor effects can cause headache or optic nerve compression with visual field impairment.

B. Laboratory Findings

Initial laboratory studies may show hyponatremia or hypoglycemia. Fasting hypoglycemia may be present with secondary hypoadrenalism, hypothyroidism, or GH deficiency. Hyponatremia can be caused by hypothyroidism or hypoadrenalism. Patients with lymphocytic hypophysitis frequently have elevated serum antinuclear or anticytoplasmic antibodies. Patients with hypopituitarism without an established etiology should be screened for hemochromatosis with a serum ferritin or iron and transferrin saturation.

Male hypogonadotropic hypogonadism is diagnosed by drawing blood before 10 AM after an overnight fast in men without an acute or subacute illness. Affected men have a low fasting serum total or free serum testosterone with a low or normal serum LH. A serum PRL is also obtained, since hyperprolactinemia of any cause can result in hypogonadism.

Female hypogonadotropic hypogonadism is suspected in nonpregnant women with amenorrhea or oligomenorrhea, who do not have acute illness, hyperthyroidism, or hyperandrogenism. The serum estradiol is low and the serum FSH is low or normal. In nonpregnant women, a serum PRL is obtained, since hyperprolactinemia of any cause can result in hypogonadism. In postmenopausal women, the absence of an elevated serum FSH (in a woman not taking estrogen replacement) indicates gonadotropin deficiency.

Central hypothyroidism is diagnosed with a low serum free thyroxine (FT_4) in the setting of pituitary disease. The serum TSH can be low, normal, or even mildly elevated (oddly). Central hypothyroidism can emerge when patients begin GH replacement, so thyroid levels must be monitored in that setting. Patients undergoing pituitary surgery should be assessed for central hypothyroidism preoperatively and again 6 weeks postoperatively.

Central adrenal insufficiency is diagnosed after withholding corticosteroid replacement for at least 18–24 hours. Blood is drawn at 8–9 AM for baseline plasma ACTH and serum cortisol. A serum cortisol less than 3 mcg/dL (80 nmol/L) usually indicates adrenal insufficiency, whereas an 8–9 AM serum cortisol higher than 15 mcg/dL (400 nmol/L) usually excludes adrenal insufficiency. For 8–9 AM cortisol levels between 3 and 15 mcg/dL, a cosyntropin test is often required. For the cosyntropin test, patients should hold any corticosteroid replacement for at least 18–24 hours. At 8–9 AM, blood is drawn for serum cortisol, ACTH, and dehydroepiandrosterone (DHEA); then cosyntropin (synthetic $ACTH_{1-24}$) 0.25 mg is administered intramuscularly or intravenously. Another serum cortisol is obtained 45 minutes after the cosyntropin injection; a stimulated serum cortisol of less than 20 mcg/dL (550 nmol/L) indicates probable adrenal insufficiency. With gradual pituitary damage and early in the course of ACTH deficiency, patients can have a stimulated serum cortisol of 20 mcg/dL or more (550 nmol/L) but a baseline 8 AM serum cortisol of 5 mcg/dL or less (138 nmol/L), which is suspicious for adrenal insufficiency. The baseline serum ACTH level is low or normal in secondary hypoadrenalism, distinguishing it from primary adrenal disease. Serum DHEA is a proxy for ACTH; levels are usually low in patients with secondary adrenal deficiency, helping confirm the diagnosis. Hyponatremia may occur, especially when ACTH and TSH deficiencies are both present.

For patients with signs of secondary adrenal insufficiency (hyponatremia, hypotension, pituitary tumor) but borderline cosyntropin test results, treatment can be instituted empirically and the test repeated at a later date. Patients undergoing pituitary surgery with normal preoperative adrenal function should have an individualized clinical approach to postoperative corticosteroid replacement until ACTH-adrenal function can be retested postoperatively.

GH deficiency in adults is difficult to diagnose, since GH secretion is normally pulsatile and serum GH levels are normally undetectable for much of the day. Also, adults (particularly men) physiologically tend to produce less GH when they are over age 50 or have abdominal obesity. Therefore, pathologic GH deficiency is often inferred by symptoms of GH deficiency in the presence of pituitary destruction or other pituitary hormone deficiencies. GH deficiency is present in 96% of patients with three or more other pituitary hormone deficiencies and a low serum IGF-1. While GH stimulates the production of IGF-1, the serum IGF-1 level is neither a sensitive (about 50%) nor specific test for GH deficiency in adults. While very low serum IGF-1 levels (less than 84 mcg/L) are usually indicative of GH deficiency, they also occur in malnutrition, prolonged fasting, oral estrogen, hypothyroidism, uncontrolled diabetes mellitus, and liver failure. In GH deficiency (but also in most adults over age 40), exercise-stimulated serum GH levels remain at less than 5 ng/mL and usually fail to rise.

Provocative GH stimulation testing to help diagnose adult GH deficiency has a sensitivity of only 66%. Therefore, a therapeutic trial of GH therapy should be considered for symptomatic patients who have either a serum IGF-1 less than 84 mcg/L or three other pituitary hormone deficiencies.

Provocative GH-stimulation tests are sometimes indicated or required for insurance coverage of GH therapy. In the absence of a serum IGF-1 level less than 84 mcg/L or multiple other pituitary hormone deficiencies, provocative GH-stimulation testing may be indicated for the following patients: (1) young adult patients who have completed GH therapy for childhood GH deficiency and have achieved maximal linear growth; (2) patients who have a hypothalamic or pituitary tumor or who have received surgery or radiation therapy to these areas; and (3) patients who have had prior head trauma, cerebrovascular accident, or encephalitis. When required, such testing usually entails measuring serum GH following provocative stimuli. **The single-dose oral macimorelin (Macrilen) GH stimulation test** involves the oral administration of macimorelin (a GH secretogogue) to a fasting individual at a dose of 0.5 mg/kg body weight. Blood samples for GH are drawn immediately prior to administration and then at 30, 45, 60, and 90 minutes afterward. A maximum serum GH level below 5.1 ng/mL suggests GH deficiency with 92% sensitivity and 96% specificity. **The glucagon stimulation test** is a practical alternative to traditional provocative GH stimulation testing to diagnose pathologic GH deficiency or functional GH deficiency due to aging or obesity. It should not be given to patients who are malnourished or who have not eaten for over 48 hours. Side effects are usually mild, but nausea or headache occurs in about 20% of patients. Glucagon 1.0 mg (or 1.5 mg if greater than 200 lbs [90 kg]) is administered intramuscularly to patients who have not eaten for 8–9 hours. Serum GH is measured before the injection and every 30 minutes for 4 hours. In patients with GH deficiency, the maximum serum GH is usually less than 3 mcg/L. The test is quite sensitive (95%), but much less specific, mostly due to obesity. Therefore, for overweight or obese individuals (body mass index [BMI] is 25 kg/m^2 or more), GH deficiency is considered likely if the stimulated GH is below 1 ng/mL. Do not administer glucagon to patients who are malnourished or during a prolonged fast. Mild nausea or headache occurs in 20%. Late hypoglycemia can occur after glucagon, so patients are advised to eat immediately following completion of the test.

C. Imaging

MRI may also show hypoplasia or agenesis of the olfactory bulbs in 75% of cases of Kallmann syndrome and in 8% of patients with normosmic hypogonadotropic hypogonadism. MRI may show a distinct lesion in the pituitary, infundibulum, or hypothalamus. However, for hypophysitis, MRI may show only some generalized pituitary enlargement or thickening of the pituitary stalk. The hypophysitis associated with immune checkpoint inhibitor chemotherapy can appear on MRI as either a distinct mass or a diffusely enlarged pituitary. MRI is not warranted in cases of functional hypopituitarism associated with severe obesity, drugs, or nutritional disorders.

▶ Differential Diagnosis

The failure to enter puberty may simply reflect delayed puberty, also known as constitutional delay in growth and puberty. Secondary adrenal insufficiency may persist for many months following high-dose corticosteroid therapy and may also be seen with inhaled or topical corticosteroid therapy.

Reversible, second hypothyroidism with suppression of TSH and T$_4$ can be caused by severe illness, hyperthyroxinemia, and administration of triiodothyronine (Cytomel), mitotane, or bexarotene, resulting in temporary central hypothyroidism. Corticosteroids or megestrol reversibly suppress endogenous ACTH and cortisol secretion.

GH deficiency occurs normally with aging and physiologically with obesity (reversible with sufficient weight loss). Very low serum IGF-1 levels can be seen with prolonged fasting, malnutrition, liver failure, hypothyroidism, and uncontrolled diabetes mellitus.

▶ Complications

Among patients with craniopharyngiomas, diabetes insipidus is found in 16% preoperatively and in 60% postoperatively. Hyponatremia often presents abruptly during the first 2 weeks following pituitary surgery. Visual field impairment may occur. Hypothalamic damage may result in morbid obesity as well as cognitive and emotional problems. Conventional radiation therapy for intracranial disorders can result in an increased incidence of small vessel ischemic strokes, second tumors and damaged hypothalamic-pituitary function.

Patients with untreated hypoadrenalism and a stressful illness may become febrile and comatose and die of hyponatremia and shock.

Adults with GH deficiency have experienced an increased cardiovascular morbidity. Rarely, acute hemorrhage may occur in large pituitary tumors, manifested by rapid loss of vision, headache, and evidence of acute pituitary failure (pituitary apoplexy) requiring emergency decompression of the sella.

▶ Treatment

The therapy for hypopituitarism is lifetime hormone replacement.

A. Corticosteroid Replacement

Most patients do well with oral hydrocortisone 10–25 mg in the morning and 5–15 mg in the late afternoon. There is considerable variation in corticosteroid requirements, so corticosteroid dosing and timing are tailored to each individual. Patients with partial ACTH deficiency (basal morning serum cortisol above 8 mg/dL [220 mmol/L]) require hydrocortisone replacement in lower doses of about 5 mg orally twice daily or even 10 mg every morning. Some patients feel poorly despite hydrocortisone replacement; they may feel better with the substitution of prednisone (2–7.5 mg/day orally) or methylprednisolone (2–6 mg/day orally), given in divided doses. Fludrocortisone is not required. To determine the optimal corticosteroid replacement dosage, it is necessary to monitor patients carefully for clinical signs of over- or under-replacement. A white blood cell (WBC) count with a differential can be useful, since a relative neutrophilia and lymphopenia can indicate corticosteroid over replacement, and vice versa. Additional corticosteroid must be given during stress, eg, infection, trauma, or surgical procedures. For mild illness or mild-moderate surgical stress, corticosteroid doses are doubled or tripled. For severe illness, trauma, or major surgical stress, hydrocortisone 100 mg is given intravenously, followed by 200 mg daily, given as either a continuous intravenous infusion or as 50 mg boluses given every 6 hours intravenously or intramuscularly and then reduced to usual doses as the stress subsides. Patients with adrenal insufficiency are advised to wear a medical alert bracelet describing their condition and treatment.

Patients with secondary adrenal insufficiency due to treatment with corticosteroids require their usual daily dose of corticosteroid during surgery and acute illness; supplemental hydrocortisone is not usually required.

B. Thyroid Hormone Replacement

Levothyroxine is given to correct hypothyroidism only after the patient is assessed for cortisol deficiency or is already receiving corticosteroids. The typical maintenance dose is about 1.6 mcg/kg body weight, averaging 125 mcg daily with a wide range of 25–300 mcg daily. Assessment of serum TSH is useless for monitoring patients with hypopituitarism. The optimal replacement dose of levothyroxine is determined clinically by raising or lowering the dose, according to the patient's symptoms and clinical examination, until an optimal dose is found. In patients receiving clinically optimal levothyroxine replacement, serum FT_4 levels are usually in the mid to high-normal range. Some patients do not feel clinically euthyroid until they receive levothyroxine in doses at which the serum FT_4 levels are mildly elevated; however, serum T_3 or FT_3 levels should be in the low-normal range. During pregnancy, clinical status and serum FT_4 or total T_4 levels need to be monitored frequently, since higher doses of levothyroxine are usually required.

C. Gonadotropin Replacement

Hypogonadotropic hypogonadism often develops in patients with hyperprolactinemia and usually resolves with its treatment. See Male Hypogonadism and Female Hypogonadism.

Women with panhypopituitarism have profound androgen deficiency caused by the combination of both secondary hypogonadism and adrenal insufficiency. When serum DHEA levels are less than 400 ng/mL, women may also be treated with compounded USP-grade DHEA 50 mg/day orally. DHEA therapy tends to increase pubic and axillary hair and may modestly improve libido, alertness, stamina, and overall psychological well-being.

For men with oligospermia, human chorionic gonadotropin (hCG) (equivalent to LH) may be given at a dosage of 2000–3000 units intramuscularly three times weekly and testosterone replacement discontinued. The dose of hCG is adjusted to normalize serum testosterone levels. After 6–12 months of hCG treatment, if the sperm count remains low, hCG injections are continued along with injections of follitropin beta (synthetic recombinant FSH) or urofollitropins (urine-derived FSH). An alternative for patients with an intact pituitary is the use of leuprolide (GnRH analog) by intermittent subcutaneous infusion. With treatment, testicular volumes increase within 5–12 months, and some spermatogenesis occurs in most cases. With persistent treatment and the use of intracytoplasmic sperm injection for some cases, the pregnancy success rate is about 70%. Men often feel better during hCG therapy than during testosterone replacement. Therefore, some men may elect to continue hCG therapy long term.

Clomiphene, 25–50 mg/day orally, can sometimes stimulate men's own pituitary gonadotropins (when his pituitary is intact), thereby increasing testosterone and sperm production. For fertility induction in females, ovulation may be induced with clomiphene, 50–100 mg/day orally for 5 days every 2 months. Ovulation induction with FSH and hCG can induce multiple births and should be used only by those experienced with their administration.

D. Human Growth Hormone (hGH) Replacement

Symptomatic adults with GH deficiency may be treated with a subcutaneous recombinant human growth hormone (rhGH, somatropin) injections starting at a dosage of about 0.2 mg/day (0.6 international units/day), administered three times weekly. The dosage of rhGH is increased every 2–4 weeks by increments of 0.1 mg (0.3 international units) until side effects occur or a sufficient salutary response and a normal serum IGF-1 level are achieved. In adults, if the desired effects (eg, improved energy and mentation, reduction in visceral adiposity) are not seen within 3–6 months at maximum tolerated dosage, rhGH therapy is discontinued. Therapy with hGH can bring out central hypothyroidism, so serum FT_4 levels require monitoring when beginning hGH therapy.

During pregnancy, rhGH may be safely administered to women with hypopituitarism at their usual pregestational dose during the first trimester, tapering the dose during the second trimester, and discontinuing rhGH during the third trimester.

Oral estrogen replacement reduces hepatic IGF-1 production. Therefore, prior to commencing rhGH therapy, oral estrogen should be changed to transdermal or transvaginal estradiol.

Treatment of adult GH deficiency usually improves the patient's overall quality of life, with better emotional sense of well-being, increased muscle mass, and decreased visceral fat and waist circumference. Long-term treatment with rhGH does not appear to affect mortality.

Side effects of rhGH therapy may include peripheral edema, hand stiffness, arthralgias and myalgias, paresthesias, carpal tunnel syndrome, tarsal tunnel syndrome, headache, pseudotumor cerebri, gynecomastia, hypertension, and proliferative retinopathy. Treatment with rhGH can also cause sleep apnea, insomnia, dyspnea, sweating, and fatigue. Side effects usually remit promptly after a sufficient reduction in dosage. Therapy with rhGH does not increase the risk of any malignancy or the regrowth of pituitary or brain neoplasms; serum IGF-1 levels should be kept in the normal range.

GH should not be administered during critical illness, since administration of very high doses of rhGH increased mortality in patients receiving intensive care. *There is currently no proven role for GH replacement for the physiologic GH deficiency that is seen with abdominal obesity or normal aging.*

E. Other Treatment

Selective transsphenoidal surgery is usually performed to resect non-prolactinoma pituitary masses and Rathke cleft cysts that cause local symptoms or hypopituitarism. Such surgery reverses hypopituitarism in a minority of cases. Patients with lymphocytic hypophysitis have been treated with corticosteroid therapy and other immunosuppressants without much response and without reversing hypopituitarism.

▶ Prognosis

Hypopituitarism resulting from a pituitary tumor may be reversible with dopamine agonists for prolactinomas (see Prolactinoma, below) or with careful selective resection of the tumor. Spontaneous recovery from hypopituitarism associated with pituitary stalk thickening has been reported. Patients can also recover from functional hypopituitarism. Spontaneous reversal of idiopathic isolated hypogonadotropic hypogonadism occurs in about 10% of patients after several years of hormone replacement therapy (HRT). However, hypopituitarism is usually permanent, and long-term HRT is ordinarily required.

Patients with hypopituitarism have an increased mortality risk, particularly women and those in whom diagnosis was made at a younger age, who have a craniopharyngioma, or who required transcranial surgery or radiation therapy. There is also an increased risk of death from infections with adrenal crisis in patients with untreated secondary insufficiency. Some pituitary tumors are locally invasive. In patients who have received pituitary radiation therapy, there is an increased risk of a second intracranial neoplasm and small-vessel stroke. Asymptomatic Rathke cleft cysts may not require surgery but do require endocrine, ophthalmic, and scan surveillance.

Functionally, most patients with hypopituitarism do very well with hormone replacement. Men with infertility who are treated with hCG/FSH or GnRH are likely to resume spermatogenesis if they have a history of sexual maturation, descended testicles, and a baseline serum inhibin B level over 60 pg/mL. Women under age 40 years, with infertility due to hypogonadotropic hypogonadism, can usually have successful ovulation induction.

Diri H et al. Sheehan's syndrome: new insights into an old disease. Endocrine. 2016 Jan;51(1):22–31. [PMID: 26323346]

Fleseriu M et al. Hormonal replacement in hypopituitarism in adults: an Endocrine Society clinical practice guideline. J Clin Endocrinol Metab. 2016 Nov;101(11):3888–921. [PMID: 27736313]

Garcia JM et al. Macimorelin as a diagnostic test for adult GH deficiency. J Clin Endocrinol Metab. 2018 Aug 1;103(8):3083–93. [PMID: 29860473]

Gordon MB et al. Trends in growth hormone stimulation testing and growth hormone dosing in adult growth hormone deficiency patients: results from the ANSWER program. Endocr Pract. 2016 Apr;22(4):396–405. [PMID: 26574788]

Joshi MN et al. Immune checkpoint inhibitor-related hypophysitis and endocrine dysfunction: clinical review. Clin Endocrinol (Oxf). 2016 Sep;85(3):331–9. [PMID: 26998595]

Molitch ME. Diagnosis and treatment of pituitary adenomas: a review. JAMA. 2017 Feb 7;317(5):516–24. [PMID: 28170483]

CENTRAL DIABETES INSIPIDUS

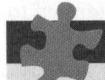

ESSENTIALS OF DIAGNOSIS

► Antidiuretic hormone (ADH) deficiency with polyuria (2–20 L/day) and polydipsia.

► Hypernatremia occurs if fluid intake is inadequate.

► General Considerations

Central diabetes insipidus is an uncommon disease caused by a deficiency in vasopressin (antidiuretic hormone [ADH]) from the posterior pituitary.

Primary central diabetes insipidus (without an identifiable lesion noted on MRI of the pituitary and hypothalamus) accounts for about one-third of all cases of diabetes insipidus. Familial diabetes insipidus occurs as a dominant genetic trait with symptoms developing at about 2 years of age. Diabetes insipidus also occurs in Wolfram syndrome, a rare autosomal recessive disorder that is also known by the acronym DIDMOAD (diabetes insipidus, type 1 diabetes mellitus, optic atrophy, and deafness). Central diabetes insipidus may also be idiopathic or due to autoimmunity against hypothalamic arginine vasopressin (AVP)-secreting cells. Reversible central diabetes insipidus can occur during chemotherapy with temozolomide and in the myelodysplastic preleukemic phase of acute myelogenous leukemia.

Secondary central diabetes insipidus is due to damage to the hypothalamus or pituitary stalk by tumor, hypophysitis, infarction, hemorrhage, anoxic encephalopathy, surgical or accidental trauma, infection (eg, encephalitis, tuberculosis, syphilis), or granulomas (sarcoidosis or Langerhans cell granulomatosis). Cancer immune therapy with the anti-PD-L1 monoclonal antibody avelumab has been reported to cause reversible central diabetes insipidus. Metastases to the pituitary are more likely to cause diabetes insipidus (33%) than are pituitary adenomas (1%).

► Clinical Findings

A. Symptoms and Signs

The symptoms of the disease are intense thirst, especially with a craving for ice water, with the volume of ingested fluid varying from 2 L to 20 L daily, and polyuria, with large urine volumes and low urine specific gravity (usually less than 1.006 with ad libitum fluid intake). The urine is otherwise normal. Partial diabetes insipidus presents with less intense symptoms and should be suspected in patients with enuresis. Most patients with diabetes insipidus are able to maintain fluid balance by continuing to ingest large volumes of water. However, in patients without free access to water or with a damaged hypothalamic thirst center and altered thirst sensation, diabetes insipidus may present with hypernatremia and dehydration. Diabetes insipidus is aggravated by administration of high-dose corticosteroids, which increases renal free water clearance.

B. Laboratory Findings

Diagnosis of central diabetes insipidus is a clinical one; there is no single diagnostic laboratory test. Evaluation should include a 24-hour urine collection for volume and creatinine. A urine volume of less than 2 L/24 h (in the absence of hypernatremia) rules out diabetes insipidus. The patient can be tested during ad libitum fluid intake. A random urine is tested for osmolality. Blood testing includes plasma vasopressin and serum glucose, urea nitrogen, calcium, potassium, sodium, and uric acid.

With central diabetes insipidus and primary polydipsia, the plasma AVP level is usually low (below 1 pg/mL), while the urine osmolarity is also low (less than 300 mOsm/L). With nephrogenic diabetes insipidus, the plasma AVP level is normal or elevated (more than 2.5 pg/mL), while the urine osmolarity is low (less than 300 mOsm/L). Hyperuricemia occurs in many patients with central diabetes insipidus, since reduced vasopressin stimulation of the renal V1 receptor causes a reduction in the renal tubular clearance of urate.

A supervised "vasopressin challenge test" may be done: Desmopressin acetate 0.05–0.1 mL (5–10 mcg) intranasally (or 1 mcg subcutaneously or intravenously) is given, with measurement of urine volume for 12 hours before and 12 hours after administration. A serum sodium is obtained baseline, 12 hours after the desmopressin, and immediately if symptoms of hyponatremia develop. Patients with central diabetes insipidus notice a distinct reduction in thirst and polyuria; serum sodium usually remains normal. The dosage of desmopressin is doubled if the response is marginal. In patients with primary polydipsia, a desmopressin challenge causes no significant reduction in polydipsia, but does reduce polyuria that caused hyponatremia. Patients with nephrogenic diabetes insipidus show no response in polydipsia or urine volume.

Another test to distinguish central diabetes insipidus from primary polydipsia involves the carefully supervised hypertonic 3% saline-stimulated measurement of plasma copeptin, the C-terminal fragment of pre-pro-arginine vasopressin. Hypertonic 3% saline is administered intravenously as a 250 mL bolus, followed by a continuous infusion rate of 0.15 mL/kg/min. Plasma sodium is measured stat every 30 minutes; when the plasma sodium level reaches 150 mmol/L, blood is drawn for plasma copeptin. A level 4.9 pmol/L or less helps confirm the diagnosis of central diabetes insipidus.

C. Imaging

Distinguishing central diabetes insipidus from primary polydipsia usually requires an MRI of the pituitary and hypothalamus. The normal posterior "bright spot" seen on the MRI T1-weighted imaging is undetectable or small with central diabetes insipidus. MRI can also detect pathology responsible for central diabetes insipidus.

▶ Differential Diagnosis

Central diabetes insipidus must be distinguished from polyuria caused by psychogenic polydipsia, diabetes mellitus, Cushing syndrome, hypercalcemia, hypokalemia, and nocturnal polyuria of Parkinson disease.

Vasopressinase-induced diabetes insipidus may be seen in the last trimester of pregnancy, associated with oligohydramnios, preeclampsia, or liver dysfunction, and in the puerperium. Maternal circulating vasopressin is destroyed by placental vasopressinase; however, synthetic desmopressin is unaffected.

Nephrogenic diabetes insipidus is caused by unresponsiveness of the kidney tubules to the normal secretion of vasopressin. A congenital form is familial and transmitted as an X-linked trait; it is caused by defective expression of renal vasopressin V2 receptors or vasopressin-sensitive water channels. Adults often also have hyperuricemia. Acquired forms are usually less severe and occur in pyelonephritis, renal amyloidosis, myeloma, potassium depletion, Sjögren syndrome, sickle cell anemia, chronic hypercalcemia, or recovery from acute tubular necrosis. Certain drugs (eg, corticosteroids, diuretics, demeclocycline, lithium, foscarnet, or methicillin) may induce nephrogenic diabetes insipidus.

▶ Complications

If water is not readily available, the excessive output of urine will lead to severe dehydration. Patients with an impaired thirst mechanism are very prone to hypernatremia, as are those with impaired mentation who forget to take their desmopressin. Excessive desmopressin acetate can induce water intoxication and hyponatremia.

▶ Treatment

Mild cases of diabetes insipidus require no treatment other than adequate fluid intake. Reduction of aggravating factors (eg, corticosteroids) will improve polyuria.

Desmopressin acetate is the treatment of choice for central diabetes insipidus and for vasopressinase-induced diabetes insipidus associated with pregnancy or the puerperium. Desmopressin acetate (100 mcg/mL solution) is given intranasally every 12–24 hours as needed for thirst and polyuria. It may be administered via metered-dose nasal inhaler containing 0.1 mL (10 mcg/spray) or via a calibrated rhinal tube. The starting dose is one metered-dose spray or 0.05–0.1 mL every 12–24 hours, and the dose is then individualized according to response. Desmopressin nasal may cause rhinitis or conjunctivitis. If the generic preparation is ineffective, switching to the desmopressin brand may provide relief.

Oral desmopressin, 0.1- and 0.2-mg tablets, is given in a starting dose of 0.05 mg twice daily and increased to a maximum of 0.4 mg every 8 hours, if required. Sublingual desmopressin, 60, 120, or 250 mcg, is not available in the United States; hyponatremia has been reported with this formulation. Oral desmopressin is particularly useful for patients in whom rhinitis or conjunctivitis develops from the nasal preparation. Gastrointestinal symptoms, asthenia, and mild increases in hepatic enzymes can occur with the oral preparation.

Desmopressin can also be given intravenously, intramuscularly, or subcutaneously in doses of 1–4 mcg every 12–24 hours as needed.

Desmopressin may cause hyponatremia, but this is uncommon if minimum effective doses are used and the patient allows thirst to occur every 1–2 days. Desmopressin can sometimes cause agitation, emotional changes, and depression with an increased risk of suicide. Patients should be monitored by family, friends, and medical staff when desmopressin therapy is started.

▶ Prognosis

Central diabetes insipidus after pituitary surgery or head trauma usually remits after days to weeks but may be permanent if the hypothalamus or upper pituitary stalk is damaged.

Chronic central diabetes insipidus is ordinarily more an inconvenience than a dire medical condition. Treatment with desmopressin allows normal sleep and activity. Hypernatremia can occur, especially when the hypothalamic thirst center is damaged, but diabetes insipidus does not otherwise reduce life expectancy, and the prognosis is that of the underlying disorder.

Ananthakrishnan S. Diabetes insipidus during pregnancy. Best Pract Res Clin Endocrinol Metab. 2016 Mar;30(2):305–15. [PMID: 27156766]

Fenske W et al. A copeptin-based approach in the diagnosis of diabetes insipidus. N Engl J Med. 2018 Aug 2;379(5):428–39. [PMID: 30067922]

Robertson GL. Diabetes insipidus: differential diagnosis and management. Best Pract Res Clin Endocrinol Metab. 2016 Mar; 30(2):205–18. [PMID: 27156759]

Zhao C et al. Anti-PD-L1 treatment induced central diabetes insipidus. J Clin Endocrinol Metab. 2018 Feb 1;103(2):365–9. [PMID: 29220526]

ACROMEGALY & GIGANTISM

ESSENTIALS OF DIAGNOSIS

▸ Pituitary tumor.

▸ **Gigantism** before closure of epiphyses.

▸ **Acromegaly:** excessive growth of hands, feet, jaw, internal organs.

▸ Amenorrhea, hypertension, headaches, visual field loss, weakness.

▸ Soft, doughy, sweaty handshake.

▸ Elevated serum IGF-1.

▸ General Considerations

GH exerts much of its growth-promoting effects by stimulating the release of IGF-1 from the liver and other tissues.

Acromegaly is nearly always caused by a pituitary adenoma. Most are macroadenomas (over 1 cm in diameter). These tumors may be locally invasive, particularly into the cavernous sinus. Less than 1% are malignant. Acromegaly is usually sporadic but may rarely be familial, with less than 3% being due to multiple endocrine neoplasia (MEN) types 1 or 4. Acromegaly may also be seen rarely in McCune-Albright syndrome and Carney complex. Acromegaly is very occasionally caused by ectopic secretion of GHRH or GH secreted by a lymphoma, hypothalamic tumor, bronchial carcinoid, or pancreatic tumor.

▸ Clinical Findings

A. Symptoms and Signs

Excessive GH causes tall stature and gigantism if it occurs in youth, before closure of epiphyses. Afterward, acromegaly develops. The hands enlarge and a doughy, moist handshake is characteristic. The fingers widen, causing patients to enlarge their rings. Carpal tunnel syndrome is common. The feet also grow, particularly in shoe width. Facial features coarsen since the bones and sinuses of the skull enlarge; hat size increases. The mandible becomes more prominent, causing prognathism and malocclusion. Tooth spacing widens. Older photographs of the patient can be a useful comparison.

Macroglossia occurs, as does hypertrophy of pharyngeal and laryngeal tissue; this causes a deep, coarse voice and sometimes makes intubation difficult. Obstructive sleep apnea may occur. A goiter may be noted. Hypertension (50%) and cardiomegaly are common. At diagnosis, about 10% of acromegalic patients have a dilated left ventricle and heart failure with reduced ejection fraction. Weight gain is typical, particularly of muscle and bone. Insulin resistance is usually present and frequently causes diabetes mellitus (30%). Arthralgias and degenerative arthritis occur. Overgrowth of vertebral bone can cause spinal stenosis. Colon polyps are common, especially in patients with skin papillomas. The skin may also manifest hyperhidrosis, thickening, cystic acne, skin tags, and acanthosis nigricans.

GH-secreting pituitary tumors usually cause some degree of hypogonadism, either by cosecretion of PRL or by direct pressure upon normal pituitary tissue. Decreased libido and erectile dysfunction are common in men and irregular menses or amenorrhea in women. Women who become pregnant have an increased risk of gestational diabetes and hypertension. Secondary hypothyroidism sometimes occurs; hypoadrenalism is unusual. Headaches are frequent. Temporal hemianopia may occur as a result of the optic chiasm being impinged by a suprasellar growth of the tumor.

B. Laboratory Findings

For screening purposes, a random serum IGF-1 can be obtained. If it is normal for age, acromegaly is ruled out.

For further evaluation, the patient should be fasting for at least 8 hours (except for water), not be acutely ill, and not have exercised on the day of testing. Assay for the following: serum GH, IGF-1 (increased and usually over five times normal in acromegalic patients), PRL (cosecreted by many GH-secreting tumors), glucose (diabetes mellitus is common in acromegaly), liver enzymes and serum creatinine or urea nitrogen (liver failure or kidney disease can misleadingly elevate GH), serum calcium (to exclude hyperparathyroidism), serum inorganic phosphorus (frequently elevated), serum free T_4, and TSH (secondary hypothyroidism is common in acromegaly; primary hypothyroidism may increase PRL). Acromegaly is excluded if any serum GH is less than 1 mcg/L; however, many normal individuals can have a serum GH above this level. Therefore, the glucose suppression test is usually performed. Glucose syrup (100 g) is administered orally, and serum GH is measured 60 minutes afterward; acromegaly is excluded if the serum GH is suppressed to below 0.4 mcg/L with an ultrasensitive GH assay. The serum IGF-1 and glucose-suppressed GH are usually complementary tests; however, disparities between the two occur in up to 30% of patients.

C. Imaging

MRI shows a pituitary tumor in over 90% of acromegalic patients. MRI is generally superior to CT scanning, especially in the postoperative setting. Radiographs of the skull may show an enlarged sella and thickened skull. Radiographs may also show tufting of the terminal phalanges of the fingers and toes. A lateral view of the foot shows increased thickness of the heel pad.

Differential Diagnosis

Active acromegaly must be distinguished from familial coarse features, large hands and feet, and isolated prognathism and from inactive ("burned-out") acromegaly in which there has been a spontaneous remission due to infarction of the pituitary adenoma. GH-induced gigantism must be differentiated from familial tall stature and from aromatase deficiency.

Misleadingly high serum GH levels can be caused by exercise or eating just prior to the test; acute illness or agitation; liver failure or kidney disease; malnourishment; diabetes mellitus; or concurrent treatment with oral estrogens, beta-blockers, or clonidine. Acromegaly can be difficult to diagnose during pregnancy, since the placenta produces GH and commercial GH assays may not be able to distinguish between pituitary and placental GH. During normal adolescence, serum IGF-1 is usually elevated and GH may fail to be suppressed.

Complications

Complications include hypopituitarism, hypertension, glucose intolerance or frank diabetes mellitus, cardiac enlargement, heart failure, and colon polyps. Arthritis of hips, knees, and spine can be troublesome as can carpal tunnel syndrome. Cord compression may occur. Visual field defects may be severe and progressive. Acute loss of vision or cranial nerve palsy may occur if the tumor undergoes spontaneous hemorrhage and necrosis (pituitary apoplexy).

Treatment

A. Pituitary Microsurgery

Transsphenoidal pituitary microsurgery removes the adenoma while preserving anterior pituitary function in most patients. Transsphenoidal surgery is usually well tolerated, but complications occur in about 12% of patients, including infection, cerebrospinal fluid (CSF) leak, and hypopituitarism.

Postoperatively, GH levels fall immediately. Fluid and electrolyte disturbances occur in most patients; diabetes insipidus can occur within 2 days postoperatively but is usually mild and self-correcting. Hyponatremia can occur abruptly 4–13 days postoperatively in 21% of patients; symptoms may include nausea, vomiting, headache, malaise, or seizure. It is treated with free water and hypotonic fluid restriction. It is prudent to monitor serum sodium levels postoperatively. Diaphoresis and carpal tunnel syndrome often improve within a day after surgery.

Corticosteroids are administered perioperatively and tapered to replacement doses over 1 week; hydrocortisone is discontinued and a cosyntropin stimulation test is performed about 6 weeks after surgery. At that time, the patient is screened for secondary hypothyroidism (by a serum FT_4) and secondary hypogonadism.

B. Medications

Acromegalic patients with an incomplete biochemical remission after pituitary surgery may benefit from medical therapy with dopamine agonists, somatostatin analogs, tamoxifen, or pegvisomant.

Cabergoline is the oral dopamine agonist of choice. It is most successful for tumors that secrete both PRL and GH but can also be effective for patients with normal serum PRL levels. Cabergoline will shrink one-third of acromegaly-associated pituitary tumors by more than 50%. It appears to be safe during pregnancy. The initial dose is 0.25 mg orally twice weekly, which is gradually increased to a maximum dosage of 1 mg twice weekly (based on serum GH and IGF-1 levels). Side effects of cabergoline include nausea, fatigue, constipation, abdominal pain, and dizziness.

Octreotide and **lanreotide** are long-acting somatostatin analogs that are given by monthly subcutaneous injection. They can achieve serum GH levels under 2 ng/mL in 79% of patients and normal serum IGF-1 levels in 53% of patients.

Tamoxifen is a selective estrogen receptor modulator (SERM) that may be particularly useful for persistent acromegaly in men and in women who are postmenopausal or who have had breast cancer. Tamoxifen (20–40 mg orally daily) does not reduce serum GH levels but reduces serum IGF-1 levels in 82% of patients and normalizes serum IGF-1 levels in 47%. Serum testosterone levels increase in men.

Pegvisomant, a GH receptor antagonist, is given by daily subcutaneous injection. It blocks hepatic IGF-1 production but does not shrink GH-secreting tumors. Pegvisomant therapy produces symptomatic relief and normalizes serum IGF-1 levels in over 90% of patients. Patients need to be monitored carefully for growth of the pituitary tumor with visual field examinations, GH levels, and MRI scanning of the pituitary.

C. Stereotactic Radiosurgery

Acromegalic patients who do not achieve a complete remission with transsphenoidal surgery or medical therapy may be treated with one or a combination of three types of stereotactic radiosurgery: linear accelerator (eg, Cyberknife), gamma knife radiosurgery, and proton beam radiosurgery. Following any pituitary radiation therapy, patients are advised to take lifelong daily low-dose aspirin because of the increased risk of small-vessel stroke. Stereotactic radiosurgery to pituitary tumors causes anterior hypopituitarism in 35–60% of patients within 5 years, so patients must have regular monitoring of their pituitary function.

Prognosis

Acromegaly is usually chronic and progressive unless treated. Spontaneous remissions are rare but have been reported following clinical or subclinical apoplexy (hemorrhage) within the tumor. Patients with acromegaly have increased morbidity and mortality from cardiovascular disorders and progressive acromegalic symptoms. Those who are treated and have a random serum GH under 1.0 ng/mL or a glucose-suppressed serum GH under 0.4 ng/mL with a normal age-adjusted serum IGF-1 level have reduced morbidity and mortality.

Transsphenoidal pituitary surgery achieves a remission in about 70% of patients followed over 3 years. In patients with tumors smaller than 2 cm in diameter and GH levels below 50 ng/mL, transsphenoidal pituitary surgery is successful in 80%. Extrasellar extension of the pituitary tumor, particularly cavernous sinus invasion, reduces the likelihood of surgical cure.

Adjuvant medical therapy is successful in treating patients who are not cured by pituitary surgery. Postoperatively, normal pituitary function is usually preserved. Soft tissue swelling regresses but bone enlargement is permanent. Hypertension frequently persists despite successful surgery. Conventional radiation therapy (alone) produces a remission in about 40% of patients by 2 years and 75% of patients by 5 years after treatment. Gamma knife or cyberknife radiosurgery reduces GH levels an average of 77%, with 20% of patients having a full remission after 12 months. Proton beam radiosurgery produces a remission in about 70% of patients by 2 years and 80% of patients by 5 years. Radiation therapy eventually produces some degree of hypopituitarism in most patients. Conventional radiation therapy may cause some degree of organic brain syndrome and predisposes to small strokes. Patients must receive lifelong follow-up, with regular monitoring of serum GH and IGF-1 levels. Serum GH levels over 5 ng/mL and rising IGF-1 levels usually indicate a recurrent tumor. Most pregnant women with acromegaly do not have an increase in the size of the pituitary tumor and neonatal outcome is unaffected.

Giustina A et al. Expert consensus document: a consensus on the medical treatment of acromegaly. Nat Rev Endocrinol. 2014 Apr;10(4):243–8. [PMID: 24566817]

Katznelson L et al. Acromegaly: An Endocrine Society clinical practice guideline. J Clin Endocrinol Metab. 2014 Nov; 99(11):3933–51. [PMID: 25356808]

Lim DS et al. The role of combination medical therapy in the treatment of acromegaly. Pituitary. 2017 Feb;20(1):136–48. [PMID: 27522663]

Melmed S. New therapeutic agents for acromegaly. Nat Rev Endocrinol. 2016 Feb;12(2):90–8. [PMID: 26610414]

HYPERPROLACTINEMIA

ESSENTIALS OF DIAGNOSIS

▶ **Women:** Oligomenorrhea, amenorrhea; galactorrhea; infertility.

▶ **Men:** Hypogonadism; decreased libido and erectile dysfunction; infertility.

▶ Elevated serum PRL; PRL is normally elevated during pregnancy.

▶ CT or MRI may show a pituitary adenoma.

Table 26–1. Causes of hyperprolactinemia.

Physiologic Causes	Pharmacologic Causes	Pathologic Causes
Exercise	Amoxapine	Acromegaly
Familial (mutant prolactin receptor)	Amphetamines	Chronic chest wall stimulation (thoracotomy, augmentation or reduction mammoplasty, mastectomy, herpes zoster, mammoplasty, chest acupuncture, nipple rings, etc)
Idiopathic	Anesthetic agents	
Macroprolactin ("big prolactin")	Antipsychotics (conventional and atypical)	
Nipple stimulation	Androgens	
Neonatal	Butyrophenones	
Pregnancy	Cimetidine and ranitidine (not famotidine or nizatidine)	Hypothalamic or pituitary stalk damage
Sleep (REM phase)	Cocaine	Hypothyroidism
Stress (trauma, surgery)	Domperidone	Liver disease
Suckling	Estrogens	Multiple sclerosis and other demyelinating diseases
	Hydroxyzine	
	Licorice (real)	
	Locaserin	Optic neuromyelitis
	MAO inhibitors	Pituitary stalk damage
	Methyldopa	Prolactin-secreting tumors
	Metoclopramide	
	Opioids	Pseudocyesis (false pregnancy)
	Nicotine	
	Phenothiazines	Kidney failure (especially with zinc deficiency)
	Protease inhibitors	Spinal cord lesions
	Progestins	Systemic lupus erythematosus
	Reserpine	
	Selective serotonin reuptake inhibitors	
	Tricyclic antidepressants	
	Verapamil	

MAO, monoamine oxidase; REM, rapid eye movement.

▶ General Considerations

The causes of hyperprolactinemia are shown in Table 26–1. In acromegaly, there may be cosecretion of GH and PRL. Hyperprolactinemia (without a pituitary adenoma) may also be familial. PRL-secreting pituitary tumors are more common in women than in men and are usually sporadic but may rarely be familial as part of MEN type 1 or 4. Most are microadenomas (smaller than 1 cm in diameter) that do not grow even with pregnancy or oral contraceptives. However, some giant prolactinomas (over 3 cm in diameter) can spread into the cavernous sinuses and suprasellar areas; rarely, they may erode the floor of the sella to invade the paranasal sinuses.

▶ Clinical Findings

A. Symptoms and Signs

Hyperprolactinemia may cause hypogonadotropic hypogonadism and reduced fertility. Men usually have diminished libido and erectile dysfunction that may not respond to testosterone replacement; gynecomastia sometimes occurs. The diagnosis of a prolactinoma is often delayed in men, such that pituitary adenomas may grow and present with late manifestations of a pituitary macroprolactinoma (diameter 10 mm or larger).

About 90% of premenopausal women with prolactinomas experience amenorrhea, oligomenorrhea, or infertility. Estrogen deficiency can cause decreased vaginal lubrication, irritability, anxiety, and depression. Galactorrhea (lactation in the absence of nursing) is common. During pregnancy, clinically significant enlargement of a microprolactinoma (diameter smaller than 10 mm) occurs in less than 3%; clinically significant enlargement of a macroprolactinoma occurs in about 30%.

Pituitary prolactinomas may cosecrete GH and cause acromegaly. Large tumors may cause headaches, visual symptoms, and pituitary insufficiency.

Aside from pituitary tumors, some women secrete an abnormal form of PRL that appears to cause peripartum cardiomyopathy. Suppression of PRL secretion with dopamine agonists can reverse the cardiomyopathy.

B. Laboratory Findings

Evaluate for conditions known to cause hyperprolactinemia, particularly pregnancy (serum hCG), hypothyroidism (serum FT_4 and TSH), kidney disease (blood urea nitrogen [BUN] and serum creatinine), cirrhosis (liver tests), and hyperparathyroidism (serum calcium). Men are evaluated for hypogonadism with serum total and free testosterone, LH, and FSH. Women who have amenorrhea are assessed for hypogonadism with serum estradiol, LH, and FSH. Patients with pituitary macroadenomas larger than 3 cm in diameter should have PRL measured on serial dilutions of serum, since certain immunoradiometric assay assays may otherwise report falsely low titers, the "high-dose hook effect." Patients with macroprolactinomas or manifestations of possible hypopituitarism should be evaluated for hypopituitarism. Patients with hyperprolactinemia who are relatively asymptomatic and have no apparent cause for hyperprolactinemia should have an assay for macroprolactinemia, which is an increased circulating level of a high molecular weight PRL that is biologically inactive but is detected on assays.

C. Imaging

Patients with hyperprolactinemia not induced by drugs, hypothyroidism, or pregnancy should be examined by pituitary MRI. Small prolactinomas may be demonstrated, but clear differentiation from normal variants is not always possible. In the event that a woman with a macroprolactinoma becomes pregnant and elects not to take dopamine agonists during her pregnancy, MRI is usually not performed since the normal pituitary grows during pregnancy. However, if visual-field defects or other neurologic symptoms develop in a pregnant woman, a limited MRI study should be done, focusing on the pituitary without gadolinium contrast.

▶ Differential Diagnosis

The differential diagnosis for galactorrhea includes the small amount of breast milk that can normally be expressed from the nipple in many parous women. Nipple stimulation from nipple rings, chest surgery, or acupuncture can cause galactorrhea; serum PRL levels may be normal or minimally elevated. Some women can have idiopathic galactorrhea with normal serum PRL levels. Normal breast milk may be various colors besides white. However, bloody galactorrhea requires evaluation for breast cancer.

Other pituitary lesions can produce hyperprolactinemia by damaging the hypothalamus or pituitary stalk, thereby reducing the amount of dopamine reaching pituitary lactotrophes that produce PRL unless inhibited by dopamine. About 40% of nonfunctional pituitary macroadenomas produce some degree of hyperprolactinemia. These and other lesions and malignancies can be misdiagnosed as prolactinomas. One distinguishing characteristic is that the serum PRL is usually only marginally elevated in the latter tumors, whereas with pituitary macroprolactinomas the serum PRL typically exceeds 100 mcg/L.

Pregnant women have high serum PRL levels, with physiological hyperplastic enlargement of the pituitary on MRI. Increased pituitary size is a normal variant in young women. Primary hypothyroidism can cause hyperprolactinemia and hyperplasia of the pituitary that can be mistaken for a pituitary adenoma. Macroprolactinemia occurs in 3.7% of the general population and accounts for 10–25% of all cases of hyperprolactinemia; pituitary MRI shows a nonpathological abnormality in 22% of such patients.

▶ Treatment

Medications known to increase PRL should be stopped if possible (Table 26–1). Hyperprolactinemia due to hypothyroidism is corrected by levothyroxine.

Women with microprolactinomas who have amenorrhea or are desirous of contraception may safely take estrogen replacement or oral contraceptives—there is minimal risk of stimulating enlargement of the microadenoma. Patients with infertility and hyperprolactinemia may be treated with a dopamine agonist in an effort to improve fertility. Women with amenorrhea who elect to receive no treatment have an increased risk of developing osteoporosis; such women require periodic bone densitometry.

Pituitary macroprolactinomas have a higher risk of progressive growth, particularly during estrogen or testosterone HRT or during pregnancy. Therefore, patients with macroprolactinomas should not be treated with HRT unless they are in remission with dopamine agonist medication or surgery.

Pregnant women with macroprolactinomas should continue to receive treatment with dopamine agonists throughout the pregnancy to prevent tumor growth. If dopamine agonists are not used during pregnancy in a woman with a macroprolactinoma, visual field testing is required in each trimester. Measurement of PRL is not useful surveillance for tumor growth due to the fact that PRL increases greatly during normal pregnancy.

A. Dopamine Agonists

Dopamine agonists (cabergoline, bromocriptine, or quinagolide) are the initial treatment of choice for patients with giant prolactinomas and those with hyperprolactinemia desiring restoration of normal sexual function and fertility. Even cystic prolactinomas respond to dopamine agonists; in one report, median cyst volume was reduced by 83% and chiasmal compression resolved in four of five cases. Cabergoline is the most effective and usually the best-tolerated ergot-derived dopamine agonist. The beginning dosage is 0.25 mg orally once weekly for 1 week, then 0.25 mg twice weekly for the next week, then 0.5 mg twice weekly. Further dosage increases may be required monthly, based on serum PRL levels, up to a maximum of 1.5 mg twice weekly. Bromocriptine (1.25–20 mg/day orally) is an alternative. Women who experience nausea with oral preparations may find relief with deep vaginal insertion of cabergoline or bromocriptine tablets; vaginal irritation sometimes occurs. Quinagolide (Norprolac; not available in the United States) is a non–ergot-derived dopamine agonist for patients intolerant or resistant to ergot-derived medications; the starting dosage is 0.075 mg/day orally, increasing as needed and tolerated to a maximum of 0.6 mg/day. Patients whose tumor is resistant to one dopamine agonist may be switched to another in an effort to induce a remission.

Dopamine agonists are given at bedtime to minimize side effects of fatigue, nausea, dizziness, and orthostatic hypotension. These symptoms usually improve with dosage reduction and continued use. Erythromelalgia is rare. In doses used for prolactinomas, dopamine agonists have not caused valvulopathy. Dopamine agonists can cause a variety of psychiatric side effects that are not dose related and may take weeks to resolve once the drug is discontinued.

Because dopamine agonists usually restore fertility promptly, many pregnancies have resulted; no increased risk of miscarriage or teratogenicity has been noted. However, women with microadenomas may have treatment withdrawn during pregnancy and may safely breastfeed postpartum without dopamine agonist therapy. Macroadenomas may enlarge significantly during pregnancy; if therapy is withdrawn, patients must be monitored with serum PRL determinations and computer-assisted visual fields. Women with macroprolactinomas who have responded to dopamine agonists may safely receive oral contraceptives as long as they continue receiving dopamine agonist therapy.

B. Surgical Treatment

Transsphenoidal pituitary surgery may be urgently required for large tumors undergoing apoplexy or those severely compromising visual fields. It is also used electively for patients who do not tolerate or respond to dopamine agonists. Transsphenoidal pituitary surgery is generally well tolerated, with a mortality rate of less than 0.5%. For pituitary microprolactinomas, skilled neurosurgeons are successful in normalizing PRL in 87% of patients and some patients prefer surgery to lifetime therapy with dopamine agonists.

Complications, such as CSF leakage, meningitis, stroke, or visual loss, occur in about 3% of cases; sinusitis, nasal septal perforation, or infection complicates about 6.5% of transsphenoidal surgeries. Diabetes insipidus can occur within 2 days postoperatively but is usually mild and self-correcting. Hyponatremia can occur abruptly 4–13 days postoperatively in 21% of patients; symptoms may include nausea, vomiting, headache, malaise, or seizure. It is treated with free water and hypotonic fluid restriction.

C. Stereotactic Radiosurgery

Stereotactic radiosurgery is seldom required for prolactinomas, since they usually respond to cabergoline or surgery. It is reserved for patients with macroadenomas that are growing despite treatment with dopamine agonists.

D. Chemotherapy

Some patients with aggressive pituitary macroadenomas or carcinomas are not surgical candidates and do not respond to dopamine agonists or radiation therapy. A small percentage of patients with aggressive tumors respond to temozolomide (150–200 mg/m^2 orally daily for 5 days of each 28-day cycle); after three cycles, treatment efficacy is determined by PRL measurement and MRI scanning.

▶ Prognosis

Pituitary prolactinomas generally respond well to dopamine agonist therapy. Ninety percent of patients with prolactinomas experience a fall in serum PRL to 10% or less of pretreatment levels and about 80% of treated patients achieve a normal serum PRL level. Shrinkage of a pituitary adenoma occurs early, but the maximum effect may take up to 1 year. Nearly half of prolactinomas—even massive tumors—shrink more than 50%. During pregnancy, growth of a pituitary prolactinoma occurs in 2.7% of women with a microprolactinoma and in 22.9% of those with a macroprolactinoma. If cabergoline is stopped after 2 years of therapy, hyperprolactinemia recurs in 68% of patients with idiopathic hyperprolactinemia, 79% with microprolactinomas, and 84% with macroprolactinomas.

The 10-year recurrence rate is 13% for pituitary microadenomas after transsphenoidal surgery; pituitary function can be preserved in over 95% of cases. However, the surgical success rate for macroprolactinomas is much lower, and the complication rates are higher.

Faje A et al. Dopamine agonists can reduce cystic prolactinomas. J Clin Endocrinol Metab. 2016 Oct;101(10):3709–15. [PMID: 27459530]

Losa M et al. Temozolomide therapy in patients with aggressive pituitary adenomas or carcinomas. J Neurooncol. 2016 Feb; 126(3):519–25. [PMID: 26614517]

Rutkowski MJ et al. Medical versus surgical treatment of prolactinomas: an analysis of treatment outcomes. Expert Rev Endocrinol Metab. 2018 Jan;13(1):25–33. [PMID: 30063440]

Samson SL et al; AACE Neuroendocrine and Pituitary Scientific Committee; American College of Endocrinology (ACE). Clinical relevance of macroprolactin in the absence or presence of true hyperprolactinemia. Endocr Pract. 2015 Dec; 21(12):1427–35. [PMID: 26642103]

Wong A et al. Update on prolactinomas. Part 1: Clinical manifestations and diagnostic challenges. J Clin Neurosci. 2015 Oct; 22(10):1562–7. [PMID: 26256063]

Wong A et al. Update on prolactinomas. Part 2: Treatment and management strategies. J Clin Neurosci. 2015 Oct;22(10): 1568–74. [PMID: 26243714]

DISEASES OF THE THYROID GLAND

THYROIDITIS

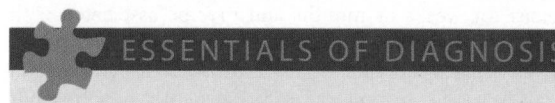

ESSENTIALS OF DIAGNOSIS

Autoimmune thyroiditis (Hashimoto)

▸ Most common thyroiditis.

▸ Antithyroperoxidase or antithyroglobulin antibodies usually high.

▸ Often progresses to hypothyroidism.

Painful subacute thyroiditis

▸ Hallmark is tender thyroid gland with painful dysphagia.

▸ Elevated erythrocyte sedimentation rate (ESR).

▸ Low antithyroid antibodies distinguish it from autoimmune thyroiditis.

Infectious thyroiditis

▸ Severe, painful thyroid gland.

▸ Febrile with leukocytosis and elevated ESR.

Riedel thyroiditis

▸ Most often in middle age or older women.

▸ Usually part of a systemic fibrosing syndrome.

▸ General Considerations

Autoimmune thyroiditis is the most common thyroid disorder in the United States. Cell-mediated autoimmunity is present with T-lymphocytes invading the thyroid gland, giving the microscopic appearance of "lymphocytic thyroiditis." Humoral autoimmunity, with detectable serum antithyroid antibodies, is present in most but not all affected patients. This condition is also known as "Hashimoto thyroiditis." Elevated serum levels of antithyroid antibodies (antithyroperoxidase or antithyroglobulin antibodies, or both) are detectable in the general population in 3% of men and 13% of women. Women over the age of 60 years have a 25% incidence of elevated serum levels of antithyroid antibodies, yet thyroid dysfunction develops in only a small subset of such individuals. However, 1% of the population has serum antithyroid antibody titers greater than 1:640, and they are at particular risk for thyroid dysfunction. The incidence of autoimmune thyroiditis varies by kindred, race, and sex. It is commonly familial. In the United States, elevated levels of antithyroid antibodies are found in 14.3% of whites, 10.9% of Mexican Americans, and 5.3% of blacks.

Childhood or occupational exposure to head-neck external beam radiation increases the lifetime risk of autoimmune thyroiditis. Women with gonadal dysgenesis (Turner syndrome) have a 15% incidence of thyroiditis by age 40 years. Thyroiditis is also commonly seen in patients with hepatitis C. Subclinical thyroiditis is extremely common; autopsy series have found focal thyroiditis in about 40% of women and 20% of men.

Dietary iodine supplementation (especially when excessive) increases the risk of autoimmune thyroiditis. Certain drugs can trigger autoimmune thyroiditis, including tyrosine kinase inhibitors, denileukin diftitox, alemtuzumab, interferon-alpha, interleukin-2, thalidomide, lenalidomide, lithium, amiodarone, and immune checkpoint inhibitors.

Autoimmune thyroiditis often progresses to hypothyroidism, which may be linked to thyrotropin receptor–blocking antibodies, detected in 10% of patients with Hashimoto thyroiditis. Hypothyroidism is more likely to develop in smokers than in nonsmokers, possibly due to the thiocyanates in cigarette smoke. High serum levels of thyroid peroxidase antibody also predict progression from subclinical to symptomatic hypothyroidism. Although the hypothyroidism is usually permanent, up to 11% of patients experience a remission after several years. Autoimmune thyroiditis is the most common cause for hyperthyroidism (Graves disease) and most patients with Graves disease have concomitant antithyroid antibodies.

Autoimmune thyroiditis is sometimes associated with other endocrine deficiencies as part of autoimmune polyendocrine syndrome type 2 (APS-II). Adults with APS-II are prone to autoimmune thyroiditis, type 1 diabetes mellitus, autoimmune gonadal failure, hypoparathyroidism, and adrenal insufficiency. Thyroiditis is frequently associated with other autoimmune conditions: pernicious anemia, Sjögren syndrome, vitiligo, inflammatory bowel disease, celiac disease, and gluten sensitivity. It is less commonly associated with alopecia areata, hypophysitis, encephalitis, myocarditis, primary pulmonary hypertension, and membranous nephropathy.

Painless postpartum thyroiditis is an acute autoimmune thyroiditis that occurs soon after delivery in 7.2% of women. The affected thyroid releases stored thyroid hormone, resulting in transient hyperthyroidism (that may be mild and undiagnosed), followed by hypothyroidism. Most women recover normal thyroid function. Women in whom postpartum thyroiditis develops have a 70% chance of recurrence after subsequent pregnancies. It occurs most commonly in women who have high levels of antithyroperoxidase antibody in the first trimester of pregnancy or immediately after delivery. It is also more common in women with preexistent type 1 diabetes mellitus, other autoimmunity, or a family history of Hashimoto thyroiditis.

Painless sporadic subacute thyroiditis is a form of autoimmune thyroiditis that is similar to painless postpartum thyroiditis, except that it is not related to pregnancy. It is caused by a release of stored thyroid hormone and accounts for about 1% of cases of thyrotoxicosis. It is followed by hypothyroidism that may or may not resolve spontaneously.

Painful subacute thyroiditis—also called de Quervain thyroiditis, granulomatous thyroiditis, and giant cell thyroiditis—is relatively common. Its hallmark is a tender thyroid gland associated with painful dysphagia. Low-grade fever is common. The ESR is often elevated. Multinucleated giant cells are found on histology. Some patients also have antithyroid antibodies. Like painless subacute thyroiditis, most affected patients have transient hyperthyroidism, followed by hypothyroidism. Painful subacute thyroiditis is likely caused by a viral infection and often follows an upper respiratory tract infection. Its incidence peaks in the summer. It affects both sexes, but young and middle-aged women are most commonly affected.

Infectious (suppurative) thyroiditis, a nonviral infection of the thyroid gland, is quite rare among immunocompetent patients, since the thyroid is resistant to infection due to its vasculature, encapsulation, and high iodine content. Congenital pyriform sinus fistulas are a cause for recurrent infectious thyroiditis. While infectious thyroiditis is usually bacterial, mycobacterial, fungal, and parasitic infections can occur, particularly in immunosuppressed individuals. In affected patients who are appropriately treated, when immunosuppression is reduced, the patient may experience an immune reconstitution inflammatory syndrome (IRIS) from residual antigens triggering the normal immune response.

Riedel thyroiditis, also called invasive fibrous thyroiditis, Riedel struma, woody thyroiditis, ligneous thyroiditis, and invasive thyroiditis, is the rarest form of thyroiditis. It is found most frequently in middle-aged or elderly women and is usually part of a multifocal systemic fibrosis syndrome. It may occur as a thyroid manifestation of IgG_4-related systemic disease.

▶ Clinical Findings

A. Symptoms and Signs

In **autoimmune thyroiditis**, the thyroid gland may be diffusely enlarged, firm, and finely nodular. One thyroid lobe may be asymmetrically enlarged, raising concerns about neoplasm. Although patients may complain of neck tightness, pain and tenderness are not usually present. Other patients have no palpable goiter and no neck symptoms. About 10% of cases are atrophic, the gland being fibrotic, particularly in elderly women.

Symptoms and signs are mostly related to ambient levels of thyroid hormone. There may be hyperthyroidism caused by destructive release of thyroid hormones (followed by hypothyroidism), or hyperthyroidism caused by increased synthesis of thyroid hormones (Graves disease). Affected patients may have combinations of these presentations. For example, a patient with hypothyroidism might later develop hyperthyroidism that can wax and wane.

Depression and chronic fatigue are more common in such patients, even after correction of hypothyroidism. About one-third of patients have mild dry mouth (xerostomia) or dry eyes (keratoconjunctivitis sicca) related to Sjögren syndrome. Associated myasthenia gravis is usually of mild severity, mainly affecting the extraocular muscles and having a relatively low incidence of detectable AChR Ab or thymic disease. Associated celiac disease or gluten intolerance can produce fatigue or depression, sometimes in the absence of gastrointestinal symptoms.

Postpartum thyroiditis is typically manifested by hyperthyroidism that begins 1–6 months after delivery and persists for only 1–2 months. Then, hypothyroidism tends to develop beginning 4–8 months after delivery.

In painless sporadic thyroiditis, thyrotoxic symptoms are usually mild; a small, nontender goiter may be palpated in about 50% of such patients. The course is similar to postpartum thyroiditis.

Subacute thyroiditis presents with an acute, usually painful enlargement of the thyroid gland, often with dysphagia. The pain may radiate to the ears. Patients usually have a low-grade fever and fatigue. The manifestations may persist for weeks or months and may be associated with malaise. If there is no pain, it is called silent thyroiditis. Thyrotoxicosis develops in 50% of affected patients and tends to last for several weeks. Subsequently, hypothyroidism develops that lasts 4–6 months. Normal thyroid function typically returns within 12 months, but persistent hypothyroidism develops in 5% of patients.

Patients with **infectious thyroiditis** usually are febrile and have severe pain, tenderness, redness, and fluctuation in the region of the thyroid gland. In **Riedel thyroiditis**, thyroid enlargement is often asymmetric; the gland is stony hard and adherent to the neck structures, causing signs of compression and invasion, including dysphagia, dyspnea, pain, and hoarseness. Related conditions include retroperitoneal fibrosis, fibrosing mediastinitis, sclerosing cervicitis, subretinal fibrosis, and sclerosing cholangitis.

B. Laboratory Findings

In **Hashimoto thyroiditis** with clinically evident disease, there are usually increased circulating levels of antithyroperoxidase (90%) or antithyroglobulin (40%) antibodies. However, some patients with autoimmune thyroiditis have no detectable antithyroid antibodies. In patients with thyroiditis caused by immune checkpoint inhibitors, most have no detectable antithyroid antibodies. Antithyroid antibodies decline during pregnancy and are often undetectable in the third trimester. Once Hashimoto thyroiditis has been diagnosed, monitoring of these antibody levels is not helpful. The serum TSH level is elevated if thyroid hormone is not released in adequate amounts by the thyroid gland. High serum antithyroperoxidase antibody concentrations are found in only 50% of patients with painless sporadic thyroiditis.

Patients with Hashimoto thyroiditis have a 15% incidence of having serum antibodies (IgA tissue transglutaminase [tTG] antibody) associated with celiac disease, and at least 5% have clinically significant celiac disease. Seronegative gluten sensitivity is even more common.

In **subacute thyroiditis,** the ESR is markedly elevated while antithyroid antibody titers are low, distinguishing it from autoimmune thyroiditis. In **infectious (suppurative) thyroiditis,** both the leukocyte count and ESR are usually elevated.

With hyperthyroidism due to Hashimoto thyroiditis or subacute thyroiditis, serum FT_4 levels tend to be proportionally higher than T_3 levels, since the hyperthyroidism is due to the passive release of stored thyroid hormone, which is predominantly T_4; this is in contrast to Graves disease and toxic nodular goiter, where T_3 is relatively more elevated. Because T_4 is less active than T_3, the hyperthyroidism seen in thyroiditis is usually less severe. Serum levels of TSH are suppressed in hyperthyroidism due to thyroiditis.

C. Imaging

The ultrasound in cases of Hashimoto thyroiditis typically shows a gland with characteristic diffuse heterogeneous density and reduced echogenicity. It helps distinguish thyroiditis from multinodular goiter or thyroid nodules that are suspicious for malignancy. It is also helpful in guiding FNA biopsy of small suspicious thyroid nodules. Color flow Doppler ultrasonography can help distinguish thyroiditis from Graves disease; in thyroiditis, vascularity is normal or reduced vascularity, whereas in Graves disease, the thyroid gland is hypervascular.

Radioiodine (RAI) uptake and scan can help distinguish thyroiditis from Graves disease; subacute thyroiditis exhibits a very low RAI uptake. However, RAI uptake may be normal or high with uneven uptake on the scan in chronic Hashimoto thyroiditis (euthyroid or hypothyroid); scanning is not useful in diagnosis.

[18F] Fluorodeoxyglucose positron emission tomography (18FDG-PET) scanning frequently shows diffuse thyroid uptake of isotope in cases of thyroiditis. In fact, of 18FDG-PET scans done for any reason, about 3% show such uptake. However, discrete thyroid nodules can also be discovered on 18FDG-PET scanning; these nodules are known as "thyroid PET incidentalomas" and 50% are malignant.

D. Fine-Needle Aspiration Biopsy

Patients with autoimmune thyroiditis who have a thyroid nodule should have an ultrasound-guided FNA biopsy, since the risk of papillary thyroid cancer is about 8% in such nodules. When infectious (suppurative) thyroiditis is suspected, an FNA biopsy with Gram stain and culture is required. FNA biopsy is usually not required for subacute thyroiditis but shows characteristic giant multinucleated cells.

▶ Complications

Autoimmune thyroiditis may lead to hypothyroidism or transient thyrotoxicosis. Hyperthyroidism may develop, either due to the emergence of Graves disease or due to the release of stored thyroid hormone, which is caused by inflammation. Variably termed "hashitoxicosis" or "painless sporadic thyroiditis," it is known as postpartum painless thyroiditis when it occurs in women after delivery. Perimenopausal women with high serum levels of antithyroperoxidase antibodies have a higher relative risk of depression, independent of ambient thyroid hormone levels.

In the suppurative forms of thyroiditis, any of the complications of infection may occur. Subacute and chronic thyroiditis are complicated by the effects of pressure on the neck structures: dyspnea and, in Riedel struma, vocal cord palsy. Papillary thyroid carcinoma or thyroid lymphoma may rarely be associated with chronic thyroiditis and must be considered in the diagnosis of uneven painless enlargements that continue despite treatment; such patients require FNA biopsy.

▶ Differential Diagnosis

Thyroiditis must be considered in the differential diagnosis of all types of goiters, especially if enlargement is rapid. The very low RAI uptake in subacute thyroiditis with elevated T_4 and T_3 is helpful. Thyroid autoantibody tests have been helpful in the diagnosis of Hashimoto thyroiditis, but the tests are not specific (positive in patients with multinodular goiters, malignancy [eg, thyroid carcinoma, lymphoma], and concurrent Graves disease). The subacute and suppurative forms of thyroiditis may resemble any infectious process in or near the neck structures. Chronic thyroiditis may resemble thyroid carcinoma, especially if the enlargement is uneven and if there is pressure on surrounding structures; both disorders may be present in the same gland.

▶ Treatment

A. Autoimmune (Hashimoto) Thyroiditis

If hypothyroidism is present, levothyroxine should be given in the usual replacement doses (0.05–0.2 mg orally daily) (See Hypothyroidism & Myxedema, below). In patients with a large goiter and normal or elevated serum TSH, an attempt is made to shrink the goiter by administering levothyroxine in doses sufficient to drive the serum TSH below the reference range while maintaining clinical euthyroidism. Suppressive doses of T_4 tend to shrink the goiter an average of 30% over 6 months. If the goiter does not regress, lower replacement doses of levothyroxine may be given. If the thyroid gland is only minimally enlarged and the patient is euthyroid, regular observation is in order, since hypothyroidism may develop subsequently—often years later.

Dietary supplementation with selenium 200 mcg/day reduces serum levels of antithyroperoxidase antibodies. However, whether selenium supplementation improves clinical outcome is unknown.

B. Subacute Thyroiditis

All treatment is empiric and must be continued for several weeks. Recurrence is common. The drug of choice is aspirin, which relieves pain and inflammation. Thyrotoxic symptoms are treated with propranolol, 10–40 mg every 6 hours. Iodinated contrast agents cause a prompt fall in serum T_3 levels and a dramatic improvement in thyrotoxic symptoms. Ipodate sodium (Bilivist, Oragrafin) or iopanoic acid (Telepaque) is given orally in doses of 500 mg orally daily until serum FT_4 levels return to normal. Transient hypothyroidism is treated with T_4 (0.05–0.1 mg orally daily) if symptomatic.

C. Infectious Thyroiditis

Treatment is with antibiotics and with surgical drainage when fluctuation is marked. Immunocompromised individuals are particularly at risk and coccidioidomycosis thyroiditis has been reported. Surgical thyroidectomy may be required.

D. Riedel Thyroiditis

The treatment of choice is tamoxifen, 20 mg orally twice daily, which must be continued for years. Tamoxifen can induce partial to complete remissions in most patients within 3–6 months. Its mode of action appears to be unrelated to its antiestrogen activity. Short-term corticosteroid treatment may be added for partial alleviation of pain and compression symptoms. Surgical decompression usually fails to permanently alleviate compression symptoms; such surgery is difficult due to dense fibrous adhesions, making surgical complications more likely. Rituximab may be useful for Riedel thyroiditis that is refractory to tamoxifen and corticosteroids.

► Prognosis

Autoimmune (Hashimoto) thyroiditis is occasionally associated with other autoimmune disorders (celiac disease, diabetes mellitus, Addison disease, pernicious anemia, etc). In general, however, patients with Hashimoto thyroiditis have an excellent prognosis, since the condition either remains stable for years or progresses slowly to hypothyroidism, which is easily treated. Although 80% of women with postpartum thyroiditis subsequently recover normal thyroid function, permanent hypothyroidism eventually develops in about 50% within 7 years, more commonly in women who are multiparous or who have had a spontaneous abortion. In subacute thyroiditis, spontaneous remissions and exacerbations are common; the disease process may smolder for months. Papillary thyroid carcinoma carries a relatively good prognosis when it occurs in patients with Hashimoto thyroiditis.

Hu S et al. Multiple nutritional factors and the risk of Hashimoto's thyroiditis. Thyroid. 2017 May;27(5):597–610. [PMID: 28290237]

Ranganath R et al. de Quervain's thyroiditis: a review of experience with surgery. Am J Otolaryngol. 2016 Nov–Dec; 37(6):534–7. [PMID: 27686396]

Wichman J et al. Selenium supplementation significantly reduces thyroid autoantibody levels in patients with chronic autoimmune thyroiditis: a systematic review and meta-analysis. Thyroid. 2016 Dec;26(12):1681–92. [PMID: 27702392]

HYPOTHYROIDISM & MYXEDEMA

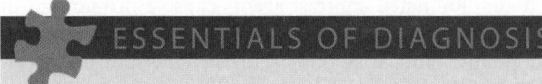
ESSENTIALS OF DIAGNOSIS

- ► Hashimoto thyroiditis is the most common cause of hypothyroidism.
- ► Fatigue, cold intolerance, constipation, weight change, depression, menorrhagia, hoarseness.
- ► Dry skin, bradycardia, delayed return of deep tendon reflexes.
- ► FT_4 level is usually low.
- ► TSH elevated in primary hypothyroidism.

► General Considerations

Hypothyroidism is common, affecting over 1% of the general population and about 5% of individuals over age 60 years. About 85% of affected individuals are women. Thyroid hormone deficiency affects almost all body functions. The degree of severity ranges from mild and unrecognized hypothyroid states to striking myxedema. Maternal hypothyroidism during pregnancy results in offspring with IQ scores that are an average 7 points lower than those of euthyroid mothers. Congenital hypothyroidism occurs in about 1:4000 births; untreated, it causes cretinism with permanent cognitive impairment.

Hypothyroidism may be due to failure or resection of the thyroid gland itself or deficiency of pituitary TSH. The condition must be distinguished from the functional hypothyroidism that occurs in severe nonthyroidal illness, which does not require treatment with levothyroxine. Hashimoto thyroiditis is the most common cause of hypothyroidism. A hypothyroid phase also occurs in subacute (de Quervain) viral thyroiditis following initial hyperthyroidism.

Goiter may be present with thyroiditis, iodide deficiency, genetic thyroid enzyme defects, drug goitrogens (lithium, iodide, propylthiouracil or methimazole, sulfonamides, amiodarone, interferon-alpha, interferon-beta, interleukin-2), food goitrogens in iodide-deficient areas (eg, turnips, cassavas) or, rarely, peripheral resistance to thyroid hormone or infiltrating diseases (eg, cancer, sarcoidosis). Goiter is often absent in patients with autoimmune thyroiditis. Goiter is also usually absent when hypothyroidism is due to destruction of the gland by head-neck or chest-shoulder radiation therapy or ^{131}I therapy. Thyroidectomy causes hypothyroidism; after hemithyroidectomy, hypothyroidism develops in 22% of patients.

Amiodarone, because of its high iodine content, causes clinically significant hypothyroidism in about 15–20% of patients as well as thyrotoxicosis (see Amiodarone-induced thyrotoxicosis, below). Hypothyroidism occurs most often in patients with preexisting autoimmune thyroiditis and in patients who are not iodine-deficient. The T_4 level is low or low-normal, and the TSH is elevated, usually over 20 milli-international units/L. Another 17% of patients taking amiodarone are asymptomatic with normal serum T_4 levels despite elevations in serum TSH; they can be closely monitored without levothyroxine therapy. Low-dose amiodarone is less likely to cause hypothyroidism. Patients with coronary insufficiency who have amiodarone-induced symptomatic hypothyroidism are treated with just enough levothyroxine to relieve symptoms. Hypothyroidism usually resolves over several months if amiodarone is discontinued. Hypothyroidism may also develop in patients with a high iodine intake from other sources, especially if they have underlying lymphocytic thyroiditis. Some malignancies overexpress thyroid hormone inactivating enzyme (type 3 deiodinase) and cause "consumptive hypothyroidism." This has occurred with large hemangiomas or a heavy tumor burden of colon cancer, basal cell cancer, fibrous tumors, or gastrointestinal stromal tumors (GISTs).

Chemotherapeutic agents that can cause silent thyroiditis include the following: tyrosine kinase inhibitors, denileukin diftitox, alemtuzumab, interferon-alpha, interleukin-2, thalidomide, and lenalidomide. Immune checkpoint inhibitors include pembrolizumab, ipilimumab, tremelimumab, and atezolizumab. This usually starts with hyperthyroidism (often unrecognized) and then progresses to hypothyroidism. Radioiodine-based targeted radioisotope therapy can also cause hypothyroidism.

Chronic hepatitis C is associated with an increased risk of autoimmune thyroiditis, with 21% of affected patients having antithyroid antibodies and 13% having hypothyroidism. Oral direct-acting anti–hepatitis C agents do not increase the risk of thyroid dysfunction that has been seen with interferon.

▶ Clinical Findings

A. Symptoms and Signs

1. Common manifestations—Mild hypothyroidism often escapes detection without a screening serum TSH. Patients typically have nonspecific symptoms of hypothyroidism that include weight gain, fatigue, lethargy, depression, weakness, dyspnea on exertion, arthralgias or myalgias, muscle cramps, menorrhagia, constipation, dry skin, headache, paresthesias, cold intolerance, carpal tunnel syndrome, and Raynaud syndrome. Physical findings can include bradycardia; diastolic hypertension; thin, brittle nails; thinning of hair; peripheral edema; puffy face and eyelids; and skin pallor or yellowing (carotenemia). Delayed relaxation of deep tendon reflexes may be present. Patients often have a palpably enlarged thyroid (goiter) that arises due to elevated serum TSH levels or the underlying thyroid pathology.

2. Less common manifestations—Less common symptoms of hypothyroidism include diminished appetite and weight loss, hoarseness, decreased sense of taste and smell, and diminished auditory acuity. Some patients may complain of dysphagia or neck discomfort. Although most menstruating women have menorrhagia, some women have scant menses or amenorrhea. Physical findings may include thinning of the outer halves of the eyebrows; thickening of the tongue; hard pitting edema; and effusions into the pleural and peritoneal cavities as well as into joints. Galactorrhea may also be present. Cardiac enlargement ("myxedema heart") and pericardial effusions may occur. Psychosis "myxedema madness" can occur from severe hypothyroidism or from toxicity of other drugs whose metabolism is slowed in hypothyroidism. Hypothermia and stupor or myxedema coma, which is often associated with infection (especially pneumonia), may develop in patients with severe hypothyroidism.

Some hypothyroid patients with Hashimoto thyroiditis have symptoms that are not due to hypothyroidism but rather to conditions associated with Hashimoto thyroiditis; these include Addison disease, hypoparathyroidism, diabetes mellitus, pernicious anemia, Sjögren syndrome, vitiligo, biliary cirrhosis, gluten sensitivity, and celiac disease.

B. Laboratory Findings

Hypothyroidism is a common disorder and thyroid function tests should be obtained for any patient with its nonspecific symptoms or signs. The single best screening test for hypothyroidism is the serum TSH (Table 26–2). The normal reference range for ultrasensitive TSH levels is generally 0.4–4.0 milli-international units/L. Over 95% of normal adults have serum TSH concentrations under 3.0 milli-international units/L. However, there is considerable controversy about what represents "normal," such that each laboratory uses a slightly different range. The normal range of TSH varies with age; for example, the reference range for elderly patients is higher than the reference range for younger patients.

Table 26–2. Appropriate use of thyroid tests.

	Test	Comment
For screening	Serum thyroid-stimulating hormone (TSH)	Most sensitive test for primary hypothyroidism and hyperthyroidism
	Free thyroxine (FT_4)	Excellent test
For hypothyroidism	Serum TSH	High in primary and low in secondary hypothyroidism
	Antithyroperoxidase and antithyroglobulin antibodies	Elevated in Hashimoto thyroiditis
For hyperthyroidism	Serum TSH	Suppressed except in TSH-secreting pituitary tumor or pituitary hyperplasia (rare)
	Triiodothyronine (T_3) or free triiodothyronine (FT_3)	Elevated
	^{123}I uptake and scan	Increased uptake; diffuse versus "hot" foci on scan
	Antithyroperoxidase and antithyroglobulin antibodies	Elevated in Graves disease
	Thyroid-stimulating immunoglobulin (TSI)	Usually (65%) positive in Graves disease
For thyroid nodules	Fine-needle aspiration (FNA) biopsy	Best diagnostic method for thyroid cancer
	^{123}I uptake and scan	Cancer is usually "cold"; less reliable than FNA biopsy
	^{99m}Tc scan	Vascular versus avascular
	Ultrasonography	Useful to assist FNA biopsy. Useful in assessing the risk of malignancy (multinodular goiter or pure cysts are less likely to be malignant). Useful to monitor nodules and patients after thyroid surgery for carcinoma.

In primary hypothyroidism, the serum TSH is increased in a reflex effort to stimulate the failing gland, while the serum FT$_4$ is low or low-normal. Other laboratory abnormalities can include hypoglycemia or anemia (with normal or increased mean corpuscular volume). Hyponatremia due to syndrome of inappropriate ADH secretion (SIADH) or decreased glomerular filtration rate is common. Additional frequent findings include increased serum levels of LDL cholesterol, triglycerides, lipoprotein (a), liver enzymes, creatine kinase, or PRL. Semen analysis shows an increase in abnormal sperm morphology. In patients with autoimmune thyroiditis, titers of antibodies against thyroperoxidase and thyroglobulin are high; serum antinuclear antibodies may be present but are not usually indicative of lupus.

Subclinical hypothyroidism is defined as the state of having a normal serum FT$_4$ with a serum TSH that is above the reference range. It occurs most often in persons aged 65 years or older, in whom the prevalence is 13%. Subclinical hypothyroidism is often transient and the TSH normalizes spontaneously in about 35% of cases within 2 years. The likelihood of TSH normalization is higher in patients without antithyroid antibodies and those with a marginally elevated serum TSH. The term "subclinical" is somewhat misleading, since it does not refer to patients' symptoms but rather refers only to serum hormone levels; in fact, such patients can have subtle manifestations of hypothyroidism (eg, fatigue, depression, hyperlipidemia) that may improve with a trial of levothyroxine replacement. Patients without such symptoms do not require levothyroxine therapy but must be monitored regularly for the emergence of symptoms.

A retrospective analysis of 1954 patients aged 65 years and older with subclinical hypothyroidism found a threshold serum TSH above 6.38 milli-international units/L was associated with increased mortality; however, it is uncertain whether levothyroxine therapy reduces mortality risk in this group.

C. Imaging

Radiologic imaging is usually not necessary for patients with hypothyroidism. However, on CT or MRI, a goiter may be noted in the neck or in the mediastinum (retrosternal goiter). An enlarged thymus is frequently seen in the mediastinum in cases of autoimmune thyroiditis. On MRI, the pituitary is often quite enlarged in primary hypothyroidism, due to hyperplasia of TSH-secreting cells, which is reversible following thyroid therapy; concomitant hyperprolactinemia can lead to the mistaken diagnosis of a TSH-secreting or PRL-secreting pituitary adenoma.

▶ Differential Diagnosis

The differential diagnosis for subclinical hypothyroidism includes antibody interference with the serum TSH assay, macro-TSH, sleep deprivation, exercise, recovery from nonthyroidal illness, acute psychiatric emergencies, and other conditions and medications that can cause a low serum T$_4$ or high serum TSH in the absence of hypothyroidism (Table 26–3).

Euthyroid sick syndrome should be considered in patients without known thyroid disease who are found to

Table 26–3. Factors that may cause aberrations in laboratory tests that may be mistaken for primary hypothyroidism.[1]

Low Serum T$_4$ or T$_3$	High Serum TSH
Acute psychiatric problems	Acute psychiatric illness (transient) (14%)
Cirrhosis	Anti-mouse antibodies
Familial thyroid-binding globulin deficiency	Antithyrotropin (TSH) antibodies
Laboratory error	Anti-TSH receptor antibodies
Nephrotic syndrome	Autoimmune disease (assay interference)
Severe illness	
Drugs	Drugs
Androgens	Amphetamines
Antiseizure drugs	Atypical antipsychotics
Carbamazepine	Dopamine agonists
Phenobarbitol	Heroin
Phenytoin	Phenothiazines
Asparaginase	Elderly (especially women) (11%)
Carbamazepine (T$_4$)	Exercise before testing
Chloral hydrate	Following prolonged primary hypothyroidism
Corticosteroids	
Diclofenac (T$_3$)	Heterophile antibodies
Didanosine	Laboratory error
Fenclofenac	Macro-thyrotropin
5-Fluorouracil	Nonadherence to thyroid replacement therapy
Halofenate	
Imatinib	Pituitary TSH hypersecretion
Mitotane	Recovery from acute nonthyroidal illness (transient)
Naproxen (T$_3$)	
Nicotinic acid	Strenuous exercise (acute)
Oxcarbazepine	Sleep deprivation (acute)
Phenobarbital	TSH resistance
Phenytoin (T$_4$ as low as 2 mcg/dL)	
Salicylates in large doses (T$_3$ and T$_4$)	
Sertraline	
Stavudine	
T$_3$ therapy (T$_4$)	

[1]True primary hypothyroidism may coexist.
T$_4$, levothyroxine; T$_3$, triiodothyronine; TSH, thyroid-stimulating hormone.

have a low serum FT$_4$ with a serum TSH that is not elevated. This syndrome can be seen in patients with severe illness, caloric deprivation, or major surgery. Serum TSH tends to be suppressed in severe nonthyroidal illness, making the diagnosis of concurrent primary hypothyroidism quite difficult, although the presence of a goiter suggests the diagnosis.

The clinician must decide whether such severely ill patients (with a low serum T$_4$ but no elevated TSH) might have hypothyroidism due to hypopituitarism. Patients without symptoms of prior brain lesion or hypopituitarism are very unlikely to suddenly develop hypopituitarism during an unrelated illness. Patients with diabetes insipidus, hypopituitarism, or other signs of a central nervous system (CNS) lesion may be given T$_4$ empirically.

Patients receiving prolonged dopamine infusions can develop true secondary hypothyroidism caused by dopamine's direct suppression of TSH-secreting cells.

Complications

Patients with severe hypothyroidism have an increased susceptibility to bacterial pneumonia. Megacolon has been described in long-standing hypothyroidism. Organic psychoses with paranoid delusions may occur ("myxedema madness"). Rarely, adrenal crisis may be precipitated by thyroid therapy. Hypothyroidism is a rare cause of infertility, which may respond to thyroid replacement. Untreated hypothyroidism during pregnancy often results in miscarriage. Preexistent coronary artery disease and heart failure may be exacerbated by levothyroxine therapy.

Myxedema crisis refers to severe, life-threatening manifestations of hypothyroidism. Myxedema crisis particularly affects elderly women and can occur spontaneously in severely hypothyroid patients with prolonged exposure to the cold, with resultant hypothermia. It can also be induced by a stroke, heart failure, infection (particularly pneumonia), or trauma. Metabolism of drugs is slowed in hypothyroidism and myxedema crisis is often precipitated by the administration of sedatives, antidepressants, hypnotics, anesthetics, or opioids. The drugs further impair cognition and respiratory drive and can precipitate respiratory arrest. Affected patients have impaired cognition, ranging from confusion to somnolence to coma (myxedema coma). Convulsions and abnormal CNS signs may occur. Patients have profound hypothermia, hypoventilation, hyponatremia, hypoglycemia, hypoxemia, hypercapnia, and hypotension. Rhabdomyolysis and acute kidney injury may occur. The mortality rate is high.

Treatment

Before beginning therapy with thyroid hormone, the hypothyroid patient requires at least a clinical assessment for adrenal insufficiency and angina. The presence of either condition requires further evaluation and management.

A. Treatment for Hypothyroidism

Synthetic levothyroxine is the preferred preparation for treating hypothyroid patients. However, some clinicians prescribe mixtures of levothyroxine and triiodothyronine for certain patients. Otherwise healthy young and middle-aged adults with hypothyroidism may be treated initially with levothyroxine in average doses of about 1.6 mcg/kg/day. Lower doses can be used for very mild hypothyroidism, while full doses are given for more symptomatic hypothyroidism. During pregnancy, women with mild hypothyroidism may be treated with initial levothyroxine doses of about 75–100 mcg daily. Pregnant women with overt hypothyroidism or myxedema should be treated immediately with levothyroxine at full replacement doses of 1.6 mcg/kg/day (about 100–150 mcg daily). Thyroid function testing is repeated every 4–6 weeks during pregnancy, with levothyroxine doses being adjusted to normalize the serum TSH and restore euthyroidism. For initial titration, the levothyroxine dosage may be increased according to clinical response and serum TSH, measuring serum TSH every 4–6 weeks and trying to keep the serum TSH level between 0.4 milli-international units/L and 2.0 milli-international units/L. However, patients receiving levothyroxine replacement, with serum TSH levels within the reference range, have higher average levels of LDL cholesterol compared to matched euthyroid controls. Also, some treated patients continue to have subjective symptoms suggestive of mild hypothyroidism, despite normal serum TSH levels. Such patients may benefit from a carefully increased dose of levothyroxine. Bedtime levothyroxine administration results in somewhat higher serum T_4 and lower TSH levels than morning administration. Therefore, the administration timing for levothyroxine should be kept constant. After beginning daily administration, significant increases in serum T_4 levels are seen within 1–2 weeks, and near-peak levels are seen within 3–4 weeks.

Patients with stable coronary artery disease or those who are over age 60 years are treated with smaller initial doses of levothyroxine, 25–50 mcg orally daily; higher initial doses may be used if such patients are severely hypothyroid. The dose can be increased by 25 mcg every 1–3 weeks until the patient is euthyroid. Ideally, patients with hypothyroidism and unstable coronary artery disease or uncontrolled atrial fibrillation should begin levothyroxine replacement following medical or interventional therapy.

Myxedema crisis requires larger initial doses of levothyroxine intravenously, since myxedema itself can interfere with intestinal absorption of oral levothyroxine. Levothyroxine sodium 500 mcg is given intravenously as a loading dose, followed by 50–100 mcg intravenously daily; the lower dose is given to patients with suspected coronary artery disease. In patients with myxedema coma, liothyronine (T_3, Triostat) can be given intravenously with a loading dose of 10–20 mcg, followed by 10 mcg every 4–6 hours for the first 48 hours. The hypothermic patient is warmed only with blankets, since faster warming can precipitate cardiovascular collapse. Hypoglycemic patients are given 5% dextrose intravenously. Hyponatremic patients with a serum sodium 120–130 mEq/mL are administered 0.9% NaCl intravenously, while patients with a serum sodium below 120 mEq/mL are treated with boluses of 100 mL of 3% NaCl intravenously with intravenous furosemide 20–40 mg to promote water diuresis; serum sodium levels must be followed closely and boluses of 3% NaCl can be repeated about every 6 hours until the serum sodium rises to 120 mmol/L or higher. When giving intravenous saline to myxedematous patients, care must be taken to avoid fluid overload.

Patients with hypercapnia require mechanical assistance with ventilation. Opioid medications must be stopped or used in very low doses. Infections must be detected and treated aggressively. Patients in whom concomitant adrenal insufficiency is suspected are treated with hydrocortisone, 100 mg intravenously, followed by 25–50 mg every 8 hours.

B. Monitoring and Optimizing Treatment of Hypothyroidism

Regular clinical and laboratory monitoring is critical to determine the optimal levothyroxine dose for each patient. The initial goal should be to normalize the serum TSH within 1–2 months of commencing thyroid replacement therapy. The patient should be prescribed sufficient levothyroxine to restore a clinically euthyroid state; this can usually be attained by maintaining the serum TSH, FT_4, and

FT$_3$ within their reference ranges. However, when patients take levothyroxine replacement in doses sufficient to normalize serum TSH levels, their serum FT$_3$ levels are lower and serum FT$_4$ levels are higher, on average, than matched euthyroid individuals not taking levothyroxine. Perhaps for that reason, a significant number of patients taking levothyroxine continue to feel hypothyroid while taking levothyroxine, despite having a normal serum TSH. Unless contraindicated by unstable angina, such patients may be carefully administered a slightly higher dose of levothyroxine that suppresses the serum TSH while achieving clinical euthyroidism and a serum FT$_3$ near the low-normal range. For most patients with hypothyroidism, an ideal stable maintenance dose of levothyroxine can usually be found.

Different levothyroxine preparations vary in their bioavailability by up to 14% and such differences may have a subtle but significant clinical impact. It is optimal for patients to consistently take the same manufacturer's brand of levothyroxine.

Pregnancy usually increases the levothyroxine dosage requirement; an increase in levothyroxine requirement has been noted as early as the fifth week of pregnancy. Adequate levothyroxine is critical to the health of the fetus. Therefore, it is prudent to increase levothyroxine dosages by approximately 20–30% as soon as pregnancy is confirmed. The fetus is at least partially dependent on maternal T$_4$ for its CNS development—particularly in the second trimester. By mid-pregnancy, women require an average of 47% increase in their levothyroxine dosage. Postpartum, levothyroxine replacement requirement ordinarily returns to prepregnancy level.

Decreased levothyroxine dose requirements occur in women after delivery, after bilateral oophorectomy or natural menopause, after cessation of oral estrogen replacement, or during therapy with GnRH agonists. Levothyroxine dosage may need to be titrated downward for patients who start taking teduglutide for short bowel syndrome.

1. Elevated serum TSH level—This usually indicates underreplacement with levothyroxine. However, before increasing the T$_4$ dosage, it is important to confirm that the patient is taking the levothyroxine as directed and does not have coronary insufficiency.

Increased levothyroxine dosage requirements (low serum T$_4$ levels) can occur with drugs that increase the hepatic metabolism of levothyroxine (Table 26–3). Amiodarone can increase or decrease levothyroxine dose requirements. Malabsorption of levothyroxine can be caused by coadministration of binding substances, such as iron (eg, in multivitamins); fiber; raloxifene; sucralfate; aluminum hydroxide antacids; sevelemer; orlistat; soy milk; bile acid–binding resins (cholestyramine and colesevelam); and calcium, magnesium, and soy protein supplements.

Proton pump inhibitors interfere slightly with the absorption of levothyroxine. Gastrointestinal disorders can interfere with levothyroxine absorption, including celiac disease, inflammatory bowel disease, lactose intolerance, *Helicobacter pylori* gastritis, and atrophic gastritis. Nephrotic syndrome can increase the required dose of oral levothyroxine. Women with hypothyroidism may require increased doses of levothyroxine after commencing oral estrogen therapy.

Serum TSH may be elevated transiently in acute psychiatric illness, with antipsychotics and phenothiazines, and during recovery from nonthyroidal illness. Autoimmune disease can cause false elevations of TSH by interfering with the assay. Very rarely, a high TSH can be caused by a thyrotropin-secreting pituitary tumor or hyperplasia.

2. Normal serum TSH level—Most patients may be given levothyroxine in doses sufficient to achieve a serum TSH in the low-normal range. However, for patients with coronary artery disease or recurrent atrial fibrillation, it may be prudent to administer lower doses of levothyroxine to keep their serum TSH in the high-normal range or even at a slightly elevated level.

About 10% of otherwise healthy treated hypothyroid patients (taking levothyroxine with a normal serum TSH) continue to have hypothyroid-type symptoms, such as lethargy, weight gain, depression, or cognitive problems. An even larger percentage has been found to have subtle but significantly reduced psychological wellbeing, compared to gender-matched and age-matched euthyroid controls. Such patients must be assessed for concurrent conditions, such as an adverse drug reaction, Addison disease, depression, hypogonadism, anemia, celiac disease, or gluten sensitivity. If such conditions are not present or are treated and hypothyroid-type symptoms persist, a serum T$_3$ or free T$_3$ level is often helpful. Low serum T$_3$ levels may reflect inadequate peripheral deiodinase activity to convert inactive T$_4$ to active T$_3$. Such patients may be given a careful clinical trial of a slightly higher dose of levothyroxine that results in a low serum TSH and a low-normal serum T$_3$ or free T$_3$.

For such patients, some clinicians have found success with other strategies, such as using desiccated natural porcine thyroid preparations containing both T$_4$ and T$_3$ (eg, Armour Thyroid, Nature-Throid, NP Thyroid). For product conversion purposes, 100 mcg of levothyroxine is equivalent to about 65 mg (1 grain) of desiccated thyroid. The use of desiccated thyroid preparations has been discouraged by several professional medical societies, but some patients prefer them.

3. Low or suppressed serum TSH level—A serum TSH level below the reference range (adults 0.4–4.0 milli-international units/L) is either "low" (0.1–0.39 milli-international units/L) or "suppressed" (less than 0.1 milli-international units/L). Clinically euthyroid patients receiving levothyroxine who have "low" TSH levels do not have increased morbidity. However, a "suppressed" serum TSH often indicates overreplacement with levothyroxine, and such patients may have symptoms of hyperthyroidism and have an increased risk for atrial fibrillation, osteoporosis, and clinical hyperthyroidism. When the serum TSH is suppressed, the dosage of levothyroxine is reduced. However, some patients feel unmistakably hypothyroid while taking the reduced dose of levothyroxine and have low serum T$_3$ or free T$_3$ levels. For such patients, a higher levothyroxine dose may be resumed with close surveillance for atrial fibrillation, osteoporosis, and manifestations of subtle hyperthyroidism. A suppressed serum TSH can also occur with hypopituitarism, severe nonthyroidal illness, and certain medications (eg, nonsteroidal anti-inflammatory drugs [NSAIDs], opioids, nifedipine, verapamil, and high-dose [short-term] corticosteroids).

Prognosis

Patients with mild hypothyroidism caused by Hashimoto thyroiditis have a remission rate of 11%. Hypothyroidism caused by interferon-alpha resolves within 17 months of stopping the drug in 50% of patients. With levothyroxine treatment of hypothyroidism, striking transformations take place both in appearance and mental function. Return to a normal state is usually the rule, but relapses will occur if treatment is interrupted. However, untreated patients with myxedema crisis have a mortality rate approaching 100%; even with optimal treatment, the mortality rate is 20–50%.

When to Refer

- Difficulty titrating levothyroxine replacement to normal TSH or clinically euthyroid state.
- Any patient with significant coronary artery disease needing levothyroxine therapy.

When to Admit

- Suspected myxedema crisis.
- Hypercapnia.

De Groot L et al. Management of thyroid dysfunction during pregnancy and postpartum: An Endocrine Society clinical practice guideline. J Clin Endocrinol Metab. 2012 Aug;97(8): 2543–65. [PMID: 22869843]

Elnaggar MN et al. Amiodarone-induced thyroid dysfunction: a clinical update. Exp Clin Endocrinol Diabetes. 2018 Jun; 126(6):333–41. [PMID: 29558786]

Jonklaas J et al. Guidelines for the treatment of hypothyroidism: prepared by the American Thyroid Association Task Force on Thyroid Hormone Replacement. Thyroid. 2014 Dec;24(12): 1670–751. [PMID: 25266247]

McAninch EA et al. Systemic thyroid hormone status during levothyroxine therapy in hypothyroidism: a systemic review and meta-analysis. J Clin Endocrinol Metab. 2018 Dec; 103(12):4533–42. [PMID: 30124904]

Okosieme O et al. Management of primary hypothyroidism: statement by the British Thyroid Association executive committee. Clin Endocrinol (Oxf). 2016 Jun;84(6):799–808. [PMID: 26010808]

Peeters RP. Subclinical hypothyroidism. N Engl J Med. 2017 Jun 29; 376(26):2556–65. [PMID: 28657873]

Salomo LH et al. Myxoedema coma: an almost forgotten, yet still existing cause of multiorgan failure. BMJ Case Rep. 2014 Jan 30;2014:2013203223. [PMID: 24481020]

HYPERTHYROIDISM (Thyrotoxicosis)

ESSENTIALS OF DIAGNOSIS

▶ Sweating, weight loss or gain, anxiety, palpitations, loose stools, heat intolerance, menstrual irregularity.

▶ Tachycardia; warm, moist skin; stare; tremor.

▶ Graves disease is most common cause of hyperthyroidism; palpable goiter (sometimes with bruit) seen in most patients; ophthalmopathy also common.

▶ Suppressed TSH in primary hyperthyroidism; usually increased T_4, FT_4, T_3, FT_3.

General Considerations

The term "thyrotoxicosis" refers to the clinical manifestations associated with elevated serum levels of T_4 or T_3 that are excessive for the individual (hyperthyroidism). Serum TSH levels are suppressed in primary hyperthyroidism. However, certain drugs and conditions can affect laboratory tests and lead to the erroneous diagnosis of hyperthyroidism in euthyroid individuals (Table 26–4). The causes of hyperthyroidism are many and diverse, as described below.

A. Graves Disease

Graves disease (known as Basedow disease in Europe) is the most common cause of thyrotoxicosis. It is an autoimmune disorder affecting the thyroid gland, characterized by an increase in synthesis and release of thyroid hormones; autoantibodies known as thyroid-stimulating immunoglobulins (TSI) or TSH receptor antibodies bind to the TSH receptor in thyroid cell membranes and stimulate the gland to hyperfunction.

Table 26–4. Factors that can cause aberrations in laboratory tests that may be mistaken for spontaneous clinical primary hyperthyroidism.[1]

High Serum T_4 or T_3	Low Serum TSH
Laboratory error	Laboratory error
Collection vial contains gel barrier for T_3	Autonomous thyroid or thyroid nodule
Acute psychiatric problems (30%)	Biotin supplements
Acute medical illness (eg, acute intermittent porphyria)	Corticosteroid administration (acute)
Acute or chronic active hepatitis, primary biliary cirrhosis	Drugs
AIDS (increased thyroid-binding globulin)	Amphetamines
Autoimmunity	Calcium channel blockers (nifedipine, verapamil)
Familial thyroid-binding abnormalities	Dopamine
Familial resistance to thyroid (Refetoff syndrome)	Dopamine agonists
Pregnancy: morning sickness, hyperemesis gravidarum	Thyroid hormone
Drugs	Elderly euthyroid
Amiodarone	hCG-secreting trophoblastic tumors
Amphetamines	Hypopituitarism
Biotin supplements	Nonthyroidal illness (severe)
Clofibrate	Pregnancy (especially with morning sickness)
Estrogens (oral)	Suppression after recent therapy for hyperthyroidism
Heparin (dialysis method)	TSH variants not detected by commercial assays
Heroin	
Methadone	
Perphenazine	
Tamoxifen	
Thyroid hormone therapy (excessive or factitious)	

[1]True clinical hyperthyroidism may coexist.
hCG, human chorionic gonadotropin; T_4, levothyroxine; T_3, triiodothyronine; TSH, thyroid-stimulating hormone.

Graves disease is much more common in women than in men (8:1), and its onset is usually between the ages of 20 and 40 years. It may be accompanied by infiltrative ophthalmopathy (Graves exophthalmos) and, less commonly, by infiltrative dermopathy (pretibial myxedema). The thymus gland is typically enlarged and serum antinuclear antibody levels are usually elevated. Many patients with Graves disease have a family history of either Graves disease or autoimmune (Hashimoto) thyroiditis.

Dietary iodine supplementation can trigger Graves disease. An increased incidence of Graves disease occurs in countries that have embarked on national programs to fortify commercial salt with potassium iodide; the increase in Graves disease lasts about 4 years. Similarly, patients being treated with potassium iodide or amiodarone (which contains iodine) have an increased risk of developing Graves disease.

Chemotherapy with immune checkpoint inhibitors (ipilimumab, pembrolizumab, tremelimumab, and atezolizumab) can precipitate Graves disease, which must be distinguished from hyperthyroidism from destructive autoimmune thyroiditis (silent thyroiditis), which can be caused by these same medications.

Patients with Graves disease have an increased risk of other systemic autoimmune disorders, including Sjögren syndrome, celiac disease, pernicious anemia, Addison disease, alopecia areata, vitiligo, type 1 diabetes mellitus, hypoparathyroidism, myasthenia gravis, and cardiomyopathy.

B. Toxic Multinodular Goiter and Thyroid Nodules

Autonomous hyperfunctioning thyroid nodules that produce hyperthyroidism are known as toxic multinodular goiter (Plummer disease) and are more prevalent among older adults and in iodine-deficient regions. A single hyperfunctioning nodule can also produce hyperthyroidism. Toxic multinodular goiter and Graves disease may sometimes coexist in the same gland (Marine-Lenhart syndrome). Thyroid cancer is found in about 4.7% of patients with toxic multinodular goiter.

C. Postpartum, Subacute, and Silent Thyroiditis

These conditions cause thyroid inflammation with release of stored hormone. They all produce a variable triphasic course: variable hyperthyroidism is followed by transient euthyroidism, and progresses to hypothyroidism.

Postpartum thyroiditis refers to autoimmune thyroiditis that occurs in the first 12 months postpartum and occasionally after miscarriages. See Thyroiditis, above. About 22% of affected women experience hyperthyroidism followed by hypothyroidism, whereas 30% of such women have isolated thyrotoxicosis and 48% have isolated hypothyroidism. The thyrotoxic phase typically occurs 2–6 weeks postpartum and lasts 2–3 months. Over 80% have antithyroid antibodies. Most women progress to a hypothyroid phase that usually lasts a few months but that can be permanent.

Subacute thyroiditis is also known as "de Quervain" or "granulomatous" thyroiditis. It is typically caused by various viral infections. Women are affected four times more frequently than men. Patients typically experience a viral upper respiratory infection and develop an enlarged and extremely painful thyroid. About 50% of affected patients experience a symptomatic thyrotoxic phase that lasts 3–6 weeks. It is important to differentiate subacute thyroiditis from infectious (suppurative bacterial) thyroiditis. About 10% remain hypothyroid after 1 year. The recurrence rate is 1–4%.

Silent thyroiditis is also known as subacute lymphocytic thyroiditis or "Hashitoxicosis." It can occur spontaneously; women are affected four times more frequently than men. About 50% have antithyroid antibodies. Silent thyroiditis can also be caused by chemotherapeutic agents (such as tyrosine kinase inhibitors; denileukin diftitox; alemtuzumab; interferon-alpha; interleukin-2; and immune checkpoint inhibitors). Other drugs can cause silent thyroiditis, including lithium and amiodarone. In those with spontaneous silent thyroiditis, about 10–20% remain hypothyroid after 1 year. There is a recurrence rate of 5–10%; this rate is higher in Japan.

D. Medication-Induced Hyperthyroidism

1. Amiodarone-induced thyrotoxicosis—Amiodarone is 37% iodine by weight. The half-life of amiodarone and its metabolites is about 100 days. In the short term, amiodarone normally increases the serum TSH, though usually not over 20 milli-international units/L (see Thyroiditis, above). Serum T_4 and FT_4 rise about 40% and may become frankly elevated in clinically euthyroid patients. Meanwhile, serum T_3 levels decline. Due to these short-term changes, it is best to not check thyroid function tests during the first 3 months of therapy with amiodarone, unless clinically indicated. After about 3 months, the serum TSH usually normalizes. Since serum T_4 levels can be misleadingly high, the serum TSH level must be suppressed to diagnose amiodarone-induced thyrotoxicosis. With amiodarone-induced thyrotoxicosis, the serum T_3 or FT_3 is usually high or high-normal. In the United States, amiodarone causes thyrotoxicosis in about 3% of patients taking the drug. In Europe and iodine-deficient geographic areas, amiodarone induces thyrotoxicosis in about 20%. Thyrotoxicosis can occur suddenly at any time during treatment and may even develop several months after it has been discontinued. The manifestations of amiodarone-induced thyrotoxicosis can be missed, particularly since amiodarone tends to cause bradycardia. Therefore, thyroid function tests (TSH, FT_4, T_3) should be checked before starting amiodarone, again at 3–6 months, and then every 6 months (or sooner if clinically indicated).

Amiodarone-induced thyrotoxicosis is categorized as type 1 or type 2; about 27% are mixed type 1–2. Type 1 is caused by the *active* production of excessive thyroid hormone. Type 2 is caused by thyroiditis with the *passive* release of stored thyroid hormone.

2. Iodine-induced hyperthyroidism—This is also known as Jod-Basedow disease. The recommended iodine intake for nonpregnant adults is 150 mcg/day. Higher iodine intake can precipitate hyperthyroidism in patients with nodular goiters, autonomous thyroid nodules, or asymptomatic Graves disease, and less commonly in patients with no detectable underlying thyroid disorder. Common sources of excess iodine include intravenous iodinated radiocontrast dye, certain foods (eg, kelp, nori), topical iodinated antiseptics (eg, povidine iodine), and medications (eg, amiodarone or potassium iodide). Intravenous iodinated radiocontrast dye can rarely induce a painful, destructive subacute thyroiditis, similar to type 2 amiodarone-induced thyrotoxicosis.

3. Tyrosine kinase inhibitors—Silent thyroiditis that releases stored thyroid hormone, resulting in hyperthyroidism, develops in about 3.2% of patients receiving chemotherapy with tyrosine kinase inhibitors (eg, axitinib, sorafenib, sunitinib). While this hyperthyroidism may be subclinical, thyrotoxic crisis has been reported. Hypothyroidism usually follows hyperthyroidism and overall occurs in 19% of patients taking these drugs.

4. Immune checkpoint inhibitor cancer therapy—Immune checkpoint inhibitor therapy directed against either PD-1/PD-L1 or CTLA-4/B7-1/B7-2 can be effective against certain malignancies but frequently precipitates autoimmune adverse reactions. Thyroid autoimmunity commonly causes thyroiditis, hypothyroidism (primary or secondary), or hyperthyroidism from either passive release of thyroid hormone or active production of thyroid hormone (Graves disease), in whom ophthalmopathy has been observed.

E. Pregnancy, hCG-Secreting Trophoblastic Tumors, and Testicular Choriocarcinoma

Human chorionic gonadotropin (hCG) can bind to the thyroid's TSH receptors, so very high levels of serum hCG, particularly during the first 4 months of pregnancy, may cause sufficient receptor activation to cause hyperthyroidism. About 18% of pregnant women have a low serum TSH during pregnancy, but only about 10% of such women have clinical hyperthyroidism that requires treatment. Pregnant women are more likely to have hCG-induced thyrotoxicosis if they have high levels of serum asialo-hCG, a subfraction of hCG that has a greater affinity for TSH receptors. Such women are also more likely to suffer from hyperemesis gravidarum. This condition must be distinguished from true Graves disease in pregnancy, which usually predates conception and may be associated with high serum levels of TSI and antithyroid antibodies or with exophthalmos.

High levels of hCG can also cause thyrotoxicosis in some cases of pregnancies with gestational trophoblastic disease (molar pregnancy, choriocarcinoma). Some such pregnancies have produced thyrotoxic crisis. Men have developed hyperthyroidism from high levels of serum hCG secreted by a testicular choriocarcinoma.

F. Rare Causes of Hyperthyroidism

Thyrotoxicosis factitia is due to intentional or accidental ingestion of excessive amounts of exogenous thyroid hormone. Struma ovarii refers to thyroid tissue contained in about 3% of ovarian dermoid tumors and teratomas. Pituitary TSH hypersecretion by a pituitary thyrotrophe tumor or hyperplasia can rarely cause hyperthyroidism. Serum

TSH is elevated or inappropriately normal in the presence of true thyrotoxicosis. Pituitary hyperplasia may be detected on an MRI as a pituitary enlargement without a discrete adenoma being visible. Metastatic functioning thyroid carcinoma can cause hyperthyroidism in patients with a heavy tumor burden. Recombinant human thyroid-stimulating hormone (rhTSH) can rarely induce hyperthyroidism when it is given prior to radioiodine therapy or scanning for metastatic differentiated thyroid cancer.

► Clinical Findings

A. Symptoms and Signs

Thyrotoxicosis due to any cause can produce nervousness, restlessness, heat intolerance, increased sweating, palpitations, pruritus, fatigue, muscle weakness, muscle cramps, frequent bowel movements, weight change (usually loss), or menstrual irregularities. There may be fine resting finger tremors, moist warm skin, fever, hyperreflexia, fine hair, and onycholysis. Angina or atrial fibrillation may also be present, sometimes in the absence of other thyrotoxic symptoms **(apathetic hyperthyroidism).** Women with **postpartum thyroiditis** are often asymptomatic or experience only minor symptoms, such as palpitations, heat intolerance, and irritability. Chronic thyrotoxicosis may cause osteoporosis. Even subclinical hyperthyroidism (suppressed serum TSH with normal FT_4) may increase the risk of nonvertebral fractures. Clubbing and swelling of the fingers (acropachy) develop rarely. Tetany is a rare presenting symptom; hyperthyroidism causes an increased renal excretion of magnesium, resulting in functional hypoparathyroidism and hypocalcemia.

Thyroid examination in patients with Graves disease usually reveals a diffusely enlarged thyroid, frequently asymmetric, often with a bruit. However, there may be no palpable thyroid enlargement. The thyroid gland in subacute thyroiditis is usually moderately enlarged and tender. There is often dysphagia and pain that can radiate to the jaw or ear. In patients with toxic multinodular goiter, the thyroid usually has palpable nodules. Patients with silent thyroiditis or postpartum thyroiditis have either no palpable goiter or a small, nontender goiter. **Cardiopulmonary manifestations** of thyrotoxicosis commonly include a forceful heartbeat, premature atrial contractions, and sinus tachycardia. Patients often have exertional dyspnea. Atrial fibrillation or atrial tachycardia occurs in about 8% of patients with thyrotoxicosis, more commonly in men, older adults, and those with ischemic or valvular heart disease. The ventricular response from the atrial fibrillation may be difficult to control. Thyrotoxicosis itself can cause a thyrotoxic cardiomyopathy, and the onset of atrial fibrillation can precipitate heart failure. Echocardiogram reveals pulmonary hypertension in 49% of patients with hyperthyroidism; of these, 71% have pulmonary artery hypertension while 29% have pulmonary venous hypertension. Even "subclinical hyperthyroidism" increases the risk for atrial fibrillation and overall mortality. Hemodynamic abnormalities and pulmonary hypertension are reversible with restoration of euthyroidism.

Thyrotoxic crisis or "storm" is an extreme form of severe thyrotoxicosis that is an immediate threat to life. It may be triggered by stressful illness, thyroid surgery, or RAI administration. Its manifestations typically include marked agitation or delirium, very high fever, severe tachycardia, vomiting, diarrhea, and dehydration. Cardiac arrhythmias, heart failure, and myocardial infarction are possible complications.

Eye manifestations that occur with hyperthyroidism of any etiology include: upper eyelid retraction, lid lag with downward gaze, and a staring appearance. See Thyroid Eye Disease, Chapter 7. Thyroid-associated ophthalmopathy with exophthalmos is clinically apparent in 20–40% of patients with Graves disease and some cases of amiodarone-induced thyrotoxicosis. Aggravation of Graves eye disease has occurred after treatment with radioiodine or during therapy with thiazolidinediones (eg, pioglitazone). About 5–10% of patients experience more severe exophthalmos, with the eye being pushed forward by increased retro-orbital fat and eye muscles that have been thickened by lymphocytic infiltration. Such patients can experience diplopia from extraocular muscle entrapment. The severity of eye disease is not closely correlated with the severity of thyrotoxicosis.

Exophthalmometry should be performed on all patients with Graves disease to document their degree of exophthalmos and detect progression of orbitopathy. The protrusion of the eye beyond the orbital rim is measured with a prism instrument (Hertel exophthalmometer). Maximum normal eye protrusion varies between kindreds and races, being about 24 mm for blacks, 20 mm for whites, and 18 mm for Asians.

It is important to determine whether thyroid-associated orbitopathy is in an acute stage of inflammation versus a stable "burned out" stage with exophthalmos. It is also important to distinguish active eye disease from congenital proptosis or asymmetry in orbital protrusion.

Graves dermopathy (pretibial myxedema) occurs in about 3% of patients with Graves disease. It usually affects the pretibial region, but can also affect the dorsal forearms and wrists and dorsum of the feet. It is more common in patients with high levels of serum TSI and severe Graves ophthalmopathy. Glycosaminoglycans accumulation and lymphoid infiltration occur in affected skin, which becomes erythematous with a thickened, rough texture. Elephantiasis of the legs is a rare complication.

Thyroid acropachy is an extreme and unusual manifestation of Graves disease. It presents with digital clubbing, swelling of fingers and toes, and radiographic findings of periostitis involving phalangeal and metacarpal bones. Extremity skin can become very thickened, resembling elephantiasis. Thyroid acropachy is ordinarily associated with ophthalmopathy and thyroid dermopathy. Most affected patients are smokers.

Hyperthyroidism during pregnancy has a prevalence of about 0.2%. It may commence before conception or emerge during pregnancy, particularly the first trimester. Pregnancy can have a beneficial effect on the thyrotoxicosis of Graves disease, with decreasing antibody titers and decreasing serum T_4 levels as the pregnancy advances; about 30% of affected women experience a remission by late in the second trimester. However, undiagnosed or undertreated hyperthyroidism in pregnancy carries an increased risk of miscarriage, preeclampsia-eclampsia, preterm delivery, abruptio placenta, maternal heart failure, and thyrotoxic crisis (thyroid storm) (see Thyroid Disease, Chapter 19). Such thyrotoxic crisis can be precipitated by trauma, infection, surgery, or delivery and confers a fetal/maternal mortality rate of about 25%.

Hypokalemic periodic paralysis occurs in about 15% of Asian or Native American men with thyrotoxicosis. It usually presents abruptly with symmetric flaccid paralysis (and few thyrotoxic symptoms), often after intravenous dextrose, oral carbohydrate, or vigorous exercise. Attacks last 7–72 hours.

B. Laboratory Findings

Serum FT_4, T_3, FT_3, T_4, thyroid resin uptake, and FT_4 index are all usually increased. Sometimes the FT_4 level may be normal but with an elevated serum T_3 (T_3 toxicosis). The severity of the elevation of serum FT_4 and FT_3 levels does not always correlate with the severity of thyrotoxic manifestations; patients with thyrotoxic crisis tend to have serum thyroid levels that are not significantly higher than those with less pronounced symptoms. Serum T_3 can be misleadingly elevated when blood is collected in tubes using a gel barrier, which causes certain immunoassays to report falsely elevated serum total T_3 levels in 24% of normal patients. Serum T_4 or T_3 can be elevated in other nonthyroidal conditions (Table 26–4).

Serum TSH is suppressed in hyperthyroidism (except in the very rare cases of pituitary inappropriate secretion of thyrotropin). Serum TSH may be misleadingly low in other nonthyroidal conditions (Table 26–4). The term "**subclinical hyperthyroidism**" is used to describe asymptomatic individuals with a low serum TSH but normal serum levels of FT_4 and T_3.

Hyperthyroidism can cause hypercalcemia, increased liver enzymes, increased alkaline phosphatase, anemia, and decreased neutrophils. Hypokalemia and hypophosphatemia occur in thyrotoxic periodic paralysis. Hyperthyroidism also increases urinary magnesium excretion, which can lead to hypomagnesemia, resulting in functional hypoparathyroidism with hypocalcemia.

Problems of diagnosis occur in patients with acute psychiatric disorders; about 30% of these patients have elevated serum T_4 levels without clinical thyrotoxicosis. The TSH is not usually suppressed, distinguishing psychiatric disorder from true hyperthyroidism. T_4 levels return to normal gradually.

In **Graves disease**, serum TSI (TSHrAb) is usually detectable (65%). Antithyroperoxidase or antithyroglobulin antibodies are usually elevated but are nonspecific. Serum antinuclear antibodies are also usually elevated without any evidence of SLE or other rheumatologic disease.

With **subacute thyroiditis**, patients often have an increased WBC, ESR, and C-reactive protein. About 25% have antithyroid antibodies (usually in low titer) and serum TSI (TSHrAb) levels are normal. Patients with iodine-induced hyperthyroidism also have undetectable serum TSI (or TSHrAb), an absence of serum antithyroperoxidase antibodies, and an elevated urinary iodine concentration. In thyrotoxicosis factitia, serum thyroglobulin levels are low, distinguishing it from other causes of hyperthyroidism.

With **hyperthyroidism during pregnancy**, women have an elevated serum total T_4 and FT_4 while the TSH is suppressed. However, about 18% of normal pregnant women have a low serum TSH. An apparent lack of full TSH suppression in hyperthyroidism can be seen due to misidentification of hCG as TSH in certain assays. The serum FT_4 assay is difficult in pregnancy. Although the serum T_4 is elevated in most pregnant women, values over 20 mcg/dL (257 nmol/L) are encountered only in hyperthyroidism. On treatment, serum total T_4 levels during pregnancy should be kept at about 1.5 × the pre-pregnancy level. The T_3 resin uptake, which is low in normal pregnancy because of high thyroxine-binding globulin (TBG) concentration, is normal or high in thyrotoxic persons.

Since high levels of T_4 and FT_4 are normally seen in patients taking **amiodarone, a** suppressed TSH must be present along with a greatly elevated T_4 (greater than 20 mcg/dL [257 nmol/L]) or T_3 (greater than 200 ng/dL [3.1 nmol/L]) in order to diagnose hyperthyroidism. In type 1 amiodarone-induced thyrotoxicosis, the presence of proptosis and serum TSI (TSHrAb) is diagnostic. In type 2 amiodarone-induced thyrotoxicosis, serum levels of interleukin-6 (IL-6) are usually quite elevated.

C. Radioisotope Uptake and Imaging

Note: *All radioisotope testing is contraindicated during pregnancy or breastfeeding.*

Radioiodine (RAI) uptake and scanning can be helpful in determining the cause of hyperthyroidism. RAI uptake and scanning is not necessary for diagnosis in patients with obvious Graves disease who have elevated serum TSI or associated Graves ophthalmopathy. Women should ideally have the RAI scan extended to include the pelvis in order to screen for concomitant struma ovarii (rare). A high RAI uptake is seen in Graves disease and toxic nodular goiter. Patients with type 1 amiodarone-induced thyrotoxicosis have RAI uptake that is usually detectable. A low RAI uptake is also characteristic of iodine-induced hyperthyroidism and thyroiditis (subacute, silent, or postpartum), distinguishing them from Graves disease. In type 2 amiodarone-induced thyrotoxicosis, thyroid RAI uptake is usually below 3%.

Patients with Graves disease have increased or normal uptake of **technetium (Tc-99m) pertechnetate**, whereas those with thyrotoxicosis from thyroiditis (silent, subacute, postpartum) have reduced uptake. Technetium (Tc-99m) pertechnetate mimics radioiodine scanning but is more convenient, costs less, and confers less radiation exposure.

Thyroid ultrasound can be helpful in patients with hyperthyroidism, particularly in patients with palpable thyroid nodules. Thyroid ultrasound shows a variably heterogeneous, hypoechoic gland in thyroiditis. Color flow Doppler sonography is helpful to distinguish type 1 amiodarone-induced thyrotoxicosis (normal to increased blood flow velocity and vascularity) from type 2 amiodarone-induced thyrotoxicosis (reduced vascularity).

99mTc-sestamibi scanning usually shows normal or increased uptake with type 1 amiodarone-induced thyrotoxicosis and decreased uptake in type 2.

MRI and CT scanning of the orbits are the imaging methods of choice to visualize Graves ophthalmopathy affecting the extraocular muscles. Imaging is required only in severe or unilateral cases or in euthyroid exophthalmos that must be distinguished from orbital pseudotumor, tumors, and other lesions.

▶ Differential Diagnosis

True thyrotoxicosis must be distinguished from those conditions that elevate serum T_4 and T_3 or suppress serum TSH without affecting clinical status (see Table 26–4). Serum TSH is commonly suppressed in early pregnancy and only about 10% of pregnant women with a low TSH have clinical hyperthyroidism.

Some states of hypermetabolism without thyrotoxicosis—notably severe anemia, leukemia, polycythemia, cancer, and pheochromocytoma—rarely cause confusion. Acromegaly may also produce tachycardia, sweating, and thyroid enlargement. Appropriate laboratory tests will easily distinguish these entities.

The differential diagnosis for thyroid-associated ophthalmopathy includes an orbital tumor (eg, lymphoma) or pseudotumor. Ocular myasthenia gravis is another autoimmune condition that occurs more commonly in Graves disease but is usually mild, often with unilateral eye involvement. Acetylcholinesterase receptor antibody (AChR Ab) levels are elevated in only 36% of such patients, and a thymoma is present in 9%.

Diabetes mellitus and Addison disease may coexist with thyrotoxicosis and can aggravate the weight loss, fatigue, and muscle weakness seen with hyperthyroidism.

▶ Complications

Hypercalcemia, osteoporosis, and nephrocalcinosis may occur in hyperthyroidism. Decreased libido, erectile dysfunction, diminished sperm motility, and gynecomastia may be noted in men. Other complications include cardiac arrhythmias and heart failure, thyroid crisis, ophthalmopathy, dermopathy, and thyrotoxic hypokalemic periodic paralysis.

▶ Treatment

A. Treatment of Graves Disease

1. Propranolol—Propranolol is generally used for symptomatic relief of tachycardia, tremor, diaphoresis, and anxiety until the hyperthyroidism is resolved. It is the initial treatment of choice for thyrotoxic crisis and effectively treats thyrotoxic hypokalemic periodic paralysis. Propranolol has no effect on thyroid hormone secretion. Treatment is usually begun with propranolol ER 60 mg orally once or twice daily, with dosage increases every 2–3 days to a maximum daily dose of 320 mg. Propranolol ER is initially given every 12 hours for patients with severe hyperthyroidism, due to accelerated metabolism of the propranolol; it may be given once daily as hyperthyroidism improves.

2. Thiourea drugs—Methimazole or propylthiouracil is generally used for young adults or patients with mild thyrotoxicosis, small goiters, or fear of isotopes. See Treatment of Hyperthyroidism during Pregnancy-Planning, Pregnancy, and Lactation, below. Elderly patients usually respond particularly well. These drugs are also useful for preparing hyperthyroid patients for surgery and elderly patients for RAI treatment. When thiourea therapy is discontinued, there is a high recurrence rate for hyperthyroidism (about 50%). A better likelihood of long-term remission is seen in patients with small goiters, mild hyperthyroidism, those requiring small doses of thiourea, and those with serum TSI (TSHrAb) less than 2 milli-units/L. Patients whose antithyroperoxidase and antithyroglobulin antibodies remain low after 2 years of therapy have been reported to have only a 10% rate of relapse. Some clinicians advocate RAI or surgery for patients with Graves disease who continue to require thiourea therapy after 1 year. However, there should be no rush to discontinue thiourea therapy that may be continued long term for patients who are tolerating it well.

All patients receiving thiourea therapy must be informed of the danger of agranulocytosis or pancytopenia and the need to stop the drug and seek medical attention immediately with the onset of any infection or unusual bleeding. Agranulocytosis (defined as an absolute neutrophil count below 500/mcL) or pancytopenia usually occurs abruptly in about 0.4% of patients taking either methimazole or propylthiouracil. Over 70% of agranulocytosis cases occur within the first 60 days and nearly 85% within 90 days of commencing therapy, but continued long-term vigilance for this side effect is required. About half the cases are discovered because of fever, pharyngitis, or bleeding, but the other cases are discovered with routine complete blood counts. There is a genetic tendency to develop agranulocytosis with thiourea therapy; if a close relative has had this adverse reaction, other therapies should be considered. Agranulocytosis generally remits spontaneously with discontinuation of the thiourea and during antibiotic treatment. Recovery has not been improved by filgrastim (granulocyte colony-stimulating factor [G-CSF]). Surveillance of the WBC can be done when blood is drawn to check thyroid levels during the first few months of treatment. Such surveillance may be helpful, since some cases of agranulocytosis occur gradually and many cases may be discovered while the patient is still asymptomatic.

Other side effects common to thiourea drugs include pruritus, allergic dermatitis, nausea, and dyspepsia. Antihistamines may control mild pruritus without discontinuation of the drug. Since the two thiourea drugs are similar, patients who have a major allergic reaction to one should not be given the other.

The patient may become clinically hypothyroid for 2 weeks or more before TSH levels rise, the pituitary gland having been suppressed by the preceding hyperthyroidism. Therefore, the patient's changing thyroid status is best monitored clinically and with serum FT_4 levels. Rapid growth of the goiter usually occurs if prolonged hypothyroidism is allowed to develop; the goiter may sometimes become massive but usually regresses rapidly with reduction or cessation of thiourea therapy or with thyroid hormone replacement.

A. Methimazole—Except during the first trimester of pregnancy, methimazole is generally preferred over propylthiouracil, since methimazole is more convenient to use and is less likely to cause fulminant hepatic necrosis. Methimazole therapy is also less likely to cause ^{131}I treatment failure. Methimazole is given orally in initial doses of 30–60 mg once daily. Some patients with very mild hyperthyroidism may respond well to smaller initial doses of methimazole (10–20 mg daily). Methimazole may also be administered twice daily to reduce the likelihood of gastrointestinal upset. Rare complications peculiar to methimazole include serum sickness, cholestatic jaundice, alopecia, nephrotic syndrome, hypoglycemia, and loss of taste. Methimazole use in pregnancy has been associated with an increased risk of major fetal anomalies (4.1% vs 2.1% in controls). If methimazole is used during pregnancy or breastfeeding, the dose should not exceed 20 mg daily. The dosage is reduced as manifestations of hyperthyroidism resolve and as the FT_4 level falls toward normal. For patients receiving ^{131}I therapy, methimazole is discontinued 4 days prior to receiving the ^{131}I and is resumed at a lower dose 3 days afterward to avoid recurrence of hyperthyroidism. Following ^{131}I therapy, the dose of methimazole is gradually reduced according to frequent thyroid function testing; most patients are able to discontinue methimazole within 1–3 months following RAI therapy.

B. Propylthiouracil—Initially, propylthiouracil is given orally in doses of 300–600 mg daily in four divided doses. The dosage and frequency of administration are reduced as symptoms of hyperthyroidism resolve and the FT_4 level approaches normal. Rare complications peculiar to propylthiouracil include arthritis, lupus, aplastic anemia, thrombocytopenia, and hypoprothrombinemia. With propylthiouracil, acute hepatitis occurs rarely and is treated with prednisone. Acute liver failure occurs in about 1 in 10,000 patients, making this a second-line drug, usually reserved for pregnancy, since it is not known to cause fetal anomalies. During pregnancy, the dose of propylthiouracil is kept below 200 mg/day to avoid goitrous hypothyroidism in the infant; the patient may be switched to methimazole in the second trimester.

3. Iodinated contrast agents—These agents provide effective temporary treatment for thyrotoxicosis of any cause. Iopanoic acid (Telepaque) or ipodate sodium (Bilivist, Oragrafin) is given orally in a dosage of 500 mg twice daily for 3 days, then 500 mg once daily. These agents inhibit peripheral 5′-monodeiodination of T_4, thereby blocking its conversion to active T_3. Within 24 hours, serum T_3 levels fall an average of 62%. For patients with Graves disease, methimazole is begun first to block iodine organification; the next day, ipodate sodium or iopanoic acid may be added. The iodinated contrast agents are particularly useful for patients who are symptomatically very thyrotoxic. They offer a therapeutic option for patients with T_4 overdosage, subacute thyroiditis, and amiodarone-induced thyrotoxicosis; for those intolerant to thioureas; and for newborns with thyrotoxicosis (due to maternal Graves disease). Treatment periods of 8 months or more are possible, but efficacy tends to wane with time. In Graves disease, thyroid RAI uptake may be suppressed during treatment but typically returns to pretreatment uptake by 7 days after discontinuation of the drug, allowing ^{131}I treatment.

4. Lithium carbonate—Thioureas are greatly preferred over lithium for the medical treatment of hyperthyroidism in Graves disease. However, lithium may be used effectively in cases of methimazole or propylthiouracil-induced hepatic toxicity or leukopenia, while the patient receives supportive treatment. The regimen for lithium carbonate is 500–750 mg/day orally in divided doses. Lithium should not be used during pregnancy. Most patients require concurrent treatment with propranolol and sometimes prednisone.

5. Radioactive iodine (^{131}I, RAI)—The administration of ^{131}I is an excellent method of destroying overactive thyroid tissue (either diffuse or toxic nodular goiter). Adolescent and adult patients who have been treated with RAI in adulthood do not have an increased risk of subsequent thyroid cancer, leukemia, or other malignancies. Children born to parents previously treated with ^{131}I show no increase in rates of congenital abnormalities.

Precautions: Because radiation is harmful to the fetus and children, *RAI should not be given to pregnant or lactating women or to mothers who lack childcare. Women are advised to avoid pregnancy for at least 4 months following ^{131}I therapy. A pregnancy test should be obtained within 48 hours before therapy for any woman with childbearing potential. Men have been found to have abnormal spermatozoa for up to 6 months following ^{131}I therapy and are advised to use contraceptive methods during that time.*

Patients may receive ^{131}I while being symptomatically treated with propranolol ER, which is then reduced in dosage as hyperthyroidism resolves. A higher rate of ^{131}I treatment failure has been reported in patients with Graves disease who have been receiving methimazole or propylthiouracil. However, therapy with ^{131}I will usually be effective if the methimazole is discontinued at least 3–4 days before RAI therapy and if the therapeutic dosage of ^{131}I is adjusted (upward) according to RAI uptake on the pretherapy scan. Prior to ^{131}I therapy, patients are instructed against receiving intravenous iodinated contrast and should consume a low-iodine diet.

The presence of Graves ophthalmopathy is a relative contraindication to ^{131}I therapy. Following ^{131}I treatment for hyperthyroidism, Graves ophthalmopathy appears or worsens in 15% of patients (23% in smokers and 6% in nonsmokers) and improves in none, whereas during treatment with methimazole, ophthalmopathy worsens in 3% and improves in 2% of patients. Among patients receiving prednisone following ^{131}I treatment, preexistent ophthalmopathy worsens in none and improves in 67%. Therefore, patients with Graves ophthalmopathy who are to be treated with radioiodine should be considered for prophylactic prednisone (20–40 mg/day) for 2 months following administration of ^{131}I, particularly in patients who have severe orbital involvement.

Smoking increases the risk of having a flare in ophthalmopathy following ^{131}I treatment and also reduces the effectiveness of prednisone treatment. Patients who smoke are strongly encouraged to quit prior to RAI treatment. Smokers receiving RAI should be considered for prophylactic prednisone (see above).

FT_4 levels may sometimes drop within 2 months after ^{131}I treatment, but then rise again to thyrotoxic levels, at which time thyroid RAI uptake is low. This phenomenon is caused by a release of stored thyroid hormone from injured thyroid cells and does not indicate a treatment failure. In fact, serum FT_4 then falls abruptly to hypothyroid levels.

There is a high incidence of hypothyroidism in the months to years after ^{131}I, even when low activities are given. Patients with Graves disease treated with ^{131}I also have an increased lifetime risk of developing hyperparathyroidism, particularly when radioiodine therapy was administered in childhood or adolescence. Lifelong clinical follow-up is mandatory, with measurements of serum TSH, FT_4, and calcium when indicated.

6. Thyroid surgery—Surgery may be indicated for patients with Graves disease who do not wish to have radioiodine therapy, for those with an intolerance to thioureas, and women planning pregnancy in the near future. The surgical procedure of choice is a total resection of one lobe and a subtotal resection of the other lobe, leaving about 4 g of thyroid tissue (Hartley–Dunhill operation). Total thyroidectomy of both lobes poses an increased risk of hypoparathyroidism and damage to the recurrent laryngeal nerves. See below for surgical treatment of Graves disease during pregnancy.

Patients are ordinarily rendered euthyroid preoperatively with a thiourea drug. Propranolol ER is given orally at initial doses of 60–80 mg twice daily and increased every 2–3 days until the heart rate is less than 90 beats per minute. Propranolol is continued until the serum T_3 (or free T_3) is normal preoperatively. If a patient undergoes surgery while thyrotoxic, larger doses of propranolol are given perioperatively to reduce the likelihood of thyroid crisis. Ipodate sodium or iopanoic acid (500 mg orally twice daily) may be used in addition to a thiourea to accelerate the decline in serum T_3. The patient should be euthyroid by the time of surgery.

To reduce thyroid vascularity preoperatively, the patient may be treated for 3–10 days preoperatively with oral potassium iodide 25–50 mg (eg, ThyroShield 65 mg/mL, 0.5 mL, or SSKI 1 g/mL, 1 drop) three times daily. However, preoperative potassium iodide often increases the volume of the thyroid, so the requirement for preoperative potassium iodide for Graves disease is debatable. Preoperative iodide supplementation is not recommended prior to surgery for multinodular goiter. Alternatively, iodinated radiocontrast agents (eg, iopanoic acid 500 mg orally twice daily) may be given for 1 week preoperatively.

Surgical morbidity includes possible damage to a recurrent laryngeal nerve, with resultant vocal cord paralysis. If both recurrent laryngeal nerves are damaged, airway obstruction may develop, and the patient may require intubation and tracheostomy. Hypoparathyroidism also occurs; serum calcium levels must be checked postoperatively. Patients should be admitted for thyroidectomy surgery for at least an overnight observation period.

B. Treatment of Toxic Solitary Thyroid Nodules

Toxic solitary thyroid nodules are usually benign but may rarely be malignant. If a nonsurgical therapy is elected, the nodule should be evaluated with a fine-needle aspiration

(FNA) biopsy. **Medical therapy** for hyperthyroidism caused by a single hyperfunctioning thyroid nodule may be treated symptomatically with propranolol ER and methimazole or propylthiouracil, as in Graves disease (see above). Patients who tolerate methimazole well may elect to continue it for long-term therapy. The dose of methimazole should be adjusted to keep the TSH slightly suppressed, so the risk of TSH-stimulated growth of the nodule is reduced. **Surgery** is usually recommended for patients under age 40 years, for healthy older patients with toxic solitary thyroid nodules, and for nodules that are suspicious for malignancy. Patients are made euthyroid with a thiourea preoperatively and given several days of iodine, ipodate sodium, or iopanoic acid before surgery. Postoperative hypothyroidism usually resolves spontaneously, but permanent hypothyroidism occurs in about 14% of patients by 6 years after surgery. **Radioiodine (^{131}I) therapy** may be offered to patients with a toxic solitary nodule who are over age 40 or in poor health. A pregnancy test should be obtained within 48 before therapy for any premenopausal woman. RAI should not be given to women with Graves disease within 3 months prior to a planned conception. If the patient has been receiving methimazole preparatory to ^{131}I, the TSH should be kept slightly suppressed in order to reduce the uptake of ^{131}I by the normal thyroid. Nevertheless, permanent hypothyroidism occurs in about one-third of patients by 8 years after ^{131}I therapy. The nodule remains palpable in 50% and may grow in 10% of patients after ^{131}I.

C. Treatment of Toxic Nodular Goiter

Medical therapy for patients with toxic nodular goiter consists of propranolol ER (while hyperthyroid) and a thiourea, as in Graves disease. Thioureas (methimazole or propylthiouracil) reverse hyperthyroidism but do not shrink the goiter. There is a 95% recurrence rate if the drug is stopped.

Surgery is the definitive treatment for patients with large toxic nodular goiter, following therapy with a thiourea to render them euthyroid. Surgery is particularly indicated to relieve pressure symptoms or for cosmetic indications. Patients with toxic nodular goiter are not treated preoperatively with potassium iodide. Total or near-total thyroidectomy is recommended, since surgical pathology reveals unsuspected differentiated thyroid cancer in 18.3% of cases.

Radioiodine (RAI, ^{131}I) therapy may be used to treat patients with toxic nodular goiter. See **Precautions** for RAI use, above. Any suspicious nodules should be evaluated beforehand for malignancy with FNA cytology. Patients are rendered euthyroid with methimazole, which is stopped 3–4 days before a repeat RAI therapy.

Meanwhile, the patient follows a low-iodine diet in order to enhance the thyroid gland's uptake of RAI, which may be relatively low in this condition (compared to Graves disease). Relatively high doses of ^{131}I are usually required; hypothyroidism or recurrent thyrotoxicosis typically occurs, so patients must be monitored closely. Peculiarly, in about 5% of patients with diffusely nodular toxic goiter, the administration of ^{131}I therapy may induce Graves disease. Also, Graves eye disease has occurred rarely following ^{131}I therapy for multinodular goiter.

D. Treatment of Hyperthyroidism from Thyroiditis

Patients with thyroiditis (subacute, postpartum, or silent) are treated with propranolol during the hyperthyroid phase, which usually subsides spontaneously within weeks to months. For symptomatic relief, begin propranolol ER 60–80 mg twice daily and increase every 3 days until the heart rate is less than 90 beats per minute. Ipodate sodium or iopanoic acid, 500 mg orally daily, promptly corrects elevated T_3 levels and is continued for 15–60 days until the serum FT_4 level normalizes. Thioureas are ineffective, since thyroid hormone production is actually low in this condition. Patients are monitored carefully for the development of hypothyroidism and treated with levothyroxine as needed. With subacute thyroiditis, pain can usually be managed with NSAIDs and corticosteroids, but opioid analgesics are sometimes required.

E. Treatment of Hyperthyroidism During Pregnancy-Planning, Pregnancy, and Lactation

Both men and women with Graves disease who are planning pregnancy should not have RAI treatment within about 4 months of conception. Women who are planning to become pregnant are encouraged to consider definitive therapy with RAI or surgery well before conception. See **Precautions** for RAI use, above. Dietary iodine must not be restricted for such women. There is an increased risk of fetal anomalies associated with methimazole in the first trimester. Therefore, women who are being treated with a thiourea should be treated with propylthiouracil through the first trimester and then switched to methimazole (see Thiourea drugs, above). Thiourea should be given in the smallest dose possible, permitting mild subclinical hyperthyroidism to occur, since it is usually well tolerated. About 30% of women with Graves disease experience a remission by the late second trimester.

Both propylthiouracil and methimazole cross the placenta and can induce hypothyroidism, with fetal TSH hypersecretion and goiter. Fetal ultrasound at 20–32 weeks gestation can visualize any fetal goiter, allowing fetal thyroid dysfunction to be diagnosed and treated. Thyroid hormone administration to the mother does not prevent hypothyroidism in the fetus, since T_4 and T_3 do not freely cross the placenta. Fetal hypothyroidism is rare if the mother's hyperthyroidism is controlled with small daily doses of propylthiouracil (50–150 mg/day orally) or methimazole (5–15 mg/day orally). Serum total T_4 levels during pregnancy should be kept at about $1.5 \times$ the prepregnancy level. Maternal serum TSI levels over 500% at term predict an increased risk of neonatal Graves disease in the infant.

Subtotal thyroidectomy is indicated for pregnant women with Graves disease or for fertile women of reproductive age who are sexually active and decline contraceptives, under the following circumstances: (1) severe adverse reaction to thioureas; (2) high dosage requirement for thioureas (methimazole greater than or equal to 30 mg/day or propylthiouracil greater than or equal to 450 mg/day); or (3) uncontrolled hyperthyroidism due to nonadherence to thiourea therapy. Surgery is best performed during the second trimester.

Both methimazole and propylthiouracil are secreted in breast milk, but not in amounts that affect the infant's thyroid hormone levels. No adverse reactions to these drugs (eg, rash, hepatic dysfunction, leukopenia) have been reported in breast-fed infants. Recommended doses are less than or equal to 20 mg orally daily for methimazole and less than or equal to 450 mg orally (in divided doses) daily for propylthiouracil. It is recommended that the medication be taken just after breastfeeding.

F. Treatment of Amiodarone-Induced Thyrotoxicosis

Patients with either type 1 or type 2 amiodarone-induced thyrotoxicosis require treatment with propranolol ER for symptomatic relief and methimazole 30 mg orally daily. After two doses of methimazole, iopanoic acid or sodium ipodate may be added to the regimen to further block conversion of T_4 to T_3; the recommended dosage for each is 500 mg orally twice daily for 3 days, followed by 500 mg once daily until thyrotoxicosis is resolved. If iopanoic acid or sodium ipodate is not available, the alternative is potassium perchlorate; it is given in doses of less than or equal to 1000 mg daily (in divided doses) for a course not to exceed 30 days in order to avoid the complication of aplastic anemia. Amiodarone may be withdrawn but this does not have a significant therapeutic impact for several months because of its long half-life. For patients with type 1 amiodarone-induced thyrotoxicosis, therapy with ^{131}I may be successful, but only for those with sufficient RAI uptake. Patients with clear-cut type 2 amiodarone-induced thyrotoxicosis are usually also treated with prednisone at an initial dose of about 0.5–0.7 mg/kg orally daily; that dose of prednisone is continued for about 2 weeks and then slowly tapered and finally withdrawn after about 3 months. Subtotal thyroidectomy should be considered for patients with amiodarone-induced thyrotoxicosis that is resistant to treatment.

G. Treatment of Complications

1. Thyroid-associated orbitopathy—[131]I treatment can "flare" thyroid-associated orbitopathy (see Radioactive iodine, above). Thyroid-associated orbitopathy can also be aggravated by thiazolidinediones (eg, pioglitazone, rosiglitazone); these oral diabetic agents should be avoided or withdrawn in patients with Graves disease. Patients with mild orbitopathy may be treated with selenium 100 mcg orally twice daily, which may slow its progression.

For active thyroid-associated orbitopathy, therapy with intravenous methylprednisolone, begun promptly, is superior to oral prednisone. Methylprednisolone is given in intravenous pulses, 500 mg weekly for 6 weeks, and then 250 mg weekly for 6 weeks. Oral prednisone, if chosen for treatment, must be given promptly in doses of 40–60 mg/day orally, with dosage reduction over several weeks. Higher initial prednisone doses of 80–120 mg/day are used when there is optic nerve compression. Prednisone alleviates acute eye symptoms in 64% of nonsmokers but in only 14% of smokers.

Patients with corticosteroid-resistant acute Graves ophthalmopathy may also be treated with monoclonal antibody drugs that reduce immune-mediated inflammation.

Teprotumumab, an experimental drug, or tocilizumab are administered intravenously, whereas rituximab may be given by retro-orbital injections.

Progressive active exophthalmos may be treated with retrobulbar radiation therapy over 2 weeks to the extraocular muscles, avoiding the cornea and lens. Prednisone in high doses is given concurrently. Patients who respond well to orbital radiation include those with signs of acute inflammation, recent exophthalmos (less than 6 months), or optic nerve compression. Patients with chronic proptosis and orbital muscle restriction respond less well. Retrobulbar radiation does not cause cataracts or tumors; however, it can cause radiation-induced retinopathy (usually subclinical) in about 5% of patients overall, mostly in patients with diabetes.

For severe cases, orbital decompression surgery may save vision, though diplopia often persists postoperatively. General eye protective measures include wearing glasses to protect the protruding eye and taping the lids shut during sleep if corneal drying is a problem. Methylcellulose drops and gels ("artificial tears") may also help. Tarsorrhaphy or canthoplasty can frequently help protect the cornea and provide improved appearance. Hypothyroidism and hyperthyroidism must be treated promptly.

2. Cardiac complications—

A. Sinus tachycardia—Treatment consists of treating the thyrotoxicosis. A beta-blocker such as propranolol is used in the interim unless there is an associated cardiomyopathy.

B. Atrial fibrillation—Hyperthyroidism must be treated immediately. Other drugs, including digoxin, beta-blockers, and anticoagulants, may be required. Electrical cardioversion is unlikely to convert atrial fibrillation to normal sinus rhythm while the patient is thyrotoxic. Spontaneous conversion to normal sinus rhythm occurs in 62% of patients with return of euthyroidism, but that likelihood decreases with age. Following conversion to euthyroidism, there is a 60% chance that atrial fibrillation will recur, despite normal thyroid function tests. Those with persistent atrial fibrillation may have elective cardioversion following anticoagulation 4 months after resolution of hyperthyroidism.

(1) Digoxin—Digoxin is used to slow a fast ventricular response to thyrotoxic atrial fibrillation; it must be used in larger than normal doses. Digoxin doses are reduced as hyperthyroidism is corrected.

(2) Beta-blockers—Beta-blockers may also reduce the ventricular rate, but they must be used with caution—particularly in patients with heart failure with reduced ejection fraction—since their negative inotropic effect may precipitate overt heart failure. Therefore, an initial trial of a short-duration beta-blocker should be considered, such as esmolol intravenously. If a beta-blocker is used, doses of digoxin must be reduced.

(3) Anticoagulants—The doses of warfarin required in thyrotoxicosis are smaller than normal because of an accelerated plasma clearance of vitamin K–dependent clotting factors. Higher warfarin doses are usually required as hyperthyroidism subsides. Dabigatran malabsorption has been reported in thyrotoxicosis-induced diarrhea.

C. Heart failure—Thyrotoxicosis can cause high-output heart failure due to extreme tachycardia, cardiomyopathy, or both. Very aggressive treatment of the hyperthyroidism is required in either case.

Heart failure may also occur as a result of low-output dilated cardiomyopathy. It is uncommon and may be caused by an idiosyncratic severe toxic effect of hyperthyroidism upon certain hearts. Cardiomyopathy may occur at any age and without preexisting cardiac disease. See Chapter 10 for treatment of heart failure and dilated cardiomyopathy. The patient should be rendered euthyroid. However, the heart failure usually persists despite correction of the hyperthyroidism.

D. Apathetic hyperthyroidism—Apathetic hyperthyroidism may present with angina pectoris. Treatment is directed at reversing the hyperthyroidism as well as providing standard antianginal therapy. PCI or CABG can often be avoided by prompt diagnosis and treatment.

3. Thyroid crisis or "storm"—A thiourea drug is given (eg, methimazole, 15–25 mg orally every 6 hours, or propylthiouracil, 150–250 mg orally every 6 hours). Ipodate sodium (500 mg/day orally) can be helpful if begun 1 hour after the first dose of thiourea. Iodide is given 1 hour later as potassium iodide (10 drops three times daily orally). Propranolol is given (cautiously in the presence of heart failure; see above) in a dosage of 0.5–2 mg intravenously every 4 hours or 20–120 mg orally every 6 hours. Hydrocortisone is usually given in doses of 50 mg orally every 6 hours, with rapid dosage reduction as the clinical situation improves. Aspirin is avoided since it displaces T_4 from thyroxine-binding globulin (TBG), raising FT_4 serum levels. Definitive treatment with ^{131}I or surgery is delayed until the patient is euthyroid.

4. Hyperthyroidism from postpartum thyroiditis—Propranolol ER is given during the hyperthyroid phase followed by levothyroxine during the hypothyroidism phase.

5. Graves dermopathy—Treatment involves application of a topical corticosteroid (eg, fluocinolone) with nocturnal plastic occlusive dressings. Compression stockings may improve any associated edema.

6. Thyrotoxic hypokalemic periodic paralysis—Sudden symmetric flaccid paralysis, along with hypokalemia and hypophosphatemia, can occur with hyperthyroidism despite few, if any, of the classic signs of thyrotoxicosis. It is most prevalent in Asian and Native Americans with hyperthyroidism and is 30 times more common in men than women. Therapy with oral propranolol, 3 mg/kg in divided doses, normalizes the serum potassium and phosphate levels and reverses the paralysis within 2–3 hours. No intravenous potassium or phosphate is ordinarily required. Intravenous dextrose and oral carbohydrate aggravate the condition and are to be avoided. Therapy is continued with propranolol, 60–80 mg orally every 8 hours (or sustained-action propranolol ER daily at equivalent daily dosage), along with a thiourea drug such as methimazole to treat the hyperthyroidism.

7. Thyroid acropachy—This rare complication of Graves disease is often mild and may not require therapy. More severe cases are treated with systemic immunosuppressant therapy that may include intravenous immune globulin and rituximab.

▶ **Prognosis**

Mild or subclinical **Graves disease** may sometimes subside spontaneously. Graves disease that presents in early pregnancy has a 30% chance of spontaneous remission before the third trimester. The ocular, cardiac, and psychological complications can become serious and persistent even after treatment. Permanent hypoparathyroidism and vocal cord palsy are risks of surgical thyroidectomy. Recurrences are common following thiourea therapy but also occur after low-dose ^{131}I therapy or subtotal thyroidectomy. With adequate treatment and long-term follow-up, the results are usually good. However, despite treatment for their hyperthyroidism, women experience an increased long-term risk of death from thyroid disease, cardiovascular disease, stroke, and fracture of the femur. Posttreatment hypothyroidism is common. It may occur within a few months or up to several years after RAI therapy or subtotal thyroidectomy. Malignant exophthalmos has a poor prognosis unless treated aggressively. Patients with thyrotoxic crisis have a high mortality rate despite treatment.

Subclinical hyperthyroidism generally subsides spontaneously. Progression to symptomatic thyrotoxicosis occurs at a rate of 1–2% per year in patients without a goiter and at a rate of 5% per year in patients with a multinodular goiter. Most patients do well without treatment and the serum TSH usually reverts to normal within 2 years. Most such patients do not have accelerated bone loss. However, if a baseline bone density shows significant osteopenia, bone densitometry may be performed periodically. In persons over age 60 years, serum TSH is suppressed (less than 0.1 milli-international units/L) in 3% and mildly low (0.1–0.4 milli-international units/L) in 9%. The chance of developing atrial fibrillation is 2.8% yearly in elderly patients with very low TSH and 1.1% yearly in those with mildly low TSH. Asymptomatic persons with very low TSH are monitored closely but are not treated unless atrial fibrillation or other manifestations of hyperthyroidism develop.

▶ **When to Admit**

- Thyroid crisis.
- Hyperthyroidism-induced atrial fibrillation with severe tachycardia.
- Thyroidectomy.

Bartalena L et al. The 2016 European Thyroid Association/European Group on Graves' Orbitopathy guidelines for the management of Graves' orbitopathy. Eur Thyroid J. 2016 Mar; 5(1):9–26. [PMID: 27099835]

Burch HB et al. Management of Graves disease: a review. JAMA. 2015 Dec;314(23):2544–54. [PMID: 26670972]

De Leo S et al. Hyperthyroidism. Lancet. 2016 Aug 27; 388(10047):906–18. [PMID: 27038492]

Kravets I. Hyperthyroidism: diagnosis and treatment. Am Fam Physician. 2016 Mar;93(5):363–70. [PMID: 26926973]

Pallais JC et al. Case records of the Massachusetts General Hospital. Case 38-2015. A 21-year-old man with fatigue and weight loss. N Engl J Med. 2015 Dec;373(24):2358–69. [PMID: 26650156]

Ross DS et al. 2016 American Thyroid Association guidelines for diagnosis and management of hyperthyroidism and other causes of thyrotoxicosis. Thyroid. 2016 Oct;26(10):1343–421. [PMID: 27521067]

Smith TJ et al. Graves' disease. N Engl J Med. 2016 Oct 30; 375(16):1552–63. [PMID: 27797318]

Smith TJ et al. Teprotumumab for thyroid-associated ophthalmopathy. N Engl J Med. 2017 May 4;376(1):174–61. [PMID: 28467880]

THYROID NODULES & MULTINODULAR GOITER

ESSENTIALS OF DIAGNOSIS

▶ Single or multiple thyroid nodules are commonly palpated by the patient or clinician or discovered incidentally on imaging studies.

▶ Thyroid function tests recommended.

▶ FNA cytology for thyroid nodules 1 cm or larger in diameter or for smaller nodules when prior head-neck or chest-shoulder radiation.

▶ Ultrasound guidance improves FNA diagnosis for palpable and nonpalpable nodules.

▶ Clinical follow-up required.

▶ General Considerations

Thyroid nodules are extremely common. Palpable nodules occur in 4–7% of all adults in the United States. They are much more common in women than men and become more prevalent with age. About 90% of palpable thyroid nodules are benign adenomas, colloid nodules, or cysts, but some are primary thyroid malignancies or (less frequently)

metastatic malignancy. The general use of scanning also incidentally detects nonpalpable thyroid nodules. On MRI, incidental small thyroid nodules are found in about 50% of adults. Thyroid nodules 1 cm or larger in diameter warrant follow-up and further testing for function and malignancy. An occasional nodule smaller than 1 cm in diameter requires follow-up if it has high-risk characteristics on ultrasound or if the patient is at high-risk for thyroid cancer due to prior head-neck radiation therapy during childhood. Thyroid nodules that are incidentally discovered with increased standard uptake value (SUV) on ^{18}FDG-PET scanning have a 33% risk for being malignant and require FNA cytology.

Most patients with a thyroid nodule are euthyroid, but there is a high incidence of hypothyroidism or hyperthyroidism. Patients with multiple thyroid nodules have the same overall risk of thyroid cancer as patients with solitary nodules. The risk of a thyroid nodule being malignant is higher in men and among patients with a history of head-neck radiation, total body radiation for bone marrow transplantation, exposure to radioactive fallout as a child or teen, a family history of thyroid cancer or a thyroid cancer syndrome (eg, Cowden syndrome, multiple endocrine neoplasia type 2, familial polyposis, Carney syndrome), or a personal history of another malignancy. The risk of malignancy is also higher for large solitary nodules and if there is hoarseness or vocal fold paralysis, adherence to the trachea or strap muscles, cervical lymphadenopathy. The presence of Hashimoto thyroiditis does not reduce the risk of malignancy; a nodule of 1 cm or larger in a gland with thyroiditis carries an 8% chance of malignancy.

▶ Clinical Findings

Table 26–5 illustrates the approach to the evaluation of thyroid nodules based on the index of suspicion for malignancy.

Table 26–5. Clinical evaluation of thyroid nodules.[1]

Clinical Evidence	Low Index of Suspicion	High Index of Suspicion
History	Family history of goiter; residence in area of endemic goiter	Previous therapeutic radiation of head, neck, or chest; hoarseness
Physical characteristics	Older women; soft nodule; multinodular goiter	Young adults, men; solitary, firm nodule; vocal cord paralysis; enlarged lymph nodes; distant metastatic lesions
Serum factors	High titer of anti-thyroperoxidase antibody; hypothyroidism; hyperthyroidism	Elevated serum calcitonin
Fine-needle aspiration biopsy	Colloid nodule or adenoma	Papillary carcinoma, follicular lesion, medullary or anaplastic carcinoma
Scanning techniques		
Uptake of ^{123}I	Hot nodule	Cold nodule
Ultrasonogram	Cystic lesion	Solid lesion
Radiograph	Shell-like calcification	Punctate calcification
Response to levothyroxine therapy	Regression after 0.05–0.1 mg/day for 6 months or more	Increase in size

[1]Clinically suspicious nodules should be evaluated with fine-needle aspiration biopsy.

A. Symptoms and Signs

Most small thyroid nodules cause no symptoms. They may sometimes be detected only by having the patient swallow during careful inspection and palpation of the thyroid.

A thyroid nodule or multinodular goiter can grow to become visible and of concern to the patient. Particularly large nodular goiters can become a cosmetic embarrassment. Nodules can grow large enough to cause discomfort, hoarseness, or dysphagia. Nodules that cause ipsilateral recurrent laryngeal nerve palsy are more likely to be malignant. Retrosternal large multinodular goiters can cause dyspnea due to tracheal compression. Large substernal goiters may cause superior vena cava syndrome, manifested by facial erythema and jugular vein distention that progress to cyanosis and facial edema when both arms are kept raised over the head.

Depending on their cause, goiters and thyroid nodules may be associated with hypothyroidism (Hashimoto thyroiditis, endemic goiter) or hyperthyroidism (Graves disease, toxic nodular goiter, subacute thyroiditis, and thyroid cancer with metastases).

B. Laboratory Findings

A serum TSH and FT_4 determine if the thyroid is hyperfunctioning. Patients with a subnormal serum TSH must have a radionuclide (^{123}I or ^{99m}Tc pertechnetate) thyroid scan to examine whether the nodule is hyperfunctioning; hyperfunctioning nodules are usually benign but not reliably so. Very high levels of antithyroperoxidase antibodies and antithyroglobulin antibodies are found in Hashimoto thyroiditis. However, thyroiditis frequently coexists with malignancy, so suspicious nodules should always be biopsied. Serum calcitonin is obtained if a medullary thyroid carcinoma is suspected in a patient with a family history of medullary thyroid carcinoma or MEN types 2 or 3.

C. Imaging

Neck ultrasonography should be performed (see Fine-Needle Aspiration of Thyroid Nodules, below). Malignant nodules are more likely to grow more than 2 mm/year. Ultrasonography is preferred over CT and MRI. CT scanning is helpful for larger thyroid nodules and multinodular goiter; it can determine the degree of tracheal compression and the degree of extension into the mediastinum.

RAI (^{123}I or ^{131}I) scans are not helpful for assessing whether a thyroid nodule is benign or malignant. Hyperfunctioning (hot) nodules are ordinarily benign (but may rarely be malignant). RAI uptake and scanning is helpful mainly for assessing the etiology of hyperthyroidism (eg, hyperfunctioning nodule).

D. Incidentally Discovered Thyroid Nodules

Thyroid nodules are frequently discovered as an incidental finding, with an incidence that depends on the imaging modality: Ultrasound, about 30% (20% are larger than 1 cm in diameter); MRI, 50%; CT, 13%; and ^{18}FDG-PET, 2%. When MRI, CT, and ^{18}FDG-PET detect a thyroid nodule, an ultrasound is performed to better determine the nodule's risk for malignancy and the need for FNA cytology, and to establish a baseline for ultrasound follow-up. The malignancy risk is about 13–17% for nodules discovered incidentally on CT, MRI, or ultrasound and 25–50% for nodules discovered incidentally by ^{18}FDG-PET. However, most such malignancies are very low grade. For incidentally discovered thyroid nodules of borderline concern, follow-up thyroid ultrasound in 3–6 months may be helpful; growing lesions should be assessed with FNA cytology or resected.

E. Fine-Needle Aspiration of Thyroid Nodules

FNA is the best method to assess a thyroid nodule for malignancy. FNA can be done while patients continue taking anticoagulants or aspirin. For multinodular goiters, the four largest nodules (1 cm or larger in diameter) are usually biopsied to minimize the risk of missing a malignancy.

Thyroid nodules are classified for malignancy risk according to their appearance on ultrasound. High-risk nodules (80% malignancy risk) have microcalcifications, irregular margins, extrathyroidal extension, extrusion of soft tissue into a calcified rim, or are taller than wide; such nodules require FNA if they are 1 cm or larger in diameter. Intermediate-risk nodules (15% malignancy risk) are hypoechoic and solid; they also usually require FNA if they are 1 cm or larger in diameter. Low-risk nodules (7% malignancy risk) are partially cystic with eccentric solid areas; they require biopsy if they are 1.5 cm or larger in diameter. Very low-risk nodules (below 3% malignancy risk) are those that are spongiform or simple cysts; FNA is optional if they are 2 cm or larger in diameter. Using ultrasound guidance for FNA biopsy improves the diagnostic accuracy for both palpable and nonpalpable thyroid nodules. FNA cytology is typically reported using The Bethesda System for Reporting Thyroid Cytopathology (TBSRTC), which divides results into six categories:

1. **Nondiagnostic or unsatisfactory:** The malignancy risk is 1–4%. The usual management is a repeat FNA under ultrasound guidance.

2. **Benign:** The malignancy risk is about 2.5%. The usual management is clinical follow-up with palpation or ultrasound at 6- to 18-month intervals.

3. **Atypia of undetermined significance (AUS):** The malignancy risk is about 14%, higher with sonographic features of malignancy. The usual management is clinical correlation and a repeat FNA.

4. **Suspicious for follicular neoplasm (SFN) or follicular neoplasm (FN):** The malignancy risk is about 25%, higher when Hürthle cells are present and in patients over age 50. The usual management is usually direct surgical lobectomy.

5. **Suspicious for malignancy (SFM):** The malignancy risk is about 70%. The usual management is usually direct thyroid lobectomy or near-total thyroidectomy.

6. **Malignant:** The malignancy risk is about 99%. The usual management is a near-total thyroidectomy.

Treatment

All thyroid nodules, including those that are benign, need to be monitored by regular periodic palpation and ultrasound about every 6 months initially. After several years of stability, yearly examinations are sufficient. Thyroid nodules should be rebiopsied if growth occurs. A toxic multinodular goiter and hyperthyroidism may develop in patients who have had exposure to large amounts of iodine, either orally (eg, amiodarone) or intravenously (eg, radiographic contrast). Therefore, excessive iodine intake should be minimized. Patients found to have hyperthyroidism may have a RAI uptake and scan, especially if ^{131}I is a therapeutic consideration.

Managing thyroid nodules and multinodular goiter is the treatment of hyperthyroidism, if present, with thioureas, propranolol, surgery, or RAI (see Hyperthyroidism treatment of toxic nodular goiter, above).

A. Levothyroxine Suppression Therapy

Patients with nodules larger than 2 cm and elevated or normal TSH levels may be considered for TSH suppression with levothyroxine (starting doses of 50 mcg orally daily). Levothyroxine suppression therapy is not recommended for small benign thyroid nodules if the serum TSH level is normal. Levothyroxine suppression therapy is more successful in iodine-deficient areas of the world. Long-term levothyroxine suppression of TSH tends to keep nodules from enlarging but only 20% shrink more than 50%. Thyroid nodule size increased in 29% of patients treated with levothyroxine versus 56% of patients not receiving levothyroxine. Levothyroxine suppression also reduces the emergence of new nodules: 8% with levothyroxine and 29% without levothyroxine. Levothyroxine suppression therapy is not usually given to patients with ischemic heart disease, since it increases the risk for angina and atrial fibrillation. Levothyroxine suppression causes a small loss of bone density, particularly in postmenopausal women if the serum TSH is suppressed to less than 0.05 milli-international units/L. Such patients are advised to have bone density testing every 3–5 years. For patients with a low baseline TSH level, levothyroxine should not be administered, since that is an indication of autonomous thyroid secretion; levothyroxine will be ineffective and could cause thyrotoxicosis.

Levothyroxine suppression needs to be carefully monitored, since it carries a 17% risk of inducing hyperthyroidism. All patients receiving levothyroxine suppression therapy should have serum TSH levels monitored at least annually, with the levothyroxine dose adjusted to keep the serum TSH mildly suppressed (between 0.1 milli-international units/L and 0.8 milli-international units/L).

B. Surgery

Total thyroidectomy is required for thyroid nodules that are malignant on FNA biopsy. More limited thyroid surgery is indicated for benign nodules with indeterminate or suspicious cytologic test results, compression symptoms, discomfort, or cosmetic embarrassment. Surgery may also be used to remove hyperfunctioning "hot" thyroid adenomas or toxic multinodular goiter causing hyperthyroidism.

C. Percutaneous Ethanol Injection

Percutaneous ethanol injection can shrink pure cysts; the success rate is 80%, although it must often be repeated. Percutaneous ethanol injection can also be used to shrink biopsy-proven benign nodules. While complications occur in about 9%, serious or permanent complications are rare. Thyroid cysts can be aspirated, but cystic fluid recurs in 75% of patients.

D. Radioiodine (^{131}I) Therapy

Radioactive ^{131}I is a treatment option for hyperthyroid patients with toxic thyroid adenomas, multinodular goiter, or Graves disease. See **Precautions** for RAI use, above. Therapy with ^{131}I shrinks benign nontoxic thyroid nodules by an average of 40% by 1 year and 59% by 2 years after ^{131}I therapy. Nodules that shrink after ^{131}I therapy generally remain palpable and become firmer; they may develop unusual cytologic characteristics on FNA biopsy. [131]I therapy may be used to shrink large multinodular goiters but may rarely induce Graves disease. Hypothyroidism may occur years after ^{131}I therapy, so it is advisable to assess thyroid function every 3 months for the first year, every 6 months thereafter, and immediately for symptoms of hypothyroidism or hyperthyroidism.

Prognosis

Benign thyroid nodules may involute but usually persist or grow slowly. About 90% of thyroid nodules will increase their volume by 15% or more over 5 years; about 11% of nodules increase their volume by more than 50% on follow-up. Growth is more common with multinodular goiter and larger nodules and in men; nodules are less likely to grow when they are solitary or cystic and when patients are over age 60. Multinodular goiters tend to persist or grow slowly. Cytologically benign nodules that grow are unlikely to be malignant; in one series, only 1 of 78 rebiopsied nodules was found to be malignant. The risk of a given thyroid nodule being malignant decreases with age. Iodine supplementation in iodine-deficient areas does not usually shrink established goiters. Patients with very small (less than 1 cm diameter), incidentally discovered, nonpalpable thyroid nodules that have a benign ultrasound appearance require no FNA cytology and only yearly palpation and clinical follow-up, whereas such small nodules that have a slightly suspicious ultrasound appearance may require FNA cytology or thyroid ultrasound every 1–2 years.

Angell TE et al. Differential growth rates of benign vs. malignant thyroid nodules. J Clin Endocrinol Metab. 2017 Dec 1; 102(12):4642–7. [PMID: 29040691]

Cohen RN et al. Management of adult patients with thyroid nodules and differentiated thyroid cancer. JAMA. 2017 Jan 24;317(4):434–5. [PMID: 28118436]

Durante C et al. The diagnosis and management of thyroid nodules: a review. JAMA. 2018 Mar 6;319(9):914–24. [PMID: 29509871]

Straccia P et al. A meta-analytic review of the Bethesda System for Reporting Thyroid Cytopathology: has the rate of malignancy in indeterminate lesions been underestimated? Cancer Cytopathol. 2015 Dec;123(12):713–22. [PMID: 26355876]

THYROID CANCER

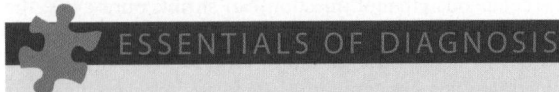

ESSENTIALS OF DIAGNOSIS

▶ Painless swelling in region of thyroid.

▶ Thyroid function tests usually normal.

▶ Possible history of childhood irradiation to head and neck region.

▶ Positive thyroid FNA cytology.

▶ General Considerations

The incidence of differentiated (papillary and follicular) thyroid carcinomas increases with age (Table 26–6). The overall female:male ratio is 3:1. The yearly incidence of thyroid cancer has been increasing in the United States, with the number of cases diagnosed annually reaching 52,000, probably as a result of the wider use of ultrasound, CT, MRI, and PET that incidentally find small thyroid malignancies. Thyroid cancer mortality has been stable, accounting for about 2000 deaths in the United States annually. Clearly, the increasing incidence of thyroid cancer has been mainly due to incidentally found tumors; however, some true increase in cancer incidence is possible. In routine autopsy series, thyroid papillary microcarcinoma (10 mm diameter or smaller) is found with the surprising frequency of 11.5%. Most thyroid cancers remain microscopic and indolent. However, larger thyroid cancers (palpable or greater than or equal to 1 cm in diameter) are more malignant and require treatment.

Pure papillary (and mixed papillary-follicular) carcinoma comprises about 80% of all thyroid cancers. It usually presents as a single thyroid nodule, but it can arise out of a multinodular goiter. Papillary thyroid carcinoma is commonly multifocal within the gland, with other foci usually arising de novo rather than representing intraglandular metastases. The tumor involves both lobes in 30% of patients.

Papillary thyroid carcinoma is generally the least aggressive thyroid malignancy. It tends to grow slowly and often remains confined to the thyroid and regional lymph nodes for years. In about 80% of patients, there are microscopic metastases to cervical lymph nodes. However, the malignancy may become more aggressive, especially in patients over age 45 years, and most particularly in older adults. The cancer may invade the trachea and local muscles and may spread to the lungs.

Exposure to head and neck radiation therapy poses a particular threat to children who then have an increased lifetime risk of developing thyroid cancer, including papillary carcinoma. These cancers may emerge between 10 and 40 years after exposure, with a peak occurrence 20–25 years later.

Papillary thyroid carcinoma can occur in familial syndromes as an autosomal dominant trait, caused by loss of various tumor suppressor genes.

Microscopic "micropapillary" carcinoma (1 mm or smaller and invisible on thyroid ultrasound) is a variant of normal, being found in 24% of thyroidectomies performed for benign thyroid disease when 2-mm sections were carefully examined. Thus, the overwhelming majority of these microscopic foci never become clinically significant. The surgical pathology report of such a tiny papillary carcinoma does not justify aggressive measures. All that may be required is yearly follow-up with palpation of the neck and mild TSH suppression by thyroxine.

Follicular thyroid carcinoma and its variants (eg, Hürthle cell carcinoma) account for about 14% of thyroid malignancies; follicular carcinomas are generally more aggressive than papillary carcinomas. Most follicular thyroid carcinomas avidly absorb iodine, making possible diagnostic scanning and treatment with ^{131}I after total thyroidectomy. The follicular histopathologic features that are associated with a high risk of metastasis and recurrence are poorly differentiated and Hürthle cell (oncocytic) variants. The latter variants do not take up RAI.

Medullary thyroid carcinoma represents 2–3% of thyroid cancers. About one-third of cases are sporadic, one-third are familial, and one-third are associated with MEN type 2A or 2B. Medullary thyroid carcinoma is often caused by an activating mutation of the *ret* protooncogene on chromosome 10. Mutation analysis of the *ret* protooncogene exons 10, 11, 13, 14, and 16 detects most mutations causing MEN 2A and MEN 2B and the mutations causing

Table 26–6. Some characteristics of thyroid cancer.

	Papillary	Follicular	Medullary	Anaplastic
Incidence	Most common	Common	Uncommon	Uncommon
Average age	42	50	50	57
Females	70%	72%	56%	56%
Invasion				
Juxtanodal	+++++	+	++++++	+++
Blood vessels	+	+++	+++	+++++
Distant sites	+	+++	++	++++
^{123}I uptake	+	++++	0	0
10-year disease-specific survival	97%	92%	78%	7.3%

familial medullary thyroid carcinoma. These germline mutations can be detected by DNA analysis of peripheral WBCs. Therefore, discovery of a medullary thyroid carcinoma makes genetic analysis mandatory. If a gene defect is discovered, related family members must have genetic screening for that specific gene defect. When a family member with MEN 2 or 3 or familial medullary thyroid carcinoma does not have an identifiable *ret* protooncogene mutation, gene carriers may still be identified using family linkage analysis. Even when no gene defect is detectable, family members should have thyroid surveillance every 6 months. Medullary thyroid carcinoma arises from thyroid parafollicular cells that can secrete calcitonin, prostaglandins, serotonin, ACTH, corticotropin-releasing hormone (CRH), and other peptides. These peptides can cause symptoms and can be used as tumor markers.

Anaplastic thyroid carcinoma represents about 2% of thyroid cancers. It usually presents in an older patient as a rapidly enlarging mass in a multinodular goiter. It is the most aggressive thyroid carcinoma and metastasizes early to surrounding nodes and distant sites. This tumor does not concentrate iodine.

Other thyroid malignancies together represent about 3% of thyroid cancers. Primary thyroid lymphomas are most commonly diffuse large B-cell lymphomas (50%), mucosa-associated lymphoid tissue lymphoma (23%), or mixed type; other types include follicular, small lymphocytic, and Burkitt lymphoma and Hodgkin disease. Thyroidectomy is rarely required. Other cancers may sometimes metastasize to the thyroid, particularly bronchogenic, breast, and renal carcinomas and malignant melanoma.

► Clinical Findings

A. Symptoms and Signs

Thyroid carcinoma usually presents as a palpable, firm, nontender nodule in the thyroid. Most thyroid carcinomas are asymptomatic, but large thyroid cancers can cause neck discomfort, dysphagia, or hoarseness (due to pressure on the recurrent laryngeal nerve). **Papillary thyroid cancer** presents with palpable lymph node involvement in 10%; it may invade the trachea and local muscles. Occult metastases to the lung occur in 10–15%. **Follicular thyroid carcinoma** commonly metastasizes to neck nodes, bones, and lung, but nearly every organ can be involved. Metastatic functioning differentiated thyroid carcinoma can sometimes secrete enough thyroid hormone to produce thyrotoxicosis.

Medullary thyroid carcinoma typically metastases to local nodes and adjacent muscle and trachea as well as mediastinal lymph nodes. Eventually, metastases may appear in the bones, lungs, adrenals, or liver. Medullary thyroid carcinoma frequently causes flushing and persistent diarrhea (30%), which may be the initial clinical feature. Patients with metastases often experience fatigue as well as other symptoms. Cushing syndrome develops in about 5% of patients from secretion of ACTH or CRH.

Anaplastic thyroid carcinoma is more apt to be advanced at the time of diagnosis, presenting with signs of pressure or invasion of surrounding tissue, resulting in dysphagia, hoarseness, or recurrent laryngeal nerve palsy. Patients may also have dyspnea with metastases to the lungs. **Lymphoma** usually presents as a rapidly enlarging, painful mass arising out of a multinodular or diffuse goiter due to autoimmune thyroiditis, with which it may be confused microscopically. About 20% of cases have concomitant hypothyroidism.

B. Laboratory Findings

FNA biopsy is discussed in Thyroid Nodules, above. Thyroid function tests are generally normal unless there is concomitant thyroiditis. Follicular carcinoma may secrete enough T_4 to suppress TSH and cause clinical hyperthyroidism.

Serum thyroglobulin is high in most metastatic papillary and follicular tumors, making this a useful marker for recurrent or metastatic disease. Caution must be exercised for the following reasons: (1) Circulating antithyroglobulin antibodies can cause erroneous thyroglobulin determinations. However, declining levels of antithyroglobulin antibodies are a good prognostic sign after treatment. (2) Thyroglobulin levels may be misleadingly elevated in thyroiditis, which often coexists with carcinoma. (3) Certain thyroglobulin assays falsely report the continued presence of thyroglobulin after total thyroidectomy and tumor resection, causing undue concern about possible metastases. Therefore, unexpected detectable thyroglobulin levels post-thyroidectomy should prompt a repeat assay in another reference laboratory.

Serum calcitonin levels are usually elevated in medullary thyroid carcinoma, making this a marker for metastatic disease. However, serum calcitonin may be elevated in many other conditions, such as thyroiditis; pregnancy; kidney disease; hypergastrinemia; hypercalcemia; and other malignancies, particularly neuroendocrine tumors (including pheochromocytomas, carcinoid tumors) and carcinomas of the lung, pancreas, breast, and colon. Serum calcitonin and carcinoembryonic antigen (CEA) determinations should be obtained before surgery, then regularly in postoperative follow-up: every 4 months for 5 years, then every 6 months for life. In patients with extensive metastases, serum calcitonin should be measured in the laboratory with serial dilutions. Calcitonin levels remain elevated in patients with persistent tumor but also in some patients with apparent cure or indolent disease. Therefore, serum calcitonin levels greater than 250 ng/L (73 pmol/L) or rising levels of calcitonin are the best indication for recurrence or metastatic disease. Serum CEA levels are also usually elevated with medullary thyroid carcinoma, making this a useful second marker; however, it is not specific for this cancer.

C. Imaging

1. Ultrasound of the neck—Ultrasound of the neck should be performed on all patients with thyroid cancer for the initial diagnosis and for follow-up. Ultrasound is useful in determining the size and location of the malignancy as well as the location of any neck metastases.

2. Radioactive iodine scanning—RAI (^{131}I or ^{123}I) thyroid and whole-body scanning is used after thyroidectomy for differentiated thyroid cancer utilizing the protocol described later. (See Radioactive Iodine (^{131}I) Therapy for Differentiated Thyroid Cancer, later.) Medullary thyroid cancer does not avidly uptake RAI.

3. CT and MRI scanning—CT scanning may demonstrate metastases and is particularly useful for localizing and monitoring lung metastases but is less sensitive than ultrasound for detecting metastases within the neck. Medullary carcinoma in the thyroid, nodes, and liver may calcify, but lung metastases rarely do so. MRI is particularly useful for imaging bone metastases.

4. PET scanning—PET scanning is especially helpful for detecting thyroid cancer metastases that do not have sufficient iodine uptake to be visible on RAI scans. Metastases are best detected using ^{18}FDG-PET whole-body scanning. The sensitivity of ^{18}FDG-PET scanning for differentiated thyroid cancer is enhanced if the patient is hypothyroid or receiving thyrotropin, which increases the metabolic activity of differentiated thyroid cancer. Patients with medullary thyroid cancer are monitored with MRI and ^{18}FDG PET/CT scanning. ^{68}Ga PET is usually inferior to ^{18}FDG PET and other imaging for locating medullary thyroid cancer.

▶ Differential Diagnosis

RAI uptake occurs in many different tissues and can be mistaken for metastatic differentiated thyroid carcinoma. Head-neck RAI uptake is seen in normal thyroid, salivary glands, nasal mucosa, thyroglossal duct remnants, and sinusitis.

Negative RAI scans are common in early metastatic differentiated thyroid carcinoma. Unfortunately, negative RAI scans also occur frequently with more advanced metastatic thyroid carcinoma, making it more difficult to detect and to distinguish from nonthyroidal neoplasms. An elevated serum thyroglobulin in patients with a clear RAI scan should arouse suspicion for metastases that are not avid for radioiodine. Medullary thyroid carcinoma does not concentrate iodine.

▶ Complications

Hyperthyroidism can develop in patients with a heavy tumor burden. One-third of medullary thyroid carcinomas secrete serotonin and prostaglandins, producing flushing and diarrhea. The management of patients with medullary carcinomas may be complicated by the coexistence of pheochromocytomas or hyperparathyroidism.

▶ Treatment of Differentiated Thyroid Carcinoma

A. Surgical Treatment

Surgical removal is the treatment of choice for thyroid carcinomas. Neck ultrasound is obtained preoperatively, since suspicious cervical lymphadenopathy is detected in about 25%.

For differentiated papillary and follicular carcinoma larger than 1 cm diameter, total thyroidectomy is performed with limited removal of cervical lymph nodes. Surgery consists of a thyroid lobectomy for an indeterminate "follicular lesion" that is 4 cm diameter or smaller. If malignancy is diagnosed on pathology intraoperatively, a completion thyroidectomy is performed. For indeterminate follicular lesions larger than 4 cm diameter that are at higher risk for being malignant, a bilateral thyroidectomy is performed as the initial surgery. Higher-risk lesions include those with an FNA biopsy that shows marked atypia or that are suspicious for papillary carcinoma and those that occur in patients with a history of radiation exposure or a family history of thyroid carcinoma.

For biopsies that are diagnostic of malignancy, surgery involves lobectomy alone for papillary thyroid carcinomas smaller than 1 cm in diameter in patients under age 45 years who have no history of head and neck irradiation and no evidence of lymph node metastasis on ultrasonography. Other patients should have a total or near total thyroidectomy. The advantage of near-total thyroidectomy for differentiated thyroid carcinoma is that multicentric foci of carcinoma are more apt to be resected. Also, there is less normal thyroid tissue to compete with cancer for ^{131}I administered later for scans or treatment. A central neck lymph node dissection is performed at the time of thyroidectomy for patients with nodal metastases that are clinically evident. A lateral neck dissection is performed for patients with biopsy-proven lateral cervical lymphadenopathy. Metastases to the brain are best treated surgically, since treatment with radiation or RAI is ineffective. Levothyroxine is prescribed in doses of 0.05–0.1 mg orally daily immediately postoperatively. About 2–4 months after surgery, patients require reevaluation and often ^{131}I therapy.

Permanent injury to one recurrent laryngeal nerve occurs in between 1–2% and 7% of patients, depending on the experience of the surgeon. Temporary recurrent laryngeal nerve palsies occur in another 5% but often resolve within 6 months. After total thyroidectomy, temporary hypoparathyroidism occurs in 20% and becomes permanent in about 2%. The incidence of hypoparathyroidism may be reduced if accidentally resected parathyroids are immediately autotransplanted into the neck muscles. Thyroidectomy requires at least an overnight hospital admission, since late bleeding, airway problems, and tetany can occur. *Ambulatory thyroidectomy is potentially dangerous and should not be done.* Following surgery, staging (Table 26–7) should be done to help determine prognosis and to plan therapy and follow-up.

In pregnant women with thyroid cancer, surgery is usually delayed until after delivery, except for fast-growing tumors that may be resected after 24 weeks gestation; there has been no difference in survival or tumor recurrence rates in women who underwent surgery during or after their pregnancy. Differentiated thyroid carcinoma does not behave more aggressively during pregnancy. However, compared to nonpregnant women, there is a higher risk of complications in pregnant women undergoing thyroid surgery.

B. Active Surveillance for Papillary Thyroid Microcarcinoma

Most papillary thyroid microcarcinomas that are less than 1 cm in diameter are indolent with an excellent prognosis. Therefore, for microcarcinomas, an ongoing active

Table 26–7. Staging and prognosis for patients with papillary thyroid carcinoma using MACIS scoring.

Total Score[1] - Stage	Percentage of Patients with Papillary Thyroid Carcinoma	20-Year Survival
< 6.0 = Stage I	74.2%	96–99%
6.0–6.99 = Stage II	8.5%	68–89%
7.0–7.99 = Stage III	9.2%	55–56%
≥ 8.0 = Stage IV	8.1%	17–24%

[1]Total score = 3.1 × age (if aged ≤ 39 years) *or* 0.08 × age (if aged ≥ 40 yr) + 0.3 × tumor size (cm, if not completely resected), +1 (if locally invasive), +3 (if distant metastases).
MACIS, metastases, age, complete resection, invasion, size.

surveillance protocol used in some medical centers is to perform a clinical examination and neck ultrasound every 6 months. Such conservative management may be particularly warranted for patients who have a limited life expectancy, a high surgical risk, or very low-risk tumors.

C. Levothyroxine Suppression for Differentiated Thyroid Cancer

Patients who have had a thyroidectomy for differentiated thyroid cancer must take levothyroxine replacement for life. Oral levothyroxine should be given in doses that suppress serum TSH without causing clinical thyrotoxicosis. Serum TSH should be suppressed below 0.1 milli-international units/L for patients with stage II disease and below 0.05 milli-international units/L for patients with stage 3–4 disease. (See Table 26–7.) Although patients receiving levothyroxine suppression therapy (TSH less than 0.05 milli-international units/L) are at risk for a lower bone density than age-matched controls, the adverse effect upon bone density and fracture risk is relatively minor for patients who remain clinically euthyroid. Nevertheless, patients receiving levothyroxine suppression therapy should have periodic bone densitometry.

D. Radioactive Iodine (^{131}I) Therapy for Differentiated Thyroid Cancer

There are two reasons to treat patients with ^{131}I after thyroidectomy: (1) thyroid remnant ablation for patients at high risk for recurrence and (2) treatment of metastatic thyroid cancer. ^{131}I is usually administered 2–4 months after surgery. However, the indications and optimal activity (dose) for ^{131}I therapy for differentiated thyroid cancer remain controversial since there is an overwhelmingly good prognosis for most patients with differentiated thyroid cancer.

Before receiving ^{131}I therapy, patients should follow a low-iodine diet for at least 2 weeks. Patients must not be given amiodarone or intravenous radiologic contrast dyes containing iodine. Despite restriction of dietary iodine, differentiated thyroid cancer frequently lacks sufficient radioiodine avidity to allow RAI therapy.

1. RAI thyroid remnant ablation—A low activity[1] of 30 mCi (1.1 GBq) ^{131}I is given for "remnant ablation" of residual normal thyroid tissues after surgery for differentiated thyroid cancer. This small amount of ^{131}I is given to patients with no known lymph node involvement who are at low risk for metastases. However, ^{131}I remnant ablation is not required for patients with low-risk stage I papillary thyroid carcinomas or carcinomas that are smaller than 1 cm in diameter (whether unifocal or multifocal), except for patients with unfavorable histopathology (tall-cell, columnar cell, insular cell, Hürthle cell, or diffuse sclerosing subtypes).

2. RAI treatment of metastases—Therapy with ^{131}I improves survival and reduces recurrence rates for patients with stage III–IV cancer and those with stage II cancer having gross extrathyroidal extension. RAI therapy is also given to patients with stage II cancer who have distant metastases, a primary tumor larger than 4 cm in diameter, or primary tumors 1–4 cm diameter with lymph node metastases or other high-risk features. Brain metastases do not usually respond to ^{131}I and are best resected or treated with gamma knife radiosurgery. A post-therapy whole-body scan is performed 2–10 days after ^{131}I therapy. About 70% of small lung metastases resolve following ^{131}I therapy; however, larger pulmonary metastases have only a 10% remission rate.

Staging with RAI scanning or ^{18}FDG-PET/CT scanning assists with determining the activity of ^{131}I to be administered. Treatment protocols vary among institutions. Generally, patients with higher-risk stage I cancer or stage II cancer are treated with ^{131}I activities of 50–100 mCi (1.8–3.7 GBq). Patients with stage III–IV cancers typically receive ^{131}I activities of 100–150 mCi (3.7–5.5 GBq). Repeated treatments may be required for persistent radioiodine-avid metastatic disease. Patients with differentiated thyroid carcinoma who have little or no uptake of RAI into metastases (about 35% of cases) should not be treated with ^{131}I. Patients with asymptomatic, stable, radioiodine-resistant metastases should receive levothyroxine to suppress serum TSH and should be carefully monitored for tumor progression.

Some patients have elevated serum thyroglobulin levels but a negative whole-body radioiodine scan and a negative neck ultrasound. In such patients, an ^{18}F-FDG PET/CT scan is obtained. If all scans are negative, the patient has a good prognosis and empiric therapy with ^{131}I is not useful.

Activities of ^{131}I over 100 mCi (3.7 GBq) can cause gastritis, temporary oligospermia, sialadenitis, and xerostomia. Therapy with ^{131}I can cause neurologic decompensation in patients with brain metastases; such patients are treated with prednisone 30–40 mg orally daily for several days before and after ^{131}I therapy. Cumulative doses of ^{131}I over 500 mCi (18.5 GBq) can cause infertility, pancytopenia (4%), and leukemia (0.3%). Pulmonary fibrosis can occur in patients with diffuse lung metastases after receiving cumulative ^{131}I activities over 600 mCi (22 GBq). The kidneys excrete RAI, so patients receiving dialysis require only 20% of the usual ^{131}I activity.

---

[1]The amount of radioiodine radioactivity given in a procedure is referred to as radioactivity or "activity" and is expressed as Curies (Ci) or Becquerels (Bq), whereas the term "dose" is reserved to describe the amount of radiation absorbed by a given organ or tumor and is expressed as Gray (Gy) or radiation-absorbed dose (RAD).

3. Recombinant human TSH (rhTSH)-stimulated ^{131}**I therapy**—Recombinant human thyroid-stimulating hormone (rhTSH, Thyrogen) is given to increase the sensitivity of serum thyroglobulin for residual cancer and to increase the uptake of ^{131}I into residual thyroid tissue (thyroid remnant "ablation") or cancer. Thyrogen must be kept refrigerated and is administered according to the following protocol: Levothyroxine replacement is held for 2 days before rhTSH and for 3 days afterward. For 2 consecutive days, rhTSH (0.9 mg/day, reconstituted with 0.2 mL sterile saline) should be administered intragluteally (not intravenously). On the third day, blood is drawn: serum TSH is assayed to confirm that it is greater than 30 milli-units/L; serum hCG is measured in reproductive-age women to exclude pregnancy; and serum thyroglobulin is measured as a tumor marker. RAI is then administered at the prescribed activity (see above).

Thyrogen should not be administered to patients with an intact thyroid gland because it can cause severe thyroid swelling and hyperthyroidism. Hyperthyroidism can also occur in patients with significant metastases or residual normal thyroid. Other side effects include nausea (11%) and headache (7%). Thyrotropin has caused neurologic deterioration in 7% of patients with CNS metastases.

4. Thyroid-withdrawal stimulated ^{131}**I therapy**—Thyroid withdrawal is sometimes used because of its lower cost, despite the discomforts of becoming hypothyroid. Levothyroxine is withdrawn for 14 days and the patient is allowed to become hypothyroid; high levels of endogenous TSH stimulate the uptake of RAI and production of thyroglobulin by thyroid cancer or residual thyroid. Just prior to ^{131}I therapy, the following blood tests are obtained: serum TSH to confirm it is greater than 30 milli-units/L, serum hCG in reproductive-age women to screen for pregnancy, and serum thyroglobulin as a tumor marker. Three days after ^{131}I therapy, levothyroxine therapy may be resumed at full replacement dose.

5. Side effects and contraindications to ^{131}**I therapy**—National Cancer Institute surveillance data for thousands of patients with thyroid cancer indicate that patients with differentiated thyroid cancer, treated with only surgery, have a 5% increased risk of developing a second non-thyroid malignancy. Patients with thyroid cancer who received ^{131}I therapy have a slightly increased risk of developing a second non-thyroid malignancy (especially leukemia and lymphoma). The risk of second cancers peaks about 5 years following ^{131}I therapy.

Sialadenitis and xerostomia are potential side effects, particularly in women, older-age patients, patients with a prior history of sialadenitis, and patients with autoimmune diseases associated with Sjögren syndrome. See **Precautions** about RAI use, above.

E. Other Therapies for Differentiated Thyroid Cancer

Patients with osteolytic metastases to bone from differentiated thyroid cancer may be treated with one of two anti-bone resorptive drugs: (1) zoledronic acid, 4 mg intravenously; or (2) denosumab, 120 mg subcutaneously.

The frequency and duration of therapy are individualized according to each patient's symptoms and response. These drugs must be used judiciously; there is an increased risk of atypical femur fractures and osteonecrosis of the jaw with prolonged therapy with either drug.

Patients with aggressive differentiated thyroid cancers may have metastases that are refractory to RAI therapy. Recurrence in the neck may be treated with surgical debulking and external beam radiation therapy. Patients with RAI-refractory differentiated thyroid cancer metastases that are advanced and rapidly progressive may be treated with certain tyrosine kinase inhibitors. Vandetanib and sunitinib induce partial responses in about 40%, while lenvatinib induces partial responses in about 65%; however, median progression-free survival has been only about 18 months and all tyrosine kinase inhibitors can cause serious adverse reactions, so the patient and clinician must decide whether this chemotherapy is worthwhile.

▶ Treatment of Other Thyroid Malignancies

Anaplastic thyroid carcinoma is treated with local resection and radiation. Lovastatin has been demonstrated to cause differentiation and apoptosis of anaplastic thyroid carcinoma cells in vitro, but clinical studies are lacking. Anaplastic thyroid carcinoma does not respond to ^{131}I therapy and is resistant to most chemotherapy. Anaplastic thyroid cancers with mTOR mutations may be inhibited by everolimus.

Medullary thyroid carcinoma is best treated with surgery for the primary tumor and metastases. Patients with a ret protooncogene mutation should have a prophylactic total thyroidectomy, ideally by age 6 years (MEN 2A) or at age 6 months (MEN 2B). Medullary thyroid carcinoma does not respond to ^{131}I therapy and is relatively resistant to chemotherapy. Patients should be monitored closely, with serum calcitonin levels checked about every 3 months. Since medullary thyroid carcinoma can be indolent, patients should be considered for chemotherapy only if they have rapidly progressive metastases, as evidenced by a doubling time of serum calcitonin or CEA doubling time is within 2 years. Scanning with ^{18}FDG-PET is also useful for identifying rapidly progressive metastases. Vandetanib and cabozantinib are approved for use against rapidly progressive metastatic medullary thyroid carcinoma; both require close observation to avoid toxicity. Vandetanib should usually not be administered to patients with cardiac disease or a prolonged QT interval. Cabozantinib should usually not be administered to patients with small bowel or large bowel disease or prior radiation to the neck or mediastinum, since it increases the risk for gastrointestinal perforation and tracheoesophageal fistula. Patients with medullary thyroid carcinoma and diabetes should not receive diabetic therapy with glucagon-like peptide-1 (GLP-1) agonists because they may stimulate the growth of medullary thyroid carcinoma.

Thyroid mucosa-associated lymphoid tissue lymphomas have a low risk of recurrence after simple thyroidectomy. Patients with other thyroid lymphomas are best treated with external radiation therapy; chemotherapy is added for extensive lymphoma (Table 39–2).

External beam radiation therapy may be delivered to bone metastases, especially those that are without radioiodine uptake or are RAI-refractory. Local neck radiation therapy may also be given to patients with anaplastic thyroid carcinoma. Brain metastases can be treated with gamma knife radiosurgery.

► **Follow-Up**

Most differentiated thyroid carcinoma recurs within the first 5–10 years after thyroidectomy. While lifetime monitoring is recommended, the follow-up protocol can be tailored to the staging and aggressiveness of the malignancy. All patients require at least a yearly thyroid ultrasound and serum thyroglobulin level (while taking levothyroxine). Patients at higher risk usually require at least two annual consecutively negative stimulated serum thyroglobulin determinations less than 1 ng/mL and normal RAI scans (if done) and neck ultrasound scans before they are considered to be in remission. The first surveillance occurs with stimulated postoperative serum thyroglobulin, ^{131}I therapy, and post-therapy scanning about 2–4 months after surgery. At 9–12 months postoperatively, patients may receive another stimulated serum thyroglobulin and RAI scan. Patients need not have repeated ^{131}I therapies if persistent RAI uptake is confined to the thyroid bed and if neck ultrasounds appear normal and stimulated serum thyroglobulin levels remain less than 2 ng/mL. Patients with differentiated thyroid carcinoma must be monitored long term for recurrent or metastatic disease. Further radioiodine or other scans may be required for patients with more aggressive differentiated thyroid cancer, prior metastases, rising serum thyroglobulin levels, or other evidence of metastases.

1. Serum TSH suppression—Patients with differentiated thyroid cancer are treated with levothyroxine doses that are sufficient to suppress the serum TSH below the normal range. For intermediate- or high-risk patients, the serum TSH should be suppressed below 0.1 milli-international units/L, while the target TSH for low-risk patients is 0.1–0.5 milli-international units/mL. Patients who are considered cured should nevertheless be treated with sufficient levothyroxine to keep the serum TSH less than 2 milli-international units/L. Follow-up must include physical examinations and laboratory testing to ensure that patients remain clinically euthyroid with serum TSH levels in the target range. To achieve suppression of serum TSH, the required dose of levothyroxine may be such that serum FT_4 levels may be slightly elevated; in that case, measurement of serum T_3 or free T_3 can be useful to ensure the patient is not frankly hyperthyroid. Thyrotoxicosis can be caused by over-replacement with levothyroxine or by the growth of functioning metastases.

2. Serum thyroglobulin—Thyroglobulin is produced by normal thyroid tissue and by most differentiated thyroid carcinomas. It is only after a total or near-total thyroidectomy and ^{131}I remnant ablation that thyroglobulin becomes a useful tumor marker for patients with differentiated papillary or follicular thyroid cancer, particularly for patients who do not have serum antithyroglobulin antibodies.

Detectable thyroglobulin levels do not necessarily indicate the presence of residual or metastatic thyroid cancer. Conversely, baseline serum thyroglobulin levels are insensitive markers for disease recurrence. However, baseline or stimulated serum thyroglobulin levels 2 ng/mL or higher indicate the need for a repeat neck ultrasound and further scanning with RAI or [18]FDG-PET. If serum thyroglobulin levels remain 2 ng/mL or higher in the presence of normal scanning, it is prudent to repeat the serum thyroglobulin in a national reference laboratory. In one series of patients with differentiated thyroid cancer following thyroidectomy, there was a 21% incidence of metastases in patients with serum thyroglobulin less than 1 ng/mL (while receiving levothyroxine for TSH suppression). Therefore, *baseline* serum thyroglobulin levels are inadequately sensitive and *stimulated* serum thyroglobulin measurements should be used and *always* with neck ultrasound. The usefulness of routinely doing a radioiodine scan in low-risk patients is controversial but continues to be done in many centers during stimulation following either rhTSH or thyroid hormone withdrawal.

3. Neck ultrasound—Neck ultrasound should be used in all patients with thyroid carcinoma to supplement neck palpation; it should be performed preoperatively, 3 months postoperatively, and regularly thereafter. Ultrasound is more sensitive for lymph node metastases than either CT or MRI scanning. Small inflammatory nodes may be detected postoperatively and do not necessarily indicate metastatic disease, but follow-up is necessary. Ultrasound-guided FNA biopsy should be performed on suspicious lesions.

4. Radioactive iodine (RAI: [131]I or ^{123}I) neck and whole-body scanning—Despite its limitations, RAI scanning has traditionally been used to detect metastatic differentiated thyroid cancer and to determine whether the cancer is amenable to treatment with [131]I. RAI scanning is particularly useful for high-risk patients and those with persistent antithyroglobulin antibodies that make serum thyroglobulin determinations unreliable.

The ^{131}I radioisotope may be used in scanning activities provided it is given less than 2 weeks before scheduled ^{131}I treatment to avoid "stunning" metastases such that they take up less of the RAI therapy activity. Alternatively, the ^{123}I radioisotope may also be used and does not stun tumors; it allows single-photon emission computed tomography (SPECT) to better localize metastases. Initial RAI scanning is typically performed about 2–4 months following surgery for differentiated thyroid carcinoma.

About 65% of metastases are detectable by RAI scanning but only after optimal preparation. Patients should ideally have a total or near-total thyroidectomy, since any residual normal thyroid competes for RAI with metastases, which are less avid for iodine. It is reasonable to perform a rhTSH-stimulated scan and thyroglobulin level 2–3 months after the initial neck surgery; if the scan is negative and the serum thyroglobulin is less than 2 ng/mL, low-risk patients may not require further scanning but should continue to be monitored with neck ultrasound and serum thyroglobulin levels every 6–12 months. For higher-risk patients, the rhTSH-stimulated thyroglobulin and RAI scan may be repeated about 1 year after surgery and then again if warranted. Serum thyroglobulin and radioiodine scanning are stimulated by either rhTSH or thyroid hormone withdrawal according to the protocols described above for ^{131}I treatment.

The combination of rhTSH-stimulated scanning and thyroglobulin levels detects a thyroid remnant or cancer with a sensitivity of 84%. However, the presence of antithyroglobulin antibodies renders the serum thyroglobulin determination uninterpretable. In about 21% of low-risk patients, rhTSH stimulates serum thyroglobulin to above 2 ng/mL; such patients have a 23% risk of local neck metastases and a 13% risk of distant metastases. The rhTSH-stimulated radioiodine neck and whole-body scan detects only about half of these metastases because they are small or not avid for iodine. Some patients have persistent radioiodine uptake in the neck on diagnostic scanning but have no visible tumor on neck ultrasound; such patients do not require additional radioiodine therapy, especially if the serum thyroglobulin level is very low.

5. Positron emission tomography scanning—^{18}FDG-PET scanning is particularly useful for detecting thyroid cancer metastases in patients with a detectable serum thyroglobulin (especially serum thyroglobulin levels greater than 10 ng/mL and rising) who have a normal whole-body RAI scan and an unrevealing neck ultrasound. It is also sensitive for detecting metastases from medullary thyroid carcinoma. Diabetic patients with serum glucose less than 200 mg/dL (11.2 mmol/L) may be scanned, since the tracer acts like glucose in the body. ^{18}FDG-PET scanning can be combined with a CT scan; the resultant ^{18}FDG-PET/CT fusion scan is 60% sensitive for detecting metastases that are not visible by other methods. This scan is less sensitive for small brain metastases. ^{18}FDG-PET scanning detects the metabolic activity of tumor tissue; for differentiated thyroid carcinoma, this scan is more sensitive when the patient's thyroid cancer is stimulated with rhTSH (Thyrogen). One problem with ^{18}FDG-PET scanning is its lack of specificity. False-positives can occur with benign hepatic tumors, sarcoidosis, radiation therapy, suture granulomas, reactive lymph nodes, or inflammation at surgical sites that can persist for months.

6. Other scanning—Thallium-201 (^{201}Tl) scans may be useful for detecting metastatic differentiated thyroid carcinoma when the ^{131}I scan is normal but serum thyroglobulin is elevated. MRI scanning is particularly useful for imaging metastases in the brain, mediastinum, or bones. CT scanning is useful for imaging and monitoring pulmonary metastases.

▶ **Prognosis**

Papillary thyroid carcinoma has an overall mortality rate of 3%. It is best staged using the MACIS (metastasis, age, completeness of resection, invasion, size) scoring system (Table 26–7). ^{18}FDG-PET scanning independently predicts survival, with patients having few PET-avid metastases and low SUV$_{max}$ (highest image-pixel standardized uptake value) having a generally good prognosis, particularly for adults under age 45 years. Unlike other forms of cancer, patients with papillary thyroid carcinoma who have palpable lymph node metastases do not have a particularly increased mortality rate; however, their risk of local recurrence is increased.

The following characteristics imply a worse prognosis: age over 45 years, male sex, bone or brain metastases, macronodular (greater than 1 cm) pulmonary metastases, and lack of ^{131}I uptake into metastases. Younger patients with pulmonary metastases tend to respond better to ^{131}I therapy than do older adults. Certain papillary histologic types are associated with a higher risk of recurrence and reduced survival: tall cell, columnar cell, and diffuse sclerosing types tend to be more aggressive than classic papillary thyroid cancer; the best prognosis has been with the follicular variant of papillary thyroid cancer. Brain metastases are detected in 1%; they reduce median survival to 12 months, but the patient's prognosis is improved by surgical resection.

Patients with **follicular thyroid carcinoma** have a cancer mortality rate that is 3.4 times higher than patients with papillary carcinoma. The Hürthle cell variant of follicular carcinoma is even more aggressive. Both follicular carcinoma and its Hürthle cell variant tend to present at a more advanced stage than papillary carcinoma. However, at a given stage, the different types of differentiated thyroid carcinoma have a similar prognosis. Patients with primary tumors larger than 1 cm in diameter who undergo limited thyroid surgery (subtotal thyroidectomy or lobectomy) have a 2.2-fold increased mortality over those having total or near-total thyroidectomies. Patients who have not received ^{131}I ablation have mortality rates that are increased twofold by 10 years and threefold by 25 years (over those who have received ablation). The risk of cancer recurrence is twofold higher in men than in women and 1.7-fold higher in multifocal than in unifocal tumors.

Patients with a normal ^{18}FDG-PET scan have a 98% 5-year survival, while those having more than 10 metastases have a 20% 5-year survival. Those with a SUV$_{max}$ of 0.1-4.6 have a 5-year survival of 85%, while those with a SUV$_{max}$ greater than 13.3 have a 5-year survival of 20%. Patients with only local metastases have a 5-year survival of 95%, while those with regional (supraclavicular, mediastinal) metastases have a 5-year survival of 70%, and those with distant metastases have a 5-year survival of 35%.

Medullary thyroid carcinoma is more aggressive than differentiated thyroid cancer but is typically fairly indolent. However, medullary thyroid carcinoma with a somatic *RET* codon M918T mutation is the most aggressive medullary thyroid carcinoma and has a poorer prognosis. The overall 10-year survival rate is 90% when the tumor is confined to the thyroid, 70% for those with metastases to cervical lymph nodes, and 20% for those with distant metastases. When postoperative serum calcitonin levels are below 150 pg/mL (44 pmol/L), residual disease is likely confined to the neck, whereas when postoperative serum calcitonin levels are above 500 pg/mL (146 pmol/L), distant metastases are likely. Patients with sporadic disease usually have lymph node involvement noted at the time of diagnosis, whereas distal metastases may not be noted for years. For patients who have metastases to lymph nodes, modified radical neck dissection is recommended. Familial cases and those associated with MEN 2A tend to be less aggressive; the 10-year survival rate is higher, in part due to earlier detection. Patients with metastatic medullary thyroid carcinoma whose serum calcitonin doubling time is over 2 years also have a relatively good prognosis.

Medullary thyroid carcinoma that is seen in MEN 2B (MEN 3) is more aggressive, arises earlier in life, and carries a worse overall prognosis, especially when associated with a germline *M918T* mutation. Older adults tend to have more aggressive medullary thyroid carcinomas. Women with medullary thyroid carcinoma who are under age 40 years have a better prognosis. A better prognosis is also obtained in patients undergoing total thyroidectomy and neck dissection; radiation therapy reduces recurrence in patients with metastases to neck nodes. The mortality rate is increased 4.5-fold when primary or metastatic tumor tissue stains heavily for myelomonocytic antigen M-1. Conversely, tumors with heavy immunoperoxidase staining for calcitonin are associated with prolonged survival even in the presence of significant metastases.

Anaplastic thyroid carcinoma carries a 1-year survival rate of about 10% and a 5-year survival rate of about 5%. Patients with fully localized tumors on MRI have a better prognosis.

Localized thyroid lymphoma carries a 5-year survival of nearly 100%. Those with disease outside the thyroid have a 63% 5-year survival. However, the prognosis is better for those with mucosa-associated lymphoid tissue lymphoma compared to diffuse large B-cell lymphoma. Patients presenting with stridor, pain, laryngeal nerve palsy, or mediastinal extension tend to fare worse.

Banerjee M et al. Treatment-free survival in patients with differentiated thyroid cancer. J Clin Endocrinol Metab. 2018 Jul 1;103(7):2720–7. [PMID: 29788217]

Bibbins-Domingo K et al. Screening for thyroid cancer: US Preventive Services Task Force recommendation statement. JAMA. 2017 May 9;317(18):1882–7. [PMID: 28492905]

Cabanillas ME et al. Thyroid cancer. Lancet. 2016 Dec 3; 388(10061):2783–95. [PMID: 27240885]

Haugen BR et al. 2015 American Thyroid Association management guidelines for adult patients with thyroid nodules and differentiated thyroid cancer. Thyroid. 2016 Jan;26(1):1–133. [PMID: 26462967]

Nixon IJ et al. Management of invasive differentiated thyroid cancer. Thyroid. 2016 Sep;26(9):1156–66. [PMID: 27480110]

Takano T. Natural history of thyroid cancer. Endocr J. 2017 Mar 31;64(3):237–44. [PMID: 28154351]

Wells SA Jr et al. Revised American Thyroid Association guidelines for the management of medullary thyroid carcinoma. Thyroid. 2015 Jun;25(6):567–610. [PMID: 25810047]

IODINE DEFICIENCY DISORDER & ENDEMIC GOITER

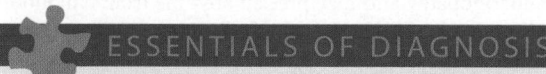

ESSENTIALS OF DIAGNOSIS

► Common in regions with low-iodine diets.

► High rate of congenital hypothyroidism and cretinism.

► Goiters may become multinodular and enlarge.

► Most adults with endemic goiter are euthyroid; however, some are hypothyroid or hyperthyroid.

► General Considerations

The daily minimum dietary requirement for iodine is 150 mcg/day in nonpregnant adults and 250 mcg/day for pregnant or lactating women. Mild-to-moderate and sometimes severe iodine deficiency exists in 30 countries. An estimated 1.9 billion people have insufficient iodine intake. Severe iodine deficiency increases the risk of miscarriage and stillbirth. Cretinism occurs in about 0.5% of live births in iodine-deficient areas. Moderate iodine deficiency during gestation and infancy can cause manifestations of hypothyroidism, deafness, short stature, and lowers a child's intelligence quotient by 10–15 points. Even mild-to-moderate iodine deficiency appears to impair a child's perceptual reasoning and global cognitive index.

Although iodine deficiency is the most common cause of endemic goiter, there are other natural goitrogens, including certain foods (eg, sorghum, millet, maize, cassava), mineral deficiencies (selenium, iron, zinc), and water pollutants, which can themselves cause goiter or aggravate a goiter proclivity caused by iodine deficiency. In iodine-deficient patients, smoking can induce goiter growth. Pregnancy aggravates iodine deficiency and can increase the size of thyroid nodules and cause new nodules. Some individuals are particularly susceptible to goiter owing to congenital partial defects in thyroid enzyme activity.

► Clinical Findings

A. Symptoms and Signs

Endemic goiters may become multinodular and very large. Growth often occurs during pregnancy and may cause compressive symptoms.

Substernal goiters are usually asymptomatic but can cause tracheal compression, respiratory distress and failure, dysphagia, superior vena cava syndrome, gastrointestinal bleeding from esophageal varices, palsies of the phrenic or recurrent laryngeal nerves, or Horner syndrome. Cerebral ischemia and stroke can result from arterial compression or thyrocervical steal syndrome. Substernal goiters can rarely cause pleural or pericardial effusions. The incidence of significant malignancy is less than 1%.

Some patients with endemic goiter may become hypothyroid. Others may become thyrotoxic as the goiter grows and becomes more autonomous, especially if iodine is added to the diet.

B. Laboratory Findings

The serum T_4 and TSH are generally normal. TSH falls in the presence of hyperthyroidism if a multinodular goiter has become autonomous in the presence of sufficient amounts of iodine for thyroid hormone synthesis. TSH rises with hypothyroidism. Thyroid RAI uptake is usually elevated, but it may be normal if iodine intake has improved. Serum levels of antithyroid antibodies are usually either undetectable or in low titers. Serum thyroglobulin is often elevated above 13 mcg/L. Urine iodine concentrations are low.

Differential Diagnosis

Endemic goiter must be distinguished from all other forms of nodular goiter that may coexist in an endemic region.

Prevention

The minimum dietary requirement for iodine is about 50 mcg daily, with optimal iodine intake being 150–300 mcg daily. Iodized salt contains iodine at about 20 mg per kg salt. Other sources of iodine include commercial bread, milk, and seafood. Initiating iodine supplementation in an iodine-deficient area greatly reduces the emergence of new goiters but causes an increased frequency of hyperthyroidism during the first year. One iodine-depleted area was Pescopagano, Italy, where 46% of adults had goiters. Salt was iodized (30 mg of potassium iodate per kg salt) and made available in 1985. After 15 years, the incidence of goiter declined to 23%. However, the prevalence of Hashimoto thyroiditis rose from 3.5% to 14.5% after 15 years of iodine supplementation.

Treatment

Iodine supplementation has not proven effective for treating adults with large multinodular goiter due to iodine deficiency and actually increases their risk of developing thyrotoxicosis. Thyroidectomy may be required for cosmesis, compressive symptoms, or thyrotoxicosis. There is a high goiter recurrence rate in iodine-deficient geographic areas, so near-total thyroidectomy is preferred when surgery is indicated. Certain patients may be treated with ^{131}I for large compressive goiters.

Complications

Dietary iodine supplementation increases the risk of autoimmune thyroid dysfunction, which may cause hypothyroidism or hyperthyroidism. Excessive iodine supplementation increases the risk of goiter. Suppression of TSH by administering levothyroxine carries the risk of inducing hyperthyroidism, particularly in patients with autonomous multinodular goiters; therefore, levothyroxine suppression should not be started in patients with a low TSH level. Treating patients with ^{131}I for large multinodular goiter may shrink the gland; however, Graves disease develops in some patients 3–10 months following therapy.

Doggui R et al. Iodine deficiency: physiological, clinical and epidemiological features, and pre-analytical considerations. Ann Endocrinol (Paris). 2015 Feb;76(1):59–66. [PMID: 25613936]

Niwattisaiwong S et al. Iodine deficiency: clinical implications. Cleve Clin J Med. 2017 Mar;84(3):236–44. [PMID: 28322679]

Zimmerman MB et al. Iodine deficiency and thyroid disorders. Lancet Diabetes Endocrinol. 2015 Apr;3(4):286–95. [PMID: 25591468]

▼ DISEASES OF THE PARATHYROIDS

Parathyroid hormone (PTH) increases osteoclastic activity in bone, increases the renal tubular reabsorption of calcium, and stimulates the synthesis of 1,25-dihydroxycholecalciferol by the kidney. Meanwhile, PTH inhibits the reabsorption of phosphate and bicarbonate by the renal tubule. All of these effects cause a net increase in serum calcium.

HYPOPARATHYROIDISM & PSEUDOHYPOPARATHYROIDISM

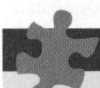

ESSENTIALS OF DIAGNOSIS

- ▶ Tetany, carpopedal spasms, tingling of lips and hands, cramps, irritability.
- ▶ Chvostek sign and Trousseau phenomenon.
- ▶ Hypocalcemia with low serum PTH; serum phosphate high; alkaline phosphatase normal; urine calcium excretion reduced.
- ▶ Serum magnesium may be low.

General Considerations

Acquired hypoparathyroidism is most commonly caused by anterior neck surgery, occurring after total thyroidectomy in about 25% of patients transiently, and in about 4% of patients permanently. The risk of permanent postoperative hypoparathyroidism can be reduced during thyroid surgery by taking parathyroid glands with suspected vascular damage and autotransplanting them into the sternocleidomastoid muscle. Permanent hypoparathyroidism may occur after the resection of multiple parathyroid adenomas. It also occurs transiently after the surgical removal of a single parathyroid adenoma for primary hyperparathyroidism due to suppression of the remaining normal parathyroids and accelerated remineralization of the skeleton. This is known as "hungry bone syndrome." In such cases, hypocalcemia can be quite severe, particularly in patients with preoperative hyperparathyroid bone disease and vitamin D or magnesium deficiency. *All patients undergoing thyroidectomy or parathyroidectomy must be observed closely overnight.* Neck irradiation is a rare cause of hypoparathyroidism.

Autoimmune hypoparathyroidism may be isolated or combined with other endocrine deficiencies. Autoimmune polyendocrine syndrome type I (APS-I) is also known as autoimmune polyendocrinopathy-candidiasis-ectodermal dystrophy (APECED). In APS-I, mucocutaneous candidiasis appears in the newborn period. Hypoparathyroidism is the most frequent and often the only endocrine deficiency. Addison disease is the next most common autoimmune endocrinopathy and may present anytime from childhood to young adulthood. Hypothyroidism, type 1 diabetes, or pituitary deficiency as well as cataracts, uveitis, alopecia, or vitiligo can also develop. Autoimmune gastrointestinal manifestations are also common. Fat malabsorption occurs in 20% of patients with APS-I; treatment of hypocalcemia can be challenging in patients with APS-I, since vitamin D_3 is fat-soluble. Hypoparathyroidism can also occur in SLE caused by antiparathyroid antibodies.

Parathyroid deficiency may also be the result of damage from heavy metals such as copper (Wilson disease) or iron (hemochromatosis, transfusion hemosiderosis), granulomas, Riedel thyroiditis, tumors, or infection.

Magnesium deficiency causes functional hypoparathyroidism. Hypomagnesemia is most commonly caused by alcoholism, diuretics, intestinal malabsorption, and proton pump inhibitors. Hypomagnesemia can also be caused by aminoglycosides, amphotericin, pentamidine, and epithelial growth factor inhibitors (panitumumab, cetuximab). Although mild hypomagnesemia stimulates PTH secretion, more severe hypomagnesemia (below 1.2 mg/dL) inhibits PTH secretion. Hypomagnesemia also causes resistance to PTH in bone and renal tubules. Correction of hypomagnesemia results in rapid disappearance of the condition.

Hypermagnesemia also suppresses PTH secretion. Hypermagnesemia occurs most commonly in patients with kidney dysfunction who take magnesium-containing antacids, laxatives, or dietary supplements.

~ Symptomatic hypoparathyroidism may be precipitated by a proton pump inhibitor, since absorption of calcium decreases with reduced stomach acidity.

Congenital hypoparathyroidism causes hypocalcemia beginning in infancy. However, it may not be diagnosed for many years. Since hypoparathyroidism can be familial, screening is suggested for family members of any patient with idiopathic hypoparathyroidism.

▶ Clinical Findings

A. Symptoms and Signs

Manifestations of hypocalcemia vary from subtle to life-threatening. Patients have a reduced quality of life, with fatigue; irritability; depression; anxiety; cognitive impairment or "brain fog"; lethargy; and paresthesias in the circumoral area, hands, and feet. More severe manifestations include muscle weakness or cramps, carpopedal spasm, convulsions, tetany, laryngospasm and stridor. Chronic hypocalcemia with hyperphosphatemia can cause calcifications in soft tissues, such as joints, skin, and arteries. Brain calcifications in the basal ganglia and cerebral cortex can cause parkinsonian symptoms or choreoathetosis. However, some patients with chronic hypocalcemia are asymptomatic, even with very low levels of serum calcium.

Chvostek sign (facial muscle contraction on tapping the facial nerve in front of the ear) is positive, and Trousseau phenomenon (carpal spasm after application of a sphygmomanometer cuff) is present. Cataracts may occur; the nails may be thin and brittle; the skin is dry and scaly, at times with fungus infection (candidiasis), and there may be loss of eyebrows; and deep tendon reflexes may be hyperactive. Pseudotumor cerebri with papilledema and elevated CSF pressure is occasionally seen. Teeth may be defective if the onset of the disease occurs in childhood.

B. Laboratory Findings

Serum calcium is low, serum phosphate high, urinary calcium low, and alkaline phosphatase normal. Serum calcium is largely bound to albumin. In patients with hypoalbuminemia, the serum ionized calcium may be determined; it should be 4.6–5.3 mg/dL (1.15–1.32 mmol/L).

Alternatively, the serum calcium level can be corrected for serum albumin level as follows:

$$\text{"Corrected" serum } Ca^{2+} = \text{Serum } Ca^{2+} \text{mg/dL} + (0.8 \times [4.0 - \text{Albumin g/dL}])$$

Serum PTH levels are usually low or not elevated in the presence of hypocalcemia. Serum magnesium levels should always be measured. Serum calcium should not be determined within 24 hours following intravenous gadolinium, since gadolinium interferes with the colorimetric calcium assay, thereby causing artefactual hypocalcemia.

C. Imaging

Radiographs or CT scans of the skull may show basal ganglia calcifications. The bones may appear denser than normal and the bone mineral density is usually increased. Cutaneous calcification may occur.

D. Other Examinations

Slit-lamp examination may show early posterior lenticular cataract formation. The electrocardiogram (ECG) may show heart block, have a prolonged QTc interval, and there may be T wave abnormalities in the presence of hypocalcemia. Patients with chronic hypoparathyroidism tend to have increased bone mineral density, particularly in the lumbar spine.

▶ Complications

Acute tetany with stridor, especially if associated with vocal cord palsy, may lead to respiratory obstruction requiring tracheostomy. There may be associated autoimmunity causing celiac disease, pernicious anemia, or Addison disease. Ossification of the paravertebral ligaments may occur with nerve root compression; surgical decompression may be required. Seizures are common in untreated patients. Overtreatment with vitamin D and calcium may produce nephrocalcinosis and impairment of kidney function. Hypocalcemia can also cause heart failure and dysrhythmias.

▶ Differential Diagnosis

Paresthesias, muscle cramps, or tetany due to respiratory alkalosis, in which the serum calcium is normal, can be confused with hypocalcemia. In fact, hyperventilation tends to accentuate hypocalcemic symptoms.

Hypocalcemia may be caused by certain drugs: loop diuretics, plicamycin, phenytoin, foscarnet, denosumab, and bisphosphonates. In addition, hypocalcemia may be seen in cases of rapid intravascular volume expansion or due to chelation from transfusions of large volumes of citrated blood. Hypocalcemia may also be due to malabsorption of calcium, magnesium, or vitamin D; patients do not always have diarrhea. It is also observed in patients with acute pancreatitis. Hypocalcemia may develop in some patients with certain osteoblastic metastatic carcinomas (especially breast, prostate) instead of the expected hypercalcemia. Hypocalcemia with hyperphosphatemia (simulating hypoparathyroidism) is seen in azotemia, but may also be caused by large doses of intravenous, oral, or rectal phosphate preparations and by chemotherapy of responsive lymphomas or leukemias.

Hypocalcemia with hypercalciuria may be due to a familial syndrome involving a mutation in the calcium-sensing receptor; such patients have serum PTH levels that are in the normal range, distinguishing it from hypoparathyroidism. It is transmitted as an autosomal dominant disorder. Such patients are hypercalciuric; treatment with calcium and vitamin D may cause nephrocalcinosis.

Congenital pseudohypoparathyroidism is a group of disorders characterized by hypocalcemia due to resistance to PTH. Subtypes are caused by different mutations involving the renal PTH receptor, the receptor's G protein, or adenylyl cyclase.

▶ **Treatment**

A. Prophylaxis Against Severe Postoperative Hypocalcemia

Post-thyroidectomy hypocalcemia can be detected early by closely monitoring serum PTH and calcium. If the serum calcium falls below 8.0 mg/dL (2.0 mmol/L) with a serum PTH below 10–15 pg/mL (1.0–1.5 pmol/L) after thyroid or parathyroid surgery, the patient is at high risk for hypocalcemia and can be prophylactically treated with calcitriol and oral calcium. Calcitriol is typically given orally in doses of 0.25–1 mcg twice daily. Prophylactic elemental calcium is given orally as calcium carbonate (with meals) 500–1000 mg twice daily.

B. Emergency Treatment for Acute Hypocalcemia (Hypoparathyroid Tetany)

1. Airway—Be sure an adequate airway is present.

2. Intravenous calcium gluconate—Calcium gluconate, 10–20 mL of 10% solution intravenously, may be given *slowly* until tetany ceases. Ten to 50 mL of 10% calcium gluconate may be added to 1 L of 5% glucose in water or saline and administered by slow intravenous drip. The rate should be adjusted so that the serum calcium is maintained in the range of 8–9 mg/dL (2–2.25 mmol/L).

3. Oral calcium—Calcium salts should be given orally as soon as possible to supply 1–2 g of calcium daily. Liquid calcium carbonate, 500 mg/5 mL, contains 40% calcium and may be especially useful. The dosage is 1–3 g calcium orally daily; it should be given with meals.

4. Vitamin D preparations—(Table 26–8.) Therapy should be started as soon as oral calcium is begun. The active metabolite of vitamin D, 1,25-dihydroxycholecalciferol (calcitriol), has a very rapid onset of action and is not long-lasting if hypercalcemia occurs. It is of great use in the treatment of acute hypocalcemia. Therapy is commenced at a dosage of 0.25 mcg orally each morning with upward dosage titration to near normocalcemia. Ultimately, doses of 0.5–2 mcg/day are usually required.

5. Magnesium—If hypomagnesemia (serum magnesium less than 1.8 mg/dL or less than 0.8 mmol/L) is present, it must be corrected to treat the resulting hypocalcemia. For critical hypomagnesemia (serum magnesium less than 1.0 mg/dL or less than 0.45 mmol/L), 50% magnesium sulfate solution (5 g/10 mL) is diluted in 250 mL 0.9% saline or 5% dextrose in water and given by an intravenous infusion of 5 g over 3 hours, with further dosing based on serum magnesium levels. Long-term oral magnesium replacement may be given as magnesium oxide 500 mg (60% elemental magnesium) tablets, one to three times daily.

C. Maintenance Treatment of Hypoparathyroidism

Patients with mild hypoparathyroidism may require no therapy but need close monitoring for manifestations of hypocalcemia. Therapy is ordinarily required for patients with symptomatic hypocalcemia or serum calcium levels below 8.0 mg/dL (2 mmol/L).

Vitamin D, calcium, and magnesium therapy: Patients with hypoparathyroidism have a reduced renal tubular reabsorption of calcium and are thus prone to hypercalciuria and kidney stones if the serum calcium is normalized with calcium and vitamin D therapy. Therefore, the goal is to maintain the serum calcium in a slightly low but asymptomatic range of 8–8.6 mg/dL (2–2.15 mmol/L). It is prudent to monitor urine calcium with "spot" urine determinations and keep the level below 30 mg/dL (7.5 mmol/L), if possible. Hypercalciuria may respond to oral hydrochlorothiazide, 25 mg daily, usually given with a potassium supplement. Serum magnesium should be monitored and kept in the normal range with supplemental magnesium, if required. Serum phosphate should also be monitored and the serum calcium × phosphate product kept below 55 mg²/dL² (4.4 mmol²/L²).

Calcium supplements can be given in doses of 800–1000 mg orally daily. Calcium carbonate 1 g contains 400 mg of elemental calcium and should be given with meals;

Table 26–8. Vitamin D preparations used in the treatment of hypoparathyroidism.

	Available Preparations	Daily Dose	Duration of Action
Ergocalciferol, ergosterol (vitamin D₂, calciferol)	50,000 international units capsules; 8000 international units/mL oral solution	2000–200,000 units	1–2 weeks
Cholecalciferol (vitamin D₃)	50,000 international units capsules, not available commercially in United States; may be compounded	10,000–50,000 units	4–8 weeks
Calcitriol (Rocaltrol)	0.25 and 0.5 mcg capsules; 1 mcg/mL oral solution; 1 mcg/mL for injection	0.25–4 mcg	½–2 weeks

calcium citrate 1 g contains 211 mg of elemental calcium, but can be given any time and causes less gastrointestinal intolerance. Calcium lactate (13% elemental calcium) and calcium gluconate (9% elemental calcium) are other options for calcium supplementation.

Vitamin D is generally required for patients with chronic hypoparathyroidism (Table 26–8). Monitoring of serum calcium at regular intervals (at least every 3–4 months) is recommended. Calcitriol, a short-acting preparation, is given in doses that range from 0.25 mcg/day to 2.0 mcg orally daily. Ergocalciferol (vitamin D_2) is derived from plants; the usual dose ranges from 25,000 to 150,000 units/day. It is stored in fat, giving it a long duration of action. If toxicity develops, hypercalcemia—treatable with hydration and prednisone—may persist for weeks after it is discontinued. Despite this risk, ergocalciferol usually produces a more stable serum calcium level than do the shorter-acting preparations.

PTH is effective for treating patients with hypoparathyroidism but is restricted to patients whose hypocalcemia cannot be adequately treated with calcium and vitamin D analogs (see above). Recombinant human parathyroid hormone (rhPTH) is an 84-amino acid polypeptide that is identical to native PTH (1–84). It is FDA approved and marketed as NATPARA as an adjunct to calcium and vitamin D analogs to control symptomatic hypocalcemia in patients with hypoparathyroidism. It must be given by subcutaneous injection every 1–2 days. Although rhPTH can normalize serum calcium levels in patients with severe hypocalcemia, there have been no controlled studies indicating that rhPTH is superior to conventional therapy in reversing the fatigue and muscle weakness often reported by these patients. Side effects of rhPTH include nausea, vomiting, diarrhea, arthralgias, and paresthesias. Also, osteosarcoma has occurred in rats receiving very high-dose PTH. The FDA requires that prescribers be certified before prescribing the drug and that patients and prescribers formally acknowledge the risk of osteosarcoma. rhPTH is expensive, which limits its use.

Transplantation of cryopreserved parathyroid tissue, removed during prior surgery, restores normocalcemia in about 23% of cases.

Hypoparathyroidism in pregnancy presents special challenges. Maternal hypocalcemia can adversely affect the skeletal development of the fetus and cause compensatory hyperparathyroidism in the newborn. Maternal hypercalcemia can suppress fetal parathyroid development, resulting in neonatal hypocalcemia. This requires very close clinical and biochemical monitoring during pregnancy.

Caution: Phenothiazine drugs should be administered with caution, since they may precipitate extrapyramidal symptoms in hypocalcemic patients. Furosemide should be avoided, since it may worsen hypocalcemia.

▶ Prognosis

Patients with mild hypoparathyroidism generally do well. Periodic serum calcium levels are required, since changes may call for modification of the treatment schedule. Hypercalcemia that develops in patients with seemingly stable, treated hypoparathyroidism may be a presenting sign of Addison disease.

Despite optimal therapy, patients with moderate-to-severe hypoparathyroidism have been reported to have an overall reduced quality of life. Chronically affected patients frequently develop calcifications in their kidneys and basal ganglia. They have an increased risk of calcium kidney stones and kidney dysfunction as well as seizures, mood and psychiatric disorders, and a reduced overall sense of well-being. Therapy with rhPTH may prevent or improve these manifestations.

Brandi ML et al. Management of hypoparathyroidism: summary statement and guidelines. J Clin Endocrinol Metab. 2016 Jun; 101(6):2273–83. [PMID: 26943719]

Büttner M et al. Quality of life in patients with hypoparathyroidism receiving standard treatment: a systematic review. Endocrine. 2017 Oct;58(1):14–20. [PMID: 28822059]

Cianferotti L et al. Pseudohypoparathyroidism. Minerva Endocrinol. 2018 Jun;43(2):156–67. [PMID: 29125274]

Clarke BL et al. Epidemiology and diagnosis of hypoparathyroidism. J Clin Endocrinol Metab. 2016 Jun;101(6):2284–99. [PMID: 26943720]

Mannstadt M et al. Hypoparathyroidism. Nat Rev Dis Primers. 2017 Aug 31;3:17055. [PMID: 28857066]

Winer KK. Does PTH replacement therapy improve quality of life in patients with chronic hypoparathyroidism? J Clin Endocrinol Metab. 2018 Jul 1;103(7):2752–5. [PMID: 29897557]

HYPERPARATHYROIDISM

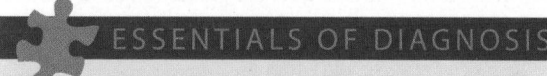
ESSENTIALS OF DIAGNOSIS

- ▶ Often found incidentally by routine blood testing.
- ▶ Renal calculi, polyuria, hypertension, constipation, fatigue, mental changes.
- ▶ Bone pain; rarely, cystic lesions and pathologic fractures.
- ▶ Elevated PTH, serum and urine calcium, and urine phosphate; serum phosphate low to normal; alkaline phosphatase normal to elevated.

▶ General Considerations

Primary hyperparathyroidism is the most common cause of hypercalcemia, with a prevalence of 1000 to 4000 cases per 1 million persons. It occurs at all ages but most commonly in the seventh decade and in women (74%). Before age 45, the prevalence is similar in men and women. It is more prevalent in blacks, followed by whites, then other races.

Parathyroid glands vary in number and location and ectopic parathyroid glands have been found within the thyroid gland, high in the neck or carotid sheath, in the retroesophageal space, and within the thymus or mediastinum. Hyperparathyroidism is caused by hypersecretion of PTH, usually by a single parathyroid adenoma (80%), and less commonly by hyperplasia of two or more parathyroid glands (20%), or carcinoma (less than 1%). However, when hyperparathyroidism presents before age 30 years, there is a higher incidence of multiglandular disease (36%) and parathyroid carcinoma (5%). The size of the parathyroid adenoma correlates with the serum PTH level.

Hyperparathyroidism is familial in about 10% of cases; hyperparathyroidism presenting before age 45 has a higher chance of being familial. Parathyroid hyperplasia may arise in MEN types 1, 2 (2A), and 4. (See Table 26–12.) In MEN 1, multiglandular hyperparathyroidism is usually the initial manifestation and ultimately occurs in 90% of affected individuals. Hyperparathyroidism in MEN 2 (2A) is less frequent than in MEN 1 and is usually milder.

Hyperparathyroidism results in the excessive excretion of calcium and phosphate by the kidneys. PTH stimulates renal tubular reabsorption of calcium; however, hyperparathyroidism causes hypercalcemia and an increase in calcium in the glomerular filtrate that overwhelms tubular reabsorption capacity, resulting in hypercalciuria. At least 5% of renal calculi are associated with this disease. Diffuse parenchymal calcification (nephrocalcinosis) is seen less commonly. Hyperparathyroidism causes demineralization of cortical bone and a gain of trabecular bone. Severe, chronic hyperparathyroidism can cause pathologic fractures, and cystic bone lesions throughout the skeleton, a condition known as osteitis fibrosa cystic.

Parathyroid carcinoma is a rare cause of hyperparathyroidism, accounting for less than 1% of hyperparathyroidism. There is typically a palpable neck mass (75%). However, some cases present with smaller tumors, less severe hypercalcemia, and benign-appearing histologic features. Local recurrence is the rule if surgical margins are positive. Distant metastases arise most commonly in the lungs but also in bones, liver, brain, and mediastinum. Although parathyroid carcinoma is typically indolent, an increasing tumor burden is associated with critically severe hypercalcemia and death.

Secondary and tertiary hyperparathyroidism usually occurs in patients with chronic kidney disease, in which hyperphosphatemia and decreased renal production of 1,25-dihydroxycholecalciferol ($1,25[OH]_2D_3$) initially produce a decrease in ionized calcium. The parathyroid glands are stimulated (secondary hyperparathyroidism) and may enlarge, becoming autonomous (tertiary hyperparathyroidism). The bone disease seen in this setting is known as renal osteodystrophy (see Disorders of Mineral Metabolism, Chapter 22). Hypercalcemia often occurs after kidney transplant. Secondary hyperparathyroidism predictably develops in patients with a deficiency in vitamin D. Serum calcium levels are typically in the normal range, but may rise to become borderline elevated with time, with tertiary hyperparathyroidism due to parathyroid glandular hyperplasia.

▶ Clinical Findings

A. Symptoms and Signs

In the developed world, hypercalcemia is typically discovered incidentally by routine chemistry panels. Many patients are asymptomatic or have mild symptoms that may be elicited only upon questioning. Parathyroid adenomas are usually so small and deeply located in the neck that they are almost never palpable; when a mass is palpated, it usually turns out to be an incidental thyroid nodule.

Symptomatic patients are said to have problems with "bones, stones, abdominal groans, psychic moans, with fatigue overtones."

1. Skeletal manifestations—Low bone density is typically most prominent at the distal one-third of the radius, a site of mostly cortical bone. Lumbar (trabecular) spine bone density is often spared and is higher compared to the distal radius. Hip bones are a mixture of trabecular and cortical bone, and femur bone density tends to be midway between the lumbar spine and distal radius. Postmenopausal women are prone to asymptomatic vertebral fractures. Although significant bone demineralization is uncommon in mild hyperparathyroidism, osteitis fibrosa cystica may present as pathologic fractures or as "brown tumors" or cysts of the jaw. More commonly, patients experience arthralgias and bone pain, particularly involving the legs.

2. Hypercalcemia manifestations—Mild hypercalcemia may be asymptomatic. However, hypercalcemia of hyperparathyroidism usually causes a variety of manifestations whose severity is not entirely predictable by the level of serum calcium or PTH. In fact, patients with only mild hypercalcemia can have significant symptoms, particularly depression, constipation, and bone and joint pain. **Neuromuscular** manifestations include paresthesias, muscle cramps and weakness, and diminished deep tendon reflexes. **Central nervous system** manifestations include malaise, headache, fatigue, intellectual weariness, insomnia, irritability, and depression. Patients may have cognitive impairment that can vary from intellectual weariness to more severe disorientation, psychosis, or stupor. **Cardiovascular** symptoms include hypertension, palpitations, prolonged P-R interval, shortened Q-T interval, bradyarrhythmias, heart block, asystole, and sensitivity to digitalis. **Kidney** manifestations include polyuria and polydipsia, caused by hypercalcemia-induced nephrogenic diabetes insipidus. Among all patients with newly discovered hyperparathyroidism, calcium-containing renal calculi have occurred or are detectable in about 18%. Patients with asymptomatic hyperparathyroidism have a 7% incidence of asymptomatic calcium nephrolithiasis, compared to 1.6% incidence in age-matched controls. **Gastrointestinal** symptoms include anorexia, nausea, heartburn, vomiting, abdominal pain, weight loss, constipation, and obstipation. Pancreatitis occurs in 3%. Pruritus may be present. Calcium may precipitate in the corneas ("band keratopathy"), in extravascular tissues (calcinosis), and in small arteries, causing small vessel thrombosis and skin necrosis (calciphylaxis).

3. Normocalcemic primary hyperparathyroidism—Patients with normocalcemic primary hyperparathyroidism generally have few symptoms. However, on average, such patients have a slightly more atherogenic lipid panel and higher blood pressures (systolic blood pressure 10 mm Hg higher and diastolic blood pressure 7 mm Hg higher) than controls. Also, affected patients can have very subtle symptoms, such as mild fatigue, that may not be appreciated as abnormal.

4. Hyperparathyroidism during pregnancy—Pregnant women having mild hyperparathyroidism with a serum calcium below 11.0 mg/dL (less than 2.75 mmol/L) generally tolerate pregnancy well with normal outcomes. However, the majority of women with more severe hypercalcemia during pregnancy experience complications such as nephrolithiasis, hyperemesis, pancreatitis, muscle weakness, and cognitive changes. Hypercalcemic crisis may occur, especially postpartum. About 80% of fetuses experience complications of maternal hyperparathyroidism, including fetal demise, preterm delivery, and low birth weight. Newborns have hypoparathyroidism that can be permanent. Hypocalcemia in the infant can present with tetany even 2–3 months after delivery.

5. Parathyroid carcinoma—Hyperparathyroidism with a large neck mass, or vocal fold paralysis from recurrent laryngeal nerve palsy, raises concern for parathyroid carcinoma. *FNA biopsy is not recommended because it may seed the biopsy tract with tumor and cytologic distinction between benign and malignant tumors is problematic.* Parathyroid carcinoma is more frequent in patients with hyperparathyroidism–jaw tumor (HP-JT) syndrome as well as patients with MEN 1 and MEN 2A. Therefore, patients should have genetic testing.

B. Laboratory Findings

The hallmark of primary hyperparathyroidism is hypercalcemia, with the serum adjusted total calcium greater than 10.5 mg/dL (2.6 mmol/L). The adjusted total calcium = measured serum calcium in mg/dL + [0.8 × (4.0 − patient's serum albumin in g/dL)]. Serum ionized calcium levels are elevated (above 1.36 mmol/L).

To confirm the diagnosis of hyperparathyroidism, an assessment of urinary calcium excretion is recommended, particularly for patients with mild hyperthyroidism. In primary hyperparathyroidism the urine calcium excretion may be high or normal: 100–300 mg/day (25–75 mmol/day). However, low urine calcium excretions (below 100 mg/day [25 mmol/day]) in the absence of thiazide diuretics, occurs in only 4% of cases of primary hyperthyroidism and raises the differential diagnosis of familial hypocalciuric hypercalcemia.

The serum phosphate is often less than 2.5 mg/dL (0.8 mmol/L). In primary hyperparathyroidism, there is an excessive loss of phosphate in the urine in the presence of hypophosphatemia (25% of cases). A serum calcium:phosphate (Ca/P) ratio above 2.5 (mg/dL) or above 2.17 (mmol/L) helps confirm the diagnosis of primary hyperparathyroidism. The alkaline phosphatase is elevated only if bone disease is present. The plasma chloride and uric acid levels may be elevated. Vitamin D deficiency is common in patients with hyperparathyroidism, and it is prudent to screen for vitamin D deficiency with a serum 25-OH vitamin D determination. Serum 25-OH vitamin D levels below 20 mcg/L (50 nmol/L) can aggravate hyperparathyroidism and its bone manifestations.

Elevated serum levels of intact PTH confirm the diagnosis of hyperparathyroidism. Parathyroid carcinoma must always be suspected in patients with a serum calcium of 14.0 mcg/dL (3.5 mmol/L) or more and a serum PTH 5 or more times the upper limit of normal.

Patients with low bone density who have an elevated serum PTH but a normal serum calcium must be evaluated for causes of secondary hyperparathyroidism (eg, vitamin D or calcium deficiency, hyperphosphatemia, chronic kidney disease). In the absence of secondary hyperparathyroidism, patients with an elevated serum PTH but normal serum calcium are determined to have normocalcemic hyperparathyroidism. Such individuals require monitoring, since hypercalcemia develops in about 19% of patients over 3 years of follow-up.

Genetic testing is recommended for patients with documented primary hyperparathyroidism who are younger than age 40 or who have multiglandular disease or a family history of hyperparathyroidism.

C. Imaging

Parathyroid imaging is not necessary for the diagnosis of hyperparathyroidism. Imaging is performed for most patients prior to parathyroid surgery and is particularly important for patients who have had prior neck surgery. The visualization of an apparent parathyroid adenoma helps secure the diagnosis when there is occasional diagnostic difficulty and often allows for minimally invasive surgery.

Ultrasound of the neck should scan the neck from the mandible to the superior mediastinum in an effort to locate ectopic parathyroid adenomas. Ultrasound has a sensitivity of 79% for single adenomas but only 35% for multiglandular disease.

Sestamibi scintigraphy with ^{99m}Tc-sestamibi and single-photon emission computed tomography (SPECT) is most useful for localizing parathyroid adenomas. However, false-positive scans are common, caused by thyroid nodules, thyroiditis, or cervical lymphadenopathy. Sestamibi-SPECT imaging improves sensitivity for single parathyroid adenomas. Small benign thyroid nodules are discovered incidentally in nearly 50% of patients with hyperparathyroidism who have imaging with ultrasound or MRI.

^{18}**F-flurocholine PET/MRI** is a useful scan for patients with primary hyperparathyroidism and negative or discordant localization imaging on neck ultrasound and sestamibi scanning. In a small study, the sensitivity of this scan was 90%, with a 100% positive predictive value.

Conventional CT and MRI imaging are not usually required prior to a first neck surgery for hyperparathyroidism. However, a four-dimensional CT (4D-CT), with the fourth dimension referring to time, captures the rapid uptake and washout of contrast from parathyroid adenomas; it is particularly useful for preoperative imaging when ultrasonography and sestamibi scans are negative. It can also be helpful for patients who have had prior neck surgery and for those with ectopic glands. In such patients, 4D-CT has a sensitivity of 88%, versus 54% for sestamibi SPECT and 21% for ultrasound. However, 4D-CT delivers more radiation to the thyroid and so is used mostly for older patients. MRI may also be useful for repeat neck operations and when ectopic parathyroid glands are suspected. MRI shows better soft tissue contrast than CT.

Noncontrast-enhanced CT scanning of the kidneys should be considered in all patients with hyperparathyroidism to determine whether calcium-containing stones are present. For patients with apparently asymptomatic hyperparathyroidism, the presence or absence of calcium nephrolithiasis can be a deciding factor about whether to have parathyroidectomy surgery.

Bone density measurements by dual energy x-ray absorptiometry (DXA) are helpful in determining the amount of bone loss in patients with hyperparathyroidism. Bone loss occurs mostly in long bones, and DXA should ideally include three areas: lumbar spine, hip, and distal radius.

Bone radiographs are usually normal and are not required to make the diagnosis of hyperparathyroidism.

▶ Complications

Pathologic long bone fractures are a complication of hyperparathyroidism. Urinary tract infection due to stone and obstruction may lead to kidney disease and uremia. If the serum calcium level rises rapidly, clouding of sensorium, kidney disease, and rapid precipitation of calcium throughout the soft tissues may occur. Peptic ulcer and pancreatitis may be intractable before surgery. Insulinomas or gastrinomas may be associated, as well as pituitary tumors (MEN type 1). Pseudogout may complicate hyperparathyroidism both before and after surgical removal of tumors. Hypercalcemia during gestation produces neonatal hypocalcemia.

In tertiary hyperparathyroidism due to chronic kidney disease, high serum calcium and phosphate levels may cause disseminated calcification in the skin, soft tissues, and arteries (calciphylaxis); this can result in painful ischemic necrosis of skin and gangrene, cardiac arrhythmias, and respiratory failure. The actual serum levels of calcium and phosphate have not correlated well with calciphylaxis, but a calcium (mg/dL) × phosphate (mg/dL) product over 70 is usually present.

▶ Differential Diagnosis

Artefactual hypercalcemia is common, so a confirmatory serum calcium level should be drawn after an overnight fast along with a serum protein, albumin, and triglyceride while ensuring that the patient is well-hydrated. Hypercalcemia may be due to high serum protein concentrations; in the presence of very high or low serum albumin concentrations, an adjusted serum calcium or a serum ionized calcium is more dependable than the total serum calcium concentration. Hypercalcemia may also be seen with dehydration.

Hypercalcemia of malignancy occurs most frequently with breast, lung, pancreatic, uterine, and renal cell carcinoma, and paraganglioma. Most of these tumors secrete PTH-related protein (PTHrP) that has tertiary structural homologies to PTH and causes bone resorption and hypercalcemia similar to those caused by PTH. Serum PTH levels are low or low-normal while serum PTHrP levels are elevated; phosphate is often low. Other tumors can secrete excessive 1,25 (OH)$_2$ vitamin D$_3$, particularly lymphoproliferative and ovarian malignancies. The clinical features of malignant hypercalcemia can closely simulate hyperparathyroidism.

Pseudohyperparathyroidism of pregnancy presents with hypercalcemia during pregnancy. It is caused by hypersensitivity of the breasts to PRL. The breasts become abnormally enlarged and secrete excessive amounts of PTHrP that causes hypercalcemia. Treatment with dopamine agonists reverses the hypercalcemia.

Plasma cell myeloma causes hypercalcemia in older individuals. Many other hematologic cancers, such as monocytic leukemia, T cell leukemia and lymphoma, and Burkitt lymphoma, have also been associated with hypercalcemia.

Sarcoidosis and other granulomatous disorders, such as tuberculosis, berylliosis, histoplasmosis, coccidioidomycosis, leprosy, and foreign-body granuloma, can cause hypercalcemia. Sarcoid granulomas can secrete PTHrP, but granulomas secrete 1,25(OH)$_2$D$_3$ and serum levels of 1,25(OH)$_2$D$_3$ are usually elevated in the presence of hypercalcemia. However, in hypercalcemia with disseminated coccidiomycosis, serum 1,25(OH)$_2$D$_3$ levels may not be elevated. Serum PTH levels are usually low.

Excessive calcium or vitamin D ingestion can cause hypercalcemia, especially in patients who concurrently take thiazide diuretics, which reduce urinary calcium loss. Hypercalcemia is reversible following withdrawal of calcium and vitamin D supplements. If hypercalcemia persists, the possibility of associated hyperparathyroidism should be considered. In vitamin D intoxication, hypercalcemia may persist for several weeks. Serum levels of 25-hydroxycholecalciferol (25[OH]D$_3$) are helpful to confirm the diagnosis. A brief course of corticosteroid therapy may be necessary if hypercalcemia is severe.

Familial hypocalciuric hypercalcemia (FHH) is an uncommon autosomal dominant inherited disorder. Three different loss-of-function germline mutations have been recognized as causative. Reduced function of the calcium-sensing receptor (CaSR) causes the parathyroid glands to falsely "sense" hypocalcemia and inappropriately release excessive amounts of PTH. The renal tubule CaSRs are also affected, causing hypocalciuria.

FHH was previously termed "benign FHH" and thought to be asymptomatic. However, FHH can sometimes present with neonatal severe primary hyperparathyroidism with serum calcium levels as high as 12 mg/dL and hyperparathyroidism and rickets-like bone disease with rib fractures in the newborn period. In adulthood, patients with hypercalcemia due to FHH are either asymptomatic or have nonspecific complaints such as fatigue, weakness, or cognitive issues. Recurrent pancreatitis can occur.

FHH is characterized by a mildly elevated serum calcium that is usually below 11.0 mg/dL (2.75 mmol/L) and a low urine calcium excretion that is usually less than 50 mg/24 h (13 mmol/24 h). Serum PTH levels are usually normal or minimally elevated. Serum phosphate levels are normal. About 4% of patients with true hyperparathyroidism can have a low urine calcium (below 100 mg/day). Therefore, FHH is most reliably confirmed with genetic testing for FHH gene mutations. These patients do not normalize their hypercalcemia after subtotal parathyroid removal and should not be subjected to surgery. Cinacalcet, a calcimimetic, has provided successful therapy for several reported patients.

Prolonged immobilization at bed rest commonly causes hypercalcemia, particularly in adolescents, critically ill patients, and patients with extensive Paget disease of bone. Hypercalcemia develops in about one-third of acutely ill patients being treated in intensive care units, particularly patients with acute kidney injury. Serum calcium elevations are typically mild but may reach 15 mg/dL (3.75 mmol/L). Serum PTH levels are usually slightly elevated, consistent with mild hyperparathyroidism but may be suppressed or normal.

Rare causes of hypercalcemia include untreated adrenal insufficiency. Modest hypercalcemia is occasionally seen in patients taking thiazide diuretics or lithium; such patients may have an inappropriately nonsuppressed PTH level with hypercalcemia. Hyperthyroidism causes increased turnover of bone and occasional hypercalcemia. Bisphosphonates can increase serum calcium in 20% and serum PTH becomes high in 10%, mimicking hyperparathyroidism. Hypercalcemia may also occur following liver transplantation. Other causes of hypercalcemia are shown in Table 21–8.

► Treatment

A. "Asymptomatic" Primary Hyperparathyroidism

Patients with mild hyperparathyroidism should be considered "asymptomatic" only after very close questioning. Many patients may not realize they have manifestations, such as cognitive slowing, having become accustomed to such symptoms over years. It is important to assess blood pressure, kidney function with a serum BUN and creatinine, and to determine the presence of nephrolithiasis or nephrocalcinosis by radiography, ultrasonography, or CT scan of the kidneys. Truly asymptomatic patients may be closely monitored and advised to keep active, avoid immobilization, and drink adequate fluids. For postmenopausal women with hyperparathyroidism, estrogen replacement therapy reduces serum calcium by an average of 0.75 mg/dL (0.19 mmol/L) and slightly improves bone density. For patients with hypercalciuria (more than 400 mg daily) or calcium nephrolithiasis, hydrochlorthiazide may be used in doses of 12.5–25 mg daily to reduce calciuria; however, serum calcium must be monitored carefully.

Affected patients should avoid large doses of thiazide diuretics, vitamin A, and calcium-containing antacids or supplements. Serum calcium and albumin are checked at least twice yearly, kidney function and urine calcium once yearly, and three-site bone density (distal radius, hip, and spine) every 2 years. Rising serum calcium should prompt further evaluation and determination of serum PTH levels.

If it is not clear whether a patient with primary hyperparathyroid is symptomatic, it is reasonable to consider a trial of medical therapy with cinacalcet.

B. Medical Measures

1. Fluids—Hypercalcemia is treated with a large fluid intake unless contraindicated. Severe hypercalcemia requires hospitalization and intensive hydration with intravenous saline.

2. CaSR activators—Cinacalcet hydrochloride is a calcimimetic agent that binds to sites of the parathyroid glands' extracellular CaSRs to increase the glands' affinity for extracellular calcium, thereby decreasing PTH secretion. Cinacalcet may be used as the initial therapy for patients with hyperparathyroidism or for failed surgical parathyroidectomy. For mild hypercalcemia, an initial dose of 15 mg (one-half of a 30-mg tablet) is advisable with weekly monitoring of serum calcium and an increased dose every 2 weeks if hypercalcemia persists until the patient becomes normocalcemic, which is successful in 73% of patients. Patients with parathyroid carcinoma and severe hypercalcemia are treated with cinacalcet in addition to zoledronic acid. For parathyroid cancer, cinacalcet is administered in doses of 30 mg orally twice daily, increased progressively to 60 mg twice daily, then 90 mg twice daily to a maximum of 90 mg every 6–8 hours. Cinacalcet is usually well tolerated but may cause nausea and vomiting, which are usually transient. Hypocalcemia has occurred, even at 30 mg/day. About 50% of azotemic patients with secondary or tertiary hyperparathyroidism have hypercalcemia that is resistant to vitamin D analogs; cinacalcet is given orally in starting doses of 30 mg daily to a maximum of 250 mg daily, with dosage adjustments to keep the serum PTH in the range of 150–300 pg/mL (15.8–31.6 pmol/L). Etelcalcetide also activates the parathyroid glands' CaSR and reduces hypercalcemia in dialysis patients; it is given intravenously at the end of hemodialysis sessions, thereby avoiding the gastrointestinal side effects of cinacalcet.

3. Bisphosphonates—Intravenous bisphosphonates are potent inhibitors of bone resorption and can temporarily treat the hypercalcemia of hyperparathyroidism. Pamidronate in doses of 30–90 mg (in 0.9% saline) is administered intravenously over 2–4 hours. Zoledronic acid 5 mg is administered intravenously over 15–20 minutes. These drugs cause a gradual decline in serum calcium over several days that may last for weeks to months. Such intravenous bisphosphonates are used generally for patients with severe hyperparathyroidism in preparation for surgery. Oral bisphosphonates, such as alendronate, are not effective for treating the hypercalcemia or hypercalciuria of hyperparathyroidism. However, oral alendronate has been shown to improve bone mineral density in the lumbar spine and hip (not distal radius) and may be used for asymptomatic patients with hyperparathyroidism who have a low bone mineral density. It may also be combined with cinacalcet for the medical treatment of osteoporosis in patients with persistent hyperparathyroidism.

4. Denosumab—For patients with severe hypercalcemia due to parathyroid carcinoma, denosumab 120 mcg subcutaneously monthly may be effective. However, high-dose denosumab increases the risk of jaw osteonecrosis and serious infections.

5. Vitamin D and vitamin D analogs—

A. Primary hyperparathyroidism—For patients with vitamin D deficiency, vitamin D replacement may be beneficial to patients with hyperparathyroidism. Aggravation of hypercalcemia does not ordinarily occur. Serum PTH levels may fall with vitamin D replacement in doses of 800–2000 international units daily or more to achieve serum 25-OH vitamin D levels 30 ng/mL or more (50 nmol/L or more).

B. Secondary and tertiary hyperparathyroidism associated with azotemia—Calcitriol, given orally or intravenously after dialysis, suppresses parathyroid hyperplasia of kidney disease. For patients with normal serum calcium levels, it is given orally in starting doses of 0.25 mcg on alternate days or daily. Calcitriol often causes hypercalcemia, so that serum levels of calcium and phosphate must be monitored to ensure that the serum $Ca^{2+} \times PO_4^3$ product remains no greater than 70. If the product exceeds 70, the dose of calcitriol is decreased or the patient is switched to therapy with vitamin D analogs or cinacalcet.

The vitamin D analogs paricalcitol and doxercalciferol suppress PTH secretion and cause less hypercalcemia than calcitriol. The doses are adjusted to keep serum PTH levels in the range of 150–300 pg/mL (15.9–31.8 pmol/L). Paricalcitol is administered intravenously during dialysis three times weekly in starting doses of 0.04–0.1 mcg/kg to a maximum dose of 0.24 mcg/kg three times weekly. Alternatively, paricalcitol may be administered orally at doses of 1–2 mcg daily for serum PTH levels 100–500 pg/mL (10.5–53.7 pmol/L) or 2–4 mcg daily for serum PTH levels greater than 500 pg/mL (53.7 pmol/L). Dialysis patients receiving paricalcitol have improved survival compared with patients receiving calcitriol. Doxercalciferol is administered intravenously three times weekly during hemodialysis to patients with azotemic secondary hyperparathyroidism in starting doses of 4 mcg three times weekly to a maximum dose of 18 mcg three times weekly. Alternatively, doxercalciferol may be administered orally three times weekly at dialysis, starting with 10 mcg three times weekly at dialysis to a maximum of 60 mcg/wk.

6. Other measures—Estrogen replacement reduces hypercalcemia slightly in postmenopausal women with hyperparathyroidism. Similarly, oral raloxifene (60 mg/day) may be given to postmenopausal women with hyperparathyroidism; it reduces serum calcium an average of 0.4 mg/dL (0.1 mmol/L), while having an anti-estrogenic effect on breast tissue. Beta-blockers, such as propranolol, may also be useful for preventing the adverse cardiac effects of hypercalcemia. Parathyroid carcinoma metastases may be treated with radiofrequency ablation or arterial embolization.

C. Surgical Parathyroidectomy

Parathyroidectomy is recommended for patients with hyperparathyroidism who are symptomatic or who have nephrolithiasis or bone disease. During pregnancy, parathyroidectomy is performed in the second trimester for women who are symptomatic or have a serum calcium above 11 mg/dL (2.75 mmol/L).

Some patients with seemingly asymptomatic hyperparathyroidism may be surgical candidates for other reasons such as (1) serum calcium 1 mg/dL (0.25 mmol/L) above the upper limit of normal with urine calcium excretion greater than 50 mg/24 h (off thiazide diuretics), (2) urine calcium excretion greater than 400 mg/day (10 mmol/day), (3) creatinine clearance less than 60 mL/min, (4) nephrolithiasis or nephrocalcinosis, (5) cortical bone density (wrist, hip, or distal radius) indicating osteoporosis (T score below –2.5) or previous fragility bone fracture, (6) relative youth (under age 50 years), (7) difficulty ensuring medical follow-up, or (8) pregnancy.

Surgery for patients with "asymptomatic" hyperparathyroidism may improve bone mineral density and confer modest benefits in social and emotional well-being and overall quality of life in comparison to similar patients being monitored without surgery. Cognitive function may benefit with improvements in nonverbal abstraction and memory.

Preoperative parathyroid imaging has been used in an attempt to allow unilateral minimally invasive neck surgery (see Imaging, above). The reported success rates vary considerably. Even in patients with concordant sestamibi and ultrasound scans, and an intraoperative PTH drop of more than 50%, hyperparathyroidism may persist postoperatively in up to 15% of patients.

Without preoperative localization studies, bilateral neck exploration is usually advisable for the following: (1) patients with a family history of hyperparathyroidism, (2) patients with a personal or family history of MEN, and (3) patients wanting an optimal chance of success with a single surgery. Patients undergoing unilateral neck exploration can have the incision widened for bilateral neck exploration if two abnormal glands are found or if the serum quick PTH level falls by less than 63% within 10 minutes of the parathyroid resection. Parathyroid glands are often supernumerary (five or more) or ectopic (eg, intrathyroidal, carotid sheath, mediastinum). The optimal surgical management for patients with MEN type 1 is subtotal parathyroidectomy that usually results in a cure, although recurrent hyperparathyroidism develops in 18% and the rate of postoperative hypoparathyroidism is high.

Intraoperative quick serum PTH monitoring is helpful. Serum PTH levels that fall greater than 63% within 10 minutes of a parathyroid adenoma resection indicates a high likelihood that the surgery will be curative.

Intraoperative near-infrared autofluorescence spectroscopy imaging may improve intraoperative localization of parathyroid glands in primary hyperparathyroidism, particularly when preoperative localization studies have been negative or discrepant.

Parathyroid hyperplasia is commonly seen with secondary or tertiary hyperparathyroidism associated with uremia. Cinacalcet is an alternative to surgery. When surgery is performed, a subtotal parathyroidectomy is optimal; three and one-half glands are usually removed, and a metal clip is left to mark the location of residual parathyroid tissue.

Parathyroid carcinoma surgery consists of en bloc resection of the tumor and ipsilateral thyroid lobe with care to avoid rupturing the tumor capsule. If the surgical margins are not clear of tumor, postoperative neck radiation therapy may be given. Local and distant metastases may be debulked or irradiated. Preoperative MRI scanning is required to delineate the tumor. Zoledronic acid or denosumab is given preoperatively. Severe hypercalcemia requires multiple medical measures, including hydration, furosemide, cinacalcet, zoledronic acid, or denosumab. Patients with refractory metastases may receive combined chemotherapy with dacarbazine-based chemotherapy that has produced short-term remissions but with adverse effects.

Complications—Serum PTH levels fall below normal in 70% of patients within hours after successful surgery, commonly causing hypocalcemic paresthesias or even tetany. Hypocalcemia tends to occur the evening after surgery or on the next day. Therefore, frequent postoperative monitoring of serum calcium (or serum calcium plus albumin) is advisable beginning the evening after surgery. Once hypercalcemia has resolved, liquid or chewable calcium carbonate is given orally to reduce the likelihood of hypocalcemia. Symptomatic hypocalcemia is treated with larger doses of calcium; calcitriol (0.25–1 mcg daily orally) may be added, with the dosage depending on symptom severity. Magnesium salts are sometimes required postoperatively, since adequate magnesium is required for functional recovery of the remaining suppressed parathyroid glands.

In about 12% of patients having successful parathyroid surgery, PTH levels rise above normal (while serum calcium is normal or low) by 1 week postoperatively. This secondary hyperparathyroidism is probably due to "hungry bones" and is treated with calcium and vitamin D preparations. Such therapy is usually needed only for 3–6 months but is required long term by some patients.

Hyperthyroidism commonly occurs immediately following parathyroid surgery. It is caused by release of stored thyroid hormone during surgical manipulation of the thyroid. In symptomatic patients, short-term treatment with propranolol may be required for several days.

Prognosis

Patients with symptomatic hyperparathyroidism usually experience worsening disease (eg, nephrolithiasis) unless they have treatment. Conversely, the majority of completely asymptomatic patients with a serum calcium below 11.0 mg/dL (2.75 mmol/L) remain stable with follow-up. However, worsening hypercalcemia, hypercalciuria, and reductions in cortical bone mineral density develop in about one-third of asymptomatic patients. Therefore, asymptomatic patients must be monitored carefully and treated with oral hydration and mobilization.

Surgical removal of apparently single sporadic parathyroid adenomas is successful in 94%. Patients with MEN 1 undergoing subtotal parathyroidectomy may experience long remissions, but hyperparathyroidism frequently recurs. Despite treatment for hyperparathyroidism, patients remain at increased risk for all-cause mortality, cardiovascular disease, renal calculi, and kidney dysfunction. These increased risks are likely the residuals of pretreatment hypertension and nephrolithiasis.

Spontaneous cure due to necrosis of the tumor has been reported but is exceedingly rare. The bones, in spite of severe cyst formation, deformity, and fracture, will heal if hyperparathyroidism is successfully treated. The presence of pancreatitis increases the mortality rate. Acute pancreatitis usually resolves with correction of hypercalcemia, whereas subacute or chronic pancreatitis tends to persist. Significant kidney damage may progress even after removal of a parathyroid adenoma.

Parathyroid carcinoma is associated with 5- and 10-year survival rates of 78% and 49%, respectively. A better prognosis is associated with clear surgical margins and no detectable metastases postoperatively. Conversely, positive surgical margins or metastases predict a very poor 5-year survival. The prognosis is also poorer for nonfunctioning parathyroid carcinoma and those tumors that carry a *CDC73* mutation, loss of fibromin, or loss of CaSR expression. Repeat surgical debulking procedures may improve survival. Aggressive medical management can also prolong life. Metastases are relatively radiation-resistant, but additional therapies such as radiofrequency ablation or arterial embolization may be palliative.

When to Refer

Refer to parathyroid surgeon for parathyroidectomy.

When to Admit

Patients with severe hypercalcemia for intravenous hydration.

Babwah F et al. Normocalcaemic primary hyperparathyroidism: a pragmatic approach. J Clin Pathol. 2018 Apr;71(4):291–7. [PMID: 29437827]

Bilezikian JP. Primary hyperparathyroidism. J Clin Endocrinol Metab. 2018 Nov 1;103(11):3993–4004. [PMID: 30060226]

Cetani F et al. Update on parathyroid carcinoma. J Endocrinol Invest. 2016 Jun;39(6):595–606. [PMID: 27001435]

Khan AA et al. Primary hyperparathyroidism: review and recommendations on evaluation, diagnosis, and management. A Canadian and international consensus. Osteoporos Int. 2017 Jan;28(1):1–19. [PMID: 27613721]

Madeo B et al. Serum calcium to phosphorous (Ca/P) ratio is a simple, inexpensive, and accurate tool in the diagnosis of primary hyperparathyroidism. JBMR Plus. 2017 Nov 2; 2(2):109–17. [PMID: 30283895]

Marx SJ. Familial hypocalciuric hypercalcemia as an atypical form of primary hyperparathyroidism. J Bone Miner Res. 2018 Jan;33(1):27–31. [PMID: 29115694]

Stephen AE et al. Indications for surgical management of hyperparathyroidism: a review. JAMA Surg. 2017 Sep 1;152(9):878–82. [PMID: 28658490]

METABOLIC BONE DISEASE

The term "metabolic bone disease" denotes those conditions producing diffusely decreased bone density and diminished bone strength. It is categorized by histologic appearance: osteoporosis (bone matrix and mineral both decreased) and osteomalacia (bone matrix intact, mineral decreased). Osteoporosis and osteomalacia often coexist in the same patient.

OSTEOPOROSIS

ESSENTIALS OF DIAGNOSIS

▶ Fracture propensity of spine, hip, pelvis, and wrist from depletion of bone matrix with subsequent demineralization.

▶ Asymptomatic until a fracture has occurred.

▶ Serum PTH, calcium, phosphorus, and alkaline phosphatase usually normal.

▶ Serum 25-hydroxyvitamin D levels often low as a comorbid condition.

General Considerations

Osteoporosis is a skeletal disorder characterized by a loss of bone osteoid that reduces bone integrity and bone strength, predisposing to an increased risk of fracture. In the United States, osteoporosis causes over 1.5 million fractures annually, most commonly vertebral fractures, followed by hip fractures (300,000 annually) and pelvic fractures. In the United States, at least 20% of men and women over age 50 years have one or more fractured vertebrae. White women age 50 years and older (who do not receive estrogen replacement) have a 46% risk of sustaining an osteoporotic fracture during the remainder of their lives. Vertebral fractures are the most common fracture; they are associated with increased mortality, pain, and spinal kyphosis, although they are usually diagnosed incidentally on radiographs or CT scanning. Hip fractures are also associated with increased mortality, pain, reduced independence, and diminished quality of life.

The frequency of fragility fractures varies with ethnicity, sex, and age. The lifetime risk of hip fracture in the United States is 15.8% in white women and 6.0% in white men, 8.5% in Hispanic women and 3.8% in Hispanic men, and 2.4% in Chinese women and 1.9% in Chinese men. Blacks also have a lower risk for fracture due to higher bone mineral density and hip morphology that is less fracture-prone. There is much less ethnic variability for vertebral fractures. The prevalence of vertebral fractures in women older than 65 years is 70% for white women, 68% for Japanese women, 55% for Mexican women, and 50% in African American women.

Osteoporosis can be caused by a variety of factors (Table 26–9). The most common causes include aging, sex hormone deficiency, alcoholism, smoking, long-term proton pump inhibitor therapy, and high-dose corticosteroid administration. Hypogonadal men frequently develop osteoporosis. Anti-androgen therapy for prostate cancer can cause osteoporosis, and such men should be monitored with bone densitometry.

Table 26–9. Causes of osteoporosis.[1]

Aging	Genetic disorders
Hormone deficiency	Aromatase deficiency
Estradiol (women)	Collagen disorders
Testosterone (men)	Ehlers-Danlos syndrome
Hormone excess	Homocystinuria
Cushing syndrome or	Hypophosphatasia
corticosteroid	Idiopathic juvenile and adult
administration	osteoporosis
Hyperparathyroidism	Marfan syndrome
Thyrotoxicosis	Osteogenesis imperfecta
Alcoholism	Miscellaneous conditions
Immobilization and	Anorexia nervosa
microgravity	Celiac disease
Malignancy, especially plasma	Copper deficiency
cell myeloma	Diabetes mellitus
Tobacco	(uncontrolled)
Medications (long-term)	Hyponatremia (chronic)
Aromatase inhibitors	Inflammatory bowel disease
Heparin	Liver disease (chronic)
Pioglitazone	Mastocytosis (systemic)
Proton pump inhibitors	Protein-calorie malnutrition
Selective serotonin reuptake	Rheumatoid arthritis
inhibitors	Vitamin C deficiency
SGLT2 inhibitors	
Vitamin A excess, vitamin D	
excess	

[1]See Table 26–10 for causes of osteomalacia.

▶ **Clinical Findings**

A. Symptoms and Signs

Osteoporosis is usually asymptomatic until fractures occur. It may present as backache of varying degrees of severity or as a spontaneous fracture or collapse of a vertebra. Loss of height is common. Once osteoporosis is identified, a directed history and physical examination must be performed to determine its cause (Table 26–9).

B. Laboratory Findings

The objective for laboratory testing is to screen for secondary causes of osteoporosis or concomitant osteomalacia. For primary osteoporosis, the BUN, creatinine, albumin, serum calcium, phosphate, and PTH are normal. The alkaline phosphatase is usually normal but may be slightly elevated, especially following a fracture. A low serum alkaline phosphatase (below 40 units/L in adults) may indicate hypophosphatasia. A complete blood count is obtained and is usually normal; for patients with anemia, further screening is required, including a serum protein electrophoresis to screen for myeloma and intestinal malabsorption screening, where indicated. Vitamin D deficiency is very common and serum determination of 25-hydroxyvitamin D should be obtained for every individual with low bone density. Serum 25-hydroxyvitamin D levels below 20 ng/mL (50 nmol/L) are considered frank vitamin D deficiency. Lesser degrees of vitamin D insufficiency (serum 25-hydroxyvitamin D levels in the range of 20–30 ng/mL [50–75 nmol/L]) may also slightly increase the risk for hip fracture. Testing for thyrotoxicosis and hypogonadism may be required. If intestinal malabsorption is suspected, appropriate screening should be performed. Celiac disease may be screened for with serum tissue transglutaminase antibody determinations.

C. Bone Densitometry

Dual-energy x-ray absorptiometry (DXA) is used to determine the bone density of the lumbar spine, hip, and distal radius. Bone densitometry should be performed on all patients who are at risk for osteoporosis or osteomalacia, including all postmenopausal women aged 65 years and older and all men aged 70 years and older. DXA screening should also be considered for younger postmenopausal women with elevated risk, especially women with early menopause and those with a family history of osteoporosis. It should also be performed in younger patients who have had pathologic fractures or radiographic evidence of diminished bone density. DXA delivers negligible radiation, and the measurements are quite accurate. However, DXA cannot distinguish osteoporosis from osteomalacia; in fact, both are often present. Also, the bone mineral density does not directly measure bone quality and is only fairly successful at predicting fractures. Vertebral bone mineral density may be misleadingly high in compressed vertebrae and in patients with extensive arthritis. DXA also overestimates the bone mineral density of taller persons and underestimates the bone mineral density of smaller persons.

Bone mineral density is typically expressed in g/cm^2, for which there are different normal ranges for each bone and for each type of DXA-measuring machine. The "T score" is a simplified way of reporting bone density in which the patient's bone mineral density is compared to the young normal mean and expressed as a standard deviation score. The World Health Organization has established criteria for defining osteoporosis based upon the T score:

T score ≥ –1.0: Normal.

T score –1.0 to –2.5: Osteopenia ("low bone density").

T score < –2.5: Osteoporosis.

T score < –2.5 with a fracture: Severe osteoporosis.

It is prudent to obtain DXA bone density measurements at two or three sites, including total lumbar spine and total hip. DXA bone density of the non-dominant distal radius is helpful for patients with hyperparathyroidism, for men receiving androgen deprivation therapy, and for patients with conditions causing other DXA measurement artifacts. Such artifacts can be caused by hip arthroplasties, spinal orthopedic hardware, severe spinal arthritis, or lumbar vertebral compression fractures; in such patients, only noncompressed vertebrae are relevant. Any bone density classification is somewhat arbitrary and there really is no bone mineral density fracture threshold; instead, the fracture risk increases about twofold for each standard deviation drop in bone mineral density. Surveillance DXA bone densitometry is recommended for postmenopausal women and elderly men with a frequency according to their T scores: obtain DXA every 5 years for T scores –1.0 to –1.5, every 3–5 years for scores –1.5 to –2.0, and every 1–2 years for scores under –2.0.

The "Z score" is used to express bone density in premenopausal women and young adult men. The Z score is a statistical term expressing an individual's bone density as standard deviation from age-matched, race-matched, and sex-matched means.

Pharmacologic treatment is recommended for patients with a spontaneous hip or vertebral fracture or a T score in any location less than or equal to –2.5.

Fracture Risk Assessment Tool (FRAX) was developed by the World Health Organization to better predict an individual's 10-year risk of hip or other major osteoporotic fracture. It is particularly useful for treatment decisions in patients with osteopenia and takes into consideration age, sex, ethnicity, bone mineral density, and other risk factors. Treatment is recommended for individuals with osteopenia (T score between –1.0 and –2.5) with a computed 10-year hip fracture risk of at least 3% or a 10-year risk of any major fracture of at least 20%. However, the FRAX model has limitations, only considering femoral neck bone mineral density and not considering vertebral bone mineral density. Also, FRAX does not consider the *dose* of exposure to corticosteroids, alcohol, smoking, or an individual's proclivity to falls; treatment decisions must always be individualized. FRAX is available for use online at http://www.shef.ac.uk/FRAX/.

▶ Differential Diagnosis

Osteopenia and fractures can be caused by osteomalacia and bone marrow neoplasia such as myeloma or metastatic bone disease. These conditions coexist in many patients and cannot be distinguished with bone densitometry.

▶ Prevention & Treatment

A. Nonpharmacologic Measures

For prevention and treatment of osteoporosis, the diet should be adequate in protein, total calories, calcium, and vitamin D. Pharmacologic corticosteroid (oral, parenteral, or inhaled) should be reduced or discontinued if possible. Cigarette smoking cessation is strongly urged. Excessive alcohol intake must be avoided. Exercise is strongly recommended to increase both bone density and strength, thereby reducing the risk of fractures due to frailty falls. Walking increases the bone density at both the spine and hip. Resistance exercise increases spine density. The patient must choose an enjoyable exercise regimen to facilitate long-term compliance. Other fall prevention measures include adequate home lighting, handrails on stairs, handholds in bathrooms, and physical therapy training in fall prevention and balance exercises. Patients who have weakness or balance problems must use a cane or a walker; rolling walkers should have a brake mechanism. Medications that cause orthostasis, dizziness, or confusion should be avoided.

B. Pharmacologic Measures

Generally, treatment is indicated for all patients with osteoporosis (DXA T scores below –2.5), women with previous fragility fractures of the hip or vertebra, or a DXA T score between –2.5 and –1.0 with FRAX-determined (see above) 10-year hip fracture risk greater than 3% or major osteoporotic fracture risk greater than 20%.

1. Vitamin D and calcium—Deficiency of vitamin D or calcium causes osteomalacia, rather than osteoporosis, but they often coexist and cannot be distinguished by DXA bone densitometry; it is crucial to ensure sufficient vitamin D and calcium intake. Recommended daily vitamin D intake of 600–800 units/day is difficult to achieve by diet (unless high in fish) and sun exposure, particularly during winter months and for patients with intestinal malabsorption or during prolonged hospitalization or nursing home care. Oral vitamin D_3 (cholecalciferol) is given either as a universal supplement of 800–2000 units/day or in doses titrated to achieve 25-hydroxvitamin D (25-OHD) serum levels greater than or equal to 20 ng/mL (50 nmol/L) for most of the population. However, the 25-OHD serum levels should be maintained at 30 ng/mL (75 nmol/L) or higher for those "at risk": pregnant women, older adults, and those with osteoporosis or fragility fractures. There are early observational data of adverse outcomes (increased heart disease and all-cause mortality) at 25-OHD serum levels greater than 50 ng/mL (125 nmol/L), so the optimal therapeutic range for 25-OHD serum levels appears to about 30–50 ng/mL (75–125 nmol/L).

A total elemental calcium intake at least 1000 mg/day is recommended for all adults and 1200 mg/day for postmenopausal women and men older than 70 years. Most healthy individuals do not require calcium supplementation, and 74% of cohort studies showed no association between dietary calcium intake and fracture risk. Other studies have reported that associated calcium supplementation (1 g/day or more) showed no reduced risk for hip or forearm fractures and a mere 14% reduction in vertebral fractures. Calcium supplements are generally reserved for patients with intestinal malabsorption or calcium-deficient diets that do not include dairy products, dark leafy greens, sardines, tofu, or fortified foods. Calcium citrate does not require acid for absorption and is preferred for patients receiving acid blockers. Calcium carbonate should be taken with food to enhance calcium absorption. Calcium supplements are usually taken along with vitamin D_3, and many commercial supplements contain the combination.

Some reports have indicated that calcium supplements increase the risk of myocardial infarction. However, the Women's Health Initiative found that 7 years of vitamin D and calcium supplementation did not increase cardiovascular disease but did increase the risk of nephrolithiasis by 13%. Taking calcium supplements with meals can reduce the risk of nephrolithiasis. Although calcium supplements are usually tolerated, some patients experience intestinal bloating and constipation.

2. Sex hormones—Sex hormone replacement can prevent osteoporosis in hypogonadal women and men but is not an effective therapy for established osteoporosis. Low-dose transdermal systemic estrogen prevents osteoporosis in women with hypogonadism (see Hormone Replacement Therapy). Testosterone replacement therapy prevents osteoporosis in men with severe testosterone deficiency (see Male Hypogonadism).

3. Bisphosphonates—Bisphosphonate therapy is indicated for patients with a pathologic spine fracture or a low-impact hip fracture, and for patients with osteoporosis, defined as a DXA T score of –2.5 or less in the spine, total hip, or femoral neck. They are also indicated for patients with osteopenia (DXA T score between –2.5 and –1.5) and a FRAX-determined (see above) 10-year hip fracture risk greater than 3% or major osteoporotic fracture risk greater than 20%. Bisphosphonates all work similarly, inhibiting osteoclast-induced bone resorption. They increase bone density significantly and all reduce the incidence of vertebral fractures; all but ibandronate have been demonstrated to also reduce the risk of nonvertebral fractures. Bisphosphonates have also been effective in preventing corticosteroid-induced osteoporosis. To ensure intestinal absorption, oral bisphosphonates must be taken in the morning with at least 8 oz of plain water at least 40 minutes before consumption of anything else. The patient must remain upright after taking bisphosphonates to reduce the risk of esophagitis. No dosage adjustments are required for patients with creatinine clearances above 35 mL/min. There has been little experience giving bisphosphonates to patients with severe kidney disease; if given, the dose would need to be greatly reduced and serum phosphate levels monitored. Bone density falls in 18% of patients during their first year of treatment with bisphosphonates, but 80% of such patients gain bone density with continued bisphosphonate treatment. The half-life of bisphosphonates in bone is about 10 years. Therefore, after 3 years, a DXA bone densitometry may be obtained. If the patient's T score has risen above –2.5 and the patient has a relatively low fracture risk, the bisphosphonate may be discontinued.

However, for patients with continued osteoporosis and a high fracture risk, the bisphosphonate may be continued another 2 years. The usual treatment course with bisphosphonates is 3–5 years due to the increasing risk of atypical femoral fractures after that time.

Alendronate is administered orally once weekly as either a 70-mg standard tablet (Fosamax) or a 70-mg effervescent tablet (Binosto). The effervescent tablet must be dissolved in 4 oz plain water over at least 5 minutes and stirred 10 seconds before drinking; it is easier to swallow for some patients and may reduce esophageal injury, but there have been no studies comparing it to standard alendronate tablets. **Risedronate** (Actonel) may be given once monthly as a 150-mg tablet. Risedronate is favored for women of childbearing age, since it has a shorter half-life and less bone retention than other bisphosphonates. Both medications reduce the risk of vertebral and nonvertebral fractures, but alendronate appears to be superior to risedronate in preventing nonvertebral fractures. **Ibandronate sodium** (Boniva) is taken once monthly in a dose of 150 mg orally. It reduces the risk of vertebral fractures but not nonvertebral fractures; its effectiveness has not been directly compared with other bisphosphonates. Oral bisphosphonates can cause nausea, chest pain, and hoarseness. Erosive esophagus can occur, particularly in patients with hiatal hernia and gastroesophageal reflux. Although no increased risk of esophageal cancer has been conclusively demonstrated, the FDA recommends that oral bisphosphonates not be used by patients with Barrett esophagus.

For patients who cannot take oral bisphosphonates, intravenous bisphosphonates are available. **Zoledronic acid** (Reclast) is a third-generation bisphosphonate and a potent osteoclast inhibitor. It can be given every 12 months in doses of 5 mg intravenously over at least 15–30 minutes. **Pamidronate** (Aredia) can be given in doses of 30–60 mg by slow intravenous infusion in normal saline solution every 3–6 months.

Bisphosphonate therapy can cause side effects that are collectively known as the acute-phase response. Such a response occurs in 42% of patients following the first infusion of zoledronic acid and usually starts within the first few days following the infusion. Among patients receiving their first infusion of zoledronic acid, these adverse side effects have included fever, chills, or flushing (20%); musculoskeletal pain (20%); nausea, vomiting, or diarrhea (8%); nonspecific symptoms, such as fatigue, dyspnea, edema, headache, or dizziness (22%); and ocular inflammation (0.6%). Intravenous zoledronic acid has caused seizures that may be idiosyncratic or due to hypocalcemia. The acute-phase response tends to diminish with time. Symptoms are transient, lasting several days and usually resolving spontaneously but typically recurring with subsequent doses. Symptoms may be treated with acetaminophen or NSAIDs. Loratadine may reduce musculoskeletal pain. For patients experiencing a severe acute-phase response with zoledronic acid, intravenous pamidronate can be substituted for subsequent treatment. In addition, patients who experience an especially severe acute-phase response can be given prophylactic corticosteroids and ondansetron prior to subsequent bisphosphonate infusions.

Osteonecrosis of the jaw is a rare complication of bisphosphonate therapy for osteoporosis. A painful, necrotic, nonhealing lesion of the jaw occurs, particularly after tooth extraction. It occurs twice as frequently in the mandible compared to the maxilla. The risk is increased with older age, in women, and in patients concomitantly receiving chemotherapy or corticosteroid therapy. About 95% of jaw osteonecrosis cases have occurred with intravenous high-dose therapy with zoledronic acid or pamidronate for patients with osteolytic metastases. Only about 5% of cases have occurred in patients receiving oral bisphosphonates or once-yearly bisphosphonate infusions for osteoporosis. The incidence of osteonecrosis is estimated to be about 1:100,000 patients treated for osteoporosis with oral bisphosphonates and 1:100 patients being treated for cancer with intravenous bisphosphonates. The risk for osteonecrosis of the jaw with dental surgery can be approximated with a serum level of C-telopeptide, a fragment of collagen released during bone remodeling. Bisphosphonates reduce C-telopeptide levels. Serum C-telopeptide levels greater than or equal to 150 pg/mL are associated with a minimal risk of osteonecrosis, whereas C-telopeptide levels 100–149 pg/mL are associated with a moderate risk, and C-telopeptide levels less than 100 pg/mL are associated with a high risk for osteonecrosis. Patients receiving bisphosphonates must receive regular dental care and try to avoid dental extraction. Ideally, elective dental surgery should be completed before starting bisphosphonates. If dental surgery is required, bisphosphonate therapy is ordinarily stopped 3 months before the surgery and may be resumed about 1 month afterward if the bone has healed.

Atypical low-impact "chalkstick" fractures of the femoral shaft are a rare complication of bisphosphonate therapy. In more than 52,000 postmenopausal women taking bisphosphonates for 5 years or longer, a subtrochanteric fracture occurred in 0.22% during the subsequent 2 years; 27% of such fractures were bilateral. About 70% of affected patients have had prodromal thigh pain prior to the fracture. The risk for atypical femoral fractures is particularly increased among Asian women and among patients taking high-dose corticosteroids and those receiving bisphosphonate treatment for more than 5 years. Teriparatide may be helpful to promote healing of such fractures. Despite this rare complication, the overall risk of hip fracture is reduced among patients taking bisphosphonates for up to 5 years.

In patients taking bisphosphonates, hypercalcemia is seen in 20% and serum PTH levels increase above normal in 10%, mimicking primary hyperparathyroidism. Hypocalcemia occurs frequently, resulting in secondary hyperparathyroidism; such patients may be treated with oral calcium salt supplements (500–1000 mg/day) and with oral vitamin D_3 (starting at 1000 units/day).

4. Denosumab—Denosumab (Prolia) is a monoclonal antibody that inhibits the proliferation and maturation of preosteoclasts into mature osteoclast bone-resorbing cells. It does this by binding to the osteoclast receptor activator of nuclear factor-kappa B ligand (RANKL). It is indicated for treatment of osteoporosis, major fragility fractures, or osteopenia with a high FRAX score in both men and women. It is also used for patients with high fracture risk who are receiving sex hormone suppression therapy for breast cancer or prostate cancer. Treatment reduces vertebral fractures by 68% and reduces hip fractures by 40%. Denosumab is administered in doses of 60 mg subcutaneously every 6 months. Unlike bisphosphonates, denosumab can be given to patients with severe kidney disease. It has been relatively well tolerated, with an 8% incidence of flu-like symptoms. It can decrease serum calcium and should not be administered to patients with hypocalcemia. Other side effects include hypercholesterolemia, eczema and dermatitis, new malignancies, and pancreatitis. Denosumab may also increase the risk of serious infections, so it is not recommended for patients receiving high-dose corticosteroid therapy, whose risk of infection is already high. *In women with childbearing potential, denosumab should be used with great caution and with birth control, since denosumab has caused fetal teratogenicity in animal studies.* With prolonged use, denosumab predisposes to atypical femoral fractures and osteonecrosis of the jaw and is additive to bisphosphonates in that regard. As with bisphosphonates, denosumab is usually administered for a 3- to 5-year course.

Compared to oral bisphosphonates, denosumab appears to be slightly superior at improving bone mineral density of the spine, total femur, and femoral neck and at reducing fracture risk after 2 years of therapy. Compared to intravenous zoledronic acid, denosumab has been somewhat superior at increasing bone mineral density at the total femur and femoral neck, but the two have similar efficacy at improving spine bone mineral density.

5. PTH analogs—**Teriparatide** (Forteo) and **abaloparatide** (Tymlos) are analogs of PTH and PTHrP, respectively. These analogs are anabolic agents that stimulate the production of new collagenous bone matrix, particularly in vertebral trabecular bone that must be mineralized. Patients receiving teriparatide or abaloparatide must have sufficient intake of vitamin D and calcium. When given in a sequence with an antiresorptive agent, the preferred sequence is to first give a course of PTH/PTHrP analog therapy followed by a bisphosphonate or denosumab.

Teriparatide is administered subcutaneously in doses of 20 mg daily, whereas abaloparatide is given subcutaneously in doses of 80 mg daily. When administered to patients with osteoporosis for 2 years, these drugs dramatically improve bone density in most bones except the distal radius. They may also be used to promote healing of atypical femoral chalkstick fractures associated with bisphosphonate therapy. The recommended dose should not be exceeded, since both drugs have caused osteosarcoma in rats when administered long-term in very high doses. Due to the potential risk for osteosarcoma, patients are excluded from receiving teriparatide or abaloparatide if they have an increased risk of osteosarcoma due to the following: Paget disease of bone, unexplained elevations in serum alkaline phosphatase, prior radiation therapy to bones, open epiphyses, or a past history of osteosarcoma or chondrosarcoma. Side effects may include injection site reactions, orthostatic hypotension, arthralgia, muscle cramps, depression, or pneumonia. Hypercalcemia can occur and manifest as nausea, constipation, asthenia, or muscle weakness. These drugs are approved for only a 2-year course of treatment.

Teriparatide and abaloparatide should not be used for patients with hypercalcemia. Similarly, they should be used with caution in patients if they are also taking corticosteroids and thiazide diuretics along with oral calcium supplementation because hypercalcemia may develop.

Following a 2-year course of teriparatide or abaloparatide, bisphosphonates should be considered in order to retain the improved bone density. Alternatively, for very severe osteoporosis, these drugs may be administered along with denosumab; combined treatment for 2 years is more effective than any other single therapy.

6. Selective estrogen receptor modulators (SERMs)— SERMs can prevent osteoporosis but are not effective therapy for established osteoporosis. **Raloxifene** 60 mg/day orally may be taken by postmenopausal women in place of estrogen for prevention of osteoporosis. Bone density increases about 1% over 2 years in postmenopausal women versus 2% increases with estrogen replacement. It reduces the risk of vertebral fractures by about 40% but does not appear to reduce the risk of nonvertebral fractures. Raloxifene produces a reduction in LDL cholesterol, but not the rise in high-density lipoprotein (HDL) cholesterol seen with estrogen. It has no direct effect on coronary plaque. Unlike estrogen, raloxifene does not reduce hot flushes; in fact, it often intensifies them. It does not relieve vaginal dryness. Unlike estrogen, however, raloxifene does not cause endometrial hyperplasia, uterine bleeding, or cancer, nor does it cause breast soreness. The risk of breast cancer is reduced 76% in women taking raloxifene for 3 years. Since it is a potential teratogen, it is relatively contraindicated in women capable of pregnancy. Raloxifene increases the risk for thromboembolism and should not be used by women with such a history. Leg cramps can also occur. **Tamoxifen** is another SERM that is commonly administered to women for up to 5 years after resection of breast cancer that is estrogen receptor positive. **Bazedoxifene** is a SERM that is available as a fixed-dose combination medication with conjugated estrogens (dose: 0.45 mg/20 mg [Duavee]). It is FDA approved for the prevention of osteoporosis in postmenopausal women with an intact uterus. However, unlike raloxifene, it has not been shown to reduce the risk of breast cancer. Women taking this combination medication long-term experience an increased risk of thromboembolic events.

7. Calcitonin—Nasal salmon calcitonin is used primarily for its analgesic effect for the pain of acute osteoporotic vertebral compression fractures. It is ineffective for chronic pain. Its analgesic effect may be seen within 2–4 weeks. If it appears to be effective for analgesia, it is continued for up to 3 months. A nasal spray of calcitonin-salmon (Miacalcin) is available that contains 2200 units/mL in 2-mL metered-dose bottles. The usual dose is one puff (0.09 mL, 200 international units) once daily, alternating nostrils. Nasal symptoms such as rhinitis and epistaxis occur commonly; other less common adverse reactions include flu-like symptoms, allergy, arthralgias, back pain, headache, and hypocalcemia. Salmon calcitonin is available in an injectable form that can be used when the nasal formulation is not tolerated due to local reactions; it is used for up to 3

months for vertebral fracture pain in doses of 100 international units subcutaneously or intramuscularly every 1–2 days. Salmon calcitonin is no longer used long-term as an anti-osteoporosis therapy, since other available therapies are much more effective. Also, while long-term calcitonin therapy reduces the risk of breast cancer, it increases the risk of liver cancer.

8. Orthopedic surgery—Percutaneous vertebroplasty or kyphoplasty may be considered for patients with vertebral compression fractures who fail conservative pain management. However, no prospective randomized study has adequately compared the effectiveness of these orthopedic procedures compared to conservative therapy.

▶ **Prognosis**

Osteoporosis should ideally be prevented, since it can be only partially reversed. Measures noted above are reasonably effective in preventing and treating osteoporosis and reducing fracture risk.

Black DM et al. Clinical practice. Postmenopausal osteoporosis. N Engl J Med. 2016 Jan 21;374(3):254–62. [PMID: 26789873]

Bone HG et al. ACTIVExtend: 24 months of alendronate after 18 months of abaloparatide or placebo for postmenopausal osteoporosis. J Clin Endocrinol Metab. 2018 Aug 1;103(8):2949–57. [PMID: 29800372]

Buckley L et al. Glucocorticoid-induced osteoporosis. N Engl J Med. 2018 Dec 27;379(26):2547–56. [PMID: 30586507]

Curry SJ et al. Screening for osteoporosis to prevent fractures: US Preventive Services Task Force Recommendation Statement. JAMA. 2018 Jun 6;319(24):2521–31. [PMID: 29946735]

Ensrud KE et al. Osteoporosis. Ann Intern Med. 2017 Aug 1;167(3):ITC17–32. Erratum in: Ann Intern Med. 2017 Oct 3;167(7):528. [PMID: 28761958]

Grossman DC et al. Vitamin D, calcium, or combined supplementation for the primary prevention of fractures in community-dwelling adults: US Preventive Services Task Force Recommendation Statement. JAMA. 2018 Apr 17;319(15):1592–9. [PMID: 29677309]

Lyu H et al. Comparison of denosumab vs. bisphosphonates in osteoporosis patients: a meta-analysis of randomized controlled trials. J Clin Endocrinol Metab. 2019 May 1;104(5):1753–65. [PMID: 30535289]

Qaseem A et al. Treatment of low bone density or osteoporosis to prevent fractures in men and women: a clinical practice guideline update from the American College of Physicians. Ann Intern Med. 2017 Jun 6;166(11):818–39. [PMID: 28492856]

RICKETS & OSTEOMALACIA

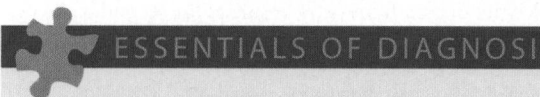
ESSENTIALS OF DIAGNOSIS

▶ Low bone density from defective mineralization.

▶ Caused by deficiency in calcium, phosphorus, or low alkaline phosphatase.

▶ **Rickets:** defective bone mineralization in childhood or adolescence before epiphyseal fusion.

▶ **Osteomalacia:** defective bone mineralization in adults with fused epiphyses.

► Painful proximal muscle weakness (especially pelvic girdle); bone pain.

► Low 25-hydroxy-vitamin D (25-OHD), hypocalcemia, hypocalciuria, hypophosphatemia, secondary hyperparathyroidism.

► Classic radiologic features may be present.

General Considerations

Defective mineralization of the growing skeleton in childhood causes permanent bone deformities (rickets). Defective skeletal mineralization in adults is known as osteomalacia. It is caused by any condition that results in inadequate calcium or phosphate mineralization of bone osteoid.

Etiology (Table 26–10)

A. Vitamin D Deficiency and Resistance

Vitamin D deficiency is the most common cause of osteomalacia; its incidence is increasing throughout the world as a result of diminished exposure to sunlight caused by urbanization, automobile and public transportation, modest clothing, and sunscreen use. About 36% of adults in the United States are deficient in vitamin D.

Vitamin D deficiency is most commonly caused by insufficient sunlight exposure from living at high latitudes,

Table 26–10. Causes of osteomalacia.[1]

Vitamin disorders
  Insufficient sunlight exposure
  Kidney: chronic kidney disease, nephrotic syndrome, kidney
    transplantation
  Liver disease
  Nutritional deficiency of vitamin D
  Malabsorption: aging, excess wheat bran, bariatric surgery,
    pancreatic enzyme deficiency, orlistat
  Vitamin D–dependent rickets type I
  Phenytoin, carbamazepine, valproate, or barbiturate therapy
    (long-term)
Dietary calcium deficiency
Phosphate deficiency
  Adefovir therapy
  Fanconi syndrome, renal tubular acidosis, and alcoholism
  Intestinal malabsorption
  Nutritional deficiency of phosphorus
  Phosphate-binding antacid therapy
  Renal loss
  Tumoral hypophosphatemic osteomalacia
  X-linked hypophosphatemic rickets
  Other disorders, including paraproteinemias, glycogen
    storage diseases, neurofibromatosis, Wilson disease
Inhibitors of mineralization
  Aluminum
  Bisphosphonates
Disorders of bone matrix
  Axial osteomalacia
  Hypophosphatasia
  Fibrogenesis imperfecta

[1]See Table 26–9 for causes of osteoporosis.

winter season, institutionalization, wearing sun protection, or very modest dressing. Other risk factors for vitamin D deficiency include the following: pregnant women, infants breastfed exclusively, age over 65 years, obesity, dark skin, malnutrition, and intestinal malabsorption. Orlistat causes fat and vitamin D malabsorption. Cholestyramine binds bile acids necessary for vitamin D absorption. Patients with severe nephrotic syndrome lose large amounts of vitamin D–binding protein in the urine.

Anticonvulsants (eg, phenytoin, carbamazepine, valproate, phenobarbital) inhibit the hepatic production of 25-OHD and sometimes cause osteomalacia. Phenytoin can also directly inhibit bone mineralization.

Vitamin D–dependent rickets type I is caused by a rare autosomal recessive disorder with a defect in the renal enzyme 1-alpha-hydroxylase leading to defective synthesis of $1,25(OH)_2D$. It presents in childhood with rickets and alopecia; osteomalacia develops in adults with this condition unless treated with oral calcitriol in doses of 0.5–1 mcg daily.

Vitamin D–dependent rickets type II (better known as hereditary $1,25[OH]_2$D-resistant rickets) is caused by a genetic defect in the $1,25(OH)_2D$ receptor. Patients have hypocalcemia with childhood rickets and adult osteomalacia. Alopecia is common. These patients respond variably to oral calcitriol in very large doses (2–6 mcg daily).

B. Deficient Calcium Intake

The total daily consumption of calcium should be at least 1000 mg daily. Patients who have deficient calcium intake develop rickets (childhood) or osteomalacia (adulthood) despite sufficient vitamin D. A nutritional deficiency of calcium can occur in any severely malnourished patient. Some degree of calcium deficiency is common in older adults, since intestinal calcium absorption declines with age. Ingestion of excessive wheat bran also causes calcium malabsorption.

C. Phosphate Deficiency

Osteomalacia develops in patients with hypophosphatemia due to lack of sufficient phosphate to mineralize bone osteoid. Such patients typically have musculoskeletal pain, muscle weakness, and are prone to fractures.

1. Genetic disorders—Fibroblast growth factor-23 (FGF23) is a phosphaturic factor (phosphatonin) that is secreted by bone osteoblasts in response to elevated serum phosphate levels. Families with autosomal dominant hypophosphatemic rickets have a gain-of-function mutation in the gene encoding FGF23, which makes it resistant to proteolytic cleavage. In X-linked hypophosphatemic rickets, there is a mutation in the gene encoding PHEX endopeptidase, which fails to cleave FGF23. An autosomal recessive form of hypophosphatemic rickets is caused by mutations in DMP1, a transcription factor that regulates FGF23 production in bone. All three conditions have high serum FGF23 levels causing hypophosphatemia and bone mineral depletion.

2. Tumor-induced osteomalacia—A variety of mesenchymal tumors (87% benign) secrete FGF23 and cause marked hypophosphatemia due to renal phosphate wasting.

Such tumors are usually phosphaturic mesenchymal tumors (70%); other tumors include hemangiopericytomas, osteosarcomas, and giant cell tumors. The condition is characterized by hypophosphatemia, excessive phosphaturia, reduced or normal serum $1,25(OH)_2D$ concentrations, and osteomalacia. Serum levels of FGF23 are elevated. Such tumors are often small and difficult to find, frequently lying in extremities.

3. Other causes of hypophosphatemia—Osteomalacia from hypophosphatemia can be caused by severe intestinal malabsorption or poor nutrition. Tenofovir therapy (tenofovir disoproxil fumarate more so than tenofovir alafenamide) can cause renal phosphate wasting and hypophosphatemia. Severe hypophosphatemia can occur with refeeding after starvation. Hypophosphatemia can also be caused by chelation of phosphate in the gut by aluminum hydroxide antacids, calcium acetate (Phos-Lo), or sevelamer hydrochloride (Renagel). Excessive renal phosphate losses are also seen in proximal renal tubular acidosis and Fanconi syndrome.

D. Aluminum Toxicity

Bone mineralization is inhibited by aluminum. Osteomalacia may occur in patients receiving long-term renal hemodialysis with tap water dialysate or from aluminum-containing antacids used to reduce phosphate levels.

E. Hypophosphatasia

Hypophosphatasia must not be confused with hypophosphatemia. Hypophosphatasia refers to a severe deficiency of bone alkaline phosphatase. It is a rare genetic cause of osteomalacia that is commonly misdiagnosed as osteoporosis.

F. Fibrogenesis Imperfecta Ossium

This rare condition sporadically affects middle-aged patients, who present with progressive bone pain and pathologic fractures. Bones have a dense "fishnet" appearance on radiographs. Serum alkaline phosphatase levels are elevated. Some patients have a monoclonal gammopathy, indicating a possible plasma cell dyscrasia causing an impairment in osteoblast function and collagen disarray. Remission has been reported after repeated courses of melphalan, corticosteroids, and vitamin D analog over 3 years.

► Clinical Findings

The clinical manifestations of osteomalacia depend on the underlying cause, severity, and the age at onset.

Neonates and young children with hypocalcemia may have spasms and convulsions. Older children and adolescents can have bone pain and muscle weakness and may develop the skeletal deformities of classic rickets, such as delayed longitudinal growth, deformities at epiphyses leading to thickened wrists and ankles, and bowing of the legs as well as bowed legs or knock-knees (adolescents). Kyphoscoliosis or lumbar lordosis is common. Thickening at the costochondral joints can cause widening of the chest and deformities known as a "rachitic rosary."

In adults, osteomalacia is initially asymptomatic. Then, nonspecific complaints that include fatigue, reduced endurance and muscle strength, and pain in the bones involving their shoulders ribs, low back, and thighs develop. Pathologic fractures can occur with little or no trauma.

Hypocalcemia causes a reduced quality of life, with fatigue, irritability, depression, anxiety, cognitive impairment, lethargy, and paresthesias in the circumoral area, hands, and feet. More severe manifestations include muscle weakness or cramps, carpopedal spasm, convulsions, tetany, laryngospasm, and stridor. Hypophosphatemia can cause severe major muscle weakness, reduced endurance, dysphagia, diplopia, cardiomyopathy, and respiratory muscle weakness. Patients may also have impaired cognition.

► Diagnostic Tests

Serum is obtained for calcium, albumin, phosphate, alkaline phosphatase, PTH, and 25-OHD determinations. Vitamin D *deficiency* is defined as a serum 25-OHD less than 20 ng/mL (50 nmol/L). Vitamin D *insufficiency* is defined as a serum 25-OHD between 20 ng/mL and 30 ng/mL (50–75 nmol/L). Patients in whom clinically severe osteomalacia develops typically have had chronic *severe vitamin D deficiency* (serum 25-OHD under 10 ng/mL or 25 nmol/L).

$1,25(OH)_2D_3$ may be low even when $25(OH)D_2$ levels are normal. In one series of biopsy-proved osteomalacia, alkaline phosphatase was elevated in 94% of patients; the calcium or phosphorus was low in 47% of patients; $25(OH)D_3$ was low in 29% of patients; and urinary calcium was low in 18% of patients. Pseudofractures were seen in 18% of patients. Radiographs may show diagnostic features. Bone densitometry helps document the degree of osteopenia.

Genetic testing can confirm the diagnosis of autosomal dominant hypophosphatemic rickets (*FGF23*), X-linked hypophosphatemic rickets (*PHEX*), and autosomal recessive hypophosphatemic rickets (*DMP1*).

Patients with apparent tumor-induced osteomalacia with hypophosphatemia require localization studies. Whole-body scanning with somatostatin analogs ^{68}Ga-DOTATOC PET/CT is the preferred imaging technique in this condition, detecting about 90% of tumors in small series.

Patients with hypophosphatasia have low serum levels of alkaline phosphatase (below 40 units/L in adults and below 20 units/L in severe cases). To confirm the diagnosis of hypophosphatasia in patients with a low serum alkaline phosphatase, a 24-hour urine is assayed for phosphoethanolamine, a substrate for tissue-nonspecific alkaline phosphatase whose excretion is always elevated in patients with hypophosphatasia. The diagnosis is further confirmed with genetic testing for mutations in the *ALPL* gene.

► Differential Diagnosis

Osteomalacia often coexists with osteoporosis. The relative contribution of the two entities to diminished bone density may not be apparent until treatment, since a dramatic rise in bone density is often seen with therapy for osteomalacia. Phosphate deficiency must be distinguished from hypophosphatemia seen in hyperparathyroidism.

▶ Prevention & Treatment

Humans naturally receive about 90% of their vitamin D from sunlight. To obtain adequate sunshine vitamin D, the face, arms, hands, or back must have sun exposure without sunscreen for 15 minutes at least twice weekly. In sunlight-deprived individuals (eg, veiled women, confined patients, or residents of higher latitudes during winter), vitamin D_3, 1000 international units daily, should be given prophylactically. Patients receiving long-term phenytoin therapy should also receive vitamin D_3 supplementation. The main natural food source of vitamin D is fish, particularly salmon, mackerel, cod liver oil, and sardines or tuna canned in oil. Most commercial cow's milk is fortified with vitamin D at about 400 international units (10 mcg) per quart; however, yogurt and cottage cheese may contain little to no vitamin D_3.

Many vitamin supplements contain plant-derived vitamin D_2, which has variable biologic availability. Over-the-counter multivitamin/mineral supplements contain variable amounts of vitamin D, and vitamin D toxicity has occurred from two different multivitamins sold in the United States. Therefore, it is prudent to recommend that patients take a dedicated vitamin D_3 supplement from a reliable manufacturer.

Frank vitamin D deficiency can be treated with ergocalciferol (D_2), 50,000 international units orally once weekly for 8 weeks. Some patients require long-term supplementation with D_2 of up to 50,000 international units weekly. The danger of high-dose D_2 therapy is that some patients may mistakenly take it daily. The alternative is to treat vitamin D–deficient patients with daily cholecalciferol D_3 at doses of at least 2000 international units daily. The recommended maximum daily dose of vitamin D_3 is 4000 international units/day for children and 10,000 international units/day for adults, with such high daily doses sometimes being required for patients with obesity, intestinal malabsorption, or following gastric bypass surgery. Some patients with severe malabsorption may require oral doses of 25,000–100,000 international units of vitamin D_3 daily. Some patients with steatorrhea respond better to oral 25(OH)D_3 (calcifediol), 50–100 mcg/day. Serum levels of 25-OHD should be monitored, and the dosage of vitamin D adjusted to maintain serum 25-OHD levels above 30 ng/mL. The Endocrine Society has recommended a preferred target range of serum 25-OHD of 40–60 ng/mL.

Beyond increasing the intestinal absorption of calcium, vitamin D supplementation may improve muscle strength and reduce fall risk, factors that reduce the risk of bone fracture.

The addition of calcium supplements to vitamin D is probably not necessary for the prevention of osteomalacia in the majority of otherwise well-nourished patients. However, patients with malabsorption or poor nutrition should receive calcium supplementation: calcium citrate (eg, Citracal), 0.4–0.6 g elemental calcium per day, or calcium carbonate (eg, OsCal, Tums), 1–1.5 g elemental calcium per day. Calcium supplements are best administered with meals.

In hypophosphatemic rickets or osteomalacia, nutritional deficiencies are corrected, aluminum-containing antacids are discontinued, and patients with renal tubular acidosis are given bicarbonate therapy. In patients with sporadic adult-onset hypophosphatemia, hyperphosphaturia, and low serum 1,25(OH)$_2$D levels, a search is conducted for occult tumors; whole-body MRI scanning may be required.

For those with X-linked or idiopathic hypophosphatemia and hyperphosphaturia, oral phosphate supplements must be given long term. Calcitriol, 0.25–0.5 mcg/day, is given also to improve the impaired calcium absorption caused by the oral phosphate. Oral phosphate causes diarrhea at higher doses, and many patients do not achieve normal serum phosphate levels. If necessary, recombinant human growth hormone (rhGH) may be added to the above regimen to reduce phosphaturia. The hypophosphatemia of autosomal dominant hypophosphatemic rickets has been reported to resolve with high-dose dietary iron supplementation.

Patients with hypophosphatasia may be treated with asfotase alfa (Strensiq), which is administered subcutaneously in doses of 2 mg/kg three times weekly; adverse effects include injection site reactions, lipodystrophy ectopic calcifications, and hypersensitivity reactions. Patients have also been treated with teriparatide with improvement in bone pain and fracture healing.

Gonciulea AR et al. Fibroblast growth factor 23-mediated bone disease. Endocrinol Metab Clin North Am. 2017 Mar;46(1):19–39. [PMID: 28131132]

Holick MF. The vitamin D deficiency pandemic: approaches for diagnosis, treatment and prevention. Rev Endocr Metab Disord. 2017 Jun;18(2):153–65. [PMID: 28516265]

Kilim HP et al. Optimizing calcium and vitamin D intake through diet and supplements. Cleve Clin J Med. 2018 Jul; 85(7):543–50. [PMID: 30004379]

Minisola S et al. Tumour-induced osteomalacia. Nat Rev Dis Primers. 2017 Jul 13;3:17044. [PMID: 28703220]

Mornet E. Hypophosphatasia. Metabolism. 2018 May;82:142–55. [PMID: 28939177]

PAGET DISEASE OF BONE
(Osteitis Deformans)

ESSENTIALS OF DIAGNOSIS

▶ Often asymptomatic.

▶ Bone pain may be the first symptom.

▶ Kyphosis, bowed tibias, large head, deafness, and frequent fractures.

▶ Serum calcium and phosphate normal; elevated alkaline phosphatase and urinary hydroxyproline.

▶ Dense, expanded bones on radiographs.

▶ General Considerations

Paget disease of bone is manifested by one or more bony lesions having high bone turnover and disorganized osteoid formation. The involved bone first has increased osteoclast activity, causing lytic lesions in bone that may progress at about 1 cm/year. Increased osteoblastic activity follows, producing a high rate of disorganized bone formation. Involved bones become vascular, weak, and deformed. Eventually, there appears to be a final burned-out phase with markedly reduced bone cell activity and abnormal bones that may be enlarged with skeletal deformity.

The prevalence of Paget disease has declined by about 36% over the past 20 years, yet it is the second most common bone disease after osteoporosis. In the United States, Paget disease affects 3% of whites over age 55 years, with its prevalence increasing with age. It is uncommon in Africa, Asia, and Scandinavia. Usually diagnosed in patients over age 40 years, its prevalence doubles with each decade thereafter, reaching an incidence of about 10% after age 80. About 20% of cases are symptomatic, but most cases are discovered incidentally during radiology imaging or because of incidentally discovered elevations in serum alkaline phosphatase.

The cause of Paget disease is unknown. About 20% of cases are familial and transmitted as an autosomal dominant trait with incomplete penetrance. Mutations in the *SQSTM1* gene have been discovered in about 35% of patients with familial Paget disease and in 7% of patients with apparently sporadic Paget disease.

► Clinical Findings

A. Symptoms and Signs

Paget disease is often mild and asymptomatic. Only 27% of affected individuals are symptomatic at the time of diagnosis. Paget disease involves multiple bones (polyostotic) in 72% and only a single bone (monostotic) in 28%. It occurs most commonly in the pelvis, vertebrae, femur, humerus, and skull. The affected bones are typically involved simultaneously, and the disease tends not to involve additional bones during its course. Pain, often described as aching and deep and often worse at night, is the usual first symptom. It may occur in the involved bone or in an adjacent joint, which can be involved with degenerative arthritis. Paget disease typically first affects long bones proximally and then advances distally, with bone pain at the osteolytic front being aggravated by weight bearing. Joint surfaces (such as the knee) can be involved and cause arthritic pain. The bones can become soft, leading to bowed tibias, kyphosis, and frequent "chalkstick" fractures with slight trauma. If the skull is involved, the patient may report headaches and an increased hat size; the finding of dilated scalp veins, present in half such patients, is known as the "scalp vein sign." Involvement of the petrous temporal bone frequently damages the cochlea and causes hearing loss (mixed sensorineural and conductive) and occasionally tinnitus or vertigo. Increased vascularity over the involved bones causes increased warmth and can cause vascular "steal" syndromes.

B. Laboratory Findings

Serum alkaline phosphatase is usually markedly elevated. However, some patients with monostotic involvement may have normal serum alkaline phosphatase levels. A serum bone-specific alkaline phosphatase is usually high and is useful for patients with a normal serum alkaline

phosphatase and to distinguish the source of an elevated alkaline phosphatase as being from bone (rather than liver). However, bone alkaline phosphatase is less useful for following the effectiveness of therapy. Other useful measures for bone turnover are serum N-terminal propeptide of type 1 collagen (NTx) and serum beta C-terminal propeptide of type 1 collagen (betaCTx). However, such bone turnover markers may overestimate or underestimate the response to treatment. Serum calcium may be elevated, particularly if the patient is at bed rest. A serum 25-OH vitamin D determination should be obtained to screen for vitamin D deficiency, which can also present with an increased serum alkaline phosphatase and bone pain.

C. Imaging

On radiographs, the initial lesions are typically osteolytic, with focal radiolucencies ("osteoporosis circumscripta") in the skull or advancing flame-shaped lytic lesions in long bones. Bone lesions may subsequently become sclerotic and have a mixed lytic and sclerotic appearance. The affected bones eventually become thickened and deformed. Technetium-99m pyrophosphate bone scans are helpful in delineating activity of bone lesions even before any radiologic changes are apparent.

► Differential Diagnosis

Certain rare familial types of sclerosing bone dysplasias share phenotypic homologies with Paget disease of bone. The differential diagnosis also includes myelofibrosis, intramedullary osteosclerosis, Erdheim-Chester disease, Langerhans cell histiocytosis, and sickle cell disease.

Paget disease must be differentiated from primary bone lesions such as osteogenic sarcoma, plasma cell myeloma, and fibrous dysplasia and from secondary bone lesions such as osteitis fibrosa cystica and metastatic carcinoma to bone. Fibrogenesis imperfecta ossium is a rare symmetric disorder that can mimic the features of Paget disease; serum alkaline phosphatase is likewise elevated. This condition may be associated with paraproteinemias.

► Complications

If immobilization occurs, hypercalcemia and renal calculi may develop. With severe polyostotic disease, the increased vascularity may give rise to high-output heart failure. Arthritis frequently develops in joints adjacent to involved bone.

Extensive skull involvement may cause cranial nerve palsies from impingement of the neural foramina. Skull involvement can also cause a vascular steal syndrome with somnolence or ischemic neurologic events; the optic nerve may be affected, resulting in loss of vision. Jaw involvement can cause the teeth to spread intraorally and become misaligned. Vertebral collapse can cause compression of spinal cord or spinal nerves, resulting in radiculopathy or paralysis. Vertebral involvement can also cause a vascular steal syndrome with paralysis. Surgery for fractured long bones is often complicated by excessive blood loss from these vascular lytic lesions.

A sarcoma or giant cell tumor may develop in longstanding lesions but is rare (less than 1%). Sarcomatous change is suggested by a marked increase in bone pain, sudden rise in alkaline phosphatase, and appearance of a new lytic lesion.

▶ Treatment

Asymptomatic patients may require only clinical surveillance and no treatment. However, treatment should be considered for asymptomatic patients who have significant involvement of the skull, long bones, or vertebrae. Patients must be monitored carefully before, during, and after treatment with clinical examinations and serial serum alkaline phosphatase determinations.

Bisphosphonates are used to treat patients with Paget disease. Zoledronic acid is the treatment of choice. Administered intravenously as a single 5-mg dose, it normalizes the serum alkaline phosphatase in 89% of patients by 6 months and in 98% by 2 years.

Zoledronic acid should be administered prior to total arthroplasty for a Paget-involved joint in order to reduce the risk of intraoperative hemorrhaging and loosening of the prosthesis postoperatively. Zoledronic acid should also be administered before osteotomy for severe bowing of a lower extremity caused by Paget disease. For patients with paraplegia due to vertebral involvement, intravenous zoledronic acid should be given while neurosurgical consultation is obtained.

Patients frequently experience a paradoxical increase in pain at sites of disease soon after commencing bisphosphonate therapy; this is the "first dose effect" and the pain usually subsides with further treatment. Following intravenous zoledronic acid, patients frequently experience fever, fatigue, myalgia, bone pain, and ocular problems. Serious side effects are rare but include seizures, uveitis, and acute kidney disease. Asthma may occur in aspirin-sensitive patients. Hypocalcemia is common and may be severe, especially if intravenous bisphosphonates are given along with loop diuretics. Therefore, it is advisable to administer calcium and vitamin D supplements, especially during the first 2 weeks following treatment. Any vitamin D deficiency should be corrected before prescribing a bisphosphonate.

Oral bisphosphonate regimens are inferior to intravenous zoledronic acid for therapy of Paget disease. However, if they are given, to prevent esophageal complications, oral bisphosphonates should be taken with 8 oz of plain water only; they are relatively contraindicated in patients with a history of esophagitis, esophageal stricture, dysphagia, hiatal hernia, or achalasia.

▶ Prognosis

The prognosis is good, but relapse can occur after an initial successful treatment with bisphosphonate. By 6.5 years after initial therapy, the recurrence rate is 12.5% after treatment with zoledronic acid and 62% after risedronate. Therefore, patients must be monitored long term, measuring serum alkaline phosphatase at least yearly. In general, the prognosis is worse the earlier in life the disease starts. Fractures usually heal well. In the severe forms, marked deformity, intractable pain, and high-output heart failure occur if not treated with bisphosphonates. Osteosarcoma

that arises at sites of Paget disease results in a 2-year survival of only 25%.

Corral-Gudino L et al. Bisphosphonates for Paget's disease of bone in adults. Cochrane Database Syst Rev. 2017 Dec 1; 12:CD004956. [PMID: 29192423]
Cundy T. Paget's disease of bone. Metabolism. 2018 Mar;80:5–14. [PMID: 28780255]
Paul Tuck S et al. Adult Paget's disease of bone: a review. Rheumatology (Oxford). 2017 Dec 1;56(12):2050–9. [PMID: 28339664]

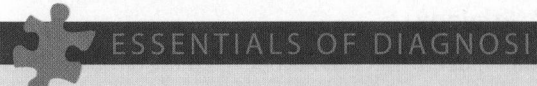

▼ DISEASES OF THE ADRENAL CORTEX

PRIMARY ADRENAL INSUFFICIENCY (Addison Disease)

ESSENTIALS OF DIAGNOSIS

▶ Weakness, vomiting, diarrhea; abdominal pain, arthralgias; amenorrhea.

▶ Sparse axillary hair; increased skin pigmentation, especially of creases, pressure areas, and nipples.

▶ Hypotension, small heart.

▶ Hyponatremia; potassium, calcium, and BUN elevated; mild anemia and relative neutropenia, lymphocytosis, and eosinophilia.

▶ Plasma ACTH level elevated; cosyntropin unable to stimulate serum cortisol to 20 mcg/dL (550 nmol/L) or more.

▶ **Acute adrenal crisis:** above manifestations become critical, with fever, shock, confusion, coma, death.

▶ General Considerations

Primary adrenal insufficiency (Addison disease) is caused by dysfunction or absence of the adrenal cortices. It is distinct from secondary adrenal insufficiency caused by deficient secretion of ACTH.

Addison disease is an uncommon disorder with a prevalence of about 140 per million and an annual incidence of about 5 cases per million in the United States. Addison disease is characterized by a chronic deficiency of cortisol. Serum ACTH and alpha-MSH levels are consequently elevated, causing pigmentation that ranges from none to strikingly dark. Patients with destruction of the adrenal cortices or with classic 21-hydroxylase deficiency also have mineralocorticoid deficiency, typically with hyponatremia, volume depletion, and hyperkalemia. In contrast, mineralocorticoid deficiency is not present in patients with familial corticosteroid deficiency and Allgrove syndrome.

Acute adrenal (addisonian) crisis is an emergency caused by insufficient cortisol. Crisis may occur in the course of treatment of chronic adrenal insufficiency, or it may be the presenting manifestation of adrenal insufficiency. Acute adrenal crisis is more commonly seen in primary adrenal insufficiency than in secondary adrenal insufficiency.

Adrenal crisis may occur in the following situations: (1) during stress (eg, infection, trauma, surgery, hyperthyroidism, or prolonged fasting) in a patient with latent or treated adrenal insufficiency; (2) following sudden withdrawal of adrenocortical hormone in a patient with chronic insufficiency or in a patient with temporary insufficiency due to suppression by exogenous corticosteroids or megestrol; (3) following bilateral adrenalectomy or removal of a functioning adrenal tumor that had suppressed the other adrenal gland; (4) following sudden destruction of the pituitary gland (pituitary necrosis), or when thyroid hormone is given to a patient with adrenal insufficiency; (5) following injury to both adrenals (by trauma, hemorrhage, anticoagulant therapy, thrombosis, infection or, rarely, metastatic carcinoma); and (6) following administration of intravenous etomidate (used for rapid anesthesia induction or intubation).

▶ Etiology

Autoimmunity is the most common cause of Addison disease in industrialized countries, accounting for about 90% of spontaneous cases. With such autoimmunity, adrenal function decreases over several years as it progresses to overt adrenal insufficiency. Over half the cases of autoimmune Addison disease occur as part of autoimmune polyendocrine syndrome (APS-I), also known as APECED syndrome. APS-I is caused by a defect in T cell–mediated immunity inherited as an autosomal recessive trait. APS-I usually presents in early childhood with mucocutaneous candidiasis, followed by hypoparathyroidism and dystrophy of the teeth and nails; Addison disease usually appears by age 15 years. Partial or late expression of the syndrome is common. A varied spectrum of associated diseases may be seen in adulthood, including hypogonadism, hypothyroidism, pernicious anemia, alopecia, vitiligo, hepatitis, malabsorption, and Sjögren syndrome.

Tuberculosis is the most common infection of the adrenals. Coccidioidomycosis, histoplasmosis, cytomegalovirus infection, and syphilitic gummas are rare causes and usually occur in immunocompromised patients.

Infections of the adrenal glands, particularly with cytomegalovirus, are found in nearly half of patients with untreated HIV at autopsy. However, a much lower percentage have clinical Addison disease. The diagnosis of adrenal insufficiency in HIV patients is often problematic. A cortisol resistance syndrome has been described in patients with HIV, and a revision of normal range for the cosyntropin test for these patients has been advocated (normal peak cortisol over 22 mcg/dL). Also, isolated hyperkalemia occurs commonly in HIV patients, particularly during therapy with pentamidine; this is usually due to isolated hypoaldosteronism and responds to mineralocorticoid (fludrocortisone) therapy alone.

Bilateral adrenal hemorrhage may occur with sepsis, heparin-associated thrombocytopenia, anticoagulation, or the antiphospholipid antibody syndrome. It may occur in association with major surgery or trauma, presenting about 1 week later with pain, fever, and shock. It may also occur spontaneously and present with flank pain. Meningococcemia may be associated with purpura and adrenal insufficiency secondary to adrenal infarction (Waterhouse-Friderichsen syndrome).

Adrenoleukodystrophy is an X-linked peroxisomal disorder causing accumulation of very long-chain fatty acids in the adrenal cortex, testes, brain, and spinal cord. It may present at any age and accounts for one-third of cases of Addison disease in boys. Aldosterone deficiency occurs in 9%. Hypogonadism is common.

Rare causes of adrenal insufficiency include lymphoma, metastatic carcinoma, scleroderma, amyloidosis, and hemochromatosis.

Congenital adrenal insufficiency occurs in several conditions. Familial corticosteroid deficiency is an autosomal recessive disease that is caused by mutations in the adrenal ACTH receptor (melanocortin 2 receptor, MC2R). It is characterized by isolated cortisol deficiency and ACTH resistance and may present with neonatal hypoglycemia, frequent infections, and dark skin pigmentation. Triple A (Allgrove) syndrome is caused by a mutation in the *AAAS* gene that encodes a protein known as ALADIN (*a*lachrima, *a*chalasia, a*d*renal *i*nsufficiency, *n*eurologic disorder). Cortisol deficiency usually presents in infancy but may not occur until the third decade of life. Congenital adrenal hypoplasia causes adrenal insufficiency due to absence of the adrenal cortex; patients may also have hypogonadotropic hypogonadism, myopathy, and high-frequency hearing loss.

Congenital adrenal hyperplasia is caused by various genetic defects in the enzymes responsible for steroid synthesis. Due to defective cortisol synthesis, patients have variable degrees of adrenal insufficiency and increased levels of ACTH that causes hyperplasia of the adrenal cortex. The most common enzyme defect is *P450c21 (21-hydroxylase deficiency)*. Patients with severely defective P450c21 (classic congenital adrenal hyperplasia) manifest a deficiency of mineralocorticoids (salt wasting) in addition to deficient cortisol and excessive androgens. Hypertension commonly develops in older adult patients. Testicular adrenal rests can be found in 44% of men with the condition. Women with milder enzyme defects have adequate cortisol, but develop hirsutism in adolescence or adulthood and are said to have "late-onset" congenital adrenal hyperplasia.

Drugs that cause primary adrenal insufficiency include mitotane and abiraterone acetate.

▶ Clinical Findings

A. Symptoms and Signs

The onset of symptoms can occur suddenly but usually develops gradually over months or years. The diagnosis is often delayed, since many early symptoms are nonspecific. Nearly all patients complain of fatigue, reduced stamina, weakness, anorexia, and weight loss. Abdominal pain, nausea, and vomiting eventually develop in most patients; diarrhea can occur. Fevers and lymphoid tissue hyperplasia may also occur. Patients often have significant pain: arthralgias, myalgias, chest pain, abdominal pain, back pain, leg pain, or headache. Psychiatric symptoms include anxiety, irritability and depression. Cerebral edema can cause headache, vomiting, gait disturbance, and intellectual dysfunction that may progress to coma. Hypoglycemia can occur and worsen the patient's weakness and mental functioning. Patients often have salt craving. Blood pressure is usually low and orthostatic; about 90% have systolic blood pressures under 110 mm Hg; blood pressure over 130 mm Hg is rare. Hypotension is aggravated by dehydration caused by nausea or vomiting.

Skin hyperpigmentation eventually occurs in most patients due to increased pituitary secretion of alpha-MSH (melanocyte-stimulating hormone). Skin hyperpigmentation varies among affected patients (eg, from none to increased freckling to diffuse darkening that resembles a suntan or a bronze appearance). Sun-exposed areas darken the most, but nonexposed areas darken as well. Hyperpigmentation is often especially prominent over the knuckles, elbows, knees, posterior neck, palmar creases, gingival mucosa, and vermilion border of the lips. Nail beds may develop longitudinal pigmented bands. Nipples and areolas tend to darken. The skin also darkens in pressure areas, such as the belt or brassiere lines and the buttocks. Skin folds and new scars may also become pigmented. Conversely, patches of autoimmune vitiligo can be found in about 10% of patients. Scant axillary and pubic hair typically develops in women.

In pregnancy, undiagnosed adrenal insufficiency is rare, since the condition tends to cause anovulation and reduced fertility. In the first trimester, symptoms such as fatigue, nausea, vomiting, abdominal pain, and orthostasis are typically attributed to the pregnancy, thus delaying the diagnosis. Worse, the increased skin pigmentation of adrenal insufficiency may be mistaken for chloasma (melasma). Undiagnosed adrenal insufficiency can cause intrauterine growth retardation and fetal loss. Pregnant women with undiagnosed adrenal insufficiency can experience shock from adrenal crisis, particularly during the first trimester, concurrent illness, labor, or postpartum.

Patients with preexistent type 1 diabetes experience more frequent hypoglycemia with the onset of adrenal insufficiency, such that their insulin dosage must be reduced.

Acute adrenal crisis is an immediate threat to life. Nausea, vomiting, fever, dehydration, and profound hypotension progresses to life-threatening shock that does not fully respond to intravenous fluids and vasopressors.

B. Laboratory Findings

The WBC count typically shows moderate neutropenia, lymphocytosis, and eosinophilia (total eosinophil count over 300/mcL). Among patients with chronic adrenal insufficiency, the serum sodium is usually low (88%) and the potassium usually elevated (64%). However, patients with vomiting or diarrhea may not be hyperkalemic. Fasting hypoglycemia is common. Hypercalcemia may be present.

A plasma cortisol less than 3 mcg/dL (83 nmol/L) at 8 AM is diagnostic, especially if accompanied by simultaneous elevation of the plasma ACTH level greater than 200 pg/mL (44 pmol/L). The diagnosis is confirmed by a simplified cosyntropin stimulation test: (1) Synthetic $ACTH_{1-24}$ (cosyntropin), 0.25 mg, is given intramuscularly. (2) Serum cortisol is obtained 45 minutes after cosyntropin is administered. Normally, serum cortisol rises to at least 20 mcg/dL (550 pmol/L), whereas patients with adrenal insufficiency have stimulated serum cortisol levels less than 20 mcg/dL (550 pmol/L). For patients receiving corticosteroid

treatment, hydrocortisone must not be given for at least 8 hours before the test. Other corticosteroids (eg, prednisone, dexamethasone) do not interfere with specific assays for cortisol. Cosyntropin is usually well tolerated, but infrequent (less than 5%) side effects have included hypersensitivity reactions with nausea, headache, dizziness, dyspnea, palpitations, flushing, edema, and local injection site reactions. Cosyntropin may be administered during pregnancy; however, the test may lack sensitivity, since adrenal ACTH-responsiveness increases during pregnancy.

Serum DHEA levels are less than 1000 ng/mL (350 nmol/L) in 100% of patients with adrenal insufficiency but also in about 15% of the population, so the test is very sensitive but not specific.

One or more serum anti-adrenal antibodies are found in about 50% of cases of autoimmune Addison disease. Serum is assayed for four different anti-adrenal antibodies with the following sensitivities: cytoplasmic antibodies (26%), 21-hydroxylase antibodies (21%), 17-hydroxylase antibodies (21%), and side-chain cleavage antibodies (16%). Antibodies to thyroid (45%) and other tissues may also be present.

Salt-wasting congenital adrenal hyperplasia due to 21-hydroxylase deficiency is usually diagnosed at birth in females due to ambiguous genitalia. Males and patients with milder enzyme defects may present later. The diagnosis of adrenal insufficiency is made as above. The specific diagnosis requires elevated serum levels of 17-OH progesterone.

Elevated plasma renin activity (PRA) indicates the presence of depleted intravascular volume and the need for fludrocortisone administration. Serum epinephrine levels are low in patients with adrenal insufficiency, since these patients do not have the high local concentrations of cortisol that are required to induce the enzyme PNMT in adrenal medulla for the synthesis of epinephrine from norepinephrine.

Young men with idiopathic Addison disease are screened for X-linked adrenoleukodystrophy by determining plasma very long-chain fatty acid levels; affected patients have high levels.

In acute adrenal crisis, blood, sputum, or urine cultures may be positive if bacterial infection is the precipitating cause.

C. Imaging

When adrenal insufficiency is not clearly autoimmune, a CT scan of the adrenal glands should be obtained. Small, noncalcified adrenals are seen in autoimmune Addison disease. The adrenals are enlarged in about 85% of cases related to metastatic or granulomatous disease. Adrenal calcifications occur in about 50% of cases of tuberculous Addison disease but are also seen with hemorrhage, fungal infection, pheochromocytoma, and melanoma.

▶ Differential Diagnosis

Patients with ACTH deficiency have normal mineralocorticoid production and do not develop hyperkalemia. Patients with secondary adrenal insufficiency (see Hypopituitarism) lack ACTH and have normal to decreased skin pigmentation that has been described as "alabaster skin." This contrasts with the increased skin pigmentation in patients with Addison disease. Hemochromatosis also causes bronze skin hyperpigmentation, but hemochromatosis may in fact be the cause of Addison disease. Acute adrenal insufficiency must be distinguished from other causes of shock (eg, septic, hemorrhagic, cardiogenic).

The constitutional symptoms may be mistaken for occult cancer, anorexia nervosa, or emotional stress. Acute adrenal insufficiency must be distinguished from an acute abdomen in which neutrophilia is the rule, whereas in adrenal insufficiency there is lymphocytosis and eosinophilia. The neurologic manifestations of Allgrove syndrome and adrenoleukodystrophy (especially in women) may mimic multiple sclerosis. Hyperkalemia can be caused by hyporeninemic hypoaldosteronism related to type IV renal tubular acidosis. Hyperkalemia is also seen with gastrointestinal bleeding, rhabdomyolysis, hyperkalemic paralysis, and some drugs (eg, angiotensin-converting enzyme [ACE] inhibitors, spironolactone, and drospirenone).

Hyponatremia is seen in many other conditions (eg, hypothyroidism, diuretic use, heart failure, cirrhosis, vomiting, diarrhea, severe illness, or major surgery) (Figure 21–1). Nearly 40% of critically ill patients have low serum cortisol levels due to low serum albumin levels, such that their total serum cortisol levels may be low but their serum free cortisol levels are normal.

► Complications

Any of the complications of the underlying disease (eg, tuberculosis) are more likely to occur in adrenal insufficiency, and intercurrent infections may precipitate an acute adrenal crisis. Associated autoimmune diseases are common (see above).

► Treatment

A. General Measures

Patients with adrenal insufficiency (and family members) must be thoroughly educated about adrenal insufficiency. Patients are advised to wear a medical alert bracelet or medal reading, "Adrenal insufficiency—takes hydrocortisone." They need to be provided with a dose escalation schedule for increased corticosteroids for illness, accidents, or prior to minor surgical procedures and for increased fludrocortisone for hot weather or prolonged strenuous exercise. Corticosteroids and fludrocortisone must be prescribed in liberal amounts with automatic refills to avoid the patient's running out of medication. It is also advisable to prescribe a routine antiemetic such as ondansetron ODT 8-mg tablets to be taken every 8 hours for nausea. Parenteral hydrocortisone (Solu-Cortef) 100 mg is also prescribed for patient self-injection in the event of vomiting. Patients must also receive advance instructions to seek medical attention at an emergency facility immediately in the event of vomiting or severe illness. All infections should be treated immediately and vigorously, with hydrocortisone administered at appropriately increased doses.

B. Specific Therapy

Replacement therapy should include corticosteroids with mineralocorticoids for primary adrenal insufficiency. In mild cases, corticosteroids alone may be adequate.

1. Corticosteroid replacement therapy—Maintenance therapy for most patients with Addison disease involves 15–30 mg of hydrocortisone orally daily in two or three divided doses (eg, 10 mg at 7 AM, 10 mg at 1 PM, and 5 mg at 7 PM). Some patients respond better to prednisone or methylprednisolone in doses of about 3–6 mg daily in divided doses. Adjustments in dosage are made according to the clinical response. The corticosteroid dose should be kept at the lowest level at which the patient feels clinically well.

Plenadren MR (5- or 20-mg modified-release tablets) is a once-daily dual-release preparation of hydrocortisone that may be administered in the morning (usual dose range is 20–30 mg daily). It is not available in the United States but is available in Canada and elsewhere.

A proper corticosteroid dose usually results in clinical improvement, a normal WBC count differential, and no manifestations of Cushing syndrome. Serum ACTH levels vary substantially and should not be used to determine dosing. *Increased corticosteroid dosing* is required in circumstances of infection, trauma, surgery, stressful diagnostic procedures, or other forms of stress. Rifampin use increases the clearance of hydrocortisone and necessitates increased dosing of hydrocortisone by up to 50%. During the third trimester of pregnancy, corticosteroid requirements are higher, so usual corticosteroid doses are increased by 50%. For severe stress of major illness, surgery, or delivery, a maximum stress dose of hydrocortisone is given as 50–100 mg intravenously or intramuscularly, followed by 50 mg every 6 hours. Lower doses, oral or parenteral, are used for less severe stress. For immunizations that are given with an adjuvant, such as varicella zoster (Shingrix), there is sufficient local inflammation that an increased dose of hydrocortisone is recommended for 4–5 days following the immunization. The dose is reduced back to normal as the stress subsides. *Decreased corticosteroid dosing* is required when medications are prescribed that inhibit corticosteroid metabolism by blocking the isoenzyme CYP34A, particularly the antifungals ketoconazole or itraconazole, the antidepressant nefazodone, anti-HIV protease inhibitors, and cobicistat.

2. Mineralocorticoid replacement therapy—**Fludrocortisone acetate** has a potent sodium-retaining effect. The dosage is 0.05–0.3 mg orally daily or every other day. In the presence of postural hypotension, hyponatremia, or hyperkalemia, the dosage is increased. Similarly, in patients with fatigue, an elevated PRA indicates the need for a higher replacement dose of fludrocortisone. If edema, hypokalemia, or hypertension ensues, the dose is decreased. During treatment with hydrocortisone with maximum doses appropriate for stress, fludrocortisone replacement is not required. Some patients cannot tolerate fludrocortisone and must substitute NaCl tablets to replace renal sodium loss.

DHEA is given to some women with adrenal insufficiency. In a double-blind clinical trial, women taking DHEA 50 mg orally each morning experienced an improved sense of well-being, increased muscle mass, and a reversal in bone loss at the femoral neck. DHEA replacement did not improve fatigue, cognitive problems, or sexual dysfunction; however, its placebo effect may be significant in that regard. Older women who receive

DHEA should be monitored for androgenic effects. Because over-the-counter preparations of DHEA have variable potencies, it is best to have the pharmacy formulate this with pharmaceutical-grade micronized DHEA.

3. Treatment of acute adrenal crisis—If acute adrenal crisis is suspected but the diagnosis of adrenal insufficiency is not yet established, blood is drawn for routine emergency laboratory tests and blood cultures, as well as serum cortisol and ACTH levels. Without waiting for the results, treatment is initiated *immediately* with hydrocortisone phosphate or hydrocortisone sodium succinate 100–300 mg intravenously along with saline solution. Thereafter, hydrocortisone is continued as intravenous infusions of 50–100 mg every 6 hours for the first day. The dosage may then be reduced according to the clinical picture and laboratory test results.

Since bacterial infection frequently precipitates acute adrenal crisis, broad-spectrum antibiotics should be administered empirically while waiting for the results of initial cultures (Table 30–5). The patient must also be treated for electrolyte abnormalities, hypoglycemia, and dehydration, as indicated.

When the patient is able to take food by mouth, hydrocortisone is administered orally in doses of 10–20 mg every 6 hours, and the dosage is reduced to maintenance levels as needed. Most patients ultimately require hydrocortisone twice daily (10–20 mg in the morning; 5–10 mg in the evening). Mineralocorticoid replacement is not needed when large amounts of hydrocortisone are being given, but as its dose is reduced, it is usually necessary to add fludrocortisone acetate, 0.05–0.2 mg orally daily. Some patients never require fludrocortisone or become edematous at doses of more than 0.05 mg once or twice weekly. Once the crisis has passed, the patient must be evaluated to assess the degree of permanent adrenal insufficiency and to establish the cause, if possible.

Prognosis

The life expectancy of patients with Addison disease is reasonably normal, as long as they are compliant with their medications and knowledgeable about their condition. However, one retrospective Swedish study of 1675 patients with Addison disease found an unexpected increase in all-cause mortality, mostly from cardiovascular disease, malignancy, and infection. Adrenal crisis can occur in patients who stop their medication or who experience stress such as infection, trauma, or surgery without appropriately higher doses of corticosteroids. Patients who take excessive doses of corticosteroid replacement can develop Cushing syndrome, which imposes its own risks.

Some patients feel residual fatigue, despite corticosteroid and mineralocorticoid replacement. This may be due, in part, to the inadequacy of oral replacement to duplicate cortisol's normal circadian rhythm. Also, patients with Addison disease are deficient in epinephrine, but replacement epinephrine is not available. Fatigue may also be an indication of suboptimal dosing of medication, electrolyte imbalance, or concurrent hypothyroidism or diabetes mellitus.

Rapid treatment is usually lifesaving in acute adrenal crisis. However, if adrenal crisis is unrecognized and untreated, shock that is unresponsive to fluid replacement and vasopressors can result in death.

Bensing S et al. Epidemiology, quality of life and complications of primary adrenal insufficiency: a review. Eur J Endocrinol. 2016 Sep;175(3):R107–16. [PMID: 27068688]

Bornstein SR et al. Diagnosis and treatment of primary adrenal insufficiency: an Endocrine Society clinical practice guideline. J Clin Endocrinol Metab. 2016 Feb;101(2):364–89. [PMID: 26760044]

Cadegiani FA et al. Adrenal fatigue does not exist: a systematic review. BMC Endocr Disord. 2016 Aug 24;16(1):48. Erratum in: BMC Endocr Disord. 2016 Nov 16;16(1):63. [PMID: 27557747]

Esposito D et al. Primary adrenal insufficiency: managing mineralocorticoid replacement therapy. J Clin Endocrinol Metab. 2018 Feb 1;103(2):376–87. [PMID: 29156052]

Hahner S. Acute adrenal crisis and mortality in adrenal insufficiency: still a concern in 2018! Ann Endocrinol (Paris). 2018 Jun;79(3):164–6. [PMID: 29716733]

Hellesen A et al. Autoimmune Addison's disease—an update on pathogenesis. Ann Endocrinol (Paris). 2018 Jun;79(3):157–63. [PMID: 29631795]

CUSHING SYNDROME (Hypercortisolism)

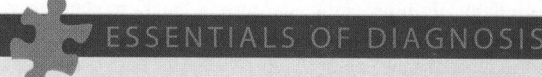

ESSENTIALS OF DIAGNOSIS

▸ Central obesity, muscle wasting, hirsutism, purple striae.

▸ Psychological changes.

▸ Osteoporosis, hypertension, poor wound healing.

▸ Hyperglycemia, leukocytosis, lymphocytopenia, hypokalemia.

▸ Elevated serum cortisol and urinary free cortisol. Lack of normal suppression by dexamethasone.

General Considerations

The term Cushing "syndrome" refers to the manifestations of excessive corticosteroids, commonly due to supraphysiologic doses of corticosteroid drugs and rarely due to spontaneous production of excessive cortisol by the adrenal cortex.

Cases of spontaneous Cushing syndrome are rare, with an incidence of 2.6 new cases yearly per million population in the United States. About 68% of cases are due to Cushing "disease," caused by a benign ACTH-secreting pituitary adenoma that is typically smaller than 5 mm and usually located in the anterior pituitary (94%); however, about 6% of such adenomas are ectopic in locations such as the cavernous sinus, sphenoid sinus, ethmoid sinus, or posterior pituitary. Cushing disease is at least three times more frequent in women than men.

About 7% of cases are due to nonpituitary ACTH-secreting neuroendocrine neoplasms that produce ectopic ACTH. Ectopic locations include the lungs (55%), pancreas (9%), mediastinum-thymus (8%), adrenal (6%), gastrointestinal tract (5%), thyroid (4%), and other sites (13%).

About 15% of cases are due to ACTH from a source that cannot be initially located.

About 25% of cases are due to excessive autonomous secretion of cortisol by the adrenals. Cortisol secretion is independent of ACTH and plasma ACTH levels are usually low or low-normal. Most such cases are due to a unilateral adrenal tumor. Benign adrenal adenomas are generally small and produce mostly cortisol; adrenocortical carcinomas are usually large when discovered and can produce excessive cortisol as well as androgens but may be nonsecretory. ACTH-independent macronodular adrenal hyperplasia can also produce hypercortisolism due to the adrenal cortex cells' abnormal stimulation by hormones such as catecholamines, arginine vasopressin, serotonin, hCG/LH, or gastric inhibitory polypeptide; in the latter case, hypercortisolism may be intermittent and food-dependent and plasma ACTH levels may not be completely suppressed.

▶ Clinical Findings

A. Symptoms and Signs

The manifestations of Cushing syndrome vary considerably. Early in the course of the disease, patients frequently complain of nonspecific symptoms, such as fatigue or reduced endurance but may have few, if any, of the physical stigmata described below. Central obesity with a plethoric "moon face," "buffalo hump," supraclavicular fat pads, protuberant abdomen, and thin extremities eventually develop in most patients with Cushing syndrome. Muscle atrophy causes weakness, with difficulty standing up from a seated position or climbing stairs. Patients may also experience backache, headache, hypertension, osteoporosis, avascular necrosis of bone, acne, superficial skin infections, and oligomenorrhea or amenorrhea in women or erectile dysfunction in men. Patients may have thirst and polyuria (with or without glycosuria), renal calculi, glaucoma, purple striae (especially around the thighs, breasts, and abdomen), and easy bruisability. Unusual bacterial or fungal infections are common. Wound healing is impaired. Mental symptoms may range from diminished ability to concentrate to increased lability of mood to frank psychosis. Patients are susceptible to opportunistic infections. Hyperpigmentation is common with ectopic ACTH-secreting neoplasms but not with pituitary Cushing disease.

Adrenal carcinomas usually have gross metastases by the time of diagnosis. Microscopic metastases are not visible by scanning but can be inferred from the presence of detectable cortisol levels following removal of the primary adrenal tumor in patients with a cortisol-secreting carcinoma and Cushing syndrome. The ENSAT staging system is used: stage 1 is a localized tumor 5 cm or smaller; stage 2 is a localized tumor larger than 5 cm; stage 3, tumor with local metastases; and stage 4, tumor with distant metastases.

B. Laboratory Findings

Glucose tolerance is impaired as a result of insulin resistance. Polyuria is present as a result of increased free water clearance; diabetes mellitus with glycosuria may worsen it. Patients with Cushing syndrome often have leukocytosis with relative granulocytosis and lymphopenia. Hypokalemia may be present, particularly in cases of ectopic ACTH secretion.

1. Diagnostic tests for hypercortisolism—Testing for hypercortisolism involves determining whether the following characteristics of Cushing syndrome are present: (1) lack of cortisol diurnal variation, (2) reduced suppressibility of cortisol by dexamethasone, (3) increased cortisol production rate, and (4) suppression of plasma ACTH by hypercortisolism from an adrenal nodule. Conflicting results are common.

Late-night (10–11 PM) salivary cortisol determinations are particularly useful, particularly for ACTH-dependent hypercortisolism. Late-night salivary cortisol levels are normally 150 ng/dL (4.0 nmol/L) or less. Late-night salivary cortisol levels that are consistently greater than 250 ng/dL (7.0 nmol/L) are considered very abnormal. The late-night salivary cortisol test has a relatively high sensitivity and specificity for Cushing syndrome.

The **overnight dexamethasone suppression test** is an easy screening test for hypercortisolism and is particularly sensitive for mild ACTH-independent hypercortisolism from an adrenal nodule. Dexamethasone 1 mg is given orally at 11 PM and serum is collected for cortisol determination at 8 AM the next morning; a cortisol level less than 1.8 mcg/dL (50 nmol/L, high-performance liquid chromatography [HPLC] assay) excludes Cushing syndrome with some certainty. However, 8% of established patients with pituitary Cushing disease have dexamethasone-suppressed cortisol levels less than 2 mcg/dL (55 nmol/L). Antiseizure drugs (eg, phenytoin, phenobarbital, primidone) and rifampin accelerate the metabolism of dexamethasone, causing a lack of cortisol suppression by dexamethasone. Estrogens—during pregnancy or as oral contraceptives or HRT—may also cause lack of dexamethasone suppressibility.

A **24-hour urinary free cortisol and creatinine** is usually used to confirm hypercortisolism in patients with a high late-night salivary cortisol or an abnormal dexamethasone suppression test. A high 24-hour urine free cortisol (greater than 50 mcg/day or 140 nmol/day in adults), or free cortisol to creatinine ratio of greater than 95 mcg cortisol/g creatinine, helps confirm hypercortisolism. However, many patients with mild hypercortisolism have a urinary free cortisol that is misleadingly within the reference range when measured by liquid chromatography-tandem mass spectrometry. A misleadingly high urine free cortisol excretion occurs with high fluid intake. In pregnancy, urine free cortisol is increased, while 17-hydroxycorticosteroids remain normal and diurnal variability of serum cortisol is normal. Carbamazepine and fenofibrate cause false elevations of urine free cortisol when determined by HPLC.

2. Diagnostic tests for the source of hypercortisolism— Once hypercortisolism is confirmed, a plasma ACTH and plasma DHEAS are obtained. A plasma ACTH below 6 pg/mL (1.3 pmol/L), with a low serum DHEAS, indicates a probable adrenal tumor, whereas higher levels are produced by pituitary or ectopic ACTH-secreting tumors. Certain ACTH assays suffer interference and report low-normal plasma ACTH levels in patients with

ACTH-independent hypercortisolism. Serum dehydroepi-androsterone sulfate (DHEAS) levels can be used as a proxy for ACTH, since DHEAS secretion is ACTH-dependent; levels below the reference range and particularly below 40 mcg/dL (1.1 mcmol/L) imply ACTH-independent hypercortisolism.

C. Imaging

In ACTH-independent Cushing syndrome, CT of the adrenals usually detects a mass lesion, which is most often an adrenal adenoma. Adrenocortical carcinomas can usually be distinguished from benign adrenal adenomas since they are generally larger (average 11 cm diameter) and many have metastases that are visible on preoperative scans.

In ACTH-dependent Cushing syndrome, MRI of the pituitary demonstrates a pituitary lesion in about 50% of cases. Premature cerebral atrophy is often noted. When the pituitary MRI is normal or shows a tiny (less than 5 mm diameter) irregularity that may be incidental, selective catheterization of the inferior petrosal sinus veins draining the pituitary is performed. ACTH levels in the inferior petrosal sinus that are more than twice the simultaneous peripheral venous ACTH levels are indicative of pituitary Cushing disease. Inferior petrosal sinus sampling is also done during ovine CRH (oCRH or Acthrel) administration, which ordinarily causes the ACTH levels in the inferior petrosal sinus to be over three times the peripheral ACTH level when the pituitary is the source of ACTH.

When inferior petrosal sinus ACTH concentrations are not above the requisite levels, a search for an ectopic source of ACTH is undertaken. Location of ectopic sources of ACTH begins with CT scanning of the chest and abdomen, with special attention to the lungs (for carcinoid or small cell carcinomas), the thymus, the pancreas, and the adrenals. In patients with ACTH-dependent Cushing syndrome, chest masses should not be assumed to be the source of ACTH, since opportunistic infections are common, so it is prudent to biopsy a chest mass to confirm the pathologic diagnosis prior to resection.

For Cushing syndrome due to ectopic ACTH, CT scanning fails to detect the source of ACTH in about 34% of cases. In such cases, the most sensitive (82%) scanning technique is whole-body imaging with ^{68}Ga-somatostatin receptor-PET/CT (^{68}Ga-DOTATOTATE-PET/CT). The next most sensitive (58%) scanning technique is whole-body imaging with ^{18}F-DOPA-PET/CT.

▶ Differential Diagnosis

Alcoholic patients can have hypercortisolism and many clinical manifestations of Cushing syndrome. Pregnant women have elevated serum ACTH levels, increased urine free cortisol, and high serum cortisol levels due to high serum levels of cortisol-binding globulin. Critically ill patients frequently have hypercortisolism, usually with suppression of serum ACTH. Depressed patients also have hypercortisolism that can be nearly impossible to distinguish biochemically from Cushing syndrome but without clinical signs of Cushing syndrome. Cushing syndrome can

be misdiagnosed as anorexia nervosa (and vice versa) owing to the muscle wasting and extraordinarily high urine free cortisol levels found in anorexia. Patients with severe obesity frequently have an abnormal dexamethasone suppression test, but the urine free cortisol is usually normal, as is diurnal variation of serum cortisol. Patients with familial cortisol resistance have hyperandrogenism, hypertension, and hypercortisolism without actual Cushing syndrome. Excessive ingestion of gamma-hydroxybutyric acid (GHB, sodium oxybate) can also induce ACTH-dependent Cushing syndrome that resolves after the drug is stopped.

Some adolescents develop violaceous striae on the abdomen, back, and breasts; these are known as "striae distensae" and are not indicative of Cushing syndrome. Patients receiving antiretroviral therapy for HIV-1 infection frequently develop partial lipodystrophy with thin extremities and central obesity with a dorsocervical fat pad ("buffalo hump") causing pseudo-Cushing syndrome. Patients with familial partial lipodystrophy type I develop central obesity and moon facies, along with thin extremities due to atrophy of subcutaneous fat. However, these patients' muscles are strong and may be hypertrophic, distinguishing this condition from Cushing syndrome.

▶ Treatment

Patients must receive treatment for cortisol-dependent comorbidities, including osteoporosis, psychiatric disorders, diabetes mellitus, hypertension, hypokalemia, muscle weakness, and infections. Bone densitometry is recommended for all patients and treatment is commenced for patients with osteoporosis.

A. Surgical Therapy

Pituitary Cushing disease is best treated with transsphenoidal selective resection of the pituitary adenoma. With an experienced pituitary neurosurgeon, remission rates range from 80% to 90%. Postoperative hyponatremia occurs frequently, so serum sodium should be monitored frequently for the first 2 weeks postoperatively. The patient should be screened for secondary hypothyroidism with a serum free T_4 within 1–2 weeks after surgery. After successful pituitary surgery, the rest of the pituitary usually returns to normal function; however, the pituitary corticotrophs remain suppressed and require 6–36 months to recover normal function. Therefore, patients receive empiric replacement-dose hydrocortisone postoperatively. Postoperative secondary adrenal insufficiency is a mark of successful pituitary surgery; screening may include a morning serum cortisol 8 hours following the prior evening dose of hydrocortisone. The cosyntropin test becomes abnormal by 2 weeks following successful pituitary surgery. Patients with secondary adrenal insufficiency and their families require patient education about the condition and must continue corticosteroid replacement until a cosyntropin stimulation test is normal. A pituitary MRI is obtained about 3 months postoperatively and repeated as indicated for clinical evidence of recurrent Cushing disease or Nelson syndrome, the progressive enlargement of ACTH-secreting pituitary tumors following bilateral adrenalectomy.

Cushing disease may persist after pituitary surgery, particularly when there has been cavernous sinus involvement. After apparent successful pituitary surgery, Cushing disease recurs in 16% after a mean of 38 months. Patients must have repeated evaluations for recurrent Cushing disease for years postoperatively. For patients with persistent or recurrent Cushing disease, repeat transsphenoidal pituitary surgery may be warranted if the recurrent tumor is visible and deemed resectable. Otherwise, bilateral laparoscopic adrenalectomy is usually the best treatment option, particularly for patients with very severe disease, since it renders an immediate remission in a condition with significant morbidity and mortality. Residual or recurrent ACTH-secreting pituitary tumors may also be treated with stereotactic radiosurgery, which normalizes urine free cortisol in 70% of patients within a mean of 17 months, compared with a 23% remission rate with conventional radiation therapy. Pituitary radiosurgery can also be used to treat Nelson syndrome.

Ectopic ACTH-secreting tumors should be surgically resected. If the tumor cannot be localized or is metastatic, laparoscopic bilateral adrenalectomy is usually recommended. Medical treatment with an oral combination of mitotane (3–5 g/24 h), ketoconazole (0.4–1.2 g/24 h), and metyrapone (3–4.5 g/24 h) often suppresses the hypercortisolism.

Metastatic ACTH-producing tumors that are visible with Octreoscan or ^{68}Ga-DOTATATE-PET imaging have somatostatin receptors. Such tumors may respond to therapy with somatostatin analogs; pasireotide LAR (60 mg intramuscularly every 28 days) or octreotide LAR (30–40 mg intramuscularly every 28 days) slows progression of the malignancy and reduces ACTH secretion in up to half such patients. Potassium-sparing diuretics are often helpful. Radionuclide therapy with several cycles of ^{177}Lu-DOTATATE has produced remissions in some patients.

Patients who are successfully surgically treated for Cushing syndrome typically develop "cortisol withdrawal syndrome," even when given replacement corticosteroids for adrenal insufficiency. Manifestations can include hypotension, nausea, fatigue, arthralgias, myalgias, pruritus, and flaking skin. Increasing the hydrocortisone replacement to 30 mg orally twice daily can improve these symptoms; the dosage is then reduced slowly as tolerated.

Benign adrenal adenomas may be resected laparoscopically if they are smaller than 6 cm in diameter; cure is achieved in most patients. However, most patients experience prolonged secondary adrenal insufficiency. Patients with bilateral adrenal macronodular hyperplasia usually require bilateral adrenalectomies and an evaluation for Carney complex that can be confirmed with a genetic evaluation for activating mutations in the gene *PRKAR1A* or genetic changes at chromosome 2p16.

Adrenocortical carcinomas are resected surgically. If the adrenocortical carcinoma was functional, postoperative secondary adrenal insufficiency is a good prognostic sign, with an increased chance that the tumor was completely resected without metastases; however, detectable postoperative cortisol levels predict metastases, even if no metastases are visible on scans. Patients with secretory adrenocortical carcinomas are usually treated with mitotane postoperatively, particularly if metastases are visible or cortisol is detectable postoperatively. Patients with nonsecretory metastatic adrenocortical carcinomas have also responded to mitotane. Mitotane is typically given for 2–5 years postoperatively. It is given orally with meals, beginning with 0.5 g twice daily, increasing to 1 g twice daily within 2 weeks, with subsequent increased doses every 2–3 weeks to reach serum levels of 14–20 mcg/mL. Unfortunately, only half the patients are able to reach these levels due to side effects. Mitotane can cause hypogonadism and can suppress TSH and cause hypothyroidism. Mitotane often causes primary adrenal insufficiency. Replacement hydrocortisone or prednisone should be started when mitotane doses reach 2 g daily. The replacement dose of oral hydrocortisone starts at 15 mg in the morning and 10 mg in the afternoon but must often be doubled or tripled because mitotane increases cortisol metabolism and cortisol binding globulin levels; the latter can artifactually raise serum cortisol levels. Combined chemotherapy with etoposide, doxorubicin, cisplatin, and mitotane (EDP-M) appears to be the most effective regimen for recurrent or metastatic adrenocortical carcinoma.

B. Medical Therapy

For patients with Cushing syndrome who decline surgery or for whom surgery has been unsuccessful, mineralocorticoid hypertension can be treated with spironolactone, eplerenone, and dihydropyridine calcium channel blockers. Women with hyperandrogenism may be treated with flutamide. Cabergoline, 0.5–3.5 mg orally twice weekly, reduced hypercortisolemia in 40% of patients with Cushing disease in one small study. Pasireotide, a multireceptor-targeting somatostatin analog, is a treatment option for refractory ACTH-secreting pituitary tumors causing Cushing disease or Nelson syndrome. Ketoconazole inhibits adrenal steroidogenesis and is another treatment option when given in doses of about 200 mg orally every 6 hours; however, it is marginally effective and can cause liver toxicity. Metyrapone can suppress hypercortisolism; required median oral daily doses are 1250–1500 mg/day in divided doses. It may be combined with ketoconazole. Metyrapone also may be used for patients with secretory adrenocortical carcinoma whose hypercortisolism is not fully controlled with mitotane.

► Prognosis

The manifestations of Cushing syndrome regress with time, but patients may have residual cognitive or psychiatric impairment, muscle weakness, osteoporosis, and sequelae from vertebral fractures. Continued impaired quality of life is more common in women compared to men. Younger patients have a better chance for full recovery.

Patients with Cushing syndrome from a benign adrenal adenoma experience a 5-year survival of 95% and a 10-year survival of 90%, following a successful adrenalectomy. Patients with Cushing disease from a pituitary adenoma experience a similar survival if their pituitary surgery is successful, which can be predicted if the postoperative nonsuppressed serum cortisol is less than 2 mcg/dL (55 nmol/L). Following successful treatment, overall mortality remains particularly higher for patients with older age at diagnosis, higher preoperative ACTH concentrations, and longer duration of hypercortisolism.

Patients who have a complete remission after transsphenoidal surgery have about a 15–20% chance of recurrence over the next 10 years. Patients with failed pituitary surgery may require pituitary radiation therapy, which has its own morbidity. Laparoscopic bilateral adrenalectomy may be required. Recurrence of hypercortisolism may occur as a result of growth of an adrenal remnant stimulated by high levels of ACTH. The prognosis for patients with ectopic ACTH-producing tumors depends on the aggressiveness and stage of the particular tumor. Patients with ACTH of unknown source have a 5-year survival rate of 65% and a 10-year survival rate of 55%.

In patients with adrenocortical carcinoma, 5-year survival rates of treated patients have correlated with the ENSAT stage. For stage 1, the 5-year survival was 81%; for stage 2, 61%; for stage 3, 50%; and for stage 4, 13%. In patients with stage 1 or 2 disease, long-term survival does occur. Improved survival has been associated with younger age, resection of the primary tumor, stage at diagnosis, and adjuvant treatment with mitotane.

▶ Complications

Following bilateral adrenalectomy for Cushing disease, a pituitary adenoma may enlarge progressively (Nelson syndrome), causing local destruction (eg, visual field impairment, cranial nerve palsy) and hyperpigmentation. Following successful therapy for Cushing syndrome, secondary adrenal insufficiency occurs and requires long-term corticosteroid replacement. Five years after successful surgery, secondary hypoadrenalism resolves in about 58% of patients with pituitary Cushing disease, 82% of those with ectopic ACTH, and only 38% of those who had an adrenal tumor.

▶ When to Refer

Dexamethasone suppression test is abnormal.

▶ When to Admit

- Transsphenoidal hypophysectomy.
- Adrenalectomy.
- Resection of ectopic ACTH-secreting tumor.

Findling JW et al. Diagnosis of endocrine disease: differentiation of pathologic/neoplastic hypercortisolism (Cushing's syndrome) from physiologic/non-neoplastic hypercortisolism (formerly known as pseudo-Cushing's syndrome). Eur J Endocrinol. 2017 May;176(5):R205–16. [PMID: 28179447]

Loriaux DL. Diagnosis and differential diagnosis of Cushing's Syndrome. N Engl J Med. 2017 Apr 13;376(15):1451–9. [PMID: 28402781]

Nieman LK et al. Treatment of Cushing's syndrome: an Endocrine Society clinical practice guideline. J Clin Endocrinol Metab. 2015 Aug;100(8):2807–31. [PMID: 26222757]

Pappachan JM et al. Cushing's syndrome: a practical approach to diagnosis and differential diagnoses. J Clin Pathol. 2017 Apr; 70(4):350–9. [PMID: 28069628]

Valassi E et al. Diagnostic tests for Cushing's syndrome differ from published guidelines: data from ERCUSYN. Eur J Endocrinol. 2017 May;176(5):613–24. [PMID: 28377460]

Wang S et al. Prognostic factors of adrenocortical carcinoma: an analysis of the Surveillance Epidemiology and End Results (SEER) database. Asian Pac J Cancer Prev. 2017 Oct;18(10): 2817–23. [PMID: 29072424]

PRIMARY ALDOSTERONISM

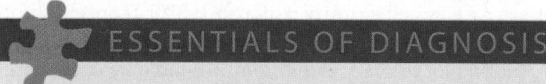

ESSENTIALS OF DIAGNOSIS

▶ Hypertension may be severe or drug-resistant.

▶ Hypokalemia (in minority of patients) may cause polyuria, polydipsia, muscle weakness.

▶ Low plasma renin; elevated plasma and urine aldosterone levels.

▶ General Considerations

Primary aldosteronism (hyperaldosteronism) refers to an inappropriately high aldosterone secretion that does not suppress adequately with sodium loading. Most affected patients have hypertension, although some may be normotensive. Primary aldosteronism is common and is believed to account about 8% of cases of stage 2 (mild) hypertension and about 13% of cases of stage 3 (moderate) hypertension. It should be suspected with early-onset hypertension or stroke before age 50 years (or both). It may be difficult to distinguish primary aldosteronism from cases of low renin essential hypertension, with which it may overlap. Patients of all ages may be affected, but the peak incidence is between 30 years and 60 years. Excessive aldosterone production increases sodium retention and suppresses plasma renin. It increases renal potassium excretion, which can lead to hypokalemia. Cardiovascular events are more prevalent in patients with aldosteronism (35%) than in those with essential hypertension (11%).

Primary aldosteronism may be caused by a unilateral aldosterone-producing adrenal cortical adenoma (Conn syndrome, 25%) that is more common in women with a 2:1 ratio, peaking between ages 30 and 50. However, primary aldosteronism is more commonly caused by adrenal cortical hyperplasia (75%) that is more common in men with a 4:1 ratio, peaking between ages 50 and 60. It is important to distinguish the two, since a unilateral aldosteronoma (Conn syndrome) may be cured by surgical resection, whereas patients with bilateral adrenal hyperplasia are treated medically.

▶ Clinical Findings

A. Symptoms and Signs

Primary aldosteronism is the most common cause of refractory hypertension in youths and middle-aged adults. Patients have hypertension that is typically moderate but may be severe. Some patients have only diastolic hypertension, without other symptoms and signs. Edema is rarely seen in primary aldosteronism. Hypokalemia can produce muscle weakness, paresthesias with frank tetany, headache, polyuria, and polydipsia.

B. Laboratory Findings

Plasma potassium should be determined in hypertensive individuals. However, hypokalemia, once thought to be the hallmark of hyperaldosteronism, is present in only 37% of affected patients: 50% of those with an aldosterone-producing adenoma and 17% of those with adrenal hyperplasia. An elevated serum bicarbonate (HCO_3) concentration indicates metabolic alkalosis and is commonly present.

Testing for primary aldosteronism should be done for all hypertensive patients with any of the following: (1) sustained hypertension above 150/100 mm Hg on 3 different days; (2) hypertension resistant to three conventional antihypertensive drugs, including a diuretic; (3) controlled blood pressure requiring four or more antihypertensive drugs; (4) hypokalemia, whether spontaneous or diuretic induced; (5) personal or family history of early-onset hypertension or cerebrovascular accident at age 40 or younger; (6) first-degree relative with primary aldosteronism; (7) presence of an adrenal mass; and (8) low PRA.

For at least 2 weeks prior to testing, patients should have any hypokalemia corrected and then consume a diet high in NaCl (more than 6 g/day) and ideally withhold certain medications: all diuretics, ACE inhibitors, ARBs (stimulate PRA); beta-blockers, clonidine, NSAIDs (suppress PRA); oral estrogens and oral contraceptives should also ideally be held. Medications that are allowed include slow-release verapamil, hydralazine, terazosin, and doxazosin.

For blood testing, the patient should be out of bed for at least 2 hours and seated for 15–60 minutes before the blood draw, which should preferably be obtained between 8 AM and 10 AM. The blood should be drawn slowly with a syringe and needle (rather than a vacutainer) at least 5 seconds after tourniquet release and without fist clenching. Plasma potassium, rather than the routine serum potassium, should be measured in cases of unexpected hyperkalemia, with the separation of plasma from cells within 30 minutes of collection. Plasma potassium levels must be normal, since hypokalemia suppresses aldosterone. For practical purposes, the same blood draw can be used for simultaneous assays for plasma potassium, serum aldosterone, and PRA or direct renin assay (DRA). Patients with primary aldosteronism have a suppressed PRA that is below or near 1.0 ng/mL/h or DRA less than 0.36 ng/mL. PRA of 1.0 ng/mL/h (12.8 pmol/L/min) is equivalent to a DRA of 5.2 ng/mL (8.2 milli-international units/L). Suppressed PRA or DRA with a serum aldosterone concentration greater than 15 ng/dL (416 pmol/L) indicates probable primary hyperaldosteronism. Serum aldosterone (ng/dL) to PRA (ng/mL/h) ratios less than 24 exclude primary aldosteronism; ratios between 24 and 30 are indeterminate; ratios between 30 and 67 are suspicious; a ratio above 64 helps confirm the diagnosis of primary aldosteronism. In patients with a suppressed PRA or DRA plus a serum aldosterone of 20 ng/day or higher, the diagnosis of primary

hyperaldosteronism is confirmed. To further confirm the diagnosis and for patients with a suppressed PRA or DRA but lower serum aldosterone levels, a 24-hour urine is collected in an acidified container for aldosterone, cortisol, and creatinine; urine aldosterone greater than 12 mcg/24 h (33 nmol/24 h) confirms primary aldosteronism with 93% specificity.

Genetic testing is recommended for patients with confirmed primary aldosteronism by age 20 years and those with a family history of primary aldosteronism or stroke at young age (under age 40). The testing is for familial corticosteroid remediable aldosteronism.

C. Imaging

Some patients with undiagnosed primary aldosteronism are incidentally found to have an adrenal nodule (incidentaloma) during abdominal or chest imaging. All patients with biochemically confirmed primary aldosteronism require a thin-section CT scan of the adrenals to screen for a rare adrenal carcinoma. In the absence of a large adrenal carcinoma, adrenal CT scanning cannot reliably distinguish unilateral from bilateral aldosterone excess, having both a sensitivity and specificity of 78% for unilateral aldosteronism. Therefore, the decision to perform a unilateral adrenalectomy should not be based solely on the adrenal CT scan. Adrenal vein sampling is often required.

D. Adrenal Vein Sampling

Unfortunately, bilateral selective adrenal vein sampling is invasive, expensive, not widely available, and often unsuccessful. The procedure (and surgery) may not be required for patients whose blood pressure is well controlled with spironolactone or eplerenone and for those with familial hyperaldosteronism. It is indicated only if surgery is contemplated in order to direct the surgeon to the correct adrenal gland. Adrenal vein sampling is probably not required in patients who have a classic adrenal adenoma (Conn syndrome), which is characterized by spontaneous hypokalemia and a unilateral adrenal adenoma 10 mm or larger in diameter on CT.

Before this procedure, the patient must be properly prepared (see Laboratory Findings). However, patients with a persistently suppressed PRA may continue mineralocorticoid blockade. Lateralization is present when the aldosterone:cortisol ratio from one adrenal vein is at least four times that from the opposite adrenal vein.

Aldosterone hypersecretion that is lateralized to one adrenal usually indicates that adrenal has a unilateral aldosteronoma or hyperplasia, particularly when aldosterone secretion from the contralateral adrenal is suppressed, in which case unilateral surgery improves hypertension in 96%. Adrenal vein sampling has a sensitivity of 95% and a specificity of 100% but only when performed by an experienced radiologist. This procedure entails a 0.6% risk of major complications.

▶ Differential Diagnosis

The differential diagnosis of primary aldosteronism includes other causes of hypokalemia (see Chapter 21) in patients with essential hypertension, especially diuretic therapy; chronic depletion of intravascular volume stimulates renin secretion and secondary hyperaldosteronism.

Real (black) licorice (derived from anise) or anise-flavored drinks (sambuca, pastis) contain glycyrrhizinic acid, which has a metabolite that inhibits the enzyme that normally inactivates cortisol in the renal tubule. Oral contraceptives may increase aldosterone secretion in some patients. Renal vascular disease can cause severe hypertension with hypokalemia but PRA is high. Excessive adrenal secretion of other corticosteroids (besides aldosterone), certain congenital adrenal enzyme disorders, and primary cortisol resistance may also cause hypertension with hypokalemia. The differential diagnosis also includes Liddle syndrome, an autosomal dominant cause of hypertension and hypokalemia resulting from excessive sodium absorption from the renal tubule; renin and aldosterone levels are low.

Complications

Cardiovascular complications occur more frequently in primary aldosteronism than in idiopathic hypertension. Following unilateral adrenalectomy for Conn syndrome, suppression of the contralateral adrenal may result in temporary postoperative hypoaldosteronism, characterized by hyperkalemia and hypotension.

Treatment

The **unilateral adrenal adenoma** of Conn syndrome is usually treated by laparoscopic adrenalectomy. During pregnancy, such surgery is best performed during the second trimester. However, long-term medical therapy is an option for unilateral hyperaldosteronism, if adequate blood pressure control can be maintained.

Bilateral adrenal hyperplasia is best treated with medical therapy. Medical treatment must include a potassium-sparing diuretic, particularly spironolactone, eplerenone, or amiloride. Spironolactone is the most effective drug but also has antiandrogen activity and men frequently experience breast tenderness, gynecomastia, or reduced libido; it is given at initial doses of 12.5–25 mg orally once daily; the dose may be titrated upward to 200 mg daily. Spironolactone might lead to undervirilization of male infants and is contraindicated in pregnancy; reproductive-age women are cautioned to use contraception during therapy. Eplerenone is favored during pregnancy (FDA pregnancy category B) and for men, since it does not have antiandrogen effects; it must be taken orally in doses of 25–50 mg twice daily. Blood pressure must be monitored daily when beginning these anti-mineralocorticoid medications; significant drops in blood pressure have occurred when these drugs are added to other antihypertensives. Other antihypertensive drugs may be required, particularly amlodipine, and ACE inhibitors or ARBs. Corticosteroid-remediable aldosteronism is very rare, but may respond well to suppression with low-dose corticosteroids.

Prognosis

The hypertension is reversible in about two-thirds of cases but persists or returns despite surgery in the remainder.

The prognosis is much improved by early diagnosis and treatment. Only 2% of aldosterone-secreting adrenal tumors are malignant.

Funder JW et al. The management of primary aldosteronism: case detection, diagnosis, and treatment: an Endocrine Society clinical practice guideline. J Clin Endocrinol Metab. 2016 May;101(5):1889–916. [PMID: 26934393]

Kline G et al. Adrenal venous sampling for primary aldosteronism: laboratory medicine best practice. J Clin Pathol. 2017 Nov; 70(11):911–6. [PMID: 28893861]

Velema M et al; SPARTACUS investigators. Quality of life in primary aldosteronism: a comparative effectiveness study of adrenalectomy and medical treatment. J Clin Endocrinol Metab. 2018 Jan 1;103(1):16–24. [PMID: 29099925]

Vilela LAP et al. Diagnosis and management of primary aldosteronism. Arch Endocrinol Metab. 2017 May–Jun;61(3):305–12. [PMID: 28699986]

Williams TA et al. Management of endocrine disease: diagnosis and management of primary aldosteronism: the Endocrine Society guideline 2016 revisited. Eur J Endocrinol. 2018 Jul; 179(1):R19–29. [PMID: 29674485]

PHEOCHROMOCYTOMA & PARAGANGLIOMA

ESSENTIALS OF DIAGNOSIS

▶ "Attacks" of headache, perspiration, palpitations, anxiety. Multisystem crisis.

▶ **Hypertension:** sustained but often paroxysmal, especially during surgery or delivery; may be orthostatic.

▶ Elevated plasma free metanephrines. Normal serum T_4 and TSH.

General Considerations

Both pheochromocytomas and non–head-neck paragangliomas are rare tumors of the sympathetic nervous system. Pheochromocytomas arise from the adrenal medulla and usually secrete both epinephrine and norepinephrine. Paragangliomas ("extra-adrenal pheochromocytomas") arise from sympathetic paraganglia and often metastasize. About 50% of paragangliomas secrete norepinephrine; the rest are nonfunctional or secrete only dopamine, normetanephrine, or serum chromogranin A (CgA). Tumoral secretion of norepinephrine or neuropeptide Y cause hypertension. Excessive epinephrine causes tachyarrhythmias. These tumors may be located in either or both adrenals or anywhere along the sympathetic nervous chain, and sometimes in the mediastinum, heart, or bladder.

These tumors are particularly dangerous and deceptive and cause death in at least one-third of patients prior to diagnosis. They account for less than 0.4% of hypertension cases. The incidence is higher in children and patients with moderate to severe hypertension, particularly in the presence of suspicious symptoms of headache, significant palpitations, or diaphoretic episodes. Over 10% of cases are discovered incidentally on imaging studies. They account for about 4% of adrenal incidentalomas. The yearly incidence is 2 to 4 new cases per million. However, many cases are undiagnosed during life, since the prevalence of pheochromocytomas and paragangliomas in autopsy series is 1 in 2000.

Nonsecretory paragangliomas arise in the head or neck, particularly in the carotid body, jugular-tympanic region, or vagal body; only about 4% secrete catecholamines. They often arise in patients who have *SDHD*, *SDHC*, or *SDHB* germline mutations.

About 35% of patients with pheochromocytomas or paragangliomas harbor a germline mutation in 1 of at least 16 known susceptibility genes that predispose to the tumor, usually in an autosomal dominant manner with incomplete penetrance. Thorough genetic testing is recommended for all patients with these tumors.

Pheochromocytoma eventually develops in about 30% of patients with **von Hippel–Lindau (VHL) disease type 2;** it can present as early as age 5 years or later in adulthood. Pheochromocytomas in patients with VHL are usually adrenal, less likely to be malignant (3.5%), and more likely to be bilateral. About 25% of patients with VHL-1–related pheochromocytomas are asymptomatic and normotensive at diagnosis. The condition is also associated with hemangiomas of the retina, cerebellum, brainstem, and spinal cord; hyperparathyroidism; pancreatic cysts; endolymphatic sac tumors; cystadenomas of the adnexa or epididymis; pancreatic neuroendocrine tumors; and renal cysts, adenomas, and carcinomas; inheritance is autosomal dominant.

MEN 2 (MEN 2A) is associated with pheochromocytomas, hyperparathyroidism, cutaneous lichen amyloidosis, and medullary thyroid carcinoma. Pheochromocytomas are often silent in MEN 2; at diagnosis, only about 50% have symptoms and fewer are hypertensive. The lack of symptoms may be due to earlier diagnosis through yearly screening of mutation carriers. **MEN 3 (MEN 2B)** may be familial, but usually arises from a de novo *ret* mutation; MEN 3 is associated with pheochromocytoma (50%), aggressive medullary thyroid carcinoma, mucosal neuromas, and Marfan-like habitus.

von Recklinghausen neurofibromatosis type 1 (NF-1) is associated with an increased risk of pheochromocytomas/paragangliomas as well as cutaneous neurofibromas, optic and brainstem gliomas, astrocytomas, vascular anomalies, hamartomas, malignant nerve sheath tumors, and smooth-bordered café au lait spots.

Familial paraganglioma can be caused by mutations in the genes encoding succinate dehydrogenase (SDH) subunits A, B, C, or D. Patients with such germline mutations are more apt to have bilateral pheochromocytomas or multicentric paragangliomas; they are also prone to pulmonary chondromas and gastric stromal sarcomas.

Pheochromocytomas are also more common in patients with Carney triad, Beckwith-Wiedemann syndrome, Sturge-Weber syndrome, and tuberous sclerosis.

► Clinical Findings

A. Symptoms and Signs

Pheochromocytomas can be lethal unless they are diagnosed and treated appropriately. Catastrophic hypertensive crisis and fatal cardiac arrhythmias can occur spontaneously or may be triggered by needle biopsy or manipulation of the mass, intravenous contrast dye or glucagon injection, vaginal delivery, trauma, anesthesia, or surgery (both unrelated to the tumor or for its removal). Exercise, bending, lifting, or emotional stress can trigger paroxysms. Bladder paragangliomas may present with paroxysms during micturition. Certain drugs can precipitate attacks: decongestants, amphetamines, cocaine, epinephrine, corticosteroids, fluoxetine and other selective serotonin reuptake inhibitors (SSRIs), metoclopramide, monoamine oxidase (MAO) inhibitors, caffeine, nicotine, and ionic intravenous contrast.

Manifestations are variable, but typically include hypertension (81%) that may be paroxysmal or sustained, headache (60%), palpitations (60%), or diaphoresis (52%). About 58% of patients have episodic nonspecific "spells." Other symptoms include anxiety (often with a sense of impending doom), weakness/fatigue, dyspnea, nausea/vomiting, tremor, dizziness, chest pain, abdominal pain, paresthesias, or constipation. Vasospasm during an attack can cause Raynaud syndrome, mottled cyanosis, or facial pallor. As the attack subsides, facial flushing and drenching sweats can occur. Epinephrine secretion by an adrenal pheochromocytoma can cause episodic tachyarrhythmias and sometimes orthostatic hypotension or even syncope. Cardiac manifestations include acute coronary syndrome, cardiomyopathy, heart failure, and potentially fatal dysrhythmias. Catecholamine-induced cardiomyopathy can present with shock. Confusion, psychosis, paresthesias, seizures, transient ischemic attacks, or stroke may occur with cerebrovascular vasoconstriction or hemorrhagic stroke. Aneurysms may dissect. Abdominal pain, nausea, vomiting, and even ischemic bowel can occur. Patients may experience increased appetite, loss of weight, numbness, or fevers. During pregnancy, pheochromocytomas can produce hypertension and proteinuria, mimicking eclampsia; vaginal delivery can produce hypertensive crisis followed by postpartum shock. A minority of patients are normotensive and asymptomatic, particularly when the tumor is nonsecretory or discovered at an early stage.

Pheochromocytomas can also rarely produce other "ectopic" peptide hormones, resulting in Cushing syndrome (ACTH), Verner-Morrison syndrome (VIP), or hypercalcemia (PTHrP). **Multisystem crisis** can occur, with manifestations of severe hypertension or hypotension, acute respiratory distress syndrome (ARDS), cardiomyopathy with acute heart failure, kidney dysfunction, liver failure, and death. Multisystem crisis can occur spontaneously, or it may be provoked by surgery, vaginal delivery, or treatment of metastatic disease.

B. Laboratory Findings

Pheochromocytomas are rare tumors, but they are deadly, and a missed diagnosis can be catastrophic. However, less than 1% of biochemical evaluations in patients with suspicious symptoms lead to a diagnosis of pheochromocytoma. More commonly, testing yields misleading minor elevations in tumor markers, particularly when levels are less than three times the upper limit of normal (Table 26–11).

Plasma fractionated free metanephrines is the most sensitive test for secretory pheochromocytomas and paragangliomas. However, plasma levels of free metanephrines

Table 26–11. Factors that can cause misleading catecholamine or metanephrine results.[1]

Drugs	Foods	Conditions
Acetaminophen[2]	Bananas[3]	Age (children and older adults)[4]
Aldomet[2]	Caffeine[3]	
Amphetamines[3]	Coffee[2]	Alcoholism
Anesthetics (local)[4]	Curry leaves[2]	Amyotrophic lateral sclerosis[3]
Bronchodilators[3]	Peppers[2]	
Buspirone[2]	Pineapples[3]	Anxiety[3,4]
Captopril[2]	Walnuts[3]	Brain lesions[3]
Cimetidine[2]		Carcinoid[3]
Cocaine[3]		Drug withdrawal (narcotic, alcohol, clonidine)[3,4]
Codeine[2]		
Contrast media (meglumine acetrizoate, meglumine diatrizoate)[5]		Eclampsia[3]
		Emotion (severe)[3,4]
Cyclobenzaprine		Essential hypertension[3]
Decongestants[3]		
Ephedrine and epinephrine[3]		Exercise (vigorous)[3,4]
		Guillain-Barré syndrome[3]
Fenfluramine[6]		
Halothane anesthesia[4]		Hypoglycemia[3]
Isoproterenol[3]		Kidney dysfunction[3,4,6]
Labetalol[2,3]		
Levodopa[2]		Lead poisoning[3]
Mandelamine[2]		Myocardial infarction (acute)[3]
Methenamine[6]		
Mesalamine[2]		Pain (severe)[3]
Metoclopramide[2]		Porphyria (acute)[3]
Monoamine oxidase inhibitors[4]		Psychosis (acute)[3]
		Quadriplegia
Nitroglycerin[3]		Sleep apnea[3,4]
Phenothiazines[3,4]		Winter[4]
Phenoxybenzamine[2,3]		
Serotonin-norepinephrine reuptake inhibitors (SNRIs): desvenlafaxine, duloxetine, levomilnacipran, venlafaxine,[3]		
Smoking[4]		
Sulfasalazine[2]		
Tricyclic antidepressants[2,3]		

[1]Note that assays for metanephrine using tandem mass spectroscopy (MS/MS) are not prone to interference from drugs or foods, except those that increase catecholamine excretion.
[2]May cause confounding peaks for catecholamines or metanephrines with an HPLC-ECD chromatogram.
[3]Increases measured catecholamine excretion.
[4]Increases plasma and urinary normetanephrine and metanephrine.
[5]May decrease urine metanephrine excretion.
[6]Decreases measured catecholamine excretion.

fluctuate and are lower when the patient is supine than when ambulatory. For practicality, the blood specimen is usually obtained after the patient sits quietly in the laboratory for at least 15 minutes. The test is 97% sensitive, so normal levels rule out pheochromocytoma and paraganglioma with some certainty. The exceptions are patients who are being monitored because they harbor a germline mutation for familial pheochromocytoma; such patients with a pheochromocytoma are often asymptomatic early-on and frequently have normal testing or only mild elevations in plasma metanephrines. However, for other patients with severe hypertension or "spells" caused by a pheochromocytoma, plasma fractionated free metanephrines are ordinarily at least three times the upper limit of normal. For less dramatic elevations in plasma metanephrines, patients are retested while lying supine in a quiet room for 30–90 minutes before the blood is drawn. False-positive test results should be particularly suspected when the ratio of normetanephrine to norepinephrine is less than 0.52 or the ratio of metanephrine to epinephrine is less than 4.2. In such cases, it is best to repeat biochemical testing under optimal conditions, eg, after eliminating potentially interfering drugs. Most patients with elevated plasma fractionated free metanephrines require confirmation with a 24-hour urine for fractionated metanephrines and creatinine.

Urinary fractionated metanephrines and creatinine effectively confirms most pheochromocytomas that were detected by elevated plasma fractionated free metanephrines. A 24-hour urine specimen is usually obtained, although an overnight or shorter collection may be used; patients with pheochromocytomas generally have more than 2.2 mcg of total metanephrine per milligram of creatinine, and more than 135 mcg total catecholamines per gram creatinine. Urinary assay for total metanephrines is about 97% sensitive for detecting functioning pheochromocytomas.

Plasma fractionated catecholamines may be helpful to confirm whether an adrenal tumor is a secretory pheochromocytoma. The test may also be useful for normotensive patients with a paraganglioma; the tumor may secrete only dopamine, which can be followed as a tumor marker.

Serum CgA is elevated in about 85% of patients with pheochromocytoma or paraganglioma and the levels correlate with tumor size, being higher in patients with metastatic disease. Serum CgA must be assayed in the fasting state, since levels rise after meals. Misleading elevated CgA levels also occur in patients with azotemia or hypergastrinemia, and in those treated with corticosteroids or proton pump inhibitors. Serum CgA is not specific for pheochromocytoma, so its measurement is not very useful for the initial diagnosis.

Clonidine suppression testing can help distinguish whether elevated plasma free normetanephrine levels are physiologic or indicative of pheochromocytoma. Plasma fractionated free metanephrines are measured before the administration of clonidine (0.3 mg orally) and 3 hours afterward. A fall of plasma normetanephrine into the normal range or a fall of greater than 40% from baseline helps rule out the presence of a tumor.

Hyperglycemia is present in about 35% of patients but is usually mild. Proteinuria is present in about 10–20% of patients. Leukocytosis is common. Erythrocytosis or eosinophilia can occur. The ESR is sometimes elevated. PRA may be increased by catecholamines.

C. Imaging

1. CT and MRI scanning—When an adrenal pheochromocytoma is suspected, a noncontrast CT scan of the abdomen is performed, with thin sections through the adrenals. If an adrenal mass is present, another CT is immediately performed, infusing nonionic contrast with a "washout" protocol. Pheochromocytomas are usually avid for contrast and about 80% of tumors retain greater than 40% of contrast after 15 minutes. Glucagon should not be used during scanning, since it can provoke hypertensive crisis.

MRI scanning has the advantage of not requiring intravenous contrast dye; its lack of radiation makes it the imaging of choice during pregnancy and childhood and for serial imaging. Both CT and MRI scanning have a sensitivity of about 90% for adrenal pheochromocytoma and a sensitivity of 95% for adrenal tumors over 0.5 cm in diameter. However, both CT and MRI are less sensitive for detecting recurrent tumors, metastases, and extra-adrenal paragangliomas. If no adrenal tumor is found, the scan is extended to include the entire abdomen, pelvis, and chest.

2. Nuclear imaging—No single nuclear imaging modality is 100% sensitive for pheochromocytoma or paraganglioma. Positron emission tomography (PET) imaging gives crisper imaging than scintigraphy. Nuclear imaging is usually combined with volumetric imaging (CT or MRI) to determine the precise size and location of tumors. ^{68}Ga-**DOTATOC-PET** scanning is the most sensitive scan, detecting about 90% of pheochromocytomas, paragangliomas, and metastases. However, it is not entirely specific for these tumors.

^{18}FDG-PET scanning detects about 54% of metastases but is more sensitive for patients with *SDHB* germline mutations. However, ^{18}FDG-PET scanning is not specific for pheochromocytoma or paraganglioma.

^{123}I-MIBG whole-body scintigraphy can lateralize and confirm adrenal pheochromocytomas with a sensitivity of over 90%, but is only about 67% sensitive for extra-adrenal (paraganglioma) tumors and metastases and is also less sensitive for MEN 2– or MEN 3–related pheochromocytomas. ^{123}I-MIBG scintigraphy is also less sensitive for particularly aggressive tumors. Prior to the scan, the patient is given KI to competitively inhibit the uptake of free ^{123}I into the thyroid. Also, drugs that reduce ^{123}I-MIBG uptake should be avoided: tricyclic antidepressants and cyclobenzaprine (6 weeks); and amphetamines, decongestants, cocaine, phenothiazines, haloperidol, labetalol, and serotonin and norepinephrine reuptake inhibitors (2 weeks). Drug interference is suspected in negative ^{123}I-MIBG scans that do not show normal uptake in salivary glands.

▶ Differential Diagnosis

Certain conditions mimic pheochromocytoma: thyrotoxicosis, labile essential hypertension, myocarditis, glomerulonephritis or other renal lesions, eclampsia, acute intermittent porphyria, hypogonadal vascular instability (hot flushes),

anxiety attacks, cocaine or amphetamine use, and clonidine withdrawal. Patients taking nonselective MAO inhibitor antidepressants can have hypertensive crisis after eating foods that contain tyramine. Patients with erythromelalgia can have hypertensive crises. Renal artery stenosis can cause severe hypertension and may coexist with pheochromocytoma. Plasma fractionated free metanephrines can be elevated in sleep apnea or with stressful illness. On CT scan, adrenal pheochromocytomas must be distinguished from adrenal adenomas and other masses. ^{123}I-MIBG scintigraphy uptake in the adrenal glands can be physiologic uptake and can sometimes occur in benign adrenal adenomas.

▶ Complications

All of the complications of severe hypertension may be encountered. In addition, a catecholamine-induced cardiomyopathy may develop. Severe heart failure and cardiovascular collapse may develop in patients during a paroxysm. Sudden death may occur due to cardiac arrhythmia. ARDS and multisystem crisis can occur acutely and thus the initial manifestation of pheochromocytoma may be hypotension or even shock. Hypertensive crises with sudden blindness or cerebrovascular accidents are not uncommon.

After removal of the tumor, a state of severe hypotension and shock (resistant to epinephrine and norepinephrine) may ensue with precipitation of acute kidney injury or myocardial infarction. Hypotension and shock may occur from spontaneous infarction or hemorrhage of the tumor.

Pheochromocytomas and paragangliomas may metastasize. Cells can also be seeded within the peritoneum, either spontaneously or as a complication during surgical resection. Such seeding of the abdomen can result in multifocal recurrent intra-abdominal tumors, a condition known as pheochromocytomatosis.

▶ Medical Treatment

Patients must receive adequate treatment for hypertension and tachyarrhythmias prior to surgery for pheochromocytoma/paraganglioma. Patients are advised to measure their blood pressures daily and immediately during paroxysms. Some patients with pheochromocytoma or paraganglioma are not hypertensive and do not require preoperative antihypertensive management. Alpha-blockers or calcium channel blockers can be used, either alone or in combination. Blood pressure should be controlled before cardioselective beta-blockers are added for control of tachyarrhythmias. Normotensive patients with pheochromocytoma or sympathetic paraganglioma do not require preoperative alpha blockade, which increases their requirement for vasopressors and colloid after the tumor resection.

Alpha-blockers are typically administered in preparation for surgery. Phenoxybenzamine is a long-acting nonselective alpha-blocker with a half-life of 24 hours; it is given initially in a dosage of 10 mg orally every 12 hours, increasing gradually by about 10 mg/day about every 3 days until hypertension is controlled. Maintenance doses range from 10 mg/day to 120 mg/day. Doxazosin (half-life 22 hours), a selective alpha-1-blocker, may also be used in doses of 2–32 mg daily. Preoperative preparation with phenoxybenzamine reduces intraoperative hypertension but may increase the post-resection risk of hypotension compared to patients given a preoperative selective alpha-1-blocker. Optimal alpha-blockade is achieved when supine arterial pressure is below 140/90 mm Hg or as low as possible for the patient to have a standing arterial pressure above 80/45 mm Hg.

Calcium channel blockers (nifedipine ER or nicardipine ER) are very effective and are usually added to alpha-blockers, but may be used alone. Nifedipine ER is initially given orally at a dose of 30 mg/day, increasing the dose gradually to a maximum of 60 mg twice daily. Calcium channel blockers are superior to phenoxybenzamine for long-term use, since they cause less fatigue, nasal congestion, and orthostatic hypotension. However, they should not be used for patients with severe heart failure. For acute hypertensive crisis (systolic blood pressure higher than 170 mm Hg) a nifedipine 10-mg capsule may be chewed and swallowed. Nifedipine is quite successful for treating acute hypertension in patients with pheochromocytoma/paraganglioma, even at home; it is reasonably safe as long as the blood pressure is carefully monitored.

Beta-blockers (eg, metoprolol XL) are often required after institution of alpha-blockade or calcium channel blockade. The use of a beta-blocker as initial antihypertensive therapy has resulted in an "unopposed alpha" status that causes paradoxical worsening of hypertension. Labetalol has combined alpha- and beta-blocking activity and is an effective agent, but can cause paradoxical hypertension if used as the initial antihypertensive agent. Labetalol can also interfere with catecholamine determinations in some laboratories and reduces the tumor's uptake of radioisotopes, such that it must be discontinued for at least 4–7 days before ^{123}I-MIBG or ^{18}FDG-PET scanning or therapy with high-dose ^{131}I-MIBG.

Surgical Treatment

Surgical removal of pheochromocytomas or abdominal paragangliomas is the treatment of choice. For surgery, a team approach—endocrinologist, anesthesiologist, and surgeon—is critically important. Laparoscopic surgery is preferred, but large and invasive tumors require open laparotomy. Patients with small familial or bilateral pheochromocytomas may undergo selective resection of the tumors, sparing the adrenal cortex; however, there is a recurrence rate of 10% over 10 years.

Prior to surgery, blood pressure control should be maintained for a minimum of 4–7 days or until optimal cardiac status is established. The ECG should be monitored until it becomes stable. (It may take a week or even months to correct ECG changes in patients with catecholamine myocarditis, and it may be prudent to defer surgery until then in such cases.) Patients must be very closely monitored during surgery to promptly detect sudden changes in blood pressure or cardiac arrhythmias.

Intraoperative severe hypertension is managed with continuous intravenous nicardipine (a short-acting calcium channel blocker), 2–6 mcg/kg/min, or nitroprusside, 0.5–10 mcg/kg/min. Prolonged nitroprusside administration can cause cyanide toxicity. Tachyarrhythmia is treated with intravenous atenolol (1 mg boluses), esmolol, or lidocaine.

Autotransfusion of 1–2 units of blood at 12 hours preoperatively plus generous intraoperative volume replacement reduces the risk of postresection hypotension and shock caused by desensitization of the vascular alpha-1-receptors. Shock is treated with intravenous saline or colloid and high doses of intravenous norepinephrine. Intravenous 5% dextrose is infused postoperatively to prevent hypoglycemia.

Detecting & Managing Metastatic Pheochromocytoma & Paraganglioma

Surgical histopathology for pheochromocytoma and paraganglioma cannot reliably determine whether a tumor is malignant. Only the presence of metastases defines malignancy. Therefore, all pheochromocytomas and paragangliomas must be approached as possibly malignant. It is essential to recheck blood pressure and plasma fractionated metanephrine levels about 4–6 weeks postoperatively, at least every 6 months for 5 years, then once yearly for life and immediately if hypertension, suspicious symptoms, or metastases become evident.

Metastases from a pheochromocytoma or paraganglioma are visible in only about 35% when the primary tumor is discovered. The other 65% of metastases emerge clinically an average of 5.5 years (range 0.3 and 53 years) after the initial diagnosis. Since some metastases are indolent, it is important to tailor treatment to each individual according to their tumor's aggressiveness. Most surgeons resect the main tumor and larger metastases (debulking). Asymptomatic, indolent metastases may be kept under close surveillance without treatment.

A. Chemotherapy

Various chemotherapy regimens have been used, but there have been no controlled clinical trials to prove the effectiveness of one regimen over another or whether any regimen actually improves overall survival. The most common chemotherapy regimen combines intravenous cyclophosphamide, vincristine, and dacarbazine over 2 days in cycles that are repeated every 3 weeks (Table 39–3). About one-third of patients experience some degree of temporary remission. Sunitinib, a tyrosine kinase inhibitor, can also produce remissions, given orally in doses of 50 mg/day for 4 weeks on and then 2 weeks off; alternatively, a dose of 37.5 mg/day can be given continuously. Another chemotherapy regimen uses temozolomide, 250 mg/day orally for 5 days, repeating the cycle every 28 days; this is usually the best-tolerated chemotherapy and is particularly effective for metastatic pheochromocytoma or paraganglioma in patients with *SDHB* germline mutations. Each chemotherapy regimen has toxicities.

Metyrosine reduces catecholamine synthesis but does not impede the progressive growth of metastases; the initial metyrosine dosage is 250 mg four times daily, increased daily by increments of 250–500 mg to a maximum of 4 g/day. Metyrosine causes CNS side effects and crystalluria; hydration must be ensured.

B. Targeted Radioisotope Therapy

1. ^{131}I-MIBG—About 60% of patients with metastatic pheochromocytoma or paraganglioma have tumors with sufficient uptake of ^{123}I-MIBG on diagnostic scanning to allow for therapy with high-activity ^{131}I-MIBG. Azedra ([131]Idobenguanine) is a no-carrier-added formulation that is FDA-approved for treating patients with metastatic pheochromocytoma or paraganglioma. Medications that reduce MIBG uptake must be avoided, particularly labetalol, phenothiazines, tricyclics, and sympathomimetics. Myelodysplastic syndrome and leukemia can develop several years after ^{131}I-MIBG therapy, with the risk proportional to the cumulative amount of isotope. ARDS and multisystem failure occur rarely after ^{131}I-MIBG therapy, particularly in patients with pretreatment proteinuria.

2. Peptide receptor radionuclide treatment (PRRT)—This therapy uses a radioisotope-tagged somatostatin analog against neuroendocrine tumors that express somatostatin receptors. ^{177}Lu-DOTATATE (Lutathera) is FDA-approved for treating patients with metastatic gastroenteropancreatic neuroendocrine tumors (GEP-NETs); it is being used off-label and on protocol to treat patients with metastatic pheochromocytoma and paraganglioma tumors, 90% of which are avid for PRRT.

C. Treatment for Bone Metastases

Patients with significant osteolytic bone metastases may be treated with external beam radiation therapy, which is often helpful in relieving pain and stabilizing local osseous disease. Patients with vertebral metastases and spinal cord compression require surgical decompression and kyphoplasty. Intravenous zoledronic acid or subcutaneous denosumab may also be administered to patients with osteolytic bone metastases.

► Prognosis

A pheochromocytoma or sympathetic paraganglioma is considered malignant if metastases are present, but metastases may take many years to become clinically evident. Therefore, lifetime surveillance is recommended. Malignancy is more likely for larger tumors and for paragangliomas. The prognosis is good for patients with pheochromocytomas that are resected before causing cardiovascular damage. Hypertension usually resolves after successful surgery, but may persist or return in 25% of patients despite successful surgery. In such cases, biochemical reevaluation is required to detect a possible second or metastatic pheochromocytoma.

The surgical mortality is under 3% with the use of laparoscopic surgical techniques, intraoperative monitoring, and preoperative blood pressure control with alpha-blockers or calcium channel blockers.

Patients with metastatic pheochromocytoma or paraganglioma have an extremely variable prognosis. Some metastases are extremely indolent and may not progress or may present clinically for several decades after the primary tumor diagnosis. Metastases from head-neck paragangliomas are particularly slow-growing. However, some of these tumors are extremely aggressive. Rapid disease progression has been associated with male sex, older age, larger primary tumor size, dopamine hypersecretion, failure to undergo primary tumor resection, very high tumor burden, and metastases that are visible at the time of primary tumor diagnosis.

Casey RT et al. Clinical and molecular features of renal and pheochromocytoma/paraganglioma tumor association syndrome (RAPTAS): case series and literature review. J Clin Endocrinol Metab. 2017 Nov 1;102(11):4013–22. [PMID: 28973655]

Hamidi O et al. Malignant pheochromocytoma and paraganglioma: 272 patients over 55 years. J Clin Endocrinol Metab. 2017 Sep 1;102(9):3296–305. [PMID: 28605453]

Lenders JW et al. Pheochromocytoma and paraganglioma: an Endocrine Society clinical practice guideline. J Clin Endocrinol Metab. 2014 Jun;99(6):1915–42. [PMID: 24893135]

Plouin PF et al. European Society of Endocrinology clinical practice guidelines for long term follow-up of patients operated on for a phaeochromocytoma or a paraganglioma. Eur J Endocrinol. 2016 May;175(5):G1–10. [PMID: 27048283]

Pourian M et al. Does this patient have pheochromocytoma? A systematic review of clinical signs and symptoms. J Diabetes Metab Disord. 2016 Mar 31;15:1–12. [PMID: 27034920]

INCIDENTALLY DISCOVERED ADRENAL MASSES

Adrenal incidentalomas are defined as adrenal nodules that are discovered incidentally on up to 4% of abdominal CT or MRI scans obtained for other reasons. Although the overwhelming majority of adrenal incidentalomas are benign adrenal adenomas, it is always necessary to determine whether such masses are malignant or pheochromocytomas and whether they secrete excessive cortisol or aldosterone. Patients with an adrenal nodule and any possible manifestation of hypercortisolism should be screened for Cushing syndrome with a plasma ACTH, serum cortisol, and serum DHEAS; patients with a low or low-normal ACTH, a suppressed DHEAS, or a high cortisol should then be assessed with a 1-mg dexamethasone suppression test (see Cushing syndrome). Patients with hypertension are screened for primary aldosteronism with a PRA and serum aldosterone (see Primary Aldosteronism). Most adrenal incidentalomas should be assessed for pheochromocytoma, particularly when their diameter exceeds 3 cm, density exceeds 10 HU, and in patients with hypertension or suspicious symptoms; screening is done with plasma fractionated free metanephrines.

When an adrenal incidentaloma larger than 4 cm in diameter is detected in a patient without a history of malignancy, it should be resected, unless it is an unmistakably benign myelolipoma, hemorrhage, or adrenal cyst. Masses 3–4 cm in diameter may be resected if they have suspicious features (heterogeneity or irregularity). Smaller adrenal incidentalomas are usually observed after endocrine testing. A noncontrast CT scan can determine the density of the mass; adrenal incidentalomas with a density less than 10 HU on CT are unlikely to be a pheochromocytoma or metastasis. For small adrenal incidentalomas with a density of greater than or equal to 10 HU, an adrenal intravenous contrast "washout" CT scan may be obtained; the density of the adrenal incidentaloma in HU is calculated 60 seconds after contrast and again 15 minutes after contrast; a reduction (washout) of 40% or more is consistent with a benign adrenal adenoma. However, adrenal washout studies are only suggestive and about 20% of pheochromocytomas have adrenal washout of 40% or more; so, if the adrenal incidentaloma is not clinically a pheochromocytoma and not resected, a follow-up CT of the adrenals in 6–12 months is recommended to look for growth.

Bourdeau I et al. Management of endocrine disease: differential diagnosis, investigation and therapy of bilateral adrenal incidentalomas. Eur J Endocrinol. 2018 Aug;179(2):R57–67. [PMID: 29748231]

Gendy R et al. Incidental adrenal masses—a primary care approach. Aust Fam Physician. 2017 Jun;46(6):385–90. [PMID: 28609594]

Loscalzo J et al. Case 8-2018: a 55-year-old woman with shock and labile blood pressure. N Engl J Med. 2018 Mar 15;378(11):1043–53. [PMID: 29539275]

Mayo-Smith WW et al. Management of incidental adrenal masses: a white paper of the ACR incidental findings committee. J Am Coll Radiol. 2017 Aug;14(8):1038–44. [PMID: 28651988]

GASTROENTEROPANCREATIC NEUROENDOCRINE TUMORS (GEP-NETS) & CARCINOID TUMORS

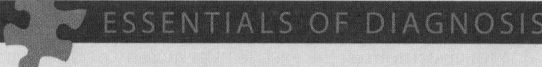

ESSENTIALS OF DIAGNOSIS

► GEP-NETs are neuroendocrine tumors that originate in the gastrointestinal tract.

► About 60% GEP-NETs are nonsecretory or secretory without clinical manifestations; they may be detected incidentally or may present with weight loss, abdominal pain, or jaundice.

► Carcinoid tumors arise from the intestines or lung, secrete serotonin, and may metastasize.

► General Considerations

GEP-NETs are a subset of neuroendocrine tumors (NETs) that arise from the stomach, intestines, or endocrine pancreas.

The reported incidence of GEP-NETs has increased to about 37 per million yearly in the United States due to the incidental detection of small tumors on abdominal scans. About 40% are functional, producing hormones that also serve as tumor markers, important for diagnosis and follow-up. At presentation, 65% of GEP-NETs are unresectable or metastatic. Up to 25% of GEP-NETs are associated with one of four different inherited disorders: MEN 1, von Hippel-Lindau disease (VHL),

neurofibromatosis 1 (NF-1), and tuberous sclerosis complex (TSC). In MEN 1, GEP-NETs are usually gastrinomas, carcinoids, or nonfunctioning tumors and are a common cause of death. In VHL, GEP-NETs are usually benign and multiple.

Insulinomas are the most common functional type of GEP-NET and are usually small, intrapancreatic, and benign (90%) and secrete excessive amounts of insulin. Insulinomas also produce proinsulin and C-peptide. Insulinomas are solitary in 95% of sporadic cases but are multiple in about 90% of cases arising in MEN 1. (See Chapter 27.)

Gastrinomas secrete excessive quantities of the hormone gastrin (as well as "big" gastrin). About 50% of gastrinomas are malignant and metastasize to the liver. Gastrinomas are typically found in the duodenum (49%), pancreas (24%), or lymph nodes (11%). Sporadic gastrinoma is rarely suspected at the onset of symptoms; typically, there is a 5-year delay in diagnosis. About 22% of gastrinomas arise in patients with MEN 1, who usually present at a younger age, often with multiple tumors; hyperparathyroidism can occur many years before or after the discovery of a gastrinoma.

Glucagonomas are rare and usually malignant, despite their benign histologic appearance. They usually arise as a large intrapancreatic tumor with 60% having liver metastases apparent by the time of diagnosis. Besides glucagon, they usually secrete additional hormones, including gastrin.

Somatostatinomas are very rare and usually single. They arise in the pancreas (50%) or small intestine. They secrete somatostatin.

VIPomas are very rare and usually single intrapancreatic tumors with metastases usually evident (80%) at diagnosis. They produce vasoactive intestinal polypeptide (VIP).

CCKomas are rare tumors of the endocrine pancreas that secrete cholecystokinin.

Carcinoid tumors can arise from the small bowel (53%, particularly terminal ileum), colon (12%), esophagus through duodenum (6%), or lung (bronchial carcinoid [5%]). About 20% of cases present with metastases without a known primary location. Carcinoids are multiple in about 28% of cases. Although tumors are usually indolent, metastases are common, particularly to liver, lymph nodes, and peritoneum.

► Clinical Findings

A. Symptoms and Signs

Nonfunctioning tumors typically present with mass effect and metastases, such as pancreatitis, jaundice, abdominal pain, or weight loss.

Insulinomas secrete insulin and present with the symptoms of fasting hypoglycemia. (See Chapter 27.)

Gastrinomas usually present with peptic ulcer disease—abdominal pain (75%), heartburn (44%), bleeding (25%)—or weight loss (17%) (Zollinger-Ellison syndrome). Endoscopy usually shows hyperplastic gastric rugae (94%).

Glucagonomas usually present with weight loss caused by glucagon-stimulated protein hepatic gluconeogenesis and related protein catabolism. Other common manifestations include diarrhea, nausea, peptic ulcer, hypoaminoacidemia, or necrolytic migratory erythema, known as "glucagonoma syndrome." Diabetes mellitus develops in about 35% of patients. The median survival is 34 months after diagnosis.

Somatostatinomas can present with a classic triad of symptoms: diabetes mellitus due to its inhibition of insulin and glucagon secretion; cholelithiasis due to its inhibition of gallbladder motility; and steatorrhea due to its inhibition of pancreatic exocrine function. Diarrhea, hypochlorhydria, and anemia can also occur.

VIPomas present with profuse *w*atery *d*iarrhea (unremitting), *h*ypokalemia, and *a*chlorhydria ("WDHA"), the so-called Verner-Morrison syndrome.

CCKomas may present with liver metastases and symptoms of diarrhea, peptic ulcer disease, and weight loss. Patients have elevated serum levels of cholecystokinin and CgA.

Carcinoid tumors can produce "carcinoid syndrome": episodes of abdominal pain, diarrhea, bronchospasm, and weight loss. Dry skin and flushing typically affect the upper chest, neck, and face and lasts from 30 seconds to 30 minutes, although flushing with bronchial carcinoids can persist for days. Although abdominal pain and diarrhea may occur at the same time as flushing, they usually occur at other times. Flushing can be unprovoked or precipitated by exercise, anesthesia, emotional stimuli, or foods (bananas, tomatoes, cheese, kiwi, eggplant, and alcohol). However, the full-blown carcinoid syndrome occurs with only about 10% of tumors. Other manifestations include carcinoid heart disease caused by endocardial fibrotic plaques. Tumor-induced fibrosis can also occur in the retroperitoneum causing ureteral obstruction or in the penis causing Peyronie disease. Pellagra (glossitis, confusion, dry skin), which results from the conversion of tryptophan (a precursor to niacin) to serotonin by tumor cells, may develop in affected patients with widespread metastases.

Bronchial carcinoids secrete serotonin and can produce carcinoid syndrome even without hepatic metastases. Foregut carcinoids secrete serotonin that is metabolized by the liver and produce carcinoid syndrome only when they have metastasized to the liver. Appendiceal carcinoids are typically discovered incidentally during appendectomy; hemicolectomy is required if the tumor is 2 cm or larger or has unfavorable histopathology. Cecal carcinoids often present with intestinal obstruction or intestinal bleeding. Hindgut carcinoids rarely produce serotonin and do not cause carcinoid syndrome.

Ectopic hormones can be secreted by GEP-NETs. Ectopic ACTH secretion from bronchial carcinoids or pancreatic neuroendocrine tumors (pNETs) can produce Cushing syndrome.

B. Laboratory Findings

About 40% of GEP-NETs are functional, producing hormones that serve as tumor markers, which are important for diagnosis and follow-up. For carcinoid tumors, serum serotonin may be elevated along with urinary 5-hydroindoleacetic acid (5-HIAA). Additionally, serum CgA may be elevated in neuroendocrine tumors and can be another useful tumor marker.

C. Imaging

Localization of noninsulinoma GEP-NETs and their metastases is best done with PET scanning with ^{68}Ga-DOT-ATATE, a radiolabeled somatostatin analog; it is extremely sensitive. ^{111}In-pentreotide (Octreoscan) detects about 75% of noninsulinomas. ^{18}F-DOPA PET/CT may also be helpful in detecting occult carcinoid tumors. MRI scanning is more useful than CT for imaging and following hepatic metastases.

For insulinomas, preoperative localization studies are less successful and have the following sensitivities: ultrasonography 25%, CT 25%, endoscopic ultrasonography 27%, transhepatic portal vein sampling 40%, and arteriography 45%. Nearly all insulinomas can be successfully located at surgery by the combination of intraoperative palpation (sensitivity 55%) and ultrasound (sensitivity 75%). An abdominal CT scan is usually obtained, but extensive preoperative localization procedures, especially with invasive methods, are not required. Tumors may be located in the pancreatic head or neck (57%), body (15%), or tail (19%) or in the duodenum (9%). MRI is used to screen members of kindreds with genetic syndromes that predispose them to GEP-NETs.

▶ Treatment

Surgery is the primary initial treatment for all types of GEP-NETs and is a reasonable option even for patients with stage IV disease. The aggressiveness of the surgery may vary from conservative debulking to radical resection and even liver transplantation.

With gastrinomas, the gastric hyperacidity of Zollinger-Ellison syndrome is treated with a proton pump inhibitor at quadruple the usual doses. Proton pump inhibitors increase serum gastrin, which would otherwise be useful as a tumor marker for gastrinoma recurrence after surgical resection.

Tumor visualization on octreotide scanning indicates that they may respond to long-acting preparations of somatostatin analogs, including lanreotide (Somatuline Depot) and octreotide (Sandostatin LAR Depot). Subcutaneous injections of Octreotide LAR 20–30 mg are required every 4 weeks. Treatment improves symptoms in patients with functioning tumors and also appears to improve progression-free survival in patients with either functioning or nonfunctioning GEP-NETs. Enlarging hepatic metastases may be embolized with ^{90}Y-labeled resin or glass microspheres. For patients with progressive metastatic disease, chemotherapy improves progression-free survival when added to somatostatin analog therapy (Table 39–2).

▶ Prognosis

The prognosis for patients with GEP-NETs is variable, depending on the tumor grade and stage. Patients with well or moderately well differentiated GEP-NETs (Ki-67, a marker for cellular proliferation, less than 20%) have a much better survival than those with poorly differentiated tumors. Smaller tumors without detectable metastases have a much lower chance of recurrence after surgery. However, most patients with GEP-NETs are stage IV with hepatic metastases by the time of diagnosis. Nevertheless, low-grade metastases may be indolent or slow-growing and may respond to octreotide or lanreotide. The overall prognosis for patients with GEP-NETs is much better than that for adenocarcinomas that arise from the same organs. The prognosis is worse for patients with serum pancreastatin levels above 500 pmol/L, since it correlates with the amount of hepatic metastases.

The surgical complication rate for GEP-NETs is about 40%, with patients commonly developing fistulas and infections. Extensive pancreatic resection may cause diabetes mellitus. The overall 5-year survival is higher with functional tumors (77%) than with nonfunctional ones (55%) and higher with benign tumors (91%) than with malignant ones (55%). For patients with gastrinomas, the 5-, 10-, and 20-year survival rates with MEN 1 are 94%, 75%, and 58%, respectively, while the survival rates for patients with sporadic gastrinomas are 62%, 50%, and 31%, respectively.

Cives M et al. Treatment strategies for metastatic neuroendocrine tumors of the gastrointestinal tract. Curr Treat Options Oncol. 2017 Mar;18(3):14. [PMID: 28286921]

Dasari A et al. Trends in the incidence, prevalence, and survival outcomes in patients with neuroendocrine tumors in the United States. JAMA Oncol. 2017 Oct 1;3(10):1335–42. [PMID: 28448665]

Howe JR et al. The surgical management of small bowel neuroendocrine tumors: consensus guidelines of the North American Neuroendocrine Tumor Society. Pancreas. 2017 Jul;46(6):715–31. [PMID: 28609357]

Raphael MJ et al. Principles of diagnosis and management of neuroendocrine tumours. CMAJ. 2017 Mar 13;189(10):E398–404. [PMID: 28385820]

Strosberg JR et al. North American Neuroendocrine Tumor Society consensus guidelines for surveillance and medical management of midgut neuroendocrine tumors. Pancreas. 2017 Jul;46(6):707–14. [PMID: 28609356]

MULTIPLE ENDOCRINE NEOPLASIA (MEN)

MEN TYPES 1–4

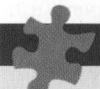 ESSENTIALS OF DIAGNOSIS

► **MEN 1:** tumors of the parathyroid glands, endocrine pancreas and duodenum, anterior pituitary, adrenal, thyroid; carcinoid tumors; lipomas and facial angiofibromas.

► **MEN 2 (MEN 2A):** medullary thyroid cancers, hyperparathyroidism, pheochromocytomas, Hirschsprung disease.

► **MEN 3 (MEN 2B):** medullary thyroid cancers, pheochromocytomas, Marfan-like habitus, mucosal neuromas, intestinal ganglioneuroma, delayed puberty.

► **MEN 4:** tumors of the parathyroid glands, anterior pituitary gland, adrenal gland, ovary, testicle, kidney.

Syndromes of MEN are inherited as autosomal dominant traits that cause a predisposition to the development of tumors of two or more different endocrine glands (Table 26–12). MEN syndromes are caused by different germline mutations and tumors arising when certain additional somatic mutations occur in predisposed organs. Patients with MEN should have genetic testing so that their first-degree relatives may then be tested for the specific mutation.

1. MEN 1

Multiple endocrine neoplasia type 1 (MEN 1, Wermer syndrome) is a tumor syndrome with a prevalence of 2–10 per 100,000 persons in the United States. About 90% of affected patients harbor a detectable germline mutation in the *menin* gene.

Table 26–12. Multiple endocrine neoplasia (MEN) syndromes: incidence of tumor types.

Tumor Type	MEN 1	MEN 2 (MEN 2A)	MEN 3 (MEN 2B)	MEN 4
Parathyroid	95%	20–50%	Rare	Common
Pancreatic	54%			Common
Pituitary	42%			Common
Medullary thyroid carcinoma		> 90%	80%	
Pheochromocytoma	Rare	20–35%	60%	
Mucosal and gastrointestinal ganglioneuromas		Rare	> 90%	
Subcutaneous lipoma	30%			
Adrenocortical adenoma	30%			Common
Thoracic carcinoid	15%			
Thyroid adenoma	55%			Common
Facial angiofibromas and collagenomas	85%			

The presentation of MEN 1 is quite variable, even in the same kindred. Affected patients are prone to many different tumors, particularly involving the parathyroids, endocrine pancreas and duodenum, and anterior pituitary (Table 26–12). The initial biochemical manifestations (usually hypercalcemia) can often be detected as early as age 14–18 years in patients with a MEN 1 gene mutation, although clinical manifestations usually present in the third or fourth decade.

Hyperparathyroidism is the first clinical manifestation of MEN 1 in two-thirds of affected patients, but it may present at any time of life.

GEP-NETs and carcinoids occur in up to 70% of patients with MEN 1. The GEP-NETs may secrete only pancreatic polypeptide or be nonsecretory altogether (20–55%). **Gastrinomas** occur in about 40% of patients with MEN 1. Concurrent hypercalcemia, due to hyperparathyroidism in MEN 1, stimulates gastrin and worsens gastric acid secretion; control of the hypercalcemia often reduces serum gastrin levels and gastric acid secretion. Carcinoid tumors can arise in the lung or abdomen and can metastasize, especially to the liver.

Insulinomas occur in about 10% of patients with MEN 1. Extrapancreatic neuroendocrine tumors are common in MEN 1, are frequently malignant, and include carcinoid tumors usually in foregut locations (69%), such as the lung, thymus, duodenum, or stomach.

Pituitary adenomas are the presenting tumor in 29% of patients with MEN 1 and eventually are found in about 42% of patients with MEN 1. About 42% of such pituitary adenomas are nonsecretory. While nonsecretory pituitary microadenomas (less than 1 cm diameter and detected on routine MRI screening) are usually indolent, about 25% of nonsecretory pituitary adenomas are macroadenomas (1 cm or more in diameter) and more aggressive.

Adrenal adenomas or hyperplasia occur in about 40% of patients with MEN 1 and 50% are bilateral. They are generally benign and nonfunctional. These adrenal lesions are ACTH-independent.

Thymic neuroendocrine tumors occur in 3.4% of affected patients, mostly in males, with a 10-year survival of 25%. Lung neuroendocrine tumors occur in 13%, with a 10-year survival of 71%.

Benign thyroid adenomas or multinodular goiter occurs in about 55% of MEN 1 patients. Patients may undergo a thyroidectomy at the time of parathyroidectomy.

Nonendocrine tumors occur commonly in MEN 1, particularly small head-neck angiofibromas (85%) and lipomas (30%). Collagenomas are common (70%), presenting as firm dermal nodules. Affected patients may also be more prone to meningiomas, breast cancer, colorectal cancers, prostate cancer, and malignant melanomas.

Overall, patients with MEN 1 have an increased mortality rate with a mean life expectancy of only 55 years.

2. MEN 2 (MEN 2A)

Multiple endocrine neoplasia type 2 (MEN 2A, Sipple syndrome) is a rare autosomal-dominant tumor syndrome that arises in patients with a germline gain-of-function *ret* protooncogene mutation. Genetic testing identifies about 95% of affected individuals.

Medullary thyroid carcinoma (greater than 90%); **hyperparathyroidism** (30%), with hyperplasia or adenomas of multiple parathyroid glands developing in most cases; **pheochromocytomas** (30%), which are often bilateral and frequently asymptomatic; and **Hirschsprung disease** may develop. No patients with MEN 2 should receive therapy for diabetes with glucagon-like peptide 1 (GLP 1) agonists that may increase the risk for medullary thyroid carcinoma. Before any surgical procedure, MEN 2 (2A) carriers should be screened for pheochromocytoma (see above) and for medullary thyroid carcinoma.

3. MEN 3 (MEN 2B)

Multiple endocrine neoplasia type 3 (MEN 2B) is a familial, autosomal dominant multiglandular syndrome that is also caused by a germline gain-of-function mutation of the *ret* protooncogene. MEN 3 (2B) is characterized by mucosal neuromas (in more than 90% of affected patients) with bumpy and enlarged lips and tongue, Marfan-like habitus (75% of cases), and adrenal pheochromocytomas (60%) that are rarely malignant and often bilateral. Patients also have intestinal abnormalities (75%) such as intestinal ganglioneuromas, skeletal abnormalities (87%), and delayed puberty (43%). Medullary thyroid carcinoma (80%) is aggressive and presents early in life.

4. MEN 4

Multiple endocrine neoplasia type 4 (MEN 4) is a rare autosomal-dominant familial tumor syndrome caused by germline mutations in the gene *CDKN1B*. Affected patients are particularly prone to adenomas of the pituitary and parathyroid glands and neuroendocrine tumors of the pancreas. Unlike patients with MEN 1, those with MEN 4 are also appear to be prone to adrenal tumors, renal tumors, testicular cancer, and neuroendocrine cervical carcinoma.

OTHER SYNDROMES OF MULTIPLE ENDOCRINE NEOPLASIA

Patients with **Carney complex** develop adrenocortical nodular hyperplasia, pituitary adenomas, thyroid tumors, gonadal Sertoli cell tumors, and cardiac myxomas. With **McCune-Albright syndrome,** precocious puberty (particularly girls) develops due to gonadal hypersecretion. Multiple adrenal nodules can rarely cause Cushing syndrome. Hyperthyroidism results from autonomously functioning thyroid nodules. Acromegaly is caused by GH-secreting pituitary tumors. Patients also have fibrous dysplasia of bones and hypophosphatemia, and bone fractures are common. Sudden death has been reported. **Type 2 von Hippel Lindau (VHL) syndrome** is associated with pheochromocytomas, pancreatic/duodenal neuroendocrine tumors, hyperparathyroidism, and pituitary tumors as well as hemangiomas and renal cell carcinomas. **Hypoxia inducible factor 2A (HIF2A) germline mutations** predispose to pheochromocytomas, pancreatic/duodenal somatostatinomas, as well as erythrocytosis and retinal abnormalities. **Neurofibromatosis type 1 (NF-1)** is associated with pheochromocytomas and pancreatic/duodenal somatostatinomas as well as neurofibromas and hypothalamic hamartomas.

Grajo JR et al. Multiple endocrine neoplasia syndromes: a comprehensive imaging review. Radiol Clin North Am. 2016 May;54(3):441–51. [PMID: 27153782]

Hyde SM et al. Genetics of multiple endocrine neoplasia type 1/multiple endocrine neoplasia type 2 syndromes. Endocrinol Metab Clin North Am. 2017 Jun;46(2):491–502. [PMID: 28476233]

Marx SJ. Recent topics around multiple endocrine neoplasia Type 1. J Clin Endocrinol Metab. 2018 Apr;103(4):1296–301. [PMID: 29897580]

van Leeuwaarde RS et al. Impact of delay in diagnosis in outcomes in MEN1: results from the Dutch MEN1 Study Group. J Clin Endocrinol Metab. 2016 Mar;101(3):1159–65. [PMID: 26751192]

DISEASES OF THE TESTES & MALE BREAST

MALE HYPOGONADISM

ESSENTIALS OF DIAGNOSIS

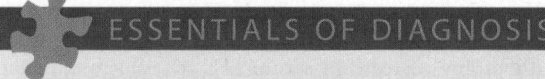

▶ Diminished libido and erections.

▶ Fatigue, depression, reduced exercise endurance.

▶ Decreased growth of body hair.

▶ Testes small or normal in size.

▶ Low serum total testosterone or free testosterone.

▶ Serum LH and FSH are low or normal in hypogonadotropic hypogonadism; they are high in testicular failure (hypergonadotropic hypogonadism).

General Considerations

Male hypogonadism is caused by deficient testosterone secretion by the testes. It may be classified according to whether it is due to (1) insufficient gonadotropin secretion by the pituitary (hypogonadotropic); (2) pathology in the testes themselves (hypergonadotropic); or (3) both (Table 26–13). Partial male hypogonadism may be difficult to distinguish from the physiologic reduction in serum testosterone seen in normal aging, obesity, and illness.

Etiology

A. Hypogonadotropic Hypogonadism (Low Testosterone With Normal or Low LH)

A deficiency in FSH and LH may be isolated or associated with other pituitary hormonal abnormalities. (See Hypopituitarism.) Hypogonadotropic hypogonadism can be primary, defined as failure to enter puberty by age 14, with causes including isolated hypogonadotropic hypogonadism, hypopituitarism, or simple constitutional delay of growth and puberty; or it can be acquired, with causes listed in Table 26–13. Genetic conditions (eg, Kallmann syndrome or *PROKR2* mutations, X-linked congenital adrenal hypoplasia, 17-ketosteroid reductase deficiency, Prader-Willis syndrome) account for about 40% of cases of isolated, and apparently idiopathic, acquired hypogonadotropic

Table 26–13. Causes of male hypogonadism.

Hypogonadotropic (Low or Normal LH)	Hypergonadotropic (High LH)
Aging	Aging
Alcohol	Antitumor chemotherapy
Chronic illness	Autoimmunity
Congenital syndromes	Anorchia (bilateral)
Constitutional delay of growth and puberty	Idiopathic
	Klinefelter syndrome
Cushing syndrome	Leprosy
Drugs	Lymphoma
Estrogen	Male climacteric
GnRH agonist (leuprolide)	Myotonic dystrophy
Ketoconazole	Noonan syndrome
Marijuana	Orchiectomy (bilateral or unilateral)
Prior androgens	Orchitis
Spironolactone	Radiation or radioisotope therapy
Granulomatous diseases	Sertoli cell-only syndrome
Hemochromatosis	Testicular trauma
Hypopituitarism	Tuberculosis
Hypothalamic or pituitary tumors	Uremia
Hypothyroidism, hyperthyroidism	Viral infections (mumps)
Idiopathic	
Kidney disease	
Lymphocytic hypophysitis	
Major medical or surgical illnesses	
Malnourishment	
Obesity (BMI > 30 kg/m²)	

BMI, body mass index; GnRH, gonadotropin-releasing hormone; LH, luteinizing hormone.

hypogonadism with a serum testosterone level less than 150 ng/dL (5.2 nmol/L).

Partial male hypogonadotropic hypogonadism is defined as a serum testosterone in the range of 150–300 ng/dL (5.2–10.4 nmol/L). The main causes of acquired partial male hypogonadotropic hypogonadism include obesity, poor health, or normal aging, such that it is termed **age-related hypogonadism**. Spermatogenesis is usually preserved.

B. Hypergonadotropic Hypogonadism (Testicular Failure With High LH)

A failure of the testicular Leydig cells to secrete adequate testosterone causes a rise in LH and FSH. Acquired conditions that can cause testicular failure are listed in Table 26–13. Male hypergonadotropic hypogonadism can also be caused by XY gonadal dysgenesis, partial 17-ketosteroid reductase deficiency and a congenital partial deficiency in the steroidogenic enzyme CYP17 (17-hydroxylase). CYP17 may be deliberately inhibited by abiraterone acetate, a drug for prostate cancer. In men who have had a unilateral orchiectomy for cancer, the remaining testicle frequently fails, even in the absence of radiation or chemotherapy.

Klinefelter syndrome (47,XXY and its variants) is the most common chromosomal abnormality among males, with an incidence of about 1:500 (see Chapter 40). Although puberty occurs at the normal time, the degree of virilization is variable. Serum testosterone is usually low and gonadotropins are elevated. Other common findings include tall stature and abnormal body proportions that are unusual for hypogonadal men (eg, height more than 3 cm greater than arm span).

XY gonadal dysgenesis describes several conditions that result in the failure of the testes to develop normally. *SRY* is a gene on the Y chromosome that initiates male sexual development. Mutations in *SRY* result in testicular dysgenesis. Affected individuals lack testosterone, which results in sex reversal: female external genitalia with a blind vaginal pouch, no uterus, and intra-abdominal dysgenetic gonads. Affected individuals appear as normal girls until their lack of pubertal development and amenorrhea leads to the diagnosis. Intra-abdominal rudimentary testes have an increased risk of developing a malignancy and are usually resected.

C. Androgen Insensitivity

Partial resistance to testosterone is a rare condition in which phenotypic males have variable degrees of apparent hypogonadism, hypospadias, cryptorchism, and gynecomastia. Serum testosterone levels are normal.

▶ **Clinical Findings**

A. Symptoms and Signs

Hypogonadism that is congenital or acquired during childhood presents as delayed puberty. Men with acquired hypogonadism have variable manifestations, known as "testosterone deficiency syndrome." Most men experience decreased libido. Others complain of erectile dysfunction, poor morning erection, or hot sweats. Men often have depression, fatigue, or decreased ability to perform vigorous physical activity. The presenting complaint may also be infertility, gynecomastia, headache, fracture, or other symptoms related to the cause or result of the hypogonadism. The patient's history often gives a clue to the cause (Table 26–13).

Physical signs associated with hypogonadism may include decreased body, axillary, beard, or pubic hair, but only after years of severe hypogonadism. Men with hypogonadism lose muscle mass and gain weight due to an increase in subcutaneous fat. Examination should include measurements of arm span and height. Testicular size should be assessed with an orchidometer (normal volume is about 10–25 mL; normal length is usually over 6 cm). Testicular size may decrease but usually remains within the normal range in men with postpubertal hypogonadotropic hypogonadism, but it may be diminished with testicular injury or Klinefelter syndrome. The testes must also be carefully palpated for masses, since Leydig cell tumors may secrete estrogen and present with hypogonadism. The testicles must be carefully examined for evidence of trauma, infiltrative lesions (eg, lymphoma), or infection (eg, leprosy, tuberculosis).

B. Laboratory Findings

The evaluation for hypogonadism begins with a morning (before 10 AM) serum testosterone and free testosterone

measurement. In men with low serum testosterone levels, testing is repeated in order to confirm the diagnosis. Serum testosterone levels are considered low if they are confirmed to be less than 240 ng/dL (8.3 nmol/L). For men ages 18–69, serum free testosterone levels are considered low if they are confirmed to be less than 35 pg/mL (120 pmol/L) or less than 30 pg/mL (100 pg/L) for men ages 70 and over.

Normal ranges for serum testosterone have been derived from nonfasting morning blood specimens, which tend to be the highest of the day. Later in the day, serum testosterone levels can be 25–50% lower. Therefore, a serum testosterone drawn fasting or late in the day may be misleadingly below the "reference range."

Serum testosterone levels in men are highest at age 20–30 years and slightly lower at age 30–40 years. After age 40, serum total testosterone declines variably by an average of 1–2% annually; serum free testosterone levels decline even faster, since sex hormone binding globulin increases with age. Serum levels of free testosterone are lower in men aged 40–70 compared with younger men, without any increase in serum LH. A problem with the diagnosis of age-related hypogonadism is that most laboratories provide reference ranges for testosterone that are derived from young men and may not provide age-adjusted reference ranges for serum testosterone and free testosterone. The main conditions that contribute to the general decline in serum testosterone with aging include obesity, illness, and opioids. After age 70, LH levels tend to rise, indicating a contribution of primary gonadal dysfunction with advancing age. Testing for serum free testosterone is especially important for detecting hypogonadism in elderly men, who generally have high levels of sex hormone binding globulin. A low serum testosterone or free testosterone should be verified with a repeat morning nonfasting assay, along with serum LH and PRL levels. Serum LH levels are high in patients with hypergonadotropic hypogonadism but low or inappropriately normal in men with hypogonadotropic hypogonadism or normal aging. High serum estradiol levels are seen in men with obesity-related hypogonadotropic hypogonadism.

Testosterone stimulates erythropoiesis in men, causing the normal red blood count range to be higher in men than in women; mild anemia is common in men with hypogonadism. For men with longstanding severe male hypogonadism, osteoporosis is common, so a bone densitometry is recommended.

1. Hypogonadotropic hypogonadism—A serum PRL determination is obtained to screen for a pituitary prolactinoma and other pituitary/hypothalamic lesions, but serum PRL may be elevated for many other reasons (see Table 26–1). The serum estradiol level may be elevated in patients with cirrhosis and in rare cases of estrogen-secreting tumors (testicular Leydig cell tumor or adrenal carcinoma). Men with no discernible definite cause for hypogonadotropic hypogonadism should be screened for hemochromatosis. Men with hypogonadotropic hypogonadism should have an MRI of the pituitary/hypothalamus to search for a mass lesion in presence of one or more of the following: (1) severe hypogonadism (serum testosterone below 150 ng/mL or 5.2 nmol/L), (2) elevated serum PRL, (3) other pituitary hormone deficiencies, or (4) symptoms of a mass lesion (headaches or visual field deficits).

2. Hypergonadotropic hypogonadism—Men with hypergonadotropic hypogonadism have low serum testosterone levels with a compensatory increase in FSH and LH. Klinefelter syndrome can be confirmed by karyotyping or by measurement of leukocyte XIST. Testicular biopsy is usually reserved for younger patients in whom the reason for primary hypogonadism is unclear.

► Treatment

Testosterone replacement is reasonable for boys who have not entered puberty by age 14 years. It is also beneficial for most men with primary testicular failure (hypergonadotropic hypogonadism). Testosterone replacement or gonadal stimulation therapy is also warranted for men with severe hypogonadotropic hypogonadism of any etiology with serum testosterone levels less than 150 ng/mL (5.2 nmol/L). Testosterone therapy should also be considered for men with low or low-normal serum testosterone or free testosterone, along with elevated serum LH levels. For other men without elevated serum LH levels and an average of at least two morning serum total testosterone levels below 275 ng/dL (9.5 nmol/L, "physiologic hypogonadism"), a trial of testosterone therapy may be considered, particularly if they have at least three of the following six symptoms: erectile dysfunction, poor morning erection, low libido, depression, fatigue, and inability to perform vigorous activity. Testosterone replacement should be continued only if they clearly derive clinical benefit from therapy. Therapy can be adjusted with an aim to improve clinical symptoms while maintaining normal serum levels of testosterone or free testosterone. Men with physiologic low-normal serum testosterone levels above 325 ng/dL (11.3 nmol/L) are unlikely to benefit from testosterone therapy.

Testosterone replacement or stimulation therapy carries certain risks. Therefore, testosterone therapy should only be given to men who have a documented low serum total or free testosterone. Testosterone therapy should not be given to men with active breast cancer or prostate cancer. It is also prudent to monitor the hematocrit and lipid profile of men receiving testosterone, since therapy can cause erythrocytosis and hyperlipidemia. Testosterone therapy can also cause gynecomastia. Testosterone therapy is not given to men with untreated sleep apnea or heart failure.

Drug interactions can occur. Testosterone should be administered cautiously to men receiving coumadin, since the combination can increase the INR and risk of bleeding. Similarly, testosterone therapy can increase serum levels of cyclosporine, tacrolimus, and tolvaptan. Testosterone can predispose to hypoglycemia in diabetic men receiving insulin or oral hypoglycemic agents, so close monitoring of blood sugars is advisable during initiation of testosterone therapy.

Oral androgen therapy with methyltestosterone is not advisable due to the potential for causing liver tumors, peliosis hepatis, and cholestatic jaundice.

Men with severe osteoporosis may require treatment with bisphosphonates and vitamin D, in addition to testosterone replacement therapy.

A. Therapies for Male Hypogonadism

1. Testosterone topical gels—Topical testosterone is usually applied once daily in the morning after showering. One or two fingers are used to apply the gel evenly to skin. Afterwards, the hands should be washed. Topical testosterone should not be applied to the breast or genitals. The gel should be allowed to air-dry (about 10 minutes) before dressing. Before close contact with women or children, a shirt must be worn or the areas of application washed with soap and water to prevent transfer of testosterone to them. The patient should avoid swimming, showering, or washing the application area for at least 2 hours following application.

Testosterone topical generic 1% gel is available in packets (12.5 mg/1.25 g, 25 mg/2.5 g, or 50 mg/5g) or tubes (50 mg/5 g). The recommended dose is 50–100 mg daily. Testosterone topical generic 2% gel is available in a gel pump (10 mg/0.5 g actuation). The recommended dose is 40–70 mg daily. Androgel 1% gel is available in 2.5-g packets (25 mg testosterone) and 5-g packets (50 mg testosterone) and in a pump that dispenses 12.5 mg testosterone per pump actuation: the recommended dose is 50–100 mg applied daily to the shoulders. Androgel 1.6% gel is available in a pump that dispenses 20.25 mg testosterone per pump actuation; the recommended dose is 40.5–81 mg daily. Testim 1% gel is available in 5-g tubes (50 mg testosterone); the recommended dose is 50–100 mg applied daily. Fortesta 2% gel is available in a pump that dispenses 10 mg testosterone per pump actuation; the recommended dose is 40–70 mg daily. Testogel is distributed in 5-g sachets (50 mg testosterone); this brand is not available in the United States. Testim, Fortesta, and Testogel may be applied to shoulders, upper arms, or abdomen. Axiron 2% solution is available in a pump that dispenses 30 mg per actuation; the recommended dose is 30–60 mg applied to each axilla daily. Vogelxo is a 1% testosterone gel that is available in packets or tubes (50 mg/5 g) or a gel pump (12.5 mg/1.25 g); it is applied to the shoulders in doses of 50–100 mg once daily.

The serum testosterone level should be determined about 14 days after starting therapy; if the level remains below normal or the clinical response is inadequate, the daily dose may be increased to 1.5 to 2 times the initial dose. Unfortunately, serum testosterone levels vary considerably during the day after topical testosterone gel application, such that a single serum testosterone level may not accurately reflect the average serum testosterone for that individual.

2. Transdermal testosterone patches—Testosterone transdermal systems (skin patches) are applied to nongenital skin. Androderm (2 or 4 mg/day) patches may be applied at bedtime in doses of 4–8 mg; it adheres tightly to the skin and may cause skin irritation.

3. Parenteral testosterone—The dose and injection intervals are adjusted according to the patient's clinical response and serum testosterone levels drawn just before the next injection is due. A target serum testosterone level of 500 ng/dL (17.3 nmol/L) is suggested. **Testosterone cypionate** has been in use for decades; it is an intramuscular testosterone formulation that is available in solutions containing 200 mg/mL. Its main advantage is low cost. The usual dose is 200 mg every 2 weeks or 300 mg every 3 weeks. It is usually injected into the gluteus medius muscle in the upper lateral buttock, alternating sides. The injection technique must include sterile precautions and draw-back prior to injection to ensure against intravenous injection, which can result in pulmonary oil embolism.

Testosterone pellets (Testopel) are a very long-lasting depot testosterone formulation that is available as individual vials containing a single 75 mg implantable pellet in each vial. With sterile technique, the skin of the upper-outer buttock is anesthetized with lidocaine; using a trochar, the pellets are injected subcutaneously in doses of 150–450 mg every 3–6 months as an in-office procedure.

Testosterone undecanoate (Aveed, Nebido) is a long-lasting depot testosterone formulation. Its use is restricted to qualified health care facilities. It is usually injected into the gluteus medius muscle in the upper lateral buttock, alternating sides. Care must be taken to avoid intravascular injection by pulling back on the syringe plunger before injection; if any blood appears in the syringe, the needle is withdrawn and the syringe is discarded. Testosterone undecanoate (Aveed) is formulated as individual vials containing 750 mg/3 mL oily solution for intramuscular injection. The initial injection of 750 mg is followed by another 750 mg injection 4 weeks later and maintenance doses of 750 mg every 10 weeks. Testosterone undecanoate (Nebido) is formulated as individual vials containing 1000 mg/4 mL oily solution for intramuscular injection. The initial injection of 1000 mg is followed by another 1000 mg injection 6 weeks later and maintenance doses of 1000 mg every 12 weeks. A serum testosterone level is measured before the fourth dose; if the serum testosterone remains low, the dosing interval is shortened to every 10 weeks.

Caution: Testosterone undecanoate injections have caused serious pulmonary oil microembolism reactions that present with cough, dyspnea, tight throat, chest pain, and syncope. Anaphylaxis can also occur. *Patients must be observed in the health care setting for 30 minutes after the injection in order to provide appropriate medical care for the complication.*

4. Buccal testosterone—Testosterone buccal tablets (Striant) are placed between the upper lip and gingivae. One or two 30-mg tablets are thus retained and changed every 12 hours. They should not be chewed or swallowed.

5. Testosterone nasal gel—Intranasal gel testosterone (Natesto) is self-administered by a metered-dose nasal pump: one pump actuation (5.5 mg) into each nostril three times daily. The nasal pump needs to be primed by inverting it and pressing the pump 10 times before it is used the first time. It should not be used concurrently with intranasal sympathomimetic decongestants. Adverse effects include nasopharyngitis, sinusitis, bronchitis, epistaxis, nasal discomfort, and headache.

6. Oral methyltestosterone—Oral testosterone supplementation is available as methyltestosterone 10-mg tablets. The usual dose is 10–50 mg daily, given either once daily or in divided doses. Oral methyltestosterone can produce

acute hepatitis and chronic high-dose use can cause peliosis hepatis, cholestatic hepatitis, and hepatocellular carcinoma. Therefore, its use is not recommended, and it is no longer available in some countries.

7. Clomiphene citrate—Men with functional hypogonadotropic hypogonadism usually respond well to clomiphene citrate that is administered orally in doses that are titrated to achieve the desired clinical response with a serum testosterone level of about 500 ng/dL (17.3 nmol/L). Treatment with clomiphene is commenced with 25 mg on alternate days and increased to 50 mg on alternate days if necessary, with a maximum dose of 50 mg daily. Serum testosterone levels usually normalize while spermatogenesis usually improves.

8. Gonadotropins—Patients with hypogonadotropic hypogonadism may require therapy with gonadotropins, particularly to induce fertility. Men may receive hCG 1000 units subcutaneously three times weekly for 6 months; if the semen analysis shows inadequate sperm, FSH 75 units subcutaneously three times weekly is added. Many men prefer long-term therapy with hCG over testosterone therapy, but cost is an issue.

9. Weight loss—When hypogonadotropic hypogonadism is due to morbid obesity, significant weight loss will improve serum testosterone levels. The rise in serum testosterone is proportionate to the weight loss. Although diet-induced weight loss is beneficial, bariatric surgery has been much more effective and serum testosterone levels may normalize after dramatic weight loss.

B. Benefits of Testosterone Replacement Therapy

Testosterone therapy given for the indications listed under Treatment, above, usually benefits men with low serum testosterone and at least three manifestations of hypogonadism. Testosterone therapy can improve overall mood, sense of well-being, sexual desire, and erectile function. It also increases physical vigor and muscle strength. Testosterone replacement also improves exercise endurance and stair climbing ability. Long-term testosterone replacement causes significant weight loss and a reduction in waist circumference. After 2 years of testosterone replacement, muscle mass increases about 4.5%, while fat mass decreases by about 9.1%. Appropriate testosterone replacement therapy also appears to improve longevity.

C. Risks of Testosterone Replacement or Stimulation Therapy

Testosterone therapy does not appear to significantly increase the risk of prostate cancer or benign prostatic hypertrophy above that of normal men, as long as serum testosterone levels are maintained in the normal reference range on therapy. However, testosterone therapy is contraindicated in the presence of active prostate cancer. Hypogonadal men who have had a prostatectomy for low-grade prostate cancer, and who have remained in complete remission for several years, may have testosterone therapy given cautiously while monitoring serum PSA levels.

Erythrocytosis develops in some men who are treated with testosterone. Erythrocytosis is more common with intramuscular injections of testosterone enanthate than with transcutaneous testosterone. However, no increase in the incidence of thromboembolic events has been reported.

Testosterone therapy tends to aggravate sleep apnea in older men, likely through CNS effects. Surveillance for sleep apnea is recommended during testosterone therapy and a formal evaluation is recommended for all high-risk patients with snoring, obesity, partner's report of apneic episodes, nocturnal awakening, unrefreshing sleep with daytime fatigue, or hypertension.

Men who are treated with testosterone frequently experience some increase in acne that is usually mild and tolerated; topical antiacne therapy or a reduction in testosterone replacement dosage may be required. Increases in intraocular pressure have occurred during testosterone therapy. During the initiation of testosterone replacement therapy, gynecomastia develops in some men, which usually is mild and tends to resolve spontaneously; switching from testosterone injections to testosterone transdermal gel may help this condition.

D. Risks of Performance-Enhancing Anabolic Steroids

Performance-enhancing agents, particularly androgenic anabolic steroids, are used by up to 2% of young athletes and by 20–65% of power sport athletes. They are often used as part of a "stacking" polypharmacy that may include nandrolone decanoate, dimethandrolone, testosterone propionate, or testosterone enanthate. These androgens are usually illegal and often contaminated by toxic substances and can produce toxic hepatitis, dependence, aggression, depression, dyslipidemias, gynecomastia, acne, male pattern baldness, hepatitis, thromboembolism, and cardiomyopathy. Shared needles may transmit hepatitis or HIV. Arsenic contamination has been reported to cause multiorgan failure and death.

▶ Prognosis of Male Hypogonadism

If hypogonadism is due to a pituitary lesion, the prognosis is that of the primary disease (eg, tumor, necrosis). The prognosis for restoration of virility is good if testosterone is given. In one large study, cardiovascular risk was reduced in hypogonadal men over age 40 who were receiving testosterone replacement therapy to maintain serum testosterone levels within the normal reference range.

Budoff MJ et al. Testosterone treatment and coronary artery plaque volume in older men with low testosterone. JAMA. 2017 Feb 21;317(7):708–16. [PMID: 28241355]

Cheetham TC et al. Association of testosterone replacement with cardiovascular outcomes among men with androgen deficiency. JAMA Intern Med. 2017 Apr;177(4):491–9. [PMID: 28241244]

Dubruyne FM et al. Testosterone treatment is not associated with increased risk of prostate cancer or worsening of lower urinary tract symptoms: prostate health outcomes in the Registry of Hypogonadism in Men. BJU Int. 2017 Feb;119(2):216–24. [PMID: 27409523]

Grossmann M et al. A perspective on middle-aged and older men with functional hypogonadism: focus on holistic management. J Clin Endocrinol Metab. 2017 Mar;102(3):1067–75. [PMID: 28359097]

Mohler ER 3rd et al. The effect of testosterone on cardiovascular biomarkers in the testosterone trials. J Clin Endocrinol Metab. 2018 Feb 1;103(2):681–8. [PMID: 29253154]

Petering RC et al. Testosterone therapy: review of clinical applications. Am Fam Physician. 2017 Oct 1;96(7):441–9. [PMID: 29094914]

Travison TG et al. Harmonized reference ranges for circulating testosterone levels in men of four cohort studies in the United States and Europe. J Clin Endocrinol Metab. 2017 Apr 1;102(4): 1161–73. [PMID: 28324103]

CRYPTORCHISM

Cryptorchidism is found in 1–2% of males after 1 year of age but must be distinguished from retractile testes, which require no treatment. Infertility or subfertility occurs in up to 75% of men with bilateral cryptorchism and in 50% of men with unilateral cryptorchism. Some patients have underlying hypogonadism, including hypogonadotropic hypogonadism.

For a testis that is not palpable, it is important to locate the testis and bring it into the scrotum or prove its absence. About one-third of nonpalpable testes are located within the inguinal canal, one-third are intra-abdominal, and one-third are absent. Ultrasound can detect an inguinal testis. If ultrasound is negative, MRI is performed to locate the testis.

The lifetime risk of testicular neoplasia is 0.002% in normal males. The risk of malignancy is higher for cryptorchid testes (0.06%) and for intra-abdominal testes (5%). Orchiopexy decreases the risk of neoplasia when performed before 10 years of age. Orchiectomy after puberty is an option for intra-abdominal testes.

Berger C et al. Nonpalpable testes: ultrasound and contralateral testicular hypertrophy predict the surgical access, avoiding unnecessary laparoscopy. J Pediatr Urol. 2018 Apr;14(2):163. e1–7. [PMID: 29199091]

Schneuer FJ et al. Association between male genital anomalies and adult male reproductive disorders: a population-based data linkage study spanning more than 40 years. Lancet Child Adolesc Health. 2018 Oct;2(10):736–43. [PMID: 30236382]

GYNECOMASTIA

 ESSENTIALS OF DIAGNOSIS

▶ Palpable enlargement of the male breast, often asymmetric or unilateral.

▶ **Glandular gynecomastia:** typically tender.

▶ **Fatty gynecomastia:** typically nontender.

▶ Must be distinguished from carcinoma or mastitis.

Table 26–14. Causes of gynecomastia.

Physiologic causes	Drugs (partial list) (cont.)
Aging	Antipsychotics (first- and
Neonatal period, puberty	second-generation)
Obesity	Antiretroviral agents
Endocrine diseases	Calcium channel blockers (rare)
Androgen insensitivity	Chorionic gonadotropin
syndrome	Cimetidine
Aromatase excess syndrome	Clomiphene
(sporadic or familial)	Diazepam
Diabetic lymphocytic mastitis	Digitalis preparations
Hyperprolactinemia	Dutasteride
Hyperthyroidism	Estrogens (oral or topical)
Klinefelter syndrome	Ethionamide
Male hypogonadism	Famotidine (rare)
(primary or secondary)	Fenofibrate (rare)
Partial 17-ketosteroid	Finasteride
reductase deficiency	GnRH analogs
Systemic diseases	Growth hormone
Chronic liver disease	Hydroxyzine
Chronic kidney disease	Isoniazid
Hansen disease	Ketoconazole
Neurologic disorders	Lavender (topical)
Refeeding after starvation	Marijuana
Spinal cord injury	Methadone
Neoplasms	Methotrexate (rare)
Adrenal tumors	Methyldopa
Bronchogenic carcinoma	Metoclopramide
Carcinoma of the breast	Metronidazole
Ectopic hCG: CNS germinoma,	Omeprazole (rare)
lung, hepatocellular,	Opioids
gastric, renal carcinomas	Phenothiazines
Pituitary prolactinoma	Progestins
Testicular hCG-secreting	Proton pump inhibitors
tumors	(uncommon)
Drugs (partial list)	Ranitidine (rare)
Alcohol	Soy ingestion
Alkylating chemotherapeutic	Statins (rare)
agents	Spironolactone (common)
Amiodarone	Sunitinib
Anabolic steroids	Tea tree oil (topical)
Androgens (testosterone)	Tricyclics
Anti-androgens	Verapamil

GnRH, gonadotropin-releasing hormone.

General Considerations

Gynecomastia is defined as the presence of palpable glandular breast tissue in males. Pubertal gynecomastia develops in about 60% of boys; the swelling usually subsides spontaneously within a year. It is particularly common in teenagers who are very tall or overweight. The causes are multiple and diverse (Table 26–14). About 20% of adult gynecomastia is caused by drug therapy. It can develop in HIV-infected patients treated with antiretroviral therapy, especially in men receiving efavirenz or didanosine; breast enlargement resolves spontaneously in 73% of patients within 9 months. Gynecomastia develops in about 50% of athletes who abuse androgens and anabolic steroids. Fatty pseudogynecomastia is common among elderly men, particularly when there is associated weight gain. However,

true glandular gynecomastia can be the first sign of a serious disorder in older men (Table 26–14).

Clinical Findings

A. Symptoms and Signs

The male breasts must be palpated carefully to distinguish firm true glandular gynecomastia from softer fatty pseudogynecomastia in which only adipose tissue is felt. The breasts are best examined both seated and supine. Using the thumb and forefinger as pincers, the subareolar tissue is compared to nearby adipose tissue. Fatty tissue is usually diffuse and nontender. True glandular enlargement beneath the areola may be tender. Pubertal gynecomastia is characterized by tender discoid enlargement of breast tissue 2–3 cm in diameter beneath the areola. The following characteristics are worrisome for malignancy: asymmetry; location not immediately below the areola; unusual firmness; or nipple retraction, bleeding, or discharge. The examination must also include an assessment of masculinization, examination of the testes for size and masses, and examination of the penis for hypospadias.

B. Laboratory Findings

In the presence of true glandular gynecomastia, a laboratory assessment should include liver biochemical tests, serum BUN, and creatinine. Endocrine testing, including serum testosterone, free testosterone, LH, FSH, is obtained to determine whether primary or secondary hypogonadism or androgen resistance may be present. Primary hypogonadism is characterized by a low serum testosterone with a high LH. Secondary hypogonadism is present in men with a low serum testosterone with a low or normal serum LH. High serum testosterone levels plus high LH levels characterize partial androgen insensitivity syndrome. A serum PRL is obtained to screen for hyperprolactinemia and pituitary/hypothalamic lesions. Serum beta-hCG and estradiol levels are obtained to screen for malignancy-associated gynecomastia. Detectable levels of beta-hCG implicate a testicular tumor (germ cell or Sertoli cell) or other malignancy (usually lung or liver). Increased serum estradiol levels may result from testicular tumors, increased beta-hCG, liver disease, obesity, adrenal tumors (rare), true hermaphroditism (rare), or aromatase gene gain-of-function mutations (rare). Serum TSH and FT_4 levels are also obtained to screen for hyperthyroidism and hypothyroidism. A karyotype for Klinefelter syndrome is obtained in men with persistent gynecomastia without obvious cause.

C. Imaging and Biopsy

Investigation of unclear cases should include bilateral mammography and a chest CT to search for bronchogenic or metastatic carcinoma. Benign mammographic findings make malignancy very unlikely. Suspicious mammographic findings require ultrasound examination that includes the axilla. Needle biopsy with cytologic examination may be performed on suspicious male breast lesions to distinguish gynecomastia from benign lesions (pseudogynecomastia, lipoma, posttraumatic hematoma/fat necrosis, epidermal inclusion cyst), lymphoma, and male breast cancer. Male breast cancer and gynecomastia may coexist.

Men with a high serum hCG or estradiol levels should have the test confirmed with repeat testing. Confirmed increased levels warrant a testicular ultrasound. If the testicular ultrasound is normal, high serum estradiol levels may warrant a CT of the adrenals; high serum hCG levels may warrant additional CT scanning to detect rare hCG-secreting carcinomas of the lung, mediastinum, liver, stomach, or kidney.

▶ Treatment

Pubertal gynecomastia often resolves spontaneously within 1–2 years. Drug-induced gynecomastia resolves after the offending drug is removed (eg, spironolactone stopped, with substitution of eplerenone). Patients with painful or persistent gynecomastia may be treated with medical therapy, usually for 9–12 months. Generally, it is prudent to treat patients for gynecomastia only when it is a continuing troubling problem.

Selective estrogen receptor modulator (SERM) therapy is effective for true glandular gynecomastia. Raloxifene, 60 mg orally daily, may be somewhat more effective than tamoxifen, 10–20 mg orally daily.

Aromatase inhibitor (AI) therapy is also reasonably effective; anastrozole reduces breast volume significantly over 6 months in adolescents given in a dose of 1 mg orally daily. Serum estradiol levels fall slightly while serum testosterone levels rise. Long-term AI therapy in adolescents is not recommended because of the possibility of inducing osteoporosis and of delaying epiphyseal fusion, which could cause an increase in adult height.

Testosterone therapy for men with hypogonadism may improve or worsen preexistent gynecomastia.

Radiation therapy has been used prophylactically to prevent gynecomastia in men with prostate cancer being treated with antiandrogen therapy. Low-dose prophylactic radiation therapy reduces its incidence from 71% to 28%. Existing gynecomastia improves in 33% with radiation therapy. However, the long-term breast and other cancer risks of such radiation are unknown.

Surgical correction is reserved for patients with persistent or severe gynecomastia.

Ali SN et al. Which patients with gynaecomastia require more detailed investigation? Clin Endocrinol (Oxf). 2018 Mar; 88(3):360–3. [PMID: 29193251]

Chau A et al. Male breast: clinical and imaging evaluations of benign and malignant entities with histologic correlation. Am J Med. 2016 Aug;129(8):776–91. [PMID: 26844632]

MacDonald SM et al. Case records of the Massachusetts General Hospital. Case 32-2016. A 20-year-old man with gynecomastia. N Engl J Med. 2016 Oct 20;375(16):1567–79. [PMID: 27797319]

Sansone A et al. Gynecomastia and hormones. Endocrine. 2017 Jan;55(1):37–44. [PMID: 27145756]

Wibowo E et al. Tamoxifen in men: a review of adverse events. Andrology. 2016 Sep;4(5):776–88. [PMID: 27152880]

HIRSUTISM & VIRILIZATION

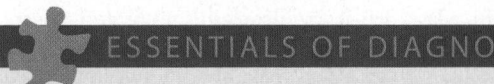

ESSENTIALS OF DIAGNOSIS

▶ Hirsutism, acne, menstrual disorders.

▶ Virilization: muscularity, androgenic alopecia, deepening voice, clitoromegaly.

▶ Rarely, a palpable pelvic tumor.

▶ Urinary 17-ketosteroids, serum DHEAS and androstenedione elevated in adrenal disorders; variable in others.

▶ Serum testosterone is often elevated.

▶ General Considerations

Hirsutism is defined as cosmetically unacceptable terminal hair growth that appears in women in a male pattern. Significant hirsutism affects about 5–10% of non-Asian women of reproductive age and over 40% of women at some point during their life. The amount of hair growth deemed unacceptable depends on a woman's ethnicity and familial and cultural norms. Virilization is defined as the development of male physical characteristics in women, such as pronounced muscle development, deep voice, male pattern baldness, and more severe hirsutism.

▶ Etiology

Hirsutism may be idiopathic or familial or be caused by the following disorders: polycystic ovary syndrome (PCOS), ovarian hyperthecosis, steroidogenic enzyme defects, neoplastic disorders; or rarely by medications, acromegaly, or ACTH-induced Cushing disease.

A. Idiopathic or Familial

Most women with hirsutism or androgenic alopecia have no detectable hyperandrogenism. Patients often have a strong familial predisposition to hirsutism that may be considered normal in the context of their genetic background. Such patients may have elevated serum levels of androstenediol glucuronide, a metabolite of dihydrotestosterone that is produced by skin in cosmetically unacceptable amounts.

B. Polycystic Ovary Syndrome (PCOS, Hyperthecosis, Stein-Leventhal Syndrome)

PCOS is a common functional disorder of the ovaries of unknown etiology (see Chapter 18). It accounts for at least 50% of all cases of hirsutism associated with elevated serum testosterone levels. It is familial and transmitted as a complex polygenic disorder whose phenotypic expression may involve both protective and susceptible genomic variants.

A diagnosis of PCOS must meet three criteria: (1) androgen excess with clinical hyperandrogenism or elevated serum free or total testosterone; (2) ovarian dysfunction with oligoanovulation or polycystic ovary morphology;

and (3) absence of other causes of testosterone excess or anovulation such as pregnancy, thyroid dysfunction, 21-hydroxylase deficiency, neoplastic testosterone secretion, Cushing syndrome, or hyperprolactinemia.

Affected women usually have signs of hyperandrogenism, including hirsutism, acne, or male-pattern thinning of scalp hair; this persists after natural menopause. However, women of East Asian ancestry are less likely to exhibit hirsutism. Most women also have elevated serum testosterone or free testosterone levels. About 70% of affected women have polycystic ovaries on pelvic ultrasound and 50% have oligomenorrhea or amenorrhea with anovulation. Of note, about 30% of women with PCOS do *not* have cystic ovaries and 25–30% of normal menstruating women *have* cystic ovaries.

Obesity and high serum insulin levels (due to insulin resistance) contribute to the syndrome in 70% of women. The serum LH:FSH ratio is often greater than 2.0. Both adrenal and ovarian androgen hypersecretion are commonly present.

C. Steroidogenic Enzyme Defects

Congenital adrenal steroidogenic enzyme defects result in reduced cortisol secretion with a compensatory increase in ACTH that causes adrenal hyperplasia. The most common enzyme defect is 21-hydroxylase deficiency, with a prevalence of about 1:18,000.

Partial deficiency in adrenal 21-hydroxylase can present in women as hirsutism. About 2% of patients with adult-onset hirsutism have been found to have a partial defect in adrenal 21-hydroxylase. The condition is more common in Ashkenazi Jews, Yupic Alaskans, and natives of La Reunion Island. The phenotypic expression is delayed until adolescence or adulthood; such patients do not have salt wasting. Polycystic ovaries and adrenal adenomas are more likely to develop in these women.

D. Neoplastic Disorders

Ovarian tumors are uncommon causes of hirsutism (0.8%) and include arrhenoblastomas, Sertoli-Leydig cell tumors, dysgerminomas, and hilar cell tumors. Adrenal carcinoma is a rare cause of Cushing syndrome and hyperandrogenism that can be quite virilizing. Pure androgen-secreting adrenal tumors occur very rarely; about 50% are malignant.

E. Rare Causes of Hirsutism & Virilization

Acromegaly and ACTH-induced Cushing syndrome are rare causes of hirsutism and virilization. Porphyria cutanea tarda can cause periorbital hair growth in addition to dermatitis in sun-exposed areas. Maternal virilization during pregnancy may occur as a result of a luteoma of pregnancy, hyperreactio luteinalis, or polycystic ovaries. In postmenopausal women, diffuse stromal Leydig cell hyperplasia is a rare cause of hyperandrogenism. Acquired hypertrichosis lanuginosa is manifested by the appearance of diffuse fine lanugo hair growth on the face and body along with stomatologic symptoms; the disorder is usually associated with an internal malignancy, especially colorectal cancer, and

may regress after tumor removal. Pharmacologic causes include minoxidil, cyclosporine, phenytoin, anabolic steroids, interferon, cetuximab, diazoxide, and certain progestins.

▶ Clinical Findings

A. Symptoms and Signs

Modest androgen excess from any source increases sexual hair (chin, upper lip, abdomen, and chest) and increases sebaceous gland activity, producing acne. Menstrual irregularities, anovulation, and amenorrhea are common. If androgen excess is pronounced, defeminization (decrease in breast size, loss of feminine adipose tissue) and virilization (frontal balding, muscularity, clitoromegaly, and deepening of the voice) occur. Virilization points to the presence of an androgen-producing neoplasm.

Hirsutism is quantitated using the Ferriman-Gallwey score in which hirsutism is graded from 0 (none) to 4 (severe) in nine areas of the body with a maximum possible score of 36. Scores below 8 are considered mild hirsutism and normal variants. Scores of 8–15 indicate moderate hirsutism. Scores over 15 indicate severe hirsutism. Of note, the normal score is lower in Asian women and higher in Mediterranean women. The Endocrine Society's Ferriman-Gallwey hirsutism scoring system (https://education.endocrine.org/ferriman-gallwey-hirsutism-system) is recommended.

A pelvic examination may disclose clitoromegaly or ovarian enlargement that may be cystic or neoplastic. Hypertension may be present in Cushing syndrome, adrenal 11-hydroxylase deficiency, or cortisol resistance syndrome.

B. Laboratory Testing and Imaging

Serum androgen testing is mainly useful to screen for rare occult adrenal or ovarian neoplasms. Testing is warranted for women with moderate to severe hirsutism, mild hirsutism with menstrual disturbances, and women with worsening hirsutism despite therapy.

Serum is assayed for total testosterone and free testosterone. A serum testosterone level greater than 200 ng/dL (6.9 nmol/L) or free testosterone greater than 40 ng/dL (140 pmol/L) indicates the need for a manual pelvic examination and ultrasound. If that is negative, an adrenal CT scan is performed. A serum androstenedione level greater than 1000 ng/dL (34.9 nmol/L) also points to an ovarian or adrenal neoplasm.

Patients with a serum DHEAS greater than 700 mcg/dL (35 nmol/L) have an adrenal source of androgen. This usually is due to adrenal hyperplasia and rarely to adrenal carcinoma. Patients with any clinical signs of Cushing syndrome should receive a screening test.

Screening for nonclassical "late-onset" congenital adrenal hyperplasia (CAH) due to 21-hydroxylase deficiency is warranted for women with (1) high serum testosterone or free testosterone levels and (2) hirsutism with normal serum testosterone levels who are at high risk for CAH due to having a family history of hirsutism or being a member of a high-risk ethnic group (eg, Ashkenazi Jews, Croatians,

Iranians, Yupik Inuit). The evaluation requires an early morning blood draw for serum 17-hydroxyprogesterone, ideally during the follicular (early) phase of the menstrual cycle or on a random day for women with irregular menses or amenorrhea. Patients with congenital adrenal hyperplasia usually have a baseline 17-hydroxyprogesterone level greater than 300 ng/dL (9.1 nmol/L). Serum levels of FSH and LH are elevated if amenorrhea is due to ovarian failure. An LH:FSH ratio greater than 2.0 is common in patients with PCOS. On abdominal ultrasound, about 25–30% of normal young women have polycystic ovaries, so the appearance of ovarian cysts on ultrasound is not helpful. Pelvic ultrasound or MRI usually detects virilizing tumors of the ovary. However, small virilizing ovarian tumors may not be detectable on imaging studies; selective venous sampling for testosterone may be used for diagnosis in such patients.

► Treatment

Any drugs causing hirsutism (see above) should be stopped. Any underlying medical causes of hirsutism (eg, Cushing syndrome, acromegaly) should be treated.

A. Surgery

Androgenizing tumors of the adrenal or ovary are resected laparoscopically. Postmenopausal women with severe hyperandrogenism should undergo laparoscopic bilateral oophorectomy (if CT scan of the adrenals and ovaries is normal), since small hilar cell tumors of the ovary may not be visible on scans. Women with classic salt-wasting congenital adrenal hyperplasia and infertility or treatment-resistant hyperandrogenism may be treated with laparoscopic bilateral adrenalectomy.

B. Laser and Topical Treatments

Laser therapy (photoepilation) can be a very effective treatment for facial hirsutism, particularly for women with dark hair and light skin. For women of color, a longer-wavelength laser such as Nd:YAG or diode laser given with skin cooling is used. In such women, laser removal of facial hair significantly improves their appearance and quality of life. Repeated laser treatments are usually required. Accidental eye injuries have been reported; eye shields should be used during treatments. Laser therapy is not recommended for Middle Eastern and Mediterranean women with facial hirsutism, since they have a particularly increased risk of paradoxical hypertrichosis with laser therapy.

Local treatment of facial hirsutism is by shaving or depilatories, waxing, electrolysis, or bleaching. Eflornithine (Vaniqa) 13.9% topical cream retards hair growth when applied twice daily to unwanted facial hair; improvement is noted within 4–8 weeks. Eflornithine may be used during laser therapy for a more dramatic response. However, local skin irritation may occur. Hirsutism returns with discontinuation, unless it is given with laser therapy.

Topical minoxidil may be used to treat androgenic alopecia and is mildly effective when applied to the scalp twice daily. Only the 2% formulation is FDA approved for women.

C. Medications

Oral contraceptives are warranted as an initial therapy for women with hirsutism who are not actively pursuing pregnancy. To reduce the risk of deep venous thrombosis, particularly in women who are obese or over age 39 years, an oral contraceptive with a low-dose of estradiol (20 mcg) is recommended, with a progestin having a relatively low risk of venous thrombosis (norethindrone, norgestimate, levonorgestrel); nevertheless, such oral contraceptives confer over 2-fold increased risk of deep venous thrombosis. Also, levonorgestrel causes insulin resistance, so its use is problematic in women with polycystic ovary syndrome. Oral contraceptives that contain particularly antiandrogenic progestins such as desogestrel (Azurette, Kariva), drospirenone (Yaz, Gianvi), norgestimate (Ortho Tri-Cyclen Lo), or cyproterone acetate (Diane 35, not available in United States) more effectively reduce hirsutism and acne; however, such antiandrogenic oral contraceptives confer a 4-fold risk of deep venous thrombosis, such that their use is discouraged in high-risk patients. Oral contraceptives for hirsutism are given daily and a favored formulation contains norethindrone 1 mg with ethinyl estradiol 20 mcg.

Cyproterone acetate is a unique progestin that is used to treat women with hirsutism worldwide, except in the United States, where it is not FDA-approved. Cyproterone acetate blocks androgen receptors as well as 5-alpha-reductase activity while also suppressing testosterone levels. It is typically prescribed as an oral contraceptive in a dose of 2 mg with ethinyl estradiol 35 mcg.

The risk for arterial thrombosis is increased by 50–100% for all combined oral contraceptives. For this reason, combined oral contraceptives are relatively contraindicated for women who are predisposed to thromboembolism, such as women who are smokers or who have migraines, women who are obese, those with hypertension or a personal history of thromboembolism. Metabolic syndrome and hypertriglyceridemia are seen, particularly with antiandrogenic progestins.

Spironolactone is effective for reducing hirsutism, acne, and androgenic alopecia in women and is a first-line medical strategy for these women. It may be taken in doses of 100–200 mg orally daily (taken as a single dose or in two divided doses) on days 5–25 of the menstrual cycle or daily if used concomitantly with an oral contraceptive. Spironolactone is contraindicated in pregnancy, so reproductive-age women must use reliable contraception during this therapy. Hyperkalemia is an uncommon side effect, but serum potassium should be checked 1 month after beginning therapy or after dosage increases. Spironolactone should be avoided or used cautiously in women who are prone to hyperkalemia, including women with kidney disease or who are taking an ACE inhibitor or ARB for hypertension. Spironolactone should not be given with an oral contraceptive containing drospirenone because the progestin has an anti-mineralocorticoid effect that predisposes to hyperkalemia. Trimethoprim-sulfamethoxazole should not be taken along with high-dose spironolactone. Trimethoprim has potassium-sparing diuretic effects and combining it with spironolactone increases the risk of severe hyperkalemia and sudden death. Side effects of spironolactone include breast tenderness, menstrual irregularity, headaches, nausea, and fatigue, which may improve with continued treatment or dose reduction; paradoxical scalp hair loss has been reported at higher doses. If necessary, metformin can be added and may enhance the anti-hirsutism effect of low-dose spironolactone.

Flutamide and **bicalutamide** inhibit testosterone binding to androgen receptors and also suppress serum testosterone. These drugs can rarely cause severe hepatotoxicity with liver failure. Also, exposure during pregnancy causes fetal malformations and disorders of sexual development in male infants. Therefore, the use of these drugs for hirsutism is discouraged. They should only be used as a last resort for women with severe hirsutism/virilization and only with strict contraceptive precautions and very close monitoring for hepatic toxicity. Flutamide is given orally in a dosage of 250 mg twice daily for the first year and then 125–250 mg/day for maintenance. Flutamide decreases cortisol renal clearance and corticosteroid replacement doses (eg, in congenital adrenal hyperplasia) should be reduced when flutamide is added. Bicalutamide is given in a dosage of 50 mg once daily.

Finasteride inhibits 5-alpha-reductase, the enzyme that converts testosterone to active dihydrotestosterone in the skin. It provides inconsistent reduction in hirsutism and androgenic alopecia over 6 months. Also, this drug causes pseudohermaphroditism in male infants if mistakenly taken during pregnancy. Therefore, the use of finasteride for hirsutism is strongly discouraged.

Metformin alone is ineffective in improving hirsutism, but can enhance the anti-hirsutism effect of spironolactone. Metformin therapy is usually given orally with meals and is started at a dose of 500 mg/day with breakfast for 1 week, then increased to 500 mg with breakfast and dinner. If this dose is clinically insufficient but tolerated, the dose may be increased to 850–1000 mg twice daily. The most common side effects are dose-related gastrointestinal upset and diarrhea or constipation. Metformin appears to be nonteratogenic. Although metformin reduces insulin resistance, it does not cause hypoglycemia in nondiabetic patients. Metformin is contraindicated in severe kidney or liver disease. **GLP-1 agonist** therapy reduced weight and serum testosterone levels in women with PCOS in one short-term study. However, an effect on hirsutism has not been demonstrated clinically.

Simvastatin can reduce hirsutism in women with PCOS. In one study, simvastatin 20 mg orally daily was given to women receiving an oral contraceptive for PCOS. Besides improving their serum lipid profiles, women receiving simvastatin had greater decreases in hirsutism and serum free testosterone levels than the women receiving an oral contraceptive alone. Atorvastatin also reduced serum testosterone by an average of 25% in women with PCOS.

Glucocorticoid replacement is necessary for women with classical congenital adrenal hyperplasia (21-hydroxylase deficiency) with hirsutism and adrenal insufficiency that requires glucocorticoid and mineralocorticoid replacement. However, women with partial "late onset" 21-hydroxylase deficiency are not cortisol deficient and do not require glucocorticoid replacement. Also, glucocorticoids are ineffective in reducing hirsutism in these women. However, such women may require replacement doses of glucocorticoids (prednisone, methylprednisolone) to normalize menses and for ovulation induction. Dexamethasone is not recommended due to its potency and risk of causing iatrogenic Cushing syndrome.

GnRH agonist therapy has been successful in treating postmenopausal women with severe ovarian hyperandrogenism when laparoscopic oophorectomy is contraindicated or declined by the patient.

Barrionuevo P et al. Treatment options for hirsutism: a systematic review and network meta-analysis. J Clin Endocrinol Metab. 2018 Apr;103(4):1258–64. [PMID: 29522176]

Bellver J et al; Group of interest in Reproductive Endocrinology (GIER) of the Spanish Fertility Society (SEF). Polycystic ovary syndrome throughout a woman's life. J Assist Reprod Genet. 2018 Jan;35(1):25–39. [PMID: 28951977]

El-Maouche D et al. Congenital adrenal hyperplasia. Lancet. 2017 Nov 11;390(10108):2194–210. [PMID: 28576284]

Goodman NF et al; American Association of Clinical Endocrinologists (AACE); American College of Endocrinology (ACE); Androgen Excess and PCOS Society (AES). Guide to the best practices in the evaluation and treatment of polycystic ovary syndrome—Part 1. Endocr Pract. 2015 Nov;21(11):1291–300. [PMID: 26509855]

Goodman NF et al; American Association of Clinical Endocrinologists (AACE); American College of Endocrinology (ACE); Androgen Excess and PCOS Society (AES). Guide to the best practices in the evaluation and treatment of polycystic ovary syndrome—Part 2. Endocr Pract. 2015 Dec;21(12):1415–26. [PMID: 26642102]

Martin KA et al. Evaluation and treatment of hirsutism in premenopausal women: an Endocrine Society clinical practice guideline. J Clin Endocrinol Metab. 2018 Apr 1;103(4):1233–57. [PMID: 29522147]

Moretti C et al. Combined oral contraception and bicalutamide in polycystic ovary syndrome and severe hirsutism—a double-blind RTC. J Clin Endocrinol Metab. 2018 Mar 1;103(3):824–38. [PMID: 29211888]

▼ AMENORRHEA & MENOPAUSE

PRIMARY AMENORRHEA

Menarche ordinarily occurs between ages 11 and 15 years (average in the United States: 12.7 years) (see also Chapter 18). The failure of any menses to appear is termed "primary amenorrhea," and evaluation is commenced (1) at age 14 years if neither menarche nor any breast development has occurred or if height is in the lowest 3%, or (2) at age 16 years if menarche has not occurred.

▶ Etiology of Primary Amenorrhea

The differential diagnoses for primary amenorrhea include hypothalamic-pituitary causes, hyperandrogenism, ovarian causes (gonadal dysgenesis, Müllerian dysgenesis), disorders of sexual development (pseudohermaphroditism), uterine causes, and pregnancy.

A. Hypothalamic-Pituitary Causes (With Low or Normal FSH)

The most common cause of primary amenorrhea is a variant of normal known as constitutional delay of growth and puberty, which accounts for about 30% of delayed puberty cases. There is a strong genetic basis for this condition; over 50% of girls with it have a family history of delayed puberty. However, constitutional delay of growth and puberty is a diagnosis of exclusion.

A genetic deficiency of GnRH and gonadotropins may be isolated or associated with other pituitary deficiencies or diminished olfaction (Kallmann syndrome). Hypothalamic lesions, particularly craniopharyngioma, may be present. Pituitary tumors may be nonsecreting or may secrete PRL or GH. Cushing syndrome may be caused by corticosteroid treatment, a cortisol-secreting adrenal tumor, or an ACTH-secreting pituitary tumor. Hypothyroidism can delay adolescence. Head trauma or encephalitis can cause gonadotropin deficiency. Primary amenorrhea may also be caused by severe illness, vigorous exercise (eg, ballet dancing, running), stressful life events, dieting, or anorexia nervosa; however, these conditions should not be assumed to account for amenorrhea without a full endocrinologic evaluation.

B. Uterine Causes (With Normal FSH)

Müllerian agenesis (Mayer-Rokitansky-Küster-Hauser syndrome) results in a missing uterus and variable degrees of upper vaginal hypoplasia. It is the most common cause of permanent primary amenorrhea. Affected women have intact ovaries and undergo an otherwise normal puberty. Such women ovulate and fertility is possible with in vitro fertilization and surrogacy.

An imperforate hymen is occasionally the reason for the absence of visible menses.

C. Hyperandrogenism (With Low or Normal FSH)

Polycystic ovaries and ovarian tumors can secrete excessive testosterone. Excess testosterone can also be secreted by adrenal tumors or by adrenal hyperplasia caused by steroidogenic enzyme defects such as P450c21 deficiency (salt-wasting) or P450c11 deficiency (hypertension). Androgenic steroid abuse may also cause this syndrome.

D. Ovarian Causes (With High FSH)

Gonadal dysgenesis (Turner syndrome and variants) is a frequent cause of primary amenorrhea. Autoimmune ovarian failure is another cause. Rare deficiencies in certain ovarian steroidogenic enzymes are causes of primary hypogonadism without virilization: 3-beta-hydroxysteroid dehydrogenase deficiency (adrenal insufficiency with low serum 17-hydroxyprogesterone) and P450c17 deficiency (hypertension and hypokalemia with high serum 17-hydroxyprogesterone). Deficiency in P450 aromatase (P450arom) activity produces female hypogonadism associated with polycystic ovaries, tall stature, osteoporosis, and virilization.

E. 46 XY Disorders of Sexual Development (Pseudohermaphroditism)

Complete androgen insensitivity syndrome is caused by homozygous inactivating mutations in the androgen receptor. 46 XY individuals with complete androgen insensitivity syndrome are born with completely normal external female genitalia, although some may have labial or inguinal swellings due to cryptorchid testes. Affected individuals are phenotypic girls and experience normal breast development at puberty, but fail to develop sexual hair and have primary amenorrhea.

Partial androgen insensitivity syndrome in 46 XY individuals results in variable degrees of ambiguous genitalia. Newborns have micropenis, hypospadias, and bifid scrotum.

F. Pregnancy (With High hCG)

Pregnancy may be the cause of primary amenorrhea even when the patient refutes having had sexual intercourse.

▶ Clinical Findings

A. Symptoms and Signs

Patients with primary amenorrhea require a thorough history and physical examination to look for signs of the conditions noted above. Headaches or visual field abnormalities implicate a hypothalamic or pituitary tumor. Signs of pregnancy may be present. Blood pressure elevation, acne, and hirsutism should be noted. Short stature may be seen with an associated GH or thyroid hormone deficiency. Short stature with manifestations of gonadal dysgenesis indicates Turner syndrome. Olfactory deficits are seen in Kallmann syndrome. Obesity and short stature may be signs of Cushing syndrome. Tall stature may be due to eunuchoidism or acromegaly. Hirsutism or virilization suggests excessive testosterone.

An external pelvic examination plus a rectal examination should be performed to assess hymen patency and the presence of a uterus.

B. Laboratory and Radiologic Findings

The initial endocrine evaluation should include serum determinations of FSH, LH, PRL, testosterone, TSH, FT_4, and beta-hCG (pregnancy test). Patients who are virilized or hypertensive require serum electrolyte determinations and further hormonal evaluation (see Hirsutism & Virilization, above). MRI of the hypothalamus and pituitary is used to evaluate teens with primary amenorrhea and low or normal FSH and LH—especially those with high PRL levels. Pelvic duplex/color sonography is very useful. Girls who have a normal uterus and high FSH without the classic features of Turner syndrome may require a karyotype to diagnose X chromosome mosaicism.

▶ Treatment

Treatment of primary amenorrhea is directed at the underlying cause. Girls with permanent hypogonadism are treated with HRT.

Batista RL et al. Androgen insensitivity syndrome: a review. Arch Endocrinol Metab. 2018 Mar–Apr;62(2):227–35. [PMID: 29768628]

Choussein S et al. Mullerian dysgenesis: a critical review of the literature. Arch Gynecol Obstet. 2017 Jun;295(6):1369–81. [PMID: 28434104]

Gomez-Lobo V et al; North American Society for Pediatric and Adolescent Gynecology. Disorders of sexual development in adult women. Obstet Gynecol. 2016 Nov;128(5):1162–73. [PMID: 27741188]

SECONDARY AMENORRHEA & MENOPAUSE

Secondary amenorrhea is defined as the absence of menses for 3 consecutive months in women who have passed menarche. Menopause is defined as the terminal episode of naturally occurring menses; it is a retrospective diagnosis, usually made after 6 months of amenorrhea.

▶ **Etiology**

The causes of secondary amenorrhea include pregnancy, hypothalamic-pituitary causes, hyperandrogenism, uterine causes, premature ovarian failure, and menopause.

A. Pregnancy (High hCG)

Pregnancy is the most common cause for secondary amenorrhea in premenopausal women. The differential diagnosis includes rare ectopic secretion of hCG by a choriocarcinoma or bronchogenic carcinoma.

B. Hypothalamic-Pituitary Causes (With Low or Normal FSH)

The hypothalamus must release GnRH in a pulsatile manner for the pituitary to secrete gonadotropins. GnRH pulses occurring more than once per hour favor LH secretion, while less frequent pulses favor FSH secretion. In normal ovulatory cycles, GnRH pulses in the follicular phase are rapid and favor LH synthesis and ovulation; ovarian luteal progesterone is then secreted that slows GnRH pulses, causing FSH secretion during the luteal phase. Most women with hypothalamic amenorrhea have a persistently low frequency of GnRH pulses.

Secondary "hypothalamic" amenorrhea may be caused by stressful life events such as school examinations or leaving home. Such women usually have a history of normal sexual development and irregular menses since menarche. Amenorrhea may also be the result of strict dieting, vigorous exercise, organic illness, or anorexia nervosa. Intrathecal infusion of opioids causes amenorrhea in most women. These conditions should not be assumed to account for amenorrhea without a full physical and endocrinologic evaluation. Young women in whom the results of evaluation and progestin withdrawal test are normal have noncyclic secretion of gonadotropins resulting in anovulation. Such women typically recover spontaneously but should have regular evaluations and a progestin withdrawal test about every 3 months to detect loss of estrogen effect.

PRL elevation due to any cause may cause amenorrhea. Pituitary tumors or other lesions may cause hypopituitarism. Corticosteroid excess of any cause suppresses gonadotropins.

C. Hyperandrogenism (With Low-Normal FSH)

Elevated serum levels of testosterone can cause hirsutism, virilization, and amenorrhea. In PCOS, GnRH pulses are persistently rapid, favoring LH synthesis with excessive androgen secretion; reduced FSH secretion impairs follicular maturation. Progesterone administration can slow the GnRH pulses, thus favoring FSH secretion that induces follicular maturation. Rare causes of secondary amenorrhea include adrenal P450c21 deficiency, ovarian or adrenal malignancies, and Cushing syndrome. Anabolic steroids also cause amenorrhea.

D. Uterine Causes (With Normal FSH)

Infection of the uterus commonly occurs following delivery or D&C but may occur spontaneously. Endometritis due to tuberculosis or schistosomiasis should be suspected in endemic areas. Endometrial scarring may result, causing amenorrhea (Asherman syndrome). Such women typically continue to have monthly premenstrual symptoms. The vaginal estrogen effect is normal.

E. Early and Premature Menopause (With High FSH)

Early menopause refers to primary ovarian failure that occurs before age 45. It affects approximately 5% of women. About 1% of women experience **premature menopause** that is defined as ovarian failure before age 40; about 30% of such cases are due to autoimmunity against the ovary. X chromosome mosaicism accounts for 8% of cases of premature menopause. Other causes include surgical bilateral oophorectomy, radiation therapy for pelvic malignancy, and chemotherapy. Women who have undergone hysterectomy are prone to premature ovarian failure even though the ovaries were left intact. Myotonic dystrophy, galactosemia, and mumps oophoritis are additional causes. Early or premature menopause is frequently familial. Ovarian failure is usually irreversible.

F. Normal Menopause (With High FSH)

Normal menopause refers to primary ovarian failure that occurs after age 45. "Climacteric" is defined as the period of natural physiologic decline in ovarian function, generally occurring over about 10 years. By about age 40 years, the remaining ovarian follicles are those that are the least sensitive to gonadotropins. Increasing titers of FSH are required to stimulate estradiol secretion. Estradiol levels may actually rise during early climacteric.

The normal age for menopause in the United States ranges between 48 and 55 years, with an average of about 51.5 years. Serum estradiol levels fall and the remaining estrogen after menopause is estrone, derived mainly from peripheral aromatization of adrenal androstenedione. Such peripheral production of estrone is enhanced by obesity and liver disease. Individual differences in estrone levels partly explain why the symptoms noted above may be minimal in some women but severe in others.

▶ **Clinical Findings**

A. Symptoms and Signs

See Chapter 18 for symptoms and signs of the menopausal syndrome. Women with premature menopause (before age 45 years), compared to women with normal menopause, have an 50% increased risk of coronary disease, a 23% increased risk for stroke, and a 12% increased overall mortality.

A careful pelvic examination is useful to check for uterine or adnexal enlargement and to obtain a Papanicolaou smear and a vaginal smear for assessment of estrogen effect.

B. Laboratory Findings

1. Premature amenorrhea

An elevated hCG overwhelmingly indicates pregnancy; false-positive testing may occur very rarely with ectopic hCG secretion (eg, choriocarcinoma or bronchogenic carcinoma). Further laboratory evaluation for women who are not pregnant includes serum PRL, FSH and LH (both elevated in menopause), and TSH. Hyperprolactinemia or hypopituitarism (without obvious cause) should prompt an MRI study of the pituitary region. Routine testing of kidney and liver function (BUN, serum creatinine, bilirubin, alkaline phosphatase, and alanine aminotransferase) is also performed. A serum testosterone level is obtained in hirsute or virilized women. Patients with manifestations of hypercortisolism receive a 1-mg overnight dexamethasone suppression test for initial screening. Nonpregnant women without any laboratory abnormality may receive a 10-day course of a progestin (eg, medroxyprogesterone acetate, 10 mg/day); absence of withdrawal menses typically indicates a lack of estrogen or a uterine abnormality.

2. Typical menopause

—No laboratory testing is required to diagnose menopause, when amenorrhea occurs at the expected age. The expected age of menopause correlates with a woman's mother's age at menopause and varies among different kindreds and ethnic groups. An elevated serum FSH with a low or low-normal serum estradiol helps confirm the diagnosis.

▶ Treatment

See Menopausal Syndrome, Chapter 18. Women with night sweats should sleep in a cool room and avoid the use of down comforters. They can try avoiding triggers for hot flushes, such as smoking, alcohol, caffeine, and hot spicy foods. Slow, deep breathing can ameliorate hot flushes. **Aerobic training** for 50 minutes four times weekly reduced all menopausal symptoms except vaginal dryness in a randomized controlled trial. **Clinical hypnosis** reduced hot flushes over 12 weeks in one study. Acupuncture may help alleviate symptoms in some women. Vaginal lubricants can be used daily or 2 hours prior to intercourse.

A. Non-Estrogen Medications

For women with severe hot flushes who cannot take estrogen, SSRIs may offer modest relief effective within a week; escitalopram (10–20 mg/day) can reduce hot flushes significantly, but must not be used by women taking tamoxifen for breast cancer, since it inhibits its metabolism to its active metabolite. Venlafaxine extended release (75 mg/day) may also be effective and does not have a drug interaction with tamoxifen. Sexual dysfunction has not been as significant with the latter drugs when used for vasomotor symptoms,

compared to their use for depression. Gabapentin is also quite effective in oral doses titrated up to 200–800 mg every 8 hours. Side effects such as drowsiness, fatigue, dizziness, and headache, which are most pronounced during the first 2 weeks of therapy, often improve within 4 weeks. An herb, black cohosh, may possibly relieve hot flushes. Tamoxifen and raloxifene offer bone protection but aggravate hot flushes. Women with low serum testosterone levels may experience hypoactive sexual desire disorder that may respond to low-dose testosterone replacement.

B. Estrogen Replacement Therapy

Overall survival is improved among women who begin HRT before age 60 or within 10 years of menopause. However, no survival advantage was found in older women, according to a meta-analysis of 43 randomized controlled trials. Specifically, HRT does not increase the risk of cardiac death or stroke. Breast cancer risk is increased among women taking combined daily estrogen and progestin HRT. Women taking estrogen alone have been variably found to have a decreased risk (Women's Health Initiative, WHI) or an increased risk of breast cancer (California Teachers' Study). Venous thromboembolic disease and stroke are increased by oral but not transdermal estrogen. Osteoporosis risk is reduced by even low-dose systemic estrogen replacement.

In light of these considerations, estrogen replacement is most commonly prescribed for women in early menopause, when symptoms are worst and the benefits are greatest. Transdermal estrogen is favored over oral therapy to reduce the risk of thromboembolism. In women with an intact uterus, estrogen replacement without a progestin risks endometrial hypertrophy and dysfunctional uterine bleeding. The addition of a progestin, however, increases the risk of breast cancer. Therefore, only the smallest effective dose of estrogen should be used to avoid the need for progestins or use them in lower doses or intermittently. Also, progestin may be delivered directly to uterus with progesterone-eluting intrauterine devices. The decision to prescribe menopausal hormonal therapy and its type and duration are dictated by individual symptoms, risk profile, and personal preferences, while considering potential benefits and risks.

1. Benefits of HRT

—Estrogen replacement is the best treatment for hot flushes and sweats and eliminates these symptoms or improves them by more than 70%, usually within a month. Vaginal moisture is improved and libido is enhanced in some women. Estradiol vaginal rings can improve symptoms of an overactive bladder and vaginal dryness. Sleep disturbances are common in menopause and can be reversed with estrogen replacement. Some women notice a mild impairment in memory and cognitive function at menopause that may improve with HRT that is commenced soon after menopause. HRT does not reduce the risk of Alzheimer dementia. However, shortterm transdermal estradiol has been demonstrated to slightly improve memory in women with existent mild to moderate Alzheimer disease. Estrogen replacement may also improve the joint pains, generalized body pain, and reduced physical function experienced by some women at the time of menopause. Women with perimenopausal depression typically experience a significantly improved mood and overall sense of well-being with estrogen replacement. Estrogen replacement does not prevent facial skin wrinkling; however, it may improve facial skin moisture and thickness, reducing seborrhea and atrophy.

Estrogen replacement prevents postmenopausal osteoporosis. The WHI study found that women who received estrogen therapy experienced a reduced number of hip fractures (six fewer fractures/year per 10,000 women) compared with placebo. Even "microdose" transdermal estradiol (0.014 mg/day) preserves bone density.

Women aged 50–59 years in the WHI who received estrogen alone developed significantly lower CT coronary calcium scores (a marker for coronary atherosclerosis) than women receiving placebo. In the California Teachers Study, HRT in women under age 60 was associated with a dramatic 46% reduction in all-cause mortality, particularly cardiovascular disease. This association of HRT and lower mortality may suffer from self-selection bias. Nevertheless, there appears to be a survival advantage of HRT that requires longer-term administration (more than 5 years) to become apparent. The survival advantage is particularly strong for women under age 60 and diminishes with age; no reduction in mortality was noted in the group of women aged 85–94 years. The reduction in cardiovascular disease among younger postmenopausal women taking HRT may be explained by the reduction in serum levels of atherogenic lipoprotein(a) with HRT, with or without a progestin. Improvement in serum HDL cholesterol is greatest with unopposed estrogen but is also seen with the addition of a progestin.

A. Estrogen replacement without progestin (unopposed HRT)—The WHI study reported that postmenopausal women taking unopposed estrogen had a *reduction in breast cancer risk*, whereas the California Teachers' Study reported an *increase in breast cancer risk* among such women. Unopposed estrogen replacement improves glycemic control in women with type 2 diabetes mellitus. Perimenopause-related depression is improved by unopposed estrogen replacement; the addition of a progestin may negate this effect. A 20-year study of 8801 women living in a retirement community found that estrogen use was associated with improved survival. Age-adjusted mortality rates were 56.4 (per 1000 person-years) among nonusers and 50.4 among women who had used estrogen for 15 years or longer.

B. Estrogen replacement therapy with progestins (combined HRT)—Women receiving conventional-dose daily conjugated estrogen and medroxyprogesterone acetate (0.625 mg and 2.5 mg, respectively) for an average of 5.6 years, experienced a lower risk of developing diabetes mellitus (3.5%) versus those taking a placebo (4.2%).

2. Risks of HRT—Oral estrogen increases the risk of arterial and venous thrombotic events in a dose-dependent manner, although the absolute risk is small. The WHI study found that women who received long-term conventional oral combined HRT had an increased risk of deep venous thrombosis (3.5 per 1000 person-years) compared with

women receiving placebo (1.7 per 1000 person-years). Oral estrogen also increases the risk of ischemic stroke by about 30%. Oral estrogen causes a particularly increased risk for thromboembolic disease among older women and those with increased stroke proclivity (current smokers and those with hypertension, atrial fibrillation, prior thromboembolic event). Long-term use of oral conjugated estrogens in women over age 65 has been associated with poorer cognitive performance, perhaps due to small strokes. Transdermal or vaginal estrogen administration avoids this risk. Urinary stress incontinence appears to be increased by conventional-dose oral estrogen replacement, whereas topical vaginal estrogen may have a beneficial effect. Estrogen replacement may cause mastalgia that typically responds to dose reduction. Estrogen replacement also appears to increase the risk of seizures in women with epilepsy. Estrogen can stimulate the growth of untreated large pituitary prolactinomas. Oral estrogen and SERMs also increase the risk of gastroesophageal reflux disease. Oral HRT can increase the size of hepatic hemangiomas, but significant enlargement is uncommon. Conventional doses of estrogen carry higher risks than lower doses. The risks for HRT also depend on whether estrogen is administered alone (unopposed HRT) or with a progestin (combined HRT).

A. Estrogen replacement without progestin (unopposed HRT)—The California Teachers' Study reported an *increased breast cancer risk* among such women while the WHI study reported that postmenopausal women taking unopposed estrogen had a *reduced breast cancer risk*. Women taking lower-dose unopposed estrogen therapy would be expected to have a lower long-term risk of breast cancer compared to women taking high-dose estrogens.

Conventional-dose unopposed conjugated estrogen replacement (0.625–1.25 mg daily) increases the risk of endometrial hyperplasia and dysfunctional uterine bleeding, which often prompts patients to stop the estrogen. However, lower-dose unopposed estrogen confers a much lower risk of dysfunctional uterine bleeding. Recurrent dysfunctional bleeding necessitates a pelvic examination and possibly an endometrial biopsy. There has been considerable concern that unopposed estrogen replacement might increase the risk for endometrial carcinoma. However, a Cochrane Database Review found no increased risk of endometrial carcinoma in a review of 30 randomized controlled trials. Therefore, lower-dose unopposed estrogen replacement does not appear to confer any significant increased risk for endometrial cancer.

Long-term conventional-dose unopposed estrogen increases the mortality risk from ovarian cancer, although the absolute risk is small. The annual age-adjusted ovarian cancer death rates for women taking estrogen replacement for 10 years or longer are 64:100,000 for current users, 38:100,000 for former users, and 26:100,000 for women who had never taken estrogen. Lower-dose estrogen replacement is believed to confer a negligible increased risk for ovarian cancer.

The risk of stroke among women taking a conventional dose of unopposed estrogen is increased; the risk is about 44 strokes per 10,000 person-years versus about 32 per

10,000 person-years in women taking placebo. Transdermal or transvaginal estrogen is not thought to increase the risk of stroke.

Oral estrogens can cause hypertriglyceridemia, particularly in women with preexistent hyperlipidemia, rarely resulting in pancreatitis. Postmenopausal estrogen therapy also slightly increases the risk of gallstones and cholecystitis. These side effects may be reduced or avoided by using transdermal or vaginal estrogen replacement.

B. Estrogen replacement with a progestin (combined HRT)—Long-term conventional-dose oral combined HRT increases breast density and the risk for abnormal mammograms (9.4% versus 5.4% for placebo). There is also a higher risk of breast cancer (8 cases per 10,000 women/year versus 6.5 cases per 10,000 women/year for placebo); the increased risk of breast cancer is highest shortly after menopause (about 2 cases per 1000 women annually). This increased risk for breast cancer appears to mostly affect relatively thin women with a BMI less than 24.4. The Iowa Women's Health Study reported an increase in breast cancer with HRT only in women consuming more than 1 oz of alcohol weekly. No accelerated risk of breast cancer has been seen in users of HRT who have benign breast disease or a family history of breast cancer. Women in whom new-onset breast tenderness develops with combined HRT have an increased risk of breast cancer, compared with women without breast tenderness.

The Women's Health Initiative Mental Study (WHIMS) followed the effect of combined conventional-dose oral HRT on cognitive function in women 65–79 years old. HRT did not protect these older women from cognitive decline. In fact, they experienced an increased risk for severe dementia at a rate of 23 more cases/year for every 10,000 women over age 65 years. It is unknown whether this finding applies to younger postmenopausal women.

In the WHI study, women receiving conventional-dose combined oral HRT experienced an increased risk of stroke (31 strokes per 10,000 women/year versus 26 strokes per 10,000 women/year for placebo). Stroke risk was also increased by hypertension, diabetes, and smoking.

Women taking combined oral estrogen–progestin replacement do not experience an increased risk of ovarian cancer. They do experience a slightly increased risk of developing asthma.

Progestins may cause moodiness, particularly in women with a history of premenstrual dysphoric disorder. Cycled progestins may trigger migraines in certain women. Many other adverse reactions have been reported, including breast tenderness, alopecia, and fluid retention. Contraindications to the use of progestins include thromboembolic disorders, liver disease, breast cancer, and pregnancy.

3. HRT agents—Hormone replacement needs to be individualized. Ideally, in women with an intact uterus, very low-dose transdermal estradiol may be used alone or with intermittent progestin or a progesterone-eluting intrauterine device, in order to reduce the risk of endometrial hyperplasia, while avoiding the need for daily oral progestin. Vaginal estrogen can be added if low-dose systemic estradiol replacement is insufficient to relieve symptoms of vulvovaginal atrophy. Women who have had a hysterectomy may receive transdermal estrogen at whatever is the lowest dose that adequately relieves symptoms. However, some women cannot find sufficient relief with transdermal estradiol and must use an oral preparation.

A. Transdermal estradiol—Estradiol can be delivered systemically with different systems of skin patches, mists, or gels. Transdermal estradiol works for most women, but some women have poor transdermal absorption. If a woman has a skin reaction to an estradiol patch, then a gel or mist may be tried at different doses until the ideal formulation is found.

(1) Estradiol patches mixed with adhesive—These systems tend to cause minimal skin irritation. Generic estradiol transdermal is available as a patch that is replaced biweekly (0.025, 0.0375, 0.05, 0.075, 0.1 mg/day) or weekly (0.025, 0.0375, 0.05, 0.06, 0.075, 0.1 mg/day). Brand products include: Vivelle-Dot (0.025) or Minivivelle (0.0375, 0.05, 0.075, or 0.1 mg/day) or Alora (0.025, 0.05, 0.075, or 0.1 mg/day), replaced twice weekly; Climara (0.025, 0.0375, 0.05, 0.06, 0.075, or 0.1 mg/day), replaced weekly; and Menostar (0.014 mg/day), replaced weekly. This type of estradiol skin patch can be cut in half and applied to the skin without proportionately greater loss of potency. Minivivelle patches are the smallest.

(2) Estradiol mists and gels—Evamist is available as a topical mist dispenser that dispenses 1.53 mg estradiol/spray; 1–3 sprays are applied to the inner forearm daily; a single daily spray may provide sufficiently low-dose estradiol to possibly obviate the need for daily progestin in women with an intact uterus. EstroGel 0.06% is available in a metered-dose pump that dispenses 1.25 g gel per actuation (dose: half to 2 actuations/day). Elestrin 0.06% is available in a metered-dose pump that dispenses 0.87 g gel per activation (dose: half to 2 actuations/day). These gels are applied daily to one arm from the wrist to the shoulder after bathing. Divigel 0.1% gel (0.25, 0.5, 1 g/packet) is applied to the upper thigh daily. Estrasorb 2.5% is available in 1.74-g pouches (4.35 mg estradiol); 1–2 pouches of lotion are applied to the thigh/calf daily. To avoid spreading topical estradiol to others, the hands should be washed and precautions taken to avoid prolonged skin contact with children. Application of sunscreen prior to estradiol gel has been reported to *increase* the transdermal absorption of estradiol.

(3) Estradiol patches with progestin mixed with adhesive—These preparations mix estradiol with either norethindrone acetate or levonorgestrel. Combipatch (0.05 mg E with 0.14 mg norethindrone acetate daily or 0.05 mg E with 0.25 mg norethindrone acetate daily) is replaced twice weekly. Climara Pro (0.045 mg E with 0.015 mg levonorgestrel daily) is replaced once weekly. The addition of a progestin reduces the risk of endometrial hyperplasia, but breakthrough bleeding occurs commonly. The combined patch increases the risk of breast cancer. Scalp hair loss, acne, weight gain, skin reactions, and poor skin adherence have been reported with these patches.

B. Oral estrogen—

(1) Oral estrogen-only preparations—These preparations include conjugated equine estrogens that are available

as Premarin (0.3, 0.45, 0.625, 0.9, and 1.25 mg), conjugated plant-derived estrogens (eg, Menest, 0.3, 0.625, and 2.5 mg), and conjugated synthetic estrogens that are available as Cenestin (0.3, 0.45, 0.625, 0.9, and 1.25 mg) and Enjuvia (0.3, 0.45, 0.625, 0.9, and 1.25 mg). Other preparations include estradiol (0.5, 1, and 2 mg), and estropipate (0.75, 1.5, and 3 mg).

(2) Oral estrogen plus progestin preparations—Conjugated equine estrogens with medroxyprogesterone acetate is available as Prempro (0.3/1.5, 0.45/1.5, 0.625/2.5, and 0.625 mg/5 mg); conjugated equine estrogens for 14 days cycled with conjugated equine estrogens plus medroxyprogesterone acetate for 14 days is available as Premphase (0.625/0, then 0.625 mg/5 mg); estradiol with norethindrone acetate (0.5/0.1 and 1 mg/0.5 mg); ethinyl estradiol with norethindrone acetate is available as Femhrt (2.5/0.5 and 5 mcg/1 mg) and Jinteli (5 mcg/1 mg); estradiol with drospirenone is available as Angeliq (0.5 mg/0.25 mg, and 1.0 mg/0.5 mg); estradiol with norgestimate is available as Prefest (estradiol 1 mg/day for 3 days, alternating with 1 mg estradiol/0.09 mg norgestimate daily for 3 days). Oral contraceptives can also be used for combined HRT.

C. Vaginal Estrogen—Vaginal estrogen is intended to deliver estrogen directly to local tissues and is moderately effective in reducing symptoms of urogenital atrophy, while minimizing systemic estrogen exposure. Some estrogen is absorbed systemically and can relieve menopausal symptoms. Vaginal estrogen can be used without a break at low doses or in women who have had a hysterectomy. To reduce the risk of endometrial proliferation and dysfunctional bleeding, manufacturers recommend that these preparations be used for only 3–6 months and for only 3 out of every 4 weeks in women with an intact uterus, since vaginal estrogen can cause endometrial proliferation. However, most clinicians use them for longer periods and without cycling. Vaginal estrogen can be administered in three different ways: creams, tablets, and rings.

(1) Estrogen vaginal creams—These creams are administered intravaginally with a measured-dose applicator daily for 2 weeks for atrophic vaginitis, then administered one to three times weekly. Available preparations include *conjugated equine estrogens,* which is available as Premarin Vaginal (0.625 mg/g cream), dosed as 0.25–2 g cream administered vaginally one to three times weekly. *Estradiol* is available as Estrace Vaginal (0.1 mg/g cream), 1 g cream administered vaginally one to two times weekly.

(2) Estradiol vaginal tablets and softgel inserts—*Vagifem and Yuvafem* (generic equivalent) are available as 10 mcg tablets. *Imvexxy* is a softgel vaginal insert (4 mcg or 10 mcg estradiol in a coconut oil base). Either preparation can be administered intravaginally daily for 2 weeks for atrophic vaginitis, then twice weekly.

(3) Estradiol vaginal rings—These rings are inserted manually into the upper third of the vagina, worn continuously, and replaced every 3 months. Only a small amount of the released estradiol enters the systemic circulation. Vaginal rings do not usually interfere with sexual intercourse. If a ring is removed or descends into the introitus, it may be washed in warm water and reinserted. *Estring* (2 mg estradiol/ring) releases 17-beta-estradiol 7.5 mcg/day

with only 8% entering the systemic circulation, resulting in mean serum estradiol concentrations of only about 10 pg/mL; it is most effective for local vaginal symptoms. *Femring* releases estradiol acetate that is quickly hydrolyzed to estradiol and is available in two strengths: 12.4 mg/ring releases estradiol acetate 0.05 mg/day or 24.8 mg/ring releases estradiol acetate 0.1 mg/day, resulting in mean serum estradiol concentrations of about 40 pg/mL and 80 pg/mL, respectively; it is effective for both systemic and local vaginal symptoms. Both rings are replaced every 90 days. For women with postmenopausal urinary urgency and frequency, even the low-dose Estring can successfully reduce urinary symptoms.

(4) Estradiol with progestin vaginal rings—The available preparation is NuvaRing that releases a mixture of ethinyl estradiol 0.015 mg/day and etonogestrel 0.12 mg/day. It is a contraceptive vaginal ring that is placed in the vagina on or before day 5 of the menstrual cycle, left for 3 weeks, removed for 1 week, and then replaced.

D. Estradiol Injections—Parenteral estradiol should be used only for particularly severe menopausal symptoms when other measures have failed or are contraindicated. Estradiol cypionate (Depo-Estradiol 5 mg/mL) may be administered intramuscularly in doses of 1–5 mg every 3–4 weeks. Estradiol valerate (20 or 40 mg/mL) may be administered intramuscularly in doses of 10–20 mg every 4 weeks. Women with an intact uterus should receive progestin for the last 10 days of each cycle.

E. Oral Progestins—For a woman with an intact uterus, long-term conventional-dose unopposed systemic estrogen therapy can cause endometrial hyperplasia, which typically results in dysfunctional uterine bleeding and might rarely lead to endometrial cancer. Progestin therapy transforms proliferative into secretory endometrium, causing a possible menses when given intermittently or no bleeding when given continuously.

The type of progestin preparation, its dosage, and the timing of administration may be tailored to the given situation. Progestins may be given daily, monthly, or at longer intervals. When given episodically, progestins are usually administered for 7- to 14-day periods. Bedtime administration may improve sleep. Some women find that progestins produce adverse effects, such as irritability, nausea, fatigue, or headache; long-term progestins given with estrogen replacement increase the risk for breast cancer.

Oral progestins are available in different formulations: Micronized progesterone (100 mg and 200 mg/capsule), medroxyprogesterone (2.5, 5.0, and 10 mg/tablet), norethindrone acetate (5 mg/tablet), and norethindrone (0.35 mg/tablet). Topical progesterone (20–50 mg/day) may reduce hot flushes in women who are intolerant to oral HRT. It may be applied to the upper arms, thighs, or inner wrists daily. It may be compounded as micronized progesterone 250 mg/mL in a transdermal gel. Its effects upon the breast and endometrium are unknown. Progesterone is also available as vaginal gels (eg, Prochieve, 4% = 45 mg/applicatorful, and 8% = 90 mg/applicatorful) that are typically given for secondary amenorrhea and administered vaginally every other day for six doses.

F. VAGINAL PROGESTERONE—Vaginal progesterone minimizes dysfunctional uterine bleeding while reducing systemic progesterone exposure. Crinone and Prochieve are available as a 4% and 8% gel with 45 mg and 90 mg per applicatorful, respectively. Endometrin comes as a 100 mg vaginal insert. Administered twice weekly with daily estrogen, most women experience no endometrial hypertrophy or dysfunctional uterine bleeding.

G. PROGESTIN-RELEASING INTRAUTERINE DEVICES—Intrauterine devices that release progestins can be useful for women receiving ERT, since they can reduce the incidence of dysfunctional uterine bleeding and endometrial carcinoma without exposing women to the significant risks of systemic progestins. The Mirena intrauterine device releases levonorgestrel and is inserted into the uterus by a clinician within 7 days of the onset of menses. It is equally effective at reducing endometrial hyperplasia as cycled medroxyprogesterone acetate and is associated with less hirsutism. It remains effective for up to 5 years. Parous women are generally better able to tolerate the Mirena intrauterine device than nulliparous women.

H. SELECTIVE ESTROGEN RECEPTOR MODULATORS—SERMs (eg, raloxifene, ospemifene, tamoxifen) are an alternative to estrogen replacement for hypogonadal women at risk for osteoporosis who prefer not to take estrogens because of their contraindications (eg, breast or uterine cancer) or side effects (see Osteoporosis, above). Raloxifene (Evista) does not reduce hot flushes, vaginal dryness, skin wrinkling, or breast atrophy; it does not improve cognition. However, in doses of 60 mg/day orally, it inhibits bone loss without stimulating effects upon the breasts or endometrium. Raloxifene does not stimulate the endometrium and actually reduces the risk of endometrial carcinoma, so concomitant progesterone therapy is not required. Another advantage to raloxifene is that it reduces the risk of invasive breast cancer by about 50%. Raloxifene slightly increases the risk of venous thromboembolism (though less so than tamoxifen), so it should not be used by women at prolonged bed rest or otherwise prone to thrombosis. Ospemifene (Osphena) is a SERM that has unique estrogen-like effects on the vaginal epithelium and is indicated for the treatment of postmenopausal dyspareunia when other therapies are ineffective. Given orally in doses of 60 mg/day, it commonly aggravates hot flushes but has an estrogenic effect upon bone and slows bone loss in menopause. It does not usually cause endometrial hypertrophy. Ospemifene has unknown long-term effects upon the breast.

Tibolone (Livial) is a SERM whose metabolites have mixed estrogenic, progestogenic, and weak androgenic activity. It is comparable to HRT for the treatment of climacteric-related complaints. It does not appear to significantly stimulate proliferation of breast or endometrial tissue. It depresses both serum triglycerides and HDL cholesterol. Long-term studies are lacking. It is not available in the United States.

I. ANDROGEN REPLACEMENT THERAPY IN WOMEN—In premenopausal women, serum testosterone levels decline with age. Between 25 and 45 years of age, women's testosterone levels fall 50%. After natural menopause, the ovaries remain a significant source for testosterone and serum testosterone levels do not fall abruptly. In contrast, very low serum testosterone levels are found in women after bilateral oophorectomy, autoimmune ovarian failure, or adrenalectomy, and in hypopituitarism. Testosterone deficiency contributes to hot flushes, loss of sexual hair, muscle atrophy, osteoporosis, and diminished libido, also known as hypoactive sexual desire disorder (see Chapter 25). Selected women may be treated with low-dose testosterone. Methyltestosterone can be compounded into capsules and taken orally in doses of 1.25–2.5 mg daily. Testosterone can also be compounded as a cream containing 1 mg/mL, with 1 mL applied to the abdomen daily. Methyltestosterone also is available combined with esterified estrogens: 1.25 mg methyltestosterone/0.626 mg esterified estrogens or 2.5 mg methyltestosterone/1.25 mg esterified estrogens. The latter formulations are convenient but carry the same disadvantages as oral estrogen—particularly an increased risk of thromboembolism.

Women receiving androgen therapy must be monitored for the appearance of any acne or hirsutism, and serum testosterone levels are determined periodically if women feel that they are benefitting and long-term testosterone therapy is instituted. Side effects of low-dose testosterone therapy are usually minimal but may include erythrocytosis, emotional changes, hirsutism, acne, an adverse effect on lipids, and potentiation of warfarin anticoagulation therapy. Testosterone therapy tends to reduce both triglyceride and HDL cholesterol levels. Hepatocellular neoplasms and peliosis hepatis, rare complications of oral androgens at higher doses, have not been reported with oral methyltestosterone doses of 2.5 mg or less daily.

Vaginal androgen is an option for postmenopausal women who are experiencing vaginal dryness and reduced sexual satisfaction. It is also an option for women who cannot use systemic or vaginal estrogen due to breast cancer. Testosterone cream 150–300 mcg (formulated) is administered vaginally daily for 2 weeks and then three times weekly. It improves sexual satisfaction while reducing vaginal dryness and dyspareunia without increasing systemic estrogen or testosterone levels. Prasterone 0.5% vaginal (Intrarosa) is a formulation of DHEA that is available as a 6.5 mg tablet that is inserted vaginally nightly at bedtime. It is indicated for relief of moderate to severe dyspareunia of menopause. However, it is contraindicated in women with breast cancer.

Caution: *Androgens should not be given to women with liver disease or during pregnancy or breastfeeding.* Testosterone replacement therapy for women should be used judiciously, since long-term prospective clinical trials are lacking. An analysis of the Nurses' Health Study found that women who had been taking conjugated equine estrogens plus methyltestosterone experienced an increased risk of breast cancer, so breast cancer screening is recommended.

Committee on Gynecologic Practice. Committee Opinion No. 698: Hormone therapy in primary ovarian insufficiency. Obstet Gynecol. 2017 May;129(5):e134–41. [PMID: 28426619]

Davis SR et al. Intravaginal testosterone improves sexual satisfaction and vaginal symptoms associated with aromatase inhibitors. J Clin Endocrinol Metab. 2018 Nov 1;103(11):4145–54. [PMID: 30239842]

Gordon CM et al. Functional hypothalamic amenorrhea: an Endocrine Society clinical practice guideline. J Clin Endocrinol Metab. 2017 May 1;102(5):1413–39. [PMID: 28368518]

Grossman DC et al. Hormone therapy for the primary prevention of chronic conditions in postmenopausal women: US Preventive Services Task Force Recommendation Statement. JAMA. 2017 Dec 12;318(22):2224–33. [PMID: 29234814]

Moreno AC et al. Genitourinary syndrome of menopause in breast cancer survivors: treatments are available. Cleve Clin J Med. 2018 Oct;85(10):760–6. [PMID: 30289755]

Muka T et al. Association of age at onset of menopause and time since onset of menopause with cardiovascular outcomes, intermediate vascular traits, and all-cause mortality: a systematic review and meta-analysis. JAMA Cardiol. 2016 Oct; 1(7):767–76. [PMID: 27627190]

TURNER SYNDROME (Gonadal Dysgenesis)

ESSENTIALS OF DIAGNOSIS

► Short stature with normal GH levels.

► Primary amenorrhea or early ovarian failure.

► Epicanthal folds, webbed neck, short fourth metacarpals.

► Renal and cardiovascular anomalies.

Turner syndrome comprises a group of X chromosome disorders that are associated with spontaneous abortion, primary hypogonadism, short stature, and other phenotypic anomalies (Table 26–15). It affects 1–2% of fetuses, of which about 97% abort, accounting for about 10% of all spontaneous abortions. Nevertheless, it affects about 1 in every 2500 live female births. Patients with the classic syndrome (about 50% of cases) lack one of the two X chromosomes (45,XO karyotype). About 12% of patients harbor mosaicism for Y chromosome sequences. Other patients with Turner syndrome have X chromosome abnormalities, such as ring X or Xq (X/abnormal X) or X chromosome deletions affecting all or some somatic cells (mosaicism, XX/XO).

1. Classic Turner Syndrome (45,XO Gonadal Dysgenesis)

► Clinical Findings

A. Symptoms and Signs

Features of Turner syndrome are variable and may be subtle in girls with mosaicism. Turner syndrome may be diagnosed in infant girls at birth, since they tend to be small and may exhibit severe lymphedema. Evaluation for childhood short stature often leads to the diagnosis. Girls and women with Turner syndrome have an increased risk of aortic coarctation and bicuspid aortic valves; these cardiac abnormalities are more common in patients with a webbed neck. Typical manifestations in adulthood include short stature, hypogonadism, webbed neck, high-arched palate,

Table 26–15. Manifestations of Turner syndrome.

Short stature (98%)	Coarctation (14%) and cystic medial necrosis of the aorta
Head and neck features	
High-arched palate (35%)	Hypertension (50%, idiopathic or due to coarctation or kidney disease)
Low posterior hairline (40%)	
Micrognathia (60%)	
Pterygium colli (40% webbed neck)	Partial anomalous pulmonary venous return (18%)
Eye abnormalities	Gastrointestinal disorders
Cataracts, corneal opacities	Achlorhydria
Epicanthal folds (20%), strabismus (15%), ptosis (10%)	Celiac disease (8%)
	Colon carcinoma
Gonadal abnormalities	Hepatic transaminases elevated (65%)
Gonadal dysgenesis (primary amenorrhea 80%) or early ovarian failure (20%)	Inflammatory bowel disease (3%)
	Telangiectasias with bleeding
Skeletal and extremity abnormalities	Kidney abnormalities (60%)
Broad (shield) chest (30%) with wide-spaced hypoplastic nipples	Horseshoe kidney (10%), duplication or abnormal positioning of renal pelvis or ureters (15%)
Cubitus valgus of arms (50%) and knock knees (35%)	CNS disorders
Lymphedema of hands and feet (30%)	Emotional immaturity (40%)
Madelung wrist deformity (5%)	Learning disabilities and ADHD (40%)
Osteopenia (65%)	Sensorineural hearing loss
Scoliosis (10%)	Skin and nail disorders
Short fourth metacarpals (40%)	Hyperconvex nails
Ear abnormalities	Keloid formation
Conductive hearing loss (30%) and recurrent otitis media (60%)	Pigmented nevi
	Associated conditions
Low-set and posteriorly rotated ears	Diabetes mellitus (10%) or glucose intolerance (35%)
Cardiovascular anomalies	Dyslipidemia
Aortic dilation or aneurysm (25% with bicuspid aortic valve)	Hashimoto thyroiditis (37%)
	Hyperuricemia
	Neuroblastoma (1%)
Bicuspid aortic valve (30%) with aortic stenosis or regurgitation	Obesity
	Rheumatoid arthritis

ADHD, attention deficit/hyperactivity disorder; CNS, central nervous system.

wide-spaced nipples, hypertension, and kidney abnormalities (Table 26–15). Emotional disorders are common. Affected women are also more prone to autoimmune disease, particularly thyroiditis, inflammatory bowel disease, and celiac disease.

Hypogonadism presents as "delayed adolescence" (primary amenorrhea, 80%) or early ovarian failure (20%); girls with 45,XO Turner (blood karyotyping) who enter puberty are typically found to have mosaicism if other tissues are karyotyped.

B. Laboratory Findings

Hypogonadism is confirmed in girls who have high serum levels of FSH and LH. A blood karyotype showing 45,XO (or X chromosome abnormalities or mosaicism) establishes the diagnosis. GH and IGF-1 levels are normal.

C. Imaging

A transthoracic ultrasound and MRI scan of the chest and abdomen should be done in all patients with Turner syndrome to determine whether cardiac, aortic, and renal abnormalities are present.

▶ Treatment

For short stature, GH therapy should be started early, ideally by age 4–6 and before age 12 years. GH is given subcutaneously in doses of 50 mcg/kg/day or 4.5 international units/m²/day; the GH dose is titrated to keep the serum IGF-I levels within 3 SD above the mean for age. Rarely, GH treatment causes pseudotumor cerebri. The oral androgen oxandrolone (0.03–0.05 mg/kg/day) is added after age 10 for girls whose growth is inadequate with GH therapy alone. After age 12 years, estrogen therapy is begun with low doses of transdermal estradiol, with a gradual increase in dose over 2–3 years. Progesterone is added after 2 years of estrogen therapy or if menstrual bleeding occurs. For girls age 12 years or older with Turner mosaicism and spontaneous menses, early oocyte retrieval and cryopreservation should be considered, while weighing the risks of pregnancy.

▶ Complications & Surveillance

Women with Turner syndrome have a reduced life expectancy due in part to their increased risk of diabetes mellitus (types 1 and 2), hypertension, dyslipidemia, and osteoporosis. Patients are prone to keloid formation after surgery or ear piercing. Annual surveillance should include a blood pressure determination and laboratory evaluations that include a serum TSH, liver enzymes, BUN, creatinine, and fasting serum lipids and glucose. Celiac disease screening (serum TTG IgA Ab) is warranted every 2–5 years for school-age girls and then whenever indicated clinically. Audiology exams are recommended every 1–5 years. Bone mineral densitometries should be measured periodically for women over age 18 years.

Bicuspid aortic valves are common and are associated with an increased risk of infective endocarditis, aortic valvular stenosis or regurgitation, and ascending aortic root dilation and dissection. The risk of aortic dissection is increased more than 100-fold in women with Turner syndrome, particularly those with pronounced neck webbing and shield chest. Patients with aortic root enlargement are usually treated with beta-blockade and serial imaging.

About 5% of women with Turner syndrome experience natural pregnancy and even more can become pregnant with oocyte donation. Such pregnancies are very high-risk, with increased fetal morbidity and preeclampsia. During pregnancy, women with Turner syndrome have a 2% risk of aortic dissection or rupture, so they require close monitoring with repeated echocardiography; those with aortic root diameter 4 cm or more are delivered by elective caesarean section, whereas those with an aortic root diameter less than 4 cm may deliver vaginally.

Partial anomalous pulmonary vein connections can lead to left-to-right shunting of blood. Adults with Turner syndrome also have a high incidence of ECG abnormalities, such as long QT syndrome.

Patients with the classic 45,XO karyotype have a high risk of renal structural abnormalities, whereas those with 46 X/abnormal X are more prone to malformations of the urinary collecting system.

2. Turner Syndrome Variants

A. 46,X (Abnormal X) Karyotype

Patients with small distal short arm deletions of the X chromosome (Xp-) that include the *SHOX* gene often have short stature and skeletal abnormalities but have a low risk of ovarian failure. Transmission of Turner syndrome from mother to daughter can occur. There may be an increased risk of trisomy 21 in the conceptuses of women with Turner syndrome. Patients with deletions of the long arm of the X chromosome (distal to Xq24) often have amenorrhea without short stature or other features of Turner syndrome. Abnormalities or deletions of other genes located on both the long and short arms of the X chromosome can produce gonadal dysgenesis with few other somatic features.

B. 45,XO/46,XX and 45,XO/46,XY Mosaicism

45,XO/46,XX mosaicism results in a modified form of Turner syndrome. Such girls tend to be taller and may have more gonadal function and fewer other manifestations of Turner syndrome.

45,XO/46,XY mosaicism can produce some manifestations of Turner syndrome. Patients may have ambiguous genitalia or male infertility with an otherwise normal phenotype. Germ cell tumors, such as gonadoblastomas and seminomas, develop in about 10% of patients with 45,XO/46,XY mosaicism; most such tumors are benign.

Cintron D et al. Effect of estrogen replacement therapy on bone and cardiovascular outcomes in women with Turner syndrome: a systematic review and meta-analysis. Endocrine. 2017 Feb;55(2):366–75. [PMID: 27473099]

Gravholt CH et al; International Turner Syndrome Consensus Group. Clinical practice guidelines for the care of girls and women with Turner syndrome: proceedings from the 2016 Cincinnati International Turner Syndrome Meeting. Eur J Endocrinol. 2017 Sep;177(3):G1–70. [PMID: 28705803]

▼ CLINICAL USE OF CORTICOSTEROIDS

Prolonged treatment with high-dose corticosteroids causes toxic effects that can be life threatening. Besides oral and parenteral administration, transdermal and inhaled corticosteroids have some systemic absorption and can cause similar adverse effects. Patients should be thoroughly informed of the major possible side effects of treatment: insomnia, cognitive and personality changes, weight gain with central obesity, skin thinning and bruising, striae, muscle weakness, polyuria, renal calculi, diabetes mellitus, glaucoma, cataracts, sex hormone suppression, candidiasis,

Table 26–16. Management of patients receiving systemic corticosteroids.

Recommendations for prescribing
- Do not administer systemic corticosteroids unless absolutely indicated or more conservative measures have failed.
- Keep dosage and duration of administration to the minimum required for adequate treatment.

Monitoring recommendations
- Screen for tuberculosis with a purified protein derivative (PPD) test or chest radiograph before commencing long-term corticosteroid therapy.
- Screen for pregnancy in reproductive age women; recommend contraceptive measures.
- Screen for diabetes mellitus before treatment and every 3–4 months.
- Teach patient about the symptoms of hyperglycemia.
- Screen for hypertension before treatment and every 3–4 months.
- Screen for glaucoma and cataracts before treatment, 3 months after treatment inception, and then at least yearly.
- Monitor plasma potassium for hypokalemia and treat as indicated.
- Obtain bone densitometry before treatment and then periodically. Treat osteoporosis.
- Weigh daily. Use dietary measures to avoid obesity and optimize nutrition.
- Measure height frequently to document the degree of axial spine demineralization and compression.
- Watch for fungal or yeast infections of skin, nails, mouth, vagina, and rectum, and treat appropriately.
- With dosage reduction, watch for signs of adrenal insufficiency or corticosteroid withdrawal syndrome.

Patient information
- Prepare the patient and family for possible adverse effects on mood, memory, and cognitive function.
- Inform the patient about other possible side effects, particularly weight gain, osteoporosis, and aseptic necrosis of bone.
- Counsel to avoid smoking and excessive ethanol consumption.

Prophylactic measures
- Institute a vigorous physical exercise and isometric regimen tailored to each patient's abilities or disabilities.
- Administer calcium (1 g elemental calcium) and vitamin D_3, 400–800 units orally daily.
  - Check spot morning urine for calcium; alter dosage to keep urine calcium concentration < 30 mg/dL (< 7.5 mmol/L).
  - If the patient is receiving thiazide diuretics, check for hypercalcemia, and administer only 500 mg elemental calcium daily.
- If the patient has preexistent osteoporosis or has been receiving corticosteroids for ≥ 3 months, consider prophylaxis:
  - Bisphosphonate such as alendronate (70 mg every week orally), zoledronic acid (5 mg every year intravenously) for up to 3–5 years;
  Or
  - Teriparatide, 20 mcg subcutaneously daily for up to 2 years
- Avoid prolonged bed rest that will accelerate muscle weakness and bone mineral loss. Ambulate early after fractures.
- Avoid elective surgery, if possible. Vitamin A in a daily dose of 20,000 units orally for 1 week may improve wound healing, but it is not prescribed in pregnancy.
- Fall prevention strategies: walking assistance (cane, walker, wheelchair, handrails) when required due to weakness or balance problems; avoid activities that could cause falls or other trauma.
- For ulcer prophylaxis, if administering corticosteroids with nonsteroidal anti-inflammatory drugs, prescribe a proton pump inhibitor (not required for corticosteroids alone). Avoid large doses of antacids containing aluminum hydroxide (many popular brands) because aluminum hydroxide binds phosphate and may cause a hypophosphatemic osteomalacia that can compound corticosteroid osteoporosis.
- Treat hypogonadism.
- Treat infections aggressively. Consider unusual pathogens.
- Treat edema as indicated.

and opportunistic infections. Prolonged high-dose corticosteroids also increase the risk of hypertension, dyslipidemia, myocardial infarction, stroke, atrial fibrillation or flutter, and heart failure. Gastric ulceration is more common with high-dose corticosteroids, particularly when patients take NSAIDs concurrently. Prolonged oral, inhaled, intravenous, or high-dose topical corticosteroid therapy commonly suppresses pituitary ACTH secretion, causing secondary adrenal insufficiency. High-dose inhaled corticosteroids predispose to oral thrush and pulmonary nontuberculous mycobacterial infection. To reduce risks, the dosage and duration of corticosteroid administration must be minimized. Immediately following inhaled corticosteroids, proper mouth-washing and gargling can reduce systemic absorption.

Most corticosteroids (dexamethasone, prednisone, hydrocortisone, deflazacort, budesonide) are metabolized by the enzyme CYP34A. When drugs that inhibit CYP34A

are administered along with even modest doses of corticosteroids (oral, inhaled, intravenous), the blood levels of the corticosteroids rise and can cause iatrogenic Cushing syndrome and secondary adrenal insufficiency. Medications that strongly inhibit CYP34A include itraconazole, ketoconazole, and nefazodone. Other strong CYP34A inhibitors include protease inhibitors and cobicistat that is an antiretroviral booster for the treatment of patients with HIV.

In pregnancy, corticosteroids taken by the mother are transmitted across the placenta to the fetus, causing adverse effects on fetal growth and development as well as childhood cognition and behavior. Therefore, women who are to receive high-dose corticosteroids should be screened for pregnancy and counseled to use contraception.

Osteoporotic fractures (especially vertebral) ultimately occur in about 40% of patients receiving long-term corticosteroid therapy. Osteoporotic fractures can occur even in patients receiving long-term corticosteroid therapy at relatively low doses (eg, 5–7.5 mg prednisone daily). The risk of vertebral fractures increases 14-fold and the risk of hip fractures increases 3-fold. Patients at increased risk for corticosteroid osteoporotic fractures include those who are over age 60 or who have a low body mass index, pretreatment osteoporosis, a family history of osteoporosis, or concurrent disease that limits mobility. Avascular necrosis of bone (especially hips) develops in about 15% of patients who receive corticosteroids at high doses (eg, prednisone 15 mg daily or more) for more than 1 month with cumulative prednisone doses of 10 g or more.

Bisphosphonates (eg, alendronate) prevent the development of osteoporosis among patients receiving prolonged courses of corticosteroids (Table 26–16). For patients who are unable to tolerate oral bisphosphonates (due to esophagitis, hiatal hernia, or gastritis), parenteral bisphosphonates can be used. Denosumab inhibits bone resorption, but may increase the risk of infection compared to bisphosphonates; so, the use of denosumab is not recommended for patients receiving high-dose corticosteroid therapy who are already at an increased risk for infection.

The PTH/PTHrP analogs teriparatide and abaloparatide are anabolic agents that are also effective against corticosteroid-induced osteoporosis. They can be given for a 2-year course and increase bone density more effectively than bisphosphonates. For patients who are currently receiving corticosteroid therapy, however, these analogs increase the risk of hypercalcemia and must be used with great caution; they are most useful for patients with osteoporosis who have stopped high-dose corticosteroid therapy. Following a 2-year course of therapy with these analogs, bone loss and fractures occur quickly after discontinuation, so such therapy is usually followed by bisphosphonate therapy in patients with a history of fracture or osteoporosis by bone densitometry. (See Osteoporosis.) It is wise to follow an organized treatment plan such as the one outlined in Table 26–16.

Bandoli G et al. A review of systemic corticosteroid use in pregnancy and the risk of select pregnancy and birth outcomes. Rheum Dis Clin North Am. 2017 Aug;43(3):489–502. [PMID: 28711148]

Buckley L et al. 2017 American College of Rheumatology guideline for the prevention and treatment of glucocorticoid-induced osteoporosis. Arthritis Rheumatol. 2017 Aug; 69(8):1521–37. [PMID: 28585373]

Buckley L et al. Glucocorticoid-induced osteoporosis. N Engl J Med. 2018 Dec 27;379(26):2547–56. [PMID: 30586507]

Paragliola RM et al. Treatment with synthetic glucocorticoids and the hypothalamus-pituitary-adrenal axis. Int J Mol Sci. 2017 Oct;18(10):2201. [PMID: 29053578]

Saag KG et al. Denosumab versus risedronate in glucocorticoid-induced osteoporosis: a multicentre, randomised, double-blind, active-controlled, double-dummy, non-inferiority study. Lancet Diabetes Endocrinol. 2018 Jun;6(6):445–54. [PMID: 29631782]

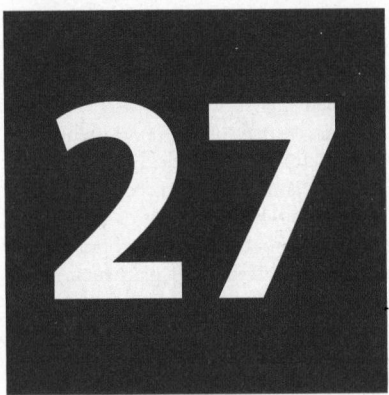

Diabetes Mellitus & Hypoglycemia

Umesh Masharani, MB, BS, MRCP (UK)

DIABETES MELLITUS

Type 1 diabetes

▸ Polyuria, polydipsia, and weight loss associated with random plasma glucose of 200 mg/dL (11.1 mmol/L) or more.

▸ Plasma glucose of 126 mg/dL (7.0 mmol/L) or more after an overnight fast, documented on more than one occasion.

▸ Ketonemia, ketonuria, or both.

▸ Islet autoantibodies are frequently present.

Type 2 diabetes

▸ Many patients are over 40 years of age and obese.

▸ Polyuria and polydipsia. Ketonuria and weight loss are uncommon at time of diagnosis. Candidal vaginitis in women may be an initial manifestation. Many patients have few or no symptoms.

▸ Plasma glucose of 126 mg/dL or more after an overnight fast on more than one occasion. Two hours after 75 g oral glucose, diagnostic values are 200 mg/dL (11.1 mmol) or more.

▸ HbA$_{1c}$ 6.5% or more.

▸ Hypertension, dyslipidemia, and atherosclerosis are often associated.

▸ Epidemiologic Considerations

An estimated 30.3 million people (9.4%) in the United States have diabetes mellitus, of which approximately 1.5 million have type 1 diabetes and most of the rest have type 2 diabetes. A third group designated as "other specific types" by the American Diabetes Association (ADA) (Table 27–1) number in the thousands.

▸ Classification & Pathogenesis

Diabetes mellitus is a syndrome with disordered metabolism and inappropriate hyperglycemia due to either a deficiency of insulin secretion or to a combination of insulin resistance and inadequate insulin secretion to compensate for the resistance.

A. Type 1 Diabetes Mellitus

This form of diabetes is due to pancreatic islet B cell destruction predominantly by an autoimmune process in over 95% of cases (type 1A) and idiopathic in less than 5% (type 1B). The rate of pancreatic B cell destruction is quite variable, being rapid in some individuals and slow in others. It occurs at any age but most commonly arises in children and young adults with a peak incidence before school age and again at around puberty. It is a catabolic disorder in which circulating insulin is virtually absent, plasma glucagon is elevated, and the pancreatic B cells fail to respond to all insulinogenic stimuli. Type 1 diabetes is usually associated with ketosis in its untreated state. Exogenous insulin is therefore required to reverse the catabolic state, prevent ketosis, reduce the hyperglucagonemia, and reduce blood glucose.

1. Immune-mediated type 1 diabetes mellitus (type 1A)— Approximately one-third of the disease susceptibility is due to genes and two-thirds to environmental factors. Genes that are related to the HLA locus contribute about 40% of the genetic risk. About 95% of patients with type 1 diabetes possess either HLA-DR3 or HLA-DR4, compared with 45–50% of white controls. *HLA-DQ* genes are even more specific markers of type 1 susceptibility, since a particular variety *(HLA-DQB1*0302)* is found in the DR4 patients with type 1, while a "protective" gene *(HLA-DQB1*0602)* is often present in the DR4 controls. The other important gene that contributes to about 10% of the genetic risk is found at the 5′ polymorphic region of the insulin gene. Mutations in genes associated with T cell tolerance can also cause autoimmune diabetes. The autoimmune regulatory gene *(AIRE)* product regulates the expression of several proteins in the thymus causing the deletion of self-reactive T cells. Type 1 diabetes mellitus as well as other autoimmune disorders (autoimmune polyglandular syndrome 1) develop in 20% of individuals with homozygote mutations in *AIRE*. Most patients with type 1 diabetes mellitus have circulating antibodies to islet cells (ICA), glutamic acid decarboxylase 65 (GAD65), insulin (IAA), tyrosine phosphatase IA2 (ICA-512), and zinc transporter 8 (ZnT8) at the

Table 27–1. Other specific types of diabetes mellitus.

Genetic defects of pancreatic B cell function
    MODY 1 (HNF-4alpha); rare
    MODY 2 (glucokinase); less rare
    MODY 3 (HNF-1alpha); accounts for two-thirds of all MODY
    MODY 4 (PDX1); very rare
    MODY 5 (HNF-1beta); very rare
    MODY 6 (neuroD1); very rare
    Mitochondrial DNA
Genetic defects in insulin action
    Type A insulin resistance
    Leprechaunism
    Rabson-Mendenhall syndrome
    Lipoatrophic diabetes
Diseases of the exocrine pancreas
Endocrinopathies
Drug- or chemical-induced diabetes
Other genetic syndromes (Down, Klinefelter, Turner, others)
    sometimes associated with diabetes

MODY, maturity-onset diabetes of the young; PDX1, pancreatic duodenal homeobox 1.

time the diagnosis is made (Table 27–2). These antibodies facilitate screening for an autoimmune cause of diabetes, particularly screening siblings of affected children, as well as adults with atypical features of type 2 diabetes mellitus. Also, low levels of anti-insulin antibodies develop in almost all patients once they are treated with insulin.

Family members of diabetic probands are at increased lifetime risk for developing type 1 diabetes mellitus. A child whose mother has type 1 diabetes has a 3% risk of developing the disease and a 6% risk if the child's father has it. The risk in siblings is related to the number of HLA haplotypes that the sibling shares with the diabetic proband. If one haplotype is shared, the risk is 6% and if two haplotypes are shared, the risk increases to 12–25%. The highest risk is for identical twins, where the concordance rate is 25–50%.

Some patients with a milder expression of type 1 diabetes mellitus initially retain enough B cell function to avoid ketosis, but as their B cell mass diminishes later in life, dependence on insulin therapy develops. Islet cell antibody surveys among northern Europeans indicate that up to 15% of "type 2" diabetic patients may actually have this

Table 27–2. Diagnostic sensitivity and specificity of autoimmune markers in patients with newly diagnosed type 1 diabetes mellitus.

	Sensitivity	Specificity
Islet cell antibodies (ICA)	44–100%	96%
Glutamic acid decarboxylase (GAD65)	70–90%	99%
Insulin (IAA)	40–70%	99%
Tyrosine phosphatase (IA-2)	50–70%	99%
Zinc transporter 8 (ZnT8)	50–70%	99%

mild form of type 1 diabetes (latent autoimmune diabetes of adulthood; LADA). Evidence for environmental factors playing a role in the development of type 1 diabetes include the observation that the disease is more common in Scandinavian countries and becomes progressively less frequent in countries nearer and nearer to the equator. Also, the risk for type 1 diabetes increases when individuals who normally have a low risk emigrate to the Northern Hemisphere. For example, Pakistani children born and raised in Bradford, England, have a higher risk for developing type 1 diabetes compared with children who lived in Pakistan all their lives.

Which environmental factor is responsible for the increased risk is not known. Breastfeeding in the first 6 months of life appears to be protective. There is accumulating evidence that improvements in public health and reduced infections (especially parasitic) lead to immune system dysregulation and development of autoimmune disorders such as asthma and type 1 diabetes.

Check point inhibitor immunotherapies for advanced malignancies, such as nivolumab, pembrolizumab, and ipilimumab, can precipitate autoimmune disorders, including type 1 diabetes. Patients receiving these drugs should be monitored for the development of diabetes.

2. Idiopathic type 1 diabetes mellitus (type 1B)—Approximately 5% of subjects have no evidence of pancreatic B cell autoimmunity to explain their insulinopenia and ketoacidosis. This subgroup has been classified as "idiopathic type 1 diabetes" and designated as "type 1B." Although only a minority of patients with type 1 diabetes fall into this group, most of these individuals are of Asian or African origin. About 4% of the West Africans with ketosis-prone diabetes are homozygous for a mutation in *PAX-4* (*Arg133Trp*)—a transcription factor that is essential for the development of pancreatic islets.

B. Type 2 Diabetes Mellitus

This represents a heterogeneous group of conditions that used to occur predominantly in adults, but it is now more frequently encountered in children and adolescents. Circulating endogenous insulin is sufficient to prevent ketoacidosis but is inadequate to prevent hyperglycemia in the face of increased needs owing to tissue insensitivity (insulin resistance).

Genetic and environmental factors combine to cause both the insulin resistance and the beta cell loss. Most epidemiologic data indicate strong genetic influences, since in monozygotic twins over 40 years of age, concordance develops in over 70% of cases within a year whenever type 2 diabetes develops in one twin. So far, more than 30 genetic loci have been associated with an increased risk of type 2 diabetes. A significant number of the identified loci appear to code for proteins that have a role in beta cell function or development. One of the genetic loci with the largest risk effect is *TCF7L2*. This gene codes for a transcription factor involved in the WNT signaling pathway that is required for normal pancreatic development.

Early in the disease process, hyperplasia of pancreatic B cells occurs and probably accounts for the fasting hyperinsulinism and exaggerated insulin and proinsulin responses to glucose and other stimuli. With time, chronic deposition of amyloid in the islets may combine with inherited genetic defects progressively to impair B cell function.

Obesity is the most important environmental factor causing insulin resistance. The degree and prevalence of obesity varies among different racial groups with type 2 diabetes. While obesity is apparent in no more than 30% of Chinese and Japanese patients with type 2, it is found in 60–70% of North Americans, Europeans, or Africans with type 2 and approaches 100% of patients with type 2 among Pima Indians or Pacific Islanders from Nauru or Samoa.

Visceral obesity, due to accumulation of fat in the omental and mesenteric regions, correlates with insulin resistance; subcutaneous abdominal fat seems to have less of an association with insulin insensitivity. There are many patients with type 2 diabetes who, while not overtly obese, have increased visceral fat; they are termed the "metabolically obese." Exercise may affect the deposition of visceral fat as suggested by CT scans of Japanese wrestlers, whose extreme obesity is predominantly subcutaneous. Their daily vigorous exercise program prevents accumulation of visceral fat, and they have normal serum lipids and euglycemia despite daily intakes of 5000–7000 kcal and development of massive subcutaneous obesity.

C. Other Specific Types of Diabetes Mellitus

1. Maturity-onset diabetes of the young (MODY)—This subgroup of monogenic disorders is characterized by noninsulin requiring diabetes with autosomal dominant inheritance and an age at onset of 25 years or younger. Patients are nonobese, and their hyperglycemia is due to impaired glucose-induced secretion of insulin. Six types of MODY have been described (Table 27–1). Except for MODY 2, in which a glucokinase gene is defective, all other types involve mutations of a nuclear transcription factor that regulates islet gene expression. Patients younger than 30 years with endogenous insulin production (urinary C-peptide/creatinine ratio of 0.2 nmol/mmol or higher) and negative autoantibodies are candidates for genetic screening for MODY. The enzyme glucokinase is a rate-limiting step in glycolysis and determines the rate of adenosine triphosphate (ATP) production from glucose and the insulin secretory response in the beta cell. MODY 2, due to glucokinase mutations, is usually quite mild, associated with only slight fasting hyperglycemia and few if any microvascular diabetic complications. MODY 3, due to mutations in hepatic nuclear factor 1 alpha is the most common form, accounting for two-thirds of all MODY cases. Initially, patients with MODY 3 are responsive to sulfonylurea therapy but the clinical course is of progressive beta cell failure and eventual need for insulin therapy. Mutations in both alleles of glucokinase present with more severe neonatal diabetes. Mutation in one allele of the pancreatic duodenal homeobox 1 (PDX1) causes diabetes usually at a later age (~ 35 years) than other forms of MODY; mutations in both alleles of PDX1 cause pancreatic agenesis.

2. Diabetes mellitus associated with a mutation of mitochondrial DNA—Since sperm do not contain mitochondria, only the mother transmits mitochondrial genes to her offspring. Diabetes due to mutations of mitochondrial DNA occurs in less than 2% of patients with diabetes. The most common cause is the A3243G mutation in the gene coding for the tRNA (Leu, UUR). Diabetes usually develops in these patients in their late 30s, and characteristically, they also have hearing loss (maternally inherited diabetes and deafness [MIDD]).

3. Wolfram syndrome—Wolfram syndrome is an autosomal recessive neurodegenerative disorder first evident in childhood. It consists of diabetes insipidus, diabetes mellitus, optic atrophy, and deafness, hence the acronym DIDMOAD. It is due to mutations in a gene named *WFS1*, which encodes a 100.3 KDa transmembrane protein localized in the endoplasmic reticulum. Cranial diabetes insipidus and sensorineural deafness develop during the second decade in 60–75% of patients. Ureterohydronephrosis, neurogenic bladder, cerebellar ataxia, peripheral neuropathy, and psychiatric illness develop later in many patients.

4. Autosomal recessive syndromes—Homozygous mutations in a number of pancreatic transcription factors, *NEUROG3, PTF1A, RFX6,* and *GLI-similar 3 (GLIS3)*, cause neonatal or childhood diabetes. Homozygous *PTF1A* mutations result in absent pancreas and cerebellar atrophy; *NEUROG3* mutations cause severe malabsorption and diabetes before puberty. Homozygous mutations in *RFX6* cause the Mitchell-Riley syndrome characterized by absence of all islet cell types apart from pancreatic polypeptide cells, hypoplasia of the pancreas and gallbladder, and intestinal atresia. *GLIS3* gene plays a role in transcription of insulin gene, and homozygous mutations cause neonatal diabetes and congenital hypothyroidism. The gene *EIF2AK3* encodes PKR-like ER kinase (PERK), which controls one of the pathways of the unfolded protein response. Absence of PERK leads to inadequate response to ER stress and accelerated beta cell apoptosis. Patients with mutation in this gene have neonatal diabetes, epiphyseal dysplasia, developmental delay, and liver and kidney dysfunction (Wolcott-Rallison syndrome).

5. Diabetes mellitus secondary to other causes—Endocrine tumors secreting growth hormone, glucocorticoids, catecholamines, glucagon, or somatostatin can cause glucose intolerance (Table 27–3). In the first four of these situations, peripheral responsiveness to insulin is impaired. With excess of glucocorticoids, catecholamines, or glucagon, increased hepatic output of glucose is a contributory factor; in the case of catecholamines, decreased insulin release is an additional factor in producing carbohydrate intolerance, and with somatostatin, inhibition of insulin secretion is the major factor. Diabetes mainly occurs in individuals with underlying defects in insulin secretion, and hyperglycemia typically resolves when the hormone excess is resolved.

High-titer anti-insulin receptor antibodies that inhibit insulin binding cause a clinical syndrome characterized by severe insulin resistance, glucose intolerance or diabetes mellitus, and acanthosis nigricans. These patients usually have other autoimmune disorders. There are reports of spontaneous remission or remission with cytotoxic therapy.

Table 27–3. Secondary causes of hyperglycemia.

Hyperglycemia due to tissue insensitivity to insulin
  Hormonal tumors (acromegaly, Cushing syndrome, glucagonoma, pheochromocytoma)
  Pharmacologic agents (corticosteroids, sympathomimetic drugs, niacin)
  Liver disease (cirrhosis, hemochromatosis)
  Muscle disorders (myotonic dystrophy)
  Adipose tissue disorders (lipodystrophy, truncal obesity)
  Insulin receptor disorders (acanthosis nigricans syndromes, leprechaunism)
Hyperglycemia due to reduced insulin secretion
  Hormonal tumors (somatostatinoma, pheochromocytoma)
  Pancreatic disorders (pancreatitis, hemosiderosis, hemochromatosis)
  Pharmacologic agents (thiazide diuretics, phenytoin, pentamidine, calcineurin inhibitors)

Many medications are associated with carbohydrate intolerance or frank diabetes (Table 27–3). The medications act by decreasing insulin secretion or by increasing insulin resistance or both. Cyclosporine and tacrolimus impair insulin secretion; sirolimus principally increases insulin resistance. These agents contribute to the development of new-onset diabetes after transplantation. Corticosteroids increase insulin resistance but may also have an effect on beta cell function; in a case control study and a large population cohort study, oral corticosteroids doubled the risk for development of diabetes. Thiazide diuretics and beta-blockers modestly increase the risk for diabetes. Treating the hypokalemia due to thiazides may reverse the hyperglycemia. Atypical antipsychotics, particularly olanzapine and clozapine, are associated with increased risk of glucose intolerance. These medications cause weight gain and insulin resistance but may also impair beta cell function; an increase in rates of diabetic ketoacidosis (DKA) has been reported.

Chronic pancreatitis or subtotal pancreatectomy reduces the number of functioning B cells and can result in a metabolic derangement very similar to that of genetic type 1 diabetes except that a concomitant reduction in pancreatic A cells may reduce glucagon secretion so that relatively lower doses of insulin replacement are needed.

Insulin Resistance Syndrome (Metabolic Syndrome)

Twenty-five percent of the general nonobese, nondiabetic population has insulin resistance of a magnitude similar to that seen in type 2 diabetes. These insulin-resistant nondiabetic individuals are at much higher risk for developing type 2 diabetes than insulin-sensitive persons. These individuals also have a cluster of abnormalities termed **metabolic syndrome** that significantly increases their risk of atherosclerotic disease: elevated plasma triglycerides and small, dense, low-density lipoproteins (LDLs); lower high-density lipoproteins (HDLs); higher blood pressure; hyperuricemia; abdominal obesity; prothrombotic state with increased levels of plasminogen activator inhibitor type 1 (PAI-1); and proinflammatory state with increased levels of proinflammatory cytokines such as IL-6 and TNF-alpha.

It has been postulated that hyperinsulinemia and insulin resistance play a direct role in these metabolic abnormalities, but supportive evidence is inconclusive. The main value of grouping these disorders as a syndrome, however, is to remind clinicians that the therapeutic goals are not only to correct hyperglycemia but also to manage the elevated blood pressure and dyslipidemia that result in increased cerebrovascular and cardiac morbidity and mortality in these patients.

American Diabetes Association. Standards of medical care in diabetes—2019. Diabetes Care. 2019 Jan;42(Suppl):S1–204. [PMID: 30559243]

Thompson AE. JAMA patient page. Hypoglycemia. JAMA. 2015 Mar 24–31;313(12):1284. [PMID: 25803359]

Clinical Findings

A. Symptoms and Signs

1. Type 1 diabetes—A characteristic symptom complex of hyperosmolality and hyperketonemia from the accumulation of circulating glucose and fatty acids typically presents in patients with type 1 diabetes. Increased urination and thirst are consequences of osmotic diuresis secondary to sustained hyperglycemia. The diuresis results in a loss of glucose as well as free water and electrolytes in the urine. Blurred vision often develops as the lenses are exposed to hyperosmolar fluids.

Weight loss despite normal or increased appetite is a common feature of type 1 when it develops subacutely. The weight loss is initially due to depletion of water, glycogen, and triglycerides; thereafter, reduced muscle mass occurs as amino acids are diverted to form glucose and ketone bodies. Loss of subcutaneous fat and muscle wasting are features of more slowly developing insulin deficiency. Lowered plasma volume produces symptoms of postural hypotension, which is a serious prognostic sign. Total body potassium loss and the general catabolism of muscle protein contribute to the weakness.

Paresthesias may be present at the time of diagnosis, particularly when the onset is subacute. They reflect a temporary dysfunction of peripheral sensory nerves, which clears as insulin replacement restores glycemic levels closer to normal, suggesting neurotoxicity from sustained hyperglycemia.

When absolute insulin deficiency is of acute onset, the above symptoms develop abruptly. Ketoacidosis exacerbates the dehydration and hyperosmolality by producing anorexia and nausea and vomiting, interfering with oral fluid replacement.

The patient's level of consciousness can vary depending on the degree of hyperosmolality. When insulin deficiency develops relatively slowly and sufficient water intake is maintained, patients remain relatively alert and physical findings may be minimal. When vomiting occurs in response to worsening ketoacidosis, dehydration progresses and compensatory mechanisms become inadequate to keep serum osmolality below 320–330 mOsm/L. Under these circumstances, stupor or even coma may occur. The fruity breath odor of acetone further suggests the diagnosis of DKA.

2. Type 2 diabetes—While increased urination and thirst may be presenting symptoms in some patients with type 2 diabetes, many other patients have an insidious onset of hyperglycemia and are asymptomatic initially. This is particularly true in obese patients, whose diabetes may be detected only after glycosuria or hyperglycemia is noted during routine laboratory studies. Occasionally, when the disease has been occult for some time, patients with type 2 diabetes may have evidence of neuropathic or cardiovascular complications at the time of presentation. Chronic skin infections are common. Generalized pruritus and symptoms of vaginitis are frequently the initial complaints of women. Diabetes should be suspected in women with chronic candidal vulvovaginitis as well as in those who have delivered babies larger than 9 lb (4.1 kg) or have had polyhydramnios, preeclampsia, or unexplained fetal losses. Balanoposthitis (inflammation of the foreskin and glans in uncircumcised males) may occur.

Many patients with type 2 diabetes are overweight or obese. Even those who are not significantly obese often have characteristic localization of fat deposits on the upper segment of the body (particularly the abdomen, chest, neck, and face) and relatively less fat on the appendages, which may be quite muscular. This centripetal fat distribution is characterized by a high waist circumference; a waist circumference larger than 40 inches (102 cm) in men and 35 inches (88 cm) in women is associated with an increased risk of diabetes. Some patients may have acanthosis nigricans, which is associated with significant insulin resistance; the skin in the axilla, groin, and back of neck is hyperpigmented and hyperkeratotic (Figure 27–1). Mild hypertension is often present in obese patients with diabetes. Eruptive xanthomas on the flexor surface of the limbs and on the buttocks and lipemia retinalis due to hyperchylomicronemia can occur in patients with uncontrolled type 2 diabetes who also have a familial form of hypertriglyceridemia.

Hyperglycemic hyperosmolar coma can also be present; in these cases, patients are profoundly dehydrated, hypotensive, lethargic, or comatose but without Kussmaul respirations.

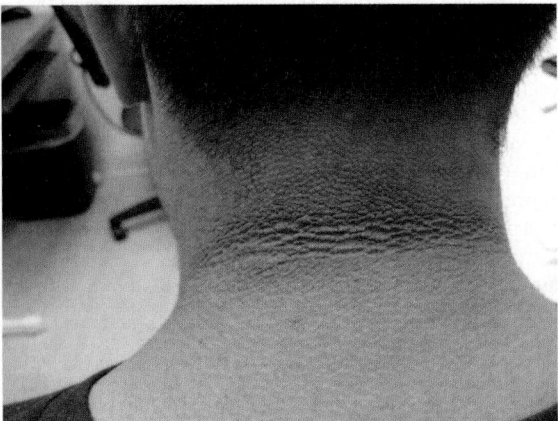

▲ **Figure 27–1.** Acanthosis nigricans of the nape of the neck, with typical dark and velvety appearance. (Used, with permission, from Umesh Masharani, MB, BS, MRCP [UK].)

B. Laboratory Findings

1. Urine glucose—A convenient method to detect glucosuria is the paper strip impregnated with glucose oxidase and a chromogen system (Clinistix, Diastix), which is sensitive to as little as 100 mg/dL (5.5 mmol) glucose in urine. A normal renal threshold for glucose as well as reliable bladder emptying is essential for interpretation.

Nondiabetic glycosuria (renal glycosuria) is a benign asymptomatic condition wherein glucose appears in the urine despite a normal amount of glucose in the blood, either basally or during a glucose tolerance test. Its cause may vary from mutations in the *SGLT2* gene coding for sodium-glucose transporter 2 (familial renal glycosuria) to one associated with dysfunction of the proximal renal tubule (Fanconi syndrome, chronic kidney disease), or it may merely be a consequence of the increased load of glucose presented to the tubules by the elevated glomerular filtration rate (GFR) during pregnancy. As many as 50% of pregnant women normally have demonstrable sugar in the urine, especially during the third and fourth months. This sugar is practically always glucose except during the late weeks of pregnancy, when lactose may be present.

2. Urine and blood ketones—Qualitative detection of ketone bodies can be accomplished by nitroprusside tests (Acetest or Ketostix). Although these tests do not detect beta-hydroxybutyric acid, which lacks a ketone group, the semiquantitative estimation of ketonuria thus obtained is nonetheless usually adequate for clinical purposes. Many laboratories measure beta-hydroxybutyric acid, and there are meters available (Precision Xtra; Nova Max Plus) for patient use that measures beta-hydroxybutyric acid levels in capillary glucose samples. Beta-hydroxybutyrate levels greater than 0.6 mmol/L require evaluation. Patients with levels greater than 3.0 mmol/L, equivalent to very large urinary ketones, require hospitalization.

3. Plasma or serum glucose—The glucose concentration is 10–15% higher in plasma or serum than in whole blood because structural components of blood cells are absent. A plasma glucose level of 126 mg/dL (7 mmol/L) or higher on more than one occasion after at least 8 hours of fasting is diagnostic of diabetes mellitus (Table 27–4). Fasting plasma glucose levels of 100–125 mg/dL (5.6–6.9 mmol/L) are associated with increased risk of diabetes (impaired fasting glucose tolerance).

4. Oral glucose tolerance test—If the fasting plasma glucose level is less than 126 mg/dL (7 mmol/L) when diabetes is nonetheless suspected, then a standardized oral glucose tolerance test may be done (Table 27–4). In order to optimize insulin secretion and effectiveness, especially when patients have been on a low-carbohydrate diet, a minimum of 150–200 g of carbohydrate per day should be included in the diet for 3 days preceding the test. The patient should eat nothing after midnight prior to the test day. On the morning of the test, patients are then given 75 g of glucose in 300 mL of water. The glucose load is consumed within 5 minutes. The test should be performed in the morning because there is some diurnal variation in oral glucose tolerance, and patients should not smoke or be active during the test.

Table 27–4. Criteria for the diagnosis of diabetes.

	Normal Glucose Tolerance	Impaired Glucose Tolerance	Diabetes Mellitus[2]
Fasting plasma glucose mg/dL (mmol/L)	< 100 (5.6)	100–125 (5.6–6.9)	≥ 126 (7.0)
Two hours after glucose load[1] mg/dL (mmol/L)	< 140 (7.8)	≥ 140–199 (7.8–11.0)	≥ 200 (11.1)
HbA$_{1c}$ (%)	< 5.7	5.7–6.4	≥ 6.5

[1]Give 75 g of glucose dissolved in 300 mL of water after an overnight fast in persons who have been receiving at least 150–200 g of carbohydrate daily for 3 days before the test.
[2]A fasting plasma glucose ≥ 126 mg/dL (7.0 mmol) or HbA$_{1c}$ of ≥ 6.5% is diagnostic of diabetes if confirmed by repeat testing. A fasting plasma glucose ≥ 126 mg/dL (7.0 mmol) and HbA$_{1c}$ ≥ 6.5% on the *same sample* is also diagnostic of diabetes.

Blood samples for plasma glucose are obtained at 0 and 120 minutes after ingestion of glucose. An oral glucose tolerance test is normal if the fasting venous plasma glucose value is less than 100 mg/dL (5.6 mmol/L) and the 2-hour value falls below 140 mg/dL (7.8 mmol/L). A fasting value of 126 mg/dL (7 mmol/L) or higher or a 2-hour value of greater than 200 mg/dL (11.1 mmol/L) is diagnostic of diabetes mellitus. Patients with 2-hour value of 140–199 mg/dL (7.8–11.1 mmol/L) have impaired glucose tolerance. False-positive results may occur in patients who are malnourished, bedridden, or afflicted with an infection or severe emotional stress.

5. Glycated hemoglobin (hemoglobin A$_1$) measurements—Office-based immunoassays for HbA$_{1c}$ using capillary blood give a result in about 9 minutes and this allows for nearly immediate feedback to the patients regarding their glycemic control.

Since HbA$_{1c}$ circulates within red blood cells whose life span lasts up to 120 days, it generally reflects the state of glycemia over the preceding 8–12 weeks, thereby providing an improved method of assessing diabetic control. The HbA$_{1c}$ value, however, is weighted to more recent glucose levels (previous month) and this explains why significant changes in HbA$_{1c}$ are observed with short-term (1 month) changes in mean plasma glucose levels. Measurements should be made in patients with either type of diabetes mellitus at 3- to 4-month intervals. In patients monitoring their own blood glucose levels, HbA$_{1c}$ values provide a valuable check on the accuracy of monitoring. In patients who do not monitor their own blood glucose levels, HbA$_{1c}$ values are essential for adjusting therapy. The A$_{1c}$ Derived Average Glucose Study reported that the relationship between average glucose in the previous 3 months and HbA$_{1c}$ was $(28.7 \times HbA_{1c}) - 46.7$. There is, however, substantial individual variability; for HbA$_{1c}$ values between 6.9% and 7.1%, the glucose levels range from 125 mg/dL to 205 mg/dL (6.9–11.4 mmol/L; 95% CIs). For HbA$_{1c}$ of 6%,

the mean glucose levels range from 100 mg/dL to 152 mg/dL (5.5–8.5 mmol/L); and for 8% they range from 147 mg/dL to 217 mg/dL (8.1–12.1 mmol/L). For this reason, caution should be exercised in estimating average glucose levels from measured HbA$_{1c}$.

The accuracy of HbA$_{1c}$ values can be affected by hemoglobin variants or traits. In patients with high levels of hemoglobin F, immunoassays give falsely low values of HbA$_{1c}$. The National Glycohemoglobin Standardization Program website (www.ngsp.org) has information on the impact of frequently encountered hemoglobin variants and traits on the results obtained with the commonly used HbA$_{1c}$ assays.

Any condition that shortens erythrocyte survival or decreases mean erythrocyte age (eg, recovery from acute blood loss, hemolytic anemia) will falsely lower HbA$_{1c}$ irrespective of the assay method used. Intravenous iron and erythropoietin therapy for treatment of anemia in chronic kidney disease also falsely lower HbA$_{1c}$ levels. Alternative methods such as fructosamine should be considered for these patients. Vitamins C and E are reported to falsely lower test results possibly by inhibiting glycation of hemoglobin. Conditions that increase erythrocyte survival such as splenectomy for hereditary spherocytosis will falsely raise HbA$_{1c}$ levels. Iron deficiency anemia is also associated with higher HbA$_{1c}$ levels.

HbA$_{1c}$ is endorsed by the ADA as a diagnostic test for type 1 and type 2 diabetes (Table 27–4). A cutoff value of 6.5% (48 mmol/mol) was chosen because the risk for retinopathy increases substantially above this value. The advantages of using the HbA$_{1c}$ to diagnose diabetes is that there is no need to fast; it has lower intraindividual variability than the fasting glucose test and the oral glucose tolerance test; and it provides an estimate of glucose control for the preceding 2–3 months. People with HbA$_{1c}$ levels of 5.7–6.4% (39–46 mmol/mol) should be considered at high risk for developing diabetes (prediabetes). The diagnosis should be confirmed with a repeat HbA$_{1c}$ test, unless the patient is symptomatic with plasma glucose levels greater than 200 mg/dL (11.1 mmol/L). This test is not appropriate to use in populations with high prevalence of hemoglobinopathies or in conditions with increased red cell turnover. Also, the testing is performed using a National Glycohemoglobin Standardization Program (NGSP) certified method and standardized to the Diabetes Control and Complication Trial assay. In the European Union, the tests are standardized to the International Federation of Clinical Chemistry (IFCC), which defines HbA$_{1c}$ as mmol glycated hexapeptide per mol (glycated and non-glycated hexapeptides) and reported as mmol HbA$_{1c}$/mol Hb. The conversion factor for NGSP and IFCC results is NGSP (USA) result = (0.09148*IFCC result) + 2.152. There is worldwide consensus that HbA$_{1c}$ should be reported in both NGSP (%) and IFCC (mmol/mol) units.

6. Serum fructosamine—Serum fructosamine is formed by nonenzymatic glycosylation of serum proteins (predominantly albumin). Since serum albumin has a much shorter half-life than hemoglobin, serum fructosamine generally reflects the state of glycemic control for only the preceding 1–2 weeks. Reductions in serum albumin (eg, nephrotic state, protein-losing enteropathy, or hepatic disease) will lower the serum fructosamine value. When abnormal hemoglobins or hemolytic states affect the interpretation of glycohemoglobin or when a narrower time frame is required, such as for ascertaining glycemic control at the time of conception in a diabetic woman who has recently become pregnant, serum fructosamine assays offer some advantage. Normal values vary in relation to the serum albumin concentration and are 200–285 mcmol/L when the serum albumin level is 5 g/dL. HbA_{1c} values and serum fructosamine are highly correlated. Serum fructosamine levels of 300, 367, and 430 mcmol/L approximate to HbA_{1c} values of 7%, 8%, and 9%, respectively. Substantial individual variability exists, though, when estimating the likely HbA_{1c} value from the fructosamine measurement.

7. Self-monitoring of blood glucose—Capillary blood glucose measurements performed by patients themselves, as outpatients, are extremely useful. In type 1 patients in whom "tight" metabolic control is attempted, they are indispensable. A large number of blood glucose meters are available. All are accurate, but they vary with regard to speed, convenience, size of blood samples required, reporting capability, and cost. Popular models include those manufactured by LifeScan (One Touch), Bayer Corporation (Breeze, Contour), Roche Diagnostics (Accu-Chek), and Abbott Laboratories (Precision, FreeStyle). These blood glucose meters are relatively inexpensive, ranging from $20 to $80 each. Test strips remain a major expense, costing about $.25 to $1.50 apiece. Each glucose meter also comes with a lancet device and disposable 26- to 33-gauge lancets. Most meters can store from 100 to 1000 glucose values in their memories and have capabilities to download the values into a computer or smartphone. Some meters are designed to communicate with a specific insulin pump. Contour Next Link meter, for example, communicates with the MiniMed Medtronic pump. The accuracy of data obtained by home glucose monitoring does require education of the patient in sampling and measuring procedures as well as in properly calibrating the instruments.

The clinician should be aware of the limitations of the self-monitoring glucose systems. The strips have limited lifespans and improper storage (high temperature; open vial) can affect their function. Patients should also be advised not to use expired strips. Increases or decreases in hematocrit can decrease or increase the measured glucose values. Meters and the test strips are calibrated over the glucose concentrations ranging from 60 mg/dL (3.3 mmol/L) to 160 mg/dL (8.9 mmol/L) and the accuracy is not as good for higher and lower glucose levels. When the glucose is less than 60 mg/dL (3.3 mmol/L), the difference between the meter and the laboratory value may be as much as 20%. Glucose oxidase–based amperometric systems underestimate glucose levels in the presence of high oxygen tension. This may be important in the critically ill who are receiving supplemental oxygen; under these circumstances, a glucose dehydrogenase–based system may be preferable. Glucose-dehydrogenase pyrroloquinoline quinone (GDH-PQQ) systems may report falsely high glucose levels in patients who are receiving parenteral products containing nonglucose sugars such as maltose, galactose, or xylose or their metabolites. Some meters have been approved for measuring glucose in blood samples obtained at alternative sites such as the forearm and thigh. There is, however, a 5- to 20-minute lag in the glucose response on the arm with respect to the glucose response on the finger. Forearm blood glucose measurements could therefore result in a delay in detection of rapidly developing hypoglycemia. Impaired circulation to the fingers (for example, in patients with Raynaud disease) will artificially lower fingerstick glucose measurements (pseudohypoglycemia).

8. Continuous glucose monitoring systems—Increasing number of patients, especially those with type 1 diabetes are using continuous glucose monitoring systems. These systems, manufactured by Medtronic MiniMed, DexCom systems, and Abbott Diagnostics, involve inserting a subcutaneous sensor (rather like an insulin pump cannula) that measures glucose concentrations continuously in the interstitial fluid for 7–14 days. The DexCom and MiniMed systems transmit glucose data wirelessly to smartphones or to the screens of insulin pumps. Directional arrows indicate rate and direction of change of glucose levels, and alerts can be set for dangerously low or high glucose values. The FreeStyle Libre (Abbott Diagnostics) sensor system requires the patient to hold a reading device or a smartphone close to the sensor patch for about a second to see the real time glucose value. The MiniMed system requires calibration with periodic fingerstick glucose levels, which is not necessary for the Dexcom and Freestyle Libre systems. A 6-month randomized controlled study of type 1 patients showed that adults (25 years and older) using these continuous glucose monitoring systems had improved glycemic control without an increase in the incidence of hypoglycemia. A randomized controlled study of continuous glucose monitoring during pregnancy showed improved glycemic control in the third trimester, lower birth weight, and reduced risk of macrosomia. The individual glucose values are not that critical—what matters is the direction and the rate at which the glucose is changing, allowing the user to take corrective action. The wearer also gains insight into the way particular foods and activities affect their glucose levels. The other main benefit is the low glucose alert warning. The MiniMed insulin pump can be programmed to automatically suspend insulin delivery for up to 2 hours when the glucose levels on its continuous glucose monitoring device falls to a preset level and the patient does not respond to the alert. This insulin suspension feature has been shown to reduce the amount of time patients are in the hypoglycemic range at night. Many of these systems are covered by insurance. The initial cost is about $800 to $1000, and the sensor, which has to be changed every 7 to 14 days, costs $35 to $60; the out-of-pocket expense is about $4000 annually.

9. Lipoprotein abnormalities in diabetes—Circulating lipoproteins are just as dependent on insulin as is the plasma glucose. In type 1 diabetes, moderately deficient control of hyperglycemia is associated with only a slight elevation of LDL cholesterol and serum triglycerides and little if any change in HDL cholesterol. Once the hyperglycemia is corrected, lipoprotein levels are generally normal.

However, in patients with type 2 diabetes, a distinct "diabetic dyslipidemia" is characteristic of the insulin resistance syndrome. Its features are a high serum triglyceride level (300–400 mg/dL [3.4–4.5 mmol/L]), a low HDL cholesterol (less than 30 mg/dL [0.8 mmol/L]), and a qualitative change in LDL particles, producing a smaller dense particle whose membrane carries supranormal amounts of free cholesterol. These smaller dense LDL particles are more susceptible to oxidation, which renders them more atherogenic. Measures designed to correct the obesity and hyperglycemia, such as exercise, diet, and hypoglycemic therapy, are the treatment of choice for diabetic dyslipidemia, and in occasional patients in whom normal weight was achieved, all features of the lipoprotein abnormalities cleared. Since primary disorders of lipid metabolism may coexist with diabetes, persistence of lipid abnormalities after restoration of normal weight and blood glucose should prompt a diagnostic workup and possible pharmacotherapy of the lipid disorder. Chapter 28 discusses these matters in detail.

Selph S et al. Screening for type 2 diabetes mellitus: a systematic review for the U.S. Preventive Services Task Force. Ann Intern Med. 2015 Jun 2;162(11):765–76. [PMID: 25867111]

▶ Clinical Trials in Diabetes

Findings of the Diabetes Control and Complications Trial and of the United Kingdom Prospective Diabetes Study have confirmed the beneficial effects of improved glycemic control in both type 1 and type 2 diabetes.

The Diabetes Control and Complications Trial (DCCT), a long-term therapeutic study involving 1441 patients with type 1 diabetes mellitus, reported that "near" normalization of blood glucose resulted in a delay in the onset and a major slowing of the progression of established microvascular and neuropathic complications of diabetes during a follow-up period of up to 10 years. Multiple insulin injections (66%) or insulin pumps (34%) were used in the intensively treated group, who were trained to modify their therapy in response to frequent glucose monitoring. The conventionally treated groups used no more than two insulin injections, and clinical well-being was the goal with no attempt to modify management based on HbA_{1c} determinations or the glucose results.

In half of the patients, a mean hemoglobin A_{1c} of 7.2% (normal: less than 6%) and a mean blood glucose of 155 mg/dL (8.6 mmol/L) were achieved using intensive therapy, while in the conventionally treated group HbA_{1c} averaged 8.9% with an average blood glucose of 225 mg/dL (12.5 mmol/L). Over the study period, which averaged 7 years, there was an approximately 60% reduction in risk between the two groups in regard to diabetic retinopathy, nephropathy, and neuropathy. The intensively treated group also had a nonsignificant reduction in the risk of macrovascular disease of 41% (95% CI, –10% to 68%). Intensively treated patients had a threefold greater risk of serious hypoglycemia as well as a greater tendency toward weight gain. However, there were no deaths definitely attributable to hypoglycemia in any persons in the DCCT study, and no evidence of posthypoglycemic cognitive damage was detected.

Subjects participating in the DCCT study were subsequently enrolled in a follow-up observational study, the Epidemiology of Diabetes Interventions and Complications (EDIC) study. Even though the between-group differences in mean HbA_{1c} narrowed over 4 years, the group assigned to intensive therapy had a lower risk of retinopathy at 4 years, microalbuminuria at 7 to 8 years, and impaired GFR (less than 60 mL/min/1.73 m²) at 22 years of continued study follow-up. Moreover, by the end of the 11-year follow-up period, the intensive therapy group had significantly reduced their risk of any cardiovascular disease events by 42% (95% CI, 9% to 23%; $P = 0.02$). Thus, it seems that the benefits of good glucose control persist even if control deteriorates at a later date.

The general consensus of the ADA is that intensive insulin therapy associated with comprehensive self-management training should become standard therapy in patients with type 1 diabetes mellitus after the age of puberty. Exceptions include those with advanced chronic kidney disease and older adults since in these groups the detrimental risks of hypoglycemia outweigh the benefits of tight glycemic control.

The United Kingdom Prospective Diabetes Study (UKPDS), a multicenter study, was designed to establish, in type 2 diabetic patients, whether the risk of macrovascular or microvascular complications could be reduced by intensive blood glucose control with oral hypoglycemic agents or insulin and whether any particular therapy was of advantage.

Intensive treatment with either sulfonylureas, metformin, combinations of those two, or insulin achieved mean HbA_{1c} levels of 7%. This level of glycemic control decreased the risk of microvascular complications (retinopathy and nephropathy) in comparison with conventional therapy (mostly diet alone), which achieved mean levels of HbA_{1c} of 7.9%. Weight gain occurred in intensively treated patients except when metformin was used as monotherapy. No adverse cardiovascular outcomes were noted regardless of the therapeutic agent. In the overweight or obese subgroup, metformin therapy was more beneficial than diet alone in reducing the number of cases that progressed to diabetes as well as decreasing the number of patients who suffered myocardial infarctions and strokes. Hypoglycemic reactions occurred in the intensive treatment groups, but only one death from hypoglycemia was documented during 27,000 patient-years of intensive therapy.

Tight control of blood pressure (median value 144/82 mm Hg vs 154/87 mm Hg) substantially reduced the risk of microvascular disease and stroke but not myocardial infarction. In fact, reducing blood pressure by this amount had substantially greater impact on microvascular outcomes than that achieved by lowering HbA_{1c} from 7.9% to 7%. An epidemiologic analysis of the UKPDS data did show that every 10 mm Hg decrease in updated mean systolic blood pressure was associated with 11% reduction in risk for myocardial infarction. More than half of the patients needed two or more medications for adequate therapy of their hypertension, and there was no demonstrable advantage of angiotensin-converting enzyme (ACE) inhibitor therapy over therapy with beta-blockers with regard to diabetes end points. Use of a calcium channel blocker added to both treatment groups appeared to be safe over the long term in this diabetic population despite some controversy in the literature about its safety in patients with diabetes.

Like the DCCT trialists, the UKPDS researchers performed post-trial monitoring to determine whether there were long-term benefits of having been in the intensively treated glucose and blood pressure arms of the study. The intensively treated group had significantly reduced risk of myocardial infarction (15%, $P = 0.01$) and death from any cause (13%, $P = 0.007$) during the follow-up period. The subgroup of overweight or obese subjects who were initially randomized to metformin therapy showed sustained reduction in risk of myocardial infarction and death from any cause in the follow-up period. Unlike the sustained benefits seen with glucose control, there were no sustained benefits from having been in the more tightly controlled blood pressure group. Both blood pressure groups were at similar risk for microvascular events and diabetes-related end points during the follow-up period.

Thus, the follow-up of the UKPDS type 2 diabetes cohort showed that, as in type 1 diabetes, the benefits of good glucose control persist even if control deteriorates at a later date. Blood pressure benefits, however, last only as long as the blood pressure is well controlled.

▶ Treatment Regimens

A. Diet

A well-balanced, nutritious diet remains a fundamental element of therapy. There is no specific recommendation on the percentage of calories that should come from carbohydrate, protein, and fat. The macronutrient proportions should be individualized based on the patient's eating patterns, preferences, and metabolic goals. In general, most patients with diabetes consume about 45% of their total daily calories in the form of carbohydrates, 25–35% in the form of fat, and 10–35% in the form of protein. In patients with type 2 diabetes, limiting the carbohydrate intake and substituting some of the calories with monounsaturated fats, such as olive oil, rapeseed (canola) oil, or the oils in nuts and avocados, can lower triglycerides and increase HDL cholesterol. A Mediterranean-style eating pattern (a diet supplemented with walnuts, almonds, hazelnuts, and olive oil) has been shown to improve glycemic control and lower combined endpoints for cardiovascular events and stroke. In those patients with obesity and type 2 diabetes, weight reduction by caloric restriction is an important goal of the diet (see Chapter 29). Patients with type 1 diabetes or type 2 diabetes who take insulin should be taught "carbohydrate counting," so they can administer their insulin bolus for each meal based on its carbohydrate content.

The current recommendations for saturated fats and dietary cholesterol intake for people with diabetes are the same as for the general population. Saturated fats should be limited to less than 10% of daily calories and dietary cholesterol intake should be less than 300 mg/day. For those patients with kidney disease, dietary protein should be maintained at the recommended daily allowance of 0.8 g/kg/day. Exchange lists for meal planning can be obtained from the American Diabetes Association and its affiliate associations or from the American Dietetic Association (http://www.eatright.org), 216 W. Jackson Blvd., Chicago, IL 60606 (312-899-0040).

1. Dietary fiber—Plant components such as cellulose, gum, and pectin are indigestible by humans and are termed dietary "fiber." Insoluble fibers such as cellulose or hemicellulose, as found in bran, tend to increase intestinal transit and may have beneficial effects on colonic function. In contrast, soluble fibers such as gums and pectins, as found in beans, oatmeal, or apple skin, tend to retard nutrient absorption rates so that glucose absorption is slower and hyperglycemia may be slightly diminished. Although its recommendations do not include insoluble fiber supplements such as added bran, the ADA recommends food such as oatmeal, cereals, and beans with relatively high soluble fiber content as staple components of the diet in diabetics. High soluble fiber content in the diet may also have a favorable effect on blood cholesterol levels.

2. Glycemic index—The glycemic index of a carbohydrate containing food is determined by comparing the glucose excursions after consuming 50 g of test food with glucose excursions after consuming 50 g of reference food (white bread):

$$\text{Glycemic index} = \frac{\text{Blood glucose area under the curve (3h) for test food}}{\text{Blood glucose area under the curve (3h) for reference food}} \times 100$$

Eating low glycemic index foods results in lower glucose levels after meals. Low glycemic index foods have values of 55 or less and include many fruits, vegetables, grainy breads, pasta, and legumes. High glycemic index foods have values of 70 or greater and include baked potato, white bread, and white rice. Glycemic index is lowered by presence of fats and protein when food is consumed in a mixed meal. Even though it may not be possible to accurately predict the glycemic index of a particular food in the context of a meal, it is reasonable to choose foods with low glycemic index.

3. Artificial and other sweeteners—Saccharin (Sweet N Low), sucralose (Splenda), acesulfame potassium (Sweet One), and rebiana (Truvia) are "artificial" sweeteners that can be used in cooking and baking. Aspartame (NutraSweet) lacks heat stability, so it cannot be used in cooking. None of these sweeteners raise blood glucose levels.

Fructose represents a "natural" sugar substance that is a highly effective sweetener, induces only slight increases in plasma glucose levels, and does not require insulin for its metabolism. However, because of potential adverse effects of large amounts of fructose on raising serum cholesterol, triglycerides, and LDL cholesterol, it does not have any advantage as a sweetening agent in the diabetic diet. This does not preclude, however, ingestion of fructose-containing fruits and vegetables or fructose-sweetened foods in moderation.

Sugar alcohols, also known as polyols or polyalcohol, are commonly used as sweeteners and bulking agents. They occur naturally in a variety of fruits and vegetables but are also commercially made from sucrose, glucose, and starch. Examples are sorbitol, xylitol, mannitol, lactitol, isomalt, maltitol, and hydrogenated starch hydrolysates (HSH). They are not as easily absorbed as sugar, so they do not raise blood glucose levels as much. Therefore, sugar alcohols are often used in food products that are labeled as "sugar free," such as chewing gum, lozenges, hard candy, and sugar-free ice cream. However, if consumed in large quantities, they will raise blood glucose and can cause bloating and diarrhea.

B. Medications for Treating Hyperglycemia

The medications for treating type 2 diabetes are listed in Table 27–5.

1. Medications that primarily stimulate insulin secretion by binding to the sulfonylurea receptor on the beta cell—

A. SULFONYLUREAS—The primary mechanism of action of the sulfonylureas is to stimulate insulin release from pancreatic B cells.

Sulfonylureas are used in patients with type 2 but not type 1 diabetes, since these medications require functioning pancreatic B cells to produce their effect on blood glucose. Sulfonylureas are metabolized by the liver and apart from acetohexamide, whose metabolite is more active than the parent compound, the metabolites of all the other sulfonylureas are weakly active or inactive. The metabolites are excreted by the kidney and, in the case of the second-generation sulfonylureas, partly excreted in the bile.

Hypoglycemia is a common adverse reaction with the sulfonylureas. Weight gain is also common, especially in the first year of use. The mechanisms of the weight gain include improved glucose control and increased food intake in response to hypoglycemia.

Idiosyncratic reactions are rare, with skin rashes or hematologic toxicity (leukopenia, thrombocytopenia) occurring in less than 0.1% of users.

(1) First-generation oral sulfonylureas (tolbutamide, tolazamide, acetohexamide, chlorpropamide)—Tolbutamide is probably best administered in divided doses (eg, 500 mg before each meal and at bedtime); however, some patients require only one or two tablets daily with a maximum dose of 3000 mg/day. Tolbutamide has a relatively short duration of effect (about 6–10 hours). Because of its short duration of action, which is independent of kidney function, tolbutamide is relatively safe to use in kidney disease. Prolonged hypoglycemia has been reported rarely with tolbutamide, mostly in patients receiving antibacterial sulfonamides (sulfisoxazole), phenylbutazone for arthralgias, or the oral azole antifungal medications to treat candidiasis. These medications apparently compete with tolbutamide for oxidative enzyme systems in the liver, resulting in maintenance of high levels of unmetabolized, active sulfonylurea in the circulation.

Tolazamide, acetohexamide, and chlorpropamide are rarely used. Chlorpropamide has a prolonged biologic effect, and severe hypoglycemia can occur especially in older adults as their renal clearance declines with aging. Its other side effects include alcohol-induced flushing and hyponatremia due to its effect on vasopressin secretion and action.

(2) Second-generation sulfonylureas (glyburide, glipizide, gliclazide, glimepiride)—Glyburide, glipizide, gliclazide, and glimepiride are 100–200 times more potent than tolbutamide. These medications should be used with caution in patients with cardiovascular disease or in elderly patients, in whom prolonged hypoglycemia would be especially dangerous.

The usual starting dose of glyburide is 2.5 mg/day, and the average maintenance dose is 5–10 mg/day given as a single morning dose; maintenance doses higher than 20 mg/day are not recommended. Some reports suggest that 10 mg is a maximum daily therapeutic dose, with 15–20 mg having no additional benefit in poor responders and doses over 20 mg actually worsening hyperglycemia. A "Press Tab" formulation of "micronized" glyburide—easy to divide in half with slight pressure if necessary—is available. Glyburide is metabolized in the liver and the metabolic products of glyburide have hypoglycemic activity.

Glyburide has few adverse effects other than its potential for causing hypoglycemia, which at times can be prolonged. Flushing has rarely been reported after ethanol ingestion. It does not cause water retention, as chlorpropamide does, but rather slightly enhances free water clearance. Glyburide should not be used in patients with liver failure and chronic kidney disease because of the risk of hypoglycemia. Elderly patients are at particular risk for hypoglycemia even with relatively small daily doses.

The recommended starting dose of glipizide is 5 mg/day, with up to 15 mg/day given as a single daily dose before breakfast. When higher daily doses are required, they should be divided and given before meals. The maximum dose recommended by the manufacturer is 40 mg/d, although doses above 10–15 mg probably provide little additional benefit in poor responders and may even be *less* effective than smaller doses. For maximum effect in reducing postprandial hyperglycemia, glipizide should be ingested 30 minutes before meals, since rapid absorption is delayed when the medication is taken with food.

At least 90% of glipizide is metabolized in the liver to inactive products, and 10% is excreted unchanged in the urine. Glipizide therapy should therefore not be used in patients with liver failure. Because of its lower potency and shorter duration of action, it is preferable to glyburide in elderly patients and for those patients with kidney disease. Glucotrol-XL provides extended release of glipizide during transit through the gastrointestinal tract with greater effectiveness in lowering prebreakfast hyperglycemia than the shorter-duration immediate-release standard glipizide tablets. However, this formulation appears to have sacrificed its lower propensity for severe hypoglycemia compared with longer-acting glyburide without showing any demonstrable therapeutic advantages over glyburide.

Table 27–5. Drugs for treatment of type 2 diabetes mellitus.

Drug	Tablet Size	Daily Dose	Duration of Action
Sulfonylureas			
Acetohexamide (Dymelor) (not available in United States)	250 and 500 mg	0.25–1.5 g as single dose or in two divided doses	8–24 hours
Chlorpropamide (Diabinese)	100 and 250 mg	0.1–0.5 g as single dose	24–72 hours
Gliclazide (not available in United States)	80 mg	40–80 mg as single dose; 160–320 mg as divided dose	12 hours
Glimepiride (Amaryl)	1, 2, and 4 mg	1–4 mg once a day is usual dose; 8 mg once a day is maximal dose	Up to 24 hours
Glipizide			
(Glucotrol)	5 and 10 mg	2.5–40 mg as a single dose or in two divided doses 30 minutes before meals	6–12 hours
(Glucotrol XL)	2.5, 5, and 10 mg	2.5 to 10 mg once a day is usual dose; 20 mg once a day is maximal dose	Up to 24 hours
Glyburide			
(Dia Beta, Micronase)	1.25, 2.5, and 5 mg	1.25–20 mg as single dose or in two divided doses	Up to 24 hours
(Glynase)	1.5, 3, and 6 mg	1.5–12 mg as single dose or in two divided doses	Up to 24 hours
Tolazamide (Tolinase)	100, 250, and 500 mg	0.1–1 g as single dose or in two divided doses	Up to 24 hours
Tolbutamide (Orinase)	250 and 500 mg	0.5–2 g in two or three divided doses	6–24 hours
Meglitinide Analogs			
Mitiglinide (available in Japan)	5 and 10 mg	5 or 10 mg three times a day before meals	2 hours
Repaglinide (Prandin)	0.5, 1, and 2 mg	0.5 to 4 mg three times a day before meals	3 hours
D-Phenylalanine Derivative			
Nateglinide (Starlix)	60 and 120 mg	60 or 120 mg three times a day before meals	4 hours
Biguanides			
Metformin (Glucophage)	500, 850, and 1000 mg	1–2.5 g; 1 tablet with meals two or three times daily	4 hours
Metformin, extended release (Glucophage XR)	500, 750, and 1000 mg	500–2000 mg once a day	Up to 24 hours
Thiazolidinediones			
Pioglitazone (Actos)	15, 30, and 45 mg	15–45 mg daily	Up to 24 hours
Rosiglitazone (Avandia)	2, 4, and 8 mg	4–8 mg daily (can be divided)	Up to 24 hours
Alpha-Glucosidase Inhibitors			
Acarbose (Precose)	25, 50, and 100 mg	25–100 mg three times a day just before meals	4 hours
Miglitol (Glyset)	25, 50, and 100 mg	25–100 mg three times a day just before meals	4 hours
Voglibose (not available in United States)	0.2 and 0.3 mg	0.2–0.3 mg three times a day just before meals	4 hours
GLP-1 Receptor Agonists			
Dulaglutide (Trulicity)	0.75-, 1.5-mg single-dose pen or prefilled syringe	0.75 mg subcutaneously once weekly. Dose can be increased to 1.5 mg if necessary.	1 week
Exenatide (Byetta)	1.2 mL and 2.4 mL prefilled pens delivering 5 mcg and 10 mcg doses	5 mcg subcutaneously twice a day within 1 hour of breakfast and dinner. Increase to 10 mcg subcutaneously twice a day after about a month **AVOID** if CrCl < 30 mL/min	6 hours
Exenatide, long-acting release (Byetta LAR, Bydureon)	2 mg (powder)	Suspend in provided diluent and inject subcutaneously.	1 week
Liraglutide (Victoza)	Prefilled, multi-dose pen that delivers doses of 0.6 mg, 1.2 mg, or 1.8 mg	0.6 mg subcutaneously once a day (starting dose). Increase to 1.2 mg after a week if no adverse reactions. Dose can be further increased to 1.8 mg, if necessary.	24 hours

(continued)

Table 27–5. Drugs for treatment of type 2 diabetes mellitus. (continued)

Drug	Tablet Size	Daily Dose	Duration of Action
GLP-1 Receptor Agonists (cont.)			
Lixisenatide (Adlyxin, Lyxumia)	3-mL prefilled pens delivering 10- or 20-mcg doses	10 mcg daily. Increase to 20 mcg daily after 2 weeks.	24 hours
Semaglutide (Ozempic)	Prefilled pens delivering 0.25 mg or 0.5 mg; and 1 mg	0.25 mg weekly for 1 month and increase to 0.5 mg weekly if no adverse reactions. Dose can be further increased to 1 mg weekly	1 week
DPP-4 Inhibitors			
Alogliptin (Nesina)	6.25, 12.5, and 25 mg	25 mg once daily; CrCl 30–59 mL/min: 12.5 mg daily; CrCl < 30 mL/min: 6.25 mg daily.	24 hours
Linagliptin (Tradjenta)	5 mg	5 mg daily	24 hours
Saxagliptin (Onglyza)	2.5 and 5 mg	2.5 mg or 5 mg once daily. CrCl ≤ 50 mL/min or if also taking drugs that are strong CYP3A4/5 inhibitors such as ketoconazole: 2.5 mg daily.	24 hours
Sitagliptin (Januvia)	25, 50, and 100 mg	100 mg once daily; CrCl 30–50 mL/min: 50 mg once daily; CrCl < 30 mL/min: 25 mg once daily	24 hours
Vildagliptin (Galvus) (not available in United States)	50 mg	50 mg once or twice daily. **AVOID** if CrCl ≤ 60 mL/min or AST/ALT three times upper limit of normal	24 hours
SGLT2 Inhibitors			
Canagliflozin (Invokana)	100 and 300 mg	100 mg daily is usual dose. 300-mg dose can be used if normal eGFR, resulting in lowering the HbA_{1c} an additional ~ 0.1–0.25%. **AVOID** if eGFR < 45 mL/min/1.72 m^2.	24 hours
Dapagliflozin (Farxiga)	5 and 10 mg	10 mg daily.	24 hours
Empagliflozin (Jardiance)	10 and 25 mg	10 mg daily. 25-mg dose can be used if necessary.	24 hours
Ertugliflozin (Steglatro)	5 and 15 mg	5 mg daily. 15 mg dose can be used if necessary	24 hours
Others			
Bromocriptine (Cycloset)	0.8 mg	0.8 mg daily. Increase weekly by 1 tablet until maximal tolerated dose of 1.6–4.8 mg daily.	24 hours
Colesevelam (Welchol)	625 mg	3 tablets twice a day	24 hours
Pramlintide (Symlin)	5-mL vial containing 0.6 mg/mL; also available as prefilled pens. Symlin pen 60 or Symlin pen 120 (subcutaneous injection)	For insulin-treated type 2 patients, start at 60-mcg dose three times a day (10 units on U100 insulin syringe). Increase to 120 mcg three times a day (20 units on U100 insulin syringe) if no nausea for 3–7 days. Give immediately before meal. For type 1 patients, start at 15 mcg three times a day (2.5 units on U100 insulin syringe) and increase by increments of 15 mcg to a maximum of 60 mcg three times a day, as tolerated. To avoid hypoglycemia, lower insulin dose by 50% on initiation of therapy.	2 hours

AST/ALT, aspartate aminotransferase/alanine aminotransferase; CrCl, creatinine clearance by estimated glomerular filtration rate.

Gliclazide (not available in the United States) is another intermediate duration sulfonylurea with a duration of action of about 12 hours. The recommended starting dose is 40–80 mg/day with a maximum dose of 320 mg. Doses of 160 mg and above are given as divided doses before breakfast and dinner. The medication is metabolized by the liver; the metabolites and conjugates have no hypoglycemic effect. An extended release preparation is available.

Glimepiride has a long duration of effect with a half-life of 5 hours allowing once or twice daily dosing. Glimepiride achieves blood glucose lowering with the lowest dose of any sulfonylurea compound. A single daily dose of 1 mg/day has been shown to be effective, and the maximal recommended dose is 8 mg. It is completely metabolized by the liver to relatively inactive metabolic products.

B. Meglitinide analogs—Repaglinide is structurally similar to glyburide but lacks the sulfonic acid-urea moiety. It acts by binding to the sulfonylurea receptor and closing the adenosine triphosphate (ATP)-sensitive potassium channel. It is rapidly absorbed from the intestine and then undergoes complete metabolism in the liver to inactive biliary products, giving it a plasma half-life of less than 1 hour. The medication therefore causes a brief but rapid pulse of insulin. The starting dose is 0.5 mg three times a day 15 minutes before each meal. The dose can be titrated to a maximum daily dose of 16 mg. Like the sulfonylureas, repaglinide can be used in combination with metformin. Hypoglycemia is the main side effect. Like the sulfonylureas, repaglinide causes weight gain. Metabolism is by cytochrome P450 3A4 isoenzyme, and other medications that induce or inhibit this isoenzyme may increase or inhibit (respectively) the metabolism of repaglinide. The medication may be useful in patients with kidney impairment or in older adults.

Mitiglinide is a benzylsuccinic acid derivative that binds to the sulfonylurea receptor and is similar to repaglinide in its clinical effects. It is approved for use in Japan.

C. D-Phenylalanine derivative—Nateglinide stimulates insulin secretion by binding to the sulfonylurea receptor and closing the ATP-sensitive potassium channel. It is rapidly absorbed from the intestine, reaching peak plasma levels within 1 hour. It is metabolized in the liver and has a plasma half-life of about 1.5 hours. Like repaglinide, it causes a brief rapid pulse of insulin, and when given before a meal it reduces the postprandial rise in blood glucose. For most patients, the recommended starting and maintenance dose is 120 mg three times a day before meals. Use 60 mg in patients who have mild elevations in HbA_{1c}. Like the other insulin secretagogues, its main side effects are hypoglycemia and weight gain.

2. Medications that primarily lower glucose levels by their actions on the liver, muscle, and adipose tissue—

A. Metformin—Metformin is the first-line therapy for patients with type 2 diabetes. It can be used alone or in conjunction with other oral agents or insulin in the treatment of patients with type 2 diabetes. It is ineffective in patients with type 1 diabetes.

Metformin's therapeutic effects primarily derive from the increasing hepatic adenosine monophosphate-activated protein kinase activity, which reduces hepatic gluconeogenesis and lipogenesis. Metformin has a half-life of 1.5–3 hours and is not bound to plasma proteins or metabolized, being excreted unchanged by the kidneys.

The current recommendation is to start metformin at diagnosis. A side benefit of metformin therapy is its tendency to improve both fasting and postprandial hyperglycemia and hypertriglyceridemia in obese patients with diabetes without the weight gain associated with insulin or sulfonylurea therapy. Patients with chronic kidney disease should not be given this medication because failure to

excrete it would produce high blood and tissue levels of metformin that could stimulate lactic acid overproduction. In the United States, metformin use is not recommended at or above a serum creatinine level of 1.4 mg/dL in women and 1.5 mg/dL in men. In the United Kingdom, the recommendations are to review metformin use when the serum creatinine exceeds 130 mcmol/L (1.5 mg/dL) or the estimated glomerular filtration rate (eGFR) falls below 45 mL/min/1.73 m^2. The medication should be stopped if the serum creatinine exceeds 150 mcmol/L (1.7 mg/dL) or the eGFR is below 30 mL/min/1.73 m^2. Patients with liver failure or persons with excessive alcohol intake should not receive this medication because of the risk of lactic acidosis.

The maximum dosage of metformin is 2550 mg, although little benefit is seen above a total dose of 2000 mg. It is important to begin with a low dose and increase the dosage very gradually in divided doses—taken with meals—to reduce minor gastrointestinal upsets. A common schedule would be one 500-mg tablet three times a day with meals or one 850- or 1000-mg tablet twice daily at breakfast and dinner. Up to 2000 mg of the extended-release preparation can be given once a day. Lower doses should be used in patients with eGFRs between 30 and 45 mL/min/1.73 m^2. Lower doses should also be used in the elderly who have reduced renal functional reserve and are at higher risk for acute kidney injury.

The most frequent side effects of metformin are gastrointestinal symptoms (anorexia, nausea, vomiting, abdominal discomfort, diarrhea), which occur in up to 20% of patients. These effects are dose-related, tend to occur at onset of therapy, and often are transient. However, in 3–5% of patients, therapy may have to be discontinued because of persistent diarrheal discomfort. Patients switching from immediate-release metformin to comparable dose of extended-release metformin may experience fewer gastrointestinal side effects.

Hypoglycemia does not occur with therapeutic doses of metformin, which permits its description as a "euglycemic" or "antihyperglycemic" medication rather than an oral hypoglycemic agent. Dermatologic or hematologic toxicity is rare. Metformin interferes with the calcium dependent absorption of vitamin B_{12}-intrinsic complex in the terminal ileum; vitamin B_{12} deficiency can occur after many years of metformin use. Periodic screening with vitamin B_{12} levels should be considered, especially in patients with peripheral neuropathy or if a macrocytic anemia develops. Increased intake of dietary calcium may prevent the metformin-induced B_{12} malaborption.

Lactic acidosis has been reported as a side effect but is uncommon with metformin in contrast to phenformin. Almost all reported cases have involved persons with associated risk factors that should have contraindicated its use (kidney, liver, or cardiorespiratory insufficiency and alcoholism). Acute kidney injury can occur rarely in certain patients receiving radiocontrast agents. Metformin therapy should therefore be temporarily halted on the day of radiocontrast administration and restarted a day or two later after confirmation that kidney function has not deteriorated.

B. Thiazolidinediones—Two medications of this class, rosiglitazone and pioglitazone, are available for clinical use. These medications sensitize peripheral tissues to insulin. They bind the nuclear receptor peroxisome proliferator-activated receptor gamma (PPAR-gamma) and affect the expression of a number of genes. Like the biguanides, this class of medications does not cause hypoglycemia.

Both rosiglitazone and pioglitazone are effective as monotherapy and in combination with sulfonylureas or metformin or insulin, lowering HbA_{1c} by 1–2%. When used in combination with insulin, they can result in a 30–50% reduction in insulin dosage, and some patients can come off insulin completely. The dosage of rosiglitazone is 4–8 mg daily and of pioglitazone, 15–45 mg daily, and the medications do not have to be taken with food. Rosiglitazone is primarily metabolized by the CYP 2C8 isoenzyme and pioglitazone is metabolized by CYP 2C8 and CYP 3A4.

The combination of a thiazolidinedione and metformin has the advantage of not causing hypoglycemia. Patients inadequately managed on sulfonylureas can do well on a combination of sulfonylurea and rosiglitazone or pioglitazone.

These medications have some additional effects apart from glucose lowering. Rosiglitazone therapy is associated with increases in total cholesterol, LDL cholesterol (15%), and HDL cholesterol (10%). There is a reduction in free fatty acids of about 8–15%. The changes in triglycerides are generally not different from placebo. Pioglitazone in clinical trials lowered triglycerides (9%) and increased HDL cholesterol (15%) but did not cause a consistent change in total cholesterol and LDL cholesterol levels. A prospective randomized comparison of the metabolic effects of pioglitazone and rosiglitazone showed similar effects on HbA_{1c} and weight gain. Small prospective studies have demonstrated that treatment with these medications leads to improvements in the biochemical and histologic features of nonalcoholic fatty liver disease. The thiazolidinediones also may limit vascular smooth muscle proliferation after injury, and there are reports that pioglitazone can reduce neointimal proliferation after coronary stent placement. In one double-blind, placebo-controlled study, rosiglitazone was shown to be associated with a decrease in the ratio of urinary albumin to creatinine excretion.

Safety concerns and some troublesome side effects limit the use of this class of medication. Rosiglitazone use declined when a meta-analysis of 42 randomized clinical trials suggested that this medication increases the risk of angina pectoris or myocardial infarction; the European Medicines Agency suspended the use of rosiglitazone in Europe. In the United States, the FDA established a restricted distribution program. A subsequent large prospective clinical trial (the RECORD study) failed to confirm the meta-analysis finding and the restrictions were lifted in the United States.

Edema occurs in about 3–4% of patients receiving monotherapy with rosiglitazone or pioglitazone. The edema occurs more frequently (10–15%) in patients receiving concomitant insulin therapy and may result in heart failure. The medications are contraindicated in diabetic individuals with New York Heart Association class III and IV cardiac status. Thiazolidinediones have also been reported as being associated with new onset or worsening macular edema. Apparently, this is a rare side effect, and most of these patients also had peripheral edema. The macular edema resolved or improved once the medication was discontinued.

Troglitazone, the first medication in this class, was withdrawn from clinical use because of medication-associated fatal liver failure. Although rosiglitazone and pioglitazone have not been reported to cause liver injury, the FDA recommends that they should not be used in patients with clinical evidence of active liver disease or pretreatment elevation of the alanine aminotransferase (ALT) level that is 2.5 times greater than the upper limit of normal. Liver biochemical tests should be performed on all patients prior to initiation of treatment and periodically thereafter.

An increase in fracture risk in women (but not men) has been reported with both rosiglitazone and pioglitazone. The fracture risk is in the range of 1.9 per 100 patient-years with the thiazolidinedione compared to 1.1 per 100 patient-years on comparison treatment. In at least one study of rosiglitazone, the fracture risk was increased in premenopausal as well as postmenopausal women.

Other side effects include anemia, which occurs in 4% of patients treated with these medications; it may be due to a dilutional effect of increased plasma volume rather than a reduction in red cell mass. Weight gain occurs, especially when the medication is combined with a sulfonylurea or insulin. Some of the weight gain is fluid retention, but there is also an increase in total fat mass. Clinical studies have reported conflicting results regarding an association of bladder cancer with pioglitazone use. A 10-year observational cohort study of patients taking pioglitazone failed to find an association with bladder cancer. A large multipopulation pooled analysis (1.01 million persons over 5.9 million person-years) also failed to find an association between cumulative exposure of pioglitazone or rosiglitazone and incidence of bladder cancer. Another population-based study, however, generating 689,616 person-years of follow-up did find that pioglitazone but not rosiglitazone was associated with an increased risk of bladder cancer.

3. Medications that affect absorption of glucose— Alpha-glucosidase inhibitors competitively inhibit the alpha-glucosidase enzymes in the gut that digest dietary starch and sucrose. Two of these medications—acarbose and miglitol—are available for clinical use in the United States. Voglibose, another alpha-glucosidase inhibitor is available in Japan, Korea, and India. Acarbose and miglitol are potent inhibitors of glucoamylase, alpha-amylase, and sucrase but have less effect on isomaltase and hardly any on trehalase and lactase.

A. Acarbose—The recommended starting dose of acarbose is 50 mg twice daily, gradually increasing to 100 mg three times daily. For maximal benefit on postprandial hyperglycemia, acarbose should be given with the first mouthful of food ingested. In diabetic patients, it reduces postprandial hyperglycemia by 30–50%, and its overall effect is to lower the HbA_{1c} by 0.5–1%.

The principal adverse effect, seen in 20–30% of patients, is flatulence. This is caused by undigested carbohydrate reaching the lower bowel, where gases are produced by bacterial flora. In 3% of cases, troublesome diarrhea occurs. This gastrointestinal discomfort tends to discourage excessive carbohydrate consumption and promotes improved compliance of type 2 patients with their diet prescriptions. When acarbose is given alone, there is no risk of hypoglycemia. However, if combined with insulin or sulfonylureas, it might increase the risk of hypoglycemia from these agents. A slight rise in hepatic aminotransferases has been noted in clinical trials with acarbose (5% vs 2% in placebo controls, and particularly with doses greater than 300 mg/day). The levels generally return to normal on stopping the medication.

B. Miglitol—Miglitol is similar to acarbose in terms of its clinical effects. It is indicated for use in diet- or sulfonylurea-treated patients with type 2 diabetes. Therapy is initiated at the lowest effective dosage of 25 mg three times a day. The usual maintenance dose is 50 mg three times a day, although some patients may benefit from increasing the dose to 100 mg three times a day. Gastrointestinal side effects occur as with acarbose. The medication is not metabolized and is excreted unchanged by the kidney. Miglitol should not be used in end-stage chronic kidney disease, when its clearance would be impaired.

4. Incretins—Oral glucose provokes a threefold to fourfold higher insulin response than an equivalent dose of glucose given intravenously. This is because the oral glucose causes a release of gut hormones, principally glucagon-like peptide 1 (GLP-1) and glucose-dependent insulinotropic polypeptide (GIP1), that amplify the glucose-induced insulin release. This "incretin effect" of GLP-1 secretion (but not GIP1 secretion) is reduced in patients with type 2 diabetes and when GLP-1 is infused in patients with type 2 diabetes, it stimulates insulin secretion and lowers glucose levels. GLP-1, unlike the sulfonylureas, has only a modest insulin stimulatory effect at normoglycemic concentrations. This means that GLP-1 has a lower risk for hypoglycemia than the sulfonylureas.

In addition to its insulin stimulatory effect, GLP-1 also has a number of other pancreatic and extrapancreatic effects. It suppresses glucagon secretion and so may ameliorate the hyperglucagonemia that is present in people with diabetes and improve postprandial hyperglycemia. GLP-1 acts on the stomach delaying gastric emptying; the importance of this effect on glucose lowering is illustrated by the observation that antagonizing the deceleration of gastric emptying markedly reduces the glucose lowering effect of GLP-1. GLP-1 receptors are present in the central nervous system and may play a role in the anorectic effect of the drugs. Type 2 diabetic patients undergoing GLP-1 infusion are less hungry; it is unclear whether this is mainly due to a deceleration of gastric emptying or whether there is a central nervous system effect as well.

A. GLP-1 receptor agonists—GLP-1's half-life is only 1–2 minutes. It is rapidly proteolyzed by dipeptidyl peptidase 4 (DPP-4) and by other enzymes, such as endopeptidase 24.11, and is also cleared quickly by the kidney. The native peptide, therefore, cannot be used therapeutically. Five GLP-1 receptor agonists with longer half-lives, exenatide, liraglutide, dulaglutide, lixisenatide, and semaglutide, are available for clinical use.

(1) Dosages and pharmacokinetics—Exenatide (Exendin 4) is a GLP-1 receptor agonist isolated from the saliva of the Gila monster (a venomous lizard) that is more resistant to DPP-4 action and cleared by the kidney. Its half-life is 2.4 hours, and its glucose lowering effect is about 6 hours. Exenatide is dispensed as two fixed-dose pens (5 mcg and 10 mcg). It is injected 60 minutes before breakfast and before dinner. Patients with type 2 diabetes should be prescribed the 5 mcg pen for the first month and, if tolerated, the dose can then be increased to 10 mcg twice a day. The medication is not recommended in patients with eGFR less than 30 mL/min. In clinical trials, adding exenatide therapy to patients with type 2 diabetes already taking metformin or a sulfonylurea, or both, further lowered the HbA_{1c} value by 0.4% to 0.6% over a 30-week period. These patients also experienced a weight loss of 3–6 pounds. Exenatide LAR is a once-weekly preparation that is dispensed as a powder (2 mg). It is suspended in the provided diluent just prior to injection. In comparative clinical trials, the long-acting drug lowers the HbA_{1c} level a little more than the twice daily drug. Low-titer antibodies against exenatide develop in over one-third (38%) of patients, but the clinical effects are not attenuated. High-titer antibodies develop in a subset of patients (~6%), and in about half of these cases, an attenuation of glycemic response has been seen.

Liraglutide is a soluble fatty acid acylated GLP-1 analog. The half-life is approximately 12 hours, allowing the medication to be injected once a day. The dosing is initiated at 0.6 mg daily, increased after 1 week to 1.2 mg daily. Some patients may benefit from increasing the dose to 1.8 mg. In clinical trials lasting 26 and 52 weeks, adding liraglutide to the therapeutic regimen (metformin, sulfonylurea, thiazolidinedione) of patients with type 2 diabetes further lowered the HbA_{1c} value. Depending on the dose and design of the study, the HbA_{1c} decline was in the range of 0.6% to 1.5%. The patients had sustained weight loss of 1–6 pounds. Liraglutide at a dose of 3 mg daily has been approved for weight loss.

In a postmarketing multinational study of 9340 patients with type 2 diabetes with known cardiovascular disease, the addition of liraglutide was associated with a lower primary composite outcome of death from cardiovascular causes, nonfatal myocardial infarction, or nonfatal stroke (hazard ratio 0.87, $P = 0.01$). Patients taking liraglutide had lower HbA_{1c} levels, weight loss of 2.3 kg, lower systolic blood pressure, and fewer episodes of severe hypoglycemia.

Dulaglutide consists of two GLP-1 analog molecules covalently linked to an Fc fragment of human IgG_4. The GLP-1 molecule has amino acid substitutions that resist DPP-4 action. The half-life of dulaglutide is about 5 days. The usual dose is 0.75 mg weekly by subcutaneous injection. The maximum recommended dose is 1.5 mg weekly. Dulaglutide monotherapy and combination therapy lowers HbA_{1c} by about 0.7% to 1.6%. Weight loss ranged from 2 pounds to 7 pounds.

Lixisenatide is a synthetic analog of exendin 4 (deletion of a proline and addition of 6 lysines to the C-terminal region) with a half-life of 3 hours. It is dispensed as two fixed-dose pens (10 mcg and 20 mcg). The 10-mcg dose is injected once daily before breakfast for the first 2 weeks, and if tolerated, the dose is then increased to 20 mcg daily. Its clinical effect is about the same as exenatide with HbA_{1c} lowering in the 0.4–0.6% range. Weight loss ranges from 2 pounds to 6 pounds. Antibodies to lixisenatide occur frequently (70%) and ~ 2.4% with the highest antibody titers have attenuated glycemic response.

Semaglutide is a synthetic analog of GLP-1 with a drug half-life of about 1 week. It has an alpha-aminoisobutyric acid substitution at position 8 that makes the molecule resistant to DPP4 action and a C-18 fatty di-acid chain attached to lysine at position 26 that binds to albumin, which accounts for the drug's long half-life. Semaglutide is dispensed as two pens: one pen delivers a 0.25-mg or 0.5-mg dose and the other pen delivers a 1-mg dose. The recommended dosing is 0.25 mg weekly for 4 weeks and if tolerated the dose is then increased to 0.5 mg per week. The 1-mg per week dose can provide additional glucose lowering effect. Semaglutide monotherapy and combination therapy lowers HbA_{1c} from 1.5% to 1.8%. An increase in diabetic retinopathy was observed in the semaglutide treated group in one of the clinical trials. It is thought that this might have been secondary to the rapid glucose lowering with the drug.

(2) Adverse effects of GLP-1 receptor agonists—The most frequent adverse reactions of the GLP-1 receptor agonists are nausea (11–40%), vomiting (4–13%), and diarrhea (9–17%). The reactions are more frequent at the higher doses. In clinical trials about 1–5% of participants withdrew from the studies because of the gastrointestinal symptoms.

The GLP-1 receptor agonists have been associated with increased risk of pancreatitis. The pancreatitis was severe (hemorrhagic or necrotizing) in 6 instances, and 2 of these patients died. In the liraglutide and dulaglutide clinical trials, there were 13 and 5 cases of pancreatitis in the drug-treated groups versus 1 and 1 case in the comparator groups, respectively. This translates to about 1.4–2.2 vs 0.6–0.9 cases of pancreatitis per 1000 patient-years. *Patients taking GLP-1 receptor agonists should be advised to seek immediate medical care if they experience unexplained persistent severe abdominal pain.*

There have been rare reports of acute kidney injury in patients taking exenatide. Some of these patients had pre-existing kidney disease, and others had one or more risk factors for kidney disease. A number of the patients reported nausea, vomiting, and diarrhea, and it is possible that these side effects caused volume depletion and contributed to the development of the kidney injury. For this reason, the GLP-1 receptors agonists should be prescribed cautiously in patients with kidney impairment.

GLP-1 receptor agonists stimulate C-cell neoplasia and cause medullary thyroid carcinoma in rats. Human C-cells express very few GLP-1 receptors, and the relevance to human therapy is unclear. The medications, however, should not be used in patients with personal or family history of medullary thyroid carcinoma or multiple endocrine neoplasia (MEN) syndrome type 2.

B. DPP-4 INHIBITORS—An alternate approach to the use of GLP-1 receptor agonists is to inhibit the enzyme DPP-4 and prolong the action of endogenously released GLP-1 and GIP. Four oral DPP-4 inhibitors, sitagliptin, saxagliptin, linagliptin, and alogliptin, are available in the United States for the treatment of type 2 diabetes. An additional DPP-4 inhibitor, vildagliptin, is available in Europe. Other DPP-4 inhibitors—gemigliptin, anagliptin, teneligliptin, trelagliptin, omarigliptin, evogliptin, and gosogliptin—have been approved outside the United States and European Union (Korea, India, Thailand, Japan, Russia, and several South American countries).

Sitagliptin, when used alone or in combination with other diabetes medications, lowers HbA_{1c} by approximately 0.5%. The usual dose of sitagliptin is 100 mg once daily, but the dose is reduced to 50 mg daily if the calculated creatinine clearance is 30–50 mL/min and to 25 mg for clearances less than 30 mL/min. Unlike exenatide, sitagliptin does not cause nausea or vomiting. It also does not result in weight loss. Saxagliptin, when added to the therapeutic regimen (metformin, sulfonylurea, thiazolidinedione) of patients with type 2 diabetes, further lowered the HbA_{1c} value by about 0.7–0.9%. The dose is 2.5 mg or 5 mg orally once a day. The 2.5-mg dose should be used in patients with calculated creatinine clearance less than 50 mL/min. The medication is weight neutral.

Alogliptin lowers HbA_{1c} by about 0.5–0.6% when added to metformin, sulfonylurea, or pioglitazone. The usual dose is 25 mg orally daily. The 12.5-mg dose is used in patients with calculated creatinine clearance of 30 to 60 mLs/min; and 6.25 mg for clearance less than 30 mL/min. Linagliptin lowers HbA_{1c} by about 0.4–0.6% when added to metformin, sulfonylurea, or pioglitazone. The dose is 5 mg orally daily, and, since it is primarily excreted unmetabolized via the bile, no dose adjustment is needed in patients with kidney disease. Vildagliptin lowers HbA_{1c} by about 0.5–1% when added to the therapeutic regimen of patients with type 2 diabetes. The dose is 50 mg once or twice daily.

5. Sodium-glucose co-transporter 2 inhibitors—Glucose is freely filtered by the kidney glomeruli and is reabsorbed in the proximal tubules by the action of sodium-glucose co-transporters (SGLT). Sodium-glucose co-transporter 2 (SGLT2) accounts for about 90% of glucose reabsorption and its inhibition causes glycosuria in people with diabetes, lowering plasma glucose levels. The SGLT2 inhibitors canagliflozin, dapagliflozin, empagliflozin, and ertugliflozin are approved for clinical use in the United States. These agents reduce the threshold for glycosuria from a plasma glucose threshold of about a 180 mg/dL to about 40 mg/dL; and lower HbA_{1c} by 0.5–1% when used alone or in combination with other oral agents or insulin. The efficacy is higher at higher HbA_{1c} levels when more glucose is excreted as a result of SGLT2 inhibition. The loss of calories results in modest weight loss of 2–5 kg.

The usual dose of canagliflozin is 100 mg daily but up to 300 mg daily can be used in patients with normal kidney function. The dose of dapagliflozin is 10 mg daily but 5 mg daily is the recommended initial dose in patients with hepatic failure. The usual dosage of empagliflozin is 10 mg daily but a higher dose of 25 mg daily can be used. The recommended starting dose of ertugliflozin is 5 mg, but the dose can be increased to 15 mg daily if additional glucose lowering is needed.

In a postmarketing multinational study of 7020 patients with type 2 diabetes with known cardiovascular disease, the addition of empagliflozin was associated with a lower primary composite outcome of death from cardiovascular causes, nonfatal myocardial infarction, or nonfatal stroke (hazard ratio 0.86, $P = 0.04$). The mechanisms regarding the benefit remain unclear. Weight loss, lower blood pressure, and diuresis may have played a role since there were fewer deaths from heart failure in the treated group whereas the rates of myocardial infarction were unaltered. A similar multinational study was performed with the addition of canagliflozin. This was a study of 10,142 patients with type 2 diabetes with known or at increased risk for cardiovascular disease. The canagliflozin treated group had a lower primary composite outcome of death from cardiovascular causes, nonfatal myocardial infarction, or nonfatal stroke (hazard ratio 0.86, $P = 0.02$). Both empagliflozin and canagliflozin showed benefit in terms of progression of albuminuria and kidney injury, possibly by lowering glomerular hyperfiltration. In type 2 diabetes patients with diabetic kidney disease (eGFR 30 to less than 90 mL/min/1.73 m^2 and urine albumin excretion more than 300 mg/g creatinine), canagliflozin has been shown to prevent progression to end-stage renal disease.

As might be expected, the efficacy of the SGLT2 inhibitors is reduced in chronic kidney disease. They can also increase creatinine and decrease eGFR, especially in patients with kidney impairment. Canagliflozin is contraindicated in patients with eGFR less than 45 mL/min/1.73 m^2. The main side effects are increased incidence of genital mycotic infections and urinary tract infections affecting ~8–9% of patients. There have also been reports of cases of pyelonephritis and septicemia requiring hospitalization. The glycosuria can cause intravascular volume contraction and hypotension.

The multinational study with canagliflozin showed an increased risk of amputations, especially of the toes (hazard ratio 1.97, 95 % CI 1.41–2.75). It is not known if this is a class effect or an adverse effect specific to this agent.

Canagliflozin has been reported to cause a decrease in bone mineral density at the lumbar spine and the hip. In a pooled analysis of eight clinical trials (mean duration 68 weeks), a 30% increase in fractures was observed in patients taking canagliflozin. It is likely that the effect on the bones is a class effect and not restricted to canagliflozin. All the SGLT2 inhibitors cause a modest increase in LDL cholesterol levels (3–8%). Also, in clinical trials, patients taking dapagliflozin had higher rates of breast cancer (nine cases vs none in comparator arms) and bladder cancer (10 cases vs 1 in placebo arm). These cancer rates exceeded the expected rates in age-matched reference diabetes population.

Cases of DKA have been reported with off-label use of SGLT2 inhibitors in patients with type 1 diabetes. Type 1 patients are taught to give less insulin if their glucose levels are not elevated. SGLT2 inhibitors lower glucose levels by changing the renal threshold and not by insulin action. Type 1 patients taking an SGLT2 inhibitor, because the glucose levels are not elevated, may either withhold or reduce their insulin doses to such a degree as to induce ketoacidosis. SGLT2 inhibitors should not be used in patients with type 1 diabetes and in those patients labeled as having type 2 diabetes but who are very insulin deficient and ketosis-prone.

6. Others—Pramlintide is a synthetic analog of islet amyloid polypeptide (IAPP or amylin). When given subcutaneously, it delays gastric emptying, suppresses glucagon secretion, and decreases appetite. It is approved for use both in type 1 diabetes and in insulin-treated type 2 diabetes. In 6-month clinical studies with type 1 and insulin-treated type 2 patients, those taking the medication had an approximately 0.4% reduction in HbA$_{1c}$ and about 1.7 kg weight loss compared with placebo. The HbA$_{1c}$ reduction was sustained for 2 years but some of the weight was regained. The medication is given by injection immediately before the meal. Hypoglycemia can occur, and it is recommended that the short-acting or premixed insulin doses be reduced by 50% when the medication is started. Since the medication slows gastric emptying, recovery from hypoglycemia can be a problem because of delay in absorption of fast-acting carbohydrates. Nausea was the other main side effect, affecting 30–50% of persons, but tended to improve with time. In patients with type 1 diabetes, the initial dose of pramlintide is 15 mcg before each meal and titrated up by 15-mcg increments to a maintenance dose of 30 mcg or 60 mcg before each meal. In patients with type 2 diabetes, the starting dose is 60 mcg premeals increased to 120 mcg in 3 to 7 days if no significant nausea occurs.

Bromocriptine, a dopamine 2 receptor agonist, has been shown to modestly lower HbA$_{1c}$ by 0.1–0.5% when compared to baseline and 0.4–0.5% compared to placebo. The tablet dose is 0.8 mg and the daily dose is 2 (1.6 g) to 6 (4.8 mg) tablets as tolerated. Common side effects are nausea, vomiting, dizziness, and headache.

Colesevelam, the bile acid sequestrant, when added to metformin or sulfonylurea or insulin, lowered HbA$_{1c}$ 0.3–0.4% when compared to baseline and 0.5–0.6% compared to placebo. HbA$_{1c}$ lowering, however, was not observed in a single monotherapy clinical trial comparing colesevelam to placebo. Colesevelam use is associated with ~20% increase in triglyceride levels. Other adverse effects include constipation and dyspepsia.

With their modest glucose lowering and significant side effects, using bromocriptine or colesevelam to treat diabetes is not recommended.

7. Medication combinations—Several medication combinations are available in different dose sizes, including glyburide and metformin (Glucovance); glipizide and metformin (Metaglip); repaglinide and metformin (PrandiMet); rosiglitazone and metformin (Avandamet); pioglitazone and metformin (ACTOplusMet); rosiglitazone and glimepiride (Avandaryl); pioglitazone and glimepiride (Duetact); sitagliptin and metformin (Janumet); saxagliptin and metformin XR (Kombiglyze XR); linagliptin and metformin (Jentadueto); alogliptin and metformin (Kazano); alogliptin and pioglitazone (Oseni); dapagliflozin and metformin (Xigduo); canagliflozin and metformin (Invokamet); empagliflozin and metformin (Synjardy); empagliflozin and linagliptin (Glyxambi);

Table 27–6. Summary of bioavailability characteristics of the insulins.

Insulin Preparations	Onset of Action	Peak Action	Effective Duration
Insulins lispro, aspart,[1] glulisine	5–15 minutes	1–1.5 hours	3–4 hours
Human regular	30–60 minutes	2 hours	6–8 hours
Human NPH	2–4 hours	6–7 hours	10–20 hours
Insulin glargine	0.5–1 hour	Flat	~24 hours
Insulin detemir	0.5–1 hour	Flat	17 hours
Insulin degludec	0.5–1.5 hours	Flat	More than 42 hours
Technosphere inhaled insulin	5–15 minutes	1 hour	3 hours

[1]Insulin aspart formulated with niacinamide has an ~10-minute faster onset of action.

ertugliflozin and metformin (Segluromet); ertugliflozin and sitagliptin (Steglujan); insulin degludec and liraglutide (Xultophy); and insulin glargine and lixisenatide (Soliqua). These medication combinations, however, limit the clinician's ability to optimally adjust dosage of the individual medications and for that reason are not recommended.

C. Insulin

Insulin is indicated for type 1 diabetes as well as for type 2 diabetic patients with insulinopenia whose hyperglycemia does not respond to diet therapy either alone or combined with other hypoglycemic medications.

1. Characteristics of available insulin preparations—
Human insulin is dispensed as either regular (R) or NPH (N) formulations. Six analogs of human insulin—three rapidly acting (insulin lispro, insulin aspart, insulin glulisine) and three long-acting (insulin glargine, insulin detemir, and insulin degludec)—are approved by the FDA for clinical use. Commercial insulin preparations differ with respect to the time of onset and duration of their biologic action (Table 27–6). All currently available insulins contain less than 10 ppm of proinsulin and are labeled as "purified." These purified insulins preserve their potency, so that refrigeration is recommended but not crucial. During travel, reserve supplies of insulin can be readily transported for weeks without losing potency if protected from extremes of heat or cold. All the insulins in the United States are available in a concentration of 100 units/mL (U100) and dispensed in 10-mL vials or 0.3-mL cartridges or prefilled disposable pens. Several insulins are available at higher concentrations: insulin glargine, 300 units/mL (U300); insulin degludec, 200 units/mL (U200); insulin lispro, 200 units/mL (U200); and regular insulin, 500 units/mL (U500).

2. Insulin preparations—See Table 27–7. The rapidly acting insulin analogs and the long-acting insulins are designed for subcutaneous administration, while regular insulin can also be given intravenously.

A. SHORT-ACTING INSULIN PREPARATIONS—

*(1) Regular insulin—*Regular insulin is a short-acting soluble crystalline zinc insulin whose effect appears within 30 minutes after subcutaneous injection and lasts 5–7 hours when usual quantities are administered.

Intravenous infusions of regular insulin are particularly useful in the treatment of DKA and during the perioperative management of patients with diabetes who require insulin. For markedly insulin-resistant persons who would otherwise require large volumes of insulin solution, a U500 preparation of human regular insulin is available both in a vial form and a disposable pen. A U500 insulin syringe should be used if the vial form is dispensed. U500 regular insulin is much more expensive than the U100 concentration and is rarely needed. There is a U300 preparation of insulin glargine, a U200 preparation of insulin lispro, and a U200 preparation of insulin degludec.

*(2) Rapidly acting insulin analogs—*Insulin lispro (Humalog) is an insulin analog where the proline at

Table 27–7. Insulin preparations available in the United States.[1]

Rapidly acting human insulin analogs
    Insulin lispro (Humalog, Lilly)
    Insulin aspart (Novolog, FiAsp, Novo Nordisk)
    Insulin glulisine (Apidra, Sanofi Aventis)
Short-acting regular insulin
    Regular insulin (Lilly, Novo Nordisk)
    Technosphere inhaled regular insulin (Afrezza)
Intermediate-acting insulins
    NPH insulin (Lilly, Novo Nordisk)
Premixed insulins
    70% NPH/30% regular (70/30 insulin—Lilly, Novo Nordisk)
    70% NPL/25% insulin lispro (Humalog Mix 75/25—Lilly)
    50% NPL/50% insulin lispro (Humalog Mix 50/50—Lilly)
    70% insulin aspart protamine/30% insulin aspart (Novolog Mix 70/30—Novo Nordisk)
    70% insulin degludec/30 insulin aspart (Ryzodeg, Novo Nordisk)
Long-acting human insulin analogs
    Insulin glargine (Lantus (U100), Toujeo (U300), Sanofi Aventis; Basaglar (U100), Lilly)
    Insulin detemir (Levemir, Novo Nordisk)
    Insulin degludec (Tresiba, Novo Nordisk)

[1]All insulins available in the United States are recombinant human or human insulin analog origin. All the above insulins are dispensed at U100 concentration. There is an additional U500 preparation of regular insulin; U300 preparation of insulin glargine; U200 preparation of insulin lispro; U200 preparation of insulin degludec. NPH, neutral protamine Hagedorn.

position B28 is reversed with the lysine at B29. Insulin aspart (Novolog) is a single substitution of proline by aspartic acid at position B28. In insulin glulisine (Apidra) the asparagine at position B3 is replaced by lysine and the lysine in position B29 by glutamic acid. These three analogs have less of a tendency to form hexamers, in contrast to human insulin. When injected subcutaneously, the analogs quickly dissociate into monomers and are absorbed very rapidly, reaching peak serum values in as soon as 1 hour—in contrast to regular human insulin, whose hexamers require considerably more time to dissociate and become absorbed. The amino acid changes in these analogs do not interfere with their binding to the insulin receptor, with the circulating half-life, or with their immunogenicity, which are all identical with those of human regular insulin. An insulin aspart formulation (FiAsp) that contains niacinamide (vitamin B_3) has a more rapid initial absorption and its onset of action is about 10 minutes faster than the standard insulin aspart formulation. Because of this more rapid onset of action, the 1-hour (but not 2-hour) postprandial glucose excursions are lower compared to the standard formulation.

Clinical trials have demonstrated that the optimal times of preprandial subcutaneous injection of comparable doses of the rapidly acting insulin analogs and of regular human insulin are 20 minutes and 60 minutes, respectively, before the meal. While this more rapid onset of action has been welcomed as a great convenience by diabetic patients who object to waiting as long as 60 minutes after injecting regular human insulin before they can begin their meal, patients must be taught to ingest adequate absorbable carbohydrate early in the meal to avoid hypoglycemia during the meal. Another desirable feature of rapidly acting insulin analogs is that their duration of action remains at about 4 hours irrespective of dosage. This contrasts with regular insulin, whose duration of action is prolonged when larger doses are used.

The rapidly acting analogs are also commonly used in pumps. In a double-blind crossover study comparing insulin lispro with regular insulin in insulin pumps, persons using insulin lispro had lower HbA_{1c} values and improved postprandial glucose control with the same frequency of hypoglycemia. In the event of pump failure, however, users of the rapidly acting insulin analogs will have more rapid onset of hyperglycemia and ketosis.

While insulin aspart has been approved for intravenous use (eg, in hyperglycemic emergencies), there is no advantage in using insulin aspart over regular insulin by this route. A U200 concentration of insulin lispro is available in a disposable prefilled pen. The only advantage of the U200 over the U100 insulin lispro preparation is that it delivers the same dose in half the volume.

B. Long-acting Insulin Preparations—

(1) NPH (neutral protamine Hagedorn or isophane) insulin—NPH is an intermediate-acting insulin whose onset of action is delayed to 2–4 hours, and its peak response is generally reached in about 6–7 hours. The onset of action is delayed by combining 2 parts soluble crystalline zinc insulin with 1 part protamine zinc insulin. This produces equivalent amounts of insulin and protamine, so that neither is present in an uncomplexed form ("isophane"). Because its duration of action is often less than 24 hours (with a range of 10–20 hours), most patients require at least two injections daily to maintain a sustained insulin effect. Occasional vials of NPH insulin have tended to show unusual clumping of their contents or "frosting" of the container, with considerable loss of bioactivity. This instability is rare and occurs less frequently if NPH human insulin is refrigerated when not in use and if bottles are discarded after 1 month of use.

(2) Insulin glargine—In this insulin, the asparagine at position 21 of the insulin A chain is replaced by glycine and two arginines are added to the carboxyl terminal of the B chain. The arginines raise the isoelectric point of the molecule closer to neutral making it more soluble in an acidic environment. In contrast, human insulin has an isoelectric point of pH 5.4. Insulin glargine is a clear insulin, which, when injected into the neutral pH environment of the subcutaneous tissue, forms microprecipitates that slowly release the insulin into the circulation. This insulin lasts for about 24 hours without any pronounced peaks and is given once a day to provide basal coverage. This insulin cannot be mixed with the other human insulins because of its acidic pH. When this insulin was given as a single injection at bedtime to type 1 patients in clinical trials, fasting hyperglycemia was better controlled with less nocturnal hypoglycemia when compared to NPH insulin.

A more concentrated form of insulin glargine (U300) is available as an insulin pen. In pharmacodynamic studies in type 1 patients, the U300 compared to the U100 preparation had approximately 5 hours longer duration of action. In clinical trials in type 1 patients, U300 use did not result in better control or reduce the rates of hypoglycemia. Although limited clinical data suggest that insulin glargine is safe in pregnancy, it is not approved for this use.

(3) Insulin detemir—In this insulin analog, the threonine at position B30 has been removed and a 14-C fatty acid chain (tetradecanoic acid) is attached to the lysine at position 29 by acylation. Its prolonged action is due to dihexamerization and binding of hexamers and dimers to albumin at the injection site as well as binding of the monomer via its fatty acid side chain to albumin in the circulation. The affinity of insulin detemir is fourfold to fivefold lower than that of human soluble insulin and therefore the U100 formulation of insulin detemir has an insulin concentration of 2400 nmol/mL compared with 600 nmol/mL for NPH. The duration of action for insulin detemir is about 17 hours at therapeutically relevant doses. It is recommended that the insulin be injected once or twice a day to achieve a stable basal coverage. It has been approved for use during pregnancy.

(4) Insulin degludec—In this insulin analog, the threonine at position B30 has been removed, and the lysine at position B29 is conjugated to hexdecanoic acid via a gamma-L-glutamyl spacer. In the vial, in the presence of phenol and zinc, the insulin is in the form of dihexamers but when injected subcutaneously, it self associates into large multihexameric chains consisting of thousands of dihexamers. The chains slowly dissolve in the subcutaneous tissue and insulin monomers are steadily released into the systemic circulation. The half-life of insulin degludec is 25 hours. Its onset of action is in 30–90 minutes and its duration of action is more than 42 hours. It is recommended that the insulin be injected once or twice a day to achieve a stable basal coverage. Insulin degludec is available in two concentrations, U100 and U200, and dispensed in prefilled disposable pens.

C. Mixed insulin preparations—Patients with type 2 diabetes can sometimes achieve reasonable glucose control with just prebreakfast and predinner injections of mixtures of short acting and NPH insulins. The regular insulin or rapidly acting insulin analog is withdrawn first, then the NPH insulin and then injected immediately. Stable premixed insulins (70% NPH and 30% regular) are available as a convenience to patients who have difficulty mixing insulin because of visual problems or impairment of manual dexterity (Table 27–7). Premixed preparations of insulin lispro and NPH insulins are unstable; stability is achieved by replacing the NPH insulin with NPL (neutral protamine lispro). This insulin has the same duration of action as NPH insulin. Premixed combinations of NPL and insulin lispro (75% NPL/25% insulin lispro mixture [Humalog Mix 75/25] and 50% NPL/50% insulin lispro mixture [Humalog Mix 50/50]) are available for clinical use. Similarly, a 70% insulin aspart protamine/30% insulin aspart (NovoLog Mix 70/30) is available. The main advantages of these mixtures are that they can be given within 15 minutes of starting a meal and they are superior in controlling the postprandial glucose rise after a carbohydrate rich meal. These benefits have not translated into improvements in HbA_{1c} levels when compared with the usual 70% NPH/30% regular mixture. The longer-acting insulin analogs, insulin glargine and insulin detemir, cannot be mixed with either regular insulin or the rapidly acting insulin analogs. Insulin degludec, however, can be mixed and is available as 70% insulin degludec/30% insulin aspart and is injected once or twice a day.

3. Methods of insulin administration—

A. Insulin syringes and needles—Plastic disposable syringes are available in 1-mL, 0.5-mL, and 0.3-mL sizes. The "low-dose" 0.3-mL syringes are popular because many patients with diabetes do not take more than 30 units of insulin in a single injection except in rare instances of extreme insulin resistance. Three lengths of needles are available: 6 mm, 8 mm, and 12.7 mm. Long needles are preferable in obese patients to reduce variability of insulin absorption. The needles are of 28, 30, and 31 gauges. The 31-gauge needles are almost painless. "Disposable" syringes may be reused until blunting of the needle occurs (usually after three to five injections). Sterility adequate to avoid infection with reuse appears to be maintained by recapping syringes between uses. Cleansing the needle with alcohol may not be desirable since it can dissolve the silicone coating and can increase the pain of skin puncturing.

B. Sites of injection—Any part of the body covered by loose skin can be used, such as the abdomen, thighs, upper arms, flanks, and upper buttocks. Preparation with alcohol is not required prior to injection as long as the skin is clean.

Rotation of sites is recommended to avoid delayed absorption when fibrosis or lipohypertrophy occurs from repeated use of a single site. Regular insulin is absorbed more rapidly when injected in the deltoid or abdomen compared to thighs and buttocks. Exercise can increase absorption when the injection site is adjacent to the exercise muscle. For most patients, the abdomen is the recommend region for injection because it provides adequate area in which to rotate sites. The effect of anatomic regions appears to be much less pronounced with the analog insulins.

C. Insulin pen injector devices—Insulin pens eliminate the need for carrying insulin vials and syringes. Cartridges of insulin lispro and insulin aspart are available for reusable pens (Novo Nordisk, and Owen Mumford). Disposable prefilled pens are also available for regular insulin (U100 and U500), insulin lispro, insulin aspart, insulin glulisine, insulin detemir, insulin glargine, insulin degludec, NPH, 70% NPH/30% regular, 75% NPL/25% insulin lispro, 50% NPL/50% insulin lispro, 70% insulin aspart protamine/30% insulin aspart, and 70% insulin degludec/30% insulin aspart. Pen needles are available in 29, 31, and 32 gauges and 4-, 5-, 6-, 8-, and 12.7-mm lengths (Novofine; BD).

D. Insulin pumps—In the United States, Medtronic MiniMed, Insulet, and Tandem make battery operated continuous subcutaneous insulin infusion (CSII) pumps. These pumps are small (about the size of a pager) and easy to program. They offer many features, including the ability to set a number of different basal rates throughout the 24 hours and to adjust the time over which bolus doses are given. They also are able to detect pressure build-up if the catheter is kinked. The catheter connecting the insulin reservoir to the subcutaneous cannula can be disconnected, allowing the patient to remove the pump temporarily (eg, for bathing). Ominpod (Insulet Corporation) is an insulin infusion system in which the insulin reservoir and infusion set are integrated into one unit (pod), so there is no catheter (electronic patch pump). The pod, placed on the skin, delivers subcutaneous basal and bolus insulin based on wirelessly transmitted instructions from a personal digital assistant. The great advantage of continuous subcutaneous insulin infusion (CSII) is that it allows for establishment of a basal profile tailored to the patient allowing for better overnight and between meals glucose control. The ability to adjust the basal insulin infusion makes it easier for the patient to manage glycemic excursions that occur with exercise. The pumps have software that can assist the patient to calculate boluses based on glucose reading and carbohydrates to be consumed. They keep track of the time elapsed since last insulin bolus and the patient is reminded of this when he or she attempts to give additional correction bolus before the effect of the previous bolus has worn off ("insulin on board" feature). This feature reduces the risk of overcorrecting and subsequent hypoglycemia.

CSII therapy is appropriate for patients with type 1 diabetes who are motivated, mechanically inclined, educated about diabetes (diet, insulin action, treatment of hypoglycemia and hyperglycemia), and willing to monitor their blood glucose four to six times a day. Known complications of CSII include ketoacidosis, which can occur when insulin delivery is interrupted, and skin infections. Another disadvantage is its cost and the time demanded of the clinician and staff in initiating therapy. Almost all patients use rapid-acting insulin analogs in their pumps.

V-go (Valeritas) is a mechanical patch pump designed specifically for people with type 2 diabetes who use a basal/bolus insulin regimen. The device is preset to deliver one of three fixed and flat basal rates (20, 30, or 40 units) for 24 hours (at which point it must be replaced) and there is a button that delivers two units per press to help cover meals.

E. Closed loop systems—Algorithms have been devised to use glucose data from the continuous glucose monitoring systems to automatically deliver insulin by continuous subcutaneous insulin infusion pump. These closed loop systems (artificial pancreas) have been shown in short-term clinical studies to improve nighttime glucose control and reduce the risk of nocturnal hypoglycemia. The FDA-approved MiniMed 670 G closed loop system uses glucose data from a sensor to automatically adjust basal insulin doses every 5 minutes, targeting a sensor glucose level of 120 mg/dL (6.7 mmol/L). Insulin delivery is suspended when the sensor glucose level falls below or is predicted to fall below target level. The glucose target can be adjusted up to 150 mg/dL (8.3 mmol/L) for physical activity. The patient is still responsible for bolusing insulin for meals and snacks. Successful use of this closed loop system requires the patient to be proficient at using both the insulin pump and continuous glucose monitor.

F. Inhaled insulin—Technosphere insulin (Afrezza) is a dry-powder formulation of recombinant human regular insulin that can be inhaled. It consists of 2- to 2.5-mcm crystals of the excipient fumaryl diketopiperazine that provide large surface area for adsorption of proteins like insulin. The technosphere insulin is rapidly absorbed with peak insulin levels reached in 12–15 minutes and declining to baseline in 3 hours; the median time to maximum effect with inhaled insulin is approximately 1 hour and declines to baseline by about 3 hours. In contrast, the median time to maximum effect with subcutaneous insulin lispro is about 2 hours and declines to baseline by 4 hours. In clinical trials, technosphere insulin combined with basal insulin was as effective in glucose lowering as rapid-acting insulin analogs combined with basal insulin. It is formulated as a single-use, color-coded cartridge delivering 4, 8, or 12 units immediately before the meal. The manufacturer provides a dose conversion table; patients injecting up to 4 units of rapid-acting insulin analog should use the 4-unit cartridge. Those injecting 5 to 8 units should use the 8-unit cartridge. If the dose is 9–12 units of rapid-acting insulin premeal then one 4-unit cartridge and one 8-unit cartridge or one 12-unit cartridge should be used. The inhaler is about the size of a referee's whistle.

The most common adverse reaction of the inhaled insulin is a cough, affecting about 27% of patients. A small decrease in pulmonary function (forced expiratory volume in 1 second [FEV_1]) is seen in the first 3 months of use, which persists over 2 years of follow-up. Inhaled insulin is contraindicated in smokers and patients with chronic lung disease, such as asthma and chronic obstructive pulmonary disease. Spirometry should be performed to identify potential lung disease prior to initiating therapy. During clinical trials, there were two cases of lung cancer in patients who were taking inhaled insulin and none in the comparator-treated patients. All the patients in whom lung cancer developed had a history of prior cigarette smoking. There were also two cases of squamous cell carcinoma of the lung in nonsmokers exposed to inhaled insulin; these cases occurred after completion of the clinical trials. Cases of lung cancer were also reported in cigarette smokers using a previously available inhaled insulin preparation (Exubera). The incidence rate in the Exubera treated group was 0.13 per 1000 patient-years and 0.03 per 1000 patient-years in the comparator-treated group.

D. Transplantation

1. Pancreas transplantation—All patients with end-stage kidney disease and type 1 diabetes who are candidates for a kidney transplant should be considered potential candidates for a pancreas transplant. Eligibility criteria include age younger than 55 and minimal cardiovascular risk. Contraindications include noncorrectable coronary artery disease, extensive peripheral vascular disease, and significant obesity (weight greater than 100 kg). The pancreas transplant may occur at the same time as kidney transplant or after kidney transplant. Patients undergoing simultaneous pancreas and kidney transplantation have an 83% chance of pancreatic graft survival at 1 year and 69% at 5 years. Solitary pancreatic transplantation in the absence of a need for kidney transplantation is considered only in those rare patients who do not respond to all other insulin therapeutic approaches and who have frequent severe hypoglycemia, or who have life-threatening complications related to their lack of metabolic control. Solitary pancreas transplant graft survival is 78% at 1 year and 54% at 5 years.

2. Islet transplantation—Total pancreatectomy is curative for severe pain syndrome associated with chronic pancreatitis. The pancreatectomy, however, results in surgical diabetes. Harvesting islets from the removed pancreas and autotransplanting them into the liver (via portal vein) can prevent the development of diabetes or result in "mild" diabetes (partial islet function) that is easier to manage. Since the islets are autologous no immunosuppression is required. The number of islets transplanted is the main predictor of insulin independence.

People with type 1 diabetes can become insulin independent after receiving islets isolated from a donor pancreas (alloislet transplant). The islets are infused into the portal vein using a percutaneous transhepatic approach, and they lodge in the liver releasing insulin in response to physiologic stimuli. Long-term immunosuppression is necessary to prevent allograft rejection and to suppress the autoimmune process that led to the disease in the first place. Insulin independence for more than 5 years has been demonstrated in patients who got anti-CD3 antibody or anti-thymocyte globulin induction immunosuppression and calcineurin inhibitors, mTor inhibitors, and mycophenolate mofetil as maintenance immunosuppression. One major limitation is the need for more than one islet infusion to achieve insulin independence. This is because of significant loss of islets during isolation and the period prior to engraftment. Widespread alloislet transplantation will depend on improving insulin independence rates with one infusion and also demonstrating that the long-term outcomes are as good as those of pancreas transplant alone.

DeFronzo RA et al. Renal, metabolic and cardiovascular considerations of SGLT2 inhibition. Nat Rev Nephrol. 2017 Jan; 13(1):11–26. [PMID: 27941935]

Nauck M. Incretin therapies: highlighting common features and differences in the modes of action of glucagon-like peptide-1 receptor agonists and dipeptidyl peptidase-4 inhibitors. Diabetes Obes Metab. 2016 Mar;18(3):203–16. [PMID: 26489970]

Qaseem A et al. Oral pharmacologic treatment of type 2 diabetes mellitus: a clinical practice guideline update from the American College of Physicians. Ann Intern Med. 2017 Feb 21;166(4): 279–90. [PMID: 28055075]

▶ Steps in the Management of the Diabetic Patient

A. Diagnostic Examination

An attempt should be made to characterize the diabetes as type 1 or type 2 or other specific types such as MODY, based on the clinical features present and on whether or not ketonuria accompanies the glycosuria. Features that suggest end-organ insulin insensitivity to insulin, such as visceral obesity, acanthosis nigricans, or both, must be identified. The family history should document not only the incidence of diabetes in other members of the family but also the age at onset, association with obesity, the need for insulin, and whether there were complications. For the occasional patient, measurement of GAD65, IAA, ICA 512, and zinc transporter 8 antibodies can help distinguish between type 1 and type 2 diabetes (Table 27–2). Many patients with newly diagnosed type 1 diabetes still have significant endogenous insulin production, and C peptide levels do not reliably distinguish between type 1 and type 2 diabetes. Other factors that increase cardiac risk, such as smoking history, presence of hypertension or hyperlipidemia, or oral contraceptive pill use, should be recorded.

Laboratory diagnosis of diabetes should document fasting plasma glucose levels above 126 mg/dL (7 mmol/L) or postprandial values consistently above 200 mg/dL (11.1 mmol/L) or HbA_{1c} of at least 6.5% and whether ketonuria accompanies the glycosuria. An HbA_{1c} measurement is also useful for assessing the effectiveness of future therapy. Baseline values include fasting plasma triglycerides, total cholesterol and HDL cholesterol, electrocardiography, kidney function studies, peripheral pulses, and neurologic, podiatric, and ophthalmologic examinations to help guide future assessments.

B. Patient Education (Self-Management Training)

Since diabetes is a lifelong disorder, education of the patient and the family is probably the most important obligation of the clinician who provides care. The best persons to manage a disease that is affected so markedly by daily fluctuations in environmental stress, exercise, diet, and infections are the patients themselves and their families. The "teaching curriculum" should include explanations by the clinician or nurse of the nature of diabetes and its potential acute and chronic hazards and how they can be recognized early and prevented or treated. Self-monitoring of blood glucose should be emphasized, especially in insulin-requiring diabetic patients, and instructions must be given on proper testing and recording of data.

Patients taking insulin should have an understanding of the actions of basal and bolus insulins. They should be taught to determine whether the basal dose is appropriate and how to adjust the rapidly acting insulin dose for the carbohydrate content of a meal. Patients and their families and friends should be taught to recognize signs and symptoms of hypoglycemia and how to treat low glucose reactions. Strenuous exercise can precipitate hypoglycemia, and patients must therefore be taught to reduce their insulin dosage in anticipation of strenuous activity or to take supplemental carbohydrate. Injection of insulin into a site farthest away from the muscles most involved in the exercise may help ameliorate exercise-induced hypoglycemia, since insulin injected in the proximity of exercising muscle may be more rapidly mobilized. Exercise training also increases the effectiveness of insulin, and insulin doses should be adjusted accordingly. Infections can cause insulin resistance, and patients should be instructed on how to manage the hyperglycemia with supplemental rapidly acting insulin.

Advice on personal hygiene, including detailed instructions on foot and dental care, should be provided. All infections (especially pyogenic ones) provoke the release of high levels of insulin antagonists, such as catecholamines or glucagon, and thus bring about a marked increase in insulin requirements. Patients who are taking oral agents may decompensate and temporarily require insulin. Patients should be told about community agencies, such as Diabetes Association chapters, that can serve as a continuing source of instruction.

Finally, vigorous efforts should be made to persuade patients with newly diagnosed diabetes who smoke to give up the habit, since large vessel peripheral vascular disease and debilitating retinopathy are less common in nonsmoking diabetic patients.

C. Therapy

Treatment must be individualized on the basis of the type of diabetes and specific needs of each patient. However, certain general principles of management can be outlined for hyperglycemic states of different types.

1. Type 1 diabetes—Traditional once- or twice-daily insulin regimens are usually ineffective in type 1 patients without residual endogenous insulin. In these patients, information and counseling based on the findings of the DCCT, which showed that near normalization of blood glucose in patients with type 1 diabetes resulted in a delay in the onset and a major slowing of the progression of established microvascular and neuropathic complications of diabetes, should be provided about the advantages of taking multiple injections of insulin in conjunction with self–blood glucose monitoring. If near-normalization of blood glucose is attempted, at least four measurements of capillary blood glucose and three or four insulin injections are necessary.

A combination of rapidly acting insulin analogs and long-acting insulin analogs allows for more physiologic insulin replacement. The rapidly acting insulin analogs have been advocated as a safer and much more convenient alternative to regular human insulin for preprandial use. However, because of their relatively short duration (no more than 3–4 hours), the rapidly acting insulin analogs need to be combined with longer-acting insulins to provide basal coverage and avoid hyperglycemia prior to the next meal. In addition to carbohydrate content of the meal, the effect of simultaneous fat ingestion must also be considered a factor in determining the rapidly acting insulin analog dosage required to control the glycemic increment during and just after the meal. With low-carbohydrate content and high-fat intake, there is an increased risk of hypoglycemia from insulin lispro within 2 hours after the meal. Table 27–8 illustrates a regimen with a rapidly acting insulin analog and insulin detemir or insulin glargine that might be appropriate for a 70-kg person with type 1 diabetes eating meals providing standard carbohydrate intake and moderate to low fat content.

Insulin glargine or insulin degludec is usually given once in the evening to provide 24-hour coverage. There are occasional patients in whom insulin glargine does not seem to last for 24 hours, and in such cases it needs to be given twice a day. Insulin detemir may also need to be given twice a day to get adequate 24-hour basal coverage. Alternatively, small doses of NPH (~3–4 units) can be given with each meal to provide daytime basal coverage with a larger dose at night. Unlike the long-acting insulin analogs, NPH can be mixed in the same syringe as the insulin lispro, insulin aspart, and insulin glulisine.

CSII by portable battery-operated "open loop" devices currently provides the most flexible approach, allowing the setting of different basal rates throughout the 24 hours and permitting bolus dose adjustments by as little as 0.05-unit increments. The 24-hour basal dosage is usually based on age and body weight. An adolescent might need as much as 0.4 unit/kg/day; young adult (less than 25 years), 0.35 unit per/kg/day; and older adults, 0.25 unit/kg/day. For example, a 70-kg, 30-year-old man may require a basal rate of 0.7 unit per hour throughout the 24 hours with the exception of 3 AM to 8 AM, when 0.8 unit per hour might be appropriate (given the "**dawn phenomenon**"—reduced tissue sensitivity to insulin between 5 AM and 8 AM). The meal bolus varies based on the time of day and the person's age. Adolescents and young adults usually require 1 unit for about 10 g of carbohydrate. Older adults usually require about 1 unit for 15 g of carbohydrate. The correction factor—how much insulin is needed to lower glucose levels by 50 mg/dL—can be calculated from the insulin-to-carbohydrate ratios. For example, if 1 unit is required for 15 g of carbohydrate, then 1 unit will lower glucose levels by 50 mg/dL. If 1.5 units of insulin are required for 15 g of carbohydrate (that is, 1 unit for 10 g carbohydrate), then 1.5 units of insulin will lower glucose levels by 50 mg/dL (that is, 1 unit will lower glucose level by 33 mg/dL). For a 70-kg 30-year-old man, bolus ratios of 1 unit for 12–15 g of carbohydrate plus 1 unit for 50 mg/dL of blood glucose over a target value of 120 mg/dL would be reasonable starting point. Further adjustments to basal and bolus dosages would depend on the results of blood glucose monitoring. One of the more difficult therapeutic problems in managing patients with type 1 diabetes is determining the proper adjustment of insulin dose when the prebreakfast blood glucose level is high. Occasionally, the prebreakfast hyperglycemia is due to the **Somogyi effect,** in which nocturnal hypoglycemia leads to a surge of counterregulatory hormones to produce high blood glucose levels by 7 AM. However, a more common cause for prebreakfast hyperglycemia is the waning of circulating insulin levels by the morning.

The diagnosis of the cause of prebreakfast hyperglycemia can be facilitated by self-monitoring of blood glucose at 3 AM in addition to the usual bedtime and 7 AM measurements (Table 27–9). This is required for only a few nights, and when a particular pattern emerges from monitoring blood glucose levels overnight, appropriate therapeutic measures can be taken. The Somogyi effect can be treated by eliminating the dose of intermediate insulin at dinnertime and giving it at a lower dosage at bedtime or by supplying more food at bedtime. When a waning insulin level is the cause, then either increasing the evening dose or shifting it from dinnertime to bedtime (or both) can be effective. A bedtime dose either of insulin glargine or insulin detemir provides more sustained overnight insulin levels than human NPH and may be effective in managing refractory prebreakfast hyperglycemia. If this fails, insulin pump therapy may be required.

Table 27–8. Examples of intensive insulin regimens using rapidly acting insulin analogs (insulin lispro, aspart, or glulisine) and insulin detemir, or insulin glargine or degludec in a 70-kg man with type 1 diabetes.[1-3]

	Pre-breakfast	Pre-lunch	Pre-dinner	At Bedtime
Rapidly acting insulin analog	5 units	4 units	6 units	
Insulin detemir[3]	6–7 units			8–9 units
OR				
Rapidly acting insulin analog	5 units	4 units	6 units	—
Insulin glargine or degludec[3]		—		15–16 units

[1]Assumes that patient is consuming approximately 75 g carbohydrate at breakfast, 60 g at lunch, and 90 g at dinner.

[2]The dose of rapidly acting insulin can be raised by 1 or 2 units if extra carbohydrate (15–30 g) is ingested or if premeal blood glucose is > 170 mg/dL (9.4 mmol/L).

[3]Insulin glargine or insulin detemir must be given as a separate injection.

Table 27–9. Prebreakfast hyperglycemia: classification by blood glucose and insulin levels.

	Blood Glucose (mg/dL [mmol/L])			Free Immunoreactive Insulin (microunit/mL)		
	10:00 PM	3:00 AM	7:00 AM	10:00 PM	3:00 AM	7:00 AM
Somogyi effect	90 [5]	40 [2.2]	200 [11.1]	High	Slightly high	Normal
Dawn phenomenon	110 [6.1]	110 [6.1]	150 [8.3]	Normal	Normal	Normal
Waning of insulin dose plus dawn phenomenon	110 [6.1]	190 [10.6]	220 [12.2]	Normal	Low	Low
Waning of insulin dose plus dawn phenomenon plus Somogyi effect	110 [6.1]	40 [2.2]	380 [21.1]	High	Normal	Low

2. Type 2 diabetes—Therapeutic recommendations are based on the relative contributions of beta cell insufficiency and insulin insensitivity in individual patients. The possibility that the individual patient has a specific etiologic cause for their diabetes should always be considered, especially when the patient does not have a family history of type 2 diabetes or does not have any evidence of central obesity or insulin resistance. Such patients should be evaluated for other types of diabetes such as LADA or MODY (Table 27–1). Patients with LADA should be prescribed insulin when the disease is diagnosed and treated like patients with type 1 diabetes. It is also important to note that many patients with type 2 diabetes mellitus have a progressive loss of beta cell function and will require additional therapeutic interventions with time.

A. Weight reduction—One of the primary modes of therapy in the obese patient with type 2 diabetes is weight reduction. Normalization of glycemia can be achieved by weight loss and improvement in tissue sensitivity to insulin. A combination of caloric restriction, increased exercise, and behavior modification is required if a weight reduction program is to be successful. Understanding the risks associated with the diagnosis of diabetes may motivate the patient to lose weight.

For selected patients, medical or surgical options for weight loss should be considered. Orlistat, phentermine/topiramate, lorcaserin, naltrexone/extended-release bupropion, and high-dose liraglutide (3 mg daily) are weight loss medications approved for use in combination with diet and exercise (see Chapter 29).

Bariatric surgery (Roux-en-Y, gastric banding, gastric sleeve, biliopancreatic diversion/duodenal switch) typically results in substantial weight loss and improvement in glucose levels. A meta-analysis examining the impact of bariatric surgery on patients with diabetes and BMI of 40 kg/m^2 or greater noted that 82% of patients had resolution of clinical and laboratory manifestations of diabetes in the first 2 years after surgery and 62% remained free of diabetes more than 2 years after surgery. The improvement was most marked in the procedure that caused the greatest weight loss (biliopancreatic diversion/duodenal switch). There was, however, a high attrition of patients available for follow-up, and there was little information about different ethnic types. Weight regain does occur after bariatric surgery, and it can be expected that 20–25% of the lost

weight will be regained over 10 years. The impact of this weight gain on diabetes recurrence depends principally on the degree of beta cell dysfunction.

Nonobese patients with type 2 diabetes frequently have increased visceral adiposity—the so-called metabolically obese normal weight patient. There is less emphasis on weight loss, but exercise remains an important aspect of treatment.

B. Glucose-lowering agents—Figure 27–2 outlines the treatment approach based on the consensus algorithm proposed by the American Diabetes Association and the European Association for the Study of Diabetes. The current recommendation is to start metformin therapy at diagnosis and not wait to see whether the patient can achieve target glycemic control with weight management and exercise. See discussion of the individual medications, above.

When diabetes is not well controlled with initial therapy (usually metformin), then a second agent should be added. Sulfonylureas have been available for many years and their use in combination with metformin is well established. They do, however, have the propensity of causing hypoglycemia and weight gain. In patients who experience hyperglycemia after a carbohydrate-rich meal (such as dinner), a short-acting secretagogue (repaglinide or nateglinide) before meals may suffice to get the glucose levels into the target range. Patients with severe insulin resistance may be candidates for pioglitazone. Patients who are very concerned about weight gain may benefit from a trial of GLP-1 receptor agonist or DPP-4 inhibitor or SGLT2 inhibitor. Presence of cardiovascular disease should be considered; liraglutide, empagliflozin, and canagliflozin have been shown to have improved cardiovascular outcomes. If two agents are inadequate, then a third agent is added, although data regarding efficacy of such combined therapy are limited.

When the combination of oral agents (and injectable GLP-1 receptor agonists) fails to achieve euglycemia in patients with type 2 diabetes, then insulin treatment should be instituted. Various insulin regimens may be effective. One proposed regimen is to continue the oral combination therapy and then simply add a bedtime dose of NPH or long-acting insulin analog (insulin glargine or insulin detemir) to reduce excessive nocturnal hepatic glucose output and improve fasting glucose levels. If the patient does not achieve target glucose levels during the day, then daytime insulin treatment can be initiated. A convenient

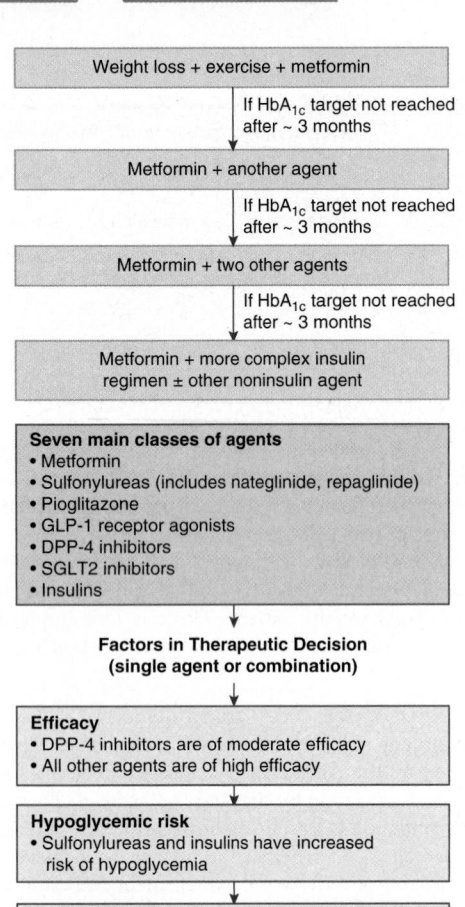

Weight loss + exercise + metformin

↓ If HbA_{1c} target not reached after ~ 3 months

Metformin + another agent

↓ If HbA_{1c} target not reached after ~ 3 months

Metformin + two other agents

↓ If HbA_{1c} target not reached after ~ 3 months

Metformin + more complex insulin regimen ± other noninsulin agent

Seven main classes of agents
• Metformin
• Sulfonylureas (includes nateglinide, repaglinide)
• Pioglitazone
• GLP-1 receptor agonists
• DPP-4 inhibitors
• SGLT2 inhibitors
• Insulins

Factors in Therapeutic Decision (single agent or combination)

Efficacy
• DPP-4 inhibitors are of moderate efficacy
• All other agents are of high efficacy

Hypoglycemic risk
• Sulfonylureas and insulins have increased risk of hypoglycemia

Effect on weight
• Metformin and DPP-4 inhibitors are weight neutral
• GLP-1 receptor agonists and SGLT2 inhibitors promote weight loss
• Sulfonylureas, insulins, and pioglitazone are associated with weight gain

Major side effects
• Metformin can cause lactic acidosis
• Pioglitazone is associated with fluid retention, fracture risk, and possibly bladder cancer
• GLP-1 receptor agonists are associated with nausea, vomiting and pancreatitis
• DPP-4 inhibitors may be associated with pancreatitis
• SGLT2 inhibitors can cause urinary tract infections; genital mycotic infections; dehydration; cannot use in renal impairment

Cost
• All agents except metformin and sulfonylureas are expensive
• Insulins are expensive if the additional cost of monitoring is taken into consideration

Cardiovascular and renal effects
• Metformin, liraglutide, semaglutide, empagliflozin, and canagliflozin have known cardiovascular benefits
• SGLT2 inhibitors reduce the risk of kidney disease in patients with diabetic nephropathy

▲ **Figure 27–2.** Algorithm for the treatment of type 2 diabetes based on the 2018 recommendations of the consensus panel of the American Diabetes Association/European Association for the Study of Diabetes.

insulin regimen under these circumstances is a split dose of 70/30 NPH/regular mixture (or Humalog Mix 75/25 or NovoLogMix 70/30) before breakfast and before dinner. If this regimen fails to achieve satisfactory glycemic goals or is associated with unacceptable frequency of hypoglycemic episodes, then a more intensive regimen of multiple insulin injections can be instituted as in patients with type 1 diabetes. Metformin principally reduces hepatic glucose output, and it is reasonable to continue with this medication when insulin therapy is instituted. Pioglitazone, which improves peripheral insulin sensitivity, can be used together with insulin but this combination is associated with more weight gain and peripheral edema. The sulfonylureas, the GLP-1 receptor agonists, and the DPP-4 inhibitors also have been shown to be of continued benefit. Weight-reducing interventions should continue even after initiation of insulin therapy and may allow for simplification of the therapeutic regimen in the future.

D. Acceptable Levels of Glycemic Control

A reasonable aim of therapy is to approach normal glycemic excursions without provoking severe or frequent hypoglycemia. Table 27–10 summarizes blood glucose and HbA_{1c} goals for different patient groups. The UKPDS study demonstrated that blood pressure control was as significant or more significant than glycemic control in patients with type 2 diabetes regarding the prevention of microvascular as well as macrovascular complications.

American Diabetes Association. Standards of Medical Care in Diabetes-2018. Diabetes Care. 2018;41(Suppl 1):S1–159.

Jin J. JAMA patient page. Starting insulin treatment for diabetes. JAMA. 2014 Jun 11;311(22):2347. [PMID: 24915279]

Mingrone G et al. Bariatric surgery versus conventional medical therapy for type 2 diabetes. N Engl J Med. 2012 Apr 26; 366(17):1577–85. [PMID: 22449317]

Switzer SM et al. Intensive insulin therapy in patients with type 1 diabetes mellitus. Endocrinol Metab Clin North Am. 2012 Mar; 41(1):89–104. [PMID: 22575408]

The Diabetes Control and Complications Trial Research Group. The effect of intensive treatment of diabetes on the development and progression of long-term complications in insulin-dependent diabetes mellitus. N Engl J Med. 1993 Sep 30; 329(14):977–86. [PMID: 8366922]

UK Prospective Diabetes Study (UKPDS) Group. Intensive blood-glucose control with sulphonylureas or insulin compared with conventional treatment and risk of complications in patients with type 2 diabetes (UKPDS 33). Lancet. 1998 Sep 12;352(9131):837–53. [PMID: 9742976]

E. Complications of Insulin Therapy

1. Hypoglycemia—Hypoglycemic reactions are the most common complications that occur in patients with diabetes who are treated with insulin. The signs and symptoms of hypoglycemia may be divided into those resulting from stimulation of the autonomic nervous system and those from neuroglycopenia (insufficient glucose for normal central nervous system function). When the blood glucose falls to around 54 mg/dL (3 mmol/L), the patient starts to experience both sympathetic (tachycardia, palpitations,

Table 27–10. Glycemic targets for different groups of patients with diabetes.

	Blood Glucose Targets (mg/dL [mmol/L])	HbA$_{1c}$ Target (% [mmol/mol])
Nonpregnant healthy adults	Premeal glucose 90–130 (5–7.2) 1-hour peak < 180 (10) 2-hour peak < 150 (8.3)	< 7 (53). Aim for < 6.5 (48) if it can be achieved without significant hypoglycemia or polypharmacy
Pregnancy	Premeal glucose ≤ 95 (5.3) 1-hour peak ≤ 140 (7.8) 2-hour peak ≤ 120 (6.7)	6–6.5 (42–48). Aim for < 6 (42) if possible without significant hypoglycemia
Older adults Healthy	Premeal 90–130 (5–7.2) Bedtime 90–150 (5–8.3)	< 7.5 (58)
Frail with limited life expectancy	Premeal 100–180 (5.6–10) Bedtime 110–200 (6.1–11.1)	< 8.5 (69)
History of severe hypoglycemia	Premeal 90–150 (5–8.3) Bedtime 100–180 (5.6–10)	< 8 (64)
Hospitalized patient	140–180 (7.8–10)	—
CKD	Glycemic targets in CKD are the same as those without CKD. HbA$_{1c}$ and fructosamine values may not be accurate in end-stage renal disease and greater reliance should be placed on the home glucose measurements	
Children and adolescents	Premeal glucose 90–130 (5–7.2) Bedtime/overnight 90–150 (5–8.3)	< 7.5 (58)

CKD, chronic kidney disease.

sweating, tremulousness) and parasympathetic (nausea, hunger) nervous system symptoms. If these autonomic symptoms are ignored and the glucose levels fall further (to around 50 mg/dL [2.8 mmol/L]), then neuroglycopenic symptoms appear, including irritability, confusion, blurred vision, tiredness, headache, and difficulty speaking. A further decline in glucose can then lead to loss of consciousness or even a seizure. With repeated episodes of hypoglycemia, there is adaptation, and autonomic symptoms do not occur until the blood glucose levels are much lower and so the first symptoms are often due to neuroglycopenia. This condition is referred to as "hypoglycemic unawareness." It has been shown that hypoglycemic unawareness can be reversed by keeping glucose levels high for a period of several weeks. Except for sweating, most of the sympathetic symptoms of hypoglycemia are blunted in patients receiving beta-blocking agents. Though not absolutely contraindicated, these medications must be used with caution in patients with diabetes who require insulin, and beta-1-selective blocking agents are preferred.

Hypoglycemia can occur in a patient taking sulfonylureas, repaglinide, and nateglinide, particularly if the patient is elderly, has kidney or liver disease, or is taking certain other medications that alter metabolism of the sulfonylureas (eg, phenylbutazone, sulfonamides, or warfarin). It occurs more frequently with the use of long-acting sulfonylureas than when shorter-acting agents are used. Otherwise, hypoglycemia in insulin-treated patients with diabetes occurs as a consequence of three factors: behavioral issues, impaired counterregulatory systems, and complications of diabetes.

Behavioral issues include injecting too much insulin for the amount of carbohydrates ingested. Drinking alcohol in excess, especially on an empty stomach, can also cause hypoglycemia. In patients with type 1 diabetes, hypoglycemia can occur during or even several hours after exercise, and so glucose levels need to be monitored and food and insulin adjusted. Some patients do not like their glucose levels to be high, and they treat every high glucose level aggressively. These individuals who "stack" their insulin—that is, give another dose of insulin before the first injection has had its full action—can develop hypoglycemia.

Counterregulatory issues resulting in hypoglycemia include impaired glucagon response, sympatho-adrenal responses, and cortisol deficiency. Patients with diabetes of greater than 5 years in duration lose their glucagon response to hypoglycemia. As a result, they are at a significant disadvantage in protecting themselves against falling glucose levels. Once the glucagon response is lost, their sympatho-adrenal responses take on added importance. Unfortunately, aging, autonomic neuropathy, or hypoglycemic unawareness due to repeated low glucose levels further blunts the sympatho-adrenal responses. Occasionally, Addison disease develops in persons with type 1 diabetes mellitus; when this happens, insulin requirements fall significantly, and unless insulin dose is reduced, recurrent hypoglycemia will develop.

Complications of diabetes that increase the risk for hypoglycemia include autonomic neuropathy, gastroparesis, and end-stage chronic kidney disease. The sympathetic nervous system is an important system alerting the individual that the glucose level is falling by causing symptoms of tachycardia, palpitations, sweating, and tremulousness.

Failure of the sympatho-adrenal responses increases the risk of hypoglycemia. In addition, in patients with gastroparesis, if insulin is given before a meal, the peak of insulin action may occur before the food is absorbed causing the glucose levels to fall. Finally, in end-stage chronic kidney disease, hypoglycemia can occur presumably because of decreased insulin clearance as well as loss of renal contribution to gluconeogenesis in the postabsorptive state.

To prevent and treat insulin-induced hypoglycemia, the diabetic patient should carry glucose tablets or juice at all times. For most episodes, ingestion of 15 grams of carbohydrate is sufficient to reverse the hypoglycemia. The patient should be instructed to check the blood glucose in 15 minutes and treat again if the glucose level is still low. A parenteral glucagon emergency kit (1 mg) should be provided to every patient with diabetes who is receiving insulin therapy. Family or friends should be instructed how to inject it subcutaneously or intramuscularly into the buttock, arm, or thigh in the event that the patient is unconscious or refuses food. The medication can occasionally cause vomiting, and the unconscious patient should be turned on his or her side to protect the airway. The glucagon mobilizes glycogen from the liver, raising the blood glucose by about 36 mg/dL (2 mmol/L) in about 15 minutes. After the patient recovers consciousness, additional oral carbohydrate should be given. People with diabetes receiving hypoglycemic medication therapy should also wear an identification MedicAlert bracelet or necklace or carry a card in his or her wallet (1-800-ID-ALERT, www.medicalert.org).

Medical personnel treating severe hypoglycemia can give 50 mL of 50% glucose solution by rapid intravenous infusion. If intravenous access is not available, 1 mg of glucagon can be injected intramuscularly.

2. Immunopathology of insulin therapy—At least five molecular classes of insulin antibodies are produced during the course of insulin therapy in diabetes, including IgA, IgD, IgE, IgG, and IgM. With the switch to human and purified pork insulin, the various immunopathologic syndromes such as insulin allergy, immune insulin resistance, and lipoatrophy have become quite rare since the titers and avidity of these induced antibodies are generally quite low.

A. Insulin allergy—Insulin allergy, or immediate-type hypersensitivity, is a rare condition in which local or systemic urticaria is due to histamine release from tissue mast cells sensitized by adherence of anti-insulin IgE antibodies. In severe cases, anaphylaxis results. When only human insulin has been used from the onset of insulin therapy, insulin allergy is exceedingly rare. Antihistamines, corticosteroids, and even desensitization may be required, especially for systemic hypersensitivity. There have been case reports of successful use of insulin lispro in those rare patients who have a generalized allergy to human insulin or insulin resistance due to a high titer of insulin antibodies.

B. Immune insulin resistance—A low titer of circulating IgG anti-insulin antibodies that neutralize the action of insulin to a small extent develops in most insulin-treated patients. With the old animal insulins, a high titer of circulating antibodies sometimes developed, resulting in extremely high insulin requirements—often more than 200 units daily. This is now rarely seen with the switch to human or highly purified pork insulins and has not been reported with the analogs.

C. Lipodystrophy—Atrophy of subcutaneous fatty tissue leading to disfiguring excavations and depressed areas may rarely occur at the site of injection. This complication results from an immune reaction, and it has become rarer with the development of human and highly purified insulin preparations. Lipohypertrophy, on the other hand, is a consequence of the pharmacologic effects of insulin being deposited in the same location repeatedly. It can occur with purified insulins as well. Rotation of injection sites will prevent lipohypertrophy.

International Hypoglycaemia Study Group. Minimizing hypoglycemia in diabetes. Diabetes Care. 2015 Aug;38(8):1583–91. [PMID: 26207052]

▶ Chronic Complications of Diabetes

Late clinical manifestations of diabetes mellitus include a number of pathologic changes that involve small and large blood vessels, cranial and peripheral nerves, the skin, and the lens of the eye. These lesions lead to hypertension, end-stage chronic kidney disease, blindness, autonomic and peripheral neuropathy, amputations of the lower extremities, myocardial infarction, and cerebrovascular accidents. These late manifestations correlate with the duration of the diabetic state subsequent to the onset of puberty. In type 1 diabetes, end-stage chronic kidney disease develops in up to 40% of patients, compared with less than 20% of patients with type 2 diabetes. Proliferative retinopathy ultimately develops in both types of diabetes but has a slightly higher prevalence in type 1 patients (25% after 15 years' duration). In patients with type 1 diabetes, complications from end-stage chronic kidney disease are a major cause of death, whereas patients with type 2 diabetes are more likely to have macrovascular diseases leading to myocardial infarction and stroke as the main causes of death. Cigarette use adds significantly to the risk of both microvascular and macrovascular complications in diabetic patients.

A. Ocular Complications

1. Diabetic cataracts—Premature cataracts occur in diabetic patients and seem to correlate with both the duration of diabetes and the severity of chronic hyperglycemia. Nonenzymatic glycosylation of lens protein is twice as high in diabetic patients as in age-matched nondiabetic persons and may contribute to the premature occurrence of cataracts.

2. Diabetic retinopathy—There are two main categories of diabetic retinopathy: nonproliferative and proliferative (see Chapter 7). Diabetic macular edema can occur at any stage. **Nonproliferative ("background") retinopathy** represents the earliest stage of retinal involvement by diabetes and is characterized by such changes as microaneurysms, dot hemorrhages, exudates, and retinal edema. The prevalence of nonproliferative retinopathy in patients with type 2 diabetes is 60% after 16 years.

Proliferative retinopathy involves the growth of new capillaries and fibrous tissue within the retina and into the vitreous chamber. It is a consequence of small vessel occlusion, which causes retinal hypoxia; this in turn stimulates new vessel growth. New vessel formation may occur at the optic disk or elsewhere on the retina. Prior to proliferation of new capillaries, a preproliferative phase often occurs in which arteriolar ischemia is manifested as cotton-wool spots (small infarcted areas of retina). Vision is usually normal until vitreous hemorrhage or retinal detachment occurs.

Proliferative retinopathy can occur in both types of diabetes but is more common in type 1, developing about 7–10 years after onset of symptoms, with a prevalence of 25% after 15 years' duration. Vision-threatening retinopathy virtually never appears in type 1 patients in the first 3–5 years of diabetes or before puberty. Up to 20% of patients with type 2 diabetes have retinopathy at the time of diagnosis, because many were probably diabetic for an extensive period of time before diagnosis. Annual consultation with an ophthalmologist should be arranged for patients who have had type 1 diabetes for more than 3–5 years and for all patients with type 2 diabetes. Chapter 7 describes the treatment of retinopathy and macular edema. There is no contraindication to using aspirin in patients with proliferative retinopathy.

3. Glaucoma—Glaucoma occurs in approximately 6% of persons with diabetes. It is responsive to the usual therapy for open-angle disease. Neovascularization of the iris in patients with diabetes can predispose to closed-angle glaucoma, but this is relatively uncommon except after cataract extraction, when growth of new vessels has been known to progress rapidly, involving the angle of the iris and obstructing outflow.

B. Diabetic Nephropathy

Diabetic nephropathy is initially manifested by albuminuria; subsequently, as kidney function declines, urea and creatinine accumulate in the blood (see Chapter 22). Conventional 24-hour urine collections, in addition to being inconvenient for patients, also show wide variability of albumin excretion, since several factors such as sustained erect posture, dietary protein, and exercise tend to increase albumin excretion rates. For these reasons, an albumin-creatinine ratio in an early morning spot urine collected upon awakening is preferable. In the early morning spot urine, a ratio of albumin (mcg/L) to creatinine (mg/L) of less than 30 mcg/mg creatinine is normal, and a ratio of 30–300 mcg/mg creatinine suggests abnormal microalbuminuria. At least two early morning spot urine collections over a 3- to 6-month period should be abnormal before a diagnosis of microalbuminuria is justified. Short-term hyperglycemia, exercise, urinary tract infections, heart failure, and acute febrile illness can cause transient albuminuria and so testing for microalbuminuria should be postponed until resolution of these problems.

Subsequent end-stage chronic kidney disease can be predicted by persistent urinary albumin excretion rates exceeding 30 mcg/mg creatinine. Glycemic control as well as a protein diet of ~0.8 g/kg/day may reduce both the hyperfiltration and the elevated microalbuminuria in patients in the early stages of diabetes and those with incipient diabetic nephropathy. Antihypertensive therapy also decreases microalbuminuria. Evidence from some studies supports a specific role for ACE inhibitors in reducing intraglomerular pressure in addition to their lowering of systemic hypertension. An ACE inhibitor (captopril, 50 mg twice daily) in normotensive diabetic patients impedes progression to proteinuria and prevents the increase in albumin excretion rate. Since microalbuminuria has been shown to correlate with elevated *nocturnal* systolic blood pressure, it is possible that "normotensive" diabetic patients with microalbuminuria have slightly elevated systolic blood pressure during sleep, which is lowered during antihypertensive therapy. This action may contribute to the reported efficacy of ACE inhibitors in reducing microalbuminuria in "normotensive" patients.

If treatment is inadequate, then the disease progresses with proteinuria of varying severity occasionally leading to nephrotic syndrome with hypoalbuminemia, edema, and an increase in circulating LDL cholesterol, as well as progressive azotemia. In contrast to all other kidney disorders, the proteinuria associated with diabetic nephropathy does not diminish with progressive end-stage chronic kidney disease (patients continue to excrete 10–11 g daily as creatinine clearance diminishes). As end-stage chronic kidney disease progresses, there is an elevation in the renal threshold at which glycosuria appears.

Diabetic patients with normal kidney function do not appear to be at increased risk for contrast nephropathy. If a contrast study is considered essential, patients with a serum creatinine of 1.5–2.5 mg/dL should be adequately hydrated before the procedure. Hydration with saline has been the cornerstone of contrast nephropathy prevention: intravenous saline 1 mL/kg/h is started 12 hours before the procedure and continued for 12 hours afterward. Radiographic contrast material should not be given to a patient with a serum creatinine greater than 3 mg/dL unless the potential benefit outweighs the high risk of acute kidney injury.

C. Diabetic Neuropathy

Diabetic neuropathies are the most common complications of diabetes, affecting up to 50% of older patients with type 2 diabetes.

1. Peripheral neuropathy—

A. DISTAL SYMMETRIC POLYNEUROPATHY—This is the most common form of diabetic peripheral neuropathy where loss of function appears in a stocking-glove pattern and is due to an axonal neuropathic process. Longer nerves are especially vulnerable, hence the impact on the foot. Both motor and sensory nerve conduction is delayed in the peripheral nerves, and ankle jerks may be absent.

Sensory involvement usually occurs first and is generally bilateral, symmetric, and associated with dulled perception of vibration, pain, and temperature. The pain can range from mild discomfort to severe incapacitating symptoms. The sensory deficit may eventually be of sufficient degree to prevent patients from feeling pain. Patients who have a sensory neuropathy should therefore be examined

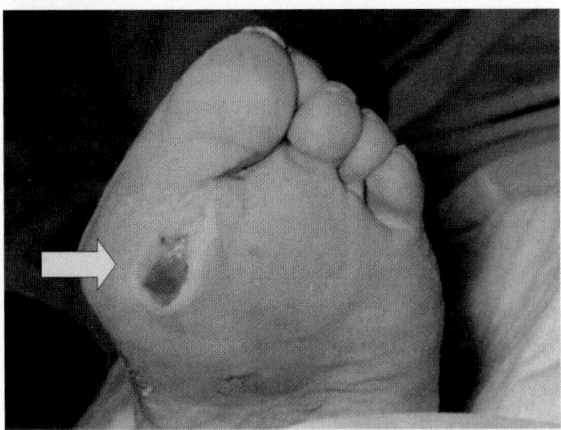

▲ **Figure 27–3.** Diabetic foot ulcer over head of first metatarsal (arrow). (Used, with permission, from Dean SM, Satiani B, Abraham WT. *Color Atlas and Synopsis of Vascular Diseases.* McGraw-Hill, 2014.)

with a 5.07 Semmes-Weinstein filament and those who cannot feel the filament must be considered at risk for unperceived neuropathic injury.

The denervation of the small muscles of the foot results in clawing of the toes and displacement of the submetatarsal fat pads anteriorly. These changes, together with the joint and connective tissue changes, alter the biomechanics of the foot and increase plantar pressures. This combination of decreased pain threshold, abnormally high foot pressures, and repetitive stress (such as from walking) can lead to calluses and ulcerations in the high-pressure areas such as over the metatarsal heads (Figure 27–3). Peripheral neuropathy, autonomic neuropathy, and trauma also predisposes to the development of Charcot arthropathy. An acute case of Charcot foot arthropathy presents with pain and swelling, and if left untreated, leads to a "rocker bottom" deformity and ulceration. The early radiologic changes show joint subluxation and periarticular fractures. As the process progresses, there is frank osteoclastic destruction leading to deranged and unstable joints particularly in the midfoot. Not surprisingly, the key issue for the healing of neuropathic ulcers in a foot with good vascular supply is mechanical unloading. In addition, any infection should be treated with debridement and appropriate antibiotics; healing duration of 8–10 weeks is typical. Occasionally, when healing appears refractory, platelet-derived growth factor (becaplermin [Regranex]) should be considered for local application. A post-marketing epidemiologic study showed increased cancer deaths in patients who had used three or more tubes of becaplermin on their leg or feet ulcers, resulting in a "black box" warning on the medication label. Once ulcers are healed, therapeutic footwear is key to preventing recurrences. Custom molded shoes are reserved for patients with significant foot deformities. Other patients with neuropathy may require accommodative insoles that distribute the load over as wide an area as possible. Patients with foot deformities and loss of their protective threshold should get regular care from a podiatrist. Patients should be educated on appropriate

footwear and those with loss of their protective threshold should be instructed to inspect their feet daily for reddened areas, blisters, abrasions, or lacerations.

In some patients, hypersensitivity to light touch and occasionally severe "burning" pain, particularly at night, can become physically and emotionally disabling. Nortriptyline or desipramine in doses of 25–150 mg/day orally may provide dramatic relief for pain from diabetic neuropathy, often within 48–72 hours. This rapid response is in contrast to the 2 or 3 weeks required for an antidepressive effect. Patients often attribute the benefit to having a full night's sleep. Mild to moderate morning drowsiness is a side effect that generally improves with time or can be lessened by giving the medication several hours before bedtime. This medication should not be continued if improvement has not occurred after 5 days of therapy. Amitriptyline, 25–75 mg orally at bedtime, can also be used but has more anticholinergic effects. Tricyclic antidepressants, in combination with fluphenazine (3 mg daily in three divided doses) have been shown in two studies to be efficacious in painful neuropathy, with benefits unrelated to relief of depression. Gabapentin (900–1800 mg orally daily in three divided doses) has also been shown to be effective in the treatment of painful neuropathy and should be tried if the tricyclic medications prove ineffective. Pregabalin, a congener of gabapentin, has been shown in an 8-week study to be more effective than placebo in treating painful diabetic peripheral neuropathy. However, this medication was not compared with an active control. Also, because of its abuse potential, it has been categorized as a schedule V controlled substance. Duloxetine (60–120 mg), a serotonin and norepinephrine reuptake inhibitor, is approved for the treatment of painful diabetic neuropathy. Capsaicin, a topical irritant, is effective in reducing local nerve pain; it is dispensed as a cream (Zostrix 0.025%, Zostrix-HP 0.075%) to be rubbed into the skin over the painful region two to four times daily. Gloves should be used for application since hand contamination could result in discomfort if the cream comes in contact with eyes or sensitive areas such as the genitalia. Application of a 5% lidocaine patch over an area of maximal pain has been reported to be of benefit. It is approved for treatment of postherpetic neuralgia.

Diabetic neuropathic cachexia is a syndrome characterized by a symmetric peripheral neuropathy associated with profound weight loss (up to 60% of total body weight) and painful dysesthesias affecting the proximal lower limbs, the hands, or the lower trunk. Treatment is usually with insulin and analgesics. The prognosis is generally good, and patients typically recover their baseline weight with resolution of the painful sensory symptoms within 1 year.

B. ISOLATED PERIPHERAL NEUROPATHY—Involvement of the distribution of only one nerve ("mononeuropathy") or of several nerves ("mononeuropathy multiplex") is characterized by sudden onset with subsequent recovery of all or most of the function. This neuropathology has been attributed to vascular ischemia or traumatic damage. Cranial and femoral nerves are commonly involved, and motor abnormalities predominate. The patient with cranial nerve involvement usually has diplopia and single third, fourth, or sixth nerve weakness on examination but the pupil is spared. A full recovery of function occurs in 6–12 weeks. Diabetic amyotrophy presents with onset of severe pain in the front of the thigh. Within a few days or weeks of the onset of pain, weakness and wasting of the quadriceps develops. As the weakness appears, the pain tends to improve. Management includes analgesia and improved diabetes control. The symptoms improve over 6–18 months.

2. Autonomic neuropathy—Neuropathy of the autonomic system occurs principally in patients with diabetes of long duration. It affects many diverse visceral functions including blood pressure and pulse, gastrointestinal activity, bladder function, and erectile dysfunction. Treatment is directed specifically at each abnormality.

Involvement of the gastrointestinal system may be manifested by nausea, vomiting, postprandial fullness, reflux or dysphagia, constipation or diarrhea (or both), and fecal incontinence. Gastroparesis should be considered in type 1 diabetic patients in whom unexpected fluctuations and variability in their blood glucose levels develops after meals. Metoclopramide has been of some help in treating diabetic gastroparesis. It is given in a dose of 10 mg orally three or four times a day, 30 minutes before meals and at bedtime. Drowsiness, restlessness, fatigue, and lassitude are common adverse effects. Tardive dyskinesia and extrapyramidal effects can occur, especially when used for longer than 3 months, and the FDA has cautioned against the long-term use of metoclopramide.

Erythromycin appears to bind to motilin receptors in the stomach and has been found to improve gastric emptying over the short term in doses of 250 mg three times daily, but its effectiveness seems to diminish over time. In selected patients, injections of botulinum toxin into the pylorus can reduce pylorus sphincter resistance and enhance gastric emptying. Gastric electrical stimulation has been reported to improve symptoms and quality of life indices in patients with gastroparesis refractory to pharmacologic therapy.

Diarrhea associated with autonomic neuropathy has occasionally responded to broad-spectrum antibiotic therapy (such as rifaximin, metronidazole, amoxicillin/clavulanate, ciprofloxacin, or doxycycline), although it often undergoes spontaneous remission. Refractory diabetic diarrhea is often associated with impaired sphincter control and fecal incontinence. Therapy with loperamide, 4–8 mg daily, or diphenoxylate with atropine, two tablets up to four times a day, may provide relief. In more severe cases, tincture of paregoric or codeine (60-mg tablets) may be required to reduce the frequency of diarrhea and improve the consistency of the stools. Clonidine has been reported to lessen diabetic diarrhea; however, its usefulness is limited by its tendency to lower blood pressure in these patients who already have autonomic neuropathy, resulting in orthostatic hypotension. Constipation usually responds to stimulant laxatives such as senna.

Incomplete emptying of the bladder can sometimes occur. Bethanechol in doses of 10–50 mg orally three times a day has occasionally improved emptying of the atonic urinary bladder. Catheter decompression of the distended bladder has been reported to improve its function, and considerable benefit has been reported after surgical severing of the internal vesicle sphincter.

Use of Jobst fitted stockings, tilting the head of the bed, and arising slowly from the supine position can be helpful in treating symptoms of orthostatic hypotension. When such measures are inadequate, then treatment with fludrocortisone 0.1–0.2 mg orally daily can be considered. This medication, however, can result in supine hypertension and hypokalemia. Midodrine (10 mg orally three times a day), an alpha-agonist, can also be used.

Erectile dysfunction can result from neurologic, psychological, or vascular causes, or a combination of these causes. Sildenafil (Viagra), vardenafil (Levitra), and tadalafil (Cialis) have been shown in placebo-controlled clinical trials to improve erections in response to sexual stimulation. The recommended dose of sildenafil for most patients is one 50-mg tablet taken approximately 1 hour before sexual activity. The peak effect is at 1.5–2 hours, with some effect persisting for 4 hours. Patients with diabetes mellitus using sildenafil reported 50–60% improvement in erectile function. The maximum recommended dose is 100 mg. The recommended dose of both vardenafil and tadalafil is 10 mg. The doses may be increased to 20 mg or decreased to 5 mg based on efficacy and side effects. Tadalafil has been shown to improve erectile function for up to 36 hours after dosing. Low doses are available for daily use. In clinical trials, only a few adverse effects have been reported—transient mild headache, flushing, dyspepsia, and some altered color vision. Priapism can occur with these medications, and patients should be advised to seek immediate medical attention if an erection persists for longer than 4 hours. These phosphodiesterase type 5 (PDE5) inhibitors potentiate the hypotensive effects of nitrates and their use is contraindicated in patients who are concurrently using organic nitrates in any form. Caution is advised for men who have suffered a heart attack, stroke, or life-threatening arrhythmia within the previous 6 months; men who have resting hypotension or hypertension; and men who have a history of heart failure or have unstable angina. Rarely, a decrease in vision or permanent visual loss has been reported after PDE5 inhibitor use.

Intracorporeal injection of vasoactive medications causes penile engorgement and erection. Medications most commonly used include papaverine alone, papaverine with phentolamine, and alprostadil (prostaglandin E_1). Alprostadil injections are relatively painless, but careful instruction is essential to prevent local trauma, priapism, and fibrosis. Intraurethral pellets of alprostadil avoid the problem of injection of the medication.

External vacuum therapy (Erec-Aid System) is a non-surgical treatment consisting of a suction chamber operated by a hand pump that creates a vacuum around the penis. This draws blood into the penis to produce an erection that is maintained by a specially designed tension ring inserted around the base of the penis and which can be kept in place for up to 20–30 minutes. While this method is generally effective, its cumbersome nature limits its appeal.

Surgical implants of penile prostheses remain an option for those patients in whom the nonsurgical approaches are ineffective.

D. Cardiovascular Complications

1. Heart disease—Microangiopathy occurs in the heart and may explain the etiology of congestive cardiomyopathies in diabetic patients who do not have demonstrable coronary artery disease. More commonly, however, heart disease in patients with diabetes is due to coronary atherosclerosis. Myocardial infarction is three to five times more common in diabetic patients and is the leading cause of death in patients with type 2 diabetes. Cardiovascular disease risk is increased in patients with type 1 diabetes as well, although the absolute risk is lower than in patients with type 2 diabetes. Premenopausal women who normally have lower rates of coronary artery disease lose this protection once diabetes develops. The increased risk in patients with type 2 diabetes reflects the combination of hyperglycemia, hyperlipidemia, abnormalities of platelet adhesiveness, coagulation factors, hypertension, oxidative stress, and inflammation. Large intervention studies of risk factor reduction in diabetes are lacking, but it is reasonable to assume that reducing these risk factors would have a beneficial effect. Lowering LDL cholesterol reduces first events in patients without known coronary disease and secondary events in patients with known coronary disease. These intervention studies included some patients with diabetes, and the benefits of LDL cholesterol lowering was apparent in this group. The National Cholesterol Education Program clinical practice guidelines have designated diabetes as a coronary risk equivalent and have recommended that patients with diabetes should have an LDL cholesterol goal of less than 100 mg/dL (2.6 mmol/L). Lowering LDL cholesterol to 70 mg/dL (1.8 mmol/L) may have additional benefit and is a reasonable target for most patients with type 2 diabetes who have multiple risk factors for cardiovascular disease.

Aspirin at a dose of 81–325 mg daily is effective in reducing cardiovascular morbidity and mortality in patients who have a history of myocardial infarction or stroke (secondary prevention). For primary prevention, a 2018 randomized study of 15,480 persons with diabetes but no evident cardiovascular disease observed that 100 mg aspirin reduced the first vascular event of myocardial infarction, stroke or transient ischemic attack or death from vascular event (excluding intracranial hemorrhage) (rate ratio 0.88; 95% confidence interval 0.79 to 0.97). There were, however, more major bleeding events, especially gastrointestinal, in the aspirin group (rate ratio 1.29; 95% confidence interval 1.09 to 1.52). Thus, for primary prevention, the use of aspirin should only be considered for patients with high cardiovascular risk and low bleeding risk and generally not for adults older than 70 years. Based on the Early Treatment Diabetic Retinopathy Study (ETDRS), there does not appear to be a contraindication to aspirin use to achieve cardiovascular benefit in diabetic patients who have proliferative retinopathy. Aspirin also does not seem to affect the severity of vitreous/preretinal hemorrhages or their resolution.

2. Hypertension—The ADA also recommends lowering systolic blood pressure to less than 140 mm Hg and diastolic pressure to less than 90 mm Hg in patients with diabetes. The systolic target of 130 mm Hg or less and diastolic target of 80 mm Hg or less are recommended for the younger patient if they can be achieved without undue treatment burden. The Systolic Blood Pressure Intervention Trial (SPRINT) reported that treating to a systolic blood pressure of less than 120 mm Hg reduced cardiovascular events by 25% and death from cardiovascular causes by 43% during 3.26 years of follow-up. People with diabetes, however, were excluded from this study, and it is unclear if the results are applicable to this population. Patients with type 2 diabetes who already have cardiovascular disease or microalbuminuria should be considered for treatment with an ACE inhibitor. More clinical studies are needed to address the question of whether patients with type 2 diabetes who do not have cardiovascular disease or microalbuminuria would specifically benefit from ACE inhibitor treatment.

3. Peripheral vascular disease—Atherosclerosis is markedly accelerated in the larger arteries. It is often diffuse, with localized enhancement in certain areas of turbulent blood flow, such as at the bifurcation of the aorta or other large vessels. Clinical manifestations of peripheral vascular disease include ischemia of the lower extremities, erectile dysfunction, and intestinal angina.

The incidence of **gangrene of the feet** in patients with diabetes is 30 times that in age-matched controls. The factors responsible for its development, in addition to peripheral vascular disease, are small vessel disease, peripheral neuropathy with loss of both pain sensation and neurogenic inflammatory responses, and secondary infection. In two-thirds of patients with ischemic gangrene, pedal pulses are not palpable. In the remaining one-third who have palpable pulses, reduced blood flow through these vessels can be demonstrated by plethysmographic or Doppler ultrasound examination. Prevention of foot injury is imperative. Agents that reduce peripheral blood flow such as tobacco should be avoided. Control of other risk factors such as hypertension is essential. Beta-blockers are relatively contraindicated because of presumed negative peripheral hemodynamic consequences but data that support this are lacking. Cholesterol-lowering agents are useful as adjunctive therapy when early ischemic signs are detected and when dyslipidemia is present. Patients should be advised to seek immediate medical care if a diabetic foot ulcer develops. Improvement in peripheral blood flow with endarterectomy and bypass operations is possible in certain patients.

E. Skin and Mucous Membrane Complications

Chronic pyogenic infections of the skin may occur, especially in poorly controlled diabetic patients. Candidal infection can produce erythema and edema of intertriginous areas below the breasts, in the axillas, and between the fingers. It causes vulvovaginitis in women with chronically uncontrolled diabetes who have persistent glucosuria and is a frequent cause of pruritus. While antifungal creams containing miconazole or clotrimazole offer immediate relief of vulvovaginitis, recurrence is frequent unless glucosuria is reduced.

In some patients with type 2 diabetes, poor glycemic control can cause a severe hypertriglyceridemia, which can present as eruptive cutaneous xanthomas and pancreatitis. The skin lesions appear as yellow morbilliform eruptions 2–5 mm in diameter with erythematous areolae. They occur on extensor surfaces (elbows, knees, buttocks) and disappear after triglyceride levels are reduced.

Necrobiosis lipoidica diabeticorum is usually located over the anterior surfaces of the legs or the dorsal surfaces of the ankles. They are oval or irregularly shaped plaques with demarcated borders and a glistening yellow surface and occur in women two to four times more frequently than in men. Pathologically, the lesions show degeneration of collagen, granulomatous inflammation of subcutaneous tissues and blood vessels, capillary basement membrane thickening and obliteration of vessel lumina. The condition is associated with type 1 diabetes, although it can occur in patients with type 2 diabetes, and also in patients without diabetes. First-line therapy includes topical and subcutaneous corticosteroids. Improving glycemic control may help the condition.

"**Shin spots**" are not uncommon in adults with diabetes. They are brownish, rounded, painless atrophic lesions of the skin in the pretibial area.

F. Bone and Joint Complications

Long-standing diabetes can cause progressive stiffness of the hand secondary to contracture and tightening of skin over the joints (diabetic cheiroarthropathy), frozen shoulder (adhesive capsulitis), carpal tunnel syndrome, and Dupuytren contractures. These complications are believed to be due to glycosylation of collagen and perhaps other proteins in connective tissue. There may also be an inflammatory component.

Data on bone mineral density and fracture risk in people with diabetes are contradictory. Patients with type 2 diabetes do appear to be at increased risk for nonvertebral fractures. Women with type 1 diabetes have an increased risk of fracture when compared with women without diabetes. Other factors, such as duration of diabetes, and diabetes complications, such as neuropathy and kidney disease, likely affect both the bone mineral density and fracture risk.

Diffuse idiopathic skeletal hyperostosis (DISH) is characterized by ossification of the anterior longitudinal ligaments of the spine and various extraspinal ligaments. It causes stiffness and decreased range of spinal motion. The peripheral joints most commonly affected are the metacarpophalangeal joints, elbows, and shoulders. Diabetes, obesity, hypertension, and dyslipidemia are risk factors for this condition.

Hyperuricemia and acute and tophaceous gout are more common in type 2 diabetes.

Bursitis, particularly of the shoulders and hips, occurs more frequently than expected in patients with diabetes.

ASCEND Study Collaborative Group et al. Effects of aspirin for primary prevention in persons with diabetes mellitus. N Engl J Med. 2018 Oct 8;379(16):1529–39. [PMID: 30146931]
Chin JA et al. Diabetes mellitus and peripheral vascular disease: diagnosis and management. Clin Podiatr Med Surg. 2014 Jan; 31(1):11–26. [PMID: 24296015]

Gregg EW et al. Changes in diabetes-related complications in the United States, 1990–2010. N Engl J Med. 2014 Apr 17; 370(16):1514–23. [PMID: 24738668]
Razmaria AA. Diabetic neuropathy. JAMA Patient Page. JAMA. 2015 Nov 24;314(20):2202. [PMID: 26599195]
Stitt AW et al. The progress in understanding and treatment of diabetic retinopathy. Prog Retin Eye Res. 2016 Mar;51:156–86. [PMID: 26297071]
Waanders F et al. Current concepts in the management of diabetic nephropathy. Neth J Med. 2013 Nov;71(9):448–58. [PMID: 24218418]
Wright JT Jr et al; SPRINT research group. A randomized trial of intensive versus standard blood-pressure control. N Engl J Med. 2015 Nov 26;373(22):2103–16. [PMID: 26551272]

▶ Special Situations

A. Diabetes Management in the Hospital

Most patients with diabetes are hospitalized for reasons other than their diabetes. Indeed, up to 10–15% of all hospitalized patients have diabetes. It is challenging using outpatient oral therapies or insulin regimens in the hospital because patients are not eating as usual; they are often fasting for procedures; clinical events increase adverse reactions associated with diabetes medicines, eg, thiazolidinediones can cause fluid retention and worsen heart failure; metformin should not be used in patients with significant chronic kidney or liver disease, or those getting contrast for radiographic studies. Subcutaneous or intravenous insulin therapy is frequently substituted for other diabetes medicines because the insulin dose can be adjusted to match changing inpatient needs and it is safe to use insulin in patients with heart, kidney, and liver disease.

Surgery represents a stress situation during which most of the insulin antagonists (eg, catecholamines, growth hormone, and corticosteroids) are mobilized. In the diabetic patient, this can lead to a worsening of hyperglycemia and perhaps even ketoacidosis. The aim of medical management of people with diabetes during the perioperative period is to minimize these stress-induced changes. Recommendations for management depend both on the patient's usual diabetic regimen and on the type of surgery (major or minor) to be done (see also Chapter 3).

For people with diabetes controlled with diet alone, no special precautions must be taken unless diabetic control is markedly disturbed by the procedure. If this occurs, small doses of short-acting insulin as needed will correct the hyperglycemia.

Patients taking oral agents should not take them on the day of surgery. If there is significant hyperglycemia, small doses of short-acting insulin are given as needed. If this approach does not provide adequate control, an insulin infusion should be started in the manner indicated below. The oral agents can be restarted once the patient is eating normally after the operation. It is important to order a postoperative serum creatinine level to ensure adequate kidney function prior to restarting metformin therapy.

Patients taking insulin represent the only serious challenge to management of diabetes when surgery is necessary. However, with careful attention to changes in the clinical or laboratory picture, glucose control can be

Table 27–11. Recommendations for management of insulin-treated diabetes during surgery.

Type of Diabetes	Minor Surgical Procedures (< 2 hours; eating afterward)	Major Surgical Procedures (> 2 hours; invasion of body cavity; not eating immediately after recovery)
Type 1: Patients using basal bolus insulin regimen or insulin pump	Patients using pump should discontinue the pump the evening before procedure and take 24-hour basal insulin. On day of procedure, start 5% dextrose; monitor blood glucose and give subcutaneous short-acting insulin every 4 or 6 hours	Start insulin infusion on morning of procedure and transition back to usual regimen when eating
Type 2: Patients using basal bolus insulin regimen; twice daily premixed insulin	No insulin on the day of operation. Start 5% dextrose infusion; monitor fingerstick blood glucose and give subcutaneous short-acting insulin every 4 or 6 hours	Same regimen as minor procedure If control is not satisfactory, start intravenous insulin infusion

managed successfully. The protocol used to control the glucose depends on the kind of diabetes (type 1 or type 2); whether it is minor surgery (lasting less than 2 hours and patient eating afterwards) or major surgery (lasting more than 2 hours, with invasion of a body cavity, and patient not eating afterwards); and the preoperative insulin regimen (basal bolus or premixed insulin twice a day or premeal bolus only or regular insulin before meals and NPH at bedtime). Patients with type 1 diabetes must be receiving some insulin to prevent the development of DKA. Many patients with type 2 diabetes who are taking insulin do well perioperatively without insulin for a few hours. Ideally, patients with diabetes should undergo surgery early in the morning. Table 27–11 summarizes the approach for these patients.

One insulin infusion method adds 10 units of regular insulin to 1 L of 5% dextrose in 0.45% saline, and this is infused intravenously at a rate of 100–180 mL/h. This gives the patient 1–1.8 units of insulin per hour which, except in the most severe cases, generally keeps the blood glucose within the range of 100–250 mg/dL (5.5–13.9 mmol/L). The infusion may be continued for several days, if necessary. Perioperatively, plasma glucose or blood glucose should be determined every 2–4 hours to be sure metabolic control is adequate. If it is not, adjustments in the ratio of insulin to dextrose in the intravenous solution can be made.

An alternative method consists of separate infusions of insulin and glucose delivered by pumps to permit independent adjustments of each infusion rate, depending on hourly variation of blood glucose values. There are a number of different algorithms available for insulin infusions (see http://www.hospitalmedicine.org).

After surgery, when the patient has resumed an adequate oral intake, subcutaneous administration of insulin can be resumed and intravenous administration of insulin and dextrose can be stopped 30 minutes after the first subcutaneous dose. Insulin needs may vary in the first several days after surgery because of continuing postoperative stresses and because of variable caloric intake. In this situation, multiple doses of short-acting insulin plus some long-acting basal insulin, guided by blood glucose determinations, can keep the patient in acceptable metabolic control.

In the **intensive care units (ICUs),** glucose levels are controlled most frequently using insulin infusions. Patients receiving total parenteral nutrition can have insulin added to the bag. Standard total parenteral nutrition contains 25% dextrose so an infusion rate of 50 mL/h delivers 12.5 g of dextrose per hour.

Based on the evidence available, ICU patients with diabetes and new-onset hyperglycemia with blood glucose levels above 180 mg/dL (10 mmol/L) should be treated with insulin, aiming for target glucose levels between 140 mg/dL (7.8 mmol/L) and 180 mg/dL (10 mmol/L). In the ICU setting, aiming for blood glucose levels close to 100 mg/dL (5.6 mmol/L) is not beneficial and may even be harmful. When patients leave the ICU, target glucose values between 100 mg/dL (5.6 mmol/L) and 180 mg/dL (10 mmol/L) may be appropriate, although this view is based on clinical observations rather than conclusive evidence.

On the **general surgical and medical inpatient services,** most patients are treated with subcutaneous insulin regimens. Limited cross-sectional and prospective studies suggest that the best glucose control is achieved on a combination of basal and bolus regimen with 50% of daily insulin needs provided by intermediate- or long-acting insulins. Standardized order sets can reduce errors, and they often include algorithms for recognition and treatment of hypoglycemia (see http://ucsfinpatientdiabetes.pbworks.com for examples).

The morbidity and mortality in diabetic patients are twice those of nondiabetic patients. Those with new-onset hyperglycemia (ie, those without a preadmission diagnosis of diabetes) have even higher mortality—almost eightfold that of nondiabetic patients in one study. These observations have led to the question of whether tight glycemic control in the hospital improves outcomes.

Kansagara D et al. Intensive insulin therapy in hospitalized patients: a systematic review. Ann Intern Med. 2011 Feb 15; 154(4):268–82. [PMID: 21320942]

B. Pregnancy and the Diabetic Patient

See Chapter 19. Tight glycemic control with normal HbA$_{1c}$ levels is very important during pregnancy. Early in pregnancy, poor control increases the risk of spontaneous abortion and congenital malformations. Late in pregnancy, poor control can result in polyhydramnios, preterm labor, stillbirth, and fetal macrosomia with its associated problems. Diabetes complications can impact both maternal and fetal health. Diabetic retinopathy can first develop during pregnancy or retinopathy that is already present can worsen. Diabetic women with microalbuminuria can have worsening albuminuria during pregnancy and are at higher risk for preeclampsia. Aspirin can reduce the risk of preeclampsia and should be prescribed after 12 weeks of gestation. Patients who have preexisting kidney failure (prepregnancy creatinine clearance less than 80 mL/min) are at high risk for further decline in kidney function during the pregnancy, and this may not reverse after delivery. Diabetic gastroparesis can severely exacerbate the nausea and vomiting of pregnancy and some patients may require fluid and nutritional support.

Although there is evidence that glyburide is safe during pregnancy, the current practice is to control diabetes with insulin therapy. Every effort should be made, utilizing multiple injections of insulin or a continuous infusion of insulin by pump, to maintain near-normalization of fasting and preprandial blood glucose values while avoiding hypoglycemia.

Regular and NPH insulin and the insulin analogs lispro, aspart, and detemir are labeled pregnancy category B. Insulin glargine, glulisine, and degludec are labeled category C because of lack of clinical safety data. A small study using insulin glargine in 32 pregnancies did not reveal any problems.

Unless there are fetal or maternal complications, diabetic women should be able to carry the pregnancy to full-term, delivering at 38 to 41 weeks. Induction of labor before 39 weeks may be considered if there is concern about increasing fetal weight. See Chapter 19 for further details.

Blumer I et al. Diabetes and pregnancy: an endocrine society clinical practice guideline. J Clin Endocrinol Metab. 2013 Nov; 98(11):4227–49. [PMID: 24194617]

Prognosis

The DCCT showed that the previously poor prognosis for as many as 40% of patients with type 1 diabetes is markedly improved by optimal care. DCCT participants were generally young and highly motivated and were cared for in academic centers by skilled diabetes educators and endocrinologists who were able to provide more attention and services than are usually available. Improved training of primary care providers may be beneficial.

For type 2 diabetes, the UKPDS documented a reduction in microvascular disease with glycemic control, although this was not apparent in the obese subgroup. Cardiovascular outcomes were not improved by glycemic control, although antihypertensive therapy showed benefit in reducing the number of adverse cardiovascular complications as well as in reducing the occurrence of microvascular disease among hypertensive patients. In patients with visceral obesity, successful management of type 2 diabetes

remains a major challenge in the attempt to achieve appropriate control of hyperglycemia, hypertension, and dyslipidemia. Once safe and effective methods are devised to prevent or manage obesity, the prognosis of type 2 diabetes with its high cardiovascular risks should improve considerably.

In addition to poorly understood genetic factors relating to differences in individual susceptibility to development of long-term complications of hyperglycemia, it is clear that in both types of diabetes, the diabetic patient's intelligence, motivation, and awareness of the potential complications of the disease contribute significantly to the ultimate outcome.

When to Refer

- All patients should receive self-management education when diabetes is diagnosed and at intervals thereafter. The instructional team should include a registered dietitian and registered nurse; they must be Certified Diabetes Educators (CDEs).
- Patients with type 1 diabetes should be comanaged by an endocrinologist and a primary care provider.
- Patients with type 2 diabetes should be referred to an endocrinologist if treatment goals are not met or if the patient requires an increasingly complex regimen to maintain glycemic control.
- Patients with type 2 diabetes should be referred to an ophthalmologist or optometrist for a dilated eye examination when the diabetes is diagnosed, and patients with type 1 diabetes should be referred 5 years after the diagnosis is made.
- Patients with peripheral neuropathy, especially those with loss of protective threshold (unable to detect 5.07 Semmes-Weinstein filament) or structural foot problems, should be referred to a podiatrist.
- Referrals to other specialists may be required for management of chronic complications of diabetes.

Academy of Nutrition and Dietetics. https://www.eatright.org
American Association of Diabetes Educators. https://www.diabeteseducator.org/
American Diabetes Association. http://www.diabetes.org
American Diabetes Association. Standards of Medical Care in Diabetes—2015. Diabetes Care. 2015 Jan;38(Suppl 1):S11–90. [PMID: 25537706]
Juvenile Diabetes Research Foundation. https://www.jdrf.org

DIABETIC COMA

Coma may be due to a variety of causes not directly related to diabetes. Certain causes directly related to diabetes require differentiation: (1) Hypoglycemic coma resulting from excessive doses of insulin or oral hypoglycemic agents. (2) Hyperglycemic coma associated with either severe insulin deficiency (DKA) or mild to moderate insulin deficiency (hyperglycemic hyperosmolar state). (3) Lactic acidosis associated with diabetes, particularly in patients with diabetes stricken with severe infections or with cardiovascular collapse.

DIABETIC KETOACIDOSIS

ESSENTIALS OF DIAGNOSIS

▸ Hyperglycemia greater than 250 mg/dL (13.9 mmol/L).

▸ Metabolic acidosis with blood pH < 7.3; serum bicarbonate less than 15 mEq/L.

▸ Serum positive for ketones.

▸ General Considerations

Diabetic ketoacidosis (DKA) may be the initial manifestation of type 1 diabetes or may result from increased insulin requirements in type 1 diabetes patients during the course of infection, trauma, myocardial infarction, or surgery. It is a life-threatening medical emergency with a mortality rate just under 5% in individuals under 40 years of age, but with a more serious prognosis in older adults, who have mortality rates over 20%. The National Data Group reports an annual incidence of five to eight episodes of DKA per 1000 diabetic persons. Ketoacidosis may develop in patients with type 2 diabetes when severe stress such as sepsis or trauma is present. DKA is one of the more common serious complications of insulin pump therapy, occurring in approximately 1 per 80 patient-months of treatment. Many patients who monitor capillary blood glucose regularly ignore urine ketone measurements, which signals the possibility of insulin leakage or pump failure before serious illness develops. Poor compliance, either for psychological reasons or because of inadequate education, is one of the most common causes of recurrent DKA.

▸ Clinical Findings

A. Symptoms and Signs

The appearance of DKA is usually preceded by a day or more of polyuria and polydipsia associated with marked fatigue, nausea, and vomiting. If untreated, mental stupor ensues that can progress to coma. Drowsiness is fairly common, but frank coma only occurs in about 10% of patients. On physical examination, evidence of dehydration in a stuporous patient with rapid deep breathing and a "fruity" breath odor of acetone strongly suggests the diagnosis. Hypotension with tachycardia indicates profound fluid and electrolyte depletion, and mild hypothermia is usually present. Abdominal pain and even tenderness may be present in the absence of abdominal disease. Conversely, cholecystitis or pancreatitis may occur with minimal symptoms and signs.

B. Laboratory Findings

Typically, the patient with moderately severe DKA has a plasma glucose of 350–900 mg/dL (19.4–50 mmol/L), serum ketones at a dilution of 1:8 or greater or beta-hydroxybutyrate more than 4 nmol/L, hyperkalemia (serum potassium level of 5–8 mEq/L), slight hyponatremia (serum sodium of approximately 130 mEq/L), hyperphosphatemia (serum phosphate level of 6–7 mg/dL [1.9–2.3 mmol/L]), and elevated blood urea nitrogen and serum creatinine levels (Table 27–12). Acidosis may be severe (pH ranging from 6.9 to 7.2 and serum bicarbonate ranging from 5 mEq/L to 15 mEq/L); PCO_2 is low (15–20 mm Hg) related to compensatory hyperventilation. Fluid depletion is marked, typically about 100 mL/kg.

The difference between venous and arterial pH is 0.02 to 0.15 pH units and venous and arterial bicarbonate is 1.88 mEq/L. These small differences will not affect either the diagnosis or the management of DKA, and there is no need to collect arterial blood for measuring the acid-base status.

The hyperkalemia occurs despite total body potassium depletion because of the shift of potassium from the intracellular to extracellular spaces that occurs in systemic acidosis. The average total body potassium deficit resulting from osmotic diuresis, acidosis, and gastrointestinal losses is about 3–5 mEq/kg. Similarly, despite the elevated serum phosphate, total body phosphate is generally depleted. Serum sodium is generally reduced due to loss of sodium

Table 27–12. Laboratory diagnosis of coma in diabetic patients.

	Urine Glucose	Urine Ketones	Plasma Glucose	Plasma Bicarbonate	Plasma Ketones
Related to Diabetes					
Hypoglycemia	0[1]	0 or +	Low	Normal	0
Diabetic ketoacidosis	++++	++++	High	Low	++++
Hyperglycemic hyperosmolar state coma	++++	0	High	Normal or slightly low	0
Lactic acidosis	0 or +	0 or +	Normal or low or high	Low	0 or +
Unrelated to Diabetes					
Alcohol or other toxic drugs	0 or +	0 or +	May be low	Normal or low[2]	0 or +
Cerebrovascular accident or head trauma	+ or 0	0	Often high	Normal	0
Uremia	0 or +	0	High or normal	Low	0 or +

[1]Leftover urine in bladder might still contain glucose from earlier hyperglycemia.
[2]Alcohol can elevate plasma lactate as well as keto acids to reduce pH.

ions (7–10 mEq/kg) by polyuria and vomiting and because severe hyperglycemia shifts intracellular water into the interstitial compartment. For every 100 mg/dL of plasma glucose, serum sodium decreases by 1.6 mEq/L (5.56 mmol/L). The decrease in serum sodium may be greater when patients have more severe hyperglycemia (greater than 400 mg/dL, 22.2 mmol/L) and a correction factor of 2.4 mEq/L may be used. Hypertriglyceridemia should be considered if the corrected sodium is very low. Serum osmolality can be directly measured by standard tests of freezing point depression or can be estimated by calculating the molarity of sodium, chloride, and glucose in the serum. A convenient method of estimating effective serum osmolality is as follows (normal values in humans are 280–300 mOsm/kg):

$$mOsm/kg = 2\,[\text{measured Na}^+] + \frac{\text{Glucose (mg/dL)}}{18}$$

These calculated estimates are usually 10–20 mOsm/kg lower than values measured by standard cryoscopic techniques. Central nervous system depression or coma occurs when the effective serum osmolality exceeds 320–330 mOsm/L. Coma in a diabetic patient with a lower osmolality should prompt a search for cause of coma other than hyperosmolality (see Table 27–12 and Chapter 24).

Ketoacidemia represents the effect of insulin lack at multiple enzyme loci. Insulin lack associated with elevated levels of growth hormone, catecholamines, and glucagon contributes to increases in lipolysis from adipose tissue and in hepatic ketogenesis. In addition, reduced ketolysis by insulin-deficient peripheral tissues contributes to the ketoacidemia. The only true "keto" acid present is acetoacetic acid which, along with its by-product acetone, is measured by nitroprusside reagents (Acetest and Ketostix). The sensitivity for acetone, however, is poor, requiring over 10 mmol/L, which is seldom reached in the plasma of ketoacidotic patients—although this detectable concentration is readily achieved in urine. Thus, in the plasma of ketotic patients, only acetoacetate is measured by these reagents. The more prevalent beta-hydroxybutyric acid has no ketone group and is therefore not detected by conventional nitroprusside tests. This takes on special importance in the presence of circulatory collapse during DKA, wherein an increase in lactic acid can shift the redox state to increase beta-hydroxybutyric acid at the expense of the readily detectable acetoacetic acid. Bedside diagnostic reagents are then unreliable, suggesting no ketonemia in cases where beta-hydroxybutyric acid is a major factor in producing the acidosis. Combined glucose and ketone meters (Precision Xtra, Nova Max Plus) that measure blood beta-hydroxybutyrate concentration on capillary blood are available. Many clinical laboratories also offer direct blood beta-hydroxybutyrate measurement.

Nonspecific elevations of serum amylase and lipase occurs in about 16–25% of cases of DKA, and an imaging study may be necessary if the diagnosis of acute pancreatitis is being seriously considered. Leukocytosis as high as 25,000/mcL with a left shift may occur with or without associated infection. The presence of an elevated or even a normal temperature can suggest the presence of an infection, since patients with DKA are generally hypothermic if uninfected.

▶ **Treatment**

Patients with mild DKA are alert and have pH levels between 7.25 and 7.30 and beta-hydroxybutyrate levels of 3–4 mmol/L; those with moderate ketoacidosis are either alert or little drowsy and have pH levels between 7.0 and 7.24 and beta-hydroxybutyrate levels of 4–8 mmol/L; and those with severe ketoacidosis are stuporose and have a pH < 7.0 and beta-hydroxybutyrate levels of greater than 8 mmol/L. Those with mild ketoacidosis can be treated in the emergency department, but those with moderate or severe ketoacidosis require admission to the ICU or stepdown unit. Therapeutic goals are to restore plasma volume and tissue perfusion, reduce blood glucose and osmolality toward normal, correct acidosis, replenish electrolyte losses, and identify and treat precipitating factors. Gastric intubation is recommended in the comatose patient to prevent vomiting and aspiration that may occur as a result of gastric atony, a common complication of DKA. An indwelling catheter may also be necessary. In patients with preexisting heart or kidney failure or those in severe cardiovascular collapse, a central venous pressure catheter should be inserted to evaluate the degree of hypovolemia and to monitor subsequent fluid administration.

A comprehensive flow sheet that includes vital signs, serial laboratory data, and therapeutic interventions (eg, fluids, insulin) should be meticulously maintained by the clinician responsible for the patient's care. Plasma glucose should be recorded hourly and electrolytes and pH at least every 2–3 hours during the initial treatment period. Bedside glucose meters should be used to titrate the insulin therapy. The patient should not receive sedatives or opioids in order to avoid masking signs and symptoms of impeding cerebral edema.

A. Fluid Replacement

In most patients, the fluid deficit is 4–5 L. Initially, 0.9% saline solution is the solution of choice to help reexpand the contracted vascular volume and should be started in the emergency department as soon as the diagnosis is established. The saline should be infused rapidly to provide 1 L/h over the first 1–2 hours. After the first 2 L of fluid have been given, the intravenous infusion should be at the rate of 300–400 mL/h. Use 0.9% ("normal") saline unless the serum sodium is greater than 150 mEq/L, when 0.45% ("half normal") saline solution should be used. The volume status should be very carefully monitored. Failure to give enough volume replacement (at least 3–4 L in 8 hours) to restore normal perfusion is one of the most serious therapeutic shortcomings adversely influencing satisfactory recovery. Excessive fluid replacement (more than 5 L in 8 hours) may contribute to acute respiratory distress syndrome or cerebral edema. When blood glucose falls to approximately 250 mg/dL (13.9 mmol/L), the fluids should be changed to a 5% glucose-containing solution to maintain serum glucose in the range of 250–300 mg/dL (13.9–16.7 mmol/L). This will prevent the development of hypoglycemia and will also reduce the likelihood of cerebral edema, which could result from too rapid decline of blood glucose.

B. Insulin Replacement

Immediately after initiation of fluid replacement, regular insulin can be given intravenously in a loading dose of 0.1 unit/kg as a bolus to prime the tissue insulin receptors. Following the initial bolus, intravenous doses of insulin as low as 0.1 unit/kg/h are continuously infused or given hourly as an intramuscular injection; this is sufficient to replace the insulin deficit in most patients. A prospective randomized study showed that a bolus dose is not required if patients are given hourly insulin infusion at 0.14 unit/kg. Replacement of insulin deficiency helps correct the acidosis by reducing the flux of fatty acids to the liver, reducing ketone production by the liver, and also improving removal of ketones from the blood. Insulin treatment reduces the hyperosmolality by reducing the hyperglycemia. It accomplishes this by increasing removal of glucose through peripheral utilization as well as by decreasing production of glucose by the liver. This latter effect is accomplished by direct inhibition of gluconeogenesis and glycogenolysis as well as by lowered amino acid flux from muscle to liver and reduced hyperglucagonemia.

The insulin infusion should be "piggy-backed" into the fluid line so the rate of fluid replacement can be changed without altering the insulin delivery rate. If the plasma glucose level fails to fall at least 10% in the first hour, a repeat loading dose (0.1 or 0.14 unit/kg) is recommended. Rarely, a patient with immune insulin resistance is encountered, and this requires doubling the insulin dose every 2–4 hours if hyperglycemia does not improve after the first two doses of insulin. The insulin dose should be adjusted to lower the glucose concentration by about 50–70 mg/dL/h (2.8–3.9 mmol/L). If clinical circumstances prevent use of insulin infusion, then the insulin can be given intramuscularly. An initial 0.15 unit/kg of regular insulin is given intravenously, and at the same time, the same size dose is given intramuscularly. Subsequently, regular insulin is given intramuscularly hourly at a dose of 0.1 unit/kg until the blood glucose falls to around 250 mg/dL, when the insulin can be given subcutaneously. Patients who normally take insulin glargine or insulin detemir can be given their usual maintenance doses during initial treatment of their DKA. The continuation of their subcutaneous basal insulins means that lower doses of intravenous insulin will be needed, and there will be a smoother transition from intravenous insulin infusion to the subcutaneous regimen.

C. Potassium

Total body potassium loss from polyuria and vomiting may be as high as 200 mEq. However, because of shifts of potassium from cells into the extracellular space as a consequence of acidosis, serum potassium is usually normal to slightly elevated prior to institution of treatment. As the acidosis is corrected, potassium flows back into the cells, and hypokalemia can develop if potassium replacement is not instituted. If the patient is not uremic and has an adequate urinary output, potassium chloride in doses of 10–30 mEq/h should be infused during the second and third hours after beginning therapy as soon as the acidosis starts to resolve. Replacement should be started sooner if the initial serum potassium is inappropriately normal or low and should be delayed if serum potassium fails to respond to initial therapy and remains above 5 mEq/L, as in cases of chronic kidney disease. Occasionally, a patient may present with a serum potassium level less than 3.5 mEq/L, in which case insulin therapy should be delayed until the potassium level is corrected to greater than 3.5 mEq/L. An ECG can be of help in monitoring the patient's potassium status: High peaked T waves are a sign of hyperkalemia, and flattened T waves with U waves are a sign of hypokalemia. Foods high in potassium content should be prescribed when the patient has recovered sufficiently to take food orally. Tomato juice has 14 mEq of potassium per 240 mL, and a medium-sized banana provides about 10 mEq.

D. Sodium Bicarbonate

The use of sodium bicarbonate in management of DKA has been questioned since clinical benefit was not demonstrated in one prospective randomized trial and because of the following potentially harmful consequences: (1) development of hypokalemia from rapid shift of potassium into cells if the acidosis is overcorrected; (2) tissue anoxia from reduced dissociation of oxygen from hemoglobin when acidosis is rapidly reversed (leftward shift of the oxygen dissociation curve); and (3) cerebral acidosis resulting from lowering of cerebrospinal fluid pH. It must be emphasized, however, that these considerations are less important when very severe acidosis exists. Therefore, it is recommended that bicarbonate be administered in DKA if the arterial blood pH is 7.0 or less, with careful monitoring to prevent overcorrection. One or two ampules of sodium bicarbonate (one ampule contains 44 mEq/50 mL) should be added to 1 L of 0.45% saline with 20 mEq KCl or to 400 mL of sterile water with 20 mEq KCl and infused over 1 to 2 hours. (**Note:** Addition of sodium bicarbonate to 0.9% saline would produce a markedly hypertonic solution that could aggravate the hyperosmolar state already present.) It can be repeated until the arterial pH reaches 7.1, but *it should not be given if the pH is 7.1 or greater* since additional bicarbonate would increase the risk of rebound metabolic alkalosis as ketones are metabolized. Alkalosis shifts potassium from serum into cells, which could precipitate a fatal cardiac arrhythmia.

E. Phosphate

Phosphate replacement is seldom required in treating DKA. However, if severe hypophosphatemia of less than 1 mg/dL (0.32 mmol/L) develops during insulin therapy, a small amount of phosphate can be replaced per hour as the potassium salt. Three randomized studies, though, in which phosphate was replaced in patients with DKA did not show any apparent clinical benefit from phosphate administration. Moreover, attempts to use potassium phosphate as the sole means of replacing potassium have led to a number of reported cases of severe hypocalcemia with tetany. To minimize the risk of inducing tetany from too-rapid replacement of phosphate, the average deficit of 40–50 mmol of phosphate should be replaced intravenously at a rate *no greater than 3–4 mmol/h* in a 60- to 70-kg person. A stock solution (Abbott) provides a mixture of 1.12 g KH_2PO_4 and 1.18 g K_2HPO_4 in a 5-mL single-dose vial (this equals 22 mmol of potassium and 15 mmol of phosphate). One-half of this vial (2.5 mL) should be added to 1 L of either 0.45% saline or 5% dextrose in water. Two liters of this solution, infused at a rate of 400 mL/h, will correct the phosphate deficit at the optimal rate of 3 mmol/h while providing 4.4 mEq of potassium per hour. (Additional potassium should be administered as potassium chloride to provide a total of 10–30 mEq of potassium per hour, as noted above.) If the serum phosphate remains below 2.5 mg/dL (0.8 mmol/L) after this infusion, a repeat 5-hour infusion can be given.

F. Hyperchloremic Acidosis During Therapy

Because of the considerable loss of keto acids in the urine during the initial phase of therapy, substrate for subsequent regeneration of bicarbonate is lost and correction of the total bicarbonate deficit is hampered. A portion of the bicarbonate deficit is replaced with chloride ions infused in large amounts as saline to correct the dehydration. In most patients, as the ketoacidosis clears during insulin replacement, a hyperchloremic, low-bicarbonate pattern emerges with a normal anion gap. This is a relatively benign condition that reverses itself over the subsequent 12–24 hours once intravenous saline is no longer being administered. Using a balanced electrolyte solution with a pH of 7.4 and 98 mEq/L chloride instead of normal saline (pH ~ 5.5; chloride 154 mEq/L) similar to serum in chloride concentration and pH during resuscitation instead of normal saline has been reported to prevent the hyperchloremic acidosis.

G. Treatment of Associated Infection

Antibiotics are prescribed as indicated (Table 30–5). Cholecystitis and pyelonephritis may be particularly severe in these patients.

H. Transition to Subcutaneous Insulin Regimen

Once the DKA is controlled and the patient is awake and able to eat, subcutaneous insulin therapy can be initiated. The patient with type 1 diabetes may have persistent significant tissue insulin resistance and may require a total daily insulin dose of approximately 0.6 unit/kg. The amount of insulin required in the previous 8 hours can also be helpful in estimating the initial insulin doses. Half the total daily dose can be given as a long-acting basal insulin and the other half as short-acting insulin premeals. The patient should receive subcutaneous basal insulin and rapid-acting insulin analog with the first meal and the insulin infusion discontinued an hour later. The overlap of the subcutaneous insulin action and insulin infusion is necessary to prevent relapse of the DKA. In patients with preexisting diabetes,

giving their basal insulin by subcutaneous injection at initiation of treatment simplifies the transition from intravenous to subcutaneous regimen. The increased insulin resistance is only present for a few days, and it is important to reduce both the basal and bolus insulins to avoid hypoglycemia. A patient with new-onset type 1 diabetes usually still has significant beta cell function and may not need any basal insulin and only very low doses of rapid-acting insulin before meals after recovery from the ketoacidosis. Patients with type 2 diabetes and DKA due to severe illness may initially require insulin therapy but can often transition back to oral agents during outpatient follow-up.

► Prognosis

Low-dose insulin infusion and fluid and electrolyte replacement combined with careful monitoring of patients' clinical and laboratory responses to therapy have dramatically reduced the mortality rates of DKA to less than 5%. However, this complication remains a significant risk in the aged who have mortality rates greater than 20% and in patients in profound coma in whom treatment has been delayed. Acute myocardial infarction and infarction of the bowel following prolonged hypotension worsen the outlook. A serious prognostic sign is end-stage chronic kidney disease, and prior kidney dysfunction worsens the prognosis considerably because the kidney plays a key role in compensating for massive pH and electrolyte abnormalities. Symptomatic cerebral edema occurs primarily in the pediatric population. Risk factors for its development include severe baseline acidosis, rapid correction of hyperglycemia, and excess volume administration in the first 4 hours. Onset of headache or deterioration in mental status during treatment should lead to consideration of this complication. Intravenous mannitol at a dosage of 1–2 g/kg given over 15 minutes is the mainstay of treatment. Excess crystalloid infusion can precipitate pulmonary edema. Acute respiratory distress syndrome is a rare complication of treatment of DKA.

After recovery and stabilization, patients should be instructed on how to recognize the early symptoms and signs of ketoacidosis. Urine ketones or capillary blood beta-hydroxybutyrate should be measured in patients with signs of infection or in insulin pump-treated patients when capillary blood glucose remains unexpectedly and persistently high. When heavy ketonuria and glycosuria persist on several successive examinations, supplemental rapid acting insulin should be administered and liquid foods such as lightly salted tomato juice and broth should be ingested to replenish fluids and electrolytes. The patient should be instructed to contact the clinician if ketonuria persists, and especially if there is vomiting and inability to keep down fluids. Recurrent episodes of severe ketoacidosis often indicate poor compliance with the insulin regimen, and these patients will require intensive counseling.

Savage MW et al. Joint British Diabetes Societies guideline for the management of diabetic ketoacidosis. Diabet Med. 2011 May;28(5):508–15. [PMID: 21255074]

HYPERGLYCEMIC HYPEROSMOLAR STATE

ESSENTIALS OF DIAGNOSIS

▶ Hyperglycemia greater than 600 mg/dL (33.3 mmol/L).

▶ Serum osmolality greater than 310 mOsm/kg.

▶ No acidosis; blood pH > 7.3.

▶ Serum bicarbonate greater than 15 mEq/L.

▶ Normal anion gap (less than 14 mEq/L).

▶ General Considerations

This second most common form of hyperglycemic coma is characterized by severe hyperglycemia in the absence of significant ketosis, with hyperosmolality and dehydration. It occurs in patients with mild or occult diabetes, and most patients are typically middle-aged to elderly. Accurate figures are not available as to its true incidence, but from data on hospital discharges it is rarer than DKA even in older age groups. Underlying chronic kidney disease or heart failure is common, and the presence of either worsens the prognosis. A precipitating event such as infection, myocardial infarction, stroke, or recent operation is often present. Certain medications such as phenytoin, diazoxide, corticosteroids, and diuretics have been implicated in its pathogenesis, as have procedures associated with glucose loading such as peritoneal dialysis.

▶ Pathogenesis

A partial or relative insulin deficiency may initiate the syndrome by reducing glucose utilization of muscle, fat, and liver while inducing hyperglucagonemia and increasing hepatic glucose output. With massive glycosuria, obligatory water loss ensues. If a patient is unable to maintain adequate fluid intake because of an associated acute or chronic illness or has suffered excessive fluid loss, marked dehydration results. As the plasma volume contracts, kidney function becomes impaired, limiting the urinary glucose losses and exacerbating the hyperglycemia. Severe hyperosmolality develops that causes mental confusion and finally coma. It is not clear why ketosis is virtually absent under these conditions of insulin insufficiency, although reduced levels of growth hormone may be a factor, along with portal vein insulin concentrations sufficient to restrain ketogenesis.

▶ Clinical Findings

A. Symptoms and Signs

Onset may be insidious over a period of days or weeks, with weakness, polyuria, and polydipsia. The lack of features of ketoacidosis may retard recognition of the syndrome and delay therapy until dehydration becomes more profound than in ketoacidosis. Reduced intake of fluid is not an uncommon historical feature, due to either inappropriate lack of thirst, nausea, or inaccessibility of fluids to elderly, bedridden patients. A history of ingestion of large quantities of glucose-containing fluids, such as soft drinks or orange juice, can occasionally be obtained. Lethargy and confusion develop as serum osmolality exceeds 310 mOsm/kg, and convulsions and coma can occur if osmolality exceeds 320–330 mOsm/kg. Physical examination confirms the presence of profound dehydration in a lethargic or comatose patient without Kussmaul respirations.

B. Laboratory Findings

Severe hyperglycemia is present, with blood glucose values ranging from 800 mg/dL to 2400 mg/dL (44.4 mmol/L to 133.2 mmol/L) (Table 27–12). In mild cases, where dehydration is less severe, dilutional hyponatremia as well as urinary sodium losses may reduce serum sodium to 120–125 mEq/L, which protects to some extent against extreme hyperosmolality. However, as dehydration progresses, serum sodium can exceed 140 mEq/L, producing serum osmolality readings of 330–440 mOsm/kg. Ketosis and acidosis are usually absent or mild. Prerenal azotemia is the rule, with serum urea nitrogen elevations over 100 mg/dL (35.7 mmol/L) being typical.

▶ Treatment

A. Fluid Replacement

Fluid replacement is of paramount importance in treating nonketotic hyperglycemic coma. The onset of hyperosmolarity is more insidious in elderly people without ketosis than in younger individuals with high serum ketone levels, which provide earlier indicators of severe illness (vomiting, rapid deep breathing, acetone odor, etc). Consequently, diagnosis and treatment are often delayed until fluid deficit has reached levels of 6–10 L.

If hypovolemia is present as evidenced by hypotension and oliguria, fluid therapy should be initiated with 0.9% saline. In all other cases, 0.45% saline appears to be preferable as the initial replacement solution because the body fluids of these patients are markedly hyperosmolar. As much as 4–6 L of fluid may be required in the first 8–10 hours. Careful monitoring of the patient is required for proper sodium and water replacement. An important end point of fluid therapy is to restore urinary output to 50 mL/h or more. Once blood glucose reaches 250 mg/dL (13.9 mmol/L), fluid replacement should include 5% dextrose in either water, 0.45% saline solution, or 0.9% saline solution. The rate of dextrose infusion should be adjusted to maintain glycemic levels of 250–300 mg/dL (13.9–16.7 mmol/L) in order to reduce the risk of cerebral edema.

B. Insulin

Less insulin may be required to reduce the hyperglycemia in nonketotic patients as compared to those with diabetic ketoacidotic coma. In fact, fluid replacement alone can reduce hyperglycemia considerably by correcting the hypovolemia, which then increases both glomerular filtration and renal excretion of glucose. Insulin treatment should therefore be delayed unless the patient has significant ketonemia (beta-hydroxybutyrate more than 1 mmol/L). Start the insulin infusion rate at 0.05 unit/kg/h (bolus is not needed) and titrate to lower blood glucose levels by 50–70 mg/dL per hour (2.8–3.9 mmol/L/h). Once the patient has stabilized and the blood glucose falls to around 250 mg/dL (13.9 mmol/L), insulin can be given subcutaneously.

C. Potassium

With the absence of acidosis, there may be no initial hyperkalemia unless associated end-stage chronic kidney disease is present. This results in less severe total potassium depletion than in DKA, and less potassium replacement is therefore needed. However, because initial serum potassium is usually not elevated and because it declines rapidly as a result of insulin's effect on driving potassium intracellularly, it is recommended that potassium replacement be initiated earlier than in ketotic patients, assuming that no chronic kidney disease or oliguria is present. Potassium chloride (10 mEq/L) can be added to the initial bottle of fluids administered if the patient's serum potassium is not elevated.

D. Phosphate

If severe hypophosphatemia (serum phosphate less than 1 mg/dL [0.32 mmol/L]) develops during insulin therapy, phosphate replacement can be given as described for ketoacidotic patients (at 3 mmol/h).

► Prognosis

The severe dehydration and low output state may predispose the patient to complications such as myocardial infarction, stroke, pulmonary embolism, mesenteric vein thrombosis, and disseminated intravascular coagulation. Fluid replacement remains the primary approach to the prevention of these complications. Low-dose heparin prophylaxis is reasonable but benefits of routine anticoagulation remain doubtful. Rhabdomyolysis is a recognized complication and should be looked for and treated.

The overall mortality rate of hyperglycemic hyperosmolar state coma is more than ten times that of DKA, chiefly because of its higher incidence in older patients, who may have compromised cardiovascular systems or associated major illnesses and whose dehydration is often excessive because of delays in recognition and treatment. (When patients are matched for age, the prognoses of these two hyperglycemic emergencies are reasonably comparable.) When prompt therapy is instituted, the mortality rate can be reduced from nearly 50% to that related to the severity of coexistent disorders.

After the patient is stabilized, the appropriate form of long-term management of the diabetes must be determined. Insulin treatment should be continued for a few weeks but patients usually recover sufficient endogenous insulin secretion to make a trial of diet or diet plus oral agents worthwhile. When the episode occurs in a patient who has known diabetes, then education of the patient and caregivers should be instituted. They should be taught how to recognize situations (nausea and vomiting, infection) that predispose to recurrence of the hyperglycemic, hyperosmolar state, as well as detailed information on how to prevent the escalating dehydration that culminates in hyperosmolar coma (small sips of sugar-free liquids, increase in usual hypoglycemic therapy, or early contact with the clinician).

Fayfman M et al. Management of hyperglycemic crises: diabetic ketoacidosis and hyperglycemic hyperosmolar state. Med Clin North Am. 2017 May;101(3):587–606. [PMID: 28372715]

Scott AR; Joint British Diabetes Societies (JBDS) for Inpatient Care; JBDS hyperosmolar hyperglycaemic guidelines group. Management of hyperosmolar hyperglycaemic state in adults with diabetes. Diabet Med. 2015 Jun;32(6):714–24. [PMID: 25980647]

LACTIC ACIDOSIS

ESSENTIALS OF DIAGNOSIS

► Severe metabolic acidosis with compensatory hyperventilation.

► Blood pH < 7.30.

► Serum bicarbonate less than 15 mEq/L.

► Anion gap greater than 15 mEq/L.

► Absent serum ketones.

► Serum lactate greater than 5 mmol/L.

► General Considerations

Lactic acidosis is characterized by accumulation of excess lactic acid in the blood. Normally, the principal sources of this acid are the erythrocytes (which lack enzymes for aerobic oxidation), skeletal muscle, skin, and brain. Conversion of lactic acid to glucose and its oxidation principally by the liver but also by the kidneys represent the chief pathways for its removal. Hyperlactatemia and acidosis occur when lactate production exceeds lactate consumption. Causes include tissue hypoxia (global or local), disorders that increase epinephrine levels (severe asthma with excess beta-adrenergic agonist use, cardiogenic or hemorrhagic shock, pheochromocytoma), and drugs that impair oxidative phosphorylation (antiretroviral agents and propofol). Most cases of metformin-associated lactic acidosis occur in patients in whom there were contraindications to the use of metformin, in particular kidney failure. Metformin levels are usually greater than 5 mcg/L when metformin is implicated as the cause of lactic acidosis. Other causes of lactic acidosis include several inborn errors of metabolism and the MELAS syndrome (mitochondrial encephalopathy, lactic acidosis, and stroke-like episodes). D-lactic acidosis can occur in patients with short bowel syndrome when unabsorbed carbohydrates are presented as substrate for fermentation by colonic bacteria.

Clinical Findings

A. Symptoms and Signs

The main clinical feature of lactic acidosis is marked hyperventilation. When lactic acidosis is secondary to tissue hypoxia or vascular collapse, the clinical presentation is variable, being that of the prevailing catastrophic illness. However, in the idiopathic, or spontaneous, variety, the onset is rapid (usually over a few hours), blood pressure is normal, peripheral circulation is good, and there is no cyanosis.

B. Laboratory Findings

Plasma bicarbonate and blood pH are quite low, indicating the presence of severe metabolic acidosis. Ketones are usually absent from plasma and urine or at least not prominent. The first clue may be a high anion gap (serum sodium minus the sum of chloride and bicarbonate anions [in mEq/L] should be no greater than 15). A higher value indicates the existence of an abnormal compartment of anions. If this cannot be clinically explained by an excess of keto acids (diabetes), inorganic acids (uremia), or anions from medication overdosage (salicylates, methyl alcohol, ethylene glycol), then lactic acidosis is probably the correct diagnosis. (See also Chapter 21.) In the absence of azotemia, hyperphosphatemia may be a clue to the presence of lactic acidosis for reasons that are not clear. The diagnosis is confirmed by a plasma lactic acid concentration of 5 mmol/L or higher (values as high as 30 mmol/L have been reported). Normal plasma values average 1 mmol/L, with a normal lactate/pyruvate ratio of 10:1. This ratio is greatly exceeded in lactic acidosis.[1]

Treatment

Aggressive treatment of the precipitating cause of lactic acidosis is the main component of therapy, such as ensuring adequate oxygenation and vascular perfusion of tissues. Empiric antibiotic coverage for sepsis should be given after culture samples are obtained in any patient in whom the cause of the lactic acidosis is not apparent (Table 30–5).

Alkalinization with intravenous sodium bicarbonate to keep the pH above 7.2 has been recommended by some in the emergency treatment of lactic acidosis; as much as 2000 mEq in 24 hours has been used. However, there is no evidence that the mortality rate is favorably affected by administering bicarbonate, and its use remains controversial. Hemodialysis may be useful in cases where large sodium loads are poorly tolerated and in cases associated with metformin toxicity.

Prognosis

The mortality rate of spontaneous lactic acidosis is high. The prognosis in most cases is that of the primary disorder that produced the lactic acidosis.

DeFronzo R et al. Metformin-associated lactic acidosis: current perspectives on causes and risk. Metabolism. 2016 Feb; 65(2):20–9. [PMID: 26773926]

THE HYPOGLYCEMIC STATES

Spontaneous hypoglycemia in adults is of two principal types: fasting and postprandial. Symptoms begin at plasma glucose levels in the range of 60 mg/dL (3.3 mmol/L) and impairment of brain function at approximately 50 mg/dL (2.8 mmol/L). Fasting hypoglycemia is often subacute or chronic and usually presents with neuroglycopenia as its principal manifestation; postprandial hypoglycemia is relatively acute and is often heralded by symptoms of neurogenic autonomic discharge (sweating, palpitations, anxiety, tremulousness).

Differential Diagnosis (Table 27–13)

Fasting hypoglycemia may occur in certain endocrine disorders, such as hypopituitarism, Addison disease, or myxedema; in disorders related to liver malfunction, such as acute alcoholism or liver failure; and in instances of end-stage chronic kidney disease, particularly in patients requiring dialysis. These conditions are usually obvious, with hypoglycemia being only a secondary feature. When fasting hypoglycemia is a primary manifestation developing in adults without apparent endocrine disorders or inborn metabolic diseases from childhood, the principal diagnostic possibilities include (1) hyperinsulinism, due to either pancreatic B cell tumors, iatrogenic or surreptitious administration of insulin or sulfonylurea; and (2) hypoglycemia due to extrapancreatic tumors.

Postprandial (reactive) hypoglycemia may be seen after gastrointestinal surgery and is particularly associated with the dumping syndrome after gastrectomy and Roux-en-Y gastric bypass surgery. Occult diabetes very occasionally presents with postprandial hypoglycemia. Rarely, it occurs

Table 27–13. Common causes of hypoglycemia in adults.[1]

Fasting hypoglycemia
Pancreatic B cell tumor
Surreptitious administration of insulin or sulfonylureas
Extrapancreatic tumors
Postprandial hypoglycemia
Alimentary
Noninsulinoma pancreatogenous hypoglycemia syndrome
Functional
Occult diabetes mellitus
Alcohol-related hypoglycemia
Immunopathologic hypoglycemia
Idiopathic anti-insulin antibodies (which release their bound insulin)
Antibodies to insulin receptors (which act as agonists)
Drug-induced hypoglycemia

[1]In the absence of clinically obvious endocrine, kidney, or liver disorders and exclusive of diabetes mellitus treated with hypoglycemic agents.

---

[1]In collecting samples, it is essential to rapidly chill and separate the blood in order to remove red cells, whose continued glycolysis at room temperature is a common source of error in reports of high plasma lactate. Frozen plasma remains stable for subsequent assay.

with islet cell hyperplasia—the so-called noninsulinoma pancreatogenous hypoglycemia syndrome.

Alcohol-related hypoglycemia is due to hepatic glycogen depletion combined with alcohol-mediated inhibition of gluconeogenesis. It is most common in malnourished individuals with excessive alcohol intake but can occur in anyone who is unable to ingest food after an acute alcoholic episode followed by gastritis and vomiting.

Immunopathologic hypoglycemia is an extremely rare condition in which anti-insulin antibodies or antibodies to insulin receptors develop spontaneously.

HYPOGLYCEMIA DUE TO PANCREATIC B CELL TUMORS

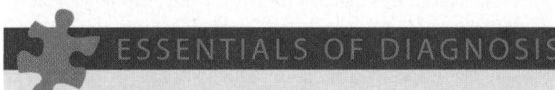

ESSENTIALS OF DIAGNOSIS

▶ Hypoglycemic symptoms—often neuroglycopenic (confusion, blurred vision, anxiety, convulsions).

▶ Immediate recovery upon administration of glucose.

▶ Blood glucose less than 45 mg/dL (2.5 mmol/L) with a serum insulin level of 6 microunits/mL or more.

▶ General Considerations

Fasting hypoglycemia in an otherwise healthy, well-nourished adult is rare and is most commonly due to an adenoma of the islets of Langerhans. Ninety percent of such tumors are single and benign, but multiple adenomas can occur as well as malignant tumors with functional metastases. Adenomas may be familial, and multiple adenomas have been found in conjunction with tumors of the parathyroids and pituitary (MEN type 1 [MEN 1]). It has been reported that about 30% of sporadic insulinoma tumors have a somatic mutation in the YY1 gene (T372R) that encodes the transcriptional repressor YY1. Over 99% of insulinomas are located within the pancreas and less than 1% in ectopic pancreatic tissue.

▶ Clinical Findings

A. Symptoms and Signs

The most important prerequisite to diagnosing an insulinoma is simply to consider it, particularly in relatively healthy-appearing persons who have fasting hypoglycemia associated with some degree of central nervous system dysfunction such as confusion or abnormal behavior. A delay in diagnosis can result in unnecessary treatment for psychomotor epilepsy or psychiatric disorders and may cause irreversible brain damage. In long-standing cases, obesity can result as a consequence of overeating to relieve symptoms.

The so-called Whipple triad is characteristic of hypoglycemia regardless of the cause. It consists of (1) a history of hypoglycemic symptoms, (2) an associated low plasma glucose level (40–50 mg/dL), and (3) relief of symptoms upon ingesting fast-acting carbohydrates in approximately 15 minutes. The hypoglycemic symptoms in insulinoma often develop in the early morning or after missing a meal. Occasionally, they occur after exercise.

Patients typically complain of neuroglycopenic symptoms such as blurred vision or diplopia, headache, feelings of detachment, slurred speech, and weakness. Personality and mental changes vary from anxiety to psychotic behavior, and neurologic deterioration can result in convulsions or coma. Hypoglycemic unawareness is very common and adrenergic symptoms of palpitations and sweating may be blunted. With the ready availability of home blood glucose–monitoring systems, patients sometimes present with documented fingerstick blood glucose levels in 40s and 50s at time of symptoms. Access to diabetic medications (sulfonylureas or insulin) should be explored—does a family member have diabetes, or does the patient or family member work in the medical field? Medication-dispensing errors should be excluded—has the patient's prescription medication changed in shape or color? Patients with insulinoma or factitious hypoglycemia usually have a normal physical examination.

B. Laboratory Findings

B cell adenomas do not reduce secretion of insulin in the presence of hypoglycemia, and the critical diagnostic test is to demonstrate inappropriately elevated serum insulin, proinsulin, and C-peptide levels, at a time when plasma glucose level is below 45 mg/dL.

The diagnostic criteria for insulinoma after a 72-hour fast are listed in Table 27–14. Other causes of hyperinsulinemic hypoglycemia include factitious administration of insulin or sulfonylureas. Factitious use of insulin will result in suppression of endogenous insulin secretion and low C-peptide levels. In patients who have injected insulin, the insulin/C-peptide ratio (pmol/L) will be greater than 1. An elevated circulating proinsulin level in the presence of fasting hypoglycemia is characteristic of most B cell adenomas

Table 27–14. Diagnostic criteria for insulinoma after a 72-hour fast.

Laboratory Test	Result
Plasma glucose	< 45 mg/dL (2.5 mmol/L)
Plasma insulin (RIA)[1]	≥ 6 microunits/mL (36 pmol/L)
Plasma insulin (ICMA)[1]	≥ 3 microunits/mL (18 pmol/L)
Plasma C-peptide	≥ 200 pmol/L (0.2 nmol/L, 0.6 ng/mL)
Plasma proinsulin	≥ 5 pmol/L
Beta-hydroxybutyrate	≤ 2.7 mmol/L
Sulfonylurea screen (including repaglinide and nateglinide)	Negative

[1]Conversion factors: insulin microunit/mL × 6.0 = pmol/L; C-peptide ng/mL × 0.333 = nmol/L

ICMA, immunochemiluminometric assays; RIA, radioimmunoassay.

and does not occur in factitious hyperinsulinism. Thus, C-peptide levels (by immunochemiluminometric assays [ICMA]) of greater than 200 pmol/L and proinsulin levels (by radioimmunoassay [RIA]) of greater than 5 pmol/L are characteristic of insulinomas. In patients with insulinoma, plasma beta-hydroxybutyrate levels are suppressed to 2.7 mmol/L or less. No single hormone measurement (insulin, proinsulin, C-peptide) is 100% sensitive and specific for the diagnosis of insulinoma, and insulinoma cases have been reported with insulin levels below 3 microunits/mL (ICMA assay) or proinsulin level below 5 pmol/L. These hormonal assays are also not standardized between laboratories, and there can be significant variation in the results. Therefore, the diagnosis should be based on multiple biochemical parameters.

In patients with epigastric distress, a history of renal calculi, or menstrual or erectile dysfunction, a serum calcium, gastrin, or prolactin level may be useful in screening for MEN 1 associated with insulinoma.

C. Diagnostic Tests

If the history is consistent with episodic spontaneous hypoglycemia, patients should be given a home blood glucose monitor and advised to monitor blood glucose levels at the time of symptoms and before consumption of carbohydrates, if this can be done safely. Patients with insulinomas frequently report fingerstick blood glucose levels between 40 mg/dL (2.2 mmol/L) and 50 mg/dL (2.8 mmol/L) at the time of symptoms. The diagnosis, however, cannot be made based on a fingerstick blood glucose. It is necessary to have a low laboratory glucose concomitantly with elevated plasma insulin, proinsulin, and C-peptide levels and a negative sulfonylurea screen. When patients give a history of symptoms after only a short period of food withdrawal or with exercise, then an outpatient assessment can be attempted. The patient should be brought by a family member to the office after an overnight fast and observed in the office. Activity such as walking should be encouraged and fingerstick blood glucose measured repeatedly during observation. If symptoms occur or fingerstick blood glucose is below 50 mg/dL (2.8 mmol/L) then samples for plasma glucose, insulin, C-peptide, proinsulin, sulfonylurea screen, serum ketones, and antibodies to insulin should be sent. If outpatient observation does not result in symptoms or hypoglycemia and if the clinical suspicion remains high, then the patient should undergo an inpatient supervised 72-hour fast. A suggested protocol for the supervised fast is shown in Table 27–15.

In 30% of patients with insulinoma, the blood glucose levels often drop below 45 mg/dL (2.5 mmol/L) after an overnight fast, but some patients require up to 72 hours to develop symptomatic hypoglycemia. However, the term "72-hour fast" is actually a misnomer in most cases since the fast should be immediately terminated as soon as symptoms appear and laboratory confirmation of hypoglycemia is available. In normal male subjects, the blood glucose does not fall below 55–60 mg/dL (3.1–3.3 mmol/L) during a 3-day fast. In contrast, in normal premenopausal women who have fasted for only 24 hours, the plasma glucose may fall normally to such an extent that it can reach

Table 27–15. Suggested hospital protocol for supervised fast in diagnosis of insulinoma.

(1) Place intravenous cannula and obtain baseline plasma glucose, insulin, proinsulin, beta-hydroxybutyrate, and C-peptide measurements at onset of fast.

(2) Permit only calorie-free and caffeine-free fluids and encourage supervised activity (such as walking).

(3) Obtain fingerstick glucose measurements every 4 hours until values < 60 mg/dL are obtained. Then increase the frequency of fingersticks to each hour, and when capillary glucose value is < 45 mg/dL send a venous blood sample to the laboratory for plasma glucose.[1] Check frequently for manifestations of neuroglycopenia.

(4) At 48 hours into the fast, send venous blood sample for plasma glucose, insulin, proinsulin, C-peptide, beta-hydroxybutyrate, and sulfonylurea measurement.

(5) If symptoms of hypoglycemia occur **or** if a laboratory value of serum glucose is < 45 mg/dL, or if 72 hours have elapsed, then conclude the fast with a final blood sample for plasma glucose,[1] insulin, proinsulin, C-peptide, beta-hydroxybutyrate, and sulfonylurea measurements. Then give oral fast-acting carbohydrate followed by a meal. If the patient is confused or unable to take oral agents, then administer 50 mL of 50% dextrose intravenously over 3 to 5 minutes. Do not conclude a fast based simply on a capillary blood glucose measurement—wait for the laboratory glucose value—unless the patient is very symptomatic and it would be dangerous to wait.

[1]Glucose sample should be collected in sodium fluoride containing tube on ice to prevent glycolysis and the plasma separated immediately upon receipt at the laboratory. Arrange for the laboratory to run the glucose samples "stat."

values as low as 35 mg/dL (1.9 mmol/L). In these cases, however, the women are not symptomatic, presumably owing to the development of sufficient ketonemia to supply energy needs to the brain. Insulinoma patients, on the other hand, become symptomatic when plasma glucose drops to subnormal levels, since inappropriate insulin secretion restricts ketone formation. Moreover, the demonstration of a nonsuppressed insulin level of 3 microunits/mL or more using a ICMA assay (greater than 6 microunits/mL using an RIA assay) in the presence of hypoglycemia suggests the diagnosis of insulinoma. If hypoglycemia does not develop in a male patient after fasting for up to 72 hours—and particularly when this prolonged fast is terminated with a period of moderate exercise—insulinoma must be considered an unlikely diagnosis.

Stimulation with pancreatic B cell secretagogues such as tolbutamide, glucagon, or leucine has been devised to demonstrate exaggerated and prolonged insulin secretion in the presence of insulinomas. However, because insulin-secreting tumors have a wide range of granule content and degrees of differentiation, they are variably responsive to these secretagogues; and a negative response does not necessarily rule out an insulinoma. For these reasons, stimulation tests are not recommended in the diagnostic workup of insulinoma.

An oral glucose tolerance test is of no value in the diagnosis of insulin-secreting tumors. HbA_{1c} levels may be low but there is considerable overlap with normal patients and no particular value is diagnostic.

D. Preoperative Localization of B Cell Tumors

After the diagnosis of insulinoma has been unequivocally made by clinical and laboratory findings, studies to localize the tumor should be initiated. The focus of attention should be directed to the pancreas since that is where virtually all insulinomas originate. Ectopic cases are very rare.

Because of the small size of these tumors (averaging 1.5 cm in diameter in one large series), imaging studies do not necessarily identify all of them. A pancreatic dual phase helical CT scan with thin section can identify 82–94% of the lesions. MRI scans with gadolinium can be helpful in detecting a tumor in 85% of cases. One case report suggests that diffusion-weighted MRI can be useful for detecting and localizing small insulinomas, especially for those with no hypervascular pattern. ^{111}In-octreotide scans for insulinomas, which typically express somatostatin receptor type 3, are positive in only 50–70% of cases. Newer PET/CT scans, using gallium-labeled somatostatin analogs such as DOTA-1-NaI3-octreotide (DOTA-NOC), which have a higher affinity for somatostatin receptor subtypes 2, 3, and 5, have been reported to be useful in localizing the tumors. Insulinomas express GLP-1 receptors, and radiolabeled GLP-1 receptor agonists such as Lys(40)(Ahx-hydrazinonicotinamide [HYNIC]-[(99m)Tc]NH(2)]-exendin-4 for SPECT/CT have also been reported to visualize the tumors. The imaging study used will depend on local availability and local radiologic skill. If the imaging study is normal, then an endoscopic ultrasound should be performed. In experienced hands, about 80–90% of tumors can be detected with this procedure. Fine-needle aspiration of the identified lesion can be attempted to confirm the presence of a neuroendocrine tumor. If the tumor is not identified or the imaging result is equivocal, then the patient should undergo selective calcium-stimulated angiography, which has been reported to localize the tumor to a particular region of the pancreas approximately 90% of the time. In this test, angiography is combined with injections of calcium gluconate into the gastroduodenal, splenic, and superior mesenteric arteries, and insulin levels are measured in the hepatic vein effluent. The procedure is performed after an overnight fast. Calcium gluconate 10% solution diluted to a volume of 5 mL with 0.95% saline is bolused into the selected artery at a dose of 0.0125 mmol calcium/kg (0.005 mmol calcium/kg for obese patients). Small samples of blood (5 mL) are taken from the hepatic effluent at times 0, 30, 60, 90, 120, and 180 seconds after the calcium injection. Fingerstick blood glucose levels are measured at intervals and a dextrose infusion is maintained throughout the procedure to prevent hypoglycemia. Calcium stimulates insulin release from insulinomas but not normal islets, and so a step-up from baseline in insulin levels at 30 or 60 seconds (twofold or greater) regionalizes the source of the hyperinsulinism to the head of the pancreas for the gastroduodenal artery, the uncinate process for the superior mesenteric artery, and the body and tail of the pancreas for the splenic artery calcium infusions. A less than twofold elevation of insulin in the 120-second sample may represent effects of recirculating calcium and is not considered a positive localization. In a single insulinoma, the response is in one artery alone unless the tumor resides in an area fed by two arteries or if there are multiple insulinomas (eg, in MEN 1).

Patients who have diffuse islet hyperplasia (the noninsulinoma pancreatogenous hypoglycemia syndrome) will have positive responses in multiple arteries. Because diazoxide may interfere with this test, it should be discontinued for at least 48–72 hours before sampling. Patients should be closely monitored during the procedure to avoid hypoglycemia (as well as hyperglycemia, which could affect insulin gradients). These studies combined with careful intraoperative ultrasonography and palpation by a surgeon experienced in insulinoma surgery identifies up to 98% of tumors.

▶ Treatment

The treatment of choice for insulin-secreting tumors is surgical resection. While waiting for surgery, patients should be given oral diazoxide. Divided doses of 300–400 mg/day usually suffice, although an occasional patient may require up to 800 mg/day. Side effects include edema due to sodium retention, gastric irritation, and mild hirsutism. Hydrochlorothiazide, 25–50 mg daily, can be used to counteract the sodium retention and edema as well potentiate diazoxide's hyperglycemic effect.

In patients with a single benign pancreatic B cell adenoma, 90–95% have a successful cure at the first surgical attempt when intraoperative ultrasound is used by a skilled surgeon. Diazoxide should be administered on the day of the surgery because it reduces the risk of hypoglycemia during surgery. Typically, it does not mask the glycemic rise indicative of surgical cure. Blood glucose should be monitored throughout surgery, and 5% or 10% dextrose infusion should be used to maintain euglycemia. In cases where the diagnosis has been established but no adenoma is located after careful palpation and use of intraoperative ultrasound, it is no longer advisable to blindly resect the body and tail of the pancreas, since a nonpalpable tumor missed by ultrasound is most likely embedded within the fleshy head of the pancreas that is left behind with subtotal resections. Most surgeons prefer to close the incision and schedule a selective arterial calcium stimulation with hepatic venous sampling to locate the tumor site prior to a repeat operation. Laparoscopy using ultrasound and enucleation has been successful with a single tumor of the body or tail of the pancreas, but open surgery remains necessary for tumors in the head of the pancreas.

In patients with inoperable functioning islet cell carcinoma with and without hepatic metastasis and in approximately 5–10% of MEN 1 cases when subtotal removal of the pancreas has failed to produce cure, the treatment approach is the same as for other types of pancreatic neuroendocrine tumors (pNETs). Diazoxide is the treatment of choice in preventing hypoglycemia. Frequent carbohydrate feedings (every 2–3 hours) can also be helpful, although weight gain can become a problem. Somatostatin analogs, octreotide or lanreotide, should be considered if diazoxide is ineffective or if there is tumor progression. Surgery or embolization (bland, chemo- and radio-) or thermal ablation (radiofrequency, microwave, and cryoablation) can be used to reduce tumor burden and also provide symptomatic relief. Chemotherapy regimens that can be considered include combination of streptozocin, 5–fluorouracil, and doxorubicin; capecitabine and oxaliplatin;

and capecitabine and temozolomide. Targeted therapies against multiple steps in PI3K/AKT/mTor pathway have been shown to be helpful. Everolimus, an inhibitor of mTor, is approved for treatment of advanced pNETs. Sunitinib, a monoclonal antibody against VEGF receptors 2 and 3, PDGFR alpha and beta, and c-kit, has been shown to slow growth of pNETs. Treatment with radioisotopes (indium-111 or yttrium-90 or lutetium-177) linked to a somatostatin analog have been reported to show benefit in a proportion of patients.

Cryer PE et al. Evaluation and management of adult hypoglyce-mic disorders: an Endocrine Society Clinical Practice Guideline. J Clin Endocrinol Metab. 2009 Mar;94(3):709–28. [PMID: 19088155]

Mathur A et al. Insulinoma. Surg Clin North Am. 2009 Oct; 89(5):1105–21. [PMID: 19836487]

NONISLET CELL TUMOR HYPOGLYCEMIA

These rare causes of hypoglycemia include mesenchymal tumors such as retroperitoneal sarcomas, hepatocellular carcinomas, adrenocortical carcinomas, and miscellaneous epithelial-type tumors. The tumors are frequently large and readily palpated or visualized on CT scans or MRI.

In many cases the hypoglycemia is due to the expression and release of an incompletely processed insulin-like growth factor 2 (IGF-2) by the tumor.

The diagnosis is supported by laboratory documentation of serum insulin levels below 5 microunit/mL with plasma glucose levels of 45 mg/dL (2.5 mmol/L) or lower. Values for growth hormone and IGF-1 are also decreased. Levels of IGF-2 may be increased but often are "normal" in quantity, despite the presence of the immature, higher-molecular-weight form of IGF-2, which can be detected only by special laboratory techniques.

Not all the patients with nonislet cell tumor hypoglyce-mia have elevated pro-IGF-2. Ectopic insulin production has been described in bronchial carcinoma, ovarian carcinoma, and small cell carcinoma of the cervix. Hypoglycemia due to IGF-1 released from a metastatic large cell carcinoma of the lung has also been reported. GLP-1–secreting tumors (ovarian and pNETs) can also cause hypoglycemia by stimulating insulin release from normal pancreatic islets.

The prognosis for these tumors is generally poor, and surgical removal should be attempted when feasible. Dietary management of the hypoglycemia is the mainstay of medical treatment, since diazoxide is usually ineffective.

Bodnar TW et al. Management of non-islet-cell tumor hypogly-cemia: a clinical review. J Clin Endocrinol Metab. 2014 Mar; 99(3):713–22. [PMID: 24423303]

POSTPRANDIAL HYPOGLYCEMIA

1. Hypoglycemia Following Gastric Surgery

Hypoglycemia sometimes develops in patients who have undergone gastric surgery (eg, gastrectomy, vagotomy, pyloroplasty, gastrojejunostomy, Nissan fundoplication,

Billroth II procedure, and Roux-en-Y), especially when they consume foods containing high levels of readily absorbable carbohydrates. This late dumping syndrome occurs about 1–3 hours after a meal and is a result of rapid delivery of high concentration of carbohydrates in the proximal small bowel and rapid absorption of glucose. The hyperinsulinemic response to the high carbohydrate load causes hypoglycemia. Excessive release of gastrointestinal hormones such as GLP-1 likely play a role in the hyperin-sulinemic response. The symptoms include lightheaded-ness, sweating, confusion and even loss of consciousness after eating a high carbohydrate meal. To document hypo-glycemia, the patient should consume a meal that leads to symptoms during everyday life. An oral glucose tolerance test is not recommended because many normal persons have false-positive test results. There have been case reports of insulinoma and noninsulinoma pancreatoge-nous hypoglycemia syndrome in patients with hypoglyce-mia post Roux-en-Y surgery. It is unclear how often this occurs. A careful history may identify patients who have a history of hypoglycemia with exercise or missed meals, and these individuals may require a formal 72-hour fast to rule out an insulinoma.

Treatment for secondary dumping includes dietary mod-ification, but this may be difficult to sustain. Patients can try more frequent meals with smaller portions of less rapidly digested carbohydrates. Alpha-glucosidase therapy may be a useful adjunct to a low carbohydrate diet. Octreotide 50 mcg administered subcutaneously two or three times a day 30 minutes prior to each meal has been reported to improve symptoms due to late dumping syndrome. Treatment with exendin 9-39, a GLP-1 receptor agonist, may prevent post gastric bypass hypoglycemia. Various surgical procedures to delay gastric emptying have been reported to improve symp-toms but long-term efficacy studies are lacking.

2. Functional Alimentary Hypoglycemia

Patients have symptoms suggestive of increased sympa-thetic activity, including anxiety, weakness, tremor, sweat-ing or palpitations after meals. Physical examination and laboratory tests are normal. It is not recommended that patients with symptoms suggestive of increased sympa-thetic activity undergo either a prolonged oral glucose tol-erance test or a mixed meal test. Instead, the patients should be given home blood glucose monitors (with memories) and instructed to monitor fingerstick glucose levels at the time of symptoms. Only patients who have symptoms when their fingerstick blood glucose is low (less than 50 mg/dL) and who have resolution of symptoms when the glucose is raised by eating rapidly released carbo-hydrate need additional evaluation. Patients who do not have evidence for low glucose levels at time of symptoms are generally reassured by their findings. Counseling and support should be the mainstays in therapy, with dietary manipulation only an adjunct.

3. Occult Diabetes

This condition is characterized by a delay in early insulin release from pancreatic B cells, resulting in initial exaggeration of hyperglycemia during a glucose tolerance test. In response to this hyperglycemia, an exaggerated insulin release produces a late hypoglycemia 4–5 hours after ingestion of glucose. These patients are often obese and frequently have a family history of diabetes mellitus.

Patients with this type of postprandial hypoglycemia often respond to reduced intake of refined sugars with multiple, spaced, small feedings high in dietary fiber. In the obese, treatment is directed at weight reduction to achieve ideal weight. These patients should be considered to have prediabetes or early diabetes (type 1 or 2) and advised to have periodic medical evaluations.

4. Autoimmune Hypoglycemia

Patients with autoimmune hypoglycemia have early postprandial hyperglycemia followed by hypoglycemia 3–4 hours later. The hypoglycemia is attributed to a dissociation of insulin-antibody immune complexes, releasing free insulin.

The disorder is associated with methimazole treatment for Graves disease, although it can also occur in patients treated with various other sulfhydryl-containing medications (captopril, penicillamine) as well as other drugs such as hydralazine, isoniazid, and procainamide. In addition, it has been reported in patients with autoimmune disorders such as rheumatoid arthritis, systemic lupus erythematosus, and polymyositis as well as in plasma cell myeloma (formerly multiple myeloma) and other plasma cell dyscrasias where paraproteins or antibodies cross-react with insulin. There is also an association with the HLA class II alleles (DRB1*0406, DQA1*0301, and DQB1*0302). These alleles are 10 to 20 times more common in Japanese and Korean populations, which explains why the disorder has been reported mostly in Japanese patients.

High titers of insulin autoantibodies, usually IgG class, can be detected. Insulin, proinsulin, and C-peptide levels may be elevated, but the results may be erroneous because of the interference of the insulin antibodies with the immunoassays for these peptides.

In most cases, the hypoglycemia is transient and usually resolves spontaneously within 3–6 months of diagnosis, particularly when the offending medications are stopped. The most consistent therapeutic benefit in management of this syndrome has been achieved by dietary treatment with small, frequent low-carbohydrate meals. Prednisone (30–60 mg orally daily) has been used to lower the titer of insulin antibodies.

Lupsa BC et al. Autoimmune forms of hypoglycemia. Medicine (Baltimore). 2009 May;88(3):141–53. [PMID: 19440117]

FACTITIOUS HYPOGLYCEMIA

Factitious hypoglycemia may be difficult to document. A suspicion of self-induced hypoglycemia is supported when the patient is associated with the health professions or has access to insulin or sulfonylurea medications taken by a diabetic member of the family. The triad of hypoglycemia, high immunoreactive insulin, and suppressed plasma C-peptide immunoreactivity is pathognomonic of exogenous insulin administration. Insulin and C-peptide are secreted in a 1:1 molar ratio. A large fraction of the endogenous insulin is cleared by the liver, whereas C-peptide, which is cleared by the kidney, has a lower metabolic clearance rate. For this reason, the molar ratio of insulin and C-peptide in a hypoglycemic patient should be less than 1.0 in cases of insulinoma and is greater than 1.0 in cases of exogenous insulin administration. When sulfonylureas, repaglinide, and nateglinide are suspected as a cause of factitious hypoglycemia, a plasma level of these medications to detect their presence may be required to distinguish laboratory findings from those of insulinoma.

HYPOGLYCEMIA DUE TO INSULIN RECEPTOR ANTIBODIES

Hypoglycemia due to insulin receptor autoantibodies is an extremely rare syndrome; most cases have occurred in women often with a history of autoimmune disease. Almost all of these patients have also had episodes of insulin-resistant diabetes and acanthosis nigricans. Their hypoglycemia may be either fasting or postprandial and is often severe and is attributed to an agonistic action of the antibody on the insulin receptor. Balance between the antagonistic and agonistic effects of the antibodies determines whether insulin-resistant diabetes or hypoglycemia occurs. Hypoglycemia was found to respond to corticosteroid therapy but not to plasmapheresis or immunosuppression.

Kim CH et al. Autoimmune hypoglycemia in a type 2 diabetic patient with anti-insulin and insulin receptor antibodies. Diabetes Care. 2004 Jan;27(1):288–9. [PMID: 14694017]

MEDICATION-INDUCED HYPOGLYCEMIA

A number of medications apart from the sulfonylureas can occasionally cause hypoglycemia. Common offenders include the fluoroquinolones such as gatifloxacin and levofloxacin, pentamidine, quinine, ACE inhibitors, salicylates and beta-adrenergic blocking agents. The fluoroquinolones, particularly gatifloxacin, have been associated with both hypoglycemia and hyperglycemia. It is thought that the drug acts on the ATP sensitive potassium channels in the beta cell. Hypoglycemia is an early event, and hyperglycemia occurs several days into therapy. Intravenous pentamidine is cytotoxic to beta cells and causes acute hyperinsulinemia and hypoglycemia followed by insulinopenia and hyperglycemia. Fasting patients taking noncardioselective beta-blockers can have an exaggerated hypoglycemic response to starvation. The beta-blockade inhibits fatty acids and gluconeogenesis substrate release and reduces plasma glucagon response. Therapy with ACE inhibitors increases the risk of hypoglycemia in patients who are taking insulin or sulfonylureas presumably because these drugs increase sensitivity to circulating insulin by increasing blood flow to the muscle. Some opioids cause hypoglycemia. Tramadol use has been associated with increased risk of hospitalization for hypoglycemia. Methadone overdose has also been reported to cause hypoglycemia and a rapid dose escalation of methadone in cancer patients can lower glucose levels.

Ethanol-associated hypoglycemia may be due to hepatic alcohol dehydrogenase activity depleting NAD. The resultant change in the redox state—increase in NADH to NAD$^+$ ratio—causes a partial block at several points in the gluconeogenic pathway. With prolonged starvation, glycogen reserves become depleted within 18–24 hours and hepatic glucose output becomes totally dependent on gluconeogenesis. Under these circumstances, a blood concentration of ethanol as low as 45 mg/dL (9.8 mmol/L) can induce profound hypoglycemia by blocking gluconeogenesis. Neuroglycopenia in a patient whose breath smells of alcohol may be mistaken for alcoholic stupor. Prevention consists of adequate food intake during ethanol ingestion.

Therapy consists of glucose administration to replenish glycogen stores until gluconeogenesis resumes.

When sugar-containing soft drinks are used as mixers to dilute alcohol in beverages (gin and tonic, rum and cola), there seems to be a greater insulin release than when the soft drink alone is ingested and a tendency for more of a late hypoglycemic overswing to occur 3–4 hours later. Prevention would consist of avoiding sugar mixers while ingesting alcohol and ensuring supplementary food intake to provide sustained absorption.

Vue MH et al. Drug-induced glucose alterations part 1: drug-induced hypoglycemia. Diabetes Spectrum. 2011 Aug; 24(3):171–7.

Lipid Disorders

Michael J. Blaha, MD, MPH

Robert B. Baron, MD, MS

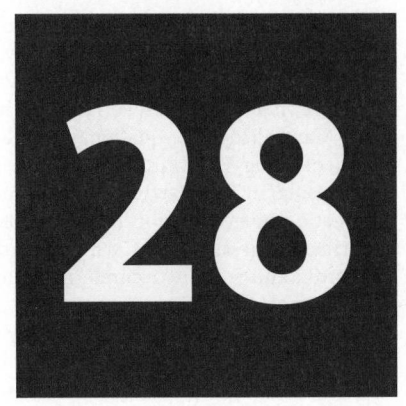

The "Lipid Hypothesis" of cardiovascular disease (CVD)—stating that cholesterol is causal in the development of atherosclerotic cardiovascular disease (ASCVD) and that lowering of cholesterol is associated with lower cardiovascular event rates—is generally accepted throughout the medical community. For patients with known CVD (secondary prevention), studies have shown that cholesterol lowering leads to a consistent reduction in total mortality and in recurrent cardiovascular events in men and women; other studies have documented lowered mortality and events in middle-aged and older patients. Among patients without CVD (primary prevention), the data are generally consistent, with rates of cardiovascular events, heart disease mortality, and all-cause mortality differing among studies. Treatment guidelines have been designed to assist clinicians in selecting patients for cholesterol-lowering therapy based on their overall risk of developing CVD.

There are several genetic disorders that provide insight into the pathogenesis of lipid-related diseases. **Familial hypercholesterolemia,** rare in the homozygous state (about one per million), causes markedly high low-density lipoprotein (LDL) levels and early CVD. The most common genetic defects involve absent or defective LDL receptors, resulting in unregulated LDL metabolism, genetic mutations of apolipoprotein B, or gain of function in proprotein convertase subtilisin/kexin type 9 (PCSK9), a protein that regulates breakdown of LDL receptors. Patients with two abnormal genes (homozygotes) have extremely high levels—up to eight times normal—and present with atherosclerotic disease in childhood. Homozygotes may require liver transplantation or plasmapheresis to correct their severe lipid abnormalities. Those with one defective gene (heterozygotes) have LDL concentrations twice normal; persons with this condition may develop CVD in their 30s or 40s.

Another rare condition is caused by an abnormality of lipoprotein lipase, the enzyme that enables peripheral tissues to take up triglyceride from chylomicrons and very-low-density lipoprotein (VLDL) particles. Patients with this condition, one cause of **familial chylomicronemia syndrome,** have marked hypertriglyceridemia with recurrent pancreatitis and hepatosplenomegaly in childhood.

Numerous other genetic abnormalities of lipid metabolism are named for the abnormality noted when serum is electrophoresed (eg, dysbetalipoproteinemia) or from combinations of lipid abnormalities in families (eg, familial combined hyperlipidemia).

▶ When to Refer

- Known genetic lipid disorders.
- Striking family history of hyperlipidemia or premature atherosclerosis.
- Extremely high serum LDL cholesterol or triglycerides, or extremely low serum high-density lipoprotein (HDL) cholesterol.

Bruikman CS et al. Molecular basis of familial hypercholesterolemia. Curr Opin Cardiol. 2017 Feb 4. [Epub ahead of print] [PMID: 28169949]

Khera AV et al. Diagnostic yield and clinical utility of sequencing familial hypercholesterolemia genes in patients with severe hypercholesterolemia. J Am Coll Cardiol. 2016 Jun 7; 67(22):2578–89. [PMID: 27050191]

LIPID FRACTIONS & THE RISK OF CORONARY HEART DISEASE

In serum, cholesterol is carried primarily on three different lipoproteins—the VLDL, LDL, and HDL molecules. Total cholesterol equals the sum of these three components:

$$\text{Total cholesterol} = \text{HDL cholesterol} + \text{VLDL cholesterol} + \text{LDL cholesterol}$$

Using these assumptions, the Friedewald equation states that LDL cholesterol can be estimated as:

$$\underset{\text{(mg/dL)}}{\text{LDL cholesterol}} = \underset{\text{(mg/dL)}}{\text{Total cholesterol}} - \underset{\text{(mg/dL)}}{\text{HDL cholesterol}} - \frac{\text{Triglycerides (mg/dL)}}{5}$$

When using SI units, the formula becomes

$$\underset{\text{(mmol/L)}}{\text{LDL cholesterol}} = \underset{\text{(mmol/L)}}{\text{Total cholesterol}} - \underset{\text{(mmol/L)}}{\text{HDL cholesterol}} - \frac{\text{Triglycerides (mmol/L)}}{2.2}$$

Modern research has questioned several of the assumptions underlying the Friedewald equation, particularly the assumption that VLDL is always best estimated as triglycerides/5, which is inaccurate when triglycerides are above 150 mg/dL and when LDL cholesterol is less than 70 mg/dL. Therefore, many commercial laboratories have switched to the Martin/Hopkins equation, which uses a flexible factor for deriving VLDL from triglycerides (as opposed to always using 5). The Martin/Hopkins equation reduces the systematic underestimation of LDL cholesterol when triglycerides are greater than 150 mg/dL and LDL is less than 70 mg/dL, and is more accurate in estimating LDL from nonfasting blood specimens.

Non-HDL cholesterol is increasingly recognized as an important measure of the total quantity of apolipoprotein B–containing atherogenic lipid particles. Non-HDL cholesterol is calculated as: total cholesterol – HDL cholesterol. Advantages of non-HDL cholesterol are that it is less sensitive to fasting status and it is a better predictor of cardiovascular risk compared to LDL cholesterol.

Lipoprotein(a), a subfraction of LDL that is largely genetically determined, has also been recognized as a casual factor in atherosclerosis. Lipoprotein(a) may be useful to measure in patients with a strong family history or with early signs of early ASCVD.

It is difficult to assign a "normal" range for serum lipids. This is because our cholesterol values are vastly higher than our evolutionary ancestors and because mean values vary across the world. In Western populations, cholesterol values are about 20% higher than in Asian populations and exceed 300 mg/dL (7.76 mmol/L) in nearly 5% of adults. About 10% of adults have LDL cholesterol levels above 200 mg/dL (5.17 mmol/L).

Quispe R et al. Accuracy of low-density lipoprotein cholesterol estimation at very low levels. BMC Med. 2017 Apr 20;15(1):83. [PMID: 28427464]
Sathiyakumar V et al. Fasting versus nonfasting and low-density lipoprotein cholesterol accuracy. Circulation. 2018 Jan 2; 137(1):10–9. [PMID: 29038168]

THERAPEUTIC EFFECTS OF LOWERING CHOLESTEROL

Reducing cholesterol levels in healthy middle-aged men without coronary heart disease (CHD) (in **primary prevention studies**) reduces their risk in direct proportion to the reduction in LDL cholesterol. Treated adults have statistically significant and clinically important reductions in the rates of myocardial infarctions, strokes, new cases of angina, and need for coronary artery bypass procedures. The West of Scotland Study showed a 31% decrease in myocardial infarctions in middle-aged men treated with pravastatin compared with placebo. The Air Force/Texas Coronary Atherosclerosis Prevention Study (AFCAPS/TexCAPS) study showed similar results with lovastatin. As with any primary prevention interventions, large numbers of healthy patients need to be treated to prevent a single event. The numbers of patients needed to treat (NNT) to prevent one nonfatal myocardial infarction or one coronary artery disease death in these two studies were 46 and 50, respectively. The Anglo-Scandinavian Cardiac Outcomes Trial (ASCOT) study of atorvastatin in persons with hypertension and other risk factors but without CHD demonstrated a 36% reduction in CHD events. The Justification for the Use of Statins in Prevention: An Intervention Trial Evaluating Rosuvastatin (JUPITER) study showed a 44% reduction in a combined end point of myocardial infarction, stroke, revascularization, hospitalization for unstable angina, or death from cardiovascular causes in both men and women. The NNT for 1 year to prevent one event was 169. The Heart Outcomes Prevention Evaluation (HOPE-3) trial of rosuvastatin showed a 24% reduction in cardiovascular events. The NNT over 5.6 years was 91.

Primary prevention studies have found a less consistent effect on total mortality. The West of Scotland study found a 20% decrease in total mortality, tending toward statistical significance. The AFCAPS/TexCAPS study with lovastatin showed no difference in total mortality. The Antihypertensive and Lipid-Lowering Treatment to Prevent Heart Attack Trial (ALLHAT-LLT) also showed no reduction either in all-cause mortality or in CHD events when pravastatin was compared with usual care. Subjects treated with atorvastatin in the ASCOT study had a 13% reduction in mortality, but the result was not statistically significant. This study, however, was stopped early due to the marked reduction in CHD events. The JUPITER trial demonstrated a statistically significant 20% reduction in death from any cause. The NNT for 1 year was 400. The HOPE-3 trial showed a 7% reduction in all-cause mortality, but the result was not statistically significant.

In **secondary prevention studies** among patients with established CVD, the benefits of cholesterol lowering are clearer. Major studies with statins have shown significant reductions in cardiovascular events, cardiovascular deaths, and all-cause mortality in men and women with coronary artery disease. The NNT to prevent a non-fatal myocardial infarction or a coronary artery disease death in these studies was between 12 and 34. Aggressive cholesterol lowering with these agents causes regression of atherosclerotic plaques in some patients, reduces the progression of atherosclerosis in saphenous vein grafts, and can slow or reverse carotid artery atherosclerosis. Results with other classes of medications, particularly those with little effect on LDL or the LDL receptor, have been less consistent. For example, patients treated with gemfibrozil had fewer cardiovascular events, but there was no benefit in all-cause mortality when compared with placebo. The benefits and adverse effects of cholesterol lowering may be specific to each type of drug; the clinician cannot assume that the effects of new drugs with novel mechanisms of action will generalize to other classes of medication.

The disparities in results between primary and secondary prevention studies highlight a critical aspect of clinical cholesterol lowering. The net benefits from cholesterol lowering depend on the underlying risk of ASCVD as well as the competing risks of other diseases. In middle-aged patients with atherosclerosis and high cholesterol, morbidity and mortality rates are high, and measures that reduce cholesterol-related risk are more likely to provide a robust net benefit to the patient. In older patients with little atherosclerosis and lower cholesterol levels, there may be no meaningful net benefit to cholesterol lowering.

Blaha MJ. Personalizing treatment: between primary and secondary prevention. Am J Cardiol. 2016 Sep 15;118(6 Suppl): 4A–12A. [PMID: 27620358]

Collins R et al. Interpretation of the evidence for the efficacy and safety of statin therapy. Lancet. 2016 Nov 19;388(10059): 2532–61. Erratum in: Lancet. 2017 Feb 11;389(10069):602. [PMID: 27616593]

Driver SL et al. Fasting or nonfasting lipid measurements: it depends on the question. J Am Coll Cardiol. 2016 Mar 15; 67(10):1227–34. [PMID: 26965545]

Grundy SM et al. 2018 AHA/ACC/AACVPR/AAPA/ABC/ ACPM/ADA/AGS/APhA/ASPC/NLA/PCNA guideline on the management of blood cholesterol: executive summary. Circulation. 2018 Nov 10. [Epub ahead of print] [PMID: 30565953]

Navarese EP et al. Association between baseline LDL-C level and total and cardiovascular mortality after LDL-C lowering: a systematic review and meta-analysis. JAMA. 2018 Apr 17; 319(15):1566–79. [PMID: 29677301]

Silverman MG et al. Association between lowering LDL-C and cardiovascular risk reduction among different therapeutic interventions: a systematic review and meta-analysis. JAMA. 2016 Sep 27;316(12):1289–97. [PMID: 27673306]

Svatikova A et al. Cholesterol management in the era of PCSK9 inhibitors. Curr Cardiol Rep. 2017 Sep;19(9):83. [PMID: 28779284]

Vallejo-Vaz AJ et al. Low-density lipoprotein cholesterol lowering for the primary prevention of cardiovascular disease among men with primary elevations of low-density lipoprotein cholesterol levels of 190 mg/dL or above: analyses from the WOSCOPS (West of Scotland Coronary Prevention Study) 5-year randomized trial and 20-year observational follow-up. Circulation. 2017 Nov 14;136(20):1878–91. [PMID: 28877913]

Yusuf S et al; HOPE-3 Investigators. Cholesterol lowering in intermediate-risk persons without cardiovascular disease. N Engl J Med. 2016 May 26];374(21):2021–31. [PMID: 27040132]

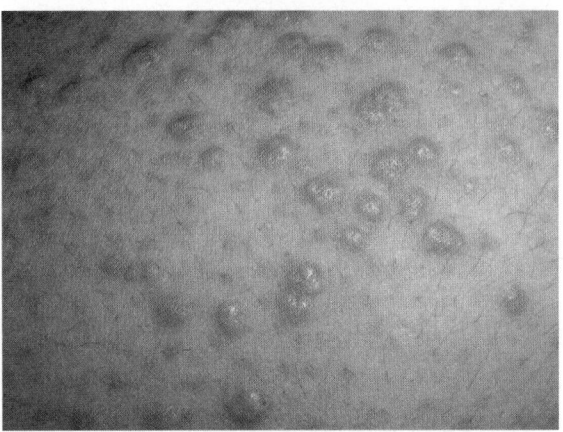

▲ **Figure 28–1.** Eruptive xanthomas on the arm of a man with untreated hyperlipidemia and diabetes mellitus. (Used, with permission, from Richard P. Usatine, MD, in Usatine RP, Smith MA, Mayeaux EJ Jr, Chumley H. *The Color Atlas of Family Medicine,* 2nd ed. McGraw-Hill, 2013.)

a preventive screening strategy. Extremely high levels of chylomicrons or VLDL particles (triglyceride level above 1000 mg/dL or 10 mmol/L) result in the formation of **eruptive xanthomas** (Figure 28–1) (red-yellow papules, especially on the buttocks). High LDL concentrations result in **tendinous xanthomas** on certain tendons (Achilles, patella, back of the hand). Such xanthomas usually indicate one of the underlying genetic hyperlipidemias. **Lipemia retinalis** (cream-colored blood vessels in the fundus) is seen with extremely high triglyceride levels (above 2000 mg/dL or 20 mmol/L).

SECONDARY CONDITIONS THAT AFFECT LIPID METABOLISM

Several factors, including drugs, can influence serum lipids. These are important for two reasons: abnormal lipid levels (or changes in lipid levels) may be the presenting sign of some of these conditions, and correction of the underlying condition may obviate the need to treat an apparent lipid disorder. Thyroid disease, particularly hypothyroidism, is associated with a high LDL. Poorly controlled diabetes mellitus and alcohol use, in particular, are commonly associated with high triglyceride levels that decline with improvements in glycemic control or reduction in alcohol use, respectively. Thus, secondary causes of high blood lipids should be considered in each patient with a lipid disorder before lipid-lowering therapy is started. In most instances, special testing is not needed: a history and physical examination are sufficient.

CLINICAL PRESENTATIONS

Most patients with high cholesterol levels have no specific symptoms or signs. The vast majority of patients with lipid abnormalities are detected by the laboratory, either as part of the workup of a patient with CVD or as part of

SCREENING & TREATMENT OF HIGH BLOOD CHOLESTEROL

While screening of all children for cholesterol disorders remains controversial, all adults should have their lipids checked before middle age. Patients with CVD and diabetes deserve the most scrutiny of their lipids since these patients are at the highest risk for suffering additional manifestations in the near term and thus have the most to gain from lipid lowering. In such patients, a complete lipid profile (serum total cholesterol, HDL cholesterol, and triglyceride levels) should be obtained. Additional risk reduction measures for atherosclerosis are discussed in Chapter 10; lipid lowering should be just one aspect of a program to reduce the progression and effects of atherosclerosis.

The best screening and treatment strategy for adults who do not have ASCVD is less clear. Several algorithms have been developed to guide the clinician in treatment decisions, but management decisions must always be individualized based on the patient's risk to maximize net benefit.

The 2018 American Heart Association/American College of Cardiology (AHA/ACC)/Multi-specialty guidelines recommend screening of all adults aged 20 years or older for high blood cholesterol. The 2016 United States Preventive Services Task Force (USPSTF) guidelines recommend beginning at age 20 years only if there are other cardiovascular risk factors such as tobacco use, diabetes, hypertension, obesity, or a family history of premature CVD. For men without other risk factors, screening is recommended beginning at age 35 years. For women and for men aged 20 to 35 without increased risk, the USPSTF makes no recommendation for or against routine screening for lipid disorders. Although there is no established interval for screening, screening can be repeated every 5 years for those with average or low risk and more often for those whose levels are close to therapeutic thresholds.

Individuals without CVD should have their 10-year risk of CVD calculated. Although those with LDL cholesterol greater than 190 mg/dL (4.91 mmol/L) are recommended for treatment independent of their 10-year risk of CVD, all other patients are recommended for treatment based on their overall cardiovascular risk. While other calculators (such as SCORE or QRISK) may be more appropriate for other parts of the world, the best method for estimating 10-year risk in the United States is the Pooled Cohort Equations. First introduced in the 2013 ACC/AHA guidelines, the Pooled Cohort Equations include separate equations for white and black patients and estimate the 10-year risk of heart attack, stroke, and cardiovascular death. This represents an improvement over older Framingham 10-year calculator, which includes CHD but not stroke risk. The ACC/AHA risk estimator can be found at http://www.cvriskcalculator.com/, and mobile apps are available for download. While it has been shown to overestimate risk in some modern populations, including those with at least moderate socioeconomic status, the ACC/AHA risk estimator remains an excellent starting point for a risk discussion. Recalibrated versions of the calculator are available for countries across the world.

The 2018 AHA/ACC/Multi-specialty guidelines identify a set of **"risk-enhancing factors"** that might influence a clinician and patient to favor cholesterol-lowering treatment. Table 28–1 lists these risk-enhancing factors that may be considered, particularly for patients at borderline to intermediate risk (5–20% 10-year cardiovascular risk).

Importantly, the 2018 AHA/ACC/Multi-specialty guidelines also identify the **coronary artery calcium score** as the single best test for risk stratification. The coronary calcium score is a simple noncontrast cardiac-gated CT scan that takes about 10–15 minutes to do, is associated with approximately 1 mSv of radiation, and costs between $75 and $300. As opposed to the risk-enhancing factors, which may incline a clinician and patient toward treatment, the coronary artery calcium score may also help identify patients who are unlikely to benefit from cholesterol-lowering therapy. For example, when the coronary artery calcium score is zero in the absence of smoking or diabetes, the patient is low risk and less likely to receive net benefit from therapy; instead, the calcium artery calcium score can be repeated in 5 years. The USPSTF does not endorse calcium scoring as a screening test; rather the test should be reserved for situations in which additional data will inform shared decision making and potentially change a therapeutic decision.

Statins are nearly always the first-line therapy. Treatment decisions are based on the presence of clinical CVD

Table 28–1. Risk-enhancing factors that help identify patients who may benefit most from lipid-lowering therapy: 2018 AHA/ACC/Multi-specialty guidelines.

Family history of premature disease (males, age < 55 years; females, age < 65 years)
Primary hypercholesterolemia (LDL cholesterol, 160–189 mg/dL [4.1–4.8 mmol/L]; non–HDL cholesterol, 190–219 mg/dL [4.9–5.6 mmol/L])
Metabolic syndrome
Chronic kidney disease (not end-stage renal disease)
Chronic inflammatory conditions, such as psoriasis, rheumatoid arthritis, or HIV/AIDS
History of preeclampsia or of premature menopause before age 40 years
High-risk race/ethnicities (eg, South Asian ancestry)
Persistently high triglycerides ≥ 175 mg/dL
Elevated high-sensitivity C-reactive protein (≥ 2.0 mg/L)
Elevated lipoprotein(a) (≥ 50 mg/dL or ≥ 125 nmol/L)
Elevated apolipoprotein B (≥ 130 mg/dL)
Ankle brachial index < 0.9

or diabetes, LDL cholesterol greater than 190 mg/dL (4.91 mmol/L), patient age, and the estimated 10-year risk of developing CVD. The 2018 AHA/ACC/Multi-specialty guidelines define four groups of patients who benefit from statin medications: (1) individuals with clinical ASCVD; (2) individuals with primary elevation of LDL cholesterol greater than 190 mg/dL (4.91 mmol/L); (3) individuals aged 40–75 with diabetes and LDL greater than or equal to 70 mg/dL (1.81 mmol/L); and (4) individuals aged 40–75 without clinical ASCVD or diabetes, with LDL 70–189 mg/dL (1.81–4.91 mmol/L), and estimated 10-year CVD risk of 7.5% or higher.

Ezetimibe and PCSK9 inhibitors have the strongest recommendations as second-line therapy for patients with (1) CVD whose LDL on statin therapy remains above the 70 mg/dL treatment threshold or (2) possible familial hypercholesterolemia with baseline LDL greater than 190 mg/dL (4.91 mmol/L) whose LDL remains above the 100 mg/dL treatment threshold. In high-risk patients, ezetimibe therapy is favored, while in very high-risk patients, PCSK9 inhibitor therapy should be considered.

Screening & Treatment in Women

The foregoing screening and treatment guidelines are designed for both men and women. Meta-analysis of studies including women with known heart disease has found that statins prevent recurrent myocardial infarctions in women. Although most experts recommend application of the same primary prevention guidelines for women as for men, clinicians should be aware of the uncertainty in this area. Estimating the 10-year cardiovascular risk is particularly important in women since a larger percentage of women than men will have estimated 10-year cardiovascular risks below 7.5% per year and thus be advised not to take statins unless their LDL is very high (greater than 190 mg/dL [4.91 mmol/L]).

Screening & Treatment in Older Patients

Meta-analysis of evidence relating cholesterol to CVD in older adults suggests that cholesterol is a weak risk factor for CVD for persons over age 75 years. Clinical trials have rarely included such individuals. One exception is the Prospective Study of Pravastatin in the Elderly at Risk (PROSPER). In this study, elderly patients with CVD (secondary prevention) benefited from statin therapy, whereas those without CVD (primary prevention) did not. The 2018 AHA/ACC/Multi-specialty guidelines suggest continuing statin treatment in patients over age 75 who have CVD. The guidelines, however, suggest selectively treating patients over the age of 75 who do not have evidence of CVD. Individual patient decisions to discontinue statin therapy should be based on overall functional status and life expectancy, comorbidities, and patient preference and should be made in context with overall therapeutic goals and end-of-life decisions.

Bell DA et al. Progress in the care of familial hypercholesterolaemia: 2016. Med J Aust. 2016 Sep 5;205(5):232–6. [PMID: 27581271]

Catapano AL et al. 2016 ESC/EAS Guidelines for the Management of Dyslipidaemias: the Task Force for the Management of Dyslipidaemias of the European Society of Cardiology (ESC) and European Atherosclerosis Society (EAS) developed with the special contribution of the European Association for Cardiovascular Prevention & Rehabilitation (EACPR). Atherosclerosis. 2016 Oct;253:281–344. [PMID: 27594540]

Chang Y et al. Dyslipidemia management update. Curr Opin Pharmacol. 2017 Apr;33:47–55. [PMID: 28527325]

Chaudhary R et al. PCSK9 inhibitors: a new era of lipid lowering therapy. World J Cardiol. 2017 Feb 26;9(2):76–91. [PMID: 28289523]

Greenland P et al. Coronary calcium score and cardiovascular risk. J Am Coll Cardiol. 2018 Jul 24;72(4):434–47. [PMID: 30025580]

Grundy SM et al. 2018 AHA/ACC/AACVPR/AAPA/ABC/ACPM/ADA/AGS/APhA/ASPC/NLA/PCNA guideline on the management of blood cholesterol: executive summary. Circulation. 2018 Nov 10. [Epub ahead of print] [PMID: 30565953]

Khera AV et al. Diagnostic yield and clinical utility of sequencing familial hypercholesterolemia genes in patients with severe hypercholesterolemia. J Am Coll Cardiol. 2016 Jun 7; 67(22):2578–89. [PMID: 27050191]

Miedema MD et al. Statin eligibility, coronary artery calcium, and subsequent cardiovascular events according to the 2016 United States Preventive Services Task Force (USPSTF) statin guidelines: MESA (Multi-Ethnic Study of Atherosclerosis). J Am Heart Assoc. 2018 Jun 13;7(12):e008920. [PMID: 29899017]

Ogura M. PCSK9 inhibition in the management of familial hypercholesterolemia. J Cardiol. 2018 Jan;71(1):1–7. [PMID: 28784313]

Page MM et al. PCSK9 in context: a contemporary review of an important biological target for the prevention and treatment of atherosclerotic cardiovascular disease. Diabetes Obes Metab. 2018 Feb;20(2):270–82. [PMID: 28736830]

U.S. Preventive Services Task Force; Bibbins-Domingo K et al. Screening for lipid disorders in children and adolescents: U.S. Preventive Services Task Force recommendation statement. JAMA. 2016 Aug 9;316(6):625–33. [PMID: 27532917]

U.S. Preventive Services Task Force; Bibbins-Domingo K et al. Statin use for the primary prevention of cardiovascular disease in adults: U.S. Preventive Services Task Force recommendation statement. JAMA. 2016 Nov 15;316(19):1997–2007. [PMID: 27838723]

TREATMENT OF HIGH LDL CHOLESTEROL

Reduction of LDL cholesterol with statins is just one part of a program to reduce the risk of CVD. Other measures—including diet, exercise, smoking cessation, hypertension control, diabetes control, and antithrombotic therapy—are also of central importance. For example, exercise (and weight loss) may reduce the LDL cholesterol and increase the HDL.

The use of medications to raise the HDL cholesterol has not been demonstrated to provide additional benefit. For example, cholesteryl ester transfer protein inhibitors are a class of medicines being investigated to raise HDL levels; however, agents in this class have not been shown to be effective in so doing. The addition of niacin to statins has also been carefully studied in the AIM-HIGH study and the HPS2-THRIVE study in patients at high risk for CVD and shown not to produce any further benefit (ie, to decrease parameters of cardiovascular risk).

Zeman M et al. Niacin in the treatment of hyperlipidemias in light of new clinical trials: has niacin lost its place? Med Sci Monit. 2015 Jul 25;21:2156–62. [PMID: 26210594]

Diet Therapy

Studies of nonhospitalized adults have reported only modest cholesterol-lowering benefits of dietary therapy, typically in the range of a 5–10% decrease in LDL cholesterol, and even less over the long term. The effect of diet therapy, however, varies considerably among individuals; some patients will have striking reductions in LDL cholesterol—up to a 25–30% decrease—whereas others will have clinically important increases. Thus, the results of diet therapy should be assessed about 4 weeks after initiation.

Several nutritional approaches to diet therapy are available. Most Americans currently eat over 35% of calories as fat, of which 15% is saturated fat. A traditional cholesterol-lowering diet recommends reducing total fat to 25–30% and saturated fat to less than 7% of calories, with complete elimination of trans fats. These diets replace fat, particularly saturated fat, with carbohydrate. Other diet plans, including the Dean Ornish Diet, the Pritikin Diet, and most vegetarian diets, restrict fat even further. Low-fat, high-carbohydrate diets may, however, result in insulin resistance and reductions in HDL cholesterol.

An alternative strategy is the Mediterranean diet, which maintains total fat at approximately 35–40% of total calories but replaces saturated fat with monounsaturated fat such as that found in canola oil and in olives, peanuts, avocados, and their oils. This diet is equally effective at lowering LDL cholesterol, and is less likely to lead to reductions in HDL cholesterol. Several studies have suggested that this diet may also be associated with reductions in endothelial dysfunction, insulin resistance, and markers of vascular inflammation and may result in better resolution of the metabolic syndrome than traditional cholesterol-lowering diets. A clinical trial demonstrated reduced cardiovascular events in persons on a Mediterranean diet supplemented with additional nuts or extra-virgin olive oil compared to persons on a less intensive standard Mediterranean diet.

Other dietary changes may also result in beneficial changes in blood lipids. Soluble fiber, such as that found in oat bran or psyllium, may reduce LDL cholesterol by 5–10%. Plant stanols and sterols can reduce LDL cholesterol by 10%. Intake of garlic, soy protein, vitamin C, and pecans may also yield modest reductions of LDL cholesterol. Because oxidation of LDL cholesterol is a potential initiating event in atherogenesis, diets rich in antioxidants, found primarily in fruits and vegetables, may be helpful (see Chapter 29). Studies have suggested that when all of these elements are combined into a single dietary prescription, the impact of diet on LDL cholesterol may approach that of statin medications, lowering LDL cholesterol by close to 30%.

Abdelhamid AS et al. Polyunsaturated fatty acids for the primary and secondary prevention of cardiovascular disease. Cochrane Database Syst Rev. 2018 Jul 18;7:CD012345. [PMID: 30019767]

Burke MF et al. Review of cardiometabolic effects of prescription omega-3 fatty acids. Curr Atheroscler Rep. 2017 Nov 7; 19(12):60. [PMID: 29116404]

Chalvon-Demersay T et al. A systematic review of the effects of plant compared with animal protein sources on features of metabolic syndrome. J Nutr. 2017 Mar;147(3):281–92. [PMID: 28122929]

Eckel RH et al. 2013 AHA/ACC Guideline on lifestyle management to reduce cardiovascular risk: a report of the American College of Cardiology/American Heart Association Task Force on Practice Guidelines. Circulation. 2014 Jun 24; 129(25 Suppl 2):S76–99. [PMID: 24222015]

Estruch R et al; PREDIMED Study Investigators. Primary prevention of cardiovascular disease with a Mediterranean diet supplemented with extra-virgin olive oil or nuts. N Engl J Med. 2018 Jun 21;378(25):e34. [PMID: 29897866]

Grundy SM et al. 2018 AHA/ACC/AACVPR/AAPA/ABC/ ACPM/ADA/AGS/APhA/ASPC/NLA/PCNA guideline on the management of blood cholesterol: executive summary. Circulation. 2018 Nov 10. [Epub ahead of print] [PMID: 30565953]

Hooper L et al. Reduction in saturated fat intake for cardiovascular disease. Cochrane Database Syst Rev. 2015 Jun 10; (6):CD011737. [PMID: 26068959]

Khera AV et al. Genetic risk, adherence to a healthy lifestyle, and coronary disease. N Engl J Med. 2016 Dec 15;375(24):2349–58. [PMID: 27959714]

Lu M et al. Effects of low-fat compared with high-fat diet on cardiometabolic indicators in people with overweight and obesity without overt metabolic disturbance: a systematic review and meta-analysis of randomised controlled trials. Br J Nutr. 2018 Jan;119(1):96–108. [PMID: 29212558]

Schwingshackl L et al. Effects of oils and solid fats on blood lipids: a systematic review and network meta-analysis. J Lipid Res. 2018 Sep;59(9):1771–82. [PMID: 30006369]

▶ Pharmacologic Therapy

There are seven types of medications to consider in patients who require drug treatment of an elevated cholesterol. As discussed above, statins are the cornerstone of nearly all medical regimens, and current guidelines define four groups of patients who benefit from statin medications. The evidence is then strongest for ezetimibe and

Table 28–2. Indications for high-intensity and moderate-intensity statins: recommendations of the 2018 AHA/ACC/Multi-specialty guidelines.

Indications	Treatment Recommendation
Presence of clinical ASCVD	High-intensity statin **or** moderate-intensity statin if over age 75 years
Primary elevation of LDL cholesterol ≥ 190 mg/dL (4.91 mmol/L)	High-intensity statin
Age 40–75 years[1] Presence of diabetes LDL ≥ 70 mg/dL (1.81 mmol/L)	Moderate-intensity statin **or** high-intensity statin if 10-year CVD risk ≥ 7.5% or other risk-enhancing criteria[1]
Aged 40–75 years No clinical ASCVD or diabetes LDL 70–189 mg/dL (1.81–4.91 mmol/L) Estimated 10-year CVD risk ≥ 7.5% or coronary artery calcium > 0 and > 75th percentile	Treat with moderate- to high-intensity statin

[1]Diabetes duration > 10 years, microalbuminuria, chronic kidney disease, and ankle brachial index < 0.9 favor aggressive treatment even for patients age 20–39 years.
AHA/ACC, American Heart Association/American College of Cardiology; ASCVD, atherosclerotic cardiovascular disease; CVD, cardiovascular disease; HDL, high-density lipoprotein; LDL, low-density lipoprotein.

PCSK9 inhibitors, with less evidence for cholesterol absorption inhibitors, fibrates, and niacin, with strong emerging randomized controlled trial evidence for select omega-3 fatty acid preparations.

A. Statins (Hydroxymethylglutaryl-Coenzyme A [HMG-CoA] Reductase Inhibitors)

The statins (HMG-CoA reductase inhibitors) work by inhibiting the rate-limiting enzyme in the formation of cholesterol. Cholesterol synthesis in the liver is reduced, with a compensatory increase in hepatic LDL receptors (presumably so that the liver can take more of the cholesterol that it needs from the blood) and a reduction in the circulating LDL cholesterol level by 50% or more at the highest doses. There are also modest increases in HDL levels, substantial decreases in triglyceride levels, and marked reductions in high-sensitivity C-reactive protein levels.

The 2018 AHA/ACC/Multi-specialty guidelines divide statins into two categories: "high-intensity" and "moderate-intensity" statins (Table 28–2). High-intensity statins lower LDL cholesterol by approximately 50%. Examples include high-dose atorvastatin 40–80 mg/day and rosuvastatin 20–40 mg/day (Table 28–3). Moderate-intensity statins lower LDL cholesterol by approximately 30–50%. Examples include simvastatin 20–40 mg/day, pravastatin

Table 28–3. Effects of selected lipid-modifying drugs (listed alphabetically).

Drug	Lipid-Modifying Effects			Initial Daily Dose	Maximum Daily Dose	Cost for 30 Days of Treatment With Dose Listed[1]
	LDL	HDL	Triglyceride			
Alirocumab (Praluent)	−45 to −60%	±	±	75 mg once every 2 weeks	150 mg once every 2 weeks	$1344.00 (75 mg every 2 weeks)
Atorvastatin (Lipitor)	−25 to −40%	+5 to 10%	↓↓	10 mg once	80 mg once	$15.75 (20 mg once)
Cholestyramine (Questran, others)	−15 to −25%	+5%	±	4 g twice a day	24 g divided	$21.00 (8 g divided)
Colesevelam (WelChol)	−10 to −20%	+10%	±	625 mg, 6–7 tablets once	625 mg, 6–7 tablets once	$749.52 (6 tablets once)
Colestipol (Colestid)	−15 to −60%	+5%	±	5 g twice a day	30 g divided	$235.82 (10 g divided)
Evolocumab (Repatha)	−50 to −60%	±	±	140 mg once every 2 weeks	420 mg once monthly	$1340.59 (140 mg every 2 weeks)
Ezetimibe (Zetia)	−20%	+5%	±	10 mg once	10 mg once	$308.43 (10 mg once)
Fenofibrate (Tricor, others)	−10 to −15%	+15 to 25%	↓↓	48 mg once	145 mg once	$37.20 (145 mg once)
Fenofibric acid (Trilipix)	−10 to −15%	+15 to 25%	↓↓	45 mg once	135 mg once	$160.20 (135 mg once)
Fluvastatin (Lescol)	−20 to −30%	+5 to 10%	↓	20 mg once	40 mg once	$113.40 (20 mg once)
Gemfibrozil (Lopid, others)	−10 to −15%	+15 to 20%	↓↓	600 mg once	1200 mg divided	$71.40 (600 mg twice a day)
Lomitapide (Juxtapid)[2,3]	−40 to −50%[4]	−7%[4]	↓↓	5 mg once	60 mg once	$44,390.40 (any dose)
Lovastatin (Mevacor, others)	−25 to −40%	+5 to 10%	↓	10 mg once	80 mg divided	$63.00 (20 mg once)
Mipomersen (Kynamro)[2,3]	−20 to −25%[5]	+11%[5]	↓	200 mg subcutaneously once weekly	200 mg subcutaneously once weekly	$36,532.96 (200 mg weekly)
Niacin (OTC, Niaspan)	−15 to −25%	+25 to 35%	↓↓	100 mg once	3–4.5 g divided	$9.00 (1.5 g twice a day, OTC) $449.40 (2 g Niaspan)
Omega-3 fatty acid ethyl esters (Lovaza)			↓↓	4 g once	4 g once	$348.76 (4 g daily)
Omega-3 fatty acid icosapent ethyl (Vascepa)			↓↓	2 g twice	2 g twice	$334.30 (2 g twice day)
Pitavastatin (Livalo, Zypitamag)	−30 to 40%	+10 to 25%	↓↓	2 mg once	4 mg once	$331.50 (2 mg once)
Pravastatin (Pravachol)	−25 to −40%	+5 to 10%	↓	20 mg once	80 mg once	$75.00 (20 mg once)
Rosuvastatin (Crestor)	−40 to −50%	+10 to 15%	↓↓	10 mg once	40 mg once	$43.20 (20 mg once)
Simvastatin (Zocor, others)	−25 to −40%	+5 to 10%	↓↓	5 mg once	80 mg once	$6.00 (10 mg once)

[1]Average wholesale price (AWP, for AB-rated generic when available) for quantity listed. Source: IBM Micromedex Red Book (electronic version) IBM Watson Health, Greenwood Village, CO, USA. Available at https://www.micromedexsolutions.com (cited April 25, 2019). AWP may not accurately represent the actual pharmacy cost because wide contractual variations exist among institutions.
[2]Restricted to patients with homozygous familial hypercholesterolemia.
[3]FDA Black Box warning regarding hepatotoxicity.
[4]62% of patients also received plasma lipoprotein apheresis.
[5]No plasma lipoprotein apheresis allowed in clinical trial.
HDL, high-density lipoprotein; LDL, low-density lipoprotein; ± variable, if any; others, indicates availability of less expensive generic preparations; OTC, over the counter.

40–80 mg/day, and lovastatin 40 mg/day, as well as low-dose atorvastatin 10–20 mg/day and rosuvastatin 5–10 mg/day. All statins are given once daily in the morning or evening.

Statin-associated muscle aches, with normal serum creatine kinase levels, occur in up to 10% of patients, and often such patients can tolerate the statin upon rechallenge. More serious, but very uncommon, muscle disease includes myositis and rhabdomyolysis, with moderate and marked elevations of serum creatine kinase levels, respectively. Such muscle disease occurs more often when the statin is taken with niacin or a fibrate, as well as with erythromycin, antifungal medications, nefazodone, or cyclosporine. Simvastatin at the highest approved dose (80 mg) is associated with an elevated risk of muscle injury or myopathy; this dose should be used only in patients who have been taking simvastatin at a lower dose for longer than 1 year without muscle toxicity. Liver disease, with elevations of serum transaminases, is another side effect of statin therapy and is again more common in patients who are also taking fibrates or niacin. Manufacturers of statins recommend monitoring liver enzymes before initiating therapy and as clinically indicated thereafter. Liver failure can occur but is extremely uncommon. Finally, statin therapy is associated with mild gastrointestinal symptoms and a 10% increase in risk of developing diabetes mellitus.

B. Ezetimibe

Ezetimibe inhibits the intestinal absorption of dietary and biliary cholesterol across the intestinal wall by inhibiting a cholesterol transporter. The dose of ezetimibe is 10 mg/day orally. Ezetimibe reduces LDL cholesterol between 15% and 20% when used as monotherapy, reduces high-sensitivity C-reactive protein, and can further reduce LDL in patients taking statins in whom the therapeutic goal has not been reached. While beneficial effects of ezetimibe monotherapy on cardiovascular outcomes are available from only a large open-label trial, the double-blind IMPROVE-IT trial showed that adding ezetimibe to a statin resulted in a small incremental 5–10% relative risk reduction in cardiovascular outcomes. At the end of 7 years of study, patients taking ezetimibe-simvastatin had a 2% absolute reduction in cardiovascular events compared to patients taking simvastatin alone. Current guidelines recommend adding ezetimibe therapy to maximally tolerated statin therapy in patients at high risk for CVD whose LDL cholesterol remains above the treatment threshold of 70 mg/dL.

C. Proprotein Convertase Subtilisin/Kexin Type 9 (PCSK9) Inhibitors

PCSK9 inhibitors are fully human monoclonal antibodies that inhibit PCSK9-mediated LDL-receptor degradation and lower LDL cholesterol levels by 50–60% and lipoprotein(a) by up to 20–30%. Two agents, alirocumab and evolocumab, are approved for use in the United States for patients with familial hypercholesterolemia or CVD who require additional lowering of LDL cholesterol. The medications are injected subcutaneously every 2–4 weeks.

No significant increase in adverse events has been observed compared to placebo. The FOURIER (Further Cardiovascular Outcomes Research with PCSK9 Inhibition in Subjects with Elevated Risk) trial compared evolocumab with placebo in 27,564 patients with established atherosclerotic disease already taking statin therapy; participants were monitored for a median of 2.2 years. LDL cholesterol was reduced by 59%. Patients receiving the evolocumab plus statin had a 15% reduction in the primary composite endpoint of cardiovascular death, myocardial infarction, stroke, hospital admission for unstable angina, or coronary revascularization and a 20% reduction in the secondary outcome of cardiovascular death, myocardial infarction, or stroke. The ODYSSEY-OUTCOMES study randomized 18,924 patients with recent acute coronary syndrome to alirocumab or placebo, demonstrating a 15% reduction in the primary composite cardiovascular endpoint and a 15% reduction in all-cause mortality in secondary statistical testing after median 2.8-year follow-up.

However, despite encouraging results from multiple clinical trials, initial cost-effectiveness models suggested that PCSK9 inhibitors were not cost-effective. After marked price reductions in 2018 and 2019, PCSK9 inhibitors are closer to being cost-effective; however, guidelines suggest that their relatively high cost must still remain part of the consideration regarding their use. Current guidelines recommend addition of PCSK9 inhibitors to statins at maximally tolerated doses in patients at very high risk for CVD when on-treatment LDL cholesterol remains above 70 mg/dL (or above 100 mg/dL in patients with familial hypercholesterolemia). Patients considered to be at very high-risk for CVD include those with recent acute coronary syndrome within 12 months; multiple prior myocardial infarctions or strokes; significant unrevascularized coronary artery disease; and polyvascular disease (coronary plus cerebrovascular or peripheral vascular disease).

D. Bile Acid–Binding Resins

The bile acid–binding resins include cholestyramine, colesevelam, and colestipol. In the pre-statin era, treatment with these agents reduced the incidence of coronary events in middle-aged men by about 20%, with no significant effect on total mortality. The resins work by binding bile acids in the intestine. The resultant reduction in the enterohepatic circulation causes the liver to increase its production of bile acids, using hepatic cholesterol to do so. Thus, hepatic LDL receptor activity increases, with a decline in plasma LDL levels. The triglyceride level tends to increase slightly in some patients treated with bile acid–binding resins; these resins should be used with caution in patients with elevated triglycerides and probably not at all in patients who have triglyceride levels above 500 mg/dL. The clinician can anticipate a reduction of 15–25% in the LDL cholesterol level, with insignificant effects on the HDL level.

These agents often cause gastrointestinal symptoms, such as constipation and gas. They may interfere with the absorption of fat-soluble vitamins (thereby complicating the management of patients receiving warfarin) and may bind other drugs in the intestine. Concurrent use of psyllium may ameliorate the gastrointestinal side effects.

E. Omega-3 Fatty Acid Preparations

Omega-3 fatty acids are essential fatty acids that must be consumed in the diet and are a prominent feature of Mediterranean-style diets. In pharmacologic doses, omega-3 fatty acid preparations can lower triglycerides by up to 30%, with modest reductions in apolipoprotein-B–containing lipoproteins and high-sensitivity C-reactive protein. Pharmacologic therapy should be differentiated from dietary omega-3 fatty acid supplements. The former is an FDA-approved product usually given at a much higher dose; dietary supplements are variable and not currently regulated.

There is weak evidence that omega-3 fatty acids reduce myocardial infarctions, though with no reduction in total or cardiovascular mortality. Omega-3 ethyl esters have not been associated with cardiovascular event reduction when added to statin therapy. In contrast, icosapent ethyl, which is a highly purified eicosapentaenoic acid (EPA) only preparation, was shown to reduce cardiovascular deaths, nonfatal myocardial infarctions, nonfatal strokes, coronary revascularizations, and unstable angina by 25% in statin-treated patients with triglycerides greater than 135 mg/dL in the 8179 person REDUCE-IT randomized clinical trial. The mechanism of icosapent ethyl is not yet clear but likely involves multiple mechanisms beyond lipid lowering, including antiplatelet activity, anti-inflammatory activity, and arrhythmia prevention.

F. Fibric Acid Derivatives

The fibrates are peroxisome proliferative-activated receptor-alpha (PPAR-alpha) agonists that result in significant reductions of plasma triglycerides and increases in HDL cholesterol. They reduce LDL levels by about 10–15% (although the result is quite variable) and triglyceride levels by about 40% and raise HDL levels by about 15–20%. The fibric acid derivatives or fibrates approved for use in the United States are gemfibrozil and fenofibrate. Ciprofibrate and bezafibrate are also available for use internationally.

Gemfibrozil monotherapy reduced CHD rates in hypercholesterolemic middle-aged men free of coronary disease in the Helsinki Heart Study. The effect was observed only among those who also had lower HDL cholesterol levels and high triglyceride levels. In a Veteran Affairs study, gemfibrozil monotherapy was also shown to reduce cardiovascular events in men with existing CHD whose primary lipid abnormality was a low HDL cholesterol. There was no effect on all-cause mortality.

However, fibrates have not been shown to reduce cardiovascular events in all statin-treated patients with CVD or diabetes. For example, in the ACCORD study, addition of fenofibrate to statin in patients with diabetes and mild triglyceride elevations resulted in no benefit.

The usual dose of gemfibrozil is 600 mg once or twice a day. Side effects include cholelithiasis, hepatitis, and myositis. The incidence of the latter two conditions may be higher among patients also taking other lipid-lowering

agents. Fenofibrate, 48–145 mg daily, can be used and has slightly fewer side effects than gemfibrozil. Resins are the only lipid-modifying medication considered safe in pregnancy.

G. Niacin (Nicotinic Acid)

Niacin was the first lipid-lowering agent that was associated with a reduction in total mortality. Long-term follow-up of a secondary prevention trial in middle-aged men with previous myocardial infarction disclosed that about half of those who had been previously treated with niacin had died, compared with nearly 60% of the placebo group. This favorable effect on mortality was not seen during the trial itself, though there was a reduction in the incidence of recurrent coronary events. A meta-analysis of 10 randomized trials using niacin in the pre-statin era showed a 27% reduction in cardiovascular events.

Niacin reduces the production of VLDL particles, with secondary reduction in LDL and increases in HDL cholesterol levels. The average effect of full-dose niacin therapy is a 15–25% reduction in LDL cholesterol and a 25–35% increase in HDL cholesterol. Full doses are required to obtain the LDL effect, but the HDL effect is observed at lower doses, eg, 1 g/day. Niacin also reduces triglycerides and can lower lipoprotein(a) (Lp[a]) levels. Intolerance to niacin is common; only 50–60% of patients can take full doses. Niacin causes a prostaglandin-mediated flushing that patients may describe as "hot flashes" or pruritus. It can be decreased with aspirin (81–325 mg/day) or other nonsteroidal anti-inflammatory agents taken an hour before niacin dosing. Extended-release niacin is better tolerated by most patients. Niacin can also exacerbate gout and peptic ulcer disease. Although niacin may increase blood sugar in some patients, clinical trials have shown that it can be safely used in diabetic patients.

In two large clinical trials, AIM-HIGH and HPS2-THRIVE, extended-release niacin did not reduce cardiovascular events when added to statin therapy in high-risk patients.

▶ Treatment Algorithms

For patients who require a lipid-modifying medication, an HMG-CoA reductase inhibitor (statin) is recommended. In patients with CVD, this should generally be at its maximally tolerated dose.

Combination therapy is indicated for (1) patients with familial hypercholesterolemia with on-treatment LDL cholesterol that is above 100 mg/dL and (2) patients with existing CVD with on-treatment LDL cholesterol that remains above 70 mg/dL. Patients with homozygous familial hypercholesterolemia may need plasmapheresis and/or special lipid-lowering therapies uniquely approved for this population (Table 28–3). Patients with heterozygous familial hypercholesterolemia may need two or more medications to get below the treatment threshold, while those with CVD less commonly need multiple medications. The 2018 AHA/ACC/Multi-specialty guidelines recommend addition of ezetimibe in high-risk patients, while reserving PCSK9

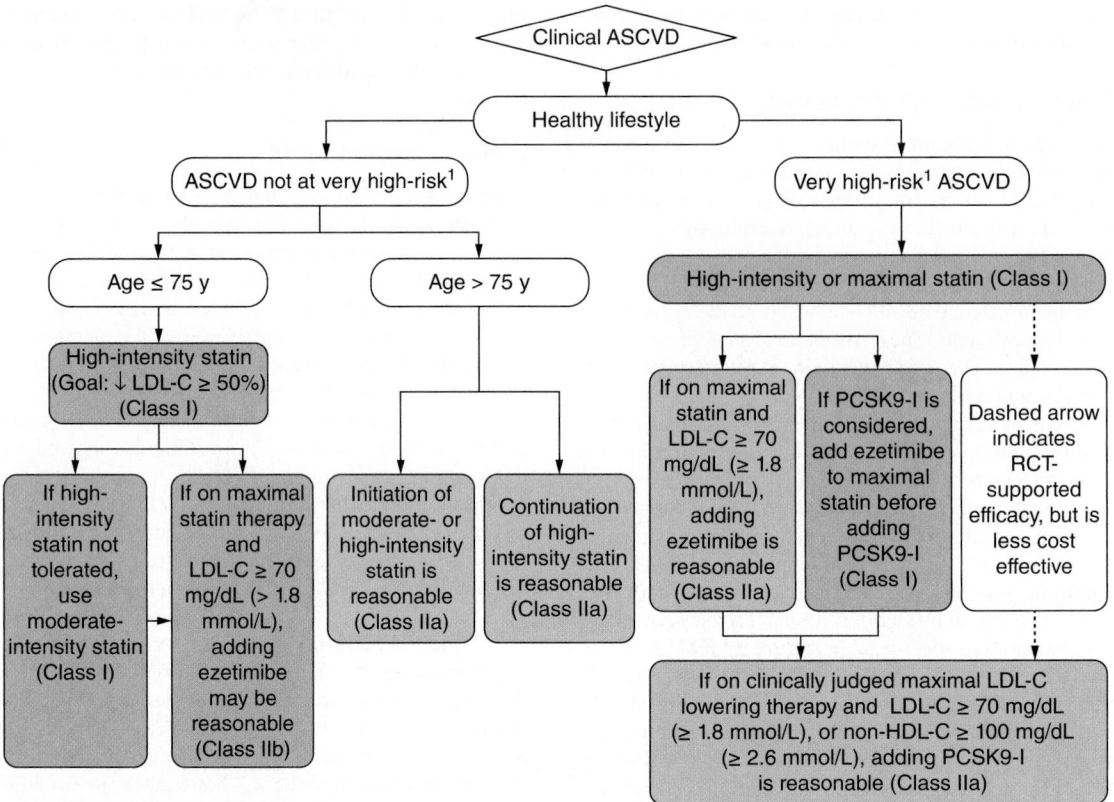

¹Very high-risk groups include patients with recent acute coronary syndrome within 12 months; multiple prior myocardial infarctions or strokes; significant unrevascularized coronary artery disease; and polyvascular disease (coronary + cerebrovascular or peripheral vascular)
(Class I = Strong recommendation [benefit >>> risk]; Class IIa = Moderately strong recommendation [benefit >> risk]; Class IIb = Weak recommendation [benefit > risk])
HDL-C, high-density lipoprotein cholesterol; LDL-C, low-density lipoprotein cholesterol; PCSK9-I, proprotein convertase subtilisin/kexin type 9 inhibitor; RCT, randomized controlled trial.

▲ **Figure 28–2.** Clinical treatment algorithm for patients with atherosclerotic cardiovascular disease (ASCVD). (Used, with permission, from Grundy SM et al. 2018 AHA/ACC/AACVPR/AAPA/ABC/ACPM/ADA/AGS/APhA/ASPC/NLA/PCNA Guideline on the Management of Blood Cholesterol: Executive Summary. Circulation. 2018 Nov 10. [Epub ahead of print]. © 2018 American Heart Association, Inc.)

inhibitor therapy for very high-risk patients or those taking maximally tolerated statins and ezetimibe with LDL cholesterol still not below 70 mg/dL (Figure 28–2).

Bhatt DL et al; REDUCE-IT Investigators. Cardiovascular risk reduction with icosapent ethyl for hypertriglyceridemia. N Engl J Med. 2019 Jan 3;380(1):11–22. [PMID: 30415628]

Cannon CP et al; IMPROVE-IT Investigators. Ezetimibe added to statin therapy after acute coronary syndromes. N Engl J Med. 2015 Jun 18;372(25):2387–97. [PMID: 26039521]

Cholesterol Treatment Trialists' (CTT) Collaboration. Efficacy and safety of LDL-lowering therapy among men and women: meta-analysis of individual data from 174,000 participants in 27 randomised trials. Lancet. 2015 Apr 11;385(9976):1397–405. [PMID: 25579834]

Grundy SM et al. 2018 AHA/ACC/AACVPR/AAPA/ABC/ ACPM/ADA/AGS/APhA/ASPC/NLA/PCNA guideline on the management of blood cholesterol: executive summary. Circulation. 2018 Nov 10. [Epub ahead of print] [PMID: 30565953]

Hovingh GK et al. Identification and management of patients with statin-associated symptoms in clinical practice: a clinician survey. Atherosclerosis. 2016 Feb;245:111–7. [PMID: 26717273]

HPS2-THRIVE Collaborative Group. Effects of extended-release niacin with laropiprant in high-risk patients. N Engl J Med. 2014 Jul 17;371(3):203–12. [PMID: 25014686]

Karmali KN et al. Drugs for primary prevention of atherosclerotic cardiovascular disease: an overview of systematic reviews. JAMA Cardiol. 2016 Jun 1;1(3):341–9. [PMID: 27438118]

Kazi DS et al. Cost-effectiveness of PCSK9 inhibitor therapy in patients with heterozygous familial hypercholesterolemia or atherosclerotic cardiovascular disease. JAMA. 2016 Aug 16; 316(7):743–53. [PMID: 27533159]

Mark DB et al. PCSK9 inhibitors and the choice between innovation, efficiency, and affordability. JAMA. 2017 Aug 22; 318(8):711–2. [PMID: 28829851]

Rosenson RS et al. Optimizing cholesterol treatment in patients with muscle complaints. J Am Coll Cardiol. 2017 Sep 5;70(10): 1290–301. [PMID: 28859793]

Sabatine MS et al. Clinical benefit of evolocumab by severity and extent of coronary artery disease. Circulation. 2018 Aug 21; 138(8):756–66. [PMID: 29626068]

Schwartz GG et al; ODYSSEY OUTCOMES Committees and Investigators. Alirocumab and cardiovascular outcomes after acute coronary syndrome. N Engl J Med. 2018 Nov 29; 379(22):2097–107. [PMID: 30403574]

Tice JA et al. Proprotein convertase subtilisin/kexin type 9 (PCSK9) inhibitors for treatment of high cholesterol levels: effectiveness and value. JAMA Intern Med. 2016 Jan 1; 176(1):107–8. [PMID: 26662572]

Wiggins BS et al. Recommendations for management of clinically significant drug-drug interactions with statins and select agents used in patients with cardiovascular disease: a scientific statement from the American Heart Association. Circulation. 2016 Nov 22;134(21):e468–95. [PMID: 27754879]

HIGH BLOOD TRIGLYCERIDES

Patients with very high levels of serum triglycerides (greater than 1000 mg/dL) are at risk for pancreatitis. The pathophysiology is not certain, since pancreatitis never develops in some patients with very high triglyceride levels. Most patients with congenital abnormalities in triglyceride metabolism present in childhood; hypertriglyceridemia-induced pancreatitis first presenting in adults is more commonly due to an acquired problem in lipid metabolism.

Although there are no clear triglyceride levels that predict pancreatitis, most clinicians treat fasting levels above 500 mg/dL (5 mmol/L). The risk of pancreatitis may be more related to the triglyceride level following consumption of a fatty meal. Because postprandial increases in triglyceride are inevitable if fat-containing foods are eaten, fasting triglyceride levels in persons prone to pancreatitis should be kept well below that level.

The primary therapy for high triglyceride levels is dietary, avoiding alcohol, simple sugars, refined starches, and saturated and trans fatty acids, and restricting total calories. Control of secondary causes of high triglyceride levels may also be helpful. In patients with fasting triglycerides greater than or equal to 500 mg/dL (5 mmol/L) despite adequate dietary compliance—and certainly in those with a previous episode of pancreatitis—therapy with a triglyceride-lowering drug (eg, statins, fibric acid derivative, omega-3-acid ethyl esters, or niacin) is indicated. Combinations of these medications may also be used.

Currently, drug treatment for patients with triglycerides greater than 150 mg/dL (1.5 mmol/L) is reserved for those with established CVD with well-controlled LDL cholesterol on maximally tolerated therapy with statins or other agents. Currently, data are strongest for icosapent ethyl.

Bhatt DL et al; REDUCE-IT Investigators. Cardiovascular risk reduction with icosapent ethyl for hypertriglyceridemia. N Engl J Med. 2019 Jan 3;380(1):11–22. [PMID: 30415628]

Chaudhry R et al. Pharmacological treatment options for severe hypertriglyceridemia and familial chylomicronemia syndrome. Expert Rev Clin Pharmacol. 2018 Jun;11(6):589–98. [PMID: 29842811]

Dallinga-Thie GM et al. Triglyceride-rich lipoproteins and remnants: targets for therapy? Curr Cardiol Rep. 2016 Jul;18(7):67. [PMID: 27216847]

Karalis DG. A review of clinical practice guidelines for the management of hypertriglyceridemia: a focus on high dose omega-3 fatty acids. Adv Ther. 2017 Feb;34(2):300–23. [PMID: 27981496]

Klempfner R et al. Elevated triglyceride level is independently associated with increased all-cause mortality in patients with established coronary heart disease: twenty-two-year follow-up of the Bezafibrate Infarction Prevention Study and Registry. Circ Cardiovasc Qual Outcomes. 2016 Mar;9(2):100–8. [PMID: 26957517]

Rygiel K. Hypertriglyceridemia—common causes, prevention and treatment strategies. Curr Cardiol Rev. 2018 Mar 14; 14(1):67–76. [PMID: 29366425]

Valdivielso P et al. Current knowledge of hypertriglyceridemic pancreatitis. Eur J Intern Med. 2014 Oct;25(8):689–94. [PMID: 25269432]

Wiesner P et al. Triglycerides: a reappraisal. Trends Cardiovasc Med. 2017 Aug;27(6):428–32. [PMID: 28438398]

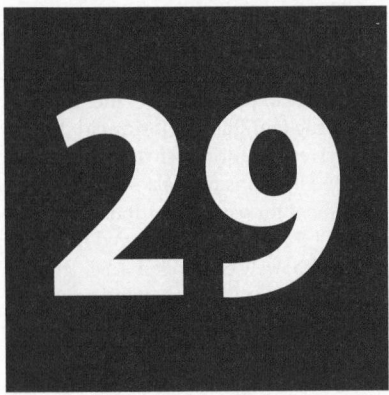

Nutritional Disorders

Katherine H. Saunders, MD

Leon I. Igel, MD, FACP, FTOS

Robert B. Baron, MD, MS

NUTRITIONAL DISORDERS

PROTEIN–ENERGY MALNUTRITION

ESSENTIALS OF DIAGNOSIS

► Decreased intake of energy or protein, increased nutrient losses, or increased nutrient requirements.

► **Kwashiorkor:** caused by protein deficiency.

► **Marasmus:** caused by combined protein and energy deficiency.

► Protein loss correlates with weight loss: 35–40% total body weight loss is usually fatal.

General Considerations

Protein–energy malnutrition occurs as a result of a relative or absolute deficiency of energy and protein. It may be primary, due to inadequate food intake, or secondary, as a result of other illness. For most developing nations, primary protein–energy malnutrition remains among the most significant health problems. It occurs in two distinct syndromes. **Kwashiorkor,** caused by a deficiency of protein in the presence of adequate energy, is typically seen in weaning infants at the birth of a sibling in areas where foods containing protein are insufficient. **Marasmus,** caused by combined protein and energy deficiency, is seen where adequate quantities of food are simply not available.

In industrialized societies, protein–energy malnutrition is most often secondary to other diseases. **Kwashiorkor-like secondary protein–energy malnutrition** occurs primarily in association with hypermetabolic acute illnesses such as trauma, burns, and sepsis. **Marasmus-like secondary protein–energy malnutrition** typically results from chronic diseases such as chronic obstructive pulmonary disease (COPD), heart failure, cancer, or AIDS. These two syndromes are estimated to be present in at least 20% of hospitalized patients. A substantially greater number of patients have risk factors that could result in them. In both syndromes, protein–energy malnutrition is caused either by decreased intake of energy and protein or by increased nutrient losses related to the underlying illness. For example, diminished energy intake may result from poor dentition or various gastrointestinal disorders. Increased nutrient losses result from malabsorption, diarrhea, and glycosuria. Increased nutrient requirements occur with fever, surgery, neoplasia, and burns.

Clinical Findings

Clinical manifestations of protein–energy malnutrition range from mild growth retardation and weight loss to a number of distinct clinical syndromes. In the developing world, children manifest marasmus and kwashiorkor. In industrialized nations, clinical manifestations of secondary protein–energy malnutrition are affected by the patient's nutritional status prior to illness, illness resulting in the protein and energy deficiency, and degree of the deficiency.

Progressive wasting that begins with weight loss and proceeds to more severe cachexia typically develops in most patients with marasmus-like secondary protein–energy malnutrition. In the most severe form of this disorder, most body fat stores disappear and muscle mass decreases, most noticeably in the temporalis and interosseous muscles. Laboratory studies may be unremarkable—serum albumin, for example, may be normal or slightly decreased, rarely decreasing to less than 2.8 g/dL (28 g/L). In contrast, owing to its rapidity of onset, kwashiorkor-like secondary protein–energy malnutrition may develop in patients with normal subcutaneous fat and muscle mass or, if the patient has obesity, even in patients with excess fat and muscle. The serum protein level, however, typically declines and the serum albumin is often less than 2.8 g/dL (28 g/L). Dependent edema, ascites, or anasarca may develop. As with primary protein–energy malnutrition, combinations of the marasmus-like and kwashiorkor-like syndromes can occur simultaneously, typically in patients with progressive chronic disease in whom a superimposed acute illness develops.

Treatment

The treatment of severe protein–energy malnutrition is a slow process requiring great care. Initial efforts should be directed at correcting fluid and electrolyte abnormalities and infections. Of particular concern are depletion of potassium, magnesium, and calcium and acid–base abnormalities. The second phase of treatment is directed at repletion of protein, energy, and micronutrients. Treatment is started with modest quantities of protein and calories calculated based on the patient's actual body weight. Adult patients are given 1 g/kg of protein and 30 kcal/kg of calories. Concomitant administration of vitamins and minerals is obligatory. Either the enteral or parenteral route can be used, although the former is preferable. Enteral fat and lactose are withheld initially. Patients with less severe protein–calorie undernutrition can be given calories and protein simultaneously with the correction of fluid and electrolyte abnormalities. Similar quantities of protein and calories are recommended for initial treatment.

Patients treated for protein–energy malnutrition require close follow-up. In adults, both calories and protein are advanced as tolerated, adults to 1.5 g/kg/day of protein and 40 kcal/kg/day of calories.

Patients who are refed too rapidly may develop a number of untoward clinical sequelae. During refeeding, circulating potassium, magnesium, phosphorus, and glucose move intracellularly and can result in low serum levels of each. The administration of water and sodium with carbohydrate refeeding can result in heart failure in persons with depressed cardiac function. Enteral refeeding can lead to malabsorption and diarrhea due to abnormalities in the gastrointestinal tract.

Refeeding edema is a benign condition to be differentiated from heart failure. Changes in renal sodium reabsorption and poor skin and blood vessel integrity result in the development of dependent edema without other signs of heart disease. Treatment includes reassurance, elevation of the dependent area, and modest sodium restriction. Diuretics are usually ineffective, may aggravate electrolyte deficiencies, and should not be used.

The prevention and early detection of protein–energy malnutrition in hospitalized patients require awareness of its risk factors and early symptoms and signs. Patients at risk require formal assessment of nutritional status and close observation of dietary intake, body weight, and nutritional requirements during the hospital stay.

Guyonnet S et al. Screening for malnutrition in older people. Clin Geriatr Med. 2015 Aug;31(3):429–37. [PMID: 26195101]

Marshall S. Why is the skeleton still in the hospital closet? A look at the complex aetiology of protein-energy malnutrition and its implications for the nutrition care team. J Nutr Health Aging. 2018;22(1):26–9. [PMID: 29300418]

Marshall S et al. A systematic review and meta-analysis of the criterion validity of nutrition assessment tools for diagnosing protein-energy malnutrition in the older community setting (the MACRo study). Clin Nutr. 2018 Dec;37(6 Pt A):1902–12. [PMID: 29102322]

McClave SA et al. Guidelines for the provision and assessment of nutrition support therapy in the adult critically ill patient: Society of Critical Care Medicine (SCCM) and American Society for Parenteral and Enteral Nutrition (A.S.P.E.N.). J Parenter Enteral Nutr. 2016 Feb;40(2):159–211. [PMID: 26773077]

Pereira GF et al. Malnutrition among cognitively intact, non-critically ill older adults in the emergency department. Ann Emerg Med. 2015 Jan;65(1):85–91. [PMID: 25129819]

Zha Y et al. Protein nutrition and malnutrition in CKD and ESRD. Nutrients. 2017 Feb 27;9(3):208. [PMID: 28264439]

OBESITY

ESSENTIALS OF DIAGNOSIS

▶ Excess adipose tissue; body mass index (BMI) greater than 30.

▶ Upper body obesity (abdomen and flank) of greater health consequence than lower body obesity (buttocks and thighs).

▶ Many associated comorbid conditions, including diabetes mellitus, hypertension, hyperlipidemia, heart disease, stroke, and sleep apnea.

▶ Definition & Measurement

Obesity is a multifactorial, chronic disease characterized by an accumulation of visceral and subcutaneous fat. Obesity predisposes to a wide variety of comorbid conditions. The **BMI** correlates with excess adipose tissue. It is calculated by dividing body weight in kilograms by height in meters squared. The National Institutes of Health (NIH) defines a normal BMI as 18.5–24.9. Overweight is defined as BMI 25–29.9. Class I obesity is 30–34.9, class II obesity is 35–39.9, and class III obesity is BMI greater than or equal to 40. Upper body obesity (excess fat around the waist and flank) is a greater health hazard than lower body obesity (fat in the thighs and buttocks). Patients with obesity and increased abdominal circumference (greater than 102 cm or 40 inches in men and 88 cm or 35 inches in women) or high waist–hip ratios (greater than 1.0 in men and 0.85 in women) have a greater risk of weight-related comorbid conditions and early death than patients with the same BMI and lower ratios. Furthermore, visceral fat within the abdominal cavity is more hazardous to health than subcutaneous fat around the abdomen. US survey data demonstrate that almost 40% of Americans have obesity.

▶ Etiology

Both genetic and environmental factors contribute to the development of obesity. Twin studies have demonstrated that genetics account for 50–90% of the variation in BMI. Only a small percentage of human obesity is thought to be due to single gene mutations. Most human obesity develops from the interactions of multiple genes, environmental factors, and behavior. The rapid increase in obesity in the last several decades points to major roles for environmental and behavioral factors in its development.

Medical Evaluation of the Patient with Obesity

Historical information should be obtained about age at onset, recent weight changes, family history of obesity, occupational history, eating and exercise behavior, cigarette and alcohol use, previous weight loss experience, and psychosocial factors including assessment for depression and eating disorders.

Physical examination should assess the BMI, degree and distribution of body fat, overall nutritional status, and signs of secondary causes of obesity. Less than 1% of patients with obesity have an identifiable secondary cause of obesity. Hypothyroidism and Cushing syndrome are important examples that can be diagnosed by physical examination, laboratory testing, and imaging studies in patients with unexplained recent weight gain. Such patients require endocrinologic evaluation (see Chapter 26). All patients with obesity should be assessed for weight-related comorbid conditions. Blood pressure, waist circumference, fasting glucose, comprehensive metabolic profile, lipid panel, and hemoglobin A_{1c} should be measured as well as other laboratory tests as clinically indicated.

Treatment

Weight loss of 5–10% body weight is sufficient for clinically relevant improvements in many risk factors among patients with obesity and risk reduction appears to be dose-related. Magnitude of weight loss at 1 year is strongly associated with improvements in many parameters including blood sugar, blood pressure, triglycerides, and high-density lipoprotein (HDL) cholesterol. Successful treatment of obesity requires a multidisciplinary approach to counteract the body's resistance to weight loss. Diet, physical activity, and behavioral modifications are the cornerstones of weight management. Many **dietary strategies** can be effective for weight loss. Recommendations should be tailored to a patient's preferences as dietary adherence is associated with greater weight loss and greater reductions in cardiac risk factors. Dietary instructions should emphasize intake of a variety of predominantly "unprocessed" foods, with special attention to limiting foods that provide large amounts of calories without other nutrients, ie, sugary drinks, fast food, junk food and sweets. A Mediterranean diet can be a good option for patients at high cardiovascular risk, since it has been shown to reduce the incidence of major cardiovascular events. A low-glycemic-index diet can curb hunger and decrease cravings by reducing blood sugar fluctuations. Meal replacement diets can also be used effectively to achieve weight loss. Registered dietitians can provide dietary education and customize diet plans.

Long-term changes in eating behavior are required to maintain weight loss and formal **behavior modification** programs are available. It is important to emphasize planning and self-monitoring, including weighing at regular intervals and keeping a food log to track caloric intake. Self-monitoring not only aids in behavioral change but also provides the practitioner with additional data from which to tailor recommendations. Patients can learn to recognize "eating cues" (emotional, situational, etc) and how to avoid or control them. As weight maintenance can be more challenging than initial weight loss, it is important that patients continue self-monitoring and regular follow up to ensure long-term adherence to their treatment plan.

Exercise offers several advantages for patients trying to lose weight and maintain weight loss. Aerobic exercise directly increases daily energy expenditure and is particularly useful for long-term weight maintenance. Exercise also preserves lean body mass and partially prevents the decrease in basal energy expenditure (BEE) resulting from weight loss. Compared to no treatment, exercise alone results in small amounts of weight loss. Exercise plus diet results in slightly greater weight loss than diet alone. A greater intensity of exercise is associated with a greater amount of weight loss. Up to 1 hour of moderate exercise per day is associated with long-term weight maintenance in individuals who have successfully lost weight.

The American College of Sports Medicine recommends 150 minutes of moderate-intensity aerobic physical activity (such as tennis or brisk walking) per week, 75 minutes of vigorous-intensity aerobic exercise (such as jogging or swimming laps) per week, or an equivalent combination of moderate- and vigorous-intensity aerobic activity. Episodes should last at least 10 minutes and, if possible, be spread out throughout the week. Weight resistance is also recommended at least twice per week. Exercise physiologists, physical therapists, and trainers can provide additional support for patients.

Medications can have unpredictable and variable effects on patients' weight, so it is important to review patients' medication regimens and balance the benefits of treatment against the probability of weight gain. Multiple medications are associated with weight gain, including corticosteroids, contraceptives and other hormonal agents as well as certain antidiabetic, antihypertensive, antidepressant, antipsychotic, antiepileptic, and antihistamine agents. Table 29–1 provides an overview of weight-gaining medications as well as potential alternatives. When possible, clinicians should prescribe weight-neutral or weight loss–promoting medications. If there are no alternatives, weight gain can be prevented or lessened by selecting the lowest dose needed to produce clinical efficacy for the shortest duration necessary.

Weight loss achieved by lifestyle modifications alone is often limited and difficult to maintain. As a result, patients may require antiobesity medications, bariatric surgery, devices, or endoscopic bariatric therapies to achieve and maintain clinically significant weight loss.

Antiobesity medications (Table 29–2) can be considered in patients with a BMI 30 or higher or a BMI 27 or higher with weight-related comorbidities. Since obesity is a chronic disease, most medications for weight loss are approved for long-term treatment. Medications approved for weight management should be viewed as additions to diet and exercise for patients who have been unsuccessful with lifestyle changes alone. The six most widely prescribed antiobesity medications approved by the FDA are phentermine, orlistat, phentermine/topiramate extended release (ER), lorcaserin, naltrexone sustained-release (SR)/bupropion SR, and liraglutide 3.0 mg. Table 29–2 provides an overview of these medications.

Table 29–1. Medications and their effects on weight.

Drug Class	Result: Weight Gain	Result: Weight Neutral (or Minor Weight Gain)	Result: Weight Loss
Antidiabetics	Insulin Meglitinides Sulfonylureas Thiazolidinediones	Alpha-glucosidase inhibitors Bromocriptine Colesevelam DPP-4 inhibitors	GLP-1 agonists Metformin Pramlintide SGLT2 inhibitors
Antihypertensives	Alpha-adrenergic blockers Beta-adrenergic blockers (atenolol, metoprolol, nadolol, propranolol)	ACE inhibitors ARBs Beta-adrenergic blockers (carvedilol, nebivolol) Calcium channel blockers Thiazides	
Antidepressants	Lithium MAOIs Mirtazapine SSRIs (paroxetine) Tricyclic antidepressants (amitriptyline, desipramine, doxepin, imipramine, nortriptyline)	SSRIs (fluoxetine, sertraline)	Bupropion
Antipsychotics	Clozapine Olanzapine Quetiapine Risperidone	Aripiprazole Lurasidone Ziprasidone	
Antiepileptics	Carbamazepine Gabapentin Pregabalin Valproic acid	Lamotrigine Levetiracetam Phenytoin	Topiramate Zonisamide
Contraceptives	Medroxyprogesterone acetate	Barrier methods IUDs Surgical sterilization	
Antihistamines	First-generation antihistamines	Second- and third-generation antihistamines	
Steroids	Glucocorticoids	Inhaled steroids Topical steroids	

ACE, angiotensin-converting enzyme; ARBs, angiotensin II receptor blockers; DPP-4, dipeptidyl peptidase-4; GLP-1, glucagon-like peptide-1; IUD, intrauterine device; MAOI, monoamine oxidase inhibitor; NSAIDs, nonsteroidal anti-inflammatory drugs; SGLT2, sodium-glucose co-transporter 2; SSRI, selective serotonin reuptake inhibitor.
(Adapted, with permission, from Igel LI et al. Practical use of pharmacotherapy for obesity. Gastroenterology. 2017 May;152(7):1765–79. Copyright © 2017 AGA Institute. Published by Elsevier, Inc.)

Phentermine is the most commonly prescribed adrenergic agonist and antiobesity medication in the United States; other adrenergic agonists include diethylpropion, benzphetamine, and phendimetrazine. In a 28-week randomized controlled trial, participants taking phentermine 15 mg daily lost an average of 6.0 kg compared with 1.5 kg among those assigned to placebo. The recommended dosage of phentermine is up to 37.5 mg daily, but the dosage should be individualized to achieve response with the lowest effective dose.

Orlistat works in the gastrointestinal tract to inhibit intestinal lipase, thus reducing dietary fat absorption. Not unexpectedly, it may cause diarrhea, gas, and cramping and perhaps reduced absorption of fat-soluble vitamins. Orlistat is associated with a 5.8 kg weight loss after 4 years compared to 3.0 kg with placebo. The recommended dose is 120 mg (Xenical, prescription-strength) or 60 mg (Alli, over-the-counter) three times a day with each main meal containing fat.

Lorcaserin, a selective serotonin 2C receptor agonist available at a dose of 10 mg orally twice daily or 20 mg ER once daily, is associated with 5.8% weight loss compared to 2.2% with placebo at 52 weeks. In the CAMELLIA-TIMI 61 trial, which enrolled a high-risk population of persons with obesity and overweight, lorcaserin facilitated sustained weight loss without a higher rate of major cardiovascular events compared to placebo.

The combination of **phentermine** and **topiramate ER** (3.75 mg/23 mg orally daily for 14 days, then 7.5 mg/46 mg orally daily, to a maximum dosage of 15 mg/92 mg orally daily) targets two different weight-regulation mechanisms simultaneously. In a 56-week clinical trial, participants taking 15/92 mg lost significantly more weight (9.8 kg) than those assigned to 7.5/46 mg (7.8 kg) or placebo (1.2 kg). The FDA requires a Risk Evaluation and Mitigation Strategy to inform women of reproductive potential and prescribers about a potential increased risk of orofacial clefts

Table 29-2. Medications tested in clinical trials for treatment of obesity.

Medication	Mechanism, Dosage, and Available Formulations	Trial and Duration	Trial Arms	Weight Loss (%)	Most Common Adverse Events	Good Candidates	Poor Candidates
Phentermine (Adipex,[1] Ionamin,[2] Lomaira[3]) Schedule IV controlled substance NOTE: approved for short-term use (up to 3 months)	Adrenergic agonist 8–37.5 mg daily (8 mg dose can be prescribed up to three times daily) Capsule, tablet	Aronne LJ et al.[4] 28 weeks	15 mg daily	6.06*	Dry mouth, insomnia, dizziness, irritability	Younger patients who need assistance with appetite suppression	Patients with uncontrolled hypertension, active or unstable coronary disease, hyperthyroidism, glaucoma, anxiety, insomnia, or general sensitivity to stimulants. Patients with a history of drug abuse or recent MAOI use. Patients who are pregnant
			7.5 mg daily	5.45*			
			Placebo (topiramate ER and phentermine/topiramate ER arms excluded)	1.71			
Orlistat (Alli,[5] Xenical[6])	Lipase inhibitor 60–120 mg three times daily with meals Capsule	XENDOS[7] 208 weeks	120 mg three times daily	9.6 (week 52)* 5.25 (week 208)*	Fecal urgency, oily stool, flatus with discharge, fecal incontinence	Patients with hypercholesterolemia and/or constipation who can limit their intake of dietary fat	Patients with malabsorption syndromes or other GI conditions that predispose to GI upset/diarrhea. Patients who cannot modify the fat content of their diets. Patients who are pregnant
			Placebo	5.61 (week 52) 2.71 (week 208)			
Phentermine/ Topiramate Extended Release (Qsymia)[8] Schedule IV controlled substance	Adrenergic agonist/ neurostabilizer 3.75/23–15/92 mg daily (dose titration) Capsule	EQUIP[9] 56 weeks	15/92 mg daily	10.9*	Paresthesias, dizziness, dysgeusia, insomnia, constipation, dry mouth	Younger patients who need assistance with appetite suppression	Patients with uncontrolled hypertension, active or unstable coronary disease, hyperthyroidism, glaucoma, anxiety, insomnia, or general sensitivity to stimulants. Patients with a history of drug abuse or recent MAOI use. Patients with a history of nephrolithiasis. Patients who are pregnant or trying to conceive
			3.75/23 mg daily	5.1*			
			Placebo	1.6			
		CONQUER[10] 56 weeks	15/92 mg daily	9.8*			
			7.5/46 mg daily	7.8*			
			Placebo	1.2 (weeks 0–56)			
		SEQUEL[11] 108 weeks (52-week extension of CONQUER trial)	15/92 mg daily	10.5*			
			7.5/46 mg daily	9.3*			
			Placebo	1.8 (weeks 0-108)			

Drug	Mechanism and Dose	Trial	Dose	% Weight Loss	Common Side Effects	Patients Who Would Benefit	Contraindications
Lorcaserin (Belviq, Belviq XR)[12] Schedule IV controlled substance	Serotonin (5-HT)$_{2C}$ receptor agonist 10 mg twice daily or 20 mg extended release daily. Tablet	BLOOM[13] 52 weeks	10 mg twice daily Placebo	5.8* 2.2	Headache, dizziness, fatigue, nausea, dry mouth, constipation	Patients who would benefit from appetite suppression	Patients on other serotonin-modulating medications, and patients with known cardiac valvular disease Patients who are pregnant
		BLOSSOM[14] 52 weeks	10 mg twice daily 10 mg daily Placebo	5.8* 4.7* 2.8			
		BLOOM-DM[15] 52 weeks	10 mg twice daily 10 mg daily Placebo	4.5* 5.0* 1.5			
Naltrexone/Bupropion Sustained-Release (Contrave)[16]	Opioid receptor antagonist/dopamine and norepinephrine reuptake inhibitor 8/90 mg daily to 16/180 mg twice daily. Tablet	COR-I[17] 56 weeks	16/180 mg twice daily 8/180 mg twice daily Placebo	6.1* 5.0* 1.3	Nausea, vomiting, constipation, headache, dizziness, insomnia, dry mouth	Patients who describe cravings for food and/or addictive behaviors related to food; patients who are trying to quit smoking, reduce alcohol intake, and/or who have concomitant depression	Patients with uncontrolled hypertension, uncontrolled pain, recent MAOI use, history of seizures, or any condition that predisposes to seizure, such as anorexia/bulimia nervosa, abrupt discontinuation of alcohol, benzodiazepines, barbiturates, or antiepileptic drugs Patients who are pregnant
		COR-II[18] 56 weeks	16/180 mg twice daily Placebo	6.4* 1.2			
		COR-BMOD[19] 56 weeks	16/180 mg twice daily Placebo	9.3* 5.1			
		COR-DIABETES[20] 56 weeks	16/180 mg twice daily Placebo	5.0* 1.8			
Liraglutide 3.0 mg (Saxenda)[21]	GLP-1 receptor agonist 0.6 to 3.0 mg daily. Prefilled pen for subcutaneous injection	SCALE Obesity and Prediabetes[22] 56 weeks	3.0 mg daily Placebo	8.0* 2.6	Nausea, vomiting, diarrhea, constipation, dyspepsia, abdominal pain	Patients who report inadequate meal satiety, and/or have type 2 diabetes, prediabetes, or impaired glucose tolerance Patients requiring use of concomitant psychiatric medications	Patients with a history of pancreatitis, personal/family history of MTC or MEN2 Patients with an aversion to needles Patients who are pregnant
		SCALE Diabetes[23] 56 weeks	3.0 mg daily 1.8 mg daily Placebo	6* 4.7* 2.0			
		SCALE Maintenance[24] 56 weeks (after initial ≥ 5% weight loss with low-calorie diet)	3.0 mg daily Placebo	6.2* 0.2			

(continued)

Table 29–2. Medications tested in clinical trials for treatment of obesity. (continued)

*P < 0.001 vs. placebo

[1]Adipex [package insert]. Tulsa, OK: Physicians Total Care, Inc; 2012.

[2]Ionamin [package insert]. Rochester, NY: Celltech Pharmaceuticals, Inc; 2006.

[3]Lomaira [package insert]. Newtown, PA: KVK-TECH, INC; 2016.

[4]Aronne LJ et al. Evaluation of phentermine and topiramate versus phentermine/topiramate extended-release in obese adults. Obesity (Silver Spring). 2013;21(11):2163–71.

[5]Alli [package insert]. Moon Township, PA: GlaxoSmithKline Consumer Healthcare, LP; 2015.

[6]Xenical [package insert]. South San Francisco, CA: Genentech USA, Inc; 2015.

[7]Torgerson JS et al. XENical in the prevention of diabetes in obese subjects (XENDOS) study: a randomized study of orlistat as an adjunct to lifestyle changes for the prevention of type 2 diabetes in obese patients. Diabetes Care. 2004;27(1):155–61.

[8]Qsymia [package insert]. Mountain View, CA: VIVUS, Inc; 2012.

[9]Allison DB et al. Controlled-release phentermine/topiramate in severely obese adults: a randomized controlled trial (EQUIP). Obesity (Silver Spring). 2012;20(2):330–42.

[10]Gadde KM et al. Effects of low-dose, controlled-release, phentermine plus topiramate combination on weight and associated comorbidities in overweight and obese adults (CONQUER): a randomized, placebo-controlled, phase 3 trial. Lancet. 2011;377(9774):1341–52.

[11]Garvey WT et al. Two-year sustained weight loss and metabolic benefits with controlled-release phentermine/topiramate in obese and overweight adults (SEQUEL): a randomized, placebo-controlled, phase 3 extension study. Am J Clin Nutr. 2012;95(2):297–308.

[12]Belviq [package insert]. Zofingen, Switzerland: Arena Pharmaceuticals; 2012.

[13]Smith SR et al. Multicenter, placebo-controlled trial of lorcaserin for weight management. N Engl J Med. 2010;363(3):245–56.

[14]Fidler MC et al. A one-year randomized trial of lorcaserin for weight loss in obese and overweight adults: the BLOSSOM trial. J Clin Endocrinol Metab. 2011;96(10):3067–77.

[15]O'Neil PM et al. Randomized placebo controlled clinical trial of lorcaserin for weight loss in type 2 diabetes mellitus: the BLOOM-DM study. Obesity (Silver Spring). 2012;20(7):1426–36.

[16]Contrave [package insert]. Deerfield, IL: Takeda Pharmaceuticals America, Inc; 2014.

[17]Greenway FL et al. Effect of naltrexone plus bupropion on weight loss in overweight and obese adults (COR-I): a multicentre, randomised, double-blind, placebo-controlled, phase 3 trial. Lancet. 2010;376(9741):595–605.

[18]Apovian CM et al. A randomized, phase 3 trial of naltrexone SR/bupropion SR on weight and obesity-related risk factors (COR-II). Obesity (Silver Spring). 2013;21(5):935–43.

[19]Wadden TA et al. Weight loss with naltrexone SR/bupropion SR combination therapy as an adjunct to behavior modification: the COR-BMOD trial. Obesity (Silver Spring). 2011;19(1):110–20.

[20]Hollander P et al. Effects of naltrexone sustained-release/bupropion sustained-release combination therapy on body weight and glycemic parameters in overweight and obese patients with type 2 diabetes. Diabetes Care. 2013;36(12):4022–9.

[21]Saxenda [package insert]. Plainsboro, NJ: Novo Nordisk; 2014.

[22]Pi-Sunyer X et al. A randomized, controlled trial of 3.0 mg of liraglutide in weight management. N Engl J Med. 2015;373(1):11–22.

[23]Davies MJ et al. Efficacy of liraglutide for weight loss among patients with type 2 diabetes: the SCALE Diabetes randomized clinical trial. JAMA. 2015;314(7):687–99.

[24]Wadden TA et al. Weight maintenance and additional weight loss with liraglutide after low-calorie-diet induced weight loss: the SCALE Maintenance randomized study. Int J Obes (Lond). 2013;37(11):1443–51.

GI, gastrointestinal; GLP-1, glucagon-like peptide-1; MAOI, monoamine oxidase inhibitor; MEN2, multiple endocrine neoplasia syndrome type 2; MTC, medullary thyroid carcinoma; XR, extended release.

Adapted, with permission, from Saunders KH et al. Obesity pharmacotherapy. Med Clin North Am. 2018 Jan;102(1):135–48. Copyright © Elsevier, Inc.

in infants exposed to the medication during the first trimester of pregnancy.

The combination of **naltrexone SR** and **bupropion SR** (8 mg/90 mg, increasing from 1 tablet orally daily by 1 additional daily tablet each week to a maximum of 2 tablets twice daily) reduces both appetite and food cravings by targeting two areas of the brain: the arcuate nucleus of the hypothalamus and the mesolimbic dopamine reward circuit. Naltrexone 32 mg/bupropion 360 mg is associated with a 6.1% reduction in body weight compared to 1.3% with placebo after 56 weeks. As with all antidepressants, bupropion carries a black box warning related to a potential increase in suicidality among younger patients during the early phase of treatment. Two cardiovascular outcome trials were terminated early.

Liraglutide, an injectable glucagon-like peptide-1 receptor agonist, is approved at a dose of 0.6 mg subcutaneously daily, increasing by 0.6 mg daily each week to a maximum of 3 mg subcutaneously daily. Liraglutide was initially FDA approved in 2010 for the treatment of type 2 diabetes at doses up to 1.8 mg subcutaneously daily. Liraglutide 3.0 mg subcutaneously daily is associated with 6.0% weight loss compared to 2.0% with placebo after 56 weeks. Thyroid C-cell tumors were found in rodents given supratherapeutic doses of liraglutide, but there is no evidence of liraglutide causing C-cell tumors in humans. Liraglutide 1.8 mg subcutaneously daily has been approved for cardiovascular risk reduction in patients with type 2 diabetes at elevated cardiovascular risk and a cardiovascular outcomes trial of liraglutide 3.0 mg is being conducted in patients with obesity.

Bariatric surgery is the most effective treatment for obesity. The three most common bariatric procedures in the United States are the sleeve gastrectomy, the Roux-en-Y gastric bypass, and the laparoscopic adjustable gastric band. Bariatric surgery can be considered in patients with a BMI 40 or higher or with a BMI 35 or higher plus one or more obesity-related complications who are motivated to lose weight but have not achieved sufficient weight loss to address health goals following lifestyle modification, with or without pharmacotherapy. Long-term medical follow up, lifestyle changes, and adherence to a vitamin regimen are crucial to the success of bariatric surgery; however, some patients have difficulty maintaining weight loss and regain some portion of the lost weight.

Sleeve gastrectomy involves removing approximately 70% of the stomach along the greater curvature. The pyloric valve and the small intestine remain intact. The fundus of the stomach, which secretes ghrelin, a hormone that stimulates appetite, is removed. Sleeve gastrectomy is associated with approximately 25% total body weight loss after 1 year. Because this procedure is mainly restrictive, there is a lower risk of nutritional deficiencies. In general, sleeve gastrectomy is associated with fewer complications than both the Roux-en-Y gastric bypass and laparoscopic adjustable gastric band. Early adverse events include bleeding, leakage along the staple line, stenosis, and vomiting. Late complications include gastroesophageal reflux, nutritional deficiencies, and stomach expansion, leading to decreased restriction. Unlike the other two procedures, sleeve gastrectomy is not reversible.

The **Roux-en-Y gastric bypass** attaches a small pouch created from the proximal stomach to the jejunum, thus bypassing the remainder of the stomach, duodenum, and most of the jejunum. Roux-en-Y gastric bypass is associated with approximately 30–35% total body weight loss at 2 years and greater improvements in comorbid disease markers compared to the two other procedures. Roux-en-Y gastric bypass is associated with a lower rate of gastroesophageal reflux than sleeve gastrectomy and can even alleviate gastroesophageal reflux in patients who have it. Roux-en-Y gastric bypass is often recommended over sleeve gastrectomy for patients with mild or moderate type 2 diabetes because it leads to greater long-term remission; however, both procedures have low efficacy for type 2 diabetes remission among patients with limited pancreatic beta cell reserve. Early adverse events associated with Roux-en-Y gastric bypass include obstruction, stricture, leak, and failure of the staple partition of the upper stomach. Late adverse events include nutritional deficiencies and anastomosis ulceration. Dumping syndrome can develop at any time. Roux-en-Y gastric bypass is technically a reversible procedure; however, it is generally only reversed in extreme circumstances.

The **laparoscopic adjustable gastric band** is an inflatable device that is placed around the fundus of the stomach to create a small pouch. This procedure is associated with 15% total body weight loss at 2 years. Laparoscopic adjustable gastric band is reversible and less invasive than the other two procedures, but it is associated with more complications than sleeve gastrectomy and Roux-en-Y gastric bypass. The most common adverse events include nausea, vomiting, obstruction, band erosion or migration, and esophageal dysmotility leading to acid reflux.

► When to Refer

- Patients with a BMI greater than or equal to 30 or a BMI greater than or equal to 27 with weight-related comorbidities may be referred to an obesity medicine specialist.

- Patients with a BMI greater than or equal to 40 (or greater than or equal to 35 with obesity-related morbidities) who have not achieved sufficient weight loss to address health goals following behavioral treatment, with or without pharmacotherapy, may be referred to a bariatric surgeon.

Courcoulas AP et al. Seven-year weight trajectories and health outcomes in the Longitudinal Assessment of Bariatric Surgery (LABS) Study. JAMA Surg. 2018 May 1;153(5):427–34. [PMID: 29214306]

Igel LI et al. Practical use of pharmacotherapy for obesity. Gastroenterology. 2017 May;152(7):1765–79. [PMID: 28192104]

Jakobsen GS et al. Association of bariatric surgery vs medical obesity treatment with long-term medical complications and obesity-related comorbidities. JAMA. 2018 Jan 16;319(3): 291–301. [PMID: 29340680]

LeBlanc EL et al. Behavioral and pharmacotherapy weight loss interventions to prevent obesity-related morbidity and mortality in adults. Updated evidence report and systematic review for the US Preventive Services Task Force. JAMA. 2018 Sep 18;320(11):1172–91. [PMID: 30326501]

Reges O et al. Association of bariatric surgery using laparoscopic banding, Roux-en-Y gastric bypass, or laparoscopic sleeve gastrectomy vs usual care obesity management with all-cause mortality. JAMA. 2018 Jan 16;319(3):279–90. [PMID: 29340677]

Ryan DH et al. Guideline recommendations for obesity management. Med Clin North Am. 2018 Jan;102(1):49–63. [PMID: 29156187]

Saunders KH et al. Devices and endoscopic bariatric therapies for obesity. Curr Obes Rep. 2018 Jun;7(2):162-71. [PMID: 29667157]

Saunders KH et al. Obesity pharmacotherapy. Med Clin North Am. 2018 Jan;102(1):135–48. [PMID: 29156182]

US Preventive Services Task Force. Behavioral weight loss interventions to prevent obesity-related morbidity and mortality in adults. US Preventive Services Task Force Recommendation Statement. JAMA. 2018 Sep 18;320(11):1163–71. [PMID: 30326502]

EATING DISORDERS

ANOREXIA NERVOSA

ESSENTIALS OF DIAGNOSIS

▶ Disturbance of body image and intense fear of becoming fat.

▶ Weight loss leading to body weight 15% below expected.

▶ In females, absence of three consecutive menstrual cycles.

General Considerations

Anorexia nervosa typically begins in the years between adolescence and young adulthood. Ninety percent of patients are female, most of middle and upper socioeconomic status.

The prevalence of anorexia nervosa is greater than previously suggested. Many adolescent girls have features of the disorder without the severe weight loss.

The cause of anorexia nervosa is not known. Although multiple endocrinologic abnormalities exist in these patients, most authorities believe they are secondary to malnutrition and not primary disorders. Most experts favor a primary psychiatric origin, but no hypothesis explains all cases. The patient characteristically comes from a family whose members are highly goal-oriented. The parents may be directive and concerned with slimness and physical fitness, and family conversation often centers around dietary matters. One theory holds that the patient's refusal to eat is an attempt to regain control of one's body in defiance of parental control. The patient's unwillingness to inhabit an "adult body" may also represent a rejection of adult responsibilities and the implications of adult interpersonal relationships. Patients are often perfectionistic in behavior and exhibit obsessional personality characteristics.

Clinical Findings

A. Symptoms and Signs

Patients with anorexia nervosa may exhibit severe emaciation and may complain of cold intolerance or constipation. Amenorrhea is almost always present. Bradycardia, hypotension, and hypothermia may be present in severe cases. Examination demonstrates loss of body fat, dry and scaly skin, and increased lanugo body hair. Parotid enlargement and edema may also occur.

B. Laboratory Findings

Laboratory findings are variable but may include anemia, leukopenia, electrolyte abnormalities, and elevations of blood urea nitrogen (BUN) and serum creatinine. Serum cholesterol levels are often increased. Endocrine abnormalities include depressed levels of luteinizing and follicle-stimulating hormones and impaired response of luteinizing hormone to luteinizing hormone-releasing hormone.

Diagnosis & Differential Diagnosis

The diagnosis is based on weight loss to a body weight 15% below expected, distorted body image, fear of weight gain or of loss of control over food intake and, in females, absence of at least three consecutive menstrual cycles. Other medical or psychiatric illnesses that can account for anorexia and weight loss must be excluded.

Behavioral features required for the diagnosis include intense fear of developing obesity, disturbance of body image, and refusal to exceed a minimal normal weight.

The differential diagnosis includes endocrine and metabolic disorders (eg, panhypopituitarism, Addison disease, hyperthyroidism, and diabetes mellitus); gastrointestinal disorders (eg, Crohn disease and gluten enteropathy); chronic infections (eg, tuberculosis); cancers (eg, lymphoma); and rare central nervous system disorders (eg, hypothalamic tumor).

Treatment

The goal of treatment is restoration of normal body weight and improvement in psychological difficulties. Hospitalization may be necessary. Treatment programs conducted by experienced teams are successful in about two-thirds of cases, restoring normal weight and menstruation. The remainder continue to experience difficulties with eating behaviors and psychiatric problems. About 2% to 6% of patients die of the complications of the disorder or commit suicide.

Various treatment methods have been used without clear evidence of superiority of one over another. Supportive care by clinicians and family is probably the most important feature of therapy. Cognitive-behavioral therapy, intensive psychotherapy, and family therapy may be tried. A variety of medications including tricyclic antidepressants, selected serotonin reuptake inhibitors (SSRIs), and lithium carbonate are effective in some cases; however, clinical trial results have been disappointing. Patients with severe malnutrition must be hemodynamically stabilized and may require enteral or parenteral feeding. Forced feedings should be reserved for life-threatening situations, since the goal of treatment is to reestablish normal eating behavior.

When to Refer

- Adolescents and young adults with otherwise unexplained profound weight loss should be evaluated by a psychiatrist.
- All patients with diagnosed anorexia nervosa should be co-managed with a psychiatrist.

When to Admit

- Signs of hypovolemia, major electrolyte disorders, and severe protein–energy malnutrition.
- Failure to improve with outpatient management.

Dalle Grave R et al. Cognitive behavioral therapy for anorexia nervosa: an update. Curr Psychiatry Rep. 2016 Jan;18(1):2. [PMID: 26689208]

Hay PJ et al. Individual psychological therapy in the outpatient treatment of adults with anorexia nervosa. Cochrane Database Syst Rev. 2015 Jul 27;(7):CD003909. [PMID: 26212713]

Hirst RB et al. Anorexia nervosa and bulimia nervosa: a meta-analysis of executive functioning. Neurosci Biobehav Rev. 2017 Dec;83:678–90. [PMID: 28851577]

Khalsa SS et al. What happens after treatment? A systematic review of relapse, remission, and recovery in anorexia nervosa. J Eat Disord. 2017 Jun 14;5:20. [PMID: 28630708]

McElroy SL et al. Psychopharmacologic treatment of eating disorders: emerging findings. Curr Psychiatry Rep. 2015 May; 17(5):35. [PMID: 25796197]

Treasure J. Applying evidence-based management to anorexia nervosa. Postgrad Med J. 2016 Sep;92(1091):525–31. [PMID: 26944338]

Westmoreland P et al. Medical complications of anorexia nervosa and bulimia. Am J Med. 2016 Jan;129(1):30–7. [PMID: 26169883]

BULIMIA NERVOSA

ESSENTIALS OF DIAGNOSIS

- ► Uncontrolled episodes of binge eating at least twice weekly for 3 months.
- ► Recurrent inappropriate compensation to prevent weight gain such as self-induced vomiting, laxatives, diuretics, fasting, or excessive exercise.
- ► Overconcern with weight and body shape.

General Considerations

Bulimia nervosa is the episodic uncontrolled ingestion of large quantities of food followed by recurrent inappropriate compensatory behavior to prevent weight gain, such as self-induced vomiting, diuretic or cathartic use, strict dieting, or vigorous exercise.

Like anorexia nervosa, bulimia nervosa is predominantly a disorder of young, white, middle- and upper-class women. It is more difficult to detect than anorexia, and some studies have estimated that the prevalence may be as high as 19% in college-aged women.

Clinical Findings

Patients with bulimia nervosa typically consume large quantities of easily ingested high-calorie foods, usually in secrecy. Some patients may have several such episodes a day over multiple days; others report regular and persistent patterns of binge eating. Binging is usually followed by vomiting, cathartics, or diuretics and accompanied by feelings of guilt or depression. Periods of binging may be followed by intervals of self-imposed starvation. Body weight may fluctuate but generally is within 20% of desirable weight.

Some patients with bulimia nervosa also have a cryptic form of anorexia nervosa with significant weight loss and amenorrhea. Family and psychological issues are generally similar to those of patients with anorexia nervosa. Bulimic patients, however, have a higher incidence of premorbid obesity, greater use of cathartics and diuretics, and more impulsive or antisocial behavior. Menstruation is usually preserved.

Medical complications are numerous. Gastric dilatation and pancreatitis have been reported after binges. Vomiting can result in poor dentition, pharyngitis, esophagitis, aspiration, and electrolyte abnormalities. Cathartic and diuretic abuse can also cause electrolyte abnormalities or dehydration. Constipation is common.

Treatment

Treatment of bulimia nervosa requires supportive care and psychotherapy. Individual, group, family, and behavioral therapy have all been utilized. Antidepressant medications may be helpful. The best results have been with fluoxetine and other SSRIs. Although death from bulimia is rare, the long-term psychiatric prognosis in severe bulimia is worse than that in anorexia nervosa.

When to Refer

All patients with diagnosed bulimia should be co-managed with a psychiatrist.

Linardon J et al. Psychotherapy for bulimia nervosa on symptoms of depression: a meta-analysis of randomized controlled trials. Int J Eat Disord. 2017 Oct;50(10):1124–36. [PMID: 28804915]

Palavras MA et al. The efficacy of psychological therapies in reducing weight and binge eating in people with bulimia nervosa and binge eating disorder who are overweight or obese—a critical synthesis and meta-analyses. Nutrients. 2017 Mar 17;9(3):299. [PMID: 28304341]

Westmoreland P et al. Medical complications of anorexia nervosa and bulimia. Am J Med. 2016 Jan;129(1):30–7. [PMID: 26169883]

DISORDERS OF VITAMIN METABOLISM

THIAMINE (B₁) DEFICIENCY

ESSENTIALS OF DIAGNOSIS

▶ Most common in patients with chronic alcoholism.

▶ Early symptoms of anorexia, muscle cramps, paresthesias, irritability.

▶ Advanced syndromes of high-output heart failure ("wet beriberi"), peripheral nerve disorders, and Wernicke-Korsakoff syndrome ("dry beriberi").

General Considerations

Most thiamine deficiency in the United States is due to chronic alcoholism, with poor dietary intake of thiamine and impaired thiamine absorption, metabolism, and storage. Thiamine deficiency is also associated with malabsorption, dialysis, and other causes of chronic protein–calorie undernutrition. Thiamine deficiency can be precipitated in patients with marginal thiamine status given intravenous dextrose solutions.

Clinical Findings

Early manifestations of thiamine deficiency include anorexia, muscle cramps, paresthesias, and irritability. Advanced deficiency primarily affects the cardiovascular system ("wet beriberi") or the nervous system ("dry beriberi"). Wet beriberi occurs in thiamine deficiency accompanied by severe physical exertion and high carbohydrate intake. Dry beriberi occurs in thiamine deficiency accompanied by inactivity and low-calorie intake.

Wet beriberi is characterized by marked peripheral vasodilation resulting in high-output heart failure with dyspnea, tachycardia, cardiomegaly, pulmonary edema, and peripheral edema with warm extremities mimicking cellulitis.

Dry beriberi involves both the peripheral and the central nervous systems. Peripheral nerve involvement is typically a symmetric motor and sensory neuropathy with pain, paresthesias, and loss of reflexes. The legs are affected more than the arms. Central nervous system involvement results in Wernicke-Korsakoff syndrome. Wernicke encephalopathy consists of nystagmus progressing to ophthalmoplegia, truncal ataxia, and confusion. Korsakoff syndrome includes amnesia, confabulation, and impaired learning.

Diagnosis

In most instances, the clinical response to empiric thiamine therapy is used to support a diagnosis of thiamine deficiency. The most commonly used biochemical tests measure thiamine concentration directly, while other assays measure erythrocyte transketolase activity and urinary thiamine excretion. Normal thiamine values typically range from 70 nmol/L to 180 nmol/L.

Treatment

Thiamine deficiency is treated with large parenteral doses of thiamine. Fifty to 100 mg/day is administered intravenously for the first few days, followed by daily oral doses of 5–10 mg/day. All patients should simultaneously receive therapeutic doses of other water-soluble vitamins. Although treatment results in complete resolution in half of patients (one-fourth immediately and another one-fourth over days), the other half obtain only partial resolution or no benefit.

When to Refer

Patients with signs of dry beriberi or Wernicke-Korsakoff syndrome should be referred to a neurologist. Patients with signs of wet beriberi should be referred to a cardiologist.

THIAMINE TOXICITY

There is no known toxicity of thiamine.

DiNicolantonio JJ et al. Thiamine and cardiovascular disease: a literature review. Prog Cardiovasc Dis. 2018 May - Jun;61(1):27-32. [PMID: 29360523]

Kröll D et al. Wernicke encephalopathy: a future problem even after sleeve gastrectomy? A systematic literature review. Obes Surg. 2016 Jan;26(1):205–12. [PMID: 26476834]

Isenberg-Grzeda E et al. Wernicke-Korsakoff syndrome in patients with cancer: a systematic review. Lancet Oncol. 2016 Apr;17(4):e142–8. [PMID: 27300674]

Scalzo SJ et al. Wernicke-Korsakoff syndrome not related to alcohol use: a systematic review. J Neurol Neurosurg Psychiatry. 2015 Dec;86(12):1362–8. [PMID: 25589780]

RIBOFLAVIN (B₂) DEFICIENCY

Clinical Findings

Riboflavin deficiency almost always occurs in combination with deficiencies of other vitamins. Dietary inadequacy, interactions with a variety of medications, alcoholism, and other causes of protein–calorie undernutrition are the most common causes of riboflavin deficiency.

Manifestations of riboflavin deficiency include cheilosis, angular stomatitis, glossitis, seborrheic dermatitis, weakness, corneal vascularization, and anemia.

Diagnosis

Riboflavin deficiency can be confirmed by measuring the riboflavin-dependent enzyme erythrocyte glutathione reductase. Activity coefficients greater than 1.2–1.4 are suggestive of riboflavin deficiency. Urinary riboflavin excretion and serum levels of plasma and red cell flavins can also be measured.

Treatment

Riboflavin deficiency is usually treated empirically when the diagnosis is suspected. It is easily treated with foods such as meat, fish, and dairy products or with oral preparations of the vitamin. Administration of 5–15 mg/day until clinical findings are resolved is usually adequate. Riboflavin can also be given parenterally, but it is poorly soluble in aqueous solutions.

RIBOFLAVIN TOXICITY

There is no known toxicity of riboflavin.

Manole A et al. Clinical, pathological and functional characterization of riboflavin-responsive neuropathy. Brain. 2017 Nov 1; 140(11):2820–37. [PMID: 29053833]
Saedisomeolia A et al. Riboflavin in human health: a review of current evidences. Adv Food Nutr Res. 2018;83:57–81. [PMID: 29477226]

NIACIN DEFICIENCY

▶ General Considerations

"Niacin" is a generic term for nicotinic acid and other derivatives with similar nutritional activity. Unlike most other vitamins, niacin can be synthesized from the amino acid tryptophan. Niacin is an essential component of the co-enzymes nicotinamide adenine dinucleotide (NAD) and nicotinamide adenine dinucleotide phosphate (NADP), which are involved in many oxidation-reduction reactions. The major food sources of niacin are proteins containing tryptophan and numerous cereals, vegetables, and dairy products.

Historically, niacin deficiency occurred when corn, which is relatively deficient in both tryptophan and niacin, was the major source of calories. Currently, niacin deficiency is more commonly due to alcoholism and nutrient–drug interactions. Niacin deficiency can also occur in inborn errors of metabolism. Niacin in the form of nicotinic acid is used therapeutically for the treatment of hypercholesterolemia and hypertriglyceridemia. Niacinamide (the form of niacin usually used to treat niacin deficiency) does not exhibit the lipid-lowering effects of nicotinic acid.

▶ Clinical Findings

As with other B vitamins, early manifestations of niacin deficiency are nonspecific—anorexia, weakness, irritability, mouth soreness, glossitis, stomatitis, and weight loss. More advanced deficiency results in the classic triad of pellagra: dermatitis, diarrhea, and dementia. The dermatitis is symmetric, involving sun-exposed areas. Skin lesions are dark, dry, and scaling. The dementia begins with insomnia, irritability, and apathy and progresses to confusion, memory loss, hallucinations, and psychosis. The diarrhea can be severe and may result in malabsorption due to atrophy of the intestinal villi. Advanced pellagra can result in death.

▶ Diagnosis

In early deficiency, diagnosis requires a high index of suspicion and attempts at confirmation of niacin deficiency. Niacin metabolites, particularly N-methylnicotinamide, can be measured in the urine. Low levels suggest niacin deficiency but may also be found in patients with generalized under-nutrition. Serum and red cell levels of NAD and NADP are also low but are similarly nonspecific. In advanced cases, the diagnosis of pellagra can be made on clinical grounds.

▶ Treatment

Niacin deficiency can be effectively treated with oral niacin, usually given as nicotinamide (10–150 mg/day).

NIACIN TOXICITY

At the high doses of niacin used to treat hyperlipidemia, side effects are common. These include cutaneous flushing (partially prevented by pretreatment with aspirin, 81–325 mg/day, and use of extended-release preparations) and gastric irritation. Elevation of liver enzymes, hyperglycemia, and gout are less common untoward effects.

Goldie C et al. Niacin therapy and the risk of new-onset diabetes: a meta-analysis of randomised controlled trials. Heart. 2016 Feb; 102(3):198–203. [PMID: 26370223]
Superko HR et al. Niacin and heart disease prevention: engraving its tombstone is a mistake. J Clin Lipidol. 2017 Nov–Dec; 11(6):1309–17. [PMID: 28927896]

VITAMIN B$_6$ DEFICIENCY

Vitamin B$_6$ deficiency most commonly occurs as a result of alcoholism or interactions with medications, especially isoniazid, cycloserine, penicillamine, and oral contraceptives. A number of inborn errors of metabolism and other pyridoxine-responsive syndromes, particularly pyridoxine-responsive anemia, are not clearly due to vitamin deficiency but commonly respond to high doses of the vitamin. Patients with common variable immunodeficiency may have concomitant vitamin B$_6$ deficiency.

▶ Clinical Findings

Vitamin B$_6$ deficiency results in clinical symptoms similar to those of other B vitamin deficiencies, including mouth soreness, glossitis, cheilosis, weakness, and irritability. Severe deficiency can result in peripheral neuropathy, anemia, and seizures.

▶ Diagnosis

The diagnosis of vitamin B$_6$ deficiency can be confirmed by measurement of pyridoxal phosphate in blood. Normal levels vary per laboratory but are typically greater than 5.0 ng/mL.

▶ Treatment

Vitamin B$_6$ deficiency can be effectively treated with vitamin B$_6$ supplements (10–20 mg/day orally). Some patients taking medications that interfere with pyridoxine metabolism (such as isoniazid) may need doses as high as 50–100 mg/day orally to prevent vitamin B$_6$ deficiency. This is particularly true for patients who are more likely to have diets marginally adequate in vitamin B$_6$, such as older patients, patients with alcoholism, or patients with lower socioeconomic status. Inborn errors of metabolism and pyridoxine-responsive syndromes often require doses up to 600 mg/day orally.

VITAMIN B₆ TOXICITY

A sensory neuropathy, at times irreversible, occurs in patients receiving large doses of vitamin B₆ (200–2000 mg/day).

Van Arsdale S et al. Pyridoxine deficiency after solid organ transplant. Prog Transplant. 2017 Sep;27(3):251–6. [PMID: 29187089]

VITAMIN B₁₂ & FOLATE

Vitamin B₁₂ (cobalamin) and folate are discussed in Chapter 13.

VITAMIN C (Ascorbic Acid) DEFICIENCY

Most cases of vitamin C deficiency seen in the United States are due to dietary inadequacy in patients with lower socioeconomic status, older patients, and patients with chronic alcoholism. Patients with chronic illnesses such as cancer and chronic kidney disease and individuals who smoke cigarettes are also at risk.

▶ Clinical Findings

Early manifestations of vitamin C deficiency are nonspecific and include malaise and weakness. In more advanced stages, the typical features of scurvy develop. Manifestations include perifollicular hemorrhages, perifollicular hyperkeratotic papules, petechiae and purpura, splinter hemorrhages, bleeding gums, hemarthroses, and subperiosteal hemorrhages. Anemia is common, and wound healing is impaired. The late stages of scurvy are characterized by edema, oliguria, neuropathy, intracerebral hemorrhage, and death.

▶ Diagnosis

The diagnosis of advanced scurvy can be made clinically on the basis of the skin lesions in the proper clinical situation. Atraumatic hemarthrosis is also highly suggestive. The diagnosis can be confirmed with decreased plasma ascorbic acid levels, typically below 0.2 mg/dL.

▶ Treatment

Adult scurvy can be treated with ascorbic acid 300–1000 mg/day orally. Improvement typically occurs within days.

VITAMIN C TOXICITY

Very large doses of vitamin C can cause gastric irritation, flatulence, or diarrhea. Oxalate kidney stones are of theoretical concern because ascorbic acid is metabolized to oxalate, but stone formation has not been frequently reported. Vitamin C can also confound common diagnostic tests by causing false-negative results for some fecal occult blood tests and both false-negative and false-positive results for urine glucose.

Al-Khudairy L et al. Vitamin C supplementation for the primary prevention of cardiovascular disease. Cochrane Database Syst Rev. 2017 Mar 16;3:CD011114. [PMID: 28301692]
Gabb G et al. Scurvy not rare. Aust Fam Physician. 2015 Jul; 44(7):438–40. [PMID: 26922826]
Granger M et al. Dietary vitamin C in human health. Adv Food Nutr Res. 2018;83:281–310. [PMID: 29477224]
Hagel AF et al. Plasma concentrations of ascorbic acid in a cross section of the German population. J Int Med Res. 2018 Jan; 46(1):168–74. [PMID: 2876008]
Monacelli F et al. Vitamin C, aging and Alzheimer's disease. Nutrients. 2017 Jun 27;9(7):670. [PMID: 28654021]

VITAMIN A DEFICIENCY

▶ Clinical Findings

Vitamin A deficiency is one of the most common vitamin deficiency syndromes, particularly in developing countries. In many such regions, it is the most common cause of blindness. In the United States, vitamin A deficiency is usually due to fat malabsorption syndromes or mineral oil laxative abuse and occurs most commonly in older adults and individuals of lower socioeconomic status.

Night blindness is the earliest symptom. Dryness of the conjunctiva (xerosis) and the development of small white patches on the conjunctiva (Bitot spots) are early signs. Ulceration and necrosis of the cornea (keratomalacia), perforation, endophthalmitis, and blindness are late manifestations. Xerosis and hyperkeratinization of the skin and loss of taste may also occur.

▶ Diagnosis

Abnormalities of dark adaptation are strongly suggestive of vitamin A deficiency. Serum levels below the normal range of 30–65 mg/dL are commonly seen in advanced deficiency.

▶ Treatment

Night blindness, poor wound healing, and other signs of early deficiency can be effectively treated with vitamin A 30,000 international units orally daily for 1 week. Advanced deficiency with corneal damage calls for administration of 20,000 international units/kg orally for at least 5 days. The potential antioxidant effects of beta-carotene can be achieved with supplements of 25,000–50,000 international units of beta-carotene.

VITAMIN A TOXICITY

Excess intake of beta-carotene (hypercarotenosis) results in staining of the skin a yellow-orange color but is otherwise benign. Skin changes are most marked on the palms and soles, while the scleras remain white, clearly distinguishing hypercarotenosis from jaundice.

Excessive vitamin A (hypervitaminosis A), on the other hand, can be quite toxic. Chronic toxicity usually occurs after ingestion of daily doses of over 50,000 international units/day for more than 3 months. Early manifestations include dry, scaly skin, hair loss, mouth sores, painful hyperostoses, anorexia, and vomiting. More serious findings include hypercalcemia; increased intracranial pressure with papilledema, headaches, and decreased cognition; and hepatomegaly, occasionally progressing to cirrhosis. Excessive vitamin A is also related to increased risk of hip fracture. Acute toxicity can result from ingestion of massive doses of vitamin A, such as in drug overdoses or consumption of polar bear liver. Manifestations include nausea, vomiting, abdominal pain, headache, papilledema, and lethargy.

The diagnosis can be confirmed by elevations of serum vitamin A levels. The only treatment is withdrawal of vitamin A from the diet. Most symptoms and signs improve rapidly.

Benn CS et al. An enigma: why vitamin A supplementation does not always reduce mortality even though vitamin A deficiency is associated with increased mortality. Int J Epidemiol. 2015 Jun;44(3):906–18. [PMID: 26142161]

Lu Z et al. Rapid diagnostic testing platform for iron and vitamin A deficiency. Proc Natl Acad Sci U S A. 2017 Dec 19; 114(51): 13513–8. [PMID: 29203653]

VITAMIN D

Vitamin D is discussed in Chapter 26.

VITAMIN E DEFICIENCY

▶ Clinical Findings

Clinical deficiency of vitamin E is most commonly due to severe malabsorption or abetalipoproteinemia in adults and chronic cholestatic liver disease, biliary atresia, or cystic fibrosis in children. Manifestations of deficiency include areflexia, disturbances of gait, decreased vibration and proprioception, and ophthalmoplegia.

▶ Diagnosis

Plasma vitamin E levels can be measured; normal levels are 0.5–0.7 mg/dL or higher. Since vitamin E is normally transported in lipoproteins, the serum level should be interpreted in relation to circulating lipid levels.

▶ Treatment

The optimum therapeutic dose of vitamin E has not been clearly defined. Large doses, often administered parenterally, can be used to improve the neurologic complications seen in abetalipoproteinemia and cholestatic liver disease. Several trials of supplemental vitamin E have shown slower cognitive decline in patients with Alzheimer disease. Vitamin E supplementation may also provide benefit in patients with nonalcoholic fatty liver disease.

VITAMIN E TOXICITY

Clinical trials have suggested an increase in all-cause mortality with high dose (400 international units/day or more) vitamin E supplements. Large doses of vitamin E can also increase the vitamin K requirement and can result in bleeding in patients taking oral anticoagulants.

Lloret A et al. The effectiveness of vitamin E treatment in Alzheimer's disease. Int J Mol Sci. 2019 Feb 18;20(4). [PMID: 30781638]

Okebukola PO et al. Vitamin E supplementation in people with cystic fibrosis. Cochrane Database Syst Rev. 2017 Mar 6; 3:CD009422. [PMID: 28262916]

VITAMIN K

Vitamin K is discussed in Chapter 14.

DIET THERAPY

In consultation with a registered dietician, specific therapeutic diets can be designed to facilitate the medical management of most common illnesses. Diet therapy is a difficult process, though, and not all patients are able to adhere to dietary recommendations. Requesting the patient to record dietary intake for 3–5 days may provide useful insight into the patient's motivation as well as providing nutrient information about the current diet.

Therapeutic diets can be divided into three groups: (1) diets that alter the consistency of food, (2) diets that restrict or otherwise modify dietary components, and (3) diets that supplement dietary components.

DIETS THAT ALTER CONSISTENCY

▶ Clear Liquid Diet

This diet provides adequate water, 500–1000 kcal as simple sugar, and some electrolytes. It is fiber free and requires minimal digestion or intestinal motility.

A clear liquid diet is useful for patients with resolving postoperative ileus, acute gastroenteritis, partial intestinal obstruction, and as preparation for diagnostic gastrointestinal procedures. It is commonly used as the first diet for patients who have been taking nothing by mouth for long periods. Because of the low calorie and minimal protein content of the clear liquid diet, it is used only for short periods.

▶ Full Liquid Diet

The full liquid diet provides adequate water and can be designed to provide adequate calories and protein. Vitamins and minerals—especially folic acid, iron, and vitamin B_6—may be inadequate and should be provided in the form of supplements. Dairy products and soups are used to supplement clear liquids. Commercial oral supplements can also be incorporated into the diet or used alone.

This diet is low in residue and can be used in many instances instead of the clear liquid diet described above—especially in patients with difficulty chewing or swallowing, with partial obstructions, or in preparation for some diagnostic procedures. Full liquid diets are commonly used following clear liquid diets to advance diets in patients who have been taking nothing by mouth for long periods.

Soft Diets

Soft diets are designed for patients unable to chew or swallow hard or coarse food. Tender foods are used, and most raw fruits and vegetables as well as coarse breads and cereals are eliminated. Soft diets are commonly used to assist in progression from full liquid diets to regular diets in postoperative patients, in patients who are too weak or those whose dentition is too poor to handle a regular diet, in head and neck surgical patients, in patients with esophageal strictures, and in other patients who have difficulty with chewing or swallowing.

The soft diet can be designed to meet all nutritional requirements.

DIETS THAT RESTRICT NUTRIENTS

Diets can be designed to restrict (or eliminate) virtually any nutrient or food component. The most commonly used restricted diets are those that limit sodium, fat, carbohydrate, and protein. Other restrictive diets include gluten restriction in gluten enteropathy, potassium and phosphate reduction in chronic kidney disease, and various elimination diets for food allergies.

Sodium-Restricted Diets

Low-sodium diets are useful in the management of hypertension and in conditions in which sodium retention and edema are prominent features, particularly heart failure, chronic liver disease, and chronic kidney disease. Sodium restriction may be beneficial with or without diuretic therapy. When used in conjunction with diuretics, sodium restriction allows lower dosage of the diuretic medication and may prevent side effects. Potassium excretion, in particular, is directly related to distal renal tubule sodium delivery, and sodium restriction will decrease diuretic-related potassium losses.

Typical American diets contain 4–6 g (175–260 mEq) of sodium per day. A no-added-salt diet contains approximately 3 g (132 mEq) of sodium per day. Further restriction can be achieved with diets of 2 or 1 g of sodium per day. Diets with more severe restriction are poorly accepted by patients and are rarely used. Current Institute of Medicine guidelines recommend 2.3 g of sodium per day, which is approximately 1 teaspoon of salt.

Dietary sodium includes sodium naturally occurring in foods, sodium added during food processing, and sodium added by the consumer during cooking and at the table. About 80% of the current US dietary intake is from processed and pre-prepared foods. Diets designed for 2.3 g of sodium per day require elimination of most processed foods, added salt, and foods with particularly high sodium content. Many patients with mild hypertension will achieve significant reductions in blood pressure (approximately 5 mm Hg diastolic) with this degree of sodium restriction.

Diets allowing 1 g of sodium require further restriction of commonly eaten foods. Special "low-sodium" products are available to facilitate such diets. These diets are difficult for most people to follow and are generally reserved for hospitalized patients, most commonly those with severe liver disease and ascites.

Fat-Restricted Diets & Low-Saturated-Fat Diets

Traditional fat-restricted diets are useful in the treatment of fat malabsorption syndromes. Such diets will improve the symptoms of diarrhea with steatorrhea independently of the primary physiologic abnormality by limiting the quantity of fatty acids that reach the colon. The degree of fat restriction necessary to control symptoms must be individualized. Patients with severe malabsorption can be limited to 40–60 g of fat per day. Diets containing 60–80 g of fat per day can be designed for patients with less severe abnormalities.

Fat-restricted diets that specifically restrict saturated fats are the mainstay of dietary treatment of hyperlipidemia with elevated low-density lipoprotein cholesterol (see Chapter 28). Similar diets are often recommended for the prevention of coronary artery disease (see Chapter 10). The large Women's Health Initiative Dietary Modification Trial, however, did not show any significant benefit of a low-fat diet on weight control or prevention of cardiovascular disease or cancer. In contrast, a study of Mediterranean diets, supplemented by nuts or extra-virgin olive oil, did demonstrate a reduction in cardiovascular events.

The aim of low-fat diets is to restrict total fat to less than 30% of calories and to achieve a normal body weight by caloric restriction and increased physical activity. Saturated fat is restricted to 7% of calories. Saturated fat and total fat can be restricted further, but studies suggest that more extreme restriction offers little further advantage in overall modification of serum lipids. Low-fat diets can be augmented with the addition of plant stanols and sterols and with soluble dietary fiber to further reduce serum lipids.

Carbohydrate-Restricted Diets

Low carbohydrate diets restrict carbohydrate intake to at most 50–100 g/day (sometimes even lower). The consumption of foods that contain higher protein and fat with a lower carbohydrate content has been shown to promote satiety. Carbohydrate-restricted diets, including low glycemic index diets (see Chapter 27), can be particularly helpful for patients with type 2 diabetes and other forms of insulin resistance to reduce both blood sugar and weight. There have been several studies investigating the efficacy of low-fat versus low-carbohydrate diets for weight loss with no clear benefit of one versus the other.

Protein-Restricted Diets

Protein-restricted diets are most commonly used in patients with hepatic encephalopathy due to chronic liver disease and in patients with advanced chronic kidney disease to slow the progression of early disease and to decrease symptoms of uremia in more severe disease. Patients with selected inborn errors of amino acid metabolism and other abnormalities resulting in hyperammonemia also require restriction of protein or of specific amino acids.

Protein restriction is intended to limit the production of nitrogenous waste products. Energy intake must be adequate to facilitate the efficient use of dietary protein.

Proteins must be of high biologic value and be provided in sufficient quantity to meet minimal requirements. For most patients, the diet should contain at least 0.6 g/kg/day of protein. Patients with encephalopathy who do not respond to this degree of restriction are unlikely to respond to more severe restriction.

DIETS THAT SUPPLEMENT NUTRIENTS

▶ High-Fiber Diet

Dietary fiber is a diverse group of plant constituents that is resistant to digestion by the human digestive tract. Guidelines suggest that men should eat 30–38 g/day and women 21–25 g/day. Typical US diets, however, contain about half of that amount. Epidemiologic evidence has suggested that populations consuming greater quantities of fiber have a lower incidence of certain gastrointestinal disorders, including diverticulitis and, in some studies, colon cancer and a lower risk of cardiovascular disease. A meta-analysis of 22 studies suggested that each 7 g of dietary fiber was associated with a 9% decrease in first cardiovascular event.

Diets high in dietary fiber (21–38 g/day) are also commonly used in the management of a variety of gastrointestinal disorders, particularly irritable bowel syndrome and recurrent diverticulitis. Diets high in fiber, particularly soluble fiber, may also be useful to reduce blood sugar in patients with diabetes and to reduce cholesterol levels in patients with hypercholesterolemia. Good sources of soluble fiber are oats, nuts, seeds, legumes, and most fruits. Foods with insoluble fiber include whole wheat, brown rice, other whole grains, and most vegetables. For some patients, the addition of psyllium seed (2 tsp per day) or natural bran (one-half cup per day) may be a useful adjunct to increase dietary fiber.

▶ High-Potassium Diets

Potassium-supplemented diets are used most commonly to compensate for potassium losses caused by diuretics. Although potassium losses can be partially prevented by using lower doses of diuretics, concurrent sodium restriction, and potassium-sparing diuretics, some patients require additional potassium to prevent hypokalemia. High-potassium diets may also have a direct antihypertensive effect. Typical American diets contain about 3 g (80 mEq) of potassium per day. High-potassium diets commonly contain 4.5–7 g (120–180 mEq) of potassium per day.

Most fruits, vegetables, and their juices contain high concentrations of potassium. Supplemental potassium can also be provided with potassium-containing salt substitutes (up to 20 mEq in one-quarter tsp) or as potassium chloride in solution or capsules, but this is rarely necessary if the above measures are followed to prevent potassium losses and to supplement dietary potassium.

▶ High-Calcium Diets

Additional intake of dietary calcium has been recommended for the prevention of postmenopausal osteoporosis, the prevention and treatment of hypertension, and the prevention of colon cancer. The Women's Health Initiative, however, suggested that calcium and vitamin D supplementation did not prevent fractures or colon cancer. Observational studies have also suggested that calcium supplements, especially when taken without vitamin D, may be associated with an increased risk of coronary heart disease. The recommended dietary allowance for the total calcium intake (from food and supplements) in adults ranges from 1000 mg/day to 1200 mg/day. Average American daily intakes are approximately 700 mg/day.

Dairy products are the primary dietary sources of calcium in the United States. An 8-ounce glass of milk, for example, contains approximately 300 mg of calcium. Patients with lactose intolerance who cannot tolerate liquid dairy products may be able to use lactose-free milk, take supplemental lactase enzyme supplements, or tolerate nonliquid products such as yogurt and aged cheeses. Leafy green vegetables and canned fish with bones also contain high concentrations of calcium, although the latter is also high in sodium.

Dinu M et al. A heart-healthy diet: recent insights and practical recommendations. Curr Cardiol Rep. 2017 Aug 24;19(10):95. [PMID: 28840462]

Estruch R et al; PREDIMED Study Investigators. Primary prevention of cardiovascular disease with a Mediterranean diet supplemented with extra-virgin olive oil or nuts. N Engl J Med. 2018 Jun 21;378(25):e34. [PMID: 29897866]

Gardner CD et al. Effect of low-fat vs low-carbohydrate diet on 12-month weight loss in overweight adults and the association with genotype pattern or insulin secretion: the DIET-FITS randomized clinical trial. JAMA. 2018 Feb 20;319(7):667–79. Errata in: JAMA. 2018 Apr 3;319(13):1386; JAMA. 2018 Apr 24;319(16):1728. [PMID: 29466592]

Rehm CD et al. Dietary intake among US adults, 1999–2012. JAMA. 2016 Jun 21;315(23):2542–53. [PMID: 27327801]

▼ NUTRITIONAL SUPPORT

Nutritional support is the provision of nutrients to patients who cannot meet their nutritional requirements by eating standard diets. Nutrients may be delivered enterally, using oral nutritional supplements, nasogastric and nasoduodenal feeding tubes, and tube enterostomies, or parenterally, using lines or catheters placed in peripheral or central veins, respectively. Current nutritional support techniques permit adequate nutrient delivery to most patients. Nutrition support should be utilized, however, only if it is likely to improve the patient's clinical outcome. The financial costs and risks of side effects must be balanced against the potential advantages of improved nutritional status in each clinical situation.

INDICATIONS FOR NUTRITIONAL SUPPORT

The precise indications for nutritional support remain controversial. Most authorities agree that nutritional support is indicated for at least four groups of adult patients: (1) those with inadequate bowel syndromes, (2) those with severe prolonged hypercatabolic states (eg, due to extensive burns, multiple trauma, mechanical ventilation), (3) those requiring prolonged therapeutic bowel rest, and (4) those with severe protein–calorie undernutrition with a treatable disease who have sustained a loss of over 25% of body weight.

It has been difficult to prove the efficacy of nutritional support in the treatment of most other conditions. In most cases it has not been possible to show a clear advantage of treatment by means of nutritional support over treatment without such support.

The American Society for Parenteral and Enteral Nutrition (ASPEN) has published recommendations for the rational use of nutritional support. The recommendations emphasize the need to individualize the decision to begin nutritional support, weighing the risks and costs against the benefits to each patient. They also reinforce the need to identify high-risk malnourished patients by nutritional assessment.

► Nutritional Support Methods

Selection of the most appropriate nutritional support method involves consideration of gastrointestinal function, the anticipated duration of nutritional support, and the ability of each method to meet the patient's nutritional requirements. The method chosen should meet the patient's nutritional needs with the lowest risk and lowest cost possible. For most patients, enteral feeding is safer and cheaper and offers significant physiologic advantages. An algorithm for selection of the most appropriate nutritional support method is presented in Figure 29–1.

Prior to initiating specialized enteral nutritional support, efforts should be made to supplement food intake. Attention to patient food preferences, timing of meals in relation to diagnostic procedures and required medications, and the use of foods brought to the hospital by family and friends can often increase oral intake. Patients unable to eat enough at regular mealtimes to meet nutritional requirements can be given **oral supplements** as snacks or to replace low-calorie beverages. Oral supplements of differing nutritional composition are available for the purpose of individualizing the diet in accordance with specific clinical requirements. Fiber and lactose content, caloric density, protein level, amino acid profiles, vitamin K, and calcium can all be modified as necessary.

Patients unable to take adequate oral nutrients who have functioning gastrointestinal tracts and who meet the criteria for nutritional support are candidates for **liquid artificial nutrition ("tube feedings")**. Small-bore feeding tubes are placed via the nose into the stomach or duodenum. Patients able to sit up in bed who can protect their airways can be fed into the stomach. Because of the increased risk of aspiration, patients who cannot adequately protect their airways should be fed nasoduodenally (though, as noted below, this may not prevent all aspirations, particularly if the pylorus is patulous). Feeding tubes can usually be passed into the duodenum by leaving an extra length of tubing in the stomach and placing the patient in the right decubitus position. Metoclopramide, 10 mg intravenously, can be given 20 minutes prior to insertion and continued every 6 hours thereafter to facilitate passage through the pylorus. Occasionally, patients will require fluoroscopic or endoscopic guidance to insert the tube distal to the pylorus. Placement of nasogastric and, particularly, nasoduodenal tubes should be confirmed radiographically before delivery of feeding solutions.

Liquid artificial nutrition can also be accomplished by placing tubes directly into the gastrointestinal tract using **tube enterostomies**. Most tube enterostomies are placed in patients who require long-term enteral nutritional support. Gastrostomies have the advantage of allowing bolus feedings, while jejunostomies require continuous infusions. Gastrostomies—like nasogastric feeding—should be used only in patients at low risk for aspiration. Gastrostomies can also be placed percutaneously with the aid of endoscopy. These tubes can then be advanced into the jejunum. Tube enterostomies can also be placed surgically.

Patients who require nutritional support but whose gastrointestinal tracts are nonfunctional should receive **parenteral nutritional support**. Most patients receive parenteral feedings via a central vein—most commonly the subclavian vein. Peripheral veins can be used in some patients, but this

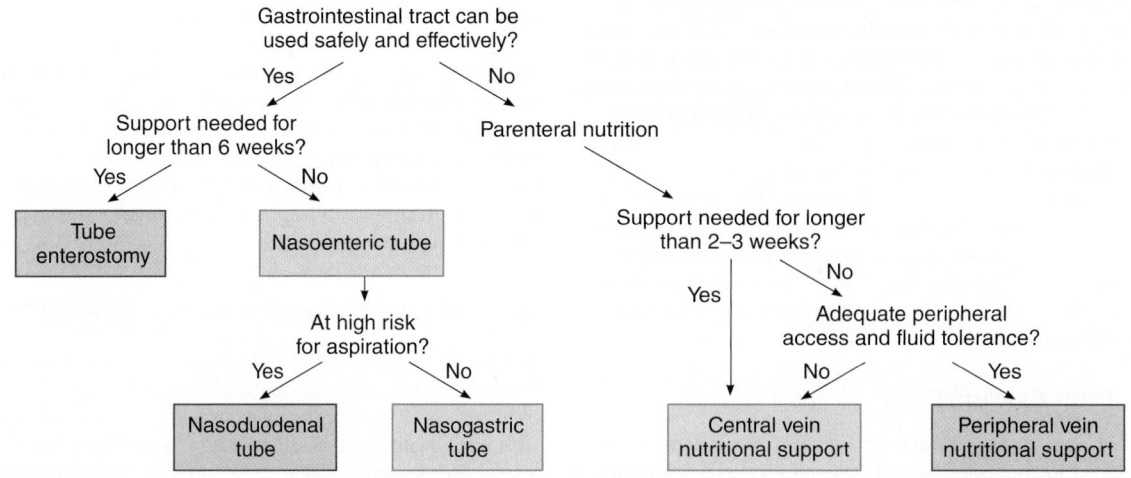

▲ **Figure 29–1.** Nutritional support method decision tree.

is rarely tolerated for more than a few weeks because of the high osmolality of parenteral solutions.

Peripheral vein nutritional support is most commonly used in patients with nonfunctioning gastrointestinal tracts who require immediate support but whose clinical status is expected to improve within 1–2 weeks, allowing enteral feeding. Peripheral vein nutritional support is administered via standard intravenous lines. Solutions should always include lipid and dextrose in combination with amino acids to provide adequate nonprotein calories. Serious side effects are infrequent, but there is a high incidence of phlebitis and infiltration of intravenous lines.

Central vein nutritional support is delivered via intravenous catheters placed percutaneously using aseptic technique. Proper placement in the superior vena cava is documented radiographically before the solution is infused. Catheters must be carefully maintained by experienced nursing personnel and used solely for nutritional support to prevent infection and other catheter-related complications.

NUTRITIONAL REQUIREMENTS

Each patient's nutritional requirements should be determined independently of the method of nutritional support. In most situations, solutions of equal nutrient value can be designed for delivery via enteral and parenteral routes, but differences in absorption must be considered. A complete nutritional support solution must contain water, energy, amino acids, electrolytes, vitamins, minerals, and essential fatty acids.

▶ Water

For most patients, water requirements can be calculated by allowing 1500 mL for the first 20 kg of body weight plus 20 mL for every kilogram over 20. Additional losses should be replaced as they occur. For average-sized adult patients, fluid needs are about 30–35 mL/kg, or approximately 1 mL/kcal of energy required.

▶ Energy

Energy requirements can be estimated by one of three methods: (1) by using standard equations to calculate BEE plus additional calories for activity and illness, (2) by applying a simple calculation based on calories per kilogram of body weight, or (3) by measuring energy expenditure with indirect calorimetry.

BEE can be estimated by the **Harris–Benedict equation**: for men, BEE = 666 + (13.7 × weight in kg) + (5 × height in cm) – (6.8 × age in years). For women, BEE = 655 + (9.5 × weight in kg) + (1.8 × height in cm) – (4.7 × age in years). For undernourished patients, actual body weight should be used; for patients with obesity, ideal body weight should be used. For most patients, an additional 20–50% of BEE is administered as nonprotein calories to accommodate energy expenditures during activity or relating to the illness. Occasional patients are noted to have energy expenditures greater than 150% of BEE.

Energy requirements can be estimated also by multiplying actual body weight in kilograms (for patients with obesity, ideal body weight) by 30–35 kcal.

Both of these methods provide imprecise estimates of actual energy expenditures, especially for the markedly underweight, overweight, and critically ill patient. Studies using indirect calorimetry have demonstrated that as many as 30–40% of patients will have measured expenditures 10% above or below estimated values. For a more accurate determination of energy expenditure, indirect calorimetry can be used.

▶ Protein

Protein and energy requirements are closely related. If adequate calories are provided, most patients can be given 0.8–1.2 g of protein per kilogram per day. Patients undergoing moderate to severe stress should receive up to 1.5 g/kg/day. As in the case of energy requirements, actual weights should be used for normal and underweight patients and ideal weights for patients with significant obesity.

Patients who are receiving protein without adequate calories will catabolize protein for energy rather than utilizing it for protein synthesis. Thus, when energy intake is low, excess protein is needed for nitrogen balance. If both energy and protein intakes are low, extra energy will have a more significant positive effect on nitrogen balance than extra protein.

▶ Electrolytes & Minerals

Requirements for sodium, potassium, and chloride vary widely. Most patients require 45–145 mEq/day of each. The actual requirement in individual patients will depend on the patient's cardiovascular, renal, endocrine, and gastrointestinal status as well as measurements of serum concentration.

Patients receiving enteral nutritional support should receive adequate vitamins and minerals according to the recommended daily allowances. Most premixed enteral solutions provide adequate vitamins and minerals as long as adequate calories are administered.

Patients receiving parenteral nutritional support require smaller amounts of minerals: calcium, 10–15 mEq/day; phosphorus, 15–20 mEq per 1000 nonprotein calories; and magnesium, 16–24 mEq/day. Most patients receiving nutritional support do not require supplemental iron because body stores are adequate. Iron nutrition should be monitored closely by following the hemoglobin concentration, mean corpuscular volume, and iron studies. Parenteral administration of iron is associated with a number of adverse effects and should be reserved for iron-deficient patients unable to take oral iron.

Patients receiving parenteral nutritional support should be given the trace elements zinc (about 5 mg/day) and copper (about 2 mg/day). Patients with diarrhea will require additional zinc to replace fecal losses. Additional trace elements—especially chromium, manganese, and selenium—are provided to patients receiving long-term parenteral nutrition.

Parenteral vitamins are provided daily. Standardized multivitamin solutions are currently available to provide adequate quantities of vitamins A, B_{12}, C, D, E, thiamine, riboflavin, niacin, pantothenic acid, pyridoxine, folic acid, and biotin. Vitamin K is not given routinely but administered when the prothrombin time becomes abnormal.

► Essential Fatty Acids

Patients receiving nutritional support should be given 2–4% of their total calories as linoleic acid to prevent essential fatty acid deficiency. Most prepared enteral solutions contain adequate linoleic acid. Patients receiving parenteral nutrition should be given at least 250 mL of a 20% intravenous fat (emulsified soybean or safflower oil) about two or three times a week. Intravenous fat can also be used as an energy source in place of dextrose.

ENTERAL NUTRITIONAL SUPPORT SOLUTIONS

Most patients who require enteral nutritional support can be given commercially prepared enteral solutions (Table 29–3). Nutritionally complete solutions have been designed to provide adequate proportions of water, energy, protein, and micronutrients. Nutritionally incomplete solutions are also available to provide specific macronutrients (eg, protein, carbohydrate, and fat) to supplement complete solutions for patients with unusual requirements or to design solutions that are not available commercially.

Table 29–3. Enteral solutions.

Complete
Blenderized (eg, Compleat Regular, Compleat Modified[1])
Whole protein, lactose-containing (eg, Carnation Instant Breakfast)
Whole protein, lactose-free, low-residue:
1 kcal/mL (eg, Ensure, Isocal, Osmolite, Nutren 1.0,[1] Sustacal, Resource)
1.5 kcal/mL (eg, Ensure Plus, Comply, Nutren 1.5, Resource Plus)
2 kcal/mL (eg, Isocal HN, Magnacal, TwoCal HN)
High-nitrogen: > 15% total calories from protein (eg, Ensure HN, Osmolite HN,[1] Replete, Isocal HN,[1] Isosource HN,[1])
Whole protein, lactose-free, high-residue:
1 kcal/mL (eg, Jevity,[1] Nutren 1.0 with fiber,[1] Fibersource HN)
Chemically defined peptide- or amino acid–based (eg, Peptamen,[1] Vital HN, AlitraQ, Tolerex, Vivonex TEN)
"Disease-specific" formulas
Advanced chronic kidney disease: with essential amino acids (eg, Amin-Aid, Magnacal, Nepro, Nepro Carb Steady, Suplena, Travasorb Renal, Novasource Renal, Renalcal)
Type 2 diabetes: with lower carbohydrate content (eg, Glucerna, Glucerna Select, Glucerna 1.2, Glucerna 1.5, Glytrol, Diabetisource AC)
Malabsorption: with medium-chain triglycerides (eg, Portagen,[1] Travasorb MCT)
Respiratory failure: with > 50% calories from fat (eg, Pulmocare, NutriVent, Nutren Pulmonary)
Hepatic encephalopathy: with high amounts of branched-chain amino acids (eg, Hepatic-Aid II, Nutri-Hep)
Wound healing: with high protein content (eg, Promote, Replete)
Incomplete (modular)
Protein (eg, ProMod, Propac); protein supplements (eg, ProStat Sugar Free, Beneprotein, Unjury)
Carbohydrate (eg, Polycose, SolCarb)
Fat (eg, MCT Oil, Microlipid)

Nutritionally complete solutions are characterized as follows: (1) by osmolality (isotonic or hypertonic), (2) by lactose content (present or absent), (3) by the molecular form of the protein component (intact proteins; peptides or amino acids), (4) by the quantity of protein and calories provided, and (5) by fiber content (present or absent). For most patients, isotonic solutions containing no lactose or fiber are preferable. Such solutions generally contain moderate amounts of fat and intact protein. Most commercial isotonic solutions contain 1000 kcal and about 37–45 g of protein per liter.

Solutions containing hydrolyzed proteins or crystalline amino acids and with no significant fat content are called elemental solutions, since macronutrients are provided in their most "elemental" form. These solutions have been designed for patients with malabsorption, particularly pancreatic insufficiency and limited fat absorption. Elemental diets are extremely hypertonic and often result in more severe diarrhea. Their use should be limited to patients who cannot tolerate isotonic solutions.

Although formulas have been designed for specific clinical situations—solutions containing primarily essential amino acids (for advanced chronic kidney disease), medium-chain triglycerides (for fat malabsorption), more fat (for respiratory failure and CO_2 retention), and more branched-chain amino acids (for hepatic encephalopathy and severe trauma)—they have not been shown to be superior to standard formulas for most patients.

Enteral solutions should be administered via continuous infusion, preferably with an infusion pump. Isotonic feedings should be started at full strength at about 25–33% of the estimated final infusion rate. Feedings can be advanced by similar amounts every 12 hours as tolerated. Hypertonic feedings should be started at half strength. The strength and the rate can then be advanced every 6 hours as tolerated.

COMPLICATIONS OF ENTERAL NUTRITIONAL SUPPORT

Minor complications of enteral nutritional support occur in 10–15% of patients. Gastrointestinal complications include diarrhea (most common), inadequate gastric emptying, emesis, esophagitis, and occasionally gastrointestinal bleeding. Diarrhea associated with enteral nutritional support may be due to intolerance to the osmotic load or to one of the macronutrients (eg, fat, lactose) in the solution. Patients being fed in this way may also have diarrhea from other causes (as side effects of antibiotics or other drugs, associated with infection, etc), and these possibilities should always be investigated in appropriate circumstances.

Mechanical complications of enteral nutritional support are potentially the most serious. Of particular importance is aspiration. All patients receiving nasogastric tube feedings are at risk for this life-threatening complication. Limiting nasogastric feedings to those patients who can adequately protect their airway and careful monitoring of patients being fed by tube should limit these serious complications to 1–2% of cases. Minor mechanical complications are common and include tube obstruction and dislodgment.

Metabolic complications during enteral nutritional support are common but are easily managed in most cases. The most important problem is hypernatremic dehydration, most commonly seen in elderly patients given excessive protein intake who are unable to respond to thirst. Abnormalities of potassium, glucose, CO_2 production, and acid–base balance may also occur.

Feinberg J et al. Nutrition support in hospitalised adults at nutritional risk. Cochrane Database Syst Rev. 2017 May 19; 5:CD011598. [PMID: 28524930]

Lewis SR et al. Enteral versus parenteral nutrition and enteral versus a combination of enteral and parenteral nutrition for adults in the intensive care unit. Cochrane Database Syst Rev. 2018 Jun 8;6:CD012276. [PMID: 29883514]

Reintam Blaser A et al. Early enteral nutrition in critically ill patients: ESICM clinical practice guidelines. Intensive Care Med. 2017 Mar;43(3):380–98. [PMID: 28168570]

Shi J et al. Effect of combined parenteral and enteral nutrition versus enteral nutrition alone for critically ill patients: a systematic review and meta-analysis. Medicine (Baltimore). 2018 Oct;97(41):e11874. [PMID: 30313021]

Yao H et al. Enteral versus parenteral nutrition in critically ill patients with severe pancreatitis: a meta-analysis. Eur J Clin Nutr. 2018 Jan;72(1):66–8. [PMID: 28901335]

Zhang G et al. The effect of enteral versus parenteral nutrition for critically ill patients: a systematic review and meta-analysis. J Clin Anesth. 2018 Dec;51:62–92. [PMID: 30098572]

PARENTERAL NUTRITIONAL SUPPORT SOLUTIONS

Parenteral nutritional support solutions can be designed to deliver adequate nutrients to most patients. The basic parenteral solution is composed of dextrose, amino acids, and water. Electrolytes, minerals, trace elements, vitamins, and medications can also be added. Most commercial solutions contain the monohydrate form of dextrose that provides 3.4 kcal/g. Crystalline amino acids are available in a variety of concentrations, so that a broad range of solutions can be made up that will contain specific amounts of dextrose and amino acids as required.

Typical solutions for central vein nutritional support contain 25–35% dextrose and 2.75–6% amino acids depending upon the patient's estimated nutrient and water requirements. These solutions typically have osmolalities in excess of 1800 mOsm/L and require infusion into a central vein. A typical formula for patients without organ failure is shown in Table 29–4.

Solutions with lower osmolalities can also be designed for infusion into peripheral veins. Typical solutions for peripheral infusion contain 5–10% dextrose and 2.75–4.25% amino acids. These solutions have osmolalities between 800 and 1200 mOsm/L and result in a high incidence of thrombophlebitis and line infiltration. These solutions will provide adequate protein for most patients but inadequate energy. Additional energy must be provided in the form of emulsified soybean or safflower oil. Such intravenous fat solutions are currently available in 10% and 25% solutions providing 1.1 and 2.2 kcal/mL, respectively. Intravenous fat solutions are isosmotic and well tolerated by peripheral veins.

Table 29–4. Typical parenteral nutrition solution (for stable patients without organ failure).

Dextrose (3.4 kcal/g)	25%
Amino acids (4 kcal/g)	6%
Na^+	50 mEq/L
K^+	40 mEq/L
Ca^{2+}	5 mEq/L
Mg^{2+}	8 mEq/L
Cl^-	60 mEq/L
P	12 mEq/L
Acetate	Balance
MVI-12 (vitamins)	10 mL/day
MTE (trace elements)	5 mL/day
Fat emulsion 20%	250 mL five times a week
Typical rate	Day 1: 30 mL/h
	Day 2: 60 mL/h
By day 2, solution provides:	Calories: 1925 kcal total
	Protein: 86 g
	Fat: 19% of total kcal
	Fluid: 1690 mL

Typical patients are given 200–500 mL of a 20% solution each day. As much as 60% of total calories can be administered in this manner.

Intravenous fat can also be provided to patients receiving central vein nutritional support. In this instance, dextrose concentrations should be decreased to provide a fixed concentration of energy. Intravenous fat has been shown to be equivalent to intravenous dextrose in providing energy to spare protein. Intravenous fat is associated with less glucose intolerance, less production of carbon dioxide, and less fatty infiltration of the liver and has been increasingly utilized in patients with hyperglycemia, respiratory failure, and liver disease. Intravenous fat has also been increasingly used in patients with large estimated energy requirements. The maximum glucose utilization rate is approximately 5–7 mg/min/kg. Patients who require additional calories can be given them as fat to prevent excess administration of dextrose. Intravenous fat can also be used to prevent essential fatty acid deficiency. The optimal ratio of carbohydrate and fat in parenteral nutritional support has not been determined.

Infusion of parenteral solutions should be started slowly to prevent hyperglycemia and other metabolic complications. Typical solutions are given initially at a rate of 50 mL/h and advanced by about the same amount every 24 hours until the desired final rate is reached.

Burden S et al. The impact of home parenteral nutrition on the burden of disease including morbidity, mortality and rate of hospitalisations. Clin Nutr ESPEN. 2018 Dec;28:222–7. [PMID: 30390885]

Derenski K et al. Parenteral nutrition basics for the clinician caring for the adult patient. Nutr Clin Pract. 2016 Oct;31(5):578–95. [PMID: 27440772]

Elke G et al. Enteral versus parenteral nutrition in critically ill patients: an updated systematic review and meta-analysis of randomized controlled trials. Crit Care. 2016 Apr 29; 20(1): 117. [PMID: 27129307]

Kirby DF et al. Overview of home parenteral nutrition: an update. Nutr Clin Pract. 2017 Dec;32(6):739–52. [PMID: 29035672]

Kovacevich DS et al. American Society for Parenteral and Enteral Nutrition guidelines for the selection and care of central venous access devices for adult home parenteral nutrition administration. JPEN J Parenter Enteral Nutr. 2019 Jan; 43(1):15–31. [PMID: 30339287]

Russell MK et al. Supplemental parenteral nutrition: review of the literature and current nutrition guidelines. Nutr Clin Pract. 2018 Jun;33(3):359–69. [PMID: 29878557]

COMPLICATIONS OF PARENTERAL NUTRITIONAL SUPPORT

Complications of central vein nutritional support occur in up to 50% of patients. Although most are minor and easily managed, significant complications will develop in about 5% of patients. Complications of central vein nutritional support can be divided into catheter-related complications and metabolic complications.

Catheter-related complications can occur during insertion or while the catheter is in place. Pneumothorax, hemothorax, arterial laceration, air emboli, and brachial plexus injury can occur during catheter placement. The incidence of these complications is inversely related to the experience of the physician performing the procedure but will occur in at least 1–2% of cases even in major medical centers. Each catheter placement should be documented by chest radiograph prior to initiation of nutritional support.

Catheter thrombosis and catheter-related sepsis are the most important complications of indwelling catheters. Patients with indwelling central vein catheters in whom fever develops without an apparent source should have their lines changed over a wire or removed immediately, the tip quantitatively cultured, and antibiotics begun empirically. Quantitative tip cultures and blood cultures will help guide further antibiotic therapy. Catheter-related sepsis occurs in 2–3% of patients even if maximal efforts are made to prevent infection.

Metabolic complications of central vein nutritional support occur in over 50% of patients (Table 29–5). Most are minor and easily managed, and termination of support is seldom necessary.

McCleary EJ et al. Parenteral nutrition and infection risk in the intensive care unit: a practical guide for the bedside clinician. Nutr Clin Pract. 2016 Aug;31(4):476–89. [PMID: 27317614]

Santacruz E et al. Infectious complications in home parenteral nutrition: a long-term study with peripherally inserted central catheters, tunneled catheters, and ports. Nutrition. 2019 Feb; 58:89–93. [PMID: 30391696]

PATIENT MONITORING DURING NUTRITIONAL SUPPORT

Every patient receiving enteral or parenteral nutritional support should be monitored closely. Formal nutritional support teams composed of a physician, a nurse, a dietitian, and a pharmacist have been shown to decrease the rate of complications.

Patients should be monitored both for the adequacy of treatment and to prevent complications or detect them early when they occur. Because estimates of nutritional requirements are imprecise, frequent reassessment is necessary. Daily intakes should be recorded and compared with estimated requirements. Body weight, hydration status, and overall clinical status should be followed. Patients who do not appear to be responding as anticipated can be evaluated for nitrogen balance by means of the following equation:

$$\text{Nitrogen balance} = \frac{24\text{-hour protein intake (g)}}{6.25} - \left(\frac{24\text{-hour urinary nitrogen (g)}}{} + 4 \right)$$

Table 29–5. Metabolic complications of parenteral nutritional support.

Complication	Common Causes	Possible Solutions
Hyperglycemia	Too rapid infusion of dextrose, "stress," corticosteroids	Decrease glucose infusion; insulin; replacement of dextrose with fat
Hyperosmolar nonketotic dehydration	Severe, undetected hyperglycemia	Insulin, hydration, potassium
Hyperchloremic metabolic acidosis	High chloride administration	Decrease chloride
Azotemia	Excessive protein administration	Decrease amino acid concentration
Hyperphosphatemia, hypokalemia, hypomagnesemia	Extracellular to intracellular shifting with refeeding	Increase solution concentration
Liver enzyme abnormalities	Lipid trapping in hepatocytes, fatty liver	Decrease dextrose
Acalculous cholecystitis	Biliary stasis	Oral fat
Zinc deficiency	Diarrhea, small bowel fistulas	Increase concentration
Copper deficiency	Biliary fistulas	Increase concentration

Patients with positive nitrogen balances can be continued on their current regimens; patients with negative balances should receive moderate increases in calorie and protein intake and then be reassessed. Monitoring for metabolic complications includes daily measurements of electrolytes; serum glucose, phosphorus, magnesium, calcium, and creatinine; and BUN until the patient is stabilized. Once the patient is stabilized, electrolytes, phosphorus, calcium, magnesium, and glucose should be obtained at least twice weekly. Red blood cell folate, zinc, and copper should be checked at least once a month.

Lewis SR et al. Enteral versus parenteral nutrition and enteral versus a combination of enteral and parenteral nutrition for adults in the intensive care unit. Cochrane Database Syst Rev. 2018 Jun 8;6:CD012276. [PMID: 29883514]

McClave SA et al. ACG Clinical Guideline: nutrition therapy in the adult hospitalized patient. Am J Gastroenterol. 2016 Mar; 111(3):315–34. [PMID: 26952578]

McClave SA et al. Guidelines for the provision and assessment of nutrition support therapy in the adult critically ill patient: Society of Critical Care Medicine (SCCM) and American Society for Parenteral and Enteral Nutrition (A.S.P.E.N.). J Parenter Enteral Nutr. 2016 Feb;40(2):159–211. [PMID: 26773077]

Reintam Blaser A et al; ESICM Working Group on Gastrointestinal Function. Early enteral nutrition in critically ill patients: ESICM clinical practice guidelines. Intensive Care Med. 2017 Mar; 43(3):380–98. [PMID: 28168570]

Shi J et al. Effect of combined parenteral and enteral nutrition versus enteral nutrition alone for critically ill patients: a systematic review and meta-analysis. Medicine (Baltimore). 2018 Oct;97(41):e11874. [PMID: 30313021]

30

Common Problems in Infectious Diseases & Antimicrobial Therapy

Peter V. Chin-Hong, MD

B. Joseph Guglielmo, PharmD

FEVER OF UNKNOWN ORIGIN (FUO)

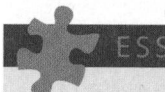 ESSENTIALS OF DIAGNOSIS

▶ Illness of at least 3 weeks in duration.

▶ Fever over 38.3°C on several occasions.

▶ Diagnosis has not been made after three outpatient visits or 3 days of hospitalization.

▶ General Considerations

The intervals specified in the criteria for the diagnosis of FUO are arbitrary ones intended to exclude patients with protracted but self-limited viral illnesses and to allow time for the usual radiographic, serologic, and cultural studies to be performed. The criteria for FUO are met when a diagnosis has not been made after three outpatient visits or 3 days of hospitalization.

The recently added categories of FUO include complications of current health care scenarios: (1) **Hospital-associated FUO** refers to the hospitalized patient with fever of 38.3°C or higher on several occasions, due to a process not present or incubating at the time of admission, in whom initial cultures are negative and the diagnosis remains unknown after 3 days of investigation (see Health Care–Associated Infections below); (2) **neutropenic FUO** includes patients with fever of 38.3°C or higher on several occasions with less than 500 neutrophils per microliter in whom initial cultures are negative and the diagnosis remains uncertain after 3 days (see Chapter 2 and Infections in the Immunocompromised Patient, below); (3) **HIV-associated FUO** pertains to HIV-positive patients with fever of 38.3°C or higher who have been febrile for 4 weeks or more as an outpatient or 3 days as an inpatient, in whom the diagnosis remains uncertain after 3 days of investigation with at least 2 days for cultures to incubate (see Chapter 31). Although not usually considered

separately, **FUO in solid organ transplant recipients** and **FUO in the returning traveler** are common scenarios, each with a unique differential diagnosis, and are also discussed in this chapter.

For a general discussion of fever, see the section on fever and hyperthermia in Chapter 2.

A. Common Causes

Most cases represent unusual manifestations of common diseases and not rare or exotic diseases—eg, tuberculosis, endocarditis, gallbladder disease, and HIV (primary infection or opportunistic infection) are more common causes of FUO than Whipple disease or familial Mediterranean fever.

B. Age of Patient

In adults, infections (25–40% of cases) and cancer (25–40% of cases) account for the majority of FUOs. In children, infections are the most common cause of FUO (30–50% of cases) and cancer a rare cause (5–10% of cases). Autoimmune disorders occur with equal frequency in adults and children (10–20% of cases), but the diseases differ. Juvenile rheumatoid arthritis is particularly common in children, whereas systemic lupus erythematosus, granulomatosis with polyangiitis (formerly Wegener granulomatosis), and polyarteritis nodosa are more common in adults. Still disease, giant cell arteritis, and polymyalgia rheumatica occur exclusively in adults. In adults over 65 years of age, multisystem immune-mediated diseases such as temporal arteritis, polymyalgia rheumatica, sarcoidosis, rheumatoid arthritis, and granulomatosis with polyangiitis account for 25–30% of all FUOs.

C. Duration of Fever

The cause of FUO changes dramatically in patients who have been febrile for 6 months or longer. Infection, cancer, and autoimmune disorders combined account for only 20% of FUOs in these patients. Instead, other entities such as granulomatous diseases (granulomatous hepatitis, Crohn disease, ulcerative colitis) and factitious fever become important causes. One-fourth of patients who say they have been febrile for 6 months or longer actually have no true fever or underlying disease. Instead, the usual normal circadian variation in temperature (temperature 0.5–1°C higher in the afternoon than in the morning) is interpreted as abnormal. Patients with **episodic** or **recurrent fever** (ie, those who meet the criteria for FUO but have fever-free periods of 2 weeks or longer) are similar to those with **prolonged fever**. Infection, malignancy, and autoimmune disorders account for only 20–25% of such fevers, whereas various miscellaneous diseases (Crohn disease, familial Mediterranean fever, allergic alveolitis) account for another 25%. Approximately 50% of cases remain undiagnosed but have a benign course with eventual resolution of symptoms.

D. Immunologic Status

In the neutropenic patient, fungal infections and occult bacterial infections are important causes of FUO. In the patient taking immunosuppressive medications (particularly organ transplant patients), cytomegalovirus (CMV) infections are a frequent cause of fever, as are fungal infections, nocardiosis, *Pneumocystis jirovecii* pneumonia, and mycobacterial infections.

E. Classification of Causes of FUO

Most patients with FUO will fit into one of five categories.

1. Infection—Both systemic and localized infections can cause FUO. Tuberculosis and endocarditis are the most common systemic infections associated with FUO, but mycoses, viral diseases (particularly infection with Epstein-Barr virus and CMV), toxoplasmosis, brucellosis, Q fever, cat-scratch disease, salmonellosis, malaria, and many other less common infections have been implicated. Primary infection with HIV or opportunistic infections associated with AIDS—particularly mycobacterial infections—can also present as FUO. The most common form of localized infection causing FUO is an occult abscess. Liver, spleen, kidney, brain, and bone abscesses may be difficult to detect. A collection of pus may form in the peritoneal cavity or in the subdiaphragmatic, subhepatic, paracolic, or other areas. Cholangitis, osteomyelitis, urinary tract infection, dental abscess, or paranasal sinusitis may cause prolonged fever.

2. Neoplasms—Many cancers can present as FUO. The most common are lymphoma (both Hodgkin and non-Hodgkin) and leukemia. Posttransplant lymphoproliferative disorders may also present with fever. Other diseases of lymph nodes, such as angioimmunoblastic lymphoma and Castleman disease, can also cause FUO. Primary and metastatic tumors of the liver are frequently associated with fever, as are renal cell carcinomas. Atrial myxoma is an often forgotten neoplasm that can result in fever. Chronic lymphocytic leukemia and multiple myeloma are rarely associated with fever, and the presence of fever in patients with these diseases should prompt a search for infection.

3. Autoimmune disorders—Still disease, systemic lupus erythematosus, cryoglobulinemia, and polyarteritis nodosa are the most common causes of autoimmune-associated FUO. Giant cell arteritis and polymyalgia rheumatica are seen almost exclusively in patients over 50 years of age and are nearly always associated with an elevated erythrocyte sedimentation rate (greater than 40 mm/h).

4. Miscellaneous causes—Many other conditions have been associated with FUO but less commonly than the foregoing types of illness. Examples include thyroiditis, sarcoidosis, Whipple disease, familial Mediterranean fever, recurrent pulmonary emboli, alcoholic hepatitis, drug fever, and factitious fever.

5. Undiagnosed FUO—Despite extensive evaluation, the diagnosis remains elusive in 15% or more of patients. Of these patients, the fever abates spontaneously in about 75% with no diagnosis; in the remainder, more classic manifestations of the underlying disease appear over time.

► Clinical Findings

Because the evaluation of a patient with FUO is costly and time-consuming, it is imperative to first document the presence of fever. This is done by observing the patient while the temperature is being taken to ascertain that fever is not factitious (self-induced). Associated findings that accompany fever include tachycardia, chills, and piloerection. A thorough history—including family, occupational, social (sexual practices, use of injection drugs), dietary (unpasteurized products, raw meat), exposures (animals, chemicals), and travel—may give clues to the diagnosis. Repeated physical examination may reveal subtle, evanescent clinical findings essential to diagnosis.

A. Laboratory Tests

In addition to routine laboratory studies, blood cultures should always be obtained, preferably when the patient has not taken antibiotics for several days, and should be held by the laboratory for 2 weeks to detect slow-growing organisms. Cultures on special media are requested if *Legionella, Bartonella*, or nutritionally deficient streptococci are possible pathogens. "Screening tests" with immunologic or microbiologic serologies ("febrile agglutinins") are of low yield and should *not* be done. If the history or physical examination suggests a specific diagnosis, specific serologic tests with an associated fourfold rise or fall in titer may be useful. Because infection is the most common cause of FUO, other body fluids are usually cultured, ie, urine, sputum, stool, cerebrospinal fluid, and morning gastric aspirates (if one suspects tuberculosis). Direct examination of blood smears may establish a diagnosis of malaria or relapsing fever (*Borrelia*).

B. Imaging

All patients with FUO should have a chest radiograph. Studies such as sinus CT, upper gastrointestinal series with small bowel follow-through, barium enema, proctosigmoidoscopy, and evaluation of gallbladder function are reserved for patients who have symptoms, signs, or a history that suggest disease in these body regions. CT scan of the abdomen and pelvis is also frequently performed and is particularly useful for looking at the liver, spleen, and retroperitoneum. When the CT scan is abnormal, the findings often lead to a specific diagnosis. A normal CT scan is not quite as useful; more invasive procedures such as biopsy or exploratory laparotomy may be needed. The role of MRI in the investigation of FUO has not been evaluated. In general, however, MRI is better than CT for detecting lesions of the nervous system and is useful in diagnosing various vasculitides. Ultrasound is sensitive for detecting lesions of the kidney, pancreas, and biliary tree. Echocardiography should be used if one is considering endocarditis or atrial myxoma. Transesophageal echocardiography is more sensitive than surface echocardiography for detecting valvular lesions, but even a negative transesophageal study does not exclude endocarditis (10% false-negative rate). The usefulness of radionuclide studies in diagnosing FUO is variable. Some experts use positron emission tomography (PET) in conjunction with CT scans early in the investigation of FUO. However, more studies are needed before this practice can be more fully integrated into clinical practice. Theoretically, a gallium or PET scan would be more helpful than an indium-labeled white blood cell scan because gallium and fluorodeoxyglucose may be useful for detecting infection, inflammation, and neoplasm whereas the indium scan is useful only for detecting infection. Indium-labeled immunoglobulin may prove to be useful in detecting infection and neoplasm and can be used in the neutropenic patient. It is not sensitive for lesions of the liver, kidney, and heart because of high background activity. In general, radionuclide scans are plagued by high rates of false-positive and false-negative results that are not useful when used as screening tests and, if done at all, are limited to those patients whose history or examination suggests local inflammation or infection.

C. Biopsy

Invasive procedures are often required for diagnosis. Any abnormal finding should be aggressively evaluated: Headache calls for lumbar puncture to rule out meningitis; skin rash should be biopsied for cutaneous manifestations of collagen vascular disease or infection; and enlarged lymph nodes should be aspirated or biopsied for neoplasm and sent for culture. Bone marrow aspiration with biopsy is a relatively low-yield procedure (15–25%; except in HIV-positive patients, in whom mycobacterial infection is a common cause of FUO), but the risk is low and the procedure should be done if other less invasive tests have not yielded a diagnosis, particularly in persons with hematologic abnormalities. Liver biopsy will yield a specific diagnosis in 10–15% of patients with FUO and should be considered in any patient with abnormal liver tests even if the liver is normal in size. CT scanning and MRI have decreased the need for exploratory laparotomy; however, surgical visualization and biopsies should be considered when there is continued deterioration or lack of diagnosis.

► Treatment

Although an empiric course of antimicrobials is sometimes considered for FUO, it is *rarely* helpful and may impact infectious diseases diagnoses (eg, by reducing the sensitivity of blood cultures).

► When to Refer

- Any patient with FUO and progressive weight loss and other constitutional signs.
- Any immunocompromised patient (eg, transplant recipients and HIV-infected patients).
- Infectious diseases specialists may also be able to coordinate and interpret specialized testing (eg, Q fever serologies) with outside agencies, such as the US Centers for Disease Control and Prevention.

► When to Admit

- Any patient who is rapidly declining with weight loss where hospital admission may expedite workup.
- If FUO is present in immunocompromised patients, such as those who are neutropenic from recent chemotherapy or those who have undergone transplantation (particularly in the previous 6 months).

Loizidou A et al. Fever of unknown origin in cancer patients. Crit Rev Oncol Hematol. 2016 May;101:125–30. [PMID: 26995082]
Mulders-Manders CM et al. Long-term prognosis, treatment, and outcome of patients with fever of unknown origin in whom no diagnosis was made despite extensive investigation: a questionnaire based study. Medicine (Baltimore). 2018 Jun; 97(25):e11241. [PMID: 29924054]
Takeuchi M et al. Nuclear imaging for classic fever of unknown origin: meta-analysis. J Nucl Med. 2016 Dec;57(12):1913–9. [PMID: 27339873]
Zhai YZ et al. Clinical analysis of 215 consecutive cases with fever of unknown origin: A cohort study. Medicine (Baltimore). 2018 Jun;97(24):e10986. [PMID: 29901588]

INFECTIONS IN THE IMMUNOCOMPROMISED PATIENT

ESSENTIALS OF DIAGNOSIS

► Fever and other symptoms may be blunted because of immunosuppression.

► A contaminating organism in an immunocompetent individual may be a pathogen in an immunocompromised one.

► The interval since transplantation and the degree of immunosuppression can narrow the differential diagnosis.

► Empiric broad-spectrum antibiotics may be appropriate in high-risk patients whether or not symptoms are localized.

► General Considerations

Immunocompromised patients have defects in their natural defense mechanisms resulting in an increased risk for infection. In addition, infection is often severe, rapidly progressive, and life threatening. Organisms that are not usually problematic in the immunocompetent person may be important pathogens in the compromised patient (eg, *Staphylococcus epidermidis, Corynebacterium jeikeium, Propionibacterium acnes, Bacillus* species). Therefore, culture results must be interpreted with caution, and isolates should not be disregarded as solely contaminants. Although the type of immunodeficiency is associated with specific infectious disease syndromes, any pathogen can cause infection in any immunosuppressed patient at any time. Thus, a systematic evaluation is required to identify a specific organism.

A. Impaired Humoral Immunity

Defects in humoral immunity are often congenital, although hypogammaglobulinemia can occur in multiple myeloma, chronic lymphocytic leukemia, small lymphocyte lymphoma, and in patients who have undergone splenectomy. Patients with ineffective humoral immunity lack opsonizing antibodies and are at particular risk for infection with *encapsulated organisms*, such as *Haemophilus influenzae, Neisseria meningitides*, and *Streptococcus pneumoniae*. Although rituximab is normally thought of as being linked to impaired cellular immunity, it has been associated with the development of *Pneumocystis jirovecii* infection and progressive multifocal leukoencephalopathy (PML) as well as with hepatitis B reactivation.

B. Granulocytopenia (Neutropenia)

Granulocytopenia is common following hematopoietic cell transplantation ("stem cell transplantation") and among patients with solid tumors—as a result of myelosuppressive chemotherapy—and in acute leukemias. The risk of infection begins to increase when the absolute granulocyte count falls below *1000/mcL*, with a dramatic increase in frequency and severity when the granulocyte count falls below 100/mcL. The infection risk is also increased with a rapid rate of decline of neutrophils and with a prolonged period of neutropenia. The granulocytopenic patient is particularly susceptible to infections with gram-negative enteric organisms, *Pseudomonas*, gram-positive cocci (particularly *Staphylococcus aureus, S epidermidis*, and viridans streptococci), *Candida, Aspergillus*, and other fungi that have recently emerged as pathogens such as *Trichosporon, Scedosporium, Fusarium*, and the mucormycoses.

C. Impaired Cellular Immunity

Patients with cellular immune deficiency encompass a large and heterogeneous group, including patients with HIV infection (see Chapter 31); patients with lymphoreticular malignancies, such as Hodgkin disease; and patients receiving immunosuppressive medications, such as corticosteroids, cyclosporine, tacrolimus, and other cytotoxic medications. This latter group—those who are immunosuppressed as a result of medications—includes patients who have undergone solid organ transplantation, many patients receiving therapy for solid tumors, and patients receiving prolonged high-dose corticosteroid treatment (eg, for asthma, temporal arteritis, systemic lupus erythematosus). Patients taking tumor necrosis factor (TNF) inhibitors, such as etanercept and infliximab, are also included in this category. Patients with cellular immune dysfunction are susceptible to infections by a large number of organisms, particularly ones that replicate intracellularly. Examples include bacteria, such as *Listeria, Legionella, Salmonella*, and *Mycobacterium;* viruses, such as herpes simplex, varicella, and CMV; fungi, such as *Cryptococcus, Coccidioides, Histoplasma*, and *Pneumocystis;* and protozoa, such as *Toxoplasma*.

D. Hematopoietic Cell Transplant Recipients

The length of time it takes for complications to occur in hematopoietic cell transplant recipients can be helpful in determining the etiologic agent. In the **early (preengraftment) posttransplant period (days 1–21),** patients will become severely neutropenic for 7–21 days. Patients are at risk for gram-positive (particularly catheter-related) and gram-negative bacterial infections, as well as herpes simplex virus, respiratory syncytial virus, and fungal infections. In contrast to solid organ transplant recipients, the source of fever is unknown in 60–70% of hematopoietic cell transplant patients. **Between 3 weeks and 3 months posttransplant,** infections with CMV, adenovirus, *Aspergillus*, and *Candida* are most common. *P jirovecii* pneumonia is possible, particularly in patients who receive additional immunosuppression for treatment of graft-versus-host disease. Patients continue to be at risk for infectious complications **beyond 3 months following transplantation,** particularly those who have received allogeneic transplantation and those who are taking immunosuppressive therapy for chronic graft-versus-host disease. Varicella-zoster is common, and *Aspergillus* and CMV infections are increasingly seen in this period as well.

E. Solid Organ Transplant Recipients

The length of time it takes for infection to occur following solid organ transplantation can also be helpful in determining the infectious origin. **Immediate postoperative infections** often involve the transplanted organ. Following lung transplantation, pneumonia and mediastinitis are particularly common; following liver transplantation, intra-abdominal abscess, cholangitis, and peritonitis may be seen; after kidney transplantation, urinary tract infections, perinephric abscesses, and infected lymphoceles can occur.

Most infections that occur in the **first 2–4 weeks posttransplant** are related to the operative procedure and to hospitalization itself (wound infection, intravenous catheter infection, urinary tract infection from a Foley catheter) or are related to the transplanted organ. In rare instances, donor-derived infections (eg, West Nile virus, tuberculosis) may present during this time period. Compensated organ transplants obtained abroad through "medical tourism" can introduce additional risk of infections, which vary by country and by transplant setting. Infections that occur **between the first and sixth months** are often related to immunosuppression. During this period, reactivation of viruses, such as herpes simplex, varicella-zoster, and CMV is quite common. Opportunistic infections with fungi (eg, *Candida, Aspergillus, Cryptococcus, Pneumocystis*), *Listeria monocytogenes, Nocardia*, and *Toxoplasma* are also common. **After 6 months,** if immunosuppression has been reduced to maintenance levels, infections that would be expected in any population occur. Patients with poorly functioning allografts receiving long-term immunosuppression therapy continue to be at risk for opportunistic infections.

F. Tumor Necrosis Factor Inhibitor Recipients

Patients taking TNF inhibitors have specific defects that increase risk of bacterial, mycobacterial (particularly tuberculosis), viral (HBV reactivation and HCV progression), and fungal infections (*Pneumocystis*, molds, and endemic mycoses). Infection risk may be highest shortly after therapy is initiated (within the first 3 months) and with a higher dose of medications.

G. Recipients of Other Biologics

In addition to TNF inhibitors, other biologics target a variety of immunologic pathways that are involved in immunologic mediated disease and in cancer replication. Disruption of these pathways include, but are not limited to impact on B cells, T cells, complement and leukocytes. This may result in not only serious infections, but the development of autoimmune disease and malignancies as well. Some medications have been observed to have specific associations with opportunistic infections (eg, natalizumab and PML, or eculizumab and meningococcal disease). Other biologics such as chimeric antigen receptor T cells may have unintended infectious risks that are currently unknown, or may have adverse effects that mimic infection (eg, cytokine release syndrome). As more biologics are developed and used, clinicians must remain vigilant for the possibility of serious infectious disease risk.

H. Other Immunocompromised States

A large group of patients who are not specifically immunodeficient are at increased risk for infection due to debilitating injury (eg, burns or severe trauma), invasive procedures (eg, chronic central intravenous catheters, Foley catheters, dialysis catheters), central nervous system dysfunction (which predisposes patients to aspiration pneumonia and decubitus ulcers), obstructing lesions (eg, pneumonia due to an obstructed bronchus, pyelonephritis due to nephrolithiasis, cholangitis secondary to cholelithiasis), and use of broad-spectrum antibiotics. Patients with diabetes mellitus have alterations in cellular immunity, resulting in mucormycosis, emphysematous pyelonephritis, and foot infections.

► Clinical Findings

A. Laboratory Findings

Routine evaluation includes complete blood count with differential, chest radiograph, and blood cultures; urine and respiratory cultures should be obtained if indicated clinically or radiographically. Any focal complaints (localized pain, headache, rash) should prompt imaging and cultures appropriate to the site.

Patients who remain febrile without an obvious source should be evaluated for viral infection (serum CMV antigen test or polymerase chain reaction), abscesses (which usually occur near previous operative sites), candidiasis involving the liver or spleen, or aspergillosis. Serologic evaluation may be helpful if toxoplasmosis or an endemic fungal infection (coccidioidomycosis, histoplasmosis) is a possible cause. Antigen-based assays may be useful for the diagnosis of aspergillosis (detected by galactomannan level in serum or bronchoalveolar lavage fluid), or other invasive fungal disease, including *Pneumocystis* infection (serum [1 → 3]-beta-D-glucan level).

B. Special Diagnostic Procedures

Special diagnostic procedures should also be considered. The cause of pulmonary infiltrates can be easily determined with simple techniques in some situations—eg, induced sputum yields a diagnosis of *Pneumocystis* pneumonia in 50–80% of AIDS patients with this infection. In other situations, more invasive procedures may be required (bronchoalveolar lavage, transbronchial biopsy, open lung biopsy). Skin, liver, or bone marrow biopsy may be helpful in establishing a diagnosis. Next generation DNA-sequencing analysis is an increasingly used and validated option for diagnosis of infectious diseases in immunocompromised persons.

► Differential Diagnosis

Transplant rejection, organ ischemia and necrosis, thrombophlebitis, and lymphoma (posttransplant lymphoproliferative disease) may all present as fever and must be considered in the differential diagnosis.

► Prevention

While prophylactic antimicrobial medications are used commonly, the optimal medications or dosage regimens are debated. *Hand washing is the simplest and most effective means of decreasing hospital-associated infections,* especially in the compromised patient. Invasive devices such as central and peripheral lines and Foley catheters are potential sources of infection. Some centers use laminar airflow isolation or high-efficiency particulate air (HEPA) filtering in hematopoietic cell transplant patients. Rates of infection and episodes of febrile neutropenia, but not mortality, are decreased if colony-stimulating factors are used (typically in situations where the risk of febrile neutropenia is 20% or higher) during chemotherapy or during stem-cell transplantation.

A. *Pneumocystis* & Herpes Simplex Infections

Trimethoprim-sulfamethoxazole (TMP-SMZ), one double-strength tablet orally three times a week, one double-strength tablet twice daily on weekends, or one single-strength tablet daily for 3–6 months, is frequently used to prevent *Pneumocystis* infections in transplant patients. In patients allergic to TMP-SMZ, dapsone, 50 mg orally daily or 100 mg three times weekly, is recommended. Glucose-6-phosphate dehydrogenase (G6PD) levels should be assessed before dapsone is instituted. Acyclovir prevents herpes simplex infections in bone marrow and solid organ transplant recipients and is given to seropositive patients who are not receiving ganciclovir or valganciclovir for

CMV prophylaxis. The usual dose is 200 mg orally three times daily for 4 weeks (hematopoietic cell transplants) to 12 weeks (other solid organ transplants).

B. CMV

No uniformly accepted approach has been adopted for prevention of CMV. Prevention strategies often depend on the serologic status of the donor and recipient and the organ transplanted, which determines the level of immunosuppression after transplant. In solid organ transplants (liver, kidney, heart, lung), the greatest risk of developing CMV disease is in seronegative recipients who receive organs from seropositive donors. These high-risk patients usually receive oral valganciclovir, 900 mg daily for 3–6 months (longer in lung transplant recipients). Other solid organ transplant recipients (seropositive recipients) are at lower risk for developing CMV disease, but still usually receive oral valganciclovir for 3 months. The lowest-risk group for the development of CMV disease is in seronegative patients who receive organs from seronegative donors. Typically, no CMV prophylaxis is used in this group. Ganciclovir and valganciclovir also prevent herpes virus reactivation. Because immunosuppression is increased during periods of rejection, patients treated for rejection usually receive CMV prophylaxis during rejection therapy. Alternatively, in a preemptive approach, patients can be monitored without specific prophylaxis by having blood sampled weekly to look for CMV by polymerase chain reaction techniques. If CMV is detected, then therapy is instituted with oral valganciclovir, 900 mg orally twice daily for a minimum of 2–3 weeks.

Recipients of hematopoietic cell transplants are more severely immunosuppressed than recipients of solid organ transplants, are at greater risk for developing serious CMV infection (usually CMV reactivation), and thus usually receive more aggressive prophylaxis. Like in solid organ transplant recipients, two approaches have been used: *universal prophylaxis* or *preemptive therapy*. In the former, all high-risk patients (seropositive patients who receive allogeneic transplants) may receive oral valganciclovir, 900 mg daily to day 100. However, valganciclovir is associated with significant bone marrow toxicity. Letermovir is being used increasingly, and it is not associated with bone marrow toxicity. Universal prophylaxis may be costly. Because of the possibility of bone marrow toxicity and the expense, many clinicians traditionally preferred the preemptive approach over the universal prophylaxis approach for recipients of hematopoietic stem cell transplants. However, while this preemptive approach is effective, it does miss a small number of patients in whom CMV disease would have been prevented had prophylaxis been used. Other preventive strategies include use of CMV-negative or leukocyte-depleted blood products for CMV-seronegative recipients.

C. Other Organisms

Routine decontamination of the gastrointestinal tract to prevent bacteremia in the neutropenic patient is not recommended. The use of prophylactic antibiotics in the afebrile, asymptomatic neutropenic patient is debated, although many centers have adopted this strategy. Rates of bacteremia are decreased, but overall mortality is not affected

and emergence of resistant organisms takes place. Use of intravenous immunoglobulin is reserved for the small number of patients with severe hypogammaglobulinemia following hematopoietic stem cell transplantation and should not be routinely administered to all transplant patients.

Prophylaxis with antifungal agents to prevent invasive mold (primarily *Aspergillus*) and yeast (primarily *Candida*) infections is routinely used, but the optimal agent, dose, and duration are also debated. Lipid-based preparations of amphotericin B, aerosolized amphotericin B, intravenous and oral fluconazole or voriconazole, and oral posaconazole solution and tablets are all prophylactic options in the neutropenic patient. Because voriconazole is superior to amphotericin for documented *Aspergillus* infections and because posaconazole prophylaxis (compared with fluconazole) has been shown to result in fewer cases of invasive aspergillosis among allogeneic stem cell transplant recipients with graft-versus-host disease, one approach to prophylaxis is to use oral fluconazole (400 mg/day) for patients at low risk for developing fungal infections (those who receive autologous stem cell transplants) and oral voriconazole (200 mg twice daily) or oral posaconazole (200 mg suspension three times daily or 300 mg [three 100-mg tablets] sustained-release tablets once daily) for those at high risk (allogeneic transplants, graft-versus-host disease) at least until engraftment (usually 30 days). In solid organ transplant recipients, the risk of invasive fungal infection varies considerably (1–2% in liver, pancreas, and kidney transplants and 6–8% in heart and lung transplants). Whether universal prophylaxis or observation with preemptive therapy is the best approach has not been determined. Although fluconazole is effective in preventing yeast infections, emergence of fluconazole-resistant *Candida* and molds (*Fusarium, Aspergillus, Mucor*) has raised concerns about its routine use as a prophylactic agent in the general solid organ transplant population. However, liver transplant recipients with additional risk factors, such as having undergone a choledochojejunostomy, having had a high transfusion requirement or having developed kidney disease, may benefit from abbreviated postoperative *Candida* prophylaxis.

Given the high risk of reactivation of tuberculosis in patients taking TNF inhibitors, all patients should be screened for latent tuberculosis infection (LTBI) with a tuberculin skin test or an interferon-gamma release assay prior to the start of therapy. If LTBI is diagnosed, treatment with the TNF inhibitors should be delayed until treatment for LTBI is completed. There is also a marked risk of reactivation of hepatitis B and hepatitis C in patients taking TNF inhibitors; patients should also be screened for these viruses when TNF inhibitor treatment is being considered. Providers should also ensure that patients' vaccinations are up-to-date before starting TNF inhibitors therapy.

▶ Treatment

A. General Measures

Because infections in the immunocompromised patient can be rapidly progressive and life-threatening, diagnostic procedures must be performed promptly, and empiric therapy is usually instituted.

While reduction or discontinuation of immunosuppressive medication may jeopardize the viability of the transplanted organ, this measure may be necessary if the infection is life-threatening. Hematopoietic growth factors (granulocyte and granulocyte-macrophage colony-stimulating factors) stimulate proliferation of bone marrow stem cells, resulting in an increase in peripheral leukocytes. These agents shorten the period of neutropenia and have been associated with reduction in infection.

B. Specific Measures

Antimicrobial medication therapy ultimately should be tailored to culture results. While combinations of antimicrobials are used with the intent of providing synergy or preventing resistance, the primary reason for empiric combination therapy is broad-spectrum coverage of all likely pathogens.

Empiric therapy is often instituted at the earliest sign of infection in the immunosuppressed patient because prompt therapy favorably affects outcome. The antibiotic or combination of antibiotics used depends on the degree of immune compromise and the site of infection. For example, in the febrile neutropenic patient, an *algorithmic approach* to therapy is often used. Febrile neutropenic patients should be empirically treated with broad-spectrum agents active against selected gram-positive bacteria, *Pseudomonas aeruginosa*, and other aerobic gram-negative bacilli (such as cefepime 2 g every 8 hours intravenously). The addition of vancomycin, 10–15 mg/kg/dose intravenously every 12 hours, should be considered in those patients with suspected infection due to methicillin-resistant *Staphylococcus aureus* (MRSA), *S epidermidis*, enterococcus, and resistant viridans streptococci. Continued neutropenic fever necessitates broadening of antibacterial coverage from cefepime to agents such as imipenem 500 mg every 6 hours or meropenem 1 g every 8 hours intravenously with or without tobramycin 5–7 mg/kg intravenously every 24 hours. Antifungal agents (such as voriconazole, 200 mg intravenously or orally every 12 hours, or caspofungin, 50 mg daily intravenously) should be added if fevers continue after 5–7 days of broad-spectrum antibacterial therapy. Regardless of whether the patient becomes afebrile, *therapy is continued until resolution of neutropenia*. Failure to continue antibiotics through the period of neutropenia has been associated with increased morbidity and mortality.

Patients with fever and low-risk neutropenia (neutropenia expected to persist for less than 10 days, no comorbid complications requiring hospitalization, and cancer adequately treated) can be treated with oral antibiotic regimens, such as ciprofloxacin, 750 mg every 12 hours, plus amoxicillin-clavulanic acid, 500 mg every 8 hours. Antibiotics are continued as long as the patient is neutropenic even if a source is not identified. In the organ transplant patient with interstitial infiltrates, the main concern is infection with *Pneumocystis* or *Legionella* species, so that empiric treatment with a macrolide or fluoroquinolone (*Legionella*) and TMP-SMZ, 15 mg/kg/day orally or intravenously, based on trimethoprim component (*Pneumocystis*) would be reasonable in those patients not receiving TMP-SMZ prophylaxis. If the patient does not respond to empiric treatment, a decision must be made to add more antimicrobial agents or perform invasive procedures (see above) to make a specific diagnosis. By making a definite diagnosis, therapy can be specific, thereby reducing selection pressure for resistance and superinfection.

▶ When to Refer

- Any immunocompromised patient with an opportunistic infection.
- Patients with potential drug toxicities and drug interactions related to antimicrobials where alternative agents are sought.
- Patients with latent tuberculosis, HBV, and HCV infection in whom therapy with TNF inhibitors is planned.

▶ When to Admit

Immunocompromised patients who are febrile, or those without fevers in whom an infection is suspected, particularly in the following groups: solid-organ or hematopoietic stem cell transplant recipient (particularly in the first 6 months), neutropenic patients, patients receiving TNF inhibitors, and transplant recipients who have had recent rejection episodes (including graft-versus-host disease).

Beyar-Katz O et al. Empirical antibiotics targeting gram-positive bacteria for the treatment of febrile neutropenic patients with cancer. Cochrane Database Syst Rev. 2017 Jun 3;6:CD003914. [PMID: 28577308]

Bonnafous P et al. Fatal outcome after reactivation of inherited chromosomally integrated HHV-6A (iciHHV-6A) transmitted through liver transplantation. Am J Transplant. 2018 Jun; 18(6):1548–51. [PMID: 29316259]

Fung M et al. Plasma cell-free DNA Next-generation sequencing to diagnose and monitor infections in allogeneic hematopoietic stem cell transplant patients. Open Forum Infect Dis. 2018 Nov 16;5(12):ofy301. [PMID: 30581881]

Hamandi B et al. Voriconazole and squamous cell carcinoma after lung transplantation: a multicenter study. Am J Transplant. 2018 Jan;18(1):113–24. [PMID: 28898527]

Maertens JA et al. Isavuconazole versus voriconazole for primary treatment of invasive mould disease caused by *Aspergillus* and other filamentous fungi (SECURE): a phase 3, randomised-controlled, non-inferiority trial. Lancet. 2016 Feb 20; 387(10020):760–9. [PMID: 26684607]

Marty FM et al. Letermovir prophylaxis for cytomegalovirus in hematopoietic-cell transplantation. N Engl J Med. 2017 Dec 21; 377(25):2433–44. [PMID: 29211658]

Patterson TF et al. Executive summary: practice guidelines for the diagnosis and management of aspergillosis: 2016 update by the Infectious Diseases Society of America. Clin Infect Dis. 2016 Aug 15;63(4):433–42. [PMID: 27481947]

Reese PP et al. Twelve-month outcomes after transplant of hepatitis C-infected kidneys into uninfected recipients: a single-group trial. Ann Intern Med. 2018 Sep 4;169(5):273–81. [PMID: 30083748]

Vallabhaneni S et al. Investigation of the first seven reported cases of *Candida auris*, a globally emerging invasive, multidrug-resistant fungus—United States, May 2013–August 2016. MMWR Morb Mortal Wkly Rep. 2016 Nov 11;65(44): 1234–7. [PMID: 27832049]

HEALTH CARE–ASSOCIATED INFECTIONS

ESSENTIALS OF DIAGNOSIS

▶ Health care–associated infections are acquired during the course of receiving health care treatment for other conditions.

▶ Hospital-associated infections are a subset of health care–associated infections defined as those not present or incubating at the time of hospital admission and developing 48 hours or more after admission.

▶ Most health care–associated infections are preventable.

▶ Hand washing is the most effective means of preventing health care–associated infections and should be done routinely even when gloves are worn.

▶ General Considerations

Worldwide, approximately 10% of patients acquire a health care–associated infection, resulting in prolongation of the hospital stay, increase in cost of care, and significant morbidity and mortality. The most common infections are urinary tract infections, usually associated with Foley catheters or urologic procedures; bloodstream infections, most commonly from indwelling catheters but also from secondary sites, such as surgical wounds, abscesses, pneumonia, the genitourinary tract, and the gastrointestinal tract; pneumonia in intubated patients or those with altered levels of consciousness; surgical wound infections; MRSA infections; and *Clostridioides difficile* colitis.

Some general principles are helpful in preventing, diagnosing, and treating health care–associated infections:

1. Many infections are a direct result of the use of *invasive devices* for monitoring or therapy, such as intravenous catheters, Foley catheters, shunts, surgical drains, catheters placed by interventional radiology for drainage, nasogastric tubes, and orotracheal or nasotracheal tubes for ventilatory support. *Early removal of such devices reduces the possibility of infection.*

2. Patients in whom health care–associated infections develop are often critically ill, have been hospitalized for extended periods, and have received several courses of broad-spectrum antibiotic therapy. As a result, health care–associated infections are often due to *multidrug resistant pathogens* and differ from those encountered in community-acquired infections. For example, *S aureus* and *S epidermidis* (a frequent cause of prosthetic device infection) are often resistant to methicillin and most cephalosporins (ceftaroline is active against MRSA) and require vancomycin for therapy; *Enterococcus faecium* resistant to ampicillin and vancomycin; gram-negative infections caused by *Pseudomonas, Citrobacter, Enterobacter, Acinetobacter, Stenotrophomonas,* extended-spectrum beta-lactamases (ESBL)–producing *E coli,* and *Klebsiella* may be resis-

tant to most antibacterials. When choosing antibiotics to treat the seriously ill patient with a health care–associated infection, antimicrobial history and the "local ecology" must be considered. In the most seriously ill patients, broad-spectrum coverage with vancomycin and a carbapenem with or without an aminoglycoside is recommended. Once a pathogen is isolated and susceptibilities are known, the most narrow-spectrum, least toxic, most cost-effective regimen should be used.

Widespread use of antimicrobial medications contributes to the selection of drug-resistant organisms; thus, *every effort should be made to limit the spectrum of coverage and unnecessary duration.* All too often, unreliable or uninterpretable specimens are obtained for culture that result in unnecessary use of antibiotics. The best example of this principle is the diagnosis of line-related or bloodstream infection in the febrile patient. To avoid unnecessary use of antibiotics, thoughtful consideration of culture results is mandatory. A positive wound culture without signs of inflammation or infection, a positive sputum culture without pulmonary infiltrates on chest radiograph, or a positive urine culture in a catheterized patient without symptoms or signs of pyelonephritis are all likely to represent *colonization,* not infection.

▶ Clinical Findings

A. Symptoms and Signs

Catheter-associated infections have a variable presentation, depending on the type of catheter used (peripheral or central venous catheters, nontunneled or tunneled). Local signs of infection may be present at the insertion site, with pain, erythema, and purulence. Fever is often absent in uncomplicated infections and if present, may indicate more disseminated disease such as bacteremia, cellulitis and septic thrombophlebitis. Often signs of infection at the insertion site are absent.

1. Fever in an intensive care unit patient—Fever complicates up to 70% of patients in intensive care units, and the etiology of the fever may be infectious or noninfectious. Common infectious causes include catheter-associated infections, hospital-acquired and ventilator-associated pneumonia (see Chapter 9), surgical site infections, urinary tract infections, and sepsis. Clinically relevant sinusitis is relatively uncommon in the patient in the intensive care unit.

An important noninfectious cause is thromboembolic disease. Fever in conjunction with refractory hypotension and shock may suggest sepsis; however, adrenal insufficiency, thyroid storm, and transfusion reaction may have a similar clinical presentation. Drug fever is difficult to diagnose and is usually a diagnosis of exclusion unless there are other signs of hypersensitivity, such as a typical maculopapular rash (most common with beta-lactams).

2. Fever in the postoperative patient—Postoperative fever is very common and noninfectious fever resolves spontaneously. Timing of the onset of the fever in relation to the surgical procedure may be of diagnostic benefit.

A. IMMEDIATE FEVER (IN THE FIRST FEW HOURS AFTER SURGERY)—Immediate fever can be due to medications that were given perioperatively, to surgical trauma, or to infections that were present before surgery. Necrotizing fasciitis due to group A streptococci or mixed organisms may present in this period. Malignant hyperthermia is rare and presents 30 minutes to several hours following inhalational anesthesia and is characterized by extreme hyperthermia, muscle rigidity, rhabdomyolysis, electrolyte abnormalities, and hypotension. Aggressive cooling and dantrolene are the mainstays of therapy. Aspiration of acidic gastric contents during surgery can result in a chemical pneumonitis (**Mendelson syndrome**) that develops rapidly, is transient, and does not require antibiotics. Fever due to surgical trauma usually resolves in 2–3 days; however, it may be longer in more complicated operative cases and in patients with head trauma.

B. Acute fever (within 1 week of surgery)—Acute fever is usually due to common causes of hospital-associated infections, such as ventilator-associated pneumonia (including aspiration pneumonia in patients with decreased gag reflex) and line infections. Noninfectious causes include alcohol withdrawal, gout, pulmonary embolism, and pancreatitis. Atelectasis following surgery is commonly invoked as a cause of postoperative fever but *there is no good evidence to support a causal association between the presence or degree of atelectasis and fever.*

C. Subacute fever (at least 1 week after surgery)—Surgical site infections commonly present at least 1 week after surgery. The type of surgery that was performed predicts specific infectious etiologies. Patients undergoing cardiothoracic surgery may be at higher risk for pneumonia and deep and superficial sternal wound infections. Meningitis without typical signs of meningismus may complicate neurosurgical procedures. Postoperative deep abdominal abscesses may require drainage.

B. Laboratory Findings

Blood cultures are universally recommended, and chest radiographs are frequently obtained. A properly prepared sputum Gram stain and semi-quantitative sputum cultures may be useful in selected patients where there is a high pretest probability of pneumonia but multiple exclusion criteria probably limit generalizability in most patients, such as immunocompromised patients and those with drug resistance. Other diagnostic strategies will be dictated by the clinical context (eg, transesophageal echocardiogram in a patient with *S aureus* bacteremia).

Any fever in a patient with a central venous catheter should prompt the collection of blood. The best method to evaluate bacteremia is to gather *at least two peripherally obtained blood cultures*. Blood cultures from unidentified sites, a single blood culture from any site, or a blood culture through an existing line will often be positive for coagulase-positive staphylococci, particularly *S epidermidis*, often resulting in the inappropriate use of vancomycin. Unless two separate venipuncture cultures are obtained—not through catheters—interpretation of results is impossible, and unnecessary therapy often results. Each "pseudobacteremia" increases laboratory costs, antibiotic use, and length of stay. Microbiologic evaluation of the removed catheter can sometimes be helpful, but only in addition to

(not instead of) blood cultures drawn from peripheral sites. The **differential time to positivity** measures the difference in time that cultures simultaneously drawn through a catheter and a peripheral site become positive. A positive test (at least 120 minutes' difference in time) supports a catheter-related bloodstream infection, while a negative test suggests catheters may be retained.

► Complications

Complications such as septic thrombophlebitis, endocarditis, or metastatic foci of infection (particularly with *S aureus*) may be suspected in patients with persistent bacteremia and fever despite removal of the infected catheter. Additional studies such as venous Doppler studies, transesophageal echocardiogram, and chest radiographs may be indicated, and 4–6 weeks of antibiotics may be needed. In the case of septic thrombophlebitis, anticoagulation with heparin is also recommended if there are no contraindications.

► Differential Diagnosis

Although most fevers are due to infections, about 25% of patients will have fever of noninfectious origin, including drug fever, nonspecific postoperative fevers (tissue damage or necrosis), hematoma, pancreatitis, pulmonary embolism, myocardial infarction, and ischemic bowel disease.

► Prevention

The concept of universal precautions emphasizes that all patients are treated as though they have a potential blood-borne transmissible disease, and thus all body secretions are handled with care to prevent spread of disease. Body substance isolation requires use of gloves whenever a health care worker anticipates contact with blood or other body secretions. *Even though gloves are worn, health care workers should routinely wash their hands, since it is the easiest and most effective means of preventing hospital-associated infections.* Application of a rapid drying, alcohol-based antiseptic is simple, takes less time than traditional hand washing with soap and water, is more effective at reducing hand colonization, and promotes compliance with hand decontamination. For prevention of transmission of *C difficile* infection, hand washing is more effective than alcohol-based antiseptics. Consequently, even after removing gloves, providers should always wash hands in cases of proven or suspected *C difficile* infection.

Peripheral intravenous lines should be replaced no more frequently than every 3–4 days. Some clinicians replace only when clinically indicated or if the line was put in emergently. Arterial lines and lines in the central venous circulation (including those placed peripherally) can be left in place indefinitely and are changed or removed when they are clinically suspected of being infected, when they are nonfunctional, or when they are no longer needed. Using sterile barrier precautions (including cap, mask, gown, gloves, and drape) is recommended while inserting central venous catheters. Antibiotic-impregnated (minocycline plus rifampin or chlorhexidine plus silver sulfadiazine) venous catheters reduce line infections. Silver alloy–impregnated Foley catheters reduce the incidence of catheter-associated bacteriuria, but not consistently catheter-associated urinary tract infections. Best practices to prevent ventilator-associated pneumonia include avoiding intubation if possible, minimizing and daily interruption of sedation, pooling/draining of subglottic secretions above the tube cuff, and elevating the head of the bed. Silver-coated endotracheal tubes may reduce the incidence of ventilator-associated pneumonia but has limited impact on hospital stay duration or mortality, so they are not generally recommended. Catheter-related urinary tract infections and intravenous catheter-associated infections are not Medicare-reimbursable conditions in the United States. Preoperative skin preparation with chlorhexidine and alcohol (versus povidone-iodine) reduces the incidence of infection following surgery. Another strategy that can prevent surgical-site infections is the identification and treatment of S aureus nasal carriers with 2% mupirocin nasal ointment and chlorhexidine soap. Daily bathing of ICU patients with chlorhexidine-impregnated washcloths versus soap and water results in lower incidence of health care–associated infections and colonization. Selective decontamination of the digestive tract with nonabsorbable or parenteral antibiotics, or both, may prevent hospital-acquired pneumonia and decrease mortality but is in limited use because of the concern of the development of antibiotic resistance. Prevention bundles (implementing more than one intervention concomitantly) are commonly used as a practical strategy to enhance care in the healthcare setting.

Attentive nursing care (positioning to prevent pressure injuries, wound care, elevating the head during tube feedings to prevent aspiration) is critical in preventing hospital-associated infections. In addition, monitoring of high-risk areas by hospital epidemiologists is critical in the prevention of infection. Some guidelines advocate rapid screening (active surveillance cultures) for MRSA on admission to acute care facilities among certain subpopulations of patients (eg, those recently hospitalized, admission to the intensive care unit, patients undergoing hemodialysis). However, outside the setting of an MRSA outbreak, it is not clear whether this strategy decreases the incidence of hospital-associated MRSA infections.

Vaccines, including hepatitis A, hepatitis B, and the varicella, pneumococcal, and influenza vaccinations, are important adjuncts. (See section below titled Immunization Against Infectious Diseases.)

▶ Treatment

A. Fever in an Intensive Care Unit Patient

Unless the patient has a central neurologic injury with elevated intracranial pressure or has a temperature higher than 41°C, there is less physiologic need to maintain euthermia. Empiric broad-spectrum antibiotics (see Table 30–5) are recommended for neutropenic and other immunocompromised patients and in patients who are clinically unstable.

B. Catheter-Associated Infections

Factors that inform treatment decisions include the type of catheter, the causative pathogen, the availability of alternate catheter access sites, the need for ongoing intravascular access, and the severity of disease.

In general, catheters should be removed if there is purulence at the exit site; if the organism is S aureus, gram-negative rods, or Candida species; if there is persistent bacteremia (more than 48 hours while receiving antibiotics); or if complications, such as septic thrombophlebitis, endocarditis, or other metastatic disease exist. Central venous catheters may be exchanged over a guidewire provided there is no erythema or purulence at the exit site and the patient does not appear to be septic. Methicillin-resistant, coagulase-negative staphylococci are the most common pathogens; thus, empiric therapy with vancomycin, 15 mg/kg/dose intravenously twice daily, should be given assuming normal kidney function. Empiric gram-negative coverage should be used in patients who are immunocompromised or who are critically ill (see Table 30–5).

Antibiotic treatment duration depends on the pathogen and the extent of disease. For uncomplicated bacteremia, 5–7 days of therapy is usually sufficient for coagulase-negative staphylococci, even if the original catheter is retained. Fourteen days of therapy is generally recommended for uncomplicated bacteremia caused by gram-negative rods, Candida species, and S aureus. **Antibiotic lock therapy** involves the instillation of supratherapeutic concentrations of antibiotics with heparin in the lumen of catheters. The purpose is to achieve adequate concentrations of antibiotics to kill microbes in the biofilm. Antibiotic lock therapy can be used for catheter-related bloodstream infections caused by both gram-positive and gram-negative bacterial pathogens and when the catheter is being retained in a salvage situation.

▶ When to Refer

- Any patient with multidrug-resistant infection.
- Any patient with fungemia or persistent bacteremia.
- Patients with multisite infections.
- Patients with impaired or fluctuating kidney function for assistance with dosing of antimicrobials.
- Patients with refractory or recurrent C difficile colitis.

Baur D et al. Effect of antibiotic stewardship on the incidence of infection and colonization with antibiotic-resistant bacteria and Clostridium difficile infection: a systematic review and meta-analysis. Lancet Infect Dis. 2017 Sep;17(9):990–1001. [PMID: 28629876]

Cortegiani A et al. Antifungal agents for preventing fungal infections in non-neutropenic critically ill patients Cochrane Database Syst Rev. 2016 Jan 16;(1):CD004920. [PMID: 26772902]

Dare RK et al. Health care-acquired viral respiratory diseases. Infect Dis Clin North Am. 2016 Dec;30(4):1053–70. [PMID: 27816139]

Harris PNA et al; MERINO Trial Investigators and the Australasian Society for Infectious Disease Clinical Research Network (ASID-CRN). Effect of piperacillin-tazobactam vs meropenem on 30-day mortality for patients with E coli or Klebsiella pneumoniae bloodstream infection and ceftriaxone resistance: a randomized clinical trial. JAMA. 2018 Sep 11; 320(10):984–94. [PMID: 30208454]

Kalil AC et al. Management of adults with hospital-acquired and ventilator-associated pneumonia: 2016 clinical practice guidelines by the Infectious Diseases Society of America and the American Thoracic Society. Clin Infect Dis. 2016 Sep 1; 63(5):e61–111. [PMID: 27418577]

Kao D et al. Effect of oral capsule- vs colonoscopy-delivered fecal microbiota transplantation on recurrent *Clostridium difficile* infection: a randomized clinical trial. JAMA. 2017 Nov 28;318(20):1985–93. [PMID: 29183074]

McDonald LC et al. Clinical practice guidelines for *Clostridium difficile* infection in adults and children: 2017 update by the Infectious Diseases Society of America (IDSA) and Society for Healthcare Epidemiology of America (SHEA). Clin Infect Dis. 2018 Mar 19;66(7):e1–48. [PMID: 29462280]

Wilcox MH et al; MODIFY I and MODIFY II Investigators. Bezlotoxumab for prevention of recurrent *Clostridium difficile* infection. N Engl J Med. 2017 Jan 26;376(4):305–17. [PMID: 28121498]

INFECTIONS OF THE CENTRAL NERVOUS SYSTEM

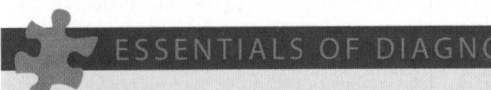

ESSENTIALS OF DIAGNOSIS

▶ Central nervous system infection is a medical emergency.

▶ Symptoms and signs common to all central nervous system infections include headache, fever, sensorial disturbances, neck and back stiffness, positive Kernig and Brudzinski signs, and cerebrospinal fluid abnormalities.

General Considerations

Infections of the central nervous system can be caused by almost any infectious agent, including bacteria, mycobacteria, fungi, spirochetes, protozoa, helminths, and viruses.

Etiologic Classification

Central nervous system infections can be divided into several categories that usually can be readily distinguished from each other by cerebrospinal fluid examination as the first step toward etiologic diagnosis (Table 30–1).

A. Purulent Meningitis

Patients with bacterial meningitis usually seek medical attention within hours or 1–2 days after onset of symptoms. The organisms responsible depend primarily on the age of the patient as summarized in Table 30–2. The diagnosis is usually based on the Gram-stained smear (positive in 60–90%) or culture (positive in over 90%) of the cerebrospinal fluid.

B. Chronic Meningitis

The presentation of chronic meningitis is less acute than purulent meningitis. Patients with chronic meningitis usually have a history of symptoms lasting weeks to months. The most common pathogens are *Mycobacterium tuberculosis*, atypical mycobacteria, fungi (*Cryptococcus, Coccidioides, Histoplasma*), and spirochetes (*Treponema pallidum* and *Borrelia burgdorferi*). The diagnosis is made by culture or in some cases by serologic tests (cryptococcosis, coccidioidomycosis, syphilis, Lyme disease).

C. Aseptic Meningitis

Aseptic meningitis—a much more benign and self-limited syndrome than purulent meningitis—is caused principally by viruses, especially herpes simplex virus and the enterovirus group (including coxsackieviruses and echoviruses). Infectious mononucleosis may be accompanied by aseptic meningitis. Leptospiral infection is also usually placed in

Table 30–1. Typical cerebrospinal fluid findings in various central nervous system diseases.

Diagnosis	Cells/mcL	Glucose (mg/dL)	Protein (mg/dL)	Opening Pressure
Normal	0–5 lymphocytes	45–85[1]	15–45	70–180 mm H$_2$O
Purulent meningitis (bacterial)[2] community-acquired	200–20,000 polymorphonuclear neutrophils	Low (< 45)	High (> 50)	Markedly elevated
Granulomatous meningitis (mycobacterial, fungal)[3]	100–1000, mostly lymphocytes[3]	Low (< 45)	High (> 50)	Moderately elevated
Spirochetal meningitis	100–1000, mostly lymphocytes[3]	Normal	High (> 50)	Normal to slightly elevated
Aseptic meningitis, viral meningitis, or meningoencephalitis[4]	25–2000, mostly lymphocytes[3]	Normal or low	High (> 50)	Slightly elevated
"Neighborhood reaction"[5]	Variably increased	Normal	Normal or high	Variable

[1]Cerebrospinal fluid glucose must be considered in relation to blood glucose level. Normally, cerebrospinal fluid glucose is 20–30 mg/dL lower than blood glucose, or 50–70% of the normal value of blood glucose.
[2]Organisms in smear or culture of cerebrospinal fluid; counterimmunoelectrophoresis or latex agglutination may be diagnostic.
[3]Polymorphonuclear neutrophils may predominate early.
[4]Viral isolation from cerebrospinal fluid early; antibody titer rise in paired specimens of serum; polymerase chain reaction for herpesvirus.
[5]May occur in mastoiditis, brain abscess, epidural abscess, sinusitis, septic thrombus, brain tumor. Cerebrospinal fluid culture results usually negative.

Table 30–2. Initial antimicrobial therapy for purulent meningitis of unknown cause.

Population	Usual Microorganisms	Standard Therapy
18–50 years	*Streptococcus pneumoniae, Neisseria meningitidis*	Vancomycin[1] **plus** ceftriaxone[2]
Over 50 years	*S pneumoniae, N meningitidis, Listeria monocytogenes*, gram-negative bacilli, group B *Streptococcus*	Vancomycin[1] **plus** ampicillin,[3] **plus** ceftriaxone[2]
Impaired cellular immunity	*L monocytogenes*, gram-negative bacilli, *S pneumoniae*	Vancomycin[1] **plus** ampicillin[3] **plus** cefepime[4]
Postsurgical or posttraumatic	*Staphylococcus aureus, S pneumoniae*, aerobic gram-negative bacilli, coagulase-negative staphylococci,[5] diphtheroids (eg, *Propionibacterium acnes*)[5] (uncommon)	Vancomycin[1] **plus** cefepime[4]

[1]Given to cover highly penicillin- or cephalosporin-resistant pneumococci. The dose of vancomycin is 15 mg/kg/dose intravenously every 8 hours. Vancomycin trough levels should be maintained at > 15 mcg/mL. Stopped if the causative organism is susceptible to ceftriaxone.
[2]Ceftriaxone can often be used safely in meningitis patients with a history of penicillin allergy (aztreonam can be considered for empiric coverage of gram-negative bacilli in patients with serious penicillin and cephalosporin allergy). The usual dose of ceftriaxone is 2 g intravenously every 12 hours. If the organism is sensitive to penicillin, 3–4 million units intravenously every 4 hours are given.
[3]In severely ill patients, ampicillin is used when *L monocytogenes* infection is a consideration. For confirmed infection due to *L monocytogenes*, gentamicin is sometimes added to ampicillin. (For patients allergic to penicillin, trimethoprim-sulfamethoxazole [TMP-SMZ] in a dosage of 15–20 mg/kg/day of TMP in 3 or 4 divided doses can be considered.) The dose of ampicillin is usually 2 g intravenously every 4 hours.
[4]Cefepime is given in a dose of 2–3 g intravenously every 8 hours.
[5]Primarily associated with presence of hardware.

the aseptic group because of the lymphocytic cellular response and its relatively benign course. This type of meningitis also occurs during secondary syphilis and disseminated Lyme disease. Prior to the routine administration of measles-mumps-rubella (MMR) vaccines, mumps was the most common cause of viral meningitis. Drug-induced aseptic meningitis has been reported with nonsteroidal anti-inflammatory drugs, sulfonamides, and certain monoclonal antibodies.

D. Encephalitis

Encephalitis (due to herpesviruses, arboviruses, rabies virus, flaviviruses [West Nile encephalitis, Japanese encephalitis], and many others) produces disturbances of the sensorium, seizures, and many other manifestations. Patients are more ill than those with aseptic meningitis. Cerebrospinal fluid may be entirely normal or may show some lymphocytes and, in some instances, (eg, herpes simplex) red cells as well. Influenza has been associated with encephalitis, but the relationship is not clear. An autoimmune form of encephalitis associated with N-methyl-D-aspartate receptor antibodies should be suspected in younger patients with encephalitis and associated seizures, movement disorders, and psychosis.

E. Partially Treated Bacterial Meningitis

Previous effective antibiotic therapy given for 12–24 hours will decrease the rate of positive cerebrospinal fluid Gram stain results by 20% and culture by 30–40% but will have little effect on cell count, protein, or glucose. Occasionally, previous antibiotic therapy will change a predominantly polymorphonuclear response to a lymphocytic pleocytosis, and some of the cerebrospinal fluid findings may be similar to those seen in aseptic meningitis.

F. Neighborhood Reaction

As noted in Table 30–1, this term denotes a purulent infectious process in close proximity to the central nervous system that spills some of the products of the inflammatory process—white blood cells or protein—into the cerebrospinal fluid. Such an infection might be a brain abscess, osteomyelitis of the vertebrae, epidural abscess, subdural empyema, or bacterial sinusitis or mastoiditis.

G. Noninfectious Meningeal Irritation

Carcinomatous meningitis, sarcoidosis, systemic lupus erythematosus, chemical meningitis, and certain medications—nonsteroidal anti-inflammatory drugs, OKT3, TMP-SMZ, and others—can also produce symptoms and signs of meningeal irritation with associated cerebrospinal fluid pleocytosis, increased protein, and low or normal glucose. Meningismus with normal cerebrospinal fluid findings occurs in the presence of other infections such as pneumonia and shigellosis.

H. Brain Abscess

Brain abscess presents as a space-occupying lesion; symptoms may include vomiting, fever, change of mental status, or focal neurologic manifestations. When brain abscess is suspected, a CT scan should be performed. If positive, lumbar puncture should *not* be performed since results rarely provide clinically useful information and herniation can occur. The bacteriology of brain abscess is usually polymicrobial and includes *S aureus*, gram-negative bacilli, streptococci, and mouth anaerobes (including anaerobic streptococci and *Prevotella* species).

I. Health Care–Associated Meningitis

This infection may arise as a result of invasive neurosurgical procedures (eg, craniotomy, internal or external ventricular catheters, external lumbar catheters), complicated head trauma, or hospital-acquired bloodstream infections. Outbreaks have been associated with contaminated epidural or paraspinal corticosteroid injections. In general, the microbiology is distinct from community-acquired meningitis, with gram-negative organisms (eg, *Pseudomonas*), *S aureus*, and coagulase-negative staphylococci and, in the outbreaks associated with contaminated corticosteroids, mold and fungi (*Exserohilum rostratum* and *Aspergillus fumigatus*) playing a larger role.

▶ Clinical Findings

A. Symptoms and Signs

The classic triad of fever, stiff neck, and altered mental status has a low sensitivity (44%) for bacterial meningitis. However, nearly all patients with bacterial meningitis have at least two of the following symptoms—fever, headache, stiff neck, or altered mental status.

B. Laboratory Tests

Evaluation of a patient with suspected meningitis includes a blood count, blood culture, lumbar puncture followed by careful study and culture of the cerebrospinal fluid, and a chest film. The fluid must be examined for cell count, glucose, and protein, and a smear stained for bacteria (and acid-fast organisms when appropriate) and cultured for pyogenic organisms and for mycobacteria and fungi when indicated. Latex agglutination tests can detect antigens of encapsulated organisms (*S pneumoniae, H influenzae, N meningitidis*, and *Cryptococcus neoformans*) but are rarely used except for detection of *Cryptococcus* or in partially treated patients. Polymerase chain reaction (PCR) testing of cerebrospinal fluid has been used to detect bacteria (*S pneumoniae, H influenzae, N meningitidis, M tuberculosis, B burgdorferi*, and *Tropheryma whipplei*) and viruses (herpes simplex, varicella-zoster, CMV, Epstein-Barr virus, and enteroviruses) in patients with meningitis. The greatest experience is with PCR for herpes simplex, varicella-zoster, and JC virus. These tests are very sensitive (greater than 95%) and specific. In addition to its use in meningitis, molecular methods such as PCR and next-generation sequencing are being used increasingly for the diagnosis of encephalitis, transverse myelitis, and brain abscess. In general, molecular diagnostic tests may provide a more sensitive and rapid alternative to traditional culture and serology methods. However, it is difficult to ascertain the true sensitivity of many molecular tests for CNS infections given the absence of a gold standard. In some cases, tests to detect several organisms may not be any more sensitive than culture (or serology), but the real value is the rapidity with which results are available, ie, hours compared with days or weeks.

C. Lumbar Puncture and Imaging

Since performing a lumbar puncture in the presence of a space-occupying lesion (brain abscess, subdural hematoma,

subdural empyema, necrotic temporal lobe from herpes encephalitis) may result in brainstem herniation, a CT scan is performed *prior to* lumbar puncture if a space-occupying lesion is suspected on the basis of papilledema, seizures, or focal neurologic findings. Other indications for CT scan are an immunocompromised patient or moderately to severely impaired level of consciousness. If delays are encountered in obtaining a CT scan and bacterial meningitis is suspected, blood cultures should be drawn and antibiotics and corticosteroids administered even before cerebrospinal fluid is obtained for culture to avoid delay in treatment (Table 30–1). *Antibiotics given within 4 hours before obtaining cerebrospinal fluid probably do not affect culture results.* MRI with contrast of the epidural injection site and surrounding areas is recommended (sometimes repeatedly) for those with symptoms following a possibly contaminated corticosteroid injection to exclude epidural abscess, phlegmon, vertebral osteomyelitis, discitis, or arachnoiditis.

▶ Treatment

Although it is difficult to prove with existing clinical data that early antibiotic therapy improves outcome in bacterial meningitis, prompt therapy is still recommended. In purulent meningitis, the identity of the causative microorganism may remain unknown or doubtful for a few days and initial antibiotic treatment as set forth in Table 30–2 should be directed against the microorganisms most common for each age group.

The duration of therapy for bacterial meningitis varies depending on the etiologic agent: *H influenzae*, 7 days; *N meningitidis*, 3–7 days; *S pneumoniae*, 10–14 days; *L monocytogenes*, 14–21 days; and gram-negative bacilli, 21 days.

For adults with pneumococcal meningitis, dexamethasone 10 mg administered intravenously 15–20 minutes before or simultaneously with the first dose of antibiotics and continued every 6 hours for 4 days decreases morbidity and mortality. Patients most likely to benefit from corticosteroids are those infected with gram-positive organisms (*Streptococcus pneumoniae* or *S suis*), and those who are HIV negative. It is unknown whether patients with meningitis due to *N meningitidis* and other bacterial pathogens benefit from the use of adjunctive corticosteroids. Increased intracranial pressure due to brain edema often requires therapeutic attention. Hyperventilation, mannitol (25–50 g intravenously as a bolus), and even drainage of cerebrospinal fluid by repeated lumbar punctures or by placement of intraventricular catheters have been used to control cerebral edema and increased intracranial pressure. Dexamethasone (4 mg intravenously every 4–6 hours) may also decrease cerebral edema.

Therapy of brain abscess consists of drainage (excision or aspiration) in addition to 3–4 weeks of systemic antibiotics directed against organisms isolated. An empiric regimen often includes metronidazole, 500 mg intravenously or orally every 8 hours, plus ceftriaxone, 2 g intravenously every 12 hours, with or without vancomycin, 10–15 mg/kg/dose intravenously every 12 hours. Vancomycin trough serum levels should be greater than 15 mcg/mL in such patients. In cases where abscesses are smaller than 2 cm, where there are multiple abscesses that cannot be drained, or if an abscess is located in an area where significant neurologic sequelae would result from drainage, antibiotics for 6–8 weeks can be used without drainage.

In addition to antibiotics, in cases of health care–associated meningitis associated with an external intraventricular catheter, the probability of cure is increased if the catheter is removed. In infections associated with internal ventricular catheters, removal of the internal components and insertion of an external drain is recommended. After collecting cerebrospinal fluid, epidural aspirate, or other specimens for culture, empiric antifungal therapy with voriconazole as well as routine empiric treatment for other pathogens (as above) is recommended until the specific cause of the patient's central nervous system or parameningeal infection has been identified. In addition, early consultation with a neurosurgeon is recommended for those found to have an epidural abscess, phlegmon, vertebral osteomyelitis, discitis, or arachnoiditis to discuss possible surgical management (eg, debridement).

Therapy of other types of meningitis is discussed elsewhere in this book (fungal meningitis, Chapter 36; syphilis and Lyme borreliosis, Chapter 34; tuberculous meningitis, Chapter 33; herpes encephalitis, Chapter 32).

▶ When to Refer

- Patients with acute meningitis, particularly if culture negative or atypical (eg, fungi, syphilis, Lyme disease, *M tuberculosis*), or if the patient is immunosuppressed.
- Patients with chronic meningitis.
- All patients with brain abscesses and encephalitis.
- Patients with suspected hospital-acquired meningitis (eg, in patients who have undergone recent neurosurgery or epidural or paraspinal corticosteroid injection).
- Patients with recurrent meningitis.

▶ When to Admit

- Patients with suspected acute meningitis, encephalitis, and brain or paraspinous abscess should be admitted for urgent evaluation and treatment.
- There is less urgency to admit patients with chronic meningitis; these patients may be admitted to expedite diagnostic procedures and coordinate care, particularly if no diagnosis has been made in the outpatient setting.

McGill F et al. Acute bacterial meningitis in adults. Lancet. 2016 Dec 17;388(10063):3036–47. [PMID: 27265346]

Prasad K et al. Corticosteroids for managing tuberculous meningitis. Cochrane Database Syst Rev. 2016 Apr 28;4:CD002244. [PMID: 27121755]

Tunkel AR et al. 2017 Infectious Diseases Society of America's clinical practice guidelines for healthcare-associated ventriculitis and meningitis. Clin Infect Dis. 2017 Mar 15;64(6):e34–65. [PMID: 28203777]

Wilson M et al. Emerging diagnostic and therapeutic tools for central nervous system infections. JAMA Neurol. 2016 Dec 1; 73(12):1389–90. [PMID: 27695862]

ANIMAL & HUMAN BITE WOUNDS

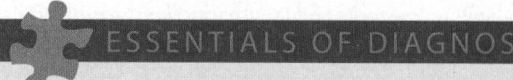

ESSENTIALS OF DIAGNOSIS

- ▶ Cat and human bites have higher rates of infection than dog bites.
- ▶ Hand bites are particularly concerning for the possibility of closed-space infection.
- ▶ Antibiotic prophylaxis indicated for noninfected bites of the hand and hospitalization required for infected hand bites.
- ▶ All infected wounds need to be cultured to direct therapy.

▶ General Considerations

About 1000 dog bite injuries require emergency department attention each day in the United States, most often in urban areas. Dog bites occur most commonly in the summer months. Biting animals are usually known by their victims, and most biting incidents are provoked (ie, bites occur while playing with the animal or after surprising the animal while eating or waking it abruptly from sleep). Failure to elicit a history of provocation is important, because *an unprovoked attack raises the possibility of rabies.* Human bites are usually inflicted by children while playing or fighting; in adults, bites are associated with alcohol use and closed-fist injuries that occur during fights.

The animal inflicting the bite, the location of the bite, and the type of injury inflicted are all important determinants of whether they become infected. Cat bites are more likely to become infected than human bites—between 30% and 50% of all cat bites become infected. Infections following human bites are variable. Bites inflicted by children rarely become infected because they are superficial, and bites by adults become infected in 15–30% of cases, with a particularly high rate of infection in closed-fist injuries. Dog bites, for unclear reasons, become infected only 5% of the time. Bites of the head, face, and neck are less likely to become infected than bites on the extremities. "Through and through" bites (eg, involving the mucosa and the skin) have an infection rate similar to closed-fist injuries. Puncture wounds become infected more frequently than lacerations, probably because the latter are easier to irrigate and debride.

The bacteriology of bite infections is polymicrobial. Following dog and cat bites, over 50% of infections are caused by aerobes and anaerobes and 36% are due to aerobes alone. Pure anaerobic infections are rare. *Pasteurella* species are the single most common isolate (75% of infections caused by cat bites and 50% of infections caused by dog bites). Other common aerobic isolates include streptococci, staphylococci, *Moraxella*, and *Neisseria;* the most common anaerobes are *Fusobacterium, Bacteroides, Porphyromonas,* and *Prevotella.* The median number of isolates following human bites is four (three aerobes and one anaerobe). Like dog and cat bites, infections caused by most human bites are a mixture of aerobes and anaerobes (54%) or are due to aerobes alone (44%). Streptococci and *S aureus* are the most common aerobes. *Eikenella corrodens* (found in up to 30% of patients), *Prevotella*, and *Fusobacterium* are the most common anaerobes. Although the organisms noted are the most common, innumerable others have been isolated—including *Capnocytophaga* (dog and cat), *Pseudomonas*, and *Haemophilus*—emphasizing the point that *all infected bites should be cultured* to define the microbiology.

HIV can be transmitted from bites (either from biting or receiving a bite from an HIV-infected patient) but has rarely been reported.

► Treatment

A. Local Care

Vigorous cleansing and irrigation of the wound as well as debridement of necrotic material are the most important factors in decreasing the incidence of infections. Radiographs should be obtained to look for fractures and the presence of foreign bodies. Careful examination to assess the extent of the injury (tendon laceration, joint space penetration) is critical to appropriate care.

B. Suturing

If wounds require closure for cosmetic or mechanical reasons, suturing can be done. However, one should never suture an infected wound, and wounds of the hand should generally not be sutured since a closed-space infection of the hand can result in loss of function.

C. Prophylactic Antibiotics

Prophylaxis is indicated in high-risk bites and in high-risk patients. *Cat bites in any location and hand bites by any animal, including humans, should receive prophylaxis.* Individuals with certain comorbidities (diabetes, liver disease) are at increased risk for severe complications and should receive prophylaxis even for low-risk bites, as should patients without functional spleens who are at increased risk for overwhelming sepsis (primarily with *Capnocytophaga* species). Amoxicillin-clavulanate (Augmentin) 500 mg orally three times daily for 5–7 days is the regimen of choice. For patients with serious allergy to penicillin, a combination of clindamycin 300 mg orally three times daily together with one of the following is recommended for 5–7 days: doxycycline 100 mg orally twice daily, or double-strength TMP-SMZ orally twice daily, or a fluoroquinolone (ciprofloxacin 500 mg orally twice daily or levofloxacin 500–750 mg orally once daily). Moxifloxacin, a fluoroquinolone with good aerobic and anaerobic activity, may be suitable as monotherapy at 400 mg orally once daily for 5–7 days. Agents such as dicloxacillin, cephalexin, macrolides, and clindamycin should not be used alone because they lack activity against *Pasteurella* species. TMP-SMZ has poor activity against anaerobes and should only be used in combination with clindamycin.

Because the risk of HIV transmission is so low following a bite, routine postexposure prophylaxis is *not* recommended. Each case should be evaluated individually and consideration for prophylaxis should be given to those who present within 72 hours of the incident, the source is known to be HIV infected, and the exposure is high risk.

D. Antibiotics for Documented Infection

For wounds that are infected, antibiotics are clearly indicated. How they are given (orally or intravenously) and the need for hospitalization are individualized clinical decisions. The most commonly encountered pathogens require treatment with ampicillin-sulbactam (Unasyn), 1.5–3.0 g intravenously every 6–8 hours; or amoxicillin-clavulanate (Augmentin), 500 mg orally three times daily; or with ertapenem, 1 g intravenously daily. For the patient with severe penicillin allergy, a combination of clindamycin 600–900 mg intravenously every 8 hours plus a fluoroquinolone (ciprofloxacin, 400 mg intravenously every 12 hours; levofloxacin, 500–750 mg intravenously once daily) or TMP-SMZ (10 mg/kg of trimethoprim daily in two or three divided doses) is indicated. Duration of therapy is usually 2–3 weeks unless complications such as septic arthritis or osteomyelitis is present; if these complications are present, therapy should be extended to 4 and 6 weeks, respectively.

E. Tetanus and Rabies

All patients must be evaluated for the need for tetanus (see Chapter 33) and rabies (see Chapter 32) prophylaxis.

► When to Refer

- If septic arthritis or osteomyelitis is suspected.
- For exposure to bites by dogs, cats, reptiles, amphibians, and rodents.
- When rabies is a possibility.

► When to Admit

- Patients with infected hand bites.
- Deep bites, particularly if over joints.

Bula-Rudas FJ et al. Human and animal bites. Pediatr Rev. 2018 Oct;39(10):490–500. [PMID: 30275032]

Edens MA et al. Mammalian bites in the emergency department: recommendations for wound closure, antibiotics, and postexposure prophylaxis. Emerg Med Pract. 2016 Apr;18(4):1–20. [PMID: 27104678]

Smith HR et al. Predicting serious complications and high cost of treatment of tooth-knuckle injuries: a systematic literature review. Eur J Trauma Emerg Surg. 2016 Dec;42(6):701–10. [PMID: 27363840]

Wilde H et al. Worldwide rabies deaths prevention—a focus on the current inadequacies in postexposure prophylaxis of animal bite victims. Vaccine. 2016 Jan 4;34(2):187–9. [PMID: 26626211]

SEXUALLY TRANSMITTED DISEASES

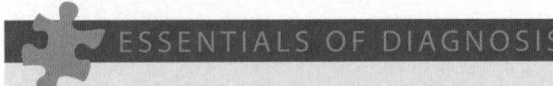

ESSENTIALS OF DIAGNOSIS

► All sexually transmitted diseases (STDs) have subclinical or latent periods, and patients may be asymptomatic.

► Simultaneous infection with several organisms is common.

► All patients who seek STD testing should be screened for syphilis and HIV.

> ▶ Partner notification and treatment are important to prevent further transmission and reinfection of the index case.

▶ General Considerations

The most common STDs are gonorrhea,* syphilis,* human papillomavirus (HPV)–associated condyloma acuminatum, chlamydial genital infections,* herpesvirus genital infections, trichomonas vaginitis, chancroid,* granuloma inguinale, scabies, louse infestation, and bacterial vaginosis (among women who have sex with women). However, shigellosis*; hepatitis A, B, and C*; amebiasis; giardiasis*; cryptosporidiosis*; salmonellosis*; and campylobacteriosis may also be transmitted by sexual (oral-anal) contact, especially in men who have sex with men. Ebola virus and Zika virus have both been associated with sexual transmission. Both homosexual and heterosexual contact are risk factors for the transmission of HIV (see Chapter 31). All STDs have *subclinical* or *latent phases* that play an important role in long-term persistence of the infection or in its transmission from infected (but largely asymptomatic) persons to other contacts. Simultaneous infection by several different agents is common.

Infections typically present in one of several ways, each of which has a defined differential diagnosis, which should prompt appropriate diagnostic tests.

A. Genital Ulcers

Common etiologies include herpes simplex virus, primary syphilis, and chancroid. Other possibilities include lymphogranuloma venereum (see Chapter 33), granuloma inguinale caused by *Klebsiella granulomatis* (see Chapter 33), as well as lesions caused by infection with Epstein-Barr virus and HIV. Noninfectious causes are Behçet disease (see Chapter 20), neoplasm, trauma, drugs, and irritants.

B. Urethritis With or Without Urethral Discharge

The most common infections causing urethral discharge are *Neisseria gonorrhoeae* and *Chlamydia trachomatis*. *N gonorrhoeae* and *C trachomatis* are also frequent causes of prostatitis among sexually active men. Other sexually transmitted infections that can cause urethritis include *Mycoplasma genitalium* and, less commonly, *Ureaplasma urealyticum* and *Trichomonas vaginalis*. Noninfectious causes of urethritis include reactive arthritis with associated urethritis.

C. Vaginal Discharge

Common causes of vaginitis are bacterial vaginosis (caused by overgrowth of anaerobes such as *Gardnerella vaginalis*), candidiasis, and *T vaginalis* (see Chapter 18). Less common infectious causes of vaginitis include HPV-associated condylomata acuminata and group A streptococcus. Noninfectious causes are physiologic changes related to the menstrual cycle, irritants, and lichen planus. Even though *N gonorrhoeae* and *C trachomatis* are frequent causes of cervicitis, they *rarely* produce vaginal discharge.

---

*Reportable to public health authorities.

▶ Screening & Prevention

All persons who seek STD testing should undergo routine screening for HIV infection, using rapid HIV testing (if patients may not follow up for results obtained by standard methods) or nucleic acid amplification followed by confirmatory serology (if primary HIV infection may be a possibility) as indicated. Patients in whom certain STDs have been diagnosed and treated (chlamydia or gonorrhea, and trichomonas in women) are at a high risk for reinfection and should be encouraged to be rescreened for STDs at 3 months following the initial STD diagnosis.

Asymptomatic patients often request STD screening at the time of initiating a new sexual relationship. Routine HIV testing and hepatitis B serology testing should be offered to all such patients. In sexually active women who have not been recently screened, cervical Papanicolaou testing and nucleic acid amplification testing of a urine specimen for gonorrhea and chlamydia are recommended. Among men who have sex with men, additional screening is recommended for syphilis; hepatitis A; urethral, pharyngeal, and rectal gonorrhea; as well as urethral and rectal chlamydia. Nucleic acid amplification testing is recommended for gonorrhea or chlamydia. There are no recommendations to screen heterosexual men for urethral chlamydia, but this could be considered in STD clinics, adolescent clinics, or correctional facilities. The periodicity of screening thereafter depends on sexual risk, but most screening should be offered at least annually to sexually active adults (particularly to those 25 years old and under). Clinicians should also evaluate transgender men and women for STD screening, based on current anatomy and behaviors practiced. If not immune, hepatitis B vaccination is recommended for all sexually active adults, and hepatitis A vaccination in men who have sex with men. Persons between the ages of 9 and 26 should be routinely offered vaccination against HPV (9-valent).

The risk of developing an STD following a sexual assault is difficult to accurately ascertain given high rates of baseline infections and poor follow-up. Victims of assault have a high baseline rate of infection (*N gonorrhoeae*, 6%; *C trachomatis*, 10%; *T vaginalis*, 15%; and bacterial vaginosis, 34%), and the risk of acquiring infection as a result of the assault is significant, but is often lower than the pre-existing rate (*N gonorrhoeae*, 6–12%; *C trachomatis*, 4–17%; *T vaginalis*, 12%; syphilis, 0.5–3%; and bacterial vaginosis, 19%). Victims should be evaluated within 24 hours after the assault, and nucleic acid amplification tests for *N gonorrhoeae* and *C trachomatis* should be performed. Vaginal secretions are obtained for *Trichomonas* wet mount and culture, or point-of-care testing. If a discharge is present, if there is itching, or if secretions are malodorous, a wet mount should be examined for *Candida* and bacterial vaginosis. In addition, a blood sample should be obtained for immediate serologic testing for syphilis, hepatitis B, and HIV. Follow-up examination for STDs should be repeated within 1–2 weeks, since concentrations of infecting organisms may not have been sufficient to produce a positive test at the time of initial examination. If prophylactic treatment was given (may include postexposure hepatitis B vaccination without hepatitis B immune globulin; treatment for chlamydial, gonorrheal, or trichomonal infection; and emergency contraception), tests should be repeated only if the victim has symptoms. If prophylaxis was not administered, the individual should be seen in 1 week so that any positive tests can be treated. Follow-up serologic testing for syphilis and HIV infection should be performed in 6, 12, and 24 weeks if the initial tests are negative. The usefulness of presumptive therapy is controversial, with some feeling that all patients should receive it and others that it should be limited to those in whom follow-up cannot be ensured or to patients who request it.

Although seroconversion to HIV has been reported following sexual assault when this was the only known risk, this risk is believed to be low. The likelihood of HIV transmission from vaginal or anal receptive intercourse when the source is known to be HIV positive is 1 per 1000 and 5 per 1000, respectively. Although prophylactic antiretroviral therapy has not been studied in this setting, the Department of Health and Human Services recommends the prompt institution of postexposure prophylaxis with antiretroviral therapy if the person seeks care within 72 hours of the assault, the source is known to be HIV positive, and the exposure presents a substantial risk of transmission.

In addition to screening asymptomatic patients with STDs, other strategies for preventing further transmission include evaluating sex partners and administering preexposure vaccination of preventable STDs to individuals at risk; other strategies include the consistent use of male and female condoms and male circumcision. Adult male circumcision has been shown to decrease the transmission of HIV by 50%, and of herpes simplex virus and HPV by 30% in heterosexual couples in sub-Saharan Africa. For each patient, there are one or more sexual contacts who require diagnosis and treatment. Prompt treatment of contacts by giving antibiotics to the index case to distribute to all sexual contacts (**patient-delivered therapy**) is an important strategy for preventing further transmission and to prevent reinfection of the index case.

Note that vaginal spermicides and condoms containing nonoxynol-9 provide no additional protection against STDs. Early initiation of antiretroviral therapy in HIV-infected individuals can prevent HIV acquisition in an uninfected sex partner. Also, preexposure prophylaxis with a once-daily pill containing emtricitabine plus tenofovir disoproxil fumarate (TDF) has been shown to be effective in preventing HIV infection among high-risk men who have sex with men, heterosexual women and men, transgender women, and persons who inject drugs.

When to Refer

- Patients with a new diagnosis of HIV.
- Patients with persistent, refractory, or recurrent STDs, particularly when drug resistance is suspected.

Marcus JL et al. Risk compensation and clinical decision making—the case of HIV preexposure prophylaxis. N Engl J Med. 2019 Feb 7;380(6):510–2. [PMID: 30726699]

Price JC et al. Sexually acquired hepatitis C infection in HIV-uninfected men who have sex with men using pre-exposure prophylaxis against HIV. J Infect Dis. 2019 Apr 16;219(9):1373–76. [PMID: 30462305]

Rodger AJ et al; PARTNER Study Group. Sexual activity without condoms and risk of HIV transmission in serodifferent couples when the HIV-positive partner is using suppressive antiretroviral therapy. JAMA. 2016 Jul 12;316(2):171–81. [PMID: 27404185]

Sonawane K et al. Oral human papillomavirus infection: differences in prevalence between sexes and concordance with genital human papillomavirus infection, NHANES 2011 to 2014. Ann Intern Med. 2017 Nov 21;167(10):714–24. [PMID: 29049523]

Unemo M et al. Sexually transmitted infections: challenges ahead. Lancet Infect Dis. 2017 Aug;17(8):e235–79. [PMID: 28701272]

Wiesenfeld HC. Screening for *Chlamydia trachomatis* infections in women. N Engl J Med. 2017 Feb 23;376(8):765–73. [PMID: 28225683]

INFECTIONS IN PERSONS WHO INJECT DRUGS

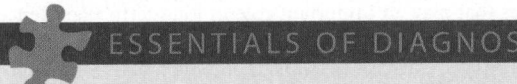

ESSENTIALS OF DIAGNOSIS

- ▶ Common infections that occur with greater frequency in persons who inject drugs include:
  - Skin infections, aspiration pneumonia, tuberculosis.
  - Hepatitis A, B, C, D; STDs; HIV/AIDS.
  - Pulmonary septic emboli, infective endocarditis.
  - Osteomyelitis and septic arthritis.

General Considerations

There is a high incidence of infection among drug users, particularly among people who inject drugs. Increased risk of infection is likely associated with poor hygiene and colonization with potentially pathogenic organisms, contamination of drugs and equipment, increased sexual risk behaviors, and impaired immune defenses. The use of parenterally administered recreational drugs has increased enormously in recent years, fueled in part by an epidemic of prescription opioid misuse and abuse. More than 2 million persons in North America are estimated to have used injection drugs in the past year.

Skin infections are associated with poor hygiene and use of nonsterile technique when injecting drugs. *S aureus* (including community-acquired methicillin-resistant strains) and oral flora (streptococci, *Eikenella, Fusobacterium, Peptostreptococcus*) are the most common organisms, with enteric gram-negatives generally more likely seen in those who inject into the groin. Cellulitis and subcutaneous abscesses occur most commonly, particularly in association with subcutaneous ("skin-popping") or intramuscular injections and the use of cocaine and heroin mixtures (probably due to ischemia). Myositis, clostridial myonecrosis, and necrotizing fasciitis occur infrequently but are life-threatening. Wound botulism in association with black tar heroin occurs sporadically but often in clusters.

Aspiration pneumonia and its complications (lung abscess, empyema, brain abscess) result from altered consciousness associated with drug use. Mixed aerobic and anaerobic mouth flora are usually involved.

Tuberculosis also occurs in persons who use drugs, and infection with HIV has fostered the spread of tuberculosis in this population. Morbidity and mortality rates are increased in HIV-infected individuals with tuberculosis. Classic radiographic findings are often absent; tuberculosis is suspected in any patient with infiltrates who does not respond to antibiotics.

Hepatitis is very common among persons who inject drugs and is transmissible both by the parenteral (hepatitis B, C, and D) and by the fecal-oral route (hepatitis A). Multiple episodes of hepatitis with different agents can occur.

Pulmonary septic emboli may originate from venous thrombi or right-sided endocarditis.

STDs are not directly related to drug use, but the practice of exchanging sex for drugs has resulted in an increased frequency of STDs. Syphilis, gonorrhea, and chancroid are the most common.

HIV/AIDS has a high incidence among persons who inject drugs and their sexual contacts and among the offspring of infected women (see Chapter 31).

Infective endocarditis in persons who inject drugs is most commonly caused by *S aureus*, *Candida* (usually *C albicans* or *C parapsilosis*), *Enterococcus faecalis*, other streptococci, and gram-negative bacteria (especially *Pseudomonas* and *Serratia marcescens*). See Chapter 33.

Other vascular infections include septic thrombophlebitis and mycotic aneurysms. Mycotic aneurysms resulting from direct trauma to a vessel with secondary infection most commonly occur in femoral arteries and less commonly in arteries of the neck. Aneurysms resulting from hematogenous spread of organisms frequently involve intracerebral vessels and thus are seen in association with endocarditis.

Osteomyelitis and **septic arthritis** involving vertebral bodies, sternoclavicular joints, the pubic symphysis, the sacroiliac joints, and other sites usually results from hematogenous distribution of injected organisms or septic venous thrombi. Pain and fever precede radiographic changes, sometimes by several weeks. While *S aureus*—often methicillin-resistant—is most common, *Serratia*, *Pseudomonas*, *Candida* (often not *C albicans*), and other pathogens rarely encountered in spontaneous bone or joint disease are found in persons who inject drugs.

▶ Treatment

A common and difficult clinical problem is management of a person known to inject drugs who presents with fever. In general, after obtaining appropriate cultures (blood, urine, and sputum if the chest radiograph is abnormal), empiric therapy is begun. If the chest radiograph is suggestive of a community-acquired pneumonia (consolidation), therapy for outpatient pneumonia is begun with ceftriaxone, 1 g intravenously every 24 hours, plus either azithromycin

(500 mg orally or intravenously every 24 hours) or doxycycline (100 mg orally or intravenously twice daily). If the chest radiograph is suggestive of septic emboli (nodular infiltrates), therapy for presumed endocarditis is initiated, usually with vancomycin 15 mg/kg/dose every 12 hours intravenously (due to the high prevalence of MRSA and the possibility of enterococcus). If the chest radiograph is normal and no focal site of infection can be found, endocarditis is presumed. While awaiting the results of blood cultures, empiric treatment with vancomycin is started. If blood cultures are positive for organisms that frequently cause endocarditis in drug users (see above), endocarditis is presumed to be present and treated accordingly. If blood cultures are positive for an organism that is an unusual cause of endocarditis, evaluation for an occult source of infection should go forward. In this setting, a transesophageal echocardiogram may be quite helpful since it is 90% sensitive in detecting vegetations and a negative study is strong evidence against endocarditis. If blood cultures are negative and the patient responds to antibiotics, therapy should be continued for 7–14 days (oral therapy can be given once an initial response has occurred). In every patient, careful examination for an occult source of infection (eg, genitourinary, dental, sinus, gallbladder) should be done. Given the intersecting epidemics of opioid use disorder and the infectious complications that arise, clinicians must also be prepared to integrate treatment of opioid use disorder whenever possible.

▶ When to Refer

- Any patient with suspected or proven infective endocarditis.
- Patients with persistent bacteremia.

▶ When to Admit

- Persons who inject drugs with fever.
- Patients with abscesses or progressive skin and soft tissue infection that require debridement.

Hartman L et al. Opiate injection-associated infective endocarditis in the southeastern United States. Am J Med Sci. 2016 Dec;352(6):603–8. [PMID: 27916215]

Ip EJ et al. Infectious disease, injection practices, and risky sexual behavior among anabolic steroid users. AIDS Care. 2016 Mar; 28(3):294–9. [PMID: 26422090]

Jackson KA et al. Invasive methicillin-resistant *Staphylococcus aureus* infections among persons who inject drugs—six sites, 2005–2016. MMWR Morb Mortal Wkly Rep. 2018 Jun 8; 67(22):625–8. [PMID: 29879096]

Schranz AJ et al. Trends in drug use-associated infective endocarditis and heart valve surgery, 2007 to 2017: a study of statewide discharge data. Ann Intern Med. 2018 Dec 4. [Epub ahead of print] [PMID: 30508432]

Springer SA et al. Integrating treatment at the intersection of opioid use disorder and infectious disease epidemics in medical settings: a call for action after a national academies of sciences, engineering, and medicine workshop. Ann Intern Med. 2018 Sep 4;169(5):335–6. [PMID: 30007032]

ACUTE INFECTIOUS DIARRHEA

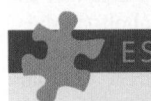

ESSENTIALS OF DIAGNOSIS

▶ **Acute diarrhea:** lasts less than 2 weeks

▶ **Chronic diarrhea:** lasts longer than 2 weeks.

▶ **Mild diarrhea:** 3 or fewer stools per day.

▶ **Moderate diarrhea:** 4 or more stools per day with local symptoms (abdominal cramps, nausea, tenesmus).

▶ **Severe diarrhea:** 4 or more stools per day with systemic symptoms (fever, chills, dehydration).

▶ General Considerations

Acute diarrhea can be caused by a number of different factors, including emotional stress, food intolerance, inorganic agents (eg, sodium nitrite), organic substances (eg, mushrooms, shellfish), medications, and infectious agents (including viruses, bacteria, and protozoa) (Table 30–3). From a diagnostic and therapeutic standpoint, it is helpful to classify infectious diarrhea into syndromes that produce inflammatory or bloody diarrhea and those that are noninflammatory, nonbloody, or watery. In general, the term "**inflammatory diarrhea**" suggests colonic involvement by invasive bacteria or parasites or by toxin production. Patients complain of frequent bloody, small-volume stools, often associated with fever, abdominal cramps, tenesmus, and fecal urgency. Common causes of this syndrome include *Shigella*, *Salmonella*, *Campylobacter*, *Yersinia*, invasive strains of *Escherichia coli*, and other Shiga-toxin-producing strains of *E coli* (STEC), *Entamoeba histolytica*, and *C difficile*. Tests for fecal leukocytes or the neutrophil marker lactoferrin are frequently positive, and definitive etiologic diagnosis requires stool culture. **Noninflammatory diarrhea** is generally milder and is caused by viruses or toxins that affect the small intestine and interfere with salt and water balance, resulting in large-volume watery diarrhea, often with nausea, vomiting, and cramps. Common causes of this syndrome include viruses (eg, rotavirus, norovirus, astrovirus, enteric adenoviruses), vibriones *(Vibrio cholerae, Vibrio parahaemolyticus)*, enterotoxin-producing *E coli, Giardia lamblia*, cryptosporidia, and agents that can cause food-borne gastroenteritis. In developed countries, viruses (particularly norovirus) are an important cause of hospitalizations due to acute gastroenteritis among adults.

The term "food poisoning" denotes diseases caused by toxins present in consumed foods. When the incubation period is short (1–6 hours after consumption), the toxin is usually *preformed*. Vomiting is usually a major complaint, and fever is usually absent. Examples include intoxication from *S aureus* or *Bacillus cereus*, and toxin can be detected in the food. When the incubation period is longer—between 8 hours and 16 hours—the organism is present in the food and *produces toxin after being ingested*. Vomiting is less prominent, abdominal cramping is frequent, and

fever is often absent. The best example of this disease is that due to *Clostridium perfringens*. Toxin can be detected in food or stool specimens.

The inflammatory and noninflammatory diarrheas discussed above can also be transmitted by food and water and usually have incubation periods between 12 and 72 hours. *Cyclospora*, cryptosporidia, and *Isospora* are protozoans capable of causing disease in both immunocompetent and immunocompromised patients. Characteristics of disease include profuse watery diarrhea that is prolonged but usually self-limited (1–2 weeks) in the immunocompetent patient but can be chronic in the compromised host. Epidemiologic features may be helpful in determining etiology. Recent hospitalization or antibiotic use suggests *C difficile*; recent foreign travel suggests *Salmonella, Shigella, Campylobacter, E coli*, or *V cholerae*; undercooked hamburger suggests STEC; outbreak in long-term care facility, school, or cruise ship suggests norovirus (including newly identified strains, eg, GII.4 Sydney); and fried rice consumption is associated with *B cereus* toxin. Prominent features of some of these causes of diarrhea are listed in Table 30–3.

▶ Treatment

A. General Measures

In general, *most cases of acute gastroenteritis are self-limited and do not require therapy other than supportive measures.* Treatment usually consists of replacement of fluids and electrolytes and, very rarely, management of hypovolemic shock and respiratory compromise. In mild diarrhea, increasing ingestion of juices and clear soups is adequate. In more severe cases of dehydration (postural light-headedness, decreased urination), oral glucose-based rehydration solutions can be used (Ceralyte, Pedialyte).

B. Specific Measures

In immunocompetent adults, empiric antimicrobial therapy for bloody diarrhea while waiting for results is recommended only with the following circumstances: (1) documented fever, abdominal pain, bloody diarrhea, and bacillary dysentery (frequent scant bloody stools, fever, abdominal cramps, tenesmus) presumptively due to *Shigella*; and (2) returning travelers with a temperature of at least 38.5°C or signs of sepsis.

Either a fluoroquinolone or azithromycin should be used as empiric antimicrobial therapy for bloody diarrhea. Empiric antibacterial treatment should be considered in immunocompromised people with severe illness and bloody diarrhea. Loperamide may be given to immunocompetent adults with acute watery diarrhea, but should be avoided with *Shigella* infection or in suspected or proven toxic megacolon. Therapeutic recommendations for specific agents can be found elsewhere in this book.

Bányai K et al. Viral gastroenteritis. Lancet. 2018 Jul 14; 392(10142):175–86. [PMID: 30025810]

Beinortas T et al. Comparative efficacy of treatments for *Clostridium difficile* infection: a systematic review and network meta-analysis. Lancet Infect Dis. 2018 Sep;18(9):1035–44. [PMID: 30025913]

Table 30–3. Acute bacterial diarrheas and "food poisoning" (listed in alphabetical order).

Organism	Incubation Period	Vomiting	Diarrhea	Fever	Associated Foods	Diagnosis	Clinical Features and Treatment
Bacillus cereus (diarrheal toxin)	10–16 hours	±	+++	–	Toxin in meats, stews, and gravy.	Clinical. Food and stool can be tested for toxin.	Abdominal cramps, watery diarrhea, and nausea lasting 24–48 hours. Supportive care.
Bacillus cereus (preformed toxin)	1–8 hours	+++	±	–	Reheated fried rice causes vomiting or diarrhea.	Clinical. Food and stool can be tested for toxin.	Acute onset, severe nausea and vomiting lasting 24 hours. Supportive care.
Campylobacter jejuni	2–5 days	±	+++	+	Raw or undercooked poultry, unpasteurized milk, water.	Stool culture on special medium.	Fever, diarrhea that can be bloody, cramps. Usually self-limited in 2–10 days. Treat with azithromycin or fluoroquinolones for severe disease. May be associated with Guillain-Barré syndrome.
Clostridium botulinum	12–72 hours	±	–	–	Clostridia grow in anaerobic acidic environment eg, canned foods, fermented fish, foods held warm for extended periods.	Stool, serum, and food can be tested for toxin. Stool and food can be cultured.	Diplopia, dysphagia, dysphonia, respiratory embarrassment. Treatment requires clear airway, ventilation, and intravenous polyvalent antitoxin (see text). Symptoms can last for days to months.
Clostridioides difficile	Usually occurs after 7–10 days of antibiotics. Can occur after a single dose or several weeks after completion of antibiotics.	–	+++	++	Associated with antibacterial drugs; clindamycin and beta-lactams most commonly implicated. Fluoroquinolones associated with hypervirulent strains.	Stool tested for toxin.	Abrupt onset of diarrhea that may be bloody; fever. Vancomycin 125 mg orally four times per day or fidaxomicin 200 mg twice daily for 10 days recommended over metronidazole.
Clostridium perfringens	8–16 hours	±	+++	–	Clostridia grow in rewarmed meat and poultry dishes and produce an enterotoxin.	Stools can be tested for enterotoxin or cultured.	Abrupt onset of profuse diarrhea, abdominal cramps, nausea; vomiting occasionally. Recovery usual without treatment in 24–48 hours. Supportive care; antibiotics not needed.
Enterohemorrhagic *Escherichia coli*, including Shiga-toxin–producing *E coli* strains (STEC)	1–8 days	+	+++	–	Undercooked beef, especially hamburger; unpasteurized milk and juice; raw fruits and vegetables.	Shiga-toxin–producing *E coli* can be cultured on special medium. Other toxins can be detected in stool.	Usually abrupt onset of diarrhea, often bloody; abdominal pain. In adults, it is usually self-limited to 5–10 days. In children, it is associated with hemolytic-uremic syndrome (HUS). Antibiotic therapy may increase risk of HUS. Plasma exchange may help patients with STEC-associated HUS.
Enterotoxigenic *E coli* (ETEC)	1–3 days	±	+++	±	Water, food contaminated with feces.	Stool culture. Special tests required to identify toxin-producing strains.	Watery diarrhea and abdominal cramps, usually lasting 3–7 days. In travelers, fluoroquinolones shorten disease.

(continued)

Table 30-3. Acute bacterial diarrheas and "food poisoning" (listed in alphabetical order). (continued)

Organism	Incubation Period	Vomiting	Diarrhea	Fever	Associated Foods	Diagnosis	Clinical Features and Treatment
Noroviruses and other caliciviruses	12–48 hours	++	+++	+	Shellfish and fecally contaminated foods touched by infected food handlers.	Clinical diagnosis with negative stool cultures. PCR available on stool.	Nausea, vomiting (more common in children), diarrhea (more common in adults), fever, myalgias, abdominal cramps. Lasts 12–60 hours. Supportive care.
Rotavirus	1–3 days	++	+++	+	Fecally contaminated foods touched by infected food handlers.	Immunoassay on stool.	Acute onset, vomiting, watery diarrhea that lasts 4–8 days. Supportive care.
Salmonella species	1–3 days	–	++	+	Eggs, poultry, unpasteurized milk, cheese, juices, raw fruits and vegetables.	Routine stool culture.	Gradual or abrupt onset of diarrhea and low-grade fever. No antimicrobials unless high risk (see text) or systemic dissemination is suspected, in which case give a fluoroquinolone. Prolonged carriage can occur.
Shigella species (mild cases)	24–48 hours	±	+	+	Food or water contaminated with human feces. Person to person spread.	Routine stool culture.	Abrupt onset of diarrhea, often with blood and pus in stools, cramps, tenesmus, and lethargy. Stool cultures are positive. Therapy depends on sensitivity testing, but the fluoroquinolones are most effective. Do not give opioids. Often mild and self-limited.
Staphylococcus (preformed toxin)	1–8 hours	+++	±	±	Staphylococci grow in meats, dairy, and bakery products and produce enterotoxin.	Clinical. Food and stool can be tested for toxin.	Abrupt onset, intense nausea and vomiting for up to 24 hours, recovery in 24–48 hours. Supportive care.
Vibrio cholerae	24–72 hours	+	+++	–	Contaminated water, fish, shellfish, street vendor food.	Stool culture on special medium.	Abrupt onset of liquid diarrhea in endemic area. Needs prompt intravenous or oral replacement of fluids and electrolytes. Tetracyclines and azithromycin shorten excretion of vibrios.
Vibrio parahaemolyticus	2–48 hours	+	+	±	Undercooked or raw seafood.	Stool culture on special medium.	Abrupt onset of watery diarrhea, abdominal cramps, nausea and vomiting. Recovery is usually complete in 2–5 days.
Yersinia enterocolitica	24–48 hours	±	+	+	Undercooked pork, contaminated water, unpasteurized milk, tofu.	Stool culture on special medium.	Severe abdominal pain (appendicitis-like symptoms), diarrhea, fever. Polyarthritis, erythema nodosum in children. If severe, give tetracycline or fluoroquinolone. Without treatment, self-limited in 1–3 weeks.

PCR, polymerase chain reaction.

DuPont HL. Persistent diarrhea: a clinical review. JAMA. 2016 Jun 28;315(24):2712–23. [PMID: 27357241]

Nelson RL et al. Antibiotic treatment for *Clostridium difficile*-associated diarrhoea in adults. Cochrane Database Syst Rev. 2017 Mar 3;3:CD004610. [PMID: 28257555]

Shane AL et al. 2017 Infectious Diseases Society of America clinical practice guidelines for the diagnosis and management of infectious diarrhea. Clin Infect Dis. 2017 Nov 29;65(12): e45–80. [PMID: 29053792]

INFECTIOUS DISEASES IN THE RETURNING TRAVELER

ESSENTIALS OF DIAGNOSIS

▸ Most infections are common and self-limited.

▸ Identify patients with transmissible diseases that require isolation.

▸ The incubation period may be helpful in diagnosis.

▸ Less than 3 weeks following exposure may suggest dengue, leptospirosis, and yellow fever; more than 3 weeks suggest typhoid fever, malaria, and tuberculosis.

▸ General Considerations

The differential diagnosis of fever in the returning traveler is broad, ranging from self-limited viral infections to life-threatening illness. The evaluation is best done by identifying whether a particular syndrome is present, then refining the differential diagnosis based on an exposure history. The travel history should include directed questions regarding geography (rural versus urban, specific country visited), time of year, animal or arthropod contact, unprotected sexual intercourse, ingestion of untreated water or raw foods, historical or pretravel immunizations, and adherence to malaria prophylaxis.

▸ Etiologies

The most common infectious causes of fever—excluding simple causes such as upper respiratory infections, bacterial pneumonia and urinary tract infections—in returning travelers are malaria (see Chapter 35), diarrhea (see next section), and dengue (see Chapter 32). Others include mononucleosis (associated with Epstein-Barr virus or cytomegalovirus), respiratory infections, including seasonal influenza, influenza A/H1N1 "swine" influenza, and influenza A/H5N1 or A/H7N9 "avian" influenza (see Chapter 32); leptospirosis (see Chapter 34); typhoid fever (see Chapter 33); and rickettsial infections (see Chapter 32). Foreign travel is increasingly recognized as a risk factor for colonization and disease with resistant pathogens, such as ESBL-producing gram-negative organisms. Systemic febrile illnesses without a diagnosis also occur commonly, particularly in travelers returning from sub-Saharan Africa or Southeast Asia.

A. Fever and Rash

Potential etiologies include dengue, Ebola, Chikungunya, and Zika viruses, viral hemorrhagic fever, leptospirosis, meningococcemia, yellow fever, typhus, *Salmonella typhi*, and acute HIV infection.

B. Pulmonary Infiltrates

Tuberculosis, ascaris, *Paragonimus*, and *Strongyloides* can all cause pulmonary infiltrates.

C. Meningoencephalitis

Etiologies include *N meningitidis*, leptospirosis, arboviruses, rabies, and (cerebral) malaria.

D. Jaundice

Consider hepatitis A, yellow fever, hemorrhagic fever, leptospirosis, and malaria.

E. Fever Without Localizing Symptoms or Signs

Malaria, typhoid fever, acute HIV infection, rickettsial illness, visceral leishmaniasis, trypanosomiasis, and dengue are possible etiologies.

F. Traveler's Diarrhea

See next section.

▸ Clinical Findings

Fever and rash in the returning traveler should prompt blood cultures and serologic tests based on the exposure history. The workup of a pulmonary infiltrate should include the placement of a PPD or use of an interferon-gamma release assay, examination of sputum for acid-fast bacilli and possibly for ova and parasites. Patients with evidence of meningoencephalitis should receive lumbar puncture, blood cultures, thick/thin smears of peripheral blood, history-guided serologies, and a nape biopsy (if rabies is suspected). Jaundice in a returning traveler should be evaluated for hemolysis (for malaria), and the following tests should be performed: liver biochemical tests, thick/thin smears of peripheral blood, and directed serologic testing. The workup of traveler's diarrhea is presented in the following section. Finally, patients with fever but no localizing signs or symptoms should have blood cultures performed. Routine laboratory studies usually include complete blood count with differential, electrolytes, liver biochemical tests, urinalysis, and blood cultures. Thick and thin peripheral blood smears should be done (and repeated in 12–24 hours if clinical suspicion remains high) for malaria if there has been travel to endemic areas. Other studies are directed by the results of history, physical examination, and initial laboratory tests. They may include stool for ova and parasites, chest radiograph, HIV test, and specific serologies (eg, dengue, leptospirosis, rickettsial disease, schistosomiasis, *Strongyloides*). Bone marrow biopsy to diagnose typhoid fever could be helpful in the appropriate patient.

When to Refer

Travelers with fever, particularly if immunocompromised.

When to Admit

Any evidence of hemorrhage, respiratory distress, hemodynamic instability, and neurologic deficits.

Hahn WO et al. Malaria in the traveler: how to manage before departure and evaluate upon return. Med Clin North Am. 2016 Mar;100(2):289–302. [PMID: 26900114]

Polen KD et al. Update: interim guidance for preconception counseling and prevention of sexual transmission of Zika virus for men with possible Zika virus exposure—United States, August 2018. MMWR Morb Mortal Wkly Rep. 2018 Aug 10;67(31):868–71. [PMID: 30091965]

Rasmussen SA et al. Zika virus and birth defects—reviewing the evidence for causality. N Engl J Med. 2016 May 19;374(20):1981–7. [PMID: 27074377]

Rello J et al. Management of infections in critically ill returning travellers in the intensive care unit—II: Clinical syndromes and special considerations in immunocompromised patients. Int J Infect Dis. 2016 Jul;48:104–12. [PMID: 27134159]

Sanford CA et al. Illness in the returned international traveler. Med Clin North Am. 2016 Mar;100(2):393–409. [PMID: 26900121]

Thwaites GE et al. Approach to fever in the returning traveler. N Engl J Med. 2017 Feb 9;376(6):548–60. [PMID: 28177860]

Vasievich MP et al. Got the travel bug? A review of common infections, infestations, bites, and stings among returning travelers. Am J Clin Dermatol. 2016 Oct;17(5):451–62. [PMID: 27344566]

TRAVELER'S DIARRHEA

ESSENTIALS OF DIAGNOSIS

- ► Usually a benign, self-limited disease occurring about 1 week into travel.

- ► Prophylaxis *not* recommended unless there is a comorbid disease (inflammatory bowel syndrome, HIV, immunosuppressive medication).

- ► Single-dose therapy of a fluoroquinolone usually effective if significant symptoms develop.

General Considerations

Whenever a person travels from one country to another—particularly if the change involves a marked difference in climate, social conditions, or sanitation standards and facilities—diarrhea may develop within 2–10 days. Bacteria cause 80% of cases of traveler's diarrhea, with enterotoxigenic *E coli*, *Shigella* species, and *Campylobacter jejuni* being the most common pathogens. Less common are *Aeromonas*, *Salmonella*, noncholera vibriones, *E histolytica*, and *G lamblia*. Contributory causes include unusual food and drink, change in living habits, occasional viral infections (adenoviruses or rotaviruses), and change in bowel flora. Chronic watery diarrhea may be due to amebiasis or giardiasis or, rarely, tropical sprue.

Clinical Findings

A. Symptoms and Signs

There may be up to ten or even more loose stools per day, often accompanied by abdominal cramps and nausea, occasionally by vomiting, and rarely by fever. The stools are usually watery and not associated with fever when caused by enterotoxigenic *E coli*. With invasive bacterial pathogens (*Shigella*, *Campylobacter*, *Salmonella*), stools can be bloody and fever may be present. The illness usually subsides spontaneously within 1–5 days, although 10% remain symptomatic for 1 week or longer, and symptoms persist for longer than 1 month in 2%. Traveler's diarrhea is also a significant risk factor for developing irritable bowel syndrome.

B. Laboratory Findings

In patients with fever and bloody diarrhea, stool culture is indicated, but in most cases, cultures are reserved for those who do not respond to antibiotics.

Prevention

A. General Measures

Avoidance of fresh foods and water sources that are likely to be contaminated is recommended for travelers to developing countries, where infectious diarrheal illnesses are endemic.

B. Specific Measures

Because not all travelers will have diarrhea and because most episodes are brief and self-limited, the currently recommended approach is to *provide the traveler with a supply of antimicrobials*. Prophylaxis is recommended for those with significant underlying disease (inflammatory bowel disease, AIDS, diabetes mellitus, heart disease in older adults, conditions requiring immunosuppressive medications) and for those whose full activity status during the trip is so essential that even short periods of diarrhea would be unacceptable.

Prophylaxis is started upon entry into the destination country and is continued for 1 or 2 days after leaving. For stays of more than 3 weeks, prophylaxis is not recommended because of the cost and increased toxicity. For prophylaxis, several oral antimicrobial once-daily regimens are effective, such as ciprofloxacin, 500 mg, or rifaximin, 200 mg. Bismuth subsalicylate is effective but turns the tongue and the stools black and can interfere with doxycycline absorption, which may be needed for malaria prophylaxis; it is rarely used.

Treatment

For most individuals, the affliction is short-lived, and symptomatic therapy with loperamide is all that is required, provided the patient is not systemically ill (fever 39°C or higher) and does not have dysentery (bloody stools), in which case antimotility agents should be avoided. Packages of oral rehydration salts to treat dehydration are available over the counter in the United States (Infalyte, Pedialyte, others) and in many foreign countries.

When treatment is necessary, in areas where toxin-producing bacteria are the major cause of diarrhea (Latin America and Africa), loperamide (4 mg oral loading dose, then 2 mg after each loose stool to a maximum of 16 mg/day) with a single oral dose of ciprofloxacin (750 mg), levofloxacin (500 mg), or ofloxacin (200 mg), cures most cases of traveler's diarrhea. If diarrhea is associated with bloody stools or persists despite a single dose of a fluoroquinolone, 1000 mg of azithromycin should be taken. In pregnant women and in areas where invasive bacteria more commonly cause diarrhea (Indian subcontinent, Asia, especially Thailand where fluoroquinolone-resistant *Campylobacter* is prevalent), azithromycin is the medication of choice. Rifaximin, a nonabsorbable agent, is also approved for therapy of traveler's diarrhea at a dose of 200 mg orally three times per day or 400 mg twice a day for 3 days. Because luminal concentrations are high, but tissue levels are insufficient, it should not be used in situations where there is a high likelihood of invasive disease (eg, fever, systemic toxicity, or bloody stools).

When to Refer

- Cases refractory to treatment.
- Persistent infection.
- Immunocompromised patient.

When to Admit

Patients who are severely dehydrated or hemodynamically unstable should be admitted to the hospital.

Eckbo EJ et al. New tools to test stool: managing travelers' diarrhea in the era of molecular diagnostics. Infect Dis Clin North Am. 2019 Mar;33(1):197–212. [PMID: 30712762]
Giddings SL et al. Traveler's diarrhea. Med Clin North Am. 2016 Mar;100(2):317–30. [PMID: 26900116]

ANTIMICROBIAL THERAPY

SELECTED PRINCIPLES OF ANTIMICROBIAL THERAPY

Specific steps (outlined below) are required when considering antibiotic therapy for patients. Medications within classes, medications of first choice, and alternative medications are presented in Table 30–4.

Table 30–4. Medication of choice for suspected or documented microbial pathogens (listed in alphabetical order, within classes).

Suspected or Proved Etiologic Agent	Medication(s) of First Choice	Alternative Medication(s)
Gram-Negative Cocci		
Moraxella catarrhalis	Cefuroxime, amoxicillin-clavulanic acid	Ceftriaxone, cefuroxime axetil, a fluoroquinolone,[1] a macrolide,[2] a tetracycline,[3] TMP-SMZ[4]
Neisseria gonorrhoeae (gonococcus)	Ceftriaxone + azithromycin or doxycycline	Cefixime + azithromycin or doxycycline[5]
Neisseria meningitidis (meningococcus)	Penicillin[6]	Ceftriaxone, ampicillin
Gram-Positive Cocci		
Enterococcus faecalis	Ampicillin ± gentamicin[7]	Vancomycin ± gentamicin
Enterococcus faecium	Vancomycin ± gentamicin[7]	Linezolid,[8] quinupristin-dalfopristin,[8] daptomycin,[8] tigecycline,[8] tedizolid,[8] oritavancin[8]
Streptococcus, hemolytic, groups A, B, C, G	Penicillin[6]	Macrolide,[2] a cephalosporin,[9] vancomycin, clindamycin
Staphylococcus, methicillin-resistant	Vancomycin	TMP-SMZ,[4] doxycycline, minocycline, linezolid,[8] tedizolid,[8] daptomycin,[8] televancin,[8] dalbavancin,[8] oritavancin,[8] ceftaroline, delafloxacin
Staphylococcus, methicillin-susceptible	Penicillinase-resistant penicillin[10]	Vancomycin, a cephalosporin,[9] clindamycin, amoxicillin-clavulanic acid, ampicillin-sulbactam
Streptococcus pneumoniae[11] (pneumococcus)	Penicillin[6]	Macrolide,[2] a cephalosporin,[9] vancomycin, clindamycin, a tetracycline,[3] respiratory fluoroquinolones[1]
Viridans streptococci	Penicillin[6]	Cephalosporin,[9] vancomycin
Gram-Negative Rods		
Acinetobacter	Imipenem, meropenem	Tigecycline, minocycline, doxycycline, aminoglycosides,[12] colistin
Bacteroides, gastrointestinal strains	Metronidazole	Ampicillin-sulbactam, piperacillin-tazobactam, ertapenem
Brucella	Doxycycline + rifampin[3]	TMP-SMZ[4] ± gentamicin; ciprofloxacin + rifampin
Burkholderia mallei (glanders)	Streptomycin + tetracycline[3]	Chloramphenicol + streptomycin

(continued)

Table 30–4. Medication of choice for suspected or documented microbial pathogens (listed in alphabetical order, within classes). (continued)

Suspected or Proved Etiologic Agent	Medication(s) of First Choice	Alternative Medication(s)
Gram-Negative Rods (cont.)		
Burkholderia pseudomallei (melioidosis)	Ceftazidime	Tetracycline,[3] TMP-SMZ,[4] amoxicillin-clavulanic acid, imipenem or meropenem
Campylobacter jejuni	Azithromycin	A fluoroquinolone[1]
Enterobacter	Ertapenem, imipenem, meropenem, cefepime	Aminoglycoside, a fluoroquinolone,[1] TMP-SMZ[4]
Escherichia coli (uncomplicated outpatient urinary infection)	Nitrofurantoin, fosfomycin	Fluoroquinolones,[1] TMP-SMZ,[4] oral cephalosporin
Escherichia coli (sepsis)[13]	Cefotaxime, ceftriaxone	Ertapenem[13] imipenem[13] or meropenem,[13] aminoglycosides,[12] aztreonam, ticarcillin-clavulanate, piperacillin-tazobactam, ceftazidime-avibactam,[13] ceftolozane-tazobactam,[13,14] meropenem/vaborbactam[15]
Haemophilus (respiratory infections, otitis)	Ampicillin-clavulanate	Doxycycline, azithromycin, ceftriaxone, cefuroxime, cefuroxime axetil, TMP-SMZ[4]
Haemophilus (serious infection)	Ceftriaxone	Aztreonam
Helicobacter pylori	Proton pump inhibitor (PPI), clarithromycin, amoxicillin, and metronidazole	PPI, clarithromycin, and amoxicillin **or** metronidazole
Klebsiella[13]	Ceftriaxone	TMP-SMZ,[4] aminoglycoside,[12] ertapenem,[13] imipenem[13] or meropenem,[13] a fluoroquinolone,[1] aztreonam, ticarcillin-clavulanate, piperacillin-tazobactam, ceftazidime-avibactam,[13] ceftolozane-tazobactam,[13,14] meropenem/vaborbactam[15]
Legionella species (pneumonia)	Azithromycin, or fluoroquinolones[1] ± rifampin	Doxycycline ± rifampin
Prevotella, oropharyngeal strains	Clindamycin	Metronidazole
Proteus mirabilis	Ampicillin	An aminoglycoside,[12] TMP-SMZ,[4] a fluoroquinolone,[1] a cephalosporin[9]
Proteus vulgaris and other species (*Morganella, Providencia*)	Ceftriaxone	Aminoglycoside,[12] ertapenem, imipenem or meropenem, TMP-SMZ,[4] a fluoroquinolone[1]
Pseudomonas aeruginosa	Piperacillin-tazobactam or ceftazidime or cefepime, or imipenem or meropenem or doripenem or aztreonam ± aminoglycoside[12]	Ciprofloxacin (or levofloxacin) ± piperacillin-tazobactam; ciprofloxacin (or levofloxacin) ± ceftazidime; ciprofloxacin (or levofloxacin) ± cefepime; ceftazidime-avibactam[13]; ceftolozane-tazobactam[13]
Salmonella (bacteremia)	Ceftriaxone	A fluoroquinolone[1]
Serratia	Carbapenem	TMP-SMZ,[4] aminoglycosides,[12] a fluoroquinolone,[1] ceftriaxone
Shigella	Azithromycin, ciprofloxacin, or ceftriaxone	TMP-SMZ[4]
Vibrio (cholera, sepsis)	A tetracycline[3]	TMP-SMZ,[4] a fluoroquinolone[1]
Yersinia pestis (plague)	Streptomycin ± a tetracycline[3]	Chloramphenicol, TMP-SMZ[5]
Gram-Positive Rods		
Actinomyces	Penicillin[6]	Tetracycline,[3] clindamycin
Bacillus (including anthrax)	Penicillin[6]	A macrolide,[2] a fluoroquinolone[1]
Clostridium (eg, gas gangrene, tetanus)	Penicillin[6]	Metronidazole, clindamycin, imipenem, or meropenem
Corynebacterium diphtheria	Macrolide[2]	Penicillin[6]
Corynebacterium jeikeium	Vancomycin	Linezolid
Listeria	Ampicillin ± aminoglycoside[12]	TMP-SMZ[4]

(continued)

Table 30–4. Medication of choice for suspected or documented microbial pathogens (listed in alphabetical order, within classes). (continued)

Suspected or Proved Etiologic Agent	Medication(s) of First Choice	Alternative Medication(s)
Acid-Fast Rods		
Mycobacterium avium complex	Clarithromycin or azithromycin + ethambutol, ± rifabutin	Amikacin, ciprofloxacin
Mycobacterium fortuitum-chelonei	Cefoxitin + clarithromycin	Amikacin, rifampin, sulfonamide, doxycycline, linezolid
Mycobacterium kansasii	INH + rifampin ± ethambutol	Clarithromycin, azithromycin, ethionamide, cycloserine
Mycobacterium leprae	Dapsone + rifampin ± clofazimine	Minocycline, ofloxacin, clarithromycin
Mycobacterium tuberculosis[16]	Isoniazid (INH) + rifampin + pyrazinamide ± ethambutol	Other antituberculous drugs (see Tables 9–14 and 9–15)
Nocardia	TMP-SMZ[4]	Minocycline, imipenem or meropenem, linezolid
Spirochetes		
Borrelia burgdorferi (Lyme disease)	Doxycycline, amoxicillin, cefuroxime axetil	Ceftriaxone, penicillin, azithromycin
Borrelia recurrentis (relapsing fever)	Doxycycline[3]	Penicillin[6]
Leptospira	Penicillin[6]	Doxycycline,[3] ceftriaxone
Treponema pallidum (syphilis)	Penicillin[6]	Doxycycline, ceftriaxone
Treponema pertenue (yaws)	Penicillin[6]	Doxycycline
Mycoplasmas	Azithromycin or doxycycline	A fluoroquinolone[1]
Chlamydiae		
C pneumoniae	Doxycycline[3]	Azithromycin, a fluoroquinolone[1,17]
C psittaci	Doxycycline	Chloramphenicol
C trachomatis (urethritis or pelvic inflammatory disease)	Doxycycline or azithromycin	Levofloxacin, ofloxacin
Rickettsiae	Doxycycline[3]	Chloramphenicol, a fluoroquinolone[1]

[1]Fluoroquinolones include ciprofloxacin, levofloxacin, moxifloxacin, and others. Gemifloxacin, levofloxacin, and moxifloxacin, the so-called respiratory fluoroquinolones, demonstrate the most reliable activity against penicillin-resistant S pneumoniae and other respiratory infection pathogens. Delafloxacin is predictably active against methicillin-resistant S aureus (MRSA).

[2]Azithromycin is the preferred macrolide due to increased safety profile and minimal drug interaction potential.

[3]All tetracyclines have similar activity against most microorganisms. Minocycline (the most active tetracycline) and doxycycline are more active than tetracycline against S aureus.

[4]TMP-SMZ is a mixture of 1 part trimethoprim and 5 parts sulfamethoxazole.

[5]Test of cure required if ceftriaxone not used.

[6]Penicillin G is preferred for parenteral injection; penicillin V for oral administration.

[7]Addition of gentamicin indicated only for severe enterococcal infections (eg, endocarditis, meningitis).

[8]Linezolid, tedizolid, daptomycin, televancin, dalbavancin, and oritavancin should be reserved for the treatment of vancomycin-resistant isolates or in patients intolerant of vancomycin.

[9]Most intravenous cephalosporins (with the exception of ceftazidime) are active against streptococci and staphylococci.

[10]Parenteral nafcillin or oxacillin; oral dicloxacillin, cloxacillin, or oxacillin.

[11]Infections caused by isolates with intermediate resistance may respond to high dose penicillin or ceftriaxone or the respiratory fluoroquinolones (gemifloxacin, levofloxacin, and moxifloxacin). Infections caused by highly penicillin-resistant isolates should be treated with vancomycin. Penicillin-resistant pneumococci are often resistant to macrolides, tetracyclines, and TMP-SMZ.

[12]Aminoglycosides—gentamicin, tobramycin, amikacin, netilmicin—should be chosen on the basis of local patterns of susceptibility.

[13]Extended beta-lactamase–producing (ESBL) isolates should be treated with a carbapenem. If a carbapenem cannot be used, ceftazidime-avibactam or possibly ceftolozane-tazobactam can be considered.

[14]Ceftolozane-tazobactam and occasionally ceftazidime-avibactam may be active against multidrug-resistant P aeruginosa.

[15]Consider in cases of infection due to carbapenemase-producing Enterobacteriaceae.

[16]Resistance is common and susceptibility testing must be performed.

[17]Ciprofloxacin has inferior antichlamydial activity compared with levofloxacin or ofloxacin.

±, alone or combined with.

A. Etiologic Diagnosis

Based on the organ system involved, the organism causing infection can often be predicted. See Tables 30–5 and 30–6.

B. "Best Guess"

Select an empiric regimen that is likely to be effective against the suspected pathogens.

C. Laboratory Control

Specimens for laboratory examination should be obtained before institution of therapy to determine susceptibility.

D. Clinical Response

Based on clinical response and other data, the laboratory reports are evaluated and then the desirability of changing the regimen is considered. If the specimen was obtained from a normally sterile site (eg, blood, cerebrospinal fluid, pleural fluid, joint fluid), the recovery of a microorganism in significant amounts is meaningful even if the organism recovered is different from the clinically suspected agent, and this may force a change in treatment. Isolation of unexpected microorganisms from the respiratory tract, gastrointestinal tract, or surface lesions (sites that have a complex flora) may represent colonization or contamination, and cultures must be critically evaluated before medications are abandoned that were judiciously selected on a "best guess" basis.

E. Drug Susceptibility Tests

Some microorganisms are predictably inhibited by certain medications; if such organisms are isolated, they need not be tested for drug susceptibility. For example, all group A hemolytic streptococci are inhibited by penicillin. Other organisms (eg, enteric gram-negative rods) are variably susceptible and generally require susceptibility testing whenever they are isolated. *Organisms that once had predictable susceptibility patterns are now associated with resistance and require testing.* Examples include the pneumococci, which may be resistant to multiple medications (including penicillin, macrolides, and TMP-SMZ); the enterococci, which may be resistant to penicillin, aminoglycosides, and vancomycin; and ESBL producing–*E coli* resistant to third-generation cephalosporins and fluoroquinolones.

When culture and susceptibility results have been finalized, clinicians must use the most narrow-spectrum agent and the shortest duration possible to decrease the selection pressure for antibacterial resistance.

Antimicrobial drug susceptibility tests may be performed on solid media as disk diffusion tests, in broth, in tubes, in wells of microdilution plates, or as E-tests (strips with increasing concentration of antibiotic). The latter three methods yield results expressed as MIC (minimal inhibitory concentration). In most infections, the MIC is the appropriate in vitro test to guide selection of an antibacterial agent. When there appear to be marked discrepancies between susceptibility testing and clinical response, the following possibilities must be considered:

1. Selection of an inappropriate medication, medication dosage, or route of administration.
2. Failure to drain a collection of pus or to remove a foreign body.
3. Failure of a poorly diffusing drug to reach the site of infection (eg, central nervous system) or to reach intracellular phagocytosed bacteria.
4. Superinfection in the course of prolonged chemotherapy.
5. Emergence of drug resistance in the original pathogen or superinfection with a new more resistant organism.
6. Participation of two or more microorganisms in the infectious process, of which only one was originally detected and used for medication selection.
7. Inadequate host defenses, including immunodeficiencies and diabetes mellitus.
8. Noninfectious causes, including drug fever, malignancy, and autoimmune disease.

F. Promptness of Response

Response depends on a number of factors, including the patient (immunocompromised patients respond slower than immunocompetent patients), the site of infection (deep-seated infections such as osteomyelitis and endocarditis respond more slowly than superficial infections such as cystitis or cellulitis), the pathogen (virulent organisms such as *S aureus* respond more slowly than viridans streptococci; mycobacterial and fungal infections respond slower than bacterial infections), and the duration of illness (in general, the longer the symptoms are present, the longer it takes to respond). Thus, depending on the clinical situation, persistent fever and leukocytosis several days after initiation of therapy may not indicate improper choice of antibiotics but may be due to the natural history of the disease being treated. In most infections, either a bacteriostatic or a bactericidal agent can be used. In some infections (eg, infective endocarditis and meningitis), a bactericidal agent should be used. When potentially toxic medications (eg, aminoglycosides, flucytosine) are used, serum levels of the medication are measured to minimize toxicity and ensure appropriate dosage. In patients with altered renal or hepatic clearance of medications, the dosage or frequency of administration must be adjusted; it is best to measure levels in older adults, in morbidly obese patients, or in those with altered kidney function when possible and adjust therapy accordingly.

G. Duration of Antimicrobial Therapy

Generally, effective antimicrobial treatment results in reversal of the clinical and laboratory parameters of active infection and marked clinical improvement. However, varying periods of treatment may be required for cure. Key factors include (1) the type of infecting organism (bacterial infections generally can be cured more rapidly than fungal or mycobacterial ones), (2) the location of the process (eg, endocarditis and osteomyelitis require prolonged therapy), and (3) the immunocompetence of the patient.

Table 30–5. Examples of initial antimicrobial therapy for acutely ill, hospitalized adults pending identification of causative organism (in alphabetical order).

Suspected Clinical Diagnosis	Likely Etiologic Diagnosis	Medication of Choice
Brain abscess	Mixed anaerobes, pneumococci, streptococci	Ceftriaxone, 2 g intravenously every 12 hours **plus** metronidazole, 500 mg orally every 8 hours **plus** vancomycin, 15 mg/kg intravenously every 8 hours
Endocarditis, acute (including injection drug user)	S aureus, E faecalis, viridans streptococci	Vancomycin, 15 mg/kg/dose intravenously every 12 hours
Fever in neutropenic patient receiving cancer chemotherapy	S aureus, Pseudomonas, Klebsiella, E coli	Cefepime, 2 g intravenously every 8 hours
Intra-abdominal sepsis (eg, postoperative, peritonitis, cholecystitis)	Gram-negative bacteria, Bacteroides, anaerobic bacteria, enterococcus	Piperacillin-tazobactam, 4.5 g intravenously every 6 hours, **or** ertapenem, 1 g every 24 hours
Meningitis, bacterial, age > 50, community-acquired	Pneumococcus, meningococcus, Listeria monocytogenes,[1] gram-negative bacilli, group B Streptococcus	Ampicillin, 2 g intravenously every 4 hours, **plus** ceftriaxone, 2 g intravenously every 12 hours, **plus** vancomycin, 15 mg/kg intravenously every 8 hours
Meningitis, bacterial, community-acquired	Streptococcus pneumoniae (pneumococcus),[2] Neisseria meningitidis (meningococcus)	Ceftriaxone, 2 g intravenously every 12 hours,[1] **plus** vancomycin, 15 mg/kg intravenously every 8 hours
Meningitis, postoperative (or posttraumatic)	S aureus, gram-negative bacilli, coagulase-negative staphylococci, diphtheroids (eg, Propionibacterium acnes) (uncommon) pneumococcus (in posttraumatic)	Vancomycin, 15 mg/kg intravenously every 8 hours, **plus** cefepime, 3 g intravenously every 8 hours[3]
Osteomyelitis	S aureus, secondarily gram-negative aerobes	Vancomycin 15 mg/kg intravenously every 8 hours **plus** ceftriaxone 2 g intravenously every 24 hours
Pneumonia, acute, community-acquired, non-ICU hospital admission	Pneumococci, M pneumoniae, Legionella, C pneumoniae	Ceftriaxone, 1 g intravenously every 24 hours or ampicillin, 2 g intravenously every 6 hours) **plus** azithromycin, 500 mg intravenously every 24 hours; **or** a respiratory fluoroquinolone[4] alone
Pneumonia, postoperative or nosocomial	S aureus, mixed anaerobes, gram-negative bacilli	Cefepime, 2 g intravenously every 8 hours; **or** ceftazidime, 2 g intravenously every 8 hours; **or** piperacillin-tazobactam, 4.5 g intravenously every 6–8 hours; **or** imipenem, 500 mg intravenously every 6 hours; **or** meropenem, 1 g intravenously every 8 hours **plus** tobramycin, 5–7 mg/kg intravenously every 24 hours; **or** ciprofloxacin, 400 mg intravenously every 12 hours; **or** levofloxacin, 500 mg intravenously every 24 hours **plus** vancomycin, 15 mg/kg/dose intravenously every 12 hours
Pyelonephritis with flank pain and fever (recurrent urinary tract infection)	E coli, Klebsiella, Enterobacter, Pseudomonas	Ceftriaxone, 1 g intravenously every 24 hours; **or** if culture results confirm susceptibility, ciprofloxacin, 400 mg intravenously every 12 hours (500 mg orally); **or** levofloxacin, 500 mg once daily (intravenously/orally)
Septic arthritis	S aureus, N gonorrhoeae	Ceftriaxone, 1–2 g intravenously every 24 hours
Septic thrombophlebitis (eg, IV tubing, IV shunts)	S aureus, gram-negative aerobic bacteria	Vancomycin, 15 mg/kg/dose intravenously every 12 hours, **plus** ceftriaxone, 1 g intravenously every 24 hours

[1]TMP-SMZ can be used to treat Listeria monocytogenes in patients allergic to penicillin in a dosage of 15–20 mg/kg/day of TMP in three or four divided doses.
[2]Including penicillin nonsusceptible isolates.
[3]Cefepime 3 g is a higher dose than sometimes recommended in order to optimize treatment of Pseudomonas and Enterobacter.
[4]Levofloxacin 750 mg/day, moxifloxacin 400 mg/day.

Table 30–6. Examples of empiric choices of antimicrobials for adult outpatient infections (in alphabetical order).

Suspected Clinical Diagnosis	Likely Etiologic Agents	Medications of Choice	Alternative Medications
Acute sinusitis	*Streptococcus pneumoniae, Haemophilus influenzae, Moraxella catarrhalis*	Augmentin,[1] 875 mg orally twice daily for 10 days	For patients allergic to penicillin, doxycycline, 100 mg twice daily for 10 days
Aspiration pneumonia	Mixed oropharyngeal flora, including anaerobes	Clindamycin, 300 mg orally four times daily for 10–14 days	Amoxicillin 500 mg orally three times daily for 10–14 days
Cystitis	*Escherichia coli, Staphylococcus saprophyticus, Klebsiella pneumoniae, Proteus* species, other gram-negative rods or enterococci	Nitrofurantoin monohydrate macrocrystals 100 mg twice daily for 5–7 days (unless pregnant); fosfomycin 3 g orally as a single dose	Cephalexin, 500 mg orally four times daily for 7 days, for uncomplicated cystitis. Due to increasing bacterial resistance, TMP-SMZ and fluoroquinolones are **not** recommended as first-line therapy for empiric treatment
Erysipelas, impetigo, cellulitis, ascending lymphangitis	Group A *Streptococcus*	Penicillin V, 500 mg orally four times daily for 7–10 days	Cephalexin, 500 mg orally four times daily for 7–10 days; **or** azithromycin, 500 mg on day 1 and 250 mg on days 2–5
Furuncle with surrounding cellulitis	*Staphylococcus aureus*	Dicloxacillin, 500 mg orally four times daily for 7–10 days for MSSA. For CA-MRSA: TMP-SMZ[2] one double-strength tablet twice daily for 7–10 days; **or** clindamycin 300 mg orally three times daily for 7–10 days	Cephalexin, 500 mg orally four times daily for 7–10 days for MSSA. For CA-MRSA, doxycycline is a reasonable alternative
Gastroenteritis	*Salmonella, Shigella, Campylobacter, Entamoeba histolytica*	See footnote 3	
Otitis media	*S pneumoniae, H influenzae, M catarrhalis*	Amoxicillin, 500 mg–1 g orally three times daily for 10 days	Amoxicillin-clavulanate,[1] 875 mg orally twice daily; **or** cefuroxime, 500 mg orally twice daily; **or** cefpodoxime, 200–400 mg daily; **or** doxycycline, 100 mg twice daily
Pelvic inflammatory disease	*Neisseria gonorrhoeae, Chlamydia trachomatis,* anaerobes, gram-negative rods	Ceftriaxone 250 mg intramuscularly once plus doxycycline 100 mg orally twice daily for 14 days +/– metronidazole 500 mg orally twice daily for 14 days; **or** cefoxitin 2 g intramuscularly once plus probenecid 1 g orally once, plus doxycycline 100 mg orally twice daily for 14 days +/– metronidazole 500 mg orally twice daily for 14 days	
Pharyngitis	Group A *Streptococcus*	Penicillin V, 500 mg orally four times daily, **or** amoxicillin, 500 mg–1 g orally three times daily, for 10 days	For patients with history of mild penicillin allergy, cephalexin, 500 mg orally four times daily for 10 days; for patients with IgE-mediated reaction, clindamycin, 300 mg orally four times daily for 10 days; **or** azithromycin, 500 mg on day 1 and 250 mg on days 2–5
Pneumonia	*S pneumoniae, Mycoplasma pneumoniae, Legionella pneumophila, Chlamydophila pneumoniae*	Doxycycline, 100 mg orally twice daily	Amoxicillin, 1.0 g orally three times daily plus azithromycin 500 mg orally on day 1 and 250 mg on days 2–5. A respiratory fluoroquinolone[4] for patients at high risk for infection due to resistant pneumococci

(continued)

Table 30–6. Examples of empiric choices of antimicrobials for adult outpatient infections (in alphabetical order). (continued)

Suspected Clinical Diagnosis	Likely Etiologic Agents	Medications of Choice	Alternative Medications
Pyelonephritis	*E coli, K pneumoniae, Proteus* species, *S saprophyticus*	Fluoroquinolones[5] for 7 days if prevalence of resistance among uropathogens is < 10%	TMP-SMZ,[2] one double-strength tablet twice daily for 7–14 days for susceptible pathogens. Oral beta-lactams are less effective than fluoroquinolones or TMP-SMZ
Urethritis, epididymitis	*N gonorrhoeae, C trachomatis*	Ceftriaxone, 250 mg intramuscularly once **plus** azithromycin (or doxycycline) for *N gonorrhoeae*; azithromycin 1 g orally once, **or** doxycycline, 100 mg orally twice daily for 7 days, for *C trachomatis*	Cefixime 400 mg orally once for *N gonorrhoeae*[6]
Syphilis			
Early syphilis (primary, secondary, or latent of < 1 year's duration)	*Treponema pallidum*	Benzathine penicillin G, 2.4 million units intramuscularly once	Doxycycline, 100 mg orally twice daily for 2 weeks. Ceftriaxone 1–2 g intravenously once daily for 10–14 days
Latent syphilis of > 1 year's duration or cardiovascular syphilis	*T pallidum*	Benzathine penicillin G, 2.4 million units intramuscularly once a week for 3 weeks (total: 7.2 million units)	Doxycycline, 100 mg orally twice daily, for 4 weeks
Neurosyphilis	*T pallidum*	Aqueous penicillin G, 18–24 million units/day intravenously for 10–14 days	

[1]Amoxicillin-clavulante is available as a combination of amoxicillin, 250 mg, 500 mg, or 875 mg, plus 125 mg of clavulanic acid. Augmentin XR is a combination of amoxicillin 1 g and clavulanic acid 62.5 mg.

[2]TMP-SMZ is a fixed combination of 1 part trimethoprim and 5 parts sulfamethoxazole. Single-strength tablets: 80 mg TMP, 400 mg SMZ; double-strength tablets: 160 mg TMP, 800 mg SMZ.

[3]The diagnosis should be confirmed by culture before therapy. *Salmonella* gastroenteritis does not require therapy. For susceptible *Shigella* isolates, give ciprofloxacin, 500 mg orally twice daily for 5 days. For *Campylobacter* infection, give azithromycin, 1 g orally times one dose, or ciprofloxacin, 500 mg orally twice daily for 5 days. For *E histolytica* infection, give metronidazole, 750 mg orally three times daily for 5–10 days, followed by diiodohydroxyquinoline (not available in United States), 650 mg orally three times daily for 3 weeks.

[4]Fluoroquinolones with activity against *S pneumoniae*, including penicillin-resistant isolates, include gemifloxacin (not available in United States) (320 mg orally once daily), levofloxacin (500–750 mg orally once daily), and moxifloxacin (400 mg orally once daily). Use fluoroquinolones as drug of choice if recent antibiotic use within 3 months or comorbidities present.

[5]Fluoroquinolones and dosages include ciprofloxacin, 500 mg orally twice daily; ofloxacin, 400 mg orally twice daily; levofloxacin, 500 mg orally daily.

[6]Test of cure recommended if ceftriaxone is not used.

CA-MRSA, community-acquired methicillin-resistant *Staphylococcus aureus*; MRSA, methicillin-resistant *S aureus*; MSSA, methicillin-sensitive *S aureus*; TMP-SMZ, trimethoprim-sulfamethoxazole.

H. Adverse Reactions and Toxicity

These include hypersensitivity reactions, direct toxicity, superinfection by drug-resistant microorganisms, and drug interactions. If the infection is life-threatening and treatment cannot be stopped, the reactions are managed symptomatically or another medication is chosen that does not cross-react with the offending one (Table 30–4). If the infection is less serious, it may be possible to stop all antimicrobials and monitor the patient closely.

I. Route of Administration

Intravenous therapy is preferred for acutely ill patients with serious infections (eg, endocarditis, meningitis, sepsis, severe pneumonia) when dependable levels of antibiotics are required for successful therapy. Certain medications (eg, doxycycline, fluconazole, voriconazole, rifampin, metronidazole, TMP-SMZ, and fluoroquinolones) are so well absorbed that they generally can be administered orally in seriously ill—but not hemodynamically unstable—patients.

Food does not significantly influence the bioavailability of most oral antimicrobial agents. However, the tetracyclines (particularly tetracycline) and the quinolones chelate multivalent cations resulting in decreased oral bioavailability. Posaconazole suspension should always be administered with food.

A major complication of intravenous antibiotic therapy is infection due to the manipulation of the intravenous catheter. Peripheral catheters are changed every 48–72 hours to decrease the likelihood of catheter-associated infection, and antimicrobial-coated central venous catheters (minocycline and rifampin, chlorhexidine and sulfadiazine) have been associated with a decreased incidence of these infections. Most of these infections present with local signs of infection (erythema, tenderness) at the insertion site. In a patient with fever who is receiving intravenous therapy, the catheter must always be considered a potential source. Small-gauge (20–23F) peripherally inserted silicone or polyurethane catheters (Per Q Cath, A-Cath, Ven-A-Cath, and others) are associated with a low infection rate and can be maintained for 3–6 months without replacement. Such catheters are ideal for long-term outpatient antibiotic therapy.

J. Cost of Antibiotics

The cost of these agents can be substantial. In addition to acquisition costs and monitoring costs (drug levels, liver biochemical tests, electrolytes, etc), the cost of treating adverse reactions, the cost of treatment failure and superinfection, and the costs associated with drug administration must be considered.

Chua KP et al. Appropriateness of outpatient antibiotic prescribing among privately insured US patients: ICD-10-CM based cross sectional study. BMJ. 2019 Jan 16;364:k5092. [PMID: 30651273]

Tamma PD et al. Association of adverse events with antibiotic use in hospitalized patients. JAMA Intern Med. 2017 Sep 1; 177(9):1308–15. [PMID: 28604925]

HYPERSENSITIVITY

▶ Penicillin Allergy

All penicillins are cross-sensitizing and cross-reacting. Skin tests using penicilloyl-polylysine and undegraded penicillin can identify most individuals with IgE-mediated reactions (hives, bronchospasm). In those patients with positive reaction to skin tests, the incidence of subsequent immediate severe reactions associated with penicillin administration is high. A history of a penicillin reaction in the past is often *not* reliable. Only a small proportion (less than 5%) of patients with a stated history of penicillin allergy experience an adverse reaction when challenged with the medication. The decision to administer penicillin or related medications (other beta-lactams) to patients with an allergic history depends on the severity of the reported reaction, the severity of the infection being treated, and the availability of alternative medications. For patients with a history of severe reaction (anaphylaxis), alternative medications should be used. In the rare situations when there is a strong indication for using penicillin (eg, syphilis in pregnancy) in allergic patients, desensitization can be performed. If the reaction is mild (nonurticarial rash), the patient may be rechallenged with penicillin or may be given another beta-lactam antibiotic.

Allergic reactions include anaphylaxis, serum sickness (urticaria, fever, joint swelling, angioedema 7–12 days after exposure), skin rashes, fever, interstitial nephritis, eosinophilia, hemolytic anemia, other hematologic disturbances, and vasculitis. The incidence of hypersensitivity to penicillin is estimated to be 1–5% among adults in the United States. Life-threatening anaphylactic reactions are very rare (0.05%). Ampicillin produces maculopapular skin rashes more frequently than other penicillins, but many ampicillin (and other beta-lactam) rashes are not allergic in origin. The nonallergic ampicillin rash usually occurs after 3–4 days of therapy, is maculopapular, is more common in patients with coexisting viral illness (especially Epstein-Barr infection), and resolves with continued therapy. The maculopapular rash may or may not reappear with rechallenge. Beta-lactams can induce nephritis with primary tubular lesions associated with anti-basement membrane antibodies.

If the intradermal test described below is negative, desensitization is not necessary, and a full dose of the penicillin may be given. If the test is positive, alternative medications should be strongly considered. If that is not feasible, desensitization is necessary.

Patients with a history of allergy to penicillin are also at an increased risk for having a reaction to cephalosporins or carbapenems. A common approach to these patients is to assess the severity of the reaction. If an IgE-mediated reaction to penicillin can be excluded by history, a cephalosporin can be administered. When the history justifies concern about an immediate-type reaction, penicillin skin testing should be performed. If the test is negative, the cephalosporin or carbapenem can be given. If the test is positive, there is a 5–10% chance of cross reactivity with cephalosporins, and the decision whether to use cephalosporins depends on the availability of alternative agents and the severity of the infection. While carbapenems historically have been considered highly cross reactive with penicillins, the cross reactivity appears to be minimal (1%).

Leis JA et al. Point-of-care beta-lactam allergy skin testing by antimicrobial stewardship programs: a pragmatic multicenter prospective evaluation. Clin Infect Dis. 2017 Oct 1;65(7): 1059–65. [PMID: 28575226]

MacFadden DR et al. Impact of reported beta-lactam allergy on inpatient outcomes: a multicenter prospective cohort study. Clin Infect Dis. 2016 Oct 1;63(7):904–10. [PMID: 27402820]

Sacco KA et al. Clinical outcomes following inpatient penicillin allergy testing: a systematic review and meta-analysis. Allergy. 2017 Sep;72(9):1288–96. [PMID: 28370003]

IMMUNIZATION AGAINST INFECTIOUS DISEASES

RECOMMENDED IMMUNIZATION FOR ADULTS

Immunization is one of the most important tools (along with sanitation) used to prevent morbidity and mortality from infectious diseases. In general, the administration of most vaccinations induces a durable antibody response (**active immunity**). In contrast, **passive immunization** occurs when preformed antibodies are given (eg, immune globulin from pooled serum), resulting in temporary protection which is a less durable response. The two variants of active immunization are **live attenuated vaccines** (which are believed to result in an immunologic response more like natural infection), and **inactivated or killed vaccines.**

The schedule of vaccinations varies based on the risk of the disease being prevented by vaccination, whether a vaccine has been given previously, the immune status of the patient (probability of responding to vaccine) and safety of the vaccine (live versus killed product, as well as implications for the fetus in pregnant women). Recommendations for healthy adults as well as special populations based on medical conditions are summarized in Table 30–7, which can be accessed online at https://www.cdc.gov/vaccines/schedules.

1. Healthy Adults

Vaccination recommendations are made by the Advisory Committee on Immunization Practices (ACIP) of the US Centers for Disease Control and Prevention (Table 30–7).

2. Pregnant Women

Given the uncertainty of risks to the fetus, vaccination during pregnancy is generally avoided with the following exceptions: tetanus (transfer of maternal antibodies across the placenta is important to prevent neonatal tetanus), diphtheria, and influenza. Live vaccines are avoided during pregnancy.

Influenza can be a serious infection if acquired in pregnancy, and *all pregnant women should be offered influenza (inactivated) vaccination.* The live attenuated (intranasal) influenza vaccine is *not* recommended during pregnancy.

3. HIV-Infected Adults

HIV-infected patients have impaired cellular and B cell responses. Inactivated or killed vaccinations can generally be given without any consequence, but the recipient may not be able to mount an adequate antibody response. Live or attenuated vaccines are generally avoided with some exceptions (ie, in patients with CD4$^+$ T lymphocytes greater than 200 cells/mcL). Guidelines for vaccinating HIV-infected patients have been issued jointly by the Centers for Disease Control and Prevention, the US National Institutes of Health, and the HIV Medical Association of the Infectious Diseases Society of America. Timing of vaccination is important to optimize response. If possible, vaccination should be given early in the course of HIV disease or following immune reconstitution.

4. Hematopoietic Cell Transplant Recipients

Hematopoietic cell transplant (HCT) recipients have varying rates of immune reconstitution following transplantation, depending on (1) the type of chemotherapy or radiotherapy used pretransplant (in autologous HCT), (2) the preparative regimen used for the transplant, (3) whether graft-versus-host disease is present, and (4) the type of immunosuppression used posttransplantation (in allogeneic HCT). Vaccines may not work immediately in the posttransplant period. B cells may take 3–12 months to return to normal posttransplant, and naïve T cells that can respond to new antigens appear only 6–12 months posttransplant. B cells of posttransplant patients treated with rituximab may take up to 6 months to fully recover after the last dose of the medication. Vaccines are therefore administered 6–12 months following transplantation with a minimum of 1 month between doses to maximize the probability of response.

5. Solid Organ Transplant Recipients

Solid organ transplant recipients demonstrate a broad spectrum of immunosuppression, depending on the reason for and type of organ transplantation and the nature of the immunosuppression (including T-cell-depleting agents during treatment of organ rejection). These factors affect the propensity for infection posttransplantation and the ability to develop antibody responses to vaccination. In many cases, the time between placing a patient on a transplant list and undergoing the transplantation takes months or years. Providers should take this opportunity to ensure that indicated vaccines are given during this pretransplant period to *optimize antibody responses.* If this is not possible, most experts give vaccines 3–6 months following transplantation. Live vaccines are contraindicated in the posttransplant period.

RECOMMENDED IMMUNIZATIONS FOR TRAVELERS

Individuals traveling to other countries frequently require immunizations in addition to those routinely recommended and may benefit from chemoprophylaxis against various diseases. Vaccinations against yellow fever and meningococcus are the only ones required by certain countries. These and other travel-specific vaccines are listed at http://wwwnc.cdc.gov/travel/destinations/list.

Various vaccines can be given simultaneously at different sites. Some, such as cholera, plague, and typhoid vaccine, cause significant discomfort and are best given at different times. In general, live attenuated vaccines (measles, mumps, rubella, yellow fever, and oral typhoid vaccine) should not be given to immunosuppressed individuals or household members of immunosuppressed people or to pregnant women. Immunoglobulin should not be given for 3 months before or at least 2 weeks after live virus vaccines, because it may attenuate the antibody response.

Chemoprophylaxis of malaria is discussed in Chapter 35.

VACCINE SAFETY

Most vaccines are safe to administer. In general, it is recommended that the use of live vaccines be avoided in immunocompromised patients, including pregnant women. Vaccines are generally not contraindicated in the following situations: mild, acute illness with low-grade

Table 30–7. Recommended adult immunization schedule—United States, 2019.

Recommended Adult Immunization Schedule by Age Group United States, 2019

Vaccine	19–21 years	22–26 years	27–49 years	50–64 years	≥65 years
Influenza inactivated (IIV) or Influenza recombinant (RIV) *or*	1 dose annually				
Influenza live attenuated (LAIV)	1 dose annually				
Tetanus, diphtheria, pertussis (Tdap or Td)	1 dose Tdap, then Td booster every 10 yrs				
Measles, mumps, rubella (MMR)	1 or 2 doses depending on indication (if born in 1957 or later)				
Varicella (VAR)	2 doses (if born in 1980 or later)				
Zoster recombinant (RZV) *(preferred)* *or*				2 doses	
Zoster live (ZVL)				1 dose	
Human papillomavirus (HPV) Female	2 or 3 doses depending on age at initial vaccination				
Human papillomavirus (HPV) Male	2 or 3 doses depending on age at initial vaccination				
Pneumococcal conjugate (PCV13)				1 dose	
Pneumococcal polysaccharide (PPSV23)	1 or 2 doses depending on indication				1 dose
Hepatitis A (HepA)	2 or 3 doses depending on vaccine				
Hepatitis B (HepB)	2 or 3 doses depending on vaccine				
Meningococcal A, C, W, Y (MenACWY)	1 or 2 doses depending on indication, then booster every 5 yrs if risk remains				
Meningococcal B (MenB)	2 or 3 doses depending on vaccine and indication				
Haemophilus influenzae type b (Hib)	1 or 3 doses depending on indication				

Recommended vaccination for adults who meet age requirement, lack documentation of vaccination, or lack evidence of past infection

Recommended vaccination for adults with an additional risk factor or another indication

No recommendation

Recommended Adult Immunization Schedule by Medical Condition and Other Indications United States, 2019

Vaccine	Pregnancy	Immuno-compromised (excluding HIV infection)	HIV infection CD4 count <200	HIV infection CD4 count ≥200	Asplenia, complement deficiencies	End-stage renal disease, on hemodialysis	Heart or lung disease, alcoholism[1]	Chronic liver disease	Diabetes	Health care personnel[2]	Men who have sex with men
IIV or RIV	1 dose annually										
LAIV	CONTRAINDICATED	CONTRAINDICATED	CONTRAINDICATED	CONTRAINDICATED	CONTRAINDICATED	CONTRAINDICATED	PRECAUTION	PRECAUTION	PRECAUTION	or 1 dose annually	or 1 dose annually
Tdap or Td	1 dose Tdap each pregnancy	1 dose Tdap, then Td booster every 10 yrs									
MMR	CONTRAINDICATED	CONTRAINDICATED	CONTRAINDICATED	1 or 2 doses depending on indication							
VAR	CONTRAINDICATED	CONTRAINDICATED	CONTRAINDICATED	2 doses							
RZV (preferred)	DELAY				2 doses at age ≥50 yrs						
or ZVL	CONTRAINDICATED	CONTRAINDICATED	CONTRAINDICATED	1 dose at age ≥60 yrs							
HPV Female	DELAY	3 doses through age 26 yrs			2 or 3 doses through age 26 yrs						
HPV Male		3 doses through age 26 yrs			2 or 3 doses through age 21 yrs					2 or 3 doses through age 26 yrs	
PCV13					1 dose						
PPSV23					1, 2, or 3 doses depending on age and indication						
HepA							2 or 3 doses depending on vaccine				
HepB							2 or 3 doses depending on vaccine				
MenACWY		1 or 2 doses depending on indication, then booster every 5 yrs if risk remains									
MenB	PRECAUTION	2 or 3 doses depending on vaccine and indication									
Hib		3 doses HSCT[3] recipients only			1 dose						

Legend:
- Recommended vaccination for adults who meet age requirement, lack documentation of vaccination, or lack evidence of past infection
- Recommended vaccination for adults with an additional risk factor or another indication
- Precaution—vaccine might be indicated if benefit of protection outweighs risk of adverse reaction
- Delay vaccination until after pregnancy if vaccine is indicated
- Contraindicated—vaccine should not be administered because of risk for serious adverse reaction
- No recommendation

1. Precaution for LAIV does not apply to alcoholism. 2. See notes for influenza; hepatitis B; measles, mumps, and rubella; and varicella vaccinations. 3. Hematopoietic stem cell transplant.

(continued)

Table 30–7. Recommended adult immunization schedule—United States, 2019. (continued)

NOTES

***Haemophilus influenzae* type b vaccination**

Special situations

- Anatomical or functional asplenia (including sickle cell disease): 1 dose Hib if previously did not receive Hib; if elective splenectomy, 1 dose Hib, preferably at least 14 days before splenectomy
- Hematopoietic stem cell transplant (HSCT): 3-dose series Hib 4 weeks apart starting 6–12 months after successful transplant, regardless of Hib vaccination history

Hepatitis A vaccination

Routine vaccination

- Not at risk but want protection from hepatitis A (identification of risk factor not required): 2-dose series HepA (Havrix 6–12 months apart or Vaqta 6–18 months apart [minimum interval: 6 months]) or 3-dose series HepA-HepB (Twinrix at 0, 1, 6 months [minimum intervals: 4 weeks between doses 1 and 2, 5 months between doses 2 and 3])

Special situations

- At risk for hepatitis A virus infection: 2-dose series HepA or 3-dose series HepA-HepB as above
  - Chronic liver disease
  - Clotting factor disorders
  - Men who have sex with men
  - Injection or non-injection drug use
  - Homelessness
  - Work with hepatitis A virus in research laboratory or nonhuman primates with hepatitis A virus infection
  - Travel in countries with high or intermediate endemic hepatitis A
  - Close personal contact with international adoptee (e.g., household, regular babysitting) in first 60 days after arrival from country with high or intermediate endemic hepatitis A (administer dose 1 as soon as adoption is planned, at least 2 weeks before adoptee's arrival)

Hepatitis B vaccination

Routine vaccination

- Not at risk but want protection from hepatitis B (identification of risk factor not required): 2- or 3-dose series HepB (2-dose series Heplisav-B at least 4 weeks apart [2-dose series HepB only applies when 2 doses of Heplisav-B are used at least 4 weeks apart] or 3-dose series Engerix-B or Recombivax HB at 0, 1, 6 months [minimum intervals: 4 weeks between doses 1 and 2, 8 weeks between doses 2 and 3, 16 weeks between doses 1 and 3]) or 3-dose series HepA-HepB (Twinrix at 0, 1, 6 months [minimum intervals: 4 weeks between doses 1 and 2, 5 months between doses 2 and 3])

Special situations

- At risk for hepatitis B virus infection: 2-dose (Heplisav-B) or 3-dose (Engerix-B, Recombivax HB) series HepB, or 3-dose series HepA-HepB as above
  - Hepatitis C virus infection
  - Chronic liver disease (e.g., cirrhosis, fatty liver disease, alcoholic liver disease, autoimmune hepatitis, alanine aminotransferase [ALT] or aspartate aminotransferase [AST] level greater than twice upper limit of normal)
  - HIV infection
  - Sexual exposure risk (e.g., sex partners of hepatitis B surface antigen (HBsAg)-positive persons; sexually active persons not in mutually monogamous relationships, persons seeking evaluation or treatment for a sexually transmitted infection, men who have sex with men)
  - Current or recent injection drug use
  - Percutaneous or mucosal risk for exposure to blood (e.g., household contacts of HBsAg-positive persons; residents and staff of facilities for developmentally disabled persons; health care and public safety personnel with reasonably anticipated risk for exposure to blood or blood-contaminated body fluids; hemodialysis, peritoneal dialysis, home dialysis, and predialysis patients; persons with diabetes mellitus age younger than 60 years and, at discretion of treating clinician, those age 60 years or older)
  - Incarcerated persons
  - Travel in countries with high or intermediate endemic hepatitis B

Human papillomavirus vaccination

Routine vaccination

- Females through age 26 years and males through age 21 years: 2- or 3-dose series HPV vaccine depending on age at initial vaccination; males age 22 through 26 years may be vaccinated based on individual clinical decision (HPV vaccination routinely recommended at age 11–12 years)
- Age 15 years or older at initial vaccination: 3-dose series HPV vaccine at 0, 1–2, 6 months (minimum intervals: 4 weeks between doses 1 and 2, 12 weeks between doses 2 and 3, 5 months between doses 1 and 3; repeat dose if administered too soon)

- Age 9 through 14 years at initial vaccination and received 1 dose, or 2 doses less than 5 months apart: 1 dose HPV vaccine
- Age 9 through 14 years at initial vaccination and received 2 doses at least 5 months apart: HPV vaccination complete, no additional dose needed
- If completed valid vaccination series with any HPV vaccine, no additional doses needed

Special situations

- Immunocompromising conditions (including HIV infection) through age 26 years: 3-dose series HPV vaccine at 0, 1–2, 6 months as above
- Men who have sex with men and transgender persons through age 26 years: 2- or 3-dose series HPV vaccine depending on age at initial vaccination as above
- Pregnancy through age 26 years: HPV vaccination not recommended until after pregnancy; no intervention needed if vaccinated while pregnant; pregnancy testing not needed before vaccination

Influenza vaccination

Routine vaccination

- Persons age 6 months or older: 1 dose IIV, RIV, or LAIV appropriate for age and health status annually
- For additional guidance, see www.cdc.gov/flu/professionals/index.htm

Special situations

- Egg allergy, hives only: 1 dose IIV, RIV, or LAIV appropriate for age and health status annually
- Egg allergy more severe than hives (e.g., angioedema, respiratory distress): 1 dose IIV, RIV, or LAIV appropriate for age and health status annually in medical setting under supervision of health care provider who can recognize and manage severe allergic conditions
- Immunocompromising conditions (including HIV infection), anatomical or functional asplenia, pregnant women, close contacts and caregivers of severely immunocompromised persons in protected environment, use of influenza antiviral medications in previous 48 hours, with cerebrospinal fluid leak or cochlear implant: 1 dose IIV or RIV annually (LAIV not recommended)
- History of Guillain-Barré syndrome within 6 weeks of previous dose of influenza vaccine: Generally should not be vaccinated

Measles, mumps, and rubella vaccination

Routine vaccination

- No evidence of immunity to measles, mumps, or rubella: 1 dose MMR
- Evidence of immunity: Born before 1957 (except health care personnel [see below]), documentation of receipt of MMR, laboratory evidence of immunity or disease (diagnosis of disease without laboratory confirmation is not evidence of immunity)

Special situations

- Pregnancy with no evidence of immunity to rubella: MMR contraindicated during pregnancy; after pregnancy (before discharge from health care facility), 1 dose MMR
- Non-pregnant women of childbearing age with no evidence of immunity to rubella: 1 dose MMR
- HIV infection with CD4 count ≥200 cells/µL for at least 6 months and no evidence of immunity to measles, mumps, or rubella: 2-dose series MMR at least 4 weeks apart; MMR contraindicated in HIV infection with CD4 count <200 cells/µL
- Severe immunocompromising conditions: MMR contraindicated
- Students in postsecondary educational institutions, international travelers, and household or close personal contacts of immunocompromised persons with no evidence of immunity to measles, mumps, or rubella: 1 dose MMR if previously received 1 dose MMR, or 2-dose series MMR at least 4 weeks apart if previously did not receive any MMR
- Health care personnel born in 1957 or later with no evidence of immunity to measles, mumps, or rubella: 2-dose series MMR at least 4 weeks apart for measles or mumps, or at least 1 dose MMR for rubella; if born before 1957, consider 2-dose series MMR at least 4 weeks apart for measles or mumps, or 1 dose MMR for rubella

Meningococcal vaccination

Special situations for MenACWY

- Anatomical or functional asplenia (including sickle cell disease), HIV infection, persistent complement component deficiency, eculizumab use: 2-dose series MenACWY (Menactra, Menveo) at least 8 weeks apart and revaccinate every 5 years if risk remains
- Travel in countries with hyperendemic or epidemic meningococcal disease, microbiologists routinely exposed to Neisseria meningitidis: 1 dose MenACWY
- First-year college students who live in residential housing (if not previously vaccinated at age 16 years or older) and military recruits: 1 dose MenACWY

Special situations for MenB

- Anatomical or functional asplenia (including sickle cell disease), persistent complement component deficiency, eculizumab use, microbiologists routinely exposed to Neisseria meningitidis: 2-dose series MenB-4C (Bexsero) at least 1 month apart, or 3-dose series MenB-FHbp (Trumenba) at 0, 1–2, 6 months (if dose 2 was administered at least 6 months after dose 1, dose 3 not needed); MenB-4C and MenBFHbp are not interchangeable (use same product for all doses in series)
- Pregnancy: Delay MenB until after pregnancy unless at increased risk and vaccination benefit outweighs potential risks
- Healthy adolescents and young adults age 16 through 23 years (age 16 through 18 years preferred) not at increased risk for meningococcal disease: Based on individual clinical decision, may receive 2-dose series MenB-4C at least 1 month apart, or 2-dose series MenB-FHbp at 0, 6 months (if dose 2 was administered less than 6 months after dose 1, administer dose 3 at least 4 months after dose 2); MenB-4C and MenB-FHbp are not interchangeable (use same product for all doses in series)

(continued)

Table 30–7. Recommended adult immunization schedule—United States, 2019. (continued)

Pneumococcal vaccination

Routine vaccination

- Age 65 years or older (immunocompetent): 1 dose PCV13 if previously did not receive PCV13, followed by 1 dose PPSV23 at least 1 year after PCV13 and at least 5 years after last dose PPSV23
  - Previously received PPSV23 but not PCV13 at age 65 years or older: 1 dose PCV13 at least 1 year after PPSV23
  - When both PCV13 and PPSV23 are indicated, administer PCV13 first (PCV13 and PPSV23 should not be administered during same visit)

Special situations

- Age 19 through 64 years with chronic medical conditions (chronic heart [excluding hypertension], lung, or liver disease; diabetes), alcoholism, or cigarette smoking: 1 dose PPSV23
- Age 19 years or older with immunocompromising conditions (congenital or acquired immunodeficiency [including B- and T-lymphocyte deficiency, complement deficiencies, phagocytic disorders, HIV infection], chronic renal failure, nephrotic syndrome, leukemia, lymphoma, Hodgkin disease, generalized malignancy, iatrogenic immunosuppression [e.g., drug or radiation therapy], solid organ transplant, multiple myeloma) or anatomical or functional asplenia (including sickle cell disease and other hemoglobinopathies): 1 dose PCV13 followed by 1 dose PPSV23 at least 8 weeks later, then another dose PPSV23 at least 5 years after previous PPSV23; at age 65 years or older, administer 1 dose PPSV23 at least 5 years after most recent PPSV23 (note: only 1 dose PPSV23 recommended at age 65 years or older)
- Age 19 years or older with cerebrospinal fluid leak or cochlear implant: 1 dose PCV13 followed by 1 dose PPSV23 at least 8 weeks later; at age 65 years or older, administer another dose PPSV23 at least 5 years after PPSV23 (note: only 1 dose PPSV23 recommended at age 65 years or older)

Tetanus, diphtheria, and pertussis vaccination

Routine vaccination

- Previously did not receive Tdap at or after age 11 years: 1 dose Tdap, then Td booster every 10 years

Special situations

- Previously did not receive primary vaccination series for tetanus, diphtheria, and pertussis: 1 dose Tdap followed by 1 dose Td at least 4 weeks after Tdap, and another dose Td 6–12 months after last Td (Tdap can be substituted for any Td dose, but preferred as first dose); Td booster every 10 years thereafter
- Pregnancy: 1 dose Tdap during each pregnancy, preferably in early part of gestational weeks 27–36
- For information on use of Tdap or Td as tetanus prophylaxis in wound management, see www.cdc.gov/mmwr/volumes/67/rr/rr6702a1.htm

Varicella vaccination

Routine vaccination

- No evidence of immunity to varicella: 2-dose series VAR 4–8 weeks apart if previously did not receive varicella-containing vaccine (VAR or MMRV [measles-mumps-rubella-varicella vaccine] for children); if previously received 1 dose varicella-containing vaccine: 1 dose VAR at least 4 weeks after first dose
  - Evidence of immunity: U.S.-born before 1980 (except for pregnant women and health care personnel [see below]), documentation of 2 doses varicella-containing vaccine at least 4 weeks apart, diagnosis or verification of history of varicella or herpes zoster by a health care provider, laboratory evidence of immunity or disease

Special situations

- Pregnancy with no evidence of immunity to varicella: VAR contraindicated during pregnancy; after pregnancy (before discharge from health care facility), 1 dose VAR if previously received 1 dose varicella-containing vaccine, or dose 1 of 2-dose series VAR (dose 2: 4–8 weeks later) if previously did not receive any varicella-containing vaccine, regardless of whether U.S.-born before 1980
- Health care personnel with no evidence of immunity to varicella: 1 dose VAR if previously received 1 dose varicella-containing vaccine, or 2-dose series VAR 4–8 weeks apart if previously did not receive any varicella-containing vaccine, regardless of whether U.S.-born before 1980
- HIV infection with CD4 count ≥200 cells/μL with no evidence of immunity: Consider 2-dose series VAR 3 months apart based on individual clinical decision; VAR contraindicated in HIV infection with CD4 count <200 cells/μL
- Severe immunocompromising conditions: VAR contraindicated

Zoster vaccination

Routine vaccination

- Age 50 years or older: 2-dose series RZV 2–6 months apart (minimum interval: 4 weeks; repeat dose if administered too soon) regardless of previous herpes zoster or previously received ZVL (administer RZV at least 2 months after ZVL)
- Age 60 years or older: 2-dose series RZV 2–6 months apart (minimum interval: 4 weeks; repeat dose if administered too soon) or 1 dose ZVL if not previously vaccinated (if previously received ZVL, administer RZV at least 2 months after ZVL); RZV preferred over ZVL

Special situations

- Pregnancy: ZVL contraindicated; consider delaying RZV until after pregnancy if RZV is otherwise indicated
- Severe immunocompromising conditions (including HIV infection with CD4 count <200 cells/μL): ZVL contraindicated; recommended use of RZV under review

Table 30–8. Adverse effects and contraindications to commonly used vaccines in adults (listed in alphabetical order).

Vaccine	Adverse Effects	Contraindications[1]
Haemophilus influenzae Type b (Hib)	Minimal Consist mainly of pain at the injection site	Any severe allergic reaction (eg, anaphylaxis) after a previous dose or to a vaccine component.
Hepatitis A	Minimal Consist mainly of pain at the injection site	Any severe allergic reaction (eg, anaphylaxis) after a previous dose or to a vaccine component.
Hepatitis B	Minimal Consist mainly of pain at the injection site	Any severe allergic reaction (eg, anaphylaxis) after a previous dose or to a vaccine component.
Human papillomavirus	Minimal Consist mainly of mild to moderate localized pain, erythema, swelling Systemic reactions, mainly fever, seen in 4% of recipients	Any severe allergic reaction (eg, anaphylaxis) after a previous dose or to a vaccine component.
Influenza (intramuscular inactivated and intranasal live attenuated vaccines)	**Intramuscular, inactivated vaccine:** Local reactions (erythema and tenderness) at the site of injection are common, but fevers, chills, and malaise (which last in any case only 2–3 days) are rare. **Either inactivated or live attenuated vaccine:** A potential association between Guillain-Barré syndrome (3000–6000 cases per year in the United States, usually following respiratory infections) and vaccination with intramuscular, inactivated influenza vaccine has been reported (possibly, 1–2 persons per million persons vaccinated), but this rate is lower than the risk of the syndrome developing after influenza itself (given that approximately 750 persons per million adults are hospitalized annually with influenza, and many more cases remain as outpatients). Influenza vaccination may be associated with multiple false-positive serologic tests to HIV, HTLV-1, and hepatitis C, but it is self-limited, lasting 2–5 months.	Contraindication to both inactivated and live attenuated vaccine: History of Guillain-Barré syndrome, especially within 6 weeks of receiving a previous influenza vaccine. Any severe allergic reaction (eg, anaphylaxis) after a previous dose or to a vaccine component, including egg protein.[2] Intranasal, live attenuated vaccine [FluMist] should not be used in: • People 50 years of age and over • Immunosuppressed individuals and those on immunosuppressive therapy • Household members of immunosuppressed individuals • Health care workers, or others with close contact with immunosuppressed persons • Presence of reactive airway disease (eg, asthma) or chronic underlying metabolic (eg, kidney), pulmonary, or heart diseases (use intramuscular inactivated vaccine) • Pregnancy[3] It is recommended that salicylates should be avoided for 6 weeks following vaccination (to prevent Reye syndrome).
Measles, mumps, and rubella (MMR)[4]	Fever will develop in about 5–15% of unimmunized individuals, and a mild rash will develop in about 5% 5–12 days after vaccination. Fever and rash are self-limited, lasting only 2–3 days. Local swelling and induration are particularly common in individuals previously vaccinated with inactivated vaccine.	Pregnancy[5] Known severe immunodeficiency (eg, from hematologic and solid cancers, receipt of chemotherapy, congenital immunodeficiency, long-term immunosuppressive therapy [eg, > 2 weeks of prednisone 20 mg daily or higher]), other disease- or therapy-related immune suppression, or patients with HIV infection who are severely immunocompromised. May be used in asymptomatic HIV-infected individuals whose CD4 count is > 200/mcL. Severe allergic reaction (eg, anaphylaxis) to a previous dose or to a vaccine component (eg, neomycin or to related agents such as streptomycin).
Meningococcal, oligosaccharide conjugate; (MCV4 or MenACWY [Menactra, Menveo]; meningococcal polysaccharide conjugate MPSV4 [Menomune]); meningococcal group B, recombinant (MenB [Bexsero, Trumenba])	Minor reactions (fever, redness, swelling, erythema, pain) occur slightly more commonly with MCV4. Major reactions are rare. A potential association between Guillain-Barré syndrome (3000–6000 cases per year in the United States, usually following respiratory infections) and vaccination with MCV4 has been reported, but current recommendations favor continued use of MCV4, since the benefits of preventing the serious consequences of meningococcal infection outweigh the theoretical risk of Guillain-Barré syndrome.	Any severe allergic reaction (eg, anaphylaxis) to a previous dose or to a vaccine component (eg, persons with history of adverse reaction to diphtheria toxoid should not receive meningococcal oligosaccharide conjugate and polysaccharide conjugate vaccines since the protein conjugate used in them is diphtheria toxoid).

(continued)

Table 30–8. Adverse effects and contraindications to commonly used vaccines in adults (listed in alphabetical order). (continued)

Vaccine	Adverse Effects	Contraindications[1]
Pneumococcal conjugate (PCV13 [Prevnar]); Pneumococcal polysaccharide (PPSV23) [Pneumovax])	Mild local reactions (erythema and tenderness) occur in up to 50% of recipients, but systemic reactions are uncommon. Similarly, revaccination at least 5 years after initial vaccination is associated with mild self-limited local but not systemic reactions.	Any severe allergic reaction (eg, anaphylaxis) after a previous dose or to a vaccine component (eg, for PCV13 to any vaccine containing diphtheria toxoid).
Tetanus, diphtheria, and pertussis (DTP, Tdap); tetanus, diphtheria (Td)	Minimal Consist mainly of pain at the injection site	Any severe allergic reaction (eg, anaphylaxis) after a previous dose or to a vaccine component. For pertussis-containing vaccines: any history of unexplained encephalopathy (eg, coma, decreased level of consciousness, or prolonged seizures) within 7 days of administration of a previous dose of Tdap or diphtheria and tetanus toxoids and pertussis (DTP) or diphtheria and tetanus toxoids and acellular pertussis (Tdap) vaccine.
Varicella	Can occur as late as 4–6 weeks after vaccination. Tenderness and erythema at the injection site are seen in 25%, fever in 10–15%, and a localized maculopapular or vesicular rash in 5%; a diffuse rash, usually with five or fewer vesicular lesions, develops in a smaller percentage. Spread of virus from vaccinees to susceptible individuals is possible, but the risk of such transmission even to immunocompromised patients is small, and disease, when it develops, is mild and treatable with acyclovir.	Known severe immunodeficiency (eg, from hematologic and solid cancers, receipt of chemotherapy, congenital immunodeficiency, long-term immunosuppressive therapy [eg, > 2 weeks of prednisone 20 mg daily or higher; other immunosuppressive medications], other disease- or therapy-related immune suppression, or patients with HIV infection who are severely immunocompromised). Pregnancy. Severe allergic reaction (eg, anaphylaxis) after a previous dose or to a vaccine component (eg, neomycin). For theoretic reasons, it is recommended that salicylates should be avoided for 6 weeks following vaccination (to prevent potential for Reye syndrome).
Zoster	Mild and limited to local reactions Although it is theoretically possible to transmit the virus to susceptible contacts, no such cases have been reported.	Known severe immunodeficiency (eg, from hematologic and solid cancers, receipt of chemotherapy, congenital immunodeficiency, long-term immunosuppressive therapy [eg, > 2 weeks of prednisone 20 mg daily or higher; other immunosuppressive medications], other disease- or therapy-related immune suppression, or patients with HIV infection who are severely immunocompromised. May be used in asymptomatic HIV-infected individuals whose CD4 count is > 200/mcL. Pregnancy. Any severe allergic reaction (eg, anaphylaxis) after a previous dose or to a vaccine component (eg, gelatin or neomycin).

[1]Adapted from Centers for Disease Control and Prevention. Contraindications and precautions to commonly used vaccines in adults. General recommendations on immunization: recommendations of the Advisory Committee on Immunization Practices, 2019. https://www.cdc.gov/vaccines/hcp/acip-recs/general-recs/contraindications.html; and from Hamborsky J et al (editors). Appendix A. Epidemiology and prevention of vaccine preventable diseases. 13th edition. Washington, DC, Public Health Foundation, 2015. Available at www.cdc.gov/vaccines/pubs/pinkbook/index.html.

[2]The vaccine has typically been prepared using embryonated chicken eggs. However, a new vaccine using mammalian cell culture is now FDA approved.

[3]The inactivated influenza vaccine can be given during any trimester.

[4]MMR vaccine can be safely given to patients with a history of egg allergy even when severe.

[5]Although vaccination of pregnant women is *not* recommended, with the currently available RA27/3 vaccine strain, the congenital rubella syndrome does not occur in the offspring of those inadvertently vaccinated during pregnancy or within 3 months before conception.

fevers (less than 40.5°C); concurrent antibiotic therapy; soreness or redness at the site; and family history of adverse reactions to vaccinations. Absolute contraindications to vaccines are rare (Table 30–8).

Centers for Disease Control and Prevention (CDC). Adult immunization schedules—United States, 2019. https://www .cdc.gov/vaccines/schedules/index.html

Centers for Disease Control and Prevention (CDC). Health Information for International Travel. https://wwwnc.cdc.gov/ travel/page/yellowbook-home

Centers for Disease Control and Prevention (CDC). Vaccine safety. https://www.cdc.gov/vaccinesafety/index.html

Grohskopf LA et al. Prevention and control of seasonal influenza with vaccines: recommendations of the Advisory Committee on Immunization Practices—United States, 2018–19 Influenza Season. MMWR Recomm Rep. 2018 Aug 24;67(3):1–20. [PMID: 30141464]

Kim DK et al. Advisory Committee on Immunization Practices recommended immunization schedule for adults aged 19 years or older—United States, 2019. MMWR Morb Mortal Wkly Rep. 2019 Feb 8;68(5):115–8. [PMID: 30730868]

Leidner AJ et al. Cost-effectiveness of adult vaccinations: a systematic review. Vaccine. 2019 Jan 7;37(2):226–34. [PMID: 30527660]

MacNeil JR et al. Recommendations for use of meningococcal conjugate vaccines in HIV-infected persons—Advisory Committee on Immunization Practices, 2016. MMWR Morb Mortal Wkly Rep. 2016 Nov 4;65(43):1189–94. [PMID: 27811836]

Paules CI et al. Chasing seasonal influenza—the need for a universal influenza vaccine. N Engl J Med. 2018 Jan 4;378(1):7–9. [PMID: 29185857]

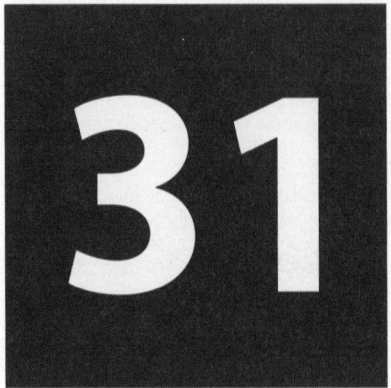

31

HIV Infection & AIDS

Mitchell H. Katz, MD

► Modes of transmission: sexual contact with an infected person, parenteral exposure to infected blood (transfusion or needle sharing), perinatal exposure.

► Prominent systemic complaints: sweats, diarrhea, weight loss, and wasting.

► Opportunistic infections due to diminished cellular immunity—often life-threatening.

► Aggressive cancers, particularly non-Hodgkin lymphoma.

► Neurologic manifestations, including dementia, aseptic meningitis, and neuropathy.

General Considerations

The Centers for Disease Control and Prevention (CDC) AIDS case definition (Table 31–1) includes opportunistic infections and malignancies that rarely occur in the absence of severe immunodeficiency (eg, *Pneumocystis* pneumonia, central nervous system lymphoma). It also classifies persons as having AIDS if they have positive HIV serology and certain infections and malignancies that can occur in immunocompetent hosts but that are more common among persons infected with HIV (pulmonary tuberculosis, invasive cervical cancer). Several nonspecific conditions, including dementia and wasting (documented weight loss)—in the presence of a positive HIV serology—are considered AIDS. The definition includes criteria for both definitive and presumptive diagnoses of certain infections and malignancies. Finally, persons with positive HIV serology who have ever had a CD4 lymphocyte count below 200 cells/mcL or a CD4 lymphocyte percentage below 14% are considered to have AIDS. Inclusion of persons with low CD4 counts as AIDS cases reflects the recognition that immunodeficiency is the defining characteristic of AIDS. The choice of a cutoff point at 200 cells/mcL is supported by several cohort studies showing that AIDS will develop within 3 years in over 80% of persons with counts

below this level in the absence of effective antiretroviral therapy. The prognosis of persons with HIV/AIDS has dramatically improved due to the development of effective antiretroviral treatment. One consequence is that fewer persons with HIV ever develop an infection or malignancy or have a low enough CD4 count to classify them as having AIDS, which means that the CDC definition has become a less useful measure of the impact of HIV/AIDS in the United States. Conversely, persons in whom AIDS had been diagnosed based on a serious opportunistic infection, malignancy, or immunodeficiency may now be markedly healthier, with high CD4 counts, due to the use of antiretroviral treatment. Therefore, the Social Security Administration as well as most social service agencies focus on functional assessment for determining eligibility for benefits rather than the simple presence or absence of an AIDS-defining illness.

Epidemiology

The modes of transmission of HIV are similar to those of hepatitis B, in particular with respect to sexual, parenteral, and vertical transmission. Although certain sexual practices (eg, receptive anal intercourse) are significantly riskier than other sexual practices (eg, oral sex), it is difficult to quantify per-contact risks. The reason is that studies of sexual transmission of HIV show that most people at risk for HIV infection engage in a variety of sexual practices and have sex with multiple persons, only some of whom may actually be HIV infected. Thus, it is difficult to determine which practice with which person actually resulted in HIV transmission.

Nonetheless, the best available estimates indicate that the risk of HIV transmission with receptive anal intercourse is between 1:100 and 1:30, with insertive anal intercourse 1:1000, with receptive vaginal intercourse 1:1000, with insertive vaginal intercourse 1:10,000, and with receptive fellatio with ejaculation 1:1000. The per-contact risk of HIV transmission with other behaviors, including receptive fellatio without ejaculation, insertive fellatio, and cunnilingus, is not known.

A number of cofactors are known to increase the risk of HIV transmission during a given encounter, including the

Table 31–1. CDC AIDS case definition for surveillance of adults and adolescents.

Definitive AIDS Diagnoses (with or without laboratory evidence of HIV infection)

1. Candidiasis of the esophagus, trachea, bronchi, or lungs.

2. Cryptococcosis, extrapulmonary.

3. Cryptosporidiosis with diarrhea persisting longer than 1 month.

4. Cytomegalovirus disease of an organ other than liver, spleen, or lymph nodes.

5. Herpes simplex virus infection causing a mucocutaneous ulcer that persists longer than 1 month; or bronchitis, pneumonitis, or esophagitis of any duration.

6. Kaposi sarcoma in a patient younger than 60 years of age.

7. Lymphoma of the brain (primary) in a patient younger than 60 years of age.

8. *Mycobacterium avium* complex or *Mycobacterium kansasii* disease, disseminated (at a site other than or in addition to lungs, skin, or cervical or hilar lymph nodes).

9. *Pneumocystis jirovecii* pneumonia.

10. Progressive multifocal leukoencephalopathy.

11. Toxoplasmosis of the brain.

Definitive AIDS Diagnoses (with laboratory evidence of HIV infection)

1. Coccidioidomycosis, disseminated (at a site other than or in addition to lungs or cervical or hilar lymph nodes).

2. HIV encephalopathy.

3. Histoplasmosis, disseminated (at a site other than or in addition to lungs or cervical or hilar lymph nodes).

4. Isosporiasis with diarrhea persisting longer than 1 month.

5. Kaposi sarcoma at any age.

6. Lymphoma of the brain (primary) at any age.

7. Other non-Hodgkin lymphoma of B cell or unknown immunologic phenotype.

8. Any mycobacterial disease caused by mycobacteria other than *Mycobacterium tuberculosis*, disseminated (at a site other than or in addition to lungs, skin, or cervical or hilar lymph nodes).

9. Disease caused by extrapulmonary *M tuberculosis*.

10. Salmonella (nontyphoid) septicemia, recurrent.

11. HIV wasting syndrome.

12. CD4 lymphocyte count below 200 cells/mcL or a CD4 lymphocyte percentage below 14%.

13. Pulmonary tuberculosis.

14. Recurrent pneumonia.

15. Invasive cervical cancer.

Presumptive AIDS Diagnoses (with laboratory evidence of HIV infection)

1. Candidiasis of esophagus: (a) recent onset of retrosternal pain on swallowing; and (b) oral candidiasis.

2. Cytomegalovirus retinitis. A characteristic appearance on serial ophthalmoscopic examinations.

3. Mycobacteriosis. Specimen from stool or normally sterile body fluids or tissue from a site other than lungs, skin, or cervical or hilar lymph nodes, showing acid-fast bacilli of a species not identified by culture.

4. Kaposi sarcoma. Erythematous or violaceous plaque-like lesion on skin or mucous membrane.

5. *Pneumocystis jirovecii* pneumonia: (a) a history of dyspnea on exertion or nonproductive cough of recent onset (within the past 3 months); and (b) chest film evidence of diffuse bilateral interstitial infiltrates or gallium scan evidence of diffuse bilateral pulmonary disease; and (c) arterial blood gas analysis showing an arterial oxygen partial pressure of less than 70 mm Hg or a low respiratory diffusing capacity of less than 80% of predicted values or an increase in the alveolar-arterial oxygen tension gradient; and (d) no evidence of a bacterial pneumonia.

6. Toxoplasmosis of the brain: (a) recent onset of a focal neurologic abnormality consistent with intracranial disease or a reduced level of consciousness; and (b) brain imaging evidence of a lesion having a mass effect or the radiographic appearance of which is enhanced by injection of contrast medium; and (c) serum antibody to toxoplasmosis or successful response to therapy for toxoplasmosis.

7. Recurrent pneumonia: (a) more than one episode in a 1-year period; and (b) acute pneumonia (new symptoms, signs, or radiologic evidence not present earlier) diagnosed on clinical or radiologic grounds by the patient's clinician.

8. Pulmonary tuberculosis: (a) apical or miliary infiltrates and (b) radiographic and clinical response to antituberculous therapy.

presence of ulcerative or inflammatory sexually transmitted diseases, trauma, menses, and lack of male circumcision.

The risk of acquiring HIV infection from a needlestick with infected blood is approximately 1:300. Factors known to increase the risk of transmission include depth of penetration, hollow bore needles, visible blood on the needle, and advanced stage of disease in the source. The risk of HIV transmission from a mucosal splash with infected blood is unknown but is assumed to be significantly lower.

The risk of acquiring HIV infection from illicit drug use with sharing of needles from an HIV-infected source is estimated to be 1:150. Use of clean needles markedly decreases the chance of HIV transmission, but does not eliminate it if other drug paraphernalia are shared (eg, cookers).

When blood transfusion from an HIV-infected donor occurs, the risk of transmission is 95%. Fortunately, since 1985, blood donor screening using the HIV enzyme-linked immunosorbent assay (ELISA) has been universally practiced in the United States. Also, persons who have recently engaged in unsafe behaviors (eg, sex with a person at risk for HIV, injection drug use) are not allowed to donate. This essentially eliminates donations from persons who are HIV infected but have not yet developed antibodies (ie, persons in the "window" period). HIV antigen and viral load testing have been added to the screening of blood to further lower the chance of HIV transmission. With these precautions, the chance of HIV transmission with receipt of blood transfusion in the United States is about 1:1,000,000. Between 13% and 40% of children born to HIV-infected mothers contract HIV infection when the mother has not received treatment or when the child has not received perinatal HIV prophylaxis. The risk is higher with vaginal than with cesarean delivery, higher among mothers with high viral loads, and higher among those who breastfeed their children. The combination of prenatal HIV testing and counseling, antiretroviral treatment for infected mothers during pregnancy and for the infant immediately after birth, scheduled cesarean delivery when the mother has a viral load of greater than 1000 copies/mL, and avoidance of breastfeeding has reduced the rate of perinatal transmission of HIV to less than 2% in the United States and Europe.

HIV has not been shown to be transmitted by respiratory droplet spread, by vectors such as mosquitoes, or by casual nonsexual contact. Saliva, sweat, stool, and tears are not considered infectious fluids.

Since the epidemic began in the early 1980s, a total of 1,232,346 Americans have been diagnosed with AIDS. There are an estimated 1.1 million adults and adolescents in the United States living with HIV, 15% of whom are undiagnosed. Young people (age 13 to 24) are the most likely to not know they are infected (51%). In 2016, 39,782 Americans were newly diagnosed with HIV infection. Gay and bisexual men accounted for most of the new diagnoses (67%), and among them, black/African-American men accounted for more new diagnoses (10,223) than Latinos (7425) or whites (7390). Between 2011 and 2015, new HIV diagnoses decreased by 10% among white gay and bisexual males, but increased 4% among African-American gay and bisexual males, and 14% among Latino gay and bisexual men. Heterosexual contacts accounted for 24% (9578) of new HIV diagnoses, women accounted for 19% (7529) and

injection drug users for 9% (3425) of new HIV diagnoses, including gay and bisexual men who inject drugs. In 2016, African Americans and Latinos were disproportionately hard hit by the epidemic. Though representing 12% of the US population, African Americans accounted for 44% of new HIV diagnoses (17,528 cases). Latinos, who represent about 18% of the US population, accounted for 25% of new HIV diagnoses (9766 cases).

In general, the progression of HIV-related illness is similar in men and women. However, there are some important differences. Women are at risk for gynecologic complications of HIV, including recurrent candidal vaginitis, pelvic inflammatory disease, and cervical dysplasia. Violence directed against women, pregnancy, and frequent occurrence of drug use and poverty all complicate the treatment of HIV-infected women.

Worldwide there are an estimated 36.9 million persons infected with HIV, with heterosexual spread being the most common mode of transmission for men and women. The reason for the greater risk for transmission with heterosexual intercourse in Africa and Asia than in the United States may relate to cofactors such as general health status, the presence of genital ulcers, relative lack of male circumcision, the number of sexual partners, and different HIV serotypes. It is estimated that in 2016, 19.5 million persons infected with HIV were receiving treatment (53%), up from 17.1 million in 2015.

Centers for Disease Control and Prevention. HIV in the United States and Dependent Areas. Updated January 29, 2019. https://www.cdc.gov/hiv/statistics/overview/ataglance.html

DiNenno EA et al. Recommendations for HIV screening of gay, bisexual, and other men who have sex with men—United States, 2017. MMWR Morb Mortal Wkly Rep. 2017 Aug 11; 66(31):830–2. [PMID: 28796758]

Katz IT et al. The global HIV/AIDS epidemic: What will it take to get to the finish line? [editorial] JAMA. 2018 Mar 20; 319(11):1094–5. [PMID: 29509836]

Mitsch A et al. Age-associated trends in diagnosis and prevalence of infection with HIV among men who have sex with men—United States, 2008–2016. MMWR Morb Mortal Wkly Rep. 2018 Sep 21;67(37):1025–31. [PMID: 30235184]

World Health Organization. Number of people (all ages) living with HIV: estimates by WHO region. Updated 2019. https://www.who.int/gho/hiv/epidemic_status/cases_all_text/en/

▶ **Pathophysiology**

Clinically, the syndromes caused by HIV infection are usually explicable by one of three known mechanisms: immunodeficiency, autoimmunity, and allergic and hypersensitivity reactions.

A. Immunodeficiency

Immunodeficiency is a direct result of the effects of HIV upon immune cells as well as the indirect impact of a generalized state of inflammation and immune activation due to chronic viral infection. A spectrum of infections and neoplasms is seen, as in other congenital or acquired immunodeficiency states. Two remarkable features of HIV immunodeficiency are the low incidence of certain infections such as listeriosis and aspergillosis and the frequent occurrence of certain neoplasms such as lymphoma or Kaposi sarcoma. This latter complication has been seen primarily in men who have sex with men (MSM) or in bisexual men, and its incidence steadily declined through the first 15 years of the epidemic. A herpesvirus (KSHV or HHV-8) is the cause of Kaposi sarcoma.

B. Autoimmunity/Allergic and Hypersensitivity Reactions

Autoimmunity can occur as a result of disordered cellular immune function or B lymphocyte dysfunction. Examples of both lymphocytic infiltration of organs (eg, lymphocytic interstitial pneumonitis) and autoantibody production (eg, immunologic thrombocytopenia) occur. These phenomena may be the only clinically apparent disease or may coexist with obvious immunodeficiency. Moreover, HIV-infected individuals appear to have higher rates of allergic reactions to unknown allergens as seen with eosinophilic pustular folliculitis ("itchy red bump syndrome") as well as increased rates of hypersensitivity reactions to medications (for example, the fever and sunburn-like rash seen with trimethoprim-sulfamethoxazole reactions).

▶ Clinical Findings

The complications of HIV-related infections and neoplasms affect virtually every organ. The general approach to the HIV-infected person with symptoms is to evaluate the organ systems involved, aiming to diagnose treatable conditions rapidly. As can be seen in Figure 31–1, the CD4 lymphocyte count result enables the clinician to focus on the diagnoses most likely to be seen at each stage of immunodeficiency. Certain infections may occur at any CD4 count, while others rarely occur unless the CD4 lymphocyte count has dropped below a certain level. For example, a patient with a CD4 count of 600 cells/mcL, cough, and fever may have a bacterial pneumonia but would be very unlikely to have *Pneumocystis* pneumonia.

A. Symptoms and Signs

Many individuals with HIV infection remain asymptomatic for years even without antiretroviral treatment, with a mean time of approximately 10 years between infection and development of AIDS. When symptoms occur, they may be remarkably protean and nonspecific. Since virtually all the findings may be seen with other diseases, a combination of complaints is more suggestive of HIV infection than any one symptom.

Physical examination may be entirely normal. Abnormal findings range from completely nonspecific to highly specific for HIV infection. Those that are specific for HIV infection include hairy leukoplakia of the tongue, disseminated Kaposi sarcoma, and cutaneous bacillary angiomatosis. Generalized lymphadenopathy is common early in infection.

The specific presentations and management of the various complications of HIV infection are discussed under the Complications section below.

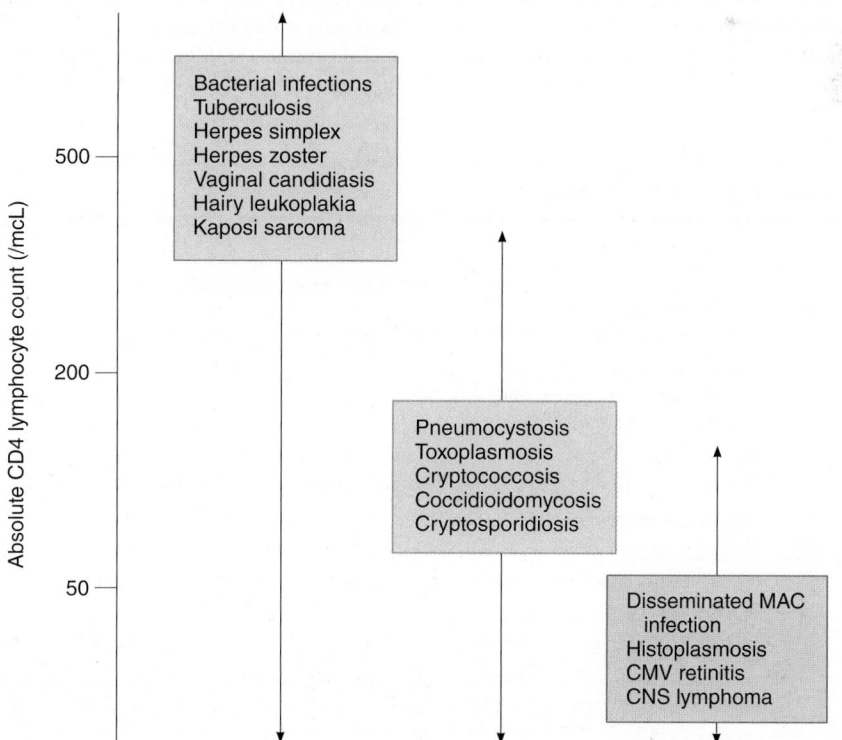

▲ **Figure 31–1.** Relationship of CD4 count to development of opportunistic infections. MAC, *Mycobacterium avium* complex; CMV, cytomegalovirus; CNS, central nervous system.

Henn A et al. Primary HIV infection: clinical presentation, testing, and treatment. Curr Infect Dis Rep. 2017 Sep 7; 19(10):37. [PMID: 28884279]

B. Laboratory Findings

Specific tests for HIV include antibody and antigen detection (Table 31–2). Conventional HIV antibody testing is done by ELISA. Positive specimens are then confirmed by a different method (eg, Western blot). The sensitivity of screening serologic tests is greater than 99.9%. The specificity of positive results by two different techniques approaches 100% even in low-risk populations. False-positive screening tests may occur as normal biologic variants or in association with recent influenza vaccination or other disease states, such as connective tissue disease. These are usually detected by negative confirmatory tests. Antibodies will be detectable with current screening serologic tests in 95% of persons within 6 weeks after infection.

Rapid HIV antibody tests of blood or oral fluid provide results within 10–20 minutes and can be performed in clinician offices, including by personnel without laboratory training and without a Clinical Laboratory Improvement Amendment (CLIA)–approved laboratory. Persons who test positive on a rapid test should be told that they may be HIV-infected or their test may be falsely reactive. Standard testing (ELISA with Western blot confirmation) should be performed to distinguish these two possibilities. Rapid testing is particularly helpful in settings where a result is needed immediately (eg, a woman in labor who has not recently been tested for HIV) or when the patient is unlikely to return for a result. Rapid HIV home tests that allow the testers to learn their status privately by simply swabbing along their gum lines are also available (www.oraquick.com).

Nonspecific laboratory findings with HIV infection may include anemia, leukopenia (particularly lymphopenia), and thrombocytopenia in any combination, elevation of the erythrocyte sedimentation rate, polyclonal hypergammaglobulinemia, and hypocholesterolemia. Cutaneous anergy is common.

The absolute CD4 lymphocyte count is the most widely used marker to provide prognostic information and to guide therapy decisions (Table 31–2). As counts decrease, the risk of serious opportunistic infection over the subsequent 3–5 years increases (Figure 31–1). There are many limitations to using the CD4 count, including diurnal variation, depression with intercurrent illness, and intra-laboratory and interlaboratory variability. Therefore, the trend is more important than a single determination. The frequency of performance of counts depends on the patient's health status and whether or not they are receiving antiretroviral treatment. All patients regardless of CD4 count should be offered antiretroviral treatment; CD4 counts should be monitored every 3–6 months in patients taking antiretroviral treatment consistently. Initiation of *Pneumocystis jirovecii* prophylactic therapy is recommended when the CD4 count drops below 200 cells/mcL, and initiation of *Mycobacterium avium* prophylaxis is recommended when the CD4 count drops below 75–100 cells/mcL. Some studies suggest that the percentage of CD4 lymphocytes is a more reliable indicator of prognosis than the absolute counts because the percentage does not depend on calculating a manual differential. While the CD4 count measures immune dysfunction, it does not provide a measure of how actively HIV is replicating in the body. **HIV viral load** tests assess the level of viral replication and provide useful prognostic information that is independent of the information provided by CD4 counts.

Table 31–2. Laboratory findings with HIV infection.

Test	Significance
HIV enzyme-linked immunosorbent assay (ELISA)	Screening test for HIV infection. Of ELISA tests 50% are positive within 22 days after HIV transmission; 95% are positive within 6 weeks after transmission. Sensitivity greater than 99.9%; to avoid false-positive results, repeatedly reactive results must be confirmed with Western blot.
Western blot	Confirmatory test for HIV. Specificity when combined with ELISA greater than 99.99%. Indeterminate results with early HIV infection, HIV-2 infection, influenza vaccine, autoimmune disease, pregnancy, and recent tetanus toxoid administration.
HIV rapid antibody test	Screening test for HIV. Produces results in 10–20 minutes. Can be performed by personnel with limited training. Positive results must be confirmed with standard HIV tests (ELISA and Western blot).
Complete blood count	Anemia, neutropenia, and thrombocytopenia common with advanced HIV infection.
Absolute CD4 lymphocyte count	Most widely used predictor of HIV progression. Risk of progression to an AIDS opportunistic infection or malignancy is high with CD4 less than 200 cells/mcL in the absence of treatment.
CD4 lymphocyte percentage	Percentage may be more reliable than the CD4 count. Risk of progression to an AIDS opportunistic infection or malignancy is high with percentage less than 14% in the absence of treatment.
HIV viral load tests	These tests measure the amount of actively replicating HIV virus. Correlate with disease progression and response to antiretroviral medications. Best tests available for diagnosis of acute HIV infection (prior to seroconversion); however, caution is warranted when the test result shows low-level viremia (ie, less than 500 copies/mL) as this may represent a false-positive test.

Differential Diagnosis

HIV infection may mimic a variety of other medical illnesses. Specific differential diagnosis depends on the mode of presentation. In patients presenting with constitutional symptoms such as weight loss and fevers, differential considerations include cancer, chronic infections such as tuberculosis and endocarditis, and endocrinologic diseases such as hyperthyroidism. When pulmonary processes dominate the presentation, acute and chronic lung infections must be considered as well as other causes of diffuse interstitial pulmonary infiltrates. When neurologic disease is the mode of presentation, conditions that cause mental status changes or neuropathy—eg, alcoholism, liver disease, kidney dysfunction, thyroid disease, and vitamin deficiency—should be considered. If a patient presents with headache and a cerebrospinal fluid pleocytosis, other causes of chronic meningitis enter the differential. When diarrhea is a prominent complaint, infectious enterocolitis, antibiotic-associated colitis, inflammatory bowel disease, and malabsorptive syndromes must be considered.

Complications

A. Systemic Complaints

Fever, night sweats, and weight loss are common symptoms in HIV-infected patients and may occur without a complicating opportunistic infection. Patients with persistent fever and no localizing symptoms should nonetheless be carefully examined, and evaluated with a chest radiograph (*Pneumocystis* pneumonia can present without respiratory symptoms), bacterial blood cultures if the fever is greater than 38.5°C, serum cryptococcal antigen, and mycobacterial cultures of the blood. Sinus CT scans should be considered to evaluate occult sinusitis. If these studies are normal, patients should be observed closely. Antipyretics are useful to prevent dehydration.

Bolduc P et al. Care of patients with HIV infection: medical complications and comorbidities. FP Essent. 2016 Apr;443: 16–22. [PMID: 27092563]

Chu C et al. HIV-associated complications: a systems-based approach. Am Fam Physician. 2017 Aug 1;96(3):161–9. [PMID: 28762691]

1. Weight loss and wasting syndrome—Weight loss is a particularly distressing complication of long-standing HIV infection. Patients typically have disproportionate loss of muscle mass, with maintenance or less substantial loss of fat stores. The mechanism of HIV-related weight loss is not completely understood but appears to be multifactorial.

A. PRESENTATION—AIDS patients frequently suffer from anorexia, nausea, and vomiting, all of which contribute to weight loss by decreasing caloric intake. In some cases, these symptoms are secondary to a specific infection, such as viral hepatitis. In other cases, however, evaluation of the symptoms yields no specific pathogen, and it is assumed to be due to a primary effect of HIV. Malabsorption also plays a role in decreased caloric intake. Patients may suffer diarrhea from infections with bacterial, viral, or parasitic agents.

Exacerbating the decrease in caloric intake, many AIDS patients have an increased metabolic rate. This increased rate has been shown to exist even among asymptomatic HIV-infected persons, but it accelerates with disease progression and secondary infection. AIDS patients with secondary infections also have decreased protein synthesis, which makes maintaining muscle mass difficult.

B. MANAGEMENT—Several strategies have been developed to slow AIDS wasting. In the long term, nothing is as effective as antiretroviral treatment, since it treats the underlying HIV infection. In the short term, effective fever control decreases the metabolic rate and may slow the pace of weight loss, as does treating the underlying opportunistic infection. Food supplementation with high-calorie drinks may enable patients with not much appetite to maintain their intake. Selected patients with otherwise good functional status and weight loss due to unrelenting nausea, vomiting, or diarrhea may benefit from total parenteral nutrition (TPN). It should be noted, however, that TPN is more likely to increase fat stores than to reverse the muscle wasting process.

Two pharmacologic approaches for increasing appetite and weight gain are the progestational agent **megestrol acetate** liquid suspension (400–800 mg orally daily in divided doses) and the antiemetic agent **dronabinol** (2.5–5 mg orally three times a day), but neither of these agents increases lean body mass. Side effects from megestrol acetate are rare, but thromboembolic phenomena, edema, nausea, vomiting, and rash have been reported. Euphoria, dizziness, paranoia, and somnolence and even nausea and vomiting have been reported in 3–10% of patients using dronabinol. Dronabinol contains only one of the active ingredients in marijuana, and many patients report better relief of nausea and improvement of appetite with **medical cannabis** (administered via smoking, vaporization, essential oils, or cooked in food). In the United States, 33 states have legalized medical marijuana, and 10 states and the District of Columbia have legalized recreational (nonmedical) use. However, the use and sale of marijuana are still illegal under federal law.

Two regimens that have resulted in increases in lean body mass are growth hormone and anabolic steroids. **Growth hormone** at a dose of 0.1 mg/kg/day (up to 6 mg) subcutaneously for 12 weeks has resulted in modest increases in lean body mass. Treatment with growth hormone can cost as much as $10,000 per month. **Anabolic steroids** also increase lean body mass among HIV-infected patients. They seem to work best for patients who are able to do weight training. The most commonly used regimens are testosterone enanthate or testosterone cypionate (100–200 mg intramuscularly every 2–4 weeks). Testosterone transdermal system (apply 5 mg system each evening) and testosterone gel (1%; apply a 5-g packet [50 mg testosterone] to clean, dry skin daily) are also available. The anabolic steroid oxandrolone (20 mg orally in two divided doses) has also been found to increase lean body mass.

Badowski ME et al. Dronabinol oral solution in the management of anorexia and weight loss in AIDS and cancer. Ther Clin Risk Manag. 2018 Apr 6;14:643–51. [PMID: 29670357]

2. Nausea—Nausea leading to weight loss is sometimes due to esophageal candidiasis. Patients with oral candidiasis and nausea should be empirically treated with an oral antifungal agent. Patients with weight loss due to nausea of unclear origin may benefit from use of antiemetics prior to meals (prochlorperazine, 10 mg three times daily; metoclopramide, 10 mg three times daily; or ondansetron, 8 mg three times daily). Dronabinol (5 mg three times daily) or medical cannabis can also be used to treat nausea. Depression and adrenal insufficiency are two potentially treatable causes of weight loss.

Hall VP. Common gastrointestinal complications associated with human immunodeficiency virus/AIDS: an overview. Crit Care Nurs Clin North Am. 2018 Mar;30(1):101–7. [PMID: 29413205]

B. Pulmonary Disease

1. *Pneumocystis* pneumonia—(See also Chapter 36.) *P jirovecii* pneumonia is the most common opportunistic infection associated with AIDS. *Pneumocystis* pneumonia may be difficult to diagnose because the symptoms—fever, cough, and shortness of breath—are nonspecific. Furthermore, the severity of symptoms ranges from fever and no respiratory symptoms through mild cough or dyspnea to frank respiratory distress.

Hypoxemia may be severe, with a PO_2 less than 60 mm Hg. The cornerstone of diagnosis is the chest radiograph. Diffuse or perihilar infiltrates are most characteristic, but only two-thirds of patients with *Pneumocystis* pneumonia have this finding. Normal chest radiographs are seen in 5–10% of patients with *Pneumocystis* pneumonia, while the remainder have atypical infiltrates. Apical infiltrates are commonly seen among patients with *Pneumocystis* pneumonia who have been receiving aerosolized pentamidine prophylaxis. Large pleural effusions are uncommon with *Pneumocystis* pneumonia; their presence suggests bacterial pneumonia, other infections such as tuberculosis, or pleural Kaposi sarcoma.

Definitive diagnosis can be obtained in 50–80% of cases by Wright-Giemsa stain or direct fluorescence antibody (DFA) test of induced sputum. Sputum induction is performed by having patients inhale an aerosolized solution of 3% saline produced by an ultrasonic nebulizer. Patients should not eat for at least 8 hours and should not use toothpaste or mouthwash prior to the procedure since they can interfere with test interpretation. The next step for patients with negative sputum examinations in whom *Pneumocystis* pneumonia is still suspected should be bronchoalveolar lavage. This technique establishes the diagnosis in over 95% of cases.

In patients with symptoms suggestive of *Pneumocystis* pneumonia but with negative or atypical chest radiographs and negative sputum examinations, other diagnostic tests may provide additional information in deciding whether to proceed to bronchoalveolar lavage. Elevation of serum lactate dehydrogenase occurs in 95% of cases of *Pneumocystis* pneumonia, but the specificity of this finding is at best 75%. A serum beta-glucan test is a more sensitive and specific test for *Pneumocystis* pneumonia compared with serum lactate dehydrogenase and may avoid more invasive tests when used in the appropriate clinical setting. Either a normal diffusing capacity of carbon monoxide (DL_{CO}) or a high-resolution CT scan of the chest that demonstrates no interstitial lung disease makes the diagnosis of *Pneumocystis* pneumonia very unlikely. In addition, a CD4 count greater than 250 cells/mcL within 2 months prior to evaluation of respiratory symptoms makes a diagnosis of *Pneumocystis* pneumonia unlikely; only 1–5% of cases occur above this CD4 count level (Figure 31–1). This is true even if the patient previously had a CD4 count lower than 200 cells/mcL but has had an increase with antiretroviral treatment. Pneumothoraces can be seen in HIV-infected patients with a history of *Pneumocystis* pneumonia.

Trimethoprim-sulfamethoxazole is the preferred treatment of *Pneumocystis* pneumonia (Table 31–3). In addition to specific anti-*Pneumocystis* treatment, corticosteroid therapy has been shown to improve the course of patients with moderate to severe *P jirovecii* pneumonia (PaO_2 less than 70 mm Hg on room air or alveolar-arterial O_2 gradient greater or equal to 35 mm Hg) when administered within 72 hours of the start of anti-*Pneumocystis* treatment. It should be started as early as possible after initiation of treatment, using prednisone 40 mg orally twice daily for days 1–5, 40 mg daily for days 6–10, and 20 mg daily for days 11–21 (for patients who cannot take oral medication, intravenous methylprednisolone can be substituted at 75% of the dose). The mechanism of action is presumed to be a decrease in alveolar inflammation.

Huang YS et al. Treatment of *Pneumocystis jirovecii* pneumonia in HIV-infected patients: a review. Expert Rev Anti Infect Ther. 2017 Sep;15(9):873–92. [PMID: 28782390]

Limonta S et al. Lung ultrasound in the management of pneumocystis pneumonia: a case series. Int J STD AIDS. 2019 Feb; 30(2):188–93. [PMID: 30236043]

Maartens G et al. Development of a clinical prediction rule to diagnose *Pneumocystis jirovecii* pneumonia in the World Health Organization's algorithm for seriously ill HIV-infected patients. South Afr J HIV Med. 2018 Jul 23;19(1):851. [PMID: 30167340]

US Department of Health and Human Services. Guidelines for the prevention and treatment of opportunistic infections in HIV-infected adults and adolescents. https://aidsinfo.nih.gov/guidelines

2. Other infectious pulmonary diseases—

A. PRESENTATION—Other infectious causes of pulmonary disease in AIDS patients include bacterial, mycobacterial, and viral pneumonias. Community-acquired pneumonia is the most common cause of pulmonary disease in HIV-infected persons. An increased incidence of pneumococcal pneumonia with septicemia and *Haemophilus influenzae* pneumonia has been reported. *Pseudomonas aeruginosa* is an important respiratory pathogen in advanced disease and, more rarely, pneumonia from *Rhodococcus equi* infection can occur. The incidence of infection with *Mycobacterium tuberculosis* has markedly increased in metropolitan areas because of HIV infection as well as homelessness.

Table 31–3. Treatment of AIDS-related opportunistic infections and malignancies.[1]

Infection or Malignancy	Treatment	Complications[2]
Pneumocystis jirovecii infection[3]	Preferred regimen: Trimethoprim-sulfamethoxazole, 15 mg/kg/day (based on trimethoprim component) intravenously or one double-strength tablet orally three times a day for 21 days. Add prednisone when PaO$_2$ < 70 mm Hg on room air or alveolar-arterial O$_2$ gradient > 35 mm Hg: 40 mg orally twice a day on days 1–5, 40 mg orally daily on days 6–10, 20 mg orally daily on days 11–21	Nausea, neutropenia, anemia, hepatitis, rash, Stevens-Johnson syndrome
	Pentamidine, 3–4 mg/kg/day intravenously for 21 days plus prednisone when indicated as above	Hypotension, hypoglycemia, anemia, neutropenia, pancreatitis, hepatitis
	Primaquine, 30 mg/day orally, and clindamycin, 600 mg every 8 hours orally, for 21 days plus prednisone when indicated as above	Primaquine: hemolytic anemia in G6PD-deficient patients,[3] methemoglobinemia, neutropenia, colitis Clindamycin: rash, nausea, abdominal pain, colitis
	Not recommended for severe disease: Trimethoprim, 15 mg/kg/day orally in three divided doses, with dapsone, 100 mg/day orally, for 21 days,[3] plus prednisone when indicated as above	Nausea, rash, hemolytic anemia in G6PD[3]-deficient patients; methemoglobinemia (weekly levels should be less than 10% of total hemoglobin)
	Not recommended for severe disease: Atovaquone, 750 mg orally twice daily with food for 21 days, plus prednisone when indicated as above	Rash, elevated aminotransferases, anemia, neutropenia
Mycobacterium avium complex infection	Clarithromycin, 500 mg orally twice daily with ethambutol, 15 mg/kg/day orally (maximum, 1 g). May also add:	Clarithromycin: hepatitis, nausea, diarrhea Ethambutol: hepatitis, optic neuritis
	Rifabutin, 300 mg orally daily	Rash, hepatitis, uveitis
Toxoplasmosis	Preferred regimen: Pyrimethamine, 200 mg orally as loading dose, followed by 50 mg daily (weight ≤ 60 kg) or 75 mg daily (weight > 60 kg), combined with sulfadiazine, 1000 mg orally four times daily (weight ≤ 60 kg) or 1500 mg orally four times daily (weight > 60 kg) and leucovorin 10–25 mg orally daily for at least 6 weeks. Longer courses are necessary for extensive disease or incomplete clinical or radiographic resolution. Maintenance therapy with pyrimethamine 25–50 mg orally plus sulfadiazine 2000–4000 mg in two to four divided doses plus leucovorin 10–25 mg orally daily. Long-term treatment should be maintained until immune reconstitution with antiretroviral treatment occurs.	Pyrimethamine: leukopenia, anorexia, vomiting Sulfadiazine: nausea, vomiting, Stevens-Johnson syndrome
	For patients who are intolerant of sulfa who cannot be desensitized: Substitute clindamycin 600 mg intravenously or orally every 6 hours for the sulfadiazine in the above regimen	Pyrimethamine: leukopenia, anorexia, vomiting Clindamycin: rash, nausea, abdominal pain, colitis
	If pyrimethamine not available: Trimethoprim-sulfamethoxazole, 10 mg/kg/day (based on trimethoprim component)	Nausea, neutropenia, anemia, hepatitis, rash, Stevens-Johnson syndrome
Non-Hodgkin lymphoma	Combination chemotherapy (eg, EPOCH with rituximab and G-CSF) Central nervous system disease: Radiation treatment with dexamethasone for edema	Nausea, vomiting, anemia, neutropenia, thrombocytopenia, cardiac toxicity (with doxorubicin)
Cryptococcal meningitis	Preferred regimen: Liposomal amphotericin B, 3–4 mg/kg/day intravenously, with flucytosine, 25 mg/kg/dose orally four times daily for 2 weeks (adjust dose for kidney function), then fluconazole, 400 mg orally daily for 8 weeks, then 200 mg orally daily to complete 1 year of therapy	Liposomal amphotericin: fever, chills, hypokalemia, kidney disease Flucytosine: bone marrow suppression, kidney disease, hepatitis Fluconazole: hepatitis
	Amphotericin B, 0.7 mg/kg/day intravenously, with flucytosine, 25 mg/kg/dose orally four times daily for 2 weeks (adjust dose for kidney function), then fluconazole, 400 mg orally daily for 8 weeks, then 200 mg orally daily to complete 1 year of therapy	Amphotericin: fever, chills, hypokalemia, kidney disease Flucytosine: bone marrow suppression, kidney disease, hepatitis Fluconazole: hepatitis

(continued)

Table 31–3. Treatment of AIDS-related opportunistic infections and malignancies.[1] (continued)

Infection or Malignancy	Treatment	Complications[2]
	Fluconazole, used alone, is inferior to amphotericin B as induction therapy; it is recommended only for patients who cannot tolerate or do not respond to the preferred regimen above. If used for primary induction therapy, give fluconazole, 1200 mg orally daily for 2 weeks, then 400 mg orally daily for 8 weeks, then 200 mg orally daily to complete 1 year of therapy. Give with flucytosine, 25 mg/kg/dose orally four times daily for > 2 weeks (adjust dose for kidney function).	Hepatitis
Cytomegalovirus retinitis (immediate sight-threatening)	Preferred regimen: Intravitreal ganciclovir (2 mg/injection) or foscarnet (2.4 mg/injection) for 1–4 doses for 7–10 days plus valganciclovir, 900 mg orally twice a day with food for 14–21 days followed by 900 mg daily (maintenance)	Neutropenia, anemia, thrombocytopenia
	Ganciclovir, 10 mg/kg/day intravenously in two divided doses for 14 days, followed by 5 mg/kg daily or valganciclovir 900 mg orally daily (maintenance)	Neutropenia (especially when used concurrently with zidovudine), anemia, thrombocytopenia Adjust ganciclovir dose for kidney function
	Foscarnet, 60 mg/kg intravenously every 8 hours or 90 mg/kg intravenously every 12 hours for 14–21 days, followed by 90–120 mg/kg once daily	Nausea, hypokalemia, hypocalcemia, hyperphosphatemia, azotemia Adjust foscarnet dose for kidney function
	Cidofovir, 5 mg/kg/week intravenously for 2 weeks, then 5 mg/kg every other week with probenecid 2 g orally 3 hours before dose, 1 g orally 2 hours after dose, and 1 g orally 8 hours after dose	Nephrotoxicity (to reduce likelihood, pre- and post-saline hydration, along with probenecid), neutropenia Avoid in patients with sulfa allergy because of cross hypersensitivity with probenecid
Esophageal candidiasis or recurrent vaginal candidiasis	Fluconazole, 100–200 mg orally daily for 14–21 days for esophageal disease and > 7 days for recurrent vaginal disease	Hepatitis, development of azole resistance
Herpes simplex infection	Acyclovir, 400 mg orally three times daily for 5–10 days; or acyclovir, 5 mg/kg intravenously every 8 hours for severe cases	Resistant herpes simplex with long-term therapy
	Famciclovir, 500 mg orally twice daily for 5–10 days	Nausea
	Valacyclovir, 1 g orally twice daily for 5–10 days	Nausea
	Foscarnet, 40 mg/kg intravenously every 8 hours, for acyclovir-resistant cases	Nausea, hypokalemia, hypocalcemia, hyperphosphatemia, azotemia Adjust foscarnet dose for kidney function
Herpes zoster	Preferred regimen: Valacyclovir, 1000 mg orally three times daily for 7–10 days	Nausea
	Preferred regimen: Famciclovir, 500 mg orally three times daily for 7–10 days	Nausea
	Acyclovir, 800 mg orally five times daily for 7–10 days. Intravenous therapy at 10 mg/kg every 8 hours for extensive cutaneous or visceral disease until clinical improvement, then switch to oral therapy to complete a 10- to 14-day course. For ocular involvement, consult an ophthalmologist immediately.	Nausea
Kaposi sarcoma		
Mild to moderate	Initiation or optimization of antiretroviral treatment	Side effects of antiretroviral treatment
Advanced disease	Combination chemotherapy (eg, daunorubicin, bleomycin, vinblastine)	Bone marrow suppression, cardiac toxicity (with daunorubicin), fever

[1]Recommendations drawn from Centers for Disease Control and Prevention. Guidelines for the prevention and treatment of opportunistic infections in HIV-infected adults and adolescents. November 29, 2018. Downloaded from https://aidsinfo.nih.gov/guidelines on December 30, 2018.

[2]List of complications is not exhaustive.

[3]Prior to use of primaquine or dapsone, check glucose-6-phosphate dehydrogenase (G6PD) level in black patients and those of Mediterranean origin.

EPOCH, etoposide, prednisolone, vincristine (Oncovin), cyclophosphamide, doxorubicin (hydroxydaunomycin); G-CSF, granulocyte-colony stimulating factor (filgrastim).

Tuberculosis occurs in an estimated 4% of persons in the United States who have AIDS. Patients with active tuberculosis and CD4 counts above 350 cells/mcL are likely to present with upper lobe and hilar and paratracheal adenopathy findings similar to persons uninfected with HIV. With advanced immunodeficiency, lower lobe, middle lobe, interstitial and miliary infiltrates are more common, along with mediastinal adenopathy and extrapulmonary involvement. Although a purified protein derivative (PPD) test or an **interferon gamma release assay** (**IGRA,** including the QuantiFERON and T-SPOT tests) should be performed on all HIV-infected persons in whom a diagnosis of tuberculosis is being considered, the lower the CD4 cell count, the greater the likelihood of falsely negative PPD or IGRA test results or of indeterminate IGRA test results. Because "anergy" skin test panels do not accurately classify those patients who are infected with tuberculosis but unreactive to the PPD, they are not recommended.

B. MANAGEMENT—Treatment of HIV-infected persons with active tuberculosis is similar to treatment of HIV-uninfected tubercular individuals. However, rifampin should not be given to patients receiving a boosted protease inhibitor (PI) regimen. In these cases, rifabutin may be substituted, but it may require dosing modifications depending on the antiretroviral regimen. Multidrug-resistant tuberculosis has been a major problem in several metropolitan areas of the developed world, and reports from South Africa of "extremely resistant" tuberculosis in AIDS patients are a growing global concern. Noncompliance with prescribed antituberculous medications is a major risk factor. Several of the reported outbreaks appear to implicate nosocomial spread. The emergence of medication resistance makes it essential that antibiotic sensitivities be performed on all positive cultures. Medication therapy should be individualized. Patients with multidrug-resistant *M tuberculosis* infection should receive at least three medications to which their organism is sensitive. Atypical mycobacteria can cause pulmonary disease in AIDS patients with or without preexisting lung disease and responds variably to treatment. Making a distinction between *M tuberculosis* and atypical mycobacteria requires culture of sputum specimens. If culture of the sputum produces acid-fast bacilli, definitive identification may take several weeks using traditional techniques. DNA probes allow for presumptive identification usually within days of a positive culture. While awaiting definitive diagnosis, clinicians should err on the side of treating patients as if they have *M tuberculosis* infection. In cases in which the risk of atypical mycobacteria is very high (eg, a person without risk for tuberculosis exposure with a CD4 count under 50 cells/mcL—see Figure 31–1), clinicians may wait for definitive diagnosis if the person is smear-negative for acid-fast bacilli, clinically stable, and not living in a communal setting. Isolation of cytomegalovirus (CMV) from bronchoalveolar lavage fluid occurs commonly in AIDS patients but does not establish a definitive diagnosis. Diagnosis of CMV pneumonia requires biopsy; response to treatment is poor. Histoplasmosis, coccidioidomycosis, and cryptococcal disease as well as more common respiratory viral infections should also be considered in the differential diagnosis of unexplained pulmonary infiltrates.

Almeida A et al. Community-acquired pneumonia in HIV-positive patients: an update on etiologies, epidemiology and management. Curr Infect Dis Rep. 2017 Jan;19(1):2. [PMID: 28160220]

Centers for Disease Control and Prevention. Tuberculosis treatment of persons living with HIV. Updated August 11, 2016. https://www.cdc.gov/tb/topic/treatment/tbhiv.htm

Hu Z et al. Radiological characteristics of pulmonary cryptococcosis in HIV-infected patients. PLoS One. 2017 Mar 16; 12(3):e0173858. [PMID: 28301552]

Limper AH et al. Fungal infections in HIV/AIDS. Lancet Infect Dis. 2017 Nov;17(11):e334–43. [PMID: 28774701]

Mangalore RP et al. Treatment of disseminated histoplasmosis in advanced HIV using itraconazole with increased bioavailability. Int J STD AIDS. 2018 Aug 16;9(14):1448–50. [PMID: 30114999]

Pettit AC. Treatment of drug-susceptible tuberculosis among people living with human immunodeficiency virus infection: an update. Curr Opin HIV AIDS. 2018 Nov;13(6):469–77. [PMID: 30222609]

Scott L et al. Diagnosis of opportunistic infections: HIV co-infections—tuberculosis. Curr Opin HIV AIDS. 2017 Mar; 12(2):129–38. [PMID: 28059955]

Skolnik K et al. Cryptococcal lung infections. Clin Chest Med. 2017 Sep;38(3):451–64. [PMID: 28797488]

Tiberi S et al. The cursed duet today: tuberculosis and HIV-coinfection. Presse Med. 2017 Mar;46(2 Pt 2):e23–39. [PMID: 28256380]

3. Noninfectious pulmonary diseases—

A. PRESENTATION—Noninfectious causes of lung disease include Kaposi sarcoma, non-Hodgkin lymphoma, interstitial pneumonitis, and increasingly, in the current antiretroviral treatment era, lung cancer. In patients with known Kaposi sarcoma, pulmonary involvement complicates the course in approximately one-third of cases. However, pulmonary involvement is rarely the presenting manifestation of Kaposi sarcoma. Non-Hodgkin lymphoma may involve the lung as the sole site of disease, but more commonly involves other organs as well, especially the brain, liver, and gastrointestinal tract. Both of these processes may show nodular or diffuse parenchymal involvement, pleural effusions, and mediastinal adenopathy on chest radiographs.

Nonspecific interstitial pneumonitis may mimic *Pneumocystis* pneumonia. Lymphocytic interstitial pneumonitis seen in lung biopsies has a variable clinical course. Typically, these patients present with several months of mild cough and dyspnea; chest radiographs show interstitial infiltrates. Many patients with this entity undergo transbronchial biopsies in an attempt to diagnose *Pneumocystis* pneumonia. Instead, the tissue shows interstitial inflammation ranging from an intense lymphocytic infiltration (consistent with lymphoid interstitial pneumonitis) to a mild mononuclear inflammation.

B. MANAGEMENT—Corticosteroids may be helpful in some cases refractory to antiretroviral treatment.

Ranjit S et al. Recent advances in cancer outcomes in HIV-positive smokers. F1000Res. 2018 Jun 11;7. [PMID: 29946425]

Sigel K et al. Lung cancer in persons with HIV. Curr Opin HIV AIDS. 2017 Jan;12(1):31–8. [PMID: 27607596]

Thao C et al. Non-infectious pulmonary disorders in HIV. Expert Rev Respir Med. 2017 Mar;11(3):209–20. [PMID: 28128006]

Triplette M et al. Non-infectious pulmonary diseases and HIV. Curr HIV/AIDS Rep. 2016 Jun;13(3):140–8. [PMID: 27121734]

4. Sinusitis—

A. Presentation—Chronic sinusitis can be a frustrating problem for HIV-infected patients. Symptoms include sinus congestion and discharge, headache, and fever. Some patients may have radiographic evidence of sinus disease on sinus CT scan in the absence of significant symptoms.

B. Management—HIV-infected patients with purulent drainage should be treated for possible *H influenzae* with amoxicillin-potassium clavulanate (500 mg orally three times a day) (see Chapter 8). A 7-day course of pseudo-ephedrine 60 mg twice daily may be helpful in decreasing congestion. Prolonged treatment (3–6 weeks) with an antibiotic and guaifenesin (600 mg orally twice daily) is sometimes necessary. For patients not responding to amoxicillin-potassium clavulanate, levofloxacin may be tried (400 mg orally daily). In patients with advanced immunodeficiency, *Pseudomonas* infections should be suspected, especially if there is not a response to first-line antibiotics. Some patients may require referral to an otolaryngologist for sinus drainage and culture for possible fungal infection (*Aspergillus, Histoplasma capsulatum*).

Elansari R et al. *Histoplasma capsulatum* sinusitis: possible way of revelation to the disseminated form of histoplasmosis in HIV patients: case report and literature review. Int J Surg Case Rep. 2016;24:97–100. [PMID: 27227446]

Humphrey JM et al. Invasive *Aspergillus* sinusitis in human immunodeficiency virus infection: case report and review of the literature. Open Forum Infect Dis. 2016 Jul 26;3(3):ofw135. [PMID: 27800523]

C. Central Nervous System Disease

Central nervous system disease in HIV-infected patients can be divided into intracerebral space-occupying lesions, encephalopathy, meningitis, and spinal cord processes. Many of these complications have declined markedly in prevalence in the era of effective antiretroviral treatment. Cognitive declines, however, may be more common in HIV patients, especially as they age (older than 50 years), even those who are taking fully suppressive antiretroviral treatment.

Bowen LN et al. HIV-associated opportunistic CNS infections: pathophysiology, diagnosis and treatment. Nat Rev Neurol. 2016 Oct 27;12(11):662–74. [PMID: 27786246]

1. Toxoplasmosis—Toxoplasmosis is the most common CNS space-occupying lesion in HIV-infected patients. Headache, focal neurologic deficits, seizures, or altered mental status may be presenting symptoms. The diagnosis is usually made presumptively based on the characteristic appearance of cerebral imaging studies in an individual known to be seropositive for *Toxoplasma*. Typically, toxoplasmosis appears as multiple contrast-enhancing lesions on CT scan. Lesions tend to be peripheral, with a predilection for the basal ganglia.

Single lesions are atypical of toxoplasmosis. When a single lesion has been detected by CT scanning, MRI scanning may reveal multiple lesions because of its greater sensitivity. If a patient has a single lesion on MRI and is neurologically stable, clinicians may pursue a 2-week empiric trial of toxoplasmosis therapy. A repeat scan should be performed at 2 weeks. If the lesion has not diminished in size, biopsy of the lesion should be performed. A positive *Toxoplasma* serologic test does not confirm the diagnosis because many HIV-infected patients have detectable titers without having active disease. Conversely, less than 3% of patients with toxoplasmosis have negative titers. Therefore, negative *Toxoplasma* titers in an HIV-infected patient with a space-occupying lesion should be a cause for aggressively pursuing an alternative diagnosis. The preferred treatment of toxoplasmosis is with pyrimethamine and sulfadiazine (Table 31–3). If pyrimethamine is not available, patients can be treated with trimethoprim-sulfamethoxazole.

Basavaraju A. Toxoplasmosis in HIV infection: an overview. Trop Parasitol. 2016 Jul–Dec;6(2):129–35. [PMID: 27722101]

Mahmoudi S et al. Early detection of *Toxoplasma gondii* infection by using a interferon gamma release assay: a review. Exp Parasitol. 2017 Jan;172:39–43. [PMID: 27988201]

Martin-Iguacel R et al. Incidence, presentation and outcome of toxoplasmosis in HIV infected in the combination antiretroviral therapy era. J Infect. 2017 Sep;75(3):263–73. [PMID: 28579301]

2. Central nervous system lymphoma—Primary non-Hodgkin lymphoma is the second most common CNS space-occupying lesion in HIV-infected patients. Symptoms are similar to those with toxoplasmosis. While imaging techniques cannot distinguish these two diseases with certainty, lymphoma more often is solitary. Other less common lesions should be suspected if there is preceding bacteremia, positive tuberculin test, fungemia, or injection drug use. These include bacterial abscesses, cryptococcomas, tuberculomas, and *Nocardia* lesions.

Stereotactic brain biopsy should be strongly considered if lesions are solitary or do not respond to toxoplasmosis treatment, especially if they are easily accessible. Diagnosis of lymphoma is important because many patients benefit from treatment (radiation therapy). Although a positive polymerase chain reaction (PCR) assay of cerebrospinal fluid for Epstein–Barr virus DNA is consistent with a diagnosis of lymphoma, the sensitivity and specificity of the test are not high enough to obviate the need for a brain biopsy.

Brandsma D et al. Primary CNS lymphoma in HIV infection. Handb Clin Neurol. 2018;152:177–86. [PMID: 29604975]

Yang M et al. Diagnostic accuracy of SPECT, PET, and MRS for primary central nervous system lymphoma in HIV patients: a systematic review and meta-analysis. Medicine (Baltimore). 2017 May;96(19):e6676. [PMID: 28489744]

3. HIV-associated dementia and neurocognitive

disorders—Patients with HIV-associated dementia typically have difficulty with cognitive tasks (eg, memory, attention), exhibit diminished motor function, and have emotional or behavioral problems. Patients may first notice a deterioration in their handwriting. The manifestations of dementia may wax and wane, with persons exhibiting periods of lucidity and confusion over the course of a day. The diagnosis of HIV-associated dementia is one of exclusion based on a brain imaging study and on spinal fluid analysis that excludes other pathogens. Neuropsychiatric testing is helpful in distinguishing patients with dementia from those with depression. Many patients improve with effective antiretroviral treatment. However, slowly progressive neurocognitive deficits may still develop in patients taking antiretroviral treatment as they age.

Metabolic abnormalities may also cause changes in mental status: hypoglycemia, hyponatremia, hypoxia, and drug overdose are important considerations in this population. Other less common infectious causes of encephalopathy include progressive multifocal leukoencephalopathy (discussed below), CMV, syphilis, and herpes simplex encephalitis.

Calcagno A et al. Treating HIV infection in the central nervous system. Drugs. 2017 Feb;77(2):145–57. [PMID: 28070871]
Eggers C et al; German Association of Neuro-AIDS und Neuro-Infectiology (DGNANI). HIV-1-associated neurocognitive disorder: epidemiology, pathogenesis, diagnosis, and treatment. J Neurol. 2017 Aug;264(8):1715–27. [PMID: 28567537]
Trunfio M et al. Diagnostic accuracy of new and old cognitive screening tools for HIV-associated neurocognitive disorders. HIV Med. 2018 Aug;19(7):455–64. [PMID: 29761877]
Vera JH et al. PET brain imaging in HIV-associated neurocognitive disorders (HAND) in the era of combination antiretroviral therapy. Eur J Nucl Med Mol Imaging. 2017 May;44(5):895–902. [PMID: 28058461]

4. Cryptococcal meningitis—Cryptococcal meningitis

typically presents with fever and headache. Less than 20% of patients have meningismus. Diagnosis is based on a positive latex agglutination test of serum that detects cryptococcal antigen (or "CRAG") or positive culture of spinal fluid for *Cryptococcus*. Seventy to 90% of patients with cryptococcal meningitis have a positive serum CRAG. Thus, a negative serum CRAG test makes a diagnosis of cryptococcal meningitis unlikely and can be useful in the initial evaluation of a patient with headache, fever, and normal mental status. The preferred treatment is liposomal amphotericin with flucytosine (Table 31–3).

Eshun-Wilson I et al. Early versus delayed antiretroviral treatment in HIV-positive people with cryptococcal meningitis. Cochrane Database Syst Rev. 2018 Jul 24;7:CD009012. [PMID: 30039850]
Maziarz EK et al. Cryptococcosis. Infect Dis Clin North Am. 2016 Mar;30(1):179–206. [PMID: 26897067]
Recio R et al. Cryptococcus neoformans meningoencephalitis. N Engl J Med. 2018 Jul 19;379(3):281. [PMID: 30021095]
Tenforde MW et al. Treatment for HIV-associated cryptococcal meningitis. Cochrane Database Syst Rev. 2018 Jul 25;7: CD005647. [PMID: 30045416]

Williamson PR et al. Cryptococcal meningitis: epidemiology, immunology, diagnosis and therapy. Nat Rev Neurol. 2017 Jan; 13(1):13–24. [PMID: 27886201]

5. Meningococcal meningitis—HIV-infected persons are at

increased risk for meningococcal disease. Treatment is the same as in uninfected persons. Therefore, the Advisory Committee on Immunization Practices recommends the meningococcal conjugate vaccine (serogroups A, C, W, and Y) for all HIV-infected persons aged 2 months or older.

Harris CM et al. Meningococcal disease in patients with human immunodeficiency virus infection: a review of cases reported through active surveillance in the United States, 2000–2008. Open Forum Infect Dis. 2016 Dec 20;3(4):ofw226. [PMID: 28018927]
MacNeil JR et al. Recommendations for use of meningococcal conjugate vaccines in HIV-infected persons—Advisory Committee on Immunization Practices, 2016. MMWR Morb Mortal Wkly Rep. 2016 Nov 4;65(43):1189–94. [PMID: 27811836]

6. HIV meningitis and HIV myelopathy—HIV meningitis,

characterized by lymphocytic pleocytosis of the spinal fluid with negative culture, is common early in HIV infection. Spinal cord function may also be impaired in HIV-infected individuals. HIV myelopathy presents with leg weakness and incontinence. Spastic paraparesis and sensory ataxia are seen on neurologic examination. Myelopathy is usually a late manifestation of HIV disease, and most patients will have concomitant HIV encephalopathy. Pathologic evaluation of the spinal cord reveals vacuolation of white matter. Because HIV myelopathy is a diagnosis of exclusion, symptoms suggestive of myelopathy should be evaluated by lumbar puncture to rule out CMV polyradiculopathy (described below) and an MRI or CT scan to exclude epidural lymphoma.

Levin SN et al. HIV and spinal cord disease. Handb Clin Neurol. 2018;152:213–27. [PMID: 29604979]

7. Progressive multifocal leukoencephalopathy (PML)—

PML is a viral infection of the white matter of the brain seen in patients with very advanced HIV infection. It typically results in focal neurologic deficits such as aphasia, hemiparesis, and cortical blindness. Imaging studies are strongly suggestive of the diagnosis if they show nonenhancing white matter lesions without mass effect. Extensive lesions may be difficult to differentiate from the changes caused by HIV. Several patients have stabilized or improved after the institution of effective antiretroviral treatment, and due to wide use of antiretroviral treatment, PML is now rarely seen.

Grebenciucova E et al. Progressive multifocal leukoencephalopathy. Neurol Clin. 2018 Nov;36(4):739–50. [PMID: 30366552]
Harel A et al. Successful treatment of progressive multifocal leukoencephalopathy with recombinant interleukin-7 and maraviroc in a patient with idiopathic CD4 lymphocytopenia. J Neurovirol. 2018 Oct;24(5):652–5. [PMID: 29987583]

D. Peripheral Nervous System

A. Presentation—Peripheral nervous system syndromes include inflammatory polyneuropathies, sensory neuropathies, and mononeuropathies.

An **inflammatory demyelinating polyneuropathy** similar to Guillain-Barré syndrome occurs in HIV-infected patients, usually prior to frank immunodeficiency. The syndrome in many cases improves with plasmapheresis, supporting an autoimmune basis of the disease. CMV can cause an ascending polyradiculopathy characterized by lower extremity weakness and a neutrophilic pleocytosis on spinal fluid analysis with a negative bacterial culture. Transverse myelitis can be seen with herpes zoster or CMV.

Peripheral neuropathy is common among HIV-infected persons. Patients typically complain of numbness, tingling, and pain in the lower extremities. Symptoms are disproportionate to findings on gross sensory and motor evaluation. Beyond HIV infection itself, the most common cause is prior antiretroviral treatment with stavudine or didanosine. Although not used commonly in Western countries, stavudine is still being used in resource-limited settings through national antiretroviral treatment programs. Caution should be used when administering these agents to patients with a history of peripheral neuropathy. Unfortunately, medication-induced neuropathy is not always reversed when the offending agent is discontinued. Patients with advanced disease may also develop peripheral neuropathy even if they have never taken antiretroviral treatment. Evaluation should rule out other causes of sensory neuropathy such as alcoholism, thyroid disease, vitamin B_{12} deficiency, and syphilis.

B. Management—Treatment of peripheral neuropathy is aimed at symptomatic relief. Patients should be initially treated with gabapentin (start at 300 mg at bedtime and increase to 300–900 mg orally three times a day) or other co-analgesics for neuropathic pain (see Chapter 5). Opioid analgesics should be avoided because the condition tends to be chronic and patients are likely to become dependent on these agents without significant improvement in their well-being.

Mochan A et al. CIDP [chronic inflammatory demyelinating polyradiculoneuropathy] in a HIV endemic population: a prospective case series from Johannesburg, South Africa. J Neurol Sci. 2016 Apr 15;363:39–42. [PMID: 27000218]

E. Rheumatologic and Bone Manifestations

Arthritis, involving single or multiple joints, with or without effusion, has been commonly noted in HIV-infected patients. Involvement of large joints is most common. Although the cause of HIV-related arthritis is unknown, most patients will respond to nonsteroidal anti-inflammatory medications. Patients with a sizable effusion, especially if the joint is warm or erythematous, should have the joint aspirated, followed by culture of the fluid to rule out suppurative arthritis as well as fungal and mycobacterial disease.

Several rheumatologic syndromes, including reactive arthritis, psoriatic arthritis, sicca syndrome, and systemic lupus erythematosus, have been reported in HIV-infected patients (see Chapter 20). However, it is unclear if the prevalence is greater than in the general population. Cases of avascular necrosis of the femoral heads have been reported sporadically, generally in the setting of advanced disease with long-standing infection and in patients receiving long-term antiretroviral treatment. The etiology is not clear but is probably multifactorial in nature.

Osteoporosis and osteopenia appear to be more common in HIV-infected patients with chronic infection and perhaps associated with long-term use of antiretroviral treatment. Vitamin D deficiency appears to be quite common among HIV-infected populations and monitoring vitamin D levels and replacement therapy for detected deficiency are recommended. Bone mineral density scans for postmenopausal women and for men over the age of 50 is also recommended.

Moran CA et al. Bone loss in HIV infection. Curr Treat Options Infect Dis. 2017 Mar;9(1):52–67. [PMID: 28413362]
Parperis K et al. Rheumatic diseases in HIV-infected patients in the post-antiretroviral therapy era: a tertiary care center experience. Clin Rheumatol. 2019 Jan;38(1):71–6. [PMID: 29619587]
Walker-Bone K et al. Assessment and management of musculoskeletal disorders among patients living with HIV. Rheumatology (Oxford). 2017 Oct 1;56(10):1648–61. [PMID: 28013196]

F. Myopathy

Myopathies are infrequent in the era of effective antiretroviral treatment but can be related to either HIV infection or antiretroviral treatment, particularly with use of zidovudine (azidothymidine [AZT]). Proximal muscle weakness is typical, and patients may have varying degrees of muscle tenderness. Given its long-term toxicities, zidovudine is no longer recommended when alternative treatments are available.

G. Retinitis

In HIV-infected patients, complaints of visual changes must be evaluated immediately by an ophthalmologist familiar with the manifestations of HIV disease. **CMV retinitis,** characterized by perivascular hemorrhages and white fluffy exudates, is the most common retinal infection in AIDS patients and can be rapidly progressive. In contrast, cotton wool spots, which are also common in HIV-infected patients, are benign, remit spontaneously, and appear as small indistinct white spots without exudation or hemorrhage. Other rare retinal processes include other herpesvirus infections or toxoplasmosis. Choice of treatment for CMV retinitis (Table 31–3) depends on severity and location of lesions, and the patient's overall condition and circumstances.

Heiden D et al. Active cytomegalovirus retinitis after the start of antiretroviral therapy. Br J Ophthalmol. 2019 Feb;103(2):157–60. [PMID: 30196272]
Port AD et al. Cytomegalovirus retinitis: a review. J Ocul Pharmacol Ther. 2017 May;33(4):224–34. [PMID: 28355091]

H. Oral Lesions

A. PRESENTATION—The presence of oral candidiasis or hairy leukoplakia is significant for several reasons. First, these lesions are highly suggestive of HIV infection in patients who have no other obvious cause of immunodeficiency. Second, several studies have indicated that patients with candidiasis have a high rate of progression to AIDS even with statistical adjustment for CD4 count.

Hairy leukoplakia is caused by the Epstein-Barr virus. The lesion is not usually troubling to patients and sometimes regresses spontaneously. Hairy leukoplakia is commonly seen as a white lesion on the lateral aspect of the tongue. It may be flat or slightly raised, is usually corrugated, and has vertical parallel lines with fine or thick ("hairy") projections (Figure 8–6). **Oral candidiasis** can be bothersome to patients, many of whom report an unpleasant taste or mouth dryness. The two most common forms of oral candidiasis seen are pseudomembranous (removable white plaques) (Figure 31–2A) and erythematous (red friable plaques) (Figure 31–2B).

B. MANAGEMENT—Treatment of oral candidiasis is with topical agents such as clotrimazole 10-mg troches (one troche four or five times a day). Patients with candidiasis who do not respond to topical antifungals can be treated with fluconazole (50–100 mg orally once a day for 3–7 days). **Angular cheilitis**—fissures at the sides of the mouth—is usually due to *Candida* as well (Figure 31–2B) and can be treated topically with ketoconazole cream (2%) twice a day.

Gingival disease is common in HIV-infected patients and is thought to be due to an overgrowth of microorganisms. It usually responds to professional dental cleaning and chlorhexidine rinses. A particularly aggressive gingivitis or periodontitis will develop in some HIV-infected patients; these patients should be given antibiotics that cover anaerobic oral flora (eg, metronidazole, 250 mg four times a day for 4 or 5 days) and referred to oral surgeons with experience with these entities.

Aphthous ulcers (Figure 31–3) are painful and may interfere with eating. They can be treated with fluocinonide (0.05% ointment mixed 1:1 with plain Orabase and applied six times a day to the ulcer). For lesions that are difficult to reach, patients should use dexamethasone swishes (0.5 mg in 5 mL elixir three times a day). The pain of the ulcers can be relieved with use of an anesthetic spray (10% lidocaine). Other lesions seen in the mouths of HIV-infected patients include **Kaposi sarcoma** (usually on the hard palate) and **warts**.

Batavia AS et al. Diagnosis of HIV-associated oral lesions in relation to early versus delayed antiretroviral therapy: results from the CIPRA HT001 Trial. PLoS One. 2016 Mar 1;11(3): e0150656. [PMID: 26930571]

de Almeida VL et al. Impact of highly active antiretroviral therapy on the prevalence of oral lesions in HIV-positive patients: a systematic review and meta-analysis. Int J Oral Maxillofac Surg. 2017 Nov;46(11):1497–504. [PMID: 28684301]

Greenspan JS et al. Hairy leukoplakia; lessons learned: 30-plus years. Oral Dis. 2016 Apr;22(Suppl 1):120–7. [PMID: 27109280]

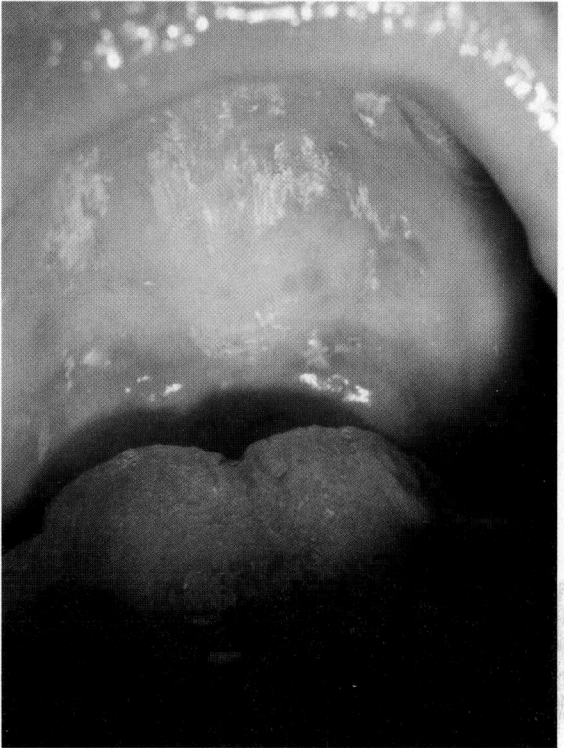
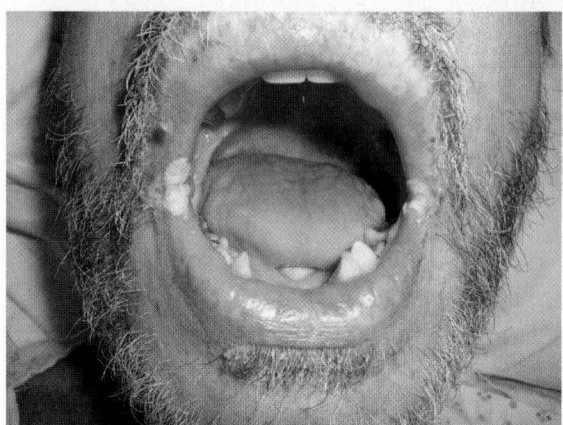

▲ **Figure 31–2.** Oral candidiasis. **A:** The pseudomembranous form of oral candidiasis is the most common; the white plaques over the hard palate raise the suspicion of underlying HIV/AIDS. They can be scraped off with a tongue blade, placed on a slide, and mixed with potassium hydroxide solution to make the diagnosis of *Candida albicans*. **B:** This man with HIV-AIDS has the (less common) erythematous form of oral candidiasis. The patient also has perlèche or angular cheilitis (*Candida* infection at the corners of the mouth). (Used, with permission, from Richard P. Usatine, MD, in Usatine RP, Smith MA, Mayeaux EJ Jr, Chumley H. *The Color Atlas of Family Medicine,* 2nd ed. McGraw-Hill, 2013.)

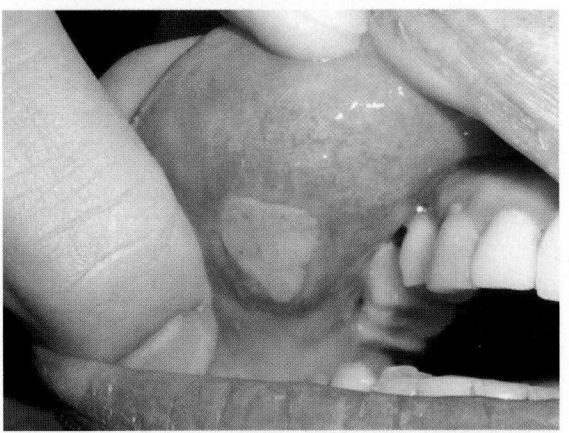

▲ **Figure 31–3.** Recurrent oral aphthous stomatitis. A 58-year-old man presented with a 1-year history of recurrent painful sores in his mouth. He had lost 20 pounds over the year because it hurt so much to eat. The ulcers, which had a red base and were covered with a central white membrane, occurred in different locations—on his tongue, gums, inner lips, and buccal mucosa (shown here). HIV-AIDS is an underlying systemic disease that can be documented on work-up of such patients. (Used, with permission, from Richard P. Usatine, MD, in Usatine RP, Smith MA, Mayeaux EJ Jr, Chumley H. *The Color Atlas of Family Medicine,* 2nd ed. McGraw-Hill, 2013.)

Millsop JW et al. Oral candidiasis. Clin Dermatol. 2016 Jul–Aug; 34(4):487–94. [PMID: 27343964]

Nittayananta W. Oral fungi in HIV: challenges in antifungal therapies. Oral Dis. 2016 Apr;22(Suppl 1):107–13. [PMID: 27109279]

I. Gastrointestinal Manifestations

1. Candidal esophagitis—(See also Chapter 15.) Esophageal candidiasis is a common AIDS complication. In a patient with characteristic symptoms, empiric antifungal treatment is begun with fluconazole (100–200 mg orally daily for 14–21 days). Improvement in symptoms should be apparent within 1–2 days of antifungal treatment. If there is no improvement, further evaluation to identify other causes of esophagitis (herpes simplex, CMV) is recommended.

O'Rourke A. Infective oesophagitis: epidemiology, cause, diagnosis and treatment options. Curr Opin Otolaryngol Head Neck Surg. 2015 Dec;23(6):459–63. [PMID: 26371605]

2. Hepatic disease—

A. Presentation—Autopsy studies have demonstrated that the liver is a frequent site of infections and neoplasms in HIV-infected patients. However, many of these infections are not clinically symptomatic. Mild elevations of alkaline phosphatase and aminotransferases are often noted on routine chemistry panels. **Mycobacterial disease, CMV,**
hepatitis B virus, hepatitis C virus, and **lymphoma** cause liver disease and can present with varying degrees of nausea, vomiting, right upper quadrant abdominal pain, and jaundice. Sulfonamides, imidazole medications, antituberculous medications, pentamidine, clarithromycin, and didanosine have also been associated with hepatitis. All nucleoside reverse transcriptase inhibitors cause lactic acidosis, which can be fatal. Lactic acidosis, however, occurs most commonly when didanosine is used with stavudine; this combination is no longer recommended in antiretroviral treatment regimens. HIV-infected patients with chronic hepatitis may have more rapid progression of liver disease because of the concomitant immunodeficiency or hepatotoxicity of antiretroviral treatment. Percutaneous liver biopsy may be helpful in diagnosing liver disease, but some common causes of liver disease (eg, *M avium* complex, lymphoma) can be determined by less invasive measures (eg, blood culture, biopsy of a more accessible site).

B. Management—With patients living longer as a result of advances in antiretroviral treatment, advanced liver disease and hepatic failure due to chronic active hepatitis B and/or C are increasing causes of morbidity and mortality. HIV-infected individuals who are coinfected with hepatitis B should be treated with antiretroviral regimens that include medications with activity against both viruses (tenofovir disoproxil fumarate [TDF] or tenofovir alafenamide [TAF], lamivudine, or emtricitabine). Entecavir may be used if HIV viral load is suppressed; otherwise, its use can lead to lamivudine/emtricitabine-resistant HIV. It is important to be extremely cautious about discontinuing these medications in coinfected patients as sudden discontinuation could lead to a fatal flare of hepatitis B infection.

Hepatitis C is more virulent in persons with HIV and should be treated using the new HCV direct-acting antivirals (Table 16–6). Prior to treatment, the patient's HCV viral load and HCV genotype should be determined. Depending on the genotype and the proposed treatment regimen, HCV resistance testing is recommended. For example, HCV resistance testing is recommended for patients with genotype 1a (the most common hepatitis C genotype in the United States) who are being considered for treatment with elbasvir/grazoprevir because substitutions in certain amino acid positions confer resistance. Because the appropriate treatment regimen depends on genotype, resistance profile, whether the patient is treatment naïve or not, as well as whether or not the patient has cirrhosis (and, if so, whether it is compensated or decompensated), clinicians should check the guidelines of the AASLD/IDSA (see website in references below) to see the recommended regimens (see also Tables 16–6 and 16–7). Costs of the different regimens vary by purchaser, and many clinicians choose the least expensive of the recommended regimens.

Although the recommended regimens are the same for HIV-infected patients, potential drug interactions with antiretroviral treatment may complicate treatment. Clinicians should check the guidelines of the AASLD/IDSA and US Department of Health and Human Services or the guidelines of the University of Liverpool (see references below) to determine interactions between proposed hepatitis C regimen and HIV regimen.

Liver transplants have been performed successfully in HIV-infected patients. This strategy is most likely to be successful in persons who have CD4 counts greater than 100 cells/mcL and nondetectable viral loads.

American Association for the Study of Liver Diseases and Infectious Diseases Society of America. HCV guidance (AASLD/IDSA): Recommendations for testing, managing, and treating hepatitis C. 2017 Sep 21. https://www.hcvguidelines.org

Singh KP et al. HIV-hepatitis B virus co-infection: epidemiology, pathogenesis, and treatment. AIDS. 2017 Sep 24;31(15):2035–52. [PMID: 28692539]

University of Liverpool. HEP drug interactions. https://www.hep-druginteractions.org

US Department of Health and Human Services. Guidelines for the prevention and treatment of opportunistic infections in HIV-infected adults and adolescents, March 28, 2019. https://aidsinfo.nih.gov/guidelines/html/4/adult-and-adolescent-opportunistic-infection/0

3. Biliary disease—**Cholecystitis** presents with manifestations similar to those seen in immunocompetent hosts, but is more likely to be acalculous. **Sclerosing cholangitis** and **papillary stenosis** have also been reported in HIV-infected patients. Typically, the syndrome presents with severe nausea, vomiting, and right upper quadrant pain. Liver enzymes generally show alkaline phosphatase elevations disproportionate to elevation of the aminotransferases. Although dilated ducts can be seen on ultrasound, the diagnosis is made by endoscopic retrograde cholangiopancreatography, which reveals intraluminal irregularities of the proximal intrahepatic ducts with "pruning" of the terminal ductal branches. Stenosis of the distal common bile duct at the papilla is commonly seen. CMV, *Cryptosporidium*, and microsporidia are thought to play inciting roles in this syndrome, but these conditions are rarely seen unless the patient is suffering with very advanced HIV-related immunodeficiency.

4. Enterocolitis—

A. Presentation—**Enterocolitis** is a common problem in HIV-infected individuals. Organisms known to cause enterocolitis include bacteria (*Campylobacter*, *Salmonella*, *Shigella*), viruses (CMV, adenovirus), and protozoans (*Cryptosporidium*, *Entamoeba histolytica*, *Giardia*, *Isospora*, microsporidia). HIV itself may cause enterocolitis. Several of the organisms causing enterocolitis in HIV-infected individuals also cause diarrhea in immunocompetent persons. However, HIV-infected patients tend to have more severe and more chronic symptoms, including high fevers and severe abdominal pain that can mimic acute abdominal catastrophes. Bacteremia and concomitant biliary involvement are also more common with enterocolitis in HIV-infected patients. Relapses of enterocolitis following adequate therapy have been reported with both *Salmonella* and *Shigella* infections.

Because of the wide range of agents known to cause enterocolitis, a stool culture and multiple stool examinations for ova and parasites (including modified acid-fast staining for *Cryptosporidium*) should be performed. Those patients who have *Cryptosporidium* in one stool with improvement in symptoms in less than 1 month should not be considered to have AIDS, as *Cryptosporidium* is a cause of self-limited diarrhea in HIV-negative persons. More commonly, HIV-infected patients with *Cryptosporidium* infection have persistent enterocolitis with profuse watery diarrhea.

B. Management—To date, no consistently effective treatments have been developed for *Cryptosporidium* infection. The most effective treatment of cryptosporidiosis is to improve immune function through the use of effective antiretroviral treatment. The diarrhea can be treated symptomatically with diphenoxylate with atropine (one or two tablets orally three or four times a day). Those who do not respond may be given paregoric with bismuth (5–10 mL orally three or four times a day). Octreotide in escalating doses (starting at 0.05 mg subcutaneously every 8 hours for 48 hours) has been found to ameliorate symptoms in approximately 40% of patients with cryptosporidia or idiopathic HIV-associated diarrhea, although the benefit is often short-lived.

Patients with a negative stool examination and persistent symptoms should be evaluated with colonoscopy and biopsy. Patients whose symptoms last longer than 1 month with no identified cause of diarrhea are considered to have a presumptive diagnosis of **AIDS enteropathy.** Patients may respond to institution of effective antiretroviral treatment. Upper endoscopy with small bowel biopsy is not recommended as a routine part of the evaluation.

Wang RJ et al. Widespread occurrence of *Cryptosporidium* infections in patients with HIV/AIDS: epidemiology, clinical feature, diagnosis, and therapy. Acta Trop. 2018 Nov;187:257–63. [PMID: 30118699]

5. Other disorders—Two other important gastrointestinal abnormalities in HIV-infected patients are **gastropathy** and malabsorption. It has been documented that some HIV-infected patients do not produce normal levels of stomach acid and therefore are unable to absorb medications that require an acid medium. This decreased acid production may explain, in part, the susceptibility of HIV-infected patients to *Campylobacter*, *Salmonella*, and *Shigella*, all of which are sensitive to acid concentration. There is no evidence that *Helicobacter pylori* is more common in HIV-infected persons.

A **malabsorption** syndrome occurs commonly in AIDS patients. It can be due to infection of the small bowel with *M avium* complex, *Cryptosporidium*, or microsporidia.

Logan C et al. HIV and diarrhoea: what is new? Curr Opin Infect Dis. 2016 Oct;29(5):486–94. [PMID: 27472290]

J. Endocrinologic Manifestations

Hypogonadism is probably the most common endocrinologic abnormality in HIV-infected men. The adrenal gland is also a commonly afflicted endocrine gland in patients with AIDS. Abnormalities demonstrated on autopsy include infection (especially with CMV and *M avium* complex), infiltration with Kaposi sarcoma, and injury from hemorrhage and presumed autoimmunity. The prevalence of clinically significant adrenal insufficiency is low. Patients with suggestive symptoms should undergo a cosyntropin stimulation test.

Although frank deficiency of cortisol is rare, an isolated defect in mineralocorticoid metabolism may lead to salt-wasting and hyperkalemia. Such patients should be treated with fludrocortisone (0.1–0.2 mg orally daily).

AIDS patients appear to have abnormalities of thyroid function tests different from those of patients with other chronic diseases. AIDS patients have been shown to have high levels of triiodothyronine (T_3), thyroxine (T_4), and thyroid-binding globulin and low levels of reverse triiodothyronine (rT_3). The causes and clinical significance of these abnormalities are unknown.

Gomes AR et al. Prevalence of testosterone deficiency in HIV-infected men under antiretroviral therapy. BMC Infect Dis. 2016 Nov 3;16(1):628. [PMID: 27809804]

Jasuja GK et al. Use of testosterone in men infected with human immunodeficiency virus in the Veterans Healthcare System. AIDS Care. 2018 Oct;30(10):1207–14. [PMID: 29557189]

Lachâtre M et al. HIV and hypogonadism: a new challenge for young-aged and middle-aged men on effective antiretroviral therapy. AIDS. 2017 Jan 28;31(3):451–3. [PMID: 28081039]

Mirza FS et al. Endocrinological aspects of HIV infection. J Endocrinol Invest. 2018 Aug;41(8):881–99. [PMID: 29313284]

Wong N et al. Hypogonadism in the HIV-infected man. Curr Treat Options Infect Dis. 2017;9(1):104–16. [PMID: 28344518]

K. Skin Manifestations

The skin manifestations that commonly develop in HIV-infected patients can be grouped into viral, bacterial, fungal, neoplastic, and nonspecific dermatitides.

1. Viral dermatitides—

A. HERPES SIMPLEX INFECTIONS—These infections occur more frequently, tend to be more severe, and are more likely to disseminate in AIDS patients than in immunocompetent persons. Because of the risk of progressive local disease, all herpes simplex attacks should be treated for 5–10 days with acyclovir (400 mg orally three times a day), famciclovir (500 mg orally twice daily), or valacyclovir (500 mg orally twice daily) (Table 31–3). To avoid the complications of attacks, many clinicians recommend suppressive therapy for HIV-infected patients with a history of recurrent herpes. Options for suppressive therapy include acyclovir (400 mg orally twice daily), famciclovir (250 mg orally twice daily), and valacyclovir (500 mg orally daily). Long-term suppressive herpes prophylaxis with acyclovir does not reduce HIV transmission between heterosexual men and women from developing countries.

Andrei G et al. The anti-HIV drug tenofovir, a reverse transcriptase inhibitor, also targets the herpes simplex virus (HSV) DNA polymerase. J Infect Dis. 2018 Feb 14;217(5):790–801. [PMID: 29186456]

B. HERPES ZOSTER—This is a common manifestation of HIV infection (Figure 31–4). Patients with herpes zoster infections should be treated for 7–10 days with famciclovir

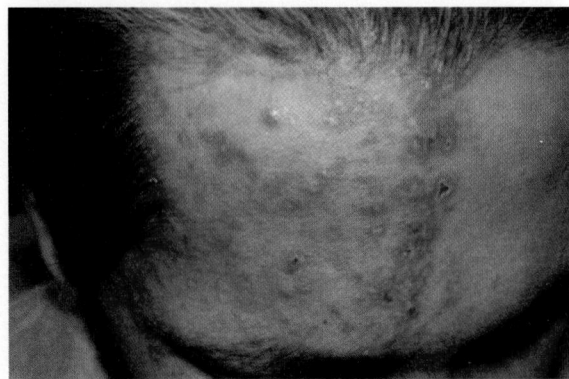

▲ **Figure 31–4.** Herpes zoster. A painful vesicular eruption developed over the right forehead in this 44-year-old HIV-positive man. Herpes zoster was diagnosed clinically and confirmed by a positive direct fluorescent antibody test on fluid from one of the vesicles. (Used, with permission, from Usatine RP, Smith MA, Mayeaux EJ Jr, Chumley H. *The Color Atlas of Family Medicine,* 2nd ed. McGraw-Hill, 2013.)

(500 mg orally three times a day) or valacyclovir (500 mg three times a day). Acyclovir can also be used, but it requires very frequent dosing (800 mg orally four or five times per day for 7 days). Vesicular lesions should be cultured if there is any question about their origin, since herpes simplex responds to much lower doses of acyclovir. Disseminated zoster and cases with ocular involvement should be treated with intravenous (10 mg/kg every 8 hours for 7–10 days) rather than oral acyclovir. The recombinant zoster vaccine (Shingrix, two doses administered 2–6 months apart) can be given to HIV-infected patients. Because it is not a live virus like the previous zoster vaccine (Zostavax), it is not contraindicated in patients with immune deficiency but, based on other vaccines, HIV-infected patients are likely to develop more robust immune response to the vaccine when their CD4 count is greater than 200/mcL. The long-term benefit of Shingrix in preventing shingles in HIV-infected persons has yet to be established.

Dooling KL et al. Recommendations of the Advisory Committee on Immunization Practices for use of herpes zoster vaccines. MMWR Morb Mortal Wkly Rep. 2018 Jan 26;67(3):103–8. [PMID: 29370152]

C. MOLLUSCUM CONTAGIOSUM—This infection is caused by a pox virus and is seen in HIV-infected patients, as in other immunocompromised patients. The characteristic umbilicated fleshy papular lesions have a propensity for spreading widely over the patient's face and neck and should be treated with topical liquid nitrogen.

Martin P. Interventions for molluscum contagiosum in people infected with human immunodeficiency virus: a systematic review. Int J Dermatol. 2016 Sep;55(9):956–66. [PMID: 26991246]

van der Wouden JC et al. Interventions for cutaneous molluscum contagiosum. Cochrane Database Syst Rev. 2017 May 17;5: CD004767. [PMID: 28513067]

2. Bacterial dermatitides—

A. **STAPHYLOCOCCAL INFECTION**—*Staphylococcus* is the most common bacterial cause of skin disease in HIV-infected patients; it usually presents as **folliculitis, superficial abscesses (furuncles), or bullous impetigo.** These lesions should be treated aggressively since sepsis can occur. Folliculitis is initially treated with topical clindamycin or mupirocin, and patients may benefit from regular washing with an antibacterial soap such as chlorhexidine. Intranasal mupirocin has been used successfully for staphylococcal decolonization in other settings. In HIV-infected patients with recurrent staphylococcal infections, weekly intranasal mupirocin should be considered in addition to topical care and systemic antibiotics. Abscesses often require incision and drainage. Patients may need anti-staphylococcal antibiotics as well. Due to high frequency of methicillin-resistant *Staphylococcus aureus* (MRSA) skin infections in HIV-infected populations, lesions should be cultured prior to initiating empiric antistaphylococcal therapy. Recommendations for empiric treatment are either (1) trimethoprim-sulfamethoxazole (one double-strength tablet orally twice daily) with or without clindamycin (500 mg orally three times daily); or (2) doxycycline (100 mg orally twice daily) with close follow-up.

Hemmige V et al. Predictors of skin and soft tissue infections in HIV-infected outpatients in the community-associated methicillin resistant *Staphylococcus aureus* era. Eur J Clin Microbiol Infect Dis. 2015 Feb;34(2):339–47. [PMID: 25213720]

Sabbagh P et al. The global and regional prevalence, burden, and risk factors for methicillin-resistant *Staphylococcus aureus* colonization in HIV-infected people: a systematic review and meta-analysis. Am J Infect Control. 2019 Mar;47(3):323–33. [PMID: 30170767]

B. **BACILLARY ANGIOMATOSIS**—It is caused by two closely related organisms: *Bartonella henselae* and *Bartonella quintana*. The epidemiology of these infections suggests zoonotic transmission from fleas of infected domestic cats. The most common manifestation is raised, reddish, highly vascular skin lesions (Figure 31–5) that can mimic the lesions of Kaposi sarcoma. Fever is a common manifestation of this infection; involvement of bone, lymph nodes, and liver has also been reported. The infection responds to doxycycline, 100 mg orally twice daily, or erythromycin, 250 mg orally four times daily. Therapy is continued for at least 14 days, and patients who are seriously ill with visceral involvement may require months of therapy.

Mantis J et al. Cat-scratch disease in an AIDS patient presenting with generalized lymphadenopathy: an unusual presentation with delayed diagnosis. Am J Case Rep. 2018 Aug 2;19:906–11. [PMID: 30068900]

Markowicz M et al. Bacillary angiomatosis presenting with facial tumor and multiple abscesses: a case report. Medicine (Baltimore). 2016 Jul;95(28):e4155. [PMID: 27428207]

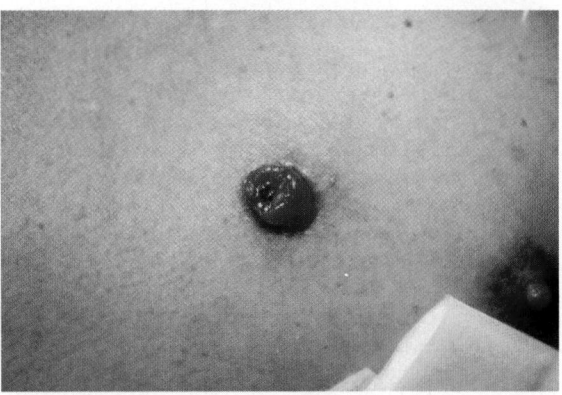

▲ **Figure 31–5.** Bacillary angiomatosis. Bacillary angiomatosis is a systemic infection caused by *Bartonella* species. Its cutaneous lesions appear as scattered papules and nodules (like the one shown here) or as abscesses. In HIV-infected patients, bacillary angiomatosis most often occurs when the CD4 count is below 200/mcL. It can be treated with antibiotics. (Reproduced, with permission, from Usatine RP, Moy RL, Tobinick EL, Siegel DM. *Skin Surgery: A Practical Guide.* Mosby, 1998. Copyright © Elsevier.)

3. Fungal rashes—

A. **RASHES DUE TO DERMATOPHYTES AND *CANDIDA***—Most **fungal rashes** afflicting AIDS patients are due to dermatophytes and *Candida*. While particularly common in the inguinal region, they may occur anywhere on the body. Fungal rashes generally respond well to topical clotrimazole (1% cream twice a day) or ketoconazole (2% cream twice a day).

B. **SEBORRHEIC DERMATITIS**—This is more common in HIV-infected patients. Scrapings of seborrhea have revealed *Malassezia furfur* (*Pityrosporum ovale*), implying that the seborrhea is caused by this fungus. Consistent with the isolation of this fungus is the clinical finding that seborrhea responds well to topical clotrimazole (1% cream) as well as hydrocortisone (1% cream).

Forrestel AK et al. Diffuse HIV-associated seborrheic dermatitis—a case series. Int J STD AIDS. 2016 Dec; 27(14):1342–5. [PMID: 27013615]

4. Neoplastic dermatitides—See Chapter 6 and the Kaposi sarcoma section below.

5. Nonspecific dermatitides—

A. **XEROSIS**—This condition presents in HIV-infected patients with severe pruritus. The patient may have no rash, or nonspecific excoriations from scratching. Treatment is with emollients (eg, absorption base cream) and antipruritic lotions (eg, camphor 9.5% and menthol 0.5%).

B. **PSORIASIS**—Psoriasis can be very severe in HIV-infected patients. Phototherapy and etretinate (0.25–9.75 mg/kg/day orally in divided doses) may be used for recalcitrant cases in consultation with a dermatologist.

L. HIV-Related Malignancies

Four cancers are currently included in the CDC classification of AIDS: Kaposi sarcoma, non-Hodgkin lymphoma, primary lymphoma of the brain, and invasive cervical carcinoma. Epidemiologic studies have shown that between 1973 and 1987, among single men in San Francisco, the risk of Kaposi sarcoma increased more than 5000-fold and the risk of non-Hodgkin lymphoma more than 10-fold. The increase in incidence of malignancies is probably a function of impaired cell-mediated immunity. In the current treatment era, cancers not classified as AIDS-related, such as lung cancer, are being increasingly diagnosed in aging HIV-infected individuals despite optimal antiretroviral treatment treatment. Cohort studies suggest that HIV-infected adults are at increased risk for a variety of cancers compared to age-matched uninfected populations. Mortality secondary to malignancies represents an increasing cause of death in HIV-infected populations.

Bender Ignacio R et al. Evolving paradigms in HIV malignancies: review of ongoing clinical trials. J Natl Compr Canc Netw. 2018 Aug;16(8):1018–26. [PMID: 30099376]

Hessol NA et al. Incidence of first and second primary cancers diagnosed among people with HIV, 1985–2013: a population-based, registry linkage study. Lancet HIV. 2018 Nov;5(11): e647–55. [PMID: 30245004]

Kelly H et al; ART and HPV Review Group. Association of antiretroviral therapy with high-risk human papillomavirus, cervical intraepithelial neoplasia, and invasive cervical cancer in women living with HIV: a systematic review and meta-analysis. Lancet HIV. 2018 Jan;5(1):e45–58. [PMID: 29107561]

Shiels MS et al. Projected cancer incidence rates and burden of incident cancer cases in HIV-infected adults in the United States through 2030. Ann Intern Med. 2018 Jun 19;168(12):866–73. [PMID: 29801099]

Valanikas E et al. Cancer prevention in patients with human immunodeficiency virus infection. World J Clin Oncol. 2018 Sep 14;9(5):71–3. [PMID: 30254961]

1. Kaposi sarcoma—

A. Presentation—Lesions may appear anywhere; careful examination of the eyelids, conjunctiva, pinnae, palate, and toe webs is mandatory to locate potentially occult lesions. In light-skinned individuals, Kaposi lesions usually appear as purplish, nonblanching lesions that can be papular or nodular (Figure 31–6). In dark-skinned individuals, the lesions may appear browner. In the mouth, lesions are most often palatal papules, though exophytic lesions of the tongue and gingivae may also be seen. Kaposi lesions may be confused with other vascular lesions such as angiomas and pyogenic granulomas. Kaposi sarcoma lesions can occur shortly after initiating antiretroviral treatment, especially in patients starting antiretroviral treatment who have advanced immunodeficiency. In this situation, Kaposi sarcoma is likely to be an immune reconstitution reaction (see Inflammatory Reactions below). Kaposi sarcoma can also cause visceral disease (eg, gastrointestinal, pulmonary).

B. Management—Patients with mild to moderate forms of Kaposi sarcoma do not require specific treatment as

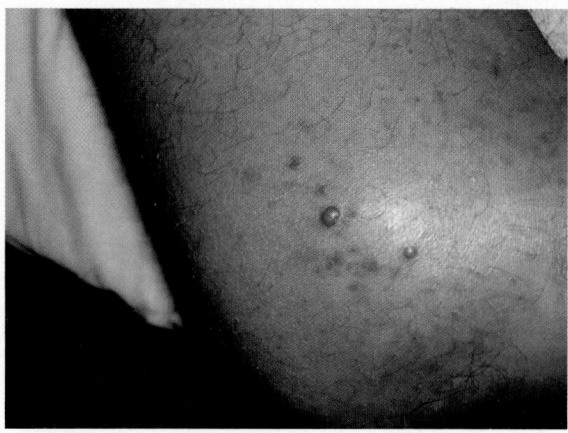

▲ **Figure 31–6.** Kaposi sarcoma. A 35-year-old man presented with several reddish-purple papular lesions on his elbow. When these were diagnosed on shave biopsy as Kaposi sarcoma (KS), he was tested and found to be positive for HIV. He was begun on systemic treatment with combination antiretroviral therapy and topical treatment with alitretinoin gel and the KS lesions eventually resolved. (Used, with permission, from Heather Wickless, MD, in Usatine RP, Smith MA, Mayeaux EJ Jr, Chumley H. *The Color Atlas of Family Medicine,* 2nd ed. McGraw-Hill, 2013.)

the lesions usually resolve with effective antiretroviral treatment. However, it should be noted that the lesions may flare when antiretroviral treatment is first initiated—probably as a result of an immune reconstitution process. Advanced disease is treated with combination chemotherapy (Table 31–3).

Franco JB et al. Regression of human immunodeficiency virus-associated oral Kaposi sarcoma with combined antiretroviral therapy: a case report and literature review. Head Neck. 2019 Feb;41(2):E21–5. [PMID: 30552825]

Gonçalves PH et al. HIV-associated Kaposi sarcoma and related diseases. AIDS. 2017 Sep 10;31(14):1903–16. [PMID: 28609402]

Liu Z et al. The world-wide incidence of Kaposi's sarcoma in the HIV/AIDS era. HIV Med. 2018 May;19(5):355–64. [PMID: 29368388]

2. Non-Hodgkin lymphoma—

A. Presentation—Non-Hodgkin lymphomas in HIV-infected persons tends to be very aggressive. These malignancies are usually of B cell origin and characterized as diffuse large-cell tumors. Over 70% of the malignancies are extranodal.

B. Management—The prognosis of patients with systemic non-Hodgkin lymphoma depends primarily on the degree of immunodeficiency at the time of diagnosis. Patients with high CD4 counts do markedly better than those diagnosed at a late stage of illness. Patients with primary central nervous system lymphoma are treated with radiation. Response to treatment is good, but prior to the availability of antiretroviral treatment, most patients died within a few months after diagnosis due to their underlying disease. Systemic disease is treated with combination chemotherapy (eg, EPOCH [etoposide, prednisolone, vincristine, cyclophosphamide, doxorubicin]) with rituximab. Granulocyte colony-stimulating factor (G-CSF; filgrastim) is used to maintain white blood counts.

Cingolani A et al; ICONA Foundation Study group. Survival and predictors of death in people with HIV-associated lymphoma compared to those with a diagnosis of lymphoma in general population. PLoS One. 2017 Oct 31;12(10):e0186549. [PMID: 29088223]

Oishi N et al. Head and neck lymphomas in HIV patients: a clinical perspective. Int Arch Otorhinolaryngol. 2017 Oct; 21(4):399–407. [PMID: 29018505]

Qian L et al. Advances in the treatment of newly diagnosed primary central nervous system lymphomas. Blood Res. 2017 Sep; 52(3):159–66. [PMID: 29043230]

Re A et al. Early consolidation with high-dose therapy and autologous stem cell transplantation is a feasible and effective treatment option in HIV-associated non-Hodgkin lymphoma at high risk. Bone Marrow Transplant. 2018 Feb; 53(2):228–30. [PMID: 28991244]

3. Hodgkin disease—Although Hodgkin disease is not included as part of the CDC definition of AIDS, studies have found that HIV infection is associated with a fivefold increase in the incidence of Hodgkin disease. HIV-infected persons with Hodgkin disease are more likely to have mixed cellularity and lymphocyte depletion subtypes of Hodgkin disease and to seek medical attention at an advanced stage of disease.

Lawal IO et al. The role of F-18 FDG PET/CT in evaluating the impact of HIV infection on tumor burden and therapy outcome in patients with Hodgkin lymphoma. Eur J Nucl Med Mol Imaging. 2017 Nov;44(12):2025–33. [PMID: 28660348]

Sorigué M et al. HIV-infection has no prognostic impact on advanced-stage classical Hodgkin lymphoma. AIDS. 2017 Jun 19;31(10):1445–9. [PMID: 28358739]

4. Anal dysplasia and squamous cell carcinoma—These lesions have been strongly correlated with previous infection by human papillomavirus (HPV) and have been noted in HIV-infected men and women. Although many of the infected MSM report a history of anal warts or have visible warts, a significant percentage have silent papillomavirus infection. Cytologic (using Papanicolaou smears) and papillomavirus DNA studies can easily be performed on specimens obtained by anal swab. Because of the risk of progression from dysplasia to cancer in immunocompromised patients, some experts suggest that annual anal swabs for cytologic examination should be done in all HIV-infected persons. An anal Papanicolaou smear is performed by rotating a moistened Dacron swab about 2 cm into the anal canal. The swab is immediately inserted into a cytology bottle. However, there is no evidence that screening for anal cancer with Papanicolaou smears decreases the incidence of invasive cancer.

HPV also appears to play a causative role in **cervical dysplasia** and **neoplasia**. The incidence and clinical course of cervical disease in HIV-infected women are discussed below.

Cajas-Monson LC et al. Expectant management of high-grade anal dysplasia in people with HIV: long-term data. Dis Colon Rectum. 2018 Dec;61(12):1357–63. [PMID: 30346366]

Douaiher J et al. Multidisciplinary approach to the management and treatment of anal dysplasia. Clin Colon Rectal Surg. 2018 Nov;31(6):361–7. [PMID: 30397395]

Gonçalves JCN et al. Accuracy of anal cytology for diagnosis of precursor lesions of anal cancer: systematic review and meta-analysis. Dis Colon Rectum. 2019 Jan;62(1):112–20. [PMID: 30451747]

Oette M et al. HIV-associated anal dysplasia and anal carcinoma. Oncol Res Treat. 2017;40(3):100–5. [PMID: 28253522]

M. Gynecologic Manifestations

Vaginal candidiasis, cervical dysplasia and neoplasia, and pelvic inflammatory disease are more common in HIV-infected women than in uninfected women. These manifestations also tend to be more severe when they occur in association with HIV infection. Therefore, HIV-infected women need frequent gynecologic care. **Vaginal candidiasis** may be treated with topical agents or a single dose of oral fluconazole (150 mg) (see Chapter 36). Recurrent vaginal candidiasis should be treated with fluconazole (100–200 mg) for at least 7 days.

The incidence of **cervical dysplasia** in HIV-infected women is 40%. Because of this finding, recommended screening for HIV-infected women is more extensive than for uninfected women (see Chapter 18). For women younger than age 30 years, a Papanicolaou smear should be performed within a year of the onset of sexual activity, but no later than age 21 years. If normal, Papanicolaou smears should be performed yearly. After three negative examinations, screening should be done every 3 years. HPV DNA testing of the cervical specimen is not recommended for women younger than age 30 years.

For women age 30 and older, screening should continue beyond age 65 unlike the general population. There are two accepted screening protocols, one using cytology alone, the other using cytology with HPV DNA cotesting. A Papanicolaou smear is done when HIV is diagnosed and every 12 months thereafter and after three negative examinations, ongoing screening should be performed every 3 years. Alternatively, a Papanicolaou smear with cotesting for HPV DNA can be performed when HIV is diagnosed or starting when patients are age 30 years old. If Papanicolaou is normal and HPV test is negative, then the next screening should be in 3 years.

The management of abnormal Papanicolaou tests and positive HPV tests is the same in infected women as in uninfected women. Treatment should follow the consensus guidelines in the references below.

While **pelvic inflammatory disease** appears to be more common in HIV-infected women, the bacteriology of this condition appears to be the same as among HIV-uninfected women. HIV-infected women with pelvic inflammatory disease should be treated with the same regimens as uninfected women (see Chapter 18).

Dreyer G. Clinical implications of the interaction between HPV and HIV infections. Best Pract Res Clin Obstet Gynaecol. 2018 Feb;47:95–106. [PMID: 28958633]

Ghebre RG et al. Cervical cancer control in HIV-infected women: past, present and future. Gynecol Oncol Rep. 2017 Jul 21; 21:101–8. [PMID: 28819634]

N. Coronary Artery Disease

HIV-infected persons are at higher risk for coronary artery disease than age- and sex-matched controls. Part of this increase in coronary artery disease is due to changes in lipids caused by antiretroviral agents (see Treatment section on Antiretroviral Therapy below), especially stavudine and several of the PIs. However, some of the risk appears to be due to HIV infection, independent of its therapy. It is important that clinicians pay close attention to this issue because myocardial infarctions tend to present at a younger age in HIV-infected individuals than in HIV-uninfected individuals. HIV-infected patients with symptoms of coronary artery disease such as chest pain or dyspnea should be rapidly evaluated. Clinicians should aggressively treat conditions that result in increased risk of heart disease, especially smoking, hypertension, hyperlipidemia, obesity, diabetes mellitus, and sedentary lifestyle.

Ballocca F et al. Cardiovascular disease in patients with HIV. Trends Cardiovasc Med. 2017 Nov;27(8):558–63. [PMID: 28779949]

Currier JS. Management of long-term complications of HIV disease: focus on cardiovascular disease. Top Antivir Med. 2018 Apr;25(4):133–7. [PMID: 29689541]

Maggi P et al. Cardiovascular risk and dyslipidemia among persons living with HIV: a review. BMC Infect Dis. 2017 Aug 9; 17(1):551. [PMID: 28793863]

Manga P et al. HIV and nonischemic heart disease. J Am Coll Cardiol. 2017 Jan 3;69(1):83–91. [PMID: 28057254]

O. Inflammatory Reactions (Immune Reconstitution Inflammatory Syndromes)

With initiation of antiretroviral treatment, some patients experience **inflammatory reactions** that appear to be associated with immune reconstitution as indicated by a rapid increase in CD4 count. These inflammatory reactions may present with generalized signs of fevers, sweats, and malaise with or without more localized manifestations that usually represent unusual presentations of opportunistic infections. For example, vitreitis has developed in patients with CMV retinitis after they have been treated with antiretroviral treatment.

M avium can present as focal even suppurative lymphadenitis or granulomatous masses in patients receiving antiretroviral treatment. Tuberculosis may paradoxically worsen with new or evolving pulmonary infiltrates and lymphadenopathy. PML and cryptococcal meningitis may also behave atypically. Clinicians should be alert to these syndromes, which are most often seen in patients who have

initiated antiretroviral treatment in the setting of advanced disease and who show rapid increases in CD4 counts with treatment. The diagnosis of **immune reconstitution inflammatory syndrome (IRIS)** is one of exclusion and can be made only after recurrence or new opportunistic infection has been ruled out as the cause of the clinical deterioration. Management of IRIS is conservative and supportive with use of corticosteroids only for severe reactions. Most authorities recommend that antiretroviral treatment be continued unless the IRIS reaction is life-threatening.

Hammoud DA et al. Increased metabolic activity on 18F-fluorodeoxyglucose positron emission tomography-computed tomography in human immunodeficiency virus-associated immune reconstitution inflammatory syndrome. Clin Infect Dis. 2019 Jan 7;68(2):229–38. [PMID: 30215671]

Shahani L et al. Therapeutics targeting inflammation in the immune reconstitution inflammatory syndrome. Transl Res. 2016 Jan;167(1):88–103. [PMID: 26303886]

▶ Prevention

A. Primary Prevention

Until vaccination is a reality, prevention of HIV infection will depend on HIV testing and counseling, including precautions regarding sexual practices and injection drug use, initiation of antiretroviral treatment as a prevention tool for transmission to others, preexposure and postexposure use of antiretroviral treatment, perinatal management including antiretroviral treatment of the mother, screening of blood products, and infection control practices in the health care setting.

1. HIV testing and counseling—Primary care clinicians should routinely obtain a sexual history and provide risk factor assessment of their patients. Because approximately 15% of the HIV-infected persons in the United States do not know they are infected, the US Preventive Services Task Force recommends that clinicians screen for HIV infection in adolescents and adults ages 15 to 65 years. Younger adolescents and older adults who are at increased risk should also be screened. Clinicians should review the risk factors for HIV infection with the patient and discuss safer sex and safer needle use as well as the meaning of a positive test. Although the CDC recommends "opt-out" testing in medical settings, some states require specific written consent. For persons whose test results are positive, it is critically important that they be connected to ongoing medical care. Many public health systems advocate for initiating care and treatment the same day that someone tests positive if appropriate resources are available (see C. Antiviral Treatment, below). Referrals for partner-notification services, social services, mental health services, and HIV-prevention services should also be provided. Prevention interventions focused on the importance of HIV-infected persons not putting others at risk have been successful.

For patients whose test results are negative, clinicians should review safer sex and needle use practices, including counseling not to exchange bodily fluids unless they are in a long-term mutually monogamous relationship with someone who has tested HIV antibody-negative and has not engaged in unsafe sex, injection drug use, or other HIV risk behaviors for at least 6 months prior to or at any time since the negative test.

To prevent sexual transmission of HIV, only latex or polyurethane condoms should be used, along with a water-soluble lubricant. Although nonoxynol-9, a spermicide, kills HIV, it is contraindicated because in some patients it may cause genital ulcers that could facilitate HIV transmission. Patients should be counseled that condoms are not 100% effective. They should be made familiar with the use of condoms, including, specifically, the advice that condoms must be used every time, that space should be left at the tip of the condom as a receptacle for semen, that intercourse with a condom should not be attempted if the penis is only partially erect, that men should hold on to the base of the condom when withdrawing the penis to prevent slippage, and that condoms should not be reused. Although anal intercourse remains the sexual practice at highest risk for transmitting HIV, seroconversions have been documented with vaginal and oral intercourse as well. Therefore, condoms should be used when engaging in these activities. Women as well as men having sex with men should understand how to use condoms to be sure that their partners are using them correctly. Partners of HIV-infected women should use latex or polyurethane barriers such as dental dams (available at dental supply stores) to prevent direct oral contact with vaginal secretions. Several randomized trials in Africa demonstrated that male circumcision significantly reduced HIV incidence in men, but there are a number of barriers to performing widespread circumcisions among men in Africa.

Persons using injection drugs should be cautioned never to share needles or other drug paraphernalia. When sterile needles are not available, bleach does appear to inactivate HIV and should be used to clean needles.

2. Antiretroviral treatment for decreasing transmission of HIV to others—Besides preventing progression of HIV disease, effective antiretroviral treatment likely decreases the risk of HIV transmission between sexual partners. Among serodiscordant couples, stably suppressing HIV with antiretroviral treatment almost completely eliminates the risk of HIV transmission to the uninfected partner. Although HIV-negative persons in stable long-term partnerships with HIV-infected persons represent only one group of at-risk persons, theoretically increasing the use of antiretroviral treatment among the population of HIV-infected persons could decrease community-wide transmission of HIV. Despite major improvements in effectiveness and tolerability of antiretroviral treatment, only about 60% of HIV-infected persons in the United States are virally suppressed. Persons in whom the HIV virus has been "undetectable" for a prolonged period have virtually no chance of *sexually* transmitting HIV. Still, because of the possibility of variations in measured viral load, and not knowing whether their partners are virally suppressed, and the possibility of transmission through blood, all HIV-infected persons should practice safer sex and not share needles so as to avoid the possibility of transmitting HIV.

Centers for Disease Control and Prevention. National Center for HIV/AIDS, Viral Hepatitis, STD, and TB Prevention, March 11, 2019. https://www.cdc.gov/nchhstp/default.htm

Kalapila AG et al. Antiretroviral therapy for prevention of human immunodeficiency virus infection. Med Clin North Am. 2016 Jul;100(4):927–50. [PMID: 27235622]

Marrazzo JM. HIV prevention: opportunities and challenges. Top Antivir Med. 2017 Dec/Jan;24(4):123–6. [PMID: 28208119]

Saag MS et al. Antiretroviral drugs for treatment and prevention of HIV infection in adults: 2018 recommendations of the International Antiviral Society—USA Panel. JAMA. 2018 Jul 24;320(4):379–96. [PMID: 30043070]

3. Preexposure antiretroviral treatment prophylaxis—Several large randomized double-blind placebo-controlled trials demonstrated that administering emtricitabine/TDF (Truvada) can reduce the risk of sexual transmission of HIV among uninfected individuals at high risk for infection; one study was of HIV-negative men and transgender women who have sex with men, and two studies were of heterosexual HIV-discordant couples. Preexposure tenofovir has also been shown to reduce HIV infection among injection drug users from Thailand. In addition, real-world studies of men who have sex with men, where adherence with emtricitabine/TDF has been high, have found **preexposure prophylaxis (PrEP)** to be highly effective in preventing HIV infection. Emtricitabine/TAF (Descovy) is under study for PrEP, but is not currently recommended because of questions of whether it has as good penetration into genital fluids.

Who should be prescribed PrEP is not a simple question. PrEP is best thought of as one "option" for HIV prevention, rather than as the only option. Whether it is the "best" option depends on three things: (1) the likelihood that a person will have HIV-infected partners or use the needles of infected persons, (2) whether there is a better option available to prevent HIV, and (3) the patient's ability to take a daily medication. CDC guidelines recommend offering PrEP to persons at "substantial risk" for HIV. Risk for HIV is a combination of the likelihood of having a partner who is HIV-infected and the likelihood that the behavior (eg, type of intercourse, shared needles) transmits HIV. Men who have sex with men, and transgender male-to-females are the groups with the highest HIV seroprevalence in the United States, and they are likely to have partners who are known to be or at risk for being HIV-infected. Those who have receptive anal intercourse have the highest risk of HIV because the behavior is much more efficient at transmitting HIV than other sexual practices. Heterosexual drug users are also at high risk for HIV-infection if they do not consistently use clean needles or if they trade drugs for sex. It can be hardest to assess the risk of heterosexual non-drug users because it requires assessing the likelihood that their partners have HIV risks such as being bisexual men or using injection drugs. Factors known to increase the risk of HIV transmission and therefore make PrEP a good choice for particular groups of patients are shown in Table 31–4.

Table 31–4. Recommendations for preexposure prophylaxis (PrEP) of HIV infection.

Patients for whom PrEP should be considered as an option for HIV prevention
Sexually active homosexual and bisexual men, male-to-female transgender persons, and heterosexuals and bisexual women who are likely to have partners with HIV risks
Injection drug users
Factors that increase the likelihood that PrEP is a good option
Patient has receptive anal intercourse
Patient has a known HIV-infected partner
Patient has a history of sexually transmitted diseases
Patient has a high number of sex partners
Patient is a commercial sex worker
Patient with inconsistent or no condom use
Patient who is sharing needles or related paraphernalia ("works")
Initial assessment before prescribing PrEP
HIV antibody test to confirm HIV negative
Symptom review to exclude primary HIV infection (eg, no history of acute illness with fever and rash in prior month)
STD tests: syphilis; gonorrhea (at risk site-specific); and chlamydia (at risk site-specific)
Serum creatinine and eGFR[1]
Confirm immunity to HBV or vaccinate if nonimmune[2]
Pregnancy test
Discuss risks, including that PrEP is not 100% effective, does not protect against other STDs, and may have side effects
Counsel patients to use latex or polyurethane condoms and clean needles, in addition to PrEP
Assess substance use and offer treatment, if needed
Discuss importance of daily medication adherence
PrEP prescription
Emtricitabine/TDF daily (Truvada) 1 tablet orally daily, initially for 90 days
Follow-up assessment
HIV antibody test every 3 months
Serum creatinine every 6 months
Pregnancy test every 3 months
STD tests: syphilis, gonorrhea (at risk site-specific); and chlamydia (at risk site-specific)
Assess and support daily medication adherence
Reinforce benefits of using latex or polyurethane condoms and clean needles with PrEP
Assess substance use and offer treatment, if needed

[1]Emtricitabine/TDF is contraindicated if creatinine clearance < 60 mL/min.
[2]HBV-infected persons may experience HBV reactivation and liver damage if emtricitabine/TDF is stopped.
eGFR, estimated glomerular filtration rate; HBV, hepatitis B virus; STD, sexually transmitted disease; TDF, tenofovir diproxil fumarate.
PrEP checklists for providers and patients are available at https://www.cdc.gov/hiv/risk/prep/index.html (Last updated November 1, 2018).

How does PrEP compare to other options for preventing HIV? Latex or polyurethane condoms are an excellent choice for preventing sexual transmission of HIV because they are inexpensive, have no side effects, and prevent other sexually transmitted diseases and pregnancy. However, for a variety of reasons, people do not always use condoms even when taught to do so. In addition, condoms break or slip on occasion, so even persons who always use

condoms may want the extra protection of PrEP if they have a known HIV-infected partner. History of sexually transmitted diseases is proof of unprotected sex and increases the likelihood that PrEP is a good option for a patient.

Finally, for PrEP to be effective, patients have to be willing to take it. Taking one pill right before sex would not be expected to offer protection because the medicine would not have adequate drug levels in the body. Maximum concentrations are achieved in various locations in the body at different treatment intervals: in blood, maximum levels are achieved after 20 days of daily dosing; in rectal tissue, after 7 days; in cervicovaginal tissue, after 20 days. Study participants who took at least 4 daily doses in a week were protected almost as well as those who took the drug every day, indicating that missed doses do not render the treatment ineffective; however, adherence to daily dosing is the safest method.

Recommendations on initial and follow-up assessments are shown in Table 31–4. Emtricitabine/TDF is contraindicated for persons with kidney disease (creatinine clearance less than 60 mL) because of the small risk of kidney toxicity with TDF. Decreases in bone mineral density have been documented in persons taking emtricitabine/TDF for PrEP at 24 weeks; whether this decrease will have clinical significance is unknown. In someone with osteoporosis or at high risk for osteoporosis, clinical judgement would be needed to assess whether the benefits of emtricitabine/TDF justified the risks of worsening bone density. If emtricitabine/TAF is found to be effective as PrEP, it would be a good alternative to emtricitabine/TDF for patients with kidney disease or osteoporosis since TAF appears to have less effect on the kidney and bone than TDF.

Substantial increases in sexually transmitted diseases have also been seen in persons taking PrEP, indicating the importance of regular follow-up in patients using PrEP. Some patients are reluctant to use insurance to cover the cost of the medication for fear of revealing that they are at risk for HIV; without insurance, the cost is high. Compassionate use programs are available from the medication manufacturer for low-income uninsured persons.

Buchbinder SP. Maximizing the benefits of HIV preexposure prophylaxis. Top Antivir Med. 2018 Apr;25(4):138–42. [PMID: 29689539]

Jenness SM et al. Impact of the Centers for Disease Control's HIV preexposure prophylaxis guidelines for men who have sex with men in the United States. J Infect Dis. 2016 Dec 15; 214(12):1800–7. [PMID: 27418048]

Seidman D et al. Integrating preexposure prophylaxis for human immunodeficiency virus prevention into women's health care in the United States. Obstet Gynecol. 2016 Jul;128(1):37–43. [PMID: 27275793]

4. Postexposure prophylaxis for sexual and drug use exposures to HIV—The goal of **postexposure prophylaxis** is to reduce or prevent local viral replication prior to dissemination such that the infection can be aborted. Although there is no proof that administration of antiretroviral medications following a sexual or parenteral drug use exposure reduces the likelihood of infection, there is suggestive data from animal models, perinatal experience, and a case-control study of health care workers who experienced a needle stick.

Treatment of persons who have been exposed to HIV should be within 72 hours, but sooner is better. All exposed persons should first receive HIV testing to exclude the possibility that they are already infected. If rapid tests are not available, treatment should begin pending the results of a standard HIV test.

The choice of antiretroviral agents and the duration of treatment are the same as those for exposures that occur through the occupational route; the preferred regimen is tenofovir 300 mg with emtricitabine 200 mg daily with raltegravir 400 mg twice a day. In contrast to those with occupational exposures, some individuals may present very late after exposure. Because the likelihood of success declines with length of time from HIV exposure, treatment is not recommended after more than 72 hours after exposure. In addition, because the psychosocial issues involved with postexposure prophylaxis for sexual and drug use exposures are complex, it should be offered with prevention counseling. Counseling should focus on how to prevent future exposures. Individuals with ongoing risk for HIV infection should be considered candidates for PrEP. Clinicians needing more information on postexposure prophylaxis for occupational or nonoccupational exposures should contact the National Clinicians' Post-Exposure Prophylaxis Hotline (1-888-448-4911; http://nccc.ucsf.edu/clinician-consultation/pep-post-exposure-prophylaxis/).

Centers for Disease Control and Prevention. HIV/AIDS, HIV Risk and Prevention, Post-Exposure Prophylaxis. Update, May 23, 2018. https://www.cdc.gov/hiv/risk/pep/index.html

Inciarte A et al; STRIBPEP Study Group. Tenofovir disoproxil fumarate/emtricitabine plus ritonavir-boosted lopinavir or cobicistat-boosted elvitegravir as a single-tablet regimen for HIV post-exposure prophylaxis. J Antimicrob Chemother. 2017 Oct 1;72(10):2857–61. [PMID: 29091217]

Mayer KH et al. Optimal HIV postexposure prophylaxis regimen completion with single tablet daily elvitegravir/cobicistat/tenofovir disoproxil fumarate/emtricitabine compared with more frequent dosing regimens. J Acquir Immune Defic Syndr. 2017 Aug 15;75(5):535–9. [PMID: 28696345]

O'Donnell S et al. Missed opportunities for HIV prophylaxis among emergency department patients with occupational and nonoccupational body fluid exposures. Ann Emerg Med. 2016 Sep;68(3):315–23. [PMID: 27112264]

Scholten M et al. To prescribe, or not to prescribe: decision making in HIV-1 post-exposure prophylaxis. HIV Med. 2018 Oct; 19(9):645–53. [PMID: 29993176]

5. Prevention of perinatal transmission of HIV—Prevention of perinatal transmission of HIV begins by offering HIV counseling and testing to all women who are pregnant or considering pregnancy. HIV-infected women who are pregnant should start antiretroviral treatment with at least three medications. Recommended regimens are zidovudine and lamivudine with either ritonavir-boosted lopinavir or ritonavir-boosted atazanavir. Cesarean delivery should be planned if HIV viral load is greater than 1000 copies/mL near the time of delivery. Zidovudine should be given to the infant after birth for 6 weeks. When possible, breastfeeding should be avoided.

Davies N et al. Global and national guidance for the use of pre-exposure prophylaxis during peri-conception, pregnancy and breastfeeding. Sex Health. 2018 Nov;15(6):501–12. [PMID: 30447703]

Heffron R et al. PrEP as peri-conception HIV prevention for women and men. Curr HIV/AIDS Rep. 2016 Jun;13(3):131–9. [PMID: 26993627]

Seidman DL et al. Offering pre-exposure prophylaxis for HIV prevention to pregnant and postpartum women: a clinical approach. J Int AIDS Soc. 2017 Mar 8;20(Suppl 1):24–30. [PMID: 28361503]

6. Prevention of HIV transmission in health care settings—In health care settings, universal body fluid precautions should be used, including use of gloves when handling body fluids and the addition of gown, mask, and goggles for procedures that may result in splash or droplet spread, and use of specially designed needles with sheath devices to decrease the risk of needle sticks. Because transmission of tuberculosis may occur in health care settings, all patients with cough should be encouraged to wear masks. Hospitalized HIV-infected patients with cough should be placed in respiratory isolation until tuberculosis can be excluded by chest radiograph and sputum smear examination.

Epidemiologic studies show that needle sticks occur commonly among health care professionals, especially among surgeons performing invasive procedures, inexperienced hospital housestaff, and medical students. Efforts to reduce needle sticks should focus on avoiding recapping needles and use of safety needles whenever doing invasive procedures under controlled circumstances. The risk of HIV transmission from a needle stick with blood from an HIV-infected patient is about 1:300. The risk is higher with deep punctures, large inoculum, and source patients with high viral loads. The risk from mucous membrane contact is too low to quantitate.

Health care professionals who sustain needle sticks should be counseled and offered HIV testing as soon as possible. HIV testing is done to establish a negative baseline for worker's compensation claims in case there is a subsequent conversion. Follow-up testing is usually performed at 6 weeks, 3 months, and 6 months. With the patient's permission, their blood can be tested for HIV antibody and HIV viral load.

A case-control study by the CDC indicates that administration of zidovudine following a needle stick decreases the rate of HIV seroconversion by 79%. Therefore, providers should be offered antiretroviral treatment as soon as possible after exposure and continued for 4 weeks. The preferred regimen is TDF 300 mg with emtricitabine 200 mg (Truvada) daily with raltegravir 400 mg twice a day. Providers who have exposures to persons who are likely to have antiretroviral medication resistance (eg, persons receiving therapy who have detectable viral loads) should have their therapy individualized, using at least two medications to which the source is unlikely to be resistant. Because reports have noted hepatotoxicity due to nevirapine in this setting, this agent should be avoided. Unfortunately, there have been documented cases of seroconversion following potential parenteral exposure to HIV despite prompt use of zidovudine prophylaxis.

Counseling of the provider should include "safer sex" guidelines.

Centers for Disease Control and Prevention. Human Immuno-deficiency Virus (HIV) in Healthcare Settings. https://www.cdc.gov/hai/organisms/hiv/hiv.html

7. Prevention of transmission of HIV through blood or blood products—Current efforts in the United States to screen blood and blood products have lowered the risk of HIV transmission with transfusion of a unit of blood to 1:1,000,000. Use of blood and blood products should be judicious, with patients receiving the least amount necessary, and patients should be encouraged to donate their own blood prior to elective procedures.

8. HIV vaccine—Primate model data have suggested that development of a protective vaccine may be possible, but clinical trials in humans have been disappointing. Only one vaccine trial has shown any degree of efficacy. In this randomized, double-blind, placebo-controlled trial, a recombinant canarypox vector vaccine plus two booster injections of a recombinant gp120 vaccine reduced the risk of HIV among a primarily heterosexual population in Thailand, but efficacy was too low (31%) for widespread use. A mosaic HIV vaccine resulted in a strong immune response among adult humans and protection against infection with an HIV-like virus in rhesus monkeys. The vaccine is currently being studied in a phase IIB trial in sub-Saharan Africa.

Barouch DH et al. Evaluation of a mosaic HIV-1 vaccine in a multicentre, randomized, double-blind, placebo-controlled, phase 1/2a clinical trial (APPROACH) and in rhesus monkeys (NHP 13-19). Lancet. 2018 Jul 21;392(10143):232–43. [PMID: 30047376]
Fauci AS. Viewpoint: An HIV vaccine is essential for ending the HIV/AIDS pandemic. JAMA. 2017 Oct 24;318(16):1535–6. [PMID: 29052689]
Lyon J. Hunt for an HIV vaccine intensifies. JAMA. 2017 Jun 27; 317(24):2475. [PMID: 28654994]
Pavlakis GN et al. A new step towards an HIV/AIDS vaccine. Lancet. 2018 Jul 21;392(10143):192–4. [PMID: 30047374]

B. Secondary Prevention

In the era prior to the development of effective antiretroviral treatment, cohort studies of individuals with documented dates of seroconversion demonstrate that AIDS developed within 10 years in approximately 50% of untreated seropositive persons. With currently available treatment, progression of disease has been markedly decreased. In addition to antiretroviral treatment, prophylactic regimens can prevent opportunistic infections and improve survival. Prophylaxis and early intervention prevent several infectious diseases, including tuberculosis and syphilis, which are transmissible to others. Recommendations for screening tests, vaccinations, and prophylaxis are listed in Table 31–5.

1. Tuberculosis—Because of the increased occurrence of tuberculosis among HIV-infected patients, all such individuals should undergo an intradermal **PPD test** or an **interferon-gamma release assay (IGRA)** blood test at baseline and yearly thereafter if they remain at risk of exposure (eg, incarcerated, living in congregate settings). Those with a positive PPD (defined for HIV-infected patients as greater than 5 mm of induration) or a positive IGRA assay (results that are reported as positive and not negative or indeterminate) should be clinically evaluated for active tuberculosis, including by a chest radiograph. Patients with an infiltrate in any location, especially if accompanied by mediastinal adenopathy, should have sputum sent for acid-fast staining. Patients with active tuberculosis should be treated as outlined in Chapter 9 (see Tables 9–14 and 9–15). Patients with a positive PPD or IGRA assay, a normal chest radiograph, or negative sputum sample for active tuberculosis infection are classified as having latent tuberculosis infection. Patients with latent tuberculosis infection who have not been previously treated for (active or latent) tuberculosis should receive isoniazid (300 mg orally daily or twice weekly) with pyridoxine (50 mg orally daily) for 9 months. In patients with advanced immunodeficiency, both the PPD and IGRA assay are more likely to be falsely negative or (for IGRA assay) indeterminant. Therefore, it may be worth retesting patients with initially low CD4 counts once they have received antiretroviral treatment and have immune reconstitution (CD4 count greater than or equal to 200 cells/mcL).

Jacobson KR. Tuberculosis. Ann Intern Med. 2017 Feb 7; 166(3):ITC17–32. [PMID: 28166561]
Khan PY et al. Transmission of drug-resistant tuberculosis in HIV-endemic settings. Lancet Infect Dis. 2019 Mar;19(3): e77–e88. [PMID: 30554996]
Peters JS et al. Advances in the understanding of *Mycobacterium tuberculosis* transmission in HIV-endemic settings. Lancet Infect Dis. 2019 Mar;19(3):e65–e76. [PMID: 30554995]

2. Syphilis—Because of the increased number of cases of syphilis among MSM, including those who are HIV-infected, all such men should be screened for syphilis by a rapid plasma reagin (RPR) or Venereal Disease Research Laboratories (VDRL) test every 6 months. Increases of syphilis cases among HIV-infected persons are of particular concern because these individuals are at increased risk for reactivation of syphilis and progression to tertiary syphilis despite standard treatment. Because the only widely available tests for syphilis are serologic and because HIV-infected individuals are known to have disordered antibody production, there is concern about the interpretation of these titers. This concern has been fueled by a report of an HIV-infected patient with secondary syphilis and negative syphilis serologic testing. Furthermore, HIV-infected individuals may lose fluorescent treponemal antibody absorption (FTA-ABS) reactivity after treatment for syphilis, particularly if they have low CD4 counts. Thus, in this population, a nonreactive treponemal test does not rule out a past history of syphilis. In addition, persistence of treponemes in the spinal fluid after one dose of benzathine penicillin has been demonstrated in HIV-infected patients with primary and secondary syphilis. Therefore, the CDC has recommended an aggressive diagnostic approach to HIV-infected patients with reactive RPR or VDRL tests of longer than 1 year (or unknown) duration.

Table 31–5. Health care maintenance and monitoring of HIV-infected individuals.

For all HIV-infected individuals:
CD4 counts every 3–6 months (can decrease to every 12 months if viral load suppressed on antiretroviral treatment for 2 years and CD4 count greater than 300 cells/mcL)
Viral load tests every 3–6 months and 1 month following a change in therapy
Genotypic resistance testing at baseline and if viral load not fully suppressed and patient taking antiretroviral treatment
Complete blood count, chemistry profile, transaminases and total bilirubin, at baseline and every 3–6 months
Urinalysis at baseline and annually during antiretroviral treatment (every 6 months if antiretroviral treatment regimen includes TDF)
Fasting glucose or hemoglobin A_{1c} at baseline and annually during antiretroviral treatment
Fasting lipid panel at baseline, 4–8 weeks after starting or changing an antiretroviral treatment regimen that affects lipids, and annually for everyone over 40 years of age
PPD or interferon-gamma release assay (IGRA) at baseline and annually if at high risk for exposure to persons with active TB
INH for those with positive PPD or IGRA, normal chest radiograph, and no history of treatment for active or latent TB
RPR or VDRL at entry and periodically based on sexual activity
Toxoplasma IgG serology at baseline
Hepatitis serologies: hepatitis A antibody, hepatitis B surface antigen, hepatitis B surface antibody, hepatitis B core antibody, hepatitis C antibody
Pneumococcal vaccine
Meningococcal vaccine
Herpes zoster vaccine[1]
Inactivated influenza vaccine annually in season
Hepatitis A vaccine for those without immunity to hepatitis A
Hepatitis B vaccine for those who are hepatitis B surface antigen and antibody negative. (Use 40 mcg formulation at 0, 1, and 6 months; repeat if no immunity 1 month after three-vaccine series.)
Combined tetanus, diphtheria, pertussis vaccine
Human papillomavirus vaccine for HIV-infected women age 26 years or less
Haemophilus influenzae type b vaccination
Bone mineral density monitoring for postmenopausal women and men 50 years of age or older
Papanicolaou smears annually; if three smears are negative, can switch to longer intervals (see Complications, Section M. Gynecologic Manifestations)
Consider anal swabs for cytologic evaluation
For HIV-infected individuals with CD4 less than 200 cells/mcL:
Pneumocystis jirovecii prophylaxis (see Treatment, Section B. Prophylactic Treatment of Complications of HIV Infection)
For HIV-infected individuals with CD4 less than 75 cells/mcL:
Mycobacterium avium complex prophylaxis (see Treatment, Section A. Complications of HIV Infection)
For HIV-infected individuals with CD4 less than 50 cells/mcL:
Consider CMV prophylaxis

[1]Consider in patients age > 50 years with history of varicella immunity and T cells > 200 cells/mcL.

BUN, blood urea nitrogen; CMV, cytomegalovirus; IgG, immunoglobulin G; IGRA, interferon gamma release assay; INH, isoniazid; PPD, purified protein derivative; RPR, rapid plasma reagin; TB, tuberculosis; TDF, tenofovir diproxil fumarate; VDRL, Venereal Disease Research Laboratories.

All such patients should have a lumbar puncture with cerebrospinal fluid cell count and cerebrospinal fluid VDRL. Those with a normal cerebrospinal fluid evaluation are treated as having late latent syphilis (benzathine penicillin G, 2.4 million units intramuscularly weekly for 3 weeks) with follow-up titers. Those with a pleocytosis or a positive cerebrospinal fluid-VDRL test are treated as having neurosyphilis (aqueous penicillin G, 2–4 million units intravenously every 4 hours, or procaine penicillin G, 2.4 million units intramuscularly daily, with probenecid, 500 mg four times daily, for 10 days) followed by weekly benzathine penicillin G 2.4 million units intramuscularly for 3 weeks. Some clinicians take a less aggressive approach to patients who have low titers (less than 1:8), a history of having been treated for syphilis, and a normal neurologic examination. Close follow-up of titers is mandatory if such a course is taken. For a more detailed discussion of this topic, see Chapter 34.

Cantor AG et al. Screening for syphilis: updated evidence report and systematic review for the U.S. Preventive Services Task Force. JAMA. 2016 Jun 7;315(21):2328–37. [PMID: 27272584]
Hook EW 3rd. Syphilis. Lancet. 2017 Apr 15;389(10078):1550–7. [PMID: 27993382]
U.S. Preventive Services Task Force (USPSTF), Bibbins-Domingo K et al. Screening for syphilis infection in nonpregnant adults and adolescents: U.S. Preventive Services Task Force Recommendation Statement. JAMA. 2016 Jun 7;315(21):2321–7. [PMID: 27272583]

3. Immunizations—HIV-infected individuals should receive immunizations as outlined in Table 31–5. Patients without evidence of hepatitis B surface antigen or surface antibody should receive hepatitis B vaccination, using the 40-mcg formulation; the higher dose is to increase the chance of developing protective immunity. If the patient does not have immunity 1 month after the three-shot series, then the series should be repeated. HIV-infected persons should also receive the standard inactivated vaccines such as tetanus and diphtheria boosters that would be given to uninfected persons. Most live vaccines, such as yellow fever vaccine, should be avoided. Measles vaccination, while a live virus vaccine, appears relatively safe when administered to HIV-infected individuals and should be given if the patient has never had measles or been adequately vaccinated. The new recombinant adjuvanted herpes zoster vaccine (Shingrix), two doses 2–6 months apart, is recommended for HIV-infected persons with CD4 counts greater than 200 cells/mcL. However, it is not known if it is efficacious in preventing herpes zoster in this population.

Catherine FX et al. Hepatitis B virus vaccination in HIV-infected people: a review. Hum Vaccin Immunother. 2017 Jun 3;13(6): 1–10. [PMID: 28267387]

4. Other measures—A randomized study found that multivitamin supplementation decreased HIV disease progression and mortality in HIV-infected women in Africa. However, supplementation is unlikely to be as effective in well-nourished populations.

HIV-infected individuals should be counseled with regard to the importance of practicing safer sex even with other HIV-infected persons because of the possibility of contracting a sexually transmitted disease, such as gonorrhea or syphilis. There is also the possibility of transmission of a particularly virulent or a drug-resistant strain between HIV-infected persons. Substance abuse treatment should be recommended for persons who are using recreational drugs. They should be warned to avoid consuming raw meat, eggs, or shellfish to avoid infections with *Toxoplasma*, *Campylobacter*, and *Salmonella*. HIV-infected patients should wash their hands thoroughly after cleaning cat litter or should forgo this household chore to avoid possible exposure to toxoplasmosis. To reduce the likelihood of infection with *Bartonella* species, patients should avoid activities that might result in cat scratches or bites. Although the data are not conclusive, many clinicians recommend that HIV-infected persons—especially those with low CD4 counts—drink bottled water instead of tap water to prevent cryptosporidia infection.

Because of the emotional impact of HIV infection and subsequent illness, many patients will benefit from supportive counseling.

Treatment

Treatment for HIV infection can be broadly divided into the following categories: (1) prophylaxis for opportunistic infections, malignancies, and other complications of HIV infection; (2) treatment of opportunistic infections, malignancies, and other complications of HIV infection; and (3) treatment of the HIV infection itself with combination antiretroviral treatment.

A. Prophylaxis for Complications of HIV Infection

In general, decisions about prophylaxis of opportunistic infections are based on the CD4 count, recent HIV viral load, and a history of having had the infection in the past. In the era prior to antiretroviral treatment, patients who started taking prophylactic regimens were maintained on them indefinitely. However, studies have shown that in patients with robust improvements in immune function—as measured by increases in CD4 counts above the levels that are used to initiate treatment—prophylactic regimens can safely be discontinued.

Because individuals with advanced HIV infection are susceptible to a number of opportunistic pathogens, the use of agents with activity against more than one pathogen is preferable.

1. Prophylaxis against *Pneumocystis* pneumonia—Patients with CD4 counts below 200 cells/mcL, a CD4 lymphocyte percentage below 14%, or weight loss or oral candidiasis should be offered primary prophylaxis for *Pneumocystis* pneumonia. Patients with a history of *Pneumocystis* pneumonia should receive secondary prophylaxis until their viral load is undetectable and they have maintained a CD4 count of 200 cells/mcL or more while receiving antiretroviral treatment for longer than 3 months. Regimens for *Pneumocystis* prophylaxis are given in Table 31–6.

2. Prophylaxis against *M avium* complex infection—Patients whose CD4 counts fall to below 75–100 cells/mcL should be given prophylaxis against *M avium* complex infection. Clarithromycin (500 mg orally twice daily) and azithromycin (1200 mg orally weekly) have both been shown to decrease the incidence of disseminated *M avium* complex infection by approximately 75%, with a low rate of breakthrough of resistant disease. The azithromycin regimen is generally preferred based on high compliance and low cost. Prophylaxis against *M avium* complex infection may be discontinued in patients whose CD4 counts rise above 100 cells/mcL in response to antiretroviral treatment for longer than 3 months.

3. Prophylaxis against toxoplasmosis—Toxoplasmosis prophylaxis is desirable in patients with a positive IgG toxoplasma serology and CD4 counts below 100 cells/mcL. Trimethoprim-sulfamethoxazole (one double-strength tablet daily) offers good protection against toxoplasmosis, as does a combination of pyrimethamine, 25 mg orally once a week, plus dapsone, 50 mg orally daily, plus leucovorin, 25 mg orally once a week. A glucose-6-phosphate dehydrogenase (G6PD) level should be checked prior to dapsone therapy, and a methemoglobin level should be checked at 1 month. Prophylaxis can be discontinued when the CD4 cells have increased to greater than 200 cells/mcL for more than 3 months.

B. Treatment of Complications of HIV Infection

Treatment of common AIDS-related complications is detailed above and in Table 31–3. In the era prior to the use of antiretroviral treatment, patients required lifelong treatment for many infections, including CMV retinitis, toxoplasmosis, and cryptococcal meningitis. However, among patients who have a good response to antiretroviral treatment, maintenance therapy for some opportunistic infections can be terminated. For example, in consultation with

Table 31–6. *Pneumocystis jirovecii* prophylaxis, in order of preference.

Medication	Dose	Side Effects	Limitations
Trimethoprim-sulfamethoxazole	One double-strength tablet three times a week to one tablet daily	Rash, neutropenia, hepatitis, Stevens-Johnson syndrome	Hypersensitivity reaction is common but, if mild, it may be possible to treat through.
Dapsone	50–100 mg orally daily or 100 mg two or three times per week	Anemia, nausea, methemoglo-binemia, hemolytic anemia	Less effective than above. Glucose-6-phosphate dehydrogenase (G6PD) level should be checked prior to therapy. Check methemoglobin level after 1 month of treatment.
Atovaquone	1500 mg orally daily with a meal	Rash, diarrhea, nausea	Less effective than suspension trimethoprim-sulfamethoxazole; equal efficacy to dapsone, but more expensive.
Aerosolized pentamidine	300 mg monthly	Bronchospasm (pretreat with bronchodilators); rare reports of pancreatitis	Apical *P jirovecii* pneumonia, extrapulmonary *P jirovecii* infections, pneumothorax.

an ophthalmologist, maintenance treatment for CMV infection can be discontinued when persons receiving anti-retroviral treatment have had a sustained increase in CD4 count to greater than 100 cells/mcL for at least 3–6 months. Similar results have been observed in patients with *M avium* complex bacteremia, who have completed a year or more of therapy for *M avium* complex and have an increase in their CD4 count to 100 cells/mcL for greater than 6 months while receiving antiretroviral treatment. Cessation of secondary prophylaxis for *Pneumocystis* pneumonia is described above.

Treating patients with repeated episodes of the same opportunistic infection can pose difficult therapeutic challenges. For example, patients with second or third episodes of *Pneumocystis* pneumonia may have developed allergic reactions to standard treatments with a prior episode. Fortunately, there are several alternatives available for the treatment of *Pneumocystis* infection. Trimethoprim with dapsone and primaquine with clindamycin are two combinations that often are tolerated in patients with a prior allergic reaction to trimethoprim-sulfamethoxazole and intravenous pentamidine. Patients in whom second episodes of *Pneumocystis* pneumonia develop while taking prophylaxis tend to have milder courses.

Adjunctive Treatments—Epoetin alfa (erythropoietin) is approved for use in HIV-infected patients with anemia, including those with anemia secondary to zidovudine use. As zidovudine is rarely used now, especially at high doses, the use of epoetin alfa has also decreased. An erythropoietin level less than 500 milli-units/mL should be demonstrated before starting therapy. The starting dose of epoetin alfa is 8000 units subcutaneously three times a week. Hypertension is the most common side effect.

Human G-CSF (filgrastim) and granulocyte-macrophage colony-stimulating factor (GM-CSF [sargramostim]) have been shown to increase the neutrophil counts of HIV-infected patients. Because of the high cost of this therapy,

the dosage should be closely monitored and minimized, aiming for a neutrophil count of 1000/mcL. When the medication is used for indications other than cytotoxic chemotherapy, one or two doses at 5 mcg/kg per week subcutaneously are usually sufficient.

C. Antiretroviral Therapy

The availability of agents that in combination suppress HIV replication (Table 31–7) has had a profound impact on the natural history of HIV infection. Indeed, with the advent of effective antiretroviral treatment, the life expectancy of HIV-infected persons approaches that of uninfected persons when treatment is initiated early in the course of the disease and maintained.

The recognition that HIV damages the immune system from the beginning of infection, even when the damage is not easily measured by conventional tests, combined with the greater potency, the improved side-effect profile, and the decreased pill burden of modern HIV regimens, have led to the recommendation to start treatment for all HIV-infected persons regardless of CD4 count. The START trial demonstrated that immediate treatment is associated with a greater than 50% reduction in risk for serious illness or death, compared to delaying treatment until the CD4 count falls below 350 cells/mcL.

Rapid initiation programs have been created, where treatment can be started on the same day that patients test positive for HIV, so patients can start receiving treatment promptly and avoid being lost to follow-up. To do this, the clinic must have sufficient resources, medical and non-medical, to help patients cope with these major events in a short time. Also, 5–20% of patients in developed countries who are treatment-naïve have a virus that is resistant to some medications; therefore, if treatment is started before the results of resistance testing are available, a nonnucleoside reverse transcriptase inhibitor (NNRTI) should not be used. Recommended regimens for initiating treatment

Table 31–7. Antiretroviral therapy agents by class (alphabetical order within class).

Medication	Dose	Common Side Effects	Special Monitoring[1]	Cost[2]	Cost/Month
Nucleoside Reverse Transcriptase Inhibitors (NRTIs)					
Abacavir (Ziagen)	300 mg orally twice daily	Rash, fever—if occur, rechallenge may be fatal	No special monitoring	$9.64/300 mg	$578.56
Didanosine (Videx)	400 mg orally daily (enteric-coated capsule) for persons greater or equal to 60 kg 250 mg orally daily (enteric-coated capsule) for persons 30–59 kg	Peripheral neuropathy, pancreatitis, dry mouth, hepatitis	Bimonthly neurologic questionnaire for neuropathy, potassium, amylase, bilirubin, triglycerides	$12.29/400 mg	$368.72
Emtricitabine (Emtriva)	200 mg orally once daily	Skin discoloration palms/soles (mild)	No special monitoring	$21.46/200 mg	$643.82
Lamivudine (Epivir)	150 mg orally twice daily or 300 mg daily	Rash, peripheral neuropathy	No special monitoring	$7.16/150 mg	$429.60
Stavudine (Zerit)	40 mg orally twice daily for persons ≥ 60 kg 30 mg orally twice daily for persons < 60 kg	Peripheral neuropathy, hepatitis, pancreatitis	Monthly neurologic questionnaire for neuropathy, amylase	$6.85/40 mg	$410.70
Zidovudine (AZT) (Retrovir)	600 mg orally daily in two divided doses	Anemia, neutropenia, nausea, malaise, headache, insomnia, myopathy	CBC with differential 4–8 weeks after starting AZT	$0.90/300 mg	$54.00
Nucleotide Reverse Transcriptase Inhibitors (NRTI)					
Tenofovir alafenamide (TAF)/ emtricitabine (Descovy)	25 mg of TAF with 200 mg of emtricitabine once daily	Nephrotoxicity; hepatoxicity (if HBsAg positive, HBV exacerbation after discontinuation); bone resorption	Creatinine at baseline, at 2–8 weeks, then every 3–6 months; urinalysis and urine glucose and protein at baseline and repeated as clinically indicated; HBsAg, liver enzymes at baseline at 2–8 weeks, every 3–6 months, continue for months after discontinuation; consider bone densitometry	$70.32/tablet	$2109.48
Tenofovir (TDF) (Viread)	300 mg orally once daily	Kidney dysfunction, bone resorption, gastrointestinal distress	Creatinine at baseline, at 2–8 weeks, every 3–6 months; urinalysis and urine glucose and protein at baseline and repeated as clinically indicated; consider bone densitometry	$38.51/300 mg	$1155.30
Nonnucleoside Reverse Transcriptase Inhibitors (NNRTIs)					
Delavirdine (Rescriptor)	400 mg orally three times daily	Rash	No special monitoring	$2.97/200 mg	$533.89
Doravirine	100 mg daily	Headache, fatigue, abdominal pain	No special monitoring	$55.20/100 mg	$1656.00

(continued)

Table 31–7. Antiretroviral therapy agents by class (alphabetical order within class). (continued)

Medication	Dose	Common Side Effects	Special Monitoring[1]	Cost[2]	Cost/Month
Nonnucleoside Reverse Transcriptase Inhibitors (NNRTIs) (cont.)					
Efavirenz (Sustiva)	600 mg orally daily	Neurologic disturbances, rash, hepatitis	No special monitoring	$37.26/600 mg	$1117.80
Etravirine (Intelence)	200 mg orally twice daily	Rash, peripheral neuropathy	No special monitoring	$13.57/100 mg	$1628.02
Nevirapine (Viramune)	200 mg orally daily for 2 weeks, then 200 mg orally twice daily	Rash	No special monitoring	$10.83/200 mg	$649.80
Rilpivirine (Edurant)	25 mg daily	Depression, rash	No special monitoring	$44.60/25 mg	$1338.13
Protease Inhibitors (PIs)					
Atazanavir (Reyataz)	400 mg orally once daily or 300 mg atazanavir with 100 mg ritonavir daily	Hyperbilirubinemia	Bilirubin level every 3–4 months	$27.80/200 mg or $52.20/300 mg	$1668.00 (plus cost of ritonavir) $1566.00 (plus cost of ritonavir)
Atazanavir/cobicistat (Evotaz)	300 mg of atazanavir with 150 mg of cobicistat orally once daily	Hyperbilirubinemia	Bilirubin level every 3–4 months	$64.22/tablet	$1926.56
Darunavir/cobicistat (Prezcobix)	800 mg of darunavir and 150 mg of cobicistat orally once daily	Rash	No special monitoring	$72.27/tablet	$2167.96
Darunavir/ritonavir (Prezista/Norvir)	**PI-experienced patients:** 600 mg of darunavir and 100 mg of ritonavir orally twice daily **For PI-naïve patients:** 800 mg of darunavir and 100 mg of ritonavir orally daily	Rash	No special monitoring	$33.79/600 mg (darunavir) $9.26/100 mg (ritonavir) $67.59/800 mg (darunavir)	$2027.40 (plus cost of ritonavir) $2027.70 (plus cost of ritonavir)
Fosamprenavir (Lexiva)	**For PI-experienced patients:** 700 mg orally twice daily and 100 mg of ritonavir orally twice daily **For PI-naïve patients:** 1400 mg orally twice daily or 1400 mg orally once daily and 200 mg of ritonavir orally once daily	Gastrointestinal, rash	No special monitoring	$20.83/700 mg	$1249.86/700 mg (plus cost of ritonavir) $2499.72/1400 mg (plus cost of ritonavir)
Indinavir (Crixivan)	800 mg orally three times daily	Renal calculi	Bilirubin level every 3–4 months	$3.05/400 mg	$548.12
Lopinavir/ritonavir (Kaletra)	400 mg/100 mg orally twice daily	Diarrhea	No special monitoring	$10.24/200 mg (Kaletra)	$1228.97
Nelfinavir (Viracept)	750 mg orally three times daily or 1250 mg twice daily	Diarrhea	No special monitoring	$4.86/250 mg or $12.14/625 mg	$1456.80 (for either dose)
Ritonavir (Norvir)	600 mg orally twice daily or in lower doses (eg, 100 mg orally once or twice daily) for boosting other PIs	Gastrointestinal distress, peripheral paresthesias	No special monitoring	$9.26/100 mg	$3333.60 ($555.60 in lower doses)

(continued)

Table 31–7. Antiretroviral therapy agents by class (alphabetical order within class). (continued)

Medication	Dose	Common Side Effects	Special Monitoring[1]	Cost[2]	Cost/Month
Protease Inhibitors (PIs) (cont.)					
Saquinavir hard gel (Invirase)	1000 mg orally twice daily with 100 mg of ritonavir orally twice daily	Gastrointestinal distress	No special monitoring	$12.02/500 mg	$1442.09 (plus cost of ritonavir)
Tipranavir/ritonavir (Aptivus/Norvir)	500 mg of tipranavir and 200 mg of ritonavir orally twice daily	Gastrointestinal, rash	No special monitoring	$16.73/250 mg (tipranavir) $9.26/100 mg (ritonavir)	$2007.58 (plus cost of ritonavir)
Entry Inhibitors					
Enfuvirtide (Fuzeon)	90 mg subcutaneously twice daily	Injection site pain and allergic reaction	No special monitoring	$71.71/90 mg	$4302.67
Maraviroc (Selzentry)	150 mg orally twice daily or 300 mg orally twice daily	Cough, fever, rash	No special monitoring	$31.12 (for either dose)	$1867.44 (for either dose)
Integrase Inhibitors					
Bictegravir	50 mg orally daily. No longer marketed as a single agent; used in antiretroviral combination (Table 31–8)	Diarrhea, nausea, headache	No special monitoring	No longer marketed as a single agent	No longer marketed as a single agent
Dolutegravir (Tivicay)	Treatment-naïve or integrase-naïve patients: 50 mg daily. When administered with efavirenz, fosamprenavir/ritonavir, tipranavir/ritonavir, or rifampin: 50 mg twice daily. When administered to integrase-experienced patients with suspected integrase resistance: 50 mg twice daily.	Hypersensitivity, insomnia, fatigue, headache, rash	No special monitoring	$69.62/50 mg	$2088.59/50 mg daily or $4177.18/ 50 mg twice daily
Elvitegravir	No longer marketed as a single agent; used in antiretroviral combinations (Table 31–8)	Diarrhea, headache	No special monitoring	No longer marketed as a single agent	No longer marketed as a single agent
Raltegravir (Isentress)	400 mg orally twice daily	Diarrhea, nausea, headache	No special monitoring	$30.00/400 mg	$1800.00

[1]Standard monitoring is complete blood count (CBC) and differential, basic chemistries, serum aminotransferases and total bilirubin every 3–6 months, urinalysis at baseline and annually during antiretroviral treatment, fasting glucose or hemoglobin A_{1c} at baseline and annually during antiretroviral treatment, and fasting lipid profile at baseline, 4–8 weeks after starting an antiretroviral treatment regimen that affects lipids, and annually for everyone over 40 years of age.

[2]Average wholesale price (AWP, for AB-rated generic when available) for quantity listed. Source: IBM Micromedex Red Book (electronic version) IBM Watson Health, Greenwood Village, CO, USA. Available at https://www.micromedexsolutions.com (cited April 25, 2019). AWP may not accurately represent the actual pharmacy cost because wide contractual variations exist among institutions.

before resistance testing results are available include (1) dolutegravir/TAF or TDF/emtricitabine (or lamivudine), (2) bictegravir/TAF/emtricitabine, or (3) boosted darunavir/TAF or TDF/emtricitabine (or lamivudine). Also, patients requiring abacavir as part of their regimen, should not start treatment prior to the results of HLA-B*5701 allele testing.

Once a decision to initiate therapy has been made, several important principles should guide therapy. First, because medication resistance to antiretroviral agents develops in HIV-infected patients, a primary goal of therapy should be complete suppression of viral replication as measured by the serum viral load. Therapy that achieves undetectable viral load has been shown to provide a durable response to the therapy. To achieve this and maintain virologic control over time, combination therapy with at least three medications from at least two different classes is necessary. Partially suppressive combinations should be avoided. Similarly, if toxicity develops, it is preferable to change the offending medication rather than reduce individual doses. Exceptions to the three-drug rule from at least two different classes are emerging. A combination of dolutegravir plus lamivudine has been shown to be noninferior to dolutegravir plus TDF and emtricitabine as initial therapy in patients with HIV viral load of less than 500,000 copies/mL. In April 2019, the FDA approved Dovato, a complete, once-daily, single-tablet combination of dolutegravir 50 mg and lamivudine 300 mg. A second exception is the coformulation of dolutegravir and rilpivirine (Juluca); this combination is FDA approved as an alternative treatment for patients who have been successfully virally suppressed for at least 6 months, have no history of treatment failure, and are not resistant to either of the two component agents.

The presence of an acute opportunistic infection in most cases does not preclude the initiation of antiretroviral treatment. Randomized trials compared early initiation of antiretroviral treatment (within 2 weeks of starting treatment for an opportunistic infection or tuberculosis) with antiretroviral treatment that was deferred until after treatment of the opportunistic infection was completed (6 weeks after its start); results demonstrated that early initiation reduced death or AIDS progression by 50%. The reduced progression rates were related to more rapid improvements in CD4 counts in patients with advanced immunodeficiency. Furthermore, IRIS and other adverse events were no more frequent in the early antiretroviral treatment arm.

Several randomized studies have also demonstrated improved clinical outcomes in HIV/tuberculosis coinfected patients who initiate antiretroviral treatment early in the setting of active treatment for tuberculosis and whose CD4 counts are less than 50 cells/mcL. The exception to early antiretroviral treatment in the setting of active infections may be in patients with a CNS-associated infection, such as cryptococcal or tuberculosis meningitis. Several studies from low-income countries have shown high mortality rates with early antiretroviral treatment initiation in this setting.

For hospitalized patients, initiating treatment in patients with opportunistic infections requires close coordination between inpatient and outpatient clinicians to ensure that treatment is continued once patients are discharged.

D. Choosing an Antiretroviral Treatment Regimen

Although the ideal combination of medications has not yet been defined for all possible clinical situations, optimal regimens can be better understood after a review of the available agents. These medications can be grouped into five major categories: nucleoside and nucleotide reverse transcriptase inhibitors (NRTIs); nonnucleoside reverse transcriptase inhibitors (NNRTIs); protease inhibitors (PI); entry inhibitors, which include a fusion inhibitor and CCR5 antagonists; and integrase inhibitors.

1. Nucleoside and nucleotide reverse transcriptase inhibitors (NRTI)—There are currently eight NRTI agents available (counting TDF and TAF as separate agents) for use. The choice of which agent to use depends primarily on the patient's prior treatment experience, results of resistance testing, medication side effects, other underlying conditions, and convenience of formulation. However, most clinicians use fixed-dose combinations (see Table 31–8) of either emtricitabine/TDF, emtricitabine/TAF, or abacavir/lamivudine (ABC/lamivudine), all of which can be given once a day. Abacavir should be given only to HLA-B*5701-negative persons. In patients with viral loads greater than 100,000 copies/mL, ABC/lamivudine was less effective than emtricitabine/TDF when combined with efavirenz or

ritonavir-boosted atazanavir. However, ABC/lamivudine appears to be equally efficacious as emtricitabine/TDF in patients with viral loads greater than 100,000 copies/mL when combined with dolutegravir or raltegravir. In some studies, abacavir increased risks of myocardial infarction, and therefore should be avoided in patients at high risk for cardiovascular disease. Zidovudine/lamivudine (AZT/lamivudine) is usually reserved for second- or third-line regimens because of toxicity and dosing schedule. Of the available agents, zidovudine is the most likely to cause anemia. Zidovudine and didanosine are the most likely to cause neutropenia. Stavudine is the most likely to cause lipoatrophy (loss of fat in the face, extremities, and buttocks) and should no longer be used; zidovudine is the next most likely agent to cause lipoatrophy. Didanosine is the most likely to cause peripheral neuropathy. Emtricitabine, TDF, TAF, and lamivudine have activity against hepatitis B. Didanosine, emtricitabine, TDF, TAF, and lamivudine can be administered once daily. Information specific to each medication is given below and in Table 31–7.

A. ZIDOVUDINE—Zidovudine was the first approved antiviral medication for HIV infection. It is administered at a dose of 300 mg orally twice daily. A combination of zidovudine 300 mg and lamivudine 150 mg (Combivir) is available. Approximately 40% of patients experience subjective side effects that usually remit within 6 weeks. The common dose-limiting side effects are anemia and neutropenia, which require ongoing laboratory monitoring. Long-term use has been associated with lipoatrophy.

B. LAMIVUDINE—Lamivudine is a safe and well-tolerated agent. The dosage is 150 mg orally twice daily or 300 mg orally once a day. The dose should be reduced in patients with chronic kidney disease. There are no significant side effects with lamivudine; it has activity against hepatitis B, though HBV resistance to it is an increasing problem.

C. EMTRICITABINE—Emtricitabine is dosed at 200 mg orally once daily. Emtricitabine also has activity against hepatitis B. Its dosage should be reduced in patients with chronic kidney disease.

D. ABACAVIR—Abacavir is dosed at 300 mg orally twice daily. Prior to initiation of abacavir, patients should undergo testing for HLA typing. Those with the B*5701 allele should not be treated with abacavir because the likelihood of a hypersensitivity reaction developing is high; the reaction is characterized by a flu-like syndrome with rash and fever that worsens with successive doses. Unfortunately, the absence of this allele does not guarantee that the patient will avoid the hypersensitivity reaction. Individuals in whom the hypersensitivity reaction develops *should not* be rechallenged with this agent because subsequent hypersensitivity reactions can be fatal. Abacavir has also been associated with an increased risk of myocardial infarction in some cohort studies, generally in patients who have underlying risks for cardiovascular disease. Consequently, abacavir should not be used in such patients if effective alternative nucleoside or nucleotide analog agents exist. Abacavir is usually prescribed as a fixed-dose combination pill with lamivudine for use as a once-daily pill (Epzicom; Table 31–8).

Table 31–8. Fixed-dose antiretroviral combinations (alphabetical order by brand name).

Name	Components	Dosing and Special Considerations	Cost per Month
Atripla	TDF 300 mg Emtricitabine 200 mg Efavirenz 600 mg	One pill daily constitutes a complete antiretroviral treatment regimen.	$3429.06
Biktarvy	Emtricitabine 200 mg TAF 25 mg Bictegravir 50 mg	One pill daily constitutes a complete antiretroviral treatment regimen. One of the recommended initial treatment regimens.	$3707.99
Complera	TDF 300 mg Emtricitabine 200 mg Rilpivirine 25 mg	One pill daily constitutes complete antiretroviral treatment regimen. Only for patients with HIV viral load less than 100,000/mL.	$3374.56
Delstrigo	TDF 300 mg Lamivudine 300 mg Doravirine 100 mg	One pill daily constitutes a complete antiretroviral treatment regimen.	$2520.00
Descovy	TAF 25 mg Emtricitabine 200 mg	One pill daily along with an NNRTI, protease inhibitor, integrase inhibitor, or maraviroc (entry inhibitor). The difference between Descovy and Truvada is that Descovy has a different form of tenofovir (TAF) that appears to be safer than the form of tenofovir (TDF) in Truvada because TAF has less effect on kidney function and bone mineral density. Descovy is not approved for use as PrEP.	$2109.48
Dovato	Dolutegravir 50 mg Lamivudine 300 mg	One pill daily constitutes a complete antiretroviral treatment regimen in adults with no antiviral treatment and no known substitutions associated with resistance to either component.	$2754.00
Epzicom	Abacavir 600 mg Lamivudine 300 mg	One pill daily along with an NNRTI, protease inhibitor, integrase inhibitor, or maraviroc (entry inhibitor).	$1550.05
Genvoya	TAF 10 mg Emtricitabine 200 mg Elvitegravir 150 mg Cobicistat 150 mg	One pill daily constitutes a complete antiretroviral treatment regimen. Although it contains four medications, one component (cobicistat) is a medication booster only. The only difference between Stribild and Genvoya is that Genvoya has a different form of tenofovir (TAF) that appears to be safer than tenofovir TDF with less effect on kidney function and bone mineral density.	$3707.99
Juluca	Dolutegravir 50 mg Rilpivirine 25 mg	One pill daily with a meal for patients who have been virologically suppressed (viral load < 50 copies/mL) on a stable antiretroviral treatment regimen for 6 months or more and no history of treatment failure or resistance to dolutegravir or rilpivirine.	$3249.54
Odefsey	TAF 25 mg Emtricitabine 200 mg Rilpivirine 25 mg	One pill daily constitutes a complete antiretroviral treatment regimen. Only for patients with no history of HIV viral load greater or equal to 100,000 copies/mL or replacement of stable antiretroviral regimen in patients fully suppressed for more than 6 months, with no history of treatment failure, and with no known resistance to components of the drug combination.	$3374.56
Stribild	TDF 300 mg Emtricitabine 200 mg Elvitegravir 150 mg Cobicistat 150 mg	One pill daily constitutes a complete antiretroviral treatment regimen. Although it contains four medications, one component (cobicistat) is a medication booster only.	$3889.68
Symtuza	TAF 10 mg Emtricitabine 200 mg Darunavir 800 mg Cobicistat 150 mg	One pill daily constitutes a complete antiretroviral treatment regimen. Although it contains four medications, one component (cobicistat) is a medication booster only. One of the recommended initial treatment regimens.	$4466.71
Triumeq	Abacavir 600 mg Lamivudine 300 mg Dolutegravir 50 mg	One pill constitutes a complete antiretroviral treatment regimen. One of the recommended initial treatment regimens.	$3467.23
Trizivir	Abacavir 300 mg Lamivudine 150 mg Zidovudine 300 mg	One tablet twice daily with an NNRTI, protease inhibitor, integrase inhibitor, or maraviroc (entry inhibitor). Although it contains three medications it *does not* constitute a complete antiretroviral treatment regimen.	$1931.64
Truvada	TDF 300 mg Emtricitabine 200 mg	One pill daily with an NNRTI, protease inhibitor, integrase inhibitor, or maraviroc (entry inhibitor). TDF is the most commonly used NRTI backbone.	$2109.48

NNRTI, non-nucleoside reverse transcriptase inhibitor (eg, delavirdine, efavirenz, etravirine, nevirapine, rilpivirine); NRTI, nucleoside/nucleotide reverse transcriptase inhibitor (eg, abacavir, didanosine, emtricitabine, lamivudine, stavudine, tenofovir, zidovudine); PrEP, preexposure prophylaxis; TAF, tenofovir alafenamide; TDF, tenofovir disoproxil fumarate.

Average wholesale price (AWP, for AB-rated generic when available) for quantity listed. Source: IBM Micromedex Red Book (electronic version) IBM Watson Health, Greenwood Village, CO, USA. Available at https://www.micromedexsolutions.com (cited April 25, 2019). AWP may not accurately represent the actual pharmacy cost because wide contractual variations exist among institutions.

Abacavir is also formulated with zidovudine and lamivudine in a single pill (Trizivir, one tablet orally twice daily; Table 31–8). Trizivir is not recommended as solo treatment for HIV because it is not as efficacious as combining two nucleoside/nucleotide analogs with a ritonavir-boosted PI, an NNRTI, or an integrase inhibitor.

E. TENOFOVIR—Tenofovir is the only licensed nucleotide analog. It comes in two forms: tenofovir disoproxil fumarate (TDF) and tenofovir alafenamide (TAF). TDF is available for use both in the form of a single pill at an oral dose of 300 mg once daily and as an oral fixed-dose combination pill with emtricitabine 200 mg (Truvada; Table 31–8) once daily. Several other single-tablet once-a-day complete regimens include TDF (Atripla, Complera, Stribild) (Table 31–8). Tenofovir is active against hepatitis B, including isolates that have resistance to lamivudine. TDF is associated with a clinically modest loss of kidney function, a small increased risk of acute renal injury, and increased rate of bone resorption. It should not be used in patients at risk for kidney disease or without dose adjustment in those with creatinine clearance below 60 mL/min or in those with or at risk for osteopenia/osteoporosis. For these patients, TAF is the better choice.

TAF attains higher levels in cells with a much lower plasma level. For this reason, it appears to cause less harm to kidneys and less bone resorption. It is not available as a single agent but is available in a combination tablet with emtricitabine (Descovy, Table 31–8). Single-tablet once-a-day regimens that include TAF (Genvoya and Odefsey) are also available (Table 31–8). TAF should not be used with rifamycins.

Because of concern regarding nephrotoxicity for both TDF and TAF, it is recommended that the serum creatinine be checked at baseline, at 2–8 weeks, and then every 3–6 months and that a urinalysis and urine glucose and protein be checked at baseline and monitored periodically as clinically indicated.

F. DIDANOSINE—The most convenient formulation of didanosine is the enteric-coated capsule. For adults weighing at least 60 kg, the dose is one 400-mg enteric-coated capsule orally daily; for those 30–59 kg, the dose is one 250-mg enteric-coated capsule orally daily. Didanosine should be taken on an empty stomach.

Didanosine has been associated with pancreatitis. The incidence of pancreatitis with didanosine is 5–10%—of fatal pancreatitis, less than 0.4%. Patients with a history of pancreatitis, as well as those taking other medications associated with pancreatitis (including trimethoprim-sulfamethoxazole and intravenous pentamidine) are at higher risk for this complication. Other common side effects with didanosine include a dose-related, reversible, painful peripheral neuropathy, which occurs in about 15% of patients, and dry mouth. Fulminant hepatic failure and electrolyte abnormalities, including hypokalemia, hypocalcemia, and hypomagnesemia, have been reported in patients taking didanosine. Because of the side-effect profile, didanosine is rarely used today.

2. Nonnucleoside reverse transcriptase inhibitors—NNRTIs inhibit reverse transcriptase at a site different from that of the nucleoside and nucleotide agents described above. The major advantage of NNRTIs is that four of them (efavirenz, rilpivirine, doravirine, and nevirapine) have potencies comparable to that of PI (next section), at least for patients with viral loads under 100,000 copies/mL—with lower pill burden and fewer side effects. Unlike PI, they do not appear to cause lipodystrophy; patients with cholesterol and triglyceride elevations who are switched from a PI to an NNRTI may have improvement in their lipids. The resistance patterns of NNRTIs are distinct from those of the PI. Because these agents may cause alterations in the clearance of PIs, dose modifications may be necessary when these two classes of medications are administered concomitantly. There is a high degree of cross-resistance among the "first-generation" NNRTIs, such that resistance to one medication in this class uniformly predicts resistance to other medications. However, the "second-generation" NNRTI etravirine appears to have consistent antiviral activity in patients with prior exposure and resistance to nevirapine, efavirenz, or delavirdine. In particular, the *K103N* mutation does not appear to have an impact on etravirine (or rilpivirine). There is no therapeutic reason for using more than one NNRTI at the same time.

A. EFAVIRENZ—The major advantages of efavirenz are that it can be given once daily in a single dose (600 mg orally) and is available in a once-daily fixed-dose combination with TDF and emtricitabine in a single pill (Atripla; Table 31–8). The major side effects are rash and psychiatric/neurologic complaints, with patients reporting symptoms ranging from lack of concentration and strange dreams to delusions and mania. These side effects tend to wane over time, usually within a month or so; however, there are some patients who cannot tolerate these effects, especially if they persist longer than a month. Participant level data from four randomized trials of efavirenz regimens versus non-efavirenz containing regimens found increased suicidality (hazard ratio of 2.6) among those taking efavirenz. Administration of efavirenz with food, especially fatty food, may increase its serum levels and consequent neurotoxicity. Therefore, it should be taken on an empty stomach; taking before bedtime may also reduce patients' experience of neuropsychiatric symptoms.

B. DORAVIRINE—Dosed at 100 mg orally daily, this drug can be taken with or without food. Two 48-week Phase III studies showed that, in previously untreated individuals, doravirine, when used with two NRTIs resulted in similar levels of viral suppression as efavirenz plus two NRTIs or darunavir/ritonavir plus two NRTIs. It is also available as a single-pill combination with TDF and lamivudine (Delstrigo; Table 31–8). It is well tolerated. In cases of virologic failure, NNRTI cross-resistance may develop.

C. RILPIVIRINE—This medication, dosed at 25 mg once daily, is equal in efficacy to efavirenz in patients with HIV viral loads below 100,000 copies/mL. Rilpivirine should not be used in patients with baseline viral loads of 100,000 copies/mL or greater or those with CD4 counts below 200 cells/mcL because of greater risk of viral failure. As is true of efavirenz, rilpivirine is available in a once-daily fixed-dose combination with TDF and emtricitabine (Complera; Table 31–8) and with TAF and emtricitabine

(Odefsey; Table 31–8) to be taken with a meal. It is also available in a two-drug regimen with dolutegravir (Juluca, Table 31–8). Proton pump inhibitors should not be given with rilpivirine. Rilpivirine has fewer neurologic side effects than efavirenz.

D. Nevirapine—The dose of nevirapine is 400 mg orally daily (extended release), but it is initiated at a dose of 200 mg once a day to decrease the incidence of rash, which is as high as 40% when full doses are begun immediately. If rash develops while the patient is taking 200 mg daily, liver enzymes should be checked and the dose should not be increased until the rash resolves. Patients with mild rash and no evidence of hepatotoxicity can continue to be treated with nevirapine. Nevirapine should not be used in treatment-naïve women with CD4 counts greater than 250 cells/mcL or in males with CD4 counts greater than 400 cells/mcL because they have greater risk of hepatotoxicity. In general, because of the risk of fatal hepatotoxicity, nevirapine should be used only when there is not a better alternative.

E. Delavirdine—Of the available NNRTIs, delavirdine is used the least largely because of its inconvenient dosing and pill burden compared with the other available NNRTIs. Unlike nevirapine and efavirenz, delavirdine inhibits P450 cytochromes rather than inducing these enzymes. This means that delavirdine can act like ritonavir and boost other antiretrovirals, although delavirdine is not as potent as ritonavir in this capacity. The dosage is 400 mg orally three times a day. The major side effect is rash.

F. Etravirine—Etravirine is an NNRTI approved for the treatment of patients with prior NNRTI intolerance or resistance. Etravirine has been shown to be effective even when some degree of NNRTI resistance is present, making it a true "second-generation" medication in this class. Etravirine dosage is one 200-mg tablet twice daily. It should be used with a PI and an NRTI and not just with two NRTIs. The most common side effects are nausea and rash; rarely, the rash can be severe (toxic epidermal necrolysis). Patients with signs of severe rash or hypersensitivity reactions should immediately discontinue the medication. Prior rash due to treatment with one of the other NNRTIs does not make rash more likely with etravirine. Etravirine should not be taken by people with severe liver disease or administered with tipranavir/ritonavir, fosamprenavir/ritonavir, atazanavir/ritonavir, full-dose ritonavir, or PI without low-dose ritonavir.

3. Protease inhibitors—Ten PIs—indinavir, nelfinavir, ritonavir, saquinavir, amprenavir, fosamprenavir, lopinavir (in combination with ritonavir), atazanavir, darunavir, and tipranavir—are available. PIs are potent suppressors of HIV replication and are administered as part of a combination regimen.

All of the PIs—to differing degrees—are metabolized by the cytochrome P450 system, and each can inhibit and induce various P450 isoenzymes. Therefore, medication interactions are common and difficult to predict. Clinicians should consult the product inserts before prescribing PIs with other medications. Medications such as rifampin that are known to induce the P450 system should be avoided.

The fact that the PIs are dependent on metabolism through the cytochrome P450 system has led to the use of ritonavir to boost the medication levels of saquinavir, lopinavir, indinavir, atazanavir, tipranavir, darunavir, and amprenavir, allowing use of lower doses and simpler dosing schedules of these PIs. A second boosting agent, cobicistat, is coformulated with the PI atazanavir (Evotaz) and darunavir (Prescobix). Similar to ritonavir, cobicistat also inhibits liver enzymes that metabolize other HIV medications.

In fact, guidelines recommend that all PI-containing regimens except nelfinavir use boosting if possible.

When choosing which PI to use, prior patient experience, resistance patterns, side effects, and ease of administration are the major considerations. The first three PIs to be developed—indinavir, saquinavir, and ritonavir (as single agents)—are now rarely used because of the superiority of the second generation of PIs. Amprenavir has been almost entirely replaced by its prodrug, fosamprenavir. Unfortunately, all PIs, with the exception of unboosted atazanavir have been linked to a constellation of metabolic abnormalities, including elevated cholesterol levels, elevated triglyceride levels, insulin resistance, diabetes mellitus, and changes in body fat composition (eg, buffalo hump, abdominal obesity). The lipid abnormalities and body habitus changes are referred to as **lipodystrophy.** Although lipodystrophy is commonly associated with PIs, it has been seen also in HIV-infected persons who have never been treated with these agents. In particular, the lipoatrophy effects seen in patients receiving antiretroviral treatment appears to be more related to the nucleoside toxicity and in particular to the thymidine analogs (stavudine and zidovudine).

Of the different manifestations of lipodystrophy, the dyslipidemias that occur are of particular concern because of the likelihood that increased levels of cholesterol and triglycerides will result in increased prevalence of heart disease. All patients taking PIs or NRTIs should have fasting serum cholesterol, low-density lipoprotein (LDL) cholesterol, and triglyceride levels performed every 12 months. Clinicians should assess for coronary heart disease risk (see Chapter 28) and consider initiating dietary changes or medication therapy (or both). PIs inhibit statin metabolism. Lovastatin and simvastatin should be avoided. In general, the least interaction is with pravastatin (20 mg daily orally). Atorvastatin (10 mg daily orally) or rosuvastatin (5 mg/day orally initially; maximum 10 mg/day) may also be used cautiously. Fish oil (3000 mg daily) combined with exercise and dietary counseling has been found to decrease triglyceride levels by 25%. Patients with persistently elevated fasting serum triglyceride levels of 500 mg/dL or more who do not respond to dietary intervention should be treated with gemfibrozil (600 mg twice daily prior to the morning and evening meals). PIs are associated with abnormalities in cardiac conduction, especially prolongation of the PR interval.

A. Indinavir—Indinavir is usually dosed at 800 mg twice daily in combination with 100 mg of ritonavir twice daily. Nausea and headache are common complaints with this medication. Indinavir crystals are present in the urine in approximately 40% of patients; this results in clinically apparent nephrolithiasis in about 15% of patients receiving indinavir. Lower urinary tract symptoms and acute kidney injury also have been reported. Patients taking this medication should be instructed to drink at least 48 ounces of fluid a day to ensure adequate hydration in an attempt to limit these complications. Mild indirect hyperbilirubinemia is also commonly observed in patients taking indinavir but is not an indication for discontinuation of the medication.

B. SAQUINAVIR—Saquinavir is formulated only as a hard-gel capsule (Invirase). It should be used only with ritonavir (1000 mg of hard-gel saquinavir with 100 mg of ritonavir orally twice daily). The most common side effects with saquinavir are diarrhea, nausea, dyspepsia, and abdominal pain.

C. RITONAVIR—Use of this potent PI at full dose (600 mg orally twice daily) has been limited by its inhibition of the cytochrome P450 pathway causing a large number of drug-drug interactions and by its frequent side effects of fatigue, nausea, and paresthesias. However, it is widely used in lower dose (eg, 100 mg daily to 100 mg twice daily) as a booster of other PIs.

D. NELFINAVIR—Nelfinavir is the only PI for which ritonavir boosting is not recommended. Unboosted nelfinavir is generally not as potent as a boosted PI regimen (eg, lopinavir plus ritonavir). The dose of nelfinavir is 1250 mg orally twice daily. Diarrhea is a side effect in 25% of patients taking nelfinavir, but this symptom may be controlled with over-the-counter antidiarrheal agents in most patients.

E. AMPRENAVIR—Amprenavir has efficacy and side effects similar to those of other PIs. Common side effects are nausea, vomiting, diarrhea, rash, and perioral paresthesia. The dose is 1200 mg orally twice daily. The concentration of amprenavir decreases when coadministered with ethinyl estradiol; therefore, amprenavir should be used with circumspection in the treatment of transgender persons requiring high-dose estrogen.

F. FOSAMPRENAVIR—Fosamprenavir is a prodrug of amprenavir. Its major advantage over using amprenavir is a much lower pill burden. For PI-naïve patients, it can be dosed at 1400 mg orally twice daily (four capsules a day) or at 1400 mg orally daily (two capsules) with ritonavir 200 mg orally daily (two capsules) or at 700 mg orally with ritonavir 100 mg orally twice daily. Patients previously treated with a PI should receive 700 mg orally with ritonavir 100 mg orally twice daily. Side effects are similar to those with amprenavir—most commonly gastrointestinal distress and hyperlipidemia. As with amprenavir, the concentration of fosamprenavir decreases when coadministered with ethinyl estradiol; therefore, fosamprenavir should be used with circumspection in the treatment of transgender persons requiring high-dose estrogen.

G. LOPINAVIR/R—Lopinavir/r is lopinavir (200 mg) coformulated with a low dose of ritonavir (50 mg) to maximize the bioavailability of lopinavir. It has been shown to be more effective than nelfinavir when used in combination with stavudine and lamivudine. The usual dose is lopinavir 400 mg with ritonavir 100 mg (two tablets) orally twice daily with food. When given along with efavirenz or nevirapine, a higher dose (600 mg/150 mg—three tablets) is usually prescribed. The most common side effect is diarrhea, and lipid abnormalities are frequent. Because of these side effects, lopinavir/r has fallen off the list of medications recommended as part of first-line treatment regimens.

H. ATAZANAVIR—Atazanavir is available alone and coformulated with cobicistat (Evotaz). Atazanavir can be dosed as 400 mg (two 200-mg capsules) daily with food or it can be dosed as 300 mg in combination with 100 mg of ritonavir once daily with food. When coformulated with cobicistat, it is dosed at 300-mg atazanavir and 150-mg cobicistat. The most common side effect is mild hyperbilirubinemia that resolves with discontinuation of the medication. Nephrolithiasis and cholelithiasis have also been reported with this PI. Both tenofovir and efavirenz lower the serum concentration of atazanavir. Therefore, when either of these two medications is used with atazanavir, it should be boosted by administering ritonavir or given coformulated with cobicistat. Proton pump inhibitors are contraindicated in patients taking atazanavir because atazanavir requires an acidic pH to remain in solution.

I. TIPRANAVIR—Tipranavir is the only nonpeptidic PI approved by the US Food and Drug Administration (FDA). Because of its unique structure, it is active against some strains of HIV that are resistant to other PIs. It is dosed with ritonavir (two 250-mg capsules of tipranavir with two 100-mg capsules of ritonavir orally twice daily with food). The most common side effects are nausea, vomiting, diarrhea, fatigue, and headache. Tipranavir/ritonavir has been also associated with liver damage and should be used very cautiously in patients with underlying liver disease. Reports of intracranial hemorrhage in patients taking tipranavir-containing regimens have raised additional safety concerns about this potent PI. Because it is a sulfa-containing medication, its use should be closely monitored in patients with sulfa allergy.

J. DARUNAVIR—Darunavir has impressive antiviral activity in the setting of significant PI resistance and in treatment-naïve patients. It is formulated by itself and coformulated with cobicistat (Prezcobix). When formulated without cobicistat it requires boosting with ritonavir. For initial treatment of HIV or for treatment-experienced patients without darunavir-related resistance mutations, daily dosing is 800 mg of darunavir with 100 mg of ritonavir or with 150 mg of cobicistat. Darunavir 800 mg is also available in a coformulated tablet with emtricitabine, TAF, and cobicistat (Symtuza, Table 31–8). It has been approved for use by the FDA and the European Commission. For patients with prior PI treatment experience or PI resistance (with mutations known to impact darunavir), darunavir should be dosed at 600 mg orally twice daily, with ritonavir, 100 mg orally twice daily. Darunavir has a safety profile similar to other PIs, such as ritonavir-boosted lopinavir, but is generally better tolerated. Like tipranavir, darunavir is a sulfa-containing medication, and its use should be closely monitored in patients with sulfa allergy.

4. Entry inhibitors—

A. ENFUVIRTIDE—Enfuvirtide (Fuzeon) is known as a fusion inhibitor; it blocks the entry of HIV into cells by blocking the fusion of the HIV envelope to the cell membrane. The addition of enfuvirtide to an optimized antiretroviral regimen improved CD4 counts and lowered viral loads in heavily pretreated patients with multidrug-resistant HIV. Unfortunately, resistance develops rapidly in patients receiving nonsuppressive treatment. The dose is 90 mg by subcutaneous injection twice daily; unfortunately, painful injection site reactions develop in most patients, which makes long-term use problematic.

B. MARAVIROC—Maraviroc is a CCR5 co-receptor antagonist. Medications in this class prevent the virus from entering uninfected cells by blocking the CCR5 co-receptor. Before starting therapy, a viral tropism assay should be performed because this class of entry inhibitors is only active against "CCR5-tropic virus." This form of the HIV-1 virus tends to predominate early in infection, while so-called dual/mixed tropic virus (which utilizes either R5 or CXCR4 co-receptors) emerges later as infection progresses. Approximately 50–60% of previously treated HIV-infected patients have circulating CCR5-tropic HIV. The medication has been shown to be effective in HIV-infected persons with ongoing viral replication despite being heavily treated and who have CCR5-tropic virus. The dose of maraviroc is 150–300 mg orally twice daily, based on the other medications the patient is taking at the time—in combination with a ritonavir boosted PI, 150 mg daily of maraviroc has been used successfully. Common side effects are cough, fever, rash, musculoskeletal problems, abdominal pain, and dizziness; however, maraviroc is generally well tolerated with limited impact on serum lipids.

5. Integrase inhibitors—

Integrase inhibitors slow HIV replication by blocking the HIV integrase enzyme needed for the virus to multiply. They are now the preferred regimens for initiating therapy because of the combination of efficacy, ease of administration, and low incidence of side effects. Four integrase inhibitors are currently available: raltegravir, elvitegravir, dolutegravir and bictegravir. A fifth agent, cabotegravir, currently in phase III testing, can be coformulated with rilpivirine in a long-acting injectable form; it may prove to be an effective two-drug antiretroviral treatment regimen for patients successfully suppressed on a three-drug regimen. Clinical trials of available integrase inhibitors reveal a consistent pattern of more rapid decline in viral load compared with more standard PI/r or NNRTI-based regimens. Integrase inhibitors are effective (when combined with other active medications) in the treatment of HIV-infected patients with documented resistance to each of the three main classes of antiretroviral medications (nucleoside analogs, PIs, NNRTIs). Avoid administering integrase inhibitors with antacids or other medications with divalent cations (Ca^{2+}, Mg^{2+}, Al^{2+}, Fe^{2+}) because chelation of the integrase inhibitor by the cation reduces absorption. When these medications must be taken with integrase inhibitors, consult a pharmacist to determine the best separation of times of administration.

A. RALTEGRAVIR—The dose of raltegravir is 400 mg orally twice daily. It has been found to be superior to efavirenz and ritonavir-boosted darunavir and ritonavir-boosted atazanavir. It is the recommended integrase inhibitor for pregnant women. Common side effects are diarrhea, nausea, and headache, but overall, it is well tolerated and has the additional advantage over PI-based regimens and efavirenz-based regimens in that it appears to have little impact on lipid profiles or glucose metabolism.

B. ELVITEGRAVIR—Elvitegravir is not manufactured as a single agent. It can be prescribed in a once-a-day combination pill (Stribild) that contains 125 mg of elvitegravir and 150 mg of cobicistat, a boosting agent, along with standard doses of TDF and emtricitabine (Table 31–8). Stribild has been shown to be noninferior to two preferred first-line regimens: Atripla and boosted atazanavir with emtricitabine/ TDF. The main side effect of Stribild is an increase in serum creatinine levels that has been shown to be related to the cobicistat inhibition of tubular secretion of creatinine by the kidney and is thought to be nonpathologic and reversible. However, because of this effect, Stribild is recommended in patients with estimated creatinine clearance greater than 70 mL/min. A urine analysis should be done at baseline and at initial follow-up to look for proteinuria and glycosuria, which are signs of tubulopathy. Diarrhea and rash may also occur, although overall the medication is well tolerated. Elvitegravir is also coformulated with emtricitabine and TAF along with cobicistat boosting in a single once-a-day pill (Genvoya, Table 31–8). Since TAF appears to have fewer side effects than TDF, this is likely to become the preferred elvitegravir regimen.

C. DOLUTEGRAVIR—Dolutegravir shows excellent potency and tolerability and is dosed once a day in most circumstances. It has been shown to be superior to efavirenz and darunavir. Unlike elvitegravir, dolutegravir does not require a boosting agent and has fewer drug-drug interactions. Similar to cobicistat, it inhibits tubular secretion of creatinine by the kidney, resulting in small increases in serum creatinine levels. The standard dosage used in treatment-naïve, integrase-naïve patients is 50 mg/day. It is available combined with abacavir and lamivudine in a single once a day tablet (Triumeq, Table 31–8). In patients receiving efavirenz, fosamprenavir/ritonavir, tipranavir/ ritonavir, or rifampin, the dose should be increased to 50 mg twice daily. It should also be dosed at 50 mg twice daily in integrase-experienced patients in whom integrase resistance is suspected. Indeed, when combined with other active medications, it has been shown to provide some activity in patients with integrase resistance who have not responded to prior raltegravir- or elvitegravir-containing regimens. Dolutegravir has demonstrated impressive results in clinical trials of treatment-naïve patients, in terms of effectiveness, tolerability, and high barrier to resistance, when compared with the more standard NNRTI, boosted PI, and raltegravir-containing regimens. Dolutegravir is coformulated in combination with rilpivirine (Juluca, Table 31–8) for use as a once-a-day (to be taken with a meal) treatment for patients who are virologically suppressed (viral load less than 50 copies/mL) on a stable regimen for at least 6 months, with no history of treatment failures or resistance to either of the two agents.

D. Bictegravir—Bictegravir is dosed once daily, does not require boosting, and has a high barrier to resistance. It is dosed at 50 mg daily. It has been shown to be noninferior to dolutegravir. It is not available as a single agent but is marketed as a fixed-dose combination of bictegravir with emtricitabine and TAF.

6. Ibalizumab—A novel treatment for HIV, ibalizumab is a monoclonal antibody that blocks the entry of HIV into the CD4 cell by blocking the CD4 receptor. Given as an intravenous infusion therapy along with other oral HIV medications, it is used as rescue therapy for patients with multidrug-resistant HIV that is not controlled by other treatments.

7. Constructing an initial regimen—Consensus guidelines of the International Antiviral Society—USA Panel recommend starting antiretroviral treatment with one of three integrase inhibitor–containing regimens (Table 31–9). For the two regimens that use tenofovir, the TAF form is recommended due to less kidney and bone toxicity. All three regimens are available as a single once a day pill.

Studies have shown dolutegravir/abacavir/lamivudine to be superior to efavirenz/TDF/emtricitabine and have shown dolutegravir to be superior to ritonavir-boosted darunavir (both combined with either abacavir/lamivudine or TDF/emtricitabine). A network meta-analysis adjusting for NRTI backbone found that dolutegravir had superior efficacy in suppressing viral load compared with regimens containing ritonavir-boosted atazanavir, ritonavir-boosted darunavir, efavirenz, or ritonavir-boosted lopinavir. Discontinuation due to adverse events was also statistically lower in the dolutegravir regimens.

The drug combinations incorporating the integrase inhibitor raltegravir have done well in comparative studies. Among treatment-naïve patients, raltegravir in combination with TDF/emtricitabine is as effective as efavirenz/TDF/emtricitabine for daily treatment and has fewer side effects. In a 5-year follow-up to the double-blind trial, the raltegravir arm outperformed the efavirenz combination regimen largely due to better long-term tolerability. Furthermore, the CD4 response appeared better in patients treated with the raltegravir combination.

Neural tube defects have been reported in the offspring of women taking dolutegravir at conception, so the drug should be avoided in women who may become pregnant. For now, raltegravir is the integrase inhibitor recommended for women who are already pregnant. Elvitegravir/cobicistat and other drugs boosted with cobicistat should not be used during pregnancy and neither should bictegravir (because of lack of data regarding adverse effects). Recommended drugs in pregnancy include atazanavir/ritonavir, darunavir/ritonavir, efavirenz, and rilpivirine.

For patients who cannot take an integrase inhibitor, alternative regimens are recommended (Table 31–9).

Resistance testing should be performed prior to starting antiretroviral treatment. Of newly infected persons in some urban areas of the United States, 8–10% have NNRTI resistance (primarily *K103N*). Patients with NNRTI resistance would not be expected to respond fully to an efavirenz-based regimen. The most important determinant of treatment efficacy is adherence to the regimen. Therefore, it is vitally important that the regimen chosen be one to which the patient can easily adhere (Figure 31–7). In general, patients are more compliant with medication regimens (Table 31–9) that offer a complete regimen in one pill that needs to be taken only once or twice a day, do not require special timing with regard to meals, can be taken at the same time as other medications, do not require refrigeration or special preparation, and do not have bothersome side effects. Given the high level of effectiveness of recommended regimens, patients for whom the viral load does not fully suppress are likely noncompliant. Pharmacists and other specially trained clinicians can be very effective in helping patients improve their adherence by taking the time to understand why patients miss their medications and problem solve (eg, take medicine at same time every day, keep a supply in the car or at work in case they forget). For certain populations (eg, unstably housed individuals), specially tailored programs that include medication dispensing are needed.

E. Monitoring Antiretroviral Treatment

1. Goals of monitoring antiretroviral treatment—Monitoring of antiretroviral treatment (Figure 31–7) has two goals: evaluate for toxicity and measure efficacy using objective markers to determine whether to maintain or change regimens. Laboratory evaluation for toxicity depends on the specific medications in the combination but generally should be done approximately every 3–4 months once a patient is on a stable regimen. Patients who are intolerant of their initial regimen should be changed to one of the other initial recommended or alternative regimens in Table 31–9. The second aspect of monitoring is to measure objective markers of efficacy. The CD4 cell count and HIV viral load should be repeated 1–2 months after the initiation or change of antiretroviral regimen and every 3–6 months thereafter in clinically stable patients. With integrase regimens, approximately 80% of patients will have undetectable HIV viral load at 1 month. All patients should have undetectable viral loads by 3 months; if not, the usual problem is compliance (see next section). (Patients receiving antiretroviral treatment with undetectable viral load for 2 years and CD4 counts 300 cells/mcL or more may need CD4 testing only every 12 months.)

2. The challenge of compliance—In a patient who is adherent to an effective regimen, viral loads should be undetectable within 4–12 weeks. For patients in whom viral loads are not suppressed or who have viral rebound after suppression, the major question facing the clinician is whether the patient is nonadherent or has resistance to the regimen, or both. The issue is complicated because many patients report being more compliant than they really are. Patients who are having trouble adhering to their treatment should receive counseling on how to better comply with their treatment. In patients who are adherent or who have missed enough doses to make resistance possible,

Table 31–9. Recommended and alternative initial antiretroviral regimens and other commonly used three-drug regimens[1] (alphabetical order).

Regimen	Advantages	Disadvantages
Recommended Initial Regimens		
Bictegravir + TAF + emtricitabine (Bictarvy)	Single pill once-a-day regimen Low risk of resistance Noninferior to dolutegravir	Less experience than with dolutegravir
Dolutegravir + abacavir + lamivudine[2] (Triumeq)	Single pill once-a-day regimen Low risk of resistance Superior to Atripla Dolutegravir plus either abacavir/lamivudine or emtricitabine/TDF is superior to darunavir/ritonavir plus either of the NRTI backbones	Abacavir should be used only in HLA-B*5701-negative persons When used in patients with integrase resistance or combined with certain other medications, requires twice-a-day dosing
Dolutegravir (50 mg daily) + emtricitabine/TAF	Has activity in some patients with integrase resistance Once-a-day regimen	No single tablet available When used in patients with integrase resistance or combined with certain other medications, requires twice-a-day dosing
Other Integrase Inhibitor Regimens		
Emtricitabine/TAF/elvitegravir with cobicistat boosting (Genvoya)	Single tablet once-a-day regimen Excellent response across broad range of CD4 and viral loads	Lower barrier to resistance than bictegravir and dolutegravir Cobicistat boosting causes similar drug-drug interactions as ritonavir; increases in serum creatinine (nonpathologic) No dosage adjustment with estimated creatinine clearance > 30 mL/min
Emtricitabine/TDF/elvitegravir with cobicistat boosting (Stribild)	Single tablet once-a-day regimen Excellent response across broad range of CD4 and viral loads	Cobicistat boosting causes similar drug-drug interactions as ritonavir; increases in serum creatinine (nonpathologic) Requires estimated creatinine clearance ≥ 70 mL/min.
Raltegravir (400 mg twice daily) + emtricitabine + TAF or TDF	Superior to Atripla over 5 years of follow-up (when studied with TDF form of tenofovir)	Lower barrier to resistance than bictegravir and dolutegravir Requires twice-a-day dosing No single tablet available
Alternative Initial Regimens for Patients Who Cannot Take an Integrase Inhibitor		
Darunavir (800 mg daily) with cobicistat + emtricitabine + TAF or TDF	Single table once-a-day regimen (with TAF)	Cobicistat boosting causes similar drug-drug interactions as ritonavir; increases in serum creatinine (nonpathologic)
Darunavir (800 mg daily) with ritonavir (100 mg daily) boosting + emtricitabine + TAF or TDF	Potent boosted PI Can be given once daily Limited risk of resistance with poor adherence	Not available as a single tablet May cause rash in patients with sulfa allergy Ritonavir boosting required Has metabolic side effects
Efavirenz/emtricitabine/TDF (Atripla)	Single tablet once-a-day regimen Longest-term clinical experience Highly effective across broad range of initial CD4 counts and viral loads	Avoid in patients with transmitted K103N resistance Neuropsychiatric symptoms common and can be persistent
Rilpivirine/emtricitabine/TDF (Complera) or with emtricitabine/TAF (Odefsey)	Single tablet once-a-day regimen Noninferior to Atripla in patients with baseline viral load < 100,000/mcL Limited metabolic side effects	Requires taking with a meal Cannot be used with proton pump inhibitors Use only in patients with viral loads < 100,000 copies/mL and CD4 counts > 200 cells/mcL Do not use in patients with viral loads > 100,000 copies/mL or CD4 counts < 200 cells/mcL

[1]These recommended and alternative initial regimens are drawn from Saag MS et al. Antiretroviral drugs for treatment and prevention of HIV infection in adults: 2018 recommendations of the International Antiviral Society—USA Panel. JAMA. 2018;320(4):379–96.
[2]Usual medication doses are supplied when not part of a fixed-dose preparation.
TAF, tenofovir alafenamide; TDF, tenofovir disoproxil fumarate.

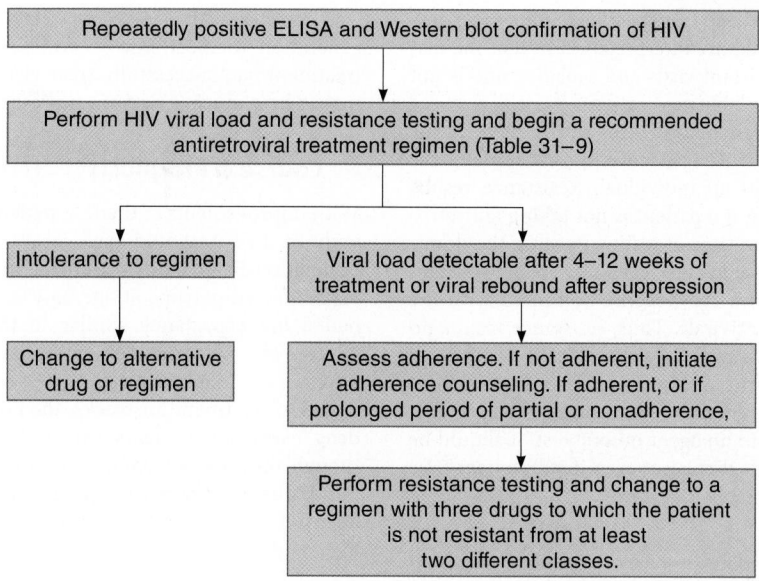

▲ **Figure 31–7.** Approach to monitoring initial and subsequent antiretroviral therapy.

resistance testing should be performed. Based on the results of resistance testing, and assessment of the patient's ability to comply with complicated regimens or to tolerate predictable side effects, the clinician should prescribe a combination of three medications to which there is no or only minimal resistance.

Once antiretroviral treatment has been initiated, it is not advisable to stop the therapy unless there is a compelling reason (eg, toxicity, poor adherence, etc). So-called drug holidays or structured treatment interruptions have been shown to increase risk of AIDS-related complications, increase CD4 declines, and increase morbidity from non–AIDS-related complications (eg, myocardial infarctions and liver failure) and are not recommended.

3. The challenge of medication resistance—HIV-1 medication resistance limits the ability to fully control HIV replication and remains an important cause for antiretroviral regimen failure. Resistance has been documented for all currently available antiretrovirals including the newer classes of fusion inhibitor, CCR5 inhibitors, and integrase inhibitors. Although HIV medication resistance has been common historically, reports suggest that the degree of high-level resistance is declining in the past few years, which is likely related to better tolerated, easier to use, and more efficacious antiretroviral agents. Resistance also occurs in patients who are antiretroviral treatment-naïve, but who have been infected with a medication resistant strain—primary resistance or transmitted medication resistance. Cohort studies of antiretroviral treatment-naïve patients entering care in North America and Western Europe show that roughly 10–12% (and as high as 25%) of recently infected individuals have been infected with a medication-resistant strain of HIV-1.

In addition to being performed as part of a standard baseline, resistance testing is also recommended for patients who are receiving antiretroviral treatment and have suboptimal viral suppression (ie, viral loads greater than 200 copies/mL). Both genotypic and phenotypic tests are commercially available and in randomized controlled studies their use has been shown to result in improved short-term virologic outcomes compared to making treatment choices without resistance testing. Furthermore, multiple retrospective studies have conclusively demonstrated that resistance tests provide prognostic information about virologic response to newly initiated therapy that cannot be gleaned from standard clinical information (ie, treatment history, examination, CD4 count, and viral load tests).

Because of the complexity of resistance tests, many clinicians require expert interpretation of results. In the case of genotypic assays, results may show that the mutations that are selected for during antiretroviral treatment are medication-specific or contribute to broad cross-resistance to multiple medications within a therapeutic class. An example of a medication-specific mutation for the reverse transcriptase inhibitors would be the *M184V* mutation that is selected for by lamivudine or emtricitabine therapy—this mutation causes resistance only to those two medications. Conversely, the thymidine analog mutations ("TAMs") of *M41L*, *D67N*, *K70R*, *L210W*, *T215Y/F*, and *T219Q/K/E* are selected for by either zidovudine or stavudine therapy, but cause resistance to all the medications in the class and often extend to the nucleotide inhibitor tenofovir when three or more of these TAMs are present. Further complicating the interpretation of genotypic tests is the fact that some mutations that cause resistance to one medication can actually make the virus that contains this mutation more sensitive to another medication. The *M184V* mutation, for example, is associated with increased sensitivity to zidovudine, stavudine, and tenofovir. The most common mutations associated with medication resistance and cross-resistance patterns for NRTIs, NNRTIs, PIs, and integrase inhibitors can be found at https://hivdb.stanford.edu (see specific references below). Phenotypic tests also require interpretation in that the distinction between a resistant virus and sensitive one is not fully defined for all available medications.

Both methods of resistance testing are limited by the fact that they may measure resistance in only some of the viral strains present in an individual. Resistance results may also be misleading if a patient is not taking antiretroviral medications at the time of testing because the dominant virus is likely the wild-type, even if there are resistant viruses in the body that can become dominant with the selective pressure of antivirals. Thus, resistance results do not replace a careful history of what medications a patient has taken in the past and for how long. Also, the results of resistance testing should be viewed cumulatively—ie, if resistance is reported to an agent on one test, it should be presumed to be present thereafter even if subsequent tests do not give the same result.

Stanford University HIV Drug Resistance Database Home Page (https://hivdb.stanford.edu/) provides Genotypic Resistance Interpretation Algorithm, HIVdb Program, version 8.8, February 13, 2019 (https://hivdb.stanford.edu/hivdb/by-mutations/); Genotype-Phenotype Correlations (https://hivdb.stanford.edu/pages/genotype-phenotype.html); Genotype-Treatment Correlations (https://hivdb.stanford.edu/pages/genotype-rx.html); Genotype-Clinical Outcome Correlations (https://hivdb.stanford.edu/pages/genotype-clinical.html)

F. Constructing Alternative Antiretroviral Treatment Regimens

In designing second-line regimens for patients with resistance to initial therapy, the goal is to identify three medications from at least two different classes to which the virus is not resistant. Even without resistance testing, certain forms of cross-resistance between medications within a class can be assumed. For example, the resistance patterns of lopinavir/ritonavir and indinavir are overlapping, and patients with virus resistant to these agents are unlikely to respond to nelfinavir or saquinavir even though they have never received treatment with these agents. Similarly, the resistance patterns of nevirapine and efavirenz are overlapping—as are the resistance patterns between raltegravir and elvitegravir.

In constructing regimens, toxicities should be nonoverlapping and agents that are either virologically antagonistic or incompatible in terms of drug-drug interactions should be avoided. For example, the combination of stavudine plus didanosine should be avoided, since there is increased risk of toxicities, in particular in pregnant women because of the increased risk of lactic acidosis, which can be fatal. Moreover, the nucleoside pair of zidovudine and stavudine should be avoided because of increased toxicity and the potential for antagonism that results from intracellular competition for phosphorylation. The combination of didanosine with tenofovir should be avoided because of observed declines in CD4 counts. Etravirine should not be used with boosted tipranavir because of drug-drug interactions. Lamivudine and emtricitabine are essentially the same medication and so are not used together.

Given the availability of new class medications and new generation medications, a combination of antiretroviral treatment can successfully treat virtually all patients—no matter how much resistance is present.

► Course & Prognosis

With improvements in therapy, patients who are compliant with treatment should have near normal life spans. A population-based study conducted in Denmark found that HIV-infected persons at age 25 years without hepatitis C had a life expectancy similar to that of an uninfected 25-year-old. Unfortunately, not all HIV-infected persons have access to treatment. Studies consistently show less access to treatment for blacks, the homeless, and injection drug users. For patients whose disease progresses even though they are receiving appropriate treatment, meticulous palliative care must be provided (see Chapter 5), with attention to pain control, spiritual needs, and family (biologic and chosen) dynamics.

► When to Refer

- HIV-infected patients in whom viral loads cannot be fully suppressed on one of the initial recommended regimens should be referred to specialists.

- Specialty consultation is particularly important for those patients with detectable viral loads on antiretroviral treatment; those intolerant of standard medications; those in need of systemic chemotherapy; and those with complicated opportunistic infections, particularly when invasive procedures or experimental therapies are needed.

► When to Admit

Patients with opportunistic infections who are acutely ill (eg, who are febrile, who have had rapid change of mental status, or who are in respiratory distress) or who require intravenous medications.

Cahn P et al; GEMINI Study Team. Dolutegravir plus lamivudine versus dolutegravir plus tenofovir disoproxil fumarate and emtricitabine in antiretroviral-naive adults with HIV-1 infection (GEMINI-1 and GEMINI-2): week 48 results from two multicentre, double-blind, randomised, non-inferiority, phase 3 trials. Lancet. 2019 Jan 12;393(10167):143–55. Erratum in: Lancet. 2018 Nov 28. [PMID: 30420123]

Emu B et al. Phase 3 study of ibalizumab for multidrug-resistant HIV-1. N Engl J Med. 2018 Aug 16;379(7):645–54. [PMID: 30110589]

Gallant J et al. Bictegravir, emtricitabine, and tenofovir alafenamide versus dolutegravir, abacavir, and lamivudine for initial treatment of HIV-1 infection (GS-US-380-1489): a double-blind, multicenter, phase 3 randomised controlled non-inferiority trial. Lancet. 2017 Nov 4;390 (10107):2063–72. [PMID: 28867497]

Johnson SC. Antiretroviral therapy for HIV infection: when to initiate therapy, which regimen to use, and how to monitor patients on therapy. Top Antivir Med. 2016 Dec–2017 Jan; 23(5):161–7. [PMID: 27398769]

Kalapila AG et al. Antiretroviral therapy for prevention of human immunodeficiency virus infection. Med Clin North Am. 2016 Jul;100(4):927–50. [PMID: 27235622]

Kanters S et al. Comparative efficacy and safety of first-line antiretroviral therapy for the treatment of HIV infection: a systematic review and network meta-analysis. Lancet HIV. 2016 Nov; 3(11):e510–20. [PMID: 27658869]

Kanters S et al. Comparative efficacy and safety of second-line antiretroviral therapy for treatment of HIV/AIDS: a systematic review and network meta-analysis. Lancet HIV. 2017 Oct; 4(10):e433–441. [PMID: 28784426]

Molina JM et al; DRIVE-FORWARD Study Group. Doravirine versus ritonavir-boosted darunavir in antiretroviral-naive adults with HIV-1 (DRIVE-FORWARD): 48-week results of a randomised, double-blind, phase 3, non-inferiority trial. Lancet HIV. 2018 May;5(5):e211–20. [PMID: 29592840]

Orkin C et al. Nucleoside reverse transcriptase inhibitor-reducing strategies in HIV treatment: assessing the evidence. HIV Med. 2018 Jan;19(1):18–32. [PMID: 28737291]

Orkin C et al; DRIVE-AHEAD Study Group. Doravirine/lamivudine/tenofovir disoproxil fumarate is non-inferior to efavirenz/emtricitabine/tenofovir disoproxil fumarate in treatment-naive adults with human immunodeficiency virus-1 infection: week 48 results of the DRIVE-AHEAD trial. Clin Infect Dis. 2019 Feb 1; 68(4):535–44. [PMID: 30184165]

Psichogiou M et al. Recent advances in antiretroviral agents: potent integrase inhibitors. Curr Pharm Des. 2017; 23(18):2552–67. [PMID: 28356041]

Saag MS et al. Antiretroviral drugs for treatment and prevention of HIV infection in adults: 2018 recommendations of the International Antiviral Society-USA Panel. JAMA. 2018 Jul 24; 320(4):379–96. [PMID: 30043070]

Sax PE et al. Coformulated bictegravir, emtricitabine, and tenofovir alafenamide versus dolutegravir, abacavir, and lamivudine for initial treatment of HIV-1 infection (GS-US-380-1490): a double-blind, multicenter, phase 3 randomised controlled non-inferiority trial. Lancet. 2017 Nov 4;390(10107):2073–82. [PMID: 28867499]

Tieu HV et al. CROI 2018: Advances in antiretroviral therapy. Top Antivir Med. 2018 May;26(1):40–53. [PMID: 29727296]

U.S. Department of Health and Human Services. Guidelines for the prevention and treatment of opportunistic infections in HIV-infected adults and adolescents. Last updated March 28, 2019. https://aidsinfo.nih.gov/contentfiles/lvguidelines/adult_oi.pdf

U.S. Department of Health and Human Services. Guidelines for the use of antiretroviral agents in HIV-1-infected adults and adolescents. Last updated February 15, 2019. https://aidsinfo.nih.gov/ContentFiles/lvguidelines/AdultandAdolescentGL.pdf

U.S. Food and Drug Administration. FDA Drug Safety Communication: interactions between certain HIV or hepatitis C drugs and cholesterol-lowering statin drugs can increase the risk of muscle injury. https://www.fda.gov/Drugs/DrugSafety/ucm293877.htm

Wang H et al. The efficacy and safety of tenofovir alafenamide versus tenofovir disoproxil fumarate in antiretroviral regimens for HIV-1 therapy: meta-analysis. Medicine (Baltimore). 2016 Oct;95(41):e5146. [PMID: 27741146]

32

Viral & Rickettsial Infections

Wayne X. Shandera, MD

Eva Clark, MD, PhD

VIRAL DISEASES

HUMAN HERPESVIRUSES

1. Herpesviruses 1 & 2

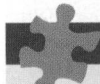

ESSENTIALS OF DIAGNOSIS

► Spectrum of illness: stomatitis, urogenital lesions, Bell palsy, encephalitis.

► Variable intervals between exposure and clinical disease, since herpes simplex virus (HSV) causes both primary (often subclinical) and reactivation disease.

► General Considerations

HSV-1 and HSV-2 affect primarily the oral and genital areas, respectively. Asymptomatic shedding of either virus is common, but it is more common with HSV-2 and from genital areas, with most infected individuals shedding virus at least once a month, which may be responsible for transmission. Asymptomatic HSV-2–infected individuals shed the virus less often than those with symptomatic infection. Clinical disease typically indicates reactivation. Total and subclinical shedding of HSV-2 virus decrease after the first year of initial infection, although viral shedding continues for years thereafter.

Although HSV-2 is the most common cause of genital ulcers in the developed world, epidemiologic studies show that HSV-1 is a more common cause of both genital and oral lesions than HSV-2 in young women in the United States. Most HSV-2–infected persons in the United States are unaware that they are infected.

HSV-2 seropositivity increases the risk of HIV acquisition (it is threefold higher among persons who are HSV-2 seropositive than among those who are HSV-2 seronegative), and HSV-2 reactivates more often in advanced HIV infection. HIV replication is increased by interaction with HSV proteins. Suppression of HSV-2 decreases HIV-1 plasma levels and genital tract shedding of HIV, which can contribute to a reduction in the sexual transmission of HIV-1.

► Clinical Findings

A. Symptoms and Signs

1. Mucocutaneous disease—See Chapter 6 for HSV-1 mucocutaneous disease ("herpes labialis" or "gingivostomatitis"). Digital lesions (whitlows) (Figure 32–1) are an occupational hazard in medicine and dentistry. Contact sports (eg, wrestling) are associated with outbreaks of skin infections ("herpes gladiatorum").

Vesicles form moist ulcers after several days and epithelialize over 1–2 weeks if untreated. Primary infection is usually more severe than recurrences but may be asymptomatic. Recurrences often involve fewer lesions, tend to be labial, heal faster, and are induced by stress, fever, infection, sunlight, chemotherapy (eg, fludarabine, azathioprine), or other undetermined factors.

HSV-2 lesions largely involve the genital tract, with the virus remaining latent in the presacral ganglia (see Chapter 6). Occasionally, lesions arise in the perianal region or on the buttocks and upper thighs. Dysuria, cervicitis, and urinary retention may occur in women. Urethritis may occur in men. Proctitis and extensive, ulcerating, weeping sacral lesions may be presenting symptoms in HIV-infected persons with CD4 cytopenia. Large ulcerations and atypical lesions suggest drug-resistant isolates.

2. Ocular disease—HSV can cause uveitis, keratitis, blepharitis, and keratoconjunctivitis (see Chapter 7). Lesions limited to the epithelium usually heal without affecting vision, whereas stromal involvement can cause uveitis, scarring, and eventually blindness. HSV is the second most common cause, after VZV, of acute retinal necrosis.

3. Neonatal and congenital infection—Both herpesviruses rarely infect the fetus and induce congenital malformations (organomegaly, bleeding, and central nervous system [CNS] abnormalities). The global rate of neonatal herpes is estimated to be about 10 cases per 100,000 live births. Maternal infection during the third trimester is associated with the highest risk of neonatal transmission, but about 70% of these infections are asymptomatic or unrecognized. Neonatal transmission during delivery, however, is more common than intrauterine infection. Invasive fetal monitoring and vacuum or forceps delivery increase the risk of herpesvirus transmission.

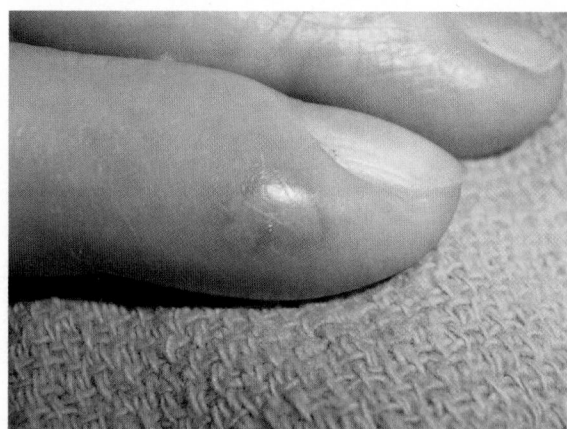

▲ **Figure 32–1.** Herpetic whitlow. (Used, with permission, from Richard P. Usatine, MD, in Usatine RP, Smith MA, Mayeaux EJ Jr, Chumley H. *The Color Atlas of Family Medicine*, 2nd ed. McGraw-Hill, 2013.)

4. CNS disease—Traditionally, herpes simplex encephalitis is associated with HSV-1 infection and aseptic meningitis with HSV-2 infection. Both viruses, however, can cause encephalitis (and in one report, simultaneously). Encephalitis presents with nonspecific symptoms: a flu-like prodrome, followed by headache, fever, behavioral and speech disturbances, and focal or generalized seizures. The temporal lobe is often involved. Untreated disease and presentation with coma carry a high mortality. Ischemic stroke, although infrequent, can complicate the course of HSV meningitis or encephalitis. Many survivors suffer neurologic sequelae, which are observed more frequently among patients with HSV-1 infection. Both HSV-1 and HSV-2 can cause mild, nonspecific neurologic symptoms and are also associated with benign recurrent lymphocytic (Mollaret) meningitis.

5. Disseminated infection—Disseminated HSV infection occurs in the setting of immunosuppression, either primary or iatrogenic, or rarely with pregnancy. In disseminated disease, skin lesions are not always present. Disseminated skin lesions are a particular complication in patients with atopic eczema (eczema herpeticum) and burns. Pneumonia can occur regardless of immune status.

6. Bell palsy—HSV-1 is a cause of Bell palsy (facial nerve paralysis).

7. Esophagitis and proctitis—HSV-1 can cause esophagitis in immunocompromised patients, particularly those with AIDS. The lesions are smaller and deeper than those observed in patients with cytomegalovirus (CMV) esophagitis or with other herpesviruses known to cause esophagitis in immunocompromised persons. Proctitis occurs mainly in men who have sex with men.

8. Erythema multiforme—Herpes simplex viruses and certain drugs are a leading cause of erythema multiforme minor ("herpes-associated erythema multiforme") and of the more severe condition Stevens-Johnson syndrome/toxic epidermal necrolysis (see also Chapter 6).

9. Other—HSV is the cause of approximately 1% of cases of acute liver failure, particularly in pregnant women and immunosuppressed patients. The mortality of such rare fulminant hepatitis is nearly 75%. An HSV lower respiratory tract infection of unknown clinical significance is common in mechanically ventilated patients. Evidence suggests that this finding is usually an indicator rather than the cause of a poor clinical condition. HSV-1 pneumonia is associated with high morbidity in patients with solid tumors. HSV-1 is reported to be a cause of perinephric abscess, febrile neutropenia, chronic urticaria, and esophagitis and enteritis in systemic lupus erythematosus. HSV is also associated with *Helicobacter pylori*–negative upper gastrointestinal tract ulcers.

B. Laboratory Findings

1. Mucocutaneous disease—See Chapter 6.

2. Ocular disease—Herpes keratitis is diagnosed by branching (dendritic) ulcers that stain with fluorescein. The extent of epithelial injury in herpes keratitis correlates well with polymerase chain reaction (PCR) positivity. Uveitis from HSV is often diagnosed clinically, although PCR assays on anterior chamber aspirated material may assist in making the diagnosis.

3. Encephalitis and recurrent meningitis—Cerebrospinal fluid (CSF) pleocytosis is common, with a similar increase in the number of red cells although CSF findings may be atypical in immunosuppressed patients. HSV real-time DNA PCR of the CSF is a rapid, sensitive, and specific tool for early diagnosis and can be included in a multiple rapid array panel. Viral detection by this method can be used if the clinical picture is consistent, especially if initial studies are negative. Antibodies to HSV in CSF can confirm the diagnosis but appear late in disease. Viral culture shows a sensitivity of only 10%. MRI scanning is often a useful adjunct showing increased signal in the temporal and frontal lobes. Temporal lobe seizure foci may be shown on electroencephalograms (EEGs).

4. Esophagitis, proctitis, and other gastrointestinal disease—Esophagitis is diagnosed by endoscopic biopsy with real-time PCR and cultures. Proctitis may be diagnosed by rectal swab for PCR, culture, or both. Complicated cases may require biopsy. Concomitant hepatitis and colitis have been reported with herpes simplex.

5. Pneumonia—Pneumonia is diagnosed by clinical, pathologic, and radiographic findings. The CT findings include diffuse or multifocal areas of ground-glass attenuation or consolidative changes or both and are best confirmed by using high-resolution CT techniques.

▶ **Treatment & Prophylaxis**

Medications that inhibit replication of HSV-1 and HSV-2 include trifluridine and vidarabine (both for keratitis), acyclovir and related compounds, foscarnet, and cidofovir (Table 32–1). Agents under study include helicase-primase inhibitors (amprenavir, fosamprenavir, and pritelivir) with promising preliminary (phase II) data.

Table 32–1. Agents for viral infections.[1]

Drug	Dosing[2]	Spectrum	Toxicities
Acyclovir	HSV and VZV infections: 200–800 mg orally five times daily; 250–500 mg/m² intravenously every 8 hours for 7 days Acute herpes encephalitis: 10 mg/kg intravenously every 8 hours for 14–21 days	HSV, VZV	Neurotoxic reactions, reversible kidney dysfunction, local reactions
Baloxavir	40 mg dose if patient is 40 to < 80 kg 80 mg if patient is 80 kg or more Only use for patients 12 years and older	Influenza A and B strains	Diarrhea and bronchitis
Cidofovir	5 mg/kg intravenously weekly for 2 weeks, then every other week	CMV	Neutropenia, kidney disease, ocular hypotonia
Famciclovir	500 mg orally three times daily for 7 days for acute VZV; 250 mg three times daily for 7–10 days for genital or cutaneous HSV-1/HSV-2 infection; 125 mg twice daily for 5 days for recurrences (500 mg twice daily for 7 days if HIV-infected)	HSV, VZV	Early angioedema; later rarely, gastrointestinal symptoms, headaches, rashes
Foscarnet	Induction: 90 mg/kg intravenously (90- to 120-minute infusion) every 12 hours or 60 mg/kg intravenously (minimum 1-hour infusion) every 8 hours over 2–3 weeks depending on clinical response Maintenance: 90–120 mg/kg intravenously (2-hour infusion) once daily	CMV, HSV resistant to acyclovir, VZV, HIV-1	Nephrotoxicity, genital ulcerations, calcium disturbances
Ganciclovir	Induction: 5 mg/kg intravenously every 12 hours for 14–21 days Maintenance: 6 mg/kg/day intravenously for 5 days each week	CMV	Neutropenia, thrombocytopenia, CNS side effects
Idoxuridine	Topical, 0.1% every 1–2 hours for 3–5 days (not available in the United States)	HSV keratitis	Local reactions
Interferon alfa-2b	HBV infection: 10 million international units subcutaneously three times weekly or 5 million units daily[1] Condylomata: 1 million international units intralesionally in up to five warts three times weekly for 3 weeks	HBV, HCV, HPV	Influenza-like syndrome, myelosuppression, neurotoxicity
Interferon alfa-n3	Refractory or recurring external condylomata acuminata: 0.05 mL (250,000 international units) per wart intralesionally twice weekly for up to 8 weeks; 0.5 mL (2.5 million international units) is the maximum dose per treatment session	HPV, HCV	Local reactions Influenza-like syndrome, myelosuppression, neurotoxicity
Oseltamivir	75 mg orally twice daily for 5 days	Influenza A and B	Dose needs to be adjusted for kidney dysfunction
Palivizumab	15 mg/kg intramuscularly every month in RSV season	RSV	Upper respiratory infection symptoms
Penciclovir	Topical 1% cream every 2 hours for 4 days	HSV	Local reactions
Peramivir	Intravenous, 600-mg single dose	Uncomplicated influenza A	Nausea, vomiting, diarrhea, neutropenia
Ribavirin	RSV infection: one vial (6 g) dissolved and delivered through a Small Particle Aerosol Generator (SPAG-2) over a continuous 12- to 18-hour period daily for 5 consecutive days	RSV, severe influenza A or B, Lassa fever	Wheezing, hemolytic anemia
Trifluridine	Topical, 1% drops every 2 hours to 9 drops/day	HSV keratitis	Local reactions
Valacyclovir	Acute VZV: 1 g orally three times daily for 7 days Primary genital HSV-1/HSV-2 infection: 1 g twice daily for 10 days Recurrent genital HSV-1/HSV-2 infection: 500 mg twice daily for 3 days Suppressive therapy: 1 g daily; 500 mg if fewer than 9 recurrences/year (Dose depends on immune status and number of recurrences.)	VZV, HSV	Thrombotic thrombocytopenic purpura or hemolytic-uremic syndrome in AIDS
Valganciclovir	900 mg orally twice daily for 3 weeks; 900 mg daily as maintenance	CMV	See ganciclovir
Zanamivir	5 mg inhalations twice daily for 5 days	Uncomplicated influenza A and B	Bronchospasm in patients with asthma

Sources: Data from Drugs.com and Lexicomp Online.
[1]Agents used exclusively in the management of HIV infection and AIDS are found in Chapter 31. Agents used in the management of HBV and HCV infections are found in Chapter 16.
[2]Dosing varies considerably by indication and may require adjustment based on patient's clinical state and type of viral infection. Consultation with a pharmacist is recommended.
CMV, cytomegalovirus; CNS, central nervous system; CSF, cerebrospinal fluid; HBV, hepatitis B virus; HCV, hepatitis C virus; HPV, human papillomavirus; HSV, herpes simplex virus; RSV, respiratory syncytial virus; VZV, varicella-zoster virus.

A. Mucocutaneous Disease

See Chapter 6.

B. Keratitis and Uveitis

For the treatment of acute epithelial keratitis, oral antiviral agents such as valacyclovir or famciclovir are first-line therapies (see Chapter 7). The usage of topical corticosteroids may exacerbate the infection, although systemic corticosteroids may help with selected cases of stromal infection. Long-term treatment (more than 1 year) with acyclovir at a dosage of 800 mg/day orally decreases recurrence rates of keratitis, conjunctivitis, or blepharitis due to HSV.

Uveitis is best managed with oral systemic (not topical) acyclovir, although HSV resistance among HIV-infected patients is reported because of the diversity of the HSV quasispecies often present.

C. Neonatal Disease

Counseling (but not serologic screening) should be offered to pregnant mothers. The use of maternal antenatal suppressive therapy with acyclovir (typically, 400 mg orally three times daily) beginning at 36 weeks' gestation decreases the presence of detectable HSV, the rates of recurrence at delivery, and the need for cesarean delivery. Cesarean delivery is recommended for pregnant women with active genital lesions or typical prodromal symptoms.

D. Encephalitis and CNS Meningitis

Because of the need for rapid treatment to decrease mortality and neurologic sequelae, intravenous acyclovir (10 mg/kg every 8 hours for 10 days or more, adjusting for kidney disease) should be started in those patients with suspected HSV encephalitis, stopping only if another diagnosis is established. If the PCR of CSF is negative but clinical suspicion remains high, treatment should be continued for 10 days because the false-negative rate for PCR can be as high as 25% (especially in children) and acyclovir is relatively nontoxic. HSV viral load does not appear to correlate with outcome of meningitis, and it is not recommended to follow viral load over time.

Long-term neurologic sequelae of HSV encephalitis are common, and late pediatric relapse is recognized. Acyclovir resistance in a case of herpes simplex encephalitis is reported. Aseptic meningitis may also require a course of intravenous acyclovir or valacyclovir. Long-term oral prophylaxis with valacyclovir, however, does not appear to prevent recurrences of aseptic meningitis with HSV-2.

E. Disseminated Disease

Disseminated disease responds best to parenteral acyclovir when treatment is initiated early.

F. Bell Palsy

Prednisolone, 25 mg orally twice daily for 10 days started within 72 hours of onset, significantly increases the rate of recovery. Data on antiherpes antiviral agents are equivocal and therefore HSV assays are not routinely recommended; according to one study, valacyclovir (but not acyclovir), 1 g orally daily for 5 days, plus corticosteroid therapy may be beneficial if started within 7 days of symptom onset. In patients with severe or complete facial paralysis, such antiviral therapy is often administered but without proof of efficacy.

G. Esophagitis and Proctitis

Patients with esophagitis should receive either intravenous acyclovir (5–10 mg/kg every 8 hours) or oral acyclovir (400 mg five times daily) through resolution of symptoms, typically 3–5 days; however, longer treatment may be necessary for immunosuppressed patients. Maintenance therapy for AIDS patients is also with acyclovir (400 mg orally three to five times daily). Proctitis is treated with similar dosages and usually responds within 5 days.

H. Erythema Multiforme

Suppressive therapy with oral acyclovir (400 mg twice a day for 6 months) decreases the recurrence rate of HSV-associated erythema multiforme. Valacyclovir (500 mg orally twice a day) may be effective in cases unresponsive to acyclovir.

▶ Prevention

Besides antiviral suppressive therapy (see Erythema multiforme, above and in Chapter 6), prevention also requires counseling and the use of condom barrier precautions during sexual activity. Disclosure to sexual partners of HSV-seropositive status is associated with about a 50% reduction in HSV-2 acquisition. Male circumcision is associated with a lower incidence of acquiring HSV-2 infection.

Preventing spread to hospital staff and other patients from cases with mucocutaneous, disseminated, or genital disease requires isolation and usage of hand washing and gloving–gowning precautions. Staff with active lesions (eg, whitlows) should not have contact with patients. There is no approved herpes vaccine.

Birkmann A et al. HSV antivirals—current and future treatment options. Curr Opin Virol. 2016 Jun;18:9–13. [PMID: 26897058]

McQuillan G et al. Prevalence of herpes simplex virus type 1 and type 2 in persons aged 14–49: United States, 2015–2016. NCHS Data Brief. 2018 Feb;(304):1–8. [PMID: 29442994]

Quenelle DC et al. Efficacy of pritelivir and acyclovir in the treatment of herpes simplex virus infections in a mouse model of herpes simplex encephalitis. Antiviral Res. 2018 Jan;149:1–6. [PMID: 29113740]

US Preventive Services Task Force. Serologic screening for genital herpes infection: US Preventive Services Task Force recommendation statement. JAMA. 2016 Dec 20;316(23):2525–30. [PMID: 27997659]

Workowski KA et al; Centers for Disease Control and Prevention. Sexually transmitted diseases treatment guidelines, 2015. MMWR Recomm Rep. 2015 Jun 5;64(RR-03):1–137. Erratum in: MMWR Recomm Rep. 2015 Aug 28;64(33):924. [PMID: 26042815]

2. Varicella (Chickenpox) & Herpes Zoster (Shingles)

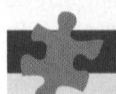

ESSENTIALS OF DIAGNOSIS

► **Varicella rash:** pruritic, centrifugal, papular changing to vesicular ("dew drops on a rose petal"), pustular, and finally crusting.

► **Zoster rash:** tingling, pain, eruption of vesicles in a dermatomal distribution, evolving to pustules and then crusting.

General Considerations

Varicella-zoster virus (VZV), or HHV-3, disease manifestations include chickenpox (varicella) and shingles (herpes zoster). Chickenpox generally presents during childhood; has an incubation period of 10–20 days (average 2 weeks); and is highly contagious, spreading by inhalation of infective droplets or contact with lesions.

The incidence and severity of herpes zoster ("shingles"), which affects up to 25% of persons during their lifetime, increases with age due to an age-related decline in immunity against VZV. More than half of all patients in whom herpes zoster develops are older than 60 years, and the incidence of herpes zoster reaches 10 cases per 1000 patient-years by age 80 (by which time 50% are infected with VZV). The annual incidence in the United States of 1 million cases is increasing as the population ages. Populations at increased risk for varicella-zoster–related diseases include immunosuppressed persons and persons receiving biologic agents.

► Clinical Findings

A. Varicella

1. Symptoms and signs—Fever and malaise are mild in children and more marked in adults. The pruritic rash begins prominently on the face, scalp, and trunk, and later involves the extremities (Table 32–2). Maculopapules change within a few hours to vesicles that become pustular and eventually form crusts (Figures 32–2 and 32–3). New lesions may erupt for 1–5 days, so that different stages of

Table 32–2. Diagnostic features of some acute exanthems.

Disease	Prodromal Signs and Symptoms	Nature of Eruption	Other Diagnostic Features	Laboratory Tests
Atypical measles	Same as measles.	Maculopapular centripetal rash, becoming confluent.	History of measles vaccination.	Measles antibody present in past, with titer rise during illness.
Chikungunya fever	2–4 (sometimes 1–12) days, fever, headaches, abdominal complaints, myalgias, arthralgias.	Maculopapular, centrally distributed, pruritus, can be bullous with sloughing in children, occasional facial edema and petechiae.	History of mosquito bites, epidemiologic factors.	ELISA-based IgM or IgG (fourfold increase in titers); PCR and cultures are infrequently available.
Eczema herpeticum	None.	Vesiculopustular lesions in area of eczema.		Herpes simplex virus isolated in cell culture. Multinucleate giant cells in smear of lesion.
Ehrlichiosis	Headache, malaise.	Rash in one-third, similar to Rocky Mountain spotted fever.	Pancytopenia, elevated liver biochemical tests.	Polymerase chain reaction, immunofluorescent antibody.
Enterovirus infections	1–2 days of fever, malaise.	Maculopapular rash resembling rubella, rarely papulovesicular or petechial.	Aseptic meningitis.	Virus isolation from stool or cerebrospinal fluid; complement fixation titer rise.
Erythema infectiosum (erythrovirus)	None. Usually in epidemics.	Red, flushed cheeks; circumoral pallor; maculopapules on extremities.	"Slapped face" appearance.	White blood cell count normal.
Exanthema subitum (HHV-6, 7; roseola)	3–4 days of high fever.	As fever falls, pink maculopapules appear on chest and trunk; fade in 1–3 days.		White blood cell count low.
Infectious mononucleosis (EBV)	Fever, adenopathy, sore throat.	Maculopapular rash resembling rubella, rarely papulovesicular.	Splenomegaly, tonsillar exudate.	Atypical lymphocytes in blood smears; heterophile agglutination (Monospot test).
Kawasaki disease	Fever, adenopathy, conjunctivitis.	Cracked lips, strawberry tongue, maculopapular polymorphous rash, peeling skin on fingers and toes.	Edema of extremities. Angiitis of coronary arteries.	Thrombocytosis, electrocardiographic changes.

(continued)

Table 32–2. Diagnostic features of some acute exanthems. (continued)

Disease	Prodromal Signs and Symptoms	Nature of Eruption	Other Diagnostic Features	Laboratory Tests
Measles (rubeola)	3–4 days of fever, coryza, conjunctivitis, and cough.	Maculopapular, brick red; begins on head and neck; spreads downward and outward, in 5–7 days rash brownish, desquamating. See Atypical measles, above.	Koplik spots on buccal mucosa.	White blood cell count low. Virus isolation in cell culture. Antibody tests by hemagglutination inhibition or neutralization.
Meningococcemia	Hours of fever, vomiting.	Maculopapules, petechiae, purpura.	Meningeal signs, toxicity, shock.	Cultures of blood, cerebrospinal fluid. White blood cell count high.
Rocky Mountain spotted fever	3–4 days of fever, vomiting.	Maculopapules, petechiae, initial distribution centripetal (extremities to trunk, including palms).	History of tick bite.	Indirect fluorescent antibody; complement fixation.
Rubella	Little or no prodrome.	Maculopapular, pink; begins on head and neck, spreads downward, fades in 3 days. No desquamation.	Lymphadenopathy, postauricular or occipital.	White blood cell count normal or low. Serologic tests for immunity and definitive diagnosis (hemagglutination inhibition).
Scarlet fever	One-half to 2 days of malaise, sore throat, fever, vomiting.	Generalized, punctate, red; prominent on neck, in axillae, groin, skin folds; circumoral pallor; fine desquamation involves hands and feet.	Strawberry tongue, exudative tonsillitis.	Group A beta-hemolytic streptococci in cultures from throat; antistreptolysin O titer rise.
Smallpox	Fever, malaise, prostration.	Maculopapules to vesicles to pustules to scars (lesions develop at the same pace).	Centrifugal rash; fulminant sepsis in small percentage of patients, gastrointestinal and skin hemorrhages.	Contact CDC[1] for suspicious rash; EM and gel diffusion assays.
Typhus	3–4 days of fever, chills, severe headaches.	Maculopapules, petechiae, initial distribution centrifugal (trunk to extremities).	Endemic area, lice.	Complement fixation.
Varicella (chickenpox)	0–1 day of fever, anorexia, headache.	Rapid evolution of macules to papules, vesicles, crusts; all stages simultaneously present; lesions superficial, distribution centripetal.	Lesions on scalp and mucous membranes.	Specialized complement fixation and virus neutralization in cell culture. Fluorescent antibody test of smear of lesions.

[1]https://www.cdc.gov/smallpox/index.html
CDC, Centers for Disease Control and Prevention; EBV, Epstein-Barr virus; ELISA, enzyme-linked immunosorbent assay; EM, electron microscopy; HHV, human herpesvirus; Ig, immunoglobulin; PCR, polymerase chain reaction.

the eruption are usually present simultaneously. The crusts slough in 7–14 days. The vesicles and pustules are superficial and elliptical, with slightly serrated borders. Pitted scars are frequent. Although the disease is often mild, complications (such as secondary bacterial infection, pneumonitis, and encephalitis) occur in about 1% of cases and often lead to hospitalization.

Varicella is more severe in older patients and immunocompromised persons. In the latter, atypical presentations, including widespread dissemination in the absence of skin lesions, are often described. After the primary infection, the virus remains dormant in cranial nerve sensory ganglia and spinal dorsal root ganglia. Latent VZV will reactivate as herpes zoster in about 10–30% of persons. There is a small increased risk of Guillain-Barré syndrome for at least 2 months after an acute herpes zoster attack.

2. Laboratory findings—Diagnosis is usually made clinically, with confirmation by direct immunofluorescent antibody staining or PCR of scrapings from lesions, both of which are more sensitive than culture. Multinucleated giant cells are usually apparent on a Tzanck smear of material from the vesicle base. Leukopenia and subclinical transaminase elevation are often present, and

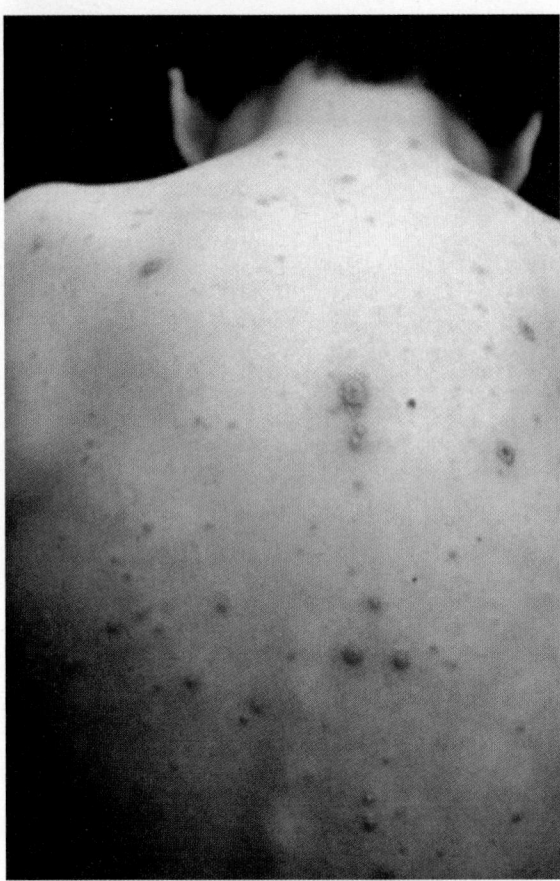

▲ **Figure 32–2.** Primary varicella (chickenpox) skin lesions. (Public Health Image Library, CDC.)

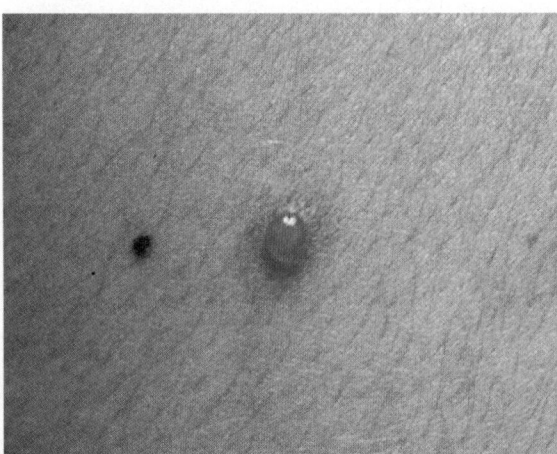

▲ **Figure 32–3.** Chickenpox (varicella) with classic "dew drop on rose petal" appearance. (Used, with permission, from Richard P. Usatine, MD, in Usatine RP, Smith MA, Mayeaux EJ Jr, Chumley H. *The Color Atlas of Family Medicine*, 2nd ed. McGraw-Hill, 2013.)

thrombocytopenia occasionally occurs. Although elevation of varicella IgM is occasionally used to diagnose a primary VZV infection, the assay has poor performance and is generally not recommended. The exception is that varicella antibody tested in the CSF is useful for identifying CNS involvement if VZV vasculopathy is suspected but CSF VZV DNA PCR is negative. A varicella skin test and interferon-gamma enzyme-linked immunospot (ELISPOT) can screen for VZV susceptibility.

B. Herpes Zoster

Herpes zoster ("**shingles**") usually occurs among adults, but cases are reported among infants and children. Shingles incidence rises markedly with age because of immunosenescence and loss of specific immunity to VZV, with rates of 8 to 12 per 1000 person-years in individuals older than 80 years. Skin lesions resemble those of chickenpox. Pain is often severe and commonly precedes the appearance of rash. Lesions follow a dermatomal distribution, with thoracic and lumbar roots being the most common. In most cases, a single unilateral dermatome is involved, but occasionally, neighboring and distant areas are involved. Lesions on the tip of the nose, inner corner of the eye, and root and side of the nose (Hutchinson sign) indicate involvement of the trigeminal nerve (herpes zoster ophthalmicus). Facial palsy and lesions of the external ear with or without tympanic membrane involvement, vertigo and tinnitus, or deafness signify geniculate ganglion involvement (Ramsay Hunt syndrome or herpes zoster oticus). Shingles is a particularly common and serious complication among immunosuppressed patients.

▶ Complications

A. Varicella

Secondary bacterial skin superinfections, particularly with group A *Streptococcus* and *Staphylococcus aureus*, are the most common complications. Cellulitis, erysipelas, and scarlet fever are described. Bullous impetigo and necrotizing fasciitis are less often seen. Other associations with varicella include epiglottitis, necrotizing pneumonia, osteomyelitis, septic arthritis, epidural abscess, meningitis, endocarditis, pancreatitis, giant cell arteritis, inflammatory bowel disease, and purpura fulminans. Toxic shock syndrome can also develop.

Interstitial VZV pneumonia is more common in adults (especially smokers, HIV-infected patients, and pregnant women) and may result in acute respiratory distress syndrome (ARDS). After healing, numerous densely calcified lesions are seen throughout the lung fields on chest radiographs.

Historically, neurologic complications developed in about 1 in 2000 children. Cerebellar ataxia occurs at a frequency of 1:4000 in the young. A limited course and complete recovery are the rule. Encephalitis is similarly infrequent, occurs mostly in adults, and is characterized by delirium, seizures, and focal neurologic signs. The rates for both mortality and long-term neurologic sequelae are about 10%. Ischemic strokes in the wake of acute VZV infection present at a mean of 4 months after rashes and may be due to an associated vasculitis. Multifocal encephalitis, ventriculitis, myeloradiculitis, arterial aneurysm formation, and arteritis are also described in immunosuppressed, especially HIV-infected, patients.

Clinical hepatitis is uncommon and mostly presents in the immunosuppressed patient but can be fulminant and fatal. Reye syndrome (fatty liver with encephalopathy) also complicates varicella (and other viral infections, especially influenza B virus), usually in childhood, and is associated with aspirin therapy (see Influenza, below).

When contracted during the first or second trimesters of pregnancy, varicella carries a very small risk of congenital malformations, including cicatricial lesions of an extremity, growth retardation, microphthalmia, cataracts, chorioretinitis, deafness, and cerebrocortical atrophy. If varicella develops around the time of delivery, the newborn is at risk for disseminated disease.

B. Herpes Zoster

Postherpetic neuralgia occurs in 60–70% of patients who have herpes zoster and are older than 60 years. The pain can be prolonged and debilitating. Risk factors for postherpetic neuralgia include advanced age, female sex, the presence of a prodrome, and severity of rash or pain but not family history.

Other complications include the following: (1) bacterial skin superinfections; (2) herpes zoster ophthalmicus, which occurs with involvement of the trigeminal nerve, is a sight-threatening complication (especially when it involves the iris), and is a marker for stroke over the ensuing year (Hutchinson sign is a marker of ocular involvement in the HIV-positive population); (3) rarely, unilateral ophthalmoplegia; (4) involvement of the geniculate ganglion of cranial nerve VII as well as cranial nerves V, VIII, IX, and X; (5) aseptic meningitis; (6) peripheral motor neuropathy; (7) transverse myelitis; (8) encephalitis; (9) acute cerebellitis; (10) stroke; (11) vasculopathy; (12) acute retinal necrosis; (13) progressive outer retinal necrosis (largely among HIV infected persons); (14) temporal arteritis; and (15) sacral meningoradiculitis (Elsberg syndrome). VZV is a major cause of Bell palsy in patients who are HSV seronegative.

Diagnosis of neurologic complications requires the detection of VZV DNA in CSF or the detection of VZV DNA in tissue. Diagnosis by examination of saliva may be possible. Zoster sine herpete (pain without rash) can also be associated with most of the above complications.

▶ Treatment

A. General Measures

In general, patients with varicella should be isolated until primary lesions have crusted. The skin is kept clean. Pruritus can be relieved with antihistamines, calamine lotion, and colloidal oatmeal baths. Fever can be treated with acetaminophen (not aspirin). Fingernails can be closely cropped to avoid skin excoriation and infection.

B. Antiviral Therapy

1. Varicella—Uncomplicated disease in otherwise healthy children and adolescents does not require antiviral therapy. Acyclovir, 20 mg/kg (up to 800 mg per dose) orally four times daily for 5–7 days, should be given within the first 24 hours after the onset of varicella rash and should be considered for patients older than 12 years, secondary household contacts (disease tends to be more severe in secondary cases), patients with chronic cutaneous and cardiopulmonary diseases, and children receiving long-term therapy with salicylates (to decrease the risk of Reye syndrome). Acyclovir hastens defervescence and healing of lesions but does not impact complication rates. Experience with valacyclovir and famciclovir in these settings is scant and while these agents are often used, their use is not FDA-approved in the United States. Nonsteroidal anti-inflammatory drug (NSAID) use in varicella-infected children appears to be associated with an increase in bacterial infections.

In immunocompromised patients, in pregnant women during the third trimester, and in patients with extracutaneous disease (encephalitis, pneumonitis), antiviral therapy with high-dose acyclovir (30 mg/kg/day in three divided doses intravenously for at least 7 days) should be started once the diagnosis is suspected. Corticosteroids may be useful in the presence of pneumonia. Prolonged prophylactic acyclovir is important to prevent VZV reactivation in profoundly immunosuppressed patients.

2. Herpes zoster—For uncomplicated herpes zoster, valacyclovir or famciclovir is preferable to acyclovir due to dosing convenience and higher drug levels in the body (Table 32–1). Therapy should start within the first 72 hours of the onset of the lesions and be continued for 7 days or until the lesions crust over. Amenamevir is an oral helicase-primase inhibitor given as a single dose that was approved to treat shingles in Japan in 2017 but is not yet available in the United States. Antiviral therapy reduces the duration of herpetic lesions and associated episodes of acute pain but does not in all studies decrease the risk of postherpetic neuralgia. Corticosteroids (a tapering course starting at 60 mg/day, for 2–3 weeks) are safe in immunocompetent patients and may be useful in the acute management of disease to hasten the resolution of acute lesions. Corticosteroids do not prevent the development of postherpetic neuralgia.

Intravenous acyclovir is used for extradermatomal complications of zoster. Adjunctive therapy may be considered in retinal disease (foscarnet) and acute herpes zoster (sorivudine, a topical antiviral). In cases of prolonged or repeated acyclovir use, immunosuppressed patients may require a switch to foscarnet due to the development of acyclovir-resistant VZV infections. VZV associated with the Ramsay Hunt syndrome is more resistant to antiviral therapy.

C. Treatment of Postherpetic Neuralgia

Once established, postherpetic neuralgia is difficult to treat, and less than half of patients achieve adequate pain relief. This condition may respond to neuropathic pain agents such as gabapentin or lidocaine patches. Tricyclic antidepressants, opioids, and capsaicin cream are also widely used and effective. The epidural injection of corticosteroids and local anesthetics appears to modestly reduce herpetic pain at 1 month but, as with oral corticosteroids, is not effective for prevention of long-term postherpetic neuralgia. There is reported success using transcutaneous electrical nerve stimulation.

Prognosis

The total duration of varicella from onset of symptoms to disappearance of crusts rarely exceeds 2 weeks. Fatalities are rare except in immunosuppressed patients.

Herpes zoster resolves in 2–6 weeks. Antibodies persist longer and at higher levels than with primary varicella. Eye involvement with herpes zoster necessitates periodic future examinations.

Prevention

Health care workers should be screened for varicella and vaccinated if seronegative. Patients with active varicella or herpes zoster are promptly separated from seronegative patients. For patients with varicella, airborne and contact isolation is recommended, whereas for those with zoster, contact precautions are sufficient. For immunosuppressed patients with zoster, precautions should be the same as if the patient had varicella. Exposed serosusceptible patients should be placed in isolation and exposed serosusceptible employees should stay away from work for 8–21 days after exposure. Health care workers with zoster should receive antiviral agents during the first 72 hours of disease and withdraw from work until lesions are crusted. The need for postexposure prophylaxis should be assessed.

A. Varicella

1. Vaccination—Universal childhood vaccination against varicella is effective. The varicella vaccine is live and attenuated, safe, and over 98.1% effective when given after 13 months of age. A single antigen live attenuated vaccine (VARIVAX, VARILRIX) or a quadrivalent measles, mumps, rubella, and varicella (MMRV) vaccine (ProQuad) is available (the combination is immunogenic). The first dose of the single antigen vaccine should be administered at 12–18 months of age and the second at 4–6 years. Alternatively, the MMRV vaccine can be given as a first dose at 12–15 months of age and the second dose before elementary school entry. Aspirin should be avoided for at least 6 weeks after vaccination because of the risk of Reye syndrome. The single antigen vaccine is safe and well tolerated, but the quadrivalent MMRV vaccine is associated with a small risk of febrile seizures 5–12 days after vaccination among infants aged 12–23 months. Because of this risk, the Centers for Disease Control and Prevention (CDC) recommends using separate varicella and measles, mumps, and rubella (MMR) vaccines for the first dose in children younger than 48 months old. Rashes, when secondary to the varicella vaccine, appear 15–42 days after vaccination. Rare cases of keratitis are associated with zoster and varicella vaccines.

For serosusceptible individuals older than 13 years, two doses of varicella vaccine (single antigen) administered 4–8 weeks apart are recommended. For those who received a single dose in the past, a catch-up second dose is advised, especially in the epidemic setting (where it is effective when it can be given during the first 5 days postexposure). Household contacts of immunocompromised patients should adhere to these recommendations. Susceptible pregnant women (who should not be vaccinated with live varicella or zoster vaccines during pregnancy) need to receive the first dose of single antigen vaccine before discharge after delivery and the second dose 4–8 weeks later. The Advisory Committee on Immunization Practices (ACIP) recommends administration of the single agent varicella vaccine as two doses 3 months apart to HIV-infected children aged 12 months or older with CD4 lymphocyte percentage greater than 15% and adolescents and adults with CD4 lymphocyte counts 200 cells/mcL or higher.

The vaccine may also be given to patients with impaired humoral immunity, to patients receiving corticosteroids, to pediatric oncology patients receiving chemotherapy, and to patients with juvenile rheumatoid arthritis who receive methotrexate. Patients receiving high doses of corticosteroids for over 2 weeks may be vaccinated a month after discontinuation of the therapy. Patients with leukemia, lymphoma, or other malignancies whose disease is in remission and who have not undergone chemotherapy for at least 3 months may be vaccinated. Kidney and liver transplant patients should be vaccinated if they are susceptible to varicella.

The incidence of varicella in the United States is significantly reduced with the varicella vaccine. Although uncommon, the varicella vaccine, like any of the live varicella-zoster vaccines, has the potential to reactivate and cause clinical disease. It is thought that vaccination against varicella provides less protection against future zoster than does natural varicella infection. The incidence of varicella-associated group A streptococcal infection and varicella neurologic complications are both diminished with the advent of varicella vaccination.

The FDA no longer maintains a registry for exposed pregnant women because of the low rate of such incidents and the general safety of varicella vaccines. Incidents can be reported to Merck (877-888-4231) or through the Vaccine Adverse Events Registry System Vaccine (https://vaers.hhs.gov/index).

2. Postexposure—Postexposure vaccination is recommended for unvaccinated persons without other evidence of immunity. Varicella-zoster immune globulin available in the United States only as VariZIG should be considered for susceptible exposed patients (for up to 10 days after exposure but as soon as feasible) who cannot receive the vaccine, including immunosuppressed patients, neonates from mothers with varicella around the time of delivery, exposed premature infants born from serosusceptible mothers at greater than 28 weeks of gestation, neonates born at less than 28 weeks of gestation regardless of maternal serostatus, and nonimmune pregnant women. No controlled studies have evaluated the use of acyclovir in this setting. VariZIG is given by intramuscular injection in a dosage of 125 international units/10 kg, to a maximum of 625 international units with a weight-based (2-kg cutoff) minimum dose of 62.5 or 125 international units), with a repeat identical dose in 3 weeks if a high-risk patient remains exposed. VariZIG has no place in therapy of established disease; however, it reduces severity of varicella in high-risk children or adults (ie, those with impaired immunity, pregnant women, and infants exposed peripartum) if given within 4 days of exposure. Varicella vaccination should be delayed at least 5 months after VariZIG administration. If VariZIG is not available, standard pooled intravenous immunoglobulin (IVIG) (400 mg/kg given in one dose) can be given. Acyclovir (40–80 mg/kg) for 5 days or the varicella vaccine (if not contraindicated) can also be given as postexposure prophylaxis within 3 days of exposure. Either of these options offers an efficacy of 70–85% compared to 90% efficacy for VariZIG.

Further information may be obtained by calling the Centers for Disease Control and Prevention's Immunization Information Hotline (800-232-2522).

B. Herpes Zoster

Shingrix, HZ/su (GlaxoSmithKline Biologics), an adjuvanted recombinant subunit vaccine, was approved in 2017 by the FDA for VZV and is recommended for individuals 50 years of age and older. Unlike the older live attenuated VZV vaccine (ZOSTAVAX, see below), Shingrix is particularly effective in reducing the incidence of herpes zoster infection and postherpetic neuralgia in adults 70 years of age and older; immunosenescence to the vaccine does not appear to occur in older patients. It can also be used in immunosuppressed patients. Two doses of the vaccine given 2 months apart had 97% efficacy in preventing herpes zoster. Shingrix also appears to be safe in HIV-infected persons with CD4 counts above 50 cells/mcL, recipients of autologous stem cell transplants, and adults with autoimmune disease taking immunosuppressive therapy.

The older live attenuated VZV vaccine, ZOSTAVAX (19,400 plaque forming units [pfu] of Oka/Merck strain) contains at least 14 times the concentration of varicella virus found in VARIVAX. It is recommended for persons 60 years and older because it reduces the incidence of herpes zoster by 33–55% in the first 3 years after vaccination and reduces the incidence of postherpetic neuralgia by 55–67%. The efficacy of ZOSTAVAX wanes over time, from 69% in the first year after vaccination to 45% by the third year.

Even if the person has had a prior episode of herpes zoster, either of the two zoster vaccines has efficacy and can be administered. No specific recommendations exist regarding how long to wait between a zoster outbreak and administering the vaccine; the CDC recommends waiting at least until the outbreak has resolved. The attenuated VZV vaccine is safe, but only moderately immunogenic among HIV-infected persons with a CD4 count of at least 200 cells/mcL. Decreased efficacy occurs in patients older than 70, and this vaccine should not be given to immunosuppressed persons. Nonetheless, hematologic oncology patients taking anti-CD20 monoclonal antibodies may be successfully vaccinated. An increased risk of herpes zoster during a 6-week interval following vaccination is reported among patients taking immunosuppressant medications. This vaccine provides protection for about 3 years.

Concurrent administration of the adjuvanted recombinant subunit vaccine or the live attenuated VZV vaccine with pneumococcal vaccine is safe. If a varicella vaccine is mistakenly administered to an adult instead of a live attenuated zoster vaccine, the dose should be considered invalid and the patient should be administered a dose of zoster vaccine at the same visit. The zoster vaccine cannot be used in children in place of varicella vaccine; if the vaccine is accidentally given to a child, the event should be reported to the CDC.

Cunningham AL et al; ZOE-70 Study Group. Efficacy of the herpes zoster subunit vaccine in adults 70 years of age or older. N Engl J Med. 2016 Sep 15;375(11):1019–32. [PMID: 27626517]

Eberhardson M et al. Safety and immunogenicity of inactivated varicella-zoster virus vaccine in adults with autoimmune disease: a phase 2, randomized, double-blind, placebo-controlled clinical trial. Clin Infect Dis. 2017 Oct 1;65(7): 1174–82. [PMID: 29126292]

Grillo AP et al. Keratitis in association with herpes zoster and varicella vaccines. Drugs Today (Barc). 2017 Jul;53(7):393–7. [PMID: 28837183]

Han Y et al. Corticosteroids for preventing postherpetic neuralgia. Cochrane Database Syst Rev. 2013 Mar 28;3:CD005582. [PMID: 23543541]

Walker JL et al. Effectiveness of herpes zoster vaccination in an older United Kingdom population. Vaccine. 2018 Apr 19; 36(17):2371–7. [PMID: 29555217]

3. Epstein-Barr Virus & Infectious Mononucleosis

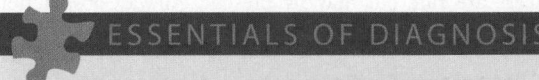

ESSENTIALS OF DIAGNOSIS

► Malaise, fever, and (exudative) sore throat.

► Palatal petechiae, lymphadenopathy, splenomegaly, and, occasionally, a maculopapular rash.

► Positive heterophile agglutination test (Monospot).

► Atypical large lymphocytes in blood smear; lymphocytosis.

► **Complications:** hepatitis, myocarditis, neuropathy, encephalitis, airway obstruction from adenitis, hemolytic anemia, thrombocytopenia.

► General Considerations

Epstein-Barr virus (EBV, or human herpes virus-4 [HHV-4]) is one of the most ubiquitous human viruses, infecting more than 95% of the adult population worldwide and persisting for the lifetime of the host. Infectious mononucleosis is a common manifestation of EBV and may occur at any age. In the United States the incidence of EBV infection is declining although prevalence of EBV remains high for those aged 12–19 years. In the developing world, infectious mononucleosis occurs at younger ages and tends to be less symptomatic. Rare cases in older adults occur usually without the full symptomatology. EBV is largely transmitted by saliva but can also be recovered from genital secretions. Saliva may remain infectious during convalescence, for 6 months or longer after symptom onset. The incubation period lasts several weeks (30–50 days). Patients with immunodeficiency disorders are at risk for the full spectrum of EBV-associated disorders.

Clinical Findings

A. Symptoms and Signs

Fever, sore throat, fatigue, malaise, anorexia, and myalgia typically occur in the early phase of the illness. Physical findings include lymphadenopathy (discrete, nonsuppurative, slightly painful, especially along the posterior cervical chain), transient bilateral upper lid edema (Hoagland sign), and splenomegaly (in up to 50% of patients and sometimes massive). A maculopapular or occasionally petechial rash occurs in less than 15% of patients unless ampicillin is given (in which case rash was thought to occur in more than 90% of patients; however, recent data indicates that the incidence of drug hypersensitivity is much lower than previously reported). Conjunctival hemorrhage, exudative pharyngitis, uvular edema, tonsillitis, or gingivitis may occur and soft palatal petechiae may be noted. Complications of acute disease are more common among older adults.

Other manifestations include hepatitis, interstitial pneumonitis (sometimes with pleural involvement), cholestasis, gastritis, kidney disease (mostly interstitial nephritis), epiglottitis, and nervous system involvement in 1–5% (mononeuropathies and occasionally aseptic meningitis, encephalitis, cerebellitis, peripheral and optic neuritis, transverse myelitis, or Guillain-Barré syndrome). Vaginal ulcers are rare but may be present. Airway obstruction from lymph node enlargement can occur.

B. Laboratory Findings

An initial phase of granulocytopenia is followed within 1 week by lymphocytic leukocytosis (greater than 50% of all leukocytes) with atypical lymphocytes (larger than normal mature lymphocytes, staining more darkly, and showing vacuolated, foamy cytoplasm and dark nuclear chromatin) comprising more than 10% of the leukocyte count. Hemolytic anemia, with antibodies, occurs occasionally as does thrombocytopenia (at times marked and life-threatening).

Diagnosis is made based on characteristic manifestations and serologic evidence of infection (the heterophile sheep cell agglutination [HA] antibody tests or the correlated mononucleosis spot test [Monospot]). These tests usually become positive within 4 weeks after onset of illness and are specific but often not sensitive in early illness. Heterophile antibodies may be absent in young children and in as many as 20% of adults. During acute illness, there is a rise and fall in immunoglobulin M (IgM) antibody to EB virus capsid antigen (VCA) and a rise in immunoglobulin G (IgG) antibody to VCA, which persists for life. Antibodies (IgG) to EBV nuclear antigen (EBNA) appear after 4 weeks of onset and also persist. Absence of IgG and IgM VCA or the presence of IgG EBNA should make one reconsider the diagnosis of acute EBV infection.

PCR for EBV DNA is useful in the evaluation of malignancies associated with EBV. For instance, detection of EBV DNA in CSF shows a sensitivity of 90% and specificity of nearly 100% for the diagnosis of primary CNS lymphoma in patients with AIDS.

Differential Diagnosis

CMV infection, toxoplasmosis, acute HIV infection, secondary syphilis, HHV-6 infection, rubella, and drug hypersensitivity reactions may be indistinguishable from infectious mononucleosis due to EBV, but exudative pharyngitis is usually absent and the heterophile antibody tests are negative. With acute HIV infection, rash and mucocutaneous ulceration are common but atypical lymphocytosis is much less common. Heterophile-negative infectious mononucleosis with nonsignificant lymphocytosis (especially if rash or mucocutaneous ulcers are present) should prompt investigation for acute HIV infection. CMV, toxoplasmosis and, on occasion, EBV can cause heterophile-negative infectious mononucleosis with atypical lymphocytosis. Mycoplasma infection may also present as pharyngitis, though lower respiratory symptoms usually predominate. A hypersensitivity syndrome induced by carbamazepine or phenytoin may mimic infectious mononucleosis.

The differential diagnosis of acute exudative pharyngitis includes gonococcal and streptococcal infections, and infections with adenovirus and herpes simplex. Head and neck soft tissue infections (pharyngeal and tonsillar abscesses) may occasionally be mistaken as the lymphadenopathy of mononucleosis.

Complications

Secondary bacterial pharyngitis can occur and is often streptococcal. Splenic rupture (0.5–1%) is a rare but dramatic complication, and a history of preceding trauma can be elicited in 50% of the cases. Acalculous cholecystitis, fulminant hepatitis with massive necrosis, pericarditis and myocarditis are also infrequent complications.

Treatment

A. General Measures

Over 95% of patients with acute EBV-associated infectious mononucleosis recover without specific antiviral therapy. Treatment is symptomatic with NSAIDs or acetaminophen and warm saline throat irrigations or gargles three or four times daily. Acyclovir decreases viral shedding but shows no clinical benefit. Corticosteroid therapy, although widespread, is not recommended in uncomplicated cases; its use is reserved for impending airway obstruction from enlarged lymph nodes, hemolytic anemia, and severe thrombocytopenia. The value of corticosteroid therapy in impending splenic rupture, pericarditis, myocarditis, and nervous system involvement is less well established. If a throat culture grows beta-hemolytic streptococci, a 10-day course of penicillin or azithromycin is indicated. Ampicillin and amoxicillin are avoided because of the frequent association with rash, although one recent study indicates that the incidence of drug hypersensitivity is much lower than previously reported.

EBV infections in solid organ transplant recipients are difficult to prevent and treat, although recent data suggest possible utility of pretransplant rituximab for high-risk transplant recipients. The role of antiviral prophylaxis for preventing posttransplantation EBV infection and sequelae, including posttransplant lymphoproliferative disorders

(PTLD) in patients who are donor organ EBV-positive and recipient negative (the main risk factor for both early PTLD [less than 1 year posttransplantation] and late PTLD [more than 1 year]). One recent retrospective study indicated that prophylaxis with acyclovir, valacyclovir, ganciclovir, or valganciclovir delayed primary EBV infection at 100 days posttransplant. A decreased incidence of late-onset PTLD and EBV-related neoplasias in treated patients was also noted. Finally, new therapies are being developed to protect hematopoietic stem cell transplant recipients from many viruses, including EBV.

B. Treatment of Complications

Hepatitis, myocarditis, and encephalitis are treated symptomatically. Rupture of the spleen requires splenectomy and is most often caused by deep palpation of the spleen or vigorous activity. Patients should avoid contact or collision sports for at least 4 weeks to decrease the risk of splenic rupture (even if splenomegaly is not detected by physical examination, which can be insensitive).

▶ Prognosis & Prevention

In uncomplicated cases, fever disappears in 10 days and lymphadenopathy and splenomegaly in 4 weeks. The debility sometimes lingers for 2–3 months.

Death is uncommon and is usually due to splenic rupture, hypersplenic phenomena (severe hemolytic anemia, thrombocytopenic purpura), or encephalitis.

4. Other EBV-Associated Syndromes

EBV viral antigens are found in more than 90% of patients with endemic (African) Burkitt lymphoma and nasopharyngeal carcinoma (among whom quantified EBV DNA can be used to follow disease). Risk factors for Burkitt lymphoma include a history of malaria (which may decrease resistance to EBV infection) while risk factors for nasopharyngeal carcinoma include long-term heavy cigarette smoking and seropositive EBV serologies (VCA and deoxyribonuclease [DNase]). VCA-IgA in peripheral blood is a sensitive and specific predictor for nasopharyngeal carcinoma in an endemic area.

Among Hodgkin lymphoma patients, EBV seropositivity is common when the disease is found in the developing world or is associated with HIV infection, when pathologic specimens show mixed cellularity, and when patients are younger than 10 years or older than 45 years at onset of the lymphoma. The EBV-seropositive have a worse prognosis for early stages of Hodgkin lymphoma.

Chronic EBV infection is associated with aberrant cellular immunity (a low frequency of EBV-specific CD8+ T cells), an X-linked lymphoproliferative syndrome (Duncan disease), lymphomatoid granulomatosis, and a fatal T-cell lymphoproliferative disorder in children.

EBV is an important trigger for hemophagocytic lymphohistiocytosis among immunodeficient patients and causes B-cell lymphomas (such as primary CNS lymphoma in HIV-infected individuals), natural killer/T-cell lymphoma, and posttransplant lymphoproliferative disorders. CD30 and EBV viral loads are prognostic markers for EBV-associated lymphoproliferative disease. PTLD are commonly associated with EBV, especially in children. EBV-naïve patients who receive a donor organ from an EBV-infected donor are at the highest risk for the development of PTLD. EBV serostatus, however, is not associated with overall survival among patients with PTLD. Decreasing the iatrogenic immunosuppression given to prevent graft rejection is the initial step in managing such patients, while rituximab (CD20 monoclonal antibody) is effective in treating more than two-thirds of cases. Oral mucocutaneous ulcerative disease in the HIV-infected may be due to EBV.

Age is a major determinant of the type of tumor associated with EBV. T and NK cell lymphoma caused by chronic active EBV infections are more frequent in childhood while peripheral T-cell lymphomas and diffuse large B-cell lymphomas are more common in older patients due to waning immunity. EBV is also associated with leiomyomas in children with AIDS and with nasal T-cell lymphomas.

▶ When to Admit

Presence of severe complications of EBV disease including the following:

- Acute meningitis, encephalitis, or Guillain-Barré syndrome.
- Severe thrombocytopenia; significant hemolysis.
- Potential splenic rupture.
- Airway obstruction from severe adenitis.
- Pericarditis.
- Abdominal findings mimicking an acute abdomen.

Linke-Serinsöz E et al. Human immunodeficiency virus (HIV) and Epstein-Barr virus (EBV) related lymphomas, pathology view point. Semin Diagn Pathol. 2017 Jul;34(4):352–63. [PMID: 28506687]

Myriam BD et al. Prognostic significance of Epstein-Barr virus (EBV) infection in Hodgkin lymphoma patients. J Infect Chemother. 2017 Mar;23(3):121–30. [PMID: 28034523]

Okamoto A et al. The prognostic significance of EBV DNA load and EBER status in diagnostic specimens from diffuse large B-cell lymphoma patients. Hematol Oncol. 2017 Mar; 35(1):87–93. [PMID: 26177728]

Shabani M et al. Primary immunodeficiencies associated with EBV-induced lymphoproliferative disorders. Crit Rev Oncol Hematol. 2016 Dec;108:109–27. [PMID: 27931829]

Ville S et al. Impact of antiviral prophylaxis in adults Epstein-Barr virus-seronegative kidney recipients on early and late post-transplantation lymphoproliferative disorder onset: a retrospective cohort study. Transpl Int. 2018 May;31(5):484–94. [PMID: 29057508]

5. Cytomegalovirus Disease

ESSENTIALS OF DIAGNOSIS

- ▶ Mononucleosis-like syndrome.
- ▶ Frequent pathogen seen in transplant populations.
- ▶ Diverse clinical syndromes in HIV (retinitis, esophagitis, pneumonia, encephalitis).

General Considerations

Most cytomegalovirus (CMV) infections are asymptomatic. After primary infection, the virus remains latent in most body cells. Seroprevalence in adults of Western developed countries is about 60–80% but is higher in developing countries. The virus can be isolated from a variety of tissues under nonpathogenic conditions. Transmission occurs through sexual contact, breastfeeding, blood products, or transplantation; it may also occur person-to-person (eg, day care centers) or be congenital. Serious disease occurs primarily in immunocompromised persons, including those with inflammatory bowel disease.

There are three recognizable clinical syndromes: (1) perinatal disease and CMV inclusion disease, (2) diseases in immunocompetent persons, and (3) diseases in immunocompromised persons. Congenital CMV infection is the most common congenital infection in developed countries (about 0.6% of live births, with higher rates in underdeveloped areas and among lower socioeconomic groups). Transmission is much higher from mothers with primary disease than those with reactivation (40% vs 0.2–1.8%). About 10% of infected newborns will be symptomatic with CMV inclusion disease.

In immunocompetent persons, acute CMV infection is the most common cause of the mononucleosis-like syndrome with negative heterophile antibodies. In critically ill immunocompetent adults, CMV reactivation is associated with prolonged hospitalization and death. CMV appears to be involved in the malignant manifestations of glioblastoma multiforme.

In immunocompromised persons, solid organ and bone marrow transplant patients are at highest risk for a year after allograft transplantation (but especially during the first 100 days afterward) and in particular when graft-versus-host disease is present or when the donor is CMV seropositive and the recipient is seronegative. Depending on the serostatus of the donor and recipient, disease may present as primary infection or reactivation. The risk of CMV disease is proportionate to the degree of immunosuppression and manifestations may differ by the cause. CMV may contribute to transplanted organ dysfunction, which often mimics organ rejection. CMV retinitis may develop after solid organ or bone marrow transplantation. CMV disease in HIV-infected patients (retinitis, serious gastrointestinal disease) occurs most prominently when the CD4 count is less than 50 cells/mcL and can be a marker for increased mortality. Antiretroviral therapy (ART) reduces the frequency of retinitis and may reverse active disease. Patients with immune recovery with CD4 cell count greater than 100 cells/mcL show decreased mortality. CMV retinitis associated with intravitreal delivery of corticosteroids (injections or implants) or systemic anti-TNF antibodies is also described. Occasionally, CMV retinitis presents in immunocompetent persons. Serious gastrointestinal CMV disease also occurs after organ transplantation, cancer chemotherapy, or corticosteroid therapy. CMV may exist alongside other pathogens, such as *Cryptosporidium*, in up to 15% of patients with AIDS cholangiopathy. CMV pneumonitis occurs in transplant recipients (mainly bone marrow and lung) with a mortality rate up to 60–80%, and less often in AIDS patients. CMV pneumonitis in hematologic malignancies (eg, lymphoma) is increasingly reported. Neurologic CMV in patients with advanced AIDS is usually associated with disseminated CMV infection.

Clinical Findings

A. Symptoms and Signs

1. Perinatal disease and CMV inclusion disease—CMV inclusion disease in infected newborns is characterized by hepatitis, thrombocytopenia, microcephaly, periventricular CNS calcifications, mental retardation, and motor disability. Hearing loss develops in more than 50% of infants who are symptomatic at birth. Most infected neonates are asymptomatic, but neurologic deficits may ensue later in life, including hearing loss in 15% and mental retardation in 10–20%. Perinatal infection acquired through breastfeeding or blood products typically shows a benign clinical course.

2. Disease in immunocompetent persons—Acute CMV infection is characterized by fever, malaise, myalgias, arthralgias, and splenomegaly. Exudative pharyngitis or cervical lymphadenopathies are uncommon, but cutaneous rashes (including the typical maculopapular rash after exposure to ampicillin) are common. The mean duration of symptoms is 7–8 weeks. Complications include mucosal gastrointestinal damage, encephalitis, severe hepatitis, thrombocytopenia (on occasion, refractory), the Guillain-Barré syndrome, pericarditis, and myocarditis. A mononucleosis-like syndrome due to CMV can also occur post splenectomy, often years later and associated with a protracted fever, marked lymphocytosis, and impaired anti-CMV IgM response.

3. Disease in immunocompromised persons—Distinguishing between CMV infection (with evidence of CMV replication) and CMV disease (evidence for systemic symptoms or organ invasion by pathologic diagnosis) is important. In addition to patients infected with HIV, those who have undergone transplantation (solid organ or hematopoietic stem cell) show a wide spectrum of disease including gastrointestinal (eg, acute cholecystitis), kidney, and CNS disease, as outlined above. CMV viral loads serve as an important predictor of disease presence.

A. CMV RETINITIS—A funduscopic examination reveals neovascular, proliferative lesions ("pizza-pie" retinopathy). Immune restoration with ART is associated with CMV vitritis and cystoid macular edema.

B. GASTROINTESTINAL AND HEPATOBILIARY CMV—Esophagitis presents with odynophagia. Gastritis can occasionally cause bleeding, and small bowel disease may mimic inflammatory bowel disease or may present as ulceration or perforation. Colonic CMV disease causes diarrhea, hematochezia, abdominal pain, fever, and weight loss and may mimic inflammatory bowel disease. CMV hepatitis commonly complicates liver transplantation and appears to be increased in those with hepatitis B or hepatitis C viral infection.

C. **Respiratory CMV**—CMV pneumonitis is characterized by cough, dyspnea, and relatively little sputum production. Concomitant infection with *Pneumocystis jirovecii* occurs among patients regardless of HIV status.

D. **Neurologic CMV**—Neurologic syndromes associated with CMV include polyradiculopathy, transverse myelitis, ventriculoencephalitis (suspected with ependymitis), and focal encephalitis. These manifestations are more prominent in patients with advanced AIDS in whom the encephalitis has a subacute onset.

B. Laboratory Findings

1. Mothers and newborns—Pregnant women should be tested for CMV viremia every 3 months if found to be seropositive during the first trimester. Congenital CMV disease is confirmed by presence of the virus in amniotic fluid or an IgM assay from fetal blood. Amniocentesis is less reliable before 21 weeks of gestation (due to inadequate fetal urinary development and release into the amniotic fluid), but amniocentesis is attendant with greater risk when performed after 21 weeks of gestation. PCR assays of dried blood samples from newborns, micro-enzyme-linked immunosorbent assay (ELISA), shell-vial culture, or culture of urine, saliva, or blood specimens obtained during the first 3 weeks of life are used to diagnose congenital CMV infection.

2. Immunocompetent persons—The acute mononucleosis-like syndrome is characterized by initial leukopenia; within 1 week, it is followed by absolute lymphocytosis with atypical lymphocytes. Abnormal liver biochemical tests are common in the first 2 weeks of the disease (often 2 weeks after the fever). Detection of CMV DNA, specific IgM, or a fourfold increase of specific IgG levels support the diagnosis of acute infection.

3. Immunocompromised persons—CMV retinitis is diagnosed on the basis of the characteristic ophthalmoscopic findings. In HIV-infected patients, negative CMV serologies lower the possibility of the diagnosis but do not eliminate it. Cultures alone are of little use in diagnosing AIDS-related CMV infections, since viral shedding of CMV is common. Detection of CMV by quantitative DNA PCR should be used to diagnose CNS infection since cultures are not specific for disease.

Detection of CMV by quantitative DNA PCR is also used in posttransplant patients to guide both treatment and prevention and should be interpreted in the context of clinical and pathologic findings. CMV viral loads are internationally standardized and have replaced conventional CMV antigenemia tests in many settings. The PCR is sensitive in predicting clinical disease. Serial PCR should be performed and compared using the same specimen type (ie, whole blood or plasma). To assist in the diagnosis CMV pneumonia, bronchoalveolar lavage fluid can be tested to quantify CMV viral load. Rapid shell-vial cultures detect early CMV antigens with fluorescent antibodies in 24–48 hours. Shell-vial cultures are more useful on bronchoalveolar lavage fluid than in routine blood monitoring. CMV colitis can occur in the absence of a detectable viremia.

C. Imaging

The chest radiographic findings of CMV pneumonitis are consistent with interstitial pneumonia.

D. Biopsy

Tissue confirmation is especially useful in diagnosing CMV pneumonitis and CMV gastrointestinal disease; the diagnosis of colonic CMV disease is made by mucosal biopsy showing characteristic CMV histopathologic findings of intranuclear ("owl's eye") and intracytoplasmic inclusions. In situations where histopathologic or immunohistochemical findings are not seen but CMV colitis is suspected, CMV DNA PCR can be used to identify additional cases.

▶ **Treatment**

In immunocompetent persons, CMV infection is usually self-limited, and no specific antiviral therapy is needed. In immunocompromised persons, treatment of CMV disease is necessary. Treatment of **CMV retinitis** is discussed in Chapter 7. The role of ART in HIV infections in reducing the need for CMV antiviral agents is essential. Because recurrence occurs even at high CD4 cell counts, ongoing ophthalmologic surveillance is necessary. CMV disease in patients with solid organ transplants, AIDS, and invasive end-organ disease is typically treated initially with intravenous ganciclovir (recommended dose is 5 mg/kg every 12 hours, although this needs to be adjusted for kidney function) until two CMV PCRs 1 week apart are negative (usually 14–21 days). Oral valganciclovir (900 mg every 12 hours), which also needs to be adjusted for kidney function, is an acceptable alternative in patients with non–life-threatening disease.

Pneumonia due to CMV in hematopoietic stem cell transplant recipients is treated even more aggressively, with 5 mg/kg of ganciclovir intravenously every 12 hours for 21 days followed by 5 mg/kg daily for 3–4 weeks plus CMV immunoglobulin (500 mg/kg) or CMV immunoglobulin (150 mg/kg) twice per week for 2 weeks and then once weekly for an additional 4 weeks.

Reduction of immunosuppression should be attempted when possible (especially for muromonab, azathioprine, or mycophenolate mofetil). Secondary prophylaxis is typically maintained until immune restoration (with two CD4 T-cell counts greater than 100 cells/mcL present for at least 6 months in the setting of HIV infection). Prolonged prophylaxis may be necessary in other immunosuppressed patients, such as those receiving TNF inhibitors.

Foscarnet and cidofovir are reserved for treatment of resistant infections. Other agents that may be useful in resistant CMV infections include CMV immunoglobulin, leflunomide, sirolimus-based therapy, artesunate, and adoptive immunotherapy. New anti-CMV drugs under development include brincidofovir and maribavir.

▶ **Prevention**

A major source of CMV for pregnant women is their own young children, particularly those in childcare. These women can decrease their risk of contracting primary CMV just before pregnancy or during pregnancy by practicing hand hygiene after changing diapers and after contact with respiratory secretions; avoiding kissing young children on the face; and avoiding sharing utensils, food, and cleansing objects that have been in contact with children's secretions.

ART is effective in preventing CMV infections in HIV-infected patients. Primary prevention is best accomplished by good hand hygiene and use of barrier methods during sexual contacts with persons who are members of high-prevalence groups (ie, men who have sex with men, injection drug users, and those who have exposure to children in child care).

The use of leukocyte-depleted blood products effectively reduces the incidence of CMV disease in patients who have undergone transplantation. Prophylactic and preemptive strategies (eg, antiviral agents only when antigen detection or PCR assays show evidence of active CMV replication) appear equally effective in preventing invasive disease and mortality after hematopoietic stem cell transplant. The appropriate management of transplant patients is based on the serostatus of the donor and the recipient. All effective anti-CMV agents can serve as prophylactic agents for CMV-seropositive transplants or for CMV-seronegative recipients of CMV-positive organ transplants, although starting CMV prophylaxis 14 days after transplant may help reduce late-onset CMV end-organ disease. The typical dose for valganciclovir prophylaxis is 450 mg orally twice daily, although a recent prospective trial in kidney transplant recipients indicated that prophylaxis with low-dose valganciclovir (450 mg/day, three times a week for 6 months) seemed to be effective. Acyclovir may also be used. Recommended duration of CMV prophylaxis in posttransplant patients and in other immunocompromised patients varies by the type of transplant. Letermovir is useful in prophylaxis against CMV infections in adult allogenic hematopoietic stem cell transplant recipients. It is given as 480 mg orally daily with dose adjustments for cyclosporine administration and for advanced kidney dysfunction (less than a creatinine clearance of 10 mL/min). Major side effects reported to date include cough, diarrhea, headache, nausea, stomach pain, weakness, and vomiting.

CMV immune globulin may also be useful in reducing the incidence of bronchiolitis obliterans in the bone marrow transplant population and is used in some centers as part of the prophylaxis in kidney, liver, and lung transplantation patients. CMV immune globulin as prophylaxis is not recommended in hematopoietic stem cell transplant recipients.

▶ When to Refer

- AIDS patients with retinitis, esophagitis, colitis, hepatobiliary disease, or encephalitis.
- Organ and hematopoietic stem cell transplants with suspected reactivation CMV.

▶ When to Admit

- Escalating CMV viral load at the onset of illness.
- Risk of colonic perforation.

- Evaluation of unexplained, advancing encephalopathy.
- Initiation of treatment with intravenous anti-CMV agents.

Boekh M et al. Valganciclovir for the prevention of complications of late cytomegalovirus infection after allogeneic hematopoietic cell transplantation: a randomized trial. Ann Intern Med. 2015 Jan 6;162(1):1–10. [PMID: 25560711]

Liu J et al. Patients with refractory cytomegalovirus (CMV) infection following allogeneic hematopoietic stem cell transplantation are at high risk for CMV disease and non-relapse mortality. Clin Microbiol Infect. 2015 Dec;21(12):1121.e9–15. [PMID: 26093077]

Marty FM et al. Letermovir prophylaxis for cytomegalovirus in hematopoietic-cell transplantation. N Engl J Med. 2017 Dec 21;377(25):2433–44. [PMID: 29211658]

Nanmoku K et al. Prevention of late-onset cytomegalovirus infection and disease in donor-positive/recipient-negative kidney transplant recipients using low-dose valganciclovir. Transplant Proc. 2018 Jan–Feb;50(1):124–9. [PMID: 29407294]

US Department of Health and Human Services (HHS). AIDSinfo. Guidelines for the prevention and treatment of opportunistic infections in HIV-infected adults and adolescents. Cytomegalovirus. 2017 Jan 17. https://aidsinfo.nih.gov/guidelines/html/4/adult-and-adolescent-opportunistic-infection/337/cytomegalovirus-disease

6. Human Herpesviruses 6, 7, & 8

HHV-6 is a B-cell lymphotropic virus that is the principal cause of exanthema subitum (roseola infantum, sixth disease). Primary HHV-6 infection occurs most commonly in children under 2 years of age and is a major cause of infantile febrile seizures (21% in one recent series). HHV-6 is also associated with encephalitis (symptoms may include insomnia, seizures, and hallucinations), Hashimoto thyroiditis, myocarditis, and acute liver failure. Primary infection in immunocompetent adults is not common but can produce a mononucleosis-like illness. Pathologically, HHV-6 is associated with mesial temporal sclerosis, which may lead to mesial temporal lobe epilepsy. Reactivation of HHV-6 in immunocompetent adults is rare and can present as encephalitis. Imaging studies in HHV-6 encephalitis typically show lesions in the hippocampus, amygdala, and limbic structures.

Infection during pregnancy and congenital transmission is recognized. Most cases of reactivation occur in immunocompromised persons. Reactivation is associated with graft rejection, graft-versus-host disease, and bone marrow suppression in transplant patients and with encephalitis and pneumonitis in AIDS patients. In recipients of hematopoietic stem cell transplants, HHV-6 may cause fever. It is also associated with an HHV-6–induced encephalitis (diagnosed with multiplex PCR assays) that is correlated strongly with umbilical cord hematopoietic cell transplants (although HHV-6 is not associated with survival in such patients and surveillance for the virus may not be needed).

HHV-6 is on occasion also associated with drug-induced hypersensitivity syndromes. HHV-6 may cause fulminant hepatic failure and acute decompensation of chronic liver disease in children. Purpura fulminans and corneal inflammation are reported with HHV-6 infection. Two variants (A and B) of HHV-6 have been identified. HHV-6B is the predominant strain found in both normal and immunocompromised persons. Ganciclovir, cidofovir, and foscarnet (but not acyclovir) appear to be clinically active against HHV-6. Adoptively transferred virus-specific T cell therapy is also being developed for treatment of HHV-6 infections in hematopoietic stem cell transplant recipients.

HHV-7 is a T-cell lymphotropic virus that is associated with roseola seizures and, rarely, encephalitis, even in immunocompetent adults. Pregnant women are often infected. Infection with HHV-7 is synergistic with CMV in kidney transplant recipients.

HHV-8 (see also Chapter 31) is associated with Kaposi sarcoma, multicentric Castleman disease, and primary effusion (body cavity) lymphoma. HHV-8 infection is endemic in Africa; transmission seems to be primarily horizontal in childhood from intrafamilial contacts and continues through adulthood possibly by nonsexual routes.

Komaroff AL et al. Summary of the 9th international conference on human herpesviruses 6 and 7 (HHV-6A, HHV-6B, and HHV-7). J Med Virol. 2016 Dec;88(12):2038–43. [PMID: 27124385]

Mohammadpour Touserkani F et al. HHV-6 and seizure: a systematic review and meta-analysis. J Med Virol. 2017 Jan; 89(1):161–9. [PMID: 27272972]

Riva N et al. Acute human herpes virus 7 (HHV-7) encephalitis in an immunocompetent adult patient: a case report and review of literature. Infection. 2017 Jun;45(3):385–8. [PMID: 28386807]

Sultanova A et al. Association of active human herpesvirus-6 (HHV-6) infection with autoimmune thyroid gland diseases. Clin Microbiol Infect. 2017 Jan;23(1):50.e1–5. [PMID: 27693656]

Tzannou I et al. Off-the-shelf virus-specific T cells to treat BK virus, human herpesvirus 6, cytomegalovirus, Epstein-Barr virus, and adenovirus infections after allogeneic hematopoietic stem-cell transplantation. J Clin Oncol. 2017 Nov 1; 35(31):3547–57. [PMID: 28783452]

MAJOR VACCINE-PREVENTABLE VIRAL INFECTIONS

1. Measles

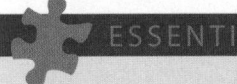

ESSENTIALS OF DIAGNOSIS

► Exposure 7–18 days before onset of prodrome in an unvaccinated patient.

► Prodrome: fever, coryza, cough, conjunctivitis, malaise, irritability, photophobia, Koplik spots.

► Rash: brick red, maculopapular; appears 3–4 days after onset of prodrome; begins on the face and proceeds "downward and outward," affecting the palms and soles last.

► Leukopenia.

General Considerations

Measles is a reportable acute systemic paramyxoviral infection transmitted by direct contact with infectious droplets or by airborne spread. It is highly contagious with communicability greatest during the preeruptive and catarrhal stages but continues 4 days after the appearance of rash.

Measles elimination is defined as the absence of endemic measles virus transmission in an area for 12 months or longer. Measles remains a major cause internationally of mortality with nearly 90,000 estimated deaths per year.

Between 2000 and 2016, the annual incidence of measles decreased by 87%, although in recent years the global tally of cases has increased, with the World Health Organization (WHO) estimating 7 million infections for 2016, the year with most recently compiled complete data. The WHO previously considered measles eradicated in the Americas. Major outbreaks, however, continue throughout the world (countries with over 1000 suspected cases in 2019 include Bangladesh, Cameroon, Chad, China, the Democratic Republic of the Congo, Georgia, Kazakhstan, Kyrgyzstan, India, Indonesia, Japan, Madagascar, Malaysia, Myanmar, Nigeria, the Philippines, Russian, Thailand, the Ukraine, and possibly Venezuela) and in the United States.

Most measles cases in the United States are due to either travel to endemic areas or exposure to individuals who have not been vaccinated against measles. A large 2015 outbreak at a California Disney theme park developed into a multistate outbreak involving 147 people. A 2017 outbreak in New York included 17 reported cases among unvaccinated Orthodox Jews and developed into a tristate outbreak. Additionally, 65 confirmed cases were identified in 2017 in a Somali-American community from Minnesota due to a decline in MMR vaccination coverage. The 2019 outbreak of measles includes 704 cases documented between January 1, 2019 and April 26, 2019 in 13 outbreaks occurring in 22 states with major outbreaks in California, New Jersey, New York, and Washington State. Previously, the highest number of reported measles cases was 667 in 27 states in 2014 followed by 372 in 2018. Intentional undervaccination continues to undermine measles elimination programs.

► Clinical Findings

A. Symptoms and Signs

The incubation period for measles is 10–14 days. The illness starts with a prodromal phase manifested by high-grade fever (often as high as 40–40.6°C), malaise, coryza (nasal obstruction, sneezing, and sore throat resembling upper respiratory infections), persistent cough, and conjunctivitis (redness, swelling, photophobia, and discharge). These symptoms intensify over 2–4 days before onset of the rash and peak on the first day of the rash. The fever persists through the early rash (about 5–7 days) (Table 32–2).

The characteristic measles rash appears on the face and behind the ears. Initial lesions are pinhead-sized papules that coalesce to form a brick red, irregular, blotchy maculopapular rash. The rash spreads to the trunk and extremities, including the palms and soles. It lasts for 3–7 days and fades in the same manner it appeared. Other findings include pharyngeal erythema, tonsillar exudate, moderate generalized lymphadenopathy and, at times, splenomegaly.

Koplik spots (small, irregular, and red with whitish center on the mucous membranes) are pathognomonic of measles (Figure 32–4). They appear about 2 days before the rash and last 1–4 days as tiny "table salt crystals" on the palatal or buccal mucosa opposite the molars.

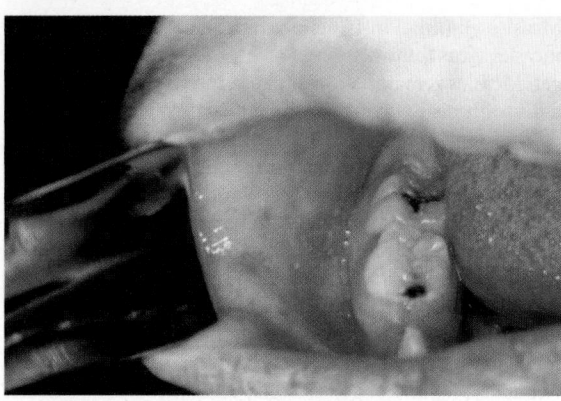

▲ **Figure 32–4.** Very small, bright red spots on the buccal mucosa indicative of Koplik spots. (Public Health Image Library, CDC.)

B. Laboratory Findings

Leukopenia is usually present unless secondary bacterial complications exist. A lymphocyte count under 2000/mcL is a poor prognostic sign. Thrombocytopenia is common. Proteinuria is often observed.

Detection of IgM measles antibodies with ELISA or a fourfold rise in serum hemagglutination inhibition antibody supports the diagnosis. IgM assays can be falsely negative the first few days of infection and falsely positive in the presence of rheumatoid factor or with acute rubella, erythrovirus (formerly parvovirus B19), or HHV-6 infection.

Measles virus is technically difficult to culture. Real-time reverse transcriptase-PCR (RT-PCR), available from the CDC and some public health laboratories, can help establish a diagnosis promptly.

▶ Differential Diagnosis

Measles is usually diagnosed clinically but may be mistaken for Kawasaki disease and other exanthematous infections (Table 32–2). Frequent difficulty in establishing a diagnosis suggests that measles may be more prevalent than is recognized.

▶ Complications

A. Respiratory Tract Disease

Early in the course of the disease, bronchopneumonia or bronchiolitis due to the measles virus may occur in up to 5% of patients and result in serious respiratory difficulties. Bronchiectasis may occur in up to a quarter of nonvaccinated children. The incidence of severe respiratory disease may be increased among immunocompromised children and pregnant women.

B. Central Nervous System

Postinfectious encephalomyelitis occurs in 0.05–0.1% of cases, with higher rates occurring in adolescents. It is an acute demyelinating disease that usually starts 3–7 days after the rash. Seizures, coma, and other neurologic symptoms and signs may develop. Treatment is symptomatic and supportive. Virus isolation from the CNS is uncommon. There is

an appreciable mortality (10–20%) and morbidity (33% of survivors are left with neurologic deficits).

Measles inclusion body encephalitis is another form of neurologic complication that results in neurologic deterioration and death within months of the acute illness among patients with impaired cellular immunity. Treatment is supportive, including stopping immunosuppressants when feasible. Interferon and ribavirin are variably successful.

Subacute sclerosing panencephalitis is a very rare, and fatal CNS complication that occurs 5–15 years after infection. It is characterized by progressive deterioration of motor and cognitive function leading to death. It is more common in boys of rural backgrounds who are infected with measles before 2 years of age.

C. Other Complications

Immediately following measles, secondary bacterial infection, particularly cervical adenitis, otitis media (the most common complication), and pneumonia, occurs in about 15% of patients. Keratoconjunctivitis is a serious complication that caused blindness before the widespread use of measles vaccine and vitamin A supplementation. Diarrhea and protein-losing enteropathy (prodromal rectal Koplik spots may occur) are significant complications among malnourished children, although the mortality associated with diarrhea is primarily 1 week prior to and 4 weeks after the measles rash, with no longer-term mortality shown with measles-associated diarrhea. Some data implicate the measles virus in the pathogenesis of rheumatoid arthritis.

▶ Treatment

Treatment is symptomatic, including antipyretics and fluids as needed. Vitamin A supplementation for children reduces pediatric morbidity and measles-associated mortality. Data are less substantial for adult supplementation, although many advocate megadose vitamin A at the time of delivery in order to boost infant levels of the vitamin.

Measles virus is susceptible to ribavirin and other antivirals in vitro. Ribavirin is used in selected severe cases of pneumonitis, but insufficient data prevent recommending antiviral use. Zinc has a role in the maintenance of normal immune functions, but routine zinc supplementation to children with measles is not recommended, again for lack of data.

▶ Prognosis

It is estimated that 20.4 million deaths were prevented by use of measles vaccination. In the United States, the case fatality rate is around 2 per 1000 reported cases, with deaths principally due to respiratory and neurologic complications. Deaths in the developing world are mainly related to acute diarrhea and protein-losing enteropathy. Pregnant women with measles may be at increased risk for death. Historically famines are particularly associated with high measles mortality.

▶ Prevention

Because measles is highly contagious, the vaccine coverage rates must exceed 95% to prevent outbreaks. Illness confers permanent immunity. One vaccine dose is about 93% effective. Two doses of vaccine are estimated to be 97% protective.

Migrants and asylum seekers are thought to be at higher risk because their antibody levels often are lower than needed for adequate protection. The CDC currently recommends that all individuals embarking on international travel assure that they have been vaccinated. Infants under 1 year of age should have a first dose with boosters at 12–15 months and at age 4–6, children 1 year or older should receive two doses separated by 28 days, and teens and adults without evidence of immunity similarly should receive two doses separated by 28 days.

Vaccine site reactions appear to differ by the manufacturer.

In the United States, based on the 2016 National Immunization Survey, 91.1% of children aged 19–35 months received one or more doses of MMR and 90.9% of adolescents aged 13–17 years received two or more doses. These data suggest considerable geographic disparity. Clustering of unvaccinated individuals increases the likelihood of an outbreak.

At 6 months of age, more than 99% of infants of vaccinated women and 95% of infants of naturally immune women lose maternal antibodies. The susceptibility to measles is 2.4-fold higher if the vaccine is given prior to 15 months (with impact of waning maternal antibody levels). Thus, in the United States, children receive their first vaccine dose at 12–15 months of age. The second dose is given at age 4–6 years, prior to school entry. For individuals born before 1957, herd immunity is assumed. All adults born after 1957, without evidence of immunity should receive at least one dose of MMR vaccine. Persons at high risk for measles exposure (teachers, health care workers, post–high school students, travelers to developing countries) should receive two vaccination doses at least 28 days apart. Immigrants and refugees should be screened and vaccinated if necessary. Combination MMRV vaccines may be used in place of the traditional MMR vaccine.

MMR and MMRV vaccine should not be administered to pregnant women, patients with anaphylactic reactions to neomycin, and patients with known primary or acquired immunodeficiency. Asymptomatic patients living with HIV with CD4 counts higher than 200 cells/mcL should receive MMR vaccine but not MMRV (without a varicella component) vaccine.

Repeated studies fail to show an association between vaccination and autism. MMR vaccine can cause fever and transient rash. Severe allergic reactions are rare. Quadrivalent MMRV vaccine is associated with an increased risk of febrile seizures that appears to be age-related; the risk is highest when MMRV is given to infants between 12 and 23 months of age. Postimmunization seizures appear in whole genome studies to be associated with an interferon receptor and a measles receptor. Immune thrombocytopenia is a documented side effect. Rare cases of postimmunization encephalitis are reported.

In case of an outbreak, when susceptible individuals are exposed to measles, MMR vaccine can prevent disease if given within 3 days of exposure. Immunoglobulin should be administered within 6 days of exposure in any high-risk person exposed to measles, followed by active immunization 3 months later. All infants less than 1 year of age should receive intramuscular immunoglobulin (0.5 mL/kg, maximum dose 15 mL). For infants between 6 months and 12 months, MMR vaccination with repeat at 15 months can be given in place of intramuscular immunoglobulin. Pregnant women and severely immunocompromised persons who are exposed to active measles cases should receive IVIG (400 mg/kg).

Patients with measles should be isolated for 4 days after the onset of rash. In the hospital setting, patients with measles should be placed under air-borne precautions.

An aerosolized measles vaccine remains under study. Future vaccines for a variety of infectious agents may utilize measles vectors, thereby augmenting immunity to measles.

▶ **When to Refer**

- Any suspect cases should be reported to public health authorities.
- HIV infection.
- Pregnancy.

▶ **When to Admit**

- Meningitis, encephalitis, or myelitis.
- Severe pneumonia.
- Diarrhea that significantly compromises fluid or electrolyte status.

Ceccarelli G et al; Sanitary Bureau of the Asylum Seekers Center of Castelnuovo di Porto. Susceptibility to measles in migrant population: implication for policy makers. J Travel Med. 2018 Jan 1;25(1). [PMID: 29232456]

Jackson BD et al. Available studies fail to provide strong evidence of increased risk of diarrhea mortality due to measles in the period 4–26 weeks after measles rash onset. BMC Public Health. 2017 Nov 7;17(Suppl 4):783. [PMID: 29143685]

Lo NC et al. Public health and economic consequences of vaccine hesitancy for measles in the United States. JAMA Pediatr. 2017 Sep 1;171(9):887–92. [PMID: 28738137]

Moss WJ. Measles. Lancet. 2017 Dec 2;390(10111):2490–502. [PMID: 28673424]

Orenstein WA et al. Measles and Rubella Global Strategic Plan 2012–2020 midterm review report: background and summary. Vaccine. 2018 Jan 11;36(Suppl 1):A35–42. [PMID: 29307368]

Trentini F et al. Measles immunity gaps and the progress towards elimination: a multi-country modelling analysis. Lancet Infect Dis. 2017 Oct;17(10):1089–97. [PMID: 28807627]

Willame C et al. Pain caused by measles, mumps, and rubella vaccines: a systematic literature review. Vaccine. 2017 Oct 9; 35(42):5551–8. [PMID: 28893478]

2. Mumps

ESSENTIALS OF DIAGNOSIS

▶ Exposure 12–25 days before onset.

▶ Painful, swollen salivary glands, usually parotid.

▶ Frequent involvement of testes, pancreas, and meninges in unvaccinated individuals.

▶ Mumps can occur in appropriately vaccinated persons in highly vaccinated communities.

General Considerations

Mumps is a paramyxoviral disease spread by respiratory droplets. Children are most commonly affected; however, in outbreaks, infection can affect patients in their second or third decades of life. Mumps can spread rapidly in congregate settings, such as colleges and schools. The incubation period is 12–25 days (average, 16–18 days). The mumps virus spreads through direct contact with respiratory secretions or saliva or infected surfaces. Transmission can also be airborne or via droplets. Up to one-third of affected individuals have subclinical infection, which is still transmissible. Despite high vaccination rates, several mumps outbreaks were reported over the past few years in an increasing number. In 2016 and 2017, mumps cases surged to about 6000/year, with the largest outbreak occurring at a college in northwest Arkansas, which involved 3000 cases. A combination of factors contributes to outbreaks, including efficacy of vaccines; waning individual immunity; and crowded conditions, which promote transmission.

Clinical Findings

A. Symptoms and Signs

Mumps is more serious in adults than in children and appears to occur more commonly in males. Parotid tenderness and overlying facial edema (Figure 32–5) are the most common physical findings and typically develop within 48 hours of the prodromal symptoms. Usually, one parotid gland enlarges before the other, but unilateral parotitis occurs in 25% of patients. The parotid duct (orifice of Stensen) may be red and swollen. Trismus may result from parotitis. The parotid glands return to normal within 1 week. Involvement of other salivary glands (submaxillary and sublingual) occurs in 10% of cases. Fever and malaise

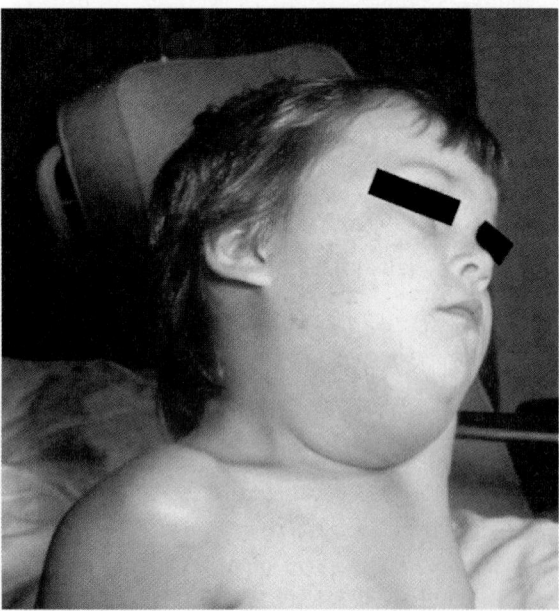

▲ **Figure 32–5.** **Mumps.** (Public Health Image Library, CDC.)

are variable but often minimal in young children. The entire course of mumps rarely exceeds 2 weeks.

The testes are the most common extra salivary disease site in adults. High fever, testicular swelling, and tenderness (unilateral in 75% of cases) denote orchitis, which usually develops 7–10 days after the onset of parotitis. In recent outbreaks in the United States, complications from mumps were rare; 3.3–10% of adolescent and adult males developed orchitis (which occurred less frequently in persons who have received two doses of vaccine). Lower abdominal pain and ovarian enlargement suggest oophoritis, which is usually unilateral and occurs in less than 1% of postpubertal women.

Other rare complications, occurring in less than 1% of cases, are meningitis, encephalitis, Guillain-Barré syndrome, hearing loss, priapism or testicular infarction from orchitis, pancreatitis, thyroiditis, keratitis, neuritis, hepatitis, myocarditis, thrombocytopenia, migratory arthralgias, and nephritis. No mumps-related deaths have occurred in the United States in recent outbreaks. A rare cause of mumps is iodine exposure in medical procedures ("iodide mumps").

Some epidemiologic studies have suggested an association between mumps and risk of type 1 diabetes mellitus. Further studies do not provide evidence of this association.

B. Laboratory Findings

Mild leukopenia with relative lymphocytosis may be present. Elevated serum amylase usually reflects salivary gland involvement rather than pancreatitis. Mild kidney injury is found in up to 60% of patients.

The characteristic clinical picture usually suffices for diagnosis. An elevated serum IgM is considered diagnostic. Repeat testing 2–3 weeks after the onset of symptoms is recommended if the first assay is negative because the rise in IgM may be delayed, especially in vaccinated persons. A fourfold rise in complement-fixing antibodies to mumps virus in paired serum IgG also confirms infection. Anti-mumps IgM and IgG in the CSF can confirm the diagnosis of meningitis. Nucleic acid amplification techniques, such as real-time RT-PCR, are more sensitive than viral cultures and are available from some commercial laboratories, selected state laboratories, and the CDC. Diagnostic yield is highest if collected during the first 3 days of illness. Confirmatory diagnosis of mumps is also made by isolating the virus preferably from a swab of the duct of the parotid or other affected salivary gland. The virus can also be isolated from CSF early in aseptic meningitis. Vaccinated persons may shed virus for shorter periods of time compared to those who are unvaccinated.

Differential Diagnosis

Swelling of the parotid gland may be due to calculi in the parotid ducts, tumors, or cysts. Other causes include sarcoidosis, cirrhosis, diabetes, bulimia, pilocarpine usage, and Sjögren syndrome. Parotitis may be produced by pyogenic organisms (eg, *S aureus*, gram-negative organisms [particularly in debilitated individuals with poor oral intake]), drug reaction (phenothiazines, propylthiouracil), and other viruses (HIV, influenza A, parainfluenza, EBV infection, coxsackieviruses, adenoviruses, HHV-6). Swelling of the parotid gland must be differentiated from inflammation of the lymph nodes located more posteriorly and inferiorly than the parotid gland.

Treatment

Treatment is symptomatic. Topical compresses may relieve parotid discomfort. Some clinicians advocate IVIG for complicated disease (eg, thrombocytopenia), although its definitive role is unproven. There is no specific treatment for orchitis.

Prevention

Vaccination is the most effective way to prevent mumps.

Monovalent mumps vaccine is no longer available in the United States. Mumps vaccine is now administered as combined vaccine in MMR or MMRV vaccine. The vaccination schedule, indications, and contraindications are described in the measles section. The mumps vaccine component of the MMR is less effective than the measles and rubella components. One dose is 78% (range: 49–92%) protective. Two doses of the vaccine are 88% (range: 66–95%) effective. Rare reported complications of mumps vaccination include immune thrombocytopenic purpura and aseptic meningitis.

A 2017 study, evaluating the effect of a third dose of MMR vaccine after a mumps outbreak, showed that the attack rate was significantly lower among students who received a third dose compared with two doses, especially if the second dose was given more than 13 years prior to the outbreak. The CDC recommends a third dose of vaccine in case of an outbreak.

The patient should be isolated. For outbreak control, the most important step is to vaccinate all susceptible individuals. MMR vaccine is not effective in preventing the disease in unvaccinated patients who already have been exposed to the virus. In the healthcare setting, the following steps should be taken: implement droplet and standard precaution, isolate patients until swelling subsides (about 9 days from onset), and provide vaccination to healthcare workers with no evidence of immunity.

When to Refer

Any suspect cases should be reported to public health authorities.

When to Admit

- Trismus; meningitis; encephalitis; myocarditis; pancreatitis.
- Severe testicular pain; priapism.
- Severe thrombocytopenia.

Bockelman C et al. Mumps: an emergency medicine-focused update. J Emerg Med. 2018 Feb;54(2):207–14. [PMID: 29110978]
Cardemil CV et al. Effectiveness of a third dose of MMR vaccine for mumps outbreak control. N Engl J Med. 2017 Sep 7; 377(10):947–56. [PMID: 28877026]

Marin M et al. Recommendation of the Advisory Committee on Immunization Practices for use of a third dose of mumps virus-containing vaccine in persons at increased risk for mumps during an outbreak. MMWR Morb Mortal Wkly Rep. 2018 Jan 12;67(1):33–8. [PMID: 29324728]
Perez-Vilar S et al; WHO Global Vaccine Safety-Multi Country Collaboration. Enhancing global vaccine pharmacovigilance: proof-of-concept study on aseptic meningitis and immune thrombocytopenic purpura following measles-mumps containing vaccination. Vaccine. 2018 Jan 8;36(3):347–54. [PMID: 28558983]

3. Rubella

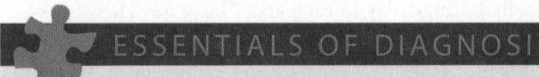

ESSENTIALS OF DIAGNOSIS

- Exposure 14–21 days before onset.
- No prodrome in children, mild prodrome in adults; mild symptoms (fever, malaise, coryza) coincide with, or precede by up to 5 days, the eruption of rash.
- Posterior cervical and postauricular lymphadenopathy 5–10 days before rash.
- Fine maculopapular rash of 3 days' duration; face to trunk to extremities.
- Leukopenia, thrombocytopenia.

General Considerations

Rubella is a systemic disease caused by a togavirus transmitted by inhalation of infective droplets. It is moderately communicable. Infection usually confers permanent immunity. The incubation period is 14–21 days. The disease is transmissible from 1 week before the rash appears until 15 days afterward.

The last cases of endemic rubella and congenital rubella syndrome were reported in 2009 from the Americas region. Each year in the United States, fewer than 10 cases of rubella are reported, all of which are due to the arrival of infected persons from other countries. In 2015, the WHO declared the Americas region free of rubella and congenital rubella syndrome. Some European countries are facing a challenge with lower immunization coverage among refugees and migrants. Worldwide, cases are decreasing due to widespread implementation of rubella-containing vaccines; as of 2016, the vaccine was added to the national vaccine schedule in 152 of 194 (78%) countries, though it is important to note that extensive variation in the rate of national coverage exists. On the other hand, the number of cases of congenital rubella syndrome remains high, particularly in Africa and Southeast Asia. The increase in congenital rubella syndrome may be secondary to an increase in surveillance and reporting of congenital rubella cases. The WHO set a goal to eliminate rubella in at least five of the six WHO regions (all but the Western Pacific region, which includes China) by 2020, although plans for rubella control are inadequate in 42 countries, especially in Africa and the Eastern Mediterranean regions.

Clinical Findings

A. Postnatal Rubella

Rubella is a common childhood disease; the majority of the cases are asymptomatic. The clinical picture of rubella is difficult to distinguish from other viral illnesses, such as infectious mononucleosis, measles, echovirus infections, and coxsackievirus infections. Fever and malaise, usually mild, accompanied by tender suboccipital adenitis, may precede the eruption by 1 week. Early posterior cervical and postauricular lymphadenopathy is common. A fine, pink maculopapular rash appears and fades from the face, trunk, and extremities in rapid progression (2–3 days), usually lasting 1 day in each area (Table 32–2).

B. Congenital Rubella

The principal importance of rubella lies in its devastating effects on the fetus in utero causing fetal death, preterm delivery, and teratogenic effects. The severity of symptoms is directly related to the gestational age; fetal infection during the first trimester leads to congenital rubella in at least 80% of fetuses; however, an infection during the fourth month can lead to 10% risk of a single congenital defect. In the second trimester of pregnancy, deafness is the primary complication.

C. Laboratory Findings

When rubella is suspected, the diagnosis requires serologic confirmation. Diagnosis of acute rubella infection is based on elevated IgM antibody, fourfold or greater rise in IgG antibody titers, or isolation of the virus. Serosensitivity to rubella is thought to change with subsequent pregnancies, although data from Hong Kong (lower immunity) and the United Kingdom (higher immunity) differed in their findings.

IgM is detectable in 50% of persons on day 1 of the rash but in most on day 5 after rash onset. Antibody testing can be performed on sera or saliva. An isolated IgM-positive test does not necessarily imply acute infection. IgM antibodies can persist after an infection or could be false-positive due to cross-reactivity with other antigens such as EBV, CMV, erythrovirus, and rheumatoid factor. This distinction is very important to make when infection is suspected in pregnancy. High-avidity anti-rubella IgG assays can distinguish between recent and remote infection. Low-avidity IgG is observed in acute rubella infections and lasts up to 3 months postinfection. After 3 months, low-avidity antibodies are replaced by high-avidity antibodies indicating remote infection.

The CDC can test for virus by RT-PCR from throat swabs, oral fluids, or nasopharyngeal secretions. The timing of sample collection is important and is best if collected within the first 3 days of an acute illness and within 3 months in case of congenital rubella syndrome. After 3 months of age, up to 50% of infants with congenital rubella syndrome will not shed the virus.

Complications

Complications of rubella are rare. Polyarticular arthritis and arthralgia occur more commonly in adult women; involve the fingers, wrists, and knees; and usually subside within 7 days but may persist for weeks. Hemorrhagic manifestations due to thrombocytopenia and vascular damage occur more commonly in children, unlike other complications. Hepatitis has been reported. Encephalitis, another rare complication, occurs more commonly in adults and has a high mortality rate.

Treatment

Rubella infection, including complications, is treated symptomatically.

Prevention

Patients with rubella should be isolated for 7 days after rash onset.

In the United States, monovalent rubella vaccine is no longer produced. Live attenuated rubella virus vaccine is primarily given as combination with the MMR vaccine or in combination with MMRV vaccine. It is recommended that the first dose be given between 12 months and 15 months. The second dose is given between age 4 and 6 years, prior to school entry. More details on scheduling, side effects, and contraindications are explained in the measles section. It is important that girls are immune to rubella prior to menarche. In the United States, about 80% of 20-year-old women are immune to rubella.

Rubella vaccine is safe and highly efficacious; a single dose of MMR vaccine is about 97% effective at preventing rubella.

The immune status of pregnant women should be evaluated because antibody titers fall in about 10% of vaccinated individuals within 12 years of vaccination. There is no evidence of adverse outcomes with MMR immunization of pregnant women, yet it is still recommended that women avoid pregnancy for at least 3 months after vaccination. Opportunities should be made available to vaccinate all women of childbearing age.

The administration of live vaccines to immunocompromised patients is controversial. In patients receiving immunosuppressive therapy as well as in patients who have undergone solid organ or bone marrow transplantation, seroconversion is higher to rubella compared with measles, mumps, and varicella. In addition, response to live attenuated vaccines may be lessened due to presence of antibodies from IVIG or other blood products. Safety is another concern when administering live attenuated vaccines to immunocompromised patients. Because MMR vaccine is contraindicated in solid organ transplant recipients, current evidence recommends that seronegative patients receive one or two doses of the MMR vaccine at least 4 weeks prior to solid organ transplantation. Patients who have undergone bone marrow transplant lose antigen-specific antibodies and should be revaccinated regardless of their vaccination history. The revised guidelines recommend MMR and varicella vaccines be given to seronegative patients without graft-versus-host disease 2 years after hematopoietic stem cell transplantation.

Prognosis

Rubella is a mild illness and rarely lasts more than 3–4 days. Congenital rubella has a high fetal mortality rate, and the associated congenital defects are largely permanent.

When to Refer

- Pregnancy.
- Meningitis/encephalitis.
- Significant vaccination reactions.
- Any suspect cases should be reported to public health authorities.

Croce E et al. Safety of live vaccinations on immunosuppressive therapy in patients with immune-mediated inflammatory diseases, solid organ transplantation or after bone-marrow transplantation—a systematic review of randomized trials, observational studies and case reports. Vaccine. 2017 Mar 1; 35(9):1216–26. [PMID: 28162821]

Hinman AR. Measles and rubella eradication. Vaccine. 2018 Jan 2;36(1):1–3. [PMID: 29183733]

Khanal S et al. Progress toward rubella and congenital rubella syndrome control—south-east Asia region, 2000–2016. MMWR Morb Mortal Wkly Rep. 2018 Jun 1;67(21):602–6. [PMID: 29851943]

Lao TT et al. Prior pregnancy and antenatal rubella sero-negativity-evidence of persistent maternal immunologic alteration? Am J Reprod Immunol. 2017 Sep;78(3). [PMID: 28653441]

Mipatrini D et al. Vaccinations in migrants and refugees: a challenge for European health systems. A systematic review of current scientific evidence. Pathog Glob Health. 2017 Mar; 111(2):59–68. [PMID: 28165878]

Snell LB et al. Screening for potential susceptibility to rubella in an antenatal population: a multivariate analysis. J Med Virol. 2017 Sep;89(9):1532–8. [PMID: 28370103]

World Health Organization. Rubella (CRS) reported cases: WHO vaccine-preventable diseases: monitoring system 2017 global summary. Updated 2018 Sep 21. http://apps.who.int/immunization_monitoring/globalsummary/timeseries/tsincidencecrs.html

4. Poliomyelitis

ESSENTIALS OF DIAGNOSIS

- ► Incubation period 7–14 days from exposure.
- ► Headache, stiff neck, fever, vomiting, sore throat.
- ► Lower motor neuron lesion (flaccid paralysis) with decreased deep tendon reflexes and muscle wasting.

General Considerations

Poliomyelitis virus, an enterovirus, is highly contagious through fecal-oral route, especially during the first week of infection. There are three wild poliovirus serotypes; however, only wild poliovirus type 1 has remained endemic since 2012. Pakistan and Afghanistan currently are the only countries with endemic wild type poliovirus transmission. In 2017, there were only 22 cases of wild type polio (14 in Afghanistan and 8 in Pakistan), and as of October 2018, only 20 cases of polio in these two endemic countries have been reported. In 2017, there were 96 vaccine-derived poliovirus infections, and as of October 2018, 68 vaccine-derived poliovirus cases (most of these type 2) had been

reported in five countries, including The Democratic Republic of the Congo, Niger, Nigeria, Papa New Guinea, and Somalia.

Cases of acute flaccid paralysis resembling polio with residual weakness are increasingly being reported throughout Africa (20 countries), the Eastern Mediterranean region (5 countries), intermittently in Europe (Germany and France), and the United States (a California outbreak in 2012–2014, surge in 2018).

In 2018, an increase in acute flaccid paralysis was noted in the United States, with 80 confirmed cases between January 1, 2018, and November 1, 2018. All but one of the 2018 cases (79, 99%) had a preceding viral illness in the month before presentation of neurologic signs. These signs most commonly involved the upper limbs (38, 47.5%) or all four limbs (23, 28.8%). The most commonly associated viruses (among 50 with virus isolation) were enterovirus A71 and enterovirus D68. In all instances, poliomyelitis was ruled out but an exact etiology for the acute flaccid paralysis was not always determined.

Clinical Findings

A. Symptoms and Signs

At least 95% of infections are asymptomatic. Patients who become symptomatic can present with abortive poliomyelitis, nonparalytic poliomyelitis, or paralytic poliomyelitis. **Post-poliomyelitis syndrome** is the constellation of symptoms that affect polio survivors and is not infectious.

1. Abortive poliomyelitis—Nonspecific symptoms of this minor illness include fever, headache, vomiting, diarrhea, constipation, and sore throat lasting 2–3 days.

2. Nonparalytic poliomyelitis—In addition to the above symptoms, signs of meningeal irritation and muscle spasm occur in the absence of frank paralysis.

3. Paralytic poliomyelitis—Characterized as a flaccid asymmetric paralysis affecting mostly the proximal muscles of the lower extremities; the febrile period is present over 2–3 days. Sensory loss is very rare. Paralytic poliomyelitis is divided into two forms, which may coexist: (1) spinal poliomyelitis involving the muscles innervated by the spinal nerves, and (2) bulbar poliomyelitis involving the muscles supplied by the cranial nerves (especially nerves IX and X) and of the respiratory and vasomotor centers. The most life-threatening aspect of bulbar poliomyelitis is respiratory paralysis. The incidence of paralytic poliomyelitis is higher when infections are acquired later in life.

4. Post-poliomyelitis syndrome—The syndrome presents with signs of chronic and new denervation. The most frequent symptoms are progressive muscle limbs paresis with muscle atrophy, with fasciculations and fibrillation during rest activity. The restless leg syndrome is also reported.

B. Laboratory Findings

The virus may be recovered from throat washings (early) and stools (early and late) and PCR of washings, stool, or CSF can also facilitate diagnosis. CSF findings include the following: (1) normal or slightly increased pressure and protein, (2) glucose is not decreased, and (3) white blood cells usually number less than 500/mcL and are principally lymphocytes after the first 24 hours. CSF findings are normal in 5% of patients. Neutralizing and complement-fixing antibodies appear during the first or second week of illness. Serologic testing cannot distinguish between wild type and vaccine-related virus infections.

Differential Diagnosis

Acute inflammatory polyneuritis (Guillain-Barré syndrome), Japanese encephalitis virus infection, West Nile virus infection, and tick paralysis may resemble poliomyelitis. In Guillain-Barré syndrome (see Chapter 24), the weakness is more symmetric and ascending in most cases, but the Miller Fisher variant of Guillain-Barré is similar to bulbar poliomyelitis. Paresthesia is uncommon in poliomyelitis but common in Guillain-Barré syndrome. The CSF usually has high protein content but normal cell count in Guillain-Barré syndrome. Acute flaccid paralysis resembling polio with residual weakness are increasingly recognized with no evidence of polio infection. Enterovirus is isolated in some of these cases.

Treatment

In the acute phase of paralytic poliomyelitis, patients should be hospitalized. In cases of respiratory weakness or paralysis, intensive care is needed. Intensive physiotherapy may help recover some motor function with paralysis. Attention to psychological disorders in longstanding disease is also important.

Immunodeficient individuals have prolonged excretion of poliovirus leading to virus circulation and threatening the polio eradication efforts. Pocapavir, an experimental capsid inhibitor antiviral agent, was tested in healthy adults given monovalent live oral poliovirus vaccine (OPV) type 1 and was shown to be safe and effective in reducing the duration of viral excretion in stool, but resistance emerged in 44% of treated participants in this study.

Immune modulators, such as prednisone, interferon, and IVIG, do not show any clear benefit in the treatment of post-poliomyelitis syndrome.

Prognosis

The death-to-case ratio for paralytic polio ranges between 2% and 30%, depending on age. Bulbar poliomyelitis carries a mortality rate of up to 75%.

Prevention

Given the epidemiologic distribution of poliomyelitis and the continued concern about vaccine-associated disease with the trivalent live OPV, the inactive (Salk) parenteral vaccine is currently used in the United States for all four recommended doses (at ages 2 months, 4 months, 6–18 months, and at 4–6 years). Inactivated vaccine is also routinely used elsewhere in the developed world where one dose is often administered, although immunogenicity is improved with additional doses.

Because most of circulating vaccine-derived poliovirus and vaccine-associated poliomyelitis are live OPV type 2, the WHO replaced worldwide the trivalent live OPV (containing types 1, 2, and 3) with the bivalent live OPV (type 1 and 3) in 2016. The goal is to replace all live OPV with inactive parenteral vaccination to eliminate poliovirus circulation. The advantages of oral vaccination are the ease of administration, low cost, effective local gastrointestinal and circulating immunity, and herd immunity. Monovalent OPV type 2 (mOPV2) as well as the trivalent OPV are used for control in countries with vaccine-derived type 2 outbreaks.

Routine immunization of adults in the United States is no longer recommended because of the low incidence of the disease. Vaccination should be considered for adults not vaccinated within the prior decade who are exposed to poliomyelitis or who plan to travel to endemic areas and adults engaged in high-risk activities (eg, laboratory workers handling stools).

When to Refer

Any suspicious cases should be referred to public health authorities.

Collett MS et al. Antiviral activity of pocapavir in a randomized, blinded, placebo-controlled human oral poliovirus vaccine challenge model. J Infect Dis. 2017 Feb 1;215(3):335–43. [PMID: 27932608]

Khan F et al. Progress toward polio eradication—worldwide, January 2016–March 2018. MMWR Morb Mortal Wkly Rep. 2018 May 11;67(18):524–8. [PMID: 29746452]

McCarthy KA et al. The risk of type 2 oral polio vaccine use in post-cessation outbreak response. BMC Med. 2017 Oct 4; 15(1):175. [PMID: 28974220]

McKay SL et al. Increase in acute flaccid myelitis—United States, 2018. MMWR Morb Mortal Wkly Rep. 2018 Nov 16;67(45): 1273–5. [PMID: 30439867]

Messacar K et al. Acute flaccid myelitis: a clinical review of US cases 2012–2015. Ann Neurol. 2016 Sep;80(3):326–38. [PMID: 27422805]

Pastuszak Ż et al. Post-polio syndrome. Cases report and review of literature. Neurol Neurochir Pol. 2017 Mar–Apr;51(2): 140–5. [PMID: 28209439]

World Health Organization. Global Polio Eradication Initiative. Polio today. http://polioeradication.org/polio-today

OTHER NEUROTROPIC VIRUSES

1. Rabies

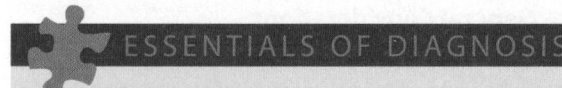

ESSENTIALS OF DIAGNOSIS

► History of animal bite.
► Paresthesias, hydrophobia, rage alternating with calm.
► Convulsions, paralysis, thick tenacious saliva.

General Considerations

Rabies is a viral (rhabdovirus) encephalitis transmitted by infected saliva that enters the body by an animal bite or an open wound. Worldwide, over 17 million cases of animal bites are reported every year, and it is estimated that about 60,000 deaths annually are attributable to rabies. Rabies is endemic in over 150 countries; on the basis of interviews, it is estimated that over 40% of the world's population lives in areas without rabies surveillance. Most cases of rabies occur in rural areas of Africa and Asia. India has the highest incidence, accounting for 36% of global deaths (http://www.who.int/rabies/epidemiology/en/). In developing countries, more than 90% of human cases and 99% of human deaths from rabies are secondary to bites from infected dogs. Rabies among travelers to rabies-endemic areas is usually associated with animal injuries (including dogs in North Africa and India, cats in the Middle East, and nonhuman primates in sub-Saharan Africa and Asia), with most travel-associated cases occurring within 10 days of arrival. Rare but related viruses are the Australian lyssavirus, transmitted by bats including one referred to as the black flying fox, and which has caused 3 deaths over the last 20 years, and the European lyssavirus, with cases from Germany and the United Kingdom.

In the United States, domestically acquired rabies cases are rare (approximately 92% of cases are associated with wildlife) but probably underreported. Reports largely from the East Coast show an increase in rabies among cats, with about 1% of tested cats showing rabies seropositivity. The annual caseload in the United States is 1–3 cases (https://www.cdc.gov/rabies/location/usa/surveillance/human_rabies.html). Surveillance for animal rabies in 2015 showed 5508 cases occurring in 49 states and Puerto Rico. Wildlife reservoirs, with each species having its own rabies variant(s), follow a unique geographic distribution in the United States: raccoons on the East Coast; skunks in the Midwest, Southwest, and California; and foxes in the Southwest and in Alaska. However, some areas have all three wildlife reservoirs (eg, the hill country of Texas). Hawaii is the only rabies-free state to date. Most of Western Europe and much of Oceania is rabies-free.

Raccoons, bats, and skunks account for 84% of the rabid animals found in the United States; other rabid animals include foxes, cats, cattle, and dogs. Rodents and lagomorphs (eg, rabbits) are unlikely to spread rabies because they cannot survive the disease long enough to transmit it (woodchucks and groundhogs are exceptions). Wildlife epizootics present a constant public health threat in addition to the danger of reintroducing rabies to domestic animals. Vaccination is the key to controlling rabies in small animals and preventing rabies transmission to human beings.

The virus enters the salivary glands of dogs 5–7 days before their death from rabies, thus limiting their period of infectivity. Less common routes of transmission include contamination of mucous membranes with saliva or brain tissue, aerosol transmission, and corneal transplantation. Recognized mutations in rabies virus proteins can subvert the host immune system. Transmission through solid organ and vascular segment transplantation from donors with unrecognized infection is also reported. A number of transplantation-associated cases are reported, including two clusters in the United States. Postexposure prophylaxis can be administered in these patients and may prevent development of disease.

The incubation period may range from 10 days to many years but is usually 3–7 weeks depending in part on the distance of the wound from the CNS. The virus travels in the nerves to the brain, multiplies there, and then migrates along the efferent nerves to the salivary glands. Rabies virus infection forms cytoplasmic inclusion bodies similar to Negri bodies. These Negri bodies are thought to be the sites of viral transcription and replication.

▶ Clinical Findings

A. Symptoms and Signs

While there is usually a history of animal bite, bat bites may not be recognized. The prodromal syndrome consists of pain at the site of the bite in association with fever, malaise, headache, nausea, and vomiting. The skin is sensitive to changes of temperature, especially air currents (aerophobia). Percussion myoedema (a mounding of muscles after a light pressure stimulus) can be present and persist throughout the disease. The CNS stage begins about 10 days after the prodrome and may be either encephalitic ("furious") or paralytic ("dumb"). The encephalitic form (about 80% of the cases) produces the classic rabies manifestations of delirium alternating with periods of calm, extremely painful laryngeal spasms on attempting drinking (hydrophobia), autonomic stimulation (hypersalivation), and seizures. In the less common paralytic form, an acute ascending paralysis resembling Guillain-Barré syndrome predominates with relative sparing of higher cortical functions initially. Both forms progress relentlessly to coma, autonomic nervous system dysfunction, and death.

B. Laboratory Findings

Biting animals that appear well should be quarantined and observed for 10 days. Sick or dead animals should be tested for rabies. A wild animal, if captured, should be sacrificed and the head shipped on ice to the nearest laboratory qualified to examine the brain for evidence of rabies virus. When the animal cannot be examined, raccoons, skunks, bats, and foxes should be presumed to be rabid.

Direct fluorescent antibody testing of skin biopsy material from the posterior neck (where hair follicles are highly innervated) has a sensitivity of 60–80%.

Quantitative RT-PCR, nucleic acid sequence-based amplification, direct rapid immunohistochemical test, and viral isolation from the CSF or saliva are advocated as definitive diagnostic assays. Antibodies can be detected in the serum and the CSF. Pathologic specimens often demonstrate round or oval eosinophilic inclusion bodies (Negri bodies) in the cytoplasm of neuronal cells, but the finding is neither sensitive nor specific. MRI signs are diffuse and nonspecific.

▶ Treatment & Prognosis

Management requires intensive care with attention to the airway, maintenance of oxygenation, and control of seizures. Universal precautions are essential. Corticosteroids are of no use. Survival is rare, and data are insufficient to provide estimate of success.

If postexposure prophylaxis (discussed below) is given expediently, before clinical signs develop, it is nearly 100% successful in prevention of disease. Once the symptoms have appeared, death almost inevitably occurs after 7 days, usually from respiratory failure. Most deaths occur in persons with unrecognized disease who do not seek medical care or in individuals who do not receive postexposure prophylaxis. The very rare cases in which patients recover without intensive care are referred to as "abortive rabies."

Prevention

Immunization of household dogs and cats and active immunization of persons with significant animal exposure (eg, veterinarians) are important. The most important decisions, however, concern animal bites. Animals that are frequent sources of infection to travelers are dogs, cats, and nonhuman primates.

In the developing world, education, surveillance, and animal (particularly dog) vaccination programs (at recurrent intervals) are preferred over mass destruction of dogs, which is followed typically by invasion of susceptible feral animals into urban areas. In some Western European countries, campaigns of oral vaccination of wild animals led to the elimination of rabies in wildlife.

A. Local Treatment of Animal Bites and Scratches

Thorough cleansing, debridement, and repeated flushing of wounds with soap and water are important. Rabies immune globulin or antiserum should be given as stated below. Wounds caused by animal bites should not be sutured.

B. Postexposure Immunization

The decision to treat should be based on the circumstances of the bite, including the extent and location of the wound, the biting animal, the history of prior vaccination, and the local epidemiology of rabies. *Any contact or suspect contact with a bat, skunk, or raccoon is usually deemed a sufficient indication to warrant prophylaxis.* Consultation with state and local health departments is recommended. Postexposure treatment including both immune globulin and vaccination should be administered as promptly as possible when indicated.

For patients who had not received rabies vaccination prior to possible exposure, the optimal form of **passive immunization** is human rabies immune globulin (HRIG; 20 international units/kg), administered once. As much as possible of the full dose should be infiltrated around the wound, with any remaining injected intramuscularly at a site distant from the wound. Finger spaces can be safely injected without development of a compartment syndrome. If HRIG is not available and appropriate tests for horse serum sensitivity are done, equine rabies antiserum (40 international units/kg) can be used.

Two vaccines are licensed and available for use in humans in the United States: a human diploid cell vaccine (HDCV, Immovax) and a purified chick embryo cell vaccine (PCEC, RabAvert). There are several postexposure

prophylaxis strategies. The most commonly used one is the "abbreviated Essen" strategy, where either of the current vaccines is given as four intramuscular injections of 1 mL in the deltoid or, in small children, into the anterolateral thigh muscles on days 0, 3, 7, and 14 after exposure. (The fifth dose at 28 days after exposure is no longer recommended except among immunosuppressed patients.) The vaccine should not be given in the gluteal area due to suboptimal response. An alternative intramuscular vaccination strategy that takes only 1 week, with injections on days 0, 3, and 7 after exposure with a Vero cell vaccine (Verorab) is reportedly successful in achieving adequate neutralizing titers at days 14 and 28 in a study from Thailand; this vaccine is not currently available in the United States.

The WHO supports an intradermal vaccination strategy using Verorab and the inactivated rabies virus vaccine Rabipur (an alternative formulation of the PCEC [purified chick embryo cell]) (0.1 mL per intradermal injection) for regions of the world where vaccine is in short supply; either vaccine can be given at two sites on days 0, 3, 7, and 28.

Rabies vaccines and HRIG should never be given in the same syringe or at the same site. Allergic reactions to the vaccine are rare and include a report of sudden unilateral sensorineural hearing loss and immune thrombocytopenic purpura, although local reactions (pruritus, erythema, tenderness) occur in about 25% and mild systemic reactions (headaches, myalgias, nausea) in about 20% of recipients. Intradermal vaccines appear to be better tolerated than intramuscular vaccines, especially among young children. Adverse reactions to HRIG seem to be more frequent in women and rare in young children. The vaccines are commercially available or can be obtained through health departments.

In patients with history of past vaccination, the need for HRIG is eliminated (HRIG is in short supply worldwide), but postexposure vaccination is still required. The vaccine should be given 1 mL in the deltoid twice (on days 0 and 3). Neither the passive nor the active form of postexposure prophylaxis is associated with fetal abnormalities and thus pregnancy is not considered a contraindication to vaccination. Peripartum rabies transmission occurs but is rare. Neonates may also receive both forms of postexposure prophylaxis at birth.

The WHO has a program to eliminate dog-transmitted human rabies by 2030.

C. Preexposure Immunization

Preexposure prophylaxis with three injections of human diploid cell vaccine intramuscularly (1 mL on days 0, 7, and 21 or 28) is recommended for persons at high risk for exposure: veterinarians (who should have rabies antibody titers checked every 2 years and be boosted with 1 mL intramuscularly); animal handlers; laboratory workers; Peace Corps workers; and travelers with stays over 1 month to remote areas in endemic countries in Africa, Asia, and Latin America. An intradermal route is also available (0.1 mL on days 0, 7, and 21 over the deltoid) but not in the United States. Immunosuppressive illnesses and agents including corticosteroids as well as antimalarials—in particular chloroquine—may diminish the antibody response.

A single-dose booster at 10 years after initial immunization increases the level of antibody titers. Unfortunately, data from travel services indicate that only a small proportion of travelers with anticipated lengthy stays in rabies-impacted areas receive the vaccine as recommended.

▶ When to Refer

Suspicion of rabies requires contact with public health personnel to initiate appropriate passive and active prophylaxis and observation of suspect cases.

▶ When to Admit

- Respiratory, neuromuscular, or CNS dysfunction consistent with rabies.
- Patients with suspect rabies require initiation of therapy until the disease is ruled out in suspect animals, and this requires coordination of care based on likelihood of patient compliance, availability of inpatient and outpatient facilities, and response of local public health teams.

Alberer M et al. Safety and immunogenicity of a mRNA rabies vaccine in healthy adults: an open-label, non-randomised, prospective, first-in-human phase 1 clinical trial. Lancet. 2017 Sep 23;390(10101):1511–20. [PMID: 28754494]

Davis BM et al. Everything you always wanted to know about rabies virus (but were afraid to ask). Annu Rev Virol. 2015 Nov;2(1):451–71. [PMID: 26958924]

2. Arbovirus Encephalitides

ESSENTIALS OF DIAGNOSIS

- ▶ Fever, malaise, stiff neck, sore throat, and vomiting, progressing to stupor, coma, and convulsions.
- ▶ Upper motor neuron lesion signs: exaggerated deep tendon reflexes, absent superficial reflexes, and spastic paralysis.
- ▶ CSF opening pressure and protein are often increased with lymphocytic pleocytosis.

▶ General Considerations

The arboviruses are arthropod-borne viral pathogens carried by mosquitoes or ticks that produce clinical manifestations in humans. The **mosquito-borne pathogens** include togaviruses (causing Western, Eastern, and Venezuelan equine encephalitis), flaviviruses (causing West Nile fever, St. Louis encephalitis, Japanese encephalitis, and Murray Valley encephalitis; dengue, Zika, and yellow fever can present with encephalitis), bunyaviruses (the California serogroup of viruses, including the Jamestown Canyon [seen largely in Northern states] and the La Crosse viruses [seen in the upper Midwest and mid-Atlantic primarily]), and the alphavirus chikungunya. The **tick-borne** causes of encephalitis include the flavivirus of the Powassan encephalitis (North American Northeast and Great Lakes), tick-borne encephalitis virus (Europe and Asia), and the

Colorado tick fever reovirus. Only those viruses causing primarily encephalitis in the United States are discussed here. The most commonly encountered arboviruses from 2017 in the United States are West Nile virus (2097 cases, 89% of arboviral neuroinvasive disease), Jamestown Canyon virus (75 cases), the La Crosse virus (63 cases), and Powassan virus (34 cases). Rare causes of domestic arboviruses were St. Louis encephalitis virus (11 cases) and eastern equine encephalitis virus disease (5 cases, 3 via organ transplantation).

West Nile virus is the leading cause of domestically acquired arboviral disease in the United States. West Nile virus disease is a nationally notifiable condition. Among the 2291 cases of domestic arboviral disease from 2017, cases were reported to the CDC from 48 states and the District of Columbia, 1425 (68%) were classified as neuroinvasive disease, and 32% were classified as non-neuroinvasive disease. Most cases are identified in Texas and California. Asymptomatic seroconversion is the norm and is not reported. Epidemiologic studies from the Dallas-Fort Worth area show consistency through time of the percentage of neuroinvasive disease.

Outbreaks with West Nile infection tend to occur between mid-July and early September. Climatic factors, including elevated mean temperatures and rainfall, correlate with increased West Nile infection. West Nile virus circulates between mosquitoes (mainly *Culex* species) and birds. In case of West Nile virus outbreak, infected birds develop high levels viremia that lead to substantial avian mortality and a high incidence of mosquito infection. Infected mosquitoes bite and infect people and other mammals. However, humans and other mammals are "dead end" hosts, since they do not transmit the virus on to other biting mosquitoes; only dengue and Venezuelan equine encephalitis viruses produce viremias high enough to allow continued transmission to other mosquitoes and ticks between humans and vectors. Human-to-human transmission is usually related to blood transfusion and organ transplantation. Since 2003, all blood donations in the United States are screened with nucleic acid amplification assays for West Nile virus. Eastern equine encephalitis is now also shown to be transmitted by organ transplantation.

▶ Clinical Findings

A. Symptoms and Signs

West Nile virus infection has an incubation period of 2–14 days. The infection is symptomatic in no more than 10% of the cases; of those, about 10% progress to neuroinvasive disease, including meningitis, encephalitis, and flaccid paralysis. The case fatality rate is about 10%.

Symptoms include acute febrile illness, and a nonpruritic maculopapular rash is variably present. Meningitis is indistinguishable from other viral meningitis. West Nile virus encephalitis presents with fever and altered mental status. Other signs include tremors, seizures, cranial nerve palsies, and pathologic reflexes. Acute flaccid (poliomyelitis-like) paralysis, which is asymmetric and can involve facial and respiratory muscles, is a well-known complication and is less commonly seen with other arboviruses infection. West Nile virus can also present as Guillain-Barré syndrome with radiculopathy. The disease manifestations associated with West Nile virus infection are strongly age-dependent: the acute febrile syndrome and mild neurologic symptoms are more common in the young, aseptic meningitis and poliomyelitis-like syndromes are seen in middle-aged persons, and frank encephalopathy is seen more often in older adults. All forms of disease tend to be severe in immunocompromised persons in whom neuroinvasive manifestations and associated high mortality are more apt to develop. Other risk factors for development of neuroinvasive disease and increased mortality include black race, diabetes, chronic kidney disease, and hepatitis C virus infection.

Host genetic variation in the interferon response pathway is associated with both risk for symptomatic West Nile virus infection and increased likelihood of West Nile virus disease progression.

B. Laboratory Findings

The peripheral white blood cell count is usually normal. Usually a CSF lymphocytic pleocytosis is present, and polymorphonuclear cells predominate early. The diagnosis of arboviral encephalitides depends on serologic tests. For West Nile virus, an IgM capture ELISA in serum or CSF is almost always positive by the time the disease is clinically evident, and the presence of IgM in CSF indicates neuroinvasive disease. Documentation of a fourfold increase in acute/convalescent IgG titers is confirmatory for all arboviruses. Antibodies to arboviruses persist for life, and the presence of IgG in the absence of a rising titer of IgM may indicate past exposure rather than acute infection. Serologic tests are available commercially and through local and state health departments. Cross-reactivity exists among the different flaviviruses, so a plaque reduction assay may be needed to definitively distinguish between West Nile fever, St. Louis encephalitis, and others. PCR assays (available through state laboratories and the CDC) can be used to detect viral RNA in serum, CSF, or tissue early after illness onset and may be particularly useful in immunocompromised patients with abnormal antibody responses. Individuals with chronic symptoms after West Nile virus infection may show persistent kidney infection for up to 6 years with West Nile virus RNA present in urine. Blood products are best screened using nucleic acid assays. MRI of the brain may reveal leptomeningeal, basal ganglia, thalamic, or periventricular enhancement.

▶ Differential Diagnosis

Mild forms of encephalitis must be differentiated from aseptic meningitis, lymphocytic choriomeningitis, and nonparalytic poliomyelitis.

Severe forms of arbovirus encephalitides are to be differentiated from other causes of viral encephalitis (HSV, mumps virus, poliovirus or other enteroviruses, HIV), encephalitis accompanying exanthematous diseases of childhood (measles, varicella, infectious mononucleosis, rubella), encephalitis following vaccination or infection (a demyelinating type seen after rabies, measles, pertussis

vaccination), toxic encephalitis (from drugs, poisons, or bacterial toxins such as *Shigella dysenteriae* type 1), Reye syndrome, and severe forms of stroke, brain tumors, brain abscess, autoimmune processes such as lupus cerebritis, and intoxications. In the California Encephalitis Project, anti-*N*-methyl-D-aspartate receptor (anti-NMDAR) encephalitis is a more common cause of encephalitis than viral diseases, especially in the young, with 65% of cases of encephalitis due to anti-NMDAR occurring among patients 18 or younger.

▶ Complications

Bronchial pneumonia, urinary retention and infection, prolonged weakness, and pressure injuries may occur. Retinopathy occurs in 24% of patients with a history of West Nile virus infection and is associated with increased risk in those with encephalitis. Few studies suggest that West Nile virus infection can persist in the kidneys, but in a subset of patients following West Nile virus infection, kidney infection may lead to progressive renal pathology.

▶ Treatment

Although specific antiviral therapy is not available for most causative entities, vigorous supportive measures can be helpful. Some studies suggest improved outcomes with the use of IVIG enriched with West Nile virus antibody; however, a randomized, controlled trial of IVIG did not show a benefit.

▶ Prognosis

Although most infections are mild or asymptomatic, the prognosis is always guarded, especially at the extremes of age. Most fatalities occur with neuroinvasive disease. Most patients with non-neuroinvasive West Nile virus disease or West Nile virus meningitis recover completely, but a syndrome of fatigue, malaise, and weakness can linger for weeks or months. Patients who recover from West Nile virus encephalitis or poliomyelitis often have residual neurologic deficits. The recovery of persons with severe neurologic compromise may take 6 months or longer. The sequelae of West Nile virus infection include a poliomyelitis-like syndrome, cognitive complaints, movement disorders, epilepsy, and depression; and they may become apparent late in the course of what appears to be a successful recovery.

Another entity, nonprimary infection, characterized by elevated serum IgG, absent serum IgM, and occasional detection of West Nile virus RNA in blood or CSF, is associated with underlying psychiatric disorders, hospitalization during times not associated with peak West Nile transmission, fever, and increased in-hospital mortality.

The long-term prognosis is generally better for Western equine than for Eastern equine or St. Louis encephalitis.

▶ Prevention

Mosquito avoidance (repellents, protective clothing, and insecticide spraying) is effective prevention. Laboratory precautions are indicated for handling all these pathogens. No human vaccine is currently available for the arboviruses prevalent in North America. A chimeric live attenuated West Nile virus vaccine is tested in phase I clinical trials and is shown to be safe and immunogenic in healthy adults.

Berlin D et al. Eastern equine encephalitis. Pract Neurol. 2017 Oct;17(5):387–91. [PMID: 28754695]

Burakoff A et al. West Nile virus and other nationally notifiable arboviral diseases—United States, 2016. MMWR Morb Mortal Wkly Rep. 2018 Jan 12;67(1):13–7. [PMID: 29324725]

Curren EJ et al. West Nile virus and other nationally notifiable arboviral diseases—United States, 2017. MMWR Morb Mortal Wkly Rep. 2018 Oct 19;67(41):1137–42. [PMID: 30335737]

Lyons JL et al. Case 34-2017. A 76-year old man with fever, weight loss, and weakness. N Engl J Med. 2017 Nov 9; 377(19):1878–86. [PMID: 29117489]

Yeung MW et al. Health-related quality of life in persons with West Nile virus infection: a longitudinal cohort study. Health Qual Life Outcomes. 2017 Oct 23;15(1):210. [PMID: 29061146]

3. Japanese Encephalitis

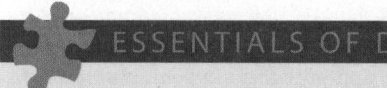

ESSENTIALS OF DIAGNOSIS

► Most important vaccine-preventable cause of encephalitis in the Asia-Pacific region.

► The virus is transmitted by mosquitoes, especially *Culex* species.

► Wide symptom spectrum; most infections asymptomatic.

General Considerations

The Japanese encephalitis virus is a flavivirus akin to those causing West Nile infection and St. Louis encephalitis. It is the most common cause of encephalitis in East Asia with over 68,000 estimated annual cases and up to 20,400 annual deaths. It is geographically contained to East Asia. Most cases occur in the summer and late fall, although in tropical and subtropical areas transmission occurs throughout the year. Major outbreaks every 2–15 years often correlate with patterns of agricultural development. The virus is transmitted by mosquitoes, especially *Culex* species. Areas with high endemicity tend to be warm-temperate, semitropical or tropical areas with high annual rainfalls. Wading birds (such as herons) and pigs more commonly sustain the infection as reservoirs in nature, since the viremia in humans is transient and not usually high enough to sustain transmission. In endemic countries, Japanese encephalitis is primarily a disease of children. Travelers to major urban areas for less than 1 month are at minimal risk for Japanese encephalitis. Transmission by blood transfusion is documented.

Clinical Findings

A. Symptoms and Signs

The median incubation period is 5–15 days. Most persons asymptomatically seroconvert. The 1% of patients in whom disease develops report sudden-onset headaches, nausea, and vomiting, followed by mental status changes, parkinsonian movement disorders, and in a smaller percentage, seizures, typically in children.

Japanese encephalitis most closely resembles St. Louis encephalitis and West Nile encephalitis, although epidemiologic data readily distinguish these infections in most instances. The clinical course is less severe in patients with a history of dengue virus infection.

B. Laboratory Findings and Diagnosis

The disease should be suspected in persons with symptoms of CNS infection who recently visited or who reside in an endemic area.

Common laboratory abnormalities include leukocytosis, mild anemia, and hyponatremia. CSF typically has a mild to moderate pleocytosis with a lymphocytic predominance, slightly elevated protein, and normal glucose.

Diagnosis is confirmed by finding anti-Japanese encephalitis IgM in CSF or serum using ELISA. Definitive diagnosis requires fourfold increase in virus-specific IgG confirmed by plaque reduction neutralization assay. Because of low levels of viremia in humans, RT-PCR is not recommended.

In severe disease, brain imaging reveals thalamic lesions, with the hippocampus, midbrain, basal ganglia, and cerebral cortex affected to varying degrees.

Complications

A variety of cognitive, neurologic, and psychiatric complications, including memory impairment and intellectual impairment in adults and children, are recognized to occur in as many as 50% of survivors and to persist at least 1–2 years after the acute infection. Rare reported complications include the opsoclonus myoclonus syndrome and the Kasabach-Merritt phenomenon of consumptive coagulopathy. The mortality is reportedly as high as 30%.

Treatment

Treatment is supportive, including antipyretics, analgesics, bed rest, and fluids. Corticosteroids may be needed for rare complications, such as the opsoclonus myoclonus syndrome.

Prevention

Using mosquito repellents; wearing long sleeves, long pants, and socks; and using air-conditioned facilities and bed nets are essential means of protection.

In the United States, inactivated Vero-cell culture-derived Japanese encephalitis vaccine (IXIARO) is licensed for the prevention of Japanese encephalitis in persons 2 months of age and older. Travelers who plan to spend more than 1 month in rural East Asia during Japanese encephalitis virus transmission season should receive the vaccine. Primary vaccination requires two doses administered 28 days apart, to be completed more than 1 week before travel. For adults, a booster dose is recommended in case of potential reexposure or of continued risk for infection if the primary series of the vaccine was administered over a 1 year before.

Four effective types of vaccine against Japanese encephalitis are available worldwide, including live attenuated and inactivated vaccines. The risk of serious reactions, including potential encephalitis, with live vaccines is low and decreases with age. Rare reported neurologic reactions are not definitively associated with vaccination. There are no studies about the safety of IXIARO in pregnant women. Therefore, administration of this vaccine to pregnant women should be deferred, unless the risk of infection outweighs the risk of vaccine complications.

Cheng VCC et al. Japanese encephalitis virus transmitted via blood transfusion, Hong Kong, China. Emerg Infect Dis. 2018 Jan;24(1). [PMID: 29043965]

Hills SL et al. Japanese encephalitis. In: Centers for Disease Control and Prevention. Chapter 3 (83): Infectious Diseases Related to Travel. CDC Health Information for International Travel 2018. New York: Oxford University Press, 2018. https://wwwnc.cdc.gov/travel/yellowbook/2018/infectious-diseases-related-to-travel/japanese-encephalitis

Sunwoo JS et al. Clinical characteristics of severe Japanese encephalitis: a case series from South Korea. Am J Trop Med Hyg. 2017 Aug;97(2):369–75. [PMID: 28829730]

World Health Organization. Japanese encephalitis: fact sheet No. 386. December 2015. http://www.who.int/mediacentre/factsheets/fs386/en/

4. Tick-Borne Encephalitis

ESSENTIALS OF DIAGNOSIS

► Flaviviral encephalitis found in Eastern, Central, and occasionally Northern Europe and Asia.

► Transmitted via ticks or ingestion of unpasteurized milk.

► Long-term neurologic sequelae in 2–25% of cases.

► Therapy is largely supportive.

► Prevention: avoid tick exposure, pasteurize milk, and vaccinate.

General Considerations

Tick-borne encephalitis (TBE) is a flaviviral infection caused by TBE virus with three subtypes: European, Siberian, and Far Eastern. The principal reservoirs and vectors for TBE virus are ticks with small rodents as the amplifying host; humans are an accidental host. The vectors for most cases are *Ixodes ricinus* (European subtype) and *Ixodes persulcatus* (Siberian and Far Eastern subtype). Infection results from tick bites during outdoor activities in forested areas, predominantly in the late spring through fall. Ingestion of unpasteurized milk from viremic livestock (goats, sheep, and cattle) is also a recognized mode of transmission. Transmission by transplantation of solid organs is reported leading to fatal outcomes. TBE is endemic in certain parts of Europe (reported recent foci include northeastern France and Bulgaria) and Asia (principally China but a few cases from Japan as well). The number of cases reported annually fluctuates significantly depending on surveillance, human activities, socioeconomic factors, ecology, and climate. Modeling studies from Prague suggests several superimposed cycles of variable year duration. The incubation period is 7–14 days for tick-borne exposures but only 3–4 days for milk ingestion.

Powassan virus is the only North American member of the tick-borne encephalitides. Its vector is several *Ixodes* species ticks. Most cases occur in older men (median age, 62; all deaths have occurred in persons over age 50), primarily from Northeast and North Central states (especially Minnesota, New York, and Wisconsin). Most reported cases are neuroinvasive with presentations including acute encephalitis and aseptic meningitis. The incubation period can range from 1 to 5 weeks, although pinpointing the date of actual exposure is often difficult.

Clinical Findings

A. Symptoms and Signs

Most cases are subclinical, and many resemble an influenza-like syndrome with 2–10 days of fever (usually with malaise, headache, and myalgias). In some cases, the disease is biphasic where the initial flu-like period is followed by a 1- to 21-day symptom-free interval followed by a second phase with fevers and neurologic symptoms (cases from Asia appear not to show this biphasic pattern). The neurologic manifestations range from febrile headache to aseptic meningitis and encephalitis with or without myelitis (preferentially of the cervical anterior horn) and spinal paralysis (usually flaccid). A myeloradiculitic form can also develop but is less common. Peripheral facial palsies, sometimes bilateral, tend to occur infrequently late in the course of infection, usually after encephalitis and usually are associated with a favorable outcome within 30–90 days. The main sequela of disease is paresis. Other causes of long-term morbidity include protracted cognitive dysfunction and persistent spinal nerve paralysis. The **post-encephalitic syndrome** is characterized by headache, difficulties concentrating, balance disorders, dysphasia, hearing defects, and chronic fatigue. A progressive motor neuron disease and partial continuous epilepsy are complications. Longstanding psychiatric complications are reported and include attention deficits, slowness of thought and learning impairment, depression, lability, and mutism.

Mortality in TBE is usually a consequence of brain edema or bulbar involvement.

B. Laboratory Findings and Diagnosis

Leukocytosis and neutrophilia are common. Abnormal CSF findings include an inconsistent pleocytosis that may persist for up to 4 months. Hyponatremia is more commonly seen than with other viral encephalitides. Neuroimaging might show hyperintense lesions in the thalamus, brainstem, and basal ganglia, and cerebral atrophy.

When neurologic symptoms develop, the TBE virus is typically no longer detectable in blood and CSF samples. Virus detection by RT-PCR in ticks from TBE patients, if available, can help with the diagnosis. TBE virus IgM and IgG are detected by ELISA when neurologic symptoms occur.

Cross-reactivity with other flaviviruses or a vaccinated state may require confirmation by detection of TBE virus–specific antibodies by plaque-reduction neutralization tests.

Differential Diagnosis

The differential diagnosis includes other causes of aseptic meningitis, such as enteroviral infections; poliomyelitis (no longer reported from Eastern Europe); herpes simplex encephalitis; and a variety of tick-borne pathogens, including tularemia, the rickettsial diseases, babesiosis, Lyme disease, and other flaviviral infections. Coinfections are documented with *Anaplasma*, *Babesia*, and *Borrelia* infections.

Treatment

There is no specific antiviral treatment, and therapy is largely supportive.

Prognosis

The three subtypes of TPE have different prognoses. The European subtype is usually milder with up to 2% mortality and 30% neuroinvasive disease. The Siberian subtype is associated with 3% mortality and chronic, progressive disease. The Far Eastern subtype is usually more severe with up to 40% mortality and higher likelihood of neurologic involvement. All three subtypes are more severe among elderly adults compared with children. Coinfection with *Borrelia burgdorferi* (the agent of Lyme disease; transmitted by the same tick vector) may result in more severe disease.

Prevention

There is no available TBE vaccine in the United States. There are four different inactivated TBE virus vaccines for adults and children licensed in Europe (two in Austria and Germany and two in Russia) and one available in China. The vaccine is safe and effective and should provide cross-protection against all three TBE virus subtypes. The initial vaccination schedule requires two to three doses given over 6 or more months with boosters every 1–5 years, the interval dependent on the vaccine and national guidelines. Breakthrough TBE in vaccinated individuals is reported, especially among recipients who are over 50 years of age and among persons who are immunosuppressed, such as those receiving anti-TNF therapy or methotrexate, indicating the need for a modified immunization strategy in such patients. Neuritis and neuropathies of peripheral nerves (plexus neuropathy—paresis of lower limb muscles, polyradiculopathy) are recognized complications of TBE vaccination.

The low popular support for the vaccine in endemic countries is responsible for limited abilities to control the disease. Other prevention recommendations include avoidance of tick exposure and pasteurization of cow and goat milk.

Fischer M et al. Tickborne encephalitis. In: Centers for Disease Control and Prevention. Chapter 3 (83): *CDC Health Information for International Travel 2018*. New York: Oxford University Press, 2018. https://wwwnc.cdc.gov/travel/yellowbook/2018/infectious-diseases-related-to-travel/tickborne-encephalitis

Krow-Lucal ER et al. Powassan virus disease in the United States, 2006–2016. Vector Borne Zoonotic Dis. 2018 Jun;18(6):286–90. [PMID: 29652642]

Velay A et al. A new hot spot for tick-borne encephalitis (TBE): a marked increase of TBE cases in France in 2016. Ticks Tick Borne Dis. 2018 Jan;9(1):120–5. [PMID: 28988602]

Yoshii K et al. Tick-borne encephalitis in Japan, Republic of Korea and China. Emerg Microbes Infect. 2017 Sep 20; 6(9):e82. [PMID: 28928417]

5. Lymphocytic Choriomeningitis

ESSENTIALS OF DIAGNOSIS

▶ "Influenza-like" prodrome of fever, chills, and cough, followed by a meningeal phase.

▶ Aseptic meningitis: stiff neck, headache, vomiting, lethargy.

▶ CSF: slight increase of protein, lymphocytic pleocytosis (500–3000/mcL).

▶ Complement-fixing antibodies within 2 weeks.

General Considerations

The lymphocytic choriomeningitis virus is an arenavirus (related to the pathogen causing Lassa fever, discussed below) that primarily infects the CNS. Its main reservoir is the house mouse (*Mus musculus*). Other rodents (such as rats, guinea pigs, and even pet hamsters), monkeys, dogs, and swine are also potential reservoirs. The infected animal sheds lymphocytic choriomeningitis virus in nasal secretions, urine, and feces; transmission to humans probably occurs through aerosolized particles and mucosal exposure, percutaneous inoculation, direct contact, or animal bites. The disease in humans is underdiagnosed and occurs most often in autumn. The lymphocytic choriomeningitis virus is typically not spread person to person, although vertical transmission is reported, and it is considered to be an under-recognized teratogen. Rare cases related to solid organ transplantation and autopsies of infected individuals are also reported. All reported cases were donor derived. Outbreaks are uncommon, and usually occur in laboratory settings among those workers with significant rodent exposure.

The ubiquitous nature of its reservoir and the large distribution of the reported cases suggest a widespread geographic risk of lymphocytic choriomeningitis virus infection. Serologic surveys in the southern and eastern United States suggest past infection in approximately 3–5% of those tested, although later data from upstate New York showed less than 1% seroprevalence. Infection risk can be reduced by limiting contact with pet rodents and rodent trappings.

Clinical Findings

A. Symptoms and Signs

The incubation period is 8–13 days to the appearance of systemic manifestations and 15–21 days to the appearance of meningeal symptoms. Symptoms are biphasic, with a prodromal illness characterized by fever, chills, headache, myalgia, cough, and vomiting, occasionally with lymphadenopathy and maculopapular rash. After 3–5 days the fever subsides only to return after 2–4 days alongside the meningeal phase, characterized by headache, nausea and vomiting, lethargy, and variably present meningeal signs. Arthralgias can develop late in the course. Transverse myelitis, deafness, Guillain-Barré syndrome, and transient and permanent hydrocephalus are reported. Lymphocytic choriomeningitis virus is a well-known, albeit underrecognized, cause of congenital infection frequently complicated with obstructive hydrocephalus and chorioretinitis. In fetuses and newborns with ventriculomegaly or other abnormal neuroimaging findings, screening for congenital lymphocytic choriomeningitis may be considered; mothers are asymptomatic half the time. In over one-third of cases, rodent exposure is reported retrospectively. Occasionally, a syndrome resembling the viral hemorrhagic fevers is described in transplant recipients of infected organs and in patients with lymphoma.

B. Laboratory Findings

Leukocytosis or leukopenia and thrombocytopenia may be initially present. During the meningeal phase, CSF analysis frequently shows lymphocytic pleocytosis (total count is often 500–3000/mcL) alongside a slight increase in protein, while a low to normal glucose is seen in at least 25%. The virus may be recovered from the blood and CSF by mouse inoculation. Complement-fixing antibodies appear during or after the second week. Detection of specific IgM by ELISA is widely used. Detection of lymphocytic choriomeningitis virus by PCR is available in research settings.

► Differential Diagnosis

The influenza-like prodrome and latent period may distinguish this from other aseptic meningitides, and bacterial and granulomatous meningitis. A history of exposure to mice or other potential vectors is an important diagnostic clue.

► Treatment

Treatment is supportive. In several survivors of transplant-associated outbreaks, ribavirin (which is effective against other arenaviruses) has been used successfully along with decreasing immunosuppression.

► Prognosis

Complications and fatalities are rare in the general population. The illness usually lasts 1–2 weeks, though convalescence may be prolonged. Lymphocytic choriomeningitis in solid organ transplant recipients is associated with a poor prognosis; of reported cases, the mortality rate is more than 80%.

► Prevention

Pregnant women should be advised of the dangers to their unborn children inherent in exposure to rodents.

Aebischer O et al. Lymphocytic choriomeningitis virus infection induced by percutaneous exposure. Occup Med (Lond). 2016 Mar;66(2):171–3. [PMID: 26416845]

Talley P et al. Notes from the field: lymphocytic choriomeningitis virus meningoencephalitis from a household rodent infestation—Minnesota, 2015. MMWR Morb Mortal Wkly Rep. 2016 Mar 11;65(9):248–9. Erratum in: MMWR Morb Mortal Wkly Rep. 2016;65(11):295. [PMID: 26963688]

6. Prion Diseases

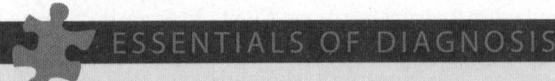

ESSENTIALS OF DIAGNOSIS

- ► Rare in humans.
- ► Cognitive decline.
- ► Myoclonic fasciculations, ataxia, visual disturbances, pyramidal and extrapyramidal symptoms.
- ► Variant form presents in younger persons with prominent psychiatric or sensory symptoms.
- ► Specific EEG patterns.

► General Considerations

The transmissible spongiform encephalopathies are a group of fatal neurodegenerative diseases affecting humans and animals. They are caused by proteinaceous infectious particles or prions. These agents show slow replicative capacity and long latent intervals in the host. They induce the conformational change ("misfolding") of a normal brain protein (prion protein; PrP[C]) into an abnormal isoform (PrP[Sc]) that accumulates and causes neuronal vacuolation (spongiosis), reactive proliferation of astrocytes and microglia, and, in some cases, the deposition of beta-amyloid oligomeric plaques.

Prion disease can be hereditary, sporadic, or transmissible in humans. Hereditary disorders are caused by germ line mutations in the PrP[C] gene causing familial Creutzfeldt–Jakob disease (fCJD), Gerstmann-Sträussler-Scheinker syndrome (GSS), and fatal familial insomnia. Another uncommon hereditary disorder is PrP systemic amyloidosis.

Sporadic Creutzfeldt-Jakob disease (sCJD) is the most common of the human prion diseases, accounting for approximately 85% of cases; it has no known cause. Transmissible prion disease is described only for kuru and Creutzfeldt-Jakob disease in its iatrogenic (iCJD) and variant (vCJD) form. Iatrogenic transmission of CJD is associated with prion contaminated human corneas, dura mater grafts, growth hormone, gonadotropins, stereotactic electroencephalography, electrodes, and neurosurgical instruments. Abnormal prion proteins have been detected in the nasal mucosa and urine of patients with Creutzfeldt-Jakob disease, raising health concerns about possibility of transmission.

Kuru, once prevalent in central New Guinea, is now rare, a decline in prevalence that started after the abandonment of cannibalism in the late 1950s (a protective allele of the PrP gene is now identified at codon 127).

More than 200 cases of vCJD (bovine spongiform encephalopathy [BSE] or "mad cow disease") were reported in the United Kingdom since the first documented cases there in the mid-1990s. It is far less common in North America, with only four cases reported in the United States (the last one in 2015) and two deaths in Canada from definite or probable vCJD. Of the US-reported cases, none are confirmed to have acquired the disease locally (two of them acquired the infection in the United Kingdom, one in Saudi Arabia, one possibly in a Middle Eastern or Eastern European country). This disease is characterized by its bovine-to-human transmission through ingestion of meat from cattle infected with BSE. There is no animal-to-animal spread of BSE, and milk and its derived products are not considered infectious. Reports of secondary transmission of vCJD due to blood transfusions from asymptomatic donors are reported in the United Kingdom. Although iCJD and vCJD are not associated with a known PrP gene mutation, a polymorphism in codon 129 is prevalent and seems to determine susceptibility and expression of clinical disease.

The overall annual incidence of prion disease worldwide is approximately 1–2/1 million person-years. In the United States, among the 4085 cases reported through September 18, 2018, to the US National Prion Disease Pathology Surveillance Center, 3656 (89.5%) were sporadic, 400 (9.8%) familial, 12 (0.3%) iatrogenic, and 4 (0.1%) vCJD.

A **chronic wasting disease** also due to a transmissible spongiform encephalopathic agent is occurring among deer, elk, and moose and has been reported from 24 states including most of Wyoming and parts of Colorado but present in the East and South as well. Although there are no documented of transmission to humans, the CDC recommends refraining from killing bizarrely acting animals, not handling or eating roadkill, and wearing gloves when dressing wild game. Testing for the virus in game animals may be useful, but its efficacy is not established.

▶ Clinical Findings

A. Symptoms and Signs

Both sCJD and fCJD usually present in the sixth or seventh decade of life, whereas the iCJD form tends to occur in a much younger population. Clinical features of these three forms of disease usually involve mental deterioration (dementia, behavioral changes, loss of cortical function) that is progressive over several months, as well as myoclonus and extrapyramidal (hypokinesia) and cerebellar manifestations (ataxia, dysarthria). Finally, coma ensues, usually associated with an akinetic state and less commonly decerebrate/decorticate posturing. Like iCJD, vCJD usually affects younger patients (averaging ~28 years), but the duration of disease is longer (about 1 year). The degree of organ involvement is often extensive, and the clinical symptoms are unique, mainly characterized by prominent psychiatric and sensory symptoms.

B. Laboratory Findings

CJD should be considered as a diagnosis in the proper clinical scenario, in the absence of alternative diagnoses after routine investigations. Abnormalities in CSF are subtle and rarely helpful. The detection of 14-3-3 protein in the CSF is helpful for the diagnosis of sCJD but not in vCJD and fCJD. Its sensitivity and specificity are widely variable among different studies and may be increased with use of tau protein assays. CSF detection of total PrP can differentiate CJD from atypical Alzheimer disease with 82% sensitivity and 91% specificity.

A blood-based assay and PCR in CSF may help with the diagnosis of vCJD with high specificity but 71% sensitivity. The assay as well as 14-3-3 protein assay and a "quaking induced conversion" assay are all available through the National Prion Disease Surveillance Center at Case Western University in Cleveland. Other referral laboratories with variable availability of assays include state health departments, academic centers, and the National Prion Clinics in the United Kingdom. It is also recognized that the presence of a variant with low titers ("very low peripheral prion colonization") in peripheral tissue, including frequently biopsied tonsillar tissue, may be responsible for the underrecognition of vCJD.

Probable diagnosis requires the presence of rapidly progressive dementia plus two of four clinical features (myoclonus, visual or cerebellar signs, pyramidal/extrapyramidal signs, and akinetic mutism) as well as a positive laboratory assay (typical EEG, positive 14-3-3 CSF assay with duration under 2 years) and MRI high signal in the caudate and/or putamen on diffusion-weighted imaging (DWI) or fluid-attenuated inversion recovery (FLAIR) imaging. In sCJD, the EEG typically shows a pattern of paroxysms with high voltages and slow waves, while the MRI is characteristic for bilateral areas of increased signal intensity, predominantly in the caudate and putamen. An MRI can improve early diagnosis of sCJD because clinical findings are often missed. When an experienced neuroradiologist or a prion disease expert reviews the MRI, diagnostic sensitivity of MRI for sCJD increases to 91%.

▶ Differential Diagnosis

Autoimmune encephalitis can have a similar clinical picture. The presence of high titer autoantibodies (eg, to the NMDA receptor) in the CSF is consistent with autoimmune encephalitis.

▶ Treatment & Prevention

There is no specific treatment for CJD. Once symptoms appear, the infection invariably leads to death. Flupirtine (an analgesic drug) is sometimes useful in slowing the associated cognitive decline but does not affect survival. Quinacrine (mepacrine) was evaluated as an oral treatment option but was not shown to improve survival for people with sCJD. Antibodies against PrP is also proposed as a therapeutic strategy. Studies are in progress to identify epitopes for vaccine development, but no promising candidates exist to date.

Iatrogenic CJD can be prevented by limiting patient exposure to potentially infectious sources as mentioned above. Prevention of vCJD relies on monitoring livestock for possible infection. The American Red Cross does not accept blood donations from persons with a family history of CJD or with a history of dural grafts or pituitary-derived growth hormone injections.

An international referral and database for CJD is available at http://www.cjdsurveillance.com.

Reference centers are available at Case Western Reserve University in the United States and the University College London Hospitals in the United Kingdom.

Annus Á et al. Prion diseases: new considerations. Clin Neurol Neurosurg. 2016 Nov;150:125–32. [PMID: 27656779]
Bardelli M et al. A bispecific immunotweezer prevents soluble PrP oligomers and abolishes prion toxicity. PLoS Pathog. 2018 Oct 1;14(10):e1007335. [PMID: 30273408]
Giles K et al. Developing therapeutics for PrP prion diseases. Cold Spring Harb Perspect Med. 2017 Apr 3;7(4). pii: a023747. [PMID: 28096242]

7. Progressive Multifocal Leukoencephalopathy (PML)

PML is a rare demyelinating CNS disorder caused by the reactivation of the JC virus (John Cunningham virus or JCV). This polyomavirus usually causes its primary infection during childhood with about 80% of adults typically being seropositive. The virus remains latent in the kidneys, lymphoid tissues, epithelial cells, peripheral blood leukocytes, bone marrow, and possibly brain until reactivation occurs and symptoms become evident. This reactivation is usually seen in adults with impaired cell-mediated immunity, especially AIDS patients (5–10% of whom develop PML), as well as those with idiopathic CD4 lymphopenia syndrome. It is also reported among those with lymphoproliferative and myeloproliferative disorders; in those with granulomatous, inflammatory, and rheumatic diseases (systemic lupus erythematosus and rheumatoid arthritis in particular); in those who have undergone solid and hematopoietic cell transplantation; and occasionally in those who have other medical states, including cirrhosis and kidney disease.

Diagnostic criteria that use clinical, imaging, pathologic, and virologic manifestations of JCV are available from the American Academy of Neurology.

Medication-associated PML is described with the use of natalizumab, rituximab, infliximab (one case), azathioprine with corticosteroids (one case), and mycophenolate mofetil. Natalizumab, a monoclonal antibody used in the treatment of multiple sclerosis, is associated with the risk of PML developing in 4 per 1000 treated patients, with the rate increasing with duration of therapy. The risk of clinical PML appears to increase up to 36 months of therapy and levels off thereafter. The mean interval between use of the drug to the diagnosis of PML is 5.5 months. The virus is detected in the CSF of up to one-half of all patients treated with natalizumab. An immune reconstitution inflammatory state (IRIS) may follow cessation of natalizumab or other monoclonal antibody therapy, although the JCV presence and the residual neurologic deficits may not clear for years after therapy is stopped. The risk of developing PML associated with rituximab is at least 1 in 25,000 exposed patients with cases reported in various autoimmune conditions treated with rituximab (systemic lupus erythematosus,

rheumatoid arthritis, multiple sclerosis). Although the exact relationship between latent JCV and frank PML remains unclear, higher JC viral loads are detected among patients who are immunosuppressed and among those who have HIV infection with lower CD4 counts.

Smoking is reportedly associated with an increased risk of PML.

▶ Clinical Findings

A. Symptoms and Signs

JCV causes lytic infection of oligodendrocytes in the white matter and symptoms presenting subacutely reflect the diverse areas of CNS involvement. Symptoms include altered mental status, aphasia, ataxia, hemiparesis or hemiplegia, and visual field disturbances. Seizures occur in about 18%. Involvement of cranial nerves and the cervical spine is rare.

B. Laboratory Findings

Quantitative PCR for JCV in CSF is used for diagnosis in patients with compatible clinical and radiologic findings. Persistent JC viremia and increasing urinary JCV DNA may be predictive of PML. An anti-JCV IgG was higher 6 months before diagnosis but was not predictive of PML in a cohort of HIV-infected persons.

MRI of the brain shows multifocal areas of white matter demyelination without mass effect or, usually, contrast enhancement. These findings may not be distinguishable from IRIS. Increased uptake of methionine with concomitant decreased uptake of fluorodeoxyglucose in positron emission tomography may be helpful for diagnosis. In HIV-infected patients, a syndrome of cerebellar degeneration is described.

▶ Treatment & Prevention

Limiting the immunosuppressed state without inducing an IRIS represents the mainstay of therapy for PML. Treatment of HIV with ART reduces the incidence of PML, improves the clinical symptoms, reverses some of the radiographic abnormalities, and improves the 1-year mortality rate, regardless of baseline CD4 count. Immune recovery can induce worsening of the clinical picture in a small number of cases. Immune reconstitution syndromes do not alter mortality but are associated with a form of PML called non-determined leukoencephalopathy associated with a chemokine polymorphism. Significant neurologic sequelae to PML infections are the rule and deficits may persist for years.

Decreasing immunosuppression in non-AIDS patients with PML (eg, multiple sclerosis or transplant patients) is also important. Cidofovir may be beneficial in non–AIDS-related cases, while corticosteroids may be useful with immune reconstitution. Because the JCV infects cells through serotonin receptors, some clinicians recommend the use of risperidone and mirtazapine. Anecdotal reports show that premature stopping of natalizumab in multiple sclerosis may itself lead to IRIS states. Plasma exchange, which theoretically reduces the plasma level of agents associated with PML, may be useful in natalizumab-associated PML but is associated with a high risk of IRIS. In kidney transplant patients, a preinduction regimen with IVIG and rituximab and transplantation with lymphocyte-depleted cells appears to reduce the risk of PML. Similarly, titers of JC antibody are not shown to significantly increase prior to clinical onset of PML.

Loignon M et al. Treatment options for progressive multifocal leukoencephalopathy in HIV-infected persons: current status and future directions. Expert Rev Anti Infect Ther. 2016;14(2):177–91. [PMID: 26655489]

Major EO et al. JC viremia in natalizumab-treated patients with multiple sclerosis. N Engl J Med. 2013 Jun 6;368(23):2240–1. [PMID: 23738566]

8. Human T-Cell Lymphotropic Virus (HTLV)

HTLV-1 and -2 are retroviruses that infect CD4 and CD8 T cells, respectively, where they persist as a lifelong latent infection. HTLV-1 currently infects approximately 20 million individuals worldwide. It is endemic to many regions in the world including southern Japan, the Caribbean, much of sub-Saharan Africa, South America, Eastern Europe, and Oceania. The Caribbean basin and southwestern Japan show the highest prevalence of infection (4–37%). Conversely, HTLV-2 is mainly found in native populations of South (1–58%), Central (8–10%), and North America (2–13%) as well as African pygmy tribes. In some areas of Africa (eg, Malawi), HTLV-2 seroprevalence is higher than HTLV-1 seroprevalence.

In the United States, studies done in blood donors show a seroprevalence of HTLV-1 of 0.005% and HTLV-2 of 0.014%, a decline since the early 1990s. The virus is transmitted horizontally (sex), vertically (intrauterine, peripartum, and prolonged breastfeeding), and parenterally (injection drug use and blood transfusion). Hence, a higher prevalence is seen among injection drug users. Coinfection with HIV-1 occurs but is often underrecognized. Transmission via organ transplant has been reported. Disease may flare when biologic agents are used for rheumatoid conditions.

▶ **Clinical Findings**

A. Symptoms and Signs

HTLV-1 infection is associated with HTLV-1 adult T-cell lymphoma/leukemia (ATL) and HTLV-1 associated myelopathy/tropical spastic paraparesis (HAM/TSP). In contrast, HTLV-2 is significantly less pathogenic, with few reported cases of HAM/TSP as well as other neurologic manifestations. The causative association of HTLV-1 with ATL, attributed to the virally encoded oncoprotein *tax*, is well established. The lifetime risk of developing ATL among seropositive persons is estimated to be 3% in women and 7% in men, with an incubation period of at least 15 years. The mean age at diagnosis of ATL is 40–50 years in Central and South America and 60 years in Japan.

ATL clinical syndromes may be classified as chronic, acute (leukemic), smoldering, or lymphomatous. A primary cutaneous tumor is also described and shows a worse

prognosis compared with the smoldering type. Clinical features of ATL include diffuse lymphadenopathy, maculopapular skin lesions that may evolve into erythroderma, a bronchoalveolar disorder, organomegaly, lytic bone lesions, and hypercalcemia. Opportunistic infections, such as *P jirovecii* pneumonia and cryptococcal meningitis, are common.

HAM/TSP, associated with both HTLV-1 and HTLV-2, develops in 0.3–4% of seropositive individuals and is more common in women and in older individuals. A chronic inflammation of the spinal cord leads to intense and progressive motor weakness and symmetric spastic paraparesis, bilateral facial palsies, falls, nociceptive low back pain, and paraplegia with hyperreflexia. Bladder and sexual disorders (eg, dyspareunia, erectile dysfunction), sensory disturbances, and constipation are also common. Both viruses can also induce motor abnormalities, such as leg weakness, impaired tandem walk, and vibration sense, without overt HTLV-associated myelopathy.

HTLV-1 seropositivity is associated with an increased risk of tuberculosis, *Strongyloides stercoralis* hyperinfection, crusted scabies, and infective dermatitis. Inflammatory states associated with HTLV-1 infection include arthropathy, recurrent facial palsies, polymyositis, uveitis, and sicca, but inconsistently Sjögren syndrome, vasculitis, cryoglobulinemia, infiltrative pneumonitis, and ichthyosis. Bronchioloalveolar carcinoma is increased in frequency in the presence of HTLV-1.

HTLV-2 appears to cause a myelopathy that is milder and slower to progress than HAM. All-cause and cancer mortality are higher among HTLV-2 seropositive patients.

HTLV-1/HIV coinfection is associated both with higher CD4 counts and a higher risk of HAM.

B. Laboratory Findings

The peripheral smear can show atypical lymphoid cells with basophilic cytoplasm and convoluted nuclei (flower cells) but the diagnostic standard is evidence of clonal integration of the proviral DNA genome into tumor cell. The identification of HTLV-1 antibodies supports the diagnosis. Serum neopterin levels may indicate disease activity. An HTLV-1 provirus load in peripheral blood mononuclear cells and CSF cells and an HTLV-1 mRNA load are proposed as markers of HAM risk and progression. HTLV positivity is associated with erythrocytosis, lymphocytosis (HTLV-2), and thrombocytosis (HTLV-1).

▶ **Treatment, Prevention, & Prognosis**

No vaccine or antiviral therapy currently exists for the prevention and treatment of HTLV infections.

Management of ATL consists mainly of chemotherapy, with allogeneic stem cell transplantation and the use of monoclonal antibodies (anti-CCR4 and anti-CD25). A chemotherapy regimen in Japan using eight different agents shows a higher response rate than traditional biweekly CHOP (40% vs 25%). Combination therapy with interferon-alpha has been used with success. Nivolumab is being studied as a novel therapy. Prophylaxis against infections is needed in ATL because patients show a profound immunodeficiency. Patients who are coinfected with HIV-1 and HTLV reportedly do respond to ART for HIV.

HAM is treated with a variety of immune-modulating agents (including corticosteroids) without consistent results. Combination therapy with antiretrovirals does not show benefit, although several trials evaluating raltegravir alone or in combination with zidovudine are underway. Interferon-alpha may be of some efficacy. A significant response is reported with the combined regimen of prednisolone, pegylated interferon, and sodium valproate. Clinical trials also are currently underway to assess the efficacy of pentoxifylline, cyclosporine, and the retinoid tamibarotene in the treatment of HAM. Small, uncontrolled studies suggest plasmapheresis results in improvement in gait and sensory disturbance among some patients and improvement in muscle pain with pulsed methylprednisolone. In general, however, no agent is effective.

Screening of the blood supply for HTLV-1 is required in the United States. There is significant cross-reactivity between HTLV-1 and HTLV-2 by serologic studies, but PCR can distinguish the two. Improved assays to screen organ donors for HTLV-1 and -2 infections are needed, although such screening is not currently required.

Boostani R et al. Triple therapy with prednisolone, pegylated interferon and sodium valproate improves clinical outcome and reduces human T-cell leukemia virus type 1 (HTLV-1) proviral load, tax and HBZ mRNA expression in patients with HTLV-1-associated myelopathy/tropical spastic paraparesis. Neurotherapeutics. 2015 Oct;12(4):887–95. [PMID: 26174324]

Kabiri M et al. The novel immunogenic chimeric peptide vaccine to elicit potent cellular and mucosal immune responses against HTLV-1. Int J Pharm. 2018 Oct 5;549(1-2):404–14. [PMID: 30075250]

Khan MY et al. HTLV-1 associated neurological disorders. Curr Top Med Chem. 2017;17(12):1320–30. [PMID: 28017149]

Terada Y et al. Treatment of rheumatoid arthritis with biologics may exacerbate HTLV-1-associated conditions: a case report. Medicine (Baltimore). 2017 Feb;96(6):e6021. [PMID: 28178142]

VIRAL HEMORRHAGIC FEVERS

1. Ebola Viral Disease (EVD)

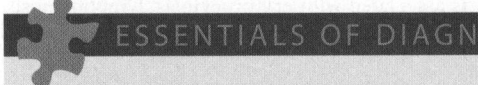

ESSENTIALS OF DIAGNOSIS

▸ **Early stage EVD:** a nonspecific febrile illness.

▸ **Later stage EVD:** severe gastrointestinal symptoms, then neurologic symptoms and hypovolemic shock.

▸ Hemorrhagic manifestations are late manifestations.

▸ Uveitis is a prominent ocular finding.

▸ Travel and contact history from an Ebola-affected country raise suspicion.

▸ Virus is detected with a real-time RT-PCR.

▸ General Considerations

Genus *Ebolavirus* is a single-stranded RNA virus in the Filoviridae family. Four different species of *Ebolavirus* have been identified to cause human disease. Fruit bats are possible reservoir for *Ebolavirus*. Zoonotic transmission to humans occurs via contact with the reservoir or an infected primate. *Ebolavirus* can continue to be transmitted among humans who have direct contact with infected body fluids. To acquire EVD, the virus must enter the body via mucous membranes, nonintact skin, sexual intercourse, breastfeeding, or needlesticks. Traditional burial practices in Africa (which entail considerable contact with the corpse) and unprotected direct care of persons with EVD are associated with highest transmission risk. *Ebolavirus* has been detected in semen up to 9 months after recovery from infection.

EVD has a 2–21-day incubation period. Prior to manifestation of symptoms, *Ebolavirus* is not transmissible. Even at symptom onset, the risk of transmission is low but increases over time.

The first Ebola outbreak occurred in 1976 as a simultaneous epidemic in the Democratic Republic of Congo and South Sudan. Subsequent outbreaks were confined to the Democratic Republic of Congo, Uganda, and Sudan until March 2014 when the first Ebola case in West Africa was identified in Guinea. *Zaire ebolavirus* was the associated species. This Ebola outbreak grew to be larger than all prior Ebola outbreaks combined. The number of EVD cases spread rapidly; there were at least 10 affected countries, especially Guinea, Liberia, and Sierra Leone. Many cases and deaths in these countries occurred among healthcare workers. In the United States, 11 persons were treated for Ebola. Most were healthcare workers who were evacuated to the United States and 4 patients were diagnosed in the United States. Sierra Leone contained its last EVD outbreak as of March 2016. Guinea was declared free of EVD transmission in June 2016. Liberia declared the end of its last outbreak in June 2016. The WHO reports that the West African Ebola outbreak was associated with 28,616 cases and 11,310 deaths during the approximately 2-year interval of the outbreak between March 2014 and March 2016.

Two outbreaks were reported in May and August of 2018, both in the Democratic Republic of Congo (where outbreaks also were reported in 2014 and 2017), and while the isolates from the two outbreaks were both the same species, complete genetic homogeneity between the isolates was not present. As of December 11, 2018, 505 probable and confirmed cases (and 296 deaths) were reported from 12 health zones in the two provinces of the Democratic Republic of Congo impacted with EVD, including 51 cases (and 17 deaths) among health care workers. In total, 10 outbreaks of Ebola have occurred in Africa since 1976.

▸ Clinical Findings

A. Symptoms and Signs

At symptom onset, early-stage EVD most typically presents as a nonspecific febrile illness. Along with fever, patients tend to experience headache, weakness, dizziness, malaise, fatigue, myalgia, and arthralgia. After 3–5 days, patients with later stage EVD may develop abdominal pain, severe nausea, vomiting, and diarrhea accompanying the febrile illness. This stage of the illness may continue for a week during which time neurologic symptoms gain prominence. Encephalitis is commonly observed and manifested as confusion, slowed cognition, agitation, and occasional seizures. Shock develops in most patients, but hemorrhagic manifestations develop in only 1–5% of patients. Respiratory symptoms are not typical for EVD, although interstitial pneumonia and respiratory failure are reported.

B. Laboratory Findings

During the first few days of symptoms, diagnosis may be made via several modalities, including antigen-capture ELISA, IgM ELISA, RT-PCR, or virus isolation. Blood samples obtained within the first 3 days of illness and tested by RT-PCR should be repeated if results are negative and clinical symptoms and signs persist. RNA levels peak a median of 7 days after illness onset. Later in the disease course or after recovery, IgM and IgG serologic tests may be sent. After about 10 days, IgM antibodies begin to develop, and, after approximately 2 weeks, an IgG antibody response develops. Postmortem diagnosis may be made by using immunohistochemistry, RT-PCR, or virus isolation.

Given that filoviruses infect dendritic cells and then hepatocytes and renal cortical cells, laboratory findings typically include a low platelet count (and a thrombotic thrombocytopenic purpura syndrome has been postulated with the probable cause multifactorial), leukopenia, and transaminitis (aspartate aminotransferase [AST] greater than alanine aminotransferase [ALT]). Additional observed laboratory abnormalities include hypoalbuminemia, electrolytes imbalance, and increased serum creatinine level. Elevated blood urea nitrogen, AST, and creatinine upon presentation are associated with higher mortality.

▶ Differential Diagnosis

The differential diagnosis varies with the stage of illness. Early-stage EVD is commonly mistaken for malaria, typhoid, and other viral illnesses. As gastrointestinal symptoms develop, health providers should also consider viral hepatitis, toxins, leptospirosis, and rickettsial diseases. In later stage EVD, bacterial, viral, and parasitic illnesses, including cholera and, in children, rotavirus infection can present with severe gastroenteritis and shock. Encephalitis must be differentiated from the confusion associated with uremia. Hemorrhagic manifestations raise suspicion for EVD but could be due to leukemia, thrombotic thrombocytopenic purpura, hemolytic-uremic syndrome, or disseminated intravascular coagulation. Travel and contact history are crucial when considering the differential diagnosis in areas where Ebola is not endemic.

▶ Complications

Hypovolemic shock and multiorgan failure are the most common complications of EVD. Hemorrhage can occur in late stages. Rhabdomyolysis is reported frequently and may explain many of the associated laboratory abnormalities. Coinfections with malaria or bacteria (or both) are important considerations and can occur before presentation and during treatment of EVD. The virus is known to persist in immunologically privileged sites, such as the CNS, eye, and testes; however, viral relapse is uncommon. Post-EVD musculoskeletal pain, headache, auditory symptoms, and ocular symptoms (uveitis being the most common ocular finding) may develop. EVD survivors exhibit high rates of neuropsychological long-term sequelae including depression, anxiety, and posttraumatic stress disorder.

▶ Treatment

Treatment is supportive. Several studies have shown that intravenous fluids can reduce the mortality rates to less than 50%. Despite the wide availability of oral rehydration salts, mortality approximates 70% in endemic areas. In these studies, the amount of intravenous fluid replacement was relatively less than what would be used in countries with developed health systems. Among patients treated in the United States or Europe, almost all received intravenous fluids, electrolyte supplementation, and empiric antibiotic therapy. Invasive or noninvasive mechanical ventilation and continuous renal replacement therapy are necessary in many cases. This increased level of care likely contributed to the decreased mortality (19%) among these patients. The use of individual air-conditioned biosecure cubicles is preferred to the burdensome protective equipment used during the 2014 West African outbreaks and allows for more time spent with patients.

There are no approved medications for the treatment of EVD, although five agents were available for compassionate use in a Congolese EVD outbreak. Administration of convalescent plasma does not result in improved survival. Several drugs have advanced to clinical trials; however, some trials were terminated due to low enrollment or lack of efficacy. The tested monoclonal antibodies were MAb114 (a first-generation agent isolated from a survivor of the 1995 outbreak in the Congo), ZMapp, and REGN-EB3. ZMapp is an antiviral monoclonal antibody combination developed against *Zaire ebolavirus*. ZMapp showed some therapeutic benefit, but many of these patients received multiple agents and were not part of randomized controlled trials. The PREVAIL II study evaluated ZMapp for treatment of EVD and found it to be safe and well tolerated but failed to establish efficacy due to low enrollment numbers. REGN-EB3 is given as a single dose, does not require freezing, and shows efficacy in nonhuman primates, including reduction in mortality.

The two antivirals utilized in a recent outbreak were the nucleotide analog remdesivir (GS-5734) and the RNA-dependent RNA polymerase inhibitor favipiravir. Mathematical models show a high likelihood of efficacy for both agents against EVD if given within 3–4 days of infection, and the efficacy of remdesivir is theoretically 100% while that of favipiravir is 60%. Both agents are effective in nonhuman primates and one study in man found favipiravir to be effective in patients with low to moderate viremia.

Aside from supportive treatment and experimental therapeutics, patients typically receive empiric antimalarial agents in endemic areas and broad-spectrum antibiotics.

Prognosis

Children under 5 years of age and adults older than 40 have a high risk of death from EVD. Pregnancy is a risk factor for severe illness and death. In the 2014–2016 outbreak, the average maternal mortality was 86%. Immunosuppressed patients had shorter incubation time, rapid progression of disease, and poor outcomes. A higher baseline viral load was strong predictor of mortality. In general, poor overall medical care confers a poor prognosis. Among survivors, protective antibodies persist for at least 10 years.

Prevention

Risk reduction should focus on preventing wildlife to human transmission and reducing human to human transmission by surveillance, early detection and isolation of cases, contact tracing, containment measures (disinfection, hygiene, and sanitation), strict droplet and contact precautions in health care setting, and reduction of sexual transmission in Ebola survivors. The WHO recommends that men avoid sexual activity or use barrier protection during intercourse for 12 months from onset of symptoms or until their semen tests negative twice for Ebola virus.

The experimental recombinant vesicular stomatitis virus (rVSV)-based vaccine expressing *Zaire ebolavirus* (ZEBOV) glycoprotein is found to be highly effective in disease prevention after 10 days from receiving the vaccine. Side effects, such fever, myalgia, chills, fatigue, headaches, and oligo-arthritis, developed in most of the persons who received the vaccine. A phase III clinical trial to evaluate the safety and immunogenicity of rVSV-ZEBOV has shown promising results (most study participants have persistent antibody levels at 1 year; NCT02503202). A chimpanzee type 3 adenovirus vector vaccine is also under evaluation (NCT03140774). More than 12,000 persons were vaccinated with the glycoprotein vaccine in the most recent Congolese outbreak. Final efficacy data for this and the earlier Equateur outbreaks in the Democratic Republic of Congo are pending.

Risk stratification may be useful in deciding when and to whom to administer antiviral postexposure prophylaxis. A high-risk exposure is defined as penetrating sharps injury from used device or through contaminated gloves or clothing, direct contact with an infected patient (alive or deceased) or their bodily fluids with broken skin or mucous membranes such as eyes, nose, or mouth. The ZEBOV vaccine was used in the setting of postexposure prophylaxis among healthcare workers and found to be effective, but the evidence is limited to case series. In addition, the vaccine designed against *Zaire ebolavirus* might not be effective for infection with other species. The vaccine-mediated immunity requires an average of 10 days to develop and might not be fast enough in certain cases to prevent infection.

Current studies focus on isolation of cross-reactive monoclonal antibodies across Ebola virus species. The use of different preparations of combination monoclonal antibodies (ZMapp and MIL-77E) as postexposure prophylaxis during the West African outbreak failed to show statistical significance, and the conclusion was that the benefit was modest, at best. Newer forms of monoclonal antibodies include virus-like particles (VLP), mucin-deleted glycoproteins, and bispecific binding proteins (which bind Ebola proteins as well as those of related viruses such as the Sudan virus). The use of antiviral agents in postexposure prophylaxis is another alternative that, to date, also shows no clear survival benefit. The agent brincidofovir, for example, was not studied further because of inadequate sample size in Liberia.

When to Admit

Persons living in or returning from a country with high rates of Ebola transmission should be monitored for 21 days and admitted to a health care facility when symptoms meeting the WHO case definition of a suspected EVD case develop, in accordance with the screening protocol designated by the respective country's governmental health decision-making body.

Centers for Disease Control and Prevention (CDC). MMWR Ebola reports. http://www.cdc.gov/mmwr/ebola_reports. html

Damon IK et al. New tools in the Ebola arsenal. N Engl J Med. 2018 Nov 22;379(21):1981–3. [PMID: 30281389]

Fischer WA 2nd et al. Ebola virus disease: an update on postexposure prophylaxis. Lancet Infect Dis. 2018 Jun;18(6): e183–e192. [PMID: 29153266]

Kennedy SB et al; PREVAIL I Study Group. Phase 2 placebo-controlled trial of two vaccines to prevent Ebola in Liberia. N Engl J Med. 2017 Oct 12;377(15):1438–47. [PMID: 29020589]

Mendoza EJ et al. The ongoing evolution of antibody-based treatments for Ebola virus infection. Immunotherapy. 2017 Mar;9(5):435–50. [PMID: 28357917]

Shantha JG et al. An update on ocular complications of Ebola virus disease. Curr Opin Ophthalmol. 2017 Nov;28(6):600–6. [PMID: 28872492]

Wong G et al. From bench to almost bedside: the long road to a licensed Ebola virus vaccine. Expert Opin Biol Ther. 2018 Feb;18(2):159–73. [PMID: 29148858]

World Health Organization. Ebola virus disease. https://www.who.int/ebola

2. Other Hemorrhagic Fevers

This diverse group of illnesses results from infection with one of several single-stranded RNA viruses (members of the families Arenaviridae, Bunyaviridae, Filoviridae, and Flaviviridae). Flaviviruses, such as the pathogens causing dengue and yellow fever, and Filoviridae, causing EVD, are discussed in separate sections.

Lassa fever is a rodent-associated disease caused by an Old-World *arenavirus*. Rodents shed the virus in urine and droppings and transmit the virus to humans either by direct contact with these materials, ingestion, or inhalation of aerosolized particles. Lassa fever is mostly endemic in West Africa. Other arenaviruses include the Junin virus (cause of Argentinian hemorrhagic fever) and the Lujo virus. Lujo virus was first described in 2008 in Zambia where it caused a small cluster of nosocomial infections.

The bunyaviruses include hantaviruses (discussed separately). **Crimean Congo hemorrhagic fever** (CCHF) is a disease transmitted from ticks and livestock. Human-to-human transmission can occur in the community or hospital setting by contact with infected body secretions.

The geographic distribution is widespread with cases reported from Africa, Asia, the Middle East, and Eastern Europe, with increased incidence recently in the East Mediterranean region. Butchers and slaughterhouse workers in southeastern Iran are at high risk for infection with the CCHF pathogen. Turkey reported the largest outbreak yet in 2002, with nearly 10,000 recorded cases.

Rift Valley fever is transmitted from livestock animals, infected mosquitoes, and flies. To date, there is no human-to-human transmission. Risk factors for acquiring Rift Valley fever include working with abortive animal tissue; slaughtering, skinning, or sheltering animals; and drinking unpasteurized milk. Rift Valley fever causes outbreaks in Africa, Madagascar, and the Arabian Peninsula.

A new bunyavirus, a phlebovirus, was identified in 2010 in central and northeastern China and was named for its symptoms: **severe fever with thrombocytopenia syndrome (SFTS) virus**. STFS is transmitted by tick bite (Ixodidae family, including the newly discovered tick *Haemaphysalis longicornis*, which is found in Asia as well as among animals [rarely humans] in the eastern United States). It may also be transmitted between humans through direct contact with infected blood or secretions. Another virus (**Heartland virus**), identified in the United States, is similar to the SFTS virus. Transmission occurs via the Lone Star tick (*Amblyomma americanum*). The virus appears to be amplified in deer and raccoons. In the United States, most cases are reported from the Midwest and southern states.

▶ Clinical Findings

A. Symptoms and Signs

The incubation period varies between species, ranging from 2 to 21 days. The clinical symptoms in the early phase of a viral hemorrhagic fever are indistinguishable from other viral illnesses. Due to lack of specific symptoms on presentation, viral hemorrhagic fevers are an important cause to consider in fever of unknown origin in children in endemic areas. The late phase is more specific and is characterized by organ failure, altered mental status, and hemorrhage. Exanthems and mucosal lesions can occur.

In advanced stages, significant edema, pleural effusion, and fewer hemorrhagic manifestations compared with EVD can develop in patients with Lassa fever and Lujo virus infection. Hearing loss in various degrees is the most common complication of Lassa fever infection. Mortality in pregnant patients during the third trimester and fetal mortality are very high.

CCHF has more prominent hemorrhagic manifestations. Patients have red eyes, flushed face, red throat, and petechiae that progress to severe uncontrollable bleeding. Severe headaches are common in CCHF and correlate with the severity of vascular damage, vasodilatation, and cytokine release.

Rift Valley fever disease can present with three distinct syndromes: (1) ocular disease; retinitis is the most common complication and permanent vision loss develops in 1–10% of patients; (2) meningoencephalitis occurs in less than 1% of cases; these patients have headache, coma, or seizures 1–4 weeks after initial symptoms and a low mortality but a high morbidity with neurologic deficits that can be severe; and (3) a hemorrhagic fever form in which patients present 2–4 days after illness and show evidence of severe liver impairment and later hemorrhages; the hemorrhagic state occurs in less than 1% of patients, but the case-fatality ratio of such patients reaches about 50%.

B. Laboratory Findings

Laboratory features usually include thrombocytopenia, leukopenia (although with Lassa fever leukocytosis is noted), anemia, elevated liver biochemical tests, and abnormalities consistent with disseminated intravascular coagulation.

Special care should be taken for handling clinical specimens of suspected cases. Laboratory personnel should be warned about the diagnostic suspicion, and the CDC must be contacted for guidance. The diagnosis may be made by antigen detection (by ELISA), culture of the virus (the "gold standard" for Lassa virus diagnosis), PCR, or demonstration of a fourfold rise in antibody titer. CCHF is best diagnosed with an IgM serology, although IgG ELISA or immunofluorescence and quantitative RT-PCR are nearly as effective. Isolation of the viruses in culture requires a biosafety level 4 laboratory. Serologic assays are attendant with early false-negative and late false-positive assays.

▶ Differential Diagnosis

The differential diagnosis for hemorrhagic fever includes meningococcemia or other septicemias, Rocky Mountain spotted fever, dengue, typhoid fever, and malaria. SFTS differential diagnosis includes anaplasmosis, hemorrhagic fever with renal syndrome, or leptospirosis. The likelihood of acquiring hemorrhagic fevers among travelers is low.

▶ Treatment & Prevention

Patients should be placed in private rooms with standard contact and droplet precautions. Barrier precautions to prevent contamination of skin or mucous membranes should also be adopted by the caring personnel. Airborne precautions should be considered in patients with significant pulmonary involvement or undergoing procedures that stimulate cough.

Supportive care is the mainstay of therapy. There is no approved antiviral medication, but ribavirin is shown to be effective in vitro and in vivo against certain viruses (Lassa virus, CCHF, and Rift Valley fever pathogens). Early diagnosis and management can reduce mortality.

The efficacy for postexposure ribavirin in the management of Lassa fever, other arenaviruses, or CCHF remains anecdotal. The antitrypanosomal agent suramin may be effective against the Rift Valley fever virus. Sorafenib, a tyrosine kinase inhibitor approved for treatment of renal cell and hepatocellular carcinoma, has antiviral activity against Rift Valley fever virus. A combination of monoclonal antibodies that cross-react with the glycoproteins of Lassa virus have been tested in macaques with promising results.

An inactivated vaccine is available for Rift Valley fever but is not licensed and is not commercially available. There are no vaccines approved for other viruses causing viral hemorrhagic fever. A DNA vaccine against CCHF is developed and shows high humoral immune responses with significant protection in mouse models. A vaccine is also under development in Argentina for Argentinian hemorrhagic fever.

▶ When to Admit

- Persons with symptoms of any hemorrhagic fever and who have been in possible endemic area should be isolated for diagnosis and symptomatic treatment.

- Isolation is particularly important because diseases due to some of these agents, such as Lassa virus, are highly transmissible to health care workers.

Al-Abri SS et al. Current status of Crimean-Congo haemorrhagic fever in the World Health Organization Eastern Mediterranean Region: issues, challenges, and future directions. Int J Infect Dis. 2017 May;58:82–9. [PMID: 28259724]

Fill MA et al. Novel clinical and pathologic findings in a Heartland virus-associated death. Clin Infect Dis. 2017 Feb 15; 64(4):510–2. [PMID: 27927857]

Houlihan C et al. Lassa fever. BMJ. 2017 Jul 12;358:j2986. [PMID: 28701331]

Mire CE et al. Human-monoclonal-antibody therapy protects nonhuman primates against advanced Lassa fever. Nat Med. 2017 Oct;23(10):1146–9. [PMID: 28869611]

Raabe V et al. Laboratory diagnosis of Lassa fever. J Clin Microbiol. 2017 Jun;55(6):1629–37. [PMID: 28404674]

Silvas JA et al. The emergence of severe fever with thrombocytopenia syndrome virus. Am J Trop Med Hyg. 2017 Oct; 97(4):992–6. [PMID: 28820686]

3. Dengue

> ### ESSENTIALS OF DIAGNOSIS

- ▶ Incubation period 7–10 days.

- ▶ Sudden onset of high fever, chills, severe myalgias and arthralgias, headache, and retroorbital pain.

- ▶ Severe dengue is defined by the presence of plasma leakage, hemorrhage, or organ involvement.

- ▶ Signs of hemorrhage such as ecchymoses, gastrointestinal bleeding, and epistaxis appear later in the disease.

▶ General Considerations

Dengue virus belongs to the genus *Flavivirus* and has four distinct serotypes that can cause infection. Infection with one serotype does not confer immunity to the other serotypes. Dengue is transmitted primarily from human to human by the bite of the *Aedes* mosquito. Healthcare-associated transmission (needlestick or mucocutaneous exposure) and vertical transmission occur rarely. WHO reports that dengue is currently endemic in 128 countries, mostly in tropical and subtropical regions with 3.9 billion persons at risk for infection. An estimated 390 million cases of dengue fever occur annually (with 96 million manifesting clinical disease including at least 500,000 with severe disease and up to 20,000 deaths). The surge of cases is associated with climatic factors, travel, and urbanization. Thus, along with malaria, dengue is one of the two most common vector-borne diseases of humans. Dengue is also the second overall cause of a febrile illness (after malaria and excluding common upper respiratory viral infections) in travelers returning from developing countries.

There are several factors that contribute to intermittent outbreaks in these regions, including the season of the year when rainfall is optimal for mosquito breeding, presence of a large population with no previous immunity to the specific serotype, and frequent contact between people and the vector.

In the United States, even though dengue is endemic in Northern Mexico and the *Aedes* mosquito is common in the southern states, outbreaks are uncommon. Most cases occur in travelers, immigrants, or inhabitants of US territories that are endemic to the dengue virus. Puerto Rico experiences periodic large outbreaks. In 2015 and 2016, an outbreak of locally acquired cases of dengue fever was reported from Hawaii where 264 dengue patients were identified with 46 (17.4%) of the cases among children; all cases were serotype 1.

The incubation period is usually 7–10 days. When the virus is introduced into susceptible populations, usually by viremic travelers from endemic countries, epidemic attack rates range from 50% to 70%.

▶ Clinical Findings

A. Symptoms and Signs

A history of travel to a dengue-endemic area within 14 days of symptom onset is helpful in establishing a diagnosis. Most infected patients are asymptomatic. Only 20% develop symptoms ranging from mild disease (dengue fever) to severe hemorrhagic fever to fatal shock (dengue shock syndrome). In 2009, the WHO classified dengue as the following: dengue without warning signs; dengue with warning signs; and severe dengue.

After the incubation period, the febrile phase begins abruptly with nonspecific symptoms, high fever, chills, facial flushing, malaise, retroorbital eye pain, generalized body pain, and arthralgia. Some patients might have maculopapular rash, sore throat, and conjunctival injection. Not all patients have all symptoms or fever. Mild hemorrhagic manifestations can be seen. Most of the patients will recover, and fever is usually cleared by day 8.

A subset of patients, especially those with suboptimally controlled type 2 diabetes, may progress to severe dengue, which is defined by the presence of plasma leakage, hemorrhage, or organ involvement. Hematocrit drop may be the earliest sign and an indicator of the severity of plasma leakage. Pleural effusion and ascites can develop and may be detected by lateral decubitus chest radiograph or ultrasound before clinical detection. Increasing liver size, persistent vomiting, and severe abdominal pain are indications of plasma leakage. Signs of hemorrhage such as ecchymoses, gastrointestinal bleeding, and epistaxis appear. Severe organ involvement may develop, such as hepatitis, encephalitis, and myocarditis.

Shock develops in patients when a critical volume of plasma is lost through leakage. Decrease in the level of consciousness, hypothermia, hypoperfusion resulting in metabolic acidosis, progressive organ impairment, and disseminated intravascular coagulation leading to severe hemorrhage should raise concern for shock. Acute kidney injury in dengue largely occurs with shock syndrome and shows a high mortality.

B. Laboratory Findings

Leukopenia is characteristic, and elevated transaminases are found frequently in dengue fever. Thrombocytopenia, fibrinolysis, and hemoconcentration occur more often in the hemorrhagic form of the disease. In other forms of disease, especially in children, anemia is more common. The erythrocyte sedimentation rate (ESR) is often normal in most cases.

The nonspecific nature of the illness mandates laboratory verification for diagnosis, usually with IgM and IgG ELISAs after the febrile phase. Virus is recovered from the blood by PCR or detection of the specific viral protein NS1 by ELISA during the first few days of infection. Immunohistochemistry for antigen detection in tissue samples and dried blood spots can also be used. Thrombocytopenia in remote settings can be assessed with a tourniquet cuff test.

▶ Differential Diagnosis

Distinguishing between dengue and other causes of febrile illness in endemic areas is difficult. Fevers due to dengue are more often associated with neutropenia and thrombocytopenia and with myalgias, arthralgias/arthritis, and lethargy among adults. Chikungunya is more apt to develop a chronic arthritis. The arboviral encephalitides require additional epidemiologic information and serologic data to make the diagnosis. Influenza and malaria are easily confused early in disease, although the rhinitis and malaise should help distinguish influenza, and the cyclicity of fevers and presence of splenomegaly should suggest malaria.

▶ Complications

Usual complications include pneumonia, bone marrow failure, hepatitis, iritis, retinal hemorrhages and maculopathy, orchitis, and oophoritis. Neurologic complications (such as encephalitis, Guillain-Barré syndrome, phrenic neuropathy, subdural hematoma, cerebral vasculitis, and transverse myelitis) are less common. Acute disseminated encephalomyelitis has been linked with infection and vaccination. Bacterial superinfection can occur. Oral complications include acute gingivitis, palatal bleeding, tongue plaques, xerostomia, and rarely osteonecrosis of the jaw.

Maternal infection poses a risk of hemorrhage in both the mother and the infant if infection occurs near term. Severe dengue is a risk factor for obstetric complications, cesarean delivery, fetal distress, and maternal morbidity

▶ Treatment

There are no specific therapeutic options for the clinical management of dengue besides supportive care. Treatment entails the appropriate use of volume replacement, blood products, and vasopressors. Acetaminophen is recommended for analgesic and antipyretic treatment. NSAID usage should be minimized and preferably avoided to decrease the risk of gastritis and bleeding, particularly in patients with a predilection for hemorrhage or when there are abnormalities in platelet, liver function, or clotting factors.

Platelet counts do not usefully predict clinically significant bleeding. Platelet transfusions may be considered for severe thrombocytopenia (less than 10,000/mcL) or when there is evidence of bleeding. However, benefit in the absence of bleeding may not be observed, and harm may be caused by delay in count recovery. Monitoring vital signs and blood volume may help in anticipating the complications of dengue hemorrhagic fever or shock syndrome.

Repurposed drugs, such as chloroquine, statins, and balapiravir, are being explored for the treatment of dengue, although none has shown clear therapeutic benefit. New research is focusing on monoclonal antibodies as a therapeutic option as well as drugs including peptide agents that target structural and nonstructural proteins of dengue virus essential to its replication.

▶ Prognosis

Although fatalities occur with severe disease, the estimated mortality (2.5% of severe cases) appears to be diminishing, likely due to improved recognition of the disease and wider availability of supportive treatment. Causes of death include hemorrhagic fever (seen with recurrent disease) and occasionally fulminant hepatitis. Thrombocytopenia and acute hepatitis are predictors of severe dengue and higher mortality. Acute kidney injury in dengue shock syndrome portends poor prognosis. In general, the more advanced forms of disease (hemorrhagic fever and shock) occur more often in Asia than in Americas. Comorbidities of cardiovascular disease, diabetes, stroke, pulmonary disease, kidney disease, and older age are associated with more severe dengue.

▶ Prevention

Preventive measures should be encouraged, such as control of mosquitoes by screening and insect repellents including long-lasting insecticides, particularly during early morning and late afternoon exposures. Screening blood transfusions for dengue is of increasing importance, especially in endemic areas.

Dengvaxia, a recombinant, live, attenuated, tetravalent dengue vaccine (CYD-TDV), is the first vaccine to be approved and is now licensed for use by 19 regulatory authorities. Trials evaluating the efficacy of this vaccine reported overall 60% efficacy; however, efficacy was lower in younger age groups, seronegative individuals at the time of vaccination, and those infected with dengue serotype 2. The vaccine is given as a 0-, 6-, and 12-month series. Serious side effects were no more common than in placebo recipients. Vaccination is indicated for those between ages 9 and 45 years. Some investigators recommend limiting the vaccine to those who have prior exposure because of immune enhancement, and recommend community vaccination only when serosurveys document seropositivity levels of at least 70%. Pregnant women and immunosuppressed persons should not be vaccinated.

Chew MF et al. Peptides as therapeutic agents for dengue virus. Int J Med Sci. 2017 Oct 15;14(13):1342–59. [PMID: 29200948]

Lee IK et al. Diabetic patients suffering dengue are at risk for development of dengue shock syndrome/severe dengue: emphasizing the impacts of co-existing comorbidity(ies) and glycemic control on dengue severity. J Microbiol Immunol Infect. 2018 Jan 31. [Epub ahead of print] [PMID: 30146413]

Machain-Williams C et al. Maternal, fetal, and neonatal outcomes in pregnant dengue patients in Mexico. Biomed Res Int. 2018 Jan 21;2018:9643083. [PMID: 29607328]

Muller DA et al. Clinical and laboratory diagnosis of dengue virus infection. J Infect Dis. 2017 Mar 1;215(Suppl 2):S89–95. [PMID: 28403441]

Robinson ML et al. Dengue vaccines: implications for dengue control. Curr Opin Infect Dis. 2017 Oct;30(5):449–54. [PMID: 28719400]

Sridhar S et al. Effect of dengue serostatus on dengue vaccine safety and efficacy. N Engl J Med. 2018 Jul 26;379(4):327–40. [PMID: 29897841]

World Health Organization. Dengue and severe dengue. 2018 Sep 13. https://www.who.int/en/news-room/fact-sheets/detail/dengue-and-severe-dengue

World Health Organization. Dengue vaccine: WHO position paper, September 2018—Recommendations. Vaccine. 2018 Nov 10. [Epub ahead of print] [PMID: 30424888]

4. Hantaviruses

ESSENTIALS OF DIAGNOSIS

► Transmitted by rodents and cause two clinical syndromes.

► **Hemorrhagic fever with renal syndrome (HFRS):** mild to severe illness.

► **Hantavirus pulmonary syndrome (HPS):** 40% mortality rate.

General Considerations

Hantaviruses are enveloped RNA bunyaviruses naturally hosted in rodents, moles, and shrews. Hantavirus infection in humans can cause several disease syndromes. HFRS is primarily caused by Dobrava-Belgrade virus, Puumala virus, Seoul virus, and Hantaan virus in Asia and Europe; these viruses are called Old World hantaviruses. Nephropathia epidemica is a milder form of HFRS. Puumala virus is the most prevalent pathogen and is present throughout Europe. The HPS, also known as hantavirus cardiopulmonary syndrome, is caused mainly by Sin Nombre virus and Andes virus, the New World Hantaviruses in Americas. While they share many clinical features, a specific strain is not associated with a specific syndrome and overlap is seen between the syndromes.

A total of 728 cases of hantavirus infection were reported between 1993 and January 27, 2017. A total of 33 cases were reported in 2017 and 3 cases were reported in 2018.

Aerosols of virus-contaminated rodent urine and feces are thought to be the main vehicle for transmission to humans. Person-to-person transmission is observed only with the Andes virus. Occupation is the main risk factor for transmission of all hantaviruses: animal trappers, forestry workers, laboratory personnel, farmers, and military personnel are at highest risk. Climate change appears to be impacting the incidence of hantavirus infection mainly through effects on reservoir ecology.

Clinical Findings

A. Symptoms and Signs

Vascular leakage is the hallmark of the disease for both syndromes, with kidneys being the main target with variants associated with HFRS and the lungs with variants associated with HPS.

HFRS manifests as mild, moderate, or severe illness depending on the causative strain. A 2- to 3-week incubation period is followed by a protracted clinical course, typically consisting of five distinct phases: febrile period, hypotension, oliguria, diuresis, and convalescence phase. Various degrees of renal involvement are usually seen, occasionally with frank hemorrhage. Disseminated intravascular coagulation and thromboembolic phenomena are recognized complications. Pulmonary edema is not typically seen but when present usually occurs in the final stages of disease (oliguric and diuretic phase). Encephalitis and pituitary involvement are rare findings with hantavirus infection, although a few cases are reported with Puumala virus. Patients may have persistent hematuria, proteinuria, or hypertension up to 35 months after infection. Smoking appears to exacerbate the viremia with the Puumula variant of HFRS.

The clinical course of HPS is divided into a febrile prodrome, a cardiopulmonary stage, oliguric and diuretic phase, followed by convalescence. A 14- to 17-day incubation period is followed by a prodromal phase, typically lasting 3–6 days, that is associated with myalgia; malaise; abdominal pain along with nausea, vomiting, and diarrhea; headache; chills; and fever of abrupt onset. An ensuing cardiopulmonary phase is characterized by the acute onset of pulmonary edema. In this stage, cough is generally present, abdominal pain and symptoms as above may dominate the clinical presentation, and in severe cases, significant myocardial depression occurs. Acute kidney injury and myositis may occur. Sequelae include neuropsychological impairments in some HPS survivors.

B. Laboratory Findings

Laboratory features include hemoconcentration and elevation in lactate dehydrogenase, serum lactate, and hepatocellular enzymes. Early thrombocytopenia and leukocytosis (as high as 90,000 cells/mcL in HPS) are seen in both HFRS and HPS. In HPS, immunoblasts (activated lymphocytes with plasmacytoid features) can be seen in blood, lungs, kidneys, bone marrow, liver, and spleen.

An indirect fluorescent assay and enzyme immunoassay are available for detection of specific IgM or low-avidity IgG virus-specific antibodies. A quantitative RT-PCR is available; however, the viremia of human hantavirus infections is short-term, and therefore, viral RNA cannot be readily detected in the blood or urine of patients unless for the more readily detected early viremia of the Andes variant.

A plaque reduction neutralization test remains a gold standard serologic assay and distinguishes between the different hantavirus species, although cross reaction between Old and New World viruses exist. This test needs to be performed in a laboratory with appropriate biosafety (level 3).

▶ Differential Diagnosis

The differential diagnosis of the acute febrile syndrome seen with HFRS or early HPS includes scrub typhus, leptospirosis, and dengue. HPS requires differentiation from other respiratory infections caused by such pathogens as *Legionella*, *Chlamydia*, and *Mycoplasma*. Coxsackievirus infection should also be considered in the differential diagnosis.

▶ Treatment

Treatment is mainly supportive. Cardiorespiratory support with vasopressors is frequently needed; extracorporeal membrane oxygenation may be required in severe cases of HPS. Intravenous ribavirin is used in HFRS (Hantaan virus) with some success in decreasing the severity of the kidney injury. Its effectiveness in HPS, however, is not established.

▶ Prevention

Because infection is thought to occur by inhalation of rodent waste, prevention is aimed at eradication of rodents in houses and avoidance of exposure to rodent excreta, including forest service facilities. While inactivated vaccines have been used in the past in Korea and China, there is currently no commercially available vaccine and the WHO does not recommend preventive vaccination.

▶ Prognosis

The outcome is highly variable depending on severity of disease. HPS is a more severe disease than HFRS, with a mortality rate of about 40%. In Sin Nombre virus infections, the persistence of elevated IgG titers correlates with a favorable outcome.

de St Maurice A et al. Exposure characteristics of hantavirus pulmonary syndrome patients, United States, 1993–2015. Emerg Infect Dis. 2017 May;23(5):733–9. [PMID: 28418312]
Szabó R. Antiviral therapy and prevention against hantavirus infections. Acta Virol. 2017;61(1):3–12. [PMID: 28105849]

5. Yellow Fever

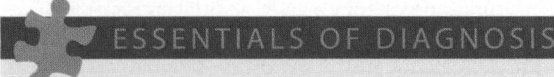

ESSENTIALS OF DIAGNOSIS

- ▶ Endemic area exposure: tropical and subtropical South America and Africa.
- ▶ Sudden onset of severe headache, aching in legs, and tachycardia.
- ▶ Brief (1 day) remission, followed by bradycardia, hypotension, jaundice, hemorrhagic tendency.
- ▶ Albuminuria, leukopenia, bilirubinemia.

▶ General Considerations

Yellow fever is a zoonotic flavivirus infection transmitted by *Aedes* mosquitoes bite. There are three types of transmission cycles: sylvatic (or jungle; humans working or travelling in the forest are bitten by infected mosquitoes), intermediate (most common type of outbreak in Africa; mosquitoes infect both monkeys and people leading to outbreaks in separate villages), and urban (seen in large epidemics; infected mosquitoes transmit the virus from person to person). Elevated temperatures and increased rainfall are major determinants of transmission.

Yellow fever occurs in 47 endemic countries in Africa and in Central and South America. Around 90% of cases reported every year occur in sub-Saharan Africa. Adults and children are equally susceptible, though attack rates are highest among adult males because of their work habits. Modeling data from Africa in 2013 estimates the annual case load is 84,000 to 170,000 annual cases with 29,000 to 60,000 deaths. The number of susceptible vaccinees worldwide is estimated to be between 394 million and 473 million.

▶ Clinical Findings

A. Symptoms and Signs

Most persons have no illness or only mild illness. The incubation period is 3–6 days in persons in whom symptoms develop.

1. Mild form—Symptoms are malaise, headache, fever, retroorbital pain, nausea, vomiting, and photophobia. Relative bradycardia, conjunctival injection, and facial flushing may be present.

2. Severe form—Severe illness develops in about 15%. Initial symptoms are similar to the mild form, but brief fever remission lasting hours to a few days is followed by a "period of intoxication" manifested by fever and relative bradycardia (Faget sign), hypotension, jaundice, hemorrhage (gastrointestinal, nasal, oral), and delirium that may progress to coma.

B. Laboratory Findings

Leukopenia, elevated liver enzymes, and bilirubin can occur. Proteinuria is present and usually disappears completely with recovery. Bleeding dyscrasias with elevated prothrombin and partial thromboplastin times, decreased platelet count, and presence of fibrin-split products, can also occur.

In the early stages of the disease (up to 10 days), diagnosis is confirmed if yellow fever virus RNA is detected by RT-PCR in blood from a person with no history of recent yellow fever vaccination. PCR determinants are now available that distinguish between wild type virus and vaccine-associated strains.

In later stages, serologic diagnosis can be made by using ELISA to measure IgM 3 days after the onset of symptoms; however, yellow fever vaccine and other flaviviruses, including dengue, West Nile, and Zika viruses, may give a false-positive ELISA test result. Thus, the presence of yellow fever virus–specific IgM antibody and negative ELISA panel for other relevant flaviviruses confirm the diagnosis.

If ELISA is positive for other flaviviruses, the more specific plaque reduction neutralization assay should be done in reference laboratories, which measures the titer of the neutralizing antibodies in the serum toward the infecting virus.

Differential Diagnosis

It may be difficult to distinguish yellow fever from other viral hepatidites, malaria, leptospirosis, louse-borne relapsing fever, dengue, and other hemorrhagic fevers on clinical evidence alone. Albuminuria is a constant feature in yellow fever patients, and its presence helps differentiate yellow fever from other viral hepatidites. Serologic confirmation is often needed.

Treatment

No specific antiviral therapy is available. Treatment is directed toward symptomatic relief and management of complications.

Prognosis

The mortality rate of the severe form is 20–50%, with death occurring most commonly between the sixth and the tenth days. Convalescence is prolonged, including 1–2 weeks of asthenia. Infection confers lifelong immunity to those who recover.

Prevention

The yellow fever vaccine, which is derived from the live attenuated 17D strain (with substrains 17D-204 and 17DD similar in efficacy and side effects) and currently given as a single dose for a lifetime, is the most effective way to prevent and control disease. A single dose of vaccine in the past was considered to provide lifelong immunity. While the 10-year booster dose is no longer recommended for most people, persistent seropositivity at 8 years post vaccination is only 85%. Thus, at-risk groups with waning immunity and high probability of exposure may consider receiving a second dose of vaccine after 10 years (these groups are listed at https://www.cdc.gov/yellowfever/healthcareproviders/vaccine-info.html).

Yellow fever vaccine is recommended for persons aged over 9 months who are traveling to or living in areas at risk for yellow fever virus transmission. This vaccine should never be given to children under 6 months old due to their higher risk of developing encephalitis related to the vaccine. WHO recommends that all endemic countries should include yellow fever vaccine in their national immunization programs.

The vaccine is contraindicated in persons with severe egg allergies or who are severely immunocompromised, including patients with primary immunodeficiencies, HIV infection with CD4+ count below 200/mcL, thymus disorder with abnormal immune function, malignant neoplasms, transplantation, or immunosuppressive and immunomodulatory therapies. The vaccine should probably not be given to patients over 60 years of age nor should it be given to breastfeeding women. It should be administered at least 24 hours apart from the measles vaccine. Pregnant women should receive the vaccine only if they cannot defer travel to endemic areas (Chapter 30). Clinicians should be aware of rare but frequently fatal vaccine-induced reactions, including anaphylaxis, yellow fever vaccine–associated viscerotropic disease, and yellow fever vaccine–associated neurologic disease.

A 2017 initiative, the Eliminate Yellow Fever program, is composed of 50 organizations and is designed to increase surveillance and control in 40 countries of Africa and the Americas in an attempt to reach a billion at-risk individuals with seroprotection by 2026.

The best personal protective measures are to avoid mosquito bites. If not in an endemic area, the patient should be isolated from mosquitoes to prevent transmission, since blood in the acute phase is potentially infectious.

Barrett ADT. Yellow fever live attenuated vaccine: a very successful live attenuated vaccine but still we have problems controlling the disease. Vaccine. 2017 Oct 20;35(44):5951–5. [PMID: 28366605]

Eliminate Yellow fever Epidemics (EYE): a global strategy, 2017–2026. Wkly Epidemiol Rec. 2017 Apr 21;92(16): 193–204. [PMID: 28429585]

Litvoc MN et al. Yellow fever. Rev Assoc Med Bras (1992). 2018 Feb;64(2):106–13. [PMID: 29641667]

Vasconcelos PF. Single shot of 17D vaccine may not confer lifelong protection against yellow fever. Mem Inst Oswaldo Cruz. 2018 Feb;113(2):135–7. [PMID: 29185596]

World Health Organization. Yellow fever. https://www.who.int/csr/disease/yellowfev

World Health Organization. Yellow fever in Africa and the Americas, 2017. Wkly Epidemiol Rec. 2018 Aug 10;93 (32):409–16. https://apps.who.int/iris/bitstream/handle/10665/273782/WER9332.pdf

OTHER SYSTEMIC VIRAL DISEASES

1. Zika Virus

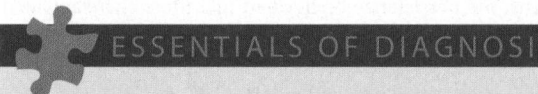

ESSENTIALS OF DIAGNOSIS

▶ Most infected persons asymptomatically seroconvert.

▶ Clinical symptoms are akin to those of chikungunya virus infection but with less arthritis.

▶ Complications include microcephaly and ocular complications in infants born to mothers infected during pregnancy as well as Guillain-Barré.

▶ There is no effective antiviral or vaccine.

General Considerations

Zika virus is a flavivirus, akin to the viruses that cause dengue fever, Japanese encephalitis, and West Nile infection.

The virus was noted in Africa and Asia during the 1950s–1980s, but first spread beyond those two continents during 2007 when an outbreak occurred in Yap State, Federated States of Micronesia. A large outbreak occurred in

French Polynesia in 2013. A smaller outbreak occurred on Easter Island during 2014. The virus then spread to the Western hemisphere and was first noted in northeastern Brazil in 2015. Zika virus then spread rapidly throughout the Americas, including the United States and worldwide http://www.who.int/csr/disease/zika/en/. Despite distinct lineages, Zika virus exists as only one serotype.

Aedes species mosquitoes, particularly *Aedes aegypti*, are primarily responsible for transmission of Zika virus. The biodistribution of the species largely determines the area of prevalence for Zika virus. *Aedes* species mosquitoes are found primarily in the southeastern United States, but one species *Aedes albopictus* (the Asian tiger mosquito known to sequester in tires) may be seen as far north as Pennsylvania and New Jersey. Rarely, a few other mosquito species including *Anopheles* and *Culex* may be competent for the Zika virus. Sexual transmission is reported from males and females to partners via vaginal, anal, or oral sex. Vertical transmission from pregnant woman to fetus is prominent. Transmission via platelet transfusion is also reported.

Since the onset of the first reported cases in the United States in 2015, the number of reported Zika cases is over 43,000, with 37,286 symptomatic cases from US territories (largely Puerto Rico) and 5728 cases from US states. The territorial cases are largely locally acquired and the US state cases are largely travel-acquired (with 231 of the 5728 US cases acquired via local transmission and 55 via sexual, bloodborne, or unknown routes). As of October 31, 2018, the US states reported 45 cases, with California (12) and New York (8) having the highest numbers. The number of annual cases is diminishing markedly in the United States with a peak in 2016 of 4897 travel-associated cases and 224 locally acquired cases (Florida, 218; Texas, 6).

► Clinical Findings

A. Symptoms and Signs

The incubation period is about 10 days. Symptoms include acute onset fever, maculopapular rash that is usually pruritic, nonpurulent conjunctivitis, and arthralgias, the latter mimicking the symptoms of the chikungunya virus. Rash may outlast the fever but is not always present. Symptoms last up to 7 days. Most infections are asymptomatic. Viral infections most often confused with Zika include dengue and chikungunya virus infections.

B. Laboratory Findings and Diagnostic Studies

The CDC recommends that persons with symptoms of Zika infection be tested if they live in or have traveled recently to an area with active transmission, as well as all pregnant women who have lived in or visited affected regions.

Diagnosis is made by detecting viral RNA or neutralizing antibody, IgM 4 days or more after symptom onset or IgG after 7 days or more. The Trioplex real-time RT-PCR assay, which detects Zika virus, chikungunya virus, and dengue virus RNA, and the Zika MAC-ELISA, which detects Zika virus IgM antibodies, are available in some laboratories. The real-time RT-PCR detects the virus in blood or urine and should be performed within 2 weeks of illness onset. Matched serum and urine specimens should be tested simultaneously. Although not routinely recommended, RT-PCR can be performed on amniotic fluid, CSF, and placental tissue. A positive real-time RT-PCR test definitively makes the diagnosis of Zika virus infection and does not require additional confirmatory testing. A negative test does not exclude the presence of the virus in other tissues and does not rule out infection. Persons with negative tests should undergo further testing for Zika virus IgM antibody and other arboviral infections.

Persons being tested 14 days or more after symptom onset should be tested for IgM and neutralizing antibodies. Asymptomatic pregnant women should be tested for IgM 2 to 12 weeks, and on occasion longer, after travel to an area with Zika activity or if they have had sexual contact with a man with confirmed Zika virus infection. In areas with active Zika transmission, asymptomatic pregnant women should be tested for IgM antibody as part of routine obstetric care. RT-PCR testing is recommended for pregnant women more than 2 weeks after exposure who test positive for Zika IgM antibody. Persistent Zika virus RNA in serum has been reported in pregnancy. The Zika MAC-ELISA can be performed on serum or CSF. Neutralizing antibodies can cross-react with dengue and other flaviviruses, so samples testing positive should be sent to public health laboratories for confirmation. Pregnant women with confirmed or suspected Zika virus infection (positive IgM antibodies not yet confirmed to be due to Zika infection) may be monitored by serial ultrasounds at 3- to 4-week intervals, assessing fetal anatomy and growth. With a declining prevalence of Zika virus infection, positive antibody tests run the risk of more likely being false-positives and thus the need for the outlined assessments exists.

► Complications

Two neurologic complications are of particular concern: (1) congenital microcephaly, often associated with brain calcifications and other abnormalities, first noted during the outbreak in Brazil and subsequently recognized to have occurred in French Polynesia as well; and (2) Guillain-Barré syndrome, first noted during the outbreak in French Polynesia. A Brazilian/European meta-analysis shows the rate of Guillain-Barré syndrome to be about 1.32%. Other congenital anomalies, including arthrogryposis among infected fetuses and infants, and spontaneous abortions are also observed. Rare deaths related to Zika virus infection are reported.

Ocular findings in Zika, reported in those congenitally infected, include focal macular pigment mottling, chorioretinal atrophy (especially in the macular area), congenital glaucoma with optical nerve hypoplasia, and optic disk abnormalities.

As with Ebola virus, the Zika virus can persist in semen for months; in the male reproductive tract the prostate gland and the testes are the presumed reservoirs. Persistence does not appear to occur in the female reproductive tract.

► Treatment

There are no antivirals approved for treatment of Zika virus. Sofosbuvir, which is FDA-approved to treat hepatitis C, another flavivirus, shows some ability to inhibit Zika replication and infection in vitro and in mice and appears to also be synergistic with interferon-alpha and with interferon-beta. Sofosbuvir also prevents vertical transmission in a mouse model. Aspirin and NSAIDs are avoided during illness caused by the flavivirus dengue because of its propensity to cause hemorrhage. Zika virus infections, however, do not appear to be associated with major hemorrhagic complications.

Prevention

The most effective means is environmental control of mosquitoes and removal of areas where water is stagnant or builds up. Such measures include screens on houses; removal of old tires and debris from endemic areas of infection; and movement toward better living conditions, including air conditioning in impoverished areas. Because of the association between microcephaly and Zika virus infection during pregnancy, pregnant women are advised to avoid travel to areas where Zika virus is circulating (http://www.who.int/csr/disease/zika/information-for-travelers/en/). Guidelines for testing of pregnant women potentially exposed are available through the CDC. Infected individuals should refrain from blood donations for several months.

No approved vaccine against Zika virus exists. Over 40 vaccines are under study globally and 3 have entered clinical trials, including inactivated virus vaccines, VLP, recombinant viral vaccines, and DNA vaccines. Monoclonal antibodies appear to provide some relief.

Barbi L et al. Prevalence of Guillain-Barré syndrome among Zika virus infected cases: a systematic review and meta-analysis. Braz J Infect Dis. 2018 Mar–Apr;22(2):137–41. [PMID: 29545017]

Bullard-Feibelman KM et al. The FDA-approved drug sofosbuvir inhibits Zika virus infection. Antiviral Res. 2017 Jan; 137:134–40. [PMID: 27902933]

Chibueze EC et al. Zika virus infection in pregnancy: a systematic review of disease course and complications. Reprod Health. 2017 Feb 28;14(1):28. [PMID: 28241773]

de Paula Freitas B et al. Zika virus and the eye. Curr Opin Ophthalmol. 2017 Nov;28(6):595–9. [PMID: 28795959]

Halstead SB. Achieving safe, effective, and durable Zika virus vaccines: lessons from dengue. Lancet Infect Dis. 2017 Nov;17(11):e378–82. [PMID: 28711586]

Silva JVJ Jr et al. Current status, challenges and perspectives in the development of vaccines against yellow fever, dengue, Zika and chikungunya viruses. Acta Trop. 2018 Jun;182:257–63. [PMID: 29551394]

Stassen L et al. Zika virus in the male reproductive tract. Viruses. 2018 Apr 16;10(4):E198. [PMID: 29659541]

Wang Q et al. Monoclonal antibodies against Zika virus: therapeutics and their implications for vaccine design. J Virol. 2017 Sep 27;91(20):e01049–17. [PMID: 28768876]

2. Chikungunya Fever

Chikungunya ("that which bends up" in the Bantu language Kimakonde) fever is an alphavirus infection transmitted to humans by *A aegypti* and *A albopictus* and is considered a classic "arthritogenic" virus. The virus originated with two strains, one in West Africa and the other in East/Central/ Southern Africa. In 2013, the first autochthonous case of chikungunya reported in the western hemisphere occurred on Saint Martin in the Caribbean, with isolates derivative of the East/Central/South Africa strains. Despite these differences, only one serotype exists.

For 2018, the CDC reports 75 travel-associated cases in 22 states and Puerto Rico (with the largest number of reports from California, New York, New Jersey, and Texas). The territory of Puerto Rico reports the only current locally acquired cases, with five cases as of October 30, 2018. Chikungunya virus prevalence is ubiquitous in endemic countries in Africa, the Americas, Asia, and Europe.

Among naïve populations, attack rates are often as high as 50%. On Saint Martin, 39% of infections were asymptomatic. Vertical transmission is documented if the mother is viremic during parturition, and transmission does not appear to occur throughout pregnancy as it does with Zika virus. Infectious virus was isolated from saliva, although transmission from oral secretions is not observed among humans. Endemicity of *A aegypti* in the Americas and the introduction of *A albopictus* into Europe and the New World raise concern for further extension of the epidemic. Case reports show that chikungunya virus may coinfect patients with yellow fever virus, plasmodia, Zika virus, and dengue virus.

Clinical Findings

A. Symptoms and Signs

After an incubation period of 1–12 days (estimated median 3), there is abrupt onset of fever; headache; intestinal complaints, including diarrhea, vomiting, or abdominal pain; myalgias; and arthralgias/arthritis affecting small, large, and axial joints. The simultaneous involvement of more than 10 joints and the presence of tenosynovitis (especially in the wrist) are characteristic. The stooped posture of patients gives the disease its name. Joint symptoms persist for 4 months in 33% and linger for years in about 10%. A centrally distributed pigmented or pruritic maculopapular rash is reported in 10–40% of patients; it can be bullous with sloughing in children. Mucosal disease occurs in about 15%. Facial edema and localized petechiae are reported. Neurologic complications, including encephalitis, myelopathy, peripheral neuropathy, Guillain-Barré syndrome, myeloneuropathy, and myopathy, are usually found in persons younger than 5 or older than 49 years. Encephalitis occurred in 8.6 per 100,000 persons infected in La Réunion during 2005–2006 with 17% mortality and increased risk of encephalitis among those older than 65 years. Hemorrhagic fever–like presentations are unusual. Coinfection with other respiratory viruses and with dengue is common. Some of the neuropathology may be immune-mediated, and these cases are usually in those over age 20 and associated with longer latencies and better outcomes. Death is rare and usually related to underlying comorbidities.

B. Laboratory Findings

Diagnosis is made epidemiologically and clinically. Mild leukopenia occurs as does thrombocytopenia, which

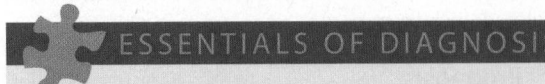
is seldom severe. Elevated inflammatory markers do not correlate well with the severity of arthritis. Radiographs of affected joints are normal during the acute phase. Bone lesions are visible in some patients with chronic symptoms.

Serologic confirmation requires elevated IgM titers or fourfold increase in convalescent IgG levels using an ELISA. RT-PCR and ELISA are commercially available; no ELISA kit is FDA-cleared. Culture techniques (viral isolation in insect or mammalian cell lines or by inoculation of mosquitoes or mice) require BSL-3 containment. Directions on submitting specimens for testing may be obtained from the CDC Arboviral Diseases Branch, 970-221-6400. Suspected cases in the United States should be promptly reported to public health authorities. The differential diagnosis includes other tropical febrile diseases, such as malaria, leishmaniasis, or dengue.

Complications & Prognosis

Common complications of chikungunya fever are long-term weakness, asthenia, myalgia, arthralgia, and arthritis, noted to be present in 25–66.5% of cases at 1 year. Risk factors for long-term arthralgias include the existence of such symptoms at 4 months after onset of disease and age over 35 years. Persons with preexisting arthritis are also at increased risk for prolonged symptoms after chikungunya infection with polyarthralgias occasionally lasting for years. Nasal skin necrosis is rarely reported. The Guillain-Barré syndrome is reported from the French West Indies during an outbreak in 2014, and more recently from New Delhi, India. Comorbid conditions, including hypertension, diabetes, and cardiac diseases, may contribute to severe outcomes; although in some series, patients with significant neurologic complications do not show comorbidities. Severe outcomes and higher mortality are reported among more recent Brazilian cases.

Treatment & Prevention

Treatment is supportive with NSAIDs and corticosteroids. Chloroquine may be useful for managing refractory arthritis. Chronic disease may require disease modifying antirheumatic drugs, such as the reports from La Réunion where methotrexate was associated with a positive response. No licensed vaccine exists, although at least 18 vaccines are in trials including inactivated and live attenuated vaccines. At this time, prevention relies on avoidance of mosquito vectors.

Badawi A et al. Prevalence of chronic comorbidities in Chikungunya: a systematic review and meta-analysis. Int J Infect Dis. 2018 Feb;67:107–13. [PMID: 29277382]

Brito CAA. Alert: severe cases and deaths associated with chikungunya in Brazil. Rev Soc Bras Med Trop. 2017 Sep–Oct; 50(5):585–9. [PMID: 29160503]

Mehta R et al. The neurological complications of chikungunya virus: a systematic review. Rev Med Virol. 2018 May;28(3):e1978. [PMID: 29671914]

Sales GMPG et al. Treatment of chikungunya chronic arthritis: a systematic review. Rev Assoc Med Bras (1992). 2018 Jan;64(1): 63–70. [PMID: 29561944]

3. Colorado Tick Fever

ESSENTIALS OF DIAGNOSIS

▶ Onset 1–19 days (average, 4 days) following tick bite.

▶ Fever, chills, myalgia, headache, prostration.

▶ Leukopenia, thrombocytopenia.

▶ Second attack of fever after remission lasting 2–3 days.

General Considerations

Colorado tick fever is a reportable biphasic, febrile illness caused by a reovirus infection transmitted by *Dermacentor andersoni* tick bite. About five cases occur annually, largely among men over age 40. The disease is limited to the western United States and Canada and is most prevalent during the tick season (March to November). There is a discrete history of tick bite or exposure in 90% of cases. The virus infects the marrow erythrocyte precursors. Blood transfusions can be a vehicle of transmission.

Clinical Findings

A. Symptoms and Signs

The incubation period is 3–6 days, rarely as long as 19 days. The onset is usually abrupt with a high fever. Severe myalgia, headache, photophobia, anorexia, nausea and vomiting, and generalized weakness are prominent. Physical findings are limited to an occasional faint rash. The acute symptoms resolve within a week. Remission is followed in 50% of cases by recurrent fever and a full recrudescence lasting 2–4 days. In an occasional case, there may be three bouts of fever.

The differential diagnosis includes influenza, Rocky Mountain spotted fever, numerous other viral infections, and, in the right setting, relapsing fevers.

B. Laboratory Findings

Leukopenia with a shift to the left and atypical lymphocytes occurs, reaching a nadir 5–6 days after the onset of illness. Thrombocytopenia may occur. An RT-PCR assay may be used to detect early viremia. Detection of IgM by capture ELISA or plaque reduction neutralization is possible after 2 weeks from symptom onset and is the most frequently used diagnostic tool.

Complications

Aseptic meningitis (particularly in children), encephalitis, and hemorrhagic fever occur rarely. Malaise may last weeks to months. Fatalities are very uncommon. Rarely, spontaneous abortion or multiple congenital anomalies may complicate Colorado tick fever infection acquired during pregnancy.

Treatment

No specific treatment is available. Ribavirin has shown efficacy in an animal model. Antipyretics are used, although salicylates should be avoided due to potential bleeding with the thrombocytopenia seen in patients with Colorado tick fever.

► Prognosis

The disease is usually self-limited and benign.

► Prevention

Tick avoidance is the best prevention. The tick season is primarily from March to November, and the ticks mostly live at high altitudes (over 7000 feet) in sagebrush.

Kadkhoda K et al. Case report: a case of Colorado tick fever acquired in southwestern Saskatchewan. Am J Trop Med Hyg. 2018 Mar;98(3):891–3. [PMID: 29363458]

Yendell SJ et al. Colorado tick fever in the United States, 2002–2012. Vector Borne Zoonotic Dis. 2015 May;15(5):311–6. [PMID: 25988440]

COMMON VIRAL RESPIRATORY INFECTIONS

1. Respiratory Syncytial Virus (RSV) & Other Paramyxoviruses

ESSENTIALS OF DIAGNOSIS

► RSV is a major cause of morbidity and mortality at the extremes of age (younger than 5 and older than 65).

► Treatment is largely supportive.

► No active vaccination for RSV is available.

► General Considerations

Respiratory syncytial virus (RSV) is a paramyxovirus that causes annual outbreaks during the wintertime with usual onset of pulmonary symptoms between mid-October and early January in the continental United States (excluding Florida). Outside the United States, RSV usually peaks during wet months in areas with high annual precipitation and during cooler months in hot and dry areas. It occurs earlier in urban areas.

There are two major subtypes, A and B, and it appears that the A subtype is associated with disease severity. RSV is the leading cause of hospitalization in US children, with annual hospitalization rates of 6 per 1000 children younger than 5 years. Globally, the annual RSV hospitalization rates are 4 per 1000 children less than 5 years old, 19 among children less than 1 year old, 20 among children less than 6 months old, and 64 among premature children less than 1 year. Prematurity is a major risk factor for severe disease. Early RSV bronchiolitis in children, along with a family history of asthma, are associated with persistence of airway reactivity later in life.

RSV also causes upper and lower respiratory tract infection in adults, with the virus entering through contact with mucous membranes. RSV occurs with increasing severity in those with comorbid conditions, older adults (accounting for a rate of 4 per 1000 hospitalizations and 14,000 deaths annually), persons with severe combined immunodeficiency, and patients after lung or bone marrow transplantation (because CD8 T cells are not available for viral clearance). An interleukin-1 receptor polymorphism is shown to be associated with more severe bronchiolitis. Recurrences occur throughout life. The average incubation period is 5 days. Up to 10% of disease classified as invasive pneumococcal disease is thought to be RSV or influenza.

In immunocompromised patients, such as bone marrow transplant recipients, serious pneumonia can occur, and outbreaks with a high mortality rate (greater than 70%) are reported.

Other paramyxoviruses important in human disease include human metapneumovirus, parainfluenza virus, and Nipah virus.

Human metapneumovirus is a ubiquitous seasonal virus circulating during late winter to early spring. It is divided into subgroups A and B. Metapneumovirus accounted for 7.3% of childhood (younger than 16 years old) pneumonia in a Norwegian series of 3650 patients in which RSV accounted for 28.7%. Clinical presentations range from mild upper respiratory tract infections to severe lower respiratory tract infections (eg, bronchiolitis, croup, and pneumonia). Lower respiratory tract (sometimes severe) infections have been observed among immunocompromised and elderly adults, especially residents of nursing homes. In lung transplant recipients, human metapneumovirus is a common cause of respiratory illness and is thought to increase the risk of acute and chronic graft rejection. Ribavirin appears to be well tolerated in lung transplant recipients with metapneumovirus infection.

Human parainfluenza viruses (HPIVs) are commonly seen in children and are the most common cause of laryngotracheitis (croup). Four different serotypes are described, and they differ in their clinical presentations as well as epidemiology. HPIV-1 and HPIV-2 are responsible for croup. HPIV-3 is associated with bronchiolitis and pneumonia. HPIV-4 is a less frequently reported pathogen. Reinfections are common throughout life. HPIVs can also cause severe disease in older individuals, immunocompromised persons, and patients with chronic illnesses.

Nipah virus is a highly virulent paramyxovirus first described in 1999. Cases are concentrated mainly in Southeast Asia (Malaysia, Singapore, Bangladesh, and India). Fruit bats are identified as the natural host of the virus. An outbreak of 14 cases, 8 fatal, occurred in Bangladesh associated with drinking date palm sap between 2010 and 2014. Direct pig-human, cow-human, human-human, and nosocomial transmission are reported. Nipah virus causes acute encephalitis with a high fatality rate (67–92%), although respiratory symptoms are also described. Cranial nerve palsies, encephalopathy, and dystonia are among neurologic sequelae (15–32%) seen in infected individuals. Relapses occurring weeks and months after initial infection are described (3.4–7.5%).

Clinical Findings

A. Symptoms and Signs

In RSV bronchiolitis, proliferation and necrosis of bronchiolar epithelium develop, producing obstruction from sloughed epithelium and increased mucus secretion. Signs of infection include low-grade fever, tachypnea, and wheezes. Apnea is a common presenting symptom. Hyperinflated lungs, decreased gas exchange, and increased work of breathing are present. Pulmonary hemorrhage is reported. In children, RSV is globally the most common cause of acute lower respiratory infection and also a common cause of acute and recurrent otitis media. In patients with Down syndrome, RSV develops at a later age and is associated with more protracted hospitalizations.

B. Laboratory Findings

A rapid diagnosis of RSV infection is made by viral antigen identification of nasal washings using an ELISA or immunofluorescent assay, but PCR-based rapid tests are increasingly used. Multiplex assays in conjunction with influenza A and B tests are available commercially. RSV viral load assay values at day 3 of infection may correlate with requirement of intensive care and respiratory failure in children.

Human metapneumovirus is best diagnosed by PCR. Tests for rapid detection of viral antigens with immunofluorescence or ELISA, and PCR techniques are also widely available for detection of HPIV. Culture may also be used. ELISA (serum and CSF) and PCR (urine and respiratory secretions but not blood) are both used for Nipah virus infection diagnosis.

Treatment & Prevention

Treatment of RSV consists of supportive care, including hydration, humidification of inspired air, antibiotic therapy (to reduce other respiratory morbidity), and ventilatory support as needed. Neither bronchodilating agents nor corticosteroids have demonstrated efficacy in bronchiolitis although individual patients with significant bronchospasm or history of asthma might respond to them. Oral antiviral agents remain under study.

The use of aerosolized ribavirin or RSV-enriched IVIG, or both, can be considered in high-risk patients, such as those with a history of bone marrow transplantation, and appears to lessen mortality. The prophylactic monoclonal antibody palivizumab, while recommended for and effective in high-risk infants (premature infants less than 32 weeks' gestational age, as well as infants with congenital heart and lung diseases and Down syndrome), is not of proven efficacy among adults with RSV.

A 2017 clinical trial studied the administration of palivizumab to preterm infants to prevent long-term sequelae; palivizumab did not suppress the onset of atopic asthma but did result in a significantly lower incidence of recurrent wheezing. Azithromycin therapy during RSV infection has been shown to reduce the probability of recurrent wheezing during the subsequent year by approximately 50%.

No RSV vaccine is currently commercially available.

Prevention in hospitals entails rapid diagnosis, hand washing contact isolation, and perhaps passive immunization. (Passive immunization is costly but is associated with improved antiviral titers in hematologic stem cell transplant recipients). The use of conjugated pneumococcal vaccination appears to decrease the incidence of concomitant pneumonia associated with viral infections in children in some countries. Viral shedding averages 11 days and correlates inversely with age and directly with severity of infection.

Therapeutic modalities for human metapneumovirus and parainfluenza virus infections under investigation include intravenous ribavirin administration.

Clayton BA. Nipah virus: transmission of a zoonotic paramyxovirus. Curr Opin Virol. 2017 Feb;22:97–104. [PMID: 28088124]
Falsey AR et al. Compassionate use experience with high-titer respiratory syncytical virus (RSV) immunoglobulin in RSV-infected immunocompromised persons. Transpl Infect Dis. 2017 Apr;19(2). [PMID: 28054734]
Noveroske DB et al. Local variations in the timing of RSV epidemics. BMC Infect Dis. 2016 Nov 11;16(1):674. [PMID: 27835988]
Stein RT et al. Respiratory syncytial virus hospitalization and mortality: systematic review and meta-analysis. Pediatr Pulmonol. 2017 Apr;52(4):556–69. [PMID: 27740723]

2. Seasonal Influenza

> ### ESSENTIALS OF DIAGNOSIS
>
> ▶ Cases usually in epidemic pattern.
> ▶ Onset with fever, chills, malaise, cough, coryza, and myalgias.
> ▶ Aching, fever, and prostration out of proportion to catarrhal symptoms.
> ▶ Leukopenia.

General Considerations

Influenza (an orthomyxovirus) is a highly contagious disease transmitted by the respiratory route in humans. Transmission occurs primarily by droplet nuclei rather than fomites or direct contact. There are three types of influenza viruses that infect humans. While type A can infect a variety of mammals (humans, swine, horses, etc) and birds, types B and C almost exclusively infect humans. Type A viruses are further divided into subtypes based on the hemagglutinin (H) and the neuraminidase (N) expressed on their surface. There are 18 subtypes of hemagglutinin and 11 subtypes of neuraminidase.

Annual epidemics usually appear in the fall or winter in temperate climates. Up to 5 million cases of severe influenza are estimated by the WHO to occur annually, with up to 0.5 million annual deaths. Influenza epidemics affect 10–20% of the global population on average each year and are typically the result of minor antigenic variations of the virus, or antigenic drift, which occur often in influenza A virus.

On the other hand, pandemics—associated with higher mortality—appear at longer and varying intervals (decades) as a consequence of major genetic reassortment of the virus (antigenic shift) or adaptation of an avian or swine virus to humans (as with the pandemic H1N1 virus of 1918). (https://www.who.int/influenza/surveillance_monitoring/updates/latest_update_GIP_surveillance/en/).

The highly pathogenic avian influenza subtypes are discussed in the next section. The novel swine-origin influenza A (pandemic H1N1) virus emerged in Mexico in 2009 and quickly spread throughout North America and the world causing a pandemic. This virus originated from triple-reassortment of North American swine, human, and avian virus lineages and Eurasian swine virus lineages and replaced the previous H1N1 seasonal virus.

▶ Clinical Findings

A. Symptoms and Signs

Type A and B seasonal influenza viruses produce clinically indistinguishable infections, whereas type C usually causes mild illness. The incubation period is 1–4 days. In unvaccinated persons, uncomplicated influenza often begins abruptly. Symptoms range widely from nearly asymptomatic to a constellation of systemic symptoms (including fever, chills, headache, malaise, and myalgias) and respiratory symptoms (including rhinorrhea, congestion, pharyngitis, hoarseness, nonproductive cough, and substernal soreness). Gastrointestinal symptoms and signs may occur, particularly among young children with influenza B virus infections. Fever lasts 1–7 days (usually 3–5). Elderly patients especially may present with lassitude and confusion, often without fever or respiratory symptoms. Signs include mild pharyngeal injection, flushed face, and conjunctival redness. Moderate enlargement of the cervical lymph nodes and tracheal tenderness may be observed. The presence of fever (higher than 38.2°C) and cough during influenza season is highly predictive of influenza infection in those older than 4 years.

B. Laboratory Findings

Rapid influenza diagnostic tests for detection of influenza antigens from nasal or throat swabs are widely available, highly specific, and produce fast results but have low sensitivity leading to high false-negative results. Not all commercial rapid influenza diagnostic tests can differentiate between influenza A and influenza B, and none of the available rapid influenza diagnostic tests can provide information on influenza A subtypes. Newer digital immunoassays and rapid nucleic acid amplification tests are more sensitive than traditional rapid influenza diagnostic tests; however, the sensitivity of newer PCR techniques is compromised early in the season during low prevalence periods. A nasopharyngeal swab, nasal aspirate, combined nasopharyngeal swab with oropharyngeal swab, or material from a bronchoalveolar lavage can be tested for any influenza strain. When influenza pneumonia is suspected, lower respiratory tract specimens should be collected and tested for influenza viruses by RT-PCR or the above assays.

▶ Differential Diagnosis

The differential diagnoses for influenza-like infections include a variety of viral respiratory infections (parainfluenza, RSV, atypical dengue, adenovirus, enterovirus, coronavirus) or other viral infections (flavivirus, CMV, EBV, acute HIV infection), as well as bacterial infections such as mycobacterial infection (atypical pneumonia), pertussis, and Legionnaire disease. Epidemiologic factors can suggest Legionnaire (elderly smokers). Chronicity of cough may suggest adenovirus, mycobacterial, or pertussis infection. Leukocytosis and lymphadenopathy are more often seen with CMV and EBV. Distinguishing influenza from dengue requires attention to rhinitis (influenza) and thrombocytopenia (dengue).

▶ Complications

Hospitalization or ICU admission for influenza is often a consequence of diffuse viral pneumonitis with severe hypoxemia and sometimes shock. Patients with asthma, residents of nursing homes and long-term care facilities, adults aged 65 years or older, persons who are morbidly obese, and persons with underlying medical conditions (pulmonary, renal, cardiovascular, hepatic, hematologic, neurologic and neurodevelopmental conditions; and immune-deficient conditions, such as HIV, diabetes, and cirrhosis) are at high risk for complications. Infection during pregnancy increases the risk for hospitalization and may be associated with severe illness, sepsis, pneumothorax and respiratory failure, spontaneous abortion, preterm labor, and fetal distress.

Influenza causes necrosis of the respiratory epithelium, increased adherence of bacteria to infected cells, and ciliary dysfunction, which predispose to secondary bacterial infections due to pneumococci, staphylococci, or *Haemophilus* spp. In turn, bacterial enzymes (eg, proteases, trypsin-like compounds, and streptokinase) activate influenza viruses. Frequent complications are acute sinusitis, otitis media, purulent bronchitis, and pneumonia.

Cardiovascular diseases are a complication of influenza infection, in particular among older adults, and influenza is postulated to be a significant trigger for myocardial infarction, cerebrovascular disease, and sudden death. Several studies suggest that influenza vaccination has protective effect against major adverse cardiovascular events. Neurologic complications, including seizures and encephalopathy, may occur. Encephalopathic complications of influenza are uncommon.

Reye syndrome (fatty liver with encephalopathy) is a rare and severe complication of influenza (usually B type) and other viral diseases (especially varicella), particularly in young children. It consists of rapidly progressive hepatic failure and encephalopathy, and there is a 30% mortality rate. The pathogenesis is unknown, but the syndrome is associated with aspirin use in the management of viral infections.

▶ Treatment

Treatment is supportive. Antiviral therapy should be considered for all persons with acute illness, in particular those at high risk for developing complications who have a suggestive clinical presentation or with laboratory-confirmed influenza. Clinical trials show a reduction in the duration of symptoms, hospital admissions, as well as secondary complications, such as otitis, sinusitis, or pneumonia, but not mortality when using these agents. Maximum benefit is expected with the earliest initiation of therapy. Although the benefit of antiviral therapy after 48 hours of illness is reduced, it should be initiated if the patient is hospitalized or critically ill. Benefit has been noted up to 4–5 days into illness.

The antiviral treatment of choice should be based on the susceptibility of the circulating virus. Currently, since high levels of resistance to the adamantanes (amantadine and rimantadine) persist among seasonal H1N1 and H3N2 influenza A viruses and these agents are not effective against influenza B viruses, amantadine and rimantadine are not recommended for treatment.

Three neuraminidase inhibitors are FDA approved for treatment of influenza A and B: oral oseltamivir, inhaled zanamivir, and intravenous peramivir. The CDC recommends treatment with oral oseltamivir (75 mg twice daily for 5 days) as the drug of choice for patients of any age, pregnant women, and patients who are hospitalized or have complicated infection. Absorption of oral oseltamivir is considered reliable, except in patients with impaired gastric motility or gastrointestinal bleeding.

Inhaled zanamivir (10 mg, 2 inhalations twice daily for 5 days) is indicated for uncomplicated acute influenza in patients 7 years and older, is relatively contraindicated among persons with asthma because of the risk of bronchospasm, and is not formulated for use in mechanically ventilated patients. Inhaled zanamivir lacks efficacy in pneumonia, probably due to poor bioavailability in the peripheral lungs.

Intravenous peramivir (600 mg in single dose) is used for outpatient treatment of uncomplicated infection in patients 18 years and older and is recommended when there is a concern about inadequate oral absorption of oseltamivir. The efficacy of peramivir in patients with severe illness and in patients with influenza B is not well established. Some studies demonstrated that repeated doses for up to 5 days of intravenous peramivir is safe, effective and shorten the duration of influenza illness.

Resistance to neuraminidase inhibitors (oseltamivir, zanamivir, and peramivir) can occur during or after prolonged use in immunocompromised patients, particularly in persons who have undergone hematopoietic stem cell transplant. Intravenous zanamivir is an investigational drug that could be requested for clinical use if there is a concern for oseltamivir-resistant influenza strain. Laninamivir is a long-acting inhaled neuraminidase inhibitor used for the treatment of seasonal influenza, including infection caused by oseltamivir-resistant virus. It is licensed in Japan and South Korea and is currently in phase III clinical trials in the United States.

Baloxavir (a selective inhibitor of influenza cap-dependent endonuclease that is given as a single oral dose) was approved by the FDA in 2018 for treatment of uncomplicated influenza A and B infections. Baloxavir is given as 40 mg or 80 mg orally once daily depending on weight (the higher dose for persons 80 kg or more) and should be given within the first 48 hours of infection. Its side effects include diarrhea and bronchitis, and to date, its effects in patients older than 65 years or younger than 12 years are not established. Baloxavir's unique mechanism of action will likely make it useful as part of multidrug therapy for resistant disease. For complicated disease, especially in immunosuppressed patients, the combination of oseltamivir, amantadine, and ribavirin appears to produce faster viral clearance but no definite clinical improvement.

The first class of organosilanes have potent antiviral activity against influenza A viruses that are resistant to amantadine and oseltamivir. Dapivirine, an FDA-approved HIV nonnucleoside reverse transcriptase inhibitor, has broad-spectrum antiviral against multiple strains of influenza A and B viruses. Iminosugars are also under study. Updated advice is available at http://www.cdc.gov/flu/index.htm.

► Prognosis

The duration of the uncomplicated illness is 1–7 days, and the prognosis is excellent in healthy, nonelderly adults. Hospitalization typically occurs in those with underlying medical disease, at the extremes of age, and in pregnant women. Most fatalities are due to bacterial pneumonia although exacerbations of other disease processes, in particular cardiac diseases, occur. Pneumonia resulting from influenza has a high mortality rate among pregnant women and persons with a history of rheumatic heart disease. Mortality among adults hospitalized with influenza ranges from 4% to 8%, although higher mortality (greater than 10–15%) may be seen during pandemics and among immunocompromised individuals. At least 64% of pneumonia and influenza deaths occurred among elderly persons in the United States, who comprised only 15% of the population.

If the fever recurs or persists for more than 4 days with productive cough and white cell count over 10,000/mcL, secondary bacterial infection should be suspected. Pneumococcal pneumonia is the most common secondary infection, and staphylococcal pneumonia is the most serious. Major complications include viral myocarditis and viral encephalitis.

► Prevention

Annual administration of influenza vaccine is the most effective measure for preventing influenza and its complications. Seasonal influenza vaccines can reduce influenza hospitalizations by an estimated 61%. Vaccination of healthcare workers is associated with decreased mortality among hospitalized patients and those in long-term care facilities. Vaccination prevents influenza illness among pregnant women and their infants during the first months of life.

The ACIP and the American College of Obstetricians and Gynecologists' Committee recommend annual influenza vaccination for all persons over 6 months of age with no contraindications. Vaccination is emphasized for high-risk groups and their contacts and caregivers.

Several Cochrane database analyses have analyzed the efficacy of the influenza vaccines in select populations.

The studied groups include patients with COPD (a documented reduction in exacerbations with inactivated vaccine), the elderly (where vaccination shows some efficacy), adults with cancer (weak evidence, some lower mortality and influenza-related outcomes), healthy adults (established efficacy with inactivated vaccine, but only modest effects in pregnant women and newborns), and healthy children (where both live and inactivated vaccines lower the rate of influenza infections).

Other reviews establish the efficacy and safety of influenza vaccination in patients with rheumatoid arthritis, asthma, or myasthenia gravis, and elderly nursing home patients. The obese have an impaired response to the influenza vaccine.

Multiple influenza vaccine products are licensed in the United States and available from different manufacturers. These include inactivated influenza vaccines (standard- or high-dose, trivalent [IIV3] or quadrivalent [IIV4], adjuvanted or unadjuvanted), recombinant vaccines (trivalent [RIV3] or quadrivalent [RIV4]), and live attenuated influenza vaccine (LAIV4). All trivalent vaccines contain antigens from one strain each of influenza A (H1N1), influenza A (H3N2), and influenza B. Quadrivalent vaccines include an additional influenza B strain. The CDC does not endorse one influenza vaccine product over another, although each influenza vaccine product has different age indications and contraindications. The CDC publishes its annual influenza recommendations in the late summer (www.cdc.gov/mmwr).

LAIV4 use, not recommended by the CDC for the last two seasons due to concerns about its effectiveness against influenza viruses in prior years, is currently considered an acceptable option for groups in whom it is indicated. The efficacy of including the fourth A/Slovenian strain is as yet unknown.

Adults over the age of 18 years, including pregnant women, can receive any influenza vaccine, with few exceptions. Patients 65 years or older should receive a high-dose trivalent inactivated influenza vaccine containing four times more hemagglutinin than standard dose, or Fluad, a trivalent inactivated influenza vaccine that contains an adjuvant (MF59), which enhances the immune response to the vaccine. Fluzone intradermal inactivated quadrivalent vaccine is equally immunogenic and safe but more expensive than the intramuscular vaccine and is not recommended for persons older than 65 years. Adults older than 65 years can use any IIV or RIV intramuscular vaccine; in a large randomized trial, high-dose IIV3 showed superior efficacy over standard-dose IIV3 and may provide better protection. Some data suggest intradermal vaccination is more effective than intramuscular vaccination in the elderly. The herpes zoster vaccine can be safely coadministered with the seasonal influenza vaccines in patients over 50 years of age, with similar immunogenicity.

For patients with cancer, chemotherapeutic regimens containing rituximab show persistent perturbations of B-cell and Ig synthesis, and these modifications decrease humoral responses to the influenza vaccine. Adjuvanted vaccine is efficacious but has resulted in brief disease exacerbation in persons with psoriatic arthritis taking TNF-alpha inhibitors.

Vaccination is contraindicated for persons with a history of severe allergic reaction to influenza. Precautions should be taken if patients report a history of Guillain-Barré syndrome 6 weeks following an influenza vaccine and if patients have a moderate to severe acute illness with or without fever until clinical improvement. Persons with a history of egg allergy with hives only may receive any recommended influenza vaccine. Those with more severe allergic reactions to eggs may receive any recommended vaccine under close observation in a health care facility under the supervision of a provider with experience treating severe allergic reactions. Only the recombinant vaccine is completely egg-free.

Additional vaccine information can be found at http://www.cdc.gov/flu/professionals/vaccination/index.htm.

When antiviral chemoprophylaxis is used, it prevents 70–90% of influenza infections. Chemoprophylaxis is not routinely recommended and is not recommended prior to exposure to prevent development of resistance. Chemoprophylaxis may be considered for persons at increased risk for complications from infection who are exposed to an infected patient within 2 weeks of vaccination, for persons unlikely to respond to vaccination because of immunosuppression after exposure to an infected person, for persons for whom vaccination is contraindicated and who are at high risk for complications after exposure to an infected person, and for prevention of infection in residents of institutions during an outbreak. Alternatively, a person can be monitored closely, and antiviral therapy initiated at the first onset of symptoms after exposure. Initiation of chemoprophylaxis is not recommended more than 48 hours after exposure. Patients taking chemoprophylaxis should seek urgent medical care if an influenza-like illness develops.

Chemoprophylaxis against influenza A and B is accomplished with daily administration of the neuraminidase inhibitors oseltamivir (75 mg/day, oral) or zanamivir (10 mg/day, inhaled) to continue through 7 days after last known exposure. For outbreak control in long-term care facilities and hospitals, a minimum of 2 weeks is recommended, including in vaccinated persons if the seasonal vaccine is not well matched to the circulating strain, to continue until 1 week after identification of the last known case. Zanamivir should not be given as chemoprophylaxis to asthmatic persons, nursing home residents, or children younger than 5 years.

Breakthrough infections with influenza occur with neuraminidase inhibitors (in a study with zanamivir) and with vaccination. The efficacy of chemoprophylaxis is proven for individuals and households but not community settings.

Hand hygiene and surgical facemasks appear to prevent household transmission of influenza virus isolates when implemented within 36 hours of recognition of symptoms in an index patient. Such nonpharmaceutical interventions assist in mitigating the spread of pandemic and interpandemic influenza to nonvaccinated persons. In one study, patients with seasonal H1N1 influenza infection were infectious from 1 day before to about 7 days following illness onset. Children and immunosuppressed persons exhibit prolonged viral shedding and may be infectious longer. Winter school breaks during periods of high influenza transmission appear to decrease rates of visits to primary care practitioners for influenza illness among children and adults.

The data are not currently sufficient to modify statin usage for influenza vaccination. There may be, however, some impaired effectiveness against the H3N2 influenza A component of vaccines from the immunomodulatory effects of statins.

Any hospital patient in whom the infection is suspected should be isolated in an individual room with standard and droplet precautions. CDC guidelines recommend the equivalent of N95 masks for aerosol generating procedures (eg, bronchoscopy, elective intubation, suctioning, administering nebulized medications). For such procedures, an airborne infection isolation room can be used, with air exhausted directly outside or recirculated after filtration by a high efficiency particulate air (HEPA) filter. Strict adherence to hand hygiene with soap and water or an alcohol-based hand sanitizer and immediate removal of gloves and other equipment after contact with respiratory secretions is essential. Precautions should be maintained until 7 days from symptom onset or until 24 hours after symptom resolution, whichever is longer. Postexposure prophylaxis or close monitoring and early treatment should be considered for close contacts of patients who are at high risk for complications of influenza and may be considered for health care personnel, public health workers, or first responders who experienced a recognized, unprotected close contact exposure to a person with influenza virus infection during that person's infectious period.

A regimen of dose sparing vaccination (to 3.5 mcg) is advocated by some providers to address the extreme shortage of influenza vaccine, particularly in developing world countries, with adequate vaccination against all components except H3N2, where there is reduced seroconversion.

▶ When to Admit

- Limited availability of supporting services.
- Pneumonia or decreased oxygen saturation.
- Changes in mental status.
- Consider with pregnancy.

Beigel JH et al; IRC003 Study Team. Oseltamivir, amantadine, and ribavirin combination antiviral therapy versus oseltamivir monotherapy for the treatment of influenza: a multicentre, double-blind, randomised phase 2 trial. Lancet Infect Dis. 2017 Dec;17(12):1255–65. [PMID: 28958678]

Centers for Disease Control and Prevention (CDC). FluView: a weekly U.S. influenza surveillance report. https://www.cdc.gov/flu/weekly

Cochrane Library. Influenza: evidence from Cochrane Reviews. https://www.cochranelibrary.com/collections/doi/10.1002/14651858.SC000006/full

Domnich A et al. Effectiveness of MF59-adjuvanted seasonal influenza vaccine in the elderly: a systematic review and meta-analysis. Vaccine. 2017 Jan 23;35(4):513–20. [PMID: 28024956]

Gravenstein S et al. Comparative effectiveness of high-dose versus standard-dose influenza vaccination on numbers of US nursing home residents admitted to hospital: a cluster-randomised trial. Lancet Respir Med. 2017 Sep;5(9):738–46. [PMID: 28736045]

Green WD et al. Obesity impairs the adaptive immune response to influenza virus. Ann Am Thorac Soc. 2017 Nov;14(Supplement 5):S406–9. [PMID: 29161078]

Grohskopf LA et al. Update: ACIP Recommendations for the use of quadrivalent Live Attenuated Influenza Vaccine (LAIV4)—United States, 2018–19 influenza season. MMWR Morb Mortal Wkly Rep. 2018 Jun 8;67(22):643–5. [PMID: 29879095]

Hayden FG et al; Baloxavir Marboxil Investigators Group. Baloxavir marboxil for uncomplicated influenza in adults and adolescents. N Engl J Med. 2018 Sep 6;379(10):913–23. [PMID: 30184455]

McLean HQ et al. Effect of statin use on influenza vaccine effectiveness. J Infect Dis. 2016 Oct 15;214(8):1150–8. [PMID: 27471318]

Merckx J et al. Diagnostic accuracy of novel and traditional rapid tests for influenza infection compared with reverse transcriptase polymerase chain reaction: a systematic review and meta-analysis. Ann Intern Med. 2017 Sep 19;167(6):394–409. [PMID: 28869986]

Ortiz JR et al. Influenza immunization of pregnant women in resource-constrained countries: an update for funding and implementation decisions. Curr Opin Infect Dis. 2017 Oct;30(5):455–62. [PMID: 28777109]

Schwarz TF et al. Immunogenicity and safety of an adjuvanted herpes zoster subunit vaccine coadministered with seasonal influenza vaccine in adults aged 50 years or older. J Infect Dis. 2017 Dec 12;216(11):1352–61. [PMID: 29029224]

Talbot HK. Influenza in older adults. Infect Dis Clin North Am. 2017 Dec;31(4):757–66. [PMID: 28911829]

Uyeki TM. Influenza. Ann Intern Med. 2017 Sep 5;167(5):ITC33–48. [PMID: 28869984]

Vajo Z et al. Dose sparing and the lack of a dose-response relationship with an influenza vaccine in adult and elderly patients—a randomized, double-blind clinical trial. Br J Clin Pharmacol. 2017 Sep;83(9):1912–20. [PMID: 28378403]

3. Avian Influenza

ESSENTIALS OF DIAGNOSIS

- ▶ Most human cases occur after exposure to infected poultry.
- ▶ Clinically indistinguishable from seasonal influenza.
- ▶ Epidemiologic factors assist in diagnosis.
- ▶ Rapid antigen assays confirm diagnosis but do not distinguish avian from seasonal influenza.

▶ General Considerations

Zoonotic influenza viruses are distinct from human seasonal influenza viruses and do not easily transmit between humans. In addition, a number of viral genetic changes are required for adaptation to humans. For avian influenza viruses, birds are the natural hosts. Around the world and in North America, avian influenza A outbreaks occur in poultry from time to time (including a 2016 outbreak in Dubois County, Indiana, with avian but no human cases), and the virus has become endemic in poultry in some countries, mostly in Southeast Asia and Egypt. Occasionally, avian influenza viruses may infect humans or other mammals, including domestic cats and dogs. Illness in humans ranges from mild disease to rapid progressive severe disease and death depending on the subtype.

The primary risk factor for human infection is direct or indirect exposure to infected live or dead poultry or contaminated environments, such as live bird markets. Slaughtering and handling carcasses of infected poultry are also risk factors.

The emergence of H5, H7, and H9 avian influenza virus subtypes in humans raises concern that the virus may undergo genetic reassortment or mutations in some of the genes and develop greater human-to-human transmissibility with the potential to produce a global pandemic. All fatal avian influenza virus infections acquire their internal gene segments from H9N2 viruses, the most widespread avian influenza subtype.

Human infections with H5N1 viruses have been reported to WHO from 16 countries, the first report in the Americas was in Canada in 2014, and approximately 60% of the cases have died. Infection with H7N9 avian influenza virus was first reported in China in 2013. Since then, many cases have been reported around the world with an average case fatality rate of 40%. Infections with other H7 avian influenza viruses (H7N2, H7N3, and H7N7) have occurred sporadically around the world. Rare human cases of influenza H9N2 are also reported.

► Clinical Findings

A. Symptoms and Signs

Distinguishing avian influenza from regular influenza is difficult. History of exposure to dead or ill birds or live poultry markets in the prior 10 days, recent travel to Southeast Asia or Egypt, or contact with known cases should be investigated. Patients infected by H5N1 or H7N9 avian influenza A viruses have an aggressive clinical course. The symptoms and signs include fever followed by lower respiratory symptoms (cough, dyspnea). Upper respiratory tract symptoms are less common. Gastrointestinal symptoms are reported more frequently in H5N1 infections. Conjunctivitis is reported in influenza H7 infections. Other systems can also be involved leading to neurologic manifestations (encephalopathy, seizure) and liver impairment. Prolonged febrile states and generalized malaise are common. Respiratory failure, multiorgan dysfunction, and septic shock are the usual cause of death. Bacterial superinfections are reported.

For human infections with H7N7 and N9B2 avian influenza virus infections, most cases have been mild with a few cases hospitalized and very few reports of deaths resulting from infection.

B. Laboratory Findings

Current commercial rapid antigen tests are not optimally sensitive or specific for detection of H5N1 influenza and should not be the definitive test for influenza. More sensitive RT-PCR assays are available through many hospitals and state health departments. Diagnostic yield can be improved by early collection of samples, preferably within 7 days of illness onset. Throat swabs or lower respiratory specimens (such as tracheal aspirate or bronchoalveolar lavage fluid) may provide higher yield of detection than nasal swabs. When highly pathogenic strains, such as H5N1 influenza virus infections, are suspected, extreme care in the handling of these samples must be observed during preliminary testing. Positive samples must then be forwarded to the appropriate public health authorities for further investigation (eg, culture) in laboratories with the adequate level of biosafety (level 3).

► Treatment

Persons with severe illness and confirmed and probable cases with mild disease should receive treatment as soon as possible. The current first-line recommendation is to use the neuraminidase inhibitor oseltamivir, 75 mg orally twice daily for 5 days administered within 48 hours from onset of illness. Longer courses of therapy (eg, 10 days) should be considered in hospitalized patients with severe illness and persistent viral shedding. Data are lacking for use of inhaled zanamivir or peramivir for severe avian influenza. Overall oseltamivir, by modeling, is associated with a 49% reduction in mortality from H5N1 avian influenza virus infections. As with seasonal influenza, enteric oseltamivir is well absorbed in critically ill persons without gastric stasis, known malabsorption, or gastrointestinal bleeding. Daily intravenous peramivir (600 mg, reduced to 200 mg for kidney dysfunction) for a minimum of 5 days and a maximum of 10 or more days (depending on severity of illness) or zanamivir (10 mg inhaled daily for 10 days) may be considered in such patients. Combination therapy with amantadine or rimantadine (in countries where H5N1 influenza virus A strains are likely to be susceptible to adamantanes) may be considered in patients with pneumonia or progressive disease. Resistance of avian H5N1 influenza strains to amantadine and rimantadine is present in most geographic areas. Resistance to neuraminidase inhibitors (oseltamivir, zanamivir, and peramivir) can occur with H5NA and H7N9 avian–infected patients. Successful treatment with administration of convalescent plasma is reported.

► Prevention

The most effective method of prevention is avoidance of exposure. Persons who work with poultry should practice good hand hygiene and use appropriate personal protective equipment. These workers should also be vaccinated against seasonal influenza, since this can reduce the likelihood of coinfection with avian and seasonal influenza. Persons should avoid visiting live poultry markets when able and should avoid contact with ill birds. No risk exists for acquiring avian influenza through the consumption of well-cooked poultry products. The US government bans the importation of poultry from infected areas. Culling of animals has been effective in ending outbreaks of highly pathogenic avian influenza but is difficult with H7-infected poultry because most are asymptomatic. Policies regarding closure of live poultry markets during avian epidemics are controversial.

Persons with exposure should monitor themselves for 10 days after the last known exposure and should seek prompt medical attention if new fever or respiratory symptoms develop. Postexposure prophylaxis is not recommended in persons working with noninfected birds or who used appropriate personal protective equipment while working with infected birds. For persons with exposure to infected persons, postexposure prophylaxis is recommended for household and family members and may be considered for health care personnel with close unprotected contact. Postexposure prophylaxis regimens include 75 mg of oseltamivir orally or 10 mg inhaled zanamivir twice daily for 5 or 10 days from the last known exposure, depending on the length of the exposure. Careful surveillance for human cases and prudent stockpiling of medications with establishment of an infrastructure for dissemination are essential modalities of control. Nonpharmacologic means of control include masks, social distancing, quarantine, travel limitations, and infrastructure development, particularly for emergency departments.

Current vaccines do not provide cross-protection against strains of the H5, H7, and H9 influenza viruses. The United States government has prepandemic stockpiles of adjuvanted H5N1 vaccines and H7N9 vaccines that are not available to the public. The highly diverse genetic nature and the rapid evolution of the avian influenza viruses has resulted in the emergence of viruses that are distinct from stockpiled vaccines. New vaccine development is ongoing to generate vaccines against H7N9 and H5N1 with broadened protection against unmatched strains. Some of these vaccines are under study in preclinical and clinical trials; however, no vaccines are currently commercially available for humans.

Because the potential for pandemic influenza for many of the new reassortment viruses is not fully known, continued surveillance is essential, and stockpiling of vaccines, adjuvant, and medications (oseltamivir and zanamivir) is warranted at the public health level.

Hassan AO et al. Adenovirus vector-based multi-epitope vaccine provides partial protection against H5, H7, and H9 avian influenza viruses. PLoS One. 2017 Oct 12;12(10):e0186244. [PMID: 29023601]

Pitisuttithum P et al. Safety and immunogenicity of a live attenuated influenza H5 candidate vaccine strain A/17/turkey/Turkey/05/133 H5N2 and its priming effects for potential pre-pandemic use: a randomised, double-blind, placebo-controlled trial. Lancet Infect Dis. 2017 Aug;17(8):833–42. [PMID: 28533093]

Sun X et al. Stockpiled pre-pandemic H5N1 influenza virus vaccines with AS03 adjuvant provide cross-protection from H5N2 clade 2.3.4.4 virus challenge in ferrets. Virology. 2017 Aug;508:164–9. [PMID: 28554058]

4. Middle East Respiratory Syndrome–Coronavirus (MERS-CoV)

ESSENTIALS OF DIAGNOSIS

▶ Mild, moderate, or severe respiratory illness.

▶ Travel to endemic area, including Saudi Arabia, United Arab Emirates, Qatar, and Jordan, within 14 days before symptom onset.

▶ Contact with camels reported in many cases.

▶ Fever, cough, and dyspnea.

▶ CDC can assist with real-time PCR using serum and respiratory samples, or serology.

▶ Supportive treatment; mortality 36% to 45%.

▶ General Considerations

Middle East respiratory syndrome (MERS) is a syndrome associated with a coronavirus similar to the cause of severe acute respiratory syndrome (SARS). Patients with MERS have had a history of residence or travel in the Middle East, in particular Saudi Arabia, or contact with such patients. The virus is probably transmitted through direct or indirect contact of mucous membranes with infectious respiratory droplets. The virus is shed in stool, but the role of fecal-oral transmission is unknown. The earliest cases were identified in 2012 in the Kingdom of Saudi Arabia, and 75% of all cases have occurred there. Additional cases have occurred throughout the Middle East, Africa, and Europe, with a reported death rate of 36% (http://www.who.int/emergencies/mers-cov/en/). So-called super-spreaders are often responsible for propagating the pathogen in the early stages of an outbreak.

Person-to-person transmission can occur within families; hospital-associated cases comprise 25% of cases. The median incubation period is 5 days (range, 2–14) with the mean age of 50 (range 9 months to 99 years) and 65% occurring among men. Over 90% of patients have an underlying medical condition, including diabetes mellitus (68%), hypertension (34%), or chronic heart or kidney disease. Those with diabetes, kidney disease, chronic lung disease, or other immunocompromising conditions likely are at highest risk for severe disease.

Camels appear to be the principal reservoir, and several studies show that contact with dromedary herds of camels is greater among cases than controls. Raw camel milk is considered a potential source. Persons who work with camels are more likely to have antibody evidence of past infection.

▶ Clinical Findings

A. Symptoms and Signs

MERS is an acute respiratory syndrome, with the most common symptoms being fever (98%), cough (83%), and dyspnea (72%). Chills and rigors are common (87%). Gastrointestinal symptoms may occur, with diarrhea being most common (26%), followed by nausea and abdominal pain, and may precede respiratory symptoms. Mild and asymptomatic cases are reported.

B. Laboratory Findings and Imaging

Hematologic findings in the largest series to date include thrombocytopenia (36%), lymphopenia (34%), and lymphocytosis (11%). Moderate elevations in lactate dehydrogenase (49%), AST (15%), and ALT (11%) are recognized. Chest radiograph abnormalities are nearly universal and include increased bronchovascular markings, patchy infiltrates or consolidations, interstitial changes, opacities (reticular and nodular) and pleural effusions, and total lung opacification. Ground-glass opacities and consolidation are most commonly seen. The findings mimic those of many other causes of pneumonia.

Serum serologies and RT-PCR are available through CDC (contact information below, on MMWR reference site). Highest viral loads are found in lower respiratory tract specimens, including bronchoalveolar lavage fluid, sputum, and tracheal aspirates. These samples are preferred for diagnosis. The CDC recommends sending lower respiratory tract specimens, nasopharyngeal and oropharyngeal swabs, and serum for testing. In confirmed cases, serial sample collection (perhaps every 2–4 days) from multiple sites is recommended to increase understanding of virus shedding kinetics. In cases in which symptom onset occurred more than 14 days prior and symptoms are ongoing, serum should be sent to the CDC for serologic testing and the above specimens should be sent for RT-PCR.

C. Case Definition

A patient with severe illness shows the following characteristics: fever (38°C, 100.4°F or higher) and pneumonia or ARDS (based on clinical or radiologic evidence); and either history of travel in or near the Arabian Peninsula within 14 days before symptom onset; or close contact with a symptomatic traveler in whom fever and acute respiratory illness (not necessarily pneumonia) developed within 14 days after traveling in or near the Arabian Peninsula (above); or is a member of a cluster of patients with severe acute respiratory illness (eg, fever and pneumonia requiring hospitalization) of unknown etiology in which MERS-CoV is being evaluated, in consultation with state and local health departments.

In milder illness, patients have fever and symptoms of respiratory illness (not necessarily pneumonia; eg, cough, shortness of breath) and history of having close contact with a confirmed MERS case as well as a history of being in a health care facility (as a patient, worker, or visitor) within 14 days of symptom onset in a country or territory within the Arabian Peninsula in which recent health care–associated cases of MERS have been identified.

Of note, fever may not be present in certain patients, including the very young, elderly persons, immunosuppressed individuals, or those taking certain medications.

▶ Complications

Respiratory failure is such a common complication that in a series from Saudi Arabia, 89% of patients required intensive care and mechanical ventilation. Patients with MERS-CoV appear to advance faster to respiratory failure than do those with SARS.

▶ Treatment

Respiratory support is essential. No vaccine or known antiviral therapy exists to combat MERS. Current therapies are adapted from SARS treatments, which include broad-spectrum antibiotics, corticosteroids, interferons, ribavirin, lopinavir-ritonavir, or mycophenolate mofetil. A small retrospective study found improved survival at 14 days with ribavirin and interferon-alpha but not at 28 days.

▶ Prognosis

The overall mortality rate of identified cases is about 36%. Advanced age is associated with a poor prognosis.

▶ Prevention

Isolation and quarantine of cases is authorized by CDC. Strict infection control measures are essential as well as care and management of household contacts and hospital workers engaged in the care of patients. Travelers to Saudi Arabia (including the many pilgrims to the holy sites) should practice frequent hand washing and avoid contact with those who have respiratory symptoms. Evaluation of patients with suspect symptoms within 14 days of return from Saudi Arabia is essential. Because healthcare workers engaged in procedures that involve contact with respiratory droplets are at risk, isolation of high-risk patients is essential, as are simple hygienic measures. Control measures, including quarantining in the home for high-risk exposed persons and the use of facemasks for preventing hospital-acquired infections, are important. Assisting public health authorities with case reporting and surveillance is essential.

Camel workers including slaughterhouse and market workers, veterinarians, and racing personnel should wear facial protection and protective clothing and practice good personal hygiene, including frequent hand washing after touching animals. Family members of such personnel should not be exposed to work paraphernalia including clothing and shoes and workers should shower at the site of employment rather than the home. Avoid direct contact with camels (who may be asymptomatic but who can transmit the virus though nasal or ocular discharge, milk, urine, and feces). All infected animals should be kept off the market, including their meat products, and buried or destroyed.

Arabi YM et al. Middle East Respiratory Syndrome. N Engl J Med. 2017 Feb 9;376(6):584–94. [PMID: 28177862]

Das KM et al. Acute Middle East respiratory syndrome coronavirus: temporal lung changes observed on the chest radiographs of 55 patients. AJR Am J Roentgenol. 2015 Sep; 205(3):W267–74. [PMID: 26102309]

Rabaan AA et al. A review of candidate therapies for Middle East respiratory syndrome from a molecular perspective. J Med Microbiol. 2017 Sep;66(9):1261–74. [PMID: 28855003]

ADENOVIRUS INFECTIONS

▶ General Considerations

At least 60 serotypes of adenovirus are currently described and these are members of 7 species classified A–G. About half of these subgroups produce a variety of clinical syndromes. Adenoviruses show a worldwide distribution and occur throughout the year. These infections are usually self-limited or clinically inapparent and occur most commonly among infants, young children, and military recruits. However, these infections may cause significant morbidity and mortality in immunocompromised persons, such as HIV-infected persons and COPD patients, as well as in patients who have undergone solid organ and hematopoietic stem cell transplantation or cardiac surgery or in those who have received cancer chemotherapy. A few cases of donor-transmitted adenoviral infection have been reported in past years. An outbreak with adenovirus type 55 was reported in 2017 from a neurosurgical unit in China.

Adenoviruses, although a common cause of human disease, also receive particular recognition through their role as vectors in gene therapy and vaccine development.

► **Clinical Findings**

A. Symptoms and Signs

The incubation period is 4–9 days. Clinical syndromes of adenovirus infection, often overlapping, include the following. The common cold (see Chapter 8) is characterized by rhinitis, pharyngitis, and mild malaise without fever. Conjunctivitis is often present. Nonstreptococcal exudative pharyngitis is characterized by fever lasting 2–12 days and accompanied by malaise and myalgia. Lower respiratory tract infection may occur, including bronchiolitis, suggested by cough and rales, or pneumonia. Types 1, 2, 3, 4, and 7 commonly cause acute respiratory disease and atypical pneumonia; coinfections or serial infections are documented to occur. Infections are especially severe in Native American children. Adenovirus type 14 is increasingly reported as a cause of severe and sometimes fatal pneumonia in those with chronic lung disease but is also seen in healthy young adults and military recruit outbreaks. Viral or bacterial coinfections occur with adenovirus in 15–20% of cases. Pharyngoconjunctival fever is manifested by fever and malaise, conjunctivitis (often unilateral), mild pharyngitis, and cervical adenitis. Epidemic keratoconjunctivitis (transmissible person-to-person, most often types 8, 19, and 37) occurs in adults and is manifested by bilateral conjunctival redness, pain, tearing, and an enlarged preauricular lymph node (multiple types may be involved in a single outbreak). Type 53 (a D adenovirus) was the cause of a 2017 outbreak in a Los Angeles County Eye Clinic. Keratitis may lead to subepithelial opacities (especially with the above types).

Sexually transmitted genitourinary ulcers and urethritis may be caused by types 2, 8, and 37. Adenoviruses also cause acute gastroenteritis (types 40 and 41), mesenteric adenitis, acute appendicitis, rhabdomyolysis, and intussusception. Rarely, they are associated with encephalitis, meningitis, acute respiratory distress syndrome (ARDS), acute flaccid paralysis, and pericarditis. Adenovirus is commonly identified in endomyocardial tissue of patients with myocarditis and dilated cardiomyopathy. Risk factors associated with severity of infection include youth, chronic underlying infections, recent transplantation, and serotypes 5 or 21.

Hepatitis (type 5 adenovirus), pneumonia, and hemorrhagic cystitis (types 11 and 34) tend to develop in infected liver, lung, or kidney transplant recipients, respectively. Disease states that may develop in hematopoietic stem cell transplant patients include hepatitis, pneumonia, diarrhea, hemorrhagic cystitis, tubulointerstitial nephritis, colitis, and encephalitis.

B. Laboratory Findings and Imaging

Antigen detection assays including direct fluorescence assay or enzyme immunoassay are rapid and show sensitivity of 40–60% compared with viral culture (considered the standard). Samples with negative rapid assays require PCR assays or viral cultures for diagnosis. Quantitative real-time rapid-cycle PCR is useful in distinguishing disease from colonization, especially in hematopoietic stem cell transplant patients. Multiplex nucleic acid amplification assays can test for multiple respiratory viruses simultaneously with increased sensitivity. Adenovirus differs from other viral and bacterial respiratory infections seen on chest CT imaging, appearing as a multifocal consolidation or ground-glass opacity without airway inflammatory findings.

► **Treatment & Prognosis**

Treatment is symptomatic. Ribavirin or cidofovir is used in immunocompromised individuals with occasional success, although cidofovir is attendant with significant renal toxicity. Brincidofovir, the lipid-conjugated prodrug of cidofovir, has better oral bioavailability, is better tolerated, and achieves higher intracellular concentrations of active drug than cidofovir but currently is only available through compassionate use policies. A 2017 study of brincidofovir showed efficacy in controlling adenovirus in pediatric hematopoietic cell transplant patients. IVIG is also used in immunocompromised patients and can be used in combination with other therapies, but data are still limited. Reduced immunosuppression is often required. Typing of isolates is useful epidemiologically and in distinguishing transmission from endogenous reactivation. Topical steroids or tacrolimus may be used to treat adenoviral keratoconjunctivitis. Complications of adenovirus pneumonia in children include bronchiolitis obliterans. Deaths are reported on occasion.

The control of epidemic adenoviral conjunctivitis is often difficult and requires meticulous attention to hand hygiene, use of disposable gloves, sterilization of equipment (isopropyl alcohol is insufficient, recommendations of manufacturers are preferred), cohorting of cases, and furloughing of employees. Treatment with a combination of povidone-iodine 1.0% eyedrops and dexamethasone 0.1% eyedrops four times a day can reduce symptoms and expedite recovery.

Vaccines are not available for general use. Use of live oral vaccines containing attenuated type 4 and type 7 was reinstated in military personnel in 2013 and has been associated with significant decrease in adenoviral disease.

Hiwarkar P et al; United Kingdom Paediatric Bone Marrow Transplant Group. Brincidofovir is highly efficacious in controlling adenoviremia in pediatric recipients of hematopoietic cell transplant. Blood. 2017 Apr 6;129(14):2033–7. [PMID: 28153824]

Kovalyuk N et al. Treatment of adenoviral keratoconjunctivitis with a combination of povidone-iodine 1.0% and dexamethasone 0.1% drops: a clinical prospective controlled randomized study. Acta Ophthalmol. 2017 Dec;95(8):e686–92. [PMID: 28342227]

Tzannou I et al. Off-the-shelf virus-specific T cells to treat BK virus, human herpesvirus 6, cytomegalovirus, Epstein-Barr virus, and adenovirus infections after allogeneic hematopoietic stem-cell transplantation. J Clin Oncol. 2017 Nov 1;35(31): 3547–57. [PMID: 28783452]

OTHER EXANTHEMATOUS VIRAL INFECTIONS

1. *Erythroparvovirus* Infections

Primate erythroparvovirus 1, more commonly known as parvovirus B19, infects human erythroid precursor cells. It is quite widespread (by age 15 years about 50% of children have detectable IgG), and its transmission occurs through respiratory secretions and saliva, through the placenta (vertical transmission with 30–50% of pregnant women nonimmune), and through administration of blood products. The incubation period is 4–14 days. Chronic forms of the infection can occur. Bocavirus, another erythroparvovirus, is a cause of winter acute respiratory disease in children and adults.

▶ Clinical Findings

A. Symptoms and Signs

Parvovirus B19 causes several syndromes and manifests differently in various populations.

1. Children—In children, an exanthematous illness ("fifth disease," erythema infectiosum) is characterized by a fiery red "slapped cheek" appearance, circumoral pallor, and a subsequent lacy, maculopapular, evanescent rash on the trunk and limbs. Eosinophilic cellulitis (Well syndrome) is also reported with parvovirus B19, as are microvesicular eruptions and atypical rashes. Parvovirus B19 is also one of the most common causes of myocarditis in childhood.

2. Immunocompromised patients—A transient aplastic crisis and pure red blood cell aplasia may occur. Bone marrow aspirates reveal absence of mature erythroid precursors and characteristic giant pronormoblasts. The parvovirus B19 gene is detected in 16–19% of acute leukemia and chronic myeloid leukemia patients.

3. Adults—A limited nonerosive symmetric polyarthritis that mimics lupus erythematosus and rheumatoid arthritis, which may in some cases be a type II mixed cryoglobulinemia, can develop in middle-aged persons (especially women). Rashes, especially facial, are less common in adults.

Chloroquine and its derivatives exacerbate parvovirus B19–associated anemia and are linked with significantly lower hematocrit in hospital admissions in malaria endemic areas. Rare reported presentations include myocarditis with infarction, constrictive pericarditis, chronic dilated cardiomyopathy (although a 2016 analysis from the Netherlands dispute some cardiac findings), Hashimoto thyroiditis, hepatitis, pneumonitis, neutropenia, thrombocytopenia, a lupus-like syndrome, glomerulonephritis, CNS vasculitis, papular-purpuric "gloves and socks" syndrome, complications of drug hypersensitivity, and a chronic fatigue syndrome. A subclinical infection is documented among patients with sickle cell disease. Other CNS manifestations of parvovirus B19 include encephalitis, meningitis, stroke (usually in sickle cell anemia patients with aplastic crises), and peripheral neuropathy (brachial plexitis and carpal tunnel syndrome) with occasional chronic residua.

The symptoms of parvovirus B19 infection can mimic those of autoimmune states such as lupus, systemic sclerosis, antiphospholipid syndrome, or vasculitis. A more specific entity named relapsing symmetric seronegative synovitis with edema was reported in two cases to be associated serologically with parvovirus B19 infection.

In pregnancy, premature labor, hydrops fetalis, and fetal loss are reported sequelae. Pregnant women with a recent exposure or with suggestive symptoms should be tested for the disease and carefully monitored if results are positive.

A serosurvey from France suggests parvovirus B19 infection may occur more commonly in patients with schizophrenia.

B. Laboratory Findings

The diagnosis is clinical (Table 32–2) but may be confirmed by either an elevated titer of IgM anti-parvovirus B19 antibodies in serum or with PCR in serum or bone marrow. By the time common presenting symptoms manifest, in particular a rash or polyarthropathy in an immunocompetent patient, the viremia may have cleared but IgM antibodies are likely present. In immunocompromised patients, RT-PCR is the optimal test. Autoimmune antibodies (antiphospholipid and antineutrophil cytoplasmic antibodies) can be present and are thought to be a consequence of molecular mimicry. False-positive serologies also occur in the presence of recent IVIG and anti–B-cell therapy. Also, remnant parvovirus B19, from tissue and serum, is thought to explain some false-positive findings. Assays on marrow tissue are indicated only if a marrow is deemed necessary for other hematologic reasons.

▶ Treatment

Treatment in healthy persons is symptomatic (NSAIDs are used to treat arthralgias, and transfusions are used to treat transient aplastic crises). In immunosuppressed patients including those infected with HIV, IVIG is very effective in the short-term reduction of anemia. Relapses tend to occur about 4 months after administration of IVIG. There is no reduction in encephalitic complications with IVIG. Intrauterine blood transfusion can be considered in severe fetal anemia, although such transfusions have been linked to impaired neurologic development.

▶ Prevention & Prognosis

Several nosocomial outbreaks are documented. In these cases, standard containment guidelines, including hand washing after patient exposure and avoiding contact with pregnant women, are paramount.

The prognosis is generally excellent in immunocompetent individuals. In immunosuppressed patients, persistent anemia may require prolonged transfusion dependence. Remission of parvovirus B19 infection in AIDS patients may occur with ART, though the immune reconstitution inflammatory syndrome is also reported.

Puttarakasa K et al. Parvovirus B19V non-structural protein NS1 induces dsDNA autoantibodies and end organ damage in non-autoimmune mice. J Infect Dis. 2019 Apr 16;219(9):1418–29. [PMID: 30346568]

Verdonschot J et al. Relevance of cardiac parvovirus B19 in myo-carditis and dilated cardiomyopathy: review of the literature. Eur J Heart Fail. 2016 Dec;18(12):1430–41. [PMID: 27748022]

Wolfromm A et al. Spectrum of adult parvovirus B19 infection according to the underlying predisposing condition and pro-posals for clinical practice. Br J Haematol. 2015 Jul;170(2):192–9. [PMID: 25920561]

2. Poxvirus Infections

Among the poxviruses causing disease in humans, the fol-lowing are the most clinically important: variola/vaccinia, molluscum contagiosum, orf and paravaccinia, and monkeypox.

1. Variola/vaccinia—Smallpox (variola) was a highly con-tagious disease associated with high mortality and dis-abling sequelae. Its manifestations include severe headache, acute onset of fever, prostration and a rash characterized by uniform progression from macules to papules to firm, deep-seated vesicles or pustules. The synchronous progres-sion in smallpox readily differentiates lesions from those of varicella (see also Chapter 6).

Complications of smallpox include bacterial superin-fections (cellulitis and pneumonia), encephalitis, and kera-titis with corneal ulcerations (risk factor for blindness). Effective vaccination led to its global elimination by 1979 and routine vaccination stopped in 1985. Recommenda-tions to destroy remaining samples of this virus have not been acted upon thus far, and significant concern exists for potential misuse of these repositories in military or terror-ist activities.

Smallpox should be considered, in concordance with the CDC Smallpox Response Plan (https://www.cdc.gov/smallpox/bioterrorism-response-planning/community/index.html), in any patient with fever and a characteristic rash for which other etiologies—such as herpes infections (eczema herpeticum may be differentiated from suspect smallpox by appropriate serologic stains and clinical appearance), erythema multiforme, drug reactions, or other infections—are unlikely. Patients with suspected infection should be placed in airborne and contact isola-tion and the official agency contacted (CDC Poxvirus and Rabies Branch help desk may be reached at 404-639-4129 and the Director's Emergency Operation Center at 770-488-7100).

Guidelines regarding smallpox vaccination are available at https://www.cdc.gov/smallpox/vaccine-basics/index.html.

2. Molluscum contagiosum—Molluscum contagiosum is caused by a molluscipox virus that may be transmitted sexually or by other close contact. The disease is mani-fested by pearly, raised, umbilicated skin nodules sparing the palms and soles. Keratoconjunctivitis can occur. Most ocular lesions are typical umbilicated dome-shaped lesions, but a variety of atypical ocular lesions are reported often in immunocompetent patients, more often in females and young adults (mean age 19).

There may be an association with atopic dermatitis or eczema. Marked and persistent lesions in AIDS patients respond readily to combination ART. Treatment options include destructive therapies (curettage, cryotherapy, can-tharidin, 10–15% hydrogen peroxide, and keratolytics, among others), immunomodulators (imiquimod, cimeti-dine, and *Candida* antigen), and antiviral agents (topical cidofovir is effective anecdotally in refractory cases; brin-cidofovir, an agent under investigation for treating other viral infections, has shown some efficacy). No treatment is uniformly effective, and multiple courses of therapy are often needed. One meta-analysis recommends natural reso-lution of lesions if normal immunity can be restored. Cryp-tococcal skin lesions can mimic molluscum contagiosum.

3. Orf and paravaccinia—Orf (contagious pustular derma-titis, or ecthyma contagiosa) and paravaccinia (milker's nodules) are occupational diseases acquired by contact with sheep/goats and cattle, respectively. Household meat processing and animal slaughter have been implicated as risk factors. A new poxvirus akin to parapoxviruses was reported in 2015 in two patients from rural Tennessee and Missouri (the latter had also traveled to Tanzania). Orf is a common infection in sheep, goats, and deer. Thus, it is found worldwide, and farmers, veterinarians, and hunters are considered high-risk populations. It progresses through six clinically distinct dermatologic stages and lesions usu-ally heal in 3–6 weeks without scarring. The use of nonpo-rous gloves for persons handling animals is recommended, especially if the persons are immunosuppressed. Molecular tests are used to confirm clinical diagnosis. Although there is no specific treatment, Orf anecdotally responds to imiquimod. A live vaccine is available for animals.

4. Monkeypox—First identified in 1970, monkeypox is enzootic in the rain forests of equatorial Africa and pres-ents in humans as a syndrome similar to smallpox. The incubation period is about 13 days (range, 6–28 in a recent Central African Republic outbreak) and limited person-to-person spread occurs. African mortality rates vary from 3% to 11% depending on the immune status of the patient. Secondary attack rates appear to be about 10%. Since 2016, confirmed cases of monkeypox have occurred in Central African Republic, Democratic Republic of the Congo, Liberia, Nigeria, and Sierra Leone and in captive chimpan-zees in Cameroon. Risk factors identified from the Demo-cratic Republic of Congo include being bitten by rodents, working as a hunter, and being male over 18 years of age. Confusion with smallpox and varicella occurs; however, both lymphadenopathy (seen in up to 90% of unvaccinated persons) and a febrile prodrome are prominent features in monkeypox infection. The monkeypox rash is distin-guished by its deep-seated and well-circumscribed nature, lesions at the same stage of development (unlike varicella but like smallpox), and its centrifugal progression (includ-ing palms and soles). Suspected cases should be placed on standard, contact, and droplet precautions; local and state public health officials and the CDC should be notified for assistance with confirmation of the diagnosis (by electron microscopy, viral culture, ELISA, PCR, and a GeneXpert assay referred to as MPX/OPX [monkeypox/orthopox]). There are no standard or optimized guidelines for the clini-cal management of monkeypox. Cidofovir is effective in vitro against monkeypox, and its less toxic prodrug brincidofovir may be useful as well. Vaccinia immune globulin can be used in selected cases.

Other general precautions that should be taken are avoidance of contact with rodents from endemic areas (whose illness is manifested by alopecia, rash, and ocular or nasal discharge), appropriate care and isolation of humans exposed to such animals within the prior 3 weeks, and veterinary examination and investigation of suspect animals through health departments. Vaccinia immunization is effective against monkeypox and is recommended for those involved in the investigation of the outbreak and for health care workers caring for those infected with monkeypox if no contraindication exists (outlined above). Postexposure vaccination is also advised for documented contacts of infected persons or animals. US federal agencies prohibit the importation of African rodents.

5. Novel orthopoxviruses—Two cases in the country of Georgia with a novel orthopox virus occurred in 2013 with a third diagnosed serologically from 2010. All cases had animal contact, cattle for two, and serologic data showed possible associations with rodents and shrews as well as cattle. None had been vaccinated for smallpox. Another novel orthopoxvirus was identified in a patient who had undergone kidney transplantation in North America in 2015.

Centers for Disease Control and Prevention (CDC). Updated interim CDC guidance for use of smallpox vaccine, cidofovir, and vaccinia immune globulin (VIG) for prevention and treatment in the setting of an outbreak of monkeypox infections. http://www.cdc.gov/ncidod/monkeypox/treatmentguidelines.htm

Chittick G et al. Short-term clinical safety profile of brincidofovir: a favorable benefit-risk proposition in the treatment of smallpox. Antiviral Res. 2017 Jul;143:269–77. [PMID: 28093339]

Durski KN et al. Emergence of monkeypox—west and central Africa, 1970–2017. MMWR Morb Mortal Wkly Rep. 2018 Mar 16;67(10):306–10. [PMID: 29543790]

Grosenbach DW et al. Oral tecovirimat for the treatment of smallpox. N Engl J Med. 2018 Jul 5;379(1):44–53. [PMID: 29972742]

Teixidó C et al. Efficacy and safety of topical application of 15% and 10% potassium hydroxide for the treatment of Molluscum contagiosum. Pediatr Dermatol. 2018 May;35(3):336–42. [PMID: 29479727]

van der Wouden JC et al. Interventions for cutaneous molluscum contagiosum. Cochrane Database Syst Rev. 2017 May 17;5:CD004767. [PMID: 28513067]

VIRUSES & GASTROENTERITIS

Viruses are responsible for at least 30–40% of cases of infectious diarrhea in the United States. These agents include rotaviruses; caliciviruses, including noroviruses such as Norwalk virus; astroviruses; enteric adenoviruses; and, less often, toroviruses, coronaviruses, picornaviruses (including the Aichi virus), and pestiviruses. Rotaviruses and noroviruses are responsible for most nonbacterial cases of gastroenteritis.

Rotaviruses are reoviruses with eight species and significant animal reservoirs. They are the leading worldwide cause of dehydrating gastroenteritis in very young children and are associated with significant morbidity and mortality. Each year, over 400,000 children die of rotavirus infection worldwide. Children aged 6 months to 2 years are the most affected, although adults are affected occasionally as well. By age 5, virtually every child has been infected with this pathogen. The diverse set of rotaviruses (classified by glycoproteins and protease-sensitive proteins [G-type and P-type antigens], which segregate independently) results in a constellation of phenotypes, although only about four of these are responsible for over 90% of disease. Rotavirus infections follow an endemic pattern, especially in the tropics and low-income countries, but they peak during the winter in temperate regions. The virus is transmitted by fecal-oral route and can be shed in feces for up to 3 weeks in severe infections. In outbreak settings (eg, day care centers), the virus is ubiquitously found in the environment, and secondary attack rates are between 16% and 30% (including household contacts). Nosocomial outbreaks are reported.

The disease is usually mild and self-limiting. A 2- to 3-day prodrome of fever and vomiting is followed by nonbloody diarrhea (up to 10–20 bowel movements per day) lasting for 1–4 days. It is thought that systemic disease occurs rarely, and unusual reported presentations include cerebellitis and pancreatitis. Patients with gastroenteritis are not routinely tested for rotavirus because the results do not alter treatment. Oral and intravenous rehydration solutions are the primary treatment options, but effective adjunctive therapies include specific probiotics (eg, *Lactobacillus* GG or *Saccharomyces boulardii*), nitazoxanide, diosmectite, or racecadotril. Adjunctive therapies such as oral odansetron shorten the median duration of diarrhea and hospitalization. Local intestinal immunity gives protection against successive infection.

Vaccines have been highly successful in reducing the global burden of rotavirus. Currently they are recommended for infants older than 6 weeks but younger than 2 years; studies are underway to assess the safety and efficacy of starting vaccination in the newborn period. Several rotavirus vaccines exist, and two are available in the United States: a live, oral, pentavalent human-bovine reassortment rotavirus vaccine (PRV, RotaTeq; to be given at 2, 4, and 6 months of age) and a live, oral attenuated monovalent human rotavirus vaccine (HRV, Rotarix; to be given at 2 and 4 months of age). The vaccines showed 85–98% efficacy against severe rotavirus gastroenteritis in trials based in the Americas and Europe. Reduced efficacy (50–64%) has been noted in studies conducted in Asia and Africa. One advantage of these vaccines is the evidence of heterotypic immunity (prevention against rotavirus strains not included in the vaccine). Accordingly, some data from the Americas suggest that rotavirus vaccination confers herd immunity to children under 1 year of age.

Vaccine coverage is inadequate in the United States for rotavirus (74.6% in the 2016 National Immunization Study), particularly among the poor. National immunization programs of over 80 countries include rotavirus vaccine, and the different rotavirus vaccines are available commercially in 100 countries.

Effectiveness of live oral rotavirus vaccines is reduced in low-resource settings.

With the control of rotavirus, noroviruses, such as Norwalk virus (one of a variety of small round viruses divided into 6 genogroups [3 causing disease in man] and at least 25 genotypes), are now the major cause of diarrhea globally. Noroviruses are a leading cause of food-borne disease in the United States (with food handlers largely responsible and associated foods most often leafy vegetables, fruits/nuts, and mollusks) and are significantly associated with military deployment as well as travel-associated and nosocomial infections.

Norovirus gastroenteritis is responsible for up to 20% of all diarrhea in both children and adults and an estimated 800 deaths annually in the United States and 200,000 deaths globally. The efficacy of the rotavirus vaccination has increased the percentage of gastroenteritis caused by norovirus. The noroviruses appear to evolve by antigenic drift (similar to influenza). While 90% of young adults show serologic evidence of past infection, no long-lasting protective immunity develops, and reinfections are common.

Outbreak environments include long-term care facilities (nursing homes in particular), restaurants, hospitals, schools, day care centers, vacation destinations (including cruise ships), and military bases. Persons at particular risk are younger individuals, older adults, those who are institutionalized, and those who are immunosuppressed. A strain that began in Australia (GII.4 Sydney) is responsible for increasing proportions of US cases. The GII.4 Sydney strain was the main cause of all cruise ship norovirus infections between 2008 and 2014. It was also the predominant cause of acute gastroenteritis in the 2016–2017 season in the United States. Although transmission is usually fecal-oral, airborne, person-to-person, and waterborne transmission are also documented. A short incubation period (24–48 hours), a short symptomatic illness (12–60 hours, but up to 5 days in hospital-associated cases), a high frequency (greater than 50%) of vomiting, and absence of bacterial pathogens in stool samples are highly predictive of norovirus gastroenteritis.

RT-PCR of stool samples is used for diagnostic and epidemiologic purposes. Several licensed multiple pathogen platform assays are available, but they are expensive and interpretation of the cause of illness in a given patient may be difficult. Treatment options are similar to rotavirus (see above) and rely mostly on oral and intravenous rehydration. Deaths are rare in the developed world, and the more common associated diseases are aspiration pneumonia, septicemia, and necrotizing enterocolitis.

Outbreak control for both rotavirus and norovirus infections include strict adherence to general hygienic measures. Despite the promise of alcohol-based sanitizers for the control of pathogen transmission, such cleansers may be relatively ineffective against the noroviruses compared with antibacterial soap and water, reinforcing the need for new hygienic agents against this prevalent group of viruses. Cohorting of sick patients, contact precautions for symptomatic hospitalized patients, exclusion from work of symptomatic staff until symptom resolution (or 48–72 hours after this for norovirus disease), and proper decontamination procedures are crucial.

Bines JE et al. Human neonatal rotavirus vaccine (RV3-BB) to target rotavirus from birth. N Engl J Med. 2018 Feb 22; 378(8):719–30. [PMID: 29466164]

Hagbom M. Ondansetron treatment reduces rotavirus symptoms—a randomized double-blinded placebo-controlled trial. PLoS One. 2017 Oct 27;12(10):e0186824. [PMID: 29077725]

Isanaka S et al. Efficacy of a low-cost, heat-stable oral rotavirus vaccine in Niger. N Engl J Med. 2017 Mar 23;376(12):1121–30. [PMID: 28328346]

Leroux-Roels G et al. Safety and immunogenicity of different formulations of norovirus vaccine candidate in healthy adults: a randomized, controlled, double-blind clinical trial. J Infect Dis. 2018 Jan 30;217(4):597–607. [PMID: 29140444]

ENTEROVIRUSES THAT PRODUCE SEVERAL SYNDROMES

The most famous enterovirus, the poliomyelitis virus, is discussed above under Major Vaccine-Preventable Viral Infections. Other clinically relevant enteroviral infections are discussed in this section.

1. Coxsackievirus Infections

Coxsackievirus infections cause several clinical syndromes. As with other enteroviruses, infections are most common during the summer. Two groups, A and B, are defined either serologically or by mouse bioassay. There are more than 50 serotypes.

▶ Clinical Findings

A. Symptoms and Signs

The clinical syndromes associated with coxsackievirus infection are summer grippe; herpangina; epidemic pleurodynia; aseptic meningitis and other neurologic syndromes; acute nonspecific pericarditis; myocarditis; hand, foot, and mouth disease; epidemic conjunctivitis; and other syndromes.

1. Summer grippe (A and B)—A febrile illness, principally of children, summer grippe usually lasts 1–4 days. Minor upper respiratory tract infection symptoms are often present.

2. Herpangina (A2–6, 10; B3)—There is sudden onset of fever, which may be as high as 40.6°C, sometimes with febrile convulsions. Other symptoms are headache, myalgia, and vomiting. The sore throat is characterized early by petechiae or papules on the soft palate that ulcerate in about 3 days and then heal. Treatment is symptomatic.

3. Epidemic pleurodynia (Bornholm disease) (B1–5)—Pleuritic pain is prominent. Tenderness, hyperesthesia, and muscle swelling are present over the area of diaphragmatic attachment. Other findings include headache, sore throat, malaise, nausea, and fever. Orchitis and aseptic meningitis occur in less than 10% of patients. Most patients are ill for 4–6 days.

4. Aseptic meningitis (A and B) and other neurologic syndromes—Fever, headache, nausea, vomiting, stiff neck, drowsiness, and CSF lymphocytosis without chemical abnormalities may occur, and pediatric clusters of group B (especially B5) meningitis are reported. Focal encephalitis and transverse myelitis are reported with coxsackievirus group A and acute flaccid paralysis with group B in India. Disseminated encephalitis occurs after group B infection, and acute flaccid paralysis is reported with both coxsackievirus groups A and B.

5. Acute nonspecific pericarditis (B types)—Sudden onset of anterior chest pain, often worse with inspiration and in the supine position, is typical. Fever, myalgia, headache, and pericardial friction rub appear early and these symptoms are often transient. Evidence for pericardial effusion on imaging studies is often present, and the occasional patient has a paradoxical pulse. Electrocardiographic evidence of pericarditis is often present. Relapses may occur.

6. Myocarditis (B1–5)—Heart failure in the neonatal period secondary to in utero myocarditis and over 20% of adult cases of myocarditis and dilated cardiomyopathy are associated with group B (especially B3) infections.

7. Hand, foot, and mouth disease (A5, 6, 10, 12, and 16, B5)—This disease is sometimes epidemic and is characterized by stomatitis, a vesicular rash on hands and feet, nail dystrophies, and onychomadesis (nail shedding) (Figure 32–6). Enterovirus 71 is also a causative agent of usually more severe disease. A16 disease is usually mild. A6 may be atypical but is usually self-limited. Rare fatalities are reported among surveillance programs in China.

8. Epidemic conjunctivitis—As with enterovirus 70, the A24 variant of coxsackievirus is associated with acute epidemic hemorrhagic conjunctivitis in tropical areas with outbreaks reported in southern China, Pakistan, southern Sudan, the Comoros, Uganda, Cuba, and Thailand. It is also reported as a cause of corneal endothelitis after cataract surgery.

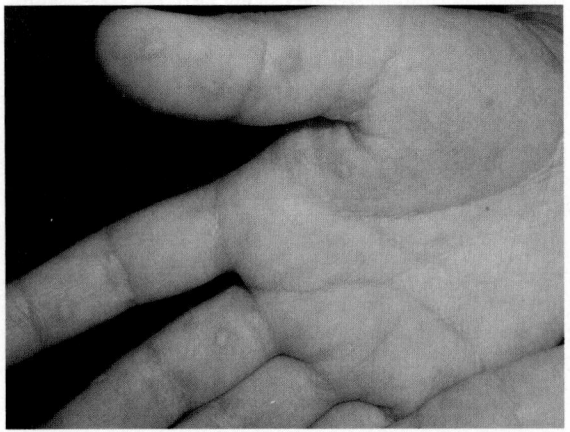

▲ **Figure 32–6.** Typical flat, gray, oval vesicular lesions on the ventral hand and fingers. (Used, with permission, from Richard P. Usatine, MD, in Usatine RP, Smith MA, Mayeaux EJ Jr, Chumley H. *The Color Atlas of Family Medicine,* 3rd ed. McGraw-Hill, 2019.)

9. Other syndromes associated with coxsackievirus infections—These include rhabdomyolysis, fulminant neonatal hepatitis (occurs rarely), pancreatitis with concomitant hepatitis and myocarditis (A4), glomerulopathy (group B infections), onychomadesis (B1), neonatal hemophagocytic lymphohistocytosis (B1), types 1 and 2 diabetes mellitus (mainly group B infections), and thyroid disease (group B4), although definitive causality is not established. A pathogenic role in primary Sjögren syndrome and acute myocardial infarction has also been proposed for group B coxsackievirus infections. A report of confirmed infective endocarditis due to coxsackievirus B2 in a patient with a prosthetic cardiac device suggests that viral etiologies of culture-negative infective endocarditis should be considered.

B. Laboratory Findings

Routine laboratory studies show no characteristic abnormalities. Neutralizing antibodies appear during convalescence. The virus may be isolated from throat washings or stools inoculated into suckling mice. Viral culture is expensive, labor intensive, and requires several days for results. A PCR test for enterovirus RNA is available and, although it cannot identify the serotype, may be useful, particularly in cases of meningitis.

▶ **Treatment & Prognosis**

Treatment is symptomatic. Except for meningitis, myocarditis, pericarditis, diabetes, and rare illnesses such as pancreatitis or poliomyelitis-like states, the syndromes caused by coxsackieviruses are benign and self-limited. Two controlled trials showed a potential clinical benefit with pleconaril for patients with enteroviral meningitis although the compassionate use of this medication has stopped (clinicians can contact Schering Plough for updates). There are anecdotal reports of success with IVIG in severe disease. Vaccines against the most common etiologic agents in a given country have been developed, but simultaneous circulation of more than one virus make coxsackievirus vaccines based on a single agent relatively ineffective.

Aswathyraj S et al. Hand, foot and mouth disease (HFMD): emerging epidemiology and the need for a vaccine strategy. Med Microbiol Immunol. 2016 Oct;205(5):397–407. [PMID: 27406374]

Esposito S et al. Hand, foot and mouth disease: current knowledge on clinical manifestations, epidemiology, aetiology and prevention. Eur J Clin Microbiol Infect Dis. 2018 Mar; 37(3):391–8. [PMID: 29411190]

Greninger AL et al. A novel outbreak enterovirus D68 strain associated with acute flaccid myelitis cases in the USA (2012–14): a retrospective cohort study. Lancet Infect Dis. 2015 Jun; 15(6):671–82. [PMID: 25837569]

2. Echovirus Infections

Echoviruses are enteroviruses that produce several clinical syndromes, particularly in children. Infection is most common during summer. Among reported specimens, death ensues in about 3%. Males younger than 20 years are more commonly infected than other persons.

Over 30 serotypes of echoviruses are recognized and the most common serotypes for disease are types 6, 9, 11, 19, and 30. Most can cause aseptic meningitis, which may be associated with a rubelliform rash. Transmission is primarily fecal-oral. Hand washing is an effective control measure in outbreaks of aseptic meningitis. Outbreaks related to fecal contamination of water sources, including drinking water and swimming and bathing pools, were reported previously.

Besides meningitis, other conditions associated with echoviruses range from common respiratory diseases and epidemic diarrhea to myocarditis, a hemorrhagic obstetric syndrome, keratoconjunctivitis, severe hepatitis with coagulopathy, leukocytoclastic vasculitis, encephalitis with sepsis, interstitial pneumonitis, pleurodynia, hemophagocytic syndromes (in children with cancer), sudden deafness, encephalitis, acute flaccid paralysis (a leading cause in India), optic neuritis, uveitis, and septic shock. Echoviruses and enteroviruses are also a common cause of nonspecific exanthems.

As with other enterovirus infections, diagnosis is best established by correlation of clinical, epidemiologic, and laboratory evidence. Cytopathic effects are produced in tissue culture after recovery of virus from throat washings, blood, or CSF. An enterovirus PCR of the CSF can assist in the diagnosis and is associated with a shorter duration of hospitalization in febrile neonates. Fourfold or greater rises in antibody titer signify systemic infection.

Treatment is usually symptomatic, and the prognosis is excellent, though there are reports of mild paralysis after CNS infection. In vitro data suggest some role for amantadine or ribavirin, but clinical studies supporting these findings are not available.

From a public health standpoint, clustered illnesses, such as among travelers swimming in sewage-infested seawater, suggest point-source exposure. Prevention of fecal-oral contamination and maintenance of pool hygiene through chlorination and pH control are important public health control measures.

Iwasaki J et al. Lower anti-echovirus antibody responses in children presenting to hospital with asthma exacerbations. Clin Exp Allergy. 2015 Oct;45(10):1523–30. [PMID: 25640320]

3. Enteroviruses 68, 70, 71, & Related Agents

Several distinct clinical syndromes are described in association with enteroviruses.

Enterovirus D68 (EV-D68) is a unique enterovirus that shares epidemiologic characteristics with human rhinovirus and is typically associated with respiratory illness. Several clusters are reported from the Netherlands, Japan, the Philippines, and Thailand. An outbreak throughout the United States was reported during 2014–2015. The outbreak was also associated with cases of acute flaccid myelitis but not definitively linked thus far. The virus is implicated also in aseptic meningitis and encephalitis.

Enterovirus 70 (EV-70), a ubiquitous virus first identified in 1969 and responsible for abrupt bilateral eye discharge and subconjunctival hemorrhage with occasional systemic symptoms, is most commonly associated with acute hemorrhagic conjunctivitis.

Enterovirus 71 (EV-71) almost always occurs in the Asia-Pacific region and is associated with hand, foot, and mouth disease (HFMD), which can be severe or even fatal, herpangina as well as a form of epidemic encephalitis associated on occasion with pulmonary edema, and acute flaccid paralysis often mimicking poliomyelitis. A recombinant virus (between EV-71 and coxsackievirus A16) caused an outbreak of HFMD in Fuyang, China, in 2008. In Taiwan, 29% of EV-71 cases in children are asymptomatic. There is an association reported between gastrointestinal enterovirus infection and type 1 diabetes.

Human enteroviruses are neurotropic. They may have a role in amyotrophic lateral sclerosis. EV-D68 has been reported in a case of fatal meningitis/encephalitis. A number of nonpolio type C enteroviruses are associated with polio-like syndromes, and surveillance for these is most active in China. Enterovirus infection of the pancreas can trigger cell-mediated autoimmune destruction of beta cells resulting in diabetes. Enterovirus myocarditis can be a serious infection in neonates, complicated by cardiac dysfunction and arrhythmias.

Mortality is especially high in EV-71–associated brainstem encephalitis, which is often complicated by pulmonary edema, particularly when it occurs in children younger than 5 years. A complication is autonomic nervous system dysregulation, which may precede the pulmonary edema. Because of lower herd immunity, HFMD tends to infect the very young (under age 5) in nonendemic areas. Clinical and epidemiologic findings aided by isolation of the suspect agent from conjunctival scraping for EV-70; vesicle swabs, body secretions, or CSF for EV-71; and respiratory secretions for D68 facilitate diagnosis of these enteroviral entities. Enzyme immunoassays and complement fixation tests show good specificity but poor sensitivity (less than 80%). RT-PCR may increase the detection rate in enterovirus infections and is useful in the analysis of CSF samples among patients with meningitis and of blood samples among infants with a sepsis-like illness.

Treatment of these entities remains largely symptomatic. A study in China showed that recombinant human interferon-alpha1b in EV-71–associated hand, foot, and mouth disease was associated with decreased fever duration, healing time of typical skin or oral mucosal lesions, and EV-71 viral load. There is anecdotal success in managing myocarditis with immunoglobulins.

The major complication associated with EV-70 is the rare development of an acute neurologic illness with motor paralysis akin to poliomyelitis. Treatment of acute flaccid paralysis related to EV-71 with IVIG does not appear to improve neurologic outcomes. Attention-deficit with hyperactivity occurs in about 20% with confirmed infection.

EV-D68 requires supportive care with particular attention to respiratory support. The CDC's National Enterovirus Surveillance System should receive reports of disease at wnix@cdc.gov.

Household contacts, especially children under 6 months of age, are at particular risk for EV-71 acquisition. A commercial disinfectant, Virkon S at 1–2% application, appears to reduce infectivity of fomites. A stage-based supportive treatment for EV-71 infections, recognizing the potential for late-onset CNS disease and cardiopulmonary failure is important. There is no commercially available EV-71 vaccine in the United States, although vaccines produced in China appear to be successful against EV-71–associated hand, foot, and mouth disease and herpangina. Decreases in antibody titers suggest booster doses of these vaccines may be needed.

Enterovirus 72 (EV-72) is another term for hepatitis A virus (see Chapter 16). Enterovirus EV-104A is related to rhinoviruses and associated with respiratory illness in reports from Italy and Switzerland.

Bauer L et al. Direct-acting antivirals and host-targeting strategies to combat enterovirus infections. Curr Opin Virol. 2017 Jun; 24:1–8. [PMID: 28411509]

Greninger AL et al. A novel outbreak enterovirus D68 strain associated with acute flaccid myelitis cases in the USA (2012–14): a retrospective cohort study. Lancet Infect Dis. 2015 Jun;15(6):671–82. [PMID: 25837569]

Huang X et al. Clinical efficacy of therapy with recombinant human interferon α1b in hand, foot, and mouth disease with enterovirus 71 infection. PLoS One. 2016 Feb 16;11(2): e0148907. [PMID: 26882102]

Wallace SS et al. Impact of enterovirus testing on resource use in febrile young infants: a systematic review. Hosp Pediatr. 2017 Feb;7(2):96–102. [PMID: 28082417]

Zhu W et al. Correlates of protection for inactivated enterovirus 71 vaccine: the analysis of immunological surrogate endpoints. Expert Rev Vaccines. 2017 Sep;16(9):945–9. [PMID: 28548626]

4. Human Parechovirus Infection (HPeV)

HPeV is 1 of 19 genotypes among a distinct genus of picornaviruses and causes a wide variety of disease in humans, especially in infants. The pathogen mainly affects small children during the summer and early fall, although disease can also occur in older adults. Cases are reported worldwide. HPeV3 is the most commonly reported isolate in the United States. Clinical presentation is mainly driven by gastrointestinal and respiratory illness, although otitis, neonatal sepsis, fever without a detectable source, gastroenteritis, flaccid paralysis, myalgias (which may be epidemic), diffuse maculopapular and palmar-plantar rashes, aseptic meningitis, intracranial hemorrhage, seizures, pericarditis, and an acute disseminated encephalitis are described in the literature.

HPeV6 typically affects individuals older than 20 years. HPeV3 is responsible for meningitis/encephalitis, neonatal sepsis (13% of late-onset neonatal sepsis [between 4 and 120 days of life] in one series was due to parechovirus) and was reported in association with necrotizing enterocolitis and hepatitis. It is the most common cause of neonatal meningitis and is the picornavirus most often found in CSF samples of CNS-related infections in very young children. CSF parameters include a normal count in over 90% and an abnormal protein in less than 50%. CNS infection may be seen with HPeV4 as well. Respiratory and gastrointestinal illnesses are seen with types HPeV4–HPeV6, HPeV10, and HPeV13-HPeV15.

Treatment is largely supportive and rapid identification of the viral antigen by PCR in stools, respiratory samples, and CSF may decrease use of unnecessary antibiotics and shorten hospital stay, although current PCR assays are not always sufficiently sensitive to exclude parechoviruses.

Intravenous immunoglobulin was anecdotally successful in one case of parechovirus dilated cardiomyopathy and maternal antibodies to parechovirus type 3 are protective. Reported complications of neonatal cerebral infections include learning disabilities, epilepsy, and cerebral palsy. Because intrafamilial transmission is well documented, it may help isolate the affected children.

Abedi GR et al. Enterovirus and parechovirus surveillance—United States, 2014–2016. MMWR Morb Mortal Wkly Rep. 2018 May 11;67(18):515–8. [PMID: 29746455]

Aizawa Y et al. Human parechovirus type 3 infection: an emerging infection in neonates and young infants. J Infect Chemother. 2017 Jul;23(7):419–26. [PMID: 28511987]

RICKETTSIAL DISEASES

TYPHUS GROUP

1. Epidemic (Louse-Borne) Typhus

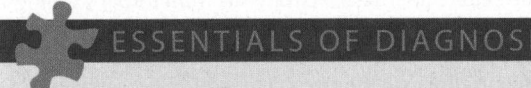

ESSENTIALS OF DIAGNOSIS

- ▶ Prodrome of headache, then chills and fever.
- ▶ Severe, intractable headaches, prostration, persisting high fever.
- ▶ Macular rash appearing on days 4–7 on the trunk and in the axillae, spreading to the rest of the body but sparing the face, palms, and soles.
- ▶ Diagnosis confirmed by complement fixation, microagglutination, or immunofluorescence.

▶ General Considerations

Epidemic louse-borne typhus is caused by *Rickettsia prowazekii*, an obligate parasite of the body louse *Pediculus humanus* (other lice were thought not to contribute although a 2018 report from Turkey suggests *P humanus capitus* may transmit *R prowazekii*) (Table 32–3). Transmission is favored by crowded, unsanitary living conditions, famine, war, or any circumstances that predispose to heavy infestation with lice. After biting a person infected with *R prowazekii*, the louse becomes infected by the organism, which persists in the louse gut and is excreted in its feces. When the same louse bites an uninfected individual, the feces enter the bloodstream when the person scratches the itching wound. Dry, infectious louse feces may also enter via the respiratory tract. Cases can be acquired by travel to pockets of infection (eg, central and northeastern Africa, Central and South America). Outbreaks have been reported from Peru, Burundi, Ethiopia, Turkey, and Russia and are associated with migration of peoples as well as with refugee camps where crowding and poor hygiene may occur. Because of aerosol transmissibility, *R prowazekii* is considered a possible bioterrorism agent. In the United States, cases occur among the homeless, refugees, and the unhygienic, most often in the winter.

Table 32–3. Rickettsial diseases.

Disease	Rickettsial Pathogen	Geographic Areas of Prevalence	Insect Vector	Mammalian Reservoir	Travel Association
Typhus Group					
Epidemic (louse-borne) typhus	*Rickettsia prowazekii*	South America, Northeastern and Central Africa	Louse	Humans, flying squirrels	Rare
Endemic (murine) typhus	*Rickettsia typhi*	Worldwide; small foci (United States: southeastern Gulf Coast)	Flea	Rodents, opossums	Often
Scrub Typhus Group					
Scrub typhus	*Orientia tsutsugamushi*	Southeast Asia, Japan, Australia, Western Siberia	Mite[1]	Rodents	Often
Spotted Fever Group					
Rocky Mountain spotted fever	*Rickettsia rickettsii*	Western hemisphere; United States (especially mid-Atlantic coast region)	Tick[1]	Rodents, dogs, porcupines	Rare
California flea rickettsiosis	*Rickettsia felis*	Worldwide	Flea	Cats, opossums	
Mediterranean spotted fever, Boutonneuse fever, Kenya tick typhus, South African tick fever, Indian tick typhus	*Rickettsia conorii*	Africa, India, Mediterranean regions	Tick[1]	Rodents, dogs	Often
Queensland tick typhus	*Rickettsia australis*	Eastern Australia	Tick[1]	Rodents, marsupials	Rare
Siberian Asian tick typhus	*Rickettsia sibirica*	Siberia, Mongolia	Tick[1]	Rodents	Rare
African tick bite fever	*Rickettsia africae*	Rural sub-Saharan Africa, Eastern Caribbean	Tick[1]	Cattle	Often
Lymphangitis-associated rickettsiosis	*R sibirica mongolitimonae*	Europe, Africa, Mongolia	Tick[1]	Unknown	Unknown
Tick-borne lymphadenopathy/ Dermacentor-borne necrosis erythema lymphadenopathy/scalp eschar neck lymphadenopathy	*R slovaca, R raoultii, Candidatus R rioja*	Europe	Tick	Unknown	Occasional
Transitional Group					
Rickettsialpox	*Rickettsia akari*	United States, Korea, former USSR	Mite[1]	Mice	Occasional
Other					
Ehrlichiosis and anaplasmosis, human Monocytic	*Ehrlichia chaffeensis, Anaplasma equi, Ehrlichia canis*	Southeastern United States	Tick[1]	Dogs	Occasional
Granulocytic	*Anaplasma phagocytophilum, Ehrlichia ewingii, Ehrlichia muris eauclairensis[2] Neorickettsia sennetsu[2]*	Northeastern United States and upper Midwest (*E muris eauclairensis*) Southeast Asia (*N sennetsu*)	Tick[1]	Rodents, deer, sheep	Occasional
Q fever	*Coxiella burnetii*	Worldwide	None[3]	Cattle, sheep, goats	Occasional

[1]Also serve as arthropod reservoirs by maintaining rickettsiae through transovarian transmission.
[2]Limited data available on exact cell involved in pathogenesis.
[3]Human infection results from inhalation of dust.

R prowazekii can survive in lymphoid and adipose (in endothelial reservoirs) tissues after primary infection, and years later, produce recrudescence of disease (Brill-Zinsser disease) without exposure to infected lice. This phenomenon can serve as a point source for future outbreaks.

An extrahuman reservoir of *R prowazekii* in the United States is flying squirrels, *Glaucomys volans*. Transmission to humans can occur through their ectoparasites, known as sylvatic typhus, usually causing atypical mild disease. A case of recrudescent (Brill-Zinsser) disease 11 years after disease acquired by contact with flying squirrels is reported. Foci of sylvatic typhus are found in the eastern United States and are reported to occur in Brazil, Ethiopia, and Mexico.

Clinical Findings

A. Symptoms and Signs

Prodromal malaise, cough, headache, backache, arthralgia, myalgia, and chest pain begin after an incubation period of 10–14 days, followed by an abrupt onset of chills, high fever, and prostration, with flu-like symptoms progressing to delirium and stupor. The headache is severe, and the fever is prolonged (Table 32–2).

Other findings consist of conjunctivitis, mild vitritis, retinal lesions, optic neuritis, and hearing loss from neuropathy of the eighth cranial nerve, abdominal pain, and often splenomegaly. Flushed faces and macular rash (that may become confluent) appear; the rash appears first in the axillae and then over the trunk, spreading to the extremities on the fifth or sixth day of illness but sparing the palms of hands and soles of feet. In severely ill patients, the rash becomes hemorrhagic, and hypotension becomes marked. Pneumonia, thromboses, vasculitis with major vessel obstruction and gangrene, circulatory collapse, myocarditis, uremia, and seizure may occur. Improvement begins 13–16 days after onset with a rapid drop of fever and typically a spontaneous recovery.

Brill-Zinsser disease has a more gradual onset than primary *R prowazekii* infection; fever and rash are of shorter duration, and the disease is milder.

B. Laboratory Findings

The white blood cell count is variable. Thrombocytopenia, elevated liver enzymes, proteinuria, and hematuria commonly occur. Serum obtained 5–12 days after onset of symptoms usually shows specific antibodies for *R prowazekii* antigens as demonstrated by complement fixation, microagglutination, or immunofluorescence. In primary rickettsial infection, early antibodies are IgM; in recrudescence (Brill-Zinsser disease), early antibodies are predominantly IgG. A PCR test exists, but its availability is limited.

C. Imaging

Radiographs of the chest may show patchy consolidation.

Differential Diagnosis

The prodromal symptoms and the early febrile stage lack enough specificity to permit diagnosis in nonepidemic situations. The rash is sufficiently distinctive for diagnosis, but it may be absent in up to 50% of cases or may be difficult to observe in dark-skinned persons. A variety of other acute febrile diseases should be considered, including typhoid fever, meningococcemia, and measles.

Treatment

Treatment consists of doxycycline 100 mg orally twice daily for 7–10 days or for at least 3 days after the fever subsides. A single dose of 200 mg of doxycycline may be effective; however, some patients may relapse. Chloramphenicol is considered less effective than doxycycline, but it is still the drug of choice in pregnancy.

Prognosis

The prognosis depends greatly on the patient's age and immune status. The mortality rate is 10% in the second and third decades but in the past, it reached 60% in the sixth decade. Brill-Zinsser disease is rarely fatal.

Prevention

Prevention consists of louse control with insecticides, particularly by applying chemicals to clothing or treating it with heat, and frequent bathing.

A deloused and bathed typhus patient is not infectious. The disease is not transmitted from person to person. Patients are infectious from the lice during the febrile period and perhaps 2–3 days after the fever returns to normal.

No vaccine is available for the prevention of *R prowazekii* infection.

Centers for Disease Control and Prevention (CDC). Typhus Fevers. https://www.cdc.gov/typhus/healthcare-providers/index.html

Ulutasdemir N et al. The epidemic typhus and trench fever are risk for public health due to increased migration in southeast of Turkey. Acta Trop. 2018 Feb;178:115–8. [PMID: 29126839]

2. Endemic (Murine) Typhus

Rickettsia typhi, a ubiquitous pathogen recognized on all continents, is transmitted from rat to rat through the rat flea (Table 32–3). Serosurveys of animals show high prevalence of antibodies to *R typhi* in opossums, followed by dogs and cats. Humans usually acquire the infection in an urban or suburban setting when bitten by an infected flea. Rare human cases in the developed world occur in travelers, usually to Southeast Asia, Africa, or the Mediterranean area, although other pockets of infection are also known to occur in the Andes and the Yucatán. In the United States, the related *Rickettsia felis* cases (now a spotted fever rickettsia, discussed below) are mainly reported from Texas and southern California.

Clinical Findings

A. Symptoms and Signs

The presentation is nonspecific, including fever, headache, myalgia, and chills. Relative bradycardia is reported. Maculopapular rash occurs in around 50% of cases; it is concentrated on the trunk, mostly sparing the palms and soles, and fades rapidly.

The illness may be associated with maternal death, miscarriage, preterm birth, and low birth weight if acquired early during pregnancy.

B. Laboratory Findings

Serologic confirmation may be necessary for differentiation, with complement-fixing or immunofluorescent antibodies detectable within 15 days after onset, with specific *R typhi* antigens. A fourfold rise in serum antibody titers between the acute and the convalescent phase is diagnostic. It is important to note that *R typhi* antigens frequently cross-react with those of *R prowazekii*. The PCR can distinguish between these two infections depending on the sample type, the timing of sample collection, bacterial load, and severity of disease. During the first week of illness, PCR is the most sensitive test if samples are taken before doxycycline administration.

Differential Diagnosis

The most common entity in the differential diagnosis is Rocky Mountain spotted fever, usually occurring after rural exposure and with a different rash (centripetal versus centrifugal for epidemic or endemic typhus).

Complications

The most common complication is pulmonary, in the form of pneumonia, followed by pleural effusion and respiratory failure. Other complications include neurologic (peripheral facial paralysis, meningismus, ataxia, seizures), acute kidney injury, and multiorgan failure. Rare complications include ocular findings, disseminated intravascular coagulation, and hemophagocytosis syndrome. Anemia, thrombocytopenia, leukopenia, hyponatremia, and elevated levels of liver enzymes commonly occur.

Treatment

Doxycycline 100 mg orally twice daily for 7–10 days (or until the patient is afebrile for 48 hours) is the drug of choice, except during pregnancy. Ciprofloxacin (500–750 mg orally twice a day) and ampicillin (500 mg orally three times a day) are reportedly successful in pregnant women. Azithromycin is frequently used but is not associated with improved fetal outcomes.

Prevention

Preventive measures are directed at control of rats and ectoparasites (rat fleas) with insecticides, rat poisons, and rat-proofing of buildings.

Prognosis

Endemic typhus is usually a self-limited disease. A large case series from Texas reported a fatality rate of 0.4%.

Paris DH et al. State of the art of diagnosis of rickettsial diseases: the use of blood specimens for diagnosis of scrub typhus, spotted fever group rickettsiosis, and murine typhus. Curr Opin Infect Dis. 2016 Oct; 29(5):433–9. [PMID: 27429138]

Pieracci EG et al. Fatal Flea-borne typhus in Texas: a retrospective case series, 1985–2015. Am J Trop Med Hyg. 2017 May; 96(5):1088–93. [PMID: 28500797]

Tsioutis C et al. Clinical and laboratory characteristics, epidemiology, and outcomes of murine typhus: a systematic review. Acta Trop. 2017 Feb;166:16–24. [PMID: 27983969]

3. Scrub Typhus (Tsutsugamushi Fever)

ESSENTIALS OF DIAGNOSIS

▶ Exposure to mites in endemic South and East Asia, the western Pacific (including Korea), and Australia.

▶ Black eschar at site of the bite, with regional and generalized lymphadenopathy.

▶ High fever, relative bradycardia, headache, myalgia, and a short-lived macular rash.

▶ Frequent pneumonitis, encephalitis, and myocarditis.

General Considerations

Scrub typhus is caused by *Orientia tsutsugamushi*, which is a parasite of rodents and is transmitted by larval trombiculid mites (chiggers). Multiple strains exist and are associated with geographic areas. The disease is endemic in Korea; China; Taiwan; Japan; Pakistan; India (where it is reported to be the leading cause of acute febrile illness in central India); Thailand (where scrub typhus is also the leading cause of acute undifferentiated fever); Malaysia; Vietnam; Laos; and Queensland, Australia (Table 32–3), which form an area known as the "tsutsugamushi triangle." Scrub typhus is a cause of acute febrile illness in India and China and is a recognized cause of fever of unknown origin. Cases are also reported in the Middle East, Kenya, and South America. Transmission is often more common at higher altitudes. The mites live on vegetation (grass and brush) but complete their maturation cycle by biting humans who encounter infested vegetation. Risk factors in China include female sex, age between 60 and 69 years, and farming. Therefore, the disease is more common in rural areas, but urban cases have also been described. Vertical transmission occurs, and blood transfusions may transmit the pathogen as well. Rare occupational transmission via inhalation is documented among laboratory workers. Cases among travelers to endemic areas are increasingly recognized.

Clinical Findings

A. Symptoms and Signs

After a 1- to 3-week incubation period, malaise, chills, severe headache, and backache develop. At the site of the bite, a papule evolves into a flat black eschar (the groin and the abdomen being the most common sites followed by the chest and axilla), which is a helpful finding for diagnosis but was only described in 19% of patients in a South Korean series of scrub typhus. The regional lymph nodes are commonly enlarged and tender, and sometimes a more generalized adenopathy occurs. Fever rises gradually during the first week of infection, and the rash is usually macular and primarily on the trunk area. The rash can be fleeting or more severe, peaking at 8 days but lasting up to 21 days after onset of infection. Relative bradycardia, defined as an increase in heart rate of fewer than 10 beats/min for a 1-degree Celsius increase in temperature, frequently accompanies scrub typhus infection. The occurrence of relative bradycardia has no effect on clinical outcome. Gastrointestinal symptoms, including nausea, vomiting, and diarrhea, occur in nearly two-thirds of patients and correspond to the presence of superficial mucosal hemorrhage, multiple erosions, or ulcers in the gastrointestinal tract. Acute kidney injury and other renal abnormalities are frequently present.

Severe complications, such as pneumonitis, myocarditis, encephalitis or aseptic meningitis, peritonitis, granulomatous hepatitis, hemophagocytic syndrome, immune thrombocytopenia, disseminated intravascular coagulation, cerebrovascular hemorrhage or infarction, cranial nerve palsies, parkinsonian symptoms, ARDS, or hemophagocytosis, may develop during the second or third week. An attack confers prolonged immunity against homologous strains and transient immunity against heterologous strains. Heterologous strains produce mild disease if infection occurs within a year after the first episode.

B. Laboratory Findings

Thrombocytopenia and elevation of liver enzymes, bilirubin, and creatinine are common. Indirect immunofluorescent assay and indirect immunoperoxidase assays are the gold standard for scrub typhus diagnosis. These tests are expensive and have limited availability. An ELISA detecting *Orientia* specific antibodies in serum is available. PCR (from the eschar or blood) is the most sensitive diagnostic test but remains positive even after initiation of treatment. Culture of the organism from blood obtained in the first few days of illness is another diagnostic modality but requires a specialized biological safety level 3 laboratory. It is suggested to combine IgM detection by ELISA and conventional PCR to improve the diagnosis of scrub typhus.

▶ Differential Diagnosis

Leptospirosis, typhoid, dengue, malaria, Q fever, hemorrhagic fevers, tuberculous meningitis, and other rickettsial infections should be considered. The headache may mimic trigeminal neuralgia. Scrub typhus is a recognized cause of obscure tropical fevers, especially in children. The presence of an eschar, lymphocytosis, and elevated C-reactive protein (CRP) helped distinguish scrub typhus from dengue in a Northern Thai study.

▶ Treatment & Prognosis

Without treatment, fever subsides spontaneously after 2 weeks, but the mortality rate may be 10–30%. The treatment of choice is doxycycline (100 mg orally twice daily) or minocycline (100 mg intravenously twice daily) until there is evidence of clinical improvement for at least 3 days after the fever subsides. Shorter duration of therapy is associated with relapse. Alternative therapy for pregnant women and patients with doxycycline allergy include chloramphenicol, although chloramphenicol- and tetracycline-resistant strains have been reported from Southeast Asia. Azithromycin is shown to be as effective as doxycycline with fewer side effects, but it is more expensive. Azithromycin may not prevent poor fetal outcomes in infected pregnant women.

Poor prognostic factors include hypotension requiring vasopressors, ICU care, age over 60 years, absence of an eschar (making the diagnosis difficult), pregnancy, and laboratory findings such as leukocytosis or hypoalbuminemia. Most patients recover without neurologic sequelae.

▶ Prevention

Mite control with repeated application of long-acting miticides and, less so, rodent control can make endemic areas safe. Insect repellents on clothing and skin as well as protective clothing are effective preventive measures. Although chemoprophylaxis with doxycycline has been used, the CDC does not recommend prophylaxis with antibiotics for asymptomatic travelers. No effective vaccines are available.

Lee HS et al. Central nervous system infection associated with *Orientia tsutsugamushi* in South Korea. Am J Trop Med Hyg. 2017 Oct;97(4):1094–8. [PMID: 28820719]

Lee SC et al. Comparative effectiveness of azithromycin for treating scrub typhus: a PRISMA-compliant systematic review and meta-analysis. Medicine (Baltimore). 2017 Sep;96(36):e7992. [PMID: 28885357]

Rajan SJ et al. Scrub typhus in pregnancy: maternal and fetal outcomes. Obstet Med. 2016 Dec; 9(4):164–6. [PMID: 27829876]

Shelke YP et al. Spectrum of infections in acute febrile illness in central India. Indian J Med Microbiol. 2017 Oct–Dec;35(4):480–4. [PMID: 29405137]

Wangrangsimakul T et al. Causes of acute undifferentiated fever and the utility of biomarkers in Chiangrai, northern Thailand. PLoS Negl Trop Dis. 2018 May 31;12(5).e0006477. [PMID: 29852003]

Zhao M et al. Comparison of minocycline and azithromycin for the treatment of mild scrub typhus in northern China. Int J Antimicrob Agents. 2016 Sep;48(3):317–20. [PMID: 27449540]

SPOTTED FEVERS

1. Rocky Mountain Spotted Fever

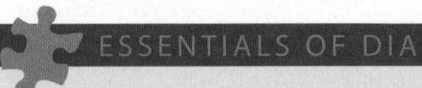

ESSENTIALS OF DIAGNOSIS

- ▶ Exposure to tick bite in an endemic area.
- ▶ Influenza-like prodrome followed by fever, severe headache, and myalgias; occasionally, delirium and coma.
- ▶ Red macular rash appears between days 2 and 6 of fever, first on the wrists and ankles and then spreading centrally; it may become petechial.
- ▶ Mortality over 70% in untreated patients.
- ▶ Serial serologic examinations by indirect fluorescent antibody confirm the diagnosis retrospectively.

General Considerations

Despite its name, most cases of Rocky Mountain spotted fever (RMSF) occur outside the Rocky Mountain area. More than half of the cases are from five states: North Carolina, Tennessee, Oklahoma, Missouri, and Arkansas. RMSF is endemic in Central and South America with a small fatal familial cluster reported from Panama (Table 32–3). Native Americans are at high risk for infection. The causative agent, *R rickettsii*, is transmitted to humans by the bite of ticks, including the Rocky Mountain wood tick, *Dermacentor andersoni*, in the western United States, and the American dog tick, *D variabilis*, in the eastern United States. Several hours of contact between the tick and the human host are required for transmission. The brown dog tick, *Rhipicephalus sanguineus*, is a vector in eastern Arizona and responsible for many Native American cases. Epidemic RMSF, as described in Arizona and Mexico, is associated with massive local infestations of the brown dog tick in domestic dogs, which may explain why the incidence of RMSF in the three most highly affected communities in an Arizona epidemic from 2003 to 2012 was 150 times the US national average. Other hard-bodied ticks transmit the organism in the southern United States and in Central and South America and are responsible for transmitting it among rodents, dogs, porcupines, and other animals. Human cases reemerged in Mexico in 2008 after decades of quiescence (since the 1940s). In 2015, northern Mexico reported a total of 1129 RMSF cases including 188 deaths, mostly in Sonora, Mexico.

There are 25 genotypes of *R rickettsii* in four different groups, and potential genomic-clinical correlations are underway. Several other rickettsial species cause mild, nonlethal infections in the United States, including *R parkeri*, *R phillipi*, and *R massiliae*. These are discussed in the "tick typhus" section.

In the United States, the estimated annual incidence of RMSF is as high as seven cases per million persons (primarily occurring from April through September), with a higher incidence among children and men. Better diagnostic capacity and improved surveillance are thought responsible for the changing epidemiology.

A Brazilian spotted fever with higher mortality than RMSF is thought to be due to a virulent strain of *R rickettsii*. A host of spotted fever species have been identified from human patients over the last 20 years throughout the world including species from China (*Rickettsia* sp. XY99), Slovakia (*R slovaca*), Morocco (*R aeschlimannii*), Sicily (*R massiliae*), China, and Egypt (*R sibirica monolitimonae*).

Clinical Findings

A. Symptoms and Signs

RMSF can cause severe multiorgan dysfunction and fatality rates of up to 73% if left untreated, making it the most serious rickettsial disease. Two to 14 days (mean, 7 days) after the bite of an infectious tick, symptoms begin with the abrupt onset of high fever, chills, headache, nausea and vomiting, myalgias, restlessness, insomnia, and irritability. The characteristic rash (faint macules that progress to maculopapules and then petechiae) appears between days

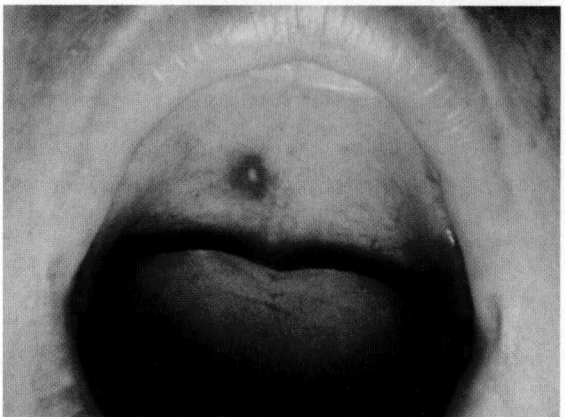

▲ **Figure 32–7.** Hard palate lesion caused by Rocky Mountain spotted fever. (Public Health Image Library, CDC.)

2 and 6 of fever. It initially involves the wrists and ankles, spreading *centrally* to the arms, legs, and trunk over the next 2–3 days. Involvement of the palms and soles is characteristic. Facial flushing, conjunctival injection, and hard palate lesions (Figure 32–7) may occur. In about 10% of cases, however, no rash or only a minimal rash is seen. Cough and pneumonitis may develop, and delirium, lethargy, seizures, stupor, and coma may also appear in more severe cases. Splenomegaly, hepatomegaly, jaundice, myocarditis (which may mimic an acute coronary syndrome), adrenal hemorrhage, polyarticular arthritis, or uremia is occasionally present. ARDS and necrotizing vasculitis, when present, are of greatest concern.

A group of four cases of RMSF in pregnant women from Sonora, Mexico, in 2015–2016, three of whom sustained spontaneous abortions, is a reminder of the grave risk of this infection for pregnant women and their fetuses.

B. Laboratory Findings

Thrombocytopenia, hyponatremia, elevated aminotransferases, and hyperbilirubinemia are common. CSF may show hypoglycorrhachia and mild pleocytosis. Disseminated intravascular coagulation is observed in severe cases. Diagnosis during the acute phase of the illness can be made by immunohistologic or PCR demonstration of *R rickettsii* in skin biopsy specimens (or cutaneous swabs of eschars or skin lesions). Performing such studies as soon as skin lesions become apparent and before antibiotics commence maximizes sensitivity.

Serologic studies confirm the diagnosis, but most patients do not mount an antibody response until the second week of illness. The indirect fluorescent antibody test is most commonly used.

Differential Diagnosis

The diagnosis is challenging because early symptoms resemble those of many other infections. The classic triad of fever, rash, and tick bite is rarely recognized, with up to 40% of patients not recalling a tick bite. Moreover, the rash may be confused with that of measles, typhoid, and ehrlichiosis, or—most importantly—meningococcemia. Blood cultures and examination of CSF establish the latter. Coinfections may mask the diagnosis. Some spotted fever rickettsioses may also mimic RMSF but will not be detected by routine serologic testing for RMSF.

Treatment & Prognosis

Treatment with doxycycline at similar doses and duration as for epidemic typhus (100 mg orally twice daily for 4–10 days) is recommended. Similarly, chloramphenicol (50–100 mg/kg/day in four divided doses, orally or intravenously for 4–10 days) is the preferred alternative during pregnancy. Patients usually defervesce within 48–72 hours, and therapy should be continued for at least 3 days after defervescence occurs.

The reported mortality rate for treated patients in the United States is about 3–5%. The following features are associated with increased mortality: (1) infection in older adults or Native Americans; (2) the presence of atypical clinical features (absence of headache, no history of tick attachment, gastrointestinal symptoms) and underlying chronic diseases; and (3) a delay in initiation of appropriate antibiotic therapy. The usual cause of death is pneumonitis with respiratory or cardiac failure. A fulminant form of RMSF can be seen in patients with glucose-6-phosphate dehydrogenase deficiency. Sequelae may include seizures, encephalopathy, peripheral neuropathy, paraparesis, bowel and bladder incontinence, cerebellar and vestibular dysfunction, hearing loss, and motor deficits.

Unfavorable prognostic factors for mortality from a 2017 Brazilian series of spotted fever cases included male sex, shock, seizures, and hypotension, and favorable prognostic factors were urban exposure, recognition of a tick, and lymphadenopathy. Recent Mexican cases were more severe among children under 10 years of age and among the very poor.

Prevention

Protective clothing, tick-repellent chemicals, and the removal of ticks at frequent intervals are helpful measures. The effectiveness of aggressive campaigns to decrease ticks in the community is under investigation in Native American communities with high RMSF attack rates. Prophylactic therapy after a tick bite is not recommended.

Álvarez-Hernández G et al. Rocky Mountain spotted fever in Mexico: past, present, and future. Lancet Infect Dis. 2017 Jun; 17(6):e189–96. [PMID: 28365226]

Erickson T et al. Evidence of locally acquired spotted fever group rickettsioses in Southeast Texas, 2008–2016. Zoonoses Public Health. 2018 Nov;65(7):897–901. [PMID: 30152119]

Licona-Enriquez JD et al. Rocky Mountain spotted fever and pregnancy: four cases from Sonora, Mexico. Am J Trop Med Hyg. 2017 Sep;97(3):795–8. [PMID: 28722584]

2. Tick Typhus (Rickettsial Fever)

The term "tick typhus" denotes a variety of spotted rickettsial fevers, often named by their geographic location (eg, Mediterranean spotted fever, Queensland tick typhus, Oriental spotted fever, African tick bite fever, Siberian tick typhus, North Asian tick typhus) or by morphology (eg, boutonneuse fever). These illnesses are caused by various rickettsial organisms (eg, *R africae*, *R australis*, *R conorii*, *R japonica*, *R massiliae*, *R parkeri*, *R sibirica*, and *R 364D*) and are transmitted by various tick species. Lymphangitis-associated rickettsiosis (LAR), caused by *R sibirica mongolitimonae*, was first described in 1996 and has been reported in Europe only thus far, including a small outbreak in Spain (Table 32–3). Dogs and wild animals, usually rodents and even reptiles, may serve as reservoirs for rickettsial fevers. Travel is a risk factor for disease, particularly among elderly ecotourists. In a series of 280 international travelers with rickettsial disease, the most common cause was spotted fever rickettsiosis (231 cases, 82.5% of the total) followed by scrub typhus (16, 5.7%).

Tick-borne rickettsioses are the main source of rickettsia infections in Europe and cause a syndrome similar to that seen in Mediterranean spotted fever. Newer recognized species include *R helvetica*, *R monacensis*, *R massiliae*, and *R aeschlimannii*. Another described syndrome is tick-borne lymphadenopathy/Dermacentor-borne-necrosis-erythema-lymphadenopathy/scalp eschar neck lymphadenopathy associated with *R slovaca*, *Candidatus R rioja*, and *R raoultii* and characterized by tick bite, eschar on the scalp, and cervical lymphadenopathy.

The pathogens usually produce an eschar or black spot (tâche noire) at the site of the tick bite that may be useful in diagnosis, though spotless boutonneuse fever occurs. Symptoms include fever, headache, myalgias, and rash. Painful lymphadenopathy or lymphangitis may also occur. Rarely, papulovesicular lesions may resemble rickettsialpox. Endothelial injury produces perivascular edema and dermal necrosis. Regional adenopathy, disseminated lesions, kidney disease, splenic rupture, and focal hepatic necrosis are observed. Neurologic manifestations, including encephalitis, internuclear ophthalmoplegia, coronary involvement, and the hemophagocytic syndrome, are rare.

The diagnosis is clinical, with serologic or PCR (culture can be used but is less sensitive than either) of the buffy coat of blood, or an eschar if one is available, used for confirmation. Treatment should be started upon clinical suspicion since delayed therapy is the usual cause of increased morbidity. Oral treatment with doxycycline (100 mg twice daily) or chloramphenicol (50–75 mg/kg/day in four divided doses) for 7–10 days is indicated. Caution is advised with the use of ciprofloxacin because it is associated with a poor outcome and increases the severity of disease in Mediterranean spotted fever. The combination of azithromycin and rifampin is effective and safe in pregnancy. Prevention entails protective clothing, repellents, and inspection for and removal of ticks.

Formerly classified as an endemic or murine typhus, the cat-flea typhus, caused by *R felis* is more properly classified as a spotted fever. The causative agent has been linked to the cat flea and opossum exposure. While the diseases appear to be ubiquitous, most cases in the United States (southern Texas and California, and possibly Hawaii) occur in the spring and summer. Treatment is the same as for other rickettsial fevers.

Cases of non-rickettsiae–associated spotted fever tend to have a better prognosis than due those due to *R rickettsiae* infection. Treatment for non-rickettsiae–associated spotted fever as well as *R rickettsiae* infection is with tetracycline, and there is some laboratory evidence that these organisms may be less responsive to macrolides.

de Oliveira SV et al. Predictive factors for fatal tick-borne spotted fever in Brazil. Zoonoses Public Health. 2017 Nov; 64(7):e44–50. [PMID: 28169507]

Erickson T et al. Newly recognized pediatric cases of typhus group rickettsiosis, Houston, Texas, USA. Emerg Infect Dis. 2017 Dec;23(12):2068–71. [PMID: 29148369]

Nelson K et al. A 2015 outbreak of flea-borne rickettsiosis in San Gabriel Valley, Los Angeles County, California. PLoS Negl Trop Dis. 2018 Apr 20;12(4):e0006385. [PMID: 29677221]

Portillo A et al. Rickettsioses in Europe. Microbes Infect. 2015 Nov–Dec;17(11–12):834–8. [PMID: 26384814]

RICKETTSIALPOX

Rickettsialpox is an acute, self-limiting, febrile illness caused by *Rickettsia akari*, a parasite of mice, transmitted by the mite *Liponyssoides sanguineus* (Table 32–3). Because rickettsialpox has features of both the typhus group and of the spotted fever group of rickettsia, it falls into its own "transitional" category. *R akari* infections are reported globally. Seroprevalence studies among injection drug users in Baltimore show seropositivity as high as 16%. In New York, its association with poverty is very strong. The illness has also been found in farming communities. Crowded conditions and mouse-infested housing allow transmission of the pathogen to humans. The classic triad of fever, rash, and eschar is found in 99% of cases. The primary lesion is a painless red papule that appears at variable times but on the average a week after a mite bite. The lesion often vesiculates and forms a black eschar.

The onset of symptoms—chills, fever, headache, photophobia, and disseminated aches and pains—is sudden. The fever may be followed by a widespread papular eruption 2–4 days later, with an average of 30–40 lesions that spare the palms and soles. The interval from vesiculation to crust formation is about 10 days. Early lesions may resemble those of chickenpox (typically vesicular versus papulovesicular in rickettsialpox). Pathologic findings include dermal edema, subepidermal vesicles, and at times a lymphocytic vasculitis.

Transient leukopenia and thrombocytopenia and acute hepatitis can occur. A fourfold rise in serum antibody titers to rickettsial antigen, detected by complement fixation or indirect fluorescent assays, is diagnostic and available through the CDC. Conjugated anti-rickettsial globulin can identify antigen in punch biopsies of skin lesions. PCR detection of rickettsial DNA in fresh tissue also appears of value. *R akari* can also be isolated from eschar biopsy specimens.

Treatment consists of oral doxycycline (100 mg twice daily) for 2–5 days or until defervescence. The disease is usually mild and self-limited without treatment, but occasionally, severe symptoms may require hospitalization. Control requires the elimination of mice from human habitations and insecticide applications.

OTHER RICKETTSIAL & RICKETTSIAL-LIKE DISEASES

1. Ehrlichiosis & Anaplasmosis

ESSENTIALS OF DIAGNOSIS

▶ Infection of monocyte or granulocyte by tick-borne gram-negative bacteria.

▶ Nine-day incubation period; clinical disease ranges from asymptomatic to life-threatening.

▶ Malaise, nausea, fever, and headaches.

▶ US cases of ehrlichiosis typically occur in men aged 60–69 years; US cases of anaplasmosis typically occur in men aged over 40 years; both occur in the summer, with different geographic areas of prevalence.

▶ Excellent response to therapy with tetracyclines.

▶ General Considerations

Human ehrlichiosis and anaplasmosis are endemic in the United States.

Ehrlichia chaffeensis (Table 32–3), the most common species infecting humans, is seen primarily in the south-central United States (especially Arkansas, Missouri, Oklahoma, and New York). *Ehrlichia ewingii* causes human granulocytic ehrlichiosis similar to anaplasmosis and constitutes almost 10% of ehrlichiosis cases; most cases in the United States are reported from the Midwest and Southeast. A new species of *Ehrlichia* isolated in 2009 is referred to as *Ehrlichia muris eauclairensis* and is seen in the upper Midwestern United States. Human granulocytic anaplasmosis is caused by *Anaplasma phagocytophilum;* most cases in the United States are reported from New England, New York, Minnesota, and Wisconsin. Increasingly, anaplasmosis is being reported from Asia, South Korea, Mongolia, China (where a new species is identified, *Anaplasma capra*), and Northern Europe.

In North America, the major tick-borne rickettsial disease vectors for these pathogens are (1) the Lone Star tick (*Amblyomma americanus*), which is the vector for *E chaffeensis* and *E ewingii;* (2) the black-legged tick (*Ixodes scapularis*), which is a vector for *B burgdorferi* (Lyme disease), *Babesia microti* (babesiosis), and *A phagocytophilum* (anaplasmosis), and a possible vector for *E muris eauclairensis;* and (3) the western black-legged tick (*Ixodes pacificus*), which is a vector for *A phagocytophilum* along the Pacific coast of the United States. Vectors for European and Asian cases are not reported to date. The principal reservoirs for human monocytic ehrlichiosis and human granulocytic anaplasmosis are the white tail deer and the white-footed mouse, respectively. Other mammals are implicated as well. Transfusion-transmitted anaplasmosis has been reported.

CDC reports indicate that the incidences of human monocytic ehrlichiosis, granulocytic ehrlichiosis and, in particular, anaplasmosis are increasing; cases are reportable to local and state health departments. Because more than one agent may coexist in the same area, cases of human ehrlichiosis and anaplasmosis may be reported as "human ehrlichiosis/anaplasmosis undetermined" in the absence of species identification.

Neorickettsia sennetsu is a related rickettsial pathogen that causes rare infection in Southeast Asia among populations who consume raw fish.

The case fatality rate is 1% with *E chaffeensis* infections and 0.3% among cases of human anaplasmosis. Contrary to earlier reports, most recent cases of *E ewingii* infection have occurred among immunocompetent patients. No deaths have been reported from either *E ewingii* or *E muris euclairensis*.

► Clinical Findings

A. Symptoms and Signs

Clinical disease of human monocytic ehrlichiosis ranges from mild to life-threatening. Typically, after a 1- to 2-week incubation period and a prodrome consisting of malaise, rigors, and nausea, high fever and headache develop. A pleomorphic rash may occur. Presentation in immunosuppressed patients (including transplant patients) and older patients tends to be more severe. Rare serious sequelae include acute respiratory failure and ARDS; neurologic complications, the most common being meningoencephalitis and aseptic meningitis; acute kidney disease (which may mimic thrombotic thrombocytopenic purpura); hemophagocytic syndrome; and multiorgan failure.

The clinical manifestations of human granulocytic ehrlichiosis and anaplasmosis are similar to those seen with human monocytic ehrlichiosis. Rash, however, is infrequent. If a rash is present, coinfection with other tick-borne diseases or an alternative diagnosis should be suspected. Persistent fever and malaise are reported to occur for 2 or more years. Reported complications of anaplasmosis include leukopenia, thrombocytopenia, and cerebral infarction.

Coinfection with anaplasmosis and Lyme disease or babesiosis may occur, but the clinical manifestations (including fever and cytopenias) are more severe with anaplasmosis than with Lyme disease. A spirochete, *Borrelia miyamotoi*, may mimic anaplasmosis in its clinical manifestations.

B. Laboratory Findings

Diagnosis can be made by the history of tick exposure followed by a characteristic clinical presentation. Leukopenia, absolute lymphopenia, thrombocytopenia, and transaminitis occur often. Thrombocytopenia occurs more often than leukopenia in human granulocytic ehrlichiosis. Examination of peripheral blood with Giemsa stain may reveal characteristic intraleukocytic vacuoles (morulae) in up to 20% of patients. An indirect fluorescent antibody assay is available through the CDC and requires acute and convalescent sera. A PCR assay can be helpful for making the diagnosis early in the disease course. PCR assay is most sensitive in the first week of illness and can be used as a confirmatory test.

► Treatment & Prevention

Treatment for human ehrlichiosis and anaplasmosis is with doxycycline, 100 mg twice daily (orally or intravenously) for 10–14 days or until 3 days of defervescence. Rifampin is an alternative in pregnant women. Treatment should not be withheld while awaiting confirmatory serology when suspicion is high. Lack of clinical improvement and defervescence 48 hours after doxycycline initiation suggests an alternate diagnosis. Some patients may continue to have headache, weakness, and malaise for weeks despite adequate treatment. Tick control is the essence of prevention.

Centers for Disease Control and Prevention (CDC). Ehrlichiosis: epidemiology and statistics. Last reviewed 2019 Feb 11.https://www.cdc.gov/ehrlichiosis/stats/index.html

Centers for Disease Control and Prevention (CDC). Anaplasmosis: epidemiology and statistics. Last reviewed 2019 Feb 19. https://www.cdc.gov/anaplasmosis/stats/index.html

2. Q Fever (*Coxiella burnetti* Infection)

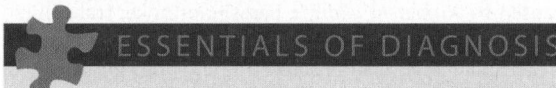
ESSENTIALS OF DIAGNOSIS

► Exposure to sheep, goats, cattle, or their products; some infections are laboratory acquired.

► Acute or chronic febrile illness: headache, cough, prostration, and abdominal pain.

► Pneumonitis, hepatitis, or encephalopathy; less often, endocarditis, vascular infections, or chronic fatigue syndrome.

► A common cause of culture-negative endocarditis.

► General Considerations

Q fever, a reportable and significantly underestimated disease in the United States, is caused by the gram-negative intracellular coccobacillus *C burnetii*. *Coxiella* infections occur globally, mostly in cattle, sheep, and goats, in which they cause mild or subclinical disease (Table 32–3). In these animals, reactivation of the infection occurs during pregnancy and causes abortions or low birth weight offspring. *Coxiella* is resistant to heat and drying and remains infective in the environment for months.

Human infection occurs via inhalation of aerosolized bacteria (in dust or droplets) from feces, urine, milk, or products of conception of infected animals. Ingestion and skin penetration are other recognized routes of transmission. A major outbreak in the Netherlands during 2007–2010 was thought to be due inhalation of aborted cattle products of conception associated with changes in breeding practices. There is a known occupational risk for animal handlers, slaughterhouse workers, veterinarians, laboratory workers, and other workers exposed to animal products. In the United States, over 60% of cases do not report an exposure to potentially infectious animals, but cases are more than twice as likely as non-cases to report drinking raw milk.

Human-to-human transmission does not seem to occur, but maternal-fetal infection can occur and infection after liver transplant is reported.

Clinical Findings

A. Symptoms and Signs

Asymptomatic infection is common. For the remaining cases, a febrile illness develops after an incubation period of 2–3 weeks, usually accompanied by headache, relative bradycardia, prostration, and muscle pains. The clinical course may be acute, chronic (duration 6 months or longer), or relapsing. Pneumonia and granulomatous hepatitis are the predominant manifestations in the acute form (and these may vary in incidence geographically), whereas other less common manifestations include skin rashes (maculopapular or purpuric), fever of unknown origin, myocarditis, pericarditis, aortic aneurysms, aseptic meningitis, encephalitis, orchitis, iliopsoas abscess, spondylodiscitis, tenosynovitis, granulomatous osteomyelitis (more often seen in children), and regional (mediastinal) or diffuse lymphadenopathies.

It has been recommended that the term "chronic Q fever" be abandoned to avoid confusion and be replaced with "persistent focalized infections." The most common presentation in patients with persistent focalized infections is culture-negative endocarditis. Risk factors for endocarditis are the immunocompromised state, presence of preexisting valvular conditions, male sex, and age above 40 years. Valvular prosthesis (mechanical or bioprosthesis) represents the most important risk factor. In series of post-cardiac surgery patients with culture-negative endocarditis, Q fever is often the most common cause (about 40% of cases).

The clinical manifestations of endocarditis are nonspecific with fever, night sweats, and weight loss. Rarely, urticaria, edema, erythema nodosum, and arthralgias are reported. Sudden cardiac insufficiency, stroke, or other embolic and mycotic aneurysms can also develop. Vascular infections, particularly of the aorta (causing mycotic aneurysms) and of graft prostheses, are the second most common presentation and are associated with a high mortality (25%). A post–Q fever chronic fatigue syndrome (1 year after acute infection with chronic symptoms) is controversial and of unknown pathophysiology. Cognitive behavioral therapy is effective in reducing fatigue severity in patients with Q fever fatigue syndrome; long-term treatment with doxycycline has not been shown to be effective.

New infection or reactivation of Q fever can occur in pregnant women and is associated with spontaneous abortions, intrauterine growth retardation, intrauterine fetal death, and premature delivery. *C burnetii* infection during the first trimester can cause oligohydramnios.

B. Laboratory Findings

Laboratory examination during the acute phase may show elevated liver biochemical tests and occasional leukocytosis. Patients with acute Q fever usually produce antibodies to *C burnetii* phase II antigen (phase II antigens are formed in vitro from deleted avirulent mutants and are empirically more commonly seen in acute disease, whereas phase I antigens, seen in nature and laboratory infections, are found in the IgG form in chronic disease). A fourfold rise between acute and convalescent sera by indirect immunofluorescence is diagnostic of the infection. Real-time PCR for *C burnetii* DNA is helpful only in early diagnosis of Q fever. *C burnetii* DNA becomes undetectable in serum as serologic responses develop. The positive predictive value of antibodies to phase II antigens in acute disease is at most 65%, and considerable intertest variability exists with phase 2 antigens. Diagnostic tests combining PCR with ELISA (Immuno-PCR) improve the sensitivity and specificity during the first 2 weeks after the onset of symptoms.

While persistent infection can be diagnosed based on serologic tests done at 3- and 6-month intervals (with an IgG titer against phase I antigen of 1:1600 or greater), the sensitivity of such serologies is often low, and the diagnosis of Q fever is often made clinically. An automated epifluorescence assay has greater than 95% sensitivity for the detection of phase I antigens in persistent infection. *C burnetii*–specific interferon-gamma, interferon-gamma/ IL-2 ratio has a sensitivity of 79% and a specificity and 97% for the diagnosis of persistent infection.

Diagnosis of Q fever endocarditis is often made at the time of valve replacement with PCR of tissue samples. *C burnetii* may also be isolated from affected valves using the shell-vial technique.

C. Imaging

Radiographs of the chest can show patchy pulmonary infiltrates. All patients with acute Q fever should be screened for underlying valvular disease with echocardiography. Initial imaging and follow-up with serial 18-FDG PET/CT scan may be helpful in identifying chronic infection and monitoring treatment response.

Differential Diagnosis

Viral, mycoplasma, and bacterial pneumonias; viral hepatitis; brucellosis; Legionnaire disease; murine or scrub typhus; Kawasaki disease; tuberculosis; psittacosis; and other animal-borne diseases can have similar clinical presentations to Q fever. Q fever should be considered in cases of unexplained fevers with negative blood cultures in association with embolic or cardiac disease. Cases of Q fever can mimic autoimmune disease. Coinfection with typhus and leptospirosis is reported.

Treatment & Prognosis

Doxycycline is the most effective drug against *C burnetii*; there are rare reports of doxycycline resistance. Isolates remain susceptible to levofloxacin, moxifloxacin, and to a lesser extent ciprofloxacin. No resistance to sulfamethoxazole-trimethoprim is reported to date.

For acute infection, treatment with doxycycline (100 mg orally twice daily) for 14 days or at least 3 full days after defervescence is recommended. Even in untreated patients, the mortality rate is usually low, except when endocarditis develops.

There are no clear guidelines on the treatment of persistent *C burnetii* infections. To date, there is no antibiotic that has bactericidal effect against *C burnetii*. Most experts recommend a combination oral therapy with doxycycline (100 mg twice a day) plus a quinolone, rifampin, or hydroxychloroquine for approximately 18 months for native valve endocarditis and 24 months for prosthetic valve endocarditis.

Serologic responses can be monitored during and after completion of therapy and treatment can be extended in the absence of favorable serologic response. The general variability of serologic data, however, limits their usefulness and providers usually rely on clinical criteria. Patients should be monitored for at least 5 years due to risk of relapse.

For patients with endocarditis, clinical cure is possible without valve replacement. Heart valve replacement is not associated with better survival, except in the group of patients with a valvular prosthesis. Given the difficulty in treating endocarditis, transthoracic echocardiography is recommended to screen for predisposing valvulopathy in all patients with acute Q fever, and the same therapy for 1 year should be offered in the presence of valvulopathy. In addition, patients undergoing routine valve surgery should have routine Q fever serologies in endemic countries and appropriate treatment if tests are positive for Q fever.

All infected pregnant women should be given long-term trimethoprim-sulfamethoxazole (320/1600 mg orally for the duration of pregnancy, but not beyond 32 weeks' gestation) to prevent the obstetric complications.

In retrospective studies, an increased risk of diffuse B-cell lymphoma and follicular lymphoma was found in patients with Q fever compared with the general population. Patients with persistent focalized infections were at higher risk for lymphadenitis and progression to lymphoma.

► Prevention

Prevention is based on detection of the infection in livestock, with reduction of contact with infected and parturient animals or contaminated dust; special care when working with animal tissues; and effective pasteurization of milk. A whole-cell Q fever vaccine is available in Australia for persons with high-risk exposures, although there are reports of vaccine failure more than 15 days after vaccination.

The organism is highly transmissible to laboratory workers and culture techniques require a biosafety level 3 setting. *C burnetii* is a category B bioterrorism agent. In the setting of a bioterrorist attack, postexposure prophylaxis with doxycycline 100 mg orally twice a day for 5–7 days should be administered within 8–12 days of exposure. Pregnant women may take trimethoprim-sulfamethoxazole as an alternative.

Eldin C et al. From Q fever to *Coxiella burnetii* infection: a paradigm change. Clin Microbiol Rev. 2017 Jan;30(1):115–90. [PMID: 27856520]

Jang YR et al. Molecular detection of *Coxiella burnetii* in heart valve tissue from patients with culture-negative infective endocarditis. Medicine (Baltimore). 2018 Aug;97(34):e11881. [PMID: 30142785]

Keijmel SP et al. Effectiveness of long-term doxycycline treatment and cognitive-behavioral therapy on fatigue severity in patients with Q fever fatigue syndrome (Qure Study): a randomized controlled trial. Clin Infect Dis. 2017 Apr 15;64(8): 998–1005. [PMID: 28329131]

KAWASAKI DISEASE

ESSENTIALS OF DIAGNOSIS

► Fever, conjunctivitis, oral mucosal changes, rash, cervical lymphadenopathy, peripheral extremity changes.
► Elevated ESR and CRP levels.
► Risk for coronary arteritis and aneurysms.

► General Considerations

Kawasaki disease is a worldwide multisystem disease. It is also known as the "mucocutaneous lymph node syndrome." It occurs mainly in children between the ages of 3 months and 5 years but can occur occasionally in adults as well. Kawasaki disease occurs most often in Asians or native Pacific Islanders. Its incidence in Japan is twice that of the United States, and it occurs among siblings at twice the incidence of cases and at higher rates among parents of cases. These findings plus the known seasonality (higher incidence in winter and early spring) and occasional epidemic pattern of cases point to the inadequate current understanding of the etiology of this disease.

It is an acute, self-limiting, mucocutaneous vasculitis characterized by the infiltration of vessel walls with mononuclear cells and later by IgA secreting plasma cells that can result in the destruction of the tunica media and aneurysm formation. The cause of Kawasaki disease remains unknown. Epidemiologic studies show an increased risk with advanced maternal age, mother of foreign birth, maternal group B *Streptococcus* colonization, and early infancy hospitalization for a bacterial illness. Genetic factors are considered to play an important role in the pathogenesis of the disease. Ongoing analyses identify many gene polymorphisms, which significantly correlate with Kawasaki disease susceptibility (at least 23 to disease, and 10 to the presence of coronary aneurysms).

► Clinical Findings

A clinical diagnosis of classic or "complete" Kawasaki disease requires the presence of at least 5 days of fever, usually high-grade (over 39°C to 40°C) and four of the following five criteria: (1) bilateral nonexudative conjunctivitis (begins shortly after the onset of fever), (2) oral changes (erythema and cracking of lips, strawberry tongue, and erythema of oral and pharyngeal mucosa; ulcers and pharyngeal exudates are not consistent with Kawasaki disease), (3) peripheral extremity changes (erythema and edema of the hands and feet in the acute phase, and/or periungual desquamation within 2 to 3 weeks after the onset of fever), (4) polymorphous rash, and (5) cervical lymphadenopathy (larger than 1.5 cm diameter, usually unilateral; least common of the clinical features). The revised case definition allows the diagnosis on day 4 in the presence of more than four principal clinical criteria, particularly when redness and swelling of the hands and feet are present.

A diagnosis of atypical or "incomplete" Kawasaki disease could be diagnosed in patients with unexplained fever and fewer than four principal criteria if accompanied by compatible laboratory or findings of aneurysms detected by echocardiography or angiography.

Laboratory findings in the acute phase typically include leukocytosis with neutrophilic predominance, anemia, and an elevated ESR and CRP. High platelet counts are characteristic but occur in the second week. N-terminal moiety of B-type natriuretic peptide (NT-proBNP), likely indicative of myocardial involvement, may be elevated in some patients with Kawasaki disease.

Major complications include arteritis and aneurysms of the coronary vessels. The arteritis begins 6–8 days after the onset of disease, occurs in about 25% of untreated patients, and occasionally causes myocardial infarction. Coronary complications are more common among patients older than 6 years or younger than 1 year of age; males; and those unresponsive to IVIG, who received a smaller dose of IVIG, or did not receive treatment within 10 days of symptom onset. While myocarditis can be found in all patients with Kawasaki disease on histologic specimens and is prominent during the acute stage, only a small percentage of patients are clinically symptomatic.

Cardiac complications include left ventricular dysfunction, which usually normalizes promptly with IVIG therapy, and mitral regurgitation, which occurs early and does not appear to persist. Noninvasive diagnosis of coronary complications can be made with CT coronary angiography (the most sensitive test), magnetic resonance angiography, or transthoracic echocardiography (advocated for early screening). Kawasaki shock syndrome is a complication, with an estimated incidence of 7%, possibly caused by decrease in peripheral vascular resistance, myocarditis with or without myocardial ischemia, and capillary leakage.

The multisystemic findings of Kawasaki disease show it to be a systemic disease that affects medium-sized arteries of multiple organs, causing elevations in serum transaminases, interstitial pneumonitis, abdominal pain, vomiting, diarrhea, gallbladder hydrops, pancreatitis, lymphadenopathy, hypoalbuminemia, arrhythmias, aseptic meningitis, acute encephalopathy with biphasic seizures and late reduced diffusion, retinal and choroidal detachment, pulmonary complications (effusions, empyema, pneumothorax), hemophagocytic lymphohistiocytosis syndrome, and pyuria. CSF pleocytosis with a mononuclear cell predominance, normal glucose levels, and protein levels is seen in one-third of children who undergo lumbar puncture.

Other diseases with similar presentation that should be considered include measles in unimmunized children as well as other viral infections, such as adenovirus, scarlet fever, and toxic shock syndrome; rickettsial infections; or leptospirosis and drug hypersensitivity reactions.

▶ Treatment & Prevention

All patients meeting the diagnostic criteria for Kawasaki disease (complete and incomplete), including patients with recurrent Kawasaki disease, should be treated as soon as the diagnosis is suspected to reduce inflammation and arterial damage.

A single dose of IVIG should be given in the first 10 days of the illness. Patients in whom the diagnosis was made later than the tenth day may still benefit from IVIG treatment if they have elevated inflammatory markers (ESR or CRP), with persistent fever or have coronary artery aneurysms. When IVIG treatment is not given, coronary artery aneurysms occur in 20% of children. Even when treated with IVIG within the first 10 days of illness, coronary artery aneurysms still develop in 5% of patients. Rare cases of aseptic meningitis are reported with IVIG. Coombs-positive hemolytic anemia, especially in individuals with AB blood type and anaphylactic reactions to immunoglobulins with selective IgA deficiency are other complications associated with IVIG administration.

Although aspirin does not lower the frequency of development of coronary abnormalities, it has important anti-inflammatory activity and antiplatelet activity. Concomitant aspirin with IVIG should be started at 80–100 mg/kg/day orally (divided into four doses and not exceeding 4 g/day) until the patient is afebrile for 48 hours and then reduced to 3–5 mg/kg/day until markers of acute inflammation normalize. Since ibuprofen antagonizes the irreversible platelet inhibition induced by aspirin, it should be avoided when aspirin is given.

The use of corticosteroids for children with Kawasaki disease is controversial. According to the most recent published guidelines by the American Heart Association, single-dose pulse methylprednisolone should not be used routinely for patients with Kawasaki disease. A course of corticosteroid therapy with tapering over 2–3 weeks could be considered in addition to IVIG and aspirin for patients at high-risk for not responding to IVIG.

Resistant Kawasaki disease, defined as having recrudescent or persistent fever at least 36 hours after the end of the first IVIG infusion when no other source of fever is found, develops in about 10–20% of patients. The Egami score is a predictor used in Japan to help determine who will respond to IVIG, although the scoring system has been shown to have lower utility in US cases. The presence of coronary artery abnormalities on the initial echocardiogram and their presence before day 5 of fever predict nonresponse to IVIG in one Israeli study.

Options for refractory cases include a second dose of IVIG, high-dose pulse corticosteroids over 3 days with or without a subsequent oral taper course, longer oral tapering course of corticosteroids over 2–3 weeks together with IVIG and aspirin, infliximab, the anti-inflammatory interleukin 1 receptor antagonist anakinra, low-dose methotrexate, and cyclosporine. Immunomodulatory monoclonal antibody therapy and cytotoxic agents, or (rarely) plasma exchange should be considered only in highly refractory cases in which other therapy has failed.

The most common serious complication in the acute phase is thrombotic occlusion of a coronary artery aneurysm leading to myocardial infarction or sudden death. An echocardiogram is recommended within 1–2 weeks and 4–6 weeks after treatment for uncomplicated patients. More frequent imaging is recommended for patients with significant and evolving coronary artery abnormalities. Anticoagulation with warfarin or low-molecular-weight heparin is indicated, along with aspirin, in patients with rapidly expanding coronary artery aneurysms. Aspirin, a second antiplatelet agent, and anticoagulation with warfarin, low-molecular-weight heparin, or direct-acting oral anticoagulants (which need further study in this population) may be considered for patients with large or giant aneurysms (at least 8 mm) (which correlate with delay in diagnosis) and a recent history of coronary artery thrombosis. If myocardial infarction occurs, therapy with thrombolytics, percutaneous coronary intervention, coronary artery bypass grafts, and even cardiac transplantation should be considered. Manifestations of coronary artery aneurysms can occur as late as in the third or fourth decade of life with a study showing a prevalence of 5% coronary sequelae from Kawasaki disease among young adults evaluated with angiography. Calcified coronary aneurysms on CT scans are less likely to regress.

▶ Prognosis

The reported recurrence rate is 3% in one study from Japan. The highest risk of recurrence occurs in the first 2 years after the first episode. The mortality peaks between 15 and 45 days after the onset of fever, at the time of coronary artery vasculitis, thrombocytosis, and a hypercoagulable state.

Over the long-term, the risk for clinical cardiac events in patients with no coronary artery abnormalities is similar to the general population. For patients in whom coronary artery abnormalities developed, the risk for cardiac complications, such as thrombosis, stenosis, myocardial infarction, and death, ranges between 1% and 48%. Follow-up is especially needed among the subset of patients with neutropenia who have been treated with IVIG. The administration of IVIG is shown to improve left ventricular function. The AHA recommends risk stratification based on the assessment of coronary luminal dimensions by echocardiogram, under cardiologic supervision. The frequency of clinical follow-up, diagnostic testing, reproductive counseling, indications for medical therapy (beta-blockers, statins), and thromboprophylaxis (aspirin and anticoagulation) depends on the individual's risk assessment.

▶ When to Refer

All cases of Kawasaki disease merit referral to specialists.

Denby KJ et al. Management of Kawasaki disease in adults. Heart. 2017 Nov;103(22):1760–9. [PMID: 28751537]

Dhanrajani A et al. Revisiting the role of steroids and aspirin in the management of acute Kawasaki disease. Curr Opin Rheumatol. 2017 Sep;29(5):547–52. [PMID: 28661936]

Kone-Paut I et al. The use of interleukin 1 receptor antagonist (anakinra) in Kawasaki disease: A retrospective cases series. Autoimmun Rev. 2018 Aug;17(8):768–74. [PMID: 29885546]

Qiu H et al. Delayed intravenous immunoglobulin treatment increased the risk of coronary artery lesions in children with Kawasaki disease at different status. Postgrad Med. 2018 May;130(4):442–7. [PMID: 29745742]

Special Issue—Kawasaki Disease. Int J Rheum Dis. 2018 Jan;21(1):1–356.

Xie X et al. The roles of genetic factors in Kawasaki disease: a systematic review and meta-analysis of genetic association studies. Pediatr Cardiol. 2018 Feb;39(2):207–25. [PMID: 29098351]

Bacterial & Chlamydial Infections

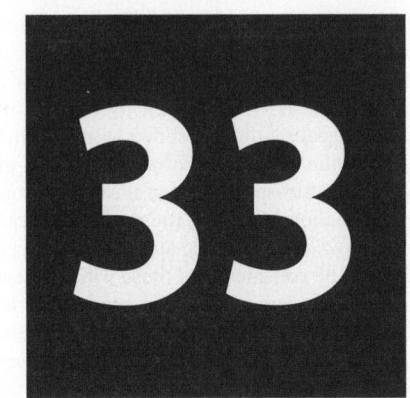

33

Bryn A. Boslett, MD

Brian S. Schwartz, MD

INFECTIONS CAUSED BY GRAM-POSITIVE BACTERIA

STREPTOCOCCAL INFECTIONS

1. Pharyngitis

> **ESSENTIALS OF DIAGNOSIS**

> ▶ Abrupt onset of sore throat, fever, malaise, nausea.

> ▶ Throat red and edematous, with or without exudate; cervical nodes tender.

> ▶ Diagnosis confirmed by culture of throat.

▶ General Considerations

Group A beta-hemolytic streptococci (*Streptococcus pyogenes*) are the most common bacterial cause of pharyngitis. Transmission occurs by droplets of infected secretions. Group A streptococci producing erythrogenic toxin may cause scarlet fever in susceptible persons.

▶ Clinical Findings

A. Symptoms and Signs

"**Strep throat**" is characterized by a sudden onset of fever, sore throat, pain on swallowing, tender cervical adenopathy, malaise, and nausea. The pharynx, soft palate, and tonsils are red and edematous. There may be a purulent exudate. The **Centor clinical criteria** for the diagnosis of streptococcal pharyngitis are temperature greater than 38°C, tender anterior cervical adenopathy, lack of a cough, and pharyngotonsillar exudate.

The rash of **scarlet fever** (also called scarletina) is diffusely erythematous and resembles a sunburn, and superimposed fine red papules give the skin a sandpaper consistency; it is most intense in the groin and axillas. It blanches on pressure, may become petechial, and fades in 2–5 days, leaving a fine desquamation. The face is flushed, with circumoral pallor, and the tongue is coated with enlarged red papillae (strawberry tongue).

B. Laboratory Findings

Leukocytosis with neutrophil predominance is common. Throat culture onto a single blood agar plate has a sensitivity of 80–90%. Rapid diagnostic tests based on detection of streptococcal antigen are slightly less sensitive than culture. Clinical criteria, such as the Centor criteria, are useful for identifying patients in whom a rapid antigen test or throat culture is indicated. Patients who meet two or more of these criteria merit further testing. When three of the four are present, laboratory sensitivity of rapid antigen testing exceeds 90%. When only one criterion is present, streptococcal pharyngitis is unlikely. In high-prevalence settings or if clinical suspicion for streptococcal pharyngitis is high, a negative antigen test or culture should be confirmed by a follow-up culture.

▶ Complications

Suppurative complications include sinusitis, otitis media, mastoiditis, peritonsillar abscess, and cervical lymphadenitis.

Nonsuppurative complications are rheumatic fever and glomerulonephritis. Rheumatic fever may follow recurrent episodes of pharyngitis beginning 1–4 weeks after the onset of symptoms. Glomerulonephritis follows a single infection with a nephritogenic strain of streptococcus group A (eg, types 4, 12, 2, 49, and 60), more commonly on the skin than in the throat, and begins 1–3 weeks after the onset of the infection. These complications are more common in children.

▶ Differential Diagnosis

Streptococcal sore throat resembles (and cannot be reliably distinguished clinically from) pharyngitis caused by viruses such as adenoviruses, Epstein-Barr virus, or other bacteria such as *Fusobacterium necrophorum* and *Arcanobacterium haemolyticum* (which also may cause a rash). Pharyngitis and lymphadenopathy are common findings in acute HIV infection. Generalized lymphadenopathy, splenomegaly, atypical lymphocytosis, and a positive serologic test distinguish mononucleosis from streptococcal pharyngitis. Diphtheria is characterized by a pseudomembrane; oropharyngeal candidiasis shows white patches of exudate and less erythema; and necrotizing ulcerative gingivostomatitis (Vincent fusospirochetal gingivitis or stomatitis) presents with shallow ulcers in the mouth. *Neisseria gonorrhoeae, Chlamydia trachomatis,* and primary herpes simplex virus should be considered in those with risk factors. Retropharyngeal abscess or bacterial epiglottitis should be considered when odynophagia and difficulty in handling secretions are present and when the severity of symptoms is disproportionate to findings on examination of the pharynx. *F necrophorum* causes pharyngitis at a similar rate as group A beta-hemolytic streptococci in adolescents and young adults. *F necrophorum* pharyngitis is associated with Lemierre syndrome, suppurative thrombophlebitis of the internal jugular vein, bacteremia, and metastatic infections. Early recognition and treatment of this syndrome is important.

▶ Treatment

Antimicrobial therapy has a modest effect on resolution of symptoms and primarily is administered for prevention of complications. Antibiotic therapy can be safely delayed until the diagnosis is established on the basis of a positive antigen test or culture. Empiric therapy usually is not a cost-effective approach to the management of most adults with pharyngitis because the prevalence of streptococcal pharyngitis is likely to be no more than 10–20% in typical clinical settings. The positive predictive value of clinical criteria is low. Since macrolides are not reliable against *F necrophorum* infection, adolescents or young adults with pharyngitis and unconfirmed streptococcal infection should be given penicillin or amoxicillin preferentially at the doses listed below. If the pharyngitis does not resolve quickly, symptoms worsen, or unilateral neck swelling develops, clinicians should consider suppurative complications such as peritonsillar abscess and Lemierre syndrome.

A. Benzathine Penicillin G

Benzathine penicillin G, 1.2 million units intramuscularly as a single dose, is optimal therapy.

B. Penicillin VK

Penicillin VK, 250 mg orally four times daily or 500 mg orally twice daily for 10 days, is effective.

C. Amoxicillin

Amoxicillin, 1000 mg orally once daily or 500 mg orally twice daily for 10 days, is another option.

D. Cephalosporins

Cephalexin, 500 mg orally twice daily for 10 days, cefdinir, 300 mg orally twice daily for 5–10 days or 600 mg orally once daily for 10 days, cefadroxil, 1000 mg orally once daily for 10 days, and cefpodoxime, 100 mg orally twice

daily for 5–10 days, should be reserved for penicillin-allergic patients who do not have immediate-type hypersensitivity.

E. Macrolides

Erythromycin, 500 mg orally four times a day, or azithromycin, 500 mg orally once daily for 5 days, is an alternative for the penicillin-allergic patient. Macrolides are less effective than penicillins and are considered second-line agents. Macrolide-resistant strains almost always are susceptible to clindamycin, a suitable alternative to penicillins; a 10-day course of 300 mg orally three times daily is effective.

▶ Prevention of Recurrent Rheumatic Fever

Effectively controlling rheumatic fever depends on identification and treatment of primary streptococcal infection and secondary prevention of recurrences. Patients who have had rheumatic fever should be treated with a continuous course of antimicrobial prophylaxis for at least 5 years. Effective regimens are erythromycin, 250 mg orally twice daily, or penicillin G, 500 mg orally daily.

▶ When to Refer

Patients with peritonsillar or retropharyngeal abscess should be referred to an otolaryngologist.

▶ When to Admit

- Odynophagia resulting in dehydration.
- Suspected or known epiglottitis.

Karthikeyan G et al. Acute rheumatic fever. Lancet. 2018 Jul 14; 392(10142):161–74. Erratum in: Lancet. 2018 Sep 8; 392(10150):820. [PMID: 30025809]

Shulman ST et al. Clinical practice guideline for the diagnosis and management of group A streptococcal pharyngitis: 2012 update by the Infectious Diseases Society of America. Clin Infect Dis. 2012 Nov 15;55(10):1279–82. [PMID: 23091044]

van Driel ML et al. Different antibiotic treatments for group A streptococcal pharyngitis. Cochrane Database Syst Rev. 2016 Sep 11;9:CD004406. [PMID: 27614728]

2. Streptococcal Skin Infections

Group A beta-hemolytic streptococci are not normal skin flora. Streptococcal skin infections result from colonization of normal skin by contact with other infected individuals or by preceding streptococcal respiratory infection.

▶ Clinical Findings

A. Symptoms and Signs

Erysipelas is a painful superficial cellulitis that frequently involves the face. It is well demarcated from the surrounding normal skin. It affects skin with impaired lymphatic drainage, such as edematous lower extremities or wounds (Figure 33–1).

Impetigo is a focal, vesicular, pustular lesion with a thick, amber-colored crust with a "stuck-on" appearance (see Chapter 6).

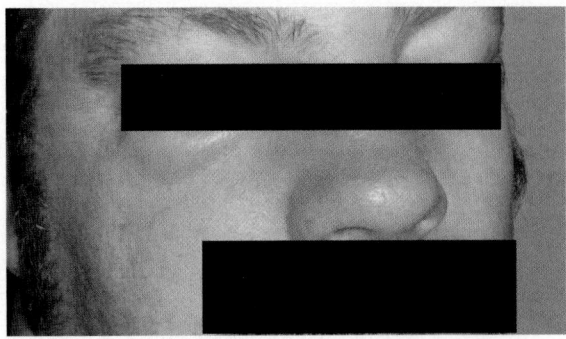

▲ **Figure 33–1.** Erysipelas of the central face that responded well to oral antibiotic therapy. (Used, with permission, from Ernesto Samano Ayon, MD, in Usatine RP, Smith MA, Mayeaux EJ Jr, Chumley H. *The Color Atlas of Family Medicine,* 2nd ed. McGraw-Hill, 2013.)

B. Laboratory Findings

Cultures obtained from a wound or pustule are likely to grow group A streptococci. Blood cultures are occasionally positive.

▶ Treatment

Parenteral antibiotics are indicated for patients with facial erysipelas or evidence of systemic infection. Penicillin, 2 million units intravenously every 4 hours, is the drug of choice. However, staphylococcal infections may at times be difficult to differentiate from streptococcal infections. In practice, initial therapy for patients with risk factors for

Staphylococcus aureus (eg, injection drug use, diabetes mellitus, wound infection) should cover this organism. Either nafcillin, 1–2 g every 4–6 hours intravenously, or cefazolin, 1 g intravenously or intramuscularly every 8 hours, is a reasonable choice. In the patient at risk for methicillin-resistant *S aureus* infection or with a serious penicillin allergy (ie, anaphylaxis), vancomycin, 1 g intravenously every 12 hours, or daptomycin, 4 mg/kg intravenously daily, should be used (Table 33–1).

Patients who do not require parenteral therapy may be treated with amoxicillin, 500 mg three times daily or 875 mg twice daily for 7–10 days. A first-generation oral cephalosporin, eg, cephalexin, 500 mg four times daily, or clindamycin, 300 mg orally three times daily, is an alternative to amoxicillin. In patients with recurrent cellulitis of the leg, maintenance therapy (for at least 1 year) with penicillin, 250 mg orally twice daily, may reduce relapses.

Cranendonk DR et al. Cellulitis: current insights into pathophysiology and clinical management. Neth J Med. 2017 Nov; 75(9):366–78. [PMID: 29219814]
Stevens DL et al. Practice guidelines for the diagnosis and management of skin and soft tissue infections: 2014 update by the Infectious Diseases Society of America. Clin Infect Dis. 2014 Jul 15;59(2):147–59. [PMID: 24947530]

3. Other Group A Streptococcal Infections

Arthritis, pneumonia, empyema, endocarditis, and necrotizing fasciitis are relatively uncommon infections that may be caused by group A streptococci. Toxic shock–like syndrome also occurs.

Table 33–1. Empiric treatment of common skin and soft tissue infections (SSTIs).

SSTI Type	Common Pathogens	Treatment

Purulent (abscess, furuncle, carbuncle, cellulitis with purulence)	*Staphylococcus aureus*	Incision and drainage is the primary treatment
		Consider the addition of antibiotics in select situations[1]
		Oral antibiotic regimens
		    Cephalexin 500 mg four times daily *or* dicloxacillin 500 mg four times daily
		    Clindamycin 300–450 mg three or four times daily[2] *or* one double-strength tablet of trimethoprim-sulfamethoxazole twice daily[2] *or* doxycycline 100 mg twice daily[2]
		Intravenous antibiotic regimens[3]
		    Cefazolin 1 g three times daily *or* nafcillin 1–2 g four to six times daily
		    Vancomycin 1 g twice daily[2] *or* daptomycin 4 mg/kg once daily[2]

Nonpurulent (cellulitis, erysipelas)	Beta-hemolytic streptococci (*S aureus* less likely)	**Oral antibiotic regimens**
		    Cephalexin 500 mg four times daily *or* dicloxacillin 500 mg four times daily
		    Clindamycin 300–450 mg three or four times daily[2] *or* amoxicillin 875 mg twice daily *plus* one double-strength tablet of trimethoprim-sulfamethoxazole twice daily[2]
		Intravenous antibiotic regimens[3]
		    Cefazolin 1 g three times daily *or* nafcillin 1–2 g four to six times daily
		    Vancomycin 1 g twice daily[2] *or* daptomycin 4 mg/kg once daily

[1]Antibiotic therapy should be given in addition to incision and drainage for purulent skin and soft tissue infections if the patient has any of the following: severe or extensive disease, symptoms and signs of systemic illness, purulent cellulitis/wound infection, comorbidities and extremes of age, abscess in area difficult to drain or on face/hand, associated septic phlebitis, or lack of response to incision and drainage alone.
[2]Regimens with activity against methicillin-resistant *S aureus.*
[3]Other regimens approved by the FDA for treatment of complicated skin and soft tissue infections include tigecycline 100 mg intravenously once followed by 50 mg intravenously twice a day, ceftaroline 600 mg twice a day for 7–14 days, dalbavancin 1 g intravenously on day 1 and then 500 mg intravenously on day 8, oritavancin as a single intravenous dose of 1200 mg, and telavancin 10 mg/kg intravenously once daily for 7–14 days.

Arthritis generally occurs in association with cellulitis. In addition to intravenous therapy with penicillin G, 2 million units every 4 hours (or cefazolin or vancomycin in doses recommended above for penicillin-allergic patients), frequent percutaneous needle aspiration should be performed to remove joint effusions. Open surgical drainage may be necessary in many cases.

Pneumonia and **empyema** often are characterized by extensive tissue destruction and an aggressive, rapidly progressive clinical course associated with significant morbidity and mortality. High-dose penicillin and chest tube drainage are indicated for treatment of empyema. Vancomycin is an acceptable substitute in penicillin-allergic patients.

Group A streptococci can cause **endocarditis** in rare instances. Endocarditis should be treated with 4 million units of penicillin G intravenously every 4 hours for 4–6 weeks. Vancomycin, 1 g intravenously every 12 hours, is recommended for persons allergic to penicillin.

Necrotizing fasciitis is a rapidly spreading infection involving the fascia of deep muscle. The clinical findings at presentation may be those of severe cellulitis, but the presence of systemic toxicity and severe pain, which may be followed by anesthesia of the involved area due to destruction of nerves as infection advances through the fascial planes, is a clue to the diagnosis. Surgical exploration is mandatory when the diagnosis is suspected. Early and extensive debridement is essential for survival.

Any streptococcal infection—and necrotizing fasciitis in particular—can be associated with **streptococcal toxic shock syndrome**, typified by invasion of skin or soft tissues, acute respiratory distress syndrome, and kidney failure. Persons who are very young, older adults, and those with underlying medical conditions are at particularly high risk for invasive disease. Bacteremia occurs in most cases. Skin rash and desquamation may not be present. Mortality rates can be up to 80%. The syndrome is due to elaboration of pyrogenic erythrotoxin (which also causes **scarlet fever**), a superantigen that stimulates massive release of inflammatory cytokines believed to mediate the shock. A beta-lactam, such as penicillin, remains the drug of choice for treatment of serious streptococcal infections, but clindamycin, which is a potent inhibitor of toxin production, should also be administered at a dose of 600 mg every 8 hours intravenously for invasive disease, especially in the presence of shock. Intravenous immune globulin can be considered for streptococcal toxic shock syndrome for possible therapeutic benefit from specific antibody to streptococcal exotoxins in immune globulin preparations. Many dosing regimens have been used, including 0.5 g/kg once daily for 5–6 days or a single dose of 2 g/kg with a repeat dose at 48 hours if the patient remains unstable.

Outbreaks of invasive disease have been associated with colonization by invasive clones that can be transmitted to close contacts who, though asymptomatic, may be a reservoir for disease. Tracing contacts of patients with invasive disease is controversial.

Gunderson CG et al. Do patients with cellulitis need to be hospitalized? A systematic review and meta-analysis of mortality rates of inpatients with cellulitis. J Gen Intern Med. 2018 Sep; 33(9):1553–60. [PMID: 30022408]

Kadri SS et al. Impact of intravenous immunoglobulin on survival in necrotizing fasciitis with vasopressor-dependent shock: a propensity score-matched analysis from 130 US hospitals. Clin Infect Dis. 2017 Apr 1;64(7):877–85. [PMID: 28034881]

Stevens DL et al. Necrotizing soft-tissue infections. N Engl J Med. 2017 Dec 7;377(23):2253–65. [PMID: 29211672]

4. Non–Group A Streptococcal Infections

Non–group A hemolytic streptococci (eg, groups B, C, and G) produce a spectrum of disease similar to that of group A streptococci. The treatment of infections caused by these strains is similar to group A streptococci.

Group B streptococci are an important cause of sepsis, bacteremia, and meningitis in the neonate. Antepartum screening to identify carriers and peripartum antimicrobial prophylaxis are recommended in pregnancy. This organism, part of the normal vaginal flora, may cause septic abortion, endometritis, or peripartum infections and, less commonly, cellulitis, bacteremia, and endocarditis in adults. Treatment of infections caused by group B streptococci is with either penicillin or vancomycin in doses recommended for group A streptococci. Because of in vitro synergism, some experts recommend the addition of low-dose gentamicin, 1 mg/kg every 8 hours.

Viridans streptococci, which are nonhemolytic or alpha-hemolytic (ie, producing a green zone of hemolysis on blood agar), are part of the normal oral flora. Although these strains may produce focal pyogenic infection, they are most notable as the leading cause of native valve endocarditis.

Group D streptococci include *Streptococcus gallolyticus* (*bovis*) and the enterococci. *S gallolyticus* (*bovis*) is a cause of endocarditis in association with bowel neoplasia or cirrhosis and is treated like viridans streptococci.

Baddour LM et al. Infective endocarditis in adults: diagnosis, antimicrobial therapy, and management of complications: a scientific statement for healthcare professionals from the American Heart Association. Circulation. 2015 Oct 13; 132(15):1435–86. Erratum in: Circulation. 2015 Oct 27; 132(17):e215. [PMID: 26373316]

Kim SL et al. Distribution of streptococcal groups causing infective endocarditis: a descriptive study. Diagn Microbiol Infect Dis. 2018 Jul;91(3):269–72. [PMID: 29567126]

ENTEROCOCCAL INFECTIONS

Two species, *Enterococcus faecalis* and *Enterococcus faecium*, are responsible for most human enterococcal infections. Enterococci cause wound infections, urinary tract infections, bacteremia, and endocarditis. Infections caused by penicillin-susceptible strains should be treated with ampicillin 2 g every 4 hours or penicillin 3–4 million units every 4 hours; if the patient is penicillin-allergic, vancomycin 15 mg/kg every 12 hours intravenously can be given. If the patient has endocarditis or meningitis, gentamicin 1 mg/kg every 8 hours intravenously should be added to the regimen for a duration of 2–3 weeks in order to achieve the bactericidal activity that is required to cure these infections.

In cases of endocarditis, ceftriaxone 2 g every 12 hours may be given instead of gentamicin in combination with the ampicillin.

Resistance to vancomycin, penicillin, and gentamicin is common among enterococcal isolates, especially *E faecium*; it is essential to determine antimicrobial susceptibility of isolates. Infection control measures that may be indicated to limit their spread include isolation, barrier precautions, and avoidance of overuse of vancomycin and gentamicin. Consultation with an infectious diseases specialist is strongly advised when treating infections caused by resistant strains of enterococci. Quinupristin/dalfopristin and linezolid are approved by the FDA for treatment of infections caused by vancomycin-resistant strains of enterococci. Daptomycin, tigecycline, tedizolid, and oritavancin are not approved by the FDA for the treatment for vancomycin-resistant strains of enterococci, although they are frequently active in vitro.

Quinupristin/dalfopristin is not active against strains of *E faecalis* and should be used only for infections caused by *E faecium*. The dose is 7.5 mg/kg intravenously every 8–12 hours. Phlebitis and irritation at the infusion site (often requiring a central line) and an arthralgia-myalgia syndrome are relatively common side effects. Linezolid, an oxazolidinone, is active against both *E faecalis* and *E faecium*. The dose is 600 mg twice daily, and both intravenous and oral preparations are available. Its two principal side effects are thrombocytopenia and bone marrow suppression; however, peripheral neuropathy, optic neuritis, and lactic acidosis have been observed with prolonged use (typically greater than 6 weeks) due to mitochondrial toxicity. Emergence of resistance has occurred during therapy with both quinupristin/dalfopristin and linezolid.

Baddour LM et al. Infective endocarditis in adults: diagnosis, antimicrobial therapy, and management of complications: a scientific statement for healthcare professionals from the American Heart Association. Circulation. 2015 Oct 13; 132(15):1435–86. Erratum in: Circulation. 2015 Oct 27; 132(17):e215. [PMID: 26373316]

Britt NS et al. Comparative effectiveness and safety of standard-, medium-, and high-dose daptomycin strategies for the treatment of vancomycin-resistant enterococcal bacteremia among Veterans Affairs patients. Clin Infect Dis. 2017 Mar 1; 64(5):605–13. [PMID: 28011602]

PNEUMOCOCCAL INFECTIONS

1. Pneumococcal Pneumonia

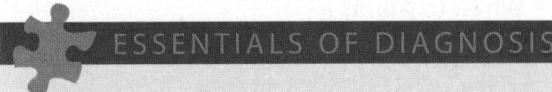

ESSENTIALS OF DIAGNOSIS

- ► Productive cough, fever, rigors, dyspnea, early pleuritic chest pain.
- ► Consolidating lobar pneumonia on chest radiograph.
- ► Gram-positive diplococci on Gram stain of sputum.

General Considerations

Pneumococcus is the most common cause of community-acquired pyogenic bacterial pneumonia. Alcoholism, asthma, HIV infection, sickle cell disease, splenectomy, and hematologic disorders are predisposing factors. Mortality rates remain high in cases of advanced age, multilobar disease, hypoxemia, extrapulmonary complications, and bacteremia.

Clinical Findings

A. Symptoms and Signs

Presenting symptoms and signs include high fever, productive cough, occasional hemoptysis, and pleuritic chest pain. Rigors may occur initially but are uncommon later in the course. Bronchial breath sounds are an early sign.

B. Laboratory Findings

Pneumococcal pneumonia classically is a lobar pneumonia with radiographic findings of consolidation and occasionally effusion. However, differentiating it from other pneumonias is not possible radiographically or clinically because of significant overlap in presentations. Diagnosis requires isolation of the organism in culture, although the Gram stain appearance of sputum can be suggestive. Sputum and blood cultures, positive in 60% and 25% of cases of pneumococcal pneumonia, respectively, should be obtained prior to initiation of antimicrobial therapy in patients who are admitted to the hospital. A good-quality sputum sample (less than 10 epithelial cells and greater than 25 polymorphonuclear leukocytes per high-power field) shows gram-positive diplococci in 80–90% of cases. A rapid urinary antigen test for *Streptococcus pneumoniae*, with sensitivity of 70–80% and specificity greater than 95%, can assist with early diagnosis.

Complications

Parapneumonic (sympathetic) effusion is common and may cause recurrence or persistence of fever. These sterile fluid accumulations need no specific therapy. Empyema occurs in 5% or less of cases and is differentiated from sympathetic effusion by the presence of organisms on Gram-stained fluid or positive pleural fluid cultures.

Pneumococcal pericarditis is a rare complication that can cause tamponade. Pneumococcal arthritis also is uncommon. Pneumococcal endocarditis usually involves the aortic valve and often occurs in association with meningitis and pneumonia (sometimes referred to as Austrian or Osler triad). Early heart failure and multiple embolic events are typical.

Treatment

A. Specific Measures

Initial antimicrobial therapy for pneumonia is empiric (see Table 9–9) pending isolation and identification of the causative agent. Once *S pneumoniae* is identified as the infecting pathogen, any of several antimicrobial agents may be used depending on the clinical setting, community patterns of penicillin resistance, and susceptibility of the particular isolate. Uncomplicated pneumococcal pneumonia (ie, arterial PO_2 greater than 60 mm Hg, no coexisting medical problems, and single-lobe disease without signs of extrapulmonary infection) caused by penicillin-susceptible strains of pneumococcus may be treated on an outpatient basis with amoxicillin, 750 mg orally twice daily for 7–10 days. Cephalosporins including cefpodoxime, 200 mg orally twice daily, and cefdinir, 300 mg twice daily, may also be used. For penicillin-allergic patients, alternatives are azithromycin, one 500-mg dose orally on the first day and 250 mg for the next 4 days; clarithromycin, 500 mg orally twice daily for 10 days; doxycycline, 100 mg orally twice daily for 10 days; levofloxacin, 750 mg orally for 5 days; or moxifloxacin, 400 mg orally for 7–14 days. Patients should be monitored for clinical response (eg, less cough, defervescence within 2–3 days) because pneumococci have become increasingly resistant to penicillin and the second-line agents.

Parenteral therapy is generally recommended for the hospitalized patient at least until there has been clinical improvement. Aqueous penicillin G, 2 million units intravenously every 4 hours, or ceftriaxone, 1 g intravenously every 24 hours, is effective for strains that are penicillin-susceptible (ie, strains for which the minimum inhibitory concentration [MIC] of penicillin is 2 mcg/mL or less for non-CNS specimens). For serious penicillin allergy or infection caused by a highly penicillin-resistant strain, vancomycin, 1 g intravenously every 12 hours, is effective. Alternatively, a respiratory fluoroquinolone (eg, levofloxacin, 750 mg) can be used. The total duration of therapy is not well defined but 5 days is appropriate for patients who have an uncomplicated infection and demonstrate a good clinical response. Corticosteroid use remains controversial in community-acquired pneumonia and should not be administered routinely.

B. Treatment of Complications

Pleural effusions developing after initiation of antimicrobial therapy usually are sterile, and thoracentesis need not be performed if the patient is otherwise improving. Thoracentesis is indicated for an effusion present prior to initiation of therapy and in the patient who has not responded to antibiotics after 3–4 days. Chest tube drainage may be required if pneumococci are identified by culture or Gram stain, especially if aspiration of the fluid is difficult.

Echocardiography should be done if pericardial effusion is suspected. Patients with pericardial effusion who are responding to antibiotic therapy and have no signs of tamponade may be monitored and treated with indomethacin, 50 mg orally three times daily, for pain. In patients with increasing effusion, unsatisfactory clinical response, or evidence of tamponade, pericardiocentesis will determine whether the pericardial space is infected. Infected fluid must be drained either percutaneously (by tube placement or needle aspiration), by placement of a pericardial window, or by pericardiectomy. Pericardiectomy eventually may be required to prevent or treat constrictive pericarditis.

Endocarditis should be treated for 4 weeks with 3–4 million units of penicillin G every 4 hours intravenously; ceftriaxone, 2 g once daily intravenously; or vancomycin, 15 mg/kg every 12 hours intravenously. Mild heart failure due to valvular regurgitation may respond to medical therapy, but moderate to severe heart failure is an indication for prosthetic valve implantation, as are systemic emboli or large friable vegetations as determined by echocardiography.

C. Penicillin-Resistant Pneumococci

Resistance breakpoints for parenterally administered penicillin and high-dose oral amoxicillin (2 g twice daily) are as follows: susceptible, penicillin MIC of 2 mcg/mL or less; intermediate, MIC of 4 mcg/mL; resistant, MIC of 8 mcg/mL or more. Note, however, that these breakpoints do not apply to orally administered penicillin, which are the same as for use of penicillin in treatment of meningitis. In cases of pneumococcal pneumonia where the isolate has a penicillin MIC greater than 2 mcg/mL, cephalosporin cross-resistance is common, and a non–beta-lactam antimicrobial, such as vancomycin, 1 g intravenously every 12 hours, or a fluoroquinolone with enhanced gram-positive activity (eg, levofloxacin, 750 mg intravenously or orally once daily, or moxifloxacin, 400 mg intravenously or orally once daily), is recommended. Penicillin-resistant strains of pneumococci may be resistant to macrolides, trimethoprim-sulfamethoxazole, and chloramphenicol, and susceptibility must be documented prior to their use. All blood and cerebrospinal fluid isolates should still be tested for resistance to penicillin. There has been no change to the penicillin susceptibility breakpoint for pneumococcal isolates causing meningitis, nor any change in treatment recommendations.

▶ Prevention

See Chapter 30 for discussion of pneumococcal vaccines. All patients should have screening for smoking cessation.

▶ When to Refer

- All patients with suspected pneumococcal endocarditis or meningitis to an infectious disease specialist.
- Extensive disease.
- Seriously ill patient with pneumonia, particularly in the setting of comorbid conditions (eg, liver disease).
- Progression of pneumonia or failure to improve on antibiotics.

▶ When to Admit

- All patients in whom pneumococcal endocarditis or meningitis is suspected or documented should be admitted for observation and empiric therapy.
- All patients with pneumococcal pneumonia that is multilobar or associated with significant hypoxemia.
- Failure of outpatient pneumonia therapy, including inability to maintain oral intake and medications.
- Exacerbations of underlying disease (eg, heart failure) by pneumonia that would benefit from hospitalization.

Galán-Ros J et al. Bacteremic pneumococcal pneumonia in adults. Arch Bronconeumol. 2018 Jan;54(1):54–5. [PMID: 28757279]

Uranga A et al. Duration of antibiotic treatment in community-acquired pneumonia: a multicenter randomized clinical trial. JAMA Intern Med. 2016 Sep 1;176(9):1257–65. [PMID: 27455166]

Wunderink RG et al. Advances in the causes and management of community acquired pneumonia in adults. BMJ. 2017 Jul 10; 358:j2471. [PMID: 28694251]

2. Pneumococcal Meningitis

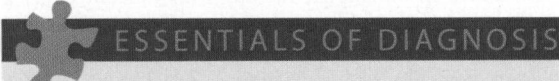

ESSENTIALS OF DIAGNOSIS

▶ Fever, headache, altered mental status.

▶ Meningismus.

▶ Gram-positive diplococci on Gram stain of cerebrospinal fluid.

General Considerations

S pneumoniae is the most common cause of meningitis in adults. Head trauma with cerebrospinal fluid leaks, sinusitis, and pneumonia may precede it.

Clinical Findings

A. Symptoms and Signs

The onset is rapid, with fever, headache, meningismus, and altered mentation. Pneumonia may be present. Compared with meningitis caused by the meningococcus, pneumococcal meningitis lacks a rash. Obtundation, focal neurologic deficits, and cranial nerve palsies are more prominent features and may lead to long-term sequelae.

B. Laboratory Findings

The cerebrospinal fluid typically has greater than 1000 white blood cells per microliter, over 60% of which are polymorphonuclear leukocytes; the glucose concentration is less than 40 mg/dL (2.22 mmol/L), or less than 50% of the simultaneous serum concentration; and the protein usually exceeds 150 mg/dL (1500 mg/L) (see Chapter 30). Not all cases of meningitis will have these typical findings, and alterations in cerebrospinal fluid cell counts and chemistries may be surprisingly minimal, overlapping with those of aseptic meningitis.

Gram stain of cerebrospinal fluid shows gram-positive cocci in 80–90% of cases, and in untreated cases, blood or cerebrospinal fluid cultures are almost always positive.

Treatment

Antibiotics should be given as soon as the diagnosis is suspected. If lumbar puncture must be delayed (eg, while awaiting results of an imaging study to exclude a mass lesion), the patient should be treated empirically for presumed meningitis with intravenous ceftriaxone, 2 g, plus vancomycin, 15 mg/kg, plus dexamethasone, 0.15 mg/kg administered concomitantly after blood cultures (positive in 50% of cases) have been obtained. Once susceptibility to penicillin has been confirmed, penicillin, 24 million units intravenously daily in six divided doses, or ceftriaxone, 2 g every 12 hours intravenously, is continued for 10–14 days in documented cases.

The best therapy for penicillin-resistant strains is not known. Penicillin-resistant strains (MIC greater than 0.06 mcg/mL) are often cross-resistant to the third-generation cephalosporins as well as other antibiotics. Susceptibility testing is essential to proper management of this infection. If the MIC of ceftriaxone or cefotaxime is 0.5 mcg/mL or less, single-drug therapy with either of these cephalosporins is likely to be effective; when the MIC is 1 mcg/mL or more, treatment with a combination of ceftriaxone, 2 g intravenously every 12 hours, plus vancomycin, 30 mg/kg/day intravenously in two or three divided doses, is recommended. If a patient with a penicillin-resistant organism is slow to respond clinically, repeat lumbar puncture may be indicated to assess bacteriologic response.

Dexamethasone administered with antibiotic to adults has been associated with a 60% reduction in mortality and a 50% reduction in unfavorable outcomes. It is recommended that dexamethasone be given immediately prior to or concomitantly with the first dose of appropriate antibiotic and continued in those with pneumococcal disease every 6 hours thereafter for a total of 4 days. The effect of dexamethasone on outcome of meningitis caused by penicillin-resistant organisms is not known.

Costerus JM et al. Community-acquired bacterial meningitis. Curr Opin Infect Dis. 2017 Feb;30(1):135–41. [PMID: 27828810]

Mora Carpio AL et al. Pneumococcal bacteremia and meningitis. N Engl J Med. 2018 Nov 22;379(21):2063. [PMID: 30462944]

STAPHYLOCOCCUS AUREUS INFECTIONS

1. Skin & Soft Tissue Infections

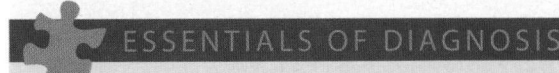

ESSENTIALS OF DIAGNOSIS

▶ Localized erythema with induration and purulent drainage.

▶ Abscess formation.

▶ Folliculitis commonly observed.

▶ Gram stain of pus shows gram-positive cocci in clusters; cultures usually positive.

General Considerations

Approximately one-quarter of people are asymptomatic nasal carriers of *S aureus*, which is spread by direct contact. Carriage often precedes infection, which occurs as a consequence of disruption of the cutaneous barrier or impairment of host defenses. *S aureus* tends to cause more purulent skin infections than streptococci, and abscess formation is common. The prevalence of methicillin-resistant strains in many communities is high and should influence antibiotic choices when antimicrobial therapy is needed.

▶ **Clinical Findings**

A. Symptoms and Signs

S aureus skin infections may begin around one or more hair follicles, causing folliculitis; may become localized to form boils (or furuncles); or may spread to adjacent skin and deeper subcutaneous tissue (ie, a carbuncle) (Figure 33–2). Deep abscesses involving muscle or fascia may occur, often in association with a deep wound or other inoculation or injection. Necrotizing fasciitis, a rare form of *S aureus* skin and soft tissues infection, has been reported with community strains of methicillin-resistant *S aureus*.

B. Laboratory Findings

Cultures of the wound or abscess material will almost always yield the organism. In patients with systemic signs of infection, blood cultures should be obtained because of potential bacteremia, endocarditis, osteomyelitis, or metastatic seeding of other sites. Patients who are bacteremic should have blood cultures taken early during therapy to exclude persistent bacteremia, an indicator of severe or complicated infection.

▶ **Treatment**

Proper drainage of abscess fluid or other focal infections is the mainstay of therapy. Incision and drainage alone is highly effective for the treatment of most uncomplicated cutaneous abscesses. A small benefit can be obtained from the addition of antimicrobials following incision and drainage. In areas where methicillin resistance among community *S aureus* isolates is high, recommended oral

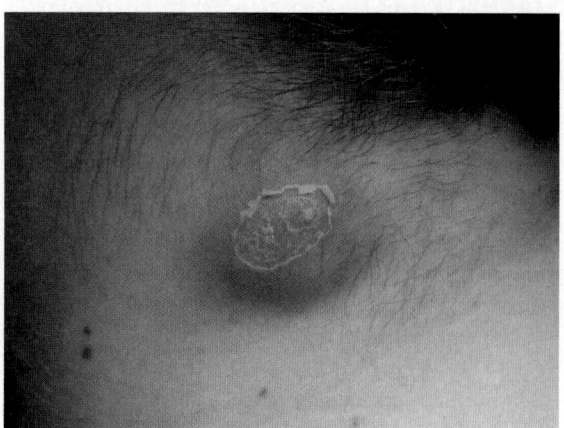

▲ **Figure 33–2.** Methicillin-resistant *Staphylococcus aureus* (MRSA) abscess of the neck. (From Edward Wright, MD; reproduced, with permission, from Usatine RP, Smith MA, Mayeaux EJ Jr, Chumley H, Tysinger J. *The Color Atlas of Family Medicine.* McGraw-Hill, 2009.)

antimicrobials agents include clindamycin, 300 mg three times daily; trimethoprim-sulfamethoxazole, given in two divided doses based on 5–10 mg/kg/day of the trimethoprim component; or doxycycline or minocycline, 100 mg twice daily. When the risk of methicillin resistance is low or methicillin susceptibility has been confirmed by testing of the isolate, consider dicloxacillin or cephalexin, 500 mg four times a day (see Table 33–1). Seven days of treatment are sufficient in most cases.

For complicated infections with extensive cutaneous or deep tissue involvement or fever, initial parenteral therapy is often indicated. When methicillin resistance rates are high (above 10%), empiric therapy with vancomycin, 1 g intravenously every 12 hours, is a drug of choice. Cefazolin 1 g intravenously or intramuscularly or a penicillinase-resistant penicillin such as nafcillin or oxacillin in a dosage of 1.5 g every 6 hours intravenously is preferred for infections caused by methicillin-susceptible isolates. Total duration of therapy for soft tissue infections depends on clinical response and effectiveness of drainage/debridement. Courses of 7 days with early transition to oral therapy are effective in many cases.

Linezolid is FDA approved for treatment of skin and skin-structure infections as well as hospital-acquired pneumonia caused by methicillin-resistant strains of *S aureus* and clinically is as effective as vancomycin for these indications. The dose is 600 mg orally or intravenously twice a day for 10–14 days. Its considerable cost makes it an unattractive choice for most routine outpatient infections, and its safety in treatment courses lasting longer than 2–3 weeks is not well characterized. Tedizolid (an oxazolidinone, like linezolid) is also approved for treating skin and soft tissue infection at a dose of 200 mg orally once daily for 6 days. Other drugs FDA approved for treating skin and soft tissue infections include daptomycin, 4 mg/kg intravenously once daily for 7–14 days; tigecycline (a glycylcycline class antimicrobial), 100 mg intravenously once followed by 50 mg intravenously twice a day for 5–14 days; ceftaroline (a novel cephalosporin with activity against methicillin-resistant *S aureus*), 600 mg twice a day for 7–14 days; dalbavancin (a lipoglycopeptide), a single intravenous dose of 1500 mg; oritavancin (a lipoglycopeptide), a single intravenous dose of 1200 mg; telavancin (a lipoglycopeptide), 10 mg/kg intravenously once daily for 7–14 days; and delafloxacin, 450 mg orally or 300 intravenously twice daily for 5–14 days. Telavancin is also approved for the treatment of hospital-acquired *S aureus* pneumonia but has been associated with nephrotoxicity.

Khan A et al. Current and future treatment options for community-associated MRSA infection. Expert Opin Pharmacother. 2018 Apr;19(5):457–70. [PMID: 29480032]

Moran GJ et al. Effect of cephalexin plus trimethoprim-sulfamethoxazole vs cephalexin alone on clinical cure of uncomplicated cellulitis: a randomized clinical trial. JAMA. 2017 May 23;317(20):2088–96. [PMID: 28535235]

Pullman J et al; PROCEED Study Group. Efficacy and safety of delafloxacin compared with vancomycin plus aztreonam for acute bacterial skin and skin structure infections: a Phase 3, double-blind, randomized study. J Antimicrob Chemother. 2017 Dec 1;72(12):3471–80. [PMID: 29029278]

Talan DA et al. Trimethoprim-sulfamethoxazole versus placebo for uncomplicated skin abscess. N Engl J Med. 2016 Mar 3; 374(9):823–32. [PMID: 26962903]

2. Osteomyelitis

S aureus causes approximately 60% of all cases of osteomyelitis. Osteomyelitis may be caused by direct inoculation, eg, from an open fracture or as a result of surgery; by extension from a contiguous focus of infection or open wound; or by hematogenous spread. Long bones and vertebrae are the usual sites. Epidural abscess is a common complication of vertebral osteomyelitis and should be suspected if fever and severe back or neck pain are accompanied by radicular pain or symptoms or signs indicative of spinal cord compression (eg, incontinence, extremity weakness, pathologic extremity reflexes).

▶ Clinical Findings

A. Symptoms and Signs

The infection may be acute, with abrupt development of local symptoms and systemic toxicity, or indolent, with insidious onset of vague pain over the site of infection, progressing to local tenderness and constitutional symptoms (fever, malaise, anorexia, night sweats). Fever is absent in one-third or more of cases. Back pain is often the only symptom in vertebral osteomyelitis and may be associated with an epidural abscess and spinal cord compression. Draining sinus tracts occur in chronic infections or infections of foreign body implants.

B. Laboratory Findings

The diagnosis is established by isolation of *S aureus* from the blood, bone, or a contiguous focus of a patient with symptoms and signs of focal bone infection. Blood culture will be positive in approximately 60% of untreated cases. Bone biopsy and culture are indicated if blood cultures are sterile. Inflammatory markers (C-reactive protein, erythrocyte sedimentation rate) are typically elevated.

C. Imaging

Bone scan and gallium scan, each with a sensitivity of approximately 95% and a specificity of 60–70%, are useful in identifying or confirming the site of bone infection. Plain bone films early in the course of infection are often normal but will become abnormal in most cases even with effective therapy. Spinal infection (unlike malignancy) traverses the disk space to involve the contiguous vertebral body. CT is more sensitive than plain films and helps localize associated abscesses. MRI is slightly less sensitive than bone scan, but has a specificity of 90%. It is indicated when epidural abscess is suspected in association with vertebral osteomyelitis. ^{18}F-FDG-PET/CT may be useful in diagnosis of vertebral osteomyelitis as well as the detection of other metastatic sites of infection.

▶ Treatment

Prolonged therapy is required to cure staphylococcal osteomyelitis. Durations of 4–6 weeks or longer are recommended.

Intravenous therapy is preferred, particularly during the acute phase of the infection for patients with systemic toxicity. Cefazolin, 2 g every 8 hours, or alternatively, nafcillin or oxacillin, 9–12 g/day in six divided doses, are the drugs of choice for infection with methicillin-sensitive isolates. Patients with infections due to methicillin-resistant strains of *S aureus* or who have severe penicillin allergies should be treated with vancomycin, 30 mg/kg/day intravenously divided in two or three doses. Doses should be adjusted to achieve a vancomycin trough level of 15–20 mcg/mL. In patients with *S aureus* isolates susceptible to a fluoroquinolone and rifampin, that combination has been shown to be effective if given for 4 weeks following 2 weeks of induction therapy with an intravenous agent as above. Consultation with an infectious diseases specialist is recommended. The role of newer agents, such as daptomycin or linezolid, remains to be defined.

Surgical treatment is often indicated under the following circumstances: (1) staphylococcal osteomyelitis with associated epidural abscess and spinal cord compression, (2) other abscesses (psoas, paraspinal), (3) extensive disease, or (4) recurrent or persistent infection despite standard medical therapy. Follow-up imaging may not be needed in patients who demonstrate improvement in symptoms and normalization of inflammatory markers.

Berbari EF et al. 2015 Infectious Diseases Society of America (IDSA) clinical practice guidelines for the diagnosis and treatment of native vertebral osteomyelitis in adults. Clin Infect Dis. 2015 Sep 15;61(6):e26–46. [PMID: 26229122]

Bernard L et al; Duration of Treatment for Spondylodiscitis (DTS) study group. Antibiotic treatment for 6 weeks versus 12 weeks in patients with pyogenic vertebral osteomyelitis: an open-label, non-inferiority, randomised, controlled trial. Lancet. 2015 Mar 7;385(9971):875–82. [PMID: 25468170]

Kouijzer IJE et al. The diagnostic value of ^{18}F-FDG-PET/CT and MRI in suspected vertebral osteomyelitis—a prospective study. Eur J Nucl Med Mol Imaging. 2018 May;45(5):798–805. [PMID: 29256136]

3. Staphylococcal Bacteremia

S aureus readily invades the bloodstream and infects sites distant from the primary site of infection. Whenever *S aureus* is recovered from blood cultures, the possibility of endocarditis, osteomyelitis, or other metastatic deep infection must be considered. Bacteremia that persists for more than 48–96 hours after initiation of therapy is strongly predictive of worse outcome and complicated infection. Given the relatively high risk of infective endocarditis in patients with *S aureus* bacteremia, transesophageal echocardiography is recommended for most patients as a sensitive and cost-effective method for excluding underlying endocarditis. However, transthoracic echocardiography may be sufficient in select patients considered to be at low risk for endocarditis, namely those who meet all the following criteria: (1) no permanent intracardiac device, (2) sterile follow-up blood cultures within 4 days after the initial set, (3) no hemodialysis dependence, (4) nosocomial acquisition of *S aureus* bacteremia, and (5) no clinical signs of infective endocarditis or secondary foci of infection.

Empiric therapy of staphylococcal bacteremia should be with vancomycin, 15–20 mg/kg/dose intravenously every 8–12 hours, or daptomycin 6 mg/kg/day intravenously until results of susceptibility tests are known. If the *S aureus* isolate is methicillin-susceptible, treatment should be narrowed to cefazolin, 2 g every 8 hours, or nafcillin or oxacillin, 2 g intravenously every 4 hours. Cefazolin is as effective as nafcillin or oxacillin and has been associated with fewer adverse events during treatment. In patients with methicillin-resistant *S aureus*, treatment should be with vancomycin, 15–20 mg/kg/dose intravenously every 8–12 hours. Maintaining a vancomycin trough concentration of 15–20 mcg/mL may improve outcomes and is recommended. Daptomycin 6 mg/kg/day is also an FDA-approved option as long as the patient does not require treatment for concomitant *S aureus* pneumonia. The addition of rifamycins to standard antimicrobial therapy has not been shown to be beneficial in the absence of indwelling prosthetic material and is associated with more adverse events. Duration of therapy for *S aureus* bacteremia is 4–6 weeks of antibiotic therapy but a subset of patients with uncomplicated infection may be able to be treated for 14 days. A patient with uncomplicated bacteremia must meet all the following criteria: (1) infective endocarditis has been excluded, (2) no implanted prostheses are present, (3) follow-up blood cultures drawn 2–4 days after the initial set are sterile, (4) the patient defervesces within 72 hours of initiation of effective antibiotic therapy, and (5) no evidence of metastatic infection is present on examination. When present at the time of diagnosis, central venous catheters should be removed. Vancomycin treatment failures are relatively common, particularly for complicated bacteremia and among infections involving foreign bodies. Improved outcomes have been demonstrated when consultation is obtained with an infectious diseases specialist and should be considered in all cases of *S aureus* bacteremia.

Li J et al. β-Lactam therapy for methicillin-susceptible *Staphylococcus aureus* bacteremia: a comparative review of cefazolin versus antistaphylococcal penicillins. Pharmacotherapy. 2017 Mar; 37(3):346–60. [PMID: 28035690]

Liu C et al. Clinical practice guidelines by the Infectious Diseases Society of America for the treatment of methicillin-resistant *Staphylococcus aureus* infections in adults and children. Clin Infect Dis. 2011 Feb 1;52(3):e18–55. [PMID: 21208910]

Rao SN et al. Treatment outcomes with cefazolin versus oxacillin for deep-seated methicillin-susceptible *Staphylococcus aureus* bloodstream infections. Antimicrob Agents Chemother. 2015 Sep;59(9):5232–8. Erratum in: Antimicrob Agents Chemother. 2015 Nov;59(11):7159. [PMID: 26077253]

4. Toxic Shock Syndrome

S aureus produces toxins that cause three important entities: "scalded skin syndrome" in children, toxic shock syndrome in adults, and enterotoxin food poisoning. Toxic shock syndrome is characterized by abrupt onset of high fever, vomiting, and watery diarrhea. Sore throat, myalgias, and headache are common. Hypotension with kidney and heart failure is associated with a poor outcome. A diffuse macular erythematous rash and nonpurulent conjunctivitis are common, and desquamation, especially of palms and soles, is typical during recovery (Figure 33–3). Fatality rates may be

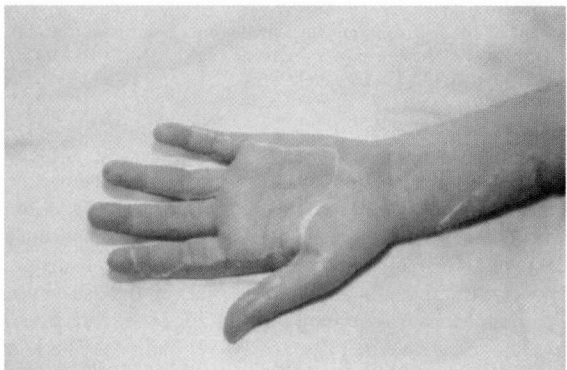

▲ **Figure 33–3.** Marked desquamation due to toxic shock syndrome, which develops late in the disease. (Public Health Image Library, CDC.)

as high as 15%. Although originally associated with tampon use, any focus (eg, nasopharynx, bone, vagina, rectum, abscess, or wound) harboring a toxin-producing *S aureus* strain can cause toxic shock syndrome. Classically, blood cultures are negative because symptoms are due to the effects of the toxin and not systemic infection. Other entities associated with toxic shock include invasive group A streptococcal infection and certain *Clostridium* species (*C perfringens*, *C sordellii*).

Important aspects of treatment include rapid rehydration, targeted antimicrobials (antistaphylococcal therapy when *S aureus* is implicated), management of kidney or heart failure, and addressing sources of toxin, eg, removal of tampon or drainage of abscess. Intravenous clindamycin, 900 mg every 8 hours, is often added to inhibit toxin production. Intravenous immune globulin may be considered, although there are limited data compared with streptococcus toxic shock syndrome.

5. Infections Caused by Coagulase-Negative Staphylococci

Coagulase-negative staphylococci are an important cause of infections of intravascular and prosthetic devices and of wound infection following cardiothoracic surgery. These organisms infrequently cause infections such as osteomyelitis and endocarditis in the absence of a prosthesis. Most human infections are caused by *Staphylococcus epidermidis*, *S haemolyticus*, *S hominis*, *S warnerii*, *S saprophyticus*, *S saccharolyticus*, and *S cohnii*. These common hospital-acquired pathogens are less virulent than *S aureus*, and infections caused by them tend to be more indolent.

Because coagulase-negative staphylococci are normal inhabitants of human skin, it is difficult to distinguish infection from contamination, the latter perhaps accounting for three-fourths of blood culture isolates. Infection is more likely if the patient has a foreign body (eg, sternal wires, prosthetic joint, prosthetic cardiac valve, pacemaker, intracranial pressure monitor, cerebrospinal fluid shunt, peritoneal dialysis catheter) or an intravascular device in place. Purulent or serosanguineous drainage, erythema, pain, or tenderness at the site of the foreign body or device suggests infection. Joint instability and pain are signs of prosthetic joint infection. Fever, a new murmur, instability of the prosthesis, or signs of systemic embolization are evidence of prosthetic valve endocarditis.

Infection is also more likely if the same strain is consistently isolated from two or more blood cultures (particularly if samples were obtained at different times) and from the foreign body site. Contamination is more likely when a single blood culture is positive or if more than one strain is isolated from blood cultures. The antimicrobial susceptibility pattern and speciation are used to determine whether one or more strains have been isolated.

Whenever possible, the intravascular device or foreign body suspected of being infected should be removed. However, removal and replacement of some devices (eg, prosthetic joint, prosthetic valve, cerebrospinal fluid shunt) can be a difficult or risky procedure, and it may sometimes be preferable to treat with antibiotics alone with the understanding that the probability of cure is reduced and that surgical management may eventually be necessary.

Coagulase-negative staphylococci are commonly resistant to beta-lactams and multiple other antibiotics. For patients with normal kidney function, vancomycin, 1 g intravenously every 12 hours, is the treatment of choice until susceptibility to penicillinase-resistant penicillins or other agents has been confirmed. Duration of therapy has not been established for relatively uncomplicated infections, such as those secondary to intravenous devices, which may be eliminated by simply removing the device. Infection involving bone or a prosthetic valve should be treated for 6 weeks. A combination regimen of vancomycin plus rifampin, 300 mg orally twice daily, plus gentamicin, 1 mg/kg intravenously every 8 hours, is recommended for treatment of prosthetic valve endocarditis caused by methicillin-resistant strains.

Baddour LM et al. Infective endocarditis in adults: diagnosis, antimicrobial therapy, and management of complications: a scientific statement for healthcare professionals from the American Heart Association. Circulation. 2015 Oct 13; 132(15):1435–86. Erratum in: Circulation. 2015 Oct 27; 132(17):e215. [PMID: 26373316]

Tan EM et al. Outcomes in patients with cardiovascular implantable electronic device infection managed with chronic antibiotic suppression. Clin Infect Dis. 2017 Jun 1;64(11):1516–21. [PMID: 28329125]

CLOSTRIDIAL DISEASES

1. Clostridial Myonecrosis (Gas Gangrene)

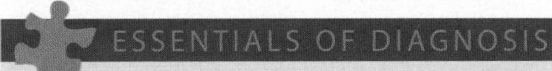
ESSENTIALS OF DIAGNOSIS

> ► Sudden onset of pain and edema in an area of wound contamination.
> ► Prostration and systemic toxicity.
> ► Brown to blood-tinged watery exudate, with skin discoloration of surrounding area.

> ► Gas in the tissue by palpation or radiograph.
> ► Gram-positive rods in culture or smear of exudate.

► General Considerations

Gas gangrene or clostridial myonecrosis is produced by any one of several clostridia (*Clostridium perfringens, C ramosum, C bifermentans, C histolyticum, C novyi*, etc). Trauma and injection drug use are common predisposing conditions. Toxins produced in devitalized tissues under anaerobic conditions result in shock, hemolysis, and myonecrosis.

► Clinical Findings

A. Symptoms and Signs

The onset is usually sudden, with rapidly increasing pain in the affected area, hypotension, and tachycardia. Fever is present, but is not proportionate to the severity of the infection. In the last stages of the disease, severe prostration, stupor, delirium, and coma occur.

The wound becomes swollen, and the surrounding skin is pale. There is a foul-smelling brown, blood-tinged serous discharge. As the disease advances, the surrounding tissue changes from pale to dusky and finally becomes deeply discolored, with coalescent, red, fluid-filled vesicles. Gas may be palpable in the tissues.

B. Laboratory Findings

Gas gangrene is a clinical diagnosis, and empiric therapy is indicated if the diagnosis is suspected. Radiographic studies may show gas within the soft tissues, but this finding is not sensitive nor specific. The smear shows absence of neutrophils and the presence of gram-positive rods. Anaerobic culture confirms the diagnosis.

► Differential Diagnosis

Other bacteria can produce gas in infected tissue, eg, enteric gram-negative organisms, or anaerobes.

► Treatment

Adequate surgical debridement and exposure of infected areas are essential, with radical surgical excision often necessary. Penicillin, 2 million units every 3 hours intravenously, is an effective adjunct. Clindamycin may decrease the production of bacterial toxin, and some experts recommend the addition of clindamycin, 600–900 mg every 8 hours intravenously, to penicillin. Hyperbaric oxygen therapy has been used empirically, but must be used in conjunction with administration of an appropriate antibiotic and surgical debridement.

De Prost N et al. Therapeutic targets in necrotizing soft tissue infections. Intensive Care Med. 2017 Nov;43(11):1717–9. [PMID: 28474117]

Stevens DL et al. Practice guidelines for the diagnosis and management of skin and soft tissue infections: 2014 update by the Infectious Diseases Society of America. Clin Infect Dis. 2014 Jul 15;59(2):147–59. [PMID: 24947530]

Yang Z et al. Interventions for treating gas gangrene. Cochrane Database Syst Rev. 2015 Dec 3;12:CD010577. [PMID: 26631369]

2. Tetanus

ESSENTIALS OF DIAGNOSIS

- ► History of wound and possible contamination.
- ► Jaw muscle stiffness ("lock jaw"), then spasms (trismus).
- ► Stiffness of the neck and other muscles, dysphagia, irritability, hyperreflexia.
- ► Finally, painful convulsions precipitated by minimal stimuli.

General Considerations

Tetanus is caused by the neurotoxin tetanospasmin, elaborated by *C tetani*. Spores of this organism are ubiquitous in soil and may germinate when introduced into a wound. Tetanospasmin interferes with neurotransmission at spinal synapses of inhibitory neurons. As a result, minor stimuli result in uncontrolled spasms, and reflexes are exaggerated. The incubation period is 5 days to 15 weeks, with the average being 8–12 days.

Most cases occur in unvaccinated individuals. Persons at risk are older adults, migrant workers, newborns, and injection drug users. While puncture wounds are particularly prone to causing tetanus, any wound, including bites or decubiti, may become colonized and infected by *C tetani*.

Clinical Findings

A. Symptoms and Signs

The first symptom may be pain and tingling at the site of inoculation, followed by spasticity of the muscles nearby. Stiffness of the jaw, neck stiffness, dysphagia, and irritability are other early signs. Hyperreflexia develops later, with spasms of the jaw muscles (trismus) or facial muscles and rigidity and spasm of the muscles of the abdomen, neck, and back. Painful tonic convulsions precipitated by minor stimuli are common. Spasms of the glottis and respiratory muscles may cause acute asphyxia. The patient is awake and alert throughout the illness. The sensory examination is normal. The temperature is normal or only slightly elevated.

B. Laboratory Findings

The diagnosis of tetanus is made clinically.

Differential Diagnosis

Tetanus must be differentiated from various acute central nervous system (CNS) infections such as meningitis.

Trismus may occasionally develop with the use of phenothiazines. Strychnine poisoning should also be considered.

Complications

Airway obstruction is common. Urinary retention and constipation may result from spasm of the sphincters. Respiratory arrest and cardiac failure are late, life-threatening events.

Prevention

Tetanus is preventable by *active* immunization (see Table 30–7). For primary immunization of adults, Td (tetanus and diphtheria toxoids vaccine) is administered as two doses 4–6 weeks apart, with a third dose 6–12 months later. For one of the three doses, Tdap (tetanus toxoid, reduced-dose diphtheria toxoid, acellular pertussis vaccine) should be substituted for Td. Booster Td doses are given every 10 years or at the time of major injury if it occurs more than 5 years after a dose; a single dose of Tdap is preferred to Td for wound management if the patient has not been previously vaccinated with Tdap. Women should receive Tdap with each pregnancy, preferably between 27 and 36 weeks, with immunization at 27–30 weeks associated with the highest antibody concentrations.

Passive immunization should be used in nonimmunized individuals and those whose immunization status is uncertain whenever a wound is contaminated or likely to have devitalized tissue; tetanus immune globulin, 250 units, is given intramuscularly. Active immunization with tetanus toxoid vaccine is started concurrently. Table 33–2 provides a guide to prophylactic management.

Treatment

A. Specific Measures

Human tetanus immune globulin, 500 units, should be administered intramuscularly within the first 24 hours of presentation. Whether intrathecal administration has any additional benefit is controversial. An unblinded, randomized trial comparing intramuscular tetanus immune globulin to intramuscular plus intrathecal tetanus immune globulin found clinical benefit in the intrathecal group. However, the exact immunoglobulin preparation was not specified and the total dose was 4000 units. Tetanus does not produce natural immunity, and a full course of immunization with tetanus toxoid should be administered once the patient has recovered.

B. General Measures

Debridement of wounds should be undertaken if implicated as the source. Metronidazole, 7.5 mg/kg administered intravenously or orally every 6 hours (maximum 4 g daily), is preferred and should be administered to all patients. Penicillin, 20 million units intravenously daily in divided doses, is an alternative. Minimal stimuli can provoke spasms, so the patient should be placed at bed rest and monitored under the quietest conditions possible. Sedation, paralysis with curare-like agents, and mechanical

Table 33–2. Guide to tetanus prophylaxis in wound management.

History of Absorbed Tetanus Toxoid	Clean, Minor Wounds		All Other Wounds[1]	
	Tdap or Td[2]	TIG[3]	Tdap or Td[2]	TIG[3]
Unknown or < 3 doses	Yes	No	Yes	Yes
3 or more doses	No[4]	No	No[5]	No

[1]Such as, but not limited to, wounds contaminated with dirt, feces, soil, saliva, etc; puncture wounds; avulsions; and wounds resulting from missiles, crushing, burns, and frostbite.
[2]Td indicates tetanus toxoid and diphtheria toxoid vaccine, adult form. Tdap indicates tetanus toxoid, reduced diphtheria toxoid, and acellular pertussis vaccine, which may be substituted as a single dose for Td. Unvaccinated individuals should receive a complete series of three doses, one of which is Tdap.
[3]Human tetanus immune globulin, 250 units intramuscularly.
[4]Yes if more than 10 years have elapsed since last dose.
[5]Yes if more than 5 years have elapsed since last dose. (More frequent boosters are not needed and can enhance side effects.) Tdap has been safely administered within 2 years of Td vaccination, although local reactions to the vaccine may be increased.

ventilation are often necessary. Enteral nutritional support should be given early.

Prognosis

High mortality rates are associated with a short incubation period, early onset of convulsions, and delay in treatment. Contaminated lesions about the head and face are more dangerous than wounds on other parts of the body.

Healy CM et al. Association between third-trimester Tdap immunization and neonatal pertussis antibody concentration. JAMA. 2018 Oct 9;320(14):1464–70. [PMID: 30304426]

3. Botulism

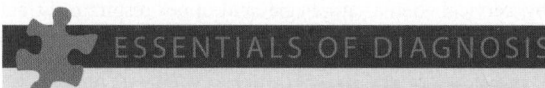

ESSENTIALS OF DIAGNOSIS

- ► Recent ingestion of home-canned or smoked foods; recovery of toxin in serum or food.
- ► Injection drug use.
- ► Diplopia, dry mouth, dysphagia, dysphonia, and muscle weakness progressing to respiratory paralysis.
- ► Pupils are fixed and dilated in most cases.

General Considerations

Botulism is a paralytic disease caused by botulinum toxin, which is produced by *Clostridium botulinum*, a ubiquitous, strictly anaerobic, spore-forming bacillus found in soil. Four toxin types—A, B, E, and F—cause human disease. Botulinum toxin is extremely potent and is classified by the CDC as a high-priority agent because of its potential for use as an agent of bioterrorism. Naturally occurring botulism exists in three forms: food-borne botulism, infant botulism, or wound botulism. Food-borne botulism is caused by ingestion of pre-formed toxin present in canned, smoked, or vacuum-packed

foods such as home-canned vegetables, smoked meats, and vacuum-packed fish. Commercial foods have been associated with outbreaks of botulism. Infant botulism (associated with ingestion of honey) and wound botulism (often occurs in association with injection drug use) result from organisms present in the gut or wound that secrete toxin.

Clinical Findings

A. Symptoms and Signs

Twelve to 36 hours after ingestion of the toxin, visual disturbances appear, particularly diplopia and loss of accommodation. Ptosis, cranial nerve palsies with impairment of extraocular muscles, and fixed dilated pupils are characteristic signs. The sensory examination is normal. Other symptoms are dry mouth, dysphagia, and dysphonia. Nausea and vomiting may be present, particularly with type E toxin. The sensorium remains clear and the temperature normal. Paralysis progressing to respiratory failure and death may occur unless mechanical assistance is provided.

B. Laboratory Findings

Toxin in foods and patients' serum can be demonstrated by mouse inoculation and identified with specific antiserum.

Differential Diagnosis

Because the clinical presentation of botulism is so distinctive and the differential diagnosis limited, botulism once considered is not easily confused with other diseases. Cranial nerve involvement may be seen with vertebrobasilar insufficiency, the C. Miller Fisher variant of Guillain-Barré syndrome, myasthenia gravis, or any basilar meningitis (infectious or carcinomatous). Intestinal obstruction or other types of food poisoning are considered when nausea and vomiting are present.

Treatment

If botulism is suspected, the practitioner should contact the state health authorities or the CDC for advice and help with procurement of equine serum heptavalent botulism antitoxin and for assistance in obtaining assays for toxin in serum, stool, or food. Skin testing is recommended to exclude hypersensitivity to the antitoxin preparation. Antitoxin should be administered as early as possible, ideally within 24 hours of the onset of symptoms or signs, to arrest progression of disease; its administration should not be delayed for laboratory confirmation of the diagnosis. Respiratory failure is managed with intubation and mechanical ventilation. Parenteral fluids or alimentation should be given while swallowing difficulty persists. The removal of unabsorbed toxin from the gut may be attempted. Any remnants of suspected foods should be assayed for toxin. Persons who might have eaten the suspected food must be located and observed.

Adalja AA et al. Clinical management of potential bioterrorism-related conditions. N Engl J Med. 2015 Mar 5;372(10):954–62. [PMID: 25738671]

Schulte M et al. Effective and rapid treatment of wound botulism, a case report. BMC Surg. 2017 Oct 26;17(1):103. [PMID: 29073888]

ANTHRAX

ESSENTIALS OF DIAGNOSIS

▶ Epidemiologic setting: exposure to animals or animal hides or potential exposure from bioterrorism.

▶ A painless cutaneous black eschar on exposed skin, with marked surrounding edema and vesicles.

▶ Nonspecific flu-like symptoms that rapidly progress to extreme dyspnea and shock; mediastinal widening and pleural effusions on chest radiograph.

▶ General Considerations

Naturally occurring anthrax is a disease of sheep, cattle, horses, goats, and swine. *Bacillus anthracis* is a gram-positive spore-forming aerobic rod. Spores—not vegetative bacteria—are the infectious form of the organism. These are transmitted to humans from contact with contaminated animals, animal products, or animal hides, or from soil by inoculation of broken skin or mucous membranes; by inhalation of aerosolized spores; or, rarely, by ingestion resulting in cutaneous, inhalational, or gastrointestinal forms of anthrax, respectively. Inhalation of aerosolized spores that were deliberately placed in the mail as an act of bioterrorism occurred in the United States in 2001. Spores germinate into vegetative bacteria that multiply locally in cutaneous and gastrointestinal anthrax but may also disseminate to cause systemic infection. Inhaled spores are ingested by pulmonary macrophages and carried via lymphatics to regional lymph nodes, where they germinate. The bacteria rapidly multiply within the lymphatics, causing a hemorrhagic lymphadenitis. Invasion of the bloodstream leads to overwhelming sepsis, killing the host.

▶ Clinical Findings

A. Symptoms and Signs

1. Cutaneous anthrax—This occurs within 2 weeks after exposure to spores; there is no latency period for cutaneous disease as there is with inhalational anthrax. The initial lesion is an erythematous papule, often on an exposed area of skin that vesiculates and then ulcerates and undergoes necrosis, ultimately progressing to a purple to black eschar. The eschar typically is painless; pain indicates secondary bacterial infection. The surrounding area is edematous and vesicular but not purulent. Regional adenopathy, fever, malaise, headache, and nausea and vomiting may be present. The infection is self-limited in most cases, but hematogenous spread with sepsis or meningitis may occur.

2. Inhalational anthrax—Illness occurs in two stages, beginning on average 10 days after exposure, but may have a latent onset 6 weeks after exposure. Nonspecific viral-like symptoms such as fever, malaise, headache, dyspnea, cough, and congestion of the nose, throat, and larynx are characteristic of the initial stage. Anterior chest pain is an early symptom of mediastinitis. Within hours to a few days, progression to the fulminant stage of infection occurs in which symptoms or signs of overwhelming sepsis predominate. Delirium, obtundation, or findings of meningeal irritation suggest an accompanying hemorrhagic meningitis.

3. Gastrointestinal anthrax—Fever, diffuse abdominal pain, rebound abdominal tenderness, vomiting, constipation, and diarrhea occur 2–5 days after ingestion of food products contaminated with anthrax spores. The primary lesion is ulcerative, producing emesis that may be blood-tinged or coffee-grounds and stool that may be blood-tinged or melenic. Bowel perforation can occur. The oropharyngeal form of the disease is characterized by local lymphadenopathy, cervical edema, dysphagia, and upper respiratory tract obstruction.

B. Laboratory Findings

Laboratory findings are nonspecific. The white blood cell count initially may be normal or modestly elevated, with polymorphonuclear predominance and an increase in immature forms. Pleural fluid from patients with inhalational anthrax is typically hemorrhagic with few white cells. Cerebrospinal fluid from meningitis cases is also hemorrhagic. Gram stain of pleural fluid, cerebrospinal fluid, unspun blood, blood culture, or fluid from a cutaneous lesion may show the characteristic boxcar-shaped encapsulated rods in chains.

The diagnosis is established by isolation of the organism from culture of the skin lesion (or fluid expressed from it), blood, or pleural fluid—or cerebrospinal fluid in cases of meningitis. In the absence of prior antimicrobial therapy, cultures are invariably positive. Cultures obtained after initiation of antimicrobial therapy may be negative. If anthrax is suspected on clinical or epidemiologic grounds, immunohistochemical tests (eg, to detect capsular antigen), polymerase chain reaction assays, and serologic tests (useful for documenting past cutaneous infection) are available through the CDC and should be used to establish the diagnosis. Any suspected case of anthrax should be immediately reported to the CDC so that an investigation can be conducted.

C. Imaging

The chest radiograph is the most sensitive test for inhalational disease, being abnormal (though the findings can be subtle) initially in every case of bioterrorism-associated disease. Mediastinal widening due to hemorrhagic lymphadenitis, a hallmark feature of the disease, was present in 70% of the bioterrorism-related cases. Pleural effusions were present initially or occurred over the course of illness in all cases, and approximately three-fourths had pulmonary infiltrates or signs of consolidation.

▶ Differential Diagnosis

Cutaneous anthrax, despite its characteristic appearance, can be confused with a variety of other also uncommon or rare conditions such as ecthyma gangrenosum, rat-bite fever, ulceroglandular tularemia, plague, glanders, rickettsialpox, orf (parapoxvirus infection), or cutaneous mycobacterial infection. Inhalational anthrax must be differentiated from mediastinitis due to other bacterial causes, fibrous mediastinitis due to histoplasmosis, coccidioidomycosis, atypical or viral pneumonia, silicosis, sarcoidosis, and other causes of mediastinal widening (eg, superior vena cava syndrome or aortic aneurysm or dissection). Gastrointestinal anthrax shares clinical features with a variety of common intra-abdominal disorders, including bowel obstruction, perforated viscus, peritonitis, gastroenteritis, and peptic ulcer disease.

▶ Treatment

Strains of *B anthracis* (including the strain isolated in the bioterrorism cases) are susceptible in vitro to penicillin, amoxicillin, chloramphenicol, clindamycin, imipenem, doxycycline, ciprofloxacin (as well as other fluoroquinolones), macrolides, rifampin, and vancomycin. *B anthracis* may express beta-lactamases that confer resistance to cephalosporins and penicillins. For this reason, penicillin or amoxicillin is not recommended for use as a single agent in treatment of disseminated disease. Based on results of animal experiments and because of concern for engineered drug resistance in strains of *B anthracis* used in bioterrorism, ciprofloxacin is considered the drug of choice for treatment and for prophylaxis following exposure to anthrax spores. Other fluoroquinolones with activity against gram-positive bacteria (eg, levofloxacin, moxifloxacin) are likely to be just as effective as ciprofloxacin. Doxycycline is an alternative first-line agent. Combination therapy with at least one additional agent is recommended for inhalational or disseminated disease and in cutaneous infection involving the face, head, and neck or associated with extensive local edema or systemic signs of infection, eg, fever, tachycardia, and elevated white blood cell count. Single-drug therapy is recommended for prophylaxis following exposure to spores.

The required duration of therapy is poorly defined. In naturally occurring disease, treatment for 7–10 days for cutaneous disease and for at least 2 weeks following clinical response for disseminated, inhalational, or gastrointestinal infection have been standard recommendations. Because of concern about relapse from latent spores acquired by inhalation of aerosol in bioterrorism-associated cases, the initial recommendation was treatment for 60 days.

Several monoclonal antibodies are FDA approved as adjunctive treatments for inhalation anthrax. Raxibacumab is a human monoclonal antibody directed against the protective antigen component of lethal toxin and is used for treatment of inhalation anthrax in combination with recommended antibacterial treatments. Obiltoxaximab is another toxin-targeting monoclonal antibody and is given in combination with antibacterial drugs. A vaccine is also available for postexposure prophylaxis (and preexposure prophylaxis). This vaccine is administered at 0, 2, and 4 weeks postexposure combined with antimicrobial therapy.

▶ Prevention

In 2001, the CDC offered one of two options for postal workers receiving prophylaxis for exposure to contaminated mail: (1) antibiotics for 100 days (fearing that even with 60 days of treatment late relapses might occur) or (2) vaccination with an investigative agent (three doses administered over a 1-month period) in conjunction with 40 days of antibiotic administration to cover the time required for a protective antibody response to develop. Insufficient information exists to favor one recommendation over the other.

An FDA-approved vaccine is available for persons at high risk for exposure to anthrax spores. The vaccine is cell-free antigen prepared from an attenuated strain of *B anthracis*. Multiple injections over 18 months and an annual booster dose are required to achieve and maintain protection. Existing supplies have been reserved for vaccination of military personnel. Raxibacumab and obiltoxaximab are approved for prevention of inhalation anthrax when other treatments are not available or appropriate.

▶ Prognosis

The prognosis in cutaneous infection is excellent. Death is unlikely if the infection has remained localized, and lesions heal without complications in most cases. By contrast, the reported mortality rate for gastrointestinal and inhalational infections is up to 85%. Yet, the experience with bioterrorism-associated inhalational cases in which six of eleven victims survived suggests a somewhat better outcome with modern supportive care and antibiotics provided that treatment is initiated before the patient has progressed to the fulminant stage of disease. No cases of anthrax have occurred among the several thousand individuals receiving antimicrobial prophylaxis following exposure to spores.

Adalja AA et al. Clinical management of potential bioterrorism-related conditions. N Engl J Med. 2015 Mar 5;372(10):954–62. [PMID: 25738671]

Bower WA et al; Centers for Disease Control and Prevention (CDC). Clinical framework and medical countermeasure use during an anthrax mass-casualty incident. MMWR Recomm Rep. 2015 Dec 4;64(4):1–22. [PMID: 26632963]

Hou AW et al. Obiltoxaximab: adding to the treatment arsenal for *Bacillus anthracis* infection. Ann Pharmacother. 2017 Oct; 51(10):908–13. [PMID: 28573869]

DIPHTHERIA

ESSENTIALS OF DIAGNOSIS

▶ Tenacious gray membrane at portal of entry in pharynx.

▶ Sore throat, nasal discharge, hoarseness, fever.

▶ Myocarditis, neuropathy.

▶ Culture confirms the diagnosis.

General Considerations

Diphtheria is an acute infection caused by *Corynebacterium diphtheriae* that usually attacks the respiratory tract but may involve any mucous membrane or skin wound. The organism is spread chiefly by respiratory secretions. Exotoxin produced by the organism is responsible for myocarditis and neuropathy.

Clinical Findings

A. Symptoms and Signs

Nasal, laryngeal, pharyngeal, and cutaneous forms of diphtheria occur. Nasal infection produces few symptoms other than a nasal discharge. Laryngeal infection may lead to upper airway and bronchial obstruction. In pharyngeal diphtheria, the most common form, a tenacious gray membrane covers the tonsils and pharynx. Mild sore throat, fever, and malaise are followed by toxemia and prostration.

Myocarditis and neuropathy are the most common and most serious complications. Myocarditis causes cardiac arrhythmias, heart block, and heart failure. The neuropathy usually involves the cranial nerves first, producing diplopia, slurred speech, and difficulty in swallowing.

B. Laboratory Findings

The diagnosis is made clinically but can be confirmed by culture of the organism.

Differential Diagnosis

Diphtheria must be differentiated from streptococcal pharyngitis, infectious mononucleosis, adenovirus or herpes simplex infection, Vincent angina, pharyngitis due to *Arcanobacterium haemolyticum*, and candidiasis. A presumptive diagnosis of diphtheria should be made on clinical grounds without waiting for laboratory verification, since emergency treatment is needed.

Prevention

Active immunization with diphtheria toxoid is part of routine childhood immunization with appropriate booster injections. The immunization schedule for adults is the same as for tetanus (see Table 30–7). Women should receive Tdap with each pregnancy, preferably between 27 and 36 weeks.

Susceptible persons exposed to diphtheria should receive a booster dose of diphtheria toxoid (or a complete series if previously unimmunized), as well as a course of penicillin or erythromycin.

Treatment

Removal of membrane by direct laryngoscopy or bronchoscopy may be necessary to prevent or alleviate airway obstruction. Antitoxin, which is prepared from horse serum, must be given in all cases when diphtheria is suspected. For mild early pharyngeal or laryngeal disease, the dose is 20,000–40,000 units; for moderate nasopharyngeal disease, 40,000–60,000 units; for severe, extensive, or late (3 days or more) disease, 80,000–100,000 units. Diphtheria equine antitoxin can be obtained from the CDC.

Either penicillin, 250 mg orally four times daily, or erythromycin, 500 mg orally four times daily, for 14 days is effective therapy, although erythromycin is slightly more effective in eliminating the carrier state. Azithromycin or clarithromycin is probably as effective as erythromycin. The patient should be isolated until three consecutive cultures at the completion of therapy have documented elimination of the organism from the oropharynx. Contacts to a case should receive erythromycin, 500 mg orally four times daily for 7 days, to eradicate carriage.

Liang JL et al. Prevention of pertussis, tetanus, and diphtheria with vaccines in the United States: recommendations of the Advisory Committee on Immunization Practices (ACIP). MMWR Recomm Rep. 2018 Apr 27;67(2):1–44. [PMID: 29702631]

McMillan M et al. Safety of tetanus, diphtheria, and pertussis vaccination during pregnancy: a systematic review. Obstet Gynecol. 2017 Mar;129(3):560–73. [PMID: 28178054]

LISTERIOSIS

ESSENTIALS OF DIAGNOSIS

▶ Ingestion of contaminated food product.

▶ Undifferentiated fever in a pregnant woman in her third trimester.

▶ Altered mental status and fever in an elderly or immunocompromised patient.

▶ Obtain blood and cerebrospinal fluid cultures to confirm the diagnosis.

General Considerations

Listeria monocytogenes is a facultative, motile, gram-positive rod that is capable of invading several cell types and causes intracellular infection. Most cases of infection caused by *L monocytogenes* are sporadic, but outbreaks have been traced to eating contaminated food, including unpasteurized dairy products, hot dogs, delicatessen meats, cantaloupes, and ricotta cheese. Outbreaks have been associated with significant morbidity and mortality in infected persons.

▶ Clinical Findings

Five types of infection are recognized:

(1) **Infection during pregnancy**, usually in the last trimester, is a mild febrile illness without an apparent primary focus and may resolve without specific therapy. However, approximately one in five pregnancies complicated by listeriosis result in spontaneous abortion or stillbirth and surviving infants are at risk for clinical neonatal listeriosis.

(2) **Granulomatosis infantisepticum** is a neonatal infection acquired in utero, characterized by disseminated abscesses, granulomas, and a high mortality rate.

(3) **Bacteremia** with or without sepsis syndrome is an infection of neonates or immunocompromised adults. The presentation is of a febrile illness without a recognized source.

(4) **Meningitis** caused by *L monocytogenes* affects infants under 2 months of age as well as older adults, ranking third after pneumococcus and meningococcus as common causes of bacterial meningitis. Cerebrospinal fluid shows a *neutrophilic* pleocytosis. Adults with meningitis are often immunocompromised, and cases have been associated with HIV infection and therapy with tumor necrosis factor (TNF) inhibitors such as infliximab.

(5) **Focal infections**, including adenitis, brain abscess, endocarditis, osteomyelitis, and arthritis, occur rarely.

▶ Prevention

At-risk patients (eg, pregnant women) should avoid unpasteurized milk products. Smoked seafoods, cold cuts, hot dogs, and meat spreads also carry risk. Thoroughly cook animal source food and wash raw vegetables.

▶ Treatment

Ampicillin, 8–12 g/day intravenously in four to six divided doses (the higher dose for meningitis), is considered the treatment of choice. Gentamicin, 5 mg/kg/day intravenously once or in divided doses, is synergistic with ampicillin against *Listeria* in vitro and in animal models, and the use of combination therapy may be considered during the first few days of treatment to enhance eradication of organisms. In patients with penicillin allergies, trimethoprim-sulfamethoxazole has excellent intracellular and cerebrospinal fluid penetration and is considered an appropriate alternative. The dose is 10–20 mg/kg/day intravenously of the trimethoprim component. Mortality and morbidity rates still are high. Therapy should be administered for at least 2–3 weeks. Longer durations—between 3 and 6 weeks—have been recommended for treatment of meningitis, especially in immunocompromised persons.

Jackson BR et al; Centers for Disease Control and Prevention (CDC). Notes from the field: listeriosis associated with stone fruit—United States, 2014. MMWR Morb Mortal Wkly Rep. 2015 Mar 20;64(10):282–3. [PMID: 25789745]

Madjunkov M et al. Listeriosis during pregnancy. Arch Gynecol Obstet. 2017 Aug;296(2):143–52. [PMID: 28536811]
Salama PJ et al. Learning from listeria: safer food for all. Lancet. 2018 Jun 9;391(10137):2305–6. [PMID: 29900862]

INFECTIVE ENDOCARDITIS

ESSENTIALS OF DIAGNOSIS

- ▶ Fever.
- ▶ Preexisting organic heart lesion.
- ▶ Positive blood cultures.
- ▶ Evidence of vegetation on echocardiography.
- ▶ Evidence of systemic emboli.

▶ General Considerations

Endocarditis is a bacterial or fungal infection of the valvular or endocardial surface of the heart. The clinical presentation depends on the infecting organism and the valve or valves that are infected. More virulent organisms—*S aureus* in particular—tend to produce a more rapidly progressive and destructive infection. Endocarditis caused by more virulent organisms often presents as an acute febrile illnesses and is complicated by early embolization, acute valvular regurgitation, and myocardial abscess formation. Viridans strains of streptococci, enterococci, other bacteria, yeasts, and fungi tend to cause a more subacute picture.

Predisposing valvular abnormalities include rheumatic involvement of any valve, bicuspid aortic valves, calcific or sclerotic aortic valves, hypertrophic subaortic stenosis, mitral valve prolapse, and a variety of congenital disorders such as ventricular septal defect, tetralogy of Fallot, coarctation of the aorta, or patent ductus arteriosus. Rheumatic disease is no longer the major predisposing factor in developed countries. Regurgitation lesions are more susceptible than stenotic ones.

The initiating event in native valve endocarditis is colonization of the valve by bacteria or yeast that gain access to the bloodstream. Transient bacteremia is common during dental, upper respiratory, urologic, and lower gastrointestinal diagnostic and surgical procedures. It is less common during upper gastrointestinal and gynecologic procedures. Intravascular devices are increasingly implicated as a portal of access of microorganisms into the bloodstream. A large proportion of cases of *S aureus* endocarditis are attributable to health care–associated bacteremia.

Native valve endocarditis is usually caused by *S aureus*, viridans streptococci, enterococci, or HACEK organisms (an acronym for *Haemophilus aphrophilus* [now *Aggregatibacter aphrophilus*], *Actinobacillus actinomycetemcomitans* [now *Aggregatibacter actinomycetemcomitans*], *Cardiobacterium hominis*, *Eikenella corrodens*, and *Kingella* species). Streptococcal species formerly accounted for the majority of native valve endocarditis cases; *S aureus* is now the leading cause. Gram-negative organisms and fungi account for a small percentage.

In injection drug users, *S aureus* accounts for over 60% of all endocarditis cases and for 80–90% of cases in which the tricuspid valve is infected. Enterococci and streptococci comprise the balance in about equal proportions. Gram-negative aerobic bacilli, fungi, and unusual organisms may cause endocarditis in injection drug users.

The microbiology of **prosthetic valve endocarditis** also is distinctive. Early infections (ie, those occurring within 2 months after valve implantation) are commonly caused by staphylococci—both coagulase-positive and coagulase-negative—gram-negative organisms, and fungi. In late prosthetic valve endocarditis, streptococci are commonly identified, although coagulase-negative and coagulase-positive staphylococci still cause many cases.

▶ Clinical Findings

A. Symptoms and Signs

Virtually all patients have fever at some point in the illness, although it may be very low grade (less than 38°C) in elderly individuals and in patients with heart failure or kidney failure. Rarely, there may be no fever at all.

The duration of illness typically is a few days to a few weeks. Nonspecific symptoms are common. The initial symptoms and signs of endocarditis may be caused by direct arterial, valvular, or cardiac damage. Although a changing regurgitant murmur is significant diagnostically, it is the exception rather than the rule. Symptoms also may occur as a result of embolization, metastatic infection or immunologically mediated phenomena. These include cough; dyspnea; arthralgias or arthritis; diarrhea; and abdominal, back, or flank pain.

The characteristic peripheral lesions—petechiae (on the palate or conjunctiva or beneath the fingernails), sub-ungual ("splinter") hemorrhages (Figure 33–4), Osler nodes (painful, violaceous raised lesions of the fingers, toes, or feet) (Figure 33–5), Janeway lesions (painless erythematous lesions of the palms or soles), and Roth spots (exudative lesions in the retina)—occur in about 25% of patients. Strokes and major systemic embolic events are present in about 25% of patients and tend to occur before or within the first week of antimicrobial therapy. Hematuria and proteinuria may result from emboli or immunologically mediated glomerulonephritis, which can cause kidney dysfunction.

B. Imaging

Chest radiograph may show evidence for the underlying cardiac abnormality and, in right-sided endocarditis, pulmonary infiltrates. The electrocardiogram is nondiagnostic, but new conduction abnormalities suggest myocardial abscess formation. Echocardiography is useful in identifying vegetations and other characteristic features suspicious for endocarditis and may provide adjunctive information about the specific valve or valves that are infected. The sensitivity of transthoracic echocardiography is between 55% and 65%; it cannot reliably rule out endocarditis but may confirm a clinical suspicion. Transesophageal echocardiography is 90% sensitive in detecting vegetations and

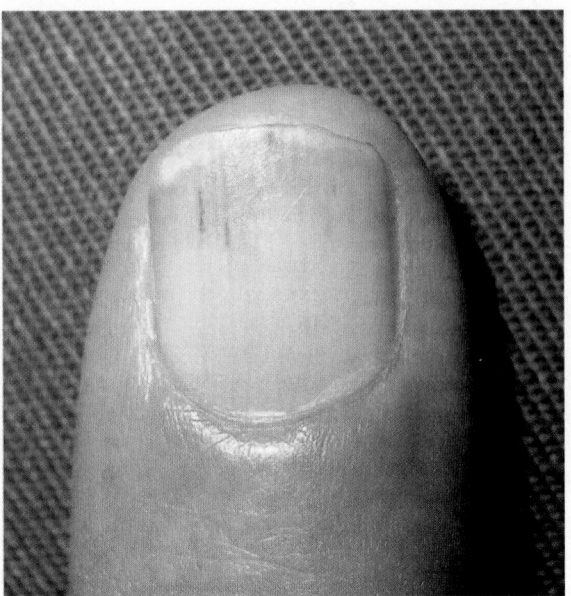

▲ **Figure 33–4.** Splinter hemorrhages appearing as red lineal streaks under the nail plate and within the nail bed, in endocarditis, psoriasis, and trauma. (Reproduced, with permission, from Richard P. Usatine, MD.)

is particularly useful for identifying valve ring abscesses as well as prosthetic valve endocarditis.

C. Diagnostic Studies

1. Blood cultures—Three sets of blood cultures are recommended before starting antibiotics to maximize microbiologic diagnosis. To maximize the yield of blood cultures, adequate volume is important. Each culture bottle should be filled with 10 mL of blood since half of adults have less than 1 colony forming unit of bacteria per mL blood. The yield of bacteria may be up to 5% higher for every additional milliliter collected. Optimal yield is with two or three sets of cultures from different sites. There is no difference in yield if blood is collected simultaneously or several hours apart.

Approximately 5% of cases will be culture-negative, usually attributable to administration of antimicrobials prior to cultures. If antimicrobial therapy has been administered prior to obtaining cultures and the patient is clinically stable, it is reasonable to withhold antimicrobial therapy for 2–3 days so that appropriate cultures can be obtained. Culture-negative endocarditis may also be due to organisms that require special media for growth (eg, *Legionella*, *Bartonella*, *Abiotrophia* species, formerly referred to as nutritionally deficient streptococci), organisms that do not grow on artificial media (*Tropheryma whipplei*, or pathogens of Q fever or psittacosis), or those that may require prolonged incubation (eg, *Brucella*, anaerobes, HACEK organisms). *Bartonella quintana* is an important cause of culture-negative endocarditis.

2. Modified Duke criteria—The Modified Duke criteria are useful for the diagnosis of endocarditis. Major criteria met. If fewer criteria are found, or a sound alternative explanation for illness is identified, or the patient's febrile illness has resolved within 4 days, endocarditis is unlikely.

Complications

The course of infective endocarditis is determined by the degree of damage to the heart, by the site of infection (right-sided versus left-sided, aortic versus mitral valve), by the presence of metastatic foci of infection, by the occurrence of embolization, and by immunologically mediated processes. Destruction of infected heart valves is especially common and precipitous with *S aureus*, but can occur with any organism and can progress even after bacteriologic cure. The infection can also extend into the myocardium, resulting in abscesses leading to conduction disturbances, and involving the wall of the aorta, creating sinus of Valsalva aneurysms.

Peripheral embolization to the brain and myocardium may result in infarctions. Embolization to the spleen and kidneys is also common. Peripheral emboli may initiate metastatic infections or may become established in vessel walls, leading to mycotic aneurysms. Right-sided endocarditis, which usually involves the tricuspid valve, causes septic pulmonary emboli, occasionally with infarction and lung abscesses.

Prevention

The American Heart Association recommends antibiotic prophylaxis for infective endocarditis in a relatively small group of patients with predisposing congenital or valvular anomalies (Table 33–3) undergoing select dental procedures, operations involving the respiratory tract, or operations of infected skin, skin structure, or musculoskeletal

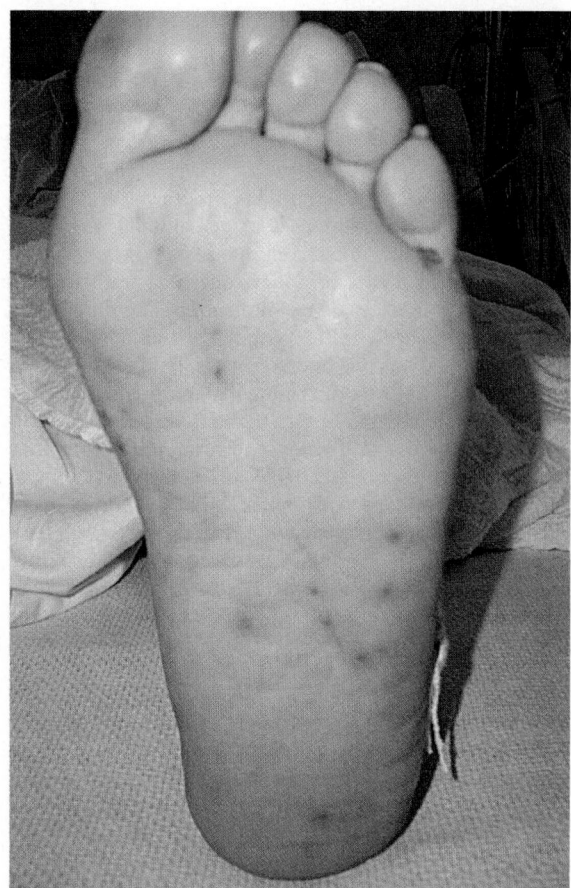

▲ **Figure 33–5.** Osler node causing pain within the pulp of the big toe and multiple painless flat Janeway lesions over the sole of the foot. (Used, with permission, from David A. Kasper, DO, MBA, in Usatine RP, Smith MA, Mayeaux EJ Jr, Chumley H, Tysinger J. *The Color Atlas of Family Medicine.* McGraw-Hill, 2009.)

include (1) two positive blood cultures for a microorganism that typically causes infective endocarditis or persistent bacteremia, or a single positive blood culture for *Coxiella burnetii* or anti–phase 1 IgG antibody titer greater than or equal to 1:800; and (2) evidence of endocardial involvement documented by echocardiography showing definite vegetation, myocardial abscess, new partial dehiscence of a prosthetic valve, or new valvular regurgitation (increase or change in murmur is not sufficient). Minor criteria include the presence of a predisposing condition; fever of 38°C or higher; vascular phenomena, such as cutaneous hemorrhages, aneurysm, systemic emboli, or pulmonary infarction; immunologic phenomena, such as glomerulonephritis, Osler nodes, Roth spots, or rheumatoid factor; and positive blood cultures not meeting the major criteria or serologic evidence of an active infection. A definite diagnosis can be made with 80% accuracy if two major criteria, one major criterion and three minor criteria, or five minor criteria are fulfilled. A possible diagnosis of endocarditis is made if one major and one minor criterion or three minor criteria are

Table 33–3. Cardiac conditions with high risk of adverse outcomes from endocarditis for which prophylaxis with dental procedures is recommended.[1,2]

Prosthetic cardiac valve
Previous infective endocarditis
Congenital heart disease (CHD)[3]
Unrepaired cyanotic CHD, including palliative shunts and conduits
Completely repaired congenital heart defect with prosthetic material or device, whether placed by surgery or by catheter intervention, during the first 6 months after the procedure[4]
Repaired CHD with residual defects at the site or adjacent to the site of a prosthetic patch or prosthetic device
Cardiac transplantation recipients in whom cardiac valvulopathy develops

[1]Reproduced, with permission, from Wilson W et al. Prevention of infective endocarditis. Circulation. 2007 Oct 9;116(15):1736–54. Copyright © 2007 American Heart Association, Inc.
[2]See Table 33–5 for prophylactic regimens.
[3]Except for the conditions listed above, antibiotic prophylaxis is no longer recommended for other forms of CHD.
[4]Prophylaxis is recommended because endothelialization of prosthetic material occurs within 6 months after procedure.

Table 33–4. Recommendations for administration of bacterial endocarditis prophylaxis for patients according to type of procedure.[1]

Prophylaxis Recommended	Prophylaxis Not Recommended
Dental procedures All dental procedures that involve manipulation of gingival tissue or the periapical region of the teeth or perforation of the oral mucosa **Respiratory tract procedures** Only respiratory tract procedures that involve incision of the respiratory mucosa **Procedures on infected skin, skin structure, or musculoskeletal tissue**	**Dental procedures** Routine anesthetic injections through noninfected tissue, taking dental radiographs, placement of removable prosthodontic or orthodontic appliances, adjustment of orthodontic appliances, placement of orthodontic brackets, shedding of deciduous teeth, and bleeding from trauma to the lips or oral mucosa **Gastrointestinal tract procedures** **Genitourinary tract procedures**

[1]Reproduced, with permission, from Wilson W et al. Prevention of infective endocarditis. Circulation. 2007 Oct 9;116(15):1736–54. Copyright © 2007 American Heart Association, Inc.

tissue (Table 33–4). Current antimicrobial recommendations are given in Table 33–5.

▶ **Treatment**

Empiric regimens for endocarditis while culture results are pending should include agents active against staphylococci, streptococci, and enterococci. Vancomycin 1 g every 12 hours intravenously plus ceftriaxone 2 g every 24 hours provides appropriate coverage pending definitive diagnosis; consultation with an infectious disease expert is strongly recommended when initiating treatment.

A. Viridans Streptococci

For penicillin-susceptible viridans streptococcal endocarditis (ie, MIC 0.1 mcg/mL or less), penicillin G, 18 million units intravenously either continuously or in four to six equally divided doses, or ceftriaxone, 2 g intravenously once daily for 4 weeks, is recommended. The duration of therapy can be shortened to 2 weeks if gentamicin, 3 mg/kg intravenously every 24 hours, is used with penicillin or ceftriaxone. The 2-week regimen is reasonable and can be considered in patients with uncomplicated endocarditis, rapid response to therapy, and no underlying kidney disease. For the patient unable to tolerate penicillin or ceftriaxone, vancomycin, 15 mg/kg intravenously every 12 hours for 4 weeks, is given with a desired trough level of 10–15 mcg/mL. Prosthetic valve endocarditis is treated with a 6-week course of penicillin or ceftriaxone and the clinician can consider adding 2 weeks of gentamicin at the start of therapy.

Viridans streptococci relatively resistant to penicillin (ie, MIC greater than 0.12 mcg/mL but less than or equal to 0.5 mcg/mL) should be treated for 4 weeks. Penicillin G, 24 million units intravenously either continuously or in four to six equally divided doses, is combined with gentamicin, 3 mg/kg intravenously every 24 hours for the first 2 weeks. Ceftriaxone may be a reasonable alternative treatment option for isolates that are susceptible to ceftriaxone. In the patient with IgE-mediated allergy to penicillin, vancomycin alone, 15 mg/kg intravenously every 12 hours for 4 weeks, should be administered. Prosthetic valve endocarditis

Table 33–5. American Heart Association recommendations for endocarditis prophylaxis for dental procedures for patients with cardiac conditions.[1–3]

Oral	Amoxicillin	2 g 1 hour before procedure
Penicillin allergy	Clindamycin	600 mg 1 hour before procedure
	or	
	Cephalexin	2 g 1 hour before procedure (contraindicated if there is history of a beta-lactam immediate hypersensitivity reaction)
	or	
	Azithromycin or clarithromycin	500 mg 1 hour before procedure
Parenteral	Ampicillin	2 g intramuscularly or intravenously 30 minutes before procedure
Penicillin allergy	Clindamycin	600 mg intravenously 1 hour before procedure
	or	
	Cefazolin	1 g intramuscularly or intravenously 30 minutes before procedure (contraindicated if there is history of a beta-lactam immediate hypersensitivity reaction)

[1]Data from the American Heart Association. Circulation. 2007 Oct 9;116(15):1736–54.
[2]For patients undergoing respiratory tract procedures involving incision of respiratory tract mucosa to treat an established infection or a procedure on infected skin, skin structure, or musculoskeletal tissue known or suspected to be caused by S aureus, the regimen should contain an anti-staphylococcal penicillin or cephalosporin. Vancomycin can be used to treat patients unable to tolerate a beta-lactam or if the infection is known or suspected to be caused by a methicillin-resistant strain of S aureus.
[3]See Table 33–3 for list of cardiac conditions.

is treated with a 6-week course of penicillin or ceftriaxone plus gentamicin as above.

Endocarditis caused by viridans streptococci with an MIC greater than 0.5 mcg/mL or by nutritionally deficient streptococci should be treated the same as enterococcal endocarditis.

B. Other Streptococci

Endocarditis caused by *S pneumoniae, S pyogenes* (group A streptococcus), or groups B, C, and G streptococci is unusual. *S pneumoniae* sensitive to penicillin (MIC less than 0.1 mcg/mL) can be treated with penicillin 18 million units intravenously either continuously or in four to six equally divided doses or cefazolin 6 g intravenously either continuously or in three equally divided doses, or ceftriaxone 2 g daily intravenously for 4 weeks. High-dose penicillin (24 million units) or a third-generation cephalosporin may be required for the treatment of endocarditis (without meningitis) caused by strains resistant to penicillin (MIC greater than 0.1 mcg/mL). The addition of vancomycin and rifampin to ceftriaxone may be considered in patients with *S pneumoniae* strains with cefotaxime MIC greater than 2 mcg/mL. Group A streptococcal infection can be treated with penicillin or ceftriaxone for 4–6 weeks. Groups B, C, and G streptococci tend to be more resistant to penicillin than group A streptococci, and some experts have recommended adding gentamicin, 3 mg/kg intravenously every 24 hours, to penicillin for the first 2 weeks of a 4- to 6-week course. Endocarditis caused by *S gallolyticus (bovis)* is associated with liver disease, especially cirrhosis, and gastrointestinal abnormalities, especially colon cancer. Colonoscopy should be performed to exclude the latter.

C. Enterococci

For enterococcal endocarditis, penicillin or ampicillin alone is inadequate. One recommended regimen is ampicillin, 2 g intravenously every 4 hours, or penicillin G, 18–30 million units intravenously continuously or in six equally divided doses plus gentamicin, 1 mg/kg intravenously every 8 hours. The second recommended regimen is ampicillin (2 g intravenously every 4 hours) plus ceftriaxone 2 g intravenously every 12 hours. The recommended duration of therapy is 4–6 weeks (the longer duration for patients with symptoms for more than 3 months, relapse, or prosthetic valve endocarditis). The combination of ampicillin plus ceftriaxone is recommended for patients with creatinine clearance less than 50 mL/min or whose enterococcal isolates are resistant to gentamicin. In patients intolerant of penicillin and ampicillin or who have enterococcal isolate resistant to these agents, vancomycin plus gentamicin can be used.

Endocarditis caused by strains resistant to penicillin and vancomycin are difficult to treat and should always be managed in consultation with an infectious diseases specialist.

D. Staphylococci

For methicillin-susceptible *S aureus* isolates, nafcillin or oxacillin, 12 g intravenously daily given continuously or in four to six divided doses or cefazolin, 6 g intravenously daily given continuously or in three divided doses for 6 weeks, is the preferred therapy. In cases of brain abscess resulting from methicillin-susceptible *S aureus* endocarditis, nafcillin should be used instead of cefazolin. For patients with history of immediate type hypersensitivity to beta-lactams, a desensitization protocol should be undertaken. For patients with a history of nonanaphylactoid reactions to penicillins, cefazolin should be used. Patients who are infected with methicillin-resistant *S aureus* or who are unable to tolerate beta-lactam therapy should receive vancomycin, 30 mg/kg/day intravenously divided in two or three doses, to achieve a goal trough level of 15–20 mcg/kg, or daptomycin intravenously at greater than or equal to 8 mg/kg/day. Aminoglycoside combination regimens are not recommended. The effect of rifampin with antistaphylococcal drugs is variable, and its routine use is not recommended.

Because coagulase-negative staphylococci—a common cause of prosthetic valve endocarditis—are routinely resistant to methicillin, beta-lactam antibiotics should not be used for this infection unless the isolate is demonstrated to be susceptible. A combination of vancomycin, 30 mg/kg/day intravenously divided in two or three doses for 6 weeks; rifampin, 300 mg every 8 hours for 6 weeks; and gentamicin, 3 mg/kg intravenously every 8 hours for the first 2 weeks, is recommended for prosthetic valve infection. If the organism is sensitive to methicillin, either nafcillin or oxacillin or cefazolin can be used in combination with rifampin and gentamicin. Combination therapy with nafcillin or oxacillin (vancomycin or daptomycin for methicillin-resistant strains), rifampin, and gentamicin is also recommended for treatment of *S aureus* prosthetic valve infection.

E. HACEK Organisms

HACEK organisms are slow-growing, fastidious gram-negative coccobacilli or bacilli (*H aphrophilus* [now *A aphrophilus*], *A actinomycetemcomitans, C hominis, E corrodens,* and *Kingella* species) that are normal oral flora and cause less than 5% of all cases of endocarditis. They may produce beta-lactamase, and thus the treatment of choice is ceftriaxone (or another third-generation cephalosporin), 2 g intravenously once daily for 4 weeks. Prosthetic valve endocarditis should be treated for 6 weeks. In the penicillin-allergic patient, experience is limited, but fluoroquinolones have in vitro activity and should be considered.

F. Culture-Negative Endocarditis

Failure to culture microorganisms from patients with suspected infective endocarditis may be due to infection from organisms not recovered in routine microbiology testing or previous administration of antimicrobial agents before blood cultures were obtained. These cases must be managed with the assistance of an infectious disease specialist. Pathogens that are not able to be cultured by commonly used techniques include *Bartonella* species, *Chlamydia* species, *Brucella* species, and *Tropheryma whipplei.* Serologic testing should be performed in patients who have epidemiologic risk factors for these infections. Treatment should be directed at likely pathogens while awaiting serologic results; treatment of patients given prior antimicrobials before cultures were obtained must also consider likely pathogens.

G. Role of Surgery

While many cases can be successfully treated medically, operative management is frequently required. Acute heart failure unresponsive to medical therapy is an indication for valve replacement even if active infection is present. Infections unresponsive to appropriate antimicrobial therapy after 7–10 days (ie, persistent fevers, positive blood cultures despite therapy) are more likely to be eradicated if the valve is replaced. Surgery is nearly always required for cure of fungal endocarditis and is more often necessary with highly resistant bacteria. It is also indicated when the infection involves the sinus of Valsalva or produces septal abscesses. Recurrent infection with the same organism prompts an operative approach, especially with infected prosthetic valves. Continuing embolization presents a difficult problem when the infection is otherwise responding; surgery may be the proper approach. Particularly challenging is a large and fragile vegetation demonstrated by echocardiography in the absence of embolization. Most clinicians favor an operative approach with vegetectomy and valve repair if the patient is a good candidate. Operation without delay may be considered in patients with endocarditis and an ischemic stroke who have an indication for surgery. If not urgent or if intracranial hemorrhage is present, a delay of at least 4 weeks should be considered. Embolization after bacteriologic cure does not necessarily imply recurrence of endocarditis.

H. Role of Anticoagulation

Anticoagulation is contraindicated in native valve endocarditis because of an increased risk of intracerebral hemorrhage from mycotic aneurysms or embolic phenomena. The role of anticoagulant therapy during prosthetic valve endocarditis is more controversial. Reversal of anticoagulation may result in thrombosis of the mechanical prosthesis, particularly in the mitral position. Conversely, anticoagulation during active prosthetic valve endocarditis caused by *S aureus* has been associated with fatal intracerebral hemorrhage. One approach is to discontinue anticoagulation during the septic phase of *S aureus* prosthetic valve endocarditis. In patients with *S aureus* prosthetic valve endocarditis complicated by a CNS embolic event, anticoagulation should be discontinued for the first 2 weeks of therapy. Indications for anticoagulation following prosthetic valve implantation for endocarditis are the same as for patients with prosthetic valves without endocarditis (eg, nonporcine mechanical valves and valves in the mitral position).

▶ Response to Therapy

If infection is caused by viridans streptococci, enterococci, or coagulase-negative staphylococci, defervescence occurs in 3–4 days on average; with *S aureus* or *Pseudomonas aeruginosa*, fever may persist for longer. Blood cultures should be obtained every 1–2 days to document sterilization.

Other causes of persistent fever are myocardial or metastatic abscess, sterile embolization, superimposed hospital-acquired infection, and drug reaction. Most relapses occur within 1–2 months after completion of therapy. Obtaining one or two blood cultures during this period is prudent.

▶ When to Refer

- Consider consulting an infectious diseases specialist in all cases of suspected infective endocarditis.
- Consult a cardiac surgeon in the situations mentioned in the Role of Surgery section above to prevent further embolic disease, heart failure, and other complications including death.

▶ When to Admit

Patients with infective endocarditis should be hospitalized for expedited evaluation and treatment.

Baddour LM et al. Infective endocarditis in adults: diagnosis, antimicrobial therapy, and management of complications: a scientific statement for healthcare professionals from the American Heart Association. Circulation. 2015 Oct 13; 132(15):1435–86. Erratum in: Circulation. 2015 Oct 27; 132(17):e215. [PMID: 26373316]

Vincent LL et al. Infective endocarditis: update on epidemiology, outcomes and management. Curr Cardiol Rep. 2018 Aug 16; 20(10):86. [PMID: 30117004]

Wilson W et al. Prevention of infective endocarditis: guidelines from the American Heart Association: a guideline from the American Heart Association Rheumatic Fever, Endocarditis, and Kawasaki Disease Committee, Council on Cardiovascular Disease in the Young, and the Council on Clinical Cardiology, Council on Cardiovascular Surgery and Anesthesia, and the Quality of Care and Outcomes Research Interdisciplinary Working Group. Circulation. 2007 Oct 9; 116(15):1736–54. [PMID: 17446442]

INFECTIONS CAUSED BY GRAM-NEGATIVE BACTERIA

BORDETELLA PERTUSSIS INFECTION (Whooping Cough)

ESSENTIALS OF DIAGNOSIS

- ▶ Predominantly in infants under age 2 years; adolescents and adults are reservoirs of infection.
- ▶ Two-week prodromal catarrhal stage of malaise, cough, coryza, and anorexia.
- ▶ Paroxysmal cough ending in a high-pitched inspiratory "whoop."
- ▶ Absolute lymphocytosis, often striking; culture confirms diagnosis.

▶ General Considerations

Pertussis is an acute infection of the respiratory tract caused by *B pertussis* that is transmitted by respiratory droplets. The incubation period is 7–17 days. Half of all cases occur before age 2 years. Neither immunization nor disease confers lasting immunity to pertussis. Consequently, adults are an important reservoir of the disease.

Clinical Findings

The symptoms of classic pertussis last about 6 weeks and are divided into three consecutive stages. The catarrhal stage is characterized by its insidious onset, with lacrimation, sneezing, and coryza, anorexia and malaise, and a hacking night cough that becomes diurnal. The paroxysmal stage is characterized by bursts of rapid, consecutive coughs followed by a deep, high-pitched inspiration (whoop). The convalescent stage begins 4 weeks after onset of the illness with a decrease in the frequency and severity of paroxysms of cough. The diagnosis often is not considered in adults, who may not have a typical presentation. Cough persisting more than 2 weeks is suggestive. Infection may also be asymptomatic.

The white blood cell count is usually 15,000–20,000/mcL (rarely, as high as 50,000/mcL or more), 60–80% of which are lymphocytes. The diagnosis is established by isolating the organism from nasopharyngeal culture. A special medium (eg, Bordet-Gengou agar) must be requested. Polymerase chain reaction assays for diagnosis of pertussis may be available in some clinical or health department laboratories.

Prevention

Acellular pertussis vaccine is recommended for all infants, combined with diphtheria and tetanus toxoids (DTaP). Infants and susceptible adults with significant exposure should receive prophylaxis with an oral macrolide. In recognition of their importance as a reservoir of disease, vaccination of adolescents and adults against pertussis is recommended (see Table 30–7 and www.cdc.gov/vaccines/schedules). Adolescents aged 11–18 years (preferably between 11 and 12 years of age) who have completed the DTP or DTaP vaccination series should receive a single dose of either Tdap product instead of Td (tetanus and diphtheria toxoids vaccine) for booster immunization against tetanus, diphtheria, and pertussis. Adults of all ages (including those older than age 64 years) should receive a single dose of Tdap. In addition, pregnant women should receive a dose of Tdap during each pregnancy regardless of prior vaccination history, ideally between 27 and 36 weeks of gestation, in order to maximize the antibody response of the woman and the passive antibody transfer to the infant. For any woman who was not previously vaccinated with Tdap and for whom the vaccine was not given during her pregnancy, Tdap should be administered immediately postpartum. The CDC has eliminated the recommendation that a 2-year period window is needed between receiving the Td and Tdap vaccines based on data showing that there is not an increased risk of adverse events.

Treatment

Antibiotic treatment should be initiated in all suspected cases. Treatment options include erythromycin, 500 mg

four times a day orally for 7 days; azithromycin, 500 mg orally on day 1 and 250 mg for 4 more days; or clarithromycin, 500 mg orally twice daily for 7 days. Trimethoprim-sulfamethoxazole, 160 mg–800 mg orally twice a day for 7 days, also is effective. Treatment shortens the duration of carriage and may diminish the severity of coughing paroxysms. These same regimens are indicated for prophylaxis of contacts to an active case of pertussis that are exposed within 3 weeks of the onset of cough in the index case.

DeSilva M et al. Tdap vaccination during pregnancy and microcephaly and other structural birth defects in offspring. JAMA. 2016 Nov 1;316(17):1823–5. [PMID: 27802536]

Nguyen VTN et al. Pertussis: the whooping cough. Prim Care. 2018 Sep;45(3):423–31. [PMID: 30115332]

Winter K et al. Effectiveness of prenatal versus postpartum tetanus, diphtheria, and acellular pertussis vaccination in preventing infant pertussis. Clin Infect Dis. 2017 Jan 1;64(1):3–8. [PMID: 27624955]

OTHER *BORDETELLA* INFECTIONS

Bordetella bronchiseptica is a pleomorphic gram-negative coccobacillus causing kennel cough in dogs. On occasion it causes upper and lower respiratory infection in humans, principally HIV-infected patients. Infection has been associated with contact with dogs and cats, suggesting animal-to-human transmission. Treatment of *B bronchiseptica* infection is guided by results of in vitro susceptibility tests.

MENINGOCOCCAL MENINGITIS

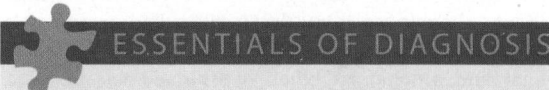

ESSENTIALS OF DIAGNOSIS

▶ Fever, headache, vomiting, delirium, convulsions.

▶ Petechial rash of skin and mucous membranes in many.

▶ Neck and back stiffness and positive Kernig and Brudzinski signs are characteristic.

▶ Purulent spinal fluid with gram-negative intracellular and extracellular diplococci.

▶ Culture of cerebrospinal fluid, blood, or petechial aspiration confirms the diagnosis.

General Considerations

Meningococcal meningitis is caused by *Neisseria meningitidis* of groups A, B, C, Y, and W-135, among others. Meningitis due to serogroup A is uncommon in the United States. Serogroup B generally causes sporadic cases. Serogroup C meningococcus is the most common cause of epidemic disease in the United States. Up to 40% of persons are nasopharyngeal carriers of meningococci, but disease develops in relatively few of these persons. Infection is transmitted by droplets. The clinical illness may take the form of meningococcemia (a fulminant form of septicemia without meningitis), meningococcemia with meningitis, or meningitis. Recurrent meningococcemia with fever, rash, and arthritis is seen rarely in patients with certain terminal complement deficiencies. Asplenic patients are also at risk.

Clinical Findings

A. Symptoms and Signs

High fever, chills, nausea, vomiting, and headache as well as back, abdominal, and extremity pains are typical. Rapidly developing confusion, delirium, seizures, and coma occur in some. On examination, nuchal and back rigidity are typical. Positive Kernig and Brudzinski signs (Kernig sign is pain in the hamstrings upon extension of the knee with the hip at 90-degree flexion; Brudzinski sign is flexion of the knee in response to flexion of the neck) are specific but not sensitive findings. A petechial rash appearing in the lower extremities and at pressure points is found in most cases. Petechiae may vary in size from pinpoint lesions to large ecchymoses or even skin gangrene that may later slough.

B. Laboratory Findings

Lumbar puncture typically reveals a cloudy or purulent cerebrospinal fluid, with elevated pressure, increased protein, and decreased glucose content. The fluid usually contains greater than 1000 cells/mcL, with polymorphonuclear cells predominating and containing gram-negative intracellular diplococci. The absence of organisms in a Gram-stained smear of the cerebrospinal fluid sediment does not rule out the diagnosis. The capsular polysaccharide can be demonstrated in cerebrospinal fluid or urine by latex agglutination; this is useful in partially treated patients, though sensitivity is 60–80%. The organism is usually demonstrated by smear and culture of the cerebrospinal fluid, oropharynx, blood, or aspirated petechiae.

Disseminated intravascular coagulation is an important complication of meningococcal infection and is typically present in toxic patients with ecchymotic skin lesions.

Differential Diagnosis

Meningococcal meningitis must be differentiated from other meningitides. In small infants and in older adults, fever or stiff neck is often missing, and altered mental status may dominate the picture.

Rickettsial, echovirus, and, rarely, other bacterial infections (eg, staphylococcal infections, scarlet fever) also cause petechial rash.

Prevention

Four meningococcal vaccines are available. There are two vaccines with coverage against meningococcal serogroups A, C, Y, and W-135 and two with coverage against meningococcal serogroup B. The two vaccines effective for meningococcal serogroups A, C, Y, and W-135 are the meningococcal polysaccharide vaccine (MPSV4) indicated for vaccination of persons over age 55 and the conjugate vaccine (MCV4) indicated for persons aged 2–55 years. The two vaccines against meningococcal serogroup B are MenB-FHbp and MenB-4C are approved for persons aged 10–25 years and are not interchangeable.

The Advisory Committee on Immunization Practices recommends immunization with a dose of MCV4 for preadolescents aged 11–12 with a booster at age 16 (see www.cdc.gov/vaccines/schedules/hcp/child-adolescent.html). For ease of program implementation, persons aged 21 years or younger should have documentation of receipt of a dose of MCV4 not more than 5 years before enrollment to college. If the primary dose was administered before the sixteenth birthday, a booster dose should be administered before enrollment. Vaccine is also recommended as a two-dose primary series administered 2 months apart for persons aged 2 through 54 years with persistent complement deficiency, persons with functional or anatomic asplenia, and for adolescents with HIV infection. All other persons at increased risk for meningococcal disease (eg, military recruits, microbiologists, or travelers to an epidemic or highly endemic country) should receive a single dose. One of the meningococcal serogroup B vaccines may be administered to persons 10 years of age or older who are at increased risk for meningococcal disease. These persons include those with persistent complement component deficiencies; persons with anatomic or functional asplenia; microbiologists routinely exposed to isolates of *Neisseria meningitidis*; and persons identified to be at increased risk because of a serogroup B meningococcal disease outbreak. Vaccination of persons aged 16–23 years may provide short-term protection against most strains of serogroup B meningococcal disease.

Eliminating nasopharyngeal carriage of meningococci is an effective prevention strategy in closed populations and to prevent secondary cases in household or otherwise close contacts. Rifampin, 600 mg orally twice a day for 2 days, ciprofloxacin, 500 mg orally once, or one intramuscular 250-mg dose of ceftriaxone is effective. Cases of fluoroquinolone-resistant meningococcal infections have been identified in the United States. However, ciprofloxacin remains a recommended empiric agent for eradication of nasopharyngeal carriage. School and work contacts ordinarily need not be treated. Hospital contacts receive therapy only if intense exposure has occurred (eg, mouth-to-mouth resuscitation). Accidentally discovered carriers without known close contact with meningococcal disease do not require prophylactic antimicrobials.

Treatment

Blood cultures must be obtained and intravenous antimicrobial therapy started immediately. This may be done prior to lumbar puncture in patients in whom the diagnosis is not straightforward and for those in whom MR or CT imaging is indicated to exclude mass lesions. Aqueous penicillin G is the antibiotic of choice (24 million units/24 h intravenously in divided doses every 4 hours). The prevalence of strains of *N meningitidis* with intermediate resistance to penicillin in vitro (MICs 0.1 to 1 mcg/mL) is increasing, particularly in Europe. At what level of resistance penicillin treatment failure can occur is not known. Penicillin-intermediate strains thus far remain fully susceptible to ceftriaxone and other third-generation cephalosporins used to treat meningitis, and these should be effective alternatives to penicillin. In penicillin-allergic patients or those in whom *Haemophilus influenzae* or gram-negative meningitis is a consideration, ceftriaxone, 2 g intravenously every 12 hours, should be used. Treatment should be continued in full doses by the intravenous route until the patient is afebrile for 5 days. Shorter courses—as few as 4 days if ceftriaxone is used—are also effective.

▶ When to Admit

All patients with suspected meningococcal infection including meningitis and meningococcemia should be admitted for evaluation and empiric intravenous antibiotic therapy.

Di Caprio G et al. Increased rate of penicillin non-susceptible strains of *N. meningitidis* in Naples, Italy. J Chemother. 2017 Dec;29(6):389–90. [PMID: 28728477]

MacNeil JR et al. Use of serogroup B meningococcal vaccines in adolescents and young adults: recommendations of the Advisory Committee on Immunization Practices, 2015. MMWR Morb Mortal Wkly Rep. 2015 Oct 23;64(41):1171–6. [PMID: 26492381]

INFECTIONS CAUSED BY *HAEMOPHILUS* SPECIES

H influenzae and other *Haemophilus* species may cause sinusitis, otitis, bronchitis, epiglottitis, pneumonia, cellulitis, arthritis, meningitis, and endocarditis. Nontypeable strains are responsible for most disease in adults. Alcoholism, smoking, chronic lung disease, advanced age, and HIV infection are risk factors. *Haemophilus* species colonize the upper respiratory tract in patients with chronic obstructive pulmonary disease and frequently cause purulent bronchitis.

Beta-lactamase–producing strains are less common in adults than in children. For adults with sinusitis, otitis, or respiratory tract infection, oral amoxicillin, 750 mg twice daily for 10–14 days, is adequate. For beta-lactamase–producing strains, use of the oral fixed-drug combination of amoxicillin, 875 mg, with clavulanate, 125 mg, is indicated. For the penicillin-allergic patient, oral cefuroxime axetil, 250 mg twice daily; or a fluoroquinolone (ciprofloxacin, 500 mg orally twice daily; levofloxacin, 500–750 mg orally once daily; or moxifloxacin, 400 mg orally once daily) for 7 days is effective. Azithromycin, 500 mg orally once followed by 250 mg daily for 4 days, is preferred over clarithromycin when a macrolide is the preferred agent. Trimethoprim-sulfamethoxazole (160/800 mg orally twice daily) can be considered, but resistance rates have been reported to be up to 25%.

In the more seriously ill patient (eg, the toxic patient with multilobar pneumonia), ceftriaxone, 1 g/day intravenously, is recommended pending determination of whether the infecting strain is a beta-lactamase producer. A fluoroquinolone (see above for dosages) can be used for the penicillin-allergic patients for a 10- to 14-day course of therapy.

Epiglottitis is characterized by an abrupt onset of high fever, drooling, and inability to handle secretions. An important clue to the diagnosis is complaint of a severe sore throat despite an unimpressive examination of the pharynx. Stridor and respiratory distress result from laryngeal obstruction. The diagnosis is best made by direct visualization of the cherry-red, swollen epiglottis at laryngoscopy. Because laryngoscopy may provoke laryngospasm and obstruction, especially in children, it should be performed in an intensive care unit or similar setting, and only at a time when intubation can be performed promptly. Ceftriaxone, 1 g intravenously every 24 hours for 7–10 days, is the drug of choice. Trimethoprim-sulfamethoxazole or a fluoroquinolone (see above for dosage) may be used in the patient with serious penicillin allergy.

Meningitis, rare in adults, is a consideration in the patient who has meningitis associated with sinusitis or otitis. Initial therapy for suspected *H influenzae* meningitis should be with ceftriaxone, 4 g/day in two divided doses, until the strain is proved not to produce beta-lactamase. Meningitis is treated for at least 7 days. Dexamethasone, 0.15 mg/kg intravenously every 6 hours, may reduce the incidence of long-term sequelae, principally hearing loss.

Brouwer MC et al. Epidemiology of community-acquired bacterial meningitis. Curr Opin Infect Dis. 2018 Feb;31(1):78–84. [PMID: 29176349]

Sriram KB et al. Nontypeable *Haemophilus influenzae* and chronic obstructive pulmonary disease: a review for clinicians. Crit Rev Microbiol. 2018 Mar;44(2):125–42. [PMID: 28539074]

INFECTIONS CAUSED BY *MORAXELLA CATARRHALIS*

M catarrhalis is a gram-negative aerobic coccus morphologically and biochemically similar to *Neisseria*. It causes sinusitis, bronchitis, and pneumonia. Bacteremia and meningitis have also been reported in immunocompromised patients. The organism frequently colonizes the respiratory tract, making differentiation of colonization from infection difficult. If *M catarrhalis* is the predominant isolate, therapy is directed against it. *M catarrhalis* typically produces beta-lactamase and therefore is usually resistant to ampicillin and amoxicillin. It is susceptible to amoxicillin-clavulanate, ampicillin-sulbactam, trimethoprim-sulfamethoxazole, ciprofloxacin, and second- and third-generation cephalosporins.

LEGIONNAIRES DISEASE

ESSENTIALS OF DIAGNOSIS

▶ Patients are often immunocompromised, smokers, or have chronic lung disease.

▶ Scant sputum production, pleuritic chest pain, toxic appearance.

▶ Chest radiograph: focal patchy infiltrates or consolidation.

▶ Gram stain of sputum: polymorphonuclear leukocytes and no organisms.

General Considerations

Legionella infection ranks among the three or four most common causes of community-acquired pneumonia and is considered whenever the etiology of a pneumonia is in question. Legionnaires disease is more common in immunocompromised persons, in smokers, and in those with chronic lung disease. Outbreaks have been associated with contaminated water sources, such as showerheads and faucets in patient rooms and air conditioning cooling towers.

Clinical Findings

A. Symptoms and Signs

Legionnaires disease is one of the atypical pneumonias, so called because a Gram-stained smear of sputum does not show organisms. However, many features of Legionnaires disease are more like typical pneumonia, with high fevers, toxic appearance, pleurisy, and grossly purulent sputum. Nausea, vomiting, and diarrhea may be prominent. There may be relative bradycardia. Classically, this pneumonia is caused by *Legionella pneumophila*, though other species can cause identical disease.

B. Laboratory Findings

There may be hyponatremia, hypophosphatemia, elevated liver enzymes, and elevated creatine kinase. Culture of *Legionella* species has a 80–90% sensitivity. Dieterle silver staining of tissue, pleural fluid, or other infected material is also a reliable method for detecting *Legionella* species. Direct fluorescent antibody stains and serologic testing such as urinary antigen are less sensitive because these will detect only *L pneumophila* serotype 1. In addition, making a serologic diagnosis requires that the host respond with sufficient specific antibody production.

Treatment

Azithromycin (500 mg orally once daily), clarithromycin (500 mg orally twice daily), or a fluoroquinolone (eg, levofloxacin, 750 mg orally once daily), and not erythromycin, are the drugs of choice for treatment of legionellosis because of their excellent intracellular penetration and in vitro activity, as well as desirable pharmacokinetic properties that permit oral administration and once or twice daily dosing. Duration of therapy is 10–14 days, although a 21-day course of therapy is recommended for immunocompromised patients.

Cunha BA et al. Legionnaire's disease: a clinical diagnostic approach. Infect Dis Clin North Am. 2017 Mar;31(1):81–93. [PMID: 28159178]

Del Castillo M et al. Atypical presentation of *Legionella* pneumonia among patients with underlying cancer: a fifteen-year review. J Infect. 2016 Jan;72(1):45–51. [PMID: 26496794]

GRAM-NEGATIVE BACTEREMIA & SEPSIS

Gram-negative bacteremia can originate in a number of sites, the most common being the genitourinary system, hepatobiliary tract, gastrointestinal tract, and lungs. Less common sources include intravenous lines, infusion fluids, surgical wounds, drains, and pressure injuries.

Patients with potentially fatal underlying conditions in the short term such as neutropenia or immunoparesis have a mortality rate of 40–60%; those with serious underlying diseases likely to be fatal in 5 years, such as solid tumors, cirrhosis, and aplastic anemia, die in 15–20% of cases; and individuals with no underlying diseases have a mortality rate of 5% or less.

Clinical Findings

A. Symptoms and Signs

Most patients have fevers and chills, often with abrupt onset. However, 15% of patients are hypothermic (temperature 36.4°C or less) at presentation, and 5% never develop a temperature above 37.5°C. Hyperventilation with respiratory alkalosis and changes in mental status are important early manifestations. Hypotension and shock, which occur in 20–50% of patients, are unfavorable prognostic signs.

B. Laboratory Findings

Neutropenia or neutrophilia, often with increased numbers of immature forms of polymorphonuclear leukocytes, is the most common laboratory abnormality in septic patients. Thrombocytopenia occurs in 50% of patients, laboratory evidence of coagulation abnormalities in 10%, and overt disseminated intravascular coagulation in 2–3%. Both clinical manifestations and the laboratory abnormalities are nonspecific and insensitive, which accounts for the relatively low rate of blood culture positivity (approximately 20–40%). If possible, three blood cultures from separate sites should be obtained in rapid succession before starting antimicrobial therapy. The chance of recovering the organism in at least one of the three blood cultures is greater than 95%. The false-negative rate for a single culture of 5–10 mL of blood is 30%. This may be reduced to 5–10% (albeit with a slight false-positive rate due to isolation of contaminants) if a single volume of 30 mL is inoculated into several blood culture bottles. Because blood cultures may be falsely negative, when a patient with presumed septic shock, negative blood cultures, and inadequate explanation for the clinical course responds to antimicrobial agents, therapy should be continued for 10–14 days.

Treatment

Several factors are important in the management of patients with sepsis.

A. Removal of Predisposing Factors

This usually means decreasing or stopping immunosuppressive medications and, in certain circumstances, giving granulocyte colony-stimulating factor (filgrastim; G-CSF) to the neutropenic patient.

B. Identifying the Source of Bacteremia

By simply finding the source of bacteremia and removing it (central venous catheter) or draining it (abscess), a fatal disease becomes easily treatable.

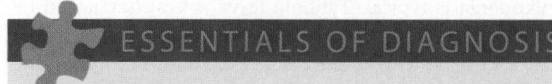

C. Supportive Measures

The use of fluids, vasopressors, and corticosteroids in septic shock are discussed in Chapter 14; management of disseminated intravascular coagulation is discussed in Chapter 13.

D. Antibiotics

Antibiotics should be given as soon as the diagnosis is suspected, since delays in therapy have been associated with increased mortality rates, particularly once hypotension develops. In general, bactericidal antibiotics should be used and given intravenously to ensure therapeutic serum levels. Penetration of antibiotics into the site of primary infection is critical for successful therapy—ie, if the infection originates in the CNS, antibiotics that penetrate the blood-brain barrier should be used—eg, third- or fourth-generation cephalosporin—but not first-generation cephalosporins or aminoglycosides, which penetrate poorly. Sepsis caused by gram-positive organisms cannot be differentiated on clinical grounds from that due to gram-negative bacteria. Therefore, initial therapy should include antibiotics active against both types of organisms.

The number of antibiotics necessary remains controversial and depends on the cause. Table 30–4 provides a guide for empiric therapy. Although a combination of antibiotics is often recommended for "synergism," combination therapy has not been shown to be superior to a single-drug regimen with any of several broad-spectrum antibiotics (eg, a third-generation cephalosporin, piperacillin-tazobactam, carbapenem). If multiple drugs are used initially, the regimen should be modified and coverage narrowed based on the results of culture and sensitivity testing.

Aillet C et al. Bacteraemia in emergency departments: effective antibiotic reassessment is associated with a better outcome. Eur J Clin Microbiol Infect Dis. 2018 Feb;37(2):325–31. [PMID: 29164361]

Rhodes A et al. Surviving Sepsis Campaign: international guidelines for management of sepsis and septic shock: 2016. Intensive Care Med. 2017 Mar;43(3):304–77. [PMID: 28101605]

SALMONELLOSIS

Salmonellosis includes infection by any of approximately 2000 serotypes of salmonellae. All *Salmonella* serotypes are members of a single species, *Salmonella enterica*. Human infections are caused almost exclusively by *S enterica* subsp *enterica*, of which three serotypes—*typhi*, *typhimurium*, and *choleraesuis*—are predominantly isolated. Three clinical patterns of infection are recognized: (1) enteric fever, the best example of which is typhoid fever, due to serotype *typhi*; (2) acute enterocolitis, caused by serotype *typhimurium*, among others; and (3) the "septicemic" type, characterized by bacteremia and focal lesions, exemplified by infection with serotype *choleraesuis*. All types are transmitted by ingestion of the organism, usually from tainted food or drink.

1. Enteric Fever (Typhoid Fever)

> ### ESSENTIALS OF DIAGNOSIS
>
> ▶ Gradual onset of malaise, headache, nausea, vomiting, abdominal pain.
>
> ▶ Rose spots, relative bradycardia, splenomegaly, and abdominal distention and tenderness.
>
> ▶ Slow (stepladder) rise of fever to maximum and then slow return to normal.
>
> ▶ Leukopenia; blood, stool, and urine cultures positive for *Salmonella*.

General Considerations

Enteric fever is a clinical syndrome characterized by gastrointestinal symptoms as well as constitutional symptoms such as fever, malaise, and headache. It may have a long incubation period (6–30 days), and the gastrointestinal symptoms may resolve but then recur. Progressive infection often evolves with delirium. Enteric fever can be caused by any *Salmonella* species, including *S typhi* (typhoid fever) and non-typhoidal strains, especially *S paratyphi* subtype A in the United States. Infection begins when organisms breach the mucosal epithelium of the intestines. Having crossed the epithelial barrier, organisms invade and replicate in macrophages in Peyer patches, mesenteric lymph nodes, and the spleen. Serotypes other than *typhi* usually do not cause invasive disease, presumably because they lack the necessary human-specific virulence factors. Bacteremia occurs, and the infection then localizes principally in the lymphoid tissue of the small intestine. Peyer patches become inflamed and may ulcerate, with involvement greatest during the third week of disease. The organism may disseminate to the lungs, gallbladder, kidneys, or CNS.

Clinical Findings

A. Symptoms and Signs

During the prodromal stage, there is increasing malaise, headache, cough, and sore throat, often with abdominal pain and constipation, while the fever ascends in a stepwise fashion. After about 7–10 days, it reaches a plateau and the patient is much more ill. There may be marked constipation, especially early, or "pea soup" diarrhea; marked abdominal distention occurs as well. If there are no complications, the patient's condition will gradually improve over 7–10 days. However, relapse may occur for up to 2 weeks after defervescence.

During the early prodrome, physical findings are few. Later, splenomegaly, abdominal distention and tenderness, relative bradycardia, and occasionally meningismus appear. The rash (rose spots) commonly appears during the second week of disease. The individual spot, found principally on the trunk, is a pink papule 2–3 mm in diameter that fades on pressure. It disappears in 3–4 days.

B. Laboratory Findings

Leukopenia is typical. Typhoid fever is best diagnosed by blood culture, which is positive in the first week of illness in 80% of patients who have not taken antimicrobials. The rate of positivity declines thereafter, but one-fourth or more of patients still have positive blood cultures in the third week. Cultures of bone marrow occasionally are positive when blood cultures are not. Stool culture is unreliable because it may be positive in gastroenteritis without typhoid fever.

▶ Differential Diagnosis

Enteric fever must be distinguished from other gastrointestinal illnesses and from other infections that have few localizing findings. Examples include tuberculosis, infective endocarditis, brucellosis, lymphoma, and Q fever. Often there is a history of recent travel to endemic areas, and viral hepatitis, malaria, or amebiasis may be in the differential.

▶ Complications

Complications occur in about 30% of untreated cases and account for 75% of deaths. Intestinal hemorrhage, manifested by a sudden drop in temperature and signs of shock followed by dark or fresh blood in the stool, or intestinal perforation, accompanied by abdominal pain and tenderness, is most likely to occur during the third week. Appearance of leukocytosis and tachycardia should suggest these complications. Urinary retention, pneumonia, thrombophlebitis, myocarditis, psychosis, cholecystitis, nephritis, osteomyelitis, and meningitis are less often observed.

▶ Prevention

Immunization is not always effective, but should be considered for household contacts of a typhoid carrier, for travelers to endemic areas, and during epidemic outbreaks. A multiple-dose oral vaccine and a single-dose parenteral vaccine are available. Their efficacies are similar, but oral vaccine causes fewer side effects. Boosters, when indicated, should be given every 5 years and 2 years for oral and parenteral preparations, respectively.

Adequate waste disposal and protection of food and water supplies from contamination are important public health measures to prevent salmonellosis. Carriers cannot work as food handlers.

▶ Treatment

A. Specific Measures

Because of increasing antimicrobial resistance, fluoroquinolones—such as ciprofloxacin 750 mg orally twice daily or levofloxacin 500 mg orally once daily, 5–7 days for uncomplicated enteric fever and 10–14 days for severe infection—are the agents of choice for treatment of salmonella infections. Ceftriaxone, 2 g intravenously for 7 days, is also effective. Although resistance to fluoroquinolones or cephalosporins occurs uncommonly, the prevalence is increasing. When an infection is caused by a multidrug-resistant strain, select an antibiotic to which the isolate is susceptible in vitro. Alternatively, increasing the dose of ceftriaxone to 4 g/day and treating for 10–14 days or using azithromycin 500 mg orally for 7 days in uncomplicated cases may be effective. In years past, ampicillin, chloramphenicol, and trimethoprim-sulfamethoxazole had been effective treatments but resistance has spread globally.

B. Treatment of Carriers

Ciprofloxacin, 750 mg orally twice a day for 4 weeks, has proved to be highly effective in eradicating the carrier state. Cholecystectomy may also achieve this goal. When the isolate is susceptible, treatment of carriage with ampicillin, trimethoprim-sulfamethoxazole, or chloramphenicol may be successful.

▶ Prognosis

The mortality rate of typhoid fever is about 2% in treated cases. Elderly or debilitated persons are likely to do worse. With complications, the prognosis is poor. Relapses occur in up to 15% of cases. A residual carrier state frequently persists in spite of therapy.

Wain J et al. Typhoid fever. Lancet. 2015 Mar 21;385(9973): 1136–45. [PMID: 25458731]

Zuckerman JN et al. Review of current typhoid fever vaccines, cross-protection against paratyphoid fever, and the European guidelines. Expert Rev Vaccines. 2017 Oct;16(10):1029–43. [PMID: 28856924]

2. *Salmonella* Gastroenteritis

By far the most common form of salmonellosis is acute enterocolitis, which can be caused by both typhoidal and non-typhoidal *Salmonella*. The incubation period is 8–48 hours after ingestion of contaminated food or liquid.

Symptoms and signs consist of fever (often with chills), nausea and vomiting, cramping abdominal pain, and diarrhea, which may be grossly bloody, lasting 3–5 days. Differentiation must be made from viral gastroenteritis, food poisoning, shigellosis, amebic dysentery, and acute ulcerative colitis. The diagnosis is made by culturing the organism from the stool. The disease is usually self-limited, but bacteremia with localization in joints or bones may occur, especially in patients with sickle cell disease.

In most cases, treatment of uncomplicated enterocolitis is symptomatic only. However, patients who are malnourished or severely ill, patients with sickle cell disease, and patients who are immunocompromised (including those who are HIV-positive) should be treated with ciprofloxacin, 500 mg orally twice a day; ceftriaxone, 1 g intravenously once daily; trimethoprim-sulfamethoxazole, 160 mg/80 mg orally twice a day; or azithromycin, 500 mg orally once daily for 7–14 days (14 days for immunocompromised patients).

Haselbeck AH et al. Current perspectives on invasive nontyphoidal Salmonella disease. Curr Opin Infect Dis. 2017 Oct; 30(5):498–503. [PMID: 28731899]

Shane AL et al. 2017 Infectious Diseases Society of America clinical practice guidelines for the diagnosis and management of infectious diarrhea. Clin Infect Dis. 2017 Nov 29;65(12): 1963–73. [PMID: 29194529]

3. *Salmonella* Bacteremia

Salmonella infection may be manifested by prolonged or recurrent fevers accompanied by bacteremia and local infection in bone, joints, pleura, pericardium, lungs, or other sites. Mycotic abdominal aortic aneurysms may also occur. Serotypes other than typhi usually are isolated. This complication of bacteremia tends to occur in immunocompromised persons, including HIV-infected individuals, who typically have bacteremia without an obvious source. Treatment is the same as for typhoid fever, plus drainage of any abscesses. In HIV-infected patients, relapse is common, and lifelong suppressive therapy may be needed. Ciprofloxacin, 750 mg orally twice a day, is effective both for therapy of acute infection and for suppression of recurrence. Incidence of infections caused by drug-resistant strains may be on the rise.

Crump JA et al. Epidemiology, clinical presentation, laboratory diagnosis, antimicrobial resistance, and antimicrobial management of invasive salmonella infections. Clin Microbiol Rev. 2015 Oct;28(4):901–37. [PMID: 26180063]
Gibani MM et al. Control of invasive salmonella disease in Africa: is there a role for human challenge models? Clin Infect Dis. 2015 Nov 1;61(Suppl 4):S266–71. [PMID: 26449941]

SHIGELLOSIS

ESSENTIALS OF DIAGNOSIS

▶ Diarrhea, often with blood and mucus.

▶ Crampy abdominal pain and systemic toxicity.

▶ White blood cells in stools; organism isolated on stool culture.

General Considerations

Shigella dysentery is a common disease, often self-limited and mild but occasionally serious. *S sonnei* is the leading cause in the United States, followed by *S flexneri*. *S dysenteriae* causes the most serious form of the illness. Shigellae are invasive organisms. The infective dose is low at 10^2–10^3 organisms. There has been a rise in strains resistant to multiple antibiotics.

Clinical Findings

A. Symptoms and Signs

The illness usually starts abruptly, with diarrhea, lower abdominal cramps, and tenesmus. The diarrheal stool often is mixed with blood and mucus. Systemic symptoms are fever, chills, anorexia and malaise, and headache. The

abdomen is tender. Sigmoidoscopic examination reveals an inflamed, engorged mucosa with punctate and sometimes large areas of ulceration.

B. Laboratory Findings

The stool shows many leukocytes and red cells. Stool culture is positive for shigellae in most cases, but blood cultures grow the organism in less than 5% of cases.

Differential Diagnosis

Bacillary dysentery must be distinguished from salmonella enterocolitis and from disease due to enterotoxigenic *Escherichia coli*, *Campylobacter*, and *Yersinia enterocolitica*. Amebic dysentery may be similar clinically and is diagnosed by finding amoebas in the fresh stool specimen. Ulcerative colitis is also an important cause of bloody diarrhea.

Complications

Temporary disaccharidase deficiency may follow the diarrhea. Reactive arthritis is an uncommon complication, usually occurring in HLA-B27 individuals infected by *Shigella*. Hemolytic-uremic syndrome occurs rarely.

Treatment

Treatment of dehydration and hypotension is lifesaving in severe cases. Recommended empiric antimicrobial therapy is either a fluoroquinolone (ciprofloxacin, 750 mg orally twice daily for 7–10 days, or levofloxacin, 500 mg orally once daily for 3 days) or ceftriaxone, 1 g intravenously once daily for 5 days. If the isolate is susceptible, trimethoprim-sulfamethoxazole, 160/80 mg orally twice daily for 5 days, or azithromycin, 500 mg orally once daily for 3 days, is also effective. High rates of resistance to amoxicillin make it a less effective treatment option.

Goulart MA et al. Shigellosis in men who have sex with men: an overlooked opportunity to counsel with pre-exposure prophylaxis for HIV. Int J STD AIDS. 2016 Nov;27(13):1236–8. [PMID: 26945593]
Puzari M et al. Emergence of antibiotic resistant Shigella species: a matter of concern. J Infect Public Health. 2018 Jul–Aug; 11(4):451–4. [PMID: 29066021]
Shane AL et al. 2017 Infectious Diseases Society of America clinical practice guidelines for the diagnosis and management of infectious diarrhea. Clin Infect Dis. 2017 Nov 29; 65(12): 1963–73. [PMID: 29194529]

GASTROENTERITIS CAUSED BY *ESCHERICHIA COLI*

E coli causes gastroenteritis by a variety of mechanisms. Enterotoxigenic *E coli* (ETEC) elaborates either a heat-stable or heat-labile toxin that mediates the disease. ETEC is an important cause of traveler's diarrhea. Enteroinvasive *E coli* (EIEC) differs from other *E coli* bowel pathogens in that these strains invade cells, causing bloody diarrhea and dysentery similar to infection with *Shigella* species. EIEC is uncommon in the United States. Neither ETEC nor EIEC strains are routinely isolated and identified from stool cultures because there is no selective medium. Antimicrobial therapy against *Salmonella* and *Shigella*, such as ciprofloxacin 500 mg orally twice daily, shortens the clinical course, but the disease is self-limited.

Shiga-toxin–producing *E coli* (STEC) infection can result in asymptomatic carrier stage, nonbloody diarrhea, hemorrhagic colitis, hemolytic-uremic syndrome, or thrombotic thrombocytopenic purpura. Although *E coli* O157:H7 is responsible for most cases of STEC infection in the United States, other STEC strains that cause severe disease (such as *E coli* O104:H4) have been reported in Europe. *E coli* O157:H7 has caused several outbreaks of diarrhea and hemolytic-uremic syndrome related to consumption of undercooked hamburger, raw flour, unpasteurized apple juice, and spinach, while *E coli* O145 was linked to the consumption of contaminated lettuce. Older individuals and young children are most affected, with hemolytic-uremic syndrome being more common in the latter group. STEC identification can be difficult and the CDC recommends that all stools submitted for routine testing from patients with acute community-acquired diarrhea be simultaneously cultured for *E coli* O157:H7 and tested with an assay that detects Shiga toxins to detect non-O157 STEC, such as *E coli* O145. Antimicrobial therapy does not alter the course of the disease and may increase the risk of hemolytic-uremic syndrome. Treatment is primarily supportive. Hemolytic-uremic syndrome or thrombotic thrombocytopenic purpura occurring in association with a diarrheal illness suggests the diagnosis and should prompt evaluation for STEC. Confirmed infections should be reported to public health officials.

Lübbert C. Antimicrobial therapy of acute diarrhoea: a clinical review. Expert Rev Anti Infect Ther. 2016;14(2):193–206. [PMID: 26641310]

Marder EP et al. Incidence and trends of infections with pathogens transmitted commonly through food and the effect of increasing use of culture-independent diagnostic tests on surveillance—Foodborne Diseases Active Surveillance Network, 10 U.S. Sites, 2013–2016. MMWR Morb Mortal Wkly Rep. 2017 Apr 21;66(15):397–403. [PMID: 28426643]

CHOLERA

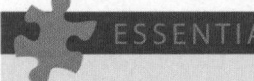

ESSENTIALS OF DIAGNOSIS

► History of travel in endemic area or contact with infected person.

► Voluminous diarrhea (up to 15 L/day).

► Characteristic "rice water stool."

► Rapid development of marked dehydration.

► Positive stool cultures and agglutination of vibrios with specific sera.

▶ General Considerations

Cholera is an acute diarrheal illness caused by certain serotypes of *Vibrio cholerae*. The disease is toxin-mediated, and

fever is unusual. The toxin activates adenylyl cyclase in intestinal epithelial cells of the small intestines, producing hypersecretion of water and chloride ion and a massive diarrhea of up to 15 L/day. Death results from profound hypovolemia. Cholera occurs in epidemics under conditions of crowding, war, and famine (eg, in refugee camps) and where sanitation is inadequate. Infection is acquired by ingestion of contaminated food or water. For over a century, cholera was rarely seen in the Western Hemisphere until an outbreak occurred in Peru, starting in the early 1990s and ending by 2001; the outbreak resulted in almost 400,000 cholera cases and more than 4000 deaths. Cholera again became a rare disease in the Western Hemisphere until late 2010, when there was a massive earthquake in Haiti followed by a cholera outbreak that resulted in thousands of deaths.

▶ Clinical Findings

Cholera is characterized by a sudden onset of severe, frequent watery diarrhea (up to 1 L/h). The liquid stool is gray; turbid; and without fecal odor, blood, or pus ("rice water stool"). Dehydration and hypotension develop rapidly. Stool cultures are positive, and agglutination of vibrios with specific sera can be demonstrated.

▶ Prevention

A vaccine is available that confers short-lived, limited protection and may be required for entry into or reentry after travel to some countries. It is administered in two doses 1–4 weeks apart. A booster dose every 6 months is recommended for persons remaining in areas where cholera is a hazard.

Vaccination programs are expensive and not particularly effective in managing outbreaks of cholera. When outbreaks occur, efforts should be directed toward establishing clean water and food sources and proper waste disposal.

▶ Treatment

Treatment is by replacement of fluids. In mild or moderate illness, oral rehydration usually is adequate. A simple oral replacement fluid can be made from 1 teaspoon of table salt and 4 heaping teaspoons of sugar added to 1 L of water. Intravenous fluids are indicated for persons with signs of severe hypovolemia and those who cannot take adequate fluids orally. Lactated Ringer infusion is satisfactory.

Antimicrobial therapy will shorten the course of illness. Antimicrobials active against *V cholerae* include tetracycline, ampicillin, chloramphenicol, trimethoprim-sulfamethoxazole, fluoroquinolones, and azithromycin. Multiple drug-resistant strains are increasingly encountered, so susceptibility testing, if available, is advisable. A single 1 g oral dose of azithromycin is effective for severe cholera caused by strains with reduced susceptibility to fluoroquinolones, but resistance is emerging to this drug as well.

Clemens JD et al. Cholera. Lancet. 2017 Sep 23;390(10101): 1539–49. [PMID: 28302312]

Wong KK et al. Recommendations of the Advisory Committee on Immunization Practices for use of cholera vaccine. MMWR Morb Mortal Wkly Rep. 2017 May 12;66(18):482–5. [PMID: 28493859]

INFECTIONS CAUSED BY OTHER *VIBRIO* SPECIES

Vibrios other than *V cholerae* that cause human disease are *Vibrio parahaemolyticus, V vulnificus,* and *V alginolyticus.* All are halophilic marine organisms. Infection is acquired by exposure to organisms in contaminated, undercooked, or raw crustaceans or shellfish and warm (greater than 20°C [82.4°F]) ocean waters and estuaries. Infections are more common during the summer months from regions along the Atlantic coast and the Gulf of Mexico in the United States and from tropical waters around the world. Oysters are implicated in up to 90% of food-related cases. *V parahaemolyticus* causes an acute watery diarrhea with crampy abdominal pain and fever, typically occurring within 24 hours after ingestion of contaminated shellfish. The disease is self-limited, and antimicrobial therapy is usually not necessary. *V parahaemolyticus* may also cause cellulitis and sepsis, though these findings are more characteristic of *V vulnificus* infection.

V vulnificus and *V alginolyticus*—neither of which is associated with diarrheal illness—are important causes of cellulitis and primary bacteremia following ingestion of contaminated shellfish or exposure to sea water. Cellulitis with or without sepsis may be accompanied by bulla formation and necrosis with extensive soft tissue destruction, at times requiring debridement and amputation. The infection can be rapidly progressive and is particularly severe in immunocompromised individuals—especially those with cirrhosis—with death rates as high as 50%. Patients with chronic liver disease and those who are immunocompromised should be cautioned to avoid eating raw oysters.

Tetracycline at a dose of 500 mg orally four times a day for 7–10 days is the drug of choice for treatment of suspected or documented primary bacteremia or cellulitis caused by *Vibrio* species. *V vulnificus* is susceptible in vitro to penicillin, ampicillin, cephalosporins, chloramphenicol, aminoglycosides, and fluoroquinolones, and these agents may also be effective. *V parahaemolyticus* and *V alginolyticus* produce beta-lactamase and therefore are resistant to penicillin and ampicillin, but susceptibilities otherwise are similar to those listed for *V vulnificus.*

Baker-Austin C et al. *Vibrio vulnificus*: new insights into a deadly opportunistic pathogen. Environ Microbiol. 2018 Feb; 20(2):423–30. [PMID: 29027375]

Wong KC et al. Antibiotic use for *Vibrio* infections: important insights from surveillance data. BMC Infect Dis. 2015 Jun 11; 15:226. [PMID: 26062903]

INFECTIONS CAUSED BY *CAMPYLOBACTER* SPECIES

Campylobacter organisms are microaerophilic, motile, gram-negative rods. Two species infect humans: *Campylobacter jejuni,* an important cause of diarrheal disease, and

C fetus subsp *fetus,* which typically causes systemic infection and not diarrhea. Dairy cattle and poultry are an important reservoir for campylobacters. Outbreaks of enteritis have been associated with consumption of raw milk. *Campylobacter* gastroenteritis is associated with fever, abdominal pain, and diarrhea characterized by loose, watery, or bloody stools. The differential diagnosis includes shigellosis, *Salmonella* gastroenteritis, and enteritis caused by *Y enterocolitica* or invasive *E coli.* The disease is self-limited, but its duration can be shortened with antimicrobial therapy. Either azithromycin, 1 g orally as a single dose, or ciprofloxacin, 500 mg orally twice daily for 3 days, is effective therapy. However, fluoroquinolone resistance among *C jejuni* isolates has been increasing, particularly in Southeast Asia, and susceptibility testing should be routinely performed.

C fetus causes systemic infections that can be fatal, including primary bacteremia, endocarditis, meningitis, and focal abscesses. It infrequently causes gastroenteritis. Patients infected with *C fetus* are often older, debilitated, or immunocompromised. Closely related species, collectively termed "campylobacter-like organisms," cause bacteremia in HIV-infected individuals. Systemic infections respond to therapy with gentamicin, chloramphenicol, ceftriaxone, or ciprofloxacin. Ceftriaxone or chloramphenicol should be used to treat infections of the CNS because of their ability to penetrate the blood-brain barrier.

Shane AL et al. 2017 Infectious Diseases Society of America clinical practice guidelines for the diagnosis and management of infectious diarrhea. Clin Infect Dis. 2017 Nov 29;65(12): 1963–73. [PMID: 29194529]

BRUCELLOSIS

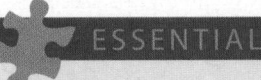

ESSENTIALS OF DIAGNOSIS

▶ History of animal exposure, ingestion of unpasteurized milk or cheese.

▶ Insidious onset: fatigability, headache, arthralgia, anorexia, sweating, irritability.

▶ Intermittent and persistent fever.

▶ Cervical and axillary lymphadenopathy; hepatosplenomegaly.

▶ Lymphocytosis, positive blood culture, positive serologic test.

▶ General Considerations

The infection is transmitted from animals to humans. *Brucella abortus* (cattle), *B suis* (hogs), and *B melitensis* (goats) are the main agents. Transmission to humans occurs by contact with infected meat (slaughterhouse workers), placentae of infected animals (farmers, veterinarians), or ingestion of infected unpasteurized milk or cheese. The incubation period varies from a few days to several weeks.

Brucellosis is a systemic infection that may become chronic. In the United States, brucellosis is very rare. Almost all US cases are imported from countries where brucellosis is endemic (eg, Mexico, Mediterranean Europe, Spain, South American countries).

▶ Clinical Findings

A. Symptoms and Signs

The onset may be acute, with fever, chills, and sweats, but more often is insidious with symptoms of weakness, weight loss, low-grade fevers, sweats, and exhaustion upon minimal activity. Headache, abdominal or back pain with anorexia and constipation, and arthralgias are also common. The chronic form may assume an undulant nature, with periods of normal temperature between acute attacks; symptoms may persist for years, either continuously or intermittently.

Fever, hepatosplenomegaly, and lymphadenopathy are the most common physical findings. Infection may present with or be complicated by specific organ involvement with signs of endocarditis, meningitis, epididymitis, orchitis, arthritis (especially sacroiliitis), spondylitis, or osteomyelitis.

B. Laboratory Findings

The organism can be recovered from cultures of blood, cerebrospinal fluid, urine, bone marrow, or other sites. Cultures are more likely to be negative in chronic cases. The diagnosis often is made by serologic testing.

▶ Differential Diagnosis

Brucellosis must be differentiated from any other acute febrile disease, especially influenza, tularemia, Q fever, mononucleosis, and enteric fever. In its chronic form it resembles Hodgkin disease, tuberculosis, HIV infection, malaria, and disseminated fungal infections such as histoplasmosis and coccidioidomycosis.

▶ Complications

The most frequent complications are bone and joint lesions such as spondylitis and suppurative arthritis (usually of a single joint), endocarditis (often culture negative), and meningoencephalitis. Less common complications are pneumonitis with pleural effusion, hepatitis, and cholecystitis.

▶ Treatment

Single-drug regimens are not recommended because the relapse rate may be as high as 50%. Combination regimens of two or three drugs are most effective. Regimens of doxycycline (200 mg/day orally for 6 weeks) plus rifampin (600 mg/day orally for 6 weeks) or streptomycin (1 g/day intramuscularly for 2 weeks) or gentamicin (240 mg intramuscularly once daily for 7 days) have the lowest recurrence rates. Longer courses of therapy may be required to prevent relapse of meningitis, osteomyelitis, or endocarditis.

Herrick JA et al. *Brucella* arteritis: clinical manifestations, treatment, and prognosis. Lancet Infect Dis. 2014 Jun;14(6):520–6. [PMID: 24480149]

Vilchez G et al. Brucellosis in pregnancy: clinical aspects and obstetric outcomes. Int J Infect Dis. 2015 Sep;38:95–100. [PMID: 26159844]

TULAREMIA

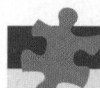

ESSENTIALS OF DIAGNOSIS

- ▶ History of contact with rabbits, other rodents, and biting ticks in summer in endemic area.
- ▶ Fever, headache, nausea, and prostration.
- ▶ Papule progressing to ulcer at site of inoculation.
- ▶ Enlarged regional lymph nodes.
- ▶ Serologic tests or culture of ulcer, lymph node aspirate, or blood confirm the diagnosis.

▶ General Considerations

Tularemia is a zoonotic infection of wild rodents and rabbits caused by *Francisella tularensis*. Humans usually acquire the infection by contact with animal tissues (eg, trapping muskrats, skinning rabbits) or from a tick or insect bite. Hamsters and prairie dogs also may carry the organism. An outbreak of pneumonic tularemia on Martha's Vineyard in Massachusetts was linked to lawn-mowing and brush-cutting as risk factors for infection, underscoring the potential for probable aerosol transmission of the organism. *F tularensis* has been classified as a high-priority agent for potential bioterrorism use because of its virulence and relative ease of dissemination. Infection in humans often produces a local lesion and widespread organ involvement but may be entirely asymptomatic. The incubation period is 2–10 days.

▶ Clinical Findings

A. Symptoms and Signs

Fever, headache, and nausea begin suddenly, and a local lesion—a papule at the site of inoculation—develops and soon ulcerates. Regional lymph nodes may become enlarged and tender and may suppurate. The local lesion may be on the skin of an extremity or in the eye. Pneumonia may develop from hematogenous spread of the organism or may be primary after inhalation of infected aerosols, which are responsible for human-to-human transmission. Following ingestion of infected meat or water, an enteric form may be manifested by gastrointestinal symptoms, stupor, and delirium. In any type of involvement, the spleen may be enlarged and tender and there may be nonspecific rashes, myalgias, and prostration.

B. Laboratory Findings

Culturing the organism from blood or infected tissue requires special media. For this reason and because cultures of *F tularensis* may be hazardous to laboratory personnel, the diagnosis is usually made serologically. A positive agglutination test (greater than 1:80) develops in the second week after infection and may persist for several years.

Differential Diagnosis

Tularemia must be differentiated from rickettsial and meningococcal infections, cat-scratch disease, infectious mononucleosis, and various bacterial and fungal diseases.

Complications

Hematogenous spread may produce meningitis, perisplenitis, pericarditis, pneumonia, and osteomyelitis.

Treatment

Streptomycin is the drug of choice for treatment of tularemia. The recommended dose is 7.5 mg/kg intramuscularly every 12 hours for 7–14 days. Gentamicin, which has good in vitro activity against *F tularensis*, is generally less toxic than streptomycin but some case series report lower treatment success rates. Doxycycline (200 mg/day orally) is also effective but has a higher relapse rate and should only be used for the less seriously ill. A variety of other agents (eg, fluoroquinolones) are active in vitro, but their clinical effectiveness is less well established.

Maurin M et al. Tularaemia: clinical aspects in Europe. Lancet Infect Dis. 2016 Jan;16(1):113–24. [PMID: 26738841]

Yanes H et al. Evaluation of in-house and commercial serological tests for diagnosis of human tularemia. J Clin Microbiol. 2018 Jan;56(1):e01440–17. [PMID: 29118164]

PLAGUE

ESSENTIALS OF DIAGNOSIS

- ▶ History of exposure to rodents in endemic area.
- ▶ Sudden onset of high fever, muscular pains, and prostration.
- ▶ Axillary, cervical, or inguinal lymphadenitis (bubo).
- ▶ Pustule or ulcer at inoculation site.
- ▶ Pneumonia or meningitis is often fatal.
- ▶ Positive smear and culture from bubo and positive blood culture.

General Considerations

Plague is an infection of wild rodents with *Yersinia pestis*, a small bipolar-staining gram-negative rod. It is endemic in California, Arizona, Nevada, and New Mexico. Worldwide, Madagascar accounts for three-quarters of the global burden. It is transmitted among rodents and to humans by the bites of fleas or from contact with infected animals. Following a fleabite, the organisms spread through the lymphatics to the lymph nodes, which become greatly enlarged

(buboes). They may then reach the bloodstream to involve all organs. When pneumonia or meningitis develops, the outcome is often fatal. The patient with pneumonia can transmit the infection to other individuals by droplets. The incubation period is 2–10 days. Because of its extreme virulence, its potential for dissemination and person-to-person transmission, and efforts to develop the organism as an agent of biowarfare, plague bacillus is considered a high-priority agent for bioterrorism.

Clinical Findings

A. Symptoms and Signs

The onset is sudden, with high fever, malaise, tachycardia, intense headache, delirium, and severe myalgias. The patient appears profoundly ill. If pneumonia develops, tachypnea, productive cough, blood-tinged sputum, and cyanosis also occur. There may be signs of meningitis. A pustule or ulcer at the site of inoculation and lymphangitis may be observed. Axillary, inguinal, or cervical lymph nodes become enlarged and tender and may suppurate and drain. With hematogenous spread, the patient may rapidly become toxic and comatose, with purpuric spots (black plague) appearing on the skin.

Primary plague pneumonia is a fulminant pneumonitis with bloody, frothy sputum and sepsis. It is usually fatal unless treatment is started within a few hours after onset.

B. Laboratory Findings

The plague bacillus may be found in smears from aspirates of buboes examined with Gram stain. Cultures from bubo aspirate or pus and blood are positive but may grow slowly. In convalescing patients, an antibody titer rise may be demonstrated by agglutination tests.

Differential Diagnosis

The lymphadenitis of plague is most commonly mistaken for the lymphadenitis accompanying staphylococcal or streptococcal infections of an extremity, sexually transmitted diseases such as lymphogranuloma venereum or syphilis, and tularemia. The systemic manifestations resemble those of enteric or rickettsial fevers, malaria, or influenza. The pneumonia resembles other bacterial pneumonias, and the meningitis is similar to those caused by other bacteria.

Prevention

Avoiding exposure to rodents and fleas in endemic areas is the best prevention strategy. Drug prophylaxis may provide temporary protection for persons exposed to the risk of plague infection, particularly by the respiratory route. Doxycycline, 100 mg twice daily for 7 days, is effective. No vaccine is available at this time.

Treatment

Therapy should be started immediately once plague is suspected. Either streptomycin (the agent with which there is greatest experience), 1 g every 12 hours intravenously, or gentamicin, administered as a 2-mg/kg loading dose, then

1.7 mg/kg every 8 hours intravenously, is effective. Alternatively, doxycycline, 100 mg orally or intravenously, may be used. The duration of therapy is 10 days. Patients with plague pneumonia are placed in strict respiratory isolation, and prophylactic therapy is given to any person who came in contact with the patient.

Burki T. Plague in Madagascar. Lancet Infect Dis. 2017 Dec; 17(12):1241. [PMID: 29173885]
Yang R. Plague: recognition, treatment, and prevention. J Clin Microbiol. 2018 Jan;56(1):e01519–17. [PMID: 29070654]

GONOCOCCAL INFECTIONS

ESSENTIALS OF DIAGNOSIS

▶ Purulent, profuse urethral discharge with dysuria, especially in men; yields positive smear.

▶ **Men:** epididymitis, prostatitis, periurethral inflammation, proctitis, pharyngitis.

▶ **Women:** cervicitis with purulent discharge, or asymptomatic, yielding positive culture; vaginitis, salpingitis, proctitis also occur.

▶ **Disseminated disease:** fever, rash, tenosynovitis, and arthritis.

▶ Gram-negative intracellular diplococci seen in a smear or cultured from the urethra, cervix, pharynx, or rectum.

General Considerations

Gonorrhea is caused by *Neisseria gonorrhoeae*, a gram-negative diplococcus typically found inside polymorphonuclear cells. It is transmitted during sexual activity and has its greatest incidence in the 15- to 29-year-old age group. The incubation period is usually 2–8 days.

Classification

A. Urethritis and Cervicitis

Initial symptoms seen in men include burning on urination and a serous or milky discharge. One to 3 days later, the urethral pain is more pronounced and the discharge becomes yellow, creamy, and profuse, sometimes blood-tinged. The disorder may regress and become chronic or progress to involve the prostate, epididymis, and periurethral glands with painful inflammation. Chronic infection leads to prostatitis and urethral strictures. Rectal infection is common in men who have sex with men. Atypical sites of primary infection (eg, the pharynx) must always be considered. Asymptomatic infection is common and occurs in both sexes.

Gonococcal infection in women often becomes symptomatic during menses. Women may have dysuria, urinary frequency, and urgency, with a purulent urethral discharge. Vaginitis and cervicitis with inflammation of Bartholin glands are common. Infection may be asymptomatic, with only slightly increased vaginal discharge and moderate cervicitis on examination. Infection may remain as a chronic cervicitis—an important reservoir of gonococci. It can progress to involve the uterus and tubes with acute and chronic salpingitis, with scarring of tubes and sterility. In pelvic inflammatory disease, anaerobes and chlamydiae often accompany gonococci. Rectal infection may result from spread of the organism from the genital tract or from anal coitus.

Nucleic acid amplification tests are the preferred method for diagnosing all types of gonorrhea given their excellent sensitivity and specificity. In women with suspected cervical infection, endocervical or vaginal swabs (clinician- or self-collected) as well as first catch AM urine specimen (later specimens have 10% reduced sensitivity) are options. In men with urethral infection, first catch AM urine is recommended. Nucleic acid amplification tests are also recommended by the CDC for oropharyngeal and rectal sites testing although they are not FDA approved for these specimen types. Gram stain of urethral or rectal discharge in men, especially during the first week after onset, shows gram-negative diplococci in polymorphonuclear leukocytes. Gram stain is less often positive in women. Cultures should still be obtained when evaluating a treatment failure to assess for antimicrobial resistance.

B. Disseminated Disease

Systemic complications follow the dissemination of gonococci from the primary site via the bloodstream. Two distinct clinical syndromes—either purulent arthritis or the triad of rash, tenosynovitis, and arthralgias—are commonly observed in patients with disseminated gonococcal infection, although overlap can be seen. The skin lesions can range from maculopapular to pustular or hemorrhagic, which tend to be few in number and peripherally located. The tenosynovitis is often found in the hands and wrists and feet and ankles. These unique findings can help distinguish among other infectious syndromes. The arthritis can occur in one or more joints and may be migratory. Gonococci are isolated by culture from less than half of patients with gonococcal arthritis. Rarely, gonococcal endocarditis or meningitis develops.

C. Conjunctivitis

The most common form of eye involvement is direct inoculation of gonococci into the conjunctival sac. In adults, this occurs by autoinoculation of a person with genital infection. The purulent conjunctivitis may rapidly progress to panophthalmitis and loss of the eye unless treated promptly. A single 1-g dose of ceftriaxone is effective.

Differential Diagnosis

Gonococcal urethritis or cervicitis must be differentiated from nongonococcal urethritis; cervicitis or vaginitis due to *Chlamydia trachomatis, Gardnerella vaginalis, Trichomonas, Candida*, and many other pathogens associated with sexually transmitted diseases; and pelvic inflammatory disease, arthritis, proctitis, and skin lesions. Often, several such pathogens coexist in a patient. Reactive arthritis (urethritis, conjunctivitis, arthritis) may mimic gonorrhea or coexist with it.

Prevention

Prevention is based on education and mechanical or chemical prophylaxis. The condom, if properly used, can reduce the risk of infection. Partner notification and referral of contacts for treatment has been the standard method used to control sexually transmitted diseases. Early treatment of contacts can halt the development of symptoms as well. Expedited treatment of sex partners by patient-delivered partner therapy is more effective than partner notification in reducing persistence and recurrence rates of gonorrhea and chlamydia.

Treatment

Therapy typically is administered before antimicrobial susceptibilities are known. The choice of which regimen to use should be based on the national prevalences of antibiotic-resistant organisms. Nationwide, strains of gonococci that are resistant to penicillin, tetracycline, or ciprofloxacin have been increasingly observed. Consequently, these drugs can no longer be considered first-line therapy. Resistance to azithromycin and to ceftriaxone has been reported. All sexual partners should be treated and tested for HIV infection and syphilis, as should the patient.

A. Uncomplicated Gonorrhea

Due to increasing resistance of *N gonorrhoeae* to cephalosporins, the CDC recommends a higher dose of intramuscular ceftriaxone in combination with a second drug (azithromycin or doxycycline) regardless of concern for possible secondary infection with chlamydia. For uncomplicated gonococcal infections of the cervix, urethra, and rectum, the recommended treatment is ceftriaxone (250 mg intramuscularly) plus azithromycin (1000 mg orally as a single dose). In cases where an oral cephalosporin is the only option, cefixime, 400 mg orally as a single dose, can be combined with azithromycin as above. When azithromycin is not an option, doxycycline at 100 mg orally twice daily for 7 days can be substituted. Fluoroquinolones are no longer recommended for treatment due to high rates of microbial resistance. Spectinomycin, 1 g intramuscularly once, may be used for the penicillin-allergic patient but is not currently available in the United States. Pharyngeal gonorrhea is also treated with ceftriaxone (250 mg intramuscularly) plus azithromycin (1000 mg orally as a single dose), but for conjunctival gonorrhea, the recommendation is for ceftriaxone (1 g intramuscularly) plus azithromycin (1000 mg orally as a single dose).

B. Treatment of Other Infections

Disseminated gonococcal infection (including arthritis and arthritis-dermatitis syndromes) should be treated with ceftriaxone (1 g intravenously daily) plus azithromycin (1000 mg orally as a single dose), until 48 hours after improvement begins, at which time therapy may be switched to cefixime (400 mg orally daily) to complete at least 1 week of antimicrobial therapy. Endocarditis should

be treated with ceftriaxone (2 g every 24 hours intravenously) for at least 4 weeks.

Pelvic inflammatory disease requires cefoxitin (2 g parenterally every 6 hours) or cefotetan (2 g intravenously every 12 hours) plus doxycycline (100 mg every 12 hours). Clindamycin (900 mg intravenously every 8 hours) plus gentamicin (administered intravenously as a 2-mg/kg loading dose followed by 1.5 mg/kg every 8 hours) is also effective. Ceftriaxone (250 mg intramuscularly as a single dose) or cefoxitin (2 g intramuscularly) plus probenecid (1 g orally as a single dose) plus doxycycline (100 mg twice a day for 14 days), with or without metronidazole (500 mg twice daily for 14 days), is an effective outpatient regimen.

De Ambrogi M. International forum on gonococcal infections and resistance. Lancet Infect Dis. 2017 Nov;17(11):1127. [PMID: 29115267]

Workowski KA et al; Centers for Disease Control and Prevention (CDC). Sexually transmitted diseases treatment guidelines, 2015. MMWR Recomm Rep. 2015 Jun 5;64(RR-03):1–137. Erratum in: MMWR Recomm Rep. 2015 Aug 28;64(33):924. [PMID: 26042815]

CHANCROID

Chancroid is a sexually transmitted disease caused by the short gram-negative bacillus *Haemophilus ducreyi*. The incubation period is 3–5 days. At the site of inoculation, a vesicopustule develops that breaks down to form a painful, soft ulcer with a necrotic base, surrounding erythema, and undermined edges. There may be multiple lesions due to autoinoculation. The adenitis is usually unilateral and consists of tender, matted nodes of moderate size with overlying erythema. These may become fluctuant and rupture spontaneously. With lymph node involvement, fever, chills, and malaise may develop. Balanitis and phimosis are frequent complications in men. Women may have no external signs of infection. The diagnosis is established by culturing a swab of the lesion onto a special medium.

Chancroid must be differentiated from other genital ulcers. The chancre of syphilis is clean and painless, with a hard base. Mixed sexually transmitted disease is very common (including syphilis, herpes simplex, and HIV infection), as is infection of the ulcer with fusiforms, spirochetes, and other organisms.

A single dose of either azithromycin, 1 g orally, or ceftriaxone, 250 mg intramuscularly, is effective treatment. Effective multiple-dose regimens are erythromycin, 500 mg orally four times a day for 7 days, or ciprofloxacin, 500 mg orally twice a day for 3 days.

Workowski KA et al; Centers for Disease Control and Prevention (CDC). Sexually transmitted diseases treatment guidelines, 2015. MMWR Recomm Rep. 2015 Jun 5;64(RR-03):1–137. Erratum in: MMWR Recomm Rep. 2015 Aug 28;64(33):924. [PMID: 26042815]

GRANULOMA INGUINALE

Granuloma inguinale is a chronic, relapsing granulomatous anogenital infection due to *Calymmatobacterium (Donovania) granulomatis*. The pathognomonic cell, found in tissue scrapings or secretions, is large (25–90 mcm) and contains intracytoplasmic cysts filled with bodies (Donovan bodies) that stain deeply with Wright stain.

The incubation period is 8 days to 12 weeks. The onset is insidious. The lesions occur on the skin or mucous membranes of the genitalia or perineal area. They are relatively painless infiltrated nodules that soon slough. A shallow, sharply demarcated ulcer forms, with a beefy-red friable base of granulation tissue. The lesion spreads by contiguity. The advancing border has a characteristic rolled edge of granulation tissue. Large ulcerations may advance onto the lower abdomen and thighs. Scar formation and healing occur along one border while the opposite border advances.

Superinfection with spirochete-fusiform organisms is common. The ulcer then becomes purulent, painful, foul-smelling, and extremely difficult to treat.

Several therapies are available. Because of the indolent nature of the disease, duration of therapy is relatively long. The following recommended regimens should be given for 3 weeks or until all lesions have healed: doxycycline, 100 mg orally twice daily; or azithromycin, 1 g orally once weekly; or ciprofloxacin, 750 mg orally twice daily; or erythromycin, 500 mg orally four times a day.

Workowski KA et al; Centers for Disease Control and Prevention (CDC). Sexually transmitted diseases treatment guidelines, 2015. MMWR Recomm Rep. 2015 Jun 5;64(RR-03):1–137. Erratum in: MMWR Recomm Rep. 2015 Aug 28;64(33):924. [PMID: 26042815]

BARTONELLA SPECIES

Bartonella species are responsible for a wide variety of clinical syndromes. **Bacillary angiomatosis**, an important manifestation of bartonellosis, is discussed in Chapter 31. A variety of atypical infections, including retinitis, encephalitis, osteomyelitis, and persistent bacteremia and endocarditis (especially consider in culture-negative endocarditis), have been described.

Trench fever is a self-limited, louse-borne relapsing febrile disease caused by *B quintana*. The disease has occurred epidemically in louse-infested troops and civilians during wars and endemically in residents of scattered geographic areas (eg, Central America). An urban equivalent of trench fever has been described among the homeless. Humans acquire infection when infected lice feces enter sites of skin breakdown. Onset of symptoms is abrupt and fever lasts 3–5 days, with relapses. The patient complains of weakness and severe pain behind the eyes and typically in the back and legs. Lymphadenopathy, splenomegaly, and a transient maculopapular rash may appear. Subclinical infection is frequent, and a carrier state is recognized. The differential diagnosis includes other febrile, self-limited states such as dengue, leptospirosis, malaria, relapsing fever, and typhus. Treatment is generally not required since spontaneous recovery occurs regularly.

Cat-scratch disease is an acute infection of children and young adults caused by *Bartonella henselae*. It is transmitted from cats to humans as the result of a scratch or bite. Within a few days, a papule or ulcer will develop at the inoculation site in one-third of patients. One to 3 weeks later, fever, headache, and malaise occur. Regional lymph nodes become enlarged, often tender, and may suppurate. Lymphadenopathy from cat scratches resembles that due to neoplasm, tuberculosis, lymphogranuloma venereum, and bacterial lymphadenitis. The diagnosis is usually made clinically. Special cultures for bartonellae, serology, or excisional biopsy, though rarely necessary, confirm the diagnosis. The biopsy reveals necrotizing lymphadenitis and is itself not specific for cat-scratch disease. Cat-scratch disease is usually self-limited, requiring no specific therapy. Encephalitis occurs rarely.

Disseminated forms of the disease—bacillary angiomatosis, peliosis hepatis, and retinitis—occur most commonly in immunocompromised patients such as persons with late stages of HIV or solid organ transplant recipients. The lesions are vasculoproliferative and histopathologically distinct from those of cat-scratch disease. Unexplained fever in patients with late stages of HIV infection is not uncommonly due to bartonellosis. *B quintana*, the agent of trench fever, can also cause bacillary angiomatosis and persistent bacteremia or endocarditis (which will be "culture-negative" unless specifically sought), the latter two entities being associated with homelessness. Due to the fastidious nature of the organism and its special growth requirements, serologic testing (eg, demonstration of a high antibody titer in an indirect immunofluorescence assay) or nucleic acid amplification tests are often required to establish a diagnosis.

The disseminated forms of the disease (bacillary angiomatosis, peliosis hepatis, and retinitis) require a prolonged course of antibiotic therapy often in combination with a second agent. Bacteremia and endocarditis can be effectively treated with a 6-week course of doxycycline (200 mg orally or intravenously in two divided doses per day) plus either gentamicin 3 mg/kg/day intravenously or rifampin 600 mg/day orally in two divided doses. Relapse may occur.

Edouard S et al. *Bartonella*, a common cause of endocarditis: a report on 106 cases and review. J Clin Microbiol. 2015 Mar; 53(3):824–9. [PMID: 25540398]

Okaro U et al. *Bartonella* species, an emerging cause of blood-culture-negative endocarditis. Clin Microbiol Rev. 2017 Jul; 30(3):709–46. [PMID: 28490579]

ANAEROBIC INFECTIONS

Anaerobic infections tend to be polymicrobial and abscesses are common. Pus and infected tissue often are malodorous. Septic thrombophlebitis and metastatic infection are frequent and may require incision and drainage. Diminished blood supply that favors proliferation of anaerobes because of reduced tissue oxygenation may interfere with the delivery of antimicrobials to the site of anaerobic infection. Cultures, unless carefully collected under anaerobic conditions, may yield negative results.

Important types of infections that are most commonly caused by anaerobic organisms are listed below. Treatment of all these infections consists of surgical exploration and judicious excision in conjunction with administration of antimicrobial drugs.

1. Head & Neck Infections

Prevotella melaninogenica (formerly *Bacteroides melaninogenicus*) and anaerobic spirochetes are commonly involved in periodontal infections. These organisms, fusobacteria, and peptostreptococci may cause chronic sinusitis, peritonsillar abscess, chronic otitis media, and mastoiditis. *F necrophorum* has been recognized as a common cause of pharyngitis in adolescents and young adults. *F necrophorum* infection has been associated with septic internal jugular thrombophlebitis (Lemierre syndrome) and causes septic pulmonary embolization. Hygiene, drainage, and surgical debridement are as important in treatment as antimicrobials. Penicillin alone is inadequate treatment for infections from oral anaerobic organisms because of increasing penicillin resistance, usually due to beta-lactamase production. Therefore, ampicillin/sulbactam 1.5–3 g intravenously every 6 hours (if parenteral therapy is required), or amoxicillin/clavulanic acid 875 mg/125 mg orally twice daily, or clindamycin can be used (600 mg intravenously every 8 hours or 300 mg orally every 6 hours). Antimicrobial treatment is continued for a few days after symptoms and signs of infection have resolved. Indolent, established infections (eg, mastoiditis or osteomyelitis) may require prolonged courses of therapy, eg, 4–6 weeks or longer.

Brook I. Spectrum and treatment of anaerobic infections. J Infect Chemother. 2016 Jan;22(1):1–13. [PMID: 26620376]

2. Chest Infections

Usually in the setting of poor oral hygiene and periodontal disease, aspiration of saliva (which contains 10^8 anaerobic organisms per milliliter in addition to aerobes) may lead to necrotizing pneumonia, lung abscess, and empyema. Polymicrobial infection is the rule, and anaerobes—particularly *P melaninogenica*, fusobacteria, and peptostreptococci—are common etiologic agents. Most pulmonary infections respond to antimicrobial therapy alone. Percutaneous chest tube or surgical drainage is indicated for empyema.

Penicillin-resistant *Bacteroides fragilis* and *P melaninogenica* are commonly isolated and have been associated with clinical failures. Clindamycin, 600 mg intravenously once, followed by 300 mg orally every 6–8 hours, is the treatment of choice for these infections. Metronidazole does not cover facultative streptococci, which often are present, and if used, a second agent that is active against streptococci, such as ceftriaxone 1 g intravenously or intramuscularly daily, should be added. Penicillin, 2 million units intravenously every 4 hours, followed by amoxicillin, 500 mg every 8 hours orally, is an alternative; however, increasing prevalence of beta-lactamase producing organisms is a concern. Moxifloxacin, 400 mg orally or intravenously once daily, may be used. Because these infections respond slowly, a prolonged course of therapy (eg, 4–6 weeks) is generally recommended.

Brook I. Spectrum and treatment of anaerobic infections. J Infect Chemother. 2016 Jan;22(1):1–13. [PMID: 26620376]

3. Central Nervous System

Anaerobes are a common cause of brain abscess, subdural empyema, or septic CNS thrombophlebitis. The organisms reach the CNS by direct extension from sinusitis, otitis, or mastoiditis or by hematogenous spread from chronic lung infections. Antimicrobial therapy—eg, ceftriaxone, 2 g intravenously every 12 hours, plus metronidazole, 500 mg intravenously every 8 hours—is an important adjunct to surgical drainage. Duration of therapy is 6–8 weeks but should be based on follow-up imaging. Some small multiple brain abscesses can be treated with antibiotics alone without surgical drainage.

Brook I. Spectrum and treatment of anaerobic infections. J Infect Chemother. 2016 Jan;22(1):1–13. [PMID: 26620376]

4. Intra-Abdominal Infections

In the colon there are up to 10^{11} anaerobes per gram of content—predominantly *B fragilis*, clostridia, and peptostreptococci. These organisms play a central role in most intra-abdominal abscesses following trauma to the colon, diverticulitis, appendicitis, or perirectal abscess and may also participate in hepatic abscess and cholecystitis, often in association with aerobic coliform bacteria. The bacteriology includes anaerobes as well as enteric gram-negative rods and on occasion enterococci. Therapy should be directed both against anaerobes and gram-negative aerobes. Agents that are active against *B fragilis* include metronidazole, chloramphenicol, moxifloxacin, tigecycline, ertapenem, imipenem, doripenem, ampicillin-sulbactam, ticarcillin-clavulanic acid, piperacillin-tazobactam, and ceftolozane/tazobactam. Resistance to cefoxitin, cefotetan, and clindamycin is increasingly encountered. Most third-generation cephalosporins have poor efficacy.

Table 33–6 summarizes the antibiotic regimens for management of moderate to moderately severe infections (eg, patient hemodynamically stable, good surgical drainage possible or established, low APACHE score, no multiple organ failure) and severe infections (eg, major peritoneal soilage, large or multiple abscesses, patient hemodynamically unstable), particularly if drug-resistant organisms are suspected. An effective oral regimen for patients able to take it is presented also.

Brook I. Spectrum and treatment of anaerobic infections. J Infect Chemother. 2016 Jan;22(1):1–13. [PMID: 26620376]
Sawyer RG et al. Trial of short-course antimicrobial therapy for intraabdominal infection. N Engl J Med. 2015 May 21; 372(21):1996–2005. [PMID: 25992746]

5. Female Genital Tract & Pelvic Infections

The normal flora of the vagina and cervix includes several species of bacteroides, peptostreptococci, group B streptococci, lactobacilli, coliform bacteria, and, occasionally, spirochetes and clostridia. These organisms commonly cause genital tract infections and may disseminate from there.

While salpingitis is often caused by gonococci and chlamydiae, tubo-ovarian and pelvic abscesses are associated

Table 33–6. Treatment of anaerobic intra-abdominal infections.

Community-onset
Oral therapy
Moxifloxacin 400 mg every 24 hours
Intravenous therapy
Moderate to moderately severe infections:
Ertapenem 1 g intravenously every 24 hours
or
Ceftriaxone 1 g intravenously every 24 hours plus metronidazole intravenously or orally, 500 mg every 8 hours. If penicillin allergic, can replace ceftriaxone with ciprofloxacin 400 mg intravenously (or 500 mg orally) every 12 hours.
Severe infections:
Imipenem 0.5 g intravenously every 6–8 hours or meropenem 1 g every 8 hours or doripenem 0.5 g every 8 hours or piperacillin/tazobactam 3.75 g every 6 hours
Health care–associated
Intravenous therapy
Imipenem 0.5 g intravenously every 6–8 hours or meropenem 1 g every 8 hours or doripenem 0.5 g every 8 hours or piperacillin/tazobactam 4.5 g every 6 hours
or
Ceftazidime or cefepime 2 g intravenously every 8 hours plus metronidazole 500 mg intravenously or orally every 8 hours

with anaerobes in most cases. Postpartum infections may be caused by aerobic streptococci or staphylococci, but anaerobes are often found, and the worst cases of postpartum or postabortion sepsis are associated with clostridia and bacteroides. These have a high mortality rate, and treatment requires both antimicrobials directed against anaerobes and coliforms (similar to treatment of anaerobic intra-abdominal infections, Table 33–6) and abscess drainage or early hysterectomy.

Brook I. Spectrum and treatment of anaerobic infections. J Infect Chemother. 2016 Jan;22(1):1–13. [PMID: 26620376]
Mackeen AD et al. Antibiotic regimens for postpartum endometritis. Cochrane Database Syst Rev. 2015 Feb 2;2:CD001067. [PMID: 25922861]

6. Bacteremia & Endocarditis

Anaerobic bacteremia usually originates from the gastrointestinal tract, the oropharynx, pressure injuries, or the female genital tract. Endocarditis due to anaerobic and microaerophilic streptococci and bacteroides originates from the same sites. Most cases of anaerobic or microaerophilic streptococcal endocarditis can be effectively treated with 12–20 million units of penicillin G intravenously daily for 4–6 weeks, but optimal therapy of other types of anaerobic bacterial endocarditis must rely on laboratory guidance. Propionibacteria, clostridia, and bacteroides occasionally cause endocarditis.

Brook I. Spectrum and treatment of anaerobic infections. J Infect Chemother. 2016 Jan;22(1):1–13. [PMID: 26620376]

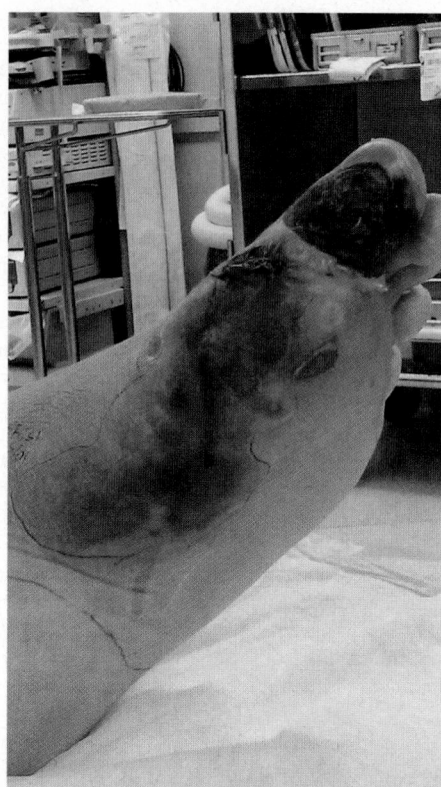

▲ **Figure 33–6.** Left foot gangrene, with plantar extension. (Used, with permission, from Dean SM, Satiani B, Abraham WT. *Color Atlas and Synopsis of Vascular Diseases.* McGraw-Hill, 2014.)

7. Skin & Soft Tissue Infections

Anaerobic infections of the skin and soft tissue usually follow trauma, inadequate blood supply, or surgery and are most common in areas that are contaminated by oral or fecal flora. These infections also occur in injection drug users and persons sustaining animal bites. There may be progressive tissue necrosis (Figure 33–6) and a putrid odor.

Several terms, such as bacterial synergistic gangrene, synergistic necrotizing cellulitis, necrotizing fasciitis, and non-clostridial crepitant cellulitis, have been used to classify these infections. Although there are some differences in microbiology among them, their differentiation on clinical grounds alone is difficult. All are mixed infections caused by aerobic and anaerobic organisms and require aggressive surgical debridement of necrotic tissue for cure.

Broad-spectrum antibiotics active against both anaerobes and gram-positive and gram-negative aerobes (eg, vancomycin plus piperacillin-tazobactam) should be instituted empirically and modified by culture results (see Table 30–5). They are given for about a week after progressive tissue destruction has been controlled and the margins of the wound remain free of inflammation.

Brook I. Spectrum and treatment of anaerobic infections. J Infect Chemother. 2016 Jan;22(1):1–13. [PMID: 26620376] de Prost N et al. Therapeutic targets in necrotizing soft tissue infections. Intensive Care Med. 2017 Nov;43(11):1717–9. [PMID: 28474117]

PROCALCITONIN

Procalcitonin is a peptide released by human cells in response to exposure to bacterial toxins and is measurable in the serum. Procalcitonin is also downregulated in the setting of viral infection. Therefore, it is more specific than C-reactive protein or white blood cell count. Procalcitonin has been studied as a marker to determine both when to start antibiotic therapy and duration of antibiotic therapy in infection. In these trials, antibiotics were safely held or withdrawn when the procalcitonin level was normal or decreasing by a substantial amount. Systematic reviews of available literature support the use of procalcitonin to guide treatment in patients presenting with acute respiratory infections and sepsis. Antibiotic consumption is significantly reduced across different clinical settings when guided by procalcitonin levels; procalcitonin can be used effectively in these settings only when used as a point of care test.

Branche AR et al. Serum procalcitonin measurement and viral testing to guide antibiotic use for respiratory infections in hospitalized adults: a randomized controlled trial. J Infect Dis. 2015 Dec 1;212(11):1692–700. [PMID: 25910632]

de Jong E et al. Efficacy and safety of procalcitonin guidance in reducing the duration of antibiotic treatment in critically ill patients: a randomised, controlled, open-label trial. Lancet Infect Dis. 2016 Jul;16(7):819–27. [PMID: 26947523]

Huang DT et al; ProACT Investigators. Procalcitonin-guided use of antibiotics for lower respiratory tract infection. N Engl J Med. 2018 Jul 19;379(3):236–49. [PMID: 29781385]

ACTINOMYCOSIS

ESSENTIALS OF DIAGNOSIS

► History of recent dental infection, abdominal trauma, or intrauterine contraception device placement.

► Chronic pneumonia or indolent cervicofacial or intra-abdominal abscess.

► Sinus tract formation.

General Considerations

Actinomyces israelii and other species of *Actinomyces* occur in the normal flora of the mouth and tonsillar crypts. They are anaerobic, gram-positive, branching filamentous bacteria (1 mcm in diameter) that may fragment into bacillary forms. When introduced into traumatized tissue and associated with other anaerobic bacteria, these actinomycetes become pathogens.

The most common site of infection is the cervicofacial area (about 60% of cases). Infection typically follows extraction of a tooth or other trauma. Lesions may develop in the gastrointestinal tract or lungs following ingestion or aspiration of the organism from its endogenous source in the mouth. Interestingly, *T whipplei*, the causative agent of Whipple disease, is an actinomycete and therefore is related to the species that cause actinomycosis.

Clinical Findings

A. Symptoms and Signs

1. Cervicofacial actinomycosis—Cervicofacial actinomycosis develops slowly. The area becomes markedly indurated, and the overlying skin becomes reddish or cyanotic. Abscesses eventually draining to the surface persist for long periods. "Sulfur granules"—masses of filamentous organisms—may be found in the pus. There is usually little pain unless there is secondary infection. Trismus indicates that the muscles of mastication are involved. Radiography may reveal bony involvement. Cervicofacial or thoracic disease may occasionally involve the CNS, most commonly brain abscess or meningitis.

2. Thoracic actinomycosis—Thoracic involvement begins with fever, cough, and sputum production with night sweats and weight loss. Pleuritic pain may be present. Multiple sinuses may extend through the chest wall, to the heart, or into the abdominal cavity. Ribs may be involved. Radiography shows areas of consolidation and in many cases pleural effusion.

3. Abdominal actinomycosis—Abdominal actinomycosis usually causes pain in the ileocecal region, spiking fever and chills, vomiting, and weight loss; it may be confused with Crohn disease. Irregular abdominal masses may be palpated. Pelvic inflammatory disease caused by actinomycetes has been associated with prolonged use of an intrauterine contraceptive device. Sinuses draining to the exterior may develop. CT scanning reveals an inflammatory mass extended to involve bone.

B. Laboratory Findings

The anaerobic, gram-positive organism may be demonstrated as a granule or as scattered branching gram-positive filaments in the pus. Anaerobic culture is necessary to distinguish actinomycetes from nocardiae because specific therapy differs for the two infections. Histopathology examination of affected tissue and bone is useful in identifying organisms that are fastidious and slow to culture.

Treatment

Penicillin G is the drug of choice. Ten to 20 million units are given via a parenteral route for 4–6 weeks, followed by oral penicillin V, 500 mg four times daily. Alternatives include ampicillin, 12 g/day intravenously for 4–6 weeks, followed by oral amoxicillin, 500 mg three times daily, or doxycycline, 100 mg twice daily intravenously or orally. Response to therapy is slow. Therapy should be continued for weeks to months after clinical manifestations have disappeared in order to ensure cure. Surgical procedures such as drainage and resection may be beneficial. With penicillin and surgery, the prognosis is good. The difficulties of diagnosis, however, may permit extensive destruction of tissue before the diagnosis is identified and therapy is started.

Könönen E et al. *Actinomyces* and related organisms in human infections. Clin Microbiol Rev. 2015 Apr;28(2):419–42. [PMID: 25788515]
Steininger C et al. Resistance patterns in clinical isolates of pathogenic *Actinomyces* species. J Antimicrob Chemother. 2016 Feb;71(2):422–7. [PMID: 26538502]
Xu Y et al. Disseminated actinomycosis. N Engl J Med. 2018 Sep 13;379(11):1071. [PMID: 30207906]

NOCARDIOSIS

Nocardia species are aerobic filamentous soil bacteria that can cause pulmonary and systemic nocardiosis. Common *Nocardia* species include members of the *Nocardia asteroides* complex and *Nocardia brasiliensis*. Bronchopulmonary abnormalities (eg, alveolar proteinosis) predispose to colonization, but infection is unusual unless the patient is also receiving systemic corticosteroids or is otherwise immunosuppressed.

► Clinical Findings

Pulmonary involvement usually begins with malaise, loss of weight, fever, and night sweats. Cough and production of purulent sputum are the chief complaints. Radiography may show infiltrates accompanied by pleural effusion. The lesions may penetrate to the exterior through the chest wall, invading the ribs.

Dissemination involves any organ. Brain abscesses and subcutaneous nodules are most frequent. Even in the absence of clinical symptoms and signs of CNS infection, clinicians should consider brain imaging in patients with nocardiosis to rule out an occult abscess.

Nocardia species are usually found as delicate, branching, gram-positive filaments. They may be weakly acid-fast, occasionally causing diagnostic confusion with tuberculosis. Identification is made by culture.

► Treatment

For isolated cutaneous infections, therapy is initiated with trimethoprim-sulfamethoxazole administered at a dosage of 5–10 mg/kg/day (based on trimethoprim) as an oral or intravenous formulation. Surgical procedures such as drainage and resection may be needed as adjunctive therapy. A higher dose of 15 mg/kg/day (based on trimethoprim) should be used for disseminated or pulmonary infections. Resistance to trimethoprim-sulfamethoxazole is increasing and initiating treatment with two drugs while awaiting antibiotic susceptibilities in cases of disseminated or severe localized disease should be considered. Alternative agents or drugs that can be given in combination with trimethoprim-sulfamethoxazole include imipenem, 500 mg intravenously every 6 hours; amikacin, 7.5 mg/kg intravenously every 12 hours; or minocycline, 100–200 mg orally or intravenously twice daily. Consultation with an infectious diseases expert is encouraged.

Response may be slow, and therapy should be continued for at least 6 months. The prognosis in systemic nocardiosis is poor when diagnosis and therapy are delayed.

Fatahi-Bafghi M. Nocardiosis from 1888 to 2017. Microb Pathog. 2018 Jan;114:369–84. [PMID: 29146497]
Takiguchi Y et al. Pulmonary nocardiosis: a clinical analysis of 30 cases. Intern Med. 2017;56(12):1485–90. [PMID: 28626172]

INFECTIONS CAUSED BY MYCOBACTERIA

NONTUBERCULOUS MYCOBACTERIAL DISEASES

About 10% of mycobacterial infections are caused by nontuberculous mycobacteria. Nontuberculous mycobacterial infections are among the most common opportunistic infections in advanced HIV disease. These organisms have distinctive laboratory characteristics, occur ubiquitously in the environment, are not communicable from person to person, and are often resistant to standard antituberculous drugs.

Egelund EF et al. Medications and monitoring in nontuberculous mycobacteria infections. Clin Chest Med. 2015 Mar; 36(1):55–66. [PMID: 25676519]
Henkle E et al. Nontuberculous mycobacteria infections in immunosuppressed hosts. Clin Chest Med. 2015 Mar; 36(1):91–9. [PMID: 25676522]

1. Pulmonary Infections

Mycobacterium avium complex (MAC) causes a chronic, slowly progressive pulmonary infection resembling tuberculosis in immunocompetent patients who typically have underlying pulmonary disease. Susceptibility testing for macrolide-resistance should be performed on clinical isolates. Treatment of nodular or bronchiectatic pulmonary disease is clarithromycin (1000 mg orally three times per week) or azithromycin (500 mg orally three times per week) plus rifampin (600 mg orally three times per week) or rifabutin (300 mg orally three times per week) plus ethambutol (25 mg/kg orally three times per week). Patients with fibrocavitary lung disease or severe nodular or bronchiectatic disease should receive three-drug therapy with clarithromycin (500–1000 mg orally daily) or azithromycin (500 mg orally daily) plus rifampin (600 mg orally daily) or rifabutin (300 mg orally daily) plus ethambutol (15 mg/kg orally daily). Therapy is continued for at least 12 months after sterilization of cultures.

M kansasii can produce clinical disease resembling tuberculosis, but the illness progresses more slowly. Most such infections occur in patients with preexisting lung disease, though 40% of patients have no known pulmonary disease. Microbiologically, *M kansasii* is similar to *M tuberculosis* and is sensitive to the same drugs except pyrazinamide, to which it is resistant. Therapy with isoniazid, ethambutol, and rifampin for 2 years (or 1 year after sputum conversion) has been successful.

Less common causes of pulmonary disease include *M xenopi*, *M szulgai*, and *M gordonae*. These organisms have variable sensitivities, and treatment is based on results of sensitivity tests. The rapid growing mycobacteria, *M abscessus, M chelonae*, and *M fortuitum*, also can cause pneumonia in the occasional patient.

Floto RA et al. US Cystic Fibrosis Foundation and European Cystic Fibrosis Society consensus recommendations for the management of non-tuberculous mycobacteria in individuals with cystic fibrosis: executive summary. Thorax. 2016 Jan; 71(1):88–90. [PMID: 26678435]

Griffith DE et al; ATS Mycobacterial Diseases Subcommittee; American Thoracic Society; Infectious Disease Society of America. An official ATS/IDSA statement: diagnosis, treatment, and prevention of nontuberculous mycobacterial diseases. Am J Respir Crit Care Med. 2007 Feb 15;175(4):367–416. [PMID: 17277290]

Jarand J et al. Long-term follow-up of *Mycobacterium avium* complex lung disease in patients treated with regimens including clofazimine and/or rifampin. Chest. 2016 May; 149(5):1285–93. [PMID: 26513209]

2. Lymphadenitis

Most cases of lymphadenitis (scrofula) in adults are caused by *M tuberculosis* and can be a manifestation of disseminated disease. In children, the majority of cases are due to nontuberculous mycobacterial species. Infection with nontuberculous mycobacteria can be successfully treated by surgical excision without antituberculous therapy.

3. Skin & Soft Tissue Infections

Skin and soft tissue infections such as abscesses, septic arthritis, and osteomyelitis can result from direct inoculation or hematogenous dissemination or may occur as a complication of surgery.

M abscessus, M chelonae, and *M fortuitum* are frequent causes of these types of infections. Most cases occur in the extremities and initially present as nodules. Ulceration with abscess formation often follows. The organisms are resistant to the usual antituberculosis drugs and may have susceptibility to clarithromycin, azithromycin, doxycycline, amikacin, cefoxitin, sulfonamides, imipenem, and ciprofloxacin. Given the multidrug-resistant nature of these organisms, obtaining antibiotic susceptibility testing is recommended. Therapy often includes surgical debridement along with at least two active antibiotics. Antibiotic therapy is usually continued for 3 months, although this must be determined based on clinical response.

M marinum infection ("swimming pool granuloma") presents as a nodular skin lesion following exposure to nonchlorinated water. The lesions respond to therapy with clarithromycin, doxycycline, minocycline, or trimethoprim-sulfamethoxazole.

M ulcerans infection (Buruli ulcer) is seen mainly in Africa and Australia and produces a large ulcerative lesion. Therapy consists of surgical excision and skin grafting.

4. Disseminated *Mycobacterium avium* Infection

MAC causes disseminated disease in immunocompromised patients, most commonly in patients in the late stages of HIV infection, when the CD4 cell count is less than 50/mcL (see Pulmonary Disease caused by Nontuberculous Mycobacteria, Chapter 9, for a discussion of the infection in immunocompetent persons). Persistent fever and weight loss are the most common symptoms. The organism can usually be cultured from multiple sites, including blood, liver, lymph node, or bone marrow. Blood culture is the preferred means of establishing the diagnosis and has a sensitivity of 98%.

Agents with proved activity against MAC are rifabutin, azithromycin, clarithromycin, and ethambutol. Amikacin and ciprofloxacin work in vitro, but clinical results are inconsistent. A combination of two or more active agents should be used to prevent rapid emergence of secondary resistance. Clarithromycin, 500 mg orally twice daily, plus ethambutol, 15 mg/kg/day orally as a single dose, with or without rifabutin, 300 mg/day orally, is the treatment of choice. Azithromycin, 500 mg orally once daily, may be used instead of clarithromycin. Insufficient data are available to permit specific recommendations about second-line regimens for patients intolerant of macrolides or those with macrolide-resistant organisms. MAC therapy may be discontinued in patients who have been treated with 12 months of therapy for disseminated MAC, who have no evidence of active disease, and whose CD4 counts exceed 100 cells/mcL for 6 months while receiving antiretroviral therapy (ART).

Antimicrobial prophylaxis of MAC prevents disseminated disease and prolongs survival. It is the standard of care to offer it to all HIV-infected patients with CD4 counts of 50/mcL or less. In contrast to active infection, single-drug oral regimens of clarithromycin, 500 mg twice daily, azithromycin, 1200 mg once weekly, or rifabutin, 300 mg once daily, are appropriate. Clarithromycin or azithromycin is more effective and better tolerated than rifabutin, and therefore preferred. Primary prophylaxis for MAC infection can be stopped in patients who have responded to antiretroviral combination therapy with elevation of CD4 counts of greater than 100 cells/mcL for 3 months.

Griffith DE et al; ATS Mycobacterial Diseases Subcommittee; American Thoracic Society; Infectious Disease Society of America. An official ATS/IDSA statement: diagnosis, treatment, and prevention of nontuberculous mycobacterial diseases. Am J Respir Crit Care Med. 2007 Feb 15;175(4):367–416. [PMID: 17277290]

Masur H et al. Prevention and treatment of opportunistic infections in HIV-infected adults and adolescents: updated guidelines from the Centers for Disease Control and Prevention, National Institutes of Health, and HIV Medicine Association of the Infectious Diseases Society of America. Clin Infect Dis. 2014 May;58(9):1308–11. [PMID: 24585567]

MYCOBACTERIUM TUBERCULOSIS INFECTIONS

Tuberculosis is discussed in Chapter 9. Further information and expert consultation can be obtained from the Curry International Tuberculosis Center at the website www.currytbcenter.ucsf.edu or by telephone, 510-238-5100.

TUBERCULOUS MENINGITIS

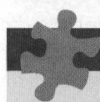

ESSENTIALS OF DIAGNOSIS

▶ Gradual onset of listlessness and anorexia.

▶ Headache, vomiting, and seizures common.

▶ Cranial nerve abnormalities typical.

▶ Tuberculosis focus may be evident elsewhere.

▶ Cerebrospinal fluid shows several hundred lymphocytes, low glucose, and high protein.

▶ General Considerations

Tuberculous meningitis is caused by rupture of a meningeal tuberculoma resulting from earlier hematogenous seeding of tubercle bacilli from a pulmonary focus, or it may be a consequence of miliary spread.

▶ Clinical Findings

A. Symptoms and Signs

The onset is usually gradual, with listlessness, irritability, anorexia, and fever, followed by headache, vomiting, convulsions, and coma. In older patients, headache and behavioral changes are prominent early symptoms. Nuchal rigidity and cranial nerve palsies occur as the meningitis progresses. Evidence of active tuberculosis elsewhere or a history of prior tuberculosis is present in up to 75% of patients.

B. Laboratory Findings

The spinal fluid is frequently yellowish, with increased pressure, 100–500 cells/mcL (predominantly lymphocytes, though neutrophils may be present early during infection), increased protein, and decreased glucose. Acid-fast stains of cerebrospinal fluid usually are negative, and cultures also may be negative in 15–25% of cases. Nucleic acid amplification tests for rapid diagnosis of tuberculosis have variable sensitivity and specificity and none are FDA approved for use in meningitis. Chest radiographs often reveal abnormalities compatible with tuberculosis but may be normal.

▶ Differential Diagnosis

Tuberculous meningitis may be confused with any other type of meningitis, but the gradual onset, the predominantly lymphocytic pleocytosis of the spinal fluid, and evidence of tuberculosis elsewhere often point to the diagnosis. The tuberculin skin test is usually (not always) positive. Fungal and other granulomatous meningitides, syphilis, and carcinomatous meningitis are in the differential diagnosis.

▶ Complications

Complications of tuberculous meningitis include seizure disorders, cranial nerve palsies, stroke, and obstructive hydrocephalus with impaired cognitive function. These result from inflammatory exudate primarily involving the basilar meninges and arteries.

▶ Treatment

Presumptive diagnosis followed by early, empiric antituberculous therapy is essential for survival and to minimize sequelae. Even if cultures are not positive, a full course of therapy is warranted if the clinical setting is suggestive of tuberculous meningitis.

Regimens that are effective for pulmonary tuberculosis are effective also for tuberculous meningitis (see Table 9–15). Rifampin, isoniazid, and pyrazinamide all penetrate into cerebrospinal fluid well. The penetration of ethambutol is more variable, but therapeutic concentrations can be achieved, and the drug has been successfully used for meningitis. Aminoglycosides penetrate less well. Regimens that do not include both isoniazid and rifampin may be effective but are less reliable and generally must be given for longer periods.

Many authorities recommend the addition of corticosteroids for patients with focal deficits or altered mental status. Dexamethasone, 0.15 mg/kg intravenously or orally four times daily for 1–2 weeks, then discontinued in a tapering regimen over 4 weeks, may be used.

Heemskerk AD et al. Intensified antituberculosis therapy in adults with tuberculous meningitis. N Engl J Med. 2016 Jan 14; 374(2):124–34. [PMID: 26760084]

Khonga M et al. Xpert MTB/RIF Ultra: a gamechanger for tuberculous meningitis? Lancet Infect Dis. 2018 Jan;18(1):6–8. [PMID: 28919337]

Prasad K et al. Corticosteroids for managing tuberculous meningitis. Cochrane Database Syst Rev. 2016 Apr 28;4:CD002244. [PMID: 27121755]

LEPROSY (Hansen Disease)

ESSENTIALS OF DIAGNOSIS

▶ Pale, anesthetic macular—or nodular and erythematous—skin lesions.

▶ Superficial nerve thickening with resultant anesthesia.

▶ History of residence in endemic area in childhood.

▶ Acid-fast bacilli in skin lesions or nasal scrapings, or characteristic histologic nerve changes.

▶ General Considerations

Leprosy (Hansen disease) is a chronic infectious disease caused by the acid-fast rod *M leprae*. The mode of transmission probably is respiratory and involves prolonged exposure in childhood. The disease is endemic in tropical and subtropical Asia, Africa, Central and South America, and the Pacific regions, and rarely seen sporadically in the southern United States.

▶ Clinical Findings

A. Symptoms and Signs

The onset is insidious. The lesions involve the cooler body tissues: skin, superficial nerves, nose, pharynx, larynx, eyes, and testicles. Skin lesions may occur as pale, anesthetic macular lesions 1–10 cm in diameter; discrete erythematous, infiltrated nodules 1–5 cm in diameter; or diffuse skin infiltration. Neurologic disturbances are caused by nerve infiltration and thickening, with resultant anesthesia, and motor abnormalities. Bilateral ulnar neuropathy is highly suggestive. In untreated cases, disfigurement due to the skin infiltration and nerve involvement may be extreme, leading to trophic ulcers, bone resorption, and loss of digits.

The disease is divided clinically and by laboratory tests into two distinct types: lepromatous and tuberculoid. The **lepromatous type** (also referred to as multibacillary leprosy) occurs in persons with defective cellular immunity. The course is progressive, with nodular skin lesions; slow, symmetric nerve involvement; abundant acid-fast bacilli in the skin lesions; and a negative lepromin skin test. In the **tuberculoid type** (paucibacillary leprosy), cellular immunity is intact and the course is more benign and less progressive, with macular skin lesions, severe asymmetric nerve involvement of sudden onset with few bacilli present in the lesions, and a positive lepromin skin test. Intermediate ("borderline") cases are frequent. Eye involvement (keratitis and iridocyclitis), nasal ulcers, epistaxis, anemia, and lymphadenopathy may occur.

B. Laboratory Findings

Laboratory confirmation of leprosy requires the demonstration of acid-fast bacilli in a skin biopsy. Biopsy of skin or of a thickened involved nerve also gives a typical histologic picture. *M leprae* does not grow in artificial media, but does grow in the foot pads of armadillos.

▶ Differential Diagnosis

The skin lesions of leprosy often resemble those of lupus erythematosus, sarcoidosis, syphilis, erythema nodosum, erythema multiforme, cutaneous tuberculosis, and vitiligo.

▶ Complications

Kidney failure and hepatomegaly from secondary amyloidosis may occur with long-standing disease.

▶ Treatment

Combination therapy is recommended for treatment of all types of leprosy. Single-drug treatment is accompanied by emergence of resistance, and primary resistance to dapsone also occurs. For borderline and lepromatous cases (ie, multibacillary disease), the World Health Organization recommends a triple oral drug regimen of rifampin, 600 mg once a month; dapsone, 100 mg daily; and clofazimine, 300 mg once a month and 50 mg daily for 12 months, although longer courses may be needed for patients with high burden of disease. For indeterminate and tuberculoid leprosy (paucibacillary disease), the recommendation is rifampin, 600 mg once a month, plus dapsone, 100 mg daily for 6 months.

Two reactional states—erythema nodosum leprosum and reversal reactions—may occur as a consequence of therapy. The reversal reaction, typical of borderline lepromatous leprosy, probably results from enhanced host immunity. Skin lesions and nerves become swollen and tender, but systemic manifestations are not seen. Erythema nodosum leprosum, typical of lepromatous leprosy, is a consequence of immune injury from antigen-antibody complex deposition in skin and other tissues; in addition to skin and nerve manifestations, fever and systemic involvement may be seen. Prednisone, 60 mg/day orally, or thalidomide, 300 mg/day orally (in the nonpregnant patient only), is effective for erythema nodosum leprosum. Improvement is expected within a few days after initiating prednisone, and thereafter the dose may be tapered over several weeks to avoid recurrence. Thalidomide is also tapered over several weeks to a 100-mg bedtime dose. Erythema nodosum leprosum is usually confined to the first year of therapy, and prednisone or thalidomide can be discontinued. Thalidomide is ineffective for reversal reactions, and prednisone, 60 mg/day, is indicated. Reversal reactions tend to recur, and the dose of prednisone should be slowly tapered over weeks to months. Therapy for leprosy should not be discontinued during treatment of reactional states.

Reibel F et al. Update on the epidemiology, diagnosis and treatment of leprosy. Med Mal Infect. 2015 Sep;45(9):383–93. [PMID: 26428602]
Van Veen NH et al. Corticosteroids for treating nerve damage in leprosy. Cochrane Database Syst Rev. 2016 May 23;(5):CD005491. [PMID: 27210895]

▼ INFECTIONS CAUSED BY CHLAMYDIAE

Chlamydiaceae is a family of obligate intracellular parasites closely related to gram-negative bacteria. They include two important genera of human pathogens—*Chlamydia*, which includes the species of *Chlamydia trachomatis*, and *Chlamydophila*, which includes the species *Chlamydophila psittaci* (formerly known as *Chlamydia psittaci*) and *Chlamydophila pneumoniae* (formerly known as *Chlamydia pneumoniae*). *C trachomatis* causes many different human infections involving the eye (trachoma, inclusion conjunctivitis), the genital tract (lymphogranuloma venereum, nongonococcal urethritis, cervicitis, salpingitis), or the respiratory tract in infants (pneumonitis). *C psittaci* causes psittacosis and *C pneumoniae* is a cause of respiratory tract infections.

CHLAMYDIA TRACHOMATIS INFECTIONS

1. Lymphogranuloma Venereum

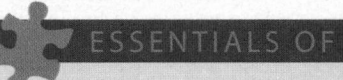

ESSENTIALS OF DIAGNOSIS

▶ Evanescent primary genital lesion.

▶ Inguinal buboes with suppuration and draining sinuses.

▶ Proctitis and rectal stricture in women or in men who have sex with men.

▶ Positive complement fixation test.

General Considerations

Lymphogranuloma venereum (LGV) is an acute and chronic sexually transmitted disease caused by *C trachomatis* types L1–L3. The disease is acquired during intercourse or through contact with contaminated exudate from active lesions. The incubation period is 5–21 days. After the genital lesion disappears, the infection spreads to lymph channels and lymph nodes of the genital and rectal areas. Inapparent infections and latent disease are not uncommon.

Clinical Findings

A. Symptoms and Signs

In men, the initial vesicular or ulcerative lesion (on the external genitalia) is evanescent and often goes unnoticed. Inguinal buboes appear 1–4 weeks after exposure, are often bilateral, and have a tendency to fuse, soften, and break down to form multiple draining sinuses, with extensive scarring. In women, the genital lymph drainage is to the perirectal glands. Early anorectal manifestations are proctitis with tenesmus and bloody purulent discharge; late manifestations are chronic cicatrizing inflammation of the rectal and perirectal tissue. These changes lead to obstipation and rectal stricture and, occasionally, rectovaginal and perianal fistulas. They are also seen with anal coitus.

B. Laboratory Findings

The complement fixation test may be positive (titers greater than 1:64), but cross-reaction with other chlamydiae occurs. Although a positive reaction may reflect remote infection, high titers usually indicate active disease. Nucleic acid detection tests are sensitive, but not FDA approved for rectal specimens and cannot differentiate LGV from non-LGV strains.

Differential Diagnosis

The early lesion of LGV must be differentiated from the lesions of syphilis, genital herpes, and chancroid; lymph node involvement must be distinguished from that due to tularemia, tuberculosis, plague, neoplasm, or pyogenic infection; and rectal stricture must be distinguished from that due to neoplasm and ulcerative colitis.

Treatment

If diagnostic testing for LGV is not available, patients with a clinical presentation suggestive of LGV should be treated empirically. The antibiotic of choice is doxycycline (contraindicated in pregnancy), 100 mg orally twice daily for 21 days. Erythromycin, 500 mg orally four times a day for 21 days, is also effective. Azithromycin, 1 g orally once weekly for 3 weeks, may also be effective.

de Vries HJ et al. 2013 European guideline on the management of lymphogranuloma venereum. J Eur Acad Dermatol Venereol. 2015 Jan;29(1):1–6. [PMID: 24661352]

Workowski KA et al; Centers for Disease Control and Prevention (CDC). Sexually transmitted diseases treatment guidelines, 2015. MMWR Recomm Rep. 2015 Jun 5;64(RR-03):1–137. Erratum in: MMWR Recomm Rep. 2015 Aug 28;64(33):924. [PMID: 26042815]

2. Chlamydial Urethritis & Cervicitis

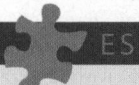
ESSENTIALS OF DIAGNOSIS

► *C trachomatis*: common cause of urethritis, cervicitis, and postgonococcal urethritis.

► Diagnosis made by nucleic acid amplification of urine or swab specimen.

General Considerations

C trachomatis immunotypes D–K are isolated in about 50% of cases of nongonococcal urethritis and cervicitis. In other cases, *Ureaplasma urealyticum* or *Mycoplasma genitalium* can be grown as a possible etiologic agent. *C trachomatis* is an important cause of postgonococcal urethritis. Coinfection with gonococci and chlamydiae is common, and postgonococcal (ie, chlamydial) urethritis may persist after successful treatment of the gonococcal component. Occasionally, epididymitis, prostatitis, or proctitis is caused by chlamydial infection. Chlamydiae are a leading cause of infertility in females in the United States.

Clinical Findings

A. Symptoms and Signs

The urethral or cervical discharge due to *C trachomatis* tends to be less painful, less purulent, and watery compared with gonococcal infection. Women infected with chlamydiae may be asymptomatic or may have symptoms and signs of cervicitis, salpingitis, or pelvic inflammatory disease. Long-term sequelae may include ectopic pregnancy and infertility.

B. Laboratory Findings

A patient with clinical signs and symptoms of urethritis or cervicitis is assumed to have chlamydial infection until proven otherwise. The diagnosis should be confirmed, whenever possible, by the FDA-approved, highly sensitive nucleic acid amplification tests for use with urine or vaginal swabs. A negative nucleic acid amplification test for chlamydia reliably excludes the diagnosis of chlamydial urethritis or cervicitis and therapy need not be administered.

C. Screening

Active screening for chlamydial infection is recommended in certain settings: pregnant women; all sexually active women 25 years of age and under; older women with risk factors for sexually transmitted diseases; and men with risk factors for sexually transmitted diseases, such as HIV-positive men or men who have sex with men.

Treatment

Recommended regimens are a single oral 1-g dose of azithromycin (preferred and safe in pregnancy), 100 mg of doxycycline orally for 7 days (contraindicated in pregnancy), or 500 mg of levofloxacin once daily for 7 days (also contraindicated in pregnancy). Presumptively administered therapy still may be indicated for some patients, such as for an individual with gonococcal infection in whom no chlamydial testing was performed or a test other than a nucleic acid amplification test was used to exclude the diagnosis, or an individual for whom a test result is pending but is considered unlikely to follow up, and for sexual contacts of documented cases. As for all patients in whom sexually transmitted diseases are diagnosed, studies for HIV and syphilis should also be performed.

Geisler WM et al. Azithromycin versus doxycycline for urogenital *Chlamydia trachomatis* infection. N Engl J Med. 2015 Dec 24; 373(26):2512–21. [PMID: 26699167]

Wiesenfeld HC. Screening for *Chlamydia trachomatis* infections in women. N Engl J Med. 2017 Feb 23;376(8):765–73. [PMID: 28225683]

Workowski KA et al; Centers for Disease Control and Prevention(CDC). Sexually transmitted diseases treatment guidelines, 2015. MMWR Recomm Rep. 2015 Jun 5; 64(RR-03): 1–137. Erratum in: MMWR Recomm Rep. 2015 Aug 28; 64(33):924. [PMID: 26042815]

CHLAMYDOPHILA PSITTACI & PSITTACOSIS (Ornithosis)

ESSENTIALS OF DIAGNOSIS

► Fever, chills, and cough; headache common.

► Atypical pneumonia with slightly delayed appearance of signs of pneumonitis.

► Contact with infected bird (psittacine, pigeons, many others) 7–15 days previously.

► Isolation of chlamydiae or rising titer of complement-fixing antibodies.

General Considerations

Psittacosis is acquired from contact with birds (parrots, parakeets, pigeons, chickens, ducks, and many others), which may or may not be ill. The history may be difficult to obtain if the patient acquired infection from an illegally imported bird.

Clinical Findings

The onset is usually rapid, with fever, chills, myalgia, dry cough, and headache. Signs include temperature-pulse dissociation, dullness to percussion, and rales. Pulmonary findings may be absent early. Dyspnea and cyanosis may occur later. Endocarditis, which is culture-negative, may occur. The radiographic findings in typical psittacosis are those of atypical pneumonia, which tends to be interstitial and diffuse in appearance, though consolidation can occur. Psittacosis is indistinguishable from other bacterial or viral pneumonias by radiography.

The organism is rarely isolated from cultures. The diagnosis is usually made serologically; antibodies appear during the second week and can be demonstrated by complement fixation or immunofluorescence. Antibody response may be suppressed by early chemotherapy.

Differential Diagnosis

The illness is indistinguishable from viral, mycoplasmal, or other atypical pneumonias except for the history of contact with birds. Psittacosis is in the differential diagnosis of culture-negative endocarditis.

Treatment

Treatment consists of giving tetracycline, 0.5 g orally every 6 hours or 0.5 g intravenously every 12 hours, for 14–21 days. Erythromycin, 500 mg orally every 6 hours, may be effective as well.

Hogerwerf L et al. *Chlamydia psittaci* (psittacosis) as a cause of community-acquired pneumonia: a systematic review and meta-analysis. Epidemiol Infect. 2017 Nov;145(15):3096–105. [PMID: 28946931]

CHLAMYDOPHILA PNEUMONIAE INFECTION

C pneumoniae causes pneumonia and bronchitis. The clinical presentation of pneumonia is that of an atypical pneumonia. The organism accounts for approximately 10% of community-acquired pneumonias, ranking second to mycoplasma as an agent of atypical pneumonia. A putative role in coronary artery disease has not held up to close scientific scrutiny.

Like *C psittaci*, strains of *C pneumoniae* are resistant to sulfonamides. Erythromycin or tetracycline, 500 mg orally four times a day for 10–14 days, appears to be effective therapy. Fluoroquinolones, such as levofloxacin (500 mg once daily for 7–14 days) or moxifloxacin (400 mg once daily for 7–14 days) are active in vitro against *C pneumoniae* and probably are effective. It is unclear if empiric coverage for atypical pathogens in hospitalized patients with community-acquired pneumonia provides a survival benefit or improves clinical outcome.

Fajardo KA et al. Pneumonia outbreak caused by *Chlamydophila pneumoniae* among US Air Force Academy cadets, Colorado, USA. Emerg Infect Dis. 2015 Jun;21(6):1049–51. [PMID: 25988545]

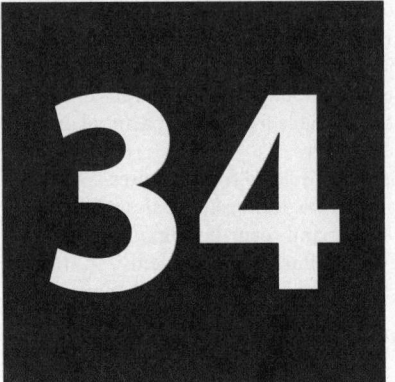

Spirochetal Infections

Susan S. Philip, MD, MPH

▼ **SYPHILIS**

NATURAL HISTORY & PRINCIPLES OF DIAGNOSIS & TREATMENT

Syphilis is a complex infectious disease caused by *Treponema pallidum*, a spirochete capable of infecting almost any organ or tissue in the body and causing protean clinical manifestations (Table 34–1). Transmission occurs most frequently during sexual contact (including oral sex). The risk of acquiring syphilis after unprotected sex with an individual with infectious syphilis is approximately 30–50%. Rarely, it can also be transmitted through nonsexual contact, blood transfusion, or via the placenta from mother to fetus (congenital syphilis).

The natural history of acquired syphilis is generally divided into two major stages: **early (infectious) syphilis** and **late syphilis.** Infectious syphilis includes primary lesions (chancre and regional lymphadenopathy) appearing during primary syphilis, secondary lesions (commonly involving skin and mucous membranes, occasionally bone, central nervous system [CNS], or liver) appearing during secondary syphilis (when dissemination of *T pallidum* produces systemic signs), relapsing lesions during early latency, and congenital lesions. The hallmark of these lesions is an abundance of spirochetes; tissue reaction is usually minimal. Late (tertiary) syphilis consists of so-called benign (gummatous) lesions involving skin, bones, and viscera; cardiovascular disease (principally aortitis); and a variety of CNS and ocular syndromes. These forms of syphilis are not contagious. The lesions contain few demonstrable spirochetes, but tissue reactivity (vasculitis, necrosis) is severe and suggestive of hypersensitivity phenomena. Between these stages are symptom-free latent phases. In early latent syphilis, which is defined as the symptom-free interval lasting up to 1 year after initial infection, infectious lesions can recur.

Public health efforts to control syphilis focus on the diagnosis and treatment of early (infectious) cases and their partners.

Most cases of syphilis in the United States continue to occur in men who have sex with men (MSM). Globally, the World Health Organization (WHO) estimates 5.6 million total incident syphilis infections occur annually, with a prevalence of 1% among pregnant women attending antenatal clinics. Preventing congenital syphilis is a major public health goal for the Centers for Disease Control and Prevention (CDC) and WHO.

COURSE & PROGNOSIS

The lesions associated with primary and secondary syphilis are self-limiting, even without treatment, and resolve with few or no residua. Ocular and otologic syphilis has been associated with permanent vision and hearing loss. Tertiary and congenital syphilis may be highly destructive and permanently disabling and may lead to death. Many experts now believe that while infection is almost never completely eradicated in the absence of treatment, most infections remain latent without sequelae, and only a small number of latent infections progress to further disease.

CLINICAL STAGES OF SYPHILIS

1. Primary Syphilis

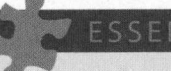 **ESSENTIALS OF DIAGNOSIS**

▶ Painless ulcer on genitalia, perianal area, rectum, pharynx, tongue, lip, or elsewhere.

▶ Fluid expressed from ulcer contains *T pallidum* by immunofluorescence or darkfield microscopy.

▶ Nontender enlargement of regional lymph nodes.

▶ Serologic nontreponemal and treponemal tests may be positive.

▶ Clinical Findings

A. Symptoms and Signs

The typical lesion is the chancre at the site or sites of inoculation, most frequently located on the penis (Figure 34–1), labia, cervix, or anorectal region. Anorectal lesions are especially common among MSM. Chancres also occur

Table 34–1. Stages of syphilis and common clinical manifestations.

Primary syphilis
    Chancre: painless ulcer with clean base and firm indurated borders
    Regional lymphadenopathy

Secondary syphilis
    Skin and mucous membranes
        Rash: diffuse (may include palms and soles), macular, papular, pustular, and combinations
        Condylomata lata
        Mucous patches: painless, silvery ulcerations of mucous membrane with surrounding erythema
    Generalized lymphadenopathy
    Constitutional symptoms
        Fever, usually low-grade
        Malaise, anorexia
        Arthralgias and myalgias
    Central nervous system
        Asymptomatic
        Symptomatic
            Meningitis
            Cranial neuropathies (II–VIII)
    Other
        Ocular: iritis, iridocyclitis
        Renal: glomerulonephritis, nephrotic syndrome
        Hepatitis
        Musculoskeletal: arthritis, periostitis

Tertiary (late) syphilis
    Late benign (gummatous): granulomatous lesion usually involving skin, mucous membranes, and bones but any organ can be involved
    Cardiovascular
        Aortic regurgitation
        Coronary ostial stenosis
        Aortic aneurysm
    Neurosyphilis
        Asymptomatic
        Meningovascular
        Tabes dorsalis
        General paresis

Note: Central nervous system involvement may occur at any stage.

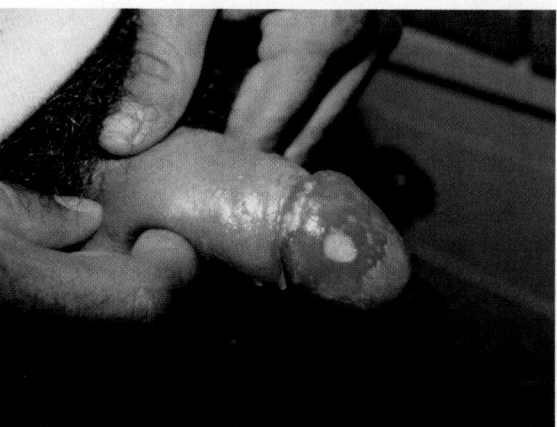

▲ **Figure 34–1.** Primary syphilis with a large chancre on the glans of the penis. The multiple small surrounding ulcers are part of the syphilis and not a second disease. (Used, with permission, from Richard P. Usatine, MD, in Usatine RP, Smith MA, Mayeaux EJ Jr, Chumley H. *The Color Atlas of Family Medicine*, 2nd ed. McGraw-Hill, 2013.)

of fresh exudate from moist lesions or material aspirated from regional lymph nodes is up to 90% sensitive for diagnosis but is usually only available in select clinics that specialize in sexually transmitted disease.

An immunofluorescent staining technique for demonstrating *T pallidum* in dried smears of fluid taken from early syphilitic lesions is also performed in only a few laboratories.

T pallidum polymerase chain reaction (PCR) is available as a "home brew" test in select research, referral, and public health laboratories and has the highest yield in primary and secondary lesions. Organisms can also be detected in blood, especially in congenital and secondary syphilis cases.

2. Serologic tests for syphilis—(Table 34–2) Serologic tests (the mainstay of syphilis diagnosis) fall into two general categories: (1) Nontreponemal tests detect antibodies to lipoidal antigens present in the host after modification

Table 34–2. Percentage of patients with positive serologic tests for syphilis.[1]

Test	Stage		
	Primary	Secondary	Tertiary
VDRL or RPR	75–85%	99–100%	40–95%
FTA-ABS, TPPA, or MHA-TP	69–100%	100%	94–98%
MHA-TP	46–89%	90–100%	NA
EIA or CIA	54–100%	100%	NA

[1]Based on untreated cases.
CIA, chemiluminescence assay; EIA, enzyme immunoassay; FTA-ABS, fluorescent treponemal antibody absorption assay; MHA-TP, microhemagglutination assay for *T pallidum*; RPR, rapid plasma reagin test; TPPA, *T pallidum* particle agglutination; VDRL, Venereal Disease Research Laboratory test.

occasionally in the oropharynx (lip, tongue, or tonsil) and rarely on the breast or finger or elsewhere. An initial small erosion appears 10–90 days (average, 3–4 weeks) after inoculation then rapidly develops into a painless superficial ulcer with a clean base and firm, indurated margins. This is associated with enlargement of regional lymph nodes, which are rubbery, discrete, and nontender. Healing occurs without treatment, but a scar may form, especially with secondary bacterial infection. Multiple chancres may be present, particularly in HIV-positive patients. Although the "classic" ulcer of syphilis has been described as nontender, nonpurulent, and indurated, only 31% of patients have this triad.

B. Laboratory Findings

1. Microscopic examination—In early (infectious) syphilis, darkfield microscopic examination by a skilled observer by *T pallidum*. (2) Treponemal tests use live or killed *T pallidum* as antigen to detect antibodies specific for pathogenic treponemes.

A. Nontreponemal antibody tests—The most commonly used nontreponemal antibody tests are the Venereal Disease Research Laboratory (VDRL) and rapid plasma reagin (RPR) tests, which measure the ability of heated serum to flocculate a suspension of cardiolipin-cholesterol-lecithin. The flocculation tests are inexpensive, rapid, and easy to perform and have therefore been commonly used for routine screening. Quantitative expression of the reactivity of the serum, based on titration of dilutions of serum, is valuable in establishing the diagnosis and in evaluating the efficacy of treatment, since titers usually correlate with disease activity. A different, enzyme immunoassay (EIA)–based screening algorithm is discussed below.

Nontreponemal tests generally become positive 4–6 weeks after infection or 1–3 weeks after the appearance of a primary lesion; they are almost invariably positive in the secondary stage. These tests are nonspecific and may be positive in patients with non–sexually transmitted treponematoses. More important, false-positive serologic reactions are frequently encountered in a wide variety of other conditions, including connective tissue diseases, infectious mononucleosis, malaria, febrile diseases, leprosy, injection drug use, infective endocarditis, old age, hepatitis C viral infection, and pregnancy. False-positive nontreponemal tests are usually of low titer and transient and may be distinguished from true positives by correlating with clinical findings and performing a treponemal specific-antibody test. False-negative results can be seen when very high antibody titers are present (**the prozone phenomenon**). If syphilis is strongly suspected and the nontreponemal test is negative, the laboratory should be instructed to dilute the specimen to detect a positive reaction.

Nontreponemal antibody titers are used to monitor the response to therapy and should decline over time. The rate of decline depends on various factors. In general, persons with repeat infections, higher initial titers, more advanced stages of disease, or those who are HIV-infected at the time of treatment have a slower seroconversion rate and are more likely to remain serofast (ie, titers decline but do not become nonreactive). The RPR and VDRL tests are equally reliable, but RPR titers tend to be higher than the VDRL. Thus, when these tests are used to follow disease activity, the same testing method should be used and preferably performed at the same laboratory.

B. Treponemal antibody tests—These tests measure antibodies capable of reacting with *T pallidum* antigens. Traditionally, they have been used to confirm a diagnosis following a positive nontreponemal test. The *T pallidum* particle agglutination (TPPA) test has been one of the most commonly used treponemal tests, along with the fluorescent treponemal antibody absorption test (FTA-ABS). Newer treponemal tests used in reverse screening algorithms include the EIA and chemiluminescence assay (CIA).

In the traditional screening algorithm, the treponemal tests are used to confirm a positive nontreponemal test. Because of their sensitivity, particularly in the late stages of the disease, treponemal tests are also of value when there is clinical evidence of syphilis, but the nontreponemal serologic test for syphilis is negative. Treponemal tests are reactive in many patients with primary syphilis and in almost all patients with secondary syphilis (Table 34–2). Although a reactive treponemal-specific serologic test remains reactive throughout a patient's life in most cases, it may (like nontreponemal antibody tests) revert to negative with adequate therapy. Final decisions about the significance of the results of serologic tests for syphilis must be based on a total clinical appraisal and may require expert consultation.

C. Enzyme immunoassay (EIA)- or chemiluminescence immunoassay (CIA)-based screening algorithms—Newer screening algorithms reverse the traditional test order and begin with an automated treponemal antibody test (eg, EIA or CIA) and then follow up with a nontreponemal test (RPR or VDRL) if the treponemal test is positive. This algorithm is faster and decreases labor costs to laboratories when compared with traditional screening.

The reverse algorithms can cause challenges in clinical management. A positive treponemal test with a negative RPR or VDRL may represent prior, treated syphilis; untreated latent syphilis; or a false-positive treponemal test. Such results should be evaluated with a second treponemal test as a "tie-breaker," but interpretation of discordant results is not yet fully standardized and a clinician may benefit from an expert opinion. Reverse algorithms are recommended by several international organizations including the International Union against Sexually Transmitted Infections (IUSTI), but the CDC still recommends the traditional algorithm.

D. Rapid treponemal tests—A single rapid point of care treponemal test is approved for use in the United States, including in outreach and other nonlaboratory settings. Other tests are available internationally and are commonly used in limited-resource settings. Sensitivity ranges from 62% to 100% and specificity from 83% to 95%.

3. Polymerase chain reaction—In the United States, there is no FDA-cleared PCR test or method for *T pallidum* PCR, but it is available as a laboratory developed test in select research, referral, and public health laboratories and has the highest yield in primary and secondary lesions. There are no standards for these tests, but PCR has many advantages as a tool for direct detection, including high sensitivity and ability to use a wide range of clinical specimen types, including cerebrospinal fluid. PCR testing of blood has low sensitivity and is not recommended.

4. Cerebrospinal fluid examination—See Neurosyphilis section.

▶ **Differential Diagnosis**

The syphilitic chancre may be confused with genital herpes, chancroid (usually painful and uncommon in the United States), lymphogranuloma venereum, or neoplasm. Any genital ulcer should be considered a possible primary syphilitic lesion. Simultaneous evaluation for herpes simplex virus types 1 and 2 using PCR or culture should also be done in these cases.

Prevention & Screening

Avoidance of sexual contact is the only completely reliable method of prevention but is an impractical public health measure. Latex or polyurethane condoms are effective but protect covered areas only. Men who have sex with men should be screened every 6–12 months, and as often as every 3 months in high-risk individuals (those who have multiple encounters with anonymous partners or who have sex in conjunction with the use of drugs). Pregnant women should be screened at the first prenatal visit and possibly again in the third trimester and at delivery if there are risk indicators, including poverty, sex work, illicit drug use, history of other sexually transmitted diseases, and residence in a community with high syphilis morbidity. Patients treated for other sexually transmitted diseases should also be tested for syphilis, and persons who have known or suspected sexual contact with patients who have syphilis should be evaluated and presumptively treated to abort development of infectious syphilis (see Treating Syphilis Contacts below).

Treatment

A. Antibiotic Therapy

Penicillin remains the preferred treatment for syphilis, since there have been no documented cases of penicillin-resistant *T pallidum* (Table 34–3). In pregnant women, penicillin is the only option that reliably treats the fetus (see below).

There are some alternatives to penicillin for nonpregnant patients, including doxycycline. There are also limited data for ceftriaxone, although optimum dose and duration are not well defined. Azithromycin has been shown to be effective in some parts of the world but should be used with caution; it should not be used at all in MSM due to demonstrated resistance. All patients treated with a non-penicillin regimen must have particularly close clinical and serologic follow-up.

B. Managing Jarisch–Herxheimer Reaction

The Jarisch–Herxheimer reaction, manifested by fever and aggravation of the existing clinical picture in the hours following treatment, is not an IgE-mediated immunologic reaction. It is most common in early syphilis, particularly secondary syphilis where it can occur in 66% of cases.

The reaction may be blunted by simultaneous administration of antipyretics, although no proven method of prevention exists. In cases with increased risk of morbidity due to the Jarisch–Herxheimer reaction (including CNS or cardiac involvement and pregnancy), consultation with an infectious disease expert is recommended. Patients should be reminded that the reaction does not signify an allergy to penicillin.

C. Local Measures (Mucocutaneous Lesions)

Local treatment is usually not necessary. No local antiseptics or topical antibiotics should be applied to a suspected syphilitic lesion until specimens for microscopy have been obtained.

Table 34–3. Recommended treatment for syphilis.[1]

Stage of Syphilis	Treatment	Alternative[2]	Comment
Early			
Primary, secondary, or early latent	Benzathine penicillin G 2.4 million units intramuscularly once	Doxycycline 100 mg orally twice daily for 14 days or Tetracycline 500 mg orally four times daily for 14 days or Ceftriaxone 1 g intramuscularly or intravenously daily for 8–10 days[3]	
Late			
Late latent or uncertain duration	Benzathine penicillin G 2.4 million units intramuscularly weekly for 3 weeks	Doxycycline 100 mg orally twice daily for 28 days or Tetracycline 500 mg orally four times a day for 28 days	No routine cerebrospinal fluid evaluation unless neurologic, otologic, or ocular abnormalities
Tertiary without neurosyphilis	Benzathine penicillin G 2.4 million units intramuscularly weekly for 3 weeks	Doxycycline 100 mg orally twice daily for 28 days or Tetracycline 500 mg orally four times a day for 28 days	Cerebrospinal fluid evaluation recommended in all patients
Neurosyphilis	Aqueous penicillin G 18–24 million units intravenously daily, given every 3–4 hours or as continuous infusion for 10–14 days	Procaine penicillin, 2.4 million units intramuscularly daily with probenecid 500 mg orally four times a day for 10–14 days or Ceftriaxone 2 g intramuscularly or intravenously daily for 10–14 days	Follow treatment with benzathine penicillin G 2.4 million units intramuscularly weekly for up to 3 weeks

[1]Penicillin is the only documented effective treatment in pregnancy, so pregnant patients with true allergy should be desensitized and treated with penicillin according to stage of disease as above.
[2]Patients treated with alternative therapies require close clinical and serologic monitoring.
[3]Fewer data for ceftriaxone treatment; optimal dose or duration not known.

D. Public Health Measures

Counsel patients with infectious syphilis to abstain from sexual activity for 7–10 days after treatment. All cases of syphilis must be reported to the appropriate local public health agency in order to identify and treat sexual contacts. In addition, all patients with syphilis who are not known to be HIV-infected should have an HIV test at the time of diagnosis. In areas of high HIV prevalence, a repeat HIV test should be performed in 3 months if the initial test result was negative.

E. Treating Syphilis Contacts

Patients who have been sexually exposed to infectious syphilis within the preceding 3 months may be infected but seronegative and thus should be treated as for early syphilis even if serologic tests are negative. Persons exposed more than 3 months previously should be treated based on serologic results; however, if the patient is unreliable for follow-up, empiric therapy is indicated.

▶ Follow-Up Care

Because treatment failures and reinfection may occur, patients treated for syphilis should be monitored clinically and serologically with nontreponemal titers every 3–6 months. In primary and secondary syphilis, titers had been expected to decrease fourfold by 12 months; however, up to 20% of patients may fail to decrease. Optimal management of these patients is unclear, but at a minimum, close clinical and serologic follow-up is indicated. In HIV-uninfected patients, an HIV test should be repeated (all patients with syphilis should have an HIV test at the time of diagnosis); a thorough neurologic history and examination should be performed and lumbar puncture considered since unrecognized neurosyphilis can be a cause of treatment failure. If symptoms or signs persist or recur after initial therapy or there is a fourfold or greater increase in nontreponemal titers, the patient has been reinfected (more likely) or the therapy failed (if a non-penicillin regimen was used). In those individuals, an HIV test should be performed, a lumbar puncture done (unless reinfection is a certainty), and re-treatment given as indicated above.

2. Secondary Syphilis

> ### ESSENTIALS OF DIAGNOSIS
>
> ▶ Generalized maculopapular skin rash.
> ▶ Mucous membrane lesions.
> ▶ Condyloma lata in moist skin areas.
> ▶ Generalized nontender lymphadenopathy.
> ▶ Fever may be present.
> ▶ Meningitis, hepatitis, osteitis, arthritis, iritis.
> ▶ Many treponemes in moist lesions by immunofluorescence or darkfield microscopy.
> ▶ Positive serologic tests for syphilis.

▶ Clinical Findings

The secondary stage of syphilis usually appears a few weeks (or up to 6 months) after development of the chancre, when dissemination of *T pallidum* produces systemic signs (fever, lymphadenopathy) or infectious lesions at sites distant from the site of inoculation. The most common manifestations are skin and mucosal lesions. The skin lesions are nonpruritic, macular, papular, pustular, or follicular (or combinations of any of these types, but generally *not* vesicular) and generalized; involvement of the palms and soles (Figure 34–2) occurs in 80% of cases. Mucous membrane lesions may include mucous patches (Figure 34–3), which can be found on the lips, mouth, throat, genitalia, and anus. Specific lesions—condylomata lata (Figure 34–4)—are fused, weeping papules on the moist areas of the skin and mucous membranes and are sometimes mistaken for genital warts. Unlike the dry skin rashes, the mucous membrane lesions are highly infectious.

Meningeal (aseptic meningitis or acute basilar meningitis), hepatic, renal, bone, and joint invasion may occur, with resulting cranial nerve palsies, jaundice,

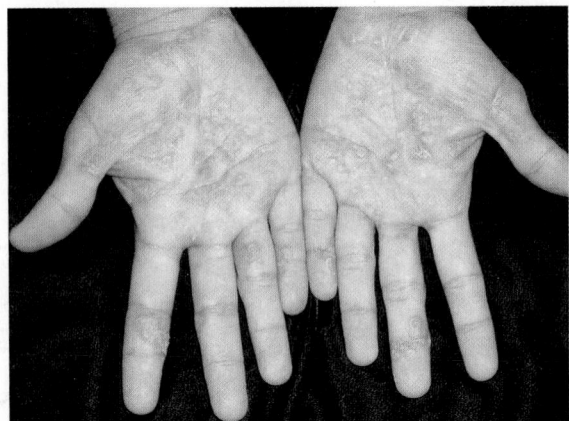

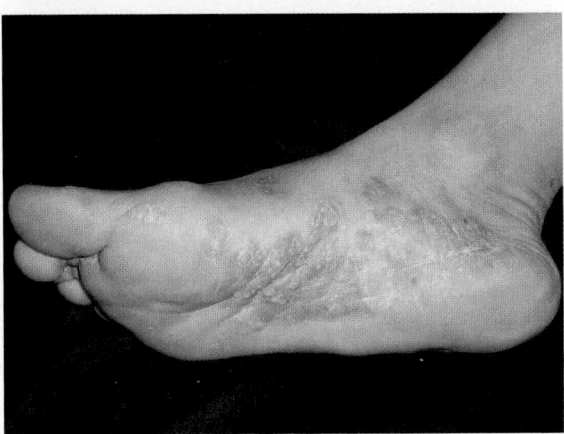

▲ **Figure 34–2.** Papular squamous eruption of the hands and feet of a woman with secondary syphilis. (Used, with permission, from Richard P. Usatine, MD, in Usatine RP, Smith MA, Mayeaux EJ Jr, Chumley H. *The Color Atlas of Family Medicine*, 2nd ed. McGraw-Hill, 2013.)

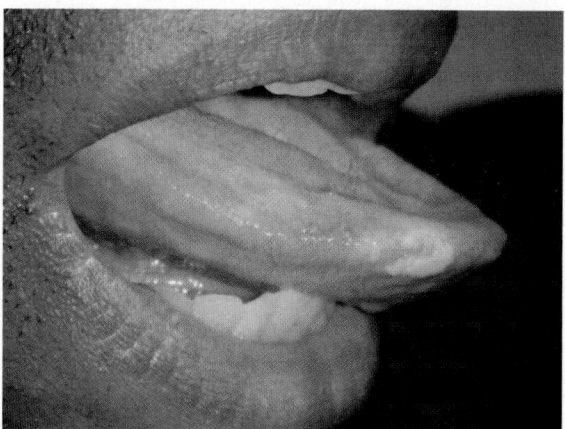

▲ **Figure 34–3.** Secondary syphilis mucous patch of the tongue. (Used with permission from Kenneth Katz, MD, MSc, MSCE.)

nephrotic syndrome, and periostitis. Alopecia (moth-eaten appearance) and uveitis may also occur.

The serologic tests for syphilis are positive in almost all cases (see Primary Syphilis and Table 34–2). The moist cutaneous and mucous membrane lesions often show *T pallidum* on darkfield microscopic examination. A transient cerebrospinal fluid (CSF) pleocytosis is seen in 40% of patients with secondary syphilis. There may be evidence of hepatitis or nephritis (immune complex type) as circulating immune complexes are deposited in blood vessel walls.

Skin lesions may be confused with the infectious exanthems, pityriasis rosea, and drug eruptions. Visceral lesions may suggest nephritis or hepatitis due to other causes.

▶ **Treatment**

Treatment is as for primary syphilis unless CNS or ocular disease or neurologic signs or symptoms are present, in which case a lumbar puncture should be performed and, if

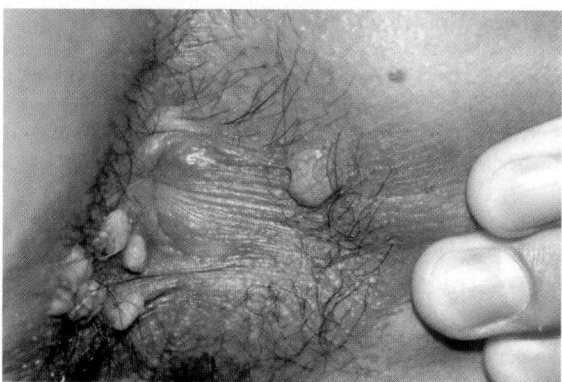

▲ **Figure 34–4.** Secondary syphilis perianal condylomata lata. (Used with permission from Joseph Engelman, MD; San Francisco City Clinic.)

positive, treatment for neurosyphilis given (Table 34–3). See Primary Syphilis for follow-up care and treatment of contacts.

3. Latent Syphilis

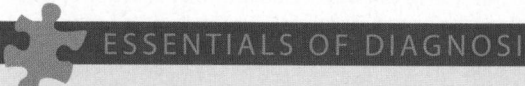

ESSENTIALS OF DIAGNOSIS

▶ **Early latent syphilis:** infection less than 1 year.
▶ **Late latent syphilis:** infection more than 1 year.
▶ No physical signs.
▶ History of syphilis with inadequate treatment.
▶ Positive serologic tests for syphilis.

▶ **General Considerations**

Latent syphilis is the clinically quiescent phase in the absence of primary or secondary lesions; the diagnosis is made by positive serologic tests. **Early latent syphilis** is defined as the first year after primary infection and may relapse to secondary syphilis if undiagnosed or inadequately treated. Relapse is almost always accompanied by a rising titer in quantitative serologic tests; indeed, a rising titer may be the first or only evidence of relapse. About 90% of relapses occur during the first year after infection.

Early latent infection can be diagnosed if there was documented seroconversion or a fourfold increase in nontreponemal titers in the past 12 months; the patient can recall symptoms of primary or secondary syphilis; or the patient had a sex partner with documented primary, secondary, or early latent syphilis.

After the first year of latent syphilis, the patient is said to be in the **late latent stage** and noninfectious to sex partners. Transmission to the fetus, however, is possible in any phase. A diagnosis of late latent syphilis is justified only when the history and physical examination show no evidence of tertiary disease or neurosyphilis. The latent stage may last from months to a lifetime.

▶ **Treatment**

Treatment of early latent syphilis and follow-up are the same as for primary syphilis unless CNS disease is present (Table 34–3). Treatment of late latent syphilis is also shown in Table 34–3. The treatment of this stage of the disease is intended to prevent late sequelae. If there is evidence of CNS involvement, a lumbar puncture should be performed and, if positive, the patient should receive treatment for neurosyphilis. Titers may not decline as rapidly following treatment compared to early syphilis. Nontreponemal serologic tests should be repeated at 6, 12, and 24 months. If titers increase fourfold or if initially high titers (1:32 or higher) fail to decrease fourfold by 12–24 months or if symptoms or signs consistent with syphilis develop, an HIV test should be repeated in HIV-uninfected patients, lumbar puncture should be performed, and re-treatment given according to the stage of the disease.

4. Tertiary (Late) Syphilis

► Infiltrative tumors of skin, bones, liver (gummas).

► Aortitis, aneurysms, aortic regurgitation.

► CNS disorders: meningovascular and degenerative changes, paresthesias, shooting pains, abnormal reflexes, dementia, or psychosis.

General Considerations

This stage may occur at any time after secondary syphilis, even after years of latency, and is rarely seen in developed countries in the modern antibiotic era. Late lesions are thought to represent a delayed hypersensitivity reaction of the tissue to the organism and are usually divided into two types: (1) a localized gummatous reaction with a relatively rapid onset and generally prompt response to therapy and (2) diffuse inflammation of a more insidious onset that characteristically involves the CNS and large arteries, may not improve despite treatment, and is often fatal if untreated. Gummas may involve any area or organ of the body but most often affect the skin or long bones. Cardiovascular disease is usually manifested by aortic aneurysm, aortic regurgitation, or aortitis. Various forms of diffuse or localized CNS involvement may occur.

Late syphilis must be differentiated from neoplasms of the skin, liver, lung, stomach, or brain; other forms of meningitis; and primary neurologic lesions.

Although almost any tissue and organ may be involved in late syphilis, the following are the most common types of involvement: skin, mucous membranes, skeletal system, eyes, respiratory system, gastrointestinal system, cardiovascular system, and nervous system.

Clinical Findings

A. Symptoms and Signs

1. Skin—Cutaneous lesions of late syphilis are of two varieties: (1) multiple nodular lesions that eventually ulcerate (lues maligna) or resolve by forming atrophic, pigmented scars and (2) solitary gummas that start as painless subcutaneous nodules, then enlarge, attach to the overlying skin, and eventually ulcerate (Figure 34–5).

2. Mucous membranes—Late lesions of the mucous membranes are nodular gummas or leukoplakia, highly destructive to the involved tissue.

3. Skeletal system—Bone lesions are destructive, causing periostitis, osteitis, and arthritis with little or no associated redness or swelling but often marked myalgia and myositis of the neighboring muscles.

4. Eyes—Late ocular lesions are gummatous iritis, chorioretinitis, optic atrophy, and cranial nerve palsies, in addition to the lesions of CNS syphilis.

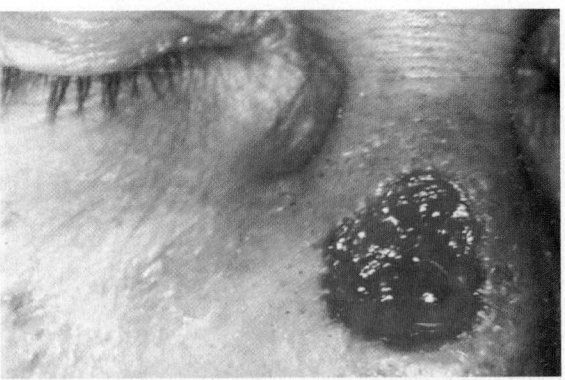

▲ **Figure 34–5.** Gumma of the nose due to long-standing tertiary syphilis. (From J. Pledger, Public Health Image Library, CDC.)

5. Respiratory system—Respiratory involvement is caused by gummatous infiltrates into the larynx, trachea, and pulmonary parenchyma, producing discrete pulmonary densities. There may be hoarseness, respiratory distress, and wheezing secondary to the gummatous lesion itself or to subsequent stenosis occurring with healing.

6. Gastrointestinal system—Gummas involving the liver may be benign but can cause cirrhosis. Gastric involvement can consist of diffuse infiltration into the stomach wall or focal lesions that endoscopically and microscopically can be confused with lymphoma or carcinoma. Epigastric pain, early satiety, regurgitation, belching, and weight loss are common symptoms.

7. Cardiovascular system—Cardiovascular lesions (10–15% of tertiary syphilitic lesions) are often progressive, disabling, and life-threatening. CNS lesions are often present concomitantly. Involvement usually starts as an arteritis in the supracardiac portion of the aorta and progresses to one or more of the following: (1) narrowing of the coronary ostia, with resulting decreased coronary circulation, angina, and acute myocardial infarction; (2) scarring of the aortic valves, producing aortic regurgitation, and eventually heart failure; and (3) weakness of the wall of the aorta, with saccular aneurysm formation (Figure 34–6) and associated pressure symptoms of dysphagia, hoarseness, brassy cough, back pain (vertebral erosion), and occasionally rupture of the aneurysm. Recurrent respiratory infections are common as a result of pressure on the trachea and bronchi.

8. Nervous system (neurosyphilis)—See next section.

Treatment

Treatment of tertiary syphilis (excluding neurosyphilis) is the same as late latent syphilis (Table 34–3); symptoms may not resolve after treatment. Positive serologic tests do not usually become negative.

The pretreatment clinical and laboratory evaluation should include neurologic, ocular, cardiovascular, psychiatric,

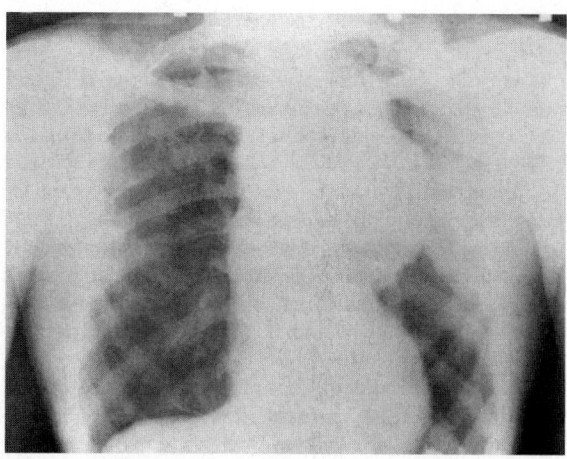

▲ **Figure 34–6.** Ascending saccular aneurysm of the thoracic aorta in tertiary syphilis. (Public Health Image Library, CDC.)

and CSF examinations. In the presence of definite CSF or neurologic abnormalities, one should treat for neurosyphilis.

5. Neurosyphilis

ESSENTIALS OF DIAGNOSIS

▶ Can occur at any stage of disease.

▶ Consider both clinical presentation and laboratory data.

▶ Carefully evaluate the neurologic examination in all patients and consider CSF evaluation for atypical symptoms or lack of decrease in nontreponemal serology titers.

▶ General Considerations

Neurosyphilis can occur at any stage of disease and can be a progressive, disabling, and life-threatening complication. Asymptomatic CSF abnormalities and meningovascular syphilis occur earlier (months to years after infection, sometimes coexisting with primary and secondary syphilis) than tabes dorsalis and general paresis (2–50 years after infection).

▶ Clinical Findings

A. Classification

1. Asymptomatic neuroinvasion—This form has been reported in up to 40% of patients with early syphilis and is characterized by spinal fluid abnormalities (positive spinal fluid serology, increased cell count, occasionally increased protein) without symptoms or signs of neurologic involvement. There are no clear data to support that these asymptomatic CSF abnormalities have clinical significance; therefore, unless treatment failure is suspected, routine CSF evaluation of asymptomatic patients is not recommended.

2. Meningovascular syphilis—This form is characterized by meningeal involvement or changes in the vascular structures of the brain (or both), producing symptoms of acute or chronic meningitis (headache, irritability); cranial nerve palsies (basilar meningitis); unequal reflexes; irregular pupils with poor light and accommodation reflexes; and when large vessels are involved, cerebrovascular accidents. The CSF shows increased cells (100–1000/mcL) and elevated protein, and may have a positive serologic test (CSF VDRL) for syphilis. The symptoms of acute meningitis are rare in late syphilis.

3. Tabes dorsalis—This is a chronic progressive degeneration of the parenchyma of the posterior columns of the spinal cord and of the posterior sensory ganglia and nerve roots. The symptoms and signs are impairment of proprioception and vibration sense, Argyll Robertson pupils (which react poorly to light but accommodate for near focus), and muscular hypotonia and hyporeflexia. Impaired proprioception results in a wide-based gait and inability to walk in the dark. Paresthesias, analgesia, or sharp recurrent pains in the muscles of the leg ("shooting" or "lightning" pains) may occur. Joint damage may occur as a result of lack of sensory innervation (Charcot joint, Figure 34–7). The CSF may have a normal or increased cell count, elevated protein, and variable results of serologic tests.

4. General paresis—This is generalized involvement of the cerebral cortex with insidious onset of symptoms. There is usually a decrease in concentrating power, memory loss, dysarthria, tremor of the fingers and lips, irritability, and mild headaches. Most striking is the change of personality; the patient may become slovenly, irresponsible, confused, and psychotic. The CSF findings resemble those of tabes dorsalis. Combinations of the various forms of neurosyphilis (especially tabes and paresis) are not uncommon.

B. Laboratory Findings

See Serologic Tests for Syphilis, above; these tests should also be performed in cases of suspected neurosyphilis.

1. Indications for a lumbar puncture—In early syphilis (primary and secondary syphilis and early latent syphilis of

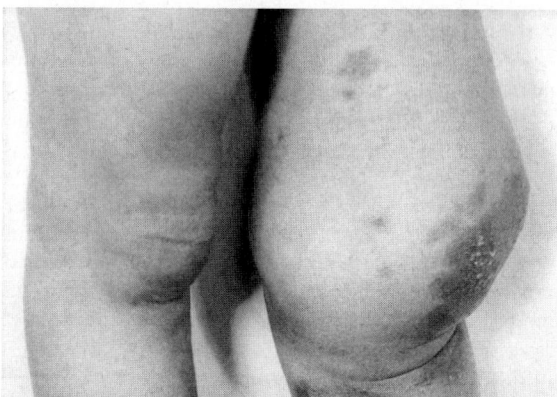

▲ **Figure 34–7.** Neuropathic arthropathy (Charcot joint) from tertiary syphilis. (From Susan Lindsley, Public Health Image Library, CDC.)

less than 1 year's duration), invasion of the CNS by *T pallidum* with CSF abnormalities occurs commonly, but clinical neurosyphilis rarely develops in patients who have received standard therapy. Thus, unless clinical symptoms or signs of neurosyphilis or ocular involvement (uveitis, neuroretinitis, optic neuritis, iritis) are present, a lumbar puncture is not routinely recommended. CSF evaluation is recommended, however, if neurologic or ophthalmologic symptoms or signs are present, if there is evidence of treatment failure (see earlier discussion), or if there is evidence of active tertiary syphilis (eg, aortitis, iritis, optic atrophy, the presence of a gumma).

2. Spinal fluid examination—CSF findings in neurosyphilis are variable. In "classic" cases, there is an elevation of total protein, lymphocytic pleocytosis, and a positive CSF reagin test. VDRL is more sensitive and preferred over RPR. The serum nontreponemal titers will be reactive in most cases. In later stages of syphilis, normal CSF analysis in the presence of infection can occur, but it is unusual. Because the CSF VDRL may be negative in 30–70% of cases of neurosyphilis, *a negative test does not exclude neurosyphilis*, while a positive test confirms the diagnosis. The CSF FTA-ABS is sometimes used; it is a highly sensitive test but lacks specificity, and a high serum titer of FTA-ABS may result in a positive CSF titer in the absence of neurosyphilis.

▶ **Treatment**

Neurosyphilis is treated with high doses of aqueous penicillin to achieve better penetration and higher levels of medication in the CSF than is possible with benzathine penicillin G (Table 34–3). There are limited data for using ceftriaxone to treat neurosyphilis as well, but because other regimens have not been adequately studied, patients with a history of an IgE-mediated reaction to penicillin may require skin testing for allergy to penicillin and, if positive, should be desensitized. Because of concerns about slowly dividing organisms that may persist after completing 10–14 days of therapy with short-acting aqueous penicillin G, many experts recommend subsequent administration of 2.4 million units of the longer-acting benzathine penicillin G intramuscularly once weekly for up to 3 weeks at the conclusion of treatment.

All patients treated for neurosyphilis should have nontreponemal serologic tests done every 3–6 months. Guidelines established by the CDC recommend spinal fluid examinations at 6-month intervals until the CSF cell count is normal; however, there are data to suggest that normalization of serum titers are an acceptable surrogate for CSF response. If the serum nontreponemal titers do not normalize, consider repeating the CSF analysis; expert consultation may be helpful in this scenario. A second course of penicillin therapy may be given if the CSF cell count has not decreased at 6 months or is not normal at 2 years.

6. Syphilis in HIV-Infected Patients

Syphilis is common among HIV-infected individuals. Some data suggest that syphilis coinfection is associated with an increase in HIV viral load and a decrease in CD4

count that normalizes with therapy; other studies have not found an association with HIV disease progression. Overall, for optimal patient care as well as prevention of transmission to partners, guidelines for the primary care of HIV-infected patients recommend at least annual syphilis screening.

Interpretation of serologic tests should be the same for HIV-positive and HIV-negative persons. If the diagnosis of syphilis is suggested on clinical grounds but nontreponemal tests are negative, consider the prozone effect caused by very high antibody titers (see nontreponemal tests, above), or try direct examination of primary or secondary lesions for spirochetes.

HIV-positive patients with primary and secondary syphilis should have careful clinical and serologic follow-up at 3-month intervals. The use of antiretroviral therapy has been associated with reduced serologic failure rates after syphilis treatment.

The diagnosis of neurosyphilis in HIV-infected patients is complicated by the fact that mild CSF abnormalities may be found in HIV infection alone. Like in HIV-uninfected patients, routine lumbar puncture is not recommended in asymptomatic patients; it should be reserved for cases in which neurologic symptoms or signs are present or there is concern for treatment failure. Following treatment, CSF white blood cell counts should normalize within 12 months regardless of HIV status, while the CSF VDRL may take longer. As discussed above, the same criteria for failure apply to HIV-positive and HIV-negative patients, and retreatment regimens are the same. Treatment in HIV-infected and HIV-uninfected patients does not differ; there is no evidence to support prolonged or enhanced treatment regimens due to HIV coinfection.

Most clinical experience in treating HIV-infected patients with syphilis is based on penicillin regimens; fewer data exist for treating the penicillin-allergic patient. Doxycycline or tetracycline regimens can be used for primary, secondary, and early latent syphilis as well as for late latent syphilis and latent syphilis of unknown duration though with caution and close follow-up (Table 34–3). For neurosyphilis, limited efficacy data exist for ceftriaxone; close clinical and serologic follow-up after treatment is essential.

7. Syphilis in Pregnancy

All pregnant women should have a nontreponemal serologic test for syphilis at the time of the first prenatal visit (see Chapter 19). In women who may be at increased risk for syphilis or for populations in which there is a high prevalence of syphilis, additional nontreponemal tests should be performed during the third trimester at 28 weeks and again at delivery. The serologic status of all women who have delivered should be known before discharge from the hospital. Seropositive women should be considered infected and should be treated unless prior treatment with fall in antibody titer is medically documented.

The only recommended treatment for syphilis in pregnancy is penicillin in dosage schedules appropriate for the stage of disease. Penicillin prevents congenital syphilis in 90% of cases, even when treatment is given late in pregnancy. Women with a history of penicillin allergy should be skin tested and desensitized if necessary. Tetracycline and doxycycline are contraindicated in pregnancy.

The infant should be evaluated immediately at birth, and, depending on the likelihood of infection, monitored for clinical and serologic manifestations in the first year of life.

► When to Refer

- Consultation with the local public health department may help obtain all prior positive syphilis serologic results and may be helpful in complicated or atypical cases.
- Early (infectious) syphilis cases may be contacted for partner notification and treatment by local public health authorities.

► When to Admit

- Pregnant women with syphilis and true penicillin allergy should be admitted for desensitization and treatment.
- Women in late pregnancy treated for early syphilis should have close outpatient monitoring or be admitted because the Jarisch–Herxheimer reaction can induce premature labor.
- Patients with neurosyphilis usually require admission for treatment with aqueous penicillin.

Hook EW 3rd. Syphilis. Lancet. 2017 Apr 15;389(10078):1550–7. [PMID: 27993382]
World Health Organization (WHO). WHO guidelines for the treatment of *Treponema pallidum* (syphilis). Geneva; 2016. [PMID: 27631046]

NON–SEXUALLY TRANSMITTED TREPONEMATOSES

A variety of treponemal diseases other than syphilis occur endemically in many tropical areas of the world. They are distinguished from disease caused by *T pallidum* by their nonsexual transmission via direct skin contact, their relatively high incidence in certain geographic areas and among children, and their tendency to produce less severe visceral manifestations. As in syphilis, skin, soft tissue, and bone lesions may develop, organisms can be demonstrated in infectious lesions with darkfield microscopy or immunofluorescence, but cannot be cultured in artificial media; the serologic tests for syphilis are positive; molecular methods such as PCR and genome sequencing are available, but not widely used in endemic areas; the diseases have primary, secondary, and sometimes tertiary stages. Treatment with 2.4 million units of benzathine penicillin G intramuscularly is generally curative in any stage of the non–sexually transmitted treponematoses. In cases of penicillin hypersensitivity, tetracycline, 500 mg orally four times a day for 10–14 days, is usually the recommended alternative. In randomized controlled trials, oral azithromycin (30 mg/kg once) was noninferior to benzathine penicillin G for the treatment of yaws in children.

YAWS (Frambesia)

Yaws is a contagious disease largely limited to tropical regions that is caused by *T pallidum* subspecies *pertenue*. It is characterized by granulomatous lesions of the skin, mucous membranes, and bone. Yaws is rarely fatal, though if untreated it may lead to chronic disability and disfigurement. Yaws is acquired by direct nonsexual contact, usually in childhood, although it may occur at any age. The "mother yaw," a painless papule that later ulcerates, appears 3–4 weeks after exposure. There is usually associated regional lymphadenopathy. Six to 12 weeks later, secondary lesions occur, which are raised papillomas and papules that weep highly infectious material appear and last for several months or years. Painful ulcerated lesions on the soles are called "crab yaws" because of the resulting gait. Late gummatous lesions may occur, with associated tissue destruction involving large areas of skin and subcutaneous tissues. The late effects of yaws, with bone change, shortening of digits, and contractions, may be confused with similar changes occurring in leprosy. CNS, cardiac, or other visceral involvement is rare. See above for therapy. The World Health Organization has set a goal of eliminating yaws by the year 2020 using mass treatment with azithromycin.

PINTA

Pinta is a non–sexually transmitted spirochetal infection caused by *T pallidum* subspecies *carateum*. It occurs endemically in rural areas of Latin America, especially in Mexico, Colombia, and Cuba, and in some areas of the Pacific. A nonulcerative, erythematous primary papule spreads slowly into a papulosquamous plaque showing a variety of color changes (slate, lilac, black). Secondary lesions resemble the primary one and appear within a year after it. These appear successively, new lesions together with older ones; are most common on the extremities; and later show atrophy and depigmentation. Some cases show pigmentary changes and atrophic patches on the soles and palms, with or without hyperkeratosis, that are indistinguishable from "crab yaws." See above for therapy.

ENDEMIC SYPHILIS (Bejel)

Endemic syphilis is an acute or chronic infection caused by *T pallidum* subspecies *endemicum*. It has been reported in a number of countries, particularly in the eastern Mediterranean area, often with local names: bejel in Syria, Saudi Arabia, and Iraq, and dichuchwa, njovera, and siti in Africa. It also occurs in Southeast Asia. The local forms have distinctive features. Moist ulcerated lesions of the skin or oral or nasopharyngeal mucosa are the most common manifestations. Generalized lymphadenopathy and secondary and tertiary bone and skin lesions are also common. Deep leg pain points to periostitis or osteomyelitis. In the late stages of disease, destructive gummatous lesions similar to those seen in yaws can develop, resulting in loss of cartilage and saber shin deformity. Cardiovascular and CNS involvement are rare. See above for therapy.

Giacani L et al. The endemic treponematoses. Clin Microbiol Rev. 2014 Jan;27(1):89–115. [PMID: 24396138]
Marks M. Advances in the treatment of yaws. Trop Med Infect Dis. 2018 Aug 29;3(3):E92. [PMID: 30274488]

SELECTED SPIROCHETAL DISEASES

RELAPSING FEVER

The infectious organisms in relapsing fever are spirochetes of the genus *Borrelia*. The infection has two forms: tick-borne and louse-borne. The main reservoir for **tick-borne** relapsing fever is rodents, which serve as the source of infection for ticks. Tick-borne relapsing fever may be transmitted transovarially from one generation of ticks to the next. Humans can be infected by tick bites or by rubbing crushed tick tissues or feces into the bite wound. Tick-borne relapsing fever is endemic, but is not transmitted from person to person. In the United States, infected ticks are found throughout the West, especially in mountainous areas, but clinical cases are uncommon in humans.

The **louse-borne** form is primarily seen in the developing world, and humans are the only reservoir. Large epidemics may occur in louse-infested populations, and transmission is favored by crowding, malnutrition, and cold climate.

▶ Clinical Findings

A. Symptoms and Signs

There is an abrupt onset of fever, chills, tachycardia, nausea and vomiting, arthralgia, and severe headache. Hepatomegaly and splenomegaly may develop, as well as various types of rashes (macular, papular, petechial) that usually occur at the end of a febrile episode. Delirium occurs with high fever, and there may be various neurologic and psychological abnormalities. The attack terminates, usually abruptly, after 3–10 days. After an interval of 1–2 weeks, relapse occurs, but often it is somewhat milder. Three to ten relapses may occur before recovery in tick-borne disease, whereas louse-borne disease is associated with only one or two relapses.

B. Laboratory Findings

During episodes of fever, large spirochetes are seen in thick and thin blood smears stained with Wright or Giemsa stain. The organisms can be cultured in special media but rapidly lose pathogenicity. The spirochetes can multiply in injected rats or mice and can be seen in their blood.

A variety of anti-*Borrelia* antibodies develop during the illness; sometimes the Weil–Felix test for rickettsioses and nontreponemal serologic tests for syphilis may also be falsely positive. Infection can cause false-positive indirect fluorescent antibody and Western blot tests for *Borrelia burgdorferi*, causing some cases to be misdiagnosed as Lyme disease. PCR assays have been developed but are not widely available.

CSF abnormalities occur in patients with meningeal involvement. Mild anemia and thrombocytopenia are common, but the white blood cell count tends to be normal.

▶ Differential Diagnosis

The manifestations of relapsing fever may be confused with malaria, leptospirosis, meningococcemia, yellow fever, typhus, or rat-bite fever.

▶ Prevention

Prevention of tick bites (as described for rickettsial diseases) and delousing procedures applicable to large groups can prevent illness. Arthropod vectors should be controlled if possible.

Postexposure prophylaxis with doxycycline 200 mg orally on day 1 and 100 mg daily for 4 days has been shown to prevent recurrent fever following tick bites in highly endemic areas.

▶ Treatment

A single dose of tetracycline or erythromycin, 0.5 g orally, or a single dose of procaine penicillin G, 600,000–800,000 units intramuscularly (adults) or 400,000 units intramuscularly (children), probably constitutes adequate treatment for louse-borne relapsing fevers; however, some experts advocate for longer courses of treatment to prevent persistent infection. In severe cases of tick-borne disease, treatment begins with penicillin G, 3 million units intravenously every 4 hours, or ceftriaxone, 1 g intravenously daily; with clinical improvement, a 10-day course can be completed with 0.5 g of tetracycline or erythromycin given orally four times daily. If CNS invasion is suspected, intravenous penicillin G or ceftriaxone should be continued for 10–14 days. Jarisch–Herxheimer reactions occur commonly following treatment and may be life-threatening, so patients should be closely monitored (see Syphilis, above). One study in patients with louse-borne relapsing fever showed that administration of anti-TNF antibodies prior to antibiotic therapy can be effective in preventing the reaction.

▶ Prognosis

The overall mortality rate is usually about 5%. Fatalities are most common in older, debilitated, or very young patients. With treatment, the initial attack is shortened and relapses are largely prevented.

Cutler SJ. Relapsing fever *Borreliae*: a global review. Clin Lab Med. 2015 Dec;35(4):847–65. [PMID: 26593261]

RAT-BITE FEVER

Rat-bite fever is an uncommon acute infectious disease caused by the treponeme *Spirillum minus* (Asia), or the bacteria *Streptobacillus moniliformis* (North America). It is transmitted to humans by the bite of a rat. Inhabitants of rat-infested dwellings, owners of pet rats, and laboratory workers are at greatest risk.

Clinical Findings

A. Symptoms and Signs

In *Spirillum* infections, the original rat bite, unless secondarily infected, heals promptly, but 1 to several weeks later the site becomes swollen, indurated, and painful; assumes a dusky purplish hue; and may ulcerate. Regional lymphangitis and lymphadenitis, fever, chills, malaise, myalgia, arthralgia, and headache are present. Splenomegaly may occur. A sparse, dusky-red maculopapular rash appears on the trunk and extremities in many cases, and there may be frank arthritis.

After a few days, both the local and systemic symptoms subside, only to reappear several days later. This relapsing pattern of fever for 3–4 days alternating with afebrile periods lasting 3–9 days may persist for weeks. The other features, however, usually recur only during the first few relapses. Endocarditis is a rare complication of infection.

B. Laboratory Findings

Leukocytosis is often present, and the nontreponemal test for syphilis is often falsely positive. The organism may be identified in darkfield examination of the ulcer exudate or aspirated lymph node material; more commonly, it is observed after inoculation of a laboratory animal with the patient's exudate or blood. It has not been cultured in artificial media.

Differential Diagnosis

Rat-bite fever must be distinguished from the rat-bite–induced lymphadenitis and rash of streptobacillary fever. Clinically, the severe arthritis and myalgias seen in streptobacillary disease are rarely seen in disease caused by *S minus*. Reliable differentiation requires an increasing titer of agglutinins against *S moniliformis* or isolation of the causative organism. Other diseases in the differential include tularemia, rickettsial disease, *Pasteurella multocida* infections, and relapsing fever.

Treatment

In acute illness, intravenous penicillin, 1–2 million units every 4–6 hours is given initially; ceftriaxone 1 g intravenously daily is another option. Once improvement has occurred, therapy may be switched to oral penicillin V 500 mg four times daily, or amoxicillin 500 mg three times daily, to complete 10–14 days of therapy. For the penicillin-allergic patient, tetracycline 500 mg orally four times daily or doxycycline 100 mg twice a day can be used.

Prognosis

The reported mortality rate of about 10% should be markedly reduced by prompt diagnosis and antimicrobial treatment.

Rahman S et al. Fever, petechiae, and joint pain. J Fam Pract. 2017 May;66(5):323–5. [PMID: 28459894]

LEPTOSPIROSIS

ESSENTIALS OF DIAGNOSIS

▶ Clinical illness can vary from asymptomatic to fatal liver and kidney disease.

▶ **Anicteric leptospirosis:** more common and milder form of the disease.

▶ **Icteric leptospirosis (Weil syndrome):** impaired kidney and liver function, abnormal mental status, and hemorrhagic pneumonia; 5–40% mortality rate.

General Considerations

Leptospirosis is an acute and sometimes severe treponemal infection that is caused by 21 species within the genus *Leptospira*. The disease is distributed worldwide, and it is among the most common zoonotic infections. The leptospires are often transmitted to humans by the ingestion of food and drink contaminated by the urine of an infected animal. The organism may also enter through minor skin lesions and probably via the conjunctiva. Cases have occurred in international travelers after swimming or rafting in contaminated water, and occupational cases occur among sewer workers, rice planters, abattoir workers, and farmers. Sporadic urban cases have been seen in the homeless exposed to rat urine.

Clinical Findings

A. Symptoms and Signs

Anicteric leptospirosis, the more common and milder form of the disease, is often biphasic. After an incubation period of 2–20 days, the initial or "septicemic" phase begins with abrupt fever to 39–40°C, chills, abdominal pain, severe headache, and myalgias, especially of the calf muscles. There may be marked conjunctival suffusion. Leptospires can be isolated from blood, CSF, and tissues. Following a 1- to 3-day period of improvement in symptoms and absence of fever, the second or "immune" phase begins; however, in severe disease the phases may appear indistinct. Leptospires are absent from blood and CSF but are still present in the kidney, and specific antibodies appear. A recurrence of symptoms is seen as in the first phase of disease with the onset of meningitis. Uveitis (which can be unilateral or bilateral and usually involves the entire uveal tract), rash, and adenopathy may occur. A rare but severe manifestation is hemorrhagic pneumonia. The illness is usually self-limited, lasting 4–30 days, and complete recovery is the rule.

Icteric leptospirosis (Weil syndrome) is the more severe form of the disease, characterized by impaired kidney and liver function, abnormal mental status, hemorrhagic pneumonia, hypotension, and a 5–40% mortality rate. Symptoms and signs often are continuous and not biphasic.

Leptospirosis with jaundice must be distinguished from hepatitis, yellow fever, rickettsial disease, and relapsing fever.

B. Laboratory Findings

The leukocyte count may be normal or as high as 50,000/mcL (0.05/L), with neutrophils predominating. The urine may contain bile, protein, casts, and red cells. Oliguria is common, and in severe cases uremia may occur. Elevated bilirubin and aminotransferases are seen in 75%, and elevated creatinine (greater than 1.5 mg/dL) (132.6 mcmol/L) is seen in 50% of cases. Serum creatine kinase is usually elevated in persons with leptospirosis and normal in persons with hepatitis. In cases with meningeal involvement, organisms may be found in the CSF during the first 10 days of illness. Early in the disease, the organism may be identified by darkfield examination of the patient's blood (a test requiring expertise since false-positives are frequent in inexperienced hands) or by culture on a semisolid medium (eg, Fletcher EMJH). Cultures take 1–6 weeks to become positive but may remain negative if antibiotics were started before culture was obtained. The organism may also be grown from the urine from the tenth day to the sixth week. Diagnosis is usually made by means of serologic tests, including the microscopic agglutination test (considered the gold standard but not widely available), and enzyme-linked immunosorbent assay (ELISA). PCR molecular diagnostics are not widely available but appear to be sensitive, specific, positive early in disease, and able to detect leptospiral DNA in blood, urine, CSF, and aqueous humor.

Complications

Myocarditis, aseptic meningitis, acute kidney injury, and pulmonary infiltrates with hemorrhage are not common but are the usual causes of death. Iridocyclitis may occur.

Prevention

The mainstay of prevention is avoidance of potentially contaminated food and water.

Prophylaxis with doxycycline (200 mg orally once a week) has been effective in trials and may be useful if a person is a high risk due to being in an area or season (eg, monsoon flooding) when exposure would be more likely. Human vaccine is used in some limited settings but is not widely available.

Treatment

Many cases are self-limited without specific treatment. Various antimicrobial medications, including penicillin, ceftriaxone, and tetracyclines, show antileptospiral activity; however, meta-analysis has not demonstrated a clear survival benefit for any antibiotic. Doxycycline (100 mg every 12 hours orally or intravenously), penicillin (eg, 1.5 million units every 6 hours intravenously), and ceftriaxone (1 g daily intravenously) are used in severe leptospirosis. Jarisch–Herxheimer reactions may occur (see Syphilis, above). Although therapy for mild disease is controversial, most clinicians treat with doxycycline, 100 mg orally twice daily, for 7 days, or amoxicillin, 50 mg/kg, divided into three doses daily. Azithromycin is also active, but clinical experience is limited.

Prognosis

Without jaundice, the disease is almost never fatal. With jaundice, the mortality rate is 5% for those under age 30 years and 40% for those over age 60 years.

When to Admit

Patients with jaundice or other evidence of severe disease should be admitted for close monitoring and may require admission to an intensive care unit.

Bourque DL et al. Illnesses associated with freshwater recreation during international travel. Curr Infect Dis Rep. 2018 May 22;20(7):19. [PMID: 29789961]

Jiménez JIS et al. Leptospirosis: report from the task force on tropical diseases by the World Federation of Societies of Intensive and Critical Care Medicine. J Crit Care. 2018 Feb;43:361–5. [PMID: 29129539]

LYME DISEASE (Lyme Borreliosis)

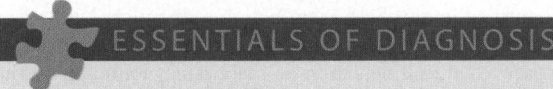

ESSENTIALS OF DIAGNOSIS

► Erythema migrans: a flat or slightly raised red lesion that expands with central clearing.

► Headache or stiff neck.

► Arthralgias, arthritis, and myalgias; arthritis is often chronic and recurrent.

General Considerations

This illness, named after the town of Old Lyme, Connecticut, is the most common tick-borne disease in the United States and Europe and is caused by genospecies of the spirochete *B burgdorferi*. Most US cases are reported from the mid-Atlantic, northeastern, and north central regions of the country. The true incidence of Lyme disease is not known for a number of reasons: (1) serologic tests are not standardized (see below); (2) clinical manifestations are nonspecific; and (3) even with reliable testing, serology is insensitive in early disease.

The tick vector of Lyme disease varies geographically and is *Ixodes scapularis* in the northeastern, north central, and mid-Atlantic regions of the United States; *Ixodes pacificus* on the West Coast; *Ixodes ricinus* in Europe; and *Ixodes persulcatus* in Asia. The disease also occurs in Australia. Mice and deer make up the major animal reservoir of *B burgdorferi*, but other rodents and birds may also be infected. Domestic animals such as dogs, cattle, and horses can also develop clinical illness, usually manifested as arthritis.

Under experimental conditions, ticks must feed for 24–36 hours or longer to transmit infections. Most cases are reported in the spring and summer months. In addition, the percentage of ticks infected varies on a regional basis. In the northeastern and midwestern United States, 15–65% of *I scapularis* ticks are infected with the spirochete; in the west, only 2% of *I pacificus* are infected. These are important epidemiologic features in assessing the likelihood that tick exposure will result in disease. Eliciting a history of brushing a tick off the skin (ie, the tick was not feeding) or removing a tick on the same day as exposure (ie, the tick did not feed long enough) decreases the likelihood that infection will develop.

Because the *Ixodes* tick is so small, the bite is usually painless and goes unnoticed. After feeding, the tick drops off in 2–4 days. If a tick is found, it should be removed immediately. The best way to accomplish this is to use fine-tipped tweezers to pull firmly and repeatedly on the tick's mouth part—not the tick's body—until the tick releases its hold. Saving the tick in a bottle of alcohol for future identification may be useful, especially if symptoms develop.

► Clinical Findings

Prior clinical description of Lyme disease divided the illness into three stages: stage 1, flu-like symptoms and a typical skin rash (erythema migrans, see Figure 6–26); stage 2, weeks to months later, facial (cranial nerve VII) palsy or meningitis; and stage 3, months to years later, arthritis. The problem with this simplified scheme is that there is a great deal of overlap, and the skin, CNS, and musculoskeletal system can be involved early or late. A more accurate classification divides disease into early and late manifestations and specifies whether disease is localized or disseminated.

A. Symptoms and Signs

1. Stage 1, early localized infection—Stage 1 infection is characterized by erythema migrans. About 1 week after the tick bite (range, 3–30 days; median 7–10 days), a flat or slightly raised red lesion appears at the site, which is commonly seen in areas of tight clothing such as the groin, thigh, or axilla. This lesion expands over several days. Although originally described as a lesion that progresses with central clearing ("bulls-eye" lesion), often there is a more homogeneous appearance or even central intensification. About 10–20% of patients either do not have typical skin lesions or the lesions go unnoticed. Most patients with erythema migrans will have a concomitant viral-like illness (the "summer flu") characterized by myalgias, arthralgias, headache, and fatigue. Fever may or may not be present. Even without treatment, the symptoms and signs of erythema migrans resolve in 3–4 weeks. Although the classic lesion of erythema migrans is not difficult to recognize, atypical forms can occur that may lead to misdiagnosis. Southern tick–associated rash illness (STARI) has a similar appearance, but it occurs in geographically distinct areas of the United States.

Completely asymptomatic disease, without erythema migrans or flu-like symptoms, can occur but is very uncommon in the United States.

2. Stage 2, early disseminated infection—Up to 50–60% of patients with erythema migrans are bacteremic and within days to weeks of the original infection, secondary skin lesions develop in about 50% of patients. These lesions are similar in appearance to the primary lesion

but are usually smaller. Malaise, fatigue, fever, headache (sometimes severe), neck pain, and generalized achiness are common with the skin lesions. Most symptoms are transient, although fatigue may persist for months. After hematogenous spread, some patients experience cardiac (4–10% of patients) or neurologic (10–15% of patients) manifestations, including myopericarditis, with atrial or ventricular arrhythmias and heart block. Neurologic manifestations include both the central and peripheral nervous systems. The most common CNS manifestation is aseptic meningitis with mild headache and neck stiffness. The most common peripheral manifestation is a cranial nerve VII neuropathy, ie, facial palsy (usually unilateral but can be bilateral, see Figure 24–1). A sensory or motor radiculopathy and mononeuritis multiplex occur less frequently. Conjunctivitis, keratitis, and, rarely, panophthalmitis can also occur. Rarely, skin involvement can be manifested as a cutaneous hypopigmented lesion called a borrelial lymphocytoma.

3. Stage 3, late persistent infection—Stage 3 infection occurs months to years after the initial infection and again primarily manifests itself as musculoskeletal, neurologic, and skin disease. In early reports, musculoskeletal complaints developed in up to 60% of patients, but with early recognition and treatment of disease, this has decreased to less than 10%. The classic manifestation of late disease is a monarticular or oligoarticular arthritis most commonly affecting the knee or other large weight bearing joints. While these joints may be quite swollen, these patients generally report less pain compared to patients with bacterial septic arthritis. Even if untreated, the arthritis is self-limited, resolving in a few weeks to months. Multiple recurrences are common but are usually less severe than the original disease. Joint fluid reflects an inflammatory arthritis with a mean white blood cell count of 25,000/mcL (0.025/L) with a predominance of neutrophils. Chronic arthritis develops in about 10% of patients. The pathogenesis of chronic Lyme arthritis may be an immunologic phenomenon rather than persistence of infection.

Rarely, the nervous system (both central and peripheral) can be involved in late Lyme disease. In the United States, a subacute encephalopathy, characterized by memory loss, mood changes, and sleep disturbance, is seen. In Europe, a more severe encephalomyelitis caused by *B garinii* is seen and presents with cognitive dysfunction, spastic paraparesis, ataxia, and bladder dysfunction. Peripheral nervous system involvement includes intermittent paresthesias, often in a stocking glove distribution, or radicular pain.

The cutaneous manifestation of late infection, which can occur up to 10 years after infection, is acrodermatitis chronicum atrophicans. It has been described mainly in Europe after infection with *B afzelii*, a genospecies that commonly causes disease in Europe but not the United States. There is usually bluish-red discoloration of a distal extremity with associated swelling. These lesions become atrophic and sclerotic with time and eventually resemble localized scleroderma. Cases of diffuse fasciitis with eosinophilia, an entity that resembles scleroderma, have been rarely associated with infection with *B burgdorferi*.

B. Laboratory Findings

The diagnosis of Lyme disease is based on both clinical manifestations and laboratory findings. **The US Surveillance Case Definition specifies a person with exposure to a potential tick habitat (within the 30 days just prior to developing erythema migrans) with (1) erythema migrans diagnosed by a physician or (2) at least one late manifestation of the disease and (3) laboratory confirmation as fulfilling the criteria for Lyme disease.**

Nonspecific laboratory abnormalities can be seen, particularly in early disease. The most common are an elevated sedimentation rate of more than 20 mm/h seen in 50% of cases, and mildly abnormal liver biochemical tests are present in 30%. The abnormal liver biochemical tests are transient and return to normal within a few weeks of treatment. A mild anemia, leukocytosis (11,000–18,000/mcL) (0.011–0.018/L), and microscopic hematuria have been reported in 10% or less of patients.

Laboratory confirmation requires serologic tests to detect specific antibodies to *B burgdorferi* in serum, preferably by ELISA and not by indirect immunofluorescence assay (IFA), which is less sensitive and specific and can cause misdiagnosis. A two-test approach is recommended for the diagnosis of active Lyme disease, with all specimens positive or equivocal by ELISA then confirmed with a Western immunoblot assay that can detect both IgM and IgG antibodies. A positive immunoblot requires that antibodies are detected against two (for IgM) or five (for IgG) specific protein antigens from *B burgdorferi*.

If a patient with suspected early Lyme disease has negative serologic studies, acute and convalescent titers should be obtained since up to 50% of patients with early disease can be antibody negative in the first several weeks of illness. A fourfold rise in antibody titer would be diagnostic of recent infection. In patients with later stages of disease, almost all are antibody positive. False-positive reactions in the ELISA and IFA have been reported in juvenile rheumatoid arthritis, rheumatoid arthritis, systemic lupus erythematosus, infectious mononucleosis, subacute infective endocarditis, syphilis, relapsing fever, leptospirosis, enteroviral and other viral illnesses, and patients with gingival disease (presumably because of cross-reactivity with oral treponemes). False-negative serologic reactions occur early in illness, and antibiotic therapy early in disease can abort subsequent seroconversion.

The diagnosis of late nervous system Lyme disease is often difficult since clinical manifestations, such as subtle memory impairment, may be difficult to document. Most patients have a history of previous erythema migrans or monarticular or polyarticular arthritis, and the vast majority have antibody present in serum. Patients with late disease and peripheral neuropathy almost always have positive serum antibody tests, usually have abnormal electrophysiology tests, and may have abnormal nerve biopsies showing perivascular collections of lymphocytes; however, the CSF is usually normal and does not demonstrate local antibody production.

Caution should be exercised in interpreting serologic tests because they are not subject to national standards, and inter-laboratory variation is a major problem. In addition, some laboratories perform tests that are entirely unreliable and should never be used to support the diagnosis of Lyme disease (eg, the Lyme urinary antigen test, immunofluorescent staining for cell wall–deficient forms of *B burgdorferi*, lymphocyte transformation tests, using PCR on inappropriate specimens such as blood or urine). Finally, testing is often done in patients with nonspecific symptoms such as headache, arthralgia, myalgia, fatigue, and palpitations. Even in endemic areas, the pretest probability of having Lyme disease is low in these patients, and the probability of a false-positive test result is greater than that of a true-positive result. For these reasons, the CDC has established guidelines for laboratory evaluation of patients with suspected Lyme disease:

1. The diagnosis of early Lyme disease is clinical (ie, exposure in an endemic area, with physician-documented erythema migrans), and does *not* require laboratory confirmation. (Tests are often negative at this stage.)

2. Late disease requires objective evidence of clinical manifestations (recurrent brief attacks of monarticular or oligoarticular arthritis of the large joints; lymphocytic meningitis, cranial neuritis [facial palsy], peripheral neuropathy or, rarely, encephalomyelitis—but *not* headache, fatigue, paresthesias, or stiff neck alone; atrioventricular conduction defects with or without myocarditis) and laboratory evidence of disease (two-stage testing with ELISA or IFA followed by Western blot, as described above).

3. Patients with nonspecific symptoms without objective signs of Lyme disease should *not* have serologic testing done. It is in this setting that false-positive tests occur more commonly than true-positive tests.

4. The role of serologic testing in nervous system Lyme disease is unclear, as sensitivity and specificity of CSF serologic tests have not been determined. However, it is rare for a patient to have positive serologic tests on CSF without positive tests on serum (see below).

5. Other tests such as the T cell proliferative assay and urinary antigen detection have not yet been studied well enough to be routinely used.

Cultures for *B burgdorferi* can be performed but are not routine and are usually reserved for clinical studies.

PCR is very specific for detecting the presence of *Borrelia* DNA, but sensitivity is variable and depends on which body fluid is tested, the stage of the disease, and collection and testing technique. In general, PCR is more sensitive than culture, especially in chronic disease but is not available in many clinical laboratories. Testing should not be done on blood or urine but has been successfully performed on synovial fluid and CSF. A negative PCR result does not rule out disease.

► Complications

Based on several observational studies, *B burgdorferi* infection in pregnant women has *not* been associated with congenital syndromes, unlike other spirochetal illnesses such as syphilis.

Some patients and advocacy groups have claimed either a post–Lyme syndrome (in the presence of positive laboratory tests and after appropriate treatment) or "chronic Lyme disease" in which tests may all be negative. Both entities include nonspecific symptoms such as fatigue, myalgias, and cognitive difficulties (see Prognosis below). Expert groups are in agreement that there are no data to support that ongoing infection is the cause of either syndrome.

▶ Prevention

There is no human vaccine currently available. Simple preventive measures such as avoiding tick-infested areas, covering exposed skin with long-sleeved shirts and wearing long trousers tucked into socks, wearing light-colored clothing, using repellents, and inspecting for ticks after exposure will greatly reduce the number of tick bites. Environmental controls directed at limiting ticks on residential property would be helpful, but trying to limit the deer, tick, or white-footed mouse populations over large areas is not feasible.

Prophylactic antibiotics following tick bites is recommended in certain high-risk situations if all of the following criteria are met: (1) a tick identified as an adult or nymphal *I scapularis* has been attached for at least 36 hours; (2) prophylaxis can be started within 72 hours of the time the tick was removed; (3) more than 20% of ticks in the area are known to be infected with *B burgdorferi*; and (4) there is no contraindication to the use of doxycycline (not pregnant, age greater than 8 years, not allergic). The medication of choice for prophylaxis is a single 200-mg dose of doxycycline. If doxycycline is contraindicated, no prophylaxis should be given and the patient should be closely monitored for early disease, since short course prophylactic therapy with other agents has not been studied, and if early disease does develop, appropriate therapy is very effective in preventing long-term sequelae. Individuals who have removed ticks (including those who have had prophylaxis) should be monitored carefully for 30 days for possible coinfections.

▶ Coinfections

Lyme disease, babesiosis (see Chapter 35), and human granulocytic anaplasmosis (formerly human granulocytic ehrlichiosis) (see Chapter 32) are endemic in similar areas of the country and are transmitted by the same tick, *I scapularis*. Coinfection with two or even all three of these organisms can occur, causing a clinical picture that is not "classic" for any of these diseases. The presence of erythema migrans is highly suggestive of Lyme disease, whereas flu-like symptoms without rash are more suggestive of babesiosis or anaplasmosis. Coinfection should be considered and excluded in patients who have persistent high fevers 48 hours after starting appropriate therapy for Lyme disease; in patients with persistent symptoms despite resolution of rash; and in those with anemia, leukopenia, or thrombocytopenia.

▶ Treatment

Present recommendations for therapy are outlined in Table 34–4. For erythema migrans, antibiotic therapy shortens the duration of rash and prevents late sequelae. Doxycycline is most commonly used and has the advantage

Table 34–4. Treatment of Lyme disease.

Manifestations	Drug and Dosage
Tick bite	No treatment in most circumstances (see text); observe
Erythema migrans[1]	Doxycycline, 100 mg orally twice daily for 10–14 days, or amoxicillin, 500 mg orally three times daily for 2–3 weeks, or cefuroxime axetil, 500 mg orally twice daily for 2–3 weeks
Neurologic disease	
Facial palsy (without meningitis)	Doxycycline, amoxicillin, or cefuroxime axetil as above for 2–3 weeks
Other central nervous system disease	Ceftriaxone, 2 g intravenously once daily, or penicillin G, 18–24 million units daily intravenously in six divided doses, or cefotaxime, 2 g intravenously every 8 hours—all for 2–4 weeks
Cardiac disease	
Atrioventricular block and myopericarditis[2]	An oral or parenteral (if more severe disease) regimen as described above can be used
Arthritis	
Oral dosage	Doxycycline, amoxicillin, or cefuroxime axetil as above for 28 days (see text)
Parenteral dosage	Ceftriaxone, cefotaxime, or penicillin G as above for 2–4 weeks
Acrodermatitis chronicum atrophicans	Doxycycline, amoxicillin, or cefuroxime axetil as above for 3 weeks
"Chronic Lyme disease" or "post-Lyme disease syndrome"	Symptomatic therapy; prolonged antibiotics are *not* recommended

[1]Patients who cannot tolerate tetracyclines or beta-lactams can be treated with azithromycin 500 mg orally daily for 10 days.
[2]Symptomatic patients, those with second- or third-degree block, and those with first-degree block with a PR interval ≥ 300 milliseconds should be hospitalized for observation.

of being active against *Anaplasma phagocytophilum* (formerly *Ehrlichia*). It has proven effective in shorter courses of 10–14 days compared to other regimens. Amoxicillin is also effective and is recommended for pregnant or lactating women and for those who cannot tolerate doxycycline. Cefuroxime axetil is as effective as doxycycline, but because of its cost, it should be considered an alternative choice for those who cannot tolerate doxycycline or amoxicillin or for those in whom the medications are contraindicated. Erythromycin and azithromycin are less effective, associated with higher rates of relapse, and are not recommended as first-line therapy.

Isolated facial palsy (without meningitis or peripheral neuropathy) can be treated with doxycycline, amoxicillin, or cefuroxime axetil for 2–3 weeks. Although therapy does not affect the rate of resolution of the cranial neuropathy, it does prevent development of late manifestations of disease.

The need for a lumbar puncture in patients with seventh nerve palsy is controversial. Some clinicians perform lumbar puncture on all patients with facial palsy and others only if there are symptoms or signs of meningitis. If meningitis is present, therapy with a parenteral antibiotic is indicated. Ceftriaxone is most commonly used, but penicillin is equally efficacious. In European countries, doxycycline 400 mg/d orally for 14 days is frequently used and is comparable in efficacy to ceftriaxone.

Patients with atrioventricular block or myopericarditis (or both) can be treated with either oral or parenteral agents for 2–3 weeks. Hospitalization and observation is indicated for symptomatic patients, those with second- or third-degree block, and those with first-degree block with a PR interval of 300 milliseconds or more. Once stabilized, hospitalized patients can be transitioned to one of the oral regimens to complete therapy.

Therapy of arthritis is difficult because some patients do not respond to any therapy, and those who do respond may do so slowly. Oral agents (doxycycline, amoxicillin, or cefuroxime axetil) are as effective as intravenous regimens (ceftriaxone, cefotaxime, or penicillin). A reasonable approach to the patient with Lyme arthritis is to start with oral therapy for 28 days. If there is partial resolution, re-treat with an additional 28 days of the same oral regimen. If arthritis persists after re-treatment, symptomatic therapy with nonsteroidal anti-inflammatory drugs is recommended. For severe refractory pain, synovectomy may be required.

Based on the limited published data, therapy of Lyme disease in pregnancy should be the same as therapy in other patients with the exception that doxycycline should not be used.

Clinicians may encounter patients with nonspecific symptoms (such as fatigue and myalgias) and positive serologic tests for Lyme disease who request (or demand) therapy for their illness. It is important in managing these patients to remember (1) that nonspecific symptoms alone are not diagnostic; (2) that serologic tests are fraught with difficulty (as noted above), and in areas where disease prevalence is low, false-positive serologic tests are much more common than true-positive tests; and (3) that parenteral therapy with ceftriaxone for 2–4 weeks is costly and has been associated with significant adverse effects, including cholelithiasis and *Clostridioides difficile* colitis. Parenteral therapy should be reserved for those most likely to benefit, ie, those with cutaneous, neurologic, cardiac, or rheumatic manifestations that are characteristic of Lyme disease.

▶ Prognosis

Most patients respond to appropriate therapy with prompt resolution of symptoms within 4 weeks. True treatment failures are thus uncommon, and in most cases re-treatment or prolonged treatment of Lyme disease is instituted because of misdiagnosis or misinterpretation of serologic results (both IgG and IgM antibodies can persist for prolonged periods despite adequate therapy) rather than inadequate therapy or response. Prolonged courses of antibiotic therapy for nonspecific symptoms that persist after completion of appropriate assessment (and treatment, if necessary) for Lyme disease is not recommended.

The long-term outcome of adult patients with Lyme disease is generally favorable, but some patients have chronic complaints. Joint pain, memory impairment, and poor functional status secondary to pain are common subjective complaints in patients with Lyme disease, but physical examination and neurocognitive testing fail to document the presence of these symptoms as objective sequelae. Similarly, in highly endemic areas, patients with a diagnosis of Lyme disease commonly complain of pain, fatigue, and an inability to perform certain physical activities when followed for several years. However, these complaints occur just as commonly in age-matched controls without a history of Lyme disease.

Immunity is not complete after Lyme disease. Reinfection, although uncommon, is predominantly seen in patients successfully treated for early disease (erythema migrans) in whom antibody titers do not develop. Clinical manifestations and serologic response are similar to an initial infection.

▶ When to Refer

Consultation with an infectious diseases specialist with experience in diagnosing and treating Lyme disease can be helpful in atypical or prolonged cases.

▶ When to Admit

Admission for parenteral antibiotics is indicated for any patient with symptomatic CNS or cardiac disease as well as those with second- or third-degree atrioventricular block, or first-degree block with a PR interval of 300 milliseconds or more.

Berende A et al. Randomized trial of longer-term therapy for symptoms attributed to Lyme disease. N Engl J Med. 2016 Mar 31;374(13):1209–20. [PMID: 27028911]

Cardenas-de la Garza JA et al. Clinical spectrum of Lyme disease. Eur J Clin Microbiol Infect Dis. 2019 Feb;38(2):201–8. [PMID: 30456435]

Protozoal & Helminthic Infections

35

Philip J. Rosenthal, MD

AFRICAN TRYPANOSOMIASIS (Sleeping Sickness)

ESSENTIALS OF DIAGNOSIS

- ► Exposure to tsetse flies; chancre at bite site uncommon.
- ► **Hemolymphatic disease:** Irregular fever, headache, joint pain, rash, edema, lymphadenopathy.
- ► **Meningoencephalitic disease:** Somnolence, severe headache, progressing to coma.
- ► Trypanosomes in blood or lymph node aspirates; positive serologic tests.
- ► Trypanosomes and increased white cells and protein in cerebrospinal fluid.

General Considerations

African trypanosomiasis is caused by the hemoflagellates *Trypanosoma brucei rhodesiense* and *Trypanosoma brucei gambiense*. The organisms are transmitted by bites of tsetse flies (genus *Glossina*), which inhabit shaded areas along streams and rivers. Trypanosomes ingested in a blood meal develop over 18–35 days in the fly; when the fly feeds again on a mammalian host, the infective stage is injected. Human disease occurs in rural areas of sub-Saharan Africa from south of the Sahara to about 30 degrees south latitude. *T b gambiense* causes West African trypanosomiasis, and is transmitted in the moist sub-Saharan savannas and forests of west and central Africa. *T b rhodesiense* causes East African trypanosomiasis, and is transmitted in the savannas of east and southeast Africa.

T b rhodesiense infection is primarily a zoonosis of game animals and cattle; humans are infected sporadically. Humans are the principal mammalian host for *T b gambiense*, but domestic animals can be infected. The number of reported cases increased from the 1960s to the 1990s and has since decreased greatly, although cases are reported

from over 20 countries. Total incidence has been estimated at less than 5000 cases per year, mostly due to *T b gambiense*, with the largest number in the Democratic Republic of the Congo. Infections are rare among travelers, including visitors to game parks.

Clinical Findings

A. Symptoms and Signs

1. West African trypanosomiasis—Chancres at the site of the bite are uncommon. After an asymptomatic period that may last for months, hemolymphatic disease presents with fever, headache, myalgias, arthralgias, weight loss, and lymphadenopathy, with discrete, nontender, rubbery nodes, referred to as Winterbottom sign when in a posterior cervical distribution. Other common signs are mild splenomegaly, transient edema, and a pruritic erythematous rash. Febrile episodes may be broken by afebrile periods of up to several weeks. The hemolymphatic stage progresses over months to meningoencephalitic disease, with somnolence, irritability, personality changes, severe headache, and parkinsonian symptoms progressing to coma and death.

2. East African trypanosomiasis—Chancres at the bite site are more commonly recognized with *T b rhodesiense* infection, with a painful lesion of 3–10 cm and regional lymphadenopathy that appears about 48 hours after the tsetse fly bite and lasts 2–4 weeks. East African disease follows a much more acute course, with the onset of symptoms usually within a few days of the insect bite. The hemolymphatic stage includes intermittent fever and rash, but lymphadenopathy is less common than with West African disease. Myocarditis can cause tachycardia and death due to arrhythmias or heart failure. If untreated, East African trypanosomiasis progresses over weeks to months to meningoencephalitic disease, somnolence, coma, and death.

B. Laboratory Findings

Diagnosis can be difficult, and definitive diagnosis requires identification of trypanosomes. Microscopic examination of fluid expressed from a chancre or lymph node may show motile trypanosomes or, in fixed specimens, parasites stained with Giemsa. During the hemolymphatic stage, detection of parasites in Giemsa-stained blood smears is common in East African disease but difficult in West African disease. Serial specimens should be examined, since parasitemias vary greatly over time. Meningoencephalitic (or second stage) disease is defined by the World Health Organization (WHO) as cerebrospinal fluid (CSF) showing at least five mononuclear cells per microliter, elevated protein, or presence of trypanosomes. Concentration techniques can aid identification of parasites in blood or CSF. Serologic tests are also available. The card agglutination test for trypanosomes (CATT) has excellent sensitivity and specificity for West African disease and can be performed in the field, but the diagnosis should be confirmed by identification of the parasites. Field-applicable immunochromatographic lateral flow rapid diagnostic tests that cost less than CATT and are simpler to perform are available; combining tests improves sensitivity and specificity. Molecular diagnostic tests, including PCR and field-friendly loop-mediated isothermal amplification (LAMP) are available, but these are not yet standardized or routinely available.

Treatment

Detection of trypanosomes is a prerequisite for treatment of African trypanosomiasis because of the significant toxicity of most available therapies. Treatment recommendations depend on the type of trypanosomiasis (Table 35–1), which is determined by geography, and stage of disease, which requires examination of CSF. Eflornithine, nifurtimox, suramin, and melarsoprol are available in the United States from the CDC Drug Service (www.cdc.gov/laboratory/drugservice).

A. West African Trypanosomiasis

1. Early stage infection—Pentamidine (4 mg/kg intramuscularly or intravenously every day or every other day for 7 days) is used to treat infection that does not involve the central nervous system (CNS). The side effects of pentamidine include immediate hypotension; tachycardia; gastrointestinal symptoms during administration; sterile abscesses; and pancreatic (hypoglycemia), liver, and kidney abnormalities. An alternate drug is eflornithine (100 mg/kg/day intravenously every 6 hours for 14 days).

Table 35–1. Treatment of African trypanosomiasis.

Disease	Stage	Treatment	
		First Line	Alternative
West African	Early	Pentamidine	Suramin Eflornithine
	CNS involvement	Eflornithine + nifurtimox	Melarsoprol
East African	Early CNS involvement	Suramin Melarsoprol	Pentamidine

CNS, central nervous system.

2. Late stage infection—The treatment of choice for CNS infection is a combination of intravenous eflornithine (400 mg/kg/day in two doses for 7 days) and oral nifurtimox (15 mg/kg/day in three doses for 10 days), which has improved efficacy and less toxicity than older regimens. Eflornithine, though less toxic than older trypanocidal drugs, can cause gastrointestinal symptoms, bone marrow suppression, seizures, and alopecia. An alternative agent is melarsoprol. Fexinidazole, a new agent, is as effective and safe as eflornithine plus nifurtimox when administered orally over 10 days; this drug has received international approval and offers an important alternative therapy.

B. East African Trypanosomiasis

Pentamidine and eflornithine are not reliably effective, and early disease is treated with suramin. The dosing regimens of suramin vary (eg, 100–200 mg test dose, then 20 mg/kg [maximum 1 g] intravenously on days 1, 3, 7, 14, and 21 or weekly for five doses). Suramin toxicities include vomiting and, rarely, seizures and shock during infusions as well as subsequent fever, rash, headache, neuropathy, and kidney and bone marrow dysfunction.

Suramin does not enter the CNS, so East African trypanosomiasis involving the CNS is treated with melarsoprol (three series of 3.6 mg/kg/day intravenously for 3 days, with 7-day breaks between the series or a 10-day intravenous course with 0.6 mg/kg on day 1, 1.2 mg/kg on day 2, and 1.8 mg/kg on days 3–10). Melarsoprol also acts against West African disease, but eflornithine plus nifurtimox is preferred due to its lower toxicity. Immediate side effects of melarsoprol include fever and gastrointestinal symptoms. The most important side effect is a reactive encephalopathy that can progress to seizures, coma, and death. To help avoid this side effect, corticosteroids are coadministered (dexamethasone 1 mg/kg/day intravenously for 2–3 days or oral prednisolone 1 mg/kg/day for 5 days, and then 0.5 mg/kg/day until treatment completion). In addition, increasing resistance to melarsoprol is a serious concern.

Prevention & Control

Individual prevention in endemic areas should include long sleeves and pants, insect repellents, and mosquito nets. Control programs focusing on vector elimination and treatment of infected persons and animals have shown good success in many areas but suffer from limited resources.

Aksoy S et al. Human African trypanosomiasis control: achievements and challenges. PLoS Negl Trop Dis. 2017 Apr 20; 11(4):e0005454. [PMID: 28426685]

Büscher P et al. Human African trypanosomiasis. Lancet. 2017 Nov 25;390(10110):2397–409. [PMID: 28673422]

Lumbala C et al. Prospective evaluation of a rapid diagnostic test for *Trypanosoma brucei gambiense* infection developed using recombinant antigens. PLoS Negl Trop Dis. 2018 Mar 28; 12(3):e0006386. [PMID: 29590116]

Mesu VKBK et al. Oral fexinidazole for late-stage African *Trypanosoma brucei gambiense* trypanosomiasis: a pivotal multicentre, randomised, non-inferiority trial. Lancet. 2018 Jan 13;391(10116):144–54. [PMID: 29113731]

AMERICAN TRYPANOSOMIASIS
(Chagas Disease)

Acute stage

▶ Inflammatory lesion at inoculation site.

▶ Fever.

▶ Hepatosplenomegaly; lymphadenopathy.

▶ Myocarditis.

▶ Parasites in blood are diagnostic.

Chronic stage

▶ Heart failure, cardiac arrhythmias.

▶ Thromboembolism.

▶ Megaesophagus; megacolon.

▶ Serologic tests are usually diagnostic.

▶ General Considerations

Chagas disease is caused by *Trypanosoma cruzi*, a protozoan parasite found only in the Americas; it infects wild animals and, to a lesser extent, humans from southern South America to the southern United States. An estimated 8–10 million people are infected, mostly in rural areas, with the highest national prevalence in Bolivia, Argentina, Paraguay, Ecuador, El Salvador, and Guatemala. Control efforts in endemic countries have decreased disease incidence to about 40,000 new infections and 12,500 deaths per year. The disease is often acquired in childhood. In many countries in South America, Chagas disease is the most important cause of heart disease. The vector is endemic in the southern United States where some animals are infected and a few instances of local transmission have been reported.

T cruzi is transmitted by reduviid (triatomine) bugs infected by ingesting blood from animals or humans who have circulating trypanosomes. Multiplication occurs in the digestive tract of the bug and infective forms are eliminated in feces. Infection in humans occurs when the parasite penetrates the skin through the bite wound, mucous membranes, or the conjunctiva. Transmission can also occur by blood transfusion, organ or bone marrow transplantation, congenital transfer, or ingestion of food contaminated with vector feces. From the bloodstream, *T cruzi* invades many cell types but has a predilection for myocardium, smooth muscle, and CNS glial cells. Multiplication causes cellular destruction, inflammation, and fibrosis, with progressive disease over decades.

▶ Clinical Findings

A. Symptoms and Signs

As many as 70% of infected persons remain asymptomatic. The **acute stage** is seen principally in children and lasts 1–2 months. The earliest findings are at the site of inoculation either in the eye—Romaña sign (unilateral edema, conjunctivitis, and lymphadenopathy)—or in the skin—a chagoma (swelling with local lymphadenopathy). Subsequent findings include fever, malaise, headache, mild hepatosplenomegaly, and generalized lymphadenopathy. Acute myocarditis and meningoencephalitis are rare but can be fatal.

An asymptomatic **latent period (indeterminate phase)** may last for life, but symptomatic disease develops in 10–30% of infected individuals, commonly many years after infection.

Chronic Chagas disease generally manifests as abnormalities in cardiac and smooth muscle. Cardiac disease includes arrhythmias, heart failure, and embolic disease. Smooth muscle abnormalities lead to megaesophagus and megacolon, with dysphagia, regurgitation, aspiration, constipation, and abdominal pain. These findings can be complicated by superinfections. In immunosuppressed persons, including AIDS patients and transplant recipients, latent Chagas disease may reactivate; findings have included brain abscesses and meningoencephalitis.

B. Diagnostic Testing

The diagnosis is made by detecting parasites in persons with suggestive findings who have resided in an endemic area. With acute infection, evaluation of fresh blood or buffy coats may show motile trypanosomes, and fixed preparations may show Giemsa-stained parasites. Concentration methods increase diagnostic yields. Trypanosomes may be identified in lymph nodes, bone marrow, or pericardial or spinal fluid. Molecular tests are highly sensitive and can be used to detect parasites in organ transplant recipients or after accidental exposure. When initial tests are unrevealing, xenodiagnosis using laboratory vectors, laboratory culture, or animal inoculation may provide a diagnosis, but these methods are expensive and slow.

Chronic Chagas disease is usually diagnosed serologically. Many different serologic assays are available, but sensitivity and specificity are not ideal; confirmatory assays are advised after an initial positive test, as is standard for blood bank testing in South America. The diagnosis of chronic disease with PCR remains suboptimal.

▶ Treatment

Treatment is inadequate because the two drugs used, benznidazole and nifurtimox, often cause severe side effects, must be used for long periods, and are ineffective against chronic infection. In acute and congenital infections, the drugs can reduce the duration and severity of infection, but cure is achieved in only about 70% of patients. During the chronic phase of infection, although parasitemia may disappear in up to 70% of patients, treatment does not clearly alter the progression of the disease. In a 2015 trial for Chagas cardiomyopathy, benznidazole significantly reduced parasite detection but not progression of cardiac disease. Nevertheless, there is general consensus that treatment should be considered in all *T cruzi*–infected persons regardless of clinical status or time since infection. In particular, treatment is recommended for acute, congenital, and reactivated infections and for children and young adults with chronic disease. Benznidazole is FDA-approved for the treatment of Chagas disease in children 2–12 years old. Both benznidazole and nifurtimox are available in the United States from the CDC Drug Service (www.cdc.gov/laboratory/drugservice).

Benznidazole is generally preferred due to better efficacy and safety profiles. It is given orally at a dosage of 5 mg/kg/day in two divided doses for 60 days. Its side effects include granulocytopenia, rash, and peripheral neuropathy. Nifurtimox is given orally in daily doses of 8–10 mg/kg in four divided doses after meals for 90–120 days. Side effects include gastrointestinal (anorexia, vomiting) and neurologic (headaches, ataxia, insomnia, seizures) symptoms, which appear to be reversible and to lessen with dosage reduction. For both drugs, some recommendations suggest higher dosing for acute infections. Patients with chronic Chagas disease may also benefit from antiarrhythmic therapy, standard therapy for heart failure, and conservative and surgical management of megaesophagus and megacolon.

▶ Prevention & Control

In South America, a major eradication program based on improved housing, use of residual pyrethroid insecticides and pyrethroid-impregnated bed curtains, and screening of blood donors has achieved striking reductions in new infections. In endemic areas and ideally in donors from endemic areas, blood should not be used for transfusion unless at least two serologic tests are negative.

Bern C. Chagas' disease. N Engl J Med. 2015 Jul 30;373(5):456–66. [PMID: 26222561]
Pérez-Molina JA et al. Chagas disease. Lancet. 2018 Jan 6; 391(10115):82–94. [PMID: 28673423]
Schijman AG. Molecular diagnosis of *Trypanosoma cruzi*. Acta Trop. 2018 Aug;184:59–66. [PMID: 29476727]

LEISHMANIASIS

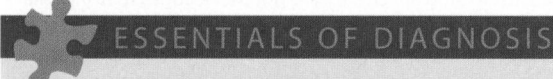

ESSENTIALS OF DIAGNOSIS

- ▶ Sand fly bite in an endemic area.
- ▶ **Visceral leishmaniasis:** irregular fever, progressive hepatosplenomegaly, pancytopenia, wasting.
- ▶ **Cutaneous leishmaniasis:** chronic, painless, moist ulcers or dry nodules.
- ▶ **Mucocutaneous leishmaniasis:** destructive nasopharyngeal lesions.
- ▶ Amastigotes in macrophages in aspirates, touch preparations, or biopsies.
- ▶ Positive culture, serologic tests, PCR, or skin test.

▶ General Considerations

Leishmaniasis is a zoonosis transmitted by bites of sand flies of the genus *Lutzomyia* in the Americas and *Phlebotomus* elsewhere. When sand flies feed on an infected host, the parasitized cells are ingested with the blood meal.

Leishmaniasis is caused by about 20 species of *Leishmania*; taxonomy is complex. Clinical syndromes are generally dictated by the infecting species, but some species can cause more than one syndrome.

The estimated annual incidence of disease has been decreasing, with current estimates of 700,000 to 1 million annual cases of cutaneous disease and 50,000–90,000 cases of visceral disease. Progress against visceral disease has been greatest on the Indian subcontinent.

Visceral leishmaniasis (kala azar) is caused mainly by *Leishmania donovani* in the Indian subcontinent and East Africa; *Leishmania infantum* in the Mediterranean, Middle East, China, parts of Asia, and Horn of Africa; and *Leishmania chagasi* in South and Central America. Other species may occasionally cause visceral disease. Over 90% of cases occur in six countries: India, Bangladesh, Nepal, Sudan, South Sudan, and Brazil. The incubation period is usually 4–6 months (range: 10 days to 24 months). Without treatment, the fatality rate reaches 90%. Early diagnosis and treatment reduce mortality to 2–5%.

About 90% of cases of cutaneous leishmaniasis occur in Afghanistan, Pakistan, Syria, Saudi Arabia, Algeria, Iran, Brazil, and Peru. **Old World cutaneous leishmaniasis** is caused mainly by *Leishmania tropica*, *Leishmania major*, and *Leishmania aethiopica* in the Mediterranean, Middle East, Africa, Central Asia, and Indian subcontinent. **New World cutaneous leishmaniasis** is caused by *Leishmania mexicana*, *Leishmania amazonensis*, and the species listed below for mucocutaneous disease in Central and South America. **Mucocutaneous leishmaniasis** (espundia) occurs in lowland forest areas of the Americas and is caused by *Leishmania braziliensis*, *Leishmania panamensis*, and *Leishmania peruviana*.

▶ Clinical Findings

A. Symptoms and Signs

1. Visceral leishmaniasis (kala azar)—Most infections are subclinical, but a small number progress to full-blown disease. A local nonulcerating nodule at the site of the sand fly bite may precede systemic manifestations but usually is inapparent. The onset of illness may be acute, within 2 weeks of infection, or insidious. Symptoms and signs include fever, chills, sweats, weakness, anorexia, weight loss, cough, and diarrhea. The spleen progressively becomes greatly enlarged, firm, and nontender. The liver is somewhat enlarged, and generalized lymphadenopathy may occur. Hyperpigmentation of skin can be seen, leading to the name kala azar ("black fever"). Other signs include skin lesions, petechiae, gingival bleeding, jaundice, edema, and ascites. As the disease progresses, severe wasting and malnutrition are seen; death eventually occurs, often due to secondary infections, within months to a few years. Post–kala azar dermal leishmaniasis may appear after apparent cure in the Indian subcontinent and Sudan. It may simulate leprosy, with hypopigmented macules or nodules developing on preexisting lesions. Viscerotropic leishmaniasis has been reported in small numbers of American military personnel in the Middle East, with mild systemic febrile illnesses after *L tropica* infections.

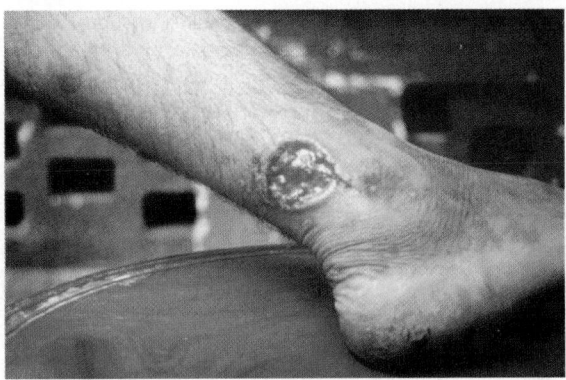

▲ **Figure 35–1.** Skin ulcer due to cutaneous leishmaniasis. Note the classic morphologic characteristics of this wound with its erythematous, nodular interior, surrounded by a raised border. (From Dr. Mae Melvin, Public Health Image Library, CDC.)

2. Old World and New World cutaneous leishmaniasis—
Cutaneous swellings appears 1 week to several months after sand fly bites and can be single or multiple. Characteristics of lesions and courses of disease vary depending on the leishmanial species and host immune response. Lesions begin as small papules and develop into nonulcerated dry plaques or large encrusted ulcers with well-demarcated raised and indurated margins (Figure 35–1). Satellite lesions may be present. The lesions are painless unless secondarily infected. Local lymph nodes may be enlarged. Systemic symptoms are uncommon, but fever, constitutional symptoms, and regional lymphadenopathy may be seen. For most species, healing occurs spontaneously in months to a few years, but scarring is common.

Leishmaniasis recidivans is a relapsing form of *L tropica* infection associated with hypersensitivity, in which the primary lesion heals centrally, but spreads laterally, with extensive scarring. Diffuse cutaneous leishmaniasis involves spread from a primary lesion, with local dissemination of nodules and a protracted course. Disseminated cutaneous leishmaniasis involves multiple nodular or ulcerated lesions, often with mucosal involvement.

3. Mucocutaneous leishmaniasis (espundia)—In Latin America, mucosal lesions develop in a small percentage of persons infected with *L braziliensis* and some other species, usually months to years after resolution of a cutaneous lesion. Nasal congestion is followed by ulceration of the nasal mucosa and septum, progressing to involvement of the mouth, lips, palate, pharynx, and larynx. Extensive destruction can occur, and secondary bacterial infection is common.

4. Infections in patients with AIDS—Leishmaniasis is an opportunistic infection in persons with AIDS. Visceral leishmaniasis can present late in the course of HIV infection, with fever, hepatosplenomegaly, and pancytopenia. The gastrointestinal tract, respiratory tract, and skin may also be involved.

B. Laboratory Findings

Identifying amastigotes within macrophages in tissue samples provides a definitive diagnosis. In **visceral leishmaniasis**, fine-needle aspiration of the spleen for culture and tissue evaluation is generally safe, and yields a diagnosis in over 95% of cases. Bone marrow aspiration is less sensitive but safer and diagnostic in most cases, and Giemsa-stained buffy coat of peripheral blood may occasionally show organisms. Cultures with media available from the CDC will grow promastigotes within a few days to weeks. Molecular assays can also be diagnostic. Serologic tests may facilitate diagnosis, but none are sufficiently sensitive or specific to be used alone. Numerous antibody-based rapid diagnostic tests are available; these have shown good specificity but limitations in sensitivity outside of India. Antigen-based rapid diagnostic tests may offer improved sensitivity. For **cutaneous lesions**, biopsies should be taken from the raised border of a skin lesion, with samples for histopathology, touch preparation, and culture. The histopathology shows inflammation with mononuclear cells. Macrophages filled with amastigotes may be present, especially early in infection. An intradermal leishmanin (Montenegro) skin test is positive in most individuals with cutaneous disease but negative in those with progressive visceral or diffuse cutaneous disease; this test is not approved in the United States. In **mucocutaneous leishmaniasis**, diagnosis is established by detecting amastigotes in scrapings, biopsy preparations, or aspirated tissue fluid, but organisms may be rare. Cultures from these samples may grow organisms. Serologic studies are often negative, but the leishmanin skin test is usually positive.

► Treatment

A. Visceral Leishmaniasis

The treatment of choice for visceral leishmaniasis on the Indian subcontinent is liposomal amphotericin B (approved by the FDA), which is generally effective and well tolerated but expensive. Standard dosing is 3 mg/kg/day intravenously on days 1–5, 14, and 21. Simpler regimens that have shown good efficacy in India include four doses of 5 mg/kg over 4–10 days and a single dose of 15 mg/kg. A single infusion of an amphotericin B lipid emulsion, which is more affordable than liposomal preparations, showed excellent efficacy, albeit lower than that of the liposomal formulation. Conventional amphotericin B deoxycholate, which is much less expensive, is also highly effective but with more toxicity. It is administered as a slow intravenous infusion of 1 mg/kg/day for 15–20 days or 0.5–1 mg/kg every second day for up to 8 weeks. Infusion-related side effects with conventional or liposomal amphotericin B include gastrointestinal symptoms, fever, chills, dyspnea, hypotension, and hepatic and renal toxicity.

Pentavalent antimonials remain the most commonly used drugs to treat leishmaniasis in most areas. Response rates are good outside India, but in India, resistance is a major problem. Two preparations are available, sodium stibogluconate in the United States and many other areas and meglumine antimonate in Latin America and francophone countries; the compounds appear to have comparable activities. In the United States, sodium stibogluconate can be obtained from the CDC Drug Service (www.cdc.gov/laboratory/drugservice). Standard dosing for either antimonial is 20 mg/kg once daily intravenously (preferred) or intramuscularly for 20 days for cutaneous leishmaniasis and 28 days for visceral or mucocutaneous disease. Toxicity increases over time, with development of gastrointestinal symptoms, fever, headache, myalgias, arthralgias, pancreatitis, and rash. Intramuscular injections can cause sterile abscesses. Monitoring should include serial ECGs, and changes are indications for discontinuation to avoid progression to serious arrhythmias.

The efficacy of amphotericin B is lower in East Africa than in Asia, and the standard treatment is a combination of sodium stibogluconate (20 mg/kg/day intravenously) plus paromomycin (15 mg/kg/day intramuscularly) for 17 days, with demonstrated excellent efficacy; liposomal amphotericin B may be considered in elderly or pregnant patients due to toxicity concerns.

Miltefosine is the first oral drug for the treatment of leishmaniasis, and it is registered in India for this indication. It initially demonstrated excellent results in India, but efficacy is decreasing due to drug resistance. It can be administered at a daily oral dose of 2.5 mg/kg in two divided doses for 28 days. A 28-day course of miltefosine (2.5 mg/kg/day) is also effective for the treatment of New World cutaneous leishmaniasis. Vomiting, diarrhea, and elevations in transaminases and kidney function studies are common, but generally short-lived, side effects.

The aminoglycoside paromomycin (11 mg/kg/day intramuscularly for 21 days) was shown to be similarly efficacious to amphotericin B for the treatment of visceral disease in India, where it is approved for this indication. It is much less expensive than liposomal amphotericin B or miltefosine. The drug is well tolerated; side effects include ototoxicity and reversible elevations in liver enzymes.

The use of drug combinations to improve treatment efficacy, shorten treatment courses, and reduce the selection of resistant parasites has been actively studied. In India, compared to a standard 30-day (treatment on alternate days) course of amphotericin, noninferior efficacy and decreased adverse events were seen with a single dose of liposomal amphotericin plus a 7-day course of miltefosine, a single dose of liposomal amphotericin plus a 10-day course of paromomycin, or a 10-day course of miltefosine plus paromomycin. As above, a combination of sodium stibogluconate and paromomycin is the standard treatment in East Africa.

B. Cutaneous Leishmaniasis

In the Old World, cutaneous leishmaniasis is generally self-healing over some months and does not metastasize to the mucosa, so it may be justified to withhold treatment in regions without mucocutaneous disease if lesions are small and cosmetically unimportant. Lesions on the face or hands are generally treated. New World leishmaniasis has a greater risk of progression to mucocutaneous disease, so treatment is more often warranted. Standard therapy is with pentavalent antimonials for 20 days, as described above. Other treatments include those discussed above for visceral disease, azole antifungals, and allopurinol. In studies in South

America, a 28-day course of miltefosine was superior to a 20-day course of meglumine antimoniate, and oral fluconazole also showed good efficacy. Topical therapy has included intralesional antimony, intralesional pentamidine, paromomycin ointment, cryotherapy, local heat, and surgical removal. Diffuse cutaneous leishmaniasis and related chronic skin processes generally respond poorly to therapy.

C. Mucocutaneous Leishmaniasis

Cutaneous infections from regions where parasites include those that cause mucocutaneous disease (eg, *L braziliensis* in parts of Latin America) should all be treated to help prevent disease progression. Treatment of mucocutaneous disease with antimonials is disappointing, with responses in only about 60% in Brazil. Other therapies listed above for visceral leishmaniasis may also be used, although they have not been well studied for this indication.

▶ Prevention & Control

Personal protection measures for avoidance of sand fly bites include use of insect repellants, fine-mesh insect netting, long sleeves and pants, and avoidance of warm shaded areas where flies are common. Disease control measures include destruction of animal reservoir hosts, mass treatment of humans in disease-prevalent areas, residual insecticide spraying in dwellings, limiting contact with dogs and other domesticated animals, and use of permethrin-impregnated collars for dogs.

Aronson N et al. Diagnosis and treatment of leishmaniasis: clinical practice guidelines by the Infectious Diseases Society of America (IDSA) and the American Society of Tropical Medicine and Hygiene (ASTMH). Clin Infect Dis. 2016 Dec 15; 63(12):1539–57. [PMID: 27941143]

Burza S et al. Leishmaniasis. Lancet. 2018 Sep 15;392(10151):951–70. [PMID: 30126638]

Kimutai R et al. Safety and effectiveness of sodium stibogluconate and paromomycin combination for the treatment of visceral leishmaniasis in eastern Africa: results from a pharmacovigilance programme. Clin Drug Investig. 2017 Mar; 37(3):259–72. [PMID: 28066878]

MALARIA

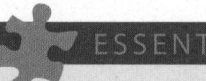 ESSENTIALS OF DIAGNOSIS

▶ Exposure to anopheline mosquitoes in a malaria-endemic area.

▶ Intermittent attacks of chills, fever, and sweating.

▶ Headache, myalgia, vomiting, splenomegaly; anemia, thrombocytopenia.

▶ Intraerythrocytic parasites identified in thick or thin blood smears or positive rapid diagnostic tests.

▶ **Falciparum malaria complications:** cerebral malaria, severe anemia, hypotension, pulmonary edema, acute kidney injury, hypoglycemia, acidosis, and hemolysis.

General Considerations

Malaria is the most important parasitic disease of humans, causing hundreds of millions of illnesses and hundreds of thousands of deaths each year. The disease is endemic in most of the tropics, including much of South and Central America, Africa, the Middle East, the Indian subcontinent, Southeast Asia, and Oceania. Transmission, morbidity, and mortality are greatest in Africa, where most deaths from malaria are in young children. Malaria is also common in travelers from nonendemic areas to the tropics. Although the disease remains a major problem, impressive advances have been made in many regions. A 2016 study estimated a 57% decrease in the malaria death rate and 37% decrease in the annual number of malaria deaths in the past 15 years. However, after marked gains, morbidity and mortality appear to have stabilized, with WHO estimates showing modest annual increases in incidence, but decreases in deaths (219 million cases and 435,000 deaths estimated in 2017); other estimates suggest greater morbidity and mortality.

Four species of the genus *Plasmodium* classically cause human malaria. *Plasmodium falciparum* is responsible for nearly all severe disease. It is endemic in most malarious areas and is by far the predominant species in Africa. *Plasmodium vivax* is about as common as *P falciparum*, except in Africa. *P vivax* uncommonly causes severe disease, although this outcome may be more common than previously appreciated. *Plasmodium ovale* and *Plasmodium malariae* are much less common causes of disease, and generally do not cause severe illness. *Plasmodium knowlesi*, a parasite of macaque monkeys, is now recognized to cause occasional illnesses, including some severe disease, in humans in Southeast Asia.

Malaria is transmitted by the bite of infected female anopheline mosquitoes. During feeding, mosquitoes inject sporozoites, which circulate to the liver, and rapidly infect hepatocytes, causing asymptomatic liver infection. Merozoites are subsequently released from the liver, and they rapidly infect erythrocytes to begin the asexual erythrocytic stage of infection that is responsible for human disease. Multiple rounds of erythrocytic development, with production of merozoites that invade additional erythrocytes, lead to large numbers of circulating parasites and clinical illness. Some erythrocytic parasites also develop into sexual gametocytes, which are infectious to mosquitoes, allowing completion of the life cycle and infection of others.

Malaria may uncommonly be transmitted from mother to infant (congenital malaria), by blood transfusion, and in nonendemic areas by mosquitoes infected after biting infected immigrants or travelers. In *P vivax* and *P ovale*, parasites also form dormant liver hypnozoites, which are not killed by most drugs, allowing subsequent relapses of illness after initial elimination of erythrocytic infections. For all plasmodial species, parasites may recrudesce following initial clinical improvement after suboptimal therapy.

In highly endemic regions, where people are infected repeatedly, antimalarial immunity prevents severe disease in most older children and adults. However, young children, who are relatively nonimmune, are at high risk for severe disease from *P falciparum* infection, and this population is responsible for most deaths from malaria. Pregnant women are also at increased risk for severe falciparum malaria. In areas with lower endemicity, individuals of all ages commonly present with uncomplicated or severe malaria. Travelers, who are generally nonimmune, are at high risk for severe disease from falciparum malaria at any age.

Clinical Findings

A. Symptoms and Signs

An acute attack of malaria typically begins with a prodrome of headache and fatigue, followed by fever. A classic malarial paroxysm includes chills, high fever, and then sweats. Patients may appear to be remarkably well between febrile episodes. Fevers are usually irregular, especially early in the illness, but without therapy may become regular, with 48-hour (*P vivax* and *P ovale*) or 72-hour (*P malariae*) cycles, especially with non-falciparum disease. Headache, malaise, myalgias, arthralgias, cough, chest pain, abdominal pain, anorexia, nausea, vomiting, and diarrhea are common. Seizures may represent simple febrile convulsions or evidence of severe neurologic disease. Physical findings may be absent or include signs of anemia, jaundice, splenomegaly, and mild hepatomegaly. Rash and lymphadenopathy are not typical in malaria, and thus suggestive of another cause of fever.

In the developed world, it is imperative that all persons with suggestive symptoms, in particular fever, who have traveled in an endemic area be evaluated for malaria. The risk for falciparum malaria is greatest within 2 months of return from travel; other species may cause disease many months—and occasionally more than a year—after return from an endemic area.

Severe malaria is characterized by signs of severe illness, organ dysfunction, or a high parasite load (peripheral parasitemia greater than 5% or greater than 200,000 parasites/mcL). It is principally a result of *P falciparum* infection because this species uniquely infects erythrocytes of all ages and mediates the sequestration of infected erythrocytes in small blood vessels, thereby evading clearance of infected erythrocytes by the spleen.

Severe falciparum malaria can include dysfunction of any organ system, including neurologic abnormalities progressing to alterations in consciousness, repeated seizures, and coma (cerebral malaria); severe anemia; hypotension and shock; noncardiogenic pulmonary edema and the acute respiratory distress syndrome; acute kidney injury due to acute tubular necrosis or, less commonly, severe hemolysis; hypoglycemia; acidosis; hemolysis with jaundice; hepatic dysfunction; retinal hemorrhages and other fundoscopic abnormalities; bleeding abnormalities, including disseminated intravascular coagulation; and secondary bacterial infections, including pneumonia and *Salmonella* bacteremia. In the developing world, severe malaria and deaths from the disease are mostly in young children, in particular from cerebral malaria and severe anemia. Cerebral malaria is a consequence of a single severe infection while severe anemia follows multiple malarial infections, intestinal helminths, and nutritional deficiencies. In a large trial of African children, acidosis, impaired consciousness, convulsions, renal impairment, and underlying chronic illness were associated with poor outcome.

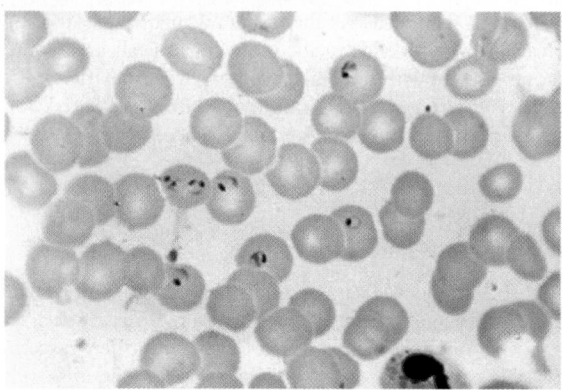

▲ **Figure 35–2.** Thin film Giemsa-stained micrograph with *Plasmodium falciparum* ring forms. (From Steven Glenn, Laboratory & Consultation Division, Public Health Image Library, CDC.)

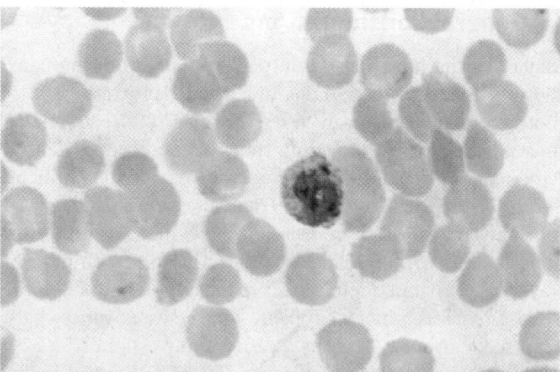

▲ **Figure 35–4.** Thin film Giemsa-stained micrograph with *Plasmodium vivax* schizont. (From Steven Glenn, Laboratory & Consultation Division, Public Health Image Library, CDC.)

Uncommon disorders resulting from immunologic responses to chronic infection are massive splenomegaly and, with *P malariae* infection, immune complex glomerulopathy with nephrotic syndrome. HIV-infected individuals are at increased risk for malaria and for severe disease, in particular with advanced immunodeficiency.

B. Laboratory Findings

Giemsa-stained blood smears remain the mainstay of diagnosis (Figures 35–2, 35–3, 35–4, and 35–5), although other routine stains (eg, Wright stain) will also demonstrate parasites. Thick smears provide efficient evaluation of large volumes of blood, but thin smears are simpler for inexperienced personnel and better for discrimination of parasite species. Single smears are usually positive in infected individuals, although parasitemias may be very low in nonimmune individuals. If illness is suspected, repeating smears at 8- to 24-hour intervals is appropriate. The severity of malaria correlates only loosely with the quantity of infecting parasites, but high parasitemias (especially greater than

10–20% of erythrocytes infected or greater than 200,000–500,000 parasites/mcL) or the presence of malarial pigment (a breakdown product of hemoglobin) in more than 5% of neutrophils is associated with a particularly poor prognosis.

A second means of diagnosis is rapid diagnostic tests to identify circulating plasmodial antigens with a simple "dipstick" format. These tests are not well standardized but are widely available. At best, they offer sensitivity and specificity near that of high-quality blood smear analysis and are simpler to perform. However, *P falciparum* lacking the most common rapid diagnostic test antigen, histidine-rich protein 2 (HRP2), has been identified in some areas, leading to concern that HRP2-based tests may miss some cases of falciparum malaria.

Serologic tests indicate history of disease but are not useful for diagnosis of acute infection. PCR and related molecular tests (eg, LAMP) are highly sensitive but not available for routine diagnosis. In immune populations, highly sensitive tests, such as PCR, have limited value because subclinical infections, which are not routinely treated, are common.

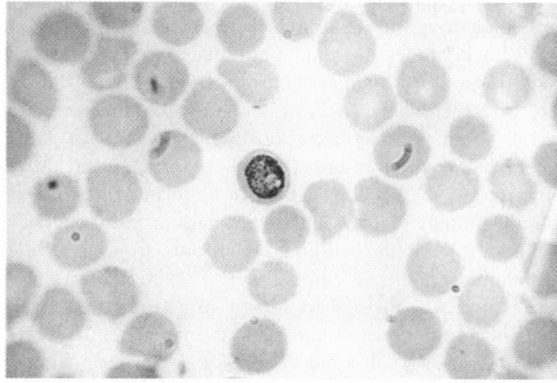

▲ **Figure 35–3.** Thin film Giemsa-stained micrograph with *Plasmodium malariae* trophozoite. (From Steven Glenn, Laboratory & Consultation Division, Public Health Image Library, CDC.)

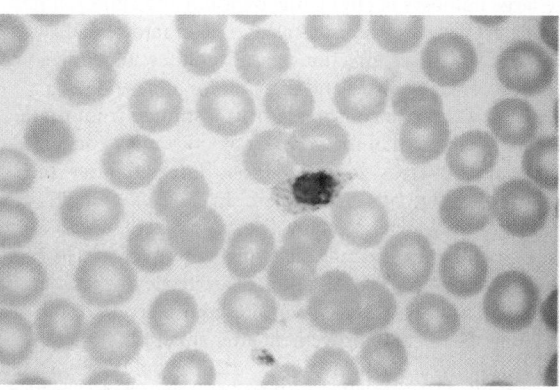

▲ **Figure 35–5.** Thin film Giemsa-stained micrograph with *Plasmodium ovale* trophozoite. (From Steven Glenn, Laboratory & Consultation Division, Public Health Image Library, CDC.)

Table 35–2. Major antimalarial drugs.

Drug	Class	Use
Chloroquine	4-Aminoquinoline	Treatment and chemoprophylaxis of infection with sensitive parasites
Amodiaquine[1]	4-Aminoquinoline	Treatment of *Plasmodium falciparum*, optimally in fixed combination with artesunate
Piperaquine[1]	4-Aminoquinoline	Treatment of *P falciparum* in fixed combination with dihydroartemisinin
Quinine	Quinoline methanol	Oral and intravenous[1] (for severe infections) treatment of *P falciparum*
Quinidine	Quinoline methanol	Intravenous therapy of severe infections with *P falciparum*
Mefloquine	Quinoline methanol	Chemoprophylaxis and treatment of infections with *P falciparum*
Primaquine, tafenoquine	8-Aminoquinoline	Radical cure and terminal prophylaxis of infections with *Plasmodium vivax* and *Plasmodium ovale*; alternative for malaria chemoprophylaxis
Sulfadoxine-pyrimethamine (Fansidar)	Folate antagonist combination	Treatment of *P falciparum*, optimally in combination with artesunate; intermittent preventive therapy
Atovaquone-proguanil (Malarone)	Quinone-folate antagonist combination	Treatment and chemoprophylaxis of *P falciparum* infection
Doxycycline	Tetracycline	Treatment (with quinine) of infections with *P falciparum*; chemoprophylaxis
Halofantrine[1]	Phenanthrene methanol	Treatment of infections with some chloroquine-resistant *P falciparum*
Lumefantrine	Amyl alcohol	Treatment of *P falciparum* malaria in fixed combination with artemether (Coartem)
Pyronaridine	Benzonaphthyridine	Treatment of *P falciparum* malaria in fixed combination artesunate
Artemisinins (artesunate, artemether, dihydroartemisinin)	Sesquiterpene lactone endoperoxides	Treatment of *P falciparum* in oral combination regimens for uncomplicated disease and parenterally for severe malaria

[1]Not available in the United States.
Modified, with permission, from Katzung BG. *Basic & Clinical Pharmacology*. 14th edition. McGraw-Hill, 2018.

Other diagnostic findings with uncomplicated malaria include thrombocytopenia, anemia, leukocytosis or leukopenia, liver function abnormalities, and hepatosplenomegaly. Severe malaria can present with the laboratory abnormalities expected for the advanced organ dysfunction discussed above.

Treatment

Malaria is the most common cause of fever in much of the tropics and in travelers seeking medical attention after return from endemic areas. Fevers are often treated presumptively in endemic areas, but ideally, treatment should follow definitive diagnosis, especially in non-immune individuals.

Symptomatic malaria is caused only by the erythrocytic stage of infection. Available antimalarial drugs (Table 35–2) act against this stage, except for primaquine, which acts principally against hepatic parasites.

A. Non-Falciparum Malaria

The first-line drug for non-falciparum malaria from most areas remains chloroquine. Due to increasing resistance of *P vivax* to chloroquine, alternative therapies are recommended when resistance is suspected, particularly for infections acquired in Indonesia, Oceania, and South America. These infections can be treated with artemisinin-based combination therapies (ACTs) or other first-line

regimens for *P falciparum* infections as discussed below. For *P vivax* or *P ovale*, eradication of erythrocytic parasites with chloroquine should be accompanied by treatment with primaquine (after evaluating for glucose-6-phosphate dehydrogenase [G6PD] deficiency; see below) to eradicate dormant liver stages (hypnozoites), which may lead to relapses with recurrent erythrocytic infection and malaria symptoms after weeks to months if left untreated. Tafenoquine, which is related to primaquine, appears to offer similar efficacy with simpler dosing, but it also engenders potential toxicity in those with G6PD deficiency, and it remains under study. *P malariae* infections need only be treated with chloroquine.

B. Uncomplicated Falciparum Malaria

P falciparum is resistant to chloroquine and sulfadoxine-pyrimethamine in most areas, with the exceptions of Central America west of the Panama Canal and Hispaniola. Falciparum malaria from other areas should not be treated with these older drugs, and decisions regarding chemoprophylaxis should follow the same geographic considerations.

ACTs, all including a short-acting artemisinin and longer-acting partner drug, are first-line therapies in nearly all endemic countries. WHO recommends six ACTs to treat falciparum malaria (Table 35–3), but the efficacy of these regimens varies. Other combination therapies are under development. Quinine generally remains effective for

Table 35–3. WHO recommendations for the treatment of uncomplicated falciparum malaria.

Regimen	Notes
Artemether-lumefantrine (Coartem, Riamet)	Coformulated, first-line therapy in many countries. Approved in the United States.
Artesunate-amodiaquine (ASAQ)	Coformulated, first-line therapy in multiple African countries.
Artesunate-mefloquine	First-line therapy in parts of Southeast Asia and South America but efficacy decreasing in parts of Thailand.
Artesunate-pyronaridine	Coformulated. Most recently approved regimen; used in some Southeast Asian countries.
Artesunate-sulfadoxine-pyrimethamine	First-line in some countries, but efficacy lower than other regimens in most areas.
Dihydroartemisinin–piperaquine	Coformulated. First-line in some Southeast Asian countries but efficacy decreasing in parts of Cambodia.

Data from World Health Organization: Guidelines for the Treatment of Malaria. World Health Organization. Geneva 2015.

falciparum malaria, but it must be taken for 7 days and is poorly tolerated, and should best be reserved for the treatment of severe malaria and for treatment after another regimen has failed (Table 35–4).

In developed countries, malaria is an uncommon but potentially life-threatening infection of travelers and immigrants, many of whom are nonimmune, so they are at risk for rapid progression to severe disease. Nonimmune individuals with falciparum malaria should generally be admitted to the hospital due to risks of rapid progression of disease. A number of options are available for the treatment of uncomplicated falciparum malaria in the United States (Table 35–4).

C. Severe Malaria

Severe malaria is a medical emergency. Parenteral treatment is indicated for severe malaria, as defined above, and with inability to take oral drugs. With appropriate prompt therapy and supportive care, rapid recoveries may be seen even in very ill individuals.

The standard of care for severe malaria is intravenous artesunate, which has demonstrated superior efficacy and better tolerability than quinine. In the United States, intravenous artesunate is available on an investigational basis through the CDC (for enrollment call 770-488-7788); if approved, the drug is provided emergently from CDC Quarantine Stations. The drug is administered in four doses of 2.4 mg/kg over 3 days, every 12 hours on day 1, and then daily. If artesunate cannot be obtained promptly, severe malaria should be treated with intravenous quinine (available in most countries but not the United States) or quinidine (available in the United States). In endemic

regions, if parenteral therapy is not available, intrarectal administration of artemether or artesunate is also effective. Patients receiving intravenous quinine or quinidine should receive continuous cardiac monitoring; if QTc prolongation exceeds 25% of baseline, the infusion rate should be reduced. Blood glucose should be monitored every 4–6 hours, and 5–10% dextrose may be coadministered to decrease the likelihood of hypoglycemia.

Appropriate care of severe malaria includes maintenance of fluids and electrolytes; respiratory and hemodynamic support; and consideration of blood transfusions, anticonvulsants, antibiotics for bacterial infections, and hemofiltration or hemodialysis. With high parasitemia (greater than 5–10%), exchange transfusion has been used, but beneficial effects have not clearly been demonstrated and it is generally no longer recommended.

D. Antimalarial Drugs

1. Chloroquine—Chloroquine remains the drug of choice for the treatment of sensitive *P falciparum* and other species of malaria parasites (Table 35–4). Chloroquine is active against erythrocytic parasites of all human malaria species. It does not eradicate hepatic stages, so it must be used with primaquine to eradicate *P vivax* and *P ovale* infections. Chloroquine-resistant *P falciparum* is widespread in nearly all areas of the world with falciparum malaria, with the exceptions of Central America west of the Panama Canal and Hispaniola. Chloroquine-resistant *P vivax* has been reported from a number of areas, most notably Southeast Asia and Oceania.

Chloroquine is the drug of choice for the treatment of non-falciparum and sensitive falciparum malaria. It rapidly terminates fever (in 24–48 hours) and clears parasitemia (in 48–72 hours) caused by sensitive parasites. Chloroquine is also the preferred chemoprophylactic agent in malarious regions without resistant falciparum malaria.

Chloroquine is usually well tolerated, even with prolonged use. Pruritus is common, primarily in Africans. Nausea, vomiting, abdominal pain, headache, anorexia, malaise, blurring of vision, and urticaria are uncommon. Dosing after meals may reduce some adverse events.

2. Amodiaquine, piperaquine, and pyronaridine—Amodiaquine is a 4-aminoquinoline that is closely related to chloroquine. Amodiaquine has been widely used to treat malaria because of its low cost, limited toxicity and, in some areas, effectiveness against chloroquine-resistant strains of *P falciparum*. Use of amodiaquine decreased after recognition of rare but serious side effects, notably agranulocytosis, aplastic anemia, and hepatotoxicity. However, serious side effects are rare with short-term use, and artesunate-amodiaquine is one of the standard ACTs recommended to treat falciparum malaria (Table 35–3). Chemoprophylaxis with amodiaquine is best avoided because of increased toxicity with long-term use.

Piperaquine is another 4-aminoquinoline that has been coformulated with dihydroartemisinin in an ACT. Piperaquine appears to be well tolerated and in combination with dihydroartemisinin to offer a highly efficacious therapy for falciparum and vivax malaria. Due to the long half-life of

Table 35–4. Treatment of malaria.

Clinical Setting	Drug Therapy[1]	Alternative Drugs
Chloroquine-sensitive *Plasmodium falciparum* and *Plasmodium malariae* infections	Chloroquine phosphate, 1 g at 0 hours, followed by 500 mg at 6, 24, and 48 hours or– Chloroquine phosphate, 1 g at 0 hours and 24 hours, then 0.5 g at 48 hours	
Plasmodium vivax and *Plasmodium ovale* infections	Chloroquine (as above), then (if G6PD normal) primaquine, 30-mg base daily for 14 days	For infections from Indonesia, Papua New Guinea, and other areas with suspected resistance: therapies listed for uncomplicated chloroquine-resistant *P falciparum* plus primaquine
Uncomplicated infections with chloroquine-resistant *P falciparum*	Coartem (artemether 20 mg, lumefantrine 120 mg), four tablets twice daily for 3 days or– Malarone, four tablets (total of 1 g of atovaquone, 400 mg of proguanil) daily for 3 days or– Quinine sulfate, 650 mg three times daily for 3–7 days Plus one of the following (when quinine given for < 7 days) Doxycycline, 100 mg twice daily for 7 days or– Clindamycin, 600 mg twice daily for 7 days	Mefloquine, 15 mg/kg once or 750 mg, then 500 mg in 6–8 hours or– Dihydroartemisinin-piperaquine[2] (dihydroartemisinin 40 mg, piperaquine 320 mg), 4 tablets daily for 3 days or– ASAQ[2] (artesunate 100 mg, amodiaquine 270 mg), two tablets daily for 3 days
Severe or complicated infections with *P falciparum*	Artesunate 2.4 mg/kg intravenously every 12 hours for 1 day, then daily[3,6]	Quinidine gluconate,[4–6] 10 mg/kg intravenously over 1–2 hours, then 0.02 mg/kg intravenously/min or– Quinidine gluconate,[4–6] 15 mg/kg intravenously over 4 hours, then 7.5 mg/kg intravenously over 4 hours every 8 hours or– Quinine dihydrochloride,[2,4–6] 20 mg/kg intravenously over 4 hours, then 10 mg/kg intravenously every 8 hours or– Artemether,[2,6] 3.2 mg/kg intramuscularly, then 1.6 mg/kg/day intramuscularly

[1]All dosages are oral and refer to salts unless otherwise indicated. See text for additional information on all agents, including toxicities and cautions. See CDC guidelines (phone: 877-FYI-TRIP; http://www.cdc.gov/malaria/) for additional information and pediatric dosing.
[2]Not available in the United States.
[3]Available in the United States only on an investigational basis through the CDC (phone: 770-488-7788).
[4]Cardiac monitoring should be in place during intravenous administration of quinidine or quinine.
[5]Avoid loading doses in persons who have received quinine, quinidine, or mefloquine in the prior 24 hours.
[6]With all parenteral regimens, change to an oral regimen as soon as the patient can tolerate it.
G6PD, glucose-6-phosphate dehydrogenase.

piperaquine (~3 weeks), dihydroartemisinin-piperaquine offers the longest period of posttreatment prophylaxis of available ACTs. However, resistance to piperaquine has emerged in southeast Asia, with consequent treatment failures of dihydroartemisinin-piperaquine in that region.

Pyronaridine is a benzonaphthyridine that was also previously used as a monotherapy to treat malaria in China and acts against many drug-resistant strains of *P falciparum*. The combination of artesunate plus pyronaridine has shown excellent efficacy against falciparum and vivax malaria and has been well tolerated, although elevated transaminases can be seen.

3. Mefloquine—Mefloquine is effective against many chloroquine-resistant strains of *P falciparum* and against other malarial species. Although toxicity is a concern, mefloquine is also a recommended chemoprophylactic drug. Resistance to mefloquine has been reported sporadically from many areas, but it appears to be uncommon except in regions of Southeast Asia with high rates of multidrug resistance (especially border areas of Thailand).

For treatment of uncomplicated malaria, mefloquine can be administered as a single dose or in two doses over 1 day. It is used in combination with artesunate as an artemisinin-based combination therapy (ACT) for falciparum malaria, although resistance limits efficacy in Southeast Asia. It should be taken with meals and swallowed with a large amount of water. Mefloquine is recommended by the CDC for chemoprophylaxis in all malarious areas except those with no chloroquine resistance (where chloroquine is preferred) and some rural areas of Southeast Asia with a high prevalence of mefloquine resistance.

Adverse effects with weekly dosing of mefloquine for chemoprophylaxis include nausea, vomiting, dizziness, sleep and behavioral disturbances, epigastric pain, diarrhea, abdominal pain, headache, rash and, uncommonly, seizures and psychosis. There is an FDA black box warning about neuropsychiatric toxicity, possibly including rare, irreversible effects. Mefloquine should be avoided in persons with histories of psychiatric disease or seizures.

Adverse effects are more common (up to 50% of treatments) with the higher dosages of mefloquine required for treatment. These effects may be lessened by splitting administration into two doses separated by 6–8 hours. Serious neuropsychiatric toxicities (depression, confusion, acute psychosis, or seizures) have been reported in less than 1 in 1000 treatments, but some authorities believe that these are more common. Mefloquine can also alter cardiac conduction, and so it should not be coadministered with quinine, quinidine, or halofantrine, and caution is required if these drugs are used to treat malaria after mefloquine chemoprophylaxis. Mefloquine is generally considered safe in young children and pregnant women.

4. Quinine and quinidine—Quinine dihydrochloride and quinidine gluconate remain first-line therapies for falciparum malaria, especially severe disease, although toxicity concerns complicate therapy (Table 35–4). Quinine acts rapidly against the four species of human malaria parasites. Quinidine, the dextrorotatory stereoisomer of quinine, is at least as effective as quinine in the treatment of severe falciparum malaria.

Resistance of *P falciparum* to quinine is common in some areas of Southeast Asia, where the drug may fail if used alone to treat falciparum malaria. However, quinine still provides at least a partial therapeutic effect in most patients.

Quinine and quinidine are effective treatments for severe falciparum malaria, although intravenous artesunate is the standard of care. The drugs can be administered in divided doses or by continuous intravenous infusion; treatment should begin with a loading dose to rapidly achieve effective plasma concentrations. Intravenous quinine and quinidine should be administered with cardiac monitoring because of their cardiac toxicity and the relative unpredictability of their pharmacokinetics. Therapy should be changed to an oral agent as soon as the patient has improved and can tolerate oral medications.

In areas without newer combination regimens, oral quinine sulfate is an alternative first-line therapy for uncomplicated falciparum malaria, although poor tolerance may limit compliance. Quinine is commonly used with a second drug (most often doxycycline) to shorten the duration of use (to 3 days) and to limit toxicity. Therapeutic dosages of quinine and quinidine commonly cause tinnitus, headache, nausea, dizziness, flushing, and visual disturbances. Hematologic abnormalities include hemolysis (especially with

G6PD deficiency), leukopenia, agranulocytosis, and thrombocytopenia. Therapeutic doses may cause hypoglycemia through stimulation of insulin release; this is a particular problem in severe infections and in pregnant patients, who have increased sensitivity to insulin. Overly rapid infusions can cause severe hypotension. ECG abnormalities (QT prolongation) are fairly common, but dangerous arrhythmias are uncommon when the drugs are administered appropriately. Quinine should not be given concurrently with mefloquine and should be used with caution in a patient who has previously received mefloquine.

5. Primaquine and tafenoquine—Primaquine phosphate, a synthetic 8-aminoquinoline, is the drug of choice for the eradication of dormant liver forms of *P vivax* and *P ovale* (Table 35–4). Primaquine is active against hepatic stages of all human malaria parasites. This action is optimal soon after therapy with chloroquine or other agents. Primaquine also acts against erythrocytic stage parasites, although this activity is too weak for the treatment of active disease, and against gametocytes. As a new strategy to lower transmission, a single low dose of primaquine in conjunction with an ACT to treat uncomplicated falciparum malaria was well tolerated and lowered transmission to mosquitoes in subjects with normal G6PD levels.

For *P vivax* and *P ovale* infections, chloroquine or other drugs are used to eradicate erythrocytic forms, and if the G6PD level is normal, a 14-day course of primaquine (52.6 mg primaquine phosphate [30 mg base] daily) is initiated to eradicate liver hypnozoites and prevent a subsequent relapse. Some strains of *P vivax*, particularly in New Guinea and Southeast Asia, are relatively resistant to primaquine, and the drug may fail to eradicate liver forms.

Standard chemoprophylaxis does not prevent a relapse of *P vivax* or *P ovale* infections, since liver hypnozoites are not eradicated by chloroquine or other standard treatments. To diminish the likelihood of relapse, some authorities advocate the use of a treatment course of primaquine after the completion of travel to an endemic area. Primaquine can also be used for chemoprophylaxis to prevent *P falciparum* and *P vivax* infection in persons with normal levels of G6PD.

Primaquine in recommended doses is generally well tolerated. It infrequently causes nausea, epigastric pain, abdominal cramps, and headache, especially when taken on an empty stomach. Rare adverse effects include leukopenia, agranulocytosis, leukocytosis, and cardiac arrhythmias. Standard doses of primaquine may cause hemolysis or methemoglobinemia (manifested by cyanosis), especially in persons with G6PD deficiency or other hereditary metabolic defects. Patients should be tested for G6PD deficiency before primaquine is prescribed. Primaquine should be discontinued if there is evidence of hemolysis or anemia and should be avoided in pregnancy.

Tafenoquine, an 8-aminoquinoline, has a much longer half-life than primaquine. These two medications share the risk of hemolysis with G6PD deficiency and probably other toxicities; tafenoquine should not be used during pregnancy or in those with G6PD deficiency. Tafenoquine is FDA-approved for patients at least 16 years of age for two indications, but with different formulations, marketed by different companies, for the two indications. To eliminate hepatic stages of *P vivax*, a single dose (Krintafel, two 150-mg tablets once daily) is taken with food soon after initiation of primary therapy (with chloroquine or other agents). For malaria chemoprophylaxis, the drug (Arakoda, two 100-mg tablets) is taken once daily for 3 days and then weekly until 1 week after the last exposure.

6. Inhibitors of folate synthesis—Inhibitors of two parasite enzymes involved in folate metabolism, dihydrofolate reductase (DHFR) and dihydropteroate synthase (DHPS), are used, generally in combination regimens, for the treatment and prevention of malaria, although the drugs are rather slow acting and now limited by resistance.

Fansidar is a fixed combination of sulfadoxine (500 mg) and pyrimethamine (25 mg). It is no longer advised for chemoprophylaxis due to rare serious side effects with long-term dosing. For treatment, advantages of sulfadoxine-pyrimethamine include ease of administration (a single oral dose) and low cost. However, resistance is now a major problem.

Sulfadoxine-pyrimethamine plus artesunate has shown efficacy for malaria treatment in some areas but is best replaced by more effective ACTs. Sulfadoxine-pyrimethamine is recommended by WHO for monthly preventive therapy in pregnant women in areas of high endemicity, although its efficacy is limited by resistance. Amodiaquine plus sulfadoxine-pyrimethamine is recommended monthly during the rainy season for chemoprophylaxis in regions of West Africa with seasonal malaria transmission and limited drug resistance. Another antifolate combination, trimethoprim-sulfamethoxazole (TMP-SMZ), is widely used to prevent coinfections in patients infected with HIV, and it offers partial protection against malaria.

7. Artemisinins—Artemisinin (qinghaosu) is a sesquiterpene lactone endoperoxide, the active component of an herbal medicine that has been used for various indications in China for over 2000 years. Analogs have been synthesized to increase solubility and improve antimalarial efficacy. The most important of these analogs are artesunate, artemether, and dihydroartemisinin. WHO encourages availability of oral artemisinins only in coformulated combination regimens.

Artemisinins act very rapidly against all erythrocytic-stage human malaria parasites. Of concern, delayed clearance of parasites and clinical failures have been seen after treatment with artesunate in parts of Southeast Asia, heralding the emergence of artemisinin resistance in this region.

Artemisinins play a vital role in the treatment of malaria, including multidrug-resistant *P falciparum* malaria. Due to their short plasma half-lives, recrudescence rates are unacceptably high after short-course therapy, leading to approved use only as initial therapy for severe malaria and in ACTs for uncomplicated malaria. The ACTs that are currently most advocated in Africa are artesunate plus amodiaquine (ASAQ) and artemether plus lumefantrine (Coartem), each of which is available as a coformulated product. Another ACT, artesunate plus mefloquine is used mostly outside of Africa; its efficacy may be declining in parts of Asia. Dihydroartemisinin-piperaquine has shown excellent efficacy and is the first-line regimen in some countries in Southeast Asia, but

efficacy has declined in Cambodia due to decreased activity of both components of the regimen. The newest approved ACT, artesunate-pyronaridine, is approved in some countries, but little used to date. Other ACTs not recommended by the WHO are available in some countries and have shown good efficacy in limited studies, including arterolane-piperaquine, artemisinin-piperaquine, and artemisinin-naphthoquine.

In studies of severe malaria, intramuscular artemether was at least as effective as intramuscular quinine, and intravenous artesunate was superior to intravenous quinine in terms of efficacy and tolerability. Thus, the standard of care for severe malaria is intravenous artesunate, when it is available, although parenteral quinine and quinidine remain acceptable alternatives. Artesunate and artemether have also been effective in the treatment of severe malaria when administered rectally, offering a valuable treatment modality when parenteral therapy is not available.

Artemisinins are very well tolerated. The most commonly reported adverse effects have been nausea, vomiting, and diarrhea, which may often be due to acute malaria, rather than drug toxicity. Neutropenia, anemia, hemolysis, and elevated levels of liver enzymes have been noted rarely. Hemolysis may occur weeks after therapy with intravenous artesunate. Artemisinins are teratogenic in animals, but with good safety seen in humans, and the importance of effectively treating malaria during pregnancy, the WHO now recommends ACTs to treat uncomplicated malaria and intravenous artesunate to treat complicated malaria during all trimesters of pregnancy.

8. Atovaquone plus proguanil (Malarone)—Atovaquone, a hydroxynaphthoquinone, is not effective when used alone, due to rapid development of drug resistance. However, Malarone, a fixed combination of atovaquone (250 mg) and the antifolate proguanil (100 mg), is highly effective for both the treatment and chemoprophylaxis of falciparum malaria, and it is approved for both indications in the United States (Table 35–4). It also appears to be active against other species of malaria parasites. Unlike most other antimalarials, Malarone provides activity against both erythrocytic and hepatic stage parasites.

For treatment, Malarone is given at an adult dose of four tablets daily for 3 days. For chemoprophylaxis, Malarone must be taken daily. It has an advantage over mefloquine and doxycycline in requiring shorter durations of treatment before and after the period at risk for malaria transmission, due to activity against liver-stage parasites. It should be taken with food.

Malarone is generally well tolerated. Adverse effects include abdominal pain, nausea, vomiting, diarrhea, headache, and rash, and these are more common with the higher dose required for treatment. Reversible elevations in liver enzymes have been reported. The safety of atovaquone in pregnancy is unknown.

9. Antibiotics—A number of antibacterials in addition to the folate antagonists and sulfonamides are slow-acting antimalarials. None of the antibiotics should be used as single agents for the treatment of malaria due to their slow rate of action.

Doxycycline is commonly used in the treatment of falciparum malaria in conjunction with quinidine or quinine, allowing a shorter and better-tolerated course of those drugs (Table 35–4). Doxycycline is also a standard chemoprophylactic drug, especially for use in areas of Southeast Asia with high rates of resistance to other antimalarials, including mefloquine. Doxycycline side effects include gastrointestinal symptoms, candidal vaginitis, and photosensitivity. The drug should be taken while upright with a large amount of water to avoid esophageal irritation. Clindamycin can be used in conjunction with quinine or quinidine in those for whom doxycycline is not recommended, such as children and pregnant women (Table 35–4). The most common toxicities with clindamycin are gastrointestinal.

10. Lumefantrine—Lumefantrine, an aryl alcohol related to halofantrine, is available only as a fixed-dose combination with artemether (Coartem or Riamet). Oral absorption is highly variable and improved when the drug is taken with food. Use of Coartem with a fatty meal is recommended. Coartem is highly effective for the treatment of falciparum malaria, but it requires twice-daily dosing. Despite this limitation, due to its reliable efficacy against falciparum malaria, Coartem is the first-line therapy for malaria in many malarious countries. Coartem is well tolerated; side effects include headache, dizziness, loss of appetite, gastrointestinal symptoms, and palpitations. Importantly, Coartem does not generally cause QT prolongation or the serious cardiac toxicity seen with halofantrine.

▶ Prevention

Malaria is transmitted by night-biting anopheline mosquitoes. Bed nets, in particular nets treated with permethrin insecticides, are heavily promoted as inexpensive means of antimalarial protection, but effectiveness varies in part due to widespread insecticide resistance. Indoor spraying of insecticides is generally highly effective in Africa but limited by resource constraints.

Extensive efforts are underway to develop a malaria vaccine, but a vaccine offering a high level of protection is not anticipated in the near future. RTS,S vaccine, which is based on a sporozoite antigen, is the most advanced vaccine candidate. Multiple clinical trials showed about 25–50% protection against malaria in children in the year after immunization, but lower levels of protection in very young children, in areas of highest malaria exposure, and over longer periods of time. Seasonal malaria immunization, using short-acting vaccines during the high transmission season, is being investigated. Other approaches under study include vaccines containing erythrocytic, liver-stage, and sexual-stage antigens, and use of radiation-attenuated or molecularly attenuated sporozoites.

When travelers from nonendemic to endemic countries are counseled on the prevention of malaria, it is imperative to emphasize measures to prevent mosquito bites (insect repellents, insecticides, and bed nets), since parasites are increasingly resistant to multiple drugs and no chemoprophylactic regimen is fully protective. Chemoprophylaxis is recommended for all travelers from nonendemic regions to endemic areas, although risks vary greatly for different locations, and some tropical areas entail no risk; specific recommendations for travel to different locales are available from the CDC (www.cdc.gov; 877-FYI-TRIP). Recommendations from the CDC include the use of chloroquine for chemoprophylaxis in the few areas with only chloroquine-sensitive malaria parasites (principally the Caribbean and Central America west of the Panama Canal), and Malarone, mefloquine, or doxycycline for other areas (Table 35–5).

Table 35–5. Drugs for the prevention of malaria in travelers.[1]

Drug	Use[2]	Adult Dosage (all oral)[3]
Chloroquine	Areas without resistant *Plasmodium falciparum*	500 mg weekly
Malarone	Areas with multidrug-resistant *P falciparum*	1 tablet (250-mg atovaquone/100-mg proguanil) daily
Mefloquine	Areas with chloroquine-resistant *P falciparum*	250 mg weekly
Doxycycline	Areas with multidrug-resistant *P falciparum*	100 mg daily
Primaquine[4]	Terminal prophylaxis of *Plasmodium vivax* and *Plasmodium ovale* infections; alternative for *P falciparum* prophylaxis	30-mg base daily: for terminal prophylaxis take for 14 days after travel; for chemoprevention begin 1–2 days before travel, take during travel and for 7 days after travel
Tafenoquine[4]	Alternative for *P falciparum* prophylaxis	200 mg once daily for 3 days and then weekly until 1 week after last exposure

[1]Recommendations may change, as resistance to all available drugs is increasing. See text for additional information on toxicities and cautions. For additional details and pediatric dosing, see CDC guidelines (phone: 800-CDC-INFO; http://wwwnc.cdc.gov/travel/). Travelers to remote areas should consider carrying effective therapy (see text) for use if a febrile illness develops, and they cannot reach medical attention quickly.
[2]Areas without known chloroquine-resistant *P falciparum* are Central America west of the Panama Canal, Haiti, Dominican Republic, Egypt, and most malarious countries of the Middle East. Malarone or mefloquine is currently recommended for other malarious areas except for border areas of Thailand, where doxycycline is recommended.
[3]For drugs other than primaquine, begin 1–2 weeks before departure (except 2 days before for doxycycline and Malarone) and continue for 4 weeks after leaving the endemic area (except 1 week for Malarone). All dosages refer to salts unless otherwise indicated.
[4]Screen for glucose-6-phosphate dehydrogenase deficiency before using primaquine.
Modified, with permission, from Katzung BG. *Basic & Clinical Pharmacology*. 14th edition. McGraw-Hill, 2018.

Primaquine and tafenoquine are also effective but not used as often. Recommendations should be checked regularly because they may change in response to changing resistance patterns and increasing experience with new drugs. In some circumstances, it may be appropriate for travelers to not use chemoprophylaxis but to carry supplies of drugs with them in case a febrile illness develops and medical attention is unavailable. Regimens for self-treatment include ACTs, Malarone, and quinine. Most authorities do not recommend routine terminal chemoprophylaxis with primaquine to eradicate dormant hepatic stages of *P vivax* and *P ovale* after travel, but this may be appropriate in some circumstances, especially for travelers with major exposure to these parasites.

Regular chemoprophylaxis is not a standard management practice in developing world populations due to the expense and potential toxicities of long-term therapy. However, the strategy of intermittent preventive therapy, whereby at-risk populations (in particular pregnant women and children) receive antimalarial therapy at set intervals, may decrease the incidence of malaria while allowing antimalarial immunity to develop. During pregnancy, intermittent preventive therapy with sulfadoxine-pyrimethamine, provided once during both the second and third trimesters, has improved pregnancy outcomes. With increasing resistance, the preventive efficacy of sulfadoxine-pyrimethamine is likely falling, and the long-acting ACT dihydroartemisinin-piperaquine is a promising replacement. In areas with seasonal malaria transmission and limited drug resistance, principally the Sahel subregion of West Africa, the policy is to administer amodiaquine and sulfadoxine-pyrimethamine to children monthly during the transmission season.

▶ Prognosis

When treated appropriately, uncomplicated malaria generally responds well, with resolution of fevers within 1–2 days and a mortality of about 0.1%. Severe malaria can commonly progress to death, but many children respond well to therapy. In the developed world, mortality from malaria is mostly in adults, and often follows extended illnesses and secondary complications long after eradication of the malarial infection. Pregnant women are at particular risk during their first pregnancy. Malaria in pregnancy also increases the likelihood of poor pregnancy outcomes, with increased prematurity, low birth weight, and mortality.

▶ When to Refer

Referral to an expert on infectious diseases or travel medicine is important with all cases of malaria in the United States, and in particular for falciparum malaria; referral should not delay initial diagnosis and therapy, since delays in therapy can lead to severe illness or death.

▶ When to Admit

- Admission for non-falciparum malaria is warranted only if specific problems that require hospital management are present.

- Patients with falciparum malaria are generally admitted because the disease can progress rapidly to severe illness; exceptions may be made with individuals who are from malaria-endemic areas, and thus expected to have a degree of immunity, who are without evidence of severe disease, and who are judged able to return promptly for medical attention if their disease progresses.

Amaratunga C et al. Dihydroartemisinin-piperaquine resistance in *Plasmodium falciparum* malaria in Cambodia: a multisite prospective cohort study. Lancet Infect Dis. 2016 Mar;16(3):357–65. [PMID: 26774243]

Ashley EA et al. Malaria. Lancet. 2018 Apr 21;391(10130):1608–21. [PMID: 29631781]

Draper SJ et al. Malaria vaccines: recent advances and new horizons. Cell Host Microbe. 2018 Jul 11;24(1):43–56. [PMID: 30001524]

Lacerda MVG et al. Single-dose tafenoquine to prevent relapse of *Plasmodium vivax* malaria. N Engl J Med. 2019 Jan 17;380(3):215–28. [PMID: 30650322]

Llanos-Cuentas A et al. Tafenoquine versus primaquine to prevent relapse of *Plasmodium vivax* malaria. N Engl J Med. 2019 Jan 17;380(3):229–41. [PMID: 30650326]

West African Network for Clinical Trials of Antimalarial Drugs (WANECAM). Pyronaridine-artesunate or dihydroartemisinin-piperaquine versus current first-line therapies for repeated treatment of uncomplicated malaria: a randomised, multicentre, open-label, longitudinal, controlled, phase 3b/4 trial. Lancet. 2018 Apr 7;391(10128):1378–90. [PMID: 29606364]

World Health Organization. *Guidelines for the treatment of malaria*, 3rd edition. Geneva, Switzerland, 2015. http://www.who.int/malaria/publications/atoz/9789241549127/en/

World Health Organization. *World Malaria Report 2018*. Geneva, Switzerland: WHO, 2018. https://www.who.int/malaria/publications/world-malaria-report-2018/en/

BABESIOSIS

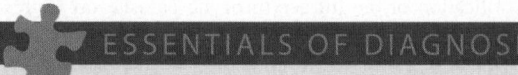
ESSENTIALS OF DIAGNOSIS

- ▶ History of tick bite or exposure to ticks.
- ▶ Fever, flu-like symptoms, anemia.
- ▶ Intraerythrocytic parasites on Giemsa-stained blood smears.
- ▶ Positive serologic tests.

▶ General Considerations

Babesiosis is an uncommon intraerythrocytic infection caused mainly by two *Babesia* species and transmitted by *Ixodes* ticks. In the United States, hundreds of cases of babesiosis have been reported, and infection is caused by *Babesia microti*, which also infects wild mammals. Most babesiosis in the United States occurs in the coastal northeast, with some cases also in the upper midwest, following the geographic range of the vector *Ixodes scapularis*, and Lyme disease and anaplasmosis, which are spread by the same vector. The incidence of the disease appears to be increasing in some areas. Babesiosis is caused by *Babesia divergens* in Europe and by *Babesia venatorum* in China. Babesiosis due to *Babesia duncani* and other Babesia-like organisms have been reported uncommonly from the western United States. Babesiosis can also be transmitted by blood transfusion, but blood supplies are not screened. A survey of a large set of blood samples from endemic regions of the United States identified ~0.4% as potentially infectious for *B microti*.

▶ Clinical Findings

A. Symptoms and Signs

Serosurveys suggest that asymptomatic infections are common in endemic areas. With *B microti* infections, symptoms appear 1 to several weeks after a tick bite; parasitemia is evident after 2–4 weeks. Patients usually do not recall the tick bite. The typical flu-like illness develops gradually and is characterized by fever, fatigue, headache, arthralgia, and myalgia. Other findings may include nausea, vomiting, abdominal pain, sore throat, depression, emotional lability, anemia, thrombocytopenia, and splenomegaly. Parasitemia may continue for months to years, with or without symptoms, and the disease is usually self-limited. Severe complications are most likely to occur in older persons or in those who have had splenectomy. Serious complications include respiratory failure, hemolytic anemia, disseminated intravascular coagulation, heart failure, and acute kidney injury. In a study of hospitalized patients, the mortality rate was 6.5%. Most recognized *B divergens* infections in Europe have been in patients who have had splenectomy. These infections progress rapidly with high fever, severe hemolytic anemia, jaundice, hemoglobinuria, and acute kidney injury, with death rates over 40%.

B. Laboratory Findings

Identification of the intraerythrocytic parasite on Giemsa-stained blood smears establishes the diagnosis (Figure 35–6). These can be confused with malaria parasites, but the morphology is distinctive. Repeated smears are often necessary because well under 1% of erythrocytes may be infected, especially early in infection, although parasitemias can exceed

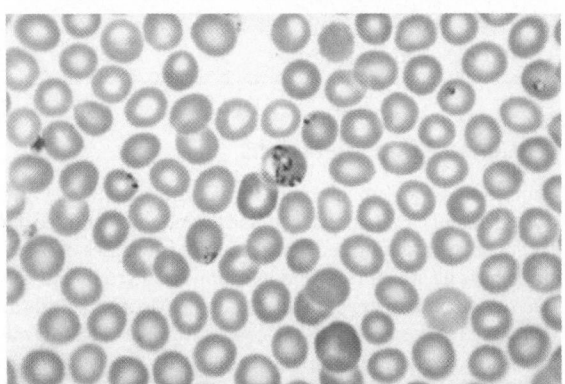

▲ **Figure 35–6.** Blood smear showing *Babesia* spp. rings with basophilic stippling. (From Dr. Mae Melvin, Public Health Image Library, CDC.)

10%. Diagnosis can also be made by PCR, which is more sensitive than blood smear. An indirect immunofluorescent antibody test for *B microti* is available from the CDC; antibody is detectable within 2–4 weeks after the onset of symptoms and persists for months.

▶ Treatment

Most patients have a mild illness and recover without therapy. Standard therapy for mild to moderate disease is a 7-day course of atovaquone (750 mg orally every 12 hours) plus azithromycin (600 mg orally once daily), which is equally effective and better tolerated than the alternative regimen, a 7-day course of quinine (650 mg orally three times daily) plus clindamycin (600 mg orally three times daily). However, there is more experience using quinine plus clindamycin, and this regimen is recommended for severe disease. Exchange transfusion has been used successfully in severely ill asplenic patients and those with parasitemia greater than 10%.

Sanchez E et al. Diagnosis, treatment, and prevention of Lyme disease, human granulocytic anaplasmosis, and babesiosis: a review. JAMA. 2016 Apr 26;315(16):1767–77. [PMID: 27115378]
Vannier EG et al. Babesiosis. Infect Dis Clin North Am. 2015 Jun; 29(2):357–70. [PMID: 25999229]

TOXOPLASMOSIS

 ESSENTIALS OF DIAGNOSIS

▶ Infection confirmed by isolation of *Toxoplasma gondii* or identification of tachyzoites in tissue or body fluids.

Primary infection

▶ Fever, malaise, headache, sore throat.

▶ Lymphadenopathy.

▶ Positive IgG and IgM serologic tests.

Congenital infection

▶ Follows acute infection of seronegative mothers and leads to CNS abnormalities and retinochoroiditis.

Infection in immunocompromised persons

▶ Reactivation leads to encephalitis, retinochoroiditis, pneumonitis, myocarditis.

▶ Positive IgG but negative IgM serologic tests.

▶ General Considerations

T gondii, an obligate intracellular protozoan, is found worldwide in humans and in many species of mammals and birds. The definitive hosts are cats. Humans are infected after ingestion of cysts in raw or undercooked meat, ingestion of oocysts in food or water contaminated by cats, transplacental transmission of trophozoites or,

including sinusitis, central nervous system infections including granulomatous encephalitis, and disseminated infections. Ocular infections with *Encephalitozoon* species cause conjunctivitis and keratitis, presenting as redness, photophobia, and loss of visual acuity.

B. Laboratory Findings

1. Cryptosporidiosis—Typically, stool is without blood or leukocytes. Diagnosis is traditionally made by detecting the organism in stool using a modified acid-fast stain; this technique is relatively insensitive, and multiple specimens should be evaluated before ruling out the diagnosis. Of note, routine evaluation for ova and parasites typically does not include a modified acid-fast stain, so this must be specifically requested in many laboratories. Various antigen detection methods, including immunofluorescence microscopy, ELISA, and immunochromatography, offer improved sensitivity and specificity, both over 90% with available assays, and these methods may be considered the optimal means of diagnosis. Molecular diagnostic panels that recognize *Cryptosporidium* and other enteropathogens in stool are available but expensive.

2. Isosporiasis—Diagnosis of isosporiasis is by examination of stool wet mounts or after modified acid-fast staining, in which the organism is clearly distinguishable from other parasites. Other stains also show the organism. Shedding of oocysts may be intermittent, so the sensitivity of stool evaluation is not high, and multiple samples should be examined. The organism may also be identified in duodenal aspirates or small bowel biopsies.

3. Cyclosporiasis—Diagnosis is made by examination of stool wet mounts or after modified acid-fast staining. Multiple specimens may need to be examined to make a diagnosis. The organism can also be identified in small bowel aspirates or biopsy specimens.

4. Sarcocystosis—Eosinophilia and elevated creatine kinase may be seen. Diagnosis is by identification of the acid-fast organisms in stool or by identification of trophozoites or bradyzoites in tissue biopsies.

5. Microsporidiosis—Diagnosis can be made by identification of organisms in specially stained stool, fluid, or tissue specimens, for example with Weber chromotrope-based stain. Electron microscopy is helpful for confirmation of the diagnosis and speciation. PCR and culture techniques are available but not used routinely.

► Treatment

Most acute infections with these pathogens in immunocompetent persons are self-limited and do not require treatment. Supportive treatment for severe or chronic diarrhea includes fluid and electrolyte replacement and, in some cases, parenteral nutrition.

1. Cryptosporidiosis—Treatment of cryptosporidiosis is challenging. No agent is clearly effective. Modest benefits have been seen in some (but not other) studies with paromomycin, a nonabsorbed aminoglycoside (25–35 mg/kg orally for 14 days has been used), and nitazoxanide (500 mg–1 g orally twice daily for 3 days in nonimmunocompromised

and 2–8 weeks in advanced AIDS patients), which is approved in the United States for this indication. Other agents that have been used with mixed success in AIDS patients with cryptosporidiosis include azithromycin, spiramycin, bovine hyperimmune colostrum, and octreotide. Reversing immunodeficiency with effective antiretroviral therapy is of greatest importance.

2. Isosporiasis—Isosporiasis is effectively treated in immunocompetent and immunosuppressed persons with TMP-SMZ (160 mg/800 mg orally two to four times daily for 10 days, with the higher dosage for patients with AIDS). An alternative therapy is pyrimethamine (75 mg orally in four divided doses) with folinic acid (10–25 mg/day orally). Maintenance therapy with low-dose TMP-SMZ (160 mg/800 mg daily or three times per week) or Fansidar (1 tablet weekly) prevents relapse in those with persistent immunosuppression.

3. Cyclosporiasis—Cyclosporiasis is also treated with TMP-SMZ (dosing as for isosporiasis). With AIDS, long-term maintenance therapy (160 mg/ 800 mg three times weekly) helps prevent relapse. For patients intolerant of TMP-SMZ, ciprofloxacin (500 mg orally twice daily for 7 days) showed efficacy, albeit with less ability to clear the organism than TMP-SMZ.

4. Sarcocystosis—For sarcocystosis, no specific treatment is established, but patients may respond to therapy with albendazole or TMP-SMZ.

5. Microsporidiosis—Treatment of microsporidiosis is complex. Infections with most species, including those causing gastrointestinal and other manifestations, should be treated with albendazole (400 mg orally twice daily for 2–4 weeks), which has activity against a number of species, but relatively poor efficacy (about 50%) against *E bieneusi*, the most common microsporidial cause of diarrhea in AIDS patients. Fumagillin, which is used to treat honeybees and fish with microsporidian infections, has shown benefit in clinical trials at a dose of 20 mg three times per day for 14 days; treatment was accompanied by reversible thrombocytopenia. As with cryptosporidiosis, the best means of controlling microsporidiosis in AIDS patients is to restore immune function with effective antiretroviral therapy. Ocular microsporidiosis can be treated with fumagillin solution (3 mg/mL); this probably should be given with concurrent systemic therapy with albendazole. Adjunctive management may include corticosteroids to decrease inflammation and keratoplasty.

► Prevention

Water purification is important for control of these infections. Chlorine disinfection is not effective against cryptosporidial oocysts, so other purification measures are needed. Immunocompromised patients should boil or filter drinking water and should consider avoidance of lakes and swimming pools. Routine precautions (hand washing, gloves, disinfection) should prevent institutional patient-to-patient spread. Optimal means of preventing microsporidial infections are not well understood, but water purification and body substance precautions for immunocompromised and hospitalized individuals are likely effective.

Checkley W et al. A review of the global burden, novel diagnostics, therapeutics, and vaccine targets for cryptosporidium. Lancet Infect Dis. 2015 Jan;15(1):85–94. [PMID: 25278220]

GIARDIASIS

ESSENTIALS OF DIAGNOSIS

► Acute diarrhea may be profuse and watery.

► Chronic diarrhea with greasy, malodorous stools.

► Abdominal cramps, distention, flatulence, and malaise.

► Cysts or trophozoites in stools.

General Considerations

Giardiasis is a protozoal infection of the upper small intestine caused by the flagellate *Giardia lamblia* (also called *Giardia intestinalis* and *Giardia duodenalis*). The parasite occurs worldwide, most abundantly in areas with poor sanitation. In developing countries, young children are very commonly infected. In the United States and Europe, the infection is the most common intestinal protozoal pathogen; the US estimate is 100,000 to 2.5 million new infections leading to 5000 hospital admissions yearly. Groups at special risk include travelers to *Giardia*-endemic areas, those who swallow contaminated water during recreation or wilderness travel, men who have sex with men, and persons with impaired immunity. Outbreaks are common in households, children's day care centers, and residential facilities, and may occur as a result of contamination of water supplies.

The organism occurs in feces as a flagellated trophozoite and as a cyst. Only the cyst form is infectious by the oral route; trophozoites are destroyed by gastric acidity. Humans are a reservoir for the pathogen; dogs, cats, beavers, and other mammals have been implicated but not confirmed as reservoirs. Under suitable moist, cool conditions, cysts can survive in the environment for weeks to months. Cysts are transmitted as a result of fecal contamination of water or food, by person-to-person contact, or by anal-oral sexual contact. The infectious dose is low, requiring as few as ten cysts. After the cysts are ingested, trophozoites emerge in the duodenum and jejunum. Epithelial damage and mucosal invasion are uncommon. Hypogammaglobulinemia, low secretory IgA levels in the gut, achlorhydria, and malnutrition favor the development of infection.

Clinical Findings

A. Symptoms and Signs

It is estimated that about 50% of infected persons have no discernable infection, about 10% become asymptomatic cyst passers, and 25–50% develop an acute diarrheal syndrome. Acute diarrhea may clear spontaneously but is commonly followed by chronic diarrhea. The incubation period is usually 1–3 weeks but may be longer. The illness may begin gradually or suddenly. Cysts may not be detected in the stool at the onset of the illness. The acute phase may last days or weeks, and is usually self-limited, although cyst excretion may be prolonged. The initial illness may include profuse watery diarrhea, and hospitalization may be required due to dehydration, particularly in young children. Typical symptoms of chronic disease are abdominal cramps, bloating, flatulence, nausea, malaise, and anorexia. Fever and vomiting are uncommon. Diarrhea is usually not severe in the chronic stage of infection; stools are greasy or frothy and foul smelling, without blood, pus, or mucus. The diarrhea may be daily or recurrent; intervening periods may include constipation. Symptoms can persist for weeks to months. Weight loss is frequent. Chronic disease can include malabsorption, including fat and protein-losing enteropathy and vitamin deficiencies.

B. Laboratory Findings

Most patients seek medical attention after having been ill for over a week, commonly with weight loss of 5 kg or more. Stool is generally without blood or leukocytes. Diagnosis is traditionally made by the identification of trophozoites or cysts in stool. A wet mount of liquid stool may identify motile trophozoites. Stained fixed specimens may show cysts or trophozoites. Sensitivity of stool analysis is not ideal, estimated at 50–80% for a single specimen and over 90% for three specimens. Sampling of duodenal contents with a string test or biopsy is no longer generally recommended, but biopsies may be helpful in very ill or immunocompromised patients. When giardiasis is suspected, antigen assays are simpler and cheaper than repeated stool examinations, but these tests will not identify other stool pathogens. Multiple tests, which identify antigens of trophozoites or cysts, are available. They are generally quite sensitive (85–98%) and specific (90–100%). Molecular diagnostic panels that recognize *Giardia* and other enteropathogens in stool are available but expensive.

Treatment

The treatments of choice for giardiasis are metronidazole (250 mg orally three times daily for 5–7 days) or tinidazole (2 g orally once). The drugs are not universally effective; cure rates for single courses are typically about 80–95%. Toxicities are as described for treatment of amebiasis, but the lower dosages used for giardiasis limit side effects. Albendazole (400 mg orally once daily for 5 days) and nitazoxanide (500 mg orally twice daily for 3 days) both appear to have similar efficacy and fewer side effects compared with metronidazole, although data are limited, and a 2016 meta-analysis suggested superiority in efficacy of tinidazole over albendazole. Nitazoxanide is generally well tolerated but may cause mild gastrointestinal side effects. Other drugs with activity against *Giardia* include furazolidone (100 mg orally four times a day for 7 days), which is about as effective as the other named drugs but causes gastrointestinal side effects, and paromomycin (500 mg orally three times a day for 7 days), which appears to have somewhat lower efficacy but unlike metronidazole, tinidazole, and furazolidone is safe in pregnancy. Symptomatic giardiasis should always be treated. Treatment of asymptomatic patients should be considered, since they can transmit the infection. With a suggestive presentation but negative diagnostic studies, an empiric course of treatment may be appropriate. Household or day care contacts with an index case should be tested and treated if infected.

Prevention

Community chlorination (0.4 mg/L) of water is relatively ineffective for inactivating cysts, so filtration is required. For wilderness or international travelers, bringing water to a boil for 1 minute or filtration with a pore size less than 1 mcm are adequate. In day care centers, appropriate disposal of diapers and frequent hand washing are essential.

Mmbaga BT et al. *Cryptosporidium* and *Giardia* infections in children: a review. Pediatr Clin North Am. 2017 Aug;64(4): 837–50. [PMID: 28734513]

TRICHOMONIASIS

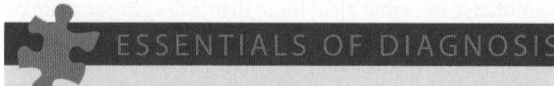

ESSENTIALS OF DIAGNOSIS

▶ **Women:** copious vaginal discharge.

▶ **Men:** nongonococcal urethritis.

▶ Motile trichomonads on wet mounts.

General Considerations

Trichomoniasis is caused by the protozoan *Trichomonas vaginalis* and is among the most common sexually transmitted diseases, causing vaginitis in women and nongonococcal urethritis in men. It can also occasionally be acquired by other means, since it can survive in moist environments for several hours.

Clinical Findings

A. Symptoms and Signs

T vaginalis is often harbored asymptomatically. For women with symptomatic disease, after an incubation period of 5 days to 4 weeks, a vaginal discharge develops, often with vulvovaginal discomfort, pruritus, dysuria, dyspareunia, or abdominal pain. Examination shows a copious discharge, which is usually not foul smelling but is often frothy and yellow or green in color. Inflammation of the vaginal walls and cervix with punctate hemorrhages are common. Most men infected with *T vaginalis* are asymptomatic, but it can be isolated from about 10% of men with nongonococcal urethritis. In men with trichomonal urethritis, the urethral discharge is generally more scanty than with other causes of urethritis.

B. Diagnostic Testing

Diagnosis is traditionally made by identifying the organism in vaginal or urethral secretions. Examination of wet mounts will show motile organisms. Tests for bacterial vaginosis (pH > 4.5, fishy odor after addition of potassium hydroxide) are often positive with trichomoniasis. Newer point-of-care antigen detection and nucleic acid probe hybridization tests and nucleic acid amplification assays offer improved sensitivity compared to wet mount microscopy and excellent specificity.

Treatment

The treatment of choice is tinidazole or metronidazole, each as a 2 g single oral dose. Tinidazole may be better tolerated and active against some resistant parasites. Toxicities of these drugs are discussed in the section on amebiasis. If the large single dose cannot be tolerated, an alternative metronidazole dosage is 500 mg orally twice daily for 1 week. A meta-analysis suggested that multiple dose regimens offer improved efficacy, although this is not standard. All infected persons should be treated, even if asymptomatic, to prevent subsequent symptomatic disease and limit spread. Treatment failure suggests reinfection, but metronidazole-resistant organisms have been reported. These may be treated with tinidazole, longer courses of metronidazole, intravaginal paromomycin, or other experimental therapies (see Chapter 18).

Gaydos CA et al. Rapid and point-of-care tests for the diagnosis of *Trichomonas vaginalis* in women and men. Sex Transm Infect. 2017 Dec;93(S4):S31–5. [PMID: 28684611]

Howe K et al. Single-dose compared with multidose metronidazole for the treatment of trichomoniasis in women: a meta-analysis. Sex Transm Dis. 2017 Jan;44(1):29–34. [PMID: 27898571]

Meites E et al. A review of evidence-based care of symptomatic trichomoniasis and asymptomatic *Trichomonas vaginalis* infections. Clin Infect Dis. 2015 Dec 15;61(Suppl 8):S837–48. [PMID: 26602621]

HELMINTHIC INFECTIONS

TREMATODE (FLUKE) INFECTIONS

SCHISTOSOMIASIS (Bilharziasis)

ESSENTIALS OF DIAGNOSIS

▶ History of freshwater exposure in an endemic area.

▶ **Acute schistosomiasis:** fever, headache, myalgias, cough, urticaria, diarrhea, and eosinophilia.

▶ **Intestinal schistosomiasis:** abdominal pain, diarrhea, and hepatomegaly, progressing to anorexia, weight loss, and features of portal hypertension.

▶ **Urinary schistosomiasis:** hematuria and dysuria, progressing to hydronephrosis and urinary infections.

▶ **Diagnosis:** characteristic eggs in feces or urine; biopsy of rectal or bladder mucosa; positive serology.

General Considerations

Schistosomiasis, which affects more than 200 million persons worldwide, leads to severe consequences in 20 million persons and about 100,000 deaths annually. The disease is caused by six species of trematode blood flukes. Five species cause intestinal schistosomiasis, with infection of mesenteric venules: *Schistosoma mansoni*, which is present in Africa, the Arabian peninsula, South America, and the Caribbean; *Schistosoma japonicum*, which is endemic in China and Southeast Asia; *Schistosoma mekongi*, which is endemic near the Mekong River in Southeast Asia; and *Schistosoma intercalatum* and *Schistosoma guineensis*, which occur in parts of Africa. *Schistosoma haematobium* causes urinary schistosomiasis, with infection of venules of the urinary tract, and is endemic in Africa and the Middle East. Transmission of schistosomiasis is focal, with greatest prevalence in poor rural areas. Control efforts have diminished transmission significantly in many areas, but high-level transmission remains common in sub-Saharan Africa and some other areas. Prevalence of infection and illness typically peaks at about 15–20 years of age.

Humans are infected with schistosomes after contact with freshwater containing cercariae released by infected snails. Infection is initiated by penetration of skin or mucous membranes. After penetration, schistosomulae migrate to the portal circulation, where they rapidly mature. After about 6 weeks, adult worms mate, and migrate to terminal mesenteric or bladder venules, where females deposit their eggs. Some eggs reach the lumen of the bowel or bladder and are passed with feces or urine, while others are retained in the bowel or bladder wall or transported in the circulation to other tissues, in particular the liver. Disease in endemic areas is primarily due to a host response to eggs, with granuloma formation and inflammation, eventually leading to fibrosis. Chronic infection can result in scarring of mesenteric or vesicular blood vessels, leading to portal hypertension and alterations in the urinary tract. In previously uninfected individuals, such as travelers with freshwater contact in endemic regions, acute schistosomiasis may occur, with a febrile illness 2–8 weeks after infection.

▶ Clinical Findings

A. Symptoms and Signs

1. Cercarial dermatitis—Following cercarial penetration, localized erythema develops in some individuals, which can progress to a pruritic maculopapular rash that persists for some days. Dermatitis can be caused by human schistosomes and, in nontropical areas, by bird schistosomes that cannot complete their life cycle in humans (swimmer's itch).

2. Acute schistosomiasis (Katayama syndrome)—A febrile illness may develop 2–8 weeks after exposure in persons without prior infection, most commonly after heavy infection with *S mansoni* or *S japonicum*. Presenting symptoms and signs include acute onset of fever; headache; myalgias; cough; malaise; urticaria; diarrhea, which may be bloody; hepatosplenomegaly; lymphadenopathy; and pulmonary infiltrates. Localized lesions may occasionally cause severe manifestations, including CNS abnormalities and death. Acute schistosomiasis usually resolves in 2–8 weeks.

3. Chronic schistosomiasis—Many infected persons have light infections and are asymptomatic, but an estimated 50–60% have symptoms and 5–10% have advanced organ damage. Asymptomatic infected children may suffer from anemia and growth retardation. Symptomatic patients with intestinal schistosomiasis typically experience abdominal pain, fatigue, diarrhea, and hepatomegaly. Over years, anorexia, weight loss, weakness, colonic polyps, and features of portal hypertension develop. Late manifestations include hematemesis from esophageal varices, hepatic failure, and pulmonary hypertension. Urinary schistosomiasis may present within months of infection with hematuria and dysuria, most commonly in children and young adults. Fibrotic changes in the urinary tract can lead to hydroureter, hydronephrosis, bacterial urinary infections and, ultimately, kidney disease or bladder cancer.

B. Laboratory Findings

Microscopic examination of stool or urine for eggs, evaluation of tissue, or serologic tests establish the diagnosis. Characteristic eggs can be identified on smears of stool or urine. The most widely used stool test is the Kato-Katz technique. Quantitative tests that yield more than 400 eggs per gram of feces or 10 mL of urine are indicative of heavy infections with increased risk of complications. Diagnosis can also be made by biopsy of the rectum, colon, liver, or bladder. Serologic tests include an ELISA available from the CDC that is 99% specific for all species, but cannot distinguish acute and past infection. Sensitivity of the test is 99% for *S mansoni*, 95% for *S haematobium*, but less than 50% for *S japonicum*. Serology is of limited use in endemic settings, but can be helpful in travelers from nonendemic regions. Point-of-care assays to detect circulating schistosome antigens in serum and urine are also available; the most widely used tests target circulating anodic and cathodic antigens. Antigen tests have better sensitivity than stool smears, especially for *S mansoni*; sensitivity is lower for *S haematobium*. Molecular tests for schistosomiasis have been developed but are not routinely used for diagnosis. In acute schistosomiasis, leukocytosis and marked eosinophilia may occur; serologic tests may become positive before eggs are seen in stool or urine. After therapy, eggs may be shed in stool or urine for months, and so the identification of eggs in fluids or tissue cannot distinguish past or active disease. With a diagnosis of schistosomiasis, evaluation for the extent of disease is warranted, including liver function studies and imaging of the liver with intestinal disease and ultrasound or other imaging studies of the urinary system in urinary disease.

▶ Treatment

Treatment is indicated for all schistosome infections. In areas where recurrent infection is common, treatment is valuable in reducing worm burdens and limiting clinical complications. The drug of choice for schistosomiasis is praziquantel. The drug is administered for 1 day at an oral dose of 40 mg/kg (in one or two doses) for *S mansoni, S haematobium, S intercalatum,* and *S guineensis* infections and a dose of 60 mg/kg (in two or three doses) for *S japonicum* and *S mekongi*. Cure rates are generally greater than 80% after a single treatment, and those not cured have marked reduction in the intensity of infection. Praziquantel is active against invading cercariae but not developing schistosomulae. Therefore, the drug may not prevent illness when given after exposure and, for recent infections, a repeat course after a few weeks may be appropriate. Praziquantel may be used during pregnancy. Resistance to praziquantel has been reported. Toxicities include abdominal pain, diarrhea, urticaria, headache, nausea, vomiting, and fever, and may be due both to direct effects of the drug and responses to dying worms. Alternative therapies are oxamniquine for *S mansoni* infection and metrifonate for *S haemotobium* infection. Both of these drugs currently have limited availability (they are not available in the United States), and resistance may be a problem. No second-line drug is available for *S japonicum* infections. The antimalarial drug artemether has activity against schistosomulae and adult worms and may be effective in chemoprophylaxis; however, it is expensive, and long-term use in malarious areas might select for resistant malaria parasites. With severe disease, use of corticosteroids in conjunction with praziquantel may decrease complications. Treatment should be followed by repeat examinations for eggs about every 3 months for 1 year after therapy, with re-treatment if eggs are seen.

► Prevention

Travelers to endemic areas should avoid freshwater exposure. Vigorous toweling after exposure may limit cercarial penetration. Chemoprophylaxis with artemether has shown efficacy but is not standard practice. Community control of schistosomiasis includes improved sanitation and water supplies, elimination of snail habitats, and intermittent treatment to limit worm burdens.

Colley DG et al. Human schistosomiasis. Lancet. 2014 Jun 28; 383(9936):2253–64. [PMID: 24698483]

Utzinger J et al. New diagnostic tools in schistosomiasis. Clin Microbiol Infect. 2015 Jun;21(6):529–42. [PMID: 25843503]

LIVER, LUNG, & INTESTINAL FLUKES

FASCIOLIASIS

Infection by *Fasciola hepatica*, the sheep liver fluke, results from ingestion of encysted metacercariae on watercress or other aquatic vegetables. Infection is prevalent in sheep-raising areas in many countries, especially parts of South America, the Middle East, and southern Europe, and it has increasingly been recognized in travelers to these areas. *Fasciola gigantica* has a more restricted distribution in Asia and Africa and causes similar findings. Eggs are passed from host feces into freshwater, leading to infection of snails, and then deposition of metacercariae on vegetation. In humans, metacercariae excyst, penetrate into the peritoneum, migrate through the liver, and mature in the bile ducts, where they cause local necrosis and abscess formation.

Two clinical syndromes are seen, related to acute migration of worms and chronic infection of the biliary tract. Symptoms related to migration of larvae present 6–12 weeks after ingestion. Typical findings are abdominal pain, fever, malaise, weight loss, urticaria, eosinophilia, and leukocytosis. Tender hepatomegaly and elevated liver biochemical tests may be seen. Rarely, migration to other organs may lead to localized disease. The symptoms of worm migration subside after 2–4 months, followed by asymptomatic infection by adult worms or intermittent symptoms of biliary obstruction, with

biliary colic and, at times, findings of cholangitis. Early diagnosis is difficult, as eggs are not found in the feces during the acute migratory phase of infection. Clinical suspicion should be based on clinical findings and marked eosinophilia in at risk individuals. CT and other imaging studies show hypodense migratory lesions of the liver. Definitive diagnosis is made by the identification of characteristic eggs in stool. Repeated examinations may be necessary. In chronic infection, imaging studies show masses obstructing the extrahepatic biliary tract. Serologic assays have sensitivity and specificity greater than 90%, but cannot distinguish between past and current infection. Antigen tests with excellent sensitivity and specificity are available in veterinary medicine and show promise for humans.

Fascioliasis is unusual among fluke infections, in that it does not respond well to treatment with praziquantel. The treatment of choice is triclabendazole, which is also used in veterinary medicine. It is not routinely available in the United States, but is available through the CDC under an investigational protocol. Standard dosing of 10 mg/kg orally in a single dose or two doses over 12 hours achieves a cure rate of about 80%, but repeat dosing is indicated if abnormal radiologic findings or eosinophilia do not resolve. Of concern, resistance to triclabendazole has been widely reported in animal infections. The second-line drug for fascioliasis is bithionol (30–50 mg/kg/day orally in three divided doses on alternate days for 10–15 days); this drug is no longer available in the United States. Treatment with either drug can be accompanied by abdominal pain and other gastrointestinal symptoms. Other potential therapies are emetine and dehydroemetine, both widely used in the past but quite toxic, and nitazoxanide. Prevention of fascioliasis involves avoidance of ingestion of raw aquatic plants.

CLONORCHIASIS & OPISTHORCHIASIS

Infection by *Clonorchis sinensis*, the Chinese liver fluke, is endemic in areas of Japan, Korea, China, Taiwan, Southeast Asia, and the far eastern part of Russia. An estimated 15 million people are infected (13 million in China); in some communities, prevalence can reach 80%. Opisthorchiasis is principally caused by *Opisthorchis felineus* (regions of the former Soviet Union) or *Opisthorchis viverrini* (Thailand, Laos, Vietnam). Clonorchiasis and opisthorchiasis are clinically indistinguishable. Parasite eggs are shed into water in human or animal feces, where they infect snails, which release cercariae, which infect fish. Human infection follows ingestion of raw, undercooked, or pickled freshwater fish containing metacercariae. These parasites excyst in the duodenum and ascend into the biliary tract, where they mature and remain for many years, shedding eggs in the bile.

Most patients harbor few parasites and are asymptomatic. An acute illness can occur 2–3 weeks after initial infection, with fever, abdominal pain, tender hepatomegaly, urticaria, and eosinophilia. The acute syndrome is difficult to diagnose, since ova may not appear in the feces until 3–4 weeks after onset of symptoms. In chronic heavy infections, findings include abdominal pain, anorexia, weight loss, and tender hepatomegaly. More serious findings can include recurrent bacterial cholangitis and sepsis, cholecystitis, liver abscess, and pancreatitis. An increased risk of cholangiocarcinoma has been documented.

Early diagnosis is presumptive, based on clinical findings and epidemiology. Subsequent diagnosis is made by finding characteristic eggs in stool or duodenal or biliary contents. The stool Kato-Katz test is widely used; performing repeated tests improves sensitivity. Imaging studies show characteristic biliary tract dilatations with filling defects due to flukes. Serologic assays for clonorchiasis with excellent sensitivity are available but cannot distinguish between past and current infection. Molecular tests have been developed but are not widely used.

The drug of choice is praziquantel, 25 mg/kg orally three times daily for 2 days, which provides cure rates over 95%. One day of treatment may be sufficient. Re-treatment may be required, especially in some areas with known decreased praziquantel efficacy. The second-line drug is albendazole (400 mg orally twice daily for 7 days), which appears to be somewhat less effective. Tribendimidine, which is approved in China, has shown efficacy for clonorchiasis similar to that of praziquantel.

PARAGONIMIASIS

Eight species of *Paragonimus* lung flukes cause human disease. The most important is *Paragonimus westermani*. *Paragonimus* species are endemic in East Asia, Oceania, West Africa, and South America, where millions of persons are infected; rare infections caused by *Paragonimus kellicotti* have occurred in North America. Eggs are released into freshwater, where parasites infect snails, and then cercariae infect crabs and crayfish. Human infection follows consumption of raw, undercooked, or pickled freshwater shellfish. Metacercariae then excyst, penetrate into the peritoneum, and pass into the lungs, where they mature into adult worms over about 2 months.

Most persons have moderate worm burdens and are asymptomatic. In symptomatic cases, abdominal pain and diarrhea develop 2 days to 2 weeks after infection, followed by fever, cough, chest pain, urticaria, and eosinophilia. Acute symptoms may last for several weeks. Chronic infection can cause cough productive of brown sputum, hemoptysis, dyspnea, and chest pain, with progression to chronic bronchitis, bronchiectasis, bronchopneumonia, lung abscess, and pleural disease. Ectopic infections can cause disease in other organs, most commonly the CNS, where disease can present with seizures, headaches, and focal neurologic findings due to parasite meningitis and to intracerebral lesions.

The diagnosis of paragonimiasis is made by identifying characteristic eggs in sputum or stool or identifying worms in biopsied tissue. Multiple examinations and concentration techniques may be needed. Serologic tests may be helpful; an ELISA available from the CDC has sensitivity and specificity more than 95%. Chest radiographs may show varied abnormalities of the lungs or pleura, including infiltrates, nodules, cavities, and fibrosis, and the findings can be confused with those of tuberculosis. With CNS disease, skull radiographs can show clusters of calcified cysts, and CT or MRI can show clusters of ring-enhancing lesions.

Treatment is with praziquantel (25 mg/kg orally three times daily for 2 days), which provides efficacy of at least 90%. Alternative therapies are bithionol and triclabendazole. As with cysticercosis, for cerebral paragonimiasis, praziquantel should generally be used with corticosteroids. Chronic infection may lead to permanent lung dysfunction and pleural disease requiring drainage procedures.

INTESTINAL FLUKES

The large intestinal fluke, *Fasciolopsis buski*, is a common parasite of pigs and humans in eastern and southern Asia. Eggs shed in stools hatch in freshwater, followed by infection of snails, and release of cercariae that encyst on aquatic plants. Humans are infected by eating uncooked plants, including water chestnuts, bamboo shoots, and watercress. Adult flukes mature in about 3 months and live in the small intestine attached to the mucosa, leading to local inflammation and ulceration. Other intestinal flukes that cause similar syndromes include *Heterophyes* (North Africa and Turkey) and *Metagonimus* (East Asia) species; these species are transmitted by undercooked freshwater fish.

Infections with intestinal flukes are often asymptomatic, although eosinophilia may be marked. In symptomatic cases, after an incubation period of 1–2 months, manifestations include epigastric pain and diarrhea. Other gastrointestinal symptoms, ileus, edema, and ascites may be seen uncommonly. Diagnosis is based on identification of characteristic eggs or adult flukes in the stool. In contrast to other fluke infections, illness more than 6 months after travel in an endemic area is unlikely. The drug of choice is praziquantel, 25 mg/kg orally as a single dose. Alternative therapies are triclabendazole and niclosamide (for most species).

Ashrafi K et al. Fascioliasis: a worldwide parasitic disease of importance in travel medicine. Travel Med Infect Dis. 2014 Nov–Dec;12(6 Pt A):636–49. [PMID: 25287722]

Blair D. Paragonimiasis. Adv Exp Med Biol. 2014;766:115–52. [PMID: 24903365]

Qian MB et al. Clonorchiasis. Lancet. 2016 Feb 20; 387(10020): 800–10. [PMID: 26299184]

CESTODE INFECTIONS

NONINVASIVE CESTODE INFECTIONS

The four major tapeworms that cause noninvasive infections in humans are the beef tapeworm *Taenia saginata*, the pork tapeworm *Taenia solium*, the fish tapeworm *Diphyllobothrium latum*, each of which can reach many meters in length, and the dwarf tapeworm *Hymenolepis nana*. *Taenia* and *Hymenolepis* species are broadly distributed, especially in the tropics; *D latum* is most prevalent in temperate regions. Other tapeworms that can cause noninvasive human disease include the rodent tapeworm *Hymenolepis diminuta*, the dog tapeworm *Dipylidium caninum*, and other *Taenia* and *Diphyllobothrium* species. Invasive tapeworm infections, including *T solium* (when infective eggs, rather than cysticerci are ingested) and *Echinococcus* species, will be discussed separately.

1. Beef Tapeworm

Infection is most common in cattle breeding areas. Humans are the definitive host. Gravid segments of *T saginata* are passed in human feces to soil, where they are ingested by grazing animals, especially cattle. The eggs then hatch to release embryos that encyst in muscle as cysticerci. Humans are infected by eating raw or undercooked infected beef. Most individuals infected with *T saginata* are asymptomatic, but abdominal pain and other gastrointestinal symptoms may be present. Eosinophilia is common. The most common presenting finding is the passage of proglottids in the stool.

2. Pork Tapeworm

T solium is transmitted to pigs that ingest human feces. Humans can be either the definitive host (after consuming undercooked pork, leading to tapeworm infection) or the intermediate host (after consuming food contaminated with human feces containing *T solium* eggs, leading to cysticercosis, which is discussed under Invasive Cestode Infections). As with the beef tapeworm, infection with *T solium* adult worms is generally asymptomatic, but gastrointestinal symptoms may occur. Infection is generally recognized after passage of proglottids. Autoinfection with eggs can progress to cysticercosis.

3. Fish Tapeworm

Infection with *D latum* follows ingestion of undercooked freshwater fish, most commonly in temperate regions. Eggs from human feces are taken up by crustaceans, these are eaten by fish, which are then infectious to humans. Infection with multiple worms over many years can occur. Infections are most commonly asymptomatic, but nonspecific gastrointestinal symptoms, including diarrhea, may occur. Diagnosis usually follows passage of proglottids. Prolonged heavy infection can lead to megaloblastic anemia and neuropathy from vitamin B_{12} deficiency, which is due to infection-induced dissociation of the vitamin from intrinsic factor and to utilization of the vitamin by worms.

4. Dwarf Tapeworm

H nana is the only tapeworm that can be transmitted between humans. Infections are common in warm areas, especially with poor hygiene and institutionalized populations. Infection follows ingestion of food contaminated with human feces. Eggs hatch in the intestines, where oncospheres penetrate the mucosa, encyst as cysticercoid larvae, and then rupture after about 4 days to release adult worms. Autoinfection can lead to amplification of infection. Infection with *H nana*, the related rodent tapeworm *H diminuta*, or the dog tapeworm *D caninum* can also follow accidental ingestion of infected insects. *H nana* are dwarf in size relative to other tapeworms but can reach 5 cm in length. Heavy infection is common, especially in children, and can be accompanied by abdominal discomfort, anorexia, and diarrhea.

Laboratory Findings

Diagnosis is usually made based on the identification of characteristic eggs or proglottids in stool. Egg release may be irregular, so examination of multiple specimens or concentration techniques may be needed.

Treatment

The treatment of choice for noninvasive tapeworm infections is praziquantel. A single dose of praziquantel (5–10 mg/kg orally) is highly effective, except for *H nana*, for which the dosage is 25 mg/kg. Treatment of *H nana* is more difficult, as the drug is not effective against maturing cysts. Therefore, a repeat treatment after 1 week and screening after therapy to document cure are appropriate with heavy infections. Therapy can be accompanied by headache, malaise, dizziness, abdominal pain, and nausea.

The alternative therapy for these infections is niclosamide. A single dose of niclosamide (2 g chewed) is effective against *D latum*, *Taenia*, and *D caninum* infections. For *H nana*, therapy is continued daily for 1 week. Niclosamide may cause nausea, malaise, and abdominal pain.

Craig P et al. Intestinal cestodes. Curr Opin Infect Dis. 2007 Oct; 20(5):524–32. [PMID: 17762788]

INVASIVE CESTODE INFECTIONS

1. Cysticercosis

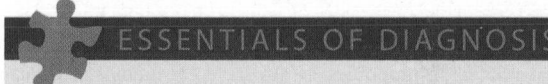

ESSENTIALS OF DIAGNOSIS

► Exposure to *T solium* through fecal contamination of food.
► Focal CNS lesions; seizures, headache.
► Brain imaging shows cysts; positive serologic tests.

General Considerations

Cysticercosis is due to tissue infection with cysts of *T solium* that develop after humans ingest food contaminated with eggs from human feces, thus acting as an intermediate host for the parasite. Prevalence is high where the parasite is endemic, in particular Mexico, Central and South America, the Philippines, and Southeast Asia. An estimated 20 million persons are infected with cysticerci yearly, leading to about 400,000 persons with neurologic symptoms and 50,000 deaths. Antibody prevalence rates up to 10% are recognized in some endemic areas, and the infection is one of the most important causes of seizures in the developing world and in immigrants to the United States from endemic countries. In Latin America, it is estimated that 0.5–1.5 million people suffer from epilepsy secondary to cysticercosis.

Clinical Findings

A. Symptoms and Signs

Neurocysticercosis can cause intracerebral, subarachnoid, and spinal cord lesions and intraventricular cysts. Single or multiple lesions may be present. Lesions may persist for years before symptoms develop, generally due to local inflammation or ventricular obstruction. Presenting symptoms include seizures, focal neurologic deficits, altered cognition, and psychiatric disease. Symptoms develop more quickly with intraventricular cysts, with findings of hydrocephalus and meningeal irritation, including severe headache, vomiting, papilledema, and visual loss. A particularly aggressive form of the disease, racemose cysticercosis, involves proliferation of cysts at the base of the brain, leading to alterations of consciousness and death. Spinal cord lesions can present with progressive focal findings.

Cysticercosis of other organ systems is usually clinically benign. Involvement of muscles can uncommonly cause discomfort and is identified by radiographs of muscle showing multiple calcified lesions. Subcutaneous involvement presents with multiple painless palpable skin lesions. Involvement of the eyes can present with ptosis due to extraocular muscle involvement or intraocular abnormalities.

B. Laboratory Findings and Imaging

Diagnosis generally requires consideration of both laboratory and imaging findings. The updated Del Brutto diagnostic criteria, which include laboratory and imaging findings, have demonstrated good sensitivity and specificity.

CSF examination may show lymphocytic or eosinophilic pleocytosis, decreased glucose, and elevated protein. Serology plays an important role in diagnosis; both antibody and antigen detection assays are available. ELISAs and related immunoblot assays have excellent sensitivity and specificity, but sensitivity is lower with only single or calcified lesions.

With neuroimaging by CT or MRI, multiple parenchymal cysts are most typically seen. Parenchymal calcification is also common. Performing both CT and MRI is ideal because CT is better for identification of calcification and MRI for smaller and ventricular lesions. Typical findings can be highly suggestive of the diagnosis.

Treatment

The medical management of neurocysticercosis has been controversial because the benefits of cyst clearance must be weighed against potential harm of an inflammatory response to dying worms. Antihelminthic therapy hastens radiologic improvement in parenchymal cysticercosis, but some randomized trials have shown that corticosteroids alone are as effective as specific therapy plus corticosteroids for controlling seizures. Overall, most authorities recommend treatment of active lesions, in particular lesions with a high likelihood of progression, such as intraventricular cysts. At the other end of the spectrum, inactive calcified lesions probably do not benefit from therapy. In addition, cysticidal therapy should be avoided if there is a high risk of hydrocephalus, as with

subarachnoid involvement. When treatment is deemed appropriate, standard therapy consists of albendazole (10–15 mg/kg/day orally for 8 days) or praziquantel (50 mg/kg/day orally for 15–30 days). Albendazole is probably preferred, since it has shown better efficacy in some comparisons and since corticosteroids appear to lower circulating praziquantel levels but increase albendazole levels. Increasing the dosage of albendazole to 30 mg/kg/day orally may improve outcomes. Combining albendazole plus praziquantel improved outcomes compared to albendazole alone in patients with multiple viable intraparenchymal cysts. Corticosteroids are usually administered concurrently, but dosing is not standardized. Patients should be observed for evidence of localized inflammatory responses. Anticonvulsant therapy is provided if needed, and shunting is performed if required for elevated intracranial pressure. Surgical removal of cysts may be helpful for some difficult cases of neurocysticercosis and for symptomatic non-neurologic disease.

Del Brutto OH et al. Revised diagnostic criteria for neurocysticercosis. J Neurol Sci. 2017 Jan 15;372:202–10. [PMID: 28017213]

Garcia HH. Neurocysticercosis. Neurol Clin. 2018 Nov; 36(4):851–64. [PMID: 30366559]

Garcia HH et al; Cysticercosis Working Group in Peru. Laboratory diagnosis of neurocysticercosis (*Taenia solium*). J Clin Microbiol. 2018 Aug 27;56(9):e00424–18. [PMID: 29875195]

White AC et al. Diagnosis and treatment of neurocysticercosis: 2017 Clinical Practice Guidelines by the Infectious Diseases Society of America (IDSA) and the American Society of Tropical Medicine and Hygiene (ASTMH). Am J Trop Med Hyg. 2018 Apr;98(4):945–66. [PMID: 29644966]

2. Echinococcosis

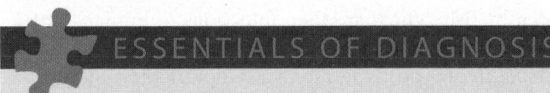

ESSENTIALS OF DIAGNOSIS

- ► History of exposure to dogs or wild canines in an endemic area.
- ► Large cystic lesions, most commonly of the liver or lung.
- ► Positive serologic tests.

General Considerations

Echinococcosis occurs when humans are intermediate hosts for canine tapeworms. Infection is acquired by ingesting food contaminated with canine feces containing parasite eggs. The principal species that infect humans are *Echinococcus granulosus*, which causes cystic hydatid disease, and *Echinococcus multilocularis*, which causes alveolar hydatid disease. *E granulosus* is transmitted by domestic dogs in areas with livestock (sheep, goats, camels, and horses) as intermediate hosts, including Africa, the Middle East, southern Europe, South America, Central Asia, Australia, New Zealand, and the southwestern United States. *E multilocularis*, which much less commonly causes human disease, is transmitted by wild canines, and endemic in northern forest areas of the Northern Hemisphere, including central Europe, Siberia, northern Japan, northwestern Canada, and western Alaska. An increase in the fox population in Europe has been associated with an increase in human cases. The disease range has also extended southward in Central Asia and China. Other species that cause limited disease in humans are endemic in South America and China.

After humans ingest parasite eggs, the eggs hatch in the intestines to form oncospheres, which penetrate the mucosa, enter the circulation, and encyst in specific organs as hydatid cysts. *E granulosus* forms cysts most commonly in the liver (65%) and lungs (25%), but the cysts may develop in any organ, including the brain, bones, skeletal muscles, kidneys, and spleen. Cysts are most commonly single. The cysts can persist and slowly grow for many years.

▶ Clinical Findings

A. Symptoms and Signs

Infections are commonly asymptomatic and may be noted incidentally on imaging studies or present with symptoms caused by an enlarging or superinfected mass. Findings may include abdominal or chest pain, biliary obstruction, cholangitis, portal hypertension, cirrhosis, bronchial obstruction leading to segmental lung collapse, and abscesses. Cyst leakage or rupture may be accompanied by a severe allergic reaction, including fever and hypotension. Seeding of cysts after rupture may extend the infection to new areas.

E multilocularis generally causes a more aggressive disease than *E granulosus*, with initial infection of the liver, but then local and distant spread commonly suggesting a malignancy. Symptoms based on the areas of involvement gradually worsen over years, with the development of obstructive findings in the liver and elsewhere.

B. Laboratory Findings

Serologic tests, including ELISA and immunoblot, offer sensitivity and specificity over 80% for *E granulosus* liver infections, but lower sensitivity for involvement of other organs. Serologic tests may also distinguish the two major echinococcal infections.

C. Imaging

Diagnosis is usually based on imaging studies, including ultrasonography, CT, and MRI. In *E granulosus* infection, a large cyst containing daughter cysts is highly suggestive of the diagnosis. In *E multilocularis* infection, imaging shows an irregular mass, often with areas of calcification.

▶ Treatment

The treatment of cystic hydatid disease is with albendazole, often with cautious surgical resection of cysts. When used alone, as in cases where surgery is not possible, albendazole (10–15 mg/kg/day orally) has demonstrated efficacy, with courses of 3 months or longer duration, in some cases with alternating cycles of treatment and rest. Mebendazole (40–50 mg/kg/day orally) is an alternative drug, and praziquantel may also be effective. In some cases, medical

therapy is begun, with surgery performed if disease persists after some months of therapy. Another approach, in particular with inoperable cysts, is percutaneous aspiration, injection, and reaspiration (PAIR). In this approach (which should not be used if cysts communicate with the biliary tract), patients receive antihelminthic therapy, and the cyst is partially aspirated. After diagnostic confirmation by examination for parasite protoscolices, a scolicidal agent (95% ethanol, hypertonic saline, or 0.5% cetrimide) is injected, and the cyst is reaspirated after about 15 minutes. PAIR includes a small risk of anaphylaxis, which has been reported in about 2% of procedures, but death due to anaphylaxis has been rare. Treatment of alveolar cyst disease is challenging, generally relying on wide surgical resection of lesions. Therapy with albendazole before or during surgery may be beneficial and may also provide improvement or even cure in inoperable cases.

Agudelo Higuita NI et al. Cystic echinococcosis. J Clin Microbiol. 2016 Mar;54(3):518–23. [PMID: 26677245]
Bhutani N et al. Hepatic echinococcosis: a review. Ann Med Surg (Lond). 2018 Nov 2;36:99–105. [PMID: 30450204]
Meinel TR et al. Vertebral alveolar echinococcosis—a case report, systematic analysis, and review of the literature. Lancet Infect Dis. 2018 Mar;18(3):e87–98. [PMID: 28807628]

INTESTINAL NEMATODE (Roundworm) INFECTIONS

ASCARIASIS

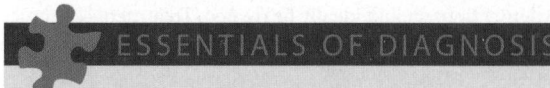

ESSENTIALS OF DIAGNOSIS

- ▶ Transient cough, urticaria, pulmonary infiltrates, eosinophilia.
- ▶ Nonspecific abdominal symptoms.
- ▶ Eggs in stool; adult worms occasionally passed.

▶ General Considerations

Ascaris lumbricoides is the most common of the intestinal helminths, causing about 800 million infections, 12 million acute cases, and 10,000 or more deaths annually. Prevalence is high wherever there is poor hygiene and sanitation or where human feces are used as fertilizer. Heavy infections are most common in children.

Infection follows ingestion of eggs in contaminated food. Larvae hatch in the small intestine, penetrate into the bloodstream, migrate to the lungs, and then travel via airways back to the gastrointestinal tract, where they develop to adult worms, which can be up to 40 cm in length, and live for 1–2 years.

▶ Clinical Findings

Most persons with *Ascaris* infection are asymptomatic. In a small proportion of patients, symptoms develop during migration of worms through the lungs, with fever, nonproductive cough, chest pain, dyspnea, and eosinophilia, occasionally with eosinophilic pneumonia. Rarely, larvae lodge ectopically in the brain, kidney, eye, spinal cord, and other sites and may cause local symptoms.

Light intestinal infections usually produce no symptoms. With heavy infection, abdominal discomfort may be seen. Adult worms may also migrate and be coughed up, be vomited, or may emerge through the nose or anus. They may also migrate into the common bile duct, pancreatic duct, appendix, and other sites, which may lead to cholangitis, cholecystitis, pyogenic liver abscess, pancreatitis, obstructive jaundice, or appendicitis. With very heavy infestations, masses of worms may cause intestinal obstruction, volvulus, intussusception, or death. Although severe manifestations of infection are uncommon, the very high prevalence of ascariasis leads to large numbers of individuals, especially children, with important sequelae. Moderate to high worm loads in children are also associated with nutritional abnormalities due to decreased appetite and food intake, and also decreased absorption of nutrients.

The diagnosis of ascariasis is made after adult worms emerge from the mouth, nose, or anus, or by identifying characteristic eggs in the feces, usually with the Kato-Katz technique. Imaging studies demonstrate worms, with filling defects in contrast studies and at times evidence of intestinal or biliary obstruction. Eosinophilia is marked during worm migration but may be absent during intestinal infection.

▶ Treatment

All infections should ideally be treated. Treatments of choice are albendazole (single 400-mg oral dose), mebendazole (single 500-mg oral dose or 100 mg twice daily for 3 days), or pyrantel pamoate (single 11-mg/kg oral dose, maximum 1 g). These drugs are all well tolerated but may cause mild gastrointestinal toxicity. They are considered safe for children above 1 year of age and in pregnancy, although use in the first trimester is best avoided. An alternative is ivermectin (single 200 mcg/kg oral dose). In endemic areas, reinfection after treatment is common. Intestinal obstruction usually responds to conservative management and antihelminthic therapy. Surgery may be required for appendicitis and other gastrointestinal complications.

TRICHURIASIS

Trichuris trichiura, the whipworm, infects about 500 million persons throughout the world, particularly in humid tropical and subtropical environments. Infection is heaviest and most frequent in children. Infections are acquired by ingestion of eggs. The larvae hatch in the small intestine and mature in the large bowel to adult worms of about 4 cm in length. The worms do not migrate through tissues.

Most infected persons are asymptomatic. Heavy infections may be accompanied by abdominal cramps, tenesmus, diarrhea, distention, nausea, and vomiting. The *Trichuris* dysentery syndrome may develop, particularly in malnourished young children, with findings resembling inflammatory bowel disease including bloody diarrhea and rectal prolapse.

Trichuriasis is diagnosed by identification of characteristic eggs and sometimes adult worms in stools. Eosinophilia is common. Treatment is typically with albendazole (400 mg/day orally) or mebendazole (200 mg/day orally), for 1–3 days for light infections or 3–7 days for heavy infections, but cure rates are lower than for ascariasis or hookworm infection. An alternative is ivermectin (200 mcg/kg orally once daily for 3 days). Oxantel pamoate (one dose of 15–30 mg/kg) has shown good efficacy in clearing infections, and randomized trials showed albendazole plus oxantel pamoate (31% cure; 96% egg reduction) to be superior to mebendazole, and albendazole plus oxantel pamoate (69% cure; 99% egg reduction) and albendazole plus ivermectin (28% cure; 95% egg reduction) to be superior to albendazole plus mebendazole. Oxantel pamoate has low efficacy against *Ascaris* and hookworm infection.

HOOKWORM DISEASE

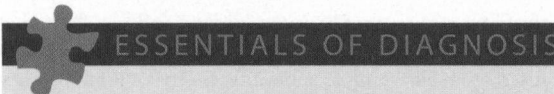

ESSENTIALS OF DIAGNOSIS

▶ Transient pruritic skin rash and lung symptoms.

▶ Anorexia, diarrhea, abdominal discomfort.

▶ Iron deficiency anemia.

▶ Characteristic eggs and occult blood in the stool.

▶ General Considerations

Infection with the hookworms *Ancylostoma duodenale* and *Necator americanus* is very common, especially in most tropical and subtropical regions. Both worms are broadly distributed. Prevalence is estimated at about 500 million, causing approximately 65,000 deaths each year. When eggs are deposited on warm moist soil they hatch, releasing larvae that remain infective for up to a week. With contact, the larvae penetrate skin and migrate in the bloodstream to the pulmonary capillaries. In the lungs, the larvae penetrate into alveoli and then are carried by ciliary action upward to the bronchi, trachea, and mouth. After being swallowed, they reach and attach to the mucosa of the upper small bowel, where they mature to adult worms. *Ancylostoma* infection can also be acquired by ingestion of the larvae in food or water. Hookworms attach to the intestinal mucosa and suck blood. Blood loss is proportionate to the worm burden.

▶ Clinical Findings

A. Symptoms and Signs

Most infected persons are asymptomatic. A pruritic maculopapular rash (ground itch) may occur at the site of larval penetration, usually in previously sensitized persons. Pulmonary symptoms may be seen during larval migration through the lungs, with dry cough, wheezing, and low-grade fever, but these symptoms are less common than with ascariasis. About 1 month after infection, as maturing worms attach to the small intestinal mucosa, gastrointestinal symptoms may develop, with epigastric pain, anorexia, and diarrhea, especially in previously unexposed individuals. Persons chronically infected with large worm burdens may have abdominal pain, anorexia, diarrhea, and findings of marked iron-deficiency anemia and protein malnutrition. Anemia can lead to pallor, weakness, dyspnea, and heart failure, and protein loss can lead to hypoalbuminemia, edema, and ascites. These findings may be accompanied by impairment in growth and cognitive development in children. Infection with the dog hookworm *Ancylostoma caninum* can uncommonly lead to abdominal pain, diarrhea, and eosinophilia, with intestinal ulcerations and regional lymphadenitis.

B. Laboratory Findings

Diagnosis is based on the demonstration of characteristic eggs in feces; concentration techniques are usually not needed. Microcytic anemia, occult blood in the stool, and hypoalbuminemia are common. Eosinophilia is common, especially during worm migration.

▶ Treatment

Treatment is with albendazole (single 400-mg oral dose) or mebendazole (100 mg orally twice daily for 3 days). Occasional adverse effects are diarrhea and abdominal pain. Pyrantel pamoate and levamisole are also effective. Anemia should be managed with iron replacement and, for severe symptomatic anemia, blood transfusion. Mass treatment of children with single doses of albendazole or mebendazole at regular intervals limits worm burdens and the extent of disease and is advocated by WHO.

STRONGYLOIDIASIS

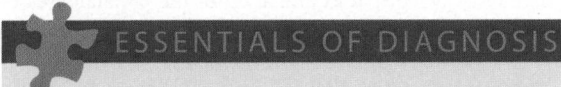

ESSENTIALS OF DIAGNOSIS

- ▶ Transient pruritic skin rash and lung symptoms.
- ▶ Anorexia, diarrhea, abdominal discomfort.
- ▶ Larvae detected in stool.
- ▶ Hyperinfection in the immunocompromised; larvae detected in sputum or other fluids.
- ▶ Eosinophilia.

▶ General Considerations

Strongyloidiasis is caused by infection with *Strongyloides stercoralis*. Although much less prevalent than ascariasis, trichuriasis, or hookworm infections, strongyloidiasis is nonetheless a significant problem, infecting tens of millions of individuals in tropical and subtropical regions. Infection is also endemic in some temperate regions of North America, Europe, Japan, and Australia. Of particular importance is the predilection of the parasite to cause severe infections in immunocompromised individuals due to its ability to replicate in humans. A related parasite, *Strongyloides fuelleborni*, infects humans in parts of Africa and New Guinea.

Among nematodes, *S stercoralis* is uniquely capable of maintaining its full life cycle both within the human host and in soil. Infection occurs when filariform larvae in soil penetrate the skin, enter the bloodstream, and are carried to the lungs, where they escape from capillaries into alveoli, ascend the bronchial tree, and are then swallowed and carried to the duodenum and upper jejunum, where maturation to the adult stage takes place. Females live embedded in the mucosa for up to 5 years, releasing eggs that hatch in the intestines as free rhabditiform larvae that pass to the ground via the feces. In moist soil, these larvae metamorphose into infective filariform larvae. Autoinfection can occur in humans, when some rhabditiform larvae develop into filariform larvae that penetrate the intestinal mucosa or perianal skin, and enter the circulation. The most dangerous manifestation of *S stercoralis* infection is the **hyperinfection syndrome**, with dissemination of large numbers of filariform larvae to the lungs and other tissues in immunocompromised individuals. Mortality with this syndrome approaches 100% without treatment and has been about 25% with treatment. The hyperinfection syndrome is seen in patients receiving corticosteroids and other immunosuppressive medications; patients with hematologic malignancies, malnutrition, or alcoholism; or persons with AIDS. The risk seems greatest for those receiving corticosteroids.

▶ Clinical Findings

A. Symptoms and Signs

As with other intestinal nematodes, most infected persons are asymptomatic. An acute syndrome can be seen at the time of infection, with a pruritic, erythematous, maculopapular rash, usually of the feet. These symptoms may be followed by pulmonary symptoms (including dry cough, dyspnea, and wheezing) and eosinophilia after a number of days, followed by gastrointestinal symptoms after some weeks, as with hookworm infections. Chronic infection may be accompanied by epigastric pain, nausea, diarrhea, and anemia. Maculopapular or urticarial rashes of the buttocks, perineum, and thighs, due to migrating larvae, may be seen. Large worm burdens can lead to malabsorption or intestinal obstruction. Eosinophilia is common but may fluctuate.

With hyperinfection large numbers of larvae can migrate to many tissues, including the lungs, CNS, kidneys, and liver. Gastrointestinal symptoms can include abdominal pain, nausea, vomiting, diarrhea, and more severe findings related to intestinal obstruction, perforation, or hemorrhage. Bacterial sepsis, probably secondary to intestinal ulcerations, is a common presenting finding. Pulmonary findings include pneumonitis, cough, hemoptysis, and respiratory failure. Sputum may contain adult worms, larvae, and eggs. CNS disease includes meningitis and brain abscesses; the CSF may contain larvae. Various presentations can progress to shock and death.

B. Laboratory Findings

The diagnosis of strongyloidiasis can be difficult, as eggs are seldom found in feces. Diagnosis is usually based on the identification of rhabditiform larvae in the stool or duodenal contents. These larvae must be distinguished from hookworm larvae, which may hatch after stool collection. Repeated examinations of stool or examination of duodenal fluid may be required for diagnosis because the sensitivity of individual tests is only about 30%. Hyperinfection is diagnosed by the identification of large numbers of larvae in stool, sputum, or other body fluids. An ELISA from the CDC offers about 90% sensitivity and specificity, but cross-reactions with other helminths may occur. Eosinophilia and mild anemia are common, but eosinophilia may be absent with hyperinfection. Hyperinfection may include extensive pulmonary infiltrates, hypoproteinemia, and abnormal liver function studies.

C. Screening

It is important to be aware of the possibility of strongyloidiasis in persons with even a distant history of residence in an endemic area, since the infection can be latent for decades. Screening of at-risk individuals for infection is appropriate before institution of immunosuppressive therapy. Screening can consist of serologic tests, with stool examinations in those with positive serologic tests, but consideration of presumptive treatment even if the stool evaluations are negative (see below).

► Treatment

Full eradication of *S stercoralis* is more important than with other intestinal helminths due to the ability of the parasite to replicate in humans. The treatment of choice for routine infection is ivermectin (200 mcg/kg orally daily for 1–2 days). Less effective alternatives are albendazole (400 mg orally twice daily for 3 days) and thiabendazole (25 mg/kg orally twice daily for 3 days). For hyperinfection, ivermectin should be administered daily until the clinical syndrome has resolved and larvae have not been identified for at least 2 weeks. Follow-up examinations for larvae in stool or sputum are necessary, with repeat dosing if the infection persists. With continued immunosuppression, eradication may be difficult, and regular repeated therapy (eg, monthly ivermectin) may be required.

ENTEROBIASIS

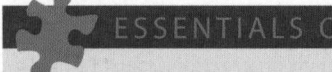

ESSENTIALS OF DIAGNOSIS

- ► Nocturnal perianal pruritus.
- ► Identification of eggs or adult worms on perianal skin or in stool.

► General Considerations

Enterobius vermicularis, the pinworm, is a common cause of intestinal infections worldwide, with maximal prevalence in school-aged children. Enterobiasis is transmitted person-to-person via ingestion of eggs after contact with the hands or perianal region of an infected individual, food or fomites

that have been contaminated by an infected individual, or infected bedding or clothing. Autoinfection also occurs. Eggs hatch in the duodenum and larvae migrate to the cecum. Females mature in about a month, and remain viable for about another month. During this time, they migrate through the anus to deposit large numbers of eggs on the perianal skin. Due to the relatively short life span of these helminths, continuous reinfection, as in institutional settings, is required, for long-standing infection.

► Clinical Findings

A. Symptoms and Signs

Most individuals with pinworm infection are asymptomatic. The most common symptom is perianal pruritus, particularly at night, due to the presence of the female worms or deposited eggs. Insomnia, restlessness, and enuresis are common in children. Perianal scratching may result in excoriation and impetigo. Many mild gastrointestinal symptoms have also been attributed to enterobiasis, but associations are not proven. Serious sequelae are uncommon. Rarely, worm migration results in inflammation or granulomatous reactions of the gastrointestinal or genitourinary tracts. Colonic ulceration and eosinophilic colitis have been reported.

B. Laboratory Findings

Pinworm eggs are usually not found in stool. Diagnosis is made by finding adult worms or eggs on the perianal skin. A common test is to apply clear cellophane tape to the perianal skin, ideally in the early morning, followed by microscopic examination for eggs. The sensitivity of the tape test is reported to be about 50% for a single test and 90% for three tests. Nocturnal examination of the perianal area or gross examination of stools may reveal adult worms, which are about 1 cm in length. Eosinophilia is rare.

► Treatment

Treatment is with single oral doses of albendazole (400 mg), mebendazole (100 mg) or pyrantel pamoate (11 mg/kg, to a maximum of 1 g). The dose is repeated in 2 weeks due to frequent reinfection. Other infected family members should be treated concurrently, and treatment of all close contacts may be appropriate when rates of reinfection are high in family, school, or institutional settings. Standard hand washing and hygiene practices are helpful in limiting spread. Perianal scratching should be discouraged. Washing of clothes and bedding should kill pinworm eggs.

Jourdan PM et al. Soil-transmitted helminth infections. Lancet. 2018 Jan 20;391(10117):252–65. [PMID: 28882382]

Nutman TB. Human infection with *Strongyloides stercoralis* and other related *Strongyloides* species. Parasitology. 2017 Mar; 144(3):263–73. [PMID: 27181117]

Palmeirim MS et al. Efficacy and safety of co-administered ivermectin plus albendazole for treating soil-transmitted helminths: a systematic review, meta-analysis and individual patient data analysis. PLoS Negl Trop Dis. 2018 Apr 27; 12(4):e0006458. [PMID: 29702653]

INVASIVE NEMATODE (Roundworm) INFECTIONS

TRICHINOSIS

 ESSENTIALS OF DIAGNOSIS

► Ingestion of inadequately cooked pork or game.
► Transient intestinal symptoms followed by fever, myalgias, and periorbital edema.
► Eosinophilia and elevated serum muscle enzymes.

General Considerations

Trichinosis (or trichinellosis) is caused worldwide by *Trichinella spiralis* and related *Trichinella* species. The disease is spread by ingestion of undercooked meat, most commonly pork in areas where pigs feed on garbage. When infected raw meat is ingested, *Trichinella* larvae are freed from cyst walls by gastric acid and pass into the small intestine. The larvae then invade intestinal epithelial cells, develop into adults, and the adults release infective larvae. These parasites travel to skeletal muscle via the bloodstream. They invade muscle cells, enlarge, and form cysts. These larvae may be viable for years. Pigs and other animals become infected by eating infected uncooked food scraps or other animals, such as rats.

The worldwide incidence of trichinosis has decreased, but human infections continue to occur sporadically or in outbreaks, with estimates of ~10,000 cases annually. In addition to undercooked pork, infections have been transmitted by ingestion of game and other animals, including bear and walrus in North America and wild boar and horse in Europe. In the United States, about 20 infections are reported annually, mostly from ingesting wild game.

Clinical Findings

A. Symptoms and Signs

Most infections are asymptomatic. In symptomatic cases, gastrointestinal symptoms, including diarrhea, vomiting, and abdominal pain, develop within the week after ingestion of contaminated meat. These symptoms usually last for less than a week but can occasionally persist for much longer. During the following week, symptoms and signs related to migrating larvae are seen. These findings include, most notably, fever, myalgias, periorbital edema, and eosinophilia. Additional findings may include headache, cough, dyspnea, hoarseness, dysphagia, macular or petechial rash, and subconjunctival and retinal hemorrhages. Systemic symptoms usually peak within 2–3 weeks, and commonly persist for about 2 months. In severe cases, generally with large parasite burdens, muscle involvement can be pronounced, with severe muscle pain, edema, and weakness, especially in the head and neck. Muscle pain may persist for months. Uncommon severe findings include myocarditis, pneumonitis, and meningoencephalitis, sometimes leading to death.

B. Laboratory Findings

The clinical diagnosis is supported by findings of elevated serum muscle enzymes (creatine kinase, lactate dehydrogenase, aspartate aminotransferase). The erthryocyte sedimentation rate is usually normal, which may help distinguish trichinosis from autoimmune myopathies. A commercial ELISA assay is available in the United States. Serologic tests become positive 2 or more weeks after infection, but cross-reactivity can be seen with other parasites. Rising antibody titers are highly suggestive of the diagnosis. Muscle biopsy can usually be avoided, but if the diagnosis is uncertain, biopsy of a tender, swollen muscle may identify *Trichinella* larvae. For maximal yield, biopsy material should be examined histologically, and a portion enzymatically digested to release larvae, but evaluation before 3 weeks after infection may not show muscle larvae. Serum and muscle biopsy analysis are available from the CDC.

Treatment

No effective specific therapy for full-blown trichinosis has been identified. However, if infection is suspected early in the course of illness, treatment with mebendazole (2.5 mg/kg orally twice daily) or albendazole (5–7.5 mg/kg orally twice daily) will kill intestinal worms and may limit progression to tissue invasion. Supportive therapy for systemic disease consists of analgesics, antipyretics, bed rest and, in severe illness, corticosteroids. Infection is prevented by cooking to a temperature of at least 71°C for at least 1 minute. Irradiation of meat is also effective in eliminating *Trichinella* larvae, but freezing is not reliable.

Gottstein B et al. Epidemiology, diagnosis, treatment, and control of trichinellosis. Clin Microbiol Rev. 2009 Jan;22(1):127–45. [PMID: 19136437]

TOXOCARIASIS

General Considerations

The dog roundworm *Toxocara canis*, the cat roundworm *Toxocara cati*, and less commonly other helminths may cause visceral larva migrans. *T canis* is highly prevalent in dogs. Humans are infected after ingestion of eggs in material contaminated by dog or other feces. Infection is spread principally by puppies and lactating females, and the eggs must be on the ground for several weeks before they are infectious. After ingestion by humans, larvae migrate to various tissues but cannot complete their life cycle.

Clinical Findings

Visceral larva migrans is seen principally in young children. Most infections are asymptomatic. The most commonly involved organs are the liver and lungs. Presentations include cough, fever, wheezing, hepatomegaly, splenomegaly, lymphadenopathy, pulmonary infiltrates, and eosinophilia. Involvement of the CNS can occur rarely, leading to eosinophilic meningitis and other abnormalities. Ocular larva migrans is a distinct syndrome, usually in children older than is typical for visceral larva migrans. Children present with visual deficits, pain, and a retinal mass, which can be confused with retinoblastoma. *Baylisascaris procyonis*, a roundworm of raccoons, can rarely cause visceral larva migrans in humans, typically with similar, but more severe manifestations than *T canis*.

The diagnosis of visceral larva migrans is suggested by the finding of eosinophilia in a child with hepatomegaly or other signs of the disease, especially with a history of exposure to puppies. The diagnosis is confirmed by the identification of larvae in a biopsy of infected tissue, usually performed when other diseases are suspected. Serologic tests may be helpful; an ELISA against a group of excreted antigens has shown good sensitivity and specificity. Molecular assays can identify specific pathogens. Most patients recover without specific therapy, although symptoms may persist for months.

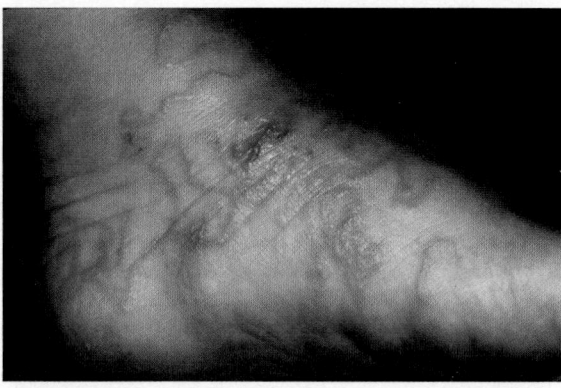

▲ **Figure 35–8.** Cutaneous larva migrans on the foot. (Used, with permission, from Richard P. Usatine, MD, in Usatine RP, Smith MA, Mayeaux EJ Jr, Chumley H. *The Color Atlas of Family Medicine,* 2nd ed. McGraw-Hill, 2013.)

 Treatment

Treatment with antihelminthics or corticosteroids may be considered in severe cases. No drugs have been proven to be effective, but albendazole (400 mg orally twice daily for 5 days), mebendazole, diethylcarbamazine, and ivermectin have been used, and albendazole has been recommended as the treatment of choice.

Chen J et al. Toxocariasis: a silent threat with a progressive public health impact. Infect Dis Poverty. 2018 Jun 13;7(1):59. [PMID: 29895324]
Ma G et al. Human toxocariasis. Lancet Infect Dis. 2018 Jan; 18(1):e14–24. [PMID: 28781085]

CUTANEOUS LARVA MIGRANS (Creeping Eruption)

Cutaneous larva migrans is caused principally by larvae of the dog and cat hookworms, *Ancylostoma braziliense* and *A caninum*. Other animal hookworms, gnathostomiasis, and strongyloidiasis may also cause this syndrome. Infections are common in warm areas, including the southeastern United States. They are most common in children. The disease is caused by the migration of worms through skin; the nonhuman parasites cannot complete their life cycles, so only cause cutaneous disease.

▶ Clinical Findings

Intensely pruritic erythematous papules develop, usually on the feet or hands, followed within a few days by serpiginous tracks marking the course of the parasite, which may travel several millimeters per day (Figure 35–8). Several tracks may be present. The process may continue for weeks, with lesions becoming vesiculated, encrusted, or secondarily infected. Systemic symptoms and eosinophilia are uncommon.

The diagnosis is based on the characteristic appearance of the lesions. Biopsy is usually not indicated.

▶ Treatment

Without treatment, the larvae eventually die and are absorbed. Mild cases do not require treatment. Thiabendazole (10% aqueous suspension) can be applied topically three times daily for 5 or more days. Systemic therapy with albendazole (400 mg orally once or twice daily for 3–5 days) or ivermectin (200 mcg/kg orally single dose) is highly effective.

Kincaid L et al. Management of imported cutaneous larva migrans: a case series and mini-review. Travel Med Infect Dis. 2015 Sep–Oct;13(5):382–7. [PMID: 26243366]

FILARIASIS

LYMPHATIC FILARIASIS

> ### ESSENTIALS OF DIAGNOSIS
>
> ▶ Episodic attacks of lymphangitis, lymphadenitis, and fever.
> ▶ Chronic progressive swelling of extremities and genitals; hydrocele; chyluria; lymphedema.
> ▶ Microfilariae in blood, chyluria, or hydrocele fluid; positive serologic tests.

▶ General Considerations

Lymphatic filariasis is caused by three filarial nematodes: *Wuchereria bancrofti*, *Brugia malayi*, and *Brugia timori*, and is among the most important parasitic diseases of man. Approximately 120 million people are infected with these organisms in tropical and subtropical countries, about a third of these suffer clinical consequences of the infections, and many are seriously disfigured. *W bancrofti* causes about 90% of episodes of lymphatic filariasis. It is transmitted by *Culex, Aedes*, and *Anopheles* mosquitoes and is widely distributed in the tropics and subtropics, including sub-Saharan Africa, Southeast Asia, the western Pacific, India, South America, and the Caribbean. *B malayi* is transmitted by *Mansonia* and *Anopheles* mosquitoes and is endemic in parts of China, India, Southeast Asia, and the Pacific. *B timori* is found only in islands of southeastern Indonesia. *Mansonella* are filarial worms transmitted by midges and other insects in Africa and South America.

Humans are infected by the bites of infected mosquitoes. Larvae then move to the lymphatics and lymph nodes, where they mature over months to thread-like adult worms, and then can persist for many years. The adult worms produce large numbers of microfilariae, which are released into the circulation, and infective to mosquitoes, particularly at night (except for the South Pacific, where microfilaremia peaks during daylight hours).

► Clinical Findings

A. Symptoms and Signs

Many infections remain asymptomatic despite circulating microfilariae. Clinical consequences of filarial infection are principally due to inflammatory responses to developing, mature, and dying worms. The initial manifestation of infection is often acute lymphangitis, with fever, painful lymph nodes, edema, and inflammation spreading peripherally from involved lymph nodes (in contrast to bacterial lymphangitis, which spreads centrally). Lymphangitis and lymphadenitis of the upper and lower extremities is common (Figure 35–9); genital involvement, including epididymitis and orchitis, with scrotal pain and tenderness, occurs principally only with *W bancrofti* infection. Acute

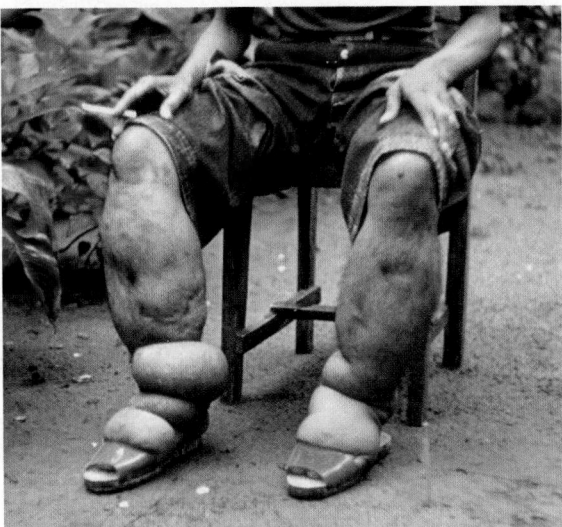

▲ **Figure 35–9.** Elephantiasis of legs due to filariasis. (Public Health Image Library, CDC.)

attacks of lymphangitis last for a few days to a week and may recur a few times per year. Filarial fevers may also occur without lymphatic inflammation.

The most common chronic manifestation of lymphatic filariasis is swelling of the extremities or genitals due to chronic lymphatic inflammation and obstruction. Extremities become increasingly swollen, with a progression over time from pitting edema, to nonpitting edema, to sclerotic changes of the skin that are referred to as elephantiasis. Genital involvement, particularly with *W bancrofti*, occurs more commonly in men, progressing from painful epididymitis to hydroceles that are usually painless but can become very large, with inguinal lymphadenopathy, thickening of the spermatic cord, scrotal lymphedema, thickening and fissuring of the scrotal skin, and occasionally chyluria. Lymphedema of the female genitalia and breasts may also occur.

Tropical pulmonary eosinophilia is a distinct syndrome principally affecting young adult males with either *W bancrofti* or *B malayi* infection, but typically without microfilaremia. This syndrome is characterized by asthmalike symptoms, with cough, wheezing, dyspnea, and low-grade fevers, usually at night. Without treatment, tropical pulmonary eosinophilia can progress to interstitial fibrosis and chronic restrictive lung disease. *Mansonella* can inhabit serous cavities, the retroperitoneum, the eye, or the skin, and cause abnormalities related to inflammation at these sites.

B. Laboratory Findings

The diagnosis of lymphatic filariasis is strongly suggested by characteristic findings of lymphangitis or lymphatic obstruction in persons with risk factors for the disease. The diagnosis is confirmed by finding microfilariae, usually in blood, but microfilariae may be absent, especially early in the disease progression (first 2–3 years) or with chronic obstructive disease. To increase yields, blood samples are obtained at about midnight in most areas, but during daylight hours in the South Pacific. Smears are evaluated by wet mount to identify motile parasites and by Giemsa staining; these examinations can be delayed until the following morning, with storage of samples at room temperature. Of note, the periodicity of microfilaremia is variable, and daytime samples may yield positive results. Microfilariae may also be identified in hydrocele fluid or chylous urine. Eosinophilia is usually absent, except during acute inflammatory syndromes. Serologic tests may be helpful but cannot distinguish past and active infections. Rapid antigen tests with sensitivity and specificity over 90% are available for detection of *W bancrofti*. These can be considered the diagnostic tests of choice and are increasingly used to guide control programs. However, cross-reactivity with *Loa loa* infections has been described. Due to potential severe toxicity, caution is appropriate before treatment with ivermectin for positive *W bancrofti* antigen tests in areas also endemic for *L loa* infection. Multiple molecular tests, including field-friendly LAMP assays, have been developed. Adult worms may also be found in lymph node biopsy specimens (although biopsy is not usually clinically indicated) or by ultrasound of a scrotal hydrocele or lymphedematous breast. When microfilaremia is lacking, especially if sophisticated techniques are not available, diagnoses may need to be made on clinical grounds.

► Treatment & Control

A. Drug Treatment

Diethylcarbamazine is the drug of choice, but it cannot cure infections due to its limited action against adult worms. Asymptomatic infection and acute lymphangitis are treated with this drug (2 mg/kg orally three times daily) for 10–14 days, leading to a marked decrease in microfilaremia. Therapy may be accompanied by allergic symptoms, including fever, headache, malaise, hypotension, and bronchospasm, probably due to release of antigens from dying worms. For this reason, treatment courses may begin with a lower dosage, with escalation over the first 4 days of treatment. Single annual doses of diethylcarbamazine (6 mg/kg orally), alone or with ivermectin (400 mcg/kg orally) or albendazole (400 mg orally) may be as effective as longer courses of diethylcarbamazine. A single dose of all three drugs cleared parasites in more than 95% of persons for 3 years and offered superior clearance compared to a single dose of diethylcarbamazine plus albendazole and noninferiority compared to three annual doses of the two-drug regimen. When onchocerciasis or loiasis is suspected, it may be appropriate to withhold diethylcarbamazine to avoid severe reactions to dying microfilariae; rather, ivermectin plus albendazole may be given, although these drugs are less active than diethylcarbamazine against adult worms. Appropriate management of advanced obstructive disease is uncertain. Drainage of hydroceles provides symptomatic relief, although they will recur. Therapy with diethylcarbamazine cannot reverse chronic lymphatic changes, but is typically provided to lower worm burdens. An interesting approach under study is to treat with doxycycline (100–200 mg/day orally for 4–6 weeks), which kills obligate intracellular *Wolbachia* bacteria, leading to death of adult filarial worms. Doxycycline was also effective at controlling *Mansonella perstans* infection, which does not respond well to standard antifilarial drugs. Secondary bacterial infections must be treated. Surgical correction may be helpful in some cases.

B. Disease Control

Avoidance of mosquitoes is a key measure; preventive measures include the use of screens, bed nets (ideally treated with insecticide), and insect repellents. Community-based treatment with single annual doses of effective drugs offers a highly effective means of control. The current WHO strategy for control includes mass treatment of at risk communities with single annual doses of diethylcarbamazine plus albendazole or, for areas with onchocerciasis, albendazole plus ivermectin; in some circumstances, more frequent dosing offers improved control.

King CL et al. A trial of a triple-drug treatment for lymphatic filariasis. N Engl J Med. 2018 Nov 8;379(19):1801–10. [PMID: 30403937]

ONCHOCERCIASIS

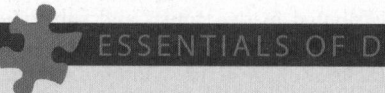

► Conjunctivitis progressing to blindness.
► Severe pruritus; skin excoriations, thickening, and depigmentation; and subcutaneous nodules.
► Microfilariae in skin snips and on slit-lamp examination; adult worms in subcutaneous nodules.

► General Considerations

Onchocerciasis, or river blindness, is caused by *Onchocerca volvulus*. An estimated 37 million persons are infected, of whom 3–4 million have skin disease, 500,000 have severe visual impairment, and 300,000 are blinded. Over 99% of infections are in sub-Saharan Africa, especially the West African savanna, with about half of cases in Nigeria and Congo. In some hyperendemic African villages, close to 100% of individuals are infected, and 10% or more of the population is blind. The disease is also prevalent in the southwestern Arabian peninsula and Latin America, including southern Mexico, Guatemala, Venezuela, Colombia, Ecuador, and northwestern Brazil. Onchocerciasis is transmitted by simulium flies (blackflies). These insects breed in fast-flowing streams and bite during the day.

After the bite of an infected blackfly, larvae are deposited in the skin, where adults develop over 6–12 months. Adult worms live in subcutaneous connective tissue or muscle nodules for a decade or more. Microfilariae are released from the nodules and migrate through subcutaneous and ocular tissues. Disease is due to responses to worms and to intracellular *Wolbachia* bacteria.

► Clinical Findings

A. Symptoms and Signs

After an incubation period of up to 1–3 years, the disease typically produces an erythematous, papular, pruritic rash, which may progress to chronic skin thickening and depigmentation. Itching may be severe and unresponsive to medications, such that more disability-adjusted life years are lost to onchocercal skin problems than to blindness. Numerous firm, nontender, movable subcutaneous nodules of about 0.5–3 cm, which contain adult worms, may be present. Due to differences in vector habits, these nodules are more commonly on the lower body in Africa but on the head and upper body in Latin America. Inguinal and femoral lymphadenopathy is common, at times resulting in a "hanging groin," with lymph nodes hanging within a sling of atrophic skin. Patients may also have systemic symptoms, with weight loss and musculoskeletal pain.

The most serious manifestations of onchocerciasis involve the eyes. Microfilariae migrating through the eyes elicit host responses that lead to pathology. Findings include punctate keratitis and corneal opacities, progressing to sclerosing keratitis and blindness. Iridocyclitis, glaucoma, choroiditis, and optic atrophy may also lead to vision loss. The likelihood of blindness after infection varies greatly based on geography, with the risk greatest in savanna regions of West Africa.

B. Diagnostic Testing

The diagnosis is made by identifying microfilariae in skin snips, by visualizing microfilariae in the cornea or anterior chamber by slit-lamp examination, by identification of adult worms in a biopsy or aspirate of a nodule or, uncommonly, by identification of microfilariae in urine. Skin snips from the iliac crest (Africa) or scapula (Americas) are allowed to stand in saline for 2–4 hours or longer, and then examined microscopically for microfilariae. Deep punch biopsies are not needed, and if suspicion persists after a skin snip is negative, the procedure should be repeated. Ultrasound may identify characteristic findings suggestive of adult worms in skin nodules. When the diagnosis remains difficult, the Mazzotti test can be used; exacerbation of skin rash and pruritus after a 50-mg dose of diethylcarbamazine is highly suggestive of the diagnosis. This test should only be used after other tests are negative, since treatment can elicit severe skin and eye reactions in heavily infected individuals. A related and safer test using topical diethylcarbamazine is also available. Eosinophilia is a common, but inconsistent finding. Antigen and antibody detection tests are under study.

▶ Treatment & Control

The treatment of choice is ivermectin, which kills microfilariae, but not adult worms, so disease control requires repeat administrations. Treatment is with a single oral dose of 150 mcg/mL, but schedules for re-treatment have not been standardized. One regimen is to treat every 3 months for 1 year, followed by treatment every 6–12 months for the suspected life span of adult worms (about 15 years). Treatment results in marked reduction in numbers of microfilariae in the skin and eyes, although its impact on the progression of visual loss remains uncertain. Toxicities of ivermectin are generally mild; fever, pruritus, urticaria, myalgias, edema, hypotension, and tender lymphadenopathy may be seen, presumably due to reactions to dying worms. Ivermectin should be used with caution in patients also at risk for loiasis, since it can elicit severe reactions including encephalopathy. As with other filarial infections, doxycycline acts against *O volvulus* by killing intracellular *Wolbachia* bacteria. A course of 100 mg/day for 4–6 weeks kills the bacteria and prevents parasite embryogenesis for at least 18 months. Doxycycline shows promise as a first-line agent to treat onchocerciasis because of its improved activity against adult worms compared to other agents and limited toxicity due to the slow action of the drug.

Protection against onchocerciasis includes avoidance of biting flies. Major efforts are underway to control insect vectors in Africa. In addition, mass distribution of ivermectin for intermittent administration at the community level is ongoing, and the prevalence of severe skin and eye disease is decreasing.

Debrah AY et al. Doxycycline leads to sterility and enhanced killing of female *Onchocerca volvulus* worms in an area with persistent microfilaridermia after repeated ivermectin treatment: a randomized, placebo-controlled, double-blind trial. Clin Infect Dis. 2015 Aug 15;61(4):517–26. [PMID: 25948064]

LOIASIS

ESSENTIALS OF DIAGNOSIS

▶ Subcutaneous swellings; adult worms migrating across the eye.

▶ Encephalitis, which may be brought on by treatment.

▶ Microfilariae in the blood.

▶ General Considerations

Loiasis is a chronic filarial disease caused by infection with *Loa loa*. The infection occurs in humans and monkeys in rainforest areas of West and central Africa. An estimated 3–13 million persons are infected. The disease is transmitted by chrysops flies, which bite during the day. Over 6–12 months after infection, larvae develop into adult worms, which migrate through subcutaneous tissues, including the subconjunctiva (leading to the term "eye worm"). Adults can live for up to 17 years.

▶ Clinical Findings

A. Symptoms and Signs

Many infected persons are asymptomatic, although they may have high levels of microfilaremia and eosinophilia. Transient subcutaneous swellings (Calabar swellings) develop in symptomatic persons. The swellings are nonerythematous, up to 20 cm in diameter, and may be preceded by local pain or pruritus. They usually resolve after 2–4 days but occasionally persist for several weeks. Calabar swellings are commonly seen around joints and may recur at the same or different sites. Visitors from nonendemic areas are more likely to have allergic-type reactions, including pruritus, urticaria, and angioedema. Adult worms may be seen to migrate across the eye, with either no symptoms or conjunctivitis, with pain and edema. The most serious complication of loiasis is encephalitis, which is most common in those with high-level microfilaremia and microfilariae in the CSF. Symptoms may range from headache and insomnia to coma and death. Encephalitis may be brought on by treatment with diethylcarbamazine or ivermectin. Other complications of loiasis include kidney disease, with hematuria and proteinuria; endomyocardial fibrosis; and peripheral neuropathy.

B. Laboratory Findings

The diagnosis is established by identifying microfilariae in blood. Blood is evaluated as for lymphatic filariasis, but for loiasis blood should be obtained during the day. The failure to find microfilariae does not rule out the diagnosis. Identification of a migrating eye worm is also diagnostic. Serologic tests may be helpful in persons from nonendemic areas who may be acutely ill without detectable microfilaremia, but such tests have limited utility for residents of endemic areas because most of them will have positive test results. Field-friendly methods, including LAMP assays and a mobile phone–based video microscope, are available to rule out high-density loiasis before administration of ivermectin for the control of other filarial infections.

▶ **Treatment**

The treatment of choice is diethylcarbamazine, which eliminates microfilariae and has some activity against adult worms. Treatment is with 8–10 mg/kg/day orally for 21 days; repeat courses may be needed. Mild side effects are common, including fever, pruritus, arthralgias, nausea, diarrhea, and Calabar swellings. These symptoms may be lessened by antihistamines or corticosteroids. Patients with large worm burdens are at greater risk for serious complications of therapy, including kidney injury, shock, encephalitis, coma, and death. Treatment with ivermectin, which is highly active against microfilariae, but not adult worms, entails a higher risk of severe reactions. To attempt to avoid these sequelae, pretreatment with corticosteroids and antihistamines, and escalating dosage of diethylcarbamazine have been used, but this strategy does not prevent encephalitis. The circulating parasite load that indicates particular risk for severe complications with therapy has been estimated at 2500/mL. Strategies to treat patients with high parasite loads include (1) no treatment; (2) apheresis, if available, to remove microfilariae prior to therapy with diethylcarbamazine; or (3) therapy with albendazole, which appears to be well tolerated due to its slow antiparasitic effects, prior to therapy with diethylcarbamazine or ivermectin. Doxycycline is not effective for loiasis.

Kamgno J et al. A test-and-not-treat strategy for onchocerciasis in *Loa loa*-endemic areas. N Engl J Med. 2017 Nov 23;377(21): 2044–52. [PMID: 29116890]
Kamgno J et al. Effect of two or six doses 800 mg of albendazole every two months on *Loa loa* microfilaraemia: a double blind, randomized, placebo-controlled trial. PLoS Negl Trop Dis. 2016 Mar 11;10(3):e0004492. [PMID: 26967331]

Mycotic Infections

Stacey R. Rose, MD
Richard J. Hamill, MD

CANDIDIASIS

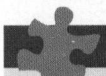

ESSENTIALS OF DIAGNOSIS

▶ Common normal flora but opportunistic pathogen.

▶ Mucosal disease, particularly vaginitis and esophagitis.

▶ Risk factors for fungemia: neutropenia, intravenous catheter, abdominal surgery, total parenteral nutrition, kidney disease, broad-spectrum antibiotics.

▶ General Considerations

Candida albicans can be cultured from the mouth, vagina, and feces of most people. Cutaneous and oral lesions are discussed in Chapters 6 and 8, respectively. The risk factors for invasive candidiasis include prolonged neutropenia, recent abdominal surgery, broad-spectrum antibiotic therapy, kidney disease, and the presence of intravascular catheters (especially when providing total parenteral nutrition). Cellular immunodeficiency predisposes to mucocutaneous disease. When no other underlying cause is found, persistent oral or vaginal candidiasis should arouse a suspicion of HIV infection.

▶ Clinical Findings

A. Mucosal Candidiasis

Esophageal involvement is the most frequent type of significant mucosal disease. Presenting symptoms include substernal odynophagia, gastroesophageal reflux, or nausea without substernal pain. Oral candidiasis, though often associated, is not invariably present. Diagnosis is best confirmed by endoscopy with biopsy and culture.

Vulvovaginal candidiasis occurs in an estimated 75% of women during their lifetime. Risk factors include pregnancy, uncontrolled diabetes mellitus, broad-spectrum antimicrobial treatment, corticosteroid use, and HIV infection. Symptoms include acute vulvar pruritus, burning vaginal discharge, and dyspareunia.

B. Candidal Funguria

Most cases of candidal funguria are asymptomatic and represent specimen contamination or bladder colonization. However, symptoms and signs of true *Candida* urinary tract infections are indistinguishable from bacterial urinary tract infections and can include urgency, hesitancy, fever, chills, or flank pain.

C. Invasive Candidiasis

Invasive candidiasis can be (1) candidemia (bloodstream infection) without deep-seated infection; (2) candidemia with deep-seated infection (typically eyes, kidney, or abdomen); and (3) deep-seated candidiasis in the absence of bloodstream infection. Varying ratios of these clinical entities depends on the predominating risk factors for affected patients (ie, neutropenia, dialysis, postsurgical). The clinical presentation of candidemia varies from minimal fever to septic shock that can resemble a severe bacterial infection. The diagnosis of invasive *Candida* infection is problematic because *Candida* species are often isolated from mucosal sites in the absence of invasive disease while blood cultures are positive only 50% of the time in invasive infection. Consecutively positive (1,3)-beta-D-glucan results may be used to guide empiric therapy in high-risk patients even in the absence of positive blood cultures.

Hepatosplenic candidiasis can occur following prolonged neutropenia in patients with underlying hematologic cancers, but this entity is less common in the era of widespread antifungal prophylaxis. Typically, fever and variable abdominal pain present weeks after chemotherapy, when neutrophil counts have recovered. Blood cultures are generally negative.

D. Candidal Endocarditis

Candidal endocarditis is a rare infection affecting patients with prosthetic heart valves or prolonged candidemia, such as with indwelling catheters. The diagnosis is established definitively by culturing *Candida* from emboli or from vegetations at the time of valve replacement.

► Treatment

A. Mucosal Candidiasis

Therapy of **esophageal candidiasis** depends on the severity of disease. If patients are able to swallow and take adequate amounts of fluid orally, fluconazole, 200–400 mg daily for 10–14 days, is recommended (Table 36–1). In the individual who is more ill or in whom esophagitis has developed while taking fluconazole, options include oral itraconazole solution, 200 mg daily; oral or intravenous voriconazole, 200 mg twice daily; intravenous amphotericin B, 0.3 mg/kg/day; intravenous caspofungin, 50 mg/day; intravenous anidulafungin, 100 mg on day 1, then 50 mg/day; or intravenous micafungin, 150 mg/day. Posaconazole tablets, 300 mg/day, may also be considered for fluconazole-refractory disease. Relapse is common with all agents

Table 36–1. Agents for systemic mycoses (listed in alphabetical order).[*]

Drug	Dosing	Renal Clearance?	CSF Penetration?	Toxicities	Spectrum of Activity
Amphotericin B	0.3–1.5 mg/kg/day intravenously	No	Poor	Rigors, fever, azotemia, hypokalemia, hypomagnesemia, renal tubular acidosis, anemia	All major pathogens except *Scedosporium*
Amphotericin B lipid complex	5 mg/kg/day intravenously	No	Poor	Fever, rigors, nausea, hypotension, anemia, azotemia, tachypnea	Same as amphotericin B, above
Amphotericin B, liposomal	3–6 mg/kg/day intravenously	No	Poor	Fever, rigors, nausea, hypotension, azotemia, anemia, tachypnea, chest tightness	Same as amphotericin B, above Preferred agent for CNS
Anidulafungin	200-mg intravenous loading dose, followed by 100 mg/day intravenously	< 1%	Poor	Diarrhea, hepatic enzyme elevations, histamine-mediated reactions	Mucosal and invasive candidiasis
Caspofungin acetate	70-mg intravenous loading dose, followed by 50 mg/day intravenously	< 50%[1]	Poor	Transient neutropenia; hepatic enzyme elevations when used with cyclosporine	Aspergillosis, mucosal and invasive candidiasis, empiric antifungal therapy in febrile neutropenia
Fluconazole	Systemic infection: 400–2000 mg/day intravenously or orally Mucosal infection: 100–200 mg/day orally	Yes	Yes	Nausea, rash, xerosis, alopecia, headache, hepatic enzyme elevations	Mucosal candidiasis (including urinary tract), cryptococcosis, histoplasmosis, coccidioidomycosis
Flucytosine (5-FC)	100–150 mg/kg/day orally in four divided doses	Yes	Yes	Leukopenia,[2] rash, diarrhea, hepatitis, nausea, vomiting	Cryptococcosis,[3] candidiasis,[3] chromomycosis
Isavuconazole	200 mg orally or intravenously every 8 hours for 6 doses (48 hours) as loading dose, followed by 200 mg/day orally or intravenously	No	Low in CSF, high in brain	Nausea, diarrhea, upper abdominal pain, dizziness	Broad range of activity including invasive aspergillosis and mucormycosis (limited data for *Mucorales*)
Itraconazole	Oral solution and capsule formulations available, both dosed at 200 mg three times daily for 3 days, then 200 mg once or twice daily thereafter[4]	No	Variable	Nausea, hypokalemia, edema, hypertension, peripheral neuropathy, exacerbation of heart failure	Histoplasmosis, coccidioidomycosis, blastomycosis, paracoccidioidomycosis, mucosal candidiasis (except urinary), sporotrichosis, aspergillosis, chromomycosis
Ketoconazole	200–800 mg/day orally in one or two doses with food or acidic beverage	No	Poor	Anorexia, nausea, suppression of testosterone and cortisol, rash, headache, hepatic enzyme elevations, hepatic failure	Nonmeningeal histoplasmosis and coccidioidomycosis, blastomycosis, paracoccidioidomycosis, mucosal candidiasis (except urinary)

(continued)

Table 36–1. Agents for systemic mycoses (listed in alphabetical order).*(continued)

Drug	Dosing	Renal Clearance?	CSF Penetration?	Toxicities	Spectrum of Activity
Micafungin sodium	100 mg/day intravenously	No	Poor	Rash, rigors, headache, phlebitis	Mucosal and invasive candidiasis, prophylaxis in hematopoietic stem cell transplantation
Posaconazole	Delayed-release tablet formulation preferred over oral solution due to more predictable absorption For delayed-release tablet or intravenous formulation: 300 mg twice daily for 2 doses (1 day) loading dose followed by 300 mg daily thereafter	No	Yes	Nausea, vomiting, abdominal pain, diarrhea, and headache	Broad range of activity including the *Mucorales*
Terbinafine	250 mg once daily orally	Yes	Poor	Nausea, abdominal pain, taste disturbance, rash, diarrhea, and hepatic enzyme elevations	Dermatophytes, sporotrichosis, chromomycosis, eumycetoma
Voriconazole[5]	Systemic infection: 6 mg/kg intravenously every 12 hours for 24 hours loading dose, followed by 4 mg/kg intravenously every 12 hours *or* 200–300 mg orally every 12 hours Mucosal infection: 200–300 mg orally every 12 hours (no loading dose required)	Yes	Yes	Transient visual disturbances, rash, photosensitivity, fluoride excess with periostitis, peripheral neuropathy, squamous cell skin cancers, hepatic enzyme elevations[4]	All major pathogens except the *Mucorales* and sporotrichosis

*General information provided, but specific dosing may vary by indication and other patient characteristics; an infectious diseases specialist should be consulted for complex cases.

[1]No dosage adjustment required for chronic kidney disease; dosage adjustment necessary with moderate to severe hepatic dysfunction.

[2]Use should be monitored with blood levels to prevent this or the dose adjusted according to creatinine clearance.

[3]In combination with amphotericin B.

[4]Oral solution preferred due to less variable absorption; capsule should be taken with food and acidic beverages to enhance absorption. For severe infections, blood levels should be measured to ensure adequate exposure.

[5]Some authorities advocate therapeutic drug monitoring in patients who are not responding to therapy. Administration with drugs that are metabolized by the cytochrome P450 system is contraindicated or requires careful monitoring of liver function. Intravenous formulation is contraindicated for patients with CrCl < 50 ml/min because of accumulation of cyclodextrin.

CNS, central nervous system; CSF, cerebrospinal fluid.

when there is underlying HIV infection without adequate immune reconstitution.

Vulvovaginal candidiasis can be treated with various topical azole preparations (eg, clotrimazole, 100-mg vaginal tablet for 7 days, or miconazole, 200-mg vaginal suppository for 3 days). The efficacy of one 150-mg oral dose of fluconazole is equivalent to topical preparations with better patient acceptance. Disease recurrence is common but can be decreased with weekly fluconazole therapy (150 mg weekly).

B. Candidal Funguria

Candidal funguria frequently resolves with discontinuance of antibiotics or removal of bladder catheters. Clinical benefit from treatment of asymptomatic candiduria has not been demonstrated, but persistent funguria should raise the suspicion of invasive infection. When symptomatic funguria persists, oral fluconazole, 200 mg/day for 7–14 days, can be used (Table 36–1).

C. Invasive Candidiasis

The 2016 guidelines for management of candidemia recommend an echinocandin such as caspofungin (loading dose of 70 mg intravenously once, then 50 mg intravenously daily), micafungin (100 mg intravenously daily), or anidulafungin (loading dose of 200 mg intravenously once, then 100 mg intravenously daily) (Table 36–1). Fluconazole (loading dose of 800 mg [12 mg/kg] intravenously, then 400 mg [6 mg/kg] intravenously daily) is an acceptable alternative for less critically ill patients without recent azole exposure. Therapy for candidemia should be continued for 2 weeks after the last positive blood culture and resolution of symptoms and signs of infection. A dilated fundoscopic examination is recommended for patients with candidemia to exclude endophthalmitis and repeat blood cultures should be drawn to demonstrate organism clearance. Susceptibility testing is recommended on all bloodstream *Candida* isolates; once patients have become clinically stable, parenteral therapy can be discontinued and treatment can be completed with oral fluconazole, 400 mg daily orally for susceptible isolates. Removal or exchange of intravascular catheters is generally recommended for patients with candidemia in whom the catheter is the suspected source of infection. Hepatosplenic candidiasis requires treatment until lesions have resolved radiographically.

Non-*albicans* species of *Candida* account for over 50% of clinical bloodstream isolates and often have resistance patterns that are different from *C albicans*. An echinocandin is recommended for treatment of *C glabrata* infection with a transition to oral fluconazole or voriconazole reserved for patients whose isolates are known to be susceptible to these agents. *C glabrata* that is resistant to azoles and echinocandins is being increasingly reported. Similarly, *Candida krusei* is generally fluconazole-resistant and so should be treated with an alternative agent, such as an echinocandin or voriconazole. Fluconazole may be optimal for *Candida parapsilosis* due to possible echinocandin resistance in such isolates. Cases of health care–associated infections due to multidrug-resistant *Candida auris* have been described from several countries, including the United States, with most cases having been treated with echinocandins plus environmental source control.

D. Candidal Endocarditis

Best results are achieved with a combination of medical and surgical therapy. Lipid formulation amphotericin B (3–5 mg/kg/day) or high-dose echinocandin (caspofungin 150 mg/day, micafungin 150 mg/day, or anidulafungin 200 mg/day) is recommended as initial therapy (Table 36–1). Step-down or long-term suppressive therapy for nonsurgical candidates may be done with fluconazole at 6–12 mg/kg/day for susceptible organisms.

E. Prevention of Invasive Candidiasis

In high-risk patients undergoing induction chemotherapy, bone marrow transplantation, or liver transplantation, prophylaxis with antifungal agents has been shown to prevent invasive fungal infections, although the effect on mortality and the preferred agent remain debated. Although the isolation of *Candida* species from mucosal sites raises the possibility of invasive candidiasis among critically ill patients, trials of empiric antifungal agents in such situations have not shown clear clinical benefit.

Ben-Ami R. Treatment of invasive candidiasis: a narrative review. J Fungi (Basel). 2018 Aug 16;4(3):E97. [PMID: 30115843]

Pappas PG et al. Clinical practice guideline for the management of candidiasis: 2016 update by the Infectious Diseases Society of America. Clin Infect Dis. 2016 Feb 15;62(4):e1–50. [PMID: 26679628]

Tsay S et al. Approach to the investigation and management of patients with *Candida auris,* an emerging multi-drug resistant yeast. Clin Infect Dis. 2018 Jan 6;66(2):306–11. [PMID: 29020224]

HISTOPLASMOSIS

ESSENTIALS OF DIAGNOSIS

- ▶ Exposure to bird and bat droppings; common along river valleys (especially the Ohio River and the Mississippi River valleys).

- ▶ Most patients asymptomatic; respiratory illness most common clinical problem.

- ▶ Disseminated disease common in AIDS or other immunosuppressed states; poor prognosis.

- ▶ Blood and bone marrow cultures and urine polysaccharide antigen are useful in diagnosis of disseminated disease.

▶ General Considerations

Histoplasmosis is caused by *Histoplasma capsulatum*, a dimorphic fungus that has been isolated from soil contaminated with bird or bat droppings in endemic areas (central and eastern United States, eastern Canada, Mexico, Central America, South America, Africa, and Southeast Asia). Infection presumably takes place by inhalation of conidia. These convert into small budding cells that are engulfed by phagocytes in the lungs. The organism proliferates and undergoes lymphohematogenous spread to other organs.

▶ Clinical Findings

A. Symptoms and Signs

Most cases of histoplasmosis are asymptomatic or mild and thus go unrecognized. Past infection is recognized by pulmonary and splenic calcification noted on incidental radiographs. Symptomatic infection may present with mild influenza-like illness, often lasting 1–4 days. Moderately severe infections are frequently diagnosed as atypical pneumonia. These patients have fever, cough, and mild central chest pain lasting 5–15 days.

Clinically evident infections occur in several forms: (1) **Acute pulmonary histoplasmosis** frequently occurs in epidemics, often when soil containing infected bird or bat droppings is disturbed. Clinical manifestations can vary from a mild influenza-like illness to severe pneumonia. The illness may last from 1 week to 6 months but is almost never fatal. (2) **Progressive disseminated histoplasmosis** is commonly seen in patients with underlying HIV infection (with CD4 cell counts usually less than 100 cells/mcL) or other conditions of impaired cellular immunity.

Disseminated histoplasmosis has also been reported in patients from endemic areas taking tumor necrosis factor (TNF)-alpha inhibitors. It is characterized by fever and multiple organ system involvement. Chest radiographs may show a miliary pattern. Presentation may be fulminant, simulating septic shock, with death ensuing rapidly unless treatment is provided. Symptoms usually consist of fever, dyspnea, cough, loss of weight, and prostration. Ulcers of the mucous membranes of the oropharynx may be present. The liver and spleen are nearly always enlarged, and all the organs of the body are involved, particularly the adrenal glands; this results in adrenal insufficiency in about 50% of patients. Gastrointestinal involvement may mimic inflammatory bowel disease. Central nervous system (CNS) invasion occurs in 5–10% of individuals with disseminated disease. (3) **Chronic pulmonary histoplasmosis** is usually seen in older patients who have underlying chronic lung disease. Chest radiographs show various lesions including complex apical cavities, infiltrates, and nodules. (4) **Complications of pulmonary histoplasmosis** include granulomatous mediastinitis characterized by persistently enlarged mediastinal lymph nodes and fibrosing mediastinitis in which an excessive fibrotic response to *Histoplasma* infection results in compromise of pulmonary vascular structures.

B. Laboratory Findings

Most patients with chronic pulmonary disease show anemia of chronic disease. Bone marrow involvement with pancytopenia may be prominent in disseminated forms. Marked lactate dehydrogenase (LD) and ferritin elevations are also common, as are mild elevations of serum aspartate aminotransferase.

With pulmonary involvement, sputum culture is rarely positive except in chronic disease; antigen testing of bronchoalveolar lavage fluid may be helpful in acute disease. The combination of a first morning urine and serum polysaccharide antigen assays has an 83% sensitivity for the diagnosis of acute pulmonary histoplasmosis. Blood or bone marrow cultures from immunocompromised patients with acute disseminated disease are positive more than 80% of the time, but may take several weeks for growth. The urine antigen assay has a sensitivity of greater than 90% for disseminated disease in immunocompromised patients and a declining titer can be used to follow response to therapy. Diagnosis of CNS disease requires antigen and antibody testing of the cerebrospinal fluid (CSF) and serum as well as urine antigen testing.

▶ Treatment

For progressive localized disease and for mild to moderately severe nonmeningeal disseminated disease in immunocompetent or immunocompromised patients, itraconazole, 200–400 mg/day orally divided into two doses, is the treatment of choice with an overall response rate of approximately 80% (Table 36–1). The oral solution is better absorbed than the capsule formulation, which requires gastric acid for absorption. Therapeutic drug monitoring of itraconazole levels should be performed to assess adequacy of drug absorption. Duration of therapy ranges from weeks to several months depending on the severity of illness. Intravenous liposomal amphotericin B, 3 mg/kg/day, is used in patients with more severe illness such as meningitis. Patients with AIDS-related histoplasmosis require lifelong suppressive therapy with itraconazole, 200 mg/day orally, although secondary prophylaxis may be discontinued if immune reconstitution occurs in response to antiretroviral therapy. Criteria for discontinuing secondary prophylaxis include 1 year of successful antifungal therapy and a CD4 cell count of greater than 150 cells/mcL and 6 months or more of antiretroviral treatment (ART). There is no clear evidence that antifungal or anti-inflammatory agents are of benefit for patients with granulomatous mediastinitis or fibrosing mediastinitis although oral itraconazole is often used. Reported outcomes in patients with fibrosing mediastinitis treated with either surgical procedures or nonsurgical intravascular interventions appear to be relatively good.

Azar MM et al. Clinical perspectives in the diagnosis and management of histoplasmosis. Clin Chest Med. 2017 Sep; 38(3):403–15. [PMID: 28797485]
Azar MM et al. Laboratory diagnostics for histoplasmosis. J Clin Microbiol. 2017 Jun;55(6):1612–20. [PMID: 28275076]

COCCIDIOIDOMYCOSIS

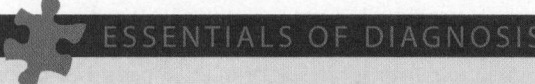

ESSENTIALS OF DIAGNOSIS

- ▶ Influenza-like illness during acute infection: malaise, fever, backache, headache, and cough.
- ▶ Erythema nodosum common with acute infection.
- ▶ Dissemination may result in meningitis, bony lesions, or skin and soft tissue abscesses.
- ▶ Chest radiograph findings vary from pneumonitis to cavitation.
- ▶ Serologic tests useful; large spherules containing endospores demonstrable in sputum or tissues.

▶ General Considerations

Coccidioidomycosis should be considered in the diagnosis of any obscure illness in a patient who has lived in or visited an endemic area. Infection results from the inhalation of arthroconidia of *Coccidioides immitis* or *C posadasii*; both organisms are molds that grow in soil in certain arid regions of the southwestern United States, in Mexico, and in Central and South America. Less than 1% of immunocompetent persons show dissemination, but among these patients, the mortality rate is high.

In HIV-infected people in endemic areas, coccidioidomycosis is a common opportunistic infection. In these patients, disease manifestations range from focal pulmonary infiltrates to widespread miliary disease with multiple organ involvement and meningitis; severity is inversely related to the extent of control of the HIV infection.

Clinical Findings

A. Symptoms and Signs

Symptoms of **primary coccidioidomycosis** occur in about 40% of infections. Symptom onset (after an incubation period of 10–30 days) is usually that of a respiratory tract illness with fever and occasionally chills. Coccidioidomycosis is a common, frequently unrecognized, etiology of community-acquired pneumonia in endemic areas.

Erythema nodosum may appear 2–20 days after onset of symptoms. Persistent pulmonary lesions, varying from cavities and abscesses to parenchymal nodular densities or bronchiectasis, occur in about 5% of diagnosed cases.

Disseminated disease occurs in about 0.1% of white and 1% of nonwhite patients. Filipinos and blacks are especially susceptible, as are pregnant women of all races. Any organ may be involved. Pulmonary findings usually become more pronounced, with mediastinal lymph node enlargement, cough, and increased sputum production. Lung abscesses may rupture into the pleural space, producing an empyema. Complicated skin and bone infections may develop. Fungemia may occur and is characterized clinically by a diffuse miliary pattern on chest radiograph and by early death. The course may be particularly rapid in immunosuppressed patients. Clinicians caring for immunosuppressed patients in endemic areas need to consider that patients may be latently infected.

Meningitis occurs in 30–50% of cases of dissemination and may result in chronic basilar meningitis. Subcutaneous abscesses and verrucous skin lesions are especially common in fulminating cases. HIV-infected persons with disseminated disease have a higher incidence of miliary infiltrates, lymphadenopathy, and meningitis, but skin lesions are uncommon.

B. Laboratory Findings

In **primary coccidioidomycosis**, there may be moderate leukocytosis and eosinophilia. Serologic testing is useful for both diagnosis and prognosis. The immunodiffusion tube precipitin test and enzyme-linked immunosorbent assay (ELISA) detect IgM antibodies and are both useful for diagnosis early in the disease process. A persistently rising IgG complement fixation titer (1:16 or more) is suggestive of disseminated disease; in addition, immunodiffusion complement fixation titers can be used to assess the adequacy of therapy. Serum complement fixation titers may be low when there is meningitis but no other disseminated disease. In patients with HIV-related coccidioidomycosis, the false-negative rate may be as high as 30%. Blood cultures are rarely positive.

Patients in whom coccidioidomycosis is diagnosed should undergo evaluation for meningeal involvement when CNS symptoms or neurologic signs are present. Demonstrable complement-fixing antibodies in spinal fluid are diagnostic of coccidioidal meningitis. These are found in over 90% of cases; *Coccidioides* antigen or (1,3)-beta-D-glucan testing may augment (not replace) CSF antibody testing. Spinal fluid findings include increased cell count with lymphocytosis and reduced glucose. Spinal fluid culture is positive in approximately 30% of meningitis cases.

C. Imaging

Radiographic findings vary, but patchy, nodular, and lobar upper lobe pulmonary infiltrates are most common. Hilar lymphadenopathy may be visible and is seen in localized disease; mediastinal lymphadenopathy suggests dissemination. There may be pleural effusions and lytic lesions in bone with accompanying complicated soft tissue collections.

Treatment

General symptomatic therapy is given as needed for disease limited to the chest with no evidence of progression. Itraconazole, 400 mg orally daily divided into two doses, or fluconazole, 200–400 mg, or higher, orally once or twice daily should be given for disease in the chest, bones, and soft tissues; however, therapy must be continued for 6 months or longer after the disease is inactive to prevent relapse (Table 36–1). Response to therapy should be monitored by following the clinical response and progressive decrease in serum complement fixation titers.

For progressive pulmonary or extrapulmonary disease, liposomal amphotericin B intravenously is used although oral azoles may be used for mild cases. Duration of therapy is determined by a declining complement fixation titer and a favorable clinical response. For meningitis, treatment usually is with high-dose oral fluconazole (400–1200 mg/day), although lumbar or cisternal intrathecal administration of amphotericin B daily in increasing doses up to 1–1.5 mg/day is used initially by some clinicians or in cases refractory to fluconazole. Systemic therapy with liposomal amphotericin B, 3–5 mg/kg/day intravenously, is generally given concurrently with intrathecal therapy, but is not sufficient alone for the treatment of meningeal disease. Once the patient is clinically stable, oral therapy with an azole, usually with fluconazole (400 mg daily) and given lifelong, is the recommended alternative to intrathecal amphotericin B therapy.

Surgical drainage is necessary for management of soft tissue abscesses, necrotic bone, and complicated pulmonary disease (eg, rupture of coccidioidal cavity).

Prognosis

The prognosis for patients with limited disease is good, but persistent pulmonary cavities may cause complications such as hemoptysis or rupture producing pyopneumothorax. Serial complement fixation titers should be performed after therapy for patients with coccidioidomycosis; rising titers warrant reinstitution of therapy because relapse is likely. Late CNS complications of adequately treated meningitis include cerebral vasculitis with stroke and hydrocephalus that may require shunting. There may be a benefit from short-term systemic corticosteroids following cerebrovascular events associated with coccidioides meningitis. Disseminated and meningeal forms still have mortality rates exceeding 50% in the absence of therapy.

Gabe LM et al. Diagnosis and management of coccidioidomycosis. Clin Chest Med. 2017 Sep;38(3):417–33. [PMID: 28797486]

Galgani JN et al. Executive summary: 2016 Infectious Diseases Society of America (IDSA) clinical practice guideline for the treatment of coccidioidomycosis. Clin Infect Dis. 2016 Sep 15;63(6):717–22. [PMID: 27559032]

PNEUMOCYSTOSIS (*Pneumocystis jirovecii* Pneumonia)

ESSENTIALS OF DIAGNOSIS

▶ Fever, dyspnea, dry cough, hypoxia.

▶ Often only slight lung physical findings.

▶ Chest radiograph: diffuse interstitial disease or normal.

▶ *P jirovecii* in sputum, bronchoalveolar lavage fluid, or lung tissue; PCR of bronchoalveolar lavage; (1,3)-beta-D-glucan in blood.

General Considerations

Pneumocystis jirovecii, the *Pneumocystis* species that affects humans, is distributed worldwide. Although symptomatic *P jirovecii* disease is rare in the general population, serologic evidence indicates that asymptomatic infections have occurred in most persons by a young age. Accumulating evidence suggests airborne transmission. Following asymptomatic primary infection, latent and presumably inactive organisms are sparsely distributed in the alveoli. De novo infection and reactivation of latent disease likely contribute to the mechanism of acute disease in older children and adults.

The overt infection is an acute interstitial plasma cell pneumonia that occurs with high frequency among two groups: (1) as epidemics of primary infections among premature infants on hospital wards in underdeveloped parts of the world, and (2) as sporadic cases among older children and adults who have an abnormal or altered cellular immunity, either due to an underlying disease process (eg, cancer, malnutrition, stem cell or organ transplantation or, most commonly, AIDS) or due to treatment with immunosuppressive medications, such as corticosteroids or cytotoxic agents.

Pneumocystis pneumonia occurs in up to 80% of AIDS patients not receiving prophylaxis and is a major cause of death. Its incidence increases in direct proportion to the fall in CD4 cells, with most cases occurring at CD4 cell counts less than 200/mcL. In non-AIDS patients receiving immunosuppressive therapy, symptoms frequently begin after corticosteroids have been tapered or discontinued.

Clinical Findings

A. Symptoms and Signs

Findings are usually limited to the pulmonary parenchyma. In the sporadic form of the disease associated with deficient cell-mediated immunity, the onset may be subacute, characterized by dyspnea on exertion and nonproductive cough. Pulmonary physical findings may be slight and disproportionate to the degree of illness and the radiologic findings; many patients have bibasilar crackles. Without treatment, the course is usually one of rapid deterioration and death. Adult patients may present with spontaneous pneumothorax, usually in patients with previous episodes or those receiving aerosolized pentamidine prophylaxis. Patients with AIDS will usually have other evidence of HIV-associated disease, including fever, fatigue, and weight loss, for weeks or months preceding the illness.

B. Laboratory Findings

Chest radiographs most often show diffuse "interstitial" infiltration, which may be heterogeneous, miliary, or patchy early in infection. There may also be diffuse or focal consolidation, cystic changes, nodules, or cavitation within nodules. Pleural effusions are not seen. About 5–10% of patients with *Pneumocystis* pneumonia have normal chest films. High-resolution chest CT scans may be quite suggestive of *P jirovecii* pneumonia, helping distinguish it from other causes of pneumonia.

Arterial blood gas determinations usually show hypoxemia with hypocapnia but may be normal; however, rapid desaturation occurs if patients exercise before samples are drawn. Serologic tests are not helpful in diagnosis; measurement of serum (1,3)-beta-D-glucan levels has good sensitivity, although specificity is compromised by being positive in other fungal infections. The organism cannot be cultured, and definitive diagnosis depends on morphologic demonstration of the organisms in respiratory specimens using specific stains, such as immunofluorescence. Polymerase chain reaction (PCR) of bronchoalveolar lavage is overly sensitive in that the test can be positive in colonized, noninfected persons but quantitative values may help with identifying infected patients, although precise cutoffs have not been established. A negative PCR from bronchoalveolar lavage rules out disease. Open lung biopsy and needle lung biopsy are infrequently done but may need to be performed to diagnose a granulomatous form of *Pneumocystis* pneumonia.

Treatment

(See Table 31–3.) It is appropriate to start empiric therapy for *P jirovecii* pneumonia if the disease is suspected clinically; however, in both AIDS patients and non-AIDS patients with mild to moderately severe disease, continued treatment should be based on a proved diagnosis because of clinical overlap with other infections, the toxicity of therapy, and the possible coexistence of other infectious organisms. Oral trimethoprim-sulfamethoxazole (TMP-SMZ) is the preferred agent because of its low cost and excellent bioavailability in both AIDS patients and non-AIDS patients with mild to moderately severe disease. Patients suffering from nausea and vomiting or intractable diarrhea should be given intravenous TMP-SMZ until they can tolerate the oral formulation. The best-studied second-line option is a combination of primaquine and clindamycin, although dapsone/trimethoprim, pentamidine, and atovaquone have also been used. Therapy should be continued with the selected medication for at least 5–10 days before considering changing agents, as fever, tachypnea, and pulmonary infiltrates persist for 4–6 days after starting treatment. Some patients have a transient worsening of their disease during the first 3–5 days, which may be related to an inflammatory response secondary to the presence of dead or dying organisms. Early addition of corticosteroids may attenuate this response (see below). Some clinicians prefer to treat episodes of AIDS-associated *Pneumocystis* pneumonia for 21 days rather than the usual 14 days recommended for non-AIDS cases.

A. Trimethoprim-Sulfamethoxazole

The dosage of TMP/SMZ is 15–20 mg/kg/day (based on trimethoprim component) given orally or intravenously daily in three or four divided doses for 14–21 days. Patients with AIDS have a high frequency of hypersensitivity reactions (approaching 50%), which may include fever, rashes (sometimes severe), malaise, neutropenia, hepatitis, nephritis, thrombocytopenia, hyperkalemia, and hyperbilirubinemia.

B. Primaquine/Clindamycin

A meta-analysis suggested that primaquine, 15–30 mg/day, plus clindamycin, 600 mg three times daily, is the best second-line therapy with superior results when compared with pentamidine. Primaquine may cause hemolytic anemia in patients with glucose-6-phosphate dehydrogenase (G6PD) deficiency.

C. Pentamidine Isethionate

The use of pentamidine has decreased as alternative agents have been studied. This medication is administered intravenously (preferred) or intramuscularly as a single dose of 3–4 mg (salt)/kg/day for 14–21 days. Pentamidine causes side effects in nearly 50% of patients. Hypoglycemia (often clinically inapparent), hyperglycemia, hyponatremia, and delayed nephrotoxicity with azotemia may occur.

D. Atovaquone

Atovaquone is FDA approved for patients with mild to moderate disease who cannot tolerate TMP-SMZ or pentamidine, but failure is reported in 15–30% of cases. Mild side effects are common, but no serious reactions have been reported. The dosage is 750 mg three times daily for 21 days. Atovaquone should be administered with a fatty meal.

E. Other Medications

Trimethoprim, 15 mg/kg/day in three divided doses daily, plus dapsone, 100 mg/day, is an alternative oral regimen for mild to moderate disease or for continuation of therapy after intravenous therapy is no longer needed.

F. Prednisone

Based on studies done in patients with AIDS, prednisone is given for moderate to severe pneumonia (when Pao_2 on admission is less than 70 mm Hg or oxygen saturation is less than 90%) in conjunction with antimicrobials. The dosage of prednisone is 40 mg twice daily orally for 5 days, then 40 mg daily for 5 days, and then 20 mg daily until therapy is completed. The role of prednisone in non-AIDS patients is less clear, although a 2018 large observational study suggested that adjunctive corticosteroids were associated with reduced mortality in non-AIDS patients with *Pneumocystis* pneumonia and severe hypoxia (Pao_2 60 mm Hg or less).

Prevention

Primary prophylaxis for *Pneumocystis* pneumonia in HIV-infected patients should be given to persons with CD4 counts less than 200 cells/mcL, a CD4 percentage below 14%, or weight loss or oral candidiasis (see Table 31–6). Primary prophylaxis is often used in patients with hematologic malignancy and transplant recipients, although the clinical characteristics of persons with these conditions who would benefit from *Pneumocystis* prophylaxis have not been clearly defined. Patients with a history of *Pneumocystis* pneumonia should receive secondary prophylaxis until they have had a durable virologic response to antiretroviral therapy for at least 3–6 months and maintained a CD4 count of greater than 200 cells/mcL.

Prognosis

In the absence of early and adequate treatment, the fatality rate for the endemic infantile form of *Pneumocystis* pneumonia is 20–50%; for the sporadic form in immunodeficient persons, the fatality rate is nearly 100%. Early treatment reduces the mortality rate to about 3% in the former and 10–20% in AIDS patients. The mortality rate in other immunodeficient patients is still 30–50%, probably because of failure to make a timely diagnosis. In immunodeficient patients who do not receive prophylaxis, recurrences are common (30% in AIDS).

Inoue N et al. Adjunctive corticosteroids decreased the risk of mortality of non-HIV pneumocystis pneumonia. Int J Infect Dis. 2019 Feb;79:109–15. [PMID: 30529109]
White PL et al. Therapy and management of *Pneumocystis jirovecii* infection. J Fungi (Basel). 2018 Nov 22;4(4):E127. [PMID: 30469526]

CRYPTOCOCCOSIS

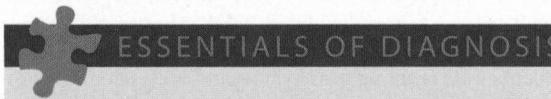

ESSENTIALS OF DIAGNOSIS

- ▶ Most common cause of fungal meningitis.
- ▶ Predisposing factors: chemotherapy for hematologic malignancies, Hodgkin lymphoma, corticosteroid therapy, transplant recipients, TNF-alpha inhibitor therapy, and HIV infection.
- ▶ Headache, abnormal mental status; meningismus seen occasionally, though rarely in HIV-infected patients.
- ▶ Demonstration of capsular polysaccharide antigen or positive culture in CSF is diagnostic.

General Considerations

Cryptococcosis is mainly caused by *Cryptococcus neoformans*, an encapsulated budding yeast that has been found worldwide in soil and on dried pigeon dung. *C gattii* is a closely related species that also causes disease in humans, although *C gattii* may affect more ostensibly immunocompetent persons. It is a major cause of cryptococcosis in the Pacific northwestern region of the United States and may result in more severe disease than *C neoformans*.

Infections are acquired by inhalation. In the lung, the infection may remain localized, heal, or disseminate. Clinically apparent cryptococcal pneumonia rarely develops in immunocompetent persons. Progressive lung disease and dissemination most often occur in the setting of cellular immunodeficiency, including underlying hematologic malignancies under treatment, Hodgkin lymphoma, long-term corticosteroid therapy, solid-organ transplant, TNF-alpha inhibitor therapy, or HIV infection.

Clinical Findings

A. Symptoms and Signs

Pulmonary disease ranges from simple nodules to widespread infiltrates leading to respiratory failure. Disseminated disease may involve any organ, but CNS disease predominates. Headache is usually the first symptom of meningitis. Confusion and other mental status changes as well as cranial nerve abnormalities, nausea, and vomiting may be seen as the disease progresses. Nuchal rigidity and meningeal signs occur about 50% of the time but are uncommon in HIV-infected patients. Communicating hydrocephalus may complicate the course. *C gattii* infection frequently presents with respiratory symptoms along with neurologic signs caused by space-occupying lesions in the CNS. Primary *C neoformans* infection of the skin may mimic bacterial cellulitis, especially in persons receiving immunosuppressive therapy such as corticosteroids. Paradoxical clinical worsening associated with improved immunologic status has been reported in HIV-positive and transplant patients with cryptococcosis; this entity has been labeled the immune reconstitution inflammatory syndrome (IRIS).

B. Laboratory Findings

Respiratory tract disease is diagnosed by culture of respiratory secretions or pleural fluid. For suspected meningeal disease, lumbar puncture is the preferred diagnostic procedure. Spinal fluid findings include increased opening pressure, variable pleocytosis, increased protein, and decreased glucose, though as many as 50% of AIDS patients have no pleocytosis. Gram stain of the CSF usually reveals budding, encapsulated fungi. Cryptococcal capsular antigen in CSF and culture together establish the diagnosis over 90% of the time. Patients with AIDS often have the antigen in both CSF and serum, and extrameningeal disease (lungs, blood, urinary tract) is common. In patients with AIDS, the serum cryptococcal antigen is also a sensitive screening test for meningitis, being positive in over 95% of cases. MRI is more sensitive than CT in finding CNS abnormalities such as cryptococcomas. Antigen testing by lateral flow assay appears to have improved sensitivity and specificity over the conventional latex agglutination test and can provide more rapid diagnostic results.

Treatment

Because of decreased efficacy, initial therapy with an azole alone is not recommended for treatment of acute cryptococcal meningitis. Liposomal amphotericin B, 3–4 mg/kg/day intravenously for 14 days, is the preferred agent for induction therapy, followed by an additional 8 weeks of fluconazole, 400 mg/day orally (Table 36–1). This regimen is quite effective, achieving clinical responses and CSF sterilization in about 70% of patients. The addition of flucytosine has been associated with improved survival, but toxicity is common. Flucytosine is administered orally at a dose of 100 mg/kg/day divided into four equal doses and given every 6 hours. Hematologic parameters should be closely monitored during flucytosine therapy, and it is important to adjust the dose for any decreases in kidney function. Fluconazole (800–1200 mg orally daily) may be given with amphotericin B when flucytosine is not available or patients cannot tolerate it. Frequent, repeated lumbar punctures or ventricular shunting should be performed to relieve high CSF pressures or if hydrocephalus is a complication. Corticosteroids should not be used. *Failure to adequately relieve raised intracranial pressure is a major cause of morbidity and mortality.* The end points for amphotericin B therapy and for switching to oral fluconazole are a favorable clinical response (decrease in temperature; improvement in headache, nausea, vomiting, and Mini-Mental State Examination scores), improvement in CSF biochemical parameters and, most importantly, conversion of CSF culture to negative.

A similar approach is reasonable for patients with cryptococcal meningitis in the absence of AIDS, though the mortality rate is higher. Therapy is generally continued until CSF cultures become negative. Maintenance antifungal therapy is important after treatment of an acute episode in HIV-related cases, since otherwise the rate of relapse is greater than 50%. Fluconazole, 200 mg/day orally, is the maintenance therapy of choice, decreasing the relapse rate approximately tenfold compared with placebo and threefold compared with weekly amphotericin B in patients whose CSF has been sterilized by the induction therapy. After successful therapy of cryptococcal meningitis, it is possible to discontinue secondary prophylaxis with fluconazole in individuals with AIDS who have had a satisfactory response to antiretroviral therapy (eg, CD4 cell count greater than 100–200 cells/mcL for at least 6 months). Among clinicians treating patients without AIDS, there has been a trend in recent years to prescribe a course (eg, 6–12 months) of fluconazole as maintenance therapy following successful treatment of the acute illness; published guidelines suggest this as an option.

Prognosis

Factors that indicate a poor prognosis include the activity of the predisposing conditions, older age, organ failure, lack of spinal fluid pleocytosis, high initial antigen titer in either serum or CSF, decreased mental status, increased intracranial pressure, and the presence of disease outside the nervous system.

Maziarz EK et al. Cryptococcosis. Infect Dis Clin North Am. 2016 Mar;30(1):179–206. [PMID: 26897067]

Mourad A et al. Present and future therapy of *Cryptococcus* infections. J Fungi (Basel). 2018 Jul 3;4(3): E79. [PMID: 29970809]

Setianingrum F et al. Pulmonary cryptococcosis: a review of pathobiology and clinical aspects. Med Mycol. 2019 Feb 1; 57(2):133–50. [PMID: 30329097]

ASPERGILLOSIS

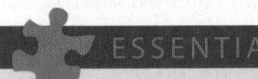

ESSENTIALS OF DIAGNOSIS

▶ Most common cause of non-candidal invasive fungal infection in transplant recipients and in patients with hematologic malignancies.

▶ Predisposing factors: leukemia, bone marrow or organ transplant, late HIV infection.

▶ Pulmonary, sinus, and CNS are most common disease sites.

▶ Detection of galactomannan by ELISA or PCR in serum or other body fluids is useful for early diagnosis and treatment.

General Considerations

Aspergillus fumigatus is the usual cause of aspergillosis, though many species of *Aspergillus* may cause a wide spectrum of disease. The lungs, sinuses, and brain are the organs most often involved. Clinical illness results either from an aberrant immunologic response or tissue invasion.

Clinical Findings

A. Symptoms and Signs

1. Allergic forms of aspergillosis—Allergic bronchopulmonary aspergillosis (ABPA) occurs in patients with preexisting asthma or cystic fibrosis who develop worsening bronchospasm and fleeting pulmonary infiltrates accompanied by eosinophilia, high levels of IgE, and IgG *Aspergillus* precipitins in the blood. Allergic aspergillus sinusitis produces a chronic sinus inflammation characterized by eosinophilic mucus and noninvasive hyphal elements.

2. Chronic aspergillosis—Chronic pulmonary aspergillosis produces a spectrum of disease that usually occurs when there is preexisting lung damage but not significant immunocompromise. Disease manifestations range from aspergillomas that develop in a lung cavity to chronic fibrosing pulmonary aspergillosis in which the majority of lung tissue is replaced with fibrosis. Long-standing (longer than 3 months) pulmonary and systemic symptoms such as cough, shortness of breath, weight loss, and malaise are common.

3. Invasive aspergillosis—Invasive aspergillosis most commonly occurs in profoundly immunodeficient patients, such as those who have undergone hematopoietic stem cell transplantation or have prolonged, severe neutropenia, but it can occur among critically ill immunocompetent patients as well. Specific risk factors in patients who have undergone a hematopoietic stem cell transplant include cytopenias, corticosteroid use, iron overload, cytomegalovirus disease, and graft-versus-host disease. Pulmonary disease is most common, with patchy infiltration leading to a severe necrotizing pneumonia. Invasive sinus disease also occurs. At any time, there may be hematogenous dissemination to the CNS, skin, and other organs. Early diagnosis and reversal of any correctable immunosuppression are essential.

B. Laboratory Findings

There is eosinophilia, high levels of total IgE, and IgE and IgG specific for *Aspergillus* in the blood of patients with ABPA.

Blood cultures have very low yield in any form of aspergillosis. Detection of galactomannan by ELISA or *Aspergillus* DNA by PCR, or both, has been used for the early diagnosis of invasive disease, though multiple determinations should be done and usefulness is decreased in patients receiving anti-mold prophylaxis (ie, voriconazole or posaconazole). Galactomannan levels and *Aspergillus* DNA PCR can be tested in serum or in bronchoalveolar lavage fluid, which may be more sensitive than serum. Higher galactomannan levels are correlated with increased mortality, and failure of galactomannan levels to fall in response to therapy portends a worse outcome. Isolation of *Aspergillus* from pulmonary secretions does not necessarily imply invasive disease, although its positive predictive value increases with more advanced immunosuppression. Therefore, a definitive diagnosis requires demonstration of *Aspergillus* in tissue or culture from a sterile site. CT scan of the chest may show characteristics quite suggestive of invasive aspergillosis (eg, "halo sign," which is a zone of diminution of ground glass around a consolidation).

Prevention

The high mortality rate and difficulty in diagnosis of invasive aspergillosis often lead clinicians to institute prophylactic therapy for patients with profound immunosuppression. The best-studied agents include voriconazole and posaconazole, although patient and agent selection criteria remain undefined. Widespread use of broad-spectrum azoles raises concern for development of invasive disease by highly resistant fungi.

Treatment

1. Allergic forms of aspergillosis—Itraconazole is the best studied agent for the treatment of allergic aspergillus sinusitis with topical corticosteroids being the cornerstone of therapy for ongoing care. For acute exacerbations of ABPA, oral prednisone is begun at a dose of 0.5 mg/kg/day and then tapered slowly over several months. Itraconazole at a dose of 200 mg orally daily for 16 weeks appears to improve pulmonary function and decrease corticosteroid requirements in these patients, although voriconazole is increasingly being used (Table 36–1).

2. Chronic aspergillosis—The most effective therapy for symptomatic aspergilloma remains surgical resection. Other forms of chronic aspergillosis are generally treated with at least 4–6 months of oral azole therapy (itraconazole 200 mg twice daily, voriconazole 200 mg twice daily, or posaconazole 300 mg daily).

3. Invasive aspergillosis—The 2016 Infectious Diseases Society of America guidelines consider voriconazole (6 mg/kg intravenously twice on day 1 and then 4 mg/kg every 12 hours thereafter) as optimal therapy for invasive aspergillosis. A randomized controlled trial did not find an overall benefit with the addition of anidulafungin (200 mg on day 1 and then 100 mg daily) to voriconazole, but among patients in whom galactomannan was detected, those who received combination therapy had better outcomes. Isavuconazole (372 mg of prodrug on days 1 and 2 and then 372 mg once daily) was equivalent to voriconazole. Alternatives include a lipid formulation of amphotericin B (3–5 mg/kg/day), caspofungin (70 mg intravenously on day 1 and then 50 mg/day thereafter), and posaconazole oral tablets (300 mg twice daily on day 1 and then 300 mg daily thereafter). Oral dosing of voriconazole at 4 mg/kg twice daily can be used for less serious infections or as a step-down strategy after intravenous therapy. Therapeutic drug monitoring should be considered for both voriconazole and posaconazole given variations in metabolism and absorption.

Surgical debridement is generally done for sinusitis, and can be useful for focal pulmonary lesions, especially for treatment of life-threatening hemoptysis and infections recalcitrant to medical therapy. The mortality rate of pulmonary or disseminated disease in the immunocompromised patient remains high, particularly in patients with refractory neutropenia.

Gago S et al. Pathophysiological aspects of *Aspergillus* colonization in disease. Med Mycol. 2019 Apr 1;57(Supplement 2):S219–227. [PMID: 30239804]

Jenks JD et al. Treatment of aspergillosis. J Fungi (Basel). 2018 Aug 19;4(3):E98. [PMID: 30126229]

Kanj A et al. The spectrum of pulmonary aspergillosis. Respir Med. 2018 Aug;141:121–31. [PMID: 30053957]

Takazono T et al. Recent advances in diagnosing chronic pulmonary aspergillosis. Front Microbiol. 2018 Aug 17;9:1810. [PMID: 30174658]

MUCORMYCOSIS

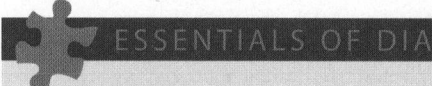

ESSENTIALS OF DIAGNOSIS

▶ Most common cause of non-*Aspergillus* invasive mold infection.

▶ Predisposing factors: poorly controlled diabetes, leukemia, transplant recipient, wound contamination by soil.

▶ Pulmonary, rhinocerebral, and skin are most common disease sites.

▶ Rapidly fatal without multidisciplinary interventions.

General Considerations

The term "mucormycosis" is applied to opportunistic infections caused by members of the genera *Rhizopus, Mucor, Lichtheimia* (formerly *Absidia*), and *Cunninghamella*. Predisposing conditions include hematologic malignancy, stem cell transplantation, solid organ transplantation, diabetic ketoacidosis, chronic kidney disease, and treatment with desferoxamine, corticosteroids, or cytotoxic drugs.

Clinical Findings

Invasive disease of the sinuses, orbits, and the lungs may occur. Necrosis is common due to hyphal tissue invasion that may manifest as ulceration of the hard palate or nasal palate or hemoptysis. Widely disseminated disease can occur. No serologic or laboratory findings assist with diagnosis, and blood cultures are unhelpful. A reverse "halo sign" (focal area of ground glass diminution surrounded by a ring of consolidation) may be seen on chest CT. Biopsy of involved tissue remains the cornerstone of diagnosis, although cultures are frequently negative. The organisms appear in tissues as broad, branching nonseptate hyphae.

Treatment

Optimal therapy of mucormycosis involves reversal of predisposing conditions (if possible), surgical debridement, and prompt antifungal therapy. A prolonged course of a lipid preparation of intravenous liposomal amphotericin B (5 mg/kg with higher doses possibly given for CNS disease) should be started early (Table 36–1). Depending on in vitro susceptibility, posaconazole 300 mg/day orally can be used after disease has been stabilized. Combination therapy with amphotericin and posaconazole is not proven but is commonly used because of the poor response to monotherapy. Other azoles are not effective. There are limited data suggesting beneficial synergistic activity when amphotericin and caspofungin are used in combination for rhino-orbital mucormycosis in diabetic patients. Despite favorable animal studies, a pilot study in humans incorporating adjunctive iron chelation therapy with deferasirox demonstrated a higher mortality rate than antifungal therapy alone. Control of diabetes and other underlying conditions, along with extensive repeated surgical removal of necrotic, nonperfused tissue, is essential. Even when these measures are introduced in a timely fashion, the prognosis remains guarded.

Sipsas NV et al. Therapy of mucormycosis. J Fungi (Basel). 2018 Jul 31;4(3):E90. [PMID: 30065232]

Skiada A et al. Challenges in the diagnosis and treatment of mucormycosis. Med Mycol. 2018 Apr 1;56(Suppl 1):93–101. [PMID: 29538730]

BLASTOMYCOSIS

Blastomycosis occurs most often in men infected during occupational or recreational activities outdoors and in a geographically limited area of the south central and midwestern United States and Canada. Disease usually occurs in immunocompetent individuals.

Chronic pulmonary infection is most common and may be asymptomatic. When dissemination takes place, lesions are most frequently seen in the skin, bones, and urogenital system.

Cough, moderate fever, dyspnea, and chest pain are common. These may resolve or progress, with purulent sputum production, pleurisy, fever, chills, loss of weight, and prostration. Radiologic studies, either chest radiographs or CT scans, usually reveal lobar consolidation or masses.

Raised, verrucous cutaneous lesions are commonly present in disseminated blastomycosis. Bones—often the ribs and vertebrae—are frequently involved. Epididymitis, prostatitis, and other involvement of the male urogenital system may occur. Although they do not appear to be at greater risk for acquisition of disease, infection in HIV-infected persons may progress rapidly, with dissemination common.

Laboratory findings usually include leukocytosis and anemia, though these are not specific. The organism is found in clinical specimens, such as expectorated sputum or tissue biopsies, as a thick-walled cell 5–20 mcm in diameter that may have a single broad-based bud. It grows readily on culture. A urinary antigen test is available, but it has considerable cross reactivity with other dimorphic fungi; it may be useful in monitoring disease resolution or progression. A serum enzyme immunoassay based on the surface protein BAD-1 has much better sensitivity and specificity than the urinary antigen test, but it is not yet commercially available.

Itraconazole, 200–400 mg/day orally for at least 6–12 months, is the therapy of choice for nonmeningeal disease, with a response rate of over 80% (Table 36–1). Liposomal amphotericin B, 3–5 mg/kg/day intravenously, is given initially for severe disease, treatment failures, or CNS involvement.

Clinical follow-up for relapse should be made regularly for several years so that therapy may be resumed or another drug instituted.

McBride JA et al. Clinical manifestations and treatment of blastomycosis. Clin Chest Med. 2017 Sep;38(3):435–49. [PMID: 28797487]

PARACOCCIDIOIDOMYCOSIS (South American Blastomycosis)

Paracoccidioides brasiliensis and *Paracoccidioides lutzii* infections have been found only in patients who have resided in South or Central America or Mexico. Long asymptomatic periods enable patients to travel far from the endemic areas before developing clinical problems. An acute form of the disease affects predominately younger patients and involves the mononuclear phagocytic system, resulting in progressive lymphadenopathy. A more chronic form affects mostly adult men and involves the lung, skin, mucous membranes, and lymph nodes. Weight loss, pulmonary complaints, or mucosal ulcerations are the most common symptoms. Extensive coalescent ulcerations may eventually result in destruction of the epiglottis, vocal cords, and uvula. Extension to the lips and face may occur. Lymph node enlargement may follow mucocutaneous lesions, eventually ulcerating and forming draining sinuses; in some patients, it is the presenting symptom. Hepatosplenomegaly may be present as well. HIV-infected patients with paracoccidioidomycosis are more likely to have extrapulmonary dissemination and a more rapid clinical disease course.

Laboratory findings are nonspecific. Serology by immunodiffusion is positive in more than 80% of cases. Complement fixation titers correlate with progressive disease and fall with effective therapy. The fungus is found in clinical specimens as a spherical cell that may have many buds arising from it. If direct examination of secretions does not reveal the organism, biopsy with Gomori staining may be helpful.

Itraconazole, 100 mg twice daily orally, is the treatment of choice and generally results in a clinical response within 1 month and effective control after 2–6 months. TMP-SMZ (480 mg/1200 mg) twice daily orally is equally effective and less costly but associated with more adverse effects and longer time to clinical cure. Amphotericin B, 0.7–1.0 mg/kg/day intravenously, is the medication of choice for severe and life-threatening infection.

Nery AF et al. Therapeutic response in adult patients with non-severe chronic paracoccidioidomycosis treated with sulfamethoxazole-trimethoprim: a retrospective study. Am J Trop Med Hyg. 2017 Aug;97(2):556–62. [PMID: 28722596]

Shikanai-Yasuda MA et al. Brazilian guidelines for the clinical management of paracoccidioidomycosis. Rev Soc Bras Med Trop. 2017 Sep–Oct;50(5):715–40. [PMID: 28746570]

SPOROTRICHOSIS

Sporotrichosis is a chronic fungal infection caused by organisms of the *Sporothrix schenckii* complex. It is worldwide in distribution; most patients have had contact with soil, sphagnum moss, or decaying wood. Infection takes place when the organism is inoculated into the skin—usually on the hand, arm, or foot, especially during gardening.

The most common form of sporotrichosis begins with a hard, nontender subcutaneous nodule. This later becomes adherent to the overlying skin and ulcerates. Within a few days to weeks, lymphocutaneous spread along the lymphatics draining this area occurs, which may result in ulceration. Cavitary pulmonary disease occurs in individuals with underlying chronic lung disease.

Disseminated sporotrichosis is rare in immunocompetent persons but may present with widespread cutaneous, lung, bone, joint, and CNS involvement in immunocompromised patients, especially those with cellular immunodeficiencies, including AIDS and alcohol abuse.

Cultures are needed to establish diagnosis. The usefulness of serologic tests is limited, but may be helpful in diagnosing disseminated disease, especially meningitis.

Itraconazole, 200–400 mg orally daily for several months, is the treatment of choice for localized disease and some milder cases of disseminated disease (Table 36–1). Terbinafine, 500 mg orally twice daily, also appears to have good efficacy in lymphocutaneous disease. Amphotericin B intravenously, 0.7–1.0 mg/kg/day, or a lipid amphotericin B preparation, 3–5 mg/kg/day are used for severe systemic infection. Surgery may be indicated for complicated pulmonary cavitary disease, and joint involvement may require arthrodesis.

The prognosis is good for lymphocutaneous sporotrichosis; pulmonary, joint, and disseminated disease respond less favorably.

Orofino-Costa R et al. Sporotrichosis: an update on epidemiology, etiopathogenesis, laboratory and clinical therapeutics. An Bras Dermatol. 2017 Sep–Oct;92(5):606–20. [PMID: 29166494]

MYCETOMA (Eumycetoma & Actinomycetoma)

Mycetoma is a chronic local, slowly progressive destructive infection that usually involves the foot; it begins in subcutaneous tissues, frequently after implantation trauma, and then spreads to contiguous structures with sinus tracts and extruding grains. Eumycetoma (also known as maduromycosis) is the term used to describe mycetoma caused by true fungi. The disease begins as a papule, nodule, or abscess that over months to years progresses slowly to form multiple abscesses and sinus tracts ramifying deep into the tissue. Secondary bacterial infection may result in large open ulcers. Radiographs may show destructive changes in the underlying bone. Causative species can often be suggested by the color of the characteristic grains and hyphal size within the infected tissues but definitive diagnosis requires culture.

The prognosis for eumycetoma is poor, though surgical debridement along with prolonged oral itraconazole therapy, 200 mg twice daily, or combination therapy including itraconazole and terbinafine may result in a response rate of 70% (Table 36–1). The various etiologic agents may respond differently to antifungal agents, so culture results are invaluable. Amputation is necessary in far advanced cases.

Relhan V et al. Mycetoma: an update. Indian J Dermatol. 2017 Jul–Aug;62(4):332–40. [PMID: 28794542]
van de Sande W et al. Closing the mycetoma knowledge gap. Med Mycol. 2018 Apr 1;56(Suppl 1):153–64. [PMID: 28992217]

OTHER OPPORTUNISTIC MOLD INFECTIONS

Fungi previously considered to be harmless colonizers, including *Pseudallescheria boydii* (*Scedosporium apiospermum*), *Scedosporium prolificans*, *Fusarium*, *Paecilomyces*, *Trichoderma longibrachiatum*, and *Trichosporon*, are now significant pathogens in immunocompromised patients. This occurs most often in patients being treated for hematopoietic malignancies and in those receiving broad-spectrum antifungal prophylaxis. Infection may be localized in the skin, lungs, or sinuses, or widespread disease may appear with lesions in multiple organs. Fusariosis should be suspected in severely immunosuppressed persons in whom multiple, painful skin lesions develop; blood cultures are often positive. Sinus infection may cause bony erosion. Infection in subcutaneous tissues following traumatic implantation may develop as a well-circumscribed cyst or as an ulcer.

Nonpigmented septate hyphae are seen in tissue and are indistinguishable from those of *Aspergillus* when infections are due to *S apiospermum* or species of *Fusarium*, *Paecilomyces*, *Penicillium*, or other hyaline molds. Spores or mycetoma-like granules are rarely present in tissue. The differentiation of *S apiospermum* and *Aspergillus* is particularly important, since the former is uniformly resistant to amphotericin B but may be sensitive to azole antifungals (eg, voriconazole). Infection by any of a number of black molds is designated as phaeohyphomycosis. These black molds (eg, *Exophiala*, *Bipolaris*, *Cladophialophora*, *Curvularia*, *Alternaria*) are common in the environment, especially on decaying vegetation. In tissues of patients with phaeohyphomycosis, the mold is seen as black or faintly brown hyphae, yeast cells, or both. Culture on appropriate medium is needed to identify the agent. Histologic demonstration of these organisms is definitive evidence of invasive infection; positive cultures must be interpreted cautiously and not assumed to be contaminants in immunocompromised hosts.

McCarthy MW et al. Recent advances in the treatment of scedosporiosis and fusariosis. J Fungi (Basel). 2018 Jun 18;4(2):E73. [PMID: 29912161]

HOUSEHOLD MOLDS

ESSENTIALS OF DIAGNOSIS

▶ Molds are very common indoors where moisture exists in enclosed spaces.

▶ Most common indoor molds are *Cladosporium*, *Penicillium*, *Aspergillus*, and *Alternaria*.

▶ People most at risk for health problems include those with allergies, asthma, and underlying immunocompromising conditions.

Molds are commonly present in homes, particularly in the presence of moisture, and patients will commonly seek assessment for whether their illness is due to molds. Invasive disease due to environmental fungi can occur in the immunocompromised patient (eg, see section on Invasive Aspergillosis), but there are no data that mold exposure can induce immune dysfunction. Similarly, the concept of toxic-mold syndrome or cognitive impairment due to inhalation of mycotoxins has not been validated despite scrutiny by expert panels. Allergic symptoms (eg, asthma, hypersensitivity pneumonitis) can be worsened by environmental mold exposure, and reduction of household mold in such patients may lead to clinical improvement. The presence of mold in the household is typically easily discernable with visual inspection or detection by odor; if present, predisposing conditions should be corrected by individuals experienced in mold remediation.

Borchers AT et al. Mold and human health: a reality check. Clin Rev Allerg Immunol. 2017 Jun;52(3):305–22. [PMID: 28299723]

ANTIFUNGAL THERAPY

Table 36–1 summarizes the major properties of currently available antifungal agents. Two different lipid-based amphotericin B formulations are used to treat systemic invasive fungal infections. Their principal advantage appears to be substantially reduced nephrotoxicity, allowing administration of much higher doses. Three agents of the echinocandin class, caspofungin acetate, anidulafungin, and micafungin sodium, are approved for use. The echinocandins have relatively few adverse effects and are useful for the treatment of invasive *Candida* infections, although resistance is beginning to emerge clinically; *C glabrata* in particular has shown resistance to this class of antifungals. Caspofungin acetate is also approved for use in refractory cases of invasive aspergillosis. Voriconazole has excellent activity against a broad range of fungal pathogens and has been FDA approved for use in invasive *Aspergillus* cases, *Fusarium* and *Scedosporium* infections, *Candida* esophagitis, deep *Candida* infections, and candidemia. Posaconazole has good activity against a broad range of filamentous fungi, including the *Mucorales*. Some experts recommend therapeutic drug monitoring in individuals with severe invasive fungal infections receiving these newer azoles because of unreliable serum levels due to either metabolic alterations as a result of genetic polymorphisms (voriconazole) or erratic absorption (posaconazole). A delayed-release tablet preparation of posaconazole provides more reliable pharmacokinetics. Isavuconazole has been approved for the treatment of aspergillosis and mucormycosis, although the data for use in the latter are scanty; it is available in an intravenous form that does not utilize the cyclodextrin carrier like previous azoles as well as an oral form with relatively reliable pharmacokinetic properties.

Nett JE et al. Antifungal agents: spectrum of activity, pharmacology, and clinical indications. Infect Dis Clin North Am. 2016 Mar; 30(1):51–83. [PMID: 26739608]

Seyedmousavi S et al. Systemic Antifungal Agents: Current Status and Projected Future Developments. In: Lion T (editor). *Human Fungal Pathogen Identification: Methods and Protocols.* Humana Press, 2017.

Disorders Related to Environmental Emergencies

Jacqueline A. Nemer, MD, FACEP

Marianne A. Juarez, MD

COLD & HEAT

The human body maintains a steady temperature through the balance of internal heat production and environmental heat loss. Heat exchange between the body and environment occurs via four common processes: radiation, evaporation, conduction, and convection. In extreme temperatures, the body's thermoregulation may fail. This results in the core body temperature moving toward the temperature of the external environment. Cold and heat exposure may cause a wide spectrum of conditions that can lead to death; the severity varies considerably among individuals. Many of these conditions are preventable with appropriate education and planning. Preventive measures must be implemented on an individual and population level.

The likelihood and severity of extreme temperature-related conditions depend on physiologic and environmental factors. Physiologic risk factors include extremes of age; cognitive impairment; poor physical conditioning, sedentary lifestyle or immobility; poor acclimatization; concurrent injury; prior temperature-related injury; and numerous underlying medical conditions, especially those affecting cognition and thermoregulation. Pharmacologic risk factors include medications, holistic or alternative treatments, illicit drugs, tobacco, and alcohol. There is a subset of medications associated with a particularly high likelihood of worsening temperature-related conditions, such as those that impact sweating and the central nervous system and those that affect cutaneous blood flow such as peripheral vasoconstrictors or vasodilators. Environmental risk factors include changing weather conditions, inadequate clothing or housing (homelessness, or housing with inadequate temperature control), and occupational or recreational exposure.

DISORDERS DUE TO HEAT

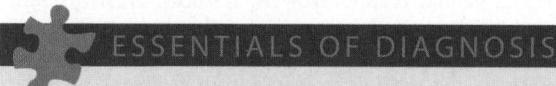

ESSENTIALS OF DIAGNOSIS

► Spectrum of preventable heat-related illnesses: heat cramps, heat exhaustion, heat syncope, and heat stroke.

► **Heat stroke:** hyperthermia with cerebral dysfunction in a patient with heat exposure.

► **Best outcome:** early recognition, initiation of rapid cooling, and avoidance of shivering during cooling.

► **Best choice of cooling method:** whichever can be instituted the fastest with the least compromise to the patient. Delays in cooling result in higher morbidity and mortality in heat stroke victims.

► General Considerations

Heat-related illnesses are among the most commonly seen environmental emergencies presenting to emergency departments. The amount of heat retained in the body is determined by internal metabolic function and environmental conditions, including temperature and humidity. Hyperthermia results from the body's inability to maintain normal internal temperature through heat loss. Hyperthermia results from either compromised heat dissipation mechanisms or abnormally high heat production. Heat loss occurs primarily through sweating and peripheral vasodilation. The direct transfer of heat from the skin to the surrounding air, by convection or conduction, occurs with diminishing efficiency as ambient temperature rises, especially above 37.2°C, at which point heat transfer reverses direction. At normal temperatures, evaporation accounts for approximately 20% of the body's heat loss, but at high temperatures it becomes the major mechanism for dissipation of heat. This mechanism diminishes as humidity rises.

Heat stress can be caused by a combination of environmental heat and metabolic heat. For children under the age of 15, heat stroke is the largest cause of non-accident–related deaths in cars. This is despite substantial campaigns and preventive devices to alert drivers to check the back seat when turning off the car. Climate change may significantly contribute to the risk of heat-related conditions.

There is a spectrum of preventable heat stress conditions, ranging from mild forms, such as heat cramps, to severe forms, such as heat stroke. Risk factors include longer duration of exertion, hot environment, insufficient acclimatization, and dehydration. Additional risk factors include skin disorders or other medical conditions that inhibit sweat production or evaporation, obesity, prolonged seizures, hypotension, reduced cutaneous blood flow, reduced cardiac output, the use of drugs that increase metabolism or muscle activity or impair sweating, and withdrawal syndromes. Illicit drugs can cause increased muscle activity and thus generate increased body heat.

Classic (nonexertional) heat-related illness may occur in any individual in a hot, relaxing environment with increased severity in individuals with the risk factors mentioned above, even despite minimal physical activity.

Heat cramping results from dilutional hyponatremia as sweat losses are replaced with water alone. **Heat exhaustion** results from prolonged strenuous activity in a hot environment without adequate water or salt intake. It is characterized by dehydration, sodium depletion, or isotonic fluid loss with accompanying cardiovascular changes.

Heat syncope or sudden collapse may result in unconsciousness from volume depletion and cutaneous vasodilation with subsequent systemic and cerebral hypotension. Exercise-associated postural hypotension is usually the cause of heat syncope and may occur during or immediately following exercise. **Heat stroke**, the hallmark of which is cerebral dysfunction with core body temperature over 40°C, presents in one of two forms: classic and exertional. **Classic (nonexertional) heat stroke** occurs in patients with impaired thermoregulatory mechanisms or in extreme environmental conditions. **Exertional heat stroke** occurs in healthy persons undergoing strenuous exertion in a hot or humid environment. Persons at greatest risk are those who are at the extremes of age, chronically debilitated, and taking medications that interfere with heat-dissipating mechanisms.

▶ **Clinical Findings**

When diagnosing and treating heat-related illnesses, use of an internal rectal, Foley, or esophageal thermometer is necessary because the skin temperature may not accurately reflect core body temperature. **Heat cramps** are painful skeletal muscle contractions and severe muscle spasms with onset during or shortly after exercise. Examination findings typically include stable vital signs; normal or slightly increased core body temperature; moist and cool skin; and tender, hard, lumpy, painful muscles that may be twitching. The diagnosis is made clinically.

Heat exhaustion is diagnosed based on symptoms and clinical findings of a core body temperature slightly elevated but less than 40°C, tachycardia, and moist skin. Symptoms are similar to those of heat syncope and heat cramps. Additional symptoms include nausea, vomiting, malaise, myalgias, hyperventilation, thirst, and weakness. Central nervous system symptoms include headache, dizziness, fatigue, anxiety, paresthesias, impaired judgment, and occasionally psychosis. Heat exhaustion may progress to heat stroke if sweating ceases and mental status declines.

Heat syncope generally occurs in the setting of prolonged vigorous physical activity or prolonged standing in a hot humid environment followed by a sudden collapse. Physical examination may reveal cool and moist skin, a weak pulse, and low systolic blood pressure.

Heat stroke is a life-threatening emergency. The hallmark of heat stroke is cerebral dysfunction when the core body temperature is over 40°C. Presenting symptoms include all findings seen in heat exhaustion with additional neurologic symptoms such as dizziness, weakness, emotional lability, confusion, delirium, blurred vision, convulsions, collapse, and unconsciousness. Physical examination findings may be variable and therefore unreliable. Exertional heat stroke may present with sudden collapse and loss of consciousness followed by irrational behavior. Sweating may not be present. Providers must be vigilant in monitoring for kidney injury, liver failure, metabolic derangements, respiratory compromise, coagulopathy, and ischemia. Initial laboratory findings are nonspecific to this condition.

▶ **Treatment**

A. Heat Cramps

The patient must be moved to a shaded, cool environment and given oral rehydration solution to replace both electrolytes and water. *Oral salt tablets are not recommended.* The patient may have to rest for at least 2 days with continued dietary supplementation before returning to work or resuming strenuous activity in the heat.

B. Heat Exhaustion

Treatment consists of moving patients to a shaded, cool environment, providing adequate fluid and electrolyte replacement, and initiating active cooling measures if necessary. Physiologic saline or isotonic glucose solution may be administered intravenously when oral administration is not appropriate. At least 48 hours of rest and rehydration are recommended.

C. Heat Syncope

Treatment consists of rest and recumbency in a shaded, cool place, and fluid and electrolyte replacement by mouth, or intravenously if necessary.

D. Heat Stroke

Initially, the patient's ABCs (airway, breathing, circulation) must be addressed and stabilized, then treatment is aimed at rapidly reducing the core body temperature within 1 hour while supporting circulation and perfusion. Patients should be observed using pulse oximetry and cardiac monitors while continuing to measure core body temperature and fluid input and output. The patient should also be observed for complications such as hypovolemic or cardiogenic shock, metabolic abnormalities, cardiac arrhythmias, coagulopathy, acute respiratory distress syndrome (ARDS), hypoglycemia, rhabdomyolysis, seizures, organ dysfunction, infection, and severe edema that can progress to a compartment syndrome. Circulatory failure in heat-related illness is mostly due to shock from relative or absolute hypovolemia. Oral or intravenous fluid administration must be provided to ensure adequate urinary output. Clinicians must also assess for and treat concurrent conditions such as infection, trauma, and drug effects.

Choice of cooling method depends on which can be instituted the fastest with the least compromise to the overall care of the patient. Evaporative cooling is preferred for nonexertional heat stroke and conductive-based cooling for exertional heat stroke. **Evaporative cooling** is a noninvasive, effective, quick, and easy way to reduce temperature. This is accomplished by placing the undressed patient in lateral recumbent position or supported in a hands-and-knees position to expose maximum skin surface to the air while the entire undressed body is sprayed with lukewarm water (20°C) and cooled by large fans circulating room air. Addition of inhaled cool air or oxygen may aid in cooling but must not be used alone. **Conductive-based cooling** involves cool fluid infusion, gastric or bladder lavage, ice packs, and immersion into ice water or cool water. When immersion in ice water or cold water is available in the field, it is the preferred method of cooling for exertional heat stroke. Ice packs are most effective when covering the whole body, as opposed to the traditional method of placing in the axilla and groin only. Intravascular heat exchange catheter systems as well as hemodialysis using cold dialysate (30–35°C) have been successful in reducing core body temperature.

Shivering must be avoided because it inhibits the effectiveness of cooling by increasing internal heat production. Medications can be used to suppress shivering including magnesium, quick-acting opioid analgesics, benzodiazepines, and quick-acting anesthetic agents. Skin massage is recommended to prevent cutaneous vasoconstriction. *Antipyretics (aspirin, acetaminophen) have no effect on environmentally induced hyperthermia and are contraindicated.* Treatment must be continued until the core body temperature drops to 39°C.

Prevention

Education is necessary to improve prevention and early recognition of heat-related disorders. Individuals may take steps to reduce personal risk factors and to gradually acclimatize to hot environments. For prevention of occupational heat-related illness, a comprehensive preventive program should assess personal risk factors, estimated wet-bulb globe temperature, workload, acclimatization status, and early symptom recognition.

Coaches, athletic trainers, athletes, and parents of young athletes must be educated about heat-related illness, specifically about prevention, risks, symptoms and signs, and treatment. Medical evaluation and monitoring should be used to identify the individuals and the weather conditions that increase the risk of heat-related disorders.

Those who are physically active in a hot environment must increase fluid consumption before, during, and after physical activities. Fluid consumption should include balanced electrolyte fluids and water. Water consumption alone may lead to electrolyte imbalance, particularly hyponatremia. *It is not recommended to have salt tablets available for use because of the risk of hypertonic hypernatremia.* Close monitoring of fluid and electrolyte intake and early intervention are recommended in situations necessitating exertion or activity in hot environments.

Prognosis

Mortality is high from heat stroke, most frequently secondary to multiorgan dysfunction. The patient is also at risk for rhabdomyolysis, ARDS, and inflammation even after temperature has normalized. Following heat stroke, immediate reexposure to ambient heat must be avoided.

When to Refer

Potential consultants include a surgeon for suspicion of compartment syndrome, nephrologist for kidney injury, and transplant surgeon for fulminant liver failure.

When to Admit

All patients with suspected heat stroke must be admitted to a hospital with intensive care capability for close monitoring.

Gaudio FG et al. Cooling methods in heat stroke. J Emerg Med. 2016 Apr;50(4):607–16. [PMID: 26525947]
Peiris AN et al. Heat stroke. JAMA patient page. 2017 Dec 26; 318(24):2503. [PMID: 29279936]
Tustin AW et al. Evaluation of occupational exposure limits for heat stress in outdoor workers—United States, 2011–2016. MMWR Morb Mortal Wkly Rep. 2018 Jul 6;67(26):733–7. [PMID: 29975679]

ACCIDENTAL SYSTEMIC HYPOTHERMIA

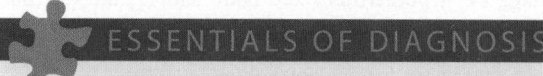

ESSENTIALS OF DIAGNOSIS

- ► Systemic hypothermia is a core body temperature below 35°C.
- ► Accurate core body temperature measurement must be obtained using a low-reading core temperature probe that measures as low as 25°C.
- ► Core body temperature must be over 32°C before terminating resuscitation efforts.
- ► Extracorporeal membrane oxygenation (ECMO) or cardiopulmonary bypass may be considered in hypothermic patients with hemodynamic instability or cardiac arrest.

General Considerations

Systemic hypothermia is defined as core body temperature below 35°C. This may be primary, from exposure to prolonged ambient, extremely low temperature, or secondary, due to thermoregulatory dysfunction. Both may be present at the same time.

Hypothermia must be considered in any patient with prolonged exposure to an ambient cold environment, especially in any patients with prior cold weather injury as well as risk factors listed in the Cold & Heat section. In prolonged or repetitive cold exposure, hypothermia ensues if the body's thermoregulatory responses become impaired.

Clinical Findings

Symptoms and signs of hypothermia are typically nonspecific and markedly variable based on the patient's underlying health and circumstances of cold exposure. Laboratory studies must assess acid-base status; electrolytes, particularly potassium and glucose; kidney, liver, and pancreas function; coagulation; and rhabdomyolysis. Inaccurate laboratory values will occur if the blood sample is warmed to 37°C for testing. All patients must be evaluated for associated conditions including hypoglycemia, trauma, infection, overdose, and peripheral cold injury.

Accurate core body temperature measurements must be obtained using a low-reading core temperature probe that measures as low as 25°C. **Stage I hypothermia** is typically seen when the core body temperature is between 32°C and 35°C and is defined by shivering and possibly poor judgment or coordination but with hemodynamic stability and a normal level of consciousness. **Stage II hypothermia** correlates with core body temperature 28–32°C. Shivering stops. Bradycardia, dilated pupils, slowed reflexes, cold diuresis, and confusion and lethargy ensue. The electrocardiogram (ECG) may reveal a J wave or Osborn wave (positive deflection in the terminal portion of the QRS complex, most notable in leads II, V_5, and V_6) (Figure 37–1). When the core body temperature is below 28°C, the likelihood of hemodynamic instability and cardiac arrest increase dramatically. **Stage III hypothermia** (core body temperature 24–28°C) is characterized by loss of consciousness but present vital signs. **Stage IV hypothermia** (core body temperature less than 24°C) is the loss of vital signs. Coma, loss of reflexes, asystole, or ventricular fibrillation may falsely lead the clinician to assume the patient is dead despite reversible hypothermia.

Treatment

Rewarming is the initial, imperative treatment for all hypothermic patients. Resuscitation begins with rapid assessment and support of airway, breathing, and circulation, simultaneously with the initiation of rewarming, and prevention of further heat loss. All cold, wet clothing must be removed and replaced with warm, dry clothing and blankets.

Mild or stage I hypothermia can be treated with passive external rewarming (ie, removing and replacing wet clothes with dry ones) or by active external rewarming. In contrast to those with more severe hypothermia, it is safe and recommended for the uninjured patient with mild hypothermia to become physically active to generate heat. **Active external rewarming** is noninvasive, highly effective, and safe for mild hypothermia. It involves applying external heat to the patient's skin. Examples include warm bedding, heated blankets, heat packs, and immersion into a 40°C bath. Warm bath immersion limits the ability to monitor the patient or treat other coexisting conditions. Patients with mild hypothermia and previous good health usually respond well to passive and active external warming.

Stage II and III hypothermia are treated as above with the addition of more aggressive rewarming strategies. This requires close monitoring of vital signs and cardiac rhythm during rewarming. Warm intravenous fluids (38–42°C) are considered minimally invasive and effective.

As hypothermia becomes more severe, there are increased complications of both hypothermia itself and of rewarming. Complications of rewarming occur as colder peripheral blood returns to central circulation. This may result in core temperature afterdrop, rewarming lactic acidosis from shunting lactate into the circulation, rewarming shock from peripheral vasodilation and hypovolemia, ventricular fibrillation, and other cardiac arrhythmias. Afterdrop can be lessened by active external rewarming of the trunk but not the extremities and by avoiding any muscle movement by the patient. Extreme caution must be taken when handling the hypothermic patient to avoid triggering potentially fatal arrhythmias in a phenomenon known as rescue collapse.

Early recognition and advance management guidelines are needed for patients with stage IV hypothermia. *For hypothermic patients in cardiac arrest, high-quality CPR must be initiated and continued until the patient's core body temperature is at least 32°C.* Below 30°C, arrhythmias and asystole may be refractory to drug therapy until the patient has been rewarmed; therefore, treatment should focus on excellent CPR technique and aggressive rewarming of the patient done in conjunction. Epinephrine or vasopressin may be given in cardiac arrest of the severely hypothermic patient. International Commission for Mountain Emergency Medicine recommends extracorporal life support as the treatment of choice for patients at high risk for hypothermic cardiac arrest. Extracorporal life support has been shown to substantially improve survival of patients with unstable circulation or cardiac arrest.

Any hypothermic patient with return of spontaneous circulation must be monitored very closely because of the high likelihood of subsequent multiorgan system failure.

When to Admit

Hypothermia patients must undergo close monitoring for potential complications. This is typically done during an inpatient admission or prolonged emergency department observation.

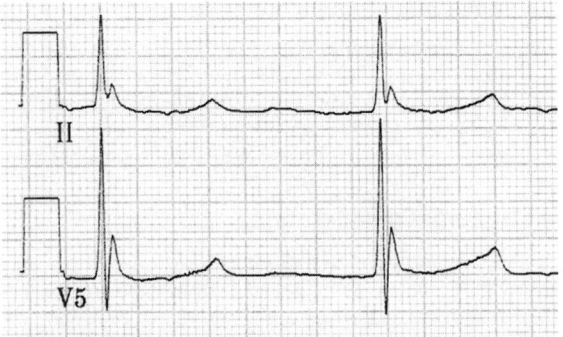

▲ **Figure 37–1.** Electrocardiogram shows leads II and V_5 in a patient whose body temperature is 24°C. Note the bradycardia and Osborn waves. These findings become more prominent as the body temperature lowers and gradually resolve with rewarming. Osborn waves have an extra positive deflection in the terminal portion of the QRS complex and are best seen in the inferior and lateral precordial leads (most notably in leads II, V_5, and V_6).

Jarosz A et al. Profound accidental hypothermia: systematic approach to active recognition and treatment. ASAIO J. 2017 May/Jun;63(3):e26–30. [PMID: 27465097]

Paal P et al. Accidental hypothermia—an update: the content of this review is endorsed by the International Commission for Mountain Emergency Medicine (ICAR MEDCOM). Scand J Trauma Resusc Emerg Med. 2016 Sep 15;24(1):111. [PMID: 27633781]

Vardon F et al. Accidental hypothermia in severe trauma. Anaesth Crit Care Pain Med. 2016 Oct;35(5):355–61. [PMID: 27185009]

Zafren K. Out-of-hospital evaluation and treatment of accidental hypothermia. Emerg Med Clin North Am. 2017 May; 35(2):261–79. [PMID: 28411927]

HYPOTHERMIA OF THE EXTREMITIES

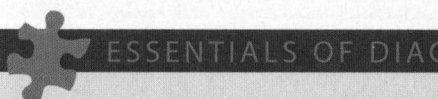

ESSENTIALS OF DIAGNOSIS

- ► "Keep warm, keep dry, and keep moving" to prevent cold-induced injury.
- ► Rewarming of the extremity suffering cold-induced injury must be performed as soon as possible after there is no risk of refreezing; exercise, rubbing, or massage must be avoided during rewarming.

► Clinical Findings

Cold exposure of the extremities produces immediate localized and then generalized vasoconstriction, which may result in a wide range of injuries. Tissue damage occurs because of ischemia and intravascular thromboses, endothelial damage, or actual freezing. Freezing (frostbite) may occur when skin temperatures drop or in the presence of wind, water, immobility, malnutrition, or vascular disease.

For all forms of cold-induced injury to an extremity, caution must be taken to avoid rubbing or massaging the injured area and to avoid applying moisture, ice, or heat. The cold-injured extremity must be protected from trauma, secondary infection, and further cold exposure.

► Prevention

"Keep warm, keep dry, and keep moving." For optimal prevention of frostbite, individuals must wear warm, dry clothing. Arms, legs, fingers, and toes must be exercised to maintain circulation. Wet clothing, socks, and shoes must be replaced with dry ones. Risk factors include underlying diseases or medications that decrease tissue perfusion and prolonged cold environmental exposure. Caution must be taken to avoid cramped positions; wet or constrictive clothing; prolonged dependency of the feet; use of tobacco, alcohol, and sedative medications; and exposure to wet, muddy ground and windy conditions.

FROSTNIP & CHILBLAIN (Erythema Pernio)

Frostnip is a mild temporary form of cold-induced injury causing local paresthesias of the involved area that completely resolve with passive external rewarming.

Chilblains or **erythema pernio** are inflammatory skin changes caused by exposure to cold without actual freezing of the tissues. These skin lesions may be red or purple papular lesions, which are painful or pruritic, with burning or paresthesias. They may be associated with edema or blistering and aggravated by warmth. With continued exposure, ulcerative or hemorrhagic lesions may appear and progress to scarring, fibrosis, and atrophy. Treatment consists of elevating and passively externally rewarming the affected part.

IMMERSION FOOT OR TRENCH FOOT

Immersion foot (or hand) is caused by prolonged immersion in cold water or mud, usually below 10°C. **Prehyperemic stage** is marked by early symptoms of cold and anesthesia of the affected area. **Hyperemic stage** follows with a hot sensation, intense burning, and shooting pains. **Posthyperemic stage** occurs with ongoing cold exposure; the affected part becomes pale or cyanotic with diminished pulsations due to vasospasm. This may result in blistering, swelling, redness, ecchymoses, hemorrhage, necrosis, peripheral nerve injury, or gangrene.

Treatment consists of air drying and gradual rewarming by exposure to air at room temperature. Affected parts are elevated to aid in removal of edema fluid. Pressure sites are protected with cushions. Bed rest is required until all ulcers have healed.

FROSTBITE

Frostbite is injury from tissue freezing and formation of ice crystals in the tissue. Most tissue destruction follows reperfusion of the frozen tissues resulting in further tissue damage. In mild cases, only the skin and subcutaneous tissues are involved. Symptoms include numbness, prickling, itching, and pallor. With increasing severity, deeper structures become involved. The skin appears white or yellow, loses elasticity, and becomes immobile. Edema, hemorrhagic blisters, necrosis, gangrene, paresthesias, and stiffness may occur.

► Treatment

A. Immediate Treatment

Evaluate and treat the patient for associated systemic hypothermia, concurrent conditions, and injury. Early use of systemic analgesics is recommended for nonfrozen injuries. Hydrate patients to avoid hypovolemia and to improve perfusion.

1. Rewarming—Rapid rewarming at temperatures slightly above normal body temperature may significantly decrease tissue necrosis and reverse the tissue crystallization. **If there is any possibility of refreezing, the frostbitten part must not be thawed.** Ideally, the frozen extremity must not be used. Rewarming is best accomplished by warm bath immersion. The frozen extremity is immersed for several minutes in a moving water bath heated to 40–42°C until the distal tip of the part being thawed flushes. Water in this temperature range feels warm but not hot to the normal hand or wrist. If warm water is not available, then passive thawing in a warm environment must be allowed. Dry heat is not recommended because it is more difficult to regulate and increases the likelihood of accidental burns. Thawing may cause tenderness and burning pain. Once the frozen part has thawed and returned to normal temperature, discontinue external heat. **In the early stage, rewarming by exercise, rubbing, or friction is contraindicated.** The patient must be kept at bed rest with the affected parts elevated and uncovered at room temperature. Avoid application of casts, occlusive dressings, or bandages. Blisters must be left intact unless signs of infection supervene.

2. Anti-infective measures and wound care—Frostbite increases susceptibility to tetanus and infection. Tetanus prophylaxis status must be verified and updated as needed. Infection risk may be reduced by aseptic wound care. Nonadherent sterile gauze and fluffy dressing must be loosely applied to wounds and cushions used for all areas of pressure. Antibiotics should not be administered empirically.

B. Medical and Surgical Treatment Options

Telemedicine may be used so that specialists can provide advice on early field treatment of cold-injured patients in remote areas, thereby improving outcomes. Clinicians must watch for evidence of compartment syndrome and need for fasciotomy. Eschar formation without evidence of infection may be conservatively treated. The underlying skin may heal spontaneously with the eschar acting as a biologic dressing. Rates of amputation have been reduced with the use of intravenous infusions of synthetic prostaglandins and of a tissue plasminogen activators, and with intra-arterial administration of a thrombolytic within 24 hours of exposure. The rate of tissue salvage decreases with every hour of delay from rewarming to thrombolytic therapy.

C. Follow-Up Care

Patient education must include ongoing care of the cold injury and prevention of future hypothermia and cold injury. Gentle, progressive physical therapy to promote circulation should be instituted as tolerated.

▶ Prognosis

Recovery from frostbite depends on the underlying comorbidities, the extent of initial tissue damage, the rewarming reperfusion injury, and the late sequelae. The involved extremity may be at increased susceptibility for discomfort and injury upon re-exposure to cold. Neuropathic sequelae include pain, numbness, tingling, hyperhidrosis, and cold sensitivity of the extremities. Nerve conduction abnormalities may persist for many years after a cold injury.

▶ When to Admit

- Management of tissue damage, comorbidities, associated injuries.
- Need for hospital-based interventions.
- Psychosocial factors that could compromise patient safety or recovery.

Handford C et al. Frostbite. Emerg Med Clin North Am. 2017 May; 35(2):281–99. [PMID: 28411928]

Heil K et al. Freezing and non-freezing cold weather injuries: a systematic review. Br Med Bull. 2016 Mar;117(1):79–93. [PMID: 26872856]

Lindford A et al. The evolution of the Helsinki frostbite management protocol. Burns. 2017 Nov;43(7):1455–63. [PMID: 28778759]

Nygaard RM et al. Time matters in severe frostbite: assessment of limb/digit salvage on the individual patient level. J Burn Care Res. 2017 Jan/Feb;38(1):53–9. [PMID: 27606554]

DROWNING

ESSENTIALS OF DIAGNOSIS

- ▶ The first requirement of rescue is immediate rescue breathing and CPR.
- ▶ Clinical manifestations include hypoxemia, pulmonary edema, and hypoventilation.
- ▶ The patient must also be assessed for hypothermia, hypoglycemia, alcohol intake, concurrent injuries, and medical conditions.

▶ General Considerations

Drowning, as defined by the World Health Organization, is the "process resulting in primary respiratory impairment from submersion in a liquid medium." Drowning may result in asphyxiation (from fluid aspiration or laryngospasm), hypoxemia, hypothermia, and acidemia. Outcomes from drowning range from life without morbidity to death. Morbidity may be immediate or delayed. A patient may be deceptively asymptomatic during the initial recovery period only to deteriorate or die as a result of acute respiratory failure within the following 12–24 hours. Disseminated intravascular coagulation may also lead to bleeding after asphyxiation from drowning.

Drowning is a leading cause of death in children and highly preventable in all ages with implementation of educational and safety measures. Clinicans must provide patient education and guidance about drowning prevention.

▶ Clinical Findings

A. Symptoms and Signs

The patient's appearance may vary from asymptomatic to marked distress with abnormal vital signs. Symptoms and signs include respiratory difficulty, chest pain, dysrhythmia, hypotension, cyanosis, and hypothermia (from cold water or prolonged submersion). The patient may experience headache, neurologic deficits, and altered level of consciousness.

B. Laboratory Findings

Metabolic acidosis is common and arterial blood gas results may be helpful in determining the degree of injury since initial clinical findings may appear benign. PaO_2 is usually decreased; $PaCO_2$ may be increased or decreased; pH is decreased. Bedside blood sugar must be checked rapidly. Other testing is based on clinical scenario.

Prevention

Education and prevention are critical given the high burden of disease from drowning.

Preventive measures must be taken to reduce morbidity and mortality from drowning. Conditions that increase risk of submersion injury include the use of alcohol, psychotropics, and other drugs, inadequate water safety skills, poor physical health, hyperventilation, sudden acute illness, acute trauma, decompression sickness, dangerous water conditions, and environmental exposures.

Treatment

A. First Aid

1. *The first requirement of rescue is immediate basic life support treatment and CPR.* At the scene, immediate airway management and measures to combat hypoxemia are critical to improve outcome.

2. Patient must be assessed for hypothermia, hypoglycemia, concurrent medical conditions, and associated trauma.

3. Rescuer must not attempt to drain water from the victim's lungs.

4. Resuscitation and basic life support efforts must be continued until core body temperature reaches 32°C.

B. Subsequent Management

1. Ensure optimal ventilation and oxygenation—The onset of hypoxemia exists even in the alert, conscious patient who appears to be breathing normally. Oxygen must be administered immediately at the highest available concentration. Oxygen saturation must be maintained at 90% or higher via some form of supplemental oxygen.

Serial physical examinations and chest radiographs must be performed to detect possible pneumonitis, atelectasis, and pulmonary edema. Bronchodilators may be used to treat wheezing. Nasogastric suctioning may be necessary to decompress the stomach.

2. Cardiovascular support—Intravascular volume status must be monitored and supported by vascular fluid replacement, vasopressors, or diuretics as needed.

3. Correction of blood pH and electrolyte abnormalities—Metabolic acidosis is present in the majority of drowning victims, but this typically corrects through adequate ventilation and oxygenation. Glycemic control improves outcome.

4. Cerebral and spinal cord injury—Central nervous system damage may progress despite apparently adequate treatment of hypoxia and shock.

5. Hypothermia—Core body temperature must be measured and managed as appropriate (see Accidental Systemic Hypothermia, above).

Course & Prognosis

As the duration of submersion lengthens, the probability of worse outcome increases. Favorable prognosis is related to a duration of submersion of less than 5 minutes. Respiratory damage is often severe in the minutes to hours following a drowning. With respiratory supportive treatment, improvements typically occur quickly over the first few days following the drowning. Long-term complications of drowning may include neurologic impairment, seizure disorder, and pulmonary or cardiac damage. Prognosis is directly correlated with the patient's age, submersion time, rapidity of prehospital resuscitation and subsequent transport to a medical facility, clinical status at time of arrival to hospital, Glasgow Coma Scale score, pupillary reactivity, and overall health assessment (APACHE II score).

When to Admit

Most patients with significant drowning or concurrent medical or traumatic conditions require inpatient monitoring following the event. This includes continuous monitoring of cardiorespiratory, neurologic, renal, and metabolic function. Pulmonary edema may not appear for 24 hours.

Idris AH et al. 2015 revised Utstein-style recommended guidelines for uniform reporting of data from drowning-related resuscitation: an ILCOR advisory statement. Resuscitation. 2017 Sep;118:147–58. [PMID: 28728893]

Quan L et al. Predicting outcome of drowning at the scene: a systematic review and meta-analyses. Resuscitation. 2016 Jul; 104:63–75. [PMID: 27154004]

Schmidt A et al. Drowning in the adult population: emergency department resuscitation and treatment. Emerg Med Pract. 2015 May;17(5):1–18. [PMID: 26301918]

THERMAL BURNS

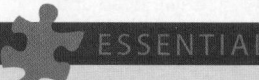
ESSENTIALS OF DIAGNOSIS

▶ Estimates of the burn location, size, and depth greatly determine treatment plan.

▶ The first 48 hours of burn care offer the greatest impact on morbidity and mortality of a burn victim.

Worldwide, burns are a common cause of injury and potential morbidity and mortality. Burn prognosis is affected by the type of environment where the burn occurred. Low-resource settings (wilderness or low-income areas) are associated with delays in and suboptimal access to standard burn treatments.

The first 48 hours after thermal burn injury offer the greatest opportunity to impact the survival of the patient. Early surgical intervention, wound care, enteral feeding, glucose control and metabolic management, infection control, and prevention of hypothermia and compartment syndrome have contributed to significantly lower mortality rates and shorter hospitalizations. Research utilizing several different well-established burn severity scores has shown the importance of patient comorbidities to the prognosis of patients with severe burn injuries.

General Considerations

A. Classification

Burns are classified by extent, depth, patient age, and associated illness or injury. Accurate estimation of burn size and depth is necessary to quantify the parameters of resuscitation.

1. Extent—In adults, the "rule of nines" (Figure 37–2) is useful for rapidly assessing the extent of a burn. It is important to view the entire patient to make an accurate assessment of skin findings on initial and subsequent examinations. One rule of thumb is that the palm of an open hand in adult patients constitutes 1% of total body surface area (TBSA). TBSA is calculated for partial- and full-thickness burns.

2. Depth—Judgment of depth of injury is difficult. **Superficial burns** may appear red or gray but will demonstrate excellent capillary refill and are not blistered initially. If the wound is blistered and appears pink and wet, this represents a **superficial partial-thickness burn**. **Deep partial-thickness burns** appear white and wet, and bleed if poked; cutaneous sensation is maintained. **Full-thickness burns** result in a loss of adnexal structures and may appear white-yellow in color, or may have a black charred appearance. This stiff, dry skin does not bleed when poked and cutaneous sensation is lost.

Deep partial-thickness and full-thickness burns are treated in a similar fashion. Both require early debridement and grafting to heal appropriately, without which the skin becomes thin and scarred.

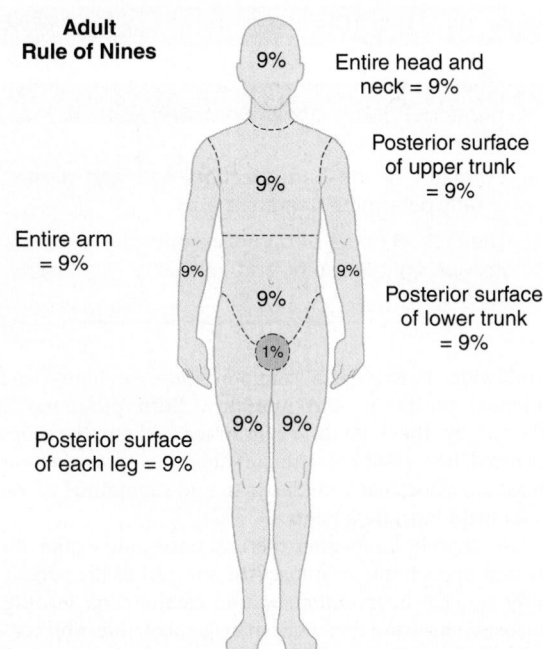

Adult Rule of Nines

Entire head and neck = 9%

9%

Posterior surface of upper trunk = 9%

9%

Entire arm = 9%

9%   9%

9%

Posterior surface of lower trunk = 9%

1%

Posterior surface of each leg = 9%

9%   9%

▲ **Figure 37–2.** Estimation of body surface area in burns.

B. Survival After Burn Injury

Transfer to a burn unit is determined by large burn size, circumferential burn, or burn involving a joint or high-risk body part, and by comorbidities. Mortality rates have been significantly reduced due to treatment advances including improvements in wound care, treatment of infection, early burn excision, skin substitute usage, and early nutritional support.

C. Associated Injuries or Illnesses

Smoke inhalation, associated trauma, and electrical injuries are commonly associated with burns. Severe burns from any source may result in similar complications (ie, infections, respiratory compromise, multiorgan dysfunction, venous thromboembolism, and gastrointestinal complications).

D. Systemic Reactions to Burn Injury

Burns greater than approximately 20% of TBSA may lead to systemic metabolic derangements requiring intensive support. The inflammatory cascade can result in shock and coagulopathy.

Treatment

A. Initial Resuscitation

1. Primary survey—Burn patients require a full trauma assessment, starting with "ABCDE" (airway, breathing, circulation, disability, exposure).

A. Airway control—Serial assessments of airway and breathing are necessary because airway compromise and ARDS may develop, particularly in those with inhalation injury.

B. Vascular access—Vascular access must be obtained on all burn patients.

C. Fluid resuscitation—Patients with burns greater than 15% of TBSA require intravascular fluid administration of large volumes of crystalloid. The most widely recognized guideline for fluid resuscitation is the **Parkland formula** (https://www.mdcalc.com/parkland-formula-burns/) in which the fluid requirement in the first 24 hours is estimated as 4 mL/kg × body weight per percent of body surface area burned. Half the calculated fluid is given in the first 8-hour period from the time of injury, not the time of arrival to medical care. The remaining fluid is delivered over the next 16 hours. An extremely large volume of fluid may be required. Crystalloid solutions alone may be insufficient to restore cardiac preload during the period of burn shock. Conversely, clinicians must watch for clinical signs of volume overload as it may lead to pulmonary complications or to a compartment syndrome from edema. Electrical burns and inhalation injury may increase the fluid requirement.

B. Management

1. Pain control—Pain control is critical in burn injury patients. Treatment is with (oral or intravenous) nonsteroidal anti-inflammatory drugs and opioids.

2. Chemoprophylaxis—

A. TETANUS IMMUNIZATION—Verify and update tetanus prophylaxis status in all burn patients. (See Chapter 33.)

B. ANTIBIOTICS—All nonsuperficial wounds need to be covered with topical antibiotics. Prophylaxis with systemic antibiotics is not indicated.

3. Surgical management—

A. ESCHAROTOMY—As tissue swelling occurs, ischemia may develop under any constricting eschar of an extremity, neck, chest, or in circumferential full-thickness burns of the trunk. Escharotomy incisions can be life- and limb-saving.

B. FASCIOTOMY—Fasciotomy is indicated for any compartment syndrome. Clinicians must frequently monitor patients for development of early signs of a compartment syndrome, particularly in those with circumferential burns.

C. DEBRIDEMENT, DRESSINGS, AND TOPICAL AND SYSTEMIC ANTIBIOTIC THERAPY—Minor burn wounds must be debrided to determine the depth of the burn and then thoroughly cleansed. Thereafter, daily wound care must consist of debridements as needed, topical antibiotics, and wound dressings. Patient compliance and adequate pain control is essential for successful outpatient treatment. The wound must be reevaluated by the treating clinician within 24–72 hours to evaluate for signs of infection.

The goal of burn wound management is to protect the wound from desiccation and avoid further injury or infection. Regular and thorough cleansing of burned areas is of critical importance. Topical antibiotics may be applied after wound cleansing. Silver sulfadiazine is no longer recommended.

It is imperative to closely monitor for and treat systemic infection, since this remains a leading cause of morbidity among patients with major burn injuries. Health care–associated infections are increasingly common.

D. WOUND MANAGEMENT—The goal of therapy after fluid resuscitation is rapid and stable closure of the wound. Wounds that do not heal spontaneously in 7–10 days (ie, deep partial-thickness or full-thickness burns) are best treated by a specialist through excision and autograft to avoid development of granulation and infection. The quality of the skin in regenerated deep partial-thickness burns is marginal because of the very thin dermis that emerges.

Cultured allogeneic keratinocyte grafts can provide rapid early coverage for superficial burn injuries. Skin substitution with cultured grafts may be life-saving for severe burns. Although the replaced dermis has nearly normal histologic dermal elements, there are no adnexal structures present, and very few, if any, elastic fibers.

E. ABDOMINAL COMPARTMENT SYNDROME—Abdominal compartment syndrome is a potentially lethal condition that may develop in severely burned patients, with mortality rates of approximately 60% despite surgical intervention. Diagnosis is confirmed by bladder pressures greater than 30 mm Hg in at-risk patients. Surgical abdominal decompression may improve ventilation and oxygen delivery but may not impact survival.

C. Patient Support

Burn patients require extensive supportive care, both physiologically and psychologically. It is important to maintain normal core body temperature and avoid hypothermia, by maintaining environmental temperature at or above 30°C, in patients with burns over more than 20% of TBSA. Burn patients are at risk for many complications such as respiratory injury, ARDS or respiratory failure unresponsive to maximal ventilatory support, sepsis, multiorgan failure, and venous thromboembolism.

Burn patients have increased metabolic and energy needs for wound healing and require careful assessment and provision of optimal nutrition. Early aggressive nutrition (by parenteral or enteral routes) reduces infections, recovery time, noninfectious complications, length of hospital stay, long-term sequelae, and mortality.

Prevention of long-term scars remains a formidable problem in seriously burned patients.

▶ Prognosis

Prognosis depends on the extent and location of the burn tissue damage, associated injuries, comorbidities, and complications. Hyperglycemia is a predictor of worse outcomes. Common complications include sepsis; gangrene requiring limb amputation; or neurologic, cardiac, cognitive, or psychiatric dysfunction. Psychiatric support may be necessary following burn injury.

▶ When to Refer

Transfer to a burn unit is indicated for large burn size (for partial-thickness burns greater than 10% of TBSA or for full-thickness burns greater than 5% of TBSA), circumferential burn, inhalation injury, or burn involving a joint or high-risk body part (face, hands, feet, genitalia), and for patients with comorbidities.

▶ When to Admit

- All severe burn patients require extensive supportive care, both physiologically and psychologically.
- Significant burns (based on location and extent).
- Patients with significant comorbidities and suboptimal home situations.
- Burn center consultation can advise which patients require transfer and which can be managed via telemedicine/telephone consultation.
- Monitoring includes vital signs, wound care, and observation for potential complications of electrolyte abnormalities, acute kidney injury, hepatic failure, cardiopulmonary compromise, hyperglycemia, and infection.

Bitter CC et al. Management of burn injuries in the wilderness: lessons from low-resource settings. Wilderness Environ Med. 2016 Dec;27(4):519–25. [PMID: 28029455]

Heng JS et al. Revised Baux score and updated Charlson comorbidity index are independently associated with mortality in burns intensive care patients. Burns. 2015 Nov;41(7):1420–7. [PMID: 26187055]

Otterness K et al. Emergency department management of smoke inhalation injury in adults. Emerg Med Pract. 2018 Mar; 20(3):1–24. [PMID: 29489306]

Porter C et al. The metabolic stress response to burn trauma: current understanding and therapies. Lancet. 2016 Oct 1; 388(10052):1417–26. [PMID: 27707498]

ELECTRICAL INJURY

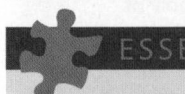

ESSENTIALS OF DIAGNOSIS

► Extent of injury is determined by the type, amount, duration, and pathway of electrical current.

► Clinical findings of death are unreliable; therefore, resuscitation efforts must be attempted before assuming the electrical injury victim is dead.

► Skin findings may be misleading and are not indicative of the degree of deeper tissue injury.

General Considerations

Electricity-induced injuries are common and yet most are preventable. These injuries occur by exposure to electrical current of low voltage, high voltage, or lightning. Electrical current type is either alternating current (AC) or direct current (DC) and is measured in volts (V). Electricity causes acute injury by direct tissue damage, muscle tetany, direct thermal injury and coagulation necrosis, and associated trauma.

Alternating current (AC) is an electric current that periodically reverses direction in a sine wave pattern and may cause muscle tetany, which prolongs the duration and amount of current exposure. AC can be low voltage or high voltage. Most households and businesses use electric power in the form of AC at **low voltages** (less than 1000 V). Low voltage electrical injuries can range from minor to significant damage and death. **High voltage** (greater than 1000 V) AC electrical injuries are often related to occupational exposure and associated with deep tissue damage and higher morbidity and mortality. **Direct current (DC)** is unidirectional electrical flow (ie, lightning, batteries, and automotive electrical systems). It is more likely to cause a single intense muscle contraction and asystole. **Lightning** differs from other high-voltage electrical shock in that lightning delivers a direct current of millions of volts in a fraction of a second.

The extent of damage from electrical injuries depends on the following factors: voltage, current type, tissue resistance, moisture, pathway, duration of exposure, associated trauma, and comorbidities. Current is the most important determinant of tissue damage. Current passes through the tissues of least resistance as energy, which produces heat and causes direct thermal injury. Tissue resistance varies throughout the body with nerve cells being the most vulnerable and bone the most resistant to electrical current.

Clinical Findings

Electrical burns are of three distinct types: flash (arcing) burns, flame (clothing) burns, and the direct heating effect of tissues by the electrical current.

Skin damage does not correlate with the degree of injury. Not all electrical injuries cause skin damage; very minor skin damage may be present with massive internal injuries. Symptoms and signs may range from very subtle to death. The presence of entrance and exit burns signifies an increased risk of deep tissue damage. Current passing through skeletal muscle can cause muscle necrosis and contractions severe enough to result in bone fracture. If the current passes through the heart or brainstem, death may be immediate due to ventricular fibrillation, asystole, or apnea.

Resuscitation must be initiated on all victims of electrical injury since clinical findings are deceptive and unreliable.

Complications

Complications include cardiac or respiratory arrest; dysrhythmias; neurologic dysfunction, such as autonomic dysfunction (resulting in pupils that are fixed, dilated, or asymmetric); altered mental status; seizures; paralysis; headache; vascular injury; tissue edema and necrosis; compartment syndrome; associated traumatic injuries (ruptured ear drums, fractures); pneumothorax; rhabdomyolysis; acute kidney injury; hypovolemia; infections; ocular complications; sepsis; gangrene; and cognitive or psychiatric dysfunction. Psychiatric support may be necessary following electrical injury.

Treatment

A. Emergency Measures

The patient must be assessed and treated as a trauma victim. The victim must be safely separated from the electrical current prior to initiation of CPR or other treatments. *Resuscitation must then be initiated since clinical findings of death are unreliable.*

B. Hospital Measures

The initial assessment involves airway, breathing, and circulation followed by a full trauma protocol. Fluid resuscitation is important to maintain adequate urinary output. Initial evaluation includes cardiac monitoring and ECG, complete blood count, electrolytes, kidney function tests, liver chemistries, creatine phosphokinase or urine myoglobin, urinalysis, and cardiac enzymes. ECG does not show typical patterns of ischemia since the electrical damage is epicardial. Victims must be evaluated for hidden injury, organ injury, blunt trauma, dehydration, skin burns, hypertension, acid-base disturbances, and neurological as well as psychological damage.

Electrical burn wounds are an underrecognized and yet devastating form of burn injury with wide-ranging and significant complications.

When electrical injury occurs, there must be a high suspicion for extensive deep tissue necrosis. Superficial skin may appear deceivingly benign, leading to a delayed or completely overlooked diagnosis of deep tissue injury.

Deep tissue necrosis leads to profound tissue swelling, which results in a high risk of a compartment syndrome. Early debridement of devitalized tissues and tetanus prophylaxis may reduce the risks of infection.

Pain management is important before, during, and after initial treatment and subsequent rehabilitation.

▶ Prognosis

Prognosis depends on the degree and location of electrical injury, initial tissue damage, associated injuries, comorbidities, and complications.

▶ When to Refer

- Specialists may be needed to perform fasciotomy for compartment syndrome, to perform debridement of devitalized tissue, or to perform microvascular reconstruction.
- Ophthalmologists should evaluate patients for possible ocular complications, and subsequent ENT physicians should evaluate for tympanic membrane rupture or hearing loss.

▶ When to Admit

Indications for hospitalization include high-voltage exposure; dysrhythmia or ECG changes; large burn; neurologic, pulmonary, or cardiac symptoms; suspicion of significant deep tissue or organ damage; transthoracic current pathway; history of cardiac disease or other significant comorbidities or injuries; and need for surgery.

Andrews CJ et al. Neurological and neuropsychological consequences of electrical and lightning shock: review and theories of causation. Neural Regen Res. 2017 May;12(5):677–86. [PMID: 28616016]

Clark AT et al. JAMA patient page. Electrical injury. JAMA. 2017 Sep 26;318(12):1198. [PMID: 28973623]

Waldmann V et al. Electrical cardiac injuries: current concepts and management. Eur Heart J. 2018 Apr 21;39(16):1459–65. [PMID: 28444167]

RADIATION EXPOSURE

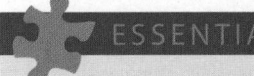

ESSENTIALS OF DIAGNOSIS

- ▶ Damage from radiation is determined by the source, type, quantity, duration, bodily location, and susceptibility and accumulation of exposures of the person.
- ▶ Clinicians and patients must be educated regarding the risks of medical diagnostic radiation. These radiation risks must be weighed against the benefits of the medical imaging needed.

▶ General Considerations

Radiation exposure may occur from environmental, occupational, medical care, accidental, or intentional causes.

The extent of damage from radiation exposure depends on the type, quantity, and duration of radiation exposure; the organs exposed; the degree of disruption to DNA; metabolic and cellular function; and the age, underlying condition, susceptibility, comorbidities, and accumulative exposures of the victim.

Radiation occurs from both nonionizing and ionizing radiation sources. **Nonionizing radiation** is low energy, resulting in injuries related to local thermal damage (ie, microwave, ultraviolet, visible light, and radiowave). **Ionizing radiation** is high energy, causing bodily damage in several ways. Ionizing radiation is either electromagnetic (ie, x-rays and gamma rays) or particulate (ie, alpha or beta particles, neutrons, and protons). Exposure may be external, internal, or both.

The International Commission on Radiological Protection (ICRP) website provides the most up-to-date recommendations for protection against ionizing radiation (http://www.icrp.org/index.asp). The World Health Organization (WHO) has published a series of guidelines on radiation emergencies (eg, see https://www.who.int/ionizing_radiation/a_e/en/). These guidelines include recommended interventions during the early, intermediate, and late emergency phases and the management of their psychosocial impact.

▶ Clinical Findings

Radiation exposure results in acute and delayed effects. Acute effects involve damage of the rapidly dividing cells (ie, the mucosa, skin, and bone marrow). This may be manifested as mucositis, nausea, vomiting, gastrointestinal edema and ulcers, skin burns, and bone marrow suppression over hours to days after exposure. Delayed effects include malignancy, reproduction abnormalities, and liver, kidney, and central nervous system and immune system dysfunction.

Clinicians must be educated to recognize and treat acute radiation sickness also referred to as **acute radiation syndrome**. Acute radiation syndrome is due to an exposure to high doses of ionizing radiation over a brief time course. The symptom onset is within hours to days depending on the dose. Symptoms include anorexia, nausea, vomiting, weakness, exhaustion, lassitude and, in some cases, prostration; these symptoms may occur singly or in combination. Dehydration, anemia, and infection may follow. The Centers for Disease Control and Prevention offers web-based information regarding acute radiation syndrome (https://www.cdc.gov/nceh/radiation/emergencies/arsphysicianfactsheet.htm).

In **acute radiation exposure**, medical care includes close monitoring of the gastrointestinal, cutaneous, hematologic, cardiopulmonary, and cerebrovascular symptoms and signs from initial exposure and over time.

▶ Therapeutic Radiation Exposure

Radiation therapy has been a successful component in the treatment of many malignancies. These radiation-treated cancer survivors have a higher risk of development of a second malignancy; obesity; and pulmonary, cardiac and thyroid dysfunction as well as an increased overall risk for chronic health conditions and mortality.

Medical Imaging Radiation Exposure

Medical imaging with ionizing radiation exposure has dramatically increased over the past few decades. Medical imaging radiation exposure is a growing concern for health care professionals and the public. With the rising use of medical imaging, there are urgent safety needs for standardization and regulation of radiation dosing in medical diagnostics and for clinician and public education about this issue.

The American College of Radiology (ACR) offers "ACR Appropriateness Criteria," which are evidence-based guidelines created by expert panels to serve as a reference for best practices for imaging decisions by health care providers (https://www.acr.org/Clinical-Resources/ACR-Appropriateness-Criteria). Clinicians and patients must carefully weigh the risks and benefits of radiation exposure when deciding on an imaging test.

Occupational & Environmental Radiation Exposure

The National Nuclear Security Administration's Radiation Emergency Assistance Center provides 24-hour access to expert consultation services over the telephone or via email (telephone: 1-865-576-1005 or email: https://orise.orau.gov/reacts/). The Centers for Disease Control and Prevention "Radiation Emergencies" website (https://www.cdc.gov/nceh/radiation/emergencies/index.htm) is a useful resource for professionals.

Treatment

Treatment is focused on decontamination, symptomatic relief, supportive care, and psychosocial support. Specific treatments focus on the dose, route, and effects of exposure.

Prognosis

Prognosis is determined by the radiation dose, duration, and frequency as well as by the underlying condition of the victim. Death is usually due to hematopoietic failure, gastrointestinal mucosal damage, central nervous system damage, widespread vascular injury, or secondary infection.

Carcinogenesis is related to the radiation type, total dose, duration, and accumulation of exposure, and to the susceptibility of the victim. The younger the victim's age at the time of exposure, the greater the risk of acute and long-term damage from radiation. Radiation-related cancer risks persist throughout the exposed person's life span.

With the increased use of ionizing radiation for medical diagnostics and treatments, there is a growing concern for the iatrogenic increase in radiation-induced cancer risks. There are age-related sensitivities to radiation; prenatal and younger age victims are more susceptible to carcinogenesis.

When to Admit

Most patients with significant ionizing radiation exposure require admission for close monitoring and supportive treatment.

Bréchignac F et al. Addressing ecological effects of radiation on populations and ecosystems to improve protection of the environment against radiation: agreed statements from a Consensus Symposium. J Environ Radioact. 2016 Jul; 158–159:21–9. [PMID: 27058410]

Carr Z et al. Using the GRADE [Grading of Recommendations Assessment, Development and Evaluation] approach to support the development of recommendations for public health interventions in radiation emergencies. Radiat Prot Dosimetry. 2016 Sep;171(1):144–55. [PMID: 27521205]

Hasegawa A et al. Health effects of radiation and other health problems in the aftermath of nuclear accidents, with an emphasis on Fukushima. Lancet. 2015 Aug 1;386(9992):479–88. [PMID: 26251393]

Kamiya K et al. Long-term effects of radiation exposure on health. Lancet. 2015 Aug 1;386(9992):469–78. [PMID: 26251392]

Oren O et al. Curbing unnecessary and wasted diagnostic imaging. JAMA. 2019 Jan 22;321(3):245–6. [PMID: 30615023]

ENVIRONMENTAL DISORDERS RELATED TO ALTITUDE

DYSBARISM & DECOMPRESSION SICKNESS

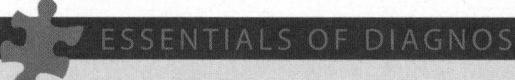

ESSENTIALS OF DIAGNOSIS

▶ Symptoms temporally related to recent altitude or pressure changes.

▶ Early recognition and prompt treatment of decompression illness are extremely important.

▶ Patient must also be assessed for hypothermia, hypoglycemia, concurrent injuries, and medical conditions.

▶ Consultation with diving medicine or hyperbaric oxygen specialist is indicated.

General Considerations

Dysbarism and decompression illness are physiologic problems that result from altitude changes and the effects of environmental pressure on the gases in the body during underwater descent and ascent. These are most likely to occur when scuba diving is followed closely by travel to high altitudes, or when the scuba diver is not adherent to the conservative dive guidelines for dive duration, course, depth, and surface times.

As a diver descends, the gases in the body compress; gases dissolve in blood and tissues. During the ascent, gases in the body expand.

Dysbarism results from barotrauma when gas compression or expansion occurs in parts of the body that are noncompressible or have limited compliance. Pulmonary overinflation syndrome is one of the most serious and potentially fatal results of barotrauma. This syndrome is due to an inappropriately rapid ascent causing alveoli rupture and air bubble extravasation into tissue planes or even the cerebral circulation.

Decompression illness occurs when the ascent is too rapid and gas bubbles form and cause damage depending on their location (ie, coronary, pulmonary, spinal or cerebral blood vessels, joints, soft tissue). Decompression illness symptoms depend on the size, number, and location of gas bubbles released (notably nitrogen). Risk of decompression illness depends on the dive details (depth, duration, number of dives, interval surface time between dives, and water conditions) as well as the diver's age, weight, physical condition, physical exertion, the rate of ascent, and the length of time between the low altitude (scuba dive) and high altitude (air travel or ground ascent). Predisposing factors include obesity, injury, hypoxia, lung or cardiac disease, right to left cardiac shunt, diver's overall health, dehydration, alcohol and medication effects, and panic attacks. Decompression illness may also occur in those who take hot showers after cold dives. There have been clinical case reports of delayed presentations of decompression illness following post-dive exercise.

Preventive measures include diver education; pre-dive medical screening and dive planning; strict adherence to dive course, timing, and depths; and a slow and controlled ascent plus proper control of buoyancy. Conservative recommendation is to avoid high altitudes (air travel or ground ascent) for at least 24 hours after surfacing from the dive, especially following multiple dives.

▶ Clinical Findings

The range of clinical manifestations varies depending on the location of the gas bubble formation or the compressibility of gases in the body. Symptom onset may be immediate, within minutes or hours (in the majority), or present up to 48 hours later. Decompression illness symptoms include pain in the joints ("the bends"); skin pruritus or burning (skin bends); cardiac symptoms (acute coronary syndrome, conduction abnormalities); spinal cord or cerebral symptoms (focal neurologic dysfunction or "dissociation" symptoms that do not follow typical distribution neuroanatomy patterns); labyrinthine decompression illness ("the staggers," central vertigo); pulmonary decompression illness ("the chokes," inspiratory pain, cough, and respiratory distress); arterial gas embolism (cerebral, pulmonary); barotrauma of the lungs, ear, and sinus; and coma and death.

Decompression illness involving the brain and spinal cord may occur by different mechanisms due to air bubbles causing arterial occlusion, venous obstruction, or in situ toxicity.

The clinician must assess for associated conditions of hypothermia, hypoglycemia, hypovolemia, drowning, trauma, envenomations, or concurrent medical conditions.

▶ Treatment

Early recognition and prompt treatment are extremely important. Decompression illness must be considered if symptoms are temporally related to recent diving or altitude or pressure changes within the past 48 hours. Continuous administration of 100% oxygen is indicated and beneficial for all patients. Hyperbaric oxygen treatment is commonly recommended for decompression illness symptoms. Immediate consultation with a diving medicine or hyperbaric oxygen specialist is indicated even if mild decompression illness symptoms resolve. Nonsteroidal anti-inflammatory drugs, acetaminophen, or aspirin may be given for pain control if there are no contraindications. *Opioids must be used very cautiously,* since these may obscure the response to recompression.

▶ When to Admit

Rapid transportation to a hyperbaric treatment facility for recompression is imperative for decompression illness. The Divers Alert Network is an excellent worldwide resource for emergency advice 24 hours daily for the management of diving-related conditions (www.diversalertnetwork.org).

Madden D et al. Intrapulmonary shunt and SCUBA diving: another risk factor? Echocardiography. 2015 Feb;32(Suppl 3): S205–10. [PMID: 25693625]

Pollock NW et al. Updates in decompression illness. Emerg Med Clin North Am. 2017 May;35(2):301–19. [PMID: 28411929]

Smart D et al. Joint position statement on persistent foramen ovale (PFO) and diving. South Pacific Underwater Medicine Society (SPUMS) and the United Kingdom Sports Diving Medical Committee (UKSDMC). Diving Hyperb Med. 2015 Jun;45(2):129–31. [PMID: 26165538]

HIGH-ALTITUDE ILLNESS

ESSENTIALS OF DIAGNOSIS

▶ The severity of the high-altitude illness is affected by the rate and height of ascent and the individual's susceptibility.

▶ Prompt recognition and medical treatment of early symptoms of high-altitude illness may prevent progression.

▶ Clinicians must assess other conditions that may coexist or mimic symptoms of high-altitude illness.

▶ Immediate descent is the definitive treatment for high-altitude cerebral edema and high-altitude pulmonary edema.

▶ General Considerations

As altitude increases, hypobaric hypoxia results due to a decrease in both barometric pressure and oxygen partial pressure. High-altitude illnesses are due to hypobaric hypoxia at high altitudes (usually greater than 2000 meters or 6562 feet). High-altitude illness includes a spectrum of disorders categorized by end-organ effects (mostly cerebral and pulmonary) and exposure duration (acute and long-term). Acute high-altitude illnesses are **acute hypoxia, acute mountain sickness (AMS), high-altitude cerebral edema (HACE),** and **high-altitude pulmonary edema (HAPE).**

Acclimatization occurs as a physiologic response to the rise in altitude and increasing hypobaric hypoxia. High-altitude illness results when the hypoxic stress is greater than the individual's ability to acclimatize. Risk factors for high-altitude illness include increased physical activity with insufficient acclimatization, inadequate education and preparation, individual susceptibility, and previous high-altitude illness. The key determinants of high-altitude illness risk and severity include both individual susceptibility factors and altitudinal factors (rapid rate and height of ascent and total change in altitude).

Individual susceptibility factors include underlying conditions such as cardiac and pulmonary dysfunction, patent foramen ovale, blood disorders, pregnancy, neurologic conditions, cigarette smoking, recent surgery, diabetes, and many other chronic medical conditions. Those with symptomatic cardiac or pulmonary disease must avoid high altitudes.

Patient assessment for high-altitude illness must also include evaluation for other conditions, which may coexist or may present in a similar manner.

1. High-Altitude–Associated Neurologic Conditions: AMS & HACE

There is a spectrum of neurologic conditions caused by high altitude, ranging from **acute mountain sickness (AMS)** to the more serious form, **high-altitude cerebral edema (HACE).** Clinicians may utilize various diagnostic tools to assess the level of cerebral impairment due to high altitude.

AMS includes symptoms such as headache (most severe and persistent symptom), lassitude, drowsiness, dizziness, chilliness, nausea and vomiting, and difficulty sleeping. Later symptoms include irritability, difficulty concentrating, anorexia, insomnia, and increased headaches.

HACE includes the severe symptoms of AMS and results from cerebral vasogenic edema and cerebral cellular hypoxia. It usually occurs at elevations above 2500 meters (8202 feet) but may occur at lower elevations. Hallmarks are altered mental status, ataxia, severe lassitude, and encephalopathy. Examination findings may include confusion, ataxia, urinary retention or incontinence, focal neurologic deficits, papilledema, and seizures. Symptoms may progress to obtundation, coma, and death.

► Treatment

Definitive treatment is immediate descent of at least 610 meters (2001 feet), and descent must continue until symptoms improve. Descent is essential if the symptoms are persistent, severe, or worsening, or if HACE or HAPE are present. If immediate descent is not possible, portable hyperbaric chambers can provide symptomatic relief, but they must not delay descent.

Initial treatment involves oxygen administration to keep the pulse oximetry S_pO_2 to greater than 90%.

Acetazolamide (250 mg twice daily) is an effective medication for both prophylaxis and treatment of mild symptoms of AMS.

Dexamethasone is given for moderate to severe AMS (4 mg orally every 6 hours). Dexamethasone is the primary treatment for HACE (8 mg once then 4 mg every 6 hours).

Acetazolamide can be added as an adjunct in severe HACE cases. In most individuals, symptoms clear within 24–48 hours. HACE treatment must continue until 24 hours after resolution of symptoms or until descent is completed. Dexamethasone should not be given for longer than 7 days.

It is imperative that the clinician also assess for other conditions that may mimic or coexist with AMS and HACE.

If HAPE symptoms and signs are present along with HACE, nifedipine or a selective phosphodiesterase inhibitor may be added for pulmonary vasodilation. The clinician must be cautious when using combinations of vasodilators.

2. Acute HAPE

HAPE is the leading cause of death from high-altitude illness. The hallmark is markedly elevated pulmonary artery pressure followed by pulmonary edema. It usually occurs at altitudes above 3000 meters (9840 feet), although it may occur at lower levels. Early symptoms may appear within 6–36 hours after arrival at a high-altitude area. These include incessant dry cough, shortness of breath disproportionate to exertion, headache, decreased exercise performance, fatigue, dyspnea at rest, and chest tightness. Recognition of the early symptoms may enable the patient to descend before incapacitating pulmonary edema develops. Strenuous exertion must be avoided. Later, wheezing, orthopnea, and hemoptysis may occur as pulmonary edema worsens.

Physical findings may include tachycardia, mild fever, tachypnea, cyanosis, prolonged respiration, rales, and rhonchi. The clinician must assess for other potential medical conditions because the clinical picture may resemble other entities. Diagnosis is usually clinical; ancillary tests are nonspecific or unavailable on site. Prompt recognition and medical attention of early symptoms of HAPE may prevent progression.

► Treatment

Immediate descent (at least 610 meters [2000 feet]) is essential, although this may not be immediately possible and may not alone improve symptoms.

The patient must be placed at rest, reclined with head elevated. Supplemental oxygen must be administered to maintain pulse oximetry reading S_pO_2 greater than 90%. Recompression in a portable hyperbaric bag will temporarily reduce symptoms if rapid or immediate descent is not possible, but must not delay descent.

Nifedipine (60 mg slow extended-release tablets daily, given in divided doses) can be used as an adjunct if the other therapies (descent, oxygen, or portable hyperbarics) are not successful or available. Selective phosphodiesterase inhibitors may be used for HAPE prevention but may also provide effective symptom relief as an alternative or if nifedipine is not available. *Administering nifedipine plus a phosphodiesterase inhibitor as pulmonary vasodilators is not recommended* because this combination may also lower the mean arterial pressure and decrease cerebral perfusion. Treatment for ARDS (see Chapter 9) is required for some patients. If neurologic symptoms are present concurrently with HAPE and do not resolve with improved oxygenation, dexamethasone may be added according to HACE treatment guidelines.

3. Subacute Mountain Sickness

This occurs most frequently in unacclimatized individuals and at high altitudes (above 4500 meters) for a prolonged period of time. Treatment consists of rest, oxygen administration, diuretics, and return to lower altitudes.

4. Chronic Mountain Sickness (Monge Disease)

This uncommon condition is seen in residents of high-altitude communities who have lost their acclimatization to such a hypobaric hypoxic environment. It is difficult to differentiate from chronic pulmonary disease.

▶ Prevention of High-Altitude Disorders

Pre-trip preventive measures include participant education, medical preparticipation evaluation, pre-trip planning, optimal physical conditioning before travel, and adequate rest and sleep the day before travel and during the trip. Preventive efforts during ascent include reduced food intake and avoidance of alcohol, tobacco, and unnecessary physical activity during travel.

Gradual ascent is the most effective way to allow acclimatization. Low-risk ascension rate is 2 or more days to arrive at 2500–3000 meters. The altitude reached during waking hours is not as important as the altitude at which the hiker sleeps. If the terrain does not allow a sleeping elevation increase below 500 meters, an extra rest day must be added before or after the increased sleep elevation more than 500 meters.

Drug prophylaxis may be prescribed for AMS and HACE if no contraindications exist. Prophylactic low-dose acetazolamide (125 mg twice daily orally) has been shown to reduce the incidence and severity of AMS and HACE when started 3 days prior to ascent and continued for 48–72 hours at high altitude. Dexamethasone is an alternative prophylactic medication for AMS and HACE.

Individuals with a past history of HAPE should use drug prophylaxis to reduce the risk of recurrence. Nifedipine started the day before ascent and continued through the fourth day at target elevation, or through the seventh day if the ascent rate was faster, is recommended. Salmeterol can be added beginning 24 hours prior to ascent. This can be used as an adjunct to nifedipine but not as monotherapy.

Phosphodiesterase inhibitors may be beneficial in the treatment of HAPE based on their physiologic effects of decreased pulmonary arterial pressures and pulmonary vasodilation.

▶ When to Admit

- All patients with HACE or HAPE must be hospitalized for further observation.
- Hospitalization must also be considered for any patient who remains symptomatic after treatment and descent.
- Pulmonary symptoms and hypoxia may be worsened by complications such as pulmonary embolism, secondary respiratory infection, bronchospasm, mucous plugging, or acute coronary syndrome.

Campbell AD et al. Risk stratification for athletes and adventurers in high-altitude environments: recommendations for preparticipation evaluation. Wilderness Environ Med. 2015 Dec; 26(4 Suppl):S30–9. [PMID: 26617376]

Jin J. JAMA patient page. Acute mountain sickness. JAMA. 2017 Nov 14;318(18):1840. [PMID: 29136446]

Luks AM et al. Acute high-altitude sickness. Eur Respir Rev. 2017 Jan 31;26(143). pii: 160096. [PMID: 28143879]

Meier D et al. Does this patient have acute mountain sickness? The Rational Clinical Examination Systematic Review. JAMA. 2017 Nov 14;318(18):1810–19. [PMID: 29136449]

Nieto Estrada VH et al. Interventions for preventing high altitude illness: Part 1. Commonly-used classes of drugs. Cochrane Database Syst Rev. 2017 Jun 27;6:CD009761. [PMID: 28653390]

SAFETY OF AIR TRAVEL & SELECTION OF PATIENTS FOR AIR TRAVEL

The medical safety of air travel depends on the nature and severity of the traveler's preflight condition and factors such as travel duration, frequency and use of inflight exercise, cabin altitude pressure, availability of medical supplies, infectious diseases of other travelers, and the presence of health care professionals on board. Air travel passengers are susceptible to a wide range of flight-related problems: pulmonary (hypoxemia, gas expansion), venous thromboembolism (VTE), infections, cardiac, gastrointestinal, ocular, immunologic, syncope, neuropsychiatric, metabolic, trauma, and illicit substance-related conditions. Air-travel risks are higher for those air travelers with preexisting medical conditions.

Hypobaric hypoxia is the underlying etiology of most serious medical emergencies in flight due to cabin altitude. Despite commercial aircraft pressurization requirements, there is significant hypoxemia, dyspnea, gas expansion, and stress in travelers.

Any form of prolonged travel involving immobilization has been associated with increased risk of VTE (referred to as "traveler's thrombosis"), although air travel has been the main focus of medical review. Risks for VTE in long-distance travelers include the following: (1) travel involving immobilization for 4 or more hours, (2) hypercoagulable disorders, and (3) acquired risks.

Air travel is not advised for anyone who is "incapacitated" or has any "unstable conditions." The Air Transport Association of America defines an **incapacitated passenger** as "one who is suffering from a physical or mental disability and who, because of such disability or the effect of the flight on the disability, is incapable of self-care; would endanger the health or safety of such person or other passengers or airline employees; or would cause discomfort or annoyance of other passengers." **Unstable conditions** include active pneumothorax, advanced pulmonary hypertension, acute worsening of an underlying lung disease, poorly controlled hypertension, dysrhythmias, angina, valvular disease, heart failure, or acute psychiatric condition; severe anemia or symptomatic sickle cell disease; recent myocardial infarction; cerebrovascular accident; poorly controlled seizure disorder; deep venous thrombosis; postsurgery, especially heart surgery (unless approved by surgeon); and any active communicable disease. Public Health Travel Restrictions have shown efficacy in preventing commercial air or international travel of persons with certain communicable diseases that pose public health threat.

▶ Pregnancy

Traveling during pregnancy is becoming more common. Pregnant travelers have unique travel-related and location-specific risks. A clinician's authorization is required if travel is essential during the ninth month of pregnancy or earlier in a complicated or high-risk pregnancy.

Long travel increases risk of VTE for the pregnant traveler. Pregnant travelers are at higher risk from infection transmission and air travel radiation exposure.

▶ Prevention

Air travel complications may be reduced by the following preventive measures: passenger prescreening, passenger education, and in-flight positioning and activity. Prescreening evaluation is recommended for all high-risk patients including preexisting requirement for oxygen, continuous positive airway pressure or ventilator support, underlying restrictive or obstructive lung disease, comorbidities worsened by hypoxemia, previous respiratory distress during air travel, recent pneumothorax, and recent (within 6 weeks) acute respiratory illness. Patients at risk for hypoxia must be assessed prior to air travel to determine if there is a need for supplemental in-flight oxygen.

Air travel education must include risk reduction measures for VTE, infectious diseases, and exacerbations of underlying medical conditions. Patients and clinicians can check the World Health Organization website for the most updated information on travel health risks and infectious diseases (https://www.who.int/ith/en/).

All long-distance travelers can reduce VTE risk by avoiding constrictive clothing, staying well-hydrated, changing position frequently, avoiding cramped position, avoiding leg crossing, engaging in frequent (at least every hour) in-flight leg stretching exercises, and walking for 5 minutes every hour. Clinicians must assess those with high risk of VTE prior to air travel to determine whether anticoagulation is indicated (see Table 14–14).

Antony KM et al. Travel during pregnancy: considerations for the obstetric provider. Obstet Gynecol Surv. 2017 Feb; 72(2):97–115. [PMID: 28218771]

Clarke MJ et al. Compression stockings for preventing deep vein thrombosis in airline passengers. Cochrane Database Syst Rev. 2016 Sep 14;9:CD004002. [PMID: 27624857]

Jungerman MR et al. Federal travel restrictions to prevent disease transmission in the United States: an analysis of requested travel restrictions. Travel Med Infect Dis. 2017 Jul–Aug;18:30–5. [PMID: 28648932]

Thibeault C et al; Aerospace Medical Association. AsMA medical guidelines for air travel: in-flight medical care. Aerosp Med Hum Perform. 2015 Jun;86(6):5723. [PMID: 26099132]

Poisoning

38

Craig Smollin, MD
Kent R. Olson, MD

Patients with drug overdoses or poisoning may initially have no symptoms or they may have varying degrees of overt intoxication. The asymptomatic patient may have been exposed to or may have ingested a lethal dose, but not yet exhibit any manifestations of toxicity. It is important to (1) quickly assess the potential danger, (2) consider gut and skin decontamination to prevent absorption, (3) treat complications if they occur, and (4) observe the asymptomatic patient for an appropriate interval.

Assess the Danger

If the drug or poison is known, its danger can be assessed by consulting a text or computerized information resource or by calling a regional poison control center. (In the United States, dialing 1-800-222-1222 will direct the call to the regional poison control center.) Assessment will usually take into account the dose ingested; the time since ingestion; the presence of any symptoms or clinical signs; preexisting cardiac, respiratory, kidney, or liver disease; and, occasionally, specific serum drug or toxin levels. Be aware that the history given by the patient or family may be incomplete or unreliable.

IMMEDIATE 24-HOUR TOXICOLOGY CONSULTATION

Call your regional poison control center
U.S. toll-free 1-800-222-1222

Observe the Patient

Asymptomatic or mildly symptomatic patients should be observed for at least 4–6 hours. Longer observation is indicated if the ingested substance is a sustained-release preparation or is known to slow gastrointestinal motility (eg, opioids, anticholinergics, aspirin) or may cause a delayed onset of symptoms (eg, acetaminophen, colchicine, hepatotoxic mushrooms). After that time, the patient may be discharged if no symptoms have developed. Before discharge, psychiatric evaluation should be performed to assess suicide risk. Intentional ingestions in adolescents should raise the possibility of unwanted pregnancy or sexual abuse.

THE SYMPTOMATIC PATIENT

In symptomatic patients, treatment of life-threatening complications takes precedence over in-depth diagnostic evaluation. Patients with mild symptoms may deteriorate rapidly, which is why all potentially significant exposures should be observed in an acute care facility. The following complications may occur, depending on the type of poisoning.

COMA

Assessment & Complications

Coma is commonly associated with ingestion of large doses of antihistamines (eg, diphenhydramine), benzodiazepines and other sedative-hypnotic drugs, ethanol, opioids, antipsychotic drugs, or antidepressants. The most common cause of death in comatose patients is respiratory failure, which may occur abruptly. Pulmonary aspiration of gastric contents may also occur, especially in victims who are deeply obtunded or convulsing. Hypoxia and hypoventilation may cause or aggravate hypotension, arrhythmias, and seizures. Thus, protection of the airway and assisted ventilation are the most important treatment measures for any poisoned patient.

Treatment

A. Emergency Management

The initial emergency management of coma can be remembered by the mnemonic *ABCD*, for *A*irway, *B*reathing, *C*irculation, and *D*rugs (dextrose, thiamine, and naloxone or flumazenil), respectively.

1. Airway—Establish a patent airway by positioning, suction, or insertion of an artificial nasal or oropharyngeal airway. If the patient is deeply comatose or if airway reflexes are depressed, perform endotracheal intubation. These airway interventions may not be necessary if the patient is intoxicated by an opioid or a benzodiazepine and responds to intravenous naloxone or flumazenil.

2. Breathing—Clinically assess the quality and depth of respiration and provide assistance if necessary with a bag-valve-mask device or mechanical ventilator. Administer supplemental oxygen, if needed. The arterial or venous blood CO_2 tension is useful in determining the adequacy of ventilation. The arterial blood PO_2 determination may reveal hypoxemia, which may be caused by respiratory depression, bronchospasm, pulmonary aspiration, or noncardiogenic pulmonary edema. Pulse oximetry provides an assessment of oxygenation, but is not reliable in patients with methemoglobinemia or carbon monoxide poisoning, unless a pulse oximetry device capable of detecting these forms of hemoglobin is used.

3. Circulation—Measure the pulse and blood pressure and estimate tissue perfusion (eg, by measurement of urinary output, skin signs, arterial blood pH). Place the patient on continuous ECG monitoring. Insert an intravenous line, and draw blood for glucose, electrolytes, serum creatinine and liver tests, and possible quantitative toxicologic testing.

4. Drugs—

A. DEXTROSE AND THIAMINE—Unless promptly treated, severe hypoglycemia can cause irreversible brain damage. Therefore, in all obtunded, comatose or convulsing patients, give 50% dextrose, 50–100 mL by intravenous bolus, unless a rapid point-of-care blood sugar test rules out hypoglycemia. In alcoholic or very malnourished patients who may have marginal thiamine stores, give thiamine, 100 mg intramuscularly or in the intravenous fluids.

B. OPIOID ANTAGONISTS—Naloxone, 0.4–2 mg intravenously or 2–4 mg by intranasal spray, may reverse opioid-induced respiratory depression and coma. It is often given empirically to any comatose patient with depressed respirations. If opioid overdose is strongly suspected, give additional doses of naloxone (up to 5–10 mg may be required to reverse the effects of potent opioids). **Note:** Naloxone has a shorter duration of action (2–3 hours) than most common opioids; repeated doses may be required, and continuous observation for at least 3–4 hours after the last dose is mandatory.

C. FLUMAZENIL—Flumazenil, 0.2–0.5 mg intravenously, repeated as needed up to a maximum of 3 mg, may reverse benzodiazepine-induced coma. **Caution:** *In most circumstances, use of flumazenil is not advised as the potential risks outweigh its benefits.* Flumazenil should **not** be given if the patient has coingested a potential convulsant drug, is a user of high-dose benzodiazepines, or has a seizure disorder because its use in these circumstances may precipitate seizures. **Note:** Flumazenil has a short duration of effect (2–3 hours), and resedation requiring additional doses may occur.

HYPOTHERMIA

▶ Assessment & Complications

Hypothermia commonly accompanies coma due to opioids, ethanol, hypoglycemic agents, phenothiazines, barbiturates, benzodiazepines, and other sedative-hypnotics and central nervous system depressants. Hypothermic patients may have a barely perceptible pulse and blood pressure.

Hypothermia may cause or aggravate hypotension, which will not reverse until the temperature is normalized.

▶ Treatment

Treatment of hypothermia is discussed in Chapter 37. Gradual rewarming is preferred unless the patient is in cardiac arrest.

HYPOTENSION

▶ Assessment & Complications

Hypotension may be due to poisoning by many different drugs, including antihypertensives, beta-blockers, calcium channel blockers, disulfiram (ethanol interaction), iron, trazodone, quetiapine, and other antipsychotic agents and antidepressants. Poisons causing hypotension include cyanide, carbon monoxide, hydrogen sulfide, aluminum or zinc phosphide, arsenic, and certain mushrooms.

Hypotension in the poisoned or drug-overdosed patient may be caused by venous or arteriolar vasodilation, hypovolemia, depressed cardiac contractility, or a combination of these effects.

▶ Treatment

Most hypotensive poisoned patients respond to empiric treatment with repeated 200 mL intravenous boluses of 0.9% saline or other isotonic crystalloid up to a total of 1–2 L; much larger amounts may be needed if the victim is profoundly volume depleted (eg, as with massive diarrhea due to *Amanita phalloides* mushroom poisoning). Monitoring the central venous pressure (CVP) can help determine whether further fluid therapy is needed. Consider bedside cardiac ultrasound or pulmonary artery catheterization (or both) to assess CVP. If fluid therapy is not successful after adequate volume replacement, give dopamine or norepinephrine by intravenous infusion.

Hypotension caused by certain toxins may respond to specific treatment. For hypotension caused by overdoses of tricyclic antidepressants or other sodium channel blockers, administer sodium bicarbonate, 50–100 mEq by intravenous bolus injection. Norepinephrine 4–8 mcg/min by intravenous infusion is more effective than dopamine in some patients with overdoses of tricyclic antidepressants or of drugs with predominantly vasodilating effects. For beta-blocker overdose, glucagon (5–10 mg intravenously) may be of value. For calcium channel blocker overdose, administer calcium chloride, 1–2 g intravenously (repeated doses may be necessary; doses of 5–10 g and more have been given in some cases). High-dose insulin (0.5–1 unit/kg/h intravenously) euglycemic therapy may also be used (see the sections Beta-Adrenergic Blockers and Calcium Channel Blockers, below). Intralipid 20% lipid emulsion has been reported to improve hemodynamics in some cases of intoxication by highly lipid-soluble drugs such as bupivacaine, bupropion, clomipramine, and verapamil. Intravenous methylene blue and extracorporeal membrane oxygenation (ECMO) have been employed in a few refractory cases; ECMO may offer temporary hemodynamic stabilization while the offending drug is eliminated.

Graudins A et al. Calcium channel antagonist and beta-blocker overdose: antidotes and adjunct therapies. Br J Clin Pharmacol. 2016 Mar;81(3):453–61. [PMID: 26344579]

Heise CW et al. Two cases of refractory cardiogenic shock secondary to bupropion successfully treated with veno-arterial extracorporeal membrane oxygenation. J Med Toxicol. 2016 Sep;12(3):301–4. [PMID: 26856351]

Laes JR et al. Improvement in hemodynamics after methylene blue administration in drug-induced vasodilatory shock: a case report. J Med Toxicol. 2015 Dec;11(4):460–3. [PMID: 26310944]

HYPERTENSION

Assessment & Complications

Hypertension may be due to poisoning with amphetamines and synthetic stimulants, anticholinergics, cocaine, performance-enhancing products (containing caffeine, phenylephrine, ephedrine, or yohimbine), monoamine oxidase (MAO) inhibitors, and other drugs.

Severe hypertension (eg, diastolic blood pressure greater than 105–110 mm Hg in a person who does not have chronic hypertension) can result in acute intracranial hemorrhage, myocardial infarction, or aortic dissection.

Treatment

Treat hypertension if the patient is symptomatic or if the diastolic pressure is higher than 105–110 mm Hg—especially if there is no prior history of hypertension.

Hypertensive patients who are agitated or anxious may benefit from a sedative (such as lorazepam, 2–3 mg intravenously) or an antipsychotic drug (eg, haloperidol or olanzapine). For persistent hypertension, administer phentolamine, 2–5 mg intravenously, or nitroprusside sodium, 0.25–8 mcg/kg/min intravenously. If excessive tachycardia is present, *add* esmolol, 25–100 mcg/kg/min intravenously, or labetalol, 0.2–0.3 mg/kg intravenously. **Caution:** Do not give beta-blockers alone, since doing so may paradoxically worsen hypertension in some cases as a result of unopposed alpha-adrenergic stimulation.

Richards JR et al. Treatment of toxicity from amphetamines, related derivatives, and analogues: a systematic clinical review. Drug Alcohol Depend. 2015 May 1;150:1–13. [PMID: 25724076]

ARRHYTHMIAS

Assessment & Complications

Arrhythmias may occur with a variety of drugs or toxins (Table 38–1). They may also occur as a result of hypoxia, metabolic acidosis, or electrolyte imbalance (eg, hyperkalemia, hypokalemia, hypomagnesemia, or hypocalcemia), or following exposure to chlorinated solvents or chloral hydrate overdose. Atypical ventricular tachycardia (torsades de pointes) is often associated with drugs that prolong the QT interval.

Table 38–1. Common toxins or drugs causing arrhythmias.[1]

Arrhythmia	Common Causes
Sinus bradycardia	Beta-blockers, calcium channel blockers, clonidine, digitalis glycosides, organophosphates
Atrioventricular block	Beta-blockers, calcium channel blockers, class Ia antiarrhythmics (including quinidine), carbamazepine, clonidine, digitalis glycosides, lithium
Sinus tachycardia	Beta-agonists (eg, albuterol), amphetamines, anticholinergics, antihistamines, caffeine, cocaine, pseudoephedrine, tricyclic and other antidepressants
Wide QRS complex	Class Ia and class Ic antiarrhythmics, phenothiazines (eg, thioridazine), potassium (hyperkalemia), propranolol, tricyclic antidepressants, bupropion, lamotrigine, diphenhydramine (severe overdose)
QT interval prolongation and torsades de pointes	Arsenic, class Ia and class III antiarrhythmics, citalopram, droperidol, lithium, methadone, pentamidine, sertraline, sotalol, and many other drugs[2]
Ventricular premature beats and ventricular tachycardia	Amphetamines, cocaine, ephedrine, caffeine, chlorinated or fluorinated hydrocarbons, digoxin, aconite (found in some Chinese herbal preparations), fluoride, theophylline. QT prolongation can lead to atypical ventricular tachycardia (torsades de pointes).

[1]Arrhythmias may also occur as a result of hypoxia, metabolic acidosis, or electrolyte imbalance (eg, hyperkalemia or hypokalemia, hypocalcemia, hypomagnesemia).
[2]https://crediblemeds.org/

Treatment

Hypoxia or electrolyte imbalance should be sought and treated. If ventricular arrhythmias persist, administer lidocaine or amiodarone at usual antiarrhythmic doses. **Note:** Wide QRS complex tachycardia in the setting of tricyclic antidepressant overdose (or diphenhydramine or class Ia antiarrhythmic drugs) should be treated with sodium bicarbonate, 50–100 mEq intravenously by bolus infusion. **Caution:** In such cases, avoid class Ia antiarrhythmic agents (eg, procainamide, disopyramide) and amiodarone, which may aggravate arrhythmias caused by tricyclic antidepressants. Torsades de pointes associated with prolonged QT interval may respond to intravenous magnesium (2 g intravenously over 2 minutes) or overdrive pacing. Treat digitalis-induced arrhythmias with digoxin-specific antibodies.

For tachyarrhythmias induced by chlorinated solvents, chloral hydrate, Freons, or sympathomimetic agents, use propranolol or esmolol (see doses given above in Hypertension section).

Al-Abri SA et al. Ventricular dysrhythmias associated with poisoning and drug overdose: a 10-year review of statewide poison control center data from California. Am J Cardiovasc Drugs. 2015 Feb;15(1):43–50. [PMID: 25567789]

Bruccoleri RE et al. A literature review of the use of sodium bicarbonate for the treatment of QRS widening. J Med Toxicol. 2016 Mar;12(1):121–9. [PMID: 26159649]

Laskowski LK et al. Start me up! Recurrent ventricular tachydysrhythmias following intentional concentrated caffeine ingestion. Clin Toxicol (Phila). 2015;53(8):830–3. [PMID: 26279469]

Paratz ED et al. The cardiac complications of methamphetamines. Heart Lung Circ. 2016 Apr;25(4):325–32. [PMID: 26706652]

SEIZURES

▶ Assessment & Complications

Seizures may be caused by many poisons and drugs, including amphetamines, antidepressants (especially tricyclic antidepressants, bupropion, and venlafaxine), antihistamines (especially diphenhydramine), antipsychotics, camphor, synthetic cannabinoids and cathinones, cocaine, isoniazid (INH), chlorinated insecticides, piperazines, tramadol, and theophylline. The onset of seizures may be delayed for up to 18–24 hours after extended-released bupropion overdose.

Seizures may also be caused by hypoxia, hypoglycemia, hypocalcemia, hyponatremia, withdrawal from alcohol or sedative-hypnotics, head trauma, central nervous system infection, or idiopathic epilepsy.

Prolonged or repeated seizures may lead to hypoxia, metabolic acidosis, hyperthermia, and rhabdomyolysis.

▶ Treatment

Administer lorazepam, 2–3 mg, or diazepam, 5–10 mg, intravenously, or—if intravenous access is not immediately available—midazolam, 5–10 mg intramuscularly. If convulsions continue, administer phenobarbital, 15–20 mg/kg slowly intravenously over no less than 30 minutes. (For drug-induced seizures, phenobarbital is preferred over phenytoin or levetiracetam.) Propofol infusion has also been reported effective for some resistant drug-induced seizures.

Seizures due to a few drugs and toxins may require antidotes or other specific therapies (as listed in Table 38–2).

Baird-Gunning J et al. Lithium poisoning. J Intensive Care Med. 2017 May;32(4):249–63. [PMID: 27516079]

Chen HY et al. Treatment of drug-induced seizures. Br J Clin Pharmacol. 2016 Mar;81(3):412–9. [PMID: 26174744]

HYPERTHERMIA

▶ Assessment & Complications

Hyperthermia may be associated with poisoning by amphetamines and other synthetic stimulants (cathinones, piperazines), atropine and other anticholinergic drugs, cocaine, salicylates, strychnine, tricyclic antidepressants, and various other medications. Overdoses of serotonin reuptake inhibitors (eg, fluoxetine, paroxetine, sertraline) or their use in a patient taking an MAO inhibitor may cause

Table 38–2. Seizures related to toxins or drugs requiring special consideration.[1]

Toxin or Drug	Comments
Methylenedioxymeth-amphetamine (MDMA; "Ecstasy")	Seizures may also be due to hyponatremia or hyperthermia.
Isoniazid	Administer pyridoxine.
Lithium	May indicate need for hemodialysis.
Organophosphates	Administer pralidoxime (2-PAM) and atropine in addition to usual anticonvulsants.
Strychnine	"Seizures" are actually spinally mediated muscle spasms and usually require neuromuscular paralysis and mechanical ventilation.
Theophylline	Seizures indicate need for hemodialysis.
Tricyclic antidepressants	Hyperthermia and cardiotoxicity are common complications of repeated seizures; paralyze early with neuromuscular blockers to reduce muscular hyperactivity.

[1]See text for dosages.

agitation, hyperactivity, myoclonus, and hyperthermia ("serotonin syndrome"). Antipsychotic agents can cause rigidity and hyperthermia (neuroleptic malignant syndrome [NMS]). (See Chapter 25.) Malignant hyperthermia is a rare disorder associated with general anesthetic agents.

Hyperthermia is a rapidly life-threatening complication. Severe hyperthermia (temperature higher than 40–41°C) can rapidly cause brain damage and multiorgan failure, including rhabdomyolysis, acute kidney injury, and coagulopathy (see Chapter 37).

▶ Treatment

Treat hyperthermia aggressively by removing the patient's clothing, spraying the skin with tepid water, and high-volume fanning. Alternatively, the patient can be placed in an ice water bath (not simply applying ice to selected surfaces). If external cooling is not rapidly effective, as shown by a normal rectal temperature within 30–40 minutes, or if there is significant muscle rigidity or hyperactivity, induce neuromuscular paralysis with a nondepolarizing neuromuscular blocker (eg, rocuronium, vecuronium). Once paralyzed, the patient must be intubated and mechanically ventilated and sedated. While the patient is paralyzed, the absence of visible muscular convulsive movements may give the false impression that brain seizure activity has ceased; bedside electroencephalography may be useful in recognizing continued nonconvulsive seizures.

Dantrolene (2–5 mg/kg intravenously) may be effective for hyperthermia associated with muscle rigidity that does not respond to neuromuscular blockade (ie, malignant hyperthermia). Bromocriptine, 2.5–7.5 mg orally daily, has been recommended for neuroleptic malignant syndrome. Cyproheptadine, 4 mg orally every hour for three or four doses, or chlorpromazine, 25 mg intravenously or 50 mg intramuscularly, has been used to treat serotonin syndrome.

Katus LE et al. Management of serotonin syndrome and neuroleptic malignant syndrome. Curr Treat Options Neurol. 2016 Sep;18(9):39. [PMID: 27469512]

Krüger BD et al. Dexmedetomidine-associated hyperthermia: a series of 9 cases and a review of the literature. Anesth Analg. 2017 Dec;125(6):1898–906. [PMID: 28763361]

Sweeney B et al. Hyperthermia and severe rhabdomyolysis from synthetic cannabinoids. Am J Emerg Med. 2016 Jan;34(1):121. e1–2. [PMID: 26143311]

Tormoehlen LM et al. Neuroleptic malignant syndrome and serotonin syndrome. Handb Clin Neurol. 2018;157:663–75. [PMID: 30459031]

Walter E et al. Drug-induced hyperthermia in critical care. J Intensive Care Soc. 2015 Nov;16(4):306–11. [PMID: 28979436]

▶ ANTIDOTES & OTHER TREATMENT

ANTIDOTES

Give an antidote (if available) when there is reasonable certainty of a specific diagnosis (Table 38–3). Be aware that some antidotes themselves may have serious side effects.

Table 38–3. Some toxic agents for which there are specific antidotes.[1]

Toxic Agent	Specific Antidote
Acetaminophen	N-Acetylcysteine
Anticholinergics (eg, atropine)	Physostigmine
Anticholinesterases (eg, organophosphate pesticides)	Atropine and pralidoxime (2-PAM)
Benzodiazepines	Flumazenil (rarely used)[2]
Carbon monoxide	Oxygen (hyperbaric oxygen of uncertain benefit)
Cyanide	Sodium nitrite, sodium thiosulfate; hydroxocobalamin
Digitalis glycosides	Digoxin-specific Fab antibodies
Heavy metals (eg, lead, mercury, iron) and arsenic	Specific chelating agents
Isoniazid	Pyridoxine (vitamin B_6)
Methanol, ethylene glycol	Ethanol (ethyl alcohol) or fomepizole (4-methylpyrazole)
Opioids	Naloxone, nalmefene
Snake venom	Specific antivenin
Sulfonylurea oral hypoglycemic drugs	Glucose, octreotide

[1]See text for indications and dosages.
[2]May induce seizures in patients with preexisting seizure disorder, benzodiazepine addiction, or concomitant tricyclic antidepressant or other convulsant overdose. If seizures occur, diazepam and other benzodiazepine anticonvulsants will not be effective. As with naloxone, the duration of action of flumazenil is short (2–3 hours) and resedation may occur, requiring repeated doses.

The indications and dosages for specific antidotes are discussed in the respective sections for specific toxins.

Dart RC et al. Expert consensus guidelines for stocking of antidotes in hospitals that provide emergency care. Ann Emerg Med. 2018 Mar;71(3):314–25. [PMID: 28669553]

Dzeshka MS et al. Direct oral anticoagulant reversal: how, when and issues faced. Expert Rev Hematol. 2017 Nov;10(11):1005–22. [PMID: 28901221]

Graudins A et al. Calcium channel antagonist and beta-blocker overdose: antidotes and adjunct therapies. Br J Clin Pharmacol. 2016 Mar;81(3):453–61. [PMID: 26344579]

Iyengar AR et al. Organophosphate-hydrolyzing enzymes as first-line of defence against nerve agent-poisoning: perspectives and the road ahead. Protein J. 2016 Dec;35(6):424–39. [PMID: 27830420]

McMartin K et al. Antidotes for poisoning by alcohols that form toxic metabolites. Br J Clin Pharmacol. 2016 Mar;81(3):505–15. [PMID: 26551875]

Schwenk M. Chemical warfare agents. Classes and targets. Toxicol Lett. 2018 Sep 1;293:253–63. [PMID: 29197625]

DECONTAMINATION OF THE SKIN

Corrosive agents rapidly injure the skin and eyes and must be removed immediately. In addition, many toxins are readily absorbed through the skin, and systemic absorption can be prevented only by rapid action.

Wash the affected areas with copious quantities of lukewarm water or saline, taking care to limit exposure to health care providers. Wash carefully behind the ears, under the nails, and in skin folds. For oily substances (eg, pesticides), wash the skin at least twice with plain soap and shampoo the hair. Specific decontaminating solutions or solvents (eg, alcohol) are rarely indicated and in some cases may paradoxically enhance absorption. For exposure to chemical warfare poisons such as nerve agents or vesicants, some authorities recommend use of a dilute hypochlorite solution (household bleach diluted 1:10 with water), but not in the eyes.

DECONTAMINATION OF THE EYES

Act quickly to prevent serious damage. Flush the eyes with copious amounts of saline or water. (If available, instill local anesthetic drops in the eye before beginning irrigation.) Remove contact lenses if present. Lift the tarsal conjunctiva to look for undissolved particles and to facilitate irrigation. Continue irrigation for 15 minutes or until each eye has been irrigated with at least 1 L of solution. If the toxin is an acid or a base, check the pH of the tears after irrigation, and continue irrigation until the pH is between 6 and 8. An amphoteric decontamination solution (Diphoterine, Prevor) is used in some countries for treatment of alkali injuries to the eye.

After irrigation is complete, perform a careful examination of the eye, using fluorescein and a slit lamp or Wood lamp to identify areas of corneal injury. Patients with serious conjunctival or corneal injury should be immediately referred to an ophthalmologist.

GASTROINTESTINAL DECONTAMINATION

Removal of ingested poisons by induced emesis or gastric lavage was a routine part of emergency treatment for decades. However, prospective randomized studies have failed to demonstrate improved clinical outcome after gastric emptying. For small or moderate ingestions of most substances, toxicologists generally recommend oral activated charcoal alone without prior gastric emptying; in some cases, when the interval after ingestion has been more than 1–2 hours and the ingestant is non–life-threatening, even charcoal is withheld (eg, if the estimated benefit is outweighed by the potential risk of pulmonary aspiration of charcoal). Exceptions are large ingestions of anticholinergic compounds and salicylates, which often delay gastric emptying, and ingestion of sustained-release or enteric-coated tablets, which may remain intact for several hours. In these cases, delayed gut decontamination may be indicated.

Gastric emptying is not generally used for ingestion of corrosive agents or petroleum distillates, because further esophageal injury or pulmonary aspiration may result. However, in certain cases, removal of the toxin may be more important than concern over possible complications. Consult a medical toxicologist or regional poison control center (1-800-222-1222) for advice.

A. Activated Charcoal

Activated charcoal effectively adsorbs almost all drugs and poisons. Poorly adsorbed substances include iron, lithium, potassium, sodium, mineral acids, and alcohols.

1. Indications—Activated charcoal can be used for prompt adsorption of drugs or toxins in the stomach and intestine. However, evidence of benefit in clinical studies is lacking. Administration of charcoal, especially if mixed with sorbitol, can provoke vomiting, which could lead to pulmonary aspiration in an obtunded patient.

2. Contraindications—Activated charcoal should not be used for comatose or convulsing patients unless it can be given by gastric tube and the airway is first protected by a cuffed endotracheal tube. It is also contraindicated for patients with ileus or intestinal obstruction or those who have ingested corrosives for whom endoscopy is planned.

3. Technique—Administer activated charcoal, 60–100 g orally or via gastric tube, mixed in aqueous slurry. Repeated doses may be given to ensure gastrointestinal adsorption or to enhance elimination of some drugs.

B. Whole Bowel Irrigation

Whole bowel irrigation uses large volumes of a balanced polyethylene glycol-electrolyte solution to mechanically cleanse the entire intestinal tract. Because of the composition of the irrigating solution, there is no significant gain or loss of systemic fluids or electrolytes.

1. Indications—Whole bowel irrigation is particularly effective for massive iron ingestion in which intact tablets are visible on abdominal radiographs. It has also been used for ingestions of lithium, sustained-release and enteric-coated tablets, and swallowed drug-filled packets.

2. Contraindications—Do not use in patients with suspected intestinal obstruction. Use with caution in patients who are obtunded or have depressed airway protective reflexes.

3. Technique—Administer a balanced polyethylene glycol-electrolyte solution (CoLyte, GoLYTELY) into the stomach via gastric tube at a rate of 1–2 L/h until the rectal effluent is clear. This may take several hours. It is most effective when patients are able to sit on a commode to pass the intestinal contents.

C. Increased Drug Removal

1. Urinary manipulation—Forced diuresis is hazardous; the risk of complications (fluid overload, electrolyte imbalance) usually outweighs its benefits. Some drugs (eg, salicylates, phenobarbital) are more rapidly excreted with an alkaline urine. To alkalinize the urine, add 100 mEq (two ampules) of sodium bicarbonate to 1 L of 5% dextrose in 0.225% saline (¼ normal saline), and infuse this solution intravenously at a rate of about 150–200 mL/h. Acidification (sometimes promoted for amphetamines, phencyclidine) is *not* very effective and is contraindicated in the presence of rhabdomyolysis or myoglobinuria.

2. Hemodialysis—The indications for dialysis are as follows: (1) known or suspected potentially lethal amounts of a dialyzable drug (Table 38–4); (2) poisoning with deep coma, apnea, severe hypotension, fluid and electrolyte or acid-base disturbance, or extreme body temperature changes that cannot be corrected by conventional measures; or (3) poisoning in patients with severe kidney, cardiac, pulmonary, or hepatic disease who will not be able to eliminate toxin by the usual mechanisms.

Table 38–4. Recommended use of hemodialysis in poisoning.

Poison	Common Indications[1]
Carbamazepine	Seizures, severe cardiotoxicity; serum level > 60 mg/L
Ethylene glycol	Acidosis, serum level > 50 mg/dL
Lithium	Severe symptoms; level > 4–5 mEq/L, especially if kidney impairment Note: dialysis of uncertain value; consult with medical toxicologist
Methanol	Acidosis, serum level > 50 mg/dL
Phenobarbital	Intractable hypotension, acidosis despite maximal supportive care
Salicylate	Severe acidosis, CNS symptoms, serum level > 100 mg/dL (acute overdose) or > 60 mg/dL (chronic intoxication)
Theophylline	Serum level > 90–100 mg/L (acute) or seizures and serum level > 40–60 mg/L (chronic)
Valproic acid	Serum level > 900–1000 mg/L or deep coma, severe acidosis

[1]See text for further discussion of indications.
CNS, central nervous system; CVVHD, continuous venovenous hemodialysis.

Continuous renal replacement therapy (including continuous venovenous hemodiafiltration and similar techniques) is of uncertain benefit for elimination of most poisons but has the advantage of gradual removal of the toxin and correction of any accompanying acidosis. Its use has been reported in the management of a variety of poisonings, including lithium intoxication.

3. Repeat-dose charcoal—Repeated doses of activated charcoal, 20–30 g orally or via gastric tube every 3–4 hours, may hasten elimination of some drugs (eg, phenytoin, carbamazepine, dapsone) by absorbing drugs excreted into the gut lumen ("gut dialysis"). However, clinical studies have failed to prove better outcome using repeat dose charcoal. Sorbitol or other cathartics should *not* be used with each dose, or else the resulting large stool volumes may lead to dehydration or hypernatremia.

Campion GH et al. Extracorporeal treatments in poisonings from four non-traditionally dialysed toxins (acetaminophen, digoxin, opioids and tricyclic antidepressants): a combined single-centre and national study. Basic Clin Pharmacol Toxicol. 2019 Mar;124(3):341–7. [PMID: 30248244]

Corcoran G et al. Use and knowledge of single dose activated charcoal: a survey of Australian doctors. Emerg Med Australas. 2016 Oct;28(5):578–85. [PMID: 27555040]

Donkor J et al. Analysis of gastric lavage reported to a statewide poison control system. J Emerg Med. 2016 Oct;51(4):394–400. [PMID: 27595368]

Ghannoum M et al. Use of extracorporeal treatments in the management of poisonings. Kidney Int. 2018 Oct;94(4):682–8. [PMID: 29958694]

Mirrakhimov AE et al. The role of renal replacement therapy in the management of pharmacologic poisonings. Int J Nephrol. 2016;2016:3047329. [PMID: 28042482]

Villarreal J et al. A retrospective review of the prehospital use of activated charcoal. Am J Emerg Med. 2015 Jan;33(1):56–9. [PMID: 25455049]

DIAGNOSIS OF POISONING

The identity of the ingested substance or substances is usually known, but occasionally a comatose patient is found with an unlabeled container or the patient is unable or unwilling to give a coherent history. By performing a directed physical examination and ordering common clinical laboratory tests, the clinician can often make a tentative diagnosis that may allow empiric interventions or may suggest specific toxicologic tests.

Physical Examination

Important diagnostic variables in the physical examination include blood pressure, pulse rate, temperature, pupil size, sweating, muscle tone, level of consciousness, and the presence or absence of peristaltic activity. Poisonings may present with one or more of the following common syndromes.

A. Sympathomimetic Syndrome

The blood pressure and pulse rate are elevated, though with severe hypertension reflex bradycardia may occur. The temperature is often elevated, pupils are dilated, and the skin is sweaty, though mucous membranes are dry. Patients are usually agitated, anxious, or frankly psychotic.

Examples: Amphetamines, cocaine, ephedrine, pseudoephedrine, synthetic cathinones and cannabinoids.

B. Sympatholytic Syndrome

The blood pressure and pulse rate are decreased and body temperature is low. The pupils are small or even pinpoint. Patients are usually obtunded or comatose.

Examples: Barbiturates, benzodiazepines and other sedative hypnotics, gamma-hydroxybutyrate (GHB), clonidine and related antihypertensives, ethanol, opioids.

C. Cholinergic Syndrome

Stimulation of muscarinic receptors causes bradycardia, miosis (constricted pupils), sweating, and hyperperistalsis as well as bronchorrhea, wheezing, excessive salivation, and urinary incontinence. Nicotinic receptor stimulation may produce initial hypertension and tachycardia as well as fasciculations and muscle weakness. Patients are usually agitated and anxious.

Examples: Carbamates, nicotine, organophosphates (including nerve agents), physostigmine.

D. Anticholinergic Syndrome

Tachycardia with mild hypertension is common, and the body temperature is often elevated. Pupils are widely dilated. The skin is flushed, hot, and dry. Peristalsis is decreased, and urinary retention is common. Patients may have myoclonic jerking or choreoathetoid movements. Agitated delirium is frequently seen, and severe hyperthermia may occur.

Examples: Atropine, scopolamine, other naturally occurring and pharmaceutical anticholinergics, antihistamines, tricyclic antidepressants.

Laboratory Tests

The following clinical laboratory tests are recommended for screening of the overdosed patient: measured serum osmolality and calculated osmol gap, electrolytes and anion gap, glucose, creatinine, blood urea nitrogen (BUN), creatine kinase, urinalysis (eg, oxalate crystals with ethylene glycol poisoning, myoglobinuria with rhabdomyolysis), and electrocardiography. Quantitative serum acetaminophen and ethanol levels should be determined in all patients with drug overdoses.

A. Osmol Gap

The osmol gap (Table 38–5) is increased in the presence of large quantities of low-molecular-weight substances, most commonly ethanol. Other common poisons associated with increased osmol gap are acetone, ethanol, ethylene glycol, isopropyl alcohol, methanol, and propylene glycol. **Note:** Severe alcoholic ketoacidosis and diabetic ketoacidosis can also cause an elevated osmol gap resulting from the production of ketones and other low-molecular-weight substances.

Table 38–5. Use of the osmol gap in toxicology.

The osmol gap (Delta osm) is determined by subtracting the calculated serum osmolality from the measured serum osmolality.
$$\text{Calculated osmolality (osm)} = 2[Na^+(mEq/L)] + \frac{Glucose\ (mg/dL)}{18} + \frac{BUN\ (mg/dL)}{2.8}$$
Delta osm = Measured osmolality – Calculated osmolality = 0 ± 10
Serum osmolality may be increased by contributions of exogenous substances such as alcohols and other low-molecular-weight substances. Since these substances are not included in the calculated osmolality, there will be a gap proportionate to their serum concentration. Contact a medical toxicologist or poison control center for assistance in calculating and interpreting the osmol gap.

Adapted, with permission, from Stone CK, Humphries RL (editors): *Current Emergency Diagnosis & Treatment*, 5th ed. McGraw-Hill, 2004.

B. Anion Gap

Metabolic acidosis associated with an elevated anion gap is usually due to an accumulation of lactic acid or other acids (see Chapter 21). Common causes of elevated anion gap in poisoning include carbon monoxide, cyanide, ethylene glycol, propylene glycol, medicinal iron, INH, methanol, metformin, ibuprofen, and salicylates. Massive acetaminophen overdose can cause early-onset anion gap metabolic acidosis.

The osmol gap should also be checked; combined elevated anion and osmol gaps suggests poisoning by methanol or ethylene glycol, though this may also occur in patients with diabetic ketoacidosis and alcoholic ketoacidosis.

C. Toxicology Laboratory Testing

A comprehensive toxicology screen is of little value in the initial care of the poisoned patient because results usually do not return in time to influence clinical management. Specific quantitative levels of certain drugs may be extremely helpful (Table 38–6), however, especially if specific antidotes or interventions (eg, dialysis) would be indicated based on the results.

Many hospitals can perform a quick but limited urine screen for "drugs of abuse" (typically these screens include only opiates, amphetamines, and cocaine, and some add benzodiazepines, barbiturates, methadone, oxycodone, phencyclidine, and tetrahydrocannabinol [marijuana]). There are numerous false-positive and false-negative results. For example, synthetic opioids, such as fentanyl, oxycodone, and methadone, are often not detected by routine opiate immunoassays.

▶ Abdominal Imaging

A plain film (or CT scan) of the abdomen may reveal radiopaque iron tablets, drug-filled condoms, or other toxic material. Studies suggest that few tablets are predictably visible (eg, ferrous sulfate, sodium chloride, calcium carbonate, and potassium chloride). Thus, the radiograph is useful only if abnormal.

Table 38–6. Specific quantitative levels and potential therapeutic interventions.[1]

Drug or Toxin	Treatment
Acetaminophen	Specific antidote (*N*-acetylcysteine) based on serum level
Carbon monoxide	High carboxyhemoglobin level indicates need for 100% oxygen, consideration of hyperbaric oxygen
Carbamazepine	High level may indicate need for hemodialysis
Digoxin	On basis of serum digoxin level and severity of clinical presentation, treatment with Fab antibody fragments (eg, DigiFab) may be indicated
Ethanol	Low serum level may suggest nonalcoholic cause of coma (eg, trauma, other drugs, other alcohols); serum ethanol may also be useful in monitoring ethanol therapy for methanol or ethylene glycol poisoning
Iron	Level may indicate need for chelation with deferoxamine
Lithium	Serum levels can guide decision to institute hemodialysis
Methanol, ethylene glycol	Acidosis, high levels indicate need for hemodialysis, therapy with ethanol or fomepizole
Methemoglobin	Methemoglobinemia can be treated with methylene blue intravenously
Salicylates	High level may indicate need for hemodialysis, alkaline diuresis
Theophylline	Immediate hemodialysis or hemoperfusion may be indicated based on serum level
Valproic acid	Elevated levels may indicate need to consider hemodialysis or L-carnitine therapy, or both

[1]Some drugs or toxins may have profound and irreversible toxicity unless rapid and specific management is provided outside of routine supportive care. For these agents, laboratory testing may provide the serum level or other evidence required for administering a specific antidote or arranging for hemodialysis.

▶ When to Refer

Consultation with a regional poison control center (1-800-222-1222) or a medical toxicologist is recommended when the diagnosis is uncertain; there are questions about what laboratory tests to order; when dialysis is being considered to remove the drug or poison; or when advice is needed regarding the indications, dose, and side effects of antidotes.

▶ When to Admit

- The patient has symptoms and signs of intoxication that are not expected to clear within a 6- to 8-hour observation period.

- Delayed absorption of the drug might be predicted to cause a later onset of serious symptoms (eg, after ingestion of a sustained-release product).

- Continued administration of an antidote is required (eg, *N*-acetylcysteine for acetaminophen overdose).

- Psychiatric or social services evaluation is needed for suicide attempt or suspected drug abuse.

Malek N et al. Common toxidromes in movement disorder neurology. Postgrad Med J. 2017 Jun;93(1100):326–32. [PMID: 28546460]

Martins SS et al. Worldwide prevalence and trends in unintentional drug overdose: a systematic review of the literature. Am J Public Health. 2015 Nov;105(11):2373. [PMID: 26451757]

Nelson LS, Hoffman RS (editors). *Goldfrank's Toxicologic Emergencies*, 11th ed. McGraw-Hill, 2019.

Olson KR (editor). *Poisoning & Drug Overdose*, 7th ed. McGraw-Hill, 2018.

Rasimas JJ et al. Assessment and management of toxidromes in the critical care unit. Crit Care Clin. 2017 Jul;33(3):521–41. [PMID: 28601133]

SELECTED POISONINGS

ACETAMINOPHEN

Acetaminophen (paracetamol in the United Kingdom, Europe) is a common analgesic found in many nonprescription and prescription products. After absorption, it is metabolized mainly by glucuronidation and sulfation, with a small fraction metabolized via the P450 mixed-function oxidase system (2E1) to a highly toxic reactive intermediate. This toxic intermediate is normally detoxified by cellular glutathione. With acute acetaminophen overdose (greater than 150–200 mg/kg, or 8–10 g in an average adult), hepatocellular glutathione is depleted and the reactive intermediate attacks other cell proteins, causing necrosis. Patients with enhanced P450 2E1 activity, such as those who chronically abuse alcohol and patients taking INH, are at increased risk for developing hepatotoxicity. Hepatic toxicity may also occur after overuse of acetaminophen—eg, as a result of taking two or three acetaminophen-containing products concurrently or exceeding the recommended maximum dose of 4 g/day for several days. The amount of acetaminophen in US oral prescription combination products (eg, hydrocodone/acetaminophen) is limited by the FDA to no more than 325 mg per tablet.

► Clinical Findings

Shortly after ingestion, patients may have nausea or vomiting, but there are usually no other signs of toxicity until 24–48 hours after ingestion, when hepatic aminotransferase levels begin to increase. With severe poisoning, fulminant hepatic necrosis may occur, resulting in jaundice, hepatic encephalopathy, acute kidney injury, and death. Rarely, massive ingestion (eg, serum levels greater than 500–1000 mg/L [33–66 mmol/L]) can cause early onset of acute coma, seizures, hypotension, and metabolic acidosis unrelated to hepatic injury.

The diagnosis after acute overdose is based on measurement of the serum acetaminophen level. Plot the serum level versus the time since ingestion on the acetaminophen nomogram shown in Figure 38–1. Ingestion of

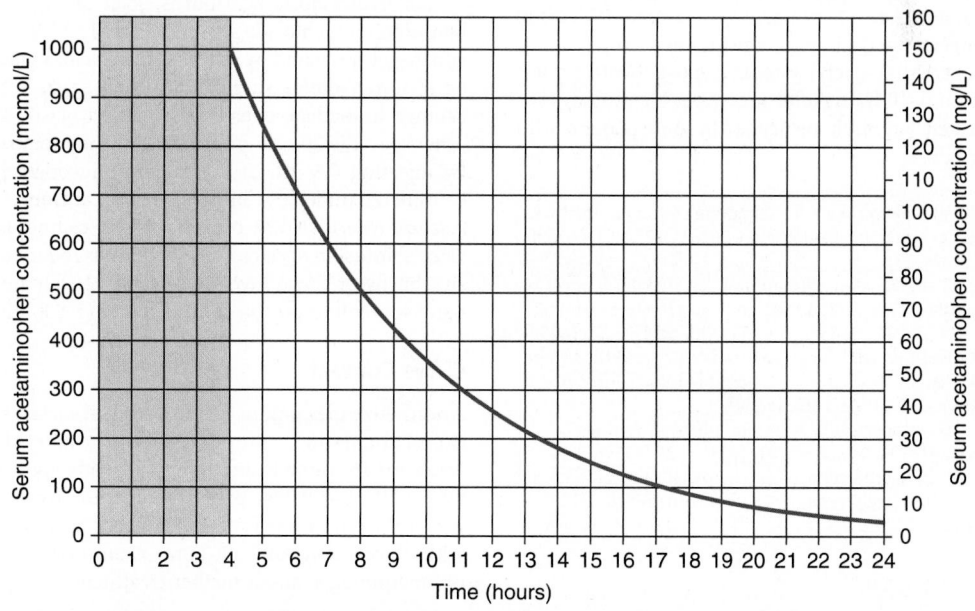

▲ **Figure 38–1.** Nomogram for prediction of acetaminophen hepatotoxicity following acute overdosage. Patients with serum levels above the line after acute overdose should receive antidotal treatment. (Adapted, with permission, from Daly FF et al. Guidelines for the management of paracetamol poisoning in Australia and New Zealand—explanation and elaboration. A consensus statement from clinical toxicologists consulting to the Australasian Poisons Information Centres. Med J Austr. 2008;188:296. © Copyright 2008 The Medical Journal of Australia. By permission from John Wiley & Sons.)

sustained-release products or coingestion of an anticholinergic agent, salicylate, or opioid drug may cause delayed elevation of serum levels, which can make it difficult to interpret the nomogram. The nomogram is also not useful after chronic or staggered overdose.

▶ Treatment

A. Emergency and Supportive Measures

Administer activated charcoal if it can be given within 1–2 hours of the ingestion. Although charcoal may interfere with absorption of the oral antidote acetylcysteine, this is not considered clinically significant.

B. Specific Treatment

If the serum or plasma acetaminophen level falls above the line on the nomogram (Figure 38–1), treatment with N-acetylcysteine is indicated; it can be given orally or intravenously. Oral treatment begins with a loading dose of N-acetylcysteine, 140 mg/kg, followed by 70 mg/kg every 4 hours. Dilute the solution to about 5% with water, juice, or soda. If vomiting interferes with oral N-acetylcysteine administration, consider giving the antidote intravenously. The conventional oral N-acetylcysteine protocol in the United States calls for 72 hours of treatment. However, other regimens have demonstrated equivalent success with 20–48 hours of treatment.

The FDA-approved 21-hour intravenous regimen of acetylcysteine (Acetadote) calls for a loading dose of 150 mg/kg given intravenously over 60 minutes, followed by a 4-hour infusion of 50 mg/kg, and a 16-hour infusion of 100 mg/kg. (If Acetadote is not available, the conventional oral formulation may also be given intravenously using a micropore filter and a slow rate of infusion. Call a regional poison control center or medical toxicologist for assistance.)

Treatment with N-acetylcysteine is most effective if it is started within 8–10 hours after ingestion. Hemodialysis is rarely indicated, but might be needed in some patients with massive overdose.

Chiew AL et al. Interventions for paracetamol (acetaminophen) overdose. Cochrane Database Syst Rev. 2018 Feb 23;2:CD003328. [PMID: 29473717]

Ghannoum M et al. Massive acetaminophen overdose: effect of hemodialysis on acetaminophen and acetylcysteine kinetics. Clin Toxicol (Phila). 2016 Jul;54(6):519–22. [PMID: 27118496]

Lucyk S. Calculated decisions: acetaminophen overdose and N-acetylcysteine (NAC) dosing. Emerg Med Pract. 2018 Apr 1; 20(4 Suppl):S3–5. [PMID: 29617550]

Park BK et al. Paracetamol (acetaminophen) poisoning. BMJ Clin Evid. 2015 Oct 19;2015:2101. [PMID: 26479248]

Wong A et al. Risk prediction of hepatotoxicity in paracetamol poisoning. Clin Toxicol (Phila). 2017 Sep;55(8):879–92. [PMID: 28447858]

ACIDS, CORROSIVE

The strong mineral acids exert primarily a local corrosive effect on the skin and mucous membranes. Symptoms include severe pain in the throat and upper gastrointestinal tract; bloody vomitus; difficulty in swallowing, breathing, and speaking; discoloration and destruction of skin and mucous membranes in and around the mouth; and shock. Severe systemic metabolic acidosis may occur both as a result of cellular injury and from systemic absorption of the acid.

Severe deep destructive tissue damage may occur after exposure to hydrofluoric acid because of the penetrating and highly toxic fluoride ion. Systemic hypocalcemia and hyperkalemia may also occur after fluoride absorption, even following skin exposure.

Inhalation of volatile acids, fumes, or gases such as chlorine, fluorine, bromine, or iodine causes severe irritation of the throat and larynx and may cause upper airway obstruction and noncardiogenic pulmonary edema.

▶ Treatment

A. Ingestion

Dilute immediately by giving a glass (4–8 oz) of water to drink. Do *not* give bicarbonate or other neutralizing agents, and do *not* induce vomiting. Some experts recommend immediate cautious placement of a small flexible gastric tube and removal of stomach contents followed by lavage, particularly if the corrosive is a liquid or has important systemic toxicity.

In symptomatic patients, perform flexible endoscopic esophagoscopy to determine the presence and extent of injury. CT scan or plain radiographs of the chest and abdomen may also reveal the extent of injury. Perforation, peritonitis, and major bleeding are indications for surgery.

B. Skin Contact

Flood with water for 15 minutes. Use no chemical antidotes; the heat of the reaction may cause additional injury.

For hydrofluoric acid burns, soak the affected area in benzalkonium chloride solution or apply 2.5% calcium gluconate gel (prepared by adding 3.5 g calcium gluconate to 5 oz of water-soluble surgical lubricant, eg, K-Y Jelly); then arrange immediate consultation with a plastic surgeon or other specialist. Binding of the fluoride ion may be achieved by injecting 0.5 mL of 5% calcium gluconate per square centimeter under the burned area. (**Caution:** *Do not use calcium chloride.*) Use of a Bier-block technique or intra-arterial infusion of calcium is sometimes required for extensive burns or those involving the nail bed; consult with a hand surgeon or poison control center (1-800-222-1222).

C. Eye Contact

Anesthetize the conjunctiva and corneal surfaces with topical local anesthetic drops (eg, proparacaine). Flood with water for 15 minutes, holding the eyelids open. Check pH with pH 6.0–8.0 test paper, and repeat irrigation, using 0.9% saline, until pH is near 7.0. Check for corneal damage with fluorescein and slit-lamp examination; consult an ophthalmologist about further treatment.

D. Inhalation

Remove from further exposure to fumes or gas. Check skin and clothing. Observe for and treat chemical pneumonitis or pulmonary edema.

Bird JH et al. Controversies in the management of caustic ingestion injury: an evidence-based review. Clin Otolaryngol. 2017 Jun; 42(3):701–8. [PMID: 28032947]

Cowan T et al. Acute esophageal injury and strictures following corrosive ingestions in a 27 year cohort. Am J Emerg Med. 2017 Mar;35(3):488–92. [PMID: 27955797]

Han HH et al. Importance of initial management and surgical treatment after hydrofluoric acid burn of the finger. Burns. 2017 Feb;43(1):e1–6. [PMID: 27650188]

Pu Q et al. Extracorporeal membrane oxygenation combined with continuous renal replacement therapy in cutaneous burn and inhalation injury caused by hydrofluoric acid and nitric acid. Medicine (Baltimore). 2017 Dec;96(48):e8972. [PMID: 29310404]

Struck MF et al. Acute emergency care and airway management of caustic ingestion in adults: single center observational study. Scand J Trauma Resusc Emerg Med. 2016 Apr 11;24:45. [PMID: 27068119]

ALKALIES

The strong alkalies are common ingredients of some household cleaning compounds and may be suspected by their "soapy" texture. Those with alkalinity above pH 12.0 are particularly corrosive. Disk (or "button") batteries are also a source. Alkalies cause liquefactive necrosis, which is deeply penetrating. Symptoms include burning pain in the upper gastrointestinal tract, nausea, vomiting, and difficulty in swallowing and breathing. Examination reveals destruction and edema of the affected skin and mucous membranes and bloody vomitus and stools. Radiographs may reveal evidence of perforation or the presence of radiopaque disk batteries in the esophagus or lower gastrointestinal tract.

▶ Treatment

A. Ingestion

Dilute immediately with a glass of water. Do *not* induce emesis. Some gastroenterologists recommend immediate cautious placement of a small flexible gastric tube and removal of stomach contents followed by gastric lavage after ingestion of liquid caustic substances, in order to remove residual material. However, others argue that passage of a gastric tube is contraindicated due to the risk of perforation or reexposure of the esophagus to the corrosive material from vomiting around the tube.

Prompt endoscopy is recommended in symptomatic patients to evaluate the extent of damage; CT scanning may also aid in assessment. If a radiograph reveals ingested disk batteries lodged in the esophagus, immediate endoscopic removal is mandatory.

The use of corticosteroids to prevent stricture formation is of no proved benefit and is definitely contraindicated if there is evidence of esophageal perforation.

B. Skin Contact

Wash with running water until the skin no longer feels soapy. Relieve pain and treat shock.

C. Eye Contact

Anesthetize the conjunctival and corneal surfaces with topical anesthetic (eg, proparacaine). Irrigate with water or saline continuously for 20–30 minutes, holding the lids open. Amphoteric solutions may be more effective than water or saline and some are available in Europe (Diphoterine, Prevor). Check pH with pH test paper and repeat irrigation for additional 30-minute periods until the pH is near 7.0. Check for corneal damage with fluorescein and slit-lamp examination; consult an ophthalmologist for further treatment.

Dohlman CH et al. Chemical burns of the eye: the role of retinal injury and new therapeutic possibilities. Cornea. 2018 Feb; 37(2):248–51. [PMID: 29135604]

Haring RS et al. Epidemiologic trends of chemical ocular burns in the United States. JAMA Ophthalmol. 2016 Oct 1; 134(10): 1119–24. [PMID: 27490908]

Wightman RS et al. Evidence-based management of caustic exposures in the emergency department. Emerg Med Pract. 2016 May;18(5):1–17. [PMID: 27074641]

AMPHETAMINES & COCAINE

Amphetamines and cocaine are widely abused for their euphorigenic and stimulant properties. Both drugs may be smoked, snorted, ingested, or injected. Amphetamines and cocaine produce central nervous system stimulation and a generalized increase in central and peripheral sympathetic activity. The toxic dose of each drug is highly variable and depends on the route of administration and individual tolerance. The onset of effects is most rapid after intravenous injection or smoking. Amphetamine derivatives and related drugs include methamphetamine ("crystal meth," "crank"), MDMA ("Ecstasy"), ephedrine ("herbal ecstasy"), and methcathinone ("cat" or "khat"). Methcathinone derivatives and related synthetic chemicals such as methylenedioxypyrovalerone (MDPV) have become popular drugs of abuse and are often sold as purported "bath salts." Amphetamine-like reactions have also been reported after use of synthetic cannabinoids (eg, "Spice" and "K2"). Nonprescription medications and nutritional supplements may contain stimulant or sympathomimetic drugs such as ephedrine, yohimbine, or caffeine (see also Theophylline & Caffeine section).

▶ Clinical Findings

Presenting symptoms may include anxiety, tremulousness, tachycardia, hypertension, diaphoresis, dilated pupils, agitation, muscular hyperactivity, and psychosis. Muscle hyperactivity may lead to metabolic acidosis and rhabdomyolysis. In severe intoxication, seizures and hyperthermia may occur. Sustained or severe hypertension may result in intracranial hemorrhage, aortic dissection, or myocardial infarction; chronic use may cause cardiomyopathy. Ischemic colitis has been reported. Hyponatremia has been reported after MDMA use; the mechanism is not known but may involve excessive water intake, syndrome of inappropriate antidiuretic hormone (SIADH), or both.

The diagnosis is supported by finding amphetamines or the cocaine metabolite benzoylecgonine in the urine. Note that many drugs can give false-positive results on the immunoassay for amphetamines, and most synthetic stimulants do not react with the immunoassay, giving false-negative results.

▶ Treatment

A. Emergency and Supportive Measures

Maintain a patent airway and assist ventilation, if necessary. Treat seizures as described at the beginning of this chapter. Rapidly lower the body temperature in patients who are hyperthermic (temperature higher than 39–40°C). Give intravenous fluids to prevent myoglobinuric kidney injury in patients who have rhabdomyolysis.

B. Specific Treatment

Treat agitation, psychosis, or seizures with a benzodiazepine such as diazepam, 5–10 mg, or lorazepam, 2–3 mg intravenously. Add phenobarbital 15 mg/kg intravenously for persistent seizures. Treat hypertension with a vasodilator drug such as phentolamine (1–5 mg intravenously) or nitroprusside, or a combined alpha- and beta-adrenergic blocker such as labetalol (10–20 mg intravenously). Do *not* administer a pure beta-blocker such as propranolol alone, as this may result in paradoxic worsening of the hypertension as a result of unopposed alpha-adrenergic effects.

Treat tachycardia or tachyarrhythmias with a short-acting beta-blocker such as esmolol (25–100 mcg/kg/min by intravenous infusion). Treat hyperthermia as described above. Treat hyponatremia as outlined in Chapter 21.

Richards JR et al. Methamphetamine use and heart failure: prevalence, risk factors, and predictors. Am J Emerg Med. 2018 Aug;36(8):1423–8. [PMID: 29307766]

Tait RJ et al. A systematic review of adverse events arising from the use of synthetic cannabinoids and their associated treatment. Clin Toxicol (Phila). 2016 Jan;54(1):1–13. [PMID: 26567470]

Vallersnes OM et al. Psychosis associated with acute recreational drug toxicity: a European case series. BMC Psychiatry. 2016 Aug 18;16:293. [PMID: 27538886]

White CM. The pharmacologic and clinical effects of illicit synthetic cannabinoids. J Clin Pharmacol. 2017 Mar;57(3): 297–304. [PMID: 27610597]

Williams MV. Cannabinoids: emerging evidence in use and abuse. Emerg Med Pract. 2018 Aug;20(8):1–20. [PMID: 30020736]

ANTICOAGULANTS

Warfarin and related compounds (including ingredients of many commercial rodenticides, the so-called superwarfarins such as brodifacoum, difenacoum, and related compounds) inhibit the normal clotting system by blocking hepatic synthesis of vitamin K–dependent clotting factors. After ingestion of "superwarfarins," inhibition of clotting factor synthesis may persist for several weeks or even months after a single dose. Newer oral anticoagulants include the direct thrombin inhibitor dabigatran and the factor Xa inhibitors apixiban, betrixaban, edoxaban, and rivaroxaban. Some of these, especially dabigatran, are largely eliminated by the kidney and may accumulate in patients with kidney dysfunction.

Excessive anticoagulation may cause hemoptysis, gross hematuria, bloody stools, hemorrhages into organs, widespread bruising, and bleeding into joint spaces.

▶ Treatment

A. Emergency and Supportive Measures

Discontinue the drug at the first sign of gross bleeding, and determine the prothrombin time (international normalized ratio, INR). The prothrombin time is increased within 12–24 hours (peak 36–48 hours) after overdose of warfarin or "superwarfarins." Note: The newer oral anticoagulants (dabigatran, apixiban, betrixaban, edoxaban, and rivaroxaban) do not predictably alter the prothrombin time; however, a normal INR suggests no significant toxicity.

If the patient has ingested an acute overdose, administer activated charcoal.

B. Specific Treatment

1. Warfarin—*In cases of warfarin and "superwarfarin" overdose, do not treat prophylactically with vitamin K*—wait for evidence of anticoagulation (elevated prothrombin time). See Table 14–21 for the management of INR above therapeutic range. Doses of vitamin K as high as 200 mg/day have been required after ingestion of "superwarfarins." Give fresh-frozen plasma, prothrombin complex concentrate, or activated factor VII as needed to rapidly correct the coagulation factor deficit if there is serious bleeding. If the patient is chronically anticoagulated and has strong medical indications for being maintained in that status (eg, prosthetic heart valve), give much smaller doses of vitamin K (1 mg orally) and fresh-frozen plasma (or both) to titrate to the desired prothrombin time. If the patient has ingested brodifacoum or a related superwarfarin, prolonged observation (over weeks) and repeated administration of large doses of vitamin K may be required.

2. Direct-acting oral anticoagulants—Vitamin K does not reverse the anticoagulant effects of the direct-acting oral anticoagulants. **Idarucizumab** has been approved by the FDA for reversal of the thrombin inhibitor dabigatran; **andexanet** is approved for reversal of the factor Xa inhibitors apixiban, edoxaban, betrixaban, and rivaroxaban. The efficacy of fresh-frozen plasma and clotting factor concentrates is uncertain.

Berling I et al. Warfarin poisoning with delayed rebound toxicity. J Emerg Med. 2017 Feb;52(2):194–6. [PMID: 27838137]

Heo YA. Andexanet alfa: first global approval. Drugs. 2018 Jul;78(10): 1049–55. Erratum in: Drugs. 2018 Aug;78(12):1285. [PMID: 29926311]

Levine M et al. Assessing bleeding risk in patients with intentional overdoses of novel antiplatelet and anticoagulant medications. Ann Emerg Med. 2018 Mar;71(3):273–8. [PMID: 29032872]

Pollack CV Jr et al. Idarucizumab for dabigatran reversal - full cohort analysis. N Engl J Med. 2017 Aug 3;377(5):431–41. [PMID: 28693366]

Zhang XY et al. Reversal of direct oral anticoagulants. Br J Hosp Med (Lond). 2017 Mar 2;78(3):165–9. [PMID: 28277769]

ANTICONVULSANTS

Anticonvulsants (carbamazepine, phenytoin, valproic acid, and many newer agents) are widely used in the management of seizure disorders and some are also used for treatment of mood disorders or pain.

Phenytoin can be given orally or intravenously. Rapid intravenous injection of phenytoin can cause acute myocardial depression and cardiac arrest owing to the solvent propylene glycol (fosphenytoin does not contain this diluent). Chronic phenytoin intoxication can occur following only slightly increased doses because of zero-order kinetics and a small toxic-therapeutic window. Phenytoin intoxication can also occur following acute intentional or accidental overdose. The overdose syndrome is usually mild even with high serum levels. The most common manifestations are ataxia, nystagmus, and drowsiness. Choreoathetoid movements have been described.

Carbamazepine intoxication causes drowsiness, stupor and, with high levels, atrioventricular block, coma, and seizures. Dilated pupils and tachycardia are common. Toxicity may be seen with serum levels over 20 mg/L (85 mcmol/L), although severe poisoning is usually associated with concentrations greater than 30–40 mg/L (127–169 mcmol/L). Because of erratic and slow absorption, intoxication may progress over several hours to days.

Valproic acid intoxication produces a unique syndrome consisting of hypernatremia (from the sodium component of the salt), metabolic acidosis, hypocalcemia, elevated serum ammonia, and mild liver aminotransferase elevation. Hypoglycemia may occur as a result of hepatic metabolic dysfunction. Coma with small pupils may be seen and can mimic opioid poisoning. Encephalopathy and cerebral edema can occur.

The newer anticonvulsants **gabapentin, levetiracetam, vigabatrin,** and **zonisamide** generally cause somnolence, confusion, and dizziness; there is one case report of hypotension and bradycardia after a large overdose of levetiracetam. **Felbamate** can cause crystalluria and kidney injury after overdose and may cause idiosyncratic aplastic anemia with therapeutic use. **Lamotrigine, topiramate,** and **tiagabine** have been reported to cause seizures after overdose; lamotrigine has sodium-channel blocking properties and may cause QRS prolongation and heart block.

▶ Treatment

A. Emergency and Supportive Measures

For recent ingestions, give activated charcoal orally or by gastric tube. For large ingestions of carbamazepine or valproic acid—especially of sustained-release formulations—consider whole bowel irrigation. Combined multiple-dose activated charcoal and whole-bowel irrigation may be beneficial in ensuring gut decontamination for selected large ingestions.

B. Specific Treatment

There are no specific antidotes. Naloxone was reported to have reversed valproic acid overdose in one anecdotal case. Carnitine (and possibly L-arginine) may be useful in patients with valproic acid–induced hyperammonemia. Consider hemodialysis for massive intoxication with valproic acid or carbamazepine (eg, carbamazepine levels greater than 60 mg/L [254 mcmol/L] or valproic acid levels greater than 800 mg/L [5544 mcmol/L]).

Alyahya B et al. Acute lamotrigine overdose: a systematic review of published adult and pediatric cases. Clin Toxicol (Phila). 2018 Feb;56(2):81–9. [PMID: 28862044]

Ghannoum M et al. Extracorporeal treatment for valproic acid poisoning: systematic review and recommendations from the EXTRIP workgroup. Clin Toxicol (Phila). 2015 Jun;53(5):454–65. [PMID: 25950372]

Mahmoud SH. Antiepileptic drug removal by continuous renal replacement therapy: a review of the literature. Clin Drug Investig. 2017 Jan;37(1):7–23. [PMID: 27587068]

Page CB et al. Cardiovascular toxicity with levetiracetam overdose. Clin Toxicol (Phila). 2016;54(2):152–4. [PMID: 26795744]

Yang X et al. Early hemoperfusion for emergency treatment of carbamazepine poisoning. Am J Emerg Med. 2018 Jun;36(6):926–30. [PMID: 29066188]

ANTIPSYCHOTIC DRUGS

Drugs in this group include "conventional" antipsychotics (eg, chlorpromazine, haloperidol, droperidol) and newer "atypical" antipsychotics (eg, risperidone, olanzapine, ziprasidone, quetiapine, aripiprazole). While conventional drugs act mainly on CNS dopamine receptors, atypical drugs also interact with serotonin receptors.

Therapeutic doses of conventional phenothiazines (particularly chlorpromazine) induce drowsiness and mild orthostatic hypotension in as many as 50% of patients. Larger doses can cause obtundation, miosis, severe hypotension, tachycardia, convulsions, and coma. Abnormal cardiac conduction may occur, resulting in prolongation of QRS or QT intervals (or both) and ventricular arrhythmias. Among the atypical agents, quetiapine is more likely to cause coma and hypotension. Hypotension is probably related to blockade of peripheral alpha-adrenergic receptors, causing vasodilatation.

With therapeutic or toxic doses, an acute extrapyramidal dystonic reaction may develop in some patients, with spasmodic contractions of the face and neck muscles, extensor rigidity of the back muscles, carpopedal spasm, and motor restlessness. This reaction is more common with haloperidol and other butyrophenones and less common with newer atypical antipsychotics. Severe rigidity accompanied by hyperthermia and metabolic acidosis ("neuroleptic malignant syndrome") may occasionally occur and is life-threatening (see Chapter 25). Atypical antipsychotics have also been associated with weight gain and diabetes mellitus, including diabetic ketoacidosis.

▶ Treatment

A. Emergency and Supportive Measures

Administer activated charcoal for large or recent ingestions. For severe hypotension, treatment with intravenous fluids and vasopressor agents may be necessary. Treat hyperthermia as outlined. Maintain cardiac monitoring.

B. Specific Treatment

Hypotension often responds to intravenous saline boluses; cardiac arrhythmias associated with widened QRS intervals on the ECG may respond to intravenous sodium bicarbonate as is given for tricyclic antidepressant overdoses. Prolongation of the QT interval and torsades de pointes is usually treated with intravenous magnesium or overdrive pacing.

For extrapyramidal signs, give diphenhydramine, 0.5–1 mg/kg intravenously, or benztropine mesylate, 0.01–0.02 mg/kg intramuscularly. Treatment with oral doses of these agents should be continued for 24–48 hours.

Bromocriptine (2.5–7.5 mg orally daily) may be effective for mild or moderate neuroleptic malignant syndrome. Dantrolene (2–5 mg/kg intravenously) has also been used for muscle rigidity but is not a true antidote. For severe hyperthermia, rapid neuromuscular paralysis is preferred.

Beach SR et al. QT prolongation, torsades de pointes, and psychotropic medications: a 5-year update. Psychosomatics. 2018 Mar-Apr;59(2):105–22. [PMID: 29275963]

Berling I et al. Prolonged QT risk assessment in antipsychotic overdose using the QT nomogram. Ann Emerg Med. 2015 Aug; 66(2):154–64. [PMID: 25639523]

Christensen AP et al. Overdoses with aripiprazole: signs, symptoms and outcome in 239 exposures reported to the Danish Poison Information Centre. Basic Clin Pharmacol Toxicol. 2018 Feb;122(2):293–8. [PMID: 28881461]

Miura N et al. Risk factors for QT prolongation associated with acute psychotropic drug overdose. Am J Emerg Med. 2015 Feb; 33(2):142–9. [PMID: 25445869]

ARSENIC

Arsenic is found in some pesticides and industrial chemicals and is used as a chemotherapeutic agent. Chronic arsenic poisoning has been associated with contaminated aquifers used for drinking water. Symptoms of acute poisoning usually appear within 1 hour after ingestion but may be delayed as long as 12 hours. They include abdominal pain, vomiting, watery diarrhea, and skeletal muscle cramps. Profound dehydration and shock may occur. In chronic poisoning, symptoms can be vague but often include pancytopenia, painful peripheral sensory neuropathy, and skin changes including melanosis, keratosis, and desquamating rash. Cancers of the lung, bladder, and skin have been reported. Urinary arsenic levels may be falsely elevated after certain meals (eg, seafood) that contain large quantities of a nontoxic form of organic arsenic.

▶ Treatment

A. Emergency Measures

After recent ingestion (within 1–2 hours), perform gastric lavage. Activated charcoal is of uncertain benefit because it binds arsenic poorly. Administer intravenous fluids to replace losses due to vomiting and diarrhea.

B. Antidote

For patients with severe acute intoxication, administer a chelating agent. The preferred drug is 2,3-dimercaptopropane-sulfonic acid (DMPS, Unithiol) (3–5 mg/kg intravenously every 4 hours); although there is no FDA-approved commercial formulation of DMPS in the United States, it can be obtained from some compounding pharmacies. An alternative parenteral chelator is dimercaprol (British anti-Lewisite, BAL), which comes as a 10% solution in peanut oil, and is given 3–5 mg/kg intramuscularly every 4–6 hours for 2 days. The side effects include nausea, vomiting, headache, and hypertension. When gastrointestinal symptoms allow, switch to the oral chelator succimer (dimercaptosuccinic acid, DMSA), 10 mg/kg every 8 hours, for 1 week. Consult a medical toxicologist or regional poison control center (1-800-222-1222) for advice regarding chelation.

Arslan B et al. Arsenic: a review on exposure pathways, accumulation, mobility and transmission into the human food chain. Rev Environ Contam Toxicol. 2017;243:27–51. [PMID: 28005215]

Dani SU et al. Chronic arsenic intoxication diagnostic score (CAsIDS). J Appl Toxicol. 2018 Jan;38(1):122–44. [PMID: 28857213]

Lu PH et al. Survival without peripheral neuropathy after massive acute arsenic poisoning: treated by 2,3-dimercaptopropane-1-sulphonate. J Clin Pharm Ther. 2017 Aug;42(4):506–8. [PMID: 28547870]

ATROPINE & ANTICHOLINERGICS

Atropine, scopolamine, belladonna, *Datura stramonium, Hyoscyamus niger,* some mushrooms, tricyclic antidepressants, and antihistamines are antimuscarinic agents with variable central nervous system effects. Symptoms of toxicity include dryness of the mouth, thirst, difficulty in swallowing, and blurring of vision. Physical signs include dilated pupils, flushed skin, tachycardia, fever, delirium, myoclonus, ileus, and flushed appearance. Antidepressants and antihistamines may also induce convulsions.

Antihistamines are commonly available with or without prescription. Diphenhydramine commonly causes delirium, tachycardia, and seizures. Massive diphenhydramine overdose may mimic tricyclic antidepressant cardiotoxic poisoning.

▶ Treatment

A. Emergency and Supportive Measures

Administer activated charcoal. External cooling and sedation, or neuromuscular paralysis in rare cases, are indicated to control high temperatures.

B. Specific Treatment

For severe anticholinergic syndrome (eg, agitated delirium), give physostigmine salicylate, 0.5–1 mg slowly intravenously over 5 minutes, with ECG monitoring; repeat as needed to a total dose of no more than 2 mg. **Caution:** Bradyarrhythmias and convulsions are a hazard with physostigmine administration, and the drug should be avoided in patients with evidence of cardiotoxic effects (eg, QRS interval prolongation) from tricyclic antidepressants or other sodium channel blockers.

Chan TY. Herbal medicines induced anticholinergic poisoning in Hong Kong. Toxins (Basel). 2016 Mar 18;8(3). [PMID: 26999208]

Dawson AH et al. Pharmacological management of anticholinergic delirium—theory, evidence and practice. Br J Clin Pharmacol. 2016 Mar;81(3):516–524. [PMID: 26589572]

Zhang XC et al. Postoperative anticholinergic poisoning: concealed complications of a commonly used medication. J Emerg Med. 2017 Oct;53(4):520–3. [PMID: 28756934]

BETA-ADRENERGIC BLOCKERS

There are a wide variety of beta-adrenergic blocking drugs, with varying pharmacologic and pharmacokinetic properties (see Table 11–9). The most toxic beta-blocker is propranolol, which not only blocks beta-1 and beta-2 adrenoceptors but also has direct membrane-depressant and central nervous system effects.

▶ Clinical Findings

The most common findings with mild or moderate intoxication are hypotension and bradycardia. Cardiac depression from more severe poisoning is often unresponsive to conventional therapy with beta-adrenergic stimulants such as dopamine and norepinephrine. In addition, with propranolol and other lipid-soluble drugs, seizures and coma may occur. Propranolol, oxprenolol, acebutolol, and alprenolol also have membrane-depressant effects and can cause conduction disturbance (wide QRS interval) similar to tricyclic antidepressant overdose.

The diagnosis is based on typical clinical findings. Routine toxicology screening does not usually include beta-blockers.

▶ Treatment

A. Emergency and Supportive Measures

Attempts to treat bradycardia or heart block with atropine (0.5–2 mg intravenously), isoproterenol (2–20 mcg/min by intravenous infusion, titrated to the desired heart rate), or an external transcutaneous cardiac pacemaker are often ineffective, and specific antidotal treatment may be necessary.

For drugs ingested within an hour of presentation (or longer after ingestion of an extended-release formulation), administer activated charcoal.

B. Specific Treatment

For persistent bradycardia and hypotension, give glucagon, 5–10 mg intravenously, followed by an infusion of 1–5 mg/h. Glucagon is an inotropic agent that acts at a different receptor site and is therefore not affected by beta-blockade. High-dose insulin (0.5–1 unit/kg/h intravenously) along with glucose supplementation has also been used to reverse severe cardiotoxicity. Membrane-depressant effects (wide QRS interval) may respond to boluses of sodium bicarbonate (50–100 mEq intravenously) as for tricyclic antidepressant poisoning. Intravenous lipid emulsion (Intralipid 20%, 1.5 mL/kg) has been used successfully in severe propranolol overdose.

Graudins A et al. Calcium channel antagonist and beta-blocker overdose: antidotes and adjunct therapies. Br J Clin Pharmacol. 2016 Mar;81(3):453–461. [PMID: 26344579]

Seegobin K et al. Severe beta blocker and calcium channel blocker overdose: role of high dose insulin. Am J Emerg Med. 2018 Apr;36(4):736.e5–6. [PMID: 29331270]

CALCIUM CHANNEL BLOCKERS

In therapeutic doses, nifedipine, nicardipine, amlodipine, felodipine, isradipine, nisoldipine, and nimodipine act mainly on blood vessels, while verapamil and diltiazem act mainly on cardiac contractility and conduction. However, these selective effects can be lost after acute overdose. Patients may present with bradycardia, atrioventricular (AV) nodal block, hypotension, or a combination of these effects. Hyperglycemia is common due to blockade of insulin release. With severe poisoning, cardiac arrest may occur.

▶ Treatment

A. Emergency and Supportive Measures

For ingested drugs, administer activated charcoal. In addition, whole bowel irrigation should be initiated as soon as possible if the patient has ingested a sustained-release product.

B. Specific Treatment

Treat symptomatic bradycardia with atropine (0.5–2 mg intravenously), isoproterenol (2–20 mcg/min by intravenous infusion), or a transcutaneous cardiac pacemaker. For hypotension, give calcium chloride 10%, 10 mL, or calcium gluconate 10%, 20 mL. Repeat the dose every 3–5 minutes. The optimum (or maximum) dose has not been established, but many toxicologists recommend raising the ionized serum calcium level to as much as twice the normal level. Calcium is most useful in reversing negative inotropic effects and is less effective for AV nodal blockade and bradycardia. High doses of insulin (0.5–1 unit/kg intravenous bolus followed by 0.5–1 unit/kg/h infusion) along with sufficient dextrose to maintain euglycemia have been reported to be beneficial, but there are no controlled studies. Infusion of Intralipid 20% lipid emulsion has been reported to improve hemodynamics in animal models and case reports of calcium channel blocker poisoning. Methylene blue (1–2 mg/kg) was reported to reverse refractory shock due to profound vasodilation in a patient with amlodipine poisoning. ECMO has been recommended for refractory shock.

Maskell KF et al. Survival after cardiac arrest: ECMO rescue therapy after amlodipine and metoprolol overdose. Cardiovasc Toxicol. 2017 Apr;17(2):223–5. [PMID: 26913719]

Rietjens SJ et al. Practical recommendations for calcium channel antagonist poisoning. Neth J Med. 2016 Feb;74(2):60–7. [PMID: 26951350]

St-Onge M et al. Experts consensus recommendations for the management of calcium channel blocker poisoning in adults. Crit Care Med. 2017 Mar;45(3):e306–15. [PMID: 27749343]

CARBON MONOXIDE

Carbon monoxide is a colorless, odorless gas produced by the combustion of carbon-containing materials. Poisoning may occur as a result of suicidal or accidental exposure to automobile exhaust, smoke inhalation in a fire, or accidental exposure to an improperly vented gas heater, generator, or other appliance. Carbon monoxide can be generated during degradation of some anesthetic gases by carbon dioxide adsorbents. Carbon monoxide avidly binds to hemoglobin, with an affinity approximately 250 times that of oxygen. This results in reduced oxygen-carrying capacity and altered delivery of oxygen to cells (see also Smoke Inhalation in Chapter 9).

► Clinical Findings

At low carbon monoxide levels (carboxyhemoglobin saturation 10–20%), victims may have headache, dizziness, abdominal pain, and nausea. With higher levels, confusion, dyspnea, and syncope may occur. Hypotension, coma, and seizures are common with levels greater than 50–60%. Survivors of acute severe poisoning may develop permanent obvious or subtle neurologic and neuropsychiatric deficits. The fetus and newborn may be more susceptible because of high carbon monoxide affinity for fetal hemoglobin.

Carbon monoxide poisoning should be suspected in any person with severe headache or acutely altered mental status, especially during cold weather, when improperly vented heating systems may have been used. Diagnosis depends on specific measurement of the arterial or venous carboxyhemoglobin saturation, although the level may have declined if high-flow oxygen therapy has already been administered, and levels do not always correlate with clinical symptoms. Routine arterial blood gas testing and pulse oximetry are not useful because they give falsely normal PaO_2 and oxyhemoglobin saturation determinations, respectively. (A specialized pulse oximetry device, the Masimo pulse CO-oximeter, is capable of distinguishing oxyhemoglobin from carboxyhemoglobin.)

► Treatment

A. Emergency and Supportive Measures

Maintain a patent airway and assist ventilation, if necessary. Remove the victim from exposure. Treat patients with coma, hypotension, or seizures as described at the beginning of this chapter.

B. Specific Treatment

The half-life of the carboxyhemoglobin (CoHb) complex is about 4–5 hours in room air but is reduced dramatically by high concentrations of oxygen. Administer 100% oxygen by tight-fitting high-flow reservoir face mask or endotracheal tube. Hyperbaric oxygen (HBO) can provide 100% oxygen under higher than atmospheric pressures, further shortening the half-life; it may also reduce the incidence of subtle neuropsychiatric sequelae. Randomized controlled studies disagree about the benefit of HBO, but commonly recommended indications for HBO in patients with carbon monoxide poisoning include a history of loss of consciousness, CoHb greater than 25%, metabolic acidosis, age over 50 years, and cerebellar findings on neurologic examination.

Bleecker ML. Carbon monoxide intoxication. Handb Clin Neurol. 2015;131:191–203. [PMID: 26563790]

Levy RJ. Anesthesia-related carbon monoxide exposure: toxicity and potential therapy. Anesth Analg. 2016 Sep;123(3):670–81. [PMID: 27537758]

Rose JJ et al. Carbon monoxide poisoning: pathogenesis, management, and future directions of therapy. Am J Respir Crit Care Med. 2017 Mar 1;195(5):596–606. Erratum in: Am J Respir Crit Care Med. 2017 Aug 1;196 (3):398–9. [PMID: 27753502]

CHEMICAL WARFARE: NERVE AGENTS

Nerve agents used in chemical warfare work by cholinesterase inhibition and are most commonly organophosphorus compounds. Agents such as **tabun** (GA), **sarin** (GB), **soman** (GD), and **VX** are similar to insecticides such as malathion but are vastly more potent. They may be inhaled or absorbed through the skin. Systemic effects due to unopposed action of acetylcholine include miosis, salivation, abdominal cramps, diarrhea, and muscle paralysis producing respiratory arrest. Inhalation also produces severe bronchoconstriction and copious nasal and tracheobronchial secretions.

► Treatment

A. Emergency and Supportive Measures

Perform thorough decontamination of exposed areas with repeated soap and shampoo washing. Personnel caring for such patients must wear protective clothing and gloves, since cutaneous absorption may occur through normal skin.

B. Specific Treatment

Give atropine in an initial dose of 2 mg intravenously and repeat as needed to reverse signs of acetylcholine excess. (Some victims have required several hundred milligrams.) Treat also with the cholinesterase-reactivating agent pralidoxime, 1–2 g intravenously initially followed by an infusion at a rate of 200–400 mg/h.

Agency for Toxic Substances and Disease Registry. Toxic Substances Portal: Medical Management Guidelines for Nerve Agents: Tabun (GA); Sarin (GB); Soman (GD); and VX. October 21, 2014. https://www.atsdr.cdc.gov/mmg/mmg.asp?id=523&tid=93

Candiotti K. A primer on nerve agents: what the emergency responder, anesthesiologist, and intensivist needs to know. Can J Anaesth. 2017 Oct;64(10):1059–70. [PMID: 28766156]

Iyengar AR et al. Organophosphate-hydrolyzing enzymes as first-line of defence against nerve agent-poisoning: perspectives and the road ahead. Protein J. 2016 Dec;35(6):424–39. [PMID: 27830420]

United States Department of Labor. Occupational Safety and Health Administration. Safety and Health Guides/Nerve Agents Guide. https://www.osha.gov/SLTC/emergencypreparedness/guides/nerve.html

CHEMICAL WARFARE: RICIN

Ricin is a naturally occurring toxin found in minute quantities in the castor bean (*Ricinus communis*). It can cause toxicity if castor beans are thoroughly chewed or blenderized, although the quantity of ricin is small and it is poorly absorbed from the gastrointestinal tract, so symptoms following castor bean ingestion are usually limited to diarrhea and abdominal pain. Less commonly, severe gastroenteritis can lead to volume depletion and advanced chronic kidney disease. On the other hand, purified ricin is extremely toxic if administered parenterally: the LD_{50} for injected ricin in animals is as low as 0.1 mcg/kg. A fatal case of suspected ricin poisoning by homicidal injection of an estimated 0.28 mg of ricin was associated with diffuse organ damage and death from cardiac failure after 2 days. Inhalation of ricin powder has not been reported in humans, but animal studies suggest it could cause hemorrhagic tracheobronchitis and pneumonia.

► Treatment

A. Emergency and Supportive Measures

After suspected ricin inhalation or exposure to powdered ricin, remove clothing and wash skin with water. Personnel caring for such patients should wear protective respiratory gear, clothing, and gloves.

B. Specific Treatment

There is no known antidote or other specific treatment. A vaccine (RiVax®) has been developed and has been granted an Orphan Drug designation by the FDA. Provide supportive care for volume loss due to gastroenteritis and cardiac and respiratory support as needed.

Centers for Disease Control and Prevention. Ricin: Diagnosis & Laboratory Guidance for Clinicians. April 4, 2018. https://emergency.cdc.gov/agent/ricin/clinicians/diagnosis.asp

Kaland ME et al. Toxalbumin exposures: 12 years' experience of U.S. poison centers. Toxicon. 2015 Jun 1;99:125–9. [PMID: 25817002]

Lopez Nunez OF et al. Ricin poisoning after oral ingestion of castor beans: a case report and review of the literature and laboratory testing. J Emerg Med. 2017 Nov;53(5):e67–71. [PMID: 28987302]

CLONIDINE & OTHER SYMPATHOLYTIC ANTIHYPERTENSIVES

Overdosage with these agents (clonidine, guanabenz, guanfacine, methyldopa) causes bradycardia, hypotension, miosis, respiratory depression, and coma. (Transient hypertension occasionally occurs after acute overdosage, a result of peripheral alpha-adrenergic effects in high doses.) Symptoms are usually resolved in less than 24 hours, and deaths are rare. Similar symptoms may occur after ingestion of topical nasal decongestants chemically similar to clonidine (oxymetazoline, tetrahydrozoline, naphazoline). Brimonidine and apraclonidine are used as ophthalmic preparations for glaucoma. Tizanidine is a centrally acting muscle relaxant structurally related to clonidine; it produces similar toxicity in overdose.

► Treatment

A. Emergency and Supportive Measures

Give activated charcoal. Maintain the airway and support respiration if necessary. Symptomatic treatment is usually sufficient even in massive overdose. Maintain blood pressure with intravenous fluids. Dopamine can also be used. Atropine is usually effective for bradycardia.

B. Specific Treatment

There is no specific antidote. Although tolazoline has been recommended for clonidine overdose, its effects are unpredictable and it should not be used. Naloxone has been reported to be successful in a few anecdotal and poorly substantiated cases.

Isbister GK et al. Adult clonidine overdose: prolonged bradycardia and central nervous system depression, but not severe toxicity. Clin Toxicol (Phila). 2017 Mar;55(3):187–92. [PMID: 28107093]

COCAINE

See Amphetamines & Cocaine.

CYANIDE

Cyanide is a highly toxic chemical used widely in research and commercial laboratories and many industries. Its gaseous form, hydrogen cyanide, is an important component of smoke in fires. Cyanide-generating glycosides are also found in the pits of apricots and other related plants. Cyanide is generated by the breakdown of nitroprusside, and poisoning can result from rapid high-dose infusions. Cyanide is also formed by metabolism of acetonitrile, a solvent found in some over-the-counter fingernail glue removers. Cyanide is rapidly absorbed by inhalation, skin absorption, or ingestion. It disrupts cellular function by inhibiting cytochrome oxidase and preventing cellular oxygen utilization.

► Clinical Findings

The onset of toxicity is nearly instantaneous after inhalation of hydrogen cyanide gas but may be delayed for minutes to hours after ingestion of cyanide salts or cyanogenic plants or chemicals. Effects include headache, dizziness, nausea, abdominal pain, and anxiety, followed by confusion, syncope, shock, seizures, coma, and death. The odor of "bitter almonds" may be detected on the victim's breath or in vomitus, though this is not a reliable finding. The venous oxygen saturation may be elevated (greater than 90%) in severe poisonings because tissues have failed to take up arterial oxygen.

► Treatment

A. Emergency and Supportive Measures

Remove the victim from exposure, taking care to avoid exposure to rescuers. For suspected cyanide poisoning due to nitroprusside infusion, stop or slow the rate of infusion. (Metabolic acidosis and other signs of cyanide poisoning usually clear rapidly.)

For cyanide ingestion, administer activated charcoal. Although charcoal has a low affinity for cyanide, the usual doses of 60–100 g are adequate to bind typically ingested lethal doses (100–200 mg).

B. Specific Treatment

In the United States, there are two available cyanide antidote regimens. The conventional cyanide antidote package (Nithiodote) contains sodium nitrite (to induce methemoglobinemia, which binds free cyanide) and sodium thiosulfate (to promote conversion of cyanide to the less toxic thiocyanate). Administer 3% sodium nitrite solution, 10 mL intravenously followed by 25% sodium thiosulfate solution, 50 mL intravenously (12.5 g). **Caution:** Nitrites may induce hypotension and dangerous levels of methemoglobin.

The other approved cyanide treatment in the United States is hydroxocobalamin (Cyanokit, EMD Pharmaceuticals), a newer and potentially safer antidote. The adult dose of hydroxocobalamin is 5 g intravenously (children's dose is 70 mg/kg). **Note:** Hydroxocobalamin causes red discoloration of skin and body fluids that may last several days and can interfere with some laboratory tests.

Hamad E et al. Case files of the University of Massachusetts Toxicology Fellowship: does this smoke inhalation victim require treatment with cyanide antidote? J Med Toxicol. 2016 Jun;12(2):192–8. [PMID: 26831054]
Parker-Cote JL et al. Challenges in the diagnosis of acute cyanide poisoning. Clin Toxicol (Phila). 2018 Jul;56(7):609–17. [PMID: 29417853]

DIETARY SUPPLEMENTS & HERBAL PRODUCTS

Unlike prescription and over-the-counter pharmaceuticals, dietary supplements do not require FDA approval, do not undergo the same premarketing evaluation of safety and efficacy as drugs, and purveyors may or may not adhere to good manufacturing practices and quality control standards. Supplements may cause illness as a result of intrinsic toxicity, misidentification or mislabeling, drug-herb reactions, or intentional adulteration with pharmaceuticals. If you suspect a dietary supplement or herbal product may be the cause of an otherwise unexplained illness, contact the FDA (1-888-463-6332) or the regional poison control center (1-800-222-1222), or consult the following online database: https://www.fda.gov/food/dietary-supplements.

Table 38–7 lists selected examples of clinical toxicity from some of these products.

Avigan MI et al. Scientific and regulatory perspectives in herbal and dietary supplement associated hepatotoxicity in the United States. Int J Mol Sci. 2016 Mar 3;17(3):331. [PMID: 26950122]
Roytman MM et al. Botanicals and hepatotoxicity. Clin Pharmacol Ther. 2018 Sep;104(3):458–69. [PMID: 29920648]
Wong LL et al. Urgent liver transplantation for dietary supplements: an under-recognized problem. Transplant Proc. 2017 Mar;49(2):322–5. [PMID: 28219592]

DIGITALIS & OTHER CARDIAC GLYCOSIDES

Cardiac glycosides paralyze the Na^+-K^+-ATPase pump and have potent vagotonic effects. Intracellular effects include enhancement of calcium-dependent contractility and shortening of the action potential duration. A number of

Table 38–7. Examples of potential toxicity associated with some dietary supplements and herbal medicines.

Product	Common Use	Possible Toxicity
Azarcon (Greta)	Mexican folk remedy for abdominal pain, colic	Contains lead
Comfrey	Gastric upset, diarrhea	Contains pyrrolizidine alkaloids, can cause hepatic veno-occlusive disease
Creatine	Athletic performance enhancement	Nausea, diarrhea, abdominal cramps; elevated serum creatinine
Ginkgo	Memory improvement, tinnitus	Antiplatelet effects, hemorrhage; abdominal pain, diarrhea
Ginseng	Immune system; stress	Decreased glucose; increased cortisol
Guarana	Athletic performance enhancement, appetite suppression	Contains caffeine: can cause tremor, tachycardia, vomiting
Kava	Anxiety, insomnia	Drowsiness, hepatitis, skin rash
Ma huang	Stimulant; athletic performance enhancement	Contains ephedrine: anxiety, insomnia, hypertension, tachycardia, seizures
Spirulina	Body building	Niacin-like flushing reaction
Yohimbine	Sexual enhancement	Hallucinations, hypertension, tachycardia
Zinc	Cold/flu symptoms	Nausea, oral irritation, anosmia

Adapted, with permission, from Table II-30 by Haller C in "Herbal and Alternative Products," In: Olson KR (ed.) *Poisoning & Drug Overdose,* 7th edition. McGraw-Hill, 2018.

plants (eg, oleander, foxglove, lily-of-the-valley) contain cardiac glycosides. Bufotenin, a cardiotoxic steroid found in certain toad secretions and used as an herbal medicine and a purported aphrodisiac, has pharmacologic properties similar to cardiac glycosides.

Clinical Findings

Intoxication may result from acute single exposure or chronic accidental overmedication, especially in patients with kidney dysfunction taking digoxin. After acute overdosage, nausea and vomiting, bradycardia, hyperkalemia, and AV block frequently occur. Patients in whom toxicity develops gradually during long-term therapy may be hypokalemic and hypomagnesemic owing to concurrent diuretic treatment and more commonly present with ventricular arrhythmias (eg, ectopy, bidirectional ventricular tachycardia, or ventricular fibrillation). Digoxin levels may be only slightly elevated in patients with intoxication from cardiac glycosides other than digoxin because of limited cross-reactivity of immunologic tests.

Treatment

A. Emergency and Supportive Measures

After acute ingestion, administer activated charcoal. Monitor potassium levels and cardiac rhythm closely. Treat bradycardia initially with atropine (0.5–2 mg intravenously) or a transcutaneous external cardiac pacemaker.

B. Specific Treatment

For patients with significant intoxication, administer digoxin-specific antibodies (digoxin immune Fab [ovine]; DigiFab). Estimation of the dose is based on the body burden of digoxin calculated from the ingested dose or the steady-state serum digoxin concentration, as described below. More effective binding of digoxin may be achieved if the dose is given partly as a bolus and the remainder as an infusion over a few hours.

1. From the ingested dose—Number of vials = approximately $1.5–2 \times$ ingested dose (mg).

2. From the serum concentration—Number of vials = serum digoxin (ng/mL) $\times$ body weight (kg) $\times 10^{-2}$. **Note:** This is based on the equilibrium digoxin level; after acute overdose, serum levels may be falsely high for several hours before tissue distribution is complete, and overestimation of the DigiFab dose is likely.

3. Empiric dosing—Empiric titration of DigiFab may be used if the patient's condition is relatively stable and an underlying condition (eg, atrial fibrillation) favors retaining a residual level of digitalis activity. Start with one or two vials and reassess the patient's clinical condition after 20–30 minutes. For cardiac glycosides other than digoxin or digitoxin, there is no formula for estimation of vials needed and treatment is entirely based on response to empiric dosing.

Note: After administration of digoxin-specific Fab antibody fragments, serum digoxin levels may be falsely elevated depending on the assay technique.

Arbabian H et al. Elderly patients with suspected chronic digoxin toxicity: a comparison of clinical characteristics of patients receiving and not receiving digoxin-Fab. Emerg Med Australas. 2018 Apr;30(2):242–8. [PMID: 29316267]

Chhabra N et al. Digoxin-specific antibody fragment dosing: a case series. Am J Ther. 2016 Nov/Dec;23(6):e1597–601. [PMID: 26057142]

Nordt SP et al. Assessment of digoxin-specific Fab fragment dosages in digoxin poisoning. Am J Ther. 2016 Jan–Feb;23(1): e63–7. [PMID: 25379735]

Roberts DM et al. Pharmacological treatment of cardiac glycoside poisoning. Br J Clin Pharmacol. 2016 Mar;81(3):488–95. [PMID: 26505271]

ETHANOL, BENZODIAZEPINES, & OTHER SEDATIVE-HYPNOTIC AGENTS

The group of agents known as sedative-hypnotic drugs includes a variety of products used for the treatment of anxiety, depression, insomnia, and epilepsy. Besides common benzodiazepines, such as lorazepam, alprazolam, clonazepam, diazepam, oxazepam, chlordiazepoxide, and triazolam, this group includes the newer benzodiazepine-like hypnotics zolpidem, zopiclone, and zaleplon, and the muscle relaxants baclofen and carisoprodol. Ethanol and other selected agents are also popular recreational drugs. All of these drugs depress the central nervous system reticular activating system, cerebral cortex, and cerebellum.

Clinical Findings

Mild intoxication produces euphoria, slurred speech, and ataxia. Ethanol intoxication may produce hypoglycemia, even at relatively low concentrations, in children and in fasting adults. With more severe intoxication, stupor, coma, and respiratory arrest may occur. Carisoprodol (Soma) commonly causes muscle jerking or myoclonus. Death or serious morbidity is usually the result of pulmonary aspiration of gastric contents. Bradycardia, hypotension, and hypothermia are common. Patients with massive intoxication may appear to be dead, with no reflex responses and even absent electroencephalographic activity. Diagnosis and assessment of severity of intoxication are usually based on clinical findings. Ethanol serum levels over 300 mg/dL (0.3 g/dL; 65 mmol/L) can produce coma in persons who are not using the drug long term, but regular users may remain awake at much higher levels.

Treatment

A. Emergency and Supportive Measures

Administer activated charcoal if the patient has ingested a massive dose and the airway is protected. Repeat-dose charcoal may enhance elimination of phenobarbital, but it has not been proved to improve clinical outcome. Hemodialysis may be necessary for patients with severe phenobarbital intoxication.

B. Specific Treatment

Flumazenil is a benzodiazepine receptor-specific antagonist; it has no effect on ethanol, barbiturates, or other sedative-hypnotic agents. If used, flumazenil is given slowly intravenously, 0.2 mg over 30–60 seconds, and repeated in

0.2–0.5 mg increments as needed up to a total dose of 3–5 mg. **Caution:** *Flumazenil should rarely be used because it may induce seizures in patients with preexisting seizure disorder, benzodiazepine tolerance, or concomitant tricyclic antidepressant or other convulsant overdose.* If seizures occur, diazepam and other benzodiazepine anticonvulsants will not be effective. As with naloxone, the duration of action of flumazenil is short (2–3 hours) and resedation may occur, requiring repeated doses.

Arens AM et al. Adverse effects from counterfeit alprazolam tablets. JAMA Intern Med. 2016 Oct 1;176(10):1554–5. [PMID: 27532131]

Penninga EI et al. Adverse events associated with flumazenil treatment for the management of suspected benzodiazepine intoxication—a systematic review with meta-analyses of randomised trials. Basic Clin Pharmacol Toxicol. 2016 Jan; 118(1):37–44. [PMID: 26096314]

GAMMA-HYDROXYBUTYRATE (GHB)

GHB is a popular drug of abuse. It originated as a short-acting general anesthetic and is occasionally used in the treatment of narcolepsy. It gained popularity among bodybuilders for its alleged growth hormone stimulation and found its way into social settings, where it is consumed as a liquid. It has been used to facilitate sexual assault ("date-rape" drug). Symptoms after ingestion include drowsiness and lethargy followed by coma with respiratory depression. Muscle twitching and seizures are sometimes observed. Recovery is usually rapid, with patients awakening within a few hours. Other related chemicals with similar effects include butanediol and gamma-butyrolactone (GBL). A prolonged withdrawal syndrome has been described in some heavy users.

► Treatment

Monitor the airway and assist breathing if needed. There is no specific treatment. Most patients recover rapidly with supportive care. GHB withdrawal syndrome may require very large doses of benzodiazepines; baclofen has also been used.

Liakoni E et al. Presentations to an urban emergency department in Switzerland due to acute γ-hydroxybutyrate toxicity. Scand J Trauma Resusc Emerg Med. 2016 Aug 31;24(1):107. [PMID: 27581664]

Lingford-Hughes A et al. Improving GHB withdrawal with baclofen: study protocol for a feasibility study for a randomised controlled trial. Trials. 2016 Sep 27;17(1):472. [PMID: 27677382]

Miró Ò et al. Intoxication by gamma hydroxybutyrate and related analogues: clinical characteristics and comparison between pure intoxication and that combined with other substances of abuse. Toxicol Lett. 2017 Aug 5;277:84–91. [PMID: 28579487]

HYPOGLYCEMIC DRUGS

Medications used for diabetes mellitus include insulin, sulfonylureas and other insulin secretagogues, alpha-glucosidase inhibitors (acarbose, miglitol), biguanides (metformin), thiazolidinediones (pioglitazone, rosiglitazone), sodium glucose transporter (SGLT2) inhibitors, and peptide analogs (pramlintide, exenatide) or enhancers (sitagliptin) (see Chapter 27). Of these, insulin and the insulin secretagogues are the most likely to cause hypoglycemia. Metformin can cause lactic acidosis, especially in patients with impaired kidney function or after intentional drug overdose. Euglycemic diabetic ketoacidosis has been reported with SGLT2 use. Table 27–5 lists the duration of hypoglycemic effect of oral hypoglycemic agents and Table 27–6 the extent and duration of various types of insulins.

► Clinical Findings

Hypoglycemia may occur quickly after injection of short-acting insulins or may be delayed and prolonged, especially if a large amount has been injected into a single area, creating a "depot" effect. Hypoglycemia after sulfonylurea ingestion is usually apparent within a few hours but may be delayed several hours, especially if food or glucose-containing fluids have been given.

► Treatment

Give sugar and carbohydrate-containing food or liquids by mouth, or intravenous dextrose if the patient is unable to swallow safely. For severe hypoglycemia, start with D50W, 50 mL intravenously (25 g dextrose); repeat, if needed. Follow up with dextrose-containing intravenous fluids (D5W or D10W) to maintain a blood glucose greater than 70–80 mg/dL.

For hypoglycemia caused by sulfonylureas and related insulin secretagogues, consider use of octreotide, a synthetic somatostatin analog that blocks pancreatic insulin release. A dose of 50–100 mcg octreotide subcutaneously every 6–12 hours can reduce the need for exogenous dextrose and prevent rebound hypoglycemia from excessive dextrose dosing.

Admit all patients with symptomatic hypoglycemia after sulfonylurea overdose. Observe asymptomatic overdose patients for at least 12 hours.

Consider hemodialysis for patients with metformin overdose accompanied by severe lactic acidosis (lactate greater than 20 mmol/L or pH < 7.0).

Elling R et al. Prolonged hypoglycemia after a suicidal ingestion of repaglinide with unexpected slow plasma elimination. Clin Toxicol (Phila). 2016;54(2):158–60. [PMID: 26692235]

Klein-Schwartz W et al. Treatment of sulfonylurea and insulin overdose. Br J Clin Pharmacol. 2016 Mar;81(3):496–504. [PMID: 26551662]

Ueda P et al. Sodium glucose cotransporter 2 inhibitors and risk of serious adverse events: nationwide register based cohort study. BMJ. 2018 Nov 14;363:k4365. [PMID: 30429124]

ISONIAZID

INH is an antibiotic used mainly in the treatment and prevention of tuberculosis. It may cause hepatitis with long-term use, especially in alcoholic patients and elderly persons. It produces acute toxic effects by competing with pyridoxal 5-phosphate, resulting in lowered brain gamma-aminobutyric acid (GABA) levels. Acute ingestion of as little as 1.5–2 g of INH can cause toxicity, and severe poisoning is likely to occur after ingestion of more than 80–100 mg/kg.

Clinical Findings

Confusion, slurred speech, and seizures may occur abruptly after acute overdose. Severe lactic acidosis—out of proportion to the severity of seizures—is probably due to inhibited metabolism of lactate. Peripheral neuropathy and acute hepatitis may occur with long-term use.

Diagnosis is based on a history of ingestion and the presence of severe acidosis associated with seizures. INH is not usually included in routine toxicologic screening, and serum levels are not readily available.

Treatment

A. Emergency and Supportive Measures

Seizures may require higher than usual doses of benzodiazepines (eg, lorazepam, 3–5 mg intravenously) or administration of pyridoxine as an antidote.

Administer activated charcoal after large recent ingestion, but with caution because of the risk of abrupt onset of seizures.

B. Specific Treatment

Pyridoxine (vitamin B_6) is a specific antagonist of the acute toxic effects of INH and is usually successful in controlling convulsions that do not respond to benzodiazepines. Give 5 g intravenously over 1–2 minutes or, if the amount ingested is known, give a gram-for-gram equivalent amount of pyridoxine. Patients taking INH are usually given 25–50 mg of pyridoxine orally daily to help prevent neuropathy.

Gray EL et al. Baseline abnormal liver function tests are more important than age in the development of isoniazid-induced hepatoxicity for patients receiving preventive therapy for latent tuberculosis infection. Intern Med J. 2016 Mar;46(3):281–7. [PMID: 26648478]

Li X et al. Liver transplantation in antituberculosis drugs-induced fulminant hepatic failure: a case report and review of the literature. Medicine (Baltimore). 2015 Dec;94(49):e1665. [PMID: 26656321]

Miyazawa S et al. Isoniazid-induced acute liver failure during preventive therapy for latent tuberculosis infection. Intern Med. 2015;54(6):591–5. [PMID: 25786447]

Skinner K et al. Isoniazid poisoning: pharmacokinetics and effect of hemodialysis in a massive ingestion. Hemodial Int. 2015 Oct;19(4):E37–40. [PMID: 25779481]

LEAD

Lead is used in a variety of industrial and commercial products, such as firearms ammunition, storage batteries, solders, paints, pottery, plumbing, and gasoline and is found in some traditional Hispanic and Ayurvedic ethnic medicines. Lead toxicity usually results from chronic repeated exposure and is rare after a single ingestion. Lead produces a variety of adverse effects on cellular function and primarily affects the nervous system, gastrointestinal tract, and hematopoietic system.

Clinical Findings

Lead poisoning often goes undiagnosed initially because presenting symptoms and signs are nonspecific and exposure is not suspected. Common symptoms include colicky abdominal pain, constipation, headache, and irritability. Severe poisoning may cause coma and convulsions. Chronic intoxication can cause learning disorders (in children) and motor neuropathy (eg, wrist drop). Lead-containing bullet fragments in or near joint spaces can result in chronic lead toxicity.

Diagnosis is based on measurement of the blood lead level. Whole blood lead levels above 5 mcg/dL warrant public health investigation. Levels between 10 and 25 mcg/dL have been associated with impaired neurobehavioral development in children. Levels of 25–50 mcg/dL may be associated with headache, irritability, and subclinical neuropathy. Levels of 50–70 mcg/dL are associated with moderate toxicity, and levels greater than 70–100 mcg/dL are often associated with severe poisoning. Other laboratory findings of lead poisoning include microcytic anemia with basophilic stippling and elevated free erythrocyte protoporphyrin.

Treatment

A. Emergency and Supportive Measures

The most critical intervention in the treatment of lead poisoning is identification of and removal from the source of exposure. For patients with encephalopathy, maintain a patent airway and treat coma and convulsions as described at the beginning of this chapter.

For recent acute ingestion, if a large lead-containing object (eg, fishing weight) is still visible in the stomach on abdominal radiograph, whole bowel irrigation, endoscopy, or even surgical removal may be necessary to prevent subacute lead poisoning. (The acidic gastric contents may corrode the metal surface, enhancing lead absorption. Once the object passes into the small intestine, the risk of toxicity declines.)

Workers with a single lead level over 60 mcg/dL (or three successive monthly levels greater than 50 mcg/dL) or construction workers with any single blood lead level above 50 mcg/dL must by federal law be removed from the site of exposure. Contact the regional office of the United States Occupational Safety and Health Administration (OSHA) for more information. Several states mandate reporting of cases of confirmed lead poisoning.

B. Specific Treatment

The indications for chelation depend on the blood lead level and the patient's clinical state. A medical toxicologist or regional poison control center (1-800-222-1222) should be consulted for advice about selection and use of these antidotes.

Note: It is impermissible under the law to treat asymptomatic workers with elevated blood lead levels in order to keep their levels under 50 mcg/dL rather than remove them from the exposure.

1. Severe toxicity—Patients with severe intoxication (encephalopathy or levels greater than 70–100 mcg/dL) should receive edetate calcium disodium (ethylenediaminetetraacetic acid, EDTA), 1500 mg/m^2/kg/day (approximately 50 mg/kg/day) in four to six divided doses or as a continuous intravenous infusion. Most clinicians also add dimercaprol (BAL), 4–5 mg/kg intramuscularly every 4 hours for 5 days, for patients with encephalopathy.

2. Less severe toxicity—Patients with less severe symptoms and asymptomatic patients with blood lead levels between 55 and 69 mcg/dL may be treated with edetate calcium disodium alone in dosages as above. An oral chelator, succimer (DMSA), is available for use in patients with mild to moderate intoxication. The usual dose is 10 mg/kg orally every 8 hours for 5 days, then every 12 hours for 2 weeks.

Angelon-Gaetz KA et al. Lead in spices, herbal remedies, and ceremonial powders sampled from home investigations for children with elevated blood lead levels—North Carolina, 2011–2018. MMWR Morb Mortal Wkly Rep. 2018 Nov 23; 67(46):1290–4. [PMID: 30462630]
Laidlaw MA et al. Lead exposure at firing ranges—a review. Environ Health. 2017 Apr 4;16(1):34. [PMID: 28376827]
Mehta V et al. Lead intoxication due to ayurvedic medications as a cause of abdominal pain in adults. Clin Toxicol (Phila). 2016 Dec 13;1–5. [PMID: 27957879]

LITHIUM

Lithium is widely used for the treatment of bipolar depression and other psychiatric disorders. The only normal route of lithium elimination is via the kidney, so patients with acute or chronic kidney disorders are at risk for accumulation of lithium resulting in gradual onset (chronic) toxicity. Intoxication resulting from chronic accidental overmedication or kidney impairment is more common and usually more severe than that seen after acute oral overdose.

▶ Clinical Findings

Mild to moderate toxicity causes lethargy, confusion, tremor, ataxia, and slurred speech. This may progress to myoclonic jerking, delirium, coma, and convulsions. Recovery may be slow and incomplete following severe intoxication. Laboratory studies in patients with chronic intoxication often reveal an elevated serum creatinine and an elevated BUN/creatinine ratio due to underlying volume contraction. The white blood cell count is often elevated. ECG findings include T-wave flattening or inversion, and sometimes bradycardia or sinus node arrest. Nephrogenic diabetes insipidus can occur with overdose or with therapeutic doses. Dysfunction of the thyroid and parathyroid glands has also been described as a result of prolonged lithium exposure.

Lithium levels may be difficult to interpret. Lithium has a low toxic:therapeutic ratio, and chronic intoxication can be seen with levels only slightly above the therapeutic range (0.8–1.2 mEq/L). In contrast, patients with acute ingestion may have transiently very high levels (up to 10 mEq/L reported) without any symptoms before the lithium fully distributes into tissues. **Note:** Falsely high lithium levels (as high as 6–8 mEq/L) can be measured if a green-top blood specimen tube (containing lithium heparin) is used for blood collection.

▶ Treatment

After acute oral overdose, consider gastric lavage or whole bowel irrigation to prevent systemic absorption (**Note:** lithium is not adsorbed by activated charcoal). In all patients, evaluate kidney function and volume status, and give intravenous saline-containing fluids as needed. Monitor serum lithium levels and seek assistance with their interpretation and the need for dialysis from a medical toxicologist or regional poison control center (1-800-222-1222). Consider hemodialysis if the patient is markedly symptomatic or if the serum lithium level exceeds 4–5 mEq/L, especially if kidney function is impaired. Continuous renal replacement therapy may be an effective alternative to hemodialysis.

Baird-Gunning J et al. Lithium poisoning. J Intensive Care Med. 2017 May;32(4):249–63. [PMID: 27516079]
Gitlin M. Lithium side effects and toxicity: prevalence and management strategies. Int J Bipolar Disord. 2016 Dec;4(1):27. [PMID: 27900734]
Gong R et al. What we need to know about the effect of lithium on the kidney. Am J Physiol Renal Physiol. 2016 Dec 1;311(6): F1168–71. [PMID: 27122541]

LSD & OTHER HALLUCINOGENS

A variety of substances—ranging from naturally occurring plants and mushrooms to synthetic substances such as phencyclidine (PCP), toluene and other solvents, dextromethorphan, and lysergic acid diethylamide (LSD)—are abused for their hallucinogenic properties. The mechanism of toxicity and the clinical effects vary for each substance.

Many hallucinogenic plants and mushrooms produce anticholinergic delirium, characterized by flushed skin, dry mucous membranes, dilated pupils, tachycardia, and urinary retention. Other plants and mushrooms may contain hallucinogenic indoles such as mescaline and LSD, which typically cause marked visual hallucinations and perceptual distortion, widely dilated pupils, and mild tachycardia. PCP, a dissociative anesthetic agent similar to ketamine, can produce fluctuating delirium and coma, often associated with vertical and horizontal nystagmus. Toluene and other hydrocarbon solvents (butane, trichloroethylene, "chemo," etc) cause euphoria and delirium and may sensitize the myocardium to the effects of catecholamines, leading to fatal dysrhythmias. Other drugs used for their psychostimulant effects include synthetic cannabinoid receptor agonists, *Salvia divinorum*, synthetic tryptamines, and phenylethylamines, and mephedrone and related cathinone derivatives. See https://www.erowid.org/psychoactives/psychoactives .shtml for descriptions of various hallucinogenic substances.

▶ Treatment

A. Emergency and Supportive Measures

Maintain a patent airway and assist respirations if necessary. Treat coma, hyperthermia, hypertension, and seizures as outlined at the beginning of this chapter. For recent large ingestions, consider giving activated charcoal orally or by gastric tube.

B. Specific Treatment

Patients with anticholinergic delirium may benefit from a dose of physostigmine, 0.5–1 mg intravenously, not to exceed 1 mg/min. Dysphoria, agitation, and psychosis associated with LSD or mescaline intoxication may respond to benzodiazepines (eg, lorazepam, 1–2 mg orally or intravenously) or haloperidol (2–5 mg intramuscularly or intravenously) or another antipsychotic drug (eg, olanzapine or ziprasidone). Monitor patients who have sniffed solvents for cardiac dysrhythmias (most commonly premature ventricular contractions, ventricular tachycardia, ventricular fibrillation); treatment with beta-blockers such as propranolol (1–5 mg intravenously) or esmolol (250–500 mcg/kg intravenously, then 50 mcg/kg/min by infusion) may be more effective than lidocaine or amiodarone.

Araújo AM et al. The hallucinogenic world of tryptamines: an updated review. Arch Toxicol. 2015 Aug;89(8):1151–73. [PMID: 25877327]
Caffrey CR et al. When good times go bad: managing 'legal high' complications in the emergency department. Open Access Emerg Med. 2017 Dec 20;10:9–23. [PMID: 29302196]

MERCURY

Mercury poisoning may occur by ingestion of inorganic mercuric salts, organic mercury compounds, or inhalation of metallic mercury vapor. Ingestion of the mercuric salts causes a burning sensation in the throat, discoloration and edema of oral mucous membranes, abdominal pain, vomiting, bloody diarrhea, and shock. Direct nephrotoxicity causes acute kidney injury. Inhalation of high concentrations of metallic mercury vapor may cause acute fulminant chemical pneumonia. Chronic mercury poisoning causes weakness, ataxia, intention tremors, irritability, and depression. Exposure to alkyl (organic) mercury derivatives from highly contaminated fish or fungicides used on seeds has caused ataxia, tremors, convulsions, and catastrophic birth defects. Nearly all fish have some traces of mercury contamination; the US Environmental Protection Agency (EPA) advises consumers to avoid swordfish, shark, king mackerel, and tilefish because they contain higher levels. Fish and shellfish that are generally low in mercury content include shrimp, canned light tuna (not albacore "white" tuna), salmon, pollock, and catfish. Dental fillings composed of mercury amalgam pose a very small risk of chronic mercury poisoning and their removal is rarely justified. Some imported skin lightening creams contain toxic quantities of mercury.

▶ Treatment

A. Acute Poisoning

There is no effective specific treatment for mercury vapor pneumonitis. Remove ingested mercuric salts by lavage and administer activated charcoal. For acute ingestion of mercuric salts, give dimercaprol (BAL) at once, as for arsenic poisoning. Unless the patient has severe gastroenteritis, consider succimer (DMSA), 10 mg/kg orally every 8 hours for 5 days and then every 12 hours for 2 weeks. Unithiol (DMPS) is a chelator that can be given orally or parenterally but is not commonly available in the United States; it can be obtained from some compounding pharmacies. Maintain urinary output. Treat oliguria and anuria if they occur.

B. Chronic Poisoning

Remove from exposure. Neurologic toxicity is not considered reversible with chelation, although some authors recommend a trial of succimer or unithiol (contact a regional poison center or medical toxicologist for advice).

Budnik LT et al. Alternative drugs go global: possible lead and/or mercury intoxication from imported natural health products and a need for scientifically evaluated poisoning monitoring from environmental exposures. J Occup Med Toxicol. 2016 Nov 8;11:49. [PMID: 27833648]
Mo T et al. Mercury poisoning caused by Chinese folk prescription (CFP): a case report and analysis of both CFP and quackery. Medicine (Baltimore). 2016 Nov;95(44):e5162. [PMID: 27858849]
Pelclova D et al. Is chelation therapy efficient for the treatment of intravenous metallic mercury intoxication? Basic Clin Pharmacol Toxicol. 2017 Jun;120(6):628–33. [PMID: 27911474]

METHANOL & ETHYLENE GLYCOL

Methanol (wood alcohol) is commonly found in a variety of products, including solvents, duplicating fluids, record cleaning solutions, and paint removers. It is sometimes ingested intentionally by alcoholic patients as a substitute for ethanol and may also be found as a contaminant in bootleg whiskey. Ethylene glycol is the major constituent in most antifreeze compounds. The toxicity of both agents is caused by metabolism to highly toxic organic acids—methanol to formic acid; ethylene glycol to glycolic and oxalic acids. Diethylene glycol is a nephrotoxic solvent that has been improperly substituted for glycerine in various liquid medications (cough syrup, teething medicine, acetaminophen), causing numerous deaths in Haiti, Panama, and Nigeria.

▶ Clinical Findings

Shortly after ingestion of methanol or ethylene glycol, patients usually appear "drunk." The serum osmolality (measured with the freezing point device) is usually increased, but acidosis is often absent early. After several hours, metabolism to toxic organic acids leads to a severe anion gap metabolic acidosis, tachypnea, confusion, convulsions, and coma. Methanol intoxication frequently causes visual disturbances, while ethylene glycol often produces oxalate crystalluria and acute kidney injury. **Note:** Point-of-care analytical devices commonly used in the emergency department may falsely measure glycolic acid (a toxic metabolite of ethylene glycol) as lactic acid.

▶ Treatment

A. Emergency and Supportive Measures

For patients presenting within 30–60 minutes after ingestion, empty the stomach by aspiration through a nasogastric tube. Charcoal is not very effective but should be administered if other poisons or drugs have also been ingested.

B. Specific Treatment

Patients with significant toxicity (manifested by severe metabolic acidosis, altered mental status, markedly elevated osmol gap, or evidence of end-organ toxicity) should undergo hemodialysis as soon as possible to remove the parent compound and the toxic metabolites. Treatment with folic acid, thiamine, and pyridoxine may enhance the breakdown of toxic metabolites.

Ethanol blocks metabolism of the parent compounds by competing for the enzyme alcohol dehydrogenase. Fomepizole (4-methylpyrazole; Antizol) blocks alcohol dehydrogenase and is much easier to use than ethanol. If started before onset of acidosis, fomepizole may be used as the sole treatment for ethylene glycol ingestion in some cases. A regional poison control center (1-800-222-1222) should be contacted for indications and dosing.

Beauchamp GA et al. Toxic alcohol ingestion: prompt recognition and management in the emergency department. Emerg Med Pract. 2016 Sep;18(9):1–20. [PMID: 27538060]

Kraut JA et al. Toxic alcohols. N Engl J Med. 2018 Jan18; 378(3):270–80. [PMID: 29342392]

Ng PCY et al. Toxic alcohol diagnosis and management: an emergency medicine review. Intern Emerg Med. 2018 Apr;13(3):375–83. Erratum in: Intern Emerg Med. 2018 Mar 22. [PMID: 29427181]

Thanacoody RH et al. Management of poisoning with ethylene glycol and methanol in the UK: a prospective study conducted by the National Poisons Information Service (NPIS). Clin Toxicol (Phila). 2016;54(2):134–40. [PMID: 26594941]

METHEMOGLOBINEMIA-INDUCING AGENTS

A large number of chemical agents are capable of oxidizing ferrous hemoglobin to its ferric state (methemoglobin), a form that cannot carry oxygen. Drugs and chemicals known to cause methemoglobinemia include benzocaine (a local anesthetic found in some topical anesthetic sprays and a variety of nonprescription products), aniline, propanil (an herbicide), nitrites, nitrogen oxide gases, nitrobenzene, dapsone, phenazopyridine (Pyridium), and many others. Dapsone has a long elimination half-life and may produce prolonged or recurrent methemoglobinemia.

▶ Clinical Findings

Methemoglobinemia reduces oxygen-carrying capacity and may cause dizziness, nausea, headache, dyspnea, confusion, seizures, and coma. The severity of symptoms depends on the percentage of hemoglobin oxidized to methemoglobin; severe poisoning is usually present when methemoglobin fractions are greater than 40–50%. Even at low levels (15–20%), victims appear cyanotic because of the "chocolate brown" color of methemoglobin, but they have normal PO_2 results on arterial blood gas determinations. Conventional pulse oximetry gives inaccurate oxygen saturation measurements; the reading is often between 85% and 90%. (A newer pulse oximetry device [Masimo Pulse CO-oximeter] is capable of estimating the methemoglobin level.) Severe metabolic acidosis may be present. Hemolysis may occur, especially in patients susceptible to oxidant stress (ie, those with glucose-6-phosphate dehydrogenase deficiency).

▶ Treatment

A. Emergency and Supportive Measures

Administer high-flow oxygen. If the causative agent was recently ingested, administer activated charcoal. Repeat-dose activated charcoal may enhance dapsone elimination.

B. Specific Treatment

Methylene blue enhances the conversion of methemoglobin to hemoglobin by increasing the activity of the enzyme methemoglobin reductase. For symptomatic patients, administer 1–2 mg/kg (0.1–0.2 mL/kg of 1% solution) intravenously. The dose may be repeated once in 15–20 minutes if necessary. Patients with hereditary methemoglobin reductase deficiency or glucose-6-phosphate dehydrogenase deficiency may not respond to methylene blue treatment. In severe cases where methylene blue is not available or is not effective, exchange blood transfusion may be necessary.

Farkas AN. Methemoglobinemia due to antifreeze ingestion. N Engl J Med. 2017 Nov 16;377(20):1993–4. [PMID: 29141168]

Kim YJ et al. Difference of the clinical course and outcome between dapsone-induced methemoglobinemia and other toxic-agent-induced methemoglobinemia. Clin Toxicol (Phila). 2016 Aug;54(7):581–4. [PMID: 27412886]

Salim SA et al. Upward trend of dapsone-induced methemoglobinemia in renal transplant community. Clin Nephrol. 2017 Sep; 88(9):156–61. [PMID: 28699887]

Sewell CR et al. A case report of benzocaine-induced methemoglobinemia. J Pharm Pract. 2017 Jan 1:897190017723211. [PMID: 28803519]

MUSHROOMS

There are thousands of mushroom species that cause a variety of toxic effects. The most dangerous species of mushrooms are *Amanita phalloides* and related species, which contain potent cytotoxins (amatoxins). Ingestion of even a portion of one amatoxin-containing mushroom may be sufficient to cause death.

The characteristic pathologic finding in fatalities from amatoxin-containing mushroom poisoning is acute massive necrosis of the liver.

▶ Clinical Findings

Amatoxin-containing mushrooms typically cause a delayed onset (8–12 hours after ingestion) of severe abdominal cramps, vomiting and profuse diarrhea, followed in 1–2 days by acute kidney injury, hepatic necrosis, and hepatic encephalopathy. Cooking the mushrooms does not prevent poisoning.

Monomethylhydrazine poisoning (*Gyromitra* and *Helvella* species) is more common following ingestion of uncooked mushrooms, as the toxin is water-soluble. Vomiting, diarrhea, hepatic necrosis, convulsions, coma, and hemolysis may occur after a latent period of 8–12 hours.

▶ Treatment

A. Emergency Measures

After the onset of symptoms, efforts to remove the toxic agent are probably useless, especially in cases of amatoxin or gyromitrin poisoning, where there is usually a delay of 8–12 hours or more before symptoms occur and patients seek medical attention. However, activated charcoal is recommended for any recent ingestion of an unidentified or potentially toxic mushroom. Administer intravenous fluids liberally to replace massive losses from vomiting and diarrhea; monitor central venous pressure, urinary output, and kidney function tests to help guide volume replacement.

B. Specific Treatment

A variety of purported antidotes (eg, thioctic acid, penicillin, corticosteroids) have been suggested for amatoxin-type mushroom poisoning, but controlled studies are lacking and experimental data in animals are equivocal. Aggressive fluid replacement for diarrhea and intensive supportive care for hepatic failure are the mainstays of treatment. Silymarin (silibinin), a derivative of milk thistle, is commonly used in Europe, but is currently commercially available in the United States only as an oral nutritional supplement. The European intravenous product (Legalon-SIL) can be obtained in the United States under an emergency IND provided by the FDA. Contact the regional poison control center (1-800-222-1222) for more information.

Liver transplant may be the only hope for survival in gravely ill patients—contact a liver transplant center early.

Bonacini M et al. Features of patients with severe hepatitis due to mushroom poisoning and factors associated with outcome. Clin Gastroenterol Hepatol. 2017 May;15(5):776–9. [PMID: 28189696]

Karvellas CJ et al; United States Acute Liver Failure Study Group. Acute liver injury and acute liver failure from mushroom poisoning in North America. Liver Int. 2016 Jul;36(7):1043–50. [PMID: 26837055]

Kim T et al. Predictors of poor outcomes in patients with wild mushroom-induced acute liver injury. World J Gastroenterol. 2017 Feb 21;23(7):1262–7. [PMID: 28275306]

OPIATES & OPIOIDS

Prescription and illicit opiates and opioids (morphine, heroin, codeine, oxycodone, fentanyl, hydromorphone, etc) are popular drugs of misuse and abuse and the cause of frequent hospitalizations for overdose. These drugs have widely varying potencies and durations of action; for example, some of the illicit fentanyl derivatives are up to 2000 times more potent than morphine. In recent years, poisonings and fatalities have been reported due to the presence of fentanyl and its derivatives in counterfeit medications and illicit drug use. All of these agents decrease central nervous system activity and sympathetic outflow by acting on opiate receptors in the brain. Tramadol is an analgesic that is unrelated chemically to the opioids but acts on opioid receptors. Buprenorphine is a partial agonist-antagonist opioid used for the outpatient treatment of opioid addiction (Table 5–8).

▶ Clinical Findings

Mild intoxication is characterized by euphoria, drowsiness, and constricted pupils. More severe intoxication may cause hypotension, bradycardia, hypothermia, coma, and respiratory arrest. Pulmonary edema may occur. Death is usually due to apnea or pulmonary aspiration of gastric contents. Methadone may cause QT interval prolongation and torsades de pointes. While the duration of effect for heroin is usually 3–5 hours, methadone intoxication may last for 48–72 hours or longer. Tramadol, dextromethorphan, and meperidine also occasionally cause seizures. With meperidine, the metabolite normeperidine is probably the cause of seizures and is most likely to accumulate with repeated dosing in patients with chronic kidney disease. Propoxyphene prolongs the QRS interval and may cause seizures; it is no longer available in the United States. Wound botulism has been associated with skin-popping, especially involving "black tar" heroin. Buprenorphine added to an opioid regimen may produce acute narcotic withdrawal symptoms. Many opioids, including fentanyl, tramadol, oxycodone, and methadone, are not detected on routine urine toxicology "opiate" screening.

▶ Treatment

A. Emergency and Supportive Measures

Protect the airway and assist ventilation. Administer activated charcoal for recent large ingestions.

B. Specific Treatment

Naloxone is a specific opioid antagonist that can rapidly reverse signs of narcotic intoxication. Although it is structurally related to the opioids, it has no agonist effects of its own. Administer 0.2–2 mg intravenously and repeat as needed to awaken the patient and maintain airway protective reflexes and spontaneous breathing. Very large doses (10–20 mg) may be required for patients intoxicated by some opioids (eg, codeine, fentanyl derivatives). **Caution:** The duration of effect of naloxone is only about 2–3 hours; repeated doses may be necessary for patients intoxicated by long-acting drugs such as methadone. Continuous observation for at least 3 hours after the last naloxone dose is mandatory.

Chou R et al. Management of suspected opioid overdose with naloxone in out-of-hospital settings: a systematic review. Ann Intern Med. 2017 Dec 19;167(12):867–75. [PMID: 29181532]

Dowell D et al. CDC Guideline for prescribing opioids for chronic pain—United States, 2016. JAMA. 2016 Apr 19; 315(15):1624–45. [PMID: 26977696]

Jones CM. Changes in synthetic opioid involvement in drug overdose deaths in the United States, 2010–2016. JAMA. 2018 May1;319(17):1819–21. [PMID: 29715347]

Rudd RA et al. Increases in drug and opioid overdose deaths—United States, 2000–2014. MMWR Morb Mortal Wkly Rep. 2016 Jan 1;64(50–51):1378–82. [PMID: 26720857]

Srivastava A et al. Primary care management of opioid use disorders: abstinence, methadone, or buprenorphine-naloxone? Can Fam Physician. 2017 Mar;63(3):200–5. [PMID: 28292795]

PESTICIDES: CHOLINESTERASE INHIBITORS

Organophosphorus and carbamate insecticides (organophosphates: parathion, malathion, etc; carbamates: carbaryl, aldicarb, etc) are widely used in commercial agriculture and home gardening and have largely replaced older, more environmentally persistent organochlorine compounds such as DDT and chlordane. The organophosphates and carbamates—also called anticholinesterases because they inhibit the enzyme acetylcholinesterase—cause an increase in acetylcholine activity at nicotinic and muscarinic receptors and in the peripheral and central nervous system. There are a variety of chemical agents in this group, with widely varying potencies. Most of them are poorly water-soluble, are often formulated with an aromatic hydrocarbon solvent such as xylene and are well absorbed through intact skin. Most chemical warfare "nerve agents" (such as GA [tabun], GB [sarin], GD [soman], and VX) are organophosphates.

Clinical Findings

Inhibition of cholinesterase results in abdominal cramps, diarrhea, vomiting, excessive salivation, sweating, lacrimation, miosis, wheezing and bronchorrhea, seizures, and skeletal muscle weakness. Initial tachycardia is usually followed by bradycardia. Profound skeletal muscle weakness, aggravated by excessive bronchial secretions and wheezing, may result in respiratory arrest and death. Symptoms and signs of poisoning may persist or recur over several days, especially with highly lipid-soluble agents such as fenthion or dimethoate.

The diagnosis should be suspected in patients who present with miosis, sweating, and hyperperistalsis. Serum and red blood cell cholinesterase activity is usually depressed at least 50% below baseline in those victims who have severe intoxication.

Treatment

A. Emergency and Supportive Measures

If the agent was recently ingested, consider gut decontamination by aspiration of the liquid using a nasogastric tube followed by administration of activated charcoal. If the agent is on the victim's skin or hair, wash repeatedly with soap or shampoo and water. Providers should take care to avoid skin exposure by wearing gloves and waterproof aprons. Dilute hypochlorite solution (eg, household bleach diluted 1:10) is reported to help break down organophosphate pesticides and nerve agents on equipment or clothing.

B. Specific Treatment

Atropine reverses excessive muscarinic stimulation and is effective for treatment of salivation, bronchial hypersecretion, wheezing, abdominal cramping, and sweating. However, it does not interact with nicotinic receptors at autonomic ganglia and at the neuromuscular junction and has no direct effect on muscle weakness. Administer 2 mg intravenously, and if there is no response after 5 minutes, give repeated boluses in rapidly escalating doses (eg, doubling the dose each time) as needed to dry bronchial secretions and decrease wheezing; as much as several hundred milligrams of atropine has been given to treat severe poisoning.

Pralidoxime (2-PAM, Protopam) is a more specific antidote that reverses organophosphate binding to the cholinesterase enzyme; therefore, it should be effective at the neuromuscular junction as well as other nicotinic and

muscarinic sites. It is most likely to be clinically effective if started very soon after poisoning, to prevent permanent binding of the organophosphate to cholinesterase. However, clinical studies have yielded conflicting results regarding the effectiveness of pralidoxime in reducing mortality. Administer 1–2 g intravenously as a loading dose and begin a continuous infusion (200–500 mg/h, titrated to clinical response). Continue to give pralidoxime as long as there is any evidence of acetylcholine excess. Pralidoxime is of questionable benefit for carbamate poisoning, because carbamates have only a transitory effect on the cholinesterase enzyme. Other, unproven therapies for organophosphate poisoning include magnesium, sodium bicarbonate, clonidine, and extracorporeal removal.

Gorecki L et al. Progress in acetylcholinesterase reactivators and in the treatment of organophosphorus intoxication: a patent review (2006–2016). Expert Opin Ther Pat. 2017 Sep; 27(9):971–85. [PMID: 28569609]

King AM et al. Organophosphate and carbamate poisoning. Emerg Med Clin North Am. 2015 Feb;33(1):133–51. [PMID: 25455666]

PETROLEUM DISTILLATES & SOLVENTS

Petroleum distillate toxicity may occur from inhalation of the vapor or as a result of pulmonary aspiration of the liquid during or after ingestion. Acute manifestations of aspiration pneumonitis are vomiting, coughing, and bronchopneumonia. Some hydrocarbons—ie, those with aromatic or halogenated subunits—can also cause severe systemic poisoning after oral ingestion. Hydrocarbons can also cause systemic intoxication by inhalation. Vertigo, muscular incoordination, irregular pulse, myoclonus, and seizures occur with serious poisoning and may be due to hypoxemia or the systemic effects of the agents. Chlorinated and fluorinated hydrocarbons (trichloroethylene, Freons, etc) and many other hydrocarbons can cause ventricular arrhythmias due to increased sensitivity of the myocardium to the effects of endogenous catecholamines.

Treatment

Remove the patient to fresh air. For simple aliphatic hydrocarbon ingestion, gastric emptying and activated charcoal are not recommended, but these procedures may be indicated if the preparation contains toxic solutes (eg, an insecticide) or is an aromatic or halogenated product. Observe the victim for 6–8 hours for signs of aspiration pneumonitis (cough, localized crackles or rhonchi, tachypnea, and infiltrates on chest radiograph). Corticosteroids are not recommended. If fever occurs, give a specific antibiotic only after identification of bacterial pathogens by laboratory studies. Because of the risk of arrhythmias, use bronchodilators with caution in patients with chlorinated or fluorinated solvent intoxication. If tachyarrhythmias occur, use esmolol intravenously 25–100 mcg/kg/min.

Chen X et al. Successful treatment of propafenone-induced cardiac arrest by calcium gluconate. Am J Emerg Med. 2017 Aug;35(8):1209.e1–2. [PMID: 28390833]

Dinsfriend W et al. Inhalant-abuse myocarditis diagnosed by cardiac magnetic resonance. Tex Heart Inst J. 2016 Jun 1; 43(3):246–8. [PMID: 27303242]

Jayanth SH et al. Glue sniffing. Med Leg J. 2017 Mar;85(1):38–42. [PMID: 27694447]

SALICYLATES

Salicylates (aspirin, methyl salicylate, bismuth subsalicylate, etc) are found in a variety of over-the-counter and prescription medications. Salicylates uncouple cellular oxidative phosphorylation, resulting in anaerobic metabolism and excessive production of lactic acid and heat, and they also interfere with several Krebs cycle enzymes. A single ingestion of more than 200 mg/kg of salicylate is likely to produce significant acute intoxication. Poisoning may also occur as a result of chronic excessive dosing over several days. Although the half-life of salicylate is 2–3 hours after small doses, it may increase to 20 hours or more in patients with intoxication.

▶ Clinical Findings

Acute ingestion often causes nausea and vomiting, occasionally with gastritis. Moderate intoxication is characterized by hyperpnea (deep and rapid breathing), tachycardia, tinnitus, and elevated anion gap metabolic acidosis. (A normal anion gap sometimes occurs due to salicylate interference with the chemistry analyzer, falsely raising the measured chloride.) Serious intoxication may result in agitation, confusion, coma, seizures, cardiovascular collapse, pulmonary edema, hyperthermia, and death. The prothrombin time is often elevated owing to salicylate-induced hypoprothrombinemia. Central nervous system intracellular glucose depletion can occur despite normal measured serum glucose levels.

Diagnosis of salicylate poisoning is suspected in any patient with metabolic acidosis and is confirmed by measuring the serum salicylate level. Patients with levels greater than 100 mg/dL (1000 mg/L or 7.2 mcmol/L) after an acute overdose are more likely to have severe poisoning. On the other hand, patients with subacute or chronic intoxication may suffer severe symptoms with levels of only 60–70 mg/dL (4.3–5 mcmol/L). The arterial blood gas typically reveals a respiratory alkalosis with an underlying metabolic acidosis.

▶ Treatment

A. Emergency and Supportive Measures

Administer activated charcoal orally. Gastric lavage followed by administration of extra doses of activated charcoal may be needed in patients who ingest more than 10 g of aspirin. The desired ratio of charcoal to aspirin is about 10:1 by weight; while this cannot always be given as a single dose, it may be administered over the first 24 hours in divided doses every 2–4 hours along with whole bowel irrigation. Give glucose-containing fluids to reduce the risk of cerebral hypoglycemia. Treat metabolic acidosis with intravenous sodium bicarbonate. This is critical because acidosis (especially acidemia, pH < 7.40) promotes greater entry of salicylate into cells, worsening toxicity. **Warning:** Sudden and severe deterioration can occur after rapid sequence intubation and controlled ventilation if the pH is allowed to fall due to hypercarbia during the apneic period.

B. Specific Treatment

Alkalinization of the urine enhances renal salicylate excretion by trapping the salicylate anion in the urine. Add 100 mEq (two ampules) of sodium bicarbonate to 1 L of 5% dextrose in 0.2% saline, and infuse this solution intravenously at a rate of about 150–200 mL/h. Unless the patient is oliguric or hyperkalemic, add 20–30 mEq of potassium chloride to each liter of intravenous fluid. Patients who are volume-depleted often fail to produce an alkaline urine (paradoxical aciduria) unless potassium is given.

Hemodialysis may be lifesaving and is indicated for patients with severe metabolic acidosis, markedly altered mental status, or significantly elevated salicylate levels (eg, greater than 100–120 mg/dL [1000–1200 mg/L or 7.2–8.6 mcmol/L] after acute overdose or greater than 60–70 mg/dL [600–700 mg/L or 4.3–5 mcmol/L] with subacute or chronic intoxication).

Juurlink DN et al. Extracorporeal treatment for salicylate poisoning: systematic review and recommendations from the EXTRIP Workgroup. Ann Emerg Med. 2015 Aug;66(2):165–81. [PMID: 25986310]

McCabe DJ et al. The association of hemodialysis and survival in intubated salicylate-poisoned patients. Am J Emerg Med. 2017 Jun;35(6):899–903. [PMID: 28438446]

Papacostas MF et al. Use of continuous renal replacement therapy in salicylate toxicity: a case report and review of the literature. Heart Lung. 2016 Sep–Oct;45(5):460–3. [PMID: 27531848]

Shively RM et al. Acute salicylate poisoning: risk factors for severe outcome. Clin Toxicol (Phila). 2017 Mar;55(3):175–80. [PMID: 28064509]

SEAFOOD POISONINGS

A variety of intoxications may occur after eating certain types of fish or other seafood. These include scombroid, ciguatera, paralytic shellfish, and puffer fish poisoning. The mechanisms of toxicity and clinical presentations are described in Table 38–8. In the majority of cases, the seafood has a normal appearance and taste (scombroid may have a peppery taste).

▶ Treatment

A. Emergency and Supportive Measures

Caution: Abrupt respiratory arrest may occur in patients with acute paralytic shellfish and puffer fish poisoning. Observe patients for at least 4–6 hours. Replace fluid and electrolyte losses from gastroenteritis with intravenous saline or other crystalloid solution.

For recent ingestions, it may be possible to adsorb residual toxin in the gut with activated charcoal, 50–60 g orally.

Table 38–8. Common seafood poisonings.

Type of Poisoning	Mechanism	Clinical Presentation
Ciguatera	Reef fish ingest toxic dinoflagellates, whose toxins accumulate in fish meat. Commonly implicated fish in the United States are barracuda, jack, snapper, and grouper.	1–6 hours after ingestion, victims develop abdominal pain, vomiting, and diarrhea accompanied by a variety of neurologic symptoms, including paresthesias, reversal of hot and cold sensation, vertigo, headache, and intense itching. Autonomic disturbances, including hypotension and bradycardia, may occur.
Scombroid	Improper preservation of large fish results in bacterial degradation of histidine to histamine. Commonly implicated fish include tuna, mahimahi, bonita, mackerel, and kingfish.	Allergic-like (anaphylactoid) symptoms are due to histamine, usually begin within 15–90 minutes, and include skin flushing, itching, urticaria, angioedema, bronchospasm, and hypotension as well as abdominal pain, vomiting, and diarrhea.
Paralytic shellfish poisoning	Dinoflagellates produce saxitoxin, which is concentrated by filter-feeding mussels and clams. Saxitoxin blocks sodium conductance and neuronal transmission in skeletal muscles.	Onset is usually within 30–60 minutes. Initial symptoms include perioral and intraoral paresthesias. Other symptoms include nausea and vomiting, headache, dizziness, dysphagia, dysarthria, ataxia, and rapidly progressive muscle weakness that may result in respiratory arrest.
Puffer fish poisoning	Tetrodotoxin is concentrated in liver, gonads, intestine, and skin. Toxic effects are similar to those of saxitoxin. Tetrodotoxin is also found in some North American newts and Central American frogs.	Onset is usually within 30–40 minutes but may be as short as 10 minutes. Initial perioral paresthesias are followed by headache, diaphoresis, nausea, vomiting, ataxia, and rapidly progressive muscle weakness that may result in respiratory arrest.

B. Specific Treatment

There is no specific antidote for paralytic shellfish or puffer fish poisoning.

1. Ciguatera—There are anecdotal reports of successful treatment of acute neurologic symptoms with mannitol, 1 g/kg intravenously, but this approach is not widely accepted.

2. Scombroid—Antihistamines such as diphenhydramine, 25–50 mg intravenously, and the H_2-blocker cimetidine, 300 mg intravenously, are usually effective.

Armstrong P et al. Ciguatera fish poisoning. N Z Med J. 2016 Oct 28;129(1444):111–4. [PMID: 27806035]

Feng C et al. Histamine (scombroid) fish poisoning: a comprehensive review. Clin Rev Allergy Immunol. 2016 Feb;50(1):64–9. [PMID: 25876709]

Mullins ME et al. Is mannitol the treatment of choice for patients with ciguatera fish poisoning? Clin Toxicol (Phila). 2017 Nov; 55(9):947–55. [PMID: 28535116]

SNAKE BITES

The venom of poisonous snakes and lizards may be predominantly neurotoxic (coral snake) or predominantly cytolytic (rattlesnakes, other pit vipers). Neurotoxins cause respiratory paralysis; cytolytic venoms cause tissue destruction by digestion and hemorrhage due to hemolysis and destruction of the endothelial lining of the blood vessels. The manifestations of rattlesnake envenomation are mostly local pain, redness, swelling, and extravasation of blood. Perioral tingling, metallic taste, nausea and vomiting, hypotension, and coagulopathy may also occur. Thrombocytopenia can persist for several days after a rattlesnake bite. Neurotoxic envenomation may cause ptosis, dysphagia, diplopia, and respiratory arrest.

► Treatment

A. Emergency Measures

Immobilize the patient and the bitten part in a neutral position. Avoid manipulation of the bitten area. Transport the patient to a medical facility for definitive treatment. Do *not* give alcoholic beverages or stimulants; do *not* apply ice; do *not* apply a tourniquet. The potential trauma to underlying tissues resulting from incision and suction performed by unskilled people is probably not justified in view of the small amount of venom that can be recovered.

B. Specific Antidote and General Measures

1. Pit viper (eg, rattlesnake) envenomation—There are two commercially available antivenins for rattlesnake envenomation (CroFab and Anavip). Depending on the severity of symptoms CroFab is administered in increments of 4–6 vials by slow intravenous drip in 250–500 mL saline. For more serious envenomation with marked local effects and systemic toxicity (eg, hypotension, coagulopathy), higher doses and additional vials may be required. The dosing of Anavip is 10 vials by slow intravenous infusion over 60 minutes initially followed by additional 10-vial increments as needed for more serious envenomations or for progression of symptoms. Monitor vital signs and the blood coagulation profile. Type and cross-match blood. The adequacy of venom neutralization is indicated by improvement in symptoms and signs, and the rate that swelling slows. Prophylactic antibiotics are not indicated after a rattlesnake bite.

2. Elapid (coral snake) envenomation—Give 1–2 vials of specific antivenom as soon as possible. **Note:** Pfizer/Wyeth no longer makes coral snake antivenom in the United States and remaining supplies are dwindling. To locate antisera for this or exotic snakes, call a regional poison control center (1-800-222-1222).

Corbett B et al. North American snake envenomation. Emerg Med Clin North Am. 2017 May;35(2):339–54. [PMID: 28411931]
Kanaan NC et al. Wilderness Medical Society practice guidelines for the treatment of pitviper envenomations in the United States and Canada. Wilderness Environ Med. 2015 Dec; 26(4):472–87. [PMID: 26433731]
Valenta J et al. Severe snakebite envenoming in intensive care. Prague Med Rep. 2016;117(4):153–63. [PMID: 27930893]

SPIDER BITES & SCORPION STINGS

Envenomation from most species of spiders in the United States causes only local pain, redness, and swelling. The more venomous black widow spiders (*Latrodectus mactans*) cause generalized muscular pains, muscle spasms, and rigidity. The brown recluse spider (*Loxosceles reclusa*) causes progressive local necrosis as well as hemolytic reactions (rare).

Stings by most scorpions in the United States cause only local pain. Stings by the more toxic *Centruroides* species (found in the southwestern United States) may cause muscle cramps, twitching and jerking, and occasionally hypertension, convulsions, and pulmonary edema. Stings by scorpions from other parts of the world are not discussed here.

▶ Treatment

A. Black Widow Spider Bites

Pain may be relieved with parenteral opioids or muscle relaxants (eg, methocarbamol, 15 mg/kg). Calcium gluconate 10%, 0.1–0.2 mL/kg intravenously, may transiently relieve muscle rigidity, though its effectiveness is unproven. *Latrodectus* antivenom is possibly more effective, but because of concerns about acute hypersensitivity reactions (horse serum–derived), it is often reserved for very young or elderly patients or those who do not respond promptly to the above measures. Horse serum sensitivity testing is required. (Instruction and testing materials are included in the antivenin kit.)

B. Brown Recluse Spider Bites

Because bites occasionally progress to extensive local necrosis, some authorities recommend early excision of the bite site, whereas others use oral corticosteroids. Anecdotal reports have claimed success with dapsone and colchicine. All of these treatments remain of unproven.

C. Scorpion Stings

No specific treatment other than analgesics is required for envenomations by most scorpions found in the United States. An FDA-approved specific antivenom is available for *Centruroides* stings.

Erickson TB et al. Arthropod envenomation in North America. Emerg Med Clin North Am. 2017 May;35(2):355–75. [PMID: 28411932]

O'Connor AD et al. Severe bark scorpion envenomation in adults. Clin Toxicol (Phila). 2018 Mar;56(3):170–4. [PMID: 28753044]
Ryan NM et al. Treatments for latrodectism—a systematic review on their clinical effectiveness. Toxins (Basel). 2017 Apr 21; 9(4):E148. [PMID: 28430165]
Santos MS et al. Clinical and epidemiological aspects of scorpionism in the world: a systematic review. Wilderness Environ Med. 2016 Dec;27(4):504–18. [PMID: 27912864]

THEOPHYLLINE & CAFFEINE

Methylxanthines, including theophylline and caffeine, are nonselective adenosine receptor antagonists. In overdose, toxicity results from the release of endogenous catecholamines with beta-1- and beta-2-adrenergic stimulation. Theophylline may cause intoxication after an acute single overdose, or intoxication may occur as a result of chronic accidental repeated overmedication or reduced elimination resulting from hepatic dysfunction or interacting drug (eg, cimetidine, erythromycin). The usual serum half-life of theophylline is 4–6 hours, but this may increase to more than 20 hours after overdose. Caffeine in energy drinks or herbal or dietary supplement products can produce similar toxicity.

▶ Clinical Findings

Mild intoxication causes nausea, vomiting, tachycardia, and tremulousness. Severe intoxication is characterized by ventricular and supraventricular tachyarrhythmias, hypotension, and seizures. Status epilepticus is common and often intractable to the usual anticonvulsants. After acute overdose (but not chronic intoxication), hypokalemia, hyperglycemia, and metabolic acidosis are common. Seizures and other manifestations of toxicity may be delayed for several hours after acute ingestion, especially if a sustained-release preparation such as Theo-Dur was taken.

Diagnosis is based on measurement of the serum theophylline concentration. Seizures and hypotension are likely to develop in acute overdose patients with serum levels greater than 100 mg/L (555 mcmol/L). Serious toxicity may develop at lower levels (ie, 40–60 mg/L [222–333 mcmol/L]) in patients with chronic intoxication. Serum caffeine levels are not routinely available in clinical practice, but in a study of 51 fatal cases the median level was 180 mg/L (range 33–567 mg/L).

▶ Treatment

A. Emergency and Supportive Measures

After acute ingestion, administer activated charcoal. Repeated doses of activated charcoal may enhance theophylline elimination by "gut dialysis." Addition of whole bowel irrigation should be considered for large ingestions involving sustained-release preparations.

Hemodialysis is effective in removing theophylline and is indicated for patients with status epilepticus or markedly elevated serum theophylline levels (eg, greater than 100 mg/L [555 mcmol/L] after acute overdose or greater than 60 mg/L [333 mcmol/L] with chronic intoxication).

B. Specific Treatment

Treat seizures with benzodiazepines (lorazepam, 2–3 mg intravenously, or diazepam, 5–10 mg intravenously) or phenobarbital (10–15 mg/kg intravenously). Phenytoin is not effective. Hypotension and tachycardia—which are mediated through excessive beta-adrenergic stimulation—may respond to beta-blocker therapy even in low doses. Administer esmolol, 25–50 mcg/kg/min by intravenous infusion, or propranolol, 0.5–1 mg intravenously.

Aggelopoulou E et al. Atrial fibrillation and shock: unmasking theophylline toxicity. Med Princ Pract. 2018;27(4):387–91. [PMID: 29936503]

Andrade A et al. Dangerous mistake: an accidental caffeine overdose. BMJ Case Rep. 2018 Jun 8;2018. [PMID: 29884665]

Ghannoum M et al. Extracorporeal treatment for theophylline poisoning: systematic review and recommendations from the EXTRIP workgroup. Clin Toxicol (Phila). 2015 May; 53(4):215–29. [PMID: 25715736]

Jones AW. Review of caffeine-related fatalities along with postmortem blood concentrations in 51 poisoning deaths. J Anal Toxicol. 2017 Apr 1;41(3):167–72. [PMID: 28334840]

TRICYCLIC & OTHER ANTIDEPRESSANTS

Tricyclic and related cyclic antidepressants are among the most dangerous drugs involved in suicidal overdose. These drugs have anticholinergic and cardiac depressant properties ("quinidine-like" sodium channel blockade). Tricyclic antidepressants produce more marked membrane-depressant cardiotoxic effects than the phenothiazines.

Newer-generation antidepressants such as trazodone, fluoxetine, citalopram, paroxetine, sertraline, bupropion, venlafaxine, and fluvoxamine are not chemically related to the tricyclic antidepressant agents and, with the exception of bupropion, do not generally produce quinidine-like cardiotoxic effects. However, they may cause seizures in overdoses and they may cause serotonin syndrome.

▶ Clinical Findings

Signs of severe intoxication may occur abruptly and without warning within 30–60 minutes after acute tricyclic overdose. Anticholinergic effects include dilated pupils, tachycardia, dry mouth, flushed skin, muscle twitching, and decreased peristalsis. Quinidine-like cardiotoxic effects include QRS interval widening (greater than 0.12 s; Figure 38–2), ventricular arrhythmias, AV block, and hypotension. Rightward-axis deviation of the terminal 40 ms of the QRS has also been described. Prolongation of the QT interval and torsades de pointes have been reported with several of the newer antidepressants. Seizures and coma are common with severe intoxication. Life-threatening hyperthermia may result from status epilepticus and anticholinergic-induced impairment of sweating. Among newer agents, bupropion and venlafaxine have been associated with a greater risk of seizures.

The diagnosis should be suspected in any overdose patient with anticholinergic side effects, especially if there is widening of the QRS interval or seizures. For intoxication by most tricyclic antidepressants, the QRS interval

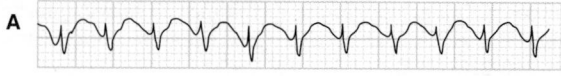
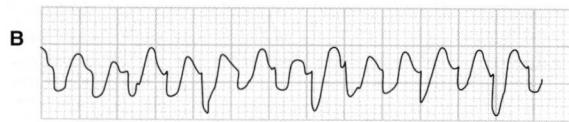
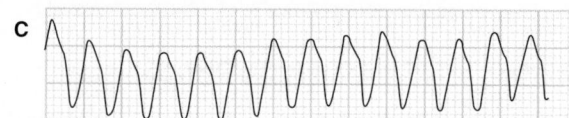

▲ **Figure 38–2.** Cardiac arrhythmias resulting from tricyclic antidepressant overdose. **A:** Delayed intraventricular conduction results in prolonged QRS interval (0.18 s). **B** and **C:** Supraventricular tachycardia with progressive widening of QRS complexes mimics ventricular tachycardia. (Reproduced, with permission, from Benowitz NL, Goldschlager N. Cardiac disturbances in the toxicologic patient. In: Haddad LM, Winchester JF [editors], *Clinical Management of Poisoning and Drug Overdose*, 3rd edition. Saunders/Elsevier, 1998. Copyright © Elsevier.)

correlates with the severity of intoxication more reliably than the serum drug level.

Serotonin syndrome should be suspected if agitation, delirium, diaphoresis, tremor, hyperreflexia, clonus (spontaneous, inducible, or ocular), and fever develop in a patient taking serotonin reuptake inhibitors.

▶ Treatment

A. Emergency and Supportive Measures

Observe patients for at least 6 hours and admit all patients with evidence of anticholinergic effects (eg, delirium, dilated pupils, tachycardia) or signs of cardiotoxicity.

Administer activated charcoal and consider gastric lavage after recent large ingestions. All of these drugs have large volumes of distribution and are not effectively removed by hemodialysis procedures.

B. Specific Treatment

Cardiotoxic sodium channel-depressant effects of tricyclic antidepressants may respond to boluses of sodium bicarbonate (50–100 mEq intravenously). Sodium bicarbonate provides a large sodium load that alleviates depression of the sodium-dependent channel. Reversal of acidosis may also have beneficial effects at this site. Maintain the pH between 7.45 and 7.50. Alkalinization does not promote excretion of tricyclic antidepressants. Prolongation of the QT interval or torsades de pointes is usually treated with intravenous magnesium or overdrive pacing. Severe cardiotoxicity in patients with overdoses of lipid-soluble drugs (eg, amitriptyline, bupropion) has reportedly responded to intravenous lipid emulsion (Intralipid), 1.5 mL/kg repeated one or two times if needed. Plasma exchange using albumin and ECMO have been reported successful in several cases.

Mild serotonin syndrome may be treated with benzodiazepines and withdrawal of the antidepressant. Moderate cases may respond to cyproheptadine (4 mg orally or via gastric tube hourly for three or four doses) or chlorpromazine (25 mg intravenously). Severe hyperthermia should be treated with neuromuscular paralysis and endotracheal intubation in addition to external cooling measures.

Bruccoleri RE et al. A literature review of the use of sodium bicarbonate for the treatment of QRS widening. J Med Toxicol. 2016 Mar;12(1):121–9. [PMID: 26159649]

Clark S et al. Rapid diagnosis and treatment of severe tricyclic antidepressant toxicity. BMJ Case Rep. 2015 Oct 14;2015: 211428. [PMID: 26468220]

Ramasubbu B et al. Serum alkalinisation is the cornerstone of treatment for amitriptyline poisoning. BMJ Case Rep. 2016 Apr 11;2016:214685. [PMID: 27068728]

Cancer

Patricia A. Cornett, MD

Sunny Wang, MD

Lawrence S. Friedman, MD

Carling Ursem, MD

Tiffany O. Dea, PharmD, BCOP

Kenneth R. McQuaid, MD

George Schade, MD

INTRODUCTION TO CANCER

Patricia A. Cornett, MD
Tiffany O. Dea, PharmD, BCOP

► Etiology

Cancer is the second most common cause of death in the United States. In 2018, an estimated 1,735,350 cases of cancer were diagnosed, and 609,640 persons died of cancer. Based on current statistics, almost 40% of Americans will be diagnosed with cancer at some point during their lifetime. Table 39–1 lists the 10 leading cancer types in men and women by site.

However, the death rates from cancer are decreasing. Compared to the 1991 cancer death rate of 215.1 per 100,000 population, the 2012 rate of 171.2 per 100,000 represents a 20% reduction in its death rate. Importantly, death rates have declined in the four most common cancer types (lung, colon-rectum, breast, and prostate). The largest declines in death rates in women have been in non-Hodgkin lymphoma and colorectal cancer and in men, in prostate and stomach cancers. Reductions in cancer mortality reflect successful implementation of a broad strategy of prevention, detection, and treatment. Due to these improvements, the number of cancer survivors is increasing. In 2015, an estimated 14.5 million people were alive in whom cancer had been previously diagnosed; that number is projected to grow to 18.9 million in 2024.

► Modifiable Risk Factors

Tobacco is the most common preventable cause of cancer death; at least 30% of all cancer deaths in the United States are directly linked to tobacco. In 2014, an estimated 167,133 cancer deaths in the United States could be directly attributed to tobacco. Clear evidence links tobacco use to at least 15 cancers. The most dramatic link is with lung cancer; 80% of lung cancer cases occur in smokers. Remarkably, almost 10% of long-term survivors of a tobacco-related cancer continue to use tobacco products, increasing their risk of yet another cancer.

The prevalence of smoking for US adults based on the 2017 National Health Interview Survey is 16% for males and 12.4% for females, which is a remarkable reduction from the 1955 peak of 57% for males and the 1965 peak of 34% for females. Cigarettes are the most common form of tobacco used in the United States, though the use of non-cigarette forms of tobacco and of electronic cigarettes is increasing. The long-term risks of electronic cigarettes are not yet determined. The use of flavoring compounds increases the attractiveness of these devices to youth with the concern that these devices will encourage youth to transition to cigarettes. In 2016, 11% of high school students in the United States reported use of electronic cigarettes in the preceding month.

Tobacco cessation directed toward the individual should start with clinician counseling. Simple, concise advice from a clinician can yield cessation rates of 10–20%. Additive strategies include more intensive counseling; nicotine replacement therapy with patches, gum, lozenges, or inhalers; and prescription medication with bupropion or varenicline (see Chapter 1).

For those Americans who do not use tobacco, the most modifiable risk factors would be nutrition and physical activity. Prudent recommendations to reduce cancer risk are to (1) avoid tobacco; (2) be physically active; (3) maintain a healthy weight; (4) consume a diet rich in fruits, vegetables, and whole grains; (5) lower consumption of saturated and trans dietary fats; (6) limit alcohol use; and (7) avoid excess sun exposure.

Another modifiable cancer risk factor is radiation from radiographic studies. A 2009 study reported that the use of computed tomography (CT) in diagnostic algorithms exposes individuals to significant radiation doses that may increase their lifetime risk of cancer. Both standardization of CT radiation doses and limiting testing have been important steps in minimizing this risk. The American Society of Hematology and American Society of Clinical Oncology have guidelines, inspired by the American Board of Internal Medicine Foundation's "Choosing Wisely" campaign, for limiting radiographic testing, particularly when used in surveillance for treated cancer patients.

Table 39–1. Estimated 10 most common cancer cases in the United States in males and females (all races).

Rank	Males Total Cases (N) = 870,970 (percent)	Females Total Cases (N) = 891,480 (percent)
1	Prostate 174,650 (20)	Breast 268,600 (30.1)
2	Lung and bronchus 116,440 (13)	Lung and bronchus 111,710 (12.5)
3	Colon and rectum 78,500 (9)	Colon and rectum 67,100 (7.5)
4	Urinary bladder 61,700 (7)	Uterine corpus 61,880 (7)
5	Melanoma 57,720 (6.5)	Melanoma 39,260 (4.4)
6	Kidney and renal pelvis 44,120 (5)	Thyroid 37,810 (4.2)
7	Non-Hodgkin lymphoma 41,090 (4.7)	Non-Hodgkin lymphoma 33,110 (3.7)
8	Oral cavity and pharynx 38,140 (4.3)	Kidney and renal pelvis 29,700 (3.3)
9	Leukemia 35,920 (4.1)	Pancreas 26,830 (3)
10	Pancreas 29,940 (3.4)	Leukemia 25,860 (2.9)
	Other sites 193,250 (22.2)	Other sites 190,220 (21.3)

Data from the American Cancer Society, 2019.

American Cancer Society. Cancer Facts & Figures 2019. https://www.cancer.org/research/cancer-facts-statistics/all-cancer-facts-figures/cancer-facts-figures-2019.html

Office of Disease Prevention and Health Promotion. Healthy People 2020. Tobacco use objectives: reduce tobacco use by adults. https://www.healthypeople.gov/2020/topics-objectives/topic/tobacco-use/objectives

Siegel RL et al. Cancer statistics, 2019. CA Cancer J Clin. 2019 Jan; 69(1):7–34. [PMID: 30620402]

Staging

The most commonly used staging system at the time of diagnosis is the TNM (Tumor, Nodes, Metastasis) system (see https://www.cancerstaging.org). Rules for staging for individual cancers are established and published by the American Joint Committee on Cancer (AJCC). The elements used for staging are tumor location, size and level of tumor invasion (T), absence or presence and extent of nodal metastases (N), and absence or presence of systemic metastases (M). Once the TNM designations have been determined, an overall stage is assigned, stage I, II, III, or IV. Clinical staging utilizes physical examination, laboratory and imaging tests as well as results from biopsies; pathologic staging relies on the results from surgery. In some instances, other classifications may be used for certain cancers such as the Ann Arbor staging system for lymphomas.

Other characteristics of cancers, not reflected in the TNM stage, may be used to indicate prognosis and guide treatment. Pathologic features seen on routine histologic examination for some cancers are very important; examples include the Gleason score for prostate cancer and the grade of sarcomas. Cancer specimens should also be sent for targeted molecular diagnostic testing, when appropriate. Examples include testing for *HER2* in breast and gastric cancer; *K-ras* and *BRAF* mutations in colorectal cancer; *BRAF* mutations in melanoma; epidermal growth factor receptor (EGFR), *K-ras* mutations, and the *ALK* fusion gene in lung cancer; and programmed death-ligand 1 (PD-L1) expression testing in a variety of cancers.

Treatment

See Primary Cancer Treatment section below. Table 39–2 outlines treatment choices by cancer type for those responsive to systemic agents, and Table 39–3 provides a listing of common chemotherapeutic agents.

Table 39–2. Treatment choices for cancers responsive to systemic agents.

Diagnosis	Initial Treatment	Other Treatments
Acute lymphoblastic leukemia (ALL)	**Induction combination chemotherapy:** Vincristine, prednisone, daunorubicin, asparaginase, intrathecal methotrexate **Consolidation combination chemotherapy:** Cyclophosphamide, vincristine, doxorubicin, dexamethasone (hyper-CVAD) alternated with cytarabine, methotrexate **Maintenance chemotherapy:** Methotrexate, 6-mercaptopurine **Philadelphia chromosome–positive ALL:** Add imatinib or dasatinib or nilotinib to above regimen	Blinatumomab, inotuzumab ozogamicin, tisagenlecleucel, liposomal vincristine, clofarabine, nelarabine (T-cell ALL), nilotinib, bosutinib, ponatinib (Philadelphia chromosome-positive ALL), autologous or allogeneic transplantation for high risk or at relapse
Acute myeloid leukemia (AML)	**Combination chemotherapy:** Cytarabine, daunorubicin or Cytarabine, idarubicin or Cytarabine, daunomycin, cladribine	Mitoxantrone, doxorubicin, fludarabine, 5-azacytidine, decitabine, clofarabine, midostaurin (*FLT3* mutation +), gemtuzumab ozogamicin (CD33+), enasidenib (*IDH2* mutation), venetoclax, glasdegib, ivosidenib (*IDH1* mutation), cladribine, gilteritinib (*FLT3* mutation)

(continued)

Table 39–2. Treatment choices for cancers responsive to systemic agents. (continued)

Diagnosis	Initial Treatment	Other Treatments
Chronic myeloid leukemia (CML)	Nilotinib or Dasatinib or Imatinib mesylate	Ponatinib, bosutinib, omacetaxine, allogeneic bone marrow transplantation
Chronic lymphocytic leukemia (CLL)	**Combination chemotherapy:** Fludarabine, cyclophosphamide, rituximab (FCR) or Bendamustine, rituximab **Single-agent chemotherapy:** Ibrutinib or obinutuzumab or ofatumumab or chlorambucil	Alemtuzumab, idelalisib, venetoclax, lenalidomide, duvelisib, acalabrutinib, pentostatin, cladribine, cyclophosphamide, vincristine, doxorubicin, prednisone
Hairy cell leukemia	Cladribine (2-chlorodeoxyadenosine)	Pentostatin, rituximab, interferon-alpha, vemu-rafenib, ibrutinib, moxetumomab pasudotox
Hodgkin lymphoma (stages III and IV)	**Combination chemotherapy:** Doxorubicin, bleomycin, vinblastine, dacarbazine (ABVD), or Doxorubicin, vinblastine, mechlorethamine, etoposide, vincristine, bleomycin, prednisone (Stanford V), or Bleomycin, etoposide, doxorubicin, cyclophosphamide, vincristine, procarbazine, prednisone (BEACOPP)	Combination chemotherapy second line: Dexamethasone, cisplatin, cytarabine (DHAP), or Etoposide, methylprednisolone, cytarabine, cisplatin (ESHAP), or Ifosfamide, carboplatin, etoposide (ICE), or Mesna, ifosfamide, mitoxantrone, etoposide (MIME); stem cell transplantation for high risk or first relapse Brentuximab vedotin, nivolumab, pembrolizumab, bendamustine, everolimus
Non-Hodgkin lymphoma (intermediate and high grade)	**Combination chemotherapy:** Cyclophosphamide, doxorubicin, vincristine, prednisone, rituximab (CHOP-R), or Etoposide, prednisone, vincristine, cyclophosphamide, doxorubicin, rituximab (dose-adjusted R-EPOCH) (for double rearrangements)	Combination chemotherapy second line: Dexamethasone, cisplatin, cytarabine (DHAP), or Etoposide, methylprednisolone, cytarabine, cisplatin (ESHAP), or Ifosfamide, carboplatin, etoposide (ICE), or Mesna, ifosfamide, mitoxantrone, etoposide (MIME); transplantation for high risk or first relapse
Non-Hodgkin lymphoma (low grade)	**Combination chemotherapy:** Bendamustine, rituximab, or Cyclophosphamide, vincristine, doxorubicin, prednisone, rituximab (CHOP-R), or Cyclophosphamide, vincristine, prednisone, rituximab (CVP-R), or Lenalidomide, rituximab	Chlorambucil, fludarabine, copanlisib, duvelisib, obinutuzumab, ^{90}Y ibritumomab tiuxetan, idelalisib, ibrutinib, belinostat (T-cell lymphoma), autologous or allogeneic transplantation
Plasma cell myeloma	**Combination chemotherapy (transplant candidates):** Bortezomib, dexamethasone, cyclophosphamide, or Bortezomib, dexamethasone, lenalidomide, or Dexamethasone, lenalidomide, or Ixazomib/lenalidomide/dexamethasone, or Carfilzomib/lenalidomide/dexamethasone Followed by autologous or miniallogeneic stem cell transplantation **Combination chemotherapy (non-transplant candidates):** Lenalidomide, dexamethasone, or Melphalan, prednisone, bortezomib, or Melphalan, prednisone, lenalidomide, or Melphalan, prednisone, thalidomide	Liposomal doxorubicin, pomalidomide, panobinostat, elotuzumab, daratumumab
Waldenström macroglobulinemia	**Plasmapheresis alone or followed by combination chemotherapy:** Bortezomib, dexamethasone, rituximab Cyclophosphamide, dexamethasone, rituximab Ibrutinib with or without rituximab Bendamustine, rituximab	Cladribine, ofatumumab, carfilzomib, fludarabine, everolimus, autologous bone marrow transplantation
Polycythemia vera	Phlebotomy, hydroxyurea, aspirin	Ruxolitinib, radiophosphorus ^{32}P, interferon-alpha

(continued)

Table 39–2. Treatment choices for cancers responsive to systemic agents. (continued)

Diagnosis	Initial Treatment	Other Treatments
Non–small cell lung cancer	**Combination chemotherapy:** Cisplatin, vinorelbine, or Cisplatin, etoposide, or Paclitaxel, carboplatin, or Cisplatin, gemcitabine (squamous histology) Cisplatin, pemetrexed (nonsquamous histology) All regimens with or without bevacizumab Erlotinib, gefitinib, osimertinib or afatinib or dacomitinib (*EGFR* mutation positive), or Crizotinib, alectinib, ceritinib, brigatinib (*ALK* mutation positive) Certitinib, crizotinib (*ROS1* rearrangement) Dabrafenib/trametinib (*BRAF* V600F mutation) Pembrolizumab (PD-L1 expression)	Docetaxel, cetuximab, pembrolizumab, nivolumab, atezolizumab, necitumumab, ramucirumab, cabozantinib (*RET* rearrangement), trastuzumab, afatinib (*HER2* mutation positive), alectinib, brigatinib, ceritinib (*ALK* rearrangement), lorlatinib (*ROS1* rearrangement)
Small cell lung cancer	**Combination chemotherapy:** Cisplatin, etoposide, or Carboplatin, etoposide, or Cisplatin, irinotecan or carboplatin, etoposide, atezolizumab	Irinotecan, cyclophosphamide, doxorubicin, vincristine, topotecan, gemcitabine, paclitaxel, bendamustine, temozolomide, nivolumab, ipilimumab
Mesothelioma	**Combination chemotherapy:** Cisplatin, pemetrexed, bevacizumab or Carboplatin, pemetrexed, with or without bevacizumab or Gemcitabine, cisplatin	Vinorelbine, nivolumab with or without ipilimumab, pembrolizumab
Head and neck cancer	**Combination chemotherapy:** Cisplatin, fluorouracil, or Paclitaxel, carboplatin, or Docetaxel, cisplatin, fluorouracil, or Cisplatin or cetuximab with radiation therapy	Methotrexate, afatinib, pembrolizumab, nivolumab
Esophageal and esophagogastric junction cancer	**Combination chemotherapy:** Cisplatin, fluorouracil, or Paclitaxel, carboplatin, or Oxaliplatin, fluorouracil, or Docetaxel, cisplatin, fluorouracil	Irinotecan, oxaliplatin, capecitabine, epirubicin, docetaxel, trastuzumab, ramucirumab (esophagogastric junction cancer), pembrolizumab
Uterine cancer	**Hormone therapy:** Progestins, tamoxifen, aromatase inhibitors, fulvestrant or **Combination chemotherapy:** Cisplatin, doxorubicin, or Docetaxel, carboplatin, or Carboplatin, paclitaxel Carboplatin, paclitaxel, trastuzumab (HER2 positive)	Liposomal doxorubicin, bevacizumab, topotecan, temsirolimus, pembrolizumab (MSI-H/dMMR)
Ovarian cancer	**Combination chemotherapy:** Paclitaxel, carboplatin with or without bevacizumab, or Docetaxel, carboplatin, or Paclitaxel, cisplatin	Gemcitabine, liposomal doxorubicin, topotecan, cyclophosphamide, etoposide, pemetrexed, olaparib, pazopanib, rucaparib, niraparib, pembrolizumab (MSI-H/dMMR)
Cervical cancer	**With radiation:** Cisplatin **Combination chemotherapy:** Cisplatin, paclitaxel with or without bevacizumab, or Cisplatin, topotecan, or Carboplatin, paclitaxel with or without bevacizumab, or Cisplatin, gemcitabine, or Topotecan, paclitaxel with or without bevacizumab	Docetaxel, ifosfamide, vinorelbine, irinotecan, mitomycin, fluorouracil, pemetrexed, bevacizumab, pembrolizumab (PD-L1+ or MSI-H/dMMR)
Breast cancer	**Adjuvant hormone therapy:** *Premenopausal:* Tamoxifen *Postmenopausal:* Aromatase inhibitors (anastrozole, letrozol, exemestane) **Adjuvant chemotherapy (without trastuzumab):** Doxorubicin, cyclophosphamide, paclitaxel, or Docetaxel, cyclophosphamide, or Doxorubicin, cyclophosphamide, or Doxorubicin, cyclophosphamide, docetaxel **Adjuvant chemotherapy (with trastuzumab):** Doxorubicin, cyclophosphamide, paclitaxel, trastuzumab with or without pertuzumab, or Docetaxel, carboplatin, trastuzumab with or without pertuzumab	Eribulin, capecitabine, mitoxantrone, cisplatin, etoposide, vinblastine, fluorouracil, ixabepilone, pertuzumab, gemcitabine, lapatinib, toremifene, fulvestrant, palbociclib, raloxifene, abemaciclib, ribociclib, olaparib

Table 39–2. Treatment choices for cancers responsive to systemic agents. (continued)

Diagnosis	Initial Treatment	Other Treatments
Choriocarcinoma (trophoblastic neoplasms)	**Single-agent chemotherapy:** Methotrexate or dactinomycin for low-risk disease **Combination chemotherapy:** Etoposide, methotrexate, dactinomycin, cyclophosphamide, vincristine (EMA-CO) for high-risk disease	Paclitaxel, cisplatin, etoposide, bleomycin, ifosfamide, gemcitabine, pembrolizumab, nivolumab
Testicular cancer	**Combination chemotherapy:** Cisplatin, etoposide (EP), or Bleomycin, etoposide, cisplatin (BEP), or Etoposide, mesna, ifosfamide, cisplatin (VIP)	Vinblastine, paclitaxel, gemcitabine, oxaliplatin Pembrolizumab (MSI-H/dMMR+)
Kidney (renal cell) cancer	**Clear cell histology** Pazopanib or sunitinib or ipilimumab and nivolumab or cabozantinib **Non–clear cell histology** Sunitinib, cabozantinib, everolimus	Interferon-alpha 2b, high-dose IL-2, axitinib, temsirolimus, bevacizumab, sorafenib, sunitinib, erlotonib, lenvatinib
Bladder cancer	**Combination chemotherapy:** Gemcitabine, cisplatin, or Methotrexate, vinblastine, doxorubicin, cisplatin (MVAC), or Cisplatin, methotrexate, vinblastine (CMV)	Atezolizumab, carboplatin, paclitaxel, docetaxel, fluorouracil, pemetrexed, pembrolizumab, durvalumab, avelumab
Prostate cancer	**Hormone therapy:** Luteinizing hormone–releasing agonist (leuprolide, goserelin, triptorelin, histrelin, degarelix) with or without an antiandrogen (flutamide, bicalutamide, nilutamide) **Chemotherapy:** Docetaxel, prednisone	Ketoconazole, abiraterone, enzalutamide, apalutamide, mitoxantrone, cabazitaxel, pembrolizumab (MSI-H or dMMR), sipuleucel-T, prednisone, radium (Ra)-223
Brain cancer (anaplastic astrocytoma and glioblastoma multiforme)	**Single-agent chemotherapy with radiation therapy:** Temozolomide	Bevacizumab, irinotecan, procarbazine, carmustine, lomustine, cyclophosphamide, etoposide
Neuroblastoma	**Combination chemotherapy:** Cyclophosphamide, doxorubicin, cisplatin, etoposide	Vincristine, topotecan, irinotecan, ifosfamide, carboplatin, 13-cis-retinoic acid, ^{131}I-MIBG, dinutuximab, autologous or allogeneic transplantation
Thyroid cancer	**Single-agent chemotherapy:** Radioiodine (^{131}I) or sorafenib, lenvatinib, vandetanib (medullary thyroid cancer) or cabozantinib (medullary thyroid cancer) **Combination chemotherapy:** Paclitaxel/carboplatin or docetaxel/doxorubicin (anaplastic carcinoma)	Sunitinib, pazopanib, doxorubicin, dacarbazine
Adrenal cancer	**Single-agent chemotherapy:** Mitotane	Doxorubicin, etoposide, cisplatin
Stomach (gastric) cancer	**Combination chemotherapy:** Epirubicin, cisplatin, fluorouracil, or Docetaxel, cisplatin, fluorouracil, or Cisplatin, fluorouracil, Fluorouracil, oxaliplatin Trastuzumab added for *HER2*-overexpressing adenocarcinomas	Capecitabine, irinotecan, paclitaxel, ramucirumab, pembrolizumab (MSI-H or dMMR tumors)
Pancreatic cancer	**Combination chemotherapy:** Gemcitabine, nab-paclitaxel, or 5-Fluorouracil, leucovorin, irinotecan, oxaliplatin (FOLFIRINOX) **Single-agent chemotherapy:** Gemcitabine	Gemcitabine, capecitabine 5-Fluorouracil, leucovorin, nanoliposomal irinotecan 5-Fluorouracil, folinic acid, oxaliplatin (FOLFOX) Pembrolizumab (MSI-H or dMMR or PD-LI positive tumors) Capecitabine
Colon cancer	**Combination chemotherapy:** Fluorouracil, leucovorin, oxaliplatin (FOLFOX), or Capecitabine, oxaliplatin (CapeOx), or Fluorouracil, leucovorin, irinotecan (FOLFIRI) each regimen with or without bevacizumab	Cetuximab, panitumumab, regorafenib, ziv-aflibercept, trifluridine/tipiracil, nivolumab, +/– ipilimumab or pembrolizumab (dMMR/MSI-H)
Rectal cancer	**Chemotherapy with radiation:** Fluorouracil or capecitabine; For adjuvant or advanced disease treatment, same regimens used with colon cancer	Cetuximab, panitumumab, regorafenib, ziv-aflibercept, trifluridine/tipiracil, nivolumab or pembrolizumab (dMMR/MSI-H)

(continued)

Table 39–2. Treatment choices for cancers responsive to systemic agents. (continued)

Diagnosis	Initial Treatment	Other Treatments
Anal cancer	**Combination chemotherapy with radiation:** Fluorouracil, mitomycin or capecitabine, mitomycin	Cisplatin, nivolumab, pembrolizumab
Carcinoid	Octreotide LAR +/- telotristat or lanreotide	Everolimus, sunitinib, ^{177}Lu-dotable (if somatostatin receptor positive imaging)
Osteogenic sarcoma	**Combination chemotherapy:** Cisplatin, doxorubicin, or Methotrexate, doxorubicin, cisplatin (MAP), or Ifosfamide, cisplatin, epirubicin	Cyclophosphamide, gemcitabine, docetaxel, etoposide, sorafenib, radium (Ra)-233, samarium (Sm)-153 (lexidronam)-ethylene diamine tetramethylene phosphate (EDTMP), topotecan, pembrolizumab (MSI-H or dMMR tumors)
Soft tissue sarcomas	**Combination chemotherapy:** Doxorubicin, dacarbazine (AD), or Doxorubicin, ifosfamide, mesna (AIM), or Mesna, doxorubicin, ifosfamide, dacarbazine (MAID), or Doxorubicin, olaratumab **Single-agent chemotherapy:** Eribulin, pazopanib; imatinib or sunitinib or regorafenib (gastrointestinal stromal tumors)	Liposomal doxorubicin, methotrexate, gemcitabine, docetaxel, temozolomide, epirubicin, pazopanib, eribulin, trabectedin; sorafenib, nilotinib, dasatinib, pazopanib, regorafenib, everolimus (gastrointestinal stromal tumors)
Melanoma	**Combination chemotherapy** (non-*BRAF* mutation): nivolumab/ipilimumab **Combination chemotherapy** (*BRAF* mutation): dabrafenib/trametinib or vemurafenib/cobimetinib or encorafenib/binimetinib **Single-agent chemotherapy** (non-*BRAF* mutation): pembrolizumab or nivolumab **Single-agent chemotherapy** (*BRAF* mutation): vemurafenib or dabrafenib	Dacarbazine, temozolomide, imatinib, paclitaxel, carboplatin, IL-2, interferon alfa-2b
Hepatocellular cancer	**Single-agent chemotherapy:** Sorafenib or lenvatinib	Regorafenib, nivolumab, ramucirumab, pembrolizumab
Kaposi sarcoma	**Single-agent chemotherapy:** Liposomal doxorubicin or liposomal daunorubicin or paclitaxel	Pomalidomide, vinorelbine, thalidomide, etoposide, gemcitabine, interferon alfa-2b, nab-paclitaxel, imatinib

MSI-H/dMMR, microsatellite instability high/deficient mismatch repair.

Table 39–3. Common cancer therapeutic agents.[1]

Chemotherapeutic Agent	Usual Adult Dosage	Adverse Effects
Alkylating Agents—Nitrogen Mustards		
Bendamustine (Treanda)	100–120 mg/m^2 intravenously every 3–4 weeks	Acute: hypersensitivity, nausea, vomiting Delayed: myelosuppression, rash, pyrexia, fatigue
Cyclophosphamide (Cytoxan)	500–1000 mg/m^2 intravenously every 3 weeks; 100 mg/m^2/day orally for 14 days every 4 weeks; various doses	Acute: nausea and vomiting Delayed: myelosuppression, alopecia, hemorrhagic cystitis, cardiotoxicity (high dose)
Ifosfamide (Ifex)	1200 mg/m^2 intravenously daily for 5 days every 3 weeks; various doses	Acute: nausea and vomiting Delayed: alopecia, myelosuppression, hemorrhagic cystitis, neurotoxicity
Melphalan (Alkeran)	0.25 mg/kg/day or 8–10 mg/m^2/day orally for 4 days every 4–6 weeks; 16 mg/m^2 intravenously every 2–4 weeks; various doses	Acute: nausea, vomiting, diarrhea, hypersensitivity (intravenously) Delayed: mucositis (intravenously), myelosuppression, increased risk of secondary malignancies

(continued)

Table 39–3. Common cancer therapeutic agents.[1] (continued)

Chemotherapeutic Agent	Usual Adult Dosage	Adverse Effects
Alkylating Agents—Platinum Analogs		
Carboplatin (Paraplatin)	Area under the curve (AUC)-based dosing use Calvert equation [Dose (mg) = AUC $\times$ (GFR + 25)] AUC = 2–7 mg/mL/min every 2–4 weeks	Acute: nausea and vomiting Delayed: myelosuppression, electrolyte disturbances, peripheral neuropathy, nephrotoxicity, hypersensitivity
Cisplatin (Platinol)	50–100 mg/m^2 intravenously every 3–4 weeks; 20 mg/m^2/day intravenously for 5 days every 3 weeks; various doses	Acute: nausea and vomiting Delayed: nephrotoxicity, ototoxicity, neurotoxicity, myelosuppression, electrolyte disturbances
Oxaliplatin (Eloxatin)	85–130 mg/m^2 intravenously every 2–3 weeks	Acute: peripheral neuropathy exacerbated by cold, nausea, vomiting, diarrhea Delayed: myelosuppression, elevated transaminases
Alkylating Agents—Triazenes		
Dacarbazine (DTIC-Dome)	375 mg/m^2 intravenously on day 1 and 15 every 4 weeks; 900–1000 mg/m^2 intravenously over 3 to 4 days; various doses	Acute: nausea, vomiting, photosensitivity Delayed: myelosuppression, anorexia, hypotension, flu-like syndrome
Procarbazine (Matulane)	60–100 mg/m^2 orally for 14 days every 4 weeks; various doses	Acute: nausea and vomiting Delayed: myelosuppression, disulfiram-like reaction, MAO inhibition, rash
Temozolomide (Temodar)	75 mg/m^2 orally daily during radiation for 42 days; 150–200 mg/m^2 orally for 5 days every 4 weeks	Acute: nausea, vomiting, constipation Delayed: myelosuppression, fatigue
Alkylating Agent—Miscellaneous		
Busulfan (Myleran)	1–8 mg orally daily; 0.8 mg/kg intravenously every 6 hours for 4 days	Acute: nausea and vomiting Delayed: myelosuppression, mucositis, rash, edema, electrolyte disturbances, hepatic veno-occlusive disease (high dose)
Chlorambucil (Leukeran)	0.1–0.2 mg/kg/day orally for 3–6 weeks; 0.4 mg/kg pulse every 4 weeks	Acute: nausea Delayed: myelosuppression, rash
Antimetabolites—Folate Antagonists		
Methotrexate (MTX; Trexall)	**Intrathecal:** 12 mg **High dose:** 1000–12,000 mg/m^2 intravenously every 2–3 weeks	Acute: nausea, vomiting, mucositis Delayed: myelosuppression, nephrotoxicity, hepatotoxicity, neurotoxicity, photosensitivity, pulmonary toxicity
Pemetrexed (Alimta)	500 mg/m^2 intravenously every 3 weeks	Acute: nausea, vomiting, diarrhea, rash Delayed: myelosuppression, fatigue, mucositis
Antimetabolites—Purine Analogs		
Cladribine (Leustatin)	0.1 mg/kg/day subcutaneously daily for 5 days or 0.09 mg/kg/day intravenously via continuous infusion for 7 days	Acute: nausea, injection site reaction Delayed: myelosuppression, immunosuppression, fever, fatigue, rash
Clofarabine (Clolar)	52 mg/m^2 intravenously daily for 5 days every 2–6 weeks (for patients < 21 years of age)	Acute: nausea, vomiting, diarrhea Delayed: myelosuppression, hepatotoxicity, nephrotoxicity, rash, capillary leak syndrome
Fludarabine (Fludara)	25 mg/m^2 intravenously for 5 days every 4 weeks	Acute: fever, nausea, vomiting Delayed: asthenia, myelosuppression, immunosuppression, neurotoxicity, anorexia
Mercaptopurine (6-MP; Purinethol)	**Induction:** 2.5–5 mg/kg/day orally **Maintenance:** 1.5–2.5 mg/kg/day orally	Acute: nausea, vomiting, diarrhea, rash Delayed: myelosuppression, immunosuppression, hepatotoxicity, mucositis
Antimetabolites—Pyrimidine Analogs		
Azacitidine (Vidaza)	75–100 mg/m^2 subcutaneously or intravenously for 7 days every 4 weeks	Acute: injection site reaction (subcutaneously), nausea, diarrhea, fever Delayed: myelosuppression, dyspnea, arthralgia

(continued)

Table 39–3. Common cancer therapeutic agents.[1] (continued)

Chemotherapeutic Agent	Usual Adult Dosage	Adverse Effects
Antimetabolites—Pyrimidine Analogs (cont.)		
Capecitabine (Xeloda)	1000–1250 mg/m² orally twice a day for 14 days every 3 weeks	Acute: nausea, vomiting, diarrhea Delayed: hand-foot syndrome, mucositis, hyperbilirubinemia, myelosuppression
Cytarabine (Ara-C, Cytosar U)	**Standard dose:** 100 mg/m²/day intravenously via continuous infusion for 7 days **High dose:** 1000–3000 mg/m² intravenously every 12 hours for 2–6 days	Acute: nausea, vomiting, rash, flu-like syndrome Delayed: myelosuppression High-dose: neurotoxicity, ocular toxicities
Decitabine (Dacogen)	15 mg/m² intravenously every 8 hours for 3 days every 8 weeks; 20 mg/m² intravenously daily for 5 days	Acute: nausea, vomiting, hyperglycemia Delayed: myelosuppression, fever, fatigue, cough
Fluorouracil (Adrucil)	400 mg/m² intravenous bolus followed by 2400 mg/m² intravenously over 46 hours every 2 weeks; 1000 mg/m² intravenously via continuous infusion for 4–5 days every 3–4 weeks; various doses	Acute: nausea, vomiting, diarrhea Delayed: myelosuppression, hand-foot syndrome, mucositis, photosensitivity, cardiotoxicity (rare)
Gemcitabine (Gemzar)	1000–1250 mg/m² intravenously on days 1 and 8 every 3 weeks or days 1, 8, 15 every 4 weeks	Acute: nausea, vomiting, rash, flu-like symptoms, fever, diarrhea Delayed: myelosuppression, edema, elevated transaminases
Antimicrotubules—Vinca Alkaloids		
Vinblastine (Velban)	6 mg/m² intravenously on days 1 and 15 every 4 weeks; various doses	Acute: constipation Delayed: myelosuppression, alopecia, bone pain, malaise
Vincristine (Oncovin)	0.5–1.4 mg/m² intravenously every 3 weeks; various doses; maximum single dose usually limited to 2 mg	Acute: constipation, nausea Delayed: peripheral neuropathy, alopecia
Vinorelbine (Navelbine)	25–30 mg/m² intravenously weekly	Acute: nausea, vomiting Delayed: myelosuppression, peripheral neuropathy, constipation, alopecia, asthenia
Antimicrotubules—Taxanes		
Cabazitaxel (Jevtana)	25 mg/m² intravenously every 3 weeks	Acute: diarrhea, nausea, vomiting, hypersensitivity Delayed: myelosuppression, peripheral neuropathy, fatigue
Docetaxel (Taxotere)	60–100 mg/m² intravenously every 3 weeks	Acute: nausea, vomiting, diarrhea, hypersensitivity, rash Delayed: myelosuppression, asthenia, peripheral neuropathy, alopecia, edema, mucositis
Paclitaxel (Taxol)	135–175 mg/m² intravenously every 3 weeks; 50–80 mg/m² intravenously weekly; various doses	Acute: diarrhea, nausea, vomiting, hypersensitivity Delayed: myelosuppression, peripheral neuropathy, alopecia, mucositis, arthralgia
Paclitaxel protein-bound (Abraxane)	100–125 mg/m² on days 1, 8, 15 every 3–4 weeks; 260 mg/m² intravenously every 3 weeks	Acute: nausea, vomiting, diarrhea Delayed: myelosuppression, peripheral neuropathy, alopecia, asthenia
Enzyme Inhibitors—Anthracyclines		
Daunorubicin (Cerubidine)	30–60 mg/m² intravenously for 3 days	Acute: nausea, vomiting, diarrhea, red/orange discoloration of urine, infusion-related reactions (liposomal products) Delayed: myelosuppression, mucositis, alopecia, hand-foot syndrome (liposomal doxorubicin), cardiotoxicity (dose related)
Doxorubicin (Adriamycin)	45–75 mg/m² intravenously every 3 weeks; various doses	
Epirubicin (Ellence)	60–120 mg/m² intravenously every 3–4 weeks	
Idarubicin (Idamycin)	10–12 mg/m² intravenously for 3 days	
Liposomal daunorubicin (Daunoxome)	40 mg/m² intravenously every 2 weeks	
Liposomal doxorubicin (Lipodox)	20–50 mg/m² intravenously every 3–4 weeks	

(continued)

Table 39–3. Common cancer therapeutic agents.[1] (continued)

Chemotherapeutic Agent	Usual Adult Dosage	Adverse Effects
Enzyme Inhibitors—Topoisomerase Inhibitors		
Etoposide (Vepesid)	50–100 mg/m^2 intravenously for 3–5 days every 3 weeks	Acute: nausea, vomiting, diarrhea, hypersensitivity, fever, hypotension Delayed: myelosuppression, alopecia, fatigue
Etoposide phosphate (Etopophos)	35–100 mg/m^2 intravenously for 3–5 days every 3–4 weeks	
Irinotecan (Camptosar)	180 mg/m^2 intravenously every other week; various doses	Acute: diarrhea, cholinergic syndrome, nausea, vomiting Delayed: myelosuppression, alopecia, asthenia
Topotecan (Hycamtin)	1.5 mg/m^2 intravenously for 5 days every 3 weeks; 2.3 mg/m^2 orally for 5 days every 3 weeks	Acute: nausea, vomiting, diarrhea Delayed: myelosuppression, alopecia, asthenia
Immunomodulatory Therapy		
Lenalidomide (Revlimid)	5–25 mg orally once daily on days 1–21 of 28-day cycle; or continuously	Acute: diarrhea, rash Delayed: myelosuppression, fatigue, venous thromboembolism, potential for birth defects
Pomalidomide (Pomalyst)	4 mg orally once daily on days 1–21 of 28-day cycle	Acute: nausea, diarrhea, dizziness Delayed: myelosuppression, fatigue, neuropathy, upper respiratory tract infections, venous thromboembolism, potential for birth defects
Thalidomide (Thalomid)	50–800 mg orally once daily	Acute: sedation, constipation, rash Delayed: edema, peripheral neuropathy, venous thromboembolism, potential for birth defects
Proteasome Inhibitors		
Bortezomib (Velcade)	1.3 mg/m^2 intravenous bolus or subcutaneously on days 1, 4, 8, 11 followed by a 10-day rest, or weekly for 4 weeks followed by 13-day rest	Acute: nausea, vomiting, diarrhea Delayed: peripheral neuropathy, fatigue, myelosuppression
Carfilzomib (Kyprolis)	20–56 mg/m^2 intravenously on days 1, 2, 8, 9, 15, 16 of a 28-day cycle or 20–70 mg/m^2 intravenously on days 1, 8, 15 of a 28-day cycle	Acute: nausea, dyspnea, diarrhea, infusion-related reaction Delayed: fatigue, myelosuppression, elevated serum creatinine
Ixazomib (Ninlaro)	4 mg orally on days 1, 8, 15 of a 28-day treatment cycle	Acute: diarrhea, constipation, nausea, vomiting Delayed: myelosuppression, peripheral neuropathy, peripheral edema, rash, hepatotoxicity (rare)
Targeted Therapy—Monoclonal Antibodies		
Ado-trastuzumab emtansine (Kadcyla)	3.6 mg/kg intravenously every 3 weeks	Acute: infusion-related reaction, nausea Delayed: fatigue, musculoskeletal pain, thrombocytopenia, cardiotoxicity, heptatotoxicity
Alemtuzumab (Campath)	3–10 mg intravenously or subcutaneously three times weekly	Acute: infusion-related reaction, nausea, vomiting, hypotension, rash Delayed: myelosuppression, immunosuppression
Atezolizumab (Tecentriq)	1200 mg intravenously every 3 weeks	Acute: infusion-related reaction Delayed: immune-mediated reactions, fatigue, decreased appetite
Bevacizumab (Avastin)	5–15 mg/kg intravenously every 2–3 weeks	Acute: infusion-related reaction Delayed: hypertension, proteinuria, wound healing complications, gastrointestinal perforation, hemorrhage
Brentuximab vedotin (Adcetris)	1.8 mg/kg intravenously every 3 weeks	Acute: infusion-related reaction, nausea, vomiting, diarrhea Delayed: myelosuppression, peripheral neuropathy, fatigue, rash, cough
Cetuximab (Erbitux)	Loading dose 400 mg/m^2 intravenously, maintenance dose 250 mg/m^2 intravenously weekly	Acute: infusion-related reaction, nausea, diarrhea Delayed: acneiform skin rash, hypomagnesemia, asthenia, paronychial inflammation, dyspnea

(continued)

Table 39–3. Common cancer therapeutic agents.[1] (continued)

Chemotherapeutic Agent	Usual Adult Dosage	Adverse Effects
Targeted Therapy—Monoclonal Antibodies (cont.)		
Daratumumab (Darzalex)	16 mg/kg intravenously weekly for weeks 1–8, every 2 weeks for weeks 9–24, and every 4 weeks from week 25 until disease progression	Acute: infusion-related reaction, nausea Delayed: myelosuppression, fatigue, upper respiratory tract infection
Elotuzumab (Empliciti)	10 mg/kg intravenously every week for the first 2 cycles and every 2 weeks thereafter	Acute: infusion-related reaction, diarrhea Delayed: fatigue, peripheral neuropathy, risk for opportunistic infections
Ipilimumab (Yervoy)	1–10 mg/kg intravenously every 3 weeks for a total of four doses	Acute: infusion-related reaction Delayed: immune-related reactions, fatigue
Nivolumab (Opdivo)	240 mg intravenously every 2 weeks or 480 mg every 4 weeks	Acute: vomiting Delayed: fatigue, musculoskeletal pain, rash, pruritus, cough, elevated transaminases
Obinutuzumab (Gazyva)	Cycle 1: 100 mg intravenously on day 1, 900 mg on day 2, 1000 mg on days 8 and 15 of a 28-day cycle; cycles 2–6: 1000 mg intravenously on day 1	Acute: infusion-related reaction, tumor lysis syndrome Delayed: myelosuppression, pyrexia, cough, musculoskeletal disorder, potential hepatitis B reactivation
Ofatumumab (Arzerra)	300 mg initial dose intravenously, followed 1 week later by 2000 mg intravenously weekly for 7 doses, followed 4 weeks later by 2000 mg intravenously every 4 weeks for four doses; or 300 mg initial dose intravenously, followed 1 week later by 1000 mg intravenously, then 1000 mg intravenously every 4 weeks	Acute: infusion-related reaction, diarrhea, nausea Delayed: neutropenia, infections, pyrexia, rash, fatigue, potential hepatitis B reactivation
Panitumumab (Vectibix)	6 mg/kg intravenously every 2 weeks	Acute: infusion-related reaction, nausea Delayed: acneiform skin rash, hypomagnesemia, asthenia, paronychia, fatigue, dyspnea
Pembrolizumab (Keytruda)	200 mg intravenously every 3 weeks	Acute: infusion-related reaction, nausea Delayed: immune-mediated reactions, fatigue, cough
Pertuzumab (Perjeta)	840 mg intravenously once followed by 420 mg intravenously every 3 weeks	Acute: infusion-related reaction, diarrhea, nausea Delayed: fatigue, alopecia, neutropenia, rash, peripheral neuropathy, cardiomyopathy
Ramucirumab (Cyramza)	8 mg/kg intravenously every 2 weeks or 10 mg/kg intravenously every 3 weeks	Acute: infusion-related reaction, hypertension, diarrhea Delayed: fatigue, neutropenia, epistaxis
Rituximab (Rituxan)	375 mg/m² intravenously weekly for 4 weeks, or every 3–4 weeks	Acute: infusion-related reaction, tumor lysis syndrome Delayed: lymphopenia, asthenia, rash, potential hepatitis B reactivation
Trastuzumab (Herceptin)	Initial dose 4 mg/kg intravenously, then 2 mg/kg intravenously weekly; or initial dose 8 mg/kg then 6 mg/kg, intravenously every 3 weeks	Acute: headache, nausea, diarrhea, infusion-related reaction Delayed: myelosuppression, pyrexia, cardiomyopathy, pulmonary toxicity (rare)
Targeted Therapy—Kinase Inhibitors		
Afatinib (Gilotrif)	40 mg orally once daily without food	Acute: diarrhea Delayed: acneiform rash, stomatitis, paronychia
Alectinib (Alecensa)	600 mg orally twice daily with food	Acute: none Delayed: myelosuppression, fatigue, edema, myalgia, dyspnea, elevated transaminases
Axitinib (Inlyta)	5–10 mg orally twice daily	Acute: diarrhea, nausea, vomiting Delayed: hypertension, fatigue, dysphonia, hand-foot syndrome, elevated transaminases
Bosutinib (Bosulif)	500–600 mg orally once daily with food	Acute: diarrhea, nausea, vomiting Delayed: myelosuppression, rash, abdominal pain, hepatotoxicity, fluid retention

(continued)

Table 39–3. Common cancer therapeutic agents.[1] (continued)

Chemotherapeutic Agent	Usual Adult Dosage	Adverse Effects
Targeted Therapy—Kinase Inhibitors (cont.)		
Ceritinib (Zykadia)	740 mg orally once daily	Acute: diarrhea, nausea, vomiting Delayed: elevated transaminases, abdominal pain, fatigue, decreased appetite
Cobimetinib (Cotellic)	60 mg orally once daily on days 1 to 21 of a 28-day cycle	Acute: diarrhea, photosensitivity reaction, nausea, vomiting Delayed: myelosuppression, hepatotoxicity, rash, cardiomyopathy (with vemurafenib)
Crizotinib (Xalkori)	250 mg orally twice daily	Acute: nausea, vomiting, diarrhea, constipation Delayed: vision disorder, edema, elevated transaminases, fatigue
Dabrafenib (Tafinlar)	150 mg orally twice daily without food	Acute: headache Delayed: hyperkeratosis, fever, hand-foot syndrome, hyperglycemia, hypophosphatemia
Dacomitinib (Vizimpro)	45 mg orally once daily	Acute: diarrhea Delayed: rash, paronychia, mucositis, cough, interstitial lung disease
Dasatinib (Sprycel)	100–180 mg orally once daily	Acute: diarrhea, nausea, vomiting Delayed: myelosuppression, fluid retention, fatigue, dyspnea, musculoskeletal pain, rash
Duvelisib (Copiktra)	25 mg orally twice daily	Acute: diarrhea Delayed: neutropenia, rash, cough (pneumonitis), upper respiratory infection, elevated transaminases
Erlotinib (Tarceva)	100 or 150 mg orally once daily without food	Acute: diarrhea, nausea, vomiting Delayed: acneiform skin rash, fatigue, anorexia, dyspnea
Everolimus (Afinitor)	10 mg orally once daily	Acute: mucositis, diarrhea, nausea Delayed: myelosuppression, fatigue, edema, hypercholesterolemia, hypertriglyceridemia, hyperglycemia
Gefitinib (Iressa)	250 mg orally once daily	Acute: diarrhea Delayed: acneiform skin rash
Ibrutinib (Imbruvica)	420 or 560 mg orally once daily	Acute: diarrhea, nausea Delayed: myelosuppression, fatigue, edema, rash, elevated serum creatinine, hemorrhage
Idelalisib (Zydelig)	150 mg orally twice daily	Acute: diarrhea, nausea Delayed: hepatotoxicity, pneumonitis, intestinal perforation, pyrexia, fatigue, neutropenia, hypertriglyceridemia, hyperglycemia
Imatinib (Gleevec)	100–800 mg orally once daily with food	Acute: nausea, vomiting, diarrhea Delayed: edema, muscle cramps, rash, myelosuppression, hepatotoxicity
Lapatinib (Tykerb)	1250 or 1500 mg orally once daily	Acute: diarrhea, nausea, vomiting Delayed: hand-foot syndrome, fatigue, hepatotoxicity (rare)
Lenvatinib (Lenvima)	24 mg orally daily	Acute: hypertension, nausea, vomiting, diarrhea Delayed: fatigue, arthralgia/myalgia, stomatitis, hand-foot syndrome
Nilotinib (Tasigna)	300 or 400 mg orally twice daily without food	Acute: nausea, vomiting, diarrhea Delayed: rash, fatigue, myelosuppression, prolonged QT interval (rare)
Osimertinib (Tagrisso)	80 mg orally once daily	Acute: diarrhea Delayed: myelosuppression, rash, dry skin, nail toxicity, cardiomyopathy (rare), QTc interval prolongation (rare)

(continued)

Table 39–3. Common cancer therapeutic agents.[1] (continued)

Chemotherapeutic Agent	Usual Adult Dosage	Adverse Effects
Targeted Therapy—Kinase Inhibitors (cont.)		
Palbociclib (Ibrance)	125 mg orally daily with food for 21 days followed by 7 days off	Acute: nausea, diarrhea, vomiting Delayed: myelosuppression, fatigue, upper respiratory infection, stomatitis, alopecia
Pazopanib (Votrient)	800 mg orally once daily without food	Acute: diarrhea, nausea, vomiting Delayed: hypertension, hair color changes, hepatotoxicity, hemorrhage
Regorafenib (Stivarga)	160 mg orally once daily with food (low-fat breakfast)	Acute: diarrhea Delayed: asthenia, hand-foot syndrome, anorexia, hypertension, mucositis, myelosuppression, hepatotoxicity
Sorafenib (Nexavar)	400 mg orally twice daily without food	Acute: diarrhea and nausea Delayed: fatigue, hand-foot syndrome, rash, hypertension, hemorrhage
Sunitinib (Sutent)	50 mg orally once daily for 4 weeks followed by 2 weeks rest; 37.5 mg orally daily	Acute: diarrhea and nausea Delayed: hypertension, hand-foot syndrome, rash, yellow discoloration of skin, fatigue, hypothyroidism, mucositis, left ventricular dysfunction, bleeding, hepatotoxicity
Temsirolimus (Torisel)	25 mg intravenously weekly	Acute: hypersensitivity, rash Delayed: myelosuppression, asthenia, hyperglycemia, hyperlipidemia, elevated serum creatinine
Trametinib (Mekinist)	2 mg orally once daily without food	Acute: rash, diarrhea Delayed: elevated transaminases, lymphedema, cardiomyopathy
Vemurafenib (Zelboraf)	960 mg orally twice daily	Acute: nausea, hypersensitivity (rare) Delayed: photosensitivity, rash, arthralgia, alopecia, fatigue, prolonged QT interval, cutaneous squamous cell carcinoma
Miscellaneous Agents		
Arsenic trioxide (Trisenox)	0.15 mg/kg intravenously daily	Acute: nausea, dizziness Delayed: acute promyelocytic leukemia differentiation syndrome, prolonged QT interval
Asparaginase *Erwinia chrysanthemi* (Erwinaze)	25,000 international units/m² intramuscularly three times weekly	Acute: hypersensitivity, nausea, vomiting Delayed: coagulation abnormalities, hepatotoxicity, pancreatitis, neurotoxicity
Bleomycin (Blenoxane)	10 units/m² intravenously on days 1 and 15 every 28 days; 30 units intravenously on days 2, 9, and 16 every 21 days	Acute: hypersensitivity, fever Delayed: skin reaction (rash, hyperpigmentation of skin, striae), mucositis, pneumonitis
Dactinomycin (Cosmegen)	15 mcg/kg or 400–600 mcg/m² intravenously daily for 5 days	Acute: nausea, vomiting Delayed: myelosuppression, mucositis, rash, diarrhea, hepatoveno-occlusive disease (rare)
Hydroxyurea (Hydrea)	20–30 mg/kg orally daily	Acute: none Delayed: myelosuppression
Mitomycin (Mutamycin)	10–20 mg/m² intravenously every 4–8 weeks; 20–40 mg intravesically	Acute: cystitis (intravesically), nausea, vomiting Delayed: myelosuppression, mucositis, anorexia
Mitoxantrone (Novantrone)	12–14 mg/m² intravenously every 3 weeks; 12 mg/m² intravenously for 2–3 days	Acute: nausea, vomiting, diarrhea, mucositis, blue-green discoloration of urine Delayed: myelosuppression, alopecia, cardiotoxicity
Omacetaxine mepe-succinate (Synribo)	Induction: 1.25 mg/m² subcutaneously twice daily for 14 days every 28 days Maintenance: 1.25 mg/m² subcutaneously twice daily for 7 days every 28 days	Acute: diarrhea, nausea, fatigue, injection site reaction Delayed: myelosuppression, infection

(continued)

Table 39–3. Common cancer therapeutic agents.[1] (continued)

Chemotherapeutic Agent	Usual Adult Dosage	Adverse Effects
Miscellaneous Agents (cont.)		
Panobinostat (Farydak)	20 mg orally per day on days 1, 3, 5, 8, 10, 12 of each 21-day cycle	Acute: diarrhea, nausea Delayed: myelosuppression, electrolyte abnormalities, infections
Tretinoin (All-Trans-Retinoic Acid, ATRA, Vesanoid)	45 mg/m² orally divided twice daily for 45–90 days or 30 days past complete remission	Acute: headache, nausea Delayed: vitamin A toxicity, retinoic acid-acute promyelocytic leukemia syndrome
Trifluridine/tipiracil (Lonsurf)	35 mg/m² based on trifluridine component orally twice daily within 1 hour of meal on days 1–5 and 8–12 (28-day cycle)	Acute: nausea, diarrhea, vomiting Delayed: myelosuppression, fatigue, anorexia
Venetoclax (Venclexta)	20 mg orally daily during week 1; 50 mg daily during week 2; 100 mg daily during week 3; 200 mg daily during week 4; then 400 mg orally daily thereafter	Acute: diarrhea, nausea, vomiting, tumor lysis syndrome Delayed: myelosuppression, upper respiratory infections, fatigue
Ziv-aflibercept (Zaltrap)	4 mg/kg intravenously every 2 weeks	Acute: diarrhea Delayed: myelosuppression, proteinuria, elevated transaminases, stomatitis, fatigue, hypertension
Antiandrogens		
Bicalutamide (Casodex)	50 mg orally once daily	Acute: none Delayed: hot flashes, back pain, asthenia
Apalutamide (Erleada)	240 mg orally daily	Acute: fatigue, diarrhea Delayed: arthralgia, hot flashes, falls, peripheral edema, seizure (rare)
Enzalutamide (Xtandi)	160 mg orally once daily	Acute: asthenia, diarrhea Delayed: hot flashes, arthralgia, peripheral edema, seizure (rare)
Flutamide (Eulexin)	250 mg orally every 8 hours	Acute: diarrhea Delayed: hot flashes, hepatotoxicity
Nilutamide (Nilandron)	300 mg orally for 30 days, then 150 mg orally once daily	Acute: none Delayed: visual disturbances (impaired adaptation to dark), hot flashes, disulfiram-like reaction
Selective Estrogen Receptor Modulators		
Tamoxifen (Nolvadex)	20–40 mg orally once daily	Acute: none Delayed: hot flashes, vaginal discharge, menstrual irregularities, arthralgia
Toremifene (Fareston)	60 mg orally once daily	Acute: nausea Delayed: hot flashes, vaginal discharge
Aromatase Inhibitors		
Anastrozole (Arimidex)	1 mg orally once daily	Acute: nausea Delayed: hot flashes, peripheral edema, asthenia, hypercholesterolemia, arthralgia/myalgia, osteoporosis
Exemestane (Aromasin)	25 mg orally once daily	
Letrozole (Femara)	2.5 mg orally once daily	
Pure Estrogen Receptor Antagonist		
Fulvestrant (Faslodex)	500 mg intramuscularly on days 1, 15, 29, then monthly	Acute: injection site reaction, nausea Delayed: hot flashes, bone pain, elevated transaminases

(continued)

Table 39–3. Common cancer therapeutic agents.[1] (continued)

Chemotherapeutic Agent	Usual Adult Dosage	Adverse Effects
LHRH Analogs		
Goserelin acetate (Zoladex)	3.6 mg subcutaneously every month; 10.8 mg subcutaneously every 3 months	Acute: injection site discomfort Delayed: hot flashes, tumor flare, edema, decreased libido, erectile dysfunction, osteoporosis
Leuprolide (Lupron)	7.5 mg intramuscularly or subcutaneously every month; 22.5 mg intramuscularly or subcutaneously every 3 months; 30 mg intramuscularly or subcutaneously every 4 months; 45 mg intramuscularly or subcutaneously every 6 months	
Triptorelin pamoate (Trelstar)	3.75 mg intramuscularly every 4 weeks; 11.25 mg intramuscularly every 12 weeks; 22.5 mg every 24 weeks	
LHRH Antagonist		
Degarelix (Firmagon)	240 mg subcutaneously once, then 80 mg subcutaneously every 28 days	Acute: injection site reaction Delayed: hot flashes, weight gain, elevated transaminases, QT prolongation
Adrenocorticosteroid		
Abiraterone (Zytiga)	1000 mg orally once daily	Acute: diarrhea, edema Delayed: adrenal insufficiency, hepatotoxicity, joint pain, hypokalemia
PARP Inhibitor		
Olaparib (Lynparza)	400 mg orally twice daily	Acute: nausea, vomiting, diarrhea Delayed: myelosuppression, elevated serum creatinine, MCV elevation, fatigue, abdominal pain
Biologic Response Modifiers		
Aldesleukin (IL-2, Proleukin)	600,000 international units/kg intravenously every 8 hours for 14 doses, repeat after 9 days rest	Acute: hypotension, nausea, vomiting, diarrhea, flu-like syndrome, capillary leak syndrome Delayed: myelosuppression, confusion, somnolence, oliguria
Interferon-alpha-2b (Intron A)	20 million international units/m^2 intravenously 5 days a week for 4 weeks, then 10 million international units/m^2 subcutaneously three times a week for 48 weeks	Acute: flu-like syndrome, nausea, vomiting, diarrhea Delayed: myelosuppression, anorexia, alopecia, depression, elevated transaminases
Sipuleucel-T (Provenge)	One dose (minimum of 50 million autologous CD54 cells) intravenously every 2 weeks for three doses	Acute: infusion-related reaction, nausea, vomiting Delayed: fatigue, back pain, arthralgia
Tisagenlecleucel (Kymriah)	One dose 0.6 to 6.0×10^8 CAR-positive viable T cells intravenously	Acute: hypersensitivity reaction, cytokine release syndrome Delayed: neurotoxicity, infections, myelosuppression, hypogammaglobulinemia

[1]For abemaciclib, acalabrutinib, altretamine, avelumab, belinostat, binimetinib, blinatumomab, brigatinib, cemiplimab-rwlc, copanlisib, denileukin diftitox, enasidenib, encorafenib, gemtuzumab ozogamicin, glasdegib, ibritumomab, inotuzumab ozogamicin, irinotecan liposome, ivosidenib, ixabepilone, ketoconazole, liposomal vincristine, lomustine, lorlatinib, mechlorethamine, midostaurin, mogamulizumab-kpkc, moxetumomab pasudotox-tdfk, niraparib, olaratumab, pentostatin, pralatrexate, ribociclib, romidepsin, rucaparib, siltuximab, talazoparib, vandetanib, and vismodegib, see Table 39–3 in *CMDT Online* at www.accessmedicine.com.

AV, atrioventricular; GFR, glomerular filtration rate; LHRH, luteinizing hormone–releasing hormone; MAO, monoamine oxidase; MCV, mean corpuscular volume; PARP, poly ADP ribose polymerase.

TYPES OF CANCER

LUNG CANCER

Sunny Wang, MD

BRONCHOGENIC CARCINOMA

ESSENTIALS OF DIAGNOSIS

▶ New cough or change in chronic cough.

▶ Dyspnea, hemoptysis, anorexia, weight loss.

▶ Enlarging nodule or mass; persistent opacity, atelectasis, or pleural effusion on chest radiograph or CT scan.

▶ Cytologic or histologic findings of lung cancer in sputum, pleural fluid, or biopsy specimen.

General Considerations

Lung cancer is the leading cause of cancer deaths in both men and women. The American Cancer Society estimates 234,030 new diagnoses and 154,050 deaths from lung cancer in the United States in 2018, accounting for approximately 13% of new cancer diagnoses and 25% of all cancer deaths.

Cigarette smoking causes 85–90% of cases of lung cancer. The causal connection between cigarettes and lung cancer is established not only epidemiologically but also through identification of carcinogens in tobacco smoke and analysis of the effect of these carcinogens on specific oncogenes expressed in lung cancer.

Other environmental risk factors for the development of lung cancer include exposure to environmental tobacco smoke, radon, asbestos, diesel exhaust, ionizing radiation, metals (arsenic, chromium, nickel, iron oxide), and industrial carcinogens. A familial predisposition to lung cancer is recognized. Certain diseases are associated with an increased risk of lung cancer, including pulmonary fibrosis, chronic obstructive pulmonary disease, and sarcoidosis.

The median age at diagnosis of lung cancer in the United States is 70; it is unusual under the age of 40. The combined relative 5-year survival rate for all stages of lung cancer is currently 19%.

There are five main histologic categories of bronchogenic carcinoma. **Squamous cell carcinomas** (23% of cases, based on US SEER data 2011–2015) arise from the bronchial epithelium and often present as intraluminal masses. They are usually centrally located and can present with hemoptysis. Squamous cell carcinomas stain for P63 and P40 on immunohistochemistry. **Adenocarcinomas** (48% of cases) arise from mucous glands or from any epithelial cell within or distal to the terminal bronchioles. They usually present as peripheral nodules or masses and stain for TTF-1 and Napsin-A on immunohistochemistry. **Adenocarcinomas in situ** (formerly **bronchioloalveolar cell carcinomas**) spread along preexisting alveolar structures (lepidic growth) without evidence of invasion. **Large cell carcinomas** (1.5% of cases) are a heterogeneous group of undifferentiated cancers that share large cells and do not fit into other categories. Large cell carcinomas are typically aggressive and have rapid doubling times. They present as central or peripheral masses. Cancers that are not better differentiated on pathologic review other than non–small cell carcinomas (NSCLC) or carcinomas not otherwise specified make up about 14% of cases. **Small cell carcinomas** (13% of cases) are tumors of bronchial origin that typically begin centrally, infiltrating submucosally to cause narrowing of the bronchus without a discrete luminal mass. They are aggressive cancers that often involve regional or distant metastasis on presentation.

For purposes of staging and treatment, bronchogenic carcinomas are divided into small cell lung cancer (SCLC) and the other four types, labeled NSCLC.

Clinical Findings

Lung cancer is symptomatic at diagnosis in a majority of patients. The clinical presentation depends on the type and location of the primary tumor, the extent of local spread, and the presence of distant metastases and any paraneoplastic syndromes.

A. Symptoms and Signs

Anorexia, weight loss, or asthenia occurs in 55–90% of patients presenting with a new diagnosis of lung cancer. Up to 60% of patients have a new cough or a change in a chronic cough; 6–31% have hemoptysis; and 25–40% complain of pain, either nonspecific chest pain or pain from bony metastases to the vertebrae, ribs, or pelvis. Local spread may cause endobronchial obstruction with atelectasis and postobstructive pneumonia, pleural effusion (12–33%), change in voice (compromise of the recurrent laryngeal nerve), superior vena cava syndrome (obstruction of the superior vena cava with supraclavicular venous engorgement), and Horner syndrome (ipsilateral ptosis, miosis, and anhidrosis from involvement of the inferior cervical ganglion and the paravertebral sympathetic chain). Distant metastases to the liver are associated with asthenia and weight loss. Brain metastases (10% in NSCLC, more common in adenocarcinoma, and 20–30% in SCLC) may present with headache, nausea, vomiting, seizures, dizziness, or altered mental status.

Paraneoplastic syndromes are patterns of organ dysfunction related to immune-mediated or secretory effects of neoplasms. These syndromes occur in 10–20% of lung cancer patients. They may precede, accompany, or follow the diagnosis of lung cancer. In patients with small cell carcinoma, the syndrome of inappropriate antidiuretic hormone (SIADH) can develop in 10–15%; in those with squamous cell carcinoma, hypercalcemia can develop in 10%. Digital clubbing is seen in up to 20% of patients at diagnosis (see Figure 6–41). Other common paraneoplastic syndromes include increased ACTH production, anemia, hypercoagulability, peripheral neuropathy, and the Lambert-Eaton myasthenic syndrome. Their recognition is important because treatment of the primary tumor may improve or resolve symptoms even when the cancer is not curable.

B. Laboratory Findings

The diagnosis of lung cancer rests on examination of a tissue or cytology specimen. **Sputum cytology** is highly specific but insensitive; the yield is highest when there are lesions in the central airways. While the diagnostic yield of **CT-guided biopsy** of peripheral nodules approaches 80–90%, the rates of pneumothorax are significant (15–30%), especially in those with emphysema. **Thoracentesis** (sensitivity 50–65%) can be used to establish a diagnosis of lung cancer in patients with malignant pleural effusions. Fine-needle aspiration (FNA) of palpable supraclavicular or cervical lymph nodes is frequently diagnostic.

Fiberoptic bronchoscopy allows visualization of the major airways, cytology brushing of visible lesions or lavage of lung segments with cytologic evaluation of specimens, direct biopsy of endobronchial abnormalities, blind transbronchial biopsy of the pulmonary parenchyma or peripheral nodules, and FNA biopsy of mediastinal lymph nodes. The use of fluorescence bronchoscopy improves the ability to identify early endobronchial lesions, and endobronchial and transesophageal endoscopic ultrasound enhance the direction and yield of FNA of mediastinal nodes. Electromagnetic navigational bronchoscopy allows bronchoscopic approaches to small peripheral nodules.

C. Imaging

Nearly all patients with lung cancer have abnormal findings on chest radiography or CT scan (Figure 39–1). These findings are rarely specific for a particular diagnosis. Interpretation of characteristic findings in isolated nodules is described in Chapter 9.

D. Special Examinations

1. Staging—Accurate staging is crucial (1) to provide the clinician with information to guide treatment, (2) to provide the patient with accurate information regarding prognosis, and (3) to standardize entry criteria for clinical trials to allow interpretation of results.

There are two essential principles of staging **NSCLC.** First, the more extensive the disease, the worse the prognosis; second, surgical resection offers the best chance for cure. Staging of NSCLC uses two integrated systems and is continuously updated. The eighth edition of the **AJCC/ Union for International Cancer Control (UICC) stage classification** for lung cancer became effective in January 2017. The **TNM international staging system** attempts a physical description of the neoplasm: T describes the size and location of the primary tumor; N describes the presence and location of nodal metastases; and M refers to the presence or absence of distant metastases. These TNM stages are grouped into summary stages I–IV, and these are used to guide therapy. Many patients with stage I and stage II disease are cured through surgery. Patients with stage IIIB and stage IV disease do not benefit from surgery

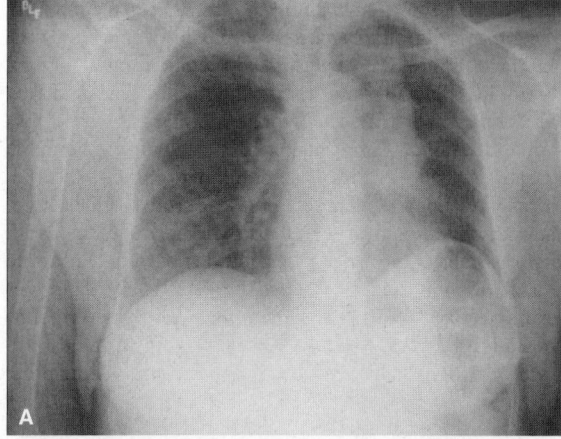

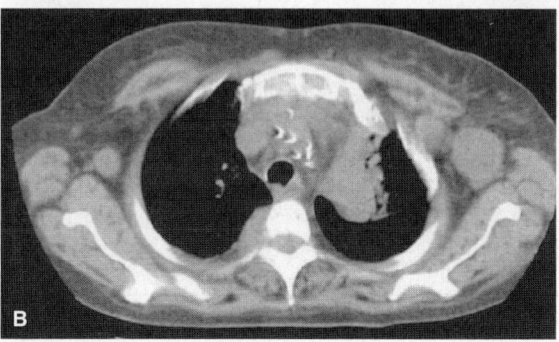

▲ **Figure 39–1.** Squamous cell carcinoma of the left lung on chest radiograph (A) and CT scan (B). (Used, with permission, from David A. Kasper, DO, MBA in Usatine RP, Smith MA, Mayeaux EJ Jr, Chumley H. *The Color Atlas of Family Medicine,* 2nd ed. McGraw-Hill, 2013.)

(Table 39–4). Patients with stage IIIA disease have locally invasive disease that may benefit from surgery in selected cases as part of multimodality therapy.

SCLC is traditionally divided into two categories: **limited disease** (30%), when the tumor is limited to the unilateral hemithorax (including contralateral mediastinal nodes); or **extensive disease** (70%), when the tumor extends beyond the hemithorax (including pleural effusion). It is also recommended to stage SCLC according to the TNM staging system.

For both SCLC and NSCLC, staging begins with a thorough history and physical examination. A complete examination is essential to exclude obvious metastatic disease to lymph nodes, skin, and bone. A detailed history is essential because the patient's performance status is a powerful predictor of disease course. All patients should have measurement of a complete blood count (CBC), serum electrolytes, calcium, creatinine, liver biochemical tests, lactate dehydrogenase, and albumin.

NSCLC patients being considered for surgery require meticulous evaluation to identify those with resectable disease. CT imaging is key for staging candidates for resection. The sensitivity and specificity of CT imaging for identifying lung cancer metastatic to the mediastinal

Table 39–4. Five-year survival rates for non–small cell lung cancer, based on TNM staging.

Stage	TNM Subset	5-Year Survival for Clinical TNM	5-Year Survival for Pathologic TNM
0	Carcinoma in situ		
1A1	T1aN0M0	92%	90%
1A2	T1bN0M0	83%	85%
IA3	T1cN0M0	77%	80%
IB	T2aN0M0	68%	73%
IIA	T2bN0M0	60%	65%
IIB	T1/T2, N1M0 T3N0M0	53%	56%
IIIA	T1/T2, N2M0 T3N1M0 T4, N0/N1, M0	36%	41%
IIIB	T1/T2, N3M0 T3/T4, N2M0	26%	24%
IIIC	T3/T4, N3M0	13%	12%
IVA	Any T, Any N, M1a/M1b	10%	—
IVB	Any T, Any N, M1c	0%	—

Data from multiple sources. Modified and reproduced, with permission, from Detterbeck FC et al. The Eighth Edition Lung Cancer Stage Classification. Chest. 2017;151(1):193–203. Copyright © Elsevier; and data from Goldstraw P et al. The IASLC Lung Cancer Staging Project: proposals for revision of the TNM stage groupings in the forthcoming (eighth) edition of the TNM classification for lung cancer. J Thorac Oncol. 2015 Sept;11(1):39–51.

lymph nodes are 57% (49–66%) and 82% (77–86%), respectively. Therefore, chest CT imaging alone does not provide definitive staging information. CT imaging helps determine where to biopsy, and how the mediastinum should be sampled.

Positron emission tomography (PET) using 2-[^{18}F] fluoro-2-deoxyglucose (FDG) is an important modality for identifying metastatic foci in the mediastinum or distant sites. The sensitivity and specificity of PET for detecting mediastinal spread of primary lung cancer depend on the size of mediastinal nodes or masses. When mediastinal lymph nodes smaller than 1 cm are present, the sensitivity and specificity of PET for tumor involvement of nodes are 74% and 96%, respectively. When CT shows lymph nodes larger than 1 cm, the sensitivity and specificity are 95% and 76%, respectively.

The combination of PET and CT imaging has improved preoperative staging compared with CT or PET alone. Whole body fusion PET-CT imaging is most useful to confirm lack of regional or metastatic disease in NSCLC patients who are candidates for surgical resection.

Disadvantages of PET imaging include limited resolution below 1 cm and false-positive scans due to sarcoidosis, tuberculosis, or fungal infections. PET-CT scans are also inadequate for evaluating brain metastases due to normal physiologic FDG uptake in the brain. Obtaining an MRI of the brain is important to rule out brain metastases in patients with SCLC and in patients with NSCLC with at least stage II disease or poorly differentiated histologies.

2. Preoperative assessment—See Chapter 3.

3. Pulmonary function testing—Many patients with NSCLC have moderate to severe chronic lung disease that increases the risk of perioperative complications as well as long-term pulmonary insufficiency following lung resection. All patients considered for surgery require spirometry. In the absence of other comorbidities, patients with good lung function (preoperative FEV_1 2 L or more) are at low risk for complications from lobectomy or pneumonectomy. High-risk patients include those with a predicted postoperative FEV_1 less than 700 mL (or less than 40% of predicted FEV_1).

4. Screening—Screening with low-dose helical CT scans has been shown to improve mortality rates for lung cancer. The National Lung Screening Trial, a multicenter randomized US trial involving over 53,000 current and former heavy smokers, showed that screening annually with low-dose helical CT for 3 years yielded a 20% relative reduction in lung cancer mortality and 6.7% reduction in all-cause mortality compared to chest radiography. Given these findings, US professional organizations, including the US Preventive Services Task Force (USPSTF), have recommended screening with low-dose helical CT for lung cancer. Smoking cessation policies and efforts should be integrated with any screening program.

▶ **Treatment**

A. Non–Small Cell Lung Carcinoma

Surgical resection offers the best chance for cure of NSCLC. Therefore, the initial approach to the patient is determined by answering two questions: (1) Is complete surgical resection technically feasible? (2) If yes, is the patient able to tolerate the surgery with acceptable morbidity and mortality? Clinical features that preclude complete resection include extrathoracic metastases or a malignant pleural effusion; or tumor involving the heart, pericardium, great vessels, esophagus, recurrent laryngeal or phrenic nerves, trachea, main carina, or contralateral mediastinal lymph nodes. Accordingly, stage I and stage II patients are treated with surgical resection where possible. Stage II and select cases of stage IB are additionally recommended to receive adjuvant chemotherapy. Stage IIIA patients have poor outcomes if treated with resection alone. They should undergo multimodality treatment that includes chemotherapy or radiotherapy, or both. Inoperable stage IIIA and stage IIIB patients treated with concurrent chemotherapy and radiation therapy have improved survival. Stage IV patients are treated with systemic therapy (targeted therapy, chemotherapy, or immunotherapy) or symptom-based palliative therapy, or both.

Surgical approach affects outcome. In 1994, the North American Lung Cancer Study Group conducted a prospective trial of stage IA patients randomized to lobectomy versus limited resection. They reported a threefold increased rate of local recurrence in the limited resection group ($P = 0.008$) and a trend toward an increase in overall death rate (increase of 30%, $P = 0.08$) and increase in cancer-related death rate (increase of 50%, $P = 0.09$), compared with patients receiving lobectomy. However, for patients who cannot tolerate lobectomy, a sublobar resection (wedge resection or segmentectomy) may be considered.

Patients with clinical stage I primary NSCLC, who are not candidates for surgery because of significant comorbidity or other surgical contraindication, are candidates for stereotactic body radiotherapy. Stereotactic body radiotherapy, which is composed of multiple non-parallel radiation beams that converge, allows the delivery of a relatively large dose of radiation to a small, well-defined target. For clinical stage I NSCLC, 3-year local control rates with stereotactic body radiotherapy exceed 90%, and large meta-analyses of nonrandomized data have shown 2-year survival at 70% and 5-year survival at 40%. Patients with locally advanced disease (stages IIIA and IIIB) who are not surgical candidates have improved survival when treated with concurrent chemotherapy and radiation therapy compared with no therapy, radiation alone, or even sequential chemotherapy and radiation.

Neoadjuvant chemotherapy consists of giving antineoplastic drugs in advance of surgery or radiation therapy. Neoadjuvant therapy is more widely used in selected patients with stage IIIA or select stage IIIB disease. Some studies suggest a survival advantage.

Adjuvant chemotherapy consists of administering antineoplastic drugs following surgery or radiation therapy. Cisplatin-containing regimens have been shown to confer an overall survival benefit in at least stage II disease and a subset of stage IB disease where primary tumor size exceeds 4 cm. The Lung Adjuvant Cisplatin Evaluation Collaborative Group, a meta-analysis of the five largest cisplatin-based adjuvant trials, reported a 5% absolute benefit in 5-year overall survival with a cisplatin-containing doublet regimen following surgery ($P = 0.005$) in patients with at least stage II disease.

For stage IIIB and stage IV NSCLC, options for therapy include targeted therapy (Table 39–3), cytotoxic chemotherapy, and immunotherapy (checkpoint inhibitors) (Table 39–2). The approach to therapy is individualized based on molecular profiling and PD-L1 testing. Molecular profiling is offered as next-generation sequencing multigene assays. The key driver mutations in lung cancer currently include *EGFR, ALK, BRAF,* and *ROS1*, but only a minority of all lung cancer cases harbor these mutations. *K-ras* mutation is more commonly found among smokers but has not been targeted effectively. Difficulties in testing may arise when only small fine-needle aspirate biopsies are obtained; to have sufficient tissue for analysis, it is recommended that clinicians obtain core biopsies. PD-L1 expression is a flawed but currently actively used biomarker to assess possible response to checkpoint inhibitor therapy (specifically, programmed death-1 [PD-1] inhibitors).

Targeted therapy has played a pivotal role in advanced NSCLC (Tables 39–2 and 39–3). Activating *EGFR* mutations are found in approximately 10–20% of the white population and 30–48% in the Asian population and are usually found among nonsmokers to light smokers, females, and persons with nonsquamous histologies (particularly adenocarcinomas). For patients with *EGFR* mutations, an EGFR tyrosine kinase inhibitor (osimertinib, erlotinib, gefitinib, or afatinib) rather than platinum-based chemotherapy is the first-line treatment. Response rates with EGFR tyrosine kinase inhibitors in patients with *EGFR* mutation are at least 70%, and median overall survival is estimated to be 21–33 months. Recent phase III data show that osimertinib (third-generation irreversible EGFR tyrosine kinase inhibitor) leads to a longer duration of response, longer progression-free survival, and lower rates of severe adverse events compared to earlier generation EGFR tyrosine kinase inhibitors. Osimertinib is FDA approved as first-line treatment of *EGFR*-mutated lung cancers. Eventual resistance to therapy still develops for patients taking osimertinib, and options for second-line therapy include platinum-based chemotherapy or chemoimmunotherapy.

Approximately 5% of all patients with NSCLC carry translocations of *ALK* resulting in novel fusion gene products with oncogenic activity. This is usually found in a comparatively younger population, with adenocarcinoma histology, and nonsmoking to light-smoking history. In a phase III trial of *ALK*-rearranged lung cancer patients, crizotinib (an ALK, cMET and ROS1 tyrosine kinase inhibitor) showed a response rate over 70% compared with a rate of 45% among those treated with standard first-line chemotherapy, and an improvement in median progression-free survival of 10.9 vs 7 months, respectively. At 1 year, however, resistance develops in most patients taking crizotinib. Second-generation ALK inhibitors (ceritinib, alectinib, and brigatinib) are recommended for *ALK*-rearranged lung cancers resistant to crizotinib. Recent randomized trials have shown that alectinib compared to crizotinib in first-line treatment of *ALK*-rearranged lung cancers has superior response rates (83% vs 75%), longer progression-free survival, and longer time to CNS progression. Alectinib is now the recommended first-line agent in *ALK*-rearranged lung cancers.

Approximately 1–2% of NSCLC harbor *ROS1* rearrangements and are usually found among nonsmokers or light smokers with lung adenocarcinomas. *ROS1* rearranged lung cancers also respond to crizotinib with response rates over 70%. *BRAF* mutations have been found in 2% of NSCLC patients and often in smokers. The combination of dabrafenib (BRAF inhibitor) and trametinib (MEK inhibitor) has shown response rates of over 60% in patients with *BRAF V600E* mutations. Finally, *K-ras* mutations are found among 25% of patients with adenocarcinomas, are associated with smoking, and indicate a poor prognosis. Unfortunately, there is still no effective targeted approach to therapy for *K-ras* mutated lung cancers.

Immune checkpoint inhibition with PD-1 or PD-L1 inhibitors (nivolumab, pembrolizumab, atezolizumab, and durvalumab) are playing highly important roles in the treatment of NSCLC (Tables 39–2 and 39–3). Checkpoint inhibitors release T cells from the inhibitory signals they receive from tumor cells via the PD-1 pathway, restoring antitumor immunity. For patients with tumors staining greater than 50% for PDL-1, pembrolizumab outperforms first-line platinum-based chemotherapy, with response rates of 45% vs 28% and median progression-free survival of 10 months vs 6 months. Recent phase III trials have shown improved survival outcomes with adding pembrolizumab to platinum-doublet chemotherapy as first-line therapy of patients with advanced NSCLC regardless of PD-L1 status. If patients received chemotherapy alone as first-line treatment, PD-1 inhibitors are recommended as second-line treatment of NSCLC, regardless of PDL-1 staining intensity. This treatment strategy yields an approximately 20% response rate, a durable response, and superior overall and progression-free survival rates compared to standard second-line chemotherapy. However, significant side effects and toxicity have been reported with PD-1 inhibitors, especially autoimmune manifestations such as hepatitis, thyroiditis, hypophysitis, colitis, pneumonitis, and type 1 diabetes mellitus. Recently, a randomized phase III trial has shown improved survival outcomes by adding durvalumab as consolidation therapy post-definitive chemoradiation for stage III NSCLCs.

If no targetable mutations are found and there is inadequate PD-L1 expression on tumor cells, patients are either offered combination immunotherapy with cytotoxic chemotherapy or cytotoxic chemotherapy alone (Table 39–2). Although not curative, chemotherapy has been shown in multiple clinical trials to provide a modest increase in overall survival in patients with stage IIIB and stage IV NSCLC compared with supportive care alone, with the median survival increased from 5 months to a range of 8–12 months and 1-year survival rate to 30–40%. Palliative chemotherapy also leads to improved quality of life and symptom control, with first-line therapy involving a platinum-based regimen.

B. Small Cell Lung Carcinoma

Response rates of SCLC to cisplatin and etoposide (Table 39–2) are excellent with 80–90% response in limited-stage disease (50–60% complete response), and 60–80% response in extensive-stage disease (15–20% complete response). However, remissions tend to be short-lived with a median duration of 6–8 months. Once the disease has recurred, median survival is 3–4 months. Overall 2-year survival is 20–40% in limited-stage disease and 5% in extensive-stage disease (Table 39–5). Modest improvement

Table 39–5. Median survival for small cell lung carcinoma following treatment.

Stage	Mean 2-Year Survival	Median Survival
Limited	20–40%	15–20 months
Extensive	5%	8–13 months

Data from multiple sources, including Van Meerbeeck JP et al. Small-cell lung cancer. Lancet. 2011 Nov 12;378(9804):1741–55.

in survival has been achieved with the addition of a checkpoint inhibitor (atezolizumab) to carboplatin and etoposide therapy in extensive stage disease. Thoracic radiation therapy improves survival in patients with limited SCLC and is given concurrently with chemotherapy. There is a high rate of brain metastasis in patients with SCLC, even following a good response to chemotherapy. Prophylactic cranial irradiation has been shown to decrease the incidence of central nervous system disease and improve survival in patients with limited-stage disease who respond to chemotherapy and a subset of patients with extensive-stage disease who have had an excellent response to chemotherapy.

C. Palliative Therapy

Photoresection with the Nd:YAG laser is sometimes performed on central tumors to relieve endobronchial obstruction, improve dyspnea, and control hemoptysis. External beam radiation therapy is also used to control dyspnea, hemoptysis, endobronchial obstruction, pain from bony metastases, obstruction from superior vena cava syndrome, and symptomatic brain metastases. Resection of a *solitary* brain metastasis improves quality of life and survival when combined with radiation therapy if there is no evidence of other metastatic disease. Stereotactic radiation therapy is offered for limited brain metastases. Repeated thoracenteses, pleurodesis, or pleurex catheter tube placement are key interventions for palliation of symptomatic malignant pleural effusions. Pain is very common in advanced disease. As patients approach the end of life, meticulous efforts at pain control are essential (see Chapter 5). In addition to standard oncologic care, early referral to a palliative care specialist is recommended in advanced disease to aid in symptom management and such palliative care can modestly improve survival.

► Prognosis

The 5-year survival rate for lung cancer is approximately 19%. Predictors of survival include the type of tumor (SCLC versus NSCLC), molecular profiling, the stage of the tumor, the patient's performance status, and weight loss in the past 6 months. Patients with targetable mutations have better overall survival when compared with those without mutations due to superior efficacy of targeted drug therapy.

Gandhi L et al; KEYNOTE-189 Investigators. Pembrolizumab plus chemotherapy in metastatic non-small-cell lung cancer. N Engl J Med. 2018 May 31;378(22):2078–92. [PMID: 29658856]

Horn L et al; IMpower133 Study Group. First-line atezolizumab plus chemotherapy in extensive-stage small-cell lung cancer. N Engl J Med. 2018 Dec 6;379(23):2220–9. [PMID: 30280641]

Paz-Ares L et al; KEYNOTE-407 Investigators. Pembrolizumab plus chemotherapy for squamous non-small-cell lung cancer. N Engl J Med. 2018 Nov 22;379(21):2040–51. [PMID: 30280635]

Peters S et al. Alectinib versus crizotinib in untreated Alk-positive non-small-cell lung cancer. N Engl J Med. 2017 Aug 31;377(9): 829–38. [PMID: 28586279]

Reck M et al; KEYNOTE-024 Investigators. Pembrolizumab versus chemotherapy for PD-L1-positive non-small-cell lung cancer. N Engl J Med. 2016 Nov 10;375(19):1823–33. [PMID: 27718847]

Siegel RL et al. Cancer statistics, 2018. CA Cancer J Clin. 2018 Jan; 68(1):7–30. [PMID: 29313949]

Soria JC et al; FLAURA Investigators. Osimertinib in untreated EGFR-mutated advanced non-small-cell lung cancer. N Engl J Med. 2018 Jan 11;378(2):113–25. [PMID: 29151359]

PULMONARY METASTASIS

Pulmonary metastasis results from the spread of an extra-pulmonary malignant tumor through vascular or lymphatic channels or by direct extension. Metastases usually occur via the pulmonary artery and typically present as multiple nodules or masses on chest radiography. The radiographic differential diagnosis of multiple pulmonary nodules also includes pulmonary arteriovenous malformation, infections (including abscesses, septic emboli, and atypical infections), sarcoidosis, rheumatoid nodules, and granulomatosis with polyangiitis. Metastases to the lungs are found in 20–55% of patients with various metastatic malignancies. Carcinomas of the kidney, breast, rectum, colon, and cervix and malignant melanoma are the most likely primary tumors.

Lymphangitic carcinomatosis denotes diffuse involvement of the pulmonary lymphatic network by primary or metastatic lung cancer, probably a result of extension of tumor from lung capillaries to the lymphatics. **Tumor embolization** from extrapulmonary cancer (renal cell carcinoma, hepatocellular carcinoma, choriocarcinoma) is an uncommon route for tumor spread to the lungs. Metastatic cancer may also present as a malignant pleural effusion.

▶ **Clinical Findings**

A. Symptoms and Signs

Symptoms are uncommon but include cough, hemoptysis and, in advanced cases, dyspnea and hypoxemia. Symptoms are more often referable to the site of the primary tumor.

B. Laboratory Findings

The diagnosis of metastatic cancer involving the lungs is usually established by identifying a primary tumor. Appropriate studies should be ordered if there is a suspicion of any primary cancer, such as breast, thyroid, testis, colorectal, or prostate, for which specific treatment is available. If the history, physical examination, and initial studies fail to reveal the site of the primary tumor, attention is better focused on the lung, where tissue samples obtained by bronchoscopy, percutaneous needle biopsy, video-assisted thoracoscopic surgery (VATS), or thoracotomy may establish the histologic diagnosis and suggest the most likely primary cancer. Occasionally, cytologic studies of pleural fluid or pleural biopsy reveals the diagnosis.

To determine a primary diagnosis, immunohistochemical staining should be done on the biopsy specimen. For example, prostate-specific antigen (PSA) and thyroglobulin staining are highly specific for prostate and thyroid cancer, respectively. Thyroid transcription factor-1 (TTF-1) and napsin-A are relatively specific for primary lung adenocarcinoma, while the former can be positive in cases of SCLC and thyroid carcinoma and the latter can be positive in papillary and clear cell renal cell carcinomas. An adenocarcinoma that demonstrates negative TTF-1 and napsin-A staining strongly suggests a nonpulmonary primary cancer. Positive estrogen receptor (ER) and progesterone receptor (PR) stains suggest primary breast cancer.

C. Imaging

Chest radiographs usually show multiple spherical densities with sharp margins. The size of metastatic lesions varies from a few millimeters (miliary densities) to large masses. The lesions are usually bilateral, pleural or subpleural in location, and more common in lower lung zones. Lymphangitic spread and solitary pulmonary nodule are less common radiographic presentations of pulmonary metastasis. CT imaging of the chest, abdomen, and pelvis may reveal the site of a primary tumor and will help determine feasibility of surgical resection of the metastatic lung tumors. PET-CT FDG scan is helpful in identifying the site of a primary cancer and identifying other areas of extrathoracic metastasis.

▶ **Treatment**

Once the diagnosis has been established, management consists of treatment of the primary neoplasm and any pulmonary complications. Surgical resection of a *solitary* pulmonary nodule is often prudent in the patient with known current or previous extrapulmonary cancer. Local resection of one or more pulmonary metastases is feasible in a few carefully selected patients with various sarcomas and carcinomas (such as testis, colorectal, and kidney). About 15–25% of metastatic solid tumor patients have metastases limited to the lungs and are surgical candidates. Surgical resection should be considered only if (1) the primary tumor is under control, (2) the patient has adequate cardiopulmonary reserve to tolerate resection, (3) all metastatic tumor can be resected, (4) effective nonsurgical approaches are not available, and (5) there is no evidence of extrathoracic metastases that are not controlled. Unfavorable prognostic factors also include shorter disease-free interval from primary tumor treatment to presentation of metastases and a larger number of metastases. Retrospective data from the International Registry of Lung Metastases report an overall 5-year survival rate of 36% and 10-year survival rate of 26% after complete resection of pulmonary metastases. Patients who are not surgical candidates but have solitary or limited metastatic disease to the lungs may be candidates for stereotactic radiotherapy, radioablation, or cryotherapy. For patients with unresectable progressive disease, chemotherapy tailored to the primary tumor can be offered, and diligent attention to palliative care is essential (see Chapter 5).

Guerrera F et al. Surgery of colorectal cancer lung metastases: analysis of survival, recurrence and re-surgery. J Thorac Dis. 2016 Jul;8(7):1764–71. [PMID: 27499967]

Handy JR et al. Expert consensus document on pulmonary metastasectomy. Ann Thorac Surg. 2019 Feb;107(2):631–49. [PMID: 30476477]

Petrella F et al. Pulmonary metastatectomy: an overview. J Thorac Dis. 2017 Oct;9(Suppl 12):S1291–8. [PMID: 29119017]

MESOTHELIOMA

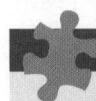

- ▶ Unilateral, nonpleuritic chest pain and dyspnea.
- ▶ Distant (more than 20 years earlier) history of exposure to asbestos.
- ▶ Pleural effusion or pleural thickening or both on chest radiographs.
- ▶ Malignant cells in pleural fluid or tissue biopsy.

General Considerations

Mesotheliomas are primary tumors arising from the surface lining of the pleura (80% of cases) or peritoneum (20% of cases). Numerous studies have confirmed the association of **malignant pleural mesothelioma** with exposure to asbestos. The lifetime risk to asbestos workers of developing malignant pleural mesothelioma is as high as 10%. The latent period between exposure and onset of symptoms ranges from 20 to 40 years. The clinician should inquire about asbestos exposure through mining, milling, manufacturing, shipyard work, insulation, brake linings, building construction and demolition, roofing materials, and other asbestos products (pipes, textiles, paints, tiles, gaskets, panels).

Clinical Findings

A. Symptoms and Signs

The average interval between onset of symptoms and diagnosis is 2–3 months; the median age at diagnosis is 72–74 years in Western countries. Symptoms include the insidious onset of shortness of breath, nonpleuritic chest pain, and weight loss. Physical findings include dullness to percussion, diminished breath sounds and, in some cases, digital clubbing.

B. Laboratory Findings

Pleural fluid is exudative and often hemorrhagic. Cytologic tests of pleural fluid are often negative. VATS biopsy is usually necessary to obtain an adequate specimen for histologic diagnosis. The histologic variants of malignant pleural mesothelioma are epithelial (50–60%), sarcomatoid (10%), and biphasic (30–40%). Since distinction from benign inflammatory conditions and metastatic adenocarcinoma may be difficult, immunohistochemical stains are important to confirm the diagnosis.

C. Imaging

Radiographic abnormalities consist of nodular, irregular, unilateral pleural thickening and varying degrees of unilateral pleural effusion. Sixty percent of patients have right-sided disease, while only 5% have bilateral involvement. CT scans demonstrate the extent of pleural involvement. PET-CT is used to help differentiate benign from malignant

pleural disease, improve staging accuracy, and identify candidates for aggressive surgical approaches.

Complications

Malignant pleural mesothelioma progresses rapidly as the tumor spreads along the pleural surface to involve the pericardium, mediastinum, and contralateral pleura. The tumor may eventually extend beyond the thorax to involve abdominal lymph nodes and organs. Progressive pain and dyspnea are characteristic. Local invasion of thoracic structures may cause superior vena cava syndrome, hoarseness, Horner syndrome, arrhythmias, and dysphagia.

Treatment

Chemotherapy is the mainstay of treatment (Tables 39–2 and 39–3), with cytoreductive surgery included in multimodality treatment only if there is localized disease that is amenable to complete macroscopic surgical resection. The optimal surgical approach is still under debate. For localized disease, surgical options include pleurectomy and decortication (surgical stripping of the pleura and pericardium from apex of the lung to diaphragm) or extrapleural pneumonectomy (a radical surgical procedure involving removal of the ipsilateral lung, parietal and visceral pleura, pericardium, and most of the hemidiaphragm). Surgical cytoreduction alone is not sufficient, and either chemotherapy or radiation therapy (or both) should be included in a multimodality approach. In advanced unresectable disease, palliative chemotherapy with cisplatin and pemetrexed can achieve response rates of 30–40%, can extend median overall survival to 12 months, and can improve quality of life. Adding bevacizumab (a monoclonal antibody to vascular endothelial growth factor [VEGF]) to cisplatin and pemetrexed has been shown to further improve overall survival. Drainage of pleural effusions, pleurodesis, radiation therapy, and even surgical resection may offer palliative benefit to some patients.

Prognosis

Most patients die of respiratory failure and complications of local extension. Median survival time from diagnosis ranges from 7 months to 17 months. Five-year survival is 5–10%. Tumors that are predominantly sarcomatoid are more resistant to therapy and have a worse prognosis, with median survivals less than 1 year. Poor prognostic features include poor performance status, non-epithelioid histology, male gender, nodal involvement, elevated lactate dehydrogenase, high white blood cell count, low hemoglobin, and high platelet count.

De Bondt C et al. Combined modality treatment in mesothelioma: a systemic literature review with treatment recommendations. Transl Lung Cancer Res. 2018 Oct;7(5):562–73. [PMID: 30450295]

de Gooijer CJ et al. Current chemotherapy strategies in malignant pleural mesothelioma. Transl Lung Cancer Res. 2018 Oct;7(5): 574–83. [PMID: 30450296]

Wald O et al. New concepts in the treatment of malignant pleural mesothelioma. Annu Rev Med. 2018 Jan 29;69:365–77. [PMID: 29029582]

Zalcman G et al; French Cooperative Thoracic Intergroup (IFCT). Bevacizumab for newly diagnosed pleural mesothelioma in the Mesothelioma Avastin Cisplatin Pemetrexed Study (MAPS): a randomised, controlled, open-label, phase 3 trial. Lancet. 2016 Apr 2;387(10026):1405–14. Erratum in: Lancet. 2016 Apr 2;387(10026):e24. [PMID: 26719230]

HEPATOBILIARY CANCERS

Lawrence S. Friedman, MD

HEPATOCELLULAR CARCINOMA

ESSENTIALS OF DIAGNOSIS

▶ Usually a complication of cirrhosis.

▶ Characteristic CT and MRI features may obviate the need for a confirmatory biopsy.

▶ General Considerations

Malignant neoplasms of the liver that arise from parenchymal cells are called hepatocellular carcinomas (accounting for 85% of liver cancers); those that originate in the ductular cells are called cholangiocarcinomas (15% or less). Rare tumors of the liver include angiosarcoma and lymphoma.

Hepatocellular carcinomas are associated with cirrhosis in 85% of cases. In Africa and most of Asia, hepatitis B virus (HBV) infection is a major etiologic factor, and a family history of hepatocellular carcinoma increases the risk synergistically. In the United States and other Western countries, incidence rates have risen rapidly (over twofold since 1978, with slowing of the rate increase since 2006 except in men ages 55–64), presumably because of the increasing prevalence of cirrhosis caused by chronic hepatitis C virus (HCV) infection and nonalcoholic fatty liver disease (NAFLD); however, incidence rates are projected to increase through 2030. In Western countries, risk factors for hepatocellular carcinoma in patients known to have cirrhosis are male gender, age greater than 55 years (although there has been an increase in the number of younger cases), Hispanic or Asian ethnicity, family history in a first-degree relative, overweight, obesity (especially in early adulthood), alcohol use (especially in combination with obesity), tobacco use, diabetes mellitus, hypothyroidism (in women), a prolonged prothrombin time, a low platelet count, and an elevated serum transferrin saturation. The risk of hepatocellular carcinoma is higher in persons with a viral rather than nonviral cause of cirrhosis and may be increased in persons with autoimmune diseases. Other associations include high levels of HBV replication; HBV genotype C; hepatitis D coinfection; elevated serum ALT levels in persons with chronic hepatitis B (in whom antiviral therapy to suppress HBV replication appears to reduce the risk); HCV genotypes 1b and 3; lack of response to antiviral therapy for HCV infection; hemochromatosis (and possibly the C282Y carrier state);

aflatoxin exposure (associated with mutation of the *TP53* gene); alpha-1-antiprotease (alpha-1-antitrypsin) deficiency; tyrosinemia; and radiation exposure. In patients with the metabolic syndrome and NAFLD, hepatocellular carcinoma may arise from a hepatocellular adenoma in the absence of cirrhosis. Evidence for an association with long-term use of oral contraceptives is inconclusive. Whereas sulfonylurea and insulin use may increase the risk of hepatocellular carcinoma, consumption of coffee, vegetables, white meat, fish, and n-3 polyunsaturated fatty acids; aspirin use; and statin and metformin use in diabetic patients appear to be protective.

The fibrolamellar variant of hepatocellular carcinoma generally occurs in young women and is characterized by a distinctive histologic picture, absence of risk factors, unique genomic profiles, and indolent course. Vinyl chloride exposure is associated with angiosarcoma of the liver. Hepatoblastoma, the most common malignant liver tumor in infants and young children, occurs rarely in adults.

▶ Clinical Findings

A. Symptoms and Signs

The presence of a hepatocellular carcinoma may be unsuspected until there is deterioration in the condition of a cirrhotic patient who was formerly stable. Cachexia, weakness, and weight loss are associated symptoms. The sudden appearance of ascites, which may be bloody, suggests portal or hepatic vein thrombosis by tumor or bleeding from a necrotic tumor.

Physical examination may show tender enlargement of the liver, occasionally with a palpable mass. In Africa, the typical presentation in young patients is a rapidly expanding abdominal mass. Auscultation may reveal a bruit over the tumor or a friction rub when the tumor has extended to the surface of the liver.

B. Laboratory Findings

Laboratory tests may reveal leukocytosis, as opposed to the leukopenia that is frequently encountered in cirrhotic patients. Anemia is common, but a normal or elevated hematocrit value may be found in up to one-third of patients owing to elaboration of erythropoietin by the tumor. Sudden and sustained elevation of the serum alkaline phosphatase in a patient who was formerly stable is a common finding. HBsAg is present in a majority of cases in endemic areas, whereas in the United States anti-HCV is found in up to 40% of cases. Alpha-fetoprotein levels are elevated in up to 70% of patients with hepatocellular carcinoma in Western countries (although the sensitivity is lower in blacks and levels are not elevated in patients with fibrolamellar hepatocellular carcinoma); however, mild elevations (10–200 ng/mL [10–200 mcg/L]) are also often seen in patients with chronic hepatitis. Serum levels of des-gamma-carboxy prothrombin are elevated in up to 90% of patients with hepatocellular carcinoma, but they may also be elevated in patients with vitamin K deficiency, chronic hepatitis, and metastatic cancer. Cytologic study of ascitic fluid rarely reveals malignant cells.

C. Imaging

Multiphasic helical CT and MRI with contrast enhancement are the preferred imaging studies for determining the location and vascularity of the tumor; MRI may be more sensitive than CT, and imaging with gadoxetic acid increases sensitivity. Lesions smaller than 1 cm may be difficult to characterize. Arterial phase enhancement of the lesion followed by delayed hypointensity ("washout") is most specific for hepatocellular carcinoma based on stringent imaging criteria with a high specificity for hepatocellular carcinoma greater than or equal to 1 cm in diameter developed by the American College of Radiology through its Liver Imaging Reporting and Data System, the Organ Procurement and Transplantation Network, and the American Association for the Study of Liver Diseases. Ultrasonography is less sensitive and more operator dependent but is used to screen for hepatic nodules in high-risk patients. Contrast-enhanced ultrasonography has a sensitivity and specificity approaching those of arterial phase helical CT but, unlike CT and MRI, cannot image the entire liver during the short duration of the arterial phase and is thus associated with false-positive results. In selected cases, endoscopic ultrasonography (EUS) may be useful. PET is under study.

D. Liver Biopsy and Staging

Liver biopsy is diagnostic, although seeding of the needle tract by tumor is a potential risk (1–3%). For lesions smaller than 1 cm, ultrasonography may be repeated every 3 months followed by further investigation of enlarging lesions. For lesions 1 cm or larger, biopsy can be deferred when characteristic arterial hypervascularity and delayed washout are demonstrated on either multiphasic helical CT or MRI with contrast enhancement (or both) in a patient with cirrhosis or if surgical resection is planned. Staging in the TNM classification includes the following definitions: T0: no evidence of primary tumor; T1a: solitary tumor less than or equal to 2 cm; T1b: solitary tumor more than 2 cm without vascular invasion; T2: solitary tumor more than 2 cm with vascular invasion or multiple tumors none more than 5 cm; T3: multiple tumors with at least one more than 5 cm; T4: single or multiple tumors of any size involving a major branch of the portal or hepatic vein or with direct invasion of adjacent organs other than the gallbladder or with perforation of the visceral peritoneum; N1: regional lymph node metastasis; M1: distant metastasis; F0: no to moderate hepatic fibrosis; F1: severe hepatic fibrosis to cirrhosis. The Barcelona Clinic Liver Cancer (BCLC) staging system is preferred and includes the Child-Pugh class, tumor stage, and liver function and has the advantage of linking overall stage with preferred treatment modalities and with an estimation of life expectancy.

▶ Screening & Prevention

Surveillance for the development of hepatocellular carcinoma is recommended in patients with chronic hepatitis B (beginning as early as age 20 in Africans, age 40 in Asians or those with a family history of hepatocellular carcinoma, and age 50 in others) or cirrhosis caused by HCV, HBV, or alcohol. There is some evidence that surveillance for hepatocellular carcinoma leads to a survival advantage over clinical diagnosis, but only a minority of cases are detected by surveillance. The standard approach is ultrasonography and alpha-fetoprotein testing every 6 months, although the value of alpha-fetoprotein screening has been questioned because of its low sensitivity. CT and MRI are considered too expensive for screening. The sensitivity of ultrasonography for detecting early hepatocellular carcinoma is only 63%. The risk of hepatocellular carcinoma in a patient with cirrhosis is 3–5% a year, and patients with tumors detected by surveillance have a less advanced stage on average and greater likelihood that treatment will prolong survival than those not undergoing surveillance, although there is controversy about whether surveillance reduces cancer-related mortality. In a population of patients with cirrhosis, over 60% of nodules smaller than 2 cm in diameter detected on a screening ultrasonography prove to be hepatocellular carcinoma. Mass vaccination programs against HBV in developing countries are leading to reduced rates of hepatocellular carcinoma. Successful treatment of hepatitis B and of hepatitis C in patients with cirrhosis also reduces the subsequent risk of hepatocellular carcinoma, and thus hepatocellular carcinoma is considered a preventable neoplasm. However, hepatocellular carcinoma may still occur after clearance of hepatitis B surface antigen or cure of HCV infection and thus may reduce the efficacy of treatment for HBV and HCV infection.

▶ Treatment

Surgical resection of a solitary hepatocellular carcinoma may result in cure if liver function is preserved (Child-Pugh class A or possibly B) and portal vein thrombosis is not present. Laparoscopic liver resection has been performed in selected cases. Treatment of underlying chronic viral hepatitis, adjuvant chemotherapy, and adaptive immunotherapy may lower postsurgical recurrence rates. Liver transplantation may be appropriate for small unresectable tumors in a patient with advanced cirrhosis, with reported 5-year survival rates of up to 75%. The recurrence-free survival may be better for liver transplantation than for resection in patients with well-compensated cirrhosis and small tumors (one tumor less than 5 cm or three or fewer tumors each less than 3 cm in diameter [Milan criteria]) and in those with expanded (University of California, San Francisco) criteria of one tumor less than or equal to 6.5 cm or three or fewer tumors less than or equal to 4.5 cm. The Extended Toronto criteria include tumor differentiation, cancer-related symptoms, confinement of tumor to the liver, and absence of vascular invasion, without regard to tumor number or size, to determine candidacy for liver transplantation, and appear to predict outcomes as well as the Milan criteria. Patients with stage 2 hepatocellular carcinoma meeting the Milan criteria receive an additional 28 points on their Model for End-Stage Liver Disease (MELD) score after 6 months on the waiting list (see Chapter 16), markedly increasing their chances of undergoing transplantation. However, liver transplantation is often impractical because of the donor organ shortage, and living donor liver transplantation may be considered in these cases. Patients with larger tumors (3–5 cm), a serum alpha-fetoprotein level of 1000 ng/mL (1000 mcg/L) or higher, or a MELD score of 20 or more have poor posttransplantation survival. In patients with a serum alpha-fetoprotein level greater than 1000 ng/mL (1000 mcg/L), downstaging by locoregional therapy to an alpha-fetoprotein level less than 500 ng/mL (500 mcg/L) improves survival following subsequent liver transplantation. Chemotherapy, hormonal therapy with tamoxifen, and long-acting octreotide have not been shown to prolong life, but transarterial chemoembolization (TACE), TACE with drug-eluting beads, transarterial chemoinfusion (TACI), and transarterial radioembolization (TARE) via the hepatic artery are palliative and may prolong survival in patients with a large or multifocal tumor in the absence of extrahepatic spread. TACI and TARE are suitable for patients with portal vein thrombosis. TARE with yttrium-90 has been shown to result in a longer time to progression than TACE. Microwave ablation, radiofrequency ablation, cryotherapy, or injection of absolute ethanol into tumors smaller than 2 cm may prolong survival in patients who are not candidates for resection and have tumors that are accessible; these interventions, as well as stereotactic body radiation therapy, may also provide a "bridge" to liver transplantation. Microwave ablation is becoming the preferred approach because it allows shorter treatment times and, like radiofrequency ablation, can be performed after TACE in select cases. Cryoablation may result in slower tumor progression than radiofrequency ablation for tumors that are 3.1–4 cm in diameter. Stereotactic body radiation therapy is also being used to treat unresectable hepatocellular carcinoma and may be effective in treating lesions larger than those treated with ablation techniques. Sorafenib (an oral multikinase inhibitor of Raf kinase, the VEGF receptor, and the platelet-derived growth factor receptor [and others]) prolongs median survival as well as the time to radiologic progression by 3 months in patients with advanced hepatocellular carcinoma; sorafenib is standard care in these patients. Lenvatinib is another oral multikinase inhibitor that is FDA approved for the same indications as sorafenib. Regorafenib is an oral multikinase inhibitor that provides a survival benefit for patients whose disease progresses despite sorafenib therapy, and nivolumab is an immune checkpoint inhibitor that has been approved for advanced hepatocellular carcinoma. Cabozantinib, another multikinase inhibitor, has been approved by the FDA for the treatment of hepatocellular carcinoma, and ramucirumab, an antibody to the VEGF receptor, is still in phase III trials. The modified Response Evaluation Criteria in Solid Tumors (mRECIST) are used to assess treatment response based on tumor shrinkage and viability after locoregional and antiangiogenic treatment. Meticulous efforts at palliative care are essential for patients in whom disease progresses despite treatment or in whom advanced tumors, vascular invasion, or extrahepatic spread are present. Severe pain may develop in such patients due to expansion of the liver capsule by the tumor and requires concerted efforts at pain management, including the use of opioids (see Chapter 5).

► Prognosis

In the United States, overall 1- and 5-year survival rates for patients with hepatocellular carcinoma are 23% and 5%, respectively. Five-year survival rates rise to 56% for patients with localized resectable disease (T1, T2, selected T3 and T4; N0; M0) but are virtually nil for those with locally unresectable or advanced disease. In patients with HCV-related hepatocellular carcinoma, the serum alpha-fetoprotein level at the time of diagnosis of cancer has been reported to be an independent predictor of mortality. Some, but not all, studies have reported an unexpectedly high rate of early tumor recurrence in patients who were cured of HCV infection with oral direct-acting antiviral agents, rather than interferon-based therapy. A serum alpha-fetoprotein level greater than or equal to 200 ng/mL (200 milli-international units/mL) or increases of greater than 15 ng/mL/month predict worse outcomes in patients awaiting liver transplantation. In patients who are not eligible for surgery, an elevated serum C-reactive protein level is associated with poor survival. Contrary to traditional opinion, the fibrolamellar variant does not have a better prognosis than conventional hepatocellular carcinoma without cirrhosis.

► When to Refer

All patients with hepatocellular carcinoma should be referred to a specialist.

► When to Admit

- Complications of cirrhosis.
- Severe pain.
- For surgery and other interventions.

European Association for the Study of the Liver. EASL Clinical Practice Guidelines: management of hepatocellular carcinoma. J Hepatol. 2018 Jul;69(1):182–236. [PMID: 29628281]

Forner A et al. Hepatocellular carcinoma. Lancet. 2018 Mar 31; 391(10127):1301–14. [PMID: 29307467]

Heimbach JK et al. AASLD guidelines for the treatment of hepatocellular carcinoma. Hepatology. 2018 Jan;67(1):358–80. [PMID: 28130846]

Marrero JA et al. Diagnosis, staging, and management of hepatocellular carcinoma: 2018 practice guidance by the American Association for the Study of Liver Diseases. Hepatology. 2018 Aug;68(2):723–50. [PMID: 29624699]

Tzartzeva K et al. Surveillance imaging and alpha fetoprotein for early detection of hepatocellular carcinoma in patients with cirrhosis: a meta-analysis. Gastroenterology. 2018 May; 154(6):1706–18. [PMID: 29425931]

CARCINOMA OF THE BILIARY TRACT

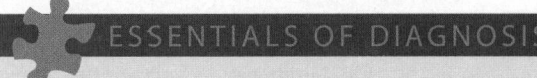

ESSENTIALS OF DIAGNOSIS

- ► Presents with obstructive jaundice, usually painless, often with dilated biliary tract.
- ► Pain is more common in gallbladder carcinoma than cholangiocarcinoma.
- ► A dilated gallbladder may be palpable (Courvoisier sign).
- ► Diagnosis by cholangiography with biopsy and brushings for cytology.

▶ General Considerations

Carcinoma of the gallbladder occurs in approximately 2% of all people operated on for biliary tract disease; the incidence, like that of carcinoma of the bile ducts, had been decreasing in the United States but may be increasing again in some Western countries because of lifestyle changes. It is notoriously insidious, and the diagnosis is often made unexpectedly at surgery. Cholelithiasis (often large, symptomatic stones) is usually present. Other risk factors are chronic infection of the gallbladder with *Salmonella typhi*, gallbladder polyps over 1 cm in diameter (particularly with hypoechoic foci on EUS), mucosal calcification of the gallbladder (porcelain gallbladder), anomalous pancreaticobiliary ductal junction, and aflatoxin exposure. Genetic factors include *K-ras* and *TP53* mutations. Spread of the cancer—by direct extension into the liver or to the peritoneal surface—may be seen on initial presentation. The TNM classification includes the following stages: Tis, carcinoma in situ; T1a, tumor invades lamina propria, and T1b, tumor invades muscle layer; T2, tumor invades perimuscular connective tissue with no extension beyond serosa (visceral peritoneum) (T2a) or into liver (T2b); T3, tumor perforates the serosa or directly invades the liver or adjacent organ or structure; T4, tumor invades the main portal vein or hepatic artery or invades two or more extrahepatic organs or structures; N1, metastasis to one to three regional lymph nodes; N2, metastasis to four or more regional lymph nodes; and M1, distant metastasis.

Carcinoma of the bile ducts (cholangiocarcinoma) accounts for 10–25% of all hepatobiliary malignancies and 3% of all cancer deaths in the United States. It is more prevalent in persons aged 50–70, with a slight male predominance, and more common in Asia. About 50% arise at the confluence of the hepatic ducts (perihilar, or so-called Klatskin, tumors), and 40% arise in the distal extrahepatic bile duct (the incidence of which has risen since 1990); the remainder are intrahepatic (the incidence of which rose dramatically from the 1970s to the early 2000s). The frequency of carcinoma in persons with a choledochal cyst has been reported to be over 14% at 20 years, and surgical excision is recommended. Most cases of cholangiocarcinoma are sporadic. There is an increased incidence of cholangiocarcinoma in patients with bile duct adenoma; biliary papillomatosis; Caroli disease; a biliary-enteric anastomosis; ulcerative colitis, especially those with primary sclerosing cholangitis; biliary cirrhosis; diabetes mellitus; hyperthyroidism; chronic pancreatitis; heavy alcohol consumption; smoking; and past exposure to Thorotrast, a contrast agent. Obesity and diabetes mellitus are risk factors for intrahepatic cholangiocarcinoma. Aspirin use is associated with a reduced risk of all types of cholangiocarcinoma, and in diabetic patients, metformin use is associated with a reduced risk of intrahepatic cholangiocarcinoma. In Southeast Asia, hepatolithiasis, chronic typhoid carriage, and infection of the bile ducts with helminths (*Clonorchis sinensis, Opisthorchis viverrini*) are associated with an increased risk of cholangiocarcinoma. Hepatitis C virus (and possibly hepatitis B virus) infection, cirrhosis, HIV infection, nonalcoholic fatty liver disease, diabetes mellitus, obesity, and tobacco smoking are risk factors for intrahepatic cholangiocarcinoma. Mixed hepatocellular carcinoma-cholangiocarcinoma is a tumor that is being increasingly recognized.

Staging for perihilar cholangiocarcinoma is as follows: Tis, carcinoma in situ/high-grade dysplasia; T1, tumor is confined to bile duct; T2, tumor invades beyond the wall of the bile duct to surrounding adipose tissue (2a) or to the adjacent liver (2b); T3, tumor invades unilateral branches of the portal vein or hepatic artery; T4, tumor invades the main portal vein or its branches bilaterally, common hepatic artery, second-order biliary radicals, and contralateral portal vein or hepatic artery; N1, metastasis to one to three regional lymph nodes; N2, metastasis to four or more regional lymph nodes; M1, distant metastasis. Staging for intrahepatic cholangiocarcinoma is as follows: T1a, solitary tumor less than or equal to 5 cm without vascular invasion; T1b, solitary tumor more than 5 cm without vascular invasion; T2, solitary tumor with intrahepatic vascular invasion or multiple tumors 5 cm or smaller with or without vascular invasion; T3, tumor perforating the visceral peritoneum; T4, tumor invades adjacent organ (except gallbladder); N1, regional lymph node metastasis; and M1, distant metastasis. Additional staging is available for distal bile duct tumors. Other staging systems consider the patient's age, performance status, tumor extent and form, perineural invasion, vascular encasement, hepatic lobe atrophy, underlying liver disease, and peritoneal metastasis.

▶ Clinical Findings

A. Symptoms and Signs

Progressive jaundice is the most common and usually the first sign of obstruction of the extrahepatic biliary system. Pain in the right upper abdomen with radiation into the back is usually present early in the course of gallbladder carcinoma but occurs later in the course of bile duct carcinoma. Anorexia and weight loss are common and may be associated with fever and chills due to cholangitis. Rarely, hematemesis or melena results from erosion of tumor into a blood vessel (hemobilia). Fistula formation between the biliary system and adjacent organs may also occur. The course is usually one of rapid deterioration, with death occurring within a few months.

Physical examination reveals profound jaundice. Pruritus and skin excoriations are common. A palpable gallbladder with obstructive jaundice usually is said to signify malignant disease (Courvoisier sign); however, this clinical generalization has been proven to be accurate only about 50% of the time. Hepatomegaly due to hypertrophy of the unobstructed liver lobe is usually present and is associated with liver tenderness. Ascites may occur with peritoneal implants.

B. Laboratory Findings

With biliary obstruction, laboratory examination reveals predominantly conjugated hyperbilirubinemia, with total serum bilirubin values ranging from 5 to 30 mg/dL. There is usually concomitant elevation of the alkaline phosphatase and serum cholesterol. AST is normal or minimally elevated. The serum CA 19-9 level is elevated in up to 85% of patients and may help distinguish cholangiocarcinoma from a benign biliary stricture (in the absence of cholangitis) but is neither sensitive nor specific.

C. Imaging

Ultrasonography and contrast-enhanced, triple-phase, helical CT may show a gallbladder mass in gallbladder carcinoma and intrahepatic mass or biliary dilatation in carcinoma of the bile ducts. CT may also show involved regional lymph nodes and atrophy of a hepatic lobe because of vascular encasement with compensatory hypertrophy of the unaffected lobe. MRI with magnetic resonance cholangiopancreatography (MRCP) and gadolinium enhancement permits visualization of the entire biliary tract and detection of vascular invasion and obviates the need for angiography and, in some cases, direct cholangiography; it is the imaging procedure of choice but may understage malignant hilar strictures. The sensitivity and image quality can be increased with use of ferumoxide enhancement. The features of intrahepatic cholangiocarcinoma on MRI appear to differ from those of hepatocellular carcinoma, with contrast washout in the latter but not the former. In indeterminate cases, PET can detect cholangiocarcinomas as small as 1 cm and lymph node and distant metastases, but false-positive results occur. The most helpful diagnostic studies before surgery are either endoscopic retrograde or percutaneous transhepatic cholangiography with biopsy and cytologic specimens, although false-negative biopsy and cytology results are common. Digital image analysis and fluorescent in situ hybridization of cytologic specimens for polysomy improve sensitivity. EUS with FNA of tumors, peroral cholangioscopy, confocal laser endomicroscopy, and intraductal ultrasonography may confirm a diagnosis of cholangiocarcinoma in a patient with bile duct stricture and an otherwise indeterminate evaluation, but FNA can result in tumor seeding and is often avoided if the tumor is potentially resectable.

▶ Treatment

In young and fit patients, curative surgery for gallbladder carcinoma may be attempted if the tumor is well localized. The 5-year survival rate for carcinoma of the gallbladder invading the lamina propria or muscularis (stage 1, T1a or 1b, N0, M0) is as high as 85% with laparoscopic cholecystectomy but drops to 60%, even with a more extended open resection, if there is perimuscular invasion (T2). The role of radical surgery for T3 and T4 tumors is debatable. If the tumor is unresectable at laparotomy, biliary-enteric bypass (eg, Roux-en-Y hepaticojejunostomy) can be performed. Carcinoma of the bile ducts is curable by surgery in less than 10% of cases. If resection margins are negative, the 5-year survival rate may be as high as 47% for intrahepatic cholangiocarcinomas, 41% for hilar cholangiocarcinoma, and 37% for distal cholangiocarcinomas, but the perioperative mortality rate may be as high as 10%. Factors predicting shorter survival for intrahepatic cholangiocarcinoma include large tumor size, multiple tumors, lymph node metastasis, and vascular invasion. Adjuvant chemotherapy with capecitabine has been shown to result in superior overall survival compared with no adjuvant therapy. Palliation can be achieved by placement of a self-expandable metal stent via an endoscopic or percutaneous transhepatic route. Covered metal stents may be more cost-effective than uncovered metal stents because of a longer duration of patency, but they are associated with a higher rate of stent migration and cholecystitis due to occlusion of the cystic duct and are not associated with longer survival. For perihilar tumors, insertion of a unilateral stent rather than bilateral stents may suffice. Plastic stents are less expensive initially, but not in the long term, because they are more prone to occlude than metal ones; they may be considered in patients expected to survive only a few months. Photodynamic therapy in combination with stent placement prolongs survival when compared with stent placement alone in patients with nonresectable cholangiocarcinoma. Endoscopic retrograde cholangiopancreatography (ERCP)–directed radiofrequency ablation, TACE, and TARE are additional emerging options. Radiotherapy may relieve pain and contribute to biliary decompression. There is limited response to chemotherapy with gemcitabine alone, but the combination of cisplatin and gemcitabine or capecitabine and gemcitabine prolongs survival in patients with locally advanced or metastatic cholangiocarcinoma. Few patients survive for more than 24 months. Although cholangiocarcinoma is generally considered to be a contraindication to liver transplantation because of rapid tumor recurrence, a 75% 5-year survival rate has been reported in patients with stage I and II perihilar cholangiocarcinoma undergoing chemoradiation and exploratory laparotomy followed by liver transplantation.

For those patients whose disease progresses despite treatment, meticulous efforts at palliative care are essential (see Chapter 5).

▶ When to Refer

All patients with carcinoma of the biliary tract should be referred to a specialist.

▶ When to Admit

- Biliary obstruction.
- Cholangitis.

Baiu I et al. JAMA patient page. Gallbladder cancer. JAMA. 2018 Sep 25;320(12):1294. [PMID: 30264121]

Brooks C et al. Role of fluorescent in situ hybridization, cholangioscopic biopsies, and EUS-FNA in the evaluation of biliary strictures. Dig Dis Sci. 2018 Mar;63(3):636–44. [PMID: 29353443]

Conio M et al. Covered versus uncovered self-expandable metal stent for palliation of primary malignant extrahepatic biliary strictures: a randomized multicenter study. Gastrointest Endosc. 2018 Aug;88(2):283–91. [PMID: 29653120]

Goldaracena N et al. Current status of liver transplantation for cholangiocarcinoma. Liver Transpl. 2018 Feb;24(2):294–303. [PMID: 29024405]

Petrick JL et al. Body mass index, diabetes and intrahepatic cholangiocarcinoma risk: the Liver Cancer Pooling Project and meta-analysis. Am J Gastroenterol. 2018 Oct;113(10):1494–505. [PMID: 30177781]

Torre LA et al. Worldwide burden of and trends in mortality from gallbladder and other biliary tract cancers. Clin Gastroenterol Hepatol. 2018 Mar;16(3):427–37. [PMID: 28826679]

CARCINOMA OF THE PANCREAS & AMPULLA OF VATER

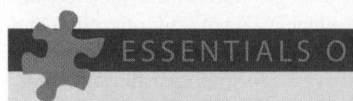

ESSENTIALS OF DIAGNOSIS

- ► Obstructive jaundice (may be painless).
- ► Enlarged gallbladder (may be painful).
- ► Upper abdominal pain with radiation to back, weight loss, and thrombophlebitis are usually late manifestations.

General Considerations

Carcinoma is the most common neoplasm of the pancreas. About 75% are in the head and 25% in the body and tail of the organ. Pancreatic carcinomas account for 2% of all cancers and 5% of cancer deaths. Ampullary carcinomas are much less common. Risk factors for pancreatic cancer include age, tobacco use (which is thought to cause 20–25% of cases), heavy alcohol use, obesity, chronic pancreatitis, diabetes mellitus, prior abdominal radiation, family history, and possibly gastric ulcer and exposure to arsenic and cadmium. New-onset diabetes mellitus after age 45 years occasionally heralds the onset of pancreatic cancer. In diabetic patients, metformin use and possibly aspirin use may reduce the risk of pancreatic cancer slightly, but insulin use and glucagon-like peptide-1-based therapy (eg, sitagliptin) may increase the risk. About 7% of patients with pancreatic cancer have a family history of pancreatic cancer in a first-degree relative, compared with 0.6% of control subjects. In 5–10% of cases, pancreatic cancer occurs as part of a hereditary syndrome, including familial breast cancer (carriers of *BRCA-2* have a 7% lifetime risk of pancreatic cancer), hereditary pancreatitis (*PSS1* mutation), familial atypical multiple mole melanoma (*p16/CDKN2A* mutation), Peutz-Jeghers syndrome (*STK11/LKB1* mutation), ataxia-telangiectasia (*ATM* mutation), and Lynch syndrome (hereditary nonpolyposis colorectal cancer [*MLH1, MSH2, MSH6* mutations]). Neuroendocrine tumors account for 1–2% of pancreatic neoplasms and may be functional (producing gastrin, insulin, glucagon, vasoactive intestinal peptide, somatostatin, growth hormone–releasing hormone, adrenocorticotropic hormone, and others) or nonfunctional. Cystic neoplasms account for only 1% of pancreatic cancers, but they are important because pancreatic cysts are common and may be mistaken for pseudocysts. A cystic neoplasm should be suspected when a cystic lesion in the pancreas is found in the absence of a history of pancreatitis. At least 15% of all pancreatic cysts are neoplasms. Serous cystadenomas (which account for 32–39% of cystic pancreatic neoplasms and also occur in patients with von Hippel-Lindau disease) are benign. However, mucinous cystic neoplasms (defined by the presence of ovarian stroma and accounting for 10–45% of cystic pancreatic neoplasms), intraductal papillary mucinous neoplasms (21–33% of cystic pancreatic neoplasms), solid pseudopapillary tumors (less than 5%,

primarily in young women), and cystic islet cell tumors (3–5%) may be malignant. Their prognoses are better than the prognosis of pancreatic adenocarcinoma, unless the cystic neoplasm is at least locally advanced.

Clinical Findings

A. Symptoms and Signs

Pain is present in over 70% of cases and is often vague, diffuse, and located in the epigastrium or, when the lesion is in the tail, located in the left upper quadrant of the abdomen. Radiation of pain into the back is common and sometimes predominates. Sitting up and leaning forward may afford some relief, and this usually indicates that the lesion has spread beyond the pancreas and is inoperable. Diarrhea, perhaps due to maldigestion, is an occasional early symptom. Migratory thrombophlebitis is a rare sign. Weight loss is a common but late finding and may be associated with depression. Occasional patients (often aged 40 years or older) present with acute pancreatitis in the absence of an alternative cause. Jaundice is usually due to biliary obstruction by a cancer in the pancreatic head. A palpable gallbladder is also indicative of obstruction by a neoplasm (Courvoisier sign), but there are frequent exceptions. A hard, fixed, occasionally tender mass may be present. In advanced cases, a hard periumbilical (Sister Mary Joseph's) nodule may be palpable.

B. Laboratory Findings

There may be mild anemia. Glycosuria, hyperglycemia, and impaired glucose tolerance or true diabetes mellitus are found in 10–20% of cases. The serum amylase or lipase level is occasionally elevated. Liver biochemical tests may suggest obstructive jaundice. Steatorrhea in the absence of jaundice is uncommon. Occult blood in the stool is suggestive of carcinoma of the ampulla of Vater (the combination of biliary obstruction and bleeding may give the stools a distinctive silver appearance). CA 19-9, with a sensitivity of 70% and a specificity of 87%, has not proven useful for early detection of pancreatic cancer; increased values are also found in acute and chronic pancreatitis and cholangitis. Plasma chromogranin A levels are elevated in 88–100% of patients with pancreatic neuroendocrine tumors (NETs).

C. Imaging

Multiphase thin-cut helical CT is generally the initial diagnostic procedure and detects a mass in over 80% of cases. CT identifies metastases, delineates the extent of the tumor, and allows percutaneous FNA for cytologic studies and tumor markers. MRI is an alternative to CT. Ultrasonography is not reliable because of interference by intestinal gas. PET is a sensitive technique for detecting pancreatic cancer and metastases, but PET-CT is not a routine staging procedure. Selective celiac and superior mesenteric arteriography may demonstrate vessel invasion by tumor, a finding that would preclude attempts at surgical resection, but it is used less commonly since the advent of multiphase helical CT. EUS is more sensitive than CT for detecting pancreatic cancer and equivalent to CT for determining nodal involvement and resectability. A normal EUS excludes pancreatic cancer. EUS may also be used to guide FNA or biopsy for tissue diagnosis, tumor markers, and DNA analysis. ERCP may clarify an ambiguous CT or MRI study by delineating the pancreatic duct system or confirming an ampullary or biliary neoplasm. MRCP appears to be at least as sensitive as ERCP in diagnosing pancreatic cancer. In some centers, pancreatoscopy or intraductal ultrasonography is used to evaluate filling defects in the pancreatic duct and assess resectability of intraductal papillary mucinous tumors. With obstruction of the splenic vein, splenomegaly or gastric varices are present, the latter detected by endoscopy, EUS, or angiography.

Cystic neoplasms can be distinguished by their appearance on CT, EUS, and ERCP and features of the cyst fluid on gross, cytologic, and genetic analysis. For example, serous cystadenomas may have a central scar or honeycomb appearance; mucinous cystadenomas are unilocular or multilocular and contain mucin-rich fluid with high carcinoembryonic antigen levels (greater than 200 ng/mL [200 mcg/L]) and *K-ras* mutations; and intraductal papillary mucinous neoplasms are associated with a dilated pancreatic duct and extrusion of gelatinous material from the ampulla.

▶ Staging

Staging of pancreatic cancer by the TNM classification includes the following definitions: Tis: carcinoma in situ; T1a: tumor limited to the pancreas, 0.5 cm or less in greatest dimension; T1b: tumor more than 0.5 cm and less than 1 cm; T1c: tumor 1–2 cm; T2: tumor limited to the pancreas, more than 2 cm and less than or equal to 4 cm in greatest dimension; T3: tumor more than 4 cm in greatest dimension; T4: tumor involves the celiac axis, superior mesenteric artery, or common hepatic artery regardless of size; N1: metastasis to one to three regional lymph nodes; N2: metastasis to four or more regional lymph nodes; M1: distant metastasis.

▶ Treatment

Abdominal exploration is usually necessary when cytologic diagnosis cannot be made or if resection is to be attempted, which includes up to 30% of patients with pancreatic carcinoma. In a patient with a localized mass in the head of the pancreas and without jaundice, laparoscopy may detect tiny peritoneal or liver metastases and thereby avoid resection in 4–13% of patients. Radical pancreaticoduodenal (Whipple) resection is indicated for cancers strictly limited to the head of the pancreas, periampullary area, and duodenum (T1, N0, M0). Five-year survival rates are 20–25% in this group and as high as 40% in those with negative resection margins and without lymph node involvement. Preoperative endoscopic decompression of an obstructed bile duct is often achieved with a plastic stent or short metal stent but does not reduce operative mortality and is associated with complications. The best surgical results are achieved at centers that specialize in the multidisciplinary treatment of pancreatic cancer. Adjuvant chemotherapy with gemcitabine, 5-fluorouracil, or gemcitabine with

capecitabine is superior to no adjuvant therapy. Gemcitabine with capecitabine has been found to be superior to gemcitabine alone. The role of adjuvant chemoradiation is controversial but often used in the United States. Neoadjuvant chemotherapy with or without radiation is increasingly being used to downstage patients and in those with resectable cancer. Common chemotherapy regimens for this purpose include FOLFIRINOX (5-fluorouracil, leucovorin, irinotecan, oxaliplatin) and gemcitabine with nanoparticle albumin-bound (nab)-paclitaxel. Chemoradiotherapy downstages about 30% of patients with locally advanced disease to allow resection. When resection is not feasible, endoscopic stenting of the bile duct is performed to relieve jaundice. A plastic stent is generally placed if the patient's anticipated survival is less than 6 months (or surgery is planned). A metal stent is preferred when anticipated survival is 6 months or greater. Whether covered metal stents designed to prevent tumor ingrowth offer an advantage over uncovered stents is uncertain because covered stents are associated with higher rates of migration and acute cholecystitis due to occlusion of the cystic duct. Surgical biliary bypass may be considered in patients expected to survive at least 6 months. Surgical duodenal bypass may be considered in patients in whom duodenal obstruction is expected to develop; alternatively, endoscopic placement of a self-expandable duodenal stent may be feasible. Chemoradiation may be used for palliation of unresectable cancer confined to the pancreas. Chemotherapy has been disappointing in metastatic pancreatic cancer, although improved response rates have been reported with FOLFIRINOX and with the combination of gemcitabine and nab-paclitaxel. In patients who have received prior chemotherapy, 5-fluorouracil and leucovorin in combination with nanoliposomal irinotecan has resulted in improved survival compared with 5-fluorouracil and leucovorin alone. Celiac plexus nerve block (under CT or endoscopic ultrasound guidance) or thoracoscopic splanchnicectomy may improve pain control.

Surgical resection is the treatment of choice for NETs, when feasible. Metastatic disease may be controlled with long-acting somatostatin analogs, interferon, chemotherapy, peptide-receptor radionuclide therapy, and chemoembolization. For potentially neoplastic cystic lesions, there is a consensus that asymptomatic incidental pancreatic cysts 2 cm or smaller are at low risk for harboring invasive carcinoma. The cysts may be monitored by imaging tests (MRI) in 1 year and then every 2 years for 5 years and perhaps longer if no changes are observed, with EUS and FNA if a cyst enlarges to 3 cm and another high-risk feature (dilated main pancreatic duct, presence of a solid component) develops. The optimal approach is uncertain, however, and other guidelines have been proposed.

Surgical resection is indicated for mucinous cystic neoplasms, symptomatic serous cystadenomas, solid pseudopapillary tumors (which have a 15% risk of malignant transformation), and cystic tumors larger than 2 cm in diameter that remain undefined after helical CT, EUS, and diagnostic aspiration. All intraductal papillary mucinous neoplasms of the main pancreatic duct should be resected, but those of branch ducts may be monitored with serial imaging if they (1) are asymptomatic and exhibit benign features; (2) have a diameter less than 3 cm (some authorities recommend a diameter 1.5 cm or smaller, but even lesions 3 cm or larger may be monitored in elderly persons with no other worrisome cyst features); and (3) lack non-enhancing mural nodules, a thick wall, an abrupt change in the caliber of the pancreatic duct with distal pancreatic atrophy, or possibly bile duct dilatation and gallbladder adenomyomatosis. Most such lesions with benign features remain stable on follow-up, but the risk of malignancy persists for at least 10 years. Moreover, the risk of pancreatic ductal carcinoma and of nonpancreatic cancers may also be increased in this group of patients. In the absence of locally advanced disease, survival is higher for malignant cystic neoplasms than for adenocarcinoma. Endoscopic resection or ablation, with temporary placement of a pancreatic duct stent, may be feasible for ampullary adenomas, but patients must be followed for recurrence.

▶ Prognosis

Carcinoma of the pancreas, especially in the body or tail, has a poor prognosis; 80–85% of patients present with advanced unresectable disease, and reported 5-year survival rates range from 2% to 5%. From 1980 to 2010, mortality from pancreatic cancer did not decrease, but it may now be starting to improve. Obesity may adversely affect mortality in Western countries. Metformin may improve survival in diabetic patients with pancreatic adenocarcinoma, and use of HMG-CoA reductase inhibitors (statins) preceding a diagnosis of pancreatic cancer may improve survival. Tumors of the ampulla have a better prognosis, with reported 5-year survival rates of 20–40% after resection; jaundice and lymph node involvement are adverse prognostic factors. In carefully selected patients, resection of cancer of the pancreatic head is feasible and results in reasonable survival. In persons with a family history of pancreatic cancer in at least two first-degree relatives, or with a genetic syndrome associated with an increased risk of pancreatic cancer, screening with EUS and helical CT or MRI/MRCP should be considered beginning at age 40–45 or 10 years before the age at which pancreatic cancer was first diagnosed in a family member.

For those patients whose disease progresses despite treatment, meticulous efforts at palliative care are essential (see Chapter 5).

▶ When to Refer

All patients with carcinoma involving the pancreas and the ampulla of Vater should be referred to a specialist.

▶ When to Admit

Patients who require surgery and other interventions should be hospitalized.

Canto MI et al. Risk of neoplastic progression in individuals at high risk for pancreatic cancer undergoing long-term surveillance. Gastroenterology. 2018 Sep;155(3):740–51. [PMID: 29803839]

Elta GH et al. ACG Clinical Guideline: diagnosis and management of pancreatic cysts. Am J Gastroenterol. 2018 Apr;113(4):464–79. [PMID: 29485131]

Khalaf N et al. Regular use of aspirin or non-aspirin nonsteroidal anti-inflammatory drugs is not associated with risk of incident pancreatic cancer in two large cohort studies. Gastroenterology. 2018 Apr;154(5):1380–90. [PMID: 29229401]

Neoptolemos JP et al. Therapeutic developments in pancreatic cancer: current and future perspectives. Nat Rev Gastroenterol Hepatol. 2018 Jun;15(6):333–48. [PMID: 29717230]

Vilas-Boas F et al. Pancreatic cystic lesions: new endoscopic trends in diagnosis. J Clin Gastroenterol. 2018 Jan;52(1):13–9. [PMID: 29087991]

ALIMENTARY TRACT CANCERS

Carling Ursem, MD

Kenneth R. McQuaid, MD

ESOPHAGEAL CANCER

ESSENTIALS OF DIAGNOSIS

▶ Progressive dysphagia to solid food.

▶ Weight loss common.

▶ Endoscopy with biopsy establishes diagnosis.

▶ General Considerations

Esophageal cancer usually develops in persons between 50 and 70 years of age. There were an estimated 17,920 new cases of esophageal cancer in 2018. The overall ratio of men to women is 3:1. There are two histologic types: squamous cell carcinoma and adenocarcinoma. Squamous cell carcinoma is common in Eastern Europe and Asia while adenocarcinoma is more common in North America and most Western European countries. In the United States, **squamous cell carcinoma** is much more common in blacks than in whites. Chronic alcohol and tobacco use are strongly associated with an increased risk of squamous cell carcinoma. **Adenocarcinoma** is more common in whites. Its incidence is increasing dramatically, and it is now more common than squamous cell carcinoma in the United States. The majority of adenocarcinomas develop as a complication of Barrett metaplasia due to chronic gastroesophageal reflux. Thus, most adenocarcinomas arise near the gastroesophageal junction. Obesity also is strongly associated with adenocarcinoma, even after controlling for gastroesophageal reflux.

▶ Clinical Findings

A. Symptoms and Signs

The majority (50–60%) of patients with esophageal cancer present with advanced, incurable disease. While early symptoms are nonspecific and subtle, over 90% eventually have solid food dysphagia, which progresses over weeks to months. Odynophagia is sometimes present. Significant weight loss is common. Local tumor extension into the tracheobronchial tree may result in a tracheo-esophageal fistula, characterized by coughing on swallowing or by pneumonia. Chest or back pain suggests mediastinal extension. Recurrent laryngeal nerve involvement may produce hoarseness. Physical examination is often unrevealing. The presence of supraclavicular or cervical lymphadenopathy or of hepatomegaly implies metastatic disease.

B. Laboratory Findings

Laboratory findings are nonspecific. Anemia related to chronic disease or occult blood loss is common. Elevated aminotransferase or alkaline phosphatase concentrations suggest hepatic or bony metastases. Hypoalbuminemia may result from malnutrition.

C. Imaging

A barium esophagogram may be the first study obtained to evaluate dysphagia. The appearance of a polypoid, obstructive, or ulcerative lesion is suggestive of carcinoma and requires endoscopic evaluation. However, even lesions believed to be benign by radiography warrant endoscopic evaluation. Chest radiographs may show adenopathy, a widened mediastinum, pulmonary or bony metastases, or signs of tracheo-esophageal fistula such as pneumonia.

D. Upper Endoscopy

Endoscopy with biopsy establishes the diagnosis of esophageal carcinoma with a high degree of reliability. In some cases, significant submucosal spread of the tumor may yield nondiagnostic mucosal biopsies. Repeat biopsy may be necessary.

► Staging

After confirmation of the diagnosis of esophageal carcinoma, the stage of the disease should be determined since doing so influences the choice of therapy. Patients should undergo evaluation with contrast CT of the chest and abdomen to look for evidence of pulmonary or hepatic metastases, lymphadenopathy, and local tumor extension. If there is no evidence of distant metastases or extensive local spread on CT, then EUS with guided FNA biopsy of suspicious lymph nodes should be performed to evaluate the locoregional stage. EUS is superior to CT in demonstrating the level of local mediastinal extension and local lymph node involvement. PET with fluorodeoxyglucose or integrated PET-CT imaging is indicated to look for regional or distant spread in patients thought to have localized disease after other diagnostic studies, prior to invasive surgery. Bronchoscopy is sometimes required in esophageal cancers above the carina to exclude tracheobronchial extension. Laparoscopy to exclude occult peritoneal carcinomatosis should be considered in patients with tumors at or near the gastroesophageal junction (see Gastric Adenocarcinoma).

► Differential Diagnosis

Esophageal carcinoma must be distinguished from other causes of progressive dysphagia, including peptic stricture, achalasia, and adenocarcinoma of the gastric cardia with esophageal involvement. Benign-appearing peptic strictures should be biopsied at presentation to exclude occult malignancy.

► Treatment

The approach to esophageal cancer depends on the tumor stage, tumor location, patient preference and functional status, and the expertise of the gastroenterologists, surgeons, oncologists, and radiation oncologists. It is helpful to classify patients into two general categories: those with early stage (curable) disease and those with advanced stage (incurable) disease.

A. Therapy for "Curable" Disease

Superficial esophageal cancers confined to the epithelium (high-grade dysplasia or carcinoma in situ [Tis]), lamina propria (T1a), or submucosal (T1b) are increasingly recognized in endoscopic screening and surveillance programs. Esophagectomy achieves high cure rates for superficial tumors but is associated with mortality (2%) and morbidity. If performed by experienced clinicians, endoscopic mucosal resection of Tis and T1a cancers achieves equivalent long-term survival with less morbidity (see Barrett Esophagus, Chapter 15). Patients with larger tumors or deeper tumors invasive to the submucosa (T1b) have higher rates of lymph node metastasis. For this reason, an esophagectomy is recommended for those with T1b tumors. If only endoscopic mucosal resection is performed, then frequent posttreatment endoscopic surveillance is required to ensure there is no residual or recurrent tumor.

1. Surgery with or without neoadjuvant chemoradiation therapy—There are multiple surgical approaches to the resection of invasive (non-superficial) but potentially "curable" esophageal cancers (stage Ib, II, IIIA, or IIIB). Accepted techniques include en bloc transthoracic excision of the esophagus with extended lymph node dissection, transhiatal esophagogastrectomy (entailing laparotomy with cervical anastomosis), and minimally invasive esophagectomy techniques. Meta-analysis data suggest equivalent oncologic outcomes from minimally invasive esophagectomy and conventional open techniques, although there are fewer postoperative complications and shorter hospital stays with the laparoscopic approach. There is general consensus that at least a D1 lymphadenectomy should be performed. However, there is much debate about whether the D2 lymphadenectomy typically performed in higher-incidence countries (such as Japan and South Korea) is superior to the D1 lymphadenectomy more commonly performed in the United States where the incidence of esophageal cancers is lower. Multiple meta-analyses have shown that regardless of surgery type, surgery at a high-volume hospital is associated with decreased perioperative mortality.

Patients with stage I tumors have high cure rates with surgery alone and do not require radiation or chemotherapy. If regional lymph node metastases have occurred (stages IIB and III), the rate of cure with surgery alone is reduced to less than 20%. Meta-analysis of trials comparing neoadjuvant (preoperative) therapy followed by surgery with surgery alone suggests a 13% absolute improvement in 2-year survival with combined therapy. Preoperative (neoadjuvant) chemoradiation therapy is recommended for stage IIA, IIB, and III tumors in fit patients. The preferred neoadjuvant chemotherapy regimen used with radiation is weekly carboplatin plus paclitaxel (Table 39–2). As an alternative, a combination of cisplatin plus 5-fluorouracil may be used along with radiation. When radiation therapy is considered, techniques that are less toxic such as intensity-modulated radiation therapy (IMRT) or proton beam therapy may be considered. Perioperative chemotherapy without radiation may also be considered for tumors of the gastroesophageal junction based on the randomized, multicenter, phase III MAGIC trial.

2. Chemotherapy plus radiation therapy without surgery—
Combined treatment with chemotherapy and radiation is superior to radiation alone and has achieved long-term survival rates in up to 25% of patients. Chemoradiation alone should be considered in patients with localized disease (stage II or IIIA) who are poor surgical candidates due to serious medical illness or poor functional status (Eastern Cooperative Oncology Group score greater than 2). Chemoradiation alone as definitive, nonsurgical therapy is more likely to achieve short-term and long-term survival in patients with squamous cell carcinoma than in patients with adenocarcinoma. This is especially true for patients with cervical esophageal cancers, which appear similar biologically to head and neck cancers.

3. Supportive care during definitive therapy—Patients with significant tumor obstruction may require local measures such as esophageal stent placement or percutaneous gastric or jejunal tube placement to maintain adequate hydration and nutrition during neoadjuvant chemoradiation or chemotherapy. Multidisciplinary consultation is required to determine the optimal procedure. Consultation with a nutritionist also is appropriate to optimize nutrition perioperatively.

B. Therapy for Incurable Disease

More than half of patients have either locally extensive tumor spread (T4b) that is unresectable or distant metastases (M1) (stage IIIC and stage IV). Surgery is not warranted in these patients. Since prolonged survival can be achieved in few patients, the primary goal is to provide relief from dysphagia and pain, optimize quality of life, and minimize treatment side effects. The optimal palliative approach depends on the presence or absence of metastatic disease, expected survival, patient preference, and institutional experience.

1. Chemotherapy or chemoradiation—Combined radiation therapy and chemotherapy may achieve palliation in two-thirds of patients but is associated with significant side effects. It should be considered for patients with locally advanced tumors without distant metastases (stage IIIC) who have good functional status and no significant medical problems, in whom prolonged survival may be achieved. Improvement in dysphagia occurs within 2–4 weeks in almost 90% of patients.

It should be noted that the systemic therapy treatment options are the same for metastatic esophageal,

gastroesophageal junction, and gastric cancers. This is true regardless of squamous cell or adenocarcinoma histology, with the exceptions noted below (Table 39–2). Combination chemotherapy may be considered in patients with metastatic disease who still have good functional status and expected survival of at least several months. Because of the decreased toxicity of two-drug regimens, they are preferred over three-drug regimens. For patients with poor functional status, single-agent therapy with a fluoropyrimidine, a taxane, or irinotecan may be used. In patients with metastatic distal esophageal and gastroesophageal junction adenocarcinomas positive for amplification of the *HER2* gene (approximately 15% of cases), addition of the monoclonal antibody trastuzumab (see Chapter 17) to chemotherapy is associated with prolonged survival. In addition, ramucirumab, a monoclonal antibody targeting the VEGF receptor-2, demonstrated a survival advantage in patients with adenocarcinoma of the gastroesophageal junction after progression on first-line therapy when used both as monotherapy and in combination with paclitaxel (Tables 39–2 and 39–3). As with all metastatic solid tumors, immunotherapy with pembrolizumab should be considered if the tumor is either microsatellite instability-high (MSI-H) or has deficient mismatch repair protein expression (dMMR). For the remainder of metastatic esophageal cancers, a PD-1 or PD-L1 targeted agent should be considered in the second-line or later setting.

2. Local therapy for esophageal obstruction—Patients with advanced esophageal cancer often have a poor functional and nutritional status. Radiation therapy alone to the area of esophageal obstruction may afford short-term relief of pain and dysphagia. Rapid palliation of dysphagia may be achieved by peroral placement of permanent expandable wire stents (alone or followed by radiation). However, placement of these stents is complicated by perforation, migration, or tumor ingrowth in up to 40% of cases. Palliative feeding tube placement may be considered for hydration and nutrition in selected cases when aligned with the patient's goals of care and overall prognosis.

▶ Prognosis

The overall 5-year survival rate of esophageal carcinoma is less than 20%. Apart from distant metastasis (M1b), the two most important predictors of poor survival are adjacent mediastinal spread (T4) and lymph node involvement. Whereas cure may be achieved in patients with regional lymph node involvement (stages IIB and III), involvement of nodes outside the chest (M1a) is indicative of metastatic disease (stage IV) that is incurable. For those patients whose disease progresses despite chemotherapy, meticulous efforts at palliative care are essential (see Chapter 5).

▶ When to Refer

- Patients should be referred to a gastroenterologist for evaluation and staging (endoscopy with biopsy, EUS) and palliative endoscopic antitumor therapy (stent).

- Patients with curable and resectable disease for whom neoadjuvant therapy may be appropriate (stage IIB or IIIA) should be referred to medical, radiation, and surgical oncologists for consideration of neoadjuvant chemotherapy, chemoradiotherapy, or surgical resection.

- Patients with metastatic disease should be referred to medical and radiation oncologists for consideration of palliative chemotherapy or chemoradiation.

- Patients with metastatic disease and obstructive tumors not amenable to or refractory to palliative radiation or stenting may require referral to an interventional radiologist, gastroenterologist, or surgeon for gastric or jejunal tube placement for liquid artificial nutrition. Early referral to palliative care services may improve symptom management in patients with advanced or metastatic disease.

▶ When to Admit

Patients with high-grade esophageal obstruction with inability to manage oral secretions or maintain hydration should be admitted. Acute complications such as perforation, bleeding, aspiration, or fistula also may require admission.

Abnet CC et al. Epidemiology of esophageal squamous cell carcinoma. Gastroenterology. 2018 Jan;154(2):360–73. Erratum in: Gastroenterology. 2018 Oct;155(4):1281. [PMID: 28823862]

Best LM et al. Non-surgical versus surgical treatment for oesophageal cancer. Cochrane Database Syst Rev. 2016 Mar 29;3:CD011498. [PMID: 27021481]

Janmaat VT et al. Palliative chemotherapy and targeted therapies for esophageal and gastroesophageal junction cancer. Cochrane Database Syst Rev. 2017 Nov 28;11:CD004063. [PMID: 29182797]

Kang YK et al. Nivolumab in patients with advanced gastric or gastro-oesophageal junction cancer refractory to, or intolerant of, at least two previous chemotherapy regimens (ONO-4538-12, ATTRACTION-2): a randomized, double-blind, placebo controlled, phase 3 trial. Lancet. 2017 Dec 2;390(10111):2461–71. [PMID: 28993052]

Klevebro F et al. A randomised clinical trial of neoadjuvant chemotherapy vs. neoadjuvant chemoradiotherapy for cancer of the oesophagus or gastro-oesophageal junction. Ann Oncol. 2016 Apr;27(4):660–7. [PMID: 26782957]

National Comprehensive Cancer Network. Clinical Practice Guidelines in Oncology. Esophageal and esophagogastric junction cancers. Version 2.2018. 2018 May 22. https://www.nccn.org/professionals/physician_gls/pdf/esophageal.pdf

Quante M et al. Insights into the pathophysiology of esophageal adenocarcinoma. Gastroenterology. 2018 Jan;154(2):406–20. [PMID: 29037468]

Vellayappan BA et al. Chemoradiotherapy versus chemoradiotherapy plus surgery for esophageal cancer. Cochrane Database Syst Rev. 2017 Aug 22;8:CD010511. [PMID: 28829911]

GASTRIC ADENOCARCINOMA

ESSENTIALS OF DIAGNOSIS

- ▶ Dyspeptic symptoms with weight loss in patients over age 40 years.

- ▶ Iron deficiency anemia: occult blood in stools.

- ▶ Abnormality detected on upper gastrointestinal series or endoscopy.

▶ General Considerations

Gastric adenocarcinoma remains the second most common cause of cancer death worldwide. However, its incidence has declined rapidly over the last 70 years, especially in Western countries, which may be attributable to changes in diet (more fruits and vegetables), food refrigeration (allowing more fresh foods and reduced salted, smoked, and preserved foods), reduced toxic environmental exposures, and a decline in *Helicobacter pylori*. The incidence of gastric cancer remains high (70/100,000) in Japan and many developing regions, including eastern Asia, Eastern Europe, Chile, Colombia, and Central America. In the United States, there were an estimated 26,240 new cases and 10,800 deaths in 2018. The incidence is higher in Asian Americans, Hispanics, African Americans, and American Indian/Alaska Natives.

There are two main histologic variants of gastric cancer: "intestinal-type" (which resembles intestinal cancers in forming glandular structures) and "diffuse" (which is poorly differentiated, has signet-ring cells, and lacks glandular formation). The incidence of **intestinal-type gastric cancer** has declined significantly, but it is still the more common type (70–80%); it occurs twice as often in men as women, primarily affects older people (mean age 63 years), and is more strongly associated with environmental factors. It is believed to arise through a gradual, multi-step progression from inflammation (most commonly due to *H pylori*), to atrophic gastritis, to intestinal metaplasia, and finally dysplasia or cancer. Chronic *H pylori* gastritis is the strongest risk factor for gastric carcinoma, increasing the relative risk 3.5- to 20-fold. It is estimated that 60–90% of cases of gastric carcinomas may be attributable to *H pylori*. Other risk factors for intestinal-type gastric cancer include pernicious anemia, a history of partial gastric resection more than 15 years previously, smoking, and diets that are high in nitrates or salt and low in vitamin C. **Diffuse gastric cancer** accounts for 20–30% of gastric cancer cases. In contrast to intestinal-type cancer, it affects men and women equally, occurs more commonly in young people, is not as strongly related to *H pylori* infection, and has a worse prognosis than intestinal-type cancer. Most diffuse gastric cancers are attributable to acquired or hereditary mutations in the genes regulating the E-cadherin cell adhesion protein. Hereditary diffuse gastric cancer accounts for 1–3% of gastric cancers. The cancer may arise at a young age, is often multifocal and infiltrating with signet ring cell histology, and confers poor prognosis. Many of these families have a germline mutation of E-cadherin *CDH1*, which is inherited in an autosomal dominant pattern and carries a greater than 60% lifetime risk of gastric cancer. Prophylactic gastrectomy should be considered in patients known to carry this mutation.

Most gastric cancers arise in the body and antrum. These may occur in a variety of morphologic types: (1) polypoid or fungating intraluminal masses; (2) ulcerating masses; (3) diffusely spreading (linitis plastica), in which the tumor spreads through the submucosa, resulting in a rigid, atonic stomach with thickened folds (prognosis dismal); and (4) superficially spreading or "early" gastric cancer—confined to the mucosa or submucosa (with or without lymph node metastases) and associated with a favorable prognosis. *HER2* amplification and overexpression is seen in 10–25% of gastric adenocarcinoma cases and is more commonly observed in intestinal histology and moderately differentiated disease. The prognostic significance of HER2 status is uncertain. Testing for microsatellite instability (MSI), deficiency in mismatch repair proteins (dMMR), and PD-L1 is recommended in advanced disease to identify tumors that may respond to immunotherapy. For gastric adenocarcinoma, MSI-H/dMMR is found in 8–16% of cases.

In contrast to the dramatic decline in cancers of the distal stomach, a rise in incidence of tumors of the gastric cardia has been noted. These tumors have demographic and pathologic features that resemble Barrett-associated esophageal adenocarcinomas (see Esophageal Cancer).

▶ Clinical Findings

A. Symptoms and Signs

Gastric carcinoma is generally asymptomatic until the disease is quite advanced. Symptoms are nonspecific and are determined in part by the location of the tumor. Dyspepsia, vague epigastric pain, anorexia, early satiety, and weight loss are the presenting symptoms in most patients. Patients may derive initial symptomatic relief from over-the-counter remedies, further delaying diagnosis. Ulcerating lesions can lead to acute gastrointestinal bleeding with hematemesis or melena. Pyloric obstruction results in postprandial vomiting. Lower esophageal obstruction causes progressive dysphagia. Physical examination is rarely helpful. Signs of metastatic spread include a left supraclavicular lymph node (Virchow node), an umbilical nodule (Sister Mary Joseph nodule), a rigid rectal shelf (Blumer shelf), and ovarian metastases (Krukenberg tumor). Guaiac-positive stools may be detectable.

B. Laboratory Findings

Iron deficiency anemia due to chronic blood loss or anemia of chronic disease is common. Liver test abnormalities, particularly elevation of alkaline phosphatase, may be present if there is metastasis to the liver. Circulating tumor markers do not have established clinical validity in screening or diagnosis of gastric cancer. However, when checked serially, tumor markers can assist in monitoring treatment response.

C. Endoscopy

Upper endoscopy should be obtained in all patients over age 60 years with new onset of epigastric symptoms (dyspepsia) and young patients with "alarm" symptoms (dysphagia, recurrent vomiting, significant weight loss), especially in immigrants from countries with a high prevalence of gastric cancer. Endoscopy with biopsies of suspicious lesions is highly sensitive for detecting gastric carcinoma. It can be difficult to obtain adequate biopsy specimens in linitis plastica lesions.

D. Imaging

Once a gastric cancer is diagnosed, preoperative evaluation with contrast CT of chest, abdomen, and pelvis and EUS is indicated to delineate the local extent of the primary tumor as well as to evaluate for nodal or distant metastases. EUS is superior to CT in determining the depth of tumor penetration and is useful for evaluation of early gastric cancers that may be removed by endoscopic mucosal resection. PET or combined PET-CT imaging is recommended for detection of distant metastasis.

▶ Screening

Because of its unproven efficacy and cost-effectiveness, screening for *H pylori* infection and treating it to prevent gastric cancer is not recommended for asymptomatic adults in the general population but may be considered in patients who have immigrated from regions with a high incidence of gastric cancer or who have a family history of gastric cancer. Because of the high incidence of gastric carcinoma in Japan, screening upper endoscopy is performed there to detect early gastric carcinoma. Approximately 40% of tumors detected by screening are early, with a 5-year survival rate of almost 90%. Screening is not recommended in the United States.

▶ Staging

Staging is defined according to the TNM system, in which T1 tumors invade the lamina propria or muscularis mucosa (T1a) or submucosa (T1b), T2 invade the muscularis propria, T3 penetrate the subserosal connective tissue, and T4 invade serosa or adjacent structures. Lymph nodes are graded as N0 if there is no involvement, and N1, N2, or N3 if there is involvement of 1–2, 3–6, or more than 7 regional nodes. M0 signifies the absence of metastatic disease and M1, its presence. Sampling of at least 15 lymph nodes is recommended during surgical staging (see Curative Surgical Resection below). A staging laparoscopy prior to definitive surgery to exclude peritoneal carcinomatosis should be considered in patients with stage T1b or greater disease without radiographic evidence of distant metastases. Pathologic review should include (1) grade of tumor, (2) histologic subtype, (3) depth of invasion, (4) whether lymphatic or vascular invasion is present, and (5) if there is known metastatic disease, the status of HER2 protein expression by immunohistochemistry or fluorescent in situ hybridization or both, along with MMR or MSI testing and possibly PD-L1 protein expression.

▶ Differential Diagnosis

Ulcerating gastric adenocarcinomas are distinguished from benign gastric ulcers by biopsies. Approximately 3% of gastric ulcers initially believed to be benign later prove to be malignant. All gastric ulcers identified at endoscopy should be biopsied to exclude malignancy. Ulcers that are suspicious for malignancy to the endoscopist or that have atypia or dysplasia on histologic examination warrant repeat endoscopy in 2–3 months to verify healing and exclude malignancy. Nonhealing ulcers should be considered for resection. Infiltrative carcinoma with thickened gastric folds must be distinguished from lymphoma and other hypertrophic gastropathies.

Treatment

A. Curative Surgical Resection

Surgical resection is the only therapy with curative potential. Laparoscopic techniques achieve similar outcomes and lower overall complication rates as open gastrectomy. After preoperative staging, about two-thirds of patients will be found to have localized disease (ie, stages I–III). In Japan and in specialized centers in the United States, endoscopic mucosal resection is performed in select patients with small (less than 1–2 cm), early (intramucosal or T1aN0) gastric cancers after careful staging with EUS. In a 2018 randomized trial in Korean patients who had endoscopic resection of early gastric cancer, there was a 50% reduction in metachronous gastric cancers over a 5-year period among patients who received treatment for *H pylori* compared with those who received a placebo. Approximately 25% of patients undergoing surgery will be found to have locally unresectable tumors or peritoneal, hepatic, or distant lymph node metastases that are incurable. The remaining patients with confirmed localized disease should undergo radical surgical resection. For adenocarcinoma localized to the distal two-thirds of the stomach, a subtotal gastrectomy should be performed. For proximal gastric cancer or diffusely infiltrating disease, total gastrectomy is necessary. The ultimate goal of surgery is obtaining negative surgical margins. Vitamin B_{12} supplementation is required after gastrectomy. For patients with localized gastric cancer that is resectable, current National Comprehensive Cancer Network (NCCN) treatment guidelines recommend gastrectomy with extended (D1), or modified regional (D2), lymph node dissection and sampling of 15 or more lymph nodes. D2 lymphadenectomy has been shown to improve disease-specific survival but is associated with increased postoperative mortality.

B. Perioperative Chemotherapy or Chemoradiation

The use of perioperative chemotherapy or adjuvant chemoradiation is associated with improved survival in patients with localized or locoregional gastric adenocarcinoma who undergo surgical resection. The choice of treatment depends on the location and extent of tumor, type of surgery, patient comorbidities and performance status, and institutional experience. Tumors arising in the gastroesophageal junction may be treated following algorithms for esophageal primary tumors. Multidisciplinary treatment decision making involving the surgeon, radiation oncologist, and medical oncologist is imperative.

C. Palliative Modalities

Many patients will be found either preoperatively or at the time of surgical exploration to have advanced disease that is not amenable to curative intent surgery due to peritoneal or distant metastases or local invasion of other organs. In some of these cases, palliative resection of the tumor nonetheless may be indicated to alleviate pain, bleeding, or obstruction. For patients with unresectable disease, a surgical diversion with gastrojejunostomy may be indicated to prevent obstruction. Alternatively, unresected tumors may be treated with endoscopic laser or stent therapy, radiation therapy, or angiographic embolization to relieve bleeding or obstruction. Chemotherapy may be considered in patients with metastatic disease who still have good functional status and expected survival of at least several months. The regimens used are the same as those discussed for esophageal and gastroesophageal junction tumors discussed above (Table 39–2).

Prognosis

The 5-year survival of gastric carcinoma is approximately 30%. However, 5-year survival in patients who undergo successful curative resection exceeds 45%. Survival is related to tumor stage, location, and histologic features. Stage I and stage II tumors resected for cure have a greater than 60% long-term survival. Patients with stage III tumors have a poor prognosis (less than 30% long-term survival) and should be considered for enrollment in clinical trials. Even with apparently localized disease, proximal tumors have a 5-year survival of less than 15%. For those whose disease progresses despite therapy, meticulous efforts at palliative care are essential (see Chapter 5).

When to Refer

- Patients with dysphagia, weight loss, protracted vomiting, iron deficiency anemia, melena, or new-onset of dyspepsia (especially if aged 55 years or older or associated with other alarm symptoms) in whom gastric cancer is suspected should be referred for endoscopy.
- Patients should be referred to a surgeon for attempt at curative resection in stage I, II, or III cancer, including staging laparoscopy if indicated.
- Prior to surgery, patients should be referred to an oncologist to determine the role for perioperative chemotherapy or adjuvant chemoradiation or chemotherapy.
- Patients who have undergone gastrectomy require consultation with a nutritionist due to propensity for malnutrition and complications, such as dumping syndrome and vitamin B_{12} deficiency, postoperatively.
- Patients with unresectable or metastatic disease should be referred to an oncologist for consideration of palliative chemotherapy or chemoradiation. Early referral to palliative care services may also be considered for symptom management in patients with advanced and metastatic disease.

When to Admit

Patients with protracted vomiting, inability to maintain hydration or nutrition, or acute bleeding.

Anandappa G et al. Emerging novel therapeutic agents in the treatment of patients with gastroesophageal and gastric adenocarcinoma. Hematol Oncol Clin North Am. 2017 Jun; 31(3):529–44. [PMID: 28501092]

Choi IJ et al. *Helicobacter pylori* treatment for the prevention of metachronous gastric cancer. N Engl J Med. 2018 May 22; 378(12):1085–95. [PMID: 29562147]

Lee YC et al. Association between *Helicobacter pylori* eradication and gastric cancer incidence: a systematic review and meta-analysis. Gastroenterology. 2016 May;150(5):1113–24. [PMID: 26836587]

Makris EA et al. Surgical considerations in the management of gastric adenocarcinoma. Surg Clin North Am. 2017 Apr; 97(2):295–316. [PMID: 28325188]

National Cancer Institute. SEER Cancer Stat Facts: Stomach Cancer, 2019. https://seer.cancer.gov/statfacts/html/stomach .html

National Comprehensive Cancer Network. Clinical Practice Guidelines in Oncology. Gastric Cancer. Version 2.2018. 2018 May 22. https://www.nccn.org/professionals/physician_gls/ pdf/gastric.pdf

Ngamruengphong S et al. Endoscopic management of early gastric adenocarcinoma and preinvasive gastric lesions. Surg Clin North Am. 2017 Apr;97(2):371–85. [PMID: 28325192]

GASTRIC LYMPHOMA

 ESSENTIALS OF DIAGNOSIS

► Symptoms of dyspepsia, weight loss, or anemia.

► Variable abnormalities on upper gastrointestinal series or endoscopy including thickened folds, ulcer, mass, or infiltrating lesions; diagnosis established by endoscopic biopsy.

► Abdominal CT and EUS required for staging.

General Considerations

Gastric lymphomas may be primary (arising from the gastric mucosa) or may represent a site of secondary involvement in patients with nodal lymphomas. Distinguishing advanced primary gastric lymphoma with adjacent nodal spread from advanced nodal lymphoma with secondary gastric spread is essential because the prognosis and treatment of primary and secondary gastric lymphomas are different. Primary gastric lymphoma is the second most common gastric malignancy, accounting for 3–5% of gastric cancers. More than 95% of these are non-Hodgkin B-cell lymphomas mainly consisting of either mucosa-associated lymphoid tissue (MALT)-type lymphoma and diffuse large B-cell lymphoma. Gastric T-cell lymphoma, which is associated with HTLV-1 infection, is rare and makes up 7% of primary gastric lymphomas.

Infection with *H pylori* is an important risk factor for the development of primary gastric lymphoma. Chronic infection with *H pylori* causes an intense lymphocytic inflammatory response that may lead to the development of lymphoid follicles. Over 90% of low-grade primary gastric MALT-type lymphomas are associated with *H pylori* infection.

Clinical Findings & Staging

The clinical presentation and endoscopic appearance of gastric lymphoma are similar to those of adenocarcinoma. Most patients have abdominal pain, weight loss, or bleeding. Patients with diffuse large B-cell lymphoma are more likely to have systemic symptoms and advanced tumor stage. At endoscopy, lymphoma may appear as an ulcer, mass, or diffusely infiltrating lesion. It tends to have horizontal infiltration as opposed to the vertical extension seen in adenocarcinoma. The diagnosis is established with endoscopic biopsy; FNA is not adequate. Since the disease can be multifocal, biopsies of both suspicious and normal-appearing areas are recommended. Biopsy specimens should be tested for *H pylori* and, if positive, for t(11;18) via PCR or FISH. EUS is the most sensitive test for determining the level of invasion and presence of perigastric lymphadenopathy and should be performed for accurate staging, if available. All patients should undergo staging with CT scanning of chest, abdomen, and pelvis. For patients with diffuse large B-cell lymphomas involving the stomach, combination PET-CT imaging, bone marrow biopsy with aspirate, tumor lysis laboratory tests, and hepatitis B and HIV serologies also may be required for staging and treatment planning (see Chapter 13).

Treatment

Treatment of primary gastric lymphomas depends on the tumor histology, grade, and stage. Marginal B-cell lymphomas of the MALT type that are low-grade and localized to the stomach wall (stage IE) or perigastric lymph nodes (stage IIE$_1$) have an excellent prognosis. Patients with primary gastric MALT-lymphoma should be tested for *H pylori* infection and treated if positive. Complete lymphoma regression after successful *H pylori* eradication occurs in approximately 75% of cases of stage IE and approximately 55% with stage IIE low-grade lymphoma. However, 95% of cancers positive for t(11;18) do not respond to antibiotics. Remission may take as long as a year, and relapse occurs in about 2% of cases per year. Restaging with endoscopy and biopsy is recommended 3 months after antibiotic treatment and 3–6 months following radiation therapy. Ultimately, endoscopic surveillance after treatment is recommended every 3–6 months for 5 years to evaluate for recurrence.

In patients whose tumors harbor specific gene translocations, including t(11;18) (API2-MALT1), t(1;14), or t(14;18), rates of remission after *H pylori* eradication are lower, and treatment with radiation may be required. Patients with localized marginal zone MALT-type lymphomas who either are not infected with *H pylori* or do not respond to eradication therapy may be treated with radiation therapy or rituximab, if not a candidate for radiation. Many patients with minimal disease after successful *H pylori* eradication may be observed closely without further therapy.

The long-term survival of low-grade MALT lymphoma for stage I is over 90% and for stage II is 35–65%. Because of a low risk of perforation with either radiation therapy or chemotherapy, surgical resection is no longer recommended. Diffuse large B-cell or other higher-grade lymphomas with secondary gastrointestinal involvement usually present at an advanced stage with widely disseminated disease and are treated according to stage and subtype of lymphoma (see Chapter 13).

Ikoma N et al. Multimodality treatment of gastric lymphoma. Surg Clin North Am. 2017 Apr;97(2):405–20. [PMID: 28325194]

Juárez-Salcedo LM et al. Primary gastric lymphoma, epidemiology, clinical diagnosis, and treatment. Cancer Control. 2018 Jan–Mar;25(1):1073274818778256. [PMID: 29779412]

GASTRIC NEUROENDOCRINE TUMORS

Gastric NETs make up less than 1% of gastric neoplasms. They may occur sporadically or secondary to chronic hypergastrinemia that results in hyperplasia and transformation of enterochromaffin cells in the gastric fundus. The majority of NETs are caused by hypergastrinemia and occur in association with either pernicious anemia (75%) (type 1) or Zollinger-Ellison syndrome (5%) (type 2). Type 1 tumors are associated with chronic atrophic gastritis, gastric achlorhydria, and secondary hypergastrinemia. Initial diagnostic workup includes serum gastrin level, upper endoscopy, and EUS. Gastrin level should be obtained 1 week after the patient has stopped taking protein pump inhibitors. For low-grade tumors (Ki-67 less than 3% or less than 2 mitoses/10 high-power fields [HPF]), somatostatin receptor–based imaging (somatostatin receptor scintigraphy or gallium-68 dotatate PET/CT) should be considered. For high-grade tumors (Ki-67 greater than 20% or greater than 20 mitoses/10 HPF), PET/CT is preferred to evaluate the extent of disease.

For patients with hypergastrinemia (suspected of type 1 or type 2 carcinoid), serum vitamin B_{12} and intrinsic factor antibody levels should be obtained to exclude pernicious anemia. Gastric NETs associated with Zollinger-Ellison syndrome occur almost exclusively in patients with multiple endocrine neoplasia type 1 (MEN 1), in which chromosomal loss of 11q13 has been reported. Gastric NETs caused by hypergastrinemia tend to be multifocal, be smaller than 1 cm, have a low potential for metastatic spread, and thus are unlikely to cause development of the carcinoid syndrome. Small lesions may be successfully treated with endoscopic resection followed by endoscopic surveillance every 6–12 months, or with observation. Antrectomy reduces serum gastrin levels and may lead to regression of small tumors. It can be considered in patients with type 1 gastric NETs to reduce recurrence risk and frequency of post-therapy monitoring. Octreotide therapy may be appropriate for patients with underlying gastrinoma and Zollinger-Ellison syndrome. Patients with tumors larger than 2 cm should undergo endoscopic or surgical resection (see Small Intestinal Adenocarcinomas below).

Type 3 gastric NETs arise sporadically, independent of gastrin production, and account for up to 20% of gastric NETs. Most sporadic gastric NETs are solitary, larger than 2 cm, and have a strong propensity for hepatic or pulmonary metastases and thus the carcinoid syndrome at initial presentation. CT or MRI should be obtained to evaluate for metastatic disease. Localized sporadic NETs should be treated with partial or total gastrectomy and regional lymphadenectomy. Advanced, low-grade gastric NETs can be monitored with serial scans, if asymptomatic. Somatostatin analogs may provide symptomatic relief for patients with functional gastric NETs. Advanced high-grade gastric neuroendocrine carcinomas are treated in a fashion similar to SCLCs.

Amair-Pinedo F et al. The treatment landscape and new opportunities of molecular targeted therapies in gastroenteropancreatic neuroendocrine tumors. Target Oncol. 2017 Dec;12(6):757–74. [PMID: 29143176]

Corey B et al. Neuroendocrine tumors of the stomach. Surg Clin North Am. 2017 Apr;97(2):333–43. [PMID: 28325190]

National Comprehensive Cancer Network. Clinical Practice Guidelines in Oncology. Neuroendocrine and Adrenal Tumors. Version 3.2018. 2018 Sep 3. https://www.nccn.org/professionals/physician_gls/pdf/neuroendocrine.pdf

GASTROINTESTINAL MESENCHYMAL TUMORS

Gastrointestinal mesenchymal tumors (which include stromal tumors, leiomyomas, and schwannomas) derive from mesenchymal stem cells and have an epithelioid or spindle cell histologic pattern, resembling smooth muscle. The most common stromal tumors are gastrointestinal stromal tumors ("GISTs"), which originate from interstitial cells of Cajal. GISTs occur throughout the gastrointestinal tract, but most commonly in the stomach (60%) and small intestine (30%). Approximately 85–90% of GISTs have mutations in *KIT*. Mesenchymal tumors may be discovered incidentally on imaging studies or endoscopy or may cause symptoms (most commonly bleeding, pain, or obstruction). At endoscopy, they appear as a submucosal mass that may have central umbilication or ulceration. EUS with guided FNA biopsy is the optimal study for diagnosing gastric mesenchymal tumors and distinguishing them from other submucosal lesions. Percutaneous biopsy may confer risk of bleeding or intra-abdominal seeding. CT of the abdomen and pelvis with contrast, MRI, and PET imaging are useful in the diagnosis and staging. PET imaging also may be useful to monitor response to treatment.

While almost all GISTs have malignant potential, the risk of developing metastasis is increased with tumor size greater than 2 cm, nongastric location, and mitotic index greater than 5 mitoses per 50 HPF. It is difficult to distinguish benign from malignant tumors by EUS appearance or by FNA. But, in general, lesions are more likely benign if they are smaller than 2 cm, have a smooth border, and have a homogeneous echo pattern on EUS. Resection settles the issue.

Surgery is recommended for all patients with tumors that are 2 cm or larger, increasing in size, have an EUS appearance suspicious for malignancy, or are symptomatic. The management of asymptomatic gastric lesions 2 cm or smaller in size depends on the EUS features. Tumors with high-risk EUS features can be surgically resected. If no high-risk features are noted, endoscopic surveillance can be performed. Because of the low but real long-term risk of malignancy, surgical resection should be considered in younger, otherwise healthy patients. However, other patients may be monitored with serial endoscopic ultrasonographic examinations or, in select cases, endoscopic resections. After complete surgical resection, GISTs recur within 5 years in over half of patients. The majority of recurrences are within the first 3 years. Adjuvant therapy with imatinib delays recurrence and prolongs survival, but it is not likely to be curative. Adjuvant imatinib is recommended for all high-risk patients for at least 1 year, though the 5-year recurrence-free survival rate is significantly better following 3 years than 1 year of such therapy (65.6% vs 47.9%). After surgical resection, patients should have surveillance with history and physical examination and CT of the abdomen and pelvis every 3–6 months. Neoadjuvant therapy with imatinib may be considered for patients with localized GIST tumors who are deemed to be at high risk for resection because of comorbidities, tumor size, or tumor location. A biopsy is required to confirm the diagnosis of GIST prior to initiation of neoadjuvant imatinib.

Untreated metastatic GIST tumors are aggressive and carry a poor prognosis. Imatinib induces disease control in up to 85% of patients with metastatic disease with a progression-free survival of 20–24 months and median overall survival of almost 5 years. Additionally, imatinib is associated with long-term survival in some patients. One study reported 18% of patients continued treatment after a median follow-up of 9 years. Imatinib-resistant tumors may respond to high-dose imatinib or to sunitinib, another multi-targeted kinase inhibitor that is approved as second-line therapy for metastatic GIST. For patients who have progressive disease after treatment with imatinib and sunitinib, the multi-targeted kinase inhibitor regorafenib can be considered.

El-Menyar A et al. Diagnosis and management of gastrointestinal stromal tumors: an up-to-date literature review. J Cancer Res Ther. 2017 Oct–Dec;13(6):889–900. [PMID: 29237949]

Heinrich MC et al. Correlation of long-term results of imatinib in advanced gastrointestinal stromal tumors with next-generation sequencing results: analysis of Phase 3 SWOG Intergroup Trial S0033. JAMA Oncol. 2017 Jul 1;3(7):944–52. [PMID: 28196207]

Schrage Y et al. Surgical management of metastatic gastrointestinal stromal tumour. Eur J Surg Oncol. 2018 Sep;44(9):1295–300. [PMID: 30131102]

Søreide K et al. Global epidemiology of gastrointestinal stromal tumours (GIST): a systematic review of population-based cohort studies. Cancer Epidemiol. 2016 Feb;40:39–46. [PMID: 26618334]

Xiong H et al. Laparoscopic surgery versus open resection in patients with gastrointestinal stromal tumors: an updated systematic review and meta-analysis. Am J Surg. 2017 Sep; 214(3):538–46. [PMID: 28412996]

MALIGNANCIES OF THE SMALL INTESTINE

1. Small Intestinal Adenocarcinomas

These are aggressive tumors that occur most commonly in the duodenum or proximal jejunum. The incidence is rare, with 10,470 new diagnoses estimated in 2018 in the United States. Overall, prognosis is poor, with 5-year survival of 85% for localized disease, 75% for regional disease, and 42% for distant disease (overall, 27% of patients are stage IV at diagnosis). The management of small intestinal adenocarcinoma is extrapolated from data available for the management of colon adenocarcinoma. The ampulla of Vater is the most common site of small bowel carcinoma. The incidence of ampullary carcinoma is increased more than 200-fold in patients with familial adenomatous polyposis. Periodic endoscopic surveillance to detect early ampullary neoplasms is therefore recommended. Ampullary carcinoma may present with jaundice due to bile duct

obstruction or bleeding. Surgical resection of early lesions is curative in up to 40% of patients.

2. Small Intestinal Lymphomas

Lymphomas may arise primarily in the gastrointestinal tract or may involve it secondarily in patients with disseminated disease. In Western countries, primary gastrointestinal lymphomas account for 5% of lymphomas and 20% of small bowel malignancies. They occur most commonly in the small intestine. There is an increased incidence of small intestinal lymphomas in patients with AIDS, Crohn disease, and those receiving immunosuppressive therapy. The most common histologic subtype is non-Hodgkin extranodal marginal zone (MALT) B-cell lymphoma. Enteropathy-associated T-cell lymphomas appear to be increasing in incidence in the United States. They are associated with the diagnosis of celiac disease. In the Middle East, lymphomas may arise in the setting of immunoproliferative small intestinal disease. Other types of intestinal lymphomas include primary intestinal follicular cell lymphoma, mantle cell lymphoma, and Burkitt lymphoma (see Chapter 13).

Presenting symptoms or signs of primary small bowel lymphoma include abdominal pain, weight loss, nausea and vomiting, distention, anemia, and occult blood in the stool. Fevers are unusual. Protein-losing enteropathy may result in hypoalbuminemia, but other signs of malabsorption are unusual. Barium radiography or CT enterography helps localize the site of the lesion. The diagnosis requires endoscopic, percutaneous, or laparoscopic biopsy. Imaging and possibly bone marrow biopsy are required to determine stage.

Treatment depends on the tumor histologic subtype and stage of disease (see Chapter 13). Surgical resection of primary intestinal lymphoma, if feasible, may be appropriate for localized tumors. In patients with limited disease (stage IE) in whom resection is performed with negative margins, the role of adjuvant chemotherapy is unclear. Locoregional radiation should be considered if surgical margins are positive. Patients with more extensive disease generally are treated according to the tumor histology.

3. Intestinal Neuroendocrine Tumors

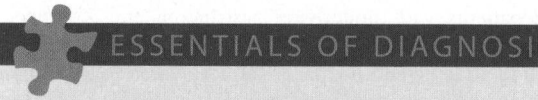

ESSENTIALS OF DIAGNOSIS

▶ Majority are asymptomatic and discovered incidentally at endoscopy or surgery.

▶ Carcinoid syndrome occurs in less than 10%; hepatic metastases are generally present.

▶ Risk of metastasis is related to tumor size and location.

▶ General Considerations

Neuroendocrine tumors account for approximately one-third of tumors arising in the small bowel. Gastrointestinal NETs most commonly occur in the small intestine (45%) but are also found in the rectum (20%), appendix (17%), and colon (11%), with the remainder occurring in the stomach (less than 10%; see Gastric Neuroendocrine Tumors above). Carcinoid tumors are well-differentiated tumors that may secrete a variety of hormones, including serotonin, somatostatin, gastrin, and substance P.

Small intestinal carcinoids most commonly arise in the distal ileum within 60 cm of the ileocecal valve. Up to 30% are multicentric. Although many carcinoids behave in an indolent fashion, the overall 5-year survival rates for patients with locoregional and metastatic small bowel carcinoids are approximately 65% and 35%, respectively. The risk of metastatic spread increases when the tumor is 1 cm or larger and when it is larger than 2 cm with invasion beyond muscularis propria. Appendiceal carcinoids are identified in 0.3% of appendectomies, usually as an incidental finding. Almost 80% of these tumors are smaller than 1 cm, and 90% are smaller than 2 cm. However, in patients with appendiceal carcinoid tumors larger than 2 cm, approximately 90% develop nodal and distant metastases; right hemicolectomy is recommended in these cases.

Rectal carcinoids are usually detected incidentally as submucosal nodules during proctoscopic examination and often locally excised by biopsy or snare polypectomy before the histologic diagnosis is known. Endorectal ultrasound is usually recommended to assess the size, presence, and depth of invasion, and presence of lymph node metastases. Rectal carcinoids smaller than 1 cm virtually never metastasize and are treated effectively with local endoscopic or transanal excision. Larger tumors are associated with the development of metastasis in 10%. Hence, a more extensive cancer resection operation is warranted in fit patients with rectal carcinoid tumors larger than 1–2 cm or with high-risk features (such as invasion of muscularis propria or evidence of nodal involvement), or both.

▶ Clinical Findings

A. Symptoms and Signs

Most lesions smaller than 1–2 cm are asymptomatic and difficult to detect by endoscopy or imaging studies. Small intestinal carcinoids may present with abdominal pain, bowel obstruction, bleeding, or bowel infarction. Appendiceal and rectal carcinoids usually are small and asymptomatic, but large lesions can cause bleeding, obstruction, or altered bowel habits. **Carcinoid syndrome** occurs in less than 10% of patients. More than 90% of patients with carcinoid syndrome have hepatic metastases, usually from carcinoids of small bowel origin. About 10% of patients with carcinoid syndrome have primary bronchial or ovarian tumors without hepatic metastases. Carcinoid syndrome is caused by tumor secretion of hormonal mediators. The manifestations include facial flushing, edema of the head and neck (especially with bronchial carcinoid), abdominal cramps and diarrhea, bronchospasm, cardiac lesions (pulmonary or tricuspid stenosis or regurgitation in 10–30%), and telangiectases.

B. Laboratory Findings

Serum chromogranin A (CgA) is elevated in the majority of NETs, although its sensitivity for small, localized carcinoid tumors is unknown. CgA is elevated in almost 90% of patients with advanced small bowel carcinoid. Urinary 5-hydroxyindoleacetic acid (5-HIAA) and platelet serotonin levels are also elevated in patients with metastatic carcinoid; however, these tests are less sensitive than CgA. There is increased urinary 5-HIAA in carcinoid syndrome; symptomatic patients usually excrete more than 25 mg of 5-HIAA per day in the urine. Because certain foods and medications can interfere with 5-HIAA levels, these should be withheld for 48 hours prior to a 24-hour urine collection.

C. Imaging

Abdominal CT may demonstrate a mesenteric mass with tethering of the bowel, lymphadenopathy, and hepatic metastasis. Abdominal CT or enterography may reveal kinking of the bowel, but because the lesion is extraluminal, the diagnosis may be overlooked for several years. Somatostatin receptor scintigraphy (OctreoScan) and gallium Ga-68 DOTATATE PET scan are routinely used in staging and can help identify diseases that may benefit from treatment with somatostatin analogs.

▶ Treatment & Outcomes

Small intestinal carcinoids generally are indolent tumors with slow spread. Patients with disease confined to the small intestine should be treated with surgical excision. There is no proven role for adjuvant therapy after complete resection. Five-year survival rates for patients with stage I and II disease are 96% and 87%, respectively. In patients with resectable disease who have lymph node involvement (stage III), the 5-year survival is 74%; however, by 25 years, less than 25% remain disease free. Even patients with metastatic disease may have an indolent course with a 5-year survival of 43%.

In patients with advanced disease, therapy historically has been deferred until the patient is symptomatic. Conventional cytotoxic chemotherapy agents do not achieve significant responses in carcinoid tumors and have not been associated with improved outcomes. For patients who are symptomatic either from tumor bulk or carcinoid syndrome, the cornerstone of therapy is typically a long-acting somatostatin analog, which inhibits hormone secretion from the carcinoid tumor. In 90% of patients, this results in dramatic relief of symptoms of carcinoid syndrome, including diarrhea or flushing, for a median period of 1 year. Thereafter, many patients stop responding to octreotide. Options at disease progression include octreotide dose escalation, or addition of everolimus, the mammalian target of rapamycin (mTOR) inhibitor. For patients with somatostatin receptor–positive disease based on imaging, another option after progression on standard dose somatostatin analog therapy is treatment with peptide receptor radionuclide therapy. Peptide receptor radionuclide therapy consists of a somatostatin analog conjugated to a radioactive isotope such as yttrium-90 or lutetium-177. In the United States, peptide receptor radionuclide therapy is specifically approved for gastroenteropancreatic NETs. Additionally, in selected patients with hepatic-dominant disease, resection of hepatic metastases may provide dramatic improvement in carcinoid syndrome symptoms.

Tumor debulking with liver-directed therapy (chemoembolization or radioembolization) may also provide symptomatic improvement in some of these patients.

Patients with advanced, poorly differentiated intestinal NETs are treated in a similar fashion to those with small cell cancers. They have a poor prognosis.

4. Small Intestine Sarcoma

Sarcomas constitute approximately 10% of small bowel neoplasms and are commonly found in the jejunum and ileum (and in a Meckel diverticulum, if present). Most arise from stromal tumors (GISTs) that stain positive for CD117; a minority arise from smooth muscle tumors (leiomyosarcomas) (see Gastrointestinal Mesenchymal Tumors above). Common symptoms of small intestine sarcoma include pain, weight loss, bleeding, and perforation. As the lesions tend to enlarge extraluminally, obstruction is rare.

Kaposi sarcoma was at one time a common complication in AIDS, but the incidence is declining with antiretroviral therapy. It can also occur in the setting of immunosuppression after organ transplant. Lesions may be present anywhere in the intestinal tract. Visceral involvement usually is associated with cutaneous disease. Most lesions are clinically silent; however, large lesions may be symptomatic. Widespread involvement may be best treated by systemic chemotherapy using single-agent therapy or combinations of pegylated-doxorubicin, paclitaxel, vincristine, bleomycin, or etoposide. Surgery or radiation may be indicated for isolated high-risk lesions.

Aparicio T et al. Small bowel adenocarcinoma. Gastroenterol Clin North Am. 2016 Sep;45(3):447–57. [PMID: 27546842]

Ecker BL et al. Efficacy of adjuvant chemotherapy for small bowel adenocarcinoma: a propensity score-matched analysis. Cancer. 2016 Mar 1;122(5):693–701. [PMID: 26717303]

Elli L et al. Use of enterosocopy for the detection of malignant and premalignant lesions of the small bowel in complicated celiac disease: a meta-analysis. Gastrointest Endosc. 2017 Aug;86(2):264–73. [PMID: 28433612]

Kim JS et al. Imaging and screening of cancer of the small bowel. Radiol Clin North Am. 2017 Nov;55(6):1273–91. [PMID: 28991566]

National Cancer Institute. SEER Cancer Stat Facts: Small Intestine Cancer, 2019. https://seer.cancer.gov/statfacts/html/smint.html

National Comprehensive Cancer Network. Clinical Practice Guidelines in Oncology. Neuroendocrine and adrenal tumors. Version 3.2018. 2018 Sep 11. https://www.nccn.org/professionals/physician_gls/pdf/neuroendocrine.pdf

Ngamruengphong S et al. Prevalence of metastasis and survival of 788 patients with T1 rectal carcinoid tumors. Gastrointest Endosc. 2019 Mar;89(3):602–6. [PMID: 30447216]

Pusceddu S et al. Update on medical treatment of small intestinal neuroendocrine tumors. Expert Rev Anticancer Ther. 2016 Sep;16(9):969–76. [PMID: 27353232]

Rondonotti E et al. Neoplastic diseases of the small bowel. Gastrointest Endosc Clin N Am. 2017 Jan;27(1):93–112. [PMID: 27908521]

Strosberg J et al; NETTER-1 Trial Investigators. Phase 3 trial of (177)Lu-Dotatate for midgut neuroendocrine tumors. N Engl J Med. 2017 Jan 12;376(2):125–35. [PMID: 28076709]

COLORECTAL CANCER

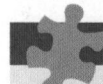

ESSENTIALS OF DIAGNOSIS

► Personal or family history of adenomatous or serrated polyps or colorectal cancer are important risk factors.
► Symptoms or signs depend on tumor location.
► **Proximal colon:** fecal occult blood, anemia.
► **Distal colon:** change in bowel habits, hematochezia.
► Diagnosis established with colonoscopy.

► General Considerations

Colorectal cancer is the second leading cause of death due to malignancy in the United States. Colorectal cancer will develop in approximately 4.2% of Americans and has a 5-year survival rate of 65%. In 2018, there were an estimated 140,250 new cases of colorectal cancer in the United States, with an estimated 50,630 deaths. Between 1996 and 2010, its mortality rate decreased by 46%. During this same period, the percentage of patients 50 years or older who were screened for colorectal cancer increased to 66%. On average, new cases have been falling 3.2% each year over the last 10 years. The colorectal cancer mortality in adults aged 20–54 years increased by 1% annually from 2004 to 2014, although the same trend was not observed in black patients.

Colorectal cancers are almost all adenocarcinomas, which tend to form bulky exophytic masses or annular constricting lesions. The majority of colorectal cancers are thought to arise from malignant transformation of an adenomatous polyp (tubular, tubulovillous, or villous adenoma) or serrated polyp (hyperplastic polyp, traditional serrated adenoma, or sessile serrated adenoma). Polyps that are "advanced" (ie, polyps at least 1 cm in size, adenomas with villous features or high-grade dysplasia, or serrated polyps with dysplasia) are associated with a greater risk of cancer. Approximately 85% of sporadic colorectal cancers arise from adenomatous polyps and have loss of function of one or more tumor suppressor genes (eg, *p53*, *APC*, or *DCC*) due to a combination of spontaneous mutation of one allele combined with chromosomal instability and aneuploidy (abnormal DNA content) that leads to deletion and loss of heterozygosity of the other allele (eg, 5q, 17q, or 18p deletion). Activation of oncogenes such as *KRAS* and *BRAF* is present in a subset of colorectal cancers with prognostic and therapeutic implications discussed further below.

Approximately 10–20% of colorectal cancers arise from serrated polyps, most of which have hypermethylation of CpG-rich promoter regions that leads to inactivation of the DNA mismatch repair gene *MLH1,* resulting in microsatellite instability, and activation of mutations of the *BRAF* gene. Serrated colon cancers have distinct clinical and pathologic characteristics, including diploid DNA content, predominance in the proximal colon, poor differentiation, and more favorable prognosis.

Up to 5% of colorectal cancers are caused by inherited germline mutations resulting in polyposis syndromes (eg, familial adenomatous polyposis) or hereditary nonpolyposis colorectal cancer (HNPCC or Lynch syndrome). These conditions are discussed further in Chapter 15.

Risk Factors

A number of factors increase the risk of developing colorectal cancer. Some of these factors include smoking, consumption of red and processed meats, alcohol intake, diabetes mellitus, physical inactivity, obesity, and history of inflammatory bowel disease. Recognition of these factors has had an impact on screening strategies. However, 75% of all cases occur in people with no known predisposing factors.

A. Age

The incidence of colorectal cancer rises sharply after age 45 years, and 90% of cases occur in persons over the age of 50 years with a median age of 68 years at the time of diagnosis. For unknown reasons, over the past two decades there has been a 50% increase in incidence among adults under age 50, although the risk remains substantially lower than in those over age 50.

B. Family History of Neoplasia

A family history of colorectal cancer is present in approximately 20% of patients with colon cancer. Hereditary factors are believed to contribute to 20–30% of colorectal cancers; however, the genes responsible for most of these cases have not yet been identified. (See Chapter 15 for discussion of inherited polyposis syndromes.) Approximately 6% of the Ashkenazi Jewish population has a missense mutation in the APC gene (APC I1307K) that confers a modestly increased lifetime risk of developing colorectal cancer (OR 1.4–1.9) but phenotypically resembles sporadic colorectal cancer rather than familial adenomatous polyposis. Genetic screening is available, and patients harboring the mutation merit more intensive screening.

A family history of colorectal cancer or adenomatous polyps is one of the most important risk factors for colorectal cancer. The risk of colon cancer is proportionate to the number and age of affected first-degree family members with colon neoplasia. People with one first-degree family member with colorectal cancer have an increased risk approximately two times that of the general population; however, the risk is almost four times if the family member was younger than 45 years when the cancer was diagnosed. Patients with two first-degree relatives have a fourfold increase, or 25–30% lifetime, risk of developing colon cancer. First-degree relatives of patients with adenomatous polyps also have a twofold increased risk for colorectal neoplasia, especially if they were younger than 60 years when the polyp was detected or if the polyp was 10 mm or larger.

C. Inflammatory Bowel Disease

The risk of adenocarcinoma of the colon begins to rise 8 years after disease onset in patients with ulcerative colitis and Crohn colitis (see Chapter 15). For this reason, initiation of surveillance with colonoscopy is recommended at 8–10 years after onset of inflammatory bowel disease symptoms.

D. Dietary and Lifestyle Factors and Chemoprevention in Colorectal Cancer Risk

In epidemiologic studies, diets rich in fats and red meat are associated with an increased risk of colorectal adenomas and cancer, whereas diets high in fruits, vegetables, and fiber are associated with a decreased risk. However, prospective studies have not shown a reduction in colon cancer or recurrence of adenomatous polyps with diets that are low in fat; are high in fiber, fruits or vegetables; or that include calcium, folate, beta-carotene, or vitamin A, C, D, or E supplements.

Low-dose aspirin has been associated with a reduced risk of colorectal adenomas and cancer in multiple studies. A 2016 USPSTF systematic review of controlled trials concluded that prolonged regular use of low-dose aspirin (81 mg/day) is associated with a 40% reduction in colorectal cancer incidence after 10 years and a 33% reduction in colorectal cancer mortality after 20 years. Because long-term aspirin use is associated with a low incidence of serious complications (gastrointestinal hemorrhage, stroke), low-dose aspirin should not be routinely administered as a chemopreventive agent without other medical indications. Persons who are not at increased risk for bleeding, have a life expectancy of at least 10 years, and are willing to take low-dose aspirin daily for at least 10 years are more likely to benefit; persons who place a higher value on its potential benefits than its potential harms may choose to take low-dose aspirin (grade C recommendation). Low-dose aspirin may also be considered in patients with a personal or family history of colorectal cancer or advanced adenomas; however, its administration does not obviate the need for colonoscopy screening and surveillance.

Retrospective analysis of randomized phase III trial data and a meta-analysis have shown that patients with higher levels of pre- and post-diagnosis physical activity experience reduced colorectal cancer–specific mortality and all-cause mortality. Maintaining a healthy body weight, a healthy diet, and a physically active lifestyle are recommended in colorectal cancer survivors.

E. Other Factors

The incidence and mortality of colon adenocarcinoma is higher in blacks than in whites. It is unclear whether this is due to genetic or socioeconomic factors (eg, diet or reduced access to medical care).

Clinical Findings

A. Symptoms and Signs

Adenocarcinomas grow slowly and may be present for several years before symptoms appear. However, some asymptomatic tumors may be detected by the presence of fecal occult blood (see Screening for Colorectal Neoplasms, below). Symptoms depend on the location of the carcinoma. Chronic blood loss from right-sided colonic cancers may cause iron deficiency anemia, manifested by fatigue and weakness. Obstruction, however, is uncommon because of the large diameter of the right colon and the liquid consistency of the fecal material. Lesions of the left colon often involve the bowel circumferentially. Because the left colon has a smaller diameter and the fecal matter is solid, obstructive symptoms may develop with colicky abdominal pain and a change in bowel habits. Constipation may alternate with periods of increased frequency and loose stools. The stool may be streaked with blood, though marked bleeding is unusual. With rectal cancers, patients note tenesmus, urgency, and recurrent hematochezia. Physical examination is usually normal except in advanced disease. The liver should be examined for hepatomegaly, suggesting metastatic spread. For cancers of the distal rectum, digital examination is necessary to determine whether there is extension into the anal sphincter or fixation, suggesting extension to the pelvic floor.

B. Laboratory Findings

A CBC should be obtained to look for anemia. Elevated liver biochemical tests, particularly the serum alkaline phosphatase, raise suspicion of metastatic disease. The serum carcinoembryonic antigen (CEA) should be measured in all patients with proven colorectal cancer but is not appropriate for screening. The CEA is not elevated in many patients with confirmed colorectal cancer; conversely, the CEA may be elevated in active smokers and those with a variety of other nonmalignant conditions. A preoperative CEA level greater than 5 ng/mL is a poor prognostic indicator. After complete surgical resection, CEA levels should normalize; persistently elevated levels suggest the presence of persistent disease and warrant further evaluation. The sensitivity of CEA for detection of recurrence ranges from 68% to 82% and its specificity from 80% to 97%. For this reason, CEA is routinely monitored at the time of adjuvant therapy and during postoperative surveillance for patients who had elevated levels before resection.

C. Colonoscopy

Colonoscopy is the required diagnostic procedure in patients with a clinical history suggestive of colon cancer or in patients with an abnormality suspicious for cancer detected on radiographic imaging. Colonoscopy permits biopsy for pathologic confirmation of malignancy.

D. Imaging

Chest, abdominal, and pelvic CT scans with contrast are required for preoperative staging. CT scans may demonstrate distal metastases but are less accurate in the determination of the level of local tumor extension (T stage) or lymphatic spread (N stage). Intraoperative assessment of the liver by direct palpation and ultrasonography can be performed to detect hepatic metastases (M stage). For rectal cancers (generally defined as tumors arising 12 cm or less proximal to the anal verge), pelvic MRI or endorectal ultrasonography is required to determine the depth of penetration of the cancer through the rectal wall (T stage) and perirectal lymph nodes (N stage), informing decisions about preoperative (neoadjuvant) chemoradiotherapy and

operative management. PET is not routinely used for staging or surveillance in colorectal cancers.

▶ Staging

The TNM system is the commonly used classification to stage colorectal cancer. Staging is important not only because it correlates with the patient's long-term survival but also because it is used to determine which patients should receive adjuvant or neoadjuvant therapy.

▶ Differential Diagnosis

The nonspecific symptoms of colorectal cancer may be confused with those of irritable bowel syndrome, diverticular disease, ischemic colitis, inflammatory bowel disease, infectious colitis, and hemorrhoids. Neoplasm must be excluded in any patient over age 40 years who reports a change in bowel habits or hematochezia or who has an unexplained iron deficiency anemia or occult blood in stool samples.

▶ Treatment

A. Surgery

Resection of the primary colonic or rectal cancer is the treatment of choice for almost all patients who have resectable lesions and can tolerate general anesthesia. For colon cancer, multiple studies demonstrate that minimally invasive, laparoscopically assisted colectomy results in similar outcomes and rates of recurrence to open colectomy. Regional dissection of at least 12 lymph nodes should be performed to determine staging, which guides decisions about adjuvant therapy.

For rectal carcinoma, preoperative (neoadjuvant) chemoradiation with 5-fluorouracil is recommended in all node-positive tumors, and in T3 and greater tumors, due to increased risk of local recurrence (see below). After neoadjuvant therapy, the operative approach depends on the level of the tumor above the anal verge, the size and depth of penetration, and the patient's overall condition. Clinical staging by endorectal ultrasound or MRI with endorectal coil is important in guiding the treatment approach. In carefully selected patients with small, mobile (less than 4 cm), well-differentiated T1 or T2 rectal tumors that are less than 8 cm from the anal verge, transanal excision may be considered. This approach avoids laparotomy and spares the rectum and anal sphincter, preserving normal bowel continence. All other patients will require either a low anterior resection with a colorectal anastomosis or an abdominoperineal resection with a colostomy, depending on how far above the anal verge the tumor is located and the extent of local tumor spread. Careful dissection of the entire mesorectum by either open or laparoscopic surgery reduces local recurrence to 5%. Although low anterior resections obviate a colostomy, they are associated with increased immediate postsurgical complications (eg, leak, dehiscence, stricture) and long-term defecatory complaints (eg, increased stool frequency, and incontinence). With unresectable rectal cancer, the patient may be palliated with a diverting colostomy. Pathology review of colorectal cancers should include testing for mismatch repair proteins for all patients. Tumors of patients with metastatic colorectal cancer should also be tested for extended *RAS* and *BRAF* mutations.

B. Systemic Chemotherapy for Colon Cancer

Chemotherapy has been demonstrated to improve overall and tumor-free survival in select patients with colon cancer depending on stage (Table 39–2).

1. Stage I—Because of the excellent 5-year survival rate (approximately 92%), no adjuvant therapy is recommended for stage I colon cancer. The 5-year survival rate of stage I rectal cancer is approximately 87%.

2. Stage II (node-negative disease)—The 5-year survival rate is approximately 87% for stage IIA disease and 63% for stage IIB disease. A significant survival benefit from adjuvant chemotherapy has not been demonstrated in most randomized clinical trials for stage II colon cancer (see discussion for stage III disease). However, otherwise healthy patients with stage II disease who are at higher risk for recurrence (perforation; obstruction; close or indeterminate margins; poorly differentiated histology; lymphatic, vascular, or perineural invasion; T4 tumors; or fewer than 12 lymph nodes sampled) may benefit from adjuvant chemotherapy. Patients whose tumors reveal microsatellite instability have a more favorable prognosis and do not benefit from 5-fluorouracil-based adjuvant therapy.

3. Stage III (node-positive disease)—With surgical resection alone, the expected 5-year survival rate is 30–50%. Postoperative adjuvant chemotherapy significantly increases disease-free survival as well as overall survival by up to 30% and is recommended for all fit patients (Table 39–2). Multiple large, well-designed studies of adjuvant therapy for stage III colorectal cancer reported a higher rate of disease-free survival at 5 years for patients treated for 6 months postoperatively with a combination of oxaliplatin, 5-fluorouracil, and leucovorin (FOLFOX) (73.3%) than with 5-fluorouracil and leucovorin (FL) alone (67.4%). Similar benefit was reported for patients treated with oxaliplatin and capecitabine (orally active fluoropyrimidine). The benefit of adding oxaliplatin to 5-fluorouracil has not been demonstrated in patients who are 70 years of age or older. A large international randomized controlled trial comparing 3 months with 6 months of adjuvant therapy found that 3 months of therapy resulted in equivalent disease-free survival for patients with earlier stage T1, T2, or T3, and N1 disease but not with more advanced T4 or N2 disease. Additionally, similar disease-free survival was seen with use of 3 months vs 6 months of capecitabine and oxaliplatin but not when infusional 5-fluorouracil plus oxaliplatin was used. The reason for the difference between regimens is currently unknown; the shorter treatment duration did result in significantly less neuropathy across regimens. For patients with high-risk disease (T4 or N2), 6 months of adjuvant chemotherapy are still recommended. The addition of a biologic agent (bevacizumab or cetuximab) to adjuvant chemotherapy does not improve outcomes.

4. Stage IV (metastatic disease)—Approximately 20% of patients have metastatic disease at the time of initial diagnosis, and an additional 30% eventually develop metastasis. A subset of these patients has limited disease that is potentially curable with surgical resection. Resection of isolated liver metastases may result in long-term (over 5 years) survival in 35–55% of cases. For those with unresectable hepatic metastases, local ablative techniques (cryosurgery, radiofrequency or microwave coagulation, embolization, hepatic intra-arterial chemotherapy) may provide long-term tumor control. A subset of patients who have isolated pulmonary metastases may undergo resection with potential cure. The majority of patients with metastatic disease do not have resectable (curable) disease. In the absence of other treatment, the median survival is less than 12 months; however, with current therapies, median survival approaches 30 months. Tumor location has been found to have a potential prognostic importance: median survival rates are 33.3 months for patients with left-sided colon cancers compared to 19.4 months for those with right-sided cancers.

The goals of therapy for patients with metastatic colorectal cancer are to slow tumor progression while maintaining a reasonable quality of life for as long as possible. Currently, either FOLFOX (the addition of oxaliplatin to 5-fluorouracil and folinic acid) or FOLFIRI (the addition of irinotecan to 5-fluorouracil and folinic acid) is the preferred first-line treatment regimen for fit patients. For convenience, oral capecitabine (instead of intravenous 5-fluorouracil and leucovorin) can be used in combination with oxaliplatin as it has similar efficacy to 5-fluorouracil; however, combination with irinotecan is not recommended due to increased toxicity (diarrhea). Addition of a biologic agent to combination chemotherapy improves response rates and overall survival and is recommended in the first-line of treatment in suitable patients. Bevacizumab is a monoclonal antibody targeting VEGF. Combination therapy with bevacizumab and FOLFOX or FOLFIRI prolongs mean survival by 2–5 months compared with either regimen alone. Cetuximab and panitumumab are monoclonal antibodies targeting EGFR. Activating codon 12 and 13 *K-ras* gene mutations downstream of EGFR are present in approximately 35% of patients with metastatic colorectal cancer and are a biomarker for nonresponse to cetuximab and panitumumab, for which reason the use of these agents is restricted to patients with tumors wild-type for *K-ras*. In stage IV patients with *K-ras* wild-type tumors, the addition of panitumumab or cetuximab to FOLFOX or FOLFIRI prolongs survival by approximately 4 months. Bevacizumab may cause serious side effects, including arterial thromboembolic events, bowel perforation, or serious bleeding, in up to 5% of patients. EGFR-targeted agents cause an acneiform rash in the majority of patients. Cetuximab is associated with severe infusion reactions in approximately 2–5%.

When disease progresses despite treatment either with FOLFOX or with FOLFIRI (often in conjunction with bevacizumab or an EGFR-targeted antibody), therapy is switched to the alternate regimen. The novel anti-angiogenic agent, aflibercept, is FDA approved for second-line treatment of colorectal cancer in combination with FOLFIRI. Palliative therapy with cetuximab or panitumumab alone or in combination with irinotecan can benefit patients with *K-ras* wild-type tumors whose disease has progressed after first-line and second-line chemotherapies. Both trifluridine/tipiracil and the multi-targeted kinase inhibitor regorafenib are FDA approved for patients with metastatic, refractory colorectal cancer after progression on standard regimens. Clinical trial participation should be considered for eligible patients who are intolerant of or ineligible for standard therapies or in whom disease has progressed.

C. Neoadjuvant and Adjuvant Therapy for Rectal Cancer

Compared with colon cancer, rectal cancer has lower long-term survival rates and significantly higher rates of local tumor recurrence with surgery alone (approximately 25%) attributed in part to the difficulty of achieving adequate surgical resection margins and to lack of serosal encasement of the rectum. When initial imaging studies suggest stage I disease, surgery may be performed first (see Surgery above). For stage II and III tumors by clinical staging (including endorectal ultrasound or pelvic MRI), preoperative chemoradiation with 5-fluorouracil or capecitabine as a radiation-sensitizing agent improves disease-free survival and decreases pelvic recurrence rate. Preoperative chemoradiation has been shown to be superior to postoperative chemoradiation with lower local recurrence and toxicity rates in the randomized, phase III CAO/ARO/AIO-94 trial. Following surgical resection with total mesorectal excision (see Surgery above), adjuvant 5-fluorouracil–based therapy (generally with the FOLFOX regimen extrapolating from its benefit in patients with similarly-staged colon cancers) is recommended for a total of approximately 6 months of perioperative therapy inclusive of neoadjuvant chemoradiation. Due to its better tolerability and potentially decreased risk of distant metastatic spread, the majority (or even the entirety) of the adjuvant FOLFOX chemotherapy can be given up-front prior to chemoradiation as "total neoadjuvant therapy," per NCCN guidelines.

▶ Follow-Up After Surgery

Patients who have undergone resections for cure are monitored closely to look for evidence of symptomatic or asymptomatic tumor recurrence that may be amenable to curative resection in a small number of patients. Patients should be evaluated every 3–6 months for 2 years and then every 6 months for a total of 5 years with history, physical examination, and laboratory surveillance, including serum CEA levels if baseline levels are elevated. The NCCN and ASCO guidelines recommend surveillance contrast CT scans of chest, abdomen, and pelvis up to every 6 months for up to 5 years post-resection in high-risk stage II and all stage III patients. Patients who had a complete preoperative colonoscopy should undergo another colonoscopy 1 year after surgical resection. Patients who did not undergo full colonoscopy preoperatively also should undergo a full colonoscopy after completion of all adjuvant therapy to exclude other synchronous colorectal neoplasms. If a colonoscopy does not detect new adenomatous polyps 1 year postoperatively, surveillance colonoscopy should be performed every 3–5 years thereafter to look for metachronous polyps or cancer. Because of the high incidence of local tumor recurrence in patients with rectal cancer,

proctoscopy surveillance of the low anterior resection anastomotic site may also be performed periodically. New onset of symptoms or a rising CEA warrants investigation with chest, abdominal, and pelvic CT and colonoscopy to look for a new primary tumor or recurrence, or metachronous metastatic disease that may be amenable to curative or palliative therapy. For patients with a rising CEA level with unrevealing CT imaging, a PET scan may be more sensitive for the detection of occult metastatic disease.

▶ Prognosis

The stage of disease at presentation is the most important determinant of 5-year survival in colon cancer: stage I, greater than 90%; stage II, 70–85%; stage III with fewer than 4 positive lymph nodes, 67%; stage III with more than 4 positive lymph nodes, 33%; and stage IV, 5–7%. For each stage, rectal cancers have a worse prognosis. For those patients whose disease progresses despite therapy, meticulous efforts at palliative care are essential (see Chapter 5).

▶ Screening for Colorectal Neoplasms

Colorectal cancer is ideal for screening because it is a common disease that is fatal in almost 50% of cases and yet is curable if detected at an earlier stage. Furthermore, most cases arise from benign adenomatous or serrated polyps that progress over many years to cancer, and removal of these polyps has been shown to prevent the majority of cancers. Colorectal cancer screening is endorsed by the USPSTF, the Agency for Health Care Policy and Research, the American Cancer Society, and every professional gastroenterology and colorectal surgery society. Although there is continued debate about the optimal cost-effective means of providing population screening, there is unanimous consent that screening of some kind should be offered to every patient over the age of 50 years. Several analyses suggest that screening is cost-effective. It is important for primary care providers to understand the relative merits of various options and to discuss them with their patients.

Only 62.6% of adults over age 50 are up-to-date with colorectal screening. Discussion and encouragement by the primary care provider are the most important factors in achieving patient compliance with screening programs. A 2018 Kaiser Permanente study reported increased participation to 82.5% through an organized screening program. Currently in the United States, the two most widely used strategies are colonoscopy every 10 years or fecal immunochemical testing (FIT) testing annually.

Recommendations for screening from the 2016 USPSTF and 2008 US Multi-Society Task Force (USMSTF) are listed in Table 39–6. Screening is recommended for all men and women 50 through 75 years of age who are at average risk for cancer. Many guidelines recommend screening for African Americans and Alaska Natives beginning at age 45. In 2018, the American Cancer Society provided a qualified recommendation for starting screening at age 45 for average-risk adults; however, other agencies do not feel that available evidence yet supports this recommendation. The potential for harm from screening must be weighed against the likelihood of benefit, especially in elderly patients with

Table 39–6. Recommendations for colorectal cancer screening,[1] including the US Preventive Services Task Force (2016) recommendations[2] and the US Multi-Society Task Force on Colorectal Cancer (2008) recommendations.[2]

Average-risk individuals ≥ 50 years old[2]
Annual fecal occult blood testing using higher sensitivity tests (Hemoccult SENSA)
Annual fecal immunochemical test (FIT)
Fecal DNA test (interval uncertain)
Flexible sigmoidoscopy every 5 years
Colonoscopy every 10 years
CT colonography every 5 years
Individuals with a family history of a first-degree member with colorectal neoplasia[3]
Single first-degree relative with colorectal cancer diagnosed at age 60 years or older: Begin screening at age 40. Screening guidelines same as average-risk individual; however, preferred method is colonoscopy every 10 years.
Single first-degree relative with colorectal cancer or advanced adenoma diagnosed before age 60 years, or two first-degree relatives: Begin screening at age 40 or at age 10 years younger than age at diagnosis of the youngest affected relative, whichever is first in time. Recommended screening: colonoscopy every 5 years.

[1]For recommendations for families with inherited polyposis syndromes or hereditary nonpolyposis colon cancer, see Chapter 15.
[2]Joint Guideline from the American Cancer Society, the US Multi-Society Task Force on Colorectal Cancer, and the American College of Radiology. Gastroenterology 2008 May;134(5):1570–95; and US Preventive Services Task Force. Screening for Colorectal Cancer: US Preventive Services Task Force Recommendation Statement. JAMA. 2016 Jun 21;315(23):2564–75.
[3]American College of Gastroenterology. Guidelines for Colorectal Cancer Screening. Am J Gastroenterol. 2009 Mar;104(3):739–50.

Table 39–7. Revised recommendations for colorectal cancer screening for average-risk individuals from the US Multi-Society Task Force on Colorectal Cancer (2017).[1]

Tier 1[2]
Colonoscopy every 10 years, or
Fecal immunochemical test (FIT) every 1 year
Tier 2[3]
CT colonography every 5 years, or
Flexible sigmoidoscopy every 5–10 years, or
Fecal FIT-fecal DNA testing every 3 years
Tier 3[3]
Colon capsule every 5 years

[1]Screening of individuals considered to be at "average risk" for colorectal cancer is recommended beginning at 50 years of age, except in African-Americans for whom beginning at 45 years of age is supported by some limited data. Since the incidence of colorectal cancer is rising in persons under age 50 years, a thorough diagnostic evaluation is recommended for younger individuals with rectal bleeding. Colorectal screening can be discontinued at 75 years of age in persons who are up-to-date with screening and who have had consistently negative screening tests (especially prior negative colonoscopy), or in individuals who have life expectancies of less than 10 years. Conversely, in persons who have no prior screening, colorectal screening can be initiated and continued to 85 years of age, depending on health and life expectancy.
[2]Colonoscopy and FIT are recommended as the cornerstones of colorectal cancer screening. In a sequential approach in which colonoscopy every 10 years is offered first, FIT done annually should be offered to patients who decline colonoscopy. "Tier 1" designation indicates that colonoscopy and FIT are recommended as the tests of choice even when multiple other options are available. A risk-stratified approach is also considered appropriate with FIT screening in patient populations estimated to have a low prevalence of advanced colonic neoplasia and colonoscopy considered more appropriate in patient populations estimated to have a high prevalence of colonic neoplasia.
[3]Tier 2 and Tier 3 tests may be offered but are considered less suitable due to various disadvantages (see text).
Note: USMSTF screening recommendations vary for individuals considered to be at "high risk" for colorectal cancer: Specifically, for individuals with a family history of colorectal cancer or advanced adenoma in a first-degree relative at age < 60 years or with these findings in two first-degree relatives at any age, screening by colonoscopy every 5 years is recommended, beginning 10 years before the age at diagnosis of the youngest relative or at age 40 years, whichever is earlier. Individuals with a single first-degree relative diagnosed with colorectal cancer or advanced adenoma at age > 60 years are recommended to undertake the "average-risk" screening options shown above but beginning at 40 years of age.
Modified, with permission, from Rex DK et al. Colorectal cancer screening: recommendations for physicians and patients from the U.S. Multi-Society Task Force on Colorectal Cancer. Am J Gastroenterol. 2017 Jul;112(7):1016–30. By permission from Springer Nature.

comorbid illnesses and shorter life expectancy. Although routine screening is not recommended in adults above age 75, it may be considered on a case-by-case basis in adults age 76 through 85 years who have excellent health and functional status. In 2017, the USMSTF issued revised, simplified recommendations in which screening tests were placed into three tiers (Table 39–7). For average-risk patients, colonoscopy every 10 years or FIT testing is preferred (Tier 1). Tier 2 tests (CT colonography every 5 years, flexible sigmoidoscopy every 5 years, or fecal FIT-fecal DNA testing every 3 years) and Tier 3 tests (colon capsule every 5 years) may be offered but are considered less suitable due to various disadvantages (discussed below).

Patients with first-degree relatives with colorectal neoplasms (cancer or adenomatous polyps) are at increased risk. Therefore, most guidelines recommend initiating screening at age 40–50 years (or 10 years younger than the familial diagnosis) in individuals with first-degree relatives with colorectal cancer or with advanced adenomas. Recommendations for screening in families with inherited cancer syndromes or inflammatory bowel disease are provided in Chapter 15. For patients at average risk for colorectal cancer, the recommendations of the USPSTF and USMSTF are discussed below.

Screening tests may be classified into two broad categories: stool-based tests and examinations that visualize the structure of the colon by direct endoscopic inspection or radiographic imaging.

A. Stool-Based Tests

1. Fecal occult blood test—Most colorectal cancers and some large adenomas result in increased chronic blood loss. A variety of tests for fecal occult blood are commercially available that have varying sensitivities and specificities for colorectal neoplasia. These include guaiac-based fecal occult blood tests (gFOBT) (eg, Hemoccult I and II and Hemoccult SENSA) that detect the pseudoperoxidase activity of heme or hemoglobin and FITs that detect human globin. In clinical trials, FITs have proven superior to gFOBT in sensitivity for detection of colorectal cancer and advanced adenomas with similar specificity. Because FITs are not affected by diet or medications and have superior accuracy, the USMSTF now recommends their use instead of gFOBT.

Several FIT kits are commercially available. These tests are highly specific for detecting human globin and therefore eliminate the need for pretest dietary restrictions. In 19 clinical studies, the pooled sensitivity and specificity of FIT for colorectal cancer in average-risk patients were 79% and 94%, respectively. The optimal interval (yearly or every 2 years) and number of stool samples (one or two) required for optimal FIT testing is as yet undetermined. Currently, annual testing of a single stool sample is recommended.

FIT testing is the preferred option for population-based screening in various European and Australian programs. In the United States, it is offered as the preferred option by many healthcare plans. For healthcare systems in which screening colonoscopy is readily available, FIT is a suitable option for patients seeking a noninvasive screening test who are willing to undertake annual fecal testing. Patients with a positive FIT test must undergo further evaluation with colonoscopy.

2. Multitarget DNA assay—Stool DNA tests measure a variety of mutated genes and methylated gene markers from exfoliated tumor cells. A newer-generation assay (Cologuard) combines a fecal DNA panel with a FIT. In a prospective comparative trial conducted in persons at average risk for colorectal cancer undergoing colonoscopy, the sensitivity for colorectal cancer for Cologuard was 92.3% vs 73.8% for FIT alone and the sensitivity for adenomas larger than 1 cm or serrated polyps for Cologuard was 42.4% vs 23.8% for FIT alone. A positive stool DNA test requires colonoscopy evaluation. Compared with FIT testing alone, FIT-fecal DNA testing has disadvantages including higher cost, lower specificity, lower cost-effectiveness, and cumbersome requirements for stool collection and mailing. Hence, the 2017 USMSTF relegated it to Tier 2, noting that it may be recommended in patients age 50–65 years who seek a noninvasive test with high-sensitivity, due to acceptable specificity in this age group.

B. Endoscopic Examinations of the Colon

1. Colonoscopy—Colonoscopy permits examination of the entire colon. In addition to detecting early cancers, colonoscopy allows removal of adenomatous polyps by biopsy or polypectomy, which is believed to reduce the risk of subsequent cancer. Over the past decade, there has been a dramatic increase in screening colonoscopy, with over 60% of US adults screened in the past 10 years. In asymptomatic individuals between 50 and 75 years of age undergoing screening colonoscopy, the prevalence of advanced colonic neoplasia is 4–11% and of colon cancer is 0.1–1%.

Although colonoscopy is believed to be the most sensitive test for detecting adenomas and cancer, it has several disadvantages. To allow adequate visualization of the entire colonic mucosa, it requires thorough bowel cleansing the evening and morning prior to the examination. To alleviate discomfort during the procedure, intravenous sedation is used for most patients, necessitating a companion to transport the patient home post-procedure. Serious complications occur uncommonly; they include perforation (0.1%), bleeding (0.25%), and death (2.9/100,000).

The skill of the operator has a major impact upon the quality of the colonoscopy examination. In several studies, the rate of colorectal cancer within 3 years of a screening colonoscopy was 0.7–0.9%, ie, approximately 1 in 110 patients. This may be attributable to polyps and early cancers that were overlooked during the colonoscopy. Polyps that are small, flat, or located behind folds are easily missed, especially if the bowel preparation is poor. Population-based case-control and cohort studies suggest that colonoscopy is associated with greater reduction in colorectal cancer incidence and mortality in the distal colon (80%) than the proximal colon (40–60%). This may be attributable to incomplete examination of the proximal colon, and differences between the proximal and distal colon that include worse bowel preparation, suboptimal colonoscopic technique, and a higher prevalence of serrated polyps and flat adenomas. To optimize diagnostic accuracy as well as patient safety and comfort, colonoscopy should be performed after optimal bowel preparation by a well-trained endoscopist who spends sufficient time (at least 7 minutes) carefully examining the colon (especially the proximal colon) while withdrawing the endoscope.

2. Flexible sigmoidoscopy—Use of a 60-cm flexible sigmoidoscope permits visualization of the rectosigmoid and descending colon. Adenomatous polyps are identified in 10–20% and colorectal cancers in 1% of patients. The finding at sigmoidoscopy of an adenomatous polyp in the distal colon increases the likelihood at least twofold that an advanced neoplasm is present in the proximal colon.

The chief disadvantage of screening with flexible sigmoidoscopy is that it requires some bowel cleansing, it may be associated with some discomfort (since intravenous sedation is not used), and it does not examine the proximal colon. The prevalence of proximal versus distal neoplasia is higher in persons older than age 65 years, in African Americans, and in women. For these reasons, the 2017 USMSTF recommendations have placed flexible sigmoidoscopy among Tier 2 tests. If chosen, flexible sigmoidoscopy should be performed every 5–10 years.

C. Radiographic and Other Imaging of the Colon

1. CT colonography—Using helical CT with computer-assisted image reconstruction, two- and three-dimensional views can be generated of the colon lumen that simulate the view of colonoscopy (virtual colonoscopy). CT colonography requires a similar bowel cleansing regimen as colonoscopy as well as insufflation of air into the colon through a rectal tube, which may be associated with discomfort. Nonetheless, this examination is performed rapidly and requires no sedation or intravenous contrast. Several large studies have compared the accuracy of virtual colonoscopy with colonoscopy for colorectal screening. Using current imaging software with multidetector helical scanners, the sensitivity is greater than 95% for the detection of cancer and greater than 84–92% for the detection of polyps 10 mm or larger. CT colonography is less sensitive than colonoscopy for the detection of polyps smaller than 1 cm, flat adenomas, and serrated polyps.

Patients undergoing screening with CT colonography should be managed appropriately. If no polyps are found, the interval for repeat screening examination is uncertain; however, 5 years may be reasonable. All patients with polyps 10 mm or larger should be referred for colonoscopy with polypectomy because of the high prevalence (30%) of advanced pathology (cancer, high-grade dysplasia, or villous features) within these polyps. The optimal management of patients with polyps less than 10 mm in size is controversial. The USMSTF currently recommends that colonoscopy with polypectomy be offered to patients with one or more 6–9 mm polyps. Patients who refuse or who have increased risk of carcinoma should undergo surveillance CT colonography in 3–5 years. At the present time, there is no consensus on the management of patients with polyps smaller than 6 mm; however, some radiologists choose not even to report these findings.

The chief disadvantages of CT colonography are the need for a bowel preparation, limited availability in many health care systems, a possible increased risk of neoplasia due to radiation exposure, and the potential for finding incidental extracolonic findings that may lead to further evaluations. The 2017 USMSTF has therefore classified this as a Tier 2 screening option (Table 39–7). CT colonography is an excellent screening option in patients who do not wish to undergo or are unsuitable for colonoscopy and in patients in whom colonoscopy could not be completed.

2. Capsule colonoscopy—Imaging of the colon can be accomplished by oral ingestion of a capsule that captures video images of the colon. Compared with colonoscopy, the colon capsule has reduced sensitivity for polyps greater than 6 mm (64% vs 84%) and for colorectal cancers (74% vs 100%). At present, it is approved by the FDA for evaluation in patients who are not suitable candidates for colonoscopy or in whom colonoscopy could not evaluate the proximal colon. In addition to its suboptimal sensitivity for neoplasia, the main disadvantages of capsule colonoscopy are its cost, need for extensive bowel preparation, lack of reimbursement by most insurance carriers, and small risk of small bowel obstruction. For these reasons, the 2017 USMSTF recommendations classified it a Tier 3 screening test, suitable for highly selected patients (Table 39–7).

3. Barium enema—Double-contrast barium enema was previously used as a screening technique because it was widely available, relatively inexpensive, and safe. However, compared to CT colonography, it is more time-consuming and difficult to perform, less comfortable, and less accurate. It can no longer be recommended for routine screening.

▶ **When to Refer**

- Patients with symptoms (change in bowel habits, hematochezia), signs (mass on abdominal examination or digital rectal examination [DRE]), or laboratory tests (iron deficiency anemia) suggestive of colorectal neoplasia should be referred for colonoscopy.

- Patients with suspected colorectal cancer or adenomatous polyps of any size should be referred for colonoscopy.

- Virtually all patients with proven colorectal cancer should be referred to a surgeon for resection. Patients with clinical stage T3 or node-positive rectal tumors (or both) also should be referred to medical and radiation oncologists preoperatively for neoadjuvant therapy. Patients with stage II, III, or IV colorectal tumors should be referred to a medical oncologist.

▶ **When to Admit**

- Patients with complications of colorectal cancer (obstruction, acute bleeding) requiring urgent evaluation and intervention.

- Patients with severe complications of chemotherapy.

- Patients with advanced metastatic disease requiring palliative care.

Inadomi J. Screening for colorectal neoplasia. N Engl J Med. 2017 Jan 12;376(2):149–56. [PMID: 28076720]

Lauby-Secretan B et al; International Agency for Research on Cancer Handbook Working Group. The IARC perspective on colorectal cancer screening. N Engl J Med. 2018 May 3;378(18):1734–40. [PMID: 29580179]

Leddin D et al. Clinical practice guideline on screening for colorectal cancer in individuals with a family history of nonhereditary colorectal cancer or adenoma: the Canadian Association of Gastroenterology Banff Consensus. Gastroenterology. 2018 Nov;155(5):1325–47. [PMID: 30121253]

Lieberman D et al. Screening for colorectal cancer and evolving issues for physicians and patients: a review. JAMA. 2016 Nov 22;316(20):2135–45. [PMID: 27893135]

Mocellin S et al. Second-line systemic therapy for metastatic colorectal cancer. Cochrane Database Syst Rev. 2017 Jan 27;1:CD006875. [PMID: 28128439]

National Comprehensive Cancer Network. Clinical Practice Guidelines in Oncology. Colon Cancer. Version 4.2018. 2018 Oct 19. https://www.nccn.org/professionals/physician_gls/pdf/colon.pdf

National Comprehensive Cancer Network. Clinical Practice Guidelines in Oncology. Rectal Cancer. Version 3.2018. 2018 Aug 7. https://www.nccn.org/professionals/physician_gls/pdf/rectal.pdf

National Institutes of Health. SEER Cancer Stat Facts: Colorectal Cancer, 2019. https://seer.cancer.gov/statfacts/html/colorect.html

Overman MJ et al. Nivolumab in patients with metastatic DNA mismatch repair-deficient or microsatellite instability-high colorectal cancer (CheckMate 142): an open-label, multicenter, phase 2 study. Lancet Oncol. 2017 Sep;18(9):1182–91. [PMID: 28734759]

Rex DK et al. Colorectal cancer screening: recommendations for physicians and patients from the U.S. Multisociety Task Force on Colorectal Cancer. Gastroenterology. 2017 Jul;153(1):307–23. [PMID: 28600072]

Robertson DJ et al. Recommendations on fecal immunochemical testing to screen for colorectal neoplasia: a consensus statement by the US Multi-Society Task Force on Colorectal Cancer. Gastrointest Endosc. 2017 Jan;85(1):2–21.e3. [PMID: 27769516]

Rusieki J et al. Colonoscopy surveillance after colorectal cancer resection. JAMA. 2017 Dec 19;318(23):2346–7. [PMID: 29260211]

Singal AG et al. Effect of colonoscopy outreach vs fecal immunochemical test outreach on colorectal cancer screening completion: a randomized clinical trial. JAMA. 2017 Sep 5; 318(9): 806–15. [PMID: 28873161]

Sinicrope FA. Lynch syndrome-associated colorectal cancer. N Engl J Med. 2018 Aug 23;379(8):764–73. [PMID: 30134129]

Sobrero A et al; TOSCA investigators. FOLFOX or CAPOX in stage II to III colon cancer: efficacy results of the Italian three or six colon adjuvant trial. J Clin Oncol. 2018 May 20;36(15):1478–85. [PMID: 29620994]

US Preventive Services Task Force; Bibbins-Domingo K et al. Screening for colorectal cancer: US Preventive Services Task Force recommendation statement. JAMA. 2016 Jun 21; 315(23):2564–75. Erratum in: JAMA. 2016 Aug 2;316(5):545. [PMID: 27304597]

Venook AP et al. Effect of first-line chemotherapy combined with cetuximab or bevacizumab on overall survival in patients with *KRAS* wild-type advanced or metastatic colorectal cancer: a randomized clinical trial. JAMA. 2017 Jun 20;317(23):2392–401. [PMID: 28632865]

Wolf AMD et al. Colorectal cancer screening for average-risk adults: 2018 guideline update from the American Cancer Society. CA Cancer J Clin. 2018 Jul;68(4):250–81. [PMID: 29846947]

CARCINOMA OF THE ANUS

The anal canal is lined from its proximal to distal extent by columnar, transitional, and non-keratinized squamous epithelium, which merges at the anal verge with the keratinized perianal skin. Tumors arising from the mucosa of the anal canal are relatively rare, comprising only 1–2% of all cancers of the anus and large intestine. Squamous cancers make up the majority of anal cancers. Anal cancer is increased among people practicing receptive anal intercourse and those with a history of anorectal warts. In over 80% of cases, HPV may be detected, suggesting that this virus is a major causal factor. In a large controlled trial, HPV vaccination of healthy men (16 to 26 years old) who have sex with men decreased the incidence of anal intraepithelial neoplasia by 50%. Women with anal cancer are at increased risk for cervical cancer (which may be due to a field effect of oncogenic HPV infection) and require gynecologic screening and monitoring. Anal cancer is increased in HIV-infected individuals, possibly due to interaction with HPV. HPV vaccine is recommended for boys and girls starting at age 11 or 12, for females aged 13 through 26 years, and in men who have sex with men up to age 26 who have not been previously vaccinated.

Bleeding, pain, and local tumor are the most common symptoms. The lesion is often confused with hemorrhoids or other common anal disorders. These tumors tend to become annular, invade the sphincter, and spread upward via the lymphatics into the perirectal mesenteric lymphatic nodes. CT or MRI scans of the abdomen and pelvis are required to identify regional lymphadenopathy or metastatic disease at diagnosis. PET imaging may be used in conjunction.

Treatment depends on the tumor location and histologic stage. Well-differentiated and small (less than 2 cm) superficial lesions of the perianal skin may be treated with wide local excision. Adenocarcinoma of the anal canal is treated in similar fashion to rectal cancer (see above), commonly by abdominoperineal resection with neoadjuvant chemoradiotherapy and adjuvant chemotherapy. The more common squamous cell cancer of the anal canal and large perianal tumors invading the sphincter or rectum are treated with combined-modality therapy that includes external radiation with simultaneous chemotherapy (5-fluorouracil plus mitomycin). Local control is achieved in approximately 80% of patients. Radical surgery (abdominoperineal resection) is reserved for patients who fail chemotherapy and radiation therapy. Metastatic disease is generally treated with 5-fluorouracil in combination with cisplatin. Checkpoint inhibitor therapy with either nivolumab or pembrolizumab has been shown in small studies to result in disease control in up to 46% of patients with chemotherapy-refractory, metastatic, or unresectable disease. The 5-year survival rate is 81% for localized tumors and approximately 30% for metastatic (stage IV) disease.

Casadei Gardini A et al. Treatment of squamous cell carcinoma of the anal canal: new strategies with anti-EGFR therapy and immunotherapy. Crit Rev Oncol Hematol. 2018 Mar;123:52–6. [PMID: 29482779]

Morris VK et al. Nivolumab for previously treated unresectable metastatic anal cancer (NCI9673): a multicentre, single-arm, phase 2 study. Lancet Oncol. 2017 Apr;18(4):446–53. [PMID: 28223062]

National Cancer Institute. SEER Cancer Stat Facts: Anal Cancer, 2019. https://seer.cancer.gov/statfacts/html/anus.html

National Comprehensive Cancer Network. Clinical Practice Guidelines in Oncology. Anal Carcinoma. Version 2.2018. 2018 Jun 8. https://www.nccn.org/professionals/physician_gls/pdf/anal.pdf

Smith CA et al. Randomized clinical trials in localized anal cancer. Surg Oncol Clin N Am. 2017 Oct;26(4):705–18. [PMID: 28923226]

CANCERS OF THE GENITOURINARY TRACT

George Schade, MD

PROSTATE CANCER

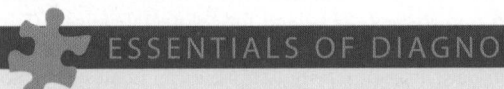

ESSENTIALS OF DIAGNOSIS

▶ Prostatic induration on DRE or elevation of PSA.

▶ Most often asymptomatic.

▶ Rarely: systemic symptoms (weight loss, bone pain).

▶ General Considerations

Prostate cancer is the most common noncutaneous cancer detected in American men and the second leading cause of cancer-related death in men. In 2018, an estimated 164,690 new cases of prostate cancer were diagnosed and

29,430 deaths resulted in the United States. However, the clinical incidence does not match the prevalence noted at autopsy, where more than 40% of men over 50 years of age are found to have prostatic carcinoma. Further, the prevalence increases with age with 30% of men aged 60–69 years and 67% of men aged 80–89 years found to have the disease at autopsy. Most such occult cancers are small and contained within the prostate gland; few are associated with regional or distant disease. Although the global prevalence of prostatic cancer at autopsy is relatively consistent, the clinical incidence varies considerably (high in North America and European countries, intermediate in South America, and low in the Far East). A 50-year-old American man has a lifetime risk of 40% for latent cancer, a 16% risk for developing clinically apparent cancer, and a 2.9% risk of death due to prostatic cancer. African-American race, family history of prostatic cancer, and history of high dietary fat intake are risk factors for prostate cancer.

► Clinical Findings

A. Symptoms and Signs

Prostate cancer may manifest as discrete nodules or areas of induration within the prostate on a DRE. However, currently most prostate cancers are detected because of elevations in serum PSA (not DRE findings).

Patients rarely present with signs of urinary retention or neurologic symptoms from epidural metastases and cord compression. Obstructive voiding symptoms are most often due to benign prostatic hyperplasia, which occurs in the same age group. Nevertheless, large or locally extensive prostatic cancers can cause obstructive voiding symptoms. Lymph node metastases can lead to lower extremity lymphedema. Because the axial skeleton is the most common site of metastases, patients may present with back pain or pathologic fractures.

B. Laboratory Findings

1. Serum tumor markers—PSA is a glycoprotein produced only by cells, either benign or malignant, of the prostate gland. The serum level is typically low and correlates with the total volume of prostate tissue and tends to increase with age. Measurement of serum PSA is useful in detecting and staging prostate cancer, monitoring response to treatment, and identifying recurrence before it becomes clinically evident. As a screening test, PSA is elevated (greater than 4.0 ng/mL [4.0 mcg/L]) in 10–15% of men. Prostate cancer will be diagnosed in approximately 18–30% of men with PSA 4.1–10 ng/mL (4.1–10 mcg/L) and 50–70% of men with PSA greater than 10 ng/mL (10 mcg/L). Patients with PSA less than 10 ng/mL usually have localized and therefore potentially curable cancers. Interestingly, approximately 20% of patients who undergo radical prostatectomy for localized prostate cancers have normal levels of PSA.

In untreated patients with prostate cancer, the level of PSA correlates with the volume and stage of disease. Whereas most organ-confined cancers are associated with PSA levels below 10 ng/mL (10 mcg/L), advanced disease (seminal vesicle invasion, lymph node involvement, or occult distant metastases) is more common in patients with PSA levels in excess of 40 ng/mL (40 mcg/L). Approximately 98% of patients with metastatic prostate cancer will have elevated PSA. However, there are rare cancers that are localized despite substantial elevations in PSA. Therefore, initial treatment decisions cannot be made on the basis of PSA testing alone. A rising PSA after therapy is usually consistent with progressive disease, either locally recurrent or metastatic.

2. Miscellaneous laboratory testing—Patients with urinary retention or with ureteral obstruction due to loco-regionally advanced prostate cancers may present with elevations in blood urea nitrogen or serum creatinine. Patients with bony metastases may have elevations in serum alkaline phosphatase or calcium. Laboratory and clinical evidence of disseminated intravascular coagulation can occur in patients with advanced prostate cancers.

3. Prostate biopsy—Transrectal ultrasound-guided biopsy is the standard method for detection of prostate cancer. The use of a spring-loaded, 18-gauge biopsy needle has allowed transrectal biopsy to be performed with minimal patient discomfort and morbidity. Local anesthesia is routinely used and increases the tolerability of the procedure. The specimen preserves glandular architecture and permits accurate grading. Prostate biopsy specimens are taken from the apex, mid-portion, and base in men who have an abnormal DRE or an elevated serum PSA, or both. Extended-pattern biopsies, including a total of at least 10 biopsies, are associated with improved cancer detection and risk stratification of patients with newly diagnosed disease. In addition, suspicious hypoechoic prostatic lesions seen on transrectal ultrasound may be targeted for biopsy. Patients with abnormalities of the seminal vesicles can have these structures specifically biopsied to identify local tumor invasion.

C. Imaging

Use of imaging should be tailored to the likelihood of advanced disease in newly diagnosed cases. Asymptomatic patients with well-differentiated to moderately differentiated cancers, thought to be localized to the prostate on DRE and **transrectal ultrasonography** and associated with modest elevations of PSA (ie, less than 10 ng/mL [10 mcg/L]), need no further imaging.

MRI allows for evaluation of the prostate as well as regional lymph nodes. The positive predictive value for detection of both capsular penetration and seminal vesicle invasion is similar for transrectal ultrasound and MRI, although newer multi-parametric MRI techniques may better stage patients considering treatment or, alternatively, active surveillance. Additionally, there is a growing role for **multi-parametric MRI** in prostate cancer diagnosis, particularly among men with previous negative prostate biopsies, to evaluate for suspicious prostatic lesions. Such lesions may then be sampled via MR-Fusion or MRI-guided biopsy. Such an approach may improve not only overall cancer detection but discovery of clinically relevant disease, and its use in routine clinical practice has increased and continues to evolve. **CT** plays little role in assessing local disease because of its inability to accurately identify or stage prostate cancers, but it is routinely used to detect regional lymphatic metastases in patients with greater than 10% risk of nodal involvement.

Conventional **radionuclide (99-technetium) bone scans** are superior to conventional plain skeletal radiographs in detecting bony metastases. Prostate cancer bony metastases tend to be multiple and most commonly occur in the axial skeleton. Men with more advanced local lesions, symptoms of metastases (eg, bone pain), high-grade disease, or elevations in PSA greater than 20 ng/mL (20 mcg/L) should undergo radionuclide bone scan. PET (eg, ^{18}F-sodium fluoride [^{18}F-NaF] PET) and ^{18}F-NaF PET/CT hybrid imaging appear to be more sensitive than conventional bone scans. A high frequency of abnormal scans with ^{18}F-NaF PET/CT resulting from degenerative joint disease, however, has resulted in a reduced enthusiasm for their use. PET imaging using fluciclovine (Axumin) has been approved for suspected cancer recurrence based on elevated PSA after prior treatment. Small molecules targeting PSMA (prostate-specific membrane antigen) also show significant promise as next-generation imaging agents (eg, ^{18}F-DCFBC (N-[N-[(S)-1,3-dicarboxypropyl]carbamoyl]-4-^{18}F-fluorobenzyl-L-cysteine), a low-molecular-weight radiotracer that targets PSMA). Intravenous urography and cystoscopy are not routinely needed to evaluate patients with prostate cancer.

Despite application of modern, sophisticated techniques, understaging of prostate cancer occurs in at least 20% of patients.

▶ Screening for Prostate Cancer

Whether screening for prostate cancer results in a decrease in its mortality rate is controversial. The screening tests currently available include DRE, PSA testing, and transrectal ultrasound. Prostate cancer detection rates using DRE alone vary from 1.5% to 7%, but unfortunately, most of these cancers are advanced (stage T3 or greater). Transrectal ultrasound should not be used as a first-line screening tool because of its expense, low specificity (and therefore high biopsy rate), and minimal improvement in detection rate when compared with the combined use of DRE and PSA testing.

PSA testing increases the detection rate of prostate cancers compared with DRE. Approximately 2–2.5% of men older than 50 years of age will be found to have prostate cancer using PSA testing compared with a rate of approximately 1.5% using DRE alone. The sensitivity, specificity, and positive predictive value of PSA and DRE are listed in Table 39–8. PSA-detected cancers are more likely to be localized compared with those detected by DRE alone. The Prostate Cancer Prevention Trial provided data demonstrating a significant risk of prostate cancer even in men with PSA less than 4.0 ng/mL (4.0 mcg/L) (Table 39–9) and a web-based calculator has been developed to estimate the risk of harboring both prostate cancer and high-grade cancer (http://riskcalc.org/PBCG).

To improve the performance of PSA as a screening test, several investigators have developed alternative methods for its use. These include establishment of age- and race-specific reference ranges, measurement of free serum and protein-bound levels of PSA (**percent free PSA**), and calculation of changes in PSA over time (**PSA velocity**).

Table 39–8. Screening for prostatic cancer: test performance.

Test	Sensitivity	Specificity	Positive Predictive Value
Abnormal PSA (> 4 ng/mL [mcg/L])	0.67	0.97	0.43
Abnormal DRE	0.50	0.94	0.24
Abnormal PSA or DRE	0.84	0.92	0.28
Abnormal PSA and DRE	0.34	0.995	0.49

DRE, digital rectal examination; PSA, prostate-specific antigen.
Modified, with permission, from Kramer BS et al. Prostate cancer screening: what we know and what we need to know. Ann Intern Med. 1993 Nov 1;119(9):914–23. Copyright © 1993 American College of Physicians. All rights reserved.

Generally, men with PSA free fractions exceeding 25% are unlikely to have prostate cancer, whereas those with free fractions less than 10% have an approximately 50% chance of having prostate cancer. Newer tests, including the Prostate Health Index (PHI) and 4kscore (https://4kscore.com), may better identify not only men at greater risk for prostate cancer but those with more aggressive disease. The frequency of PSA testing also remains a matter of debate. The traditional yearly screening approach may not be the most efficient; rather, earlier PSA testing at younger age may allow less frequent testing later as well as provide information regarding PSA velocity. Studies from the Baltimore Longitudinal Study of Aging suggest that men with PSA above the age-based median when tested between 40 and 60 years are at significantly increased risk for subsequent cancer detection over 25 years. Men with lower PSA (0.6 ng/mL [0.6 mcg/L] aged 40–50 and 0.71 ng/mL [0.71 mcg/L] aged 50–60) may require less frequent PSA tests. In addition, men with PSA velocity greater than

Table 39–9. Risk of prostate cancer in men with PSA ≤ 4.0 ng/mL (or mcg/L).

PSA Level (ng/mL [or mcg/L])	Percentage with Prostate Cancer	Percentage with High-Grade[1] Prostate Cancer
≤ 0.5	6.6	12.5
0.6–1.0	10.1	10.0
1.1–2.0	17.0	11.8
2.1–3.0	23.9	19.1
3.1–4.0	26.9	25.0

[1]High-grade cancer was defined as Gleason score ≥ 7.
Data from Thompson IM et al. Prevalence of prostate cancer among men with a prostate-specific antigen level ≤ 4.0 ng per milliliter. N Engl J Med. 2004 May 27;350(22):2239–46.

0.35 ng/mL (0.35 mcg/L) per year measured 10–15 years before diagnosis had significantly worse cancer-specific survival compared with those with lower PSA velocity. The NCCN guidelines (https://www.nccn.org/professionals/physician_gls/f_guidelines.asp) for prostate cancer early detection incorporate many of these factors (Figure 39–2). The European Association of Urology (EAU) recommends offering a baseline serum PSA to all men aged 40–45 years and subsequently initiating a risk-adapted strategy.

Two large, randomized trials question the benefit of screening men for prostate cancer. In the US Prostate, Lung, Colorectal, and Ovarian (PLCO) Cancer Screening Trial, no mortality benefit was observed after combined screening with PSA testing and DRE during 13-year follow-up. Although screening resulted in a 12% increase in prostate cancer detection, the cancer-specific mortality rate was similar in the screening and control arms (3.7 and 3.4 deaths per 10,000 person-years, respectively). Similarly, in the

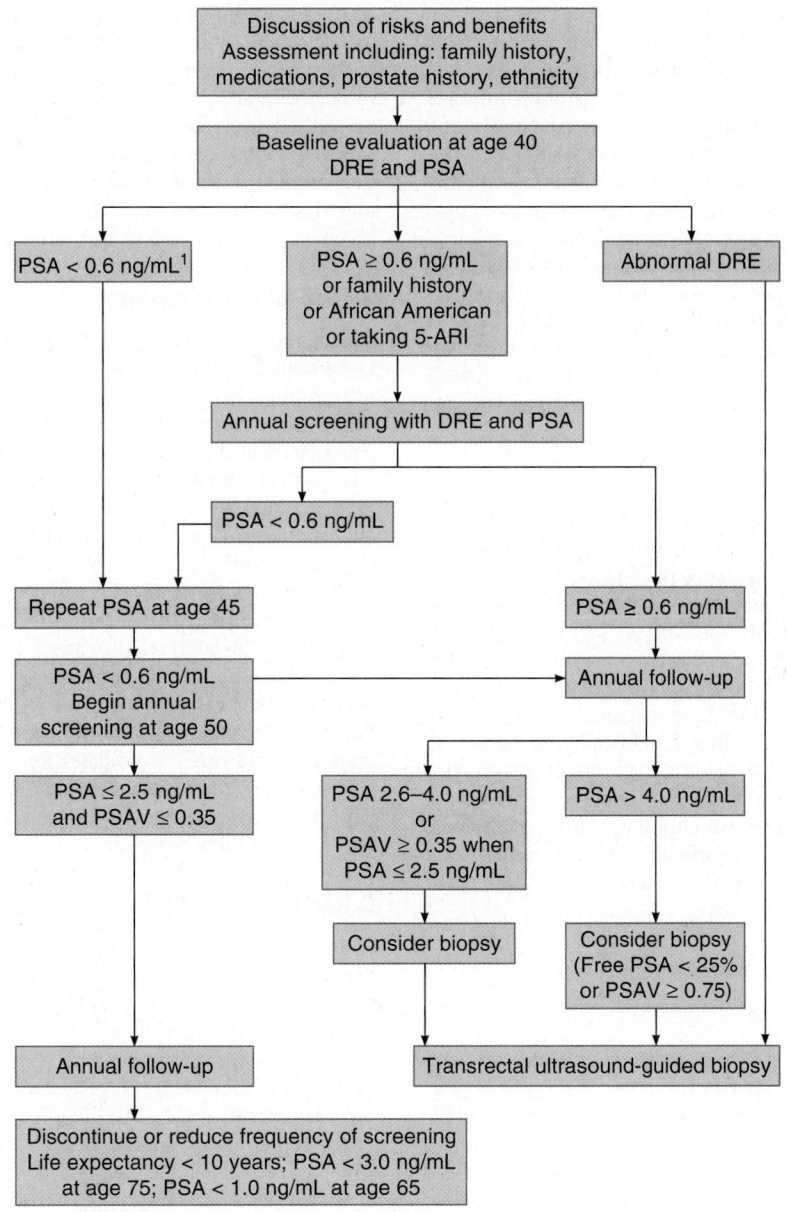

¹NCCN guidelines utilize PSA threshold of 1.0 ng/mL in men < 50 years, the 75th percentile range for this age group; the median PSA value for men 40–49 years is 0.6 ng/mL.

▲ **Figure 39–2.** An algorithm for prostate cancer early detection. DRE, digital rectal examination; 5-ARI, 5-alpha-reductase inhibitor; PSAV, PSA velocity (ng/mL/year) calculated on at least three consecutive values over at least an 18- to 24-month period. (Based on NCCN guidelines, data from the Baltimore Longitudinal Study on Aging, and Prostate Cancer Prevention Trial.)

European Randomized Study of Screening for Prostate Cancer (ERSPC) trial, the benefit of PSA screening was minimal with an absolute reduction of 1.28 prostate cancer deaths per 1000 men screened at 13-year follow-up. In 2018, the USPSTF issued a revised (Grade C) recommendation for men aged 55 to 69 years that the decision to undergo periodic PSA–based screening should be an individual one. Before deciding about screening, men should discuss its potential benefits and harms with their clinician, incorporating their own values and preferences in the decision. The revised recommendation acknowledges that, while screening offers some men a small potential benefit of reducing the chance of dying from prostate cancer, many other men will experience potential harms from screening. These include false-positive results that require additional testing and possible prostate biopsy; overdiagnosis and overtreatment; and treatment complications, such as incontinence and erectile dysfunction. In determining whether screening is appropriate in individual cases, the individual patient's family history, race/ethnicity, comorbid medical conditions, values about the benefits and harms of screening and treatment-specific outcomes, and other health needs should be considered. Clinicians should not screen men who do not express a preference for screening. For men age 70 years and older, the USPSTF recommends against PSA-based screening (Grade D recommendation).

▶ Staging

The majority of prostate cancers are adenocarcinomas. Most arise in the peripheral zone of the prostate, though a small percentage arise in the central (5–10%) and transition zones (20%) of the gland. Pathologists utilize the Gleason grading system whereby a "primary" grade is applied to the architectural pattern of malignant glands occupying the largest area of the specimen and a "secondary" grade is assigned to the next largest area of cancer. Grading is based on architectural rather than histologic criteria, and five "grades" are possible. Adding the score of the primary and secondary grades gives a Gleason score from 2 to 10. Gleason score correlates with tumor volume, pathologic stage, and prognosis. A simplified five-grade group system has been introduced by the International Society of Urological Pathologists.

▶ Treatment

A. Active Surveillance

The optimal treatment for patients with clinically localized prostate cancers remains controversial. A survival benefit of treating localized prostate cancer has not been conclusively demonstrated. Patients need to be advised of all treatment options, including active surveillance, with the specific benefits, risks, and limitations. The goal of active surveillance is to avoid treatment in men who may never require treatment while recognizing and definitively treating men harboring higher risk disease in order to balance cancer risk with the morbidity of treatment. Treatment decisions are made based on stage, PSA, and cancer grade (Gleason score) as well as the age and health of the patient.

Active surveillance alone may be effective management for appropriately selected patients, typically those with low PSA, small volume, well-differentiated cancers, and life expectancy less than 10–15 years. For such patients, active surveillance involves serial PSA levels, DREs, and periodic prostate biopsies to reassess grade and extent of cancer. Endpoints for intervention in patients on active surveillance, particularly PSA changes, have not been clearly defined and surveillance regimens remain an active area of research. Nonetheless, they are increasingly accepted by patients and clinicians with contemporary series demonstrating freedom from definitive treatment in greater than half of patients at 5 years, and risk of developing metastases and suffering cancer-specific death in less than 3% and 2%, respectively, at 10 years. Active surveillance, which is distinguished from mere observation (watchful waiting), is featured prominently in the 2018 NCCN guidelines and may be the preferred management in most men with very low risk prostate cancer. This approach is increasingly accepted and incorporated in routine clinical practice.

B. Radical Prostatectomy

During radical prostatectomy, the seminal vesicles, prostate, and ampullae of the vas deferens are removed. Refinements in technique have allowed preservation of urinary continence in most patients and erectile function in selected patients. Radical prostatectomy can be performed via open retropubic, transperineal, or laparoscopic (with or without robotic assistance) surgery. Local recurrence is uncommon after radical prostatectomy and related to pathologic stage. Organ-confined cancers rarely recur; however, cancers with adverse pathologic features (capsular penetration, seminal vesicle invasion) are associated with higher local (10–25%) and distant (20–50%) relapse rates.

Ideal candidates for radical prostatectomy include healthy patients with stages T1 and T2 prostate cancers. Patients with advanced local tumors (T4) or lymph node metastases are rarely candidates for prostatectomy alone, although the surgery is sometimes used in combination with hormonal therapy and postoperative radiation therapy for select high-risk patients.

C. Radiation Therapy

Radiation can be delivered by a variety of techniques including use of external beam radiotherapy and transperineal implantation of radioisotopes. Morbidity is limited, and the survival of patients with localized cancers (T1, T2, and selected T3) approaches 65% at 10 years. As with surgery, the likelihood of local failure correlates with technique and cancer characteristics. The likelihood of a positive prostate biopsy more than 18 months after radiation varies between 20% and 60%. Patients with local recurrence are at an increased risk of cancer progression and cancer death compared with those who have negative biopsies. Ambiguous target definitions, inadequate radiation doses, and understaging of the cancer may be responsible for the failure noted in some series. Newer techniques of radiation (implantation, conformal therapy using three-dimensional reconstruction of CT-based tumor volumes, heavy particle, charged particle, and heavy charged particle) may improve local control rates. **Three-dimensional conformal radiation** delivers a higher dose because of improved targeting and appears to be associated with greater efficacy as well as lower likelihood of adverse side effects compared with previous techniques. **Brachytherapy**—the implantation of permanent or temporary radioactive sources (palladium, iodine, or iridium) into the prostate—can be used as monotherapy in those with low-grade or low-volume malignancies or combined with external beam radiation in patients with higher-grade or higher-volume disease. The PSA may rise after brachytherapy because of prostate inflammation and necrosis. This transient elevation (PSA bounce) should not be mistaken for recurrence and may occur up to 20 months after treatment.

D. Cryosurgery

In cryosurgery, liquid nitrogen is circulated through small hollow-core needles inserted into the prostate under ultrasound guidance. The freezing process results in tissue destruction. The positive biopsy rate after cryoablation ranges between 7% and 23%.

E. Localized Disease

Although selected patients may be candidates for active surveillance based on age or health and evidence of small-volume or well-differentiated cancers, most men with an anticipated life expectancy of longer than 10 years should be considered for treatment. Newly introduced genomic tests may provide novel information to help guide treatment decisions. Both radiation therapy and radical prostatectomy result in acceptable levels of local control. A large, prospective, randomized trial compared watchful waiting with radical prostatectomy in 695 men with clinically localized and well-differentiated to moderately differentiated cancers. Radical prostatectomy significantly reduced disease-specific mortality, overall mortality, and risks of metastasis and local progression. The relative reduction in the risk of death at 23 years was 0.56 in the prostatectomy group, with the number needed to treat to avert one death (NNT) = 8 patients; the benefit was largest in men younger than age 65 years (relative risk [RR] = 0.45) and with intermediate-risk prostate cancer (RR = 0.38). Surgery also reduced the risk of metastases in older men (RR = 0.68).

F. Locally and Regionally Advanced Disease

Patients with advanced pathologic stage or positive surgical margins are at an increased risk for local and distant tumor relapse. Such patients are candidates for adjuvant therapy (radiation for positive margins and seminal vesicle invasion or androgen deprivation for lymph node metastases). Two randomized clinical trials (EORTC 22911 and SWOG 8794) have demonstrated improved progression-free and metastasis-free survival with early radiotherapy in these men, and subsequent analysis of SWOG 8794 showed improved overall survival in men receiving adjuvant radiation therapy. Evidence suggests that salvage radiotherapy after radical prostatectomy, within 2 years of PSA relapse, increases prostate cancer-specific survival in men with shorter PSA doubling time (less than 6 months).

Those with locally extensive cancers, including seminal vesicle and bladder neck invasion, are at increased risk for both local and distant relapse despite conventional therapy. A variety of investigational regimens are being tested in an effort to improve cancer outcomes in such patients. Combination therapy (androgen deprivation combined with surgery or irradiation), newer forms of irradiation, and hormonal therapy alone are being tested, as is neoadjuvant and adjuvant chemotherapy. Neoadjuvant and adjuvant androgen deprivation therapy combined with external beam radiation therapy have demonstrated improved survival compared with external beam radiation therapy alone for patients with intermediate- and high-risk disease.

G. Metastatic Disease

Since death due to prostate carcinoma is almost invariably the result of failure to control metastatic disease, research has emphasized efforts to improve control of distant disease. Most prostate carcinomas are hormone dependent and approximately 70–80% of men with metastatic prostate carcinoma will respond to various forms of androgen deprivation. **Androgen deprivation therapy** may be effective at several levels along the pituitary–gonadal axis using a variety of methods or agents (Table 39–10). Use of luteinizing hormone-releasing hormone (LHRH) agonists (leuprolide, goserelin) achieves medical castration without orchiectomy and is the most common method of reducing testosterone levels. A single LHRH antagonist (degarelix) is FDA approved and has no short-term testosterone "flare" associated with LHRH agonists. Because of its rapid onset of action, **ketoconazole** should be considered in patients with advanced prostate cancer who present with spinal cord compression, bilateral ureteral obstruction, or disseminated intravascular coagulation. Although testosterone is the major circulating androgen, the adrenal gland secretes the androgens dehydroepiandrosterone, dehydroepiandrosterone sulfate, and androstenedione. This has led to attempts to suppress both testicular and adrenal androgens in an effort to achieve better initial and longer response. Accordingly, in patients with hormone-sensitive metastatic disease, **complete androgen blockade,** combining oral **abiraterone acetate** plus **prednisone** with use of an LHRH agonist/antagonist or orchiectomy, results in superior survival compared to LHRH agonist/antagonist therapy alone. Additionally, cytotoxic chemotherapy with docetaxel plus prednisone and androgen deprivation improves survival in patients with untreated high-volume hormone-sensitive metastatic disease. Nonsteroidal antiandrogen agents may be useful in the setting of the initial treatment of non-metastatic (PSA only) disease. They act by competitively binding the receptor for dihydrotestosterone, the intracellular androgen responsible for prostate cell growth and development. A meta-analysis of trials comparing the use of either an LHRH agonist or orchiectomy alone with either in combination with an antiandrogen agent showed little benefit of combination therapy. However, patients at risk for disease-related symptoms (bone pain, obstructive voiding symptoms) should receive concurrent antiandrogens due to the initial elevation of serum testosterone that accompanies LHRH agonists. In addition to immediate side effects of androgen deprivation (sexual dysfunction and hot flashes),

Table 39–10. Androgen deprivation for prostatic cancer.

Level	Agent	Dose	Sequelae
Pituitary, hypothalamus	Diethylstilbestrol	1–3 mg orally daily	Gynecomastia, hot flushes, thromboembolic disease, erectile dysfunction
	LHRH agonists Leuprolide Goserelin Triptorelin Histrelin	Daily subcutaneous injection Monthly to quarterly depot injection Monthly depot injection Annual subcutaneous implant	Erectile dysfunction, hot flushes, gynecomastia, rarely anemia
	LHRH antagonist Degarelix	240 mg subcutaneously initial dose, then 80 mg subcutaneously monthly	Hot flushes, weight gain, erectile dysfunction, increased liver tests
Adrenal	Ketoconazole	400 mg three times orally daily	Adrenal insufficiency, nausea, rash, ataxia
	Aminoglutethimide	250 mg four times orally daily	Adrenal insufficiency, nausea, rash, ataxia
	Corticosteroid Prednisone	20–40 mg orally daily	Gastrointestinal bleeding, fluid retention
	CYP17a1 inhibitor Abiraterone	1000 mg orally daily (with prednisone 5 mg orally twice daily)	Weight gain, fluid retention, hypokalemia, hypertension
Testis	Orchiectomy		Gynecomastia, hot flushes, erectile dysfunction
Prostate cell	**Antiandrogens**		
	Flutamide	250 mg three times orally daily	No erectile dysfunction when used alone; nausea, diarrhea
	Bicalutamide	50 mg orally daily	Liver, cardiac and pulmonary toxicity
	Enzalutamide	160 mg orally daily	Seizures, dizziness, asthenia
	Cytotoxic chemotherapeutic agents		Bone marrow, skin, pulmonary, cardiac, gastrointestinal, hepatic toxicities possible
	Docetaxel	75 mg/m^2 intravenously once on day 1 of 21-day cycle (with prednisone 10 mg orally daily)	
	Cabazitaxel	20 mg/m^2 intravenously once on day 1 of 21-day cycle (with prednisone 10 mg orally daily)	

LHRH, luteinizing hormone-releasing hormone.

the chronic suppression of testosterone leads to osteoporosis and risk of fractures, cardiovascular disease and diabetes mellitus, and decreased muscle and increased fat. **Bisphosphonates** can prevent osteoporosis associated with androgen deprivation, decrease bone pain from metastases, and reduce skeletal-related events. **Denosumab**, a RANK ligand inhibitor, is approved for the prevention of skeletal-related events in patients with bone metastases from prostate cancer and also appears to delay the development of these metastases in patients with castration-resistant prostate cancer. In addition, enzalutamide definitively improves metastasis-free survival in men with nonmetastatic castrate-resistant prostate cancer and rapidly rising PSAs.

Docetaxel is the first cytotoxic chemotherapy agent to improve survival in patients with metastatic castration-resistant prostate cancer, which is defined as progressing

disease despite a castrate level of serum testosterone of less than 50 ng/dL. **Abiraterone** (which targets CYP17, a key enzyme in androgen synthesis) and **enzalutamide** (a potent androgen receptor antagonist) have both demonstrated improvement in survival in metastatic castration-resistant prostate cancer patients and can be used prior to or following docetaxel. **Sipuleucel-T,** an autologous cellular immunotherapy, is FDA approved in asymptomatic or minimally symptomatic men with metastatic castration-resistant prostate cancer. **Cabazitaxel** is a second-line taxane chemotherapy used in men who have already received docetaxel. **Radium-223 dichloride** is approved for the treatment of men with castration-resistant, symptomatic bone metastases, with significant improvements in both overall survival and time to skeletal-related events (eg, fractures and spinal cord compression).

Prognosis

The likelihood of success of active surveillance or treatment can be predicted using risk assessment tools that usually combine stage, grade, PSA level, and number and extent of positive prostate biopsies. Several web-based tools are available (eg, https://www.mskcc.org/nomograms/prostate). One of the most widely used is the **Kattan nomogram;** it incorporates cancer stage, grade, and PSA level to predict the likelihood that a patient will be disease-free after radical prostatectomy or radiation therapy.

The University of California San Francisco **CAPRA nomogram** (https://urology.ucsf.edu/research/cancer/prostate-cancer-risk-assessment-and-the-ucsf-capra-score) uses serum PSA, Gleason score, clinical stage, percent positive biopsies, and patient age in a point system to risk stratify and predict the likelihood of PSA recurrence 3 and 5 years after radical prostatectomy (Tables 39–11 and 39–12) as well as metastasis and prostate cancer-specific and overall survival. The CAPRA nomogram has been validated on large multicenter and international radical prostatectomy and radiation-treated cohorts.

The patterns of prostate cancer progression have been well defined. Small and well-differentiated cancers (Gleason grade 3) are usually confined within the prostate, whereas large-volume (greater than 4 mL) or poorly differentiated (Gleason grades 4 and 5) cancers are more often locally extensive or metastatic to regional lymph nodes or bone. Penetration of the prostate capsule by cancer is common and occurs along perineural spaces. Seminal vesicle invasion is associated with a high likelihood of regional or distant disease and disease recurrence. The most common sites of lymph node metastases are the obturator and internal iliac lymph node chains and of distant metastases, the axial skeleton.

Table 39–12. CAPRA: Probability of freedom from PSA recurrence after radical prostatectomy by CAPRA point total.

CAPRA Score	3-Year Recurrence-Free Survival (%) (95% CI)	5-Year Recurrence-Free Survival (%) (95% CI)
0–1	91 (85–95)	85 (73–92)
2	89 (83–94)	81 (69–89)
3	81 (73–87)	66 (54–76)
4	81 (69–89)	59 (40–74)
5	69 (51–82)	60 (37–77)
6	54 (27–75)	34 (12–57)
7+	24 (9–43)	8 (0–28)

PSA, prostate-specific antigen.
Source: https://urology.ucsf.edu/research/cancer/prostate-cancer-risk-assessment-and-the-ucsf-capra-score.

When to Refer

- Refer all patients to a urologist for management of localized disease or active surveillance.
- For metastatic disease, medical oncology should be consulted for consideration of systemic treatments.
- Active surveillance may be appropriate in selected patients with very low-volume, low-grade prostate cancer.
- Localized disease may be managed by active surveillance, surgery, or radiation therapy.
- Locally extensive, regionally advanced, and metastatic disease often require multimodal treatment strategies.

Table 39–11. The UCSF Cancer of the Prostate Risk Assessment (CAPRA).

Variable	Level	Points
PSA (ng/mL [or mcg/L]) at diagnosis	0–6	0
	6.1–10	1
	10.1–20	2
	20.1–30	3
	> 30	4
Gleason grade, primary/secondary	1–3/1–3	0
	1–3/4–5	1
	4–5/1–5	3
T stage	T1 or T2	0
	T3a	1
% positive biopsies (biopsy cores positive divided by the number of biopsies obtained)	< 34%	0
	≥ 34%	1
Age	< 50 years	0
	≥ 50 years	1

Source: https://urology.ucsf.edu/research/cancer/prostate-cancer-risk-assessment-and-the-ucsf-capra-score.

Barry MJ et al. Prevention of prostate cancer morbidity and mortality: primary prevention and early detection. Med Clin North Am. 2017 Jul;101(4):787–806. [PMID: 28577627]

Beer TM et al; PREVAIL Investigators. Enzalutamide in metastatic prostate cancer before chemotherapy. N Engl J Med. 2014 Jul 31;371(5):424–33. [PMID: 24881730]

Bill-Axelson A et al. Radical prostatectomy or watchful waiting in prostate cancer—29-year follow-up. N Engl J Med. 2018 Dec 13; 379(24):2319–29. [PMID: 30575473]

Cooperberg MR et al. Trends in management for patients with localized prostate cancer, 1990–2013. JAMA. 2015 Jul 7; 314(1):80–2. [PMID: 26151271]

Eggener SE et al. Prostate cancer screening. JAMA. 2015 Aug 25; 314(8):825–6. [PMID: 26305653]

Filson CP et al. Expectant management for men with early stage prostate cancer. CA Cancer J Clin. 2015 Jul–Aug;65(4):265–82. [PMID: 25958817]

Fizazi K et al. Abiraterone in metastatic prostate cancer. N Engl J Med. 2017 Oct 26;377(17):1697–8. [PMID: 29083131]

Francini E et al. Prostate cancer: developing novel approaches to castration-sensitive disease. Cancer. 2017 Jan 1;123(1):29–42. [PMID: 27802360]

Hamdy FC et al; ProtecT Study Group. 10-year outcomes after monitoring, surgery, or radiotherapy for localized prostate cancer. N Engl J Med. 2016 Oct 13;375(15):1415–24. [PMID: 27626136]

Hussain M et al. Enzalutamide in men with nonmetastatic, castration-resistant prostate cancer. N Engl J Med. 2018 Jun 28; 378(26):2465–74. [PMID: 29949494]

Jayadevappa R et al. Comparative effectiveness of prostate cancer treatments for patient-centered outcomes: a systematic review and meta-analysis (PRISMA Compliant). Medicine (Baltimore). 2017 May;96(18):e6790. [PMID: 28471976]

Litwin MS et al. The diagnosis and treatment of prostate cancer: a review. JAMA. 2017 Jun 27;317(24):2532–42. [PMID: 28655021]

National Cancer Institute. SEER Cancer Stat Facts: Prostate Cancer, 2019. https://seer.cancer.gov/statfacts/html/prost.html

Ritch CR et al. Advances in the management of castration resistant prostate cancer. BMJ. 2016 Oct 17;355:i4405. [PMID: 27754846]

Rosenkrantz AB et al. Prostate magnetic resonance imaging and magnetic resonance imaging targeted biopsy in patients with a prior negative biopsy: a consensus statement by AUA and SAR. J Urol. 2016 Dec;196(6):1613–8. [PMID: 27320841]

Sweeney CJ et al. Chemohormonal therapy in metastatic hormone-sensitive prostate cancer. N Engl J Med. 2015 Aug 20; 373(8):737–46. [PMID: 26244877]

Violette PD et al. Decision aids for localized prostate cancer treatment choice: systematic review and meta-analysis. CA Cancer J Clin. 2015 May–Jun;65(3):239–51. [PMID: 25772796]

BLADDER CANCER

ESSENTIALS OF DIAGNOSIS

- ► Gross or microscopic hematuria.
- ► Irritative voiding symptoms.
- ► Positive urinary cytology in most patients.
- ► Filling defect within bladder noted on imaging.

► General Considerations

Bladder cancer is the second most common urologic cancer; it occurs more commonly in men than women (3.1:1), and the mean age at diagnosis is 73 years. Cigarette smoking and exposure to industrial dyes or solvents are risk factors for the disease and account for approximately 60% and 15% of new cases, respectively. In the United States, almost all primary bladder cancers (98%) are epithelial malignancies, usually urothelial cell carcinomas (90%). Adenocarcinomas and squamous cell cancers account for approximately 2% and 7%, respectively. The latter is often associated with schistosomiasis, vesical calculi, or prolonged catheter use.

► Clinical Findings

A. Symptoms and Signs

Hematuria—gross or microscopic, chronic or intermittent—is the presenting symptom in 85–90% of patients with bladder cancer. Irritative voiding symptoms (urinary frequency and urgency) occur in a small percentage of patients as a result of the location or size of the cancer. Most patients with bladder cancer do not have signs of the disease because of its superficial nature. Abdominal masses detected on bimanual examination may be present in patients with large-volume or deeply infiltrating cancers. Hepatomegaly or palpable lymphadenopathy may be present in patients with metastatic disease, and lymphedema of the lower extremities results from locally advanced cancers or metastases to pelvic lymph nodes.

B. Laboratory Findings

Urinalysis reveals microscopic or gross hematuria in the majority of cases. On occasion, hematuria is accompanied by pyuria. Azotemia may be present in a small number of cases associated with ureteral obstruction. Anemia may occasionally be due to chronic blood loss or to bone marrow metastases. Exfoliated cells from normal and abnormal urothelium can be readily detected in voided urine specimens. Cytology can be useful to detect the disease initially or to detect its recurrence. Cytology is sensitive in detecting cancers of higher grade and stage (80–90%), but less so in detecting superficial or well-differentiated lesions (50%). There are numerous urinary tumor markers under investigation for screening, assessing recurrence, progression, prognosis, or response to therapy.

C. Imaging

Bladder cancers may be identified as masses within the bladder using ultrasound, CT, or MRI. However, the presence of cancer is confirmed by cystoscopy and biopsy, with imaging primarily used to evaluate the upper urinary tract and to stage more advanced lesions.

D. Cystourethroscopy and Biopsy

The diagnosis and staging of bladder cancers are made by cystoscopy and transurethral resection. If cystoscopy—performed usually under local anesthesia—confirms the presence of a bladder tumor, the patient is scheduled for transurethral resection under general or regional anesthesia. Random bladder and, on occasion, transurethral prostate biopsies are performed to detect occult disease in the bladder or elsewhere and potentially identify patients at greater risk for cancer recurrence and progression.

► Pathology & Staging

Grading is based on cellular features: size, pleomorphism, mitotic rate, and hyperchromatism. Bladder cancer staging is based on the extent (depth) of bladder wall penetration and the presence of regional or distant metastases.

The natural history of bladder cancer is based on two separate but related processes: cancer recurrence within the bladder and progression to higher-stage disease. Both are correlated with cancer grade and stage.

► Treatment

Patients with superficial cancers (Tis, Ta, T1) are treated with complete transurethral resection with selective use of a single dose intravesical chemotherapy immediately following resection. The subset of patients with carcinoma in situ (Tis) and those undergoing resection of large, high-grade, recurrent Ta lesions or T1 cancers are good candidates for additional intravesical therapy.

Patients with invasive (T2, T3) but still localized cancers are at risk for both nodal metastases and progression and require radical cystectomy or the combination of chemotherapy and selective surgery or irradiation due to the much higher risk of progression compared with patients with lower-stage lesions.

For patients with muscle invasive (T2 or greater) urothelial cell carcinoma, neoadjuvant systemic chemotherapy prior to radical cystectomy is superior to radical cystectomy alone. This is particularly important for higher-stage or bulky tumors in order to improve their surgical resectability.

A. Intravesical Chemotherapy

Immunotherapeutic or chemotherapeutic agents delivered directly into the bladder via a urethral catheter can reduce the likelihood of recurrence in those who have undergone complete transurethral resection. Most agents are administered weekly for 6–12 weeks. Efficacy may be increased by prolonging contact time to 2 hours. The use of maintenance therapy after the initial induction regimen is beneficial. Common agents include thiotepa, mitomycin, doxorubicin, valrubicin, and bacillus Calmette–Guérin (BCG), with the last being the only agent effective in reducing disease progression. Side effects of intravesical chemotherapy include irritative voiding symptoms and hemorrhagic cystitis. Patients in whom symptoms or infection develop from BCG may require antituberculous therapy.

B. Surgical Treatment

Although transurethral resection is the initial form of treatment for all bladder tumors since it is diagnostic, allows for proper staging, and controls superficial cancers, muscle-infiltrating cancers require more aggressive treatment. Partial cystectomy is indicated in selected patients with solitary lesions or those with cancer in a bladder diverticulum. Radical cystectomy entails removal of the bladder, prostate, seminal vesicles, and surrounding fat and peritoneal attachments in men and the bladder, uterus, cervix, urethra, anterior vaginal vault, and usually the ovaries in women. Bilateral pelvic lymph node dissection is performed in all patients.

Urinary diversion can be performed using a conduit of small or large bowel. However, continent forms of diversion avoid the necessity of an external appliance and can be considered in a significant number of patients.

C. Radiotherapy

External beam radiotherapy delivered in fractions over a 6- to 8-week period is generally well tolerated, but approximately 10–15% of patients will develop bladder, bowel, or rectal complications. Local recurrence is common after radiotherapy alone (30–70%) and it is therefore combined with systemic chemotherapy in an effort to reduce the need for radical cystectomy or to treat patients who are poor candidates for radical cystectomy.

D. Chemotherapy

Metastatic disease is present in 15% of patients with newly diagnosed bladder cancer, and metastases develop within 2 years in up to 40% of patients who were believed to have localized disease at the time of cystectomy or definitive radiotherapy. Cisplatin-based combination chemotherapy results in partial or complete responses in 15–45% of patients (see Table 39–2).

Combination chemotherapy has been used to decrease recurrence rates with both surgery and radiotherapy and to attempt bladder preservation in those treated with radiation. Neoadjuvant chemotherapy appears to benefit all patients with muscle-invasive disease prior to planned cystectomy. Chemotherapy should also be considered before surgery in those with bulky lesions or those suspected of having regional disease. Chemoradiation is best suited for those with T2 or limited T3 disease without ureteral obstruction. Alternatively, adjuvant chemotherapy has been used after cystectomy in patients at high risk for recurrence, such as those who have lymph node involvement or local invasion.

E. Immunotherapy

Anti–PDL-1 immunotherapy with atezolizumab is associated with response rates of 25–30% in locally advanced and metastatic bladder cancer. In many cases, however, the responses to therapy are durable. Atezolizumab has been approved as second-line therapy for urothelial cancer. Additional checkpoint inhibitors have since been approved, including the anti-PD-1 agents pembrolizumab and nivolumab and the anti-PDL-1 agents durvalumab and avelumab (Table 39–2) for patients with chemotherapy-refractory disease. Additionally, atezolizumab and pembrolizumab are approved as first-line therapy in patients with metastatic disease (PDL-1 positive tumors) or cisplatin ineligible patients (regardless of PDL-1 status).

▶ Prognosis

The frequency of recurrence and progression are correlated with grade. Whereas progression may be noted in few low-grade cancers (19–37%), it is common with poorly differentiated lesions (33–67%). Carcinoma in situ is most often found in association with papillary bladder cancers. Its presence identifies patients at increased risk for recurrence and progression.

At initial presentation, approximately 50–80% of bladder cancers are superficial: stage Ta, Tis, or T1. When properly treated, lymph node metastases and progression are uncommon in such patients and survival is excellent (81%). Five-year survival of patients with T2 and T3 disease ranges from 50% to 75% after radical cystectomy. Long-term survival for patients with metastatic disease at presentation is rare.

▶ When to Refer

- Refer all patients to a urologist. Hematuria often deserves evaluation with both upper urinary tract imaging and cystoscopy, particularly in a high-risk group (eg, older men).
- Refer when histologic diagnosis and staging require endoscopic resection of cancer.
- Metastatic urothelial cancer should be managed by a medical oncologist.

Babjuk M et al. EAU guidelines on non-muscle-invasive urothelial carcinoma of the bladder: update 2016. Eur Urol. 2017 Mar; 71(3):447–61. [PMID: 27324428]

Kamat AM et al. Bladder cancer. Lancet. 2016 Dec 3; 388(10061):2796–810. Erratum in: Lancet. 2016 Dec 3; 388(10061):2742. [PMID: 27345655]

Lee CH et al. Role of imaging in the local staging of urothelial carcinoma of the bladder. AJR Am J Roentgenol. 2017 Jun;208(6):1193–205. [PMID: 28225635]

Sternberg CN et al. ICUD-EAU International Consultation on Bladder Cancer 2012: chemotherapy for urothelial carcinoma-neoadjuvant and adjuvant settings. Eur Urol. 2013 Jan;63(1): 58–66. [PMID: 22917984]

Tripathi A et al. Immunotherapy for urothelial carcinoma: current evidence and future directions. Curr Urol Rep. 2018 Nov 7; 19(12):109. [PMID: 30406502]

CANCERS OF THE URETER & RENAL PELVIS

Cancers of the ureter and renal pelvis are rare and occur more commonly in patients who have bladder cancer, Balkan nephropathy, or Lynch syndrome, who smoke, who were exposed to Thorotrast (a contrast agent with radioactive thorium in use until the 1960s), and who have a long history of analgesic abuse. The majority are urothelial cell carcinomas. Gross or microscopic hematuria is present in most patients; flank pain secondary to bleeding and obstruction occurs less commonly. As with bladder cancers, urinary cytology is often positive. The most common signs identified at the time of CT or intravenous urography include an intraluminal filling defect, unilateral nonvisualization of the collecting system, and hydronephrosis. Ureteral and renal pelvic tumors must be differentiated from calculi, blood clots, papillary necrosis, or inflammatory and infectious lesions. On occasion, upper urinary tract lesions are accessible for biopsy, fulguration, or resection using a ureteroscope. Treatment is based on the site, size, grade, depth of penetration, and number of cancers present. Most are excised with laparoscopic or open nephroureterectomy (renal pelvic and upper ureteral lesions) or segmental excision of the ureter (distal ureteral lesions). Endoscopic resection may be indicated in patients with limited renal function or focal, low-grade, cancers. Similar to urothelial bladder cancers, use of chemotherapy prior to surgery may improve outcomes.

Aragon-Ching JB. Challenges and advances in the diagnosis, biology, and treatment of urothelial upper tract and bladder carcinomas. Urol Oncol. 2017 Jul;35(7):462–4. [PMID: 28625477]

Gregg RW et al. Perioperative chemotherapy for urothelial carcinoma of the upper urinary tract: a systematic review and meta-analysis. Crit Rev Oncol Hematol. 2018 Aug;128:58–64. [PMID: 29958631]

Kim HS et al. Immune checkpoint inhibitors for urothelial carcinoma. Investig Clin Urol. 2018 Sep;59(5):285–96. [PMID: 30182073]

Liu F et al. Laparoscopic versus open nephroureterectomy for upper urinary tract urothelial carcinoma: a systematic review and meta-analysis. Medicine (Baltimore). 2018 Aug; 97(35):e11954. [PMID: 30170392]

Nazzani S et al. Survival effect of chemotherapy in metastatic upper urinary tract urothelial carcinoma. Clin Genitourin Cancer. 2019 Feb;17(1):e97–103. [PMID: 30337106]

Rouprêt M et al. European Association of Urology guidelines on upper urinary tract urothelial carcinoma: 2017 update. Eur Urol. 2018 Jan;73(1):111–22. [PMID: 28867446]

Seisen T et al. Oncologic outcomes of kidney-sparing surgery versus radical nephroureterectomy for upper tract urothelial carcinoma: a systematic review by the EAU Non-muscle Invasive Bladder Cancer Guidelines Panel. Eur Urol. 2016 Dec; 70(6):1052–68. [PMID: 27477528]

RENAL CELL CARCINOMA

ESSENTIALS OF DIAGNOSIS

▶ Gross or microscopic hematuria.

▶ Flank pain or mass in some patients.

▶ Systemic symptoms such as fever, weight loss may be prominent.

▶ Solid renal mass on imaging.

General Considerations

Kidney (renal cell) and renal pelvis carcinomas account for 3.8% of all adult cancers. In 2018 in the United States, it is estimated that approximately 65,340 cases of renal cell carcinoma will be diagnosed and 14,970 deaths will result. Renal cell carcinoma has a peak incidence in the sixth decade of life and a male-to-female ratio of 2:1. It may be associated with a number of paraneoplastic syndromes.

Risk factors include physical inactivity, obesity, and diabetes mellitus. Cigarette smoking is the only known significant environmental risk factor. Familial causes of renal cell carcinoma have been identified (von Hippel–Lindau syndrome, hereditary papillary renal cell carcinoma, hereditary leiomyoma-renal cell carcinoma, Birt-Hogg-Dubé syndrome) and there is an association with dialysis-related acquired cystic disease and specific genetic aberrations (eg, Xp11.2 translocation), but sporadic carcinomas are far more common.

Renal cell carcinoma originates from the proximal tubule cells. Various histologic cell types are recognized (clear cell, papillary, chromophobe, collecting duct, and sarcomatoid).

Clinical Findings

A. Symptoms and Signs

Historically, 60% of patients presented with gross or microscopic hematuria. Flank pain or an abdominal mass was detected in approximately 30% of cases. The triad of flank pain, hematuria, and mass was found in only 10% of patients, and often a sign of advanced disease. Fever can occur as a paraneoplastic symptom. Symptoms of metastatic disease (cough, bone pain) occur in 20–30% of patients at presentation. Due to the widespread use of ultrasound and cross-sectional imaging, renal tumors are frequently detected incidentally in individuals with no urologic symptoms. Consequently, there has been profound stage migration toward lower stages of disease over the last 20 years. However, population mortality rates have remained stable.

B. Laboratory Findings

Contemporary studies suggest hematuria is present in less than 50% of patients. Erythrocytosis from increased erythropoietin production occurs in 5%, though anemia is more common; hypercalcemia may be present in up to 10% of patients. **Stauffer syndrome** is a reversible syndrome of hepatic dysfunction (with elevated liver tests) in the absence of metastatic disease.

C. Imaging

Solid renal masses are often first identified by abdominal ultrasonography or CT. CT and MRI scanning are the most valuable imaging tests for renal cell carcinoma. These scans confirm the character of the mass and provide valuable staging information with respect to regional lymph nodes, renal vein or vena cava tumor thrombus, and adrenal or liver metastases. CT and MRI also provide valuable information regarding the contralateral kidney (function, bilaterality of neoplasm). Chest radiographs or CT exclude pulmonary metastases. Bone scans should be performed for large tumors and in patients with bone pain or elevated serum alkaline phosphatase levels. Brain imaging should be obtained in patients with high metastatic burden or in those with neurologic deficits.

▶ Differential Diagnosis

Solid renal masses are renal cell carcinoma until proven otherwise. Other solid masses include renal angiomyolipomas (fat density usually visible by CT), renal pelvis urothelial cancers (more central location, involvement of the collecting system, positive urinary cytology), renal oncocytomas (indistinguishable from renal cell carcinoma preoperatively), renal abscesses, and adrenal tumors (superoanterior to the kidney).

▶ Treatment

Surgical extirpation is the primary treatment for localized renal cell carcinoma. Patients with a single kidney, bilateral lesions, or significant medical renal disease should be considered for partial nephrectomy. Patients harboring a small tumor with a normal contralateral kidney and good kidney function are also candidates for partial nephrectomy, while radical nephrectomy is indicated in patients with cancers larger than 7 cm and those in whom partial nephrectomy is not technically feasible. Radiofrequency and cryosurgical ablation are alternative options instead of surgery in select patients with tumors less than 3–4 cm with similar risk of metastatic progression but higher risk of local recurrence. Active surveillance is warranted in select patients (significant comorbidity, short life-expectancy) and appears safe with low risk of 5-year systemic progression. Percutaneous biopsy can provide tumor histology and grade to help guide treatment decisions.

Cytotoxic chemotherapy has no role in the treatment of metastatic renal cell carcinoma. Historically, biologic response modifiers, such as interferon-alpha and interleukin-2 produced partial response rates of 15–20% and 15–35%, respectively (Table 39–2). Responders tend to have lower tumor burdens, metastatic disease confined to the lung, and a high-performance status. Two randomized trials demonstrating a survival benefit of cytoreductive nephrectomy followed by the use of systemic therapy—specifically, interferon-alpha—compared with the use of systemic therapy alone have led to the widespread adoption of cytoreductive nephrectomy. Patients most likely to benefit from cytoreduction are those with good performance status, lung only metastases, and good prognostic features.

Presently, management strategies are based on tumor histology and patient risk (favorable, intermediate, and poor). Several targeted medications, specifically VEGF, Raf-kinase, and mTOR inhibitors, are effective (40–60% response rates) in patients with advanced kidney cancer (Table 39–2). These oral agents, which include sunitinib, pazopanib, cabozantinib, axitinib, and sorafenib, are generally well tolerated and particularly active for clear cell carcinoma. The appropriate timing and combination of these agents, with and without surgery and cytokine therapy, remain to be determined. Sunitinib is approved for adjuvant use after complete surgical resection in patients with adverse pathologic features. The mTOR inhibitors everolimus and temsirolimus are approved for use in patients with prior anti-VEGF therapy, as is the combination of lenvatinib and everolimus. Nivolumab is an approved immunotherapy for treating metastatic disease that has progressed despite antiangiogenic therapy, and the combination with ipilimumab proved superior to sunitinib in previously untreated intermediate- and poor-risk metastatic renal cell carcinoma. In 2017, the FDA granted breakthrough therapy designation to the combination of the PD-L1 inhibitor avelumab with the VEGF inhibitor axitinib (Table 39–2).

▶ Prognosis

After radical or partial nephrectomy, tumors confined to the renal capsule (T1–T2) demonstrate 5-year disease-free survivals of 90–100%. Tumors extending beyond the renal capsule (T3 or T4) and node-positive tumors have 5-year disease-free survivals of 50–60% and 0–15%, respectively. One subgroup of patients with nonlocalized disease has reasonable long-term survival, namely, those with solitary resectable metastases. In this setting, radical nephrectomy with resection of the solitary metastasis results in 5-year disease-free survival rates of 15–30%.

▶ When to Refer

- Refer patients with solid renal masses or complex cysts to a urologist for further evaluation.
- Refer patients with renal cell carcinoma to a urologic surgeon for surgical excision.
- Refer patients with metastatic disease to an oncologist and urologist.

Dey S et al. Neoadjuvant targeted molecular therapy before renal surgery. Urol Clin North Am. 2017 May;44(2):289–303. [PMID: 28411920]

Haifler M et al. Current role of renal biopsy in urologic practice. Urol Clin North Am. 2017 May;44(2):203–11. [PMID: 28411912]

Lalani AA et al. Systemic treatment of metastatic clear cell renal cell carcinoma in 2018: current paradigms, use of immunotherapy, and future directions. Eur Urol. 2019 Jan;75(1):100–10. [PMID: 30327274]

Merrill SB. Postoperative surveillance for renal cell carcinoma. Urol Clin North Am. 2017 May;44(2):313–23. [PMID: 28411922]

Motzer RJ et al; CheckMate 214 Investigators. Nivolumab plus ipilimumab versus sunitinib in advanced renal-cell carcinoma. N Engl J Med. 2018 Apr 5;378(14):1277–90. [PMID: 29562145]

Pierorazio PM et al. Management of renal masses and localized renal cancer: systematic review and meta-analysis. J Urol. 2016 Oct;196(4):989–99. [PMID: 27157369]

Sun M et al. Risk assessment in small renal masses: a review article. Urol Clin North Am. 2017 May;44(2):189–202. [PMID: 28411911]

OTHER PRIMARY TUMORS OF THE KIDNEY

Oncocytomas account for 3–5% of renal tumors, are usually benign, and are indistinguishable from renal cell carcinoma on preoperative imaging. These tumors are seen in other organs, including the adrenals, salivary glands, and thyroid and parathyroid glands.

Angiomyolipomas are rare benign tumors composed of fat, smooth muscle, and blood vessels. They are most commonly seen in patients with tuberous sclerosis (often multiple and bilateral) or in young to middle-aged women. CT scanning may identify the fat component, which is diagnostic for angiomyolipoma. Asymptomatic lesions less than 5 cm in diameter usually do not require intervention; large lesions can spontaneously bleed. Acute bleeding can be treated by angiographic embolization or, in rare cases, nephrectomy. Lesions over 5 cm are often prophylactically treated with angioembolization to reduce the risk of bleeding.

SECONDARY CANCERS OF THE KIDNEY

The kidney is not an infrequent site for metastatic disease. Of the solid tumors, lung cancer is the most common (20%), followed by breast (10%), stomach (10%), and the contralateral kidney (10%). Lymphoma, both Hodgkin and non-Hodgkin, may also involve the kidney, although it tends to appear as a diffusely infiltrative process resulting in renal enlargement rather than a discrete mass.

TESTICULAR CANCERS (Germ Cell Tumors)

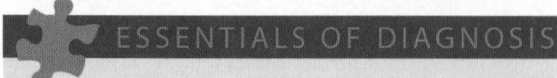

ESSENTIALS OF DIAGNOSIS

▸ Most common neoplasm in men aged 20–35 years.
▸ Patient typically discovers a painless nodule.
▸ Orchiectomy necessary for diagnosis.

▶ General Considerations

Malignant tumors of the testis are rare, with approximately five to six cases per 100,000 males reported in the United States each year. Ninety to 95 percent of all primary

testicular tumors are germ cell tumors and can be divided into two major categories: **nonseminomas,** including embryonal cell carcinoma (20%), teratoma (5%), choriocarcinoma (less than 1%), and mixed cell types (40%); and **seminomas** (35%). The lifetime probability of developing testicular cancer is 0.3% for an American male.

Approximately 5% of testicular cancers develop in a patient with a history of cryptorchism, with seminoma being the most common. However, 5–10% of these tumors occur in the contralateral, normally descended testis. The relative risk of development of malignancy is higher for the intra-abdominal testis (1:20) and lower for the inguinal testis (1:80). Placement of the cryptorchid testis into the scrotum (orchidopexy) does not alter its malignant potential but does facilitate routine examination and cancer detection.

Testicular cancer is slightly more common on the right than the left, paralleling the increased incidence of cryptorchidism on the right side. One to 2 percent of primary testicular cancers are bilateral and up to 50% of these men have a history of unilateral or bilateral cryptorchidism. Primary bilateral testicular cancers may occur synchronously or asynchronously but tend to be of the same histology. Seminoma is the most common histologic finding in bilateral *primary* testicular cancers, while malignant lymphoma is the most common bilateral testicular tumor overall.

▶ Clinical Findings

A. Symptoms and Signs

The most common symptom of testicular cancer is painless enlargement of the testis. Sensations of heaviness are not unusual. Patients are usually the first to recognize an abnormality, yet typical delay in seeking medical attention ranges from 3 to 6 months. Acute testicular pain resulting from intratesticular hemorrhage occurs in approximately 10% of cases. Ten percent of patients are asymptomatic at presentation, and 10% manifest symptoms relating to metastatic disease such as back pain (retroperitoneal metastases), cough (pulmonary metastases), or lower extremity edema (vena cava obstruction).

A discrete mass or diffuse testicular enlargement is noted in most cases. Secondary hydroceles may be present in 5–10% of cases. In advanced disease, supraclavicular adenopathy may be present, and abdominal examination may reveal a mass. Gynecomastia is seen in 5% of germ cell tumors.

B. Laboratory Findings

Several serum markers are important in the diagnosis and monitoring of testicular carcinoma, including human chorionic gonadotropin (hCG), alpha-fetoprotein, and lactate dehydrogenase. Alpha-fetoprotein is never elevated with pure seminomas, and while hCG is occasionally elevated in seminomas, levels tend to be lower than those seen with nonseminomas. Lactate dehydrogenase may be elevated with either type of tumor and is a marker for disease burden. Liver tests may be elevated in the presence of hepatic metastases, and anemia may be present in advanced disease.

C. Imaging

Scrotal ultrasound can readily determine whether a mass is intratesticular or extratesticular. Once the diagnosis of testicular cancer has been established by inguinal orchiectomy, clinical staging of the disease is accomplished by chest, abdominal, and pelvic CT scanning.

Staging

Testicular cancer is staged using the TNM system created based on extent of cancer in the testis, status of regional lymph nodes, the presence of metastases in distant lymph nodes or other viscera, and serum levels of tumor markers. Based on these features, germ cell tumors can be grouped to assign an overall stage: stage I lesion is confined to the testis; stage II demonstrates regional lymph node involvement in the retroperitoneum; and stage III indicates distant metastasis.

Differential Diagnosis

An incorrect diagnosis is made at the initial examination in up to 25% of patients with testicular tumors. Scrotal ultrasonography should be performed if any uncertainty exists with respect to the diagnosis. Although most intratesticular masses are malignant, a benign lesion—epidermoid cyst—may rarely be seen. Epidermoid cysts are usually very small benign nodules located just underneath the tunica albuginea; occasionally, however, they can be large. Testicular lymphoma is discussed below.

Treatment

Inguinal exploration with early vascular control of the spermatic cord structures is the initial intervention. If cancer cannot be excluded by examination of the testis, radical orchiectomy is warranted. Scrotal approaches and open testicular biopsies should be avoided. Further therapy depends on the histology of the tumor as well as the clinical stage.

Patients with clinical stage I **seminomas** are candidates for surveillance, single-agent carboplatin, or adjuvant radiotherapy. Stage IIa and IIb seminomas (retroperitoneal disease less than 2 cm diameter in IIa and 2–5 cm in IIb) are treated by radical orchiectomy and retroperitoneal irradiation. Retroperitoneal lymph node dissection is being studied as an alternative to radiation for stage IIa and IIb seminoma. Seminomas of stage IIc (greater than 5-cm-diameter retroperitoneal nodes) and stage III receive primary chemotherapy (etoposide and cisplatin or cisplatin, etoposide, and bleomycin) (Table 39–2). After chemotherapy, surgical resection of residual retroperitoneal nodes is warranted if the node is greater than 3 cm in diameter and positive on PET scan, since 40% will harbor residual carcinoma.

Up to 75% of clinical stage I **nonseminomas** are cured by orchiectomy alone. Selected patients who meet specific criteria may be offered surveillance after orchiectomy. These criteria are as follows: (1) cancer is confined within the tunica albuginea; (2) cancer does not demonstrate vascular invasion; (3) tumor markers normalize after orchiectomy; (4) radiographic imaging of the chest and abdomen shows no evidence of disease; and (5) the patient is reliable. Patients most likely to experience relapse on a surveillance regimen include those with predominantly embryonal cancer and those with vascular or lymphatic invasion identified in the orchiectomy specimen. Alternatives to surveillance for clinical stage I nonseminomas include adjuvant chemotherapy (bleomycin, etoposide, cisplatin) (see Table 39–2) or retroperitoneal lymph node dissection.

Following orchiectomy, patients with bulky retroperitoneal disease (greater than 5-cm nodes) or metastatic nonseminomas are treated with combination chemotherapy (cisplatin and etoposide or cisplatin, etoposide, and bleomycin) (Table 39–2). If tumor markers normalize and a residual mass greater than 1 cm persists on imaging studies, it is resected because 15–20% will harbor residual cancer and 40% will harbor teratomas. Even if patients have a complete response to chemotherapy, some clinicians advocate retroperitoneal lymphadenectomy since 10% of patients may harbor residual carcinoma and 10%, retroperitoneal teratoma. If tumor markers fail to normalize following primary chemotherapy, salvage chemotherapy is required (cisplatin, etoposide, and ifosfamide).

Postoperative active surveillance by the clinician and patient means patients are followed up every 2–6 months for the first 2 years and every 4–6 months in the third year. For nonseminomas, tumor markers are obtained at each visit, and chest radiographs and abdominal and pelvic CT scans are obtained every 4–6 months. For seminomas, serum tumor markers may be obtained (optional), chest imaging is obtained only as clinically indicated, and abdominal and pelvic CT scans are performed every 3–6 months. Follow-up continues beyond the initial 3 years; however, 80% of relapses will occur within the first 2 years. With rare exceptions, patients who relapse can be cured by chemotherapy or surgery.

Prognosis

The 5-year disease-free survival rates for stage I and IIa **seminomas** (retroperitoneal disease less than 2 cm in diameter) treated by radical orchiectomy and retroperitoneal irradiation are 98% and 92–94%, respectively. Ninety-five percent of patients with stage III disease attain a complete response following orchiectomy and chemotherapy. The 5-year disease-free survival for patients with stage I **nonseminomas** (includes all treatments) ranges from 96% to 100%. For low-volume stage II disease, a 5-year disease-free survival of 90% is expected. Patients with bulky retroperitoneal or disseminated disease treated with primary chemotherapy followed by surgery have a 5-year disease-free survival rate of 55–80%.

When to Refer

Refer all patients with solid masses of the testis to a urologist and a medical oncologist if metastatic disease is suspected.

Chovanec M et al. Management of stage I testicular germ cell tumours. Nat Rev Urol. 2016 Nov;13(11):663–73. [PMID: 27618772]

Verrill C et al; Members of the International Society of Urological Pathology Testicular Tumor Panel. Reporting and Staging of Testicular Germ Cell Tumors: The International Society of Urological Pathology (ISUP), Testicular Cancer Consultation Conference Recommendations. Am J Surg Pathol. 2017 Jun; 41(6):e22–32. [PMID: 28368923]

Williamson SR et al; Members of the ISUP Testicular Tumour Panel. The World Health Organization 2016 classification of testicular germ cell tumours: a review and update from the International Society of Urological Pathology Testis Consultation Panel. Histopathology. 2017 Feb;70(3):335–46. [PMID: 27747907]

Yadav K. Retroperitoneal lymph node dissection: an update in testicular malignancies. Clin Transl Oncol. 2017 Jul;19(7):793–8. [PMID: 28150168]

SECONDARY CANCERS OF THE TESTIS

Secondary cancers of the testis are rare. In men over the age of 50 years, lymphoma is the most common. Overall, it is the most common secondary neoplasm of the testis, accounting for 5% of all testicular cancers. It may be seen in three clinical settings: (1) late manifestation of widespread lymphoma, (2) the initial presentation of clinically occult disease, and (3) primary extranodal disease. Radical orchiectomy is indicated to make the diagnosis. Prognosis is related to the stage of disease.

Metastasis to the testis is rare. The most common primary site of origin is the prostate, followed by the lung, gastrointestinal tract, melanoma, and kidney.

CANCER COMPLICATIONS & EMERGENCIES

Patricia A. Cornett, MD

Tiffany O. Dea, PharmD, BCOP

SPINAL CORD COMPRESSION

ESSENTIALS OF DIAGNOSIS

▶ Complication of metastatic solid tumor, lymphoma, or plasma cell myeloma.

▶ Back pain is most common presenting symptom.

▶ Prompt diagnosis is essential because once a severe neurologic deficit develops, it is often irreversible.

▶ Emergent treatment may prevent or potentially reverse paresis and urinary and bowel incontinence.

▶ General Considerations

Cancers that cause spinal cord compression most commonly metastasize to the vertebral bodies, resulting in physical damage to the spinal cord from edema, hemorrhage, and pressure-induced ischemia to its vasculature. Persistent compression can result in irreversible changes to the myelin sheaths resulting in permanent neurologic impairment.

Prompt diagnosis and therapeutic intervention are essential, since the probability of reversing neurologic symptoms largely depends on the duration of symptoms. Patients who are treated promptly after symptoms appear may have partial or complete return of function and, depending on tumor sensitivity to specific treatment, may respond favorably to subsequent anticancer therapy.

▶ Clinical Findings

A. Symptoms and Signs

Back pain at the level of the tumor mass occurs in over 80% of cases and may be aggravated by lying down, weight bearing, sneezing, or coughing; it usually precedes the development of neurologic symptoms or signs. Since involvement is usually epidural, a mixture of nerve root and spinal cord symptoms often develops. Progressive weakness and sensory changes commonly occur. Bowel and bladder symptoms progressing to incontinence are late findings.

The initial findings of impending cord compression may be quite subtle, and there should be a high index of suspicion when back pain or weakness of the lower extremities develops in a cancer patient.

B. Imaging

MRI is usually the initial imaging procedure of choice in a cancer patient with new-onset back pain. If the back pain symptom is nonspecific, a whole-body PET scan with ^{18}F-2-deoxyglucose may be a useful screening procedure. Bone radiographs are neither sensitive nor specific for the evaluation of a cancer patient with back pain. When neurologic findings suggest spinal cord compression, an emergent MRI should be obtained; the MRI should survey the entire spine to define all areas of tumor involvement for treatment planning purposes.

▶ Treatment

Patients with a known cancer diagnosis found to have epidural impingement of the spinal cord should be given corticosteroids immediately. The initial dexamethasone dose is 10–100 mg intravenously followed by 4–6 mg every 6 hours intravenously or orally. Patients without a known diagnosis of cancer should have emergent surgery to relieve the impingement and obtain a pathologic specimen; preoperative corticosteroids should not be given since they might induce a tumor response and compromise the pathology results. Patients with solid tumors who have a single area of compression and who are considered candidates for surgery are best treated first with surgical decompression followed by radiation therapy. Better outcomes (ie, improved ability to ambulate and improved bladder and bowel function) occur in patients who undergo surgery followed by radiation therapy than in those who receive radiation alone. If multiple vertebral body levels are involved with cancer, fractionated radiation therapy is the preferred treatment option. Corticosteroids are generally tapered toward the end of radiation therapy. A scoring system exists for patients presenting with spinal cord metastases to identify those with poor survival times who would be best managed with supportive care or single fraction palliative radiation.

Boussios S et al. Metastatic spinal cord compression: unraveling the diagnostic and therapeutic challenges. Anticancer Res. 2018 Sep;38(9):4987–97. [PMID: 30194142]

Sodji Q et al. Management of metastatic spinal cord compression. South Med J. 2017 Sep;110(9):586–93. [PMID: 28863223]

Spratt DE et al. An integrated multidisciplinary algorithm for the management of spinal metastases: an international Spine Oncology Consortium report. Lancet Oncol. 2017 Dec; 18(12);e720–30. [PMID: 29208438]

MALIGNANT EFFUSIONS

ESSENTIALS OF DIAGNOSIS

▶ Occur in pleural, pericardial, and peritoneal spaces.

▶ Caused by direct neoplastic involvement of serous surface or obstruction of lymphatic drainage.

▶ Half of undiagnosed effusions in patients not known to have cancer are malignant.

▶ General Considerations

The development of an effusion in the pleural, pericardial, or peritoneal space may be the initial finding in a patient with cancer, or an effusion may appear during the course of disease progression. Direct involvement of the serous surface with tumor is the most frequent initiating cause of the accumulation of fluid. The most common malignancies causing pleural and pericardial effusions are lung and breast cancers; the most common malignancies associated with malignant ascites are ovarian, colorectal, stomach, and pancreatic cancers.

▶ Clinical Findings

A. Symptoms and Signs

Patients with pleural and pericardial effusions complain of shortness of breath and orthopnea. Patients with ascites complain of abdominal distention and discomfort. Cardiac tamponade causing pressure equalization in the chambers impairs both filling and cardiac output and can be life-threatening. Signs of tamponade include tachycardia, muffled heart sounds, pulsus paradoxus, and hypotension. Signs of pleural effusions include decreased breath sounds, egophony, and percussion dullness.

B. Laboratory Findings

Malignancy is confirmed as the cause of an effusion when analysis of the fluid specimen shows malignant cells in either the cytology or cell block specimen.

C. Imaging

The presence of effusions can be confirmed with radiographic studies or ultrasonography.

▶ Differential Diagnosis

The differential diagnosis of a malignant exudative pleural or pericardial effusion includes nonmalignant processes, such as infection, pulmonary embolism, heart failure, and trauma.

The differential diagnosis of malignant ascites includes similar benign processes, such as heart failure, cirrhosis, peritonitis, and pancreatic ascites.

Bloody effusions are usually due to cancer, but a bloody pleural effusion can also be due to pulmonary embolism, trauma and, occasionally, infection. Chylous pleural or ascitic fluid is generally associated with obstruction of lymphatic drainage as might occur in lymphomas.

▶ Treatment

In some cases, treatment of the underlying cancer with chemotherapy can cause regression of the effusions; however, not uncommonly, the development of an effusion is an end-stage manifestation of the cancer. In this situation, decisions regarding management are in large part dictated by the patient's symptoms and goals of care.

A. Pleural Effusion

A pleural effusion that is symptomatic may be managed initially with a **large volume thoracentesis.** With some patients, the effusion slowly reaccumulates, which allows for periodic thoracentesis when the patient becomes symptomatic. However, in many patients, the effusion reaccumulates quickly, causing rapid return of shortness of breath. For those patients, two other management options exist. **Chest tube drainage followed by pleurodesis** involves placement of a chest tube that is connected to closed water seal drainage. After lung expansion is confirmed on a chest radiograph, a sclerosing agent (such as talc slurry or doxycycline) is injected into the catheter. Patients should be premedicated with analgesics and placed in a variety of positions in order to distribute the agent throughout the pleural spaces. Occasionally, spontaneous pleurodesis will occur with drainage ceasing and the chest tube can be removed. Pleurodesis will not be successful if the lung cannot be reexpanded. These patients are better managed with the second option of **placement of an indwelling catheter** that can be drained by a family member or a visiting nurse. This procedure may also be preferable for patients with short life expectancies or for those who do not respond to pleurodesis. Chest tube drainage followed by pleurodesis or placement of an indwelling catheter have essentially equivalent outcomes in terms of cost, relief of symptoms, and other measures of quality of life.

B. Pericardial Effusion

Fluid may be removed by a needle aspiration or by placement of a catheter for more thorough drainage. As with pleural effusions, most pericardial effusions will reaccumulate. Management options for recurrent, symptomatic effusions include prolonged catheter drainage (for several days until drainage has decreased to 20–30 mL/day) or surgical intervention such as a pericardiotomy or pericardiectomy.

C. Malignant Ascites

Patients with malignant ascites not responsive to chemotherapy are generally treated with repeated large-volume paracenteses. As the frequency of drainage to maintain comfort can compromise the patient's quality of life, other alternatives include placement of a catheter or port so that the patient, family member, or visiting nurse can drain fluid as needed at home. For patients with portal hypertension from large hepatic masses, diuretics (such as spironolactone 100 mg with furosemide 20–40 mg orally daily) may be useful to decrease the need for repeated paracentesis.

Asciak R et al. Malignant pleural effusion: from diagnostics to therapeutics. Clin Chest Med. 2018 Mar;39(1):181–93. [PMID: 29433714]

Desai NR et al. Diagnosis and management of malignant pleural effusions: state of the art in 2017. J Thorac Dis. 2017 Sep;9(Suppl 10):S1111–22. [PMID: 29214068]

Ha T et al. Symptomatic fluid drainage: tunneled peritoneal and pleural catheters. Semin Intervent Radiol. 2017 Dec;34(4):337–42. [PMID: 29249857]

Thomas R et al. Effect of an indwelling pleural catheter vs. talc pleurodesis on hospitalization days in patients with malignant pleural effusion: the AMPLE randomized clinical trial. JAMA. 2017 Nov 21;318(19):1903–12. [PMID: 2916425]

HYPERCALCEMIA

ESSENTIALS OF DIAGNOSIS

▶ Usually symptomatic and severe (15 mg/dL [3.75 mmol/L] or more).

▶ Most common paraneoplastic endocrine syndrome; accounts for most inpatients with hypercalcemia.

▶ The neoplasm is clinically apparent in nearly all cases when hypercalcemia is detected.

General Considerations

Hypercalcemia affects 20–30% of cancer patients at some point during their illness. The most common cancers causing hypercalcemia are myeloma, breast carcinoma, and NSCLC. Hypercalcemia is caused by one of three mechanisms: systemic effects of tumor-released proteins, direct osteolysis of bone by tumor, or vitamin D–mediated osteoabsorption.

Clinical Findings

A. Symptoms and Signs

Symptoms and signs of hypercalcemia can be subtle; more severe symptoms occur with higher levels of hypercalcemia and with a rapid rate at which the calcium level rises. Early symptoms typically include anorexia, nausea, fatigue, constipation, and polyuria; later findings may include muscular weakness and hyporeflexia, confusion, psychosis, tremor, and lethargy.

B. Laboratory Findings

Symptoms and signs are caused by free calcium; as calcium is bound by protein in the serum, the measured serum calcium will underestimate the free or ionized calcium in patients with low albumin levels. In the setting of hypoalbuminemia, the corrected serum calcium should be calculated by one of several available formulas (eg, corrected calcium = measured calcium – measured albumin + 4). Alternatively, the free ionized calcium can be measured. When the corrected serum calcium rises above 12 mg/dL (3 mmol/L), especially if the rise occurs rapidly, sudden death due to cardiac arrhythmia or asystole may occur. The presence of hypercalcemia does not invariably indicate a dismal prognosis, especially in patients with breast cancer, myeloma, or lymphoma.

In the absence of symptoms or signs of hypercalcemia, a laboratory finding of elevated serum calcium should be retested immediately to exclude the possibility of error.

C. ECG

Electrocardiography in hypercalcemia often shows a shortening of the QT interval.

Treatment

Emergency management should begin with the initiation of intravenous fluids with 0.9% saline at 100–300 mL/h to ensure rehydration with brisk urinary output of the often volume-depleted patient. If kidney function is normal or only marginally impaired, a bisphosphonate should be given. Choices include pamidronate, 60–90 mg intravenously over 2–4 hours, zoledronic acid, 4 mg intravenously over 15 minutes, or ibandronate, 2–4 mg intravenously over 2 hours. Zoledronic acid is more potent than pamidronate and has the advantage of a shorter administration time as well as a longer duration of effect, but with repeated dosing, it is more often associated with the very uncommon but serious side effect of osteonecrosis of the jaw. Once hypercalcemia is controlled, treatment directed at the cancer should be initiated if possible. However, hypercalcemia can occur in patients with cancers that are unresponsive to treatment. In the event that the hypercalcemia becomes refractory to repeated doses of bisphosphonates, other agents that can help control hypercalcemia (at least temporarily) include calcitonin and denosumab; corticosteroids can be useful in patients with myeloma and lymphoma. Salmon calcitonin, 4–8 international units/kg given subcutaneously or intramuscularly every 12 hours, can be used in patients with severe, symptomatic hypercalcemia; its onset of action is within hours but its hypocalcemic effect wanes in 2–3 days. Denosumab, 120 mg given subcutaneously weekly for 4 weeks followed by monthly administration, is a choice for long-term management of bisphosphonate-refractory hypercalcemia or for patients with kidney dysfunction that precludes use of a bisphosphonate.

Carrick AI et al. Rapid fire: hypercalcemia. Emerg Med Clin North Am. 2018 Aug;36(3):549–55. [PMID: 30037441]

HYPERURICEMIA & TUMOR LYSIS SYNDROME

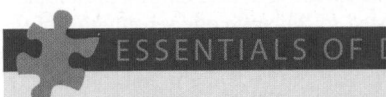

ESSENTIALS OF DIAGNOSIS

► Complication of treatment-associated tumor lysis of hematologic and rapidly proliferating malignancies.

► May be worsened by thiazide diuretics.

► Rapid increase in serum uric acid can cause acute urate nephropathy from uric acid crystallization.

► Reducing pre-chemotherapy serum uric acid is fundamental to preventing urate nephropathy.

General Considerations

Tumor lysis syndrome (TLS) is seen most commonly following treatment of hematologic malignancies, such as acute lymphoblastic leukemia and Burkitt lymphoma. However, TLS can develop from any tumor highly sensitive to chemotherapy. TLS is caused by the massive release of cellular material including nucleic acids, proteins, phosphorus, and potassium. If both the metabolism and excretion of these breakdown products are impaired, hyperuricemia, hyperphosphatemia, and hyperkalemia will develop abruptly. Acute kidney injury may then develop from the crystallization and deposition of uric acid and calcium phosphate within the renal tubules further exacerbating the hyperphosphatemia and hyperkalemia.

Clinical Findings

Symptoms of hyperphosphatemia include nausea and vomiting as well as seizures. Also, with high levels of phosphorus, co-precipitation with calcium can cause renal tubule blockage, further exacerbating the kidney injury. Hyperkalemia, due to release of intracellular potassium and impaired kidney excretion, can cause arrhythmias and sudden death.

Treatment

Prevention is the most important factor in the management of TLS. Aggressive hydration prior to initiation of chemotherapy as well as during and after completion of the chemotherapy helps keep urine flowing and facilitates excretion of uric acid and phosphorus. In addition, for patients at moderate risk for developing TLS, eg, those with intermediate-grade lymphomas and acute leukemias, allopurinol should be given before starting chemotherapy at an oral dose of 100 mg/m² every 8 hours (maximum 800 mg/day) with dose reductions for impaired kidney function. Rasburicase 0.1–0.2 mg/kg/day is given intravenously for 1–7 days to patients at high risk for developing TLS, eg, those with high-grade lymphomas or acute leukemias with markedly elevated white blood cell counts (acute myeloid leukemia, white blood cell count greater than 50,000/mcL [50,000/10⁹/L]; acute lymphoblastic leukemia, white blood cell count greater than 100,000/mcL [100,000/10⁹/L]; or chronic lymphocytic

leukemia with large lymph nodes [10 cm or larger] or nodes 5 cm or larger accompanied by white blood cell counts greater than 25,000/mcL [25,000/10⁹/L] and treated with venetoclax; or in any patient in whom hyperuricemia develops despite treatment with allopurinol). Rasburicase cannot be given to patients with known glucose 6-phosphate dehydrogenase (G6PD) deficiency nor can it be given to pregnant or lactating women. Systemic bicarbonate infusions to alkalinize the urine are not routinely recommended unless there is accompanying metabolic acidosis. In addition to the hyperuricemia, laboratory values should be monitored following initiation of chemotherapy; elevated potassium or phosphorus levels need to be promptly managed.

► When to Refer

Should urinary output drop, serum creatinine or potassium levels rise, or hyperphosphatemia persist, a nephrologist should be immediately consulted to evaluate the need for dialysis.

Dubbs SB. Rapid fire: tumor lysis syndrome. Emerg Med Clin North Am. 2018 Aug;36(3):517–25. [PMID: 30037438]

Howard SC et al. Tumor lysis syndrome in the era of novel and targeted agents in patients with hematologic malignancies: a systematic review. Ann Hematol. 2016 Mar;95(4):563–73. [PMID: 26758269]

INFECTIONS

Chapters 30 and 31 provide more detailed discussions of infections in the immunocompromised patient.

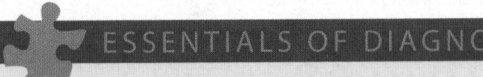

ESSENTIALS OF DIAGNOSIS

► In patients with neutropenia, infection is a medical emergency.

► Although sometimes attributable to other causes, the presence of fever, defined as a single temperature greater than 38.3°C (101°F) or a temperature of greater than 38°C (100.4°F) for longer than 1 hour, must be assumed to be due to an infection.

General Considerations

Many patients with disseminated neoplasms have increased susceptibility to infection. In some patients, this results from impaired defense mechanisms (eg, acute leukemia, Hodgkin lymphoma, plasma cell myeloma, chronic lymphocytic leukemia); in others, it results from the myelosuppressive and immunosuppressive effects of cancer chemotherapy or a combination of these factors. Complicating impaired defense mechanisms are the frequent presence of indwelling catheters, impaired mucosal surfaces, and colonization with more virulent hospital-acquired pathogens.

The source of a neutropenic febrile episode is determined in about 30% of cases through blood, urine, or sputum cultures. The bacterial organisms accounting for the majority of infections in cancer patients include gram-positive bacteria (coagulase-negative *Staphylococcus*, *Staphylococcus aureus*, *Streptococcus pneumoniae*, *Corynebacterium*, and streptococci) and gram-negative bacteria (*Escherichia coli*, *Klebsiella*, *Pseudomonas*, *Enterobacter*). Gram-positive organism infections are more common, but gram-negative infections are more serious and life-threatening. The risk of bacterial infections rises when the neutrophil count is below 500/mcL (0.5×10^9/L); the risk markedly increases when the count falls below 100/mcL (0.1×10^9/L) or when there is a prolonged duration of neutropenia, typically greater than 7 days.

▶ Clinical Findings

A thorough physical examination should be performed. Routine DREs are generally avoided unless symptoms suggest a rectal abscess or prostatitis. If a DRE is necessary, antibiotics should be administered first. Appropriate cultures (eg, blood, sputum, urine and, if indicated, cerebrospinal fluid) should always be obtained. Two sets of blood cultures should be drawn before starting antibiotics; if the patient has an indwelling catheter, one of the cultures should be drawn from the line. A chest radiograph should also be obtained.

▶ Treatment

Empiric antibiotic therapy needs to be initiated within 1 hour of presentation and following the collection of blood cultures in the febrile, neutropenic patient. The choice of antibiotics depends on a number of different factors including the patient's clinical status and any localizing source of infection. If the patient is clinically well, monotherapy with an intravenous beta-lactam with anti-*Pseudomonas* activity (cefepime, ceftazidime, imipenem/cilastatin, piperacillin/tazobactam) should be started (see Infections in the Immunocompromised Patient, Chapter 30). If the patient is clinically ill with hypotension or hypoxia, an intravenous aminoglycoside or fluoroquinolone should be added for "double" gram-negative bacteria coverage. If there is a strong suspicion of a gram-positive organism, such as from *S aureus* catheter infection, intravenous vancomycin can be given empirically. Low-risk patients may be treated with oral antibiotics and even in the outpatient setting. The Infectious Diseases Society of America (IDSA) has published recommendations for such antibiotic use. These patients must have an expected neutropenic time frame of 7 days or less and have no comorbidities or signs of hemodynamic instability, gastrointestinal symptoms, altered mental status, pulmonary problems (infiltrate, hypoxia, or underlying chronic obstructive pulmonary disease), or liver or kidney disease or impairment. Patients should receive initial doses of empiric antibacterial therapy within 1 hour of being seen and monitored for at least 4 hours before discharge. If a patient is to be treated as an outpatient, he or she must also have good support at home and easy access to returning to the hospital if the clinical status worsens. If the patient does not defervesce with the broad-spectrum oral antibiotics, then the patient should be reevaluated for inpatient management.

Antibiotics should be continued until the neutrophil count is rising and greater than 500/mcL (0.5×10^9/L) for at least 1 day and the patient has been afebrile for 2 days. If an organism is identified through the cultures, the antibiotics should be adjusted to the antibiotic sensitivities of the isolate; treatment should be continued for the appropriate period of time and at least until the neutrophil count recovers and fever resolves.

For the neutropenic patient who is persistently febrile despite broad-spectrum antibiotics, an empiric antifungal drug should be added (amphotericin B, caspofungin, itraconazole, voriconazole, or liposomal amphotericin B).

Beyar-Katz O et al. Empirical antibiotics targeting gram-positive bacteria for the treatment of febrile neutropenic patients with cancer. Cochrane Database Syst Rev. 2017 Jun 3;6:CD003914. [PMID: 28577308]

Knight T et al. Acute oncology care: a narrative review of the acute management of neutropenic sepsis and immune-related toxicities of checkpoint inhibitors. Eur J Intern Med. 2017 Nov;45:59–65. [PMID: 28993098]

Krzyzanowska MK et al. Approach to evaluation of fever in ambulatory cancer patients receiving chemotherapy: a systematic review. Cancer Treat Rev. 2016 Dec;51:35–45. [PMID: 27842279]

PRIMARY CANCER TREATMENT

Patricia A. Cornett, MD
Tiffany O. Dea, PharmD, BCOP

SYSTEMIC CANCER THERAPY

Detailed guidelines from the NCCN for cancer treatment can be found at www.nccn.org.

Use of cytotoxic drugs, hormones, antihormones, and biologic agents has become a highly specialized and increasingly effective means of treating cancer, with therapy administered and monitored by a medical oncologist or hematologist. Selection of specific drugs or protocols for various types of cancer is usually based on results of clinical trials. Increasingly, newer agents are being identified that target specific molecular pathways. Yet both initial and acquired drug resistance remains a challenge. Described mechanisms of drug resistance include impaired membrane transport of drugs, enhanced drug metabolism, mutated target proteins, and blockage of apoptosis due to mutations in cellular proteins (see Table 39–2 for suggested agents for various cancers).

TOXICITY & DOSE MODIFICATION OF CHEMOTHERAPEUTIC AGENTS

Use of chemotherapy to treat cancer is generally guided by results from clinical trials in individual tumor types. The complexity of treating cancer has increased over the last decade as more drugs, including those with more targeted mechanisms of action, have been approved by the US Food and Drug Administration (FDA) and introduced into general practice. Drug side effects and toxicities must be anticipated and carefully monitored. The short- and long-term toxicities of individual drugs are listed in Tables 39–3 and 39–13. Decisions on dose modifications for toxicities should be guided by the intent of therapy. In the palliative setting where the aim of

Table 39–13. Commonly used supportive care agents.[1]

Agent	Indication	Usual Dose	Adverse Effects
Allopurinol (Xyloprim)	Prevent hyperuricemia from tumor lysis syndrome	600–800 mg/day orally	Acute: none Delayed: rash
Dexrazoxane (Zinecard)	Prevent cardiomyopathy secondary to doxorubicin; anthracycline-induced injection site extravasation	10 times the doxorubicin dose intravenously before doxorubicin; 1000 mg/m² intravenously on days 1 and 2, then 500 mg/m² intravenously on day 3	Acute: nausea Delayed: myelosuppression, elevated transaminases
Leucovorin	Rescue after high-dose methotrexate; in combination with fluorouracil for colon cancer	10 mg/m² intravenously or orally every 6 hours; 20 mg/m² or 200–500 mg/m² intravenously before fluorouracil; various doses	Acute: nausea, vomiting, diarrhea Delayed: stomatitis, fatigue
Levoleucovorin (Fusilev)	Rescue after high-dose methotrexate; in combination with fluorouracil for colon cancer	7.5 mg intravenously every 6 hours for 10 doses; 100 mg/m² intravenously before fluorouracil	Acute: nausea, vomiting Delayed: stomatitis, diarrhea
Mesna (Mesnex)	Prevent ifosfamide-induced hemorrhagic cystitis	20% of ifosfamide dose intravenously at 0, 4, and 8 hours; various doses	Acute: nausea, vomiting Delayed: fatigue
Palifermin (Kepivance)	Prevent mucositis following chemotherapy	60 mcg/kg/day intravenously for 3 days before and 3 days after chemotherapy	Acute: none Delayed: rash, fever, elevated serum amylase, erythema, edema
Pilocarpine (Salagen)	Radiation-induced xerostomia	5–10 mg orally three times a day	Acute: flushing, sweating, nausea, dizziness Delayed: increased urinary frequency, rhinitis
Radium (Ra)-223 dichloride (Xofigo)	Symptomatic bone metastases	50 kilobecquerel/kg (1.35 micro-Curie/kg) intravenously every 4 weeks for 6 cycles	Acute: nausea, vomiting, diarrhea, peripheral edema Delayed: myelosuppression
Rasburicase (Elitek)	Prevent hyperuricemia from tumor lysis syndrome	3–6 mg intravenously once	Acute: hypersensitivity, nausea, vomiting, diarrhea, fever, headache Delayed: rash, peripheral edema
Bone-Modifying Agents			
Denosumab (Xgeva)	Osteolytic bone metastasis	120 mg subcutaneously every 4 weeks	Acute: nausea Delayed: hypocalcemia, hypophosphatemia, fatigue, osteonecrosis of the jaw
Pamidronate (Aredia)	Osteolytic bone metastasis, hypercalcemia of malignancy	90 mg intravenously every 3–4 weeks; 60–90 mg intravenously, may repeat after 7 days	Acute: nausea Delayed: dyspnea, arthralgia, bone pain, osteonecrosis of the jaw, nephrotoxicity, hypocalcemia
Zoledronic acid (Zometa)	Osteolytic bone metastasis, hypercalcemia of malignancy	4 mg intravenously every 3–4 weeks; 4 mg intravenously once, may repeat after 7 days	
Growth Factors			
Darbepoetin alfa (Aranesp)	Chemotherapy-induced anemia	2.25 mcg/kg subcutaneously weekly; 500 mcg subcutaneously every 3 weeks	
Epoetin alfa (Epogen, Procrit)	Chemotherapy-induced anemia	40,000 units subcutaneously once weekly; 150 units/kg subcutaneously three times a week	Acute: injection site reaction Delayed: hypertension, thromboembolic events, increased risk of tumor progression or recurrence
Filgrastim (Neupogen)	Febrile neutropenia prophylaxis, mobilization of peripheral stem cells	5–10 mcg/kg/day subcutaneously or intravenously once daily, treat past nadir	Acute: injection site reaction Delayed: bone pain

(continued)

Table 39–13. Commonly used supportive care agents.[1] (continued)

Agent	Indication	Usual Dose	Adverse Effects
Growth Factors (cont.)			
Pegfilgrastim (Neulasta)	Febrile neutropenia prophylaxis	6 mg subcutaneously once per chemotherapy cycle	
Sargramostim (Leukine)	Myeloid reconstitution following bone marrow transplant, mobilization of peripheral blood stem cells	250 mcg/m² intravenously daily until the absolute neutrophil count is > 1500 cells/mcL for 3 consecutive days	Acute: fever, rash, pruritus, nausea, vomiting, diarrhea, injection site reaction, dyspnea Delayed: asthenia, bone pain, mucositis, edema, arrhythmia

[1]For amifostine, samarium, strontium, filgrastim-sndz, and tbo-filgrastim, see Table 39–13 in *CMDT Online* at www.accessmedicine.com.

therapy is to improve symptoms and quality of life, lowering doses to minimize toxicity is commonly done. However, when the goal of treatment is cure, dosing frequency and intensity should be maintained whenever possible.

A CBC including a differential count, with absolute neutrophil count and platelet count, and liver and kidney tests should be obtained before the initiation of chemotherapy. In patients with normal CBCs as well as normal liver and kidney function, drugs are started at their full dose. When the intent of chemotherapy is cure, including treatment in the adjuvant setting, every attempt should be made to schedule chemotherapy on time and at full dose. A CBC with differential may be checked at mid cycle (to determine the nadir of the absolute neutrophil and platelet counts), and liver and kidney function tests should be obtained immediately before the next cycle of chemotherapy.

Dose reductions may be necessary for patients with impaired kidney or liver function depending on the clearance mechanism of the drug. For patients receiving chemotherapy for palliation, bone marrow toxicity can be managed with dose reductions or delaying the next treatment cycle. A schema for dose modification is shown in Table 39–14.

1. Bone Marrow Toxicity

A. Neutropenia

Granulocyte colony-stimulating factor (G-CSF), given as either daily subcutaneous injections (eg, filgrastim, 300 mcg or 480 mcg) or as a one-time dose (pegfilgrastim, 6 mg) beginning 24 hours after cytotoxic chemotherapy is completed, reduces the duration and severity of granulocytopenia following cytotoxic chemotherapy (Table 39–13). The American Society of Clinical Oncology and NCCN guidelines recommend primary prophylaxis with G-CSF

Table 39–14. A common scheme for dose modification of cancer chemotherapeutic agents.

Granulocyte Count (cells/mcL)	Platelet Count (/mcL)	Suggested Drug Dosage (% of Full Dose)
> 2000	> 100,000	100%
1000–2000	75,000–100,000	50%
< 2000	< 50,000	0%

when there is at least a 20% risk of febrile neutropenia or when age, medical history, and disease characteristics put the patient at high risk for complications related to myelosuppression.

B. Anemia

Erythropoiesis-stimulating agents (ESAs) ameliorate the anemia and its associated symptoms caused by cancer chemotherapy but these drugs have untoward effects, including an increased risk of thromboembolism, and possibly a decreased survival due to cancer-related deaths as well as a shortened time to tumor progression. The FDA recommends that these drugs should not be used when the intent of chemotherapy is curative. Administration of red blood cell transfusions is the alternative to managing symptomatic anemia in such patients.

ESAs can be an option in cancer patients with symptomatic anemia undergoing palliative treatment; patient preference is important in determining when to use ESAs or transfusions. When using ESAs, treatment should not be initiated until the hemoglobin is less than 10 g/dL (100 g/L) and the ESA held when the hemoglobin is greater than 12 g/dL (120 g/L). Epoetin alfa can be given subcutaneously at a dose of 40,000 units weekly or 150 units/kg three times weekly with a target hemoglobin of 11–12 g/dL (110–120 g/L). Darbepoetin alfa is given subcutaneously at a dose of 300–500 mcg every 3 weeks or 2.25 mcg weekly with the same target hemoglobin (see Table 39–13). To have maximum therapeutic effect, patients need to be iron replete. Uncontrolled hypertension is a contraindication to the use of ESAs; blood pressure must be controlled prior to initiation of this therapy.

C. Thrombocytopenia

Drug management of chemotherapy-induced thrombocytopenia is more limited. The only available drug, oprelvekin or recombinant interleukin-11, has modest activity in improving chemotherapy-related thrombocytopenia; however, it is rarely used due to the side effects of fluid retention, heart failure, and arrhythmias. Two drugs that activate the thrombopoietin receptor, romiplostim and eltrombopag, are FDA approved for use in idiopathic thrombocytopenia. Romiplostim is also approved for patients with thrombocytopenia related to interferon therapy of hepatitis C and for patients with aplastic anemia. While these agents have been used in selected cases of refractory chemotherapy-related thrombo-cytopenia with some reports of success, trials to date have not demonstrated convincing efficacy in patients with chemotherapy-induced thrombocytopenia and neither agent is FDA approved for this indication.

2. Chemotherapy-Induced Nausea & Vomiting

A number of cytotoxic anticancer drugs can induce nausea and vomiting, which can be the most anticipated and stressful side effects for patients. Chemotherapy-induced nausea and vomiting is mediated in part by the stimulation of at least two central nervous system receptors, 5-hydroxytryp-tamine subtype 3 ($5HT_3$) and neurokinin subtype 1 (NK_1). Chemotherapy-induced nausea and vomiting can be antici-patory, occurring even before chemotherapy administration; acute, occurring within minutes to hours of chemotherapy administration; or delayed until the second day and lasting up to 7 days. Chemotherapy drugs are classified into high, moderate, low, and minimal likelihoods of causing emesis (90%, 30–90%, 10–30%, less than 10%, respectively). Highly emetogenic chemotherapy drugs include carmustine, cispla-tin, cyclophosphamide (at doses over 1.5 g/m^2), dacarbazine, mechlorethamine, and streptozocin, or a combination of regularly dosed anthracyclines and cyclophosphamide. Mod-erately emetogenic chemotherapy drugs include alemtu-zumab, azacitadine, bendamustine, carboplatin, clofarabine, crizotinib, cyclophosphamide, cytarabine, daunomycin, doxorubicin, epirubicin, idarubicin, ifosfamide, irinotecan, mitotane, oxaliplatin, romidepsin, temozolomide, and vis-modegib. Low emetogenic drugs include bortezomib, bren-tuximab, capecitabine, cabozantinib, dabrafenib, dasatinib, docetaxel, erlotinib, etoposide, fludarabine, fluorouracil, gemcitabine, hydroxyurea, ipilimumab, ixabepilone, lenalid-omide, methotrexate, mitomycin, mitoxantrone, omacetax-ine, paclitaxel, pemetrexed, pomalidomide, ponatinib, temsirolimus, trametinib, and topotecan. Drugs with mini-mal risk of emesis include bevacizumab, bleomycin, cetux-imab, cladribine, decitabine, fludarabine, nivolumab, panitumumab, pembrolizumab, rituximab, temsirolimus, trastuzumab, vinblastine, vincristine, and vinorelbine.

Major advances have occurred in the development of highly effective antiemetic drugs. **Antagonists to the $5HT_3$-receptor** include alosetron, ondansetron, granisetron, dola-setron, and palonosetron, as well as tropisetron and ramosetron (neither yet available in the United States). Ondansetron can be given either intravenously (8 mg or 0.15 mg/kg) or orally (24 mg once before highly emetogenic che-motherapy, 8 mg twice daily for moderately emetogenic chemotherapy). Doses of 8 mg can be repeated parenterally or orally every 8 hours. Dosing of granisetron is 1 mg or 0.01 mg/kg intravenously or 1–2 mg orally. Dolasetron is given once as an oral 100-mg dose. Palonosetron, a long-acting $5HT_3$ with high affinity for the $5HT_3$-receptor, is given once at a dose of 0.25 mg intravenously, both for acute and delayed emesis. Where available, tropisetron is given at a dose of 5 mg either orally or intravenously and ramosetron, as a one-time 300-mcg dose intravenously. The efficacy of the $5HT_3$-blockers is improved by adding dexamethasone 10 mg once intravenously, then 4 mg orally or intravenously every 6 hours. As a class of drugs, the $5HT_3$-receptor

antagonists have the potential to cause electrocardiogram changes, including QT prolongation. Before using these agents, hypokalemia or hypomagnesemia should be cor-rected. In addition, clinicians should be cautious when using these agents in patients who are elderly, who have preexist-ing bradyarrhythmias or heart failure, or who are taking medications known to prolong the QT interval.

Aprepitant, fosaprepitant, netupitant, palonosetron, and rolapitant are **antagonists to the NK_1 receptor**. Aprepitant is given as a 125-mg oral dose followed by an 80-mg dose on the second and third day along with a $5HT_3$-receptor antag-onist (such as ondansetron or granisetron) and dexametha-sone to increase its immediate and delayed protective effect for highly emetogenic chemotherapy. Fosaprepitant, the intravenous formulation of the prodrug to aprepitant, can be given at a dose of 115 mg if followed by 2 days of aprepitant or at a dose of 150 mg if given alone. NEPA is a single-dose capsule consisting of a combination of netupitant and palo-nosetron. Rolapitant, a potent selective NK_1 receptor antag-onist, has a 7-day half-life; it is given as a one-time oral dose of 180 mg 1–2 hours before the start of moderately or highly emetogenic chemotherapy.

For highly emetogenic chemotherapy (eg, cisplatin), patients should be offered a four-drug regimen (a $5HT_3$-antagonist, dexamethasone, neurokinin-1 receptor antago-nist, and olanzapine), all given on the first day (and if used, aprepitant given again on the second and third days with decadron and olanzapine continued on days 2–4. For mod-erately emetogenic chemotherapy, standard regimens include both three-drug regimens (an NK_1 receptor antag-onist, a $5HT_3$-antagonist, and dexamethasone) or a two-drug combination ($5HT_3$-antagonist and dexamethasone). Palonosetron is the preferred $5HT_3$-blocker due to its greater affinity for the $5HT_3$-receptor and its longer half-life. For low emetogenic chemotherapy drugs, a single agent such as a $5HT_3$-antagonist or prochlorperazine or dexamethasone can be given. A 25-mg suppository form of prochlorperazine may be used for patients unable to swal-low oral medications. Another medication that is helpful for anticipatory or refractory nausea and vomiting is olan-zapine, 10 mg given orally once.

The importance of treating chemotherapy-induced nau-sea and vomiting expectantly and aggressively beginning with the first course of chemotherapy cannot be overem-phasized. Patients being treated in the clinic setting should always be given antiemetics for home use with written instructions as well as contact numbers to call for advice.

3. Gastrointestinal Toxicity

Untoward effects of cancer chemotherapy include damage to the more rapidly growing cells of the body such as the mucosal lining from the mouth through the gastrointesti-nal tract. Oral symptoms range from mild mouth soreness to frank ulcerations. Not uncommonly, mouth ulcerations will have superimposed candida or herpes simplex infec-tions. In addition to receiving cytotoxic chemotherapy, a significant risk factor for development of oral mucositis is poor oral hygiene and existing caries or periodontal dis-ease. Toxicity in the gastrointestinal tract usually manifests as diarrhea. Gastrointestinal symptoms can range from mild symptoms of loose stools to life-threatening diarrhea leading to dehydration and electrolyte imbalances. Drugs most commonly associated with causing mucositis in the mouth and the gastrointestinal tract are cytarabine, 5-fluorouracil, and methotrexate.

Patients undergoing treatment for head and neck cancer with concurrent chemotherapy and radiation therapy have a very high risk of developing severe mucositis.

Preventive strategies for oral mucositis include pretreatment dental care, particularly for all head and neck cancer patients and any cancer patient with poor dental hygiene who will be receiving chemotherapy. For patients receiving fluorouracil, simple measures such as ice chips in the mouth for 30 minutes during infusion can reduce the incidence and severity of mucositis. Once mucositis is encountered, superimposed fungal infections should be treated with topical antifungal medications (oral nystatin mouth suspensions, or clotrimazole troches) or systemic therapy (fluconazole 100–400 mg orally daily). Suspected herpetic infections can be treated with acyclovir (up to 800 mg orally five times daily) or valacyclovir (1 g orally twice daily). Mucositis may also be managed with mouthwashes; it is also important to provide adequate pain medication.

Other strategies for prevention of oral mucositis include the use of palifermin, the recombinant keratinocyte growth factor inhibitor. Prophylaxis with intravenous palifermin (60 mcg/kg/day) for patients receiving high-dose chemotherapy can reduce the incidence and duration of mucositis (Table 39–13).

Diarrhea is most associated with fluorouracil, capecitabine, and irinotecan as well as the tyrosine kinase inhibitors (dasatinib, imatinib, nilotinib, regorafenib, sorafenib, sunitinib) and epithelial growth factor inhibitors (cetuximab, erlotinib, panitumumab). Mild to moderate diarrhea can be managed with oral antidiarrheal medication (loperamide, 4 mg initially followed by 2 mg every 2–4 hours until bowel movements are formed). Occasionally, severe diarrhea will cause dehydration, electrolyte imbalances, and acute kidney injury; these patients require inpatient management with aggressive intravenous hydration and electrolyte replacement. Octreotide, 100–150 mcg subcutaneously three times daily, can be useful.

4. Skin Toxicity

Dermatologic complications from cancer chemotherapy can include hyperpigmentation (busulfan, hydroxyurea, liposomal doxorubicin), alopecia, photosensitivity, nail changes, acral erythema, and generalized rashes. Acral erythema (hand-foot syndrome), most commonly associated with administration of capecitabine, fluorouracil, and liposomal doxorubicin, manifests as painful palms or soles accompanied by erythema, progressing to blistering, desquamation, and ulceration in its worst forms. Strategies for prevention of acral erythema include oral pyridoxine, 200 mg daily, and applying cold packs to the extremities during chemotherapy administration. Agents targeting the epidermal growth factor pathway can cause an acne-like rash; the development of the rash may identify those who will respond to the drug. Inhibitors of the tyrosine kinase

pathway are also associated with a high incidence of dermatologic complications, such as rash and acral erythema.

5. Miscellaneous Drug-Specific Toxicities

The toxicities of individual drugs are summarized in Tables 39–3 and 39–13; however, several of these toxicities warrant additional mention, since they occur with frequently administered agents, and special measures are often indicated.

A. Hemorrhagic Cystitis Induced by Cyclophosphamide or Ifosfamide

Patients receiving cyclophosphamide must maintain a high fluid intake prior to and following the administration of the drug and be counseled to empty their bladders frequently. Early symptoms suggesting bladder toxicity include dysuria and increased frequency of urination. Should microscopic hematuria develop, it is advisable to stop the drug temporarily or switch to a different alkylating agent, to increase fluid intake, and to administer a urinary analgesic such as phenazopyridine. The neutralizing agent, mesna, can be used for patients in whom cystitis develops. With severe cystitis, large segments of bladder mucosa may be shed, resulting in prolonged gross hematuria. Such patients should be observed for signs of urinary obstruction and may require cystoscopy for removal of obstructing blood clots. The cyclophosphamide analog ifosfamide can cause severe hemorrhagic cystitis when used alone. However, when its use is followed by a series of doses of the neutralizing agent mesna, bladder toxicity can be prevented (Table 39–13).

B. Neuropathy Due to Vinca Alkaloids and Other Chemotherapy Drugs

Neuropathy is caused by a number of different chemotherapy drugs, the most common being vincristine. The peripheral neuropathy can be sensory, motor, autonomic, or a combination of these types. In its mildest form, it consists of paresthesias of the fingers and toes. Occasionally, acute jaw or throat pain can develop as a form of trigeminal or glossopharyngeal neuralgia. With continued vincristine therapy, the paresthesias extend to the proximal interphalangeal joints, hyporeflexia appears in the lower extremities, and significant weakness can develop. Other drugs in the vinca alkaloid class as well as the taxane drugs (docetaxel and paclitaxel) and agents to treat myeloma (bortezomib and thalidomide) cause similar toxicity. The presence of neurologic symptoms is not in itself a reason to stop therapy; the severity of the symptoms must be balanced against the goals of therapy. Usually, though, the development of moderate to severe paresthesias or motor impairment results in the decision to discontinue the drug.

Constipation is the most common symptom of autonomic neuropathy associated with the vinca alkaloids. Patients receiving these drugs should be started on mild cathartics and other agents (Table 15–4); otherwise, severe impaction may result from an atonic bowel. More serious autonomic involvement can lead to acute intestinal obstruction with signs indistinguishable from those of an acute abdomen. Bladder neuropathies are uncommon but may be severe. These two complications are absolute contraindications to continued vincristine therapy.

C. Methotrexate Toxicity

Methotrexate, a folate antagonist, is a commonly used component of regimens to treat patients with leptomeningeal disease, acute lymphoblastic leukemia, and sarcomas. Methotrexate is almost entirely eliminated by the kidney. Methotrexate toxicity affects cells with rapid turnover, including the bone marrow and mucosa resulting in myelosuppression and mucositis. Methotrexate can also damage the liver and kidney manifesting as elevated serum liver enzymes and creatinine. High-dose methotrexate, usually defined as a dose of 500 mg/m^2 or more given over 4–36 hours, would be lethal without "rescue" of the normal tissues. Leucovorin, a form of folate, will reverse the toxic effects of methotrexate and is given until serum methotrexate levels are in the safe range (less than 0.05 mmol/L). It is crucial that high-dose methotrexate and leucovorin are given precisely according to protocol as deviations of the timing of methotrexate delivery or delay in rescue can result in patient death. The dose used in intrathecal therapy is 12 mg. Lower doses of methotrexate can be problematic in patients with kidney disease who cannot clear the drug normally or in patients with effusions in which the drug distributes itself and leaks out continuously, exposing normal tissue to the drug. In a patient with kidney disease or an effusion, prolonged rescue with leucovorin is necessary.

Vigorous hydration and bicarbonate loading can help prevent crystallization of high-dose methotrexate in the renal tubular epithelium and consequent nephrotoxicity. Daily monitoring of the serum creatinine is mandatory. If possible, drugs impairing methotrexate excretion, such as aspirin, nonsteroidal anti-inflammatory drugs, amiodarone, omeprazole, penicillin, phenytoin, and sulfa, should be stopped before methotrexate administration.

D. Cardiotoxicity from Anthracyclines and Other Chemotherapy Drugs

A number of cancer chemotherapy drugs are associated with cardiovascular complications including traditional drugs such as anthracyclines as well as new targeted agents. The anthracycline drugs, including doxorubicin, daunomycin, epirubicin, and idarubicin, can produce acute (during administration), subacute (days to months following administration), and delayed (years following administration) cardiac toxicity. The most feared complication is the delayed development of heart failure. Risk factors for this debilitating toxicity include the anthracycline cumulative dose, age over 70, previous or concurrent irradiation of the chest, preexisting cardiac disease, and concurrent administration of chemotherapy drugs such as trastuzumab. The problem is greatest with doxorubicin because it is the most commonly administered anthracycline due to its major role in the treatment of lymphomas, sarcomas, breast cancer, and certain other solid tumors. Patients receiving anthracyclines should have a baseline multiple-gated (MUGA) radionuclide cardiac scan to calculate the left ventricular-ejection fraction (LVEF). If the LVEF is greater than 50%, anthracyclines can be administered; if the LVEF is less than 30%, these drugs should not be given. For patients with intermediate values, anthracyclines can be cautiously given, if necessary, at lower doses with LVEF monitoring between doses. Changes in cardiac dynamics occur in most patients by the time they have received a total dose of 300 mg/m^2 of doxorubicin. In general, patients should not receive doses in excess of 450 mg/m^2; the dose should be lower if prior chest radiotherapy has been given. The appearance of a high resting pulse may herald the appearance of overt cardiac toxicity. Unfortunately, toxicity may be irreversible and frequently fatal at total dosage levels above 550 mg/m^2. At lower doses (eg, 350 mg/m^2), the symptoms and signs of cardiac failure generally respond well to medical therapy and discontinuation of the anthracycline. Doxorubicin and daunomycin have been formulated as liposomal products; these drugs, approved for use in patients with Kaposi sarcoma and sometimes in other cancers as a substitute for the conventional anthracyclines, appear to have minimal potential for cardiac toxicity.

As molecular mechanisms for cancer have been increasingly delineated, therapies have been developed that better target these mechanisms. Therapies targeting oncogenesis pathways include (1) HER2 inhibitors (lapatinib, pertuzumab, trastuzumab); (2) VEGF signaling pathway inhibitors (afilbercept, axitinib, bevacizumab, carozantinib, lenvatinib, pazopanib, ramucirumab, regorafenib, sorafenib, sunitinib, vandertanib); (3) multitargeted tyrosine kinase inhibitors (dasatinib, nilotinib, ponatinib); (4) proteasome inhibitors (bortezomib, carfilzomib); and (5) immune checkpoint inhibitors (ipilimumab, nivolumab, pembrolizumab). Many of the pathways targeted by these drugs share a common biologic pathway in cardiac tissue. Untoward cardiac events are being increasingly reported with these agents, including arrhythmias, cardiac ischemia, myocarditis, thrombosis, and heart failure. It is important to carefully monitor patients on these drugs and aggressively manage any modifiable cardiac risk factors (smoking, hyperlipidemia, diabetes mellitus, sedentary lifestyle).

E. Cisplatin Nephrotoxicity and Neurotoxicity

Cisplatin is effective in treating testicular, bladder, head and neck, lung, and ovarian cancers. With cisplatin, the serious side effects of nephrotoxicity and neurotoxicity must be anticipated and aggressively managed. Patients must be vigorously hydrated prior to, during, and after cisplatin administration. Both kidney function and electrolytes must be monitored. Low serum magnesium, potassium, and sodium levels can develop. The neurotoxicity is usually manifested as a peripheral neuropathy of mixed sensorimotor type and may be associated with painful paresthesias. Development of neuropathy typically occurs after cumulative doses of 300 mg/m^2. Ototoxicity is a potentially serious manifestation of neurotoxicity and can progress to deafness. Amifostine, given intravenously at a dose of 910 mg/m^2 over 15 minutes prior to cisplatin, is used to protect against nephrotoxicity and neuropathy. Use of amifostine does not appear to compromise its antineoplastic effect. The second-generation platinum analog, carboplatin, is non-nephrotoxic, although it is myelosuppressive. In the setting of preexisting kidney disease or neuropathy, carboplatin is occasionally substituted for cisplatin.

F. Bleomycin Toxicity

See online text at www.accessmedicine.com/cmdt.

PROGNOSIS

Patients receiving chemotherapy for curative intent will often tolerate side effects with the knowledge that the treatment may result in eradication of their cancer. Patients receiving therapy for palliative intent often have their therapy tailored to improve quality of life while minimizing major side effects. A valuable sign of clinical improvement is the general well-being of the patient. Although general well-being is a combination of subjective (possibly partly a placebo effect) and objective factors, it nonetheless serves as a sign of clinical improvement along with improved appetite and weight gain and increased "performance status" (eg, ambulatory versus bedridden). Evaluation of factors such as activity status enables the clinician to judge whether the net effect of chemotherapy is worthwhile palliation (see Chapter 5).

Jordan K et al. Recent developments in the prevention of chemotherapy-induced nausea and vomiting (CINV): a comprehensive review. Ann Oncol. 2015 Jun;26(6):1081–90. [PMID: 25755107]

Moslehi JJ. Cardiovascular toxic effects of targeted cancer therapies. N Engl J Med. 2016 Oct;375(15):1457–67. [PMID: 27732808]

Navari RM et al. Antiemetic prophylaxis for chemotherapy-induced nausea and vomiting. N Engl J Med. 2016 Apr 7;374(14):1356–67. [PMID: 27050207]

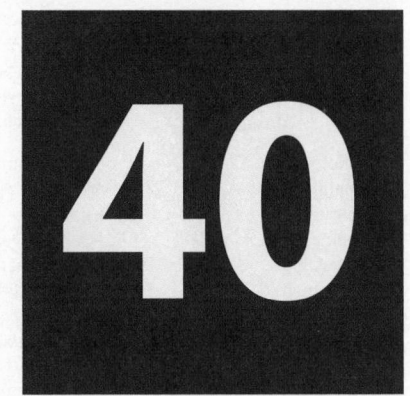

Genetic & Genomic Disorders

Reed E. Pyeritz, MD, PhD

40

ACUTE INTERMITTENT PORPHYRIA

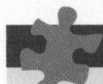

ESSENTIALS OF DIAGNOSIS

- ▶ Unexplained abdominal crisis, generally in young women.
- ▶ Acute peripheral or central nervous system dysfunction; recurrent psychiatric illnesses.
- ▶ Hyponatremia.
- ▶ Porphobilinogen in the urine during an attack.

▶ General Considerations

Though there are several different types of porphyrias, the one with the most serious consequences and the one that usually presents in adulthood is acute intermittent porphyria (AIP), which is inherited as an autosomal dominant condition, though it remains clinically silent in most patients who carry a mutation in *HMBS*. Clinical illness usually develops in women. Symptoms begin in the teens or 20s, but onset can begin after menopause in rare cases. The disorder is caused by partial deficiency of hydroxymethylbilane synthase activity, leading to increased excretion of aminolevulinic acid and porphobilinogen in the urine. The diagnosis may be elusive if not specifically considered. The characteristic abdominal pain may be due to abnormalities in autonomic innervation in the gut. In contrast to other forms of porphyria, cutaneous photosensitivity is absent in AIP. Attacks are precipitated by numerous factors, including drugs and intercurrent infections. Harmful and relatively safe drugs for use in treatment are listed in Table 40–1. Hyponatremia may be seen, due in part to inappropriate release of antidiuretic hormone, although gastrointestinal loss of sodium in some patients may be a contributing factor.

▶ Clinical Findings

A. Symptoms and Signs

Patients show intermittent abdominal pain of varying severity, and in some instances, it may so simulate acute abdomen as to lead to exploratory laparotomy. Because the origin of the abdominal pain is neurologic, there is an absence of fever and leukocytosis. Complete recovery between attacks is usual. Any part of the nervous system may be involved, with evidence for autonomic and peripheral neuropathy. Peripheral neuropathy may be symmetric or asymmetric and mild or profound; in the latter instance, it can even lead to quadriplegia with respiratory paralysis. Other central nervous system manifestations include seizures, altered consciousness, psychosis, and abnormalities of the basal ganglia. Hyponatremia may further cause or exacerbate central nervous system manifestations.

B. Laboratory Findings

Often there is profound hyponatremia. The diagnosis can be confirmed by demonstrating an increased amount of porphobilinogen in the urine during an acute attack. Freshly voided urine is of normal color but may turn dark upon standing in light and air.

Most families have different mutations in *HMBS* causing AIP. Mutations can be detected in 90% of patients and used for presymptomatic and prenatal diagnosis.

▶ Prevention

Avoidance of factors known to precipitate attacks of AIP—especially drugs—can reduce morbidity. Sulfonamides and barbiturates are the most common culprits; others are listed in Table 40–1 and on the Internet (www.drugs-porphyria.org). Starvation diets or prolonged fasting also cause attacks and so must be avoided. Hormonal changes during pregnancy can precipitate crises.

Table 40–1. Some of the "unsafe" and "probably safe" drugs used in the treatment of acute porphyrias.

Unsafe	Probably Safe
Alcohol	Acetaminophen
Alkylating agents	Amitriptyline
Barbiturates	Aspirin
Carbamazepine	Atropine
Chloroquine	Beta-adrenergic blockers
Chlorpropamide	Chloral hydrate
Clonidine	Chlordiazepoxide
Dapsone	Corticosteroids
Ergots	Diazepam
Erythromycin	Digoxin
Estrogens, synthetic	Diphenhydramine
Food additives	Guanethidine
Glutethimide	Hyoscine
Griseofulvin	Ibuprofen
Hydralazine	Imipramine
Ketamine	Insulin
Meprobamate	Lithium
Methyldopa	Naproxen
Metoclopramide	Nitrofurantoin
Nortriptyline	Opioid analgesics
Pentazocine	Penicillamine
Phenytoin	Penicillin and derivatives
Progestins	Phenothiazines
Pyrazinamide	Procaine
Rifampin	Streptomycin
Spironolactone	Succinylcholine
Succinimides	Tetracycline
Sulfonamides	Thiouracil
Theophylline	
Tolazamide	
Tolbutamide	
Valproic acid	

► Treatment

Treatment with a high-carbohydrate diet diminishes the number of attacks in some patients and is a reasonable empiric gesture considering its benignity. Acute attacks may be life-threatening and require prompt diagnosis, withdrawal of the inciting agent (if possible), and treatment with analgesics and intravenous glucose in saline and hematin. A minimum of 300 g of carbohydrate per day should be provided orally or intravenously. Electrolyte balance requires close attention. Hematin therapy should be undertaken with full recognition of adverse consequences, especially phlebitis and coagulopathy. The intravenous dosage is up to 4 mg/kg once or twice daily. Liver transplantation may provide an option for patients with disease poorly controlled by medical therapy.

► When to Refer

- For management of severe abdominal pain, seizures, or psychosis.
- For preventive management when a patient with porphyria contemplates pregnancy.
- For genetic counseling and molecular diagnosis.

► When to Admit

The patient should be hospitalized for an acute attack when accompanied by mental status changes, seizure, or hyponatremia.

Bissell DM et al. Porphyria. N Engl J Med. 2017 Aug 31;377(9): 862–72. [PMID: 28854095]

Fontanellas A et al. Emerging therapies for acute intermittent porphyria. Expert Rev Mol Med. 2016 Nov 2;18:e17. [PMID: 27804912]

O'Malley R et al. Porphyria: often discussed but too often missed. Pract Neurol. 2018 Oct;18(5):352–8. [PMID: 29540448]

Pischik E et al. An update of clinical management of acute intermittent porphyria. Appl Clin Genet. 2015 Sep 1;8:201–14. [PMID: 26366103]

Singal AK et al. Liver transplantation in the management of porphyria. Hepatology. 2014 Sep;60(3):1082–9. [PMID: 24700519]

DOWN SYNDROME

ESSENTIALS OF DIAGNOSIS

- ► Typical craniofacial features (flat occiput, epicanthal folds, large tongue).
- ► Intellectual disability.
- ► Congenital heart disease (eg, atrioventricular canal defects) in 50% of patients.
- ► Alzheimer dementia in early-to-mid adulthood.
- ► Three copies of chromosome 21 (trisomy 21) or a chromosome rearrangement that results in three copies of a region of the long arm of chromosome 21.

► General Considerations

Nearly 0.5% of all human conceptions are trisomic for chromosome 21. Because of increased fetal mortality, birth incidence of Down syndrome is 1 per 700 but varies from 1 per 1000 in young mothers to more than three times as frequent in women of advanced maternal age. The presence of a fetus with Down syndrome can be detected in many pregnancies in the first or early second trimester through screening maternal serum for alpha-fetoprotein and other biomarkers ("multiple marker screening") and by detecting increased nuchal thickness and underdevelopment of the nasal bone on ultrasonography. Prenatal diagnosis with high sensitivity and specificity can be achieved by assaying fetal DNA that is circulating in maternal blood. The chance of bearing a child with Down syndrome increases exponentially with the age of the mother at conception and begins a marked rise after age 35. By age 45 years, the odds of having an affected child are as high as 1 in 40. The risk of other conditions associated with trisomy also increases, because of the predisposition of older oocytes to nondisjunction during meiosis. There is little risk of trisomy associated with increased paternal age. However, older men do have an increased risk of fathering a child with a new autosomal dominant condition. Because there are so many distinct conditions, though, the chance of fathering an offspring with any given one is extremely small.

Clinical Findings

A. Symptoms and Signs

Down syndrome is usually diagnosed at birth on the basis of the typical craniofacial features, hypotonia, and single palmar crease. Several serious problems that may be evident at birth or may develop early in childhood include duodenal atresia, congenital heart disease (especially atrioventricular canal defects), and hematologic malignancy. The intestinal and cardiac anomalies usually respond to surgery. A transient neonatal leukemia generally responds to conservative management. The incidences of both acute lymphoblastic and myeloid leukemias are increased in childhood. Intelligence varies across a wide spectrum. Many people with Down syndrome do well in sheltered workshops and group homes, but few achieve full independence in adulthood. Other frequent complications include atlanto-axial instability, celiac disease, frequent infections due to immune deficiency, and hypothyroidism. An Alzheimer-like dementia usually becomes evident in the fourth or fifth decade. Patients with Down syndrome who survive childhood and who develop dementia have a reduced life expectancy; on average, they live to about age 55 years.

B. Laboratory Findings

Cytogenomic analysis should always be performed—even though most patients will have simple trisomy for chromosome 21—to detect unbalanced translocations; such patients may have a parent with a balanced translocation, and there will be a substantial recurrence risk of Down syndrome in future offspring of that parent and potentially that parent's relatives.

Treatment

Duodenal atresia should be treated surgically. Congenital heart disease should be treated as in any other patient. Effective treatment does no long-term harm to neurodevelopment. As yet, no medical treatment has been proven to affect the neurodevelopmental or the neurodegenerative aspects. Based on the glutamatergic hypothesis for Alzheimer disease, studies have been initiated examining the potential benefit of the N-methyl-D-aspartate receptor antagonist memantine.

When to Refer

- For comprehensive evaluation of infants to investigate congenital heart disease, hematologic malignancy, and duodenal atresia.
- For genetic counseling of the parents.
- For signs of dementia in an adult patient.

When to Admit

A young patient should be hospitalized for failure to thrive, regurgitation, or breathlessness.

Alsaied T et al. Does congenital heart disease affect neurodevelopmental outcomes in children with Down syndrome? Congenit Heart Dis. 2016 Jan–Feb;11(1):26–33. [PMID: 26914309]

Badeau M et al. Genomics-based non-invasive prenatal testing for detection of fetal chromosomal aneuploidy in pregnant women. Cochrane Database Syst Rev. 2017 Nov 10;11: CD011767. [PMID: 29125628]

Coppedè F. Risk factors for Down syndrome. Arch Toxicol. 2016 Dec;90(12):2917–29. [PMID: 27600794]

Hill M et al. Has noninvasive prenatal testing impacted termination of pregnancy and live birth rates of infants with Down syndrome? Prenat Diagn. 2017 Dec;37(13):1281–90. [PMID: 29111614]

Huiracocha L et al. Parenting children with Down syndrome: societal influences. J Child Health Care. 2017 Dec;21(4):488–97. [PMID: 29110530]

Lee P et al. The biology, pathogenesis and clinical aspects of acute lymphoblastic leukemia in children with Down syndrome. Leukemia. 2016 Sep;30(9):1816–23. [PMID: 27285583]

Neil N et al. Communication intervention for individuals with Down syndrome: systematic review and meta-analysis. Dev Neurorehabil. 2018 Jan;21(1):1–12. [PMID: 27537068]

Ross WT et al. Care of the adult patient with Down syndrome. South Med J. 2014 Nov;107(11):715–21. [PMID: 25365441]

FAMILIAL HYPERCHOLESTEROLEMIA

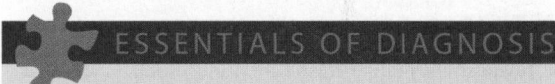

ESSENTIALS OF DIAGNOSIS

- ► Elevated serum total cholesterol and LDL cholesterol.
- ► Autosomal dominant inheritance.
- ► Mutation in *LRL*, *PCSK9*, or *APOB*.

General Considerations

Familial hypercholesterolemia (FH) is a group of autosomal dominant conditions that result in elevated low-density lipoprotein (LDL) levels in the blood. High LDL predisposes to atherosclerosis, which in turn leads to premature myocardial infarction or stroke. The incidence of these serious complications increases with age and when associated with the other common predispositions to atherosclerosis, such as smoking and hypertension. About 1 in 500 people in the United States have FH; worldwide, the prevalence is about 10 million. Only about 15% percent of people with FH are diagnosed and even fewer are treated effectively.

Clinical Findings

A. Symptoms and Signs

Yellow lipid deposits appear on tendons, especially the Achilles (tendon xanthoma).

B. Laboratory Findings

Total serum cholesterol with the LDL component is particularly high. A detailed family history and genetic testing should be obtained when individuals are younger than 40 years with an LDL level greater than 200 mg/mL and for individuals older than 40 years with a level greater than 250 mg/mL.

Prevention

In most instances, the elevated LDL is inherited as an autosomal dominant trait. An affected individual in all likelihood inherited FH from one parent, and each of his or her children has a 50/50 chance of inheriting FH. In uncommon cases, both parents have a mutation in the LDL receptor and one-quarter of their children, on average, will inherit two mutant alleles and have homozygous FH, which is a much more serious disease with manifestations in childhood.

Mutations in the following four genes can cause FH: (1) *LDLR*, which encodes the LDL receptor located on the surface of cells and responsible for moving LDL into the cell for metabolism; the most common mutant gene in FH; (2) *APOB*, which encodes a component of LDL and mutations inhibit binding to LDL receptor; (3) *PCSK9*, which encodes a protein that normally reduces production of LDL receptors, so mutations actually protect from hypercholesterolemia; and (4) *ARH*, which requires mutations in both alleles (autosomal recessive inheritance) to cause FH.

DNA analysis for mutations in all of these genes is readily available.

Treatment

Statins, usually at high doses, can reduce LDL levels, occasionally to acceptable levels. If LDL levels remain elevated, other standard medications are required. The earlier in life that treatment is begun, the better the outcome in reducing mortality from atherosclerosis. In homozygous FH, if high-dose statins do not reduce LDL sufficiently, an inhibitor of PCSK9 is a recent option. If all else fails, then plasmaphoresis is needed to reduce LDL.

Another important need in effective management is to screen relatives who are at risk, certainly by measuring LDL levels, but increasingly by identifying the mutation in the family and utilizing that for screening.

If these measures are not effective enough, treatment with an antibody that actually inhibits the product of the *PCSK9* gene can be a quite expensive adjunct to standard therapy.

When to Refer

- For comprehensive evaluation of infants for their lipid profile.
- For genetic counseling of the patient, his or her parents, siblings, and offspring.
- For signs of atherosclerotic cardiovascular disease.

When to Admit

For signs or symptoms of acute arterial occlusive events.

Ajufo E et al. Recent advances in the pharmacological management of hypercholesterolaemia. Lancet Diabetes Endocrinol. 2016 May;4(5):436–46. [PMID: 27012540]

Louter L et al. Cascade screening for familial hypercholesterolemia: practical consequences. Atheroscler Suppl. 2017 Nov;30:77–85. [PMID: 29096865]

Martin AC et al. Knowns and unknowns in the care of pediatric familial hypercholesterolemia. J Lipid Res. 2017 Sep;58(9): 1765–76. [PMID: 28701353]

Migliara G et al. Familial hypercholesterolemia: a systematic review of guidelines on genetic testing and patient management. Front Public Health. 2017 Sep 25;5:252. [PMID: 28993804]

Rosenson RS. CETP inhibition improves the lipid profile but has no effect on clinical cardiovascular outcomes in high-risk patients. Evid Based Med. 2017 Oct;22(5):184–5. [PMID: 28844064]

Sabatine MS. PCSK9 inhibitors: clinical evidence and implementation. Nat Rev Cardiol. 2019 Mar;16(3):155–65. [PMID: 30420622]

FRAGILE X MENTAL RETARDATION

> ### ESSENTIALS OF DIAGNOSIS

> ▶ Expanded trinucleotide repeat (more than 200) in the *FMR1* gene.
> ▶ **Males:** mental retardation and autism; large testes after puberty.
> ▶ **Females:** learning disabilities or mental retardation; premature ovarian failure.
> ▶ Late-onset tremor and ataxia in males and females with moderate trinucleotide repeat (55–200) expansion (premutation carriers).

Clinical Findings

A. Symptoms and Signs

This X-linked condition accounts for more cases of mental retardation in males than any condition except Down syndrome; about 1 in 4000 males is affected. The central nervous system phenotype includes autism spectrum, impulsivity and aggressiveness, and repetitive behaviors. The condition also affects intellectual function in females, although less severely and about 50% less frequently than in males. Affected (heterozygous) young women show no physical signs other than early menopause, but they may have learning difficulties, anxiety, sensory issues, or frank retardation. Affected males show macro-orchidism (enlarged testes) after puberty, large ears and a prominent jaw, a high-pitched voice, autistic characteristics, and mental retardation. Some males show evidence of a mild connective tissue defect, with joint hypermobility and mitral valve prolapse.

Women who are premutation carriers (55–200 CGG repeats) are at increased risk for premature ovarian failure and mild cognitive abnormalities. Male and female premutation carriers are at risk for mood and anxiety disorders and the development of tremor and ataxia beyond middle age (fragile-X tremor-ataxia syndrome, FXTAS). Changes in the cerebellar white matter may be evident on MRI before symptoms appear. Because of the relatively high prevalence of premutation carriers in the general population (1/130–1/600), older people in whom any of these behavioral or neurologic problems develop should undergo testing of the *FMR1* locus.

B. Laboratory Findings

The first marker for this condition was a small gap, or fragile site, evident near the tip of the long arm of the X chromosome.

Subsequently, the condition was found to be due to expansion of a trinucleotide repeat (CGG) near a gene called *FMR1*. All individuals have some CGG repeats in this location, but as the number increases beyond 52, the chances of further expansion during spermatogenesis or oogenesis increase.

Being born with one *FMR1* allele with 200 or more repeats results in mental retardation in most men, and in about 60% of women. The more repeats, the greater the likelihood that further expansion will occur during gametogenesis; this results in anticipation, in which the disorder can worsen from one generation to the next.

Prevention

DNA diagnosis for the number of repeats has supplanted cytogenetic analysis for both clinical and prenatal diagnosis. This should be done on any male or female who has unexplained mental retardation. Newborn screening based on hypermethylation of the *FMR1* gene is being considered as a means of early detection and intervention.

Treatment

Several treatments that address the imbalances in neurotransmission have been developed based on the mouse model and are in clinical trials. Valproic acid may reduce symptoms of hyperactivity and attention deficit, but standard therapies should be tried first.

When to Refer

- For otherwise unexplained mental retardation or learning difficulties in boys and girls.
- For otherwise unexplained tremor or ataxia in middle-aged individuals.
- For premature ovarian failure.
- For genetic counseling.

Hagerman RJ et al. Fragile X syndrome. Nat Rev Dis Primers. 2017 Sep 29;3:17065. [PMID: 28960184]

Kidd SA et al. Fragile X syndrome: a review of associated medical problems. Pediatrics. 2014 Nov;134(5):995–1005. [PMID: 25287458]

Niu M et al. Autism symptoms in fragile X syndrome. J Child Neurol. 2017 Sep;32(10):903–9. [PMID: 28617074]

Tassone F et al. Fragile X premutation. J Neurodev Disord. 2014;6(1):22. [PMID: 25170346]

Wheeler A et al. Implications of the *FMR1* premutation for children, adolescents, adults, and their families. Pediatrics. 2017 Jun;139(Suppl 3):S172–82. [PMID: 28814538]

GAUCHER DISEASE

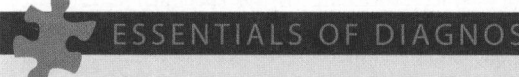

ESSENTIALS OF DIAGNOSIS

- Deficiency of beta-glucocerebrosidase.
- Anemia and thrombocytopenia.
- Enlargement of the liver and spleen.
- Pathologic fractures.

Clinical Findings

A. Symptoms and Signs

Gaucher disease has an autosomal recessive pattern of inheritance. A deficiency of beta-glucocerebrosidase causes an accumulation of sphingolipid within phagocytic cells throughout the body. Anemia and thrombocytopenia are common and may be symptomatic; both are due primarily to hypersplenism, but marrow infiltration with Gaucher cells may be a contributing factor. The abdomen can become painfully distended due to enlargement of the liver and spleen. Cortical erosions of bones, especially the vertebrae and femur, are due to local infarctions, but the mechanism is unclear. Episodes of bone pain (termed "crises") are reminiscent of those in sickle cell disease. A hip fracture in a patient of any age with a palpable spleen—especially in a Jewish person of Eastern European origin—suggests the possibility of Gaucher disease. Peripheral neuropathy may develop in patients.

Two uncommon forms of Gaucher disease, called type II and type III, involve neurologic accumulation of sphingolipid and a variety of neurologic problems. Type II is of infantile onset and has a poor prognosis. Heterozygotes for Gaucher disease are at increased risk for developing Parkinson disease.

B. Laboratory Findings

Bone marrow aspirates reveal typical Gaucher cells, which have an eccentric nucleus and periodic acid–Schiff (PAS)-positive inclusions, along with wrinkled cytoplasm and inclusion bodies of a fibrillar type. In addition, the serum acid phosphatase is elevated. Definitive diagnosis requires the demonstration of deficient glucocerebrosidase activity in leukocytes. Hundreds of mutations have been found to cause Gaucher disease and some are highly predictive of the neuronopathic forms. Thus, mutation detection, especially in a young person, is of potential value. Only four mutations in glucocerebrosidase account for more than 90% of the disease among Ashkenazi Jews, in whom the carrier frequency is 1:15.

Prevention

Gaucher disease is the most common lysosomal storage disorder. Most clinical complications can be prevented by early institution of enzyme replacement therapy. Carrier screening, especially among Ashkenazi Jews, detects those couples at 25% risk of having an affected child. Prenatal diagnosis through mutation analysis is feasible. Because of an increased risk of malignancy, especially plasma cell myeloma and other hematologic cancers, regular screening of adults with Gaucher disease is warranted.

Treatment

A recombinant form of the enzyme glucocerebrosidase (imiglucerase) for intravenous administration on a regular basis reduces total body stores of glycolipid and improves orthopedic and hematologic manifestations. Unfortunately, the neurologic manifestations of types II and III have not improved with enzyme replacement therapy. The major drawback is the exceptional cost of imiglucerase, which can exceed $300,000 per year for a severely affected adult patient. Eliglustat tartrate is an oral inhibitor of glucosylceramide synthase and reduces the compound that accumulates; while still quite expensive, this approach eliminates the need for frequent intravenous infusions. Early treatment of affected children normalizes growth and bone mineral density and improves liver and spleen size, anemia, and thrombocytopenia. In adults with thrombocytopenia due to splenic sequestration, enzyme replacement often obviates the need for splenectomy.

Biegstraaten M et al. Management goals for type 1 Gaucher disease: an expert consensus document from the European working group on Gaucher disease. Blood Cells Mol Dis. 2018 Feb;68:203–8. [PMID: 28274788]

Coutinho MF et al. Genetic substrate reduction therapy: a promising approach for lysosomal storage disorders. Diseases. 2016 Nov 9;4(4):E33. [PMID: 28933412]

Horowitz M et al. New directions in Gaucher disease. Hum Mutat. 2016 Nov;37(11):1121–36. [PMID: 27449603]

Linari S et al. Clinical manifestations and management of Gaucher disease. Clin Cases Miner Bone Metab. 2015 May–Aug; 12(2):157–64. [PMID: 26604942]

Nalysnyk L et al. Gaucher disease epidemiology and natural history: a comprehensive review of the literature. Hematology. 2017 Mar;22(2):65–73. [PMID: 27762169]

Roshan Lal T et al. The spectrum of neurological manifestations associated with Gaucher disease. Diseases. 2017 Mar 2;5(1):E10. [PMID: 28933363]

Utz J et al. Comorbidities and pharmacotherapies in patients with Gaucher disease type 1: The potential for drug-drug interactions. Mol Genet Metab. 2016 Feb;117(2):172–8. [PMID: 26674302]

DISORDERS OF HOMOCYSTEINE METABOLISM

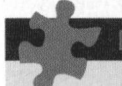

ESSENTIALS OF DIAGNOSIS

► Hyperhomocysteinemia: more vascular disease but lowering homocysteine levels is not helpful.

► Homocystinuria: Marfan-like habitus, ectopia lentis, mental retardation, thromboses.

► Elevated homocysteine in the urine or plasma.

▶ General Considerations

Patients with clinical and angiographic evidence of coronary artery disease and cerebrovascular and peripheral vascular diseases tend to have higher levels of plasma homocysteine than persons without these vascular diseases. Although this effect was initially thought to be due at least in part to heterozygotes for cystathionine beta-synthase deficiency (see below), there is little supporting evidence. Rather, an important factor leading to hyperhomocysteinemia is folate deficiency. Pyridoxine (vitamin B_6) and vitamin B_{12} are also important in the metabolism of methionine, and deficiency of any of these vitamins can lead to accumulation of homocysteine. A number of genes influence utilization of these vitamins and can predispose to deficiency. For example, having one—and especially

two—copy of an allele that causes thermolability of methylene tetrahydrofolate reductase predisposes people to elevated fasting homocysteine levels. Both nutritional and most genetic deficiencies of these vitamins can be corrected by dietary supplementation of folic acid and, if serum levels are low, vitamins B_6 and B_{12}. In the United States, cereal grains are fortified with folic acid. However, therapy with B vitamins and folate lowers homocysteine levels significantly but does not reduce the risk of either venous thromboembolism or complications of coronary artery disease. The role of lowering homocysteine as primary prevention for cardiovascular disease has received modest direct support in clinical trials. Hyperhomocysteinemia occurs with end-stage chronic kidney disease. In the general population, elevated homocysteine correlates with cognitive impairment.

▶ Clinical Findings

A. Symptoms and Signs

Homocystinuria in its classic form is caused by cystathionine beta-synthase deficiency and exhibits autosomal recessive inheritance. This results in extreme elevations of plasma and urinary homocystine levels, a basis for diagnosis of this disorder. Homocystinuria is similar in certain superficial aspects to Marfan syndrome, since patients may have a similar body habitus and ectopia lentis is almost always present. However, mental retardation is often present in homocystinuria, and the cardiovascular events are those of repeated venous and arterial thromboses whose precise cause remains obscure. Thus, the diagnosis should be suspected in patients in the second and third decades of life who have arterial or venous thromboses without other risk factors. Bone mineral density is reduced in untreated patients. Life expectancy is reduced, especially in untreated and pyridoxine-unresponsive patients; myocardial infarction, stroke, and pulmonary embolism are the most common causes of death. This condition is diagnosed by newborn screening for hypermethioninemia; however, pyridoxine-responsive infants may not be detected. In addition, homozygotes for a common mutant allele, p.I278T, show marked clinical variability, with some unaffected as adults.

B. Laboratory Findings

Although many mutations have been identified in the cystathionine beta-synthase gene (*CBS*), amino acid analysis of plasma remains the most appropriate diagnostic test. Patients should be studied after they have been off folate or pyridoxine supplementation for at least 1 week. Relatively few laboratories currently provide highly reliable assays for homocysteine. Processing of the specimen is crucial to obtain accurate results. The plasma must be separated within 30 minutes; otherwise, blood cells release the amino acid and the measurement will then be artificially elevated.

▶ Prevention

About 50% of patients have a form of cystathionine beta-synthase deficiency that improves biochemically and clinically through pharmacologic doses of pyridoxine

(50–500 mg/day) and folate (5–10 mg/day). For these patients, treatment from infancy can prevent retardation and the other clinical problems. Patients who are pyridoxine nonresponders must be treated with a dietary reduction in methionine and supplementation of cysteine, also from infancy. The vitamin betaine is also useful in reducing plasma methionine levels by facilitating a metabolic pathway that bypasses the defective enzyme.

Treatment

Patients with classic homocystinuria who have suffered venous thrombosis receive anticoagulation therapy, but there are no studies to support prophylactic use of warfarin or antiplatelet agents.

Debreceni B et al. The role of homocysteine-lowering B-vitamins in the primary prevention of cardiovascular disease. Cardiovasc Ther. 2014 Jun;32(3):130–8. [PMID: 24571382]

Kumar T et al. Homocystinuria: therapeutic approach. Clin Chim Acta. 2016 Jul 1;458:55–62. [PMID: 27059523]

Sacharow SJ et al. Homocystinuria Caused by Cystathionine Beta-Synthase Deficiency. In: Adam MP et al (editors). GeneReviews®. 2004 Jan 15 [Updated 2017 May 18]. [PMID: 20301697]

Weber DR et al. Low bone mineral density is a common finding in patients with homocystinuria. Mol Genet Metab. 2016 Mar;117(3):351–4. [PMID: 26689745]

Zeng R et al. The effect of folate fortification on folic acid-based homocysteine-lowering intervention and stroke risk: a meta-analysis. Public Health Nutr. 2015 Jun;18(8):1514–21. [PMID: 25323814]

KLINEFELTER SYNDROME

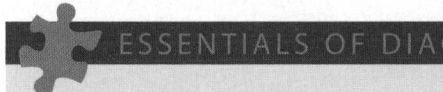

ESSENTIALS OF DIAGNOSIS

▸ Males with hypergonadotropic hypogonadism and small testes.

▸ 47,XXY karyotype.

Clinical Findings

A. Symptoms and Signs

Boys with an extra X chromosome are normal in appearance before puberty; thereafter, they have disproportionately long legs and arms, sparse body hair, a female escutcheon, gynecomastia, and small testes. Infertility is due to azoospermia; the seminiferous tubules are hyalinized. The incidence is 1 in 660 newborn males, but the diagnosis is often not made until a man is evaluated for inability to conceive. Intellectual disability is somewhat more common than in the general population. Many men with Klinefelter syndrome have language-based learning problems. However, their intelligence usually tests within the broad range of normal. As adults, detailed psychometric testing may reveal a deficiency in executive skills. The risk of osteoporosis, breast cancer, and diabetes mellitus is much higher in men with Klinefelter syndrome than in 46,XY men.

B. Laboratory Findings

Low serum testosterone is common. The karyotype is typically 47,XXY, but other sex chromosome anomalies cause variations of Klinefelter syndrome.

Prevention

Screening for cancer (especially of the breast), deep venous thrombosis, and glucose intolerance is indicated.

Treatment

Treatment with testosterone after puberty is advisable but will not restore fertility. However, men with Klinefelter syndrome have had mature sperm aspirated from their testes and injected into oocytes, resulting in fertilization. After the blastocysts have been implanted into the uterus of a partner, conception has resulted. But, men with Klinefelter syndrome do have an increased risk for aneuploidy in sperm, and therefore genomic analysis of a blastocyst should be considered before implantation.

Akcan N et al. Klinefelter syndrome in childhood: variability in clinical and molecular findings. J Clin Res Pediatr Endocrinol. 2018 Jun 1;10(2):100–7. [PMID: 29022558]

Gies I et al. Management of Klinefelter syndrome during transition. Eur J Endocrinol. 2014 Aug;171(2):R67–77. [PMID: 24801585]

Gravholt CH. Sex chromosome abnormalities. In: Rimoin DL et al (editors). *Emery and Rimoin's Principles and Practice of Medical Genetics*, 6th ed. Philadelphia: Churchill Livingstone, 2013.

Nahata L et al. Sperm retrieval in adolescents and young adults with Klinefelter syndrome: a prospective, pilot study. J Pediatr. 2016 Mar;170:260–5.e2. [PMID: 26746120]

Ross JL et al. Androgen treatment effects on motor function, cognition, and behavior in boys with Klinefelter syndrome. J Pediatr. 2017 Jun;185:193–9. [PMID: 28285751]

Skakkebæk A et al. Quality of life in men with Klinefelter syndrome: the impact of genotype, health, socioeconomics, and sexual function. Genet Med. 2018 Feb;20(2):214–22. [PMID: 28726803]

MARFAN SYNDROME

ESSENTIALS OF DIAGNOSIS

▸ Disproportionately tall stature, thoracic deformity, and joint laxity or contractures.

▸ Ectopia lentis and myopia.

▸ Aortic root dilation and dissection; mitral valve prolapse.

▸ Mutation in *FBN1*, the gene encoding fibrillin-1.

General Considerations

Marfan syndrome, a systemic connective tissue disease, has an autosomal dominant pattern of inheritance. It is characterized by abnormalities of the skeletal, ocular, and cardiovascular systems; spontaneous pneumothorax; dural ectasia; and striae atrophicae. Of most concern is disease of the ascending aorta, which begins as a dilated aortic root. Histology of the aorta shows diffuse medial degeneration. Mitral valve leaflets are also abnormal and mitral prolapse and regurgitation may be present, often with elongated chordae tendineae, which on occasion may rupture.

Clinical Findings

A. Symptoms and Signs

Affected patients are typically tall, with particularly long arms, legs, and digits (arachnodactyly). However, there can be wide variability in the clinical presentation. Commonly, scoliosis and anterior chest deformity, such as pectus excavatum, are found. Ectopia lentis is present in about half of patients; severe myopia is common and retinal detachment can occur. Mitral valve prolapse is seen in about 85% of patients. Aortic root dilation is common and leads to aortic regurgitation or dissection with rupture. To diagnose Marfan syndrome, people with an affected relative need features in at least two systems. People with no family history need features in the skeletal system, two other systems, and one of the major criteria of ectopia lentis, dilation of the aortic root, or aortic dissection. Patients with homocystinuria due to cystathionine beta-synthase deficiency also have dislocated lenses, tall, disproportionate stature, and thoracic deformity. They tend to have below normal intelligence, stiff joints, and a predisposition to arterial and venous occlusive disease. Males with Klinefelter syndrome do not show the typical ocular or cardiovascular features of Marfan syndrome and are generally sporadic occurrences in the family.

B. Laboratory Findings

Mutations in the fibrillin gene (*FBN1*) on chromosome 15 cause Marfan syndrome. Nonetheless, no simple laboratory test is available to support the diagnosis in questionable cases because related conditions may also be due to defects in fibrillin. The nature of the *FBN1* mutation has little predictive value in terms of prognosis. The pathogenesis of Marfan syndrome involves aberrant regulation of transforming growth factor (TGF)-beta activity. Mutations in either of two receptors for TGF-beta (TGFBR1 and TGFBR2) can cause conditions that resemble Marfan syndrome in terms of aortic aneurysm and dissection and autosomal dominant inheritance. Mutations in more than two dozen other genes can predispose adults to thoracic aortic aneurysm and dissection.

Prevention

There is prenatal and presymptomatic diagnosis for patients in whom the molecular defect in *FBN1* has been found.

Treatment

Children with Marfan syndrome require regular ophthalmologic surveillance to correct visual acuity and thus prevent amblyopia, and annual orthopedic consultation for diagnosis of scoliosis at an early enough stage so that bracing might delay progression. Patients of all ages require echocardiography at least annually to monitor aortic root diameter and mitral valve function. Long-term beta-adrenergic blockade, titrated to individual tolerance but enough to produce a negative inotropic effect (atenolol, 1–2 mg/kg orally daily), retards the rate of aortic dilation. While inhibition of the TGF-beta signaling pathway through angiotensin receptor blockade (ARB) in mice with Marfan syndrome is highly effective, ARB treatment in humans is no more effective than beta-adrenergic blockade. Calcium channel blockers, once used as a substitute for beta-blockade, are detrimental to the aorta. Restriction from vigorous physical exertion protects from aortic dissection. Prophylactic replacement of the aortic root with a composite graft when the diameter reaches 45–50 mm in an adult (normal: less than 40 mm) prolongs life. Earlier prophylactic surgery should be considered when there is a strong family history of aortic dissection or when the diameter of the aortic root increases more than 3–4 mm per year. A valve-sparing procedure resuspends the patient's native aortic valve inside a graft that replaces the aneurysmal sinuses of Valsalva and ascending aorta, thus avoiding the need for lifelong anticoagulation. Women with Marfan syndrome are at heightened risk for aortic dissection in the peripartum and postpartum periods. Having an aortic root dimension greater than 40 mm should prompt consideration for prophylactic, valve-sparing aortic repair before undertaking a pregnancy.

Prognosis

People with Marfan syndrome who are untreated commonly die in the fourth or fifth decade from aortic dissection or heart failure secondary to aortic or mitral regurgitation. However, because of earlier diagnosis, lifestyle modifications, beta-adrenergic blockade, and prophylactic aortic and mitral valve surgery, life expectancy has increased by several decades.

When to Refer

- For detailed ophthalmologic examination.
- For at least annual cardiologic evaluation.
- For moderate scoliosis.
- For pregnancy in a woman with Marfan syndrome.
- For genetic counseling.

When to Admit

Any patient with Marfan syndrome in whom severe or unusual chest pain develops should be hospitalized to exclude pneumothorax and aortic dissection.

Bradley TJ et al. The expanding clinical spectrum of extracardiovascular and cardiovascular manifestations of heritable thoracic aortic aneurysm and dissection. Can J Cardiol. 2016 Jan;32(1):86–99. [PMID: 26724513]

Lacro RV et al; Pediatric Heart Network Investigators. Atenolol versus losartan in children and young adults with Marfan's syndrome. N Engl J Med. 2014 Nov 27;371(22):2061–71. [PMID: 25405392]

Price J et al. Long-term outcomes of aortic root operations for Marfan syndrome: a comparison of Bentall versus aortic valve-sparing procedures. J Thorac Cardiovasc Surg. 2016 Feb;151(2):330–8. [PMID: 26704057]

Pyeritz RE. Etiology and pathogenesis of the Marfan syndrome: current understanding. Ann Cardiothorac Surg. 2017 Nov;6(6):595–8. [PMID: 29270371]

Pyeritz RE. Evaluation of the adolescent or adult with some features of Marfan syndrome. Genet Med. 2012 Jan;14(1):171–7. [PMID: 22237449]

Pyeritz RE. Recent progress in understanding the natural and clinical histories of the Marfan syndrome. Trends Cardiovasc Med. 2016 Jul;26(5):423–8. [PMID: 26908026]

Roman MJ et al. Aortic complications associated with pregnancy in Marfan syndrome: the NHLBI National Registry of Genetically Triggered Thoracic Aortic Aneurysms and Cardiovascular Conditions (GenTAC). J Am Heart Assoc. 2016 Aug 11; 5(8):e004052. [PMID: 27515814]

HEREDITARY HEMORRHAGIC TELANGIECTASIA

ESSENTIALS OF DIAGNOSIS

▶ Recurrent epistaxis.

▶ Mucocutaneous telangiectases.

▶ Visceral arteriovenous malformations (especially lung, liver, brain, bowel).

▶ Clinical Findings

A. Symptoms and Signs

Hereditary hemorrhagic telangiectasia (HHT), formerly termed "Osler-Weber-Rendu syndrome," is an autosomal dominant disorder of development of the vasculature. Epistaxis may begin in childhood or later in adolescence. Punctate telangiectases of the lips, tongue, fingers, and skin generally appear in later childhood and adolescence. Arteriovenous malformations (AVMs) can occur at any age in the brain, lungs, and liver. Bleeding from the gastrointestinal tract is due to mucosal vascular malformations and usually is not a problem until mid-adult years or later. Pulmonary AVMs can cause hypoxemia (with peripheral cyanosis, dyspnea, and clubbing) and right-to-left shunting (with embolic stroke or brain abscess). The criteria for diagnosis require presence of three of the following four features: (1) recurrent epistaxis, (2) visceral AVMs, (3) mucocutaneous telangiectases, and (4) being the near relative of a clearly affected individual. Mutation analysis can be used for presymptomatic diagnosis or exclusion of the worry of HHT.

B. Laboratory Findings

MR or CT arteriography detects AVMs. Mutations in at least five genes can cause HHT. Three have been identified, and molecular analysis to identify them is available; these mutations in *ENG*, *ALK1*, and *SMAD4* account for about 87% of families with HHT. When the familial mutation is known, molecular testing is far more cost effective than repeated clinical screening of relatives who are at risk.

▶ Prevention

Embolization of pulmonary AVMs with wire coils or other occlusive devices reduces the risk of stroke and brain abscess. Treatment of brain AVMs reduces the risk of hemorrhagic stroke. All patients with HHT with evidence of a pulmonary shunt should practice routine endocarditis prophylaxis (see Table 33–5). All intravenous lines (except those for transfusion of red blood cells and radiographic contrast) should have an air-filter to prevent embolization of an air bubble. Prenatal diagnosis through mutation detection is possible.

▶ Treatment

All patients in whom the diagnosis of HHT is considered should have an MRI of the brain with contrast. A contrast echocardiogram will detect most pulmonary AVMs when "bubbles" appear on the left side of the heart after 3–6 cardiac cycles. A positive contrast echocardiogram should be followed by a high-resolution CT angiogram for localization of pulmonary AVMs. Patients who have AVMs with a feeding artery of 2 mm diameter or greater should undergo embolization. After successful embolization of all treatable pulmonary AVMs, the CT angiogram should be repeated in 6 months and 3 years. A person with a negative contrast echocardiogram should have the test repeated every 5 years. Any person with a pulmonary AVM, even an embolized one, should utilize routine endocarditis prophylaxis. Several studies suggest that treatment with anti-estrogenic agents (eg, tamoxifen), thalidomide or its relatives, or anti-vascular endothelial growth factor agents (eg, bevacizumab) can reduce epistaxis and gastrointestinal bleeding and improve hepatic shunting. However, two randomized, controlled clinical trials of intranasal bevacizumab therapy failed to show an improvement in epistaxis.

Arizmendez NP et al. Intravenous bevacizumab for complications of hereditary hemorrhagic telangiectasia: a review of the literature. Int Forum Allergy Rhinol. 2015 Nov;5(11):1042–7. [PMID: 26202958]

Chin CJ et al. Epistaxis in hereditary hemorrhagic telangiectasia: an evidence based review of surgical management. J Otolaryngol Head Neck Surg. 2016 Jan 12;45:3. [PMID: 26754744]

Donaldson JW et al. Complications and mortality in hereditary hemorrhagic telangiectasia: a population-based study. Neurology. 2015 May 5;84(18):1886–93. [PMID: 25862798]

Dupuis-Girod S et al. Effect of bevacizumab nasal spray on epistaxis duration in hereditary hemorrhagic telangiectasia: a randomized clinical trial. JAMA. 2016 Sep 6;316(9):934–42. [PMID: 27599328]

Jackson SB et al. Gastrointestinal manifestations of Hereditary Hemorrhagic Telangiectasia (HHT): a systematic review of the literature. Dig Dis Sci. 2017 Oct;62(10):2623–30. [PMID: 28836046]

McDonald J et al. Hereditary Hemorrhagic Telangiectasia. In: Adam MP et al (editors). GeneReviews®. 2000 Jun 26 [Updated 2017 Feb 2]. [PMID: 20301525]

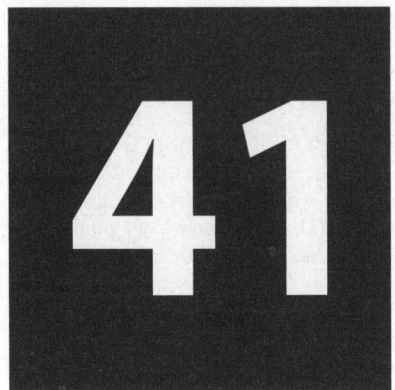

Sports Medicine & Outpatient Orthopedics

Anthony Luke, MD, MPH
C. Benjamin Ma, MD

Musculoskeletal problems account for about 10–20% of outpatient primary care clinical visits. Orthopedic problems can be classified as traumatic (ie, injury-related) or atraumatic (ie, degenerative or overuse syndromes) as well as acute or chronic. The history and physical examination are sufficient in most cases to establish the working diagnosis; the mechanism of injury is usually the most helpful part of the history in determining the diagnosis.

SHOULDER

1. Subacromial Impingement Syndrome

 ESSENTIALS OF DIAGNOSIS

▶ Shoulder pain with overhead motion.

▶ Night pain with sleeping on shoulder.

▶ Numbness and pain radiation below the elbow are usually due to cervical spine disease.

▶ General Considerations

The shoulder is a ball and socket joint. The socket is very shallow, however, which enables this joint to have the most motion of any joint. The shoulder, therefore, relies heavily on the surrounding muscles and ligaments to provide stability. The subacromial impingement syndrome describes a collection of diagnoses that cause mechanical inflammation in the subacromial space. Causes of impingement syndrome can be related to muscle strength imbalances, poor scapula control, rotator cuff tears, subacromial bursitis, and bone spurs.

With any shoulder problem, it is important to establish the patient's hand dominance, occupation, and recreational activities because shoulder injuries may present differently depending on the demands placed on the shoulder joint. For example, baseball pitchers with impingement syndrome may complain of pain while throwing. Alternatively, older adults with even full-thickness rotator cuff tears may not complain of any pain because the demands on the joint are low.

▶ Clinical Findings

A. Symptoms and Signs

Subacromial impingement syndrome classically presents with one or more of the following: pain with overhead activities, nocturnal pain with sleeping on the shoulder, or pain on internal rotation (eg, putting on a jacket or bra). On inspection, there may be appreciable atrophy in the supraspinatus or infraspinatus fossa. The patient with impingement syndrome can have mild scapula winging or "dyskinesis." The patient often has a rolled-forward shoulder posture or head-forward posture. On palpation, the patient can have tenderness over the anterolateral shoulder at the edge of the greater tuberosity. The patient may lack full active range of motion (Table 41–1) but should have preserved passive range of motion. Impingement symptoms can be elicited with the Neer and Hawkins impingement signs (Table 41–1).

B. Imaging

The following four radiographic views should be ordered to evaluate subacromial impingement syndrome: the anteroposterior (AP) scapula, the AP acromioclavicular joint, the lateral scapula (scapular Y), and the axillary lateral. The AP scapula view can rule out glenohumeral joint arthritis. The AP acromioclavicular view evaluates the acromioclavicular joint for inferior spurs. The scapula Y view evaluates the acromial shape, and the axillary lateral view visualizes the glenohumeral joint as well and for the presence of os acromiale.

MRI of the shoulder may demonstrate full- or partial-thickness tears or tendinosis. Ultrasound evaluation may demonstrate thickening of the rotator cuff tendons and tendinosis. Tears may also be visualized on ultrasound, although it is more difficult to identify partial tears from small full thickness than on MRI.

▶ Treatment

A. Conservative

The first-line treatment for impingement syndrome is usually a conservative approach with education, activity modification, and physical therapy exercises.

Table 41–1. Shoulder examination.

Maneuver	Description
Inspection	Check the patient's posture and "SEADS" (swelling, erythema, atrophy, deformity, surgical scars).
Palpation	Include important landmarks: acromioclavicular (AC) joint, long head of biceps tendon, coracoid, and greater tuberosity (supraspinatus insertion).
Range of motion testing	Check range of motion actively (patient performs) and passively (clinician performs).
Flexion	Move the arm forward as high as possible in the sagittal plane.
External rotation	Check with the patient's elbow touching their body so that external rotation occurs predominantly at the glenohumeral joint.

(continued)

Table 41–1. Shoulder examination. (continued)

Maneuver	Description
Internal rotation T8	The patient is asked to reach the thumbs as high as possible behind the spine on each side. The clinician can record the highest spinous process that the individual can reach on each side (iliac crest = L4, inferior angle of scapula = T8).
Rotator Cuff Strength Testing	
Supraspinatus (open can) test 	Perform resisted shoulder abduction at 90 degrees with slight forward flexion to around 45 degrees to test for supraspinatus tendon strength ("open can" test), or with shoulder abduction at 30 degrees and flexion to 30 degrees ("empty can" test).
External rotation 	The patient resists by externally rotating the arms with elbows at his or her side.

(continued)

Table 41–1. Shoulder examination. (continued)

Maneuver	Description
Internal rotation (lift-off test) 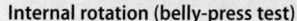	A positive "lift-off" test is the inability of the patient to hold his or her hand away from the body when reaching toward the small of the back. The clinician pushes the patient's hand toward the back while the patient resists. A positive lift-off indicates subscapularis tendon insufficiency.
Internal rotation (belly-press test) 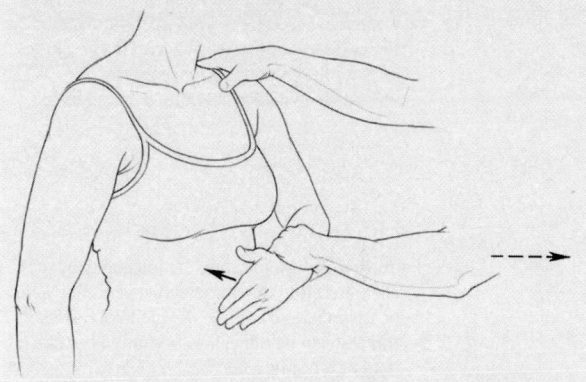	A positive "belly-press" test is the inability to hold the elbow in front of the trunk while pressing down with the hand on the belly. A positive belly-press test indicates subscapularis tendon insufficiency.
Impingement Testing	
Neer impingement sign	Perform by having the clinician flex the shoulder maximally in an overhead position. The test is positive when pain is reproduced with full passive shoulder flexion. Sensitivity is 79%; specificity is 53%.

(continued)

Table 41–1. Shoulder examination. (continued)

Maneuver	Description
Hawkins impingement sign 	Perform with the shoulder forward flexed 90 degrees and the elbow flexed at 90 degrees. The shoulder is then maximally internally rotated to impinge the greater tuberosity on the undersurface of the acromion. The test is considered positive when the patient's pain is reproduced by this maneuver. Sensitivity is 79%; specificity is 59%.
Stability Testing	
Apprehension test 	With persistent anterior instability or a recent dislocation, the patient feels pain or guards when the shoulder is abducted and externally rotated at 90 degrees. With posterior instability, the patient is apprehensive with the shoulder forward flexed and internally rotated to 90 degrees with a posteriorly directed force.
Load and shift test 	Perform to determine shoulder instability by manually translating the humeral head anteriorly and posteriorly in relation to the glenoid. However, this test can be difficult to perform when the patient is not relaxed.
O'Brien test Palm down Palm up	Performed to rule out labral cartilage tears that often occur following a shoulder subluxation or dislocation. The test involves flexing the patient's arm to 90 degrees, fully internally rotating the arm so the thumb is facing down (palm down), and adducting the arm to 10 degrees. Once positioned properly, the clinician applies downward force and asks the patient to resist. The test is then repeated in the same position except that the patient has his arm fully supinated (palm up). A positive O'Brien test for labral tear is pain deep in the shoulder with palm down more than the palm up. The O'Brien test can also be used to identify AC joint pathology. The patient would typically complain equally of pain directly over the AC joint with the palm down or up.

Impingement syndrome can be caused by muscle weakness or tear. Rotator cuff muscle strengthening can alleviate weakness or pain, unless the tendons are seriously compromised, which may cause more symptoms. Physical therapy is directed at rotator cuff muscle strengthening, scapula stabilization, and postural exercises. There is no strong evidence supporting the effectiveness of ice and NSAIDs as a prolonged therapy. In a Cochrane review, corticosteroid injections produced slightly better relief of symptoms in the short term when compared with placebo. Most patients respond well to conservative treatment.

B. Surgical

Procedures include arthroscopic acromioplasty with coracoacromial ligament release, bursectomy, or debridement or repair of rotator cuff tears. However, the value of acromioplasty alone for rotator cuff problems is not supported by evidence.

▶ When to Refer

- Failure of conservative treatment over 3 months.
- Young and active patients with impingement due to full-thickness rotator cuff tears.

McFarland EG et al. Clinical faceoff: what is the role of acromioplasty in the treatment of rotator cuff disease? Clin Orthop Relat Res. 2018 Sep;476(9):1707–12. [PMID: 30001291]

2. Rotator Cuff Tears

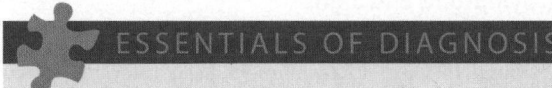

ESSENTIALS OF DIAGNOSIS

- ▶ A common cause of shoulder impingement syndrome after age 40.
- ▶ Difficulty lifting the arm with limited active range of motion.
- ▶ Weakness with resisted strength testing suggests full-thickness tears.
- ▶ Tears can occur following trauma or can be more degenerative.

▶ General Considerations

Rotator cuff tears can be caused by acute injuries related to falls on an outstretched arm or to pulling on the shoulder. It can also be related to chronic repetitive injuries with overhead movement and lifting. Partial rotator cuff tears are one of the most common reasons for impingement syndrome. Full-thickness rotator cuff tears are usually more symptomatic and may require surgical treatment. The most commonly torn tendon is the supraspinatus.

▶ Clinical Findings

A. Symptoms and Signs

Most patients complain of weakness or pain with overhead movement. Night pain is also a common complaint. The clinical findings with rotator cuff tears include those of the impingement syndrome except that with full-thickness rotator cuff tears there may be more obvious weakness noted with light resistance testing of specific rotator cuff muscles. Supraspinatus tendon strength is tested with resisted shoulder abduction at 90 degrees with slight forward flexion to around 45 degrees ("open can" test). Infraspinatus/teres minor strength is tested with resisted shoulder external rotation with shoulder at 0 degrees of abduction and elbow by side. Subscapularis strength is tested with the "lift-off" or "belly-press" tests. The affected patient usually also has positive Neer and Hawkins impingement tests (Table 41–1).

B. Imaging

Recommended radiographs are similar to impingement syndrome: AP scapula (glenohumeral), axillary lateral, supraspinatus outlet, and AP acromioclavicular joint views. The AP scapula view is useful in visualizing rotator cuff tears because degenerative changes can appear between the acromion and greater tuberosity of the shoulder. Axillary lateral views show superior elevation of the humeral head in relation to the center of the glenoid. Supraspinatus outlet views allow evaluation of the shape of the acromion. High-grade acromial spurs are associated with a higher incidence of rotator cuff tears. The AP acromioclavicular joint view evaluates for the presence of acromioclavicular joint arthritis, which can mimic rotator cuff tears, and for spurs that can cause rotator cuff injuries.

MRI is the best method for visualizing rotator cuff tears. The MR arthrogram can show partial or small (less than 1 cm) rotator cuff tears. For patients who cannot undergo MRI testing or when postoperative artifacts limit MRI evaluations, ultrasonography can be helpful.

▶ Treatment

Partial rotator cuff tears may heal with scarring. Most partial rotator cuff tears can be treated with physical therapy and scapular and rotator cuff muscle strengthening. However, research suggests that 40% of the partial-thickness tears progress to full-thickness tears in 2 years. Physical therapy can strengthen the remaining muscles to compensate for loss of strength and can have high rate of success for chronic tears. Physical therapy is also an option for older sedentary patients. On the contrary, **full-thickness rotator cuff tears** do not heal well and also have a tendency to increase in size with time. Forty-nine percent of the full-thickness tears get bigger over an average of 2.8 years. When tears get larger, they are also associated with worsening pain. Fatty infiltration is a degenerative process where muscle is being replaced by fat following injury to the rotator cuff tendons. Fatty infiltration progresses in full-thickness rotator cuff tears and it is a negative prognostic factor for successful surgical treatment. Fatty infiltration is an irreversible process so operative interventions are usually performed when the degree of infiltration is low. Most young active patients with acute, full-thickness tears should be treated with operative fixation. Full-thickness subscapularis tendon tears should undergo surgical repair since untreated tears usually lead to premature osteoarthritis (OA) of the shoulder. Nonetheless, physical therapy is indicated for atraumatic degenerative rotator cuff tears and success can be as high as 70%. That said, mid-term (5-year) outcome studies show that surgical repair of rotator cuff tears can have better outcomes than physical therapy alone.

When to Refer

- Young and active patients with full-thickness rotator cuff tears.
- Partial tears with greater than 50% involvement and with significant pain.
- Acute rotator cuff tears and loss of function.
- Older and sedentary patients with full-thickness rotator cuff tears who have not responded to nonoperative treatment.
- Full-thickness subscapularis tears.

Eljabu W et al. The natural history of rotator cuff tears: a systematic review. Arch Orthop Trauma Surg. 2015 Aug;135(8):1055–61. [PMID: 25944157]

Katthagen JC et al. Improved outcomes with arthroscopic repair of partial-thickness rotator cuff tears: a systematic review. Knee Surg Sports Traumatol Arthrosc. 2018 Jan;26(1):113–24. [PMID: 28526996]

Keener JD et al. A prospective evaluation of survivorship of asymptomatic degenerative rotator cuff tears. J Bone Joint Surg Am. 2015 Jan 21;97(2):89–98. [PMID: 25609434]

Nikolaidou O et al. Rehabilitation after rotator cuff repair. Open Orthop J. 2017 Feb 28;11:154–62. [PMID: 28400883]

Piper CC et al. Operative versus nonoperative treatment for the management of full-thickness rotator cuff tears: a systematic review and meta-analysis. J Shoulder Elbow Surg. 2018 Mar;27(3):572–6. [PMID: 29169957]

3. Shoulder Dislocation & Instability

ESSENTIALS OF DIAGNOSIS

- ▶ Most dislocations (95%) are in the anterior direction.
- ▶ Pain and apprehension with an unstable shoulder that is abducted and externally rotated.
- ▶ Acute shoulder dislocations should be reduced as quickly as possible, using manual relocation techniques if necessary.

General Considerations

The shoulder is a ball and socket joint, similar to the hip. However, the bony contours of the shoulder bones are much different than the hip. Overall, the joint has much less stability than the hip, allowing greater movement and action. Stabilizing the shoulder joint relies heavily on rotator cuff muscle strength and also scapular control. If patients have poor scapular control or weak rotator cuff tendons or tears, their shoulders are more likely to have instability. Ninety-five percent of the shoulder dislocations/instability occur in the anterior direction. Dislocations usually are caused by a fall on an outstretched and abducted arm. Patients complain of pain and feeling of instability when the arm is in the abducted and externally rotated position. Posterior dislocations are usually caused by falls from a height, epileptic seizures, or electric shocks. Traumatic shoulder dislocation can lead to instability. The rate of repeated dislocation is directly related to the patient's age: patients aged 21 years or younger have a 70–90% risk of redislocation, whereas patients aged 40 years or older have a much lower rate (20–30%). Other risks include male gender and patients with hyperlaxity. Ninety percent of young active individuals who had traumatic shoulder dislocation have labral injuries often described as Bankart lesions when the anterior inferior labrum is torn, which can lead to continued instability. Older patients (over age 55 years) are more likely to have rotator cuff tears or fractures following dislocation. Atraumatic shoulder dislocations are usually caused by intrinsic ligament laxity or repetitive microtrauma leading to joint instability. This is often seen in swimmers, gymnasts, and pitchers as well as other athletes involved in overhead and throwing sports.

Clinical Findings

A. Symptoms and Signs

For acute traumatic dislocations, patients usually have an obvious deformity with the humeral head dislocated anteriorly. The patient holds the shoulder and arm in an externally rotated position. The patient complains of acute pain and deformity that are improved with manual relocation of the shoulder. Reductions are usually performed in the emergency department. Even after reduction, the patient will continue to have limited range of motion and pain for 4–6 weeks, especially following a first-time shoulder dislocation.

Patients with recurrent dislocations can have less pain with subsequent dislocations. Posterior dislocations can be easily missed because the patient usually holds the shoulder and arm in an internally rotated position, which makes the shoulder deformity less obvious. Patients complain of difficulty pushing open a door.

Atraumatic shoulder instability is usually well tolerated with activities of daily living. Patients usually complain of a "sliding" sensation during exercises or strenuous activities such as throwing. Such dislocations may be less symptomatic and can often undergo spontaneous reduction of the shoulder with pain resolving within days after onset. The clinical examination for shoulder instability includes the apprehension test, the load and shift test, and the O'Brien test (Table 41–1). Most patients with persistent shoulder instability have preserved range of motion.

B. Imaging

Radiographs for acute dislocations should include a standard trauma series of AP and axillary lateral scapula (glenohumeral) views to determine the relationship of the humerus and the glenoid and to rule out fractures. Orthogonal views are used to identify a posterior shoulder dislocation, which can be missed easily with one AP view of the shoulder. An axillary lateral view of the shoulder can be safely performed even in the acute setting of a patient with a painful shoulder dislocation. A scapula Y view in the acute setting is insufficient to diagnose dislocation. For chronic injuries or symptomatic instability, these recommended radiographic views are helpful to identify bony injuries and Hill-Sachs lesions (indented compression fractures at the posterior-superior part of the humeral head associated with anterior shoulder dislocation). MRI is commonly used to show soft tissue injuries to the labrum and to visualize associated rotator cuff tears. MRI arthrograms better identify labral tears and ligamentous structures. Three-dimensional CT scans are used to determine the significance of bone loss.

▶ Treatment

For **acute dislocations**, the shoulder should be reduced as soon as possible. The Stimson procedure is the least traumatic method and is quite effective. The patient lies prone with the dislocated arm hanging off the examination table with a weight applied to the wrist to provide traction for 20–30 minutes. Afterward, gentle medial mobilization can be applied manually to assist the reduction. The shoulder can also be reduced with axial "traction" on the arm with "counter-traction" along the trunk. The patient should be sedated and relaxed. The shoulder can then be gently internally and externally rotated to guide it back into the socket.

Initial treatment of acute shoulder dislocations should include sling immobilization for 2–4 weeks along with pendulum exercises. Early physical therapy can be used to maintain range of motion and strengthening of rotator cuff muscles. Patients can also modify their activities to avoid active and risky sports. For patients with a traumatic incident and unilateral shoulder dislocation, a Bankart lesion is commonly present. The risk of recurrence is dependent on the age of first shoulder dislocation. Up to 70% of young patients (age less than 27 years) can have a recurrence whereas only 10% of patients older than age 40 have recurrences. However, once the patient has a second dislocation, the recurrence rate is extremely high, up to 95%, regardless of age. Operative intervention is the only treatment that has been shown to decrease recurrence. Open and arthroscopic stabilization have very similar outcomes. Repeated dislocations have been shown to increase the risk of arthritis and further bony deterioration.

The treatment of **atraumatic shoulder instability** is different than that of traumatic shoulder instability. Patients with chronic, recurrent shoulder dislocations should be managed with physical therapy and a regular maintenance program, consisting of scapular stabilization and postural and rotator cuff strengthening exercises. Activities may need to be modified. Surgical reconstructions are less successful for atraumatic shoulder instability than for traumatic shoulder instability. However, patients with recurrent dislocations have much higher incidence of bone loss or biceps pathology when compared to patients with first-time dislocations. They are also more likely to require open surgery with bone augmentation rather than arthroscopic stabilization.

▶ When to Refer

- Patients who are at risk for second dislocation, such as young patients and certain job holders (eg, police officers, firefighters, and rock climbers), to avoid recurrent dislocation or dislocation while at work.

- Patients who have not responded to a conservative approach or who have chronic instability.

Chalmers PN et al. Do arthroscopic and open stabilization techniques restore equivalent stability to the shoulder in the setting of anterior glenohumeral instability? A systematic review of overlapping meta-analysis. Arthroscopy. 2015 Feb;31(2):355–63. [PMID: 25217207]
Olds M et al. Risk factors which predispose first-time traumatic anterior shoulder dislocations to recurrent instability in adults: a systematic review and meta-analysis. Br J Sports Med. 2015 Jul;49(14):913–22. [PMID: 25900943]
Rugg CM et al. Surgical stabilization for the first-time shoulder dislocators: a multicenter analysis. J Shoulder Elbow Surg. 2018 Apr;27(4):674–85. [PMID: 29321108]

4. Adhesive Capsulitis ("Frozen Shoulder")

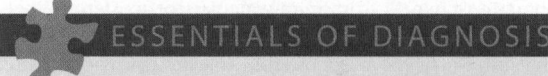

ESSENTIALS OF DIAGNOSIS

- ▶ Very painful shoulder triggered by minimal or no trauma.
- ▶ Pain out of proportion to clinical findings during the inflammatory phase.
- ▶ Stiffness during the "freezing" phase and resolution during the "thawing" phase.

▶ General Considerations

Adhesive capsulitis ("frozen shoulder") is seen commonly in patients 40 to 65 years old. It is more commonly seen in women than men, especially in perimenopausal women or in patients with endocrine disorders, such as diabetes mellitus or thyroid disease. There is higher incidence following breast cancer care (such as mastectomy). Adhesive capsulitis is a self-limiting but very debilitating disease.

▶ Clinical Findings

A. Symptoms and Signs

Patients usually present with a painful shoulder that has a limited range of motion with both passive and active movements. A useful clinical sign is limitation of movement of external rotation with the elbow by the side of the trunk

(Table 41–1). Strength is usually normal but it can appear diminished when the patient is in pain.

There are three phases: the inflammatory phase, the freezing phase, and the thawing phase. During the inflammatory phase, which usually lasts 4–6 months, patients complain of a very painful shoulder without obvious clinical findings to suggest trauma, fracture, or rotator cuff tear. During the "freezing" phase, which also usually lasts 4–6 months, the shoulder becomes stiffer and stiffer even though the pain is improving. The "thawing" phase can take up to a year as the shoulder slowly regains its motion. The total duration of an idiopathic frozen shoulder is usually about 24 months; it can be much longer for patients who have trauma or an endocrinopathy.

B. Imaging

Standard AP, axillary, and lateral glenohumeral radiographs are useful to rule out glenohumeral arthritis, which can also present with limited active and passive range of motion. Imaging can also rule out calcific tendinitis, which is an acute inflammatory process in which calcifications are visible in the soft tissue. However, adhesive capsulitis is usually a clinical diagnosis, and it does not need an extensive diagnostic workup.

▶ Treatment

Adhesive capsulitis is caused by acute inflammation of the capsule followed by scarring and remodeling. During the acute "freezing" phase, NSAIDs and physical therapy are recommended to maintain motion. There is also evidence of short-term benefit from intra-articular corticosteroid injection or oral prednisone. A randomized control trial showed that intra-articular corticosteroid injection provided better pain relief than NSAIDs in the first 8 weeks. However, no difference was seen in range of motion or pain after 12 weeks, which is similar to other noncontrolled studies. One study demonstrated improvement at 6 weeks but not 12 weeks following 30 mg of daily prednisone for 3 weeks. During the "freezing" phase, the shoulder is less painful but remains stiff. Anti-inflammatory medication is not as helpful during the "thawing" phase as it is during the "freezing" phase, and the shoulder symptoms usually resolve with time. Surgical treatments, which are rarely indicated, include manipulation under anesthesia and arthroscopic release.

▶ When to Refer

- When the patient does not respond after more than 6 months of conservative treatment.
- When there is no progress in or worsening of range of motion over 3 months.

Noten S et al. Efficacy of different types of mobilization techniques in patients with primary adhesive capsulitis of the shoulder: a systematic review. Arch Phys Med Rehabil. 2016 May;97(5):815–25. [PMID: 26284892]

Ranalletta M et al. Corticosteroid injections accelerate pain relief and recovery of function compared with oral NSAIDs in patients with adhesive capsulitis: a randomized controlled trial. Am J Sports Med. 2016 Feb;44(2):474–81. [PMID: 26657263]

Sun Y et al. Steroid injection versus physiotherapy for patients with adhesive capsulitis of the shoulder: a PRIMSA systematic review and meta-analysis of randomized controlled trials. Medicine (Baltimore). 2016 May;95(20):e3469. [PMID: 27196452]

SPINE PROBLEMS

1. Low Back Pain

ESSENTIALS OF DIAGNOSIS

- ▶ Nerve root impingement is suspected when pain is leg-dominant rather than back-dominant.
- ▶ Alarming symptoms include unexplained weight loss, failure to improve with treatment, severe pain for more than 6 weeks, and night or rest pain.
- ▶ Cauda equina syndrome is an emergency; often presents with bowel or bladder symptoms (or both).

▶ General Considerations

Low back pain remains the number one cause of disability globally and is the second most common cause for primary care visits. The annual prevalence of low back pain is 15–45%. Annual health care spending for low back and neck pain is estimated to be $87.6 billion. Low back pain is the condition associated with the highest years lived with disability. Approximately 80% of episodes of low back pain resolve within 2 weeks and 90% resolve within 6 weeks. The exact cause of the low back pain is often difficult to diagnose; its cause is often multifactorial. There are usually degenerative changes in the lumbar spine involving the disks, facet joints, and vertebral endplates (Modic changes).

Alarming symptoms for back pain caused by cancer include unexplained weight loss, failure to improve with treatment, pain for more than 6 weeks, and pain at night or rest. History of cancer and age older than 50 years are other risk factors for malignancy. Alarming symptoms for infection include fever, rest pain, recent infection (urinary tract infection, cellulitis, pneumonia), or history of immunocompromise or injection drug use. The **cauda equina syndrome** is suggested by urinary retention or incontinence, saddle anesthesia, decreased anal sphincter tone or fecal incontinence, bilateral lower extremity weakness, and progressive neurologic deficits. Risk factors for back pain due to vertebral fracture include use of corticosteroids, age over 70 years, history of osteoporosis, severe trauma, and presence of a contusion or abrasion. Back pain may also be the presenting symptom in other serious medical problems, including abdominal aortic aneurysm, peptic ulcer disease, kidney stones, or pancreatitis.

▶ Clinical Findings

A. Symptoms and Signs

The physical examination can be conducted with the patient in the standing, sitting, supine, and finally prone positions to avoid frequent repositioning of the patient. In the standing position, the patient's posture can be observed. Commonly encountered spinal asymmetries include scoliosis, thoracic kyphosis, and lumbar hyperlordosis. The active range of motion of the lumbar spine can be assessed while standing. The common directions include flexion, extension, rotation, and lateral bending. The one-leg standing extension test assesses for pain as the patient stands on one leg while extending the spine. A positive test can be caused by pars interarticularis fractures (spondylolysis or spondylolisthesis) or facet joint arthritis.

With the patient sitting, motor strength, reflexes, and sensation can be tested (Table 41–2). The major muscles in the lower extremities are assessed for weakness by eliciting a resisted isometric contraction for about 5 seconds. Comparing the strength bilaterally to detect subtle muscle weakness is important. Similarly, sensory testing to light touch can be checked in specific dermatomes for corresponding nerve root function. Knee (femoral nerve L2–4), ankle (deep peroneal nerve L4–L5), and Babinski (sciatic nerve L5–S1) reflexes can be checked with the patient sitting.

In the supine position, the hip should be evaluated for range of motion, particularly internal rotation. The straight leg raise test puts traction and compression forces on the lower lumbar nerve roots.

Finally, in the prone position, the clinician can carefully palpate each vertebral level of the spine and sacroiliac joints for tenderness. A rectal examination is required if the cauda equina syndrome is suspected. Superficial skin tenderness to a light touch over the lumbar spine, overreaction to maneuvers in the regular back examination, low back pain on axial loading of spine in standing, and inconsistency in the straight leg raise test or on the neurologic examination suggest nonorthopedic causes for the pain or malingering.

B. Imaging

In the absence of alarming "red flag" symptoms suggesting infection, malignancy, or cauda equina syndrome, most patients do not need diagnostic imaging, including radiographs, in the first 6 weeks. The Agency for Healthcare Research and Quality guidelines for obtaining lumbar radiographs are summarized in Table 41–3. Most clinicians obtain radiographs for new back pain in patients older than 50 years. If done, radiographs of the lumbar spine should include AP and lateral views. Oblique views can be useful if the neuroforamina or bone lesions need to be visualized. MRI is the method of choice in the evaluation of symptoms not responding to conservative treatment or in the presence of red flags of serious conditions.

C. Special Tests

Electromyography or nerve conduction studies may be useful in assessing patients with possible nerve root symptoms lasting longer than 6 weeks; back pain may or may not also be present. These tests are usually not necessary if the diagnosis of radiculopathy is clear.

▶ Treatment

A. Conservative

Nonpharmacologic treatments are key in the management of low back pain. Education alone improves patient satisfaction with recovery and recurrence. Patients require information and reassurance, especially when diagnostic procedures are not necessary. Discussion must include reviewing safe and effective methods of symptom control as well as how to decrease the risk of recurrence with proper lifting techniques, abdominal wall/core strengthening,

Table 41–2. Neurologic testing of lumbosacral nerve disorders.

Nerve Root	Motor	Reflex	Sensory Area
L1	Hip flexion	None	Groin
L2	Hip flexion	None	Thigh
L3	Extension of knee	Knee jerk	Knee
L4	Dorsiflexion of ankle	Knee jerk	Medial calf
L5	Dorsiflexion of first toe	Babinski reflex	First dorsal web space between first and second toes
S1	Plantar flexion of foot, knee flexors, or hamstrings	Ankle jerk	Lateral foot
S2	Knee flexors or hamstrings	Knee flexor	Back of the thigh
S2–S4	External anal sphincter	Anal reflex, rectal tone	Perianal area

Table 41–3. AHRQ criteria for lumbar radiographs in patients with acute low back pain.

| **Possible fracture** |
| Major trauma |
| Minor trauma in patients > 50 years of age |
| Long-term corticosteroid use |
| Osteoporosis |
| > 70 years of age |
| **Possible tumor or infection** |
| > 50 years of age |
| < 20 years of age |
| History of cancer |
| Constitutional symptoms |
| Recent bacterial infection |
| Injection drug use |
| Immunosuppression |
| Supine pain |
| Nocturnal pain |

AHRQ, Agency for Healthcare Research and Quality.
Adapted from Bigos S, Bowyer O, Braen G, et al. *Acute Low Back Problems in Adults.* Clinical Practice Guideline Quick Reference Guide No. 14. AHCPR Publication No. 95-0643. Rockville, MD: Agency for Health Care Policy and Research, Public Health Service, U.S. Department of Health and Human Services. December 1994.

weight loss, and smoking cessation. Tai chi, mindfulness-based stress reduction, and yoga have shown benefit for chronic low back pain patients. Exercise, psychological therapies, and multidisciplinary rehabilitation have been shown to be modestly effective for acute low back pain (strength of evidence, low).

Physical therapy exercise programs can be tailored to the patient's symptoms and pathology. A randomized controlled trial demonstrated that individualized physical therapy was clinically more beneficial than advice alone with sustained improvements at 6 months and 12 months. Strengthening and stabilization exercises effectively reduce pain and functional limitation compared with usual care. Heat and cold treatments have not shown any long-term benefits but may be used for symptomatic treatment. The efficacy of transcutaneous electrical nerve stimulation (TENS), back braces, and physical agents is unproven. Spinal manipulation, massage, and acupuncture have limited, low-strength evidence for chronic low back pain. Improvements in posture including chair ergonomics or standing desks, core stability strengthening, physical conditioning, and modifications of activities to decrease physical strain are keys for ongoing management. Radiofrequency denervation of facet joints, sacroiliac joints, or intervertebral disks did not result in clinically important improvement in chronic low back even when combined with a standardized exercise program in randomized controlled trials.

NSAIDs are effective in the early treatment of low back pain (see Chapter 20). Acetaminophen and oral corticosteroids are relatively ineffective for chronic low back. There is limited evidence that muscle relaxants provide short-term relief; since these medications have addictive potential, they should be used with care. Muscle relaxants are best used if there is true muscle spasm that is painful rather than simply a protective response. Opioids alleviate pain in the short term, but have the usual side effects and concerns of long-term opioid use (Chapter 5). Treatment of more chronic neuropathic pain with alpha-2-delta ligands (eg, gabapentin), serotonin-norepinephrine reuptake inhibitors (eg, duloxetine), or tricyclic antidepressants (eg, nortriptyline) may be helpful (Chapter 5). Epidural injections may reduce pain in the short term and reduce the need for surgery in some patients within a 1-year period but not longer. Therefore, spinal injections are not recommended for initial care of patients with low back pain without radiculopathy.

B. Surgical

Indications for back surgery include cauda equina syndrome, ongoing morbidity with no response to more than 6 months of conservative treatment, cancer, infection, or severe spinal deformity. Prognosis is improved when there is an anatomic lesion that can be corrected and symptoms are neurologic. Spinal surgery has limitations. Patient selection is very important and the specific surgery recommended should have very clear indications. Patients should understand that surgery can improve their pain but is unlikely to cure it. Surgery is not generally indicated for radiographic abnormalities alone when the patient is relatively asymptomatic. Depending on the surgery performed, possible complications include persistent pain; surgical site

pain, especially if bone grafting is needed; infection; neurologic damage; non-union; cutaneous nerve damage; implant failure; deep venous thrombosis; and death.

▶ When to Refer

- Patients with the cauda equina syndrome.
- Patients with cancer, infection, fracture, or severe spinal deformity.
- Patients who have not responded to conservative treatment.

Abdel Shaheed C et al. Efficacy, tolerability, and dose-dependent effects of opioid analgesics for low back pain: a systematic review and meta-analysis. JAMA Intern Med. 2016 Jul 1;176(7):958–68. [PMID: 27213267]

Bicket MC et al. Epidural injections in prevention of surgery for spinal pain: systematic review and meta-analysis of randomized controlled trials. Spine J. 2015 Feb 1;15(2):348–62. [PMID: 25463400]

Chou R et al. Systemic pharmacologic therapies for low back pain: a systematic review for an American College of Physicians clinical practice guideline. Ann Intern Med. 2017 Apr 4;166(7):480–92. [PMID: 28192790]

Ford JJ et al. Individualised physiotherapy as an adjunct to guideline-based advice for low back disorders in primary care: a randomised controlled trial. Br J Sports Med. 2016 Feb;50(4):237–45. [PMID: 26486585]

Hartvigsen J et al; Lancet Low Back Pain Series Working Group. What low back pain is and why we need to pay attention. Lancet. 2018 Jun 9;391(10137):2356–67. [PMID: 29573870]

Qaseem A et al. Noninvasive treatments for acute, subacute, and chronic low back pain: a clinical practice guideline from the American College of Physicians. Ann Intern Med. 2017 Apr 4;166(7):514–30. [PMID: 28192789]

2. Spinal Stenosis

ESSENTIALS OF DIAGNOSIS

- ▶ Pain is usually worse with back extension and relieved by sitting.
- ▶ Occurs in older patients.
- ▶ May present with neurogenic claudication symptoms with walking.

▶ General Considerations

OA in the lumbar spine can cause narrowing of the spinal canal. A large disk herniation can also cause stenosis and compression of neural structures or the spinal artery resulting in "claudication" symptoms with ambulation. The condition usually affects patients aged 50 years or older.

▶ Clinical Findings

Patients report pain that worsens with extension. They describe reproducible single or bilateral leg symptoms that are worse after walking several minutes and that are relieved by sitting ("neurogenic claudication"). On examination, patients often exhibit limited extension of the lumbar spine, which may reproduce the symptoms radiating down the legs. A thorough neurovascular examination is recommended (Table 41–2).

Treatment

Exercises, usually flexion-based as demonstrated by a physical therapist, can help relieve symptoms. Physical therapy showed similar results as surgical decompression in a randomized trial, though there was a 57% crossover rate from physical therapy to surgery. Facet joint corticosteroid injections can also reduce pain symptoms. While epidural corticosteroid injections have been shown to provide immediate improvements in pain and function for patients with radiculopathy, the benefits are small and only short term. Consequently, there is limited evidence to recommend epidural corticosteroids for spinal stenosis.

Surgical treatments for spinal stenosis include spinal decompression (widening the spinal canal or laminectomy), nerve root decompression (freeing a single nerve), and spinal fusion (joining the vertebra to eliminate motion and diminish pain from the arthritic joints). However, a Cochrane review showed surgery was not clearly better than nonsurgical treatment and had complication rates of 10–24% compared to 0% for nonoperative treatments. Thus, the role of surgery for spinal stenosis is limited. In one multicenter randomized trial, subgroups initially improved significantly more with surgery than with nonoperative treatment. Variables associated with greater treatment effects included lower baseline disability scores, not smoking, neuroforaminal stenosis, predominant leg pain rather than back pain, not lifting at work, and the presence of a neurologic deficit. However, long-term follow-up of the patients with symptomatic spinal stenosis who received surgery in the multicenter randomized trial showed less benefit of surgery between 4 and 8 years, suggesting that the advantage of surgery for spinal stenosis diminishes over time. A Cochrane review of 24 randomized controlled trials of treatments for lumbar spinal stenosis showed that various surgeries including decompression plus fusion and interspinous process spacers were not superior to conventional spinal decompression surgery alone.

When to Refer

- If a patient exhibits radicular or claudication symptoms for longer than 12 weeks.
- MRI or CT confirmation of significant, symptomatic spinal stenosis.
- However, surgery has not been shown to have clear benefit over nonsurgical treatment for lumbar spinal stenosis.

Chou R et al. Epidural corticosteroid injections for radiculopathy and spinal stenosis: a systematic review and meta-analysis. Ann Intern Med. 2015 Sep 1;163(5):373–81. [PMID: 26302454]

Lurie JD et al. Long-term outcomes of lumbar spinal stenosis: eight-year results of the Spine Patient Outcomes Research Trial (SPORT). Spine (Phila Pa 1976). 2015 Jan 15;40(2):63–76. [PMID: 25569524]

Zaina F et al. Surgical versus non-surgical treatment for lumbar spinal stenosis. Cochrane Database Syst Rev. 2016 Jan 29;(1):CD010264. [PMID: 26824399]

3. Lumbar Disk Herniation

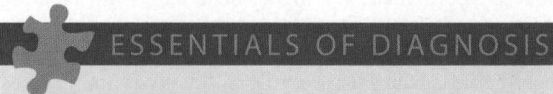

ESSENTIALS OF DIAGNOSIS

- ▶ Pain with back flexion or prolonged sitting.
- ▶ Radicular pain into the leg due to compression of neural structures.
- ▶ Lower extremity numbness and weakness.

General Considerations

Lumbar disk herniation is usually due to bending or heavy loading (eg, lifting) with the back in flexion, causing herniation or extrusion of disk contents (nucleus pulposus) into the spinal cord area. However, there may not be an inciting incident. Disk herniations usually occur from degenerative disk disease (dessication of the annulus fibrosis) in patients between 30 and 50 years old. The L5–S1 disk is affected in 90% of cases. Compression of neural structures, such as the sciatic nerve, causes radicular pain. Severe compression of the spinal cord can cause the cauda equina syndrome, a surgical emergency.

Clinical Findings

A. Symptoms and Signs

Discogenic pain typically is localized in the low back at the level of the affected disk and is worse with activity. "Sciatica" causes electric shock-like pain radiating down the posterior aspect of the leg often to below the knee. Symptoms usually worsen with back flexion such as bending or sitting for long periods (eg, driving). A significant disk herniation can cause numbness and weakness, including weakness with plantar flexion of the foot (L5/S1) or dorsiflexion of the toes (L4/L5). The cauda equina syndrome should be ruled out if the patient complains of perianal numbness or bowel or bladder incontinence.

B. Imaging

Plain radiographs are helpful to assess spinal alignment (scoliosis, lordosis), disk space narrowing, and OA changes. MRI is the best method to assess the level and morphology of the herniation and is recommended if surgery is planned.

Treatment

For an acute exacerbation of pain symptoms, bed rest is appropriate for up to 48 hours. Otherwise, first-line treatments include modified activities; NSAIDs and other analgesics; and physical therapy, including core stabilization and McKenzie back exercises. Following nonsurgical treatment for a lumbar disk for over 1 year, the incidence of low back pain recurrence is at least 40% and is predicted by longer time to initial resolution of pain. In a randomized trial, oral prednisone caused a modest improvement in function at 3 weeks, but there was no significant improvement in pain in patients with acute radiculopathy who were monitored for 1 year. The initial dose for oral prednisone is approximately 1 mg/kg once daily with tapering doses over 10–15 days. Analgesics for neuropathic pain, such as the calcium channel alpha-2-delta ligands (ie, gabapentin, pregabalin) or tricyclic antidepressants, may be helpful (see Chapter 5). Epidural and transforaminal corticosteroid injections can be beneficial. A systematic review demonstrated strong evidence that fluoroscopic-guided epidural injections gave short-term benefit (less than 6 months) in acute radicular pain for individuals. However, epidural injections have not shown any change in long-term surgery rates for disk herniations.

The severity of pain and disability as well as failure of conservative therapy were the most important reasons for surgery. A large trial has shown that patients who underwent surgery for a lumbar disk herniation achieved greater improvement than conservatively treated patients in all primary and secondary outcomes except return to work status after 4-year follow-up. Patients with sequestered fragments, symptom duration greater than 6 months, higher levels of low back pain, or who were neither working nor disabled at baseline showed greater surgical treatment effects. Microdiskectomy is the standard method of treatment with a low rate of complications and satisfactory results over 90% in the largest series. A minimally invasive technique is percutaneous endoscopic diskectomy, which involves using an endoscope to remove fragments of disk herniation (interlaminar or transforaminal approaches) under local anesthesia, although results are less successful than with microdiskectomy. Disk replacement surgery has shown benefits in short-term pain relief, disability, and quality of life compared with spine fusion surgery.

▶ When to Refer

- Cauda equina syndrome.
- Progressive worsening of neurologic symptoms.
- Loss of motor function (sensory losses can be followed in the outpatient clinic).

Gadjradj PS et al. Management of symptomatic lumbar disk herniation: an international perspective. Spine (Phila Pa 1976). 2017 Dec 1;42(23):1826–34. [PMID: 28632645]

Goldberg H et al. Oral steroids for acute radiculopathy due to a herniated lumbar disk: a randomized clinical trial. JAMA. 2015 May 19;313(19):1915–23. [PMID: 25988461]

Kerr D et al. What are long-term predictors of outcomes for lumbar disk herniation? A randomized and observational study. Clin Orthop Relat Res. 2015 Jun;473(6):1920–30. [PMID: 25057116]

Manchikanti L et al. Do epidural injections provide short- and long-term relief for lumbar disk herniation? A systematic review. Clin Orthop Relat Res. 2015 Jun;473(6):1940–56. [PMID: 24515404]

4. Neck Pain

ESSENTIALS OF DIAGNOSIS

▶ Chronic neck pain is mostly caused by degenerative joint disease; whiplash often follows a traumatic neck injury.

▶ Poor posture is often a factor for persistent neck pain.

▶ General Considerations

Most neck pain, especially in older patients, is due to mechanical degeneration involving the cervical disks, facet joints, and ligamentous structures and may occur in the setting of degenerative changes at other sites. Pain can also come from the supporting neck musculature, which often acts to protect the underlying neck structures. Posture is a very important factor, especially in younger patients. Many work-related neck symptoms are due to poor posture and repetitive motions over time. Acute injuries can also occur secondary to trauma. Whiplash occurs from rapid flexion and extension of the neck and affects 15–40% of people in motor vehicle accidents; chronic pain develops in 5–7%. Neck fractures are serious traumatic injuries acutely and can lead to OA in the long term. Ultimately, many degenerative conditions of the neck result in cervical canal stenosis or neural foraminal stenosis, sometimes affecting underlying neural structures.

Cervical radiculopathy can cause neurologic symptoms in the upper extremities usually involving the C5–C7 disks. Patients with neck pain may report associated headaches and shoulder pain. Both peripheral nerve entrapment and cervical radiculopathy, known as a "double crush" injury, may develop. Thoracic outlet syndrome, in which there is mechanical compression of the brachial plexus and neurovascular structures with overhead positioning of the arm, should be considered in the differential diagnosis of neck pain. Other causes of neck pain include rheumatoid arthritis, fibromyalgia, osteomyelitis, neoplasms, polymyalgia rheumatica, compression fractures, pain referred from visceral structures (eg, angina), and functional disorders. Amyotrophic lateral sclerosis, multiple sclerosis, syringomyelia, spinal cord tumors, and Parsonage-Turner syndrome can mimic myelopathy from cervical arthritis.

▶ Clinical Findings

A. Symptoms and Signs

Neck pain may be limited to the posterior region or, depending on the level of the symptomatic joint, may radiate segmentally to the occiput, anterior chest, shoulder girdle, arm, forearm, and hand. It may be intensified by active or passive neck motions. The general distribution of pain and paresthesias corresponds roughly to the involved dermatome in the upper extremity.

The patient's posture should be assessed, checking for shoulder rolled forward or head forward posture as well as scoliosis in the thoracolumbar spine. Patients with discogenic neck pain often complain of pain with flexion, which causes cervical disks to herniate posteriorly. Extension of the neck usually affects the neural foraminal and facet joints of the neck. Rotation and lateral flexion of the cervical spine should be measured both to the left and the right. Limitation of cervical movements is the most common objective finding.

A detailed neurovascular examination of the upper extremities should be performed, including sensory input to light touch and temperature; motor strength testing, especially the hand intrinsic muscles (thumb extension strength [C6], opponens strength (thumb to pinky) [C7], and finger abductors and adductors strength [C8–T1]); and upper extremity reflexes (biceps, triceps, brachioradialis). True cervical radiculopathy symptoms should match an expected dermatomal or myotomal distribution. The Spurling test involves asking the patient to rotate and extend the neck to one side (Table 41–4). The clinician can apply a gentle axial load to the neck. Reproduction of the cervical radiculopathy symptoms is a positive sign of nerve root compression. Palpation of the neck is best performed with the patient in the supine position where the clinician can palpate each level of the cervical spine with the muscles of the neck relaxed.

B. Imaging and Special Tests

Radiographs of the cervical spine include the AP and lateral view of the cervical spine. The odontoid view is usually added to rule out traumatic fractures and congenital abnormalities. Oblique views of the cervical spine can provide further information about arthritis changes and assess the neural foramina for narrowing. Plain radiographs can be completely normal in patients who have suffered an acute cervical strain. Comparative reduction in height of the involved disk space and osteophytes are frequent findings when there are degenerative changes in the cervical spine. Loss of cervical lordosis is commonly seen but is nonspecific.

MRI is the best method to assess the cervical spine since the soft tissue structures (such as the disks, spinal cord, and nerve roots) can be evaluated. If the patient has signs of cervical radiculopathy with motor weakness, these more sensitive imaging modalities should be obtained urgently. CT scanning is the most useful method if bony abnormalities, such as fractures, are suspected.

EMG is useful in order to differentiate peripheral nerve entrapment syndromes from cervical radiculopathy. However, sensitivity of electrodiagnostic testing for cervical radiculopathy ranges from only 50% to 71%, so a negative test does not rule out nerve root problems.

▶ Treatment

In the absence of trauma or evidence of infection, malignancy, neurologic findings, or systemic inflammation, the patient can be treated conservatively. More frequent observation of individuals in whom very severe symptoms are present early on after an injury is recommended because high pain-related disability is a predictor of poor outcome at 1 year even if individuals decline care. Ergonomics should be assessed at work and home. A course of neck stretching, strengthening, and postural exercises in physical therapy have demonstrated benefit in relieving symptoms. A soft cervical collar can be useful for short-term use (up to 1–2 weeks) in acute neck injuries. Chiropractic manual manipulation and mobilization can provide short-term benefit for mechanical neck pain. Although the rate of complications is low (5–10/million manipulations), care should be taken whenever there are neurologic symptoms present. Specific patients may respond to use of home cervical traction. NSAIDs are commonly used and opioids may be needed in cases of severe neck pain. Muscle relaxants (eg, cyclobenzaprine 5–10 mg orally three times daily) can be used short term if there is muscle spasm or as a sedative to aid in sleeping. Acute radicular symptoms can be treated with neuropathic medications (eg, gabapentin 300–1200 mg orally three times daily), and a short course of oral prednisone (5–10 days) can be considered (starting at 1 mg/kg). Cervical foraminal or facet joint injections can also reduce symptoms. Surgeries are successful in reducing neurologic symptoms in 80–90% of cases, but are still considered as treatments of last resort. Common surgeries for cervical degenerative disk disease include anterior cervical diskectomy with fusion and cervical disk arthroplasty. A meta-analysis of 18 randomized controlled trials showed that cervical disk arthroplasty was superior to anterior diskectomy and fusion for the treatment of symptomatic cervical disk disease, with better success and less reoperation rates.

Table 41–4. Spine: neck examination.

Maneuver	Description
Inspection	Check the patient's posture in the standing position. Assess for cervical hyperlordosis, head forward posture, kyphosis, scoliosis, torticollis.
Palpation	Include important landmarks: spinous process, facet joints, paracervical muscles (sternocleidomastoid, scalene muscles).
Range of motion testing	Check range of motion in the cervical spine, especially with flexion and extension. Rotation and lateral bending are also helpful to assess symmetric motion or any restrictions. Pain and radicular symptoms can be exacerbated by range of motion testing.
Neurologic examination	Check motor strength, reflexes, and dermatomal sensation in the upper (and lower if necessary) extremities.
Spurling test	Involves asking the patient to rotate and extend the neck to one side. The clinician can apply a gentle axial load to the neck. Reproduction of the cervical radiculopathy symptoms is a positive sign of nerve root compression.

► When to Refer

- Patients with severe symptoms with motor weakness.
- Surgical decompression surgery if the symptoms are severe and there is identifiable, correctable pathology.

Cohen SP et al. Advances in the diagnosis and management of neck pain. BMJ. 2017 Aug 14;358:j3221. [PMID: 28807894]
Iyer S et al. Cervical radiculopathy. Curr Rev Musculoskelet Med. 2016 Sep;9(3):272–80. [PMID: 27250042]

UPPER EXTREMITY

1. Lateral & Medial Epicondylosis

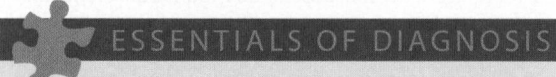

ESSENTIALS OF DIAGNOSIS

- ► Tenderness over the lateral or medial epicondyle.
- ► Diagnosis of tendinopathy is confirmed by pain with resisted strength testing and passive stretching of the affected tendon and muscle unit.
- ► Physical therapy and activity modification are more successful than anti-inflammatory treatments.

► General Considerations

Tendinopathies involving the wrist extensors, flexors, and pronators are very common complaints. The underlying mechanism is chronic repetitive overuse causing microtrauma at the tendon insertion, although acute injuries can occur as well if the tendon is strained due to excessive loading. The traditional term "epicondylitis" is a misnomer because histologically tendinosis or degeneration in the tendon is seen rather than acute inflammation. Therefore, these entities should be referred to as "tendinopathy" or "tendinosis." Lateral epicondylosis involves the wrist extensors, especially the extensor carpi radialis brevis. This is usually caused be lifting with the wrist and the elbow extended. Medial epicondylosis involves the wrist flexors and most commonly the pronator teres tendon. Ulnar neuropathy and cervical radiculopathy should be considered in the differential diagnosis.

► Clinical Findings

A. Symptoms and Signs

For lateral epicondylosis, the patient describes pain with the arm and wrist extended. For example, common complaints include pain while shaking hands, lifting objects, using a computer mouse, or hitting a backhand in tennis ("tennis elbow"). Medial epicondylosis presents with pain during motions in which the arm is repetitively pronated or the wrist is flexed. This is also known as "golfer's elbow" due to the motion of turning the hands over during the golf swing. For either, tenderness directly over the epicondyle is present, especially over the posterior aspect where the tendon insertion occurs. The proximal tendon and musculotendinous junction can also be sore. To confirm that the pain is due to tendinopathy, pain can be reproduced over the epicondyle with resisted wrist extension and third digit extension for lateral epicondylosis and resisted wrist pronation and wrist flexion for medial epicondylosis. The pain is also often reproduced with passive stretching of the affected muscle groups, which can be performed with the arm in extension. It is useful to check the ulnar nerve (located in a groove at the posteromedial elbow) for tenderness as well as to perform a Spurling test for cervical radiculopathy.

B. Imaging

Radiographs are often normal, although a small traction spur may be present in chronic cases (enthesopathy). Diagnostic investigations are usually unnecessary, unless the patient does not improve after up to 3 months of conservative treatment. At that point, a patient who demonstrates significant disability due to the pain should be assessed with an MRI or ultrasound. Ultrasound and MRI can visualize the tendon and confirm tendinosis or tears.

► Treatment

Treatment is usually conservative, including patient education regarding activity modification and management of symptoms. Ice and NSAIDs can help with pain. The mainstay of treatment is physical therapy exercises. The most important steps are to begin a good stretching program followed by strengthening exercises, particularly eccentric ones. Counterforce elbow braces might provide some symptomatic relief, although there is no published evidence to support their use. If the patient has severe or long-standing symptoms, injections can be considered. A randomized trial showed improvement with corticosteroid injection at 1 month as well as evidence of decreased tendon thickness and Doppler changes but no improvement at 3 months. Treatments such as extracorporeal shock wave therapy and other injections have not shown clear long-term benefit. Evidence on platelet-rich plasma (PRP) injections continues to accumulate and it is becoming more commonly used in practice, although it is still considered a second-line treatment. Reviews suggest that PRP and autologous blood injections both have positive benefits in lateral epicondylitis. In a randomized controlled trial comparing PRP injection to controls (n = 119), the PRP-treated patients reported 55.1% improvement in their pain scores at 12 weeks compared to 47.4% in the control patients ($P = 0.163$). More significant improvement was seen at 24 weeks; 71.5% improvement in the pain scores in the PRP-treated patients compared to 56.1% in the control patients ($P = 0.019$). (A 25% improvement of pain symptoms was considered to be clinically significant.) However, the varied methods of PRP preparations and varied post-injection recommendations for rest and physiotherapy make interpretation of various study results difficult to summarize.

► When to Refer

Patients not responding to 6 months of conservative treatment should be referred for an injection procedure (PRP or tenotomy), surgical debridement, or repair of the tendon.

Amin NH et al. Medial epicondylitis: evaluation and management. J Am Acad Orthop Surg. 2015 Jun;23(6):348–55. [PMID: 26001427]

Kwapisz A et al. Platelet-rich plasma for elbow pathologies: a descriptive review of current literature. Curr Rev Musculoskelet Med. 2018 Dec;11(4):598–606. [PMID: 30255288]

Sayegh ET et al. Does nonsurgical treatment improve longitudinal outcomes of lateral epicondylitis over no treatment? A meta-analysis. Clin Orthop Relat Res. 2015 Mar;473(3):1093–107. [PMID: 25352261]

Sirico F et al. Local corticosteroid versus autologous blood injections in lateral epicondylitis: meta-analysis of randomized controlled trials. Eur J Phys Rehabil Med. 2017 Jun;53(3):483–91. [PMID: 27585054]

2. Carpal Tunnel Syndrome

 ESSENTIALS OF DIAGNOSIS

► Pain, burning, and tingling in the distribution of the median nerve.

► Initially, most bothersome during sleep.

► Late weakness or atrophy of the thenar eminence.

► Can be caused by repetitive wrist activities.

► Commonly seen during pregnancy and in patients with diabetes mellitus or rheumatoid arthritis.

► General Considerations

An entrapment neuropathy, carpal tunnel syndrome is a painful disorder caused by compression of the median nerve between the carpal ligament and other structures within the carpal tunnel. The contents of the tunnel can be compressed by synovitis of the tendon sheaths or carpal joints, recent or malhealed fractures, tumors, tissue infiltration, and occasionally congenital syndromes (eg, mucopolysaccharidoses). The disorder may occur in fluid retention of pregnancy, in individuals with a history of repetitive use of the hands, or following injuries of the wrists. Carpal tunnel syndrome can also be a feature of many systemic diseases, such as rheumatoid arthritis and other rheumatic disorders (inflammatory tenosynovitis), myxedema, amyloidosis, sarcoidosis, leukemia, acromegaly, and hyperparathyroidism. There is a familial type of carpal tunnel syndrome in which no etiologic factor can be identified.

► Clinical Findings

A. Symptoms and Signs

The initial symptoms are pain, burning, and tingling in the distribution of the median nerve (the palmar surfaces of the thumb, the index and long fingers, and the radial half of the ring finger). Aching pain may radiate proximally into the forearm and occasionally proximally to the shoulder and over the neck and chest. Pain is exacerbated by manual activity, particularly by extremes of volar flexion or dorsiflexion of the wrist. It is most bothersome at night. Impairment of sensation in the median nerve distribution may or may not be demonstrable. Subtle disparity between the affected and opposite sides can be shown by testing for two-point discrimination or by requiring the patient to identify different textures of cloth by rubbing them between the tips of the thumb and the index finger. A Tinel or Phalen sign may be positive. A **Tinel sign** is tingling or shock-like pain on volar wrist percussion. The **Phalen sign** is pain or paresthesia in the distribution of the median nerve when the patient flexes both wrists to 90 degrees for 60 seconds. The **carpal compression test**, in which numbness and tingling are induced by the direct application of pressure over the carpal tunnel, may be more sensitive and specific than the Tinel and Phalen tests. Muscle weakness or atrophy, especially of the thenar eminence, can appear later than sensory disturbances as compression of the nerve worsens.

B. Imaging

Ultrasound can demonstrate flattening of the median nerve beneath the flexor retinaculum. Sensitivity of ultrasound for carpal tunnel syndrome is variable but estimated between 54% and 98%.

C. Special Tests

Electromyography and nerve conduction studies show evidence of sensory conduction delay before motor delay, which can occur in severe cases.

► Treatment

Treatment is directed toward relief of pressure on the median nerve. When a causative lesion is discovered, it should be treated appropriately. Otherwise, patients in whom carpal tunnel syndrome is suspected should modify their hand activities. The affected wrist can be splinted in the neutral position for up to 3 months, but a series of Cochrane reviews show limited evidence for splinting, exercises, and ergonomic positioning. Moderate evidence supported benefit from several physical therapy and electrophysical modalities (eg, ultrasound therapy and radial extracorporeal shockwave therapy). These modalities provided short-term and mid-term relief of carpal tunnel syndrome symptoms in different studies. Oral corticosteroids or NSAIDs have also shown benefit for carpal tunnel syndrome. Methylprednisolone injections were found to have more effect at 10 weeks than placebo, but the benefits diminished by 1 year.

Compared to trigger finger management, which usually includes injections, as many as 71% of patients with carpal tunnel directly undergo surgery without first getting injections. There is strong evidence that a steroid injection to the carpal tunnel is more effective in the short term than surgery. A randomized, controlled trial showed both corticosteroid injection and surgery resolved symptoms but only decompressive surgery led to resolution of neurophysiologic changes. Carpal tunnel release surgery can be beneficial if the patient has a positive electrodiagnostic test, at least moderate symptoms, high clinical probability, unsuccessful nonoperative treatment, and symptoms lasting longer than 12 months. Surgery can be done with an open approach or endoscopically, both yielding similar good improvements.

When to Refer

- If symptoms persist more than 3 months despite conservative treatment, including the use of a wrist splint.
- If thenar muscle (eg, abductor pollicis brevis) weakness or atrophy develops.

Huisstede BM et al. Carpal tunnel syndrome: effectiveness of physical therapy and electrophysical modalities. An updated systematic review of randomized controlled trials. Arch Phys Med Rehabil. 2018 Aug;99(8):1623–34. [PMID: 28942118]

Huisstede BM et al. Effectiveness of surgical and postsurgical interventions for carpal tunnel syndrome—a systematic review. Arch Phys Med Rehabil. 2018 Aug;99(8):1660–80. [PMID: 28577858]

Padua L et al. Carpal tunnel syndrome: clinical features, diagnosis, and management. Lancet Neurol. 2016 Nov;15(12):1273–84. [PMID: 27751557]

Sears ED et al. National utilization patterns of steroid injection and operative intervention for treatment of common hand conditions. J Hand Surg Am. 2016 Mar;41(3):367–73. [PMID: 26774548]

3. Dupuytren Contracture

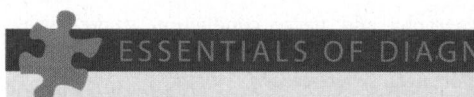

ESSENTIALS OF DIAGNOSIS

- ▶ Benign fibrosing disorder of the palmar fascia.
- ▶ Contracture of one or more fingers can lead to limited hand function.

General Considerations

This relatively common disorder is characterized by hyperplasia of the palmar fascia and related structures, with nodule formation and contracture of the palmar fascia. The cause is unknown, but the condition has a genetic predisposition and occurs primarily in white men over 50 years of age, particularly in those of Celtic descent. The incidence is higher among alcoholic patients and those with chronic systemic disorders (especially cirrhosis). It is also associated with systemic fibrosing syndrome, which includes plantar fibromatosis (10% of patients), Peyronie disease (1–2%), mediastinal and retroperitoneal fibrosis, and Riedel struma. The onset may be acute, but slowly progressive chronic disease is more common.

Clinical Findings

Dupuytren contracture manifests itself by nodular or cord-like thickening of one or both hands, with the fourth and fifth fingers most commonly affected. The patient may complain of tightness of the involved digits, with inability to satisfactorily extend the fingers, and on occasion there is tenderness. The resulting cosmetic problems may be unappealing, but in general the contracture is well tolerated since it exaggerates the normal position of function of the hand.

Treatment

Corticosteroid injection with a percutaneous needle aponeurotomy has shown some promise for Dupuytren contracture. If the palmar nodule is growing rapidly, injections of triamcinolone or collagenase into the nodule may be of benefit; the injection of collagenase *Clostridium histolyticum* lyses collagen, thereby disrupting the contracted cords. Surgical options include open fasciectomy, partial fasciectomy, or percutaneous needle aponeurotomy and are indicated in patients with significant flexion contractures. A multicenter study showed that collagenase injection and limited fasciectomy had similar improvements with contractures at the metacarpophalangeal joints, while surgery had better results for contractures involving the proximal interphalangeal joints. Splinting after surgery is beneficial. Recurrence is possible after surgery with more adverse events compared to nonoperative treatments. Compared to placebo, tamoxifen therapy produced moderate evidence of improvement before or after a fasciectomy.

When to Refer

Referral can be considered when one or more digits are affected by severe contractures, which interfere with everyday activities and result in functional limitations.

Huisstede BM et al. Effectiveness of conservative, surgical, and postsurgical interventions for trigger finger, Dupuytren disease, and De Quervain disease: a systematic review. Arch Phys Med Rehabil. 2018 Aug;99(8):1635–49. [PMID: 28860097]

Rodrigues JN et al. Surgery for Dupuytren's contracture of the fingers. Cochrane Database Syst Rev. 2015 Dec 9;(12):CD010143. [PMID: 26648251]

Zhou C et al. Collagenase *Clostridium histolyticum* versus limited fasciectomy for Dupuytren's contracture: outcomes from a multicenter propensity score matched study. Plast Reconstr Surg. 2015 Jul;136(1):87–97. [PMID: 25829153]

4. Bursitis

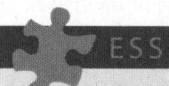

ESSENTIALS OF DIAGNOSIS

- ▶ Often occurs around bony prominences where it is important to reduce friction.
- ▶ Typically presents with local swelling that is painful acutely.
- ▶ Septic bursitis can present without fever or systemic signs.

General Considerations

Inflammation of bursae—the synovium-like cellular membranes overlying bony prominences—may be secondary to trauma, infection, or arthritic conditions such as gout, rheumatoid arthritis, or OA. Bursitis can result from infection. The two common sites are the olecranon (Figure 41–1) and prepatellar bursae; however, others include subdeltoid,

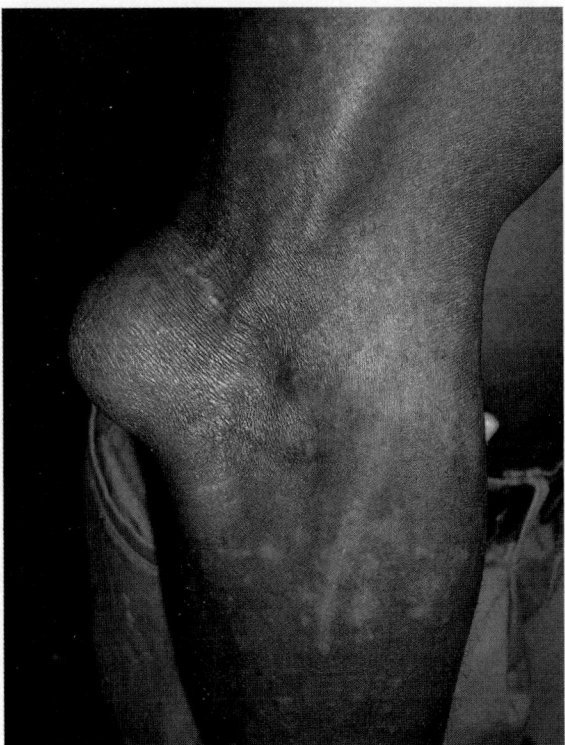

▲ **Figure 41–1.** Chronic aseptic olecranon bursitis without erythema or tenderness. (Used, with permission, from Richard P. Usatine, MD, in Usatine RP, Smith MA, Mayeaux EJ Jr, Chumley H. *The Color Atlas of Family Medicine,* 2nd ed. McGraw-Hill, 2013.)

ischial, trochanteric, and semimembranous-gastrocnemius (Baker cyst) bursae. The bursitis can be septic. Aseptic bursitis is usually afebrile.

▶ Clinical Findings

A. Symptoms and Signs

Bursitis presents with focal tenderness and swelling and is less likely to affect range of motion of the adjacent joint. Olecranon or prepatellar bursitis, for example, causes an oval (or, if chronic, bulbous) swelling at the tip of the elbow or knee and does not affect joint motion. Tenderness, erythema and warmth, cellulitis, a report of trauma, and evidence of a skin lesion are more common in septic bursitis but can be present in aseptic bursitis as well. Patients with septic bursitis can be febrile but the absence of fever does not exclude infection; one-third of those with septic olecranon bursitis are afebrile. A bursa can also become symptomatic when it ruptures. This is particularly true for Baker cyst, the rupture of which can cause calf pain and swelling that mimic thrombophlebitis.

B. Imaging

Imaging is unnecessary unless there is concern for osteomyelitis, trauma, or other underlying pathology. Ruptured

Baker cysts are imaged easily by sonography or MRI. It may be important to exclude a deep venous thrombosis, which can be mimicked by a ruptured Baker cyst.

C. Special Tests

Acute swelling and redness at a bursal site call for aspiration to rule out infection especially if the patient is either febrile (temperature more than 37.8°C) or has prebursal warmth (temperature difference greater than 2.2°C) or both. A bursal fluid white blood cell count of greater than 1000/mcL indicates inflammation from infection, rheumatoid arthritis, or gout. The bursal fluid of septic bursitis characteristically contains a purulent aspirate, fluid-to-serum glucose ratio less than 50%, white cell count more than 3000 cells/mcL, polymorphonuclear cells more than 50%, and a positive Gram stain for bacteria. Most cases are caused by *Staphylococcus aureus*; the Gram stain is positive in two-thirds.

▶ Treatment

Bursitis caused by trauma responds to local heat, rest, NSAIDs, and local corticosteroid injections. Chronic, stable olecranon bursa swelling usually does not require aspiration. Repetitive minor trauma to the olecranon bursa should be eliminated by avoiding resting the elbow on a hard surface or by wearing an elbow pad. For chronic aseptic bursitis or when there are athletic or occupational demands, aspiration with intrabursal steroid injection can be performed. Aspiration of the olecranon bursa runs the risk of creating a chronic drainage site, which can be reduced by using a "zig-zag" approach with a small needle (25-gauge if possible) and pulling the skin over the bursa before introducing it. Applying a pressure bandage may also help prevent chronic drainage. Ultrasound-guided aspiration and injection can improve the accuracy of the procedures. Treatment of a ruptured Baker cyst includes rest, leg elevation, and possibly injection of triamcinolone, 20–40 mg into the knee anteriorly (the knee compartment communicates with the cyst). However, corticosteroid injections in nonseptic bursitis have more complications and skin atrophy than simple symptomatic treatment.

Treatment for septic bursitis involves incision and drainage and antibiotics usually delivered intravenously.

▶ When to Refer

- Surgical removal of the bursa is indicated only for cases in which repeated infections occur.
- Elective removal for persistent symptoms affecting activities of daily living can be considered.

Baumbach SF et al. Prepatellar and olecranon bursitis: literature review and development of a treatment algorithm. Arch Orthop Trauma Surg. 2014 Mar;134(3):359–70. [PMID: 24305696]

Raas C et al. Treatment and outcome with traumatic lesions of the olecranon and prepatellar bursa: a literature review apropos a retrospective analysis including 552 cases. Arch Orthop Trauma Surg. 2017 Jun;137(6):823–7. [PMID: 28447166]

Reilly D et al. Olecranon bursitis. J Shoulder Elbow Surg. 2016 Jan;25(1):158–67. [PMID: 26577126]

HIP

1. Hip Fractures

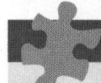

ESSENTIALS OF DIAGNOSIS

► Internal rotation of the hip is the best provocative diagnostic maneuver.

► Hip fractures should be surgically repaired as soon as possible (within 24 hours).

► Delayed treatment of hip fractures in older adults leads to increased complications and mortality.

General Considerations

Approximately 4% of the 7.9 million fractures that occur each year in the United States are hip fractures. There is a high mortality rate among older adult patients following hip fracture, with death occurring in 8–9% within 30 days and in approximately 25–30% within 1 year. Osteoporosis, female sex, height greater than 5-feet 8-inches, and age over 50 years are risk factors for hip fracture. Hip fractures usually occur after a fall. High-velocity trauma is needed in younger patients. Stress fractures can occur in athletes or individuals with poor bone mineral density following repetitive loading activities.

Clinical Findings

A. Symptoms and Signs

Patients typically report pain in the groin, though pain radiating to the lateral hip, buttock, or knee can also commonly occur. If a displaced fracture is present, the patient will not be able to bear weight and the leg may be externally rotated. Gentle logrolling of the leg with the patient supine helps rule out a fracture. Examination of the hip demonstrates pain with deep palpation in the area of the femoral triangle (similar to palpating the femoral artery). Provided the patient can tolerate it, the clinician can, with the patient supine, flex the hip to 90 degrees with the knee flexed to 90 degrees. The leg can then be internally and externally rotated to assess the range of motion on both sides. Pain with internal rotation of the hip is the most sensitive test to identify intra-articular hip pathology. Hip flexion, extension, abduction, and adduction strength can be tested.

Patients with hip stress fractures have less pain on physical examination than described previously but typically have pain with weight bearing. The Trendelenburg test can be performed to examine for weakness or instability of the hip abductors, primarily the gluteus medius muscle; the patient balances first on one leg, raising the non-standing knee toward the chest. The clinician can stand behind the patient and observe for dropping of the pelvis and buttock on the non-stance side. Another functional test is asking the patient to hop or jump during the examination. If the patient has a compatible clinical history of pain and is unable or unwilling to hop, then a stress fracture should be ruled out. The back should be carefully examined in patients with hip complaints, including examining for signs of sciatica.

Following displaced hip fractures, a thorough medical evaluation and treatment should be pursued to maximize the patients' ability to undergo operative intervention. Patients who are unable to get up by themselves may have been immobile for hours or even days following their falls. Thus, clinicians must exclude rhabdomyolysis, hypothermia, deep venous thrombosis, pulmonary embolism, and other conditions that can occur with prolonged immobilization. Delay of operative intervention leads to an increased risk of perioperative morbidity and mortality.

B. Imaging

Useful radiographic views of the hip include AP views of the pelvis and bilateral hips and frog-leg-lateral views of the painful hip. A CT scan or MRI may be necessary to identify the hip fracture pattern or to evaluate non-displaced fractures. Hip fractures are generally described by location, including femoral neck, intertrochanteric, or subtrochanteric.

Treatment

Almost all patients with a hip fracture will require surgery and may need to be admitted to the hospital for pain control while they await surgery. Surgery is recommended within the first 24 hours because studies have shown that delaying surgery 48 hours results in at least twice the rate of major and minor medical complications, including pneumonia, pressure injuries (formerly pressure ulcers), and deep venous thrombosis. High-volume centers have multidisciplinary teams (including orthopedic surgeons, internists, social workers, and specialized physical therapists) to comanage these patients, which improves perioperative medical care and expedites preoperative evaluation leading to reduced costs.

Stress fractures in active patients require a period of protected weight bearing and a gradual return to activities, although it may take 4–6 months before a return to normal activities. Femoral neck fractures are commonly treated with hemiarthroplasty or total hip replacement. This allows the patient to begin weight bearing immediately postoperatively. Peritrochanteric hip fractures are treated with open reduction internal fixation, where plate and screw construct or intramedullary devices are used. The choice of implant will depend on the fracture pattern. Since fracture fixation requires the fracture to proceed to union, the patient may need to have protected weight bearing during the early postoperative period. Dislocation, periprosthetic fracture, and avascular necrosis of the hip are common complications after surgery. Patients should be mobilized as soon as possible postoperatively to avoid pulmonary complications and pressure injuries. Supervised physical therapy and rehabilitation are important for the patient to regain as much function as possible. Unfortunately, most patients following hip fractures will lose some degree of independence. Patients with hip fracture surgery when compared with elective total hip replacement have been shown to have higher risk of in-hospital mortality.

▶ Prevention

Bone density screening can identify patients at risk for osteopenia or osteoporosis, and treatment can be planned accordingly. There is strong evidence that bisphosphonates, denosumab, and teriparatide reduce fractures compared with placebo, with relative risk reductions of 0.60–0.80 for nonvertebral fractures. Nutrition and bone health (bone densitometry, serum calcium and 25-OH vitamin D levels) should be reviewed with the patient (see Chapter 26). However, there is no evidence that increasing calcium intake prevents hip fractures. For patients with decreased mobility, systemic anticoagulation should be considered to avoid deep venous thrombosis (see Table 14–14). Fall prevention exercise programs are available for older adult patients at risk for falls and hip fractures. Hip protectors are uncomfortable and have less use in preventing fractures.

▶ When to Refer

- All patients in whom hip fracture is suspected.
- All patients with hip fracture or in whom the diagnosis is uncertain after radiographs.

Bolland MJ et al. Calcium intake and risk of fracture: systematic review. BMJ. 2015 Sep 29;351:h4580. [PMID: 26420387]

Le Manach Y et al. Outcomes after hip fracture surgery compared with elective total hip replacement. JAMA. 2015 Sep 15;314(11):1159–66. [PMID: 26372585]

Sobolev B et al; Canadian Collaborative Study of Hip Fractures. Mortality effects of timing alternatives for hip fracture surgery. CMAJ. 2018 Aug 7;190(31):E923–32. [PMID: 30087128]

Swart E et al. Dedicated perioperative hip fracture comanagement programs are cost-effective in high-volume centers: an economic analysis. Clin Orthop Relat Res. 2016 Jan;474(1):222–33. [PMID: 26260393]

2. Hip Osteoarthritis

ESSENTIALS OF DIAGNOSIS

- ▶ Pain deep in the groin on the affected side.
- ▶ Swelling.
- ▶ Degeneration of joint cartilage.
- ▶ Loss of active and passive range of motion in severe OA.

▶ General Considerations

In the United States, the prevalence of OA will grow as the number of persons over age 65 years doubles to more than 70 million by 2030. Cartilage loss and OA symptoms are preceded by damage to the collagen-proteoglycan matrix. The etiology of OA is often multifactorial, including previous trauma, prior high-impact activities, genetic factors, obesity, and rheumatologic or metabolic conditions. Femoroacetabular impingement, which affects younger active patients, is considered an early development of hip OA.

▶ Clinical Findings

A. Symptoms and Signs

OA usually causes pain in the affected joint with loading of the joint or at the extremes of motion. Mechanical symptoms—such as swelling, grinding, catching, and locking—suggest internal derangement, which is indicated by damaged cartilage or bone fragments that affect the smooth range of motion expected at an articular joint. Pain can also produce the sensation of "buckling" or "giving way" due to muscle inhibition. As the joint degeneration becomes more advanced, the patient loses active range of motion and may lose passive range of motion as well.

Patients complain of pain deep in the groin on the affected side and have problems with weight-bearing activities such as walking, climbing stairs, and getting up from a chair. They may limp and develop a lurch during their gait, leaning toward the unaffected side as they walk to reduce pressure on the arthritic hip.

B. Imaging

An anterior-posterior weight-bearing radiograph of the pelvis with a lateral view of the symptomatic hip are preferred views for evaluation of hip OA. Joint space narrowing and sclerosis suggest early OA, while osteophytes near the femoral head or acetabulum and subchondral bone cysts are more advanced changes. However, not all patients with radiographic hip OA have hip or groin pain; the converse is also true. Radiographs have low sensitivity for hip pain (sensitivity 36.7%, specificity 90.5%, positive predictive value 6.0%, and negative predictive value 98.9%). Findings of femoroacetabular impingement are commonly reported on radiograph reports with arthritic changes and anatomic variations involving the acetabulum and femoral head neck junction. After age 35, MRI of the hips already show labral changes in almost 70% of asymptomatic patients.

▶ Treatment

A. Conservative

Changes in the articular cartilage are irreversible. Therefore, a cure for the diseased joint is not possible, although symptoms or structural issues can be managed to try to maintain activity level. Conservative treatment for patients with OA includes activity modification, proper footwear, therapeutic exercises, weight loss, and use of assistive devices (such as a cane). A 2014 randomized study found that physical therapy did not lead to greater improvement in pain or function compared with sham treatment in patients with hip OA. Analgesics may be effective in some cases. Corticosteroid injections can be considered for short-term relief of pain; however, hip injections are best performed under fluoroscopic, ultrasound, or CT guidance to ensure accurate injection in the joint.

B. Surgical

Joint replacement surgeries are effective and cost-effective for patients with significant symptoms and functional limitations, providing improvements in pain, function, and quality of life. Various surgical techniques and computer-assisted navigation during operation continue to be investigated. A review of nine randomized controlled trials concluded that a direct anterior approach for hip replacement was associated with a shorter incision, lower blood loss, lower pain scores, and earlier functional recovery. However, there was no significant difference in complication rates between groups for the direct anterior or posterior approaches.

Hip resurfacing surgery is a newer joint replacement technique. Rather than use a traditional artificial joint implant of the whole neck and femur, only the femoral head is removed and replaced. Evidence to date suggests that hip resurfacing is comparable to total hip replacement and is a viable alternative for younger patients. The cumulative survival rate of this implant at 10 years is estimated to be 94%. Concerns following resurfacing surgery include the risk of femoral neck fracture and collapse of the head. In a systematic review of national databases, the average time to revision was 3.0 years for metal-on-metal hip resurfacing versus 7.8 years for total hip arthroplasty. Dislocations were more frequent with total hip arthroplasty than metal-on-metal hip resurfacing: 4.4 vs 0.9 per 1000 person-years, respectively.

Guidelines recommend prophylaxis for venous thromboembolic disease for a minimum of 14 days after arthroplasty of the hip or knee using warfarin, low-molecular-weight heparin, fondaparinux, aspirin, rivaroxaban, dabigatran, apixaban, or portable mechanical compression (see Table 14–14).

▶ When to Refer

Patients with sufficient disability, limited benefit from conservative therapy, and evidence of severe OA can be referred for joint replacement surgery.

Kim C et al. Association of hip pain with radiographic evidence of hip osteoarthritis: diagnostic test study. BMJ. 2015 Dec 2;351:h5983. [PMID: 26631296]

Nwachukwu BU et al. Arthroscopic versus open treatment of femoroacetabular impingement: a systematic review of medium- to long-term outcomes. Am J Sports Med. 2016 Apr;44(4):1062–8. [PMID: 26059179]

Wang Z et al. A systematic review and meta-analysis of direct anterior approach versus posterior approach in total hip arthroplasty. J Orthop Surg Res. 2018 Sep 6;13(1):229. [PMID: 30189881]

KNEE

1. Knee Pain

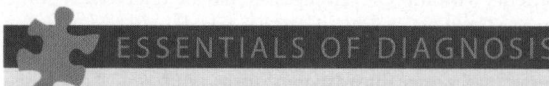

ESSENTIALS OF DIAGNOSIS

▶ Effusion can occur with intra-articular pathology (eg, OA, meniscus and cruciate ligament tears).

▶ Acute knee swelling (due to hemarthrosis) within 2 hours may indicate ligament injuries or patellar dislocation or fracture.

▶ General Considerations

The knee is the largest joint in the body and is susceptible to injury from trauma, inflammation, infection, and degenerative changes. The knee is a hinge joint. The joint line exists between the femoral condyles and tibial plateaus. Separating and cushioning these bony surfaces is the lateral and medial meniscal cartilage, which functions as a shock absorber during weight bearing, protecting the articular cartilage. The patella is a large sesamoid bone anterior to the joint. It is embedded in the quadriceps tendon, and it articulates with the trochlear groove of the femur. Poor patellar tracking in the trochlear groove is a common source of knee pain especially when the cause is atraumatic in nature. The knee is stabilized by the collateral ligaments against varus (lateral collateral ligament) and valgus (medial collateral ligament) stresses. The tibia is limited in its anterior movement by the anterior cruciate ligament (ACL) and in its posterior movement by the posterior cruciate ligament (PCL). The bursae of the knee are located between the skin and bony prominences. They act to decrease friction of tendons and muscles as they move over adjacent bony structures. Excessive external pressure or friction can lead to swelling and pain of the bursae. The prepatellar bursae (located between the skin and patella) and the pes anserine bursa (which is medial and inferior to the patella, just below the tibial plateau) are most commonly affected. Joint fluid, when excessive due to synovitis or trauma, can track posteriorly through a potential space, resulting in a popliteal cyst (also called a Baker cyst). Other structures that are susceptible to overuse injury and may cause knee pain following repetitive activity include the patellofemoral joint and the iliotibial band. OA of the knees is common after 50 years of age and can develop due to previous trauma, aging, activities, alignment issues, and genetic predisposition.

▶ Clinical Findings

A. Symptoms and Signs

Evaluation of knee pain should begin with general questions regarding duration and rapidity of symptom onset and the mechanism of injury or aggravating symptoms. Overuse or degenerative problems can occur with stress or compression from sports, hobbies, or occupation. A history of trauma, previous orthopedic problems with, or surgery to, the affected knee should also be specifically queried. Symptoms of infection (fever, recent bacterial infections, risk factors for sexually transmitted infections [such as gonorrhea] or other bacterial infections [such as staphylococcal infection]) should always be elicited.

Common symptom complaints include the following:

1. Presence of grinding, clicking, or popping with bending may be indicative of OA or the patellofemoral syndrome.
2. "Locking" or "catching" when walking suggests an internal derangement, such as meniscal injury or a loose body in the knee.

3. Intra-articular swelling of the knee or an effusion indicates an internal derangement or a synovial pathology. Large swelling may cause a popliteal (Baker) cyst. Acute swelling within minutes to hours suggests a hemarthrosis, most likely due to an ACL injury, fracture, or patellar dislocation, especially if trauma is involved.

4. Lateral "snapping" with flexion and extension of the knee may indicate inflammation of the iliotibial band.

5. Pain that is worsened with bending and walking downstairs suggests issues with the patellofemoral joint, usually degenerative such as chondromalacia of the patella or OA.

6. Pain that occurs when rising after prolonged sitting suggests a problem with tracking of the patella.

A careful history coupled with a physical examination that includes observation, palpation, and range of motion testing, as well as specific tests for particular anatomic structures is frequently sufficient to establish a diagnosis. When there is a knee joint effusion caused by increased fluid in the intra-articular space, physical examination will demonstrate swelling in the hollow or dimple around the patella and distention of the suprapatellar space.

Table 41–5 shows the differential diagnosis of knee pain, and Table 41–6 outlines possible diagnoses based on the location of pain.

B. Laboratory Findings

Laboratory testing of aspirated joint fluid, when indicated, can lead to a definitive diagnosis in most patients (see Tables 20–2 and 20–3).

C. Imaging

Knee pain is evaluated with plain (weight-bearing) radiographs and MRI most commonly, but CT and ultrasound are sometimes useful.

An acute hemarthrosis represents bloody swelling that usually occurs within the first 1–2 hours following trauma. In situations where the trauma may be activity-related and not a result of a fall or collision, the differential diagnosis most commonly includes ACL tear (responsible for more than

Table 41–5. Differential diagnosis of knee pain.

Mechanical dysfunction or disruption
Internal derangement of the knee: injury to the menisci or ligaments
Degenerative changes caused by osteoarthritis
Dynamic dysfunction or misalignment of the patella
Fracture as a result of trauma
Intra-articular inflammation or increased pressure
Internal derangement of the knee: injury to the menisci or ligaments
Inflammation or infection of the knee joint
Ruptured popliteal (Baker) cyst
Peri-articular inflammation
Internal derangement of the knee: injury to the menisci or ligaments
Prepatellar or anserine bursitis
Ligamentous sprain

Table 41–6. Location of common causes of knee pain.

Medial knee pain
Medial compartment osteoarthritis
Medial collateral ligament strain
Medial meniscal injury
Anserine bursitis (pain over the proximal medial tibial plateau)
Anterior knee pain
Patellofemoral syndrome (often bilateral)
Osteoarthritis
Prepatellar bursitis (associated with swelling anterior to the patella)
"Jumper's knee" (pain at the inferior pole of the patella)
Septic arthritis
Gout or other inflammatory disorder
Lateral knee pain
Lateral meniscal injury
Iliotibial band syndrome (pain superficially along the distal iliotibial band near lateral femoral condyle or lateral tibial insertion)
Lateral collateral ligament sprain (rare)
Posterior knee pain
Popliteal (Baker) cyst
Osteoarthritis
Meniscal tears
Hamstring or calf tendinopathy

70% in adults), fracture (patella, tibial plateau, femoral supracondylar, growth plate [physeal]), and patellar dislocation. Meniscal tears are unlikely to cause large hemarthrosis.

2. Anterior Cruciate Ligament Injury

 ESSENTIALS OF DIAGNOSIS

▶ An injury involving an audible pop when the knee buckles.

▶ Acute swelling immediately (or within 2 hours).

▶ Instability occurs with lateral movement activities and going down stairs.

▶ General Considerations

The anterior cruciate ligament (ACL) connects the posterior aspect of the lateral femoral condyle to the anterior aspect of the tibia. Its main function is to control anterior translation of the tibia on the femur. It also provides rotational stability of the tibia on the femur. ACL tears are common with sporting injuries. They can result from both contact (valgus blow to the knee) and non-contact (jumping, pivoting, and deceleration) activities. The patient usually falls down following the injury, has acute swelling and difficulty with weight bearing and complains of instability. ACL injuries are common in skiing, soccer, football, and basketball among young adolescents and middle-aged patients. Prepubertal and older patients usually sustain fractures instead of ligamentous injuries.

Clinical Findings

A. Symptoms and Signs

Acute ACL injuries usually lead to acute swelling of the knee, causing difficulty with motion. After the swelling has resolved, the patient can walk with a "stiff-knee" gait or quadriceps avoidance gait because of the instability.

Patients describe symptoms of instability while performing side-to-side maneuvers or descending stairs. Stability tests assess the amount of laxity of the knee while performing these maneuvers. The Lachman test (84–87% sensitivity and 93% specificity) is performed with the patient lying supine and the knee flexed to 20–30 degrees (Table 41–7). The clinician grasps the distal femur from

Table 41–7. Knee examination.

Maneuver	Description
Inspection	Examine for the alignment of the lower extremities (varus, valgus, knee recurvatum), ankle eversion and foot pronation, gait, SEADS.
Palpation	Include important landmarks: patellofemoral joint, medial and lateral joint lines (especially posterior aspects), pes anserine bursa, distal iliotibial band and Gerdy tubercle (iliotibial band insertion).
Range of motion testing	Check range of motion actively (patient performs) and passively (clinician performs), especially with flexion and extension of the knee normally 0–10 degrees of extension and 120–150 degrees of flexion.
Knee strength testing	Test resisted knee extension and knee flexion strength manually.
Ligament Stress Testing	
Lachman test	Performed with the patient lying supine, and the knee flexed to 20–30 degrees. The examiner grasps the distal femur from the lateral side, and the proximal tibia with the other hand on the medial side. With the knee in neutral position, stabilize the femur, and pull the tibia anteriorly using a similar force to lifting a 10–15 pound weight. Excessive anterior translation of the tibia compared with the other side indicates injury to the anterior cruciate ligament.
Anterior drawer	Performed with the patient lying supine and the knee flexed to 90 degrees. The clinician stabilizes the patient's foot by sitting on it and grasps the proximal tibia with both hands around the calf and pulls anteriorly. A positive test finds anterior cruciate ligament laxity compared with the unaffected side.

(continued)

Table 41–7. Knee examination. (continued)

Maneuver	Description
Valgus stress 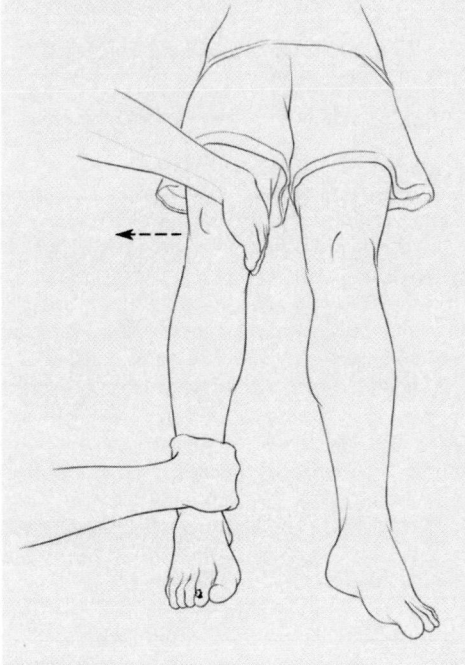 Fix ankle	Performed with the patient supine. The clinician should stand on the outside of the patient's knee. With one hand, the clinician should hold the ankle while the other hand is supporting the leg at the level of the knee joint. A valgus stress is applied at the ankle to determine pain and laxity of the medial collateral ligament. The test should be performed at both 30 degrees and 0 degrees of knee extension.
Varus stress	The patient is again placed supine. For the right knee, the clinician should be standing on the right side of the patient. The left hand of the examiner should be holding the ankle while the right hand is supporting the lateral thigh. A varus stress is applied at the ankle to determine pain and laxity of the lateral collateral ligament. The test should be performed at both 30 degrees and 0 degrees of knee flexion.

(continued)

Table 41–7. Knee examination. (continued)

Maneuver	Description
Meniscal Signs	
McMurray test	Performed with the patient lying supine. The clinician flexes the knee until the patient reports pain. For this test to be valid, it must be flexed pain-free beyond 90 degrees. The clinician externally rotates the patient's foot and then extends the knee while palpating the medial knee for "click" in the medial compartment of the knee or pain reproducing pain from a meniscus injury. To test the lateral meniscus, the same maneuver is repeated while rotating the foot internally (53% sensitivity and 59–97% specificity).
Modified McMurray 	Performed with the hip flexed to 90 degrees. The knee is then flexed maximally with internal or external rotation of the lower leg. The knee can then be rotated with the lower leg in internal or external rotation to capture the torn meniscus underneath the condyles. A positive test is pain over the joint line while the knee is being flexed and internally or externally rotated.

(continued)

Table 41–7. Knee examination. (continued)

Maneuver	Description
Thessaly test 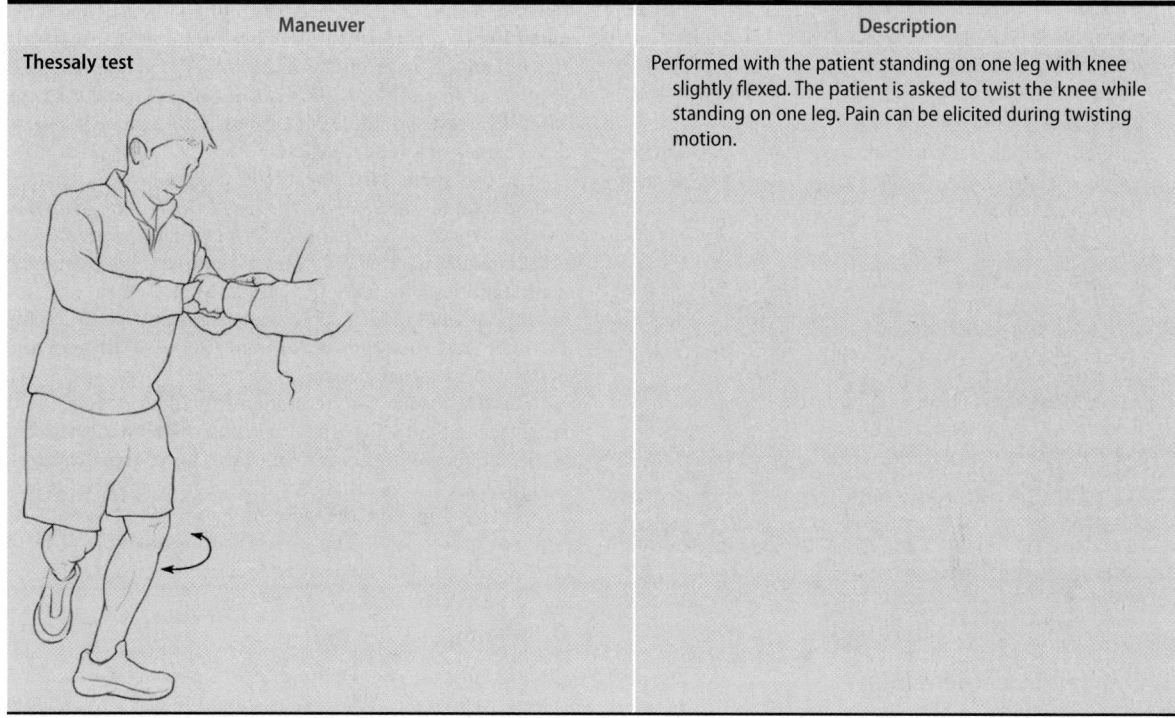	Performed with the patient standing on one leg with knee slightly flexed. The patient is asked to twist the knee while standing on one leg. Pain can be elicited during twisting motion.

SEADS, swelling, erythema, atrophy, deformity, and (surgical) scars.

the lateral side and the proximal tibia with the other hand on the medial side. With the knee in neutral position, stabilize the femur, and pull the tibia anteriorly using a similar force to lifting a 10- to 15-pound weight. Excessive anterior translation of the tibia compared with the other side indicates injury to the ACL. The anterior drawer test (48% sensitivity and 87% specificity) is performed with the patient lying supine and the knee flexed to 90 degrees (Table 41–7). The clinician stabilizes the patient's foot by sitting on it and grasps the proximal tibia with both hands around the calf and pulls anteriorly. A positive test finds ACL laxity compared with the unaffected side. The pivot shift test is used to determine the amount of rotational laxity of the knee. The patient is examined while lying supine with the knee in full extension. It is then slowly flexed while applying internal rotation and a valgus stress. The clinician feels for a subluxation at 20–40 degrees of knee flexion. The patient must remain very relaxed to have a positive test.

B. Imaging

Plain radiographs are usually negative in ACL tears but are useful to rule out fractures. A small avulsion injury can sometimes be seen over the lateral compartment of the knee ("Segond" fracture) and is pathognomonic of an ACL injury. An ACL injury that avulsed the tibial spine can be seen in radiographs. MRI is the best tool to diagnose ACL tears and associated articular and meniscal cartilage issues. It has greater than 95% sensitivity and specificity for ACL tears.

▶ Treatment

Most young and active patients will require surgical reconstruction of the ACL. Some data suggest that reconstruction within 5 months of the tear has better outcomes. However, a small randomized trial suggested that acute ACL injuries can be treated nonoperatively and delayed ACL reconstruction had similar outcomes to acute ACL reconstructions but patients for whom the reconstruction is delayed have more cartilage or meniscus problems at the time of surgery. Common surgical techniques use the patient's own tissue, usually the patellar or hamstring tendons (autograft) or a cadaver graft (allograft) to arthroscopically reconstruct the torn ACL. Different patient groups experienced improved results with specific surgical graft choices. However, allografts do have a higher failure rate when compared with autografts. Recovery from surgery usually requires 6 months.

Nonoperative treatments are usually reserved for older patients or those with a very sedentary lifestyle. Physical therapy can focus on hamstring strengthening and core stability. An ACL brace can help stability. Longitudinal studies have demonstrated that nonoperative management of an ACL tear can lead to a higher incidence of meniscus tears. Cost-analysis studies have shown that early ACL reconstruction can be more beneficial than nonoperative treatment and delayed subsequent surgeries.

When to Refer

- Almost all ACL tears should be referred to an orthopedic surgeon for evaluation.
- Individuals with instability in the setting of a chronic ACL tear (greater than 6 months) should be considered for surgical reconstruction.
- Patients with an ACL tear and associated meniscus or articular injuries may benefit from surgery to address the other injuries.

Kaeding CC et al. Risk factors and predictors of subsequent ACL injury in either knee after ACL reconstruction: prospective analysis of 2488 primary ACL reconstructions from the Moon Cohort. Am J Sports Med. 2015 Jul;43(7):1583–90. [PMID: 25899429]

Saltzman BM et al. Economic analyses in anterior cruciate ligament reconstruction: a qualitative and systematic review. Am J Sports Med. 2016 May;44(5):1329–35. [PMID: 25930672]

Sanders JO et al. Treatment of anterior cruciate ligament injuries. J Am Acad Orthop Surg. 2016 Aug;24(8):e81–3. [PMID: 27355285]

Shea KG et al. The American Academy of Orthopaedic Surgeons evidence-based guideline on management of anterior cruciate ligament injuries. J Bone Joint Surg Am. 2015 Apr 15;97(8):672–4. [PMID: 25878313]

3. Collateral Ligament Injury

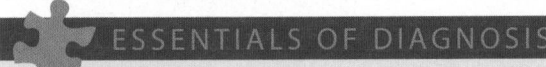

ESSENTIALS OF DIAGNOSIS

- ▶ Caused by a valgus or varus blow or stress to the knee.
- ▶ Pain and instability in the affected area.
- ▶ Limited range of motion.

General Considerations

The medial collateral ligament (MCL) is the most commonly injured ligament in the knee. It is usually injured with a valgus stress to the partially flexed knee. It can also occur with a blow to the lateral leg. The MCL is commonly injured with acute ACL injuries. The lateral collateral ligament (LCL) is less commonly injured, but this can occur with a medial blow to the knee. Since both collateral ligaments are extra-articular, injuries to these ligaments may not lead to any intra-articular effusion. Affected patients may have difficulty walking initially, but this can improve when the swelling decreases.

Clinical Findings

A. Symptoms and Signs

The main clinical findings for patients with collateral ligament injuries are pain along the course of the ligaments. The patient may have limited range of motion due to pain, especially during the first 2 weeks following the injury. The best tests to assess the collateral ligaments are the varus and valgus stress tests. The sensitivity of the tests is as high as 86–96%.

The **valgus stress test** is performed with the patient supine (Table 41–7). The clinician should stand on the outside of the patient's knee. With one hand, the clinician should hold the ankle while the other hand is supporting the leg at the level of the knee joint. A valgus stress is applied at the ankle to determine pain and laxity of the MCL. The test should be performed at both 30 degrees and at 0 degrees of knee extension.

For the **varus stress test**, the patient is again placed supine (Table 41–7). For the right knee, the clinician should be standing on the right side of the patient. The clinician's left hand should be holding the ankle while the right hand is supporting the lateral thigh. A varus stress is applied at the ankle to determine pain and laxity of the LCL. The test should be performed at both 30 degrees and at 0 degrees of knee flexion.

The test results can be graded from 1 to 3. Grade 1 is when the patient has pain with varus/valgus stress test but no instability. With grade 2 injuries, the patient has pain, and the knee shows instability at 30 degrees of knee flexion. In grade 3 injuries, the patient has marked instability but not much pain. The knee is often unstable at both 30 degrees and 0 degrees of knee flexion.

B. Imaging

Radiographs are usually nondiagnostic except for avulsion injuries. However, radiographs should be used to rule out fractures that can occur with collateral ligament injuries. Isolated MCL injuries usually do not require evaluation by MRI, but MRI should be used to evaluate possible associated cruciate ligament injuries. LCL or posterolateral corner injuries should have MRI evaluation to exclude associated injuries and to determine their significance.

Treatment

The majority of MCL injuries can be treated with protected weight bearing and physical therapy. For grade 1 and 2 injuries, the patient can usually bear weight as tolerated with full range of motion. A hinged knee brace can be given to patients with grade 2 MCL tears to provide stability. Early physical therapy is recommended to protect range of motion and muscle strength. Grade 3 MCL injuries require long leg braces to provide stability. Patients can weight-bear, but only with the knee locked in extension with a brace. The motion can then be increased with the brace unlocked. Grade 3 injuries can take up to 6–8 weeks to heal. MCL injuries rarely need surgery. LCL injuries are less common but are usually associated with other ligament injuries (such as ACL and PCL). LCL injuries do not recover well with nonoperative treatment and usually require urgent surgical repair or reconstruction.

When to Refer

- Symptomatic instability with chronic MCL tears or acute MCL tears with other ligamentous injuries.
- LCL or posterolateral corner injuries require urgent surgical repair or reconstruction (within 1 week).

Devitt BM et al. Physical examination and imaging of the lateral collateral ligament and posterolateral corner of the knee. Sports Med Arthrosc Rev. 2015 Mar;23(1):10–6. [PMID: 25545645]

Porrino J et al. An update and comprehensive review of the posterolateral corner of the knee. Radiol Clin North Am. 2018 Nov;56(6):935–51. [PMID: 30322491]

Shon OJ et al. Current concepts of posterolateral corner injuries of the knee. Knee Surg Relat Res. 2017 Dec 1;29(4):256–68. [PMID: 29172386]

4. Posterior Cruciate Ligament Injury

ESSENTIALS OF DIAGNOSIS

► Usually follows an anterior trauma to the tibia, such as a dashboard injury during a motor vehicle accident.

► The knee may freely dislocate and reduce.

► One-third of multi-ligament injuries involving the PCL have neurovascular injuries.

General Considerations

The posterior cruciate ligament (PCL) is the strongest ligament in the knee. PCL injuries usually represent significant trauma and are highly associated with multi-ligament injuries and knee dislocations. More than 70–90% of PCL injuries have associated injuries to the posterolateral corner, MCL, and ACL. Neurovascular injuries occur in up to one-third of all knee dislocations or PCL injuries. There should be high suspicion for neurovascular injuries and a thorough neurovascular examination of the limb should be performed.

Clinical Findings

A. Symptoms and Signs

Most patients with acute injuries have difficulty with ambulation. Patients with chronic PCL injuries can ambulate without gross instability but may complain of subjective "looseness" and often report pain and dysfunction, especially with bending. Clinical examinations of PCL injuries include the "sag sign"; the patient is placed supine and both hips and knees are flexed to 90 degrees. Because of gravity, the posterior cruciate ligament-injured knee will have an obvious set-off at the anterior tibia that is "sagging" posteriorly. The PCL ligament can also be examined using the **posterior drawer test;** the patient is placed supine with the knee flexed to 90 degrees. In a normal knee, the anterior tibia should be positioned about 10 mm anterior to the femoral condyle. The clinician can grasp the proximal tibia with both hands and push the tibia posteriorly. The movement, indicating laxity and possible tear of the PCL, is compared with the uninjured knee (90% sensitivity and 99% specificity). A PCL injury is sometimes mistaken for an ACL injury during the anterior drawer test since the tibia is subluxed posteriorly in a sagged position and can be abnormally translated forward, yielding a false-positive test

for an ACL injury. Pain, swelling, pallor, and numbness in the affected extremity may suggest a knee dislocation with possible injury to the popliteal artery.

B. Imaging

Radiographs are often nondiagnostic but are required to diagnose any fractures. MRI is used to diagnose PCL and other associated injuries.

Treatment

Isolated PCL injuries can be treated nonoperatively. Acute injuries are usually immobilized using a knee brace with the knee extension; the patient uses crutches for ambulation. Physical therapy can help achieve increased range of motion and improved ambulation. Many PCL injuries are associated with other injuries and may require operative reconstruction.

When to Refer

• The patient should be seen urgently within 1–2 weeks.

• If the lateral knee is also unstable with varus stress testing, the patient should be assessed for a posterolateral corner injury, which may require an urgent surgical reconstruction.

• Isolated PCL tears may require surgery if the tear is complete (grade 3) and the patient is symptomatic.

Badri A et al. Clinical and radiologic evaluation of the posterior cruciate ligament-injured knee. Curr Rev Musculoskelet Med. 2018 Sep;11(3):515–20. [PMID: 29987531]

Bedi A et al. Management of posterior cruciate ligament injuries: an evidence-based review. J Am Acad Orthop Surg. 2016 May;24(5):277–89. [PMID: 27097125]

LaPrade CM et al. Emerging updates on the posterior cruciate ligament: a review of the current literature. Am J Sports Med. 2015 Dec;43(12):3077–92. [PMID: 25776184]

5. Meniscus Injuries

ESSENTIALS OF DIAGNOSIS

► Patient may or may not report an injury.

► Joint line pain and pain with deep squatting are the most sensitive signs.

► Difficulty with knee extension suggests an internal derangement that should be evaluated urgently with MRI.

General Considerations

The menisci act as shock absorbers within the knee. Injuries to a meniscus can lead to pain, clicking, and locking sensation. Most meniscus injuries occur with acute injuries (usually in younger patients) or repeated microtrauma, such as squatting or twisting (usually in older patients).

Clinical Findings

A. Symptoms and Signs

The patient may have an antalgic (painful) gait and difficulty with squatting. He or she may complain of catching or locking of the meniscal fragment. Physical findings can include effusion or joint line tenderness. Patients can usually point out the area of maximal tenderness along the joint line. Swelling usually occurs during the first 24 hours after the injury or later. Meniscus tears rarely lead to the immediate swelling that is commonly seen with fractures and ligament tears. Meniscus tears are commonly seen in arthritic knees. However, it is often unclear whether the pain is coming from the meniscus tear or the arthritis.

Provocative tests, including the **McMurray test,** the **modified McMurray test**, and the **Thessaly test**, can be performed to confirm the diagnosis (Table 41–7). Most symptomatic meniscus tears cause pain with deep squatting and when waddling (performing a "duck walk").

B. Imaging

Radiographs are usually normal but may show joint space narrowing, early OA changes, or loose bodies. MRI of the knee is the best diagnostic tool for meniscal injuries (93% sensitivity and 95% specificity). High signal through the meniscus (bright on T2 images) represents a meniscal tear.

Treatment

Conservative treatment can be used for degenerative tears in older patients. The treatment is similar for patients with mild knee OA, including analgesics and physical therapy for strengthening and core stability. A randomized controlled trial showed that physical therapy compared to arthrosopic partial meniscectomy had similar outcomes at 6 months. However, 30% of the patients who were assigned to physical therapy alone underwent surgery within 6 months.

Randomized studies have shown that arthroscopic surgery has no benefit over sham operations in patients who have degenerative meniscal tears, especially with imaging showing signs of osteoarthritis. Another randomized controlled trial found that patients with degenerative meniscus tears but no signs of arthritis on imaging treated conservatively with supervised exercise therapy had similar outcomes to those treated with arthroscopy at 2 year follow up. There is crossover between the groups; patients can be treated with supervised exercise therapy first, and if they do not respond to nonoperative treatment, they can undergo meniscus surgeries. Acute tears in young and active patients with clinical signs of internal derangement (catching and swelling) and without signs of arthritis on imaging or patients with acute mechanical locking with a displaced meniscus can be best treated arthroscopically with meniscus repair or debridement. There is also growing evidence that untreated meniscus root tears can lead to accelerated osteoarthritic changes. Surgical treatment before cartilage breakdown is recommended for acute meniscus root injuries.

When to Refer

- If the patient has symptoms of internal derangement suspected as meniscus injury. The patient should receive an MRI to confirm the injury.
- If the patient cannot extend the knee due to a mechanical block, the patient should be evaluated as soon as possible. Certain shaped tears on MRI, such as bucket handle tears, are amenable to meniscal repair surgery.
- If the patient has not responded to physical therapy and nonoperative treatment and continues to have symptoms related to the torn meniscus.
- If the patient has MRI confirmation of acute meniscus root injuries.

Driban JB et al. Accelerated knee osteoarthritis is characterized by destabilizing meniscal tears and pre-radiographic structural disease burden. Arthritis Rheumatology. 2018 Dec 28. [Epub ahead of print] [PMID: 30592385]

Kise NJ et al. Exercise therapy versus arthroscopic partial meniscectomy for degenerative meniscal tear in middle aged patients: randomised controlled trial with two year follow-up. BMJ. 2016 Jul 20;354:i3740. [PMID: 27440192]

Mutsaerts EL et al. Surgical interventions for meniscal tears: a closer look at the evidence. Arch Orthop Trauma Surg. 2016 Mar;136(3):361–70. [PMID: 26497982]

Pache S et al. Meniscal root tears: current concepts review. Arch Bone Jt Surg. 2018 Jul;6(4):250–9. [PMID: 30175171]

6. Patellofemoral Pain

> ### ESSENTIALS OF DIAGNOSIS
>
> ► Pain experienced with bending activities (kneeling, squatting, climbing stairs).
> ► Lateral deviation or tilting of the patella in relation to the femoral groove.

General Considerations

Patellofemoral pain, also known as anterior knee pain, chondromalacia, or "runner's knee," describes any pain involving the patellofemoral joint. The pain affects any or all of the anterior knee structures, including the medial and lateral aspects of the patella as well as the quadriceps and patellar tendon insertions. The patella engages the femoral trochlear groove with approximately 30 degrees of knee flexion. Forces on the patellofemoral joint increase up to three times body weight as the knee flexes to 90 degrees (eg, climbing stairs), and five times body weight when going into full knee flexion (eg, squatting). Abnormal patellar tracking during flexion can lead to abnormal articular cartilage wear and pain. When the patient has ligamentous hyperlaxity, the patella can sublux out of the groove, usually laterally. Patellofemoral pain is also associated with muscle strength and flexibility imbalances as well as altered hip and ankle biomechanics.

▶ Clinical Findings

A. Symptoms and Signs

Patients usually complain of pain in the anterior knee with bending movements and less commonly in full extension. Pain from this condition is localized under the kneecap but can sometimes be referred to the posterior knee or over the medial or lateral inferior patella. Symptoms may begin after a trauma or after repetitive physical activity, such as running and jumping. When maltracking, palpable and sometimes audible crepitus can occur.

Intra-articular swelling usually does not occur unless there are articular cartilage defects or if OA changes develop. On physical examination, it is important to palpate the articular surfaces of the patella. For example, the clinician can use one hand to move the patella laterally, and use the fingertips of the other hand to palpate the lateral undersurface of patella. Patellar mobility can be assessed by medially and laterally deviating the patella (deviation by one-quarter of the diameter of the kneecap is consider normal; greater than one-half the diameter suggests excessive mobility). The **apprehension sign** suggests instability of the patellofemoral joint and is positive when the patient becomes apprehensive when the patella is deviated laterally. The **patellar grind test** is performed by grasping the knee superior to the patella and pushing it downward with the patient supine and the knee extended, pushing the patella inferiorly. The patient is asked to contract the quadriceps muscle to oppose this downward translation, with reproduction of pain or grinding being the positive sign for chondromalacia of the patella. There are two common presentations: (1) patients whose ligaments and patella are too loose (hypermobility); and (2) patients who have soft tissues that are too tight, leading to excessive pressure on the joint.

Evaluation of the quadriceps strength and hip stabilizers can be accomplished by having the patient perform a one-leg squat without support. Patients who are weak may display poor balance, with dropping of the pelvis (similar to a positive hip Trendelenburg sign) or excessive internal rotation of the knee medially. Normally, with a one-leg squat, the knee should align over the second metatarsal ray of the foot.

B. Imaging

Diagnostic imaging has limited use in younger patients and is more helpful in older patients to assess for OA or to evaluate patients who do not respond to conservative treatment. Radiographs may show lateral deviation or tilting of the patella in relation to the femoral groove. MRI may show thinning of the articular cartilage but is not clinically necessary, except prior to surgery or to exclude other pathology.

▶ Treatment

A. Conservative

For symptomatic relief, use of local modalities such as ice and anti-inflammatory medications can be beneficial. If the patient has signs of patellar hypermobility, physical therapy exercises are useful to strengthen the quadriceps (especially the vastus medialis obliquus muscle) to help stabilize the patella and improve tracking. There is consistent evidence that exercise therapy for patellofemoral pain syndrome may result in clinically important reduction in pain and improvement in functional ability. Lower quality research supports that hip and knee exercises are better than knee exercises alone. Strengthening the quadriceps and the posterolateral hip muscles such as the hip abductors that control rotation at the knee should be recommended. Support for the patellofemoral joint can be provided by use of a patellar stabilizer brace or special taping techniques (McConnell taping). Correcting lower extremity alignment (with appropriate footwear or over-the-counter orthotics) can help improve symptoms, especially if the patient has pronation or high-arched feet. If the patient demonstrates tight peripatellar soft tissues, special focus should be put on stretching the hamstrings, iliotibial band, quadriceps, calves, and hip flexors.

B. Surgical

Surgery is rarely needed and is considered a last resort for patellofemoral pain. Procedures performed include lateral release or patellar realignment surgery.

▶ When to Refer

Patients with persistent symptoms despite a course of conservative therapy.

Bolgla LA et al. National Athletic Trainers' Association Position Statement: management of individuals with patellofemoral pain. J Athl Train. 2018 Sep;53(9):820–36. [PMID: 30372640]

Neal BS et al. Risk factors for patellofemoral pain: a systematic review and meta-analysis. Br J Sports Med. 2019 Mar;53(5): 270–81. [PMID: 30242107]

Saltychev M et al. Effectiveness of conservative treatment for patellofemoral pain syndrome: a systematic review and meta-analysis. J Rehabil Med. 2018 May 8;50(5):393–401. [PMID: 29392329]

van der Heijden RA et al. Exercise for treating patellofemoral pain syndrome. Cochrane Database Syst Rev. 2015 Jan 20;1: CD010387. [PMID: 25603546]

7. Knee Osteoarthritis

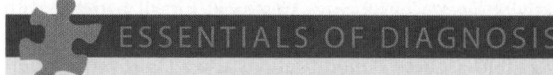

ESSENTIALS OF DIAGNOSIS

▶ Degeneration of joint cartilage.

▶ Pain with bending or twisting activities.

▶ Swelling.

▶ Loss of active and passive range of motion in severe OA.

▶ General Considerations

In the United States, the prevalence of OA will grow as the number of persons over age 65 years doubles to more than

70 million by 2030. The incidence of knee OA in the United States is 240 per 100,000 person-years.

Cartilage loss and OA symptoms are preceded by damage to the collagen-proteoglycan matrix. The etiology of OA is often multifactorial including previous trauma, prior high-impact activities, genetic factors, obesity, and rheumatologic or metabolic conditions.

Clinical Findings

A. Symptoms and Signs

OA usually causes pain in the affected joint with loading of the joint or at the extremes of motion. Mechanical symptoms—such as swelling, grinding, catching, and locking—suggest internal derangement, which is indicated by damaged cartilage or bone fragments that affect the smooth range of motion expected at an articular joint. Pain can also produce the sensation of "buckling" or "giving way" due to muscle inhibition. As the joint degeneration becomes more advanced, the patient loses active range of motion and may lose passive range of motion as well.

As the condition worsens, patients with knee OA have an increasingly limited ability to walk. Symptoms include pain with bending or twisting activities, and going up and down stairs. Swelling, limping, and pain while sleeping are common complaints with OA, especially as it progresses.

B. Imaging

The most commonly recommended radiographs include bilateral weight-bearing 45-degree bent knee posteroanterior, lateral, and patellofemoral joint views (Merchant view). Radiographic findings include diminished width of the articular cartilage causing joint space narrowing, subchondral sclerosis, presence of osteophytes, and cystic changes in the subchondral bone. MRI of the knee is most likely unnecessary unless other pathology is suspected, including ischemic osteonecrosis of the knee.

Treatment

A. Conservative

Changes in the articular cartilage are irreversible. Therefore, a cure for the diseased joint is not possible, although symptoms or structural issues can be addressed to try to maintain activity level. Conservative treatment for all patients with OA includes activity modification, therapeutic exercises, and weight loss. Lifestyle modifications also include proper footwear and avoidance of high-impact activities. Optimal exercise programs for knee OA should focus on improving aerobic capacity, quadriceps muscle strength, or lower extremity performance. Ideally, the program should be supervised and carried out three times a week.

Use of a cane in the hand opposite to the affected side is mechanically advantageous. Knee sleeves or braces provide some improvement in subjective pain symptoms most likely due to improvements in neuromuscular function. If patients have unicompartmental OA in the medial or lateral compartment, joint unloader braces are available to offload the degenerative compartment. Cushioning

footwear and appropriate orthotics or shoe adjustments are useful for reducing impact to the lower extremities.

There are several oral and intra-articular pharmacologic options. Treatments that have been studied include oral acetaminophen, diclofenac, ibuprofen, naproxen, celecoxib, and intra-articular corticosteroids and hyaluronic acid. All treatments except acetaminophen showed clinically significant improvement in pain. If a traditional NSAID is indicated, the choice should be based on cost, side-effect profile, and adherence. The cyclooxygenase (COX)-2 inhibitor celecoxib is no more effective than traditional NSAIDs; it may offer short-term, but probably not long-term, advantage in preventing gastrointestinal complications. Due to its cost and potential cardiovascular risk, celecoxib should be reserved for carefully selected patients. Topical NSAIDs or capsaicin can be effective in the treatment of OA, since they avoid many of the traditional NSAID complications. Opioids can be used appropriately in patients with severe OA (see Chapter 5). Glucosamine and chondroitin sulfate are supplements that have been widely used and marketed for OA. Despite some initial promise, the best-controlled studies indicate these supplements are ineffective as analgesics in OA. However, they have minimal side effects and may be appropriate if the patient experiences subjective benefit.

Knee joint corticosteroid injections are options to help reduce pain and inflammation and can provide short-term pain relief, usually lasting about 6–12 weeks. Viscosupplementation by injections of hyaluronic acid–based products is controversial. Because reviews suggest that viscosupplementation has a questionably clinically relevant effect size, and has an increased risk of adverse events, the American Academy of Orthopedic Surgeons has recommended that viscosupplementation should not be used in the treatment of knee OA. However, the American College of Rheumatology's 2012 OA guidelines recommend the use of intra-articular hyaluronic acid injection for the treatment of OA of the knee in adults. Platelet-rich plasma injections contain high concentration of platelet-derived growth factors, which regulate some biologic processes in tissue repair. A meta-analysis of 10 studies demonstrated that platelet-rich plasma injections reduced pain in patients with knee OA more efficiently than placebo and hyaluronic acid injections. However, 9 of the 10 studies had a high risk of bias, and the underlying mechanism of biologic healing is unknown. An FDA safety and efficacy study showed that leukocyte-poor PRP autologous conditioned plasma improved overall Western Ontario and McMaster Universities Arthritis Index scores by 78% from the baseline score after 12 months, compared to 7% for the placebo group, though the sample size was small (30 patients).

B. Surgical

Two randomized trials demonstrated that arthroscopy does not improve outcomes at 1 year over placebo or routine conservative treatment of OA. Joint replacement surgeries are effective and cost-effective for patients with significant symptoms or functional limitations, providing improvements in pain, function, and quality of life. The number of total knee arthroplasty procedures jumped 162% from 1991 to 2010, along with an increase in complications and hospital readmissions. Minimally invasive surgeries and computer-assisted navigation during operation are being investigated as methods to improve techniques (eg, accurate placement of the hardware implant) and to reduce complication rates; however, major improvements have yet to be demonstrated.

Knee realignment surgery, such as high tibial osteotomy or partial knee replacement surgery, is indicated in patients younger than age 60 with unicompartmental OA, who would benefit from delaying total knee replacement. Knee joint replacement surgery has been very successful in improving outcomes for patient with end-stage OA. Long-term series describe more than 95% survival rate of the implant at 15 years.

▶ When to Refer

Patients with sufficient disability, limited benefit from conservative therapy, and evidence of severe OA can be referred for joint replacement surgery.

Bannuru RR et al. Comparative effectiveness of pharmacologic interventions for knee osteoarthritis: a systematic review and network meta-analysis. Ann Intern Med. 2015 Jan 6;162(1): 46–54. [PMID: 25560713]

Brosseau L et al. The Ottawa panel clinical practice guidelines for the management of knee osteoarthritis. Part two: strengthening exercise programs. Clin Rehabil. 2017 May;31(5): 596–611. [PMID: 28183213]

Brosseau L et al. The Ottawa panel clinical practice guidelines for the management of knee osteoarthritis. Part three: aerobic exercise programs. Clin Rehabil. 2017 May;31(5):612–24. [PMID: 28183194]

Laudy AB et al. Efficacy of platelet-rich plasma injections in osteoarthritis of the knee: a systematic review and meta-analysis. Br J Sports Med. 2015 May;49(10):657–72. [PMID: 25416198]

Smith PA. Intra-articular autologous conditioned plasma injections provide safe and efficacious treatment for knee osteoarthritis: an FDA-sanctioned, randomized, double-blind, placebo-controlled clinical trial. Am J Sports Med. 2016 Apr; 44(4):884–91. [PMID: 26831629]

ANKLE INJURIES

1. Inversion Ankle Sprains

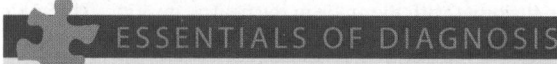

ESSENTIALS OF DIAGNOSIS

▶ Localized pain and swelling.

▶ The majority of ankle injuries involve inversion injuries affecting the lateral ligaments.

▶ Consider chronic ankle instability or associated injuries if pain persists for longer than 3 months following an ankle sprain.

▶ General Considerations

Ankle sprains are the most common sports injuries seen in outpatient clinics. Patients usually report "turning the ankle" during a fall or after landing on an irregular surface such as a hole or an opponent's foot. The most common mechanism

Table 41–8. Injuries associated with ankle sprains.

Ligaments
Subtalar joint sprain
Sinus tarsi syndrome
Syndesmotic sprain
Deltoid sprain
Lisfranc injury
Tendons
Posterior tibial tendon strain
Peroneal tendon subluxation
Bones
Osteochondral talus injury
Lateral talar process fracture
Posterior impingement (os trigonum)
Fracture at the base of the fifth metatarsal
Jones fracture
Salter fracture (fibula)
Ankle fractures

of injury is an inversion and plantar flexion sprain, which injures the anterior talofibular (ATF) ligament rather than the calcaneofibular (CF) ligament. Other injuries that can occur with inversion ankle injuries are listed in Table 41–8. Women appear to sustain an inversion injury more frequently than men. Chronic ankle instability is defined as persistent complaints of pain, swelling, and giving way in combination with recurrent sprains for at least 12 months after the initial ankle sprain. Chronic ankle instability can occur in up to 43% of ankle sprains even with physical therapy, which makes appropriate attention to acute ankle sprains important.

▶ Clinical Findings

A. Symptoms and Signs

The usual symptoms following a sprain include localized pain and swelling over the lateral aspect of the ankle, difficulty weight bearing, and limping. The patient's ankle may feel unstable. On examination, there may be swelling or bruising over the lateral aspect of the ankle. The anterior, inferior aspect below the lateral malleolus is most often the point of maximal tenderness consistent with ATF and CF ligament injuries. The swelling may limit motion of the ankle.

Special stress tests for the ankle include the **anterior drawer test**; the clinician keeps the foot and ankle in the neutral position with the patient sitting, then uses one hand to fix the tibia and the other to hold the patient's heel and draw the ankle forward. Normally, there may be approximately 3 mm of translation until an endpoint is felt. A positive test includes increased translation of one foot compared to the other with loss of the endpoint of the anterior talofibular ligament.

Another stress test is the **subtalar tilt test,** which is performed with the foot in the neutral position with the patient sitting. The clinician uses one hand to fix the tibia and the other to hold and invert the calcaneus. Normal inversion at the subtalar joint is approximately 30 degrees.

A positive test consists of increased subtalar joint inversion greater than 10 degrees on the affected side with loss of endpoint for the calcaneofibular ligament. In order to grade the severity of ankle sprains, no laxity on stress tests is considered a grade 1 injury, laxity of the ATF ligament on anterior drawer testing but a negative tilt test is a grade 2 injury, and both positive drawer and tilt tests signify a grade 3 injury. Difficulty jumping and landing within 2 weeks from the acute ankle sprain, abnormal postural or hip muscle control, or ligamentous laxity noted 8 weeks after injury are poor prognostic signs.

B. Imaging

Routine ankle radiographic views include the AP, lateral, and oblique (mortise) views. Less common views requested include the calcaneal view and subtalar view. The **Ottawa Ankle Rules** remain the best clinical prediction rules to guide the need for radiographs and have an 86–99% sensitivity and a 97–99% negative predictive value. If the patient is unable to bear weight immediately in the office setting or emergency department for four steps, then the clinician should check for (1) bony tenderness at the posterior edge of the medial or lateral malleolus and (2) bony tenderness over the navicular (medial midfoot) or at the base of the fifth metatarsal. If either malleolus demonstrates pain or deformity, then ankle radiographs should be obtained. If the foot has bony tenderness, obtain foot radiographs. An MRI is helpful when considering the associated injuries.

► Treatment

Immediate treatment of an ankle sprain follows the MICE mnemonic: *m*odified activities, *i*ce, *c*ompression, and *e*levation. Subsequent treatment involves protected weight bearing with crutches and use of an ankle stabilizer brace, especially for grade 2 and 3 injuries. Early motion is essential, and patients should be encouraged to do home exercises or physical therapy. Proprioception and balance exercises (eg, "wobble board") are useful to restore function to the ankle and prevent future ankle sprains. Regular use of an ankle support with activities can reduce the risk of lateral ankle sprains. Chronic instability can develop after acute ankle sprain in 10–20% of people and may require surgical stabilization with ligament reconstruction surgery.

► When to Refer

- Ankle fractures.
- Recurrent ankle sprains or signs of chronic ligamentous ankle instability.
- No response after more than 3 months of conservative treatment.
- Suspicion of associated injuries.

Brison RJ et al. Effect of early supervised physiotherapy on recovery from acute ankle sprain: randomised controlled trial. BMJ. 2016 Nov 16;355:i5650. [PMID: 27852621]
Czajka CM. Ankle sprains and instability. Med Clin North Am. 2014 Mar;98(2):313–29. [PMID: 24559877]

Vuurberg G et al. Diagnosis, treatment and prevention of ankle sprains: update of an evidence-based clinical guideline. Br J Sports Med. 2018 Aug;52(15):956. [PMID: 29514819]

2. Eversion ("High") Ankle Sprains

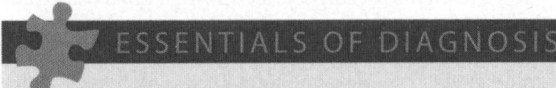

ESSENTIALS OF DIAGNOSIS

- ► Severe and prolonged pain.
- ► Limited range of motion.
- ► Mild swelling.
- ► Difficulty with weight bearing.

► General Considerations

A syndesmotic injury or "high ankle" sprain involves the anterior *tibio*fibular ligament in the anterolateral aspect of the ankle, superior to the anterior *talo*fibular (ATF) ligament. The injury mechanism often involves the foot being turned out or externally rotated and everted (eg, when being tackled). This injury is commonly missed or misdiagnosed as an ATF ligament sprain on initial visit.

► Clinical Findings

A. Symptoms and Signs

Symptoms of a high ankle sprain include severe and prolonged pain over the anterior ankle at the anterior tibiofibular ligament, worse with weight bearing. This is often more painful than the typical ankle sprain. The point of maximal tenderness involves the anterior tibiofibular ligament, which is higher than the ATF ligament. It is also important to palpate the proximal fibula to rule out any proximal syndesmotic ligament injury and associated fracture known as a "maisonneuve fracture." There is often some mild swelling in this area, and the patient may or may not have an ankle effusion. The patient usually has limited range of motion in all directions. To perform the **external rotation stress test,** the clinician fixes the tibia with one hand and grasps the foot in the other with the ankle in the neutral position. The ankle is then dorsiflexed and externally rotated, reproducing the patient's pain. (**Note:** The patient's foot should have an intact neurovascular examination before undertaking this test.)

B. Imaging

Radiographs of the ankle should include the AP, mortise, and lateral views. The mortise view may demonstrate loss of the normal overlap between the tibia and fibula, which should be at least 1–2 mm. Asymmetry in the joint space around the tibiotalar joint suggests disruption of the syndesmotic ligaments. If there is proximal tenderness in the lower leg especially around the fibula, an AP and lateral view of the tibia and fibula should be obtained to rule out a proximal fibula fracture. Radiographs during an external rotation stress test may visualize instability at the distal tibiofibular joint. MRI is the best method to visualize injury to the tibiofibular ligament and to assess status of the other ligaments and the articular cartilage.

Treatment

Whereas most ankle sprains are treated with early motion and weight bearing, treatment for a high ankle sprain should be conservative with a cast or walking boot for 4–6 weeks. Thereafter, protected weight bearing with crutches is recommended until the patient can walk pain-free. Physical therapy can start early to regain range of motion and maintain strength with limited weight bearing initially.

When to Refer

If there is widening of the joint space and asymmetry at the tibiotalar joint, the patient should be referred urgently to a foot and ankle surgeon. Severe or prolonged persistent cases that do not heal may require internal fixation to avoid chronic instability at the tibiofibular joint. Screw fixation remains the gold standard, although newer techniques with bioabsorbable constructs are emerging.

Fort NM et al. Management of acute injuries of the tibiofibular syndesmosis. Eur J Orthop Surg Traumatol. 2017 May;27(4): 449–59. [PMID: 28391516]

Kellett JJ et al. Diagnostic imaging of ankle syndesmosis injuries: a general review. J Med Imaging Radiat Oncol. 2018 Apr;62(2):159–68. [PMID: 29399975]

Yuen CP et al. Distal tibiofibular syndesmosis: anatomy, biomechanics, injury and management. Open Orthop J. 2017 Jul 31;11:670–77. [PMID: 29081864]

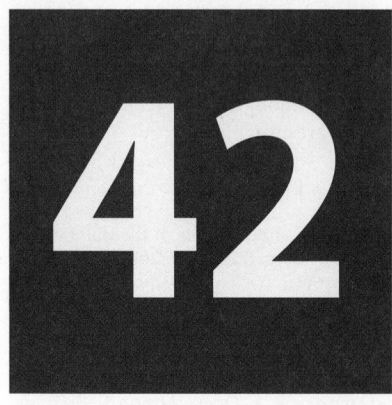

Lesbian, Gay, Bisexual, & Transgender Health

Juno Obedin-Maliver, MD, MPH, MAS

Patricia A. Robertson, MD

Kevin L. Ard, MD, MPH

Kenneth H. Mayer, MD

Madeline B. Deutsch, MD, MPH

HEALTH CARE FOR SEXUAL & GENDER MINORITY PATIENTS

Definitions & Concepts

The term **sexual and gender minorities (SGM)** refers to a broad group including lesbian women and gay men; bisexual, pansexual, and queer people; and transgender and gender non-binary people—also commonly referred to as "LGBTQ." Cisgender refers to people whose gender identity (a person's internal sense of gender) and sex assigned at birth are congruent (ie, they are not transgender). Transgender people may also be sexual minorities (ie, lesbian transgender women or gay transgender men). For the sake of expediency in this chapter, the sections on sexual minority men and women omit the term "cisgender"; however, readers of content in these sections should take into consideration that, for example, gay transgender men may have vaginal receptive sex with their cisgender male sexual partners, and therefore should be screened for contraception needs, and cisgender lesbian women may have transgender female partners who retain their penis. A growing number of people identify as pansexual, which describes an attraction to people of any gender, male, female, or on the spectrum between the two. The term queer, historically a pejorative term, has been reclaimed by many SGM people to represent someone with a sexuality or gender identity or expression that differs from that of a cisgender (ie, non-transgender), heterosexual person. Sexual orientation refers to a deep-seated sense of one's sexuality that encompasses three dimensions: identity, behavior, and desire. Sexual identities include gay or homosexual (those who are predominantly attracted to and/or sexually active with members of the same gender), bisexual (those who are attracted to and/or sexually active with both men and women), and heterosexual or straight; however, several other terms may be used, and terminology may change over time.

The three dimensions of sexual orientation—identity, behavior, and desire—do not necessarily overlap. For example, less than 50% of men who have sex with men (MSM) in one national, probability-based survey identified as gay. MSM who identify as heterosexual rather than as gay or bisexual may be more likely than their gay-identified counterparts to be married to women, foreign-born, of minority race, and of lower socioeconomic status. The incomplete overlap of identity and behavior means that clinicians cannot rely upon self-reported identity to infer sexual behavior, and vice versa. It is important to distinguish sexual orientation from their gender identity. Knowing someone's gender identity does not identify one's sexual orientation. Just as cisgender people may be sexually attracted to and have sex with people of any gender, so too can transgender men, transgender women, and non-binary people have partners of any gender. Routinely asking about sexual orientation, and when relevant for the clinical issue at hand, sexual behavior, helps build trust between the patient and clinician, ensures appropriate medical care (for example, appropriate screening tests for sexually transmitted infections [STIs] and family planning), and contributes to better health outcomes. To inquire about gender identity, the following two questions are recommended: "What is your current gender identity?" and "What sex were you assigned at birth?"

Sexual orientation may also change over time or be situational (such as during periods of limited mobility or during incarceration). People may also hide their sexual orientation from others, including clinicians, in order to avoid stigma and discrimination. Revealing one's sexual orientation is called "coming out." This process may occur at any point in life and may vary by context (for example, being "out" to family but not to coworkers).

Sexual and gender identity can be fluid throughout a person's lifetime, and the binary concept of gender is not evidence based. Some legal policies are moving to reflect this fluidity. In California, the choice of gender on legal documents is female, male, or non-binary. These choices have implications for health screening for patients who receive care in health systems with pop-up reminders for sex-specific screening examinations such as mammography or prostate examinations.

Health Disparities

Providing compassionate and informed health care for SGM patients, which include but are not limited to people who identify as lesbian, gay, bisexual, transgender, and queer, involves the acknowledgment of the negative effects on health caused by discrimination and stigma. LGBTQ people are underserved by the medical community and under-studied, with worse health outcomes compared to the heterosexual and cisgender population. One reason for these disparities is that a previous negative experience in a clinician's office influences whether the patient will repeat a visit even for an acute medical event, which can delay care and result in advanced disease. One in three transgender people report delays in seeking care due to prior discrimination, and one in five report being refused medical care due to their transgender identity. Some of the compromised health outcomes are related to limited access to the health care system due to financial issues as well as previous negative experiences in society at large. These structural issues will take time to change. However, clinicians can impact the health outcomes of LGBTQ people by ensuring that the clinical space is welcoming to people of all genders and sexual orientations (see below), obtaining comprehensive data on sexual orientation and gender identity, and being aware of the specific health needs of LGBTQ people in order to advance the health of LGBTQ patients.

The vast majority of SGM patients would like to "come out" to their clinician. Many clinicians, however, are concerned that their patients would be offended if asked about sexual orientation and identity. It is important that clinicians overcome any discomfort and ask appropriate questions of their patients. There are useful video resources to help clinicians with these issues; one example is "Acknowledging Sex and Gender" Online Training video from the University of California, San Francisco Center of Excellence for Transgender Health http://transhealth.ucsf.edu/video/story_html5.html?lms=1.

Lunn MR et al. Sociodemographic characteristics and health outcomes among lesbian, gay, and bisexual U.S. adults using Healthy People 2020 leading health indicators. LGBT Health. 2017 Aug;4(4):283–94. [PMID: 28727950]

Making Clinical Environments Welcoming to All SGM Patients

Part of serving SGM patients is to create a welcoming clinical space where each person is cared for and respected for **all** of who they are—including their sexual orientation, gender identity, and gender expression. This includes making sure that (1) senior leadership is involved; (2) nondiscrimination policies are in place, are followed, and are prominently displayed; (3) open visitation policies are concordant with patients' choice of visitors; (4) outreach and engagement efforts are made for LGBTQ patients; (5) staff receive culturally affirming training in the care of LGBTQ people; (6) processes, forms, artwork, and reading materials reflect the diversity of LGBTQ people; (7) data are collected about both sexual orientation and gender identity in an open and nonjudgmental manner; (8) patients are routinely asked about their sexual health histories; (9) clinical care and services include prevention and wellness care with family planning services and behavioral

health services available; (10) LGBTQ staff are recruited and trained; (11) preventive care is concordant with clinical practice guidelines, where applicable; and (12) if gender neutral bathrooms are not available, a posting states that patients are welcome to use either the women's or men's bathroom and the patient can determine which bathroom to use. One exercise is to look at clinic materials (ie, signs, posters, brochures, magazines, intake forms etc.) and see if materials presume heterosexual behavior and gender conformity. Often, materials discussing anatomy, sex, family planning, conception, pregnancy, and birth presume heterosexuality. If so, find or create more inclusive materials to replace them.

National LGBT Cancer Network. Cultural competency in-person trainings and on-line materials, updated 2017. https://cancer-network.org/programs/cultural-competency-training
National LGBT Education Center. Ten things: creating inclusive health care environments for LGBT people. July 2015. http://www.lgbthealtheducation.org/wp-content/uploads/Ten-Things-Brief-Final-WEB.pdf

Obtaining Sexual History From SGM Patients

The core history and physical examination is not different for SGM in comparison to other patients. Clinicians should approach each patient as an individual, using patients' preferred pronouns, using appropriate terminology, respecting the diversity of gender identity as well as the differing desires for gender affirming treatments, and performing a physical examination noting anatomic changes from any prior gender affirming treatment. As with all adolescent or adult patients, a complete medical history should include a comprehensive sexual history. Clinicians may wish to preface discussion of the patient's sexual history with a statement indicating that this information is confidential and is important in order to provide optimal health care. However, patients should not be expected to discuss their gender identity or transition unless it is relevant to the current visit. In addition, it is crucial that clinicians understand that transgender patients may have physical appearances and/or names that do not reflect their legal names or sex markers. Staff members must learn how to elicit patients' names and accepted pronouns so that these can be used consistently.

Key data to gather in a relevant sexual history include sexual function and satisfaction; number of partners if the patient is sexually active; and the gender(s) of the patient's sexual partner(s). In addition, clinicians should determine the types of sexual practices the patient engages in (for example, oral sex, insertive anal sex, and/or receptive anal sex); how often condoms are used, if at all, for the different sexual practices the patient engages in; and whether or not drugs and/or alcohol are consumed in conjunction with sex. Clinicians should also establish whether there is a history of STIs because a positive history may have implications for medical follow-up and sexual risk assessment (eg, frequency of screening, syphilis serologies, and discussion about preexposure prophylaxis [PrEP]). For example, a recent diagnosis of syphilis would indicate the need for rapid plasma reagin titer monitoring to ensure adequate treatment and would prompt consideration of PrEP due to the association of syphilis with HIV infection.

The Fenway Institute, which specializes in LGBTQ health and health care, proposes using the following statement and follow-up questions:

> "*I am going to ask you some questions about your sexual health and sexuality that I ask all my patients. The answers to these questions are important for me to know how to help keep you healthy. Like the rest of this visit, this information is strictly confidential.*"

Evidence suggests that most individuals are ready and willing to disclose to sensitive providers who make it clear the intent behind their questions. Additional questions include the following:

a. "Do you have a partner or a spouse?" or "Are you currently in a relationship?"
b. "Are you sexually active?"
c. "When was the last time you had sex?"
d. "What are the genders of your sexual partner (s)?"
e. "What body parts of yours touch which body parts of your partners?"
f. "How many sexual partners have you had during the last year?"
g. "Do you have any desires regarding sexual intimacy that you would like to discuss?"

Rather than considering this a one-time intervention, it should be thought of as a process that is assessed over time and at critical junctures and changes in health status.

The Association of American Medical Colleges (AAMC) has created a series of online videos that highlight history-taking that includes assessments of sexual orientation, gender identity, and sexual practices (https://www.aamc.org/initiatives/diversity/450606/clinicalvignettes.html); gender and sexual history taking (https://www.aamc.org/initiatives/diversity/450468/gender-and-sexual-history1.html and https://www.aamc.org/initiatives/diversity/450470/gender-and-sexual-history2.html); and ineffective history taking (https://www.aamc.org/initiatives/diversity/450472/ineffective-history-taking.html).

Centers for Disease Control and Prevention (CDC). A guide to taking a sexual history. http://www.cdc.gov/std/treatment/sexualhistory.pdf

▶ The Electronic Medical Record

Electronic medical record (EMR) systems should include functionality for the recording of gender identity and birth-assigned sex as well as chosen name and pronoun in the case of a transgender person who has not changed their legal identity documents. Chosen name and pronoun functionality should be displayed in all banners, schedules, and other viewing screens. Transgender people can be identified within the EMR that supports the data collection of gender as separate from sex assigned at birth, by

identifying those individuals whose entries for gender identity and birth sex differ. Collecting gender identity and birth assigned sex data is critical to understanding the population of people in care within a health system.

Disclosure in the EMR of a patient's sexual orientation and gender identity has been advocated in the United States by the National Academy of Medicine, the Joint Commission, and the Health Resources and Services Administration as fundamental to improving access to and quality of care for LGBTQ people. However, there are risks for LGBTQ people with having their sexual orientation and gender identity documented in the EMR. Examples of such risks include loss of employment. In 28 states in the United States, a person can be legally terminated from employment on the basis of sexual orientation, and same-sex relations are criminalized in over 72 countries. Specific issues that limit the adaptability of some medical records to the LGBTQ population are related to "sex-specific" experiences such as the inability to register a male pregnancy episode. There are "work-arounds," such as having a place for preferred name for all patients that medical assistants can routinely check before inviting a patient into an examination room. The EMR can also be used to gather answers to sensitive questions before an initial visit so that the patient can provide information privately.

Deutsch MB et al. Electronic medical records and the transgender patient: recommendations from the World Professional Association for Transgender Health EMR Working Group. J Am Med Inform Assoc. 2013 Jul–Aug;20(4):700–3. [PMID: 23631835]

Deutsch MB et al. Electronic health records and transgender patients—practical recommendations for the collection of gender identity data. J Gen Intern Med. 2015 Jun;30(6):843–7. [PMID: 25560316]

Grasso C et al. Planning and implementing sexual orientation and gender identity data collection in electronic health records. J Am Med Inform Assoc. 2019 Jan 1;26(1):66–70. [PMID: 30445621]

▶ Family Planning

A. Pregnancy Prevention

Comprehensive family planning for LGBTQ people is important to address, so that all pregnancies are intended if at all possible. Anyone with a uterus, ovaries, and fallopian tubes can potentially become pregnant if they engage in penis-in-vagina sex. This includes transgender men who are taking testosterone or still amenorrheic from testosterone. Furthermore, transgender women who have a penis and testes may still produce sperm capable of fertilizing an oocyte even if using gender affirming hormones. Since sexual orientation and gender identity do not predetermine sexual partners, all individuals should be asked about family building intentions as well as contraception if pregnancy is undesired.

The majority of lesbians have been sexually active with men at some point in their lives (85–90%), and 30% of self-identified adult lesbians are currently sexually active with men as well as with women. Fewer lesbian youth use hormonal contraception than heterosexual female youth. On multiple surveys, one of the reasons that lesbians do not follow up for gynecologic care is the assumption by the clinician that they are heterosexual, and the (insensitive) advocacy of birth control in that assumptive atmosphere about their sexuality (ie, heteronormative). On the other hand, multiple studies show that the unintended pregnancy rate of self-identified lesbian youth is higher than that of the comparison heterosexual female youth. Unintended pregnancy risk continues into adulthood with one sample from the Chicago Health and Life Experiences of Women survey reporting 24% of sexual minority women having had unintended pregnancies. The reasons for disproportionate unintended pregnancy rates have not been fully elucidated but may involve discrimination and family rejection leading to higher-risk behaviors, increased alcohol and other substance use, less effective birth control usage, and multiple sexual partners. Another reason may be attempts to prove one's "straightness" by engaging in penis-in-vagina sexual activity. If it has been determined that the patient self-identifies as a lesbian and is having (penis-in-vagina) sex with men, one suggested question might be, "Are you planning to get pregnant this year?" If the answer is no, this is an opportunity to explain that studies show a higher unintended rate of pregnancy in lesbian youth and to review effective contraception options. It is also a good time to talk about protection from STIs when having sex with men (ie, discuss condoms). As with any person engaging in penis-in-vagina sex, experts recommend additional contraceptives to condoms. Condoms are only 80% reliable in preventing pregnancy with typical use. Long-acting reversible contraceptives, which are not patient or sexual act dependent and function effectively despite alcohol or other substance use, are especially important to consider. Long-acting reversible contraceptives such as an etonogestrel subdermal implant in the arm (0.05% annual failure) or either the copper (0.8% annual failure) or levonorgestrel (0.2% annual failure) intrauterine devices are highly effective and typical use is generally equivalent to ideal use.

For transgender men and non-binary individuals who were assigned female sex at birth, contraception is important even if testosterone is being used, since testosterone is not a reliable form of contraceptive. To underscore the points, transgender men taking testosterone (even if amenorrheic) who have a uterus and ovaries and are sexually active with sperm involved should use a standard contraceptive method if they want to avoid a pregnancy. There are multiple case reports in the literature of transgender men who have unintended pregnancies while taking testosterone. Little is known about contraceptive preferences and use profiles among transgender men and non-binary people who were female sex assigned at birth. This is, however, an emerging field and new studies suggest unmet contraceptive need and diverse contraceptive method usage type, including long-acting reversible contraceptives (eg, intrauterine devices).

The AAMC has produced noteworthy videos about family counseling and coming out (https://www.aamc.org/initiatives/diversity/450466/family-counseling.html), gender and sexual history taking (https://www.aamc.org/initiatives/diversity/450468/gender-and-sexual-history1.html and https://www.aamc.org/initiatives/diversity/450470/gender-and-sexual-history2.html), and ineffective history taking (https://www.aamc.org/initiatives/diversity/450472/ineffective-history-taking.html).

Blunt-Vinti HD et al. Contraceptive use effectiveness and pregnancy prevention information preferences among heterosexual and sexual minority college women. Womens Health Issues. 2018 Jul–Aug;28(4):342–9. [PMID: 29666034]

Cipres D et al. Contraceptive use and pregnancy intentions among transgender men presenting to a clinic for sex workers and their families in San Francisco. Contraception. 2017 Feb;95(2):186–9. [PMID: 27621044]

Everett BG et al. Unintended pregnancy, depression, and hazardous drinking in a community-based sample of sexual minority women. J Womens Health (Larchmt). 2016 Sep;25(9):904–11. [PMID: 26977978]

Light A et al. Family planning and contraception use in transgender men. Contraception. 2018 Oct;98(4):266–9. [PMID: 29944875]

B. Family Building

Family building should be discussed with all patients, regardless of sexual orientation or gender identity. Options include foster-parenting or adoption (in some countries these options are not open to LGBTQ persons), co-parenting a partner's child/children, becoming pregnant, contracting with a surrogate, or step-parenting. Some fertility practices refuse to assist LGBTQ people with conception even if it is legal. The American College of Obstetricians and Gynecologists published Committee Opinion No. 749 in 2018, reaffirming their stance that no matter how a child comes into a family, all children and parents deserve equitable protections and access to available resources to maximize the health of that family unit. "Obstetricians-gynecologists should recognize the diversity in parenting desires that exists in the lesbian, gay, bisexual, transgender, queer, intersex, asexual and gender nonconforming communities and should take steps to ensure that clinical spaces are affirming and open to all parties, such that equitable and comprehensive, reproductive health care can meet the needs of these communities."

Lesbian and bisexual cisgender women have many options to consider for conception and may ask the clinician for an opinion and to guide them to resources. Many lesbian women decide to have inseminations with an unknown donor (some unknown donors sign a release so that the child may contact the donor when the child reaches 18 years old), and some lesbian women decide to involve a known sperm donor. Most sperm banks are regulated in regard to the administration of medical history forms, the testing of sperm for STIs, and the performance of genetic screening. Known donors may have risk factors but are not routinely screened. It is important for a woman to be as informed as she can be about the legal implications of each option. In some states and countries, unless the insemination with known donor sperm takes place in the office of a physician, the known donor has full legal rights as well as financial responsibilities for the offspring. In one study of 129 lesbian mothers with 77 index offspring, 77.5% of the mothers were satisfied with the type of donor chosen (36% had chosen known sperm donors, 25%

open-identity donors, and 39% unknown donors). Donor access and custody concerns were the primary themes mentioned by lesbian mothers regarding their (dis)satisfaction with the type of sperm donor they had selected.

Some lesbian women who are partnered decide to do "co–in vitro fertilization (IVF)," which is also known as "reciprocal IVF" or "co-maternity" in which one partner provides an egg, it is fertilized in the laboratory with sperm of a known or unknown donor, and then the other partner carries the pregnancy. Lactation for the nongestating mother can sometimes be induced by using a protocol that stemmed originally from the experiences of adoptive mothers who were motivated to breastfeed. Many lesbian women delay childbearing until later in life, and then the issues of fertility, pregnancy loss, and birth defects increase. Pregnancy outcomes of bisexual and lesbian women compared to heterosexually identified women include increased risk of miscarriage (odds ratio [OR] 1.77) and stillbirth (OR 2.85), as well as very preterm birth (OR 1.84).

There have been many studies on the overall outcomes of children of lesbian women, all of which have been positive when comparing their children to children raised by heterosexual parents, despite the stigma the children experience of having same-sex parents. Using the 2011–2012 National Survey of Children's Health data set from the United States, children with female same-sex parents and different-sex parents demonstrated no differences in outcomes (spouse-partner relationships, emotional difficulties, coping behaviors, and learning behavior).

Biologic options for pregnancy for cisgender gay men include conceiving with a cisgender woman who may or may not be interested in co-parenting with them, or contracting with a surrogate to carry the pregnancy after the sperm and a donor egg are fertilized and placed in the uterus of the surrogate. For transgender people, there are also options. Prior to initiation of any gender affirming hormones or gender affirming surgical procedures, a consultation with a reproductive endocrinologist to discuss fertility preservation and future genetic offspring is encouraged. Reproductive planning is often not a priority for a transitioning youth but may become a desire in the future and may also be a priority for potential grandparents. Options are limited for transgender youth who have not undergone endogenous puberty before either starting gender affirming hormones (with estrogen or testosterone) or puberty blockers and then going directly to estrogen or testosterone. The only future fertility option is either testicular or ovarian tissue cryopreservation, which is still considered experimental. For transgender women and gender non-binary individuals who were male sex assigned at birth and who have reached adulthood after endogenous puberty, sperm can be stored ideally prior to the initiation of estrogen. Of note, though some transgender women still produce sperm even after long-term estrogen exposure, it is recommended that sperm cryopreservation occur prior to hormone start because the effect on fertility is hard to quantify and coming off hormones can often be dysphoric. For transgender men and non-binary individuals who were female sex assigned at birth and have gone through endogenous puberty, next steps in genetic parentage will be predicated on the desire to carry a pregnancy and whether or not they have started gender affirming hormones. Options include penis-in-vagina sex, intravaginal insemination, intrauterine insemination, and egg cryopreservation for the individual, a partner, or surrogate to carry. Of note, if a transgender man wishes to carry a pregnancy and is using testosterone, testosterone should be stopped for the duration of the pregnancy. If a transgender man desires future genetic parentage, the consultant might recommend egg aspiration and freezing prior to the start of testosterone. If a hysterectomy is planned as part of gender affirmation, discussion of whether ovaries are left in place should occur in light of consideration of future genetic parentage as well as future hormone regulation. Although in one study in Australia, only 7% of transgender and non-binary adults had undertaken fertility preservation, 95% said that fertility preservation should be offered to all transgender and non-binary people. Participants who viewed genetic relatedness as important were more likely to have undertaken fertility preservation.

All LGBTQ persons planning a pregnancy should be encouraged to consult with a family attorney prior to conception, and if partnered, the partner needs to be aware of their rights and responsibilities. The law has not kept up with the variety of family constellations that are seen in LGBTQ families. Examples of these constellations can include two gay cisgender dads parenting together each using the same egg donor so that their children are half-siblings biologically, a lesbian couple composed of a transgender woman and cisgender woman where one mother provides the sperm and another provides the egg and carries the pregnancy, a straight cisgender dad parenting with a lesbian cisgender mom, a lesbian cisgender couple with the sperm donor being the brother of the parent who did not provide the egg so one mother is the genetically related via the egg and the other mother is the related to the child via being a biologic aunt, two cisgender lesbians each carrying a pregnancy conceived with their own eggs and using the same sperm donor so that their children are half-siblings, two gay men where one is a cisgender man and provides the sperm and one is a transgender man and provides the egg and surrogate carries the pregnancy, and so on.

Baiocco R et al. Same-sex and different-sex parent families in Italy: is parents' sexual orientation associated with child health outcomes and parental dimensions? J Dev Behav Pediatr. 2018 Sep;39(7):555–63. [PMID: 29781831]

Bos HM et al. Same-sex and different-sex parent households and child health outcomes: findings from the national survey of children's health. J Dev Behav Pediatr. 2016 Apr;37(3):179–87. [PMID: 27035692]

Carone N et al. Italian gay father families formed by surrogacy: parenting, stigmatization, and children's psychological adjustment. Dev Psychol. 2018 Oct;54(10):1904–16. [PMID: 30234340]

Everett BG et al. Sexual orientation disparities in pregnancy and infant outcomes. Matern Child Health J. 2019 Jan;23(1):72–81. [PMID: 30019158]

Gartrell NK et al. Satisfaction with known, open-identity, or unknown sperm donors: reports from lesbian mothers of 17-year-old adolescents. Fertil Steril. 2015 Jan;103(1):242–8. [PMID: 25439795]

LESBIAN & BISEXUAL WOMEN'S HEALTH SPECIFIC ISSUES

Juno Obedin-Maliver, MD, MPH, MAS
Patricia A. Robertson, MD

Cisgender lesbian and bisexual women are addressed together in this section since most medical literature does not consider the intersection of sexual orientation and gender identity deeply enough to evaluate the specific health needs and concerns of lesbian and bisexual women who are of transgender experience. In the United States, women in same-sex couples are less likely to get nonurgent medical care when needed, see a specialist, and feel that doctors spent enough time with them. Lesbian and bisexual women in the United States are also less likely to have primary care providers. This is true throughout the world with variability depending on local sociopolitical climate. In countries with more restrictive laws and policies, health disparities are likely greater. A study in Lebanon noted that significantly more sexual minority women reported having trouble accessing health care than heterosexual women, and a meta-analysis of southern African countries outlined the unique health challenges faced by sexual minority women, including social exclusion and invisibility, criminalization, and systematic homophobic sexual assault.

Gereige JD et al. The sexual health of women in Lebanon: are there differences by sexual orientation? LGBT Health. 2018 Jan;5(1):45–53. [PMID: 29130791]
Muller A et al. Making the invisible visible: a systematic review of sexual minority women's health in Southern Africa. BMC Public Health. 2016 Apr 11;16:307. [PMID: 27066890]
Obedin-Maliver J et al. Lesbian, gay, bisexual, and transgender-related content in undergraduate medical education. JAMA. 2011 Sep 7;306(9):971–7. [PMID: 21900137]

Health Disparities Affecting Lesbian & Bisexual Women

Health disparities exist across the life span for lesbian and bisexual women compared to heterosexual women. The following are increased among lesbian and bisexual women: childhood physical abuse in the home, childhood sexual abuse, substance use including alcohol and tobacco, chlamydial infection as teens and young adults, sexual assault, depression, disabilities, body mass index (BMI), intimate partner violence, threats and violence outside the home, asthma, and cardiovascular disease (CVD). Sexual dysfunction for lesbian and bisexual women is seen less often or as often as heterosexual women but is understudied and likely assessed at rates lower than among heterosexual women. A high risk of sexual dysfunction can be detected by a single question regarding sexual function: "Do you have any questions or concerns about your sexuality or sexual health?" Studies of Irish LGBTQ elders reveal concerns about residential care outside of their own home as well as respect by health professionals; similarly, there are concerns about home services for lesbian and bisexual women in Canada and the United States. Lesbian and bisexual women have fewer children available to help them as they age compared to heterosexual women. Therefore, it is critical that health care providers identify health decision makers for all patients including lesbian and bisexual women who may have more "family of choice" members versus "family of origin" members who may be estranged. This is especially important since same-sex/same-gender marriage is not allowed in many countries and is still considered socially unacceptable in many areas of the United States. To avoid conflict during critical decision-making moments, the health decision maker needs to be identified on the medical record after a private conversation with the patient. In one survey, only about 50% of same-sex couples who desired their partner to be the health decision maker had appropriate forms, and even if married, advance directives should be completed given past visitation denials. Many notable legal cases, including that of Sharon Kowalski and Karen Thompson, have documented the struggles that same-sex partners can face regarding visitation and appropriate recognition during end-of-life care or critical medical decision making when these documents have not been completed. Elder abuse screening also needs to be done, since the incidence is unknown.

Kortes-Miller K et al. Dying in long-term care: perspectives from sexual and gender minority older adults about their fears and hopes for end of life. J Soc Work End Life Palliat Care. 2018 Nov 20:1–16. [PMID: 30457453]
Reiter PL et al. HPV infection among a population-based sample of sexual minority women from USA. Sex Transm Infect. 2017 Feb;93(1):25–31. [PMID: 27165699]

Prevention of CVD

The risk of CVD is higher in sexual minority women compared with heterosexual peers. Though many studies lack objective measures such as biomarkers, a systematic review demonstrated greater CVD among sexual minority women. Ultimately this outcome seemed most influenced by societal conditions (ie, cumulative minority stress) that impact the CVD risk. In one study, lesbian and bisexual women were 14% older in vascular terms than their chronological age, which was 6% greater than that of their heterosexual counterparts and the risk was not fully explained by excessive smoking or alcohol use. When the effect of five stressful life events (physical abuse, sexual abuse and forced sex, homelessness, school expulsion, death of a parent) was compared between lesbian, gay, or bisexual (LGB) women and heterosexual women, higher cardiometabolic risk scores were found in LGB women, even after controlling for demographic factors such as socioeconomic status, health behaviors, and self-reported illness. Although many studies report similar hypertension prevalence among lesbian, bisexual, and heterosexual women, more recent work has described higher prevalence of hypertension among sexual minority women when compared with heterosexual counterparts.

The leading five modifiable risk factors for CVD are smoking, physical inactivity, obesity, elevated lipid levels, and diabetes. Three of these factors (smoking, physical inactivity, and obesity) have a higher prevalence in lesbian and bisexual women.

Caceres BA et al. A systematic review of cardiovascular disease in sexual minorities. Am J Public Health. 2017 Apr;107(4):e13–21. [PMID: 28207331]

Clark CJ et al. Disparities in long-term cardiovascular disease risk by sexual identity: The National Longitudinal Study of Adolescent to Adult Health. Prev Med. 2015 Jul;76:26–30. [PMID: 25849883]

Kinsky S et al. Risk of the metabolic syndrome in sexual minority women: results from the ESTHER study. J Womens Health (Larchmt). 2016 Aug;25(8):784–90. [PMID: 26885574]

▶ Smoking

Cigarette smoking is more common among lesbian and bisexual women than in heterosexual women. While estimates vary, the National Adult Tobacco Survey noted 22% of lesbian women and 32% of bisexual women smoke compared with 13% of heterosexual women. The National Health Interview Survey, a United States Centers for Disease Control and Prevention (CDC) sponsored and administered study, noted that lesbian and bisexual women are also heavier smokers. The tobacco industry's well-documented targeted marketing to LGBTQ groups and the use of cigarette smoking to decrease social stress are probable factors. Significant racial and ethnic differences exist with Asian and Pacific Islander lesbian and bisexual women, who have four times higher odds of smoking than heterosexual Asian and Pacific Islander women. In high school, LGB adolescents reported a higher prevalence of daily cigarette use (22%) compared with heterosexual youth (11%). Protective factors against smoking behaviors for young LGB women included connections with other LGBTQ people. Another study demonstrated that though desire to quit did not differ between sexual minority women and their heterosexual counterparts, cessation attempts did differ, suggesting that clinicians need to customize cessation interventions for sexual minority women.

Traditional smoking cessation programs and targeted LGBTQ programs are effective for LGBTQ people. A review of smoking cessation programs for LGBTI (I = intersex) people found that with cultural modifications for LGBTI people, 61% had quit at the end of interventions and this stabilized to 39% at 3–6 months. In Canada, 24 focus groups in Toronto and Ottawa detailed eight overarching themes that would be important to them in a smoking intervention: (1) be LGBTQ+ specific; (2) be accessible in terms of location, time, availability, and cost; (3) be inclusive, relatable, and highlight diversity; (4) incorporate LGBTQ+ peer support and counseling services; (5) integrate other activities beyond smoking; (6) be positive, motivational, uplifting, and empowering; (7) provide concrete coping mechanisms; and (8) integrate rewards and incentives. Other studies have corroborated that both LGBTQ-specific (such as relation to "coming out," different norms and acceptability of smoking among LGBTQ communities, or LGBTQ-related minority stress) and previously identified factors seen in other populations (such as self-efficacy around quitting) are important to support LGBTQ people in quitting smoking. The LGBTQ people in Ireland have very high tobacco use and exposure to secondhand smoke. Attention should be paid to messaging about smoking warnings because not all messages are perceived as equally effective by sexual minorities when compared with heterosexual people. Encourage patients to check with their community or online resources for smoking cessation programs and encourage participation in LGBTQ tailored programs, if available.

Baskerville NB et al. A qualitative study of tobacco interventions for LGBTQ+ youth and young adults: overarching themes and key learnings. BMC Public Health. 2018 Jan 18;18(1):155. [PMID: 29347920]

Berger I et al. Smoking cessation programs for lesbian, gay, bisexual, transgender, and intersex people: a content-based systematic review. Nicotine Tob Res. 2017 Nov 7;19(12):1408–17. [PMID: 27613909]

Fallin A et al. Smoking characteristics among lesbian, gay, and bisexual adults. Prev Med. 2015 May;74:123–30. [PMID: 25485860]

Matthews AK et al. A qualitative study of the barriers to and facilitators of smoking cessation among lesbian, gay, bisexual, and transgender smokers who are interested in quitting. LGBT Health. 2017 Feb;4(1):24–33. [PMID: 28068208]

▶ Body Weight

Data regarding obesity and overweight prevalence in lesbians and bisexual women are mixed. Many studies, though, including an analysis of over 60,000 women in the National Health Interview Survey find that being a sexual minority woman is associated with an elevated BMI compared to heterosexual women. The prevalence of obesity may not be uniform across racial and ethnic groups. The odds of obesity among lesbian women in the following groups differed when compared with heterosexual women in the same racial group: Latina lesbian women 1.39 (95% CI, 1.20, 1.61), Asian and Pacific Islander lesbian women 1.22 (95% CI, 0.76, 1.94) vs American Indian/Alaska Native lesbian women 2.06 (95% CI, 1.56, 2.70). Findings also differed between bisexual and lesbian women within racial and ethnic minority groups.

Obesity and overweight may start at a young age in lesbian and bisexual youth, and they may conceptualize their weight differently than heterosexual peers. Among adolescents in the Massachusetts Youth Risk Behavior Survey, lesbian and bisexual females were more likely to self-perceive as being of healthy weight or underweight despite being overweight or obese, and 33% engaged in hazardous weight control behaviors. A high school–based study (grades 9–12) in 22 Wisconsin schools revealed that sexual minority female youth, compared to their heterosexual counterparts, were less likely to participate in team sports, and in college, only one of three lesbian, bisexual, and queer women met national physical activity guidelines. Overweight and obesity may also develop as women age. When women were followed longitudinally, lesbian women were more at risk for developing obesity than heterosexual women. Studies of physical activity have found that while there may be greater physical activity and fitness among some sexual minority women, so is increased sedentary time. There have also been findings of differences in dietary patterns between lesbian, bisexual, and heterosexual women.

Studies about successful weight intervention programs for lesbian and bisexual women are emerging. A United

States Office on Women's Health–funded study of a 12-session intervention program targeted to lesbian and bisexual women over 60 years of age found the program to be efficacious with a 3.7% decrease in waist circumference. Further, randomized interventions using mindfulness, healthy eating, and physical activity in obese lesbian and bisexual women were effective in reducing low-density lipoprotein cholesterol and increasing healthy eating. Focus groups have identified themes related to weight for lesbian and bisexual women: aging, physical and mental health status, community norms, subgroup differences, family and partner support, and awareness and tracking of diet and physical activity. Participants expressed feeling unprepared for age-related changes to their health and voiced interest in interventions addressing these issues. Findings from focus groups included (1) a preference for interventions focusing on promoting health and full life participation rather than on weight loss only, (2) cultural norms within the lesbian community that were accepting of larger body types, (3) an increased awareness in older age that the larger body size may exacerbate chronic health problems such as knee pain, and (4) the importance of social support and group structures in initiating and maintaining healthy behaviors. Bodily norms and health ideologies are embedded and embodied in communities and navigated through the ongoing formation and configuration of communities over time.

Ingraham N. Perceptions of body size and health among older queer women of size following participation in a health programme. Cult Health Sex. 2018 Oct 8:1–14. [PMID: 30295146]
VanKim NA et al. Dietary patterns during adulthood among lesbian, bisexual, and heterosexual women in the Nurses' Health Study II. J Acad Nutr Diet. 2017 Mar;117(3):386–95. [PMID: 27889314]
Wood SM et al. Disparities in body mass index trajectories from adolescence to early adulthood for sexual minority women. J Adolesc Health. 2017 Dec;61(6):722–8. [PMID: 28935384]

Prevention of Diabetes

Lesbian and bisexual women are more likely than heterosexual women to exhibit risk factors for type 2 diabetes. In the Nurse's Health Study II, lesbian and bisexual women had a 27% higher risk of developing type 2 diabetes than heterosexual women. BMI mediated the relationship between sexual orientation and type 2 diabetes: the incidence rate ratio was completely attenuated when BMI was added to the model. Thus, efforts to prevent, detect, and manage obesity would hopefully decrease this health disparity in female sexual minorities.

Corliss HL et al. Risk of type 2 diabetes among lesbian, bisexual, and heterosexual women: findings from the Nurses' Health Study II. Diabetes Care. 2018 Jul;41(7):1448–54. [PMID: 29720541]

Prevention of Pulmonary Disease

Pulmonary disease has not been rigorously studied in lesbian or bisexual women. However, with the increased prevalence of smoking in these women compared to heterosexual women, there may be more acute respiratory illness, chronic pulmonary disease, and lung cancer—especially with increasing age. Lesbian women have a higher prevalence of lifetime and current asthma, even when statistical models are used to correct for current and past smoking, and obesity, all of which are increased in lesbian and bisexual women. Overweight or obese lesbian and bisexual women are more than seven times more likely to report current asthma and three times more likely to report lifetime asthma than lesbian and bisexual women who are not overweight or obese.

Dai H et al. Sleep deprivation and chronic health conditions among sexual minority adults. Behav Sleep Med. 2017 Jun 28:1–15. [PMID: 28657361]
Fredriksen-Goldsen KI et al. Chronic health conditions and key health indicators among lesbian, gay, and bisexual older US adults, 2013–2014. Am J Public Health. 2017 Aug;107(8):1332–8. [PMID: 28700299]

Prevention of Sexually Transmitted Infections

STIs occur in lesbian and bisexual women, but little population-based data are available to delineate precise risks. Asking about sexual *behaviors* in addition to sexual *identity* is key to identifying STI risk and advising appropriate testing, since risk may vary by specific sexual practice (eg, digital-vaginal, vaginal-vaginal, digital-anal, oral-vaginal, oral-anal contact) and the specific pathogen. Often data are mixed and inconsistent with respect to whether sources speak to infection risk by identity group or behavior. Both behavior-based risk and identity-based risk are important for assessments and interventions. We use language of identity or behavior as consistent with original research. Women who have sex with women (WSW) are noted by the CDC to have diverse sexual practices and that use of barrier protection in examined studies (eg, use of gloves, dental dams) was ubiquitously low.

Chlamydial infections were higher in 14- to 24-year-old women who reported same-sex behavior when attending family planning clinics in the US Pacific Northwest compared to women who reported exclusively heterosexual behavior. Possible explanations for this observation include differences in these groups' use of reproductive health care services, infrequent use of barrier methods to prevent STI transmission with female partners, trends toward higher-risk behaviors, and different social network characteristics. Untreated chlamydial infection places a woman's future fertility at risk due to potential fallopian tube occlusion. Some women who have a chlamydial infection do not have symptoms. Secondary sequelae of chlamydia include intra-abdominal abscesses, chronic pain, and the need for multiple surgeries. Regardless of sexual orientation, the CDC recommends annual *Chlamydia trachomatis* (and *Neisseria gonorrheae*) screening from the age of first sexual activity to the age of 25 years for all women.

It is important to ask lesbian and bisexual women about specific sexual practices, as some practices may carry a higher risk of STIs than others, although there has been little research on sexual practices and the risk of STIs in this population. Thus, inferences are drawn from heterosexual prevention of these infections. "Safer Sex Kits" have occasionally been distributed to WSW and women who have sex with women and men (WSWM) to decrease the risk of STIs, but intervention effectiveness has not been studied. These kits often include dental dams to prevent transmission of bacteria and viruses from oral sex, but the efficacy of dental dams for this function has not been studied. Female latex condoms and latex gloves may provide better protection against infectious transmission from oral sex since latex has been studied as a barrier for prevention of HIV and other STIs. Exchange of blood should be avoided as much as possible, especially in HIV-discordant lesbian couples, since viral genotype analysis has confirmed that HIV can be transmitted sexually between women. The clinician should encourage both partners in new lesbian couples to have comprehensive STI and HIV screening prior to sexual contact and recommend barrier protection for 6 months until the couple is again screened to verify that their HIV status is still negative. If the couple is consistently monogamous and HIV and other STI testing is negative, barrier precautions do not need to be continued. However, lesbian and bisexual women may not follow this advice, since many feel they are at low risk for HIV, which may be correct, but data are lacking. About 20–50% of lesbian women use sexual aids (eg, vibrators, dildos, or other sexual toys); these should not be shared with partners and should be cleaned after use. The human papillomavirus (HPV) can remain on these sexual aids for up to 24 hours after use, even after standard cleaning. Some lesbian and bisexual women are sex workers or have had sexual relationships with high-risk male sexual partners (sometimes gay male friends) and are at increased risk for STIs. Current CDC guidelines recommend that all women should be tested once in their lifetime for HIV, with testing repeated according to risk factors.

The herpes simplex virus (HSV) can be transmitted sexually between women. The same precautions regarding the transmission of HSV should be provided to lesbian, bisexual, and heterosexual women; there should be no sexual contact during any prodromal symptoms that may precede a genital herpes outbreak or during the blister stage of the outbreak. Suppression of lesions can usually be accomplished with antiviral medications, such as acyclovir or valacyclovir, if the lesions are recurrent (see Chapter 6).

There is evidence of HPV transmission between female sexual partners. Certain strains of HPV are causally related to many precancerous and cancerous lesions, including cervical dysplasia and cervical cancer (see Chapter 18). Ten percent of lesbian women have never had sex with men, yet cervical dysplasia and cervical cancer develop in some of these women. All women (including lesbian women) need cervical cancer screening, which may include Papanicolaou smears, high-risk HPV strain testing, or both, according to timetables and risk factors provided by professional society guidelines. The rate of HPV vaccination in lesbian women, though previously thought to be less than heterosexual women, has increased recently and is now equal to that of heterosexual women, yet bisexual women are vaccinated more frequently than either lesbian or heterosexual women. However, overall the HPV vaccination rate is low in adult women regardless of sexual orientation, so improvement in all groups should be the goal. Administration of the HPV vaccine is critical to the prevention of cervical cancer, and the age group to receive the HPV vaccine has now been expanded by the FDA to 45 years old. Despite recommendations that cervical cancer screening, usually Papanicolaou testing be performed regardless of sexual orientation, Papanicolaou testing varies according to identity irrespective of behavior and some studies modify screening according to identity and behavior though perhaps suboptimally. In a national probability sample of who underwent Papanicolaou testing, WSWM had the same odds of testing as WSM only, whereas women with lifetime female partners had lower odds of testing. Those who identified as bisexual also had lower odds of testing.

Trichomonas vaginalis can be transmitted easily between female sexual partners. One study of women attending an STI clinic in the United States noted that *T vaginalis* was the most common curable STI found in this population with a prevalence of 17% in WSW and 24% in WSWM.

Bacterial vaginosis is common among women and, according to the CDC, even more common among WSW. It is unknown whether bacterial vaginosis can be transmitted between women. A study from Australia found a 27% prevalence of bacterial vaginosis in women and their female partners; risk factors for bacterial vaginosis were four or more lifetime female sexual partners, a female partner with bacterial vaginosis symptoms, and smoking at least 30 cigarettes weekly. Routine screening for bacterial vaginosis, though, is not currently recommended and testing should be based on symptoms. One approach for a WSW who has symptomatic bacterial vaginosis is to treat her and not her female sexual partner. If symptoms recur, her female sexual partner(s) should be evaluated and treated with consideration of re-treating the index woman. This strategy may also be used for treatment of recurrent or hard to treat vulvovaginal candidiasis, which technically is not considered to be sexually transmitted, but anecdotally, improvement has occurred with treatment of the index patient and female partner.

Various strategies for making reproductive and sexual health clinics and providers more amenable to serving LGBTQ people were studied by a group in the United States, but the findings (such as ensuring counseling involves inclusive safe sex discussions that are relevant to LGBTQ people) have broad face validity and relevance for other regional and medical focus settings as well.

Everett BG et al. Do sexual minorities receive appropriate sexual and reproductive health care and counseling? J Womens Health (Larchmt). 2019 Jan;28(1):53–62. [PMID: 30372369]
Wingo E et al. Reproductive health care priorities and barriers to effective care for LGBTQ people assigned female at birth: a qualitative study. Womens Health Issues. 2018 Jul–Aug; 28(4):350–7. [PMID: 29661698]

Prevention of Substance Use

Substance use is higher in lesbian and bisexual women compared to heterosexual women and is especially well-documented for cigarette smoking and alcohol use. A secondary analysis of alcohol, tobacco, and other drug use among lesbian and bisexual women in the American College Health Association's National College Health Assessment revealed that bisexual women had greater odds of using alcohol, tobacco, and marijuana than heterosexual women and lesbian women. In addition, bisexual women had greater odds of using all illicit drugs (except steroids) and misusing prescription drugs than heterosexual women. Furthermore, bisexual women had greater odds of using amphetamines other than methamphetamine, sedatives, and 3,4-methylenedioxymethamphetamine (MDMA; Ecstasy) when compared to lesbian women. Lesbian women had greater odds of using tobacco, marijuana, sedatives, hallucinogens, and other illicit drugs and misusing prescription drugs than heterosexual women. This increased rate of substance use persists for bisexual women over the age of 25 but decreases for lesbian women at that time.

Multiple interventions have been initiated to decrease alcohol and other substance use in lesbian and bisexual female youth. In Canada, there were significant lower odds of binge-drinking among lesbian and bisexual youth in schools with longer-established Gay-Straight Alliances. Recommendations for improving substance use treatment for sexual minority persons include providing interventionists with training in LGBTQ cultural sensitivity. Another approach studied in the rural United States looked at training and deploying LGBTQ peer-advocates to support mental health and substance use and "bridge the gap in culturally competent care." More work is needed to study specific interventions outcomes research, however, comparing LGBTQ adapted materials with routine materials. Some LGBTQ clients in these programs find it hard to "come out" to a group that potentially includes members who may be homophobic. Sexual minority women, compared to heterosexual women, with lifetime alcohol use disorders are at heightened risk for concomitant psychiatric and drug use disorders, underscoring the need for substance abuse programs to provide access to individual counseling with mental health professionals.

Israel T et al. Development and evaluation of training for rural LGBTQ mental health peer advocates. Rural Ment Health. 2016 Jan;40(1):40–62. [PMID: 27516816]

Mereish EH et al. Sexual orientation disparities in psychiatric and drug use disorders among a nationally representative sample of women with alcohol use disorders. Addict Behav. 2015 Aug;47:80–5. [PMID: 25899096]

Schuler MS et al. Disparities in substance use behaviors and disorders among adult sexual minorities by age, gender, and sexual identity. Drug Alcohol Depend. 2018 Aug 1;189:139–46. [PMID: 29944989]

▶ Cancer Risk, Prevention, & Treatment

Very little is known about the incidence and prevalence of various cancers in lesbian and bisexual women, since sexual orientation has not been routinely included in cancer screening programs and cancer registries. However, data suggest that sexual minority women may be at a higher risk for cancer-related mortality than heterosexual counterparts. Investigators from the Women's Health Study

compared sexual minority veterans and civilians to their heterosexual counterparts and found that sexual minority women veterans had a higher risk of cancer-specific mortality. Information from the US National Health Interview Survey showed that lesbian and bisexual women have cancer risk factors, such as tobacco use, underscoring the need for vigilant screening. Since lesbian and bisexual women have barriers to accessing health care and may not see a clinician on an annual basis, any visit to a health care provider is an opportunity to check on cancer screening status (eg, colonoscopy, mammography, cervical cancer screening). There is also recognition that upon receiving a cancer diagnosis, LGBTQ people face challenges in receiving equitable care throughout the cancer care continuum and may experience cancer differently and have different needs during their care; heterosexual and sexual minority cancer survivors in the UK reported receiving different care. The US National Cancer Care Network Guidelines do not address how SGM status should be considered in site-specific guidelines. One qualitative study with SGM breast cancer survivors underscored the challenges of disclosing sexual orientation during cancer care and the importance of provider recognition that varying social networks are critical to positive experiences of care provision. The 2017 American Society for Clinical Oncology position statement recommends five action steps to enhance SGM cancer care and reduce disparities: (1) patient education and support, (2) workforce development and diversity, (3) quality improvement strategies, (4) policy solutions, and (5) research strategies. All providers need to consider whether their prevention, screening, diagnostic, treatment, and palliative approaches will be equitably experienced by lesbian and bisexual women.

Brown MT et al. Unmet support needs of sexual and gender minority breast cancer survivors. Support Care Cancer. 2018 Apr;26(4):1189–96. [PMID: 29080921]

Hudson J et al. Sexual and gender minority issues across NCCN Guidelines: results from a national survey. J Natl Compr Canc Netw. 2017 Nov;15(11):1379–82. [PMID: 29118229]

Hulbert-Williams NJ et al. The cancer care experiences of gay, lesbian and bisexual patients: a secondary analysis of data from the UK Cancer Patient Experience Survey. Eur J Cancer Care (Engl). 2017 Jul;26(4). [PMID: 28239936]

Obedin-Maliver J. Time to change: supporting sexual and gender minority people-an underserved, understudied cancer risk population. J Natl Compr Canc Netw. 2017 Nov;15(11):1305–8. [PMID: 29118223]

A. Breast Cancer

The literature has been mixed on whether lesbian and bisexual women have a slight increased risk of breast cancer compared to heterosexual women. A 2013 systemic review found the few prevalence studies of breast cancer in lesbians unreliable; however, lesbian women do have an increased prevalence of risk factors predisposing to breast cancer, including nulliparity (and decreased breastfeeding), alcohol use, obesity, and smoking. The literature is also inconsistent regarding the rate of mammography screening in lesbian women; however, a study done in Massachusetts showed that bisexual women were less likely than heterosexual women and lesbian women to adhere to mammography screening guidelines. Lesbian and bisexual women who have breast cancer may not want reconstruction at the same rate as heterosexual women and often find that breast cancer support groups focus on issues for heterosexual women (such as attractiveness to a male partner).

B. Cervical Cancer

Primary prevention of cervical cancer is essential. All people between the ages of 9 and 45 years (routine recommended age is 11 to 12 years old) should receive the HPV vaccine series. HPV can be transmitted sexually between lesbian or heterosexual partners. Cervical cancer screening, with Papanicolaou smears, primary HPV testing, or both, should be part of lesbian and bisexual women's health care at the same intervals as for heterosexual women according to national guidelines. Lesbian and bisexual women, however, receive Papanicolaou smears at a lower rate than sexually active heterosexual women, in part because many of the Papanicolaou smears are done in reproductive health clinics; lesbians who are not interested in becoming pregnant or avoiding pregnancy may not access these clinical sites. In addition, some lesbian patients as well as their health care providers mistakenly think that lesbian women do not need Papanicolaou smears. *All lesbian and bisexual women need cervical cancer screening starting at the age of 21, consistent with recommendations for cervical cancer screening for all women.*

C. Lung Cancer

Compared to heterosexual women, the rate of lung cancer is likely higher in lesbian and bisexual women compared to heterosexual women due to their increased rate of smoking. The incidence and prevalence of lung cancer, however, have not been determined in this sexual minority population.

D. Endometrial and Ovarian Cancer

Endometrial and ovarian cancer are increased among those with nulliparity, which is more likely in sexual minority women. Obesity, a known risk factor for both cancers, appears to be more prevalent among sexual minority women. Conversely, the use of oral contraceptives, which is protective against the development of both of these cancers, is lower in lesbian women than in heterosexual women. Vigilance toward and education about presenting signs and symptoms (eg, postmenopausal bleeding, early satiety, unintended weight loss) are important to detect cancers as early as possible. Neither incidence nor prevalence of endometrial or ovarian cancer has been determined in this sexual minority population.

Bazzi AR et al. Adherence to mammography screening guidelines among transgender persons and sexual minority women. Am J Public Health. 2015 Nov;105(11):2356–8. [PMID: 26378843]

Lunn MR et al. Sociodemographic characteristics and health outcomes among lesbian, gay, and bisexual U.S. adults using Healthy People 2020 leading health indicators. LGBT Health. 2017 Aug;4(4):283–94. [PMID: 28727950]

Simoni JM et al. Disparities in physical health conditions among lesbian and bisexual women: a systematic review of population-based studies. J Homosex. 2017;64(1):32–44. [PMID: 27074088]

▶ Prevention of Violence

Compared to heterosexual women, lesbian and bisexual women have higher exposures to violence throughout their lifetimes. Lifetime prevalence of sexual assault may be as high as 85%. In a study of four countries in southern Africa, nearly one-third of lesbian and bisexual women experienced forced sex and assault including "corrective rape" by men as an attempt to change the women's sexual orientation. In a study in the state of Sao Paul in Brazil, qualitative interviews were done of youth coming out to their families: The family reactions were often violent, with persecution and even expulsion from the home, which impacted their health and quality of life.

The CDC reports that 61% of bisexual women and 44% of lesbian women experience rape, physical violence, and stalking by an intimate partner. These rates are higher than similar trauma in heterosexual women (35%). Additionally, approximately 20% of bisexual women compared with 10% of heterosexual women have been raped by an intimate partner in their lifetimes. The rate of stalking experienced by bisexual women is twice that of heterosexual women and a higher percentage of bisexual women report being afraid of an intimate partner. Despite alarming rates for women of any identity, lesbian and bisexual women survivors of sexual assault and interpersonal violence may experience unique difficulties when seeking assistance. These problems include a limited understanding of interpersonal violence in the relationships of lesbian and bisexual women, stigma, and systemic inequities (such as shelters unwelcome to this population, perpetrating partners being allowed into the same shelters as the survivor of the domestic violence, "outing" someone as a psychological threat, and staff lacking cultural sensitivity and appropriate training in working with lesbian and bisexual women). Barriers to preventing LGBTQ violence include stigma, systemic discrimination, and a lack of understanding of LGBTQ intimate partner violence.

Community violence is experienced more frequently by LGBTQ persons. In-depth interviews of 19 Flemish sexual minority victims of violence revealed the use of four coping strategies: (1) avoidance, (2) assertiveness and confrontation, (3) cognitive change, and (4) social support. Applying these coping skills and actively attaching meaning to negative experiences helped victims of anti-LGBTQ violence overcome fear, embarrassment, or depressive feelings. The presence of a supportive network was important in facilitating the positive outcomes.

Braga IF et al. Family violence against gay and lesbian adolescents and young people: a qualitative study. Rev Bras Enferm. 2018;71(suppl 3):1220–7. [PMID: 29972518]

Calton JM et al. Barriers to help seeking for lesbian, gay, bisexual, transgender, and queer survivors of intimate partner violence. Trauma Violence Abuse. 2016 Dec;17(5):585–600. [PMID: 25979872]

D'haese L et al. Coping with antigay violence: in-depth interviews with Flemish LGB adults. J Sex Res. 2015;52(8):912–23. [PMID: 26010740]

Mellins CA et al. Sexual assault incidents among college undergraduates: prevalence and factors associated with risk. PLoS One. 2017 Nov 8;12(11):e0186471. Erratum in: PLoS One. 2018 Jan 25;13(1):e0192129. [PMID: 29117226]

Walters ML et al. The National Intimate Partner and Sexual Violence Survey (NISVS): 2010 Findings on Victimization by Sexual Orientation. Atlanta, GA: National Center for Injury Prevention and Control, Centers for Disease Control and Prevention. https://www.cdc.gov/violenceprevention/pdf/nisvs_sofindings.pdf

▶ Prevention of Mental Disorders

Lesbians and bisexual women have an increased risk of depression. Many of the health disparities and health risks faced by lesbians and bisexual women, such as depression and cardiovascular risk, have been attributed to Ilan Meyer's theory of minority stress. This theory proposes that individuals who identify as a sexual minority experience chronic, additive, and unique stresses stemming from living in social conditions that are characterized by prejudice and discrimination. Therefore, rather than identifying mental health problems as synonymous with a sexual minority identity or stemming from in-born association with minority sexual orientation, minority stress causes mental health challenges that stem from societal discrimination and stigma borne by individuals with minority identities (and behaviors). An examination of lesbian and bisexual women veterans from the United States Behavioral Risk Factor Surveillance System found that sexual minority women veterans were three times more likely than heterosexual women to experience "mental distress." Mortality risk from suicide is also elevated among women with same-sex partners. There is evidence from the United States National Epidemiologic Survey on Alcohol and Related Conditions–III that bisexual women had greater rates of specific psychiatric disorders than lesbians or heterosexual women. Resilience factors that are protective for mental distress and poorer mental health among lesbian, gay, bisexual, queer and questioning youth and adults in Israel included family support as well as other community-level factors, such as friends' support, LGBT connectedness, and having a steady partner. How parents react to an adolescent's "coming out" has a profound effect on their child's health outcomes. For those adolescents whose parents were supportive, there was less homelessness, depression, substance use, and unprotected sex. Interventions for building resilience can be important in achieving a reduction in anxiety and depression. There is some evidence that online friends can serve as a buffer and social support, especially for LGBTQ youth, although in-person social support appears to be more protective against victimization. However, social media can also be a place where LGBTQ youth experience bullying.

There is evidence that being in a legally recognized same-sex relationship, particularly in marriage, diminishes mental health differences between heterosexual and lesbian, gay, and bisexual persons. In contrast, psychiatric disorders increased among lesbian, gay, and bisexual persons who lived in states in the United States that enacted constitutional amendments to ban same-sex marriage compared to states that did not. One study examined the mental health of individuals living in states before (wave 1, 2001–2002) and after (wave 2, 2004–2005) the enactment of same-sex marriage bans in 2004–2005. Among LGB respondents living in states that enacted the marriage bans, the National Epidemiologic Survey on Alcohol and Related Conditions (N = 34,653), revealed that there was a significantly increased prevalence of any mood disorder (36% increase), generalized anxiety disorder (248% increase), any alcohol use disorder (42% increase), and psychiatric comorbidity (36.3%) between wave 1 and wave 2 of the survey, suggesting that living in sociopolitical environments that do not legally recognize same-sex relationships can have deleterious effects on mental health. Mental health inequities among bisexual and lesbian women are well documented. Compared to heterosexual women, both bisexual and lesbian women are more likely to report lifetime depressive disorders, with bisexual women often faring the worst on mental health outcome. Risk factors for depression, such as victimization in childhood and adulthood, are more prevalent among bisexual women. Black bisexual and black lesbian women had significantly lower odds of depression than white lesbian women, despite their higher reports of victimization in one Chicago Health and Life Experiences of Women study, an 18-year, community-based longitudinal study of sexual minority women's health. The rate of depression in Latina bisexual and lesbian women did not differ from white lesbian women.

Bostwick WB et al. Depression and victimization in a community sample of bisexual and lesbian women: an intersectional approach. Arch Sex Behav. 2019 Jan;48(1):131–41. [PMID: 29968037]

Kerridge BT et al. Prevalence, sociodemographic correlates and DSM-5 substance use disorders and other psychiatric disorders among sexual minorities in the United States. Drug Alcohol Depend. 2017 Jan 1;170:82–92. [PMID: 27883948]

Lyons A. Resilience in lesbians and gay men: a review and key findings from a nationwide Australian survey. Int Rev Psychiatry. 2015;27(5):435–43. [PMID: 26222668]

Wight RG et al. Same-sex marriage and psychological well-being: findings from the California Health Interview Survey. Am J Public Health. 2013 Feb;103(2):339–46. [PMID: 23237155]

▼ GAY & BISEXUAL MEN'S HEALTH

Kevin L. Ard, MD, MPH
Kenneth H. Mayer, MD

This section is devoted to the primary care of cisgender (that is, non-transgender) gay, bisexual, and other MSM regardless of their sexual identity. Most health-related research that focuses on MSM categorizes men based on their sexual behavior as MSM, rather than their self-reported identification as gay, bisexual, or other identities. Although sexual identity is not always congruent with sexual behavior, identity is important to recognize in order to optimize health and health care, especially when there is a difference on the basis of sexual identity (for example, gay- vs bisexual-identified men).

Demographics

The size of the MSM population in the United States is not known with certainty due to variability in the definition of sexual orientation used in surveys and the possibility that some survey respondents do not disclose nonheterosexual orientations because of concerns about discrimination. Nevertheless, based on available data, it is estimated that at least 2.2% of American adult men identify as gay, and an additional 1.4% of men identify as bisexual. The proportion of men who engage in sex with other men or experience sexual attraction to other men is estimated to be higher, with 7.3% and 6.2% of adult men reporting some same-sex attraction and sexual behavior, respectively, in one national survey.

Stigma & Discrimination

Although social acceptance of nonheterosexual orientations is increasing, gay, bisexual, and other MSM may still experience stigma and discrimination based on their sexual orientation and/or gender expression, with significant impacts on health. In one national survey of LGBT Americans, discriminatory experiences were commonly reported: 39% of respondents endorsed experiences of rejection by family or friends, 30% had been physically attacked or threatened, 23% had been treated poorly in public, and 21% reported being treated unfairly at work. These experiences may contribute to adverse health outcomes among MSM and other SGM populations. One model of how this occurs centers on the concept of minority stress. In this model, stressors (such as experiences of prejudice, expectations of rejection, the cognitive burden of deciding whether to come out in different circumstances, and internalized homophobia) lead to anxiety, depression, and maladaptive coping behaviors, including substance use disorders and condomless sexual behavior that increases the risk for HIV and STIs. In adolescents, family rejection has been linked to increased risk of depression, homelessness, suicide attempts, illegal drug use, sexual risk-taking, and HIV/STI acquisition. Avoidance of—or delays in—seeking health care due to concerns about discrimination in medical settings may also contribute to adverse health outcomes in MSM.

Copen CE et al. Sexual behavior, sexual attraction, and sexual orientation among adults aged 18–44 in the United States: data from the 2011-2013 National Survey of Family Growth. Natl Health Stat Report. 2016 Jan 7;(88):1–14. [PMID: 26766410]

Frost DM et al. Minority stress and physical health among sexual minority individuals. J Behav Med. 2015 Feb;38(1):1–8. [PMID: 23864353]

Xu F et al. Men who have sex with men in the United States: demographic and behavioral characteristics and prevalence of HIV and HSV-2 infection: results from National Health and Nutrition Examination Survey 2001–2006. Sex Transm Dis. 2010 Jun;37(6):399–405. [PMID: 20473245]

Health Disparities

Gay, bisexual, and other MSM face health disparities stemming from the biologic aspects of their sexual behavior and/or from minority stress. Because of these disparities,

MSM have been identified as a priority population for health-related research and improvement in health care by both the National Academy of Medicine and the federal government's Healthy People initiative. These health disparities are exacerbated if young MSM have experienced early life traumatic events, such as sexual abuse or familial rejection.

Institute of Medicine (US) Committee on Lesbian, Gay, Bisexual, and Transgender Health Issues and Research Gaps and Opportunities. The health of lesbian, gay, bisexual, and transgender people: building a foundation for better understanding. Washington, DC: National Academies Press (US); 2011. [PMID: 22013611]

Office of Disease Prevention and Health Promotion (ODPHP). Healthy People 2020: lesbian, gay, bisexual, and transgender health. 2016. https://www.healthypeople.gov/2020/topics-objectives/topic/lesbian-gay-bisexual-and-transgender-health

A. HIV and Other STIs

MSM account for approximately 70% of all new HIV infections in the United States, despite representing a small proportion (less than 10% by any metric) of the country's male population. The high burden of HIV infection among MSM stems in part from the efficient transmission of the virus through receptive anal intercourse, which confers a higher risk of HIV infection than other sexual activities, such as penile-vaginal and oral intercourse. Role versatility can also uniquely potentiate HIV spread among MSM, since the same person can acquire HIV via receptive intercourse and become an efficient transmitter by engaging in insertive anal intercourse with HIV-uninfected partners. The origin of disparate HIV rates between MSM and other populations is not solely biologic in origin, however, as societal stigma and psychosocial problems also contribute to sexual risk behavior among MSM. MSM of color face an increased risk of HIV; the CDC estimates that the lifetime risk of HIV infection is 1 in 2 for African American MSM and 1 in 4 for Latino MSM compared to 1 in 11 for white MSM. Racial and ethnic disparities in HIV infections among MSM do not appear to be due to differences in sexual behavior or substance use but rather factors such as lack of access to medical care, lower rates of recent HIV testing among nonwhite MSM, and assortative mixing (ie, being more likely to have sex with partners from one's own racial or ethnic group).

Beyond HIV, some STIs are more common among MSM. In 2017, 58% of primary and secondary syphilis diagnoses occurred in MSM or men who have sex with both men and women. Syphilis is associated with a high risk of subsequent HIV acquisition in MSM and may serve as a marker for individuals who could benefit from intensive HIV prevention efforts, such as the initiation of PrEP. In addition, increased cases of ocular syphilis, occasionally resulting in blindness have been reported, with a majority of cases occurring in MSM. The incidence of gonorrhea among MSM exceeds that among men who have sex with women (MSW) and has increased. MSM also are more likely than MSW to be infected with gonorrhea, including antibiotic-resistant strains. Many gonococcal infections in MSM occur at extragenital sites (ie, the pharynx or the rectum) where they may be asymptomatic, underscoring the importance of eliciting a comprehensive sexual history, including an inventory of potential anatomic exposures, in order to provide optimal health care to MSM.

MSM also face increased risks of viral hepatitis. Outbreaks of hepatitis A infection have been documented in MSM, likely due to anal sexual contact, including oral-anal exposure ("rimming") as well as insertive and receptive practices. Likewise, hepatitis B is more common among MSM than the general population; approximately 20% of MSM have evidence of either current or prior infection with hepatitis B by age 30. This highlights the importance of universal hepatitis A and B vaccination for young MSM, preferably prior to the initiation of sexual contact. Finally, although hepatitis C is generally not efficiently transmitted via sexual contact, hepatitis C infection has been identified as a problem among HIV-infected and high-risk HIV-uninfected MSM and is associated with condomless receptive anal sex, group sex, manual insertion of fingers into the rectum ("fisting"), and recent STIs, which make the rectal mucosa more susceptible to hepatitis C acquisition.

HPV infection, which can cause anogenital warts, anal dysplasia, and anal cancer, is more common among MSM than MSW. A meta-analysis estimated the prevalence of the oncogenic HPV type 16 in the anal canal to be 35.4% among HIV-infected MSM and 12.5% among MSM without HIV. Correspondingly, anal cancer incidence is higher among HIV-infected versus HIV-uninfected MSM. Studies are underway to determine the optimal frequency of screening for anal cellular atypia and follow-up high resolution anoscopy for sexually active MSM.

Enteric infections may be sexually transmitted among MSM engaging in anal sexual contact, especially oral-anal sexual contact, and should be considered in the differential diagnosis of gastrointestinal complaints. These infections include giardiasis, amebiasis, and shigellosis. In addition, *Shigella* infections are more likely to be antibiotic resistant among MSM than among other individuals.

Clusters of meningococcal disease among MSM in the United States and Europe have also been reported, particularly those frequenting sexualized environments, including saunas and bathhouses, prompting some jurisdictions to recommend meningococcal vaccination for high-risk MSM. Intimate contact with multiple partners has been identified as a risk factor for infection in some of these outbreaks.

Centers for Disease Control and Prevention (CDC). HIV among African American gay and bisexual men. 2017. https://www.cdc.gov/hiv/group/msm/bmsm.html

Centers for Disease Control and Prevention (CDC). HIV among gay and bisexual men. 2017. http://www.cdc.gov/hiv/group/msm/index.html

Nanduri S et al. Outbreak of serogroup C meningococcal disease primarily affecting men who have sex with men—Southern California, 2016. MMWR Morb Mortal Wkly Rep. 2016 Sep 9;65(35):939–40. [PMID: 27606798]

Nyitray AG et al. Incidence, duration, persistence, and factors associated with high-risk anal human papillomavirus persistence among HIV-negative men who have sex with men: a multinational study. Clin Infect Dis. 2016 Jun 1;62(11):1367–74. [PMID: 26962079]

Stall R et al. Association of co-occurring psychosocial health problems and increased vulnerability to HIV/AIDS among urban men who have sex with men. Am J Public Health. 2003 Jun;93(6):939–42. [PMID: 12773359]

Vanhommerig JW et al; MOSAIC (MSM Observational Study of Acute Infection With Hepatitis C) Study Group. Risk factors for sexual transmission of hepatitis C virus among human immunodeficiency virus-infected men who have sex with men: a case-control study. Open Forum Infect Dis. 2015 Aug 6;2(3):ofv115. [PMID: 26634219]

B. Mental Health

Likely due to minority stress (ie, growing up in non-affirming societies), MSM experience mental health disorders more commonly than other men. Whether defined by self-reported identity as gay or bisexual or behaviorally by report of sexual activity with other men, MSM have a higher lifetime prevalence of depression and anxiety disorders than men who identify as heterosexual and/or who report sexual activity only with women. Behaviorally bisexual men experience a higher burden of both depression and anxiety disorders, compared to men who engage in only homosexual behavior, in part because bisexual men may not have access to defined communities of choice, like self-identified gay men. The increased prevalence of mental health disorders among behaviorally bisexual men may also stem from dual stigmatization by both the heterosexual and gay male communities, as well as internalized stigma. Among MSM overall, anti-gay violence, community alienation, and dissatisfaction with an idealized body image have all been associated with depression.

Bostwick WB et al. Dimensions of sexual orientation and the prevalence of mood and anxiety disorders in the United States. Am J Public Health. 2010 Mar;100(3):468–75. [PMID: 19696380]

C. Substance Use

Compared to men with only female sexual partners, MSM are more likely to report lifetime recreational drug use; they are specifically more likely to have used cocaine, hallucinogens, inhalants, analgesics, and tranquilizers. In addition, men who identify as gay or bisexual are more likely to smoke cigarettes than those who identify as heterosexual. Although it is not clear that MSM are more likely than others to use methamphetamines, methamphetamine use in MSM communities has been linked to increased sexual risk behavior and transmission of hepatitis C, HIV, and other STIs. Consistent with the minority stress model, experiences of discrimination have been independently associated with substance use among MSM. Several studies have indicated that substance use programs that integrate support for minority sexual identity for MSM can result in long-term successful outcomes.

Fallin A et al. Smoking characteristics among lesbian, gay, and bisexual adults. Prev Med. 2015 May;74:123–30. [PMID: 25485860]

Hoenigl M et al. Clear links between starting methamphetamine and increasing sexual risk behavior: a cohort study among men who have sex with men. J Acquir Immune Defic Syndr. 2016 Apr 15;71(5):551–7. [PMID: 26536321]

McCabe SE et al. The relationship between discrimination and substance use disorders among lesbian, gay, and bisexual adults in the United States. Am J Public Health. 2010 Oct;100(10):1946–52. [PMID: 20075317]

▶ Preventive Care & Clinical Practice Guidelines

Clinicians can help address health disparities affecting MSM by following clinical practice guidelines that pertain to this population (Table 42–1). The CDC recommends that sexually active MSM undergo screening for HIV, syphilis, gonorrhea, and chlamydia annually and more often if the risk history warrants more frequent assessment. An HIV antibody-antigen assay is preferred for HIV screening because this test increases the sensitivity for detection of acute or recent HIV infection. Nucleic acid amplification testing (NAAT) provides optimal sensitivity for diagnosis of gonorrhea and chlamydia and can be performed on the oropharynx, rectum, urine, and urethra. Although oropharyngeal testing for chlamydia is not recommended, MSM should otherwise be screened for these infections at any of the aforementioned sites that may have been exposed during sex, regardless of condom use. First-catch urine and urethral specimens for gonorrhea and chlamydia NAAT in men provide comparable accuracy; thus, there is no advantage to the urethral swab for routine screening. Rectal swabs for NAAT can be self-collected.

The CDC also recommends that MSM be screened for chronic hepatitis B infection at least once in their lives and that they be vaccinated against hepatitis A and B. Annual hepatitis C screening with a hepatitis C antibody test is recommended for HIV-infected MSM due to the elevated incidence of this infection in this population and the advent of well-tolerated, curative therapy. HIV-uninfected MSM engaging in traumatic sexual practices, such as group sex, fisting, and any other practice that may abrade the rectal mucosa, may also benefit from annual HCV screening.

Both the CDC and the World Health Organization recommend PrEP for HIV with the fixed-dose combination of tenofovir disoproxil fumarate–emtricitabine for MSM at high risk for HIV infection (see Chapter 31). Individuals at high risk include those who engage in condomless anal sex outside of a monogamous relationship with an HIV-uninfected man; those who have recently been diagnosed with a bacterial STI; and those whose sexual partners are HIV-infected. However, the utility of PrEP is likely low in the latter scenario if the relationship is monogamous and the HIV-infected partner is consistently virologically suppressed on antiretroviral therapy, because antiretroviral therapy significantly reduces the likelihood of HIV transmission through sexual contact. PrEP has been shown in randomized controlled trials to prevent HIV infection in MSM and is addressed in more detail in Chapter 31.

Table 42–1. Clinical practice guidelines pertaining to the care of MSM.

Recommendation	Comments
Immunizations	
Human papillomavirus (quadri- or nonavalent)	Up to age 26 years
Hepatitis A and B	Consider prevaccination serologic testing if the immunization history is uncertain; vaccinate if seronegative
Meningococcal	Recommended by some jurisdictions due to outbreaks of meningococcal disease among MSM
Medications	
Preexposure prophylaxis for HIV	For MSM at high, ongoing risk of HIV infection (eg, condomless anal sex, recent STI diagnosis, HIV-infected sexual partner)
Postexposure prophylaxis for HIV	Consists of 28 days of antiretroviral medication following a discrete exposure to HIV
Screening Tests	
HIV serology	At least annually, more often if high risk
Syphilis serology	At least annually, more often if high risk
Nucleic acid amplification test for gonorrhea and chlamydia	At least annually, more often if high risk; all potentially exposed sites (oropharynx, urethra, rectum) should be screened, as indicated by the sexual history
Hepatitis C serology	Annually for HIV-infected MSM and HIV-uninfected MSM engaging in behaviors that might expose them to blood (for example, injection drug use or traumatic anal sexual practices)
Anal cytology	For HIV-infected MSM; the appropriateness of anal cytology for HIV-uninfected MSM is under study
Behavioral health (depression, substance use)	At the first clinical encounter, with follow-up screening for those who report behavioral health concerns

MSM, men who have sex with men; STI, sexually transmitted infection.

Clinicians who care for MSM should also be aware of postexposure prophylaxis (PEP), which consists of antiretrovirals started within 72 hours of a discrete exposure to HIV and taken for 28 days, and either provide PEP themselves or be able to rapidly link patients to PEP care (see Chapter 31).

While HPV immunization with the quadrivalent or nonavalent vaccines is recommended for all boys and young men up to age 21 years, vaccination is recommended for MSM up to age 26. The HIV Medicine Association (HIVMA) recommends routinely screening HIV-infected MSM for anal cancer with anal cytology; however, this approach has not yet been proven to be beneficial in a randomized controlled clinical trial. In addition, the optimal screening interval (ages at which to initiate and cease screening) and management of abnormal results are not clearly defined. Patients with abnormal anal cytology are typically referred for high-resolution anoscopy with biopsy. Colonoscopy performed for colon cancer screening is not considered a substitute for anal cytology or high-resolution anoscopy because colonoscopy does not assess for cellular abnormalities in the anal canal. Anal cytology screening of HIV-uninfected MSM is not currently recommended in any national consensus guidelines, although some clinicians perform this screening due to the elevated risk of anal cancer in these men. Large prospective studies are underway in the United States and Australia to attempt to address the questions related to optimal timing of anal HPV screening for MSM.

Finally, clinicians should ensure that MSM are offered preventive care recommended for all individuals, including smoking cessation counseling and pharmacotherapy, screening for depression, and assessment for and counseling about alcohol misuse (see Lesbian and Bisexual Women's Health, above). Some studies have found that behavioral health programs tailored specifically for MSM are more effective in promoting healthy behaviors than those that are not culturally sensitive.

Aberg JA et al. Primary care guidelines for the management of persons infected with HIV: 2013 update by the HIV Medicine Association of the Infectious Diseases Society of America. Clin Infect Dis. 2014 Jan;58(1):1–10. [PMID: 24343580]

Centers for Disease Control and Prevention (CDC). Updated guidelines for antiretroviral postexposure prophylaxis after sexual, injection-drug use, or other nonoccupational exposure to HIV—United States, 2016. MMWR Morb Mortal Wkly Rep. 2016 May 6;65(17):458. [PMID: 27149423]

Grant RM et al. Preexposure chemoprophylaxis for HIV prevention in men who have sex with men. N Engl J Med. 2010 Dec 30;363(27):2587–99. [PMID: 21091279]

Jain S et al. The transition from postexposure prophylaxis to preexposure prophylaxis: an emerging opportunity for biobehavioral HIV prevention. Clin Infect Dis. 2015 Jun 1;60(Suppl 3):S200–4. [PMID: 25972505]

McCormack S et al. Pre-exposure prophylaxis to prevent the acquisition of HIV-1 infection (PROUD): effectiveness results from the pilot phase of a pragmatic open-label randomised trial. Lancet. 2016 Jan 2;387(10013):53–60. [PMID: 26364263]

Reback CJ et al. Development of an evidence-based, gay-specific cognitive behavioral therapy intervention for methamphetamine-abusing gay and bisexual men. Addict Behav. 2014 Aug;39(8):1286–91. [PMID: 22169619]

Rodger AJ et al. Sexual activity without condoms and risk of HIV transmission in serodifferent couples when the HIV-positive partner is using suppressive antiretroviral therapy. JAMA. 2016 Jul 12;316(2):171–81. Erratum in: JAMA. 2016 Nov 15;316(19):2048. [PMID: 27404185]

TRANSGENDER HEALTH & DISEASE PREVENTION

Madeline B. Deutsch, MD, MPH

▶ Terminology

Transgender (abbr: "trans") people have a gender identity that differs from the sex they were assigned at birth. Gender identity describes a person's internal sense of gender. Sex refers to the sex assigned at birth typically by the attending medical provider, based on assessment of external genitalia. In everyday language "sex" and "gender" are used interchangeably; however, in the context of transgender people, the meanings differ. Gender expression describes the outward manner in which an individual expresses or displays gender, including choices in clothing and hairstyle, speech, and mannerisms. Gender identity and gender expression may differ; for example, a woman (transgender or non-transgender) may have an androgynous appearance, or a man (transgender or non-transgender) may have a feminine form of self-expression. Transgender people may not feel comfortable, or be unable to, outwardly express their internal felt sense of gender due to societal, work, or family pressures. Transgender people who have a well documented and persistent gender identity that differs from their sex assigned at birth and are experiencing distress as a result of this mismatch, meet the diagnostic criteria for gender dysphoria as described in the *Diagnostic and Statistical Manual of Mental Disorders*, 5th edition (*DSM-5*).

A transgender man is someone with a male gender identity and a female birth-assigned sex; a transgender woman is someone with a female gender identity and a male birth-assigned sex. A non-transgender person may be referred to as cisgender (latin root *cis* = near/next to), which refers to people whose gender identity and birth sex are the same, ie, non-transgender. Non-binary, gender nonconforming, or genderqueer describes a person whose gender identity differs from that assigned at birth but may be more complex, fluid, multifaceted, or otherwise less clearly defined than purely male or female. Non-binary people may use neutral pronouns such as "they," "them," or "their." The term transsexual is an older term that has fallen out of favor and referred specifically to a transgender person who seeks medical interventions. Other related terms include cross dresser, which describes someone who may wear clothing of the opposite gender without a clear identification with that gender, and drag, which describes cross dressing for performance purposes. For the purposes of this text, "transgender" will be inclusive of those who identify with the terms gender non-binary, nonconforming, genderqueer, and transsexual.

Sexual orientation, which describes sexual attraction and behaviors, is not directly related to gender identity.

The sexual orientation of transgender people should be described based on the lived gender; a transgender woman attracted to other women would be a lesbian, and a transgender man attracted to other men would be a gay man.

Transgender people may seek any one of a number of gender affirming medical, surgical or related interventions. Based on research demonstrating positive effects on multiple psychosocial measures, such interventions are recognized as medically necessary by the World Professional Association for Transgender Health (WPATH), an international, multidisciplinary professional organization that publishes widely recognized standards of care. Not all transgender people seek all interventions, and some may seek none; the current standard of care is to allow each transgender person to seek only those interventions they desire to affirm their own gender identity.

Cahill SR et al. Inclusion of sexual orientation and gender identity in stage 3 meaningful use guidelines: a huge step forward for LGBT health. LGBT Health. 2016 Apr;3(2):100–2. [PMID: 26698386]

Coleman E et al. Standards of Care for the Health of Transsexual, Transgender, and Gender-Nonconforming People, Version 7. Int J Transgenderism. 2012;13(4):165–232.

Deutsch MB et al. Electronic medical records and the transgender patient: recommendations from the World Professional Association for Transgender Health EMR Working Group. J Am Med Inform Assoc. 2013 Jul–Aug;20(4):700–3. [PMID: 23631835]

▶ Medical Interventions

Many, but not all, transgender people will seek gender affirming hormone therapy and/or surgery (genitals, chest, or face). Transgender women commonly seek facial hair removal and may also seek voice feminization training. Hormone therapy allows the acquisition of secondary sex characteristics more aligned with an individual's gender identity. The WPATH Standards of Care recognize that hormone therapy is within the scope of practice for primary care providers. The Standards also permit medical providers to prescribe hormone therapy under an informed consent approach without a mental health assessment if the medical provider feels comfortable making the diagnosis of gender dysphoria.

A. Feminizing Hormone Therapy

The goal of feminizing hormone therapy is the development of female secondary sex characteristics and suppression/minimization of male secondary sex characteristics. The general approach of therapy is to obtain physiologic premenopausal female range estrogen and testosterone levels through the combined use of an estrogen with an androgen blocker, and in some cases a progestagen. Clinical endpoints include breast development (often maximum Tanner stage 2/3), reduction of body hair, reduced muscle mass, and female redistribution of body fat.

The most commonly used estrogen is 17-beta estradiol, in pill, patch, or, less commonly, injected form. The choice of route is based to some degree on patient preference (Table 42–2). Transdermal estradiol has a well-established safety profile based on studies in menopausal cisgender women. Injected estradiol is the least studied route and can be associated with both supratherapeutic levels as well as cyclical levels over the dosing interval. Estrogens should be continued after gonadectomy without reduction in dose. There is no direct evidence to guide decision making regarding the discontinuation of estrogen once a patient arrives at a menopausal age, though most experts believe initiating or continuing hormone therapy in transgender women after age 50 is appropriate. Ethinyl estradiol (found in combined oral contraceptives) should be avoided due to thrombogenicity and a lack of need for suppression of ovulation.

The most commonly used anti-androgen is spironolactone, a potassium-sparing diuretic that is frequently used for female hirsutism or adult acne. Spironolactone inhibits both the synthesis of and action of testosterone. In higher doses (100–200 mg orally daily), spironolactone can lead to suppression of androgen levels into the female physiologic range. Common side effects include orthostasis and polyuria. Monitoring should include periodic assessment of kidney function and serum potassium. Other options for those who cannot tolerate spironolactone include a gonadotropin-releasing hormone (GnRH) analog, orchiectomy, or the use of a progestagen. Finasteride and dutasteride (5-alpha-reductase inhibitors) are sometimes used as an alternative; however, they have limited effects. After gonadectomy, anti-androgens can be discontinued.

No studies have been conducted on the role of progestagens in transgender women. Some believe there is benefit to breast development, mood, or libido, and there is no evidence to suggest any harm related to progestagens. Progestagens may be an effective anti-androgen, particularly cyproterone acetate, which is used widely outside the United States as the primary androgen blocker in feminizing regimens. If used, progestagens should be initiated after at least several months of estrogen plus anti-androgen.

The primary risk associated with estrogen therapy is venous thromboembolism (VTE). However, when using 17-beta estradiol at physiologic estrogen dosing, the risk is minimal. Prior studies showing 20- to 40-fold increased risk of VTE involved the use of ethinyl estradiol at doses of up to 200 mcg/day and did not control for tobacco use. More recent data found no increased risk of VTE in transgender women using transdermal 17-beta estradiol. Thus, transdermal estradiol is the preferred route for those who smoke or with risk factors for or a personal history of VTE.

Arnold JD et al. Incidence of venous thromboembolism in transgender women receiving oral estradiol. J Sex Med. 2016 Nov;13(11):1773–7. [PMID: 27671969]

Asscheman H et al. A long-term follow-up study of mortality in transsexuals receiving treatment with cross-sex hormones. Eur J Endocrinol. 2011 Apr;164(4):635–42. [PMID: 21266549]

Rosenthal SM. Approach to the patient: transgender youth: endocrine considerations. J Clin Endocrinol Metab. 2014 Dec;99(12):4379–89. [PMID: 25140398]

Wierckx K et al. Clinical review: breast development in trans women receiving cross-sex hormones. J Sex Med. 2014 May;11(5):1240–7. [PMID: 24618412]

Table 42–2. Feminizing hormone therapy.

Hormone Therapy	Dosage			Comments
	Initial, Low[1]	Initial, Typical	Maximum, Typical[2]	
Estrogen				
Estradiol oral/ sublingual	1 mg/day	2–4 mg/day	8 mg/day	If > 2 mg is recommended, dose should be divided and taken twice daily.
Estradiol transdermal	50 mcg	100 mcg	100–400 mcg	Maximum available single patch dose is 100 mcg. Frequency of change is brand and product dependent. Patients may find that more than 2 patches at a time are cumbersome.
Estradiol valerate, intramuscularly[3]	< 20 mg every 2 weeks	20 mg every 2 weeks	40 mg every 2 weeks	May divide dose into weekly injections for cyclical symptoms.
Estradiol cypionate, intramuscularly	< 2 mg every 2 weeks	2 mg every 2 weeks	5 mg every 2 weeks	May divide dose into weekly injections for cyclical symptoms.
Progestagen				
Medroxyprogesterone acetate (Provera)	2.5 mg orally each night at bedtime		5–10 mg orally each night at bedtime	
Micronized progesterone			100–200 mg each night at bedtime	
Androgen Blocker				
Spironolactone	25 mg orally daily	50 mg orally twice daily	200 mg orally twice daily	
Finasteride	1 mg orally daily		5 mg orally daily	
Dutasteride			0.5 mg orally daily	

[1]Initial low dosing for those who desire (or require due to medical history) a low dose or slow upward titration.
[2]Maximal effect does not necessarily require maximal dosing, as such maximal doses do not necessarily represent a target or ideal dose. Dose increases should be based on patient response and monitored hormone levels.
[3]Available as standard US Pharmacopia (USP) as well as compounded products.

B. Masculinizing Hormone Therapy

The goal of masculinizing hormone therapy is the development of male secondary sex characteristics, and suppression/minimization of female secondary sex characteristics. The general approach involves the use of one of several forms of parenteral testosterone using an approach similar to that in hypogonadal or agonadal cisgender men (Table 42–3). Blockade of estrogen is not needed.

Testosterone may be injected or applied as a topical gel or patch. Two studies support the use of subcutaneous (rather than intramuscular) injections, which allow the use of a smaller needle. The use of topical testosterone or using a weekly (vs biweekly) injection interval can help maintain even hormone levels in those with cyclical mood symptoms or pelvic cramping. Clinical endpoints include the development of facial hair, deepening of the voice, clitoral growth, male body fat redistribution and muscle growth, and induction of amenorrhea by 6 months.

Prior concerns of testosterone-induced hepatotoxicity were based on the use of oral methyltestosterone. There is no evidence to support a concern of hepatotoxicity in transgender men using parenteral bio-identical testosterone.

Common side effects of testosterone therapy in transgender men include acne and male pattern baldness, both of which can be approached as in cisgender men. Hemoglobin and hematocrit should be monitored, and if the levels are elevated, consider reducing testosterone dose or changing to a transdermal form or weekly injections to maintain more even levels. Polycystic ovarian syndrome and obesity have been found to be at an increased prevalence in transgender men prior to beginning testosterone therapy. Testosterone is not contraindicated in the presence of these conditions; instead, related metabolic disorders can be managed concurrently.

Baba T et al. Distinctive features of female-to-male transsexualism and prevalence of gender identity disorder in Japan. J Sex Med. 2011 Jun;8(6):1686–93. [PMID: 21477021]
Olson J et al. Subcutaneous testosterone: an effective delivery mechanism for masculinizing young transgender men. LGBT Health. 2014 Sep;1(3):165–7. [PMID: 26789709]

C. Monitoring Therapy

Hormone effects should be monitored both by clinical results as well as hormone levels, if available. Patients should be reminded that results may vary and can take up to 5 years to reach maximal effect; supraphysiologic hormone levels are not likely to enhance results but may incur

Table 42–3. Masculinizing hormone therapy.

Androgen	Initial, Low[1]	Initial, Typical	Maximum, Typical[2]	Comment
		Dosage		
Testosterone cypionate[3]	20 mg/week intramuscularly/ subcutaneously	50 mg/week intramuscularly/ subcutaneously	100 mg/week intramuscularly/ subcutaneously	For every 2-week dosing, double each dose.
Testosterone enthanate[3]	20 mg/week intramuscularly/ subcutaneously	50 mg/week intramuscularly/ subcutaneously	100 mg/week intramuscularly/ subcutaneously	
Testosterone topical gel 1%	12.5–25 mg every morning	50 mg every morning	100 mg every morning	May come in pump or packet form.
Testosterone topical gel 1.62%[4]	20.25 mg every morning	40.5–60.75 mg every morning	103.25 mg every morning	
Testosterone patch	1–2 mg every night	4 mg every night	8 mg every night	Patches come in 2-mg and 4-mg size. For lower doses, may cut patch.
Testosterone cream[5]	10 mg	50 mg	100 mg	
Testosterone axillary gel 2%	30 mg every morning	60 mg every morning	90–120 mg every morning	Comes in pump only; one pump = 30 mg.
Testosterone undecanoate[6]	N/A	750 mg intramuscularly, repeat in 4 weeks, then every 10 weeks ongoing	N/A	Requires participation in manufacturer moni- tored program.[6]

[1]Initial, low-dose regimen is recommended for genderqueer and non-binary persons.

[2]Maximum dosing does not mean maximal effect. Furthermore, these dosage ranges do not necessarily represent a target or ideal dose. Dose increases should be based on patient response and monitored hormone levels. Some patients may require less or more than this amount.

[3]Available as standard US Pharmacopia (USP) as well as compounded products.

[4]Doses of less than 20.25 mg with 1.62% gel or less than 30 mg with 2% axillary gel may be difficult, since measuring one-half of a pump or packet can present a challenge. Patients requiring doses lower than 20.25 mg and whose insurance does not cover 1% gel may require prior authorization or an appeal.

[5]Testosterone creams are prepared by individual compounding pharmacies. Specific absorption and activity varies and consultation with the individual compounding pharmacist is recommended.

[6]Testosterone undecanoate has been associated with rare cases of pulmonary oil microembolism and anaphylaxis; in the United States, the drug is available only through the AVEED Risk Evaluation and Mitigation Strategy (REMS) Program (https://www.aveedrems.com/AveedUI/ rems/preHome.action). All injections must be administered in an office or hospital setting by a trained and registered health care provider and monitored for 30 minutes afterward for adverse reactions.

risks. Note that reported laboratory reference range values may differ depending on the sex of registration of the patient; in general, clinicians should use the reference ranges driven by the current hormonal status of the patient. For example, female reference ranges will be included on automated laboratory reports of a transgender man taking testosterone while still legally registered as female. The interpreting clinician should use the male reference ranges for any tests run on this patient that have sexually dimor- phic reference ranges. Tables 42–4 and 42–5 describe gen- eral monitoring recommendations, rationales, and "sex-specific" laboratory values that may require individu- alized interpretation.

D. Long-Term Health Outcomes

Well-designed, large, long-term studies of health outcomes in transgender people are lacking. The largest existing study of mortality is in a retrospective cohort of 966 transgender women and 365 transgender men who were treated with cross-sex hormones from the Netherlands, which did not control for a number of risk factors. All-cause as well as cardiovascular, cerebrovascular, and other disease-specific mortality among transgender men did not differ from the general Dutch population of cisgender women. Among transgender women, all-cause mortality was 51% higher than cisgender men in the general Dutch population, with the overwhelming majority of the difference due to HIV, drug overdose and suicide; a 64% increased risk (95% CI 43% to 87%) in cardiovascular mortality was seen; however, no significant difference was seen for cerebrovascular mor- tality. It should be noted that this study did not control for tobacco use. Any decisions to provide hormone therapy should include a detailed informed consent discussion and consideration, including recognizing the significant risks of withholding treatment on psychological well being which can have negative impacts on physical health as well as suicidality or substance abuse.

Table 42–4. Laboratory monitoring for feminizing hormone therapy.

	Comments	Baseline	3 Months[1]	6 Months[1]	12 Months[1]	Yearly	As needed
Blood urea nitrogen/creatinine/potassium	Only if spironolactone is used	X	X	X	X	X	
Lipids		X if clinically indicated		X	X		X
Hemoglobin A$_{1c}$		X		X	X	X	
Estradiol			X	X			X
Total testosterone			X	X	X		X
Sex hormone binding globulin (SHBG)[2]			X	X	X		X
Albumin[2]			X	X	X		X
Prolactin	Only if symptomatic						X

[1]In first year of therapy only.
[2]Used to calculate bioavailable testosterone (http://www.issam.ch/freetesto.htm).

Asscheman H et al. A long-term follow-up study of mortality in transsexuals receiving treatment with cross-sex hormones. Eur J Endocrinol. 2011 Apr;164(4):635–42. [PMID: 21266549]

► Surgical Interventions

A wide range of gender-affirming surgeries are available to transgender people. These include surgeries specific to gender affirmation as well as procedures commonly performed in cisgender populations (Table 42–6).

► Cancer Risk & Screening

Several retrospective studies have not identified an increased risk of cancer in transgender people compared to birth-sex matched controls. However, because of the numerous barriers to care as well as to identifying transgender people in clinical databases, underscreening and underreporting are likely. In general, an organ-based approach to screening should be taken. There are no modifications to screening recommendations (or recommendations not to screen) for ovarian, uterine, or cervical cancer in transgender men. Breast cancer screening for transgender men who have not undergone mastectomy should be performed based on guidelines for cisgender women. The role of screening for breast cancer in transgender men who have undergone mastectomy is unknown and depends on the technique used as well as technical limitations on screening small amounts of residual breast tissue. In transgender women, breast cancer screening using guidelines for cisgender women is recommended, with the modifications starting at age 50 and only after a minimum of 5 years of lifetime estrogen exposure. Screening for prostate cancer in transgender women is complicated beyond the current debate over the utility of prostate cancer screening in cisgender men by the effects of feminizing hormones on prostatic hypertrophy and interpretation of tests of prostate-specific antigen.

Table 42–5. Laboratory monitoring for masculinizing hormone therapy.

	Comments	Baseline[1]	3 Months[2]	6 Months[2]	12 Months[2]	Yearly	As Needed
Lipids	No evidence	X		X	X	X	X
Hemoglobin A$_{1c}$ or fasting glucose		X		X	X	X	
Estradiol							X
Total testosterone			X	X	X		X
Albumin[3]			X	X	X		X
Hemoglobin and hematocrit		X	X	X	X	X	X

[1]Based on United States Prevention Services Task Force guidelines.
[2]In first year of therapy only.
[3]Used to calculate bioavailable testosterone.

Table 42–6. Procedural interventions for gender affirmation.

Surgeries specific to transgender populations
Feminizing vaginoplasty
Masculinizing phalloplasty, scrotoplasty
Metaoidioplasty (clitoral release/enlargement, may include urethral lengthening)
Masculinizing chest surgery ("top surgery")
Facial feminization procedures
Reduction thyrochondroplasty (tracheal cartilage shave)
Voice surgery
Surgeries not specific to transgender populations
Augmentation mammoplasty
Hysterectomy, oophorectomy
Orchiectomy
Vaginectomy
Other interventions
Facial hair removal
Voice modification
Genital tucking and packing
Chest binding

While screening transgender women for pituitary adenoma with serum prolactin levels has been done in the past, this is not recommended in asymptomatic patients since current guidelines for the management of incidental prolactinomas is watchful waiting. Prolactin screening should occur in transgender women with galactorrhea, visual disturbances, or a new headache pattern.

UCSF Center of Excellence for Transgender Health Guidelines for the Primary and Gender Affirming Care of Transgender and Gender Nonconforming People. http://transhealth.ucsf.edu/trans?page=protocol

Wierckx K et al. Long-term evaluation of cross-sex hormone treatment in transsexual persons. J Sex Med. 2012 Oct;9(10):2641–51. [PMID: 22906135]

Wierckx K et al. Prevalence of cardiovascular disease and cancer during cross-sex hormone therapy in a large cohort of trans persons: a case-control study. Eur J Endocrinol. 2013 Sep 13;169(4):471–8. [PMID: 23904280]

▶ **HIV**

Transgender women in the United States are 34 times more likely to be infected with HIV than the general population. This disparity is driven by a number of factors, including lack of both employment opportunities and legal protections in the workplace and elsewhere, all of which can result in survival transactional sex and sex work, and an association between unaffirmed gender identity and high-risk sexual behavior. Based on studies of hormonal contraception, gender-affirming hormone therapy is not believed to have negative interactions with antiretroviral medications, although direct studies are lacking. A subanalysis of transgender women within a larger study of HIV PrEP with a daily fixed-dose combination of tenofovir disoproxil fumarate 300 mg and emtricitabine 200 mg suggested efficacy when taken as prescribed but demonstrated poor adherence in comparison to control MSM. Such findings support the notion that HIV services and programs targeting transgender populations should be developed and implemented distinctly from those targeting MSM, and that bundling of HIV care with gender-affirming care may improve HIV outcomes.

Baral SD et al. Worldwide burden of HIV in transgender women: a systematic review and meta-analysis. Lancet Infect Dis. 2013 Mar;13(3):214–22. [PMID: 23260128]

Deutsch MB et al; iPrEx investigators. HIV pre-exposure prophylaxis in transgender women: a subgroup analysis of the iPrEx trial. Lancet HIV. 2015 Dec;2(12):e512–9. [PMID: 26614965]

Poteat T et al. HIV risk and preventive interventions in transgender women sex workers. Lancet. 2015 Jan 17;385(9964):274–86. [PMID: 25059941]

Sevelius JM. Gender affirmation: a framework for conceptualizing risk behavior among transgender women of color. Sex Roles. 2013 Jun 1;68(11–12):675–89. [PMID: 23729971]

Index

NOTE: Page numbers in **boldface** type indicate a major discussion. A *t* following a page number indicates tabular material, and *f* following a page number indicates a figure. Drugs are listed under their generic names.